HARRISON'S
PRINCIPLES OF
INTERNAL
MEDICINE

TWELFTH EDITION

VOLUME 1

EDITORS OF PREVIOUS EDITIONS

T. R. Harrison, Editor-in-Chief,
  Editions 1, 2, 3, 4, 5

W. R. Resnik, Editor,
  Editions 1, 2, 3, 4, 5

M. M. Wintrobe,
  Editor, Editions 1, 2, 3, 4, 5
  Editor-in-Chief, Editions 6, 7

G. W. Thorn,
  Editor, Editions 1, 2, 3, 4, 5, 6, 7
  Editor-in-Chief, Edition 8

R. D. Adams,
  Editor, Editions 2, 3, 4, 5, 6, 7, 8, 9, 10

P. B. Beeson,
  Editor, Editions 1, 2

I. L. Bennett, Jr.,
  Editor, Editions 3, 4, 5, 6

E. Braunwald,
  Editor, Editions 6, 7, 8, 9, 10
  Editor-in-Chief, Edition 11

K. J. Isselbacher,
  Editor, Editions 6, 7, 8, 10, 11
  Editor-in-Chief, Edition 9

R. G. Petersdorf,
  Editor, Editions 6, 7, 8, 9, 11
  Editor-in-Chief, Edition 10

J. D. Wilson,
  Editor, Editions 9, 10, 11

J. B. Martin,
  Editor, Editions 10, 11

A. S. Fauci,
  Editor, Edition 11

HARRISON'S

PRINCIPLES OF INTERNAL MEDICINE

TWELFTH EDITION

VOLUME 1

Editors

JEAN D. WILSON, M.D.
Professor of Internal Medicine, The University of Texas
Southwestern Medical Center, Dallas

EUGENE BRAUNWALD, A.B., M.D.,
M.A. (Hon.), M.D. (Hon.)
Hersey Professor of the Theory and Practice of Physic,
Harvard Medical School; Chairman, Department of Medicine,
Brigham and Women's Hospital, Boston

KURT J. ISSELBACHER, A.B., M.D.
Mallinckrodt Professor of Medicine, Harvard Medical School;
Director, Cancer Center, Massachusetts General Hospital,
Boston

ROBERT G. PETERSDORF, A.B., M.D.,
M.A. (Hon.), D.Sc. (Hon.), M.D. (Hon.),
L.H.D. (Hon.)
President, Association of American Medical Colleges,
Washington, D.C.

JOSEPH B. MARTIN, M.D., Ph.D.,
F.R.C.P.(C), M.A. (Hon.)
Professor of Neurology and Dean, School of Medicine,
University of California at San Francisco, San Francisco

ANTHONY S. FAUCI, M.D.
Director, National Institute of Allergy and Infectious Disease;
Chief, Laboratory of Immunoregulation; Director, Office of
AIDS Research, National Institutes of Health, Bethesda

RICHARD K. ROOT, M.D.
Professor of Medicine and Associate Dean for Clinical
Education, School of Medicine, University of California
at San Francisco, San Francisco

McGRAW-HILL, Inc.
Health Professions Division
New York   St. Louis   San Francisco   Colorado Springs
Auckland   Bogotá   Caracas   Hamburg   Lisbon   London
Madrid   Mexico   Milan   Montreal   New Delhi   Paris
San Juan   São Paulo   Singapore   Sydney   Tokyo   Toronto

HARRISON'S
PRINCIPLES OF INTERNAL MEDICINE
Twelfth Edition

Copyright © 1991, 1987, 1983, 1980, 1977, 1974, 1970, 1966, 1962, 1958 by
McGraw-Hill, Inc. All rights reserved. Copyright 1954, 1950 by McGraw-Hill,
Inc. All rights reserved. Copyright renewed 1978 by Maxwell Myer Wintrobe
and George W. Thorn. Printed in the United States of America. Except as
permitted under the United States Copyright Act of 1976, no part of this
publication may be reproduced or distributed in any form or by any means, or
stored in a data base or retrieval system, without the prior written permission of
the publisher.

1 2 3 4 5 6 7 8 9 0   DOW DOW   9 8 7 6 5 4 3 2 1 0

Foreign Editions
FRENCH (Eleventh Edition)—Flammarion, © 1988
GERMAN (Tenth Edition)—Schwabe and Company, Ltd., © 1986
GREEK (Eleventh Edition)—Parissianos, © 1990
ITALIAN (Twelfth Edition)—McGraw-Hill Libri Italia S.r.l. © 1992 (est.)
JAPANESE (Tenth Edition)—Hirokawa, © 1985
PORTUGUESE (Eleventh Edition)—Editora Guanabara Koogan, S.A.,
© 1988
SPANISH (Twelfth Edition)—McGraw-Hill/Interamericana de Espana,
© 1991 (est.)

This book was set in Times Roman by Monotype Composition Company.
The editors were J. Dereck Jeffers and Stuart D. Boynton. The indexer
was Irving Tullar; the production supervisor was Robert Laffler; the
designer was Marsha Cohen; R. R. Donnelley & Sons Company was
printer and binder.

Library of Congress Cataloging-in-Publication Data

Harrison's principles of internal medicine—12th ed./editors, Jean D.
  Wilson . . . [et al.]
     p.   cm.
    Also issued in 2 v.
    Includes bibliographical references.
    ISBN 0-07-070890-8 (1-vol. ed.)—ISBN 0-07-079749-8 (2-vol. set),
    0-07-070891-6 (vol. 1), 0-07-070892-4 (vol. 2)
     1. Internal medicine.   I. Harrison, Tinsley Randolph, Date.
  II. Wilson, Jean D., Date.   III. Title: Principles of internal medicine.
    [DNLM: 1. Internal Medicine.   WB 115 P957]
RC46.H333   1991
616—dc20
DLC
for Library of Congress   90-5814
                           CIP

A salute to Raymond D. Adams by the editors of Harrison's

We dedicate this twelfth edition of *Harrison's Principles of Internal Medicine* to Raymond D. Adams. Dr. Adams joined the Harrison's editorial board for preparation of the second edition, which was published in 1954. Together with the other members of the editorial board at the time, Tinsley R. Harrison, William R. Resnik, Maxwell M. Wintrobe, George W. Thorn, and Paul B. Beeson, he established *Harrison's* as a serious competitor in the field.

Ray Adams left an indelible mark on the textbook with his first contributions. He advocated what was to become the chief feature of the book, namely, the use of the introductory chapters to discuss symptoms and signs—the "Cardinal Manifestations of Disease." He argued forcibly for including diseases of the nervous system as a major component. He developed over time a systematic syndromic approach to understanding diseases of the nervous system that came to be the foundation for teaching a substantial portion of the emerging community of academic neurologists in the United States. With the assistance of his able collaborator, Maurice Victor, and other members of the neurological staff at the Massachusetts General Hospital, the section on neurology became a major instrument for teaching several generations of medical students and house officers. Because of the way that he formulated neurology as an essential component of medicine, he has had an equally important impact on the training of internists. At times the arguments over how much neurology to include in a textbook of general medicine became thunderous, leading Tinsley Harrison on one occasion to suggest (only half-facetiously) that the title be changed to *The Principles of Internal Medicine and Details of Neurology*.

The syndromic approach to diseases that affect the nervous system arose from Ray Adams' enormous personal experience with patients, an experience that continues to the present day. A complete exposition of this approach has now appeared in four editions of *Principles of Neurology*, written with Maurice Victor.

Raymond Adams was graduated from Duke University Medical School. With support from a Rockefeller fellowship he trained with James Ayer and Charles Kubik in neurology at the Massachusetts General Hospital and with Eugen Kahn in psychiatry at Yale. He returned to Boston to Harvard's service at the City Hospital as head of the Neuropathology Laboratory in 1939 where, over the course of the next decade, he made major contributions in studies of neurosyphilis, meningitis, muscle disease, and the effects of alcohol on the nervous system. He became Bullard Professor of Neuropathology at Harvard Medical School and chief of the Neurology Service at the Massachusetts General Hospital in 1951 and continued in these positions until 1978. During those years he created the leading neurological service in the country and participated in the training of a generation of academic leaders who would populate many of the university chairs of neurology in the United States and elsewhere. During this time he contributed a series of landmark studies on clinicopathologic correlations of diseases affecting the nervous system. He produced some of the first evidence for autoimmune disease of the brain and made major contributions to the understanding of developmental diseases of the nervous system. He is an expert neuropathologist and a fine neuropsychiatrist. It is difficult to find a topic in neurology that has not been advanced by the scholarship of Ray Adams.

To those who have studied under Dr. Adams and to those who have worked with him in the development of *Harrison's*, he has always been a wise and congenial colleague who demanded excellence of himself and expected it of others. His generosity, wisdom, and creativity have meant much to us, and we affectionately dedicate this volume to him.

ABBREVIATED CONTENTS

CONTENTS

PART THREE
CLINICAL PHARMACOLOGY

PART SIX
DISORDERS OF THE CARDIOVASCULAR SYSTEM

**PART SEVEN
DISORDERS OF THE RESPIRATORY SYSTEM**

**PART EIGHT
DISORDERS OF THE KIDNEY AND URINARY TRACT**

PART NINE
DISORDERS OF THE GASTROINTESTINAL SYSTEM

Section 1: Disorders of the alimentary tract

Section 2: Liver and biliary tract disease

Section 3: Disorders of the pancreas

PART TEN
DISORDERS OF THE IMMUNE SYSTEM, CONNECTIVE TISSUE, AND JOINTS

Section 1: Disorders of the immune system

PART ELEVEN
HEMATOLOGY AND ONCOLOGY

PART TWELVE
ENDOCRINOLOGY AND METABOLISM

Section 1: Endocrinology

Section 2: Disorders of intermediary metabolism

Section 3: Disorders of bone and mineral metabolism

PART THIRTEEN
NEUROLOGIC DISORDERS

Section 1: The central nervous system

Section 2: Disorders of nerve and muscle

PART FOURTEEN
PSYCHIATRY

Section 1: Psychiatric disorders

Section 2: Alcoholism and drug dependency

COLOR PLATES *After page 402*

1 Atlas of common skin lesions encountered during the physical examination of the skin
A1-1 Dermatofibroma A1-2 Acrochordon A1-3 Angiokeratomas A1-4 Café au lait macules A1-5 Acne A1-6 Dermatophytosis A1-7 Eczematous dermatitis A1-8 Localized lichenification A1-9 Melasma (chloasma) A1-10 Milia A1-11 Psoriasis A1-12 Perlèche A1-13 Acrochordon A1-14 Rosacea A1-15 Seborrheic dermatitis A1-16 Seborrheic keratosis A1-17 Senile angioma ("cherry red spot") A1-18 Senile lentigo A1-18 Senile sebaceous adenoma A1-19 Solar keratosis A1-20 Spider nevus A1-21 Tinea versicolor A1-22 Verruca vulgaris A1-23 Xanthelasma A1-24 Systemic lupus erythematosus A1-25 Necrotizing vasculitis syndrome A1-26 Glucagonoma (A) and acquired zinc deficiency (B) A1-27 Porphyria cutanea tarda A1-28 Necrobiosis lipoidica A1-29 Kaposi's sarcoma A1-30 Carcinoid A1-31 Malignant melanomas A1-32 Dysplastic melanocytic nevi A1-33 Malignant melanoma–dysplastic nevus syndrome

2 Atlas of infectious diseases
A2-1 Varicella A2-2 Measles (rubeola) A2-3 Rocky Mountain spotted fever A2-4 Rocky Mountain spotted fever A2-5 Meningococcemia A2-6 Disseminated gonococcal infection A2-7 Pseudomonas septicemia A2-8 Facial erysipelas A2-9 and A2-10 Lyme disease: erythema chronicum migrans A2-11 Secondary syphilis A2-12 Papulosquamous lesions of secondary syphilis A2-13 Macular syphilids A2-14 Molluscum contagiosum A2-15 Esthiomene A2-16 Severe primary HSV infection A2-17 Primary HSV pharyngitis A2-18 Neonatal HSV infection A2-19 Herpetic whitlow A2-20 Keratodermia blenorrhagica A2-21 Scabies excoriations A2-22 Cervicofacial actinomycosis A2-23 and A2-24 Kaposi's sarcoma

3 Atlas of endoscopic findings
A3-1 Normal esophagus A3-2 Peptic regurgitant esophagus A3-3 Ulcerated squamous cell carcinoma A3-4 Moniliasis of the esophagus A3-5 Barrett's metaplasia of the esophagus with adenocarcinoma A3-6 Normal body of the stomach with rugal folds A3-7 Benign gastric ulcer of the lesser curve A3-8 Gastric polyp A3-9 Arteriovenous malformation of the gastric mucosa A3-10 Normal pylorus A3-11 Normal duodenal bulb A3-12 Normal papilla of Vater A3-13 Periampullary carcinoma A3-14 Endoscopic papillotomy A3-15 Normal colon A3-16 Colonic adenomatous polyp A3-17 Multiple small colonic adenomatous polyps A3-18 Colon adenocarcinoma A3-19 Crohn's colitis A3-20 Severe ulcerative colitis A3-21 Kaposi's sarcoma involving the colon

4 Atlas of fundoscopic examination
A4-1 Normal optic nerve and retina A4-2 Central retinal artery occlusion A4-3 Central retinal vein occlusion A4-4 Early papilledema A4-5 Drusen of the optic nerve head A4-6 Anterior ischemic optic neuropathy A4-7 Primary optic atrophy A4-8 Angioid streaks A4-9 Retinitis pigmentosa A4-10 Band keratopathy A4-11 Glaucomatous optic disk with secondary atrophy A4-12 Diabetic retinopathy with microaneurysms A4-13 Proliferative diabetic retinopathy A4-14 Cytomegalovirus retinitis in AIDS A4-15 Retinal arteriovenous malformation in the Wyburn-Mason syndrome

5 Atlas of hematology
A5-1 Normal blood smear A5-2 Megaloblastic anemia A5-3 Liver disease A5-4 Iron-deficiency anemia A5-5 β thalassemia intermedia A5-6 Sickle cell anemia A5-7 Traumatic hemolysis A5-8 Spur cell anemia A5-9 Uremia A5-10 Hereditary spherocytosis A5-11 Immunohemolytic anemia A5-12 Myeloid metaplasia A5-13 Normal granulocyte (A); normal monocyte and lymphocyte (B) A5-14 Normal eosinophil (A); basophil (B) A5-15 Normal granulocyte precursors in marrow A5-16 Neutrophils with toxic granulation A5-17 Band with Döhle body A5-18 Hypersegmentation A5-19 Chédiak-Higashi anomaly (A); Pelger-Huet anomaly (B) A5-20 Reactive lymphocytes A5-21 Chronic granulocytic leukemia A5-22 Leukemic cell in acute promyelocytic leukemia A5-23 Chronic lymphocytic leukemia A5-24 Leukemic cells in acute lymphoblastic leukemia A5-25 Hodgkin's disease A5-26 Non-Hodgkin's nodular lymphoma A5-27 Multiple myeloma

LIST OF CONTRIBUTORS

ITAMAR B. ABRASS, M.D.
Professor of Medicine and Head, Division of Gerontology and Geriatric Medicine, University of Washington School of Medicine, Seattle

ELIAS ABRUTYN, M.D.
Professor and Assistant Chairman, Department of Medicine, Medical College of Pennsylvania; Associate Chief, Medical Service, Veterans Administration Medical Center, Philadelphia

RAYMOND D. ADAMS, B.A., M.A., M.D., M.A. (Hon.), D.Sc. (Hon.), M.D. (Hon.)
Bullard Professor of Neuropathology, Emeritus, Harvard Medical School; Consultant Neurologist and formerly Chief of Neurology Service, Massachusetts General Hospital; Emeritus Director, Eunice K. Shriver Research Center, Boston; Médicin Adjoint, L'Hôpital Cantonale de Lausanne, Lausanne

JOHN ADAMSON, M.D.
President, The New York Blood Center, New York

SETH L. ALPER, M.D., Ph.D.
Instructor in Medicine, Harvard Medical School; Section of Molecular Medicine and Nephrology, Beth Israel Hospital, Boston

ROBERT J. ANDERSON, M.D.
Professor of Medicine, University of Colorado Health Sciences Center, Denver

JACK P. ANTEL, M.D.
Professor and Chairman, Department of Neurology and Neurosurgery, McGill University; Neurologist-in-Chief, Montreal Neurological Institute and Hospital, Montreal

BARRY G.W. ARNASON, M.D.
Raymond Professor and Chairman, Department of Neurology, and Director of Brain Research Institute, University of Chicago Pritzker School of Medicine, Chicago

ARTHUR K. ASBURY, M.D.
Ruth Wagner Van Meter and J. Ray Van Meter Professor of Neurology, University of Pennsylvania School of Medicine and Hospital of the University of Pennsylvania, Philadelphia

K. FRANK AUSTEN, M.D.
Theodore Bevier Bayles Professor of Medicine, Harvard Medical School; Chairman, Department of Rheumatology and Immunology, Brigham and Women's Hospital, Boston

ROBERT AUSTRIAN, M.D., D.Sc. (Hon.)
Professor Emeritus and Chairman, Department of Research Medicine, University of Pennsylvania School of Medicine, Philadelphia

BERNARD M. BABIOR, M.D., Ph.D.
Head, Division of Biochemistry, Department of Molecular and Experimental Medicine, and Member, Division of Hematology and Oncology, Department of Medicine, Scripps Clinic and Research Foundation, La Jolla

KAMAL F. BADR, M.D.
Assistant Professor of Medicine, Vanderbilt University School of Medicine, Nashville

DONALD S. BAIM, M.D.
Associate Professor of Medicine, Harvard Medical School; Director of Invasive Cardiology, Beth Israel Hospital, Boston

M. FLINT BEAL, M.D.
Associate Professor, Harvard Medical School; Assistant Neurologist, Massachusetts General Hospital, Boston

ARTHUR L. BEAUDET, M.D.
Investigator, Howard Hughes Medical Institute; Professor of Pediatrics and Cell Biology, Baylor College of Medicine, Boston

JOHN E. BENNETT, M.D.
Head, Clinical Mycology Section, National Institute of Allergy and Infectious Diseases, National Institutes of Health, Bethesda

MICHAEL S. BERNSTEIN, M.D.
Fellow, Department of Medicine, University of California, San Francisco

DAVID R. BICKERS, M.D.
Professor and Chairman, Department of Dermatology, Case Western Reserve University School of Medicine; Director, Department of Dermatology, University Hospitals of Cleveland, Cleveland

EDWIN L. BIERMAN, M.D.
Professor of Medicine and Head, Division of Metabolism, Endocrinology, and Nutrition, University of Washington School of Medicine, Seattle

ALAN L. BISNO, M.D.
Professor of Medicine, University of Miami School of Medicine; Chief, Medical Service, Veterans Administration Medical Center, Miami

JEAN BOLOGNIA, M.D.
Assistant Professor of Dermatology, Department of Dermatology, Yale University School of Medicine, New Haven

WALTER G. BRADLEY, M.D.
Chairman and Professor of Neurology, University of Vermont College of Medicine; Chairman, Department of Neurology, University Health Center, Burlington

DAVID L. BRAFF, M.D.
Professor of Psychiatry, University of California at San Diego; Director of Psychiatry, U.C.S.D. Medical Center, San Diego

KENNETH D. BRANDT, M.D.
Professor of Medicine and Head, Rheumatology Division, Indiana University School of Medicine; Director, Indiana University Specialized Center of Research in Osteoarthritis, Indianapolis

EUGENE BRAUNWALD, A.B., M.D., M.A. (Hon.), M.D. (Hon.)
Hersey Professor of the Theory and Practice of Physic, Harvard Medical School; Chairman, Department of Medicine, Brigham and Women's Hospital, Boston

IRWIN M. BRAVERMAN, M.D.
Professor of Dermatology, Department of Dermatology, Yale University School of Medicine, New Haven

BARRY M. BRENNER, B.S., M.D., M.A. (Hon.)
Samuel A. Levine Professor of Medicine, Harvard Medical School; Senior Physician and Director, Renal Division, Brigham and Women's Hospital, Boston

KENNETH R. BRIDGES, M.D.
Assistant Professor of Medicine, Harvard Medical School; Brigham and Women's Hospital, Boston

KAREN THATCHER BRITTON, M.D., Ph.D.
Associate Professor of Psychiatry, School of Medicine, University of California at San Diego, La Jolla

MARTIN M. BROWN, M.A., M.D., M.R.C.P.
Senior Lecturer in Neurology, St. Georges Hospital Medical School, London

MICHAEL S. BROWN, M.D.
Paul J. Thomas Professor, Department of Molecular Genetics, The University of Texas Southwestern Medical Center, Dallas

ROBERT H. BROWN, JR., M.D., D.Phil.
Assistant Professor, Harvard Medical School; Associate Neurologist, Massachusetts General Hospital, Boston

H. FRANKLIN BUNN, M.D.
Professor of Medicine, Harvard Medical School; Senior Physician and Director, Hematology Research, Brigham and Women's Hospital, Boston

RONALD M. BURDE, M.D.
Professor and Chairman, Department of Ophthalmology, Ophthalmologist and Neuroophthalmologist, Albert Einstein College of Medicine, New York

JOHN BUTLER, M.D.
Professor of Medicine, University of Washington School of Medicine, Seattle

ROBERT N. BUTLER, M.D.
Chairman, Brookdale Professor of Geriatrics and Adult Development, Ritter Department of Geriatrics and Adult Development, The Mount Sinai Medical Center, New York

ALFRED E. BUXTON, M.D.
Associate Professor of Medicine, University of Pennsylvania School of Medicine; Director, Clinical Electrophysiology Laboratory, Hospital of the University of Pennsylvania, Philadelphia

EDWIN C. CADMAN, M.D.
Ensign Professor of Medicine and Chairman, Department of Medicine, Yale University Medical School, New Haven

CHARLES B. CARPENTER, M.D.
Professor of Medicine, Harvard Medical School; Director, Laboratory of Immunogenetics and Transplantation, Brigham and Women's Hospital, Boston

CHARLES C.J. CARPENTER, M.D.
Professor of Medicine, Brown University; Physician-in-Chief, The Miriam Hospital, Providence

BRUCE R. CARR, M.D.
Professor, Department of Obstetrics and Gynecology and Cecil and Ida Green Center for Reproductive Biology Sciences, The University of Texas Southwestern Medical Center, Dallas

EDWIN H. CASSEM, M.D.
Associate Professor of Psychiatry, Harvard Medical School; Acting Chief, Psychiatric Service, Massachusetts General Hospital, Boston

AGUSTIN CASTELLANOS, M.D.
Professor of Medicine, University of Miami School of Medicine; Director, Clinical Electrophysiology, Jackson Memorial Hospital, Miami

VERNE S. CAVINESS, JR., M.D., Ph.D.
Joseph and Rose Kennedy Professor of Child Neurology and Mental Retardation, Harvard Medical School; Interim Chief, Neurology Service, and Chief, Child Neurology, Massachusetts General Hospital, Boston

RICHARD CHAMPLIN, M.D.
Associate Professor of Medicine and Director, Leukemia/Bone Marrow Transplant Service, School of Medicine, University of California at Los Angeles

KEITH H. CHIAPPA, M.D.
Associate Professor of Neurology, Harvard Medical School; Director, EEG and Evoked Potentials Unit of the Clinical Neurophysiology Laboratory and Department of Neurology, Massachusetts General Hospital, Boston

JOHN S. CHILD, M.D.
Professor of Medicine, School of Medicine, University of California at Los Angeles; Associate Chief, Division of Cardiology, and Director, Adult Cardiac Imaging and Hemodynamics Laboratories, UCLA Medical Center, Los Angeles

WALLACE A. CLYDE, JR., M.D.
Professor of Pediatrics and Microbiology, University of North Carolina School of Medicine; Attending Physician, North Carolina Memorial Hospital, Chapel Hill

FREDRIC L. COE, M.D.
Professor of Medicine and Physiology and Chief, Nephrology Program, University of Chicago Pritzker School of Medicine, Chicago

ALAN S. COHEN, M.D.
Chief of Medicine and Director, Thorndike Memorial Laboratory; Conrad Wesselhoeft Professor of Medicine, Boston University School of Medicine, Boston

HARVEY R. COLTEN, M.D.
Professor and Chairman, Department of Pediatrics, Washington University School of Medicine; St. Louis Children's Hospital, St. Louis

WILSON S. COLUCCI, M.D.
Associate Professor of Medicine, Harvard Medical School; Associate Physician, Brigham and Women's Hospital, Boston

PATRICIA C. COME, M.D.
Associate Professor of Medicine, Harvard Medical School; Harvard Community Health Plan, West Roxbury

MAX D. COOPER, M.D.
Investigator, Howard Hughes Medical Institute; Professor of Medicine, Pediatrics, and Microbiology and Director, Division of Developmental and Clinical Immunology, University of Alabama at Birmingham, Birmingham

RICHARD A. COOPER, M.D.
Professor of Medicine, Executive Vice-President and Dean, Medical College of Wisconsin, Milwaukee

LAWRENCE COREY, M.D.
Professor of Laboratory Medicine and Microbiology and Head, Virology Division, University of Washington School of Medicine, Seattle

MARK A. CREAGER, M.D.
Assistant Professor of Medicine, Harvard Medical School; Director, Noninvasive Vascular Laboratory, Division of Vascular Medicine and Atherosclerosis, Brigham and Women's Hospital, Boston

RONALD G. CRYSTAL, M.D.
Chief, Pulmonary Branch, National Heart, Lung and Blood Institute, National Institutes of Health, Bethesda

JOHN J. CUSH, M.D.
Assistant Professor, Department of Internal Medicine, The University of Texas Southwestern Medical Center, Dallas

CHARLES A. CZEISLER, Ph.D., M.D.
Associate Professor of Medicine, Harvard Medical School; Associate Physician, Brigham and Women's Hospital; Director, Center for Circadian and Sleep Disorders, Boston

DAVID C. DALE, M.D.
Professor of Medicine, University of Washington School of Medicine, Seattle

THOMAS M. DANIEL, M.D.
Professor of Medicine, Case Western Reserve University, Cleveland

GILBERT H. DANIELS, M.D.
Associate Professor of Medicine, Harvard Medical School; Physician, Massachusetts General Hospital, Boston

ROBERT B. DAROFF, M.D.
Gilbert W. Humphrey Professor and Chairman, Case Western Reserve University School of Medicine; Director, Department of Neurology, University Hospitals of Cleveland; Neurology Service, Cleveland Veterans Administration Medical Center, Cleveland

JOHN R. DAVID, M.D.
John LaPorte Given Professor and Chairman, Department of Tropical Public Health, Harvard School of Public Health; Chief, Division of Tropical Medicine, Brigham and Women's Hospital, Boston

KENNETH DAVIS, M.D.
Professor of Radiology, Harvard Medical School; Director of Neuroradiology, Massachusetts General Hospital, Boston

MARC A. DICHTER, M.D., Ph.D.
Professor of Neurology, University of Pennsylvania School of Medicine, Philadelphia

JULES L. DIENSTAG, M.D.
Associate Professor of Medicine, Harvard Medical School; Associate Physician, Gastrointestinal Unit, Massachusetts General Hospital, Boston

ROBERT G. DLUHY, M.D.
Associate Professor of Medicine, Harvard Medical School; Associate Program Director of the Clinical Research Center, Brigham and Women's Hospital, Boston

RAPHAEL DOLIN, M.D.
Professor of Medicine, Microbiology and Immunology, and Head, Infectious Diseases Unit, University of Rochester School of Medicine and Dentistry, Rochester

DANIEL B. DRACHMAN, M.D.
Professor of Neurology and Neurosciences and Director, Neuromuscular Unit, The Johns Hopkins University School of Medicine, Baltimore

JEFFREY M. DRAZEN, M.D.
Professor of Medicine, Harvard Medical School; Chief, Pulmonary Division, Brigham and Women's and Beth Israel Hospitals, Boston

HENRY J. DURIVAGE, Pharm.D.
Associate Research Scientist and Director of Clinical Research, Section of Medical Oncology, Department of Internal Medicine, Yale University School of Medicine, New Haven

JOHANNA T. DWYER, D.Sc., R.D.
Professor of Medicine and Community Health, Tufts University School of Medicine; Senior Scientist, USDA Human Nutrition Research Center on Aging, Tufts University; Director, Frances Stern Nutrition Center, New England Medical Center Hospital, Boston

VICTOR J. DZAU, M.D.
William G. Irwin Professor and Chief, Division of Cardiovascular Medicine, Stanford University School of Medicine; Stanford University Hospital, Stanford

KENNETH H. FALCHUK, M.D.
Associate Professor of Medicine, Harvard Medical School; Physician, Brigham and Women's Hospital, Boston

ANTHONY S. FAUCI, M.D.
Director, National Institute of Allergy and Infectious Diseases, and Chief, Laboratory of Immunoregulation, and Director, Office of AIDS Research, National Institutes of Health, Bethesda

MURRAY J. FAVUS, M.D.
Professor of Medicine, University of Chicago Pritzker School of Medicine, Chicago

BERNARD N. FIELDS, M.D.
Adele Lehman Professor of Microbiology and Molecular Genetics, and Professor of Medicine and Chairman, Department of Microbiology and Molecular Genetics, Harvard Medical School, Boston

STUART C. FINCH, M.D.
Professor of Medicine, Robert Wood Johnson Medical School, University of Medicine and Dentistry of New Jersey, Camden

J. STEPHEN FINK, M.D.
Assistant Professor, Harvard Medical School; Assistant Neurologist, Massachusetts General Hospital, Boston

ADAM FINN, M.D.
Lecturer in Immunology, Institute of Child Health; Honorary Senior Registrar, The Hospital for Sick Children, London

DANIEL W. FOSTER, M.D.
Donald W. Seldin Distinguished Chair in Internal Medicine and Chairman, Department of Internal Medicine, The University of Texas Southwestern Medical Center, Dallas

MICHAEL M. FRANK, M.D.
Chief, Laboratory of Clinical Investigation, National Institute of Allergy and Infectious Diseases, National Institutes of Health, Bethesda

STANLEY D. FREEDMAN, M.D.
Head, Division of Infectious Diseases, Scripps Clinic and Research Foundation; Clinical Professor of Medicine, University of California at San Diego, La Jolla

BISHARA J. FREIJ, M.D.
Assistant Professor of Pediatrics, Division of Infectious Diseases, Department of Pediatrics, Georgetown University School of Medicine, Washington, D.C.

MICHAEL FREISSMUTH, M.D.
Instructor, Department of Pharmacology, University of Vienna

HARVEY M. FRIEDMAN, M.D.
Associate Professor, Department of Medicine, University of Pennsylvania School of Medicine, Philadelphia

LAWRENCE S. FRIEDMAN, M.D.
Associate Professor of Medicine and Vice Chairman of the Department of Medicine, Division of Gastroenterology and Hepatology, Thomas Jefferson University Hospital, Philadelphia

PAUL J. FRIEDMAN, M.D.
Professor of Radiology, University of California, San Diego

WILLIAM F. FRIEDMAN, M.D.
J.H. Nicholson Professor of Pediatric Cardiology and Executive Chairman, Department of Pediatrics, School of Medicine; UCLA Medical Center, Los Angeles

LAWRENCE A. FROHMAN, M.D.
Professor of Medicine, Director of Division of Endocrinology and Metabolism, University of Cincinnati College of Medicine, Cincinnati

JOHN I. GALLIN, M.D.
Director, Intramural Research Program, National Institute of Allergy and Infectious Diseases, National Institutes of Health, Bethesda

ROBERT C. GALLO, M.D.
Chief, Laboratory of Tumor Cell Biology, National Cancer Institute, National Institutes of Health, Bethesda

DONALD E. GANEM, M.D.
Associate Professor of Medicine and Microbiology, Division of Infectious Disease, Department of Medicine, University of California, San Francisco

PIERCE GARDNER, M.D.
Professor of Medicine and Associate Dean for Academic Affairs, School of Medicine, State University of New York at Stony Brook, Stony Brook

MARC B. GARNICK, M.D.
Associate Clinical Professor of Medicine, Dana-Farber Cancer Institute, Harvard Medical School; Vice President for Clinical Development, Genetics Institute, Cambridge

JAMES L. GERMAN III, M.D.
Professor (Genetics), Department of Pediatrics, Cornell University Medical College; Senior Investigator and Director, Laboratory of Human Genetics, The New York Blood Center, New York

ELOISE R. GIBLETT, M.D.
Executive Director Emeritus, Puget Sound Blood Center, Seattle

BRUCE C. GILLILAND, M.D.
Associate Dean for Clinical Affairs, University of Washington School of Medicine, Seattle

J. CHRISTIAN GILLIN, M.D.
Professor of Psychiatry, University of California at San Diego, and Director of U.C.S.D. Mental Health Research Center; Director of U.C.S.D. Fellowship in Psychopharmacology and Psychobiology, La Jolla

ALFRED G. GILMAN, M.D., Ph.D.
Raymond and Ellen Willie Professor of Molecular Neuropharmacology and Chairman, Department of Pharmacology, The University of Texas Southwestern Medical Center, Dallas

SID GILMAN, M.D.
Professor and Chairman, Department of Neurology, The University of Michigan Medical Center, Ann Arbor

RICHARD J. GLASSOCK, M.D.
Professor of Medicine, School of Medicine, University of California at Los Angeles; Chairman, Department of Medicine, Harbor-UCLA Medical Center, Torrance

ROBERT M. GLICKMAN, M.D.
Herrman L. Blumgart Professor of Medicine, Harvard Medical School; Physician-in-Chief, Beth Israel Hospital, Boston

DAVID W. GOLDE, M.D.
Professor of Medicine and Chief, Division of Hematology/Oncology, School of Medicine, University of California, Los Angeles

STEPHEN E. GOLDFINGER, M.D.
Associate Dean, Department of Continuing Education, and Associate Professor of Medicine, Harvard Medical School; Physician, Gastrointestinal Unit, Massachusetts General Hospital, Boston

PAUL GOLDHABER, D.D.S.
Dean and Professor of Periodontology, Harvard School of Dental Medicine, Boston

LEE GOLDMAN, M.D.
Professor of Medicine, Harvard Medical School; Vice-Chairman, Department of Medicine, Brigham and Women's Hospital; Chief, Division of Clinical Epidemiology, Brigham and Women's and Beth Israel Hospitals, Boston

JOSEPH L. GOLDSTEIN, M.D.
Paul J. Thomas Professor and Chairman, Department of Molecular Genetics, The University of Texas Southwestern Medical Center, Dallas

RAJ K. GOYAL, M.D.
Rabb Professor of Medicine, Harvard Medical School; Chief, Division of Gastroenterology, Beth Israel Hospital, Boston

JOHN W. GRAEF, M.D.
Associate Clinical Professor of Pediatrics, Harvard Medical School; Director, The Lead/Toxicology Clinic, The Children's Hospital, Boston

IGOR GRANT, M.D.
Professor and Acting Chairman, Department of Psychiatry, School of Medicine, University of California at San Diego, La Jolla

HARRY B. GREENBERG, M.D.
Professor of Medicine, Microbiology, and Immunology and Chief, Gastroenterology Division, Stanford University School of Medicine, Stanford

NORTON J. GREENBERGER, M.D.
Peter T. Bohan Professor and Chairman, Department of Medicine, University of Kansas School of Medicine, Kansas City

BRUCE M. GREENE, M.D.
Professor of Medicine, and Director, Division of Geographic Medicine, Department of Medicine, University of Alabama at Birmingham, Birmingham

JOHN S. GREENSPAN, Ph.D.
Professor and Chairman, Division of Oral Biology, University of California School of Dentistry, San Francisco Medical Center, San Francisco

JAMES E. GRIFFIN III, M.D.
Professor of Internal Medicine, The University of Texas Southwestern Medical Center, Dallas

J. McLEOD GRIFFISS, M.D.
Professor of Laboratory Medicine and Medicine, University of California San Francisco; Chief of Microbiology, Veterans Administration Medical Center, San Francisco

ROBERT C. GRIGGS, M.D.
Edward A. and Alma Vollertsen Rykenboer Professor of Neurophysiology, Professor of Neurology and Medicine, and Chairman, Department of Neurology, University of Rochester School of Medicine and Dentistry, University of Rochester Medical Center, Rochester

WILLIAM GROSSMAN, M.D.
Dana Professor of Medicine, Harvard Medical School; Chief, Cardiovascular Division, Beth Israel Hospital, Boston

JOHN H. GROWDON, M.D.
Associate Professor of Neurology, Harvard Medical School; Associate Neurologist and Director, Memory Disorders Unit, Massachusetts General Hospital, Boston

VLADIMIR C. HACHINSKI, M.D.
Richard and Beryl Ivey Professor and Chairman, Department of Clinical Neurological Sciences, University of Western Ontario, University Hospital, London, Ontario

BEVRA H. HAHN, M.D.
Chief of Rheumatology, University of California, Los Angeles

ROBERT I. HANDIN, M.D.
Associate Professor of Medicine, Harvard Medical School; Director, Hematology Division, Brigham and Women's Hospital, Boston

H. HUNTER HANDSFIELD, M.D.
Professor of Medicine, University of Washington School of Medicine; Director, Sexually Transmitted Disease Control Program, Seattle-King County Department of Public Health, Seattle

DONALD G. HARTER, M.D.
Senior Scientific Officer and Director, HHMI-NIH Research Scholars Program, Howard Hughes Medical Institute, Bethesda; Clinical Professor of Neurology, George Washington University School of Medicine and Health Sciences, Washington, D.C.

BARTON F. HAYNES, M.D.
Frederick M. Hanes Professor of Medicine and Chief, Division of Rheumatology and Immunology, Duke University School of Medicine, Durham

STEVEN C. HEBERT, M.D.
Associate Professor of Medicine, Harvard Medical School; Associate Physician, Brigham and Women's Hospital, Boston

CRAIG HENDERSON, M.D.
Associate Professor of Medicine, Harvard Medical School; Division of Medical Oncology, Dana-Farber Cancer Institute, Boston

FRED J. HENDLER, M.D., Ph.D.
Associate Professor of Medicine and Biochemistry, University of Louisville School of Medicine; James Graham Brown Cancer Center, Division of Hematology/Oncology, Louisville; Consulting Physician, Veterans Administration Medical Center, Dallas

FREDERICK P. HEINZEL, M.D.
Associate Professor of Medicine, Division of Infectious Disease, Department of Medicine, University of California, San Francisco

CHARLES B. HIGGINS, M.D.
Professor of Radiology and Chief, Magnetic Resonance Imaging, University of California School of Medicine, San Francisco

RAYMOND L. HINTZ, M.D.
Professor of Pediatrics and Head, Division of Pediatric Endocrinology, Stanford University School of Medicine, Stanford

MARTIN S. HIRSCH, M.D.
Associate Professor of Medicine, Harvard Medical School; Associate Physician, Infectious Diseases Unit, Massachusetts General Hospital, Boston

JAN V. HIRSCHMANN, M.D.
Associate Professor of Medicine, University of Washington School of Medicine; Assistant Chief, Medical Service, Seattle Veterans Administration Medical Center, Seattle

FRED HOCHBERG, M.D.
Associate Professor of Neurology, Harvard Medical School; Neurologist, Massachusetts General Hospital, Boston

PAUL D. HOEPRICH, M.D.
Professor of Medicine, Section of Medical Myocology, Division of Infectious and Immunologic Diseases, School of Medicine, University of California, Davis

GARY S. HOFFMAN, M.D.
Senior Investigator, Laboratory of Immunoregulation, National Institute of Allergy and Infectious Diseases, National Institutes of Health, Bethesda

JOHN H. HOLBROOK, M.D.
Professor of Internal Medicine, University of Utah School of Medicine, Salt Lake City

MICHAEL F. HOLICK, M.D., Ph.D.
Professor of Medicine, Chief of Endocrinology, and Director of the Clinical Research Center, Boston University School of Medicine, Boston

KING K. HOLMES, M.D., Ph.D.
Director, Center for AIDS and Sexually Transmitted Diseases; Professor of Medicine, University of Washington School of Medicine, Seattle

RANDALL K. HOLMES, M.D., Ph.D.
Professor and Chairman, Department of Microbiology, and Associate Dean for Academic Affairs, Uniformed Services University of the Health Sciences, Bethesda

THOMAS H. HOSTETTER, M.D.
Professor of Medicine, University of Minnesota School of Medicine; Director, Division of Renal Disease, University Hospital, Minneapolis

LYN J. HOWARD, B.M., D.Ch., F.R.C.P.
Professor of Medicine and Associate Professor of Pediatrics, and Head, Division of Clinical Nutrition, Albany Medical College, Albany

GARY W. HUNNINGHAKE, M.D.
Professor of Internal Medicine and Director, Pulmonary and Critical Care Medicine, University of Iowa College of Medicine, Iowa City

SIDNEY H. INGBAR, M.D., D.Sc. (Deceased)
Former William Bosworth Castle Professor of Medicine, Harvard Medical School; former Director, Thorndike Laboratory, Beth Israel Hospital, Boston

ROLAND H. INGRAM, Jr., M.D.
Professor and Vice-Chairman of Medicine, University of Minnesota Medical School; Chief of Medicine, Hennepin County Medical Center, Minneapolis

KURT J. ISSELBACHER, A.B., M.D.
Mallinckrodt Professor of Medicine, Harvard Medical School; Director, Cancer Center, Massachusetts General Hospital, Boston

RICHARD JACOBS, M.D., Ph.D.
Associate Clinical Professor of Medicine, Division of Infectious Disease, Department of Medicine, University of California, San Francisco

MARK E. JOSEPHSON, M.D.
Robinette Professor of Medicine (Cardiovascular Diseases), University of Pennsylvania School of Medicine; Chief, Cardiovascular Section, Hospital of the University of Pennsylvania, Philadelphia

LEWIS L. JUDD, M.D.
Director, National Institute of Mental Health, Rockville

LEE M. KAPLAN, M.D., Ph.D.
Assistant Professor of Medicine, Harvard Medical School; Assistant in Medicine, Gastrointestinal Unit, Massachusetts General Hospital, Boston

DENNIS L. KASPER, M.D.
William Ellery Channing Professor of Medicine, Harvard Medical School; Chief, Infectious Disease Division, Beth Israel Hospital, Boston

SATISH KATHPALIA, M.D.
Assistant Professor of Medicine, University of Chicago Pritzker School of Medicine; Attending Physician, Michael Reese Hospital and Medical Center, Chicago

DONALD KAYE, M.D.
Professor and Chairman, Department of Medicine, The Medical College of Pennsylvania, Philadelphia

WILLIAM N. KELLEY, M.D.
Professor of Medicine and Dean, School of Medicine, University of Pennsylvania, Philadelphia

GERALD T. KEUSCH, M.D.
Professor of Medicine, Tufts University School of Medicine; Chief, Division of Geographic Medicine and Infectious Diseases, New England Medical Center Hospital, Boston

MICHAEL B. KIMMEY, M.D.
Assistant Professor of Medicine and Director of Therapeutic Endoscopy, Division of Gastroenterology, University of Washington School of Medicine, Seattle

LOUIS V. KIRCHHOFF, M.D., M.P.H.
Assistant Professor of Medicine, Department of Internal Medicine, University of Iowa College of Medicine; Staff Physician, Veterans Administration Medical Center, Iowa City

J. PHILLIP KISTLER, M.D.
Associate Professor of Neurology, Harvard Medical School; Associate Neurologist, Massachusetts General Hospital, Boston

JOSEPH J. KLIMEK, M.D.
Associate Professor of Medicine, University of Connecticut Health Center; Acting Director, Department of Medicine, Hartford Hospital, Hartford

JAMES P. KNOCHEL, M.D.
Professor of Internal Medicine, The University of Texas Southwestern Medical Center; Chairman, Department of Medicine, Presbyterian Hospital, Dallas

HOWARD K. KOH, M.D.
Associate Professor of Dermatology, Medicine, and Public Health, Boston University Schools of Medicine and Public Health, Boston

WILLIAM J. KOVACS, M.D.
Assistant Professor of Medicine, Division of Endocrinology, Vanderbilt University School of Medicine, Nashville

KAREN KOVALOV-ST. JOHN, M.D.
Rheumatology Fellow, Indiana University School of Medicine, Indianapolis

STEPHEN M. KRANE, M.D.
Persis, Cyrus, and Marlow B. Harrison Professor of Medicine, Harvard Medical School; Physician and Chief, Arthritis Unit, Massachusetts General Hospital, Boston

J. THOMAS LaMONT, M.D.
Professor of Medicine, Boston University School of Medicine; Chief, Section of Gastroenterology, The University Hospital, Boston

LEWIS LANDSBERG, M.D.
Professor of Medicine, Harvard Medical School; Chief, Division of Endocrinology and Metabolism, Beth Israel Hospital, Boston

H. CLIFFORD LANE, M.D.
Deputy Clinical Director, National Institute of Allergy and Infectious Diseases, National Institutes of Health, Bethesda

PAUL N. LANKEN, M.D.
Associate Professor of Medicine, University of Pennsylvania School of Medicine; Medical Director, Medical Intensive Care Unit, Hospital of the University of Pennsylvania, Philadelphia

THOMAS J. LAWLEY, M.D.
Professor and Chairman, Department of Dermatology, Emory University School of Medicine, Atlanta

ALEXANDER R. LAWTON III, M.D.
Professor of Pediatrics and Microbiology, Division of Pediatrics, Immunology, and Rheumatology, Vanderbilt University School of Medicine, Nashville

J. MICHAEL LAZARUS, M.D.
Associate Professor of Medicine, Harvard Medical School; Physician, Brigham and Women's Hospital, Boston

ROBERT LEBOVICS, M.D.
Chief, Otolaryngology/Head, Neck Surgery, National Institute on Deafness and Other Communication Disorders, National Institutes of Health, Bethesda

NORMAN G. LEVINSKY, M.D.
Wade Professor and Chairman, Department of Medicine, Boston University School of Medicine; Physician-in-Chief and Director, Evans Memorial Department of Clinical Research, University Hospital, Boston

CHRISTOPHER H. LINDEN, M.D.
Assistant Professor of Medicine, University of Massachusetts Medical School; Director, Regional Poisoning Treatment Center, Worcester, Massachusetts

PETER E. LIPSKY, M.D.
Director, Harold C. Simmons Arthritis Research Center; Professor, Department of Internal Medicine, The University of Texas Southwestern Medical Center, Dallas

RICHARD M. LOCKSLEY, M.D.
Associate Professor of Medicine and Chief, Division of Infectious Disease, Department of Medicine, University of California, San Francisco

HARVEY F. LODISH, Ph.D.
Professor, Department of Biology, Massachusetts Institute of Technology; Member, Whitehead Institute for Biomedical Research, Cambridge

DAN L. LONGO, M.D.
Director, Biological Response Modifiers Program, Division of Cancer Treatment, National Cancer Institute-Frederick Cancer Research Facility, Frederick

FREDERICK H. LOVEJOY, Jr., M.D.
Professor of Pediatrics, Harvard Medical School; Associate Physician-in-Chief, The Children's Hospital, Boston

SHEILA A. LUKEHART, Ph.D.
Research Associate Professor, Department of Medicine, Division of Infectious Diseases, University of Washington School of Medicine, Seattle

ROB ROY MacGREGOR, M.D.
Professor of Medicine and Chief of Infectious Diseases Division, Department of Medicine, University of Pennsylvania School of Medicine, Philadelphia

RAYMOND MACIEWICZ, M.D.
Associate Professor of Neurology, Harvard Medical School; Associate Neurologist, Massachusetts General Hospital, Boston

JON T. MADER, M.D.
Professor of Medicine, Division of Infectious Diseases, Department of Internal Medicine, The University of Texas Medical Branch, Galveston

HENRY J. MANKIN, M.D.
Edith M. Ashley Professor of Orthopedic Surgery, Harvard Medical School; Chief, Orthopedic Services, Massachusetts General Hospital, Boston

FRANCIS E. MARCHLINSKI, M.D.
Associate Professor of Medicine, University of Pennsylvania School of Medicine; Director, Arrhythmia Evaluation Center, Hospital of the University of Pennsylvania, Philadelphia

JOSEPH B. MARTIN, M.D., Ph.D., F.R.C.P.(C), M.A.(Hon.)
Professor of Neurology and Dean, School of Medicine, University of California, San Francisco

JOEL B. MASON, M.D.
Assistant Professor of Medicine, Tufts University School of Medicine; Scientist, USDA Human Nutrition Research Center on Aging, Tufts University, Boston

HENRY MASUR, M.D.
Deputy Chief, Critical Care Medicine, Clinical Center, National Institutes of Health, Bethesda

ROBERT J. MAYER, M.D.
Associate Professor of Medicine, Harvard Medical School; Division of Medical Oncology, Dana-Farber Cancer Institute, Boston

JOHN D. McCONNELL, M.D.
Assistant Professor of Urology, The University of Texas Southwestern Medical Center, Dallas

GEORGE H. McCRACKEN, Jr., M.D.
Professor of Pediatrics and Chief, Division of Infectious Diseases, Department of Pediatrics, The University of Texas Southwestern Medical Center, Dallas

E. R. McFADDEN, Jr., M.D.
Argyl J. Beams Professor of Medicine and Director, Airway Disease Center, Case Western Reserve University School of Medicine, Cleveland

JAMES E. McGUIGAN, M.D.
Professor of Medicine and Chairman, Department of Medicine, University of Florida College of Medicine, Gainesville

NANCY K. MELLO, Ph.D.
Professor of Psychology, Department of Psychiatry (Neuroscience), Harvard Medical School, Boston; Co-Director, Alcohol and Drug Abuse Research Center, McLean Hospital, Belmont

JERRY R. MENDELL, M.D.
Professor of Neurology, Ohio State University College of Medicine, Columbus

JOHN MENDELSOHN, M.D.
Winthrop Rockefeller Chair in Medical Oncology and Chairman, Department of Medicine, Memorial Sloan-Kettering Cancer Center, New York

JACK H. MENDELSON, M.D.
Professor of Psychiatry (Neuroscience), Harvard Medical School, Boston; Co-Director, Alcohol and Drug Abuse Research Center, McLean Hospital, Belmont

URS A. MEYER, M.D.
Professor of Pharmacology and Chairman, Department of Pharmacology, Biocenter of the University of Basel, Basel, Switzerland

EDGAR L. MILFORD, M.D.
Associate Professor of Medicine, Harvard Medical School; Associate Physician, Brigham and Women's Hospital, Boston

RICHARD A. MILLER, M.D.
Assistant Professor of Medicine, University of Washington School of Medicine; Chief, Infectious Disease Division, Seattle Veterans Administration Medical Center, Seattle

JOHN D. MINNA, M.D.
Chief, NCI-Navy Medical Oncology Branch, National Cancer Institute, National Institutes of Health; Professor of Medicine, Uniformed Services University for the Health Sciences, Naval Hospital, Bethesda

JAY P. MOHR, M.D.
Sciarra Professor of Clinical Neurology, College of Physicians and Surgeons of Columbia University Neurological Institute, New York

STEPHEN A. MORSE, MSPH, Ph.D.
Director, Division of Sexually Transmitted Diseases Laboratory Research, Centers for Disease Control, Atlanta

KENNETH M. MOSER, M.D.
Professor of Medicine, School of Medicine, University of California at San Diego; Director, Pulmonary and Critical Care Division, U.C.S.D. Medical Center, La Jolla

ARNOLD M. MOSES, M.D.
Professor of Medicine and Director, Clinical Research Center, State University of New York Health Science Center; Chief, Endocrinology Section, Veterans Administration Medical Center, Syracuse

HARALAMPOS M. MOUTSOPOULOS, M.D.
Professor and Head of Medicine, Department of Internal Medicine, University of Ioannina Medical School, Ioannina, Greece

HENRY W. MURRAY, M.D.
Professor of Medicine, Cornell University School of Medicine; Chief, Infectious Diseases, The New York Hospital-Cornell Medical Center, New York

ROBERT J. MYERBURG, M.D.
Professor of Medicine and Physiology and Director, Division of Cardiology, University of Miami School of Medicine, Miami

LEE M. NADLER, M.D.
Associate Professor of Medicine, Harvard Medical School; Division of Tumor Immunology, Dana-Farber Cancer Institute, Boston

THEODORE E. NASH, M.D.
Medical Officer, Laboratory of Parasitic Diseases, National Institute of Allergy and Infectious Diseases, National Institutes of Health, Bethesda

LAURENCE NEEDLEMAN, M.D.
Assistant Professor of Radiology, Jefferson Medical College, Philadelphia

PAUL NEIMAN, M.D.
Professor of Medicine and Adjunct Professor of Pathology, University of Washington School of Medicine; Fred Hutchinson Cancer Research Center, Seattle

HAROLD C. NEU, M.D.
Professor of Medicine and Pharmacology and Chief, Division of Infectious Diseases, College of Physicians and Surgeons, Columbia University, New York

JOHN A. OATES, M.D.
Professor and Chairman, Department of Medicine, Vanderbilt University School of Medicine; Physician-in-Chief, Vandberbilt University Hospital, Nashville

JERROLD M. OLEFSKY, M.D.
Professor of Medicine and Head, Division of Endocrinology and Metabolism, School of Medicine, University of California at San Diego, La Jolla

STUART H. ORKIN, M.D.
Leland Fikes Professor of Pediatric Medicine, Harvard Medical School; Children's Hospital, Boston

ROBERT A. O'ROURKE, M.D.
Charles Conrad Brown Distinguished Professor of Medicine, University of Texas Health Science Center at San Antonio; Chief of Cardiology, University of Texas Health Science Center Teaching Hospitals, San Antonio

THOMAS D. PALELLA, M.D.
Associate Professor of Internal Medicine and Chief, Division of Rheumatology, University of Michigan Medical School, Ann Arbor

DARWIN L. PALMER, M.D.
Professor of Medicine and Chief, Division of Infectious Disease, University of New Mexico School of Medicine, Albuquerque

JOSEPH E. PARRILLO, M.D.
James B. Herrick Professor of Medicine, Rush Medical College; Chief, Section of Cardiology, Chief, Section of Critical Care Medicine, Medical Director, Rush Heart Institute, Rush-Presbyterian-St. Luke's Medical Center, Chicago

RICHARD C. PASTERNAK, M.D.
Assistant Professor of Medicine, Harvard Medical School; Director, Coronary Care Unit, Beth Israel Hospital, Boston

PETER L. PERINE, M.D.
Professor and Director, Division of Tropical Public Health, Uniformed Services University of the Health Sciences, Bethesda

ROBERT G. PETERSDORF, M.D.
President, Association of American Medical Colleges; Clinical Professor of Medicine, Georgetown University School of Medicine, Washington, D.C.

ELIOT A. PHILLIPSON, M.D.
Professor of Medicine, University of Toronto; Physician-in-Chief, Mount Sinai Hospital, Toronto

DAVID J. PIERSON, M.D.
Professor of Medicine, University of Washington School of Medicine; Medical Director of Respiratory Care, Harborview Medical Center, Seattle

JAMES J. PLORDE, M.D.
Professor of Medicine, Departments of Laboratory Medicine and Microbiology, University of Washington School of Medicine; Chief, Microbiology Laboratory, Seattle Veterans Administration Hospital, Seattle

STANLEY A. PLOTKIN, M.D.
Professor of Pediatrics and Microbiology, University of Pennsylvania; Chair, Division of Infectious Diseases, The Children's Hospital of Philadelphia, Philadelphia

FRANCIS A. PLUMMER, M.D., F.R.C.P.(C)
Associate Professor, Department of Medical Microbiology, University of Manitoba, Winnipeg

DANIEL K. PODOLSKY, M.D.
Associate Professor of Medicine, Harvard Medical School; Chief, Gastrointestinal Unit, Massachusetts General Hospital, Boston

JOHN T. POTTS, Jr., M.D.
Jackson Professor of Clinical Medicine, Harvard Medical School; Chief of the General Medical Service, Massachusetts General Hospital, Boston

LAWRIE W. POWELL, M.D.
Professor of Medicine, University of Queensland; Physician, Royal Brisbane Hospital, Brisbane, Australia

DARWIN J. PROCKOP, M.D., Ph.D.
Professor and Chairman, Department of Biochemistry, Jefferson Medical College of Thomas Jefferson University; Director, Department of Biochemistry, Jefferson Institute of Molecular Medicine, Philadelphia

AMY PRUITT, M.D.
Assistant Professor of Neurology, Harvard Medical School; Associate Neurologist, Massachusetts General Hospital, Boston

PAUL G. RAMSEY, M.D.
Associate Professor and Associate Chairman, Department of Medicine, University of Washington School of Medicine, Seattle

JOEL M. RAPPEPORT, M.D.
Professor of Medicine, Yale University School of Medicine; Director, Bone Marrow Transplantation Program, Yale New Haven Hospital, New Haven

C. GEORGE RAY, M.D.
Professor, Departments of Pathology and Pediatrics, College of Medicine, The University of Arizona Health Sciences Center, Tucson

RICHARD C. REICHMAN, M.D.
Associate Professor of Medicine, Microbiology, and Immunology, The University of Rochester Medical Center, Rochester

HERBERT Y. REYNOLDS, M.D.
J. Lloyd Huck Professor of Medicine and Chairman, Department of Medicine, The Pennsylvania State University College of Medicine; University Hospital, The Milton S. Hershey Medical Center, Hershey

STUART RICH, M.D.
Associate Professor of Medicine and Chief, Section of Cardiology, University of Illinois College of Medicine, Chicago

EDWARD P. RICHARDSON Jr., M.D.
Bullard Professor of Neuropathology, Harvard Medical School; Senior Neurologist, Massachusetts General Hospital, Boston

GARY S. RICHARDSON, M.D.
Instructor in Medicine, Harvard Medical School; Associate Physician, Brigham and Women's Hospital, Boston

HAL B. RICHERSON, M.D.
Professor of Internal Medicine and Director, Allergy-Immunology Division, University of Iowa College of Medicine, Iowa City

JAMES M. RICHTER, M.D.
Assistant Professor of Medicine, Harvard Medical School; Chief, Gastrointestinal Clinic, Massachusetts General Hospital, Boston

S. CRAIG RISCH, M.D.
Professor of Psychiatry and Director of Clinical Research Programs, Emory University, Atlanta

R. PAUL ROBERTSON, M.D.
Professor of Medicine, Director of Clinical Research Center, and Director, Diabetes Center, University of Minnesota, Minneapolis

ALLAN R. RONALD, M.D.
H. E. Sellers Professor and Head, Department of Medicine, The University of Manitoba, Winnipeg

RICHARD K. ROOT, M.D.
Professor of Medicine, Department of Medicine, and Associate Dean for Clinical Education, School of Medicine, University of California, San Francisco

ALLAN H. ROPPER, M.D.
Associate Professor of Neurology, Harvard Medical School; Associate Neurologist and Director of Neurological/Neurosurgical Intensive Care Unit, Massachusetts General Hospital, Boston

IRWIN H. ROSENBERG, M.D.
Professor of Medicine, Nutrition, and Physiology, Tufts University School of Medicine; Director, USDA Human Nutrition Research Center on Aging, Tufts University, Boston

LEON E. ROSENBERG, M.D.
Dean and C.N.H. Long Professor of Human Genetics, Medicine, and Pediatrics, Yale University School of Medicine, New Haven

DANIEL ROTROSEN, M.D.
Bacterial Diseases Section, National Institute of Allergy and Infectious Diseases, National Institutes of Health, Bethesda

JODI ROY, M.S., R.D.
Frances Stern Nutrition Center, New England Medical Center Hospital, Boston

ARTHUR H. RUBENSTEIN, M.D.
Professor and Chairman, Department of Medicine, University of Chicago Pritzker School of Medicine, Chicago

JEREMY N. RUSKIN, M.D.
Associate Professor of Medicine, Harvard Medical School; Director of Cardiac Arrhythmia Service, Massachusetts General Hospital, Boston

ARTHUR I. SAGALOWSKY, M.D.
Professor of Urology and Director of Renal Transplantation, The University of Texas Southwestern Medical Center, Dallas

JAY P. SANFORD, M.D.
President and Dean, Uniformed Services University of the Health Sciences, Bethesda

DENNIS R. SCHABERG, M.D.
Professor of Internal Medicine, The University of Michigan Medical School, Ann Arbor

I. HERBERT SCHEINBERG, M.D.
Professor of Medicine and Head, Division of Genetic Medicine, Albert Einstein College of Medicine; Attending Physician, Hospital of the Albert Einstein College of Medicine, New York

ALAN L. SCHILLER, M.D.
Irene Heinz Given and John LaPorte Given Professor and Chairman of Pathology, The Mount Sinai School of Medicine, New York

R. NEIL SCHIMKE, M.D.
Professor of Pediatrics and Internal Medicine and Director, Division of Metabolism, Endocrinology, and Genetics, The University of Kansas College of Health Sciences, Kansas City

RUDI SCHMID, M.D., Ph.D.
Professor of Medicine and Associate Dean, University of California, San Francisco

ROBERT T. SCHOOLEY, M.D.
Associate Professor of Medicine, Harvard Medical School; Assistant Physician, Infectious Disease Unit, Department of Medicine, Massachusetts General Hospital, Boston

ROBERT W. SCHRIER, M.D.
Professor and Chairman, Department of Medicine, University of Colorado School of Medicine, Denver

JOHN S. SCHROEDER, M.D.
Professor of Medicine, Cardiology Division, Stanford University School of Medicine; Stanford University Medical Center, Stanford

MARC A. SCHUCKIT, M.D.
Professor of Psychiatry, School of Medicine, University of California at San Diego; Director, Alcohol Research Center, San Diego Veterans Administration Medical Center, La Jolla

PETER H. SCHUR, M.D.
Professor of Medicine, Department of Rheumatology, Brigham and Women's Hospital, Boston

DAVID S. SEGAL, Ph.D.
Professor of Psychiatry, School of Medicine, University of California at San Diego, La Jolla

JULIAN L. SEIFTER, M.D.
Assistant Professor of Medicine, Harvard Medical School; Associate Physician, Brigham and Women's Hospital, Boston

ANDREW P. SELWYN, M.D.
Associate Professor of Medicine, Harvard Medical School; Director of Cardiac Catheterization, Brigham and Women's Hospital, Boston

BHAGWAN T. SHAHANI, M.B., B.S.
Associate Professor of Neurology, Harvard Medical School; Associate Neurologist, Massachusetts General Hospital, Boston

GORDON C. SHARP, M.D.
Department of Medicine, Division of Immunology and Rheumatology, University of Missouri-Columbia School of Medicine, Columbia

ELIZABETH M. SHORT, M.D.
Director, Division of Biomedical Research and Faculty Development, American Association of Medical Colleges, Washington, D.C.

WILLIAM SILEN, M.D.
Johnson and Johnson Professor of Surgery, Harvard Medical School; Surgeon-in-Chief, Beth Israel Hospital, Boston

FRED E. SILVERSTEIN, M.D.
Professor of Medicine, Director, Gastrointestinal Endoscopy, Division of Gastroenterology, University of Washington School of Medicine, Seattle

THOMAS L. SLAMOWITZ, M.D.
Vice Chairman of Ophthalmology and Associate Professor of Ophthalmology and Neuroophthalmology, Albert Einstein College/Montefiore Medical Center, New York

JAMES B. SNOW, Jr., M.D.
Director, National Institute on Deafness and Other Communication Disorders, National Institutes of Health, Bethesda

ARTHUR SOBER, M.D.
Associate Professor of Dermatology, Harvard Medical School; Associate Chief of Dermatology, Massachusetts General Hospital, Boston

FRANK E. SPEIZER, M.D.
Professor of Medicine, Harvard Medical School; Co-Director, Channing Laboratory, Brigham and Women's Hospital, Boston

WALTER E. STAMM, M.D.
Professor of Medicine, University of Washington School of Medicine; Head, Division of Infectious Diseases, Harborview Medical Center, Seattle

ALLEN C. STEERE, M.D.
Professor of Medicine and Chief, Division of Rheumatology, Department of Medicine, Tufts University School of Medicine, Boston, Massachusetts

ROBERT S. STERN, M.D.
Associate Professor of Dermatology, Harvard Medical School; Beth Israel Hospital, Boston

CHARLES F. STEVENS, M.D., Ph.D.
Professor of Molecular Neurobiology, Salk Institute, La Jolla

GENE H. STOLLERMAN, M.D.
Professor of Medicine, Boston University School of Medicine; Clinical Director, Bedford Division of The Geriatric Research, Educational, and Clinical Center, Veterans Administration Medical Center, Bedford

DAVID H.P. STREETEN, M.B., D. Phil, F.R.C.P.
Professor of Medicine and Head, Section of Endocrinology, State University of New York Upstate Health Science Center, Syracuse

NEIL A. SWANSON, M.D.
Professor of Dermatology, Otolaryngology, and Surgery (Plastic), Division of Plastic Surgery, Oregon Health Sciences University, Portland

ROBERT A. SWERLICK, M.D.
Department of Dermatology, Emory University School of Medicine, Atlanta

RUP TANDAN, M.D., M.R.C.P.
Assistant Professor, Department of Neurology, University of Vermont College of Medicine, Burlington

JOEL D. TAUROG, M.D.
Assistant Professor, The University of Texas Southwestern Medical Center; Southwestern Medical School, Dallas

E. DONNALL THOMAS, M.D.
Professor of Medicine, University of Washington School of Medicine; Member, Fred Hutchinson Cancer Research Center, Seattle

PHILLIP P. TOSKES, M.D.
Professor of Medicine and Chief, Division of Gastroenterology, University of Florida College of Medicine, Gainesville

MARVIN TURCK, M.D.
Professor of Medicine, University of Washington School of Medicine, Seattle

DAVID VALLE, M.D.
Professor of Pediatrics and Molecular Virology and Genetics, Johns Hopkins University School of Medicine; Investigator, Howard Hughes Medical Institute, Baltimore

MAURICE VICTOR, M.D.
Professor of Medicine (Neurology), Dartmouth Medical School, Hanover

DAVID C. WAAGNER, M.D.
Assistant Professor of Pediatrics, Department of Pediatrics, The University of Texas Health Sciences Center, Houston

JAMES F. WALLACE, M.D.
Professor of Medicine, University of Washington School of Medicine; Associate Physician-in-Chief, University Hospital, Seattle

PETER D. WALZER, M.D.
Associate Professor of Medicine, University of Cincinnati College of Medicine; Chief, Infectious Disease Service, Cincinnati Veterans Administration Medical Center, Cincinnati

JACK R. WANDS, M.D.
Associate Professor of Medicine, Harvard Medical School; Molecular Hepatology Laboratory, Cancer Center, Massachusetts General Hospital, Charlestown

LEONARD WARTOFSKY, M.D.
Professor of Medicine and Physiology, Uniformed Services University of the Health Sciences, Bethesda; Chief of Endocrinology and Metabolism, Walter Reed Army Medical Center, Washington, D.C.

STEVEN E. WEINBERGER, M.D.
Associate Professor of Medicine, Harvard Medical School; Clinical Director, Pulmonary Unit, Beth Israel Hospital, Boston

NICHOLAS J. WHITE, M.D., M.R.C.P.
Tropical Medicine Unit, Nuffield Department of Clinical Medicine, Oxford University, England; Faculty of Tropical Medicine, Mahidol University, Bangkok, Thailand

RICHARD J. WHITLEY, M.D.
Professor of Pediatrics, Microbiology, and Medicine, Department of Pediatrics, School of Medicine, The University of Alabama at Birmingham, Birmingham

GRANT R. WILKINSON, M.D.
Professor of Pharmacology, Vanderbilt University School of Medicine, Nashville

GORDON H. WILLIAMS, M.D.
Professor of Medicine, Harvard Medical School; Chief, Endocrine-Hypertension Division, Brigham and Women's Hospital, Boston

LEWIS T. WILLIAMS, Jr., M.D., Ph.D.
Associate Professor of Medicine, University of California at San Francisco School of Medicine; Cardiovascular Research Institute, Howard Hughes Medical Institute, San Francisco

JEAN D. WILSON, M.D.
Professor of Internal Medicine, The University of Texas Southwestern Medical Center, Dallas

BRUCE U. WINTROUB, M.D.
Professor and Chairman, Department of Dermatology, University of California, San Francisco

SHELDON M. WOLFF, M.D.
Endiocott Professor and Chairman, Department of Medicine, Tufts University School of Medicine; New England Medical Center, Boston

ALASTAIR J.J. WOOD, M.B., Ch.B., F.R.C.P. (Edin)
Professor of Medicine and Professor of Pharmacology, Vanderbilt University School of Medicine; Attending Physician, Vanderbilt University Hospital, Nashville

THEODORE E. WOODWARD, M.D.
Professor of Medicine Emeritus, University of Maryland School of Medicine, Baltimore

SHIRLEY H. WRAY, M.D., Ph.D., F.R.C.P.
Associate Professor of Neurology, Harvard Medical School; Director, Unit for Neurovisual Disorders, Department of Neurology, Massachusetts General Hospital, Boston

JOSHUA WYNNE, M.D.
Professor of Internal Medicine and Chief, Division of Cardiology, Wayne State University School of Medicine; Chief, Section of Cardiology, Harper Grace Hospitals, Detroit

KIM B. YANCEY, M.D.
Department of Dermatology, Uniformed Services University of the Health Sciences, Bethesda

JAMES B. YOUNG, M.D.
Associate Professor of Medicine, Harvard Medical School; Associate Physician, Beth Israel Hospital, Boston

PREFACE

In the twelfth edition of *Harrison's Principles of Internal Medicine* the editors have again attempted to incorporate the latest advances in the biology, pathophysiology, diagnosis, and treatment of disease and simultaneously to build appropriate bridges between the basic sciences and clinical medicine and emphasize the advances in medical science while retaining those facts which, while not new, remain clinically useful. Although in a preface we cannot describe all of the new and extensively updated parts of the eleventh edition, we would like to call the reader's attention to several of these:

"Introduction to Clinical Medicine" contains articles on the practice of medicine, clinical reasoning, cost awareness in medicine, and geriatric medicine.

"The Biological Basis of Disease," Part One, has been expanded and given added emphasis as the text's first major topic. It focuses on disorders affecting multiple organ systems, especially genetic diseases and disturbances of the immune system. The section provides more detailed coverage of cell growth and regulation with new chapters on normal cell growth and growth factors and on cell membranes and their receptors.

Now Part Two, "Cardinal Manifestations of Disease" remains a mainstay of this edition and serves as a comprehensive introduction to clinical medicine. Major patient symptoms, reviewed by organ system, are correlated with specific disease states—the basis of differential diagnosis. The twelfth edition contains new or rewritten chapters on chills and fever, visual disturbances, assessment of patients with disorders of cognition, disorders of sleep and circadian rhythm, prevention of cardiovascular collapse and death, and management of the resuscitated patient. The section on skin disease has been completely reorganized.

Part Three, "Clinical Pharmacology," and Part Four, "Nutrition," also have been reorganized. Chapters on clinical pharmacology review the fundamentals of clinical pharmacokinetics and individualized drug therapy. Up-to-date coverage of the physiology and pharmacology of the autonomic nervous system explores its key role in many disease states and the various ways in which drugs interact with this system. Included here as well is a new chapter on cyclic AMP and cellular messengers that work through G proteins.

Coverage of nutrition in clinical medicine encompasses nutritional requirements, the assessment of nutritional status, eating disorders such as anorexia nervosa, bulimia, and obesity, vitamin deficiency and excess, and disturbances in trace element metabolism. New discussions are featured on diet therapy and enteral and parenteral nutrition.

A primarily etiologically oriented review, Part Five, "Infectious Disease," details the latest approaches to the diagnosis, prevention, and treatment of bacterial, viral, and fungal infections and parasitic infestations. A new section focusing on commonly encountered clinical syndromes reviews septicemia and septic shock, infectious endocarditis, localized infections and abscesses, acute infectious diarrheal diseases, sexually transmitted diseases, pelvic inflammatory disease, acute urinary tract infections, infectious arthritis and osteomyelitis, and animal bite and scratch infections. Chapters on the treatment of bacterial, viral, mycotic, and parasitic infections have been grouped together and follow the section on the syndromic approach to infectious diseases.

In addition, a new chapter, "Infectious Diseases and the New Biology," accompanies major updates on host-microbe interactions, immunization, diphtheria, tetanus, botulism, meningococcal infections, salmonella infections, shigellosis, *Haemophilus* infections, cholera, Lyme disease, human retroviruses, Epstein-Barr virus, cytomegalovirus infection, leishmaniasis, trypanosomiasis, and filariasis.

"Disorders of the Organ Systems," the core of *Harrison's*, encompass Parts Six through Fourteen and include succinct accounts of the pathophysiology of major diseases—with emphasis on disease manifestations, diagnostic procedures, differential diagnosis, and treatment strategies. This comprehensive review of organ system disorders includes new chapters on therapeutic applications of cardiac catheterization, mechanical ventilatory support, endocrine tumors of the gastrointestinal tract and pancreas, cancer chemotherapy, breast cancer, benign and malignant skin lesions, gastrointestinal and pancreatic tumors, cognitive disorders, disorders of sleep and circadian rhythm, paraneoplastic diseases that affect the central nervous system, myasthenia gravis, and disorders of phosphorus and magnesium metabolism. Of particular note, the chapter on the acquired immunodeficiency syndrome has been expanded and revised to provide in-depth understanding of all aspects of this disease.

In the twelfth edition the comprehensive review of organ system disorders is complemented by a series of new chapters highlighting the impact of cellular and molecular biology on the understanding of cardiovascular, pulmonary, hematologic, renal, and neurologic disease. The impact of newer imaging techniques on diagnoses is described in chapters on the use of such techniques in diseases of the cardiovascular, pulmonary, hepatobiliary, and central nervous systems.

Finally Part Fifteen is an expanded and reorganized section on "Environmental and Occupational Hazards."

In organizing this edition of *Harrison's* the editors faced the special problem of the dual systems of laboratory nomenclature within the United States. Since July of 1988 virtually all medical journals throughout the world have utilized the International System (SI) of units for clinical laboratory values whereas most hospital laboratories in the United States use the conventional system of laboratory nomenclature. The net consequence is that the student of medicine uses one system in reading medical literature and another in dealing with patients. This dual system will probably be in operation for the indefinite future, and consequently we have decided to use both systems in the text, listing the SI units first and the conventional units in parentheses for all measurements except blood pressure, which is given only in millimeters of mercury, and for those measurements in which the numbers are the same for both systems (mmol/L or meq/L for sodium). In most instances the interconversion between SI and conventional units is straightforward. In other cases, however, the best way to convert from one system to the other is not always clearcut since there are different ways to express values in both. It is imperative that each reader consult his own laboratory for normal values. Perhaps the greatest potential danger inherent in the existence of the two systems is in the interpretation of plasma glucose and plasma calcium, but caution should be observed in the interpretation of all laboratory values.

In view of the requirements for continuing education for licensure and relicensure and of the emphasis on certification and recertification, a revision of the *PreTest Self-Assessment and Review* will appear with this edition. *PreTest Self-Assessment and Review* consists of several hundred questions based upon the textbook, along with answers and explanations for the answers. In addition, the *Companion Handbook* that was pioneered for the eleventh edition for use as a supplement to the text will be revised and updated.

One of the strengths of *Harrison's* is the close-knit relationships among the editors. Dr. Richard K. Root, Professor of Medicine and Associate Dean for Clinical Education at the University of California, San Francisco, worked together with Robert G. Petersdorf to edit the infectious disease coverage of the twelfth edition. We welcome Dr. Root as a valuable member of the editorial group.

We also wish to express our appreciation to our many associates and colleagues who as experts in their fields have helped us with constructive criticism and helpful suggestions: Raymond D. Adams, Carmen Allegra, Julian L. Ambrus, Jr., W. French Anderson, David

W. Bilheimer, Homer Boushey, George A. Bray, Barry M. Brenner, Neil A. Breslau, Michael S. Brown, William J. Burke, Harold A. Chapman, Allen W. Cheever, William W. Chin, Fred Cohen, Shaun Coughlin, George T. Curlin, Pat O. Daley, Richard T. Davey, Jr., Gregory J. Dehmer, Victor J. Dzau, Judith Falloon, Robert Fishman, Daniel W. Foster, Stephen Friend, Joseph L. Goldstein, Mark R. Green, James E. Griffin, Donald H. Harter, Jane E. Henney, Gary Hoffman, Allan Hunter, Steve Hyman, Roland H. Ingram, Jr., Seigo Izumo, Michael Jenike, Stephanie L. James, T. Scott Johnson, William S. Jordan, Jr., Lewis L. Judd, Robert E. Kalina, Robert Katzman, Joyce V. Kelly, Jeff Klein, Joseph A. Kovacs, Thomas J. Lawley, Robert S. Lebovics, John Leddy, Kenneth Luskey, James D. Marsh, Michael Matthay, Dale E. McFarlin, Steve McPhee, John Mendelsohn, John Mills, Eva J. Neer, Arthur W. Niehnuis, Frederick P. Ognibene, Steve Perkins, Dorothy Perloff, Stephen Petersdorf, Michael A. Polis, Herbert Y. Reynolds, William O. Robertson, Mark Rosenblum, Burton D. Rose, Daniel Rotrosen, Eugene H. Rubin, Walter Rubin, Kenneth Sack, Steven Schnittman, Christine E. Seidman, Julian Seifter, James H. Shelhamer, Gordon Strewler, Anthony F. Suffredini, Martin Tauber, Mark Taubman, Steven E. Weinberger, J. Woodrow Weiss, Scott Weiss, J.B. West, Peggy Wintroub, Daniel T. Wright, and Charles F. Zormuski.

This book could not have been edited without the dedicated help of our coworkers in the editorial offices of the individual editors. We are especially indebted to Patricia A. Clougherty, Hilda Gardner, Christy K. Gonzales, Brenda H. Hennis, Ann London, Joyce McKinney, Lucy A. Renzi, Kathryn A. Saxon, S. Horatio Slawson, Sandra Taylor, and Betsy Zickler.

Finally, we need to say a word of thanks to our colleagues at McGraw-Hill, J. Dereck Jeffers, Editor-in-Chief, and Stuart Boynton, Development Editor. They are an effective team who gave the editors constant encouragement and were of enormous help in the efforts involved in bringing this edition to fruition.

THE EDITORS

1 THE PRACTICE OF MEDICINE

THE EDITORS

WHAT IS EXPECTED OF THE PHYSICIAN The practice of medicine combines both science and art. The role of science in medicine is clear. Technology based on science is the foundation for the solution to many clinical problems; the dazzling advances in biochemical methodology and in biophysical imaging techniques that allow access to the remotest recesses of the body are the products of science. So too are the therapeutic maneuvers which increasingly are a major part of medical practice. Yet skill in the most sophisticated application of laboratory technology or the use of the latest therapeutic modality alone does not make a good physician. The ability to extract from a mass of contradictory physical signs and from the crowded computer printouts of laboratory data those items that are of crucial significance, to know in a difficult case whether to "treat" or to "watch," to determine when a clinical clue is worth pursuing or when to dismiss it as a "red herring," and to estimate in any given patient whether a proposed treatment entails a greater risk than the disease are all involved in the decisions which the clinician, skilled in the practice of medicine, must make many times each day. This combination of medical knowledge, intuition, and judgment is termed the *art of medicine*. It is as necessary to the practice of medicine as a sound scientific base.

The editors of the first edition of this book defined what is expected of the physician. Their words ring as true now as they did then.

No greater opportunity, responsibility, or obligation can fall to the lot of a human being than to become a physician. In the care of the suffering he needs technical skill, scientific knowledge, and human understanding. He who uses these with courage, with humility, and with wisdom will provide a unique service for his fellow man, and will build an enduring edifice of character within himself. The physician should ask of his destiny no more than this; he should be content with no less.

Tact, sympathy and understanding are expected of the physician, for the patient is no mere collection of symptoms, signs, disordered functions, damaged organs, and disturbed emotions. He is human, fearful, and hopeful, seeking relief, help and reassurance. To the physician, as to the anthropologist, nothing human is strange or repulsive. The misanthrope may become a smart diagnostician of organic disease, but he can scarcely hope to succeed as a physician. The true physician has a Shakespearean breadth of interest in the wise and the foolish, the proud and the humble, the stoic hero and the whining rogue. He cares for people.

THE PATIENT-PHYSICIAN RELATIONSHIP It may be trite to emphasize that physicians need to approach patients not as "cases" or "diseases" but as individuals whose problems all too often transcend the complaints which bring them to the doctor. Most patients are anxious and frightened. Often they go to great ends to convince themselves that illness does not exist, or unconsciously they set up elaborate defenses to divert attention from the real problem that they perceive to be serious or life-threatening. Some patients use illness to gain attention or to serve as a crutch to extricate themselves from an emotionally stressful situation; some even feign physical illness. Whatever the patient's attitude, the physician needs to consider the terrain in which an illness occurs—in terms not only of the patients themselves but also of their families and social backgrounds. All too often medical workups and records fail to include essential information about the patient's origins, schooling, job, home and family, hopes and fears. Without this knowledge it is difficult for the physician to gain rapport with the patient or to develop insight into the patient's illness. Such a relationship must be based on thorough knowledge of the patient and on mutual trust and the ability to communicate with one another.

The direct, one-to-one patient-physician relationship which traditionally has characterized the practice of medicine is changing, primarily because of the changing setting in which medicine is being practiced. Often the management of the individual patient requires the active participation of a variety of trained professional personnel as well as several physicians. In most instances, health care is a team effort. The patient can benefit greatly from such collaboration, but it is the duty of the primary physician to guide the patient through an illness. To carry out this increasingly difficult task, this physician must have some familiarity with the techniques, skills, and objectives of specialist physicians as well as colleagues in the fields allied to medicine. In giving the patient an opportunity to receive all the benefits of the important advances of science, the primary physician must, in the last analysis, retain responsibility for the major decisions concerning diagnosis and treatment.

Increasingly, patients are cared for by groups of physicians, clinics, hospitals, or health-maintenance organizations (HMOs) rather than by individual independent practitioners. There are many potential advantages in the use of such organized medical groups, but there are also drawbacks, the chief of which is a loss of the concept of a physician who is primarily and continuously responsible for the patient. It is essential, even in the group setting, that each patient have a physician who has an overview of the patient's problems and who maintains familiarity with the patient's reaction to his or her illness, to the drugs given, and to the challenges of daily living that the patient faces. Moreover, because a number of physicians may, at any one time, contribute to the care of a particular patient, accurate and detailed medical records are essential to patient care.

The modern hospital poses a particularly intimidating environment for most patients. Lying in a bed surrounded by air jets, buttons, and lights; invaded by tubes and wires; beset by the numerous members of the health care team—nurses, nurses' aides, physicians' assistants, social workers, technologists, physical therapists, medical students, house officers, attending and consulting physicians, and many others; transported to special laboratories and x-ray chambers replete with machines with blinking lights and strange sounds, it is little wonder that patients lose their sense of reality. In fact, the physician is often the only tenuous link between the patient and the real world. A strong personal relationship with the physician is essential in order to sustain the patient in such a stressful situation.

Many influences in contemporary society have the potential of leading to the impersonalization of medical care. Some of these have been mentioned already and include (1) vigorous efforts to reduce the escalating costs of health care; (2) the increasing reliance on technologic advances and computerization for many aspects of diagnosis and treatment; (3) the increased geographic mobility of both patients and physicians; (4) the growing number of "closed-system" arrangements, such as health maintenance organizations, in which the patient has little if any choice in selecting a physician; (5) the need for more than a single physician to be involved in the care of most patients who are seriously ill; and (6) an increasing reliance by patients on legal means to express their disappointments with the health care system (i.e., by malpractice litigation). Given these changes in the medical care system, maintaining the humane aspects of medical care and the empathetic qualities of the physician is a particular challenge. It is now more important than ever that the physician consider each patient to be a unique individual deserving of humane treatment, regardless of personal or financial circumstances.

The American Board of Internal Medicine has defined humanistic qualities as encompassing integrity, respect, and compassion. Availability, the expression of sincere concern, the willingness to take the time to explain all aspects of the patient's illness, and an attitude of being nonjudgmental with patients who have lifestyles, attitudes, and values different from those of the physician and which he or she may in some instances even find repugnant are just a few of the characteristics of the humane physician. Every physician will, at times, be challenged by patients who evoke strongly negative (and occasionally strongly positive) emotional responses. Physicians should be alert to their own reactions to such patients and situations and consciously monitor and control their behavior so that the patients' best interests remain the principal motivation for their actions at all times.

The famous statement of Dr. Francis Peabody is even more relevant today than when delivered more than a half century ago:

The significance of the intimate personal relationship between physician and patient cannot be too strongly emphasized, for in an extraordinarily large number of cases both the diagnosis and treatment are directly dependent on it. One of the essential qualities of the clinician is interest in humanity, for the secret of the care of the patient is in caring for the patient.

CLINICAL SKILLS   **History taking**   The written history of an illness should embody all the facts of medical significance in the life of the patient. If the history is recorded in chronologic order, recent events should be given the most attention. Likewise, if a problem-oriented approach is used, the problems that are clinically dominant should be listed first. Ideally, the narration of symptoms or problems should be in the patient's own words. However, few patients have sufficient powers of observation or recall to give a history without some guidance from the physician, who must be careful not to suggest the answers to the questions being posed. Often a symptom which has concerned a patient has little significance, while a seemingly minor complaint may be of considerable importance. Therefore, the physician must be constantly alert to the possibility that any event related by the patient, however trivial or apparently remote, may be the key to the solution of the medical problem.

An informative history is more than an orderly listing of symptoms. Something is always gained by listening to patients and noting the way in which they talk about their symptoms. Inflections of voice, facial expression, and attitude may betray important clues to the meaning of the symptoms to the patient. In listening to the history, the physician discovers not only something about the disease but also something about the patient.

With experience, the pitfalls of history taking become apparent. What patients relate for the most part consists of subjective phenomena colored by past experience. Patients obviously differ widely in their responses to the same stimuli and in their coping mechanisms. Their attitudes are variably influenced by fear of disability and death and by concern over the consequences of their illness to their families. Sometimes the accuracy of the history is affected by language or sociologic barriers, by failing intellectual powers that interfere with recall, or by disorders of consciousness that make them unaware of their illness. It is not surprising, then, that even the most careful physician may at times despair of collecting factual data and be forced to proceed with evidence that represents little more than an approximation of the truth. It is in obtaining the history that the physician's skill, knowledge, and experience are most clearly in evidence.

The family history serves several functions. First, in rare single-gene defects a positive family history of a similarly affected individual or a history of consanguinity may have important diagnostic implications. Second, in diseases of multifactorial etiology that have a familial aggregation, it may be possible to identify patients at risk for disease and to intervene prior to development of overt manifestations. For example, recent weight gain may be a more ominous development in a woman who has a family history of diabetes than in one who does not. In certain situations the family history has major implications for preventive medicine. When a diagnosis of a hereditary condition known to predispose to cancer is made, it is the physician's obligation to follow up this possibility carefully in the patient, to survey the family, and to educate them about the need for long-term follow-up.

However accurate and complete, the medical history does much more than provide facts of critical importance. The very act of taking the history provides the physician with the opportunity to establish or enhance the unique bond that is the basis for the critically important patient-physician relationship. An effort should be made to place the patient at ease, regardless of the circumstances of the encounter. The patient should, at some point, have the opportunity to tell his or her own story of the illness without frequent interruption and, when appropriate, should receive expression of interest, encouragement, and empathy from the physician. It is often enlightening to develop an appreciation of the patient's own perception of the illness, the patient's expectations of the physician and the medical care system, and the financial and social implications of the illness to the patient. The confidentiality of the patient-physician relationship should be emphasized, and the patient should be given the opportunity to identify those aspects of the history which he or she wishes not to be disclosed to anyone else.

Physical examination   Physical signs are the objective and verifiable marks of disease and represent solid, indisputable facts. Their significance is enhanced when they confirm a functional or structural change already suggested by the patient's history. At times, the physical signs may be the only evidence of disease, especially when the history has been inconsistent, confused, or lacking altogether.

The physical examination should be performed methodically and thoroughly, with due regard for the patient's comfort and modesty. Although attention has often been directed by the history to the diseased organ or part of the body, the examination must extend from head to toe in an objective search for abnormalities. Unless the examination procedure is systematic, important parts of it may be omitted, a common error even among the most skilled clinicians. The results of the examination, like the details of the history, should be recorded at the time they are elicited, not hours later when they are subject to the distortions of memory. Many inaccuracies stem from the careless practice of writing or dictating notes long after the examination has been concluded. Skill in physical diagnosis is acquired with experience, but it is not merely technique that determines success in eliciting signs. The detection of a few scattered petechiae, a faint diastolic murmur, or a small mass in the abdomen is not a question of keener eyes and ears or more sensitive fingers but of a mind alert to these findings. Skill in physical diagnosis reflects a way of thinking more than a way of doing. Physical findings are subject to change. Just because the examination is normal on one occasion does not guarantee that this will be the case on subsequent examinations. Likewise, abnormal findings may disappear in the course of illness. It is important, therefore, to repeat the physical examination as frequently as the clinical situation warrants.

Laboratory tests   The increase in the number and availability of laboratory tests has resulted in increasing reliance on these studies in the solution of clinical problems. It is essential, however, to bear in mind the limitations of such procedures, which by virtue of their impersonal quality and complexity often gain an aura of authority regardless of the fallibility of the tests themselves, of the individuals doing or interpreting them, or of their instruments. More importantly, the accumulation of laboratory data cannot relieve the physician from the responsibility of careful observation and study of the patient. Physicians also must weigh carefully the hazards and the expense involved in the laboratory procedures they order. Moreover, laboratory tests are rarely ordered and reported singly. Rather, they are produced as "batteries." Some laboratories now perform batteries of 24 and even 40 tests. The various combinations of laboratory tests are often useful. For example, they may provide the clue to such nonspecific symptoms as generalized weakness and increased fatigability by revealing abnormalities of hepatic function together with elevated levels of serum IgG which, in turn, would suggest the diagnosis of chronic liver disease. Sometimes a single abnormality, such as an elevated serum calcium, points to a specific disease, such as hyperparathyroidism.

The thoughtful use of screening tests should not be confused with indiscriminate laboratory testing. The use of screening tests is based on the fact that a group of laboratory determinations can be carried out conveniently on a single specimen of blood at relatively low cost. Biochemical measurements, together with simple laboratory examinations such as blood count, urinalysis, and sedimentation rate, often provide the major clue to the presence of a pathologic process. At the same time the physician must learn to evaluate occasional abnormalities among the screening tests that may not necessarily connote significant disease. There is nothing more wasteful and unproductive than an in-depth workup following a report of an isolated laboratory abnormality in a patient who is otherwise well. Among the more than 40 tests that are performed on many patients, one is often slightly abnormal. If there is no suspicion of an underlying illness, the test is ordinarily repeated to ensure that the abnormality does not represent a laboratory error. If the abnormality is confirmed it is important to distinguish a minor one (less than two standard deviations) from a major one (more than two standard deviations). Even in the case of the latter, the decision of whether to proceed with further workup is a test of the physician's clinical judgment.

Imaging techniques   The past two decades have seen the arrival of ultrasonography, a variety of scans that employ isotopes to visualize organs heretofore inaccessible, computed tomography with its varying permutations, magnetic resonance imaging, and position emission tomography. Aside from opening up new diagnostic vistas, this new technology benefits patients because it has frequently supplanted invasive techniques that require surgical biopsy or the insertion of tubes, wires, or catheters into the body—procedures that are often painful and sometimes risky. While the enthusiasm for noninvasive technology is understandably justified, all too often the results of these tests have not been validated properly before they are disseminated as clinical dogma. Moreover, the expense entailed in performing these imaging tests is often substantial and is not always considered when ordering them. There is no question that computed tomography has led to new insights into the problem of adrenal tumors, just as routine measurement of calcium caused a redefinition of hyperparathyroidism. Nevertheless, these examinations should be used judiciously, preferably in lieu of, not in addition to, the invasive maneuvers they are meant to replace.

THE DIAGNOSIS OF DISEASE   Clinical diagnosis requires both aspects of logic—analysis and synthesis—and the more difficult the clinical problem, the more important is a logical approach to it. Such an approach requires that the physician list carefully each problem suggested by the symptoms and physical and laboratory findings and seek answers to each. Most physicians attempt consciously or unconsciously to fit a given problem into one of a series of syndromes. *The syndrome is a group of symptoms and signs of disordered function, related to one another by means of some anatomic, physiologic, or biochemical peculiarity.* It embodies a hypothesis concerning the deranged function of an organ, organ system, or tissue. Congestive heart failure, Cushing's syndrome, and dementia

are examples. In congestive heart failure, dyspnea, orthopnea, cyanosis, dependent edema, engorged neck veins, pleural effusion, rales, and hepatomegaly are known to be connected by a single pathophysiologic mechanism—insufficiency of the cardiac pump mechanism. In Cushing's syndrome, moon facies, hypertension, diabetes mellitus, and osteoporosis are recognized effects of excess glucocorticoids acting on many target organs. In dementia, deterioration of memory, incoherent thinking, impaired language functions, visual-spatial disorientation, and faulty judgment are related to destruction of the association areas of the cerebrum.

A syndrome usually does not identify the precise cause of an illness, but it narrows the number of possibilities and often suggests certain special clinical and laboratory studies. The derangements of each organ system in humans are reducible to a relatively small number of syndromes. The diagnosis is simplified greatly if a clinical problem conforms neatly to a well-defined syndrome, because only a few diseases need to be considered in the differential diagnosis. In contrast, the search for the cause of an illness that does not conform to a syndrome is more difficult because a much greater number of diseases have to be considered. Even here an orderly approach which proceeds from symptom to sign to laboratory findings will usually result in the diagnosis.

CARING FOR THE PATIENT   Patient care begins with the development of a personal relationship between the patient and the physician. In the absence of a sense of trust and confidence on the part of the patient, the effectiveness of most therapeutic measures is diminished. In many instances, when there is confidence in the physician, reassurance is the best treatment and is all that is needed. Likewise, in those cases that do not lend themselves to easy solutions and for which no effective treatment is available, a feeling on the part of the patient that the physician is doing all that is possible is one of the most important therapeutic measures that can be provided. An important aspect of clinical decision making and patient care involves the "quality of life," a subjective assessment of what each patient values most. Such an assessment requires detailed, sometimes intimate knowledge of the patient, which can usually be obtained only through deliberate, unhurried, and often repeated conversation. In situations where complete freedom from signs and symptoms of disease is impossible, enhancement of the quality of life is the major goal of therapy.

Drug therapy   With each succeeding year, more drugs are released, every one with the hope and the promise that it is an improvement over its predecessor. Although the pharmaceutical industry must be given most of the credit for advances in drug therapy, it is also true that many new drugs have only a marginal advantage over the agents they are aimed to replace. The barrage of new information with which practitioners are deluged does little to provide a clear picture of clinical pharmacology; on the contrary, to most physicians new drugs are confusing. With some exceptions, however, the approach to a new drug should be one of caution. Unless the new agent is established beyond doubt to be a real advance, it is wiser to use well-tested and well-established agents which are efficacious and whose safety is well established.

Iatrogenic disorders   An iatrogenic disorder occurs when the deleterious effects of a therapeutic or diagnostic regimen produce pathology independent of the condition for which the regimen is given. No matter what the clinical situation, it is the responsibility of the physician to use powerful therapeutic measures wisely, with due regard to their action, potential dangers, and cost. Every medical procedure, whether diagnostic or therapeutic, has the potential for harm, but it would be impossible to afford the patient the benefits of modern scientific medicine if reasonable steps in diagnosis and therapy were withheld because of possible risks. "Reasonable" implies that the physician has weighed the pros and cons of a procedure and has concluded that it is advisable or essential for the relief of discomfort or the cure or amelioration of disease. For example, the use of glucocorticoids to arrest progressive systemic lupus erythematosus may produce Cushing's syndrome. In this instance, the benefits usually exceed the untoward side effects. However, much harm can result when the deleterious effects of a procedure or a drug exceed any possible advantages that might have been anticipated. Examples include the dangerous or fatal drug reactions that occasionally follow the use of antibiotics given for trivial respiratory infections, the gastric hemorrhage or perforation caused by glucocorticoid administration for mild arthritis, or the occurrence of fatal hepatitis that may follow needless transfusions of blood or plasma.

But the harm that a physician can do to a patient is not limited to the imprudent use of medication or procedures. Equally important are ill-considered or unjustified remarks. Many a patient has developed a cardiac neurosis because the physician ventured a grave prognosis on the basis of a misinterpreted noninvasive cardiac examination. Not only the treatment itself but the physician's words and behavior are capable of causing injury.

The physician must never become so absorbed in the disease as to forget the patient who is its victim. As the science of medicine advances, it is all too easy to become so fascinated by the manifestations of disease that the ailing person's fears and concerns about suffering and death, job and family, the cost of medical care, and the specter of economic insecurity are disregarded. Treatment of a patient consists of more than the dispassionate confrontation of a disease. It embodies also the exercise of warmth, compassion, and understanding.

Informed consent In an era of rapidly advancing technology, patients will require diagnostic and therapeutic procedures that are painful and that pose some risk. These include all surgical procedures, e.g., biopsies of tissues, endoscopy, radiographic maneuvers involving the insertion of catheters, and many others. In most hospitals and clinics, patients undergoing such procedures are required to sign a form consenting to them. More important, however, is the notion that the patient must understand clearly the risk entailed in these procedures; this is the definition of *informed consent*. It is incumbent upon the physician to explain to the patient, in a clearly understandable fashion, the procedures which he or she faces. By doing this conscientiously much of the dread of the unknown that is inherent in hospitalization will be mitigated.

Accountability Throughout the world physicians, once licensed to practice medicine, have not had to account for their actions except to their peers. In the United States, however, during the past two decades, there have been increasing demands for physicians to account for the way in which they practice medicine by meeting certain standards prescribed by federal and state governments. The hospitalization of patients whose health care is reimbursed by the government (Medicare and Medicaid) and other third parties is subjected to utilization review. This means that the physician must defend the cause for and duration of a patient's hospitalization if it falls outside certain "average" standards. In some instances a second opinion is necessary before a patient can have elective surgery. The purpose of these regulations is to contain spiraling health care costs. It is likely that this type of review will be extended to all phases of medical practice and will alter the practice of medicine even more profoundly.

Physicians also may be expected to give account of their continuing competence by mandatory continuing education, patient record audit, recertification by examination (time-limited certification), or relicensing. While these measures probably enhance the physician's factual knowledge, there is no evidence that they have a similar effect on the quality of practice.

Cost-effectiveness in medical care As the cost of medical care continues to rise, it has become necessary to establish stringent priorities in the expenditure of money for health care. In some instances, preventive measures offer the greatest return for the expenditure; outstanding examples include vaccination, immunization, reduction in accidents and occupational hazards, improved environmental control, and biochemical screening of newborns. For example, the detection of phenylketonuria by newborn screening may result in a net saving of many thousands of dollars.

As resources become more and more constrained, it will be necessary to weigh the justification of performing costly operations that provide only a limited life expectancy against the pressing need for more primary care for those persons who do not have adequate access to medical services. At the level of the individual patient it is important to minimize costly hospital admissions as far as possible, if total health care is to be provided at a cost that most can afford. This, of course, implies and depends upon a close cooperative effort between patients, their physicians, their employers, third-party carriers, and government, along with constant surveillance of those types of procedures that can be conducted safely and effectively on an ambulatory basis. Equally important in reducing total health care expenditures is the need for individual physicians to monitor both the cost and effectiveness of the drugs they prescribe. In the last analysis the medical profession should provide leadership and guidance to the public in matters of cost control, and physicians must take this responsibility seriously without being or seeming to be self-serving. It is important, however, that the socioeconomic aspects of health care delivery not be permitted to interfere with the concern of physicians for the welfare of their patients. The patient must be able to rely on the individual physician as his or her principal advocate in matters of health care.

Research and teaching The title "doctor" is derived from the Latin *docere*, "to teach," and the physician should share information and medical knowledge with others and be willing to teach what he or she has learned to colleagues as well as to students of medicine and related professions. The practice of medicine is dependent on the sum total of medical knowledge, which in turn is based on an unending chain of scientific discovery, clinical observation, analysis, and interpretation. Advances in medicine depend on the acquisition of new information, i.e., on research, which must often involve patients; improved medical care requires the transmission of this information. As part of broader societal responsibilities, the physician should encourage patients to participate in ethical and properly approved clinical investigations if they do not impose undue hazard, discomfort, or inconvenience.

Incurability and death No problem is more distressing than that presented by the patient with an incurable disease, particularly when premature death is inevitable. What should the patient and family be told, what measures should be taken to maintain life, and how is death to be defined?

Although some would argue otherwise, there is no ironclad rule that the patient must immediately be told "everything," even if the patient is an adult and the head of a family. How much the patient is told should depend upon the patient's ability and capacity to deal with the possibility of imminent death; often this capacity grows with time and, whenever possible, gradual rather than abrupt disclosure is the best strategy. This decision may also take into consideration the patient's religious beliefs, financial and business status, and to some extent the wishes of the family. The patient must be given an opportunity to talk with the physician and ask questions. Patients may find it easier to share their feelings about death with their physician, who is likely to be more objective and less emotional than family members.

One thing is certain; it is not for you to don the black cap and, assuming the judicial function, take hope away from any patient . . . hope that comes to us all.

William Osler

Even when the patient directly inquires, "Doctor, am I dying?" the physician must attempt to determine whether this is a request for information, a demand for reassurance, or even an expression of hostility. Most would agree that only open communication between the patient and the physician can resolve these questions and guide the physician in what to say and how to say it.

The physician should provide or arrange for emotional, physical, and spiritual support and must be compassionate, unhurried, and open. Pain should be adequately controlled, human dignity maintained, and isolation from family avoided. The last two in particular tend to be overlooked in hospitals, where the intrusion of life-sustaining apparatus can so easily detract from attention to the whole person and concentrate instead on the life-threatening disease. The physician must also prepare to deal with guilt feelings on the part of the family when a member becomes gravely or hopelessly ill. It is important for the doctor to reassure the family that everything possible has been done.

The President's Committee for the Study of Ethical Problems in Medicine defined death as (1) irreversible cessation of circulatory and respiratory function or (2) irreversible cessation of all functions of the entire brain, including the brainstem. Clinical and electroencephalographic criteria permit the reliable diagnosis of cerebral death. According to the criteria adopted by the staff of the Massachusetts General Hospital and the Harvard Committee on Brain Death, death occurs when all signs of receptivity and responsivity are absent, including all brainstem reflexes (pupillary reactions, ocular movement, blinking, swallowing, breathing), and the electroencephalogram is isoelectric. Occasionally, intoxications and metabolic disorders may simulate this state; hence the diagnosis requires expert evaluation. Under the aforementioned circumstances, to continue with heroic, highly costly supportive measures merely for the purpose of preserving cardiac function is against the best interests of patient, family, and society. In such instances, the dilemma of continuing care could be avoided if the medical profession, in accord with social sanction, can be brought to redefine life and death by these criteria.

A practice that has proved acceptable in many settings is as follows:

1 The diagnosis of brain death, based on the above criteria, should be corroborated by another physician and confirmed by clinical examination and EEG, repeated one or more times.
2 The family should be informed of the irreversibility of brain function but should not be requested to ratify the decision whether the medical treatment should be discontinued. An exception to this limited decision-making power of the family might apply where the patient has directed the family that he or she wishes them to make the decision.
3 The physician, after consultation with a professional colleague, may withdraw supportive measures, assuming that nothing more can be offered.
4 The possibility that such patients may become sources of organs for grafting should not enter into the aforementioned decisions, although prior to the cessation of heart action the family may be asked whether this would be their wish, or the family may suggest that organs be used for this purpose.

"Do not resuscitate" orders and cessation of therapy When carried out in a timely and expert manner, cardiopulmonary resuscitation is often useful in the prevention of sudden, unexpected death. However, unless there are reasons to the contrary it should not be carried out when it merely prolongs life in a patient with terminal, incurable disease. The decision not to resuscitate a patient and decisions about the intensity of therapy and, indeed, whether or not treatment is to be delivered at all to patients who are incurably and terminally ill must be reviewed frequently and must take into consideration any unexpected changes in the patient's condition. These decisions must also take into account both the underlying medical condition and the wishes of the patient or, if these cannot or have not been ascertained directly, those of a close relative or other surrogate who can be relied upon to transmit the patient's feelings and to be guided by the patient's best interests. The issues involving death and dying are among the most difficult in medicine. In approaching them rationally and consistently, the physician must combine the art and the science of medicine.

2 QUANTITATIVE ASPECTS OF CLINICAL REASONING

LEE GOLDMAN

The process of clinical reasoning is poorly understood but is based upon factors such as experience and learning, inductive and deductive reasoning, interpretation of evidence that itself varies in reproducibility and validity, and intuition that often is difficult to define. In an effort to improve clinical reasoning, a number of attempts have been made to analyze quantitatively the many factors involved, including defining the cognitive approaches that clinicians apply to difficult problems, devising computerized decision support systems that are designed to emulate certain features of decision making, and applying decision theory to understand how judgments should be reached. While each of these approaches has advanced the understanding of the diagnostic process, all have practical and/or theoretical problems that limit their direct applicability to the care of the individual patient.

Nevertheless, these preliminary attempts to apply the rigor and logic inherent in the quantitative method have provided significant insights into the process by which clinical reasoning is accomplished, have identified ways in which the process may be improved, and have made it possible to minimize certain features of the workup that are not cost-effective. Thus, while clinical reasoning cannot be reduced to probabilities or numbers, attempts at quantitative analysis of the process may improve the ways in which the problems of individual patients are approached and solved.

In a simplified model, quantitative clinical reasoning includes five phases. The *first* consists of an investigation of the chief complaint through key questions that are included in the history of the present illness (Table 2-1). These questions are supplemented by the past medical history and by a physical examination that emphasizes detailed investigation of potential key organ systems. In the *second* phase, the physician may select from an array of diagnostic tests, each with its own accuracy and usefulness for investigating the possibilities raised in the differential diagnosis. Since each test has its costs, and some entail risk and discomfort as well, the physician must ask whether the history and physical examination are sufficiently diagnostic before ordering tests. *Third*, the clinical data must be integrated with test results to estimate the likelihood of conditions in the differential diagnosis. *Fourth*, the comparative risks and benefits of further diagnostic and therapeutic options must be weighed to reach a recommendation for the patient. In the *fifth* and final phase, this recommendation is presented to the patient, and after appropriate discussion of the options, a therapeutic plan is initiated. Each of the five steps in this simplified model of the clinical reasoning process can be analyzed individually.

HISTORY AND PHYSICAL EXAMINATION It originally had been assumed that physicians begin investigating a patient's chief complaint by obtaining a comprehensive history, which includes many if not most of the questions included in a full review of systems, and by performing an all-inclusive physical examination. However, experienced clinicians begin to form hypotheses based on the chief complaint and on the responses to initial questioning, and they ask further questions in a sequence that allows them to evaluate the initial

TABLE 2-1 Phases of clinical reasoning and decision making

1 Investigation of the complaint by means of clinical examination (history and physical examination)
2 Ordering of diagnostic tests, each with its own intrinsic accuracy and usefulness
3 Integration of clinical findings with test results to assess diagnostic probabilities
4 Weighing of comparative risks and benefits of alternative courses of action
5 Determination of patient's preferences and development of a therapeutic plan

hypotheses and, if necessary, shorten or amend the list of possibilities. Only a limited number of diagnostic hypotheses can be entertained at any one time, and information is used to build a case for or against the most likely. In such a way, high-priority questions are selected from the almost limitless number that might be asked, and these specific questions are incorporated into the history of the present illness. Often, a key response, such as a history of melena, will be selected, a list of potential explanations for it will be formulated, and this list will then be trimmed, based on the response to more probing questions, so that a principal diagnosis can be selected and then tested. This process, termed *iterative hypothesis testing*, is an efficient approach to diagnosis and is preferable to attempts to gather every conceivable piece of information prior to formulating a differential diagnosis.

Advocacy of iterative hypothesis testing does not argue against the need for a systematic, thorough, and complete history of the present illness, past medical history, review of systems, family history, social history, and physical examination. For example, if a patient presents with abdominal pain, the physician should gather information regarding its location and quality as well as the factors that precipitate and/or relieve it. The physician then asks questions relating to the diagnoses that may be suspected based on the response to the initial questions. If the pain is suggestive of pancreatitis, the clinician would ask about alcohol intake, the use of thiazide diuretics or glucocorticosteroids, symptoms suggestive of concomitant gallbladder disease, a family history of pancreatitis, and questions aimed at uncovering the possibility of a posterior penetrating ulcer. Alternatively, if the discomfort seems more typical of reflux esophagitis, a different sequence of questions would be triggered. The use of iterative hypothesis testing encourages the physician to elicit detailed information in high-yield areas, without forgoing a systematic and thorough approach to the patient. Findings on the history and physical examination should influence each other. The history focuses the physical examination on certain organs, and findings on physical examination should encourage more detailed review of certain systems.

As physicians proceed through this reasoning process with both the history and physical examination, a variety of issues may influence the accuracy of the decision-making process. First is the potential for some historical information or physical findings to be poorly reproducible, either because the patient's responses vary or because different physicians elicit information differently or vary in the way they interpret the answers. The careful use of clear, and when possible, precise questions can increase the reproducibility and validity of the medical history, but still cannot eliminate all variability.

When assessing the reproducibility of findings on the physical examination, two observers frequently agree that an uncommon abnormality such as an enlarged spleen is not present but agree less often when one of them thinks that it is present in a patient in whom it would not usually be expected. This principle can best be demonstrated by understanding that some agreement always occurs by chance, and the likelihood of chance agreement is higher if the finding is either very common or very uncommon. For example, if two physicians each consider 90 percent of patients to be abnormal in some manner, such as having a systolic heart murmur, they will agree 81 percent of the time by chance alone. In some studies of the reproducibility of common signs and symptoms, such as an enlarged liver, actual agreement rates have not been substantially better than chance. Disagreement rates may be reduced by emphasizing physical examination skills during medical training, by looking for other correlative physical findings, and by learning how physical findings correlate with the results of diagnostic tests. Therefore, when a clinician notes an unexpected and somewhat subjective abnormality for which there may be a high rate of interobserver disagreement, such as an unexpectedly enlarged spleen, other abnormalities that may often be associated with it, such as hepatomegaly or lymphadenopathy, should be sought to increase the likelihood that the spleen would be expected to be abnormal. In some situations, ordering a

diagnostic test, such as a liver and spleen scan, to assess the finding more objectively should be considered if the test is sufficiently reliable.

These comments about the factors that limit the reproducibility and validity of the medical history and physical examination do not denigrate their critical importance in clinical reasoning. Rather, they emphasize that care and diligence in the application of these skills are necessary. For example, careful auscultation of the heart during various bedside maneuvers (see Chap. 175) has been shown to be remarkably accurate in determining the cause of systolic murmurs.

When physicians use the history and the physical examination to arrive at a diagnosis, they are rarely certain of it. Therefore, it would be better to assess the likelihood of the diagnosis in terms of probabilities. All too frequently, this probability is not expressed as an actual percentage but rather in such terms as "nearly always," "commonly," "sometimes," or "rarely." Since different physicians may assign different probabilities to the same terms, these imprecise words frequently lead to major misunderstandings among physicians or between the physician and the patient. Physicians should be as rigorous and quantitative as possible in their assessments, and when feasible, a quantitative expression of probability should be used. For example, rather than saying that it is unlikely that a radiographic pattern is indicative of a carcinoma of the colon, it would be preferable, if possible, to provide a more precise indication of the probability of carcinoma with this radiographic pattern. A 10 to 15 percent probability of carcinoma may be interpreted as "unlikely," but from a clinical perspective usually warrants further evaluation because of the serious consequences of missing a potentially resectable tumor.

Although such quantitative estimates would be desirable, they usually are not available in practice. Even experienced physicians often are unable to estimate accurately the likelihood of particular conditions. There is a tendency to overestimate the likelihood of relatively uncommon conditions, and physicians are especially poor at quantifying probabilities that are very high or very low. For example, a physician may not know whether the probability of bacterial meningitis or of another disease that could be diagnosed by a lumbar puncture in a patient with a severe headache is 1 in 20 or 1 in 2000. In both situations, the probability is low, but the decision as to whether a lumbar puncture should be performed may depend on this estimate.

As was emphasized in Chap. 1, the history and physical examination have other important purposes. They allow the physician to evaluate the emotional status of the patient and to understand how the present problems fit into the context of the patient's social and family life, and they encourage the development in the patient of confidence in the physician, which is so necessary for reaching an agreement on the coming plan of action.

DIAGNOSTIC TESTS: INDICATIONS, ACCURACY, AND USEFULNESS A diagnostic test should be ordered for specified clinical indications, be sufficiently accurate to be efficacious for such indications, and be the least expensive and/or risky of the available efficacious tests. No diagnostic test is totally accurate, and physicians often have difficulty interpreting test results. It is therefore critical to understand several commonly used terms in test analysis and epidemiology, including prevalence, sensitivity, specificity, positive predictive value, and negative predictive value (Table 2-2).

Although reports of the accuracies of diagnostic tests are commonly expressed in terms of positive and negative predictive values, these calculated values are dependent on the prevalence of the disease in the population being studied (Table 2-3). A test with a particular sensitivity and specificity has different positive and negative predictive values when used in groups of patients that have different prevalences of disease. For example, a mildly abnormal alkaline phosphatase level in a young adult with a known lymphoma suggests hepatic involvement by the tumor, i.e., it is likely to be a *true positive*, while the same alkaline phosphatase level as part of a routine screening battery of blood tests in an asymptomatic person of the same age is

TABLE 2-2 Definitions of commonly used terms in epidemiology and decision making

Test result	Disease state	
	Present	Absent
Positive	a (true positive)	b (false positive)
Negative	c (false negative)	d (true negative)

Prevalence (prior probability)	= (a+c)/(a+b+c+d) =	all patients with the disease/all patients tested
Sensitivity	= a/(a+c) =	true-positive test results/all patients with the disease
Specificity	= d/(b+d) =	true-negative test results/all patients without the disease
False-negative rate	= c/(a+c) =	false-negative test results/all patients with the disease
False-positive rate	= b/(b+d) =	false-positive test results/all patients without the disease
Positive predictive value	= a/(a+b) =	true-positive test results/all positive test results
Negative predictive value	= d/(c+d) =	true-negative test results/all patients with negative results
Overall accuracy	= (a+d)/(a+b+c+d) =	true-positive + true-negative test results/all tests

unlikely to be due to tumor, i.e., in this setting it is more likely to be a *false positive*.

Although the sensitivity and specificity of a test do not depend on the prevalence (or percentage of patients being tested who have the disease), they do depend on the spectrum of patients in whom the test is being evaluated. For example, a technetium pyrophosphate scintiscan for diagnosing myocardial infarction (Chap. 189) will appear to have a nearly perfect sensitivity and specificity if the diseased population has a history typical of myocardial infarction, electrocardiographic changes of transmural infarction, and clear-cut elevations of the MB isoenzyme of creatine kinase (CK) and the nondiseased population is composed of normal medical students. If, however, without changing the prevalence of disease in the population being tested, the spectrum of the diseased and nondiseased patients is altered by including patients with other characteristics, i.e., if the population of patients with myocardial infarction were composed principally of those with non-Q-wave infarctions and small or borderline elevations of CK-MB, while the population without acute infarction included patients with old infarcts and unstable angina pectoris, the sensitivity and specificity would change dramatically. In the latter situation, the sensitivity and specificity of the technetium pyrophosphate scintiscan are not only lower than in the first example, because the spectrum of diseased and nondiseased patients has been changed, but, more importantly, they are so low that the test has little clinical value. This example also demonstrates the methodologic problems encountered when applying data from one study to a different type of patient or when pooling data from studies of different subsets of patients.

In some situations, uncertainty about the sensitivity and specificity of the test in the type of patient being assessed may limit its clinical value. Since the physician rarely knows (or can know) the population on which every test which is ordered has been standardized, the results provide information that is far less decisive than usually thought. Furthermore, it may be quite difficult to distinguish random laboratory errors from test results that might be falsely positive or negative because of coexistence of a process that can affect the test, such as the finding of an elevated level of CK in a patient who has undergone strenuous exercise and is being evaluated for chest pain.

Because no single value or cutoff point of an individual test can be expected to have both a perfect sensitivity and a perfect specificity, it is often necessary to determine which value or cutoff point is the most appropriate to guide decision making. A graph (Fig. 2-1) of the test's *receiver operating characteristic curve*, which displays the inevitable trade-off between emphasizing a high sensitivity, such as defining an exercise electrocardiogram as abnormal if it shows ≥0.5 mm of ST-segment depression, versus emphasizing a high specificity, such as defining an exercise electrocardiogram as abnormal only if it shows ≥2.0 mm of ST-segment depression, can help the clinician understand the implications of various definitions of a "positive" test result. Such a graph demonstrates that different definitions of normal versus abnormal may be appropriate depending on whether one wishes to rule in the disease via a positive result on a test that has a high specificity or to exclude the disease via a negative result on a test that has a high sensitivity. Different tests may have different sensitivities and specificities, and better tests may have both a higher sensitivity and a higher specificity than poorer tests.

TABLE 2-3 How the positive and negative predictive values of the same test vary depending on the prior probability of disease

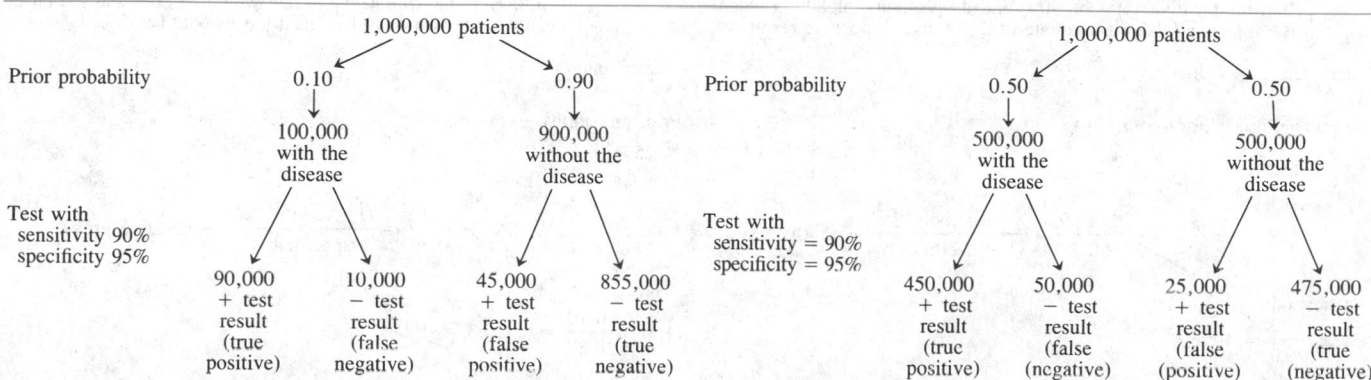

INTERPRETATION OF THE TEST RESULT WHEN 10% OF THE PATIENTS BEING TESTED HAVE THE DISEASE (PRIOR PROBABILITY = 10%)

INTERPRETATION OF THE TEST RESULT WHEN 50% OF THE PATIENTS BEING TESTED HAVE THE DISEASE (PRIOR PROBABILITY = 50%)

The probability of disease in a patient with a positive test result (positive predictive value) = 90,000/135,000 = 67%
The probability of no disease in a patient with a negative test result (negative predictive value) = 855,000/865,000 = 99%

The probability of disease in a patient with a positive test result (positive predictive value) = 450,000/475,000 = 95%
The probability of no disease in a patient with a negative test result (negative predictive value) = 475,000/525,000 = 90%

FIGURE 2-1 The inherent trade-off between sensitivity and specificity. For any diagnostic test, an increase in sensitivity will be associated with a decline in specificity. The closer this curve comes to the upper-left-hand corner, the more useful the test; the closer to the broken line, the less useful it is. When deciding on the cutoff between normal versus abnormal, one must determine what sensitivity and specificity are most useful clinically.

One example of a sensitive test is an M-mode echocardiogram to exclude severe aortic stenosis in adults: the sensitivity of this relatively inexpensive test for aortic stenosis is close to 100 percent, and a normal aortic valve echogram virtually excludes the diagnosis of severe aortic stenosis in the adult. Unfortunately, this sensitive test is not very specific, and many patients who have abnormal aortic valves on echocardiogram do not have severe aortic stenosis and require further testing (e.g., with Doppler echocardiography and perhaps cardiac catheterization) to establish the diagnosis (Chap. 188). A common example of a reasonably specific test would be an electrocardiogram to diagnose acute myocardial infarction. While the precise specificity depends on the spectrum of patients being tested, the presence of new ST-segment elevations exceeding 1.0 mm in two or more electrically contiguous leads in patients who present to an emergency room with prolonged acute chest pain consistent with myocardial ischemia is sufficiently specific, i.e., sufficiently unlikely to be a false positive, that admission to an intensive care unit is virtually always recommended. However, this test is not sensitive, and if admission to the unit were restricted to patients with this

electrocardiographic finding, almost half of patients with myocardial infarctions presenting to hospital emergency rooms would be missed.

To optimize the clinical value of a diagnostic test, it is helpful to obtain local experience with it; oftentimes, its value will differ from that reported in the literature. Reports of the efficacy of a test should emphasize its accuracy when compared to an independent standard, and the test must be evaluated in a spectrum of patients with varying severities of the disease in question and in patients who have conditions that are part of the same differential diagnosis. The reproducibility of the test should be known, and the "normal limits" of the test should be clear and appropriate. In some instances, the test or procedure required to establish the validity of a diagnostic test is so risky that only a skewed sample of patients are included in a study, as, for example, in the analysis of the usefulness of the abdominal CT scan in patients with suspected pancreatic carcinoma. If patients with "negative" CT scan results never come to laparotomy or postmortem examination, neither the sensitivity nor specificity of the CT scan for pancreatic carcinoma can be assessed. In such situations, an estimated value of the diagnostic test may be inaccurate because it has not been validated.

INTEGRATION OF CLINICAL DATA AND TEST RESULTS Although, as we have seen, neither clinical data nor test results may be entirely accurate, the integration of the two can lead to better diagnostic predictions than either alone. By knowing the probability that the patient has a particular condition before a test is performed (the prior, or pretest, probability), and by knowing the sensitivity and the specificity of the test, the posttest probability can be calculated. A common mathematical technique for integrating clinical data and a test result is the odds-likelihood form of Bayesian analysis (Table 2-4). A pretest probability can be expressed as odds (as in a horse race for example) and multiplied by the likelihood ratio (which is the sensitivity of the test divided by 1 minus the specificity of the test) to yield the posttest odds, which may be transformed back into a posttest probability. This approach can be employed in any situation in which the physician can use clinical findings to estimate a pretest diagnostic probability and integrate this with the result as well as the sensitivity and specificity of the diagnostic test. Many clinical situations may be so complex that it is not practical to estimate the prior probabilities of all likely diagnoses or to know the sensitivities and specificities of each of the tests that might be performed individually or in sequence. Nevertheless, attempts in this direction will stimulate critical thinking, expose uncertainties, and generate ideas for original investigations or a review of past experiences to

TABLE 2-4   Example of the use of Bayesian analysis to integrate the pretest probability with the test result to calculate a posttest probability

* Sensitivity = probability of a positive test result in a patient with the disease
† (1 − Specificity) = probability of a positive test result in a patient without the disease

‡ (1 − sensitivity) = probability of a negative test result in a patient with the disease.
§ Specificity = probability of a negative test result in a patient without the disease.

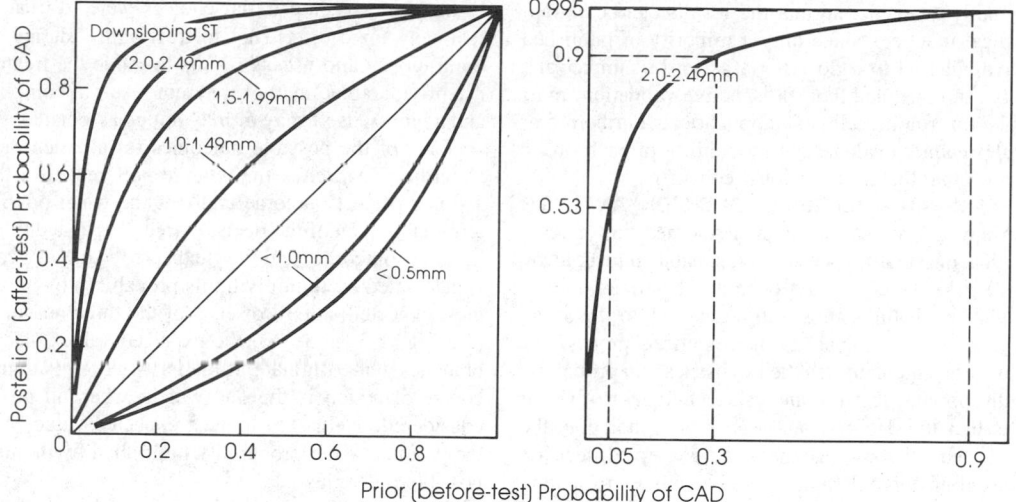

Prior (before-test) Probability of CAD

FIGURE 2-2 How the exercise tolerance test affects the probability of coronary artery disease. The before-test probability of coronary artery disease (CAD) will be modified by the result of the exercise electrocardiogram to yield a after-test probability of CAD. Note that the finding of <1 mm of ST depression will reduce the probability of CAD, whereas ≥1 mm of ST depression will increase the probability. For example, if a patient with a before-test probability of CAD of 90 percent (about that of a middle-aged man with typical anginal symptoms) had 2 to 2.49 mm on ST depression on exercise testing, the after-test probability of CAD would be 99.5 percent. In contrast the same exercise test result in a patient with 30 percent before-test probability of CAD (about that of a patient with atypical anginal symptoms) would yield an after-test probability of about 90 percent. In an asymptomatic patient, with a before-test probability of about 5 percent, the same exercise test result would yield an after-test probability of 53 percent. Thus, the same test yields different after-test probabilities in patients with different before-test probabilities. (*Adapted, with permission of the New England Journal of Medicine, from RD Rifkin, WB Hood, Bayesian analysis of electrocardiographic exercise stress testing. N Engl J Med 297:684, 1977.*)

facilitate the application of Bayesian analysis to the integration of clinical data and laboratory tests.

The results of Bayesian analyses often can be expressed in graphic form, such as the value of exercise electrocardiograms for predicting the presence of coronary artery disease (Fig. 2-2; also see Chap. 190). This series of curves also demonstrates how to consider a test whose result may be in the "gray zone" rather than clearly positive or clearly negative.

One of the key assumptions inherent in most such analyses is that the correlation between the pretest probability and the test result is no greater than expected by chance. If the diagnostic test simply duplicates information that has already been obtained by the clinical examination, it will not have any additional benefit for predicting whether or not the disease is present. For example, in trying to determine whether or not a patient with carcinoma of the colon has hepatic metastases, the finding of jaundice on physical examination should be a strong predictor. The degree of hyperbilirubinemia can also be measured, but the bilirubin level in a patient with clinical jaundice does not add substantial *independent* information to that obtained by a careful physical examination. When integrating a diagnostic test with clinical information, the test is helpful only when it adds incremental information to what can be inferred based on the history and physical examination and on prior less costly or less risky diagnostic tests. If a diagnostic test (such as a retrograde cholangiogram in the patient with hyperbilirubinemia) provides information that cannot be inferred directly, it is less likely that its results are associated with pretest probabilities to an extent greater than would be expected by chance.

A diagnostic test has an impact on the evaluation of a specific patient only if it changes the diagnostic probability to the extent that the new probability dictates a change in the diagnostic strategy or therapeutic plans or if the test serves as part of a sequence of tests that moves the probability across such a threshold. An example is a patient suspected of having a pulmonary embolism, with an estimated probability of 50 percent based on clinical data alone. A "low probability" pulmonary ventilation-perfusion scan may reduce the probability of pulmonary embolism, but if the goal is to exclude pulmonary embolism with the highest possible degree of certainty, a pulmonary angiogram would be required (Chap. 213).

Because diagnostic tests oftentimes do not provide important new information even when their results are accurate, several questions should be considered in deciding when to order diagnostic tests. First, how likely is the disease in question? Second, what would be the clinical consequences if the diagnosis were missed or if the patient were mistakenly treated for a disease that is not present? Third, what is the likelihood that the diagnostic test will change the probability sufficiently to have an effect on either diagnosis or therapy? The physician should consider the probabilities, the risks, the likelihood and costs of obtaining new information, and the adverse consequences of delay, because observation and follow-up are always among the available diagnostic options.

Since the establishment of valid diagnostic probabilities is a cornerstone to clinical reasoning, accumulated clinical experience, often in the form of computerized data banks, has been used to generate statistical approaches for improving diagnostic predictions. In such research, it is common to begin by identifying individual factors that have a univariate correlation with the diagnosis in question. Then, these univariate correlates may be included in a multivariate analysis to determine which of them are significant independent predictors of the diagnosis. Some analyses may identify the important predictive factors and then assign them "weights," which can be transformed to calculate a probability. Alternatively, the analysis may result in a limited number of categories of patients, each with a discrete probability of the diagnosis.

These quantitative approaches to the estimation of various diagnostic probabilities, which are often termed "prediction rules," are especially helpful if they are in a format that is readily usable by the clinician and if they have been validated prospectively on a sufficient number and spectrum of patients. For example, by carefully defining the key historical questions, findings on physical examination, and electrocardiographic abnormalities that might predict the probability of acute myocardial infarction among emergency department patients with chest pain, a protocol was devised and shown in prospective validation testing to have the same sensitivity as physicians for identifying infarction and at the same time to have a significantly higher specificity.

For such prediction rules to be useful to the clinician, they must be derived from relevant patient populations and use tests that are reproducible and readily available, so that the results can be extrapolated to local medical practice. Since only a minority of published prediction rules have adhered to rigid criteria as to the number and spectrum of patients examined and their prospective validation, most are not yet suitable for routine clinical application. Furthermore, many prediction rules cannot evaluate the probability of each of the diagnoses or outcomes that the clinician must consider.

COMPARING RISKS AND BENEFITS: DECISION ANALYSIS

Inherent in the concept that probabilities can guide decision making is the assumption that one can arrive at a reasonable threshold by knowing the relative risks (or costs) and benefits of various options and deciding at what probability this ratio changes to favor an alternative strategy. Decision analysis is an organized process for evaluating such situations and identifies the key issues and problems.

One problem with applying decision-analysis techniques to difficult clinical problems is that the decision analysis is no better than the data on which it is based. In some instances, an attempted decision analysis of a complex clinical problem may yield no more information than that the critical data required for the analysis are missing and that more research in the field needs to be performed. In addition, when clinicians are uncertain about diagnostic or therapeutic strategies, formal analyses may indicate that the differences in outcome among various strategies are very small. In such cases, the formal analysis may have such inherent error that it is not dependable. Even when decision analysis is potentially helpful, it may not be feasible to complete the detailed estimations and calculations within the time constraints of bedside decision making. Nevertheless, the value of the analytic approach to decision making is that it integrates available data, mandates rigorous thinking, and exposes areas of uncertainty or ignorance.

Decision analysis depicts graphically two types of issues in the decision-making process: first, the decisions (or choices) available to the physician and second, the probabilities of all of the events that may result from each decision. To illustrate how this process works, a decision analysis of whether to biopsy the brain, treat, or wait in suspected herpes encephalitis (Chap. 135) may be considered. Figure 2-3 depicts the decision tree for this problem. The square box or "node" labeled A indicates a decision that the physician must make. The circular nodes, labeled B through I, indicate where different outcomes, each of which has an estimatable probability, could occur.

In this analysis, the initial choices were to treat with vidarabine (a relatively toxic drug), not to treat with vidarabine, or to perform a brain biopsy and use its results to guide the treatment decision. The use of vidarabine may or may not result in complications of therapy, and a biopsy itself may or may not be associated with a complication.

Each of the possible outcomes for a patient is typically assigned a "utility," which is the relative preference for the outcome, where 1.0 is a perfect outcome and 0 is the worst possible outcome. Each terminal branch of the decision tree is assigned the utility corresponding to its outcome, and the "expected value" of each terminal branch is calculated by multiplying its probability by its utility. To calculate the "expected value" of each of the three possible courses of action (see Fig. 2-3, node A), the expected values of each of the terminal branches that originate from it would be summed. The preferred course of action is the one which, when all possible outcomes are considered, yields the highest expected value, which is the sum of the product of the probability multiplied by the utility for each of its possible outcomes.

In performing any decision analysis, the relevant probabilities must be known or estimated, a process that sometimes requires guesswork. Next, utilities could be assigned to each of these outcomes. A major practical limitation of decision analysis is the subjective judgment often required to estimate utilities. It is also difficult to adjust future years of life for their quality in any numerical fashion, for example, in considering how drug toxicity or the disability resulting from disease or treatment lowers the quality of future years of life.

The results and usefulness of a decision analysis depend on the probabilities and utilities that are used in the calculation, and it is imperative for decision analyses to include a *sensitivity analysis*, in which various estimates for each probability are included in the analysis to determine if the conclusions would be changed. For example, in the analysis in Fig. 2-3, some range of probabilities must be assumed for vidarabine toxicity, for serious complications of brain biopsy, and for the likelihood of false-positive or false-negative biopsy results. The authors of this particular analysis concluded that waiting, i.e., neither treating nor performing a biopsy, was the preferable course of action when the likelihood of herpes encephalitis is less than 3 percent. At probabilities between 3 and 42 percent, the analysis favored brain biopsy, but at probabilities above

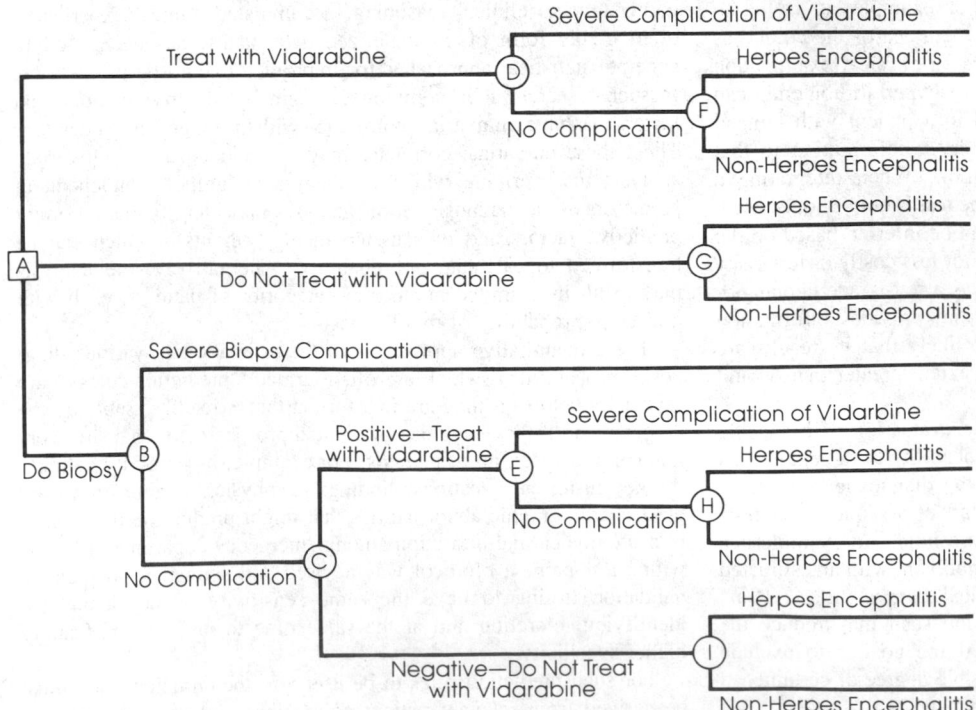

FIGURE 2-3 Decision tree for diagnosis and treatment of suspected herpes simplex encephalitis. The square node represents the decision point, and the round nodes denote chance events. See text for details. *(Reprinted with permission from M Barza, SG Pauker, The decision to biopsy, treat, or wait in suspected herpes encephalitis, Ann Intern Med 92:644, 1980.)*

42 percent, it favored immediate treatment with vidarabine. However, it is uncommon for any patient to have substantially greater than a 42 percent probability of herpes encephalitis, and hence it would be unusual for empiric vidarabine treatment ever to be preferred over brain biopsy. The authors demonstrated that these conclusions did not change when they varied the assumptions about the probabilities of several relevant events. If the conclusions of an analysis were altered by relatively minor changes in the assumptions on which it was based, the analysis would not be sufficiently reliable to become the basis for decision making.

Decision analysis sometimes demonstrates a clear and dramatic advantage with one particular option. In other circumstances, there may be little difference between two options; either option may be reasonable, or secondary issues that cannot be taken into account in the formal analysis, such as the patient's feelings about taking risks or the recent local experience with particular interventions, should be the final determinants in the decision. Physicians who perform a decision analysis therefore must determine the probabilities of each of the possible events by reviewing the pertinent patient experience at their own institution or practice, or by reviewing the pertinent literature. Even when the outcome of the analysis seems clear, the physician or the patient may believe that the situation in question is an exception to the rule. Furthermore, even the best analyses, like all clinical intuition, are based on assumptions that may be open to debate.

In the preceding example, the management of an individual patient with possible herpes encephalitis, decision analysis indicated the preferred strategy in terms of outcome but did not consider the costs at which such benefits might be achieved. In determining health policy, a formal cost-effectiveness analysis can be performed to determine how many dollars must be spent to achieve a unit of benefit, often defined as a life saved, a year of life saved, or a quality-adjusted year of life saved, in which the years are adjusted to take into account the quality of life during that time. For example, in 1990 dollars, 1 year of in-center hemodialysis can be estimated to cost about $30,000 to $35,000 per quality-adjusted year of life saved; this figure includes only the direct medical costs and not indirect costs related to issues such as time lost or travel, or any benefits in terms of a patient's ability to work. In some situations, the ability of the patient to maintain gainful employment may offset some or all of the direct medical expenses.

Although many analyses are now expressed in terms of cost-effectiveness, where dollars spent are compared to lives or years of life gained, some studies have utilized cost-benefit analyses in which a dollar value is placed on the life that is saved. For example, an analysis of the rubella vaccination, which attempted to place a dollar value on the vaccine's ability to prevent the congenital rubella syndrome and the resulting expenses, concluded that the optimal national policy would be to vaccinate all females at age 12.

ETHICS AND PATIENT INPUT In both quantitative and non-quantitative clinical reasoning, the physician must consider ethical issues as well as the patient's values and preferences. While a detailed discussion of these issues is beyond the scope of this chapter, it is important to emphasize that patients' preferences for alternate therapies may not agree with the preferences that the physicians propose on the basis of their own clinical judgment or the results of a decision-analysis approach. For example, many patients with carcinoma of the larynx may prefer radiation therapy, with a lower cure rate but a higher likelihood of maintaining speech, to extirpative surgery. It is imperative that physicians assess those characteristics of life that the patient prizes most (the elusive "quality of life") prior to basing controversial decisions solely on quantitative approaches, the physicians' own subjective impressions of the likely medical benefits, their own personal preferences, or their assumptions about the patient's preferences. Therefore, the final plan should reflect an agreement between a well-informed patient and a sympathetic physician who has detailed knowledge of the relevant medical issues and of the impact of the various possible outcomes on the specific patient.

REFERENCES

CASSIRER JP: Diagnostic reasoning. Ann Intern Med 110:893, 1989

ELSTEIN AS et al: *Medical Problem Solving. An Analysis of Clinical Reasoning.* Cambridge, Harvard University, 1978

GOLDMAN L et al: A computer protocol to predict myocardial infarction in emergency department patients with chest pain. N Engl J Med 318:797, 1988

LEMBO NJ et al: Bedside diagnosis of systolic murmurs. N Engl J Med 318:1572, 1988

MCNEIL BJ et al: Speech and survival: Trade offs between quality and quantity of life in laryngeal cancer. N Engl J Med 305:982, 1981

RANSOHOFF DF, FEINSTEIN AR: Problems of spectrum and bias in evaluating the efficacy of diagnostic tests. N Engl J Med 299:926, 1978

ROBERTS SD et al: Cost-effective care of end-stage renal disease: A billion dollar question. Ann Intern Med 92:243, 1980

SACKETT DL et al: *Clinical Epidemiology: A Basic Science for Clinical Medicine.* Boston, Little, Brown, 1985

SCHOENBAUM SC et al: Benefit-cost analysis of rubella vaccination policy. N Engl J Med 294:303, 1976

WEINSTEIN MC, FINEBERG HV: *Clinical Decision Analysis.* Philadelphia, Saunders, 1980

3 COST AWARENESS IN MEDICINE

LEE GOLDMAN

COSTS OF HEALTH CARE IN THE UNITED STATES

Health care expenditures in the United States are now about $600 billion per year. Through the 1980s, these expenditures rose at a rate of more than 10 percent per year, which exceeded the rates of inflation and of growth in the gross national product (GNP). As a consequence, the percentage of the GNP that is spent on health care increased from about 7 percent in 1970 to 9 percent in 1980 and is expected to be nearly 12 percent in 1990. As a percentage of the GNP, medical care expenditures in the United Kingdom are about five percentage points lower than in the United States. In Canada, expenditures as a percentage of GNP were similar to the United States until about 1970 but now are more than two percentage points lower.

The reasons for the increase in health care costs are multifactorial. The aging of the population and the availability of new diagnostic and therapeutic advances have increased the demand for health care. Furthermore, between 1970 and 1986, the supply of physicians in the United States increased from about 150 to 200 per 100,000 population. This increase in physicians provided Americans with easier access to medical services but raised concerns that a possible oversupply of physicians in portions of the country could contribute to an excessive escalation in costs. The costs of care are especially influenced by decisions regarding hospital admission and surgery, and by decisions affecting the use of intensive care units, life-sustaining treatments, and long-term care facilities. Efforts at cost-containment have attempted to identify unnecessary services, such as routine preoperative electrocardiograms in healthy young patients, or situations in which extraordinary expenses occur, such as in the last 6 months of life. Although some services may represent "fat" in the health care system, it is likely that any future reduction in unnecessary care may be more than counterbalanced in costs by growth in the number and age of the population and by continued advances in technology.

Despite these rising costs, an estimated 37 million Americans, or about 15% of the population, do not have health care insurance of any kind, even though nearly half are in households in which someone is employed. This lack of insurance coverage and access to health care is often blamed for the fact that the United States, despite its high expenditures on health care, ranks twentieth in the world in infant mortality and is not in the top ten in life expectancy.

HEALTH INSURANCE Traditional fee-for-service insurance reimburses the hospital and the physician for services rendered, but frequently does not cover preventive care. Even when insurance provides coverage for a service, the patient may be responsible for an initial "deductible" and a copayment, which is usually a fixed percentage of the entire amount charged.

Patients who must pay such out-of-pocket charges for some of their medical care seek less care than those whose care is fully covered by insurance. In the working poor this may result in reduced utilization of services and in an increase in the prevalence of serious disease. When adults of all socioeconomic classes lose health insurance coverage, they may use fewer medical services; as a result, their health status tends to decline.

Most alternatives to traditional fee-for-service medical care require enrolled persons to prepay a fixed premium, which, except when a relatively small copayment is required, usually covers acute, chronic, and preventive medical services, and sometimes covers medications and other health care needs. Prepaid plans have varying organizational and financial structures. Early on in their development, staff-model HMOs were among the most popular formats. In this model, groups of salaried physicians practiced physically together in one or a few central facilities to provide prepaid care. In recent years, Independent Practice Associations (IPAs) have shown the most rapid growth. IPAs provide prepaid care to the patient by contracting with office-based practitioners who agree to see patients on a prenegotiated fee schedule. To balance the normal fee-for-service incentives and control utilization, IPAs employ various forms of administrative controls and review. The rate of hospitalization can be reduced among enrollees in HMOs, and HMOs have been among the leaders in attempts to reduce hospital costs and lengths-of-stay.

REIMBURSEMENT OF HOSPITALS AND PHYSICIANS In 1983 Medicare introduced a system of prospective reimbursement using diagnosis-related groups (DRGs), whereby hospitals were paid a predetermined sum based on the patient's principal diagnosis, procedures, complications, and comorbidities regardless of the costs or charges that were actually generated by the hospital stay (Table 3-1). This reimbursement system was designed to reward hospitals for being more efficient, and hospitals could actually be paid more than their costs. In the first few years after the introduction of the DRG system, many hospitals, and especially the large teaching hospitals, reported substantial operating surpluses. In response, Medicare kept the rate of annual increase in reimbursement below the rate of increase in hospital costs, and the extra payments for teaching hospitals were reduced. By 1986, as many as one-third of all U.S. hospitals reported negative operating balances for Medicare patients. While the prospective reimbursement system has undoubtedly stimulated efficiency, it has also raised concerns about the practice of discharging patients prematurely or transferring them to other institutions if the projected cost of caring for them exceeds the expected reimbursement.

Since the introduction of federal prospective reimbursement, the

TABLE 3-1 Example of diagnosis-related groups (DRGs) for prospective payment by medicare

DRG no.	Name	Approximate average Medicare reimbursement for a large urban teaching hospital in 1989, $
89	Simple pneumonia and pleurisy with complications or comorbid conditions	5,000
121	Acute myocardial infarction with complications, discharged alive	6,500
148	Major small or large bowel procedure with complications or comorbid conditions	13,000
156	Coronary artery bypass surgery with catheterization on same admission	22,000

SOURCE: Prospective Payment Assessment Commission.

TABLE 3-2 Physician reimbursement: Traditional fee for service versus the relative value scale

Average Medicare reimbursement, 1986*	Method of calculating reimbursement	
	Traditional fee for service, $†	Relative value scale, $‡
Office visit, limited service, established patient	19	24
Initial hospital consultation, comprehensive service	81	86
Repair of inguinal hernia	503	233
Coronary artery bypass, three grafts	3652	1936

* Average relative value scale reimbursement assumes same total amount of dollars is available to reimburse the sum of all Medicare physician services.
† Defined as individual physician's customary fee for service, limited to a prevailing fee by third party insurers.
‡ Defined as service-specific reimbursement based on the resource inputs required to perform a service, including the physician's work involved and specialty differences in practice expenses and costs related to training.
SOURCE: Hsiao WC et al: *A National Study of Resource-Based Relative Value Scales for Physician Services: Final Report to the Health Care Financing Administration, No. 17-C-98795/1-03.* Boston, Harvard University School of Public Health, 1988.

number of inpatient hospital days has decreased. This reduction has been accompanied by a marked increase in ambulatory services, including a shift to the outpatient arena of services that previously were delivered only on an inpatient basis. This shift should lower the cost of delivering an individual unit of service, such as the cost of a breast biopsy, but the overall cost of medical care will rise if, for example, the breast biopsy is performed on an ambulatory basis *and* the inpatient resources that the breast biopsy patient would have used are now consumed by new services such as the treatment of a cancer patient with bone marrow transplantation.

Physician payment Methods of physician payment have also been questioned. Physician reimbursement in the United States, whether by Medicare or by private insurers, has traditionally been a direct payment based on the doctor's "usual and customary" fee. In recent years, the rate of annual increase in fees has been fixed by the payor, so that relative payments really reflect fee patterns from a decade or more ago. Because of concerns that this traditional approach had led to inequities in reimbursement and especially to underreimbursement for nonprocedural tasks such as office visits, recent analyses have considered the resource inputs of physicians' services, including time, intensity, practice costs, and the investment in training, to propose a new and fairer approach to physician reimbursement. This new proposal, which has been termed the *Relative Value Scale* (Table 3-2), is based upon the concept that payment rates for medical services should, as with other economic "goods," reflect the costs of producing those services. Using this approach, results to date suggest that procedural tasks are currently reimbursed at rates exceeding those of nonprocedural tasks that require comparable time, skill, and experience. The suggested new relative rates are similar to current fee schedules in Canada.

Proponents of changes in the reimbursement system hope that more equitable pay for cognitive tasks will reduce the incentive to perform procedures and increase the incentive for physicians to spend more time with patients, including time for discussion of issues such as health screening, health promotion, and disease prevention. Opponents of a change in the physician reimbursement system argue, among other issues, that changes in the reimbursement system may limit access and fail to take into account the extent to which patients may value some services more than others. Regardless of the outcome of this ongoing debate, the physician's diagnostic and therapeutic recommendations should be guided by the goal of providing maximal welfare for the patient, tempered by an awareness of the relative cost that must be incurred to reap this benefit.

Control of health care costs Two different approaches have been suggested to control health care costs: regulation and competition. Regulations, such as per diem rate setting, attempt to control costs by setting and enforcing practice or reimbursement standards. Other regulatory means of attempting to reduce costs include mandatory second opinions prior to elective hospitalization or surgery, but such programs usually do not save more than the costs of administration of the programs themselves. It is vital that physicians work closely with third-party payors, government agencies and commissions, and regulatory bodies such as the Joint Commission on Accreditation of Health Care Organizations that have assumed increasing responsibilities for setting reimbursement rates and for determining performance standards and conditions for payment.

The competitive approach encourages hospitals and providers to bid in a free-market atmosphere, in which consumers will presumably make rational choices based on the perceived cost and quality of the available alternatives. Insurance plans that utilize deductibles and copayments reflect this approach. It has also been proposed that physicians who practice inexpensively should be rewarded financially, but if physicians are paid to perform fewer services, the quality of care may suffer.

The reimbursement system differs in different countries. In the United Kingdom, for example, the National Health Service insurance program covers hospital and physician reimbursement on a non-fee-for-service basis, although patients can pay privately for services outside of the system. Patients often must endure long delays for nonemergency procedures. In Canada, hospitals are paid an annual lump sum, and most physicians are paid on a fee-for-service basis via a fee schedule that is negotiated between the medical societies and the provincial governments. Private insurance, by law, can cover only services such as long-term care and dental care that are not covered by public insurance. New technology has diffused less rapidly in Canada, and the rates at which many procedures are performed are lower, but may not be less optimal, than in the United States. In Canada, delays for elective services have not been a major problem, life expectancy is higher than in the United States, and the prestige and relative income of physicians is analogous to those in the United States.

COSTS AND COST-EFFECTIVENESS

The costs of medical care include direct costs, such as the salaries of health personnel, and indirect costs, such as utilities, maintenance, and mortgage payments. Some costs are fixed, i.e., they do not vary with the volume of services provided, and other costs are variable, i.e., they depend on volume. For example, consider a situation in which a new instrument to perform a blood chemistry test costs $1000 and will last for 1 year. Also assume that each individual chemical analysis has an incremental cost of $10 in reagents, personnel time, and other resource inputs. If the laboratory utilizes the instrument to analyze 100 specimens in a year, the average cost per specimen is $20 ($10 each in fixed and variable costs), but if it analyzes 10,000 specimens, the average cost per specimen is $10.10 ($0.10 in fixed costs and $10.00 in variable costs) because the fixed costs are spread over more specimens.

The charges for medical services do not necessarily correspond to the true costs of providing the services. This is in part because the costs are difficult to measure and in part because charges are usually fixed regardless of volume while costs vary with volume. Most analyses of cost and cost-effectiveness in medicine are based on charges rather than on true costs.

The net costs for a health care program include the costs of providing the program, costs that are generated by adverse side effects of treatment, and costs for treating disease that would not have occurred if the patient had not lived longer as a result of the original treatment. From these costs, the savings in health care, rehabilitation, or custodial costs due to prevention or alleviation of disease are subtracted to determine the net cost. For example, consider a program to perform mammography in women over age 40. The program would have its own direct costs related to advertising, screening, mammography, physician visits, breast biopsy, etc. Some women would have

false-positive mammograms and would receive unnecessary breast biopsies. Other women would live longer as a result of early diagnosis and treatment of breast cancer, but they might develop other illnesses, such as coronary disease, in the interim. If they developed conditions such as Alzheimer's disease, the custodial costs might be substantial. However, these costs would be countered by savings from hospitalizations for advanced cancer and by a potential increase in productive wage-earning years.

In all analyses of costs, it is important to consider *when* the costs will be incurred and *when* the effects in health benefits may be realized. Present dollars or health benefits are considered to have greater worth than a promise of future dollars or health benefits for several reasons. Other events may intercede so that a projected future cost or benefit may never occur, and there is always the possibility that money spent now will not achieve the desired effect at some time in the future. Furthermore, another illness may intervene, or there might be better ways to spend the money in the future. The principle by which future dollars and benefits are less highly valued than known immediate costs and benefits is termed *discounting*. It is independent of monetary inflation. By this concept it is preferable to spend $1000 today to prevent someone from dying today than it is to spend $1000 today in the expectation that someone will not die ten years from now.

It is unusual for any program simultaneously to achieve the greatest possible benefit and have the lowest possible cost. Instead, one usually either determines the desired benefit and then finds the lowest cost needed to achieve it or determines the resources available and then finds the greatest possible benefit that can be achieved.

Analyses of cost-effectiveness commonly examine the ratio of cost to effectiveness, i.e., the number of dollars required to save a life or a year of life. Such analyses are relevant to medicine because interventions only rarely both save lives and reduce costs. Hence, it is important to estimate the tradeoff of costs for gains in health. Two strategies with the same ratio may have quite different absolute costs and absolute benefits. For example, a program that saves 100 lives for $100,000 has the same cost effectiveness ratio as one that saves 1000 lives for $1,000,000, but the absolute costs and absolute benefits vary ten-fold. The choice between these two programs may depend on how much money is available to spend. In assessing any program, it is important to measure incremental costs and effects rather than average costs and effects. For example, consider two programs to reduce death from lung cancer. If, on average, program A costs $100,000,000 to save 100,000 years of life (average of $1000 per year of life) and program B costs $200,000,000 to save 100,100 years of life (about $2000 per year of life), the *incremental* cost of program B versus program A is $1,000,000 per year of life saved.

SOCIETAL ISSUES IN COSTS It is rare to find a medical intervention, such as measles vaccination programs, that both saves lives and reduces overall costs because the savings from disease prevention more than outweigh the expenses of the treatment itself. More commonly, medical practices that are truly of benefit also cause an associated increase in medical care costs. Among the more cost-effective examples is coronary artery bypass surgery in patients with left main coronary artery disease, which costs about $6000 per year of life saved.

The shift of services from the inpatient to the outpatient setting or from the hospital to the home generally reduces the expense of delivery of that aspect of medical care. For example, home dialysis is less expensive than dialysis in an outpatient center, which in turn is less expensive than dialysis in a hospital. Similarly, the administration of parenteral nutrition and intravenous antibiotics at home as well as home care for patients with the acquired immunodeficiency syndrome have greatly reduced the need for hospitalization for conditions in which skilled nursing care is otherwise not required. However, a byproduct of this strategy is an increased percentage of severely ill hospital inpatients, who require more intensive and expensive care than the less sick patients who otherwise might have occupied hospital beds.

To date, society has been reluctant to make ethical decisions regarding the amount of cost appropriate for any particular net benefit. Neither medicine nor society is accustomed to placing a dollar value on a life or a year of life. In many analyses, however, the annual costs of approximately $30,000 to $35,000 (in 1990 dollars) for renal dialysis for 1 year of useful life have been used as a benchmark of how much the United States is willing to spend to save a year of life, because such a program is supported with tax dollars and presumably is a reasonable reflection of national priorities.

The physician has a unique responsibility. On the one hand, the physician must serve as an advocate for the individual patient and recommend the course of action most likely to be beneficial to the patient. The overriding nature of the patient-physician relationship is the cornerstone of humane medical care. On the other hand, physicians must understand the costs as well as the benefits of medical interventions so that they can choose from among the wide range of options. The physician must serve as the advocate for providing the best options to the individual patient and should know which options are of little or no value or are more likely to do harm than good. The physician must, with the assistance and consent of the patient and the family, set priorities for the patient's management within any limits or restrictions imposed by society; such limits may be expressed, for example, in a finite number of dollars available for the treatment of a specific illness. In addition, physicians have a broad role in determining health costs. Individually and through various professional organizations, physicians have a responsibility to help set national priorities, based on their appreciation of the finite resources available for health care and their knowledge of the relative benefits and costs of various diagnostic and therapeutic options in particular types of patients.

HEALTH SCREENING Screening refers to the performance of a medical evaluation and/or diagnostic tests in asymptomatic persons in the hope that early diagnosis may lead to improved outcome. For such persons it was initially assumed that a periodic health examination, often accompanied by multiphasic diagnostic testing, is beneficial. However, there is no definitive information regarding the value of such an approach and even less information regarding which aspects yield results that are worth the costs incurred. In fact, there is no universally accepted approach to screening in the asymptomatic adult, given the uncertainties about the benefits and cost-effectiveness of each intervention. Nevertheless, the recommendations in Table 3-3 represent a reasonable set of guidelines for the periodic health assessment of asymptomatic adults.

Another issue in screening concerns the choice of which routine tests to perform in a patient who is about to undergo an operation or who is admitted to the hospital. For example, routine preoperative chest radiography is not indicated in persons without signs, symptoms, or risk factors for pulmonary or cardiac disease. Routine preoperative electrocardiography is generally recommended in any person with cardiac signs or symptoms and in men over age 40 and women over age 50, because of the age-related increase in asymptomatic cardiac disease and the likelihood that the preoperative tracing may be helpful for comparison, should any cardiac problems arise during the perioperative period. In these situations, appropriate tests must be performed to investigate specific symptoms and signs. In terms of screening tests for asymptomatic conditions, those tests and procedures that have not been performed under the guidelines in Table 3-3 normally should be performed while the patient is under medical care.

HEALTH PROMOTION AND DISEASE PREVENTION Health promotion and disease prevention require investment of time, energy, and resources, in the hope that the yield in terms of improved health warrants this investment. Unfortunately, there is limited information on the effectiveness of health promotion and disease prevention efforts. Interventions that result in a specified *relative* reduction in adverse outcomes have a greater *absolute* effect in higher-risk populations. For example, the same relative reduction in serum cholesterol will be of greater absolute benefit in persons with higher

TABLE 3-3 Guidelines for preventive medical services*

	Age of person		
	19–39 years	40–64 years	65 + years
History	Every 1 to 3 years†: diet; physical activity; tobacco, alcohol, drugs; sexual practices	Same as 19–39 years	Every year: same as 19–39 years; and also functional status and symptoms of transient ischemia attacks
Exam	Every 1 to 3 years: height, weight, blood pressure High risk: oral cavity, thyroid, breast, testes, skin	Every 1 to 3 years: height, weight, blood pressure, breast High risk: oral cavity, thyroid, skin, carotids	Every year: as for 40–64 years and also hearing and visual acuity High risk: as for 40–64 years (but every year)
Laboratory	Pap smear (every 1 to 3 years), total cholesterol High risk: fasting glucose, rubella antibodies, VDRL, urinalysis, chlamydia testing, gonorrhea culture, HIV testing, hearing, PPD, EKG, mammogram, colonoscopy	Pap smear every 1 to 3 years, mammogram (every 1 to 2 years after age 50), total cholesterol High risk: fasting glucose, VDRL, urinalysis, chlamydia testing, gonorrhea culture, HIV testing, hearing, PPD, EKG, fecal occult blood/sigmoidoscopy/colonoscopy, bone mineral content	Mammogram (every 1 to 2 years until age 75), thyroid indices (women), dipstick urinalysis, total cholesterol High risk: fasting glucose, PPD, EKG, Pap smear (every 1 to 3 years), fecal occult blood/sigmoidoscopy/colonoscopy
Special counseling	Injury prevention, dental health High risk: hemoglobin testing, skin protection from ultraviolet light	Injury prevention, dental health, skin protection from ultraviolet light, discussion of aspirin therapy in men and estrogen replacement in women	As for 40 to 64 years and also glaucoma testing
Immunizations	Tetanus-diphtheria booster every 10 years High risk: hepatitis B, pneumococcal, influenza (every year), measles-mumps-rubella	As for 19 to 39 years except not measles-mumps-rubella	Tetanus-diphtheria booster (every 10 years) influenza (every year), pneumococcal High risk: hepatitis B

* Except for the visit itself, the frequency is at clinical discretion unless otherwise specified.
† With counseling for any high-risk behaviors.
SOURCE: Adapted from U.S. Preventive Services Task Force (Guide to Clinical Preventive Services, Maryland: Williams and Wilkins, 1989), whose official report lists full details, including the definition of high-risk situations.

serum cholesterol levels or other unfavorable risk factors. In general, interventions to alter risk factors have a diminishing effect as risk factors decrease in severity.

Both patients and society commonly expect physicians to play a leadership role in health promotion and disease prevention. Patients expect and desire their physicians to make recommendations regarding physical activity, diet, and other lifestyle issues, and physicians often fail in this regard. If physicians do not become involved, patients seek advice elsewhere, risking the possibility that fads or other erroneous sources may influence their choices.

When physicians become actively involved in health promotion, patients respond frequently and make appropriate behavior changes. For example, a physician's encouragement to increase physical activity, especially if combined with explicit suggestions, is likely to lead to changes in behavior so that the time spent by the physician appears to be cost-effective. Advice by a physician that a patient should lose weight or discontinue smoking is successful in only a small minority of cases, but it is an excellent first step toward health promotion and disease prevention (Chap. 373).

Programs in the workplace or in schools can commonly achieve weight losses of 2 to 5 kg at a cost of about $10 to $30 per kilogram lost. Despite high attrition rates, group approaches, such as Weight Watchers, can also produce similar weight losses at similar costs. A physician's advice is about as effective as these programs, and it is often the physician's advice that stimulates patients to try other interventions.

Physician-directed dietary interventions commonly lower the serum cholesterol level by as much as 10 percent. Drug treatment may be more effective but is more expensive. For example, treatment with cholestyramine in men costs more than $50,000 per year of life saved except in very high risk persons. Treatment strategies for hypertension are more cost-effective; the approximate cost of screening and treating hypertension, given the average medication compliance rates, ranges from about $10,000 per year of life saved for a patient with a diastolic blood pressure of 105 mmHg or higher to about $20,000 for a person with a diastolic blood pressure of 95 to 104 mmHg.

Immunizations, including pneumococcal and influenza vaccination in elderly and high-risk patients, are effective ways to reduce disease and its associated costs. Guidelines for immunizations in adults are indicated in Table 3-3 (see also Chap. 84).

DIAGNOSTIC TESTING As detailed in Chap. 2, diagnostic tests are valuable only to the extent that they provide new, *incremental* information that cannot be obtained less expensively from the history, physical examination, or other less expensive tests. Although these tests may often be of psychological benefit in reassuring the patient or the physician, they commonly generate redundant information, often result in a needless expense, and may entail risk. For example, in the evaluation of left ventricular function, the physician must decide whether a two-dimensional echocardiogram is sufficient or whether the more precise but more expensive measurement by radionuclide ventriculography is worthwhile. The physician faces analogous choices when deciding whether to obtain both an abdominal ultrasound examination and an abdominal computed tomogram or, in a different case, whether computed tomography and magnetic resonance imaging of the head are both required.

Ideally, each test should be ordered in sequence only to the extent that it is expected to add to the data available. However, this iterative approach can be expensive in hospitalized patients, where the sequencing of tests may lead to delays in scheduling and performing them. In these situations, the expense of the additional days of waiting may more than offset the savings from possibly avoiding a particular test. Usually, careful consideration of the problem by a physician is one of the most cost-effective ways to evaluate the patient. Expert consultation may be more cost-effective and helpful than ordering more diagnostic tests. Although interventions designed to reduce test utilization have met with variable success, those that have been successful have generally included educational components, full endorsement by locally respected leaders, and frequent reinforcement.

TREATMENT CHOICES In choosing among various treatments, physicians try to enhance the likelihood of an optimal outcome. It is important to consider whether an equivalent outcome could be achieved at a lower cost. For example, generic medications may be substituted for more expensive brand-name counterparts. Similarly, outcome is not usually compromised by interventions designed to encourage the use of less expensive antibiotic regimens. Endorsement by the medical profession of restricted indications for procedures such as pacemaker implantation and tonsillectomy have led to decreased utilization without any detectable reduction in life expectancy or quality of life. Whenever possible, diagnostic and therapeutic options should be subjected to strict evaluation of both benefit and cost-effectiveness, and physicians have responsibility to assist in such evaluations and to learn from their results.

INDIVIDUALIZATION

As already stated, the physician has a moral and legal responsibility to serve as the advocate for the patient, within the limits set by society. This requires an individual approach to the patient and an understanding of how the available resources of the health care system can best be applied to the person and the problem at hand. Nevertheless, the physician and the patient must recognize that expensive medicine is not necessarily better medicine.

Special consideration revolves around the use of expensive procedures in medical care, such as liver, heart, and bone marrow transplantation. In these situations, the limited availability of donors makes it necessary to choose the best possible recipients from among a wide range of potential candidates and to "ration." Although rationing is not pleasant, physicians have often responded well in situations with limited resources. For example, when faced with a reduction in intensive care unit availability, physicians are usually successful at maintaining normal admission rates for patients who most require intensive care so that little if any adverse effects occur in those excluded from intensive care.

There is marked variability in the rates at which various procedures are performed in different geographic areas, even though there are no obvious differences in the types or ages of patients. For example, the rates of prostatectomy vary markedly in different parts of New England. To date, little difference in health care outcomes can be detected despite wide differences in the rates of various procedures. These variations may in part be related to patients' preferences and in part to differing beliefs among physicians regarding optimal medical care choices. When the records of patients who have undergone such procedures are reviewed to determine how the indications for their procedure compared to the standards recommended by experts, a substantial proportion of procedures are deemed inappropriate. However, so far there is no close correlation between the percentage of cases deemed inappropriate and the rate at which the procedure is performed in a given location. There is no definitive evidence that high rates of performance can be equated with a high rate of unnecessary use.

The variations in rates of utilization, the proportion of cases in which some procedures seem not to be necessary, and the ability of physicians to respond to situations in which rationing is necessary suggest that in many situations the quality of medical care and the likelihood of a favorable outcome can be maintained while lowering costs. Society, with the input of physicians, must exercise this role without compromising the physician's responsibility to the individual patient.

REFERENCES

CHASSIN MR et al: Does inappropriate use explain geographic variations in the use of health care services? A study of three procedures. JAMA 258:2533, 1987

DETSKY AS et al: The effectiveness of a regulatory strategy in containing hospital costs. N Engl J Med 309:151, 1983

DRUMMOND M et al: Health economics: An introduction for clinicians. Ann Intern Med 107:88, 1987

ENTHOVEN A, KRONICK R: A consumer-choice health plan for the 1990s. Universal health insurance in a system designed to promote quality and economy. N Engl J Med 320:29, 94, 1989

EVANS RG et al: Controlling health expenditures—the Canadian reality. N Engl J Med 320:571, 1989

FUCHS VR: The "competition revolution" in health care. Health Aff (Millwood) 7(3):5, 1988

GOLDBERGER AL, OKONSKI M: Utility of the routine electrocardiogram before surgery and on general hospital admission. Ann Intern Med 105:552, 1986

GOLDMAN L: Cost-effective strategies in cardiology, in *Heart Disease*, 3d ed, E Braunwald (ed). Philadelphia, Saunders, 1988, pp 1680–92

GUTERMAN S et al: The first three years of Medicare prospective payment: An overview. Health Care Financ Rev 9:67, 1988

HSIAO WC et al: Special Report. Results and policy implications of the resource-based relative-value study. N Engl J Med 319:881, 1988

ROBINSON JC, LUFT HS: Competition, regulation and hospital costs, 1982 to 1986. JAMA 260:2676, 1988

RUSSELL LB, MANNING CL: The effect of prospective payment on Medicare expenditures. N Engl J Med 320:439, 1989

SCHROEDER SA: Strategies for reducing medical costs by changing physicians' behavior. Int J Technol Assess Health Care 3:39, 1987

WEINSTEIN MC, STASON WB: Foundations of cost effectiveness analysis for health and medical practices. N Engl J Med 296:716, 1977

WENNBERG JE et al: Are hospital services rationed in New Haven or over-utilised in Boston? Lancet 1:1185, 1987

4 THE CHALLENGE OF GERIATRIC MEDICINE

ROBERT N. BUTLER

INTRODUCTION Since the beginning of this century, industrialized countries have witnessed an unprecedented increase in the absolute number and relative proportion of older persons.[1] In 1900, the average life expectancy in the United States was 47 years, and only 4 percent of the population was over 65 years of age; today's average life expectancy is 75, and 12.2 percent of Americans are over 65.

A 28-year gain in average life expectancy is quite extraordinary; in fact, it nearly equals those years of life expectancy gained between the bronze age (approximately 3000 B.C.) and 1900. This is a social achievement, not a consequence of biologic evolution. It is a function not only of medical science, but of socioeconomic progress, sanitation, and better nutrition. Approximately 80 percent of this gain is a result of marked reductions of maternal, childhood, and infant mortality rates; about 20 percent has been gained from base age 65, due to effective prevention, management, or control of hypertension, diabetes, and other chronic as well as acute diseases. It is estimated that the control of heart disease could add another 10 years of life, and the conquest of cancer could add a little more than 2 years.

These sudden, dramatic demographic changes have demanded rapid adaptation. For comparative purposes, one might note that the industrialized world is still adapting to the industrial scientific revolution initiated in the 1730s. Efforts are still underway to adapt to the separation of the family from the workplace, pollution, despoilation of the environment, and urbanization. Therefore, it should not be surprising that time is required to adjust to the major demographic changes of population aging, which, in fact, is a consequence of the industrial revolution itself. The development of social security systems and medical and health insurance in industrialized nations such as the United States, Japan, and those in Europe illustrates these social adjustments.

The development of geriatrics, particularly in Great Britain and Scandinavia, and in some measure in Japan and less so in the United States, also reflects response to current demographic trends. Demographic, epidemiologic, and socioeconomic issues have forced attention upon research into aging and encouraged new forms of health service delivery for older persons.

DEMOGRAPHICS OF AGING The dramatic rise in the number and proportion of older persons as an extraordinary historic event is important. Medicine and public health, having had their parts to play in this new, unprecedented demographic change, have assumed some of the responsibilities to help deal with the resulting challenges. In 1987, the total U.S. elderly population was 29.8 million, 12.2 percent of the country's total population. Life expectancy at age 65 increased by only 2.4 years between 1900 and 1960, but since 1960 it has increased by another 2.7 years. In 1987, those persons reaching age 65 could expect, on the average, to live another 16.9 years—18.6 years for females and 14.8 years for males.

The gradually increasing number and proportion of older persons are only partly explained by a rise in longevity; they are also due to an increased birth rate in the 1920s and after World War II. The aging of the pre-1920s group, along with the decline in the birth rate during the mid-1960s, has contributed to an increased proportion of older persons and to the rise of the median age of the U.S. population from 27.9 years in 1970 to 32.1 in 1987.

Should current fertility and immigration levels remain stable in the United States, only the over-55 age group will experience significant growth in the next century. This is apt to occur in two stages: through the year 2000, the proportion of those aged 55 and over will remain relatively stable, at approximately one in five; by 2010, due to the aging of the "baby boomers," it will rise dramatically. Over one-fourth of the U.S. population will be 55 and over, and one in seven will be at least 65. These figures will rise to one in three and one in five, respectively, by 2030 (Fig 4-1).

Since 1960, life expectancy at age 85 has increased 24 percent. Next to the baby boomer population, the 85-plus age group is growing most rapidly. Moreover, the number of centenarians has increased from 15,000 in 1980 to 25,000 in 1986 and is expected to surpass 100,000 by the year 2000. This increase in the very old makes it likely that the elderly themselves will have at least one surviving parent. Indeed, the twentieth century has seen the rise of the multigenerational family; four- and five-generation families are becoming more common. According to 1982 data, the most recent figures available from the National Center for Health Statistics, approximately 2.2 million caregivers with an average age of 57 (72 percent of whom are females) provide unpaid assistance to 1.6 million noninstitutionalized older disabled persons.

A distinct difference in life expectancy exists between the sexes. Women outlive men by an average of 6.8 years. The proportion of men to women within elderly age groups declines with age. In 1987, the over-65 group had 17.7 million women and only 12.1 million men, or 146 women for every 100 men. The upper-age ranges saw an even more marked difference. For every 100 men in the 65-to-69 age group, there were 120 women; for those 85 and over, the number of women rose to 256 for every 100 men.

This sex difference in mortality accounts for most older men being married and most older women widowed; there are at least three times as many widows as widowers. In 1988, only 23.7 percent of noninstitutionalized men aged 75 and older were widowed, compared with 66.1 percent of women in this same age group, making older women more likely to end up living alone for a longer period of time and, as a group, the ones who are especially confronted with the challenge of aging.

Diseases and accidents account for approximately 75 percent of this distinction between the sexes. In the United States, the higher male mortality rate is a result of coronary artery disease, lung cancer and emphysema associated with tobacco intake, industrial accidents and exposure to toxic chemicals, motor vehicle and other accidents, suicide, and cirrhosis of the liver. Further research is needed to determine to what extent the other 25 percent is due to differences in life-style, life stress, hormonal status, genetic make-up, immune function, and other factors.

The risk of institutionalization at age 65 is the subject of debate. Some believe that no more than 20 percent of those who live past 65 years will enter, even briefly, an institution of any kind (e.g., chronic-care hospital, home for the aged, nursing home, foster home); other projections suggest an estimated figure of closer to 40 percent. However, only 5 percent of the elderly are institutionalized at any one time. These residents tend to be very old, female, and white. Nearly 84 percent of nursing home residents are without a spouse, compared to 45 percent of the noninstitutionalized elderly. In addition, only 63 percent of older nursing-home residents have children, compared to 81 percent of the elderly living in the community.

Before 1980, most older people lived in inner-city and rural areas; since that time, however, more of the 65-and-over population has resided in the suburbs than the central cities.

EPIDEMIOLOGY OF AGING In the United States, changes in behavior during this century have resulted in different causes of death.

[1]Although age 75 is the conventional definition of a geriatric patient, age 65 is used throughout this chapter (unless noted otherwise) to designate entry into old age, for this is when many people retire and one becomes eligible for such social entitlements as Medicare.

FIGURE 4-1   Population 55 years and over by age: 1900 to 2050. (*Source: CM Teuber, Current Population Reports ser. P-23, no. 128; and G Spencer, Current Population Reports ser. P-25, no. 952.*)

In 1900, heart disease was the fourth leading cause of death, but since 1910 it has remained in the number one position. Cancer was not even among the top five causes of death until 1930, when it became number three; it has been in the number two spot since 1950. Stroke was the fifth leading cause of death from 1900 to 1930, but since 1950 it has been in third place. Accidents were not among the top five until 1950, when they became, and remain, the fourth leading cause of death. Lung disease has been the fifth leading cause of death since 1986. Since 1985, the number of suicides has increased among all age groups, but the most dramatic increase has occurred in the 75-to-84-year category.

Together, heart disease, cancer, and stroke account for 75 percent of all deaths among the elderly, 20 percent of doctor visits, 30 percent of hospital days, and 50 percent of bed-ridden days. Stroke, the third leading cause of death for this group, has been decreasing over the past 30 years, perhaps due to improved control of hypertension and better management and rehabilitation.

The average length of an older person's hospital stay has been declining, from 14.2 days in 1968 to 8.6 days in 1987. (For those under 65, the average stay is 5.4 days.) In part, this decline is a result of changing hospital regulations (DRGs), although a decrease in hospital stay occurred even prior to these changes. Most older persons are admitted to a hospital because of acute episodes of a chronic condition. In 1985, circulatory diseases accounted for 31 percent of admissions, digestive diseases for 12 percent, respiratory diseases for 11 percent, and neoplasms for 10 percent.

It is obvious that the older one gets, the more likely that illness will occur. Yet most elderly persons are in reasonably good health and able to function independently. Although acute conditions have become less frequent, chronic conditions, single and multiple, are common among the elderly, especially women. Arthritis is probably the number one, everyday quality-of-life medical problem of old age and produces immense morbidity. Although it results in relatively few deaths and only 2 percent of hospital days, it accounts for 16 percent of the days spent in bed, nearly as much as for heart disease. In fact, arthritis, hypertension, and hearing impairment, respectively, are the top three chronic conditions of the elderly.

SOCIOECONOMICS OF AGING   Negative attitudes toward older persons are common throughout U.S. culture, including the medical profession. In the latter, such prejudice probably reflects the sense of helplessness that physicians feel when required to respond to the complex needs of the older patient, coupled with the discomfort engendered by the reality of aging and proximity to dying and death.

Misconceptions and prejudices about aging must be refuted and overcome; for example, age itself does not produce senility, lack of productivity, or loss of sexual desire and ability.

Many older persons prefer to retire and do not seek work. Almost two-thirds of retirees leave the work force before age 65, largely for health reasons. There has been a steady decline in work-force participation rates. In 1900 the average male spent a little over one year, or 3 percent of his life, in retirement or in other activities outside the work force; by 1980, however, he spent 19 percent of his 70 years in retirement, or 13.6 years. In 1950, almost half of all men aged 65 and over were in the labor force; by 1987, this figure had fallen to 16 percent. Labor force participation of older women has varied only slightly: 10 percent in 1950 compared with approximately 7.4 percent in 1987. Part-time work is favored by the working public of all ages and is deemed desirable during retirement by many older persons who view their health positively.

The increase of eligibility for Social Security from age 65 to age 67, to be phased in by the year 2027, and the elimination of mandatory retirement may have only minimal impact on increasing the number of older persons in the work force, even though an estimated worker shortage is predicted in the 1990s and the next century, particularly in the service industries. Already some U.S. businesses are seeking to mainstream, hire, or rehire older workers.

Some are afraid that the increasingly older population will become unaffordable, lead to stagnation of society's productive and economic growth, and generate intergenerational conflict. While there is an increasing number of retirees compared to nonretirees, the combined total of the dependent group, defined as the young (below 18) plus the old (above 60), has decreased since 1900 and is expected to continue to decline until early into the next century, depending on immigration, when it will then begin to rise. Although working-age Americans support the young and the old, our birth rate is below the zero population growth, helping to offset the increasing number of the aged.

The support ratio has become a political issue. It has been argued that the support of the old is on the backs of the young, especially in the federal outlay of funds. However, while it is true that entitlements for the elderly are primarily supported by federal publicly funded programs, the young are supported primarily by the community, state, and private funds in the form of taxes for public education. In any case, survey data (e.g., the Louis Harris polls) show that the young, and not just the old, favor entitlements for the old. This is due partly to the fact that the young understand that they, too, will one day be old. Furthermore, such entitlements directly benefit the middle-aged children of the old by helping to relieve them of some of the financial responsibilities for their parents they might otherwise have to assume.

Older persons, as a group, enjoy a lower socioeconomic status than other adults. The median income of the elderly in 1987 was $11,854 for men and $6734 for women. Families headed by persons aged 65 and over reported a median income of $20,813. In 1986, the major source of income for older families and individuals was Social Security (35 percent), followed by asset income (24 percent), earnings (24 percent), and public and private pensions (15 percent). Social Security is a life-course protection program that provides funds for survivors and the disabled, not just persons on pensions. Indeed, 60 percent of Social Security benefits go to retirees, and 40 percent go to surviving widows and to more than 3 million children. The poverty level of older Americans is alarming. In 1987, the poverty threshold for elderly couples was $6872 and for the elderly living alone, $5447 ($132 and $104 per week, respectively). One-third of elderly Americans had total incomes below 150 percent of the poverty level; one-fifth had incomes below 125 percent of the poverty level.

Older people living alone have special problems. They tend to be aged 75 and above and are at greater risk for institutionalization. Low-income elderly are in poorer health and are more likely to suffer from chronic illness and to be functionally impaired than higher income elderly. Three-fifths of the elderly living on less than $104 per week live alone. Two-thirds of this group are widows, the primary victims of poverty among the aged.

Although older persons spend 67 percent of their income on housing (including utilities), food, and medical care, compared to 49 percent spent by younger households, one of their greatest expenditures is health care. The average per capita expenditure for acute medical care for an older person was approximately $3500 in 1987, and one-third of all the near-poor elderly were forced into poverty by medical expenses. Direct out-of-pocket health costs for the elderly average 15 percent of their income, the same amount as before Medicare and Medicaid were enacted.

According to 1984 data from the Health Care Financing Administration, Medicare covered 49 percent of all personal health care expenses for older persons. Medicare primarily provides for acute care services; care provided by hospitals accounts for 69 percent of health care. In 1984, the program paid 75 percent of hospital costs and 58 percent of physician service costs. Although spending for home health care has grown dramatically, it accounts for only 3.3 percent of Medicare benefit payments. Five percent of the elderly do not have Medicare. Since its enactment, Medicare's deductible and co-insurance requirements have increased, as has the premium. Medicaid, the federal/state program that is the principal source of financing nursing home care, accounts for 42 percent of all expenditures for nursing home care; however, only one in three older persons officially below the poverty line actually qualifies for Medicaid.

The Old Age and Survivors Insurance Trust Fund of the Social Security system is in close actuarial balance: during the next 75 years there will be no problems of insolvency. In contrast, it is estimated that the Medicare Trust Fund will be in trouble shortly after the turn of the century. The provision of new financing of long-term care is a critical issue. Some progress has been made in resolving the problem. Pending legislation reflects the government's concern with rising long-term care costs. Many large private insurers have become interested in testing and marketing long-term care, and coverage is becoming more comprehensive, inexpensive, and readily available. Several major employers, including the federal government, have been investigating long-term care insurance for their employees, and corporations are developing various programs to help workers care for aging relatives. As the elderly population continues to grow, so, too, will the need for long-term care services, both home and institutional. More pressure then will be brought to bear upon Medicaid and alternative sources of financing. Deciding the balance between private and public sectors is a major challenge for the future.

EVALUATION OF ELDERLY INDIVIDUALS   Many biologic changes over time, such as altered enzymes indicating hepatic malfunction, are now found to be connected with chronic disease and alcoholism, rather than normal aging. Numerous pathophysiologic alterations that had been attributed to the unavoidable aging process are actually results of disease, lending themselves to amelioration and even prevention. Notable examples are arteriosclerosis and senile dementia, once feared most as consequences of aging. It is also true that vulnerability to disease increases with age.

Personal-care activities—bathing, dressing, eating, getting in and out of bed and chairs, walking, going outside, and using the toilet—are known as *activities of daily living* (ADLs). *Instrumental activities of daily living* (IADLs) are home-management activities, and include preparing meals, shopping for personal items, managing money, using the telephone, and doing heavy or light housework. About one-quarter of the 65-and-over population has difficulty with one or more of the seven personal-care activities; approximately the same number has difficulty with one of the six home-management activities. Walking poses the most difficulty among the ADLs, heavy housework among the IADLs.

The geriatric patient tends to be aged 75 and over, with multiple, complex, interacting psychosocial and physical pathology, both acute and chronic. A person may enter a hospital with a kidney problem and, as a consequence of sophisticated care, leave with improved kidney function, but may barely be able to walk for numerous other reasons. To provide comprehensive care, what is required is not just a nephrologist or internist, but a team consisting of a nurse, social worker, psychiatrist, and/or neuropsychologist, among others, who are concerned with why such patients cannot walk, whether they are depressed, and how they will be able to cope outside the hospital.

The National Institutes of Health Consensus Conference defined an assessment and evaluation method that is particularly suited to older patients. It is a multidisciplinary team approach that looks at a patient functionally rather than in terms of specific organs, systems, and diseases. The American College of Physicians also argues that patients aged 75 and older need to be tested for baseline function. Geriatric assessment uncovers, describes, and explains the multiple problems of older patients, their resources and strengths, and their need for services; a coordinated care plan is then developed to focus on possible interventions. The functional assessment identifies problems that may require more detailed assessment by other medical and nonmedical professionals, including audiologists, clinical psychologists, dentists, nutritionists, occupational and physical therapists, podiatrists, and pharmacists. The assessment process provides the physician with reliable information about the patient's true ability to function independently in the community. It also identifies nonmedical issues with which a patient may need help, such as Medicaid eligibility, or community facilities with which both patient and physician may be unfamiliar, such as Meals on Wheels or respite for the caregiver. The physician also may gain insight into the patient's wishes about ultimate life support.

Numerous in-patient studies support the effectiveness of this interdisciplinary approach to management and evaluation. A Veterans Administration study revealed reduced hospital stays, less rehospitalization, and decreased mortality and morbidity rates for groups that had comprehensive assessments and received the services that were needed. Team-oriented outpatient geriatric assessment provides a promising way to deliver high-quality, satisfying care to the elderly, besides possibly decreasing health care costs.

Geriatrics requires integration throughout medicine. It need not be a practice specialty. Rather, every primary care and specialty physician must have adequate training and knowledge in the principles of geriatrics. Attention must be paid to the functional and geriatric assessment and to these interdisciplinary approaches. The definition of geriatrics implies a broad perspective that integrates all aspects of medicine, not internal medicine alone. To achieve this integration, geriatric medicine must develop the resources to pioneer innovations in diagnosis and care and to concentrate on age-related research.

REFERENCES

AMERICAN COLLEGE OF PHYSICIANS: Comprehensive functional assessment for elderly patients. Ann Intern Med 109:70, 1988

BIRREN JE et al: *Human Aging I: A Biological and Behavioral Study.* Public Health Service Publication No. 986. Washington, DC, US Government Printing Office, 1963, reprinted 1971 and 1974

BRODY JA, SCHNEIDER EL: Diseases and disorders of aging: An hypothesis. J Chron Dis 39:871, 1986

BUTLER RN: An overview of research on aging and the status of gerontology today. Milbank Mem Fund Q 61:351, 1983

————: The relation of extended life to extended employment since the passage of Social Security in 1935. Milbank Mem Fund Q 61:420, 1983

COMMONWEALTH FUND COMMISSION: Medicare's poor: Filling the gaps in medical coverage for low-income elderly Americans. New York, The Commonwealth Fund, 1987

————: Old, alone and poor: A plan for reducing poverty among elderly people living alone. New York, The Commonwealth Fund, 1987

GRANICK S, PATTERSON RD (eds): *Human Aging II: An Eleven Year Biomedical and Behavioral Study.* US Public Health Service Monograph No. (HSM) 71-9037, 1971. Reprinted 1976

HAZZARD WR et al (eds): *Principles of Geriatric Medicine and Gerontology,* 2d ed. New York, McGraw-Hill, 1990

NIH CONSENSUS DEVELOPMENT PANEL. National Institutes of Health Consensus Development Conference Statement: Geriatric assessment methods for clinical decision-making. J Am Geriatr Soc 36:342, 1988

RODIN J: Aging and health: Effects of the sense of control. Science 233:1271, 1986

ROWE JW, KAHN RL: Human aging: Usual and successful. Science 237:143, 1987

RUBENSTEIN LZ et al: Effectiveness of geriatric evaluation unit: A randomized clinical trial. N Engl J Med 311:1664, 1984

————: The Sepulveda VA geriatric evaluation unit: Data on four-year outcomes and predictors of improved patient outcomes. J Am Geriatr Soc 32:503, 1984

US SENATE SPECIAL COMMITTEE ON AGING, AMERICAN ASSOCIATION OF RETIRED PERSONS, FEDERAL COUNCIL ON THE AGING, and US ADMINISTRATION ON AGING: Aging America: Trends and projections, 1987–88. Washington, DC, U.S. Department of Health and Human Services, LR 3377 (188) D12198

WILLIAMS ME et al: How does the team approach to outpatient geriatric evaluation compare with traditional care: A report of a randomized controlled trial. J Am Geriatr Soc 35:1071, 1987

section 1 Genetics

5 GENETIC ASPECTS OF DISEASE

JOSEPH L. GOLDSTEIN / MICHAEL S. BROWN

GENETIC PRINCIPLES

More than one-fifth of the proteins (and hence genes) in each human being exist in a form that differs from the one present in the majority of the population. This remarkable genetic variability, or polymorphism, among "normal" people accounts for much of the normal variation in body traits such as height, intelligence, and blood pressure. These genetic differences also determine the ability of each individual to meet environmental challenges, including those that produce disease. All human diseases can be considered to result from an interaction between an individual's unique genetic makeup and the environment. In certain diseases, the genetic component is so overwhelming that it expresses itself in a predictable manner without a requirement for extraordinary environmental challenges. Such diseases are termed *genetic disorders*.

MOLECULAR BASIS OF GENE EXPRESSION All hereditary information is transmitted from parent to offspring through the inheritance of deoxyribonucleic acid (DNA). DNA is a linear polymer composed of purine and pyrimidine bases whose sequence ultimately determines the sequence of amino acids in every protein made by the body. The four types of bases in DNA are arranged in groups of three, each triplet forming a code word, or codon, that signifies a particular amino acid. A *gene* represents the total sequence of bases in DNA that specifies the amino acid sequence of a single polypeptide chain of a protein molecule.

Genetic information encoded in the DNA of the chromosomes is first transcribed into a *ribonucleic acid* (RNA) copy. During transcription the ribose nucleotides align themselves along the DNA according to base-pairing rules. Thus, adenine of DNA pairs with uridine of RNA, cytosine pairs with guanine, thymine pairs with adenine, and guanine pairs with cytosine. The ribose bases are joined together by RNA polymerase. The resulting *RNA transcript* forms the template for translation into the amino acid sequence of a protein. Figure 5-1 shows the DNA and mRNA code words for each of the amino acids in protein.

Figure 5-2 illustrates a schematic diagram of the genetic control of protein synthesis in higher organisms, including humans. The DNA of most genes is fragmented into discrete coding regions (exons) separated by noncoding regions (introns or intervening sequences). The *coding regions* contain the bases that specify the sequence of amino acids in the polypeptide chain. The *intervening sequences* are composed of bases that act as spacers between the coding regions; they are not translated into protein. The transcription of DNA produces a faithful copy of the entire gene sequence; thus, the RNA transcript

FIGURE 5-1 The genetic code.

Second nucleotide

		A or U		G or C		T or A		C or G		
A or **U**	**AAA** **AAG** **AAT** **AAC**	*UUU* *UUC* *UUA* *UUG*	Phe Leu	**AGA** **AGG** **AGT** **AGC**	*UCU* *UCC* *UCA* *UCG*	Ser	**ATA** **ATG** **ATT** **ATC**	*UAU* *UAC* *UAA* *UAG*	Tyr Stop	**ACA** **ACG** **ACT** **ACC**	*UGU* *UGC* *UGA* *UGG*	Cys Stop Trp	**A** or **U** **G** or **C** **T** or **A** **C** or **G**
G or **C**	**GAA** **GAG** **GAT** **GAC**	*CUU* *CUC* *CUA* *CUG*	Leu	**GGA** **GGG** **GGT** **GGC**	*CCU* *CCC* *CCA* *CCG*	Pro	**GTA** **GTG** **GTT** **GTC**	*CAU* *CAC* *CAA* *CAG*	His Gln	**GCA** **GCG** **GCT** **GCC**	*CGU* *CGC* *CGA* *CGG*	Arg	**A** or **U** **G** or **C** **T** or **A** **C** or **G**
T or **A**	**TAA** **TAG** **TAT** **TAC**	*AUU* *AUC* *AUA* *AUG*	Ile Met	**TGA** **TGG** **TGT** **TGC**	*ACU* *ACC* *ACA* *ACG*	Thr	**TTA** **TTG** **TTT** **TTC**	*AAU* *AAC* *AAA* *AAG*	Asn Lys	**TCA** **TCG** **TCT** **TCC**	*AGU* *AGC* *AGA* *AGG*	Ser Arg	**A** or **U** **G** or **C** **T** or **A** **C** or **G**
C or **G**	**CAA** **CAG** **CAT** **CAC**	*GUU* *GUC* *GUA* *GUG*	Val	**CGA** **CGG** **CGT** **CGC**	*GCU* *GCC* *GCA* *GCG*	Ala	**CTA** **CTG** **CTT** **CTC**	*GAU* *GAC* *GAA* *GAG*	Asp Glu	**CCA** **CCG** **CCT** **CCC**	*GGU* *GGC* *GGA* *GGG*	Gly	**A** or **U** **G** or **C** **T** or **A** **C** or **G**

First nucleotide (left) — *Third nucleotide* (right)

Note: The DNA codons appear in boldface type; the complementary RNA codons are in italics. A = adenine, C = cytosine, G = guanine, T = thymine, U = uridine (replaces thymine in RNA). In RNA, adenine is complementary to thymine of DNA; uridine is complementary to adenine of DNA; cytosine is complementary to guanine, and vice versa. "Stop" = termination. The amino acids are abbreviated as follows:

Ala = alanine	*Cys = cysteine*	*His = histidine*	*Met = methionine*	*Thr = threonine*
Arg = arginine	*Gln = glutamine*	*Ile = isoleucine*	*Phe = phenylalanine*	*Trp = tryptophan*
Asn = asparagine	*Glu = glutamic acid*	*Leu = leucine*	*Pro = proline*	*Tyr = tyrosine*
Asp = aspartic acid	*Gly = glycine*	*Lys = lysine*	*Ser = serine*	*Val = valine*

FIGURE 5-2 A schematic diagram of the genetic control of protein synthesis, illustrating the flow of genetic information from the base sequence of DNA to the RNA transcript (transcription) to mRNA (processing) to the polypeptide chain of a protein molecule (translation). Although DNA exists in a double-stranded form, only one of the two strands is used as a template for transcribing the RNA transcript. Solid sections represent coding regions in DNA, RNA transcript, mRNA, and amino acid sequence in polypeptide chain; dotted sections represent intervening sequences in DNA and RNA transcript.

contains altering coding and intervening sequences. The RNA transcript is edited in the nucleus before it passes into the cytoplasm. In the editing process, the intervening sequences are excised, and the coding regions are spliced together to form one continuous gene (Fig. 5-2).

After processing, the edited RNA, which is called *messenger RNA* (mRNA), leaves the nucleus and enters the cytoplasm where it becomes associated with *ribosomes* and thereby serves as a template for the ribosomal synthesis of proteins. Each of the 20 amino acids is attached in the cell cytoplasm to a specific molecule called *transfer RNA* (tRNA). Each tRNA contains a triplet sequence of purine and pyrimidine bases that is "complementary" to a specific codon in the mRNA. These tRNA molecules with their attached amino acids line up along the mRNA molecule in the precise order dictated by the genetic code. Under the action of cytoplasmic enzymes (initiation factors, elongation factors, and termination factors), peptide bonds are formed between the various amino acids, and the completed protein is released from the ribosome. For a more detailed account of the molecular basis of gene expression, see Chap. 6.

MAINTENANCE OF GENETIC DIVERSITY THROUGH TRANSMISSION AND SEGREGATION OF GENES The amount of DNA in the nucleus of each human cell is sufficient to code for more than 50,000 genes and hence to specify more than 50,000 polypeptide chains. The genes are arranged in a linear sequence of DNA that together with certain histone proteins form rod-shaped bodies called *chromosomes*. Each somatic cell contains 46 chromosomes, arranged in 23 pairs, one of each pair derived from each parent. Thus, each individual inherits two copies of each chromosome and hence two copies of each gene. The chromosomal location of the two copies of each gene is termed the *genetic locus*. When a gene occupying a genetic locus exists in two or more different forms, these alternate forms of the gene are referred to as *alleles*.

In humans, a given gene always resides at a specified genetic locus on one particular chromosome. For example, the genetic locus for the Rh blood group is on the short arm of chromosome 1; at this site there are two Rh genes, one on chromosome 1 derived from the mother and the other on chromosome 1 derived from the father. When two genes at the same genetic locus are identical, the individual is a *homozygote*. When the two genes differ (i.e., two different

alleles are present at the locus), the individual is a *heterozygote*. Each normal human is heterozygous at approximately 20 percent of genetic loci and homozygous at 80 percent. Figure 5-3 shows a map of human chromosome 1, illustrating the location of a representative sample of genes that have been assigned loci on this chromosome.

The genetic information carried on chromosomes is transmitted to daughter cells under two different sets of circumstances. One of these occurs whenever a somatic cell (i.e., a nongerm cell) divides. This process, called *mitosis*, transmits identical copies of each gene to each daughter cell, thus maintaining a uniform genetic makeup in all cells of a single individual. The other set of circumstances prevails when genetic information must be transmitted from one individual to an offspring. This process, called *meiosis*, produces germ cells (i.e., ova or spermatozoa) that possess only one copy of each parental chromosome, thus allowing for new combinations of chromosomes to occur when ovum and sperm cell fuse during fertilization.

During meiosis, the 46 chromosomes of an immature germ cell arrange themselves in 23 pairs at the center of the nucleus, each pair being composed of one chromosome derived from the mother and its homologous chromosome derived from the father. At a specified point in the meiotic process, the two partner chromosomes separate, only one of each pair going into each daughter cell, or gamete. Thus, meiosis produces gametes with a reduction in the number of chromosomes from 46 to 23, each gamete having received one chromosome from each of the 23 pairs. The assortment of the chromosomes within each pair is random so that each germ cell receives a different combination of maternal and paternal chromosomes. During the process of fertilization, the fusion of ovum and sperm cell, each of which has 23 chromosomes, produces an individual with 46 chromosomes.

The independent assortment of chromosomes into gametes during meiosis produces an enormous diversity among the possible genotypes

FIGURE 5-3 Gene map of human chromosome 1, illustrating a representative sample of the genes that have been localized to this chromosome. The black bands represent those genetic regions of the chromosome that stain brightly by a fluorescent dye such as quinacrine; the white bands are the negatively staining regions; the hatched area is a variable region that stains differently (i.e., either brightly or negatively) in the chromosomes of different individuals. Each gene is listed opposite its genetic locus on the right. (*Data provided by VA McKusick.*)

of the progeny. For each 23 pairs of chromosomes, there are 2^{23} different combinations of chromosomes that could occur in a gamete, and the likelihood that one set of parents will produce two offspring with the identical complement of chromosomes is one in 2^{23} or one in 8.4 million (assuming no monozygotic or identical twins).

RECOMBINATION Adding to the genetic diversity in humans is the phenomenon of *genetic recombination*. During meiosis, when homologous chromosomes are paired, bridges frequently form between corresponding regions of the chromosome pair. These bridges, or *chiasmata,* are regions in which the two chromosomes break at identical points along their length and subsequently rejoin, the distal segments having been switched from one homologous chromosome to another. This process is designated *crossing over*. Although no net change in the amount of genetic material occurs during crossing over, a recombination of genes does occur. For example, consider a chromosome with two loci, A and B, located at opposite ends of the same chromosome. On this particular chromosome, the A locus has a rare allele *x,* and the B locus also has a rare allele *y*. Without the phenomenon of recombination every offspring that inherited the *x* allele at the A locus would also inherit the *y* allele at the B locus. However, if recombination occurs, the A locus with the *x* allele would then be on the opposite chromosome from the B locus with the *y* allele. In this case any offspring that inherited the *x* allele at the A locus could not inherit the *y* allele at the B locus.

Crossing over occurs with great frequency in every meiosis in humans, and the resultant recombination of genes may occur at any point on a chromosome. The farther apart two genes are on the same chromosome, the greater is the likelihood that a crossing over will occur in the space between them. When two genes are on the opposite ends of a long chromosome, the probability of recombination is so great that their respective alleles are transmitted to offspring almost independently of one another, just as if the two gene loci were on different chromosomes. On the other hand, gene loci that are close together on the same chromosome are said to be *linked* so that there is a great likelihood that offspring will inherit the same combination of alleles that are present on the parental chromosome.

Several examples of *gene linkage* can be seen from the map of human chromosome 1 (Fig. 5-3). For example, the locus for the gene specifying the Rh blood group factor and the locus for the gene producing one form of the dominant trait hereditary elliptocytosis occur in close proximity on this chromosome. Thus, if a subject with hereditary elliptocytosis transmits the disease to an offspring, the offspring will usually inherit the allele that is present at the Rh locus on this chromosome. If the Rh allele happens to be a rare one in the population (such as r'), one can assume that whichever offspring inherits the r' allele at the Rh locus will also inherit the abnormal allele at the elliptocytosis locus. On the other hand, if an offspring does not exhibit the r' allele, he or she will not usually have elliptocytosis. The concept of linkage does not imply an association between any particular set of Rh alleles and the disease state elliptocytosis, rather between the two genetic loci. Thus, in different families the abnormal elliptocytosis allele may be linked to the R^1, R^0, r_2, or any other allele at the Rh locus, depending on the allele that happened to be at that locus when the elliptocytosis mutation occurred. Stated another way, the elliptocytosis locus is linked to the Rh locus in every family, but the particular Rh allele with which it is associated differs from family to family.

MUTATION Broadly defined, a *mutation* is a stable, heritable alteration in DNA. Although the causes of mutation in humans are largely unknown, a variety of environmental agents, such as radiation, viruses, and chemicals, are among the factors that are implicated. Mutations can involve a visible alteration in the structure of a chromosome, such as a deletion or translocation of a portion of a chromosome, or they can involve a minute change in one of the purine or pyrimidine bases of a single gene. Most commonly, such "point" mutations consist of the substitution of one base for another, changing the meaning of the codon containing that base, hence their designation as *missense mutations*. For example, in the gene coding

for the β chain of hemoglobin, the sixth position normally contains the nucleotide triplet CTC, which codes for the amino acid glutamic acid (Fig. 5-1). The mutation that gives rise to hemoglobin C produces a change of the first base of this triplet from cytosine to thymine, changing the triplet to TTC, which codes for lysine. On the other hand, the mutation that gives rise to hemoglobin S produces a change in the second base of the same triplet (from thymine to adenine), producing CAC, which codes for valine. Thus, in the sixth position of the β chain of hemoglobin, the normally occurring glutamic acid may be replaced with either lysine (producing hemoglobin C) or valine (producing hemoglobin S). More than 90 such single-base mutations in the hemoglobin β chain have been identified, and many of these mutations produce distinct clinical syndromes. Of all the mutations so far elucidated in humans, most involve such single-base changes.

Besides producing an amino acid substitution, a single-base substitution can also cause another abnormality in protein synthesis— premature chain termination. Three mRNA code words (UAA, UAG, and UGA) normally do not specify an amino acid but constitute the signal that the message has ended and that the protein chain should be released from the ribosome (Fig. 5-1). If a change occurs in DNA that produces one of these mRNA code words [for example, a switch in an mRNA triplet from UAU (tyrosine) to UAA (termination)], the polypeptide chain would be terminated prematurely when translation had reached that point. Such mutations, called *non-sense mutations,* produce short fragments of proteins that have reduced function.

CELLULAR MECHANISM BY WHICH MUTANT GENES PRODUCE DISEASES Critical to the understanding of heredity is the concept that the only information transmitted from generation to generation is the sequence of bases in DNA and that these sequences in turn specify only the primary structure of RNA and protein molecules. All other chemical reactions—such as the synthesis of complex lipids and carbohydrates, the formation of membranes and other cellular organelles, and the accumulation and partitioning of inorganic ions—occur as a secondary consequence of the action of specific proteins. Many of these proteins are enzymes that catalyze the biochemical conversion of one molecule into another. Others are structural proteins such as collagen and elastin, and still others are regulatory proteins that dictate how much of each enzyme and each structural protein is made.

Since proteins are the cellular molecules whose structures are encoded by genes, mutations in genes exert their deleterious effects by altering the structure of enzymes, structural proteins, or regulatory proteins. For example, in a disease such as glycogen storage disease, type I (von Gierke's disease), massive accumulation of glycogen in the liver is due not to a primary structural abnormality in the polysaccharide glycogen but to a structural abnormality in a protein, glucose-6-phosphatase, an enzyme that is required to liberate glucose so as to permit glycogen breakdown. Other examples of the biochemical mechanisms by which mutant genes alter cellular metabolism are discussed below under "Simply Inherited Disorders."

GENETIC HETEROGENEITY When two or more mutations can produce a similar clinical syndrome, genetic heterogeneity is said to exist. Hemophilia is one example of a genetically heterogeneous syndrome. A clinically similar bleeding disorder can be caused by mutations at either of two loci on the X chromosome, one leading to a deficiency of factor VIII (classic hemophilia) and the other causing a deficiency of factor IX (Christmas disease). Most, if not all, hereditary diseases, when carefully analyzed, will probably prove to be genetically heterogeneous.

Genetic heterogeneity may result from the existence of a series of different mutations at a single genetic locus (allelic mutations) or from mutations at different genetic loci (nonallelic mutations). For example, drug-induced hemolysis of red blood cells can occur in patients with several different types of allelic mutations at the glucose-6-phosphate dehydrogenase locus. On the other hand, hemophilia is an example of a syndrome in which nonallelic mutations can produce a similar clinical picture (see above).

In some cases of heterogeneity, both the genetic locus and the mode of inheritance differ. Diseases such as spastic paraplegia, Charcot-Marie-Tooth peroneal muscular atrophy, and retinitis pigmentosa are inherited as autosomal dominant traits in some families, as autosomal recessives in others, and as X-linked recessives in still others. The identification of such genetic heterogeneity in these disorders is of obvious importance for correct genetic counseling.

TAKING THE FAMILY HISTORY

The investigation of a patient with a possible genetic disorder begins with the *family history*. The first step is to obtain certain information on the *proband* or *index case* (i.e., the clinically affected person who has brought the family to attention) and on each of the *first-degree relatives* (i.e., the parents, siblings, and offspring of the proband). This information includes the given name, surname, maiden name, birth date or current age, age at death, cause of death, and name or description of any disease or defect.

The second step is to ask questions designed to survey the family for the presence of disease or defect. (1) Has any relative an identical or similar trait? (2) Has any relative a trait that is absent in the proband but is known to occur in some patients with the same disease? This question requires that the physician have some knowledge about the manifestations of the disease in question. For example, when obtaining the family history from a proband with dissecting aneurysm caused possibly by Marfan's syndrome, one should ask about the occurrence of eye abnormalities, cardiac abnormalities, and skeletal abnormalities in the relatives. (3) Has any relative a trait that is recognized to be genetically determined? The purpose of this question is to ascertain the occurrence of hereditary disease in the family even though the particular patient may not be involved. (4) Has any relative an unusual disease, or has any relative died of a rare condition? The purpose of this question is to identify a condition that might be genetically determined though not recognized as such by the informant. In addition, this question may help to identify conditions in relatives that might be etiologically related to the patient's problem. For example, a patient with pheochromocytoma should be suspected of having von Recklinghausen's disease if he or she has a brother with scoliosis and mental retardation, both of which can be manifestations of the neurofibromatosis (von Recklinghausen's) gene. (5) Is there any consanguinity in the family? This inquiry should be made directly. In addition, one should ask whether common last names appear in the families of husband-wife pairs. Consanguineous marriage may be the source of a rare autosomal recessive syndrome, and sometimes its presence in the family may not be known by the proband. (6) What is the ethnic origin of the family? Persons of various ethnic origins, such as blacks, Jews, and Greeks, have increased chances of specific genetic diseases. Table 5-1 lists examples of simply inherited disorders that are found with increased frequency in various ethnic groups.

CATEGORIES OF GENETIC DISORDERS

Genetic diseases generally fall into one of three categories: (1) *Chromosomal disorders* involve the lack, excess, or abnormal arrangement of one or more chromosomes, producing excessive or deficient genetic material. (2) *Mendelian or simply inherited disorders* are determined primarily by a single mutant gene. These disorders display inheritance patterns which can be classified into autosomal dominant, autosomal recessive, or X-linked types. (3) *Mulifactorial disorders* are caused by an interaction of multiple genes and multiple exogenous or environmental factors. Although many of these multifactorial disorders, such as essential hypertension and cleft lip and palate, are said to run in families, the inheritance pattern is complex and the risk to relatives is less than in the single-gene (mendelian) disorders. Each of these categories presents different problems with respect to causation, prevention, diagnosis, genetic counseling, and treatment.

CHROMOSOMAL DISORDERS   The karyotype of an individual (i.e., the number and structure of the chromosomes) can be ascertained from readily accessible body tissues, such as peripheral blood lymphocytes or skin, by growing them in tissue culture until active cell proliferation occurs and then preparing single cells for examination of chromosomes by microscopy. Each individual chromosome can be identified by special staining of DNA sequences, for example, by the affinity of fluorescent dyes (such as quinacrine hydrochloride) for certain chromosomal segments that can be visualized by fluorescence microscopy or by treatment with special dyes (Giemsa) and proteolytic enzymes (trypsin). These techniques produce characteristic *banding patterns* for each chromosome (Fig. 5-4).

The number of chromosomes in normal individuals is 46, of which 44 are the 22 pairs of *autosomes* and the other two are the *sex chromosomes*. Women have two X chromosomes (XX), and men have one X chromosome and one Y chromosome (XY). Each of the 22 pairs of autosomes and the two sex chromosomes can be distinguished on the basis of size, location of the centromere (which divides the chromosome into arms of equal or unequal length), and the unique banding pattern (Fig. 5-4). The relative length of the arms and the position of the centromere are used as further criteria to divide the human chromosomes into seven groups (designated A to G) (Fig. 5-4).

For a complete discussion of the etiology and clinical features of chromosomal abnormalities affecting humans, the reader is referred to Chap. 7.

TABLE 5-1   Examples of simply inherited disorders that occur with increased frequency in specific ethnic groups

Ethnic group	Simply inherited disorder
African blacks	Hemoglobinopathies, especially Hb S, Hb C, persistent Hb F, α and β thalassemias Glucose-6-phosphate dehydrogenase deficiency
Armenians	Familial Mediterranean fever
Ashkenazi Jews	Abetalipoproteinemia Bloom's syndrome Dystonia musculorum deformans (recessive form) Factor XI (PTA) deficiency Familial dysautonomia (Riley-Day syndrome) Gaucher's disease (adult form) Neimann-Pick disease Pentosuria Tay-Sachs disease
Chinese	α-Thalassemia Glucose-6-phosphate dehydrogenase deficiency Adult lactase deficiency
Eskimos	Pseudocholinesterase deficiency Adrenogenital syndrome
Finns	Congenital nephrosis Mulibrey nanism
French Canadians	Tyrosinemia
Japanese	Acatalasemia
Lebanese	Homozygous familial hypercholesterolemia
Mediterranean peoples (Italians, Greeks, Sephardic Jews)	β-Thalassemia Glucose-6-phosphate dehydrogenase deficiency Familial Mediterranean fever Glycogen storage disease, type III
Northern Europeans	Cystic fibrosis
Scandinavians	Alpha₁-antitrypsin deficiency LCAT (lecithin:cholesterol acyltransferase) deficiency
South African whites	Porphyria variegata Homozygous familial hypercholesterolemia

FIGURE 5-4 The karyotype of a normal female showing the chromosomes of a single somatic cell in the metaphase stage of cell division. The photographic images of the chromosomes have been cut out and arranged according to descending length and varying arm ratio. The chromosomes have been stained by the Giemsa technique, which allows each chromosome pair to be identified by its unique banding pattern. Chromosomes 1 to 22 are the autosomes. The sex chromosomes in this normal female are both X. The normal male has an identical karyotype except for the absence of one X chromosome and the presence instead of one Y chromosome. (*Courtesy of David H. Ledbetter.*)

SIMPLY INHERITED DISORDERS Disorders caused by the transmission of a single mutant gene show one of three simple (or mendelian) patterns of inheritance: (1) autosomal dominant, (2) autosomal recessive, or (3) X-linked. The distinction between "dominant" and "recessive" is one of convenience in pedigree analysis and does not imply a fundamental difference in genetic mechanism. The term *dominant* implies that a mutation is clinically manifest when an individual has a single dose of this mutation (or is *heterozygous* for it), while *recessive* implies that a double dose (or *homozygosity*) is required for clinical detection. Genes are never dominant or recessive; their effects, however, produce clinical patterns that are classified as dominant or recessive. Despite their overall clinical "normality," individuals who are heterozygous for "recessive" genes often have biochemical abnormalities that are demonstrable in the laboratory; on the other hand, those who are homozygous for "dominant" genes are usually more severely affected than are the heterozygotes.

With few exceptions, each of the approximately 1200 mendelian diseases is rare. However, as a group these disorders constitute an important cause of morbidity and death, accounting directly for more than 5 percent of all hospital admissions.

The genes for more than 200 simply inherited diseases have been assigned to specific chromosomes. Disease-producing genes assigned to the X chromosome outnumber those so far assigned to any single autosome. This is because assignment to the X chromosome requires only pedigree studies showing X-linked inheritance (see below). Assignment to an autosome is more complicated, requiring sophisticated techniques of somatic cell hybridization or pedigree studies showing linkage between a disease-producing gene and a "marker" gene that is known to be on a certain chromosome. Table 5-2 shows a partial list of those human genetic diseases that have been mapped to specific chromosomes.

The demonstration that a particular disease or syndrome shows one of the three mendelian patterns of inheritance implies that its pathogenesis, no matter how complex, is due to an abnormality in a single protein molecule. For example, in sickle cell anemia, the entire clinical syndrome, including such seemingly unrelated disturbances as anemia, pain crises, nephropathy, and predisposition to pneumococcal infections, are all the physiologic consequences of having thymine instead of adenine at a specific site in the gene that codes for the β chain of hemoglobin, producing a substitution of a valine

for a glutamic acid in the sixth amino acid position in the protein sequence.

In many mendelian disorders, especially in those with dominant inheritance, it is not possible to demonstrate directly the protein that is primarily altered by the mutation. In such cases (e.g., adult polycystic kidney disease and tuberous sclerosis) only the distal physiologic effects of the mutation are recognizable. Nevertheless, it is safe to assume that a single primary defect exists whenever a disease is transmitted by a single-gene mechanism and that the various manifestations of the disease all can be related to the mutational event by a more or less complicated "pedigree of causes."

TABLE 5-2 Partial list of human genetic diseases that have been mapped to specific chromosomes

Chromosome	Disease
1	Elliptocytosis
	RH erythroblastosis
	Porphyria cutanea tarda
2	Protein C deficiency
3	Protein S deficiency
	Orotic aciduria
4	Huntington's disease
5	Gardner syndrome
	Familial polyposis coli
6	Hemochromatosis
	Congenital adrenal hyperplasia (21-hydroxylase deficiency)
7	Cystic fibrosis
	Ehlers-Danlos syndrome (one form)
	Osteogenesis imperfecta (one form)
9	Galactosemia
	Nail-patella syndrome
10	Multiple endocrine neoplasia, type 2
11	Syndrome of Wilms' tumor, aniridia, gonadoblastoma, retardation
	β-Thalassemia
	Sickle cell anemia
	Acute intermittent porphyria
12	Phenylketonuria
	von Willebrand's disease
13	Retinoblastoma
	Wilson's disease
14	Nucleoside phosphorylase deficiency (immunodeficiency)
	Alpha₁-antitrypsin deficiency
15	Prader-Willi syndrome
	Tay-Sachs disease
16	α-Thalassemia
	Gout due to adenine phosphoribosyltransferase deficiency
	LCAT deficiency
17	Growth hormone deficiency (type 1A)
	von Recklinghausen neurofibromatosis
19	Familial hypercholesterolemia
	Familial type 3 hyperlipoproteinemia
	Myotonic dystrophy
	Complement C3 deficiency
20	Adenosine deaminase deficiency (immunodeficiency)
21	Alzheimer's disease
	Homocystinuria
22	Metachromatic leukodystrophy
	Hurler syndrome (mucopolysaccharidoses I)
	Scheie's syndrome (mucopolysaccharidoses V)
X	X-linked ichthyosis due to placental steroid sulfatase deficiency
	Ocular albinism
	Chronic granulomatous disease
	Duchenne muscular dystrophy
	Testicular feminization syndrome
	Phosphoglycerate kinase deficiency (hemolytic anemia)
	Fabry's disease
	Lesch-Nyhan syndrome
	Fragile site associated with X-linked mental retardation
	Color blindness
	Hemophilia A
	Glucose-6-phosphate dehydrogenase (G6PD) deficiency

SOURCE: McKusick.

TABLE 5-3 Some relatively frequent mendelian disorders affecting adults

AUTOSOMAL DOMINANT DISORDERS

Familial hypercholesterolemia
Hereditary hemorrhagic telangiectasia
Marfan's syndrome
Hereditary spherocytosis
Adult polycystic kidney disease
Huntington's chorea
Acute intermittent porphyria
Osteogenesis imperfecta tarda
von Willebrand's disease
Myotonic dystrophy
Idiopathic hypertrophic subaortic stenosis (IHSS)
Noonan's syndrome
Neurofibromatosis
Tuberous sclerosis

AUTOSOMAL RECESSIVE DISORDERS

Deafness
Albinism
Wilson's disease
Hemochromatosis
Sickle cell anemia
β-Thalassemia
Cystic fibrosis
Hereditary emphysema (alpha₁-antitrypsin deficiency)
Homocystinuria
Familial Mediterranean fever
Friedreich's ataxia
Phenylketonuria

X-LINKED DISORDERS

Hemophilia A
Glucose-6-phosphate dehydrogenase deficiency
Fabry's disease
Ocular albinism
Testicular feminization
Chronic granulomatous disease
Hypophosphatemic rickets
Color blindness

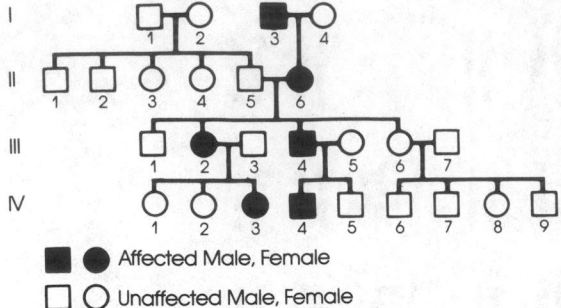

FIGURE 5-5 Pedigree pattern of an autosomal dominant trait. Note the *vertical* pattern of inheritance.

Table 5-3 lists the most commonly encountered mendelian disorders affecting adults.

Autosomal dominant disorders Dominant diseases are those manifest in the heterozygous state, that is, when only one abnormal gene (*mutant allele*) is present and the corresponding partner allele on the homologous chromosome is normal. The gene responsible for an autosomal dominant disorder is located on one of the 22 autosomes, and both males and females can be affected. Since alleles segregate independently at meiosis, there is a 1 in 2 chance that the offspring of an affected heterozygote will inherit the mutant allele and, similarly, a 1 in 2 chance of the offspring inheriting the normal allele.

Figure 5-5 shows a typical pedigree involving an autosomal dominant trait. The following features are characteristic: (1) Each affected individual has an affected parent (unless the condition arose by a new mutation or is mildly expressed in the affected parent); (2) an affected individual will bear, on the average, both normal and affected offspring in equal proportions; (3) normal children of an affected individual will have only normal offspring; (4) males and females are affected in equal proportions; (5) each sex is equally likely to transmit the condition to male and female offspring, with male-to-male transmission occurring; and (6) vertical transmission of the condition through successive generations occurs, especially when the trait does not impair reproductive capacity.

While half of the offspring of an individual with an autosomal dominant condition will inherit the disease, it is not necessarily true that each affected person must have an affected parent. In every

autosomal dominant disease a certain proportion of affected persons owe their disorder to a new mutation rather than to an inherited mutation. Since the estimated frequency of mutation is 5×10^{-6} mutations per gene per generation and since a dominant trait, by definition, requires a mutation in only one of a pair of alleles, one would expect that about 1 in 100,000 newborn persons would possess a new mutation at any given genetic locus. Many of these mutations either do not impair the function of the gene product or involve a recessive function so that the mutation is clinically silent. Others, however, cause a defective gene product that gives rise to a dominant trait. The parent in whose germ cells the mutation arose is clinically normal. Likewise, the siblings of the affected individual are normal since the mutation affects only a single germ cell. However, the affected individual transmits the disease to half of his or her children.

The proportion of patients with dominant disorders who represent new mutations is inversely proportional to the effect of the disease in question on biologic fitness. The term *biologic fitness* refers to the ability of an affected individual to produce children who survive to adult life and reproduce. In the extreme case, if a dominant mutation produced absolute infertility, then all observed cases would of necessity represent new mutations, and it would be impossible to prove the genetic transmission of the trait. In less severe disorders, as in tuberous sclerosis, the severe mental retardation reduces biologic fitness to about 20 percent of normal, and the proportion of cases due to new mutations is about 80 percent. Other examples of the relation between biologic fitness and the proportion of new mutations in dominant disorders are shown in Table 5-4.

Many new mutations appear to occur in the germ cells of fathers who are of relatively advanced age. Such a "paternal age effect" is seen, for example, in Marfan's syndrome in which the average age of fathers of sporadic or "new mutation" cases (37 years) is in excess of the mean age of fathers generally (30 years) and also in excess of the age of fathers who transmit Marfan's disease due to an inherited mutation (30 years).

Before one concludes that a dominant disorder in a given patient with unaffected parents is the result of a new mutation, it is important to consider two other possibilities: (1) that the gene may be carried by one parent in whom the disease is of low expressivity (discussed below), and (2) that extramarital paternity may have occurred. The

TABLE 5-4 Approximate percentage of patients affected by new mutations in some autosomal dominant disorders

Disorder	Percentage
Achondroplasia	80
Tuberous sclerosis	80
Neurofibromatosis	40
Marfan's syndrome	30
Myotonic dystrophy	25
Huntington's chorea	4
Adult polycystic kidney disease	1
Familial hypercholesterolemia	Very low

1 Islet Cell Adenomas
Parathyroid Adenomas
Lipomas
2 Lipomas, Kidney Stones
3 Islet Cell Adenomas
Parathyroid Adenomas
Pituitary Adenoma
Lipomas

4 Peptic Ulcer
Disease
5 Pituitary
Adenoma

FIGURE 5-6 Pedigree of a family affected with the multiple endocrine adenoma–peptic ulcer syndrome, a disorder inherited as an autosomal dominant trait. Circles denote females; squares, males. Open circles and squares denote unaffected relatives; closed circles and squares denote affected relatives. Deceased relatives are indicated by the oblique line. The age of each relative is indicated below his or her symbol. Note the marked variation in clinical expression among living affected heterozygotes.

latter is found in about 3 to 5 percent of randomly studied children in the United States.

Most autosomal dominant disorders show two characteristic features that are not usually seen in recessive syndromes: (1) *delayed age of onset* and (2) *variability in clinical expression.* Delayed age of onset is seen in disorders such as Huntington's chorea and adult polycystic kidney disease. These disorders do not manifest clinically until adult life, even though the mutant gene is present from the time of conception. Variability in clinical expression is illustrated dramatically by the multiple endocrine adenoma–peptic ulcer syndrome. Patients in the same family inheriting the same abnormal gene may have hyperplasia or neoplasia of one or more endocrine glands (including the pancreas, parathyroid glands, and pituitary gland), as well as of adipose tissue. The resulting clinical manifestations are diverse; different members of the same family may develop peptic ulcers, hypoglycemia, kidney stones, multiple lipomas of the skin, or bitemporal hemianopsia. The recognition that each family member suffers from the same genetic abnormality can be difficult, as illustrated by the family pedigree in Fig. 5-6.

Dominant mutations involve a type of gene product that produces clinical symptoms when only 50 percent of the gene product is defective. The defective genes usually do not encode enzymes, since a 50 percent deficiency of most enzymes produces no symptoms (see "Recessive Disorders" below). Rather, dominant diseases are likely to involve abnormalities in two classes of proteins: (1) those that regulate complex metabolic pathways, such as membrane receptors and rate-limiting enzymes in pathways under feedback control, and (2) key structural proteins, such as hemoglobin or collagen.

The basic biochemical defects have been identified in only a handful of the approximately 600 autosomal dominant disorders. These include familial hypercholesterolemia (abnormal cell surface receptor that binds plasma low-density lipoprotein and thereby regulates cholesterol metabolism); osteogenesis imperfecta (abnormal collagen molecule); hereditary methemoglobinemia and several hemolytic anemias due to unstable forms of hemoglobin (abnormal hemoglobin molecule); hereditary angioneurotic edema (abnormal protein inhibitor of an enzyme involved in the serum complement system); acute intermittent porphyria (abnormal enzyme that catalyzes a rate-limiting step in the heme biosynthetic pathway); and pseudohypoparathyroidism, type 1 (abnormal guanine nucleotide-binding regulatory component or G-protein of the adenylate cyclase system).

Autosomal recessive disorders Autosomal recessive conditions are clinically apparent only in the homozygous state, that is, when both alleles at a particular genetic locus are mutant. By definition, the gene responsible for an autosomal recessive disorder must be on one of the 22 autosomes; thus, both males and females can be affected.

Figure 5-7 shows a pedigree in which an autosomal recessive trait is present in the family. The following features are characteristic: (1) the parents are clinically normal; (2) only siblings are affected, and vertical transmission does not occur; and (3) males and females are affected in equal proportions.

The relative infrequency of recessive genes in the population and the requirement for two abnormal genes for clinical expression combine to create special conditions for autosomal recessive inheritance: (1) the more infrequent the mutant gene in the population, the stronger the likelihood that affected individuals are the product of consanguineous matings (see below); (2) if a husband and a wife are both carriers for the same autosomal recessive gene, 25 percent of the children will be normal, 50 percent will be heterozygous carriers, and 25 percent will be homozygous and affected with the disease; (3) if an affected individual marries a heterozygote (as may occur with consanguineous marriage), half the children will be affected, and a pedigree simulating dominant inheritance will result; and (4) if two individuals with the same recessive disease marry, all their children will be affected.

The clinical picture in autosomal recessive disorders tends to be more uniform than that of dominant diseases, and the age of onset is often early in life. As a general rule, recessive disorders are more commonly diagnosed in children, while dominant diseases are more frequently encountered in adults.

Since with recessive inheritance only one of four children in a sibship is expected to be affected, multiple cases in a family may not occur. This is especially true in a society in which small families are common. Consider, for example, 16 families in which both parents are heterozygous for the same recessive disorder. If each family has two children, 9 of the families will have no affected children, 6 will have one affected and one normal child, and only 1 of the 16 families will have two affected children. In the United States physicians usually see sporadic or isolated cases of a recessive disorder without an affected sibling to alert them to the possibility of a genetic disorder. Fortunately, because of the relatively uniform clinical picture of recessive disorders and because most can be diagnosed directly by biochemical tests, the correct diagnosis can usually be made even when no other members of a family are clinically affected.

The basic biochemical lesions underlying many autosomal recessive disorders have been identified. Of the three types of proteins in which mutations could occur (i.e., enzymes, structural proteins, and regulatory proteins), the enzymes have been the easiest to study. A mutation that destroys the catalytic activity of an enzyme generally does not impair the health of a heterozygote (i.e., an individual who has one mutant allele specifying a functionless enzyme and one

FIGURE 5-7 Pedigree pattern of an autosomal recessive trait. Note the *horizontal* pattern of inheritance.

normal allele on the partner chromosome specifying a normal enzyme). In this situation each cell in the body usually produces about 50 percent of the normal number of active enzyme molecules. However, normal regulatory mechanisms function to avert any clinical consequences of this 50 percent deficiency, and so heterozygotes usually are clinically normal. On the other hand, when an individual inherits functionless alleles at both loci specifying an enzyme, the reduction in enzyme activity is too great for a compensatory mechanism to overcome, and a disease results. For example, heterozygotes for phenylketonuria have half the normal activity of phenylalanine hydroxylase, but they are clinically asymptomatic because the body compensates for the half-normal level of the enzyme by raising the substrate concentration approximately twofold. Under these conditions a normal amount of phenylalanine can be metabolized with no symptoms. On the other hand, the homozygote for phenylketonuria has such a severe reduction in phenylalanine hydroxylase activity that enormous levels of phenylalanine and its derivatives accumulate, causing detrimental brain development. As in the case of phenylketonuria, the majority of enzyme deficiency states produce *simultaneously* both a simple accumulation of one or more metabolites preceding the enzymatic block and a deficient production of other metabolites distal to the block in the metabolic pathway.

Most of the genetic enzyme deficiencies that have been elucidated are not only inherited as recessive traits but also tend to involve enzymes that participate in catabolic pathways. Frequently these enzymes degrade organic molecules that are ingested in the diet, such as galactose (galactosemia), phenylalanine (phenylketonuria), and phytanic acid (Refsum's syndrome). A special class of such catabolic diseases is that in which the deficiency affects an acid hydrolase that occurs within lysosomes. In these *lysosomal storage disorders* the substrate, usually a complex lipid or polysaccharide, accumulates within swollen lysosomes in specific organs, giving the cells a foamy appearance. Examples of such lysosomal diseases include the mucopolysaccharidoses such as Hurler's syndrome (α-iduronidase deficiency) and the lipid storage diseases such as Gaucher's disease (glucocerebrosidase deficiency).

In general, recessive diseases are rare because the reduced biologic fitness of homozygotes acts to remove the mutant gene from the population. However, a few recessive disorders, such as cystic fibrosis and sickle cell anemia, are common. To explain this paradox, it has been postulated that the biologic fitness of heterozygotes is greater than that of noncarriers for these genes. In such a case the frequency of the gene in the population depends on the balance between the increased fitness of the relatively numerous heterozygotes and the reduced fitness of the less common homozygotes. A small selective advantage of the heterozygote over the normal results in a high gene frequency and hence a high birth frequency of homozygotes even when the disease is lethal. Thus, about 1 in 22 Caucasians is a heterozygous carrier for the genetically lethal disease cystic fibrosis, and the disease occurs in about 1 in 2000 Caucasian births. To maintain such a high gene frequency, heterozygotes for cystic fibrosis must have a definite reproductive advantage over noncarriers, but the nature of this advantage is unknown. In sickle cell anemia, another recessive disorder with high frequency among certain populations, heterozygotes appear to have increased resistance to malaria.

Inasmuch as recessive diseases require the inheritance of a mutation at the same genetic locus from each parent, when the genes are rare, the likelihood of any two parents being carriers for the same defect becomes small. However, if the parents have a common ancestor and if that ancestor was a carrier for the recessive gene, then the likelihood that two of the descendants have inherited the gene becomes relatively great. The rarer the recessive gene, the stronger the likelihood that an affected individual will have resulted from such a consanguineous mating. On the other hand, certain recessive genes are so common in the population that the likelihood of two random parents being carriers is great enough to eliminate the need for consanguinity. For common traits such as sickle cell anemia, phenylketonuria, cystic fibrosis, and Tay-Sachs disease, all of which have a high carrier frequency in certain populations, consanguinity in the parents is unusual.

In general, consanguinity is infrequent in families with recessive diseases in the United States. This is because the rate of consanguinity in the general population is low. In most of the United States (as opposed to areas with relative geographic isolation such as northern Norway and Switzerland), a disorder must indeed be rare before it is associated with an important frequency of consanguinity. For example, consanguinity is expected in a large proportion of families having children with very rare disorders such as the Laurence-Moon-Biedl syndrome and abetalipoproteinemia.

Genetic compounds represent a special type of recessively inherited disorder in which the affected individual's two mutant genes, although located at the same genetic locus, are not identical. The mutations in the paternal and maternal alleles presumably involve different alterations in the DNA of the same gene. SC hemoglobinopathy is an example of such a *heteroallelic* compound state in which individuals have a gene for sickle cell hemoglobin on one chromosome and a gene for hemoglobin C on the homologous chromosome.

X-linked disorders   The genes responsible for X-linked disorders are located on the X chromosome; therefore, the clinical risk and severity of the disease are different for the two sexes. Since a female has two X chromosomes, she may be either heterozygous or homozygous for a mutant gene, and the trait may therefore demonstrate either recessive or dominant expression. Males, on the other hand, have only one X chromosome, so they can be expected to display the full syndrome whenever they inherit the gene regardless of whether the gene behaves as a recessive or as a dominant trait in the female. Thus, the terms *X-linked dominant* or *X-linked recessive* refer only to the expression of the gene in women.

An important feature of all X-linked inheritance is the absence of male-to-male (i.e., father-to-son) transmission of the trait. This follows because a male must always contribute his Y chromosome to his sons; hence, he can never contribute his X chromosome. On the other hand, a male contributes his one X chromosome to all his daughters.

The pedigree in Fig. 5-8 illustrates the characteristic features of X-linked recessive inheritance. (1) In contrast to the vertical transmission in dominant traits (parents and children affected) and the horizontal transmission in autosomal recessive traits (siblings affected), the pedigree pattern in X-linked recessive traits tends to be oblique because of the occurrence of the trait in the sons of normal carrier sisters of affected males (uncles and nephews affected) (Fig. 5-8A); (2) male offspring of carrier women have a 50 percent chance of being affected; (3) all female offspring of affected males are carriers, and affected males do not transmit the disease to their sons (Fig. 5-8C); (4) unaffected males do not transmit the trait to any offspring; and (5) affected homozygous females occur only when an affected male fathers the child of a carrier female (Fig. 5-8B).

Examples of X-linked recessive disorders in humans include hemophilia A, nephrogenic diabetes insipidus, the Lesch-Nyhan syndrome, Duchenne form of muscular dystrophy, glucose-6-phosphate dehydrogenase deficiency, testicular feminization, and Fabry's disease. Color blindness is also inherited as an X-linked recessive trait, but it is sufficiently frequent (occurring in about 8 percent of white males) that the occurrence of homozygous color-blind females is no rarity.

X-linked dominant inheritance is illustrated by the pedigree in Fig. 5-9. Its characteristic features are as follows: (1) Females are affected about twice as often as males; (2) an affected female transmits the disorder to half of her sons and half of her daughters; (3) an affected male transmits the disorder to all his daughters and to none of his sons; and (4) the syndrome is more variable and less severe in heterozygous affected females than in hemizygous affected males. One common trait, the Xg(a+) blood group, is inherited as an X-linked dominant trait, as is vitamin D–resistant rickets (hypophosphatemic rickets).

Some rare conditions may be inherited as X-linked dominant traits

FIGURE 5-8 Pedigree patterns of an X-linked recessive trait. *A.* Note the oblique pattern of inheritance. *B.* An affected female can result from the mating of an affected male and a carrier female, as in the consanguineous marriage shown here. *C.* An affected male mating with a normal noncarrier female has all normal sons and all carrier daughters.

A

■ ● Affected Male, Female
⊙ Carrier Female
□ ○ Unaffected Male, Noncarrier Female

B

■ ● Affected Male, Female
⊙ Carrier Female
□ ○ Unaffected Male, Noncarrier Female

C

■ ● Affected Male, Female
⊙ Carrier Female
□ ○ Unaffected Male, Noncarrier Female

in which there is lethality in the hemizygous male. The characteristics of this form of inheritance are illustrated by the pedigree in Fig. 5-10: (1) The disorder occurs only in females who are heterozygous for the mutant gene; (2) an affected mother transmits the trait to half of her daughters; (3) an increased frequency of abortions occurs in affected women, the abortions representing affected male fetuses. Conditions that appear to be transmitted by this mode of inheritance include incontinentia pigmenti, focal dermal hypoplasia, orofaciodigital syndrome, and hyperammonemia due to ornithine transcarbamylase deficiency.

Expression of X-linked traits in females tends to be variable because of the phenomenon of X-chromosome inactivation. Early in embryonic development one of the two X chromosomes in each somatic cell of a female is inactivated. The inactivation process is random, so that for each cell there is an equal probability that the paternally or maternally derived X chromosome will be inactivated. The inactivated X chromosome is rendered permanently nonfunctional, so that all progeny of the initial cell inherit the same active and inactive X chromosomes. Thus, each female is a mosaic; on the average, half of her cells express the X chromosome of the father, and half express the X chromosome of the mother. If a mutation in a gene is carried on one of her X chromosomes, about one-half of the cells in each tissue will be normal and the other half will manifest the mutant phenotype. However, chance or selection of one or the other set of clones of cells may disturb these proportions in any given individual. Depending on the proportions of mutant and normal X chromosomes in each tissue, a genetically heterozygous female may either be clinically normal or have mild or severe manifestations of the disease. To illustrate, mothers of boys with the X-linked recessive Duchenne form of muscular dystrophy may occasionally show mild manifestations of the disease, such as limb girdle weakness or hypertrophied calves.

In each female cell the nonfunctional X chromosome can be visualized by several techniques. By ordinary staining, the inactivated X chromosome in metaphase appears heteropyknotic (condensed in appearance), and it replicates late in the mitotic cycle ("late-labeling" with tritiated thymidine). In nondividing cells the inactivated X chromosome can be observed as a clump of chromatin at the periphery of the nucleus—the so-called X chromatin or Barr body. In abnormal states with more than two X chromosomes such as 47, XXX, all but one of the X chromosomes are inactivated, so female cells may have multiple X chromatin bodies (see Chap. 7).

Since a single mutant allele is sufficient for the expression of X-linked recessive disorders, consanguinity does not increase the likelihood of expression in males, unlike the case in the rare autosomal recessive disorders. On the other hand, just as in the dominantly inherited disorders, new mutations can be a factor. In general, if an X-linked recessive condition reduces biologic fitness to zero, one-third of affected males will be a result of new mutations, and an

additional one-third will be born to mothers who themselves are carriers as a result of a new mutation. Thus, only one-third will come from a classic pedigree manifesting oblique transmission. An example of such a disease is the Duchenne form of muscular dystrophy in which affected hemizygous males are so severely disabled that they never reproduce. In hemophilia A, in which the biologic fitness is greater than zero, about 20 percent of affected males represent new mutations.

In families in which only one male is affected with an X-linked recessive disease and there is no other family history of the trait, it

FIGURE 5-9 Pedigree pattern of an X-linked dominant trait.

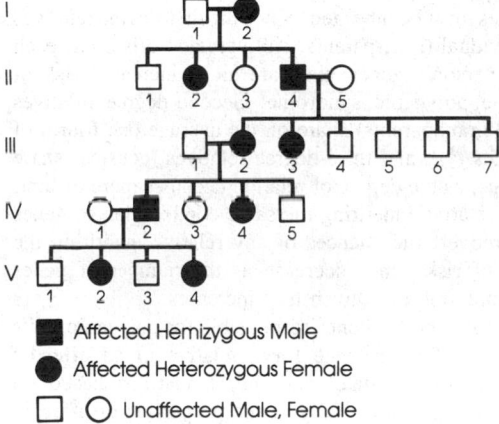

■ Affected Hemizygous Male
● Affected Heterozygous Female
□ ○ Unaffected Male, Female

FIGURE 5-10 Pedigree pattern of an X-linked dominant trait lethal in the hemizygous male.

● ○ Affected and Unaffected Female
□ Unaffected Male
⬤ Abortion

is essential for proper genetic counseling that the mother undergo biochemical tests or other relevant studies to determine whether she is a carrier. If she is a carrier, half of her daughters will be carriers and half of her sons will be affected. On the other hand, if her affected son represents a new mutation, only his daughters will inherit the gene. At present, biochemical tests can identify female carriers for several X-linked diseases including the Lesch-Nyhan syndrome, Fabry's disease, Hunter's syndrome, hemophilia, and the Duchenne form of muscular dystrophy.

The distinction between X-linked inheritance and *sex-influenced autosomal dominant inheritance* is important. Baldness is probably inherited as an autosomal dominant trait, yet it is manifested mainly in men and rarely in women. Heterozygous females express the baldness gene only when a source of testosterone becomes available as occurs with a masculinizing tumor of the ovary.

MULTIFACTORIAL GENETIC DISEASES   The common chronic diseases of adults (such as essential hypertension, coronary heart disease, diabetes mellitus, peptic ulcer disease, and schizophrenia) as well as the common birth defects (such as cleft lip and palate, spina bifida, and congenital heart disease) have been long known to ''run in families.'' They fit best into the category of *multifactorial genetic diseases*. The genetic element in these disorders rarely manifests itself in an all-or-none fashion as it does in the simply inherited (mendelian) disorders and in chromosomal aberrations. Instead, it is the interaction of multiple genes with multiple environmental factors that produces the familial aggregation.

In the multifactorial genetic diseases, there is a *polygenic component* consisting of a series of genes that interact in a cumulative fashion. An individual who inherits the right combination of these genes passes beyond a ''threshold of risk,'' at which point an *environmental component* determines whether and to what extent that person is clinically affected. In order for another individual in the same family to express the same syndrome, the same or similar combination of genes must be inherited. Since the first-degree relatives of an affected individual (i.e., parents, siblings, and offspring) each share half of that person's genes, they are all at increased risk of exhibiting the same polygenic syndrome. Second-degree relatives (uncles, aunts, and grandparents) share on the average one-fourth of an individual's genes $(\frac{1}{2})^2$, and third-degree relatives (cousins) share one-eighth $(\frac{1}{2})^3$. Thus, as the degree of relation becomes more distant, the likelihood of a relative inheriting the same combination of genes becomes less. Moreover, the chances of any relative inheriting the right combination of risk genes decrease as the number of genes required for the expression of a given trait increases.

Since the precise number of genes responsible for polygenic traits is unknown, the risk of inheritance for a relative of an affected individual is difficult to calculate, and the standard is based on empiric risk figures (i.e., a direct tally of the proportion of affected relatives in previously reported families). In contrast to the simply inherited disorders in which 25 or 50 percent of the first-degree relatives of an affected proband are at genetic risk, multifactorial genetic disorders are generally observed empirically to affect no more than 5 to 10 percent of first-degree relatives. Moreover, in contrast to mendelian traits, the recurrence risk of multifactorial conditions varies from family to family, and its estimation is significantly influenced by two factors: (1) the number of affected persons already present in the family, and (2) the severity of the disorder in the index case. The greater the number of affected relatives and the more severe their disease, the higher the risk to other relatives. For example, the risk of cleft lip in the siblings of a child with unilateral cleft lip is about 2.5 percent, but if the lesion in the index case is bilateral, the risk in the siblings rises to 6 percent. Table 5-5 lists the empiric risk figures for the familial recurrence of a number of multifactorial genetic diseases.

The hypothesis of a polygenic component in the inheritance of multifactorial diseases has been given a sound basis in recent years by the demonstration that at least one-third of all gene loci harbor polymorphic alleles that vary among individuals. Such a large degree

TABLE 5-5   Empiric risks for some common multifactorial genetic diseases affecting adults

Disorder in index case	Estimated absolute risk for first-degree relatives, %
Cleft lip and/or palate	3
Congenital heart disease	4
Coronary heart disease	8 for male relatives 3 for female relatives
Diabetes mellitus	5–10
Epilepsy	5–10
Hypertension	10
Manic-depressive psychosis	10–15
Psoriasis	10–15
Schizophrenia	15
Thyroid disease (autoimmune disorders including hyperthyroidism, thyroiditis, primary myxedema, simple goiter)	10

of variation in normal genes undoubtedly provides the substrate for variations in genetic predisposition with which environmental factors can interact. So far, the genetic loci most strikingly associated with predisposition to specific diseases are those that constitute the HLA system (also called the *major histocompatibility gene complex*) (see Chap. 14). The HLA gene complex is located on the short arm of chromosome 6. It consists of four closely linked but distinct loci (A, B, C, and D). The products of these genes are proteins that are found on the surface of body cells and that enable an individual's immune system to distinguish its own cells from those of someone else. Each HLA locus in the population consists of multiple alleles, each of which produces an immunologically distinct protein. For example, an individual may inherit any 2 of 20 alleles at the HLA-B locus.

An important observation of recent years has been the finding that certain alleles at the HLA loci predispose individuals to certain specific diseases. For example, if the B27 allele at the HLA-B locus is inherited by an individual, that person has a 121-fold greater chance of developing ankylosing spondylitis than an individual who lacks this allele (Table 5-6). Ankylosing spondylitis remains a multifactorial disease, however, because its development clearly requires one or more other factors in addition to the B27 allele. Thus, less than 15 percent of people who inherit this allele develop this disease. Table 5-6 lists some of the diseases associated with alleles at the HLA loci. Several of them are suspected to be of viral etiology, suggesting that the HLA loci may dictate the mode of expression of certain viral diseases. A more detailed discussion of the HLA system is presented in Chap. 14.

Multifactorial disorders are heterogeneous in the sense that the relative contribution of the polygenic factors (''risk genes'') and environmental factors to the etiology vary greatly from patient to patient. However, it is important to remember that among common

TABLE 5-6   Alleles at the HLA loci associated with multifactorial genetic diseases

Disease	HLA locus	Specific allele	Relative risk*
Ankylosing spondylitis	B	B27	121
Reiter's syndrome	B	B27	40
Psoriasis with arthritis	B	B27	5
Celiac disease	B	B8	10
Chronic active hepatitis	B	B8	4
Myasthenia gravis	B	B8	4
Diabetes mellitus (insulin-dependent)	DR	DR3/DR4	33
Hyperthyroidism	DR	DR3	4
Addison's disease	B	B8	7
	DR	DR4	10
Multiple sclerosis	DR	DR2	7

* *Relative risk* is the probability of the disease developing in an individual with the specific allele, divided by the probability of its development in an individual who does not possess this specific allele.

TABLE 5-7 Examples of inherited disorders involving an abnormal response to drugs

Disorder	Molecular abnormality	Mode of inheritance	Frequency	Clinical effect	Drugs producing abnormal response
Slow inactivation of isoniazid	Isoniazid acetylase in liver	Autosomal recessive	~50% of U.S. population	Polyneuritis	Isoniazid, sulfamethazine, sulfamaprine, phenelzine, dapsone, hydralazine
Suxamethonium sensitivity	Pseudocholinesterase in plasma	Autosomal recessive	Several mutant alleles; most common affects 1 in 2500	Apnea	Suxamethonium, succinylcholine
Warfarin insensitivity	? Altered receptor or enzyme in liver with increased affinity for vitamin K	Autosomal dominant	Rare	Inability to achieve anticoagulation with usual doses of drug	Warfarin
Glaucoma	Unknown	? Autosomal dominant	Common	Increased intraocular pressure	Glucocorticoids
Malignant hyperthermia	Unknown	Autosomal dominant	~1 in 20,000 anesthetized patients	Severe hyperpyrexia, muscle rigidity, death	Such anesthetics as halothane, succinylcholine, methoxyfluorane, ether, cyclopropane
Unstable hemoglobins: Hemoglobin Zurich	Arginine substitution for histidine at sixty-third position of β chain of hemoglobin	Autosomal dominant	Rare	Hemolysis	Sulfonamides
Hemoglobin H	Hemoglobin composed of four β chains	Autosomal dominant	Rare	Hemolysis	Sulfisoxazole
Glucose-6-phosphate dehydrogenase deficiency	Glucose-6-phosphate dehydrogenase in erythrocytes	X-linked recessive	$\sim 1 \times 10^8$ affected persons in world; common in persons of African, Mediterranean, Asiatic origin; multiple mutant alleles	Hemolysis	Analgesics, sulfonamides, antimalarials, nitrofurantoin, other drugs

SOURCE: ES Vesell, N Engl J Med 287:904, 1972.

phenotypes which are largely multifactorial, often a small proportion will be created by major mutant genes. For example, although coronary heart disease is usually of multifactorial etiology, about 5 percent of subjects with premature myocardial infarctions are heterozygotes for familial hypercholesterolemia, a single-gene disorder that produces atherosclerosis in the absence of any other predisposing factor. Similarly, in a small proportion of patients with other common diseases such as peptic ulcer disease or "essential" hypertension, the condition is not multifactorial but determined by a single gene, as in the multiple endocrine adenoma–peptic ulcer syndrome or the medullary thyroid carcinoma–pheochromocytoma syndrome, respectively.

INTERACTION BETWEEN SINGLE GENETIC AND ENVIRONMENTAL FACTORS

Many diseases result from an interaction between a specific genotype and a specific environmental factor. In particular, inherited single-gene mutations may produce clinically significant and often life-threatening idiosyncratic responses to certain drugs.

Table 5-7 lists the most important of these *pharmacogenetic disorders,* which encompass all the mendelian modes of inheritance. Perhaps the most common is glucose-6-phosphate dehydrogenase deficiency, an X-linked recessive trait in which a variety of drugs may precipitate a hemolytic anemia. Plasma pseudocholinesterase deficiency and hepatic transacetylase deficiency are examples of autosomal recessive traits which alter drug catabolism so that when the muscle relaxant suxamethonium or the antituberculous drug isoniazid is administered, apnea or peripheral neuropathy, respectively, may ensue. Malignant hyperthermia is an autosomal dominant trait in which acute hyperpyrexia, muscle rigidity, and hyperkalemic cardiac arrest may be induced by administration of any one of several anesthetic agents. Acute intermittent porphyria is another example of a genetic disorder that is exacerbated by drugs, such as barbiturates.

Misinterpretation of adverse drug reactions may result in serious harm to patients. In general, all unusual idiosyncratic reactions should be considered to be genetically determined until proved otherwise. Fortunately, the pharmacogenetic disorders are a group of diseases for which therapy is straightforward: avoidance of the noxious drug by patient and relatives.

In addition to drugs, other factors in the environment may aggravate specific genetic traits. Cigarette smoke may have deleterious effects on persons homozygous and possibly heterozygous for alpha$_1$-antitrypsin deficiency, who are predisposed to the development of emphysema. Patients with xeroderma pigmentosa and anhydrotic ectodermal dysplasia are unusually sensitive to sunlight and high temperatures, respectively. Avoidance of milk at an early age prevents many of the complications ordinarily seen in persons with galactosemia.

Genetic-environmental interactions are particularly important in pregnancy. Women who are affected with phenylketonuria may develop high plasma phenylalanine levels during pregnancy, and thus their offspring may suffer from a variety of phenylalanine-induced birth defects even though the offspring may not themselves have phenylketonuria. Other examples of diseases resulting from an adverse genetic relation between the mother and fetus include erythroblastosis caused by Rh incompatibility and diabetic embryopathy, a term that refers to a series of major birth defects occurring in about 5 percent of the offspring of women who are clinically diabetic during pregnancy.

REFERENCES

EMERY AEH, RIMOIN DL: *Principles and Practice of Medical Genetics,* Vols. 1 and 2. Edinburgh, Churchill Livingstone, 1983
LEWIN B: *Genes,* 3d ed. New York, Wiley, 1987
MCKUSICK VA: *Mendelian Inheritance in Man: Catalogs of Autosomal Dominant, Autosomal Recessive and X-Linked Phenotypes,* 8th ed. Baltimore, Johns Hopkins, 1988

SCRIVER CR et al: *The Metabolic Basis of Inherited Disease*, 6th ed. New York, McGraw-Hill, 1989

THOMPSON JS, THOMPSON MW: *Genetics in Medicine*, 4th ed. Philadelphia, Saunders, 1986

VOGEL F, MOTULSKY AG: *Human Genetics: Problems and Approaches*, 2d ed. Berlin, Springer-Verlag, 1986

6 MOLECULAR GENETICS AND MEDICINE

ARTHUR L. BEAUDET

The haploid human genome contains about 3×10^9 (3 billion) base pairs of DNA and is estimated to encode 30,000 to 100,000 gene products. The length of DNA frequently is quantitated in thousands of bases (kilobases, kb), e.g., the human genome is 3 million kb in length. Each individual inherits two copies of this genome, and the DNA is packaged as 23 pairs of chromosomes. Each chromosome contains a single linear duplex DNA molecule. Most of the DNA sequences that encode proteins occur as unique (single copy) sequences in the genome. Many gene products show similarities in amino acid sequence and can be viewed as members of large gene families, e.g., the globin gene family or the immunoglobulin superfamily. A large amount of DNA in the genome *appears* not to be functional. Hundreds, if not thousands, of repetitive DNA sequences of uncertain function are present in the genome; some are dispersed, and some are clustered.

If one were to print *one copy* of *one strand* of the human genome, it would fill a text 170 times the size of *Harrison's*. The analogy of the human genome to a large book can be carried further. The book can be envisioned as being bound into 46 separate volumes, each the equivalent of one chromosome. Individuals would inherit one paternal set of 23 volumes and one maternal set of 23 volumes. Sickle cell anemia would be the equivalent of changing a single letter on one page of one volume from each of the sets, while deletion of the alpha-globin gene cluster in α-thalassemia might represent the equivalent of the loss of one or two pages of text in each set. Digestion of genomic DNA with restriction enzymes, which recognize specific short DNA sequences and cut DNA at these sites, would be the equivalent of cutting the line of text each time a specific word occurred.

The human genome is extraordinarily polymorphic, but the DNA differences have a broad range of biologic significance. Beginning at the single nucleotide level, the DNA sequence for the human genome can be variable or relatively constant at a given position. As an example, a DNA base would be highly variable if 60 percent of genes in the population had an A (adenine) nucleotide at the position, 40 percent of genes had a G (guanine) nucleotide, and none had a C (cytosine) or T (thymine) nucleotide. Nucleotide positions where more than 1 percent of genes show a nonmajority sequence are designated *polymorphic sites*. Only 1 in 200 to 1 in 500 nucleotide positions qualify as polymorphic. Most nucleotide positions are relatively invariant, the vast majority having the same sequence. The remaining positions have intermediate frequencies of variation. Nucleotide sequence variation is greater in nonfunctional parts of the genome, less in regions of the genome that encode protein sequence or have other important functions. The consequence is that each copy of the human genome varies from every other copy in millions of sequence-specific ways. The nucleotide variations might be envisioned as a multimillion digit serial number embedded within each copy of the human genome. The variability in primary sequence goes beyond single-base changes to include presence or absence of whole segments of DNA. Indeed, considerable length variations occur in the human genome. Inversions of DNA sequence also occur, and translocations between chromosomes also cause DNA variation.

The second type of genetic variation involves phenotypic effect.

The alteration of a single nucleotide or single gene may have a dramatic effect. Indeed, certain DNA sequence alterations may be lethal at the stage of the gamete, fertilized egg, or preimplantation embryo. These instances in which a single alteration has a large effect on the phenotype are single-gene disorders; such disorders have been the focus of most efforts to understand human genetic disease up to the present. However, most of the nucleotide differences between human genomes do not cause any significant phenotypic effect. A continuum exists whereby variations in DNA sequence have phenotypic effects ranging from none to minuscule, to small, to moderate, to large, or to overwhelming. In many instances, multiple genetic loci may interact with each other and/or with environmental factors to produce a phenotypic effect. For example, genetic variations in lipoprotein genes, lipoprotein receptor genes, genes that influence intermediary metabolism, and other genes probably interact with diet, smoking, and additional environmental factors to determine susceptibility to atherosclerosis. Together, variations in DNA sequence and in the biologic effect caused by these differences create individuality. Individuals differ as much in DNA, biochemistry, pharmacokinetics, and susceptibility to disease as in facial appearance, fingerprints, and personality.

ANALYSIS OF THE HUMAN GENOME

Molecular analyses of medical relevance rely heavily on four strategic features: (1) the ability to clone and characterize nucleic acid sequences, (2) the specificity of nucleic acid hybridization, (3) the specificity of restriction endonucleases, and (4) the power of DNA amplification using the polymerase chain reaction (PCR). Various combinations of these capabilities are used to accomplish diverse diagnostic procedures.

MOLECULAR CLONING AND SEQUENCING The size, the complexity, and the variability of the human genome constitute barriers to the analysis of individual traits and genes. The feasibility for such analysis was greatly enhanced by the development of recombinant DNA technology. This technology allows for the analysis of one DNA fragment at a time and has provided an "index" for the human genome and made it possible to locate and isolate individual genes, segments of genes, or nucleotide sequences from the vast DNA library. One of the most powerful of these techniques, so-called cloning of DNA, makes it possible to isolate individual genes or portions of genes, to make an unlimited number of copies of such DNA fragments, to determine the nucleotide sequence of the DNA, and to transcribe and translate the genes so isolated. The various genes and gene products can then be utilized for diverse studies of gene structure and function in normal and disease states. Other recombinant DNA techniques make it possible to analyze genetic variation in individuals directly using clinical samples. Using DNA-hybridization techniques, restriction enzyme digestion, and DNA amplification, to be described below, disease traits can be analyzed both directly and by genetic linkage to polymorphic sites.

The cloning of DNA involves isolation of DNA fragments and insertion of a sequence into the nucleic acid from another biologic source (vector) for manipulation and propagation. The most widely used vectors are based on bacterial plasmids or bacteriophage such as phage λ or M13, some variations of which can accommodate DNA fragments up to 45 kb in size. In addition, vectors designed to function as yeast artificial chromosomes (YAC vectors) can be utilized for cloning DNA fragments up to hundreds of kilobases in size. Space does not allow presentation of the various methods for DNA cloning, but these are well described in Watson et al. and in Sambrook et al. For purposes of this discussion, it is adequate to point out that cDNA (DNA complementary to mRNA) clones have been isolated for hundreds of human genes. Most of these cDNAs have been cloned after characterization of the gene product to obtain amino acid sequence data or specific antibodies. Genomic DNA clones are also

HaeIII   5'-G-G|C-C-3'   HindIII   5'-A|A-G-C-T-T-3'   MstII   5'-C-C|T-N-A-G-G-3'
          3'-C-C|G-G-5'   3'-T-T-C-G-A|A-5'   3'-G-G-A-N-T|C-C-5'

FIGURE 6-1 DNA sequence specificity and nuclease activity for three restriction endonucleases. *Hae*III leaves a blunt end while the other enzymes leave single-stranded ends.

available for hundreds of human genes. In addition, many hundreds of *anonymous* genomic DNA clones are in widespread use. These anonymous DNA clones are generally of interest because they detect polymorphisms that map to a particular location in the human genome, as will be discussed below. Human genomic DNA libraries have been prepared containing most or all of the human genome in fragments of 15 to 45 kb. Radioactive, biotinylated, or otherwise modified copies of DNA can be prepared from any cloned fragment and can serve as a specific molecular *probe*. Biotinylated probes can be detected using avidin and secondary detection methods. Cloned DNA can be sequenced using manual or semiautomated methods, and the sequence of millions of base pairs of human DNA is already known, although only about 0.1 percent of the human genome was sequenced as of early 1989. If a gene or a genomic segment has been cloned, it is relatively straightforward to clone the same region from individual patients and determine the sequence for any mutation. The availability of sequence data allows for the use of the polymerase chain reaction for DNA amplification. Thus, some of the fruits of molecular cloning are the availability of probes for analytical procedures, the determination of disease mutations, and the availability of sequence data to allow for DNA amplification. Cloned DNA can also be used for production of proteins, for detection of sequences of infectious organisms, and for research activities.

NUCLEIC ACID HYBRIDIZATION Many of the steps in recombinant DNA analysis take advantage of the fact that the complementary nature of nucleic acid interaction is the result of base pairing during the synthesis of DNA and RNA (see Chap. 5). Linear pieces of double-stranded (native) DNA can be treated with heat or alkali to dissociate the two strands to yield single-stranded (denatured) DNA. The denatured DNA can be incubated under conditions that allow for nucleic acid hybridization, i.e., the recognition of two complementary strands and re-formation of double-stranded molecules by base pairing. Nucleic acid hybridization is so sensitive that a single-stranded DNA molecule can be hybridized specifically to a complementary strand of RNA or DNA present at about 1 part in 10,000. Many recombinant DNA studies involve the preparation of one radioactive or biotinylated strand of nucleic acid which is then used as a "probe" in the analysis. It is possible to identify and distinguish both fully homologous sequences and partially homologous sequences. The specificity of nucleic acid hybridization, often in combination with fractionation or amplification procedures, allows detection of a single gene among tens of thousands or of a viral sequence in the midst of other nucleic acid sequences.

A variation on nucleic acid hybridization involves the use of allele-specific oligonucleotides (ASO): The DNA probe is a synthetic, single-stranded oligonucleotide, usually 15 to 20 bases in length. The oligonucleotides are synthesized to be complementary to each of two or more sequences that represent polymorphisms or mutations in the genome. The variable nucleotide is in the midportion of the oligonucleotide. Hybridization conditions are adjusted so that the oligonucleotide detects a perfectly matched sequence but fails to hybridize if there is a single base mismatch. Allele-specific oligonucleotides can be used in combination with Southern blotting but are now more widely used in combination with DNA amplification, as described below. The majority of hybridization probes have been prepared in radioactive form, but the use of nonradioactive detection methods is likely to increase.

RESTRICTION ENDONUCLEASES The discovery in microorganisms of restriction endonucleases, commonly known as restriction enzymes, facilitated recombinant DNA manipulations. The enzymes recognize a specific oligonucleotide sequence in double-stranded DNA and cleave the DNA at this site. Many enzymes are known, each recognizing a unique DNA sequence (Fig. 6-1). Some enzymes recognize sequences only four base pairs in length. For example, the enzyme *Hae*III cleaves the sequence 5'-GGCC-3'. By convention, only one strand of DNA is printed as the recognition site, but the enzymes recognize double-stranded DNA. Other enzymes recognize sequences six base pairs in length. The enzyme *Hind*III cleaves the sequence 5'-AAGCTT-3'. Other enzymes, such as *Mst*II, recognize a seven-base-pair sequence but tolerate any base pair in the middle position. The sequence specificity of restriction enzymes is a powerful tool in dissection of large genomes. When human DNA is digested with a particular restriction enzyme, hundreds of thousands of DNA fragments are generated with remarkable reproducibility. Such fragments can vary from a few base pairs to several thousand base pairs in length, depending on the enzyme used. Restriction enzymes that recognize a sequence only four base pairs long cleave the DNA into smaller fragments than enzymes that recognize a six-base-pair sequence. With the use of multiple restriction enzymes to analyze a particular segment of DNA, it is possible to define a detailed map of restriction endonuclease cleavage sites for the region. Such a map can span a region of from several hundred to tens of thousands of base pairs of DNA. As described below, variations in the sequences of those cleavage sites can be analyzed as polymorphisms or mutations in the human genome.

SOUTHERN BLOTTING Many analyses of the human genome involve a specific application of DNA-DNA hybridization, the blotting procedure developed by E.M. Southern. For clinical analysis, *Southern blotting* (Fig. 6-2) begins with the isolation of genomic DNA from cells such as peripheral leukocytes or fetal cells. The high-molecular-weight genomic DNA is digested with a restriction enzyme to yield a series of reproducible fragments. These DNA fragments are separated by electrophoresis in agarose gels. After electrophoresis, the DNA is transferred from the gel to a membrane that binds the DNA. The membrane is treated to denature the DNA and is soaked in a solution containing a radioactive single-stranded nucleic acid probe. The probe will form a double-stranded nucleic acid complex at sites on the membrane where homologous DNA is present. The membrane is washed to remove unbound radioactivity, and regions on the membrane where homologous DNA sequences were bound are detected using x-ray film. The sensitivity of Southern blotting is achieved by splitting the DNA into small segments, fractionating the fragments, and applying a sensitive detection method to pick out specific fragments (nucleic acid hybridization). Overall, this method can detect genomic DNA fragments that represent a single gene or about 1 part in 1 million in the genome. The clinical power of Southern blotting resides in the ability it gives to analyze a tiny portion of the primary structure of human genomic DNA taken from an individual.

An analogous procedure starting with RNA for analysis has been termed *northern* (in contrast to Southern) *blotting*. In this procedure, the presence or absence of a particular mRNA as well as its approximate size can be determined. The term *immunoblotting* or *western blotting* describes a derivative procedure designed to analyze protein antigens. Proteins are separated by electrophoresis and transferred to a solid membrane through a blotting procedure. The membrane is analyzed by incubation with antibodies followed by a second step for enzymatic or radioactive detection of bound antibody. Thus, Southern blotting, northern blotting and immunoblotting or western blotting each combines a fractionation and a detection method to provide a sensitive technique for the analysis of DNA, RNA, and protein, respectively (Table 6-1).

FIGURE 6-2 Southern blotting analysis of genomic DNA.

DNA is dissociated to single-stranded DNA, an annealing temperature where oligonucleotide primers hybridize to target DNA, and a polymerization temperature for the synthetic step. The reaction is usually carried out using heat-resistant *Taq* (from *Thermus aquaticus*) polymerase such that the polymerase remains active during the

FIGURE 6-3 Polymerase chain reaction for amplification of DNA. The target DNA is shown as a solid line in cycle 1. Newly synthesized DNA is indicated by dotted lines in each cycle. Primer oligonucleotides are indicated by solid rectangles. Each DNA strand is marked with an arrow indicating 5'-to-3' orientation. The polymerase chain reaction is patented by Cetus Corporation.

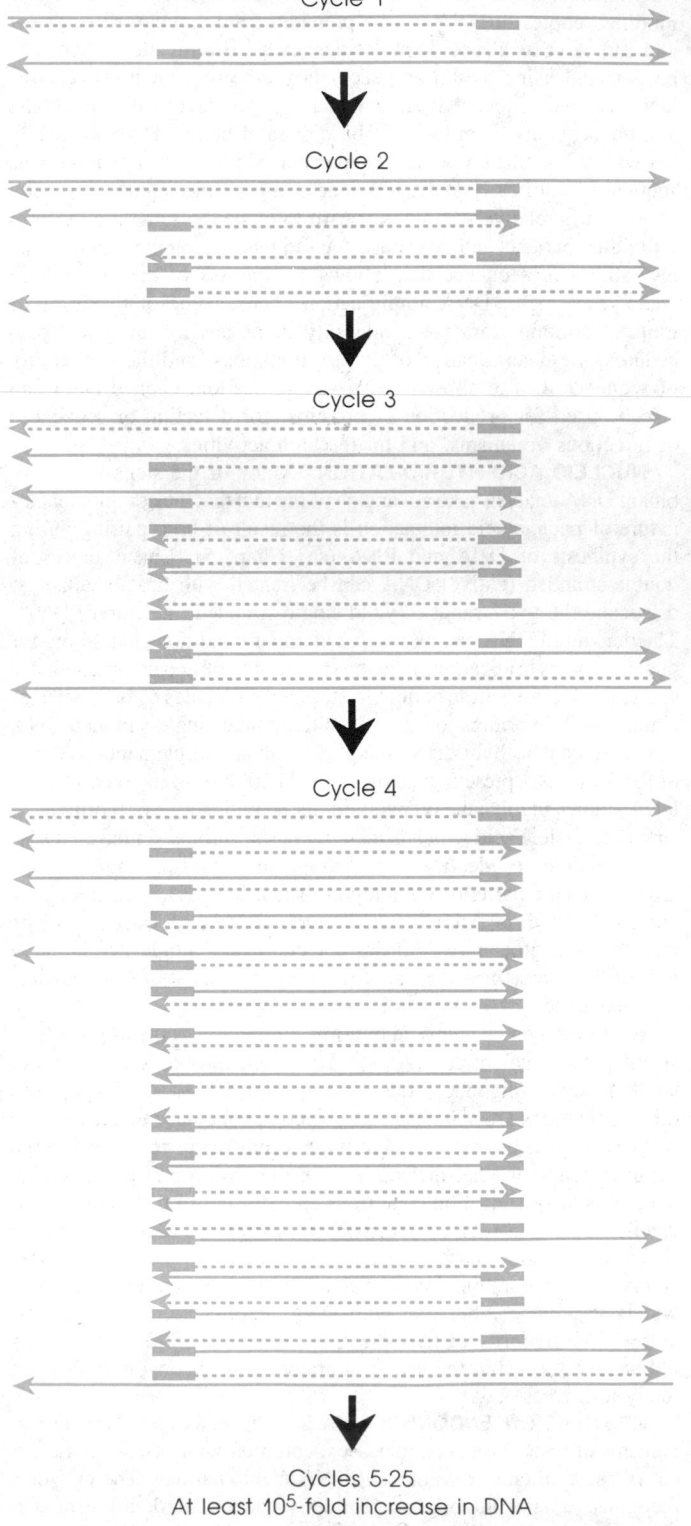

POLYMERASE CHAIN REACTION (PCR) FOR DNA AMPLIFICATION   The technique of PCR for DNA amplification is a powerful method that has had a revolutionary impact on molecular diagnosis. The method was pioneered and patented by workers at the Cetus Corporation. The technique is based on knowing the nucleic acid sequence for a region which, for a diagnostic application, is to be analyzed repeatedly. Oligonucleotide primers are prepared that are complementary to opposite strands of the DNA and are separated by up to a few hundred base pairs (Fig. 6-3). The oligonucleotide primers are incubated with the target DNA to be amplified and with a DNA polymerase that synthesizes a complementary strand in a 5'-to-3' direction. Considerable specificity is provided by the requirement that primers must lead to convergent synthesis for amplification to be effective. The reaction is subjected to a series of temperature variations including a denaturing temperature where double-stranded

TABLE 6-1   Analytical blotting procedures

Blot method	Material analyzed	Fractionation	Detection
Southern	DNA	Electrophoresis	Nucleic acid hybridization
Northern	RNA	Electrophoresis	Nucleic acid hybridization
Western or immunoblot	Protein	Electrophoresis	Immunologic

temperature cycles (usually ranging from 50 to 95°C). After a number of such cycles, typically 20 to 30 or more, hundreds of thousands of copies of the original target sequence are synthesized as depicted in Fig. 6-3. The bulk of the product is a double-stranded DNA fragment of specific length. The technique has been used to amplify and analyze DNA from a single human sperm which contains one duplex target DNA molecule. Molecular diagnosis with PCR depends on determining the presence or the absence of an amplified product, digesting the amplified product with a restriction enzyme, hybridizing the PCR product with allele-specific oligonucleotides, and direct sequencing of the PCR product, or on other methods of analysis. Many variations and modifications have been devised to take advantage of the PCR concept. These include synthesis of cDNA with reverse transcriptase followed by amplification of the cDNA. Single-stranded DNA can be synthesized by altering the ratio of the oligonucleotide primers. Research applications include preparation of recombinant DNA constructs, mutagenesis of cloned DNA, detection of rare nucleotide sequences, and detection of nucleotide sequences of infectious agents. The PCR method offers extremely rapid analysis (single day), ease of automation, relative economy, and extraordinary specificity.

A LINKAGE MAP OF THE HUMAN GENOME Linkage analysis has been used for decades to study the genetics of *Escherichia coli*, *Drosophila*, mouse, and other organisms. Although some clinically relevant linkage relationships were identified by techniques of classic genetics (e.g., that between ABO blood group and nail-patella syndrome), linkage analysis in human beings was enhanced by the advent of recombinant DNA techniques. The feasibility of human linkage analysis was revolutionized in 1978 when Kan and Dozy demonstrated genetic variation in the size of fragments generated after digestion of normal human DNA with restriction endonucleases. These restriction fragment length polymorphisms (RFLPs) are the consequence of the DNA sequence polymorphisms discussed above and are inherited according to Mendelian principles. Restriction enzyme digestion and Southern blotting made it possible to identify these polymorphisms and utilize them as genetic markers for sites within the genome. If one of the base pairs in the recognition sequence for a restriction enzyme is variable between individual copies of the genome or if there is a length variation in the DNA, there will be variation in the size of DNA fragments generated by the restriction enzyme digestion. The inheritance of a RFLP is depicted in Fig. 6-4.

A particularly informative subset of RFLPs occurs at variable number tandem repeat (VNTR) sites. These are sites of length variation in the genome where a short DNA sequence is tandemly repeated a different number of times on different chromosomes. The result is that there are many different sizes of DNA fragments, which

FIGURE 6-4 Example of restriction fragment length polymorphism (RFLP) in human DNA using Southern blotting. The solid blocks indicate segments of DNA used as probe. Parents are heterozygous and children are homozygous for the RFLP. Symbols above the arrows indicate cutting (+) or noncutting (−) by the restriction endonuclease. Numbers indicate DNA length in kilobases.

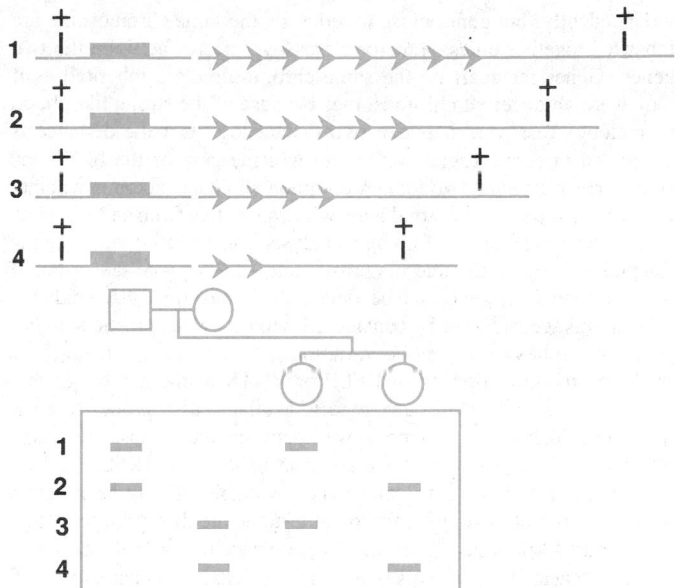

FIGURE 6-5 Example of a variable number tandem repeat (VNTR) polymorphism. Four possible alleles are indicated in the upper portion with the variable number of repeat units indicated by horizontal arrows in the DNA strand. The location of restriction enzyme sites and the DNA probe are indicated as in Fig. 6-4. Inheritance of the alleles within a family as detected by Southern blot is shown below.

can be regarded as different alleles at a VNTR site. Inheritance of a VNTR is depicted in Fig. 6-5. These polymorphic VNTR sites are informative for genetic testing and are valuable for identity testing, as in forensic or paternity analyses. In fact, PCR can be combined with ASO to detect single-base polymorphisms without relying on the fortuitous concurrence of restriction enzyme sites and polymorphisms (see below, Fig. 6-11).

Genetic linkage can be assessed between any group of markers, one of which may represent a disease mutation. The general concepts of genetic recombination and linkage are discussed in Chap. 5. For autosomal genes, each new individual inherits one copy of each chromosome from each parent. Each chromosome is a unique mosaic of polymorphic DNA sequences derived by crossing-over between grandparent chromosomes through the process of meiotic recombination (Fig. 6-6). Genes on different chromosomes are inherited

FIGURE 6-6 Depiction of two chromosomes (one in solid lines and one in dotted lines) from an individual before (*above*) and after (*below*) meiotic crossing over. The individual is heterozygous for a disease locus with a normal allele (filled square) and a disease allele (open square) and for three RFLPs with alleles *A/B*, *M/N*, and *Y/Z*. See discussion in text.

independently, but genes close together on the same chromosome are inherited together unless a meiotic crossover occurs between the two genes. Genes far apart on the same chromosome are inherited as if they were on different chromosomes because of the strong likelihood of meiotic crossovers between two distant loci. Genetic distance is expressed in centimorgans (cM) and is a measure of the likelihood of crossover between two loci. A common clinical concern is whether the disease gene or the normal gene was transmitted from an individual to the next generation. Linkage analysis can be used for prenatal diagnosis, presymptomatic diagnosis, and heterozygote detection. If the mutation in a gene can be detected directly by DNA analysis, genetic linkage need not be considered. However, diagnostic analysis frequently relies on a genetic variation near the disease locus. This often means utilization of an RFLP or VNTR as the nearby genetic marker. If the cloned disease gene is available as a probe, there is negligible likelihood of a crossover between the disease gene and RFLPs within and immediately adjacent to the gene (RFLP 1, Fig. 6-6). If the cloned disease gene is not available, it may be possible to use another cloned DNA fragment a moderate distance (perhaps a few hundred kilobases) from the disease gene. In this instance, there will be occasional crossovers between the disease locus and the RFLP (RFLP 2, Fig. 6-6). Other RFLPs may be so far from the disease locus that no linkage is demonstrable (RFLP 3, Fig. 6-6). There are on average 30 to 35 crossovers during meiosis in males and perhaps twice as many during meiosis in females. The frequency of meiotic crossing-over is not uniform along the length of the chromosomes.

With the availability of an unlimited number of DNA markers, an effort is underway to develop a detailed linkage map for the human genome. Hundreds of polymorphisms detected with specific genes and with anonymous DNA probes are being analyzed. Over 500 individuals from 40 large families are being genotyped in a collaborative effort developed by the CEPH (Centre d'Étude du Polymorphisme Humain). Detailed physical maps of the human genome are also being developed using techniques to map restriction enzyme sites over hundreds of kilobases of DNA. Major international commitments are being made to obtain a detailed map of the human genome, with the ultimate goal of determining its sequence. A short-term product of this effort is the precise mapping of many of the loci causing the more common human single-gene disorders.

REVERSE GENETICS   Most genes have been cloned by first identifying the gene product. *Reverse genetics* is a term that has been used to imply various strategies, but in this context it refers to the cloning of a gene prior to knowing the gene product. The first step in cloning a disease gene by a reverse genetic strategy is to identify

TABLE 6-2   Methods for molecular genetic diagnosis

Strategy	Southern	PCR
Direct detection of mutations		
Large DNA defects	+	+
Altered restriction site	+	+
Any mutation with allele- specific oligonucleotides	+/−*	+
Direct DNA sequencing	−	+
Linkage analysis		
RFLP or VNTR	+	+
Any sequence polymorphism with allele-specific oligonucleotide	+/−*	+

* Although Southern blotting is feasible, it would not be used in current practice.

a DNA polymorphism that is linked to the disease locus. Figure 6-7 depicts analysis for linkage to an autosomal dominant disorder using two randomly selected DNA markers, one of which has A and B alleles and resides near the disease gene on the same chromosome, and one of which has Y and Z alleles and is on a different chromosome. Inspection of the family data suggests linkage of the marker with A and B alleles to the disease locus, and analysis of sufficient pedigree data can provide conclusive evidence that a polymorphic DNA marker is near a disease gene. Analogous efforts can be applied to autosomal recessive diseases. The frequency of crossovers can be used to estimate the genetic distance between the DNA marker and the disease locus. Any DNA clone can be mapped to a chromosome. In 1983 this strategy was used to identify an anonymous (random) DNA segment linked to the Huntington's chorea locus at a distance of 3 to 5 cM on the short arm of chromosome 4. Subsequently, polyposis of the colon, cystic fibrosis, Friedreich's ataxia, adult polycystic kidney disease, neurofibromatosis, and a rare form of Alzheimer's disease have been mapped to human chromosomes 5, 7, 9, 16, 17, and 21, respectively.

With an increasingly detailed genetic map of DNA markers, it is usually possible to identify DNA markers within 1 to 2 cM of a disease gene once the gene is mapped to a chromosome. On average, a genetic distance of 1 cM is equivalent to approximately 1 megabase (1000 kb). Intensive efforts are being applied to clone disease genes once a close linkage is established. These efforts rely on long-range restriction mapping, chromosome walking by isolation of overlapping genomic clones, and chromosome hopping, which involves isolation of the ends of a genomic DNA fragment after deletion of a large intervening region. Having narrowed down the region of genomic DNA that must contain the disease gene, RNA transcripts from this region must be identified and evaluated as candidate gene products. Proof that the disease gene has been located depends on genetic and functional criteria.

STRATEGIES AND PITFALLS   Molecular genetic diagnosis can be accomplished using Southern blotting and PCR in several ways (Table 6-2). Although these are powerful techniques, there are many clinical and laboratory pitfalls. An erroneous diagnosis in an index case is a common problem, e.g., confusion of von Willebrand's disease or hemophilia B with hemophilia A. Failure to recognize nonpaternity, mislabeling of samples, and other simple errors occur. Laboratory problems such as incomplete digestion with a restriction enzyme or contamination of genomic DNA samples with cloned or amplified DNA have caused misdiagnoses.

DIAGNOSIS OF GENETIC DISEASE

MUTATIONS IN A TYPICAL GENE AND GENETIC HETEROGENEITY   A typical gene produces an mRNA that is translated into a protein (Fig. 6-8); also see Chap. 5. The end of the gene where transcription (RNA synthesis) originates is referred to as the *5′ end*, relative to the orientation of the mRNA. The site where transcription begins is referred to as the *Cap site*. At least some of the DNA sequences required for initiation and regulation of transcription are located upstream from this region (opposite from the direction of

FIGURE 6-7   Example of a search for linkage of DNA markers to an autosomal dominant disease. A and B are DNA marker alleles at one site, and Y and Z are alleles at another site. Two pairs of chromosomes are depicted for each parent. The B haplotype and the disease allele are inherited together from the father except for the last-born child in whom a crossover occurred, and the A haplotype was inherited with the disease allele.

D   Disease Allele
N   Normal Allele
■,● Disease Phenotype
□,○ Normal Phenotype

FIGURE 6-8 A typical gene encoding a protein product. Sequences included in mature mRNA (exons) are represented by open blocks with narrower regions for untranslated sequences. Introns (intervening sequences) are shown as hatched blocks.

transcription, to the left in Fig. 6-8). Many upstream regions contain sequences referred to as *TATA boxes* and *CAAT boxes,* which sequences are involved in the initiation and control of transcription. Important sequences for gene regulation may also occur even further upstream and downstream from the Cap site. The segments of DNA sequence that are retained in mature processed mRNA are called *exons.* These exons are separated by segments called *intervening sequences* (IVS) or *introns,* which initially are copied into RNA but which are spliced out in the formation of mature mRNA; i.e., the initial transcript contains an RNA copy of both introns and exons, whereas mature mRNA contains copies only of exons. Untranslated RNA sequences are present in mature mRNA and occur upstream from the protein initiator (AUG) codon and downstream from the terminator (UAA, UAG, or UGA) codon. Transcription proceeds beyond the site where mature mRNA will end. The initial RNA transcript is processed by nuclease cleavage at a poly(A) recognition site and subsequent addition of A (adenine) nucleotides to the 3' end of the mRNA.

Many types of mutation are known. The gene can be entirely deleted. The gene can be rearranged by partial deletion, insertion, or inversion of significant segments. Single-base changes in the coding region generate missense or nonsense codons that cause amino acid substitution or premature chain termination. Mutations in the initiator or terminator codon also can cause disease. In addition, mutations can cause abnormalities of mRNA splicing, usually by changing conserved sequences near intron-exon boundaries. These abnormalities of splicing usually generate mRNAs that do not produce a functional product. Mutations also can occur in control regions and in the polyadenylation signal. In addition, disease mutations may occur in parts of the genome that do not encode proteins, although there are few examples of such instances. The diversity of mutations means that detection of mutant genes at a DNA level can be quite complex.

The extent of molecular heterogeneity is exemplified by the human globin loci. Many different deletions occur in the alpha-globin and beta-globin clusters. Hundreds of single-base changes are known to cause amino acid substitutions. Molecular heterogeneity underlying β-thalassemia is particularly common, with numerous mutations causing nonsense codons, frameshift, abnormal splicing, abnormal transcription, and impaired RNA cleavage and polyadenylation (Fig. 6-9).

STRATEGIES FOR DIAGNOSIS OF MENDELIAN DISORDERS

Approaches for diagnosis of human single-gene disorders can be categorized as follows: (1) direct detection of mutations, (2) linkage analysis with negligible recombination, and (3) linkage analysis with measurable recombination. Linkage disequilibrium is of lesser importance.

Direct detection of mutations Initially, large deletions and genomic DNA rearrangements were the easiest to detect directly using Southern blotting. It is now possible to detect any mutation that occurs widely in the population if the defect is first characterized by DNA sequencing. Southern blotting is rapidly being replaced by PCR, which can be used to determine the presence or absence of a genomic DNA region, to analyze RFLPs or VNTRs, and to prepare material for analysis with ASO or direct DNA sequencing. These techniques have been widely used for human globin gene analysis. For large deletions of major portions of a globin gene cluster, Southern blotting analysis can demonstrate the presence of a homozygous defect (Fig. 6-10). Gene deletions are common causes of α-thalassemia, and prenatal diagnosis of these defects is straightforward using either cDNA or genomic DNA probes. Identification of heterozygous deletions requires either careful quantitation (dosage analysis) or demonstration of abnormal junction fragments from the deleted site. Large deletions are a less frequent cause of mutations in the beta-globin cluster, but such deletions can be demonstrated in hereditary persistance of fetal hemoglobin (Fig. 6-10) and in some forms of δβ-thalassemia.

A Southern blot of the type depicted in Fig. 6-10 would appear

FIGURE 6-9 Point mutations in β-thalassemia. The beta-globin gene is shown with numbered hatched areas representing the coding regions of exons. Boxed open areas between the exons are introns, and boxed open areas at the 5' and 3' ends of the gene are untranslated regions that appear in the messenger RNA. The various types of mutations are depicted by different symbols. *(From AH Kazazian, Jr. CD Boehm, Blood 72:1107, 1988.)*

FIGURE 6-10 Depiction of Southern blot analysis of human globin genes. Above, DNA was isolated from a normal individual and from patients with homozygous hereditary persistence of fetal hemoglobin (HPFH) or homozygous α-thalassemia. DNA was digested with the enzyme *Eco*RI. A mixed DNA probe was prepared by reverse transcription of reticulocyte globin mRNA. Below, arrows indicate *Eco*RI cut sites in the alpha- and beta-globin regions, and numbers indicate DNA fragment sizes in kilobases. *(Adapted from YW Kan, AM Dozy, Proc Natl Acad Sci USA 75:5631, 1978.)*

FIGURE 6-11 Genotype analysis of PCR amplified genomic DNA using allele-specific oligonucleotides (ASO) probes. DNA was extracted from the blood of individuals of beta-globin genotypes AA, AS, SS, SC, CC, and AC and homozygous deletion (XX). The DNA was applied to replicate filters for hybridization with ASO as follows: $β^A$ probe (19A), $β^S$ probe (19S), or $β^C$ probe (19C). *(From K Mullis et al, Cold Spring Harbor Symp Quant Biol 51:263, 1986.)*

normal in an individual with sickle cell anemia. However, many options are now available for direct detection of single-base mutations, such as that causing sickle cell anemia. One procedure for direct detection of the sickle mutation utilized a variation on Southern blotting in which the hybridization probe was a synthetic 19-base oligonucleotide that represented a perfect match for either the $β^S$ or the $β^A$ sequence, i.e., an ASO. The ASO technique can be combined with PCR for DNA amplification rather than with Southern blotting. The ASO and PCR techniques can also be combined to detect any single-base variation that must be analyzed repeatedly in the population. The ability to distinguish beta-globin genotypes is depicted in Fig. 6-11.

Another method for direct detection of the sickle cell mutation takes advantage of the fact that a variety of restriction enzymes cut the $β^A$ but not the $β^S$ sequence. A portion of the nucleotide sequence

in the $β^A$ gene is 5'-CCTGAGG-3', and the corresponding sequence in the sickle gene is 5'-CCTG*T*GG-3'. The GAG to GTG change causes the substitution of valine for glutamic acid. The restriction enzyme *Mst*II (or *Oxa*NI) cuts the sequence 5'-CCTNAGG-3' (N = any nucleotide) and hence will cut the $β^A$ but not the $β^S$ sequence at this site. Initially this strategy was combined with Southern blotting for direct detection of the sickle mutation, but restriction enzyme digestion can now be combined with PCR for rapid direct detection of the sickle mutation as depicted in Fig. 6-12. No complex equipment

FIGURE 6-12 Diagnosis of sickle cell genotype using PCR and restriction enzyme digestion. Genomic DNA was amplified to yield a 294-base pair fragment. The product was digested with the restriction enzyme *Oxa*NI which cuts the product from the normal gene but does not cut the product from the sickle gene. The DNA fragments can be detected with ethidium bromide (EtBr) or silver (Ag) stain. *(From FF Chehab et al, Nature 329:293, 1987.)*

FIGURE 6-13 Detection of deletions in the DNA isolated from Duchenne's muscular dystrophy patients using a dystrophin cDNA probe. Southern blot analysis detects deletions (absence of fragments) in five of eight patients (arrows). A junction fragment is clearly demonstrated in patient 6. *(From M Koenig et al, Cell 50:509, 1987.)*

or radioactivity need be used, and the methods can be applied in underdeveloped areas.

Another example of direct detection of mutations can be drawn from Duchenne's muscular dystrophy. Fragments of the cDNA from this very large gene can be used for Southern blotting to detect deletions in half or more of patients (Fig. 6-13). Heterozygote detection depends on dosage analysis when genomic DNA fragments are absent but is easier and more definitive when junctional DNA fragments are detected (as in patient 6 in Fig. 6-13). Certain portions of the Duchenne locus are particularly prone to deletion, and PCR

can be used to demonstrate the absence of selected portions of the gene.

Direct detection of mutations has been accomplished for numerous disorders (Table 6-3 and see Cooper and Schmidtke). A fraction of mutations for most diseases are easily detected either because they cause large DNA defects or because they alter a restriction enzyme site. Certain DNA sequences, particularly those containing methylated cytosine in CpG dinucleotides, have increased mutation rates, often leading to the loss of sites for the restriction enzymes *Msp*I or *Taq*I. Any mutant allele that is widespread in the population can be detected using PCR with ASO.

Linkage with negligible recombination The general concepts for genetic recombination and linkage are discussed earlier in this chapter and in Chap. 5. Genetic diagnosis by linkage is utilized when it is not possible to demonstrate by direct analysis the mutation or the mutant gene product. For clinical linkage analysis, it is essential that some genetic marker near the disease locus (or near the mutation if the locus is very large) be *informative*. The genetic marker is informative if an individual who is heterozygous for the disease locus is also heterozygous for the marker. Linkage analysis is appropriate when an individual carries one mutant gene and one normal gene and the goal is to determine which has been transmitted to the next generation. Most analyses can be made informative since RFLPs are frequent and since it is usually possible to identify useful polymorphisms near genes causing diseases.

A second requirement for linkage analysis is that of *phase* information between the two loci for genetic analysis. If an individual is heterozygous for a RFLP (genotype 1/2) that is tightly linked to a mutation, it must be determined whether allele 1 for the RFLP is on the chromosome with the disease gene or on the chromosome with the normal gene, assuming that allele 2 for the RFLP would be on the chromosome with the alternate gene. When the genetic marker is informative and the phase is known, genetic diagnosis can be carried out in the form of heterozygote detection, presymptomatic diagnosis, detection of lack of penetrance, and prenatal diagnosis. When the DNA probe is a portion of the gene that is mutated, crossing-over between the genetic marker (often a RFLP) and a mutation is usually negligible. Duchenne's muscular dystrophy is an exception with an extremely large gene in which crossing-over within the gene does occur at a detectable frequency.

Examples of molecular diagnosis by linkage, when there is negligible recombination between the loci, are presented in Fig. 6-14. Genetic marker data are presented as letters that might represent simple RFLP alleles or haplotypes of RFLPs. A *haplotype* is a cluster of tightly linked genetic marker information on a chromosome. Phase can usually be determined from a single index case for autosomal recessive disorders (Fig. 6-14A). Phase can also be determined for

TABLE 6-3 Examples of the role of molecular analysis for diagnosis of genetic disease

Disease	Detection of mutation*	Linkage with gene probe	Linkage with linked marker	Comments
Sickle cell anemia	+ + + +			PCR with ASO or restriction enzyme
Other globin disorders	+ + +	+		Very heterogeneous
Hemophilia A	+	+ +	+	
Phenylketonuria	+ +	+ +		
α₁-Antitrypsin ZZ	+ + + +			PCR with ASO
Familial hypercholesterolemia	+ +	+ +		Biologic tests valuable
Lesch-Nyhan syndrome	+ +	+ +		Heterozygote detection
Tay-Sachs disease	+ +	+ +		Enzyme valuable
Duchenne's muscular dystrophy	+ +	+ +		Many deletions
Retinoblastoma	+ + +	+		Inherited form
Huntington's disease			+ + +	
Myotonic dystrophy			+ + +	
Adult polycystic kidney disease			+ + +	
Fragile X syndrome			+ + +	
Cystic fibrosis			+ + +	
Neurofibromatosis			+ + +	
Polyposis of colon			+ + +	

* + = relative importance of an approach as of early 1989; the status for disorders could change rapidly. PCR, polymerase chain reactions; ASO, allele specific oligonucleotide recessive disorders in the absence of an index case if a reliable biologic or biochemical heterozygote test is available, as might occur for β-thalassemia (Fig. 6-14B). Fetuses of AA genotype are predicted to be affected in Fig. 6-14A and B. For autosomal dominant disorders, linkage phase usually cannot be determined from a single affected individual (Fig. 6-14C). Exceptions would occur in retinoblastoma or polyposis of the colon, when analysis of tumor DNA may distinguish the allele on the abnormal chromosome (often retained in the tumor) from the allele on the normal chromosome (often lost in the tumor). Linkage phase for autosomal dominant disorders can be determined from two appropriate individuals; it is not essential that both be affected (Fig. 6-14D and E). Fetuses of AB genotype are predicted to be affected in Fig. 6-14D and E. For X-linked disorders, phase information is most readily obtained from a single affected male individual (Fig. 6-14F). In general, linkage information can be used to determine the genotype of offspring of individuals of known genotype. Linkage information generally cannot be used consistently to determine the genotype of antecedents of individuals of known genotypes because of the possibility of new mutation from one generation to the next. This is exemplified by an X-linked disorder, where linkage information will not clarify whether or not the mother of an isolated affected male is a heterozygote (Fig. 6-14G). This represents an important difference between direct detection of a mutation and linkage analysis. Occasionally, linkage analysis can suggest the genotype of an antecedent. Note in Fig. 6-14G that the mutation arose on the chromosome from the unaffected maternal grandfather; the maternal grandmother and the maternal aunt of the index case do not carry the mutation, and either the mother or the index case is the recipient of the new mutation. The situation is similar in Fig. 6-14H except that the mutation is on the chromosome from the maternal grandmother and the site of the new mutation is unknown and could go back further in the family. Still by linkage analysis, the maternal aunt is not a carrier of the mutation. The

genotype of an antecedent also can be inferred when a woman has two sons with the same DNA marker, one son being affected and one son being unaffected with the X-linked disorder (Fig. 6-14I). In this instance, the mother is not a heterozygote for the X-linked disorder, although the possibility of gonadal mosaicism (i.e., some of the maternal germ cells have the new mutation) is not eliminated. Diseases where linkage analysis with negligible recombination is used for diagnosis are listed in Table 6-3.

Linkage with detectable recombination   Linkage analysis using a genetic marker that shows detectable recombination with a disease mutation has the same requirements for informativeness and phase as discussed above. However, the analysis is further complicated by the possibility of recombination at each meiosis in the family. For purposes of discussion, it is convenient to consider a genetic marker that has a recombination fraction of 0.1 with a disease mutation (Fig. 6-15). The immediate implication is that genetic diagnosis will be only 90 percent accurate using this single marker, even if complete informativeness and phase are available. The determination of phase is also complicated by the possibility of recombination. If phase is deduced from the offspring of an affected individual, a large number of offspring increases the certainty of the phase information. Continuing to assume a recombination fraction of 0.1 between a genetic marker and a disease mutation, the phase in an individual with a dominant disorder can be deduced with a probability of 0.90 from a single offspring (Fig. 6-15A) but with a probability of 0.99 if there were two identical offspring. In some families with a dominant disorder, the phase can be deduced with complete certainty from antecedent data, such as when an affected individual must have inherited the disease gene and a particular genetic marker from an affected parent (Fig. 6-15B). Fetuses of the AB genotype have probabilities of being affected of approximately 0.81 and 0.90 in Fig. 6-15A and B, respectively, since crossovers may occur in the meioses leading to conception of the fetus. For autosomal recessive

Autosomal Recessive Disorders

Autosomal Dominant Disorders

X-Linked Disorders

FIGURE 6-14   Examples of molecular diagnosis by genetic linkage with negligible recombination between the DNA probe and the disease locus. Letters indicate haplotypes for RFLPs. A and B depict autosomal recessive disorders; C through E depict autosomal dominant disorders; and F through I depict X-linked disorders. The phase is presented with the A haplotype on the same chromosome as the mutant allele in all cases in which it can be determined. (From Scriver et al, chap 1.)

Autosomal Dominant Disorders

Phase (A-M), 0.90   Phase (A-M), 1.0

A   D

X-Linked Disorders

Phase (B-M), 0.90   Phase (A-M), 1.0

C   D

FIGURE 6-15 Examples of molecular diagnosis using genetic linkage with detectable recombination between the DNA probe and the disease locus. Letters indicate haplotypes detected with RFLPs. *A* and *B* depict autosomal dominant disorders; *E* and *F* depict X-linked disorders. The probability of phase at the bottom of each panel indicates the probability that a given haplotype is on the chromosome with mutant allele (M) in the parent of the pregnancy (P). For example, phase (A-M), 0.90, in *A* indicates that the probability is 0.90 that the A haplotype is on the chromosome with a mutant allele in the father of the pregnancy. The recombination fraction is presented as 0.1 for all cases; see text for discussion. *(Modified from Scriver et al, chap 1.)*

disorders, the considerations are analogous. For X-linked disorders, phase can be deduced from offspring of heterozygous females, but more definitive phase information can often be obtained by analysis of the fathers of heterozygous females. In Fig. 6-15*C* and *D*, the same family is depicted with and without data from the maternal grandfather. If an unwise counselor (Fig. 6-15*C*) fails to obtain a sample from the maternal grandfather, the data suggest that the A marker is on the chromosome with the disease gene in the pregnant woman. The phase is known with only 90 percent certainty, and prenatal diagnosis would provide accuracy of approximately 81 percent because of the possibility of crossing-over in either of the meioses leading to the offspring of the heterozygous mother. If a wiser counselor (Fig. 6-15*D*) recognizes the absolute necessity of a sample from the maternal grandfather, the phase in the heterozygous mother becomes known with certainty, and it is evident that the affected son represents a crossover between the genetic marker and the disease mutation. Prenatal diagnosis now becomes 90 percent accurate, but, more important, the prediction of disease or nondisease has been reversed for the presence of a given marker in a male fetus. If phase is to be determined for heterozygous females based on their offspring, the accuracy of phase information increases with increasing numbers of offspring as for the autosomal disorders.

Diseases for which linkage analysis with detectable recombination is used for diagnosis are listed in Table 6-3. An example of the use of PCR to detect a RFLP for diagnosis of cystic fibrosis is shown in Fig. 6-16. An example of linkage analysis using Southern blotting

FIGURE 6-16 Use of PCR to detect a RFLP for prenatal diagnosis of cystic fibrosis. A DNA fragment was amplified at the site of an RFLP originally identified by the probe KM-19. The product was digested with the enzyme *Pst*I and the fragments detected with ethidium bromide staining. Both parents are heterozygous for the RFLP. The first fetus was predicted to be affected, and the second fetus was predicted to be a carrier.

to detect a VNTR linked to the locus for adult polycystic kidney disease is shown in Fig. 6-17.

Linkage disequilibrium Linkage disequilibrium refers to the fact that certain alleles at two or more nearby loci may be found together more often than would be predicted from their frequency in the general population. Although linkage disequilibrium occurs routinely between multiple polymorphic sites, for purposes of genetic diagnosis, this is most readily discussed in terms of a genetic marker and a disease mutation. Figure 6-18 depicts the occurrence of a disease susceptibility mutation (*Z*) at a locus where the normal allele is represented as *Y*. The mutation arises on a chromosome carrying the A allele for a nearby DNA polymorphism. With the passage of time, chromosomes carrying the A allele for the DNA haplotype and the *Z* allele for the disease locus grow to represent 10 percent of the chromosomes in the population. *Linkage disequilibrium* is the term used to describe the fact that the disease susceptibility mutation (*Z*) is found preferentially, and in this case exclusively, on chromosomes bearing the A form of the DNA polymorphism. Not all chromosomes carrying the A form of the polymorphism carry the disease susceptibility allele, but chromosomes carrying the A form of the polymorphism are associated with increased risk of disease. This model also implies that it might be possible at a future date to identify and detect directly the *Z* mutation to provide a more accurate prediction of disease susceptibility. For linkage disequilibrium to be present, the two genetic markers must be tightly linked. In addition there must be one or only a few origins for the disease mutations, or the mutations will be found randomly with different alleles for the marker site. Linkage disequilibrium can often be found using a group of close genetic markers to form a haplotype.

Linkage disequilibrium is extensive within the HLA complex, and numerous diseases are found in association with various HLA

FIGURE 6-17 Southern blotting analysis of a family affected with adult polycystic kidney disease. Alleles *C*, *D*, *G*, *J*, and *H* are detected with a linked, highly polymorphic probe. Designations above each lane refer to pedigree positions, and every person with the *C* allele also has polycystic disease. *(From ST Reeders et al, Nature 317:542, 1985; reprinted with permission.)*

kb

←4·8 C

←3·5 D
←2·9 G

←2·5 J
←2·4 H

FIGURE 6-18 Depiction of the development of linkage disequilibrium within a population of chromosomes. *A* and *B* indicate alleles for a DNA polymorphism. *Y* represents a normal allele and *Z* a disease susceptibility allele at a locus. See text for discussion.

haplotypes (see Chap. 14 in this text and Chap. 4 in Scriver et al.). For example, insulin-dependent diabetes mellitus is associated with HLA-DR3 and HLA-DR4, and susceptibility to this disease may be attributable to the presence of an aspartic acid residue in position 57 of the HLA-DQβ locus. The genotype at this position can be directly determined using PCR and allele-specific oligonucleotides. By comparison to Fig. 6-18, the HLA-DR data for diabetes could be equivalent to the A/B marker, while the aspartic acid residue could be the equivalent of the Z mutation. By analogy, DNA polymorphisms near any gene might detect linkage disequilibrium with a disease susceptibility. Using this rationale, attempts have been made to determine if certain DNA markers adjacent to the apolipoprotein genes might be associated with increased risk of atherosclerosis. If such associations are proven, they would imply that some genetic variation in the coding or regulatory portions of an apolipoprotein gene itself is responsible for the altered disease susceptibility. Ultimately these genetic variations could be used directly for assessment of disease risks.

RFLPs showing strong linkage disequilibrium with cystic fibrosis have also been identified. The DNA markers are close to the cystic fibrosis locus, and a single mutation accounts for a major proportion of the mutant genes in the population. The linkage disequilibrium information can be used for genetic counseling for cystic fibrosis (see Chap. 108 in Scriver et al.).

MOLECULAR CYTOGENETICS Recombinant DNA techniques provide a bridge between single-gene disorders and cytogenetics (see Chap. 7 in this text and Chap. 9 in Scriver et al.). Genetic alterations range in size from single-base changes to gain or loss of an entire chromosome. As an example, some patients with Duchenne's muscular dystrophy have gross cytogenetic abnormalities, some patients have large deletions of DNA detectable by molecular but not cytogenetic analysis, and presumably others have single-base changes. Patients with detectable cytogenetic abnormalities have facilitated the cloning of numerous X-linked genes, the cloning of the retinoblastoma gene, and the mapping of the locus for polyposis of the colon. Reciprocally, molecular probes have been used to define cytogenetic translocations, deletions, and insertions. DNA probes have been used to detect Y chromosome–specific sequences in 46, XX males and to demonstrate the absence of Y chromosome regions in 46, XY females.

The technique of in situ hybridization involves the use of radioactive or fluorescent DNA probes for direct annealing to chromosomal DNA in fixed tissue preparations. The technique has been used widely for mapping cloned DNA fragments to specific chromosomal regions. Clinically, the technique can be used to determine the presence or absence of a DNA segment within an abnormal chromosome; this can demonstrate whether a segment is deleted or determine the position of a DNA segment relative to a balanced translocation breakpoint. Fluorescent probes mapping to a single chromosome have been used to detect chromosomes in interphase nuclei. This technique offers the exciting possibility of automated simplified cytogenetic analysis for disorders such as Down's syndrome.

OTHER DIAGNOSTIC APPLICATIONS

MOLECULAR ONCOLOGY Just as these diagnostic techniques can be used to detect any mutation in the constitutional DNA of all cells, they can be used to detect somatic mutations in malignant cells. Southern blotting and/or PCR can be used to detect alterations affecting both dominant and recessive oncogenes. Single-base changes can be demonstrated in dominant oncogenes, e.g., substitutions in codon 12 of H-*ras* have been demonstrated in human colon and pancreatic cancer among others. Oncogenes can be shown to be amplified in numerous human tumors. Loss of heterozygosity at loci for recessive oncogenes can be shown using polymorphisms linked to these loci, e.g., loss of heterozygosity on chromosome 5q in human colon cancer. Chromosomal translocations such as those between immunoglobin loci and oncogenes can be demonstrated by Southern blotting. It is likely that molecular techniques will play an increasing role in the analysis of the basic alterations in tumor cells, in the classification and staging of tumors, and in the monitoring of therapeutic strategies.

DIAGNOSTIC VIROLOGY AND MICROBIOLOGY Virtually all microorganisms have DNA or RNA sequences that can be detected by nucleic acid hybridization techiques. As discussed above, nucleic acid hybridization is very sensitive and specific, and it can be combined with PCR to detect an extraordinarily low abundance of foreign nucleic acid sequences. Many other diagnostic procedures such as detection of infectious antigens with monoclonal antibodies and detection of human immune responses with immunoblotting can also provide rapid, sensitive, and specific diagnostic procedures. Each strategy offers special advantages. Some advantages of the detection of foreign nucleic acid sequences are as follows: (1) sequences can be detected without the delay required for the host to mount immune responses, (2) sequences can be detected without regard to passive acquisition of antibody whether by maternal transfer or by transfusion, (3) sequences can be detected even if the host fails to mount an immune response, (4) sequences can be detected even if no foreign proteins are being synthesized, and (5) the extraordinary ability of PCR to detect even a single molecule in a sample may provide the most sensitive technique in many circumstances. These techniques have been used for a broad range of viral diagnoses including cytomegalovirus, rotavirus, Epstein-Barr virus, and others. PCR has been used to detect hepatitis B sequences in serum and to detect HIV-1 sequences in peripheral blood mononuclear cells. In one study using PCR, HIV-1 sequences were detected in 100 percent of specimens from seropositive, virus culture–positive homosexual men and in 64 percent of specimens from seropositive, virus culture–negative homosexual men. DNA amplification required 3 days rather than the 3 to 4 weeks required for virus isolation.

IDENTITY TESTING Analysis with only a few highly polymorphic VNTR probes provides the ability to distinguish the genotype of virtually all individuals except identical twins. This powerful method of identification finds application in paternity testing, in settling immigration disputes, in criminal investigations, and in monitoring bone marrow transplantation. The combination of PCR with VNTR analysis is particularly powerful for forensic analysis,

FIGURE 6-19 Paternity analysis in two families using Southern blotting and two highly polymorphic VNTRs. M, mother; C, child; F, putative father; F + C, putative father and child loaded in a single lane. A ladder of marker fragments is loaded in the center and outer lanes. Each individual demonstrates two alleles with each probe. The putative father is not excluded with either probe in the family on the left. In the family on the right, the putative father is not excluded with the probe 255, but is excluded with probe 299. *(Courtesy of R Giles, GeneScreen, Inc, using Lifecodes technology; see Balazs et al.)*

since identification can be made from minuscule samples of semen, blood, hair root, skin, or other tissue. Tissue typing at the HLA loci is also feasible using molecular analysis of polymorphisms. An example of a paternity analysis using highly polymorphic VNTR probes is shown in Fig. 6-19.

THERAPEUTIC APPLICATIONS

PHARMACEUTICALS Cloned DNA sequences can be used for synthesis of proteins and peptides. The major advantages of this strategy are the ability to obtain unlimited amounts of purified products not previously available and the avoidance of contamination by pathogens. Production can be carried out in bacteria, yeast, cultured animal cells, or whole animals. Just as glucocorticoids and their synthetic derivatives have been explored for the treatment of endless numbers of human diseases, so now it will be possible to evaluate the therapeutic potential of innumerable naturally occurring and specially engineered protein products.

Bacteria do not splice eukaryotic messenger RNA properly, so the coding region is usually provided as cDNA clones or as synthetic DNA sequences. The coding region must be linked to bacterial DNA segments that control transcription and initiation of translation. The major difficulties with bacterial synthesis involve the lack of eukaryotic mechanisms for posttranslational processing. Almost all bacterial and eukaryotic proteins undergo proteolytic cleavage at the amino terminus to remove the initiator methionine, and multiple proteolytic cleavages may be involved, as in the production of various hormones from the proopiomelanocortin gene. Other forms of posttranslational modification include removal of leader sequences, carbohydrate addition, phosphorylation, acylation, formation of disulfide bridges, and vitamin K–dependent carboxylation. Improperly or incompletely processed proteins may or may not function normally and may be antigenic. These obstacles have been overcome to produce a number of human proteins that are efficacious and safe. Proteins are also being produced in yeast, and proteins that require extensive posttranslational modification may be produced in cultured animal cells. It is also feasible to create transgenic animals that will secrete large amounts of recombinant proteins into milk. These proteins could then be purified for pharmaceutical use.

Several hormones have been produced by recombinant methods, including human insulin and human growth hormone. Human insulin offers the potential advantage of reduced immunologic response in comparison to animal insulins. Growth hormone represents an instance where the natural product was in extremely short supply. Recombinant clotting factors are being evaluated for clinical use. The fact that many hemophilia patients became infected with HIV-1 again demonstrates the potential advantages of a recombinant product free of human infectious agents. Numerous recombinant cytokines such as tumor necrosis factor, interferons, interleukins, and colony-stimulating factors are being evaluated in the treatment of various diseases, primarily malignancies and AIDS. There is a suggestion that colony-stimulating factor may be efficacious in chronic granulomatous disease. Recombinant α_1-antitrypsin is being evaluated for replacement therapy for that deficiency. Thrombolytic treatment with various forms of recombinant plasminogen activator offers considerable promise in the treatment of acute myocardial infarction. Efforts are under way to engineer novel forms of recombinant plasminogen activator that might be superior to naturally occurring proteins (see Haber et al.). Recombinant erythropoietin produced in bacteria is not biologically active, whereas glycosylated erythropoietin produced in cultured mammalian cells is active. Approximately 96 recombinant proteins in some 23 different therapeutic areas are approved, undergoing clinical trials, or under development (see Copsey and Delnatte).

The value of recombinant DNA products that must function intracellularly is more tenuous. Although recombinant enzyme could be produced for replacement therapy, the problems of intracellular, tissue-specific targeting remain. For example, large amounts of α-galactosidase A and glucocerebrosidase could be produced for therapy of Fabry's disease and Gaucher's disease, respectively, but delivery systems are unproven. Proteins for which there is no mechanism for endocytosis and proteins required in the central nervous system are unlikely candidates for such replacement therapy.

VACCINES Recombinant DNA techniques make it possible to produce recombinant proteins to be used as antigens for vaccination. For example, recombinant hepatitis B surface antigen has been produced in yeast for preparation of a vaccine now in widespread use. There is great interest in the possibility for development of a recombinant vaccine for HIV, but there are significant obstacles such as the hypervariability in the envelope protein of this virus.

Another strategy for recombinant vaccine production involves the use of live recombinant vaccine such as that which might be produced with attenuated vaccinia virus (see Moss et al.). One or more antigens from a virus can be introduced into the vaccinia genome. Live vaccines offer considerable advantages in terms of efficacy, but attenuation must be monitored to reduce the risk of rare complications. Experimental animals have been protected with recombinant vaccinia viruses against diseases caused by hepatitis B, influenza, herpes simplex, rabies, Friend leukemia, Epstein-Barr, and respiratory syncytial viruses.

RESEARCH APPLICATIONS

TRANSGENIC AND MUTANT MICE   The germ-line DNA of mice can be manipulated in a variety of powerful ways (Fig. 6-20). The creation of transgenic mice typically involves microinjection of cloned DNA sequences into the male pronucleus of fertilized mouse eggs. The injected DNA becomes integrated into the mouse chromosomal DNA in a fraction of the injected cells. The transgenic DNA can be expressed in the resulting animals and can be present in the germ cells so that a series of transgenic descendant animals can be obtained. Each site of integration of foreign DNA behaves as a single Mendelian trait, and heterozygous and homozygous animals can be obtained.

Up to the present, transgenic animals have been used most widely to evaluate cis-acting regulatory DNA sequences that control tissue-specific and temporal aspects of gene expression. Putative regulatory sequences are linked to a reporter gene, which produces an easily detectable product. Using this strategy, short DNA sequences have been found to provide exquisite tissue specificity for genes such as insulin and elastase while more complex and distant regulatory sequences control the expression of globin genes. Another application of the transgenic method has involved introduction of viral or cellular oncogenes to induce tumors in animals. This opens up a variety of approaches for the study of tumor biology. A tissue-specific regulatory sequence can be linked to the SV40 T antigen to produce tumors in specific cell types. Another transgenic mouse strategy involves linking of regulatory sequences to a toxin which will selectively kill cells that express the sequence. As an example, linking of insulin regulatory sequences to diphtheria toxin can generate mice with selective absence of pancreatic beta cells. In yet another application, larger transgenic animals can be used for production of pharmaceuticals to be harvested from milk or blood.

Since integration of transgenic DNA is relatively random, it results

FIGURE 6-20   Various strategies for producing transgenic and mutant mice. DNA can be injected into the male pronucleus of fertilized mouse eggs followed by implantation in pseudopregnant mothers. Mouse embryos can be infected with retroviruses in vivo or in vitro. Transgenic mice may be mosaic, but the transgene can be recovered in nonmosaic form in the offspring of these mice. These strategies are depicted on the left. On the right, cultured embryonic stem (ES) cells can be modified by homologous or nonhomologous recombination or by retroviral infection. The modified cells can be selected and injected into a mouse blastocyst to produce a chimeric mouse with subsequent recovery of the mutation in the germ line of the offspring of the chimeric mouse.

in interruption of normal mouse genes in a certain percentage of cases. Retroviruses can also be used to infect mouse embryonic cells with the goal of relatively random insertional mutagenesis in the mouse. Mutant phenotypes can then be sought in the resulting heterozygous or homozygous mice including the identification of defects which are benign in heterozygotes but result in embryonic lethality in the homozygous state. Because the cloned DNA inserts at the site of the affected gene, it is possible to clone the gene which is associated with the mutant phenotype. Thus, it is possible to identify many new mouse mutants and to clone the relevant gene rather quickly.

The ability to carry out homologous recombination with mouse embryonic stem (ES) cells provides additional exciting opportunities. ES cells are totipotent cells that can be manipulated in culture and then reintroduced into mouse embryos. Strategies are available to use modified fragments of any cloned gene to interrupt or alter the normal mouse gene. This is achieved through homologous recombination between the cloned fragment and the mouse gene in ES cells. The genetically altered cells are often represented in the sperm of the resulting animals, and mutant mice can be obtained and bred to study heterozygotes and homozygotes. The technique will allow for creation of mouse models of many human genetic diseases. These models should be particularly valuable for studying pathogenesis and for conducting therapeutic trials. Perhaps more importantly, the ability to obtain mouse mutants for virtually any cloned gene provides an opportunity to analyze the function of the increasing number of cloned genes whose biologic roles are not delineated.

IMPACT ON BIOMEDICAL RESEARCH   Recombinant DNA techniques have revolutionized the study of biology and medicine, probably more than any technical advance since the development of the light microscope. Major advances in almost all disciplines utilize these most powerful of biologic research methods. The ability to clone and characterize virtually any gene from any organism provides for universal applicability. The ability to identify homologous genes and gene segments in bacteria, yeast, *Drosophila,* mouse, and human beings brings basic science and medicine closer together. The ability to use organisms other than humans to study genetics and function often allows for deduction of the role of a human gene by analogy. For example, the identification of classes of developmental genes (e.g., homeotic genes in *Drosophila*) has led to the identification of related genes in mouse and human beings. The ability to mutate these genes in mice is likely to clarify their function in humans and lead to the identification of human mutations. These techniques make the study of neurobiology and developmental biology in mammals particularly exciting for research.

THE PROSPECTS OF GENE REPLACEMENT THERAPY   For human genetic disorders in which the mutant gene is identified and the cloned normal gene is available, a number of strategies can be considered for gene replacement therapy. Gene replacement therapy has a major theoretical advantage over enzyme or factor replacement, since a single treatment could provide permanent correction. If the disease is caused by simple deficiency of the product, as in the case of most enzyme deficiencies and clotting disorders, any restoration of the synthesis of normal product might be beneficial, and neither normal tissue-specific expression nor precise regulation of gene expression may be an absolute requirement. For other gene products such as globins, an appropriate level of gene expression and tissue-specific expression would be critical. When a mutant gene product has a deleterious effect, elimination of the deleterious gene might be as necessary or more important than provision of a replacement gene. Initially, efforts at gene therapy should be directed at patients with serious life-threatening illness where risk-benefit ratios are acceptable.

At least three types of DNA replacement can be envisioned. In one instance, a cDNA might be inserted under the control of a foreign promoter so that the product is synthesized without proper regulation. In a second strategy, genomic DNA could include the sequences necessary for proper regulation of the level and tissue specificity of expression. Artificial "minigene" constructions that link genomic regulatory regions with cDNA may provide constructions that are of manageable size and that show proper regulation. These strategies would typically involve random insertion of DNA sequences into the chromosome, although expression of extrachromosomal sequences is also a possibility. A third strategy would utilize site-specific recombination so that the mutant region was replaced by normal DNA sequence. This approach is theoretically optimal and is feasible as the result of the achievement of homologous recombination in cultured mouse embryonic stem cells. One can at least imagine the possibility of culturing human bone marrow stem cells and selecting for clones that are corrected through homologous recombination with cloned normal DNA.

Retroviral vectors are potential agents for gene therapy. Such vectors have the ability to produce viral particles that encode foreign nucleic acid and contain mechanisms for chromosomal integration. One current strategy (Fig. 6-21) involves insertion of cDNA or minigene DNA constructions between two viral long terminal repeats (LTRs) in a plasmid vector. These constructions can be introduced into cultured cell lines that provide the viral proteins necessary to package pseudovirus particles that include the gene sequence of interest. For example, bone marrow cells could be removed from a patient with a specific defect, bone marrow stem cells could be infected with these viral particles, and the patient's bone marrow could be repopulated with his or her altered cells. Delivery to tissues such as liver would be more complex, but can be envisioned.

Alternative strategies might include packaging of DNA in liposomes, development of other viral vectors, and use of vectors that remain in an extrachromosomal state. The risk-benefit ratio for somatic gene replacement therapy must be estimated on an individual basis. Random insertion of DNA sequences into the genome is likely to have some risk for carcinogenesis. However, based on the experience with retroviruses that do not contain oncogenes, this risk might be relatively low if viral progeny are not produced in the recipient. Such risks may be acceptable in patients with life-threatening illness where no reasonable alternative therapy is available. Several human diseases are candidates for early attempts (Table 6-4). Life-threatening, recessive diseases involving bone marrow–derived cells would be excellent choices (e.g., adenosine deaminase deficiency, chronic granulomatous disease, and leukocyte adhesion deficiency), as are disorders in which extracellular products such as hormones or clotting factors might be produced in altered bone marrow cells. Dominant, neurologic disorders such as Huntington's disease appear to be the least approachable. If proper regulation of globin genes

FIGURE 6-21 One strategy for attempting somatic gene replacement therapy.

could be achieved, sickle cell anemia and thalassemia would constitute important opportunities because of the accessibility of bone marrow for in vitro treatment, because of the frequency of the diseases and because of their serious nature. Human experiments using retroviral vectors to monitor an immunotherapeutic approach to malignancy appear feasible, and this experience may guide attempts at therapy for genetic disease.

ETHICAL CONSIDERATIONS Molecular genetic diagnosis provides an increasing capacity for presymptomatic and prenatal diagnosis of disease and disease susceptibility. It is possible to diagnose a newborn infant with familial polyposis of the colon, Huntington's

TABLE 6-4 Human diseases as candidates for gene replacement therapy

Disorder	Burden of disease	Alternative treatment	Disease frequency	Requirement for tissue specificity	Regulation	Relative feasibility*
Hemoglobinopathies	Great	Transfusion, fair to poor	1 in 600 in ethnic groups	Erythroid	Required	+ + +
Lesch-Nyhan syndrome	Great	Poor	Rare	Brain, ?other	?Not essential	+ +
Adenosine deaminase and nucleoside phosphorylase deficiency	Great	Transplant, enzyme replacement, fair to good	Very rare	Bone marrow	?Not essential	+ + +
Leukocyte adhesion deficiency	Great	Transplant, fair to poor	Very rare	Bone marrow	?Not essential	+ + + +
Phenylketonuria	Small to moderate	Diet, good	1 in 11,000	Liver, ?other	?Not essential	+ +
Urea cycle disorders	Moderate to great	Diet, drug, good to poor	1 in 30,000 for all types	Liver, ?other	?Not essential	+ + +
Alpha₁ antitrypsin	Moderate	Poor, ?recombinant drug	1 in 3500	Liver, ?other	?Not essential	+ + +
Hemophilia A & B	Moderate to great	Replacement, fair	1 in 10,000 males	?Any organ, f. VIII	?Not essential	+ + + +
Lysosomal storage diseases	Great	Poor	1 in 1500 for all types	Brain for many	?Not essential	+
Familial hypercholesterolemia	Great	Diet, drug, fair	1 in 500 heterozygotes	Liver, ?other	Some importance	+ +
Cystic fibrosis	Great	Supportive, fair/poor	1 in 2500 whites	?	?	?
Duchenne's muscular dystrophy	Great	Poor	1 in 10,000 males	?Muscle	?	?Poor
Huntington's disease	Great	Poor	1 in 20,000	?Brain	?	?Poor

* Attempts to take into account requirements for regulation, accessibility of target organs, alternative treatment, and risk vs benefit.

disease, or dominant polycystic kidney disease decades before the onset of symptoms. What might be the impact of such diagnosis on the psychological development, career opportunities, and insurability of such individuals? Diagnosis of major increased susceptibility to coronary disease, diabetes, colon cancer, breast cancer, and other disorders is also likely to bring both the potential for therapeutic intervention and the risk of anxiety and discrimination. Prenatal diagnosis is now possible for diseases with a wide range of burden, such as alpha$_1$-antitrypsin deficiency, phenylketonuria, sickle cell anemia, muscular dystrophy, and familial hypercholesterolemia. Societies and individuals are divided regarding the suitability of abortion under such circumstances. Development of gene replacement therapy and other means of treating presently untreatable genetic diseases may ultimately result in a reduced utilization of abortion.

Gene replacement therapy raises other ethical considerations. Somatic gene replacement therapy requires conventional risk-benefit analyses for individual patients. So long as there is no modification of the germ-line DNA, few people have serious ethical concerns other than the question of whether such treatment is in the best interest of an individual patient. Experience with cancer chemotherapy suggests that some unintentional low level of damage to germ-line DNA might be an acceptable undesirable risk of such therapy if the patient received great benefit. In the future, it is conceivable that methods for site-specific recombination would allow replacement of mutant DNA in the germ line with normal material. If one could permanently correct the cystic fibrosis mutation, the Huntington's disease mutation, or the sickle cell mutation in the germ line of an individual and if such treatment were safe and effective, would society consider such therapeutic intervention?

REFERENCES

BALAZS I et al: Human population genetic studies of five hypervariable DNA loci. Am J Hum Genet 44:182, 1989

COOPER DN, SCHMIDTKE J: Diagnosis of genetic disease using recombinant DNA. Hum Genet 77(Suppl):66, 1987

COPSEY DN, DELNATTE SYJ (eds): *Genetically Engineered Human Therapeutic Drugs*. New York, Stockton Press, 1988

ERLICH H et al (eds): *Polymerase Chain Reaction*. Cold Spring Harbor, Cold Spring Harbor Laboratory, 1989

HABER E et al: Innovative approaches to plasminogen activator therapy. Science 243:51, 1989

Molecular Biology of Homo sapiens. Cold Spring Harbor Symp Quant Biol 51:1, 1986

MOSS R et al: Roles of vaccinia virus in the development of new vaccines. Vaccine 6:161, 1988

OU CY et al: DNA amplification for direct detection of HIV-1 in DNA of peripheral blood mononuclear cells. Science 239:295, 1988

PALMITER RD, BRINSTER RL: Germ-line transformation of mice. Annu Rev Genet 20:465, 1986

SAMBROOK J et al: *Molecular Cloning, A Laboratory Manual*, 2d ed. Cold Spring Harbor, Cold Spring Harbor Laboratory, 1989

SCRIVER CR et al (eds): *The Metabolic Basis of Inherited Disease*. New York, McGraw-Hill, 1989

WATSON JD et al: *Recombinant DNA, A Short Course*. New York, Scientific American Books, distributed by Freeman, 1983

7   CYTOGENETIC ASPECTS OF HUMAN DISEASE

JAMES GERMAN

The chromosome complement of humans, like that of other species, is guarded carefully against change; most chromosome mutations, either structural or numerical, are deleterious. Only rarely is a balanced structural rearrangement (one that results in neither deficiency nor duplication of significant chromosome segments) introduced into the population and transmitted from generation to generation. As a rule an abnormal number of autosomes results in early death, except for trisomy of the shortest chromosome. In contrast, an abnormal number of sex chromosomes is often tolerated reasonably well, although infertility or subfertility usually is present. Nevertheless, among human embryos abnormalities in chromosome structure and number are common and are, in fact, the major known cause of embryonic and early fetal wastage. However, not every fetus with an abnormal chromosome complement is aborted, and those that survive constitute the material of medical cytogenetics.

Clinical disorders resulting from chromosome imbalance present varying features including abnormal anatomic development, mental deficiency, behavioral disorders, and disturbances in growth and sexual development. Sometimes infertility, repeated abortion, or the birth of malformed children is the presenting complaint of persons with abnormal chromosome complements whose own general development is normal.

The disorders just referred to are due to chromosome imbalance that affects tissues throughout the body. In addition, change can occur in the chromosome complement in a single cell of some somatic tissue. Such a mutant cell may have a proliferative advantage over normal cells, in which case a clone bearing the abnormal chromosome complement can develop among otherwise normal cells. Although such mutant clones are in many cases clinically insignificant, they are also important in the etiology of cancer.

This chapter is addressed to those aspects of normal chromosome structure and function that constitute the basis for an understanding of the chromosome alterations in human disease. In addition, the chromosome alterations important in adult medicine and their consequences are summarized.

CHROMOSOME STRUCTURE AND FUNCTION   The human autosomes are numbered 1 through 22, and the sex chromosomes are denoted X and Y. (Figure 7-1 shows the normal human chromosome complement. In the legend of the figure several terms used in human cytogenetics are defined.) Each is recognizable microscopically by morphologic features such as relative length and position of the centromere and by staining characteristics (banding pattern). A mammalian chromosome consists of one double-stranded helix of DNA that extends from one end through the centromere to the other end.

Cell-division cycle   Chromosomes must duplicate before cell division can occur. This duplication occurs over a period of several hours prior to the onset of mitosis or meiosis in a phase of the cell cycle termed S, for synthesis of DNA (Fig. 7-2). Thus, from the completion of S to the completion of metaphase, each chromosome contains two identical double-stranded helices of DNA, and the nucleus contains four times as much DNA as a spermatozoon or ovum. During mitosis chromosomes are condensed, and the two sister chromatids can be visualized by late prophase or early metaphase (Fig. 7-1). (Metaphase is the stage in the cell-division cycle ordinarily employed for cytogenetic analysis.)

At the onset of anaphase the centromeric regions of each chromosome separate, and the two chromatids move quickly to opposite poles of the mitotic spindle. As soon as each pole receives one full complement of chromatids (now called chromosomes), a nuclear membrane—it had been disassembled late in prophase—is assembled about each cluster to complete formation of the nuclei of the two sister cells that emerge at telophase. The sister cells emerge in what is called the G_1 phase of the cell cycle, in which they remain unreplicated unless another division is to be prepared for, whereupon they enter the S phase. Cells engaged in some differentiated function ordinarily remain unreplicated.

Most normal cells in the human body are diploid; i.e., they have twice the haploid number of chromosomes, the number in a gamete (haploid = 23, diploid = 46). In the germ line, which is devoted to gamete formation, cells destined eventually to differentiate into spermatozoa or ova undergo mitotic cell cycles until they enter the two specialized divisions termed *meiosis*. In meiosis, pairing of homologous chromosomes occurs (the paternally derived chromosome 1 with the maternally derived chromosome 1, and so on), and genetic recombination takes place (see Chap. 5). At the first meiotic division

FIGURE 7-1 Normal human lymphocyte chromosomes arrested in meta-phase and stained for G bands (G standing for Giemsa). The inset shows the arrangement of chromosomes in an intact cell, and the remainder of the figure shows their ordered arrangement into a karyotype. By the time mitosis begins, each chromosome consists of two identical parts called sister chromatids and is identified by its relative length, the location of its centromere, and a distinctive sequence of bands of varying lengths and depth of staining. The number of bands visible microscopically varies from cell to cell, depending on the degree of chromosome condensation. The 300 to 400 bands seen in this particular cell can be increased to several times that number if cells with longer chromosomes are chosen for analysis, i.e., many of the bands seen here will resolve into subbands. Normally, the G-band patterns of the two chromosomes of a pair are alike, with the exception of certain polymorphic regions, examples of which are shown in Fig. 7-4.

The centromere of a chromosome divides it into a short arm (p) and a long arm (q). Numbers 13 to 15, 21, 22, and Y are called acrocentric because of the nearly terminal positions of their centromeres; the minute p of each acrocentric autosome bears a nucleolus-organizing region which often causes a secondary constriction in the metaphase chromosome (the constriction at the centromere being the primary constriction).

By standard nomenclature, this karyotype is described as 46,XY, indicating that its chromosome number is 46, its sex chromosomes are an X and a Y, and the autosomes (those besides the X and Y) number 44. The following examples show the general use of this nomenclature: A normal female karyotype is described as 46,XX. A female cell with an extra chromosome 18 (trisomic for 18) would be described as 47,XX,+18. A cell with only one sex chromosome, an X, and with deletion in the short arm of chromosome 5 would be described as 45,X,5p−. A male cell with a translocation between chromosomes 2 and 3, with breakpoints in band 13 of 2p and band 22 of 3p, would be described as t(2;3) (9q13;p22). (See also Table 7-2 footnote.)

homologous chromosomes are segregated, and the diploid chromosome number is reduced to the haploid; i.e., each cell then contains one of each of the 22 (duplicated) autosomes plus one (duplicated) sex chromosome. No S phase takes place between the first and second meiotic divisions (depicted in Fig. 7-2, right), so that at the second division, in which sister chromatids separate, emerging cells maintain the haploid number of chromosomes but are reduced in their content of DNA to half the amount of diploid G_1 cells of somatic tissues. With fertilization of an ovum by a spermatozoon, both the chromosome constitution and the DNA content of the zygote are restored to that of a G_1 somatic cell. An S period in the zygote then permits reinstitution of regular cell-division cycles characteristic of the somatic cells.

Chromosome differentiation A chromosome is differentiated along its length, and some aspects of this differentiation are resolvable, by either light or electron microscopy. The DNA is complexed with a number of proteins in a highly specific way. The DNA-protein complex together with some associated RNA is referred to as *chromatin*. The fine structure, the manner in which the DNA is compacted and interacted with proteins, and the organization of chromatin in the interphase nucleus are thought to pertain to the control of RNA production and DNA replication and perhaps to cellular differentiation as well.

The sequences of nucleotide bases in DNA that constitute the genes and that can be transcribed into messenger RNA are distributed throughout the length of the various chromosomes. (These sequences

FIGURE 7-2 Schematic representation of the mitotic and meiotic cell-division cycles, as described in the text. G_1 and G_2 = time gaps before and after S, the period in which DNA replicates. Each of these intervals is several hours in duration; together they constitute interphase. M = mitosis; I and II = the two divisions of meiosis. The DNA content of the cycling cells is indicated on the vertical axis: 1c = the content in a gamete; 2c = that in either an egg immediately postfertilization or a somatic cell emerging from mitosis; 4c = the amount in a cell which has completed chromosome duplication and is ready to enter mitosis or meiosis.

are too short to be resolved microscopically.) Over 1000 genes have been mapped to specific chromosomes, in many cases to specific regions of a chromosome. The locations of a few of the many genes of interest in clinical medicine that have been mapped are shown in Fig. 7-3.

Certain segments of at least 12 chromosomes vary in length among individuals. These segments can be delineated by their staining characteristics (Fig. 7-4). The variable segments consist of nontranscribed, highly repetitive nucleotide sequences of DNA and are transmitted from parent to child in a straightforward mendelian fashion. Techniques of molecular genetics, which are useful as an extension of the microscopic observation of human chromosomes, permit the identification and molecular definition of an even greater number of variable segments of DNA, segments that are submicroscopic. These are referred to as *restriction fragment length polymorphisms* (RFLPs). Variations in both microscopically visible and invisible segments are unassociated with detectable phenotypic effect. However, they can serve as useful cell markers in prenatal diagnosis when they lie close to or within disease-associated loci (e.g., in Duchenne's muscular dystrophy) and in determination of zygosity of twins, paternity, and survival of transplants.

Other microscopically recognizable segments in the short arms of the acrocentric autosomes are devoted to the production of ribosomal RNA and nucleoli. As mitosis progresses, these nucleolus-organizer regions tend to remain relatively uncondensed later than other regions. Consequently, at metaphase they appear understained and thereby demarcate condensed segments of chromatin distal to them on the chromosome arms—*satellites*. (Satellites are examples of the polymorphic segments just mentioned.) Several other regions that remain relatively uncondensed at metaphase and that are seen more often than the remainder of the chromatin to undergo outright disruption ("breakage") are recognizable in a low percentage of cells from some normal individuals and sometimes are called *fragile sites*. In a few cases studied the tendency for such fragile sites to be visible at metaphase is a dominantly transmitted trait. The only such region known to be of significance in relation to a human trait is one located near the distal end (the end away from the centromere) of the long arm of the X chromosome; it segregates in certain families as an X-linked trait in association with a syndrome that features mental defectiveness, a characteristic facies, and macroorchia—the

"fragile-X syndrome." (This locus is one of the mapped loci indicated in Fig. 7-3.) Other examples of segmental specialization along the chromosome include *telomeres* and *centromeres*. Telomeres, the distal termini of each arm, have some relationship to the nuclear membrane and probably are important in the maintenance of order in the interphase nucleus; centromeric regions are sites of microtubule attachment at metaphase.

A further example of chromosome differentiation is the established sequence by which various segments replicate during S; certain segments replicate early, others late. In general, late replication of a chromosome segment correlates with genetic inertness. This correlation is exemplified by one of the two X chromosomes in female cells; the chromosome inactivated by the Lyon effect is almost entirely late-replicating (see Chap. 5).

A little-understood type of chromatin is that which long has been referred to as *heterochromatin*. It is tightly condensed, not just at metaphase but throughout interphase. Such condensation of chromatin correlates positively with genetic inactivity and also with late replication. Some regions are condensed and inactive in all cells (constitutive heterochromatin), while others, for example, the X chromosome, may be either condensed and inactive or decondensed and active (facultative heterochromatin). Many chromosome imbalances that permit viability beyond intrauterine life involve chromosome segments that are rich in this apparently inactive, or inactivatable, type of chromatin, e.g., chromosomes that can be trisomic in liveborn individuals or, in the case of the X, monosomic. The activity of genes can sometimes be affected, even inactivated, if they are positioned near regions of heterochromatin, as can occur as a result of chromosome breakage and rearrangement.

Therefore, in chromosomal imbalance both the specific genetic loci and the particular types of chromatin deleted or duplicated are important. Also, the significance of a structural rearrangement probably depends on the new and abnormal positioning of structural and regulatory genes in relation to each other and to heterochromatin.

Fortunately for the cytologist, several differentiated features of the chromosome correlate with cytological artifacts that can be produced and visualized in the laboratory. A number of techniques are now in use to display a pattern of bands of various lengths and staining characteristics (Figs. 7-1 and 7-4). These patterns are identical in each chromosome 1, each chromosome 2, etc., varying only in the inert polymorphic regions mentioned above, so that they can be used in clinical cytogenetics to identify chromosomes and to detect and define structural rearrangements.

Sources of error   A large number of genetic loci must be active to produce the numerous enzymes and structural proteins required to initiate and complete a cycle. Remarkable precision and accuracy are demanded over and over in matters such as the passage of a cell from G_1 into S, orderly progression of replication, assembly of the mitotic spindle, and spindle function in segregating chromatids during mitosis. Additional loci are activated to permit a cell of the germ line to pass successfully through the complicated stages of meiotic prophase, including pairing of homologous chromosomes, genetic recombination, and then disjoining of chromosomes. Probably all these mechanisms and processes are subject to errors, some spontaneous, others promoted by some unfavorable environmental influence (e.g., Fig. 7-5) or by the presence of deleterious mutations involving one of the many steps just mentioned. Furthermore, the genetic material itself is subject to damage, and certain types of unrepaired or erroneously repaired lesions in DNA theoretically may predispose to chromosome rearrangement. Errors at many of these steps lie behind chromosome imbalance. Errors that occur in germ cells, during fertilization, and in early postfertilization divisions are important in relation to embryonic maldevelopment and infertility; errors in somatic cells are important in relation to neoplasia.

CHROMOSOME ABNORMALITIES   Mutations of a single base in a gene and deletions and duplications of chromosome segments involving even hundreds of base pairs are not visible to the cytogeneticist. In fact, for the normal chromosome banding pattern to be

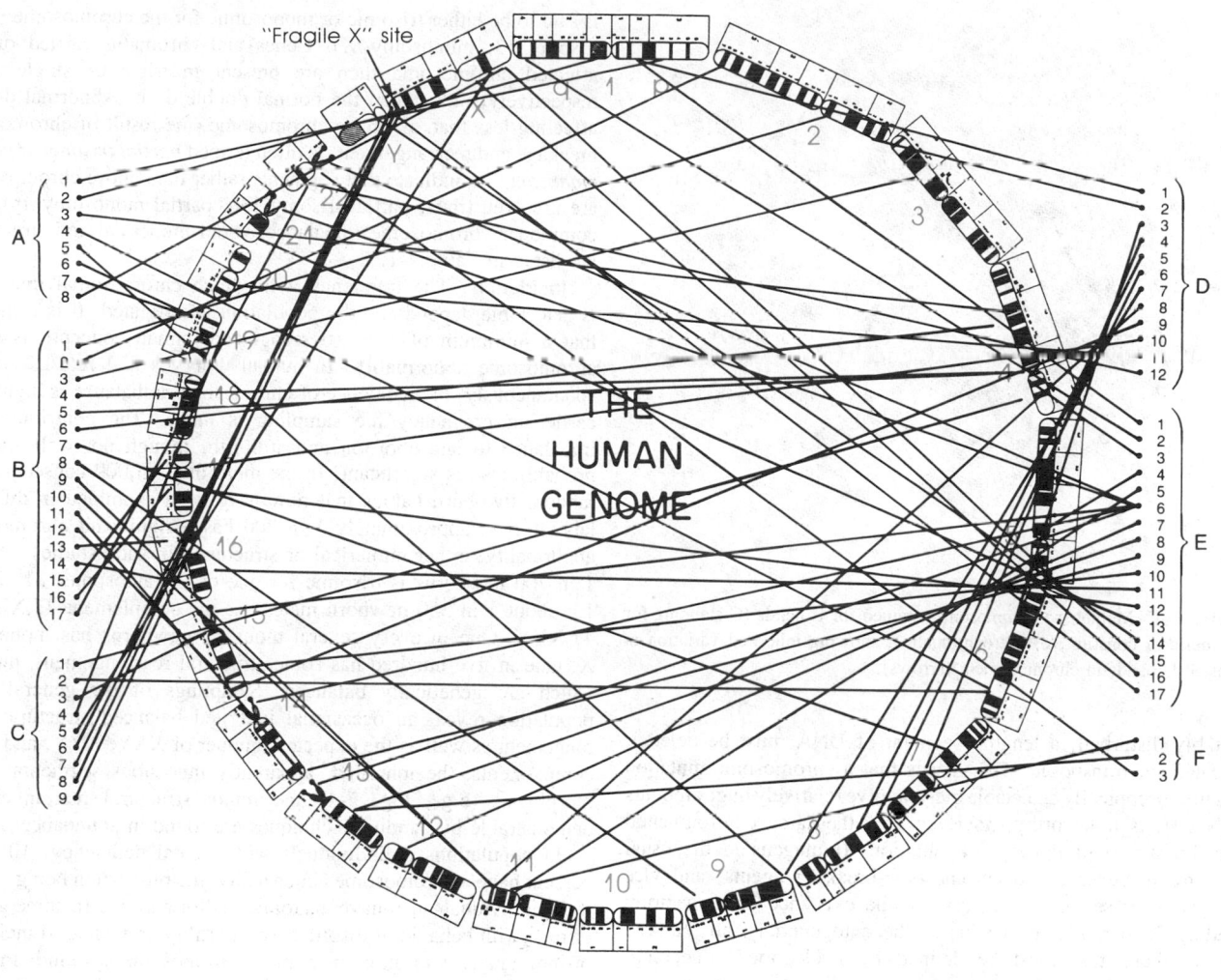

A: CELL SURFACE ANTIGENS
1 = Rhesus
2 = Duffy
3 = MNSs
4 = MHC
5 = ABO
6 = Lewis
7 = Lutheran
8 = Xg

B: DIFFERENTIATED CELL PRODUCTS
1 = Immunoglobulin kappa-light chain
2 = Glucagon
3 = Transferrin
4 = Albumin
5 = Alpha-fetoprotein
6 = Fibrinogen
7 = Collagen I
8 = Interferon (leukocyte)
9 = Insulin
10 = Hemoglobin-beta
11 = Immunoglobulin heavy chain
12 = Beta-2-microglobulin
13 = Hemoglobin-alpha
14 = Haptoglobin
15 = Myosin heavy chain
16 = Growth hormone
17 = Immunoglobulin lambda-light chain

C: GENES FOR DISEASE
1 = Huntington's chorea
2 = Congenital adrenal hyperplasia
3 = Prader-Willi syndrome
4 = Familial hypercholesterolemia
   (LDL receptor)
5 = Duchenne's muscular dystrophy
6 = Hunter's syndrome
7 = Hemophilia B
8 = Hemophilia A
9 = X-linked mental deficiency

D: CELLULAR ONCOGENES
1 = *N-ras*
2 = *N-myc*
3 = *myb*
4 = *erb B*
5 = *mos*
6 = *myc*
7 = *abl*
8 = *H-ras*
9 = *fes*
10 = *erb A*
11 = *src*
12 = *sis*

E: MISCELLANEOUS
1 = Phosphoglucomutase
2 = 5S ribosomal RNA
3 = Phosphoglucomutase-2
4 = Dihydrofolate reductase
5 = Lactate dehydrogenase A
6 = Ribosomal RNA
7 = Lactate dehydrogenase B
8 = Esterase D
9 = DNA segment D14S1
10 = Hexosaminidase-A
11 = Metallothionein
12 = Thymidine kinase
13 = Superoxide dismutase-1
14 = Testis-determining factor
15 = Steroid sulfatase
16 = DNA segment DXS7
17 = G-6-PD

F: "CANCER GENES"
1 = Wilms's tumor
2 = Retinoblastoma
3 = Meningioma

FIGURE 7-3 The 24 human chromosomes arrayed in a circle. The distinctive bands demonstrable by cytogenetic techniques are shown, with the numerical designations that were agreed upon by a series of international conferences. From the many genes that have been mapped to specific chromosome regions, a few of interest in medicine have been selected and their diverse locations indicated. In addition to the many hundreds of genes that code for enzymes and structural proteins that have been located, the map of the human genome has been blanketed with noncoding marker segments of DNA (RFLPs) for which molecular probes are available. (For a current listing of all known human gene localizations, see *Human Gene Mapping 9.*)

FIGURE 7-4 Metaphase chromosomes stained for C bands (C standing for centromeric or constitutive heterochromatin), showing inherited variation in lengths of C bands in chromosome 1 (arrows).

detectably disturbed, a lengthy segment of DNA must be deleted, duplicated, or transposed. This means that a chromosome mutation that is microscopically detectable must involve relatively huge amounts of DNA. It is noteworthy, however, that the same environmental agents known to produce point mutations (mutagens in the usual sense) are in general also chromosome-breaking agents, and vice versa. Thus, it seems safe to assume the existence of a spectrum extending from mutations visible to the cytogeneticist all the way down to those that must be defined by nucleotide sequencing. Mutations visible to the cytogeneticist ordinarily exert a more widespread effect on development than do point mutations; ordinary genes—often many of them—as well as other specialized types of chromatin whose function usually is unknown are involved in cytologically visible mutations.

If an entire chromosome is affected in an imbalance, the genome

FIGURE 7-5 Breaks and rearrangements (arrows) in metaphase chromosomes of a blood lymphocyte that received ionizing irradiation before being stimulated by phytohemagglutinin to enter S and divide.

is said to be either trisomic or monosomic for the chromosome (thus, trisomy 13, monosomy X). Genes and chromatin carried on the affected chromosome then are present in triple or single dose, respectively, rather than the normal double dose. Abnormal dosage affecting less than an entire chromosome, the result of chromosome breakage and rearrangement, is often termed *partial trisomy* or *partial monosomy*, to indicate that segments rather than entire chromosomes are involved (thus, partial trisomy 13q, partial monosomy 4p). The commoner chromosome imbalances, both numerical and structural, are listed in Table 7-1.

Incidence The frequency with which chromosomal imbalance is detectable depends on the population investigated. It is estimated that a minimum of 1 in 10 recognized human conceptions has a chromosome abnormality. In human embryos and fetuses aborted spontaneously, the incidence of chromosome imbalance is higher the earlier in pregnancy the sampling is made. The contribution of imbalance to late abortion and stillbirth, though not well studied, probably also is significant. In the more than 65,000 consecutive or random live-born babies that now have been examined in different laboratories, approximately 1 in 200 has a significant chromosome abnormality, either numerical or structural. In such studies, at least 1 in 700 newborns is trisomic for one of the autosomes 21, 18, or 13; about 1 in 350 newborn males has the complement 47,XXY or 47,XYY. One in every several thousand newborns has monosomy X. One in five hundred has some structural rearrangement, most of which are genetically balanced. Samplings of the general adult population reveal an occasional inherited balanced structural rearrangement as well as the expected number of XXY, XYY, and XXX complements; the inherited, apparently innocuous segmental polymorphisms (e.g., Fig. 7-4) and minor structural rearrangements demonstrable by banding techniques are found in abundance.

In populations of individuals with mental deficiency, 10 to 15 percent have a chromosome abnormality, the proportion being greater if the individuals also have anatomic malformations. In some groups of men with behavioral disorders or infertility an increased incidence of individuals with an extra X or Y chromosome is found. Infertile women also include many individuals with extra or missing sex chromosomes and an appreciable number with structural chromosome rearrangement; approximately one-fourth of women with primary amenorrhea have some abnormality of the X chromosome. Among infertile men and women, individuals with genes that interfere with meiosis, so-called meiotic mutants, are also found occasionally.

Numerical abnormalities Trisomy (47 chromosomes) is the most common chromosome imbalance in early spontaneous abortuses, followed by monosomy (45 chromosomes) and triploidy (69 chromosomes). The extra or missing chromosomes can be either paternal or maternal in origin, and the error in segregation of chromosomes can occur in the germ line, fertilized egg (zygote), or early embryo. Trisomy of every chromosome except the no. 1 has been observed in spontaneous abortions, trisomy 16 most frequently.

Sex chromosomal trisomy (XXY, XYY, and XXX) is compatible with intrauterine survival; in contrast, autosomal trisomy rarely permits survival to term. However, a small proportion of autosomal trisomics are live-born. For practical purposes these are only trisomy 21, 18, and 13, in decreasing frequency. Trisomies 18 and 13 cause death during infancy. Therefore trisomies of significance in adults are trisomy 21, XXY, XXX, and XYY. A few other autosomal trisomies, such as trisomy 8, have occasionally been reported, usually in mosaicism with a normal cellular component. (Mosaicism is the coexistence of multiple, genetically different populations of cells, all derived originally, however, from a single zygote.)

Autosomal monosomy is rare even among abortion material. In contrast, monosomy X (45,X) occurs in approximately 1.5 percent of recognized conceptions. It is common among spontaneously aborted human embryos (approximately 10 percent) and is present in one in every several thousand live-born babies. The reason for the death of 45,X embryos and fetuses is unknown, although developmental abnormalities doubtless contribute; cardiovascular and renal anomalies

TABLE 7-1 Common chromosome imbalances that recur in the human population and result in clinically recognizable syndromes*

Imbalance	Chromosomes affected	Karyotypes†	Clinical features‡
Monosomy	X	45,X	Turner's syndrome
Segmental deficiency—"partial monosomy"	X	46,XX,p−; 46,XX,q−; 46,X,r(X); 46,X,iso(Xp); 46,X,iso(Xq);	Turner's syndrome or some features of it
	Y	46,XY,p−; 46,XY,q−; 46,X,r(Y); 46,X,iso(Yp); 46,X,iso(Yq)	Turner's syndrome, or some features of it, sometimes with "mixed gonadal dysgenesis" when a 45,X cell line coexists
	4	46,XY,4p−	Gr, Cf, Mi, Ey, Sk, Ge, Ht, Co, Me
	5	46,XY,5p−	Cri-du-chat syndrome: Cr, Mi, Cf, Me
	8	46,XY,8q−	Langer-Gildion syndrome
	11	46,XY,11p−	WT, Ge, Me
	13	46,XY,13q−	RB, Cf, Me
	15	46,XY,15q−	Prader-Willi syndrome
	17	46,XY,17p−	Miller-Dieker syndrome
	18	46,XY,18p−	Gr, Cf, Ea, Te, Po, Sk, Ht, Me
	18	46,XY,18q−	Cf, Hy, Sk, Ey
	21	46,XY,r(21)	Cf, Hp, Ea, Me
Trisomy	X	47,XXX	Se, Me (mild), Ps
	X	47,XXY	Klinefelter's syndrome
	Y	47,XYY	Ta, Ac, Su, B; but often normal
	8	46,XY/47,XY,+8	Cf, Sk, Me (moderate)
	13	47,XY,+13	Trisomy 13 syndrome: Cp, Ey, Pd, Po, Ht, D, V, Sc, F, Ar, Me
	18	47,XY,+18	Trisomy 18 syndrome: Cf, Ea, V, F, Gr, D, He, Me
	21	47,XY,+21	Trisomy 21 syndrome (Down's syndrome)
Segmental duplication—"partial trisomy"	Y	46,X,t(X;Y)§	XX male
	9	9p+†	Cf
	22	22q+¶	Gr, Cf, Ea, Cp, Hy, Co
Chimerism	Entire complement	46,XY/46,XX	Pseudo- or true hermaphroditism; dimorphism of blood-cell-surface antigens
Triploidy	Entire complement	69,XXY	Hc, Me, Sy, Ht, Gc, D

* For complete listing, consult DeGrouchy and Turleau.
† The sex chromosome constitution might be either XY or XX, but in the example karyotypes given, XY arbitrarily is used.
‡ The clinical features given include only some of the more constant ones. Deficiency of one segment often is accompanied by duplication of another, and the phenotypic effect is the consequence of the combined imbalance. Abbreviations are defined below.
§ Translocation onto an X of a segment of the Y bearing the locus Y responsible for testicular differentiation. Random inactivation of either the normal X or the one bearing Y material determines the gonadal phenotype(s)—testis or ovary, respectively.
¶ Brought about through any of several rearrangements.
Abbreviations: Ac, acne; Ar, arrhinencephaly; B, behavior disorder; Cr, characteristically abnormal cry; Cf, characteristic craniofacial dysmorphism; Co, convulsions; Cp, cleft lip–palate; D, early death; Ea, characteristically abnormal ears; Ey, eye anomaly; F, characteristically flared, overlapping fingers; Ge, abnormality of external genitalia; Gr, severe growth deficiency; Hc, hydrocephaly; Hp, hypertonia; Ht, cardiac malformation; Hy, infantile hypotonia; Me, intellectual deficit; Mi, microcephaly; Om, omphalocele; Po, characteristically abnormal posture; Pd, polydactyly; Ps, psychotic predisposition; RB, retinoblastoma; Sc, scalp defect; Se, secondary amenorrhea; Sk, skeletal anomalies; Su, subfertility; Sy, syndactyly; Ta, tallness; Te, characteristically abnormal teeth; V, visceral anomalies; WT, Wilms's tumor with aniridia.

are common in the few that survive. In monosomy X, the missing sex chromosome can be either a Y or an X and is either paternal or maternal in origin. Often the second sex chromosome is not completely absent but is replaced by a structurally rearranged Y or X. Mosaicism is common in live-borns with monosomy X; here, tissues are populated not only by cells with a 45,X complement but by other cells, perhaps with a normal complement, either 46,XY or 46,XX, or with a complement in which the second sex chromosome is rearranged in some way.

Triploidy is rare in live-born babies and usually leads to early death, even when in a mosaicism with normal cells: 46,XY/69,XXY. The phenotypic effects of the autosomal trisomies, of 47,XXY, and of monosomy X (45,X) are characteristic and well defined so that their diagnosis usually is not difficult (see Chap. 324). The effects of the 47,XYY and 47,XXX constitutions are less striking, and therefore these complements are underdiagnosed. Mosaicism with coexistence of abnormal and normal populations of cells can cause an abnormal phenotype to approach the normal.

The mechanisms responsible for the numerical abnormalities are undefined and may be multiple. In trisomy 21 the extra chromosome is of maternal origin in 80 percent and of paternal in 20 percent of

cases. A striking but unexplained maternal age effect exists in trisomies 21, 18, 13, XXY, and XXX. Over a third of babies with trisomy 21 are born to women over 35, whereas only something over a tenth of all births occur in this group. The frequency of trisomy 21 rises from 0.5 to 0.7 per 1000 live births between ages 21 and 23 to 3.1 per 1000 at age 35, 10.5 per 1000 at age 40, and 33.6 per 1000 at age 45. After a child with trisomy 21 is born, the risk to the parents of recurrence in future pregnancies is increased to approximately 1 percent. As to the cause of monosomy X, the frequent association of the 45,X complement in mosaicism with normal complements and with structural rearrangements of the X and Y suggests that the zygote or the preimplantation embryo is often the target of a chromosome-breaking event.

Structural abnormalities Some structural chromosome rearrangements are inherited, and others represent new mutations. The cause of the new rearrangements is unknown, although they are assumed to be partly spontaneous and partly the effect of environmental agents such as mutagenic chemicals or ionizing radiation (Fig. 7-5) acting on the germ line, zygote, or early embryo. The majority of de novo rearrangements are paternal in origin.

Many of the known chromosome rearrangements have been

detected only once or a few times. Others are detected repeatedly, the same one occurring in unrelated individuals and families. For example, the commonest translocation, one that can occur either as a result of de novo mutation or by inheritance, affects one chromosome 13 and one 14 at or near their centromeres. In this translocation, only inert chromatin or functional chromatin represented elsewhere in the genome—the nucleolus-organizing regions referred to earlier—is lost from the tiny short arms. Also common is a similar translocation affecting chromosomes 14 and 21.

Chromosome complements bearing rearrangements can be genetically balanced or effectively so, thus imparting no unfavorable phenotypic effect to their bearers; about two-thirds of rearrangements detected during surveys of consecutive live-born babies are balanced. Or, the complement can be unbalanced and affect development adversely, the usual case when rearrangements are detected during surveys of spontaneous abortuses or of individuals with multiple anomalies and mental deficiency.

Some balanced rearrangements are transmitted from generation to generation without producing clinical effects. In other cases, however, they are profoundly important to members of the kindred transmitting them, by being responsible for the conception of embryos with unbalanced genomes. For example, inherited translocations involving chromosome 21 predispose to the trisomy 21 syndrome. Approximately 5 percent of live-borns with that syndrome have a translocation, and in about a fifth of those it is detectable in one of the parents. Because most babies with the trisomy 21 syndrome due to translocation are born to women under 30, a search for a translocation is important when a child with this clinical syndrome is born to young parents.

Different translocations bestow on their carriers different risks of having offspring with unbalanced rearrangements. These risks cannot be predicted on the theoretical basis. Useful empirical risk figures have been accumulated for common translocations; e.g., the 14;21 translocation bestows a 2 percent risk on a balanced male carrier and more than a 10 percent risk on a female carrier of having a child with the trisomy 21 syndrome. In contrast, the balanced carrier of a 21;21 translocation can expect only unbalanced offspring. Information of this type is indispensable to those undertaking genetic counseling in relation to chromosome disorders.

DISEASE ASSOCIATIONS Various combinations of abnormalities in malformed and defective individuals have been correlated with variations in the chromosome complement. In this way, clinical syndromes due to specific chromosome imbalances have been defined. (Many of the pediatric conditions are of little significance in adult medicine because of their lethality in infancy or early childhood.)

Autosome imbalance Of the three autosomal trisomies found in live-born babies, only trisomy 21 is compatible with survival past infancy. The phenotype produced by the presence of an extra chromosome 21, formerly known as *mongolism* but now termed the *Down syndrome* or the *trisomy 21 syndrome*, is characteristic and easily diagnosed from birth: mental deficiency, short stature, muscular hypotonia, brachycephaly, short neck, typical facies (oblique orbital fissures, flat nasal bridge, small simple or folded ears, nystagmus, mouth hanging open), narrow palate, short broad hands with incurving fifth fingers, gaps between the first and second toes, and characteristic dermatoglyphics. Additional findings may include congenital heart disease, blepharitis and conjunctivitis, Brushfield's spots of the iris, straight pubic hair, abnormal teeth, a protruding furrowed tongue, a high-arched palate, loose skin of the neck, transverse palmar creases, and hyperflexibility of the joints. Cardiac malformations lead to death in infancy in a third of individuals with trisomy 21, and other malformations and infections may also cause early death. However, subjects who survive infancy often reach adulthood, and some even old age, at which time features of Alzheimer's disease become common. The proneness to develop leukemia in affected infants is not maintained in later life. Females occasionally become pregnant, and, as expected, approximately half their children have trisomy 21.

Mosaicism of trisomy 21 with normal cells (46/47, +21) may occur in individuals with modified features of the trisomy 21 syndrome,

and it is probable that many individuals with this mosaicism go undiagnosed. The risk of such persons having trisomic children is increased, but unfortunately their mosaicism is usually detected only after they have had an affected child.

Partial trisomy, partial monosomy, or a combination of the two explains many of the instances in both children and adults of multiple developmental defects combined with mental deficiency. Sometimes a balanced autosomal translocation is detected in normally developed adults who have repeated spontaneous abortion or subnormal fertility, with or without abnormal live-born children.

Although the phenotypic effects of many of the different segmental chromosome imbalances which can occur are varied and nonspecific, the resulting anomalies sometimes compose recognizable clinical syndromes. Two examples are the following: (1) If a rearrangement causes partial trisomy of just the distal band of the long arm of 21, the clinical features composing the full syndrome associated with an extra chromosome 21 develop. (A triple dose of other segments of the long arm of chromosome 21 also produces adverse effects but not the trisomy 21 syndrome.) (2) Partial monosomy of a short segment within the short arm of chromosome 5 causes mental deficiency, a characteristic facies, and a characteristic cry during infancy. This group of signs is known as the *5p*− (five-p-minus) or *cri-du-chat syndrome*.

Additional specific syndromes produced by imbalance of many different chromosome segments now are known (Table 7-1), e.g., the 4p−, 9p partial trisomy, 13q−, and 18q− syndromes, to name a few. Furthermore, the application of high-resolution banding techniques makes possible identification of the exact band(s) deficient or duplicated. Rearrangements not previously described, partly because they were not visible without high-resolution banding or molecular cytogenetics techniques, and their corresponding clinical syndromes still are being recognized. Any of these syndromes may appear as the result either of de novo chromosome rearrangement or through formation of a genetically unbalanced gamete in a person carrying in balanced state a rearrangement affecting the segment involved.

In most individuals with chromosome imbalance, regardless of which segments are affected, a degree of phenotypic similarity is present. These recurring and nonspecific features include mental deficiency, growth deficiency, dysmorphic ears, nose, and mouth, cardiac malformations of standard types, abnormalities of dermal ridges and creases, and dysmorphic digits. (As a rule, autosomal imbalance need not be considered in the etiology of anatomic defects unaccompanied by mental deficiency.) Why similar abnormalities occur with so many different segmental imbalances is unknown, but when several such features are observed in a single individual, they can be a valuable clinical indication for cytogenetic analysis. Imbalance affecting certain segments also causes specific phenotypic changes, examples being the anomalous cry in the 5p− syndrome mentioned above, retinoblastoma, in relation to one particular band of chromosome 13, and the Prader-Willi syndrome which is often associated with a disturbance of a band near the centromere of chromosome 15. Whereas the nonspecific changes serve to call the clinician's attention to the possibility of some chromosome imbalance, the specific features can suggest the exact segment of the genome affected.

Sex chromosome imbalance (See also Chap. 324) In contrast to autosome imbalance, sex chromosome imbalance has relatively mild phenotypic effects. This is because X chromosomes beyond one in the complement of somatic cells are usually almost totally inactivated and because the Y chromosome bears relatively few genes. X-linked loci (in contrast to autosomal loci) function normally in single dose: the female is functionally hemizygous for most loci on the X through the Lyon effect; the male, with only one X chromosome, is hemizygous for X-linked genes with the exception of loci clustered in a segment at the end of Yp that is homologous to a comparable so-called pseudoautosomal segment at the end of Xp. The addition of an extra sex chromosome to the normal male or female complement has a phenotypic effect but insufficient to interfere with intrauterine survival. Since major anatomic defects are usually absent, individuals with the complements 47,XXY and 47,XYY, both of whom are males, and 47,XXX, who are females, ordinarily go unrecognized till adolescence or later, often never to be diagnosed at all.

The *Klinefelter syndrome* (Chap. 324), which in classic form consists of small testes, infertility, gynecomastia, and variable degrees of underandrogenization, sometimes with mild mental deficiency, antisocial behavior, or both, is the consequence of the addition of an extra X to the male complement: 47,XXY. The extra X interferes in some way with the survival of germ cells, and atrophy of the spermatogenic tubules and azoospermia are the consequence. Sometimes the phenotypic effects are surprisingly mild, the testicular atrophy being the only noteworthy feature in otherwise healthy and socially well-adjusted men. The mosaicism 46,XY/47,XXY sometimes occurs and may ameliorate the phenotypic effect of the extra X. More extreme phenotypic effects and mental deficiency result when more than one extra sex chromosome is added to the normal male complement: 48,XXXY or 49,XXXXY.

The phenotypic effect of 47,XYY is less well defined; although increased height, behavioral difficulties, and infertility are common, the extra Y is sometimes found in otherwise normal men. The rare complement 48,XXYY results in infertility, probably because of the extra X, as in the 47,XXY Klinefelter syndrome. The phenotype associated with 47,XXX is also poorly defined; although women with mild mental deficiency, psychosis, and menstrual abnormalities sometimes are found to have this complement, it is also sometimes detected in normal, healthy women. Further clarification is needed concerning the effects on personality and behavior of all three of the complements 47,XXY, 47,XYY, and 47,XXX.

Loss of the Y or of the second X has drastic effects on development. If it does not cause abortion, it may or may not be recognizable at birth. Loose nuchal skin folds and edema of the hands and feet in a newborn girl, with or without renal or cardiovascular anomalies, may point to the diagnosis of the 45,X complement. The *Turner syndrome* is the manifestation in subsequent life (Chap. 324): short stature, infantilism of otherwise normal female external and internal genitalia, germ-cell-free gonads referred to as gonadal streaks, and variable renal, cardiovascular, skeletal, and ectodermal anomalies. Without estrogen administration breast development remains infantile and menstruation does not occur. Although mental deficiency is not a feature, a poorly defined emotional immaturity is common.

The Turner syndrome may be the developmental consequence of several chromosome constitutions besides 45,X. Mosaicism as well as structural abnormalities affecting certain segments of a second sex chromosome, either a Y or an X, cause a spectrum of disorders at both the clinical and cytogenetic levels. A normal male or normal female cellular component may be present along with the 45,X cellular component, or one component may bear a structurally abnormal chromosome. Common abnormalities of the Y and X are isochromosome formation (one arm deleted and the other duplicated) or deletion of part or all of one arm. In some affected individuals, all cells have 46 chromosomes, with one normal X plus an abnormal Y or X, for example, 46,XXp−, deletion of a segment of the short arm of one of the X chromosomes. In others, a second or third cellular component may be present as well, for example, 45,X/46,XX/46,XXp−. Clinically pure Turner syndrome may be found in association with various combinations of these karyotypes if one of them is either monosomic or partially monosomic for X. However, when Y-bearing cells coexist with the 45,X cells, for example, 45,X/46,XY, genital ambiguity often develops, and gonads may vary from streaks to functional testes (the syndrome of *mixed gonadal dysgenesis*); here the risk of gonadal neoplasia is significant. When 46,XX cells coexist with 45,X, varying degrees of ovarian function may be maintained, including ovulation. Although the phenotype may approach a normal male or female pattern when normal and abnormal cells coexist, the effects of mosaicism are unpredictable. Thus, the clinical syndrome associated with monosomy X and structurally

abnormal Ys or Xs ranges from a predominantly male phenotype, through Turner syndrome, to an almost normal female phenotype.

Two other rare conditions deserve mention—*true hermaphroditism* and the *46,XX male* (see also Chap. 324). First, true hermaphroditism is present when testicular and ova- and follicle-containing ovarian tissue coexist in the same individual. In most cases 46,XX is the chromosome complement, and it appears normal by banding. Exceptionally, true hermaphrodites have the complement 46,XY, or chimerism 46,XY/46,XX, each of the two cellular components having been derived from a different zygote. Second, males occasionally have the complement 46,XX. As in 47,XXY men, the second X interferes with meiosis, and azoospermia results. In both the 46,XX true hermaphrodite and the 46,XX male, the rule that a Y is required for testicular differentiation appears to break down. The explanation for some XX males is that the testis-determining locus has been translocated from Yp to Xp, demonstrable not by microscopy but by molecular cytogenetics. True hermaphroditism probably is on the basis of mutation affecting the same locus.

X-linked mental deficiency In the general population more males than females are mentally deficient, and mental deficiency when familial affects males preferentially. In some such kindreds, mental deficiency segregates as an X-linked trait, and several X-linked mental deficiency syndromes are now recognized.

Although chromosome imbalance is not responsible, one cause of X-linked mental deficiency can be diagnosed by cytogenetic techniques. In a significant proportion of families in which mental deficiency is segregating, the X in the affected males and that same X in their mothers is, or can be made, recognizable cytogenetically by technical manipulations. In a variable but usually small proportion of metaphases from affected persons this phenotypically unusual X chromosome exhibits a fragile site, denoting the fragile-X syndrome. This syndrome is the most common form of X-linked mental deficiency and accounts for almost half of all cases.

Chromosome change in cancer The theory that an alteration in the chromosomal complement may cause cancer was advanced many years ago. Nevertheless, only with improved cytogenetic techniques during the past three decades and with the advent of recombinant DNA technology has firm evidence supporting the theory became available. Chromosome changes are plentiful in cancer, but this very fact—too many changes—was a major reason many rejected them as having etiologic significance. Support for the idea that chromosome alteration is involved in the etiology of human cancer comes from three sets of observations: (1) the known environmental "causes" of human cancer—carcinogenic chemicals and ionizing radiation—are also chromosome-breaking agents (Fig. 7-5); (2) several recessively inherited disorders feature increased chromosome breakage and rearrangement (Bloom's syndrome is the prototype of these disorders), and in each the risk of cancer is increased; and (3) a specific chromosome rearrangement is found in one of the major human leukemias: the so-called Philadelphia chromosome in chronic granulocytic leukemia. Thus, the known environmental and genetic causes of increased chromosome mutation all predispose to cancer, and at least one example of specificity of a chromosome mutation in a human neoplasm is available.

Now it is clear that most human cancers have chromosome complements that are altered in a microscopically detectable way. Table 7-2 lists some of those found with regularity. In the leukemias, lymphomas, and certain myeloproliferative disorders the alterations are less extensive than in solid tumors and, therefore, easier to define. As examples, in certain lymphomas chromosome 14 is often found to have undergone structural rearrangement, with the breakpoint near or in a specific region, namely, the immunoglobulin heavy chain locus; the rearrangement translocates the *myc* locus from its normal position on chromosome 8 to chromosome 14. Also, in over 95 percent of cases of chronic granulocytic leukemia (CGL) a translocation affecting chromosomes 9 and 22 is readily detected, resulting in the Philadelphia, or Ph[1] (p-h-one), chromosome, an abnormally short no. 22. If the leukemia progresses into a "blastic" phase, the

TABLE 7-2 Some of the recurring chromosome abnormalities encountered in human neoplasms

Neoplasm	Aberration	Chromosome regions affected
Leukemia		
Chronic granulocytic	Translocation	9q34 and 22q11
Acute nonlymphocytic		
M1	Translocation	9q34 and 22q11
M2	Translocation	8q22 and 21q22
M3	Translocation	15q22 and 17q11
Chronic lymphocytic	Trisomy	12
Acute lymphocytic		
L1–L2	Translocation	9q34 and 22q11
	Translocation	4q21 and 11q23
L3	Translocation	8q24 and 14q32
Lymphoma		
Burkitt's	Translocation	8q24 and 14q32
Follicular	Translocation	14q32 and 18q21
Solid tumors		
Benign		
Meningioma	Deletion or monosomy	22q
Parotid, mixed	Translocation	3p25 and 8q21
Malignant		
Ewing's sarcoma	Translocation	Bands 11q24 and 22q12
Germ cell tumors, testis	Deletion	12p
	Duplication	12q
Lung, small cell	Deletion	Bands 3p14 to 3p23
Neuroblastoma	Deletion	Bands 1p31 to 3p36
Ovary, cystadenocarcinoma	Translocation	6q21 and 14q24
Retinoblastoma	Deletion	Band 13q14
Wilms's tumor	Deletion	Band 11p13

NOTE: The FAB (French-American-British) classification of leukemias is employed above. The chromosome breakpoint and band nomenclature is that of the Paris Conference (Birth Defects: Original Articles Series VIII (7):1–46, 1971). The chromosome and chromosome-arm designation (e.g., 9q means the long arm of chromosome no. 9) appears first and is followed by the chromosome region and band on that arm (e.g., 9q34 means the fourth band in the third region of the long arm of chromosome no. 9).

already mutated karyotype evolves; certain new chromosome changes are added stepwise in a nonrandom sequence. In CGL and certain other leukemias, the chromosome changes, demonstrable either microscopically or by microscopy supplemented by molecular probes (molecular cytogenetics), may have diagnostic utility as well as considerable value in prognosis and choice of therapy.

The microscopically visible chromosome mutations that are found with regularity in human neoplasms often affect loci that play growth regulatory roles in normal cells, and in some cases the chromosome breakpoints affect known cellular oncogenes. In the examples just given, *myc* in its new position on chromosome 13 is abnormally regulated. In the Ph¹ chromosome, *abl* is translocated from its normal position on chromosome 9 into a specific region called *bcr* on chromosome 22, thereby creating a new genetic determinant; in myeloid cells, this mutant locus is transcribed, and the mRNA is translated into a novel protein that presumably plays a causative role in the autonomous growth of the neoplastic cell lineage.

Another chromosome mechanism known to be important in human neoplasia is somatic crossing-over. (Somatic crossing-over contrasts with germ line crossing-over, where recombination is legitimate.) Through crossing-over, a recessive mutation at a genetic locus concerned with growth regulation—a mutation that preexisted in a cell but remained occult because of the presence of a normal locus on the homologous chromosome—can become homozygous. The consequence of homozygosity at the mutant locus is loss of normal growth control. Such mutations were first recognized in the rare neoplasms retinoblastoma and Wilms's tumor; the loci affected were on chromosomes 13 and 11, respectively. In some cases the original (recessive) mutation consisted of outright deletion of the locus. Transmission through the germ line of such occult recessive mutations explains familial instances of those neoplasms.

Thus, chromosome mutations of at least three types constitute crucial steps in the initiation and progression of malignant neoplasia:

(1) translocations that disturb the regulation of loci concerned with growth; (2) deletion-mutation of recessive loci that play a presently obscure role in oncogenesis (e.g., the retinoblastoma locus just referred to), mutations that can either be inherited through the germ line or that occur de novo in a somatic cell; and (3) recombination yielding homozygosity for preexisting mutations affecting this last-mentioned type of locus. These mutations and their oncogenic consequences are now the subject of considerable investigation, both basic and clinical. In turn, the breakpoints in neoplasms of various types are helping identify hitherto unrecognized genetic determinants that together orchestrate normal cellular proliferation and tissue growth; thus the cytogenetics of human cancer is contributing to the understanding of normal cell biology.

Solid tumors, which generally are studied later in their natural course than neoplasms of the bone marrow, show extensive karyotypic changes, both structural and numerical. Different cells from a single tumor have similar numerical changes and structural rearrangements, but in the same direction. This apparent lack of specificity is partly due to the complexity of the karyotypic changes, however, and some chromosome alterations are specific for solid tumors (Table 7-2). The cytogenetic findings in both leukemias and solid tumors demonstrate the clonal nature of human cancer.

TECHNICAL CONSIDERATIONS Human metaphase chromosomes can be examined with light microscopy in any tissue in which sufficient cells are cycling. Preparations can therefore be made directly from almost any embryonic tissue and from adult bone marrow, lymphoid tissue, and selected malignant tissues. In searches for mosaicism, the study of multiple tissues is often required. Some tissues unlikely to contain cells in metaphase can be placed in culture, and chromosome preparations can be made from cells that reach mitosis in vitro. Blood T lymphocytes stimulated to enter cell-division cycles by phytohemagglutinin are the standard material for diagnosing constitutional chromosome imbalance in live-born individuals. Fetal tissue from aborted material can also be examined. In some myeloproliferative disorders and leukemias, unstimulated circulating blood cells divide spontaneously after a few hours in culture. Long-term cultures of fibroblasts can be derived from minute skin biopsies or from fragments of many other types of tissue, although more elaborate laboratory facilities and a longer period of time are required before cytogenetic preparations can be made. Amniotic fluid is among the sources of cells suitable for culture, and the cells, which are fetal in origin, are widely used in the prenatal diagnosis of chromosome imbalance, particularly in pregnancy in women of advanced age or who already have borne a child with a chromosome imbalance. Metaphase preparations also can be made from chorionic villi biopsied in the first trimester of pregnancy.

Meiotic chromosome preparations from testicular biopsies are sometimes useful in obscure cases of infertility. Translocations and genetically determined disturbances in meiotic pairing may be identified.

Recombinant DNA technology has been employed in conjunction with conventional cytogenetic techniques to define chromosome abnormalities in finer detail. Now that a vast number of probes for specific loci or chromosome segments have become available, molecular cytogenetics makes it possible to identify segments of chromosomes involved in rearrangements in which banding techniques had lacked the required resolution, by using molecular hybridization either to Southern blots or directly onto metaphase chromosome fixed to a slide. In prenatal diagnosis, probes for RFLPs sometimes are used to identify which chromosome has been inherited by the conceptus. This can be useful in pregnancies at risk of X-linked disease, determining in males whether the single X chromosome is the one that bears a particular undesirable locus that one of the parents is known to carry. Recombinant technology also can be useful in conditions that follow a dominant pattern of inheritance, such as Huntington's chorea, to determine whether the undesired mutant gene is present in the complement of the conceptus by discovering whether an RFLP closely linked to the mutant gene is or is not present. In a few instances, probes for undesirable mutant genes themselves or for RFLPs within the genes, are already available. Probes specific for the Y chromosome can define the sex of an embryo or fetus if a few cells can be obtained by amniocentesis or chorionic villus biopsy. They also can be of diagnostic value in obscure cases of intersex in which a Y chromosome, or a segment of the Y, is being sought. In relation to neoplasia, the use of molecular probes can identify rearrangements that affect specific chromosome regions. With the polymerase chain reaction even a small population of cells bearing some specific translocation, e.g., the Ph[1] chromosome breakpoint, can be identified.

Sometimes, metaphase, or anaphase chromosomes are analyzed to determine whether damage to the genetic material has been induced by some environmental agent (radiation, chemical, virus), or whether constitutional genomic instability is present. Cells that have proliferated in vivo and then been incubated only briefly in vitro may be used in search of evidence of damage to the genetic material of a given person or of a population (e.g., Fig. 7-5). The number of chromatid gaps, breaks, and rearrangements can be estimated directly in cells reaching their first mitosis in vitro. Another approach is to estimate the amount of in vivo damage by counting the number of exchanges that occur between sister chromatids during growth for two cell-division cycles in 5-bromodeoxyuridine. A test system less laborious than metaphase chromosome analysis, but one capable of showing that excessive chromosome breakage has occurred either in vivo or in vitro, is the determination of the proportion of nondividing cells having micronuclei. A micronucleus is produced when a chromosome fragment lacking a centromere lags at anaphase (as it will be obliged to do) and is encompassed in a separate nuclear membrane at telophase. The micronucleus assay is useful in the survey of populations for clastogen exposure, which is equivalent to mutagen and carcinogen exposure.

REFERENCES

De Grouchy J, Turleau C: *Clinical Atlas of Human Chromosomes,* 2d ed. New York, Wiley, 1984

German JL: Studying human chromosomes today. Am Sci 58:182, 1970

————: Gonadal dimorphism explained as a dosage effect of a locus on the sex chromosome, the gonad-differentiation locus (*GDL*). Am J Hum Genet 42:414, 1988

Heim S, Mitelman R: *Cancer Genetics.* New York, Alan R Liss, 1987

Human Gene Mapping 9. Ninth International Workshop on Human Gene Mapping. Cytogenet Cell Genet 46:1, 1987

McKusick VA: The human gene map. Clin Genet 27:207, 1985

Rooney DE, Czepulkowski BH (eds): *Human Cytogenetics: A Practical Approach.* Oxford and Washington, IRL Press, 1986

Schwarzacher HG: *Methods in Human Cytogenetics.* New York, Springer-Verlag, 1974

Simpson JL: *Disorders of Sexual Differentiation.* New York, Academic, 1976

8   TREATMENT AND PREVENTION OF GENETIC DISORDERS

DAVID VALLE

The complex processes of normal development and physiologic homeostasis depend on the coordinated interactions of the products of many genes working together in developmental and metabolic systems. These systems are adaptable within limits, allowing normal development and physiologic homeostasis to occur over a range of environmental conditions. For instance, the products of some 30 to 40 genes participate in blood glucose homeostasis; the result is maintenance of a relatively constant blood glucose concentration despite intermittant and highly variable ingestion of glucose precursors. Moreover, developmental and homeostatic interactions of 10,000 or so gene products are believed to be necessary for normal devel-

opment and function of the central nervous system. Mutations that reduce the adaptive capacity of these systems result in maldevelopment and/or dyshomeostasis that we recognize as genetic disease. The mutant gene may so compromise a particular developmental or homeostatic system that the system functions poorly or not at all in any environmental circumstance, thereby producing a monogenic disorder. Alternatively, the mutant gene may have modest effects under ordinary conditions but in certain environments cause maldevelopment or dyshomeostasis that we recognize as a multifactorial disorder. Thus, the role of the genes in health and disease is both central and complex. Consequently, treatment of genetic disease is both difficult and frequently less than completely effective.

TREATMENT

Effective treatment of genetic disorders requires accurate diagnosis, early intervention prior to development of irreversible tissue damage, and an understanding of the abnormal biochemistry or metabolic pathophysiology. The rapid progress in delineating the molecular basis of genetic disease has improved our capability for rapid and accurate diagnosis of monogenic disorders. Understanding of the metabolic pathophysiology is increasing at a slower rate mainly because progress in this area often requires elucidation of integrative physiology by study of the intact organism. The development of noninvasive metabolic monitoring techniques such as positron emission tomography and topical magnetic resonance spectrometry as well as new genetic technologies for the production of specific animal models of human genetic disease offers promise for progress in this area.

Approaches to treatment of genetic disease can be organized biologically proceeding from the clinical phenotype through the levels of the abnormal metabolites and dysfunctional protein to the level of the defective gene (Table 8-1).

TREATMENT OF THE CLINICAL PHENOTYPE   Treatment at the level of the clinical phenotype includes a variety of conventional medical practices such as patient education, pharmacologic interventions, and surgical procedures. It depends on a thorough understanding of the natural history of the particular disorder so that potential complications can be avoided or addressed early in the course to minimize the consequences. Although therapy at this level is not aimed at correcting the primary defect, it can markedly improve the patient's quality of life. Examples include instruction to patients with albinism or xeroderma to limit sun exposure or to patients with glucose-6-phosphate dehydrogenase deficiency to avoid the offending drugs; administration of β-blockers to Marfan syndrome patients to prevent or slow dilatation of the aortic root, anticonvulsants to patients with neurogenic disorders, or antihypertensive agents to patients with secondary hypertension; and a host of surgical interventions for patients with genetic malformations, skeletal dysplasias, and malignancies.

TREATMENT OF THE METABOLIC PHENOTYPE   Treatment at the metabolite level involves nutritional or pharmacologic approaches and is dependent on understanding the biochemical pathophysiology (Fig. 8-1). Deficient function of a mutant protein may result in a disease phenotype because a substrate accumulates to toxic levels (precursor toxicity); because the product of an alternative pathway is produced in excessive amounts (alternative pathway overflow); because of reduced formation of the reaction product or some downstream metabolite (product deficiency); or some combination of these possibilities. Although this paradigm is most easily visualized for enzymes in a metabolic pathway, it holds for virtually all proteins. The pathophysiology may involve *local* effects within the cell or tissue normally expressing the mutant protein, or it may involve *distant* biochemical effects as a consequence of pertubations of metabolite concentrations in the extracellular fluid. For example, the neurologic phenotype of Tay Sachs disease results from destruction of neurons caused by deficiency of resident hexosaminidase A whereas the mental retardation characteristic of untreated phenylketonuria due to defi-

TABLE 8-1 Some treatments for monogenic disorders

Level of treatment and method	Disorder(s)
CLINICAL PHENOTYPE	
Patient education	
Avoidance of aggravating agents (high carbohydrate diet, exposure to cold)	Periodic paralysis syndromes
Avoidance of certain drugs	Pharmacogenetic disorders, acute intermittent porphyria
Avoidance of sun exposure	Xeroderma pigmentosa, albinism
Avoidance of certain physical activity	Chondrodystrophies
Notify physician for rapid increase in size of mass or tinnitus	Neurofibromatosis
Pharmacologic	
β-Blockers	Marfan's syndrome
Anticonvulsants	Neurodegenerative disorders
Surgical	
Orthopedic reconstruction	Chondrodystrophies
Colectomy	Familial polyposis coli
Plastic reconstruction of facial malformations	Treacher-Collins syndrome, several monogenic cleft lip and/or palate syndromes
METABOLIC PHENOTYPE	
Metabolite alteration	
Substrate restriction	
Phenylalanine	Phenylketonuria
Branch chain amino acids	Maple syrup urine disease
Galactose	Galactosemia
Fructose	Hereditary fructose intolerance
Lactose	Lactase deficiency
Phytanic acid	Refsum's disease
Alternate pathway utilization	
Benzoate and phenylacetate	Urea cycle disorders
Glycine	Isovaleric acidemia
Carnitine	Organic acidosis
Cysteamine	Cystinosis
Penicillamine	Wilson's disease
Metabolic inhibition	
Allopurinol	Gout
Mevinolin	Familial hypercholesterolemia
Replacement of deficient products	
Glucose polymers (cornstarch)	Glycogen storage disease I, III
Uridine	Hereditary orotic aciduria
Glucocorticoids	Congenital adrenal hyperplasia
Thyroxine	Familial goiter
Biotin	Biotinidase deficiency
Protein alteration	
Activation of the mutant protein	
Pyridoxine (vitamin B$_6$)	Homocystinuria
Thiamine	Maple syrup urine disease
Hydroxycobalamin (vitamin B$_{12}$)	Some forms of methylmalonic acidemia
Replacement of the mutant protein	
Growth hormone	Growth hormone deficiency
Factor VIII	Classic hemophilia
Alpha$_1$-antitrypsin	Alpha$_1$-antitrypsin deficiency
Polyethylene glycol-adenosine deaminase	Adenosine deaminase deficiency
Organ transplantation	
As a source for a specific protein	
Allogeneic bone marrow	Lysosomal storage diseases, β-thalassemia
Liver	Glycogen storage disease, type I, familial hypercholesterolemia, ornithine transcarbamylase deficiency
As a protein source and replacement of damaged organ	
Liver	Alpha$_1$-antitrypsin deficiency, hepatorenal tyrosinemia
Kidney	Cystinosis

FIGURE 8-1 Pathophysiological consequences of a genetic defect in a metabolic pathway. Substrate A is converted via a series of intermediates to a final product, D. The enzymes catalyzing these reactions are indicated by the horizontal arrows. A also is converted to F in an alternative pathway. Genetic deficiency of the enzyme converting A to B (indicated by the hatched rectangle) may have pathophysiological consequences related to accumulation of A (precursor toxicity), overflow to F (alternative pathway overflow), reduced formation of D (product deficiency), or some combination of these possibilities.

ciency of hepatic phenylalanine hydroxylase is mediated by the systemic accumulation of phenylalanine.

Precursor toxicity Correction of precursor toxicity frequently involves dietary restriction of a particular substrate whose major source is nutritional. Inborn errors of amino acid and carbohydrate metabolism provide good examples of this approach. A diet restricted in the branch chain amino acids (leucine, isoleucine, valine) is effective in preventing the mental retardation associated with maple syrup urine disease caused by deficiency of branch chain ketoacid decarboxylase (see Chap. 334). Such diets should be started soon after birth, continued for life, and monitored in such a way that intake of these essential amino acids is just sufficient for normal growth. Illnesses that cause protein catabolism (e.g., those associated with intercurrent infections or trauma) periodically complicate this therapy by releasing large amounts of the offending amino acids from the breakdown of endogenous protein. These episodes may require hospitalization for administration of intravenous fluids and even dialysis. Similarly, lifetime restriction of dietary galactose in patients with galactosemia due to deficiency of galactose-1-phosphate uridyl transferase corrects growth failure, prevents cataracts, and improves intellectual outcome (see Chap. 337).

Alternate pathway utilization For some disorders alternative metabolic pathways may be utilized to remove toxic metabolites. The effectiveness of this approach is limited by the capacity of the alternate pathway and often must be combined with dietary restriction of the offending substrate. Administration of benzoate and phenylacetate to patients with inborn errors of urea metabolism is a good example of this approach. These compounds are conjugated with endogenous glycine and glutamine, forming hippurate and phenylacetylglutamine, respectively. When used in conjunction with restriction of dietary protein, this therapy reduces the accumulation of ammonia in patients with inborn errors of the urea cycle and organic acid metabolism. Similar approaches include the administration of carnitine, which conjugates with a variety of accumulated CoA esters in patients with defects of organic acid metabolism; cysteamine, which helps to eliminate excess cyctine in cystinosis; and penicillamine to reduce excessive stores of copper in Wilson's disease and iron in hemochromatosis.

Inhibition of an overactive pathway For other disorders, particularly those in which alternative pathway overflow produces a toxic level of a particular metabolite, it may be possible to prevent the accumulation by inhibiting an enzyme in the affected pathway. This approach may lead to accumulation of upstream substrates that must be well tolerated if the treatment is to be successful. For instance, in gout and other disorders in which excessive purine degradation leads to uric acid accumulation, inhibition of xanthine oxidase by allopurinol reduces uric acid production and lowers the incidence of uric acid nephropathy and gouty arthritis. Xanthine, which accumulates as a consequence, has greater aqueous solubility than uric acid and usually is well tolerated. In a similar fashion, hypercholesterolemic patients heterozygous for mutations at the low density lipoprotein receptor locus exhibit significant reductions in plasma cholesterol when treated with lovastatin, a potent inhibitor of hydroxymethylglutaryl coenzyme A reductase that catalyzes an important early and rate-limiting step in the synthesis of cholesterol.

Product deficit For disorders in which the pathophysiology involves product deficit, nutritional or pharmacologic approaches to replenishing the product can be effective if the administered material reaches the appropriate physiologic compartment. For example, many of the inborn errors in hormone biosynthesis such as the various forms of congenital adrenal hyperplasia and hereditary defects in thyroid hormone biosynthesis respond well to pharmacologic replacement of the deficient hormones. By contrast, the administration of melanin to albinos would not correct the pigment deficit in melanocytes.

TREATMENT DIRECTED TO THE PROTEIN PHENOTYPE

Therapy at the level of dysfunctional protein involves either activation of the mutant protein or replenishment of the missing protein.

Activation of the mutant protein Activation may be possible if the protein requires a vitamin cofactor and the vitamin is one that is well tolerated in pharmacologic doses. Obviously, not all mutations of a gene encoding a vitamin-dependent protein will respond. Those that do are likely to be missense mutations that either decrease the affinity of the enzyme for its cofactor or destabilize the protein in a way that can be partially overcome by substantial increments in cofactor concentration. About one-third of the cases of homocystinuria due to deficiency of the pyridoxal phosphate-requiring enzyme, cystathione-β-synthase, exhibit a significant increment in the activity when treated with pharmacologic doses (50 to 500 mg/d) of pyridoxine (vitamin B_6). The actual increase in enzyme activity may be small but suffices to improve metabolic flux in the impaired pathway. Since activation of residual activity both reduces precursor accumulation and increases product formation, knowledge of the pathophysiologic mechanism is less critical for this form of treatment.

Protein replacement therapies An alternative therapeutic approach involves replacement with an exogenous supply of the protein. To be successful, the protein must be administered directly into or eventually reach the appropriate physiologic compartment. Thus, blood proteins or proteins that traverse the vascular compartment (e.g., peptide hormones) are candidates for this approach. Other considerations include the availability, stability, and immunogenicity of the administered protein. Recombinant DNA technology can sometimes be utilized to supply sufficient amounts of the pure protein (e.g., human growth hormone and alpha$_1$ antitrypsin). Other proteins (e.g., clotting factor VIII) are available from natural sources but may eventually be produced by recombinant technology. This advance ensures an adequate supply and avoids the risk of transmission of pathologic viruses contaminating the protein purified from natural sources.

ORGAN TRANSPLANTATION

Organ transplantation is on the borderline between therapy at the level of the dysfunctional protein and gene therapy. On the one hand a transplanted organ supplies a deficient protein; on the other, the transplant tissue also brings new genetic information which, in contrast to standard models of gene therapy, is not integrated into the recipient's genome. Kidney, liver, and bone marrow transplantation are utilized for a variety of genetic diseases. The development of more effective and specific immunosuppressants (particularly cyclosporin) and the inadequacy of many less invasive therapies account, in part, for the increased utilization of this form of treatment. In some instances, the goal of transplantation is to supply the recipient with a tissue that can replace a mutant protein (e.g., liver transplant for deficiency of low density lipoprotein receptor or one of the urea cycle enzymes). For other disorders (e.g., alpha$_1$ antitrypsin deficiency or hepatorenal tyrosinemia) the transplant both provides the protein and replaces a severely damaged organ. The pathophysiologic mechanism of the disease is relevant; the physician must consider if the newly supplied protein will only be used locally or, if not, will gain access to the involved tissue(s). The long-term efficacy and consequences of organ transplantation as treatment for genetic disorders remain to be determined.

PROSPECTS FOR GENE THERAPY

Several methods are now available to introduce new, functional genetic material into mammalian cells. These methods allow consideration of a more direct approach to treatment of genetic disease, namely gene therapy or introduction of a functional gene to replace or supplement the activity of a resident defective gene. Typically, two general strategies have been considered, germline and somatic cell gene therapy, which differ in the nature of the recipient cells. In the germline model foreign DNA is introduced into the zygote or early embryo with a significant probability that the newly introduced material will contribute to the germline, i.e., be passed on to the next generation. By contrast, in somatic gene therapy models, the new genetic material is introduced only into somatic cells and is not transmitted to the germ cells. A third approach to gene therapy involves activation of endogenous genes to augment or circumvent a defective gene.

Much of the technology for germline gene therapy has been developed in work on transgenic mice. Fertilized mouse eggs are harvested from a superovulated female, microinjected with DNA molecules, and reimplanted in a pseudopregnant female. Several murine genetic diseases, including deficiency of growth hormone, myelin basic protein, and β-globin have been "treated" in this fashion with the general result that the disease phenotype is markedly ameliorated. These experiments have provided considerable information on the regulation of gene expression and the pathogenesis of genetic disease. However, the process is inefficient: only 15 to 20 percent of injected eggs produce transgenic animals, and of these only 20 to 30 percent actually express the introduced gene. Furthermore, there are appreciable risks including damage to a resident gene by the random insertion of the foreign DNA (insertional mutagenesis). In practice, availability of the molecular reagents for this approach makes prenatal diagnosis possible. The certainty of having an unaffected child as established by prenatal diagnosis is preferable to the uncertainty and risks of the transgenic approach. Thus, germline gene therapy is not applicable to human genetic disease.

Conversely, somatic gene therapy experiments will be tried for human genetic disease (Fig. 8-2). The methods for introducing the genetic material and the recipient cells will vary depending, in part, on the disease to be treated. Currently, modified retroviral vectors that allow high efficiency introduction of foreign DNA into dividing cells are favored. Bone marrow stem cells, hepatocytes, and fibroblasts are candidate recipient cells, and favorable results have been obtained in tissue culture systems. Difficulties with long-term, high-level expression of the introduced gene and with reintroduction of the recipient cells into the organism are obstacles to progress in this area. Developments in directing the introduced gene to its normal location in the genome (homologous recombination) offer promise for achieving normal regulation of the introduced gene and elimination of detrimental effects of the endogenous mutant gene. The lessons learned from more conventional therapies will apply to somatic gene therapy. The importance of early intervention, consideration of pathophysiologic mechanism(s), and the need for regulated interactions of the product of the introduced gene with other members of the involved homeostatic system are all relevant. Each disorder will have its own therapeutic requirements and problems. These considerations suggest that somatic gene therapy eventually will be useful for certain genetic diseases but is unlikely to be broadly effective.

By contrast to the first two models, activation of the expression of endogenous genes is a form of gene therapy that is already being attempted for human genetic disease. Interferon γ, a potent transcriptional regulator of several genes including those involved in X-linked chronic granulomatous disease (X-CGD), improves neutrophil function in that subset of X-CGD patients with mutations that impair a cytochrome involved in superoxide metabolism (see Chap. 81). Likewise, hydroxyurea increases the expression of the gamma globin gene in some patients with sickle cell disease, providing an alternative, nonsickling hemoglobin. The long-term efficacy of these approaches and the possible detrimental effects of administering agents that markedly affect the expression of many genes are unknown.

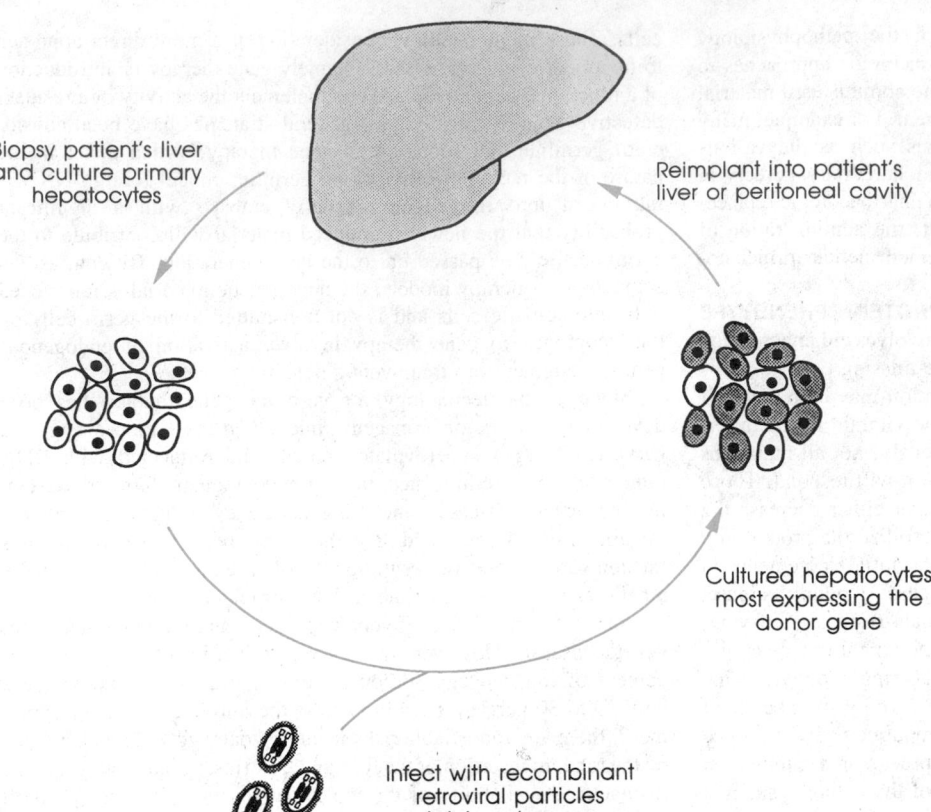

Biopsy patient's liver and culture primary hepatocytes

Reimplant into patient's liver or peritoneal cavity

Cultured hepatocytes most expressing the donor gene

Infect with recombinant retroviral particles containing donor gene

FIGURE 8-2 One model for somatic gene therapy involving retroviral-mediated gene transfer into hepatocytes.

EVALUATION OF THERAPY FOR GENETIC DISEASE

Two general questions should be posed in an evaluation of therapy for a genetic disease. First, does the treatment provide therapeutic benefit? Second, does the treatment restore the patient to full physiologic normality as if he or she did not have the disease? These questions can be asked of any disease treatment but have special significance for genetic disorders that are predictable and preventable. Studies by Costa, Scriver, and Childs evaluated the effectiveness of therapy of 351 representative monogenic disorders on three basic variables, life span, reproductive capability, and social adaptation; in their study available therapies returned life span to normal in only 15 percent, allowed reproductive capability in only 11 percent, and improved social adaptation in only 6 percent of the disorders. Only slightly better outcomes were found with a subset of 65 diseases in which the basic defect is known. Because more severe diseases are more quickly recognized, this sample may be skewed toward diseases most difficult to treat. Nevertheless, the results of therapy are worse than expected, emphasize the difficulty in developing effective therapies for genetic diseases, and highlight the need for continued work in this area. The results also underscore the value of preventive measures as therapy for genetic disease.

PREVENTION OF GENETIC DISEASE

Recognition of the limitation of therapy in genetic disease plus the predictability of the pattern of transmission of genes from one generation to the next has focused attention on prevention as the most reliable and effective means of dealing with hereditary disorders. The preventive approach includes genetic screening, counseling, and prenatal diagnosis.

GENETIC SCREENING   There are two types of genetic screening programs for autosomal recessive disorders: homozygote screening programs search for individuals who have the disorder; by contrast, heterozygote screening programs search for individuals who are carriers of a mutant gene and thus are at increased risk of having

offspring with a particular disorder. Successful homozygote screening programs require an inexpensive and reliable test, the recognition of some benefit (treatment, counseling) of early diagnosis, and education of the individuals and/or families screened so that they understand the significance of the results. The best example of such programs are the newborn screening programs. The diseases screened for vary from state to state but often include phenylketonuria, homocystinuria, maple syrup urine disease, galactosemia, cystic fibrosis, hypothyroidism, and sickle cell disease. In each instance the screening test allows early detection and the opportunity to initiate appropriate therapy prior to the onset of irreversible damage. Also, the parents of an affected individual are made aware of the risk to future offspring and have the option of prenatal diagnosis. Heterozygote screening programs are best exemplified by the program to detect carriers of Tay Sachs disease, a fatal, autosomal recessive lysosomal storage disease for which there is no effective treatment. Heterozygote screening of defined subpopulations with an increased carrier frequency (e.g., Ashkenazi Jews where the carrier frequency is approximately 1/25 as compared to approximately 1/300 in Anglo Saxons) identifies couples at risk in which both potential parents are carriers with a 25 percent chance of having an affected child. Prenatal diagnosis is possible, and the procedure provides a means for the couple to have unaffected children.

GENETIC COUNSELING   Prospective parents who seek information regarding the risk of genetic disease in their offspring may come to the physician for genetic counseling. Thus, all physicians should become familiar with the principles of medical genetics and use this knowledge to understand and counsel patients. The couples may be identified as having an increased risk for having a child with a genetic disease because of a previously affected child or other near relative. Alternatively, one or both parents may belong to a known high risk group (e.g., identified as a carrier in a heterozygote screening test), or advanced maternal age (> 35 years at the time of delivery) may be associated with increased risk of having a baby with an autosomal trisomy.

One aspect of genetic counseling involves determination of the risk for having an affected child and transmission of this information to the prospective parents so that they can make informed reproductive decisions. The first step is to determine the reliability of the diagnosis. This usually requires critical examination of existing medical data and/or additional evaluation of affected family member(s). The information is then assembled in the format of the family pedigree to determine the pattern of transmission within the particular family and to compare it with that expected for the diagnosed condition. Depending on the type of disease (monogenic, multifactorial, or chromosomal) and reliability of the diagnosis, the risk to subsequent offspring may be predicted with a degree of certainty ranging from a rough estimate to nearly perfect. The reliability of the diagnosis will be influenced by the existence of multiple etiologies for a particular phenotype and the availability of specific diagnostic tests. Molecular tests that directly and unambiguously determine the parental genotype are becoming increasingly available and allow precise prediction of the risk of recurrence and prenatal diagnosis for some monogenic disorders (see Chap. 7). For autosomal recessive and X-linked disorders in which a primary biochemical defect is known, reliable diagnosis is possible by a functional test of the gene product (e.g., assay of enzyme activity). For most autosomal dominant disorders the primary biochemical defect is not known and, thus, identification of parental genotype is subject to error resulting from heterogeneity of etiology. Availability of linked molecular markers, e.g., RFLPs, and identification of the involved genes will greatly improve the realiability and precision of counseling for some of these conditions.

Counseling for many common multifactorial disorders (e.g., diabetes, hypertension, atherosclerotic cardiovascular disease, congenital malformations, and psychiatric disorders) is imperfect and will be so until we have a better understanding of the interactions of the various genes and environmental factors that produce these diseases. In some families the etiology may involve a major contribution of a single gene, and in others a mix of multiple genes and environmental factors is the cause. In the former the risk may be predicted by a monogenic model while in the latter no simple model suffices. In these instances, the physician must resort to empiric risk estimates derived from retrospectively assembled data based on the average reproductive outcome in many different families.

Other information in addition to determining risk should be obtained prior to counseling. The prognosis and treatment of the disorder should be reviewed and the availability of prenatal diagnosis and carrier testing should be determined. Finally, the counselor must be sensitive to the emotional impact this information may have on those counseled.

During the counseling session, effective communication of the information depends on clearly expressing the essentials in language understandable to the subjects. Written notes and diagrams frequently are helpful and can be given to them at the end of the session. Finally, review at subsequent visits helps correct misconceptions and increase retention of the information. In this regard, the physician who has an established relationship with the family may have advantage over a trained counselor who meets with the subjects on only one or two occasions.

PRENATAL DIAGNOSIS Following genetic counseling, the couple at risk for having a child with a genetic disease has several options depending, in part, on the type of disorder. They may be reassured and proceed despite the risk without any subsequent monitoring. Or, they may view the risks as too high and choose to have no additional children or to adopt. Alternatively, when both parents are heterozygous for an autosomal recessive disorder, they may choose to reduce the risk by utilizing artificial insemination by donor. The magnitude of the decrease in the risk provided by this option will depend on the carrier frequency for the particular disorder in the general population. For a couple with a 1 in 4 or 25 percent chance of having a child with phenylketonuria, the risk with donor insemination will drop to 1 in 130 ($\frac{1}{2} \times \frac{1}{65}$) or less than 1 percent because the carrier frequency in the general population is 1 in 65. In the instance that mutant alleles for the gene in question are preferentially associated with particular

linked markers (linkage dysequilibrium), it may be possible to reduce the risk further by avoiding donors with the mutant-associated markers.

Finally, if the disorder can be detected antenatally, the couple may decide to proceed with reproduction and utilize prenatal diagnosis with elective abortion of affected fetuses. Because the risk of having an affected fetus ranges from a maximum of 50 percent for heterozygotes with autosomal dominant disorders to < 10 percent for nearly all chromosomal and multifactorial disorders, the great majority of pregnancies monitored by prenatal diagnosis have an unaffected fetus. This relatively low frequency of affected fetuses, together with an increase in reproductive activity which often results from the reassurance provided by the availability of prenatal diagnosis, leads to significant increases in the family size of at risk couples. Thus, in contrast to some public misconceptions, availability of prenatal diagnosis actually results in increased numbers of offspring. The indications for prenatal diagnosis are developed from a comparison of the risk of the procedures with the risk of having an affected child (Table 8-2).

Several methods for prenatal diagnosis are available (Table 8-3). Choice of a method depends on the disorder in question and on family preferences. Measurement of alpha fetoprotein (AFP) and other fetal proteins in maternal serum is noninvasive and can be used to screen for pregnancies at risk for neural tube defects (increased maternal serum AFP) and for fetal aneuploidies (decreased maternal serum AFP). It is possible by ultrasonography to visualize many fetal malformations and growth abnormalities and to monitor more invasive fetal sampling techniques with attendant reductions in the risks of the procedures. Although second trimester (15 to 16 weeks of gestation) fetal sampling by amniocentesis is the most widely used method for obtaining fetal cells, the techniques of transcervical and transabdominal chorionic villus sampling (CVS) can also be performed at 9 to 12 weeks of gestation. CVS has the advantage of allowing the diagnosis to be made earlier, and if an abortion is chosen, it will take place at a stage of pregnancy when maternal-fetal bonding is

TABLE 8-2 Major indications for prenatal diagnosis

Indication	Risk for affected fetus, %	Method of detection
Chromosomal disorders		
Advanced maternal age (>35 y)	1–10 depending on maternal age	
Parent with a balanced translocation	3–20 depending on the translocation	Chromosomal analysis of cells obtained by CVS* or amniocentesis
Previous child with chromosomal abnormality	~1	
Monogenic disorders		
Couple at risk for having a child with an inborn error of metabolism	25	Biochemical and/or molecular analysis of cells obtained by CVS or amniocentesis
Couple at risk for having a child with a monogenic disorder for which molecular markers are available	25–50	Molecular analysis of DNA obtained from cells obtained by CVS or by amniocentesis
Couple at risk for having a child with a monogenic malformation syndrome without biochemical or molecular markers	25–50	Fetal imaging by ultrasound
Malformation disorders		
Couples at risk for having a child with a neural tube defect (anencephaly or meningomyelocele) or other multifactorial malformation syndrome	1–10	Fetal imaging by ultrasound and, for neural tube defects, measurement of alpha fetoprotein and other fetal markers in amniotic fluid obtained by amniocentesis

* CVS, chorionic villus sampling

TABLE 8-3   Methods of prenatal diagnosis

Method	Stage of gestation, weeks	Sample	Fetal disorders	Risks
Maternal serum sampling	15–18	Alpha fetoprotein and other fetal proteins	Neural tube defects, aneuploidies	Negligible
Fetal ultrasonography	6–40	Image	Fetal dating, morphologic abnormalities, skeletal dysplasis	Negligible
Fetal sampling				
Chorionic villus sampling	9–12	Fetal trophoblastic tissue	Cytogenetic, biochemical, molecular	1–2% fetal loss
Amniocentesis	15–18	Amniotic fluid and cells	Cytogenetic, biochemical, molecular, neural tube defects	0.2–0.5% fetal loss
Fetal biopsy	18–20	Fetal skin	Dermatologic	~2% fetal loss
		Fetal liver	Liver-specific, enzyme deficiencies	2–5% fetal loss
		Umbilical cord, blood	Blood disorders	~2% fetal loss

less. Finally, elective abortion at 12 weeks of gestation is a 2- to 3-h outpatient procedure whereas a second trimester elective abortion requires a 1- to 3-day hospitalization. The risks of CVS are still being assessed but, in experienced hands, appear to compare well with those of amniocentesis. The tissue obtained at CVS is fetal trophoblastic tissue, expresses nearly all enzymes found in amniocytes, and provides an excellent source of fetal DNA.

REFERENCES

SCRIVER CR et al (eds): *The Metabolic Basis of Inherited Disease*, 6th ed. New York, McGraw Hill, 1989

FILKINS K, RUSSO JF (eds): New York, Marcel Dekker, 1985

FRIEDMANN T: Progress toward human gene therapy. Science 244:1275, 1989

COSTA T, SCRIVER CR, CHILDS B: The effect of mendelian disease on human health: A measurement. Am J Med Genet 21:231, 1985

section 2   Cell growth and regulation

9   GROWTH FACTORS

LEWIS T. WILLIAMS

Many diseases involve abnormalities in the rate of proliferation of cells (Table 9-1). The most obvious of these, cancer, is associated with uncontrolled cell division. A more subtle form of abnormal cell proliferation is found in atherosclerosis, a disease in which vascular smooth-muscle cells proliferate excessively, but not in a malignant fashion, and eventually obstruct blood flow. Diseases that involve nonmalignant proliferation of cells include fibroproliferative processes such as pulmonary interstitial fibrosis, and some forms of glomerulonephritis, cirrhosis, and myelofibrosis. In these processes normal tissue is replaced by fibroblasts and their extracellular products. Several of the disease syndromes are caused by inappropriately low levels of cell proliferation. Thus, in the anemia of renal disease there may be a sluggish proliferation and maturation of erythroid precursors in the bone marrow caused by the inadequate production of erythropoietin by the kidney.

One of the most important findings in the study of cell proliferation has been the recognition that both normal and abnormal proliferation of cells are under control of polypeptide growth factors that serve as intercellular messengers. In general growth factors can act in one of three ways. First, some growth factors are released into the circulation and act at a distance, essentially in the same manner as hormones. This mode of *endocrine* action is typified by erythropoietin and insulin-like growth factor 1. Second, a cell may release a factor into its local environment, perhaps into the extracellular matrix, where the factor acts on adjacent cells. This mode of action, termed *paracrine*, may be the most common way in which growth factors regulate tissue repair and embryonic development. Third, growth factors may act by *autocrine* mechanisms, in which a cell responds to a factor that the cell produces.

Growth factors were originally discovered by measuring their ability to regulate the proliferation of specific target cells in vitro. There have been three general sources for the identification and purification of most factors: serum, tissue extracts, and media

"conditioned" by cultured cells. Most of the factors described in this chapter have been purified from these sources, and amino acid sequences of small peptide fragments have been determined directly. Based on these sequences DNA probes were designed and used to isolate full-length cDNA coding sequences by hybridization screening. A similar method has been used to clone the cDNA for several growth factor receptors. An alternative approach has been to express a pool of cDNAs in cells and identify clones by measuring the activity or immunoreactivity of the expressed factor or receptor ("expression cloning"). With these methods it has been possible to express many of these molecules in large quantities. The result has been an explosion of information about the biology of growth factors and a recognition of their potential roles in diseases and therapy. The following sections include discussions of the individual factors that regulate proliferation of mesenchymal, epithelial, endothelial, and neuronal cells (Table 9-2) followed by discussions of the hematopoietic growth factors and the lymphokines.

PLATELET-DERIVED GROWTH FACTOR   Platelet-derived growth factor (PDGF) was discovered by the convergence of two lines of investigation. First, for over 50 years tissue culture workers recognized the importance of serum factors in stimulating the growth of animal cells. In retrospect, much of the growth-promoting effect of serum on fibroblasts could be attributed to the PDGF released from activated platelets. A second line of work involved factors that stimulate the proliferation of smooth-muscle cells in atherosclerotic plaques. This

TABLE 9-1   Some diseases that involve abnormal cell proliferation

Cancer	Polycystic kidney
Atherosclerosis	Scleroderma
Pulmonary fibrosis	Rheumatoid arthritis
Primary pulmonary hypertension	Ankylosing spondylitis
Neurofibromatosis	Myelodysplasia
Acoustic neuroma	Some anemias
Tuberous sclerosis	Cirrhosis
Psoriasis	Esophageal stricture
Keloid	Sclerosing cholangitis
Fibrocystic breast	Retroperitoneal fibrosis
Polycystic ovary	

TABLE 9-2 Growth factors for mesenchymal, epithelial, endothelial, and neuronal cells

Platelet-derived growth factor (PDGF AA, PDGF BB, PDGF AB)	Vascular smooth muscle, fibroblasts, glial cells, skeletal myoblasts
Epidermal growth factor family (EGF, TGF-α, vaccinia virus factor)	Epithelial cells, fibroblasts, glial cells
Transforming growth factor	Most cells
Nerve growth factor (NGF)	Sensory and sympathetic neuronal cells, some melanocytes, Schwann cells, capillary endothelial cells
Fibroblast growth factor family (basic FGF, acidic FGF, int-2 gene product, Hst/Kaposi FGF)	Endothelial cells, fibroblasts, FGF vascular smooth-muscle cells, skeletal myoblasts, neuronal cells
Keratinocyte fibroblast growth factor	Keratinocytes
Tumor necrosis factor (TNF-α, TNF-β)	Some fibroblasts, endothelial cells, T cells
Interleukin 1 (IL-1α, IL-1β)	Fibroblasts, smooth-muscle cells, T cells

work culminated in the purification of PDGF from serum and from human platelets, although other sources of this factor may be important in vivo. For example, endothelial cells are an abundant source of PDGF in blood vessels. The production and release of PDGF from these cells is closely regulated by molecules that accumulate at the site of tissue injury. PDGF is also produced by activated macrophages, mesangial cells, smooth-muscle–like cells in blood vessels, a number of embryonic cells, and several types of tumor cells.

It is likely that the main physiological roles of PDGF are in the earliest stages of embryonic development and in wound healing. In adult tissues, only a limited number of cells respond to PDGF; these include vascular smooth-muscle cells, glial cells, and fibroblasts. The ability of PDGF to stimulate the migration and proliferation of mesenchymal cells, as well as to enhance the production of extracellular matrix proteins, has suggested a role for PDGF in a number of fibroproliferative pathologic processes including atherosclerosis and restenosis following vascular angioplasty. The evidence includes the finding of a high level of expression of PDGF in atherosclerotic vessels and an unusually high number of PDGF receptors in proliferative atherosclerotic lesions biopsied during carotid endarterectomy. Further research should determine whether PDGF is involved in other nonmalignant fibroproliferative processes including glomerulonephritis, pulmonary fibrosis, myelofibrosis, keloid formation, and rheumatoid arthritis.

The possibility that PDGF plays a role in cancer was first recognized in studies of the simian sarcoma virus (SSV) that was isolated from a spontaneously occurring monkey fibrosarcoma. This virus reproducibly causes tumors when inoculated into monkeys and will also transform cells in vitro by the expression of the viral oncogene v-sis. Introduction and expression of the v-sis oncogene into appropriate fibroblast cell lines transforms the cells into tumor cells that will form solid tumors when implanted in nude mice. The discovery that the v-sis oncogene encodes a form of PDGF was revolutionary in the field of growth factors. The v-sis-encoded form of PDGF appears to activate PDGF receptors in intracellular compartments before the receptors have a chance to be fully processed and expressed at the cell surface. This autocrine activation of receptors is prevented in most normal cells by the mutually exclusive expression of either PDGF or PDGF receptors. But some human tumor cell lines express both PDGF and its receptor and therefore may utilize similar autocrine pathways. It is possible that the autocrine activation of PDGF receptors is one of several steps required to transform cells in vivo and may be a critical event in initiation of some tumors.

Future studies of the role of PDGF in disease will be based on a better understanding of the structure of the factor and its receptor. PDGF was initially purified from human platelets as a 32-kDa molecule consisting of two polypeptide chains, termed A and B, that form an AB heterodimer. Several other tissues including endothelial

cells and glial progenitor cells produce homodimeric AA or BB forms of PDGF. The biological differences between these forms are not yet clearly understood. There are at least two types of structurally related receptors for PDGF, each with a distinctive specificity pattern for binding the multiple forms of the factor. Current attempts to develop antagonists of PDGF for use in treating fibroproliferative diseases are based on molecular analysis of the structural domains that mediate the binding of PDGF to its receptors and on specific cellular reactions that are stimulated by the receptor.

EPIDERMAL GROWTH FACTOR Epidermal growth factor (EGF) was discovered by the remarkable observation that injection of extracts of mouse salivary gland into newborn mice caused precocious opening of eyelids and eruption of incisors. Using these responses as an assay, Stanley Cohen purified and characterized the polypeptide. Eyelid opening could be ascribed to epidermal growth and keratinization stimulated by EGF. Later it was shown that EGF stimulated the proliferation of epithelial cells and fibroblasts in vitro.

The biological effects of EGF are mediated by a single type of membrane receptor that is found predominantly on epithelial cells and fibroblasts. This receptor also binds and responds to at least two additional EGF-like growth factors. These include transforming growth factor alpha (TGF-α), a polypeptide first isolated from media conditioned by tumor cells, and the vaccinia virus growth factor that is encoded by a vaccinia virus gene. These three ligands are only approximately 20 percent identical in amino acid sequence. They appear to act as mitogens in vitro and differ only subtly in their ability to bind to the EGF receptor.

A major surprise in the growth factor field was the discovery that the cytoplasmic domain sequence of the EGF receptor is closely related to the sequence of a transforming gene (oncogene) of the avian erythroblastosis virus, v-erbB gene. The precise molecular mechanism by which the differences convert the normal EGF receptor into a transforming protein is not known. Acknowledging the relationship of the EGF receptor to the v-erbB oncogene, the normal cellular gene of the EGF receptor has been designated c-erbB. Another virus, the avian leukosis virus, utilizes the EGF receptor to transform cells by a different mechanism, in which expression of the EGF receptor is increased by insertion of viral sequences into the flanking regions of the receptor gene. The altered expression of this gene causes erythroblastosis.

A close relative of the EGF receptor gene is the neu proto-oncogene, which also has been designated HER-2/neu. The HER-2/neu gene is 50 percent identical to the EGF receptor gene in its coding sequence and is located on human chromosome 17. The structure of protein encoded by HER-2/neu predicts that it is a growth factor receptor, although its ligand has yet to be identified. One of the most provocative findings from studies of this gene is that the critical difference between the neu oncogene and the normal HER-2/neu gene is a single amino acid replacement in the transmembrane domain. This finding supports the hypothesis that well-defined mutations in normal growth regulatory molecules may be involved in carcinogenesis (see Chap. 10).

Other studies have suggested that there is an increased expression of the EGF receptor or the HER-2/neu gene in human cancer. For example, the HER-2/neu proto-oncogene is amplified in 25 to 30 percent of human primary breast cancers, and this alteration is predictive of disease outcome. A similar association has been reported in ovarian cancer. The concept that alterations in HER-2/neu gene expression are important in tumorigenesis has been strengthened by the observations that (1) overexpression of the normal HER-2/neu proto-oncogene can induce transformation in mouse cells in vitro and (2) that the mutated rat neu gene expressed in transgenic mice causes development of breast adenocarcinomas. Such studies may lead to improved diagnosis and therapeutic strategies for breast and ovarian cancer as well as for other tumors of epithelial cell origin.

TRANSFORMING GROWTH FACTORS A number of growth factors have been isolated from media conditioned by tumor cells. Two of these were purified on the basis of their synergistic actions in stimulating the growth of fibroblasts in soft agar, an assay often used as an index of cell "transformation." Since cancer cells grow in soft agar, the growth factors were first thought to be mitogens involved in tumorigenesis and were called *tumor growth factors*. However their main role appears to be in embryonic development and in tissue repair.

Transforming growth factor alpha (TGF-α) is a mitogen for epithelial cells and appears to mimic EGF in its ability to bind and activate EGF receptors. The major difference between TGF-α and EGF appears to be in their respective patterns of expression, especially during embryogenesis. Both of these factors have the unusual property of being synthesized as precursor proteins that have transmembrane sequences and are probably localized to the cell surface. The precursor may activate EGF receptors on adjacent cells through direct cell-cell interactions that do not involve soluble factors. This type of interaction may be especially important in organogenesis.

Transforming growth factor-beta (TGF-β) has been historically linked to TGF-α, but the functional differences between them are more apparent than their similarities. The biological activities of the TGF-β family span a confusing spectrum of celllular responses including proliferation of some cells (especially connective tissue cells), inhibition of proliferation of other cells (e.g., lymphocytes or epithelial cells), enhanced collagen and extracellular matrix production, and expression of cell adhesion molecules. Given this set of in vitro reactions, it is not surprising that when experimental animals are injected with TGF-β an exuberant granulation and fibrotic response can be seen at the site of injection within an hour. TGF-β factor may play a role in the fibrosis seen in pulmonary fibrosis, keloid formation, cirrhosis, scleroderma, rheumatoid arthritis, or proliferative vitreoretinopathy. An even more compelling case has been made for the role of TGF-β in embryonic formation of bone and cartilage. It may be possible to use TGF-β to stimulate formation of bone matrix and perhaps accelerate fracture healing. The recent finding of large amounts of TGF-β in cardiac myocytes and its increased expression during experimental myocardial infarction has suggested a role for this factor in repair of myocardial injury. There has also been considerable attention focused on the growth inhibitory effect of TGF-β. It is possible that a loss of this negative control of cell proliferation contributes to tumorigenesis.

FIBROBLAST GROWTH FACTORS
The fibroblast growth factors (FGFs) constitute a group of structurally homologous polypeptides that stimulate the proliferation of endothelial cells, fibroblasts, vascular smooth muscle cells, skeletal muscle myoblasts, and some forms of epithelial cells. They are also trophic factors for neurons. The FGFs have the unusual ability to elicit the formation of new blood vessels, a process termed angiogenesis, by stimulating endothelial cells to migrate through the vessel wall and to proliferate as capillary sprouts. While angiogenesis may be beneficial in some contexts, such as in embryonic development or in ischemic myocardium, it may have deleterious effects in a number of pathologic conditions such as diabetic retinopathy or the formation of new blood vessels required for tumors to grow beyond a certain size (tumor angiogenesis). In a sense, FGF-induced angiogenesis recapitulates the normal embryonic development of new blood vessels. In fact, FGFs are expressed at the earliest stages of vertebrate embryogenesis, suggesting that these factors have other roles in development.

The FGF family includes at least seven distinct but structurally related molecules, each encoded by a different gene. The first two FGFs (acidic and basic) were purified from tissues known to release mitogenic and angiogenic factors. Several additional FGFs (e.g., FGF-5, Kaposi sarcoma FGF, and the *int*-2 gene product) were identified by their ability to transform cells that coexpress FGF receptors. It has been shown that there are not only multiple FGFs, but also multiple forms of the FGF receptor, each with a distinctive ligand-binding domain. The therapeutic challenge is to learn how to specifically block the deleterious effects of FGFs, such as in tumor angiogenesis, or to enhance the beneficial effects, for example, in nerve regeneration or angiogenesis in ischemic tissue.

GROWTH HORMONE AND INSULIN-LIKE GROWTH FACTOR 1
Growth hormone (see Chaps. 313 and 314) produced by the pituitary gland was one of the first known growth regulatory molecules. Its important role in bone elongation in vivo was recognized by its ability to restore normal growth rates in children and in experimental animals with growth hormone deficiency. Many of the effects of growth hormone can be attributed to the stimulation of systemic release of insulin-like growth factor 1 (IGF-1) from liver. IGF-1 acts as a direct mitogen on cells containing the IGF-1 receptor, a member of the tyrosine kinase family of signal transducing molecules. Whether growth hormone has direct effects other than those mediated by the action of IGF-1 has been the subject of intense investigation. The growth hormone receptor is a molecule that is found either as a membrane receptor that lacks tyrosine kinase sequences or in a truncated soluble form without a transmembrane region that functions as a circulating growth hormone binding protein.

Interestingly there are several abnormal patterns of growth in humans that involve the growth hormone or IGF-1 systems. In Laron dwarfism there is a total absence of high-affinity growth hormone binding proteins (presumably the truncated soluble form of the receptor) in plasma and a virtual absence of hepatic growth hormone receptors. African pygmies appear to have a less severe defect in growth hormone binding protein levels. A rare syndrome of IGF-1 resistance and dwarfism involves a like reduction of IGF-1 receptors.

NERVE GROWTH FACTOR
In 1952, Rita Levi-Montalcini showed that transplants of mouse sarcoma tissue onto the chorioallantoic membrane of embryos resulted in a marked increase in the size and number of chicken sensory and sympathetic neurons. This finding could be attributed to enhanced survival of neurons which would normally degenerate during ontogenesis. The factor responsible for this process was purified and designated *nerve growth factor* (NGF) but was considered to be primarily a "survival" or "maintenance" factor rather than a mitogenic compound. Subsequently, many experiments have documented a role for NGF in neuron survival and in the targeting of sensory neurons to specific tissues. It has recently been shown that NGF has effects in the central nervous system as well as in other tissues and may be involved in a number of nonneuronal processes. Thus, NGF receptors are found on capillary endothelium cells, myoepithelium cells, perivascular cells, and mast cells.

Nerve growth factor has been isolated as a complex of noncovalently associated alpha, beta, and gamma subunits. The beta subunit is responsible for the biologic responses of NGF and binds as a dimer to the NGF receptor. Although the primary amino acid sequence of the receptor is known, little is understood about its mechanism of action since, unlike the receptors for PDGF, EGF, insulin, and IGF-1, the NGF receptor is not a tyrosine kinase. The major clinical interest in NGF has centered on the proposal that it might be useful therapeutically in promoting nerve regeneration. It is also possible that a deficiency of NGF or related factors may play a role in degenerative diseases.

GROWTH FACTORS FOR BLOOD CELLS
The control of proliferation and differentiation of blood cells are vital processes for the maintenance of adequate levels of circulating cells and for the responses of the immune system to foreign substances. This control is achieved in large part by paracrine mechanisms in which one type of cell, sensing environmental cues, releases factors that act, often at short distances, to regulate proliferation or differentiation of a second type of cell. The complex system of cell-cell interactions is maintained by the highly specific control of expression not only of the growth factors but also of their receptors in the responding cells. This is the basis of a complex network of interactions among numerous cell types in tissues such as bone marrow and lymph nodes or at sites of inflammation. While the molecular and cellular analysis of these processes has led to understanding of the general principles by which the growth and differentiation of hematopoietic cells are regulated, the terminology used in this field is confusing. Classification of these factors into hematopoietic factors and lymphokines is helpful in understanding their biological roles (see Chaps. 13 and 285).

Hematopoietic factors The first insight into the role of hematopoietic growth factors came from attempts to grow myeloid cells in culture. The culture of these cells could only be achieved in the presence of "feeder" cells that produced factors required for the growth of bone marrow-derived progenitors of each type of myeloid cell. The term *colony stimulating factor* was used to refer to the peptides that stimulated growth and maturation of granulocyte or monocyte lineages in soft agar. These assays permitted purification and characterization of the factors. Some factors, e.g., macrophage colony stimulating factor (CSF-1) appeared to be specific for one lineage whereas others, e.g., granulocyte-macrophage colony stimulating factor (GM-CSF), appeared to act on more than one lineage (Table 9-3). However, it has become apparent that initial classification of these factors by responsive cell type may be an oversimplification. For example G-CSF, which was originally thought to act exclusively on granulocytic lineages, appears to act on multiple lineages at several different stages of differentiation.

The study of myeloid cell growth factors has suggested novel approaches for the treatment of a number of diseases. The most obvious of these is the exogenous administration of growth factors to patients with cytopenia. G-CSF and GM-CSF are capable of raising blood granulocyte levels in patients with mild bone marrow suppression caused by cytotoxic drugs or who have disorders such as chronic neutropenia, myelodysplasia, aplastic anemia, AIDS, hairy cell leukemia, or cyclic hematopoiesis. The efficacy of G-CSF and GM-CSF in these syndromes does not necessarily imply that the diseases are caused by factor deficiency, but may reflect a clinically beneficial, stimulation of stem cell proliferation and differentiation in response to the exogenous factors. It is noteworthy that GM-CSF not only leads to an elevation of circulating neutrophils, eosinophils, and monocytes but also causes an increase in lymphocytes, platelets and reticulocytes, indicating the complexity of the effects of GM-CSF.

A more controversial potential use of hemopoietic growth factors is in the treatment of myeloid leukemias. This application is based on the observation that, in addition to their proliferative effects, these factors have the ability to induce differentiation of some populations of myeloid precursors. GM-CSF and G-CSF are known to induce differentiation of leukemic cells in vitro. However the obvious concern that such treatment might accelerate the progress of the disease in patients with leukemia has led to reluctance to use these factors in this setting even for treatment of cytopenias.

Erythropoietin, a factor that was studied for over 50 years before it was fully characterized, is produced primarily by the kidney but also by the liver and bone marrow macrophages. It differs from many of the hematopoietic factors and lymphokines in that it acts in vivo more as a hormone (i.e., at "long" distances) than as a local "paracrine" growth factor. When administered to patients with end-stage renal failure, it can stimulate an increase in red cell mass with relatively mild side effects of transient dyspnea, arthralgia, myalgia, flushing sensation, bone pain, or an increase in diastolic blood pressure. Erythropoietin is likely to be useful in other conditions such as anemia of chronic disease and marrow suppression induced by chemotherapy.

One of the most specific of the hemopoietic factors is the macrophage colony stimulating factor (CSF-1). This factor acts on specific monocyte receptors that are closely related structurally and, to some extent, mechanistically to the receptors for PDGF. The CSF-1 receptor appears to play a role in monocytes analogous to the role of PDGF receptors in vascular smooth muscle cells. The CSF-1 receptor also has an oncogenic form, the v-*fms* gene product, which has been found in some feline tumors. Thus the CSF-1 receptor is also known as the "c-*fms* proto-oncogene."

Lymphokines (cytokines) The search for factors that support the growth of normal lymphocytes in vitro led to the identification of a group of molecules, termed *lymphokines* or *interleukins*, that were initially believed to be specific extracellular signals between different populations of cells in the immune system (see Table 13-4). However it has become evident that neither the production nor the response to lymphokines is restricted to immunocompetent cells. Therefore the more general term *cytokine* has been used for the group of proteins. The growth and maturation of lymphocytes depends on a highly regulated pattern of expression of these factors and on their receptors in different cell populations. Activation of immune responses depends on an equally complex pattern of regulation (see Chap. 13).

Interleukin 1 (IL-1) is made by many cell types and has a diverse group of actions including a number of reactions involved in the acute phase response. It has mitogenic effects on both T-cells and vascular smooth muscle cells especially when it acts in conjunction with other growth factors. The tumor necrosis factors share many of the actions of IL-1. IL-2 plays an important role in T-cell proliferation and maturation and also enhances the cytolytic activity of a population of killer cells that may destroy tumor cells. Thus its potential use for tumor therapy is under investigation. IL-3 stimulates growth and differentiation of hematopoietic precursors of multiple cell lineages and is also a growth factor for mast cells. IL-3, IL-4, and IL-5 appear to play important roles in allergic and antiparasitic inflammatory responses.

The lymphokines are now more noted for the diversity of responses elicited by each factor than for their restricted specificity. There is much overlap in their actions, and many of them act indirectly by inducing the expression and release of other lymphokines. Most act locally as paracrine factors but some of them act as autocrine factors. For this reason the potential use of lymphokines as therapeutic agents may be complicated by numerous side effects. However understanding these important factors should provide insight into a number of diseases of the immune system.

MECHANISM OF GROWTH FACTOR ACTION The mechanism by which growth factors stimulate cells to leave a stage of quiescence, designated "G_0" in cell cycle terminology, and enter the G_1 phase that culminates in DNA synthesis (S phase) involves interactions among several cytoplasmic molecules. Although there are differences among growth factor receptors in their mechanisms of action, there are some common features. First, transcription of a group of specialized growth regulatory genes appears to be required (Fig. 9-1). Second, most growth factor receptors activate cellular kinases and the hydrolysis of phosphatidylinositol. The receptors for many growth factors, including PDGF, EGF, FGF, and IGF-1, are tyrosine kinases. The mechanism of action of this family of receptors is understood best. Upon binding ligand, the receptor phosphorylates several specific substrates on tyrosine residues. These substrates include serine/threonine kinases, phospholipase C, and phosphatidylinositol kinase. The serine/threonine kinases are thought to increase transcription of growth regulatory genes perhaps by regulating the phosphorylation state of cytoplasmic transcription factors. The enzymes phospholipase C and phosphatidylinositol kinase act on membrane phosphatidylinositol to generate diacylglycerol, which activates protein kinase C, a known regulator of gene transcription. In addition, cytoplasmic inositol phosphate second messengers are released, but their precise role in growth regulation has not been defined.

TABLE 9-3 Hematopoietic growth factors

Factor	Other nomenclature	Responsive lineage
CSF-1	MCSF, MAI-1m	Macrophage
G-CSF	MGI-1G, pluripoietin, differentiation factor	Granulocyte
GM-CSF	MGI-1GM, CSF-α, CSF-2, pluripoietin-α	Macrophage and granulocyte
IL-3	Multi-CSF-α, stem cell activating factor, hematopoietic growth factor, hematopoietin 2, burst promoting activity, mast cell growth factor	Macrophage, granulocyte, eosinophil, megakaryocyte, mast cell
Erythropoietin		Erythroid cells
Thrombopoietin		Megakaryocyte

NOTE: CSF, colony stimulating factor; MGI, macrophage growth inducer; IL, interleukin.

FIGURE 9-1 Scheme depicting the action of a tyrosine kinase growth factor receptor.

Membrane receptors other than the tyrosine kinase family of growth factor receptors may impact on some but not all of these pathways. For example, an alpha$_1$-adrenergic receptor, serotonin receptor, or angiotensin receptor, that can activate phospholipase C through guanylyl nucleotide binding proteins (see Chap. 11) may stimulate the diacylglycerol-mediated events but fail to initiate some of the other reactions that depend on tyrosine kinase. Thus under some circumstances, catecholamines, serotonin, or angiotensin might function as growth factors.

Several of the tyrosine kinase growth factor receptors as well as other cellular tyrosine kinases can be expressed as oncogenic (cancer-causing) proteins. The oncogenic forms of the nonreceptor kinases (*src, yes, fes, fps*, etc.) and of tyrosine kinase receptors (v-*erb*B, v-*fms*, and v-*kit*) stimulate growth regulatory pathways in an unregulated manner (see Chap. 10). Other oncogenes encode activated forms of the *raf* serine/threonine kinase, the *myc* and *fos* proteins, and other cellular proteins that regulate the pathways shown in Fig. 9-1. The net result of expression of an oncogene protein is that a normal growth regulatory pathway is usurped by a constitutively high activity that is independent of the presence of a growth factor.

The mechanism by which a growth factor binds to its receptor and activates the receptor is pivotal to the actions of all growth factors. The structures of the ligand binding domains of the factors and receptors are currently being studied and should yield information that would permit the design of novel growth factor agonists and antagonists. The effects of ligand binding on the receptor molecule vary among receptors. In some cases the ligand may induce receptor dimerization and formation of a cytoplasmic dimeric domain that has enhanced activity. In the case of tyrosine kinases, intermolecular receptor ''autophosphorylation'' may occur when the receptor dimerizes. Alternatively the ligand may cause the receptor to interact directly with other cellular molecules, perhaps through a conformational change induced in a cytoplasmic transmembrane domain. An understanding of these processes should lead to new approaches by which growth factor-stimulated events can be mimicked or antagonized.

REFERENCES

CARPENTER G: Receptors for epidermal growth factor and other polypeptide mitogens. Ann Rev Biochem 56:881, 1987
PAUL WE: Pleiotropy and redundancy: T cell-derived lymphokines in the immune response. Cell 57:521, 1989

SLAMON DJ et al: Studies of the HER-2/neu proto-oncogene in human breast and ovarian cancer. Science:244:707, 1989
STEWARD WP, SCARFIE JH: Clinical trials with hemopoietic growth factors. Progr Growth Factor Research 1:1, 1989
WILLIAMS LT: Signal transduction by the platelet-derived growth factor receptor. Science 243:1564, 1989

10 ONCOGENES AND NEOPLASTIC DISEASE

PAUL NEIMAN

Upon dividing, cancer cells transmit the neoplastic phenotype to daughter cells. For that reason, it has been generally assumed that the inheritance of the neoplastic phenotype is determined by specific genes. This assumption explains the great appeal of oncogenic viruses for cancer researchers. In spite of their relative genetic simplicity, these agents are capable of inducing all of the pathologic and clinical changes associated with neoplastic disease. In some cases a virus introduces into a normal cell a single gene (oncogene) whose product can initiate and maintain the neoplastic state. In the case of retroviruses, these viral oncogenes represent altered forms of cellular proto-oncogenes, which have important cellular functions in the normal state. Human homologues of some of these oncogenes appear to play a role in human cancer. This situation prompts a number of questions about the nature of oncogenes, the control of their expression, the biochemical nature of their gene products, and the mechanism of interaction with the metabolism of the host cell.

RETROVIRAL ONCOGENES Interaction of retroviruses with host cells The discovery of oncogenes was a result of study of the molecular biology of oncogenic retroviruses. Retroviruses are widespread in nature, and infection with some of them induces neoplastic disease in animals. The retroviral genome is an RNA molecule of between 8000 and 10,000 nucleotides. The distinctive feature in the life cycle of these agents is that after receptor-mediated entry of the virus into the cell the genomic RNA molecule is copied into DNA (reverse transcription) and integrated into the chromosomal DNA of the host cell (hence the name *retroviruses*) (Fig. 10-1). This integrated DNA is termed a *provirus*. The structure of typical proviruses is shown schematically in Fig. 10-2. Long terminal repeats (LTRs) containing sequences copied from both ends of viral genomic RNA are located at each end of the DNA provirus and linked directly to host DNA. These LTRs contain regulatory sequences for the expression of the genes required for viral replication: *gag*, coding for the internal structural protein; *pol*, coding for reverse transcriptase; and *env*, coding for the viral envelope glycoprotein. The regulatory sequences include signals for the initiation and termination of transcription. They usually also include powerful enhancer sequences that amplify the rate of transcription of viral genes so that proviral RNA transcripts may comprise as much as 0.1 to 1 percent of total cellular messenger RNA. The transcriptional promoter-enhancer sequences of some retroviruses function only when introduced into particular cell types, accounting for tissue-specific expression of viral genes. In other cases the activity of these enhancer sequences is regulated by steroid hormones. In contrast to many other viruses, retroviruses usually do not kill the host cell when the replicative process is completed; instead their life cycle results in the introduction and expression of exogenous genes and thus in alteration of the phenotype of the host cells.

Acute transforming retroviruses and their oncogenes Infection of animals with retroviruses encoding only the *gag, pol*, and *env* genes results in neoplastic disease after a long latent period. In contrast, acute transforming retroviruses can induce neoplastic disease in vivo in days to weeks and can transform cultured cells in vitro. The prototype of this class of viruses is the Rous sarcoma virus.

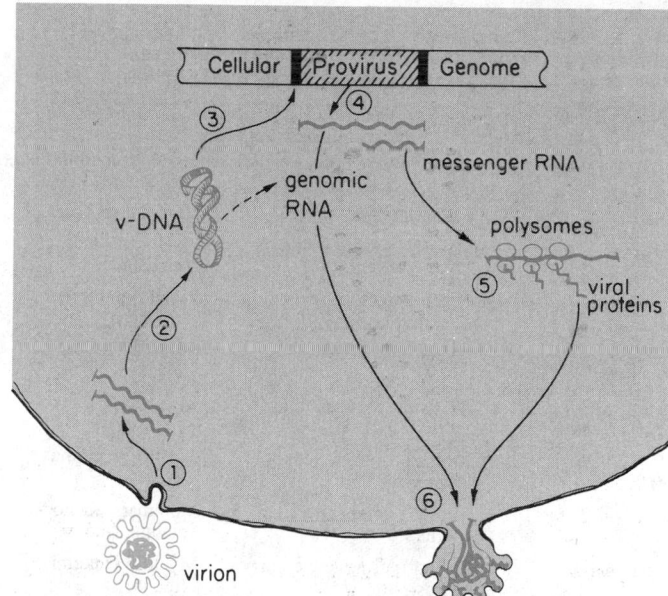

FIGURE 10-1 Replication of retroviruses. (1) Envelope glycoprotein on the surface of viral particles (virions) recognizes receptors that mediate entry into the cell and release of viral genomic RNA. (2) There are two viral RNA molecules per virion which are copied by reverse transcriptase into viral DNA molecules. (3) Some of the viral DNA molecules integrate into host chromosomal DNA at a precise point on the viral DNA molecule and a random, or near random, site on host chromosomes. (4) The integrated viral DNA copy, or provirus, is transcribed into both messenger RNA, which is translated into viral proteins on cellular polysomes (5), and full-length genomic viral RNA, which contains specific sequences serving as packaging signals for virus assembly. (6) Viral RNA and proteins are assembled into particles which bud from the cell surface. The whole process can occur without cytopathic effect on host cells.

FIGURE 10-2 Comparative structure of the proviruses of standard nondefective replication retroviruses and acute transforming retroviruses. In both cases the provirus is bounded by direct long terminal repeat sequences (LTRs), which contain essential regulatory elements including transcriptional promoters and enhancers, signals for the termination of viral RNA transcripts (poly A addition signals), and signals for integration into the host DNA. Between tne LTRs of standard retroviruses are three genes: *gag* (internal structural proteins), *pol* (reverse transcriptase), and *env* (envelope glycoprotein), which are required for infection and replication. In the acute transforming viruses, all or part of the replicative genes have been replaced by a transforming oncogene, which mediates the oncogenic properties of the virus. The most common structure is a fusion of the 5' portion of the *gag* gene with the oncogene. The standard provirus is transcribed into full-length genomic viral RNA and spliced messenger RNAs for viral proteins. The acute transforming provirus often expresses only one size RNA transcript and requires coinfection with a standard retroviral "helper" in order to replicate. The Δ*gag* symbol indicates that part of the *gag* sequence is missing because it has been deleted.

The structure of proviruses from these two classes of oncogenic agents is illustrated in Fig. 10-2. Most known acute transforming retroviruses are defective; that is, they have lost part of the genes required for replication and hence require coinfection with a standard helper retrovirus for propagation. Such defects result from the replacement of replicative genes of the virus by an oncogene that mediates the direct transforming properties of the virus. Although there is variability as to which segment of the viral genome is replaced by the oncogene, a common configuration for acute transforming retroviruses is as depicted in Fig. 10-2. In this case, the oncogene is fused to a 5' portion of the viral *gag* gene, resulting in the synthesis of a transforming protein that contains *gag* peptides at its amino terminus.

Table 10-1 lists some viral oncogenes (designated by their acronyms), the natural host species, and the types of tumors they induce. In the case of the Rous sarcoma virus, the role of the *src* gene in neoplastic transformation was established by genetic and biochemical means. Mutations that cause reversible inactivation of the *src* gene product at elevated temperature (temperature-sensitive mutations) bring about a reversal of the transformed phenotype to the normal state when infected cells are exposed to elevated temperatures. When the temperature is lowered, the cells again revert to the transformed state. Likewise, deletions of the *src* gene destroy the ability of this virus to induce acute neoplasms. Similar but less complete data exist for other viruses listed in Table 10-1. A small number of acute transforming viruses contain a second oncogene which enhances the transforming activity of the principal viral oncogene. Two important examples are *erb*A, which cooperates with *erb*B in avian erythroblastosis virus, and *ets*, which accompanies *myb* in the E-26 strain of avian myeloblastosis virus.

Almost all the acute transforming viruses can be detected in vitro by their ability to induce transformation of cultured cells. The standard assay is the formation by infected fibroblasts (or fibroblast-like cell lines) of morphologically altered cells. Some of the leukemia-inducing viruses can transform macrophages and/or hematopoietic cells in vitro.

PROTO-ONCOGENES The oncogenes of retroviruses are closely related to normal cellular genes. This relationship was deduced from the discovery of nucleotide sequence homology between the transforming oncogene of Rous sarcoma virus, v-*src* (viral-*src*), and a normal chicken gene, c-*src* (cellular-*src*). Apparently, Rous sarcoma virus originated from a recombination event between c-*src* and an ancestral standard avian retrovirus. This mechanism, recombination between a viral gene and a gene of host origin, is the apparent explanation for the formation of the transforming viruses listed in Table 10-1. The function of the normal genes and their role in nonviral tumor formation is, therefore, a subject of intense interest and investigation.

The normal forms of the oncogenes are highly conserved in nature. There are human homologues of each, and homologues of some are present in all eukaryotic organisms, including invertebrate species and yeasts. This conservation implies that these genes have vital functions in normal cells and suggests that the oncogenic potential of the genes is acquired only after functionally significant alteration (such as occurs from recombination with a retrovirus). Such genes are referred to as *proto-oncogenes*.

The nucleotide sequences of the protein coding regions of viral oncogenes differ from those of the proto-oncogenes. There are also major differences in the regulation of expression of the viral and cellular genes. For example, the normal cellular form of an oncogene can be expressed without transforming the cell, although usually at a lower level and/or in a more strictly regulated fashion than are viral oncogenes expressed from proviruses. The contributions of overexpression, altered regulation, and structural mutation to the transforming activity of viral oncogenes may all be important to degrees that vary with the individual oncogene and target cell type.

Infection with retroviruses that lack oncogenes can induce neoplastic disease in some animals after a long latent period. A common

TABLE 10-1　Viral oncogenes that cause acute transformation

Name	Virus	Tumors in vivo
AVIAN		
src	Rous sarcoma virus (RSV)	Sarcomas
yes	Y73 sarcoma virus	Sarcomas
fps/fes	Fujinami sarcoma virus	Sarcomas
ros	UR11 avian sarcoma virus	Sarcomas
erbB, erbA	Avian erythroblastosis virus (AEV)	Erythroid leukemia
myb	Avian myeloblastosis virus (AMV)	Myeloid leukemia
myc	Avian myelocytomatosis virus (MC-29)	Leukemia, endothelioma
ski	Avian SKV770 virus	Unknown
jun	Avian sarcoma virus 17	Sarcomas
crk	Avian sarcoma virus CT10	Sarcomas
sea	Avian sarcoma virus S-13	Erythroid leukemia
rel	Reticuloendotheliosis virus (REV)	Lymphomas
MOUSE		
abl	Abelson leukemia virus	B lymphomas
mos	Moloney murine sarcoma virus (MoMSV)	Sarcomas
fos	FBJ osteosarcoma virus	Osteosarcoma
raf	3611 murine sarcoma virus	Sarcomas
RAT		
Ha-ras^1	Harvey murine sarcoma virus (HaMSV)	Sarcomas, erythroid leukemia
Ki-ras^2	Kirsten murine sarcoma virus (KiMSV)	Sarcomas, erythroid leukemia
CAT		
fes/fps	Snyder Thielen feline sarcoma virus (ST-FeSV)	Sarcomas
fms	McDonough feline sarcoma virus (SM-FeSV)	Sarcomas
fgr	Gardner-Rasheed feline sarcoma virus (GR-FeSV)	Sarcomas
kit	HZ4 feline sarcoma virus (HZ4-FeSV)	Sarcomas
MONKEY		
sis	Simian sarcoma virus (SSV)	Sarcomas

TABLE 10-2　Known and putative proto-oncogenes activated in tumors by nearby integration of retroviral proviruses

Target gene or locus	Virus	Tumor
c-myc	Avian leukosis virus	B-cell lymphomas (chicken)
c-myc	Feline leukemia virus	Lymphomas (cat)
c-myb	Murine leukemia virus	Myeloid leukemia (mouse)
c-myb	Avian leukemia	B-cell lymphoma (chicken)
c-erbB	Avian leukosis virus	Erythroid leukemia (chicken)
Pim-1, Mis-1, c-myc	AKR-murine leukemia virus	T-cell lymphoma (mouse)
Mlvi-1, Mlvi-2, Mlvi-3	Moloney murine leukemia virus	T-cell lymphoma (rat)
Int-1, Int-2, Int-3	Mouse mammary tumor virus	Mammary adenocarcinoma (mouse)
Evi-1, fim-3	Friend murine leukemia virus	Myeloid leukemia (mouse)

may alter host cell behavior in humans. Infection with a different group of retroviruses, human immunodeficiency viruses (HIV), causes the acquired immunodeficiency syndrome. Normal human DNA contains sequences that appear to be proviruses and that are genetically transmitted in the germ line. Their pathologic significance is unknown.

A number of types of DNA viruses induce abnormal host cell growth through the action of viral genes that, in contrast to retroviral oncogenes, are not closely related to host cellular genes. Two important examples in humans are Epstein-Barr virus (EBV), which is implicated in both endemic African Burkitt's lymphoma and nasopharyngeal carcinoma, and certain strains of human papillomavirus (HPV) which appear to be etiologic factors in anogenital cancer. In addition, hepatitis B virus (HBV) infection is associated with hepatocellular carcinoma, and herpes simplex viruses (HSV) have been implicated by some investigators in cervical carcinoma. The mechanism of these possible oncogenic effects is at present not known.

ACTIVATION OF CELLULAR ONCOGENES IN HUMAN NEOPLASMS DETECTED BY TRANSFECTION **The transfection assay for oncogenes**　Certain established cell lines have the property of incorporating exogenous DNA into chromosomal DNA with an efficiency that makes experimental gene transfer practical in tissue culture. The transfection technique commonly involves precipitating the DNA onto the surface of the target cells with calcium phosphate. The uptake of the DNA into cells by pinocytosis follows. Some of the ingested DNA molecules are transported to the cell nucleus where they are integrated into chromosomal DNA. If the transfected DNA contains a gene that can be expressed as a dominant, selectable marker in the recipient cells, transfected cells expressing this trait can be recovered. Many of the viral oncogenes in Table 10-1 can induce transformation in this type of assay. Such transformation can be achieved either with cloned oncogene DNA or with total chromosomal DNA from cells transformed by retroviruses.

Activated cellular oncogenes can also be detected by this technique in the DNA of tumors not known to be induced by viruses. For example, DNA from chemically transformed animal cells and DNA from a variety of naturally occurring animal and human tumor cells contain transforming genes. Normal high-molecular-weight human DNA does not transform cells, while DNA from neoplastic cells in some instances may induce transformation in tissue culture and/or by outgrowth of tumors in animals receiving transfected cells.

The ras family of cellular oncogenes　Some of the transforming genes detected by transfection of cells with DNA from human tumor cells have been identified (Table 10-3). The most common oncogenes

mechanism for the oncogenic activity is the activation of cellular proto-oncogenes, as illustrated by the induction of lymphomas in the bursa of Fabricius of chickens by avian leukosis virus (ALV). In these neoplasms, a proto-oncogene called c-myc is expressed at high levels as a result of the integration of the promoter-enhancer of the ALV genome near c-myc. Table 10-2 lists cellular proto-oncogenes that are known to be activated in retrovirus-induced neoplasms of long latency. Some (myc, myb, and erbB) are homologues of known viral oncogenes. Others (Int-1, Int-2, Int-3, Pim-1, Mis-1, Mlvi-1, Mlvi-2, Mlvi-3, fim-3, and Evi-1) have not been identified as a part of the genomes of acute-transforming viruses. Their oncogenic potential, originally inferred by analogy, has been demonstrated recently in some cases by cloning and expression in experimental test systems.

HUMAN ONCOGENIC VIRUSES　Human T-cell leukemia viruses (HTLV) are retroviruses that replicate preferentially in human lymphocytes. Infection with HTLV type I is associated with the development of a specific type of adult T-cell leukemia that occurs with increased frequency in southern Japan and the Caribbean basin. In vitro infection of human T cells by HTLV-I in culture confers a capacity for growth that is independent of exogenous T-cell growth factors (immortalization). The HTLVs do not appear to contain a host cell–related oncogene. Instead, unique transacting viral regulatory genes have been shown to have oncogenic potential in animals and belong to a family of genes called *ras*. The first to be identified was the human homologue of the oncogene of Harvey murine sarcoma virus (Table 10-1) called c-*ras*^{H}, which codes for a protein of molecular weight 21,000 called p21 and is activated in a human cell line derived from bladder carcinoma. In cells transformed by Harvey sarcoma virus, p21 is expressed at high levels, and high-level expression of c-*ras*^{H} by experimental linkage of the cellular gene to viral regulatory elements is sufficient to induce cellular transformation. Nevertheless, c-*ras*^{H} is not expressed at high levels in those human tumor cell lines in which it is detectable. Instead, the ability of c-*ras* gene to transform cells is conferred by point mutations that cause amino acid changes either at amino acid positions 12, 13, or 61 of the p21 protein.

These activating mutations can be detected by techniques employing synthetic oligonucleotide probes which are convenient for screening large numbers of human tumor samples. By this approach it was found that a second member of the *ras* family is more frequently activated in human tumors, e.g., the human homologue of the transforming gene of the Kirsten murine sarcoma virus called c-*ras*^{K}. For example, about one-third of human colorectal cancers and most carcinomas of the exocrine pancreas contain mutations predominantly at codon 12. Activation of c-*ras*^{K} is also described in a variety of other human neoplasms. The protein encoded by c-*ras*^{K} is also a p21 molecule, and this activating mutation in p21 is not present in normal tissues of individuals with carcinomas containing an activated c-*ras*^{K} gene, suggesting that activation is a somatic event that occurs during tumor formation. Finally, in transfection experiments and mutational analysis of some tumors activation of a third member of this family, called *ras*^{N}, was detected. For example, mutation of *ras*^{N} occurs in 10 to 20 percent of human acute myeloid leukemias.

Fibroblast growth factor (FGF)–related oncogenes A second group of related oncogenes, called K-*fgf*, *hst*, and FGF-3, has recently been detected in some human tumor DNAs. These are highly conserved genes with extensive homology both to the known mitogens' acid and basic FGF and to the *Int*-2 proto-oncogene activated in mouse adenocarcinomas by mouse mammary tumor virus (Table 10-2). The transforming activity of these genes can be activated by overexpression. The clinical associations of abnormal expression of the FGF family are still being defined.

TABLE 10-3 Oncogenes implicated in human neoplasia

Oncogene	Tumor
By tumor DNA transfection assay:	
c-*ras*^{H}	Rare occurrence, bladder, lung, mammary carcinosarcoma
c-*ras*^{K}	About 10–20% of many types of neoplasms and most pancreatic carcinomas
c-*ras*^{N}	About 10–20% of acute myeloid leukemia, occasionally other tumors
hst-1, (K-*fgf*, FGF-3)	Stomach, colon, and liver carcinoma, Kaposi's sarcoma*
abl, *met*, *trk*, *mos*	Various individual observations†
By chromosomal translocation:	
c-*myc*	Burkitt's lymphoma (>90%), T-cell lymphoma (occasionally)
c-*abl*	Chronic myelogenous leukemia (>90%), acute lymphocytic leukemia (10–20%)
bcl-2	Follicular lymphoma (90%), diffuse lymphoma (20%)
By DNA amplification or other overexpression:	
c-*erb*B	Gliomas
*erb*B-2 (*neu*, HER-2)	Breast cancer†
hst-1, *bcl*-1, *Int*-2	Breast cancer†
N-*myc*, C-*ras*^{N}	Neuroblastoma†
N-*myc*, L-*myc*, c-*myc*	Small cell carcinoma of the lung†
By loss of heterozygosity (recessive oncogene):	
Rb-1	Retinoblastoma, breast cancer*

* Association with specific tumors and/or incidence yet to be established.
† Putative marker of poor prognosis and/or advanced disease.

ONCOGENES IMPLICATED IN HUMAN TUMOR FORMATION A major line of evidence for the activation of oncogenes during tumor formation is derived from the analysis of cytogenetic changes in human neoplasms. Most human tumors are clonal or oligoclonal, that is, composed of cell populations dominated by the progeny of single cells. The dominant cell clones of certain neoplasms are marked by consistent chromosomal abnormalities, such as reciprocal translocations between chromosomes 9 and 22 in chronic myelogenous leukemia (producing the Philadelphia chromosome, Ph^1) or between chromosomes 8 and 14 in Burkitt's lymphoma. Indeed, characteristic nonrandom chromosomal changes have been identified in many neoplasms. Genes at or near the site of the DNA rearrangements underlying these cytogenetic changes are thought to play a role in the development of the tumors. Advances in in situ hybridization and other techniques of somatic cell genetics along with molecular cloning have made it possible to locate the cytogenetic positions of a number of proto-oncogenes on human chromosomes and to demonstrate that some of these genes are located near or at the breakpoints of chromosomes that are translocated in particular tumors.

Rearrangement of the c-*myc* locus in Burkitt's lymphoma The human c-*myc* gene is located on chromosome 8. This chromosome is invariably involved in a translocation in Burkitt's lymphoma. At the DNA level the translocation involves recombination between the c-*myc* locus on chromosome 8 and an immunoglobulin gene locus, usually near a heavy chain gene on chromosome 14, less often near a light chain gene on chromosomes 2 or 22. The specific region of the breakpoint at c-*myc* on chromosome 8 differs between the sporadic, EBV-negative, American and European Burkitt's lymphoma and the endemic, EBV-positive, African form of the disease. In both types this translocation does not appear to affect the structure of the protein-coding portion of the c-*myc* locus but instead affects the regulation of its expression.

Alteration of c-*abl* by chromosomal translocation in chronic myelogenous leukemia and acute lymphoblastic leukemia The Ph^1 chromosome is present both in leukemic cells and in normal marrow cell lineages from 90 to 95 percent of patients with chronic myelogenous leukemia (CML). In this disease, the marrow and peripheral blood are thought to be populated by the progeny of a hematopoietic stem cell that retains its ability to differentiate into red cells, megakaryocytes, and granulocytes. The proliferation of granulocytes, however, is abnormal and excessive, producing the clinical manifestations of CML. Genes whose expression is altered as a consequence of the formation of the Ph^1 chromosome are strong candidates for involvement in the development of CML. The human homologue of the proto-oncogene c-*abl* (Table 10-1) is located near the breakpoint on chromosome 9 for the 9-22 translocation and is transferred to chromosome 22 in the exchange. The additional Ph^1 chromosomes that sometimes appear in blastic crisis of CML result from duplication of the original Ph^1 chromosome. Amplification of the translocation region can also occur within the Ph^1 chromosome. The protein gene product of the c-*abl* locus in CML cells is a distinct fusion product of the c-*abl* gene and a gene called *bcr* (breakpoint cluster region) at the breakpoint on chromosome 22 of the recombinant Ph^1 chromosome. This hybrid *bcr/abl* gene product is a tyrosine protein kinase of 210,000 mol wt.

The Ph^1 chromosome also appears in 5 to 20 percent of acute lymphoblastic leukemias. The 9-22 recombination event in about half of these cases is located differently than is seen in CML, and produces a distinct *bcr/abl* fusion gene associated with a high level of expression of an *abl*-derived tyrosine protein kinase of 185,000 mol wt.

Translocations in non-Hodgkin's lymphoma The most consistent cytogenetic abnormality in this group of lymphoproliferative diseases is a 14-18 translocation which joins the immunoglobulin heavy chain locus on chromosome 14 to a gene of unknown function called *bcl*-2 on chromosome 18. This event occurs in nearly 90 percent of low-grade follicular lymphomas in the United States and a smaller fraction, about 20 percent, of diffuse large cell lymphomas. Other translocations, including an 11-14 translocation at a locus called *bcl*-1 in B-cell neoplasms and 8-14 translocation in T-cell lymphomas, have been described. The latter event joins the c-*myc* locus on chromosome 8 to a T-cell receptor gene on chromosome 14.

Overexpression of proto-oncogenes in human tumors An increase in gene copy number per cell (gene amplification) can sometimes be manifested at the cytogenetic level by the formation of small chromosome-like structures called *double minute chromosomes* or by the appearance of homogeneous staining regions (HSRs) on regular chromosomes. HSRs are the result of amplification of segments of DNA within the chromosome to the extent that they are identifiable cytogenetically. As a consequence, the structure contains multiple copies of the gene(s) encoded by the DNA segment. Gene amplification in nontransformed cells can sometimes be induced by growing cells under special conditions. For example, cells containing an amplification of the dihydrofolate reductase gene, which is required for DNA replication, can be selected when cells are grown in the presence of low levels of methotrexate, an inhibitor of dihydrofolate reductase. This increase in gene copy number enhances the amount of enzyme in the cell and overcomes the effects of the inhibitor. Double minute chromosomes and HSRs are present in a variety of tumor cells, suggesting that genes critical to the growth of neoplastic cells may amplify during tumor formation.

The first amplified oncogene recognized in a human tumor cell was the c-*myc* gene, which was expressed at a high level in one case of promyelocytic leukemia, both in fresh tumor cells and in a derived cell line. Amplification of c-*myc* appears to be a rare event in this neoplasm and has not been observed in other promyelocytic leukemias. However, double minute chromosomes, amplification of c-*myc* genes, and elevated levels of c-*myc* RNA have been reported in some gastric cancers and small cell carcinomas of the lung. Human neuroblastomas are characterized by a high frequency of double minute chromosomes and HSRs. A gene called N-*myc* which is related to the c-*myc* gene is amplified and/or expressed at a high level in most neuroblastomas. This overexpression correlates with more advanced stages of the disease. Similarly amplification of N-*myc* and a third family member, L-*myc,* in small cell carcinoma of the lung correlates strongly with disease progression. A distinct relative of the *erb*B oncogene (Table 10-2) called c-*erb*B-2 (or *neu* or HER-2), originally detected as an activated transforming gene in chemically induced rat neuroglioblastoma, is amplified in 10 to about 30 percent of human breast cancers. Amplification of c-*erb*B-2 in breast cancer is reported to correlate with poor prognosis. Several oncogenes located on chromosome 11 at band q13, including *int*-2, *hst*-1, and *bcl*-1, have also been reported to be amplified in poor-prognosis breast cancer and a variety of metastatic tumors. The c-*erb*B gene is closely related to or identical with the gene for the receptor for epidermal growth factor (EGF). Amplification and rearrangement of the EGF receptor gene has also been implicated in the formation of human primary gliomas.

RECESSIVE ONCOGENES IN HUMAN NEOPLASIA Dominant oncogenes are not the only mechanism by which tumors arise. The activation of dominant oncogenes is usually a late event associated with widespread disease and metastasis, suggesting that other events may initiate malignant growth. A clue that there might be another class of oncogenes comes from epidemiologic studies of families with inherited forms of cancer. Within these families tumors that usually occur sporadically in the general population are clustered in affected family members. In the early 1970's Knudson and Comings postulated that if *both* copies of a given gene had to be altered before tumor formation occurred, these families might be at such high risk because affected members had inherited *one* altered copy in all cells. Only one further alteration in the hundreds of million cells present in a susceptible tissue would be required to initiate abnormal proliferation. Since dominant oncogenes are inappropriately activated growth stimulatory genes (that are not influenced by the remaining normal copies of the original growth stimulatory genes) it is not surprising that dominant oncogenes have never been linked to the familial cancer syndromes. It was necessary instead to infer the

FIGURE 10-3 Mechanisms of loss of the *Rb* gene function. Patients with familial retinoblastoma have one mutant *Rb* allele at conception and therefore all cells have only one wild type *Rb* gene. One single further event in the target cell, either loss of the wild type allele or generation of a second mutant, results in there being no functional *Rb* protein. Patients with sporadic retinoblastoma must undergo at least two mutational events to inactivate the two normal *Rb* alleles. (*Adapted from Friend et al 1988, N Engl J Med.*)

presence of another class of oncogenes termed "recessive oncogenes" or "antioncogenes." Unlike the dominant oncogenes that are a normal part of growth stimulatory pathways, recessive oncogenes must function normally to limit the growth of cells. When both copies are inactivated, tumors are able to occur. Additional evidence suggesting the presence of such genes came from experiments showing that fusion of normal cells with tumor cells generally leads to loss of the malignant phenotype. This would not occur if dominant oncogenes determined the transformed phenotype. However, reversion would be expected if the fusion reintroduced a normal growth-limiting gene into a tumor cell containing inactivated growth-limiting genes.

The first recessive oncogene to be isolated was the retinoblastoma gene *Rb*. It is so named because families with affected members carrying one inactivated copy of the Rb gene almost invariably present with a malignant retinoblastoma of the eye before age 3. A model of the difference between the sporadic and inherited forms of retinoblastoma is shown in Fig. 10-3. The *Rb* gene is located on a subregion of the long arm of chromosome 13 and encodes a 928-amino acid, 205-kDa nuclear phoshoprotein that binds DNA nonspecifically. Tumor formation is a result of a wide range of alterations of the gene, including deletions, point mutations, and insertions that differ for each tumor. Because of this diversity no one probe can be used to detect the alteration as is done, for example, in the detection of sickle cell disease. Nevertheless, the *Rb* gene is altered in all retinoblastoma samples that have been studied at the protein level, and it is likely that inactivation of the *Rb* gene is necessary and sufficient to induce abnormal retinal cell proliferation. Proof that the gene isolated is in fact the *Rb* gene was obtained by demonstrating that the *Rb* gene can act as a tumor suppressor and stop the growth of tumor cells that lack the normal allele.

The *Rb* gene is frequently altered in other tumors as well. Soft tissue sarcomas and osteosarcomas occur at higher frequencies in families with hereditary retinoblastoma, and these tumors frequently exhibit inactivation of the *Rb* gene. The majority of small cell lung carcinomas and bladder carcinomas also have changes at the *Rb*

TABLE 10-4 Location of potential recessive oncogenes and their association with specific tumors

Chromosome location	Associated tumors
2	Uveal melanoma
3p	Renal cell carcinoma, small cell carcinoma lung, von-Hippel Lindau
5q	Colon, leukemia
10	Gliomas, MEN type 2A
11p	Ductal breast carcinoma, Wilms' tumor, rhabdomyosarcoma
11	
13q14	Retinoblastoma, osteosarcoma, soft tissue sarcomas, small cell carcinoma lung, bladder carcinoma, ductal breast carcinoma
17p	Colon, osteosarcoma, astrocytoma
18q	Colon
22	Bilateral acoustic neurofibromatosis, meningioma

locus. However, these tumors do not occur at higher frequencies in families with hereditary retinoblastoma.

Inactivation of the *Rb* gene is due to structural alterations at the DNA level. The DNA tumor virus transforming proteins use a different mechanism and inactivate the *Rb* gene at a functional level. DNA tumor viruses (such as SV40, adenovirus, and the papilloma virus) have proteins that allow these viruses to transform cells. Mutations that prevent binding of these transforming proteins to specific cellular genes destroy their ability to carry out transformation. The Rb gene product p105 is one of the cellular proteins that bind these transforming proteins, and therefore it is believed that these DNA tumor viruses inactivate recessive oncogenes, including the *Rb* gene, as a mechanism of transformation. Thus, inactivation of recessive oncogenes is probably the way in which the human papilloma viruses potentiate cervical carcinomas.

Nine other putative recessive oncogenes have been detected. Table 10-4 shows their chromosomal location and the tumors with which they are associated. In each case their presence has been suggested in one of two ways. The strongest indications have come from linkage studies among the familial forms of these tumors. In these families there are specific chromosomal subregions that can be directly linked with a predisposition to the respective tumors. The other indications have come from comparing normal and tumor DNA for loss of specific DNA markers in the transition to the malignant phenotype. Both criteria have been met for some tumors such as bilateral acoustic

neurofibromatosis. There are tumors for which it is virtually certain that recessive oncogenes play a role. Beyond the *Rb* gene, *p53* is the only other recessive oncogene that has been isolated. It is located on chromosome 17, encodes a nuclear phosphoprotein, and is inactivated in sarcomas, brain tumors, and colon cancer.

Whereas retinal cells are transformed by the inactivation of a single recessive oncogene, this simple model will probably not apply to most other tumors. Bladder cancer, small cell carcinoma of the lung, and colon cancer undergo multiple changes, apparently including both inactivation of several recessive oncogenes and activation of dominant oncogenes within the cells. Such complexity hampers the ability to link the inactivation of specific recessive oncogenes with determinants of diagnosis and prognosis. Eventually, the recessive oncogenes are likely to define growth stimulatory pathways of the dominant oncogenes.

FUNCTIONS OF ONCOGENES Studies of the proteins encoded by the viral oncogenes and their normal cellular homologues have provided insight into the functions of these genes. The protein product of the v-*src* gene of Rous sarcoma virus acts as a tyrosine protein kinase, and the oncogenic properties of v-*src* depend upon this enzymatic activity. The viral oncogene proteins of *yes* and *fgr* (Table 10-1) and a series of cellular genes (*fyn, lyn, lck, hck*) are structurally related to the *src* protein and form a subfamily of tyrosine protein kinases. The *abl* gene product is the prototype of a second subfamily of tyrosine protein kinases which includes those encoded by *fes/fps* viral oncogenes and a human cellular gene, ARG. In addition *raf*, *mos*, and *pim*-1 viral and cellular oncogenes encode serine-threonine protein kinases. The problem has been to identify the cellular proteins that are modified by these cytoplasmic kinases and that are critical for transformation. For example, in cells transformed by Rous sarcoma virus, a number of cellular proteins are modified by the addition of phosphate groups to tyrosine residues, but a specific role for such changes in oncogenesis has not been established.

Growth factors and receptors (See also Chap. 9) An important conceptual advance has come from separate lines of research on oncogene function and growth factor function (Fig. 10-4). The proliferation and differentiation of normal cells are regulated by signals derived from the binding of growth factors to receptors on the cell surface. Three of the better characterized growth factors are platelet-derived growth factor (PDGF), which promotes the growth of connective tissue and smooth muscle cells; epidermal growth factor (EGF), which is required for optimal growth of epithelial cells in vitro; and fibroblast growth factors (acid and basic FGF), which can act as fibroblast mitogens. The receptors for PDGF and EGF are transmembrane proteins that possess a tyrosine protein kinase activity within their cytoplasmic domain that is activated by binding of PDGF or EGF (see Fig. 9-1). More recently hematopoietic and lymphoid

FIGURE 10-4 Relationships between the molecular biology of growth factors and the functions of oncogenes. Growth factors are small molecules that signal cell activation, replication, and differentiation by binding to specific receptors on the surface of target cells. As shown, a number of the proteins made by oncogenes fit into the general pathway for growth factor activity. Oncogenes may transform cells by transmitting a constitutive, unregulated signal for cell growth from their particular position in the pathway. For details see text.

growth factor genes have been isolated including those for several colony-stimulating factors and interleukins.

In addition to the FGF-related oncogenes mentioned before, a protein encoded by the viral oncogene of simian sarcoma virus, *sis*, is closely related to PDGF. In addition, the *fms* oncogene of a strain of feline sarcoma virus is an altered form of the receptor of a macrophage growth factor called colony-stimulating factors (CSF-1). As mentioned before, the *erb*B oncogene is an altered form of the receptor for EGF which can produce a transforming growth signal without normal binding to the growth factor. The cellular oncogenes c-*erb*B-2 (*neu*, HER-2), *trk*, *met*, and *ret* all have growth factor receptor–like properties. These observations have led to the postulate that the unregulated growth signal involved in neoplastic transformation might result from changes in growth factors, their receptors, or other elements in the pathway. An elaboration of this concept derives from the observation that transformed cells sometimes secrete novel growth factors as a secondary change. Examples are tumor cell growth factors alpha and beta (TGF-α and -β), which can induce transformed morphology and growth of normal cells that are reversible with removal of the growth factor. Thus, autocrine and paracrine stimulation of growth by such factors may contribute to tumorigenesis.

Ras oncogene proteins   The proteins encoded by *ras* oncogenes are associated with the inner surface of the cell membrane. They share a functional activity, the binding of guanosine triphosphate (GTP), with a family of GTP-binding or G proteins on the inner surface of the cell membrane that participate in the transmission of signals from the cell surface (see Chap. 68). Mutations that activate the transforming potential of *ras* gene alter the interaction of *ras* proteins with guanine nucleotide substrates. Thus, transforming *ras* proteins are a class of G proteins that transmit a constitutive growth signal.

Oncogene proteins in the cell nucleus   The proteins encoded by six of the oncogenes in Table 10-1, *myb, myc, ski, jun, erb*A, and *fos*, act in the cell nucleus. The normal homologue of *myb* is expressed at low levels and is cell cycle–regulated in many cell types, but is expressed at high levels independent of cell cycles in early T-cell, B-cell, and hematopoietic progenitors. Expression of *myc* family genes is elevated in many developing tissues during embryogenesis, but only c-*myc* itself is expressed in most or all lineages in postnatal life. Expression of c-*myc* and c-*fos* can be closely tied to the growth factor pathways. When growth-arrested fibroblasts are exposed to PDGF, a specific set of genes is expressed, including the proto-oncogenes c-*fos* and c-*myc*, and cellular messenger RNA and protein levels for these genes increase. Expression of c-*myc* is also enhanced in resting B and T lymphocytes after exposure to appropriate mitogens. Once cells enter the growth cycle, the expression of c-*myc* remains constant. When cells lose the ability to divide, for example, in postmitotic differentiated cells, c-*myc* expression decreases or ceases. The protein of the cellular *jun*A gene is a DNA-binding protein closely related or identical to a transcription factor for many genes called AP-1, and the c-*fos* protein has been found in nuclear protein complexes in association with AP-1. The *erb*A protein is a high-affinity nuclear receptor for thyroid hormone. This complex and rapidly evolving picture suggests that nuclear oncogenes may play pivotal roles in setting patterns of gene expression. They may function normally as regulators of cell "activation," growth, and differentiation and may be nuclear targets for growth factor–derived signals. When altered or deregulated, they may provide a constitutive drive for the uncontrolled cell growth and abnormal differentiation that characterize the neoplastic state.

EXPERIMENTAL INTRODUCTION OF ACTIVE ONCOGENES INTO CELLS   One approach to establishing experimental animal models for analysis of human tumor-associated oncogenes is to transfer activated oncogenes into normal cells in vivo and to observe the effects of these genes on development. Several different genes, such as those specifying immunoglobulin and growth hormone, have been introduced by microinjection into fertilized mouse eggs. The injected "transgenes" become integrated into the genome of progeny mice

and, in some cases, are expressed in appropriate cell types (for example, immunoglobulin transgenes are expressed predominantly in B lymphocytes).

The introduction by this technique of a T-antigen gene from the DNA tumor virus SV40 into the germ line of mice resulted in the formation of choroid plexus papillomas. Likewise, the introduction of activated *neu* (*erb*B-2, HER-2) transgenes with promoter-enhancer sequences derived from mouse mammary tumor virus into the germ line of mice uniformly caused the development of polyclonal mammary adenocarcinomas involving the entire mammary epithelium. In contrast, an analogous c-*myc* transgene acted as a predisposing factor to the development of mammary adenocarcinoma in some mice. A *myc* transgene fused to immunoglobulin-regulating elements caused pre-B-cell proliferation preceding the development of B-cell lymphomas. Transgenic mice carrying a human c-*ras*H gene with an activating mutation fused to an elastase gene regulatory element develop adenocarcinoma of the exocrine pancreas shortly after pancreatic differentiation.

Introduction into transplantable stem cells of bone marrow and lymphoid organs is done by infecting stem cells ex vivo with retrovirus-derived vectors containing the genes and then transplanting the cells into appropriately prepared hosts. The introduction of the v-*myc* gene by this technique into the stem cells of the chicken bursa induced preneoplastic proliferative lesions that precede the development of B-cell lymphomas. Introduction of hematopoietic growth factor genes, e.g., for interleukins and granulocyte-macrophage colony-stimulating factor (GM-CSF), using viral vectors into mouse marrow stem cells produces characteristic myeloproliferative changes.

ONCOGENES AND MULTISTAGED TUMORIGENESIS   Human cancer and chemically induced neoplasia in animals usually develop by a multistep process in which an abnormal preneoplastic cell type evolves into a cell population successively dominated by clones with increasingly malignant characteristics. This evolution of tumor development is thought to be preceded by a latent period, and the whole process may take a significant fraction of the life span of the affected individual. In contrast, acute transforming viruses carrying activated forms of oncogenes that are implicated in nonviral cancer appear to induce neoplasms within days or weeks, i.e., with kinetics that suggest a single-step process. This difference may be due to several factors. First, many of the viral oncogenes encode kinases with multiple cellular targets and may induce abrupt changes that would require several different mutations in more slowly evolving neoplasms. Second, expression of the viral oncogenes is driven by powerful regulatory elements (promoters and enhancers in the proviral LTRs). The transforming potential of the cellular homologues of these same genes can be activated by mechanisms that do not involve such high-level expression, for example, the point mutations at amino acids 12 or 61 of the proteins encoded by the human *ras* tumor-associated oncogenes. In these situations the concerted activity of several genes may be required to induce the same transformed phenotype that can be induced by very high level, unregulated expression of just one of the genes (as occurs with acute transforming retroviruses).

This point is illustrated by transfection experiments suggesting cooperation between oncogenes in inducing transformation of cultured fibroblasts. The activated *ras* genes from human tumor cells can transform immortalized cell lines but cannot induce full morphologic transformation of primary cell cultures. The combination of activated *myc* and *ras* gene clones, however, produces the fully transformed phenotype in primary cell cultures. Thus, in this system *myc* (and other oncogenes that do not alter these cells by themselves) can complement the transforming activation of human *ras* oncogenes. However, when powerful transcriptional enhancer sequences are engineered into the activated *ras* oncogene, this gene can itself transform primary fibroblast cultures, presumably because of a higher level of expression of the oncogene. The requirement for multiple genes in transformation may be conditioned, in part, by the level of oncogene expression, and more than one cellular oncogene may be activated in neoplasms in vivo.

IMPLICATIONS FOR CLINICAL ONCOLOGY

The clinical impact of the identification and analysis of human oncogenes and their products may be extensive, indeed, revolutionary. For example, efforts to identify and control environmental and nutritional factors that may cause or prevent cancer depend heavily on epidemiologic techniques, animal studies, and clinical trials where disease incidence and mortality are endpoints for measurement. Knowledge of the specific proto-oncogenes that are the targets of environmental carcinogens and of the nature of the changes induced may provide better methods for assessing the actual role of candidate carcinogens and for devising preventive approaches. Delineation of the molecular anatomy of neoplastic change in specific cell lineages will add new dimensions to diagnosis. Classification of disease on the basis of specific molecular changes (e.g., in CML, ALL, and non-Hodgkin's lymphomas) and detection of molecular changes associated with poor prognosis (e.g., in breast cancer) appear to hold promise for the immediate future. As the complex picture of the molecular mechanisms employed by oncogenes to transform cells is progressively revealed, it is reasonable to expect that this new knowledge will improve treatment by providing more precise and more specific means for targeting pharmacologic intervention.

REFERENCES

ALT TW et al (eds): Nuclear oncogenes, in *Current Communications in Molecular Biology*. Cold Spring Harbor Laboratory, New York, 1987

BISHOP JM: The molecular genetics of cancer. Science 235:305, 1987

DREAZEN O et al: The molecular biology of chronic myelogenous leukemia. Semin Hematol 25:35, 1988

FRIEND SH et al: Oncogenes and tumor-suppressing genes. N Engl J Med 318:618, 1988

KNUDSON AG: Hereditary cancer, oncogenes and anti-oncogenes. Cancer Res 45:1437, 1985

WEINBERG RA: The action of oncogenes in the cytoplasm and nucleus. Science 230:770, 1985

————: Finding the anti-oncogene. Sci Am 259:44, 1988

11 TRANSMEMBRANE SIGNALING BY RECEPTORS

CHARLES F. STEVENS

Our cells live in a watery world, and their life depends absolutely on the integrity of the barrier to water soluble molecules that defines the cell's boundaries, the cell membrane. Because this membrane is constructed of a phospholipid bilayer, it forms a virtually impregnable shield against the entry and exit of all hydrophilic molecules dissolved in the extracellular and intracellular aqueous environments. Although the surface membrane is necessary for the cell's existence, its very impregnability poses problems for the functioning of the cell: certain essential metabolites must, in a regulated way, be able to cross the membrane, and information about the outside environment must be communicated to the cell's interior. The first of these problems is solved by a variety of transport systems, and the second by a class of molecules, termed *receptors,* that are the subject of this chapter.

The term *receptor* is generally defined in two distinct ways. The *operational definition* identifies receptors by their binding characteristics; any cell surface molecule that binds tightly a specific molecular species is called a receptor for what is bound. "Receptors" identified in this way include a rather wide variety of functional types of molecules including such entities as cell adhesion molecules used to attach cells together and uptake proteins that transport molecules like glutamate across the surface membrane. In this chapter, the *functional definition* of receptors is used: a class of proteins residing in the cell's surface membrane that transmit information across the membrane

TABLE 11-1 The three receptor families

Receptor family	Typical receptor ligands	Primary signal	Typical signal results
Channel	Acetylcholine, glycine, GABA, glutamate	Ionic current	Voltage change in neuron
G protein coupled	Acetylcholine, GABA, norepinephrine, cholecystokinin, substance P	Activated G protein	Increased cyclic AMP levels and activation of A kinase
Tyrosine kinase	Insulin, platelet-derived growth factor	Phosphotyrosine residue	Enzyme activation leading to mitogenesis

about the presence of specific molecules outside the cell. Receptors, by this definition, are signaling molecules that inform the inside of the cell about the external environment.

Receptors fall into three categories according to their mechanism of signaling: channels, G protein–coupled receptors, and tyrosine kinases (Table 11-1). Doubtless additional categories will be added as more is learned about the relevant gene families responsible for encoding receptors. These three classes of receptors are considered in turn.

RECEPTORS INCORPORATING ION CHANNELS Four receptor channel types are now recognized, although others very likely exist. The four current classes, named by their ligand, are acetylcholine, glycine, gamma-aminobutyric acid (GABA), and glutamate receptor channels. The first three proteins have known sequences deduced from molecular genetic analysis of complementary DNA (cDNA) clones; molecular structures are not yet available for glutamate receptor channels. Within each class, a number of subclasses—perhaps half a dozen—are known.

Receptor channels are membrane-spanning proteins defined by their signaling mechanism: ligand binding induces a conformational change that opens a transmembrane aqueous pore in the receptor and permits ions to cross the membrane's lipid bilayer. The signal, then, is a voltage change produced by the ion flux; however, in one case, a type of glutamate receptor channel, a calcium ion influx and the resultant concentration change within the target cell constitute an important aspect of the signal. Which ions flow, and what voltage change occurs, depends on the channel type. Acetylcholine and glutamate receptor channels permit sodium and potassium ions to cross the membrane, and cause positive voltage changes (depolarization of the cell). One type of glutamate receptor channel, the one noted above, additionally permits a calcium ion influx. The GABA and glycine receptor channels let chloride ions permeate and, in the usual situation, produce negative voltages changes (hyperpolarization). Thus, acetylcholine and glutamate are excitatory, and GABA and glycine are inhibitory.

Receptor channels of one sort or other are universally present on neurons, where they subserve synaptic transmission. The ligand, a neurotransmitter such as acetylcholine, is released by presynaptic nerve impulses, and the receptor channels located in the postsynaptic membrane respond to the neurotransmitter to signal the arrival of the nerve impulses. Receptors of this type are found, in addition, on many other cell types such as muscle (where they function in neuromuscular transmission), secretory cells (where they are involved in excitation-secretion coupling), and lymphocytes (where they participate in the response to mitogens).

The nicotinic acetylcholine receptor channel is the best-studied example of this class. This receptor is a pentameric protein composed of four distinct subunits, each with a molecular mass on the order of 50 kDa, encoded by four different genes (Fig. 11-1). The subunits are all highly homologous and fit together like the staves of a barrel to form a membrane-spanning structure with a central pore that can be opened and closed by ligand binding–induced conformation change. Each of the subunits has an extracellular domain (where the ligand

FIGURE 11-1 Exploded view of an acetylcholine receptor channel. The subunits are thought to be arranged, as shown at the right, somewhat like staves of a barrel around a central pore through which the ion traffic flows. Each subunit is shaped much like the others even though they are encoded by separate genes. The far left part of the figure represents the four membrane-spanning peptide chains that constitute the portion of the subunit embedded in the membrane. Compare this structure with that of the G protein–coupled receptor illustrated in Fig. 68-1.

binds on one special subunit), four membrane-spanning regions, and a smaller, intracellular domain. The GABA and glycine receptor channels are proteins encoded by other membranes of the same gene superfamily and are believed to have the same general structure as the acetylcholine receptor.

A number of drugs act by disrupting channel function. For example, curare competes with acetylcholine for its binding site, strychnine similarly blocks glycine receptor channels, phencyclidine (angel dust) inhibits, by a different mechanism, the function of a subtype of glutamate receptor channel, and benzodiazepines enhance the effect of GABA on its receptor (see Chap. 346).

RECEPTORS COUPLED TO G PROTEINS   Very many receptors, dozens and possibly hundreds, are G protein coupled, with a signaling mechanism described below. These receptors, generally named according to a ligand they bind tightly, include ones that recognize peptides (e.g., β-endorphins, atrial natriuretic peptide, and chole-cystokinin), acetylcholine (muscarinic), biogenic amines (e.g., do-pamine and serotonin), amino acids (e.g., GABA and glutamate), and purines (e.g., adenosine). It should be emphasized that some of the same ligands, GABA and acetylcholine, for example, can activate both the receptor channels described above and the G protein–coupled receptors considered here. This situation can lead to terminologic confusion where two different entities have the same name. In many of these cases some further distinction is made. Thus, one speaks of GABA$_A$ and nicotinic acetylcholine receptors (channels) and also of GABA$_B$ and muscarinic acetylcholine receptors (G protein–coupled).

G protein–coupled receptors all work in basically the same way, but some variations on the general theme result finally in a very complex range of actions (see Chap. 68). In every case, ligand binding to the receptor produces a conformational change that causes an entity called a *G protein* to be converted from an inactive to an active form. The "G" in this name refers to guanosine di- or triphosphate (GDP, GTP) because activation of the G protein involves dissociating GDP and binding GTP at a special site. The active G protein then binds to a target and this leads to a final result, as described in more detail below. Much amplification of the original signal (ligand binding) occurs because a single receptor can activate many copies of a G protein, and each activated G protein can be used multiple times on its targets. A G protein remains active so long as it retains GTP in its binding site, and the active state is

terminated by an enzymatic activity of the G protein itself that converts the bound GTP into GDP (see also Chap. 68).

The complexity in action of G protein–coupled receptors arises from the fact that many distinct types of receptors can specifically activate different types of G proteins, of which about a dozen are presently recognized. These various G protein species can bind specifically to perhaps a dozen different intracellular targets. Further, different types of G proteins can exhibit antagonistic effects on their targets, thus one G protein species can stimulate whereas another can inhibit some target action. In addition, G protein targets, which are often enzymes, act on a wide range of secondary targets, and these targets can have still other sites of action so that a rather complex regulatory cascade results.

This general regulatory scheme is best understood in terms of a specific example: Norepinephrine causes the heart to beat more forcefully through the action of a G protein–coupled receptor, the beta-adrenergic receptor. An agonist binding to this receptor activates a G protein that in turn enables adenylate cyclase to convert ATP to cyclic AMP. The cyclic AMP produced by the adenylate cyclase then activates yet another enzyme, called *A kinase,* and this enzyme phosphorylates a particular membrane protein, a *calcium channel* (note that this channel is a member of a different superfamily than the receptor channels discussed above), responsible for letting calcium ions into the cardiac myocyte. The intracellular calcium ions act on the heart muscle contractile proteins to result in muscular contraction. The phosphorylated calcium channel permits more calcium ions to enter the myocyte each time the channel is turned on, and the larger influx of calcium ions produces a greater calcium concentration. This greater concentration results, by the law of mass action, in an increased activation of contractile proteins, that is, a more forceful heart beat.

In this example, the regulatory cascade has four levels. The primary target of the activated G protein is the enzyme adenylate cyclase, and this enzyme, through the cyclic AMP it produces, acts on a secondary target, the A kinase. The A kinase then phosphorylates the tertiary target, a calcium channel. This channel lets calcium ions enter in greater quantities when it is phosphorylated, and produces, by the calcium ion action on contractile proteins, the quaternary target, a stronger heart beat. Each G protein–coupled receptor acts through a regulatory cascade of this same general type. G protein actions are often hard to define, and difficult to keep straight, because the intracellular cascades have many levels, each with its own complexities.

Several generalizations can be made about the action of G protein–coupled receptors. First, the various G proteins themselves can be classified. For immediate purposes, the best classification is perhaps the simplest: Many G proteins are either stimulatory (G$_s$) or inhibitory (G$_i$) so that they constitute the accelerator and brake characteristic of all biologic regulatory systems. Second, the G proteins act, as far as is now known, on three distinct second-messenger systems: ion channels (membrane proteins responsible for electric excitability of cells), the cyclic AMP system, and the phosphoinositol (PI) turnover system. Some G proteins bind directly to certain channels to alter their function. G proteins also bind to adenylate cyclases (to make the second messenger, cyclic AMP) and to phospholipases, which break phospholipids into inositol-3-phosphate (IP3) and diacylglycerol (DAG), molecules that function as second messengers. Finally, IP3 and cyclic AMP activate kinases (designated C and A, respectively) that in turn phosphorylate various targets to alter their functions. These kinases act on a wide range of substrates and can affect cell electric excitability, activity of various enzyme systems, and expression of specific genes.

G protein–coupled receptors occur on all cell types and are especially common in the brain and gut. As might be expected, the nervous system expresses many different types of G protein–coupled receptors. The ligands for these receptors are contained in presynaptic vesicles and released by nerve activity. Although formerly ligands for all classes of receptors in the brain were called *neurotransmitters,* this term now is reserved generally for those ligands that bind to receptor channels. The ligands that bind to G protein–coupled receptors are termed *neuromodulators* to recognize that they operate through a mechanism different from that of neurotransmitters. Because the same chemical entity can bind to both receptor types, some ligands—acetylcholine, for example—are simultaneously neurotransmitters and neuromodulators.

Over a dozen G protein–coupled receptors, all members of the same gene family, have been cloned and sequenced, and more are on the way. The structures that have been determined include several adrenergic receptors, muscarinic acetylcholine receptors, serotonin receptors, peptide receptors (substance K, atrial natriuretic peptide, and angiotensin), a dopamine receptor, and rhodopsin (a photoreceptor molecule included because it is G protein–coupled and in the same gene family). In all cases, the receptors are monomeric proteins with an extracellular domain that binds ligand, an intracellular G protein–binding domain, and seven transmembrane helices. Because of the seven membrane-spanning helices, these receptors are known as members of the ''Magnificent Seven'' family. The precise nature of the conformational change that permits the G proteins to be activated has not been determined (see Chap. 68).

Many of the drugs that affect the brain—opiates and antipsychotics, for example—act on G protein–coupled receptors either as agonists or antagonists. Some G protein–coupled receptors are cellular homologues of oncogenes. (The angiotensin receptor was discovered through its homology to the *mas* oncogene and *ras* is a type of G protein.) The precise role of these signaling systems in cancer is, however, still not fully understood (see Chap. 10).

RECEPTORS WITH TYROSINE KINASE ACTIVITY Receptors in the third category phosphorylate tyrosine residues in themselves and in certain other proteins. This receptor family is usually considered to bind growth factors primarily, but some members constitute a link in the chain subserving the actions of hormones, such as insulin. Further, cell-cell interactions during development also make use of these receptors, but the mechanisms involved have not yet been extensively studied. Three main subfamilies of tyrosine kinase receptors have been identified: those related to the insulin receptor, to the epidermal growth factor (EDGF) receptor, and to the platelet-derived growth factor (PDGF) receptor (see Chap. 9).

Receptors in this family all work through tyrosine kinase activity that is enabled by ligand binding. Even now little is known about the targets for this kinase activity, nor is it understood just what these targets do. One clear target, however, is the receptor itself; these receptors autophosphorylate and thereby increase their own activity. Receptor activation often results in cell division and growth. The activated receptors affect various enzyme systems that facilitate mitogenesis and they also participate in the regulation of gene expression. The insulin receptor, of course, plays a role in normal cell function throughout life, but other related receptors are involved in determining cell fate during development.

All cells possess receptors in this class. The brain, as could be anticipated, is particularly richly endowed.

All receptors with tyrosine kinase activity have extracellular, transmembrane, and cytoplasmic domains, and all are rather large proteins with about a thousand amino acids. The extracellular domain binds agonist, characteristically quite tightly (n*M* dissociation constant), and the intracellular domain is the location of kinase activity. Unlike the receptors of the other classes described above, the tyrosine kinases appear to possess only a single membrane-spanning region. Members of the insulin receptor subfamily are composed of two distinct subunits, one of which contains the transmembrane segment and the tyrosine kinase activity, and the second of which is purely extracellular with the agonist binding site. Members of both the EDGF and PDGF families have ligand binding and tyrosine kinase activity within a single large polypeptide chain.

Although understanding of the mechanisms by which receptors of this type act is still quite limited, these molecules have attracted great interest because they are often the cellular homologues of oncogenes, and their activity promotes the expression of additional cytoplasmic oncogene homologues such as *myc* and *fos*. For example, the EDGF receptor is the cellular homologue of v-*Erb*B, and all of these receptor types belong to the same superfamily as do the *Src* and *Abl* families of oncogenes. Because of these connections, many workers believe that with increased understanding of the mechanisms through which this receptor category operates, insight into the pathogenesis of certain cancers will follow (see Chap. 10).

REFERENCES

HANKS SK et al: The protein kinase family: Conserved features and deduced phylogeny of the catalytic domains. Science 241:42, 1988

NEER EJ, CLAPHAM DE: Roles of G protein subunits in transmembrane signalling. Nature 333:129, 1988

UNWIN N et al: Arrangement of the acetylcholine receptor subunits in the resting and desensitized states, determined by cryoelectron microscopy of crystallized torpedo postsynaptic membranes. J Cell Biol 107:1123, 1988

12 BIOLOGY OF AGING

ITAMAR B. ABRASS

Over a third of patients seen by a primary-care physician are now older adults; this number will exceed 50 percent in the next century. The numbers of older adults (age 65 and older) in the United States have grown in absolute and relative terms both because of an increase in the mean life span and a decrease in birth rates. Growth in the group over age 75 is even more rapid. The result is a greater demand on the health care system (see also Chap. 4).

The gain in survival includes both active and dependent years. As mean life span has increased and maximum life span has remained unchanged, it has been widely assumed that the time of dependency will decrease as life expectancy increases. The available data do not support such an outcome. If anything, the mean prevalence of disability seems to be getting worse with time. These observations are in conflict with the widespread impression that older persons are now healthier and more active. In fact, there may be a bimodal distribution with some individuals getting healthier and others becoming more disabled as the result of survival with a problem that was previously fatal. It is important to define the factors that lead to ''successful'' aging. Delivering the needed health care and decreasing the time of disability present a challenge to both clinician and scientist.

With aging two phenomena occur: a physiologic decline and an increase in disease. Although these processes influence each other, physiologic decline occurs independently of disease.

In healthy older adults many physiologic functions are maintained in the basal resting state, but decrements in function occur in most organ systems and homeostatic mechanisms when the system is challenged or stressed. Furthermore, chronic disease of multifactorial etiology becomes more common with age. Mortality curves are exponential after the age of 30, with cardiovascular and neoplastic diseases being the commonest causes of death. However, even in the oldest, despite the prevalence of disease, the interaction of disease and physiological control mechanisms remains important. In such individuals the pathologist may identify many lesions without defining the cause of death. In fact, the cause of death may have been a relatively minor perturbation of homeostatic mechanisms.

MOLECULAR AND CELLULAR MECHANISMS OF AGING Theories of aging fall into two general categories: accumulation of damage to molecules or the regulation of specific genes.

DNA undergoes continuous change both in response to exogenous agents and intrinsic processes. Stability is maintained by the double strandedness of DNA that makes possible repair of change by specific repair enzymes. It has been proposed that biological aging is due to somatic mutagenesis, either due to greater susceptivility to mutagenesis or deficits in repair mechanisms. In fact, the longevity of different species correlates with DNA repair enzymes. However, in humans the spontaneous rate of mutagenesis is not adequate to account for the number of changes that take place, and there is no evidence that failure in repair functions causes aging.

A related theory, the error catastrophe theory, proposes that errors occur in DNA, RNA, and protein synthesis, each augmenting the other and finally culminating in an error catastrophe. Protein synthesis is considered the most likely source for age-dependent errors, since it is the final common pathway. However, increased translational errors have not been found in aging either in vivo or in vitro. Amino acid substitutions do not increase with age, although some enzyme activities may be altered by changes in posttranslational modification of proteins, such as glycosylation.

The major by-products of oxidative metabolism include superoxide radicals that can react with DNA, RNA, proteins, and lipids and lead to cellular damage and aging. Several scavenging enzymes and some small molecules, such as vitamin C and vitamin E, protect the cell from oxidative damage. There is no significant loss of scavenging enzymes in aging, and treatment with vitamins C and E does not increase longevity in experimental animals.

The most widely accepted concept of aging is that it is regulated by specific genes. Support for this hypothesis has been mostly gained from in vitro models of aging. In adulthood, cells can be divided into three categories based on their replicative capacity: continuously replicating, replicating in response to a challenge, and nonreplicating. Epidermal, gastrointestinal, and hematopoietic cells are continuously renewed; liver can regenerate in response to injury; and neurons and cardiac muscle and skeletal muscle do not regenerate.

In vitro replication is closely related to in vivo proliferation. Neurons and cardiac myocytes from adults can be maintained in culture but do not divide, whereas marrow cells, endothelial cells, and fibroblasts replicate in vitro. Since they are easily obtained from skin, fibroblasts have been the most extensively studied cell type. Although some cells replicate continuously in intact organisms, they have a finite replicative life. For fibroblasts in vitro, this is about 50 doublings. Replicative life in vitro also correlates with the age of the donor, so that the older the donor the fewer doublings. With time, doubling time increases, and ultimately cell division ceases.

When fibroblasts from younger donors are fused with nonreplicating senescent cells, DNA synthesis is inhibited in both old and young nuclei. Transient inhibition of protein synthesis immediately following fusion leads to increased DNA synthesis in both nuclei, suggesting that a protein factor in senescent cells may be involved in the inhibition of replication. When senescent cytoplasts (cells without nuclei) are fused with young, dividing cells, DNA synthesis is also depressed, suggesting that the inhibitory factor(s) is present in cytoplasm. Growth arrest both in vivo and in vitro is associated with the appearance of a specific protein that may be involved in DNA replication, and this protein is a candidate molecule for the inhibition in DNA synthesis associated with senescence.

These experiments help define the finite life span of cells in vitro but do not themselves explain aging in intact organisms, since organisms do not suddenly die because all cells stop replicating. However, factors associated with finite cell replication may indirectly influence in vivo aging. Fibroblasts aged in vitro or obtained from older adult donors are less sensitive to many growth factors at both the receptor and postreceptor levels. A decrease in these growth factors, a change in sensitivity to growth factors, and/or a slowing of the cell cycle may slow wound healing and perhaps place the older individual at greater risk for infection.

For tissues with nonreplicating cells, cell loss may lead to a permanent deficit. With aging, dopaminergic neurons are lost, impairing gait and balance and enhancing susceptibility to the side-effects of drugs. With further decrements such as ischemia or viral infection, Parkinson's disease may develop. Similar cell loss and/or functional deficits in other neurotransmitter systems may lead to autonomic dysfunction, alteration in mental function, and impairment of neuroendocrine control.

The immune system demonstrates similar phenomena with aging. Lymphocytes from older adults have a diminished proliferative response to mitogens. This diminished response may be due to a decrease in lymphokines and a decreased response to extracellular signals. As the thymus involutes postpuberty, thymic hormone (thymosins) levels decrease. With age basal and stimulated interleukin 2 (IL-2) production and responsiveness also diminish. The latter appears to be due, at least in part, to a decreased expression of IL-2 receptors. Some immune functions can be restored by the addition of these hormones to lymphocytes in vitro by their administration to intact, aged animals. The proliferative defect can also be reversed in vitro by calcium ionophores and activators of protein kinase C, suggesting that the T-cell defect may be in transduction of extracellular signals to intracellular function.

In vivo, molecular mechanisms such as those described above are believed to contribute to physiologic deficits and altered homeostatic mechanisms that predispose older individuals to dysfunction in the face of stress and disease.

PHYSIOLOGIC AGING   In assessing studies on physiologic function with age, several factors need to be considered: (1) In healthy older adults, decreases in function are usually demonstrable only under stress; (2) data generally represent means, and with aging there is usually a wide intragroup variability; and (3) most data are cross-sectional rather than longitudinal. It is also important to assess how health status was defined.

Cardiovascular   Early data suggested that cardiac output at rest declines progressively from about age 20 to age 90. However, such subjects were not screened for occult coronary artery disease. The findings are quite different when the population under scrutiny is screened for coronary artery disease with stress thallium images. In such a population, resting cardiac output in normals is unaffected by age from the 3rd to the 8th decades. Cardiac output during graded exercise is also unchanged with age. However, heart rate is decreased, and end-diastolic and end-systolic volumes increase with age. Thus, in the older subjects, cardiac output during exercise is maintained by utilization of the Frank-Starling mechanism. These individuals use reserve mechanisms to maintain cardiac output and may, therefore, be more vulnerable to decompensation when disease is superimposed.

These findings are also consistent with the concept that myocardial beta-adrenergic responsiveness decreases with age. Such changes occur in both humans and animals. Heart rate response to isoproterenol infusion decreases with age, and in animals, myocardial contractility also decreases. This deficit is related to beta-adrenergic mechanisms and not to intrinsic contractile capacity. Basal and stimulated norepinephrine levels increase with age. Whether the defect in beta-adrenergic responsiveness is due to desensitization by endogenous catecholamines or other age related phenomena is not known.

Older individuals also have decreased baroreceptor reflex sensitivity, i.e., cardiovascular responses to changes in intravascular volume are altered. Such changes may put the older patient at greater risk during rapid volume expansion and may contribute to the higher prevalence of orthostatic hypotension in older adults.

Pulmonary   Except for increases in residual volume, most pulmonary volumes are unaltered in healthy nonsmoking older adults. However, compliance increases and small airways tend to collapse as the elastic structures decrease. These changes in small airways lead to an increase in closing volumes such that by the mean age of 65 years not all the airways are opened during regular breathing in the sitting position. In the recumbent position, this phenomenon occurs by age 45. As a consequence, older individuals are more prone to develop atelectasis and pneumonia particularly when lying in bed for prolonged periods of time.

Endocrine   Aging is associated with the development of glucose intolerance. The primary defect appears to be insulin resistance, since most studies demonstrate increased insulin levels. However, abnormal regulation of insulin secretion may also be a factor, because the insulin levels may not be appropriate for the degree of hyperglycemia. The cause of this impairment in carbohydrate metabolism has not been fully defined. Body weight, activity, and dietary composition influence carbohydrate metabolism, but they are not the sole factors in the carbohydrate intolerance of aging. At the tissue level, the insulin resistance of aging appears to be at some undefined post-receptor defect since insulin receptor numbers and affinities in monocytes and adipose tissue are unaltered with age.

Although the glucose intolerance of aging is not diabetes mellitus, it may have important consequences. Even within the normal range of an oral glucose tolerance test, those at the upper range have an increased risk of coronary artery disease compared to those with the lowest levels. In healthy older adults fasting blood sugars remain in the normal range, but glycosylated hemoglobin levels rise. Similar glycosylation may occur in other structural proteins and enzymes to modify their function. Furthermore, hyperinsulinemia is an independent risk factor for atherosclerosis and may contribute to the prevalance of vascular disease in older adults.

The metabolic clearance rate of thyroid hormone decreases with age. With an intact hypothalamic-pituitary-thyroid axis, normal thyroxine levels are maintained. However, with thyroid disease, when exogenous thyroxine is administered, the replacement dose must be adjusted downward to compensate for the change in clearance.

The most marked endocrine change with aging is decrease in estrogen at the time of the menopause. Decreased estrogen causes changes in reproductive tissues, and marked alteration in bone metabolism that leads to the development of osteoporosis in those with other risk factors. It has also been hypothesized that the difference in longevity between men and women is the result of differences in atherogenesis, that this in turn is mediated by difference in lipoprotein metabolism, which in turn is determined by gender-specific sex hormone levels. At adolescence, low density lipoprotein (LDL) levels rise and high density lipoprotein (HDL) levels decline more in boys than in girls. At the menopause, LDL levels increase in women, exceeding those in men throughout the postmenopausal period. If the LDL/HDL ratio is utilized as an index of atherogenic risk, the sex differential in this ratio can account for a substantial proportion of the sex differential in atherosclerosis and, thus, for a major fraction of the sex differential in human longevity. The high male-to-female ratio of coronary heart disease mortality decreases after the menopause. Some studies have reported a reduction in the incidence of coronary heart disease and in mortality from all causes in women using postmenopausal estrogens. These benefits may be mediated by the effects of estrogen on lipoprotein metabolism. Although suggestive, these studies do not directly confirm the hypothesis related to the influence of endogenous steroids on the sex differential in longevity.

Sex hormones do not decline acutely in men as in women at the menopause. However, some studies have demonstrated a progressive decline in testosterone levels with age in men. In most individuals these levels do not reach the hypogonadal range. Although sexual activity decreases with age, it does not appear to be related directly to testosterone levels. The effects of decreasing testosterone levels on other metabolic activities have not been well defined. Muscle mass and strength decline with age, but whether testosterone contributes to this change is unclear.

Fluid and electrolytes Under normal circumstances there is no change in sodium, potassium, hydrogen ion concentration, or extracellular fluid volume with age. However, adaptive mechanisms are impaired, and acute illness is often complicated by derangements in fluid and electrolyte balance.

The response to sodium restriction is blunted. Older individuals are able to decrease sodium excretion with restriction, but the response is sluggish and the sodium deficit incurred before the decline in sodium excretion becomes maximal is greater than in younger individuals. This salt-losing tendency is contributed to by several factors: (1) nephron loss with age and a consequent increased osmotic load per nephron; (2) decrease in renin, both in the basal and stimulated state with age; and (3) diminished aldosterone levels consequent to the changes in renin.

With or without preexisting myocardial disease, older adults are at increased risk for volume expansion. They are less able to excrete an acute salt load and require a longer time to reestablish balance. These changes relate to a decrease in glomerular filtration rate and decreased baroreceptor reflex sensitivity.

Potassium handling is also altered with age, and older individuals are at increased risk for developing hyperkalemia. With a decreased glomerular filtration rate and decreased aldosterone secretion, renal potassium excretion is altered. Insulin and catecholamines modulate potassium transport into cells. With decreased insulin and beta-adrenergic responsiveness, these adaptive mechanisms are blunted.

Dehydration is a particular problem in older adults when fluid intake is limited and/or insensible loss is increased. Water conservation and urine concentrating ability are impaired. Thirst mechanisms are also impaired, compromising the adaptive response to dehydration. Combined with the salt losing tendency, hypertonic volume depletion is a common presentation.

Possibly the most serious and least-well recognized fluid and electrolyte problem in older adults is water intoxication. Basal vasopressin levels are unaltered in normal aging. However, infusion of hypertonic saline leads to a greater increase in plasma vasopressin than in younger individuals. Conversely, infusion of alcohol leads to a lesser suppression of vasopressin in older individuals. These data suggest increased osmoreceptor sensitivity in older adults with a higher "set-point" for vasopressin secretion. As a result, certain drugs as well as pulmonary and central nervous system disorders are more likely to precipitate the syndrome of inappropriate antidiuretic hormone secretion (SIADH) in older patients.

Renal In cross-sectional studies, renal blood flow, glomerular filtration rate, and creatinine clearance decrease with age. However, creatinine generation also decreases with age, and serum creatinine may not directly reflect creatinine clearance. These changes are important because it is necessary to adjust the dosage of drugs that are excreted primarily by the kidney. Longitudinal studies suggest that renal function does not deteriorate with age in all individuals; in some it remains relatively unchanged, in some it deteriorates only slightly, and in some more markedly. This is in keeping with the variability of aging, but the possibility of decrease in renal function still needs to be considered, particularly in those who are ill.

Vision and hearing Age associated changes in vision and hearing may contribute to significant functional impairment in older adults. Visual acuity may decrease due to changes in the retina or neural elements, and changes in refractive power may lead either to increased hyperopia or myopia. Loss of accommodation leads to hyperopia, and nuclear sclerosis leads to cataracts and myopia. Diminished tear secretion in older individuals, especially in postmenopausal women, may lead to dryness of the eyes, which can cause irritation and discomfort and endanger the intactness of the corneal surface.

Hearing changes occur both in the peripheral auditory system and at the level of the cerebral cortex. Loss for hearing of pure tones, particularly for higher frequencies in men, can interfere with both hearing and understanding speech. Brainstem changes may lead to problems in localizing sounds and hearing in noisy environments. Cortical changes may cause difficulty with speech and language. In summary changes in auditory function are more complex than just pure tone loss.

PROGNOSIS With changes in the environment mean life span has increased and is approaching that predicted by "ideal" survival curves. Maximum lifespan, about 120 years for humans, appears not to be changing. Newer techniques of cell and molecular biology will almost certainly define the genetic factors that determine maximum life span, but at present prospects for prolonging it are not realistic.

The molecular and cellular events that limit species longevity lead in vivo to decrements in homeostatic mechanisms and increasing vulnerability of the organism to the environment. Understanding these molecular and cellular changes and the influence of the environment on them should ultimately lead to interventions that increase mean life span and more importantly decrease disability.

REFERENCES

ARNETZ BB et al: The influence of aging on hemoglobin A_c (HbA$_{1c}$). J Gerontol 37:648, 1982

DAVIDSON MG: The effect of aging on carbohydrate metabolism. A review of the English literature and a practical approach to the diagnosis of diabetes mellitus in the elderly. Metabolism 28:688, 1979

FINCH CE: The regulation of physiological changes during mammalian aging. Quart Rev Biol 51:49, 1976

——, SCHNEIDER EL (eds): Handbook of the Biology of Aging. New York, Van Nostrand Reinhold, 1985

FINK RI et al: Mechanisms of insulin resistance in aging. J Clin Invest 71:1523, 1983

FRIEDMAN JR et al: Correlation of estimated renal function parameters versus 24-hour creatinine clearance in ambulatory elderly. J Am Geriatr Soc 37:145, 1989

GOLDSTEIN S et al: Some aspects of cellular aging. J Chron Dis 36:103, 1983

HARMAN SM et al: Pituitary-thyroid hormone economy in healthy aging men: basal indices of thyroid function and thyrotropin responses to constant infusions of thyrotropin releasing hormone. J Clin Endocrinol Metab 58:320, 1984

HAYFLICK L: Biology of aging. N Engl J Med 295:1302, 1976

HAZZARD WR: The sex differential in longevity, in Principles of Geriatric Medicine, 2d ed, WR Hazzard et al (eds). New York, McGraw-Hill, 1990, pp 37–47

HELDERMAN JH et al: The response of arginine vasopressin to intravenous ethanol and hypertonic saline in man: The impact of aging. J Gerontol 33:39, 1978

KANE RL et al: Essentials of Clinical Geriatrics, 2d ed. New York, McGraw-Hill, 1989

LEBLANC P et al: Effects of age and body position on "airway closure" in man. J Appl Physiol 28:448, 1970

LINDEMAN RD et al: Longitudinal studies on the rate of decline in renal function with age. J Am Geriatr Soc 33:278, 1985

MADER S. Hearing impairment in elderly persons. J Am Geriatr Soc 32:548, 1984

RODEHEFFER RJ et al: Exercise cardiac output is maintained with advancing age in healthy human subjects: Cardiac dilation and increased stroke volume compensate for a diminished heart rate. Circulation 69:203, 1984

ROWE JW et al: Age-related failure of volume-pressure-mediated vasopressin release. J Clin Endocrinol Metab 54:661, 1982

—— et al: Characterization of the insulin resistance of aging. J Clin Invest 71:1581, 1983

WABBA WM: Influence of aging on lung function—clinical significance of changes from age twenty. Anesth Analg 62:764, 1983

section 3 Immunology

13 THE IMMUNE SYSTEM

BARTON F. HAYNES / ANTHONY S. FAUCI

Basic research in immunology has resulted in advances in many clinical areas, ranging from allergy and rheumatology to neurology and cardiology. Monoclonal antibody technology has revolutionized the study of cell surface antigens of effector and regulatory immune cells and provided specific reagents for essentially any target molecules. The isolation, cloning, and sequencing of genes for antigen receptors on B cells, T cells, and products of the major histocompatibility locus has yielded the probes necessary to begin to understand immune effector function. These probes are being used to explain diversification of the T- and B-cell antigen repertoire, induction of self-tolerance (self-antigen nonreactivity), and regulation of immune cell growth and differentiation. Molecular biology techniques have likewise enabled production of large quantities of secreted molecules that regulate immune cell function, e.g., lymphokines from lymphocytes and monokines from monocytes.

Finally, of great significance has been the discovery of the human T-cell lymphotropic virus (HTLV) family of retroviruses (see Chap. 134) that causes forms of leukemia (HTLV type I, adult T cell leukemia) and immunodeficiency [human immunodeficiency virus (HIV), acquired immunodeficiency syndrome (AIDS)]. Analysis of the genetic mechanisms of retrovirus alteration of normal T cell growth has led to a deeper understanding of normal and abnormal immune cell growth. This understanding should bring about new and specific modes of therapy for diseases of disordered immunoregulation such as autoimmune diseases, immunodeficiency diseases, and malignant diseases of the immune system. The aim of this chapter is to provide the essentials of immunology with particular emphasis on those principles relevant to understanding at a basic level the protean clinical and laboratory manifestations of disordered immunity.

PHENOTYPE AND FUNCTION OF IMMUNE CELLS

The dual limbs of the immune system are the thymus-derived (T) lymphocyte and the bone marrow-derived or bursa-equivalent (B) lymphocyte, both of which derive from a common stem cell. Other cell types such as the monocyte-macrophage play major roles in the inductive, regulatory, and effector phases of the immune response. The principal effector and regulator cells of the immune system are T, B, and large granular lymphocytes, and monocyte-macrophages.

Nonlymphoid cells such as neutrophils, eosinophils, basophils, and tissue mast cells play roles in the inflammatory response that results from certain immune-mediated reactions and as such must be considered in the scheme of immune cell function. With the advent of monoclonal antibody technology has come the discovery of numerous functional immune cell surface molecules, which have recently been given standardized names based on the reactivity of monoclonal antibodies that bind to them (Table 13-1).

The proportion and distribution of immunocompetent cells in various tissues reflect cell traffic, homing patterns, and functional

TABLE 13-1　Surface molecules of human immune and inflammatory cells

CD group	Other names	Distribution and/or cellular function mediated by surface molecules
T LYMPHOCYTES		
CD1	T6	HLA-related molecules on cortical thymocytes and Langerhan's cells; function unknown.
CD2	T11, sheep erythrocyte receptor	T-cell adhesion and activation
CD3	T3	T-cell-receptor–associated molecules (CD3γ, δ, ϵ, ζ, η) involved in T-cell triggering.
CD4	T4	Marker of inducer-helper T cells and a subset of cytotoxic T cells; also expressed on monocytes. By binding to HLA class II antigen, facilitates antigen recognition by CD4+ cells. CD4 is the surface recognition molecule by which HIV infects CD4+ cells.
CD5	Ly1, T1	T-cell activation; present on T cells and subset of autoantibody-producing B cells.
CD7	3A1	T-cell activation; earliest marker of T lineage.
CD8	T8	Marker of suppressor and cytotoxic T cells. By binding to HLA class I molecule, facilitates CD8+ T-cell recognition of antigen.
T-cell receptor for antigen	TCR$\alpha\beta$ or TCR$\gamma\delta$	T-cell activation by antigens.

TABLE 13-1 Surface molecules of human immune and inflammatory cells (*continued*)

CD group	Other names	Distribution and/or cellular function mediated by surface molecules
B LYMPHOCYTES		
CD5	Ly1, T1	Present on autoreactive B cells.
CD9	p24	On B cells, platelets, and activated T cells; function unknown.
CD10	Common acute lymphoblastic leukemia antigen (CALLA) J-5	CD10 is the enzyme-neutral endopeptidase involved in peptide hormone inactivation; present on normal and malignant pre-B cells.
CD19	B4	On most normal and malignant B cells. B-cell activation.
CD20	B1	B-cell activation.
CD21	B2	EBV receptor on B cells; receptor for C3d component of complement.
CD23	Blast-2	Activation antigen of B cells; Fc receptor for IgE.
B cell receptor for antigen	IgM, IgD, IgA, IgG, or IgE	B-cell activation by antigen
MYELOID LINEAGES		
CD11b	MO-1, MAC-1	C3bi receptor (CR3) on monocytes, neutrophils, and dendritic cells.
CD16		Low-affinity Fc receptor for IgG on neutrophils, large granular lymphocytes, and macrophages.
CD32	p40	Fc receptor for IgG.
CD34	My10	Present on myeloid progenitor cells.
CD35		C3b receptor (CR1) present on monocytes, granulocytes, erythrocytes, B cells, dendritic cells, and renal glomerular cells.
OTHER HEMATOPOIETIC MOLECULES		
CD18	LFA-1 β chain	Adhesion molecule present on hematopoietic cells.
CD44	p80, Hermes	Homing receptor on lymphocytes; adhesion molecule on other cell types.
CD45	Leukocyte common antigen, T200	Present on most hematopoietic cell types, function unknown.
CD58	LFA-3	Endogenous ligand for T-cell CD2 molecules on erythrocytes, thymic epithelial cells, and monocytes; general adhesion molecule involved in T-cell activation.
CD54	Intracellular adhesion molecule 1 (ICAM-1)	Adhesion molecule present on multiple cell types; ligand for LFA-1 molecule; cellular receptor for rhinoviruses.

capabilities. Bone marrow is the major site of maturation of B cells, monocyte-macrophages, and granulocytes and contains pluripotent stem cells which, under the influence of various colony stimulating factors (CSF), are capable of giving rise to all hematopoietic cell types (Fig. 13-1). G-CSF stimulates the production of neutrophils; GM-CSF stimulates neutrophil, monocyte, eosinophil, erythroid and megakaryocytoid cell growth; M-CSF drives monocyte differentiation, while IL-3 (multi-CSF) drives neutrophil, monocyte, eosinophil, basophil, erythroid, and megakaryocytoid differentiation. T-cell precursors also arise from hematopoietic stem cells but leave the yolk sac, fetal liver, or bone marrow while immature and home to the thymus for completion of maturation. Mature T lymphocytes, B

lymphocytes, and monocytes enter the circulation and home to peripheral lymphoid organs (lymph nodes, spleen) and the gut associated lymphoid tissue (tonsil, Peyer's patches, and appendix) and await activation by foreign antigens. Mature myeloid effector cells (neutrophils, eosinophils, basophils) leave the bone marrow and circulate in peripheral blood as well as home to tissues to perform effector functions associated with the response to foreign antigens (Fig. 13-1).

T CELLS T lymphocytes arise from yolk sac, fetal liver, and bone marrow precursor cells that migrate to the thymus during fetal and early postnatal life. T lymphocytes differ from other immune effector cell types in that the pool of effector T cells is established in the thymus early in life and is maintained throughout life by antigen-driven expansion of long-lived T cells that reside primarily in peripheral lymph organs and recirculate in blood and lymph. Mature T lymphocytes contribute 70 percent to 80 percent of normal peripheral blood lymphocytes, 90 percent of thoracic duct lymphocytes, 30 percent to 40 percent of lymph node cells, and 20 percent to 30 percent of spleen lymphoid cells. In lymph nodes T cells occupy deep paracortical areas around B cell germinal centers and in spleen are in periarteriolar areas of white pulp (see Chap. 63). T cells are the primary effectors of cell-mediated immunity with subsets of T cells maturing into cytotoxic cells capable of lysis of virus-infected or foreign cells. T cells are also the primary regulator cells of T and B lymphocyte and monocyte function by the production of lymphokines and by direct cell contact; in addition, T cells regulate erythroid cell maturation in bone marrow.

Human T cells express cell surface proteins that mark stages of intrathymic T-cell maturation; many of these molecules mediate or augment specific T-cell functions (Table 13-1; Fig. 13-2).

T-cell maturation The earliest identifiable cells of T lineage are CD7+ pro-T cells (i.e., cells in which T-cell receptor genes are neither rearranged nor expressed); they are found in fetal liver, yolk sac, and postnatal bone marrow. In the thymus, CD7+ T-cell precursors first express the T-cell adhesion molecule CD2 and begin cytoplasmic (c) synthesis of components of the CD3 complex of T-cell-receptor–associated molecules (Fig. 13-2). Within CD7+, CD2+, and cCD3+ T-cell precursors, T-cell receptor (TCR) gene rearrangement begins; it eventuates in two T-cell lineages, expressing either TCRαβ chains or TCRγδ chains. T cells expressing the TCRαβ chains comprise the majority of peripheral T cells in blood, lymph

FIGURE 13-1 Model of hematopoietic stem cell differentiation. Multipotential hematopoietic stem cells (HSC) may give rise to more restricted progenitor cells with self-renewal capacity. Thus, lymphocyte-committed stem cells (LSC) give rise to T and B cells. Another group of hematopoietic cells, for which the immediate progenitor is a more differentiated myeloid stem cell (MSC), includes erythrocytes, megakaryocytes, and platelets as well as the granulocyte, monocyte-macrophage series; the origin of large granular lymphocytes in this schema is hypothetical. (*Adapted from MD Cooper et al.*)

FIGURE 13-2 Model of human T-cell maturation. CD7 pro-T cells migrate to the thymus and stimulate expression of CD2 molecules and the cytoplasmic (c) expression of components of the CD3 complex. CD7+/CD2+/cCD3+ pre-T cells then develop into either surface (s) CD3 TCRαβ+ cells or sCD3 TCRγδ+ cells.

node, and spleen and terminally differentiate into either CD4 or CD8 cells. Cells expressing TCRγδ chains circulate as a minor population in blood; their functions, although not fully known, have been postulated as immune surveillance at epithelial surfaces. CD1 is expressed on immature cortical thymocytes, but with functional maturity, T-cell expression of CD1 ceases and subset antigens CD4 and CD8 are reciprocally expressed. Mature CD4+ TCRαβ+ cells induce B-cell differentiation, induce CD8+ cytotoxic T-cell proliferation, produce various lymphokines, and regulate certain stages of erythropoiesis. A subset of CD4+ cells may also function as cytotoxic effector cells, recognizing foreign antigen of HLA class II. CD8+ TCRαβ+ cells function as suppressors of B-cell antibody synthesis and as cytotoxic effectors, recognizing foreign antigen of HLA class I (see Chap. 14).

T-cell maturation stages are clinically relevant in that T-cell malignancies are derived from one or another of these stages. T-cell acute lymphoblastic leukemia and lymphomas share phenotypic similarities with pro-T, pre-T, or immature T cells and thus are malignancies of immature T cells. Forms of cutaneous T-cell lymphoma (mycosis fungoides, Sézary syndrome) and the syndrome of adult T-cell leukemia (associated with HTLV-I infection) share the phenotype of mature (usually CD4+) T cells.

T-cell antigen receptors The T-cell antigen receptor is a complex of molecules consisting of an antigen-binding heterodimer of either αβ or γδ chains noncovalently linked with five CD3 subunits (γ, δ, ε, ζ, and η) (Fig. 13-3). The CD3 ζ chains are either disulfide-linked homodimers (CD3-ζ₂) or disulfide-linked heterodimers composed of one ζ chain and one η chain. TCRαβ or -γδ molecules must be associated with CD3 molecules to be inserted into the cell surface membrane, TCRα being paired with TCRβ and TCRγ being paired with TCRδ. Molecules of the CD3 complex are thought to be involved in transduction of T-cell activation signals via T-cell receptors, while TCRαβ and -γδ molecules combine to form the TCR antigen-binding site.

Foreign antigen is recognized by cell surface molecules on antigen-presenting cells such as macrophages or dendritic cells. These molecules are encoded by HLA-complex genes. Antigen-presenting cells "process" the foreign antigen and display its peptide fragments on their surfaces, where the fragments bind to TCRαβ or -γδ chains of T reactive cells. CD4 molecules act as adhesives and, by direct binding to HLA class II (DR, DQ, or DP) molecules, stabilize the interaction of TCR with the antigen. Similarly CD8 molecules stabilize the TCR-antigen interaction by direct binding to HLA class I (A, B, or C) molecules.

The α, β, γ, and δ T-cell antigen receptor molecules have amino acid sequence homology and structural similarities to immunoglobulin heavy and light chains, and like many functionally relevant molecules of immune cells (e.g., HLA, CD2, CD4, CD8) they are therefore

FIGURE 13-3 Molecules of the T-cell antigen receptor–CD3 complex. T-cell receptor (TCR) heterodimers are composed of either αβ or γδ chains. CD3 molecules are γ, δ, and ε chains and a disulfide-linked dimer of either two ζ chains or a ζη heterodimer.

members of the *immunoglobulin gene superfamily*. The TCRβ and -δ chains contains four separately encoded regions, namely the V (variable), D (diversity), J (joining) and C (constant) regions, and the TCRα and -γ chains consist of V, J, and C regions. Thus, molecules of the T-cell antigen receptor have constant and variable regions, and the genes encoding the α, β, γ, and δ chains of these molecules undergo rearrangement during T-cell maturation, culminating in synthesis of the completed molecule.

The variable region elements of α, β, γ, and δ genes, which are separate in the germline, are brought together by DNA rearrangement and deletion during differentiation of the T lymphocyte. Thus, TCR diversity is due to the large numbers of V-J combinations formed during TCR gene rearrangement.

The specificity of mature T cells is largely determined within the thymus. For example, elimination of T cells capable of reacting against autologous (self) antigens (*self tolerance*), thus preventing autoimmune reactivity, may occur there, as may positive selection for T cells that can respond to foreign antigen, i.e., immunocompetent T cells. As mentioned, T cells recognize foreign antigens in association with cell surface molecules encoded for by the major histocompatibility or HLA complex on antigen-presenting cells. Specifically, cytotoxic CD8+ T cells recognize antigens in association with autologous HLA class I (A, B, and C) molecules, and CD4+ helper and CD4+ cytotoxic T cells recognize and respond to foreign antigens bound to autologous HLA class II molecules. This ability to corecognize foreign antigen with autologous class I and II HLA molecules on antigen-presenting cells is referred to as *HLA or MHC restriction* of immune cell interactions.

Nonlymphoid cells of the thymic microenvironment play major roles in the differentiation of T cells. Thymic macrophages and dendritic cells impart to developing thymocytes HLA restriction for immune cell interactions. Thymic epithelial cells produce a variety of cytokines and thymic hormones important in T-cell activation, participate in induction of T-cell tolerance to self antigens, and drive pro-T cells (Fig. 13-2) to proliferate and differentiate.

B CELLS Mature B cells comprise 10 percent to 15 percent of human peripheral blood lymphocytes, 50 percent of splenic lymphocytes, and approximately 10 percent of bone marrow lymphocytes. B cells express on their surface intramembrane immunoglobulin molecules that function as B-cell antigen receptors. B cells also express surface receptors for the Fc region of IgG molecules as well as receptors for activated complement components (C3d, C3b). The primary function of B cells is to produce antibodies. Mature B cells are derived from bone marrow precursor cells that arise continuously

throughout life (Fig. 13-1). Like myeloid and erythroid cells, B cells are constantly replaced every few days through cell division from marrow precursor cells. However, the maturation of B lymphocytes differs from myeloid and erythroid cell lines in that B lymphocytes have antigen-dependent and antigen-independent phases of maturation (Fig. 13-4). Pre-B cells arise from precursor cells in bone marrow and are identified by the presence of cytoplasmic immunoglobulin M (cIgM) (initially IgM heavy chain followed by cytoplasmic light chain synthesis). Pre-B cells mature to immature B cells that no longer express cIgM but rather surface IgM (sIgM) molecules. Immature B cells migrate to the periphery and continue antigen-independent maturation, expressing surface IgD, diversifying the B-cell antigen repertoire, and switching the B-cell surface immunoglobulin isotype such that either surface IgM, IgG, IgA, or IgE is expressed alone with IgD. Only one Ig heavy and light chain variable region and thus only one antigen specificity is expressed by each B cell. In lymphoid organs, B cells are the principal cells in lymph node cortical germinal centers and medullary cords and in primary and secondary germinal centers in the white pulp of spleen (see Chap. 63). On contact with antigen, mature B cells in peripheral lymph nodes and spleen either terminally differentiate into antibody-secreting plasma cells or proliferate to form populations of long-lived memory B cells that are capable of interaction when rechallenged with the same antigen (Fig. 13-4).

LARGE GRANULAR LYMPHOCYTES Large granular lymphocytes (LGL) (previously called "null cells") constitute approximately 5 percent to 10 percent of peripheral blood lymphocytes, and are nonadherent, nonphagocytic cells with large azurophilic cytoplasmic granules. LGL express surface receptors for the Fc portion of IgG, and many LGL express some T-lineage markers and proliferate in response to interleukin 2 (T-cell growth factor). Functionally, LGL share features with both monocyte-macrophages and neutrophils in that subsets of LGL mediate antibody dependent cellular cytotoxicity (ADCC) and natural killer (NK) activity. ADCC is the binding of an opsonized (antibody-coated) target cell to an Fc-receptor–bearing effector cell via the Fc region of antibody resulting in lysis of the target by the effector cell. Natural killer cell activity is the nonimmune (i.e., effector cell never having had previous contact with the target), non-antibody-mediated killing of target cells, which are usually malignant cell types. Thus, LGL that mediate NK activity may play an important role in immune surveillance and destruction of cells that spontaneously undergo malignant transformation in vivo. Lymphokine-activated killer, or LAK, cells are lymphocytes that proliferate in vitro to high levels of IL-2 and develop the ability to efficiently

FIGURE 13-4 Model of B-cell differentiation. B cells undergo antigen-independent and antigen-dependent maturation stages that culminate in terminal differentiation into either antibody-secreting plasma cells or memory B cells.

kill tumor cells. LAK cells generated with IL-2 in vitro from patients with solid tumors such as renal cell carcinomas have shown promising antitumor activity in vivo when infused back into patients.

MONOCYTE-MACROPHAGES Monocytes arise from precursor cells within bone marrow (Fig. 13-1) and circulate with a half-life ranging from 1 to 3 days. Monocytes leave the peripheral circulation by marginating in capillaries and then migrating into a vast extravascular pool. Tissue macrophages arise by migration of monocytes from the circulation and by proliferation of macrophage precursors in tissue. Common locations of tissue macrophages (and some of their specialized names) are lymph node; spleen; bone marrow; perivascular connective tissue; serous cavities such as peritoneum, pleura, and synovium; skin connective tissue; lung (alveolar macrophage); liver (Kupffer cell); bone (osteoclast); and central nervous system (microglia). In addition, two types of bone-marrow–derived cells of the myeloid lineage that specialize as antigen-presenting cells are present in many tissues and are called dendritic cells (in lymph nodes, spleen, and thymus) and Langerhan's cells (in skin and thymus) (see Chap. 63).

The monocyte-macrophage system plays a major role in the expression of immune reactivity by mediation of functions such as the presentation of antigen to lymphocytes and the secretion of factors such as interleukin 1 that are central to activation of T lymphocytes. Under certain circumstances monocytes can also mediate immunoregulatory functions such as suppressor cell activity. In addition, monocyte-macrophages mediate effector functions such as destruction of antibody-coated bacteria, tumor cells, or even normal hematopoietic cells in certain types of autoimmune cytopenias. Activated macrophages can also mediate NK-like activity and eliminate cell types such as tumor cells in the absence of antibody. Monocyte-macrophages express surface receptors for a number of molecules, including the Fc region of IgG, activated complement components, and various lymphokines (macrophage inhibitory and activating factors) (Table 13-1). In addition, monocyte-macrophages express cell surface HLA class II (Ia-like) antigens and specific cell surface differentiation antigens. Finally, macrophage secretory products are more diverse than those known for any other cell of the immune system. These secretory products allow the macrophage to exert both pro- and anti-inflammatory effects and to regulate other cell types. Among monocyte-macrophage secreted products are hydrolytic enzymes, products of oxidative metabolism, tumor necrosis factor, and interleukin 1 (IL-1), also called *leukocytic pyrogen* and *lymphocyte activating factor*, which affects lymphocytes, hepatocytes, fibroblasts, synoviocytes, and cells within the hypothalamus.

NEUTROPHILS, EOSINOPHILS, AND BASOPHILS Granulocytes are present in nearly all forms of inflammation and are nonspecific amplifiers and effectors of specific responses. Unchecked accumulation and activation of granulocytes can lead to host tissue damage as seen in neutrophil- and eosinophil-mediated necrotizing vasculitis. Granulocytes are derived from stem cells in bone marrow (Fig. 13-1). Each type of granulocyte (neutrophil, eosinophil, basophil) is derived from a different subclass of progenitor cell which is stimulated to proliferate by colony-stimulating factors. During terminal maturation of granulocytes, class-specific nuclear morphology and cytoplasmic granules appear that allow for histologic identification of granulocyte type.

Neutrophils express Fc receptors for IgG and activated complement components (C3b, C3d) (Table 13-1). Upon interaction of neutrophils with immune complexes, azurophilic granules (containing myeloperoxidase, lysozyme, elastase, and other enzymes) and specific granules (containing lactoferrin, lysozyme, collagenase, and other enzymes) are released, and microbicidal superoxide radicals (O_2^-) are generated at the neutrophil surface. The generation of superoxide is thought to lead to inflammation by direct injury to tissue and cells and by alteration of macromolecules such as collagen and DNA.

Eosinophils express Fc receptors for IgG and are potent cytotoxic effector cells for various parasitic targets. Intracytoplasmic contents of eosinophils, such as major basic protein, eosinophil cationic

TABLE 13-2   Mediators released from human mast cells and basophils

Mediator	Actions
Histamine	Smooth muscle contraction, increased vascular permeability
Slow reacting substance of anaphylaxis (SRSA) (leukotriene C4, D4, E4)	Smooth muscle contraction
Eosinophil chemotactic factor of anaphylaxis (ECF-A)	Chemotactic attraction of eosinophils
Platelet activating factor	Activates platelets to secrete serotonin and other mediators; smooth muscle contraction; induce vascular permeability
Neutrophil chemotactic factor (NCF)	Chemotactic attraction of neutrophils
Leukotactic activity (leukotriene B4)	Chemotactic attraction of neutrophils
Heparin	Anticoagulant
Basophil kallikrein of anaphylaxis (BK-A)	Cleaves kininogen to form bradykinin

protein, and eosinophil-derived neurotoxin, are capable of directly damaging tissues and may be responsible in part for the organ system dysfunction in the hypereosinophilic syndromes (see Chap. 64). Since the eosinophil granule contains anti-inflammatory types of enzymes (histaminase, arylsulfatase, phospholipase D) eosinophils may downregulate or terminate ongoing inflammatory responses in normal homeostasis.

The normal functions of basophils and tissue mast cells are not completely understood; the capacity of basophil mediators to increase local delivery of antibodies and complement by increasing vascular permeability is hypothetical. Thus, the basophil is identified principally with allergic reactions and some delayed cutaneous hypersensitivity states. Certainly the promotion of increased vascular permeability by basophils is important in the genesis of inflammatory lesions in some vasculitis syndromes (see Chap. 276). Basophils express surface receptors for IgE, and upon cross linking of basophil-bound IgE by antigen, release histamine, eosinophil chemotactic factor of anaphylaxis, and neutral protease—all mediators of components of immediate (anaphylaxis) hypersensitivity responses (Table 13-2). In addition basophils express surface receptors for activated complement components (C3a, C5a), through which mediator release can be directly effected (see Chap. 267 for a discussion of tissue mast cells).

HUMORAL MEDIATORS OF IMMUNITY: IMMUNOGLOBULINS

Immunoglobulins are the products of differentiated B cells and mediate the humoral arm of the immune response. Their primary functions are to bind specifically to antigen and bring about the inactivation or removal of the offending toxin, microbe, parasite, or other foreign substance from the body. The structural basis of immunoglobulin molecule function and immunoglobulin gene organization has provided insight into the role of antibody in normal protective immunity and in unwanted immune-mediated damage by immune complexes and autoantibody formation against host determinants.

All immunoglobulins have the basic structure of two heavy and two light chains (Fig. 13-5). Immunoglobulin isotype (i.e., G, M, A, D, E) is determined by the type of heavy and light chain present. IgG and IgA isotypes can further be divided into subclasses (G1, G2, G3, G4, and A1, A2) based on specific antigenic determinants on heavy chains. The characteristics of human immunoglobulins are outlined in Table 13-3. The four chains are covalently linked by disulfide bonds. Each chain is made up of a variable (V) region and constant (C) regions (also called domains), themselves made up of homologous units of 110 amino acids. Light chains have one variable (VL) and one constant (CL) region; heavy chains have one variable

FIGURE 13-5   Schematic structure of the immunoglobulin G (IgG) molecule.

region (VH) and 3 or 4 constant (CH) regions, depending on isotype. As the name suggests, constant regions are made up of homologous sequences and share the same primary structure as all other chains of the same isotype and subclass. Constant regions are involved in biological functions of immunoglobulin molecules. The CH₂ domain of IgG and the CH₄ domain of IgM are involved with binding of the C1q portion of C1. The CH region at the carboxyterminus end of the IgG molecule, the Fc region (Fig. 13-5) binds to surface Fc receptors of macrophages, large granular lymphocytes, B cells, neutrophils, and eosinophils.

Variable regions (VL and VH) constitute the antibody-binding (Fab) region of the molecule. Within the VL and VH regions are hypervariable regions of extreme sequence variability that constitute the antigen-binding site unique to each immunoglobulin molecule. The *idiotype* is the specific region of the Fab portion of the immunoglobulin molecule to which antigen binds. Antibodies against the idiotype portion of an antibody molecule are called *anti-idiotype antibodies*. The formation of anti-idiotype antibodies in vivo during

a normal B-cell antibody response may generate a negative (or "off") signal to B cells to terminate antibody production (see "Autoimmune Disease," below).

IgG comprises approximately 75 percent of the total serum immunoglobulin. The four IgG subclasses are numbered in order of their level in serum, IgG1 being found in greatest amounts and IgG4 the least. IgG subclasses have clinical relevance in their varying ability to bind macrophage and neutrophil Fc receptors and to activate complement (Table 13-3). IgG antibodies are frequently the antibody made after rechallenge of the host with antigen (secondary antibody response). Of the immunoglobulin isotypes only IgG crosses the placenta.

IgM antibodies normally circulate as a 950,000-Da pentamer with 160,000-Da monomers joined by a molecule called the J chain, a 15,000-Da nonimmunoglobulin molecule that also effects polymerization of IgA molecules. IgM is the first immunoglobulin to appear in the immune response (primary antibody response) and is the initial type of antibody made by neonates. Membrane IgM in the monomeric form also functions as a major antigen receptor on the surface of the mature B cell. IgM is an important component of immune complexes in autoimmune diseases. For instance, IgM antibodies against IgG molecules (*rheumatoid factors*) are present in high titers in rheumatoid arthritis, other collagen diseases, and some infectious diseases (subacute bacterial endocarditis). IgM antibody binds the C1 component of complement via the CH₄ domain and thus is a potent activator of complement.

IgA comprises only 10 to 15 percent of total serum immunoglobulin but is the predominant class of immunoglobulin in secretions. IgA in secretions (tears, saliva, nasal secretions, GI tract fluid, and human milk) is in the form of secretory IgA (sIgA), a polymer consisting of two IgA monomers, a joining molecule called the J chain, and a glycoprotein called the secretory piece. Of the two IgA subclasses, IgA1 is primarily found in serum, whereas IgA2 is more prevalent in secretions. IgA fixes complement via the alternative pathway and has potent antiviral activity in man by prevention of virus binding to respiratory and gastrointestinal epithelial cells.

IgD is found in minute quantities in serum (Table 13-3) and along with IgM is a major receptor for antigen on the B-cell surface.

Present in serum in very low concentrations (Table 13-3), IgE is

TABLE 13-3   Characteristics of human immunoglobulins

Isotype	Molecular weight	Heavy chain	Light chain	Adult average serum level (mg/dL)	Half-life (days)	Complement activation Classical pathway	Complement activation Alternative pathway	Binding to cells via Fc	Other biologic properties
IgG	150,000	$\gamma_1, \gamma_2, \gamma_3, \gamma_4$	κ or λ	1250 ± 300	23.0	IgG1, IgG2, IgG3, yes; IgG4 no	IgG1, IgG2, IgG3, no; IgG4 yes	Macrophages, neutrophils, eosinophils large granular lymphocytes	Placental transfer
IgM	190,000 (950,000)*	μ	κ or λ	125 ± 50	5.1	Yes	No	Lymphocytes	Primary antibody response, rheumatoid factor
IgA	160,000 (385,000)†	α_1, α_2	κ or λ	210 ± 50	5.8	No	Yes	Lymphocytes	Antibody in mucous secretions
IgD	175,000	δ	κ or λ	4	2.8	No	Yes	None	Primary lymphocyte surface molecule
IgE	190,000	ε	κ or λ	0.03	2.5	No	Yes	Mast cells, basophils, B cells	Mediates anaphylaxis, allergy

* IgM circulates as a pentameric molecule.
† Secretory IgA is a dimer.
SOURCE: Adapted with permission from DJ Jeske, JD Capra, Immunoglobulin: Structure and Function, in *Fundamental Immunology*, WE Paul (ed), New York, Raven, 1984.

FIGURE 13-6   Schematic representation of cellular interactions involved in the generation of cell-mediated and humoral immunity. *[Adapted with permission from AS Fauci, in WN Kelly et al (eds).]*

the major class of immunoglobulin involved in arming mast cells and basophils by binding to these cells via the Fc region. Antigen crosslinking of IgE molecules on basophil and mast cell surfaces results in release of mediators of the immediate hypersensitivity response.

Similar to the genes for the T-cell antigen receptor, the heavy and light chains of immunoglobulin are each encoded by multiple genetic elements physically separated in germline DNA but brought together to create a single active gene in B cells.

The variable regions of light chains (e.g., kappa light chains) are constructed from two genes called VK and JK. These genes, though on the same chromosome, are far apart in the germline but during B lymphocyte maturation are brought close together with excision of intervening DNA sequences (gene rearrangement). There are approximately 300 VK genes and 5 JK genes resulting in the pairing of VK and JK genes to create 1500 different light chain combinations. The number of distinct kappa light chains that can be generated is increased by somatic mutations within the VK and JK genes, thus creating a large number of specificities from a limited amount of germline genetic information.

In heavy chain immunoglobulin gene rearrangement the VH domain is created by the joining of three types of germline genes called *VH, DH,* and *JH,* thus allowing for even greater diversity in the variable region of heavy chains than for light chains. (See Chap. 263 for more on generation of clonal diversity of B cells.)

CELLULAR INTERACTIONS IN REGULATION OF THE NORMAL IMMUNE RESPONSE

The net result of activation of the humoral (B-cell) and cellular (T-cell) arms of the immune system by foreign antigen is the elimination of antigen directly by effector cells or in concert with specific antibody. In addition, a series of regulatory cells are activated which modulate T-effector-cell activation and B-cell antibody production. Figure 13-6 is a simplified schematic diagram of the immune system outlining some of these cellular interactions.

MONOCYTE–T CELL INTERACTIONS   Many of the activation and regulatory effects of lymphocytes and monocytes occur via soluble mediators (Table 13-4). Monocyte-macrophages are required for optimal activation of T cells by antigens or by mitogens (nonspecific activators of lymphocytes). A soluble macrophage product, IL-1, can substitute in some cases for intact macrophages. Upon contact with antigens or mitogens, macrophages secrete IL-1, two effects of which are (1) the induction of receptors for T-cell growth factor or interleukin 2 (IL-2) on T cells and (2) the induction of IL-2 secretion. IL-2 in turn activates T cells, resulting in expansion of effector and regulatory T cells that have also been induced to express IL-2 receptors. Effector T cells mediate a variety of functions including the killing of virus-infected cells, graft rejection, graft-versus-host reaction, delayed-type hypersensitivity, and the release of lymphokines (Table 13-4).

TABLE 13-4 Selected soluble mediators of cellular and humoral immune responses

Factor	Source	Target cells	Effects
IL-1	Monocyte-macrophages, dendritic cells, large granular lymphocytes, B- and T-cell lines, endothelial cells, epidermal cells, thymic epithelial cells, fibroblasts, astrocytes	B cells, T cells, fibroblasts, synovial cells, neutrophils, macrophages, lymphocytes, large granular lymphocytes, hypothalamus	Induces fever; induces T and B cell activation; induces fibroblast, synovial cell, and endothelial cell growth; induces tissue catabolism; enhances natural killer cell activity; chemoattractant for neutrophils, macrophages, lymphocytes
IL-2	T cells	T and B cells	Induces growth of T and B cells, induces cytotoxic T cell activity, induces natural killer and lymphokine-activated killer cell activity
IL-3	T cells	Hematopoietic stem cells, erythroid and myeloid progenitor cells	Drives differentiation of erythroid, myeloid, and multipotent progenitor cells
IL-4	Activated T cells	T and B cells	Induces proliferation of B and T cells; increases IgE secretion by B cells
IL-5	T cells	B cells, eosinophils	Induces differentiation of B cells and eosinophils
IL-6	Monocytes, fibroblasts, various malignant cell lines	B cells, fibroblasts, hepatocytes	Induces B cell growth, induces HLA antigen on fibroblasts, induces production of acute-phase proteins by hepatocytes
IL-7	Bone marrow stromal cells	B-cell and T cell precursors	Promotes growth of B- and T-cell precursors
Interferon γ	T cells, large granular lymphocytes	B cells, monocytes-macrophages, large granular lymphocytes, endothelial cells, fibroblasts, epithelial cells	Augments B-cell proliferation, augments antimicrobial and tumoricidal activity of monocyte-macrophages, induces IgG Fc receptor expression on monocytes and HLA class II expression on many cell types, augments natural killer cell activity

SOURCE: Adapted with permission from O'Garra et al, Immunol Today 9:45, 1988.

T CELL–T CELL AND T CELL–B CELL INTERACTIONS The expression of immune cell function is the result of a complex series of events occurring in phases. Both T and B lymphocytes mediate immune functions, and each of these cell types, when given appropriate signals, passes through stages, from activation and induction through proliferation, differentiation, and ultimately effector functions. The effector function expressed may be at the end point of a response, such as secretion of antibody by a differentiated plasma cell, or it might serve a regulatory function that modulates other functions such as is seen with inducer or suppressor T lymphocytes, which modulate both differentiation of B cells and activation of cytotoxic T cells. As shown schematically in Fig. 13-6, upon activation by IL-1 and IL-2, regulatory T-cell subsets are generated that exert positive and negative forces on effector cells. Thus, for B cells and cytotoxic (CD4+ or CD8+) T cells, there are CD4+ inducer and CD8+ suppressor cells that either facilitate or down-regulate effector cell function. For B cells, trophic effects are mediated by a variety of cytokines, particularly T-cell–derived B-cell growth factor (BCGF or IL-4) and B-cell differentiating factor (BCDF or IL-6), which act at sequential stages of B-cell maturation, resulting in B-cell proliferation, differentiation, and ultimately antibody secretion (Table 13-4). For T cells, trophic factors include inducer T-cell secretion of IL-2. In addition, B cells themselves are capable of processing and presenting antigens to T cells.

These complex cellular and humoral interactions involve a delicate balance among positive and negative influences and ultimately result in expression of an appropriate immune response. The slightest imbalance in these immunoregulatory circuits may result in aberrant immune function leading to clinically apparent immune-mediated disease.

THE COMPLEMENT SYSTEM

The complement system is a cascading series of plasma enzymes, regulatory proteins, and proteins capable of cell lysis whose principal site of synthesis is the liver. There are two arms of the complement system (Fig. 13-7). Activation of the classical complement pathway via C1, C4, and C2 and activation of the alternative complement pathway via factor D, C3, and factor B both lead to cleavage and

activation of C3. C3 is a protein whose activation fragments, when bound to target surfaces such as bacteria and other foreign antigens, are critical for opsonization (coating by antibody and complement) in preparation for phagocytosis.

The protein fragment C3b, split from C3, is necessary for activation of the terminal complement components, C5–9. These form the so-

FIGURE 13-7 Components of the complement system. *[Adapted with permission from WE Paul, in WE Paul (ed).]*

called membrane attack complex which, when inserted into cell membranes brings about osmotic lysis of the cell.

C3b also joins with a cleavage product of factor B (called Bb) to form C3bBb, also known as the *alternative pathway C3 convertase*. Activation of the classical complement pathway results in cleavage of C4 and C2 with a resulting complex of fragments, C4b2a, also called the *classical pathway C3 convertase*. Both the classical C3 convertase (C4b2a) and the alternative pathway C3 convertase (C3bBb) function to cleave C3 to form active C3b, thus driving activation of the C5–9 membrane attack complex. The fact that C3b can combine with Bb to form the alternative C3 convertase gives rise to a potent positive feedback loop for production of C3b and thus continued activation of terminal complement components.

Activation of the classical complement pathway is by interaction of antigen and antibody to form immune complexes that bind C1q, a subunit of C1. Immunoglobulin isotypes that bind C1q and activate the classical pathway are IgM, IgG1, IgG2, and IgG3. In contrast, IgA1, IgA2, and IgD activate complement via the alternative pathway. Activation of the complement cascade via the classical pathway by IgG- or IgM-containing immune complexes is a rapid and efficient, pathway to activation of terminal components. In contrast, activation of the alternative pathway via IgA-containing immune complexes or by bacterial endotoxin is a slower and less efficient pathway to terminal component activation. Thus, the immunoglobulin isotype composition of immune complexes is a critical factor in determining complement activation and, therefore, the efficiency of clearance of immune complexes by C3-receptor-bearing cells.

In addition to the role of complement in opsonization and cell lysis, several complement component fragments are potent mediators of cell activation. C3a and C5a bind to receptors on mast cells and basophils, resulting in release of histamine and other mediators of anaphylaxis. C5a is also a potent chemoattractant for neutrophils and monocyte-macrophages (Table 13-5).

MECHANISMS OF IMMUNE DAMAGE

Several responses by the host to foreign antigen culminate in the rapid and efficient elimination of nonself substances (Table 13-6). In these scenarios the classic weapons of the immune system (T cells, B cell, macrophages) interface with cells and soluble products that are mediators of inflammatory responses (neutrophils, eosinophils, basophils, kinin and coagulation systems, and complement cascade).

There are three general phases of host defense: (1) specific and nonspecific recognition of foreign antigens mediated by T and B lymphocytes, macrophages, and the alternative complement pathway, (2) amplification of the inflammatory response with recruitment of specific and nonspecific effector cells by complement components, lymphokines and monokines, kinins, arachidonic acid metabolites, and mast cell–basophil products, and (3) macrophage, neutrophil, and lymphocyte participation in antigen destruction with ultimate removal by phagocytosis of antigen particles (by macrophages or neutrophils) or by direct cytotoxic mechanisms (involving macrophages, neutrophils, and lymphocytes). Under normal circumstances, orderly progression of host defenses through these phases results in a well-controlled immune and inflammatory response that protects the host from the offending antigen. However, regulatory dysfunction of any of the host defense systems can damage host tissue and produce clinically apparent disease.

IMMUNE COMPLEX FORMATION (TYPE III REACTION)

Clearance of antigen by immune complex formation between antigen and antibody is a highly effective mechanism of host defense. However, depending on the level of immune complexes formed and their physicochemical properties, immune complexes may or may not result in host and foreign cell damage. After antigen exposure, certain types of soluble antigen-antibody complexes freely circulate and, if not cleared by the reticuloendothelial system, can be deposited in blood vessel walls and in other tissues such as renal glomeruli.

TABLE 13-5　Biologic activities of some complement components

Component	Activity
C4a weak anaphylatoxin	Evokes histamine release from basophils and mast cells.
C3a	Anaphylatoxin; evokes histamine release from basophils and mast cells.
C5a	Anaphylatoxin; evokes histamine release from basophils and mast cells; potent chemoattractant for monocytes and neutrophils.
C3b, C3bi	Enhancement of phagocytosis by neutrophils and monocytes. Promotes immune complex binding to cells within monocyte-macrophage system, as well as neutrophils. C3b with Bb forms alternative pathway C3 convertase and amplifies alternative pathway. Promotes solubilization of immune complexes.
C5–9	Membrane attack complex; forms transmembrane channels leading to cell destruction.

SOURCE: Adapted with permission from Ruddy S: Plasma protein effectors of inflammation: Complement, in WN Kelley et al (eds).

The precise mechanisms whereby immune complexes damage tissues, particularly blood vessels, are discussed in Chaps. 268 and 276.

IgE MEDIATED ALLERGIC REACTIONS–ANAPHYLAXIS (TYPE I) Mast cells and basophils have receptors for the Fc portion of IgE, and cell-bound IgE effectively "arms" basophils and mast cells. Mediator release is triggered by antigen interaction with Fc-receptor–bound IgE; the mediators released are responsible for the pathophysiologic changes of allergic disease (Table 13-2). Mediators released from mast cells and basophils can be divided into three broad categories of action. Those which: (1) increase vascular permeability and contract smooth muscle (histamine, platelet activating factor, SRS-A, BK-A); (2) are chemotactic for or activate other inflammatory cells (ECF-A, NCF, leukotriene B4); and (3) modulate the release of other mediators (BK-A, platelet activating factor).

CYTOTOXIC REACTIONS OF ANTIBODY (TYPE II) In this type of immunologic injury, complement-fixing (C1 binding) antibodies against normal or foreign cells or tissues (IgM, IgG1, IgG2, IgG3) bind complement via the classical pathway and initiate a sequence of events similar to that initiated by immune complex deposition, resulting in cell lysis or tissue injury. Examples of type II antibody-mediated cytotoxic reactions include red cell lysis in transfusion reactions, Goodpasture's syndrome with antiglomerular basement

TABLE 13-6　Mechanisms of immunologically mediated inflammation

Mechanism type	Characteristics of inflammatory response	Clinical disease type
I Allergic (IgE-mediated)	Basophil and mast cell products leading to immediate flare-and-wheal.	Atopy, anaphylaxis
II Cytotoxic or tissue-specific antibody (IgM- or IgG-mediated)	Acute inflammation via phagocytic cells and deposition of complement in tissues, lysis or phagocytosis of target cells.	Goodpasture's syndrome, autoimmune cytopenias, anti-red cell antibodies in transfusion reactions
III Immune complex (IgG-, IgM-, IgA-mediated)	Accumulation of neutrophils, macrophages, complement components.	Systemic necrotizing vasculitis, systemic lupus erythematosus, serum sickness syndromes
IV Delayed hypersensitivity	T cell–induced mononuclear cell accumulation of regulatory and effector T cells and macrophages. Lymphokines and monokines released. Often granuloma formation.	Tuberculosis, sarcoidosis, Wegener's granulomatosis and other forms of granulomatous vasculitis

membrane antibody formation, and possibly juvenile onset diabetes mellitus with anti-islet cell antibody production.

CLASSICAL DELAYED-TYPE HYPERSENSITIVITY REACTIONS (TYPE IV) Inflammatory reactions initiated by mononuclear leukocytes and not by antibody alone have been termed delayed-type hypersensitivity reactions. The term "delayed" has been used to contrast a secondary cellular response which appears 48 to 72 h after antigen exposure to an "immediate" hypersensitivity response generally seen within 12 h of antigen challenge and initiated by basophil mediator release or preformed antibody. For example, in an individual previously infected with mycobacterium tuberculosis (TB) organisms, intradermal placement of TB purified protein derivative (PPD) as a skin test challenge results in an indurated area of skin a 48 to 72 h, indicating previous exposure to TB.

The cellular events that result in classical delayed-type hypersensitivity responses are centered around T cells, their soluble products and macrophages. In the general scheme outlined in Fig. 13-6, antigen is processed by macrophages and presented to T cells expressing a cell surface receptor specific for the antigen. Macrophage-secreted IL-1 amplifies the clonal expansion of antigen-specific T cells, and lymphokines are secreted to recruit other T cells and macrophages nonspecifically to participate in the inflammatory response. Once recruited, macrophages frequently undergo epithelioid cell transformation and form giant cells. This type of mononuclear cell infiltrate is termed *granulomatous inflammation*. Examples of diseases in which delayed-type hypersensitivity plays a major role are fungal infections (*histoplasmosis*), mycobacterial infections, chlamydial infections (*Lymphogranuloma venereum*), helminth infections (*schistosomiasis*), reactions to toxins (*berylliosis*), and hypersensitivity reactions to organic dusts (*hypersensitivity pneumonitis*). In addition, delayed-type hypersensitivity responses may play a role in *rheumatoid arthritis* and *Wegener's granulomatosis* (see Chaps. 270 and 276).

AUTOIMMUNE DISEASE Autoimmune disease is characterized by production of either antibodies that react with host tissue or immune effector T cells that are autoreactive. Since B-cell responses in man generally require inducer T cells, a B-cell autoantibody response directly implies disordered T-cell immunoregulatory control. In some instances, autoantibodies may arise by a normal T- and B-cell response activated by foreign organisms or substances that contain antigens, particularly polysaccharides, that cross react with similar polysaccharides in body tissues. Examples of clinically relevant autoantibodies are antibodies against acetylcholine receptors in myasthenia gravis; and anti-DNA, antierythrocyte, and antiplatelet antibodies in systemic lupus erythematosus.

The clonal selection theory was put forth by Burnet in 1949 to explain autoimmunity. Burnet proposed that the contact of antibody-forming cells with their respective antigens during fetal or early postnatal life lead to their elimination. Thus, in this theory self-reactive clones are avoided unless they arise in later life by somatic mutation of lymphocytes. The progeny of such mutant cells would give rise to self-reacting antibodies. As the study of autoimmunity has progressed, it has become clear that the genesis of autoimmune B and T cells is far more complex than originally thought. Certain drugs (procainamide, phenytoin) and infectious agents (Epstein-Barr virus, *Mycoplasma pneumoniae*) can elicit the production of auto antibodies to a wide array of host antigens in otherwise normal persons. Moreover, normal mice produce autoantibodies when given injections of nonspecific activators of lymphocytes (mitogens). In all of these circumstances, the autoantibodies combine with ubiquitous antigens: DNA, IgG (as the target of an IgM rheumatoid factor), phospholipids (cardiolipins), erythrocytes, lymphocytes, or cytoskeletal components (vimentin, keratins). Thus, production of autoantibodies is an inherent property of the normal immune system. The immune system controls the tendency to produce autoantibodies by a feedback network of T and B cells. It is thought that B cells normally are inhibited from terminal differentiation by suppressor T cells, a lack of inducer T cells, or both. In autoimmunity an imbalance between the two types of T cells can perturb the immunoregulatory network; this may bring about activation of autoreactive B cells.

As mentioned above in the description of immunoglobulins, the unique portion of the variable region of the immunoglobulin molecule where antigen binds is called the *idiotype*, and an antibody that reacts specifically with that region is called an *anti-idiotype antibody*. The specificity of antibody molecules and the regulation of antibody production have been probed by making rabbit antihuman idiotypic antibodies. There are also autologous anti-idiotypes (auto-anti-idiotypes) that arise during the course of the normal immune response. For example, auto-anti-idiotypes against antitetanus antibodies develop during normal immunization of humans to tetanus toxoid and may serve to deliver "off" signals to B cells secreting antitetanus antibodies. Idiotypes and auto-anti-idiotype antibodies may be an important component of the immunoregulatory network. Anti-idiotype antibodies may also be relevant to two types of autoimmunity: (1) dysfunction of the idiotype–anti-idiotype antibody system could lead to B-cell hyperreactivity by failure to generate "off" signals for B-cell differentiation, and (2) some antireceptor antibodies produced in autoimmune diseases (antiacetylcholine receptor antibodies in myasthenia gravis, anti-insulin receptor antibodies in forms of Type I diabetes mellitus, and antithyrotropin receptor antibodies in thyrotoxicosis) may be anti-idiotype antibodies made against the antibody combining site (idiotype) of an autoantibody.

Finally, genetic factors likely play a role in the genesis of autoimmune disease, either by selecting for inherent B-cell hyperreactivity and tendency toward autoantibody formation or via other unknown factors. Linkage of autoimmune diseases with known genetic loci such as the major histocompatibility complex has provoked great interest. Myasthenia gravis, thyrotoxicosis and pernicious anemia are all associated with HLB B8 (Class I) and DR3 (Class II) alloantigen expression (see Chap. 14) and are also associated with certain immunoglobulin heavy chain allotypic markers. Genetic marker systems such as HLA types and immunoglobulin heavy chain allotypic antigens may be associated with autoimmunity by making the host susceptible in some way to antiself immune cell activation. Thus, multiple genes and/or events are operative in the ultimate generation of the clinical autoimmune state.

CLINICAL EVALUATION OF IMMUNE FUNCTION Clinical assessment of immunity requires investigation of the four major components of the immune system that participate in host defense and in pathogenesis of autoimmune diseases: (1) humoral immunity (B cells), (2) cell-mediated immunity (T cells, monocytes), (3) phagocytic cells of the reticuloendothelial system (macrophages), as well as polymorphonuclear leukocytes, and (4) complement. Clinical problems that require an evaluation of immunity include chronic infections, recurrent infection, unusual infecting agents, and certain autoimmune syndromes. The type of clinical syndrome under evaluation can provide information regarding possible immune defects. Defects in cellular immunity generally result in viral, mycobacterial, and fungal infections. An extreme example of deficiency in cellular immunity is the acquired immunodeficiency syndrome (see Chap. 264). Antibody deficiencies result in recurrent bacterial infections, frequently with organisms such as *Streptococcus pneumoniae* and *Haemophilus influenzae* (see Chap. 263). Disorders of phagocyte function frequently are manifested by recurrent skin infections, often due to *Staphylococcus aureus* (see Chap. 81). Finally, deficiencies of early and late complement components are associated with autoimmune phenomena and recurrent *Neisseria* infections (Table 13-7). Table 13-8 summarizes useful initial screening tests of immune function. For evaluation of antibody-mediated immunity, measurement of total serum immunoglobulin levels, measurement of specific antibody titers to commonly administered antigens (such as tetanus toxoid), and determination of isohemagglutinin titers yield information necessary for institution of appropriate therapy. In certain cases of hypogammaglobulinemia, quantitation of B-cell markers and in vitro B-cell functional assays are of use.

For assessment of cell-mediated immunity, the total lymphocyte

TABLE 13-7 Complement deficiencies and associated diseases

Component	Associated diseases
Classical pathway	
C1q, C1r, C1s, C4	Immune complex syndromes*, pyogenic infections
C2	Immune complex syndromes*, few with pyogenic infections
C1 inhibitor	Rare immune complex disease; few with pyogenic infections
C3 and alternative pathway	
C3	Immune complex syndromes*; pyogenic infections
D	Pyogenic infections
Properdin	*Neisseria* infections
I	Pyogenic infections
H	Hemolytic uremic syndrome
Membrane attack complex	
C5	Recurrent *Neisseria* infections; immune complex disease
C6	Recurrent *Neisseria* infections; immune complex disease
C7	Recurrent *Neisseria* infections; immune complex disease
C8	Recurrent *Neisseria* infections; immune complex disease
C9	Rare *Neisseria* infections

* Immune complex syndromes include SLE and SLE-like syndromes, glomerulonephritis, and vasculitis syndromes.
SOURCE: Adapted with permission from PJ Lachmann and MJ Walport, Genetic deficiency diseases of the complement system, in GD Ross (ed), *The Immunobiology of the Complement System.* Orlando, Academic, 1986; and from JA Schifferli and DK Peters, Lancet 88, 957, 1983.

count coupled with an appropriately placed battery of intradermal skin tests provides a useful index of T-cell and macrophage response to antigens in vivo.

Anergy is the absence of an appropriate delayed-type hypersensitivity reaction and may be either general, with lack of T-cell responses to many types of antigens, or specific, with lack of T-cell responses to one antigen type. Anergy is determined by absence of reactivity in delayed-type hypersensitivity skin testing to antigens against which the patient is sensitized. For example, a battery of skin tests including *Candida*, histoplasmin, trichophytin, and mycobacterium tuberculosis antigens are placed intradermally. Most normal adult subjects should react to one of these four antigens. If there is no response on two separate occasions, the subject is said to be anergic. The causes of anergy vary in different diseases. Generalized anergy occurs in chronic fungal and TB infections and in sarcoidosis. An example of specific anergy is lack of T-cell responses to *Candida* antigen in mucocutaneous candidiasis.

Quantitation of total T cells and CD4 and CD8 T-cell subsets can be clinically useful. However, changes in the CD4/CD8 (T4/T8) ratio

TABLE 13-8 Initial screening tests of immune function

Humoral immunity
   Quantitative immunoglobulin levels, IgG, IgM, IgA, IgE
   Tests of specific antibody formation (antitetanus toxoid)
   Isohemagglutinin titer (anti-A, anti-B): measures IgM response
Cell-mediated immunity
   White blood cell count with differential: measures total lymphocyte level
   Delayed hypersensitivity skin tests: measures specific T-cell and macrophage response to antigens
Phagocytosis
   White blood cell count with differential: measures total neutrophils
   Nitroblue tetrazolium test (NBT), superoxide production: measures metabolic function
   Chemotaxis: measures cell motility
   Quantitative measurement of intracellular bacterial killing
Complement
   Total hemolytic complement (CH_{50}): quantitates complement activity
   Assay of individual complement components: defines complement component deficiencies

SOURCE: Adapted with permission from AJ Ammann, in DP Stites et al (eds).

occur in many clinical conditions and are not specific. In certain situations, such as evaluation of a transplant recipient for response to donor antigens, it is useful to measure lymphocyte activation by determination of the amount of tritiated thymidine incorporated into lymphocyte DNA in response to donor antigens and mitogens.

The evaluation of patients with recurrent cutaneous skin infections, such as Job's syndrome and chronic granulomatous disease, requires quantitation of neutrophil numbers and tests of neutrophil function. Functional neutrophil tests include NBT test, superoxide generation, chemotaxis, and quantitation of the ability of neutrophils to kill bacteria (see Chap. 81).

The total hemolytic complement (CH_{50}) determination measures the ability of a test sample of serum to lyse 50 percent of a standard suspension of sheep erythrocytes coated with rabbit antisheep erythrocyte antibody. This reaction requires the entire classical complement reaction sequence. For the classical activation pathway (C1, C4, C2) or the terminal sequence (C5–C9) the CH_{50} determination is a reliable screen for homozygous deficiencies. A normal CH_{50}, however, does not exclude heterozygous partial deficiencies of classical complement components. When the CH_{50} level is subnormal, individual complement measurements are required to determine specific component deficiency states.

REFERENCES

BUTCHER E, WEISSMAN IL: Lymphoid tissues and organs, in *Fundamental Immunology*, WE Paul (ed). New York, Raven, pp 109–127, 1984
CLARK SC, KAMEN R: The human hematopoietic colony-stimulating factors. Science 236:1229, 1987
COOPER MD, et al: Lymphocytes, in *Fundamental Immunology*, WE Paul (ed). New York, Raven, 1984
DAVIS MM: Molecular genetics of T cell antigen receptors. Hosp Practice 23:157, 1988
DENNING SM, HAYNES BF: Differentiation of human T cells. Clin Lab Med 8:1, 1988
FAUCI AS, LANE HC, VOLKMAN DJ: Activation and regulation of human immune responses. Implications in Normal and Disease States. Ann Int Med 99:61, 1983
KELLEY WN et al (eds): *Textbook of Rheumatology*, 2d ed. Philadelphia, Saunders, 1985, Chaps 2, 7, 9, and 10
MARRACK P, KAPPLER J: The T cell receptor. Science 238:1073, 1987
O'GARRA A et al: "B cell factors" are pleotropic. Immunol Today 9:45, 1988
PAUL WE: Introduction to the immune system, in *Fundamental Immunology*, WE Paul (ed). New York Raven, 1984
PLAUT, M LICHTENSTEIN LM: Cellular and chemical basis of the allergic inflammatory response in Allergy, in *Allergy Principles and Practice*, E Middleton, CE Reed, EF Ellis (eds). St. Louis, Mosby, 1978, pp 115–138
ROMAIN PL, SCHLOSSMAN SF: Human T cell subsets. Functional heterogeneity and surface recognition structures. J Clin Invest 74:1559, 1984
SHOENFELD Y, SCHWARTZ RS: Immunologic and genetic factors in autoimmune disease. New Engl J Med 312:1100, 1985
STITES DP et al (eds): *Basic and Clinical Immunology*, 5th ed. Los Gatos CA, Lange Medical Publishers, 1984

14 THE MAJOR HISTOCOMPATIBILITY GENE COMPLEX

CHARLES B. CARPENTER

Antigenic differences between members of a species are called *alloantigens*, and when these play a determining role in the rejection of allogeneic tissue grafts they are called *histocompatibility antigens*. Evolution has conserved a single closely linked region of histocompatibility genes, the products of which are prominently displayed on cell surfaces and provide a strong barrier to allotransplantation. The terms *major histocompatibility antigens* and *major histocompatibility gene complex* (MHC) refer to the gene products and genes of this chromosomal region. Many minor histocompatibility antigens, in contrast, are encoded throughout the genome. They represent weaker allotypic differences on molecules that serve a variety of functions. Structures bearing MHC antigens play a major role in immunity and in self-recognition in the differentiation of cells and tissues. Much of the evidence for MHC control of the immune response comes from work in animal models in which immune-response genes have been mapped within the mouse (H-2), rat (RT1), and guinea pig (GPLA) MHC. In humans the MHC is called *HLA*. The individual letters of HLA have various meanings, and by international agreement HLA is the logo for the human MHC.

Several generalizations can be made about the MHCs. *First*, three classes of gene products are encoded within the small [<2 cM (centimorgans)] region of the MHC. Class I molecules, expressed on virtually all cell surfaces, consist of one heavy and one light polypeptide chain and are the products of three reduplicated loci: HLA-A, HLA-B, and HLA-C. Class II molecules, restricted in expression to B lymphocytes, some monocytes, and activated T lymphocytes, consist of two polypeptide chains (α and β) of unequal length and are the products of several closely linked genes, collectively termed the HLA-D region. Class III molecules are the C4, C2, and Bf components of complement. *Second*, class I and class II molecules form complexes with immunogenic peptides (e.g., from bacteria or viruses), and they are conjointly recognized by T lymphocytes having appropriate antigen receptors. Self versus nonself discrimination in the initiation and effector phase of the immune response is thereby intimately directed by class I and II molecules. *Third*, restricted cell-to-cell interactions involving suppressor T lymphocytes are not clearly defined in humans, but HLA genes are important for some suppressor activities. *Fourth*, genes for enzyme systems having no apparent relationship to immunity are located in the region of the MHC, as are genes of importance in skeletal growth and development. *Fifth*, genes for tumor necrosis factors TNFα and TNFβ lie also within the MHC. The known loci of the HLA region on the short arm of chromosome 6 are shown in Fig. 14-1.

LOCI OF THE HLA SYSTEM Class I antigens HLA antigens of the class I type are defined serologically by human sera, principally from multiparous females, and to a limited extent by monoclonal antibodies. They are present in varying densities in most body tissues,

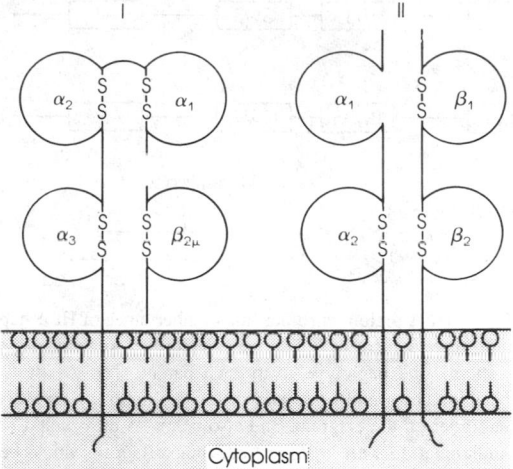

FIGURE 14-2 Schematic representation of class I and class II molecules on the cell surface. Class I molecules are composed of two polypeptide chains. The 44,000-Da heavy chain passes through the plasma membrane. Its external portion consists of three domains (α_1, α_2, α_3) formed by disulfide bonding. The beta$_2$-microglobulin ($\beta_{2\mu}$) light chain (11,500 Da) encoded by chromosome 15 is noncovalently bound to the heavy chain. Amino acid sequence homology among class I molecules is 80 to 85 percent, falling to 50 percent or less in portions of α_1 and α_2 which represent the sites of alloantigenic polymorphism. Class II molecules consist of two noncovalently associated polypeptide chains, a 34,000-Da α and a 29,000-Da β. Each chain has two domains formed by disulfide bridging (the α_1 domain lacks a sulfide bridge). (*From Carpenter and Strom.*)

FIGURE 14-1 Schematic representation of human chromosome 6, showing the location of the HLA region in the 21 region of the short arm. The HLA-A, HLA-B, and HLA-C loci encode class I heavy chains (44,000 Da), while the beta$_2$-microglobulin light chain (11,500 Da) of the class I molecule is encoded by genes of chromosome 15. HLA-D region (class II) is centromeric to the A, B, C loci, with genes for closely linked complement components C4A, C4B, Bf, and C2 in the B-D region. Two genes for tumor necrosis factor (TNFα,β) also lie between HLA-B and the complement genes (not shown). The order of the complement genes is uncertain. Each D region class II molecule is made up of an α and a β chain. They appear on the cell surface in distinct sets, DP, DQ, and DR. The numbers preceding α or β indicate that there are different genes for the chains of a given set; e.g., for DR, there are three β-chain genes. The expressed molecule may be 1$\beta\alpha$ or 3$\beta\alpha$. The 2β gene is not expressed (pseudogene). The antigens DRw52 and DRw53 are on the 3β chain, while the other DR antigens are on 1β. DRα is not polymorphic, while molecules bearing the DQ antigens have polymorphism in both α and β chains (1α1β). The other DQ set (2α2β) appears to be pseudogenes. Polymorphism in DP is confined to the 1β chain. The overall length of the HLA region is about 3 cM.

including B cells, T cells, and platelets, but not in mature red blood cells. The number of serologically defined specificities is large, and the HLA system is the most polymorphic genetic system known in humans. Three clearly defined loci are recognized within the HLA complex for class I, serologically defined (SD) HLA antigens. Each class I antigen consists of an 11,500-Da beta$_2$-microglobulin subunit and a 44,000-Da heavy chain that carries the antigenic specificities (Fig. 14-2). There are over 60 clearly defined A and B specificities, and 11 C-locus specificities are known. Antigens of the major complex are prefixed by HLA, but this may be omitted when the context is clear. Antigens tentatively accepted by the World Health Organization have a *w* after the locus designation. The number following the locus designation is the name of the antigen. The HLA antigens of African, Asian, and Oceanic peoples are less well defined at present, although they include some of the antigens commonly found in people of western European ancestry. The distribution of HLA antigens is distinctive for certain racial groups and can serve as anthropologic markers in the study of migration patterns and diseases.

Since chromosomes are paired, each individual has six serologically defined HLA-A, HLA-B, and HLA-C antigens, three from each parent. Each of these chromosomal sets is termed a *haplotype*, and by simple Mendelian inheritance one-fourth of siblings have identical haplotypes, one-half share a haplotype, and the remaining one-fourth are completely incompatible (Fig. 14-3). Evidence that this gene complex plays the major role in the transplantation response comes from the fact that haplotype-matched sibling donor-recipient combinations show excellent results in kidney transplantation, in the vicinity of 85 to 90 percent long-term survival (see Chap. 225).

Class II antigens The HLA-D region is adjacent to the class I loci on the short arm of chromosome 6 (Fig. 14-1). This region encodes a series of class II molecules, each consisting of a 29,000-Da β chain and a 34,000-Da α chain (Fig. 14-2). Incompatibility for this region, particularly concerning the DR antigens, determines the in vitro proliferative response of lymphocytes to mismatched haplotypes. This mixed lymphocyte response (MLR) is assessed by the degree of proliferation of a *mixed lymphocyte culture* (MLC) and is

Haplotypes:
a = A1, Cw3, B8, Dw3
b = A29, Cw4, Bw35, Dw1
a_r = A1, Cw3, B8, Dw1
b_r = A29, Cw4, Bw35, Dw3

Inheritance:

ab x cd

ac ad bc bd

FIGURE 14-3 HLA region, chromosome 6: inheritance of HLA haplotypes. Each chromosomal segment of linked genes is termed a haplotype, and each individual inherits one haplotype from each parent. The A, B, C, and D antigens of haplotypes a and b are shown for this hypothetical individual in chromosomal order on the diagram, and also below as they would be written in text. If individual ab were to marry cd, their offspring would be of four types only, as far as HLA is concerned. Occasionally (dotted cross) recombination occurs in the germ line (meiosis) of a parent, resulting in an altered haplotype. The frequency of recombinant children is a measure of the map distance (1 percent recombination frequency = 1 cM; see Fig. 14-1). (*From CB Carpenter, Kidney International, 14:283, 1978.*)

positive even when HLA-A, HLA-B, and HLA-C antigens are identical (Fig. 14-3). When parental recombination has occurred between HLA-B and -DR, for example, a new haplotype appears in the child, who will be identical for class I but different for class II (a versus a_r in Fig. 14-3). HLA-D antigens are defined by reference-stimulating lymphocytes that are homozygous for HLA-D and are inactivated by x-irradiation or mitomycin C to make the reaction unidirectional. There are 24 such antigens recognized by homozygous typing cells.

Attempts to define HLA-D by serology first established a series of D-related (DR) antigens expressed on class II molecules of B lymphocytes, monocytes, and activated T lymphocytes. Macrophages, dendritic cells, and skin Langerhans cells are also class II–positive. Other closely related antigen systems were soon discovered and given various local names (MB, MT, DC, SB), which have been replaced by subregion names DR, DQ, and DP. The separate identity of these sets of class II molecules is now established, and the genes for their respective α and β chains have been isolated and sequenced. The class II gene map shown in Fig. 14-1 describes a minimal number of genes and molecular sets. Although a class II molecule may be composed of a DRα from one parental haplotype and a DRβ from the other parent (transcomplementation), α and β combinations outside of each DP, DQ, DR set rarely, if ever, occur. DR, and to some extent DQ, molecules provide the stimuli for the primary mixed lymphocyte response. The secondary MLR is called the *primed lymphocyte test* (PLT) and occurs rapidly over 24 to 36 h instead of 6 to 7 days. DP alloantigens were discovered from their ability to provide PLT stimulation, although they do not produce a primary MLR. DQ and DP molecules can also be identified serologically. While B lymphocytes and activated T lymphocytes express all three sets of class II molecules, DQ antigens are not expressed on 60 to 90 percent of monocytes, which are virtually all DP- and DR-positive.

Molecular genetics Each polypeptide chain of class I and class II molecules bears several polymorphic sites in addition to the "private" antigen defined by alloantisera. In the *cell-mediated lympholysis* (CML) test the specificity of killer T cells (T_c), which arise during the proliferative events in MLR, is determined by testing upon target cells from donors other than those providing the MLR stimulus. Antigen systems defined by this method show a close but imperfect correlation with class I private antigens. Cloning of cytotoxic cells has revealed the presence of a variety of polymorphic target determinants on HLA molecules, some of which are identifiable by alloantisera or monoclonal antibodies derived from immunization of mice with human cells. Some of these reagents can be used to identify private determinants of HLA, while others are directed to more

"public" (sometimes called supertypic) determinants. One such system of public HLA-B antigens has two alleles, Bw4 and Bw6. Most HLA-B private antigens are associated with either Bw4 or Bw6. Other systems are restricted to subsets of HLA antigen groups. For example, HLA-B-bearing heavy chains carry additional sites that are common to B7, B27, Bw22, and B40 or to B5, B15, B18, and Bw35. Other types of shared antigenic determinants exist, as exemplified by a monoclonal antibody which reacts with a site shared between HLA-A and HLA-B heavy chains.

The amino acid sequence and peptide maps of several HLA molecules show that the class I hypervariable regions are clustered in the outer α_1 domain (Fig. 14-2) and the adjacent portion of α_2. Variability in the sequences of class II molecules differs from locus to locus. Remarkably, the class I α_3 domain, the class II α_2 and β_2 domains, and the portions of the CD8 (T8, Leu 2) cell surface molecule that function in T-cell interactions (see Chap. 13) all show significant amino acid sequence homologies with immunoglobulin constant regions. These findings suggest evolutionary elaboration within a family of gene products that have immune recognition functions. When genomic DNA for HLA is examined, typical exon-intron sequences of DNA have been found for class I and class II, exons having been identified for signal peptides (5′), each of the domains, a transmembrane hydrophobic segment, and a cytoplasmic segment (3′). cDNA probes are available for most of the HLA chains, and enzymatic digests have been used to study patterns of *restriction fragment length polymorphisms* (RFLP), many of which correlate with class II serologic and MLR patterns. There are 20 to 30 class I genes, however, making assessment of polymorphism by RFLP difficult. Many of these genes are not expressed (pseudogenes), while some could represent additional class I loci that are expressed only on activated T cells, and are of uncertain function. The detection of variable nucleotide sequences (tissue types) by means of the polymerase chain reaction technique is under study. This technique seeks to amplify specific segments of DNA, as defined by oligonucleotide primers, from genomic DNA. Such an approach offers the possibility of rapid HLA typing by hybridization with specific oligonucleotide probes.

Three-dimensional structure of HLA X-ray diffraction studies of the HLA-A2 molecule show a groove on the surface facing away from the cell membrane with dimensions sufficient to bind a peptide fragment 8- to 20-amino acids long, depending upon the degree of helix formation. The margins of the groove are formed by α helices, and the base is floored by a series of β strands, with the α_1 and α_2 domains contributing more or less equally to each side of the structure (Fig. 14-4). It is remarkable that the HLA variable regions and sites for alloantibody binding or cytotoxic T-cell recognition lie along the α helices that form the margins of the groove. Although class II molecules have yet to be studied to the same resolution, preliminary results suggest a similar groove formed by the α_1 and β_1 domains, and the known sequence polymorphisms would also lie along the presumed location of the groove. In brief, it appears that the site of antigen presentation by MHC molecules has been visualized. The known processing of protein antigens into smaller fragments by macrophages can now be related to the binding of certain of these fragments to class II molecules for recognition by the T-cell receptor. The phenomenon of MHC restriction, which indicates that the T cell must recognize both self-MHC and antigen, can now be viewed as the function of a single T-cell receptor that binds to both α-helical sides of the HLA groove and the peptide lying within it. Some of the polymorphism, especially on the inner surfaces of the helices and on the floor of the groove, may serve to bind the peptide fragments and possibly to alter their presentation to the T-cell receptor.

Complement (class III) Structural genes for three complement components, C4, C2, and Bf (factor B), are present in the HLA-B-D region (Fig. 14-1). There are two loci for C4, coding for C4A and C4B, formerly recognized as the Rodgers and Chido red blood cell antigens, respectively. These antigens are, in fact, adsorbed plasma C4 molecules. Other complement components are not closely linked

FIGURE 14-4 Structure of the HLA class I molecule as determined by x-ray crystallography. *A.* Shown is the face of the HLA-A2 molecule that points away from the cell surface. This ribbon diagram shows the groove that is formed by two α helices, and is supported by a floor of eight β strands. N is the amino terminal of the α_1 domain; the two small circles represent a disulfide bond. (*From PA Bjorkman et al.*) *B.* Composite display of polymorphic sites from several human and mouse class I alleles, using the HLA-A2 structure as the model. The symbols show a composite of the polymorphisms along the groove. Localization of variable amino acids and/or sites for alloantibody and/or cytotoxic T-cell recognition is shown to be along the α helices (circles). Polymorphic sites exist also in the β strands (squares). The numbers indicate the amino acid sequence. (*After PA Bjorkman et al.*)

to HLA. No crossovers have been found between the C2, Bf, and C4 loci. They are all encoded within a 100-kilobase segment between HLA-B and HLA-DR. There are two alleles of C2, four of Bf, seven of C4A, and three of C4B, plus blanks (null genes) for each locus (QO). The extensive polymorphism of complement types (complotypes) makes them useful for genetic studies. The four most common extended haplotypes found in people of western European ancestry are shown in Table 14-1. MLRs between unrelated individuals who are matched for these extended haplotypes are nonreactive, whereas reactivity is common if unrelated individuals are matched for only HLA DR and DQ. Such identical extended haplotypes may be conserved from a common ancestor.

Other sixth-chromosome genes Deficiency of steroid 21-hydroxylase, an autosomal recessive trait, results in the syndrome of congenital adrenal hyperplasia (Chaps. 317 and 324). The gene for the enzyme is localized in the HLA-B-D region. The 21-hydroxylase gene adjacent to C4A is deleted in affected individuals along with C4A (C4AQO), and the HLA-B locus gene may have been altered to convert B13 to the rare Bw47 found only in affected haplotypes. A late-onset variant of 21-hydroxylase deficiency is also linked to HLA. Congenital adrenal hyperplasia due to 11β-hydroxylase deficiency is not HLA-linked. Idiopathic hemochromatosis, an autosomal recessive disorder, is linked to HLA, as has been shown in several family studies (see Chap. 327). Although the pathogenesis of this disease is unknown, the gene that modulates gastrointestinal iron absorption is near HLA-A (Table 14-2).

Immune response genes HLA-D is analogous to the mouse H-2I region as established by studies of in vitro responses to synthetic polypeptide antigens, keyhole limpet hemocyanin, collagen, and tetanus toxoid. Presentation of antigenic fragments on the surfaces of macrophages or other cells bearing class II molecules requires conjoint recognition of a class II + antigen complex by T lymphocytes bearing the appropriate receptor(s) (see also Chap. 13). The crux of this "self + X" or "altered self" hypothesis is that in the T-dependent immune response, help from the T helper-inducer cell (T$_H$) occurs only if the appropriate class II determinant can be synthesized. The genes for the latter are Ir (immune response) genes. Since allogeneic class II determinants are perceived as already altered, the allogeneic mixed lymphocyte response represents a model for the immune system in which additional nominal antigen does not need

to be added (Fig. 14-5). Effector phases of immunity require recognition of nominal antigen together with a self structure. The latter in humans, as in mice, is the molecule bearing class I histocompatibility antigens. Human cell lines infected with influenza virus are lysed by immune cytotoxic T lymphocytes (T$_c$) only if an HLA-A- or HLA-B-locus antigen is shared between the attacking and target cells. Again, the allogeneic MLR provides a model for development of class I restricted cytotoxic T lymphocytes (Fig. 14-5). When primed cells are propagated and cloned, an array of restrictions to different class I and II molecules and epitopes can be discerned. At the level of the antigen presenting cell, for example, a given T$_H$ clone recognizes an antigenic fragment conjointly with a specific site on a class II molecule via its receptor (T$_i$). The restriction elements for some microbial antigens are DR or Dw alleles. The association of CD4-positive T cells with responses to class II antigens and of CD8-positive T cells with responses to class I antigens appears to be the result of direct interaction of CD4 and CD8 with class II

TABLE 14-1 Common extended HLA haplotypes

HLA-B	HLA-DR	Bf	C2	C4A	C4B
8	3	S	C	QO	1
7	2	S	C	3	1
57	7	S	C	6	1
44	7	F	C	3	1

TABLE 14-2 Linkage of genetic defects to HLA

	Gene location	Common haplotype found
C2 deficiency	HLA-B-D	Aw25, B18, BfS, DR2
21-OH deficiency	HLA-B-D	A3, Bw47, BfF, DR7
21-OH deficiency (late onset)	HLA-B-D,	B14, BfS, DR1
Idiopathic hemochromatosis	HLA-A	A3, B14
Paget's disease	HLA-A-D	
Spinocerebellar ataxia	HLA-A-D	
Hodgkin's disease	HLA-A-D	

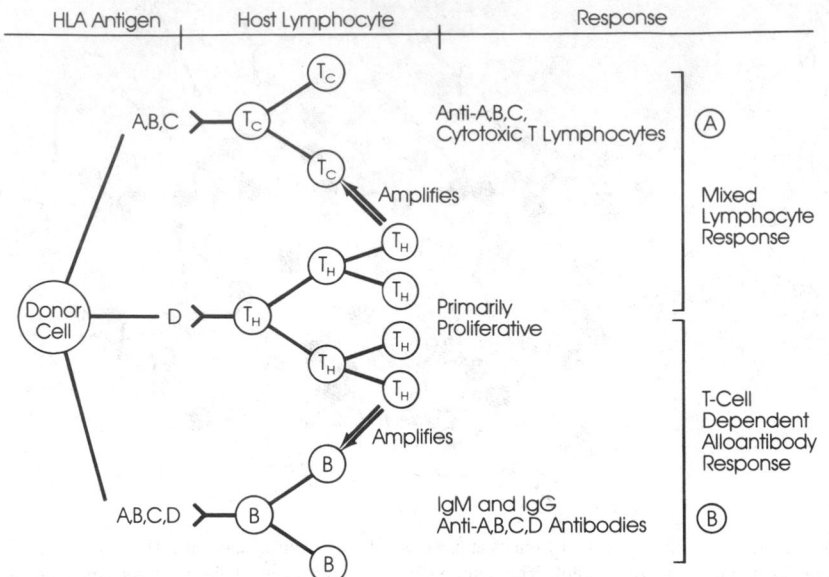

ALLOGRAFT RESPONSE

FIGURE 14-5 Schema of the relative roles of HLA-A, HLA-B, HLA-C, and HLA-D antigens in initiation of the alloimmune response and in the development of effector cells and antibodies. Two main classes of T lymphocytes recognize antigens: T_c, the precursors to the cytotoxic "killer" cells, and T_H, the helper cells for amplification of the cytotoxic response. T_H also provide help to B lymphocytes for production of a fully mature IgG response. Note that T_c generally recognize class I antigens, while the T_H signal is provided by antigens of the HLA-D region (class II). (*From CB Carpenter, Kidney International, 14:283, 1978.*)

and class I antigen-presenting molecules, respectively. Suppression of immune responses (i.e., low responder status) to cedar pollen, streptococcal antigen, and schistosomal antigen is linked to HLA-DQ as a dominant trait, suggesting the existence of immune suppressor (Is) genes. Specific allele associations with immune response (e.g., ragweed Ra5 antigen with DR2 and collagen with DR4) have also been demonstrated.

DISEASE ASSOCIATIONS If the major histocompatibility complex serves a critical natural biologic function, what might that be? One hypothesis is that it plays a role in immune surveillance against neoplastic cells that develop in the course of an individual's lifetime. The system could also play an important role in pregnancy because of the histoincompatibility that always exists between the mother and the fetus. The high degree of polymorphism may also ensure survival of the species in relation to the large numbers of microbiologic agents present in the environment. Self-tolerance which happens to cross-react with microbiologic agents would produce a high degree of susceptibility, resulting in lethal infection, whereas the polymorphism in the HLA system ensures that segments of the population recognize offending agents as foreign and initiate the appropriate response. All these hypotheses relate to the survival value of the system under selective evolutionary pressures, and there is some evidence for each of them.

Circumstantial evidence for the role of the HLA complex in immunobiology comes from the finding that a number of disease processes are positively associated with certain HLA antigens within the population. The search for such associations has been stimulated by the discovery of immune response genes linked to the H-2 complex in the mouse. Table 14-3 summarizes the most significant HLA and disease associations.

Most striking is the increased frequency of HLA-B27 in certain rheumatic diseases, particularly ankylosing spondylitis, a condition with a strong familial tendency. B27 is present in about 7 percent of people of western European ancestry, while it appears in 80 to 90 percent of patients with ankylosing spondylitis. Expressed as a relative risk, the antigen B27 confers a susceptibility to the development of ankylosing spondylitis that is 87 times that in the general population. Similarly, acute anterior uveitis, Reiter's syndrome, and reactive arthritis to at least three bacterial infections (yersinia, salmonella, and gonococcus) show a high degree of association with B27. Although the ordinary form of juvenile rheumatoid arthritis (JRA) also shows a similar association with B27, the pauciarticular form of JRA with iritis is DR5-associated. The increased incidence of B27 in psoriatic

arthritis is also significant for the central type (axial skeleton) of the disorder, while Bw38 is associated with both the central and peripheral types. Psoriasis is associated with Cw6. Patients with degenerative arthritis or gout show no alteration in antigen frequencies.

Most other disease associations are with HLA-D region antigens. Narcolepsy is virtually 100 percent associated with DR2 in both Japanese and whites. Affected individuals need inherit only a single gene dose of DR2. Although there is no apparent autoimmune component to this condition, there is speculation that an abnormality in a neurotransmitter or its receptor may be influenced by the DR2 gene or another closely linked gene. Gluten-sensitive enteropathy (celiac disease, nontropical sprue) in children and adults is associated with DR3 (relative risk = 21). The actual percentage of such patients having this antigen ranges from 63 to 96 percent compared to 22 to 27 percent of controls. The same antigen is also present in increased frequency in patients with chronic active hepatitis and in patients with dermatitis herpetiformis who also have gluten-sensitive enteropathy. Juvenile-onset insulin-dependent diabetes mellitus (type I) is associated with DR4 and DR3 and is negatively associated with DR2. Resistance to type I diabetes is strongly associated with the inheritance of aspartate at position 57 of the β chain of HLA-DQ, in linkage disequilibrium with HLA-DR2. Other amino acids at position 57, especially when HLA-DR3 or -DR4 are on the same haplotype, are associated with an increased risk of disease. Maturity-onset diabetes is not HLA-associated. A rare allele of Bf (F1) is also found in 17 to 25 percent of cases of type I diabetes. Hyperthyroidism in the United States is associated with B8, Dw3, while in Japanese populations the association is with Bw35. More extensive studies of healthy and diseased members of various races will help in clarification of which HLA markers are universal. For example, B27 is rare in healthy Japanese but is common in subjects with ankylosing spondylitis. Also, DR4 seems to be the common marker for type I diabetes in all races. Sometimes an HLA marker is clearly associated only with a subgroup within a syndrome. For example, myasthenia gravis without thymoma is more strongly B8, DR3-associated, and the association of DR2 with multiple sclerosis is strong in patients with rapidly progressive deterioration. Goodpasture's syndrome due to autoimmunity to glomerular basement membrane, idiopathic membranous glomerulonephritis, which may be an autoimmune process involving antibodies to an antigen of the glomerulus, and gold-induced membranous nephritis are strongly HLA-DR-associated.

LINKAGE DISEQUILIBRIUM Although the distribution of HLA alleles varies in racial and ethnic populations, the most salient feature

TABLE 14-3 HLA antigens and disease, showing the most highly associated antigens

Disease	Antigen	Relative risk*
RHEUMATIC		
Ankylosing spondylitis	B27	69.1
Reiter's syndrome	B27	37.0
Acute anterior uveitis	B27	8.2
Reactive arthritis (yersinia, salmonella, gonococcus)	B27	18.0
Psoriatic arthritis, central	B27	10.7
	Bw38	9.1
Psoriatic arthritis, peripheral	B27	2.0
	Bw38	6.5
Juvenile rheumatoid arthritis	B27	3.9
	DRw8	3.6
Juvenile arthritis, pauciarticular	DR5	3.3
Rheumatoid arthritis	Dw4/DR4	3.8
Sjögren's syndrome	Dw3	5.7
Systemic lupus erythematosus	DR3	2.6
Systemic lupus erythematosus (hydralazine)	DR4	5.6
GASTROINTESTINAL		
Gluten-sensitive enteropathy	DR3	11.6
Chronic active hepatitis	DR3	6.8
Ulcerative colitis	B5	3.8
HEMATOLOGIC		
Idiopathic hemochromatosis	A3	6.7
	B14	26.7
	A3, B14	90.0
Pernicious anemia	DR5	5.4
SKIN		
Dermatitis herpetiformis	Dw3	17.3
Psoriasis vulgaris	Cw6	7.5
Psoriasis vulgaris (Japanese)	Cw6	8.5
Pemphigus vulgaris (Jews)	DR4	14.6
	A10	4.8
Behçet's disease	B5	3.8
ENDOCRINE		
Type 1 diabetes mellitus	DR4	3.6
	DR3	4.8
	DR2	0.2
	BfF1	15.0
Hyperthyroidism	B8	2.5
	Dw3	3.7
Hyperthyroidism (Japanese)	Bw35	4.4
Adrenal insufficiency	Dw3	10.5
Subacute thyroiditis (de Quervain)	Bw35	13.7
Hashimoto's thyroiditis	DR5	3.2
Congenitial adrenal hyperplasia	Bw47	15.4
NEUROLOGIC		
Myasthenia gravis	B8	2.7
	DR3	2.5
Multiple sclerosis	DR2	2.7
Manic-depressive disorder	Bw16	2.3
Narcolepsy	DR2	130.0
Schizophrenia	A28	2.3
RENAL		
Idiopathic membranous glomerulonephritis	DR3	5.7
Goodpasture's syndrome (anti-GBM)	DR2	15.9
Minimal change disease (steroid response)	B12	4.2
Polycystic kidney disease	B5	2.6
IgA nephropathy	DR4	3.1
Gold nephropathy	DR3	14.0
	DR4	0.3
INFECTIOUS		
Tuberculoid leprosy (Asians)	B8	6.8
Paralytic polio	Bw16	4.3
Low vs. high response to vaccinia virus	Cw3	12.7
IMMUNODEFICIENCY		
IgA deficiency (blood donors)	DR3	13.0

* Relative risk = $\dfrac{(\% \text{ antigen-positive patients})(\% \text{ antigen-negative controls})}{(\% \text{ antigen-negative patients})(\% \text{ antigen-positive controls})}$

of population genetics of HLA antigens is the presence of linkage disequilibria among certain antigens of the A and B, B and C, and B, D, and complement loci. Linkage disequilibrium means that antigens of closely linked loci appear together more frequently than predicted by random association. The classic example is the linkage disequilibrium present between the A-locus antigen HLA-A1 and the B-locus antigen HLA-B8 in people of western European ancestry. The coincidence of A1 and B8 should be the product of their individual gene frequencies ($0.17 \times 0.11 \cong 0.02$). The observed frequency of A1 and B8 is 0.08, four times that expected, an increase of 0.06. The latter value is termed Δ (delta), and is a measure of the discequilibrium. Other A- and B locus haplotype disequilibria have been recognized and include (A3, B7), (A2, B12), (A29, B12), and (A11, Bw35). Furthermore, some D-region determinants are in linkage disequilibrium with B-locus antigens (for example, DR3 and B8), as are some B-locus and C-locus antigens. Serologically defined HLA antigens can serve as markers for the genes of an entire haplotype within a family and as markers for specific genes within a population but only where a linkage disequilibrium exists.

Linkage disequilibrium is of importance because such gene associations may have some bearing on their function. For example, selective pressures during the course of evolution may have been the major factor in the survival of certain gene combinations in a haplotype. Such a theory suggests, for example, that A1 and B8, along with certain D-region and other determinants, conferred a selective advantage in the face of epidemics such as the plague or smallpox. It would also follow that the descendants of the survivors may display susceptibility to certain diseases because their unique gene complex happens to confer an abnormal response to other environmental agents. The major difficulty with this hypothesis is the assumption that selection must work on several genes simultaneously to account for the observed Δ's; however, the need for complex interactions among the products of the several loci of the major histocompatibility complex is only beginning to be appreciated, and selection might force multiple linkage disequilibria. The conservation of certain extended haplotypes, mentioned above, supports this view.

On the other hand, the selection hypothesis is not necessary to explain linkage disequilibrium. When a population lacking certain antigens is crossed with one in which a high frequency of antigens is in equilibrium, a Δ can develop within a few generations. For example, the increasing Δ value for A1,B8 found in populations from east to west, from India to western Europe, can be explained on the basis of migration and fusion. In smaller groups, consanguinity, founder effects, and gene drift may account for disequilibria. Finally, certain linkage disequilibria could occur as a result of nonrandom crossing over during gametic meiosis, because of chromosomal segments which are either more or less likely to break. Unless there are selective pressures or restrictions in crossing over, linkage disequilibria disappear over a period of several generations. A large number of nonrandom associations occur throughout the HLA gene complex, and elucidation of the reasons for their existence may provide insight into the mechanism underlying certain disease susceptibilities.

LINKAGE AND ASSOCIATION The diseases listed in Table 14-2 are examples of HLA linkage wherein the inherited conditions are marked within families by the relevant HLA haplotypes. For C2 deficiency, 21-hydroxylase deficiency, and idiopathic hemochromatosis the mode of inheritance is recessive, with heterozygotes showing partial deficiencies. These genetic defects are also HLA-associated, with an excess of certain HLA alleles in affected unrelated individuals. Also, C2 deficiency is commonly linked to the HLA-Aw25, B18, Bfs, D/DR2 haplotype, and idiopathic hemochromatosis exhibits both linkage and strong association with HLA-A3 and -B14. The high degree of linkage disequilibria in these HLA-linked diseases may result from mutations in a single founder, and a sufficient period of time may not have passed to bring the gene pool back into equilibrium. In this view, the HLA antigens are simple markers for the linked gene. Alternatively, expression of the defect may require interaction with specific HLA alleles. This latter hypothesis would require a higher mutation rate, with defective gene expression occurring only when linked with certain HLA genes.

Paget's disease and spinocerebellar ataxia are HLA-linked autosomal dominant traits in families having multiple affected members, and Hodgkin's disease shows an HLA-linked recessive pattern of inheritance. No HLA associations have been discerned for these disorders, suggesting that there were multiple founders with mutations in linkage with different HLA alleles.

HLA linkage is readily recognized when recessive or dominant inheritance patterns are clear-cut, i.e., when expressivity is high and the process is mostly, if not entirely, determined by a single gene defect. In most of the associations HLA markers represent risk factors involving the operation and modulation of the immune response under the influence of multiple genes. An example of a polygenic immunologic disease is atopic allergy, in which the association to HLA may be evident only in individuals whose genetically controlled (non-HLA) levels of IgE production are low. Another is IgA deficiency (Table 14-3), which is HLA-DR3-associated.

CLINICAL APPLICATIONS   The clinical value of HLA typing for diagnosis of disease is limited to B27 and ankylosing spondylitis, where nevertheless there are 10 percent false-positive and false-negative rates. HLA studies are also of value in genetic counseling and early recognition of disease in families with idiopathic hemochromatosis or congenital adrenal hyperplasia due to steroid 21-hydroxylase deficiency, particularly as HLA typing can be performed upon cells obtained by amniocentesis. The high degree of polymorphism of the HLA system also makes it a powerful tool for paternity testing and other medicolegal applications. The implications for

diseases such as type I diabetes mellitus and the other diseases showing HLA associations require further study of the components of the HLA system and their role in the pathogenesis of disease. Matching for HLA antigens in allogeneic transplantation is reviewed in Chap. 225.

REFERENCES

BIDWELL J: DNA-RFLP analysis and genotyping of HLA-DR and DQ antigens. Immunol Today 9:18, 1988

BJORKMAN PA et al: Structure of the human class I histocompatibility antigen, HLA-A2. Nature 329:506, 1987

——— et al: The foreign antigen binding site and T cell recognition regions of class I histocompatibility antigens. Nature 329:512, 1987

CARPENTER CB, STROM TB: Immunobiology of renal transplantation, in *Renal Transplantation*, EL Milford et al (eds), *Contemporary Issues in Nephrology,* vol 19. New York, Churchill Livingstone, 1989

DEGOS L, DAUSSET J: Human migrations and linkage disequilibrium of HLA system. Immunogenetics 3:195, 1974

DUQUESNOY RJ, TRUCCO M: Genetic basis of cell surface polymorphism encoded by the major histocompatibility complex in humans. CRC Crit Rev Immunol 8:103, 1988

MARSH DG et al: Epidemiology and genetics of atopic allergy. N Eng J Med 305:1551, 1981

MATSUSHITA S et al: HLA linked nonresponsiveness to *Cryptomeria japonica* pollen antigen: I. Nonresponsiveness is mediated by antigen-specific suppressor T cells. J Immunol 138:109, 1987

Nomenclature for factors of the HLA system, 1987. Tissue Antigens 32:177, 1988

SASAZUKI T et al: HLA-linked gene controlling immune response and disease susceptibility. Immunol Rev 70:51, 1983

TIWARI JL, TERASAKI PI: *HLA and Disease Associations.* New York, Springer Verlag, 1985

TODD JA et al: HLA-DQ beta gene contributes to susceptibility and resistance to insulin-dependent diabetes mellitus. Nature 329:599, 1987

WHITE PC et al: HLA-linked congenital adrenal hyperplasia results from a defective gene encoding a cytochrome P-450 specific for steroid 21-hydroxylation. Proc Natl Acad Sci USA 81:7505, 1984

section 1 Pain

15 PAIN: PATHOPHYSIOLOGY AND MANAGEMENT

RAYMOND MACIEWICZ / JOSEPH B. MARTIN

Pain is the most common symptom of disease. Although the nature, location, and etiology of pain differ in each case, approximately half of all patients who visit a physician have a primary complaint of pain. For most, the correct treatment of a self-evident, limited disease process (such as a broken bone) alleviates pain. However, in some patients uncontrolled pain continues to be a major problem. In these cases, the symptom of pain requires careful assessment and evaluation to interpret its significance and to establish an approach for its effective treatment.

The evaluation of the patient with pain is frequently complex, partially because pain is a perception rather than a sensation. A person's physical state, past experience, and anticipation all influence the way pain is interpreted. For example, soldiers and athletes may deny pain despite an acute injury, while certain patients with chronic pain may continue to suffer despite the lack of an obvious source of disease. Our knowledge of pain and most of our treatments for it focus on decreasing the nociceptive sensory input; however, a patient's interpretation of a sensation, emotional response, and associated behavior are equally important factors that deserve the physician's careful attention.

ORGANIZATION OF PAIN PATHWAYS **Nociceptive afferents** Sensory stimuli of potentially tissue-damaging intensity activate free nerve endings in skin, underlying tissue, and viscera. Nociceptive signals are conveyed to the spinal cord by unmyelinated and small myelinated sensory axons. In humans, stimulation of individual small sensory axons can evoke the report of pain in the area of skin supplied by that fiber, clearly demonstrating that under certain conditions even single axons can transmit activity that is interpreted as "pain" by the brain.

Many unmyelinated nociceptive afferents exhibit "polymodal" responses. Such fibers can be activated by intense mechanical stimulation, potentially tissue-damaging thermal stimulation, and chemical stimulation by substances injected into skin. Any intense stimulus applied to normal skin can produce a "triple response" that consists of a red flush at the site of stimulation, a surrounding red flare due to arterial dilatation, and local edema caused by increased vascular permeability. Many substances likely play an important role in this response. Some of these agents are released by damaged tissue (potassium, histamine, serotonin, prostaglandins), while others enter from the circulation (bradykinin) or come from local nerve endings themselves (substance P). Certain of these substances also activate free nerve endings, and their long-lasting effects may partially explain the hypersensitivity of the skin that often follows a noxious stimulus.

Dorsal horn Sensory fibers extend distally and proximally from cells located in the segmental dorsal root ganglia. Nociceptive afferents enter the spinal cord through the dorsal root to terminate on dorsal horn neurons (Fig. 15-1A). Many of the fine afferents ending in these regions contain neuropeptides, including substance P, cholecystokinin, and somatostatin. There is increasing evidence that these peptides play an important role in normal sensory transmission. Chemical destruction of substance P fibers in animals produces analgesia in certain tests for pain, and there is also a marked decrease in substance P terminal staining in the dorsal horn in patients with congenital neuropathies that are associated with decreased sensitivity to pain.

The spinal dorsal horn can be divided into a series of layers based on cell morphology and arrangement. Neurons that process nociceptive information are found in several of these layers. Unmyelinated afferents terminate principally in layer II (the *substantia gelatinosa*), while myelinated nociceptive afferents end in layers I and V. The output neurons that project to brainstem and thalamus are found principally in layers I and V. The axons of these dorsal horn neurons form a crossed pathway that ascends in the ventrolateral quadrant of the spinal cord, the spinothalamic tract.

Spinothalamic system The axons of nociceptive dorsal horn neurons that form the spinothalamic tracts terminate in several brainstem and thalamic nuclei. The spinothalamic tract can be divided conceptually into two systems based on these connections: a direct spinothalamic system that carries sensory discriminative information about pain to thalamic levels, and a phylogenetically older spinoreticulothalamic system that terminates more diffusely in brainstem reticular nuclei.

The direct spinothalamic system that ends in the thalamus may be important for the conscious perception of nociceptive sensations. This system terminates in an orderly fashion within the *nucleus ventralis posterolateralis* (VPL). The terminal field of the spinothalamic tract in VPL overlaps the dorsal column–medial lemniscal input that relays light touch and joint sensation. The organized pattern of terminations and the convergence of light touch and pain information within VPL may be important for perception of the sensory discriminative aspects of pain, including the location, nature, and intensity of a noxious input. Consistent with this view, cells in VPL project principally to the primary somatosensory cortex.

The more diffuse spinoreticulothalamic system may mediate the autonomic and affective components of pain. Ascending spinoreticular fibers terminate at several levels of the brainstem reticular formation, forming part of a polysynaptic system that terminates in the medial thalamic nuclei (*nucleus centralis lateralis* and *nucleus parafascicularis*). Cells throughout the spinoreticulothalamic system often have large, bilateral sensory receptive fields that can include the entire body surface. These cells often respond best to noxious sensory input. Such cells are probably not involved in sensory discrimination or localization; more likely, they are important for arousal or orientation to a painful stimulus.

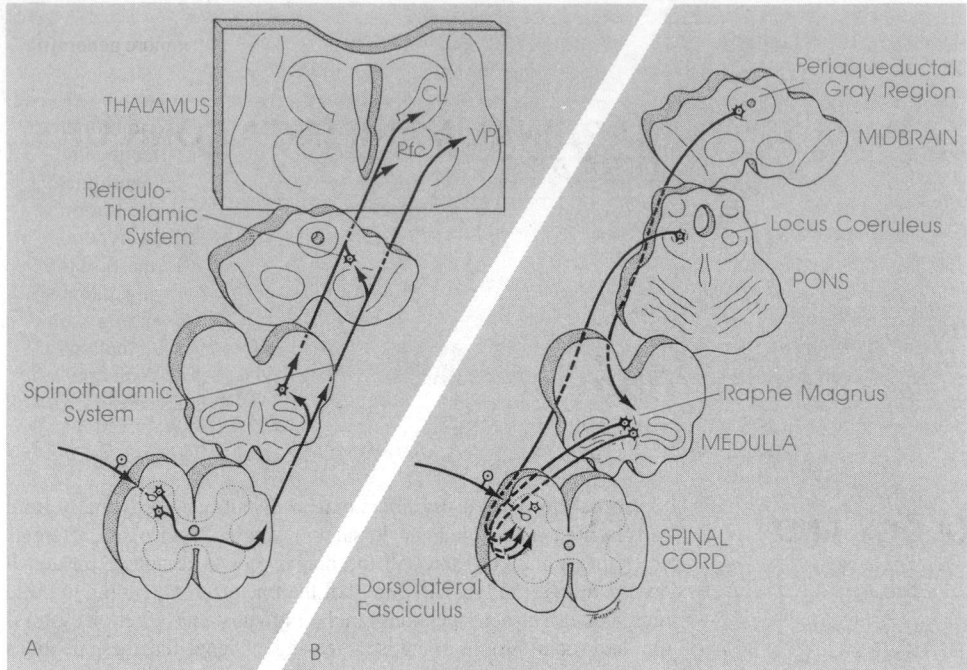

FIGURE 15-1 *A*. Ascending nociceptive pathways. The direct spinothalamic tract terminates in the nucleus ventroposterolateralis (VPL). The indirect, spinoreticulothalamic pathway relays through the brainstem reticular formation and ends in nuclei of the medial and intralaminar thalamus [nuclei parafascicularis (Pfc) and centralis lateralis (CL)]. *B*. Descending analgesia pathways. Periaqueductal gray neurons project to nucleus raphe magnus. A descending projection from raphe magnus inhibits the nociceptive responses of dorsal horn neurons. A separate inhibitory pathway from the nucleus locus coeruleus also directly ends in the dorsal horn.

Descending analgesic pathways In addition to the major ascending pain pathways outlined above, the brain contains powerful descending circuits that suppress nociceptive inputs (Fig. 15-1*B*). In animals, electrical stimulation of the midbrain periaqueductal gray region can produce generalized analgesia without other obvious sensory or motor responses. A similar system may exist in humans, as stimulation of the nearby periventricular gray is reported to relieve clinical pain. This effect appears to be at least partly mediated at the spinal level, since it can be blocked in animals by cutting pathways that carry descending projections from brainstem to dorsal horn. However, few periaqueductal gray cells project directly to the spinal cord. Instead, the descending pathway important for analgesia appears to first synapse in the midline raphe nuclei of the medulla (principally *nucleus raphe magnus*). Raphe neurons in turn project to the spinal cord, where they inhibit the nociceptive responses of dorsal horn neurons. This descending system can potentially gate the flow of nociceptive information from the level of the first synapse in the dorsal horn.

The periaqueductal gray region, the medullary raphe, and the dorsal horn all contain a high density of endogenous opiate peptides and opiate receptors. Systemic narcotic analgesics may, in part, work by activating the descending analgesia system at these sites. High densities of opiate receptors are also found in the medial thalamus and limbic forebrain; these structures may play an additional, important role in the analgesic response to and the addictive potential of systemically administered narcotics.

Biogenic amines represent another class of neurotransmitters found in the descending pathways that modulate nociception. Serotonin is contained in many of the raphe neurons that end in dorsal horn, and some serotonergic axon terminals end directly on spinothalamic tract neurons. A major descending inhibitory pathway containing norepinephrine also arises in the nucleus locus coeruleus of the pons; this system appears to inhibit the nociceptive responses of dorsal horn neurons by an alpha-adrenergic mechanism. Drugs that potentiate the central effects of biogenic amines, such as the tricyclic antidepressants, may therefore be effective analgesic adjuvants that work by enhancing the effects of these descending pathways.

EVALUATION OF THE PATIENT WITH PAIN   Somatic pain Pain usually occurs when a potentially tissue-damaging stimulus excites peripheral nociceptive afferents. When a noxious stimulus activates receptors in skin, muscle, or joint, the somatic pain that results is usually well-localized and easily described by the patient (Table 15-1). In contrast, pain of visceral origin is often poorly localized and may be referred to an area of skin supplied by the same sensory roots that innervate the diseased visceral organ. For example, myocardial pain activates visceral afferents terminating in the upper four thoracic segments of the spinal cord. This nociceptive information converges on the same neurons that receive cutaneous input from the upper thoracic dermatomes, and the reported pain is therefore frequently referred to the left shoulder and arm. In a similar fashion, the sensory innervation of cranial blood vessels terminates on brainstem trigeminal neurons that also have a cutaneous input. This convergence likely explains the referral of vascular headache pain to the ipsilateral forehead and eye.

Convergence also occurs between muscle, joint, and cutaneous nociceptive afferents. Chronic activation of these pathways can evoke referred pain, local sympathetic effects, segmental muscular contraction, and generalized postural muscle changes. This constellation of features may, with time, result in sustained changes that contribute to the development of certain chronic, painful disorders. For example, following injury or disease, many patients develop a condition of fibromyositis, with pain evoked by movement of specific muscle groups. On examination, such patients often have limitation of movement and tender muscular "trigger points" that reproduce their pain, which is often referred. Myofascial pain of this sort is often prominent in temporomandibular joint disorders, chronic cervical pain, or low back disorders. Untreated myofascial pain can frequently lead to progressive disability, loss of range of motion, and increased pain.

Both cutaneous and visceral pain are common experiences and do not always signal a disease process. The somatic pain resulting from

TABLE 15-1   Evaluation of pain

Somatic pain	Neuropathic pain
1 Nociceptive stimulus usually evident.	1 No obvious nociceptive stimulus.
2 Pain is usually well-localized; visceral pain may be referred.	2 Pain is often poorly localized.
3 Pain is similar to other somatic pains in the patient's experience.	3 Pain is unusual, dissimilar from somatic pain.
4 Pain is relieved by anti-inflammatory or narcotic analgesics.	4 Pain is only partially relieved by narcotic analgesics.

a new injury or illness is therefore generally familiar to the patient and described in the context of prior similar pains. Somatic pain due to activation of normal nociceptive mechanisms is usually effectively relieved by a brief course of an appropriate analgesic.

Neuropathic pain Pain can also result from injury to, or chronic changes in, peripheral or central somatosensory pathways. This may be due to an abnormal or disordered pattern of afferent neuronal activity that reaches the dorsal horn and more central structures. Damage to sensory pathways may also decrease the inhibitory controls that are normally activated by a peripheral input. Neuropathic pain that follows damage to sensory pathways can develop and persist without an obvious noxious input. The patient often uses unusual terms to describe the pain, emphasizing the distinction between perception of normal somatic pains and neuropathic sensations.

The sensory symptoms in neuropathic pain can be either focal or more generalized. Trauma or irritation to a peripheral nerve may result in a *neuralgia*, which is defined as pain in the distribution of a single nerve; the pain is often (but not always) accompanied by signs of nerve dysfunction, such as sensory loss or weakness of muscles innervated by the nerve. Frequently the pain consists of a background spontaneous burning or aching sensation (*dysesthesia*) that can be associated with paroxysmal jabs of sharp pain within the affected region. Despite an elevated sensory detection threshold, patients will often have an exaggerated response to a noxious stimulus (*hyperalgesia*) or to touch (*hyperesthesia*) or perceive a nonnociceptive stimulus as painful (*allodynia*). These terms for altered hypersensitivity to sensory stimuli are commonly grouped under the less specific term *hyperpathia* (see also Chap. 28).

In some forms of neuralgia (such as trigeminal neuralgia) paroxysmal, lancinating pain predominates without other signs of nerve dysfunction. In contrast, *causalgia* following nerve injury is char-acterized by a continuous, severe burning pain, allodynia, and evident sympathetic dysfunction. Pain can also be a feature of more generalized neuropathies associated with degeneration of small-caliber axons. In such cases there can be multiple locations for the pain as well as a variety of types of pain. In diffuse sensory or sensorimotor neuropathies, the pain is usually symmetric and distal, affecting the feet and, with progression, the hands. As with more focal neuralgias, the pain often consists of a spontaneous aching or burning sensation with superimposed paroxysmal jabs of pain. Allodynia and hyperalgesia are common features during acute, painful phases of the disease.

Pain may also be a debilitating symptom following damage to central somatosensory pathways. Lesions of the ascending somato-sensory pathways at the level of the cord, brainstem, thalamus, or cortex can result in a syndrome of continuous spontaneous pain that is referred to the periphery, often with superimposed sensory abnormalities as discussed above.

MANAGEMENT OF PATIENTS WITH PAIN **Moderate pain** Many acute somatic pains can be treated effectively with oral, nonnarcotic analgesics such as aspirin 650 mg or acetaminophen 650 mg orally every 4 h (Table 15-2). These drugs have few side effects, do not cause sedation, and are not associated with tolerance or dependence. Other nonsteroidal anti-inflammatory drugs (NSAIDs), such as naproxen, indomethacin, ibuprofen, or trisalicylate, are also often effective for minor or moderately severe somatic pain; however, there is little evidence that these agents are clearly better than aspirin, and aspirin is much less expensive. Acetaminophen has little anti-inflammatory action compared to aspirin and indomethacin; pain associated with inflammatory disease is therefore better managed with the latter drugs. However, the side effects of NSAIDs and aspirin, particularly dyspepsia, gastrointestinal bleeding, and inhibition of platelet aggregation can limit their usefulness in certain

---

TABLE 15-2 Drugs for relief of pain

NONNARCOTIC ANALGESICS: USUAL DOSES AND INTERVALS

Generic name	PO dose, mg	Interval	Comments
Acetylsalicylic acid	650	q 4 h	Enteric-coated preparations available
Acetaminophen	650	q 4 h	Side effects uncommon
Ibuprofen	400	q 4–6 h	Available without prescription
Naproxen	250–500	q 12 h	Delayed effects may be due to long half-life
Suprofen	200	q 6 h	Little anti-inflammatory effect
Trisalicylate	1000–1500	q 12 h	Fewer gastrointestinal or platelet effects
Indomethacin	25–50	q 8 h	Gastrointestinal side effects common

NARCOTIC ANALGESICS: USUAL DOSES AND INTERVALS

Generic name	Parenteral dose, mg	PO dose, mg	Comments
Codeine	30–60 q 4 h	30–60 q 4 h	Nausea common
Oxycodone	—	5–10 q 4–6 h	Usually available with acetominophen or aspirin
Morphine	10 q 4 h	60 q 4 h	
Morphine sustained release	90 q 12 h	Oral slow release preparation	
Hydromorphone	1–2 q 4 h	2–4 q 4 h	Shorter acting than morphine sulfate
Levorphanol	2 q 6–8 h	4 q 6–8 h	Longer acting than morphine sulfate; absorbed well PO
Methadone	10 q 6–8 h	20 q 6–8 h	Delayed sedation due to long half-life
Meperidine	75–100 q 3–4 h	300 q 4 h	Poorly absorbed PO; normeperidine a toxic metabolite

ANTICONVULSANTS

Generic name	PO dose, mg	Interval
Phenytoin	100	q 6–8 h
Carbamazepine	200–300	q 6 h
Clonazepam	1	q 6 h

TRICYCLIC ANTIDEPRESSANTS

Generic name	Uptake blockade 5HT	NE	Sedative potency	Anticholinergic potency	Orthostatic hypotension	Cardiac arrhythmia	Average dose, mg/day	Range, mg/day
Doxepin	+ +	+	High	Moderate	Moderate	Less	200	75–400
Amitriptyline	+ + + +	+ +	High	Highest	Moderate	Yes	150	75–300
Imipramine	+ + + +	+ +	Moderate	Moderate	High	Yes	200	75–400
Nortriptyline	+ + +	+ +	Moderate	Moderate	Low	Yes	100	40–150
Desipramine	+ + +	+ + + +	Low	Low	Low	Yes	150	75–300

patients; these side effects may be less common with trisalicylate and are not observed with acetaminophen.

Severe pain Narcotic analgesics are usually required for relief of severe pain. In general, patients should be treated with only one narcotic agent at a time, and therapy should be begun with an intermediate-strength narcotic such as codeine 30 mg every 4 to 6 h or oxycodone 5 mg every 4 to 6 h. In oral doses, codeine is relatively safe, potent, and well-tolerated. Aspirin or acetaminophen potentiates the analgesic effect of codeine, and so the two drugs can be used together. Oxycodone 5 mg is commonly available only in tablet form combined with aspirin or acetaminophen. Low-strength narcotic analgesics such as propoxyphene (dextropropoxyphene) or mixed agonist/antagonist drugs such as pentazocine have few indications. The analgesic effectiveness of these drugs is often little better than aspirin, and the frequency of side effects is much greater. Mixed agonist/antagonist drugs can also precipitate withdrawal in patients habituated to stronger narcotics.

If codeine 60 mg (or oxycodone 10 mg) orally every 4 h fails to provide relief, it should be discontinued, as larger doses of codeine increase the frequency of side effects without clearly adding to its analgesic effectiveness. In these situations codeine should be stopped and a higher-potency narcotic used, such as intramuscular morphine 10 mg every 4 h or oral hydromorphone 4 mg every 3 to 4 h. There is substantial variation in the effective analgesic dose and the duration of action of narcotics in individual patients. Dosages should therefore be individualized according to the patient's needs.

A variety of drugs, including antihistamines, amphetamines, and antidepressants, may enhance the analgesic effects of narcotics and can be useful in certain situations. Oral hydroxyzine 25 mg four times daily can potentiate narcotic analgesia without adding to the sedative effects. In patients who are excessively sedated by narcotics, oral dextroamphetamine 5 mg twice daily can make the patient more alert while enhancing analgesia. Benzodiazepines and phenothiazines have numerous side effects and often do not enhance analgesia; they should be used for their specific indications and not routinely.

The pharmacokinetics of narcotics are greatly influenced by disease. Hepatic cirrhosis or renal failure can enhance the bioavailability and decrease the elimination of narcotics. This is a particular problem with meperidine (pethidine). In debilitated patients receiving high doses of meperidine, the active metabolite normeperidine can accumulate, resulting in symptoms of tremor, confusion, and seizures. Morphine may be a superior drug to use when chronic, large doses of narcotics are required in debilitated patients, since the pharmacokinetics of morphine do not appear to be altered in cirrhosis.

Although side effects can result from the use of excess or inappropriate narcotics, a far more common problem is underutilization of analgesics. Hospitalized patients, including postoperative and cancer cases, frequently receive inadequate doses of narcotic analgesics. The reasons that underlie inadequate narcotic use in patients with evident painful disease are unclear. Concerns about inducing dependence and addiction in a medically ill population are largely unfounded. Similarly, concerns over respiratory depression and delayed recovery in patients on narcotics are often overstated; more often, *inadequate* analgesia in postoperative patients produces a reduction in tidal volume due to splinting and delays patient mobilization. When indicated, therefore, narcotic analgesics should be given frequently enough and in high enough doses to alleviate pain. A single narcotic medication should be offered the patient on a routine rather than on an ''as needed'' basis, with the understanding that the patient can refuse the drug if the level of analgesia is sufficient. Changes in analgesic doses and the need to taper narcotics as the acute phase of pain passes should be understood by the patient.

Chronic diseases usually cause recurrent bouts of acute pain rather than continuous discomfort. The management of acute painful exacerbations should be the same as the treatment of any new, acute pain. Analgesics should be available to the patient when pain is present, with the understanding between patient and physician that the drugs will be discontinued as the acute episode subsides.

Pain in advanced illness Patients with terminal diseases such as metastatic cancer often suffer from continuous or recurrent acute pain. For such patients, pain management is often the single most important treatment a physician can provide.

In outpatients with somatic pain due to cancer, oral codeine 30 mg or oxycodone 5 mg and acetaminophen 325 mg every 4 h may provide acceptable pain control. Patients with bony metastases often benefit from the addition of an NSAID, such as oral trisalicylate 1000 mg or naproxen 500 mg twice daily. If a total daily dose of 30 to 40 mg of oxycodone does not adequately relieve pain, the patient should be switched to a stronger narcotic such as oral hydromorphone 4 mg or levorphanol 2 mg as needed; however, there is little evidence that these drugs are more effective than oral morphine. Slow-release oral morphine preparations have little potential for abuse and can be administered every 12 h, with supplemental doses of regular oral morphine given as needed. The 12-h dosing schedule for slow-release morphine results in more continuous analgesia and often allows patients to sleep through the night without pain. Methadone also has a very long half-life and may therefore be useful in individual patients; however, the cumulative effects of methadone over many days requires careful follow-up monitoring of patients.

Essentially all patients on narcotics develop constipation. In cancer patients this can be significant, and should be anticipated.

In cancer patients an increase in pain often signals recurrence or extension of their disease. However, in some patients tolerance to medications can become an important factor. Although the underlying disease process remains essentially unchanged, increasing doses of narcotic analgesics may be necessary in such patients to maintain satisfactory analgesia. The rate at which patients clinically develop tolerance to narcotics is variable; some patients require a doubling of their dose as often as every 1 to 2 weeks. There is no absolute tolerance barrier, however, and patients tolerant to even very high doses of narcotics can still achieve analgesia by doubling or tripling their medication dosage. Although tolerance is an important issue, it should also be emphasized that most cancer patients develop tolerance only gradually, and remain responsive to relatively low doses of narcotics throughout the course of their disease.

As narcotic doses are increased, the frequency of side effects, including sedation and dysphoric reactions, may also increase. When these side effects limit the use of analgesics or require the use of continuous intravenous narcotics, surgical approaches to pain relief are worth considering. An anterolateral cordotomy can provide effective relief in patients with pain that is isolated to a single leg or hip. Touch sensation, motor power, and bladder control are all usually spared by the procedure. Cordotomy is less effective in patients with pain involving the upper extremity or involving both sides of the trunk. In evaluating patients for this procedure, the extent of disease may be as important as the location of pain. A patient with unilateral pain but evidence of bilateral or midline disease (such as extensive vertebral metastases) is not likely to get substantial relief from a cordotomy.

Spinal morphine therapy is worth considering in certain cancer patients. Morphine injections through spinal epidural or intrathecal catheters can provide substantial analgesia, potentially minimizing some of the side effects of large systemic doses of narcotic. Several systems are now available that allow patients to continue administering their own spinal morphine injections at home. The clinical indications for the use of such systems remain controversial.

For most cancer patients, however, surgical pain-relieving procedures are unnecessary. Usually a change in drug, dose, or the addition of an adjuvant analgesic can improve pain relief while minimizing adverse reactions.

Management of neuropathic pain Neuropathic pain is often a chronic disabling condition that can involve pathophysiologic changes at many levels of the nervous system. The medical management of neuropathic pain is disappointing; patients rarely achieve substantial, lasting improvement with any single therapy. For patients with neuropathic pain, conventional analgesics are only rarely effective.

The search for improved forms of treatment in such patients has resulted in a number of approaches.

ANTICONVULSANTS In patients with neuropathic pain with little or no evidence of sympathetic dysfunction, anticonvulsants and antidepressant drugs are frequently prescribed, although there is only limited evidence that such medications are effective.

Phenytoin, carbamazepine, or clonazepam may be helpful in certain patients with painful neuropathies or neuralgias. Anticonvulsants are particularly effective in treating the sharp, lancinating pains associated with focal neuralgias such as trigeminal neuralgia. They are less effective for the more constant dull, burning sensations that are a major component of conditions such as postherpetic neuralgia or diabetic neuropathy.

ANTISYMPATHETIC AGENTS In some patients, traumatic neuralgias can present with spontaneous burning pain and a disturbance in the sympathetic innervation of the affected limb. Some patients with sympathetically maintained pain ("reflex sympathetic dystrophy") may achieve substantial pain relief with a series of temporary sympathetic blocks or a surgical sympathectomy. When pain relief follows a sympathetic block, treatment with intravenous regional or systemic antisympathetic drugs such as guanethidine also may provide sustained relief in some patients.

TRICYCLIC ANTIDEPRESSANTS Antidepressant drugs are frequently used to treat pain following peripheral nerve injury. Tricyclic iminodibenzyl derivatives are the most commonly used drugs. Their pharmacologic effects include facilitation of monoamine transmission by inhibition of transmitter reuptake at the synapse and changes in pre- and postsynaptic adrenergic receptor sensitivity. The important site of action of tricyclic antidepressants for pain relief is not clear. However, they may act to potentiate the brainstem inhibition of nociceptive transmission at the level of the dorsal horn. Tricyclic antidepressants also have major effects on ascending monoaminergic systems that project into the forebrain. It seems probable that these ascending systems are also important in pain perception, although how antidepressant drugs influence sensory pathways at the level of the thalamus and cortex remains speculative.

TRANSCUTANEOUS ELECTRICAL NERVE STIMULATION (TENS) Electrical stimulation with a TENS unit applied to the painful region or over the proximal nerve may provide substantial pain relief in patients with painful nerve injuries. However, the duration of the effect is usually limited to the period of stimulation. After a period of days to months, in many patients the analgesic response to TENS habituates, and electrical stimulation may actually worsen the pain.

Management of chronic pain Unrelieved pain that has continued to be a major, disabling condition for a minimum of 6 months is usually referred to as "chronic" pain. Patients with chronic pain often present special problems in evaluation and management.

In certain pain patients, particularly those with chronic pain, there is often little correlation between the severity of active disease and the amount of pain behavior. Although restricted activity and analgesic medications are important components of the treatment of most patients with acute pain, these forms of therapy may be counterproductive in patients with chronic pain. After an extended period of inactivity due to pain, patients often become physically deconditioned. Fibromyositis is a common problem, with a loss of strength and range of motion associated with tenderness over postural muscles. Patients can become fatigued with minor efforts, and simple chores quickly exacerbate their pain. They learn to avoid activities that may be associated with pain, and become socially withdrawn. Within the family, pain often becomes a focus of attention, argument, and subtle secondary gain. In this setting, the continued use of sedating analgesic medications reinforces the sick role and often simply adds to the patient's degree of disability and progressive loss of function.

PSYCHOLOGICAL ASPECTS Several categories of psychological diagnoses can be associated with chronic pain syndromes. The two most common presentations are patients with depression and patients with somatoform disorders.

DEPRESSION Depressive symptoms are common in patients with chronic pain, and depressive illness is found in approximately 30 percent. Many pain patients deny depression and do not show a depressed affect. In such patients vegetative signs of insomnia, diminished libido, and lack of energy may be present.

The relationship between pain and depression is complex. The pain threshold is lowered in clinically depressed patients, and pain is a common complaint among patients with primary depression. Patients with pain associated with chronic somatic disease also frequently develop depressive symptoms. However, the incidence of depression defined by strict clinical criteria is not clearly different in chronic pain patients when compared to medically ill patients without pain.

In an effort to more clearly delineate the relationship between pain and depression, a subgroup of chronic pain patients with a "pain-prone" disorder has been described. Such patients tend to have a hypochondriacal preoccupation with their pain. The pain is often continuous in nature and obscure in origin. Associated with the pain complaint, the patient may have depressive symptoms of insomnia, fatigue, and despair. Pain-prone individuals have developmental histories characterized by stress and unmet dependency needs. There may be a family history of depression, alcoholism, or physical abuse. Before the onset of their pain, however, such individuals have an idealized view of themselves and their family relations, denying conflicts. They may also have compulsive work records and hold several jobs. Chronic pain in this group of individuals may be associated in part with unresolved personal or interpersonal conflicts.

Consistent with the association of pain and depression, antidepressant drugs can stabilize the sleep pattern and improve the dysphoric symptoms of patients with chronic pain. There is often a reduction in the intensity of reported pain that may be associated with a decrease in the requirement for analgesics. Antidepressants may therefore have an important role in the management of chronic pain, although it is still uncertain whether these drugs act primarily to potentiate analgesics or to relieve subclinical depression.

SOMATOFORM DISORDERS Patients with somatoform disorders have symptoms that suggest an organic disease but have no evidence of a physical disorder that might explain these symptoms. The heading "somatoform disorders" includes patients with somatization disorders, conversion disorders, hypochondriasis, or psychogenic pain disorders. Although symptoms of chronic pain are often part of the presentation of a somatoform disorder, patients with this diagnosis do not have depressive symptoms and do not usually respond to antidepressants. However, such patients seek out doctors and undergo repetitive tests to evaluate vague complaints. Anxiolytics and muscle relaxants are usually prescribed, with little or no benefit. Surgical procedures are often performed for pain relief without success.

Patients with somatoform disorders need frequent reassurance that their pain is not associated with serious illness; the management of these conditions is therefore primarily supportive. These patients should have careful follow-up from a small number of care-givers to minimize unnecessary tests and reduce the amount of medication prescribed. In this group of patients diagnosing new pains that signal true organic pathology can be a clinical challenge.

When patients with long-standing chronic pain are seen for a new evaluation, they often have unrealistic expectations of the physician. Frequently they state that none of their prior physicians was competent and that this is their last hope for relief from their suffering. A detailed medical history will often reveal poor compliance with previous treatment recommendations made by other physicians.

To avoid another treatment failure, the chronic pain patient should be evaluated by a multidisciplinary group of specialists skilled in managing chronic pain complaints. The specialists composing this group may vary, depending on the nature of the pain complaint and the resources available at an institution. At a minimum, however, a patient should receive a medical, psychological, neurologic, and physical therapy evaluation. A group approach avoids potential confrontation between patient and physician that may stall progress; it also enhances the credibility of the treatment group, increasing the likelihood of patient compliance. The goal of this evaluation is to establish a treatment plan with specific objectives. Each objective should be accomplished according to a timetable mutually agreed on by the patient and the treatment team.

In general, three main goals should be emphasized. First, drug treatment should be simplified and minimized. In many chronic pain patients, common analgesics and muscle relaxants are only minimally effective. The patient therefore tends to increase the dosage in the hope of enhancing pain relief. With the patient's understanding, the number of medications should be reduced by eliminating redundant or ineffective drugs. The dosages of the remaining medications should then be decreased systematically to a point where the patient is taking only drugs that have a definite beneficial effect with minimal side effects.

The second goal of therapy is to help the patient develop a better understanding of the pain and the factors that exacerbate it. Stress management and relaxation training may provide patients with skills to control factors that contribute to their pain. The psychological significance of the pain and its relationship to developmental or interpersonal factors may be worth exploring with individual patients. Antidepressant medications may also have a role in the management of affective symptoms in certain chronic pain patients.

The third goal of therapy should be increased mobilization and functional ability. Under the direction of a specialist in rehabilitation medicine, a program of physical treatments for pain relief (TENS, massage, etc.) should be coupled with an exercise program to increase range of motion and endurance. In some patients, vocational rehabilitation can form an important part of this program. For all patients, realistic timetables should be set for a return to self-care and independent function consistent with the patient's level of objective physical disability.

Social and interpersonal factors may perseverate pain; certain chronic pain patients are therefore refractory to treatment on an outpatient basis. Admission to an inpatient multidisciplinary pain treatment facility can provide an opportunity for an intensive program of evaluation and treatment of such patients. Standards for such inpatient units have been established by the Committee on Accreditation of Rehabilitation Facilities and the American Pain Society. Studies of the effectiveness of pain treatment units demonstrate decreased reports of pain, decreased drug use, and increased functional ability in the majority of patients completing this type of program. However, the ultimate success of such programs depends on maintained functional improvement in patients over long periods following discharge. Careful follow-up and reevaluation of patients with chronic pain is therefore an essential part of successful management.

REFERENCES

ASBURY A, FIELDS HL: Pain due to peripheral nerve damage: An hypothesis. Neurology 34:1587, 1984

BASBAUM AI, FIELDS HL: Endogenous pain control systems: Brainstem spinal pathways and endorphin circuitry. Ann Rev Neurosci 7:309, 1984

BLUMER D, HEILBRONN M: Chronic pain as a variant of depressive disease. J Nerv Ment Dis 170:381, 1982

FIELDS HL: Pain. New York, McGraw-Hill, 1987

FOLEY KM, INTRUISSI CE (eds): Opioid Analgesics in the Management of Clinical Pain. Advances in Pain Research and Therapy, vol 8. New York, Raven Press, 1986

————, PAYNE RM (eds): Current Therapy of Pain. Toronto, Decker, 1989

HACKETT TP: The pain patient: Evaluation and treatment, in Massachusetts General Hospital Handbook of General Hospital Psychiatry, TP Hackett (ed.) Boston, Massachusetts General Hospital, 1978, p 41

HANNINGTON-KIFF JG: Antisympathetic drugs in limbs, in Textbook of Pain, PD Wall, R Melzack (eds). New York, Churchill Livingstone, 1984

MACIEWICZ R, FIELDS HL: Pain pathways, in Diseases of the Nervous System, A Asbury, G McKann (eds). London, Saunders, 1985

MELZACK R (ed): Pain Measurement and Assessment. New York, Raven Press, 1983

SWEET WH, POLETTI CE: Causalgia, in Evaluation and Treatment of Chronic Pain, G Aronoff (ed). Baltimore, Urban and Schwarzenberg, 1985

TASKER RR: Deafferentation, in Textbook of Pain, PD Wall, R Melzack (eds). New York, Churchill Livingstone, 1984, p 119

TAUB A, COLLINS WF: Observations on the treatment of denervation dysesthesia with psychotropic drugs: Postherpetic neuralgia, anesthesia dolorosa, peripheral neuropathy, in Advances in Neurology, JJ Bonica (ed). New York, Raven Press, 1974, p 309

WHITE JC, SWEET WH: Pain and the Neurosurgeon—A Forty Years' Experience. Springfield, Ill., Charles C. Thomas, 1969

YAKSH TL, HAMMOND DL: Peripheral and central substrates involved in the rostrad transmission of nociceptive information. Pain 13:1, 1982

16   CHEST DISCOMFORT AND PALPITATION

LEE GOLDMAN / EUGENE BRAUNWALD

CHEST DISCOMFORT

Chest discomfort is one of the most frequent complaints for which patients seek medical attention; the potential benefit (or harm) resulting from the proper (or improper) assessment and management of the patient with this complaint is enormous. Failure to recognize a serious disorder, such as ischemic heart disease, may result in the dangerous delay of much-needed treatment, while an incorrect diagnosis of a potentially hazardous condition such as angina pectoris is likely to have harmful psychological and economic consequences and may lead to unnecessary cardiac catheterization. There is little relation between the severity of chest discomfort and the gravity of its cause. Therefore, a frequent problem in patients who complain of chest discomfort or pain is distinguishing trivial complaints from coronary artery disease and other serious disorders (Table 16-1).

PATHOPHYSIOLOGY   Discomfort due to myocardial ischemia Discomfort due to myocardial ischemia occurs when the oxygen supply to the heart is deficient in relation to the oxygen need. Oxygen consumption is closely related to the physiologic effort made during contraction, and coronary venous blood is normally much more desaturated than that draining other areas of the body. As a consequence, the removal of more oxygen from each unit of blood, which

TABLE 16-1   Some causes of chest discomfort

I Cardiac
  A Coronary artery disease
  B Aortic stenosis
  C Hypertropic cardiomyopathy
  D Pericarditis

II Vascular
  A Aortic dissection
  B Pulmonary embolism
  C Pulmonary hypertension
  D Right ventricular strain

III Pulmonary
  A Pleuritis or pneumonia
  B Tracheobronchitis
  C Pneumothorax
  D Tumor
  E Mediastinitis or mediastinal emphysema

IV Gastrointestinal
  A Esophogeal reflux
  B Esophogeal spasm
  C Mallory-Weiss tear
  D Peptic ulcer disease
  E Biliary disease
  F Pancreatitis

V Musculoskeletal
  A Cervical disk disease
  B Arthritis of the shoulder or spine
  C Costochondritis
  D Intercostal muscle cramps
  E Interscalene or hyperabduction syndromes
  F Subacromial bursitis

VI Other
  A Disorders of the breast
  B Chest wall tumors
  C Herpes zoster

is one of the adjustments commonly utilized by exercising skeletal muscle, is already employed in the heart in the basal state. Therefore, the heart must rely primarily on an increase in the coronary blood flow for obtaining additional oxygen.

The blood flow through the coronary arteries is directly proportional to the pressure gradient between the aorta and the ventricular myocardium during systole and the ventricular cavity during diastole, but is also proportional to the fourth power of the radius of the coronary arteries. A relatively slight alteration in coronary luminal diameter below a critical level can produce a large decrement in coronary flow, provided that other factors remain constant. Coronary blood flow occurs primarily during diastole, when it is unopposed by systolic myocardial compression of the coronary vessels.

When the epicardial coronary arteries are narrowed critically (>70 percent stenosis of the luminal diameter), the intramyocardial coronary arterioles dilate in an effort to maintain total flow at a level that will avert myocardial ischemia at rest. Further dilatation, which normally occurs during exercise, is therefore not possible. Hence, any condition in which increased heart rate, arterial pressure, or myocardial contractility occurs in the presence of coronary obstruction tends to precipitate anginal attacks by increasing myocardial oxygen needs in the face of a fixed oxygen supply.

By far the most frequent underlying cause of myocardial ischemia is organic narrowing of the coronary arteries secondary to coronary atherosclerosis (see also Chap. 190). A *dynamic* component of increased coronary vascular resistance, secondary to spasm of the major epicardial vessels (often near an atherosclerotic plaque) or more frequently to constriction of smaller coronary arterioles, is present in many, perhaps the majority, of patients with chronic angina pectoris. There is no evidence that systemic arterial constriction or increased cardiac contractile activity (rise in heart rate or blood pressure, or increase in contractility due to liberation of catecholamines or adrenergic activity) due to emotion can precipitate angina unless there is also organic or dynamic narrowing of the coronary vessels. Acute thrombosis superimposed on an atherosclerotic plaque is frequently the cause of unstable angina and acute myocardial infarction.

Aside from conditions which narrow the lumen of the coronary arteries, the only other frequent causes of myocardial ischemia are disorders such as valvular aortic stenosis (Chap. 188) or hypertrophic cardiomyopathy (Chap. 192), which cause a marked disproportion between the perfusion pressure and the heart's oxygen requirements. Under such conditions, the rise in left ventricular systolic pressure is not, as in hypertensive states, balanced by a corresponding elevation of aortic perfusion pressure. Recent epidemiologic studies indicate that chest pain is no more common in patients with mitral valve prolapse than in those without it.

An increase in heart rate is especially harmful in patients with coronary atherosclerosis and with aortic stenosis, because it both increases myocardial oxygen needs and shortens diastole relatively more than systole, thereby decreasing the total available perfusion time per minute. Tachycardia, a decline in arterial pressure, thyrotoxicosis, or diminution in arterial oxygen content (such as occurs in anemia or arterial hypoxia) are precipitating and aggravating factors rather than underlying causes of angina.

Discomfort due to pericarditis The visceral surface of the pericardium ordinarily is insensitive to pain, as is the parietal surface, except in its lower portion, which has a relatively small number of pain fibers carried in the phrenic nerves. The pain associated with pericarditis is believed to be due to inflammation of the adjacent parietal pleura. These observations explain why noninfectious pericarditis (e.g., that associated with uremia and with myocardial infarction) and cardiac tamponade with relatively mild inflammation are usually painless or accompanied by only mild pain, whereas infectious pericarditis, being nearly always more intense and spreading to the neighboring pleura, is usually associated with pain (Chap. 193).

Vascular causes of chest pain *Aortic dissection* develops as a result of a subintimal hematoma, which may start either because a

tear has developed in the intima of the aorta or because of bleeding into the vasa vasorum. Antegrade movement of this hematoma can compromise major branches off the aorta, just as retrograde spread can occlude a coronary artery, disrupt the aortic valve annulus, or rupture into the pericardial space.

Pulmonary emboli These commonly originate from thrombi in the venous circulation, especially in the lower extremities. Venous thrombosis is usually related to stasis or slowing of blood flow because of inactivity or impedance to venous return, to damage in the vessel wall, or to alterations in the coagulation system. When thrombi from any source embolize to the pulmonary arterial circulation, they can cause not only mechanical obstruction but also vasoconstriction and elevated pulmonary vascular resistance related to the release of humoral factors, such as histamine, serotonin, and prostaglandins. As a result, hypoxemia and, occasionally, right heart failure can ensue, and an acute fall in cardiac output can lead to sudden death. The acute pain from massive pulmonary emboli is thought to be related to pulmonary hypertension and to distention of the pulmonary artery. Infarction of a segment of the lung that is adjacent to the pleura commonly irritates the pleural surface and causes chest discomfort hours or even days later (see Chap. 213).

Other pulmonary causes of chest discomfort A variety of diseases of the lung can cause chest discomfort. Pleural pain, which is usually brief, sharp pain that is precipitated by inspiration, is very common and generally results from stretching of an inflamed parietal pleura.

Gastrointestinal causes of chest discomfort Esophageal pain includes *esophageal reflux* and *esophageal spasm*. Esophageal discomfort usually results from chemical (acid) irritation of the esophageal mucosa because of acid reflux or spasm of the esophageal muscle. Rupture of the esophagus, such as in a Mallory-Weiss tear that is caused by severe vomiting, causes severe acute chest pain (Chap. 237)

Occasionally, other gastrointestinal diseases including *peptic ulcer disease, biliary disease,* and *pancreatitis* may present with chest discomfort as well as abdominal discomfort.

Neuromusculoskeletal causes of chest discomfort Neuromusculoskeletal chest discomfort can be caused by *cervical disk disease,* because of compression of nerve roots, by *arthritis of the shoulder or spine,* or by *costochondritis,* which is an inflammation of the costochondral junctions. Inflammation of the subacromial bursa or, less commonly, the supraspinatus or deltoid tendon may cause pain that radiates to the chest. *Intercostal muscle cramps* may occur throughout the chest. Anterior scalene and hyperabduction syndromes can also cause chest discomfort.

Other causes of chest discomfort A variety of *disorders of the breast,* including inflammatory breast disease, benign and malignant tumors, and mastodynia, can cause chest discomfort, usually in association with local abnormalities of the breast. *Chest wall tumors,* including metastases from other organs or malignant disease in the ribs, can also present as chest discomfort. The pain of *herpes zoster* may antedate the typical rash by a day or more, making early diagnosis difficult (Chap. 136).

DIFFERENTIAL DIAGNOSIS The key issue in the evaluation of the patient with chest discomfort is to distinguish potentially life-threatening conditions such as coronary artery disease, aortic dissection, and pulmonary embolism from other causes of chest discomfort. Even patients who have brief episodes of pain and are otherwise in apparently excellent health may have intermittent myocardial ischemia or even recurrent pulmonary emboli.

The radiation of pain arising in the thoracic viscera can usually be explained by known neuroanatomic relationships (Chap. 15). Pain impulses which enter one cord segment may spill over and excite nearby cord segments.

The chest discomfort of myocardial ischemia, most commonly from coronary artery disease but also occasionally from the other causes of ischemia noted above, is angina pectoris. Myocardial ischemia from coronary atherosclerosis is more common in patients who have hypercholesterolemia, diabetes mellitus, hypertension, or obesity or who smoke cigarettes (Chap. 195). Toxins, including cocaine ingestion or withdrawal of chronic exposure to nitroglycerin, can cause sufficient coronary vasoconstriction to result in myocardial ischemia, and cocaine can also cause myocardial infarction.

Angina pectoris is usually described as a heaviness, pressure, or squeezing, or as a sensation of strangling or constriction in the chest, but may also be described as aching, burning, or even as indigestion. Some patients steadfastly deny pain but will admit to a discomfort or unusual feeling or may complain of difficulty in breathing.

Typically angina pectoris develops gradually during exertion, after heavy meals, and with anger, excitement, frustration, and other emotional states; it is not precipitated by coughing, respiratory movements, or other motion. When angina is induced by walking, it often forces the patient to stop or to reduce speed. Angina occurs most typically in the substernal region, anteriorly across the midthorax; it may radiate to or rarely occur alone in the interscapular region, in the arms, shoulders, teeth, and abdomen. It rarely radiates to below the umbilicus, to the back of the neck or the occiput. The more severe the attack, the greater the radiation from the substernal areas to the left arm, especially its ulnar aspect. Although the radiation of chest discomfort to the left arm increases the likelihood that myocardial ischemia or infarction is present, impulses from the skin and from visceral structures, such as the esophagus and heart, converge on a common pool of neurons in the posterior horn of the spinal cord. Their origin may be confused by the cerebral cortex; hence almost any condition capable of causing chest discomfort may induce radiation to the left arm. Also, stimulation of one of the thoracic nerves that also innervates the heart by, for example, protrusion of an intervertebral disk, may be misinterpreted as pain originating from the heart.

When the history is atypical, as is often the case, the correct diagnosis of angina pectoris may be aided by noting that the pain disappears more rapidly (usually within 5 min) and more completely when sublingual nitroglycerin is used. The demonstration that the time required for a given exercise to produce pain is consistently and considerably longer when it is undertaken within a few minutes after a sublingual nitroglycerin pill than after a placebo may, in some instances, represent powerful clinical evidence for the diagnosis of angina pectoris. Angina is rarely relieved within a few seconds of lying down, nor is it precipitated by stooping forward.

Myocardial infarction is usually associated with a discomfort similar in quality and distribution to that of angina but of longer duration (usually 30 min) and usually of greater intensity. In contrast to angina, the pain of myocardial infarction is not rapidly relieved by rest or by coronary dilator drugs and may require large doses of narcotics. It may be accompanied by diaphoresis, nausea, and hypotension (Chap. 189).

The physical examination in patients with myocardial ischemia frequently is totally normal. However, myocardial ischemia can cause a third or fourth heart sound because of an impairment of myocardial contraction or relaxation. Ischemic papillary muscle dysfunction can cause transient mitral regurgitation and its associated murmur. Myocardial infarction, and less commonly severe and generalized ischemia, can cause congestive heart failure.

The chest discomfort from myocardial ischemia that is caused by aortic stenosis, hypertrophic cardiomyopathy, and non-atherosclerotic causes of coronary artery disease is generally similar to that of angina pectoris from coronary atherosclerosis. However, the physical examination will usually reveal classic findings of an aortic systolic murmur in patients with aortic stenosis (Chap. 188) and will reveal dynamic outflow obstruction in many patients with hypertrophic cardiomyopathy (Chap. 192).

Pericarditis can cause pain in several locations (Chap. 193). Since the central part of the diaphragm receives its sensory supply from the phrenic nerve (which arises from the third to fifth cervical segments of the spinal cord), pain arising from the lower parietal pericardium and central tendon of the diaphragm is felt characteristically at the tip of the shoulder, the adjoining trapezius ridge, and the neck. Involvement of the more lateral part of the diaphragmatic pleura, supplied by branches from the sixth to ninth intercostal nerves, causes pain not only in the anterior part of the chest but also in the upper part of the abdomen or corresponding region of the back, sometimes simulating the pain of acute cholecystitis or pancreatitis.

Pericardial pain commonly has a pleuritic component, i.e., it is related to respiratory movements and aggravated by cough and/or deep inspiration, because of pleural irritation. It is sometimes brought on by swallowing, because the esophagus lies just behind the posterior portion of the heart, and is often altered by a change of bodily position, becoming sharper and more left-sided in the supine position and reduced when the patient sits upright, leaning forward. It is frequently referred to the neck and lasts longer than the pain of angina pectoris.

In some patients, however, pericardial pain may be described as a steady substernal discomfort that can mimic the pain of acute myocardial infarction. The mechanism of this steady substernal pain is not certain, but it may arise from marked inflammation of the relatively insensitive inner parietal surface of the pericardium, or from irritated afferent cardiac nerve fibers lying in the periadventitial layers of the superficial coronary arteries. Occasionally, both pleuritic and steady pain may be present simultaneously.

Patients with marked *right ventricular hypertension* may have exertional pain which is quite similar to that of angina. This discomfort probably results from relative ischemia of the right ventricle brought about by the increased oxygen needs and by the elevated intramural resistance, with reduction of the normally large systolic pressure gradient which perfuses this chamber.

The pain due to *acute dissection of the aorta* (Chap. 197) or to an expanding aortic aneurysm results from stimulation of nerve endings in the adventitia. The pain usually begins abruptly, reaches an extremely severe peak rapidly, is felt in the center of the chest and radiates to the back, lasts for hours, and requires unusually large amounts of analgesics for relief. Patients commonly describe a true pain rather that the vague discomfort that is sometimes described with myocardial ischemia. The pain is not aggravated by changes in position or respiration.

The pain resulting from *pulmonary embolism* (Chap. 213) may resemble that of acute myocardial infarction, and in massive embolism it is located substernally. In patients with smaller emboli the pain is located more laterally, is pleuritic in nature, and may be associated with hemoptysis.

Pleural pain from fibrinous pleurisy or any pneumonic process is very common. It generally results from stretching of inflamed parietal pleura and is similar in character to the pleural pain of pericarditis (see above). Pneumothorax and tumors involving the pleural space may also irritate the parietal pleura and cause pleural pain; the latter is sharp, knifelike, superficial in quality, and its aggravation by each breath and by coughing distinguishes it from the deep, dull, relatively steady pain of myocardial ischemia. Substernal discomfort also frequently occurs in the presence of *tracheobronchitis;* it is commonly described as a burning sensation accentuated by coughing.

The pain of *mediastinal emphysema* (Chap. 216) may be intense and sharp and may radiate from the substernal region to the shoulders; often a distinct crepitus is heard. The pain associated with *mediastinitis* and *mediastinal tumors* usually resembles that of pleuritis but is more likely to be maximal in the substernal region, and the associated feeling of constriction or oppression may cause confusion with myocardial infarction.

The several *abdominal disorders* which may at times mimic anginal pain may usually be suspected from the history. Esophageal pain commonly presents as a deep thoracic burning discomfort, which is the hallmark of acid-induced pain. Substernal discomfort usually suggests a hiatus hernia. Intake of aspirin, alcohol, or certain foods typically exacerbates this burning discomfort, and the discomfort may be relieved promptly by antacids or even by one or two swallows of food or water. Patients may have accompanying dysphagia, regurgitation of undigested food, or weight loss. The symptoms of a hiatus hernia tend to be exacerbated by lying down, and all forms of acid-peptic disease may be worse in the early morning when acidic secretions are not neutralized by food. Esophageal spasm, which may be induced by reflux of gastric acid into an esophagus in which the mucosa has been previously irritated, can cause a squeezing pain that may be indistinguishable from myocardial ischemia and that may even have a similar pattern of radiation. Pain resulting from gastric or duodenal ulcer (Chap. 238) is epigastric or substernal, usually commences about 1 to $1\frac{1}{2}$ h after meals, and is usually relieved in several minutes by antacids or milk.

The discomfort caused by acute cholecystitis is more commonly described as an ache, which may be epigastric or substernal. It most commonly tends to occur an hour or so after meals and not in relation to exertion.

The presence of an abdominal disorder, such as a hiatus hernia or a duodenal ulcer, does not constitute proof that the patient's chest pain is related to it. Such disorders are frequently asymptomatic and are not at all uncommon in patients who also have angina pectoris.

Musculoskeletal pain   The *costochondral and chondrosternal articulations* are the commonest sites of anterior chest pain. Objective signs in the form of swelling (Tietze's syndrome), redness, and heat are rare, but sharply localized tenderness is common. The pain may be darting and last for only a few seconds, or may be a dull ache enduring for hours or days. An associated feeling of tightness due to muscle spasm (see below) is frequent. *Pressure on the chondrosternal and costochondral junctions and on the pectoralis muscles is an essential part of the examination of every patient with chest pain* and will reproduce the pain arising from these tissues. A large percentage of patients with costochondral pain, especially those who also have minor and innocent T-wave alterations, are erroneously labeled as having coronary disease.

Pain secondary to *subacromial bursitis, biceps tendonitis,* and *arthritis of the shoulder and spine* may be precipitated by motion but not by general exertion. Pain arising in the chest wall or upper extremity may develop as a result of muscle or ligament strains brought on by unaccustomed exercise and felt in the costochondral or chondrosternal junctions or in the chest wall muscles. Other causes are *osteoarthritis* of the dorsal or thoracic spine and *ruptured cervical disk disease.* Pain in the left upper extremity and precordium may be due to compression of portions of the brachial plexus by a cervical rib or by spasm and shortening of the scalenus anticus muscle secondary to high fixation of the ribs and sternum. Deep breathing, turning or twisting of the chest, and movements of the shoulder girdle and arm may elicit and duplicate the pain of which the patient complains. The pain may be very brief, lasting only a few seconds, or aching and persist for hours. The duration is, therefore, likely to be either longer or shorter than untreated angina pectoris, which usually lasts for only a few minutes.

Emotional disorders are also common causes of chest pain. Usually, the discomfort is experienced as a sense of "tightness," sometimes called "aching," and occasionally it may be sufficiently severe as to be designated a pain of considerable magnitude. Since the discomfort has almost always the additional quality of tightness or constriction and is often localized at least in part beneath the sternum, it is not surprising that this type of discomfort is frequently confused with that of myocardial ischemia. Ordinarily, it lasts for a half hour or more, unrelated to exertion, and with slow fluctuation of intensity. The association with fatigue or emotional strain is usually clear, although this may not be volunteered by the patient. Associated hyperventilation can cause innocent changes in the T waves and ST segments, which can be confused with coronary disease.

APPROACH TO THE PATIENT WITH CHEST DISCOMFORT   A detailed and *meticulous history* of the behavior of the pain is the cornerstone of the evaluation. The location, radiation, quality, intensity, and duration of the episodes are important. Even more so is the story of the aggravating and alleviating factors. A history of intense aggravation by breathing, coughing, or other respiratory movements will usually point toward the pleura and pericardium or mediastinum as the site, although chest wall pain is likewise affected by respiratory motion. Similarly, a pain which regularly appears on rapid walking, or with other exertion such as sexual activity, and vanishes within a few minutes upon standing still suggests the diagnosis of angina pectoris, although a similar story will occasionally be obtained from patients with skeletal disorders.

While data from the history are of cardinal importance in the assessment of chest discomfort, physicians should not be misled into overreliance on any single feature. For example, acute myocardial infarction sometimes presents with pain that may be described as burning or even as sharp and may not be principally located in the substernal area.

A thorough *physical examination* can provide important clues to the cause of chest discomfort. Blood pressure should be checked in both arms if aortic dissection is being considered. Examination of the skin may reveal cyanosis, which suggests hypoxemia either from diminished cardiac output or impaired respiratory function, or xanthelasthma, which would suggest hyperlipidemia and associated coronary disease. The finding of lymphadenopathy suggests a tumor. The examination of the chest wall should include both inspection and palpation to search for costochondritis and other musculoskeletal abnormalities. Lung examination may reveal a pleural rub, signs of pneumonic consolidation, or evidence of congestive heart failure. The physical examination may be totally normal in persons with severe myocardial ischemia, but it may also demonstrate abnormalities of vital signs, a third or fourth heart sound, or mitral regurgitation from papillary muscle dysfunction. Aortic stenosis will be accompanied by its typical murmur (Chap. 188). The cardiac examination should also search for an increased pulmonic second sound that may indicate elevated pulmonary artery pressure, such as is found in pulmonary embolism, and the pericardial friction rub that strongly suggests pericarditis. A careful upper abdominal examination may be the first clue to peptic ulcer disease or cholecystitis.

Critical information can often be obtained by attempts to produce or alleviate the pain, such as with nitroglycerin. Careful palpation of the chest wall, subacromial bursa, deltoid tendon, abdomen, and other structures may be very helpful if it reproduces the chest discomfort. Shoulder and arm motion commonly reproduces pain related to these structures. However, the finding that such maneuvers can cause chest discomfort does not mean that such musculoskeletal diseases are the cause of the presenting complaint unless one can be sure that the patient's syndrome is reproduced precisely. Alternatively, the demonstration that a localized pain can be completely relieved by infiltration of a local anesthetic will be conclusive in convincing both the patient and the physician. Evaluation of the patient at the time of a spontaneous episode, such as with an electrocardiogram during pain, is also extremely helpful.

APPLICATION OF THE PRINCIPLES OF CLINICAL REASONING   The assessment of the probability of the various causes of chest pain requires the integration of multiple pieces of data, because no single clinical feature can be considered decisive. Each of the conditions that can cause chest discomfort can have varied presentations, and the diagnostic tests upon which physicians often rely can also have false-positive or false-negative results. Thus, the principles of clinical reasoning (Chap. 2) should be applied to the evaluation of the patient with chest discomfort.

History and physical examination   The information obtained from a careful medical history and physical examination can be used to develop a differential diagnosis of the causes of chest discomfort in an individual patient, to rank these diagnostic possibilities, and often to assign approximate percent probabilities to them. Although the various causes of chest discomfort have typical characteristics, these characteristics must be interpreted in light of the prior probability that a person with a given age and sex, and with a particular past medical history, would have such a cause of chest discomfort. For example, the possibility of angina pectoris as a cause of precordial or substernal discomfort must be seriously considered in a middle-aged man with coronary risk factors such as hypercholesterolemia and smoking, even if the description of the discomfort is not perfectly typical for angina pectoris. Conversely, when a 20-year old woman describes the onset of new discomfort in a way that is seemingly classic for angina pectoris, such a diagnosis is relatively unlikely because the prior probability of ischemic heart disease, given her age and sex, is so low.

Although it is not always possible to assign numerical probabilities to the various causes of chest discomfort in an individual patient, experienced clinicians either implicitly or explicitly assess the relative likelihoods of various potential explanations for any chest discomfort syndrome to help guide their future diagnostic evaluations and therapy. For example, a middle-aged or elderly man with typical characteristics for angina pectoris has about an 80 to 85 percent probability of having hemodynamically significant coronary artery disease. By comparison, the same man with a history of chest discomfort that has some characteristics that are typical for angina pectoris but other characteristics that are atypical will have a probability of important coronary disease ranging from about 30 to 60 percent. Even persons with chest pain that is decidedly unlikely to represent coronary disease still have some finite possibility of coronary disease, which may range from exceedingly unlikely in a young woman to the 10 percent range in a middle-aged man with many coronary risk factors.

Diagnostic tests   Although myocardial ischemia commonly is associated with electrocardiographic changes (Chap. 190), many patients have normal tracings between attacks, and some may even be normal during an episode of pain. However, depression of the ST segments, caused by myocardial ischemia, typically occurs during exertion and is accompanied by anginal discomfort; moreover, electrocardiographic evidence of myocardial ischemia may occur at rest and with or without accompanying chest discomfort. The finding of flat or down-sloping ST-segment depressions of 0.1 mV or greater during an attack of pain substantially increases the likelihood that the pain is anginal in origin. Exercise electrocardiography will show ischemic changes in about 50 to 80 percent of persons with symptomatic coronary disease, but also in about 10 to 15 percent of patients who do not have coronary disease. The accuracy of ambulatory ischemia monitoring in the general population is less clear. Exercise thallium scintigraphy (Chap. 177) will demonstrate a perfusion defect in about 75 to 85 percent of patients with angina pectoris and will be falsely positive in about 10 percent of patients who have chest discomfort from noncoronary causes.

The evaluation of patients with suspected pulmonary embolism should usually focus on the documentation of deep venous thrombosis (Chap. 213) and the evaluation of pulmonary perfusion with a lung scintigram and/or pulmonary arteriography (Chap. 203). Aortic dissection is often suggested by the routine chest radiograph, and the diagnosis may be established by echocardiography, computed tomography, or magnetic resonance imaging. Aortography is the definitive test, but because of its invasiveness it is usually reserved for situations in which the suspicion of dissection is moderate or high and definitive anatomic documentation or localization is needed, often because of the need to consider a surgical repair.

Esophageal or peptic-ulcer diseases can often be diagnosed by an upper gastrointestinal roentgenogram. Esophageal manometry and measurement of lower esophageal sphincter pressure are useful in identifying esophageal spasm. The Bernstein acid perfusion test, in which an attempt is made to reproduce the pain by infusing hydrochloric acid into the esophagus, can help establish acid reflux as the cause of pain (Chap. 237).

Integration of clinical data and test results   It is often useful to subdivide patients into those with an *acute* onset of a new or worsened chest pain syndrome versus those with more *chronic* pain. Acute chest pain, with a duration of minutes to hours prior to the patient's presentation to a physician, could be caused by many of the entities described in this chapter and would be especially suspicious for acute myocardial infarction, aortic dissection, pulmonary embolism, biliary colic, or acute musculoskeletal trauma. In many situations, the patient may have had prior pain that was similar to but less severe than the current discomfort; this prior pain may be an important clue to recurrent problems such as biliary colic or esophageal spasm. Some, but certainly not all, patients with acute myocardial infarctions will have had a prior history of angina pectoris.

Accumulated data from large numbers of patients who have presented to emergency departments with acute chest pain can aid the assessment of the probability that an individual is having an acute myocardial infarction. By integrating information from the history, physical examination, and electrocardiogram, such empirically derived algorithms have been able to predict which patients are having acute myocardial infarctions more accurately than are the physicians who actually saw the patients in the emergency department. For example, a person without a history of known coronary disease is unlikely to be having an acute myocardial infarction if the electrocardiogram is normal and the chest pain does not radiate to the neck or left shoulder or arm. Although no algorithm can be considered a perfect predictor that can be used in a vacuum, physicians have the opportunity to improve patient management by incorporating such information into their decision-making.

In patients with chronic or recurrent chest pain, the prior pain pattern is usually very helpful in establishing the current diagnosis. For patients with recurrent myocardial ischemia, a worsening of a stable pain pattern may herald unstable angina pectoris (Chap. 190). Unlike acute chest pain, where decision-making revolves around the need for immediate hospitalization and electrocardiographic monitoring to avoid sudden death, chronic chest pain, unless indicative of unstable angina pectoris, may be clarified by outpatient diagnostic testing, such as exercise electrocardiography and exercise thallium scintigraphy.

Although exercise electrocardiography and exercise thallium scintigraphy are of value in distinguishing between cardiac and noncardiac causes of chest discomfort, the results must be interpreted in light of the prior probability of coronary artery disease, which is the probability that the patient has coronary disease based on the presenting clinical characteristics, age, and sex (see Fig. 2-2, p. 9). Since exercise thallium scintigraphy appears to provide information that is correlated with the standard exercise electrocardiogram no more than would be expected by chance, it can provide additional independent information (Chap. 2) and further change the probability of coronary artery disease (Fig. 16-1). If absolute diagnostic knowledge is required, cardiac catheterization with coronary angiography serves as the gold standard, i.e., the test that is considered definitive regarding the presence or absence of coronary disease, even though the presence of anatomic disease does not guarantee that the coronary stenoses are causing the chest discomfort.

A sequence of consistently negative cardiologic test results reduces the probability of coronary artery disease to below 10 percent in patients with atypical chest discomfort. However, even after a normal exercise electrocardiogram and exercise thallium scintigram, the probability of coronary disease will still be about 30 percent in a patient with a typical history of angina pectoris (Fig. 16-2). By recognizing the potential change in probabilities that can be obtained with positive and negative results of the diagnostic tests that are planned, the physician can decide whether these potential changes in probability are sufficient to warrant the test. For example, the physician should commonly decide that a patient with typical angina pectoris and a positive exercise electrocardiogram does not require an exercise thallium scintigram to *diagnose* coronary disease, although under some circumstances it might aid in the estimation of the patient's subsequent prognosis.

A useful test result is commonly one that moves the likelihood of a diagnostic possibility across a threshold, so that the test result would lead to a change in management, either by influencing the decision to order additional tests or by causing a change in treatment. In the case of chest discomfort, the decisions cannot be based on a 50 percent threshold: Probabilities of coronary artery disease, pulmonary embolism, or aortic dissection that are well below 50 percent may still demand further evaluation because of the dire consequences

FIGURE 16-1 The curves show the posterior (after-test) probability as a function of the prior (before-test) probability for positive versus negative exercise thallium scintiscans, defined as a perfusion defect that is produced by exercise and resolves with rest. The before-test probability could be estimated from the clinical presentation or could be a postexercise electrocardiogram probability derived from Fig. 2-2 (p. 9). [*From L Goldman, in W Branch, Jr (ed): The Office Practice of Medicine, 2d ed, Philadelphia, Saunders, 1987.*]

seriously troubled by an occasional extrasystole. Patients with anxiety states often exhibit a lowered threshold at which disorders of rate and rhythm result in palpitation. The awareness of the heartbeat also tends to be more common at night and during introspective moments, but is less marked during activity. Patients with organic heart disease and chronic disorders of cardiac rate, rhythm, or stroke volume tend to accommodate to these abnormalities and are often less sensitive than normal persons to such events. Persistent tachycardia and/or atrial fibrillation may not be accompanied by continuous palpitation, in contrast to a sudden, brief alteration in cardiac rate or rhythm which often causes considerable subjective discomfort. Palpitation is particularly prominent when the precipitating cause for increased heart rate or contractility or arrhythmia is recent, transient, and episodic. Conversely, in emotionally well-adjusted individuals palpitation commonly becomes progressively less disconcerting as it becomes more chronic.

PATHOGENESIS OF PALPITATION Under ordinary circumstances the rhythmic heartbeat is imperceptible to the healthy individual of placid or even average temperament. Palpitation may be experienced by normal persons who have engaged in strenuous physical effort or have been aroused emotionally or sexually. This type of palpitation is physiologic and represents the normal awareness of an overactive heart—i.e., a heart that is beating at a rapid rate and with an increased contractility. Palpitation due to overactivity of the heart may also occur in certain pathologic states, e.g., fever, acute or severe anemia, or thyrotoxicosis.

When palpitation is heavy and regular, it is usually caused by an augmented stroke volume. Pathologic states, such as aortic regurgitation or a variety of hyperkinetic circulatory states (anemia, arteriovenous fistula, and thyrotoxicosis) should be considered, as well as the benign so-called idiopathic hyperkinetic heart syndrome. Palpi-

of missing one of these important diagnoses. The physician must be prepared to embark on an appropriate evaluation when the history and physical examination do not exclude these diagnoses with a reasonable degree of certainty. The degree of certainty must be determined for the individual condition and patient at hand, typically after an appropriately full and frank discussion between the patient and the physician.

PALPITATION

Palpitation is a common, disagreeable symptom which may be defined as an awareness of the beating of the heart, an awareness most commonly brought about by a change in the heart's rhythm or rate or by an augmentation of its contractility. Palpitation is not pathognomonic of any particular group of disorders; indeed, often it signifies not a primary physical disorder but rather a psychological disturbance. Even when it occurs as a more or less prominent complaint, the diagnosis of the underlying disease is made largely on the basis of other associated symptoms and data. Nevertheless, palpitation is frequently of considerable importance in the minds of patients, who fear that it may indicate heart disease. Concern is all the more pronounced in patients who have been told that they *may* have heart disease; to them palpitation may seem to be an omen of impending disaster. Since the resulting anxiety may be associated with increased activity of the autonomic nervous system, with consequent increases of the cardiac rate and rhythm and the vigor of contraction, the patient's awareness of these changes may then lead to a vicious cycle, which may ultimately be responsible for incapacitation.

Palpitation may be described by the patient in various terms, such as "pounding," "fluttering," "flopping," and "skipping," and in most cases it will be obvious that the complaint is of a sensation of disturbed heartbeat. The sensitivity to alterations in cardiac activity among different individuals varies widely. Some patients seem to be unaware of the most serious and chaotic dysrhythmias; others are

FIGURE 16-2 Approximate probability of coronary artery disease before and after noninvasive testing of a patient with typical (*A*) and atypical (*B*) angina pectoris. The percentages demonstrate how the sequential use of an exercise electrocardiogram and an exercise thallium test may affect the probability of coronary artery disease. [*From L Goldman, in W Branch, Jr (ed): The Office Practice of Medicine, 2d ed, Philadelphia, Saunders, 1987.*]

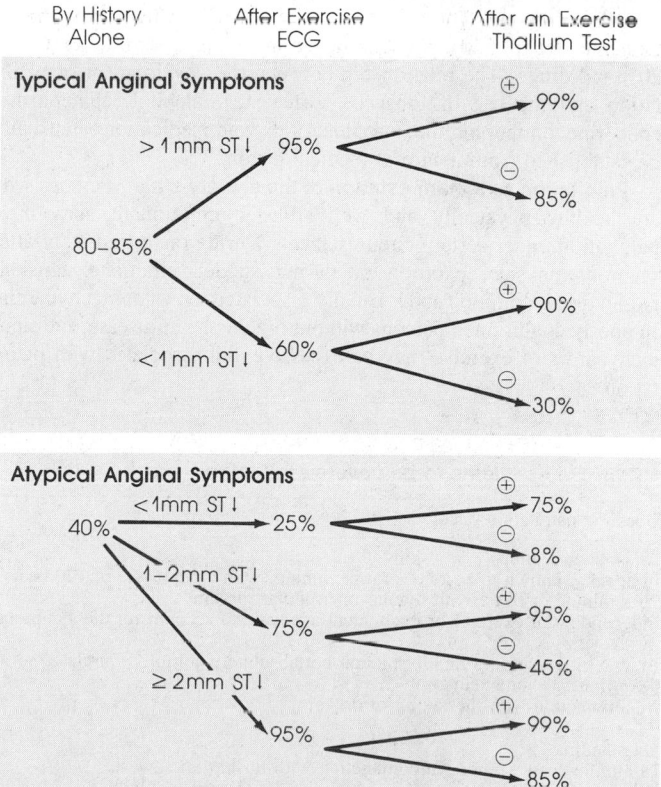

tation may also occur immediately after the onset of cardiac slowing, as with the sudden development of complete atrioventricular block, or upon the conversion from atrial fibrillation to sinus rhythm. Unusual movements of the heart within the thorax are also frequently the mechanism of palpitation. Thus, the ectopic beat and/or the compensatory pause may be appreciated, since both are associated with alterations in cardiac motion.

IMPORTANT CAUSES OF PALPITATION   (See also Chap. 185) **Extrasystoles** In most cases the diagnosis will be suggested by the patient's story. The premature contraction and postpremature beat are often described as a "flopping," or the patient may say that it feels as if "the heart were turning over." The pause following the premature contraction may be felt as an actual cessation of the heartbeat. The first ventricular contraction succeeding the pause may be felt as an unusually vigorous beat and will be described as "pounding" or "thudding."

When extrasystoles are numerous, clinical differentiation from atrial fibrillation can be made by any procedure that will bring about a definite increase in the ventricular rate. In persons without serious underlying heart disease, the extrasystoles usually diminish in frequency and then disappear at increasingly rapid heart rates, whereas the ventricular irregularity of atrial fibrillation increases.

Tachycardias These conditions, which are considered in detail in Chap. 185, are common and medically important causes of palpitation. Ventricular tachycardia, one of the most serious arrhythmias, rarely is manifested as palpitation; this may be related to the abnormal sequence, and hence impaired coordination and vigor, of ventricular contraction. If the patient is seen between attacks, the diagnosis of ectopic tachycardia and its type will have to depend on the history, but the precise diagnosis can be made only when an electrocardiogram and observations on the effect of carotid sinus pressure are made during the episode. The mode of onset and offset gives the most important lead in distinguishing sinus from one of the various forms of ectopic tachycardias. Ectopic rhythms characteristically begin instantaneously, while sinus tachycardia has a more gradual onset and ending over seconds or minutes. Continuous ambulatory (Holter) electrocardiography and asking the patient to record the time of onset and cessation of the palpitations in a diary are extremely helpful in determining the cause of this symptom.

Other causes These include thyrotoxicosis (Chap. 316), hypoglycemia (Chap. 320), pheochromocytoma (Chap. 318), fever (Chap. 20), and drugs. The relationship between the development of palpitation and the use of tobacco, coffee, tea, alcohol, epinephrine, ephedrine, aminophylline, atropine, or thyroid medication can usually be established from a careful medical history.

Palpitation as a manifestation of the anxiety state Persons who are healthy physically and well adjusted emotionally may have palpitation under certain circumstances. During or immediately after vigorous physical exertion or during sudden emotional tension, palpitation is common and is usually associated with sinus tachycardia. In poorly conditioned persons without organic heart disease, the sinus tachycardia of exercise may be excessive and associated with palpitation.

In some persons, palpitation may be one of the outstanding manifestations of an episode of acute anxiety. In others the palpitation may, with other symptoms, represent prolonged anxiety neurosis or a lifelong disorder characterized by volatile autonomic function. Whether these illnesses are simply an expression of a chronic, deep-seated anxiety state superimposed on a normal autonomic nervous system or whether they depend on instability of the autonomic nervous system is not clear. At any rate, the clinical significance of the differentiation between the transitory and the enduring forms is that the former is often dissipated by firm reassurance from the physician, whereas the latter is usually resistant even to the most thorough and expert psychiatric care. In the latter case, the patient must be treated with most carefully planned psychological support and tranquilizing medications. This chronic form of palpitation is known by various names such as *Da Costa's syndrome, soldier's heart, effort syndrome, irritable heart, neurocirculatory asthenia,* and *functional cardiovascular disease.* Aside from palpitation, the chief symptoms are those of an anxiety state.

Physical examination usually reveals the typical findings of the hyperkinetic syndrome. These include a left parasternal lift, a precordial or apical systolic murmur, a wide pulse pressure, rapidly rising pulse, and excessive perspiration. The electrocardiogram may display minor depressions of the ST junction and inversion of T waves and so occasionally lead to a mistaken diagnosis of coronary disease; this is particularly likely to occur when these findings are associated with complaints by the patients of an aching feeling of substernal tightness, commonly present in emotional stress. The presence of any kind of organic disease is one of the commonest causes of the underlying anxiety which frequently precipitates this functional syndrome. Thus, even when a patient presents undoubted objective evidence of organic cardiac disease, the possibility that a superimposed anxiety state may be responsible for the symptoms described above should be considered. Palpitation associated with organic cardiac disease is nearly always accompanied by arrhythmia or tachycardia, whereas the symptom may exist with regular rhythm and with a heart rate of 80 beats per minute or less in patients with the anxiety state. An anxiety state, in contrast to heart disease, causes a sighing type of dyspnea. Also pain localized to the apex, either brief and lancinating in character or lasting for hours or days and accompanied by hyperesthesia, is due usually to an anxiety state, not to structural cardiac disease. Giddiness due to this syndrome can usually be reproduced by hyperventilation or by change from the recumbent to the erect posture.

The *treatment* of the anxiety state with palpitation is difficult and depends on removal of the cause. In many instances a thorough examination of the heart and a statement that it is normal will suffice. Instructions to take more rather than less physical exercise will reinforce these statements. When the anxiety state is a manifestation of chronic anxiety neurosis or related emotional disorder, the symptoms are more likely to persist.

Table 16-2 summarizes the main points of information to be ascertained in the history in elucidating the significance of palpitation. The recording of an ambulatory electrocardiogram and the precise

---

TABLE 16-2 Items to be covered in history

Does the palpitation occur:	If so, suspect:
As isolated "jumps" or "skips"?	Extrasystoles
In attacks, known to be of abrupt beginning, with a heart rate of 120 beats per minute or over, with regular or irregular rhythm?	Paroxysmal rapid heart action
Independent of exercise or excitement adequate to account for the symptom?	Atrial fibrillation, atrial flutter, thyrotoxicosis, anemia, febrile states, hypoglycemia, anxiety state
In attacks developing rapidly though not absolutely abruptly, unrelated to exertion or excitement?	Hemorrhage, hypoglycemia, tumor of the adrenal medulla
In conjunction with the taking of drugs?	Tobacco, coffee, tea, alcohol, epinephrine, ephedrine, aminophylline, atropine, thyroid extract, monoamine oxidase inhibitors
On standing?	Postural hypotension
In middle-aged women, in conjunction with flushes and sweats?	Menopausal syndrome
When the rate is known to be normal and the rhythm regular?	Anxiety state

temporal correlation of the cardiac rate and rhythm with the presence of palpitation are extremely useful in the identification or exclusion of an arrhythmia if the symptom does not occur when the patient is under direct observation. The effectiveness of antiarrhythmia treatment can also be assessed objectively in this manner, without the necessity of relying only on the patient's subjective symptoms. Beta-adrenergic blockade with propranolol, beginning with 40 mg/d in divided doses, and ranging as high as 400 mg/d, or with equivalent doses of newer beta-adrenergic antagonists can be extremely effective in patients with palpitation and sinus rhythm or sinus tachycardia.

One point merits special emphasis. *As a rule palpitation produces anxiety and fear out of all proportion to its seriousness.* When the cause has been accurately determined and its significance explained to patients, their concern is often ameliorated and may disappear entirely.

REFERENCES

CONSTANT J: The clinical diagnosis of nonanginal chest pain: The differentiation of angina from nonanginal chest pain by history. Clin Cardiol 6:11, 1983

DIAMOND GA et al: Computer-assisted diagnosis in the noninvasive evaluation of patients with suspected coronary artery disease. J Am Coll Cardiol 1:444, 1983

GOLDMAN L: Atypical chest pain, in *Difficult Diagnosis*, RB Taylor (ed). Philadelphia, Saunders, 1985, p 71

GOLDMAN L et al: A computer protocol to predict myocardial infarction in emergency department patients with chest pain. N Engl J Med 318:797, 1988

GOLDSCHLAGER N: Use of the treadmill test in the diagnosis of coronary artery disease in patients with chest pain. Ann Intern Med 97:383, 1982

POZEN MW et al: A predictive instrument to improve coronary care unit admission practices in acute ischemic heart disease: A prospective multicenter clinical trial. N Engl J Med 310:1273, 1984

RIFKIN RD, HOOD WB: Bayesian analysis of electrocardiographic exercise stress testing. N Engl J Med 297:681, 1977

RUSTGI AK, CHOPRA S: Chest pain of esophageal origin. J Gen Intern Med 4:151, 1989

RUTHERFORD JD et al: Chronic ischemic heart disease, in *Heart Disease*, 3d ed, E Braunwald (ed). Philadelphia, Saunders, 1988, chap 39, p 1314

WOLF MA: Palpitations and disturbances of cardiac rhythm, in *Office Practice of Medicine*, 2d ed, WT Branch Jr (ed). Philadelphia, Saunders, 1987, chap 2, p 19

17 ABDOMINAL PAIN

WILLIAM SILEN

The correct interpretation of acute abdominal pain is one of the most challenging demands made of any physician. Since proper therapy often requires urgent action, the luxury of the leisurely approach suitable for the study of other conditions is frequently denied. Few other clinical situations demand greater experience and judgment, because the most catastrophic of events may be forecast by the subtlest of symptoms and signs. Nowhere in medicine is a meticulously executed, detailed history and physical examination of greater importance. The etiologic classification in Table 17-1, although not complete, forms a useful frame of reference for the evaluation of patients with abdominal pain.

The diagnosis of "acute or surgical abdomen" so often heard in emergency wards is not an acceptable one because of its often misleading and erroneous connotation. The most obvious of "acute abdomens" may not require operative intervention, and the mildest of abdominal pains may herald the onset of an urgently correctable lesion. Any patient with abdominal pain of recent onset requires early and thorough evaluation with specific attempts at accurate diagnosis.

SOME MECHANISMS OF PAIN ORIGINATING IN THE ABDOMEN
Inflammation of the parietal peritoneum The pain of parietal peritoneal inflammation is steady and aching in character and is located directly over the inflamed area, its exact reference being possible because it is transmitted by overlapping somatic nerves supplying the parietal peritoneum. The intensity of the pain is dependent upon the type and amount of foreign substance to which

TABLE 17-1 Some important causes of abdominal pain

I Pain originating in the abdomen
  A Parietal peritoneal inflammation
    1 Bacterial contamination, e.g., perforated appendix, pelvic inflammatory disease
    2 Chemical irritation, e.g., perforated ulcer, pancreatitis, mittelschmerz
  B Mechanical obstruction of hollow viscera
    1 Obstruction of the small or large intestine
    2 Obstruction of the biliary tree
    3 Obstruction of the ureter
  C Vascular disturbances
    1 Embolism or thrombosis
    2 Vascular rupture
    3 Pressure or torsional occlusion
    4 Sickle cell anemia
  D Abdominal wall
    1 Distortion or traction of mesentery
    2 Trauma or infection of muscles
  E Distention of visceral surfaces, e.g., hepatic or renal capsules
II Pain referred from extraabdominal sources
  A Thorax, e.g., pneumonia, referred pain from coronary occlusion
  B Spine, e.g., radiculitis from arthritis
  C Genitalia, e.g., torsion of the testicle
III Metabolic causes
  A Exogenous
    1 Black widow spider bite
    2 Lead poisoning and others
  B Endogenous
    1 Uremia
    2 Diabetic ketoacidosis
    3 Porphyria
    4 Allergic factors (C'1 esterase inhibitor deficiency)
IV Neurogenic causes
  A Organic
    1 Tabes dorsalis
    2 Herpes zoster
    3 Causalgia and others
  B Functional

the peritoneal surfaces are exposed in a given period of time. For example, the sudden release into the peritoneal cavity of a small quantity of *sterile* acid gastric juice causes much more pain than the same amount of grossly contaminated neutral fecal material. Enzymatically active pancreatic juice incites more pain and inflammation than does the same amount of sterile bile containing no potent enzymes. Blood and urine are often so bland as to go undetected if exposure of the peritoneum has not been sudden and massive. In the case of bacterial contamination, such as in pelvic inflammatory disease, the pain is frequently of low intensity early in the illness until bacterial multiplication has caused the elaboration of irritating substances.

So important is the rate at which the irritating material is applied to the peritoneum that cases of perforated peptic ulcer may be associated with entirely different clinical pictures dependent only upon the rapidity with which the gastric juice enters the peritoneal cavity.

The pain of peritoneal inflammation is invariably accentuated by pressure or changes in tension of the peritoneum, whether produced by palpation or by movement, as in coughing or sneezing. Consequently, the patient with peritonitis lies quietly in bed, preferring to avoid motion, in contrast to the patient with colic, who may writhe incessantly.

Another of the characteristic features of peritoneal irritation is tonic reflex spasm of the abdominal musculature, localized to the involved body segment. The intensity of the tonic muscle spasm accompanying peritoneal inflammation is dependent upon the location of the inflammatory process, the rate at which it develops, and the integrity of the nervous system. Spasm over a perforated retrocecal appendix or perforated ulcer into the lesser peritoneal sac may be minimal or absent because of the protective effect of overlying viscera. As in pain of peritoneal inflammation, a slowly developing process often greatly attenuates the degree of muscle spasm. Catastrophic abdominal emergencies such as a perforated ulcer have been repeatedly associated with minimal or occasionally no detectable pain or muscle spasm in obtunded, seriously ill, debilitated elderly patients or in psychotic patients.

Obstruction of hollow viscera The pain of obstruction of hollow abdominal viscera is classically described as intermittent, or colicky. Yet the lack of a truly cramping character should not be misleading, because distention of a hollow viscus may produce steady pain with only very occasional exacerbations. Although not nearly as well localized as the pain of parietal peritoneal inflammation, some useful generalities can be made concerning its distribution.

The colicky pain of obstruction of small intestine is usually periumbilical or supraumbilical and is poorly localized. As the intestine becomes progressively dilated with loss of muscular tone, the colicky nature of the pain may become less apparent. With superimposed strangulating obstruction, pain may spread in the lower lumbar region if there is traction on the root of the mesentery. The colicky pain of colonic obstruction is of lesser intensity than that of the small intestine and is often located in the infraumbilical area. Lumbar radiation of pain is common in colonic obstruction.

Sudden distention of the biliary tree produces a steady rather than colicky type of pain; hence the term *biliary colic* is misleading. Acute distention of the gallbladder usually causes pain in the right upper quadrant with radiation to the right posterior region of the thorax or to the tip of the right scapula, and distention of the common bile duct is often associated with pain in the epigastrium radiating to the upper part of the lumbar region. Considerable variation is common, however, so that differentiation between these may be impossible. The typical subscapular pain or lumbar radiation is frequently absent. Gradual dilatation of the biliary tree as in carcinoma of the head of the pancreas may cause no pain or only a mild aching sensation in the epigastrium or right upper quadrant. The pain of distention of the pancreatic ducts is similar to that described for distention of the common bile duct but in addition is very frequently accentuated by recumbency and relieved by the upright position.

Obstruction of the urinary bladder results in dull suprapubic pain, usually low in intensity. Restlessness without specific complaint of pain may be the only sign of a distended bladder in an obtunded patient. In contrast, acute obstruction of the intravesicular portion of the ureter is characterized by severe suprapubic and flank pain which radiates to the penis, scrotum, or inner aspect of the upper region of the thigh. Obstruction of the ureteropelvic junction is felt as pain in the costovertebral angle, whereas obstruction of the remainder of the ureter is associated with flank pain, which often extends into the corresponding side of the abdomen.

Vascular disturbances A frequent misconception, despite abundant experience to the contrary, is that pain associated with intraabdominal vascular disturbances is sudden and catastrophic in nature. The pain of embolism or thrombosis of the superior mesenteric artery or that of impending rupture of an abdominal aortic aneurysm certainly may be severe and diffuse. Yet just as frequently, the patient with occlusion of the superior mesenteric artery has only mild continuous diffuse pain for 2 or 3 days before vascular collapse or findings of peritoneal inflammation appear. The early, seemingly insignificant discomfort is caused by hyperperistalsis rather than peritoneal inflammation. Indeed, absence of tenderness and rigidity in the presence of continuous, diffuse pain in a patient likely to have vascular disease is quite characteristic of occlusion of the superior mesenteric artery. Abdominal pain with radiation to the sacral region, flank, or genitalia should always signal the possible presence of a rupturing abdominal aortic aneurysm. This pain may persist over a period of several days before rupture and collapse occur.

Abdominal wall Pain arising from the abdominal wall is usually constant and aching. Movement and pressure accentuate the discomfort and muscle spasm. In the case of hematoma of the rectus sheath, now most frequently encountered in association with anticoagulant therapy, a mass may be present in the lower quadrants of the abdomen. Simultaneous involvement of muscles in other parts of the body usually serves to differentiate myositis of the abdominal wall from an intraabdominal process which might cause pain in the same region.

REFERRED PAIN IN ABDOMINAL DISEASES Pain referred to the abdomen from the thorax, spine, or genitalia may prove a vexing problem in differential diagnosis, because diseases of the upper part of the abdominal cavity such as acute cholecystitis, perforated ulcer, or subphrenic abscesses are frequently associated with intrathoracic complications. A most important, yet often forgotten, dictum is that the possibility of intrathoracic disease must be considered in every patient with abdominal pain, especially if the pain is in the upper part of the abdomen. Systematic questioning and examination directed toward detecting the presence or absence of myocardial or pulmonary infarction, pneumonia, pericarditis, or esophageal disease (the intrathoracic diseases which most often masquerade as abdominal emergencies) will often provide sufficient clues to establish the proper diagnosis. Diaphragmatic pleuritis resulting from pneumonia or pulmonary infarction may cause pain in the right upper quadrant and pain in the supraclavicular area, the latter radiation to be sharply distinguished from the referred subscapular pain caused by acute distention of the extrahepatic biliary tree. The ultimate decision as to the origin of abdominal pain may require deliberate and planned observation over a period of several hours, during which time repeated questioning and examination will provide the proper explanation.

Referred pain of thoracic origin is often accompanied by splinting of the involved hemithorax with respiratory lag and decrease in excursion more marked than that seen in the presence of intraabdominal disease. In addition, apparent abdominal muscle spasm caused by referred pain will diminish during the inspiratory phase of respiration, whereas it is persistent throughout both respiratory phases if it is of abdominal origin. Palpation over the area of referred pain in the abdomen also does not usually accentuate the pain and in many instances actually seems to relieve it. The frequent coexistence of thoracic and abdominal disease may be misleading and confusing, so that differentiation might be difficult or impossible. For example, the patient with known biliary tract disease often has epigastric pain during myocardial infarction, or biliary colic may be referred to the precordium or left shoulder in a patient who has suffered previously from angina pectoris. For the explanation of the radiation of pain to a previously diseased area, see Chap. 15.

Referred pain from the spine, which usually involves compression or irritation of nerve roots, is characteristically intensified by certain motions such as cough, sneeze, or strain and is associated with hyperesthesia over the involved dermatomes. Pain referred to the abdomen from the testicles or seminal vesicles is generally accentuated by the slightest pressure on either of these organs. The abdominal discomfort is of dull aching character and is poorly localized.

METABOLIC ABDOMINAL CRISES Pain of metabolic origin may simulate almost any other type of intraabdominal disease. Here several mechanisms may be at work. In certain instances, such as hyperlipemia, the metabolic disease itself may be accompanied by an intraabdominal process such as pancreatitis, which can lead to unnecessary laparotomy unless recognized. $C'1$ esterase deficiency associated with angioneurotic edema is also often associated with episodes of severe abdominal pain. Whenever the cause of abdominal pain is obscure, a metabolic origin must always be considered. Abdominal pain is also the hallmark of familial Mediterranean fever (Chap. 278).

The problem of differential diagnosis is often not readily resolved. The pain of porphyria and of lead colic usually is difficult to distinguish from that of intestinal obstruction, because severe hyperperistalsis is a prominent feature of both. The pain of uremia or diabetes is nonspecific, and the pain and tenderness frequently shift in location and intensity. Diabetic acidosis may be precipitated by acute appendicitis or intestinal obstruction, so that if prompt resolution of the abdominal pain does not result from correction of the metabolic abnormalities, an underlying organic problem should be suspected. Black widow spider bites produce intense pain and rigidity of the abdominal muscles and of the back, an area infrequently involved in disease of intraabdominal origin.

NEUROGENIC CAUSES   Causalgic pain may occur in diseases that injure nerves of sensory type. It has a burning character and is usually limited to the distribution of a given peripheral nerve. Normal stimuli such as touch or change in temperature may be transformed into this type of pain, which is also frequently present in a patient at rest. A helpful finding is the demonstration that cutaneous pain spots are now irregularly spaced, and this may be the only indication of an old nerve lesion underlying causalgic pain. Even though the pain may be precipitated by gentle palpation, rigidity of the abdominal muscles is absent, and the respirations are not disturbed. Distention of the abdomen is uncommon, and the pain has no relationship to the intake of food.

Pain arising from spinal nerves or roots comes and goes suddenly and is of a lancinating type (see Chap. 19). It may be caused by herpes zoster, impingement by arthritis, tumors, herniated nucleus pulposus, diabetes, or syphilis. Again, it is not associated with food intake, abdominal distention, or changes in respiration. Severe muscle spasm, as in the gastric crises of tabes dorsalis, is common but is either relieved or is not accentuated by abdominal palpation. The pain is made worse by movement of the spine and is usually confined to a few dermatome segments. Hyperesthesia is very common.

Psychogenic pain conforms to none of the aforementioned patterns of disease. Here the mechanism is hard to define. The most common problem is the hysterical adolescent or young woman who develops abdominal pain; she frequently loses an appendix and other organs because of it. Ovulation or some other natural event that causes brief mild abdominal discomfort may sometimes be experienced as an abdominal catastrophe.

Psychogenic pain varies enormously in type and location but usually has no relation to meals. It is often at its onset markedly accentuated during the night. Nausea and vomiting are rarely observed, although occasionally the patient reports these symptoms. Spasm is seldom induced in the abdominal musculature and if present does not persist, especially if the attention of the patient can be distracted. Persistent localized tenderness is rare, and if found, the muscle spasm in the area is inconsistent and often absent. Restriction of the depth of respiration is the most common respiratory abnormality, but this is in the nature of a smothering or choking sensation and is part of an anxiety state (see Chap. 29). It occurs in the absence of thoracic splinting or change in the respiratory rate.

APPROACH TO THE PATIENT WITH ABDOMINAL PAIN   There are few abdominal conditions that require such urgent operative intervention that an orderly approach need be abandoned, no matter how ill the patient. Only those patients with exsanguinating hemorrhage must be rushed to the operating room immediately, but in such instances only a few minutes are required to assess the critical nature of the problem. Under these circumstances, all obstacles must be swept aside, adequate access for intravenous fluid replacement obtained, and the operation begun. Many patients of this type have died in the radiology department or the emergency room while awaiting such unnecessary examinations as electrocardiograms or films of the abdomen. *There are no contraindications to operation when massive hemorrhage is present.* Although exceedingly important, this situation fortunately is relatively rare.

Nothing will supplant an orderly, painstakingly *detailed history,* which is far more valuable than any laboratory or roentgenologic examination. This kind of history is laborious and time-consuming, making it not especially popular even though a reasonably accurate diagnosis can be made on the basis of the history alone in the majority of cases. In cases of *acute* abdominal pain, a diagnosis is readily established in most instances, whereas success is not so frequently achieved in patients with *chronic* pain. Since the irritable bowel syndrome is one of the most common causes of abdominal pain, the possibility of this diagnosis must always be kept in mind (see Chap. 242). The *chronological sequence of events* in the patient's history is often more important than emphasis on the location of pain. If the examiner is sufficiently open-minded and unhurried, asks the proper questions, and listens, the patient will often provide the diagnosis.

Careful attention should be paid to the extraabdominal regions which may be responsible for abdominal pain. An accurate menstrual history in a female patient is essential. Narcotics or analgesics should be withheld until a definitive diagnosis or a definitive plan has been formulated, because these agents often make it more difficult to secure and to interpret the history and physical findings.

In the examination, simple critical inspection of the patient, e.g., of facies, position in bed, and respiratory activity, may provide valuable clues. The amount of information to be gleaned is directly proportional to the *gentleness* and thoroughness of the examiner. Once a patient with peritoneal inflammation has been examined in a brusque manner, accurate assessment by the next examiner becomes almost impossible. For example, eliciting rebound tenderness by sudden release of a deeply palpating hand in a patient with suspected peritonitis is cruel and unnecessary. The same information can be obtained by gentle percussion of the abdomen (rebound tenderness on a miniature scale), a maneuver which can be far more precise and localizing. Asking the patient to cough will elicit true rebound tenderness without the need for placing a hand on the abdomen. Furthermore, the brusque demonstration of rebound tenderness will startle and induce protective spasm in a nervous or worried patient in whom true rebound tenderness is not present. A palpable gallbladder will be missed if palpation is so brusque that voluntary muscle spasm becomes superimposed upon involuntary muscular rigidity.

As in history taking, there is no substitute for sufficient time spent in the examination. It is important to remember that abdominal signs may be minimal but nevertheless, if accompanied by consistent symptoms, may be exceptionally meaningful when carefully assessed. Signs may be virtually or actually totally absent in cases of pelvic peritonitis, so that careful *pelvic and rectal examinations are mandatory in every patient with abdominal pain.* The presence of tenderness on pelvic or rectal examination in the absence of other abdominal signs must not lead the examiner to exclude such important operative indications as perforated appendicitis, diverticulitis, twisted ovarian cyst, and many others.

Much attention has been paid to the presence or absence of peristaltic sounds, their quality, and their frequency. Auscultation of the abdomen is probably one of the least rewarding aspects of the physical examination of a patient with abdominal pain. Severe catastrophes, such as strangulating small-intestinal obstruction or perforated appendicitis, may occur in the presence of normal peristalsis. Conversely, when the proximal part of the intestine above an obstruction becomes markedly distended and edematous, peristaltic sounds may lose the characteristics of borborygmi and become weak or absent even when peritonitis is not present. It is usually the severe chemical peritonitis of sudden onset which is associated with the truly silent abdomen. Assessment of the patient's state of hydration is important. The hematocrit and urinalysis permit an accurate estimate of the severity of dehydration, so that adequate replacement can be carried out.

Laboratory examinations may be of enormous value in the assessment of the patient with abdominal pain, yet with but a few exceptions they rarely establish a diagnosis. Leukocytosis should never be the single deciding factor as to whether or not operation is indicated. A white blood cell count greater than 20,000 per cubic millimeter may be observed with perforation of a viscus, but pancreatitis, acute cholecystitis, pelvic inflammatory disease, and intestinal infarction may be associated with marked leukocytosis. A normal white blood cell count is by no means rare in cases of perforation of abdominal viscera. The diagnosis of anemia may be more helpful than the white blood cell count, especially when combined with the history.

The urinalysis is also of great value in indicating to some degree the state of hydration or to rule out severe renal disease, diabetes, or urinary infection. Determination of the blood urea nitrogen, blood sugar, and serum bilirubin levels may also be helpful. The serum amylase determination is overrated, since in carefully controlled series of patients with proven pancreatitis where the determination has been done within the first 72 h, amylase was less than 200 Somogyi units in one-third of the cases, between 200 and 500 in another one-third of the cases, and greater than 500 in one-third. Since many diseases other than pancreatitis, e.g., perforated ulcer, strangulating intestinal obstruction, and acute cholecystitis, may be associated with very marked increase in the serum amylase, great care must be exercised in denying an operation to a patient solely on the basis of an elevated serum amylase level. The determination of the serum lipase may have a somewhat greater accuracy than the serum amylase.

Peritoneal lavage is a safe and effective diagnostic maneuver in patients with acute abdominal pain. It is of special value in patients with blunt trauma to the abdomen in whom evaluation of the abdomen may be difficult because of other multiple injuries to the spine, pelvis, or ribs and in whom blood in the peritoneal cavity produces only a very mild peritoneal reaction. The gallbladder is the only organ which may continue to seep fluid following accidental perforation, so that the region of this organ must be assiduously avoided. Determination of the pH of the aspirated fluid to ascertain the site of a perforation is misleading, because even highly acid gastric juice is rapidly buffered by peritoneal exudate.

Plain and upright or lateral decubitus roentgenograms of the abdomen may be of the greatest value. They are usually unnecessary in patients with acute appendicitis or strangulated external hernias. However, in cases of intestinal obstruction, perforated ulcer, and a variety of other conditions, films may be diagnostic. During a search for free air, the patient should be kept in the decubitus or upright position for at least 10 min before the appropriate film is taken lest a small pneumoperitoneum be missed. In rare instances, barium or water-soluble medium examination of the upper part of the gastrointestinal tract may demonstrate partial intestinal obstruction which may elude diagnosis by other means. If there is any question of obstruction of the colon, oral administration of barium sulfate should be avoided. On the other hand, barium enema is of inestimable value in cases of colonic obstruction and should be used with greater frequency where the possibility of perforation does not exist. Ultrasound recently has proved to be useful in detecting an enlarged gallbladder or pancreas, the presence of gallstones, an enlarged ovary, a tubal pregnancy, or a localized collection of fluid or pus. Radioisotopic scans (HIDA) may help differentiate acute cholecystitis from acute pancreatitis. A computed tomography scan may demonstrate an enlarged pancreas or a ruptured spleen, but it should be used only for *specific* questions such as these.

Sometimes, even under the best of circumstances with all available auxiliary aids and with the greatest of clinical skill, a definitive diagnosis cannot be established at the time of the initial examination. Nevertheless, despite lack of a clear anatomic diagnosis it may be abundantly clear to an experienced and thoughtful physician and surgeon that on clinical grounds alone operation is indicated. Should that decision be questionable, watchful waiting with repeated questioning and examination will often elucidate the true nature of the illness and indicate the proper course of action.

REFERENCES

De Dombal FT: Acute abdominal pain. Scand J Gastroenterol (Suppl) 14:29, 1979

Lee PWR: The plain x-ray in the acute abdomen: A surgeon's evaluation. Br J Surg 63:763, 1976

Leek BF: Abdominal and pelvic visceral receptors. Br Med Bull 33:163, 1977

Silen W: *Cope's Early Diagnosis of the Acute Abdomen*, 17th ed. London, Oxford Press, 1987

Staniland JR et al: Clinical presentation of acute abdomen: Study of 600 patients. Br Med J 2:393, 1972

Valman HB: Acute abdominal pain. Br Med J 282:1858, 1981

18   HEADACHE

JOSEPH B. MARTIN*

Although the term *headache* should encompass all pains located in the head, in common parlance its application is restricted to unpleasant sensations in the cranial vault. Facial, pharyngeal, laryngeal, and cervical pain, which usually signify other disorders, are described in Chaps. 19 and 360. (See also Table 18-1.)

Headache is one of the most frequent human discomforts. Its significance is often abstruse, for it may signal serious disease or represent only tension, fatigue, or a migrainous disorder. Fortunately, in most instances it reflects one of the latter, and only exceptionally does it warn of a serious intracranial abnormality. It is this dual significance, however, the benign and the potentially malignant, that requires the astute attention of the physician. A systematic approach to the headache problem necessitates a broad knowledge of the medical and surgical diseases of which it is a symptom and a clinical methodology that leaves none of the common and treatable causes unexplored.

GENERAL CONSIDERATIONS   The quality, location, duration, and time course of the headache and conditions that produce, exacerbate, or relieve it should be carefully reviewed. Unfortunately, except in special circumstances such as temporal arteritis, physical examination of the head itself is seldom useful.

The patient is rarely helpful in describing the *quality* of cephalic pain. In fact, persistent questioning on that point occasions surprise, for the patient usually assumes that the word *headache* conveys adequate information about the nature of the discomfort. Most headaches are dull, deeply located, and of aching character. Occasionally superficial burning or stinging pain localized to the skin is reported. The patient may describe tightness, pressure, or a bursting feeling, terms that may give clues to anxiety or depression.

Queries about *intensity* of pain are seldom useful, since they reflect more the patient's attitude toward the condition than the true severity. The stoical person tends to minimize discomfort, whereas the neurotic or depressed patient dramatizes it. Degree of incapacity is a better index. A severe migraine attack seldom allows performance of the day's work. The pain which awakens the patient from sleep at night, or prevents sleep, is also more likely to have a demonstrable organic basis. As a rule, the most intense cranial pains are those that accompany subarachnoid hemorrhage and meningitis, which have grave implications, or migraine and paroxysmal nocturnal *cluster* headaches, which are benign.

Data regarding *location* of the headache are often informative. If the source is in extracranial structures, as is often the case, the correspondence with the site of the pain is fairly precise. Inflammation of an extracranial artery causes pain localized to the site of the vessel. Lesions of paranasal sinuses, teeth, eyes, and upper cervical vertebrae induce a less sharply localized pain, but one that is still referred in a regional distribution that is fairly constant. Intracranial lesions in the posterior fossa cause pain in the occipital-nuchal region; it is homolateral if the lesion is one-sided. Supratentorial lesions induce frontotemporal pains, again homolateral to the lesion if it is on one side. But localization can also be uninformative or misleading. Ear pain, for example, although it may mean disease in the ear, more often is referred from other regions such as the neck, and eye pain may be referred to the occiput or cervical spine.

Duration and *time-intensity curve* of headaches both during the attack itself and in their life profile are most useful. The headache of bacterial meningitis or subarachnoid hemorrhage occurs usually in single attacks over a period of days. Single, brief, momentary (1 to 2 s) pains in the cranium (icepick-like headaches) are common but

* Revision of chapter by Raymond D. Adams and Joseph B. Martin published in the eleventh edition.

rarely indicate serious underlying disease. Classic migraine has its onset in the early morning hours or daytime, reaches a peak of severity in a half hour or so, lasts, unless treated, for several hours up to 1 to 2 days, is often accompanied by nausea or vomiting, and is terminated by sleep. A frequency of more than a single attack every few weeks is uncommon. A migraine patient having several attacks per week usually proves to have a combination of migraine and tension headaches. In contrast to this is the nightly occurrence (2 to 3 h after onset of sleep) over a period of several weeks to months of the rapidly peaking, nonthrobbing orbital, supraorbital, or temporal pain of cluster headache, which tends to dissipate within an hour. The headache of intracranial tumor can occur at any time of day or night, can interrupt sleep, varies in intensity, and lasts a few minutes to hours. The natural history is one of increasing frequency and intensity over a period of months. Tension headache, once commenced, may persist continuously for weeks or months, often waxing and waning from hour to hour or day to day.

Headache that bears a more or less constant relationship to certain biologic events and also to physical environmental changes may prove to be informative. Premenstrual headaches, most typically of migrainous or tension type, may occur as part of the premenstrual syndrome; they usually dissipate after the first day of vaginal bleeding. The headaches of cervical arthritis are most typically intense after a period of inactivity, and the first movements in the morning are both difficult and painful. Hypertensive headaches are uncommon, but like those of cerebral tumor, tend to occur on waking in the morning; excitement and tension may provoke them. Headache from infection of nasal sinuses may appear, with clocklike regularity, upon awakening and in midmorning, and is characteristically worsened by stooping and jarring of the head. Eyestrain headaches may follow prolonged use of the eyes. Anger, excitement, or irritation may initiate common migraine in certain disposed persons; this is more typical of common migraine than of classic type. Change of position, stooping, straining, cough, and sexual intercourse are each known to produce a special type of headache, described below. Exertional headaches, another well-known type, are usually benign (only 1 in 10 will have an intracranial lesion) and disappear within weeks to months.

PAIN-SENSITIVE STRUCTURES OF THE HEAD Understanding of headache has been greatly augmented by observations made during surgery of pain-sensitive structures. The following are sensitive to mechanical stimulation: (1) skin, subcutaneous tissue, muscles, arteries, and periosteum of skull; (2) tissues of the eye, ear, and nasal and sinus cavities; (3) intracranial venous sinuses and their tributary veins; (4) parts of the dura at the base of the brain and the arteries within the dura mater and pia-arachnoid; and (5) the trigeminal, glossopharyngeal, vagus, and first three cervical nerves. Interestingly, pain is practically the only sensation produced by stimulation of these structures. The bony skull, much of the pia-arachnoid and dura, and the parenchyma of the brain lack sensitivity.

Sensory stimuli from the head are conveyed to the central nervous system via the trigeminal nerves for structures above the tentorium in the anterior and middle fossae of the skull and via the first three cervical nerves for those in the posterior fossa and infradural structures. The ninth and tenth cranial nerves supply part of the posterior fossa and refer the pain to the ear and throat. The pain of intracranial disease is commonly referred to a part of the cranium lying within the areas supplied by these nerves. There may be associated local tenderness of the scalp at the site of reference. Dental or jaw pain may also have cranial reference. The pain of disease in other parts of the body is not referred to the head, although it may initiate headache by other means.

Headache can occur as a result of (1) distention, traction, or dilatation of intracranial or extracranial arteries, (2) traction or displacement of large intracranial veins or of their dural envelope, (3) compression, traction, or inflammation of cranial and spinal nerves, (4) voluntary or involuntary spasm, inflammation, and trauma to cranial and cervical muscles, and (5) meningeal irritation and raised intracranial pressure. More specifically, intracranial mass lesions cause headache only if they deform, displace, or exert traction on vessels, dural structures, or cranial nerves at the base of the brain, and this may happen long before intracranial pressure rises. Raised intracranial pressure causes headache in a bioccipital or bifrontal distribution which is rapidly relieved by lumbar puncture and lowering of the cerebrospinal fluid (CSF) pressure.

Dilatation of the extracranial, temporal, and intracranial *arteries* with stretching of surrounding sensitive structures is believed to be the mechanism of most of the pain of migraine. Extracranial, temporal, and occipital arteries, when involved in giant cell arteritis (cranial or "temporal" arteritis), a disease which usually afflicts individuals over 50 years of age, give rise to headache of dull aching and throbbing type, at first localized and then more diffuse. Characteristically it is severe and persistent over a period of weeks or months. The offending artery, strangely, is not always tender to pressure, yet section of it, as in biopsy, may relieve the pain (Chap. 276). Evolving atherosclerotic thrombosis of internal carotid, anterior, and middle cerebral arteries is sometimes accompanied by pain in the forehead or temple; with vertebral artery thrombosis the pain is postauricular, and basilar artery thrombosis causes referred pain in the occiput and sometimes the forehead.

In *infection or blockage of paranasal sinuses*, pain is usually felt over the antrum or in the forehead; with the *ethmoid* and *sphenoid sinuses*, the pain localizes around the eyes on one or both sides or in the vertex. Usually it is associated with tenderness of the skin in the same distribution. The pain may have two remarkable properties: (1) When throbbing, it may be abolished by compressing the carotid artery on the same side. (2) It tends to recur and subside at the same hours, i.e., it occurs on awakening, gradually disappears when the person is upright, and comes again in the late morning hours. The time relations are believed to yield information concerning the mechanism; morning pain is ascribed to the sinuses filling at night and its relief on arising to emptying after the erect posture has been assumed. Stooping, blowing the nose, and jarring the head intensify the pain; and inhalant sympathomimetic drugs such as phenylephrine, which reduce swelling and congestion, tend to relieve the pain. Sinus pain may persist after all purulent secretions have disappeared, probably because of persistent blockage of the draining orifices eliciting a vacuum or suction effect on the sinus wall (*vacuum sinus headaches*). The condition is relieved when aeration is restored. During air flights both earache and sinus headache tend to occur on descent, when the relative pressure in the blocked viscus falls.

Headache of ocular origin is usually located in the orbit, forehead, or temple, and has a steady, aching quality which may follow prolonged use of the eyes in close work. Ocular muscle imbalance, hyperopia, astigmatism, and impaired convergence and accommodation may give rise to sustained contraction of extraocular as well as frontal, temporal, and even occipital muscles. Raised intraocular pressure in acute glaucoma or iridocyclitis causes steady, aching pain felt in the eye. When intense, it may radiate throughout the distribution of the ophthalmic division of the trigeminal nerve. The pain of diabetic third nerve palsy, intracranial aneurysm, pituitary tumor, cavernous sinus thrombosis, and Raeder's paratrigeminal syndrome is often referred to the eye.

The *headaches accompanying disease of ligaments, muscles, and apophyseal joints* in the upper part of the spine, which are referred to occipital and upper cervical regions, are difficult to separate from the more common muscular contraction (tension) headaches. Such referred pains are especially frequent in middle and late adult life in patients with rheumatoid arthritis and cervical spondylosis and tend also to occur after whiplash injuries to the neck. If the pain is articular or synovial in origin, the first movements after being still for some hours are both stiff and painful. In fact, evocation of pain by active and passive motion of the spine should indicate traumatic or other disease of movable parts. The pain of *myofibrositis*, evidenced by tender nodules near the cranial insertion of cervical and other muscles, is more obscure (see Chap. 15). There are no pathologic data as to the nature of these vaguely palpable lesions, and it is uncertain

TABLE 18-1 Common types of headache

Type	Site	Age and sex	Clinical characteristics	Diurnal pattern	Life profile
Common migraine	Frontotemporal Uni- or bilateral	Children, young to middle-aged adults, both sexes, female > male	Throbbing and/or dull ache; worse behind one eye or ear, nausea or vomiting Headache becomes generalized	Upon awakening or later in day Duration: hours to 1–2 days	Irregular interval, weeks to months Tends to disappear in middle age and during pregnancy
Classic migraine	Same as above	Same as above	Same as above; visual prodrome common	Same as above	Same as above
Cluster, histamine headache, or migrainous neuralgia	Orbital or temporal Unilateral	Adolescent and adult males (80–90%)	Intense, nonthrobbing pain	Usually nocturnal; occurs one or more hours after falling asleep Rarely diurnal	Nightly for several weeks to months (cluster) Recurrence: years later
Tension headaches	Generalized	Children, adolescents, and adults, both sexes	Pressure (nonthrobbing); tightness Aching	Continuous, variable intensity	Recurrent episodes lasting hours to days
Meningeal irritation (meningitis, subarachnoid hemorrhage)	Generalized	Any age, both sexes	Intense, steady deep pain, may be worse in neck	Duration: days to a week or more	Single episode
Brain tumor	(See text)	Any age, both sexes	Variable in intensity May awaken patient Steady pain	Lasts minutes to hours; increasing severity	Once in a lifetime: weeks to months
Temporal arteritis	Unilateral, temporal, or occipital	Over 50 years, either sex	Persistent burning, aching	Continuous or intermittent	Persists for weeks to a few months

SOURCE: After J Patten, Neurological Differential Diagnosis, London, Harold Starke, Springer-Verlag, 1977.

whether the pain actually arises in them. They may represent only the deep tenderness felt in the region of referred pain or the involuntary secondary protective spasm of muscles. Characteristically, the pain is steady (nonthrobbing) and spreads from one to both sides of the head. Exposure to cold or draft may precipitate it. Though severe at times, it seldom prevents sleep. Massage of muscles and heat have unpredictable effects but relieve the pain in some cases.

The *headache of meningeal irritation* (infection or hemorrhage) is acute in onset, severe, generalized, deep-seated, constant, especially intense at the base of the skull, and associated with stiffness of the neck on bending forward. Dilatation and congestion of inflamed meningeal vessels are probably the main cause of the pain.

Lumbar puncture headache is characterized by a steady occipital-nuchal or bifrontal pain that comes on a few minutes after arising from a recumbent position and is relieved within a few minutes by lying down. Its cause is persistent leakage of CSF into the lumbar tissues through the needle site. The CSF pressure is low. The headache is usually increased by compression of the jugular veins and is unaffected by digital obliteration of one carotid artery. It is probable that in the upright position a low intraspinal and negative intracranial pressure exerts traction on dural attachments and dural sinuses by caudal displacement of the brain. Understandably, then, headache following cisternal puncture is rare. As soon as the leakage of CSF stops and CSF pressure is gradually restored (usually from a few days up to a week or so), the headache disappears. "Spontaneous" low-pressure headache may also follow a sneeze or strain, presumably because of rupture of the spinal arachnoid space along a nerve root.

The mechanism of the *throbbing or steady headache that accompanies febrile illnesses*, located in frontal or occipital regions or generalized, is probably vascular. It is much like histamine headache

in that it is relieved on one side by carotid artery compression and on both sides by jugular vein compression or the subarachnoid injection of saline solution. It is increased by shaking the head. It seems probable that the meningeal vessels pulsate unduly and stretch pain-sensitive structures around the base of the brain. In certain cases, however, the pain may be lessened by compression of temporal arteries, and in these cases a component of the headache seems to be derived from the walls of extracranial arteries, as in migraine.

The pain felt in *tension headaches* of patients with anxiety or depression has been alleged to be due to spasm of cranial and cervical muscles. There is, however, no direct evidence to support such a mechanism. Combinations of tension and vascular headaches give rise to "mixed headaches," which are one of the most common types of headache.

PRINCIPAL CLINICAL VARIETIES OF HEADACHE Usually there is no difficulty in diagnosing the headache of glaucoma, purulent sinusitis, bacterial meningitis, and brain tumor, and a fuller account of these special headaches will be found where these diseases are described in other sections of the book. It is when headache is chronic, recurrent, and unattended by other important signs of disease that the physician faces one of the most difficult medical problems.

The types of headache subsequently described should then be considered.

Migraine The term *migraine* refers to periodic, hemicranial, throbbing headaches often accompanied by nausea and vomiting which usually begin in childhood, adolescence, or early adult life and recur in diminishing number and intensity during advancing years. Migraine is frequent, with a prevalence of 20 to 30 percent in the population. Women are affected three times as often as men. There is a tendency for the headaches to occur during the period of

TABLE 18-1   Common types of headache (*continued*)

Provoking factors	Associated features	Treatment
Bright light, noise, tension, alcohol Dark room and sleep relieve Scalp sensitive Pressure helps	Nausea in some cases	Ergot preparation at onset Propranolol, calcium channel blockers, methysergide for prevention
Same as above	Blindness and scintillating lights Unilateral numbness Disturbed speech Vertigo Confusion	Same as above
Alcohol in some	Lacrimation, congested eye	Ergot preparation at bedtime Amitriptyline and lithium carbonate for prevention
Fatigue and nervous strain	Depression, nervousness, anxiety, insomnia	Antianxiety and antidepressant drugs
None	Neck stiff on forward bending Kernig and Brudzinski signs	For meningitis or bleeding (see text)
None Sometimes position	Papilledema Vomiting Slow mentation	Glucocorticoids Mannitol Glycerol Treatment of tumor
Scalp sensitive Tender arteries	Intermittent or permanent loss of sight Rheumatic myalgia Fever	Glucocorticoid therapy

premenstrual tension and fluid retention and to decrease during pregnancy. The immediate family history is positive for migraine in over 60 percent of cases. Migraine or vascular headaches present in one of four clinical patterns: (1) classic migraine, (2) common migraine, (3) complicated migraine, and (4) cluster headache.

Classic migraine begins with a prodrome of prominent neurologic symptoms such as visual scintillations, dazzling zigzag lines (fortification spectra), photophobia and spreading scotomas, or dizziness and tinnitus. Classic migraine may be heralded hours before the attack by premonitory symptoms, most commonly a feeling of elation, excessive energy, thirst, a craving for sweet foods, or drowsiness. At other times, there may be a slowing of mentation or a feeling of impending doom or of depression, or there may be no warning whatsoever. The disturbance of vision that commences the attack may be followed by homonymous hemianopic field defects; sometimes they are bilateral, and even total blindness may rarely occur.

In *common migraine* there is an unheralded onset of headache, often with nausea and sometimes vomiting, following the same temporal pattern but without the antecedent neurologic symptoms. Both classic and common migraine respond to ergot preparations, if administered early in the attack.

Complicated migraine refers to headaches accompanied by neurologic symptoms that may either precede or accompany the headache. Numbness and tingling of the lips, face, hand, and leg on one side may occur, sometimes in combination with an aphasic disorder. The arm and leg may become weak or paralyzed on one side, mimicking a stroke. The numbness or weakness spreads from one part of the body to another slowly over a period of minutes. Full recovery usually occurs after a period of minutes or hours. However, permanent deficits consisting of hemianopsia (lesion in distribution of the

posterior cerebral artery), hemiplegia or hemianesthesia (lesion in territory of middle cerebral artery), or ophthalmoplegia (usually third nerve lesion) may occur.

Several other neurologic syndromes have been delineated in association with complicated migraine. Bickerstaff first called attention to *basilar migraine*, in which the visual disorder and paresthesias are bilateral and are accompanied by confusion, stupor, rarely coma, aggressive outbursts, vertigo, diplopia, and dysarthria. While the full syndrome is infrequent, partial basilar syndromes are found in some 30 percent of children with migraine. Alternating hemiplegias in children have also been attributed to basilar migraine but could be due as well to alternating involvement of the middle cerebral arteries.

It is also recognized that neurologic syndromes may occur due to migraine which are not followed by headache. In children, abdominal pain and vomiting, sometimes cyclical, may occur without headache as the sole expression of migraine; the same is true of some cases of paroxysmal vertigo in children. Such *migraine equivalents* may be manifest as pain localized in the thorax, pelvis, or extremities; bouts of fever; paroxysmal vertigo; transient disturbances in mood (*psychic equivalents*). The first neurologic syndrome due to migraine may occur in late adult life in a person not previously known to have migraine. Fisher refers to these as *transient migrainous accompaniments* to distinguish them from transient cerebral ischemic attacks (TIAs).

Cluster headache, also called paroxysmal nocturnal cephalalgia, migrainous neuralgia, histamine headache, and Horton's syndrome, has a fourfold higher incidence in men than in women. It is characterized by constant, unilateral orbital pain, with onset usually within 2 or 3 h after falling asleep. It tends to occur during the phase of rapid eye movement (REM) sleep. The pain is intense and steady (nonthrobbing) with lacrimation, blocked nostril, then rhinorrhea, and sometimes miosis, ptosis, flush, and edema of cheek, all lasting approximately an hour or two. It tends to recur nightly for several weeks or a few months (hence the term *cluster*), followed by complete freedom for months or even years. The pain of a given attack may leave as rapidly as it began. Clusters may recur over the years, being possibly more likely in times of stress, prolonged strain, overwork, and with upsetting emotional experiences. Episodes of cluster headache lasting 2 to 3 weeks may recur several times over a lifetime. Often the pain involves the same orbit in each cluster. Occasionally alcohol, nitroglycerin, or tyramine-containing foods precipitate an attack. Rarely, the condition may occur in daytime and may not cluster but continue for years. The picture is so characteristic that its presentation is diagnostic, though to those unfamiliar with it the possibility of a carotid aneurysm, hemangioma, brain tumor, or sinusitis may be suggested.

The relationship of the cluster headache to migraine remains conjectural. A portion of the cases have a background of migraine, which led to the earlier designation of migrainous neuralgia, but the majority do not.

MECHANISM AND PATHOPHYSIOLOGY   A satisfactory theory of the pathophysiology of migraine has eluded clinical investigators. Certain facts appear indisputable; the symptoms of migraine are associated with changes in cerebral blood flow, presumably secondary to changes in vessel caliber; the prodromal phase with neurologic symptoms is accompanied by arteriolar constriction and decreased cerebral blood flow beginning most often in the posterior part of the brain; the decrease in cerebral blood flow in migraine proceeds at a rate of about 2 mm/min, resembling the spreading depression originally described by Leão, which is characterized by a transient self-propagating perturbation of brain electrical activity followed by hypoperfusion. The earlier assumption that the headache that follows is due to vascular dilatation has not been supported by direct measurements of cerebral blood flow during the headache phase. Regional cerebral blood flow, measured by xenon 133, shows oligemic regions of cortex during the entire migraine attack with diminished vascular reactivity to carbon dioxide, suggesting an abnormality of vascular responsivity. Between attacks of migraine, patients show normal regulation of brain circulation.

The factors that elicit these changes in cerebral blood flow are unknown. Two general hypotheses about the cause of migraine have emerged. The first is that it is due to a central nervous system neurovascular disorder that triggers alterations in vasomotor regulation. The premonitory symptoms of changes in mood, appetite, and thirst have led some to consider a central hypothalamic or brainstem disorder affecting biogenic amine regulation (norepinephrine or serotonin). The second considers migraine to be a systemic metabolic disregulation with attacks elicited secondary to intravascular events associated with changes in serotonin metabolism. Changes in platelet serotonin levels, shown to fall during the attack, accompanied by increased urinary excretion of serotonin and of 5-hydroxyindoleacetic acid support the contention that migraine is a systemic disorder. Further support for a role of serotonin comes from observations that reserpine, which triggers serotonin release, causes migraine in some patients and that antiserotonin drugs, like methysergide, show greatest success in its treatment. However, there is difficulty in understanding how changes in intravascular serotonin, which has little direct effect on vessel contraction, can induce the changes of migraine, and it is now conceded that these changes are likely secondary to a central disregulation. Lance considers the mechanism of migraine to involve changes in biogenic amine or neuropeptide neurotransmitters in the central nervous system, associated with or followed by platelet release reactions. Recent work has focused on the neurotransmitters found in nerve fibers that innervate cerebral blood vessels. Moskowitz has demonstrated that cerebral vessels are innervated by nerves that contain substance P, a peptide important for pain transmission (see Chap. 15) and also thought to be capable of eliciting local tissue reactions resembling inflammation. Other neuropeptides found in cerebral blood vessels and known to affect vascular tone include vasoactive intestinal polypeptide, neurotensin, and neuropeptide Y.

There is persistent debate concerning factors that trigger the migraine attacks. Dietary factors are important in some patients. Sensitivity to milk and wheat products is found in some patients with severe refractory migraine. Many patients learn to avoid alcohol (particularly red wine), chocolate, coffee, tea, or other agents with pharmacologically active ingredients. How these substances elicit the attacks is unknown. Some patients describe exposure to sunlight, exercise, tension, or the use of oral contraceptives as increasing the frequency and severity of migraine.

DIFFERENTIAL DIAGNOSIS   Classic migraine usually causes no difficulty in diagnosis. Difficulties arise from two sources: (1) ignorance of the fact that a progressively unfolding neurologic syndrome may be migrainous in origin, and (2) lack of appreciation that the neurologic disorder may occur without headache.

The neurologic symptoms of the migraine syndrome may resemble focal epilepsy, the clinical picture of a vascular malformation such as an angioma or aneurysm, or some other vascular disease such as a thrombotic or embolic stroke. The pace of the neurologic symptoms of migraine, rather than their character, reliably distinguishes them from epilepsy. The clinical profile of the aura of epilepsy is measured in seconds, for it depends on spreading neural excitation, in contrast to the slow progression of migraine, which is based on spreading depression of nervous tissue. Nevertheless, there are instances where episodes of coma with electroencephalogram (EEG) abnormality may be either migraine or epilepsy. Furthermore, a seizure is often followed by a generalized headache.

Ophthalmoplegic migraine always suggests a carotid aneurysm, and carotid arteriography may be necessary to exclude it. Despite many claims that vascular malformations may cause hemicranial pain occurring invariably on the same side of the head (unlike migraine), larger series of cases have shown this only rarely to be the case. Focal epilepsy, protracted headache, stiff neck and bloody CSF, a persistent neurologic deficit, and cranial bruit are indicative of a vascular type of headache associated with angioma or aneurysm.

Only in the earlier stages, when periodic throbbing headache is the sole symptom, are these conditions confused with true migraine.

Tension headache   The tension headache is usually bilateral, often with diffuse extension over the top of the cranium. Occipital-nuchal or bifrontal localization is common. Although the sensation may be described as pain, close questioning may uncover other sensations, viz., fullness, tightness, or pressure (as if the head is surrounded by a band or in a vise), on which waves of aching pain are superimposed. The onset of a given attack is more gradual than in migraine, and not infrequently a throbbing "vascular" type of headache is described. Tension headache may occur acutely under conditions of emotional duress or intense worry and lasts for hours or a day or two. More often it persists unremittingly for weeks or months. In fact, this is the only type of headache that exhibits the peculiarity of being absolutely continuous day and night for long periods of time. Although sleep may be possible, whenever the patient awakens, the headache is present; a common feature is the finding that analgesic remedies have relatively little effect in alleviating the pain. In contrast to migraine, in which pain is periodic and lifelong, with tendency to lessen in late adult years, tension headache occurs more often in middle age and may persist for many years.

It is unlikely that the origin of the pain is sustained muscle activity, since electromyographic (EMG) investigations show no changes in forehead or neck muscles. On the other hand, elicitation of headache after administration of amyl nitrite, a vasodilator, in about 50 percent of patients suggests a vascular contribution to the pain. Histamine can also cause headaches in these patients.

It is a common experience for both tension headache and common migraine to coexist in the same patient. The management of such patients may require therapy of both types of headache.

Psychological studies of groups of patients with tension headaches have revealed prominent symptoms of depression, anxiety, and, in some, hypochrondriasis. Kudrow records that 65 percent of depressed patients have this type of headache and that over 60 percent of his patients with tension headaches were depressed.

Headache of angioma and aneurysm   The temporal profile of any given attack shows the onset to be sudden or very acute, with the pain reaching a peak within minutes. Neurologic disturbances such as defects in vision, unilateral numbness, weakness, or aphasia may precede or occur after the onset of headache and outlast it. Should hemorrhage occur, the headache is often extremely severe and localizes in the occiput and neck, lasting many days in association with stiff neck. A cranial or cervical bruit and the presence of blood in the CSF establish the diagnosis. The claim that vascular malformations may give rise to migraine is probably untenable. Statistical data show migraine to be no more frequent in this group of patients than in the general population. Vascular lesions may exist for long periods of time without headache, or headache may develop many years after other manifestations such as epilepsy and hemiplegia (see Chap. 351).

Traumatic headaches   Severe, chronic, continuous, or intermittent headaches often associated with giddiness, vertigo, or tinnitus appear as the cardinal symptoms of the posttraumatic syndrome. The cause of the headache is unknown, but it is a clear-cut disorder unrelated in most instances to medicolegal issues of compensation. *Posttraumatic dysautonomic cephalalgia* is a term given by Vijayan and Dreyfus to severe, episodic, throbbing, unilateral headaches accompanied by ipsilateral mydriasis and excessive facial sweating. The condition follows injury to the neck in the region of the carotid sheath. It was postulated that the sympathetic nervous supply of the cranium had been disinhibited, and there was clinical and pharmacologic evidence of sympathetic dysfunction.

Headache and dizziness of fluctuating severity, followed by drowsiness, stupor, coma, and hemiparesis, are the usual manifestations of *chronic subdural hematoma*. The head injury may have been minor and forgotten by patient and family. The headaches are deep-seated, steady, unilateral or generalized, and respond to the usual analgesic drugs. The typical attack profile of the headache and other symptoms is one of increasing frequency and severity over several weeks or months. Diagnosis is established by computed tomography (CT), magnetic resonance imaging (MRI), or angiography (see Chap. 352).

Headaches of brain tumor Headache is the outstanding symptom of cerebral tumor. Unfortunately, the quality of the pain has no specific feature. It tends to be deep-seated, nonthrobbing (or throbbing), and aching or bursting. Attacks last a few minutes to an hour or more and occur once or many times during the day. Activity and, frequently, change in the position of the head may provoke pain, while rest in bed diminishes its frequency. Nocturnal awakening because of pain, although typical, is by no means diagnostic. Unexpected forceful (projectile) vomiting may punctuate the illness in its later stages. As the tumor grows, the pain becomes more frequent and severe; it sometimes is nearly continuous terminally. If unilateral, the headache is homolateral to the tumor in 9 out of 10 patients. Supratentorial tumors are felt anterior to the interauricular circumference of the skull; posterior fossa tumors behind this line. Bifrontal and biooccipital headache, coming on after unilateral headache, signifies the development of increased intracranial pressure.

Headaches related to medical disorders Experienced physicians are aware of many conditions in which headache figures as a dominant symptom. These include fevers of any cause, carbon monoxide exposure, chronic lung disease with hypercapnia (headaches often nocturnal), hypothyroidism, Cushing's syndrome, withdrawal of corticosteroid medication, chronic nitrite or ergot exposure, occasionally Addison's disease, aldosterone-producing adrenal tumors, use of contraceptive medications, acute rises in blood pressure, e.g., from pheochromocytoma, and acute anemia with hemoglobin below 10 g. Hypertension per se is an uncommon cause of headache.

Unusual types of headache Sharp, jabbing pains in the head (icepick-like pains) last a second or two, and have no clinical significance. They are reported in up to 3 percent of the normal population and in 46 percent of migrainous patients. The pain is usually felt in the temporal or orbital region.

Cough and exertional headache or headache brought on by stooping follows the initiating action by a few seconds and lasts a minute or two. Usually no explanation is apparent, but exceptionally it occurs in patients with arteriovenous malformations, Paget's disease of the skull, Arnold-Chiari malformation, or an intracranial tumor. In a series of 103 patients followed for 3 years or longer by Rooke, only 10 developed neurologic signs. The mechanism of this headache may be venous distention, for jugular compression induces it in some patients.

Coital headaches are generalized, often severe headaches that begin suddenly during coitus or immediately after orgasm. They are uncommon, occur more often in men than in women, and usually do not signify a serious underlying pathology. They may last minutes or hours. In the latter circumstance they must be differentiated from a subarachnoid hemorrhage due to a ruptured aneurysm.

Erythrocyanotic headache is a rare form of generalized throbbing headache which occurs in conjunction with flushing of the face and hands and numbness of the fingers (erythromelalgia). The condition has been reported in association with (1) mastocytosis (infiltration of tissues with mast cells, which elaborate histamine, heparin, and serotonin); (2) carcinoid tumors; (3) some tumors of pancreatic islets; (4) pheochromocytoma.

HEADACHE AND FACIAL PAIN The facial neuralgias are discussed in Chap. 360 (see Table 18-2).

APPROACH TO THE PATIENT WITH HEADACHE Obviously very different possibilities are raised by a patient who presents for the first time with severe headache and a patient who has had recurrent headache over a period of years. The chances of uncovering the cause in the first instance are much greater than in the second and in the former the underlying conditions (meningitis, subarachnoid hemorrhage, epidural or subdural hematoma, glaucoma, and purulent sinusitis) often are more serious. In general, severe, persistent headache with stiff neck and fever means meningitis, and the same combination without fever, subarachnoid hemorrhage. A lumbar puncture is mandatory. Acute persistent headache over a period of hours or days may occur in systemic infections such as influenza (febrile) or as a manifestation of an acute tension state. If there is a diagnosable febrile disease and no stiffness of the neck, lumbar puncture may be deferred. The first attack of migraine may also present in this way, but of course there is no fever.

In searching for the cause of recurrent headache one should investigate the status of cardiovascular and renal systems by blood pressure and urine examination, eyes by funduscopy, intraocular pressure, and refraction, the sinuses by transillumination and x-rays, the cranial arteries by palpation (and biopsy?), the cervical spine by the effect of passive movement of the head and x-rays, the nervous system by neurologic and psychological evaluation.

Hypertension, although frequent in the general population, is not often a cause of recurrent headaches. Severe hypertension with diastolic blood pressures of over 110 mmHg may be associated with headache. If headache is severe and frequent, the possibilities of underlying anxiety or tension state or a common migraine syndrome should be considered.

The adolescent with daily frontal headaches represents a special type of problem. Often the relationship of the headaches to eyestrain is unclear, and refraction of the eyes and new eyeglasses do not relieve the condition. Anxiety or tension is probably a factor in such cases, but it is difficult to be certain of a causal relationship. Some of the most persistent and inexplicable headaches, which have led to a survey by a battery of diagnostic procedures for tumor, have proved in the end to be associated with endogenous depression.

Equally puzzling is the somber, tense adult whose primary complaint is headache, or the migrainous person who in late life or at menopause begins to have daily headaches. Here it becomes important to assess mental status along the lines suggested in Chaps. 29 and 30, looking for evidence of anxiety, depression, and hypochondriasis. The quality and persistence of the headache are suggestive of the possibility of psychiatric illness. Sometimes asking the patient what is the matter may reveal suspicion and fear of brain tumor. Antidepressant drugs given as an empirical test may relieve the headache, thus clarifying the diagnosis.

The most worrisome type of patient is the one who has headache of increasing frequency and severity over a period of months or a year or so. Since an intracranial mass lesion (tumor, abscess, subdural hematoma) is a leading possibility, a complete neurologic survey, including careful inspection of optic discs, CT or MRI, and electroencephalogram, should be performed.

Every person over 50 to 55 years with severe headache of some few days' or weeks' duration should be considered as possibly having cranial arteritis (see Chap. 276). The overall incidence in patients over 50 years is 1 in 750; that of polymyalgia rheumatica in the same age group is 1 in 200. Women are more often affected than men (4:1), and there is an associated polymyalgia in 25 percent of cases. Conversely, in 50 percent of polymyalgia rheumatica patients there is a cranial arteritis. Increased sedimentation rate, fever, and anemia may occur. The findings of a thickened, tender temporal artery and claudication of jaw muscles from involvement of facial arteries are important. The disease may cause blindness and/or ophthalmoplegia but rarely involves intracranial arteries. Arterial biopsy and response to glucocorticoids establish the diagnosis.

TREATMENT The most important steps in the treatment of headache are those measures which uncover and remove the underlying disease or functional disturbance.

For the *common everyday headache* due to fatigue, acute stress, or excessive use of alcohol and tobacco, the physician advises avoidance of the offending activity or agent, and symptomatic therapy in the form of aspirin, 0.6 g, or acetaminophen, 0.6 g, given every 4 to 6 h. Chronic headaches falling into the common migraine or

TABLE 18-2　Types of facial pain

Types	Site	Clinical characteristics	Aggravating-relieving factors	Diseases	Treatment
Trigeminal neuralgia (tic douloureux)	Second or third division of trigeminal nerve, unilateral	Men : women = 1:3 Over 50 years Paroxysms (10–30 s) of stabbing, burning pain Trigger points, intermittent ache No sensory or motor paralysis	Touching face, chewing, smiling, talking, blowing nose	Idiopathic If in young adults unilateral or bilateral, multiple sclerosis Vascular anomaly Tumor of fifth cranial nerve	Carbamazepine Phenytoin Radiofrequency lesion of ganglion
Atypical facial neuralgia	Unilateral or bilateral	Predominantly female 30–50 years Continuous intolerable pain Mainly maxillary areas	None	Depressive and anxiety states Hysteria Idiopathic	Antidepressant and antianxiety medication
Supraorbital ciliary, infraorbital, sphenopalatine neuralgias	Unilateral in eye, cheek, ear, neck	Persistent, aching pain	Occasional nasal obstruction	Idiopathic Paranasal sinus disease	Decongestant nasal medication ?Nerve section and injection
Postzoster neuralgia	Unilateral Any one of trigeminal divisions	History of zoster Aching, burning pain; jabs of pain Paresthesia, slight sensory loss Dermal scars	Contact, movement	Herpes zoster	Carbamazepine, phenytoin, and antidepressants
Costen's syndrome	Unilateral, near temporomandibular joints	Elderly females Severe aching pain, intensified by chewing Tenderness over joints Malocclusion	Chewing, pressure over temporomandibular joint	Loss of teeth, rheumatoid arthritis	Bite correction and surgery
Tolosa-Hunt syndrome	Unilateral, mainly orbital	Intense sharp, aching pain; associated ophthalmoplegias of varying degree Pupil inequality, sensory loss	None	?Arteritis and granulomatous lesions	Glucocorticoids
Raeder's paratrigeminal syndrome	Unilateral, frontotemporal and maxilla	Intense sharp, aching pain Pupil inequality, sensory loss	None	Tumors, granulomatous lesions, injuries	Depends on type of lesion

SOURCE: After J Patten, Neurological Differential Diagnosis, London, Harold Starke, Springer-Verlag, 1977.

tension category are much more difficult to manage. Analgesics may alleviate the pain, but rarely abolish it. Patients commonly self-administer four to eight tablets daily of aspirin or acetaminophen for years despite acknowledging minimal benefit. Such headaches often respond to amitriptyline given in gradually increased doses to 100 to 150 mg, preferably administered as a single bedtime dose. *Premenstrual headache,* if troublesome, can often be helped by the use of a diuretic for the week preceding the menstrual period and a mixture of mild analgesic and sedative medications (aspirin or acetaminophen, 0.6 g, and barbiturate). If the headaches are severe and incapacitating, they should be treated as common migraine.

Migraine may require no treatment at all, other than an explanation of its nature to the patient and a reassurance that it will do no harm. Some patients know, or allege to know, that certain factors induce attacks, and these should be avoided. In some patients alcoholic drinks, particularly red wine, are invariably followed by a migraine. Others claim reduction of attacks of headache by an elimination diet, correction of refractive error, or by psychotherapy. Biofeedback can reduce the number of migraine attacks in some patients, and practiced relaxation is beneficial in others.

Drugs used for treatment of migraine can be separated into agents used for the acute attack and those administered for prophylaxis. Patients who experience more than three or four severe attacks each month should be considered for preventive treatment. Treatment of the neurologic aura of migraine is rarely required or possible because of its brevity. Some patients find relief with ergot preparations given orally, 1 to 3 mg held under the tongue until dissolved, or ergotamine

tartrate, 0.25 mg by intravenous injection. These treatments if given early will abort a classic migraine attack in 80 to 90 percent of patients. Sometimes the combination of caffeine, 100 mg with 1 mg ergotamine, is preferred (Cafergot or equivalent). It may be taken in the form of tablets (two at the onset of headache and a third in half an hour) or as rectal suppositories (2 mg ergotamine and 100 mg caffeine) if vomiting prevents oral administration. The acute migraine attack is managed best with an ergotamine-caffeine combination. Some patients find relief with ergotamine given orally in a dose of 1 to 3 mg. If oral administration is not tolerated because of nausea, or is ineffective, rectal administration of ergotamine is indicated. One-half suppository given at the onset of the attack followed by another half in 10 to 15 min and a whole suppository in 20 to 30 min, if necessary, is often effective. Medication should be limited to no more than two suppositories per day or four per week because of the danger of vasospasm. Ergotamine inhalation is more acceptable to some patients; one inhalation is given at the start of the attack, another in 5 min, and a third at 10 min. Inhalations should be limited to three per day or six per week. In patients who have vascular disease or are pregnant, ergot preparations must be used cautiously, if at all, because of the danger of prolonged vascular spasm.

Once the headache has become intense (after 30 min), ergot is of little help, and one must resort to codeine sulfate, 30 mg, or meperidine, 50 mg, as the only means of terminating the pain. If sleep customarily terminates the headache, 50 mg of promethazine or an equivalent drug orally is helpful; it also relieves vomiting.

In individuals with frequent migrainous attacks (more than four per month), efforts at prevention are worthwhile. Some success has been obtained with preparations of ergot, 0.5 mg, atropine, 0.3 mg, and phenobarbital, 15 mg, two or three times a day for a few weeks. Propranolol, 20 to 40 mg three times a day, has been effective in reducing the frequency and intensity of attacks in approximately one-half of cases. For the most severe forms of the disorder, methysergide in a dose of 6 to 8 mg per day given for several weeks or months has proved effective in reducing the frequency of or abolishing attacks. The main adverse effect has been retroperitoneal and pulmonary fibrosis; this complication has been reported in several dozen cases when the patient has been treated continuously for more than 6 months. Discontinuing treatment for 1 month out of every 6 has greatly reduced the incidence of this complication. Some patients benefit from tricyclic antidepressants such as doxepin or amitriptyline, which should be started in doses of 25 to 75 mg at bedtime and increased gradually every third or fourth night to 100 to 150 mg. Calcium channel blockers such as nifedipine 10 to 40 mg per day in divided doses or verapamil 80 mg given three times daily may be beneficial. Some patients experience an initial exacerbation of migraine attacks on first taking calcium channel blocking drugs, and then obtain relief. Severe attacks of common migraine lasting for several days or even weeks have been treated successfully with chlorpromazine in doses of 50 to 100 mg daily administered for 7 to 10 days. Prednisone in divided doses of 20 mg three or four times a day is also effective in some severe cases. Newer drugs with antiserotonergic effects are currently nearing approval for clinical use in migraine.

All experienced physicians appreciate the importance of helping patients rearrange their schedules so as to control the tensions and hard-driving ways of living so often a feature of migrainous patients. There is no one way of accomplishing this, but, in general, long and costly psychotherapy has not been helpful, or at least one can say there are no substantial data as to its value.

Cluster headaches have proved to be most resistant to treatment. The acute attack can be terminated with oxygen or ergotamine inhalation. However, the most effective treatment is the administration of drugs to prevent headache episodes until the cluster is over. Success has been obtained in individual cases with amitriptyline, 100 to 150 mg daily, methysergide, 6 to 8 mg per day, prednisone, 40 mg daily for 5 days then reduced to an amount necessary to control headaches, lithium carbonate in an initial dose of 250 mg three times a day, and calcium channel blockers. Histamine desensitization, originally proposed by Horton, has been little used in recent years because of inconvenience and inconsistent results. Persistent cluster headaches have also been treated effectively with indomethacin.

Hypertensive headaches respond to agents that lower blood pressure and relieve muscle tension.

Muscle tension headaches respond best to massage, relaxation, and a combination of drugs which relieve depression (e.g., amitriptyline or imipramine) and anxiety (e.g., diazepam and alprazolam). Pain-relieving medicine of non-habit-forming type (e.g., aspirin and propoxyphene hydrochloride) should be added when throbbing headache is present. Stronger analgesic medication (codeine or meperidine hydrochloride) should be avoided. Psychotherapy may be helpful in this group of patients.

The headache of the *posttraumatic syndrome* requires supportive psychotherapy in the form of reassurance and frequent explanation of its benign and transient nature, a program of increasing physical activity, and drugs which allay anxiety and depression. However, the tricyclic antidepressants are generally less effective than in the mixed tension and throbbing headaches of anxious depressions. Tender scars from scalp laceration may be novocainized repeatedly (subcutaneous injection of 5 mL of 1% procaine) with some degree of success. Settlement of litigation as soon as possible works to the patient's advantage.

Heat, massage, salicylates, and indomethacin or phenylbutazone usually effect some improvement in those arthritic diseases of the cervical spine that are associated with cervicocranial pain (see Chaps. 270 and 281). A soft collar and traction may be beneficial.

Glucocorticoid therapy is indicated in *cranial arteritis* to prevent disastrous blindness by occlusion of the ophthalmic arteries, which occurs in 50 percent of untreated patients. Prednisone should be given in full doses (40 to 60 mg per day) for at least a month and continued until all symptoms and laboratory abnormalities have disappeared. The headaches of brain tumor often respond promptly to large doses of glucocorticoids.

REFERENCES

APPENZELLER O: Migraine and cluster headache, in *Current Therapy in Neurologic Disease*, RT Johnson (ed). Philadelphia, Decker, 1987, vol 2, p 59

BICKERSTAFF ER: Basilar artery migraine. Lancet 1:15, 1961

BOGDUK N, LANCE JW: Pain and pain syndrome including headache, in *Current Neurology*, SF Appel (ed). New York, Wiley, 1981, vol 3, chap 14

CAVINESS VS, O'BRIEN P: Headache. N Engl J Med 302:446, 1980

COUCH JR, HASSANEIM RS: Platelet aggregability in migraine. Neurology 27:843, 1977

CRITCHLEY M et al (eds): *Advances in Neurology*, vol 33: *Headache: Physiopathological and Clinical Aspects*. New York, Raven Press, 1982

DIAMOND S: Prolonged benign exertional headache. Headache 22:96, 1982

EHYAI A, FENICHEL GM: Natural history of acute confusional migraine. Arch Neurol 35:368, 1978

FISHER CM: Late-life migraine accompaniment—further experience. Stroke 17:1033, 1986

GELMERS HJ: Nimodipine, a new calcium antagonist, in the prophylactic treatment of migraine. *Headache* 23:106, 1983

GREENBERG DA: Calcium channel antagonists and the treatment of migraine. Clin Neuropharmacol 9:311, 1986

HOCKADAY JM: Basilar migraine in children. Dev Med Child Neurol 21:455, 1979

JOHNS D: Benign sexual headache within a family. Arch Neurol 43:1158, 1986

KAYAN A, HOOD JD: Neuro-otological manifestations of migraine. Brain 107:1123, 1984

LAKE A et al: Biofeedback and rational-emotive therapy in the management of migraine headache. Appl Behav Anal 12:127, 1979

LANCE JW: Headache. Ann Neurol 10:1, 1981

———: Headaches related to sexual activity. J Neurol Neurosurg Psychiat 39:1226, 1976

LAURITZEN M, HANSEN AJ: Spreading depression of Leão. Possible relation to migraine pathophysiology, in *Basic Mechanisms of Headache*, vol 2: *Pain Research and Clinical Management*, J Olesen, L Edvinsson (eds). Amsterdam, Elsevier, 1988, p 439

———, OLESEN J: Regional cerebral blood flow during migraine attacks by xenon-133 inhalation and emission tomography. Brain 107:447, 1984

MEYER JS, HARDENBERG J: Clinical effectiveness of calcium entry blockers in prophylactic treatment of migraine and cluster headaches. Headache 23:266, 1983

MOSKOWITZ M: Neurobiology of vascular head pain. Ann Neurol 16:157, 1984

OLESEN J: Pathophysiological implications of migraine and symptomatology, in *Basic Mechanisms of Headache*, vol 2: *Pain Research and Clinical Management*, J Olesen, L Edvinsson (eds). Amsterdam, Elsevier, 1988, p 353

———, EDVINSSON L (eds): *Basic Mechanisms of Headache*, vol 2: *Pain Research and Clinical Management*. Amsterdam, Elsevier, 1988

PEROUTKA J: The pharmacology of calcium channel antagonists. Novel class of anti-migraine agents? Headache 23:278, 1983

RASKIN NH: Migraine, in *Diseases of the Nervous System*, AK Asbury, GM McKhann, WI McDonald (eds). Philadelphia, Saunders, 1986, p 961

SPIERINGS EL: Clinical and experimental evidence for a role of calcium entry blockers in the treatment of migraine. Ann NY Acad Sci 522:676, 1988

VIJAYAN N, DREYFUS PM: Posttraumatic dysautonomic cephalalgia: Clinical observations and treatment. Arch Neurol 32:649, 1976

VINKEN PJ, BRUYN GW (eds): *Handbook of Clinical Neurology*, vol 5: *Headache and Cranial Neuralgias*. Amsterdam, North-Holland, 1968

19   BACK AND NECK PAIN

HENRY J. MANKIN*

ANATOMY AND PHYSIOLOGY OF THE LOWER PART OF THE BACK

The bony spine is a complex structure, anatomically divisible into two parts. The anterior part consists of a series of cylindrical vertebral bodies connected to one another by the intervertebral disks and held together by the anterior and posterior longitudinal ligaments. The posterior part consists of more delicate elements that extend from the vertebral body as pedicles and broaden posteriorly to form laminae, which together with ligamentous structures form the vertebral canal. The posterior elements are joined to adjacent vertebrae by two small facetal synovial joints which allow a modest degree of motion between any two segments, but in aggregate produce a rather extensive range (Fig. 19-1). Stout transverse and spinous bony processes project laterally and posteriorly and serve as the attachments of muscles which move, support, and protect the vertebral column. The stability of the spine depends on two types of support: that provided by the bony articulations (principally by the diskal joints and the synovial articulations of the posterior elements) and a second type provided by the ligamentous (passive) and muscular (active) supporting structures. The ligamentous structures are quite strong, but because neither they nor the vertebral body–disk complexes have sufficient integral strength to resist the enormous forces acting on the column during even simple movements, voluntary and reflex contractions of the sacrospinalis, abdominal, gluteal, psoas, and hamstring muscles afford much of the stability.

The vertebral and paravertebral structures derive their innervation from the recurrent branches of the spinal nerves. Pain endings and fibers have been demonstrated in the ligaments, muscles, periosteum of bone, outer layers of annulus fibrosus, and synovium of the articular facets. The sensory fibers from these structures and the sacroiliac and lumbosacral joints join to form the sinovertebral nerves which pass via the recurrent branches of the spinal nerves of the first sacral and the fifth to first lumbar vertebrae into the gray matter of the corresponding segments of the spinal cord. Efferent fibers emerge from these segments and extend to the muscles through the same nerves.

The parts of the back that possess the greatest freedom of movement, and hence are most frequently subject to injury, are the lumbar and cervical regions. In addition to the voluntary motions required for bending, twisting, and other movements, many actions of the spine are reflex in nature and are the basis of posture.

GENERAL CLINICAL CONSIDERATIONS

TYPES OF LOW BACK PAIN   Four types of pain may be differentiated: local, referred, radicular, and that arising from secondary (protective) muscular spasm.

Local pain is caused by any pathologic process that impinges upon or irritates sensory endings. Involvement of structures which contain no sensory endings is painless. The central, medullary portion of the vertebral body may be destroyed by tumor, for example, without evocation of pain, whereas cortical fractures, or tears and distortions of the periosteum, synovial membranes, muscles, annulus fibrosus, and ligaments are often exquisitely painful. The latter structures are innervated by afferent fibers of the posterior primary rami. Although painful states are often accompanied by swelling of the affected tissues, this may not be apparent if a deep structure of

FIGURE 19-1   *Left:* Superior view of a stripped lumbar vertebra. *Right:* Lateral view of two articulated lumbar vertebrae. B = body; SC = spinal canal; IVF = intervertebral foramen; IF = inferior articular facet; SF = superior articular facet; P = pedicle; TP = transverse process; SP = spinous process; L = lamina. *(Adapted from DB Levine, in Arthritis and Allied Conditions: A Textbook of Rheumatology, 10th ed, DJ McCarty (ed), Philadelphia, Lea & Febiger, 1985.)*

the back is the site of disease. Local pain is often described as steady but may be intermittent, varying considerably with position or activity. The pain may be sharp or dull and although often diffuse is always felt in or near the affected part of the spine. Reflex splinting of the spine segments by paravertebral muscles is frequently noted, and certain movements or postures that alter the position of the injured tissues aggravate the pain. Firm pressure or percussion upon superficial structures in the region involved usually evokes tenderness, which is of aid in identifying the site of the abnormality.

Referred pain is of two types: that projected from the spine into regions lying within the area of the lumbar and upper sacral dermatomes and that projected from the pelvic and abdominal viscera to the spine. Pain due to diseases of the upper part of the lumbar spine is usually referred to the anterior aspects of the thighs and legs; that from the lower lumbar and sacral segments is referred to the gluteal regions, posterior thighs, calves, and sometimes feet. Pain of this type, although of deep, aching quality and rather diffuse, tends at times to be superficially projected. In general the referred pain parallels in intensity the local pain in the back. In other words, maneuvers that alter local pain have a similar effect on referred pain, though not with such precision and immediacy as in radicular, or "root," pain. Referred pain may be confused with pain from visceral disease, but the latter is usually described as "deep" and tends to radiate from the abdomen through to the back. Also, visceral pain is usually unaffected by movement of the spine, does not improve with recumbency, and may be modified by the activity of the involved viscus.

Radicular, or "root," *pain* has some of the characteristics of referred pain but differs in its greater intensity, distal radiation, circumscription to the territory of a root, and the factors which excite it. The mechanisms are principally distortion, stretching, irritation, and compression of a spinal root, most often central to the intervertebral foramen. In addition, it has been suggested that in patients with spinal stenosis the "lumbar claudication" pattern may be due to a relative ischemia associated with compression. Although the pain itself is often dull or aching, various maneuvers which increase the irritation of the root or stretch it may greatly intensify the pain, eliciting a lancinating quality. Nearly always the radiation of pain is from a central position near the spine to some part of the lower extremity. Cough, sneeze, and strain are characteristically evocative maneuvers; but since they may also jar or move the spine, they may aggravate local pain as well. Forward bending with the knees extended or "straight-leg raising" in disease of the lower part of the lumbar spine excites radicular pain on the basis of stretch; jugular vein compression, which raises intraspinal pressure and may cause a shift in the position of or pressure on the root, may have a similar effect. Irritation of the fourth and fifth lumbar and first sacral roots, which form the sciatic nerve, causes pain that extends mainly down the posterior aspects of the thigh, the postero- and anterolateral aspects of the leg, and into the foot—termed sciatica. Tingling, paresthesias,

* The author wishes to acknowledge the contribution of Raymond D. Adams to this chapter, which is a revision of their joint chapter in the eleventh edition.

and numbness or sensory impairment of the skin, soreness of the skin, and tenderness along the nerve usually accompany classic sciatic pain, and on physical examination, reflex loss, weakness, atrophy, fascicular twitching, and occasionally stasis edema may occur if the motor fibers of the anterior root are involved.

Pain resulting from muscular spasm is usually mentioned in relation to local pain, but the anatomic or physiologic basis is more obscure. Muscle spasm associated with many disorders of the spine can produce significant distortions of the normal posture; as a result, chronic tension in muscles may give rise to a dull and sometimes cramping ache. In this instance one can feel the tautness of the sacrospinalis and gluteal muscles and demonstrate by palpation that the pain is localized to these structures.

Other pains often of undetermined origin are sometimes described by patients with chronic disease of the lower part of the back. Unilateral symptoms of drawing, pulling, cramping sensations (without involuntary muscle spasm), tearing, throbbing, or jabbing pains, or feelings of burning or coldness are difficult to interpret but, like paresthesias and numbness, should always suggest the possibility of nerve or root disease.

In addition to assessing the character and location of the pain, one should determine the factors that aggravate and relieve it, its constancy, and its relationship to recumbency and such stereotypical movements and maneuvers as forward bending, cough, sneeze, and strain. Frequently the most important lead comes from the knowledge of the mode of onset and circumstances that initiated the pain. Inasmuch as many painful afflictions of the back are the result of injury incurred during work or in an accident, the possibility of exaggeration or prolongation of pain for purposes of compensation or other personal reasons, or because of hysteria or malingering, must always be kept in mind.

EXAMINATION OF THE LOWER PART OF THE BACK

Inspection of the normal spine shows a dorsal kyphosis and lumbar lordosis in the sagittal plane, which in some individuals may be exaggerated (swayback). In patients with spinal disorders, one should seek excessive curvature, flattening of the normal lumbar arch, presence of a gibbus (a short, sharp, kyphotic angulation usually indicative of a fracture or congenital abnormality), lateral curvature and/or rotation (scoliosis), pelvic tilt or obliquity, or asymmetry of the paravertebral or gluteal musculature. In severe sciatica, one may observe that the affected limb is held with the hip and knee flexed, presumably to reduce tension on the irritated part.

The spine, hips, and legs should be observed during certain motions, but no advantage accrues from trying to find out how much pain the patient can endure. It is more important to assess when and under what conditions the pain commences. Normally, the motion of forward bending produces flattening and reversal of the lumbar lordotic curve and exaggeration of the dorsal curve. With ruptured lumbar disks or lesions that involve the posterior ligaments, articular facets, or sacrospinalis muscle, protective reflexes prevent stretching of these structures; as a consequence, the sacrospinalis muscles remain taut and limit motion in the lumbar part of the spine, causing forward bending to occur at the hips and at the lumbar-thoracic junction. With disease principally affecting the spinal roots or the lumbosacral joints, forward bending occurs in such a way as to avoid tensing the hamstring muscles, which puts undue leverage upon the pelvis. In unilateral "sciatica," with its increased curvature toward the side of the lesion, the lumbar and lumbosacral motions are splinted, and bending is mainly at the hips; at a certain point the knee on the affected side is flexed to relieve hamstring spasm, and tilting of the pelvis occurs to slacken the lumbosacral roots and sciatic nerve.

With lumbosacral lesions and sciatica, passive lumbar flexion in the supine position causes little pain and is not limited as long as the hamstrings are relaxed and the sciatic nerve is not stretched. With lumbosacral and lumbar spine disease (e.g., arthritis), passive flexion of the hips is free, whereas flexion of the lumbar spine may be impeded and painful. Passive straight-leg raising (possible in most normal individuals up to 80 to 90° except in those who have unusually tight hamstrings), like forward bending with the knees extended in the standing posture, places the sciatic nerve and its roots under tension, thereby producing pain. It may also cause an anterior rotation of the pelvis around a transverse axis, increasing stress on the lumbosacral joint, and thus causing pain if this segment is arthritic or otherwise impaired. Consequently, in diseases of the lumbosacral joints and lumbosacral roots, this movement is limited on the affected side and to a lesser extent on the opposite side. Evocation of such a response (pain and limitation of movement during flexion of the hip when the knee is extended) is known as Lasègue's sign and is considered to be a useful test of this condition. A positive contralateral straight-leg raising sign is believed by some to be a sign of a more extensive lesion, such as an extruded disk fragment, rather than a simple prolapse or protrusion. It is important to remember, however, that the evoked pain is always referred to the diseased side, no matter which leg is flexed.

Hyperextension is best evaluated with the patient standing or lying prone. If the condition causing back pain is acute, it may be difficult to extend the spine in the standing position. A patient with lumbosacral strain or disk disease can usually extend or hyperextend the spine without aggravation of pain. If the lesion is in the upper lumbar segments or if an active inflammatory process, fracture of the vertebral body, or a very tight canal (vertebral stenosis) is present, hyperextension may be markedly limited.

Palpation and percussion of the spine are the last steps in the examination. It is preferable to palpate first those regions which are the least likely to evoke pain. At all times the examiner should know what structures are being palpated (see Fig. 19-2). Localized tenderness is seldom pronounced in disease of the spine because the involved structures are so deep that they rarely give rise to surface tenderness.

FIGURE 19-2 (1) Costovertebral angle. (2) Spinous process and interspinous ligament. (3) Region of the articular fifth lumbar to the first sacral facet (4) Dorsum of sacrum. (5) Region of iliac crest. (6) Iliolumbar angle. (7) Spinous processes of fifth lumbar to first sacral vertebrae (tenderness = faulty posture or occasionally spina bifida occulta). (8) Region between posterior superior and posterior inferior spines. Sacroiliac ligaments (tenderness = sacroiliac sprain, often tender with fifth lumbar to first sacral disk). (9) Sacrococcygeal junction (tenderness = sacrococcygeal injury, i.e., sprain or fracture). (10) Region of sacrosciatic notch (tenderness = fourth to fifth lumbar disk rupture and sacroiliac sprain). (11) Sciatic nerve trunk (tenderness = ruptured lumbar disk or sciatic nerve lesion).

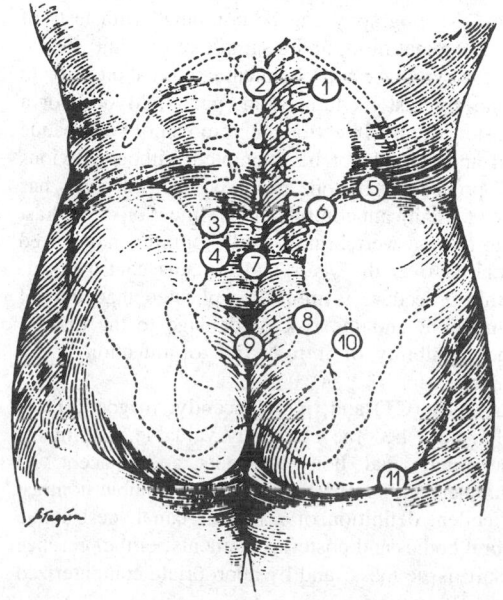

Mild superficial and poorly localized tenderness signifies only a disease process within the affected segment of the body, i.e., dermatome.

Tenderness over the costovertebral angle often indicates renal disease, adrenal disease, or an injury to the transverse processes of the first or second lumbar vertebra. Hypersensitivity on palpation of the transverse processes of the other lumbar vertebrae as well as the overlying sacrospinalis muscles may signify fracture of the transverse process or a strain of muscle attachments. Tenderness of a spinous process or aggravation of pain by the jarring of gentle percussion may be nonspecific but frequently indicates the presence of a disk lesion at the site deep to it, inflammation (as in disk space infection), or fracture. Tenderness in the region of the articular facets between the fifth lumbar and first sacral vertebrae is consistent with disease of a lumbosacral disk [Fig. 19-2 (3)]. It is also frequent in rheumatoid arthritis.

In palpation of the spinous processes, it is important to note any deviation in the lateral plane (this may be indicative of fracture or arthritis) or in the anteroposterior plane. A "step-off" forward displacement of the spinous process may be an important clue to the presence of a spondylolisthesis one segment below the displaced level.

Abdominal, rectal, and pelvic examination and assessment of the status of the peripheral vascular system are important parts of the examination of the patient with complaints in the lower back and should not be omitted. They may provide evidence for vascular, visceral, neoplastic, or inflammatory disorders which may extend to the spine or cause pain to be referred to this region. Finally, a careful neurologic examination should be performed, with special attention given to motor, reflex, and sensory changes, particularly in the lower extremities (see "Protrusion of Lumbar Intervertebral Disks," below).

SPECIAL LABORATORY PROCEDURES   Useful laboratory tests, depending on the nature of the problem and the circumstances, include a complete blood count, erythrocyte sedimentation rate (especially helpful in screening for infection or myeloma), measurement of serum calcium, phosphorus, alkaline phosphatase, acid phosphatase (the last mentioned is of importance if one suspects metastatic carcinoma from the prostate), immunoglobulin electrophoresis, and tests for rheumatoid factor. Roentgenograms of the lumbar part of the spine in the anteroposterior, lateral, and oblique planes should be obtained in every patient with low back pain and sciatica. Special spot views or stereoscopic or laminographic films may provide further information in certain cases. Bone scans are of particular aid in revealing some fractures and neoplastic and inflammatory lesions.

Examination of the spinal canal with a contrast medium is often of value, especially if a spinal cord tumor is suspected or if a patient is thought to have a disk herniation and fails to improve on a conservative regimen. Myelography can be combined with tests of dynamics of the cerebrospinal fluid, and a sample of the fluid should always be removed for cytologic and chemical examination prior to the instillation of the contrast medium (Pantopaque, Myodil, or a water-soluble contrast medium). Injection and removal of Pantopaque require special skill and should not be attempted without previous experience with the procedure. If done properly, the procedure has a very low incidence of significant complications. Injection of contrast medium directly into the intervertebral disk (diskograms) has waxed and waned in popularity over the years and remains controversial. The technique of this procedure is more complicated than that of myelographic examination, and the risk of damage to the disk or nerve roots and the possibility of introduction of infection is not inconsiderable.

Computed tomography (CT) and, more recently, magnetic resonance imaging (MRI) have become extremely valuable instruments for the study of the spinal canal, bony segments, and adjacent soft tissues. CT, if combined with instillation of water-soluble contrast media, provides excellent definition of a narrow canal, destructive lesions of the vertebral bodies and posterior elements, or the presence of a paravertebral soft tissue mass, and by appropriate computerized reconstruction techniques can also identify disk herniations, sometimes with greater accuracy than the myelogram. The MRI has in recent years virtually replaced CT for the study of the degenerate disk and its relationship to the adjacent roots. The definition of soft tissue alterations and even edema surrounding the roots is remarkable, especially with sagittal projections. The use of gadolinium to enhance regions of inflammation with MRI provides even better resolution of the defects (see Chap. 348).

Confirmation of proximal motor and sensory nerve and root disease can be obtained by nerve conduction studies, H and F responses, and electromyography (see Chap. 362).

PRINCIPAL CONDITIONS THAT GIVE RISE TO DISABLING PAIN IN THE LOWER PART OF THE BACK

CONGENITAL ANOMALIES OF THE LUMBAR SPINE   One of the most common disorders is a failure of fusion of the laminae of the neural arch (spina bifida) of one or several of the lumbar vertebrae or of the sacrum. Hypertrichosis or hyperpigmentation in the sacral area may betray the condition, but in most patients the spine defect remains entirely occult until disclosed by x-ray. The anomaly has greater potentiality for pain if accompanied by malformation of vertebral joints, and usually the pain is induced by injury. Other congenital anomalies that affect the lower lumbar vertebrae, such as asymmetric facetal joints, abnormalities of the transverse processes, sacralization of the fifth lumbar vertebra (in which L5 is firmly fixed to the sacrum), or lumbarization of the first sacral vertebra (in which the first sacral segment resembles a sixth lumbar), are rarely the cause of specific symptomatology.

Spondylolysis consists of a bony defect probably caused by trauma to a congenitally abnormal segment in the pars interarticularis (a segment near the junction of the pedicle with the lamina) of the lower lumbar area. The defect is best visualized on oblique projections or with CT. In some individuals the defect is bilateral. In the circumstance of either a single injury or repeated minor injuries, the vertebral body, pedicles, and superior articular facets slip anteriorly, leaving the posterior elements behind. This latter abnormality, known as *spondylolisthesis*, usually results in symptoms, often proportional to the degree of forward slip. The patient may complain of pain in the low back that radiating into the thighs, and a limitation of motion may be noted. Often tenderness is elicited near the segment which has "slipped" forward (most often L5 on S1 or occasionally L4 on L5), and one can feel a "step" on deep palpation of the posterior elements of the segment above the spondylolisthetic joint. In moderately severe displacements the pelvis is sometimes rotated and hip flexion limited by hamstring spasm. A variety of usually minor neurologic deficits indicative of radiculopathy may be present. In exceptionally severe degrees of spondylolisthesis the trunk may be shortened and the abdomen protuberant, both the result of the extreme forward displacement of L5 on S1.

TRAUMATIC AFFLICTIONS OF THE LOWER PART OF THE BACK Trauma constitutes the most frequent cause of acute low back pain, and such injured patients should be very carefully evaluated. In severe acute injuries which involve fracture or dislocation of the vertebral segments, the examining physician must be careful to avoid further damage. Tests of mobility and forceful manipulations should be avoided until a diagnosis has been made and adequate measures have been instituted for the proper care of the patient. A patient complaining of back pain and inability to move the legs may have a fractured spine. The neck should not be flexed, nor should the patient be allowed to sit up. (See Chap. 361 for further discussion of spinal cord injury.)

Sprains, strains, and derangements The terms lumbosacral *sprain* and *strain* are often used loosely by physicians, and do not clearly relate to a known anatomic lesion. The author prefers the term *low back derangement* or *strain* for minor, self-limited injuries usually associated with lifting a heavy object, a fall, or a sudden deceleration as may occur in an automobile accident. Occasionally, these syndromes are more chronic in nature, suggesting that diskal or arthritic factors may play a role. The patients with low back derangement are often acutely discomfited and may assume unusual postures related to spasm of the sacrospinalis muscles. The pain is usually confined to the lower back and is usually relieved by rest and analgesic medication within a few days. More extensive or longer lasting problems, formerly classified as sacroiliac strain or sprain, are now known to be due in most instances to disk disease (see below).

Vertebral fractures   Most fractures of the lumbar vertebral body result from flexion injuries and consist of anterior wedging or compression. With more severe trauma the patient may sustain a fracture dislocation, "bursting" fracture, or asymmetric fracture involving not only the body but the posterior elements. The initiating trauma which causes fractures of the vertebrae is usually a fall from a height (in which case the calcanei may also be fractured), sudden deceleration in an automobile accident, or other major violence. When fractures occur with minimal trauma (or even spontaneously), the bone is presumed to have been previously weakened by some pathologic process. Most of the time, particularly in older individuals, the cause of such an event is senile or postmenopausal osteoporosis (see Chap. 341), but there may be other underlying systemic disorders such as osteomalacia, hyperparathyroidism, hyperthyroidism, multiple myeloma, metastatic carcinoma, and a large number of local conditions that may play a role in weakening the vertebral body. Spasm of the lumbar muscles, limitation of motion of the lumbar segments, and the roentgenographic appearance of the damaged vertebra (with or without neurologic abnormalities) are the basis for the clinical diagnosis. The pain is usually immediate, though occasionally it may be delayed in onset for a few days, and the patient may develop a mild paralytic ileus or urinary retention during the acute period.

Fractures of the transverse processes are almost always associated with severe injury to the paravertebral muscles, principally the psoas. A significant retroperitoneal hemorrhage may be present (identified on CT or MRI) which can result in a marked depression in the hematocrit and, in extensive fractures, hypovolemic shock. Such injuries may be diagnosed by the finding of deep tenderness at the site of the injury, local muscle spasm on one side, and limitation of all movements which stretch the lumbar muscles. Radiologic evidence (especially CT or MRI) provides the final confirmation. Fractures of multiple transverse processes, although seemingly trivial, should be the object of considerable concern, and the patient should be carefully watched for internal hemorrhage.

Protrusion of lumbar intervertebral disks   This condition is the major cause of severe chronic or recurrent low back and leg pain. It is most likely to occur between the fifth lumbar and first sacral vertebrae, and, with lessening frequency, between the fourth and fifth lumbar, the third and fourth lumbar, the second and third lumbar, and, rarely, between the first and second lumbar vertebrae. Rare in the thoracic portion of the spine, it is next most frequent between the sixth and seventh and fifth and sixth cervical vertebrae. The cause is usually a flexion injury, but in many cases no trauma is recalled. Degeneration of the posterior longitudinal ligaments and the annulus fibrosus, which occurs in most adults of middle and advanced years, may have taken place silently or have been manifested by mild, recurrent lumbar ache. A sneeze, lurch, or other trivial movement may then cause the nucleus pulposus to prolapse, pushing the frayed and weakened annulus posteriorly. In more severe cases of disk disease, the nucleus may protrude through the annulus or become extruded to lie as a free fragment in the vertebral canal.

The fully developed syndrome of ruptured lumbar intervertebral disk consists of backache, abnormal posture, and limitation of motion of the spine (particularly flexion). Nerve root involvement is indicated by radicular pain, sensory disturbances (paresthesias, hyper- and hyposensitivity in dermatome pattern), coarse twitching and fasciculation, muscle spasms, and impairment of a tendon reflex. Motor

abnormalities (weakness and muscle atrophy) may also occur but are usually less prominent than the pain and sensory disorder. Since herniation of the intervertebral lumbar disks most often occurs between the fourth and fifth lumbar vertebrae and the fifth lumbar and first sacral vertebrae with irritation and compression of the fifth lumbar and first sacral roots, respectively, it is important to recognize the clinical characteristics of lesions of these two roots. *Lesions of the fifth lumbar root* produce pain in the region of the hip, groin, posterolateral thigh, lateral calf to the external malleolus, dorsal surface of the foot, and the first or second and third toes. Paresthesias may be in the entire territory or only in the distal parts of these territories. The tenderness is in the lateral gluteal region and near the head of the fibula. Weakness, if present, involves the extensor of the great toe and less often of the foot. The knee and ankle reflexes are seldom altered, although occasionally the ankle jerk is moderately depressed. Walking on the heels may be more difficult, because of weakness of dorsiflexion of the foot, and more uncomfortable than walking on the toes. In *lesions of the first sacral root* the pain is felt in the midgluteal region, posterior part of the thigh, posterior region of the calf to the heel, and the plantar surface of the foot and fourth and fifth toes. Tenderness is most pronounced over the midgluteal region (sacroiliac joint), posterior thigh area, and calf. Rarely it may be referred to the rectum, testicles, or labia. Paresthesias and sensory loss are mainly in the lower leg and outer toes, and weakness, if present, involves the flexor muscles of the foot and toes, abductors of the toes, and hamstring muscles. The ankle reflex is diminished or absent in the majority of cases. Walking on the toes is more difficult, because of weakness of plantar flexors, and more uncomfortable than walking on the heel. With lesions of either root there may be limitation of straight-leg raising during the acute, painful stages.

Degeneration of the intervertebral disk without frank extrusion of a fragment of disk tissue may give rise to low back pain, or the disk may herniate into the adjacent vertebral body, giving rise to a Schmorl's node, usually visualized by x-ray. Such cases often show no signs of nerve root involvement though the back pain may be referred to the thigh and leg.

The rarer *lesions of the fourth and third lumbar roots* give rise to pain in the anterior part of the thigh and knee, with corresponding sensory loss. The knee jerk is diminished or abolished. An inverted Lasègue sign (pain with hypertension of the limb in relation to the trunk, best elicited with the patient in the prone position) is often positive when the third lumbar root is affected.

The lumbar disk syndromes are usually unilateral. Occasionally with massive derangements of the disk or with the extrusion of a large, free fragment into the canal the symptoms and signs are bilateral. Often one side is affected more than the other and the pain, motor, and sensory changes may be associated with paralysis of the sphincters. The pain of lumbar disk disease is variable and may be mild or severe. There may be back pain with little or no leg pain, and occasionally the patient experiences leg pain with little or no discomfort in the back. Some patients present with evidence of multiple disk ruptures affecting both cervical and lumbar segments, suggesting a diffuse disorder of the connective tissue of the disks, possibly including both the annulus fibrosus and the nucleus pulposus.

When all components of the syndrome are present, the diagnosis is easy; when only one part is present (particularly backache), it may be difficult, especially if there has not been a clearly remembered initiating traumatic event. Since similar symptoms may occur without demonstrable disk rupture, other diagnostic procedures are required. Plain roentgenograms usually show no abnormality or at most a narrowing of the intervertebral space, sometimes more on the side of the rupture. Traction spurs, which are indicative of disk degeneration, may be present; in extreme cases, there may be a "vacuum" disk sign, in which a gas-density shadow is present in the intervertebral space, usually on lateral roentgenogram. CT transverse images with or without contrast sometimes show the herniated disk very clearly, and at times the MRI will demonstrate a remarkably sharp image of cauda equina or nerve root compression by a bulging or extruded disk fragment. Less frequently than in the past do clinicians resort to Pantopaque or soluble contrast myelography (both of which have potential complications) to demonstrate the disk herniation. The myelogram remains the most reliable of the studies, and many surgeons are loathe to consider laminectomy without such a study. Occasionally, the electromyogram is helpful in showing denervation of paravertebral and leg muscles (see Chap. 362).

It should be noted in evaluating patients with herniated disks that epidural or intradural tumors of the spinal canal may produce a syndrome similar to that of ruptured disk. These lesions may present with unremitting pain even with bed rest and predominant sphincter disturbances even early in the course (see Chap. 361).

OTHER CAUSES OF LOW BACK PAIN AND SCIATICA   In a sizable number of patients disk rupture types of symptoms occur, but the problem has a different cause. Often these patients have had multiple operations for diskogenic disease with or without arthrodesis of the lumbar vertebrae, but the pain and disability have not remitted. The indications for the original surgery may have been questionable, with only a disk bulge noted on CT, MRI, or myelogram and no definite neurologic signs. To explain these chronic pain states a number of pathologic entities have been introduced, some of uncertain status. Entrapment of one or more nerve roots may be the consequence not only of a disk rupture but also as a result of spondylotic spurs with variable stenosis of the lateral recess and intervertebral canal, hypertrophy of apophyseal facets, or a more nebulous cause.

The syndrome that is caused by spondylotic spurs and stenosis of the lateral recess and intervertebral foramen has not been clearly distinguished from that of ruptured disk. Known variously as vertebral stenosis, lumbar claudication, degenerative spinal stenosis, and narrow canal, the cause appears to be related principally to an encroachment on roots of the cauda equina by bony excrescences usually attributed to osteoarthritis but possibly related to spondylolisthesis, old trauma, Paget's disease, or a congenital abnormality of the shape or size of the canal. Many of these patients are elderly, and the pattern must be clearly distinguished from peripheral vascular claudication. The pain, often bilateral along the sciatic distribution, becomes increasingly severe with standing and walking and is relieved by a short period of rest. Although some of the patients have no physical findings, motor, reflex, and sensory changes may be present.

The *facet syndrome* is closely related to the above but tends to be unilateral. Reynolds et al. have reported 22 cases in which a lumbar monoradiculopathy had simulated a ruptured disk: 16 had an L5 radiculopathy, 3 an S1 radiculopathy, and 3 an L4 radiculopathy. Coexisting back pain was present in 15 of the cases. No disk rupture was found by myelography. At operation the spinal root was compressed against the floor or roof of the intervertebral canal by an enlarged superior or inferior facet. Foraminotomy and facetectomy relieved the symptoms in 12 of the 15 operated cases.

Lumbar adhesive arachnoiditis with radiculopathy has waxed and waned over the years as an entity employed to explain low back pain persisting after treatment. Most often it is considered in patients who have had multiple lumbar operations and myelograms and are left with backache and leg pain in combination with mild to moderate motor, sensory, and reflex changes. On surgical exploration, the arachnoidal membrane is thickened and opaque, adherent to dura, and tightly bound to pia and roots. The contrast medium during myelography does not fill the root sheaths and tends to be irregularly loculated. Disk rupture, multiple Pantopaque myelograms, operative procedures, infection, and subarachnoid hemorrhage, in various combinations, are factors that favor its development. Treatment is unsatisfactory; lysis of adhesions and intrathecal steroid therapy have been of only limited value.

In patients with persistent chronic low back pain and sciatica after failed disk surgery or due to spondylitic spurs, spondylolysis, facetal joint degeneration, or arachnoiditis, some surgeons have attributed the disability in part, at least, to "instability" of the lumbar segments, and the perpetuation of the pain to excessive or abnormal movements

of the lumbar vertebral segments. For such patients spinal fusion is occasionally advocated and can in certain circumstances provide a measure of relief. A posterior arthrodesis of the fourth and fifth lumbar segments to the sacrum may reduce motion at these parts and decrease pressure on the nerve roots associated with abnormal movements. More often than not, however, the patient continues to have pain (although often reduced in degree), and the procedure should not be regarded as a panacea. The author rarely advocates such an operative intervention, unless clear anatomic evidence exists for a mechanical problem that could be alleviated by stabilization of the spine.

ARTHRITIS   Arthritis of the spine is a major cause of backache, cervical pain, and occipital headache.

Osteoarthritis (See also Chap. 281)   This more frequent type of osteoarthritic spinal disease occurs usually in later life and may involve any part of the spine. It is most prevalent in the cervical and lumbar regions, however, and the exact location determines the localization of the symptoms. Patients often complain of pain centered in the spine that is increased by motion and is almost invariably associated with complaints of stiffness and limitation of motion. There is a notable absence of systemic symptoms such as fatigue, malaise, and fever, and the pain usually can be relieved by rest. The severity of the symptoms often bears little relation to the radiologic findings; pain may be present when there are minimal findings on an x-ray, and, conversely, marked osteophytic overgrowth with spur formation, ridging, and bridging of vertebrae can be seen in asymptomatic patients in middle and later life. Osteoarthropathic changes in the cervical spine and to a lesser extent in the lumbar spine may by their location compress roots or even the cauda equina or spinal cord, giving rise to the spondylitic form of radiculopathy or myelopathy (see Chap. 361).

Rheumatoid arthritis and ankylosing spondylitis (See also Chaps. 270 and 274)   Arthritic disease of the spine takes two distinct forms, ankylosing spondylitis (the more common) and rheumatoid arthritis.

Patients with *ankylosing spondylitis* (also called Marie-Strümpell arthritis) are usually young men who complain of mild to moderate pain which early in the course of the disease is centered in the back and on occasion radiates to the back of the thighs. The symptoms may be vague at first and the diagnosis may be overlooked for a considerable period. Although the pain is often intermittent, the finding of limitation of movement is constant and progressive and over a period of time tends to dominate the picture. Early in the course, this finding is described as "morning stiffness" or increasing stiffness after periods of inactivity, and may be present long before radiologic changes are manifest. Limitation of chest expansion, tenderness over the sternum, and decreased motion and flexion contractures of the hips may also be present early in the course. The radiologic hallmarks of the disease are periarticular destructive changes and subsequent obliteration of the sacroiliac joints, development of syndesmophytes on the margins of the vertebral bodies, followed by bridging by bone to produce the characteristic "bamboo spine." The entire spine becomes immobilized, often in a flexed position, and usually the pain then subsides. Patterns of restricted movement, indistinguishable from those of ankylosing spondylitis, may accompany Reiter's syndrome, psoriatic arthritis, and chronic inflammatory bowel diseases. Patients with these disorders rarely show the joint manifestations of peripheral rheumatoid arthritis, and seldom do they display involvement of the hips or knees. The rheumatoid factor is usually absent, but the sedimentation rate is often rapid, and many of the patients are found to have an HLA-B27 antigen.

Occasionally ankylosing spondylitis is complicated by progressively destructive vertebral lesions. This complication should be suspected whenever the pain returns, after a period of quiescence, or becomes localized. The etiology of these lesions is not known, but they may represent an exaggerated healing response to fracture or excessive production of fibrous inflammatory tissues. Rarely they may result in collapse of a segment of the spine and compression of the spinal cord. Another complication of severe ankylosing spondylitis is bilateral ankylosis of the ribs to the spine, which, coupled with a decrease in the height of axial thoracic structures, causes marked impairment of respiratory function.

Spinal rheumatoid arthritis tends to be localized to the cervical apophyseal joints and atlantoaxial articulation; the pain, stiffness, and limitation of motion are then in the neck and back of the head. Unlike ankylosing spondylitis, rheumatoid arthritis is rarely confined to the spine, and it does not lead to significant degrees of intervertebral bridging. Because of major affection of other joints, the diagnosis is relatively easy to make, but significant involvement of the neck may be overlooked. In the advanced stages of the disease, one or several of the vertebrae may be displaced anteriorly, or a synovitis of the atlantoaxial joint may damage the transverse ligament of the atlas, resulting in forward displacement of the atlas on the axis, i.e., atlantoaxial subluxation. In either instance, serious and even life-threatening compression of the spinal cord may occur gradually or suddenly (see Chaps. 270 and 361). Lateral roentgenograms in flexion and extension, performed cautiously, are sometimes necessary to visualize dislocation or subluxation.

OTHER DESTRUCTIVE DISEASES Neoplastic, infectious, and metabolic diseases Metastatic carcinoma (breast, lung, prostate, thyroid, kidney, gastrointestinal tract), multiple myeloma, and non-Hodgkin's and Hodgkin's lymphomas are the malignant tumors which most frequently involve the spine. Since the primary site may be overlooked or asymptomatic, the presenting complaint in such patients may be pain in the back. The pain tends to be constant and dull, and is often unrelieved by rest. Indeed, it may be worse at night. Radiographic changes may be absent early in the disease, but when they appear, usually are manifest as destructive lesions in one or several vertebral bodies with little or limited involvement of the disk space, even in the face of a compression fracture. A ^{99m}Tc diphosphonate bone scan is helpful in demonstrating "hot spots," indicating areas of increased blood flow and reactive bone formation associated with destructive, inflammatory, or arthritic lesions. It should be noted, however, that myeloma and sometimes metastatic thyroid carcinoma may fail to show increased activity on a bone scan.

Infection of the vertebral column is usually the result of pyogenic organisms (staphylococci or coliform bacilli) or, less commonly today, the tubercle bacilli. Patients complain of pain in the back of subacute or chronic nature that is exacerbated by motion but not materially relieved by rest. There is limitation of motion, tenderness over the spine of the involved segments, and pain with jarring of the spine, such as occurs with walking on the heels. Usually, these patients are afebrile and often do not have a leukocytosis although the erythrocyte sedimentation rate is almost invariably elevated. Radiographs may demonstrate narrowing of a disk space with erosion and destruction of the two adjacent vertebrae. A paravertebral soft tissue mass evident on contrast CT or MRI may be present, indicating an abscess, which may in the case of tuberculosis drain spontaneously at sites quite remote from the vertebral column. In addition to a bone scan, a gallium scan is sometimes helpful in identifying a soft tissue inflammatory or infectious lesion even when overt bone destruction is not visible in x-rays.

Special mention should be made of the spinal *epidural abscess* (usually staphylococcal), which necessitates urgent surgical treatment. The symptoms are a localized pain, occurring spontaneously, aggravated by percussion and palpation. The patient is febrile and usually has severe radicular complaints, often bilateral, progressing rapidly to a flaccid paraplegia (see Chap. 348). Chronic drug abusers are particularly prone to this problem. Patients with AIDS have also been noted to have increased incidence of epidural abscess and of pyogenic and granulomatous osteomyelitis.

In metabolic bone diseases (hyperparathyroidism, osteoporosis, or osteomalacia) a considerable degree of loss of bone substance may occur without any symptoms whatsoever. Many patients with such conditions do, however, complain of aching in the lumbar or thoracic area. This is most likely to occur following an injury, sometimes trivial in nature, which leads to collapse or wedging of a vertebra.

Certain movements greatly enhance the pain, while certain positions relieve it. One or more spinal roots may be involved. Paget's disease of the spine is readily identifiable on x-ray and is often painless. The disease may, however, lead to compression of the spinal cord or roots because of encroachment on the canal or foramina by the pagetoid bone. The recognition of these bone disorders is discussed in some detail elsewhere (Chaps. 341 and 344).

In general, patients thought to have neoplastic, infectious, or metabolic disease of the spine should be thoroughly evaluated by means of radiographs, bone scans, CT or MRI scans, and appropriate laboratory studies (see above).

REFERRED PAIN FROM VISCERAL DISEASE The pain of disease of the pelvic, abdominal, or thoracic viscera is often felt in the region of the spine; i.e., it is referred to the posterior parts of the spinal segment that innervates the diseased organ. Occasionally back pain may be the first and only sign. The general rule is that pelvic diseases are referred to the sacral region, lower abdominal diseases to the lumbar region (centering around the second to fourth lumbar vertebrae), and upper abdominal diseases to the lower thoracic spine (eighth thoracic to the first and second lumbar vertebrae). Characteristically local signs or stiffness of the back are not elicited, and motion may be of full range without augmentation of the pain. However, some positions, e.g., flexion of the lumbar area of the spine in the lateral recumbent position, may be more comfortable than others.

Low thoracic and upper lumbar pain in abdominal disease Peptic ulceration or tumor of the wall of the stomach and of the duodenum most typically induces pain in the epigastrium (see Chaps. 238 and 261); but if the posterior wall is involved, and particularly if there is retroperitoneal extension, the pain may be felt in the region of the spine. The pain may be central in location or more intense on one side, or it may be felt in both locations. If very intense, it may seem to encircle the body. It tends to retain the characteristics of pain from the affected organ; e.g., if due to peptic ulceration, it appears about 2 h after a meal and is relieved by food and antacids.

Diseases of the pancreas (peptic ulceration with extension to the pancreas, cholecystitis with pancreatitis, cyst, or tumor) are apt to cause pain in the back, being more to the right of the spine if the head of the pancreas is involved and to the left if the body and tail are implicated.

Diseases of retroperitoneal structures, e.g., lymphomas, sarcomas, and carcinomas, may evoke pain in the adjacent part of the spine with some tendency toward radiation to the lower part of the abdomen, groin, and anterior thighs. A secondary tumor of the iliopsoas region on one side often produces a unilateral lumbar ache with radiation toward the groin, labia, or testicle; there may also be signs of involvement of the upper lumbar spinal roots. An aneurysm of the abdominal aorta may induce pain which is localized to this region of the spine but may be felt higher or lower, depending on the location of the lesion.

The sudden appearance of obscure lumbar pain in a patient receiving anticoagulants should arouse the suspicion of retroperitoneal bleeding.

Lumbar pain with lower abdominal diseases Inflammatory diseases of segments of the colon (colitis, diverticulitis) or tumor of the colon cause pain which may be felt in the lower part of the abdomen between the umbilicus and pubis, in the midlumbar region, or in both places. If very intense, the pain may have a beltlike distribution around the body. A lesion in the transverse colon or first part of the descending colon may be central or left-sided, and its level of reference to the back is to the second to third lumbar vertebrae. If the sigmoid colon is implicated, the pain is lower, in the upper sacral region and anteriorly in the midline suprapubic region or left lower quadrant of the abdomen.

Sacral pain in pelvic (urologic and gynecologic) diseases The pelvis is seldom the site of a disease which causes obscure low back pain although gynecologic disorders may manifest themselves in this manner. Of painful pelvic lesions less than a third are due to inflammatory disease; other more hypothetical entities, such as relaxation of uterine supporting structures, retroversion of uterus, pelvic varicosities, and adnexal edema, have been largely discredited. Recently, CT, MRI, or diagnostic laparoscopy has been recommended as a valuable supplement to rectal and pelvic examinations, sigmoidoscopy, and intravenous pyelography for patients with obscure pelvic pain. The importance of psychiatric illness in the majority of undiagnosed cases has been stressed.

Menstrual pain itself may be felt in the sacral region. It is rather poorly localized, tends to radiate down the legs, and is often described as cramplike. The most important source of chronic back pain from the pelvic organs, however, is thought to be the uterosacral ligaments. Endometriosis or carcinoma of the uterus (body or cervix) may invade these structures, while malposition of the uterus may cause traction on them. The pain is localized centrally in the sacrum below the lumbosacral joint but may be more on one side than the other. In endometriosis the pain begins during the premenstrual phase and often continues until it merges with menstrual pain. Malposition of the uterus (retroversion, descensus, and prolapse) is thought by some to lead to sacral pain, especially after the patient has been standing for several hours. One may observe the effect of postural influences here as when a fibroma of the uterus pulls on the uterosacral ligaments. Carcinomatous pain due to involvement of nerve plexuses is continuous and becomes progressively more severe; it tends to be more intense at night. The primary lesion may be inconspicuous, being overlooked upon pelvic examination. Papanicolaou smears, pyelogram, and CT scan are the most useful diagnostic procedures. X-ray therapy of these tumors may produce sacral pain consequent to necrosis of tissue and injury to nerve roots. Low back pain with radiation into one or both thighs is a common phenomenon during the last weeks of pregnancy.

Chronic prostatitis, evidenced by prostatic discharge, burning and frequency of urination, and sometimes a reduction in sexual potency, may be attended by a nagging sacral ache; it may be mainly on one side, with radiation into one leg if the seminal vesicle is involved on that side. Carcinoma of the prostate with metastases to the lower part of the spine is another more common cause of sacral or lumbar pain. It may be present without urinary frequency or burning. Spinal nerves may be infiltrated by tumor cells, or the spinal cord itself may be compressed if the epidural space is invaded. The diagnosis is established by rectal examination, imaging studies and bone scans of the spine, and measurement of acid phosphatase (particularly the prostatic phosphatase fraction). Lesions of the bladder and testes are usually not accompanied by back pain. When the kidney is the site of disease, the pain is ipsilateral, being felt in the flank or lumbar region.

Visceral derangements of whatever type may intensify the pain of arthritis, and the presence of arthritis may alter the distribution of visceral pain. With disease of the spine in the lumbosacral region, for example, distention of the ampulla of the sigmoid by feces or a bout of colitis may aggravate the arthritic pain. In patients with arthritis of the cervical or thoracic spine the pain of myocardial ischemia may radiate to the back.

OBSCURE TYPES OF LOW BACK PAIN AND THE QUESTION OF PSYCHIATRIC DISEASE   The practitioner is frequently consulted by persons who complain of low back pain of obscure origin. Usually the disorder is benign in nature and results from some minor derangement, muscular strain, or diskal prolapse. This is particularly true for those lesions which are of acute onset, aggravated by motion, and relieved by rest. Considerably more difficult are patients with chronic pain, especially those who have had prior back surgery or chronic visceral disease, or those who have severe and progressive pain in which neoplasia or infection is considered.

Even when exhaustive studies have been performed, there remains a group of patients in whom no anatomic or pathologic lesion can be found. These patients generally fall into two categories: those with what might be termed "postural back pain" and those with psychiatric illness.

"Postural" back pain   Some slender asthenic young individuals complain of a vague pain in the back, diffuse in nature and most frequently noted with prolonged sitting or standing. Similarly, some obese middle-aged patients describe a discomfort in the back, either thoracic or lumbar in location. The physical examination in these patients is negative except for slack musculature and what may be best termed "poor posture." Imaging studies and laboratory evaluation usually show no abnormalities, and characteristically the pain is relieved by bed rest. Exercises to strengthen the paraspinal and abdominal muscles are sometimes therapeutic.

Psychiatric illness   Low back pain may be encountered in compensation hysteria and malingering, in chronic anxiety states or depression, and in many individuals whose symptoms and complaints do not fall within any category of psychiatric illness. It is important to be certain that pain in the back in such patients does not signify disease of the spine and adjacent structures, and all such patients should be carefully studied. However, even when organic factors are found, the pain may be exaggerated, prolonged, or woven into a pattern of invalidism or disability because of coexistent psychological factors. This is especially true when there is the possibility of secondary gain (notably compensation for a work-related injury) (see Chap. 15).

PAIN IN THE NECK AND SHOULDER

It is useful to distinguish three major categories of painful disease—of the spine, brachial plexus (thoracic outlet), and shoulder. Although pain in these three regions of the body may overlap, the patient can usually indicate the site of origin.

Cervical spine   Pain arising from the cervical spine is felt in the neck and back of the head (though it may often be projected to the shoulder, arm, and even forearm and hand), is evoked or enhanced by certain movements or positions of the neck, and is accompanied by tenderness and limitation of motions of the neck.

Osteoarthritis of the cervical spine may cause pains which radiate into the back of the head, shoulders, and arms on one or both sides of the thorax. Coincident involvement of nerve roots is manifested by paresthesias, sensory loss, weakness, or deep tendon reflex change. Should bony ridges form in the spinal canal (spondylosis) the spinal cord may be compressed (see Chap. 361). A myelogram, CT, or MRI may reveal the degree of encroachment on the spinal canal (narrowing of the canal to less than 11 mm in the anteroposterior diameter) at the level at which the spinal cord is affected. Difficulty may be experienced in distinguishing the syndrome associated with spondylosis with or without disk rupture and spinal cord compression from primary neurologic diseases (syringomyelia, amyotrophic lateral sclerosis, or tumor) with an unrelated osteoarthritis of the cervical portion of the spine, particularly at the fifth to sixth and sixth to seventh cervical vertebrae, where the disk spaces are often narrowed in the adult. The newer imaging studies such as CT or MRI are helpful in this regard. A painful injury to ligaments and muscles after an accident in which the neck is forcibly extended and flexed (e.g., "whiplash" injury to spine) may be a difficult diagnostic problem, particularly if the patient has some ostensible spurring and especially if in the course of the injury a cerebral concussion has occurred. If the pain is persistent and limited to the neck, imaging studies will sometimes prove that the problem is due to disruption of a disk, but it is often complicated by psychological factors.

Thoracic outlet   Pain resulting from abnormalities of the thoracic outlet is experienced in and around the shoulder in the supraclavicular region, or between the shoulders; is induced by the performance of certain tasks and by certain positions; and is associated with tenderness of structures above the clavicle. There may be a palpable abnormality above the clavicle (aneurysms of the subclavian artery, tumor, cervical rib). The combination of circulatory symptoms and signs referable to the lower part of the brachial plexus, manifested in the hand by obliteration of pulse when the patient holds a full breath with the head tilted back or turned (Adson's test), unilateral Raynaud's phenomenon, trophic changes in the fingers, and sensory loss over the ulnar side of the hand with or without interosseous atrophy complete the clinical picture. Roentgenograms and other imaging studies showing a cervical rib, deformed thoracic outlet, or superior sulcus tumor of the lung (Pancoast's syndrome) corroborate disease in this location. Electromyography and conduction studies along the plexus from points stimulated above and below the clavicle, and studies of arterial and venous circulation (venograms, noninvasive Doppler techniques) are especially helpful in evaluating this problem.

Shoulder Pain localized to the shoulder region is often worse at night and may be associated with local tenderness over the shoulder. The pain is characteristically aggravated by abduction, internal rotation, and extension. Most often shoulder lesions are in the form of a tendonitis or bursitis (sometimes calcific) usually affecting the supraspinatus tendon, the adjacent subdeltoid bursa, or the biceps tendon; occasionally the lesion is more extensive and consists of a rupture of the rotator cuff, in which case the patient may have weakness on abduction and forward flexion. In some such patients there is an adhesive capsulitis, leading to profound limitation of motion, designated as a "frozen shoulder." Partial cuff tears, impingement of the cuff under the acromion, and slight subluxations produce a variety of symptoms about the shoulder particularly with exercise or maintaining the arm in abduction for long periods of time. The pain of shoulder disease may at times radiate into the arm or hand, but the sensory, motor, and reflex changes which indicate disease of nerve roots, plexus, or peripheral nerves are absent.

RUPTURED CERVICAL DISKS One of the commonest causes of neck, shoulder, and arm pain is disk herniation in the lower cervical region. As with rupture of the lumbar disks, the complete syndrome includes the disorder of spinal function and evidence of neural involvement. It may develop after trauma either major or minor (sudden hyperextension of the neck, diving injuries, forceful manipulations, etc.). Virtually every patient exhibits a diminution in range of motion of the neck (often accompanied by intensification of pain). Hyperextension is the movement that most consistently aggravates the pain, although one occasionally sees patients whose principal limitation is in flexion. Rotation and lateral movements are often moderately restricted by pain. With laterally situated disk lesions between the fifth and sixth cervical vertebrae, the symptoms and signs are referred to the sixth cervical roots. The full syndrome is characterized by pain felt at the trapezius ridge, tip of the shoulder, anterior upper part of the arm, radial forearm, and often in the thumb; paresthesias and sensory impairment or hypersensitivity in the same regions; tenderness in the area above the spine of the scapula and in the supraclavicular and biceps regions; weakness in flexion of the forearm; and diminished to absent biceps and supinator reflexes (triceps retained or exaggerated). When the protruded disk lies between the sixth and seventh cervical vertebrae, the seventh cervical root is involved. Under these circumstances, in the patient with the complete syndrome, the pain is in the region of the shoulder blade, pectoral region and medial axilla, posterolateral upper arm, elbow and dorsal forearm, index and middle fingers, or all the fingers; tenderness is most pronounced over the medial aspect of the shoulder blade opposite the third to fourth thoracic spinous processes, in the supraclavicular area and triceps region; paresthesias and sensory loss are most pronounced in the second and third fingers or tips of all the fingers; weakness is seen in extension of the forearm, in the extension of the wrist, and in the hand grip; the triceps reflex is diminished to absent, and the biceps and supinator reflexes are preserved. Either of these syndromes may be incomplete in that only one of several of the typical findings (e.g., pain) is present. Usually the patient states that cough, sneeze, and downward pressure on the head in the hyperextension position exacerbate pain and that traction (even manual) tends to relieve it.

Unlike lumbar disks, the cervical ones, if large and centrally situated, may result in compression of the spinal cord (central disk,

all the cord; paracentral disk, part of the cord). The central disk is often nearly painless, and the cord syndrome may simulate a degenerative disease (amyotrophic lateral sclerosis, combined system disease). A common error is to fail to think of a ruptured disk in the cervical region in patients with obscure symptoms in the legs. The diagnosis of ruptured cervical disk should be confirmed by the same laboratory procedures that were mentioned under "Spondylosis," above.

OTHER CONDITIONS Metastases to the cervical spine are fortunately less common than to other parts of the vertebral column. They are frequently painful and the cause of disordered root function. Compression fractures or extension of the tumor posteriorly may lead to rapid development of quadriplegia.

Shoulder injuries (rotator cuff), subacromial or subdeltoid bursitis, the frozen shoulder (periarthritis or capsulitis), tendonitis, and arthritis may develop in patients who are otherwise well, but these conditions are also frequent in hemiplegics or in individuals suffering from coronary heart disease. The pain is often severe and extends toward the neck and down the arm into the hand. The dorsum of the latter may tingle without other signs of nerve involvement. Vasomotor and arthropathic changes also may occur in the hand (shoulder-hand syndrome, reflex dystrophy), and after a time, osteoporosis and atrophy of cutaneous and subcutaneous structures occur (Sudeck's atrophy or Sudeck-Leriche syndrome). These conditions fall more within the province of orthopaedics than of medicine and are not discussed here in detail. The physician, however, must know that they can often be prevented by proper exercises.

The *carpal tunnel syndrome*, with paresthesias and numbness in palmar distribution of the median nerve and aching pain which extends up into the forearm, may be mistaken for disease of the shoulder or neck. Similarly, other less common forms of nerve entrapment may involve the ulnar, radial, or median nerves and lead to a mistaken diagnosis of brachial plexus lesion or cervical syndrome. Electromyography and conduction studies are especially helpful in such conditions (Chap. 362).

MANAGEMENT OF BACK AND NECK PAIN

Without doubt the preventive aspects of back pain are important. There would be far fewer back problems if adults kept their trunk muscles in optimal condition by regular exercise such as swimming, bicycle riding, walking briskly, running, or calisthenic programs. A weight reduction diet and a regular exercise program to strengthen abdominal and paraspinal muscles is frequently very beneficial for patients with chronic low back discomfort. Morning is the ideal time since the back of the older adult tends to stiffen during the night because of inactivity. This happens regardless of whether a bed board or a stiff mattress is used. Sleeping with back hyperextended and sitting for long times in an overstuffed chair or a badly designed auto seat commonly cause difficulties for the patient with low back problems. It is estimated that pressures between disks are increased 200 percent by changing from a recumbent to a standing position and by 400 percent by sitting slumped in an easy chair. Correct sitting posture lessens this. Long trips in a car or plane without change in position put maximal strain on disk and ligamentous structures in the spine. Lifting from a position of flexed trunk, as in removing a suitcase from the trunk of a car, is dangerous (always lift with the object close to the body). Sudden strenuous activity without conditioning and warm-up also is likely to cause trouble to disks and their ligamentous envelopes (the commonest sources of back pain).

Muscular and ligamentous strains and minor disk prolapses are usually self-limited, responding to simple measures in a relatively short period of time. The basic principle of therapy is rest in a recumbent position for several days to weeks. When weight bearing is resumed, a light lumbosacral support is occasionally helpful in continuing the immobilization until the patient is restored to full health. Physical measures such as heat, cold, diathermy, or massage are of limited value; of considerably greater importance are active exercises to both reduce the spasm and improve muscle tone. Analgesic medication should be given liberally during the first few days: codeine, 30 mg, and aspirin, 0.6 g, or pentazocine, 50 mg, propoxyphene, 65 mg, or meperidine, 50 mg. Muscle relaxants are often a valuable adjunct, particularly in that such drugs as diazepam, 8 to 40 mg in divided doses, may make bed rest more tolerable. If an inflammatory component is suspected, indomethacin, 75 mg per day (in divided doses), ibuprofen, 600 mg three or four times daily, or naproxen, 375 to 500 mg once or twice daily, may be helpful.

In the treatment of a clearly diagnosed acute or chronic rupture of a lumbar or cervical disk, complete bed rest is essential, at least initially, and analgesic medication may be required. Traction is of little value in lumbar disk disease, and it is best to permit the patient to find the most comfortable position. Cervical traction with a halter may be of considerable benefit to patients with cervical disk syndrome. It can be administered with the patient in recumbency, or after sufficient improvement to allow ambulation, can be performed intermittently in the erect, slightly forward flexed position using special equipment. During the recumbent phase of treatment of lumbar disk disease, exercises to reduce spasm, muscle relaxants, and anti-inflammatory agents as described above may be of considerable value. After 2 to 3 weeks in bed, the patient can be allowed to slowly resume activities, usually with the protection of a brace or light spinal support. Exercise programs designed to increase the strength of the abdominal and paraspinal muscles are helpful at this point. The patient may suffer some minor recurrence of the pain but be able to carry on his or her usual activities, and eventually most individuals will recover. If the pain and neurologic findings do not disappear on prolonged, conservative management, or if the patient suffers frequently recurring acute episodes, surgical management may be indicated. This should always be preceded by a CT, MRI, or myelogram to localize the lesion (and rule out the presence of intra- or extradural tumors). The surgical procedure most often indicated is a hemilaminectomy with excision of the disk involved. Arthrodesis of the involved segments is indicated only in cases in which there is extraordinary instability usually related to an anatomic abnormality (such as spondylolysis) or in the cervical region when an extensive laminectomy has rendered the spine unstable. The result of conservative management of patients with diskal disease and sciatica is that approximately 80 percent improve at the end of 4 weeks regardless of whether traction, exercises, manipulation, or corset, or some combination thereof, is used. Therefore, only a small number of patients should be considered to require surgery.

Spondylosis of the cervical spine, if painful, is helped by bed rest and traction; if signs of spinal cord involvement are present, a collar to limit movement may lead to improvement. Decompressive laminectomy or anterior fusion is reserved for severe instances of the disease with advancing neurologic symptoms. The shoulder-hand syndrome may benefit from stellate ganglion blocks or ganglionectomy, but the basic treatment is physiotherapy, with or without medication, and surgical procedures are used only as measures of last resort.

The management of patients with thoracic outlet syndrome is complex and requires first a careful study to be certain that the cause of the lesion is really a mechanical encroachment of the brachial plexus in the interspace between the clavicle and first rib. Exercises to reduce the tension in this region are mainly designed to strengthen the clavicular musculature and improve posture, thus opening the outlet. Many patients benefit from change of work circumstances, and for women with pendulous breasts, a better designed brassiere is sometimes helpful. Nonsteroidal anti-inflammatory agents are sometimes beneficial, as are muscle relaxants such as diazepam. In the event that the patient's difficulties are intractable or the root compression causes neurologic deficits, exploration of the anterior scalene triangle with resection of the first rib is advocated with usually excellent results.

REFERENCES

BELL GR, PARKMAN RH: The conservative treatment of sciatica. Spine 9:54, 1984

BOGDUK N: The innervation of the lumbar spine. Spine 8:286, 1983

BRADY LP et al: An evaluation of the electromyogram in the diagnosis of lumbar disk lesion. J Bone Joint Surg 51A:539, 1969

BUCHANAN JR et al: A comparison of the risk of vertebral fracture in menopausal osteopenia and other metabolic disturbances. J Bone Joint Surg 70:704, 1988

BUNDSCHUH CV et al: Epidural fibrosis and recurrent disk herniation in the lumbar spine: MR imaging assessment. AJR 150:923, 1988

COLLIER B: Treatment for lumbar sciatic pain in posterior articular lumbar joint syndrome. Anesthesia 34:202, 1979

DEYO RA, DIEHL AK: Measuring physical and psychosocial function in patients with low back pain. Spine 8:635, 1983

FRIEDENBERG AB, MILLER WT: Degenerative disk disease of the cervical spine. J Bone Joint Surg 45A:1171, 1963

FRYMOYER JW: Back pain and sciatica. N Engl J Med 318:291, 1988

GRABIAS SL: The treatment of spinal stenosis. J Bone Joint Surg 62A:308, 1988

——, MANKIN HJ: Pain in lower back. Bull Rheum Dis 30:1040, 1980

MASARYK TJ et al: High-resolution MR imaging of sequestered lumbar intervertebral disks. AJR 150:1155, 1988

MIKHAEL MH et al: Neurologic evaluation of lateral recess syndrome. Radiology 140:97, 1981

MODIC MT et al: Imaging of degenerative disk disease. Radiology 168:177, 1988

MURPHY RW: Nerve roots and spinal nerves in degenerative disk disease. Clin Orthop 129:46, 1977

NAYLOR A: The changes in the human intervertebral disk in degeneration and nuclear prolapse. Orthop Clin North Am 2:343, 1971

PLEATMAN CW, LUKIN RR: Lumbar spinal stenosis. Semin Roentgenol 23:106, 1988

RASKIN SP: Computerized tomographic findings in lumbar disk disease. Orthopedics 5:419, 1981

REYNOLDS AV et al: Lumbar monoradiculopathy due to unilateral facet hypertrophy. Neurosurgery 10:480, 1982

ROTHMAN RC, SIMEONE F: *Lumbar Disc Disease*. Philadelphia, Saunders, 1975, pp 443–458

WILLIAMS AL et al: Computed tomography in the diagnosis of herniated nucleus pulposus. Radiology 135:95, 1980

WILSON ES, BRILL RF: Spinal stenosis: The narrow lumbar canal syndrome. Clin Orthop 122:244, 1977

section 2   Alterations in body temperature

20   CHILLS AND FEVER

RICHARD K. ROOT / ROBERT G. PETERSDORF

Body temperature is normally regulated between 35.8 and 37.2°C (96.5 and 99°F) in healthy persons, with a diurnal variation (see Chap. 377). When heat production exceeds the capacity of heat loss, as during vigorous exercise, the core body temperature may exceed 39°C (103.2°F) for variable time periods until heat is dissipated by sweating, hyperventilation, and cutaneous vasodilation. These transient physiologic elevations in core temperature must be distinguished from sustained elevations found in a number of disease states and termed *fever*. At the onset of fever an abrupt increase in core temperature can occur by means of violent muscle contractions (*rigors*) coupled with cutaneous vasoconstriction and pilocrection ("goose flesh"), a symptom complex defined as chills.

PATHOGENESIS OF FEVER   Pyrogens   Fever may be produced by many stimuli including bacteria and their endotoxins, viruses, yeasts, spirochetes, protozoa, immune reactions, progestational hormones, and drugs and synthetic polynucleotides. These substances, which have been termed collectively *exogenous pyrogens*, are both diverse and complex. Substantial evidence supports a key intermediary role in fever production for cytokines, termed *endogenous pyrogens*, which are produced by cells interacting with exogenous pyrogens. These endogenous pyrogens act centrally on thermosensitive neurons in the preoptic hypothalamus to trigger increased heat production and to decrease heat loss. The core body temperature rises until a higher stable point is reached. The temperature of the blood bathing the hypothalamus is equivalent to the new "set point," and the patient is usually flushed and warm. Defervescence occurs through activation of heat loss mechanisms, in particular sweating, until the core body temperature reaches its baseline and a new equilibrium is established. Hyperthermia from other causes is not accompanied by a resetting of the central thermostat.

The major endogenous pyrogens identified in experimental animals and humans are interleukin 1α and 1β (IL-1), and cachectin, also known as tumor necrosis factor-α (TNF). Similar in size (17-kDa glycoproteins), many actions, and highly conserved in nature, the IL-1 and TNF molecules are structurally discrete. IL-1β is the predominant species in humans (see Chap. 13). Recently, the interferons α, β, and γ (IFN-α, -β, -γ) have been shown to have pyrogenic action, although the mechanisms remain to be defined. Monocytes, macrophages, and macrophage-derived cells are major sources of IL-1 and TNF. Endothelial cells, keratinocytes, and brain astrocytes can also produce IL-1. During phagocytosis or stimulation by bacterial endotoxins, up to 5 percent of the total protein produced by macrophages consists of IL-1 and TNF. Administration of endotoxin to humans is followed by the appearance of fever and free TNF in the plasma; during severe bacterial sepsis both IL-1 and TNF may be found.

A positive feedback mechanism for IL-1 production by macrophages and endothelial cells has been demonstrated, triggered by both IL-1 and TNF. Activation of macrophages by IFN-γ can augment IL-1 and TNF production in response to other stimuli. Production of both IL-1 and TNF involves the synthesis of new specific mRNA as well as the IL-1 and TNF molecules themselves, which are then secreted by the stimulated cells. Glucocorticoids can block both the

elaboration of specific mRNA and its eventual translation into synthesis of IL-1 and TNF; release of preformed IL-1 or TNF is not affected. Prostaglandins of the E series also exert an inhibitory effect on IL-1 and TNF production. Both glucocorticoids and prostaglandin E₂ (PGE₂) appear to be important regulatory molecules for IL-1 and TNF production and action. In addition other negative regulatory molecules for IL-1 have been described, and IL-1 may downregulate its own receptors on target cells.

Once released from stimulated cells TNF and IL-1 can have actions on target cells in the immediate locale or in distal sites to which they are transported in the plasma. IL-1 that remains bound to the plasma membranes of stimulated cells also has potent biologic activity. The ability of target cells to respond to their actions is a function of specific receptors for IL-1 and TNF. Despite similarities in molecular weight, production, and in a wide variety of actions the cellular receptors for IL-1 and TNF differ, suggesting that they trigger common intracellular pathways in responding cells and tissues.

In support of this thesis, multiple actions of both compounds are mediated through the induction of arachidonate metabolism. Within the hypothalamus, IL-1 and TNF act by promoting the synthesis of prostaglandins of the E series using arachidonate released from target cell membranes. PGE₂ activates heat generating and conserving mechanisms; synthesis of cyclic adenyl monophosphate (AMP) is involved. The precise molecular mechanisms linking PGE₂ and cyclic AMP actions to "resetting" the central thermostat remain to be elucidated as do the central actions of the IFNs. Aspirin and nonsteroidal anti-inflammatory drugs (NSAIDs) are antipyretic by inhibiting cyclooxygenase activity and the synthesis of PGE₂, not by inhibiting TNF or IL-1 production. Glucocorticoids may be antipyretic through dual mechanisms involving production of IL-1 and TNF as well as inhibition of arachidonate release centrally.

GENERAL ACTIONS OF IL-1 AND TNF   Besides fever, a wide variety of actions characteristic of the acute inflammatory response can be triggered jointly by IL-1 and TNF. Many of these actions also involve arachidonate intermediates. These include myelopoiesis, release of neutrophils, and augmentation of some neutrophil functions; vasodilation and induction of cell adhesion proteins, platelet activating factor (PAF) production, and thrombomodulin expression by endothelial cells; proteolysis and glycogenolysis in muscles; mobilization of lipids from adipocytes; induction of acute phase protein synthesis and glycogenolysis in the liver; induction of fibroblast proliferation, osteoclast activation, and release of collagenase from chondrocytes; induction of slow-wave sleep activity in the brain; a variety of endocrine responses including release of ACTH, β-endorphins, growth hormone, and vasopressin from the pituitary; and the release of insulin from pancreatic cells and of cortisol and catecholamine from the adrenals. TNF and, to a lesser extent, IL-1 may contribute to the wasting (cachexia) characteristic of chronic infections and other inflammatory or neoplastic diseases by these mechanisms as well as by inhibiting appetite. In all of these actions, as well as in the production of fever, IL-1 and TNF can act synergistically or additively.

In contrast to TNF, IL-1 has major actions in triggering and amplifying the specific immune response through activating T cells and elaboration of interleukin 2 (IL-2). IL-1 also promotes B-cell proliferation (see Chap. 13). Interestingly, in vitro T-cell activation and mitogenesis as well as responses to IL-2 are enhanced at febrile body temperature, reaching an optimum at 39.5°C (103.1°F). By this means fever, as part of the inflammatory response, may exert a positive feedback on the specific immune response to infecting organisms.

Both fever and specific events mediated by IL-1 and TNF have a broad and highly integrated role in the characteristic responses to infection and/or acute inflammation. The interferons, in particular IFN-γ, may augment these responses (see Chap. 13). Some of these responses may be viewed as protective, whereas others contribute to deleterious symptoms and signs. In fact, when these responses are exaggerated or unchecked the syndrome of septicemia or septic shock (see Chap. 89) may develop. Given this complexity, it is not surprising that conflict still surrounds the need to treat fever with antipyretics and other means. While symptoms might be relieved, the cost could be interference with normally protective mechanisms, including the specific immune response and the mobilization of nutrients and cellular protective and proliferative responses necessary to promote a successful recovery.

DISEASES ACCOMPANIED BY FEVER   Omitting disorders that may involve cerebral thermoregulatory centers directly, such as brain tumors, intracranial hemorrhage or thrombosis, or heat stroke, the following disease states may be accompanied by fever:

1   All *infections* whether caused by bacteria, rickettsias, chlamydiae, viruses, or parasites (in particular protozoa) may cause fever.
2   Diseases due to *immune mechanisms* often are associated with fever. These include the connective tissue disorders, drug reactions, disorders due to other immunologic abnormalities (including immune-mediated hemolysis), and the acquired immunodeficiency syndrome (AIDS). In the latter, particular care must be taken to exclude complicating infection.
3   Diseases characterized by *vascular inflammation or thrombosis,* tissue *infarction,* or *trauma* are often accompanied by fever. These include phlebitis; the giant-cell arteridites; myocardial, pulmonary, and cerebral infarctions; crushing mechanical trauma; and rhabdomyolysis. In all cases, complicating infection must be excluded.
4   *Granulomatous disorders* such as sarcoid and granulomatous hepatitis often have fever as a major manifestation.
5   *Inflammatory bowel disease* (ulcerative colitis and Crohn's disease) as well as other intraabdominal inflammatory processes (acute pancreatitis and hepatitis) may have fever associated with them.
6   *Neoplastic disorders,* in particular those arising from the lymphoreticular or hematopoietic systems, may have fever as a prominent manifestation at the beginning or later in the course. Rarely other solid tumors (hypernephroma; carcinoma of the pancreas, lung, and bone; or hepatoma) present with fever. Fever complicating most solid tumors is usually related to widespread metastases with tumor necrosis or obstruction and infection of drainage ducts.
7   Certain *acute metabolic disorders* such as gout, porphyria, Fabry's disease, Addisonian or thyroid crises, and, rarely, pheochromocytoma are sometimes associated with fever. The pathogenesis varies from activation of the inflammatory response (e.g., gout) to alterations in thermogenesis and heat regulation (e.g., hyperthyroidism and pheochromocytoma).

ACCOMPANIMENTS OF FEVER   Systemic symptoms   The perception of fever by patients varies enormously. Some persons can tell with considerable accuracy when their body temperatures are elevated; others with chronic febrile illnesses (e.g., patients with tuberculosis) may be wholly unaware of body temperature as high as 39.9°C (103°F). Often patients may pay no attention to fever because of other unpleasant symptoms such as headache or pleuritic pain. Pain in the back, generalized myalgias, and arthralgias without arthritis are commonly associated with fever. To what extent these symptoms can be ascribed to specific infectious agents as opposed to the actions of IL-1 and TNF (e.g., muscle proteolysis) is not clear, but whatever the mechanism, many of these symptoms may be reduced or abolished with aspirin or NSAID administration.

Chills   Abrupt onset of fever with a *chill* or *rigor* is characteristic of some diseases and, in the absence of antipyretic drugs, rare in others. Although repeated rigors are typical of pyogenic infection with bacteremia, a similar pattern of fever may occur in noninfectious diseases such as vasculitis or lymphoma. A true chill, which is usually accompanied by teeth chattering and bed shaking, must be differentiated from the chilly sensations which occur in almost all fevers, particularly those in viral infections. Rarely, a true rigor occurs in viremia. Chills may be evoked or perpetuated by the intermittent administration of aspirin or other antipyretics when their action wears off or if there is an exaggerated hypothermic response. These unpleasant side effects may be minimized by administering antipyretics at 2 to 3 h intervals around the clock, rather than prescribing them only for elevations of temperature above a certain level.

Sweats   When the stimulus to fever production is removed or inhibited, for example, by the action of antipyretics, defervescence is achieved by activation of heat loss mechanisms. Diffuse sweating, sometimes soaking clothing or bedsheets, allows rapid dissipation of heat by evaporation and may add to patient discomfort. In some patients, this may be the most prominent manifestation of repetitive fevers followed by defervescence (e.g., tuberculosis).

Changes in mental status   Febrile episodes may be accompanied by obtundation, irritability, or frank delirium in some patients without evidence for central nervous system involvement by the primary disease process. This is most striking in the very old and in the very young, and in patients with other disorders such as alcoholism, cardiovascular disease, or senility. The soporific actions of TNF and IL-1 as well as release of β-endorphins may contribute to these events. The sensorium usually clears with defervescence in the absence of underlying disease of the central nervous system.

Convulsions   Infants and young children (less than age 5) may sometimes develop seizures when the temperature is elevated. A family history of epilepsy may be present, but usually febrile convulsions do not signal serious cerebral disease. When they occur, however, a primary disorder affecting the central nervous system must be excluded, as is also mandatory for patients with marked alteration in mental status.

Herpes labialis   Elevations of body temperature can activate latent herpes simplex virus (HSV) infection ("fever blisters"). For unclear reasons this is more common in acute pyogenic bacterial infections (pneumococcal, streptococcal, meningococcal), malaria, and the rickettsioses than in other infections or noninfectious causes of fever. Activation of latent HSV infection is also a manifestation of suppressed cellular immunity.

CLINICAL IMPORTANCE OF FEVER   Properly measured, the temperature is a simple, objective, and accurate indicator of a physiologic state and is much less subject to external and psychogenic stimuli than the other vital signs, such as pulse, respiratory rate, and blood pressure. For these reasons, determination of the body temperature assists in estimating the severity of an illness, its course and duration, and the effect of therapy, or even in deciding which person has an organic illness. In general, determination of rectal temperature is easily performed and most accurately reflects core body temperatures. In seriously ill patients or those in whom oral temperatures are unreliable (e.g., failure to cooperate, hyperventilation) *rectal temperature monitoring is mandatory.*

Benefit of fever   Beyond drawing attention to its cause, it has been difficult to relate more rapid resolution or decreased complications of a disease state to the presence and degree of fever. Fever therapy was used in the past to diminish the manifestations of neurosyphilis or some forms of chronic arthritis. To what extent beneficial effects could be ascribed to high core body temperature as opposed to the action of mediators of the febrile process is unclear. In vitro IL-1–mediated activation of the specific immune response is accelerated at febrile body temperatures. Similarly, minor increases of chemotactic, phagocytic, and bactericidal activity of human polymorphonuclear leukocytes have been observed. In cold-blooded animals a warm environment has been demonstrated to augment the inflammatory response.

Detrimental aspects of fever   Many of the alleged detrimental effects of fever may be due to the concurrent actions of IL-1, TNF, and other mediators at a variety of sites and may be independent of temperature elevation per se. Muscle wasting with myalgias, adipose tissue loss, other metabolic changes, and perhaps CNS alterations in febrile disorders are examples of such effects. Nevertheless, in febrile patients basal metabolism rates are increased as are cardiac output and work. Sweating may aggravate loss of salt and water. There may be general discomfort due to malaise, myalgias, headache, photophobia, or an unpleasant sensation of warmth. Fever may precipitate seizures in epileptic patients. The rigors and profuse sweats of hectic fevers are particularly unpleasant for many patients. In elderly patients, particularly those with cardiac or cerebrovascular disease, fever and its associated manifestations may be deleterious.

MANAGEMENT OF FEVER   The most important aspects of fever management should be directed at its cause. Since fever ordinarily does little harm, imposes no great discomfort, and may benefit host defense mechanisms, antipyretic drugs are rarely essential to patient welfare and may obfuscate the effect of a specific therapeutic agent or of the natural course of the disease. There are situations, however, in which lowering of the body temperature is of vital importance, e.g., heat stroke and malignant hyperthermia (see Chap. 377), epileptic seizures, or when cardiac or CNS function is impaired. Under these circumstances lowering the temperature is indicated. Cooling blankets set at hypothermic temperatures can be a highly effective means for external cooling. However, their effects may be negated if they induce further cutaneous vasoconstriction and shivering. Sponging the body surface with cool saline or water or applying cool compresses to the skin and forehead may be helpful. There is no advantage to sponging with alcohol, which, because of its pungent odor, may add to patient discomfort. When high internal temperature is combined with cutaneous vasoconstriction, as in heat stroke or malignant hyperthermia, external cooling should be combined with massage of the skin in order to promote surface vasodilation. Immediate immersion in a tub of ice water or packing with ice should be considered as a measure of last resort and can be lifesaving in patients with heat stroke if the internal body temperature is in excess of 42.2°C (108°F). In most instances cooling blankets, if available, are safer and more comfortable.

Antipyretic drugs, such as aspirin (0.650 g every 4 h) or acetaminophen (0.650 to 1.0 g every 4 h) are often employed in lowering temperature and relieving other manifestations of febrile illness. Acetaminophen is generally preferred because of its lack of adverse effects on gastric mucosa, platelet function, or the subsequent development of Reye's syndrome in some children with viral illnesses given aspirin (see Chap. 256). Candidates for antipyretic therapy include patients who are uncomfortable or those in whom fever poses a high risk, as in patients with ischemic heart disease, heart failure, febrile seizures (usually children), head injury, mental disorders, or pregnancy. Antipyretics are sometimes associated with unpleasant diaphoresis, an alarming fall in blood pressure, and the subsequent return of fever accompanied by a chill; these can be mitigated by enforcing a liberal fluid intake and by administering the drugs regularly and frequently at 2- to 3-h intervals. NSAIDs such as ibuprofen (200 mg every 6 h), indomethacin (50 mg every 6 to 8 h), or naproxen (250 mg bid) also have potent antipyretic effects and have been useful in controlling chronic fevers in patients with malignancy. Although glucocorticoids are effective antipyretics, they must be used with caution because of their tendency to precipitate abrupt falls in temperature accompanied by hypotension. The capacity of these drugs to mask other manifestations of infection and inflammation as well as potential adverse side effects constitute a relative contraindication to their use.

The discomfort of a rigor can be alleviated in many patients by the intravenous injection of calcium salts. This procedure will stop the shivering and chilliness, but has no influence on the ultimate height of the fever. Severe rigors can also be abolished with morphine sulfate (10 to 15 mg subcutaneously) or with parenteral chlorpromazine (10 to 25 mg). When this approach is employed, the patient must be carefully monitored for hypotension.

DIAGNOSTIC CONSIDERATIONS IN FEVER   In many illnesses fever is the most prominent and often the only manifestation of disease. While certain fever patterns may suggest a particular type of disease, fever per se is only an indication of a reaction to injury comparable with an elevated leukocyte count or rapid erythrocyte sedimentation rate.

Fever patterns   Fever may be intermittent, remittent, sustained, or relapsing. In *intermittent fever* the temperature falls to normal each day in an exaggeration of the circadian rhythmn. When the variation between the peak and the nadir is very large, the fever is called *hectic* or *septic*. Intermittent fevers are characteristic but not diagnostic of pyogenic infections, particularly abscesses, lymphomas, and miliary tuberculosis. In *remittent fever* the temperature falls each day, usually by morning, but does not return to normal. Most fevers are remittent and this type of febrile response is not characteristic of any disease. A *sustained fever* is characterized by persistent temperature elevation without significant diurnal variation. It is exemplified by the fever of untreated typhoid, typhus, or infectious endocarditis. With *relapsing fever* short febrile periods occur between one or several days of normal temperature. Examples of relapsing fever are the following:

Malaria (see Chap. 159), in particular that caused by infection with *Plasmodium vivax*, produces relapsing fevers at 2- to 3-day intervals. Relapsing fever caused by infection with *Borrelia* species is discussed in Chap. 131; typically 7- to 10-day febrile episodes are interspersed with 5- to 7-day afebrile periods. *Rat-bite fever* can be caused by either *Spirillum minus* or *Streptobacillus moniliformis*, both transmitted by the bite of a rat (see Chap. 98). The periodic exacerbations of fever usually follow a 7- to 10-day pattern, following a history of rat bite 1 to 10 weeks prior to the onset of symptoms. The diagnosis is made by cultures of blood, joints, or other inflamed sites or by serology.

Localized *pyogenic infections* may in rare instances produce periodic bouts of fever. The so-called Charcot's intermittent biliary fever, i.e., cholangitis with episodic biliary obstruction due to stones, is an example. Similarly, periodic ureteral obstruction due to small stones or inspissated pus may cause a relapsing fever pattern in the presence of urinary infection.

Pel-Ebstein fever—bouts of fever lasting 3 to 10 days, separated by a febrile and asymptomatic period of 3 to 10 days—is the eponym for relapsing fever occurring as a manifestation of Hodgkin's disease or other lymphomas. In some patients these cycles may be repeated for months until other manifestations of the illness become apparent. Although the pattern may suggest the nature of the underlying disease, most patients with Pel-Ebstein relapsing fever have causes other than Hodgkin's disease.

Epidemiology of fever   The diagnosis of febrile illness must take into account the epidemiologic setting. For example an acute febrile illness in southeast Asia or Africa is probably due to malaria (see Chap. 159) or one of the arboviruses (see Chap. 148); in a college student in the United States it may result from infectious mononucleosis or some other viral infection; and in a hospitalized octogenarian following prostatectomy it is probably an indication of urinary tract infection, wound infection, phlebitis from an intravenous catheter, aspiration pneumonia, or pulmonary infarction. In children, prolonged fevers are more likely to be due to infections than in adults. Travelers returning from trips to foreign countries must be evaluated for diseases indigenous to the countries visited, but they are more likely to have febrile diseases that are more common at home. Patients whose host defenses are altered by malignancy, cytotoxic or steroid therapy, or congenital or acquired immunodeficiency are more likely to have infections caused by unusual opportunistic organisms than are normal hosts.

Rare versus common diseases   Unless host defense mechanisms have been severely altered by disease or immunosuppressive therapy, fever is much more likely to be a manifestation of a common than a rare disease. On the other hand, patients with abnormal host defenses are no less prone to infections with common agents than are normal hosts. For example, while pneumococcal pneumonia is a leading cause of pulmonary infiltrates and fever in the elderly, it also is an important cause of illness in patients with AIDS, although not as frequent as *Pneumocystis carinii* (see Chap. 264).

Febrile illnesses of short duration   Acute febrile illnesses of less than 2 weeks' duration are common in medical practice. In most cases they run their course, progressing to complete recovery, and a precise diagnosis is not, nor need be, made. It is likely that the vast majority of such illnesses are infectious although short febrile episodes may be characteristic of thromboembolic disease, gout, or drug allergies in which the drug is discontinued.

Symptomatic infections with respiratory viruses are usually short-lived and self-limited. The presence of cough, coryza, and pharyngitis associated with fever supports this diagnosis (see Chap. 140). Similarly during summer months short-lived fever and malaise ("grippe") are characteristic of many enteroviral infections (see Chap. 144). It is neither practical nor cost-effective to carry out detailed diagnostic studies for these agents. In bacterial infections, however, laboratory diagnosis is simpler and can be indispensible to proper therapy.

The following characteristics, though not restricted solely to acute infections, are highly suggestive that infection is present:

1 Abrupt onset
2 High fever, i.e., 38.9 to 40.6°C (102 to 105°F) with or without chills
3 Respiratory symptoms—sore throat, cough, coryza
4 Severe malaise, with muscle or joint pain, photophobia, pain on movement of the eyes, headache
5 Nausea, vomiting, or diarrhea
6 Acute tender enlargement of the lymph nodes or spleen
7 Meningeal signs with or without spinal fluid pleocytosis
8 Dysuria, urinary frequency, and flank pain

None of the symptoms and signs listed is encountered solely in infections. Acute leukemias or vasculitis may have similar features on presentation. Nevertheless, in a given instance of acute febrile illness with some or all of the manifestations listed, the probabilities strongly favor infection.

It is desirable, of course, to establish an accurate diagnosis, and whatever steps are practicable in the circumstances to establish the cause should be taken. Cultures of the blood, urine, and other suspected sites of infection should be obtained before institution of antibacterial chemotherapy (see Chap. 80). Skin and/or serologic tests should also be carried out when indicated.

There is a tendency to rely immediately and excessively on the laboratory in ascertaining the cause of fever. In many instances, a thorough history and a complete and, if necessary, repeated physical examination along with a complete blood count (CBC) and urinalysis will provide the answer. Measurement of the erythrocyte sedimentation rate can help differentiate fevers caused by infection or inflammation from other causes. Often a little patience, in the form of watchful waiting before embarking on an expensive and extensive laboratory workup, will lead to the diagnosis.

Prolonged febrile illness   Some of the knottiest problems in medicine are posed by cases of prolonged fever in which the diagnosis remains obscure for weeks or even months. Eventually, however, the true nature of the illness usually reveals itself, since a disease which causes injury sufficient to evoke temperature elevations to 38.3°C (101°F) or higher for several weeks does not often subside without leaving some clue as to its nature. The evaluation of problems of this sort calls for skillful application of all diagnostic methods—careful history, thorough physical examination, and the carefully considered and staged use of laboratory examinations and imaging techniques.

FEVER OF UNKNOWN ORIGIN   In some, fever becomes the dominant sign or symptom in a patient's illness, and when its cause escapes detection, it is defined as a fever of unknown origin (FUO). This term should be reserved for patients who have elevations in temperature greater than 38.3°C (101°F) for a prolonged period (at least 2, and preferably, 3 weeks) and in whom the diagnosis cannot be made during at least 1 week of intensive study. These rigid criteria eliminate from this diagnostic category patients with common viral or bacterial infections, those in whom the diagnosis is obvious by simple physical and/or laboratory examination, and those whose fever is due to a sequential occurrence of etiologically unrelated diseases. An example is a patient febrile after a myocardial infarction, who then develops thrombophlebitis followed by multiple pulmonary emboli, each accompanied by recurrence of fever. Much of the confusion in the literature concerning causes of FUO is due to failure to define the criteria employed in classifying patients.

DISEASES CAUSING PROLONGED FEVERS   Table 20-1 lists some of the diseases responsible for prolonged fever.

Infections   Infections that are relatively resistant to rapid eradication by host defenses (e.g., localized pyogenic infections or intracellular infections) often pursue a chronic or subacute course. As a cause for FUO, infections account for about 30 percent, a figure that appears to be decreasing due to the common practice of administering antibiotics to any patient in whom fever persists for more than a few days. Consequently many infections may be eradicated by more or less "blind" therapy without accurate determination of their nature or location.

ABSCESSES   (See also Chap. 91) Abscesses are the most common form of bacterial infection presenting as FUO and are important because they can be cured with early diagnosis and treatment. Failure to make a diagnosis may result in a fatal or permanently disabling outcome. Intraabdominal abscesses arising in the liver or spleen, in the subphrenic space, related to a ruptured diverticulum or appendix, or in the pelvis may be associated with more fever than pain. Ultrasonography, computed tomographic (CT) scanning, or magnetic resonance imaging (MRI) have simplified the detection and localization of abscesses. In many cases percutaneous needle aspiration under imaging guidance can be employed for both diagnosis and treatment, without the need to resort to laparotomy.

RENAL INFECTION   Fever in uncomplicated pyelonephritis is usually limited to 5 to 7 days (see Chap. 95). Prolongation of fever beyond this time should suggest intra- or extrarenal obstruction or abscess. Prostate abscesses should be considered in males; sometimes there is no associated rectal pain or dysuria. Occasionally focal pyelonephritis may cause prolonged fever. Ultrasonography coupled with CT scanning will detect obstruction and abscesses with a high degree of reliability.

INTRAVASCULAR INFECTIONS   Because of a high index of suspicion, the ubiquitous use of blood cultures, and widespread application of antibiotics, which must cure some patients, bacterial endocarditis has become a rare cause of FUO. Antibiotic use or infection by highly fastidious organisms including fungi and rickettsias are important factors in "culture-negative" endocarditis (see Chap. 90). Organisms that give rise to chronic or intermittent bacteremia without prominent localizing findings include *Salmonella* (*S. typhosa, S. choleraesuis*), *Neisseria* (both gonococci and meningococci), and *Brucella*. Consideration of the epidemiologic setting, using appropriate serologic testing, and informing laboratories of the need to look for fastidious organisms in blood cultures are useful in establishing the diagnosis.

OTHER BACTERIAL INFECTIONS   These include sinusitis or mastoiditis, exacerbations of chronic or subacute osteomyelitis (in particular vertebral osteomyelitis), and retroperitoneal infection such as an aortic aneurysm filled with secondarily infected organizing clot. Enteric pathogens (including *Escherichia coli, Bacteroides*, and *Salmonella*) have been frequent isolates from patients with such infections. Blood cultures may be intermittently positive. For screening of bone infections, bone scan can demonstrate foci of increased uptake; however, the changes must be differentiated from those caused by fractures, neoplasm, or other causes of osteoblastic activity. Imaging techniques including ultrasonography, CT scan, and, if necessary, MRI can assist in establishing the diagnosis of retroperitoneal, sinus, and bone infections. Surgery is necessary for both diagnosis and therapy of infected aneurysms. In addition some patients with dissecting aneurysms have fever without infection.

TABLE 20-1   Disease entities in the United States causing prolonged fever

I Infections
  A Pyogenic infections
    1 Upper abdominal infections
      a Cholecystitis (stone), empyema of gallbladder
      b Cholangitis
      c Liver abscess
      d Lesser sac abscess
      e Subphrenic abscess
      f Splenic abscess
    2 Lower abdominal infections
      a Diverticulitis (abscess)
      b Appendicitis
    3 Pelvic inflammatory disease
      a Pelvic abscess
    4 Urinary tract infections
      a Pyelonephritis (rare)
      b Intrarenal abscess
      c Perinephric abscess
      d Ureteral obstruction
      e Prostatic abscess
    5 Sinusitis
    6 Osteomyelitis
    7 Cat-scratch fever
  B Intravascular infections
    1 Bacterial endocarditis (acute and subacute)
    2 Intravascular catheter infections
  C Bacteremias without overt primary focus
    1 Meningococcemia
    2 Gonococcemia
    3 Typhoid
    4 Vibriosis
    5 Listeriosis
    6 Brucellosis
    7 Coliform bacteremia in patients with cirrhosis
  D Granulomatous infections
    1 Tuberculosis
    2 Deep-seated fungus infections
    3 Atypical mycobacterial infections
  E Viral, rickettsial, and chlamydial infections
    1 Infectious mononucleosis
    2 Cytomegalovirus
    3 Hepatitis
    4 Group B coxsackievirus diseases
    5 Mucocutaneous lymph node syndrome (children)
    6 Human immunodeficiency virus infection (ARC, AIDS)
    7 Q fever (including endocarditis)
    8 Psittacosis
  F Parasitic diseases
    1 Amebiasis
    2 Malaria
    3 Toxoplasmosis
    4 *Pneumocystis carinii* pneumonia
    5 Trichinosis
  G Spirochetal infections
    1 Leptospirosis
    2 Relapsing fever
    3 Lyme Disease
II Neoplasms
  A Solid (localized)
    1 Kidney
    2 Lung
    3 Pancreas
    4 Liver
    5 Large Bowel
    6 Atrial myxoma
  B Metastatic
    1 From gastrointestinal tract
    2 From lung, kidneys, bone, cervix, ovary
    3 Melanoma
    4 Sarcoma
  C Tumors of the reticuloendothelial system
    1 Hodgkin's disease
    2 Non-Hodgkin's lymphoma
    3 Malignant histiocytosis
    4 Immunoblastic lymphadenopathy
    5 Lymphomatoid granulomatosis
III Connective tissue disease
  A Rheumatic fever
  B Systemic lupus erythematosus
  C Rheumatoid arthritis (particularly Still's disease)
  D Giant cell arteritis (polymyalgia rheumatica)
  E Hypersensitivity vasculitis
  F Periarteritis nodosa
  G Wegener's granulomatosis
  H Panaortitis
IV Granulomatous diseases
  A Sarcoidosis
  B Granulomatous hepatitis
  C Crohn's disease (regional enteritis)
  D Erythema nodosum
V Miscellaneous
  A Drug fever
  B Pulmonary emboli
  C Thyroiditis
  D Hemolytic states
  E Cryptic trauma with bleeding into enclosed spaces (hematomas)
  F Dissecting aneurysm
  G Whipple's disease
  H Weber-Christian Disease
VI Metabolic and inherited diseases
  A Familial Mediterranean fever
  B Hypertriglyceridemia and hypercholesterolemia with pancreatitis
  C Fabry's disease
  D Cyclic neutropenia
VII Thermoregulatory disorders
  A Central
    1 Brain tumor
    2 Cerebrovascular accident
    3 Encephalitis
  B Peripheral
    1 Hyperthyroidism
    2 Pheochromocytoma
VIII Psychogenic fevers
  A Factitious fever
  B Habitual hyperthermia
IX Undiagnosed
  A Resolved
    1 Without treatment
    2 With antibiotics
    3 With anti-inflammatory drugs
  B Recurrent
    1 Suppressed with steroids

Cat-scratch fever (see Chap. 98) may run a prolonged course with multiple systems involved. Diagnosis is made by lymph node biopsy.

IATROGENIC INFECTIONS   These include infections of catheters, arteriovenous fistulas, ventricular-peritoneal shunts, and other foreign bodies. Usually their cure requires removal of the infected material as well as antimicrobial therapy. Intravascular graft infection may give rise to prolonged bacteremia and poses a particularly difficult management problem.

GRANULOMATOUS INFECTIONS   Formation of granulomas is characteristic of chronic infection with mycobacteria and of the primary deep mycoses, particularly histoplasmosis and coccidioidomycosis (see Chap. 151). Tuberculosis (see Chap. 125) and atypical mycobacterial infections (see Chap. 127) continue to cause FUO. Reservoirs of tuberculosis exist in patients with a previous contact with an active

case, and the prevalence is higher among blacks, native Americans, southeast Asians, and natives of other countries where tuberculosis is still endemic. Symptomatic progressive disseminated infection due to *Mycobacterium avium-intracellulare* (MAI) is a common complication of AIDS (see Chap. 264) and is seen in other patients on immunosuppressive treatment, particularly in association with high-dose glucocorticoids. Most of these infections are extrapulmonary and may involve the bones, lymph nodes, genital or urinary organs, or the liver. Many of these patients are debilitated and have overwhelming mycobacterial disease. The diagnosis can be established by stain and culture of biopsy material from bone marrow, liver, lymph nodes, or other involved tissues. Granuloma formation does not occur in AIDS patients, and the number of organisms is so high that blood cultures are usually positive. Even with far-advanced disease, patients with tuberculosis may respond well to treatment with bactericidal drugs, in particular isoniazid and rifampin, making the establishment of this diagnosis imperative. In contrast, no effective treatment for progressive MAI infection is available.

VIRAL, RICKETTSIAL, AND CHLAMYDIAL INFECTIONS   Older patients with Epstein-Barr virus (EBV) or cytomegalovirus infection may have prolonged febrile illness without prominent localizing findings (see Chap. 137). Lymphadenopathy, splenomegaly, and evanescent skin rashes are variable findings. Usually atypical lymphocytosis and abnormalities of liver function tests are present. The diagnosis can be made by serology or culture. Patients with HIV infection often have periods of prolonged fever, either as a manifestation of primary infection or later as full-blown AIDS develops (see Chap. 264). While opportunistic infections are usually present in febrile AIDS patients, fever and lymphadenopathy can be manifestations of HIV infection alone.

Mucocutaneous lymph node (Kawasaki) syndrome (see Chaps. 56 or 59) affects children with a prolonged infectious mononucleosis-like illness, including aseptic meningitis and cardiac disease; a viral etiology appears likely. Psittacosis may look much like typhoid fever, and Q-fever endocarditis has been a particularly puzzling and lethal illness that must be treated both with antibiotics and valve replacement. Both infections may be diagnosed serologically, and contacts with birds, sheep, or cattle are important epidemiologic clues.

PARASITIC DISEASES   Amebiasis can present as an FUO either in the form of diffuse hepatitis or, more commonly, as liver abscesses. The diagnosis of malaria is simple when the importance of exposure to endemic areas is considered. Generalized toxoplasmosis may present with prolonged fever and lymphadenopathy. In AIDS patients or those on glucocorticoids, *carinii* pneumonia may cause prolonged fever before cough, dyspnea, hypoxemia, and chest x-ray findings appear (see Chap. 163).

SPIROCHETAL INFECTIONS   Besides relapsing fever caused by *Borrelia*, leptospirosis (see Chap. 130), secondary syphilis (see Chap. 128), and Lyme disease (see Chap. 132) can all have prolonged and occasionally relapsing fever as one of their major manifestations. Clinical suspicion of a characteristic syndrome and serologic methods are central to establishing the diagnosis in the latter three illnesses.

Neoplasms HODGKIN'S DISEASE   Fever may be the principal symptom and only objective finding early in the course of Hodgkin's disease (see Chap. 302), especially as patients with this disease who present with FUO may have only intraabdominal or retroperitoneal disease or involvement of the bone marrow. The diagnosis is usually made by biopsy or staging laparotomy. It is important to arrive at the diagnosis early because, with proper chemotherapy, prolonged remissions and even cure may be achieved.

NON-HODGKIN'S LYMPHOMA   These diseases usually present with fever, nonspecific symptoms, and lymphadenopathy which the patient recognizes. Hepatosplenomegaly, bone pain, and tenderness may be present. Primary lymphomas of the small intestine present with fever and malabsorption. The laboratory findings usually consist of anemia, leukocytosis, and sometimes atypical lymphocytosis leading to confusion with EBV infection. The diagnosis is usually made by lymph node biopsy, but biopsies can be mistaken for reactive hyperplasia or atypical lymphocytic infiltrates. Prolonged remissions can occasionally be achieved with newer chemotherapy regimens (see Chap. 302).

LYMPHOMA-LIKE SYNDROMES   Several disease entities with features similar to Hodgkin's disease have been recognized but may have a better prognosis or respond differently to steroids or antitumor agents. All may present as FUOs and they include immunoblastic lymphadenopathy, lymphomatoid granulomatosis, and acute megakaryocytic myelosis. Rarely, disseminated Kaposi's sarcoma presents with fever as a prominent manifestation. These disorders are discussed more fully in Chaps. 302 and 264.

LEUKEMIAS   It is not uncommon for acute leukemia to be mistaken for acute infection at the onset. High fever [40.6°C (105°F)] and the absence of blast cells in the peripheral blood may delay the diagnosis.

Either neutropenia or neutrophilic leukocytosis may be present, and most patients are anemic. Bone marrow aspiration and biopsy usually reveal the diagnosis (see Chap. 296), although rarely only myeloid dysplasia, a preleukemic syndrome, may be the only finding. In patients with chronic lymphatic or granulocytic leukemia, fever is most often a manifestation of concomitant infection. Similarly, before it is assumed that fever in any patient with leukemia is due to the blood dyscrasia, infection must be ruled out by appropriate tests and cultures, and attempts to treat the "most likely" pathogen must be made, particularly if the patient has neutropenia.

SOLID TUMORS   Fever is not a common occurrence in the vast majority of solid tumors, unless drainage ducts are obstructed and infection has set in or metastases with tumor necrosis have developed. Imaging techniques (ultrasound, CT, MRI) are the most useful in detecting tumor masses, which may be biopsied percutaneously or at laparotomy. Occasionally disseminated carcinomatosis with bone marrow invasion causes leukemoid reactions. Nucleated erythrocytes present in the peripheral blood smear indicate marrow injury; bone marrow biopsy makes the diagnosis. Patients are usually older and the sites of the primary tumor vary widely and include the kidney, pancreas, bowel, liver, lung, and, rarely, the uterus, ovaries, breast, or prostate.

ATRIAL MYXOMA   Patients with fever, changing heart murmurs, peripheral embolic pneumonia, and joint pains are usually suspected of having bacterial endocarditis, rheumatic fever, or occasionally some other connective tissue disease. Most intracardiac tumors are readily detected by two-dimensional echocardiography and the diagnosis should be suspected upon the finding of a pedunculated intraatrial (rarely intraventricular) mass, the occasional presence of calcification associated with negative blood cultures, or serologic tests. MRI and angiography may be needed to confirm the suspicion before surgical removal.

Connective tissue disease RHEUMATIC FEVER   Episodic outbreaks of rheumatic fever still occur in the United States and worldwide. Most victims are young and there will not be a definite history of antecedent sore throat in all patients. Similarly, serologic evidence for recent streptococcal infection may be lacking in 5 to 10 percent of patients. The diagnosis is made on clinical grounds and requires the exclusion of other connective tissue disorders or infectious diseases (see Chap. 101).

SYSTEMIC LUPUS ERYTHEMATOSUS (SLE)   The widespread availability of a variety of serologic tests has simplified the diagnosis of SLE and its variant syndromes (see Chap. 269). These disorders no longer comprise as large a part of FUO series as they once did. Fever can be either a manifestation of active lupus or due to complicating infection, particularly if steroid or cytotoxic immunosuppressive treatment is given. In the face of negative cultures or histologic evidence of infection, high titers of anti double-stranded DNA antibodies, and low serum hemolytic complement, C4 or C3 levels support a diagnosis of active SLE.

RHEUMATOID ARTHRITIS   In its classic form this disease is not difficult to recognize and high titers of serum rheumatoid factor will support the diagnosis. Some patients, usually children or young adults, may present with a seronegative version (Still's disease) in which high fever, hepatosplenomegaly, lymphadenopathy, evanescent rashes, anemia, and leukocytosis are variably present. Joint changes may not appear until late in the disease. The diagnosis is made only after prolonged observation and the exclusion of other diseases. The prognosis is generally good and patients respond well to aspirin, NSAIDs, or steroids. Other arthritis syndromes in which fever may be prominent include ankylosing spondylitis (see Chap. 274), psoriatic arthritis (see Chap. 283), and Lyme disease (see Chap. 132).

OTHER CONNECTIVE TISSUE DISEASES   These include classic periarteritis nodosa and other vasculitic syndromes that involve small and medium-sized arteries as well as the aorta and its main branches. Serologic evidence of infection with hepatitis B virus may be present in some patients but other serologic parameters of autoimmune disease are usually absent (see Chap. 276). Angiography and biopsy can be useful in establishing this diagnosis. Fever in Wegener's granulomatosis is usually due to complicating sinusitis, otitis media, or pulmonary infection. Most patients respond to treatment with steroids and cytotoxic agents.

GIANT CELL ARTERITIS (POLYMYALGIA RHEUMATICA) This is a disease of elderly persons who complain of fever, headache, and pain in the muscles and joints, particularly those of the shoulder girdle. Overt arthritis is rare. At times fever is the only symptom and there are no abnormal physical findings. The sedimentation rate is characteristically very rapid and anemia of chronic disease is present. Dramatic improvement may occur in patients with polymyalgia rheumatica (PMR) with low doses of steroids, which can be used as a therapeutic trial once other disorders are excluded. Patients with classic temporal arteritis may have a PMR syndrome as a prodrome. They may present with additional complaints of visual disturbances or jaw claudication (see Chap. 276). Swelling and tenderness of the cranial arteries are variably present, and temporal artery biopsy in the untreated state usually discloses a granulomatous vasculitis. In contrast to PMR, longer-term treatment with high doses of steroids is indicated in temporal arteritis to induce remission and prevent catastrophic complications such as blindness.

Granulomatous diseases SARCOIDOSIS Ordinarily fever is not characteristic of sarcoidosis but may be prominent in patients with arthritis, hilar lymphadenopathy, and cutaneous lesions of erythema nodosum, or in those with extensive hepatic involvement. The diagnosis is suggested by the youthful age and black race of most patients, mediastinal lymphoid enlargement with interstitial pulmonary infiltrates, and, in rare patients, infiltration of the parotid or lacrimal glands with or without uveitis or a lymphocytic meningitis. Serum angiotensin-converting enzyme activity is often increased (see Chap. 277). Noncaseating granulomas are found on biopsy of the skin, submaximal salivary glands, lymph nodes, or liver. There may be symptomatic improvement with steroid therapy although the natural history appears not to be affected.

GRANULOMATOUS HEPATITIS Patients present with fever, weight loss, variable hepatomegaly, anemia of chronic disease, and elevated alkaline phosphatase, but with relatively normal bilirubin, transaminases, and prothrombin time. Liver biopsy shows noncaseating granulomas, and specific diseases which cause this reaction must be excluded. These include tuberculosis, Hodgkin's disease, histoplasmosis, sarcoidosis, primary biliary cirrhosis, drug reactions, schistosomiasis, and berylliosis, to name only some. The fever generally subsides over a period of weeks to months and can be mitigated with glucocorticoids. In the majority of patients and certainly in all with a positive tuberculin reaction, concomitant treatment with antituberculosis medications should be given until the diagnosis of tuberculosis can be excluded.

ERYTHEMA NODOSUM These tender subcutaneous nodules (see Chap. 58) can appear with fever over extensor surfaces of the extremities as a complication of sarcoidosis, tuberculosis, histoplasmosis, coccidioidomycosis, drug reactions, inflammatory bowel disease, or rarely without precipitating cause.

Miscellaneous causes of fever DRUG FEVER This is an important cause of cryptic fever; a careful history of drug intake should be taken in every patient with unexplained fever. Fever due to allergy to an antibiotic may become superimposed on the fever of the infection for which the drug was given, resulting in a very confusing picture. Common drugs which can cause fever include sulfonamides, penicillins and cephalosporins, barbiturates, antituberculous medications, nitrofurantoin, phenytoin, procainamide, quinidine, phenolphthalein—including laxatives, allopurinol, and thioureas. Fever due to drug allergy must be distinguished from that which is a predictable part of a drug response such as amphotericin-induced fever. Fever in drug allergy may be accompanied by other manifestations of hypersensitivity, including rash, neutropenia, hemolytic anemia, eosinophilia, or thrombocytopenia or it may be the sole manifestation. Any question of drug fever can usually be resolved within several days

by discontinuing all medications. If essential, the diagnosis can be further substantiated by giving a test dose of the drug after fever has subsided, but this may result in a very unpleasant or even dangerous reaction in some patients.

MULTIPLE PULMONARY EMBOLI Symptomless thrombosis of deep calf or pelvic veins may cause prolonged febrile illness either because of thrombophlebitis or as a result of repeated pulmonary emboli. These emboli may not be manifested by pleuritic pain or hemoptysis, but cough, dyspnea, and vague thoracic discomfort are likely to be present. Lung scans, venography, and, if necessary, pulmonary angiography should reveal the diagnosis. Some patients may have nephrotic syndrome due to renal vein thrombosis. Pelvic thrombophlebitis with or without pulmonary emboli is an important cause of FUO in postpartum patients.

HEMOLYTIC EPISODES Most episodes of acute or subacute hemolysis are characterized by bouts of fever and sometimes in acute hemolytic crises by shaking chills and marked temperature elevation. The hemolysis may be due to genetic disorders such as a crisis in sickle cell disease and its variants or to immune mechanisms. Chronic hemolytic disorders, such as spherocytosis or the thalassemias, are not usually associated with fever unless there is complicating infection. Since infection is an important precipitating cause of sickle cell crisis, it must be searched for diligently and if necessary treated presumptively. Besides the appearance of sickled or fragmented erythrocytes on blood smear, the presence of hemolysis will be suggested by the rapid development of anemia without apparent bleeding, reticulocytosis, and indirect hyperbilirubinemia. Evaluation for hemoglobinopathies, glucose-6-phosphate dehydrogenase deficiency, or antibody and/or complement bound to erythrocytes will reveal the diagnosis (see Chap. 61).

CRYPTIC HEMATOMAS Accumulation of old blood in closed spaces, for instance, at sites of remote trauma, particularly in the perisplenic area, the pericardium, or retroperitoneal area, may give rise to prolonged fever. This diagnosis should be thought of in any patient receiving anticoagulants. Evacuation of the clot is usually curative. Fever commonly accompanies intraluminal dissection of the aorta.

FAMILIAL MEDITERRANEAN FEVER (See Chap. 278) This diagnosis should be suspected in patients of Armenian or Mediterranean ancestry who have short-lived episodes of fever accompanied by abdominal or pleuritic chest pain, but without evidence for infection or connective tissue disorder.

THERMOREGULATORY DISORDERS These rare disorders include central disturbances of temperature control in patients with CNS dysfunction caused by encephalitis, stroke, or hemorrhage or with unusual congenital defects affecting the hypothalamus. Such patients may have exaggerated responses in temperature during the course of other fever-producing diseases. The diagnosis is made by exclusion; some patients respond to chlorpromazine. Patients with hyperthyroidism, particularly thyroid storm or pheochromocytoma, may have episodic or sustained temperature elevations due to their hypermetabolic state. Patients taking medications that impair parasympathetic function (phenothiazines, tricyclic antidepressants, anti-Parkinsonian drugs) may develop elevated body temperatures in a warm environment; this may predispose to heat stroke (see Chap. 377).

Psychogenic fever FACTITIOUS FEVER Occasionally patients will produce either false elevations in recorded body temperature or self-administer pyrogenic substances. Typical patient groupings range from children wishing to avoid school, medically sophisticated persons (most often women), with more serious psychopathology, or malingerers with drug-seeking behavior. Clues to false elevations are a dissociation between pulse and temperature, fevers greater than 41.1°C (106°F) in adults, and the absence of chills, sweats, or tachycardia. Repeating the temperature measurement under observation or finding rectal temperatures which are substantially lower than oral will usually reveal the nature of the problem. Pyrogenic substances which may be injected include fecal material, milk or other liquids, and bacterial cultures; an inflammatory response will occur at the injection sites.

Psychopathology ranges from "borderline syndromes" to patients with serious self-mutilating behavior; the prognosis is guarded. Others, mostly young girls, falsify their temperatures as a means of asking for psychiatric help and do well with psychotherapy.

HABITUAL HYPERTHERMIA Some patients may have a body temperature range which is slightly above normal limits without apparent associated physical illness. However, if the patient is past middle age, such elevations should be viewed as indicative of organic disease unless proven otherwise. A special problem termed "habitual hyperthermia" is encountered in young females. The patient may have temperatures ranging from 37.2 to 38.0°C (99.0 to 100.5°F) regularly or intermittently for years and also a variety of complaints characteristic of psychoneurosis such as fatigability, insomnia, asthenia, vague aches, and bowel distress. Some of these individuals may have a variation of the "chronic fatigue syndrome" attributed to EBV infection (see Chap. 137). Prolonged study and observation usually fail to reveal evidence of an organic disease. Unfortunately many of these patients go from physician to physician and are subject to a variety of unpleasant, expensive, and even harmful tests, treatments, and operations. The diagnosis of this syndrome can be made with reasonable certainty after a suitable period of observation and study; if the patient can be convinced of its validity a real service will have been rendered.

Patients with FUO who remain undiagnosed These patients divide themselves into several groups. Some have a self-limited, prolonged viral infection that resembles infectious mononucleosis, cytomegalovirus, or hepatitis, but in which the causative agents are not isolated and the serologic findings are not definitive. They recover spontaneously and completely. Others appear to have responded to antibiotics and can be presumed to have had a cryptic bacterial infection. A third group has a steroid-responsive fever which resembles, but is not diagnostic of, immunologically mediated diseases. Some of these patients eventually no longer require steroids for suppression of fever, but some do not stay free of fever or other inflammatory symptoms without steroids. An occasional elderly patient may display a superannuated form of juvenile rheumatoid arthritis (Still's disease).

DIAGNOSTIC PROCEDURES IN FEVER OF UNKNOWN ORIGIN With so large a number of diagnostic possibilities, it is obvious that no single plan can be outlined for the systematic study of every problem in unexplained fever. In any given patient the history, physical examination, and, most importantly, epidemiologic setting must determine the diagnostic approach. If the features suggest infectious disease, the main dependence will be upon microbiologic methods, while in a person in the "cancer age group" with an obscure febrile disorder, the best chance of an early diagnosis may lie in x-ray studies, scans, and biopsy. Since most infectious diseases are treatable or self-limited these must be excluded first.

History Careful attention to the patient's past history and the chronologic development of symptoms may provide important leads. Places of recent residence, travel, diet, contact with domestic or wild animals and birds, preceding acute infectious diseases such as diarrheal illness or boils, and contact with persons with tuberculosis at any point in life may provide clues to infection. Localizing symptoms may provide a lead to the affected organ system. It is important to query the patient repeatedly. All too often facts of historical importance do not come to light until several interviews have been held.

Physical examination A careful search should be made for skin lesions and for petechial hemorrhages in the ocular fundi, conjunctivae, nail beds, and skin. The lymph nodes should be carefully palpated, with special attention given to the supraclavicular, axillary, and epitrochlear areas. The finding of a heart murmur may be important, particularly if it occurs in diastole. Detection of an abdominal mass may be the first lead to the diagnosis of neoplastic disease. Palpable enlargement of the spleen suggests infection, leukemia, or lymphoma and points away from a diagnosis of solid tumors. Enlargement of the liver and spleen suggests lymphoma, leukemia, chronic infection, or cirrhosis. A large liver without a palpable spleen may point to liver abscess or metastatic cancer. The rectum and the female pelvic organs may reveal masses or abscesses; the testicles may reveal tumor or tuberculosis.

Laboratory tests Patients with FUO are subjected to a large number of laboratory tests, often repeatedly and to excess. The following may be useful guidelines in the use of these tests.

HEMATOLOGY These tests are often abnormal, showing anemia, leukopenia, thrombocytopenia or thrombocytosis, and elevation in the sedimentation rate. They are rarely specific. Blood smears for morphology show many abnormalities but, by virtue of the type of patient who presents with FUO, are rarely diagnostic.

CHEMISTRY Unless specific organ dysfunction is defined, these tests are rarely useful. Tests of liver function can reveal evidence of inflammatory, obstructive, or infiltrative disease, even in the absence of specific symptoms, and are usually indicated.

IMMUNOLOGIC TESTS These are most helpful in the diagnosis of fevers caused by connective tissue disorders or, occasionally, because of secondary immune complex disease or infectious endocarditis.

MICROBIOLOGY In the initial evaluation of prolonged fever, blood cultures are indicated. However, in no instance should more than six blood cultures (which are expensive) be performed on any one patient. Smears and cultures of pus are useful but in sick patients should not delay institution of therapy. Anaerobic cultures of all abscesses should be performed. Mycobacterial cultures continue to be the mainstay in the diagnosis of acid-fast disease. Cultures and special stains or biopsies of suspected tissues are often required to diagnose disseminated fungal infections.

SEROLOGY Serologic testing is useful in Epstein-Barr virus, hepatitis A and B infection, syphilis, Lyme disease, Q fever, and occasionally cytomegalovirus infections and in amebiasis or coccidioidomycosis. Routine febrile agglutinins are rarely helpful but may reveal brucellosis.

SKIN TESTS These are rarely helpful, due to anergy or nonspecificity for acute infection. Many patients with far-advanced neoplasia are anergic. Not all patients with disseminated tuberculosis have positive tuberculin tests. Patients with disseminated histoplasmosis or coccidioidomycosis are usually skin test–negative.

Imaging techniques ROENTGENOGRAMS Chest x-rays and flat abdominal films are the most valuable films in the diagnosis of FUO. Review of earlier films, including those performed at other institutions, often turns up important clues when viewed by a fresh observer. Conversely, there is nothing to be gained by repeating earlier films that are technically satisfactory, provided such films were obtained within a reasonable period of time. Sinus and bone films are often useful. In contrast, gastrointestinal x-rays; intravenous pyelograms; oral intravenous, transhepatic, or retrograde endoscopic cholangiograms; aortograms; and lymphangiograms are helpful only if there are clues that clearly indicate the likelihood of an abnormality in the organ or organ system to be imaged. In many cases, imaging of abdominal and thoracic organs and vessels with CT scan or MRI is preferable to standard radiography.

ULTRASONOGRAPHY This technique is simple and useful to screen for abdominal, renal, retroperitoneal, or pelvic mass lesions. It is probably the method of choice for imaging the gallbladder and bilary tree and can rapidly detect renal obstruction, cardiac valve vegetations, or intracardiac masses.

COMPUTED TOMOGRAPHY SCANS CT scans are very useful in the detection of subphrenic, abdominal, and pelvic abscesses and are the most effective method for imaging the retroperitoneum, which is often the site of the cause of FUO in the form of retroperitoneal lymph nodes, tumors, abscesses, or hematomas. CT scanning is excellent for detecting space-occupying lesions in the liver and is the procedure of choice for suspected intracranial masses. MRI provides the best resolution of tissue planes of differing density and is supplanting CT scanning of the bones, spinal cord, brain, pelvis, and thoracic large vessels or where metal (e.g., surgical clips) creates obscuring artifacts.

RADIONUCLIDE SCANS Ventilation/perfusion lung scans are indicated in suspected pulmonary emboli. Bone scans may detect osseous metastases or osteomyelitis more readily than x-rays. The technetium sulfocolloid liver-spleen scan, while useful in detecting space-occupying lesions of the liver, has been largely replaced by the CT scan. Gallium scanning is subject to many false-positive and false-negative tests and has been overrated. Indium-111 leukocyte scanning may be more reliable in the diagnosis of intraabdominal abscesses, but has also produced false-positive activity in some patients with FUO.

Biopsies Often the best means of definitive diagnosis is a biopsy.

Bone marrow biopsy may be helpful not only in clarifying the histologic nature of the marrow but also for occasional demonstration of other disease processes such as metastatic carcinoma or granulomas and for culture. Bone marrow is one location where blind sampling is productive.

Needle biopsy of the liver, while often abnormal, has a low diagnostic yield. It may be particularly helpful in granulomatous diseases. It rarely yields the diagnosis if there are no abnormalities in liver function tests, ultrasonography, or CT scan.

Biopsies of other tissues that appear abnormal on physical examination or by noninvasive imaging tests are more likely to be helpful in the diagnosis than of tissues that are biopsied blindly. These include biopsies of the lung, muscle, skin, gastrointestinal mucosa, bone, and arteries. The technique of fine-needle aspiration biopsy has made percutaneous approaches safer. Occasionally, "blind biopsies" of muscle or temporal artery will yield abnormalities, but even here tenderness of the affected part makes finding an abnormality much more likely.

Lymph node biopsy is helpful in the diagnosis of many diseases, including the lymphomas, metastatic cancer, tuberculosis, cat-scratch fever, toxoplasmosis, and mycotic infections. Inguinal nodes are notoriously unsatisfactory for biopsy and are too frequently chosen because of their easy accessibility. Axillary, cervical, and supraclavicular nodes are much more likely to yield helpful information, and the node aspirated or excised need not necessarily be large.

Exploratory laparotomy In the past exploratory laparotomy has been advocated as the most definitive diagnostic maneuver in FUO but is valuable only when other investigations, including history, physical examination, noninvasive imaging techniques, and laboratory data point to the abdomen as a possible source of disease. Laparotomies are most helpful in patients with solid tumors, intraabdominal abscesses not amendable to percutaneous biopsy or aspiration, or, rarely, for granulomatous disease or vasculitis. The clues to intraabdominal disease are often subtle, but they are present nonetheless. Blind exploration of the abdomen simply because the diagnosis is obscure is not good practice, and should be discouraged.

Therapeutic trials It is common to give a trial of antibiotics to patients with unidentified febrile disorders. Occasionally, this kind of therapeutic marksmanship is sound, but in general, blind therapy does more harm than good. Undesirable features include drug toxicity, superinfection due to resistant pathogenic bacteria, and interference with accurate diagnosis by cultural methods. Furthermore, a coincidental fall in temperature not due to therapy is likely to be interpreted as response to treatment, with the conclusion that an infectious disease is present. If therapeutic trials are instituted, they should be as specific as possible. Examples are *isoniazid* and *ethambutol* or *rifampin* for tuberculosis; *metronidazole* for hepatic amebiasis; or *aspirin* for rheumatic fever. Relatively few trials with antibiotics will be successful; those with aspirin, NSAIDs, and steroids are more likely to be effective in reducing symptoms, but these drugs should be used with caution and only in patients in whom the likelihood of connective tissue disease is high and in whom granulomas, infection, and cancer have been ruled out as definitively as possible.

Prognosis in FUO The intelligent application of appropriate diagnostic maneuvers should provide the answer in approximately 90 percent of patients with prolonged obscure febrile illness. The mortality rate in patients with FUO is high among elderly patients, particularly since cancer is the most likely cause of the fever in this age group. Fortunately, most of the remaining patients respond to medical or surgical treatment or recover spontaneously. Of those who do come to autopsy (about 10 percent), fewer than half have had potentially curable disease.

A brief philosophy about patients with FUO Many patients are placed in the FUO category because attending physicians overlook, disregard, or reject an obvious clue. This statement implies no malice; it simply means that physicians, being human, are far from perfect. No algorithms or computers are likely to reverse this trend; moreover, even the new technology is not sufficiently sophisticated to sort out the causes of fever in these patients who often present in very atypical fashion.

In order to mitigate these human errors, clinicians have to work harder. This requires repeated histories and physical examinations, frequent chart reviews to look for the "clue" that is there but has not been appreciated, extensive discussion of the problem with colleagues, and last but not least, time spent in quiet contemplation of the clinical enigma. It does not mean yet another barrage of tests, some of which might be painful and all of which are likely to be expensive, or dousing the patient with more drugs, or, in the absence of corroborating data and as a last resort, subjecting the patient to exploratory surgery. Physicians who care for patients with FUO need to observe them, to talk to them, and to think about them. There are no substitutes for these simple clinical principles.

REFERENCES

Pathogenesis of fever

Beutler B, Cerami A: Cachectin: More than a tumor necrosis factor. N Engl J Med 316:379, 1987

Dinarello CA: Biology of interleukin-1. FASEB J 2:108, 1988

——— et al: New concepts in the pathogenesis of fever. Rev Infect Dis 10:168, 1988

Girardin E et al: Tumor necrosis factor and interleukin-1 in the serum of children with severe infectious purpura. N Engl J Med 319:397, 1988

Michie HR et al: Detection of circulating tumor necrosis factor after endotoxin administration. N Engl J Med 318:1481, 1988

Fever of unknown origin

Aduan RP et al: Factitious fever and self-induced infection: A report of 32 cases and review of the literature. Ann Intern Med 90:230, 1979

Datz FL, Thorne DA: Gastrointestinal tract radionuclide activity on In-111 labeled leukocyte imaging: Clinical significance in patients with fever of unknown origin. Radiology 160:635, 1986

Hall S et al: The therapeutic impact of temporal artery biopsy. Lancet ii:1217, 1983

——— et al: Takayasu arteritis: A study of 32 North American patients. Medicine 64:89, 1985

Larson EB: Adult Still's disease. Evolution of a clinical syndrome and diagnosis, treatment and follow-up of 17 patients. Medicine 63:82, 1984

——— et al: Fever of undetermined origin: Diagnosis and follow-up of 105 cases. 1970–1980. Medicine 61:269, 1982

Mackowick PA, LeMaistre CF: Drug fever: A critical appraisal of conventional concepts. Ann Intern Med 106:728, 1987

Margileth D et al: Systemic cat-scratch disease: Report of 23 patients with prolonged or recurrent severe bacterial infection. J Infect Dis 155:390, 1987

Modie MT et al: Vertebral osteomyelitis: Assessment using MR. Radiology 157:157, 1985

Simon HB, Wolff SM: Granulomatous hepatitis and prolonged fever of unknown origin: A study of 13 patients. Medicine 52:1, 1973

Wolff SM et al: Unusual etiologies of fever and their evaluation. Ann Rev Med 26:277, 1975

Fever: Treatment

Chang JC, Gross HM: Utility of naproxen in the differential diagnosis of fever of undetermined origin in patients with cancer. Am J Med 76:597, 1984

section 3   Nervous system dysfunction

21   FAINTNESS, SYNCOPE, AND SEIZURES

JOSEPH B. MARTIN / JERRY RUSKIN[1]

Episodic faintness, light-headedness, and reduced alertness are frequently difficult to distinguish, tending to shade into one another. The difference between faintness and frank syncope is often only quantitative. Types of episodic weakness, such as myasthenia gravis, cataplexy, and familial periodic paralysis, which cause striking reduction of muscular strength but no impairment of consciousness, should be set apart (see Chaps. 366 and 367). Seizures, an important cause of altered consciousness, usually differ from syncope, but in some instances distinguishing the two may be difficult. The features that distinguish seizures from syncope are discussed at the end of this chapter and in Chap. 350.

SYNCOPE AND FAINTNESS

Syncope comprises a generalized weakness of muscles, with loss of postural tone, inability to stand upright, and a loss of consciousness. The term *faintness*, in contrast, refers to lack of strength, with sensation of impending loss of consciousness (*presyncope*). At the beginning of a syncopal attack the patient is nearly always in the upright position, either sitting or standing [the Stokes-Adams attack (see Chap. 184) is exceptional in this respect]. Usually the patient is warned of the impending faint by a sense of "feeling bad." A sense of giddiness and movement or swaying of the floor or surrounding objects ensues. The senses become confused; the patient yawns or gapes, there are spots before the eyes, vision may dim, and the ears may ring. Nausea and sometimes vomiting accompany these symptoms. There is a striking pallor or ashen gray color of the face, and very often the face and body are bathed in cold perspiration. In some patients, a deliberate onset may allow time for protection against injury; in others the occurrence of syncope is sudden and without warning.

The depth and duration of unconsciousness vary. Sometimes the patient is not completely oblivious of the surroundings, or there may be profound coma with complete lack of awareness and of capacity to respond. The patient may remain in this state for seconds to minutes or even as long as half an hour. Usually the patient lies motionless with skeletal muscles relaxed, but a few clonic jerks of the limbs and face may occur shortly after the beginning of the unconsciousness. Sphincter control is usually maintained. The pulse is feeble or cannot be felt; the blood pressure may be low to undetectable; and breathing may be almost imperceptible. Once the patient is in a horizontal position, gravitation no longer hinders the flow of blood to the brain. The strength of the pulse may then improve, color begins to return to the face, breathing becomes quicker and deeper, and consciousness is regained. There is usually an immediate recovery of consciousness. Some patients may, however, be keenly aware of physical weakness, and rising too soon may precipitate another faint. In other patients, particularly those with transient tachyarrhythmias, there may be no residual symptoms

following the initial syncope. Headache and drowsiness, which, with mental confusion, are the usual sequelae of a convulsion, do not follow a syncopal attack.

ETIOLOGY   The list of causes in Table 21-1 is based on established or assumed physiologic mechanisms. The commoner types of faint are reducible to a few simple mechanisms. Syncope results from a sudden impairment of brain metabolism usually brought about by hypotension with reduction of cerebral blood flow.

Several mechanisms subserve circulatory adjustments to the upright posture. Approximately three-fourths of the systemic blood volume is contained in the venous bed, and any interference with venous return may lead to a reduction in cardiac output. Cerebral blood flow may still be maintained, as long as systemic arterial vasoconstriction

---

TABLE 21-1   Causes of recurrent weakness, faintness, and disturbances of consciousness

I Circulatory (reduced cerebral blood flow)
  A Inadequate vasoconstrictor mechanisms
    1 Vasovagal (vasodepressor)
    2 Postural hypotension
    3 Primary autonomic insufficiency
    4 Sympathectomy (pharmacologic, due to antihypertensive medications such as methyldopa and hydralazine, or surgical)
    5 Diseases of central and peripheral nervous systems, including autonomic nerves (Chap. 363)
    6 Carotid sinus syncope (see also "Bradyarrhythmias," below)
    7 Hyperbradykininemia
  B Hypovolemia
    1 Blood loss—gastrointestinal hemorrhage
    2 Addison's disease
  C Mechanical reduction of venous return
    1 Valsalva maneuver
    2 Cough
    3 Micturition
    4 Atrial myxoma, ball valve thrombus
  D Reduced cardiac output
    1 Obstruction to left ventricular outflow: aortic stenosis, hypertrophic subaortic stenosis
    2 Obstruction to pulmonary flow: pulmonic stenosis, primary pulmonary hypertension, pulmonary embolism
    3 Myocardial: massive myocardial infarction with pump failure
    4 Pericardial: cardiac tamponade
  E Arrhythmias (Chaps. 184 and 185)
    1 Bradyarrhythmias
      a Atrioventricular (AV) block (second- and third-degree), with Stokes-Adams attacks
      b Ventricular asystole
      c Sinus bradycardia, sinoatrial block, sinus arrest, sick-sinus syndrome
      d Carotid sinus syncope (see also inadequate vasoconstrictor mechanisms, above)
      e Glossopharyngeal neuralgia (and other painful states)
    2 Tachyarrhythmias
      a Episodic ventricular tachycardia with or without associated bradyarrhythmias
      b Supraventricular tachycardia without AV block
II Other causes of weakness and episodic disturbances of consciousness
  A Altered state of blood to the brain
    1 Hypoxia
    2 Anemia
    3 Diminished carbon dioxide due to hyperventilation (faintness common, syncope seldom occurs)
    4 Hypoglycemia (episodic weakness common, faintness occasional, syncope rare)
  B Cerebral
    1 Cerebrovascular disturbances (cerebral ischemic attacks, see Chap. 351)
      a Extracranial vascular insufficiency (vertebral-basilar, carotid)
      b Diffuse spasm of cerebral arterioles (hypertensive encephalopathy)
    2 Emotional disturbances, anxiety attacks, and hysterical seizures (see Chap. 29)

---

[1] A revision of the chapter by Raymond D. Adams and Joseph B. Martin in the eleventh edition.

occurs; but when this adjustment fails, serious hypotension with resultant cerebral underperfusion to less than half of normal results in syncope. Normally, the pooling of blood in the lower parts of the body is prevented by (1) pressor reflexes which induce constriction of peripheral arterioles and venules, (2) reflex acceleration of the heart by means of aortic and carotid reflexes, and (3) improvement of venous return to the heart by activity of the muscles of the limbs. Placing a normal person on a tilt table to relax the muscles and tilting upright slightly diminishes cardiac output and allows the blood to accumulate in the legs to a slight degree. This may then be followed by a slight transitory fall in systolic arterial pressure and, in patients with defective vasomotor reflexes, may be a means of producing faints.

TYPES OF SYNCOPE Vasovagal (vasodepressor) syncope This syncope is the common faint that may be experienced by normal persons; it is frequently recurrent and tends to take place during emotional stress (especially in a warm, crowded room), after an injurious, shocking accident, and during pain. Mild blood loss, poor physical condition, prolonged bed rest, anemia, fever, organic heart disease, and fasting are other factors which increase the possibility of fainting in susceptible individuals. A short premonitory phase is characterized by nausea, perspiration, yawning, epigastric distress, hyperpnea, tachypnea, weakness, confusion, tachycardia, and pupillary dilatation. Physiologically, there is first a marked fall in arterial pressure and systemic vascular resistance which is most notable in the skeletal muscular beds. Cardiac output may be within normal limits but fails to exhibit the expected increase which normally occurs with hypotension. Output declines when vagal activity leads to marked bradycardia, replacing tachycardia, resulting in further lowering of arterial pressure and reduction of cerebral perfusion. Assumption of the supine posture with elevation of the legs and removal of the offending stimulus will rapidly restore consciousness. While both components of the abnormal reflex (vasodilatation and bradycardia) are active in most patients, in some individuals one component may predominate, accounting for the range of clinical presentations of this syndrome.

Postural hypotension with syncope This type of syncope affects persons who have a chronic defect in, or variable instability of, vasomotor reflexes. The fall in blood pressure on assumption of upright posture is due to a loss of vasoconstriction reflexes in resistance and capacitance vessels of the lower extremities. Though the character of the syncopal attack differs little from that of the vasovagal or vasodepressor type, the effect of posture is its cardinal feature; sudden arising from a recumbent position or standing still are precipitating circumstances.

Postural syncope tends to occur under the following conditions:

1 In otherwise normal persons who for some unknown reason have defective postural reflexes (this may be familial). In such individuals fainting may occur when they are tilted on a table. Under such circumstances it has been found that the blood pressure at first diminishes slightly and then stabilizes at a lower level. Shortly thereafter, the compensatory reflexes suddenly fail and the arterial pressure falls precipitously.

2 In *primary autonomic insufficiency* and in the *dysautonomias*. At least three syndromes have been delineated:

ACUTE OR SUBACUTE DYSAUTONOMIA. In this disease an otherwise healthy adult or child develops over a period of a few days or weeks a partial or complete paralysis of the parasympathetic and sympathetic nervous systems. Pupillary reflexes are lost, as are lacrimation, salivation, and sweating, and there is impotence, paresis of bladder and bowel musculature, and orthostatic hypotension. The CSF protein is increased. Sensory and motor nerve fibers are demonstrably intact, but nonmedullated autonomic ones have degenerated. Recovery occurs within a few months, possibly hastened by prednisone therapy. The disease is believed to represent a variant of acute idiopathic polyneuritis, akin to Guillain-Barré syndrome.

CHRONIC POSTGANGLIONIC AUTONOMIC INSUFFICIENCY. This is a disease of middle-aged and elderly individuals who gradually develop chronic orthostatic hypotension, sometimes in conjunction with impotence and sphincter disturbances. Upon standing for 5 to 10 min, the blood pressure decreases at least 35 mmHg and the pulse pressure narrows, both without increase in pulse rate, pallor, or nausea. Men are more often affected than women. The condition is relatively benign and seemingly irreversible.

CHRONIC PREGANGLIONIC AUTONOMIC INSUFFICIENCY. In this condition orthostatic hypotension with variable anhidrosis, impotence, and sphincter disturbances is combined with a disorder of the central nervous system. The disorders include ① tremor, extrapyramidal rigidity, and akinesia (Shy-Drager syndrome); ② progressive cerebellar degeneration, some instances of which are familial; and ③ a more variable extrapyramidal and cerebellar disorder (striatonigral degeneration). These syndromes lead to disability and often death within a few years. (See Chap. 359.)

The differentiation of the chronic peripheral postganglionic and central preganglionic insufficiency is based on pathologic and pharmacologic evidence. In the postganglionic type, neurons of the sympathetic ganglia degenerate, whereas in the central type, the lateral horn cells of the thoracic spinal cord degenerate. In the postganglionic peripheral type, the resting levels of norepinephrine are subnormal because of failure to release norepinephrine from postganglionic endings, and there is hypersensitivity to injected norepinephrine. In the central type, resting levels of norepinephrine are normal. On standing, unlike the reaction in the normal individual, there is little if any rise in norepinephrine levels in either type. And in both types, the levels of plasma dopamine β-hydroxylase (the enzyme that converts dopamine to norepinephrine) are subnormal.

The distinction between the various types of orthostatic hypotension has therapeutic significance. In the peripheral postganglionic type, the most effective treatment is 9α-fluorohydrocortisone (oral dose 0.1 to 0.2 mg/d) and salt loading to increase blood volume, supplemented by mechanical devices to prevent pooling of blood in the legs and lower trunk (g suit). However, salt together with mineralocorticoids may induce serious supine hypertension, and the dose of the drug must be adjusted for this. For the central preganglionic type, there has been greater success with use of a sympathomimetic amine such as tyramine (which releases norepinephrine from intact postganglionic endings) supplemented by a monoamine oxidase inhibitor (to prevent destruction of the amine), and possibly propranolol. Levodopa has been effective in some cases. In the postganglionic type, judicious use of phenylephrine or ephedrine may be beneficial. Initial reports of the effectiveness of indomethacin in chronic orthostatic hypotension have not been substantiated.

OTHER CAUSES OF POSTURAL SYNCOPE (1) After physical deconditioning, e.g., after prolonged illness with recumbency, especially in elderly individuals with reduced muscle tone. (2) After a sympathectomy that has abolished vasopressor reflexes. (3) In diabetic, alcoholic, and other neuropathies; syringomyelia; and diseases of the nervous system which cause muscular atrophy and paralysis of vasopressor reflexes. The most common form of neurogenic orthostatic hypotension is that which accompanies diseases of the peripheral nervous system. Diabetic polyneuropathy, beriberi, amyloid polyneuropathy, and the Adie syndrome are examples. Usually the orthostatic hypotension is associated with disturbances in sweating, impotence, and sphincter difficulties. Presumably the lesion involves postganglionic, nonmedullated fibers in peripheral nerves. (4) In patients receiving antihypertensive and vasodilator drugs as well as those who may be hypovolemic because of diuretics, excessive sweating, or adrenal insufficiency.

Micturition syncope, a condition usually seen in the elderly during or after urination, particularly after arising from the recumbent position, is probably a special type of postural syncope. It has been suggested that release of intravesicular pressure causes sudden vasodilatation, augmented by standing, and that vagally mediated bradycardia is a contributory factor.

Hyperbradykininemia   Deficient kinin-inactivating enzymes with apparently normal sympathetic function may result in symptoms of faintness or syncope on assumption of upright posture. Hyperbradykininemia causes arteriolar and venular dilatation giving rise to postural hypotension and syncope with tachycardia. The pathophysiology of this condition remains uncertain. Treatment with beta-receptor antagonists has been beneficial.

Syncope of cardiac origin (cardiac syncope)   Cardiac syncope results from a sudden reduction in cardiac output, caused most commonly by a cardiac arrhythmia. In normal individuals slow ventricular rates, but above 35 to 40 beats per minute, and fast ones not exceeding 180 beats per minute do not reduce cerebral blood flow, especially if the person is in the supine position. However, changes in pulse rate outside these limits may impair cerebral circulation and function. Upright posture, cerebrovascular disease, anemia, and coronary, myocardial, or valvular disease all reduce the tolerance to alterations in rate.

High-degree atrioventricular block is one of the commonest arrhythmias that leads to fainting, and syncopal episodes associated with this arrhythmia are known as the Stokes-Adams-Morgagni syndrome. The etiology of disturbances in atrioventricular conduction is considered elsewhere (Chap. 184), but in patients with these attacks the block may be persistent or intermittent and is often preceded or followed by disturbed conduction in one or more of the three fascicles through which the ventricles are normally activated. When the block is high-grade or complete and the pacemaker below the block fails to function, syncope occurs. Stokes-Adams attacks occur usually without more than a momentary sense of weakness, the patient suddenly losing consciousness. After cardiac standstill of more than several seconds, the patient turns pale, falls unconscious, and, as in other types of fainting, may exhibit a few clonic jerks. With longer periods of asystole, the ashen gray pallor gives way to cyanosis, stertorous breathing, fixed pupils, incontinence, and bilateral Babinski signs. While recovery following a Stokes-Adams attack is usually prompt and complete, prolonged confusion and neurologic signs due to cerebral ischemia may occur in some patients, and permanent impairment of mental function may occasionally result, although focal neurologic signs are rare. Cardiac faints of this type may recur several times a day. Commonly the heart block is transitory, and the electrocardiogram taken later may not show any arrhythmia. In some patients, ventricular tachycardia or fibrillation may follow a period of asystole, resulting in syncope or sudden death.

Disorders of sinus node automaticity or sinoatrial conduction may also result in asystole or bradycardia of sufficient severity to cause presyncope or syncope. This disorder is most frequently detected with ambulatory electrocardiographic monitoring. Findings consistent with a diagnosis of sinus node dysfunction include symptomatic sinus pauses (>3 s) resulting from sinus arrest or sinoatrial block and severe unexplained sinus bradycardia (<40 beats per minute). The bradycardia-tachycardia syndrome is a common form of sinus node dysfunction in which syncope generally occurs as a result of marked sinus pauses following termination of paroxysmal supraventricular tachycardia. In occasional patients with syncope and suspected sinus node dysfunction in whom the diagnosis is not established by ambulatory ECG recording, electrophysiologic testing may be helpful in unmasking diagnostic abnormalities.

Recurrent paroxysmal tachyarrhythmias may also cause presyncope and syncope as a result of a sudden reduction in cardiac output. The magnitude of tachycardia-induced hypotension is dependent upon the interaction of several variables including the rate and mechanism of the tachycardia, the type and severity of underlying cardiac disease, the patient's posture and activity level at the onset of the tachycardia, sensitivity of the tachycardia to catecholamines, and the integrity of compensatory autonomic reflexes. Supraventricular tachyarrhythmias are not commonly associated with syncope. However, even in the absence of structural heart disease, the combination of extremely high heart rates and loss of atrial transport may impair cardiac filling and output sufficiently to cause loss of consciousness. These tachy-

cardias result most commonly from the occurrence of paroxysmal atrial flutter, atrial fibrillation, or reentry involving the atrioventricular node or accessory pathways which bypass part or all of the atrioventricular conduction system. Patients with the Wolff-Parkinson-White syndrome are susceptible to several forms of supraventricular tachycardia, the most dangerous of which is atrial fibrillation with rapid antegrade conduction to the ventricles over an accessory atrioventricular connection which may result in syncope and, in rare instances, sudden death. When supraventricular tachycardia is suspected as a cause of syncope, electrophysiologic testing is indicated to define the mechanism and pathway of the tachycardia and to facilitate the selection of an effective antiarrhythmic intervention (see also Chap. 184).

Paroxysmal ventricular tachycardia is a relatively common cause of syncope, particularly in patients with structural heart disease. Typically, the tachycardias are rapid and associated with abrupt loss of consciousness without premonitory symptoms. More often than not, the patient is unaware of palpitations, and recovery following an episode is usually prompt and complete without residual neurologic or cardiac sequelae. The occurrence of unexplained syncope in a patient with structural heart disease is a potentially ominous finding and merits careful evaluation. The presence of pathologic Q waves on the electrocardiogram indicative of a prior transmural myocardial infarction is strongly associated with ventricular tachycardia as a cause of syncope in patients with ischemic heart disease. Other forms of heart disease such as hypertrophic and dilated cardiomyopathy, right ventricular dysplasia, and the long-QT-interval syndromes are also frequently associated with paroxysmal ventricular tachycardia and syncope.

In another form of cardiac syncope the heart block is reflexive and is due to irritation of the vagus nerves. Examples of this phenomenon have been observed in patients with esophageal diverticula, mediastinal tumors, gallbladder disease, carotid sinus disease, glossopharyngeal neuralgia, and pleural and pulmonary irritation. However, in these conditions reflex bradycardia is more commonly of the sinoatrial than the atrioventricular type.

Cardiac syncope may also result from *acute massive myocardial infarction,* particularly when associated with cardiogenic shock. *Aortic stenosis* often sets the stage for exertional syncope, most commonly by limiting cardiac output in the face of peripheral vasodilatation, but sometimes during exertion, with resultant myocardial and cerebral ischemia and occasionally arrhythmias. *Idiopathic hypertrophic subaortic stenosis* may also lead to exertional syncope, because of intensified obstruction and/or ventricular arrhythmias (Chap. 192). In *primary pulmonary hypertension* a relatively fixed cardiac output and bouts of acute right ventricular failure may be associated with syncope (Chap. 191). However, vagal reflexes may be involved in this condition as well as in the syncope that occurs with *pulmonary embolism.* Ball valve thrombus in the left atrium, left atrial myxoma, or thrombosis or malfunction of a prosthetic valve may produce sudden mechanical obstruction of the circulation and syncope. *Tetralogy of Fallot* is the congenital cardiac malformation most commonly responsible for syncope. In this condition systemic vasodilatation, perhaps associated with infundibular spasm, greatly increases the right-to-left shunt and produces arterial hypoxia, which leads to syncope (Chap. 186).

Carotid sinus syncope   The carotid sinus is normally sensitive to stretch and gives rise to sensory impulses carried via the nerve of Hering, a branch of the glossopharyngeal nerve, to the medulla oblongata. Massage of one or both of the carotid sinuses, particularly in elderly persons, causes (1) a reflex cardiac slowing (sinus bradycardia, sinus arrest, or even atrioventricular block), the so-called vagal type of response, and (2) a fall of arterial pressure without cardiac slowing, the so-called depressor type of response. Both types of carotid sinus response may coexist.

Syncope due to carotid sinus sensitivity may be initiated by turning of the head to one side, by a tight collar, or, as in a few reported cases, by shaving over the region of the sinus. Spontaneous attacks may also occur. The attack nearly always begins when the patient is in an upright position, usually when standing. The period of unconsciousness seldom lasts longer than a few minutes. Full consciousness is regained immediately. Most reported cases have been in men. In a patient displaying faintness on compression of one carotid sinus, it is important to distinguish between the benign disorder (hypersensitivity of one carotid sinus) and a much more serious condition—atheromatous narrowing of the opposite carotid or of the basilar artery (see Chap. 351).

Other forms of vasovagal syncope have been described. Exceptionally intense pain of visceral origin may inhibit cardiac action through vagal stimulation, e.g., cardiac standstill during an attack of gallbladder colic, a lesion of the esophagus or mediastinum, bronchoscopy, pleural or peritoneal taps, intense vertigo from labyrinthine or vestibular disease, and needling of body cavities. Occasionally, a patient with a severe migraine attack will sustain a syncopal episode.

Vagal and glossopharyngeal neuralgia Occasionally this induces a reflex type of fainting. Again the sequence is always pain, then syncope; in this instance the pain is localized to the base of the tongue, pharynx or larynx, tonsillar area, and ear. It may be triggered by pressure at these sites. Section of the appropriate branches of the ninth or tenth cranial nerve relieves the condition. The cardiovascular effects are attributable to excitation of the dorsal motor nucleus of the vagus via collateral fibers from the nucleus of the tractus solitarius.

Tussive syncope (laryngeal vertigo) This is a rare condition that results from a paroxysm of coughing, usually in men with chronic bronchitis. After hard coughing the patient suddenly becomes weak and loses consciousness momentarily. The intrathoracic pressure becomes elevated and interferes with the venous return to the heart, as does the Valsalva maneuver (exhaling against a closed glottis).

Syncope associated with cerebrovascular disease This is usually caused by partial or complete occlusion of the large arteries in the neck. Physical activity may then critically reduce blood flow to the upper part of the brainstem, causing abrupt loss of consciousness (see Chap. 351).

PATHOPHYSIOLOGY OF SYNCOPE The loss of consciousness in each type of syncope is caused by reduction of oxygenation to those parts of the brain which subserve consciousness. There are demonstrable reductions in cerebral blood flow, cerebral oxygen utilization, and cerebrovascular resistance. If the ischemia lasts only a few minutes, there are no lasting effects on the brain. Prolonged ischemia may result in necrosis of brain tissue in the border zones of perfusion between the vascular territories of the major cerebral arteries.

In a patient with faintness or syncope attended by bradycardia, one has to distinguish that due to failure of neurogenic reflexes from that due to a cardiogenic (Stokes-Adams) attack. The electrocardiogram is decisive, but even without it, the Stokes-Adams attacks can be recognized clinically by their longer duration, by the greater constancy of the slow heart rate, by the presence of audible sounds synchronous with atrial contractions, by atrial contraction (A) waves in the jugular venous pulse, and by marked variation in intensity of the first sound, despite the regular rhythm (Chap. 184).

DIFFERENTIAL DIAGNOSIS OF CONDITIONS INVOLVING EPISODIC WEAKNESS AND FAINTNESS BUT NOT SYNCOPE
Anxiety attacks and the hyperventilation syndrome These symptoms are discussed in Chaps. 29 and 368. The giddiness of anxiety is frequently interpreted as a feeling of faintness without actual loss of consciousness. Such symptoms are not accompanied by facial pallor and are not relieved by recumbency. The diagnosis is made on the basis of the associated symptoms, and part of the attack can be reproduced by hyperventilation. Two of the mechanisms known to be involved in the attacks are reduction in carbon dioxide as the result of hyperventilation and the release of epinephrine. Hyperventilation results in hypocapnia, alkalosis, increased cerebrovascular resistance, and decreased cerebral blood flow.

Hypoglycemia When severe, hypoglycemia is usually traceable to a serious disease, such as a tumor of the islets of Langerhans or advanced adrenal, pituitary, or hepatic disease, or to excessive administration of insulin. The clinical picture is one of confusion or even a loss of consciousness. When mild, as is usually the case, hypoglycemia is often of the reactive type (Chap. 320), occurring 2 to 5 h after eating, and is not usually associated with a disturbance of consciousness. The diagnosis depends on the history and the documentation of reduced blood sugar during an attack.

Acute hemorrhage Acute hemorrhage, usually within the gastrointestinal tract, is an occasional cause of syncope. In the absence of pain and hematemesis the cause of the weakness, faintness, or even unconsciousness may remain obscure until the passage of a black stool.

Cerebral transient ischemic attacks Such attacks occur in some patients with arteriosclerotic narrowings or occlusion of the major arteries of the brain. The main symptoms vary from patient to patient and include dim vision, hemiparesis or sudden drop attacks, numbness of one side of the body, dizziness, and thick speech. In any one patient all attacks are of identical type and indicate a temporary deficit of function in a certain region of the brain due to inadequate circulation (see Chap. 351).

Hysterical fainting Fainting usually occurs under dramatic circumstances. The attack is unattended by any outward display of anxiety. The evident lack of change in pulse and blood pressure or color of the skin and mucous membranes distinguishes it from the vasodepressor faint. The diagnosis is based on the bizarre nature of the attack in a person who exhibits the general personality and behavioral characteristics of the hysteric.

Type of onset When the attack begins over the period of a few seconds, carotid sinus syncope, postural hypotension, sudden atrioventricular block, asystole, or ventricular tachycardia is likely. When the symptoms develop gradually during a period of several minutes, hyperventilation or hypoglycemia should be considered. Onset of syncope during or immediately after exertion suggests aortic stenosis, idiopathic hypertrophic subaortic stenosis or excessive bradycardia, and, in elderly subjects, postural hypotension. Exertional syncope is seen occasionally in persons with aortic insufficiency and with severe occlusive disease of cerebral arteries. In patients with ventricular standstill or ventricular fibrillation, loss of consciousness occurs several seconds later, followed rapidly by cessation of electroencephalographic activity and then often by brief clonic muscle contractions.

Position at onset of attack Epilepsy and syncopal attacks due to hypoglycemia, hyperventilation, or heart block are likely to be independent of posture. Faintness associated with a decline in blood pressure (including carotid sinus attacks) and with ectopic tachycardia usually occurs only in the sitting or standing position, whereas faintness resulting from orthostatic hypotension is apt to set in shortly after change from the recumbent to the standing position.

Associated symptoms Symptoms such as palpitation may be present when the attack is due to anxiety or hyperventilation, to ectopic tachycardia, or to hypoglycemia. Numbness and tingling in the hands and face are frequent accompaniments of hyperventilation. Genuine convulsions during the attack may occasionally occur with heart block, asystole, or ventricular tachycardia. When *duration of attack* is very brief, i.e., a few seconds to a few minutes, carotid sinus syncope or one of the several forms of postural hypotension is most likely. A duration of more than a few minutes but less than an hour suggests hypoglycemia or hyperventilation.

SPECIAL METHODS OF EXAMINATION In many patients who complain of recurrent weakness or syncope but who do not have a spontaneous attack while under observation, an attempt to reproduce attacks is of great assistance in diagnosis.

When hyperventilation is accompanied by faintness, the pattern of symptoms can be reproduced readily by having the subject breathe rapidly and deeply for 2 to 3 min. This test is often of therapeutic value also, because the underlying anxiety tends to be lessened when the patient learns that the symptoms can be produced and alleviated at will simply by controlling breathing.

Among other conditions in which the diagnosis is commonly clarified by reproducing the attacks are carotid sinus hypersensitivity (massage of one or the other carotid sinus), orthostatic hypotension and orthostatic tachycardia (observations of pulse rate, blood pressure, and symptoms in the recumbent and standing positions), and tussive syncope (by inducing the Valsalva maneuver). In all these instances the crucial point is not whether symptoms are produced (the procedures mentioned frequently induce symptoms in healthy persons) but whether the exact pattern of symptoms that occurs in the spontaneous attacks is reproduced in the artificial ones. Continuous ambulatory electrocardiographic monitoring may be extremely useful in identifying an arrhythmia responsible for the syncopal episode, particularly in patients with frequently recurring symptoms. Monitoring is most helpful if it shows that the syncopal episode is characterized by a bout of asystole, extreme bradycardia, or tachyarrhythmia.

In cases of recurrent syncope of unknown cause in which ambulatory ECG monitoring is unrevealing, the use of intracardiac electrophysiologic techniques with programmed stimulation can be helpful in detecting cardiac rhythm abnormalities and in establishing effective treatment. During stimulation, up to two-thirds of such patients can be shown to have rapid ventricular tachycardia, His bundle conduction delays, atrial flutter, sick-sinus syndrome, or hypervagotonia. The technique is particularly useful in patients with ischemic heart disease and prior myocardial infarction, a common clinical setting for recurrent ventricular tachycardia. The diagnostic yield of electrophysiologic testing is lower with patients with nonischemic heart disease and patients with structurally normal hearts than with patients with ischemic heart disease. Recently the signal-averaged surface electrocardiogram has proved to be useful in identifying patients with unexplained syncope who are likely to have ventricular tachycardia induced by electrophysiologic study.

Head-up tilt testing is a useful provocative technique for the diagnosis of vasodepressor syncope. Upright tilt to a maximum of 60 to 70° usually precipitates symptomatic hypotension or syncope within 10 to 30 min in patients with this syndrome. In normal subjects, passive tilting to 60° causes a small decrease in systolic blood pressure and an increase in diastolic blood pressure and heart rate. Recently, tilt testing has been used in conjunction with electrophysiologic testing to assess the efficacy of prophylactic pacing in selected patients with vasodepressor syncope and to evaluate the impact of posture on the hemodynamic consequences of some tachyarrhythmias.

The electroencephalogram may be helpful in differentiating syncope from seizures. In the interval between epileptic seizures it may show some degree of abnormality in 40 to 80 percent of cases. In the interval between syncopal attacks it should be normal.

TREATMENT   In most instances fainting is relatively benign. In dealing with patients who have fainted, the physician should think first of those causes of fainting that constitute a therapeutic emergency. Among them are massive internal hemorrhage and myocardial infarction, which may be painless, and cardiac arrhythmias. In elderly persons a sudden faint, without obvious cause, should arouse the suspicion of complete heart block or a tachyarrhythmia, even though all findings are negative when the patient is seen.

Patients seen during the preliminary stages of fainting or after they have lost consciousness should be placed in a position which permits maximal cerebral blood flow, i.e., with head lowered between the knees, if sitting, or in the supine position. All tight clothing and other constrictions should be loosened and the head turned so that the tongue does not fall back into the throat, blocking the airway. Peripheral irritation, such as sprinkling or dashing cold water on the face and neck or the application of cold moist towels, is helpful. If the temperature is subnormal, the body should be covered with a warm blanket. Since emesis is frequent, aspiration should be prevented. The head should be turned to the side and nothing given by mouth until the patient has regained consciousness. Patients should not be permitted to rise until the sense of physical weakness has passed and should be watched carefully for a few minutes after rising.

The *prevention* of fainting depends on the mechanisms involved. In the usual vasovagal faint of adolescents, which tends to occur in periods of emotional excitement, fatigue, hunger, etc., it is enough to advise the patient to avoid such circumstances. In postural hypotension, patients should be cautioned against arising suddenly from bed. Instead, they should first exercise their legs for a few seconds, then sit on the edge of the bed and make sure they are not light-headed or dizzy before starting to walk. Sleeping with the headposts of the bed elevated on wooden blocks 8 to 12 in high and wearing a snug elastic abdominal binder and elastic stockings are often helpful. Drugs of the ephedrine group may be useful if they do not cause insomnia. If there are no contraindications, a high intake of sodium chloride, which expands the extracellular fluid volume, may be beneficial.

In the syndrome of chronic orthostatic hypotension, special mineralocorticoid preparations (fludrocortisone acetate tablets, 0.1 to 0.2 mg/d in divided doses) have given relief in some cases. Binding of the legs (g suit) and sleeping with head and shoulders elevated are helpful.

The treatment of carotid sinus syncope involves first of all instructing the patient in measures that minimize the hazards of a fall (see below). Loose collars should be worn, and the patient should learn to turn the whole body, rather than the head alone, when looking to one side. Atropine or the ephedrine group of drugs should be used, respectively, in patients with pronounced bradycardia or hypotension during attacks. If atropine is not successful, a demand pacemaker should be inserted into the right ventricle. Radiation or surgical denervation of the carotid sinus has apparently yielded favorable results in some patients, but it is rarely necessary. Once it has been concluded that the attacks are due to a narrowing of major cerebral arteries, some of the surgical measures discussed in Chap. 351 must be considered.

The treatment of the various cardiac arrhythmias which may induce syncope is discussed in Chap. 184. The treatment of hypoglycemia is found in Chap. 320.

The chief hazard of a faint in most elderly persons is not the underlying disease but fracture or other trauma due to the fall. Therefore, patients subject to recurrent syncope should cover the bathroom floor and bathtub with rubber mats and should have as much of their home carpeted as is feasible. Especially important is the floor space between the bed and the bathroom, because faints are common in elderly persons when walking from bed to toilet. Outdoor walking should be on soft ground rather than hard surfaces, and the patient should avoid standing still, which is more likely than walking to induce an attack.

SEIZURES

A brain seizure or convulsion is defined as an abrupt alteration in cortical electrical activity manifested clinically by a change in consciousness or by a motor, sensory, or behavioral symptom. Seizures, which may be due to a variety of causes, become important in the differential diagnosis of syncope when the episode occurs with minimal or no warning and results in only a brief loss of consciousness. *Epilepsy* (discussed in Chap. 350) is the term used to describe recurrent seizures present over months or years, often with a stereotyped clinical pattern.

CLINICAL CHARACTERISTICS OF SEIZURES   A detailed account of the types of seizures, of their pathophysiology, and of their treatment is found in Chap. 350. The purpose here is to recount briefly the varieties of seizures that occur (Table 21-2), and to outline their clinical presentation, particularly with respect to their distinction from syncope. A single seizure may occur during the course of many medical illnesses; its importance derives from the fact that it signifies involvement of the central nervous system by the disease process.

Partial seizures (focal seizures)   The appearance of focal motor or sensory manifestations provides clinical documentation of the localization of the cerebral lesion. Deviation of the eyes and head to

---

TABLE 21-2 Classification of seizures

I Partial or focal seizures
   A Simple partial seizures (with motor, sensory, autonomic, or psychic signs)
   B Complex partial seizures (psychomotor or temporal lobe seizures)
   C Secondary generalized partial seizures
II Primary generalized seizures
   A Tonic clonic (grand mal)
   B Absence (petit mal)
   C Myoclonic
   D Atonic or akinetic

---

one side (aversive seizure) usually points to an irritative focus in the opposite prefrontal region. A Jacksonian seizure begins as a clonic movement in one portion of the body, often the thumb, the corner of the mouth, or the great toe, and spreads to adjacent muscular groups over a few seconds or minutes. The seizure may progress to involve the entire side or become generalized with attendant loss of consciousness. Jacksonian seizures almost always are accompanied by an abnormal interictal EEG.

Complex partial seizures (temporal lobe or psychomotor seizures) These differ from generalized motor seizures by (1) the frequent occurrence of an aura that arises from discharges in the autonomic, visceral, and olfactory portions of the temporal lobe and limbic system; and (2) the loss of awareness or contact with the environment, often associated with behavioral or complex motor movements for which the patient is amnesic after the attack. Subjective experiences of the aura include hallucinations (olfactory, gustatory, visual, or auditory), illusions (spatial distortions, shrinkage, or angulation), aberrations in cognition (déjà vu, a sense of familiarity; jamais vu, a sense of unfamiliarity; or recurrent memory), and affective changes (anxiety, fear, and, very rarely, rage). The seizure may terminate with only the subjective component or may progress to the motor phase which is often evident by repetitive motor acts like smacking the lips, swallowing, undressing, and incoherent or dysphasic speech.

The abrupt onset of complex partial seizures often indicates a disorder of the temporal lobe and its connection to the limbic system. Complete investigation in search of the cause is indicated.

Tonic-clonic (grand mal) seizure The abrupt presentation, without warning, of a generalized motor seizure is one of the commonest indications of involvement of the cerebral cortex by a disease process. Grand mal seizures usually begin with opening of the eyes and mouth, flexion and abduction of the arms, and extension of the legs. The *tonic* phase of the seizure is often heralded by contraction of the respiratory muscles resulting in a vocalization. These motor signs are followed by closure of the jaw, often with laceration of the tongue, respiratory arrest with plethora and cyanosis, and urinary, or less commonly, fecal incontinence. The tonic phase of the seizure, which usually persists for only 15 to 30 s, is followed immediately by the *clonic* phase, characterized by violent rhythmic muscular contractions affecting the whole body including the muscles of respiration. Eye movements, facial grimacing, and persistence of respiratory apnea are evident. The clonic movements subside in amplitude and frequency, and the seizure terminates, usually within 1 to 2 min. Normal respiration resumes and the patient falls asleep; arousal may occur in a few minutes but lethargy, fatigue, and postseizure (postictal) confusion are common and may persist for several hours. Postictal headache is also common.

The generalized seizure occurring in the course of a major medical illness signifies involvement of the central nervous system by the disorder and requires careful assessment and investigation. Such a seizure may accompany high fever, hyponatremia, metabolic acidosis, alcohol or drug withdrawal, and renal or liver failure, indicating the presence of a *metabolic encephalopathy*, without requiring the postulation of another separate neurologic illness. The determination that a metabolic encephalopathy may be responsible is dependent upon documentation of the systemic illness and careful attention to

the exclusion of an additional infectious, vascular, or neoplastic lesion in the nervous system. Central nervous system evaluation should include a careful history, a detailed neurologic examination searching for focal neurologic deficit, and, in many cases, electroencephalography and computed tomography (CT) scan. If infection is suspected, an examination of the cerebrospinal fluid is mandatory. Recurrent seizures (status epilepticus) indicate a serious compromise of cerebral cortical function and require vigorous treatment to prevent hypoxic damage to the brain and, following termination of the seizures, a thorough investigation of the cause.

An isolated generalized seizure occurring in an otherwise healthy, asymptomatic patient when observed by family or other bystanders is not difficult to distinguish from syncope. More difficult to assess is the circumstance of sudden loss of consciousness occurring without warning and unwitnessed by an observer or an akinetic "drop-seizure" (atypical petit mal). The latter may be indistinguishable from syncope. Postictal confusion or drowsiness, injury such as laceration of the tongue, urinary or fecal incontinence, or muscle soreness suggests that a convulsion has occurred. One common clinical presentation is the sudden occurrence of a brief clonic seizure during a minor surgical or dental procedure. The patient is usually in a seated position and the episode is considered to be due to cerebral ischemia associated with systemic hypotension and bradycardia accompanying vasovagal syncope. There are usually only two or three clonic movements, without a prior tonic phase, and recovery is rapid without postictal symptoms. Such patients should have a neurologic examination and an EEG and, if these are normal, be treated with reassurance and not given anticonvulsants. There is no evidence to indicate an underlying cerebral lesion in such patients.

Generalized seizures may be preceded by a specific warning or *aura,* and attention to these symptoms may be important in aiding in the localization of the seizure focus and can assist in distinguishing the episode from syncope. Tingling or numbness points to involvement of the parietal lobe, and visual or auditory sensations suggest occipitotemporal localization. More complex psychological and cognitive sensations may accompany temporal lobe seizures and also transient cerebral ischemic attacks (see Chap. 351), but in the latter symptoms usually persist for many minutes or hours.

Absence (petit mal) seizures Absence seizures, in contrast to grand mal, are noted for their brevity and for the degree of loss of awareness accompanied by minimal motor manifestations. They are abrupt in onset and are often evident only by a stare or cessation of ongoing behavior; they may be accompanied by fluttering of the eyelids or by a few facial twitches. Full recovery occurs in 5 to 10 s, and the episode may go unnoticed by the patient, the family, or the teacher. Loss of postural tone (atonic or akinetic seizure) with falling is uncommon but when present requires distinction from syncope. The EEG is diagnostic in such cases, consisting of three-per-second spike and wave discharges. This condition, which indicates a specific generalized disorder of cerebral electrical activity, is responsive to specific drug treatments (see Chap. 350).

DIFFERENTIAL DIAGNOSIS OF SEIZURES AND SYNCOPE
Syncope must be distinguished from disturbances of cerebral function, caused by a seizure. A seizure may occur day or night, regardless of the position of the patient; syncope rarely appears when the patient is recumbent, the only common exception being the Stokes-Adams attack. The patient's color may not change in seizures, though there may be cyanosis; pallor is an early and invariable finding in all types of syncope, except chronic orthostatic hypotension and hysteria, and it precedes unconsciousness. Seizures are often heralded by an aura, which is caused by a focal seizure discharge and hence has brain localizing significance. It is usually followed by rapid return to normal or by loss of consciousness. The onset of syncope is usually more deliberate and without aura. Injury from falling is frequent in a seizure and rare in syncope, for the reason that only in seizures are protective reflexes abolished instantaneously. Tonic-convulsive movements with upturning eyes are a feature of seizures and usually do not occur with syncope, although, as stated above, brief tonic clonic

seizure-like activity can accompany fainting episodes. The period of unconsciousness tends to be longer in seizures than in syncope. Urinary incontinence is frequent in seizures and rare in syncope. The return of consciousness is prompt in syncope, slow after a seizure. Mental confusion, headache, and drowsiness are common sequelae of seizures; physical weakness with a clear sensorium characterizes the postsyncopal state. Repeated spells of unconsciousness in a young person at a rate of several per day or month are more suggestive of epilepsy than of syncope. No one of these points will absolutely differentiate a seizure from syncope, but taken as a group and supplemented by electroencephalograms, they provide a means of distinguishing the two conditions.

REFERENCES

ALMQUIST A et al: Provocation of bradycardia and hypotension by isoproterenol and upright posture in patients with unexplained syncope. N Engl J Med 320:346, 1989

CHEN MY et al: Cardiac electrophysiologic and hemodynamic correlates of neurally mediated syncope. Am J Cardiol 63:66, 1989

DAY SC: et al: Evaluation and outcome of emergency room patients with transient loss of consciousness. Am J Med 73:15, 1982

DELGADO-ESCUETA AV et al: The treatable epilepsies (2 parts). N Engl J Med 308:1508 and 1576, 1983

DIMARCO JP et al: Approach to the patient with syncope of unknown cause. Mod Concepts Cardiovasc Dis 52:11, 1983

EAGLE KA et al: Evaluation of prognostic classifications for patients with syncope. Am J Med 79:455, 1985

ECTOR H et al: Bradycardia, ventricular pauses, syncope, and sports. Lancet 1:591, 1984

EWING DJ et al: The natural history of diabetic autonomic neuropathy. Q J Med 49:95, 1980

HICKLER R: Fainting, in Signs and Symptoms, 6th ed, RS Blacklow (ed). Philadelphia, Lippincott, 1977, chap 33

JOHNSON RH, SPAULDING JMK: Disorders of the Autonomic Nervous System. Philadelphia, Davis, 1974

KAPOOR WN et al: Diagnostic and prognostic implications of recurrences in patients with syncope. Am J Med 83:700, 1987

——— et al: A prospective evaluation and follow-up of patients with syncope. N Engl J Med 309:197, 1983

KENNY RA et al: Head-up tilt: A useful test for investigating unexplained syncope. Lancet 11:1352, 1986

LEE JE et al: Episodic unconsciousness, in Diagnostic Approaches to Presenting Syndromes, JA Barondess (ed). Baltimore, Williams & Wilkins, 1971, pp 133–167

MCLEOD JG, TUCK RR: Disorders of the autonomic nervous system. 1. Pathophysiology and clinical features. Ann Neurol 21:419, 1987

———, ———: Disorders of the autonomic nervous system. 2. Investigation and treatment. Ann Neurol 21:519, 1987

POLINSKY RJ et al: Pharmacologic distinction of different orthostatic hypotension syndromes. Neurology 31:1, 1981

RICHARDS AM et al: Syncope in aortic valvular stenosis. Lancet 1:1113, 1984

SILVERSTEIN MD et al: Patients with syncope admitted to medical intensive care units. JAMA 248:1185, 1982

STREETER DHP et al: Hyperbradykininism: A new orthostatic syndrome. Lancet 2:1048, 1972

SUTHERLAND JM, EADIE MJ: The Epilepsies, 3d ed. Edinburgh, Churchill Livingstone, 1980

WEISSLER AM, WARREN, JV: Syncope and shock, in The Heart, 4th ed, JW Hurst et al (eds). New York, McGraw-Hill, 1978, p 705

WINTERS SL et al: Signal averaging of the surface QRS complex predicts inducibility of ventricular tachycardia in patients with syncope of unknown origin: A prospective study. J Am Coll Cardiol 10:775, 1987

WRIGHT KE JR, MCINTOSH MD: Syncope: Review of pathophysiological mechanisms. Prog Cardiovasc Dis 13:580, 1971

YOUNG RR et al: Pure pandysautonomia with recovery. Description and discussion of diagnostic criteria. Brain 98:613, 1975

22 DIZZINESS AND VERTIGO

ROBERT B. DAROFF

Dizziness is a common and often vexing symptom. Patients use the term to encompass a variety of sensations including those that seem semantically appropriate (e.g., lightheadedness, fainting, spinning, giddiness, etc.) and those that are seemingly inappropriate, such as confusion, blurred vision, headache, tingling, "walking on cotton,"

etc. Moreover, some patients with gait disturbances, and no abnormal cephalic sensations, will describe their problem as "dizziness." A careful history is necessary to determine exactly what a patient who states, "Doctor, I'm dizzy," is experiencing.

After eliminating misleading symptoms such as confusion, "dizziness" usually means either *faintness* (analogous to the feelings that precede syncope) or *vertigo* (an illusory or hallucinatory sense of environmental or self-movement). In other instances, neither of these terms accurately describes a patient's symptoms, and the explanation may only become apparent when the neurologic examination reveals spasticity, parkinsonism, or other ambulation disturbances as the cause of the complaint. Operationally, dizziness is classified into four categories: (1) faintness, (2) vertigo, (3) miscellaneous head sensations, and (4) gait disturbances.

FAINTNESS Fainting (syncope) is a loss of consciousness secondary to cerebral ischemia, more specifically ischemia to the brainstem (see Chap. 21). Prior to the actual faint, there are often prodromal symptoms (*faintness*) reflecting ischemia to a degree insufficient to impair consciousness. The sequence of symptoms is reasonably stereotyped and includes increasing lightheadedness, visual blurring proceeding to blindness, and heaviness in the lower limbs progressing to postural sway. The symptoms increase in severity until consciousness is lost or the ischemia is corrected, often by assumption of the recumbent position. True vertigo almost never occurs during the presyncopal state.

The causes of faintness are described in Chap. 21 and include the multiple etiologies of decreased cardiac output, postural (orthostatic) hypotension, and mimics such as vertebrobasilar insufficiency and seizures.

VERTIGO Vertigo is a hallucination of self- or environmental movement, most commonly a feeling of spinning, usually due to a disturbance in the vestibular system. The end organs of this system, situated in the bony labyrinths of the inner ears, consist of the three semicircular canals and the otolithic apparatus (utricle and saccule) on each side. The canals transduce angular acceleration while the otoliths transduce linear acceleration and static gravitational forces, the latter providing a sense of head position in space. The neural output of the end organs is conveyed to the vestibular nuclei in the brainstem via the eighth cranial nerves. The principal projections from the vestibular nuclei are to the nuclei of cranial nerves III, IV, and VI, the spinal cord, cerebral cortex, and cerebellum. The vestibuloocular reflex (VOR) serves to maintain visual stability during head movement and depends upon direct projections from the vestibular nuclei to the sixth cranial nerve (abducens) nuclei in the pons and, via the medial longitudinal fasciculus, to the third (oculomotor) and fourth (trochlear) cranial nerve nuclei in the midbrain. These connections account for the nystagmus (to-and-fro oscillation of the eyes) which is an almost invariable accompaniment of vestibular dysfunction. The vestibulospinal pathways assist in the maintenance of postural stability. Projections to the cerebral cortex, via the thalamus, provide conscious awareness of head position and movement. The vestibular nerves and nuclei project to areas of the cerebellum (primarily the flocculus and nodulus) which modulate the VOR.

The vestibular system is one of three sensory systems subserving spatial orientation and posture; the other two are the visual system (retina to occipital cortex) and the somatosensory system that conveys peripheral information from skin, joint, and muscle receptors. The three stabilizing systems overlap sufficiently to compensate (partially or completely) for each other's deficiencies. Vertigo may represent either physiologic stimulation or pathologic dysfunction in any of the three systems.

Physiologic vertigo This occurs when (1) the brain is confronted with a mismatch among the three stabilizing sensory systems or (2) the vestibular system is subjected to unfamiliar head movements to which it has never adapted, such as in seasickness. Intersensory mismatch explains carsickness, height vertigo, and the visual vertigo most commonly experienced during motion picture chase scenes; in the latter the visual sensation of environmental movement is unaccompanied by concomitant vestibular and somatosensory movement cues. *Space sickness*, a frequent transient effect of active head movement in the weightless zero-gravity environment, is another example of physiologic vertigo.

Pathologic vertigo This results from lesions of the visual, somatosensory, or vestibular systems. Visual vertigo is caused by new or incorrect spectacles or by the sudden onset of an extraocular muscle paresis with diplopia; in either instance, central nervous system compensation rapidly counteracts the vertigo. Somatosensory vertigo, rare in isolation, is usually due to a peripheral neuropathy which reduces the sensory input necessary for central compensation when there is dysfunction of the vestibular or visual systems.

The most common cause of pathologic vertigo is vestibular dysfunction. The vertigo is frequently accompanied by nausea, jerk nystagmus, postural unsteadiness, and gait ataxia.

LABYRINTHINE DYSFUNCTION This causes severe rotational or linear vertigo with the hallucination of movement, whether of environment or self, directed away from the side of the lesion. The fast phases of nystagmus beat away from the lesion side, and the tendency to fall is toward the side of the lesion.

When the head is straight and immobile, the vestibular end organs generate a tonic resting firing frequency which is equal from the two sides. With any rotational acceleration, the anatomic positions of the semicircular canals on each side necessitate an increased firing rate from one and a commensurate decrease from the other. This change in neural activity is ultimately projected to the cerebral cortex where it is summed with inputs from the visual and somatosensory systems to produce the appropriate conscious sense of rotational movement. The end organs' response to deceleration continues for some time after cessation of prolonged rotation. The side with the initially increased firing rate decreases that rate below the steady state level and the other side increases it. A sense of rotation in the opposite direction is experienced; since there is no actual head movement, this hallucinatory sensation is *vertigo*. Any disease state that changes the firing frequency of an end organ, producing unequal neural input to the brainstem and ultimately the cerebral cortex, causes vertigo. The symptom can be conceptualized as the cortex inappropriately interpreting the abnormal neural input from the brainstem as indicating actual head rotation. Transient deficits produce short-lived symptoms. With a fixed unilateral deficit, central compensatory mechanisms ultimately diminish the vertigo. Since compensation depends upon the plasticity of connections between the vestibular nuclei and cerebellum, patients with brainstem or cerebellar disease have diminished adaptive capacity and symptoms may persist indefinitely. Compensation is always inadequate for severe fixed bilateral lesions despite normal cerebellar connections; these patients are symptomatic indefinitely.

Acute unilateral labyrinthine dysfunction is caused by infection, trauma, ischemia, and toxins (usually drugs or alcohol). Often, no specific etiology is uncovered and the nonspecific term *acute labyrinthitis* or, preferably, *acute peripheral vestibulopathy* is used to describe the event. It is impossible to determine whether a patient recovering from the first bout of vertigo will have recurrent episodes.

Schwannomas involving the eighth cranial nerve (*acoustic neuroma*) grow slowly and produce such a gradual reduction of labyrinthine output that central compensatory mechanisms usually prevent or minimize the vertigo; auditory symptoms of hearing loss and tinnitus are the most common manifestations. While lesions of the brainstem or cerebellum can cause acute vertigo, associated signs and symptoms permit distinction from a labyrinthine etiology (Table 22-1). Rarely, an acute lesion of the vestibulocerebellum may present with monosymptomatic vertigo indistinguishable from a labyrinthopathy.

Recurrent unilateral labyrinthine dysfunction, in association with signs and symptoms of cochlear disease (progressive hearing loss and tinnitus), is usually due to Ménière's disease. When auditory manifestations are absent, the term *vestibular neuronitis* denotes recurrent

TABLE 22-1 Differentiation of peripheral and central vertigo

Sign or symptom	Peripheral (labyrinth)	Central (brainstem or cerebellum)
Direction of associated nystagmus	Unidirectional; fast phase opposite lesion*	Bidirectional or unidirectional
Purely horizontal nystagmus without torsional component	Uncommon	Common
Vertical or purely torsional nystagmus	Never present	May be present
Visual fixation	Inhibits nystagmus and vertigo	No inhibition
Severity of vertigo	Marked	Often mild
Direction of spin	Toward fast phase	Variable
Direction of fall	Toward slow phase	Variable
Duration of symptoms	Finite (minutes, days, weeks) but recurrent	May be chronic
Tinnitus and/or deafness	Often present	Usually absent
Associated central abnormalities	None	Extremely common
Common causes	Infection (labyrinthitis), Ménière's, neuronitis, ischemia, trauma, toxin	Vascular or demyelinating disease, neoplasm, trauma

* In Ménière's disease, the fast phase is variable in direction.

monosymptomatic vertigo. Transient ischemic attacks of the posterior cerebral circulation (vertebrobasilar insufficiency) almost never cause recurrent vertigo without concomitant motor, sensory, cranial nerve, or cerebellar signs.

Positional vertigo is precipitated by a recumbent head position, either to the right or to the left. Benign paroxysmal positional vertigo (BPPV) is particularly common. Although the condition may be due to head trauma, usually no precipitating factors are identified. It generally abates spontaneously after weeks or months. The vertigo and accompanying nystagmus have a distinct pattern of latency, fatigability, and habituation that differs from the less common central positional vertigo (Table 22-2) due to lesions in and around the fourth ventricle. Moreover, the pattern of nystagmus in BPPV is often distinctive. The lower eye displays a large-amplitude torsional nystagmus, and the upper eye has a lesser degree of torsion combined with upbeating nystagmus. If the eyes are directed to the upper ear, the vertical nystagmus in the upper eye increases in amplitude.

Position*al* must be distinguished from position*ing* vertigo. The latter is provoked by head movement rather than head position and is an invariable feature of *all* vestibulopathies, central or peripheral. Since vertigo increases with quick head movements, patients tend to hold their heads still.

Vestibular epilepsy, vertigo secondary to temporal lobe epileptic activity, is rare, and almost always intermixed with other epileptic manifestations.

Psychogenic vertigo, usually a concomitant of agoraphobia (fear

TABLE 22-2 Benign paroxysmal positional (BPPV) and central positional vertigo

Features	BPPV	Central
Latency*	3–40 s	None: immediate vertigo and nystagmus
Fatigability†	Yes	No
Habituation‡	Yes	No
Intensity of vertigo	Severe	Mild
Reproducibility§	Variable	Good

* Time between attaining head position and onset of symptoms.
† Disappearance of symptoms with maintenance of offending position.
‡ Lessening of symptoms with repeated trials.
§ Likelihood of symptom production during any examination session.

of large open spaces, crowds, or leaving the safety of home), should be suspected in patients so "incapacitated" by their symptoms that they adopt a prolonged housebound status. Despite their discomfort, most patients with organic vertigo attempt to function. Vertigo should be accompanied by nystagmus; a psychogenic etiology is almost certain when nystagmus is absent during a vertiginous episode.

EVALUATION OF PATIENTS WITH PATHOLOGIC VESTIBULAR VERTIGO The evaluation depends upon whether a central etiology is suspected (Table 22-1). If so, computed tomography, with emphasis upon the posterior fossa, or a magnetic resonance imaging (MRI) scan of the head, is mandatory. Such an examination is rarely helpful in cases of recurrent monosymptomatic vertigo with a normal neurologic examination. Typical BPPV requires no investigation after the diagnosis is made (Table 22-2).

Vestibular function tests serve to (1) demonstrate an abnormality when the distinction between organic and psychogenic is uncertain, (2) establish the side of the abnormality, and (3) distinguish between peripheral and central etiologies. The standard test is electronystagmography (ENG) where warm and cold water (or air) is applied, in a prescribed fashion, to the tympanic membranes, and the slow phase velocities of the resultant nystagmus from the right and left ears are compared. A velocity decrease from one side indicates hypofunction ("canal paresis"). An inability to induce nystagmus with ice water denotes a "dead labyrinth." Some institutions have the capability of quantitatively determining various aspects of the vestibuloocular reflex using computer-driven rotational chairs and precise oculographic recording of eye movements.

Treatment of acute vertigo consists of bed rest and vestibular suppressant drugs such as antihistaminics (meclizine, dimenhydrinate, promethazine), centrally acting anticholinergics (scopolamine), or a tranquilizer with GABA-ergic effects (diazepam). If the vertigo persists beyond a few days, most authorities advise ambulation in an attempt to induce central compensatory mechanisms, despite the short-term discomfiture to the patient. Chronic vertigo of labyrinthine origin may be treated with a systematized exercise program to facilitate compensation.

Prophylactic measures to prevent recurrent vertigo are variably effective. Antihistamines are commonly utilized. Ménière's disease may respond to a very low salt diet (1 g per day). The unusual examples of persisting (beyond 4 to 6 weeks) BPPV respond dramatically, within 7 to 10 days, to a specific exercise program.

There are a variety of surgical procedures for all forms of refractory chronic or recurrent vertigo, but these are only rarely necessary.

MISCELLANEOUS HEAD SENSATIONS This designation is used, primarily for purposes of initial classification, to describe dizziness which is neither faintness nor vertigo. However, cephalic ischemia or vestibular dysfunction may be of such low intensity that the usual symptomatology is not clearly identified. For example, a small decrease in blood pressure or a slight vestibular imbalance may cause sensations different than distinct faintness or vertigo but which may be identified properly during provocative testing techniques. Other causes of dizziness in this category are hyperventilation syndrome, hypoglycemia, and the somatic symptoms of a clinical depression. All these patients should have normal neurologic examinations and vestibular function tests.

GAIT DISTURBANCES Some individuals with gait disorders complain of dizziness despite the absence of vertigo or other abnormal cephalic sensations. The causes include peripheral neuropathy, myelopathy, spasticity, parkinsonian rigidity, and cerebellar ataxia. In this context, the term dizziness is being used to describe disturbed mobility. There may be mild associated lightheadedness, particularly with impaired sensation from the feet or poor vision; this is known as *multiple sensory defect dizziness* and occurs in elderly individuals who complain of dizziness only during ambulation. Decreased position sense (secondary to neuropathy or myelopathy) and poor vision (from cataracts or retinal degeneration) create an overreliance on the aging vestibular apparatus. A less precise, but sometimes comforting, designation is *benign dysequilibrium of aging*.

EVALUATION OF THE DIZZY PATIENT The most important diagnostic tool is a careful history focused upon the meaning of "dizziness" to the patient. Is it faintness? Is there a sensation of spinning? If either of these is affirmed and the neurologic examination is normal, appropriate investigations for the multiple etiologies of cephalic ischemia or vestibular dysfunction are undertaken.

When the source of the dizziness is uncertain, provocative tests may be helpful. These office procedures simulate either cephalic ischemia or vestibular dysfunction. The former becomes obvious if the dizziness is duplicated during orthostatic hypotension. Further provocation involves the Valsalva maneuver, which decreases cerebral blood flow and should reproduce ischemic symptoms.

The simplest provocative test for vestibular dysfunction is rapid rotation and abrupt cessation of movement in a swivel chair. This always induces vertigo which the patients can compare to their symptomatic dizziness. The intense induced vertigo may be unlike the spontaneous symptoms, but shortly thereafter, when the vertigo has all but subsided, a lightheadedness supervenes which may be identified as "my dizziness." When this occurs, the dizzy patient, originally classified as suffering from "miscellaneous head sensations," is now properly diagnosed as having mild vertigo secondary to a vestibulopathy.

Patients with symptoms of positional vertigo should be appropriately tested (Table 22-2); positional testing is more sensitive with special spectacles that preclude visual fixation (Frenzel lenses).

A final provocative test, requiring the use of Frenzel lenses, is vigorous head shaking in the horizontal plane for about 10 s. If nystagmus develops after the shaking stops, even in the absence of vertigo, vestibular dysfunction is demonstrated. The maneuver can then be repeated in the vertical plane. If the provocative tests establish the dizziness as a vestibular symptom, the previously described evaluation of vestibular vertigo is undertaken.

Hyperventilation is the cause of dizziness in many anxious individuals; tingling of the hands and face may be absent. Two minutes of forced hyperventilation is indicated for patients with enigmatic dizziness and normal neurologic examinations. Similarly, depressive symptoms (which patients usually insist are "secondary" to the dizziness) must alert the examiner to a clinical depression as the *cause*, rather than the effect, of the dizziness.

Central nervous system disease can produce dizzy sensations of all types. Consequently, a neurologic examination is always required even if the history or provocative tests suggest a cardiac, peripheral vestibular, or psychogenic etiology. Any abnormality on the neurologic examination should prompt appropriate neurodiagnostic studies.

REFERENCES

BALOH RH et al: Benign postional vertigo: Clinical and oculographic features in 240 cases. Neurology 37:371, 1987

BARBER HO, SHARPE JA: *Vestibular Disorders*. Chicago, Year Book Medical, 1988, chaps 5, 9, 14, and 17

DELL'OSSO LF et al: Nystagmus and saccadic intrusions and oscillations, in *Clinical Ophthalmology*, TD Duane, EA Jaeger (eds). Philadelphia, Lippincott, 1988, chap 11, p 11–12, 19–20

LEIGH RJ, ZEE DS: *The Neurology of Eye Movements*. Philadelphia, Davis, 1984, chaps 2 and 9

ZEE DS: Perspectives on the pharmacotherapy of vertigo. Arch Otolarnygol 3:609, 1985

23 DISTURBANCES OF VISION AND OCULAR MOVEMENTS

SHIRLEY H. WRAY / THOMAS L. SLAMOVITS / RONALD M. BURDE

THE HUMAN VISUAL SYSTEM

The visual system functions to form color images instantly over a wide range of background illumination. In addition, the image is placed simultaneously on the foveas of both eyes producing a three-dimensional construct of the image (stereopsis).

Light entering the eye is focused first by the cornea, which has a fixed refractile power throughout adult life, and then by the lens, which can change focal length to form a sharp image on the retina. The variation in lens shape allows objects to be seen clearly at both near and far distances. Focusing an image on the retina is called *refraction,* and optical aberrations can be corrected by spectacles or contact lenses.

The lens is fully pliable at birth. It becomes more spherical when the zonules arising from the ciliary body relax, allowing an increase in its refractive power and a clear near image. With age the lens becomes less malleable, its protein changes and by the fifth decade it can no longer focus near objects. This accommodative loss (presbyopia) leads to the need for reading glasses. Progressive change in lenticular protein with age can also cause opacification and impaired vision (cataract).

The retina is a multilayered structure lining the posterior wall of the globe. Light reaches the retina after passing through the cornea, aqueous humor, lens, and vitreous humor. Light must also pass through all layers of the retina to reach the photoreceptor cells. Photoreceptors are specialized neurons whose most distal segment consists of a stack of membranes containing wavelength-specific photopigments (vitamin A congeners) connected to a neuron-specific protein. The particular photopigment and the structural anatomy of the cell (whether rod or cone) determine its function. Since each photoreceptor connects with multiple ganglion cells, the photoreceptor cell participates in more than one function.

The retina is divided into a system of rods, dealing with light detection and motion, and a system of cones, dealing with higher visual function (acuity and color perception). Rods contain one photopigment (rhodopsin) and are achromatic; cones contain one of three photopigments (red, blue, yellow) which respond to chromatic stimuli producing color vision. Incoming light is perceived by the photoreceptors as present or absent. The signals are then integrated by a network of neurons, including horizontal, bipolar, and amacrine cells, before reaching the ganglion cells. In the periphery of the retina (containing mostly rods) there is considerable convergence of information; hundreds of thousands of rods influence the response of one ganglion cell. In the foveamacular area, which subserves central vision, there is much less convergence, and for some bipolar cells there is a one-to-one relationship: one photoreceptor is connected to one bipolar cell to one ganglion cell.

Ganglion cells are of several types, each with specialized functions. Ganglion cell axons project to the brain through the optic nerve, optic chiasm, and optic tracts. The majority of axons project to the lateral geniculate body. Axon collaterals, which form proximal to the lateral geniculate body, project to pupillomotor centers in the pretectum and to ocular, sensory, and motor centers in the superior colliculus. Second-order neurons in the lateral geniculate nucleus project to the occipital cortex via the optic radiations.

The image formed by the retina is inverted and reversed. The temporal retina images the nasal visual field while the nasal retina images the temporal field. Similarly, the superior retina perceives the inferior visual field and the inferior retina the superior field.

The fovea-macula projection (papillomacular bundle) is the major ocular-cortical outflow. The central 5° of retina is subserved by 25 to 27 percent of the axons, and the central 20° by 90 percent of the axons. The temporal field axons (nasal retina), which account for 52 percent of axons in the optic nerve, cross in the chiasm to project to the contralateral lateral geniculate nucleus, where they synapse and project to the striate cortex in the occipital lobe.

CLINICAL ASSESSMENT OF DISTURBANCES OF VISION

ACUITY Acuity is a perceptual response of a subject to a stimulus of minimal magnitude. There are many different types of visual acuity in addition to that determined by the standard Snellen chart, such as resolution, orientation, motion, color, contrast sensitivity, and stereopsis. Visual disturbances are characterized by subnormal visual acuity (less than 20/20 Snellen acuity; see below) and by abnormalities of visual field, color vision, contrast sensitivity, and depth perception. A corrected visual acuity of less than 6/60 metric (20/200 conventional) bilaterally constitutes legal blindness. Refractive errors (myopia, hyperopia, astigmatism) commonly cause subnormal visual acuity and must be assessed for by measuring *best corrected* (i.e., best refracted) visual acuity. A pinhole can be used for a reasonable approximation of best corrected visual acuity. Visual acuity at distance is measured with a Snellen chart [normal 6/6 meters (20/20 feet)]. In the fractional denotation—e.g., 6/60 metric (20/200 conventional), the numerator 6 (or 20) stands for the testing distance (in meters or feet) and the denominator 60 (or 200) for the test letter's size normally seen at that denominator distance. Near acuity is measured with a near card (Jaeger chart). Bifocals or near spectacles must be worn by presbyopes (who have difficulties with accommodation) when testing near vision.

COLOR VISION Acquired color vision abnormalities in red/green perception usually imply optic neuropathy. Bedside testing may consist of gross recognition or comparison of prime colors, or the use of a series of color charts (Ishihara pseudoisochromatic or American Optical Hardy-Rand-Rittler plates). Color desaturation tests rely on a comparison of the subjective perception of a colored target (e.g., red bottle top) in the right and left eyes or in the nasal and temporal half-fields of a single eye. The test detects unilateral or hemianopic abnormalities.

CONTRAST SENSITIVITY Testing of this acuity requires manipulation of both contrast and spatial frequency by measuring the minimum contrast necessary to see patterns of various sizes. Contrast sensitivity plates (Arden or American Optical) can be used at the bedside.

STEREOPSIS There is a linear relationship between stereoacuity and Snellen visual acuity. Individuals with normal 6/6 (20/20) vision in each eye and binocular fixation (no manifest strabismus) have an average stereopsis of 40 seconds of arc. Stereoacuity is reduced with decreasing acuity down to 6/60 (20/200) at which level monocular and binocular responses become identical. The Titmus stereoacuity test is used in children and adults who have been corrected for presbyopia and is suitable for bedside use. This linearity may not exist in the presence of optic nerve damage even if visual acuity returns to normal.

VISUAL FIELDS It is possible to perform a visual field test using any perceptual stimulus. The bedside exam is performed by confrontation. Two types of "formal" field testing are in common use:

1. On *kinetic perimetry* (Goldmann, tangent screen), the patient is instructed to look at a central fixation target while test objects of varying brightness and size (white or chromatic) are moved from the periphery toward the fixation point until the patient signals that the test object is visualized. The normal field using white objects is approximately 90° temporally, 50° nasally, 50° superiorly, and 65° inferiorly. Concentric contraction of the visual field binocularly to less than 10° constitutes legal blindness.

2. On *automated static perimetry* (Humphrey, Octopus), the patient fixes on a central target in a hemisphere with a homogeneous white background, while a nonmoving light of fixed size and brightness is presented at various points in the hemisphere. Brightness is increased until the patient recognizes the presence of the stimulus above background. Thus, static perimetry measures brightness sensitivity of various retinal points.

Visual field defects are localizable on the basis of the anatomy of the visual pathway. Retinal and optic nerve lesions affect one of three types of nerve fiber bundles, leading to blind spots (scotomas) termed: (1) central/cecocentral, (2) arcuate, or (3) radial. Loss of nerve fibers between the optic nerve and macula (maculopapillary bundle) leads to central or cecocentral scotomas, i.e., involving the center of the visual field or extending between the center and the physiologic blind spot (cecum) (Fig. 23-1D and E). Temporal retinal lesions above and below the maculopapillary bundle or those involving the superotemporal or inferotemporal optic nerve affect the *arcuate* bundles and cause inferonasal or superonasal visual field defects,

FIGURE 23-1 Types of monocular visual field loss in left eye. *A.* Superior arcuate scotoma (inferior nerve fiber bundle defect). *B.* Inferior altitudinal field defect respecting the horizontal meridian (superior nerve fiber bundle defect). *C.* Enlargement of the blind spot in the left eye. *D.* Central scotoma, normal blind spot. *E.* Centrocecal scotoma. *F.* Temporal hemianopsia respecting the vertical meridian but with involvement of central vision. *G.* Generalized constriction of the visual field to 2 isopters. *H.* Nonorganic "corkscrew" field defect to 1 isopter. *(From Wray, 1985; by permission.)*

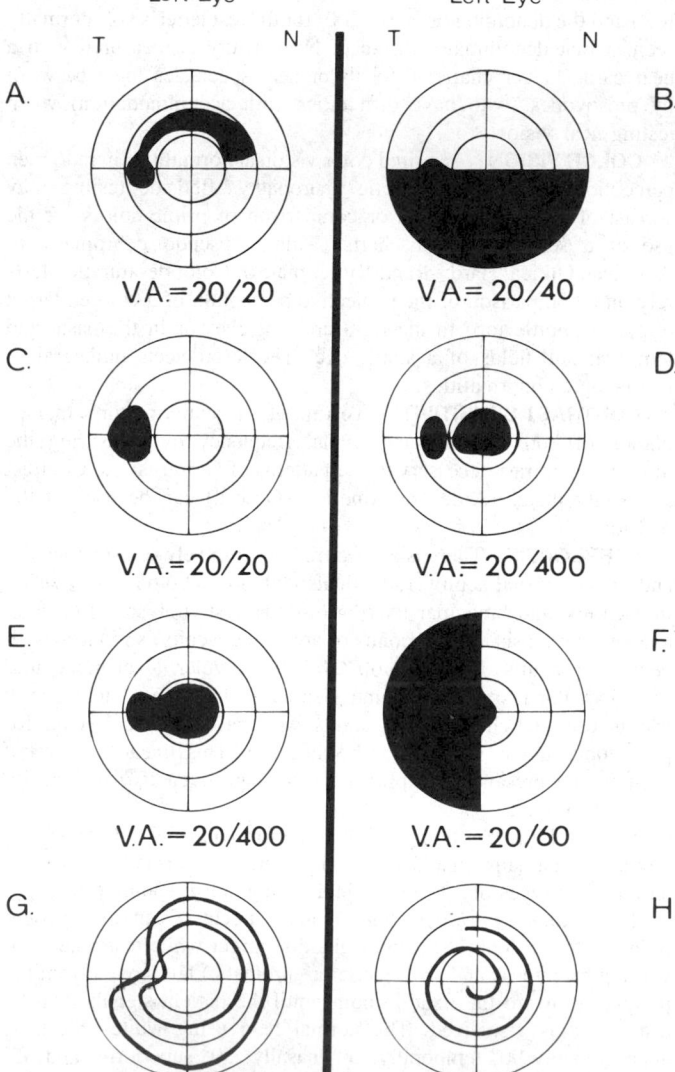

respectively. Because such field defects abut the horizontal midline, they are at times referred to as *altitudinal* (Fig. 23-1B). Lesions involving the nasal retinal or optic nerve fibers (radial nerve fiber bundle defects) lead to inferotemporal and superotemporal visual field defects that extend toward the physiologic blind spot (Fig. 23-1A).

Retinal field defects frequently correspond to lesions seen with the ophthalmoscope, i.e., areas of infarction, inflammation, or degenerative change. Macular lesions produce central scotomas. Retinitis pigmentosa usually produces constricted fields and equatorial ring scotomas.

Discrete lesions, frequently ischemic, primarily in the anterior optic nerve may produce *arcuate field defects*. Such lesions include anterior ischemic optic neuropathy, glaucoma, and optic atrophy secondary to papilledema. The central/cecocentral scotoma is a specific and common sign of optic nerve disease. It occurs in a variety of conditions both intrinsic (demyelinating, infiltrative, metabolic-toxic) and compressive in nature.

At the chiasm, the visual afferents become divided into a right and left half so that the right brain sees left visual space and the left brain sees right visual space. A discrete vertical midline is the hallmark of all visual pathway disorders at or posterior to the chiasm. A chiasmal lesion most often causes bitemporal hemianopsia (Fig. 23-2B), but several different patterns can occur: junctional scotoma, superior or inferior bitemporal quadrantanopsia, or monocular temporal hemianopsia. Each type can occur with chiasmal compression due to a pituitary tumor, craniopharyngioma, or aneurysm. Pseudochiasmal or ocular syndromes that can mimic chiasmal lesions include tilted optic discs, drug toxicity (chloroquine), sector retinitis pigmentosa, and bilateral retinal detachments. A mass in the retrochiasmatic region impinging upon or displacing the optic tract results in homonymous hemianopsia of two types: an incongruous homonymous hemianopsia or a complete homonymous hemianopsia.

Homonymous field defects due to lesions of the anterior optic radiation tend to be incongruous. Those due to damage to the radiations close to the visual cortex are congruous. (Congruity is said to be present when the edge of the field defect in each eye is identical in shape.) Depending on its site, the lesion may involve only the upper or lower fibers of the radiation and thus cause a lower or upper quadrant defect in the opposite half-field; e.g., temporal lobe radiation lesion causes "pie in the sky" (Fig. 23-2E) whereas a parietal lobe radiation lesion causes "pie on the floor" (Fig. 23-2G). A complete hemianopic defect to bilateral simultaneous visual stimulation (attention defect) may, however, be the only detectable sign of visual dysfunction in lesions of the parietal area. Left temporoparietal lesions are associated with defective recognition of visual symbols, alexia, and agraphia; lesions of the right temporoparietal area are manifested by impaired judgment of spatial relationships, as in topographic agnosia and constructional apraxia (see Chap. 32).

Destruction of the visual cortex of one occipital lobe produces a contralateral congruous homonymous hemianopsia. This is the commonest type of cortical field defect and is frequently the result of embolic occlusion of the posterior cerebral artery. Other patterns of visual loss permit precise localization of the deficit. These defects are congruous homonymous hemianopic scotoma, congruous homonymous hemianopsia sparing the temporal crescent, or, rarely, a monocular field defect due to loss of the temporal crescent, bilateral homonymous hemianopsia, bilateral altitudinal scotoma, cortical blindness, and tunnel or keyhole vision.

PUPILLARY EXAMINATION Normal pupillary responses consist of prompt, symmetric constriction (miosis) on exposure to light or on attempted near convergence. Diminished response to a direct light stimulus, combined with a normal consensual pupillary response following stimulation of the contralateral eye, is termed a relative afferent pupillary defect (RAPD). The RAPD is an important objective sign of ipsilateral optic neuropathy. The best way to elicit the RAPD is to perform a swinging flashlight test (Fig. 23-3). Anisocoria (unequal pupil size) and abnormal pupillary reflexes are two clinically

Isolated chronic pupillary dilation (mydriasis) is almost never caused by a lesion in the oculomotor nerve; it may be constitutional (physiologic, "benign"), pharmacologic (induced by local instillation of mydriatics), traumatic, or a result of a parasympathetic lesion at or distal to the ciliary ganglion (tonic pupil, Adie's pupil). The diagnostic workup utilizes changes in pupil size in response to topical agents (Table 23-1).

Unilateral mydriasis with impaired direct-light and near response, ipsilateral ptosis, and extraocular muscle paresis of the superior, medial, and inferior rectus and inferior oblique muscles constitutes an oculomotor nerve palsy. Unilateral miosis with normal direct-light response and mild ipsilateral ptosis constitutes an oculosympathetic lesion or Horner syndrome. The diagnosis of the Horner pupil can be confirmed by pharmacologic testing (Table 23-1).

Light-near dissociation (LND) of the pupillary response is bilateral and characterized by an impaired response to light with an intact response to near vision. When LND is bilateral and symmetric it occurs with dorsal midbrain lesions (hydrocephalus, pineal region

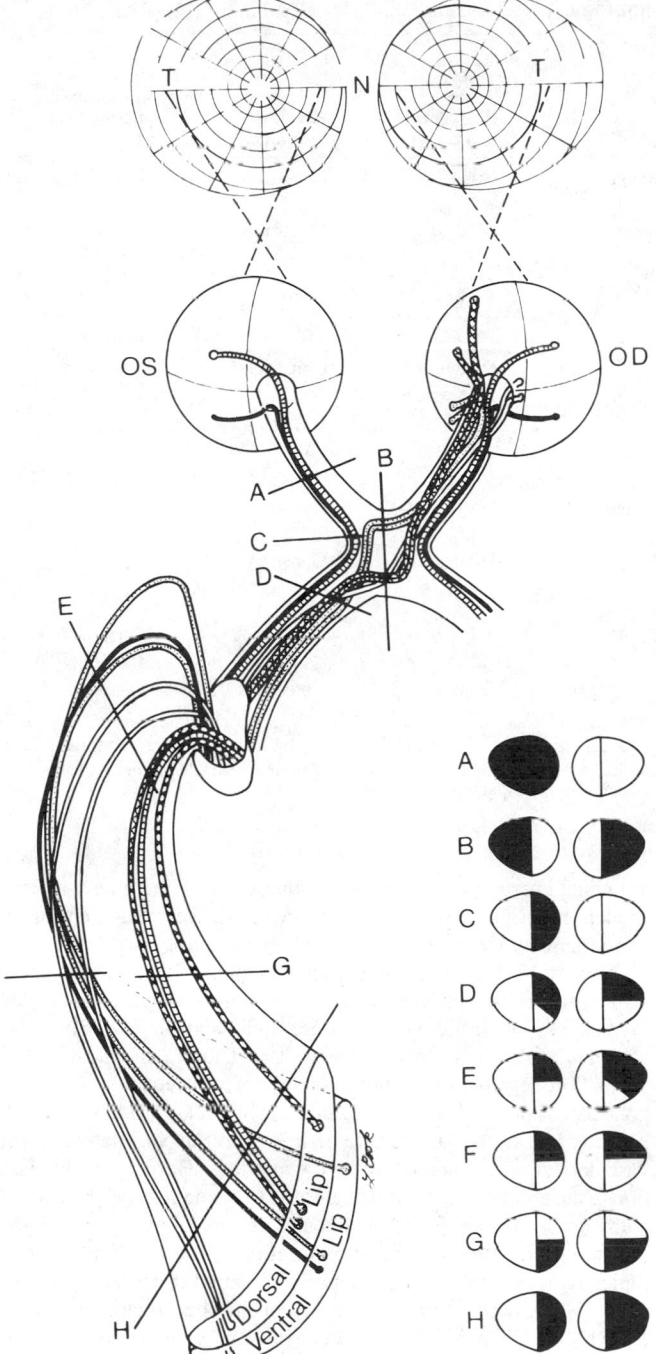

FIGURE 23-2 Nerve fiber anatomy of the visual pathways from retina to occipital cortex. The effect of the fields of vision produced by lesions at various points along the optic pathway is shown on the right. *A.* complete blindness in left eye. *B.* Bitemporal hemianopsia. *C.* Nasal hemianopsia of left eye. *D* and *E.* Right incongruous homonymous hemianopsia. *F* and *G.* Right upper and lower homonymous quadrantanopia. *H.* complete right homonymous hemianopsia. *Courtesy of DD Donaldson. (From Wray, 1985; by permission.)*

FIGURE 23-3 Swinging flashlight test demonstrating a right relative afferent pupillary defect (RAPD) in a patient with giant cell arteritis and right anterior ischemic optic neuropathy. The patient is fixating on a distant target to avoid near effort and related accommodative miosis. *A.* Pupils in a dimly lit room. *B.* Flashlight illuminates right eye, leading to minimal direct constriction of right pupil and minimal consensual constriction of left pupil. *C.* Flashlight is swung to the left eye, causing obvious pupillary constriction directly on left and consensually on right. *D.* Flashlight is again swung to right eye, leading to bilateral pupillary dilation—a result of the right optic nerve conduction deficit.

important pupillary abnormalities. Comparing pupil size in the dark and in room light and observing direct light responses help to determine whether the smaller or larger pupil is the abnormal one. With parasympathetic anisocoria, the difference in pupil size will be accentuated in room light since the affected (large) pupil constricts subnormally. With oculosympathetic paresis, the anisocoria is more marked in dim light because the affected (small) pupil dilates subnormally.

TABLE 23-1   Characteristics of pupils encountered in neuroophthalmology

	General characteristics	Responses to light and near stimuli	Room condition in which anisocoria is greater	Response to mydriatics	Response to miotics	Response to pharmacologic agents
Essential anisocoria	Round, regular	Both brisk	No change	Dilates	Constricts	Normal and rarely needed
Horner's syndrome	Small, round, unilateral	Both brisk	Darkness	Dilates	Constricts	Cocaine 4%, poor dilation; Paredrine 1%, no dilation if third-order neuron damage
Tonic pupil syndrome (Holmes-Adie syndrome)	Usually larger* in bright light; sector pupil palsy, vermiform movement Unilateral or, less often, bilateral	Absent to light, tonic to near; tonic redilation	Light	Dilates	Constricts	Pilocarpine 0.1% or 0.125% constricts; Mecholyl 2.5% constricts
Argyll Robertson pupils	Small, irregular, bilateral	Poor to light, better to near	No change	Poor	Constricts	
Midbrain pupils	Mid-dilated; may be oval; bilateral	Poor to light, better to near (or fixed to both)	No change	Dilates	Constricts	
Pharmacologically dilated pupils	Very large†, round, unilateral	Fixed‡	Light		No‡	Pilocarpine 1% will not constrict
Oculomotor palsy (nonvascular)	Mid-dilated (6–7 mm), unilateral (rarely bilateral)	Fixed	Light	Dilates	Constricts	

* Tonic pupil may appear smaller following prolonged near-effort or in dim illumination; affected pupil is initially large, but with passing time gradually becomes smaller.
† Atropinized pupils have diameters of 8 to 9 mm. No tonic, midbrain, or oculomotor palsy pupil ever is this large.
‡ Pupils may be weakly reactive, depending on interim after instillation.
SOURCE: TL Slamovits and JS Glaser in *Clinical Ophthalmology*, T Duane (ed) Vol 2, Philadelphia, Lippincott, 1988

tumors). Argyll-Robertson pupil is a special form of LND caused by syphilis; the pupils are miotic and usually irregular in shape. LND can also occur in diabetes mellitus. LND accompanied by bilaterally poor vision is generally due to anterior visual pathway disease. Unilateral LND is most commonly seen in patients with ipsilateral retinal or optic nerve disease. Bilateral pupillary enlargement with subnormal direct and near responses occurs with pharmacologic blockade, botulism, or diphtheria. Bilaterally miotic pupils are produced by the use of parasympathomimetics for glaucoma; a pontine lesion (pinpoint pontine pupils) or narcotic (heroin) overdose should be considered in a comatose patient with bilateral miosis.

OCULAR DISEASES

THE CONJUNCTIVE AND CORNEA   Diseases of the conjunctiva and cornea can produce loss of visual acuity, pain, and discharge. Examination should first be directed to the lids and lid margins as well as to the lashes. Chronic infectious processes are often characterized by scaling around the lashes or pointing of the ducts of the meibomian glands. It is to be noted that basal cell and squamous cell carcinomas often involve the lids. Evidence of discharge from the conjunctiva can frequently be observed as crusting, either nasally or temporally, on the lids.

The eyes are ordinarily white and quiet. When a patient complains of discomfort or discharge the upper and lower fornix as well as the palpebral conjunctiva should be inspected, by pulling the lower lid out and down or everting the upper lid on the tarsus. Discharge, foreign bodies, and Kaposi's sarcoma may go undetected without such an examination.

The presence of perilimbal injection is indicative of anterior uveal inflammation and such patients should be referred for ophthalmologic evaluation.

Diseases of the conjunctiva and cornea may occur as a result of direct trauma, drying associated with disorders of tearing, exposure to radiant energy (ultraviolet light, sun, and welding guns), allergens (pollen, mold), infectious agents (bacteria, viruses, fungi, and ameba) and inflammatory, metabolic, and neoplastic processes.

Neonatal infection of the cornea or conjunctiva is usually due to staphylococci or gonococci, or in some geographic areas to chlamydiae. Prophylactic silver nitrate treatment in the newborn is effective against gonococci but may itself cause a chemical conjunctivitis. Tetracycline or erythromycin ointment is equally effective for gonococcal prophylaxis. Congenital syphilis can produce interstitial keratitis late in the last decade of life, resulting in bilateral corneal vascularization, photophobia, and visual loss. Herpes simplex infections cause dendritic keratitis. Failure to recognize herpetic keratopathy and its inappropriate treatment with topical glucocorticoids can lead to corneal "melting" and perforation. Treatment with acyclovir topically or systemically can suppress herpetic keratopathy (see Chap. 135). Herpesvirus can become latent in the trigeminal ganglia, allowing recurrent keratitis to occur in some patients.

Adenovirus infection is the leading cause of keratoconjunctivitis in adults; it is usually self-limiting and benign. In sexually active young adults, inclusion conjunctivitis is common (see Chap. 155). In developing countries, trachoma and onchocerciasis are leading causes of corneal scarring and blindness.

Chronic indolent amebic ulcers of the cornea can occur in soft-contact lens wearers who have a break in the corneal epithelium; such ulcers are difficult to treat. However, this complication is rare in those who remove and clean contact lenses daily. Debilitated patients can develop keratitis due to gram-negative bacteria (*Klebsiella, Pseudomonas*) or fungi. Malnutrition and avitaminosis A can lead to conjunctival and corneal scarring with keratinization (xerosis) and severe visual loss.

Keratoconjunctivitis can also occur in patients with Stevens-Johnson syndrome (Chap. 272), Wegener's granulomatosis (Chap. 276), rheumatoid arthritis (Chap. 270), atopic dermatitis (Chap. 56), and cicatricial pemphigoid (Chap. 58). These processes are often associated with corneal ulceration. Band keratopathy is caused by corneal deposition of calcium salts, especially within the palpebral fissure (Fig. A4-10). It occurs as a result of chronic inflammation (keratouveitis) or of systemic hypercalcemia (see Chap. 340).

Corneal clouding is prominent in G_{M1} gangliosidosis (Chap. 331), in certain of the mucopolysaccharidoses (Chap. 331), and in aminoaciduria [cystinosis (Chap. 335)]. In Wilson's disease (Chap. 330) and in chronic biliary cirrhosis, copper deposits form a golden-brown ring (Kayser-Fleischer ring) (Fig. A4-16) in the cornea at the level of Descemet's membrane. Corneal drug deposition may occur following systemic use of chloroquine, phenothiazine, gold, silver, or amiodarone.

THE LENS AND CATARACTS Opacification of the normally clear and transparent crystalline lens is termed a cataract. Visual symptoms are blurred vision, glare, altered color perception, and monocular diplopia. *Congenital* cataracts occur as a complication of intrauterine rubella, herpes simplex, herpes zoster, syphilis, and cytomegalic inclusion disease. The majority are idiopathic or inherited. Acquired cataracts result from trauma, radiation, drugs, metabolic disorders, ocular inflammatory disorders, or aging (senile cataract). Cataracts develop earlier in patients with diabetes mellitus (type I and type II) and in some patients with a strong family history of cataract formation. Metabolic disorders complicated by cataract include galactosemia (Chap. 337), chronic hypercalcemic states (Chap. 340), Fabry's disease, Wilson's disease (Chap. 330), and Lowe's syndrome (Chap. 231). More than one-third of patients with myotonic dystrophy have multicolored crystalline opacities scattered throughout the lens. Cataracts may also be associated with chromosomal disorders; with the Alport, cri-du-chat, Conradi, Crouzon, and Down syndromes; and with gonadal dysgenesis. Inflammatory ocular diseases, drugs and toxic substances such as haloperidol, glucocorticoids, and iron can also cause cataracts. Cataract extraction is performed by removing the lens nucleus and cortex from within the lens capsule. In most adults, a plastic lens is then implanted within the capsule.

The zonules holding the lens may be broken in one region, allowing the lens to move eccentrically, often leaving its edge in the pupillary axis (subluxation) or totally broken, allowing the lens to move into the anterior chamber or into the vitreous cavity (luxation). The most common cause of subluxation or luxation is trauma. Others include homocystinuria (Chap. 334), Marfan's syndrome, spherophakia, and sulfite oxidase insufficiency.

UVEAL DISEASES The uvea consists of the iris and ciliary body anteriorly and the choroid posteriorly. Anatomically, the choroid has three layers of vessels and a cellular matrix including pigmented cells. Common diseases of the uvea are inflammatory or neoplastic. Inflammation can involve the iris (iritis), ciliary body (cyclitis), or choroid (choroiditis) or any combination of the three (uveitis). Uveitis causes photophobia, ocular discomfort and visual blurring. Chronic uveitis can cause cystoid macular edema with decreased central acuity, cataract formation, and secondary glaucoma. The commonest form of uveitis is idiopathic. Systemic diseases causing uveitis include pauciarticular juvenile rheumatoid arthritis (rheumatoid factor negative), juvenile nevoxanthogranuloma, rheumatoid arthritis, sarcoidosis, Lyme disease, and relapsing polychondritis. Treatment of uveitis (dependent on severity) includes cycloplegic drops and glucocorticoids (topically or systemically), and sometimes immunosuppressive drugs (chlorambucil, azathioprine, cyclophosphamide, and cyclosporin A).

Ocular malignant melanoma is a primary neoplastic disease of the choroid. Choroidal involvement also occurs as a result of metastases (lung, breast, prostate) and in association with lymphoma of the central nervous system (reticulum cell sarcoma)—conditions that are sometimes responsive to low-dose radiation.

RETINAL DISEASES Retinal abnormalities are best seen by performing a dilated fundus examination. Retinal diseases involving the macula cause distortion of straight lines (metamorphopsia), loss of central acuity, and visual field abnormalities. Nonmacular retinal disorders cause scotomata involving the peripheral or paracentral visual field, correlating with the site of retinal pathology. Retinopathies can be due to diseases of the retinal vessels, neurosensory retina, or the retinal pigment epithelium.

Retinal vasculopathies occur in many systemic conditions. In hypertensive retinopathy, the severity of retinal changes correlates closely with the level of systemic hypertension (see Chap. 196). Grade I consists of arteriolar narrowing; Grade II includes arteriovenous nicking, minimal exudation, and splinter hemorrhages; Grade III includes retinal edema, hemorrhages, and cotton-wool spots (focal ischemia in the nerve fiber layer); Grade IV includes Grade III changes plus papilledema, often with a macular star produced by deposition of cellular debris (hard exudates). Hypertensive retinopathy can be seen with all forms of hypertension—essential and secondary. Cotton-wool spots, a common feature of malignant hypertension, may also occur in anemia, leukemia, collagen vascular disease, dysproteinemia, infective endocarditis, and diabetes mellitus. They are the most common ophthalmic lesions in acquired immunodeficiency syndrome (AIDS) (see Chap. 264). Other ocular manifestations of AIDS include cytomegalovirus (CMV) retinitis (Fig. A4-14) and toxoplasmic and fungal retinal infections. Nonretinal ocular manifestations of AIDS include optic neuropathy, Kaposi's sarcoma of the conjunctiva, and orbital lymphoma.

Diabetic retinopathy is classified into two groups: (1) background retinopathy (Fig. A4-12) characterized by microaneurysms, dot-blot hemorrhages, cotton-wool spots, hard exudates, intraretinal microvascular shunt vessels, and venous beading, sometimes with related macular edema; and (2) proliferative retinopathy (Fig. A4-13) characterized by neovascularization, proliferation of fibrous tissue into the vitreous cavity, and eventually traction retinal detachments with visual loss (see Chap. 319). Panretinal photocoagulation is beneficial in maintaining vision in early proliferative retinopathy. The progression of diabetic retinopathy correlates best with the concentration of hemoglobin A_{1c}, reflecting the long-term metabolic control. The lower the hemoglobin A_{1c} concentration the slower the progression. The acute induction of so-called tight control is often associated with a short-term aggravation of the retinopathic process (e.g., insulin infusion pump or multiple injection regime).

Somewhat similar retinal vascular changes ("sea fan" proliferation) occur in sickle cell diseases (S-S, S-C, S-Thal) and in the retinopathy of prematurity. In sickle cell disease focal photocoagulation is helpful. Focal cryotherapy may be of benefit in the acute retinopathy of prematurity.

Permanent blindness occurs with *infarction* of the inner retina due to occlusion of the central retinal artery (CRA). Funduscopic examination shows rectangular "box-car" segmentation of venous blood flow and an opaque white retina due to axoplasmic stasis in ganglion cell axons. A central cherry-red spot is due to visualization of the choroid in the macular area devoid of axons (Fig. A4-2). CRA occlusion may be embolic (ipsilateral internal carotid artery, aorta, or heart) or thrombotic due to giant cell arteritis, arteriosclerosis, collagen vascular disease, or hyperviscosity states. CRA occlusion is an ophthalmic emergency. Treatment may include ballotement of the globe, retrobulbar anesthetic block, and paracentesis of aqueous humor in an attempt to move embolic material into peripheral arterioles.

Monocular transient blurring of vision (amaurosis fugax) lasting seconds to minutes may herald CRA occlusion but, more importantly, may be a precursor of a stroke. These patients require evaluation of the aortic arch and carotid circulation as well as the heart (see Chap. 351).

Central (Fig. A4-3) and branch retinal vein occlusion may occur spontaneously or in association with hypertension or elevated intraocular pressure. Venous stasis retinopathy mimics early vein occlusion with venous dilatation, hemorrhages, and cotton-wool spots; it is due to impaired retinal perfusion produced by carotid occlusive disease and Takayasu's disease. Systemic coagulopathies such as thrombocytopenia, erythematosus disseminated intravascular coagulopathy, and systemic lupus erythematosus with circulating anticoagulants (cardiolipin), may cause retinal hemorrhages, clotting in the submacular choriocapillaris, choroidal hemorrhages, and detachment of the retina. Perivenous sheathing occurs in primary retinal vasculitis (Eales disease), leukemia, and optic nerve demyelination. Fundus changes may be the mark of an abused child presenting with multiple retinal hemorrhages (subhyaloid lakes, blot and flame hemorrhages) and cotton-wool spots. This retinopathy is caused by severe shaking or choking of the child.

Retinal vascular anomalies are rare and among them are to be found retinal telangiectasia (Coat's disease), retinal angiomatosis [von Hippel-Lindau syndrome (Chap. 358)], direct arteriovenous connections [Wyburn-Mason syndrome (A4-15)], miliary aneurysms, cavernous retinal hemangiomas.

Nonvascular diseases of the retina include infections such as congenital and acquired toxoplasmosis, herpes retinitis, and *Monilia* and nematode infestations. Inflammatory diseases of the outer retina and choroid include the presumed ocular histoplasmosis syndrome, acute multifocal placoid pigment epitheliopathy, serpiginous retinopathy, "bird-shot" chorioretinopathy, multiple evanescent white dot syndrome, and neoplastic diseases such as retinoblastoma.

Retinal degenerative disease may involve the retinovitreal interface with focal capillary sclerosis and hole formation (lattice degeneration) or may appear as isolated areas of retinovitreal adhesion and vitreous liquefaction (syneresis) leading to retinal traction, retinal horseshoe-shaped tears, and detachment. Lightning-like flashes and/or an acute vitreous hemorrhage producing a spiderweb-like shadow and blurred vision may herald detachment. These patients must be examined by an ophthalmologist utilizing an indirect ophthalmoscope. Emergency surgery (laser, cryotherapy) is required to seal the tears. Degeneration of the outer retina and pigment epithelium is characteristic of retinitis pigmentosa (Fig. A4-9) which occurs in sporadic, X-linked, autosomal recessive, and autosomal dominant forms. Symptoms are loss of night vision, progressive concentric contraction of the visual field, and eventually, loss of central vision.

Multisystem disorders that cause retinal degeneration are abetalipoproteinemia (Bassen-Kornzweig syndrome, Chap. 326), neuronal ceroid lipofuscinosis (Batten-Mayou disease), Refsum's disease (Chap. 363), certain mucopolysaccharidoses, and the Kearns-Sayre syndrome (Chap. 365).

Certain lysosomal storage diseases including G_{M1} and G_{M2} gangliosidosis and the sphingolipidoses affect ganglion cell function, leading to blindness; cherry-red spots are invariably present (Chap. 331). Toxic retinopathy may follow the use of phenothiazine derivatives, especially thioridazine (Mellaril), chloroquine, and hydroxychloroquine. Long-term therapy with these agents should be monitored at regular intervals with static perimetry or kinetic perimetry with red and white targets.

DISEASES OF BRUCH'S MEMBRANE   Bruch's membrane is a multilayered structure formed by the choriocapillaris and the pigment epithelium of the retina. With aging, the pigment epithelium may accumulate intracellular material, leading to age-related macular degeneration. Visual loss is slowly progressive, associated with metamorphopsia, and rarely causes less than 6/120 (20/400) Snellen acuity. A second type of age-related macular degeneration can occur in the paramacular foveal area and cause visual loss. It results from degeneration of Bruch's membrane with the formation of large or small breaks in its integrity and subretinal neovascularization. Subsequent exudation and hemorrhage causes a further elevation of the sensory or pigment epithelium of the retina. Visual loss is often acute and catastrophic in nature, decreasing acuity to less than 6/120 (20/400) with a large central scotoma that is defined by the anatomic detachment. Laser ablation of the neovascular net may delay blindness. Angioid streaks are large breaks in Bruch's membrane (Fig. A4-8). They are associated with Paget's disease, acromegaly, pseudoxanthoma elasticum, sickle cell disease and severe myopia.

DISEASES OF THE OPTIC NERVE

The optic disc is the exit site of all retinal ganglion cell axons. The axons leave the globe in the optic nerve by passing through the lamina cribrosa. Just posterior to the lamina, the nerve fibers become myelinated. The blood supply of the nerve head is primarily derived from choroidal and posterior ciliary branches of the ophthalmic artery.

GLAUCOMA   Glaucoma is characterized by progressive field loss due to nerve damage from elevated intraocular pressure. It is an important cause of blindness worldwide and in the United States occurs in 1 to 2 percent of patients above age 60. The disease may be asymptomatic with painless, slow loss of peripheral and paracentral visual fields. Early detection depends upon a routine eye examination with intraocular pressure measurement (tonometry), funduscopy with attention to optic disc appearance, and visual field testing. In the normal eye the optic cups are symmetric and the neural rim is pink (Fig. A4-1). In glaucoma, either localized notching or generalized enlargement of the optic cup can be seen (Fig. A4-11). The rim, although thinned, remains pink until late. The central optic cup diameter can be compared to the diameter of the disc and a ratio of the horizontal and vertical dimensions can be recorded. The normal cup-disc ratio is less than 0.2 to 0.3. Vertical disparity in one or both eyes is an early sign of glaucoma. Glaucoma is often asymmetric and the finding of asymmetry of the cup-disc ratio implies glaucoma. Early visual field loss includes nonspecific constriction and small paracentral scotomas. Eventually, arcuate nerve fiber bundle defects develop with a characteristic *nasal step* (e.g., arcuate bundle defect extending to the nasal horizontal raphe forms a steplike configuration on kinetic visual field testing). The papillomacular bundle and acuity are spared until late in the disease. Intraocular pressure reflects the balance between the production and outflow of aqueous humor, and the normal range is 2.09 ± 0.33 kPa (15.8 ± 2.5 mmHg) measured by applanation tonometry. (Schiotz tonometers measure intraocular pressure by indentation of the cornea, whereas most tonometers measure by planating the corneal surface, hence applanation.)

Glaucoma is an appellation for many disease states. It results from decreased outflow of aqueous humor through the pupil, trabecular meshwork, and Schlemm's canal, leading to elevated intraocular pressure. Chronic or *primary open-angle glaucoma*, the most common of adult glaucomas, is asymptomatic and detected only by routine eye examination. It is associated with a relative obstruction to aqueous outflow through the trabecular meshwork and is of unknown cause. Treatment includes the use of topical agents including cholinergic (pilocarpine, carbachol, echothiophate) or adrenergic agonists (epinephrine, dipivefrin), or antagonists, i.e., beta-adrenergic blockers (timolol, levobunalol, betaxolol). If topical agents do not reduce the intraocular pressure satisfactorily, systemic carbonic anhydrase inhibitors (acetazolamide or methazolamide) are added. Laser trabeculoplasty or filtration surgery, to improve aqueous outflow, is indicated when medical therapy fails.

Secondary open-angle glaucoma may develop in patients with ocular inflammatory or neoplastic disease, with mature cataracts or elevated episcleral venous pressure, or during a course of long-term glucocorticoid therapy, either topical or systemic.

Angle-closure glaucoma occurs when the iris blocks egress of aqueous humor through the trabecular meshwork. In the primary form, an anatomic abnormality of the eye leads to pupillary block and obstruction of the trabecular meshwork. An acute rise in intraocular pressure occurs with dilation of the pupil causing severe eye and face pain, nausea, vomiting, colored halos around lights and loss of visual acuity. Conjunctival hyperemia, corneal edema, and a fixed mid-dilated pupil are common signs. Urgent reduction of the intraocular pressure is best accomplished by the use of hyperosmotic agents including oral glycerine and sorbitol or intravenous mannitol. Laser or surgical iridotomy is curative in most cases.

Secondary angle-closure glaucoma can occur when the lens or ciliary body becomes swollen, pushing the iris against the trabecular meshwork or sealing the iris to the trabecular meshwork as a result of the formation of a neovascular network. This process occurs in patients with diabetic retinopathy, advanced ocular ischemic syndrome due to severe occlusive carotid disease, or inflammatory adhesions (synechiae).

OPTIC NEUROPATHIES Diseases of the optic nerve cause acuity loss, subjective color and brightness desaturation, changes in contrast sensitivity, and visual field loss. There is almost always a relative afferent pupillary defect (RAPD) (Fig. 23-3). Papilledema (optic disc edema secondary to elevated intracranial pressure) and infiltration of the optic nerve sheath cause visual dysfunction late in the course of the disease. In acute optic neuropathy the optic disc may be normal or swollen. In chronic optic neuropathy the disc is swollen or pale (atrophy).

Optic neuritis most commonly afflicts patients in their twenties or thirties, women more than men, and can either be a primary demyelinating disease of unknown etiology or associated with past, present, or future manifestations of multiple sclerosis (see Chap. 356). There is acute, typically central visual loss, retrobulbar pain with eye movement, and RAPD. In the acute phase the nerve is normal (retrobulbar optic neuritis) or swollen (anterior optic neuritis or papillitis). Acute optic neuritis is generally unilateral. Bilateral recurrent bouts in the same or contralateral eye can occur, especially with multiple sclerosis.

Anterior ischemic optic neuropathy (AION) occurs most often in patients over 40 years of age. Typically sudden visual loss and altitudinal field loss occurs, i.e., a superior or inferior visual field defect with one border along the horizontal midline, associated with disc swelling due to infarction of the nerve head (Fig. A4-6). It occurs in two forms: (1) nonarteritic (median age 56 years) in which the risk factors are diabetes mellitus in younger patients and hypertension in older patients; (2) an arteritic (giant cell arteritis) variety (median age 74 years). Symptoms of giant cell arteritis (anorexia, malaise, proximal arthralgia, myalgia, headache, and jaw claudication) and an elevated erythrocyte sedimentation rate are indications for prompt systemic glucocorticoid therapy and a temporal artery biopsy. Untreated, arteritic ischemic optic neuropathy may affect the contralateral eye and cause blindness in 40 percent of cases.

Compression (intrinsic or extrinsic) of the optic nerve causes insidious progressive acuity and field loss. The disc may be normal, swollen, or atrophic (Fig. A4-7). Intrinsic tumors include optic nerve sheath meningioma and glioma. In Graves' ophthalmopathy, the optic neuropathy is due to compression of the nerve in the orbital apex by the enlarged extraocular muscles. Benign or malignant orbital tumors, metastatic lesions, tumors arising from the adjacent paranasal sinuses and middle cranial fossa, and giant pituitary adenomas can each lead to compressive optic neuropathy.

Infiltrative and toxic optic neuropathies are rare. Progressive disc swelling and visual loss characterize infiltration by inflammatory disease (sarcoidosis), infection (cryptococcosis), or neoplasia (leukemia, lymphoma, metastatic carcinoma). Toxic agents (methanol, ethambutol) cause a more acute visual loss with normal or swollen discs, whereas nutritional amblyopias are associated with a more insidious course.

Leber optic neuropathy This condition, which affects males primarily, is transmitted via female carriers through cytoplasmic DNA in the ovum (mitochondrial). It is characterized by rapid loss of central vision occurring during early adult life. Both eyes are affected either simultaneously or sequentially. The visual fields contain scotomas that are initially central and rapidly become cecocentral in location. In acute Leber optic neuropathy the ophthalmoscopic findings are (1) circumpapillary telangiectatic microangiopathy; (2) swelling of the nerve fiber layer around the disc; and (3) absence of leakage from the disc or papillary region on fluorescein angiography with arteriovenous shunting present in the area of the telangiectatic vessels. In chronic Leber optic neuropathy the optic disc is atrophic. About 15 percent of patients recover useful vision in one or both eyes many years after the ictus.

Papilledema Optic disc swelling resulting from elevated intracranial pressure (Fig. A4-4) is typically bilateral, often asymmetric, and is associated with transient visual loss lasting seconds (visual obscurations) and horizontal diplopia. Optic atrophy, impaired vision, and field loss may ensue if papilledema becomes chronic. Increased intracranial pressure may be caused by mass lesions, inflammatory disease, or idiopathic pseudotumor cerebri (benign intracranial hypertension), but the immediate obligation is to exclude an intracranial mass lesion with appropriate neuroimaging tests (see Chap. 353).

Pseudopapilledema Pseudopapilledema is usually due to congenital disc anomalies, giving rise to apparent rather than true disc swelling. Small or absent optic cups, abnormal branching of the major retinal vessels, and calcific excrescences [optic disc drusen (Fig. A4-5)] may be seen.

DISORDERS OF EYE MOVEMENT

Disorders of eye movement in the adult usually present with diplopia. The diagnostic approach to determine the cause is based on a series of specific questions and a step-by-step analysis of the eye movements to establish first whether the double vision is monocular or binocular. If diplopia is present with one eye covered, the patient has monocular diplopia. Monocular diplopia almost never signals a neurologic disorder but is most often due to an optical problem (refractive error, keratoconus, or cataract). It may be psychogenic or functional. Binocular diplopia resolves with occlusion of vision to either eye and is due to ocular misalignment, whether caused by disorders of the ocular motor nerves, of the myoneural junction (myasthenia gravis, see Chap. 366) or of the extraocular muscles themselves. Myasthenia gravis can usually be diagnosed with the edrophonium or prostigmine test. Restriction of extraocular muscle function can result from inflammation (orbital myositis), infiltration (thyroid ophthalmopathy or metastatic disease), or entrapment (blow-out fracture of the orbital floor). Restriction of movement of the globe can be confirmed with a positive forced duction test. Topical proparacaine is used to anesthetize the eye, especially over the insertion of the rectus muscles to be manipulated. While the patient looks in the direction of gaze limitation, the physician, using a cotton tipped applicator or toothed forceps, attempts to move the globe in the direction of gaze deficit. The inability to overcome the eye movement limitation signifies the presence of a restrictive process.

Once restrictive disease and myasthenia gravis are excluded, the major cause of binocular diplopia is a cranial nerve lesion. The type of binocular diplopia—horizontal, vertical, or oblique—provides clues in determining which muscle is affected. A red glass test allows a more exact documentation of the type of diplopia.

ISOLATED OCULAR MOTOR NERVE PALSIES Oculomotor nerve (third cranial nerve) The oculomotor (third nerve) nuclear complex is a compact midline structure in the rostral midbrain, containing somatic motor and visceral nuclei. Motoneurons project ipsilaterally to the medial rectus, inferior rectus, and inferior oblique muscles and contralaterally to the superior rectus muscle. One central caudal nucleus innervates the levator palpebrae superioris bilaterally. Axons from the visceral nuclei project ipsilaterally, as the preganglionic, parasympathetic outflow to the ciliary ganglion, controlling pupillary sphincter function and accommodation.

The fascicular portion of the third nerve courses through the red nucleus and ventral mesencephalon to emerge in the interpeduncular fossa. It then runs forward beneath the posterior cerebral artery and lateral to the posterior communicating artery, pierces the dura, and enters the cavernous sinus. The pupillary fibers travel superficially in the dorsomedial portion of the nerve. At the superior orbital fissure, where the nerve enters the orbit, it divides into a superior (levator, superior rectus) and inferior division (medial and inferior rectus, inferior oblique, pupillomotor fibers).

A complete third nerve lesion causes ptosis and inability to turn the eye upward, downward, or inward. At rest, the eye is deviated down and temporally. Whether the iris sphincter is involved or spared, as determined by pupillary size and reactivity, is critical in determining the appropriate workup of the patient over age 50 years.

An acute, total, isolated painful third nerve palsy with a dilated nonreactive pupil suggests aneurysm of the posterior communicating artery compressing the third nerve. Pupillary sparing (normal size and reflex response) is the hallmark of a third nerve palsy due to microinfarction as occurs in diabetes mellitus. Initial pupillary sparing can be found in 8 to 15 percent of aneurysms, but pupillary involvement usually occurs within 5 to 7 days. Prompt consideration of cerebral angiography and surgery is indicated in all third nerve palsies with pupil involvement at all ages. Patients over age 50 with an isolated oculomotor palsy in which there is pupillary sparing and without signs of subarachnoid hemorrhage can be followed expectantly.

Recovery within three to four months is common in cases of microinfarction. In compressive or traumatic oculomotor palsies, regeneration is often aberrant, consisting of activation of inappropriate muscle groups on eye movements, e.g., producing lid retraction on down gaze or pupillary constriction with adduction.

The common causes of third nerve palsies in adults are aneurysms and vascular disease (hypertension, atherosclerosis, diabetes mellitus, temporal arteritis). Trauma and tumor (pituitary tumor, cavernous sinus meningioma or metastasis) each account for 10 to 15 percent of cases. Parasellar mass lesions can cause acute onset of a third nerve palsy after only minor trauma. (A similar relation holds for fourth and sixth nerve palsies as well.) Aberrant regeneration without a history of an antecedent oculomotor palsy indicates an indolent mass lesion in the cavernous sinus.

Trochlear nerve (fourth cranial nerve)   The neurons of the fourth nerve nucleus lie dorsally in the rostral brainstem at the level of the inferior colliculi, contiguous to the caudal end of the oculomotor complex. The axons run dorsally and decussate in the anterior medullary velum (the roof of the fourth ventricle) where they are vulnerable to head trauma. The nerve exits the brainstem dorsally, crosses the superior cerebellar artery, runs forward in the cavernous sinus, and enters the orbit through the superior orbital fissure to innervate the superior oblique muscle.

A superior oblique palsy causes vertical diplopia with hypertropia and excylotorsion of the eye. Many patients compensate for this by adapting a head tilt toward the uninvolved side (i.e., a patient with a right superior oblique palsy will often have a left head tilt). Some patients who have a congenital fourth nerve palsy may be asymptomatic until later in life when the ability to fuse is lost. Such patients generally have a head tilt documented on childhood and adult photographs.

Trauma is the commonest cause of fourth nerve palsies. Vascular diseases (hypertension, atherosclerosis, diabetes mellitus) account for approximately 20 percent of cases. Miscellaneous causes include aneurysm (cavernous internal carotid artery or basilar artery), hydrocephalus, or sequelae to intracranial surgery. Management is usually conservative using vertical prism glasses or unilateral patching to alleviate symptoms. A variety of surgical procedures on the superior oblique or inferior oblique muscle can be performed if conservative treatment is unsatisfactory.

Abducens nerve (sixth nerve)   The abducens nucleus is located beneath the floor of the fourth ventricle and lateral to the midline of the pons at the junction of the pons and medulla. The genu of the facial nerve curves over the dorsal and lateral surface. The medial longitudinal fasciculus lies adjacent and medial to it. The abducens nucleus contains motor neurons that innervate the ipsilateral lateral rectus muscle and a pool of interneurons whose axons cross the midline and ascend in the medial longitudinal fasciculus to reach the contralateral oculomotor subnucleus innervating the medial rectus muscle of the opposite eye. The abducens nucleus thus participates in the control of horizontal gaze.

The fascicular portion of the sixth nerve passes ventrally, laterally, and caudally through the pons, medial to the olivary nucleus, to exit the brainstem in a groove between the pons and the medulla. The proximity of the sixth nerve nucleus and its fascicular portion to the motor nucleus of the facial nerve, facial nerve fascicle, the vestibular nucleus, and descending sympathetic fibers within the brainstem explains the association of sixth nerve deficits with a multitude of disease states.

After emerging from the brainstem, the nerve runs along the face of the bony clivus to penetrate the dura below the crest of the petrous bone to enter the cavernous sinus. The sixth nerve is not situated within the sinus wall, like the third and fourth cranial nerves, but instead lies within the body of the sinus itself. It enters the orbit through the superior orbital fissure within the annulus of Zinn to innervate the lateral rectus muscle. A sixth nerve palsy causes an inward deviation of the eye and paresis of abduction. Causes of sixth nerve palsy include infarction, aneurysm, tumor, trauma, leptomeningitis, and multiple sclerosis. However, in spite of improved diagnostic techniques, many cases of monocranial nerve palsy remain unexplained (idiopathic).

MULTIPLE OCULAR MOTOR NERVE PALSIES   The localization of lesions that cause combinations of third, fourth, or sixth nerve palsies depends upon the accurate assessment of the various combinations of associated neurologic deficits.

Lesions producing ophthalmoplegia involving the functions of more than one ocular motor nerve and associated with pain or hypesthesia in the distribution of the trigeminal nerve (fifth nerve) can be localized depending upon the extent of fifth nerve involvement. The lesion is at the superior orbital fissure or anterior cavernous sinus region, if only the first division of nerve V is involved; is at the middle to posterior cavernous sinus region, if the first (V1) and second (V2) divisions are involved; and is in the parasellar region, if all three divisions are involved. If the ipsilateral optic nerve is affected, the lesion must be in the orbital apex. Causes of these syndromes include nasopharyngeal carcinoma, granulomatous inflammatory processes (pseudotumor of the orbit or "Tolosa Hunt" syndrome), and lymphoma. Pituitary tumors, menigiomas, chordomas, and other rarer tumors can produce cavernous sinus–orbital apex syndromes. The diagnosis is aided by neuroimaging of the suspected area, including the nasopharynx.

SUPRANUCLEAR DISORDERS   The neurologic signs   The bedside diagnosis of brainstem disorders is aided by the understanding of the neuroanatomy of ocular motor control.

There are two classes of eye movements, rapid or *saccadic* movements and slow or *pursuit* movements. Both systems alter the direction of gaze (eye position in space). Rapid eye movements are used to bring new images onto the fovea. Pursuit eye movements are used to hold the object's image stationary on the moving retina.

Saccadic eye movements are tested by observation of eye movements on command, refixation saccades between two targets, and quick phases of optokinetic nystagmus and/or vestibular stimulation. Saccades and quick phases share the same immediate premotor neural circuitry within the brainstem. The descending pathways transmitting saccadic signals for gaze control are part of a corticobulbar pathway with connections between visual, frontal, and brainstem structures. All decussate in the midbrain to terminate in the contralateral pontine paramedian reticular formation (PPRF) in the brainstem, just rostral to the sixth nerve nucleus. Pursuit eye movements are tested by observation of the eyes tracking a target horizontally and vertically. Three visual cortical areas in the temporal-occipital junction are concerned with control of pursuit eye movements. They are the middle temporal and medial superior temporal cortex and the fundus of the superior temporal cortex. Pursuit pathways descend ipsilaterally to the dorsal lateral pontine nuclei, the Purkinje cells in the cerebellar flocculus, to the vestibular nuclei, and onward to the final common brainstem pathway, the PPRF.

Direct vertical gaze requires bilateral cortical activation. The rostral PPRF acts as the first brainstem center from which fibers project to the pretectal rostral interstitial nucleus of the median longitudinal fasciculus, which is the final vertical gaze center. Paralysis of horizontal and vertical gaze can be produced by lesions affecting cortical, mesencephalic, and pontine centers of their projections. Destruction of the ocular motor nuclei, fascicles, or nerves as well as myasthenia gravis can mimic a gaze palsy. Isolated upward gaze paralysis (Parinaud's syndrome) and isolated downward gaze or complete vertical gaze paralysis are produced by lesions involving the mesencephalon and pretectum. Tumors in the region of the pineal gland produce Parinaud's syndrome or the sylvian aqueduct syndrome; ocular signs include a supranuclear paralysis of upward gaze, light-near dissociation of the pupils, convergence paresis, skew deviation, and convergence retraction nystagmus. Brainstem infarction is possibly the only cause of selective paralysis of downward gaze, due to occlusion of a single perforating vessel, the posterior thalamosubthalamic paramedian artery.

Degenerative diseases e.g., progressive supranuclear palsy (see Chap. 359) may selectively or primarily involve the supranuclear structures of the brainstem. Vertical saccades are affected first, being slow and then small. Eventually there is complete loss of voluntary vertical refixations. With chronicity, the horizontal eye movements become similarly affected. Convergence may be impaired. The disease may progress to total ophthalmoplegia. Other degenerative diseases— Huntington's chorea, abetalipoproteinema, amyotrophic lateral sclerosis, and olivopontocerebellar degeneration—may be associated with a supranuclear disorder of vertical as well as horizontal gaze. Supranuclear vertical gaze disorders also occur in multiple sclerosis, Whipple's disease, syphilis, brucellosis, tetanus, encephalitis, neurofibromatosis, and tuberculoma as well as brainstem trauma, including neurosurgical procedures.

Opsoclonus is a striking disorder of saccadic eye movements reflecting the presence of unwanted saccades. It consists of involuntary, arrhythmic, multidirectional, high-amplitude, conjugate back-to-back saccades. The eye movements are usually continuous and persist during sleep. Opsoclonus can occur with encephalitis, trauma, intracranial tumors, hydrocephalus, thalamic hemorrhage, and toxic and metabolic encephalopathies. It occurs as a paraneoplastic or remote effect of neuroblastoma in children and, less commonly, of other carcinomas (ovary, lung, breast) in adults (Chap. 310).

INTERNUCLEAR OPHTHALMOPLEGIA Clinically, internuclear ophthalmoplegia (INO) is characterized by (1) paresis or paralysis of adduction of the ipsilateral eye on attempted horizontal gaze to the contralateral side, and (2) horizontal jerk nystagmus in the contralateral abducting eye. Typically convergence is intact if the lesion does not extend to the mesencephalon; gaze-evoked vertical nystagmus on upward gaze is frequent. Unilateral INO is due to the interruption of the ipsilateral medial longitudinal fasciculus (MLF), after fibers have crossed from the interneurons of the contralateral abducens nucleus projecting to the ipsilateral medial rectus subnucleus. Unilateral internuclear ophthalmoplegia is most commonly due to multiple sclerosis in young adults and to vascular infarction in the elderly. Prognosis for full recovery is good.

Bilateral INO is usually due to brainstem glioma in children and to multiple sclerosis in adults. Myasthenia gravis can mimic both unilateral and bilateral INO.

NYSTAGMUS AND OTHER ENTITIES THAT MIMIC NYSTAGMUS (See also Chap. 22) Nystagmus is a repetitive, to-and-fro movement of the eyes. *Pendular nystagmus* consists of smooth sinusoidal oscillations, and *jerk nystagmus* consists of slow drift alternating with corrective quick phases. Normal subjects develop nystagmus in response to vestibular and optokinetic stimuli.

Normally, the vestibular, optokinetic, and pursuit systems each act to hold images steady on the retina, and a neural integrator allows maintenance of eccentric positions of gaze. Disorders of these systems create nystagmus. Identification of the cause of nystagmus requires historical information—especially of drug use or alcohol abuse—and a complete ocular motor evaluation. The most important clinical types of nystagmus are discussed below and in Chap. 22.

Congenital nystagmus Congenital nystagmus is a pendular or jerk nystagmus that remains horizontal in all positions of gaze, is dampened by convergence, and is associated with better vision at near rather than far distances. Patients with congenital nystagmus often have afferent visual system dysfunction.

Labyrinthine-vestibular nystagmus Disease of the vestibular system causes constant velocity slow-phase drifts with corrective quick phases that create a "saw-tooth" jerk nystagmus. By convention, the side of the nystagmus is designated by the direction of the quick corrective saccade (fast phase). Vestibular nystagmus may be due to a peripheral or central lesion. In peripheral vestibular disease, the nystagmus is usually of mixed type. For example, in benign positional nystagmus, a mixed vertical-torsional nystagmus is common. In unilateral labyrinthine destruction, a mixed horizontal-torsional nystagmus occurs. Peripheral vestibular nystagmus is suppressed by fixation and exacerbated by changes in head position. Peripheral nystagmus if often associated with severe vertigo, nausea, vomiting, and oscillopsia. Disturbances of central vestibular connections are associated with a central imbalance between semicircular canal inputs and disruption of ascending vestibular or cerebellovestibular connections. Mixed nystagmus can be caused by peripheral labyrinthine or central vestibular disease. Purely bilateral vertical (upbeat, downbeat), torsional, or horizontal nystagmus can only occur with central vestibular disease. Central vestibular nystagmus is poorly suppressed by fixation but exacerbated or induced by changes in head position (Chap. 22).

Four forms of primary position vestibular nystagmus have anatomic localizing value: downbeat, upbeat, horizontal, and torsional nystagmus. Downbeat nystagmus in the primary position and accentuated on lateral gaze occurs with cervicomedullary junction disorders, such as Arnold-Chiari malformation and basilar invagination, and in multiple sclerosis, brainstem infarction, cerebellar atrophy, hydrocephalus, metabolic disorders, familiar periodic ataxia, or as a toxic side effect of anticonvulsant drugs. Lesions associated with primary position upbeat nystagmus are in the tegmentum of the rostral medulla and caudal pons; causes include infarction, demyelination, myelinolysis, and diffuse infiltration with glioma. Horizontal primary position nystagmus is rare and is usually due to peripheral vestibular disease.

Primary position torsional nystagmus is common in the lateral medullary syndrome. With this lesion the nystagmus may be horizontal or mixed with both torsional and vertical components. Typically the horizontal nystagmus beats away from the side of the medullary infarction with the eyes in a primary position but beats ipsilaterally when gaze is directed toward the lesion. Vertical nystagmus, if present, is usually upbeating.

Gaze-evoked nystagmus Gaze-evoked nystagmus implies a weakness in holding the eyes in an eccentric position due to a defect in the integrator in the brainstem. It is commonly caused by drugs such as sedatives or anticonvulsants. Asymmetric but conjugate horizontal gaze-evoked nystagmus occurs with unilateral cerebellar disease and cerebellopontine-angle tumors such as acoustic neuroma or meningioma.

REFERENCES

AMERICAN ACADEMY OF OPHTHALMOLOGY: *Basic and Clinical Science Course*, Sections I and II. San Francisco, 1988–1989
BURDE RM et al: *Clinical Decision in Neurophthalmology*. St. Louis, Mosby, 1985
DUANE T (ED): *Clinical Ophthalmology*. Philadelphia, Lippincott, 1988
GLASER JS: *Neuroophthalmology*. Philadelphia, Lippincott 1989
LEIGH RJ, ZEE DS: *The Neurology of Eye Movements*. Philadelphia, Davis, 1983
MILLER NR: *Walsh and Hoyt's Clinical Neuroophthalmology*, 4th ed. Baltimore, Williams & Wilkins, 1982

24 DISTURBANCES OF SMELL, TASTE, AND HEARING

JAMES B. SNOW, JR. / JOSEPH B. MARTIN

SMELL The sense of smell determines the flavor and palatability of food and drink. It serves along with the trigeminal system as a monitor of inhaled chemicals including dangerous substances such as natural gas, smoke, and air pollutants. Although qualitative sensations of smell are subserved by the olfactory neuroepithelium, many substances are capable of producing somatic sensations of coolness, warmth, and irritation through the trigeminal, glossopharyngeal, and vagal afferents in the nose, oral cavity, tongue, pharynx, and larynx. The sense of smell should be considered as one of several chemosensory systems since most chemical substances initiate olfactory, trigeminal, and taste perceptions.

The *olfactory neuroepithelium* is located in the superior part of the nasal cavities. It contains an orderly arrangement of bipolar olfactory receptor cells, microvillar cells, sustentacular cells, and basal cells. The dendritic process of the bipolar cell has a bulb-shaped knob or vesicle that projects into the mucous layer and bears six to eight cilia. The receptor sites for odorant molecules are located on the cilia. The microvillar cells are located adjacent to the receptor cells on the surface of the neuroepithelium. The sustentacular cells, unlike their counterparts in the respiratory epithelium, are not specialized to secrete mucus. Their function is unknown. The basal cells are progenitors of other cell types in the olfactory neuroepithelium including the bipolar receptor cells. There is a regular turnover of the bipolar receptor cells, which function as the primary sensory neurons. In addition with injury to the cell body or its axon, the receptor cell is replaced by a basal cell which reestablishes a central neural connection. *Hence, these primary sensory neurons are unique among sensory systems in that they are regularly replaced and regenerate after injury.*

The unmyelinated axons of the receptor cells form the fila of the olfactory nerve, pass through the cribriform plate, and terminate within spherical masses of neuropil, termed glomeruli, in the olfactory bulb. The glomeruli are a focus of a high degree of convergence of information, since many more fibers enter than leave them. The main second-order neurons are the mitral cells. The primary dendrite of each mitral cell extends into a single glomerulus. Axons of the mitral cells project along with the axons of adjacent tufted cells to the limbic system, including the anterior olfactory nucleus, the prepiriform cortex, the periamygdaloid cortex, the olfactory tubercle, the nucleus of the lateral olfactory tract, and the corticomedial nucleus of the amygdala. Cognitive awareness of smell requires stimulation of the prepiriform cortex or the amygdaloid nuclei.

Odorants are absorbed into the mucus overlying the olfactory neuroepithelium, diffuse to the cilia, and reversibly bind to membrane receptor sites. The process causes conformational changes in the receptor proteins which induce a chain of biochemical events that results in generation of action potentials in the primary neurons. Intensity appears to be coded by the amount of firing in the afferent neurons. Indeed, a clear relationship exists in humans between psychophysical measures of intensity and the magnitude of the evoked potential from the olfactory neuroepithelium. Little is known about quality coding. Individual receptor cells are responsive to a wide range of stimuli. It is thought that more than one type of receptor site is present on each cell.

Disturbances of the sense of smell Disturbances of the sense of smell are caused by conditions that interfere with the access of the odorant to the olfactory neuroepithelium (transport loss), injure the receptor region (sensory loss), or damage central olfactory pathways (neural loss).

Transport olfactory loss can result from swollen nasal mucous membrane in acute viral upper respiratory infections, herpes simplex,

viral hepatitis, bacterial rhinitis, sinusitis, and allergic rhinitis and with structural changes in the nasal cavity such as deviations of the nasal septum, polyps, and neoplasms. Nasopharyngeal tumor or lymphoma can interfere with smell perception. It is also likely that abnormalities of mucous secretion in which the olfactory cilia are immersed could result in a loss of olfactory sensitivity. Currently little is known about alterations in the mucus environment of the olfactory neuroepithelium.

Sensory olfactory losses are caused by destruction of the olfactory neuroepithelium by viral infections, neoplasms, the inhalation of toxic chemicals, drugs that affect cell turnover, and radiation therapy to the head. *Neural olfactory losses* occur in head trauma, with or without fracture of the base of the anterior cranial fossa or cribriform plate area; Parkinson's disease, Alzheimer's disease, Korsakoff's psychosis, and vitamin B_{12} deficiency; neoplasms of the anterior cranial fossa; neurosurgical procedures; administration of neurotoxic drugs (e.g., ethanol, amphetamines, topical cocaine, aminoglycosides, tetracycline, cigarette smoke); and in some congenital disorders such as Kallmann's syndrome. Other endocrine disorders, including Cushing's syndrome, hypothyroidism, and diabetes mellitus, can affect smell perception.

From the psychophysical point of view, disturbances of the sense of smell may be categorized by either the patient's complaint or the objective sensory measurements as *total anosmia* (general anosmia)—inability to detect any qualitative olfactory sensations; *partial anosmia*—ability to detect some, but not all, qualitative olfactory sensations; *specific anosmia*—loss of ability to appreciate only one or a very limited number of odorants; *total hyposmia* (general hyposmia)—decreased sensitivity to all odorants; *partial hyposmia*—decreased sensitivity to some odorants; dysosmia (cacosmia or paraosmia)—distortion in the perception of an odor, that is, the perception of an unpleasant odor when a pleasant odorant is being presented or the perception of an odor when there is no odorant in the environment; *total hyperosmia* (general hyperosmia)—increased sensitivity to all odorants; *partial hyperosmia*—increased sensitivity to some odorants; and *agnosia*—inability to classify, contrast, or identify odor sensations verbally, even though the ability to distinguish between odorants or to recognize them may be normal.

CLINICAL EVALUATION The history of the onset and development of the disturbance of the sense of smell may be of paramount importance in making an etiologic diagnosis. Unilateral anosmia is rarely a complaint. Only by separate testing of smell in each nasal cavity can it be recognized. Bilateral anosmia, on the other hand, does bring patients to medical attention. Anosmic patients usually complain of a loss of the sense of taste even though their taste thresholds may be within normal limits. In actuality, they are complaining of a loss of flavor detection, which is mainly an olfactory function. Flavor appreciation depends on the olfactory detection of volatile substances in food and beverages as well as the sense of taste. The physical examination should include a complete examination of the ears, upper respiratory tract, and head and neck. A neurologic examination emphasizing the cranial nerves is essential. Computed tomography scans of the head with enhancement is required to rule out neoplasms of the anterior cranial fossa, unsuspected fractures of the anterior cranial fossa, paranasal sinusitis, and neoplasms of the nasal cavity and paranasal sinuses.

The sensory evaluation of olfactory function is necessary for corroboration of the patient's complaint, evaluation of the efficacy of treatment, and determination of the degree of permanent impairment. The first step in the sensory evaluation is to determine the degree to which qualitative sensations are present. For this assessment, a smell identification test is used that consists of a 40-item, forced choice, microencapsulated odor, scratch-and-sniff paradigm. For example, one of the items reads, "This odor smells most like (a) chocolate, (b) banana, (c) onion, or (d) fruit punch," and the patient is instructed to answer one of the alternatives. The test is highly reliable (short-term test-retest reliability $r = 0.95$) and is sensitive to age and sex differences (Fig. 24-1). It is an accurate quantitative

FIGURE 24-1   Smell identification test. Scores for a group of male and female subjects 5 to 99 years in age are shown. *(Reprinted with permission from RL Doty et al. Copyright 1984 by the AAAS.)*

determination of the relative degree of olfactory deficit. Persons with a total loss of smell function score in the range of 7 to 19 out of 40. The average score for total anosmics is slightly higher than that expected on the basis of chance because of the inclusion of some odorants which act by trigeminal stimulation.

The second step is to establish a detection threshold for the odorant phenyl ethyl alcohol, using a graduated stimulus. Although the detection threshold usually agrees with the results of the smell identification test, in some instances patients who fail the smell identification test perform well on the threshold test. However, the reverse is much less common. Since the threshold test can be influenced by trigeminal and nonolfactory nerve clues, the results of the smell identification test are relied upon more heavily in the sensory evaluation. Sensitivity for each side of the nose is determined with a detection threshold for phenyl ethyl methyl ethyl carbinol. Nasal resistance is measured with anterior rhinomanometry for each side of the nose.

Techniques have been developed to biopsy the olfactory neuro-epithelium, but in view of the widespread degeneration of the olfactory neuroepithelium and intercalation of respiratory epithelium in the olfactory area of adults with no apparent olfactory dysfunction, biopsy material must be interpreted cautiously.

DIFFERENTIAL DIAGNOSIS   At the present time there are no psychophysical methods to differentiate sensory from neural olfactory losses. Fortunately, the history of the disease provides important clues to the cause. The leading causes of olfactory disorders are head trauma and viral infections. Head trauma is a more frequent cause of anosmia in children and young adults, and viral infections are more important causes of anosmia in older adults.

Cranial trauma is followed by uni- or bilateral impairment of smell in 5 to 10 percent of cases. Frontal injuries and fractures disrupt the cribriform plate and olfactory axons which perforate it. Sometimes there is an associated cerebrospinal fluid (CSF) rhinorrhea resulting from a tearing of the dura overlying the cribriform plate and paranasal sinuses. If the anosmia is unilateral, it is usually on the side of the CSF leak, and this fact aids in localization of the fistula. Anosmia may also follow blows to the occiput. Once traumatic anosmia develops, it is usually permanent; only about 10 percent of patients ever improve or recover. Perversion of the sense of smell may occur as a phase in the recovery process.

The occurrence of a permanent hyposmia or anosmia may follow viral infections and is called *postviral anosmia.* In this instance the sensory epithelium of the olfactory zone is destroyed by the virus and replaced by respiratory epithelial and goblet cells and scar tissue. The congenital anosmias, one type of which is associated with a

hypothalamic defect [Kallmann's syndrome, or congenital anosmia with hypogonadotropic hypogonadism (see Chap. 313)], are rare but important causes of anosmia or hyposmia. Anosmia can also occur in albinos. The receptor cells are present but hypoplastic, lack cilia, and do not project above the surrounding supporting cells.

Meningioma of the inferior frontal region is the most frequent neoplastic cause of anosmia; rarely anosmia can occur with glioma of the frontal lobe. Occasionally pituitary adenomas, craniopharyngiomas, suprasellar meningiomas, and aneurysms of the anterior part of the circle of Willis extend forward and damage olfactory structures. These tumors and hamartomas may also induce seizures with olfactory hallucinations, indicating involvement of the uncus of the temporal lobe.

Paraosmia and dysosmia, subjective distortions of olfactory perception, may occur with intranasal disease that partially impairs smell, or may represent a phase in the recovery from a neurogenic anosmia. Most paraosmic disturbances consist of disagreeable or foul odors, and they may be accompanied by distortions of taste. Dysosmia may also be a symptom in elderly patients with depression. Every article of food has an extremely unpleasant odor (cacosmia). Sensations of disagreeable taste are often noted (cacogeusia).

Olfactory hallucinations are descriptions of smelling an odor that no one else can smell. They occur in alcohol withdrawal, in which olfactory hallucinations are occasionally associated with other types of hallucinations, and in uncal seizures, which are brief and clearly related to a derangement of consciousness and other epileptic components. In other settings, olfactory hallucinations usually signify a psychiatric disease. A huge range of odors may be reported, most of them foul. Some patients perceive the smell as emanating from themselves (intrinsic); others perceive the source to be external (extrinsic). Most are associated with schizophrenia and depressive illnesses.

TREATMENT   Therapy for patients with transport olfactory losses due to allergic rhinitis, bacterial rhinitis and sinusitis, polyps, neoplasms, and structural abnormalities of the nasal cavities can be undertaken rationally and with a high chance of improvement. Allergy management, antibiotic therapy, topical and systemic glucocorticoid therapy, and operations for nasal polyps, deviation of the nasal septum, and chronic hyperplastic sinusitis are frequently effective in restoring the sense of smell.

There is no treatment with demonstrated efficacy for sensorineural olfactory losses. Fortunately spontaneous recovery often occurs. Zinc and vitamin therapy are advocated by some. Profound zinc deficiency can undoubtedly result in losses and distortion of the sense of smell, but it is not a clinical problem except in very limited geographic areas. Vitamin therapy has mainly been in the form of vitamin A. The epithelial degeneration associated with vitamin A deficiency can cause anosmia, but vitamin A deficiency is not a common clinical problem in the United States. Unfortunately at the present time there are no effective therapeutic strategies for the sensorineural disorders of the sense of smell.

TASTE   Many patients with a loss of olfactory sensitivity also complain of a loss of the sense of taste. On psychophysical testing, most of these patients have normal detection thresholds for taste. Disturbances of the sense of taste are far less frequent than disturbances of the sense of smell.

The taste receptor cells are located in the taste buds, spherical groups of cells arranged like the segments of a citrus fruit. At the surface, the taste bud has a pore into which microvilli of the receptor cells project. Taste buds have a similar appearance wherever they are located. Unlike the olfactory system the receptor cell is not the primary neuron. Instead, gustatory afferent nerve fibers contact individual taste receptor cells.

The sense of taste is mediated through the facial, glossopharyngeal, and vagal nerves. The gustatory system consists of at least five receptor populations. Taste buds are located in the foliate papillae along the lateral margin of the tongue, in the fungiform papillae throughout the dorsum of the tongue, in the circumvallate papillae at the junction of the dorsum and the base of the tongue, and in the palate, epiglottis, larynx, and esophagus. The chorda tympani branch of the facial nerve subserves taste from the anterior two-thirds of the tongue. The posterior one-third of the tongue is supplied by the lingual branch of the glossopharyngeal nerve. Afferents from the palate travel with the greater superficial petrosal nerve to the geniculate ganglion and thence via the facial nerve to the brainstem. The internal branch of the superior laryngeal nerve of the vagus nerve contains the taste afferents from the larynx including the epiglottis and esophagus.

The central connections of the nerves terminate in the brainstem in the nucleus of the tractus solitarius. The fibers of the chorda tympani and greater superficial petrosal nerves go to the cephalic portion of the nucleus. The glossopharyngeal gustatory fibers go to the middle, and the superior laryngeal nerve fibers to the caudal portion of the nucleus. The central pathway from the nucleus of the tractus solitarius projects to the ipsilateral parabrachial nuclei of the pons. Two divergent pathways project from the parabrachial nuclei. One ascends to the gustatory relay in the dorsal thalamus, synapses, and continues to the cortex of the insula. There is also evidence for a direct pathway from the parabrachial nuclei to the cortex. (Olfaction and taste appear to be unique among sensory systems in that at least some fibers bypass the thalamus.) The other pathway from the parabrachial nuclei goes to the ventral forebrain including the lateral hypothalamus, substantia innominata, central nucleus of the amygdala, and the stria terminalis.

Tastants gain access to the receptor cells through the taste pore. Four classes of taste are recognized: sweet, salt, sour, and bitter. Individual gustatory afferent fibers almost always respond to a number of different chemicals. Response patterns of gustatory afferent axons can be grouped into classes based on the stimulus chemical that produces the largest response. For example, for sucrose-best response neurons, the second-best stimulus is almost always sodium chloride. The fact that individual gustatory afferent fibers respond to a large number of different chemicals led to the *across-fiber-pattern* theory of gustatory coding, while the best-stimulus analysis led to the concept of *labeled* afferents. It appears that labeled fibers are important for establishing gross quality, but the across-fiber-pattern within a best-stimulus category, and perhaps among categories, is needed for discriminating chemicals within qualities. For example, sweetness may be carried by sucrose-best neurons, but the differentiation of sucrose and fructose may require a comparison of the relative activity among sucrose-best, salt-best, and quinine-best neurons. As with olfaction and other sensory systems, intensity appears to be encoded by the quantity of neural activity.

Disturbances of the sense of taste Disturbances of the sense of taste are caused by conditions that interfere with the access of the tastant to the receptor cells in the taste bud (transport loss), injure receptor cells (sensory loss), or damage gustatory afferent nerves and central gustatory pathways (neural loss).

Transport gustatory losses result from xerostomia due to many causes including Sjögren's syndrome, heavy metal intoxication, and bacterial colonization of the taste pore. The salivary milieu of the receptors may prove to be important to diverse causes of gustatory loss.

Sensory gustatory losses are caused by inflammatory and degenerative diseases in the oral cavity, a vast number of drugs, particularly those that interfere with cell turnover such as antithyroid and antineoplastic agents, radiation therapy to the oral cavity and pharynx, viral infections, endocrine disorders, neoplasms, and aging.

Neural olfactory losses occur with neoplasms, trauma, and operations in which the gustatory afferents are injured. Taste buds degenerate when their gustatory afferents are transected but remain when their somatosensory afferents are severed.

CLINICAL MANIFESTATIONS From the psychophysical point of view disturbances of the sense of taste may be categorized by either the patient's complaint or the objective sensory measurements as *total ageusia*—inability to detect the qualities of sweet, salt, bitter,

or sour; *partial ageusia*—ability to detect some but not all of the qualitative gustatory sensations; *specific ageusia*—inability to detect the taste quality of certain substances; *total hypoguesia*—decreased sensitivity to all tastants; *partial hypogeusia*—decreased sensitivity to some tastants; *dysgeusia*—distortion in the perception of a tastant, that is, the perception of the wrong quality when a tastant is presented or the perception of a taste when there has been no tastant ingested. Confusions of sour and bitter are common and, at times, may be semantic misunderstandings. Frequently, however, they have physiologic or pathophysiologic bases.

It may be possible to differentiate between the loss of flavor recognition in patients with olfactory losses who complain of a loss of taste as well as smell by asking if they are able to taste sweetness in sodas, saltiness in potato chips, etc.

Patients who complain of loss of taste should be evaluated psychophysically for gustatory function in addition to being evaluated for olfactory function. The first step is to perform suprathreshold whole-mouth taste testing for quality, intensity, and pleasantness perception with sucrose, citric acid, caffeine, and sodium chloride. In the quantification of the sense of taste, detection thresholds are obtained by applying graduated dilutions to the tongue quadrants or by whole-mouth sips. Finally, suprathreshold magnitude estimation may be used to shed further light on the patient's complaint. Electric taste testing (electrogustometry) is used clinically to identify taste deficits in specific quadrants of the tongue.

Biopsy of the foliate or fungiform papillae for histopathologic study of taste buds remains experimental but holds promise of shedding light on the categorization of taste disorders.

DIFFERENTIAL DIAGNOSIS As with olfaction, psychophysical methods for differentiating transport, sensory, and neural gustatory losses are not available. Once there is objective evidence of a disorder of taste, it is important to establish, as is done in other neurologic deficits, an anatomic diagnosis before proceeding to an etiologic diagnosis. The history of the disease often provides important clues to the cause. For example, absence of taste on the anterior two-thirds of the tongue associated with a facial paralysis indicates that the lesion is proximal to the point of junction of the chorda tympani branch with the facial nerve in the mastoid.

TREATMENT Therapy for gustatory losses remains limited. Artificial saliva benefits some patients with a disturbed salivary milieu. Treatment for bacterial and fungal infections of the oral cavity are appropriate and may be helpful. Withdrawal of drugs affecting cell turnover are usually helpful if the patient's general condition permits. Zinc and vitamin therapy for gustatory losses are advocated by some, but lack demonstrated efficacy. No therapeutic strategies exist for the sensorineural disorders of taste.

HEARING Hearing occurs by air conduction and bone conduction. In air conduction, sound waves reach the ear by propagation in air, enter the external auditory canal, and set the tympanic membrane in motion, which in turn moves the malleus, incus, and stapes. Movement of the footplate of the stapes causes pressure changes in the fluid-filled inner ear eliciting a traveling wave in the basilar membrane of the cochlea. The traveling wave moves from the base to the apex of the cochlea. Hairs of the hair cells of the organ of Corti, which rests on the basilar membrane, are imbedded in the tectorial membrane and are deformed by the traveling wave. A point of maximal displacement of the basilar membrane determined by the frequency of the stimulating tone occurs with each traveling wave. High-frequency tones cause maximal displacement of the basilar membrane near the base of the cochlea. As the frequency of the stimulating tone decreases, the point of maximal displacement moves toward the apex of the cochlea. Hearing by bone conduction occurs when the sounding source, in contact with the head, results in vibration of the bones of the skull including the temporal bone, producing a traveling wave in the basilar membrane.

The deformation of the hairs of the hair cells produces several bioelectric phenomena. The cochlear microphonic, an alternating current response that faithfully represents the frequency and intensity of the stimulating tone, occurs about 0.5 ms prior to the eighth nerve action potential. This latency is taken as evidence for release of an as yet unidentified neurotransmitter at the hair cell and cochlear nerve dendrite interface. Each of the cochlear nerve neurons can be activated at a frequency and intensity specific for that cell. This phenomenon of the characteristic or best frequency occurs at each point of the central auditory pathway: dorsal and ventral cochlear nuclei, trapezoid body, superior olivary complex, lateral lemniscus, inferior colliculus, medial geniculate body, and auditory cortex. At low frequencies, individual auditory nerve fibers can respond more or less synchronously with the stimulating tone. At higher frequencies, phase-locking occurs so that neurons take turns in responding to particular phases of the cycle of the sound wave. Intensity is encoded by the amount of neural activity in individual neurons, the number of neurons that are active, and the specific neurons that are activated.

Disturbances of the sense of hearing   A loss of hearing can result from lesions in the external auditory canal, middle ear, inner ear, or central auditory pathways. Lesions in the external auditory canal or the middle ear cause conductive hearing losses while lesions in the inner ear or eighth nerve cause sensorineural hearing losses.

Conductive hearing losses result from obstruction of the external auditory canal by cerumen, debris and foreign bodies, swelling of the lining of the canal, and stenosis and neoplasms of the canal. Perforations of the tympanic membrane, as in chronic otitis media, disruption of the ossicular chain, as occurs with necrosis of the long process of the incus in trauma or infection, fixation of the ossicles as in otosclerosis, and fluid, scarring, or neoplasms in the middle ear also result in conductive hearing losses. *Sensory hearing losses* are due principally to damage to the hair cells of the organ of Corti caused by intense noise, viral infections, ototoxic drugs, fractures of the temporal bone, meningitis, cochlear otosclerosis, Ménière's disease, and aging. Neural hearing losses are due mainly to cerebellar angle tumors such as acoustic neuromas, but may also result from any neoplastic, vascular, demyelinating, infectious, or degenerative disease or trauma affecting the central auditory pathways.

CLINICAL EVALUATION OF HEARING   The physical examination should evaluate the external ear canal and tympanic membrane. Careful inspection of the nose, nasopharynx, and the upper respiratory tract is indicated. The other cranial nerves should be carefully evaluated. Conductive and sensorineural hearing losses can be differentiated by comparing the threshold of hearing by air conduction with that elicited by bone conduction. Testing the hearing by air conduction is accomplished by presenting the stimulus in air. Hearing by air conduction is affected by the patency of the external auditory canal, the efficiency of the middle ear, and the integrity of the inner ear, eighth nerve, and the central auditory pathways. Testing the hearing by bone conduction is accomplished by placing an oscillator or the stem of a vibrating tuning fork in contact with the head. Hearing by bone conduction bypasses the external auditory canal and middle ear and tests the integrity of the inner ear, eighth nerve, and central auditory pathways. If air conduction thresholds are elevated and bone conduction thresholds are in the normal range, the lesion causing hearing loss is in the external auditory canal or middle ear. If both air conduction and bone conduction thresholds are elevated, the lesion is in the inner ear, eighth nerve, or central auditory pathways. Of course, conductive and sensorineural hearing losses can coexist, in which case both the air conduction and bone conduction thresholds are elevated, but in this case, air conduction thresholds are elevated more than bone conduction thresholds.

The Weber and Rinne tuning fork tests are used to differentiate conductive from sensorineural hearing losses. The Weber tuning fork test may be performed with a 256- or 512-Hz fork. The Rinne tuning fork test is most sensitive in detecting mild conductive hearing losses if a 256-Hz fork is used. Weber's test is performed by placing the stem of a vibrating tuning fork on the head in the midline and asking the patient whether the tone is heard in both ears or better in one ear than in the other. With a unilateral conductive hearing loss, the tone is perceived in the affected ear. With a unilateral sensorineural hearing

loss, the tone is perceived in the unaffected ear. Rinne's test compares the ability to hear by air conduction with the ability to hear by bone conduction. The tines of a vibrating tuning fork are held near the opening of the external auditory canal and then the stem is placed on the mastoid process. The patient is asked to indicate whether the tone is louder by air conduction or bone conduction. Normally a tone is heard louder by air conduction than by bone conduction. With a conductive hearing loss, the bone conduction stimulus is perceived as louder than the air conduction stimulus. With sensorineural hearing losses, both air and bone conduction perceptions are reduced, but the air conduction stimulus is perceived as louder, as it is in normal hearing. The combined information from the Weber and Rinne tests permits a tentative conclusion as to whether a conductive or sensorineural hearing loss is present.

Measurement of hearing   Quantification of hearing loss is obtained with an audiometer, an electronic device that allows the presentation of specific frequencies at specific intensities to each ear by either air or bone conduction. The testing is done in a sound-attenuated chamber, and masking, usually with broad-spectrum noise, is presented to the nontest ear so that responses are based on perception from the ear under test. Frequencies from 250 to 8000 Hz are used in clinical testing. The responses are measured in decibels. A decibel (dB) is equal to 10 times the logarithm of the ratio of the acoustic power required to achieve threshold in the patient to the acoustic power required to achieve threshold in a normal hearing person. An audiogram is a plot of intensity in decibels versus frequency.

The audiometric pattern of hearing loss is often of diagnostic value. Conductive hearing losses usually have a fairly equal threshold elevation for each frequency. Conductive hearing losses with a large mass component, as is often seen in middle ear effusions, have a greater elevation of thresholds in the higher frequencies. Conductive hearing losses with a large stiffness component, as in fixation of the footplate of the stapes in early otosclerosis, have a greater elevation of thresholds in the lower frequencies. In general, sensorineural hearing losses tend to have a greater threshold elevation at each higher frequency. Interesting exceptions to this generalization are noise-induced hearing loss, in which the loss at 4000 Hz is greater than it is at higher frequencies, and in Ménière's disease, particularly in the early stages of the disease, where thresholds are elevated more in lower than in higher frequencies.

Speech audiometry provides essential additional information. The *spondee threshold* is defined as the intensity at which speech is recognized as a meaningful symbol and is obtained by presenting through an audiometer two-syllable words with an equal accent on each syllable. The intensity at which the patient can repeat 50 percent of the words correctly is the spondee threshold and usually approximates the average threshold at the speech frequencies (500, 1000, and 2000 Hz). Once the spondee threshold is determined, the discrimination ability is tested by presenting one-syllable words at 25 to 40 dB above the spondee threshold. An individual with normal hearing can repeat 90 to 100 percent of the words correctly. Likewise, individuals with a conductive hearing loss do well in discrimination testing. On the other hand, patients with a sensorineural hearing loss have a loss of discrimination attributable to the loss of peripheral analysis of sound in the inner ear or eighth nerve. With a lesion in the inner ear, the discrimination is moderately affected, usually in the 50 to 80 percent range, while with neural lesions the discrimination is severely affected, often in the 0 to 50 percent range.

The discrimination testing may then be done at higher intensities than 25 to 40 dB above the spondee threshold to determine the performance-intensity function. A deterioration in discrimination ability at higher intensities suggests a lesion in the eighth nerve or central auditory pathways.

Tympanometry measures the impedance of the middle ear to sound. A sounding source and microphone are introduced into the ear canal with an airtight seal. The amount of sound that is absorbed through the middle ear or reflected from the middle ear is measured at the microphone. In conductive hearing losses, more sound is reflected than in the normal middle ear. The pressure in the ear canal can be increased or decreased from atmospheric pressure. Normally the middle ear is most compliant at atmospheric pressure. With a negative pressure in the middle ear, as with eustachian tube obstruction, the point of maximal compliance occurs with negative pressure in the ear canal. With discontinuity of the ossicular chain, no point of maximal compliance can be obtained. Tympanometry is particularly useful in the identification and diagnosis of middle ear effusions in children.

During tympanometry, an intense tone (80 dB above the hearing threshold) elicits contraction of the stapedius muscle. The change in compliance of the middle ear with contraction of the stapedius muscle can be detected. The presence or absence of this *acoustic reflex* is important in the anatomic localization of facial nerve paralysis. The presence or absence of *acoustic reflex decay* helps differentiate sensory from neural hearing losses. In neural hearing loss, the reflex adapts or decays with time.

In order to evaluate a patient with a loss of hearing the minimum audiologic assessment should include the measurement of pure tone air and bone conduction thresholds, spondee threshold, discrimination score, performance-intensity function, tympanometry, acoustic reflexes, and acoustic reflex decay. This information provides a comprehensive screening evaluation of the whole auditory system and allows one to determine whether further differentiation of a sensory (cochlear) from a neural (retrocochlear) hearing loss is indicated.

In addition to these tests, testing for recruitment, the short increment sensitivity index, tone decay, Békésy audiometry, and auditory brainstem evoked responses (ABR) help differentiate sensory from neural hearing losses. Of these, ABR is the most powerful means of differentiating the site of sensorineural hearing loss (see Chap. 349). In response to sound, five distinct waves can be recorded with computer averaging from scalp surface electrodes. Poor or absent waveforms, abnormal latency of waves, and abnormal interwave latency are evidence of lesions in the eighth nerve and brainstem. In addition, ABR is valuable in situations in which patients cannot or will not give reliable voluntary thresholds. It is also used to measure auditory function in neonates and young children and to monitor the integrity of the auditory nerve and brainstem in various clinical situations, including intraoperatively and in determination of brain death.

CLINICAL ASSESSMENT OF A COMPLAINT OF HEARING LOSS   In evaluating patients who complain of loss of hearing, associated symptoms of tinnitus, vertigo, difficulty with balance, earache, otorrhea, and aural fullness should be sought along with a careful reconstruction of the history of evolution of the hearing deficit. A sudden onset of unilateral hearing loss, with or without tinnitus, may represent a viral infection in the inner ear. Gradual progression in a hearing deficit is common with otosclerosis, noise-induced hearing loss, acoustic neuroma, or Ménière's disease. In the latter case, intermittent tinnitus and vertigo are usual. Hearing loss can occur with demyelinative lesions in the brainstem. Hearing loss is a hallmark of several genetic diseases, some with onset at birth, others occurring in children or adults (see Konigsmark for review).

Tinnitus is defined as the perception of a sound when there is no sound in the environment. It may have a buzzing, roaring, or ringing quality and may be pulsatile (synchronous with the heartbeat). Tinnitus is usually associated with a conductive or sensorineural loss of hearing. The pathophysiology of tinnitus is not well understood. The cause of the tinnitus can usually be determined by finding the cause of the associated hearing loss. Tinnitus may be the first symptom of a serious condition such as an acoustic schwannoma. Pulsatile tinnitus requires evaluation of the vascular system of the head to exclude vascular tumors such as glomus jugulare tumors, aneurysms, and stenotic lesions.

DIFFERENTIAL DIAGNOSIS   Many patients with sensorineural hearing losses should have the vestibular system evaluated with electronystagmography and caloric testing (see Chap. 22). Most patients

with conductive hearing losses should have computed tomography of the temporal tones. Patients with unilateral or asymmetric sensorineural hearing losses should have magnetic resonance imaging of the head with Gadolinium enhancement.

PREVENTION   Conductive hearing losses may be prevented by prompt and appropriate antibiotic therapy of adequate duration for acute otitis media and by reventilation of the middle ear with tympanostomy tubes in middle ear infusions lasting 6 weeks or longer. Loss of vestibular function and deafness due to aminoglycoside antibiotics can largely be prevented by careful monitoring of serum peak and trough levels. Noise-induced hearing loss can be prevented by avoidance of exposure to loud noise or by regular use of ear plugs or glycerine-filled muffs to attenuate intense sound.

TREATMENT   Most patients with conductive hearing losses can have the middle ear reconstructed using procedures such as tympanoplasty after chronic otitis media and trauma and stapedectomy for otosclerosis. Tympanostomy tubes allow the prompt return of hearing to normal in children and adults with middle ear effusions. Hearing aids are effective and well-tolerated for patients with conductive hearing losses. Patients with mild, moderate, and severe sensorineural hearing losses are regularly rehabilitated with hearing aids of varying configuration and strength. The profoundly deaf benefit from cochlear implants.

The treatment of tinnitus is particularly problematic. The frequency range and intensity of tinnitus can often be matched with the use of an audiometer. Relief of the tinnitus may be obtained by masking it with background music. Hearing aids also are helpful in tinnitus suppression, as are tinnitus maskers, devices that present a sound to the affected ear which is more pleasant to listen to than the tinnitus. The use of a tinnitus masker is often followed by several hours of inhibition of the tinnitus.

REFERENCES

ALBERTI PW, RUBEN RJ (eds): *Otologic Medicine and Surgery*. New York, Churchill Livingstone, 1988

COLE P: Upper respiratory airflow, in *The Nose: Upper Airway Physiology and the Atmospheric Environment*, DF Proctor, IB Anderson (eds). Amsterdam, Elsevier, 1982, pp 163–189

DALLOS P: *The Auditory Periphery: Biophysics and Physiology*. New York, Academic Press, 1973

DOTY RL: A review of olfactory dysfunctions in man. Am J Otolaryngol 1:57, 1979

——— et al: Smell identification ability: Changes with age. Science 226:1441, 1984

———: Presence of both odor identification and detection deficits in Alzheimer's disease. Brain Res Bull 18:597, 1987

———: Olfactory dysfunction in Parkinsonism: A general deficit unrelated to neurological signs, disease stage or disease duration. Neurology 38:1237, 1988

JERGER JR: *Modern Developments in Audiology*, 2d ed. New York, Academic Press, 1973

KONIGSMARK BW: Hereditary diseases of the nervous system with hearing loss, in *Handbook of Clinical Neurology*, PJ Vinken, GW Bruyn (eds). Elsevier, Amsterdam, 1975, vol 22, chap 23, pp 499–526

LEVINE SB, SNOW JB: Pulsatile tinnitus. Laryngoscope 97:401, 1987

LOWELL MA et al: Biopsy of human olfactory mucosa: An instrument and a technique. Arch Otolaryngol 108:247, 1982

NAKASHIMA T et al: Structure of human fetal and adult olfactory neuroepithelium. Arch Otolaryngol 110:641, 1984

NORGREN R: The gustatory system in mammals. Am J Otolaryngol 4:234, 1983

RINTELMAN WF: *Hearing Assessment*. Baltimore, Baltimore University, 1979

SNOW JB: Sudden deafness, in *Otolaryngology*, 2d ed, MM Paprella, DA Shumrick (eds). Philadelphia, Saunders, 1980, pp 1751–1767

——— et al: Central auditory imperception. Laryngoscope 87:1450, 1977

———: Clinical problems in chemosensory distrubances. Am J Otolaryngol 4:224 1983

TALAMO BR et al: Pathological changes in olfactory neurons in patients with Alzheimer's disease. Nature 337:736, 1989

25 PARALYSIS AND MOVEMENT DISORDERS

JOHN H. GROWDON / J. STEPHEN FINK[1]

Impairments of motor function may be subdivided into (1) paralysis due to lesions of corticospinal, corticobulbar, or brainstem descending (subcorticospinal) neurons, (2) abnormalities of movement and posture due to disease of the extrapyramidal motor system, (3) apraxic or nonparalytic disturbances of purposive movement due to involvement of the cerebrum, (4) abnormalities of coordination (ataxia) due to lesions in the cerebellar system, including its inputs and outputs, and (5) paralysis due to disorders of the motor unit including bulbar or spinal motor neurons, neuromuscular junction, and muscle. This chapter reviews signs and symptoms that result from lesions of lower motor neurons, descending corticospinal and other tracts, and the extrapyramidal system. It also includes consideration of apraxic disorders. The cerebellar system is discussed in Chap. 26. Signs and symptoms that result from lesions of the neuromuscular junction and muscle are discussed in Chaps. 365 and 366.

FUNCTIONAL ANATOMY OF PRINCIPAL MOTOR TRACTS AND THE MOTOR UNIT

PYRAMIDAL SYSTEM The chief element, the corticospinal tract, is the only direct connection between the cerebrum and the spinal cord. At the level of the medulla the tract contains approximately 1 million axons, far exceeding in number the 30,000 giant Betz cells of the motor cortex (area 4 of Brodmann). Thus, smaller Betz cells of area 4, cells of the adjacent precentral cortex (area 6), and those of the secondary motor cortex in the superior frontal convolution and postcentral cortex (areas 1, 2, 3, 5, and 7) all contribute to the pyramidal system. It is now known that the cells of origin of the corticospinal tract reside in cortical layer V; only 30 percent of the corticospinal and corticobulbar axons originate in area 4.

[1] The authors acknowledge the contribution to this discussion of Robert R. Young, coauthor in the 11th edition.

At the level of the internal capsule corticospinal fibers are intermingled with many others—some destined to end in the striatum, globus pallidus, substantia nigra, red nucleus, and reticular substance; others ascending from the thalamus. Fibers to the cranial nerve nuclei become separated at about the level of the midbrain, where they cross the midline to the contralateral cranial nerve nuclei. These fibers form the corticomesencephalic, corticopontine, and corticobulbar tracts and are included in the pyramidal system of motor neurons because they have functions similar to those of the corticospinal tract. The decussation of the corticospinal tract at the lower end of the medulla is variable. Most of the crossing fibers come to occupy a position in the posterolateral part of the lateral funiculus; a few cross to form an anterior funiculus. A small number of fibers, 10 to 20 percent, do not cross but descend ipsilaterally as the uncrossed corticospinal tract in the anterior funiculus of the spinal cord. Exceptionally, all of the corticospinal fibers cross; rarely, they remain uncrossed. Axons that travel in the lateral corticospinal tract terminate upon (1) neurons of the dorsal horn, (2) interneurons in the intermediate zone of spinal gray matter, and (3) motor neurons located dorsolaterally in the anterior horn. Not more than 25 percent of pyramidal tract neurons establish direct synaptic connection with anterior horn cells (Fig. 25-1). The corticospinal tract in the anterior funiculus terminates bilaterally upon motor neurons located in the ventromedial anterior horn; these neurons innervate axial muscles.

The motor area of the cerebral cortex includes that part of the precentral convolution which contains Betz cells (area 4), but it also extends anteriorly into area 6 and the secondary motor area of the superior frontal convolution and posteriorly into the anterior parietal lobe, where it overlaps the sensory areas. Physiologically the motor cortex is defined as the region of electrically excitable cortex from which isolated movements can be evoked by stimuli of minimal intensity. The muscle groups of contralateral face, arm, trunk, and leg are represented in the motor cortex, those of the face being at the lower end of the precentral convolution and those of the leg in the paracentral lobule on the medial surface of the cerebral hemisphere. The parts of the body capable of the most delicate movements have, in general, the largest cortical representation. One of the functions of the motor cortex is to synthesize simple movements into an infinite variety of finely graded, highly differentiated patterns.

VENTROMEDIAL BULBOSPINAL SYSTEM In addition to the pyramidal (corticospinal and corticobulbar) tract, the spinal gray

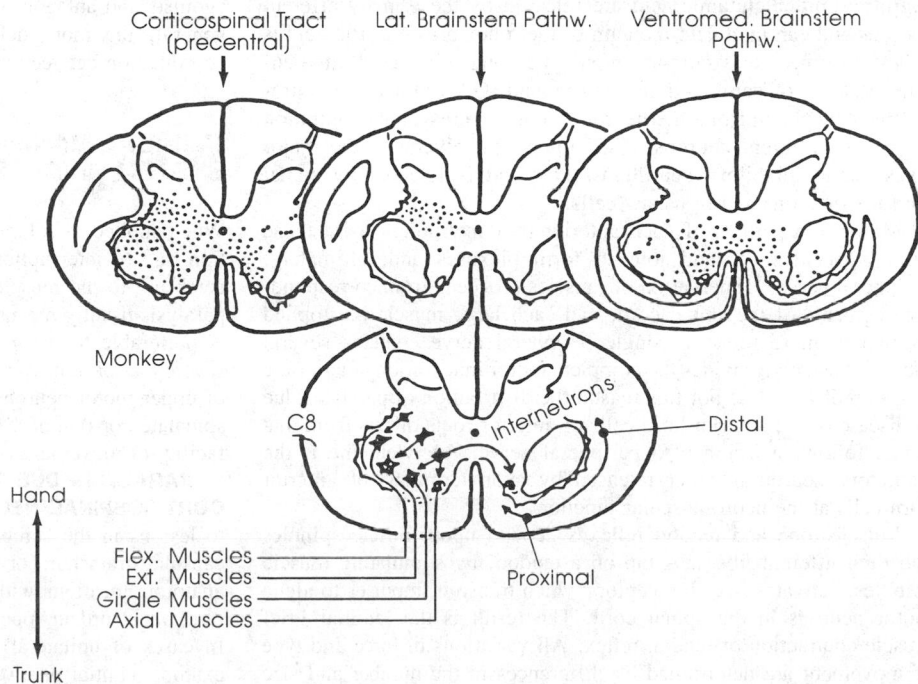

FIGURE 25-1 The distribution of terminations of cortical and brainstem descending pathways (dots) in the spinal intermediate zone and motor neuronal cell groups in rhesus monkey. Note that lateral brainstem pathways (arising from the magnocellular red nucleus and the ventrolateral pontine tegmentum) end on interneurons concerned principally with hand muscles. Ventromedial brainstem pathways (from the superior colliculus, interstitial nucleus of Cajal, pontine, medullary and mesencephalic medial reticular formation, and vestibular nuclei) end on interneurons concerned with trunkal and limb girdle muscles. [*From HGJM Kuypers, in JE Desmedt (ed). New Developments in Electromyography and Clinical Neurophysiology, Basel, Karger, 1973, vol. 3.*]

matter receives axons from two groups of descending pathways from the brainstem. Major contributions to the *ventromedial system* come from the lateral and medial vestibulospinal tracts originating in the lateral and medial vestibular nuclei, the reticulospinal tract originating in the reticular formation of the medulla and pons, and the tectospinal tract originating in the superior colliculus of the midbrain. Neurons originating in the raphe nuclei of the medulla (containing serotonin, substance P, and TRH), in the region of the locus coeruleus in the dorsal brainstem (containing norepinephrine), and in the interstitial nucleus of Cajal also contribute axons to the ventromedial brainstem descending system. These descending ventromedial axons terminate largely upon motor neurons located in the ventromedial anterior horn that innervate axial and proximal muscles; this pool of motor neurons is important in the maintenance of posture and balance. The ventromedial system is also richly collateralized in the upper and lower spinal cord.

DORSOLATERAL BULBOSPINAL SYSTEM   Neurons in the red nucleus of the midbrain contribute axons to the rubrospinal tract, which is the major component of the *dorsolateral system* of brainstem descending pathways. Like the corticospinal tract in the lateral funiculus, the dorsolateral system terminates in the lateral portion of the intermediate zone and on motor neurons located dorsolaterally in the anterior horn; these motor neurons innervate distal muscles.

FUNCTIONAL ANATOMY OF THE MOTOR UNIT   Each motor nerve cell, through extensive arborization of the terminal part of its fiber, comes into contact with hundreds of muscle fibers; together they constitute the ''motor unit.'' Motor neurons in the spinal cord gray matter are organized topographically (Fig. 25-1). Motor neurons innervating a single muscle are distributed longitudinally through two to four spinal segments. Within the anterior horn, groups of motor neurons located medially project to axial muscles, such as neck and back, whereas neurons located laterally in the anterior horn innervate the distal muscles of the limbs. There is an additional topographic representation of flexor and extensor muscles in the anterior horn; motor neurons that are located more dorsally terminate on flexor muscles, and extensor muscles are innervated by motor neurons located more ventrally. Motor neuron excitability is modulated by segmental afferent and suprasegmental descending pathways. Descending corticospinal axons are believed to release aspartic acid and glutamic acid as neurotransmitters. Afferent modulation of motor unit activity is provided, in part, by axons of dorsal root ganglia cells which innervate most lamina of the dorsal horn, the intermediate zone, and some motor neurons directly. Substance P and the excitatory neurotransmitter glutamic acid are released by the primary afferent neurons and can modulate the gain of the reflex arc. Aspartic acid is believed to mediate excitatory impulses among spinal cord interneurons. Release of gamma-aminobutyric acid (GABA) and the neuropeptide enkephalin from interneurons increases presynaptic inhibition of primary afferent neurons. The amino acid glycine is the major postsynaptic inhibitory neurotransmitter and is released by spinal cord interneurons and Renshaw cells.

Motor nerve fibers of each anterior root intermingle with those from adjacent roots and join to form plexuses and, ultimately, peripheral nerves. Innervation of muscles proceeds from corresponding segments of the spinal cord, and each large muscle is supplied by two or more roots. A single peripheral nerve contains several roots and usually provides the complete motor innervation of a muscle or group of muscles. For this reason the distribution of paralysis due to disease of the anterior horn cells or anterior roots differs from that which follows a lesion of a peripheral nerve. Acetylcholine is the excitatory neurotransmitter released by axon terminals of anterior horn cells at the neuromuscular junction.

Muscle tone and tendon reflexes depend upon muscle spindles and their afferent fibers. A tap on a tendon, by stimulating muscle spindles, activates stretch receptors which transmit impulses to alpha motor neurons in the spinal cord. The result is the familiar brief muscle contraction or tendon reflex. All variations in force and type of movement are determined by differences in the number and size

of motor units called into activity, the frequency of their firing rates, and the patterns of activity in different muscles. Feeble movements recruit few units; the number and size of motor units increase in a stereotyped fashion with stronger movements. Motor units involved in tonic contractions have muscle fibers known as type I that are rich in oxidative enzymes and mitochondria; those controlling phasic contractions innervate muscle fibers that have anaerobic metabolism (type II fibers) (see also Chap. 362). When a motor neuron becomes diseased, as in progressive muscular atrophy, its axon may manifest increased irritability and all the muscle fibers that it controls may discharge sporadically, in isolation from other units. The result of the contraction of one or several such units is a muscular twitch, or *fasciculation,* which can be observed visibly and recorded in the electromyogram (EMG). If the motor neuron or its axon is destroyed, all of the muscle fibers to which it is attached undergo profound denervation atrophy. As a result, individual muscle fibers become hypersensitive to acetylcholine and contract spontaneously, although they are unresponsive to nerve impulses. Isolated activity of individual muscle fibers is called *fibrillation;* it is so fine that it cannot be seen through the intact skin and can be recorded only as a short-duration spike potential in the EMG (see Chap. 362).

All motor activity, even of the most elementary reflex type, requires the cooperation of several muscles. Analysis of a relatively simple movement, such as clenching the fist, affords some idea of the complexity of the underlying neural arrangements. In this act the primary movement is a contraction of the flexor muscles of the fingers, the flexor digitorum sublimis and profundus, the flexor pollicis longus and brevis, and the adductor pollicis brevis. These muscles act as *agonists,* or *prime movers,* in this act. In order for flexion to be smooth and forceful, finger extensor muscles act as *antagonists* and must relax at the same rate at which the flexors contract. The muscles which flex the fingers also tend to flex the wrist; and since that weakens the grip, muscles which extend the wrist must be brought into play to prevent its flexion. The action of the wrist extensors is *synergic,* and these muscles are called synergists in this particular act. The elbow and shoulder must be stabilized by appropriate flexor and extensor muscles, which serve as *fixators.* The coordination of agonists, antagonists, synergists, and fixators involves reciprocal innervation and is managed entirely by segmental spinal mechanisms with guidance from proprioceptive input. Only the agonist movement in a voluntary act is believed to be initiated at a cortical level. There are many other basic motor activities, such as the maintenance of certain postures and stepping movements, where agonists and antagonists contract simultaneously (see Chap. 26). In general, the more delicate the movement, the more precise the coordination between agonist and antagonist muscles.

CLINICAL MANIFESTATIONS OF MOTOR SYSTEM DISEASES

When applied to voluntary muscles, *paralysis* means loss of contraction due to interruption of one or more motor pathways from the cerebrum to the muscle fiber. In everyday medical parlance, motor paralysis usually means either partial or complete loss of strength; it is preferable to use *paresis* for slight and *paralysis* or *plegia* for severe loss of motor strength. Motor paralysis may result from lesions of upper motor neurons (corticospinal, corticobulbar, or subcorticospinal neurons) or of the motor unit. In addition to weakness, impaired facility of movement is an important functional deficit.

PARALYSIS DUE TO DISEASES OF PYRAMIDAL AND SUB-CORTICOSPINAL NEURONS   Corticospinal paralysis may be due to lesions in the cerebral cortex, subcortical white matter, internal capsule, brainstem, or spinal cord. Lesions confined to one of these anatomic locations without damaging adjacent parts of the brain are rare, but afford an opportunity to assess pure pyramidal tract function. In cases of unilateral pyramidal tract damage in the medulla, for example, initial paralysis may be striking but there is a remarkable degree of recovery of motor function in the affected contralateral arm and leg, leaving only slight spasticity, an increase in phasic myotatic or tendon reflexes, and an extensor plantar reflex (Babinski's sign). The extent of recovery is surprising, and may be due to preservation of a few fibers in the pyramid or to preservation of lateral brainstem pathways. This picture of pure pyramidal tract damage is much different from the extensive deficits that generally accompany most spastic hemiplegic syndromes. In clinical practice, most lesions of the upper motor neurons interrupt descending fibers from the cerebral cortex (corticospinal, corticorubral, corticostriatal, corticopallidal, corticopontine, and corticoreticular) and from the brainstem (reticulospinal, vestibulospinal, and rubrospinal). Damage to the nonpyramidal fibers increases the degree of paralysis and accounts for dysfunction in segmental motor neurons subserving reflex, postural, and locomotor functions. In most cases, it is therefore inaccurate to refer to spastic hemiplegia as the "pyramidal syndrome."

With corticospinal lesions in humans the distribution of the paralysis varies with the lesion site, but there are certain common features. Paralysis due to a lesion of upper motor neurons always involves a group of muscles, never individual muscles. In general, hand, arm, and leg muscles are most affected after a corticospinal lesion; of the cranial musculature, only the lower face and tongue are involved to any significant degree. Whatever volitional movement remains, the maximum effort is attained more slowly than in the normal limb, fewer motor units are recruited, and the frequency of their discharge is reduced. Corticospinal paralysis never involves all the muscles on one side of the body, even with a complete hemiplegia. Movements that are invariably bilateral, such as those of the eyes, jaw, pharynx, larynx, neck, thorax, and abdomen, are usually unaffected. The cortical control of all movements is to some extent bilateral. Examples that prove this point are hemiplegias that worsen when the contralateral motor system is interrupted by disease. Corticospinal paralysis is rarely complete for long; in this respect it differs from the total and absolute paralysis due to a complete destruction of anterior horn cells and their axons. The paralyzed arm may suddenly move during yawning and stretching, and various spinal reflexes can be elicited at all times.

Acute lesions of the corticospinal and subcorticospinal motor system at lower levels, such as the cervical cord, produce a distinctive picture of total paralysis and areflexia known as *spinal shock*. After a few days to weeks flaccidity subsides, muscular tone reappears, and the affected limbs become spastic; paralysis persists unchanged. *Spasticity* is a feature of all lesions of the motor system at cerebral, capsular, midbrain, and pontine levels. Spasticity is defined as a motor disorder characterized by a velocity-dependent increase in tonic stretch reflexes ("muscle tone") with exaggerated tendon jerks, resulting from hyperexcitability of the stretch reflex; it is one component of the "upper motor neuron" syndrome. Spasticity is related to excessive activity of motor neurons that are released from inhibition consequent to lesions of the corticospinal or descending brainstem pathways. The postures of the arm and leg inform us that certain spinal neurons are more active than others. With supraspinal lesions, the arm is maintained in a pronated, flexed position and the leg in an adducted, extended position. Attempts to extend the arm or flex the leg passively will elicit increasing resistance which abruptly subsides (*clasp-knife phenomenon*). When the limb is left in the new position, the resistance reappears (*lengthening and shortening reactions*). With combined lesions of corticospinal and other suprasegmental tracts, sustained resistance to movement (*hypertonus*) is more common than the clasp-knife type of spasticity. Upper motor neuron lesions also release the nocifensive spinal flexion reflexes, including Babinski's sign, and diminish or abolish the cutaneomuscular abdominal and cremasteric reflexes. Other signs of corticospinal or upper motor neuron lesions include exaggerated stretch and cutaneous reflexes in cranial as well as in limb and trunk muscles. If the corticospinal lesions are bilateral, there is *pseudobulbar paralysis* (dysarthria, dysphonia, and dysphagia with bifacial paralysis) accompanied by forced crying and laughing. Prolonged flexor and extensor

spasms occur with lesions of the spinal cord; they are due to a release of cutaneous reflexes.

Spasticity is present with paresis as well as paralysis and can add to disturbances of voluntary movements. In general, all attempts by the patient to move the hemiparetic extremities appear to be hampered. Discrete movements of individual fingers and finely coordinated movements of the hand are lost, but voluntary control over proximal muscles is generally maintained. Synergies of movements eventually appear. For example, in the upper extremity a flexion synergy consisting of finger flexion, wrist flexion and pronation, elbow flexion, and shoulder elevation and abduction is produced in a slow, massive, stereotyped fashion upon attempted grasp of an object. Attempts to push with the hand result in a weak pronation of the hand, extension or flexion of the fingers, extension of the wrist and elbow, adduction of the upper arm, and lowering of the shoulder. In the lower extremity the extensor synergy (thigh adduction, thigh and knee extension, and plantar flexion of the toes and foot) is more powerful than the flexor synergy of hip abduction, hip and knee flexion, and dorsiflexion and inversion of toes and foot. A bias toward extensor synergy facilitates weight-bearing and walking, which are eventually achieved by nearly all hemiplegic patients. These synergies indicate that there is a diminution in voluntary anterior horn cell activation (the negative effect of a motor lesion) and excessive reflex and synergistic discharges in the same motor neuron pools (the positive effects of the lesion). Strong-willed effort to move the paretic limb may also evoke symmetric associated (mirror) movements in the normal limb.

In spasticity, where the neurons responsible for excitation of the extensor muscles of the leg and flexors of the arm are overactive, it is not known whether there is a functional excess of excitatory neurotransmitters or a deficiency of inhibitory transmitters or both. Current evidence indicates that drugs that decrease spasticity act at the spinal cord level to alter neurotransmitter function. Baclofen slows conduction in the spinal cord reflex arc, perhaps by interfering with the release of excitatory neurotransmitters, including substance P, from primary afferent neurons. Diazepam facilitates GABA-mediated presynaptic inhibition of primary afferent excitatory transmitter release.

PARALYSIS DUE TO DISEASES OF THE MOTOR UNIT Damage to the lower motor neurons can produce paresis or paralysis as a direct result of physiologic block or destruction of anterior horn cells or their axons in anterior roots and nerves. The signs and symptoms of the lower motor neuron syndrome vary according to the location of the lesion: the most important question for clinical purposes is whether sensory changes coexist with muscular weakness. The combination of flaccid areflexic paralysis and sensory loss usually indicates involvement of mixed motor and sensory nerves or damage to both anterior and posterior roots. If sensory changes are absent, the lesion must be situated in the gray matter of the spinal cord, in the anterior roots, in a purely motor branch of a peripheral nerve, or in motor axons alone. The distinction between nuclear (spinal) and anterior root (radicular) lesions may at times be impossible to make.

If all or practically all peripheral motor nerves supplying a muscle are destroyed, voluntary, postural, and reflex movements are abolished. The muscle becomes soft and yields excessively to passive stretching, a condition known as *flaccidity*. Muscle tone—the slight resistance that normal relaxed muscle offers to passive movement—is reduced (*hypotonia* or *atonia*). The denervated muscles undergo extreme atrophy, and lose 70 to 80 percent of their original bulk within 4 months. The reflex reaction of the muscle to sudden stretch, as by tapping its tendon, is lost. If only a few motor units in the muscles are affected, partial paralysis will ensue. With partial denervation, EMG evidence of fibrillations may also be obtained. Clinical features that distinguish lower motor and upper motor neuron lesions are summarized in Table 25-1.

APRAXIC OR NONPARALYTIC DISORDERS OF MOTOR FUNCTION Loss of learned movements can simulate paresis of a limb, even though the pyramidal tract and spinal cord motor units are intact. This condition is called *apraxia* and is defined as a disorder

TABLE 25-1   Differences between paralysis due to lesions of upper versus lower motor neurons

Upper motor neuron paralysis	Lower motor neuron paralysis
Muscle groups affected diffusely, never individual muscles	Individual muscles may be affected
Atrophy slight	Atrophy pronounced, 70 to 80% of total bulk
Spasticity with hyperactivity of the tendon reflexes	Flaccidity and hypotonia of affected muscles with loss of tendon reflexes
Extensor plantar reflex, Babinski's sign	Plantar reflex, if present, is of normal flexor type
Fascicular twitches not produced	Fasciculations may be present
	Electromyogram reveals reduced numbers of motor units and fibrillations

of learned movement that is not due to weakness, incoordination, sensory loss, or failure to comprehend commands. A failure to execute a designated action while retaining the ability to carry out the individual movements upon which such an act depends is the main feature of apraxia. A clinical test of motor deficits of this type is to observe a series of self-initiated actions such as using a comb, a razor, a toothbrush, or a common tool, or gesturing, e.g., waving goodbye, saluting, shaking the fist as though angry, or blowing a kiss. These actions can be normally elicited by a command or a request to imitate the examiner. Of course, failure to follow a spoken or written request may be due to an aphasia that prevents understanding of what is asked or to an agnosia that prevents recognition of the tool or object to be used. But when these difficulties are excluded, there remains a peculiar motor deficit in which the patient appears to understand but has lost the memory of how to perform a given act, especially if it is called for in an unnatural setting. The patient may have the idea of what to do but cannot translate the idea of the sequence of movements into a precise, well-executed act. An apraxic deficit may be evident both after a spoken command and in requests to imitate the gestures of the examiner. Sometimes these two conditions may be dissociated; the patient, while not aphasic, cannot execute a spoken command but can still imitate the act if it is called forth by gesture. Also, if merely given the tool, the patient may use it properly in an automatic fashion.

To understand the anatomic basis of apraxia, it is necessary to appreciate that the production of complex motor behavior results from association among several cortical brain areas. The motor response of right-handed (and most left-handed) persons to a command requires the integrity of the left parietal and temporal lobes, especially the region around the left supramarginal gyrus, and their connection with the left premotor regions for control of the right hand. Information flows through the corpus callosum from the left to the right motor cortex for control of the left side of the body. Disconnection of the supramarginal area from motor areas of the right hemisphere (most commonly by lesions of the midcallosum, dominant frontal association cortex, or posterior parietal lobe) results in apraxia of left limbs when tested by response to verbal commands. Traditionally, abnormalities in the execution of single gestures resulting from lesions of these brain areas have been referred to as *ideomotor apraxia*. The anatomic basis of *ideational apraxia*, in which the execution of a multistep activity is faulty although the constituent movements can be performed, has not been clearly delineated. Because pure disorders of these subtypes of apraxia are uncommon, and precise anatomic correlates are lacking, clinical distinctions between ideomotor and ideational apraxia are difficult to make.

EXAMINATION SCHEME FOR MOTOR PARALYSIS AND APRAXIA   The first step in examination is to inspect the paralyzed limb, taking note of its posture and whether there are signs of muscular hypertrophy, atrophy, or fascicular twitchings. Slight atrophy may be due to disuse from any cause, i.e., pain, fixation as the result of a cast, or any type of paralysis. Pronounced atrophy usually

occurs only with denervation of several weeks' or months' standing. The patient is then called upon to move each muscle group, and the power and facility of movement are graded and recorded. The examiner then determines the range of passive movement and the degree of resistance encountered moving all the joints. This provides information concerning alterations of muscle tone, i.e., hypotonia, spasticity, and rigidity. Dislocations, diseased joints, and ankyloses may also be revealed by these same maneuvers. The tendon reflexes are then tested. The usual routine is to try to elicit the jaw jerk (increased in pseudobulbar palsy) and the biceps, triceps, quadriceps, and Achilles tendon reflexes. Two cutaneous reflexes are then tested, the abdominal and plantar reflexes.

If there is no evidence of upper or lower motor neuron disease, but motor acts are nonetheless imperfectly performed, one should look for a disorder of postural control associated with cerebellar incoordination, or consider that rigidity with abnormalities of posture and movement may be due to disease of the basal ganglia. In the absence of these disorders, the possibility of an apraxic disorder may be investigated by watching the patient's own movements and those called forth by specific command and gesture.

DIFFERENTIAL DIAGNOSIS OF PARALYSIS   The diagnostic consideration of paralysis may be simplified by the following subdivisions, which relate to the location and distribution of weakness. Paralysis may result from dysfunction of upper motor neurons (corticospinal, corticobulbar, and subcorticospinal neurons) or of the motor unit (bulbar and spinal motor neurons, neuromuscular junction, and muscle). In general, the presence or absence of atrophy of muscles in a monoplegic limb can assist the clinician to arrive at an anatomic and clinical diagnosis.

Monoplegia   It is necessary to determine carefully the distribution of muscle weakness. For example, patients who complain of weakness of one extremity often have unnoticed weakness in another limb, and the condition is actually hemiplegia or paraplegia. A comprehensive physical examination should be conducted in order to determine whether there is weakness of all the muscles in a limb or only isolated muscle groups. The examination should also exclude nonparalytic conditions such as ataxia, sensory disturbances, mechanical limitation resulting from arthritis, the rigidity of parkinsonism, or pain in an extremity; such conditions are often interpreted by the patient as weakness.

PARALYSIS WITH LITTLE OR NO ATROPHY   The most frequent cause of monoplegia without muscular wasting is a lesion of the cerebral cortex; diseases that interrupt the corticospinal tract at the level of the internal capsule, brainstem, or spinal cord rarely cause monoplegia because corticospinal fibers to arm and leg are intermingled at subcortical levels. A cortical vascular lesion (thrombosis or embolus) is the commonest cause of monoplegia, but a discrete traumatic lesion, tumor, or abscess may have the same effect. Multiple sclerosis and spinal cord tumor, early in their course, may cause isolated weakness of one extremity, usually the leg. Weakness due to damage of the corticospinal and subcorticospinal system is usually accompanied by spasticity, increased reflexes, and an extensor plantar reflex (Babinski's sign). Acute traumatic or inflammatory lesions that destroy the motor tracts in the spinal cord are exceptions to this rule because immediately after damage the tendon reflexes are reduced or absent and muscle tone is flaccid (spinal shock). This does not occur in partial or slowly evolving lesions and occurs only to minimal degree, if at all, in lesions of brainstem and cerebrum. In acute diseases affecting the lower motor neurons, such as poliomyelitis, the tendon reflexes are always reduced or abolished, but atrophy may not appear for several weeks. Hence one must take into account the mode of onset and the duration of the disease in evaluating the tendon reflexes, muscle tone, and degree of atrophy before reaching an anatomic diagnosis.

PARALYSIS WITH MUSCULAR ATROPHY   Atrophy of muscles in a paralyzed limb usually indicates a lesion of some portion of the motor unit (spinal cord, spinal roots, peripheral nerve, or muscle). Disease of the neuromuscular junction is not associated with muscular atrophy.

In addition to the paralysis, reduced or abolished tendon reflexes, and decreased tone, there may be visible fasciculations. The EMG shows decreased numbers of motor units (often of large size), fasciculations at rest, and fibrillations. The location of the lesion can usually be decided by the distribution of the palsied muscles (whether the pattern is one of muscles, nerve, spinal root, or spinal cord involvement), by the associated neurologic symptoms and signs, and by special tests (cerebrospinal fluid examination, CT or magnetic resonance imaging scans of the spine, myelogram, serum muscle enzymes, EMG, and biopsy). A clinical approach to the signs and symptoms that assist the clinician in arriving at an anatomic diagnosis of diseases of the motor unit (spinal cord, spinal motor nerves, neuromuscular junction, or muscle) are described in more detail in Chaps. 362 and 363.

The anatomic pattern of paralysis with atrophy may suggest the clinical diagnosis. Atrophic monoplegia affecting the arm should suggest brachial plexus trauma in an infant; poliomyelitis in a child; and poliomyelitis, syringomyelia, amyotrophic lateral sclerosis, or neuritis of the brachial plexus in an adult. Crural monoplegia (affecting the leg) is more frequent than brachial monoplegia and may be caused by any lesion of thoracic or lumbar cord, including trauma, tumor, myelitis, or multiple sclerosis. Multiple sclerosis almost never causes atrophy, and ruptured intervertebral disk and the many varieties of neuritis rarely paralyze all or most of the muscles of a limb. Muscular dystrophy may begin in one limb, but by the time the patient is seen the typical pattern of symmetric proximal limb and trunk involvement is usually evident. A unilateral retroperitoneal tumor may paralyze the leg by implicating the lumbosacral plexus. Prolonged disuse of a limb may lead to atrophy, but this is usually not so marked as in diseases that denervate muscles. In disuse atrophy the tendon reflexes are normal, and the responses of the muscles to electric stimulation and on EMG are unaltered.

Hemiplegia Loss of strength in the arm, leg, and sometimes face on one side of the body is the most frequent distribution of paralysis in humans. With rare exceptions (a few unusual cases of poliomyelitis or motor system disease) this pattern of paralysis is due to involvement of the descending motor tracts. The site or level of the lesion that produced hemiplegia can usually be deduced from the associated neurologic findings. Diseases localized in the cerebral cortex, cerebral white matter (corona radiata), and internal capsule usually evoke weakness or paralysis of the face, arm, and leg in the side of the body contralateral to the brain lesion. The occurrence of convulsive seizures or the presence of a defect in speech (aphasia), a cortical type of sensory loss (astereognosis and loss of two-point discrimination), anosognosia, or defects in the visual fields suggest a cortical or subcortical rather than a capsular location. A pure, isolated motor hemiplegia affecting simultaneously the face, arm, and leg indicates a small discrete lesion in the posterior limb of the internal capsule, cerebral peduncle, or medullary pyramids.

Damage to the corticospinal and corticobulbar tracts in the upper portion of the brainstem will cause paralysis of the face, arm, and leg in the side opposite the lesion, plus deficits in cranial nerve function on the same side as the lesion. Some of the classic brainstem syndromes permit precise localization of the lesion, which is usually vascular. Paralysis of the oculomotor nerve on the same side as the lesion with contralateral limb paresis is known as Weber's syndrome. With low pontine lesions, an ipsilateral abducens or facial palsy combined with a contralateral weakness or paralysis of the arm and leg is the Millard-Gubler syndrome. Lesions of the lowermost part of the brainstem, i.e., in the medulla, affect the tongue and sometimes the pharynx and larynx on one side and arm and leg on the other side. Ataxic hemiplegia with or without dysarthria indicates a lesion in the contralateral basis pons. These "crossed paralyses" that are so characteristic of brainstem diseases are described in Chap. 351.

Hemiplegia that spares cranial musculature may be caused by a lesion in the lateral column of the cervical spinal cord. At this level, however, the pathologic process often induces bilateral signs, with resulting quadriparesis or quadriplegia. Homolateral paralysis, if combined with a loss of vibratory and position sense on the same side and contralateral loss of pain and temperature (Brown-Séquard syndrome), signifies disease of the spinal cord (Chap. 361).

Muscle atrophy of minor degree is often associated with hemiplegia but never reaches the proportions seen in diseases of the lower motor neurons. Atrophy secondary to upper motor neuron damage is largely due to disuse. There is an important exception to this rule: When the motor cortex and adjacent parts of the parietal lobe are damaged in infancy or childhood, the normal development of the muscles and the skeletal system in the affected limbs is retarded, and the palsied limbs and even the trunk on one side are small. Developmental atrophy does not occur, however, if the paralysis begins after puberty when the greater part of skeletal growth has been attained. In hemiplegia due to spinal cord injury, muscles at the level of the lesion may undergo atrophy if there is associated damage to anterior horn cells or ventral roots.

Vascular diseases of the cerebrum and brainstem are the most common causes of hemiplegia. Trauma (brain contusion, epidural and subdural hemorrhage) ranks second, followed by other diseases such as brain tumor, demyelinative disease, brain abcess, and encephalitis. Complications of meningitis, tuberculosis, and syphilis were common causes of hemiplegia in the past but are much less evident in current practice.

Paraplegia Paraplegia denotes a condition of weakness or paralysis of both lower extremities with sparing of the upper extremities. Paraplegia most commonly occurs in diseases of the spinal cord, spinal roots, or peripheral nerves. Among cerebral causes, parasagittal tumors and hydrocephalus cause leg weakness. If the onset is acute, it may be difficult to distinguish spinal from neural paralysis, because sudden damage to either may result in flaccidity and abolition of reflexes. As a rule, in acute spinal cord diseases the paralysis affects all muscles below a given level; often, if the white matter is extensively damaged, sensory loss below a particular level (loss of pain and temperature sense from lateral spinothalamic tracts involvement and loss of vibratory and position sense from posterior columns damage) is conjoined. Also, in bilateral disease of the spinal cord the bladder and bowel sphincters are paralyzed. Alterations of cerebrospinal fluid (dynamic block and increases in protein or cells) are frequent. In peripheral nerve diseases both sensory loss and motor loss tend to involve the distal muscles of the legs more than the proximal ones (an exception is acute idiopathic polyneuritis), and the sphincters are spared or only briefly deranged in function. Sensory loss, if present, is more likely to consist of distal impairment of touch, vibration, and position sense, with pain and temperature sense spared in many instances. The cerebrospinal fluid protein level may be normal or elevated. Studies of nerve conduction through spinal roots (F waves) are always abnormal.

Acute paraplegia most commonly occurs after trauma or in association with metastatic neoplasia. Uncommon causes of acute paraplegia include a medial pontine lesion affecting the leg fibers which are near the midline (as in pontine infarction or central pontine myelinolysis); spontaneous hematomyelia with bleeding from a vascular malformation (angioma, telangiectasis); thrombosis of a spinal artery with infarction (myelomalacia); and dissecting aortic aneurysm or atherosclerotic occlusion of nutrient spinal arteries arising from the aorta with resulting infarction (myelomalacia). Postinfectious or postvaccinal myelitis, acute demyelinative myelitis (Devic's disease if the optic nerves are affected), necrotizing myelitis, and epidural abscess or hemorrhage with spinal cord compression tend to develop somewhat more slowly over a period of hours or days, but they may have an acute onset. Poliomyelitis, in those countries where immunization is incomplete, presents as a purely motor disorder with meningitis, and must be distinguished from the other acute myelopathies.

Subacute or chronic paraplegia in adults results from such common diseases as cervical spondylosis and multiple sclerosis. Other causes are subacute combined degeneration, spinal cord tumor, ruptured cervical disk, syphilitic meningomyelitis, chronic epidural infections (fungus and other granulomatous diseases), motor system disease, and syringomyelia. Familial spastic paraparesis is a rare cause of paraplegia in which there is symmetric demyelination of the dorsolateral corticospinal tract. (See Chap. 361 for discussion of these spinal cord diseases.) The several varieties of polyneuritis, including Guillain-Barré syndrome and polymyositis, must be considered in the differential diagnosis, for they, too, may cause paraparesis. Friedreich's ataxia and familial spastic paraplegia, progressive muscular dystrophy, and the chronic varieties of polyneuritis tend to appear during late childhood and adolescence and are slowly progressive.

Paraplegia (or paraparesis) may be due to a lesion of the leg areas of the motor cortex. Arterial (anterior cerebral arteries) or venous (superior sagittal sinus and tributary cerebral veins) distribution cerebral infarction are causes of acute paraplegia; parasagittal meningioma is a cause of asymmetric chronic paraplegia. Usually other signs such as confusion, stupor, or seizures indicate the cerebral localization, and differential diagnosis is not a problem.

Quadriplegia   All that has been written about the common causes of paraplegia applies to quadriplegia except that the lesion is in the cervical rather than the thoracic or lumbar segments of the spinal cord. If it is situated in the low cervical segments and involves the anterior half of the spinal cord, as in occlusion of the anterior spinal artery, the arm paralysis may be flaccid and areflexic and the leg paralysis spastic (anterior spinal syndrome). There are only a few points of difference between the common paraplegic and quadriplegic syndromes. One of the most common causes of subacute quadriplegia is the Guillain-Barré syndrome due to inflammatory demyelination of motor neuron axons in the anterior roots. Repeated cerebral vascular accidents may lead to bilateral hemiplegia, usually accompanied by pseudobulbar palsy. An unusual cause of quadriplegia is bilateral infarctions of the medullary pyramids.

Isolated paralysis   Paralysis of isolated muscle groups usually indicates a lesion of one or more peripheral nerves. The basis for diagnosing a lesion of an individual peripheral nerve is the presence of weakness or paralysis of the muscle or group of muscles and impairment or loss of sensation in the distribution of the nerve in question (Chap. 363). Complete transection or severe injury to a peripheral nerve is usually followed by atrophy of the muscles it innervates and by loss of their tendon reflexes. Trophic changes in the skin, nails, and subcutaneous tissue may also occur. It is of considerable importance to decide whether the lesion is only a temporary one (conduction block), or whether there has been a dissolution of axonal continuity, requiring nerve regeneration for recovery.

THE BASAL GANGLIA

The basal ganglia subserve motor functions that are distinct from those attributed to the pyramidal (corticospinal) tract. The term *extrapyramidal* underscores this distinction and calls attention to a set of neurologic illnesses caused by lesions that affect the basal ganglia. In addition to motor impairments, diseases of the basal ganglia are often associated with disturbances of affect and cognition. Familiar examples of extrapyramidal disorders include Parkinson's disease, Huntington's disease, and Wilson's disease. This section reviews aspects of the anatomy, biochemistry, and physiology of the basal ganglia and describes the clinical symptoms and signs that arise from their dysfunction.

ANATOMIC CONNECTIONS AND NEURONAL TRANSMITTERS IN THE BASAL GANGLIA   The basal ganglia are paired subcortical masses of gray matter that form anatomically distinct nuclear groups. The major nuclei are the caudate and the putamen (which together are called the striatum), the internal and external segments of the globus pallidus, the subthalamic nucleus, and the substantia nigra (Fig. 25-2). The striatum receives afferent inputs from many sources, including the cerebral cortex, thalamic nuclei, brainstem raphe nuclei, and the substantia nigra. There are two anatomically and functionally distinct subdivisions of the striatum: the striosomes and the matrix. Afferents to the striosomal region originate in the frontal cortex, insula, amygdala, and midline thalamus; afferents to the matrix arise from neurons in the sensory and motor cortex, parietal-temporal-occipital association cortex, and intralaminar thalamic nuclei. Cortical neurons that project to the striatum release the excitatory amino acid glutamate. Neurons that project to the striatum from the raphe nuclei synthesize and release serotonin (5-HT). Neurons in the pars compacta of the substantia nigra synthesize and release dopamine (DA), which acts as an inhibitory neurotransmitter on striatal neurons. DA neurons in the substantia nigra pars compacta project to striosomes, whereas DA neurons in the ventral tegmental area project to the matrix. Transmitters released by thalamic projections are unknown. The striatum contains two distinct classes of cells: local circuit neurons, whose axons do not project beyond the confines of the nucleus, and other neurons whose axons project to the globus pallidus and substantia nigra. Local circuit neurons synthesize and release acetylcholine (ACh), GABA, and neuropeptides, including somatostatin and vasoactive intestinal polypeptide. Neurons in the striosomes project to the medial part of the pars compacta of the substantia nigra; the main output of the extrastriosomal matrix goes to the pallidum and pars reticulata of the substantia nigra. Striatal neurons that inhibit the pars reticulata of the substantia nigra release GABA, whereas those that

FIGURE 25-2 Simplified schematic diagram of the major neuronal connections between the basal ganglia, thalamus, and cerebral cortex. The projection from the internal segment of the globus pallidus constitutes the principal efferent pathway from the basal ganglia. Abbreviations: ext = external, int = internal, pc = pars compacta, pr = pars reticulata, cm = centromedian, va = ventroanterior, vl = ventrolateral.

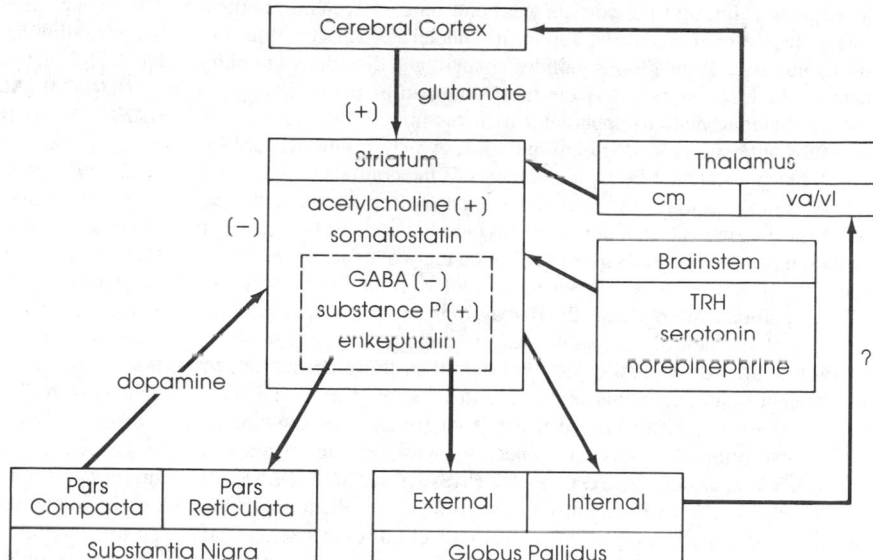

FIGURE 25-3 Schematic diagram of the excitatory and inhibitory effects of neuroregulators released by neurons in the basal ganglia pathways. The area (enclosed by dashed lines) in the striatum indicates neurons with efferent projection systems. The other striatal transmitters are present in intrinsic neurons. Plus sign (+) indicates an excitatory postsynaptic effect. Minus sign (−) indicates an inhibitory effect. Abbreviations: cm = centromedian nucleus, GABA = gamma-aminobutyric acid, TRH = thyrotropin releasing hormone, va/vl = ventroanterior and ventrolateral.

excite the pars compacta release substance P (Fig. 25-3). Transmitters released in the striatal projections to the globus pallidus include GABA, the enkephalins, and substance P.

Axons that originate in the internal segment of the globus pallidus form the main efferent projection from the basal ganglia. There is a massive projection around and through the internal capsule (the ansa and fasciculus lenticularis that pass through the fields of Forel) to the ventral anterior and ventral lateral thalamus as well as to intralaminar thalamic nuclei, including the centromedian nucleus. Chemical transmitters released by this pathway are unknown. Other efferent projections from the basal ganglia include direct dopaminergic connections from the ventral tegmental area to regions of limbic and frontal cerebral cortex; the pars reticulata of the substantia nigra also sends a projection to thalamic nuclei and to the superior colliculus.

Recent anatomic studies have clarified the cortical distribution of ascending thalamic fibers. Ventral thalamic neurons project to premotor and motor cerebral cortices; medial thalamic nuclei project primarily to prefrontal cortex. The supplementary motor cortex receives a prominent input from the basal ganglia, including a dopaminergic projection from the substantia nigra, whereas the primary motor and premotor cortex receives a major input from the cerebellum. Thus there are a series of parallel loops reciprocally linking specific basal ganglionic structures and cerebral cortical regions. Although the exact mechanism whereby these various inputs are translated into coordinated volitional acts remains uncertain, it is clear that most of the basal ganglionic and cerebellar influences on the motor system are funneled through this ventral plane of thalamic nuclei. The major cerebellar output, which exits the cerebellum through the superior cerebellar peduncle, terminates with the pallidal-thalamic fibers in the ventroanterior and ventrolateral thalamic nuclei. This region of the thalamus forms an essential link in the ascending fiber systems from both the basal ganglia and the cerebellum to the motor cortex. Despite the apparently crucial nature of these structures, lesions placed stereotactically in the ventral thalamus can abolish essential-familial tremor or the rigidity and tremor in Parkinson's disease without producing functional deficits. Ascending thalamocortical fibers pass through the internal capsule and cerebral white matter, so lesions in these parts or in the cortex may simultaneously affect both corticospinal and extrapyramidal systems.

Axons from some cortical neurons form the internal capsule (the corticobulbar and corticospinal tracts); these and others also project to the striatum. This forms a complete loop—from cerebral cortex to striatum, to globus pallidus, to thalamus, to cerebral cortex. Axons that originate in the centromedian nucleus of the thalamus project

back to the striatum, thus completing a subcortical loop from striatum to globus pallidus, to centromedian nucleus, to striatum. There is another subcortical loop between the striatum and the substantia nigra: Dopaminergic neurons in the pars compacta of substantia nigra project to the striatum, and separate striatal neurons that release GABA and substance P send projections to the pars reticulata of the substantia nigra. There are reciprocal connections between the pars reticulata and pars compacta of the substantia nigra; the pars reticulata sends projections to ventral thalamus, superior colliculus, and brainstem reticular formation structures as well. The subthalamic nucleus receives fibers from the neocortex and from the external segment of the globus pallidus; neurons within the subthalamic nucleus form reciprocal connections with the external segment of the globus pallidus and also send axons to the internal segment of the globus pallidus and pars reticulata of the substantia nigra. The neurochemicals involved in these pathways remain unknown, although GABA has been implicated.

PHYSIOLOGY OF THE BASAL GANGLIA Recordings from neurons in the globus pallidus and substantia nigra in awake, performing primates confirm the main motor function of the basal ganglia. Cells within these regions clearly participate in the initiation of movement, because they increase their firing rates before movement is observed clinically or detected by EMG. Discharges in the basal ganglia are related principally to contralateral rather than ipsilateral limb movements. Many neurons increase their firing rates during slow (ramp) movements, but some others discharge during more rapid (ballistic) movements. There is somatotopic localization of leg, arm, and face within the internal segment of the globus pallidus and pars reticulata of the substantia nigra. This observation provides a possible explanation for the occurrence of restricted dyskinesias: Focal dystonia and buccal-lingual-masticatory tardive dyskinesia may result from localized pallidal or nigral biochemical lesions that affect only regions with hand or face representation.

Although the basal ganglia are motor nuclei, it is not possible to identify a specific type of basal ganglia movement. Hypotheses about the function of the basal ganglia in human beings derive from correlations between clinical signs and sites of pathologic lesions in patients with extrapyramidal diseases. The basal ganglia are a constellation of nuclei centered around the globus pallidus, through which impulses are channeled to the thalamus and onward to the cerebral cortex (Fig. 25-2). Neurons in each satellite nucleus contribute excitatory and inhibitory impulses, and the sum of these influences on the main pathway from basal ganglia to thalamus and cerebral cortex, modified by the cerebellum, determines smooth motor function as expressed through the corticospinal and other descending cortical tracts. If one or more of the supporting nuclei is damaged, the sum of the impulses to the globus pallidus changes and disordered mobility can occur. Hemiballismus is the most dramatic of these; damage to the subthalamic nucleus apparently removes inhibitory influences on the substantia nigra and globus pallidus, which results in violent, involuntary, rotatory flinging movements of the contralateral arm and leg. Similarly, damage to the caudate nucleus often results in chorea, whereas the opposite phenomenon, akinesia, typically occurs when dopamine-producing cells in the substantia nigra degenerate, releasing the intact caudate nucleus from inhibition. Lesions restricted to the globus pallidus often cause flexion dystonia and impaired postural reflexes. The neurologic substrates of cognitive impairments in extrapyramidal diseases are more obscure than those accounting for motor abnormalities. Some of the cognitive impairments in Parkinson's disease are postulated to result from frontal lobe dysfunction due to disruption of reciprocal connections with the caudate nucleus.

NEUROPHARMACOLOGY OF THE BASAL GANGLIA: GENERAL PRINCIPLES   Transfer of information from one cell to another in the mammalian nervous system usually involves one or more chemicals released from the first neuron to a specific receptor site on a second neuron, thereby altering the biochemical and physical properties of the second neuron. These chemicals taken together are called neuroregulators. There are three distinct classes of neuroregulators: neurotransmitters, neuromodulators, and neurohormones. Neurotransmitters, such as the catecholamines, ACh, and amino acids such as glutamate and GABA, are the best known and clinically most important class of neuroregulators. They cause short-latency, brief postsynaptic effects (e.g., depolarization) close to their point of release. Neuromodulators, such as the endorphins, somatostatin, substance P, and other neuropeptides, also exert effects close to the point of release; they can enhance or diminish effects of the classic neurotransmitters. Many neurons that contain classic neurotransmitters also contain neuromodulator peptides. Substance P coexists within raphe neurons that synthesize 5-HT, for example, and vasoactive intestinal polypeptide coexists with ACh in many cortical cholinergic neurons. Neurohormones, such as vasopressin and angiotensin II, differ from other regulators because they are released into the bloodstream and are transported to remote receptors. Their effects are slow in onset and have a long duration of action. The distinction between the various classes of neuroregulators is not absolute. DA, for example, acts as a neurotransmitter in the caudate nucleus but is believed to act as a neurohormone in the hypothalamus.

Neuroregulators of the neurotransmitter class are the best-studied transmitters in the basal ganglia and the ones on which most drugs exert their effects. Neurotransmitters are synthesized in the presynaptic terminals of neurons and are stored in vesicles. Following the arrival of an electric impulse, neurotransmitters are released from the presynaptic terminal into the synaptic cleft, diffuse across the synaptic gap, and combine with specific receptor sites on the postsynaptic cell. This initiates a series of biochemical and biophysical changes; the sum of all postsynaptic excitatory and inhibitory influences determines the likelihood that a given neuron will discharge. The biogenic amines DA, norepinephrine (NE), and 5-HT are inactivated by enzymatic degradation (monamine oxidase and catechol-*O*-methyltransferase) and by uptake into the presynaptic terminals; ACh is inactivated by intrasynaptic hydrolysis. There are also receptor sites on the presynaptic terminal, called autoreceptors, and their stimulation generally causes a decrease in synthesis and release of the transmitter. The affinity of an autoreceptor for its neurotransmitter is often much greater than that of the postsynaptic receptor. Drugs that stimulate DA autoreceptors can be expected to decrease dopaminergic transmission and possibly be useful in the treatment of hyperkinetic movement disorders such as Huntington's disease and tardive dyskinesia. Receptors may be further subdivided based on response to pharmacologic agents. There are at least two separate populations of DA receptors, for example: Stimulation of D-1 sites activates adenylate cyclase, whereas D-2 receptor stimulation inhibits adenyl cyclase.

The ergot alkaloid bromocriptine, used in the treatment of Parkinson's disease, stimulates D-2 but blocks D-1 receptors; most neuroleptics block D-2 receptors.

CLINICAL MANIFESTATIONS OF LESIONS OF THE BASAL GANGLIA   Akinesia   When extrapyramidal diseases are analyzed along classic neurologic lines into primary functional deficits (negative symptoms due to loss of connectivity) and secondary release effects (positive symptoms of excessive activity), akinesia stands as a principal negative or deficit symptom. *Akinesia* refers to the inability to initiate changes in activity and to perform ordinary volitional movements rapidly and easily. The terms *bradykinesia* and *hypokinesia* are employed to describe lesser degrees of impairment. In contrast to paralysis, which is the negative symptom of corticospinal tract lesions, strength is preserved although there is a delay in achieving peak power. Akinesia is also distinct from *apraxia*, in which the command to perform a particular action never reaches the motor centers that direct the desired movement. Akinesia is the most disabling feature of Parkinson's disease. Akinetic patients display severe immobility and underactivity. They sit motionless for long periods of time without shifting postures and take double the time normally required to eat, dress, and bathe. Poverty of movement reveals itself in the loss of automatic associated motions, such as eye blinks and freely swinging arms when walking. Akinesia probably accounts for such common symptoms in Parkinson's disease as facial immobility, vocal hypophonia, micrographia, and difficulty in arising from a chair and beginning to walk. Akinesia can affect the mind as well; slowed speed of thought is called bradyphrenia. Although pathophysiologic details remain uncertain, clinical analysis of akinesia supports the hypothesis that the basal ganglia are mainly responsible for initiation and automatic execution of learned motor plans. Neuropharmacologic evidence suggests that akinesia itself results from DA deficiency.

Rigidity   *Muscle tone* is defined as the amount of resistance encountered when a relaxed limb is moved passively. In rigidity, the muscles are in continuous contraction and resistance to passive movement is constant. Rigidity secondary to extrapyramidal disorders may superficially resemble spasticity due to corticospinal tract lesions in that both produce increases in muscular tone. A few clinical guidelines provide help in distinguishing these conditions at the bedside. The distribution of increased tone often differs in rigidity and spasticity. Although rigidity is present in both flexor and extensor muscle groups, it tends to be more prominent in those that maintain a flexed posture. Rigidity is easy to detect in large muscle groups, but smaller muscles of the face, tongue, and larynx are also often affected. In contrast to rigidity, spasticity usually produces increased tone in the extensor muscles of the legs and the flexor musculature of the arms. The quality of hypertonus can also be used to distinguish the two conditions. Resistance to passive movements is constant in rigidity, accounting for terms such as "lead pipe" and "plastic" resistance. In spasticity, there may be a free interval followed classically by the clasp-knife phenomenon; muscles do not contract until they are stretched a bit, and later during stretch the augmentation in muscle tone quickly subsides. Deep tendon reflexes are normal in rigidity but increased in spastic states. Spasticity results from hyperactivity of the stretch reflex arc due to central changes but without increased sensitivity of the muscle spindle; spasticity can be abolished by sectioning posterior spinal roots. Rigidity has less relationship with hyperactivity of segmental reflex arcs and depends more upon heightened discharge of alpha motor neurons. A special type of rigidity is the cogwheel phenomenon, which is especially common in Parkinson's disease. When the hypertonic muscle is passively stretched, the resistance may be rhythmically jerky, as though the resistance of the limb were controlled by a ratchet.

Chorea   Derived from the Greek word meaning "dance," chorea refers to widespread arrhythmic movements of a forcible, rapid, jerky, restless type. Choreic movements are noted for their irregularity and variability; they are generally continuous, may be simple or quite elaborate, and affect any part of the body. They may resemble voluntary movement in complexity, but they are never combined into a coordinated act unless the patient incorporates them into a deliberate movement in order to make them less noticeable. Normal volitional movements are possible because there is no paralysis, but they may be excessively quick, poorly sustained, and deformed by choreic movements. Chorea may be generalized or limited to one side of the body. Generalized chorea is the predominant involuntary movement in Huntington's disease and in rheumatic (Sydenham's) chorea, and usually involves the face, trunk, and limbs; it is often seen with levodopa toxicity in patients with Parkinson's disease. Another common choreiform disorder, tardive dyskinesia, occurs in association with chronic neuroleptic administration. Choreic movements in this disorder are generally restricted to the buccal, lingual, and mandibular musculature, although trunk and limbs may be involved in severe cases. Sedatives such as phenobarbital or a benzodiazepine are used in treating Sydenham's chorea; neuroleptics are commonly used to suppress chorea in Huntington's disease. Drugs that increase cholinergic neurotransmission, such as phosphatidylcholine and physostigmine, have been used to suppress chorea in about 30 percent of patients with tardive dyskinesia.

A special type of paroxysmal chorea, sometimes with athetosis or dystonic features, occurs sporadically, or as an autosomal dominant disorder. These disorders usually appear during childhood or adolescence and continue throughout life; patients have paroxysms that last minutes to hours. In one special subtype, the chorea is kinesogenic, which means that it may be initiated by a sudden voluntary movement. Alcohol, hypernatremia, and phenytoin may precipitate paroxysmal chorea, especially in patients who have had Sydenham's chorea in childhood. In some cases, anticonvulsant drugs, including phenobarbital and clonazepam, and in other instances levodopa have prevented attacks.

Athetosis This term is from a Greek word meaning "unfixed" or "changeable." Athetosis is characterized by an inability to sustain the muscles of the fingers, toes, tongue or any other group of muscles in one position. The maintained posture is interrupted by continuous slow, purposeless movements. These are most pronounced in the digits and hands and consist of extension, pronation, flexion, and supination of the arm with alternating flexion and extension of the fingers. Athetotic movements are slower than those associated with chorea, but gradations are commonly seen and termed *choreoathetosis* when it is impossible to distinguish between the two. Generalized athetosis may be seen in children with static encephalopathy (cerebral palsy); it can also occur in Wilson's disease, in torsion dystonia, and following cerebral anoxia. Posthemiplegic athetosis is unilateral and occurs especially in children who have suffered a stroke. Patients whose athetosis is due to cerebral palsy or cerebral anoxia have variable degrees of additional motor deficit due to associated corticospinal tract disease. Discrete individual movements of the tongue, lips, and hands are often impossible, and attempts to perform such voluntary movements result in contraction of all the muscles in the limb and other parts of the body. Variable degrees of rigidity are generally associated with all forms of athetosis and may account for the slower quality of movement in this disorder in contrast to chorea. Treatment of athetosis is generally unsatisfactory, although some patients improve with the drugs used to suppress chorea and dystonia.

The dystonias Dystonia refers to abnormally increased muscular tone that causes fixed abnormal postures. Some patients with dystonia also have shifting postures resulting from irregular, forceful twisting movements that affect trunk and extremities and produce bizarre, grotesque movements and positions of the body. The mobile spasms of dystonia are similar to those of athetosis but are generally slower and involve axial (trunk) rather than appendicular (extremity) muscles. Dystonic movements increase during volitional motor activity, nervousness, and emotional stress; they diminish during relaxation and, like most extrapyramidal movement disorders, disappear completely during sleep. *Primary torsion dystonia*, formerly known as dystonia musculorum deformans, is frequently inherited as an autosomal dominant characteristic; families of Ashkenazic Jews with an auto-

somal recessive pattern of inheritance have been described. Spontaneous cases without family histories of dystonia are also common. Manifestations of dystonia usually begin in the first two decades of life, but adult forms are recognized. Generalized torsion spasms can also occur in children with kernicterus and after cerebral hypoxia.

The term dystonia is also used in another sense, to describe any fixed posture which may be the end result of a motor system disease. For example, dystonia secondary to a stroke (flexed arm and extended leg) is often called hemiplegic dystonia, and that associated with parkinsonism called flexion dystonia. In contrast to these permanent dystonic states, drugs such as the neuroleptics, and levodopa in patients with parkinsonism, can induce dystonic postures and spasms that subside once the offending medication is discontinued.

Secondary or *focal dystonias* are more common than torsion dystonia and include such disorders as spasmodic torticollis, writer's cramp, blepharospasm, spastic dysphonia, and Meige's syndrome. In the focal dystonias as a group, symptoms tend to be highly localized; they remain stable, and rarely spread to involve other body parts. Focal dystonias occur more frequently in adults and most often arise spontaneously without known genetic transmission or antecedent illness. Spasmodic torticollis is the most common focal dystonia. There are intermittent or continuous spasms of the sternocleidomastoid, trapezius, and other neck muscles, usually more prominent on one side than the other, that cause turning or tipping of the head. Torticollis is involuntary and cannot be inhibited, and thereby differs from habit spasm or tic. Torticollis is worse when the patient sits, stands, or walks; placing a finger to the chin or side of the jaw often alleviates the muscle imbalance. Women are affected twice as often as men; the average age of onset is 40.

Torsion dystonia is classified as an extrapyramidal disease even though no pathologic lesions have been observed in the basal ganglia or elsewhere in the brain. Development of rational therapy is further impaired by the lack of information regarding possible neurotransmitter abnormalities. Symptomatic relief is sometimes achieved with sedatives such as the benzodiazepines and high doses of anticholinergic drugs; levodopa has been helpful in some instances. Biofeedback therapy has sometimes been beneficial but psychiatric treatment is ineffectual. Blepharospasm has been successfully treated by injecting a dilute solution of botulinum toxin into periocular muscles. The toxin produces a mild neuromuscular blockade; its effect is transient and treatment must be repeated every 2 or 3 months. Preliminary reports indicate that injection of toxin into the appropriate muscle is effective treatment for torticollis, spastic dysphonia, and occupational finger dystonias. When spasmodic torticollis is severe, surgical denervation of the affected muscles (C1 to C3 bilaterally and C4 on one side) has given favorable results in most patients.

Myoclonus This is a descriptive term for very brief, involuntary, random muscular contractions. Myoclonus can occur spontaneously at rest, in response to sensory stimuli, or with voluntary movements. Myoclonus may involve a single motor unit and simulate a fasciculation, or it may simultaneously involve groups of muscles that displace the limb or distort its voluntary movement. Myoclonus is a symptom that occurs in a wide variety of generalized metabolic and neurologic disorders collectively called the myoclonias. Posthypoxic intention myoclonus is a special myoclonic syndrome that occurs as a sequel to transient cerebral anoxia such as might occur, for example, during a brief cardiorespiratory arrest. Cognitive abilities are usually preserved; however, there are signs of cerebellar dysfunction and voluntary movements are marred by action myoclonus involving the extremities, facial muscles, and even the voice. Action myoclonus deforms all movements and severely limits the patient's ability to eat, talk, write, or even walk. Myoclonus may also result from lipid storage disease, encephalitis, Creutzfeldt-Jakob disease, or metabolic encephalopathies due to respiratory failure, chronic renal failure, hepatic failure, or electrolyte imbalance. Posthypoxic intention myoclonus and idiopathic myoclonus may be treated with the 5-HT precursor 5-hydroxytryptophan (Fig. 25-4); alternative therapies include baclofen, clonazepam, and valproic acid.

L. EXT.
L. FLEX.
L. TRI.
L. BIC.
L. ACC.
L. ACC.

A   B

FIGURE 25-4 Recordings from the left arm of a patient with posthypoxic intention myoclonus (*A*) before and (*B*) during treatment with 5-hydroxytryptophan. In both, the arm was held out horizontally from the shoulder. The upper four traces are EMGs from wrist extensors, wrist flexors, triceps, and biceps. The lower two traces are from accelerometers at right angles to one another on the hand. The horizontal calibration is 1 s. *A*. The continuous, large, jerky movements during voluntary activity are produced by arrhythmic bursts of EMG activity interspersed with irregular periods of EMG silence. The former positive and latter negative abnormalities occurred synchronously in antagonistic muscle groups. *B*. Only a little irregular tremor remains, and the EMG is much more continuous. (*From JH Growdon et al, Neurology 26:1135, 1976.*)

Asterixis   Quick arrhythmic movements that occur due to brief interruptions in background tonic muscular contractions are called asterixis; in a sense, asterixis may be considered as negative myoclonus. Asterixis may be observed in any voluntary muscle during contraction but is usually demonstrated clinically as a brief lapse of posture with prompt restoration during voluntary extension of the limb with dorsiflexion of the wrist or ankle. Asterixis is characterized by 50- to 200-ms silent periods in ongoing EMG activity in all muscle groups in one limb (Fig. 25-5). This results in a downward movement of the wrist or ankle due to gravity before muscular activity resumes and restores the limb to its original position. Asterixis is commonly observed bilaterally in metabolic encephalopathies, and its description in hepatic failure accounted for the original term "liver flap." Asterixis may be caused by drugs, including all anticonvulsants and the radiographic contrast agent metrizamide. Unilateral asterixis can occur after brain lesions in the distributions of the anterior or posterior cerebral arteries. The smallest brain lesion that can cause unilateral asterixis involves structures that are destroyed during stereotactic ventrolateral thalamotomy.

Hemiballismus   Hemiballismus is a hyperkinetic movement disorder characterized by violent flinging motions in the arm contralateral to a lesion (usually vascular) in or near the subthalamic nucleus. The movements in ballism also have a rotary component at the shoulder and hip; there may be concomitant flexion and extension movements in the hand and foot as well. The involuntary motions persist throughout the day but generally attenuate during sleep. Strength and muscle tone may be slightly decreased in the affected extremities and accurate movements are impaired, but patients with hemiballismus are not paralyzed. Both experimental and clinical observations indicate that the subthalamic nucleus probably exerts a controlling influence on the globus pallidus. Damage to the subthalamic nucleus destroys this restraining influence and results in hemiballismus. The exact biochemical consequences of these lesions remain unclear, but indirect evidence suggests that there is an increase in dopaminergic tone in the remaining basal ganglia structures. Medical treatment with neuroleptic drugs given to block DA receptors are generally effective in suppressing ballismus. Surgery is reserved for refractory cases; a stereotactic lesion placed in the ipsilateral globus pallidus, thalamic fasciculus, or ventrolateral thalamus can also abolish hemiballismus

and restore normal function. Although recovery can be complete, many patients are left with variable amounts of hemichorea involving the hand and foot.

Tremor   This common symptom consists of a rhythmic oscillation of a part of the body around a fixed point. Tremors usually involve the distal parts of limbs; the head, tongue, or jaw; and rarely the trunk. There are several different types of tremor, and each has its own clinical setting, pathophysiology, and therapeutic requirements. Often several different tremors exist in the same patient and must be treated individually. In a general hospital, most patients who appear tremulous actually have asterixis as a manifestation of one or another metabolic encephalopathy. Tremors may be subdivided clinically according to their distribution, amplitude, and relationship to volitional movement.

Tremor at rest is a coarse tremor with an average rate of four to five beats per second. It is most often localized in one or both hands and, occasionally, in the jaw or tongue. It is frequently a feature of Parkinson's disease. It characteristically occurs with postural (tonic) contraction of axial and limb girdle musculature when the limb is in an attitude of repose; willed movement temporarily suppresses it (Fig. 25-6). If the proximal muscles are completely relaxed, the tremor usually disappears, but the average patient rarely achieves this state. In some cases the tremor is constant; in others it varies from time to time and may extend from one group of muscles to another as the disease progresses. In some patients with Parkinson's disease there is no tremor; in others the tremor tends to be rather gentle and more or less limited to the distal muscles, whereas in a minority of parkinsonian patients and in patients with Wilson's disease (hepatolenticular degeneration), it often has a wider range and involves proximal muscles. In many cases there is a variable degree of rigidity of a plastic type in the tremulous limb or elsewhere. Although it is

FIGURE 25-5   Asterixis recorded from the outstretched left arm of a patient with metrizamide-induced encephalopathy. The upper four EMG traces are identical to those in Fig. 25-4. The bottom trace is from an accelerometer on the dorsum of the hand. Calibration is 1 s. Note the continuous voluntary EMG interrupted at the arrow by a brief involuntary silent period in all four muscles. This silent period is followed by a lapse of posture and its jerky restitution, which is recorded by the accelerometer.

L. EXT.

L. FLEX.

L. ACC.

FIGURE 25-6 Tremor at rest in a patient with Parkinson's disease. The upper two traces are surface EMG recordings from extensors and flexors of the left wrist; the lower trace is from an accelerometer attached to the left hand. The horizontal calibration denotes 1 s. Note the tremor at rest results from alternating contractions of antagonistic muscles at approximately 5 Hz. At the arrow, the patient is asked to dorsiflex the left wrist, and the tremor at rest disappears.

a source of great embarrassment and often is deemed responsible for all of a patient's motor difficulties, this type of tremor interferes with voluntary movements surprisingly little: It is not uncommon to see a patient who has been trembling violently raise a full glass of water to the lips and drain the contents without spilling a drop. It is the combination of tremor at rest, slowness of movement, rigidity, flexed postures without true paralysis, and postural instability that constitutes Parkinson's syndrome. Often patients with Parkinson's disease also suffer from the tremor of stage fright (one of the enhanced physiologic tremors—see below) or from essential-familial tremor. Both may be exaggerated by increased levels of catecholamines in the bloodstream and may be suppressed by drugs, such as propranolol, that block beta-adrenergic receptors.

The exact pathologic anatomy of *tremor at rest* is unknown. In Parkinson's disease, the visible lesions are predominantly in the substantia nigra. In Wilson's disease, in which tremor is mixed with cerebellar ataxia, the lesions are diffuse. Elderly persons may develop resting tremor without rigidity, slowness of movement, flexed postures, or masked facies. Unlike patients with parkinsonism, individuals with this syndrome do not progress to motor disability; their tremor does not respond to anti-parkinsonian drugs. In any given case it is not predictable whether a tremor is the initial sign of Parkinson's disease. Patients with titubation and a proximal tremor at rest (rubral tremor) as a symptom of cerebellar system dysfunction can be differentiated by the presence of ataxia and dysmetria from those with Parkinson's disease.

Action tremor refers to tremors present when the limbs are active,

either when maintained in a certain position, as when outstretched, or throughout voluntary movement. Tremor amplitude may increase slightly as the action of the limbs becomes more precise, but it never approaches the degree of augmentation seen with cerebellar ataxia/dysmetria. In contrast to tremor at rest, action tremors disappear when the limbs are relaxed. Some of the action tremors are an exaggeration of normal *physiologic tremor;* such enhanced physiologic tremors are extremely common. They are experienced occasionally by all normal persons as well as by patients with essential-familial tremor or Parkinson's disease. They involve the outstretched hand as well as head, lips, and tongue. In general, they are due to a hyperadrenergic state and sometimes are iatrogenic (Table 25-2). Activation of beta$_2$ receptors in muscle alters the mechanical properties of muscle, eliciting action tremor. These alterations are reflected in discharges of muscle spindle afferents which modify the timing of activity around the stretch reflex arc and serve to augment the amplitude of preexisting physiologic tremor. Only patients without functional stretch reflex arcs are immune to these tremors. Peripherally active drugs that block beta$_2$-adrenergic receptors diminish enhanced physiologic tremors. This type of tremor is seen in numerous medical, neurologic, and psychiatric diseases and is therefore more difficult to interpret than tremor at rest.

Essential-familial tremor (Fig. 25-7) is a somewhat slower action tremor which may occur as the only neurologic abnormality either sporadically or in several members of a family. It may begin in childhood but usually comes on later and persists throughout adult life. It becomes a source of embarrassment because it suggests to the onlooker that the patient is nervous. A curious fact about this tremor is that one or two drinks of an alcoholic beverage may abolish it but it will become worse after the effects of the alcohol have worn off. Essential-familial tremors are suppressed by primidone or CNS-active beta-adrenergic blocking agents such as propranolol.

Intention tremor is an ambiguous term: The abnormal movements are certainly not intentional, and the abnormality is best described as an oscillatory ataxia generated proximally rather than as tremor. True tremors tend to affect distal musculature and the movements are more rhythmic and tend to be in one plane. Cerebellar ataxia, in which the direction of abnormal movement varies from second to second, requires for its full expression the performance of an exacting, precise, willed movement. Ataxia is absent when the limbs are inactive and during the first part of a voluntary movement, but develops as the action continues and greater precision is demanded (e.g., in touching a target such as the patient's nose or the examiner's finger). Ataxia is a jerky, arrhythmic interruption of forward progression in a voluntary motion, often with side-to-side oscillations. Ataxia continues for a fraction of a second or so after the act is completed, and may seriously interfere with the patient's performance of skilled acts. Sometimes the head is involved (titubation). This movement disorder invariably indicates disease of the cerebellar system including its connections. When the disease is very severe, every movement, even lifting a limb, causes a wide-ranging oscillation of such violence that the patient is thrown off balance. This state is occasionally seen in multiple sclerosis, Wilson's disease, and vascular, traumatic, and

TABLE 25-2 Conditions that enhance physiologic tremors

HYPERADRENERGIC STATES

Anxiety
Bronchodilators and other beta agonists
Excitement
Hypoglycemia
Hyperthyroidism
Pheochromocytoma
Peripheral metabolites of levodopa
Stage fright

POSSIBLE HYPERADRENERGIC STATES

Amphetamines
Antidepressants
Withdrawal from alcohol or opiates
Xanthines in tea and coffee

STATES OF UNCERTAIN ETIOLOGY

Glucocorticoid therapy
Exercise
Fatigue
Lithium therapy

FIGURE 25-7 Action tremor in a patient with essential-familial tremor. Recordings from the right upper extremity are with the hand actively dorsiflexed; otherwise, traces are similar to Fig. 25-4. The horizontal calibration denotes 500 ms. Note that during this action tremor, bursts of EMG activity at approximately 8 Hz occur synchronously in antagonistic muscles.

R. EXT.

R. FLEX.

R. ACC.

other lesions of the tegmentum of the midbrain and subthalamus but not of the cerebellum.

Habit spasms and tics   Many individuals develop habitual movements that persist unchanged throughout life. Common examples include sniffing, clearing the throat, protruding the chin, and pulling on the collar. These are called habit spasms. Affected individuals admit that the movements are voluntary, but that they feel compelled to make them in order to relieve tension. Habit spasms can be inhibited for a time by a willful effort but reappear when attention is diverted. In certain cases, they become so ingrained that the person is unaware of them and unable to control them. Children between 5 and 10 years of age are especially likely to have habit spasms.

Tics are characterized by stereotyped, purposeless, and irregularly repetitive movements. Gilles de la Tourette syndrome is the most common and severe form of multiple tic disorder. This syndrome is a neuropsychiatric disorder with motor and behavior abnormalities; it usually begins in the first two decades of life and affects boys four times more frequently than girls. Motor symptoms include multiple brief muscular spasms, known as convulsive tics, in the face, neck, and shoulders. Vocal tics, including grunts and barking sounds, are also common. Behavioral abnormalities include coprolalia (swearing and repeating other vile utterances) and repeating the words of others (echolalia). The cause of Tourette's syndrome is unknown, and its pathophysiology remains obscure. Treatments with neuroleptic drugs will decrease the severity and frequency of tics in 75 to 90 percent of patients with Tourette's syndrome, regardless of disease severity. The noradrenergic agonist clonidine has also been reported to suppress symptoms.

EXAMINATION AND DIFFERENTIAL DIAGNOSIS OF EXTRA-PYRAMIDAL SYNDROMES   In broad terms, all of the extrapyramidal disorders should be viewed in terms of primary deficit (negative symptoms) and of the new phenomena (abnormal postures and involuntary movements) that have appeared. The positive symptoms are ascribed to release from inhibition or disequilibrium of undamaged motor parts of the nervous system. The physician must cultivate the habit of accurately observing and describing abnormalities of movement and must not be content merely to give the condition a name or to force it into some superficial category. The fully developed extrapyramidal motor syndromes can be recognized without difficulty once the physician has become familiar with the typical pictures. A mental picture of Parkinson's disease, with its slowness of movement, poverty of facial expression, tremor at rest, and muscular rigidity, should be fixed in mind. Similarly, the gross distortions of posture found in dystonia, whether widespread in trunk muscles or involving only neck muscles as in spasmodic torticollis, should be easily recognized. Athetosis, with its instability of postures, ceaseless movements of finger and hands, and intention spasm; chorea, with its rapid and complicated movements; and myoclonus, with its abrupt movements that flit over the body, are other standard syndromes. There tends to be a mild defect in the voluntary use of the affected parts in all extrapyramidal syndromes.

Early or mild forms of these conditions, like all medical diseases, may offer special difficulties in diagnosis. Cases of Parkinson's disease, seen before the appearance of tremor, are often overlooked. Uncertainty of balance and short gait (*marche à petit pas*) in the elderly is often incorrectly attributed to loss of confidence and fear of falling. Patients may complain of being nervous and restless and describe a stiffness and aching in parts of the body. Because there is no weakness or change in reflexes, the disorder may then be considered rheumatic or even psychogenic. Parkinson's disease often begins in a hemiplegic distribution, and for this reason, the illness may be misdiagnosed as cerebral thrombosis or tumor. Facial immobility, a suggestion of a limp, mild rigidity, failure of an arm to swing naturally in walking, or loss of certain movements of cooperation will help in diagnosis at this time. Every case presenting with atypical extrapyramidal symptoms should be surveyed for Wilson's disease in order to avoid missing a treatable illness. Mild or early chorea is often mistaken for simple nervousness. Observing the patient at rest

as well as in action is critical to the diagnosis. There are instances, nonetheless, in which it is impossible to distinguish simple fidgets from early chorea, especially in children, and there are no laboratory tests to aid in the diagnosis. The first postural manifestations of dystonia may suggest hysteria, and it is only later when the fixity of the postural abnormality becomes apparent that accurate diagnosis is reached.

Motor disorders seldom appear in pure form, and extrapyramidal syndromes often coexist with lesions in the corticospinal tract or cerebellar systems. For example, syndromes such as progressive supranuclear palsy, olivopontocerebellar atrophy, or the Shy-Drager syndrome have many elements of Parkinson's disease but also have paralysis of voluntary eye movements, ataxia, apraxia, postural hypotension, or spasticity with bilateral Babinski signs. Wilson's disease usually displays tremor at rest, rigidity, slowness of movement, and flexion dystonia of the trunk, but exceptionally there are athetosis, dystonia, and intention tremor. Emotional or cognitive abnormalities may be the presenting signs in Wilson's disease. Hallervorden-Spatz disease may take the form of universal rigidity and flexion dystonia, but choreoathetosis is sometimes observed. In some forms of Huntington's disease, particularly with juvenile onset, rigidity replaces choreoathetosis. Corticospinal and various extrapyramidal disorders may be associated in patients with cerebral diplegia. Some of the neurodegenerative diseases in which corticospinal tract and basal ganglia lesions coexist are described in Chap. 359.

Anatomic and neuropathologic studies of the basal ganglia, coupled with biochemical analyses of neurotransmitter content and behavioral responses to neuropharmacologic agents, provide the basis for understanding disorders involving the basal ganglia and for guiding their treatment. Results of studies in Parkinson's disease and Huntington's disease clearly illustrate these principles. In Parkinson's disease, the DA content of the striatum is depleted owing to a loss of neurons in the substantia nigra and degeneration of their axonal projection to the striatum. As a result of decreased DA release, neurons within the striatum that synthesize ACh are released from inhibition. This results in the preponderance of cholinergic neurotransmission relative to dopaminergic transmission that accounts for most of the symptoms in Parkinson's disease. Recognition of this imbalance provides the basis for rational pharmacologic treatments. According to this formulation, drugs that increase dopaminergic neurotransmission, such as levodopa or bromocriptine, would be expected to rectify the imbalance between cholinergic and dopaminergic tone. These drugs, often prescribed in combination with anticholinergic drugs, are now standard therapy in Parkinson's disease. Excess levodopa or bromocriptine in patients with Parkinson's disease may induce a wide variety of abnormal movements that result from excessive stimulation of DA receptors in the striatum. The most frequent of these is craniofacial choreoathetosis, but more generalized choreoathetosis, facial and cervical spasms, dystonic postures, and myoclonic jerks may also occur. On the other hand, administration of drugs that block DA receptors (such as the neuroleptics) or deplete DA storage (such as reserpine or tetrabenazine) may produce a parkinsonian syndrome in an otherwise normal individual.

Huntington's disease is in many ways the clinical and pharmacologic opposite of Parkinson's disease. In Huntington's disease, characterized by personality change and dementia, gait abnormality, and chorea, there is a loss of neurons within the caudate and putamen, with resultant depletion of GABA and ACh but preserved DA content. The symptoms of chorea are believed to result from relative excess of DA compared with other transmitters in the striatum; drugs that block DA receptors, such as the neuroleptics, generally suppress chorea, whereas levodopa administration increases it. Similarly, physostigmine, given to increase cholinergic neurotransmission, may suppress chorea, whereas anticholinergic drugs enhance it.

These examples of clinical pharmacology further confirm the existence of delicate balances between excitatory and inhibitory impulses in the basal ganglia. In any one patient, the variable clinical manifestations seen during therapy are due to alterations in the neurochemical environment; the anatomic lesions remain unchanged. These examples illustrate the power of neuropharmacologic therapy in basal ganglia disease and provide the basis for optimism regarding the future ability of drugs to benefit patients with extrapyramidal movement disorders.

REFERENCES

ALEXANDER GE et al: Parallel organization of functionally segregated circuits linking basal ganglia and cortex. Ann Rev Neurosci 9:357, 1986

FAHN S et al: Classification and investigation of dystonia, in *Movement Disorders 2*. CD Marsden, S Fahn (eds). London, Butterworths, 1987, pp 332–358

GESCHWIND N: The apraxias: Neural mechanisms of disorders of learned movement. Am Sci 63:188, 1975

GRAYBIEL AM: Neuropeptides in the basal ganglia, in *Neuropeptides in Neurologic and Psychiatric Disease*, JB Martin, JD Barchas (eds). New York, Raven Press, 1986, pp 135–161

GROWDON JH, SCHEIFE RT: Medical treatment of extrapyramidal diseases, in *Update III: Harrison's Principles of Internal Medicine*. KJ Isselbacher et al (eds). New York, McGraw-Hill, 1982, pp 185–208

JAGIELLA WM, SUNG JH: Bilateral infarction of the medullary pyramids in humans. Neurology 39:21, 1989

JANKOVIC J, ORMAN J: Botulinum A toxin for cranial-cervical dystonia: A double-blind, placebo-controlled study. Neurology 37:616, 1987

KUYPERS HGJM: Anatomy of the descending pathways, in *Handbook of Physiology*, Section 1, *The Nervous System*, vol II: *Motor Control*, Part I, VB Brooks (ed). Bethesda, American Physiological Society, 1981, pp 597–666

MARSDEN CD: The mysterious motor function of the basal ganglia. Neurology 32:514, 1982

MARTIN JB: Huntington's disease: New approaches to an old problem. Neurology 34:1059, 1984

PENN RD et al: Intrathecal baclofen for severe spinal spasticity. N Engl J Med 320:1517, 1989

YOUNG RR: Treatment of spastic paresis. N Engl J Med 320:1553, 1989

26 ATAXIA AND DISORDERS OF BALANCE AND GAIT

SID GILMAN

In the assessment of patients with neurologic disorders, it is important when taking the history to inquire about posture and gait and to examine these functions routinely as part of the neurologic examination. Abnormalities of posture and gait can result from disorders affecting several levels of the nervous system, and the type of abnormality observed clinically often indicates the site affected.

NEURAL STRUCTURES REQUIRED FOR STANDING AND WALKING The structures in the central nervous system that control standing and walking are the basal ganglia, a "locomotor region" in the mesencephalon, the cerebellum, and the spinal cord. The cerebral cortex doubtless is important in many aspects of standing and walking, but in experimental animals, complete removal of the cerebral cortex during the neonatal period, preserving the basal ganglia, thalamus, and lower structures, leaves stance and locomotion essentially normal. If the cerebral cortex, basal ganglia, and thalamus are removed, leaving the mesencephalon and lower brainstem intact, standing and walking are still possible. Electrical stimulation in a region of the mesencephalon termed the "locomotor region" evokes walking motions, and the speed and form of locomotion can be modified from a slow walk to a trot or gallop with changes in stimulation strength. This region receives projections from the basal ganglia, including the subthalamic and endopeduncular nuclei and the substantia nigra.

The spinal cord contains neural circuitry that coordinates the muscles for locomotion. After experimental transection of the spinal cord in the midthoracic region, the hindlimbs maintain the capacity to perform coordinated walking movements when placed on a moving treadmill. With increased treadmill speed, walking movements can switch to simultaneous movements of the hindlimbs, as in a gallop. After a high spinal transection, both the forelimbs and the hindlimbs

can generate alternating movements and the sets of limbs remain coordinated. Thus, neural circuitry in the spinal cord can coordinate movements among all four limbs. The cerebellum controls many of the movements required for walking. Ablation of the cerebellum results in severe disorders of standing and walking.

In summary, walking is the result of integrated activity of the basal ganglia, mesencephalon, cerebellum, and spinal cord. Sensory inputs from movements of joints and muscle afferents provide important components for the control of walking. Without appropriate sensory feedback information, the pattern of walking is severely disrupted.

THE CEREBELLUM The cerebellum functions in concert with the motor cortex, basal ganglia, and many brainstem structures in executing a variety of movements. The cerebellum is needed to maintain proper posture and balance for walking and running; to perform fine voluntary movements such as those needed for writing, dressing, and eating; to carry out rapidly alternating and repetitive movements as in playing a musical instrument or working with a computer; and to coordinate smooth tracking movements of the eyes. The cerebellum controls certain properties of movements, including trajectory, velocity, and acceleration. Voluntary movements can be performed in the absence of cerebellar function, but the movements are clumsy and disorganized. The disturbances of movement from cerebellar dysfunction are termed *dyssynergia* (also *asynergia* or *ataxia*).

The cerebellum consists of a midline vermal region and two hemispheres, which are attached to the medulla, pons, and midbrain by three peduncles on each side. A layer of gray matter, the cerebellar cortex, covers the cerebellar surface and encloses an internal core of white matter. Three pairs of deep cerebellar nuclei are buried within the cerebellum. From medial to lateral these consist of the fastigial, interposed (globose and emboliform), and dentate nuclei.

The cerebellum consists of three lobes. The *flocculonodular lobe*, which is the oldest part of the cerebellum phylogenetically (archicerebellum), consists of the paired flocculi and the nodulus. This lobe receives input principally from the vestibular nuclei. The *anterior lobe*, the second oldest part (paleocerebellum), consists of vermal and paravermal structures in the anterior superior portion of the cerebellum. The anterior lobe receives input chiefly from the spinal cord. The *posterior lobe* is the largest and phylogenetically newest part of the cerebellum (neocerebellum) and is located between the other two lobes. The posterior lobe receives projections from the cerebral hemispheres via the pontine nuclei.

The cerebellar cortex contains three layers: an outermost *molecular layer*, a middle *Purkinje cell layer*, and an inner *granular layer*. The afferent fibers reaching the cerebellar cortex send collateral projections to the deep cerebellar nuclei and terminate either in the granule cell layer as *mossy fibers* or upon the dendrites of Purkinje cells as *climbing fibers*. Mossy fiber afferents are derived from the spinal cord, pontine nuclei, vestibular receptors and nuclei, trigeminal nuclei, reticular nuclei, and deep cerebellar nuclei. Climbing fiber afferents are derived exclusively from the inferior olive. Both mossy fiber and climbing fiber inputs are excitatory to the deep cerebellar nuclei and the cortex. Purkinje cells provide the only route for all information exiting from the cerebellar cortex and are inhibitory to the deep cerebellar and vestibular nuclei.

Projections to the cerebellum also originate in the locus coeruleus and the raphe nuclei of the brainstem. The afferents to the cerebellum from the locus coeruleus are noradrenergic; those from the raphe nuclei are serotonergic; and both sets of afferents are inhibitory. Several amino acids have been identified as putative neurotransmitters in the cerebellum. These include glutamate, which is used by mossy fibers and the axons of granule cells (parallel fibers); aspartate, which is used by climbing fibers; and γ-aminobutyric acid, which is used by the axons of Purkinje cells, Golgi cells, and basket cells.

The *inferior cerebellar peduncle* (*restiform body*) consists chiefly of afferent fibers. The peduncle contains a single efferent tract, the fastigiobulbar tract, which projects to the vestibular nuclei and

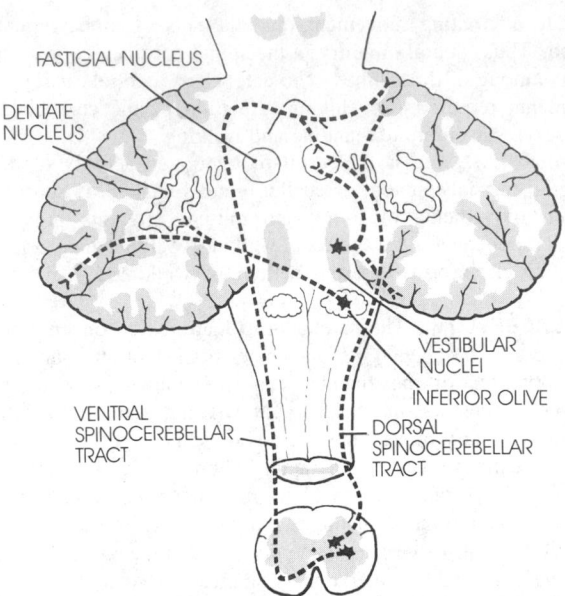

FIGURE 26-1 The central nervous system connections of the dorsal and ventral spinocerebellar tracts, the fastigial nuclei, and the vestibular nuclei. *(Adapted from S Gilman and S Winans Newman, in Manter & Gatz's Essentials of Clinical Neuroanatomy and Neurophysiology, 7th ed, Philadelphia, Davis, 1987.)*

completes a vestibular circuit through the cerebellum. Afferent fibers enter the inferior cerebellar peduncle from at least six sources (Fig. 26-1): (1) fibers from the vestibular nerve and nuclei; (2) olivocerebellar fibers from the inferior olivary nuclei; (3) the dorsal spinocerebellar tract; (4) some of the fibers from the ventral spinocerebellar tract; (5) the cuneocerebellar tract from the accessory cuneate nuclei in the medulla; and (6) reticulocerebellar fibers. *The middle cerebellar peduncle* (*brachium pontis*) consists almost entirely of crossed afferent fibers from the pontine nuclei in the gray substance of the basal part of the pons (pontocerebellar or transverse pontine fibers) (Fig. 26-2). The major projections to the pontine nuclei originate within the

FIGURE 26-2 The central nervous system connections of the dentate nucleus and interposed (emboliform and globose) nuclei. *(Adapted from S Gilman and S Winans Newman, in Manter & Gatz's Essentials of Clinical Neuroanatomy and Neurophysiology, 7th ed, Philadelphia, Davis, 1987.)*

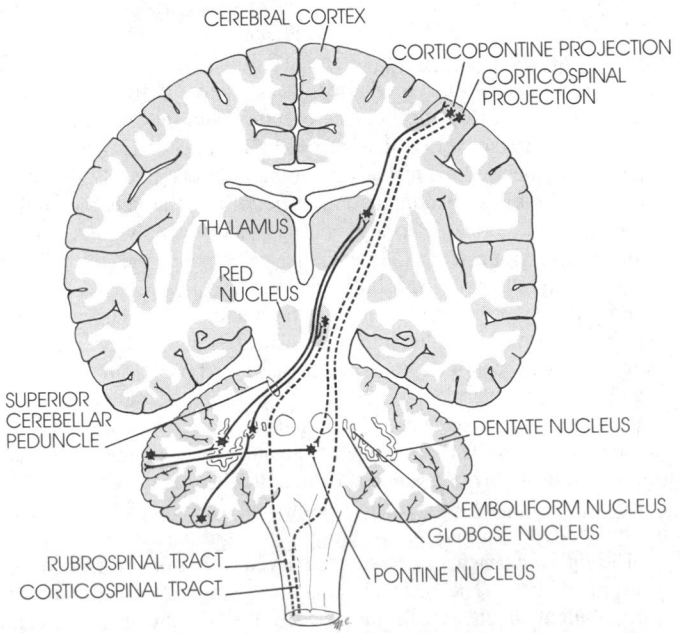

cerebral cortex. The *superior cerebellar peduncle* (*brachium conjunctivum*) consists principally of efferent projections from the cerebellum. Fibers arising in the dentate and interposed nuclei project to the reticular formation, red nucleus, and thalamus. Some of the fastigiobulbar tract fibers also run with the superior peduncle for a short distance before they enter the inferior cerebellar peduncle. The superior cerebellar peduncle contains afferent projections from the ventral spinocerebellar tract, a portion of the rostral spinocerebellar tract, and trigeminocerebellar projections.

Except for direct projections of Purkinje cells onto vestibular nuclei, the efferent pathways of the cerebellum begin with the deep nuclei. The fastigial nucleus sends fibers to the reticular and vestibular nuclei of the brainstem. These nuclei project into the spinal cord and are concerned with posture and balance. The interposed nuclei of each side of the cerebellum project axons through the superior cerebellar peduncle to the red nucleus of the contralateral side. The red nucleus sends fibers into the rubrospinal tract (Fig. 26-2), and this tract crosses the midline before descending into the spinal cord. The origin of this pathway in the interposed nuclei and the terminal portion in the spinal cord are on the same side of the body. Both the dentate and the interposed nuclei send fibers through the superior cerebellar peduncle to the contralateral ventrolateral nucleus of the thalamus. The ventrolateral nucleus relays fibers to the motor regions of the ipsilateral frontal lobe. The thalamic endings in the cerebral cortex make connection with corticospinal neurons whose efferent fibers pass through the pyramidal tract and cross to the contralateral side of the spinal cord. Thus, the origin of the cerebellothalamocortical pathway in the dentate and interposed nuclei and its termination in the spinal cord are on the same side of the body (Fig. 26-2).

For clinical purposes, a useful method of describing the cerebellum is based upon the existence of longitudinal sagittal zones. Each half of the cerebellum is subdivided into three longitudinal strips arranged from medial to lateral, including the cerebellar cortex, underlying white matter, and deep cerebellar nuclei: (1) a midline zone consisting of the vermal region with the fastigial nucleus; (2) an intermediate zone, the paravermal region, with the interposed nuclei; and (3) a lateral zone consisting of the cerebellar hemisphere with the dentate nucleus. Lesions of the midline zone cause disorders of stance and gait, truncal ataxia and titubation, and rotated or tilted postures of the head. Lesions of the lateral zone lead to disturbances in coordinated limb movement (ataxia), dysarthria, hypotonia, nystagmus, and kinetic tremor. Lesions of the intermediate zone cause symptoms characteristic of involvement of both the midline and lateral zones.

Ataxia is the result of dysmetria and decomposition of movement. *Dysmetria* is a disturbance of the trajectory or placement of a limb during active movement in which the limb falls short of its target (*hypometria*) or extends beyond its target (*hypermetria*). *Decomposition of movement* refers to errors in the sequence and speed of the component parts of a movement. The result is a lack of speed and skill in acts requiring the smoothly coordinated activity of several muscles. Movements previously fluid and accurate become halting and imprecise. *Ataxia* appears clinically as a disturbance in the rate and extent of an individual movement and commonly occurs from lesions of the cerebellum or of the sensory systems. Ataxia of gait consists of irregularities in the rate, length, and consistency of walking movements, with veering to one side or the other.

PHYSIOLOGIC RESPONSES IMPORTANT IN STANDING AND WALKING Maintenance of the upright posture results from the actions of a number of postural reflex responses: (1) local static reactions acting on individual limbs; (2) segmental static reactions linking the extremities together; and (3) general static reactions resulting from the position of the head in space. *Local static reactions* include the stretch reflex and the positive supporting reaction. The simplest *stretch reflex* is illustrated by the muscle stretch response (deep tendon reflex), a brief muscle twitch evoked by rapid stretch of the muscle's tendon. Maintenance of muscle extension results in sustained contraction of that muscle through the stretch reflex. The *positive supporting reaction*, as elucidated in animal studies, results from a light cutaneous contact of the skin of the foot and also by proprioceptive stimulation owing to stretch of the interosseous muscles. The result of these stimuli is an extensor thrust by the limb.

The *segmental static reactions* include the crossed extension reflex and interlimb coordination. In the crossed extension reflex, application of noxious stimulation to an extremity results in flexion of that limb and simultaneous extension of the contralateral limb. With stronger stimulation, the crossed extension reflex triggered from a hindlimb can induce flexion in the contralateral forelimb and extension in the ipsilateral forelimb. Thus, the whole body moves along a diagonal path through the extended contralateral hindlimb and ipsilateral forelimb, thereby removing the stimulated limb from the source of noxious stimulation. This diagonal pattern of interlimb coordination also provides postural adjustments in various situations.

The *general static reactions* consist of two general types. The first, the *tonic neck* and *labyrinthine reflexes*, function together to adjust body posture when the head moves relative to the trunk in space. The second, the *righting reflex*, is triggered by labyrinthine, neck, and visual stimuli and helps the animal to regain an upright position after a fall. The *grasp reflex* is a component of the righting reflex. Other forms of general static reactions include the placing and hopping reactions as well as adjustment of body postures during limb movements.

CLINICAL APPROACH TO DISORDERS OF EQUILIBRIUM AND GAIT When evaluating a disorder of gait, the physician should inquire whether the disturbance occurs more in the dark than in the light; whether vertigo, giddiness, or lightheadedness accompanies the disorder; and whether there is pain, numbness, tingling, or other type of paresthesias of the limbs. Inquiry should search for weakness, bowel and bladder dysfunction, and limb stiffness or rigidity. The physician should ask whether there is difficulty in the initiation or termination of walking.

Examination of stance and gait is performed best in a setting in which the physician can observe the patient walk from the front, back, and sides. The patient should rise quickly from a chair, walk normally at a slow pace, then more rapidly, and then turn around. The patient should walk on the heels, on the toes, and in tandem, placing the heel of one foot directly in front of the toes of the opposite foot, attempting to progress in a straight line. The patient should stand erect with the feet together and the head straight, first with the eyes open and then with the eyes closed to determine whether balance can be maintained (Romberg's sign). It is often helpful to observe the gait initially as the patient comes into the examining room when the patient is unaware that gait and stance are being examined.

With normal walking the body should be held erect, the head should be straight and the arms should hang loosely at the sides, each moving in rhythm with movement of the opposite leg. The shoulders and hips should be level and the arms should swing equally. The steps should be straight and equal in length. The head should not be tilted, and there should be no appreciable scoliosis or lordosis. With each step the hip and knee should flex smoothly, the ankle should dorsiflex, and the foot should clear the ground easily. The heel should strike the ground first, and the weight of the body should be transferred successively onto the sole of the foot and then onto the toes. The head and body should rotate slightly with each step without lurching or falling movements. Each person walks in a characteristic fashion that is often familial. Some people walk with the toes turned inward, others with the toes turned outward. Some people stride with large steps and others shuffle, making small steps. A person's gait is often a reflection of personality traits and can reflect shyness and timidity or aggressiveness and self-confidence.

Hemiparesis The patient with weakness of the limbs on one side of the body from a lesion of the corticospinal tract usually develops a characteristic gait disorder. The severity of the disorder depends upon the degree of weakness and stiffness of the affected limbs. The severely hemiparetic subject will stand and walk with the affected arm adducted at the shoulder and flexed at the elbow, wrist, and fingers and the affected leg stiffly extended at the hip, knee, and

ankle. There is difficulty in flexing the hip and knee and dorsiflexing the ankle. Thus, the paretic leg swings outward at the hip so that the foot does not scrape the floor. The leg is held stiffly and rotates in a semicircle, first away from and then toward the trunk in a circumduction movement. Often the upper body tilts slightly to the opposite side during the leg movement. The arm on the hemiparetic side usually swings little during walking. The loss of arm swing can be an early sign of a progressive hemiparesis. A person with a mild hemiparesis may show a gait disorder similar to that of the severely hemiparetic individual, but with a lesser degree of abnormality. In this case, a decrease in arm swing may be associated with subtle circumduction of the leg, without clear stiffness or weakness of the affected limbs.

Paraparesis Diseases of the spinal cord that affect leg function produce a characteristic gait resulting from a combination of spasticity and weakness of the lower extremities. Walking requires considerable effort and consists of slow, stiff movements at the hips and knees. The legs are usually maintained extended or slightly flexed at the hips and knees and adducted at the hips. In some people with paraparesis the legs may cross with each step, producing a scissoring motion. The steps usually are regular and short, and the patient may move the trunk from side to side, attempting to compensate for the stiff movements of the legs. The legs circumduct at the hips, and the feet scrape along the floor so that the soles of the shoes become worn at the toes.

Parkinsonism Parkinson's disease produces a characteristic posture and gait. The severely affected individual stands in a posture of flexion, with the thoracic spine bent forward, the head bent downward, the arms moderately flexed at the elbows and the legs slightly flexed at the hips and knees. The patient sits or stands with striking immobility, showing a fixed facial expression with infrequent blinking and making few automatic movements of the limbs. The patient seldom crosses the legs or adjusts body posture when seated in a chair. Although the arms are held immobile, often a tremor involves the fingers and wrists at four to five cycles per second. In some people the tremor also occurs at the elbows and even at the shoulders. In advanced cases there may be drooling and a rhythmic tremor of the jaw. The patient usually gets up slowly to walk and, with walking, the trunk bends even farther forward and the arms remain immobile at the sides of the body or become further flexed and carried a bit ahead of the body. The arms fail to swing. As forward progression begins, the legs remain bent at the hips, knees, and ankles. Characteristically, the steps are short so that the feet barely clear the ground and the soles of the feet shuffle and scrape the floor. With forward locomotion the steps become successively more rapid, and the patient may fall unless assisted (*festination*). If the patient is pushed forward or backward, compensatory flexion or extension movements of the trunk fail to occur, and the patient is forced to make a series of propulsive or retropulsive steps.

Patients with Parkinson's disease often have great difficulty in rising from a chair or walking after standing still. The individual may initiate walking with several small steps before taking longer strides. Walking may stop involuntarily with attempts to pass through a doorway or into an elevator. Parkinsonian patients at times can walk with surprising speed and dexterity for brief intervals. In times of acute emergency, as in a fire, a person previously immobile can walk rapidly or even run briefly.

Cerebellar disease Disease of the cerebellum causes difficulty in standing without support and in walking. The disorder may result from lesions intrinsic to the cerebellum or from lesions in the connecting pathways to and from the cerebellum. The difficulty is worsened by attempts to walk with a narrow base. The affected person usually stands with the legs apart, and standing may provoke *titubation*, a coarse forward and backward tremor of the trunk. Attempting to stand with the feet together provokes swaying or falling. The instability is the same whether the eyes are open or closed. The patient walks cautiously, taking steps of varying lengths, and lurches from side to side. The patient complains of difficulty with balance, is fearful of walking without support, and may insist upon holding onto objects such as a bed or chair, moving cautiously between these objects. Frequently the individual does not need to be supported; simply touching a wall or an object in the room makes it possible to walk with a greater sense of security. When a mild gait disorder is present, walking may deteriorate with attempts to walk in tandem in a straight line. This causes the patient to lose balance and, in response, to place one foot to the side to avoid falling. With unilateral lesions of the cerebellum, balance is lost toward the side of the lesion.

When disease is restricted to the midline (vermal) portions of the cerebellum, as occurs in alcoholic cerebellar degeneration, disorders of stance and gait may develop without other signs of cerebellar dysfunction such as limb ataxia or nystagmus. In contrast, disease of the cerebellar hemispheres, either unilaterally or bilaterally, often causes marked limb ataxia and nystagmus in association with a gait disorder. With a lesion confined to one cerebellar hemisphere, ipsilateral disturbances of posture and movement commonly accompany the gait disorder. The patient usually stands with the shoulder on the side of the lesion lower than the other, and there may be an accompanying scoliosis. The limbs on the side of the cerebellar lesion show diminished resistance to passive manipulation (hypotonia). On walking the patient staggers and deviates toward the affected side. This can be demonstrated by asking the patient to walk around a chair. Rotation toward the affected side results in a fall into the chair, and rotation toward the normal side causes movement away from the chair in a spiral. The affected arm and leg show marked ataxia in tests of coordinated movement such as successively touching the patient's nose and then the examiner's finger or running the heel of the affected leg down the shin of the opposite leg.

Sensory ataxia A characteristic gait disorder results from loss of sensation in the lower extremities due to disease processes in the peripheral nerves, dorsal roots, dorsal columns of the spinal cord, or medial lemnisci. The most disabling component of the sensory disorder is the loss of joint position sense, but loss of input from muscle spindle receptors, vibration detectors, and cutaneous receptors also contributes to the disability. People with sensory ataxia are unaware of the position of the lower extremities and consequently have difficulty in both standing and walking. The patient usually stands with the legs spread widely apart. The patient remains stable if asked to stand with the feet together and the eyes open, but sways and often falls (positive Romberg's sign) when the eyes are closed. The test for Romberg's sign cannot be performed if the subject is unsteady when standing with the feet together and the eyes open, as may occur with cerebellar disease.

The patient with sensory ataxia walks with the legs spread widely apart, watching the ground carefully. The legs are lifted higher than necessary at the hips and are flung forward and outward in abrupt motions. The steps vary in length, and the feet make characteristic slapping sounds as they contact the floor. The patient usually holds the body somewhat flexed at the hips, often using a cane for support. If vision is impaired or the patient attempts to walk in the dark, the gait disturbance worsens. The patient becomes unsteady and often falls when attempting to wash the face because of the temporary loss of visual compensation occurring with closure of the eyes.

Cerebral palsy This term encompasses a number of different motor abnormalities, most of them resulting from hypoxic-ischemic injury to the central nervous system in the perinatal period. The severity of the gait disturbance varies with the nature and extent of the lesion. Mild limited lesions can lead to increased deep tendon reflexes and extensor plantar responses with a slight degree of talipes equinovarus, without a clear gait disorder. More severe and extensive lesions commonly lead to bilateral hemiparesis. The patient stands and walks with a paraparetic posture and gait. The arms are adducted at the shoulders and flexed at the elbows and wrists.

Movement disorders commonly alter the gait in people with cerebral palsy. Athetosis occurs frequently and consists of slow or moderately rapid serpentine movements of the arms and legs, with postures alternating between the extremes of flexion with supination and extension with pronation. On walking, people with athetotic cerebral palsy show involuntary limb movements that are accompanied by rotary movements of the neck and frequent facial grimacing. The arms are usually flexed and the legs are extended, but asymmetric limb postures can occur with ambulation. For example, one arm may flex and supinate, and the other may extend and pronate. Asymmetric limb postures commonly occur as the head rotates from side to side. Usually when the chin turns to one side, the arm on that side extends and the opposite arm flexes.

Chorea Individuals with choreic movements often develop a characteristic gait disorder. Chorea occurs most frequently in children with Sydenham's chorea, in adults with Huntington's disease, and occasionally in adults with Parkinson's disease treated with excessive amounts of dopamine agonist medications. Choreic movements consist of intermittent rapid movements of the face, trunk, neck, and limbs. Flexion, extension, and rotary movements of the neck occur along with grimacing movements of the face, twisting movements of the trunk and limbs, and rapid piano-playing movements of the digits. Frequently, in early chorea, flexion and extension movements of the hips occur so that the individual constantly seems to be crossing and uncrossing the legs. The patient may scowl, frown, and smile involuntarily. Walking usually accentuates the choreic movements. Sudden forward or sideward thrusting movements of the pelvis and rapid twisting movements of the trunk and limbs result in a gait that resembles a series of dance steps. The steps are usually irregular in size, and the patient has difficulty walking in a straight line. The rate of progression varies from slow to rapid owing to variability in the rate and amplitude of each step.

Dystonia This is an involuntary postural and movement disorder affecting children (dystonia musculorum deformans or torsion dystonia) and adults (dystonia of adult onset). The condition may occur sporadically without known cause, as a genetic disorder, or as part of another process such as Wilson's disease. In dystonia musculorum deformans, which commonly begins in children, the first symptom often consists of an abnormal gait. Characteristically the patient will walk with one foot inverted at the ankle, placing weight on the lateral side of the foot; as the disease progresses, this problem worsens and other postural abnormalities develop. These include elevation of one shoulder, elevation of a hip, twisted postures of the trunk, and excessive flexion of the wrist and fingers of one upper limb. Intermittent spasms of the trunk and limbs may interfere with walking. Eventually torticollis, tortipelvis, lordosis, and scoliosis may supervene. In extreme cases, the patient becomes unable to walk. Adult-onset dystonia often results in a similar progression of movement disorders.

Muscular dystrophy Marked weakness of the muscles of the trunk and proximal portions of the legs causes a characteristic stance and gait. In attempting to rise from a seated position, the affected person bends forward, flexing the trunk at the hips, places the hands on the knees, and pushes the trunk upward by working the hands up the thighs. Standing occurs with exaggerated lumbar lordosis and a protuberant abdomen owing to weakness of the abdominal and paravertebral muscles. The patient walks with the legs spread widely apart and develops a waddling motion of the pelvis because of weakness of the gluteal muscles. The shoulders often slope forward, and winging of the scapulae may be seen with walking.

Frontal lobe disease Bilateral frontal lobe disease causes a characteristic gait disorder that is usually associated with dementia and frontal lobe release signs including grasp, suck, and snout reflexes. The patient characteristically stands with the feet spread widely apart and takes a first step only after a long delay. This hesitancy is followed by very small shuffling steps and then by a few steps of moderate amplitude after which time the patient freezes, unable to continue walking. The cycle then is repeated. Affected individuals usually do not show muscular weakness, abnormalities of the deep tendon reflexes, sensory changes, or extensor plantar reflex responses. Usually the patient can perform the individual limb movements required for walking if asked to mimic walking movements while lying supine. The gait disorder with frontal lobe disease is a form of apraxia, i.e., a disturbance in the performance of a motor function in the absence of weakness of the muscles required for the function.

Normal-pressure hydrocephalus Normal-pressure hydrocephalus (NPH) is a disorder characterized by dementia, gait apraxia, and urinary incontinence. Computed tomography reveals large cerebral ventricles, widening of the callosal angle, and lack of filling with cerebrospinal fluid of the subarachnoid space over the cerebral hemispheres. Injection of radioactive isotope into the lumbar subarachnoid space demonstrates pathologic reflux of the isotope into the ventricular system and inadequate penetration into the cortical subarachnoid spaces.

The gait in NPH resembles that seen in apraxia from frontal lobe disease, consisting of a series of small, shuffling steps making it appear that the feet are glued to the floor. Initiation of walking is impaired, and slow and small angular displacements of the hip, knee, and ankle joints occur along with low clearance of the foot from the floor so that the patient appears to be sliding the feet along the floor. There is continuous contraction of the antigravity muscles of the legs but low muscle activity in the calf muscles. The gait disorder in NPH is thought to result from impaired function of the frontal lobes. In about half the patients with NPH the gait is improved by surgical shunting of cerebrospinal fluid from the cerebral ventricles into the venous system.

Aging Changes in gait and difficulties with balance occur with aging. Elderly men develop forward flexion of the upper portion of the trunk with flexion of the arms and knees, decreased arm swing, and shortening of step length. Elderly women develop a waddling gait with shortening of step length. Abnormalities of gait and balance predispose the elderly to falls. About half the falls in the aged result from environmental factors, including poor illumination, stairs, and uneven or slippery surfaces. Other causes of falls include drop attacks, orthostatic hypotension, turning movements of the head, and vertigo.

Lower motor neuron disorders Diseases of the lower motor neurons or peripheral nerves characteristically cause distal limb weakness. Foot drop is a common manifestation. In the case of lower motor neuron disease, the limb weakness occurs in association with fasciculations and muscle atrophy. The patient usually cannot dorsiflex the foot and compensates by raising the knees higher than usual, thereby walking with a "steppage gait." If proximal muscles are affected, the gait also can take on a waddling quality.

Hysterical gait disorders Hysterical disorders of gait commonly appear in association with hysterical paralysis of one or more limbs. Usually the gait is bizarre, easily recognized as hysterical, and unlike any disorder of gait evoked by organic disease. In other instances, however, hysterical gait disorders may resemble organic gait disorders and can be difficult to identify. Hysterical gait disorders can occur in men or women and can appear in youth, young adulthood, and middle age.

In hysterical hemiplegia, the patient drags the affected leg along the ground behind the body and does not circumduct the leg or use it effectively to support the body weight. At times the hemiplegic leg may be pushed ahead of the patient and used mainly for support. The arm on the affected side often remains limp, hanging uselessly beside the body and does not develop the flexed posture commonly seen in hemiplegia from organic causes. The patient with hysterical hemiplegia usually shows "give way" weakness. This is tested by asking the patient to make a maximum contraction of a set of muscles in an affected limb. Initially a strong contraction may occur, but as the examiner attempts to oppose the contracting muscles, the contraction suddenly gives way. Hysterical patients also commonly contract their muscles very slowly upon request, displaying great concentration and effort to evoke the contraction. Objective signs of neurologic disease are absent; the affected limbs show normal resistance to passive manipulation, the deep tendon reflexes are equal on the two sides of the body, and the plantar responses are downgoing.

In hysterical paraplegia, the patient usually walks with one or two crutches or lies in bed with the legs maintained either completely limp or stiffly extended. The term *astasia-abasia* refers to patients who cannot stand or walk but who can carry out natural movements of the limbs when lying in bed. Some patients with hysterical paraparesis walk with seeming difficulty but show normal power and coordination when lying in bed. On walking, the hysterical person clings to the bed or the furnishings of the room. If asked to walk without support the patient may lurch forward dramatically, veering from side to side at regular intervals. The patient can manage feats of extraordinary balance to avoid falling and may assume a variety of postures, walking with the legs in stiff extension, as if the legs are granite pillars, or walking with the legs in flexion and teetering from side to side. The hysterical patient may fall with walking, but only when a nearby physician or family member can catch the patient or when soft objects are available to cushion the fall. The gait disturbance is usually dramatic when an audience is present, and the patient can display remarkable agility in the rapid postural adjustments that occur.

REFERENCES

DIETZ V et al: Afferent control of human stance and gait: Evidence for blocking of group I afferents during gait. Exp Brain Res 61:153, 1985

GILMAN S: Cerebellar deficit, in *Diseases of the Nervous System*, AK Asbury et al (eds). Philadelphia, Saunders, 1986, pp 401–422

——— et al: *Disorders of the Cerebellum*. Philadelphia, Davis, 1981

GRILLNER S: Neurobiological bases of rhythmic motor acts in vertebrates. Science 228:143, 1985

HORAK FB, NASHNER LM: Central programming of postural movements: Adaptation to altered support-surface configurations. J Neurophysiol 55:1369, 1986

KNUTSSON E, LYING-TUNELL U: Gait in normal-pressure hydrocephalus: Patterns of movement and muscle activation. Neurology 35:155, 1985

SMITH JC et al: Neural mechanisms generating locomotion studied in mammalian brainstem–spinal cord in vitro. FASEB J 2:2283, 1988

---

27 PAIN, SPASM, AND CRAMPS OF MUSCLE

ROBERT C. GRIGGS

Spontaneous or exercise-related discomfort from muscles or joints is usually benign and does not signal neuromuscular disease. Such symptoms may, however, provide clues to disabling disorders that too often evade diagnosis. The terms *pain*, *spasm*, and *cramp* are often used interchangeably by patients to describe symptoms referable to muscles. Other terms, including *aching*, *heaviness*, *stiffness*, and *rheumatism*, are also used, and usually connote less certainty about the source or localization of the discomfort. In clinical terminology, *spasm* refers to a brief, unsustained contraction of a single or multiple muscles. *Cramp* is a paroxysmal, spontaneous, prolonged, and painful contraction of one or more muscles.

SPASMS Abnormal movements of muscle may arise from abnormal electrical activity of the central nervous system mediated via the motor neuron, or occur within the muscle fiber itself. It may be difficult on clinical grounds alone to determine the precise site of origin of the abnormal motor activity. In general, movements originating in the central nervous system affect the entire side of the body, an entire limb, or a group of muscles. Central disorders may be rhythmic or intermittent; those arising in the periphery are usually random. The electroencephalogram may provide evidence for altered cortical activity in some conditions with a central nervous system etiology. The electromyogram (EMG) is less helpful because it reflects motor activity from any cause. EMG evidence of an underlying nerve disease may, however, be helpful in diagnosis (see Chap. 362), and certain abnormal muscle contractions have characteristic EMG features.

Intermittent, nonrhythmic movements of an entire limb, of the trunk, or of a portion of the face may result from cerebral seizure activity (Chap. 349) or from myoclonus (Chap. 25). Flexor and extensor spasms of an entire side or of the lower limbs result from a loss of motor inhibition within the central nervous system (Chap. 25). *Segmental myoclonus* results from focal disease within the brainstem or spinal cord that causes an abnormal discharge of groups of motor neurons. Localized vascular disease, tumor, or another lesion may be implicated.

Abnormal facial movements *Hemifacial spasm* results from paroxysmal facial nerve activity, sometimes triggered by pressure from a tortuous blood vessel adjacent to the facial nerve as it leaves the brainstem. Hemifacial spasm commonly occurs in muscles about the eye, but may also involve or spread to the entire side of the face. Symptoms are often intermittent and intensified when patients are using facial muscles in activities such as speaking. Hemifacial spasm is painless but embarrassing, especially to individuals dealing with the public. Since it is often intensified and more severe when the patient is in stressful situations, an erroneous diagnosis of tic (habit spasm) is often made. Cerebellopontine angle lesions can occasionally produce a similar disorder. Neuroradiologic investigation is indicated in patients with hemifacial spasm. Anticonvulsant medications occasionally alleviate the spasms, but surgical exploration and shielding of the facial nerve from the adjacent vessel is curative (Chap. 360).

Facial *tics* (habit spasms) are stereotyped movements of the face such as eye blinking, head turning, or grimacing that are under voluntary control but may be suppressed only by effort and anxiety on the part of the subject (see Chap. 25). Some tics are so frequently encountered as to be considered mannerisms, analogous to excessive clearing of the throat. The repetitious elevation of the eyebrows by frontalis muscle contraction is an example. Certain hereditary movement disorders such as Gilles de la Tourette syndrome are characterized by multiple tics (Chap. 25).

Synkinesias of the face result from aberrant regeneration of the facial nerve following facial paralysis from Bell's palsy or other facial nerve lesions. Nearly 50 percent of patients who recover from Bell's palsy display such movements; an example is *jaw winking*, where voluntary movements of the lower face elicit contraction of the orbicularis oculi muscle with eye closure (Chap. 360).

Trigeminal neuralgia (tic douloureux) is characterized by brief, paroxysmal, lancinating pain in one side of the face (see Chap. 360). Although the portion of the nerve involved is almost exclusively sensory, the severity of the pain causes involuntary contraction of facial muscles; hence the name tic. Abnormal movements do not occur in the absence of pain.

Facial myokymia refers to a nearly continuous, fine or coarse rippling and fascicular twitching of facial muscles. Although often benign, it may result from lesions of the pons such as a neoplasm or multiple sclerosis. Similar movements occur in motor neuron diseases such as amyotrophic lateral sclerosis or occasionally as an isolated, hereditary condition.

Abnormal limb movements No movement should be visible in totally relaxed muscles. Diseases of motor neurons or their proximal axons are often associated with *fasciculations*, the spontaneous firing of an entire motor unit. Fasciculations are visible on inspection of muscle or perceived by the patient as a pulsation or quivering within muscle. Fasciculations occur at times in most normal individuals, and unless weakness is present, are seldom of any significance. Fasciculations are normal if observed in incompletely relaxed muscles. *Myokymia*, consisting of numerous, repetitive fasciculations, may also occur in limb muscles, giving a writhing appearance. Myokymia disappears with neuromuscular blockade, proving that the activity originates in anterior horn cells or in peripheral nerve. In patients with long-standing muscle denervation and reinnervation, motor unit size enlarges and fasciculations may be so large as to produce movement of the limbs, particularly of the fingers, a condition termed

minipolymyoclonus. Similarly, the enlarged motor units of chronic denervation may be associated with a tremor of the fingers on extension.

Certain conditions are characterized by a compulsion to move the extremities. *Akathisia*, or motor restlessness, occurs in Parkinson's disease and other disorders of the basal ganglia including drug-induced movement disorders. The *restless legs syndrome* describes an uncomfortable sensation in muscles, usually in the legs and thighs, which occurs most commonly in middle-aged women. Patients feel they need to move their legs to relieve the abnormal sensation. The restless leg syndrome is frequent in uremia and may occur in other neuropathies, suggesting that the sensation is caused by an underlying neuropathy. It may also be familial, and detailed study of such patients has failed to demonstrate any evidence of neuropathy. The restless sensation may be accompanied by myoclonic jerks of muscle often occurring during sleep. These myoclonic jerks are similar to the myoclonus observed in normal individuals entering REM sleep (see Chap. 34).

These forms of muscle spasm and myoclonus are somewhat similar to a group of unusual and unexplained *startle* syndromes or *hyperexplexias* characterized by sudden jerking of limbs or occasionally of trunk muscles. Sudden noise or touch may cause a patient to jump or to fling an extremity. The cause is unknown.

SUSTAINED MUSCLE CONTRACTIONS Distinguishing central from peripheral causes of sustained muscle contraction is often difficult. Abnormal muscle contractions with increased muscle tone usually result from central nervous system disease. Thus, loss or disturbance of central nervous system inhibition may lead to abnormal muscle contraction characteristic of spasticity, rigidity, or "paratonic" rigidity. In most instances there is other evidence of central nervous system disorder (Chap. 25). Diseases of the basal ganglia, presumably resulting from altered neurotransmitter release, may lead to dystonia (Chaps. 25 and 26).

Abnormal muscle contractions may also arise from repetitive depolarization of the component portions of the motor unit: the motor neuron; the peripheral axon of the neuron; the neuromuscular junction; or muscle fibers. Electrically inactive contractions may arise from disorders of the muscle contractile system.

Motor neuron disorders *Cramp* is a term often used by patients to refer to a painful, involuntary contraction of a single muscle or a muscle group. Muscle cramps can arise from spontaneous firing of groups of anterior horn cells followed by contraction of many motor units. EMG recordings indicate that motor units fire at a rate of up to 300 per second, much higher than occurs with voluntary contraction. Cramps occur frequently in the legs in elderly patients and when severe are followed by residual tenderness and evidence of muscle fiber necrosis including elevation of serum creatine kinase. Cramps in the calf muscles are so common as to be considered normal, but more generalized cramps may be a sign of chronic disease of the motor neuron such as amyotrophic lateral sclerosis. They may be particularly troublesome during pregnancy, in patients with electrolyte disturbances (hyponatremia), and in patients on hemodialysis. When recurrent and localized to one muscle group they suggest nerve root disease. In many instances, however, it is impossible to determine the cause of cramps. Benign cramps, occurring commonly at night, may be relieved by quinine sulfate. Other causes of contractions arising from the motor neuron include *tetanus* (Chap. 105) and the *stiff-man syndrome*. In both disorders a loss of inhibitory neuronal input to anterior horn cells may result in repeated firing of motor neurons, producing severe, painful muscle contraction. A similar clinical picture may occur acutely with *strychnine poisoning*. Diazepam improves these spasms but may cause respiratory depression in doses sufficient to alleviate muscle contraction.

Peripheral nerve *Tetany* is characterized by contractions of predominantly distal muscles, particularly in the hand (carpal spasm) and feet (pedal spasm). Laryngospasm may also occur. Tetany results from increased excitability of peripheral nerves. The muscle contractions are initially painless, but if sustained may cause muscle damage with pain. Severe tetany may involve spine musculature to produce opisthotonus. Tetany is usually caused by hypocalcemia, but may occur with hypomagnesemia or severe respiratory alkalosis (see Chap. 340). Idiopathic normocalcemic tetany, *spasmophilia*, occurs in both hereditary and sporadic forms.

Muscle MYOTONIA Repetitive depolarization of muscle cells can cause muscle contraction resulting in muscle stiffness and impaired relaxation. Myotonia is usually painless, but may disable patients by interfering with fine hand movements or by slowing ambulation. Myotonic dystrophy is the commonest disorder associated with myotonia although other manifestations of the disease such as cataracts and muscle weakness are usually more symptomatic (see Chap. 365). Myotonia congenita and paramyotonia congenita are less common, but more troublesome in terms of severity of myotonia. Myotonia is often worsened by cold and characteristically is attenuated by repeated muscle activity. *Paradoxical myotonia* worsens with repeated activity and is characteristic of paramyotonia congenita; these patients also suffer from episodic and cold-induced weakness (Chap. 367). Impaired muscle relaxation that is electrically inactive is characteristic of the delayed relaxation of myxedema. This delay produces the characteristic "hung-up" ankle reflexes but is essentially asymptomatic.

CONTRACTURE Muscle contracture is a painful shortening of a muscle unassociated with muscle membrane depolarization. It occurs in disorders where a metabolic defect such as myophosphorylase deficiency limits the production of high-energy phosphates. Contractures are precipitated by exercise and are usually intensely painful. This use of the term *contracture* is confusing since the same word is used to describe the unrelated limitation of joint movement by shortening of muscle tendons seen in rheumatologic disorders, cerebral palsy, or chronic myopathies. Muscle rigidity from metabolic contracture can occur in the malignant hyperthermia syndrome, usually associated with general anesthesia (Chap. 20). In the neuroleptic malignant syndrome, muscle rigidity arises from central nervous system overactivity, and intense electrical activity is present in muscle (Chap. 20).

MUSCLE PAIN, ACHING, AND TENDERNESS Painful muscles do not always imply muscle disease. Joint and bone disease frequently produce complaints of muscle pain and may further confuse the anatomic localization of symptoms by resulting in disuse atrophy and moderate muscle weakness. Pain from disease of overlying subcutaneous tissue or fascia and of tendons may also be referred to muscle. Additionally, disease of major peripheral nerves or of their small intramuscular branches may produce both muscle pain and weakness. Muscle pain may be a major symptom in inflammatory, metabolic, endocrine, and toxic myopathies (Chaps. 364 and 365).

Muscle trauma Vigorous activity, even in conditioned athletes, may be associated with muscle and tendon tears which lead to temporary acute muscle pain, swelling, and tenderness. Rupture of muscle tendons such as the biceps or gastrocnemius muscle may produce visible muscle shortening.

The almost-pleasurable ache and fatigue of muscles after strenuous activity is separable only by degree from more severe, but still normal pain following severe, unaccustomed activity. Such symptoms are often associated with laboratory evidence of profound muscle damage including a rise in serum enzymes (creatine kinase) and widespread muscle necrosis on biopsy. Myoglobinemia and myoglobinuria may occur. Particularly likely to produce muscle pain and necrosis are certain types of exercise: brief periods of contracting a muscle while it is lengthening (eccentric contractions); and prolonged exercise such as marathon running. The point at which such symptoms become abnormal is not clear. Many patients have pain with moderate activity. Such exertional muscle pain is also characteristic of metabolic disorders of muscle including carnitine palmityl transferase deficiency and myoadenylate deaminase deficiency; deficiencies of enzymes of glycolysis are more commonly associated with contractures (see Chap. 365). The majority of patients with exertional and postexertional muscle pain do not have a definable abnormality.

Diffuse myalgias Muscle pain in the absence of muscle weakness can occur in acute infections caused by influenza and Coxsackie viruses. Fibrositis, fibromyalgia, and fibromyositis are synonyms for a disorder associated with pain and tenderness of muscle and adjacent connective tissue. Focal "trigger points" of tenderness can be identified, and systemic symptoms such as fatigue, insomnia, and depression are frequently present (see Chap. 364). Although patients often identify painful swellings, histologic evaluation discloses no abnormality of muscle or connective tissue. Symptoms may respond partially to nonsteroidal anti-inflammatory agents, but the disorder tends to be chronic and unrelenting. Patients whose symptoms persist for months or years are often considered to have a psychiatric disorder, but its nature has not been defined.

Polymyalgia rheumatica occurs in patients over age 50 and is characterized by stiffness and pain in shoulder and hip musculature. Despite symptoms of pain localized to muscles, there is convincing evidence that the disease includes a proximal, inflammatory arthritis; joint effusions are often present in knees and other peripheral joints as well. Patients often develop profound disuse atrophy of muscles and complain of weakness, giving rise to a suspicion of polymyositis. However, creatine kinase levels are usually normal, and muscle biopsy shows atrophy without evidence of muscle necrosis or inflammation. The erythrocyte sedimentation rate is elevated in most patients, and temporal arteritis may be present (see Chap. 276). Treatment with nonsteroidal anti-inflammatory agents is advocated except in patients with temporal arteritis, for whom prednisone (40 to 60 mg daily) is recommended. Patients with polymyalgia rheumatica who fail to respond to nonsteroidal anti-inflammatory agents may require low-dose prednisone (10 to 20 mg daily). Myalgias are also frequent in other rheumatologic disorders including rheumatoid arthritis, systemic lupus erythematosus, polyarteritis nodosa, scleroderma, and the mixed connective tissue syndrome. When muscle pain occurs as an early symptom, it may erroneously suggest a primary muscle disease, and the myalgia may be due to inflammatory muscle involvement that can occur in each of these conditions (see Chap. 364). Patients with polymyositis and dermatomyositis may have myalgias, although in the majority, muscle pain is lacking or minimal (Chap. 364).

EPISODIC WEAKNESS The term *weakness* is often used by a patient to describe a loss of stamina or decreased "energy." Even careful efforts at eliciting a history of true as opposed to subjective weakness may fail to distinguish the two conditions. The most helpful strategy is to ask the patient to identify whether a discrete loss of function has occurred and to elicit the circumstances in which symptoms are noted.

Weakness whether true or perceived may be due to disorders of the central or peripheral nervous system. Weakness from central nervous system disorders such as transient cerebral ischemia is usually associated with a change in level of consciousness or cognition, with increased muscle tone and muscle stretch reflexes, and often with alterations of sensation. Most neuromuscular causes of intermittent weakness are associated with normal mental function but diminished muscle tone and muscle stretch reflexes. The major causes of intermittent weakness are listed in Table 27-1. Central causes are considered in Chap. 351.

EPISODIC ASTHENIA Patients who describe intermittent "weakness" as *fatigue* and loss of *stamina* suffer from asthenia, which can be separated from true weakness by the fact that patients do not lack the ability to do a task but rather the ability to perform it repetitively. Asthenia is a major problem in many patients with serious renal, hepatic, cardiac, or pulmonary disease. Examination of such patients usually confirms their ability to do all functional activities at least once, such as rising from a knee bend, climbing stairs, or rising from a chair. Fatigue is also characteristic of relatively selective damage to central nervous system descending motor tracts, in which signs of neurologic abnormality may be minimal.

Intermittent weakness due to peripheral neuromuscular disease may result from abrupt changes in peripheral nerve function; inter-

TABLE 27-1   Causes of episodic generalized weakness

Electrolyte disturbances
   Hypokalemia: Primary aldosteronism (Conn's syndrome); barium poisoning; renal tubular acidosis; juxtaglomerular apparatus hyperplasia (Bartter's syndrome); villous adenoma of colon; alcoholism; diuretics; licorice; para-aminosalicylic acid; glucocorticoids
   Hyperkalemia: Addison's disease; chronic renal failure; hyporeninemic hypoaldosteronism; recurrent rhabdomyolysis
   Hypercalcemia
   Hypocalcemic tetany
   Hyponatremia
   Hypophosphatemia
   Hypermagnesemia
Neuromuscular junction disorders
   Myasthenia gravis
   Lambert-Eaton syndrome
Central nervous system causes
   Cataplexy and sleep paralysis associated with narcolepsy
   Multiple sclerosis
   Transient ischemic attacks
Disorders with only subjective weakness: hyperventilation, hypoglycemia

mittent destruction of muscle; alterations of electrophysiologic properties of muscle from abnormalities of blood electrolytes; and intermittent failure of neuromuscular transmission.

FAILURE OF PERIPHERAL NERVE CONDUCTION   A number of uncommon peripheral neuropathies are associated with recurrent weakness. *Hereditary liability to pressure palsies*, often termed *tomaculous* neuropathy because of the sausage-like appearance of myelin on nerve biopsy, is an autosomal dominant disorder characterized by abrupt paralysis following compression of a peripheral nerve. The paralysis is usually self-limited, lasting days to weeks. Other types of peripheral neuropathy may also predispose to the development of reversible, compressive neuropathies (see Chap. 363).

DISORDERED NEUROMUSCULAR JUNCTION TRANSMISSION   *Myasthenia gravis*, particularly in its initial manifestations, is characterized by transient weakness. Cranial muscles are usually affected first, causing double vision, ptosis, dysphagia, and dysarthria. Rarely, limb weakness may herald the onset of myasthenia gravis and in the absence of cranial muscle dysfunction may escape diagnosis for months. Diurnal variation in strength is typical, and reflexes are preserved. Other, less-common defects of the neuromuscular junction such as the Lambert-Eaton syndrome may also present with intermittent weakness (see Chap. 366).

INTERMITTENT ALTERATIONS IN ELECTROLYTES   Transient shifts in serum potassium are associated with profound alterations in muscle strength. Although the primary periodic paralyses (hypo- and hyperkalemic periodic paralysis) spring to mind in a patient with weakness and an abnormality in serum potassium, other causes of abnormal serum potassium are more frequently the cause of episodic weakness (see Chap. 367). Familial periodic paralysis seldom presents after age 30; other causes are usually present in older patients. Hypokalemic periodic paralysis may occur in patients with hyperthyroidism. Episodic weakness due to hypokalemia may occur with renal or gastrointestinal potassium loss; major causes include renal tubular acidosis, diuretic- or laxative-induced hypokalemia, primary aldosteronism, Bartter's syndrome, and villous adenoma of the colon.

Hyperkalemic weakness occurs in chronic renal or adrenal insufficiency, with hyporeninemic hypoaldosteronism, and on an iatrogenic basis from injudicious administration of oral potassium preparations alone or in combination with potassium-sparing diuretics such as triamterene, amiloride, and spironolactone. The use of potassium salts as a substitute for table salt may cause hyperkalemia in patients with impaired potassium excretion.

Other electrolyte disturbances may occasionally produce intermittent weakness as the initial clinical manifestation of a severe metabolic abnormality. These include elevation or depression of serum sodium, calcium, or magnesium as well as hypophosphatemia.

METABOLIC MUSCLE DISEASE (See Chap. 355)   A number of uncommon defects in glycogen and lipid utilization are associated with impaired energy production by muscle and cause intermittent weakness, usually accompanied by muscle pain. Carnitine palmityl transferase deficiency is one such condition. Other metabolic defects of muscle such as mitochondrial disorders and the purine nucleotide cycle defect known as myoadenylate deaminase deficiency may also cause episodic weakness. This latter disorder occurs in approximately 1 percent of the population, but inexplicably causes symptoms in a small proportion of subjects deficient in the enzyme.

Recurrent attacks of a feeling of "weakness" often occur in patients with the *hyperventilation syndrome;* such patients are, however, of normal strength when tested. Similarly, *recurrent hypoglycemic episodes* are associated with subjective weakness though hypoglycemia is uncommon as the cause of this symptom. Central nervous system disorders may cause generalized weakness without an associated alteration of consciousness. *Drop attacks* resulting from impaired blood supply to the motor pathways of the brainstem cause sudden paraparesis or quadriparesis, usually lasting only a few seconds. Patients with narcolepsy may have sudden loss of muscle strength and tone during episodes of *cataplexy*. A disorder of the reticular activating system is responsible for these episodes as well as for *sleep paralysis* that occurs as narcoleptic patients are falling asleep or awakening (see Chap. 34).

REFERENCES

BARCHI RL: The myotonic syndromes. Neurol Clin 6:473, 1988
CLARK S et al: Clinical characteristics of fibrositis. II. A "blinded," controlled study using standard psychological tests. Arthritis Rheum 28:132, 1985
JANKOVIC J, TOLOSA E (ed): Facial dyskinesias, in *Advances in Neurology*. New York, Raven Press, 1988, vol 49
LAYZER RB: Muscle pain, cramps and fatigue, in AG Engel, BQ Banker (eds), *Myology*. New York, McGraw-Hill, 1986
RIGGS JE: The periodic paralyses. Neurol Clin 6:485, 1988

28   NUMBNESS, TINGLING, AND SENSORY LOSS

ARTHUR K. ASBURY

Normal somatic sensation is a continuous process that commands considerable moment-to-moment nervous system activity. Little of the activity intrudes upon consciousness or exacts notice. In contrast, disordered sensation, particularly pains and paresthesias, may be highly intrusive, alarming, and tenacious and may dominate attention. Abnormalities of sensation tend to bring patients quickly to medical attention. When abnormal sensations are perceived as painful, medical advice is even more quickly sought. For a consideration of pain, see Chap. 15. The physician must have a framework of knowledge in order to assess abnormal sensations, estimate their likely site of origin, and recognize their implications.

POSITIVE AND NEGATIVE PHENOMENA   It is useful to divide all abnormal sensory phenomena into two great categories, positive and negative. Positive phenomena include tingling, pins-and-needles, pricking, bandlike sensations, lightning-like shooting feelings (lancinations), aching, and knifelike, twisting, drawing, pulling, tightening, burning, searing, electrical, and raw sensations. These descriptors are frequently the actual words used by patients. Such sensations may or may not be experienced as painful. It is thought that the pathophysiologic basis of positive phenomena resides in the ectopic generation of volleys of impulses at some site of lowered neural threshold along the sensory pathways, either in peripheral or central sensory fibers. Such trains of ectopically generated afferent impulses arising from sites other than normal peripheral nerve receptors determine the quality of the abnormal sensation experienced, depending upon the number, rate, and distribution of impulses and the type and function of nerve fibers in which they arise.

Positive phenomena represent heightened activity in sensory pathways; therefore they are not necessarily associated with any demonstrable sensory deficit upon examination, an important point for the examiner to bear in mind.

Negative phenomena result from loss of sensory function and are characterized by numbness, or diminution or absence of feeling in a particular distribution. Negative phenomena, in contrast to positive phenomena, are accompanied by abnormal findings on sensory examination. In disorders affecting peripheral sensation, it is estimated that at least one-half of afferent fibers innervating a given site must be lost or functionless in order for sensory deficit to be demonstrated. This estimate probably varies according to how rapidly sensory fibers have lost function. If the rate of loss is slow and chronic, lack of cutaneous feeling may be unnoticed by the patient and difficult to demonstrate on examination, even though few sensory fibers are functioning. Rapidly evolving sensory abnormality usually evokes positive phenomena of some type and is more readily recognized by patients than insidious deafferentation. Subclinical degrees of sensory dysfunction not demonstrable on clinical sensory examination may be revealed by sensory nerve conduction studies or somatosensory cerebral evoked potentials (see Chaps. 349 and 362).

Terminology Two general types of medical terms are used to characterize abnormal sensation, those referring to symptoms of which patients complain (both positive and negative phenomena) and those describing abnormalities found on examination (only negative phenomena). *Paresthesia* and *dysesthesia* are terms used to denote positive phenomena. Paresthesia carries the implication that the abnormal sensation is perceived without an apparent stimulus; whereas dysesthesia is a more general term used to describe all types of positive sensations whether stimulus-generated or not. Abnormalities on examination are denoted by *hypesthesia* or *hypoesthesia* (reduction of cutaneous sensation to a specific type of testing such as pressure, light touch, and warm or cold stimuli), *anesthesia* (complete absence of skin sensation to the same stimuli plus pinprick), and *hypalgesia* (referring to loss of pain perception, i.e., nociception, such as the pricking quality elicited by a pin). *Hyperesthesia* connotes exaggerated perception of sensations in response to mild stimuli (light touch or stroking of the skin). Similarly *allodynia* describes the situation in which an ordinarily nonpainful stimulus, once perceived, is experienced as painful, even excruciating. An example is elicitation of a painful sensation by application of a vibrating tuning fork. *Hyperalgesia* denotes an exaggerated response to a noxious stimulus, and *hyperpathia*, a broad term, encompasses the phenomena implied by hyperesthesia, allodynia, and hyperalgesia.

Disorders of deep sensation, arising from muscle spindles, tendons, and joints, deserve special comment. Normally these afferents subserve proprioception (position sense) and the moment-to-moment sense of the state of muscle contraction. If a significant number of these special nerve endings become denervated, the resulting manifestations include imbalance, particularly with eyes closed or in the dark, clumsiness of precision movements, and unsteadiness of gait, all of which is referred to as *sensory ataxia* (see Chap. 26). Other findings on examination are reduced or absent joint position and vibratory sensibility and absent deep tendon reflexes in the affected limbs. Romberg's sign is positive, which means that the patient sways or topples when asked to stand with feet close together and eyes closed.

In severe states of deafferentation involving deep sensation, the patient cannot walk or stand unaided, or even sit unsupported. Continuous, sometimes wormlike involuntary movements, called *pseudoathetosis*, of the hands and arms occur, particularly with eyes closed. Such patients are severely disabled.

Normal sensation Cutaneous afferent innervation is subserved by a rich variety of receptors, both naked endings (nociceptors and thermoreceptors) and encapsulated terminals (mechanoreceptors). Each has its own set of sensitivities to specific stimuli (see Table 28-1), size and distinctness of receptive fields, and adaptational qualities. Much of the knowledge about these receptors has come from the development of techniques to study single intact nerve fibers intraneurally in alert unanesthetized human subjects. It is possible not only to record from single nerve fibers, large or small, but also to stimulate single fibers in isolation. A single impulse, whether elicited by a natural stimulus or evoked by electrical microstimulation, in a large myelinated afferent fiber may be both perceived and localized.

Afferent fibers in peripheral nerve trunks sort themselves into topographically coherent patterns as they approach the dorsal roots and enter the dorsal horn of the spinal cord. From there, the polysynaptic projections of the smaller fibers (unmyelinated and small myelinated), which in general subserve nociception and temperature sensibility, cross and ascend in the contralateral spinothalamic tract through spinal cord, through brainstem, to the ventral posterolateral nucleus (VPL) of the thalamus, and ultimately project to the postcentral gyrus of the parietal cortex (see Chap. 15). This is the spinothalamic pathway. The larger fibers which subserve tactile and position sense and kinesthesia project rostrally in the ipsilateral posterior column of the spinal cord and finally make their first synapse in the gracile or cuneate nuclei of the lower medulla (see Fig. 28-1). The second-order neuron decussates and ascends in the medial lemniscus located medially in the medulla and in the tegmentum of the pons and midbrain, and synapses in VPL. The third-order neuron projects to parietal cortex; this system is referred to as *lemniscal*.

Although the fiber types and functions which make up the spinothalamic and lemniscal systems are relatively well known, it has been found that many other fibers, particularly those associated with touch, pressure, and position sense, ascend in a diffusely

TABLE 28-1 Human cutaneous sensory receptors*

Receptor type	Location	Activating stimulus	Afferent nerve fiber	Sensation evoked	Central pathway
Meissner's corpuscle	S	Light pressure, once or repetitive	LM	Tapping, fluttering	Lemniscal
Merkel's disk	S	Sustained pressure	LM	Sense of pressure	
Pacinian corpuscle	D	Light touch, once or repetitive	LM	Sense of vibration	
Ruffini's ending	D	Sustained, angulated pressure	LM	None, thought to be proprioceptive	
Naked ending	S	Noxious	SM	Sharp pain	Spinothalamic
Naked ending	S	Noxious	UM	Dull pain, itch	
Naked ending	S	Thermal, 34–50°C	UM	Warmth	
Naked ending	S	Thermal, range uncertain	SM	Coldness	

* LM = large myelinated fiber; SM = small myelinated fiber; UM = unmyelinated fiber; D = deep; S = superficial.
SOURCE: After Lindblom and Ochoa, 1986.

Parietal
Cortex

Neuron III

Thalamus

VPL

Midbrain

ML

Neuron II

Pons

ML

Medulla

Lower
Medulla

Medial Lemniscus
Nucleus Gracilis
Nucleus Cuneatus

Neuron I

Spinal
Cord

Posterior Column

FIGURE 28-1 Schematic diagram of lemniscal system which subserves proprioception and discriminative touch.

distributed pattern both ipsilaterally and contralaterally in the anterolateral quadrants of the spinal cord. These anatomic facts explain why an individual with a known complete lesion of the posterior columns of the spinal cord may have little sensory deficit on examination.

EXAMINATION OF SENSATION   The initial step in examination of the somatosensory system is to do the tests of primary sensation, which by convention include the sense of pain, touch, vibration, joint position, and thermal sensation, both hot and cold. These tests have gradually become codified through tradition, but they do appear to assess, if crudely, the major afferent functions and pathways (see Table 28-2). Testing of both primary sensation and cortical sensory function can be carried out in the office or at the bedside with a minimum of special equipment.

Some general principles pertain to the sensory examination. First, it should be remembered that the examiner is depending upon subjective patient response; therefore, discriminating responses depend upon the level of alertness, motivation, and intelligence of the patient and also upon the skill with which the examiner has made the task clear. In a stupefied or obtunded patient, the examiner is reduced to observing the briskness of withdrawal and the complexity of defensive movements of the patient in response to a pinch or other noxious stimulus. In the alert but uncooperative patient, it is often possible to get some idea of proprioceptive function by noting the patient's best performance in casually observed movements requiring balance and precision, but cutaneous sensation may be unexaminable.

Second, sensory examination should not be pressed if the patient is fatigued. An abbreviated survey will suffice until a more extensive examination can be carried out when the patient has rested. Third, sensory examination in a patient who has no neurologic complaints should be quite abbreviated and may consist of pin, touch, and vibration testing in the hands and feet plus evaluation of station and gait including Romberg's maneuver, which also tests the integrity of motor and cerebellar systems. Fourth, patients should be tested with their eyes closed or covered during both primary sensation and cortical sensory function examination.

Primary sensation (see Table 28-2)   The sense of pain is usually tested with a pin, asking the patient to focus on the pricking or unpleasant quality of the stimulus and not just the pressure or touch sensation elicited. Areas of hypalgesia should be mapped by proceeding from the most hypalgesic zones to less affected ones (see Figs. 28-2 and 28-3).

Temperature sensation, both to hot and to cold, is probably best tested by touching the skin for a couple of seconds with a water flask filled with water of the desired temperature, using a thermometer to verify the temperature. For most purposes, it is satisfactory if a patient can identify as warm the flask that is 35 or 36°C and as cool the one that is 28 to 32°C. Between 28 and 32°C, most individuals can distinguish temperature differences in 1°C steps. Both cold and warm should be tested because different receptors respond to each.

Touch is usually tested with a wisp of cotton or a fine camel's hair brush. In general, it is better to avoid testing touch on hairy skin because of the profusion of sensory endings which surround each hair follicle. The patients, whose eyes are covered, should be asked to say "now" each time they feel the stimulus. They may also be asked to point to the site where the stimulus was felt, although this tests not only the sense of touch but also touch localization (see cortical sensory testing below).

Joint position testing is a measure of proprioception, one of the most important functions of the sensory system. Joint position is usually tested first in the great toe and in the fingers. Patients are asked to keep their eyes closed and to relax completely the part to be examined. In the case of the great toe, one starts with the toe in

TABLE 28-2 Testing primary sensation				
Sense	Test device	Endings activated	Fiber size mediating	Central pathway*
Pain	Pinprick	Cutaneous nociceptors	Small	SpTh, also D
Temperature, heat	Flask with warm water	Cutaneous thermoreceptors for hot	Small	SpTh
Temperature, cold	Flask with cold water	Cutaneous thermoreceptors for cold	Small	SpTh
Touch	Cotton wisp, fine brush	Cutaneous mechanoreceptors, also naked endings	Large and small	Lem, also D and SpTh
Vibration	Tuning fork, 128 Hz	Mechanoreceptors, especially pacinian corpuscles	Large	Lem, also D
Joint position	Passive movement of specific joints	Joint capsule and tendon endings, muscle spindles	Large	Lem, also D

* D = diffuse ascending projections in ipsilateral and contralateral anteriolateral columns; SpTh = spinothalamic projection, contralateral; Lem = posterior column and lemniscal projection, ipsilateral.

FIGURE 28-2 Anterior view of dermatomes (left) and cutaneous areas supplied by individual peripheral nerves (right). *(Modified from MB Carpenter and J Sutin, in Human Neuroanatomy, 8th ed, Baltimore, Williams & Wilkins, 1983.)*

FIGURE 28-3 Posterior view of dermatomes (left) and cutaneous areas supplied by individual peripheral nerves (right). *(Modified from MB Carpenter and J Sutin, in Human Neuroanatomy, 8th ed, Baltimore, Williams & Wilkins, 1983.)*

a neutral position and grasps it lightly between the thumb and the forefinger on either side of the toe (not top and bottom) and then the toe is moved a few degrees either in a dorsal or a plantar direction, and the patient is asked to say whether the movement was up or down. One must make sure that the patient understands that it is the direction of movement which is being tested and not the direction the toe is pointing when it stops. A patient with absence of position sense in the part being tested will have a 50 percent error rate because only two choices are available. Answers which are consistently greater than 50 percent in error should be viewed with skepticism. If errors are made in recognizing the direction of passive movements of the toe, then passive movements of the ankle or even of the knee should be undertaken in the same way. Similarly, position sense at the proximal interphalangeal joint of the index finger may be tested, and if abnormal, other finger joints and the wrist and elbow joints should also be tested. A test of proximal joint position sense, primarily at the shoulder, can be carried out by asking the patient to bring the two index fingers together with the arms extended and the eyes closed. Normal individuals should be able to do this quite accurately with errors of a centimeter or less.

The sense of vibration is tested with a tuning fork, preferably a large one which vibrates at 128 Hz. The decay of vibration using this fork is slow enough to be of quantitative use because it requires between 15 and 20 s to decay below the threshold of perceptibility. Vibration is usually tested at bony prominences, specifically the malleoli at the ankles, the patella, the anterior iliac spine, the spinous processes of the vertebral bodies, the metacarpal-phalangeal joints (knuckles), the styloid process of the ulna, the elbow, and the acromion of the shoulder. Control sites at which to test vibration are

the sternum and on the forehead. The examiner can compare the threshold at a given site for both patient and self. A crude approximation of degree of vibratory sense loss can be made by counting the seconds that the examiner can feel the sense of vibration longer than the patient. It must be clear to the patient that it is the sense of vibration and not just the pressure of the end of the tuning fork to which attention is directed.

Cortical sensation Cortical sensory testing includes two-point discrimination, touch localization, stereognosis, graphesthesia, and bilateral simultaneous stimulation, to name the most commonly used methods. Abnormalities of these sensory tests, in the presence of normal primary sensation and an alert cooperative patient, signify a lesion of the parietal cortex or thalamocortical projections to the parietal lobe. If primary sensation is altered, it is not possible to test for these cortical discriminative functions.

Two-point discrimination is tested by special calipers whose points may be set from 2 mm to several centimeters apart and then applied simultaneously to the site to be tested. The pulp of the fingertips is a common site to test; a normal individual can distinguish about 3-mm separation of points there. One can distinguish more closely set points on the tongue and lips, but the threshold for discriminating two points may be centimeters at other sites on the body. Comparisons should always be made between analogous sites on the two sides of the body, since the deficit, with a specific parietal lesion, is likely to be hemilateral. This point holds true for all cortical sensory testing.

Touch localization is usually carried out by light pressure with the examiner's fingertip, asking the patient, whose eyes are closed, to identify the site of touch. It is usual to ask the patient to touch the same site with a fingertip. Bilateral simultaneous stimulation at analogous sites (e.g., the dorsa of both hands) can be carried out to determine whether the perception of touch is extinguished consistently on one side or the other. The phenomenon is referred to as extinction on bilateral simultaneous stimulation.

Graphesthesia means the capacity to recognize letters or numbers drawn by the examiner's fingertip on various parts of the body while the patient maintains closed eyes. The usual comparison is the palm of one hand versus the palm of the other. Numbers should be drawn large enough to occupy most of the palm. Once again, the comparison of one side to the other is of prime importance. Failure to recognize numbers or letters is termed *agraphesthesia*.

Stereognosis refers to the ability to identify common objects by palpation, recognizing their shape, texture, and size. Common standard objects are the best test objects, such as a marble, a paper clip, a small rubber ball, or coins. Patients with normal stereognosis should be able to distinguish a dime from a penny and certainly a nickel from a quarter. Patients should only be allowed to feel the object with one hand at time. If they are unable to identify it in one hand, it should be placed in the other for comparison. Individuals unable to identify common objects and coins in one hand who can do so in the other are said to have *astereognosis* of the abnormal hand. Note that the major comparison is one side of the body with the other.

Localization of sensory abnormalities   Peripheral neuropathies are generally graded, distal, and symmetric in their distribution of deficit. Although most peripheral neuropathies are pansensory and affect all modalities of sensation, selective sensory dysfunction according to nerve fiber size may occur. In small fiber neuropathies, the hallmark is burning, painful dysesthesias with reduced pinprick and thermal sensation but with sparing of proprioception, motor function, and even deep tendon jerks. Touch is variably involved, but when spared, the sensory pattern is referred to as sensory dissociation (see below). In contrast to small fiber neuropathies, large fiber neuropathies are characterized by position sense deficit, imbalance, absent tendon jerks, variable motor dysfunction, but preservation of most cutaneous sensation and few or no dysesthesias.

Paresthesias and dysesthesias may be of either peripheral nerve or spinal cord origin, and probably can arise in the brainstem, but in every instance are thought to represent abnormal showers of impulses generated from an ectopic focus or foci. By themselves, paresthesias may not be localizable, but when accompanied by other signs of neuropathy or of myelopathy, the correct site of origin may be deduced.

Dissociated sensory deficit patterns, in which pinprick and thermal sensation are lost but touch is spared, are usually a sign of spinothalamic tract involvement in the spinal cord, especially if the deficit is unilateral and has an upper level on the torso. Bilateral spinothalamic tract involvement occurs with lesions affecting the center of the spinal cord, such as happens with expansion of the central canal in hydromyelia or syringomyelia. Sensory dissociation may also occur in peripheral neuropathies in which afferent cutaneous nerve fibers of small diameter are preferentially affected. Neuropathies in which sensory dissociation may occur include leprous neuritis, hereditary sensory neuropathy, and certain cases of amyloid and diabetic polyneuropathy (see Chap. 363).

Hemisensory disturbance with tingling numbness from head to foot is usually thalamic in origin. If abrupt in onset, the thalamic lesion is likely to be due to a small stroke (lacunar infarction). Occasionally, with lesions affecting the posterolateral thalamus (VPL) or adjacent white matter, a syndrome of thalamic pain, also called Déjerine-Roussy syndrome, may ensue. This is a persistent unrelenting hemipainful state often described in dramatic terms such as "like the flesh is being torn from my limbs" or "as though that side is bathed in acid" (see Chap. 15). Harlequin patterns of sensory disturbance, in which one side of the face and the opposite side of the body are affected, localize to the lateral medulla where a small lesion may damage both the ipsilateral descending trigeminal tract and ascending spinothalamic fibers (lateral lemniscus) subserving the opposite

arm, leg, and hemitorso (see "Lateral Medulla Syndrome," Chap. 351).

With lesions of the parietal lobe, either of the cortex or subjacent white matter, the most prominent symptoms are contralateral hemineglect, hemi-inattention, and a tendency not to use the contralateral hand and arm. Tests of primary sensation are usually normal or minimally altered, but tests of cortical sensation are often severely abnormal (see Chap. 32). Dysesthesias or even a sense of numbness are unusual except in the special circumstance of focal sensory seizures. These are generally due to lesions in or near the postcentral gyrus. Symptoms of focal somatosensory seizures are usually combinations of numbness and tingling, but frequently additional, more complex sensations are present, such as a rushing feeling, a sense of warmth, a sense of movement without visible motion, or an unpleasantly dysesthetic quality. Duration of seizures is variable; they may be transient, lasting only seconds, or may persist for hours. Focal motor features (clonic jerking) may supervene, and seizures can become generalized with loss of consciousness. Likely sites of symptoms are unilaterally in the lips, face, digits, or foot, and symptoms may spread as in a Jacksonian march. On occasion, symptoms may occur in a symmetric bilateral fashion, for instance, in both hands; this results from involvement of the second sensory area (unilaterally) located in the rolandic area at and just above the Sylvian fissure.

REFERENCES

CULP W, OCHOA JL (eds): *Abnormal Nerves and Muscles as Impulse Generators.* Oxford University, New York, 1982

DYCK PJ et al: Detection thresholds of cutaneous sensation in humans, in PJ Dyck, PK Thomas, EH Lambert, RP Bunge (eds), *Peripheral Neuropathy,* 2d ed. Philadelphia, Saunders, 1984, pp 1103–1138

LINDBLOM U, OCHOA JL: Somatosensory function and dysfunction, in AK Asbury, GM McKhann, WI McDonald (eds), *Diseases of the Nervous System.* Philadelphia, Saunders, 1986, pp 283–298

MACKEL R: Single unit analysis of regenerated cutaneous afferents in man. Ann Neurol 18:165, 1985

VALLBO AB et al: Somatosensory, proprioceptive, and sympathetic activity in human peripheral nerve. Physiol Rev 59:919, 1979

<hr>

29   BEHAVIORAL AND EMOTIONAL DISTURBANCES

EDWIN H. CASSEM

Patients often seek medical attention with complaints that are difficult to ascribe to a specific clinical disorder: fatigue, tension, nervousness, listlessness, anxiety, depression. Other patients have somatic complaints—dizziness, shortness of breath, unsteadiness, or persistent pain (headache, backache, cramps)—but the intensity of the complaint is out of proportion to the physical findings, if any. The clinical challenge in such patients is to discern the contributions of emotional or psychiatric problems to the physical complaints. Some patients disclose their psychiatric disorder immediately by their complaint, as when one complains that his thoughts are being broadcast through the local television station, or another that she has lost all interest in living since shortly after the birth of her last child. Even when the patient has no complaint, clues to psychiatric disorders may be obvious, such as profuse sweating, virtual absence of eye contact, use of a handkerchief to open the door, or repeated demands for analgesic prescriptions.

When are mental and emotional disturbances "abnormal"? No person escapes stress of some sort in daily life. Anxiety or despondency may be a normal response to a threat, disappointment, or loss. When symptoms are vague and unexplained by the physical examination or laboratory assessment, and when the patient denies any psychological cause, discovery of a diagnosis that explains them may be difficult. Many of these complaints are caused by common and treatable psychiatric disorders like the anxiety and affective disorders. Another common difficulty arises when the patient has an obvious disorder, such as Parkinson's disease, appropriate treatment is prescribed that leads to significant improvement in the core symptoms of rigidity and bradykinesia, yet the patient continues to complain of exhaustion, insomnia, and inability to concentrate. In this case the patient may suffer from both Parkinson's disease and major depression and requires treatment for both conditions.

This chapter formulates an approach to the diagnosis of mental, emotional, and behavioral complaints and abnormalities. The classification of such symptoms, as defined in the *Diagnostic and Statistical Manual of Mental Disorders* (DSM III-R), is organized to ascertain whether the patient's complaints and findings meet diagnostic criteria for psychiatric disorders.

PSYCHIATRIC METHOD OF CLINICAL EVALUATION Occasionally the psychiatrist is able to approach a chief complaint with a beginning question almost the same as that asked by the neurologist, i.e., where is the lesion? That is, one can ask if the primary difficulty is in the realm of thought, of mood and feeling, or of behavior. Although not anatomic, these three areas cover the major psychiatric disorders. The delusion of the patient who complained that his thoughts were being broadcast on television, for example, is readily identifiable as a disturbance of thought, and a history and examination might swiftly confirm that his most likely diagnosis was schizophrenia. Likewise the postpartum mother might meet all the diagnostic criteria for major depression.

At present one cannot confirm either diagnosis by a laboratory test that is more reliable than the clinical diagnosis itself. In a sense, then, the psychiatrist makes a diagnosis similar to an internist's diagnostic evaluation of a systemic illness. The postpartum mother must meet five or more of the nine DSM III-R diagnostic criteria for major depression, just as a patient with bilateral, symmetric, inflammatory polyarthritis must meet seven of eleven criteria for a definite diagnosis of rheumatoid arthritis. Of the eleven criteria for rheumatoid arthritis, two are historical, four demonstrable on physical examination, and five provided by laboratory examination. Even though major mood disorders have characteristic biologic manifestations, these have yet to generate laboratory tests sufficiently useful for routine diagnostic use (see Chap. 368). Psychiatric diagnosis, therefore, remains largely a clinical effort.

Furthermore, in psychiatric diagnosis shortcuts are seldom available. A medical patient's history of cough and fever may justify a chest x-ray that confirms a diagnosis of pneumonia. Sputum can be cultured promptly, antibiotics prescribed and, on the basis of culture results, changed to more specific agents at a later time. For psychiatric disorders no x-rays or cultures can be ordered that will make the history unnecessary or indicate the psychotropic drug specific to the disorder. Hence the history and the clinical examination for a psychiatric disorder must have each step specifically addressed if the physician wishes to avoid a misdiagnosis. The steps of the psychiatric examination are outlined below.

THE PSYCHIATRIC HISTORY The salient components of the psychiatric history are summarized in Table 29-1.

PSYCHIATRIC EXAMINATION After the history has been completed, a systematic mental status examination should assess: (1) appearance and behavior; (2) flow, rate, quantity, and content of speech; (3) mood; (4) thought and perception (hallucinations, delusions, obsessions, derealization, and depersonalization); (5) orientation; (6) attention; (7) memory; and (8) judgment and insight. This examination is summarized conveniently in the Mini-Mental Status Examination (see Table 29-2). This simple examination provides a numerical score that gives both an estimate of the severity of impairment and a reference point for later comparison, as when a delirious patient begins to recover. Further elaboration on the details of the psychiatric history and examination can be found in Chap. 368.

TABLE 29-1 The psychiatric history

Chief complaint
Source of and reason for referral: why now?
History of present illness
Past psychiatric history
Family psychiatric history
Personal history: delivery, developmental milestones, school and occupational history, peer relations, psychosexual/menstrual history, service/war history, religious history, marital history
Past medical history: febrile seizures, head trauma, prolonged illness, surgery, accidents, disabilities (vision, hearing), sexually transmitted diseases
Habits: drugs, alcohol, tobacco
Current medications

FORMULATION OF THE DIAGNOSIS Proceeding in a manner similar to that for nonpsychiatric symptoms, the physician considers the medical history, the examination, and the laboratory findings and then formulates a differential diagnosis. The differential diagnosis for psychiatric symptoms has two components: (1) exclusion of organic disease and (2) the psychiatric diagnosis.

Exclusion of organic disease The physician begins the differential diagnosis by considering those medical illnesses that might give rise to the symptoms and signs elicited during examination. Dramatically disordered cognition, emotion, and behavior can occur in hypoglycemia, hypertensive encephalopathy, Wernicke's encephalopathy, hypoxemia from pulmonary failure, hepatic encephalopathy, subarachnoid hemorrhage, or drug overdose (see Chap. 30). A hypoglycemic diabetic may be mistaken initially for an inebriated alcoholic because of clouded consciousness, slurred speech, and agitated behavior.

Symptoms of depression, fatigue, insomnia, and poor concentration can be caused by drugs and medical diseases. Alcohol, antihypertensive medications (reserpine, alphamethyldopa, and beta-adrenergic blocking agents), and glucocorticoids are frequently implicated in causing depression. Cimetidine, although more often a cause of confusion, can also produce depression. Cocaine, barbiturates, and amphetamine abuse are often associated with a depressive syndrome. Hypothyroidism, hyperparathyroidism, Cushing's disease, and subcortical dementias like Huntington's and Parkinson's diseases are often heralded by depression. Anemia, hypo- and hyperglycemia, hyponatremia, hypercalcemia, hypokalemia, encephalitis, and an occult malignancy may produce symptoms of weakness and fatigue that are mistakenly ascribed to depression.

Symptoms of anxiety are defined by somatic symptoms: "butterflies" or a "knot" in the stomach, sweating, tremulousness, palpitations, flushing, breathlessness, numbness, muscular tension, dry mouth, urinary frequency. Caffeine can induce acute and chronic anxiety. Withdrawal from alcohol, barbiturates, meprobamate, and benzodiazepines can produce dramatic anxiety, occasionally progressing to a life-threatening medical emergency. Symptoms similar to anxiety can occur in hyperthyroidism, paroxysmal atrial tachycardia, mitral valve prolapse, pheochromocytoma, insulinoma, myocardial infarction, or hypoglycemia. Excess thyroid medication, sympathomimetic amines, and bronchodilators such as theophylline can produce tachycardia and anxiety. Pulmonary conditions such as asthma, obstructive pulmonary disease, and pulmonary embolism can cause breathlessness and make the patient anxious. Pulmonary edema and congestive heart failure do the same. These conditions are not often mistaken for an emotional disorder unless they are subtle—as occult, intermittent showers of pulmonary emboli may be.

Fear is a common emotion that may be produced by a complex partial seizure. Carcinoid tumor, the commonest endocrine neoplasm of the digestive tract, is of special interest because its clinical episodes of flushing and tachycardia may be triggered by intense emotion. In such a case a patient may relate that anger caused the feeling of being "on fire." Patients who receive neuroleptic medications occasionally develop akathisia, a side effect characterized by extreme restlessness, inability to remain seated (which gives the condition its name), and

TABLE 29-2   Mini-mental status examination

EXAMINATION

Patient _____
Examiner _____
Date _____

Maximum score	Score	Orientation
5	( )	What is the (year)(season)(date)(day)(month)?
5	( )	Where are we? (state)(county)(town)(hospital)(floor)
		Registration
3	( )	Name 3 objects: 1 s to say each. Then ask the patient all 3 after you have said them. Give 1 point for each correct answer. Then repeat them until he learns all 3. Count trials, and record: Trials _____
		Attention and calculation
5	( )	Serial 7s. 1 point for each correct. Stop after 5 answers. Alternative: Spell "world" backwards.
		Recall
3	( )	Ask for the 3 objects repeated above. Give 1 point for each correct.
		Language
9	( )	Name a pencil and wristwatch (2 points) Repeat the following: "No ifs, ands, or buts." (1 point) Follow a 3-stage command: "Take a paper in your right hand, fold it in half, and put it on the floor." (3 points) Read and obey the following: Close your eyes (1 point) Write a sentence (1 point) Copy design (1 point) Total score _____

Assess level of consciousness along a continuum _____

Alert   Drowsy   Stupor   Coma

INSTRUCTIONS FOR ADMINISTRATION

Orientation
Ask for the date. Then ask specifically for parts omitted, e.g., "Can you also tell me what season it is?" One point for each correct.
Ask in turn "Can you tell me the name of this hospital?" (town, country, etc.). One point for each correct.

Registration
Ask the patient if you may test his memory. Then say the names of 3 unrelated objects, clearly and slowly, about 1 s for each. After you have said all 3, ask him to repeat them. This first repetition determines his score (0–3), but keep saying them until he can repeat all 3, up to 6 trials. If he does not eventually learn all 3, recall cannot be meaningfully tested.

Attention and calculation
Ask the patient to begin with 100 and count backwards by 7. Stop after 5 subtractions (93, 86, 79, 72, 65). Score the total number of correct answers. If the patient cannot or will not perform this task, ask him to spell the word "world" backwards. The score is the number of letters in correct order: e.g., dlrow = 5, dlorw = 3.

Recall
Ask the patient if he can recall the 3 words you previously asked him to remember. Score 0–3.

Language
Naming: Show the patient a wristwatch and ask him what it is. Repeat for pencil. Score 0–2.
Repetition: Ask the patient to repeat the sentence after you. Allow only one trial. Score 0–1.
3-Stage command: Give the patient a piece of plain blank paper and repeat the command. Score 1 point for each part correctly executed.
Reading: On a blank piece of paper print the sentence "Close your eyes," in letters large enough for the patient to see clearly. Ask him to read it and do what it says. Score 1 point only if he actually closes his eyes.
Writing: Give the patient a blank piece of paper and ask him to write a sentence for you. Do not dictate a sentence, it is to be written spontaneously. It must contain a subject and verb and be sensible. Correct grammar and punctuation are not necessary.
Copying: On a clean piece of paper, draw intersecting pentagons, each side about 1 in, and ask him to copy it exactly as it is. All 10 angles must be present and 2 must intersect to score 1 point. Tremor and rotation are ignored.

Estimate the patient's level of sensorium along a continuum, from alert on the left to coma on the right.

SOURCE: Reproduced with permission from Folstein et al.

a state difficult to distinguish from anxious agitation. Failure to recognize this side effect may cause the physician to increase the dose of the neuroleptic, which only worsens the akathisia. Paradoxically, even though depression and anxiety are classified as two separate categories of psychiatric disorder, anxiety is one of the most common and most severe features of major depression. Treatment of the depression often alleviates the anxiety.

Delusions and hallucinations are the hallmark of a psychosis (see Chap. 368). Somatic delusions (that one's body is giving off a foul odor, for example), grandiose and paranoid delusions, and hallucinations (auditory, visual, olfactory, tactile), while characteristic of the major psychoses, can also occur in patients with confusional states due to medical illness or drug effects. Amphetamine and cocaine abuse may produce paranoid states. Levodopa, administered to patients with Parkinson's disease, may produce paranoid, manic, or confusional states. Lysergic acid (LSD), mescaline, phencyclidine (PCP), and other psychotomimetic agents may produce isolated hallucinations or delusions or both; PCP is particularly associated with severe confusional states marked by agitation and violence (see Chap. 372). Characteristic organic delusions are described with neurologic disorders, such as denial of blindness after bilateral occipital lobe lesions (Anton's syndrome) or the denial of hemiparesis after a parietal lobe injury. This latter lesion may be associated with the delusion that the involved side of the body has multiple limbs. Ideas of reference, e.g., a sudden intense belief that the television news commentator is referring to oneself, may be the result of a complex partial seizure. Degenerative brain disease (such as Alzheimer's disease) or toxic/metabolic disorders may be associated with psychotic manifestations, and it may be the psychotic manifestation that first leads to a consultation with the physician (see Chap. 30).

Hallucinations are often associated with organic conditions. Visual hallucinations should be considered as due to an organic etiology until proven otherwise. Alcoholic hallucinosis, as distinguished from delirium tremens, is unique in usually being *auditory*, with a paranoid theme (accusatory voices). The sensorium is clear, there is often no tremor, and it occurs during drinking, not withdrawal (see Chap. 370). It usually occurs after many years of drinking. Formed visual hallucinations have also been reported with alcohol withdrawal, digoxin and pentazocine, in viral encephalitis and Creutzfeldt-Jakob disease, and with sensory deprivation. Macropsia, micropsia (the illusion of objects expanding or shrinking in size), formed visual hallucinations, olfactory hallucinations, déjà vu or jamais vu, and amnesic episodes are symptoms common to focal epilepsy of the temporal lobe or subcortical limbic structures (see Chap. 350). Confusional states are discussed in Chap. 30.

Patients who appear "hyper"—expansive, elated, hypertalkative, egotistical, distractable, and boundlessly energetic with a decreased need for sleep—may be manifesting a lifelong personality style or be either manic or hypomanic; or they may be medically ill. If ill, the cause is either drug ingestion or brain disease. The drugs most commonly associated with manic-like symptoms are glucocorticoids and adrenocorticotropic hormone (ACTH); stimulants like cocaine, amphetamines, sympathomimetics; and excessive thyroid medication, antidepressants, and antiparkinsonian agents.

Rarely brain tumor, ACTH producing tumors, viral encephalitis (including human immunodeficiency virus infection), temporal lobe seizures, neurosyphilis, multiple sclerosis, Huntington's disease, uremia, hyperthyroidism, vitamin B_{12} deficiency, carcinoid syndrome, and dialysis dementia syndrome can cause mania. Whenever manic symptoms appear in a patient over 50 years of age who has no prior history of either mania or depression, the abnormal state is almost always *secondary* to one of the conditions listed above and not a *primary* psychiatric disorder.

Psychiatric differential diagnosis The internist cannot be expected to become an expert in psychiatric disorders. Some disorders, however, are so common that generalists not only see them frequently but see more of them than do psychiatrists. This is most often the case, for example, with major depression. Estimates suggest that up to 60 percent of depressed patients are seen by general physicians and internists and 20 percent by psychiatrists or other mental health professionals, while 20 percent consult no professional for help with their disorder. The generalist who includes depression in the differential diagnosis is in an excellent position to recognize this disorder when it appears and to treat it appropriately.

The term *neurotic*, or *psychoneurotic*, while descriptive of certain conflicts that patients carried with them from early life, is no longer a psychiatric diagnosis. Certain other terms, like *neurasthenia, psychasthenia, neurocirculatory asthenia*, and *soldier's heart* have also been eliminated from lists of psychiatric diagnoses because more precise diagnostic categories have replaced them (see DSM III-R for current usage).

Like all physicians, the psychiatrist's basic activities are diagnosis and treatment. Intuition develops with clinical experience, but even the most gifted clinician must continue to cover the basic components of the psychiatric history and examination.

REFERENCES

AMERICAN PSYCHIATRIC ASSOCIATION: *Diagnostic and Statistical Manual of Mental Disorders* (DSM III-R). Washington, DC, 1987

FOLSTEIN MF et al: "Mini-mental state," a practical method for grading the cognitive state of patients for the clinician. J Psychiatr Res 12:189, 1975

HACKETT TP, CASSEM NH (eds): *Massachusetts General Hospital Handbook of General Hospital Psychiatry*, 2d ed. Littleton, MA, PSG Publishing, 1987

KAPLAN HI, SADOCK BJ (eds): *Comprehensive Textbook of Psychiatry/V*. Baltimore, Williams & Wilkins, 1989

NICHOLI AM JR (ed): *The New Harvard Guide to Psychiatry*. Cambridge, MA, Harvard, 1988

30 ACUTE CONFUSIONAL STATES, AMNESIA, AND DEMENTIA

MARTIN M. BROWN / VLADIMIR C. HACHINSKI

The brain functions with marvelous complexity when it reasons, formulates language, or calculates. Because of this complexity and the vulnerability of neuronal function to biochemical and physiologic alterations, cognitive function is easily disturbed. The resulting syndromes are common and may result from a wide variety of conditions. Many systemic illnesses and brain diseases come to notice because of disruption of cognitive function, often without other neurologic symptoms or signs. It is important to recognize the pattern of the resulting organic neurobehavioral syndromes to avoid mistaken psychiatric diagnoses and begin appropriate management early. The examination of cognitive function is an important bedside clinical skill for the student and physician to acquire and practice so that minor degrees of confusion are not overlooked and more confused patients can be approached with confidence. Careful testing of individual components of cognitive function allows identification of specific areas of abnormality and is an essential prerequisite to establishing the diagnosis of a neurobehavioral syndrome.

SYNDROME DEFINITION

This chapter discusses the examination of cognitive function in three related syndromes—confusion, amnesia, and dementia—in which an intellectual disorder is the major presenting feature.

CONFUSION Any disorder of cognitive function may cause confusion, which can be defined as a lack of clarity and coherence of thought, perception, understanding, or action. Confusion is often the first feature of cognitive impairment noticed by relatives or the examiner. The confusion in acute confusional states and dementia reflects global or multifocal impairment of cognition and in amnesia reflects impairment of memory. Confusion may also appear to be the presenting complaint in isolated focal disorders of cognitive function such as aphasia or visuospatial agnosia (see Chap. 32), but careful examination will show that the confusion is related to a single deficit.

ACUTE CONFUSIONAL STATE The acute confusional state is a common neurobehavioral syndrome in which acute and global impairment of cognitive function is accompanied by impairment of attention and consciousness. The impairments of cognition usually include disorientation, abnormal perception, disordered reasoning, and poor memory. A wide variety of causes may be responsible.

DELIRIUM Some authors (e.g., Lipowski) use the term *delirium* as synonymous with the acute confusional state, but delirium is best reserved to describe a clinically distinct variety of acute confusional

TABLE 30-1   Clinical features of the acute confusional state and dementia compared

	Acute confusional state	Dementia
Onset	Acute	Usually insidious
Duration	Transient (hours to weeks)	Persistent (months to years)
Course	Fluctuating over hours; diurnal variation common	Stable over days
Sleep-wake cycle	Disrupted	Normal
Conscious level	Depressed	Normal
Attention	Impaired	Normal
Orientation	Impaired	Impaired
Language	Incoherent	Aphasia common
Memory		
Digit span	Shortened	Normal
Long-term memory	Impaired	Impaired
Perception	Impaired (illusions, delusions, hallucinations)	Normal early, agnosia later
Mood	Agitation or fear common	Apathy or disinhibition common
Autonomic changes	Common	Unusual
Psychomotor changes (depressed motor activity or restlessness)	Common	Uncommon
Involuntary movements	Common	Uncommon
EEG	Diffuse slow-wave activity	Mild slowing

state characterized by periods of agitation, heightened mental activity, increased wakefulness, marked readiness to respond to certain stimuli (such as sudden noises), intrusive visual hallucinations, motor hyperactivity, and autonomic stimulation. The features essential to the acute confusional state of impairment of consciousness and attention are present despite the apparent arousal (see "Consciousness," below). The agitation of delirium characteristically fluctuates and may alternate with or progress to a subdued confusional state. The clinical picture is exemplified by the excited hallucinatory state of *delirium tremens* which follows alcohol withdrawal. However, delirium may be seen in acute confusional states from any cause.

DEMENTIA   This is also a common syndrome of acquired global or multifocal impairment of cognitive function, involving decline in intellect, memory, and personality in the presence of normal consciousness. Normal alertness and attention distinguish dementia from the acute confusional state, although there are other differences (see Table 30-1). The decline in intellect usually involves all intellectual functions, but in early or limited disease, the diagnosis may be established by impairment of any three of the following spheres: language, memory, visuospatial skills, emotion, personality, or cognition. Loss of a single intellectual function such as speech or memory, however devastating, is not sufficient. Dementia is not necessarily progressive, and in some instances can be reversed or halted by appropriate treatment. It is therefore important to recognize dementia as a syndrome with many causes.

AMNESIA   This term describes an isolated disorder of memory characterized by inability to remember past events and to learn new information despite normal consciousness and attention. Like the other syndromes discussed in this chapter, amnesia has a variety of possible causes.

OBSERVABLE COMPONENTS OF COGNITION

Despite the complexity of mental activity, certain aspects can be assessed reliably at the bedside as part of the neurologic examination. A sequence of cognitive functions proceeding from the initial sensory input (the examiner's question) to motor or verbal output (the patient's response) can be distinguished, as well as a number of influences on the sequence (see Fig. 30-1).

CONSCIOUSNESS   Consciousness is the state of awareness of self and the environment and has various facets (see also Chap. 31). The *content* of consciousness represents the sum of cognitive and affective mental functions and can be assessed only by inference. *Arousal* is closely allied to the appearance of wakefulness and *alertness*, i.e., the readiness to respond to stimulation. *Attention* includes the capacity to attend selectively to relevant stimuli and to manipulate abstract ideas. Consciousness also includes the concepts of *insight* and recognition of self. *Clouding of consciousness* is an essential feature of acute confusional states and describes the mildest impairment of consciousness on the continuum from full consciousness to deep coma. In most instances clouding of consciousness involves all facets of consciousness but does not necessarily imply reduced wakefulness. In delirium the patient may appear awake or excited, but the content of consciousness, awareness of the surroundings and self, and the capacity to attend selectively to relevant stimuli are all impaired.

PERCEPTION   Perception involves conscious awareness and selection and identification of a stimulus from the environment. Even under normal conditions the perception of a stimulus depends on numerous factors, both physiologic (such as lighting) and psychological (such as mood and expectation). With clouding of consciousness attention falters, and perception becomes more subject to these influences. For example, poor vision or deafness may make the elderly more prone to misperception, and the sensory deprivation of confinement to bed or the advent of darkness often contributes to delirium. Coherent perception requires intact visuospatial or language function. Disturbances of perception are frequent in acute confusional states and include *illusions* (misperceptions of actual sensory stimuli) and *hallucinations* (perceptions experienced without apparent sensory

FIGURE 30-1   Observable components of cognition. Cognition from sensory input to verbal or motor output involves a sequence of separate but interrelated functions. The arrows indicate the influence at every stage of the level of consciousness and degree of attention, as well as the effect of mood and memory. These functions should be individually assessed at the bedside.

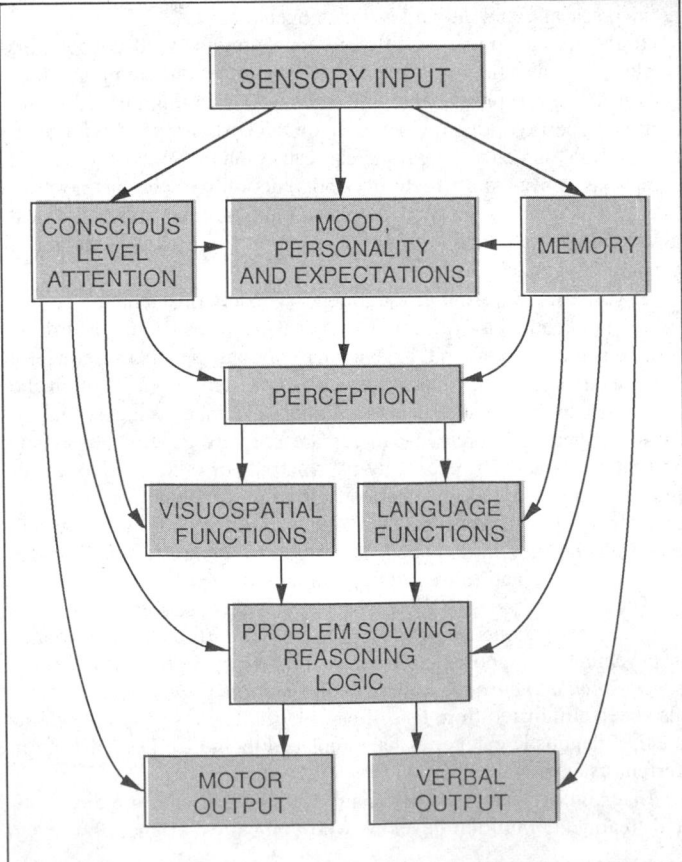

stimulation). In dementia misperception more commonly results from focal impairments of visuospatial or language function such as agnosia or aphasia.

MEMORY   Three classes of memory can be distinguished at the bedside depending on the length of recall. This distinction is important in the differentiation of acute confusional states, dementia, and amnesic syndromes. The *immediate memory* system holds information close to consciousness for a few seconds while it is used for mental activity. It can be tested by the reproduction of a string of numerals and has a finite capacity for information at around seven digits, which are retained within the span of attention for only seconds or minutes unless the information is rehearsed by internal repetition. Normal attention is therefore required for immediate memory function, and impairment of immediate memory and a shortened digit span are diagnostic features of the acute confusional syndrome. Immediate memory is relatively normal in dementia and amnesic syndromes. Immediate memory appears to be mediated by a separate system that does not necessarily lead to longer-term storage. Recall of information after a delay of a few minutes requires a process of consolidation or learning and is mediated by the *long-term* or *secondary memory* system, with almost limitless capacity and durability. In contrast to immediate memory, recall of information from long-term memory is often selected by its relevance to the individual and usually incorporates the meaning of the information rather than exact words or pictures. Clinically, *recent memory,* the recall of information presented within minutes, hours, or days, is distinguished from *remote memory,* the recall of events months or years earlier. Recent and remote memory probably both involve the same long-term memory system, but access to remote memories is less sensitive to interference (e.g., from the effect of head injury) than recent memory. Impaired recent memory is usual in dementia and acute confusional states, and is the defining feature of amnesic syndromes.

MOOD AND PERSONALITY   *Mood* refers to the prevailing emotional state, while *affect* is the emotional experience evoked by a particular stimulus. Individual reactions to any situation are closely related to underlying personality, previous experience, expectations, and degree of insight. These need to be taken into account when assessing cognitive function. The prevailing mood may have a profound affect on all aspects of cognition, especially at the extremes of the continuum of mood. Hypomania may be accompanied by illusions, flight of ideas, and extreme motor and verbal output sometimes mimicking delirium. In contrast, depression may exhibit slowing of thought, speech, and activity (psychomotor retardation) which, if severe, may be mistaken for dementia. Extreme anxiety may also interfere with the organization and coherence of thought and speech. Many diseases of the brain alter mood and affect. Frontal lobe lesions, in particular, may cause either lack of drive and initiative (abulia) with indifference to outcome or sometimes fatuous euphoria with social and sexual disinhibitions, which may interfere with cognitive function.

PROBLEM SOLVING   Thought is intangible and elusive. However, the processes of reasoning, logic, and the ability to solve problems using language or mathematics can be assessed more easily using tests of words or numbers. Disorder of these processes is an essential feature of the acute confusional states and dementia, but in contrast reasoning is intact in the amnesic syndrome, except when recent memory is required. One manifestation of defective reasoning seen in acute confusional states and sometimes in dementia is the occurrence of delusions (false beliefs maintained in spite of convincing contradictory evidence). Delusions are also seen in psychiatric illnesses such as schizophrenia but tend to be more organized and persistent than in acute confusional states.

APPROACH TO THE PATIENT WITH DISORDERS OF COGNITION

HISTORY   A careful history taken from close relatives or friends is essential to establish the first appearance of intellectual impairment

and the subsequent tempo of the disease. Was the onset over hours or days, suggesting an acute confusional state, or over months or years, making dementia a more likely diagnosis? Was there an organic precipitating event such as a head injury, or did the confusion follow an emotional crisis, suggesting a psychiatric cause or deliberate drug overdose? Questioning should include inquiries about impairment of memory, personality and mood change, and how the patient copes with work, driving, and the activities of daily life. The history should include questioning about symptoms which suggest focal pathology such as those of raised intracranial pressure (headaches, nausea, vomiting, and ataxia), strokelike events, or seizures. Attention to past medical and family history, drugs, alcohol, and toxic exposure is important (see also Chap. 347). The handedness of the patient should be determined to assess the likelihood that the left hemisphere is dominant for speech.

EXAMINATION OF COGNITIVE FUNCTION   The main focus is to establish the level of consciousness and to determine whether one or more areas of intellectual function are impaired. It is important as an initial step to determine the patient's premorbid level of intellect. A rough indicator can be obtained from the patient's profession or occupation and the amount of schooling completed. The physician is sometimes surprised to discover that a patient never learned to read or write, sometimes because of developmental dyslexia.

Examination of cognitive function needs to be adjusted according to the previous and current intellectual state, but it is useful to have a sequence of questions that the examiner has applied regularly to intellectually intact patients so as to have a good understanding of the normal range of replies. The patient's answers to questioning should be carefully recorded so that deterioration or improvement can be easily confirmed at a later evaluation. A number of pitfalls may cause the patient's intellectual function to be underestimated. Perseveration, usually a sign of frontal lobe disease, may cause the patient to repeat replies and have difficulty switching attention to a new task. Aphasia, with difficulty understanding commands or expressing the correct answer in response to questions, may cloud interpretation of the examination. The incoherence or mutism resulting from isolated expressive aphasia is commonly misinterpreted as a confusional state or dementia.

Orientation   Orientation to person, place, and time (including date, time of day, month, and year) should be tested first as a guide to the degree of amnesia and confusion. In most cases, the more severe the impairment of memory the more inaccurate the date. If the patient cannot name the place accurately, some assessment of reasoning powers can be gauged by asking the patient to identify the type of place (e.g., hospital or home).

Consciousness   Detecting clouding of consciousness requires careful observation. The normally alert individual engages in conversation or some other diversional activity, while the patient with impairment of consciousness remains quiet or engages in purposeless repetitive activities. More obtunded patients may drift into sleep when undisturbed but awaken promptly during the stimulation of questioning or physical examination. The demented patient may also lack spontaneous activity or conversation but shows normal alertness and responsiveness to questioning.

Attention   Attention is assessed during history taking. Does the patient pay attention to questions, or is the patient easily distracted, giving equal notice to relevant and irrelevant stimuli? The capacity for sustained attention and concentration can be tested by asking for sequential subtraction of 7 from 100 down to zero, but the response should be interpreted with caution, as immediate memory and mathematical ability are also required. Forward and reverse digit span are also specific tests of attention as well as of immediate memory (see below).

Abnormalities of perception   Abnormalities of perception should be sought by specific questioning about perception of the environment. The presence of hallucinations may be betrayed by the patient brushing or picking nonexistent objects off the bed covers or turning to answer an imaginary question.

Language Aphasia resulting in nonfluency of speech, hesitation, circumlocution, neologisms, or jargon is usually appreciated during routine conversation and history taking (see Chap. 33). It is also useful to ask the patient to name common and uncommon objects to assess for nominal aphasia, and to give a complex two- or three-stage conditional command to test for minor degrees of receptive dysphasia. (For example, "If I take my pen out of my pocket, please touch your left ear with your right index finger.") Agraphia should be sought by asking the patient to write his or her name and a short spontaneous sentence. Reading should be assessed using a standard text or newspaper article including an explanation of its meaning by the patient. Simple sums are given to assess mathematical skills.

Visuospatial function The most useful test of visuospatial function is to ask the patient to copy a drawing, starting with a simple object such as a five-pointed star and progressing to a more difficult object such as a three-dimensional box. Constructional apraxia, or visuospatial agnosia, results in difficulty in drawing the lines required in the correct spatial orientation or position. Other deficits of cortical function such as perseveration or visual neglect may also be revealed by this test. The visual recognition of common objects will have been tested when examining for nominal aphasia, but bedside testing for difficulty in recognition of faces (prosopagnosia) requires a newspaper or magazine containing photographs of famous people, unless individuals who should be well known to the patient can be presented without other clues such as voice to aid recognition.

Memory *Immediate memory* and attention are tested by determining *digit span*. The patient is asked to repeat a string of numerals after the examiner starting with a short string and working up to the normal digit span of six or seven consecutive numbers presented at about half-second intervals. A shorter string of numerals or a short word can be given to repeat or spell backwards. This test requires sustained attention as well as immediate memory. *Recent memory* should be assessed by asking the patient to learn the names of three common objects or a simple address. After confirming that the patient has registered the information, recall is tested after 2 and 5 min, depending on the degree of anticipated amnesia. If the patient fails to recall the information, then the severity of the amnesia can be gauged by giving the patient a clue, and if this fails, recognition can be tested by asking the patient to identify the correct answer from a choice. Recent memory for events over the last few days or weeks is assessed by asking for a description of events of personal or world importance. A relative or friend may need to corroborate the appropriateness of the description. *Remote long-term memory* can be tested by asking for items of common general knowledge such as the dates of important past events, names of important political figures, or location of major cities.

Mood and personality Judgments about personality, mood, affect, and insight should be made during history taking and examination. The appearance of the patient, content of conversation, and speed of movement provide the most useful clues to mood. Affect is signaled by language, facial expression, gestures, and posture, all of which should be studied closely. The presence of euphoria, disinhibition, or abulia should be noted.

Thought and problem solving Incoherence of reasoning and logical thought will usually have been detected during history taking or testing of language skills and mathematics. More subtle disorder of thought is sometimes revealed by asking the patient to explain the meaning of well-known proverbs or sayings.

Cognitive scales A number of scales [e.g., Blessed Dementia Scale; Mini-Mental State Examination (see Chap. 29)] have been developed to make an approximate assessment of cognitive function. These are not true psychometric tests but questionnaires that can be completed fairly quickly by untrained staff to provide a score that roughly reflects the degree of intellectual and behavioral impairment. Another scale, the Ischemic Score, helps to distinguish multi-infarct from degenerative dementia. On the whole, these scales are less useful in diagnosis than a careful cognitive examination conducted in the manner described above.

ACUTE CONFUSIONAL STATES AND DELIRIUM

Acute confusional states occur in about 10 percent of all hospitalized patients and in 30 to 50 percent of hospitalized geriatric patients; patients with dementia are particularly vulnerable.

PATHOPHYSIOLOGY *Neurologic diseases* cause confusional states in a variety of ways, including depression of consciousness level. Consciousness is normally maintained by the ascending reticular activating system in the brainstem and thalamic regions. Focal diseases (such as a brain tumor or subdural hematoma) may depress consciousness by compression of the brainstem or thalamus or by producing hydrocephalus. Many other neurologic diseases present with confusion as a result of diffuse impairment of neuronal function (e.g., concussion or encephalitis). Multifocal disease (e.g., multiple metastases or multiple infarcts) may also present with confusion if the loci of disease cause several separate deficits of cognitive function with impaired attention. Usually lesions in both hemispheres are necessary, but occasionally a single right nondominant hemispheric lesion (usually a parietal infarct) presents with an acute confusional state because of impairment of attention, which appears to be a predominant right hemisphere function.

Systemic diseases mostly result in confusion from diffuse impairment of neuronal function. This may be due to inadequate supply of oxygen (hypoxia), glucose (hypoglycemia), or other factors required for metabolism, including vitamins and hormones. In metabolic encephalopathy the mechanisms include acid-base disturbance, electrolyte imbalance, and circulating toxins (e.g., ammonia in liver failure). In systemic infections there are several possible factors, including high fever, hypoxia, dehydration, and circulating bacterial toxins. Most drug-induced confusional states result from direct interference with synaptic transmission. In delirium following drug withdrawal the excited state may result from the sudden overactivity of a previously depressed transmitter system that has developed the equivalent of denervation hypersensitivity.

In many cases of acute confusion multiple mechanisms can be identified, particularly in the elderly. Preexisting disease of the brain, blindness or deafness, age-related changes in the metabolism, and pharmacology of drugs, mild organ failure, and an unfamiliar environment may all contribute. At any age, the brain may be made more vulnerable by preexisting brain damage, sleep and sensory deprivation, or an unfamiliar environment.

CLINICAL FEATURES Because most causes of the acute confusional state affect neuronal function diffusely, all aspects of intellectual function are impaired to a lesser or greater degree (Table 30-1). The cardinal feature is *clouding of consciousness*, manifested by impaired alertness, awareness, and attention. This impairment is usually mild but can advance to coma if untreated. Depression of consciousness is distinguished from natural drowsiness by observing that the patient cannot easily be aroused. Reduced attentiveness can range from mild apathy and a failure to grasp complex details to reduced interaction with the examiner, lack of normal spontaneous comment or questions, and neglect of bodily needs. In delirium, arousal is evidenced by a readiness to respond to certain stimuli, insomnia, and excessive reactions to noise or bright lights. This is accompanied by a reduced ability to focus attention, distractibility, and inability to concentrate.

Variability in the level of arousal is a common feature of the acute confusional state. Reduced responsiveness may be interspersed with outbursts of delirium. Sleep-wake cycles are frequently disrupted or reversed, and confusion is often more marked during the night. The early symptoms of delirium often include insomnia and vivid unpleasant dreams before a frank confusional state supervenes.

Impairment of memory with reduced digit span, poor recent memory, and defective recall for distant events is an important feature. One of the earliest signs of this impairment is disorientation for time, and later, disorientation for place. Knowledge of personal identity is usually retained if the patient can understand the question. The memory deficit is characteristically patchy so that distortions of memory (para-amnesia) and partially correct information may be incorporated into confabulatory answers or delusions. When the patient recovers, partial or total amnesia for the period of confusion is usual, although isolated events, especially vivid hallucinations, may be remembered in detail.

Impairment of cognitive function leads to difficulty performing tasks requiring logic, mathematics, or spatial organization. Thought processes are slowed, although the agitated delirious patient may have flight of ideas. In all cases, thinking is disorganized and disjointed. Speech is incoherent, rambling, and often inappropriate. Comprehension of complex material is impaired, and errors in the naming of objects or in writing may be elicited.

Impaired perception may compound confusion. The patient often misperceives surroundings and attendants as those more familiar to the patient. More concrete illusions and hallucinations are common, especially following drug withdrawal and in alcoholic delirium tremens. Hallucinations are most frequently visual, but may involve any sensory modality.

Disturbances of emotion may include blunting of affect or emotional lability. Mood disturbances include dysphoria, depression, agitation, or fear, and these may be accompanied by appropriate autonomic responses. *Autonomic hyperactivity* including tachycardia, diaphoresis, and anxiety are particularly prominent with drug and alcohol withdrawal.

Psychomotor changes are common. In most patients, spontaneous motor activity is depressed, but hyperactivity and restlessness characterize delirium. Repetitive stereotyped motor behavior, such as plucking at the bed clothes or tossing from side to side, is frequent. *Involuntary movements*, including irregular tremor, asterixis, and myoclonus, are usually seen in drug withdrawal or metabolic encephalopathy. Rarely, patients show catatonic behavior.

DIFFERENTIAL DIAGNOSIS The first essential distinction to be made is whether the confusional state results from primary neurologic disease or as a complication of systemic illness. This distinction can normally be made on examination and is then supported by investigation (see Table 30-2).

Neurologic causes These can usually be recognized by the presence of focal neurologic signs in addition to disordered intellectual function. Examples include hemiparesis in *cerebral infarction*, neck stiffness in *meningitis* or *subarachnoid hemorrhage*, and gait disturbance in *hydrocephalus*. However, diffuse neurologic diseases such as *encephalitis, epileptic confusion,* or *small-vessel vasculitis* may cause no focal neurologic signs apart from the disorder of cognition. *Neoplasias* of the nervous system usually cause headache and focal signs, but midline tumors may present with a gradually evolving confusional state. Acute onset may be caused by brainstem compression or acute hydrocephalus.

Impairment of consciousness is uncommon following nonhemorrhagic *stroke* unless the stroke is large enough to cause midline mass effects. However, impairment of consciousness and confusion may occur when a cerebral ischemic event is superimposed on preexisting cerebral infarcts. *Subarachnoid hemorrhage* may present with a confusional state secondary to widespread vasospasm, and the typical history of headache may not be obtained. *Postictal confusion* after a minor seizure lasts only a few seconds and after a major seizure usually resolves within an hour unless complicated by head injury, hypoxia, or status epilepticus. However, a persistent confusional state may occur with continuous or serial minor seizures (*minor epileptic status*) (see Chap. 350). Acute confusional states may accompany *encephalitis* or *brain abscess* without systemic signs of infarction always being present.

Systemic causes Systemic causes are usually characterized by absence of focal neurologic signs apart from cognitive disorders, although minor signs such as reflex asymmetry or extensor plantar responses may be seen. An exception to this rule is occasionally seen in *hypoglycemia*, which may be accompanied in the elderly by hemiparesis. In *metabolic encephalopathy*, acidotic hyperventilation, tremor, asterixis, or myoclonus may suggest the diagnosis. *Wernicke's*

TABLE 30-2 Differential diagnosis of the acute confusional state

NEUROLOGIC (focal neurologic signs are uncommon)

Trauma
  Concussion
  Intracranial hematoma
  Subdural hematoma
Vascular disorders
  Multiple infarcts
  Right hemisphere or posterior circulation infarcts
  Hypertensive encephalopathy
  Vasculitis (e.g., systemic lupus erythematosus, polyarteritis nodosa, giant cell arteritis)
  Air and fat embolism
  Subarachnoid hemorrhage
Neoplasia
  Multiple parenchymal metastases
  Meningeal carcinomatosis
  Midline brain tumors
  Brain tumors elsewhere with brainstem compression, edema, or hydrocephalus
  Paraneoplastic syndromes (limbic encephalitis)
Infections
  Meningitis and encephalitis (viral, bacterial, fungal, protozoal)
  Multiple abscesses
  Progressive multifocal leukoencephalopathy
Inflammations
  Acute disseminated encephalomyelitis
  Postinfectious encephalitis
Epilepsy
  Postictal state
  Minor epileptic status (temporal lobe)

SYSTEMIC (focal neurologic signs are uncommon)

Substrate depletion
  Hypoglycemia
  Diffuse hypoxia
    Pulmonary
    Cardiac
    Carbon monoxide poisoning
Metabolic encephalopathy
  Diabetic ketoacidosis
  Renal failure
  Liver failure
  Electrolyte, fluid, and acid-base imbalance (especially Na^+, Ca^{2+}, Mg^{2+})
  Hereditary metabolic disease, e.g., porphyria, metachromatic leukodystrophy, mitochondrial cytopathy
Vitamin deficiency
  Thiamine (Wernicke's encephalopathy)
  Nicotinic acid (pellagra)
  B_{12} deficiency
Endocrine; over- or underactivity
  Thyroid
  Parathyroid
  Adrenal
Infection
  Septicemia
  Malaria
  Subacute bacterial endocarditis
  Focal infection, e.g., pneumonia
Thermal injuries
  hypothermia
  heat stroke
Hematologic disorders
  Hyperviscosity syndrome
  Severe anemia
Toxic causes
  Drug and alcohol intoxication (therapeutic, social, or illegal)
  Drug withdrawal, e.g., alcohol, barbiturates, narcotics
  Chemical toxins, e.g., heavy metals, organic toxins

PSYCHIATRIC

Acute mania
Depression or extreme anxiety
Schizophrenia
Hysterical fugue states

encephalopathy (see Chap. 370) should be considered in patients with a history of alcoholism or malnutrition. *Drugs* often cause confusion, especially in the elderly and those on multiple medications. *Endocrine dysfunction* (see Chap. 313 and 316) rarely causes acute confusional state but should always be considered, particularly if there is hyponatremia. *Systemic infections,* especially *septicemia* and *subacute bacterial endocarditis* can cause acute confusional states, particularly in the elderly in whom fever may not always be evident, as can meningitis or brain abscess complicating the systemic infection.

Psychiatric causes In *anxiety,* extreme *grief,* or *depression,* orientation for person and place is usually preserved, and with encouragement the patient can concentrate and improve cognitive performance. Hyperactivity, diminished need for sleep, pressure of speech, delusions, short attention span, and distractibility in *acute mania* may be confused with the hyperexcitability of delirium. Mania is characterized by a sustained elevation of mood and preservation of orientation. Hyperactivity persists throughout the manic episode in contrast to delirium, in which hyperactivity may be interspersed with somnolence. *Disassociative or hysterical disorders,* for example, psychogenic amnesia and fugue states, are usually distinguished from organic confusional states by the focal nature of the amnesia. *Acute schizophrenia* may simulate the acute confusional state, but consciousness, normal sleep-wake cycles, orientation, and attention are usually preserved (see Chap. 368).

INVESTIGATION Investigation is an urgent procedure. A *biochemical profile,* including blood sugar level, readily diagnoses the common metabolic disorders. A *blood count* detects hematologic disorders, and a neutrophilia suggests infection. If in doubt, a raised *erythrocyte sedimentation rate* supports the diagnosis of an organic disorder. *Arterial blood gas analysis* is a useful screen for hypoxia, respiratory failure, and acidosis. *Chest x-ray* and *blood and urine cultures* should be performed even if there is no fever. A complete infectious disease screen is indicated if there is a stronger suspicion of infection. *Endocrine tests* and *vitamin B_{12}* measurement may be indicated in individual patients. *Drug and toxicologic screen* are indicated for suspicion of drug overdose or toxic exposure. *Cerebrospinal fluid (CSF) examination* is mandatory in all patients with fever or neck stiffness so long as raised intracranial pressure or intracranial mass is not suspected and is also helpful in distinguishing metabolic from neurologic disease. The CSF white cell count is usually normal in metabolic disease, whereas leukocytosis implies neurologic disease, especially a central nervous system (CNS) infection. The *electroencephalogram* (EEG) is useful if the presence of encephalopathy is uncertain; it is almost always abnormal in organic causes, but does not necessarily distinguish between neurologic and systemic causes. Certain patterns may suggest metabolic disorders (particularly liver failure), encephalitis (especially herpes simplex), or epileptic status; and focal abnormalities may point to a stroke, abscess, or tumor. A *magnetic resonance imaging (MRI) or computed tomography (CT) scan* is not an emergency procedure unless examination or the EEG suggests a focal lesion, but should be considered if no systemic cause is found after initial investigation.

MANAGEMENT The patient with acute confusion state is often agitated, and before the appropriate examination and investigations can be completed, the cooperation of the patient is required. Patients can frequently be calmed by a sympathetic and friendly physician. A relative or friend can often help and should be encouraged to stay with the patient. Nursing care should be given in a well-lit, relatively quiet environment with facilities for frequent observation. Sedation is seldom required with these measures. However, in some agitated, violent, or paranoid patients parenteral medication may prevent harm to the patient or others and allow completion of the examination, investigation, or treatment. A long-acting oral or intramuscular major tranquilizer such as chlorpromazine or haloperidol is usually suitable, but for short-term sedation, such as during a CT scan, an intravenous benzodiazapine may be appropriate. The possibility that psychopharmaceutical agents may exacerbate an abnormal mental state or disguise the neurologic signs of deterioration should be borne in mind.

Management begins with identification and correction of hypoxia, hypoglycemia, hyperthermia, or dehydration. Parenteral thiamine should be given to all patients suspected of Wernicke's encephalopathy. Subsequent treatment depends on the underlying cause. If the confusional state does not quickly resolve, attention to the hydration and nutrition of the patient is required to prevent perpetuation of the confusional state.

AMNESIA

PATHOPHYSIOLOGY The anatomic basis of memory is only partly understood, but clearly involves the temporal lobes. Most lesions cause long-term memory loss without affecting immediate memory or attention. As a rule, significant amnesia occurs only after bilateral lesions of the medial temporal lobes. Unilateral lesions of the speech dominant temporal lobe cause deficits of verbal memory, and unilateral lesions of the nondominant temporal lobe result in deficits in visual or nonverbal recall, but these deficits are rarely significant in the absence of preexisting contralateral temporal lobe pathology. The minimum lesion required to produce amnesia has not been established, but involvement of limbic structures appears crucial. Cholinergic neurons may play an important role. For example, anticholinergic drugs disrupt memory storage, and cholinergic drugs may on occasion improve memory.

CLINICAL FEATURES The classic example of amnesia is *Korsakoff's syndrome,* secondary to chronic alcoholism (see Chap. 357 and Chap. 370). The cardinal feature is an inability to recall new information despite a normal level of consciousness. Immediate memory, digit span, and attention are normal. Memory of knowledge acquired before the onset of illness is relatively intact, but memory for new events is severely impaired. Patients are disoriented in place and time and incapable of recalling information for more than the duration of immediate memory. They are thus condemned to be brief visitors to the present; their inner world consists only of memories of their remote past. On first encounter, they may seem relatively normal, taking part in ward routine and engaging in conversation. Because of intact immediate memory they retain information briefly but forget as soon as they are distracted. In the pure syndrome, tests of intelligence not requiring long-term memory may be normal. Compensation is by confabulation, giving more or less plausible answers incorporating some relevant information and sometimes fantastic elaboration. Although characteristic, confabulation is not universal in Korsakoff's syndrome and may be seen in amnesia of all causes and in acute confusional states. Amnesic subjects can slowly and laboriously learn some tasks, such as tactile or visual mazes, tunes on the piano, and the use of a computer. Despite evidence that the subjects acquire and retain new skills, they do not recall learning and deny the new skills, demonstrating dramatically a disassociation between recollection and retention of information.

DIFFERENTIAL DIAGNOSIS The diagnosis of *Korsakoff's syndrome* is usually clear from its association with chronic alcoholism. It often follows an episode of Wernicke's encephalopathy, and the amnesic deficit becomes evident with recovery from the acute confusional state. Nonalcoholic causes of *thiamine deficiency* (see Chap. 357) may cause Korsakoff's syndrome. Similar clinical syndromes may occur after bilateral temporal lobe lesions resulting from *medial temporal lobectomy, head injury, herpes simplex encephalitis, strokes,* or *brain tumors. Alzheimer's disease* (see below) may also cause isolated amnesia before generalized dementia becomes evident.

Temporary amnesia is a common feature of *head injury* (see Chap. 352). The memory disturbance occurs both for events before (*retrograde amnesia*) and after (*posttraumatic amnesia*) the time of injury. *Anterograde amnesia* refers to impairment in learning new material, which accompanies posttraumatic amnesia. Almost invariably, retrograde amnesia causes permanent inability to recall the few minutes prior to the head injury, implying disruption of the immediate memory system and failure to register long-term memory. In severe head injuries retrograde amnesia may extend back for hours or weeks. With recovery, the duration of retrograde amnesia shrinks and may resolve. During retrograde amnesia, remote memory is usually accessible. The length of posttraumatic amnesia generally corresponds to the length of postconcussive confusion and may be present despite normal immediate memory and digit span. The duration of posttraumatic amnesia is an indicator of the severity of head injury, the ability to learn new material often being the last cognitive deficit to recover.

Transient global amnesia is a syndrome in which a previously well person suddenly becomes confused and amnesic. The attacks are usually spontaneous but occasionally follow immersion in cold or hot water, emotional stimuli, physical exertion, sexual intercourse, or travel in a motor vehicle. The patient appears bewildered and repeatedly asks questions about present and recent events. Orientation for person and sometimes place is preserved, but recent memory is impaired and the patient cannot recall new information after a few minutes delay. Behavior is otherwise normal and appropriate. Examination during an attack shows intact immediate memory but severe impairment of recall of recent and sometimes more distant events. General intellectual function is normal. By definition, no other neurologic signs are present. The attacks usually last 2 to 12 h. Headache, nausea, and vomiting may occur. Recovery is complete, and recurrence is unusual. The cause of transient global amnesia is a mystery. Associations with migraine-like phenomena, temporal lobe ischemia, and epilepsy have been described. The disorder is usually benign; rarely, the attack is due to an underlying temporal lobe tumor.

Brief "blanks" in memory may cause difficulties in diagnosis. Occasionally *complex partial seizures* may occur without the patient being conscious of any associated signs or loss of awareness, apart from the disruption of memory during the seizure. Amnesia may also rarely accompany *classical migraine.* A number of *drugs,* including alcohol and short-acting benzodiazepines, may impair memory and cause amnesia for events during the period of their use. *Electroconvulsive therapy* (ECT) causes temporary retrograde and anterograde amnesia.

Psychogenic amnesia for personally important memories is common, although whether this results from deliberate avoidance of unpleasant memories or from unconscious repression may be impossible to establish. This *event-specific amnesia* is particularly common after violent crimes such as homicide of a close relative but uncommon in nonviolent crimes. This type of amnesia is also associated with severe drug or alcohol intoxication and sometimes with schizophrenia. More prolonged psychogenic amnesia occurs in *fugue states* that also commonly follow severe emotional stress. The patient with a fugue state suffers from a sudden loss of personal identity and may be found wandering far from home. In contrast to organic amnesia, fugue states are associated with amnesia for personal identity and events closely associated with the personal past. At the same time, memory for other recent events and the ability to learn and use new information are preserved. The episodes usually last hours or days and occasionally weeks or months while the patient takes on a new identity. On recovery there is a residual amnesic gap for the period of the fugue.

MANAGEMENT   The cause of temporary amnesia is usually evident from the history. In patients with transient global amnesia investigations to exclude an underlying structural cause (MRI or CT), epilepsy (EEG), and vascular risk factors are appropriate. Unless the investigations are positive, reassurance is the only further measure required. The management of persistent amnesia is more demanding. Although Wernicke's encephalopathy responds to thiamine, established Korsakoff's syndrome does not, and the amnesia is usually permanent. Nevertheless, a course of thiamine should be given in newly diagnosed cases to prevent further deterioration.

DEMENTIA

Dementia is common, affecting about 4 million people in the United States alone, and is the major cause of long-term disability in old age. The prevalence of dementia increases rapidly with age, afflicting about 2 percent of the population between ages 65 and 70 and 20 percent of people above 80. With increasing longevity of the population and decreasing birth rates, the prevalence will continue to rise.

PATHOPHYSIOLOGY   Some authorities separate dementia occurring before the age of 65 (presenile dementia) from that occurring after (senile dementia). This distinction was based on the assumption that the causes were different: rare degenerations in the young and vascular disease or senescence in the elderly. Although the expression of diseases may differ at different ages, the major findings in demented patients of all ages are similar, and the distinction arbitrary.

Most diseases causing dementia are either widespread neuronal degenerations or multifocal disorders. The initial symptoms depend on where the dementing process starts, but the location and numbers of neurons lost that are required to cause dementia is difficult to establish. Aging results in a gradual loss of neurons and of brain mass, but this is not accompanied by significant intellectual decline in the absence of disease. Indeed, brain mass is a poor guide to intellectual function. Patients with a degenerative dementia in the sixth decade may have a greater brain mass than intellectually normal patients in their eighth decade. Consequently, documentation of generalized atrophy by CT scan is not a clear indication of dementia.

Dementia may result from cortical disease (e.g., Alzheimer's disease) or from disease of subcortical structures such as the basal ganglia, thalamus, and deep white matter (e.g., Huntington's disease). Cortical dementia is characterized by loss of cognitive functions such as language, perception, calculation; in contrast, subcortical dementia exhibits slowing of cognition and information processing ("bradyphrenia"), flattening of the affect, and disturbances of motivation, mood, and arousal. Memory is impaired in both types. The features of subcortical dementia also occur in cortical processes affecting the frontal lobes and probably reflect damaged projections to and from the frontal lobes.

In Alzheimer's disease, which is the commonest cause of dementia, the dementia results from loss of cortical tissue especially in the temporal and frontal lobes. This is accompanied in most cases by increased space between the gyri and enlargement of the ventricles. The histologic hallmark is the presence of numerous neurofibrillary tangles and senile plaques (see Chap. 359). Plaques and tangles are found in normal elderly brains but are increased in number in Alzheimer's disease, especially in the hippocampus and temporal lobes. The hippocampal involvement probably accounts for the memory disorder, which may be partially mediated by a reduction in cholinergic activity. The activities of other neurotransmitters including norepinephrine, serotonin, dopamine, glutamate, and somatostatin are also reduced. These changes are accompanied by reductions in cerebral blood flow and decreased metabolism of oxygen and glucose.

DIFFERENTIAL DIAGNOSIS   The causes of dementia are numerous (Table 30-3). However, a small number of diseases account for most cases. In most of the western world, Alzheimer's disease is responsible for 50 to 90 percent and vascular disease for 5 to 10 percent of cases of dementia referred to hospital. In Japan and parts of Scandinavia, vascular disease appears to be more prevalent than Alzheimer's disease, at least in hospitalized patients. Cerebral infarction contributes to intellectual loss in a further 15 percent of patients with Alzheimer's disease documented at autopsy (*mixed dementia*). Dementia attributed to ethanol abuse may account for 5 to 10 percent of cases. Metabolic disturbances, cerebral neoplasms, subdural hematoma, and normal-pressure hydrocephalus account for around 10 percent of cases, and Huntington's chorea for about 2 percent. The remainder of causes, including Creutzfeldt-Jakob disease, are rare, accounting for less than 1 percent of cases. In human immunodeficiency virus (HIV) infection, dementia is present in 30 to 40 percent of patients.

An important aim of diagnosis is to identify treatable causes of dementia. The differential diagnosis depends primarily on a careful history and examination, supported by investigation. Illnesses that cause dementia can be divided into those in which dementia is the

TABLE 30-3 Differential diagnosis of dementia

Primary dementia with no other signs
  Alzheimer's disease
  Pick's disease
  Frontal lobe degeneration
Dementia with signs of vascular disease
  Multi-infarct dementia*
  Thalamic infarction
  "Binswanger's disease"* and lacunar state*
  Vasculitis,* e.g., systemic lupus erythematosus, polyarteritis nodosa,
    granulomatous angiitis of the central nervous system, Behçet's disease
Dementia with evidence of chronic infection†
  Human immunodeficiency virus
  Syphilis*
  Papovavirus (progressive multifocal leukoencephalopathy)
  Subacute sclerosing panencephalitis
  Creutzfeldt-Jakob disease (subacute spongiform encephalopathy)
  Tuberculosis,* fungal* and protozoal infections*
  Sarcoidosis*
  Whipple's disease*
Secondary dementia with signs of the underlying neurologic condition
  Neoplasia and mass lesions
    Primary and secondary tumors*
    Carcinomatous meningitis
    Paraneoplastic encephalitis
    Chronic subdural hematoma*
    Hydrocephalus*
  Movement disorders
    Parkinson's disease
    Lewy body dementia
    Huntington's chorea
    Progressive supranuclear palsy (Steele-Richardson syndrome)
    Multisystem degeneration (Shy-Drager syndrome)
    Hereditary ataxias
  Motor neuron disease (amyotrophic lateral sclerosis)
  Multiple sclerosis
Dementia following diffuse brain damage‡
  Acute head injury
  Pugilistic dementia
  Anoxia
  Encephalitis
Endocrine disorders and vitamin deficiency
  Hypothyroidism*
  B$_{12}$ deficiency*
  Thiamine deficiency*
  Nicotinic acid deficiency* (pellagra)
  Adrenal insufficiency* and Cushing's syndrome*
  Hypo-* and hyperparathyroidism*
  Chronic hypoglycemia*
Toxic disorders
  Drug and narcotic poisoning*
  Alcoholic dementia*
  Heavy metal intoxication*
  Organic toxins*
  Dialysis dementia*
Psychiatric
  Chronic schizophrenia
  Pseudodementia*
Additional conditions to consider in adolescents or young adults
  Movement disorders
    Wilson's disease*
    Hallervorden-Spatz disease
  Tuberous sclerosis
  Progressive myoclonic epilepsy*
  Metabolic diseases, e.g., leukodystrophies, mitochondrial cytopathy,
    storage diseases, Leigh's disease, homocystinuria

---

*Condition in which treatment may reverse or prevent progression of dementia.
†Systemic, hematologic or CSF findings suggest infection except in Creutzfeldt-Jakob disease.
‡History of acute injury with depression of consciousness usual, except in pugilistic dementia.

primary manifestation of the disease (other neurologic signs are absent); those in which dementia is secondary to other neurologic disorders (additional neurologic findings are usually present); and systemic diseases in which dementia is usually associated with signs outside the central nervous system.

In the elderly, dementia must be distinguished from the minor degree of forgetfulness that accompanies aging (*benign senescent forgetfulness*); the latter is often accompanied by slowing of physical and mental agility, inability to change course, and rigidity of thinking. This is by no means universal with aging and may reflect an unidentified disease process. Benign senescent forgetfulness is not disabling in the activities of daily life and does not progress to more severe disability. The early symptoms and signs of the degenerative dementias are often indistinguishable from those of benign senescence, and it is only the young age of the patient or progression of the symptoms that allows the diagnosis of dementia to be confirmed.

Primary dementia The diagnosis of *Alzheimer's disease* is only certain at autopsy but is usually reliably suggested by the characteristic history and signs, supported by negative investigations excluding other causes of dementia. Series of well-investigated patients with dementia attributed to Alzheimer's disease always include cases with an alternative diagnosis established at autopsy. The term *dementia of Alzheimer type* is sometimes used for patients with the characteristic clinical picture and negative investigations in whom pathologic confirmation has not been obtained.

The mean duration from the onset of symptoms to death is 8 years, with a range of 2 to 15 years. The course may be more rapid in younger patients. The early features vary according to the initial brain site involved. The onset is insidious and subtle, and can rarely be pinpointed. In most cases, insight is lost early, and the patient attributes failures to old age or oversight. Some have no spontaneous complaints but become disturbed when unable to answer simple questions. The history is almost invariably given by a relative. Early loss of spontaneity and initiative is frequent. The patient may give up hobbies and lose interest in social contacts or conversation. Lapses of memory, difficulty learning new information, and failure to remember names and appointments are noticed. At this stage, the memory deficit is more likely to involve recent events. In the early stages, social graces are usually preserved, and routine behavior and simple conversation are normal, so that friends and relatives may be unaware that anything is wrong, unless the patient is tested by an unfamiliar situation or by a formal examination of cognitive function. As the disease progresses, inexplicable mistakes are made in the activities of éveryday life, and dress, appearance, and personal hygiene are neglected. Spatial disorientation may become evident, especially in unfamiliar surroundings. The patient may oscillate between apathy and unprovoked irritability or aggression.

Examination in the early stage usually shows impairment of memory for recent events with varying degrees of cognitive deficit. The patient often appears puzzled in response to questioning. Primitive reflexes such as palmomental response or suck reflex may be present.

As the disease advances, the impairments of memory, speech, and behavior become so marked that patients are unable to care for themselves, repeat questions over and over again, and fail to recognize friends and relatives. Restlessness is common especially at night, and patients become lost if allowed to wander. Delusions, paranoia, and hallucinations may occur. On examination at this stage, the patient remains alert but is disoriented to time and place and has poor memory for recent and distant events. Digit span is usually preserved. Speech lacks spontaneity and fluency and exhibits minor aphasic errors, and there is difficulty understanding complex commands. Nonfluent aphasia, especially in younger patients, may be striking. Motor and constructional apraxia and agnosia may be present. Extrapyramidal signs, including stooped posture, slow shuffling gait, generalized bradykinesia, and rigidity, are common. The tendon reflexes may be brisk, but extensor plantar responses are rare. Grasp reflexes may be elicited. In the last stage the patient is immobile, mute, and incontinent. The patient no longer recognizes relatives, and testing of cognitive function is not possible. Seizures and myoclonus may become prominent. Weight loss and a shrunken appearance may precede death, often from intercurrent infection.

Pick's disease is characterized by circumscribed cortical atrophy, usually confined to the frontal and temporal lobes, associated with a characteristic histologic appearance of degenerating neurons in the cortex, basal ganglia, and brainstem (Pick's bodies) (see Chap. 359). The age at onset and course are similar to Alzheimer's disease. Patients with Pick's disease suffer slowly progressive dementia and in the early stages may show frontal-temporal lobe features uncommon in Alzheimer's disease, including personality and emotional changes, disinhibition, lack of restraint, poor social and sexual conduct, and lack of foresight. Later, patients may appear euphoric or retreat into increasing apathy and abulia in association with nonfluent aphasia, which progresses to mutism. Comprehension of speech and spatial functions are relatively spared. Some cases of Pick's disease are indistinguishable clinically from Alzheimer's disease, and some cases of Alzheimer's disease show a frontal predominance so that the distinction may only be made at autopsy. A similar picture of *frontal lobe dementia* may occur in association with primary neuronal degeneration in the frontal and anterior temporal lobes without the neuropathologic findings of either Alzheimer's or Pick's disease.

Vascular dementia   In most instances vascular dementia results from multiple areas of discrete infarction and not from chronic diffuse ischemia. The term *multi-infarct dementia* emphasizes this distinction. The diagnosis of vascular dementia is strongly suggested by an abrupt onset, especially if there is a history of previous stroke. The course characteristically fluctuates with periods of improvement and stepwise deterioration, in contrast to the steady progression of Alzheimer's disease. Hypertension is usual in vascular dementia but rare in Alzheimer's disease. Nocturnal confusion, relative preservation of personality, emotional lability, somatic complaints, and depression are more common in vascular dementia but not diagnostic. Focal neurologic signs (other than those of the cognitive deficits) including pseudobulbar palsy, visual field deficits, hemiparesis, or extensor plantar responses may suggest vascular dementia but may also be symptomatic of other neurologic causes such as a tumor.

Multi-infarct dementia can result from all types of cerebral vascular disease but is most likely to result from recurrent bilateral cerebral embolism from the heart or carotid arteries. It can also occur following a single episode such as severe hypotension or cardiac arrest if the degree of bilateral brain damage is sufficient. Multi-infarct dementia may also result from widespread involvement of small vessels by vasculitis, from a few strategically placed large cortical infarcts, or from multiple small infarcts in subcortical structures, such as occurs in the *lacunar state* secondary to hypertensive small-vessel disease (see Chap. 351). Hypertensive or atherosclerotic disease with thickening of the perforating deep vessels and capillaries supplying the subcortical white matter may also cause *Binswanger's disease (subcortical arteriosclerotic encephalopathy)* in which dementia is associated with diffuse loss of subcortical white matter and enlargement of the underlying ventricle. In contrast to multi-infarct dementia, major stroke is unusual in Binswanger's disease, and examination shows features of subcortical dementia (see above), a characteristic small-stepped, wide-based gait (marche à petit pas), pseudobulbar palsy, and corticospinal signs.

Chronic infections   Chronic infections are important to consider, as the dementia may be treatable. Infections of the CNS are usually associated with systemic manifestations, meningeal involvement, abnormal CSF, and abnormalities on MRI or CT scan. Cerebral *syphilis* was a major cause and should still be excluded in all patients (see Chap. 128). *Human immunodeficiency virus* infection, also sexually transmitted, is an important cause of dementia in young people (see Chap. 134) but should also be considered in all patients at risk. The dementia usually occurs as a part of acquired immunodeficiency syndrome (AIDS) but may be the first manifestation. Dementia may also arise from "slow" virus infections. *Subacute sclerosing panencephalitis* causes dementia in children and occasionally in adolescents due to persistent replication of the measles virus in the brain many years after initial infection (see Chap. 355). *Creutzfeldt-Jacob disease (subacute spongiform encephalopathy)*, a rare dementia, has been transmitted by an unknown agent to animals and to humans by corneal transplantation, neurosurgical instrumentation, or injections of growth hormone extracted from human pituitaries. In most cases the route of infection is unknown. After incubating for several years, the illness occurs in middle or late life and progresses to death within months. The dementia is often combined with ataxia, corticospinal signs, abnormal movements, cortical blindness, and myoclonus (see Chap. 355). Bizarre behavior and hallucinations are sometimes striking. In contrast to most other infections of the nervous system, signs of intracranial inflammation are absent and the CSF is normal.

Neoplasia and mass lesions   *Primary or secondary brain tumors* may present with dementia, particularly slowly growing, deep, midline tumors of the corpus callosum or frontal lobe. Frontal meningiomas are the most important to consider in all patients as they are benign and the dementia potentially curable. Other curable mass lesions include *chronic subdural hematoma*. The head trauma in such cases may have been remote, trivial, or forgotten, particularly in the elderly. Diffuse primary tumors and multiple secondary tumors may also cause dementia. Features of raised intracranial pressures (such as headaches or papilledema) and focal signs apart from the cognitive disorders may be absent, although minor signs such as a grasp reflex or extensor plantar response are often present. Most causes of dementia due to mass lesions or raised intracranial pressure are easily diagnosed from the MRI or CT scan.

Malignancy arising outside the nervous system may also cause dementia through *metastatic carcinomatous meningitis* or from a *nonmetastatic paraneoplastic encephalitis* (see Chap. 353). The latter condition usually begins insidiously and progresses slowly. Depression of consciousness is absent in the early stages, and psychiatric disturbances may be striking. The CSF is usually abnormal in these conditions.

Obstructive or communicating hydrocephalus in adults characteristically presents with subacute progressive dementia and is an important treatable cause. A history of headache may be obtained, and ataxia and gait disturbance are usual. Signs of raised intracranial pressure may be absent. The diagnosis is hampered in the elderly by the difficulty of distinguishing the scan appearances of hydrocephalus due to abnormal CSF dynamics from hydrocephalus "ex vacuo" secondary to atrophy. However, the combination of dementia, urinary incontinence, and gait disorder suggests the syndrome of *normal- or low-pressure hydrocephalus*. In this condition, routine measurements of CSF pressure at lumbar puncture or ventriculography are normal, but intermittent waves of increased CSF pressure may be detected if patients are monitored for several days. Such cases may respond to ventricular drainage.

Movement disorders   A number of degenerative neurologic diseases other than the primary dementias may also cause dementia, usually as a late manifestation. Movement disorders provide the largest group, of which the most common is *idiopathic Parkinson's disease*, where dementia develops in the late stages of the disease in 15 to 30 percent (see Chap. 359). Another important cause is Huntington's chorea, partly because the diagnosis has genetic implications (see Chap. 359). In these conditions, the cause of the dementia is usually evident from the history or clinical signs of the underlying neurologic disease, but very occasionally the dementia may be the only feature.

Diffuse brain damage   In dementia secondary to *head injury, anoxia, hypoglycemia,* or *encephalitis* the cause is usually obvious from the history. The initial insult almost invariably causes loss of consciousness, and the dementia becomes evident when consciousness is regained after prolonged coma. If the patient recovers but then declines intellectually, the possibility of a secondary cause of dementia such as hydrocephalus should be considered. Repeated, less severe head trauma, such as occurs in boxers, may also lead to dementia later in life (*dementia pugilistica*, or the "punch drunk" syndrome), associated with extrapyramidal signs, dysarthria, and ataxia.

Endocrine disorders and vitamin deficiency   Imbalances sufficient to affect neuronal function usually cause an acute confusional state with disturbance of attention and consciousness, but on occasion the presentation may be more chronic and mimic dementia. These conditions are treatable and cause reversible dementia, and they must be excluded in all patients. *Hypothyroidism* is the most common endocrine condition to present with dementia.

Toxic disorders Intoxications usually present with acute confusional state, often fluctuating according to the exposure. However, chronic intoxication may result in a reversible dementia. *Drugs* are an important cause, especially in the elderly, and the medication history should be carefully reviewed. The list of potential agents is large and includes drugs of abuse, psychotherapeutic agents (including barbiturates, sleeping tablets, tranquilizers, and antidepressants), drugs used in Parkinson's disease (levodopa and anticholinergics), and anticonvulsants. *Alcohol* is the most prevalent intoxicant implicated in dementia. Chronic inebriation results in reversible intellectual impairment but may also lead to a persistent deficit. In some cases, this is pure amnesia due to Korsakoff's psychosis, but in others it is a global dementia, associated with cerebral atrophy. Factors accounting for dementia in alcoholics include vitamin deficiency, repeated head injury, anoxia or hypoglycemia during alcoholic stupor, chronic liver failure, or the rare complication of *Marchiafava-Bignami disease,* which causes widespread demyelination in the cerebral hemispheres.

Dementia in adolescents and young adults This requires consideration of a further group of conditions in addition to those already mentioned (Table 30-3). Late presentation of *Wilson's disease* is another important example of a treatable dementia and should be excluded in all patients under the age of 40. Metabolic diseases are the largest group. There is usually evidence of a systemic disorder such as a peripheral neuropathy, myopathy, retinopathy, or hepatosplenomegaly. Specific diagnosis relies on special investigation.

Pseudodementias Nonorganic causes of apparent intellectual decline are not rare, although it is probably more frequent for organic dementia to be misdiagnosed initially as a psychiatric illness. A mistaken diagnosis is particularly common in the elderly, in whom the behavioral changes of dementia may be attributed to depression. Conversely, the severely depressed patient may appear disoriented and perform poorly in all aspects of intellectual function. These deficits are caused by the psychomotor retardation, apathy, and loss of interest that accompanies depression. Such intellectual impairments may be due to reversible neurochemical changes that mimic the irreversible changes of degenerative dementias. The distinction may be difficult, but the correct diagnosis of depression is often suggested by a history of sudden onset, marked sleep disturbance, a previous history of psychiatric illness, or precipitation by an emotional event. In addition, depressed patients often complain to a greater extent about difficulties with mentation that seems justified from their performance on tests of intellectual function. In contrast, the patient with true dementia rarely complains appropriately about deficits that are obvious on examination. Dementia due to depression may also be suggested by inconsistency during the history; for example, patients may give a clear account of some topic of interest to them or recount the history and details of their personal lives reasonably well but then show inconsistent difficulties with specific questions, often failing even to attempt an answer. Variability in performance during testing, particularly improvement with encouragement, is characteristic. Negative neurologic investigation supports the diagnosis of pseudodementia but may also be found in organic dementia. The only way to confirm the diagnosis is to demonstrate improvement in intellectual functioning with appropriate psychiatric treatment (see Chap. 368).

Pseudodementias may also occur as a *hysterical phenomenon,* when amnesia is often striking. In one variety of pseudodementia (Ganser syndrome) the answers to simple questions are often inaccurate but the patient may retain a sense of the purpose of the question (''approximate'' answers) indicating that, despite the absurdity of the answer, the question is understood and the correct answer is known to the patient. In hysterical pseudodementia and the Ganser syndrome the apparent severe disturbance of intellect is not reflected in the patient's behavior. Frank simulation of dementia is rare, although the distinction between hysteria and malingering is not always clear. Intellectual impairment is a feature of *mania* and *schizophrenia;* the diagnosis is made from the accompanying thought disorder (see Chap. 368).

INVESTIGATION The age, history, and clinical findings will dictate the selection of screening tests (Table 30-4). Investigations essential in all patients are aimed at excluding reversible causes of dementia. Ideally, every patient with dementia should have an *MRI* or *CT scan* to exclude treatable intracranial pathology, especially in the presence of focal clinical signs, a history of subacute illness, or a younger age of patient. Scanning is less likely to influence management if the patient is elderly and has a long history of degenerative dementia. In Alzheimer's disease the scan may show progressive cortical atrophy and ventricular dilatation, but this is not invariable and can also be found in normal aging. The CT or MRI may show areas of low attenuation or abnormal signal in the deep white matter, particularly in the periventricular regions and centrum semiovale, referred to by the descriptive term *leuko-araiosis.* These findings are characteristic of Binswanger's disease but are not specific and can also be seen in Alzheimer's disease, in patients with cerebrovascular disease who are not demented, and in apparently normal subjects. The *electroencephalogram* may show features that support the diagnosis of Alzheimer's disease, subacute sclerosing panencephalitis, or Creutzfeldt-Jakob disease. *CSF examination* is normal in the primary degenerative dementias but may be useful if there is doubt about the diagnosis and is essential if there is a suspicion of intracranial infection. *Regional cerebral blood flow studies* (e.g., single-photon emission computed tomography) may sometimes be useful in distinguishing between frontal lobe dementias and Alzheimer's disease or in demonstrating multifocal deficits in vascular dementia. *Cerebral angiography* is rarely helpful except for the further investigation of suspected vascular dementia, vasculitis, or intracranial masses. *Neuropsychologic testing* (such as the Wechsler Adult Intelligence Scale) may help document intellectual decline or identify pseudodementia. *Meningeal and brain biopsy* may occasionally be justified when infection, vasculitis, or treatable tumor is suspected and occasionally in younger patients when etiology remains in doubt.

MANAGEMENT The initial management includes treatment of any reversible cause of dementia or superimposed confusional state. Approximately 10 percent of patients with dementia have a treatable neurologic or systemic illness, and another 10 percent have pseudodementia due to treatable psychiatric illnesses. A modifiable contributory cause such as alcoholism or hypertension is present in a further

---

TABLE 30-4   Investigation of dementia

In all cases:
    Blood count and erythrocyte sedimentation rate
    Blood sugar
    Serum electrolytes and calcium
    Liver function tests
    Thyroid function tests
    Serum B_{12} and folate
    Serology for syphilis
    Chest x-ray
    Electroencephalogram
    CT or MRI scan
In selected cases:
    CSF examination
    Neuropsychologic testing
    Human immunodeficiency virus antibodies
    Infectious diseases screen
    Autoantibody screen and immunoglobulins
    Serum copper and ceruloplasmin
    Drug and toxin screen
    Arterial blood gases
    Cerebral angiography
    Cerebral blood flow studies
In very selected cases:
    Brain biopsy
In suspected metabolic diseases:
    White cell enzyme screen
    Urinary and plasma amino acids
    Plasma pyruvate and lactate
    Urinary and fecal porphyrins
    Bone marrow, liver, nerve, muscle, or rectal biopsy

10 percent. Unfortunately, the remainder have irreversible dementia so that management aims to support the patient and the family.

The mildly demented patient may continue relatively normal activities at home but rarely at work. As the dementia progresses, more supervision is required, but the patient may still be capable of simple tasks. As the disorder deepens, the patient requires increasing help with the activities of daily life. The supervision required depends on the individual. Some fairly severely impaired patients can live alone if they have support from the community, including daily visits from family or friends, regular visits by a community nurse, the provision of meals, and help from neighbors. Many mildly demented individuals become disoriented and confused when removed to unfamiliar surroundings such as a hospital but may manage adequately in their homes.

In the early stages the patient may be helped by treatment of associated depression, anxiety, agitation, psychotic symptoms, or insomnia with appropriate psychotropic medication. However, psychotropic drugs may make demented patients more confused, requiring reduction or withdrawal of the medication. The demands on relatives caring for a severely demented patient are high, especially if the patient is restless at night and requires constant supervision to prevent wandering or personal harm. The fact that individuals may live for many years in such a state increases the burden. The situation often becomes intolerable when incontinence develops. Sleep deprivation and physical exhaustion aggravate the stress of caring for a demented relative, who may appear ungrateful, cantankerous, aggressive, or disinhibited. Sympathetic attention to the relatives of the demented is therefore important. It may help to obtain a "baby sitter" to allow the caregiver regular time off. If the caregiver can do so without undue feelings of guilt, an annual holiday while the patient is placed in a nursing home temporarily is invaluable.

Eventually, many demented patients require full-time nursing care in a residential home or hospital. Relatives should be encouraged to plan for this and should be counseled not to regard this outcome as a personal failure. In the later stages management aims at preserving the patient's dignity and comfort.

REFERENCES

Anthony JC et al: Limits of the "Mini-Mental State" as a screening test for dementia and delirium among hospital patients. Psychol Med 12:397, 1982

Blessed G et al: The association between quantitative measures of dementia and of senile change in the cerebral grey matter of elderly subjects, appendix. Br J Psychiatry 114:797, 1968

Brown MM, Hachinski VC: Vascular dementia. Curr Opinion Neurol Neurosurg 2:78, 1989

Cummings JL: Subcortical dementia: Neuropsychology, neuropsychiatry, and pathophysiology. Br J Psychiatry 149:682, 1989

—— et al: Reversible dementia: Illustrative cases, definition, and review. JAMA 243:2434, 1980

Geschwind N: Disorders of attention: A frontier in neuropsychology. Phil Trans R Soc Lond 198:173, 1982

Guberman A, Stuss D: The syndrome of bilateral paramedian thalamic infarction. Neurol 33:540, 1983

Gustafson L: Frontal lobe degeneration of non-Alzheimer type. Clinical picture and differential diagnosis. Arch Geront Geriat 6:209, 1987

Hachinski VC et al: Cerebral blood flow in dementia. Arch Neurol 32:632, 1975

Kopelman MD: Amnesia: Organic and psychogenic. Br J Psychiatry 150:428, 1987

Lipowski ZJ: Delirium (acute confusional state), in Handbook of Clinical Neurology. Amsterdam, Elsevier, 1985, vol 46, pp 523–559

Lishman WA: Organic Psychiatry: The Psychological Consequences of Cerebral Disorder, 2d ed. Oxford, Blackwell, 1987

Mesulam M et al: Acute confusional states with right middle cerebral artery infarctions. J Neurol Neursurg Psychiatry 39:84, 1976

Miller JW et al: Transient global amnesia: Clinical characteristics and prognosis. Neurol 37:733, 1987

Roman GC: Senile dementia of the Binswanger type: A vascular form of dementia in the elderly. JAMA 258:1782, 1987

Roth M, Iversen LL (eds): Alzheimer's disease and related disorders. Br Med Bull 42:1, 1986

Scholtz CL: Dementia in middle and late life. Curr Top Pathol 76:105, 1988

Wade JPH, Hachinski VC: Multi-infarct dementia, in Dementia (Medicine in Old Age). BM Pitt (ed). London, Churchill Livingstone, 1987, pp 209–228

31   COMA AND OTHER DISORDERS OF CONSCIOUSNESS

ALLAN H. ROPPER / JOSEPH B. MARTIN

Coma is a common problem in general medicine; it is estimated that up to 3 percent of admissions to the emergency ward of large municipal hospitals are due to diseases that cause a disorder of consciousness. The importance of this class of neurologic disorders points to the necessity of acquiring a systematic approach to their diagnosis and management.

The increased availability of computed tomography (CT) and magnetic resonance imaging (MRI) has resulted in an artificial focus on lesions that are radiologically detectable (e.g., hemorrhages, tumors, or hydrocephalus) in the diagnosis of coma. This approach, although at times expedient, is often imprudent because most coma is metabolic or toxic in origin. The physician confronted with an unresponsive patient should formulate a differential diagnosis based on the history and the clinical signs before leaving the bedside. Certain signs observed during general and neurologic examination allow the physician to decide which of several generic diseases is responsible for coma, thus limiting the diagnostic possibilities. A rational approach to the precise diagnosis and subsequent management can then be planned and clinical changes anticipated. The clinical approach must be coupled with knowledge of the pathologic entities that cause coma. This chapter describes a practical approach to coma based on the anatomy and physiology of consciousness, the general and neurologic examination, and CT and MRI.

Coma is epitomized by unresponsiveness and as such is easily recognized. The interesting and sometimes subtle distinctions made between coma, stupor, and drowsiness are at times clinically useful to transmit information concisely, but are largely semantic, because there is no anatomic or physiologic basis for distinguishing them except as relative degrees of unresponsiveness. A narrative description of the clinical state of the patient and of responses evoked by various stimuli, precisely as they are observed at the bedside, remains the optimal way to characterize coma and related disturbances of consciousness. Such a description is preferable to summary terms such as *semicoma* or *obtundation*, which are often ambiguous and commonly differ between observers. *Stupor*, as currently used, implies a state from which the patient can be aroused by vigorous stimuli but verbal responses are slow or absent and the patient makes some effort to avoid uncomfortable stimuli; *coma* suggests a state from which the patient cannot be aroused by stimulation, and no purposeful attempt is made to avoid painful stimuli.

Although the definition of consciousness is a psychological and philosophical matter, the distinction between *level* of consciousness, or wakefulness, and *content* of consciousness, or awareness, has physiologic significance. Wakefulness or alertness is maintained by a diffuse system of upper brainstem and thalamic neurons, the reticular activating system (RAS), and its connections to the cerebral hemispheres as a whole. Therefore, depression of either hemispheral or RAS activity may cause reduced wakefulness. Awareness is dependent on integrated and organized material thoughts, subjective experience, emotions, and mental processes, each of which resides to some extent in anatomically defined regions of the brain. The inability to maintain a coherent sequence of thoughts and actions is called *confusion* and is a disorder of content of consciousness. Reduced wakefulness often precludes evaluation of content of consciousness (for example, most stuporous patients can be said to be confused), but content of consciousness can be severely impaired, as in confusion, without affecting arousal. Confusion is used to describe a state of inattention and lack of clarity in thinking (see Chap. 30). In special cases it is accompanied by illusions (misperceptions of environmental sight, sound, or touch) or hallucinations (spontaneous endogenous perceptions). Psychiatrists often use the term *delirium* for any confusion, but delirium is usually reserved as a description for an agitated, hypersympathotonic, frequently hallucinatory state most often due to specific causes such as alcohol or drug withdrawal. Usually, the confused patient is subdued, not inclined to speak, and less active physically than usual. Many processes that ultimately lead to coma begin with confusion, and diagnostic considerations should address the primary problem as an alteration in the level of consciousness. Confusion alone generally indicates a metabolic derangement, although focal cerebral lesions that cause deficits in language, orientation, or memory may make the patient appear to be confused.

ANATOMIC CORRELATES OF CONSCIOUSNESS   A normal level of consciousness (wakefulness) depends upon activation of the cerebral hemispheres by groups of neurons located in the brainstem RAS. Both of the cerebral hemispheres, the RAS, and the connections between them must be preserved for normal consciousness. The principal causes of coma are, therefore, (1) bilateral hemispheral damage or suppression by drugs or toxins and (2) a brainstem lesion or metabolic derangement that damages or suppresses the RAS. There is some evidence that large, purely unilateral hemispheral lesions particularly on the left may cause drowsiness (though not coma) even in the absence of damage to the opposite hemisphere or RAS.

Reticular activating system   The RAS is best defined as a physiologic system, not an anatomic one. It is contained within the reticular formation, which consists of loosely grouped neurons located bilaterally in the medial tegmental gray matter of the brainstem extending from the medulla to the posterior diencephalon. These neurons have been shown in neuroanatomic studies to span long rostrocaudal distances within the reticular formation. Animal experiments and human clinical-neuropathologic observations have established that the *neurons located in the region extending from the rostral pons to the caudal diencephalon are of primary importance for maintaining wakefulness*. Lesions here that produce coma also commonly affect adjacent brainstem structures concerned with control of pupillary constriction and mechanisms for eye movements (Fig. 31-1). Abnormalities in these systems on physical examination provide signposts of brainstem damage. Lesions confined to the cerebral hemispheres do not directly affect the brainstem RAS, though secondary dysfunction of the upper brainstem may result from compression by a mass in a cerebral hemisphere.

Brainstem RAS neurons project rostrally to the cortex, primarily via "nonspecific" thalamic relay nuclei which exert a tonic influence on the activity of the cerebral cortex. Experimental work in primates suggests that the brainstem RAS indirectly affects the level of consciousness by suppressing the activity of the nonspecific nuclei. Electrical stimulation of the pontine and midbrain RAS desynchronizes the electroencephalogram (EEG), a pattern associated with behavioral arousal. Stimulation of the thalamic relay nuclei opposes this activity, resulting in synchronization and slowing of the EEG. The basis of behavioral arousal by environmental stimuli (somesthetic, auditory, and visual) depends on the rich innervation of the RAS by each sensory system.

The relay between the RAS and thalamic and cortical areas is accomplished by neurotransmitters. Of these, the influences of acetylcholine and norepinephrine on arousals have been studied most extensively. Cholinergic fibers connect the midbrain to other areas of the upper brainstem, thalamus, and cortex. These pathways are thought to mediate the clinical and EEG arousal observed after administration of cholinergic drugs such as physostigmine. Serotonin and norepinephrine also subserve important functions in the regulation of the sleep-wake cycle (see Chap. 34). Their roles in arousal and coma have not been clearly established, although the alerting effects of amphetamines are likely to be mediated by catecholamine release.

Cerebral hemispheres and consciousness   The specialized functions of the cerebral cortex in language, control of movement, and perception are regionalized (see Chaps. 30, 32, and 33). In contrast, wakefulness is related in a semiquantitative way to the total mass of functioning cortex (and RAS connections) and is not focally represented in any region of the hemispheres. Hemispheral lesions

FIGURE 31-1   Brainstem reflexes in the coma examination. Midbrain and third nerve function are tested by pupillary reaction to light, pontine function by spontaneous and reflex eye movements and corneal responses, and medullary function by respiratory and pharyngeal responses.

Reflex conjugate, horizontal eye movements are dependent upon the medial longitudinal fasciculus (MLF) interconnecting the sixth and contralateral third nerve nuclei. Eye movements are elicited by head rotation (oculocephalic reflex) or caloric stimulation of the labyrinths (oculovestibular reflex). These reflex movements are suppressed in the awake patient by the cerebral hemispheres via their connections to the brainstem.

may cause coma in one of three ways: (1) most commonly, bilateral, generalized hemispheral lesions or metabolic derangements such as occur in encephalitis, generalized epilepsy, drug ingestion, global brain ischemia, and hypoglycemia interfere with awareness in a graded fashion as more cortical territory is damaged or rendered functionally inactive; (2) rarely, enlarging masses or secondary brain swelling initially confined to one side of the brain may compress the contralateral hemisphere, effectively creating bilateral hemispheral lesions; and (3) large lesions in one or both hemispheres may compress the brainstem and diencephalic RAS causing coma indirectly. *The degree of decrease in alertness is often related to the acuteness of onset of the cortical dysfunction*.

The concept of *transtentorial herniation* with progressive brainstem compression has been used to explain neurologic signs in coma caused by supratentorial mass lesions. Herniation refers to displacement of brain tissue away from a mass, past a less mobile structure such as dura, and into a space that it normally does not occupy. Herniation suggests a degree of irreversibility because the tissue is trapped in its new location. The common herniations seen at postmortem are transfalcial (under the falx in the anterior midline), transtentorial (into the tentorial opening), and cerebellar tonsillar (into the foramen magnum). Uncal transtentorial herniation, or impaction of the uncal gyrus into the cistern between the free edge of the tentorium and lateral edge of the midbrain, causes compression of the third nerve with pupillary dilation and subsequent coma due to midbrain compression. Central transtentorial herniation denotes downward movement of the diencephalon (thalamic region) through the tentorial opening in the midline and is heralded by miotic pupils and drowsiness. In both cases, an orderly progression of rostral to caudal compression of first the midbrain, then the pons, and finally the medulla leads to the sequential appearance of neurologic signs corresponding to the level damaged, and to progressively diminished alertness. However, many patients with supratentorial masses do not follow these stereotypic patterns; an orderly progression of signs from midbrain to medulla is rarely seen in catastrophic lesions where all brainstem functions are lost almost simultaneously. Furthermore, drowsiness and stupor typically occur with moderate lateral shifts at the level of the diencephalon (3 to 8 mm) when there is only 1- to 3-mm vertical displacement of structures near the tentorial opening, and before actual downward herniation is evident on a CT or MRI scan.

PATHOPHYSIOLOGY OF COMA   The pathophysiologic basis of coma is either mechanical destruction of crucial areas of the brainstem or cerebral cortex (anatomic coma) or global disruption of brain metabolic processes (metabolic coma). Coma of metabolic origin may be produced by interruption of energy substrate delivery (hypoxia, ischemia, hypoglycemia) or by alteration of the neurophysiologic responses of neuronal membranes (drug or alcohol intoxication, epilepsy, or acute head injury).

The brain is markedly dependent on continuous blood flow and delivery of oxygen and glucose, which are consumed at rates of 3.5 mL per 100 g/min and 5 mg per 100 g/min, respectively. Brain stores of glucose provide energy for approximately 2 min after blood flow is interrupted, although consciousness is lost within 8 to 10 s. When hypoxia occurs simultaneously with ischemia, available glucose is exhausted more rapidly. Normal resting cerebral blood flow (CBF) is approximately 75 mL per 100 g/min in gray matter and 30 mL per 100 g/min in white matter (mean = 55 mL per 100 g/min). This provides for adequate metabolic supplies with a modest safety factor to accommodate most physiologic changes. When mean CBF diminishes to 25 mL per 100 g/min, the EEG becomes diffusely slowed (typical of metabolic encephalopathies), and at 15 mL per 100 g/min brain electrical activity ceases. If all other conditions such as temperature and arterial oxygenation remain normal, CBF less than 10 mL per 100 g/min causes irreversible brain damage.

Coma due to hyponatremia, hyperosmolarity, hypercapnia, and the encephalopathies of hepatic and renal failure are associated with a variety of metabolic derangements of neurons and astrocytes. The toxic effects of these conditions on the brain are not well understood, but may be multifactorial, producing impaired energy supplies, changes in resting membrane potentials, neurotransmitter abnormalities, and in some instances morphologic changes. For example, the high brain ammonia concentration associated with hepatic coma has been theorized to interfere with cerebral energy metabolism and the Na^+,K^+-ATPase pump, increase the number and size of astrocytes, result in increased concentrations of potentially toxic products of ammonia metabolism, and result in abnormalities of neurotransmitters, including possible "false" neurotransmitters, which may act competitively at monoaminergic receptor sites.

The exact cause of the encephalopathy of renal failure is also poorly understood. Unlike ammonia, urea itself does not produce nervous system toxicity. A multifactorial cause is likely, including increased permeability of the blood-brain barrier to toxic substances such as organic acids and an increase in brain calcium or cerebrospinal fluid (CSF) phosphate content.

Abnormalities of osmolarity are involved in the coma and seizures caused by several medical disorders including diabetic ketoacidosis, the nonketotic hyperosmolar state, and hyponatremia. In hyperosmolarity, brain volume is reduced while hypoosmolarity leads to brain swelling. Brain water volume correlates best with level of consciousness in hyponatremic-hypoosmolar states but other factors probably also play a role. Sodium levels below 115 mmol/L are associated with coma and convulsions, depending to some extent on the rapidity with which the hyponatremia develops. Serum osmolarity is generally above 350 mosmol/L in hyperosmolar coma.

Hypercapnia produces a diminished level of consciousness proportional to the P_{CO_2} tension in the blood and to acuteness of onset. A relationship between CSF acidosis and severity of symptoms has been established. The pathophysiology of other metabolic encephalopathies such as hypercalcemia, hypothyroidism, vitamin B_{12} deficiency, and hypothermia are incompletely understood but probably reflect multifaceted derangements of cerebral biochemistry.

Central nervous system (CNS) depressant drugs and some endogenous toxins probably produce coma by suppression of metabolic and membrane electrical activities in both the RAS and cerebral cortex. For this reason combinations of cortical and brainstem signs occur in drug overdose and other metabolic comas which may lead to a specious diagnosis of structural brainstem damage. Certain anesthetic agents also have a predilection for affecting the brainstem RAS neurons out of proportion to the cortex.

Although all metabolic derangements alter neuronal electrophysiology, the disturbance of brain electrical activity most commonly encountered in clinical practice is epilepsy. Continuous, generalized electrical discharges of the cortex may be associated with coma even in the absence of epileptic motor activity. Coma following seizures (postictal state) may be due to exhaustion of energy metabolites or be secondary to locally toxic molecules produced during the seizures. Recovery from postictal unresponsiveness occurs when neuronal metabolic balance is restored. The postictal state produces a pattern of continuous, generalized slowing of the background EEG activity similar to that of metabolic encephalopathy.

Endogenous "excitatoxins" such as glutamate released after injury have been found to cause secondary neuronal damage in experimental models of ischemia. These endogenous "neurotoxins" act to allow calcium influx into cells, a mechanism thought to lead to neuronal death. This mechanism may play a role in the genesis of coma, or at least in its neuropathologic changes, after global ischemia.

PRACTICAL APPROACH TO THE COMATOSE PATIENT   The diagnosis and acute management of coma depend on understanding the pitfalls of examining the comatose patient, an interpretation of brainstem reflexes, and the wise use of diagnostic tests. Acute respiratory and cardiovascular problems should generally be attended to prior to neurologic diagnosis. The complete medical evaluation, except for the vital signs, fundoscopy, and examination for nuchal rigidity, may be deferred until the neurologic evaluation has established the severity and nature of coma.

History   In many cases the cause of coma is immediately evident (e.g., trauma, cardiac arrest, and known drug ingestion). However, in the remainder, historical information about the onset of coma is often sparse. The most useful historical points, when obtainable, are (1) the circumstances and temporal profile of the onset of neurologic symptoms, (2) the precise details of preceding neurologic symptoms (weakness, headaches, seizures, dizziness, diplopia, or vomiting), (3) the use of drugs or alcohol, and (4) history of liver, kidney, lung, heart, or other medical disease. Telephone calls to family and observers on the scene are an important part of the initial evaluation.

Physical examination and general observations   The temperature, pulse, respiratory rate and pattern, and blood pressure should be measured. Fever suggests systemic infection, bacterial meningitis, or a brain lesion that has disturbed the temperature-regulating centers. High body temperature, 42 to 44°C, associated with dry skin should arouse the suspicion of heat stroke or anticholinergic drug intoxication. Hypothermia is observed with bodily exposure; alcoholic, barbiturate, or phenothiazine intoxication; hypoglycemia; peripheral circulatory failure; or myxedema. Hypothermia causes coma directly only when the temperature is below 31°C. Aberrant respiratory patterns that may reflect brainstem disorders are discussed below. A change of pulse rate combined with hyperventilation and hypertension may signal an increase in intracranial pressure. Marked hypertension occurs in patients with hypertensive encephalopathy, cerebral hemorrhage, and other causes of acutely increased intracranial pressure. Hypotension occurs in the coma of alcohol or barbiturate intoxication, internal hemorrhage, myocardial infarction, gram-negative bacillary septicemia, and Addisonian crisis. The funduscopic examination is useful in detecting subarachnoid hemorrhage (subhyaloid hemorrhages), hypertensive encephalopathy (exudates, hemorrhages, vessel-crossing changes), and increased intracranial pressure (papilledema). Generalized cutaneous petechiae suggest thrombotic thrombocytopenic purpura or a bleeding diathesis associated with intracerebral hemorrhage.

General neurologic assessment   An exact description of spontaneous and elicited movements in coma is of great value in establishing the level of neurologic dysfunction. The patient's state is observed first without examiner intervention. The nature of respirations, similarity to sleep, and spontaneous movements are observed. Patients who toss about, reach up toward the face, cross the midline with an arm, cross their legs, yawn, swallow, cough, or moan are closest to being awake. Adventitious movements or postures may be subtle and must be specifically sought. For example, the only sign of seizures may be small excursion twitching of a foot, finger, or facial muscle. An outturned leg at rest or lack of restless movements on one side suggests a hemiparesis.

The terms *decorticate* and *decerebrate rigidity* or "posturing" have been adapted from animal experiments to describe stereotyped tonic flexor and extensor arm movements, respectively, with extension of the legs. Spontaneous flexion of the elbows and wrists and arm supination (decortication) suggest severe bilateral damage in the hemispheres above the midbrain, while extension of the elbows and wrists with pronation (decerebration) suggests damage in the midbrain or diencephalon. Arm extension with weak leg flexion or flaccid legs has been associated with lesions in the low pons. Acute lesions, however, frequently cause limb extension regardless of location, and almost all extensor posturing becomes flexor in nature as time passes, so posturing alone cannot be depended upon to make an accurate anatomic localization. Metabolic coma, especially after acute hypoxia, may also produce vigorous spontaneous extensor (decerebrate) rigidity. Posturing may alternate or coexist with purposeful limb movements, usually reflecting subtotal damage to the motor system. Multifocal myoclonus is almost always an indication of metabolic disorder, particularly azotemia, or drug ingestion. In an awake, confused patient, asterixis is a certain sign of metabolic encephalopathy or ingestion of a drug, particularly phenytoin.

Elicited movements and level of arousal   A sequence of increasingly intense stimuli is used to determine the patient's best level of arousal and the optimal motor response of each limb. If the patient is not aroused by conversational voice, shouting should be tried. Shaking the patient is attempted next, then painful pressure on the limbs. Nasal tickle with a cotton wisp is a strong arousal stimulus. Deep pressure on the knuckles or bony prominences is the preferred and humane form of noxious stimulus. Pinching the skin over the face or chest may cause unsightly ecchymoses and is rarely necessary.

Responses to noxious stimuli should be appraised critically. Abduction avoidance movement of a limb is a purposeful, cortically derived action and denotes an intact corticospinal system to that limb. If abduction is present in all limbs, it is a reliable sign of only minimal motor dysfunction. Stereotyped posturing following stimulation of a limb indicates severe dysfunction of the corticospinal system. Adduction and flexion of the stimulated limbs may occur as reflex movements and do not imply an intact corticospinal system. Brief clonic or twitching limb movements frequently occur at the end of extensor posturing excursions and should not be mistaken for seizures.

Brainstem reflexes   Brainstem signs are a key to the localization of the causative lesion in coma (Fig. 31-1). As a rule, coma associated with normal brainstem function indicates widespread and bilateral hemispheral disease or dysfunction. The brainstem contains several intrinsic reflexes that are convenient to examine. Normal pupillary symmetry, size, shape, and reaction to light indicate intact functioning of the upper midbrain and efferent parasympathetic fibers of the third

cranial nerve responsible for pupillary constriction. (The afferent component of the light reflex utilizes the optic nerve.) Pupillary reaction should be examined with a bright diffuse light and, if absent, confirmed with a magnifying lens. Light reaction in pupils smaller than 2 mm is often difficult to appreciate. Excessive room lighting mutes pupillary reactivity. Equal and reactive round pupils (2.5 to 5 mm in diameter) usually exclude midbrain damage as the cause of coma. An enlarged (greater than 5 mm) and unreactive or poorly reactive pupil can result either from an intrinsic midbrain lesion (on the same side) or, far more commonly, can be secondary to compression of the midbrain and/or third nerve as occurs in transtentorial herniation. Unilateral pupillary enlargement usually denotes an ipsilateral mass but rarely can occur contralaterally by compression of the midbrain against the opposite tentorial margin. Oval and slightly eccentric pupils (corectopia) often accompany early midbrain–third nerve compression. Bilaterally dilated and unreactive pupils indicate severe midbrain damage, usually from secondary compression by transtentorial herniation or metabolically by ingestion of drugs with anticholinergic activity. The use of mydriatic eye drops by a previous examiner, self-administration by the patient, or direct ocular trauma may cause misleading pupillary enlargement. Reactive and bilaterally small but not pinpoint pupils (1 to 2.5 mm) are most commonly seen in metabolic encephalopathy or after deep bilateral hemispheral lesions such as hydrocephalus or thalamic hemorrhage. This has been attributed to dysfunction of sympathetic nervous system efferents emerging from the posterior hypothalamus. Profound barbiturate-induced coma may produce similar-sized pupils. Very small but reactive pupils (less than 1 mm) denote narcotic overdose but may also occur with acute, extensive bilateral pontine damage, usually from hemorrhage. The response to naloxone and the presence of reflex eye movements (see below) distinguishes these. The unilaterally small pupil of a Horner's syndrome is rare in coma but may occur ipsilateral to a large cerebral hemorrhage.

Eye movements are the foundation of physical diagnosis in coma because their examination permits exploration of a large portion of the rostrocaudal extent of the brainstem. The eyes are first observed by elevating the lids and noting the resting position and spontaneous movements of the globes. Horizontal divergence of the eyes at rest is normally observed in drowsiness. As patients either awaken or slip deeper into coma, the ocular axes become parallel again. An adducted eye at rest indicates lateral rectus paresis (weakness) due to a sixth nerve lesion and may indicate damage to the pons. However, sixth nerve paresis, often bilateral, occurs with increased intracranial pressure and is then a falsely localizing sign. An abducted eye at rest, often accompanied by ipsilateral pupillary enlargement, indicates medial rectus paresis due to third nerve paresis. With few exceptions, vertical separation of the ocular axes, or *skew deviation*, results from pontine or cerebellar lesions. In hydrocephalus with dilatation of the third ventricle, the eye globes frequently rest below the horizontal meridian. Conjugate ocular deviation at rest is discussed below.

When spontaneous eye movements are present in coma, they generally take the form of conjugate horizontal roving. This motion exonerates the midbrain and pons and has the same meaning as normal reflex eye movements (see below). Cyclic vertical downward movements are seen in specific circumstances. "Ocular bobbing" describes a brisk conjugate downward and slow upward movement of the globes in situations in which horizontal eye movement mechanisms have been disrupted and is diagnostic of bilateral pontine damage. "Ocular dipping" is a slow downward movement followed by a faster upward movement in patients with normal reflex horizontal gaze. Dipping occurs particularly in patients with diffuse anoxic damage to the cerebral cortex and may be preceded by sustained up or down gaze. The eyes may turn down and inward in thalamic and upper midbrain lesions.

Doll's-eye, or *oculocephalic*, movements are tested by moving the head from side to side or vertically, first slowly then briskly. Reflex eye movements are evoked in the opposite direction to head movement (Fig. 31-1). These responses are mediated by brainstem mechanisms originating in the labyrinths, vestibular nuclei, and cervical proprioceptors. They are normally suppressed by visual fixation mediated by the cerebral hemispheres in awake patients. The neuronal pathways for reflex horizontal eye movements require integrity of the region surrounding the sixth nerve nucleus and are yoked to the contralateral third nerve via the medial longitudinal fasciculus (MLF) (Fig. 31-1). Two disparate pieces of information can be obtained from the reflex eye movements. *First,* in coma resulting from bihemispheral disease or early metabolic or drug depression, the eyes move easily or "loosely" from side to side in a direction opposite to the direction of head turning. The ease with which the globes move toward the opposite side is a reflection of disinhibition of brainstem reflexes by damaged cerebral hemispheres. In drowsy patients, the first two or three head rotations cause opposite conjugate eye movements following which the maneuver itself usually causes arousal and the reflex movements stop. *Second,* full conjugate oculocephalic movements demonstrate the integrity of brainstem pathways extending from the high cervical spinal cord and medulla, where vestibular and proprioceptive input from head turning originates, to the midbrain, where the third nerve originates. Thus, the oculocephalic maneuver is a convenient way to demonstrate the functional integrity of a large segment of brainstem pathways and to exclude a lesion in the brainstem as the cause of coma. Lack of complete adduction indicates an ipsilateral midbrain (third nerve) lesion or, alternatively, damage to the pathways mediating reflex eye movements in the MLF (i.e., internuclear ophthalmoplegia). Third nerve damage is usually associated with an enlarged pupil and horizontal ocular divergence at rest, whereas MLF destruction shows neither. Adduction of the globes is by nature more difficult to obtain with head turning than abduction, and subtle symmetric abnormalities in the doll's-eye maneuver should be interpreted with caution.

Caloric stimulation of the vestibular apparatus (*oculovestibular* or *vestibuloocular response*) is a useful adjunct to the oculocephalic test and acts as a stronger stimulus to reflex eye movements. Irrigation of the external auditory canal with cold water causes convection currents in the endolymph of the labyrinths of the inner ear. With the head at approximately 30° elevation from the supine position, endolymph movement is induced primarily in the horizontal semicircular canals. An intact brainstem response is indicated with variable latency, by tonic deviation of both eyes (lasting 30 to 120 s) to the side of cold water irrigation. Bilateral conjugate eye movements have the same significance as full oculocephalic responses. If the cerebral hemispheres are intact, a rapid corrective conjugate movement is generated away from the side of tonic deviation. The absence of this saccadic, nystagmus-like quick phase signifies damage to the cerebral hemispheres.

Conjugate ocular deviation at rest or incomplete conjugate eye movements with head turning indicates damage in the pons on the side of the gaze paresis or frontal lobe damage on the opposite side. This phenomenon may be summarized by the phrase "the eyes look toward a hemispheral lesion and away from a brainstem lesion." It is usually possible to overcome the ocular deviation associated with frontal lobe damage by brisk head turning. Seizures may also cause aversive (opposite) eye deviation with rhythmic, jerky movements to the side of gaze. On rare occasions, the eyes may turn paradoxically away from the side of a deep hemispheral lesion ("wrong-way eyes").

A major pitfall in coma diagnosis may occur when reflex eye movements are suppressed by drugs. The eyes often move with the head as it is turned as if locked in place, thus spuriously suggesting anatomic brainstem damage. Overdoses of phenytoin, tricyclic antidepressants, and barbiturates are commonly implicated as well as, on occasion, alcohol, phenothiazines, diazepam, and neuromuscular blockers such as pancuronium. The presence of normal pupillary size and light reaction will distinguish most drug-induced coma from brainstem damage (except for pontine infarction or hemorrhage in which the pupils remain small). Small to midposition, 1- to 3-mm, nonreactive pupils may also occur with very high serum levels of barbiturates or secondary to hydrocephalus (see below).

Although the *corneal reflexes* are rarely useful alone, they may corroborate eye movement abnormalities because they also depend on the integrity of pontine pathways. By touching the cornea with a wisp of cotton, a response consisting of brief bilateral lid closure may be observed. The corneal response may be lost when the afferent fifth nerve, the efferent seventh nerve, or their reflex connections within the pons are damaged. The normal efferent response is bilateral, with closure of both eyelids. Nervous system depressant drugs diminish or eliminate the corneal responses soon after the reflex eye movements become paralyzed but before the pupils become unreactive to light.

Respiration Respiratory patterns have received much attention in coma diagnosis but are of inconsistent localizing value. Shallow, slow, but well-timed regular breathing suggests metabolic or drug depression. Rapid, deep (Kussmaul) breathing usually implies metabolic acidosis but may also occur with pontomesencephalic lesions. Cheyne-Stokes respiration in its classic cyclic form, ending with a brief apneic period, signifies mild bihemispheral damage or metabolic suppression and commonly accompanies light coma. Agonal gasps reflect bilateral lower brainstem damage and are well known as the terminal respiratory pattern of severe brain damage. In brain-dead patients, shallow respiratory-like movements with irregular, nonrepetitive back arching may be produced by hypoxia and are probably generated by the surviving cervical spinal cord and lower medulla. Other cyclic breathing variations are not usually diagnostic of specific local lesions.

COMA-LIKE SYNDROMES AND RELATED STATES The simple observation of inability to arouse a patient characterizes most comatose states. Several syndromes, however, render patients unresponsive or insensate but are considered separately because of their unusual features. The *vegetative state,* an unfortunate term, occurs in patients who were earlier comatose but whose eyelids have subsequently opened giving the appearance of being awake. There may be yawning, grunting, and random limb and head movements. These are associated with signs of extensive damage to both cerebral hemispheres, i.e., Babinski signs, decerebrate or decorticate posturing, absence of response to visual stimuli, and absent corrective nystagmus on oculovestibular testing. Autonomic nervous system functions such as cardiovascular and thermoregulatory and neuroendocrine control are preserved and may be subject to periods of overactivity. The syndrome is best viewed as a severe dementia resulting from global damage to the cerebral cortex and differs somewhat from akinetic mutism because of a complete inability to respond to commands or communicate. *Akinetic mutism* refers to a partially or fully awake patient who is immobile and silent. The state may result from hydrocephalus, from masses in the region of the third ventricle, or with lesions in the cingulate gyrus or other portions of both frontal lobes. *Abulia* is a mild form of akinetic mutism in which the patient is hypokinetic and slow to respond but generally gives correct answers. Lesions in the periaqueductal or low diencephalic regions may cause a similar state in which hypophonia is prominent. The *locked-in syndrome* (pseudocoma) describes patients who are awake but selectively deefferented, i.e., have no means of producing speech or limb, face, or pharyngeal movements. This results from infarction or hemorrhage of the ventral pons, which transects all descending corticospinal and corticobulbar pathways but spares the RAS arousal system. Vertical eye movements and lid elevation are partially preserved because these midbrain functions are outside the field of infarction in some cases of basilar artery thrombosis. Such movements can be used by the patient to signal to the examiner. A similar awake state simulating unresponsiveness may occur in severe cases of acute polyneuritis or myasthenia gravis as a result of total paralysis of limb, ocular, or bulbar musculature. Unlike basilar artery stroke, vertical eye movements are not selectively spared in these nerve and muscle diseases.

Certain psychiatric states mimic coma because they produce apparent unresponsiveness. *Catatonia* is a term for peculiar motor activities associated with major psychosis. In the typical hypomobile form catatonic patients appear awake with eyes open but make no voluntary or responsive movements, though they blink spontaneously and may not appear distressed. There may be associated "waxy flexibility" in which limbs maintain their posture when lifted by the examiner. Upon recovery, such patients have full memory of events that occurred during their catatonic stupor. Patients with *pseudocoma conversion* states (trance) have signs which indicate voluntary attempts to appear comatose. They may resist eyelid elevation, blink to threat when the lids are held open, and move the eyes concomitantly with head rotation, all signs belying brain damage.

LABORATORY EXAMINATION IN COMA   Four laboratory tests are used most frequently in the diagnosis of coma: chemical-toxicologic analysis of blood and urine, CT or MRI, EEG, and cerebral spinal fluid examination.

Chemical blood determinations are routinely made to investigate metabolic, toxic, or drug-induced encephalopathies. The major metabolic aberrations encountered in clinical practice are those of electrolytes, calcium, blood urea nitrogen (BUN), glucose, and hepatic dysfunction. Toxicologic analysis is of great value in any case of coma where the diagnosis is not immediately clear. However, the presence of exogenous drugs or toxins, especially alcohol, does not ensure that other factors, particularly head trauma, may not also contribute to the clinical state.

The notion that a normal CT scan excludes anatomic lesions as the cause of coma is erroneous. Early bilateral hemisphere infarction, small brainstem lesions, encephalitis, mechanical shearing of axons as a result of closed head trauma, absent cerebral perfusion associated with brain death, sagittal sinus thrombosis, and subdural hematomas that are isodense to adjacent brain are some of the lesions that may be overlooked by CT. Nevertheless, in coma of unknown etiology, a CT scan should be obtained early in the evaluation. In those cases in which the etiology is clinically apparent, the CT provides verification and defines the extent of the lesion. For technical reasons MRI is difficult to perform in comatose patients. It also has the disadvantage of not demonstrating hemorrhages as well as CT (see Chap. 348).

The EEG is rarely diagnostic in coma, with the occasional exceptions of coma due to ongoing clinically unrecognized seizures, herpes virus encephalitis, and Creutzfeldt-Jakob disease. The EEG, however, may suggest metabolic encephalopathy and provide important information about the general electrophysiologic state of the cortex. The amount of background slowing of the EEG is useful for gauging and following the severity of any diffuse encephalopathy. The EEG pattern of "alpha coma" is defined by widespread, invariant 8- to 12-Hz activity superficially resembling the normal alpha rhythm of waking, but which is unresponsive to environmental stimuli. Alpha coma results from either high pontine or diffuse cortical damage and is associated with a poor prognosis. Coma due to persistent epileptic discharges that are not clinically manifested may be revealed by EEG recordings. Normal alpha activity on the EEG may also alert the clinician to the "locked-in" syndrome. Evoked potential recordings (auditory and somatosensory) are currently under investigation as additional methods of coma diagnosis and monitoring.

Lumbar puncture is now used more judiciously than previously because the CT scan excludes intracerebral hemorrhages and most subarachnoid hemorrhages. The use of lumbar puncture in coma is limited to diagnosis of meningitis-encephalitis, occasional cases of subarachnoid hemorrhage, and cases with normal CT in which the origin of coma is obscure. If the CT is normal or unavailable and suspicion of meningeal infection or subarachnoid hemorrhage remains, then the CSF should be examined for white cells, microorganisms, and blood. Xanthochromia is documented by spinning the CSF in a large tube and comparing the supernatant to water. Yellow coloration indicates preexisting blood in the CSF and permits exclusion of a traumatic puncture. In addition, initial and final tubes should be inspected for a decrement in the number of erythrocytes, indicating traumatic puncture.

DIFFERENTIAL DIAGNOSIS OF COMA   In most instances, coma is part of an obvious medical problem such as known drug ingestion, hypoxia, stroke, trauma, or liver or kidney failure. Attention is appropriately focused on the primary illness. A complete listing of all diseases which cause coma would serve little purpose since it would not aid diagnosis. Some general rules, however, are helpful. Illnesses which cause sudden or acute coma are due to drug ingestion or to one of the catastrophic brain lesions—hemorrhage, trauma, hypoxia, or, rarely, acute basilar artery occlusion. Coma which appears subacutely is usually related to preceding medical or neurologic problems, including the secondary brain swelling which surrounds a preexisting lesion. Coma diagnosis, therefore, requires familiarity with the common intracerebral catastrophies. These are described in more detail in Chap. 351, but may be summarized as follows: (1) basal ganglia and thalamic hemorrhage (acute but not instantaneous onset, vomiting, headache, hemiplegia, and characteristic eye signs); (2) subarachnoid hemorrhage (instantaneous onset, severe headache, neck stiffness, vomiting, third or sixth nerve lesions, transient loss of consciousness, or sudden coma with vigorous extensor posturing); (3) pontine hemorrhage (sudden onset, pinpoint pupils, loss of reflex eye movements and corneal responses, ocular bobbing, posturing, hyperventilation, and sweating); (4) cerebellar hemorrhage (occipital headache, vomiting, gaze paresis, and inability to stand); (5) basilar artery thrombosis (neurologic prodrome or warning spells, diplopia, dysarthria, vomiting, eye movement and corneal response abnormalities, and asymmetric limb paresis). The commonest stroke, namely, infarction in the territory of the middle cerebral artery, does not cause coma acutely. The syndrome of acute hydrocephalus causing coma may accompany many intracranial catastrophes, particularly subarachnoid hemorrhage. Acute symmetric enlargement of both lateral ventricles causes headache and vomiting. Further ventricular enlargement leads to drowsiness that may progress quickly to coma, with extensor posturing of the limbs, bilateral Babinski signs, often small (1 mm diameter) nonreactive pupils, and impaired vertical oculocephalic movements.

If the history and examination are not typical for any neurologic diagnosis and metabolic or drug causes are excluded, then information obtained from CT may be used as outlined in Table 31-1. The neurologic examination remains preeminent because it allows localization of lesions to one or both hemispheres or to the brainstem (with the exceptions noted above). The CT scan is useful to focus the differential diagnosis, and because of its accuracy and general availability, the diagnoses which it facilitates are listed in the table. The majority of medical causes of coma are established without a CT or with the study being normal.

COMA AFTER HEAD TRAUMA   Concussion is a common form of transient coma which probably results from torsion of the hemispheres about the midbrain-diencephalic junction with brief interruption of RAS function. Persistent coma after head trauma presents a more complex and serious problem (Chap. 352).

EMERGENCY TREATMENT OF THE COMATOSE PATIENT   The immediate goal in acute coma is prevention of further nervous system damage. Hypotension, hypoglycemia, hypoxia, hypercapnia, and hyperthermia should be rapidly and assiduously corrected. An oropharyngeal airway is adequate to keep the pharynx open in drowsy patients who are breathing normally. Tracheal intubation is indicated if there is obvious apnea, hypoventilation, or emesis, or if the patient is liable to aspirate. Mechanical ventilation is required if the patient is apneic or hypoventilating or if there is an intracranial mass and hypocapnia is therapeutically necessary. An intravenous access is established and naloxone and dextrose administered if narcotic overdose or hypoglycemia are even remote possibilities. Thiamine is generally administered with glucose in order to prevent an exacerbation of Wernicke's encephalopathy. The veins of intravenous drug abusers may be difficult to cannulate; in such cases, naloxone can be injected sublingually through a small-gauge needle. In cases of suspected basilar thrombosis with brainstem ischemia, intravenous heparin is administered after obtaining a CT scan, keeping in mind that cerebellar and pontine hemorrhages resemble the syndrome of basilar artery occlusion. Physostigmine, when used by experienced physicians with careful monitoring, may awaken patients with anticholinergic-type

TABLE 31-1 Approach to the differential diagnosis of coma

I Normal brainstem reflexes, no lateralizing signs
  A Anatomic lesions of hemisphere found
    1 Hydrocephalus
    2 Bilateral subdural hematomas
    3 Bilateral contusions, edema, or axonal shearing of hemispheres due to closed head trauma, subarachnoid hemorrhage
  B Bilateral hemispheral dysfunction without mass lesion (CT normal)
    1 Drug-toxin ingestion (toxicologic analysis)
    2 Endogenous metabolic encephalopathy (glucose, ammonia, calcium, osmolarity, P_{O_2}, P_{CO_2}, urea, sodium)
    3 Shock, hypertensive encephalopathy
    4 Meningitis (CSF analysis)
    5 Nonherpetic viral encephalitis (CSF analysis)
    6 Epilepsy (EEG)
    7 Reye's syndrome (ammonia, increased intracranial pressure)
    8 Fat embolism
    9 Subarachnoid hemorrhage with normal CT (CSF analysis)
    10 Acute disseminated encephalomyelitis (CSF analysis)
    11 Acute hemorrhagic leukoencephalitis
    12 Advanced Alzheimer's and Creutzfeldt-Jakob disease
II Normal brainstem reflexes (with or without unilateral compressive third nerve palsy), lateralizing motor signs (CT abnormal)
  A Unilateral mass lesion found
    1 Cerebral hemorrhage (basal ganglia, thalamus)
    2 Large infarction with surrounding brain edema
    3 Herpes virus encephalitis (temporal lobe lesion)
    4 Subdural or epidural hematoma
    5 Tumor with edema
    6 Brain abscess with edema
    7 Vasculitis with multiple infarctions
    8 Metabolic encephalopathy superimposed on preexisting focal lesions (i.e., stroke)
    9 Pituitary apoplexy
  B Asymmetric signs accompanied by diffuse hemispheral dysfunction
    1 Metabolic encephalopathies with asymmetric signs (blood chemical determinations)
    2 Isodense subdural hematoma (brain scan, angiogram)
    3 Thrombotic thrombocytopenic purpura (blood smear, platelet count)
    4 Epilepsy with focal seizures or postictal state (EEG)
III Multiple brainstem reflex abnormalities
  A Anatomic lesions in brainstem found
    1 Pontine, midbrain hemorrhage
    2 Cerebellar hemorrhage, tumor, abscess
    3 Cerebellar infarction with brainstem compression
    4 Mass in hemisphere causing advanced bilateral brainstem compression
    5 Brainstem tumor or demyelination
    6 Traumatic brainstem contusion-hemorrhage (clinical signs, auditory-evoked potentials)
  D Brainstem dysfunction without mass lesion
    1 Basilar artery thrombosis causing brainstem stroke (clinical signs, angiogram)
    2 Severe drug overdose (toxicologic analysis)
    3 Brainstem encephalitis
    4 Basilar artery migraine
    5 Brain death

drug overdose, but many physicians believe that this is justified only to treat associated cardiac arrhythmias. Intravenous fluid should be carefully monitored in any serious acute nervous system illness because of the potential for exacerbating brain swelling by excess water administration. Neck injuries must not be overlooked, particularly prior to attempting the oculocephalic maneuver. Headache accompanied by fever and meningismus indicates a need for examination of the CSF to diagnose meningitis, and *lumbar puncture should not be delayed while awaiting a CT scan.*

Enlargement of one pupil usually indicates secondary midbrain compression by a hemispheral mass and demands immediate reduction of intracranial pressure. Normal saline or lactated Ringer's solution are safest because they are iso- or hyperosmolar. Therapeutic hyperventilation may be used to achieve an arterial P_{CO_2} of 3.7 to 4.2 kPa (28 to 32 mmHg). This acts rapidly to reduce intracranial pressure, but the beneficial effect rarely lasts more than 1 to 2 h. Hyperosmolar therapy with mannitol may be used simultaneously with hyperventilation in critical cases, but its effects are not apparent for several minutes. It is generally best to administer mannitol before attempting to intubate a patient with suspected impending herniation. A ventricular puncture may be necessary to decompress hydrocephalus if

medical measures fail. Virtually all patients who survive to arrive in an emergency room can be protected from further brain damage by these means until definitive therapy is possible. The use of high-dose barbiturates soon after cardiac arrest has not been shown in clinical studies to be beneficial, although they may still be useful in lowering intracranial pressure in other circumstances.

BRAIN DEATH Brain death results from total cessation of cerebral blood flow and global infarction of the brain at a time when cardiovascular and respiratory functions are preserved with artificial support. It is the only type of irrevocable loss of brain function currently recognized by law as death. Many sets of roughly equivalent criteria have been advanced for the diagnosis of brain death, and it is essential to adhere to those approved locally and recognized as standard practice. Ideal criteria are ones that are simple, conducted at the bedside, and which allow no chance of diagnostic error. Widespread cortical destruction is usually shown by unresponsiveness to the environment, midbrain damage by absent pupillary light reaction, pontine damage by absent oculovestibular and corneal reflexes, and medullary dysfunction by apnea. Some period of observation, usually 6 to 24 h, is desirable during which this state is shown to be sustained. The pupils need not be fully dilated but should not be constricted. The absence of spinal reflexes is not required since the spinal cord remains functional in many cases. Most centers use an isoelectric EEG as a confirmatory test for cortical death. The possibility of profound drug-induced or hypothermic nervous system depression should always be excluded. It is often advisable to delay clinical testing for up to 24 h if a cardiac arrest has caused brain death.

The demonstration of apnea generally requires that the P_{CO_2} be high enough to stimulate respiration. This can be safely accomplished in most patients by removal of the respirator and use of diffusion oxygenation sustained by a tracheal cannula connected to an oxygen supply. In brain-dead patients, CO_2 tension increases approximately 0.3 to 0.4 kPa/min (2 to 3 mmHg/min) during apnea. At the end of an appropriate interval, arterial P_{CO_2} should be at least above 6.6 to 8.0 kPa (50 to 60 mmHg) for the test to be valid. Large posterior fossa lesions that compress the brainstem, nervous system–depressant drugs, and profound hypothermia can simulate brain death, but adherence to recognized protocols for diagnosis will prevent these errors. Radionuclide brain scanning, cerebral angiography or transcranial Doppler measurements may be used to demonstrate the absence of cerebral blood flow in brain death. These techniques have the virtue of rapidity but are often cumbersome and have not been extensively correlated with pathologic material.

There is no implicit pressure to make the diagnosis of brain death except when organ transplantation or difficult resource allocation (intensive care) issues are involved. Although it is commonly accepted that the respirator can be disconnected from a brain-dead patient after proper explanations to the family, there is no obligation to do so, and some physicians prefer to await the inevitable cardiovascular failure that follows brain death if full medical support is omitted, usually within a week.

PROGNOSIS OF COMA Interest in predicting the outcome of coma is oriented toward allocating medical resources and limiting the support of hopeless cases. To date, no collection of clinical signs except those of brain death assuredly predicts outcome of coma. Children and young adults may have ominous early clinical findings such as abnormal brainstem reflexes and yet recover. All schemes for prognosis should, therefore, be taken as only approximate indicators, and medical judgments must be conservatively tempered by other factors such as age, underlying disease, general medical condition, and the previously expressed wishes of the patient. In an attempt to collect prognostic information from large numbers of patients with head injury, a "coma scale" scoring system has been devised which empirically has predictive value in cases of brain trauma (see Chap. 352). Major points include a 95 percent death rate in patients whose pupillary reaction or reflex eye movements were absent 6 h after onset of coma, and a 91 percent death rate if the pupils were unreactive at 24 h (though 4 percent made a good recovery).

Prognostication of nontraumatic coma is more difficult because of the heterogeneity of contributing diseases. Unfavorable signs in the first hours after admission have been reported to be the absence of any two of pupillary reaction, corneal reflex, or the oculovestibular response. One day after the onset of coma, the above signs, in addition to absence of eye opening and muscle tone, predicted death or severe disability and the same signs at 3 days strengthened the prediction of a poor outcome. In many patients precise combinations of predictive signs do not occur and coma scales lose their value. The use of evoked potentials has recently been shown to aid prognostication in head-injured and postcardiac arrest patients. Bilateral absence of cortical somatosensory evoked potentials is associated with death or a vegetative state in most cases. It may be wisest to fully support all but those patients whose extreme signs convincingly suggest a poor outcome. Medical practitioners are becoming less reluctant to withdraw support from brain-dead patients as predictions become more reliable and resources more limited.

REFERENCES

CHOI D: Glutamate neurotoxicity and diseases of the nervous system. Neuron 1:623, 1988

FINKLESTEIN S, ROPPER A: The diagnosis of coma: Its pitfalls and limitations. Heart Lung 8:1059, 1979

FISHER CM: The neurological examination of the comatose patient. Acta Neurol Scand 45 (Suppl 6):1, 1969

IVAN L, BRUCE D: Coma. Springfield, Ill, Charles C Thomas, 1982

JENNET B et al: Prognosis of patients with severe head injury. Neurosurgery 4:283, 1979

LEVY D et al: Prognosis in non-traumatic coma. Ann Intern Med 94:229, 1981

PLUM F, POSNER J: The Diagnosis of Stupor and Coma, 3d ed. Philadelphia, Davis, 1980

ROPPER AH: Coma and acutely raised intracranial pressure, in Diseases of the Nervous System, A Asbury, G McKhann, I McDonald (eds). Philadelphia, Saunders, 1986

32 SYNDROMES DUE TO FOCAL CEREBRAL LESIONS

RAYMOND D. ADAMS / MAURICE VICTOR

In addition to the general syndromes described in Chap. 30, there are many others that relate to lesions of particular parts of the cerebrum. Recognition of these constitutes irrefutable evidence that all parts of the cerebrum are not functionally equivalent. Some of the symptoms and signs that make up these syndromes have the same diagnostic value as a hemiplegia and, once identified, require the same type of clinical analysis as to cause and pathophysiologic mechanism.

These focal syndromes will be described in terms of the conventional anatomic divisions of the cerebrum, but it will be obvious that most diseases do not respect these boundaries. Hence the syndromes may overlap or occur in a number of combinations.

FRONTAL LOBES In Fig. 32-1, it is seen that the frontal lobes lie anterior to the central (rolandic) sulcus and superior to the Sylvian fissure. They consist of several functionally different parts, which are conventionally designated in the neurologic literature by numbers (according to the scheme devised by Brodmann) or by letters (according to the scheme of von Economo and Koskinas).

The posterior parts, areas 4 and 6 of Brodmann, are specifically related to motor function. There is also a supplementary motor area, located in the posterior part of the superior frontal convolution. Voluntary movement in humans depends on the integrity of these areas, and lesions in them produce a spastic paralysis of the contralateral face, arm, and leg. This is discussed in Chap. 25. A

FIGURE 32-1 Diagram to show cortical areas, numbered according to the scheme of Brodmann. The speech areas are in black, the three main ones of which are 39, 41, and 45. The zone marked by vertical stripes in the superior frontal convolution is the secondary motor area which, like Broca's area 45, if stimulated causes vocal arrest. (After Handbuch der Inneren Medizin, Berlin, Springer-Verlag, 1939.)

lesion limited more or less to the premotor area (area 6 and the supplementary motor area) is accompanied by less paralysis and more spasticity, as well as by a contralateral grasp reflex, and bilateral lesions of these parts are accompanied by a suck reflex. A lesion in area 8 of Brodmann interferes with the mechanism for turning the head and eyes contralaterally. In addition, a lesion of the left supplementary motor area can result in mutism at its onset; in time the condition resolves to a state of transcortical motor aphasia, with reduced language output and preserved repetition and naming. Ideomotor apraxia is another manifestation of area 6 lesions observed in some patients. A lesion in area 44 (Broca's area) of the dominant cerebral hemisphere, usually the left one, results in at least a temporary loss of verbal expression. A phonetic-articulatory defect (cortical dysarthria) and agrammatism, with retention of "content words," are characteristic. More extensive lesions, including adjacent insular and motor cortex, result in a more severe and persistent motor speech disorder, agraphia, and apraxia of the face, lips, and tongue (see Chap. 33). Lesions of the anterior cingulate gyrus, in the acute stages, may cause a speechless, aphonic state; with recovery, speech returns through whispering and hoarseness rather than dysarthria and aphasia, according to Brown. Lesions in the medial limbic or piriform cortex (areas 23 and 24), where the mechanisms controlling respiration, circulation, and micturition are organized bilaterally, have relatively unclear clinical effects.

The remaining parts of the frontal lobes (areas 9 to 12 of Brodmann), sometimes called the prefrontal areas, have less specific and measurable functions. In contrast to the motor areas of the frontal lobes and other areas of the brain, electrical stimulation of the prefrontal areas in humans has yielded a paucity of findings. Many patients with gunshot wounds of these areas have shown only mild and inconsistent abnormalities of behavior. Nevertheless, the following groups of symptoms have been observed in patients with large lesions of one or both of the frontal lobes and of the central white matter and the anterior part of the corpus callosum by which they are joined:

1 Lack of initiative and spontaneity in conjunction with diminished speech and with motor inactivity (apathetic, akinetic, or abulic state). Necessary daily activities are neglected. Interpersonal social reactions are reduced and shallow.

2 Change of personality, usually expressed as lack of concern over the consequences of any action and social disinhibition. Sometimes it may take the form of a childish excitement, an inappropriate joking and punning, a thoughtless impulsivity, an instability and superficiality of emotion, or irritability. The capacity for worry, anxiety, and depression (tortured self-concern) is reduced. These are especially prominent in orbital frontal lesions.

3 Slight impairment of intelligence, usually described as a lack of concentration, vacillation of attention, inability to carry out planned activity, difficulty in changing from one activity to another, or perseveration. These cognitive impairments are more prominent in dorsolateral frontal lesions. Goldstein reduced the difficulty to a loss of the capacity for abstract thinking, but the authors believe this tendency to concrete thinking to be another manifestation of abulia and perseveration. According to Luria, who views the frontal lobe as a regulating mechanism of the organism's activities, planned action is deficient with respect to steady control and goal orientation. With left frontal lesions, intelligence is reduced more (10 points on the IQ scale) than with right frontal lesions, probably because of reduced verbal skills. There is also a memory impairment, usually slight, probably because the mental strategies needed for memorization and recall are impaired.

4 A decomposition of gait and upright stance, consisting of a wide-based gait, flexed posture, and small shuffling steps, and culminating in an inability to stand (Bruns' frontal lobe ataxia or gait apraxia) accompanied by abnormal postures, reflex grasping or sucking, and incontinence of sphincters.

Some differences have been noted between the dominant (left) and right prefrontal lobes. In psychological tests, left-sided lesions impair verbal fluency and cause a greater degree of perseveration, and right-sided ones impair the learning of visual spatial patterns and cause impersistence (see Hecaen and Albert, and Luria for details).

From all the foregoing comments it should be evident that the frontal lobes do not have a unitary function, but comprise a number of interconnected functional components, each subserving a different aspect of motor function, speech, and behavior.

TEMPORAL LOBES The boundaries of the temporal lobes are illustrated in Fig. 32-1. The Sylvian fissure separates the superior surface of each temporal lobe from the frontal lobe and anterior part of the parietal lobe. Posteriorly there is no definite anatomic boundary between the temporal and the occipital and parietal lobe. The temporal lobe includes the superior, middle, and inferior temporal, fusiform, and hippocampal convolutions and the transverse convolutions of Heschl, which are the auditory receptive area on the superior surface, within the Sylvian fissure. The hippocampal convolution was once believed to be related to olfactory function, but now it is known that lesions here do not cause anosmia. Only the medial and anterior parts of the temporal lobes (uncal regions) are related to smell. The lower fibers of the geniculocalcarine pathway (from the inferior retina) swing in a wide arc over the temporal horn of the ventricle into the white matter of the temporal lobe en route to the occipital lobes, and lesions that interrupt them characteristically produce a contralateral upper homonymous quadrantanopsia. Hearing, localized in the superior surfaces of the temporal lobes (Heschl's gyri), is bilaterally represented, which accounts for the fact that both temporal lobes need to be affected to cause deafness. Loss of equilibrium has not been observed with temporal lobe lesions, although electrical stimulation (or a seizure discharge) of the superior surface of the temporal lobe, posterior to the auditory cortex, evokes vertigo. Disease in the

superior convolution of the left temporal lobe and adjacent inferior parietal lobule in right-handed individuals results in a Wernicke's aphasia. This syndrome, discussed in Chap. 33, consists of paraphasic speech or jargon aphasia and inability to read, write, repeat, or understand the meaning of spoken words.

Between the auditory and olfactory projection areas there is a large expanse of temporal lobe, subserving three specific functional systems. In the inferolateral parts (areas 20, 21, and 37) are located some of the visual-associated projections from the striate and peristriate cortex of the occipital lobes. In the superior-lateral parts (areas 22, 41, and 42) are the primary and secondary areas for acoustic perception. In the mediobasal parts are the limbic structures (amygdaloid nuclei and hippocampi) where the neural organizations for emotional and memory processes lie. Bilateral lesions of the geniculocalcarine pathways result in cortical blindness; lesions of the visual cortex of the dominant temporal lobe result in a variety of agnosias, apparently based on a loss of visual memories: recognition of written words (alexia), visual naming (anomia), loss of pattern discrimination, and possibly color recognition (achromatopsia) and object agnosia. Bilateral hippocampal/parahippocampal lesions produce a deficit in which the patient is unable to record events and information, i.e., has a loss of memory, in both its general and specific aspects (see Chap. 30). Also, the temporal lobes include a large part of the limbic system, which subserves the emotional and motivational aspects of behavior and vegetative functions ("visceral brain"). Lesions involving both the visual and limbic areas contribute to the Klüver-Bucy syndrome. This syndrome, first produced in monkeys by removal of both temporal lobes, has been observed only rarely in human beings, usually after an attack of herpes simplex encephalitis. It consists of apathy, impaired recognition of objects and persons, uncontrollable oral exploration, hypersexuality, amnesia, and bulimia. Usually the syndrome is incomplete.

Apart from aphasia, psychological studies have shown a difference between the effects of dominant and nondominant temporal lobe lesions. With dominant lesions there is impairment in learning auditorially presented verbal material; with nondominant lesions there is a failure in learning visually presented nonverbal material. In addition, about 20 percent of patients with either a right or left lobectomy have shown an alteration of personality similar to that described after lesions in the prefrontal parts of the brain (see above).

The study of patients with uncinate seizures, with the characteristic dreamy state, olfactory or gustatory hallucinations, and masticatory movements, suggests that all these functions are organized through the temporal lobes. Stimulation of the posterior parts of the temporal lobes of fully conscious epileptic patients during surgical procedures has brought to light the interesting fact that complex memories and visual and auditory images, some with strong emotional content, can be aroused. Studies of the effects of stimulation of the amygdaloid nucleus, which is in the anterior and medial part of the temporal lobe, have shed additional light on this subject. Some symptoms like those of schizophrenia and mania may be evoked. Complex emotional experiences that had occurred previously may be revived. There are also remarkable autonomic effects: the blood pressure rises, pulse increases, respirations increase in frequency and depth, and the patient looks frightened. In temporal lobe epilepsy, there may be an intensification of the patient's emotional reactions, vague preoccupation with moral and religious issues, a tendency to write excessively, and sometimes aggressiveness. Ablation of the amygdaloid nuclei has eliminated uncontrollable rage reactions in psychotic patients. Hippocampal and adjacent convolutions have been excised bilaterally, with a disastrous loss of ability to learn or to establish new memories (Korsakoff's psychosis).

The abnormalities consequent upon lesions of the temporal lobes may be summarized as follows:

1 Effects of unilateral disease of the dominant temporal lobe
  a Upper homonymous quadrantanopsia
  b Wernicke's aphasia

c Impairment in tests of verbal material presented through the auditory sense

d Dysnomia or amnesic aphasia

e Amusia (inability to name musical scores and to read and write music)

2 Effects of unilateral disease of nondominant temporal lobe

   a Upper homonymous quadrantanopsia

   b Inability to judge spatial relationships in rare cases

   c Impairment in tests of nonverbal visually presented material

   d Inability to recognize melodies and other nonlexical qualities of music

3 Effects of disease of either temporal lobe

   a Auditory illusions and hallucinations

   b Psychotic behavior (aggressivity)

   c Upper homonymous quadrantanopsia

4 Effects of bilateral disease

   a Korsakoff's amnesic defect

   b Apathy and placidity

   c Increased sexual activity ⎬ Klüver-Bucy syndrome

   d Sham rage

   e Cortical deafness

   f Loss of other unilateral functions

PARIETAL LOBES The postcentral convolution is the terminus of somatic sensory pathways from the opposite half of the body. However, destructive lesions here do not abolish cutaneous sensation but cause mainly a defect in sensory discrimination with variable impairment of primary sensation. In other words, the perception of painful, tactile, thermal, and vibratory stimuli is affected little or not at all, whereas stereognosis (ability to recognize the size, shape, and texture of objects by touch), sense of position, distinction between single and double contacts (two-point threshold), and the localization of sensory stimuli are impaired or lost (atopognosia). There is also the phenomenon of extinction, i.e., if a stimulus (tactile, painful, visual) is delivered simultaneously to corresponding parts of the body or visual fields, only the stimulus on the normal side is perceived. This type of sensory disturbance, sometimes called *cortical sensory defect,* is really a disturbance of somatic sensory perception, and is discussed in Chap. 28. Extensive lesions deep in the white matter of the parietal lobes produce an impairment of all forms of sensation contralaterally, and if these lesions encroach upon the uppermost part of the temporal lobe, there may be a contralateral homonymous hemianopsia, often incongruous and tending to be greater in the inferior quadrants. Lesions of the angular gyrus of the dominant hemisphere result in an inability to read (alexia).

Recent interest has centered more on the function of the parietal lobes in the perception of one's position in space, the interrelationships of objects in space, and the relationship of the various parts of the body to one another. Since the time of Babinski it has been known that patients with large lesions of the minor parietal lobe are often unaware of their hemiplegia and hemianesthesia. Babinski called this condition *anosognosia.* Related psychological disorders are lack of recognition of the left arm and leg, neglect of the left side of the body (as in dressing) and of external space on the left side, and constructional apraxia (an inability to perceive and construct simple figures). While all of these disorders may occur with left-sided lesions as well, they are observed less frequently, in part because the aphasia that occurs with lesions of the left hemisphere precludes adequate testing of other parietal lobe functions.

Another frequent constellation of symptoms, usually referred to as *Gerstmann's syndrome,* occurs only with lesions of the dominant parietal lobe. This consists of inability to write (agraphia), calculate (acalculia), distinguish right from left, and identify fingers (finger agnosia) and other parts of the body. This syndrome is a true *agnosia,* since it represents a defect in the formulation and use of symbolic concepts (including the significance of numbers and letters and the names of parts of the body), in which a unilateral (dominant) lesion evokes the defect bilaterally. An ideomotor apraxia may or may not

be associated. *Apraxia* and *agnosia* are discussed in Chaps. 25 and 28.

The effects of disease of the parietal lobes may be summarized as follows:

1 Effects of unilateral disease of the parietal lobe, right or left

   a Cortical sensory syndrome and sensory extinction (or total hemianesthesia with large acute lesions of white matter)

   b In children, mild contralateral hemiparesis and hemiatrophy

   c Visual inattention and sometimes anosognosia, constructional and dressing apraxias, and neglect of the opposite one-half of the body and extrapersonal space (all of these defects are observed far more frequently with right than with left parietal lesions)

   d Abolition of optokinetic nystagmus to one side

2 Effects of unilateral disease of the dominant parietal lobe (left hemisphere in right-handed patients), additional phenomena

   a Disorders of language (especially alexia)

   b Gerstmann's syndrome

   c Bimanual astereognosis (tactile agnosia)

   d Bilateral ideational or ideomotor apraxia

In all parietal lesions, if sufficiently extensive, there may be a bland mood, indifference to illness or neurologic defects, reduction in the capacity to think clearly, inattentiveness, and impaired memory.

OCCIPITAL LOBES The occipital lobes are the termini of the geniculocalcarine pathways and are essential for visual sensation and perception. Destructive lesions in one occipital lobe result in a contralateral homonymous hemianopsia, i.e., a loss of vision in part or all of the homonymous fields. Occasionally patients complain of changes in the form and contour of visually perceived objects (metamorphopsia), as well as illusory displacement of images from one side of the visual field to another (visual allesthesia), or of abnormal persistence of the visual image after the object has been removed (palinopsia). Visual illusions and elementary (unformed) hallucinations may also occur. Bilateral lesions cause "cortical" blindness, a state of blindness without change in the optic fundi or pupillary reflexes.

Lesions in Brodmann's areas 18 and 19 of the dominant hemisphere (Fig. 32-1) cause a loss of recognition of objects presented visually, despite the ability to see, at least to some degree—a state termed *visual object agnosia.* In the classic form of this disorder, individuals with intact mental powers are unable to recognize objects visually, even though by tests of visual acuity and perimetry they appear to see sufficiently well to do so; they are able to recognize objects by tactile or other nonvisual senses. In these terms, *alexia,* or inability to read, represents a visual verbal agnosia or "word blindness." Patients can see letters and words but do not know their meaning, although they can still recognize them through tactile or auditory senses. Several other types of agnosia are observed with bilateral occipital lesions: disorders of *spatial or topographic localization,* in which the patient cannot describe or find his or her way in familiar surroundings (usually due to bilateral occipitoparietal lesions); failure to identify a familiar face (*prosopagnosia*), often with achromatopsia (inferomesial occipitotemporal lesions); an inability to scan the peripheral field and to grasp an object under visual guidance, coupled with visual inattention (*Balint's syndrome,* due usually to bilateral occipitoparietal lesions); and a failure to perceive simultaneously all the elements of a scene (*simultanagnosia*). In actuality these agnosias represent the effects not of purely occipital lesions but of either occipitotemporal or occipitoparietal disconnections.

The details of these syndromes of the different lobes of the cerebrum can be found in the textbook of Adams and Victor and the monographs by Walsh and Mesulam.

CORPUS CALLOSUM AND THE DISCONNECTION SYNDROMES Considerable attention has been devoted to the study of each of the two cerebral hemispheres in isolation. This is possible only when the corpus callosum, which forms a bridge between the two hemispheres, is surgically sectioned (for epilepsy) or destroyed by infarction or tumors. From these studies emerges the well-known fact that the left hemisphere is dominant in all language functions and auditory perception and the right hemisphere is superior in spatial and visual perception. Partial lesions of the corpus callosum or of the long tracts in the cerebral white matter are found to be associated with a number of interesting syndromes (commissural and intrahemispheric) described below.

When the corpus callosum is sectioned by a surgical procedure or destroyed by an anterior cerebral artery occlusion (anterior four-fifths), the language and perceptual areas of the left hemisphere are isolated from the sensory and motor areas of the right hemisphere. These patients, if blindfolded, are then unable to match an object held in one hand with an identical object in the other hand. Further, they cannot match an object seen in the right half of the visual field with one in the left half. If given verbal commands, they perform correctly with the right hand but not with the left. Without vision, objects placed in the right hand are named correctly, but not those in the left. In lesions confined to the posterior fifth of the corpus callosum (splenium), only the visual part of the disconnection syndrome occurs. Occlusion of the left posterior cerebral artery provides the best examples of this. Infarction of the left occipital lobe causes a right homonymous hemianopsia, as a consequence of which all visual information needed for activating the speech areas of the left hemisphere must come from the right occipital lobe, across the splenium of the corpus callosum. If there is a lesion in the corpus callosum (or in other portions of the crossing fibers), the patient cannot read or name colors because the visual information cannot reach the left angular gyrus. There is no difficulty in copying words, though the patient cannot read what he or she has written (alexia without agraphia); matching colors without naming them is done without error. Apparently the visual information for activating the left motor area crosses the corpus callosum more anteriorly. A lesion that is limited to the anterior third of the corpus callosum does not result in a left-sided apraxia (a failure of the left hand to obey commands, the right one performing perfectly). A section of the entire corpus callosum does result in such an apraxia, indicating that the fiber systems connecting the left to the right motor areas cross posterior to the genu (but anterior to the splenium).

There are also intrahemispheric disconnections, of which the most important are the following:

1 *Conduction aphasia* (also called *central* aphasia). The patient has fluent but paraphasic speech and writing with nearly perfect comprehension of spoken or written language. Repetition of what is heard or read is, however, severely impaired. The lesion is presumably in the arcuate fasciculus, which connects Wernicke's area with Broca's area.

2 *Pure word deafness*. Although the patient is able to hear and identify nonverbal sounds, there is a loss of ability to comprehend spoken language. The patient's speech remains normal. The defect has been attributed to a subcortical lesion, undercutting Wernicke's area.

DIAGNOSIS AND MANAGEMENT OF PATIENTS WITH FOCAL CEREBRAL LESIONS   These involve the same principles described in Chap. 30. Special tests, mostly of the psychological type, are available for each of the focal cerebral syndromes. The investigation and care of individual patients will also be governed by the underlying disease, of course.

REFERENCES

ADAMS RD, VICTOR M: *Principles of Neurology,* 4th ed. New York, McGraw-Hill, 1989

BRODAL A: *Neurological Anatomy in Relation to Clinical Medicine,* 3d ed. New York, Oxford University Press, 1981

BROWN JW: Frontal lobe syndromes, in *Handbook of Clinical Neurology,* JAM Frederiks (ed). Amsterdam, Elsevier Science, 1985, vol 45, chap 3

DIMOND SJ: The disconnection syndromes, in *Modern Trends in Neurology,* D. Williams (ed). London, Butterworth, 1975

GESCHWIND N: Disconnection syndromes in animals and man. Brain 88:237, 585, 1965

HECAEN H, ALBERT ML: Disorders of mental functioning related to the frontal lobes, in *Modern Trends in Neurology,* D Williams (ed). London, Butterworth, 1975

HEILMAN KM, VALENSTEIN E: *Clinical Neuropsychology,* 2d ed. Oxford, Oxford University Press, 1985

LURIA AR: *The Working Brain: An Introduction to Neuropsychology.* New York, Basic Books (translation Penguin Books Ltd), 1973

MARLOWE WH et al: Complete Klüver-Bucy syndrome in man. Cortex 11:53, 1975

MESULAM M-M (ed): *Principles of Behavioral Neurology.* Philadelphia, Davis, 1985

WALSH KW: *Neuropsychology: A Clinical Approach.* London, Churchill Livingstone, 1978

---

33   DISORDERS OF SPEECH AND LANGUAGE

JAY P. MOHR

Language and speech are fundamental both to social intercourse and to intellectual life. When disordered as a consequence of disease of the brain, the loss exceeds blindness, deafness, or paralysis in gravity.

TERMS   The terms *speech* and *language* are separated here to emphasize that the two are not synonymous. A given brain lesion may affect them in different ways and degrees of severity.

The term *speech* is usually taken to mean the execution of acquired motor skills for the pronunciation of words, putting the expected emphasis on given syllables; the intonation of strings of words to make questions or statements; the grouping of words into phrases; and production of the speech "melody" that is distinctive for given languages and regional dialects. The skillful use of speech is often essential to communication. For example, the meaning of what is a sincere expression in written words may be radically altered when it is spoken in a sarcastic manner. While necessary for the communication of language, speech skills are mainly a modality by which language is conveyed from one person to another and are not themselves sufficient to produce communication. Even when speech is poorly executed (as for example in *dysarthria*), it may nonetheless permit communication.

Language has a wider connotation and refers to the selection and serial ordering of words according to rules that permit a person using one or more of the modalities of speech to modify the behavior of another, and to express that poorly understood cerebral activity termed *thinking*. Disturbances of language usage or comprehension, apart from disorders in the modalities of speech by which the words are discriminated or produced, are known broadly as *aphasia*. Since the disorder clinically encountered is rarely complete, some insist the state is better described by the term indicating a partial disturbance, namely, *dysphasia*. Because of its more common use, aphasia will be used in this chapter.

CEREBRAL DOMINANCE: RELATION TO SPEECH AND HANDEDNESS   The side dominant for language is inferred from which eye, hand, or foot is chosen preferentially for intricate, complex acts. Such preference is more complete in some persons than in others. Hereditary, anatomic and developmental factors play a role. Over 90 percent of people are right-handed. Left-handedness may be hereditary or may result from disease of the left cerebral hemisphere in early life. Left hemisphere dominance for language occurs in 95 percent of right-handed people and in 50 percent of those who are left-handed.

Anatomic differences exist between the dominant and the nondominant cerebral hemispheres. The planum temporale, a part of Wernicke's language zone, is larger in the left hemisphere in right-handed individuals. Formerly, many children were shifted at an early age from left to right (shifted sinistrals) because it is a handicap to be left-handed in a right-handed world. A disturbance in language is produced in almost all right-handers by unilateral brain damage that affects the left hemisphere. Positron emission tomography has shown the left hemisphere to be activated more for verbal tasks, the right for spatial motor tasks.

LANGUAGE DISORDERS IN MEDICAL PRACTICE

Language disorders may be divided into four categories:

1 *Aphasia* is defined as a state in which there is a loss more or less exclusively of the production and/or comprehension of speech and language from an acquired cerebral lesion.
2 *Dysarthria* is a defect in articulation usually related to poor pronunciation of consonants. These defects are pure motor disorders of the muscles of articulation in the presence of intact mental functions and may be due to flaccid or spastic paralysis, rigidity, repetitive spasms (stuttering), or ataxia.
3 *Aphonia or dysphonia* is the loss of voice due to a disease of the larynx or its innervation, causing inability to produce the basic vowel sounds.
4 *Disturbances of language* occur with diseases that produce delirium and dementia (see Chap. 30). Speech is seldom lost, and language is deranged as part of a general impairment of cerebral functions.

APHASIA As a general orientation, most lesions that lead to aphasia occur in the perisylvian regions (frontal, temporal, and parietal) of the dominant cerebral hemisphere, i.e., the left side in right-handed individuals. The anatomic site of the lesion can usually be demonstrated by computed tomography (CT scan) or magnetic resonance imaging (MRI).

Anteriorly placed sylvian lesions mainly disturb the acts of speaking. These range from mutism through impaired articulation, to disordered transitions from syllable to syllable, to abnormalities in phrasing, intonation, and melody. Lesions more posterior produce malpositioning of the tongue, lips, and other structures in the oropharynx with anticipatory errors from some syllables occurring out of sequence. Lesions grouped around the posterior sylvian fissure including the superior temporal lobe and its auditory gyri are manifested by disordered understanding of spoken words, resulting in poor repetition of speech sounds.

The language deficits that are superimposed on the speech disturbances are less well correlated with anatomic pathology. Language disturbances can be separated by pathoanatomic considerations into two large groups. Large anterior lesions involving the bulk of the frontal operculum (that region which lies above the insula) and the insula itself result in agrammatism, featuring sharply contracted sentence structure, absence of most small words, and a preservation of words serving mainly a predicative, interjectional, or substantive function. The patient may only be able to say "hi," "no," and "hello" or to use simple nouns, i.e., "ball," "top," "key." Large posterior sylvian lesions show almost the opposite, with simple speech elements missing or replaced by substitutions in which the desired response is only approximated (*paraphasias*). These latter may consist of faulty pronunciations (*literal paraphasias*) or faulty word selections (*verbal paraphasias*). Verbal paraphasias may approximate the desired word with a similarity of sound or of spelling (*formal verbal paraphasias*), such as "stock" for "stop" or by similarity of meaning (*semantic verbal paraphasias*) such as "slow" for "stop." Disturbances in understanding language, both auditory and visual speech, occur in both types of major paraphasias.

Diseases of the cerebral surface gray matter produce a more significant deficit than those confined to the white matter: tumors, located largely in the white matter, usually reach a large size before causing a speech or language deficit. Infarcts or traumatic lesions of one or more centimeters in diameter are usually associated with an evanescent deficit that fades to functional insignificance within weeks or months.

Deficits due to acute lesions are most easily demonstrated in the acute phase. Improvements over weeks to months occur in all but the largest vascular lesions, but those due to tumors show progression.

The site is more significant than the size of the lesion: the former determines the qualitative features of the deficit, while size determines the severity of the syndrome. Furthermore, deficits in speech function predominate in smaller lesions, while major disturbances in language are superimposed on the speech disturbance in the larger lesions.

Lesions well away from the sylvian region either cause no disturbance of human communicative skills or alter them only secondarily. An example of the latter is the lesion of the anterior frontal lobes, especially the medial and orbital parts, that impairs all motor activities and often results in lack of attention and responsiveness (abulia), verging on the akinetic mute state (see Chap. 32). The speech is laconic with long pauses between utterances, and there is an inability to sustain monologue and narrative. Extensive occipital lesions impair reading and reduce the utilization of all visual, lexical stimuli. Thalamic and deep cerebral lesions impair alertness and cause fluctuating states of inattention and disorientation, thereby inducing fragmentation of words (neologisms) and phrases, and protracted, uncontrollable talking (logorrhea). Strong stimulation to increase momentarily the level of awareness and alertness usually will show that such patients have intact language mechanisms.

The nondominant hemisphere provides the substratum for several types of behavior: motor responses of mimicry, social anticipation (smiling, handshaking, modesty reactions), and self-care (washing and feeding); avoidance behavior to noxious stimuli; and the capability of cross matching visually when presented simple words with pictures. It follows that tests which elicit these behaviors are no guide to functions of the hemisphere dominant for language.

Lesions of the frontal (motor) regions are generally believed to produce syndromes independent from those of the posterior (sensory) regions; the dysphasias can be classified as motor (Broca's) or sensory (Wernicke's) and can be further specified as subcortical, cortical, or transcortical in location. Subcortical lesions are believed to interfere with the main efferent or afferent projections of the cerebrum; lesions of the surface involve the "centers" themselves; transcortical lesions isolate these centers from one another or from other regions of the brain related to speech. Although an oversimplification, these basic concepts provide a rough guide for the classification of the aphasias, but they are not reliable to predict the lesion's site and size. Positron emission studies have challenged formerly popular concepts of functional connections between the major language areas.

TYPES OF APHASIA Disturbances of speech and language can result from several abnormalities. Classifications have been based upon the predominant form, the presumed physiologic or psychological bases, and the anatomy of the underlying diseases. The classification utilized here has been formulated on the basis of the anatomic localization and the clinical presentation (see Table 33-1). The prognoses are helpful in management, particularly in the choice of corrective measures in therapy. Aphasias have also been classified according to the severity of impediment to speech production and flow. *Fluent aphasias* are characterized by runs of well-articulated speech, of basically normal rhythm and flow, although lacking in language meaning. The defect is usually a lesion in the dominant parietal or temporal lobe. *Nonfluent aphasias* are characterized by slow, incorrectly articulated words and sentences. The lesion usually lies in the dominant frontal lobe.

Total (global) aphasia In total, or global, aphasia the causative lesion destroys a large part of the speech and language areas of the major cerebral hemisphere, producing a severe aphasic deficit which has the poorest prognosis for improvement of any aphasic syndrome.

Most patients with total aphasia say but a few words; they do not read or write, and they understand only a few words of the speech of others. Related signs include right hemiplegia, hemianesthesia, and homonymous hemianopsia. The alert patient may participate in common gestures of greeting, may show modesty and avoidance reactions, and is able to engage in self-help activities. The early appearance of clearly vocalized stereotyped words, such as "hi" and "yes," are often falsely encouraging signs; they may reflect the uninhibited function of the right hemisphere. After weeks or months

TABLE 33-1   Classification of aphasic disorders

	Clinical manifestations	Anatomic location	Etiology	Associated clinical symptoms
MAJOR SYNDROMES				
Global aphasia	Minimal speech, nonfluent aphasia; comprehension poor for spoken and written language	Large lesion of dominant frontal, parietal, and superior temporal lobe	Infarction in distribution of internal carotid or middle cerebral artery; trauma; tumor	Contralateral hemiplegia; hemisensory loss; hemianopsia
Broca's aphasia	Nonfluent aphasia; agrammatic sentences; poor articulation; dysprosody; may be mute	Cortical and subcortical lesion of prefrontal and frontal regions	Infarction in distribution of superior frontal branch middle cerebral artery; hemorrhage; tumor	Contralateral hemiparesis; minor or no sensory loss; no visual field disturbance; oral dyspraxia; cortical dysarthria; severe impairment in writing
Wernicke's aphasia (central or sensory aphasia)	Fluent speech; total incomprehension of spoken speech; inability to read or to repeat sounds or words; alexia, agraphia, paraphasia common	Posterior perisylvian structures of the parietal and temporal lobe	Infarction in distribution of lower division of middle cerebral artery; tumor; herpes simplex encephalitis	Parietal lobe sensory deficits; hemianopsia; no motor disturbance
MINOR CENTRAL APHASIA SYNDROMES				
Conduction aphasia	Paraphasia; difficulty in repetition of speech and in reading aloud; aware of deficit; adequate comprehension of written and spoken words	Upper bank of sylvian fissure; inferior parietal lobule	Embolic occlusion of posterior branches of middle cerebral artery	Contralateral hemihypesthesia or homonymous hemianopsia; abnormal optokinetic nystagmus
Mainly auditory (pure word deafness)	Impaired auditory comprehension; inability to repeat a sentence or write a dictation	Lesion in superior temporal gyrus	Infarction, tumor, abscess	Rarely deafness
Mainly visual (dyslexia with dysgraphia)	Visual language compromised more than auditory; cannot read or write	Parietooccipital lesion	Infarction; tumor, lobar hemorrhage	Hemianopsia
OTHER SYNDROMES				
Pure word blindness	Normal spoken language and writing, with inability to read	Left occipitostriate cortex, adjacent association cortex, and posterior corpus callosum (splenium)	Infarction in distribution of posterior cerebral artery; tumor, lobar hemorrhage	Hemianopsia
Isolation of speech areas	Parrot-like speech; echolalia	Ischemic infarction in border (watershed) zones between anterior, middle, and posterior cerebral artery distributions	Systemic hypotension or hypoxia; cardiac arrest	Decreased alertness and responsiveness; bilateral leg weakness
Amnesic-dysnomic aphasia	Inability to recall names of objects or parts of objects; difficulty with recent memory	Deep temporal lobe lesions, parahippocampal, hippocampal gyrus	Tumor; Alzheimer's disease; infarction in distribution posterior cerebral artery; herpes simplex encephalitis	Apraxia; dementia; no motor or sensory abnormalities; upper quadrantic visual field defect

the understanding of spoken speech improves slightly and a few words may be uttered.

Infarction from occlusion of the left internal carotid or the middle cerebral artery, a large hemorrhage, major tumor, or penetrating trauma is most often responsible. In the rare instances of rapid improvement, the main cause is postconvulsive paralysis, posttraumatic edema, or transitory ischemia from a fragmenting embolus. Rarely, hyperthermia, infection, or hyponatremia may transiently cause a temporary relapse of aphasia due to an old lesion.

Broca's aphasia (major motor aphasia)   This term designates a complex syndrome with severely disturbed speech and writing, accompanied by simplified grammar skills (agrammatism) in speaking and writing and a less obvious impairment in language comprehension. The syndrome results from a large lesion involving cortical and subcortical structures along the insula and superior sylvian fissure, not simply Broca's area, a circumscribed lesion in the inferior frontal convolution. CT scan may underestimate the lesion because the angle of the imaged lesion may seem to merge with the sylvian fissure.

The lesions are smaller than those causing complete aphasia and usually involve the sensorimotor rolandic region, producing an accompanying persisting hemiparesis and hemisensory syndrome. Initially, a transient ipsilateral deviation of the eyes is observed due to the frontal infarction.

In the acute phase, the entire language mechanism appears to be inactivated, and the helplessly mute, noncommunicative, and uncomprehending patient presents the syndrome of complete or global

aphasia. Within weeks to years, the disorder of comprehension abates somewhat, and this improvement exceeds that found in speaking and writing, leaving the motor speech deficits that gave the syndrome its original name.

For a time an apraxia of the lingual and oropharyngeal apparatus retards efforts to make purposeful movements. Imitation may be better performed than execution of acts on command. Certain stereotyped and simple phrases, such as "hi," "good morning," or curses are uttered more easily, and words of popular songs may be sung surprisingly well. The patient's efforts to speak and facial expressions suggest an awareness of his or her ineptitudes and mistakes, and an accompanying exasperation and despair are common.

As improvement occurs, words are enunciated slowly and laboriously, with greatly impaired melody of speech (prosody). Speech is sparse and consists mainly of nouns, transitive verbs, and important adjectives; many of the small words (articles, prepositions, conjunctions) are omitted, giving the speech an agrammatic and telegraphic character. The preservation of substantive words allows the patients to communicate despite the gross mechanical and agrammatic language difficulties. This hesitant, laconic speech has been termed nonfluent aphasia.

Most patients with Broca's aphasia have a correspondingly severe impairment in communication by writing with either hand. However, communication by writing is superior to that by speaking, suggesting a certain independence between these two acts as vehicles of language.

The syndrome is most often due to embolic occlusions of the

upper division of the left middle cerebral artery; major putaminal hypertensive hemorrhage, huge frontal lobe tumor or abscess, metastatic lesions, subdural hematoma, and encephalitis are less common causes.

Minor motor aphasia More circumscribed focal lesions along the anterior and superior sylvian operculum and insula produce remarkably discrete effects on the speech skills which may resemble major motor aphasia except for the satisfactory understanding of spoken and written words. The prognosis for nearly full recovery is excellent. Indeed, *none of these focal lesions produces significant or lasting deficits in language usage.*

Broca's area infarction affects the lower premotor cortex adjacent to the motor cortex controlling the oropharynx, larynx, and respiratory apparatus. The infarct interrupts skilled movements of these muscle groups, and the resultant dyspraxia in speech features impaired transitions between syllables in words and disruption of the melodic intonation of phrases (dysprosody). Involvement of this region alone is insufficient to produce the major syndrome referred to as Broca's aphasia. *Rolandic infarction* involves the sensorimotor cortex itself; either the syndrome of dysprosody occurs, or speech has poor articulation and lowered volume and pitch, while a nasal quality to the voice reveals the paresis of the nasopharyngeal musculature. *Postcentral, anterior parietal infarction* is associated with errors in the positioning of the oral cavity for individual sounds, syllables, and whole words; the acoustic features of the utterance are often distorted by these malpositions of the oral cavity and strike the ear as literal paraphasias.

Lesions in the more anterior parts of the dominant frontal lobe, sparing Broca's area, may also cause an aphasic disorder. Usually speech output is reduced and nonfluent, and auditory comprehension is intact. Repetition of words spoken by the examiner is preserved. This condition has been called *transcortical motor aphasia* but may be part of the broader frontal lobe syndromes in which spontaneous speech is lacking (mutism) and all motor activity is reduced (akinesia).

Most such focal lesions are due to emboli to the sequential branches of the upper division of the middle cerebral artery. Deeper, larger lesions or larger emboli involving the stem of the upper division can cause several types of deficit in a single patient, making these individual distinctions less clear and blending with the major syndrome of Broca's aphasia. Facial, lingual, and sometimes brachial paresis and ideomotor dyspraxia of the face and left, nondominant limbs commonly accompany the speech disorder. Most of these syndromes recede within weeks or months.

Wernicke's aphasia (major central or sensory aphasia) This term encompasses a range of syndromes that arise from lesions of the posterior perisylvian structures or the posterior temporal, parietal, and occipital regions supplied by the lower division of the middle cerebral artery. There is disruption of the whole array of language behavior. When restricted to the temporal lobe, the main disturbance is most evident in language tasks involving words heard; and when more parietal and occipital, in words seen.

Spoken and written efforts in communication as well as in auditory and visual comprehension are affected, a combination that justifies the term *central aphasia*. The term *sensory aphasia* was formerly used to accentuate the contrast with motor (Broca's) aphasia. Instead of the difficult articulation, faulty transitions, dysmelodic speaking, and disproportionate condensation of grammatical forms that characterize Broca's aphasia, the speech of Wernicke's aphasia is fluent, hence the name *fluent aphasia.*

In severe cases, the patient utters a series of incomprehensible syllables, makes illegible marks on a page in attempts at writing, cannot be made to repeat aloud or copy correctly at sight, and treats the examiner's attempts at written and verbal communication as if they were in a wholly unfamiliar foreign language. In less severe cases, the patient can repeat aloud and copy, but echoes the words heard with faulty pronunciation or copies the words in a slavish manner, imitating even the examiner's handwriting style, as though the test words were unfamiliar. The disturbance in language does not simply reflect a disturbance in hearing or in vision. In the mildest cases, the deficits are manifested in errors in word comprehension and usage. The patient may choose words that show approximation to the desired response, the words often belonging to the same functional class [i.e., *cow* for *pig,* but not *cow* for *yellow* (such errors are labeled *semantic verbal paraphasias*)]; or the words may be similar in sound or shape (*formal verbal paraphasias*) such as "flee" for "tree"; there may be errors in word structure, with improper tenses, prefixes, suffixes (i.e., *beautifuling*), or other errors that resemble those of normal people unfamiliar with the language in question. Some such patients pass for normal in brief or casual conversation. In its milder form or later in the course of the illness, the speech resembles that of a person tired or distracted, and the abnormality is detected only on tests of complex language function.

CT scanning and MRI are the best methods to delineate the topography of the lesion. Arteriographic findings are an unreliable basis of correlation because the vascular occlusions, most often due to cerebral embolism, frequently fail to show the embolus because it has disintegrated or drifted distally into one or more smaller branches. Radionuclide brain scanning is useful only for the largest lesions.

Minor central aphasia syndromes In time, Wernicke's aphasia improves, and a number of lesser syndromes appear. These latter, however, may be present in comparatively pure form from the beginning, when only a small, restricted lesion involves some part of the territory of the lower division of the middle cerebral artery.

The posterior sylvian region, comprising posterosuperior temporal, opercular, supramarginal, and posterior insular gyri, appears to encompass a variety of language functions. Seemingly minor changes in size and locale of the lesion are associated with important variations in the elements of Wernicke's aphasia. Depending on the location of the lesion, language behavior dependent on auditory function (hearing spoken words, echoing sounds and speech, relating the spoken to the written word, and finally repeating and writing it) may be deranged partially or completely. The same is true of language behavior dependent upon visual function, when the left posterior parietal lobe is involved. These partial syndromes are termed *conduction aphasia, pure word deafness, dyslexia with dysgraphia,* and *pure word blindness.*

CONDUCTION APHASIA: SEPARATION OF WERNICKE'S AND BROCA'S LANGUAGE AREAS The principal abnormality resembles Wernicke's aphasia. There is the same degree of paraphasia in self-initiated speech, in repeating what is heard, and in reading aloud. However, little or no difficulty is encountered in comprehending words that are heard or seen. Because the motor regions are unaffected, no element of dysarthria or dysprosody occurs. The patient is alert and unaware of the deficit. The mistakes take the form of literal paraphasia; i.e., errors in oropharyngeal positioning produce detectably different sounds from those intended. The disorder in repeating from dictation becomes more apparent when the rate of presentation of auditory material is increased, the uttered words are polysyllabic, or the words are unfamiliar, e.g., sets of nonsense syllables. Since nouns are usually the longest words in sentences, one may gain an impression that they are specifically affected.

The lesion at autopsy is located in the cortex and subcortical white matter in the upper bank of the sylvian fissure, involving the supramarginal gyrus of the inferior parietal lobule. The posterior part of the superior temporal region is occasionally affected. The usual cause is an embolus in the ascending parietal or posterior temporal branch of the middle cerebral artery. Deeper, larger lesions that interrupt the arcuate fasciculus connecting the temporal and frontal lobes may produce the syndrome, but usually they involve other pathways as well, giving rise to a more extensive speech deficit (Wernicke's aphasia or amnesic aphasia). However, these latter types of aphasia, as they regress, may resolve into conduction aphasia. More anterior insular lesions usually include some degree of Broca's aphasia.

PURE WORD DEAFNESS Instead of a disturbance confined to auditory comprehension, this syndrome is considered to be the auditory form of Wernicke's aphasia. The most obvious findings are an impaired auditory comprehension and inability to repeat what is said or to write to dictation. Spoken language is less impaired but rarely normal, and occasionally the paraphasic speech leads to an initial diagnosis of Wernicke's aphasia. By audiometric testing little defect in hearing is found. The patient frequently learns to use visual cues well enough to overcome much of the difficulty. Comprehension of visually presented material such as printed matter, although not normal, is better than auditory comprehension. When there is full preservation of reading skill, the traditional term *pure word deafness* can be applied.

In most autopsy studies the lesion is embolic, bilateral in the superior temporal gyrus, in position to damage the primary auditory cortex in the transverse gyrus of Heschl and to impair its relation to the associated areas of the superior, posterior part of the temporal lobe. The occasional unilateral lesions are localized in this part of the major (dominant) temporal lobe and encroach on those regions whose involvement precipitates the larger syndrome of Wernicke's aphasia.

DYSLEXIA WITH DYSGRAPHIA   This language disturbance is often a late sequela of the larger syndrome of Wernicke's aphasia, most evident in reading and writing. The syndrome is the visual form of Wernicke's aphasia. Errors occur in response to lexical stimuli. Auditory comprehension, while not normal, is less impaired than visual comprehension. Since conversational testing is frequently the only type of clinical evaluation in such patients, satisfactory auditory comprehension, ability to repeat aloud, and mild paraphasic errors in spontaneous speech frequently lead to a misdiagnosis of mild Wernicke's aphasia. Detailed testing of reading aloud and reading for comprehension and tests of spontaneous writing and of writing in response to dictated and visually presented material reveal a greater disturbance in these tasks.

The parietal and occipital region is usually affected. Although a discrete embolism is unusual, a small clot may pass through the more proximal territory and lodge distally. Tumors, abscess, and lobar hemorrhages usually disrupt other structures as well, and this syndrome is often a less conspicuous part of a larger clinical picture. Systemic hypotension and hypoxia may leave dyslexia with dysgraphia as a residual impairment, but more often they produce a more severe defect, described below under "Isolation of speech areas."

PURE WORD BLINDNESS   In the fully developed syndrome, the victims lose the ability to read and usually to name colors. The patient is unable to name or point to a letter or word on command. However, understanding spoken language, repetition of what is heard, writing to dictation, conversation and writing, are all intact. The condition is also sometimes termed *dyslexia without dysgraphia.* Because the victim may be unaware the deficit exists, the examiner is often required to test for its presence, rather than simply assume the complaint will be volunteered. The errors may be minimal and the defect obscured if other visual cues are available, such as the bottle on which the words Coca-Cola appear. The naming of common colors presented singly and of objects is also impaired. When the syndrome is less severe, reading is impaired mainly in the affected visual field, producing a dyslexia for the letters on the affected side of the longer words (so-called hemidyslexia).

Right homonymous hemianopsia, an amnesic defect, and a hemisensory defect on the right reflect the involvement of the left occipital lobe and its callosal decussation, the left fornix, and the left thalamus, respectively, a combination that nearly always signifies thrombosis or embolism of the left posterior cerebral artery, placing the origin of this syndrome rather remote from the main language zone supplied by the middle cerebral artery.

Autopsy usually demonstrates a lesion that destroys the left visual striate cortex (area 17) and visual association areas (18 and 19), as well as the connections of the right visual cortex and association areas with the temporoparietal region. This latter "disconnection" usually is due to interruption of the fibers passing through the posterior part (splenium) of the corpus callosum, which connect the visual

association areas of the two hemispheres. Rarely, a lesion deep in the left parietooccipital region prevents visual information from either occipital lobe from reaching the left language region. Right homonymous hemianopsia may be absent. Aside from infarction, the syndrome may occur from a primary or secondary tumor, multifocal leukoencephalopathy, or even from multiple sclerosis.

Isolation of speech areas   Following prolonged hypoxia, widespread cerebral ischemia can affect the vascular border zones linking the major cerebral arteries and their distal branches on the cerebral surfaces and spread centripetally into their adjacent territories. The central fields of supply of these arteries may be spared. In the middle cerebral artery territory, this sparing leaves largely intact the sylvian region and its speech areas. With much of the rest of the brain out of action in patients who survive such episodes, the speech mechanism can be activated by spoken words. There is parrotlike repetition of words and sounds (echolalia) and similar findings which indicate that the auditory-vocal loop is functional. Scant evidence of comprehension or self-initiated conversation is present, reflecting the widespread injury outside the speech regions. The syndrome is common following cardiac arrest.

Amnesic-dysnomic aphasia   This may be a relatively early or an isolated syndrome in patients with CNS disease. The patient has difficulty recalling names on demand, not only nouns but also adjectives and other descriptive parts of speech. There are usually pauses in speech, groping for words, and substitution of another word or phrase that conveys the meaning (circumlocution). The function of an object may be described, but its name forgotten. The difficulty applies not only to common objects seen but also to the names of things heard or felt. By contrast, other verbal tasks, including recall of the names of the letters and digits, reading, writing, spelling, etc., are far better performed.

The causative lesion is usually deep in the temporal lobe, presumably interrupting connections of sensory speech areas with the hippocampal-parahippocampal regions concerned with learning and memory (see Chap. 32). Masses such as a tumor or abscess are the most frequent causes; as they enlarge, an upper contralateral quadrantic visual field defect or Wernicke's aphasia is added. Dysnomia may be part of the syndromes produced by occlusion of the temporal branches of the posterior cerebral artery. Alzheimer's disease may begin with a dysnomic or amnesic type of aphasia; by the time the patient's difficulty is fully recognized, other disorders of speech and indifference, apathy, and abulia are conjoined. Dysnomia may also be present in confusional states caused by metabolic, infectious, intoxicative, or other acute medical illnesses, but then it has no certain localizing value.

The combination of dysnomia and major impairment of auditory comprehension with a remarkable retention of the ability to repeat what is heard is called *transcortical sensory aphasia.* The causative lesion spares the auditory cortex and Wernicke area and involves the inferior temporal cortices, particularly area 37.

DISORDERS OF ARTICULATION AND PHONATION   The highly coordinated act of speaking involves the larynx, pharynx, palate, tongue, lips, and respiratory musculature, which are innervated by the hypoglossal, vagal, facial, and phrenic nerves. Their nuclei are controlled through the corticobulbar tracts by both motor cortices and by extrapyramidal influences from the cerebellum and basal ganglia. The current of air is produced by expiration and is finely regulated by the activity of the various muscles engaged in speech. *Phonation,* or the production of vocal sounds, is a function of the larynx. Changes in the size and shape of the glottis and in the length and tension of the vocal cords are controlled by the laryngeal muscles, which transmit their vibrations to the column of air passing over the vocal cords. Sounds thus formed are modified as they pass through the nasopharynx and mouth, which act as resonators. *Articulation* consists of contractions of the tongue, lips, pharynx, and palate, which interrupt or alter the vocal sounds. Vowels are of laryngeal origin, as are some consonants, but the latter are formed for the most part during articulation. For instance, the consonants *m, b,* and *p* are labial; *l* and *t* are lingual; and *nk* and *ng* are nasoguttural.

Disorders of phonation prompt examination of the vocal cords, tongue, palate, and pharynx. Defects in articulation can be subdivided into paretic dysarthria; spastic and rigid dysarthria; and choreic, myoclonic, and ataxic dysarthria.

Aphonia   Some speech disorders involve disturbances of voice. Paresis of the respiratory movements, as in poliomyelitis and acute infectious polyneuritis, or incoordination as part of extrapyramidal disease may affect the voice because insufficient air is provided for phonation and speech. Reduced volume of speech due to limited excursion of the breathing muscles is common; the patient is unable to speak above a whisper or to shout. Whispering speech is also a feature of stupor, but strong stimulation may make the voice audible.

Paresis of both vocal cords causes complete aphonia. There is no voice, and the patient can speak only in whispers. Since the vocal cords normally separate during inspiration, their failure to do so when paralyzed may result in an inspiratory stridor. If one vocal cord is paralyzed, the voice becomes hoarse, low-pitched, and rasping. Involvement of one of the tenth cranial nerves by tumor, for example, may also cause a nasal voice because the posterior nares do not close during phonation. Consonants such as *b, p, n,* and *k* are followed by escape of air into the nasal passages. The abnormality may be less pronounced in recumbency and may increase when the head is thrown forward. Hoarseness may also be due to structural changes in the vocal cords caused by cigarette smoking, chronic inflammation, polyps, etc.

Spastic dysphonia is a poorly understood neurologic disorder similar to dystonia. Many patients, middle-aged or elderly, otherwise healthy, gradually lose the ability to speak quietly and fluently. Any effort to speak results in contraction of the speech musculature so that the voice is strained and phonation is labored. The patients are not neurotic, and psychotherapy and speech therapy are ineffective. The condition differs from the stridor caused by spasm of the laryngeal muscles in tetany. It is nonprogressive but may be combined with restricted extrapyramidal disorders such as blepharospasm and spasmodic torticollis. Surgical section of the superior laryngeal nerve on one side has been found to at least partially diminish the rigidity.

Paretic dysarthria   This disorder of articulation is due to a neural or bulbar (medullary) weakness or paralysis of the articulatory muscles (lower motor neuron paralysis). There is a special difficulty in the correct utterance of vibratives, such as *r;* the voice develops a nasal quality due to palatal weakness; as the paralysis becomes more complete, lingual and labial consonants are not pronounced. In the advanced stages, the shriveled tongue lies inert on the floor of the mouth, and the lips are relaxed and tremulous. Saliva collects in the mouth because of dysphagia and spills over the lips causing drooling. Bulbar palsy, peripheral neuropathies, and muscle diseases, including myasthenia gravis, are common causes.

Spastic and rigid dysarthria   This disorder is a supranuclear weakness of articulation. Diseases that involve the corticobulbar or subcortical tracts cause pseudobulbar palsy. In the past, the patient may have had a minor stroke affecting the corticobulbar fibers on one side; but since the bulbar muscles are probably represented in both motor cortices, there is no impairment in speech or swallowing from a unilateral lesion. Should another stroke then occur, involving the other corticobulbar tract and possibly the corticospinal tract at the pontine, midbrain, or capsular level, the patient becomes anarthric or dysarthric and dysphagic. Often the muscles of facial expression on both sides are weakened as well. Unlike bulbar paralysis due to lower neuron involvement, this condition entails no atrophy or fasciculation of the paralyzed muscles; the jaw jerk and other facial reflexes are exaggerated; the palatal reflexes are retained; emotional control is poor (pathologic laughter and crying); and sometimes breathing is periodic (Cheyne-Stokes). When the frontal operculum alone is involved, the speech deficit may be a pure dysarthria but usually without the impairment in emotional control. In the beginning, the patient may be totally anarthric and aphonic, but when improve-

ment occurs or when the patient has a milder version of the same condition, speech is notably slow, thick, and indistinct, much like that of partial bulbar paralysis.

An extrapyramidal disturbance of articulation occurs in Parkinson's syndrome. The patient speaks hastily and articulates poorly, slurring over many syllables and trailing the ends of sentences. The voice is low-pitched, monotonous, and lacking in inflection; voice volume diminishes. In advanced cases speech is almost unintelligible; only whispering is possible.

In many cases of capsular hemiplegia or partially recovered Broca's aphasia, residual dysarthria may be difficult to distinguish from a pure articulatory defect.

Choreic and myoclonic dysarthria   In chorea and myoclonus, speech may also be characteristic. Unlike the defect of pseudobulbar palsy or parkinsonism, chorea and myoclonus abruptly interrupt the pronunciation of words by the abnormal movements. Grimacing and other characteristic motor signs suggest the diagnosis.

Ataxic dysarthria   This is characteristic of acute and chronic cerebellar lesions and may be observed in multiple sclerosis, Friedreich's ataxia, cerebellar atrophy, and heat stroke. The principal speech abnormality is slowness; imprecise enunciation, monotony, and unnatural, irregular separation of the syllables of words (scanning) are additional features. Coordination of speech and respiration are poor. There may not be enough breath to utter certain words, and others may be ejaculated explosively. Myoclonic jerks involving the speech musculature may be superimposed on cerebellar ataxia in a number of diseases.

CLINICAL APPROACH TO LANGUAGE DISORDERS

DIAGNOSIS   Aphasia   Conversational testing permits quick assessment of the motor aspects of speech (praxis and prosody), apparent language formulation, and auditory comprehension. Disabilities in the purely motor aspects of speech suggest a motor aphasia, and this possibility can be pursued by tests of repeating from dictation and by tests of praxis of the oropharyngeal and respiratory apparatus. Disabilities in language formulation such as literal paraphasias with impaired comprehension are indicative of Wernicke's aphasia. Disorders confined to naming, generally without paraphasias, when other language functions (reading, writing, spelling, etc.) are adequate, are diagnostic of amnesic dysnomia.

Dyspraxia of limbs and speech musculature in response to spoken commands or to visual mimicry is generally associated with Broca's aphasia and sometimes with Wernicke's aphasia. Bilateral or unilateral homonymous hemianopsia without motor weakness is often linked with pure word blindness (alexia or dyslexia) or to amnesic-dysnomic aphasia. Bilateral hemiplegias due to extensive frontal lesions are accompanied not infrequently by pure word muteness.

When conversation shows virtually no disabilities, other tests may be revealing. Reading aloud single letters, words, and text may reveal pure word blindness, while tests of writing in this syndrome are normal. Literal and verbal paraphasic errors may appear in milder cases of Wernicke's aphasia as the patient reads aloud from text or from words in the examiner's handwriting. Similar errors occur more frequently when the patient is asked to explain the text, read aloud, or give explanations in writing. Adequacy of response channels is determined by presenting tasks that permit a response physically identical with the test stimulus, such as copying visual stimuli and repeating aloud from auditory stimuli. Inadequacy of receptive or response channels precludes further analysis of the deficit involving that channel in more complex types of tests, except in the unlikely instance that the more complex test is better performed. If reception and response channels are adequate in these initial tests, they may then be used in tests requiring all types of language function, such as writing from dictation, vocal naming of visual stimuli, matching physically dissimilar stimuli having a name in common (e.g., the word *cow* and a picture of a cow). By using the same test material as in the earlier tests, direct comparison of performances in spoken naming, written naming, and matching can be made from visual, auditory, and palpated stimuli. A performance profile can be constructed separately for each type of stimulus material tested (objects, pictures, words, letters, numbers, colors, etc.). The resultant profile can then be used to determine whether the main deficits fall across one or more input or response channels. These data provide a baseline against which later changes may be compared.

Articulatory-phonation disorders   Disturbances of articulation point to involvement of a different set of neural structures, such as the motor cortices; the corticobulbar pathways; the seventh, ninth, and tenth nuclei; the brainstem; and extrapyramidal nuclei and tracts. It may be necessary to use other neurologic findings to decide which of these are implicated. It is particularly important to distinguish between the pseudobulbar or supranuclear palsies and the bulbar palsies. The information obtained by separating these two types of dysarthria is particularly helpful in differential diagnosis.

Dysphonia should lead to an investigation of laryngeal disease, either primary or secondary to an abnormality of innervation. Inspection of the vocal cords is necessary.

TREATMENT   Except for almost pure motor defects, most patients show remarkably little concern over the sudden loss of speech. The very lesion that deprives them of speech also appears to cause a partial loss of insight into the disability. Nonetheless, as improvement occurs, many patients become discouraged. Reassurance and a positive program of speech rehabilitation are the best ways of helping the patient at this stage.

As a rule, speech therapy is not advisable in the first few days of an aphasic illness, because one does not know how lasting it will be. Also, if a global aphasia is present, the speech therapist is helpless. Under such circumstances, it is preferable to wait until some of the language function has begun to return. In milder aphasic disorders speech therapy can be begun as soon as the illness is stabilized. Although speech therapy has not been proved, in controlled studies, to be of benefit to recovery, its value in terms of support for the patient and the family needs to be emphasized.

There is no special treatment for the dysarthric disturbance of speech.

PROGNOSIS   The outcome depends on the underlying disease and the magnitude of the lesion within the speech areas. Global aphasias lasting more than a week or two usually have a bad outcome. Seldom is there enough recovery of communicative speech to permit resumption of occupation or profession. Partial aphasias frequently improve, sometimes to a gratifying degree, if of vascular or encephalitic origin. Aphasias due to embolism, whether global or restricted, may disappear in hours to days or may persist.

Most aphasias are due to vascular disease of the brain, and some degree of spontaneous improvement usually occurs over days to months after the stroke. Sometimes recovery is complete within hours or days; at times not more than a few words are regained after a year or two of assiduous speech training. Nevertheless, many experts in the field believe that speech training is worthwhile.

REFERENCES

ALBERT ML et al: *Clinical Aspects of Dysphasia.* New York, Springer-Verlag, 1981

CHASE TN et al: Wechsler adult intelligence scale performance. Cortical localization by fluorodeoxyglucose F18-positron emission tomography. Arch Neurol 41:1244, 1984

DAMASIO AR, GESCHWIND N: The neural basis of language. Ann Rev Neurosci 7:127, 1984

KEMPLER D et al: A metabolic investigation of a disconnection syndrome: Conduction aphasia. Ann Neurol 22:134, 1987

LUDLOW CL et al: Brain lesions associated with nonfluent aphasia fifteen years following penetrating head injury. Brain 109:55, 1986

METTER EJ et al: A study of Broca's aphasia by 18F-fluorodeoxyglucose positron emission tomography. Ann Neurol 22:134, 1987

MOHR JP, SIDMAN M: Aphasia: Behavioral aspects, in *American Handbook of Psychiatry,* vol 4, M Reiser (ed). New York, Basic Books, 1975, pp 279–298

PETERSEN SE et al: Position emission tomography studies of the cortical anatomy of single-word processing. Nature 331:585, 1988

POSNER MI et al: Localization of cognitive operations in the human brain. Science 240:1627, 1988

34   DISORDERS OF SLEEP AND CIRCADIAN RHYTHMS

CHARLES A. CZEISLER / GARY S. RICHARDSON / JOSEPH B. MARTIN

Disturbed sleep is among the most frequent health complaints physicians encounter. One-third of adults in the United States experience occasional or persistent sleep disturbances. Sleep deprivation or disruption of the circadian timing system can lead to serious impairment of daytime functioning. Sleep disorders may either contribute to or result from related medical or psychiatric conditions. Twenty years ago, many such complaints were treated with hypnotic medications without further diagnostic evaluation. A distinct class of sleep and arousal disorders has now been identified, and the field of sleep disorders is now an established clinical discipline. Two principal neurobiologic systems govern the sleep-wake cycle: one that actively generates sleep and sleep-related processes and another that times sleep within the 24-h day. Either intrinsic abnormalities in these systems or extrinsic disturbances (environmental, drug- or illness-related) can lead to sleep or circadian rhythm disorders.

PHYSIOLOGY OF SLEEP AND WAKEFULNESS

Most adults sleep 7 to 8 h per night, although the timing, duration, and internal structure of sleep vary among apparently healthy individuals and as a function of age. At the extremes, infants and the elderly have frequent interruptions of sleep. In the United States, individuals of intermediate age tend to have one consolidated sleep episode per day, although in some cultures sleep may be divided into a midafternoon nap and a shortened night sleep. Infants sleep more than half the day, and the elderly sleep less than half that amount. While there is a wide range of normal sleep lengths, adults with habitual sleep durations of fewer than 4 h or greater than 9 have increased mortality rates as compared to those who sleep 7 to 8 h per night.

STATES AND STAGES OF SLEEP   States and stages of human sleep are defined on the basis of characteristic patterns in three electrophysiologic parameters, the electroencephalogram (EEG), the electrooculogram (EOG—a measure of eye-movement activity), and the electromyogram (EMG). In routine sleep recordings, the EEG is recorded from a single central derivation (C3 or C4 in the 10 to 20 standard EEG nomenclature), and sleep states are defined on the basis of the EEG pattern. The EOG is recorded from electrodes placed on the outer canthus of each eye, and the EMG is recorded from the submentalis muscle of the chin. The continuous recording of this array of electrophysiologic parameters to define sleep and wakefulness is termed *polysomnography* (see Table 34-1).

Polysomnograpahic profiles define two states of sleep: (1) rapid-eye-movement (REM) sleep (also known as dreaming, paradoxical, desynchronized, or "D" sleep) and (2) non-rapid-eye-movement (NREM) sleep. NREM sleep is in turn subdivided into four stages. NREM stage 1 is the transition from wakefulness and is characterized by disappearance of the regular alpha pattern and emergence of a low-amplitude, mixed-frequency pattern, predominantly in the theta range (2 to 7 Hz) (Fig. 34-1) and slow "rolling" eye movements. The amplitude of the EMG attenuates and its variability is reduced. NREM stage 2 is defined by the occurrence of K complexes and sleep spindles superimposed upon a background activity similar to that of stage 1. K complexes are slow, high-amplitude, negative (upward) discharges followed immediately by a positive (downward) deflection. Sleep spindles are high-frequency (12 to 14 Hz) discharges lasting 0.5 to 2.0 s with a characteristic waxing-waning amplitude. Eye-movement activity is absent, and the EMG is similar to stage 1. NREM stage 3 is sleep with at least 20 percent but less than 50

TABLE 34-1   Electrophysiologic correlates of human sleep states and stages

	Electroencephalogram	Electrooculogram	Electromyogram
Wake (eyes open)	Low amplitude, mixed, (high) frequency	Rapid	High, variable
Wake (eyes closed)	Low amplitude, alpha (8–13 Hz) dominates, particularly over occipital region	Absent, but slow "rolling" eye movements	Reduced
NREM stage 1	Low amplitude, mixed frequency (alpha absent)	Slow "rolling" eye movements	Reduced
NREM stage 2	Low amplitude with addition of characteristic EEG patterns (K complexes and sleep spindles)	Absent	Reduced
NREM stage 3	Increased amplitude, decreased frequency 20–50% of record dominated by delta (0.5–2.0 Hz)	Absent	Reduced
NREM stage 4	>50% of record dominated by delta EEG activity	Absent	Reduced
REM	Low amplitude, mixed frequency	Rapid, conjugate	Absent

SOURCE: Modified from: Rechtschaffen A, Kales A (eds): *A Manual of Standardized Terminology, Technique and Scoring System for Sleep Stages of Human Subjects*. Los Angeles, UCLA Brain Information Service/Brain Research Institute, 1968.

percent high-amplitude delta (0.5 to 2 Hz) activity. Sleep spindles may persist, eye-movement activity is absent, and EMG activity persists at a reduced level. In NREM stage 4, the high-voltage, slow EEG pattern of stage 3 comprises at least 50 percent of the record. NREM stages 3 and 4 are referred to, collectively, as "slow-wave," "delta," or "deep" sleep.

FIGURE 34-1 Electroencephalogram of human sleep stages. The first trace illustrates alpha activity seen in quiet wakefulness (eyes closed) and the beta activity of an alert subject. Stage 1 theta activity is seen in the second trace; stage 2 sleep (with associated sleep spindle and K complex) in the third. The fourth and fifth traces show slow-wave (stages 3 and 4) sleep, with prominent delta activity. This synchronous activity is absent in REM sleep (sixth trace), which resembles stage 1 EEG. However, REM sleep is accompanied by rapid eye movements and muscle paralysis. (*Reproduced from Horne.*)

The second state of human sleep, REM, is characterized by a low-amplitude, mixed-frequency EEG similar to that of NREM stage 1. Superimposed are bursts of 3- to 5-Hz activity with sharp negative deflections (Fig. 34-1). The EOG shows REM indistinguishable from that seen during eyes-open wakefulness. EMG activity is absent, reflecting the characteristic descending motor paralysis of the state.

ORGANIZATION OF HUMAN SLEEP   Normal nocturnal sleep in adults displays a consistent organization from night to night (Fig. 34-2). After sleep onset, sleep usually progresses through NREM stages 1 to 4 within 45 to 60 min. Slow-wave sleep (NREM stages 3 and 4) predominates in the first third of the night and comprises 15 to 25 percent of total nocturnal sleep time in young adults. The percentage of slow-wave sleep is influenced by several factors, most notably age (see below). In addition, prior sleep deprivation increases both the rapidity with which slow-wave sleep begins and its percentage of total sleep.

After the first slow-wave sleep episode, the progression of NREM stages reverses; the first REM sleep occurs, usually not less than 80 min after sleep begins. More rapid onset of REM sleep (particularly less than 30 min) suggests pathology such as endogenous depression, narcolepsy, or circadian rhythm disorders. NREM and REM alternate through the night with an average cycle of 90 to 110 min (the "ultradian" cycle). In time the portion of each cycle composed of slow-wave sleep decreases and that of REM sleep increases. Overall, REM sleep is 20 to 25 percent of total sleep, NREM stages (1 and 2) are 50 to 60 percent (increasing in elderly subjects).

BEHAVIORAL CORRELATES OF SLEEP STATES AND STAGES
Age has a large impact on sleep state organization (Fig. 34-2). Slow-wave sleep is most prominent during childhood, decreasing sharply at puberty and across the second and third decades of life. After age 30, there is a progressive, almost linear decline in the amount of slow-wave sleep, and the amplitude of delta EEG activity comprising slow-wave sleep is reduced. In the otherwise healthy elderly, slow-wave sleep may be completely absent.

A different age profile exists for REM sleep. In infancy, REM sleep may comprise 50 percent of total sleep time, and the percentage is inversely proportional to developmental age. The amount of REM sleep falls off sharply over the first postnatal year as a mature REM-NREM cycle develops. During the rest of life into extreme old age, REM occupies a remarkably constant percentage of total sleep time.

Polysomnographic staging of sleep correlates with behavioral changes during specific states and stages. Sleep onset is associated with marked decrements in perception of both auditory and visual stimuli and lapses of consciousness. At stage 1 subjects may respond to faint auditory or visual signals without "awakening." Furthermore, although memory incorporation appears to be inhibited at the onset of NREM stage 1, subjects aroused from that stage frequently deny having been asleep. In contrast, subjective and objective assessments of sleep agree more closely for subjects awakened from NREM stage 2. This has led some investigators to define sleep onset as the

FIGURE 34-2   Plots of the stages of REM sleep (solid bars) and the four stages of NREM sleep over the course of the entire night for representative young (upper panel, age 23) and elderly (lower panel, age 68) adult men. The recording in the elderly subject illustrates the reduction of delta sleep, frequent spontaneous awakenings, early sleep onset, and early morning awakening that are characteristic features of sleep in the aged, even in the absence of specific medical or psychiatric pathology. (*From the Center for Circadian and Sleep Disorders Medicine, Brigham and Women's Hospital.*)

occurrence of the first K complex or sleep spindle suggestive of NREM stage 2 and to define NREM stage 1 as a "transitional stage." The progression of subsequent NREM stages corresponds with increasing depth of sleep as measured by threshold for arousal with a variety of auditory stimuli.

Awakenings from REM sleep are associated with recall of vivid dream imagery more than 80 percent of the time. The reliability of dream recall increases with REM periods occurring later in the night. Imagery may also be reported after NREM sleep interruptions, though these typically lack the detail and vividness of REM dreams. The incidence of NREM dream recall can be increased by selective REM sleep deprivation, suggesting that REM sleep and dreaming per se are not inexorably linked.

PHYSIOLOGIC CORRELATES OF SLEEP STATES AND STAGES
All major physiologic systems are influenced by sleep. In some cases, concomitant behavior changes such as supine posture or inactivity are the proximal causes of altered physiologic function, but in most cases the sleep state itself appears to be responsible. Changes in cardiovascular function include a decrease in blood pressure and heart rate during NREM and particularly during slow-wave sleep. During REM sleep, phasic activity (bursts of eye movements) is associated with variability in both blood pressure and heart rate mediated principally by the vagus. Cardiac dysrhythmias may occur selectively during REM sleep. Respiratory function also changes (see Chap. 217). Respiratory rate and minute ventilation decrease during NREM sleep and become variable during phasic REM sleep. The ventilatory response to carbon dioxide attenuates during NREM sleep, resulting in a higher P_{CO_2}. During REM sleep the ventilatory response to both hypercapnia and hypoxia shows marked variability. Respiratory musculature, including that responsible for upper airway patency, is hypotonic throughout sleep and more so during REM sleep, resulting in an increase in airway resistance. In addition, the cough reflex is attenuated or absent during sleep. These changes in respiratory function may be relevant to the pathogenesis of obstructive sleep apnea (OSA) and sudden infant death syndrome (SIDS) (see Chap. 217).

Endocrine function also varies with sleep. The most prominent changes are apparent in neuroendocrine parameters. Slow-wave sleep is associated with secretion of growth hormone in humans, while sleep in general is associated with augmented secretion of prolactin. Sleep has a complex effect on the secretion of luteinizing hormone (LH); during puberty sleep is associated with increased LH secretion while sleep in the mature female inhibits LH secretion in the early follicular phase of the menstrual cycle. Sleep onset (and probably slow-wave sleep) is associated with inhibition of thyroid-stimulating hormone (TSH) and of the adrenocorticotropic hormone (ACTH)–cortisol axis, an effect that is independent of the circadian rhythms in the two systems (see Fig. 34-3).

Sleep is also associated with alterations of thermoregulatory function. NREM sleep is associated with an attenuation of thermoregulatory responses to either heat or cold stress, and animal studies of thermosensitive neurons in the hypothalamus document a NREM-dependent reduction of the thermoregulatory set-point. REM sleep is associated with complete absence of thermoregulatory responsivity resulting in effective poikilothermy. However, the potential adverse impact of this failure of thermoregulation is blunted by inhibition of REM sleep by extreme ambient temperatures.

Neuroanatomy of sleep   Lesion studies in animals and neurologic diseases in humans have suggested distinct neuroanatomic sites in the generation of normal sleep and wakefulness. The studies of von Economo of patients with encephalitis lethargica suggested that the anterior hypothalamus contained a "sleep center" while the posterior hypothalamus contained a "wake center." Experimental studies in animals have variously implicated the medullary reticular formation, the thalamus, and the basal forebrain in the generation of sleep, while the brainstem reticular formation, the midbrain, the subthalamus, the thalamus, and the basal forebrain have all been suggested to play a role in the generation of wakefulness or EEG arousal (see also Chap. 31).

Despite many studies, there is little evidence for either a single, discrete "sleep center" or a single, discrete "wake center." Current hypotheses suggest that the capacity for sleep and wake generation is distributed along an axial "core" of neurons extending from the brainstem rostrally to the basal forebrain. Complex comingling of neuronal groups occurs at many points along this basal forebrain axis.

However, the neuroanatomic correlates of REM sleep appear to be more discretely localized. Specific regions in the pons are associated with each of the neurophysiologic correlates of REM sleep. Small lesions in the dorsal pons produce REM sleep without the descending muscle inhibition normally associated with that state; microinjections of carbachol into the same area produce atonia without other features of REM sleep. These experimental manipulations are mimicked by pathologic conditions in humans and animals. In narcolepsy, for example, abrupt, complete or partial paralysis (cataplexy) occurs in response to a variety of stimuli. In dogs with this condition, physostigmine, a central cholinesterase inhibitor, increases the frequency of cataplectic attacks while atropine decreases their frequency. Conversely, in REM sleep behavior disorder (see below), patients suffer from incomplete motor inhibition during REM sleep resulting in involuntary, occasionally violent movement during REM sleep.

Neurochemistry of sleep   Early experimental studies that focused on the raphe nuclei of the brainstem appeared to implicate serotonin as the primary sleep-promoting neurotransmitter, while catecholamines were considered to be responsible for wakefulness. Subsequent work has demonstrated that the raphe-serotonin system may facilitate sleep but is not necessary to its expression. The extensive pharmacology of sleep and wakefulness suggests roles for other neurotransmitters as well. The alerting influence of caffeine implicates adenosine while the hypnotic effect of benzodiazepines and barbiturates suggests a role for endogenous ligands of the GABA-receptor complex.

A variety of sleep-promoting substances have been identified.

These are principally peptides, and the hypnotic effect is commonly limited to NREM or slow-wave sleep, although peptides that increase REM sleep have also been reported. Many of these "sleep factors," including interleukin 1 and prostaglandin E_2, are immunologically active as well, suggesting a link between immune function and sleep-wake states.

PHYSIOLOGY OF CIRCADIAN RHYTHMICITY   The sleep-wake cycle is the most evident of the many 24-h rhythms in humans. Prominent daily variations also occur in endocrine, thermoregulatory, cardiac, pulmonary, renal, gastrointestinal, and cognitive functions. However, in evaluating a daily variation, it is important to distinguish between those rhythmic components passively evoked by periodic environmental or behavioral changes (e.g., the increase in blood pressure and heart rate upon assumption of the upright posture), and those actively driven by an endogenous oscillatory process (e.g., the circadian variation in plasma cortisol that persists under a variety of environmental and behavioral conditions).

The suprachiasmatic nuclei (SCN) of the hypothalamus act as the central neural pacemakers of the circadian timing system in mammals. The persistence of some rhythmicity after SCN lesions suggests that they synchronize subsidiary rhythms rather than serving as the sole source of rhythmicity. The period and phase of the endogenous neural oscillator are normally synchronized to the 24-h period of the environmental light-dark cycle. Entrainment of mammalian circadian rhythms by the light-dark cycle is mediated via the retinohypothalamic tract, a monosynaptic pathway that links the retina to the SCN.

The principal properties characterizing an endogenous circadian pacemaker are its *intrinsic period, phase, amplitude*, and *resetting capacity*. In human subjects living in controlled laboratory environments free of time cues (*free-running*), the duration of the behavioral rest-activity cycle averages 25 h. However, the rest-activity cycle often oscillates with a period that is different from that of other physiologic measures (such as body temperature, plasma cortisol, and urinary potassium). This state of "internal desynchronization" implies that the endogenous circadian pacemaker actually has a shorter period, averaging about 24.6 h. Therefore, synchronization of the endogenous circadian pacemaker to the 24-h day requires that the pacemaker be reset by about 0.6 h each day, which is normally achieved by exposure to the environmental light-dark cycle.

Exposure to light can shift the phase of the endogenous circadian pacemaker, but both the magnitude and direction of the phase shifts induced by light depend on the timing and intensity of the light. Properly timed exposure to light of sufficient intensity can, within 2 to 3 days, reset the human circadian pacemaker (presumably the SCN).

The timing and internal architecture of sleep are directly coupled to the output of the endogenous pacemaker. Spontaneous sleep duration, sleepiness, REM sleep propensity, and both the ability and the tendency to sleep vary with the circadian phase as marked by the endogenous circadian temperature cycle in humans. Sleep tendency, sleepiness, and REM sleep propensity all peak just after the nadir of the endogenous circadian temperature cycle (approximately 3 h before awakening). In addition, 85 percent of all spontaneous awakenings of subjects living in constant environmental conditions occur on the rising slope of the temperature cycle. Furthermore, there are certain times (wake maintenance zones) when it is very difficult to fall asleep, even in subjects who are sleep deprived. Misalignment of the output of the endogenous circadian pacemaker with the desired sleep-wake cycle is thought to be responsible for certain types of insomnia, as well as for the decrements of alertness and performance in night-shift workers and after jet lag.

DISORDERS OF SLEEP AND WAKEFULNESS

An international classification of sleep disorders (Table 34-2) divides these conditions into three major groups: dyssomnias, parasomnias, and medical psychiatric sleep disorders. A detailed description of

TABLE 34-2   International classification of sleep disorders

I Dyssomnias
  A Intrinsic sleep disorders
    1 Psychophysiologic insomnia
    2 Idiopathic insomnia
    3 Narcolepsy
    4 Recurrent or idiopathic hypersomnia
    5 Posttraumatic hypersomnia
    6 Sleep apnea syndromes
    7 Periodic limb movement disorder
    8 Restless legs syndrome
  B Extrinsic sleep disorders
    1 Inadequate sleep hygiene
    2 Environmental sleep disorder
    3 Altitude insomnia
    4 Adjustment sleep disorder
    5 Sleep-onset association disorder
    6 Food allergy insomnia
    7 Nocturnal eating (drinking) syndrome
    8 Drug- or alcohol-dependent sleep disorders
  C Circadian rhythm sleep disorders
    1 Time-zone change (jet-lag) syndrome
    2 Shift-work sleep disorder
    3 Delayed sleep phase syndrome
    4 Advanced sleep phase syndrome
    5 Non-24-h sleep-wake disorder
II Parasomnias
  A Arousal disorders
    1 Confusional arousals
    2 Sleepwalking
    3 Sleep terrors
  B Sleep-wake transition disorders
    1 Rhythmic movement disorder
    2 Sleep talking
    3 Nocturnal leg cramps
  C Parasomnias usually associated with REM sleep
    1 Nightmares
    2 Sleep paralysis
    3 Impaired sleep-related penile erections
    4 Sleep-related painful erections
    5 REM sleep-related cardiac arrhythmias
    6 REM sleep behavior disorder
  D Other parasomnias
    1 Sleep bruxism
    2 Sleep enuresis
    3 Nocturnal paroxysmal dystonia
III Sleep disorders associated with medical/psychiatric disorders
  A Associated with mental disorders
  B Associated with neurologic disorders
    1 Cerebral degenerative disorders
    2 Parkinsonism
    3 Fatal familial insomnia
    4 Sleep-related epilepsy
    5 Sleep-related headaches
  C Associated with other medical disorders
    1 Sleeping sickness
    2 Nocturnal cardiac ischemia
    3 Chronic obstructive pulmonary disease
    4 Sleep-related asthma
    5 Sleep-related gastroesophageal reflux
    6 Peptic ulcer disease
    7 Fibrositis syndrome

SOURCE: Modified from *International Classification of Sleep Disorders*, prepared by the Diagnostic Classification Committee, Thorpy MJ, Chairman. American Sleep Disorders Association, in press, 1990.

each of these disorders may be found in the publication of the American Sleep Disorders Association.

APPROACH TO THE PATIENT WITH A SLEEP COMPLAINT   Several general principles are useful to the physician with a patient who complains of sleep disruption. The first is recognition that the severity of the reported chronic sleep disruption (i.e., the complaint of chronic insomnia) is often exaggerated relative to objective measurement. In addition, nocturnal sleep and daytime alertness are linked in a predictable way. With the advent of objective measurements of sleep tendency (see below), quantification of the impairment of daytime alertness is a valuable adjunct in the assessment of sleep problems. As a rule, the clinical approach to a patient with disrupted sleep but without impaired daytime alertness should be conservative. Chronic treatment of isolated insomnia with hypnotic medications is rarely justified.

Laboratory investigation   In addition to the three electrophysiologic variables used to define sleep states and stages (see above), the standard clinical polysomnogram includes measures of respiration (respiratory effort, air flow, and oxygen saturation), lower extremity EMG, and ECG. Assessment of daytime functioning as an index of the adequacy of sleep can be made with the multiple sleep latency test (MSLT), which involves repeated measurement of sleep latency (time to onset of sleep) at 2-h intervals under standardized conditions during a day following quantified nocturnal sleep. The average latency across five to seven tests (administered every 2 h across the waking day) is taken as an objective measure of daytime sleep tendency. Disorders of sleep that result in pathologic, daytime somnolence can be reliably distinguished with the MSLT. In addition, the multiple measurements of sleep onset identify direct transitions from wakefulness to REM sleep that are indicative of specific pathologic conditions (e.g., narcolepsy). Finally, evaluation of penile tumescence during sleep can be used to determine whether the etiology of erectile dysfunction in a patient is psychogenic or organic (see Chap. 52).

INSOMNIA   Insomnia is a common complaint that increases in prevalence with advancing age. As many as half of people between 65 and 79 years of age complain of disturbed sleep. This may account for the fact that 40 percent of all sleeping pills are consumed by the elderly who represent only 11 percent of the general population. To reduce the number of patients dependent on hypnotics, it is important for physicians to make an effort to determine the underlying cause of insomnia before initiating treatment. Insomnia is usually subdivided into *sleep onset, sleep maintenance,* or *premature awakening* type. Transient insomnia can last up to 3 to 4 weeks; after that, it is considered chronic. It is important to note that patients often cannot estimate actual sleep time. Objective polysomnographic recording can indicate that a patient slept 6 to 7 h, even though that same patient reports having been ''up all night.''

Psychophysiologic insomnia   Persistent psychophysiologic insomnia is a behavioral disorder in which patients are preoccupied with a perceived inability to sleep at night. The sleep disturbance is often triggered by an emotionally stressful event; however, the poor sleep habits acquired during the stressful period persist long after the initial incident. Such patients become hyperaroused by their own persistent efforts to sleep, and the insomnia is a conditioned or learned response. Patients with psychophysiologic insomnia fall asleep more easily at unscheduled times (when not trying) or outside the home environment. In these cases, polysomnographic recording reveals an objective sleep disturbance, often with an abnormally long sleep latency, frequent nocturnal awakenings, and an increased amount of stage 1 transitional sleep. Behavioral therapy is often beneficial; relaxation training can improve the sleep of patients in whom anxiety is prominent. Limited use of hypnotic medications, which can serve as a catalyst for successful behavioral therapy, may be appropriate. Extrinsic factors may contribute to this condition (see below). Rigorous attention should be paid to sleep hygiene (see below) and correction of counterproductive, arousing behaviors before bedtime.

Extrinsic insomnia   A number of sleep disorders are the result of extrinsic factors that interfere with sleep. *Adjustment sleep disorder,* also called *transient situational insomnia,* can occur after a change in the sleeping environment (e.g., in an unfamiliar hotel or hospital bed) or before or after a significant life event, such as a change of occupation, loss of a loved one, illness, or anxiety over a deadline or examination. Increased sleep latency, frequent awakenings from sleep, and early morning awakening can all occur. Recovery generally occurs rapidly, certainly within 2 to 3 weeks. *Inadequate sleep hygiene* is characterized by a behavior pattern prior to sleep and/or a bedroom environment that is not conducive to sleep. On taking a careful history, physicians may learn that some insomniac patients are attempting to sleep with the television on throughout the night or are attempting to sleep just after coming home from work at midnight. Noise and/or light in the bedroom can interfere with sleep, as can a bed partner with periodic limb movements during sleep or one who snores loudly. Luminous clocks can arouse the patient, heightening anxiety about the time it has taken to fall asleep. Large meals, extensive exercise, or hot showers just before sleep may interfere with sleep onset. Patients should be counseled to develop a soporific bedtime ritual and to prepare and reserve the bedroom environment for sleeping.

Altitude Insomnia   Sleep disturbance is a common consequence of exposure to high altitude. Periodic breathing of the Cheyne-Stokes type occurs during NREM sleep about half the time at altitude, with restoration of a regular breathing pattern during REM sleep. Central rather than obstructive sleep apnea appears to be responsible, and the regularity of the respiratory pauses distinguishes this breathing pattern from central sleep apnea seen at sea level. Both hypoxia and hypocapnia are thought to be involved in the development of periodic breathing. Frequent awakenings and poor quality sleep characterize altitude insomnia, which is generally worst on the first few nights at high altitude but may persist. The duration of sleep is unchanged, but there are more arousals after sleep onset and less time in slow-wave (stages 3 and 4) sleep. Pretreatment with acetazolamide can decrease time spent in periodic breathing and substantially reduce hypoxia during sleep. Medroxyprogesterone acetate (MPA) also reduces periodic breathing but does not significantly reduce hypoxia during sleep at altitude.

Drug- or alcohol-dependent sleep disorders   Disturbed sleep can result from ingestion of a wide variety of agents. Caffeine is perhaps the most common pharmacologic cause of insomnia in sensitive patients. It produces increased latency to sleep onset, more frequent arousals during sleep, and a reduction in total sleep time for up to 8 to 14 h after ingestion. Some patients are surprised to learn that their insomnia may be related to coffee consumption; a careful history will reveal that such patients may drink 15 to 20 cups per day. As few as 3 to 5 cups of coffee can significantly disturb sleep in some patients; therefore, a 1- to 2-month caffeine withdrawal period should be attempted in patients with these symptoms. Similarly, alcohol and nicotine can interfere with sleep, although many patients use them to relax and promote sleep. Although alcohol can increase drowsiness and shorten sleep latency, even moderate amounts of alcohol increase awakenings after sleep onset by interfering with the ability of the brain to maintain sleep. In addition, alcohol ingestion prior to sleep is contraindicated in patients with sleep apnea because of the inhibitory effects of alcohol on respiration. Acutely, amphetamines and cocaine suppress REM sleep, which returns to normal with chronic use. Withdrawal leads to a REM sleep rebound. Finally, rebound insomnia associated with the acute withdrawal of hypnotics can be severe, especially following the use of benzodiazepines with a short half-life. For this reason, hypnotics should rarely be prescribed for habitual use; doses should be low to moderate, the total duration of hypnotic therapy should be limited to 2 to 3 weeks, and drug dosage should be reduced prior to withdrawal.

NARCOLEPSY   Excessive daytime sleepiness with involuntary daytime sleep episodes, disturbed nocturnal sleep, and cataplexy (sudden weakness or loss of muscle tone, often elicited by emotion) are the most common symptoms of narcolepsy. Some patients also experience muscular paralysis and/or hallucinations at sleep onset or upon awakening. The severity varies. Patients may have two to three cataplectic attacks per day or per decade, and the extent and duration of an attack may vary from a transient sagging of the jaw to flaccid paralysis of the entire voluntary musculature for 20 to 30 min.

Narcolepsy affects over 100,000 people in the United States and appears to have a genetic basis. Experiments in some canine models of narcolepsy suggest an autosomal recessive pattern of inheritance. First-degree relatives of narcoleptic patients commonly exhibit excessive daytime somnolence and have at least a hundredfold higher incidence of narcolepsy than the general population. In addition, nearly all narcoleptics are positive for the human leukocyte antigen DR2 (see Chap. 14).

Symptoms typically begin in the second decade, although the onset ranges from ages 5 to 50. An identifiable stress (e.g., sleep-wake cycle disruption, divorce, loss of a loved one) may precede symptom onset.

Diagnosis Classically, the diagnosis of narcolepsy required the presence of the "narcolepsy tetrad," consisting of (1) excessive daytime somnolence, (2) cataplexy, (3) hypnogogic hallucinations (the occurrence of vivid hallucinatory dream imagery at sleep onset), and (4) sleep paralysis (an awareness that voluntary musculature is paralyzed coincident with the onset of sleep). The last three symptoms of the tetrad are all manifestations of the abnormal REM sleep regulation inherent in the syndrome. All patients with narcolepsy have objectively verifiable daytime somnolence, but the other three symptoms are variably present. Eighty percent have cataplexy of some degree and smaller percentages report hyponogogic hallucinations and/or sleep paralysis. Other associated symptoms are useful but not specific. A history of "automatic behavior" during wakefulness (a trancelike state during which simple motor behaviors persist) serves principally to corroborate the presence of daytime somnolence but is not specific for mechanism. Patients with narcolepsy also commonly report severe disruption of nocturnal sleep, a feature that may distinguish narcolepsy from other causes of daytime somnolence.

A family history is important in the evaluation of the patient with excessive daytime somnolence. Careful observation of the children and siblings of known narcoleptics, particularly at the typical age of onset (second decade), can lead to early diagnosis. The diagnosis of narcolepsy in a patient with a suggestive history depends upon (1) objective verification of excessive daytime somnolence, typically using the MSLT after nocturnal sleep recording, and (2) documentation of abnormal REM sleep regulation as evidenced by direct wake-to-REM sleep transitions either during the nocturnal recording or on one or more of the MSLT determinations.

Treatment The treatment of narcolepsy is symptomatic. Somnolence is treated with stimulants. Amphetamine use is limited due to side effects, tolerance, and drug dependence. Methylphenidate is considered the drug of choice by most, but pemoline has a longer half-life and is associated with fewer side effects.

Treatment of cataplexy, hypnogogic hallucinations, and sleep paralysis requires the tricyclic antidepressants, which are effective, in part, because of potent REM-suppressive effects; within this class of compounds, protriptyline is most commonly used in the United States. Efficacy is limited largely by anticholinergic side effects. New compounds including viloxazine hydrochloride and fluoxetine are under evaluation.

Gamma-hydroxy-butyrate (GHB), a drug available in Europe and Canada but still under evaluation in the United States, appears to be particularly useful to reverse nocturnal sleep disruption and, perhaps as a consequence of this mechanism, may also substantially improve daytime somnolence and cataplexy. Lastly, behavioral modifications, particularly nocturnal sleep restriction and structured daytime napping, may help the narcoleptic deal with excessive daytime somnolence but are not usually a substitute for pharmacologic therapy.

SLEEP APNEA SYNDROMES Respiratory dysfunction during sleep is a common, serious cause of excessive daytime somnolence, as well as of disturbed nocturnal sleep. An estimated 2 to 5 million people in the United States stop breathing for 15 to 150 s, from a dozen to several hundred times every night during sleep. These cessations of breathing may be due to either an occlusion of the airway (*obstructive sleep apnea*), absence of respiratory effort (*central sleep apnea*), or a combination of these factors (*mixed sleep apnea*). Failure to recognize and appropriately treat these conditions may lead to serious cardiovascular complications and increased mortality. This problem is particularly prevalent in the elderly. Occult sleep-related breathing disorders may result in significant impairment of daytime alertness and functioning in otherwise healthy elderly persons. Readers are referred to Chap. 217 for a comprehensive review of the diagnosis and treatment of patients with these conditions.

DYSSOMNIA ASSOCIATED WITH LIMB MOVEMENTS Restless legs syndrome Patients with dyssomnia associated with the restless legs syndrome report an irresistible urge to move their legs when awake and inactive, especially when lying in bed just prior to sleep. This interferes with the ability to fall asleep. They report a creeping or crawling sensation deep within their calves that is only relieved by movement, particularly walking. In contrast, paresthesia secondary to peripheral neuropathy persists with activity. The severity of this chronic, idiopathic disorder may wax and wane with time and can be exacerbated by caffeine. Nearly all patients with restless legs also experience periodic limb movement disorder during sleep, although the reverse is not the case. Together, these conditions constitute the principal diagnosis in one-eighth of patients with insomnia.

Periodic limb movement disorder Periodic limb movement disorder, also known as *nocturnal myoclonus,* is the principal objective polysomnographic finding in 17 percent of patients with insomnia and 11 percent of those with excessive daytime somnolence. Stereotyped, rhythmic, 0.5- to 5.0-s extensions of the great toe and dorsiflexion of the foot recur every 20 to 40 s during NREM stages 1 and 2 sleep, in episodes lasting from minutes to hours. Most such episodes occur during the first half of the night. The disorder occurs in a wide variety of sleep disorders (including narcolepsy, sleep apnea, and various forms of insomnia) and is associated with frequent arousals and an increased number of sleep-stage transitions. However, it has not been demonstrated that these sleep disturbances lead to insomnia. In fact, periodic limb movement may be secondary to chronic sleep-wake disturbance rather than the cause of it. The incidence increases with age; 44 percent of healthy subjects over age 65 without a sleep complaint and all patients with the restless legs syndrome have periodic limb movements (see below). The pathophysiology is not well understood. Polysomnography with bilateral EMG recording of the anterior tibialis, triceps, and biceps is used to establish the diagnosis. Treatment options are limited; some patients may respond to clonazepam.

PARASOMNIAS The term *parasomnia* refers to behavioral disorders during sleep that are associated with brief or partial arousals but not with marked sleep disruption or impaired daytime alertness. The presenting complaint is usually related to the behavior itself. They are more common in children but may persist into adulthood when their occurrence may have more pathologic significance.

Sleepwalking (somnambulism) Patients affected by this disorder carry out automatic motor activities that range from minor to complex. Individuals may leave the bed, walk, urinate inappropriately, or exit from the house while remaining unconscious or uncommunicative. Arousal is difficult, and untoward or even fatal activities can occur. Sleepwalking occurs in stage 3 or 4 NREM sleep. It is most common in children and adolescents. Episodes are usually isolated but may be recurrent in 1 to 6 percent of patients. The cause is unknown, and no effective treatments have been developed.

Sleep terrors This disorder, also called *pavor nocturnus,* occurs primarily in young children during the first several hours after sleep onset, in stages 3 and 4 of NREM sleep. The child suddenly screams, exhibiting autonomic arousal with sweating, tachycardia, and hyperventilation. The individual may be difficult to arouse and rarely recalls the episode on awakening in the morning. Recurrent attacks are rare, and treatment is usually by way of reassurance of parents. Both sleep terrors and sleepwalking represent abnormalities of arousal. In contrast, *nightmares* (dream anxiety attacks) occur during REM sleep and cause full arousal, with memory for the dream-associated unpleasant episode.

REM sleep behavior disorder This disorder is a parasomnia arising from REM sleep instead of slow-wave sleep, as is characteristic of the other common parasomnias. It primarily afflicts men of middle age or older, many of whom have a history of prior neurologic disease (e.g., Guillain-Barré syndrome, dementia, subarachnoid hemorrhage). Presenting symptoms are of violent behavior during sleep, reported by a bed partner. In contrast to typical somnambulism, injury to patient or bystander is common, and, upon awakening, the patient reports vivid, often unpleasant dream imagery. The principal differential diagnosis is that of nocturnal seizures, which can be excluded with polysomnography. In REM sleep behavior disorder, seizure activity is absent, and the EEG/EOG REM sleep pattern exhibits a high-amplitude EMG. Complex, purposeful motor behavior occurs during REM sleep episodes. The pathogenesis is unclear, but the preexisting neurologic disease may have involved brainstem areas responsible for descending motor inhibition during REM sleep. In support of this hypothesis are the remarkable similarities between the REM sleep behavior disorder and the sleep of animals with bilateral lesions of the pontine tegmentum in areas controlling REM sleep motor inhibition. Treatment with clonazepam or tricyclic antidepressants has been successful in early trials.

Sleep bruxism   Bruxism is an involuntary, forceful grinding of teeth during sleep. The patient is usually unaware of the problem, and data on this parasomnia come from roommates and bed partners, alarmed by the loud grinding noise, and from dentists who see evidence of destruction of tooth enamel and dentum. The prevalence of bruxism has been estimated at 10 to 20 percent of the general population. The typical age of onset is 17 to 20 years and spontaneous remission usually occurs by age 40. Sex distribution appears to be equal.

Hypotheses about the pathophysiology suggest contributory roles for dental abnormalities, e.g., malocclusion, and for central neural mechanisms. Psychological factors may also play a role in that stress exacerbates the disorder. Treatment is dictated by the risk of dental injury. In many cases, the diagnosis is made during dental examination, damage is minor, and no treatment is indicated. In more severe cases, treatment with a rubber tooth guard is necessary to prevent permanent and disfiguring tooth injury. Psychotherapy can be useful when bruxism is a manifestation of severe stress. Useful pharmacologic therapy has not been described.

Sleep enuresis   Bedwetting, like sleepwalking and night terrors, is another parasomnia occurring during slow-wave sleep in the young. Before age 5 or 6, nocturnal enuresis should probably be considered a normal feature of development. The condition usually spontaneously improves at puberty, has a prevalence in late adolescence of 1 to 3 percent, and is rare in adulthood. The age threshold for initiation of treatment depends on parental and patient concern about the problem. Persistence of enuresis into adolescence or adulthood may reflect a variety of underlying conditions. In older patients with enuresis a distinction must be made between primary and secondary enuresis, the latter being defined as bedwetting in patients who have been fully continent for 6 to 12 months. Treatment of primary enuresis is reserved for patients of appropriate age (older than 5 or 6 years) and consists of bladder training exercises and behavioral therapy. Important causes of secondary enuresis include emotional disturbances, urinary tract infections, cauda equina lesions, epilepsy, sleep apnea, and urinary tract malformations. In the patient with secondary enuresis, underlying causes need to be eliminated. In the patient for whom enuresis may be a source of significant stress, symptomatic pharmacotherapy may be appropriate while attention is also paid to underlying causes. This is usually accomplished with oxybutynin chloride or imipramine. Intranasal desmopressin has been used in some patients.

Miscellaneous parasomnias   Other clinical entities fulfill the definition of a parasomnia in that they occur selectively during sleep and are associated with some degree of sleep disruption. Examples include *jactatio capitis nocturna* (nocturnal headbanging), sleep talking, nightmares, and nocturnal leg cramps.

SLEEP DISORDERS ASSOCIATED WITH MEDICAL/PSYCHIATRIC DISORDERS   Sleep disorders associated with mental disorders   Although some differences are present in sleep architecture and physiology in *schizophrenia* (such as a decreased amount of stage 4 sleep and a lack of augmentation of REM sleep following REM sleep deprivation), chronic schizophrenics usually sleep well. In contrast, patients with other psychiatric disorders (anxiety disorders, affective illness, obsessive-compulsive disorders, and chronic alcoholism) often sleep poorly. There is considerable heterogeneity, however, in the nature of the sleep disturbance both between conditions and among patients with the same condition.

Depression can be associated with sleep onset insomnia, sleep maintenance insomnia, and/or early morning wakefulness. However, hypersomnia occurs in some depressed patients, especially adolescents and those with seasonal (fall/winter) depression (see also Chap. 368). Indeed, sleep disturbance is an important vegetative sign of depression, and may commence before any mood changes are perceived by the patient and then return to normal at the beginning of remission. Consistent polysomnographic findings in depression include decreased REM sleep latency, lengthened first REM sleep episode, and shortened first NREM sleep episode; however, the extent of these changes varies with age and symptomatology.

In *mania* and *hypomania,* sleep latency is increased, and total sleep time can be reduced. Patients with *obsessive-compulsive disorders* have sleep disturbances similar to those of endogenously depressed patients. Finally, *chronic alcoholics* lack slow-wave sleep, have decreased amounts of REM sleep, and have frequent arousals throughout the night. This is associated with impaired daytime alertness. The sleep of chronic alcoholics remains disturbed for years after discontinuance of alcohol usage.

Sleep disorders associated with neurologic disorders   A variety of neurologic diseases result in sleep disruption through both indirect, nonspecific mechanisms (e.g., pain in cervical spondylosis or low back pain) or by impairment of central neural structures involved in the generation and control of sleep itself. Headache syndromes may show sleep-associated exacerbations (*migraine* or *cluster headache*) (see also Chap. 18). The mechanism of association between sleep and headache is unknown.

Epilepsy may also present as a sleep complaint (see also Chap. 350). Often the history is of abnormal, occasionally violent activity during sleep, and the differential diagnosis includes REM sleep behavior disorder, sleep apnea syndrome, and periodic movements of sleep (see above). Diagnosis requires nocturnal EEG recording. Other neurologic diseases associated with abnormal movements, such as *Parkinson's disease, hemiballismus, Huntington's chorea*, and *Gilles de la Tourette syndrome*, are also associated with disrupted sleep, presumably through secondary mechanisms.

Fatal familial insomnia is a rare hereditary disorder that causes bilateral degeneration of anterior and dorsomedial nuclei of the thalamus. Insomnia is a prominent early symptom. Progressively, the syndrome produces autonomic dysfunction, dysarthria, myoclonus, coma, and death. The pathogenesis of the thalamic destruction is unknown.

Sleep disorders associated with other medical disorders   A number of medical conditions are associated with disruptions of sleep. The association may be nonspecific, for example, that between sleep disruption and chronic pain from rheumatologic disorders. Attention to this association is important in that many such patients present with only sleep-associated symptoms.

Among the most prominent associations is that between sleep disruption and *asthma*. In many asthmatics there is a prominent daily variation in airway resistance, probably related to daily rhythms in catecholamine and histamine levels, which results in marked increases in asthmatic symptoms at night. In addition, treatment of asthma with theophylline-based compounds, adrenergic agonists, or glucocorticoids can independently disrupt sleep. When sleep disruption is a prominent side effect of asthma treatment, inhaled steroids (e.g., beclomethasone) that do not disrupt sleep may provide a useful alternative.

Cardiac ischemia may also be associated with sleep disruption. Variability in autonomic nervous system function during REM sleep may account for the association of sleep and angina, although this remains unproven. Patients may present with complaints of nightmares or vivid disturbing dreams, with or without awareness of the more classical symptoms of angina. *Paroxysmal nocturnal dyspnea* can also occur as a consequence of sleep-associated cardiac ischemia that causes pulmonary congestion exacerbated by recumbent posture.

Chronic obstructive pulmonary disease is also associated with sleep disruption, the pathogenesis of which is presumed to be sleep-

FIGURE 34-3 Circadian rhythms recorded during both the baseline and the constant routine in a single normal subject (age 21). The solid horizontal bar indicates lights out, and the cross-hatched bar indicates the 40-h constant routine. The solid vertical line (RW) indicates the subject's customary waketime. A harmonic regression model fitted to the temperature data is superimposed on the raw data during the constant routine, and an encircled X marks the time of the fitted minimum of the endogenous component of the temperature cycle. Note that all variables except wrist activity and growth hormone continue to show a circadian variation during the constant routine.

related exacerbation of hypoxia and hypercapnia secondary to alveolar hypoventilation. In addition, recumbent posture results in suboptimal ventilation-perfusion ratios. Other conditions associated with sleep disruption include *cystic fibrosis, menopause, hyperthyroidism, gastroesophageal reflux, chronic renal failure,* and *liver failure.*

CIRCADIAN RHYTHM SLEEP DISORDERS

A subset of patients presenting with either insomnia or hypersomnia may have a disorder of sleep *timing* rather than sleep *generation.* Disorders of sleep timing can either be organic (i.e., due to an intrinsic defect in the circadian pacemaker or its responsiveness to entraining stimuli) or environmental (i.e., due to a disruption of exposure to entraining stimuli from the environment). Regardless of etiology, the symptoms reflect the influence of the underlying circadian pacemaker on sleep-wake function. Thus, effective therapeutic approaches should aim to entrain the oscillator at an appropriate phase.

ENDOGENOUS CIRCADIAN PHASE ASSESSMENT Abnormal synchronization of the circadian pacemaker to the 24-h day can be assessed clinically by studying patients under standardized behavioral and environmental conditions. Exogenous factors (such as variations in light exposure, room temperature, activity level, posture, nutritional intake), which can evoke physiologic responses, must be held constant to assess the phase and amplitude of endogenous circadian rhythms. Patients are studied for 30 to 50 h of enforced semirecumbent wakefulness in constant indoor room light, with their daily nutritional and fluid intake equally divided into hourly snacks. During such a constant routine, the body temperature cycle serves as a reliable marker of the output of the endogenous circadian pacemaker (Fig. 34-3). In normal young men, the endogenous component of the body temperature cycle under such conditions reaches its nadir about 3 h before the habitual waketime. The technique can be used to determine whether there is an organic basis consistent with a diagnosis of delayed sleep phase syndrome, non-24-h sleep-wake schedule, or advanced sleep phase syndrome.

RAPID TIME-ZONE CHANGE (JET LAG) SYNDROME More than 60 million people experience transmeridian air travel annually, which is often associated with excessive daytime sleepiness, sleep onset insomnia, and frequent arousals from sleep, particularly in the latter half of the night. Gastrointestinal discomfort is common. The syndrome is transient, typically lasting 2 to 14 days depending on the number of time zones crossed, the direction of travel, and the traveler's age and phase-shifting capacity. Travelers who spend more time outdoors reportedly adapt more quickly than those who remain in hotel rooms, presumably due to bright (outdoor) light exposure.

SHIFT-WORK SLEEP DISORDER About 7 million workers in the United States regularly work at night, either on a permanent or rotating schedule. Studies of shift workers indicate that the circadian timing system of the average night-shift worker fails to adapt successfully to such work schedules. This leads to a misalignment between the desired work-rest schedule and the output of the pacemaker and in disturbed daytime sleep. Consequent sleep deprivation and misalignment of circadian phase produce decreased alertness and performance and cause increased safety hazards among night-shift workers. In addition, shift workers are believed to have higher rates of cardiac, gastrointestinal, and reproductive disorders.

Treatment must be aimed at minimizing both circadian disruption and sleep deprivation. The work schedule should: (1) favor a phase delay (clockwise) direction of shift rotation; (2) minimize the frequency of shift rotation so that shifts do not rotate more than once every 2 to 3 weeks; and (3) reduce the number of consecutive days worked at night from 7 (which is typical) to 4 or 5. These steps can lead to marked improvements in employee health and performance and to reduced accident rates among shift workers.

DELAYED SLEEP PHASE SYNDROME Delayed sleep phase syndrome is characterized by: (1) reported sleep onset and wake times intractably later than desired; (2) actual sleep times at nearly the same clock hours daily; and (3) essentially normal all-night polysomnography except for delayed sleep onset. Patients exhibit an abnormally delayed endogenous circadian phase, with the temperature minimum during the constant routine occurring later than normal. This delayed phase could be due to: (1) an abnormally long intrinsic period of endogenous circadian pacemaker; (2) an abnormally reduced phase-advancing capacity of the pacemaker; or (3) an irregular prior sleep-wake schedule, characterized by frequent nights when the patient chooses to remain awake well past midnight (for social, school, or work reasons). In most cases, it is difficult to distinguish among these factors, since patients with an abnormally long intrinsic period are more likely to ''choose'' such late-night activities because they are unable to sleep at that time. Patients tend to be young adults. This self-perpetuating condition can persist for years and does not usually respond to attempts to reestablish normal bedtime hours.

Patients respond to a rescheduling regimen in which bedtimes are successively delayed by about 3 h per day until the desired (and earlier) bedtime is achieved. Treatment methods involving bright-light phototherapy also show promise in these patients.

ADVANCED SLEEP PHASE SYNDROME Advanced sleep phase syndrome is the converse of the delayed sleep phase syndrome and tends to occur in the elderly. Patients with this condition report excessive daytime sleepiness during the evening hours, when they have great difficulty remaining awake, even in social settings. The patients awaken from 3 to 5 A.M. each day, often several hours before their desired wake times. Although such patients have not been studied extensively, some of these patients may benefit from bright-light phototherapy designed to reset the circadian pacemaker to a later hour.

NON-24-H SLEEP-WAKE DISORDER This condition occurs when the maximal phase-advancing capacity of the circadian pacemaker is not adequate to accommodate the difference between the 24-h geophysical day and the intrinsic period of the pacemaker in the patient. Patients affected are not able to maintain a stable phase relationship between the output of the pacemaker and the 24-h day. Such patients typically present with an incremental pattern of successive delays in sleep onsets and wake times, progressing in and out of phase with local time. When the patient's endogenous rhythms are out of phase with the local environment, insomnia coexists with excessive daytime sleepiness. Conversely, when the endogenous rhythms are in phase with the local environment, symptoms remit. The intervals of alternation between symptomatic vs. asymptomatic intervals may last several weeks to several months. Blind subjects unable to perceive light are particularly susceptible to this disorder.

MEDICAL IMPLICATIONS OF CIRCADIAN RHYTHMICITY Understanding the role of circadian rhythmicity in the pathophysiology of illness may lead to improvements in diagnosis and treatment. For example, prominent circadian variations have been reported in the incidence of *acute myocardial infarction, sudden cardiac death,* and *stroke,* the leading causes of death in the United States. Platelet aggregability is increased after arising in the early morning hours, coincident with the peak incidence of these cardiovascular events. A better understanding of the possible role of circadian rhythmicity in the acute destabilization of a chronic condition such as atherosclerotic disease could improve the understanding of the pathophysiology.

Diagnostic procedures may also be affected by the time of day at which data are collected. Examples include blood pressure, body temperature, the dexamethasone suppression test, and plasma cortisol levels. Few physicians realize the extent to which routine measures are affected by the time (or sleep/wake state) when the measurement is made.

In addition, both the toxicity and effectiveness of drugs can vary during the day. For example, more than a fivefold difference has been observed in mortality rates following administration of toxic agents to experimental animals at different times of day. Anesthetic agents are particularly sensitive to time-of-day effects.

REFERENCES

ANCH AM et al: *Sleep. A Scientific Perspective.* Englewood Cliffs, NJ, Prentice Hall, 1988

COLEMAN RM et al: Sleep-wake disorders based on a polysomnographic diagnosis: A national cooperative study. JAMA 247:997, 1982

CZEISLER CA et al: Bright light induction of strong (Type O) resetting of the human circadian pacemaker. Science 244:1328, 1989

DIAGNOSTIC CLASSIFICATION COMMITTEE, Thorpy MJ (chairman): *International Classification of Sleep Disorders.* American Sleep Disorders Association, 1990

DINGES DF, BROUGHTON RJ (eds): *Sleep and Alertness.* New York, Raven Press, 1989

FAIRBANKS DN et al (eds): *Snoring and Obstructive Sleep Apnea.* New York, Raven Press, 1987

GUILLEMINAULT C (ed): *Sleeping and Waking Disorders: Indications and Techniques.* Menlo Park, Calif, Addison-Wesley, 1982

HORNE J: *Why We Sleep: The Functions of Sleep in Humans and Other Mammals.* Oxford, Oxford University Press, 1988

KRYGER MH et al (eds): *Principles and Practice of Sleep Medicine.* Philadelphia, Saunders, 1989

LUGARESI E et al: Fatal familial insomnia and dysautonomia with selective degeneration of thalamic nuclei. N Engl J Med 315:997, 1986

LYDIC R, BIEBUYCK JF (eds): *Clinical Physiology of Sleep.* Bethesda, MD, American Physiological Society, 1988

MENDELSON WB: *Human Sleep: Research and Clinical Care.* New York, Plenum, 1987

PARKES JD: *Sleep and Its Disorders.* Philadelphia, Saunders, 1985

ROTH B: *Narcolepsy and Hypersomnia.* Basel, Karger, 1980

SCHENCK CH et al: Rapid eye movement sleep behavior disorder: A treatable parasomnia affecting older adults. JAMA 257:1786, 1987

WILLIAMS RL et al (eds): *Sleep Disorders: Diagnosis and Treatment,* 2d ed. New York, Wiley, 1988

section 4 # Alterations in circulatory and respiratory function

35 COUGH AND HEMOPTYSIS

EUGENE BRAUNWALD[1]

COUGH

Cough, one of the most frequent cardiorespiratory symptoms, is an explosive expiration which provides a means of clearing the tracheobronchial tree of secretions and foreign bodies.

MECHANISM Coughing may be initiated either voluntarily or reflexively. As a defensive reflex it has both afferent and efferent pathways. The *afferent limb* includes receptors within the sensory distribution of the trigeminal, glossopharyngeal, superior laryngeal, and vagus nerves. The *efferent limb* includes the recurrent laryngeal nerve (which causes glottic closure) and the spinal nerves (which cause contraction of the thoracic and abdominal musculature). The *sequence of a cough* includes an appropriate stimulus which initiates a deep inspiration. This is followed by glottic closure, relaxation of

---

[1] The late Gennaro M. Tisi was the senior author of this chapter in the 11th edition, and this chapter represents a revision of that work.

the diaphragm, and muscle contraction against a closed glottis so as to produce maximally positive intrathoracic and intraairway pressures. These positive intrathoracic pressures result in a narrowing of the trachea, produced by an infolding of its more compliant posterior membrane. Once the glottis opens, the combination of a large pressure differential between the airways and the atmosphere coupled with this tracheal narrowing produces flow rates through the trachea close to the speed of sound. The shearing forces which are developed aid in the elimination of mucus and foreign materials. A tracheostomy short-circuits and an endotracheal tube prevents glottic closure. Therefore, both decrease the effectiveness of the cough mechanism.

ETIOLOGY   Cough is produced by inflammatory, mechanical, chemical, and thermal stimulation of the cough receptors. *Inflammatory* stimuli are initiated by edema and hyperemia of the respiratory mucous membranes, and by irritation from exudative processes, such as postnasal drip and gastric reflux with aspiration. Such stimuli may arise either in the airways (as in laryngitis, tracheitis, bronchitis, and bronchiolitis) or in the alveoli (as in pneumonitis and lung abscess). *Mechanical* stimuli are produced by inhalation of particulate matter, such as dust particles, and by compression of the air passages and pressure or tension upon these structures. Lesions associated with airway compression may be either extramural or intramural in type. The former include aortic aneurysms, granulomas, pulmonary neoplasms, and mediastinal tumors; intramural lesions include bronchogenic carcinoma, bronchial adenoma, foreign bodies, granulomatous endobronchial involvement, and contraction of airway smooth muscle (bronchial asthma). Pressure or tension upon the air passages is usually produced by lesions associated with a decrease in pulmonary compliance. Examples of specific causes include acute and chronic interstitial fibrosis (Chap. 211), pulmonary edema, and atelectasis. *Chemical* stimuli may result from inhalation of irritant gases, including cigarette smoke and chemical fumes. Finally, *thermal* stimuli may be produced by inhalation of either very hot or cold air.

Cough is commonly associated with episodic wheezing secondary to bronchoconstriction in symptomatic patients with bronchial asthma (Chap. 204). Chronic, persistent cough may be the *sole* presenting manifestation of bronchial asthma (''cough asthma''). Such patients are characterized by (1) absence of a history of episodic wheezing and (2) no evidence of expiratory airflow obstruction by spirometry, but (3) hyperreactive airways (characteristic of asthma) when challenged with a cholinergic agent, methacholine.

DIAGNOSTIC EVALUATION   The history is the most important aspect of the evaluation. It should address the following issues:

1 Is the cough acute or chronic?
2 Is it associated with fever?
3 Is it associated with sputum? If so, what is its character?
4 Is it seasonal?
5 Does the patient have important risk factors for disease? (e.g., homosexuality, cigarette smoking, intravenous drugs, immobilization, environmental exposures?)
6 What is the past medical history?

The physical examination, chest roentgenogram, sputum examination, and screening pulmonary function studies (static lung volumes and dynamic flow rates) may then indicate a specific cause. The *history* may indicate specific diagnoses. Acute episodes of cough may be associated with such viral infections as acute tracheobronchitis or pneumonitis or with bacterial bronchopneumonia. Cough associated with an acute febrile episode and associated with hoarseness is usually produced by viral laryngotracheobronchitis. Postnasal drip is also a common cause of chronic cough.

The character of the cough may suggest the anatomic site of involvement: the patient with a ''barking'' type of cough may have epiglottal involvement (i.e., ''whooping cough'' due to *Haemophilus pertussis* infection in young children), while the cough associated with tracheal or major airway involvement is often loud and ''brassy.'' Cough associated with generalized wheezing may be produced by acute bronchospasm. The time of occurrence of a cough may indicate

a specific cause: a cough which occurs selectively at night suggests congestive heart failure; one related to meals suggests a tracheoesophageal fistula, a hiatal hernia, or an esophageal diverticulum; a cough precipitated by a change in position suggests a lung abscess or a localized area of bronchiectasis. The description of sputum or secretions produced in conjunction with the cough should include color, consistency, odor, and volume: purulent and/or large amounts of sputum suggests lung abscess and bronchiectasis; bloody sputum, bleeding (see ''Hemoptysis,'' below); frothy and pink-tinged sputum, pulmonary edema; mucoid and massive sputum, alveolar cell carcinoma.

The general *physical examination* may point to a nonpulmonary cause of cough, such as heart failure, primary nonpulmonary neoplasm, acquired immunodeficiency disease, etc. The character of the auscultatory findings may suggest the site of disease: inspiratory stridor and wheezing may be present in laryngeal disease, inspiratory and expiratory rhonchi favor tracheal and major airway involvement, coarse subcrepitant inspiratory rales may indicate interstitial fibrosis and/or edema, fine crepitant rales may indicate a process such as pneumonitis or pulmonary edema, which fills the alveoli with fluid. The *chest roentgenogram* may reveal the cause of the cough; it may show an intrapulmonary mass lesion which may be either central or peripheral (Chap. 215), an alveolar filling process which may be pneumonic or nonpneumonic, an area of honeycombing and cyst formation which may indicate an area of localized bronchiectasis, or bilateral hilar adenopathy which may indicate sarcoidosis or a lymphoma.

A careful *sputum examination* may be more enlightening than a patient's description of the character of the sputum. Examination shows whether the sputum is thin or viscid, purulent, foul-smelling, blood-tinged, or scant or copious. In pneumococcal pneumonia the sputum has a ''rusty'' color, while in *Klebsiella* pneumonia it may look like ''currant jelly.'' Gram stain and culture of deep-cough specimens may reveal a specific bacterial, fungal, or mycoplasmal causation, while sputum cytology may result in a positive diagnosis of a pulmonary neoplasm.

Bronchoscopy may reveal the cause of otherwise unexplained chronic cough. *Pulmonary function* studies (Chap. 201) may also be helpful. Significant expiratory obstruction to airflow (as determined from a forced expiratory flow maneuver), coupled with a history of cough and significant sputum production, suggests that irrespective of other lesions the patient has significant bronchitis. Decreased lung volume (as determined from the static lung volumes) suggests that a restrictive type of lung disease (Chap. 211) is present. Perhaps more important than providing a specific diagnosis, pulmonary function studies are useful in quantifying the severity of disease, its progression over time, and in assessing the efficacy of an intervention.

Two features of cough should be highlighted: (1) A cough is often so common in the cigarette smoker as to be ignored or minimized. *Any change in the nature or character of a chronic cigarette cough should initiate immediate diagnostic evaluation, with particular attention directed to detection of bronchogenic carcinoma.* (2) Female patients are inclined to swallow sputum and not to expectorate as male patients do. This tendency may lead to the incorrect conclusion that a cough in a female patient is irritative and nonproductive.

COMPLICATIONS   Three complications may be produced by the coughing mechanism: paroxysms of coughing may precipitate syncope (cough syncope, Chap. 21), and strenuous coughing may produce rupture of an emphysematous bleb, rib fractures, and costochondritis. A potential mechanism for cough syncope includes the development of markedly positive intrathoracic and alveolar pressures which decrease venous return, producing a decrease in cardiac output and resultant syncope. Although cough fractures of the ribs may occur in otherwise normal patients, their occurrence should at least raise the possibility of pathologic fractures, which are seen in multiple myeloma, osteoporosis, and osteolytic metastases.

THERAPY   Definitive treatment of cough depends on determining its precise cause and then initiating specific therapy for the underlying cause. Symptomatic therapy should be considered when the cause of the cough is idiopathic and the cough performs no useful function or represents a potential hazard to the patient. An irritative, nonproductive cough may be suppressed by an antitussive agent, such as codeine or dextromethorphan, 15 mg qid. These drugs are useful symptomatic therapy by interrupting prolonged, self-perpetuating paroxysms. However, a cough productive of significant quantities of sputum should not be suppressed, since retention of sputum in the tracheobronchial tree may interfere with the distribution of ventilation, alveolar aeration, and the ability of the lung to resist infection. When secretions are tenacious and thick, adequate hydration, expectorants, and humidification of the air with an ultrasonic nebulizer may be helpful. Ipratropium (a class of bronchodilator with antimuscarinic actions) may prove especially useful in patients with cough asthma.

HEMOPTYSIS

For purposes of definition hemoptysis includes both blood-streaked sputum and gross hemoptysis. Any patient with gross hemoptysis should be given appropriate diagnostic tests so that a specific cause may be found. The patient with blood-streaked sputum should also be studied unless one can be certain that this type of hemoptysis is due to a benign condition. Recurrent episodes of hemoptysis should not be automatically ascribed to a previously established diagnosis, such as chronic bronchiectasis or bronchitis. Such an approach may result in missing a serious but potentially treatable lesion.

ETIOLOGY AND INCIDENCE Prior to embarking upon an extensive diagnostic workup of hemoptysis, it is essential to determine that the blood is in fact coming from the respiratory tract, not from the nasopharynx or gastrointestinal tract. Distinguishing hemoptysis from hematemesis is difficult at times. In hemoptysis, the prodrome is usually a tingling in the throat or a desire to cough, the blood is coughed up, and it is usually bright-red and *frothy*; in hematemesis, the prodrome includes nausea and abdominal discomfort, the blood is vomited, and it is usually *dark red* in color. Once this point is established, the diagnostic tests for hemoptysis may proceed. Although there are numerous single case reports of diseases which have been associated with hemoptysis, Table 35-1 presents the more common disorders.

The incidence of the diagnoses listed in Table 35-1 depends upon the nature of the series reported and whether one includes both gross bleeding and blood streaking of the sputum. If both types of bleeding are included, then the major causes (approximately 60 to 70 percent) are chronic bronchitis and bronchiectasis. If the definition is restricted to gross bleeding (greater than several tablespoons) then the incidence depends upon the type of series reported. Surgical series favor the incidence of mass lesions and operable lesions (carcinoma, 20 percent; localized, segmental, or lobar bronchiectasis, 30 percent). Those

TABLE 35-1 Causes of hemoptysis

1 Inflammatory
  a Bronchitis
  b Bronchiectasis
  c Tuberculosis
  d Lung abscess
  e Pneumonia, particularly *Klebsiella*
2 Neoplastic
  a Lung cancer: squamous cell, adenocarcinoma, oat cell
  b Bronchial adenoma
3 Other
  a Pulmonary thromboembolism
  b Left ventricular failure
  c Mitral stenosis
  d Traumatic, including foreign body and lung contusion
  e Primary pulmonary hypertension; arteriovenous malformation; Eisenmenger's syndrome; pulmonary vasculitis including Wegener's granulomatosis and Goodpasture's syndrome; idiopathic pulmonary hemosiderosis; and amyloid
  f Hemorrhagic diathesis including anticoagulant therapy

from centers with a large tuberculosis population favor this condition (incidence varying between 2 and 40 percent). Combined medical-surgical series include a wider representation of those lesions which present with hemoptysis (carcinoma, 20 percent; bronchiectasis, 30 percent; bronchitis, 15 percent; other inflammatory lesions including tuberculosis, 10 to 20 percent; other lesions including the vascular, traumatic, and hemorrhagic etiologies listed in Table 35-1, 10 percent). Despite the most extensive of evaluations, 5 to 15 percent of cases entailing gross hemoptysis remain undiagnosed.

Two points should be highlighted with reference to diseases associated with hemoptysis: (1) hemoptysis is rare in metastatic carcinoma to the lung; (2) although hemoptysis may occur at some time during the course of a viral or pneumococcal pneumonia, it is usually scanty and its occurrence should always raise the question of a more serious underlying process.

DIAGNOSIS As is the case for cough, *history* is of enormous value. Recurrent, chronic hemoptysis in a young, otherwise asymptomatic female favors the diagnosis of a bronchial adenoma; recurrent hemoptysis with chronic, marked sputum production associated with ring shadows, tram lines (abnormal air bronchograms), and cyst formation on the roentgenogram suggests a diagnosis of bronchiectasis; putrid sputum production suggests a lung abscess; weight loss and anorexia in a male smoker over the age of 40 raise the possibility of a bronchogenic carcinoma; a recent history of blunt trauma to the chest suggests a lung contusion; and acute pleuritic chest pain raises the possibility of pulmonary embolism with infarction or some other pleurally based lesion (lung abscess, coccidioidomycosis cavity, and vasculitis). Several findings on the *physical examination* may also suggest a specific diagnosis: a pleural friction rub suggests those diagnoses just mentioned in connection with pleuritic pain; the findings of pulmonary hypertension raise the diagnostic possibilities of primary pulmonary hypertension, mitral stenosis, recurrent or chronic thromboembolism, and Eisenmenger's syndrome; a localized wheeze over a major lobar airway suggests an intramural lesion such as a bronchogenic carcinoma or a foreign body; systemic arteriovenous communications or the presence of a murmur over the lung fields suggest the diagnosis of Osler-Rendu-Weber disease with pulmonary arteriovenous malformation; evidence of significant expiratory obstruction to airflow coupled with sputum production suggests that whatever other lesion may be present, the patient has significant bronchitis. The *chest roentgenogram* is critical to diagnosis. The presence of ring shadows favors a diagnosis of bronchiectasis; an air-fluid level, the diagnosis of a lung abscess; and a mass lesion, the diagnosis of a central or peripheral pulmonary neoplasm. A mass lesion which may cause hemoptysis should be distinguished from an area of blood pneumonitis caused by aspiration of blood into contiguous areas.

One of the most demanding diagnostic problems is the identification of the site of bleeding in a patient with normal findings on physical examination and a normal roentgenogram of the chest. A patient with hemoptysis tends to keep the bleeding side dependent. Otherwise, gravitational drainage would cause aspiration into the noninvolved dependent lung. The patient may also be able to give a history of a burning or deep pain which may localize the side of bleeding; bronchoscopy may then be useful. This procedure generally is most helpful when the bleeding is scant, and of least help when the bleeding is massive, since blood may be aspirated into contiguous airways. Such aspiration may produce alveolar filling (i.e., a "blood pneumonitis") that may obscure the etiology of the hemoptysis on the initial chest roentgenogram. Blood pneumonitis usually clears within a week, and once clearing has occurred, a repeat chest roentgenogram may disclose the origin of the hemoptysis.

Following the history and physical examination, the diagnostic approach to a patient with hemoptysis includes whatever specialized studies and procedures are required to make a specific diagnosis. The first step is to obtain a roentgenogram. Usually computed tomography is the procedure employed next, followed by bronchoscopy. Rigid bronchoscopy permits visualization of the more central airways. It is of particular value when the source of bleeding is in this portion of the airway system, the degree of hemoptysis is massive, and selective endobronchial intubation is being considered. Fiberoptic bronchoscopy (Chap. 203) includes within the range of visualization airways as small as several millimeters in diameter. This endoscopic technique may provide definitive visual, biopsy, or cytologic information. Since direct visualization of more peripheral portions of the airway system is now possible, the indications for bronchography in the evaluation of hemoptysis are being modified. The principal indications for bronchography in such patients are (1) to establish the presence of localized bronchiectasis (including a sequestered lobe) and (2) to rule out the presence of more generalized bronchiectasis in a patient with localized disease who is regarded as a surgical candidate because of either repetitive hemoptysis or recurrent infections. The majority of patients with bronchiectasis have a normal chest roentgenogram, but the diagnosis can usually be established by computed tomography (Chaps. 202 and 203). A PPD and, if sputum is present, examination for acid-fast bacilli should be obtained. The laboratory evaluation should also rule out a bleeding disorder (Chap. 288).

THERAPY   Since hemoptysis is such an alarming symptom, there is a tendency to overtreat the patient. Usually hemoptysis is scant and will stop spontaneously without specific therapy. If the hemoptysis is substantial, the mainstays of therapy include keeping the patient calm, instituting complete bed rest, excluding unnecessary diagnostic procedures until the hemoptysis has begun to subside, and suppressing cough if it is present and an aggravating feature of the hemoptysis. The emergency care of such a patient demands that intubation and suctioning equipment be at the bedside. In patients in danger of asphyxiation by flooding of the lung contralateral to the site of hemorrhage, intubation by a technique which isolates the hemorrhaging lung and prevents contralateral aspiration of blood should be carried out. This can be accomplished by strategic location of a balloon catheter whose introduction into the bronchus in question is facilitated by direct visualization through a fiberoptic bronchoscope.

The management of potentially lethal massive hemoptysis remains controversial. The choice between a medical approach and surgical intervention hinges on the words *potentially lethal*. Massive hemoptysis, usually defined as greater than 600 to 800 mL in 24 h, is an alarming clinical situation in which asphyxiation due to aspiration of blood represents the principal threat to life. The choice between surgical and medical management relates most often to the anatomic basis for the massive hemoptysis. In patients with cavitary tuberculosis, anaerobic lung abscess, and lung cancer, the risk of mortality is far greater than when the cause of the hemoptysis is bronchitis or bronchiectasis. Operation may occasionally be necessary in the former, but virtually never in the latter group. In either case the initial management should include the conservative measures suggested above. With such management, spontaneous cessation of bleeding usually occurs. Surgical intervention should be considered in that small group of patients with a definable lesion on chest roentgenogram (i.e., cavitary disease, lung abscess, lung cancer) who have evidence of uncontrollable respiratory or hemodynamic compromise. If a patient is a surgical candidate, bronchoscopy should be performed to identify the specific site of bleeding. Otherwise bronchoscopy should be deferred for several days because of the tendency of this procedure to aggravate cough and thereby perpetuate the hemoptysis. Bronchial arterial catheterization and embolization are currently under evaluation for the nonsurgical control of massive hemoptysis, especially in patients with nonresectable lung cancer. Laser (neodymium YAG—yttrium aluminum garnet) therapy should also be considered as a palliative modality for massive hemoptysis in such patients.

REFERENCES

ADELMAN M et al: Cryptogenic hemoptysis: Clinical features, bronchoscopic findings, and natural history in 67 patients. Ann Intern Med 102:829, 1985

BOUSHEY HA et al: Medical staff conference: Evaluating and treating intractable cough. West J Med 143:223, 1985

CONLAN AA: Massive hemoptysis: Diagnostic and therapeutic implications. Surg Ann 17:337, 1985

CORRAO WMC et al: Chronic cough as the sole presenting manifestation of bronchial asthma. N Engl J Med 300:633, 1979

GROSS NJ et al: Anticholinergic, antimuscarinic bronchodilators. Am Rev Resp Dis 129:856, 1984

LEITH DE: The development of cough. Am Rev Respir Dis 131:S39, 1985

SACKNER MA: Cough, in *Textbook of Respiratory Practice*, JF Murray, JA Nadel (eds). Philadelphia, Saunders, 1988, pp 397–408

WILLIAMS MH: Management of massive hemoptysis. Pulmonary Perspectives, a publication of the American College of Chest Physicians 1:3, 1984

36 DYSPNEA AND PULMONARY EDEMA

ROLAND H. INGRAM, JR. / EUGENE BRAUNWALD

DYSPNEA

The breathing pattern is controlled by a series of higher central and peripheral mechanisms which can increase ventilation in excess of metabolic demands in conditions such as anxiety and fear, and can increase ventilation appropriate to increased metabolic demands during physical activity. A normal resting person is unaware of the act of breathing, and while he or she may become conscious of breathing during mild to moderate exertion, no discomfort is experienced. However, during and following exhausting exertion an individual may become unpleasantly aware of breathing, yet feel reasonably assured that the sensation will be transitory and is appropriate to the level of exercise. Therefore, as a cardinal symptom of diseases affecting the cardiorespiratory system, dyspnea is defined as an *abnormally uncomfortable awareness of breathing*.

Although dyspnea is not painful in the usual sense of the word, it is, like pain, involved with both the perception of a sensation and the reaction to that perception. Patients experience a number of uncomfortable sensations related to breathing and use an even larger number of verbal expressions to describe these sensations, such as "cannot get enough air," "air does not go all the way down," "smothering feeling in the chest," "tightness in the chest," "fatigue in the chest," and a "choking sensation." It may be necessary, therefore, to review meticulously the patient's history in order to ascertain whether the more abstruse descriptions do, in fact, represent dyspnea. Once it is established that a patient does have dyspnea, it is of paramount importance to define the circumstances in which it occurs and to assess associated symptoms. There are situations in which breathing appears labored but in which dyspnea does not occur. For example, the hyperventilation in association with metabolic acidemia is rarely accompanied by dyspnea. On the other hand, patients with apparently normal breathing patterns may complain of shortness of breath.

QUANTITATION OF DYSPNEA   The gradation of dyspnea may usefully be based upon the amount of physical exertion required to produce the sensation. In actual practice the major functional classifications of patients with heart or lung disease are based largely on dyspnea in relation to degree of exertion. However, in assessing the severity of dyspnea, it is important to obtain a clear understanding of the patient's general physical condition, work history, and recreational habits. For example, the development of dyspnea in a trained runner upon running 2 mi may signify a more serious disturbance than a similar degree of breathlessness in a sedentary person upon running a fraction of this distance. Another variable to consider in assessing the degree of dyspnea as an index of the severity of underlying heart or lung disease is the interindividual variation in perception. Some patients with extremely severe disease may complain of only mild dyspnea; others with mild disease may experience more severe shortness of breath. Thus, rather like variations in pain thresholds, patients have different degrees of subjective tolerance to cardiopulmonary dysfunction. There is some evidence that persons with relatively blunted ventilatory drives tolerate their disease with less dyspnea than those who have a heightened level of ventilatory responsiveness. Some patients with lung or heart disease may have such reduced capabilities due to other disease (e.g., peripheral vascular insufficiency or severe osteoarthritis of the hips or knees) that exertional dyspnea is precluded despite serious impairment of pulmonary or cardiac function.

Some patterns of dyspnea are not directly related to physical exertion. Sudden and unexpected dyspneic episodes at rest can be associated with pulmonary emboli, spontaneous pneumothorax, or anxiety. Nocturnal episodes of severe paroxysmal dyspnea are characteristic of left ventricular failure. Dyspnea upon assuming the supine posture, *orthopnea* (see below), thought to be mainly characteristic of congestive heart failure, may also occur in some patients with asthma and chronic obstruction of the airways and is a regular finding in the rare occurrence of bilateral diaphragmatic paralysis. *Trepopnea* is used to describe the unusual circumstance in which dyspnea occurs only in the left or right lateral decubitus position, most often in patients with heart disease, while *platypnea* is dyspnea which occurs only in the upright position. Both of these patterns remain to be fully explained but may be related to positional alterations in ventilation-perfusion relations (Chap. 201).

MECHANISMS OF DYSPNEA Physicians usually relate the symptom of dyspnea to a process such as obstruction of the airways or congestive heart failure and generally proceed with further diagnostic and/or therapeutic attempts, having satisfied themselves that they understand the mechanism of the dyspnea. In fact, elucidation of the *actual* mechanism(s) of dyspnea has eluded clinical investigators.

Dyspnea occurs whenever the work of breathing is excessive. Increased force generation is required of the respiratory muscles to produce a given volume change if the chest wall or lungs are less compliant or if resistance to airflow is increased. Increased work of breathing also occurs when the ventilation is excessive for the level of activity. Although an individual is more apt to become dyspneic when the work of breathing is increased, the work theory does not account for the perceptual difference between a deep breath with a normal mechanical load and a normal-sized breath with an increased mechanical load. The work might be the same with both breaths, but the normal one with the increased load will be associated with discomfort. In fact, with respiratory loading, such as adding a resistance at the mouth, there is an increase in respiratory center output, as gauged by newer indexes, that is disproportionate to the increase in work of breathing. It has been postulated that whenever the force that muscles actually generate during breathing approach some fraction of their maximal force-generating ability, which may vary among individuals, dyspnea ensues due to transduction of mechanical to neural stimuli. Such a theory would still not explain why patients who are completely paralyzed, either by cord transections or neuromuscular blockade, experience dyspnea although aided by a mechanical ventilator. It is probable, in these circumstances, that signals from the lungs and/or airways travel via the vagus nerve to the central nervous system to account for the sensation.

In all likelihood several different mechanisms operate to different degrees in the various clinical situations in which dyspnea occurs. Perhaps, in some circumstances, dyspnea is evoked by stimulation of receptors in the upper respiratory tract; in others it may originate from receptors in the lungs, airways, respiratory muscles, or some combination of those structures. In any event, dyspnea is characterized by an excessive or abnormal activation of the respiratory centers in the brainstem. This activation comes about from stimuli transmitted from or through a variety of structures and pathways including (1) intrathoracic receptors via the vagi; (2) afferent somatic nerves, particularly from the respiratory muscles and chest wall, but also from other skeletal muscles and joints; (3) chemoreceptors in the brain, aortic and carotid bodies, and elsewhere in the circulation; (4) higher (cortical) centers; and perhaps (5) afferent fibers in the phrenic nerves. In general, despite the interindividual variations described above, there is a reasonable correlation between the severity of dyspnea and the magnitude of disturbances of pulmonary or cardiac function which are responsible.

DIFFERENTIAL DIAGNOSIS Obstructive disease of airways (See also Chaps. 204 and 210) Obstruction to airflow can be present anywhere from the extrathoracic airways out to the small airways in the periphery of the lung. Large extrathoracic airway obstruction can occur acutely, as with aspiration of food or a foreign body or with angioedema of the glottis. Circumstantial evidence or testimony from witnesses should cause the physician to suspect aspiration, and an allergic history together with a few scattered hives should raise the possibility of glottic edema. The acute form of upper airway obstruction is a medical emergency. More chronic forms can occur with tumors or with fibrotic stenosis following tracheostomy or prolonged endotracheal intubation. Whether acute or chronic, the cardinal symptom is dyspnea, and the characteristic signs are stridor and retraction of the supraclavicular fossae with inspiration.

Obstruction of intrathoracic airways can occur acutely and intermittently or can be present chronically with worsening during respiratory infections. Acute intermittent obstruction with wheezing is typical of *asthma*. Chronic cough with expectoration is typical of *chronic bronchitis* and *bronchiectasis*. Most often there is a prolongation of expiration and coarse rhonchi which are generalized in chronic bronchitis and may be localized in the case of bronchiectasis. Intercurrent infection results in worsening of the cough, increased expectoration of purulent sputum, and more severe dyspnea. During such episodes the patient may complain of nocturnal paroxysms of dyspnea with wheezing relieved by cough and expectoration of sputum.

Many years of exertional dyspnea progressing to dyspnea at rest characterize the patient with predominant *emphysema* (Chap. 210). Although a parenchymal disease by definition, emphysema is invariably accompanied by obstruction of airways.

Diffuse parenchymal lung diseases (See also Chap. 211) This category includes a large number of diseases ranging from acute pneumonia to chronic disorders such as sarcoidosis and the various forms of *pneumoconiosis*. History, physical findings, and radiographic abnormalities often provide clues to the diagnosis. The patients are often tachypneic with arterial P_{CO_2} and P_{O_2} values below normal. Exertion often further reduces the arterial P_{O_2}. Lung volumes are decreased and the lungs are stiffer, i.e., less compliant than normal.

Pulmonary vascular occlusive diseases (See also Chap. 213) Repeated episodes of dyspnea at rest often occur with recurrent pulmonary emboli. A source for emboli, such as phlebitis of a lower extremity or the pelvis, is quite helpful in leading the physician to suspect the diagnosis. Arterial blood gases are almost invariably abnormal, but lung volumes are frequently normal or only minimally abnormal.

Diseases of the chest wall or respiratory muscles (See also Chap. 217) The physical examination establishes the presence of a chest wall disease such as severe kyphoscoliosis, pectus excavatum, or spondylitis. Although all three of these deformities may be associated with dyspnea, only severe kyphoscoliosis regularly interferes with ventilation sufficiently to produce chronic cor pulmonale and respiratory failure. Even though vital capacity, lung volumes, and airflow rates are normal with pectus excavatum, there is some evidence that cardiac compression from the posteriorly displaced sternum interferes with diastolic filling of the ventricle during the increased demands of exercise. Hence a cardiogenic component to the dyspnea may be present in this condition.

Both weakness and paralysis of respiratory muscles can lead to respiratory failure and dyspnea (Chap. 217), but most often the signs and symptoms of the neurologic or muscular disorder are more prominently manifested in other systems.

Heart disease In patients with cardiac disease exertional dyspnea occurs most commonly as a consequence of an elevated pulmonary capillary pressure; aside from uncommon causes such as obstructive disease of the pulmonary veins (Chap. 186), pulmonary capillary hypertension is a consequence of left atrial hypertension, which in turn may be due to left ventricular dysfunction (Chaps. 181 and 182), reduced left ventricular compliance, and mitral stenosis. The elevation of hydrostatic pressure in the pulmonary vascular bed tends to upset the Starling equilibrium (see "Pulmonary Edema," below) with resulting transudation of liquid into the interstitial space, reducing the compliance of the lungs and stimulating J (juxtacapillary) receptors in the alveolar interstitial space. When prolonged, pulmonary venous hypertension results in thickening of pulmonary vessels and an increase in perivascular cells and fibrous tissue, causing a further reduction in compliance. The competition for space between vessels, airways, and increased liquid within the interstitial space compromises the lumina of small airways, increasing the airways' resistance. Diminution in compliance and an increase in airways' resistance increase the work of breathing which, to some degree, is minimized by a reduction in tidal volume which is compensated for by an increase in frequency of respiration. In severe heart disease, usually involving elevation of both pulmonary and systemic venous pressures, hydrothorax may develop, further interfering with pulmonary function and intensifying dyspnea. In patients with heart failure and a severely diminished cardiac output, dyspnea may also be related to fatigue of the respiratory muscles as a consequence of their reduced perfusion. The metabolic acidosis characteristic of severe heart failure may play a contributory role. Dyspnea may also be associated with severe systemic and cerebral hypoxia, as occurs during exertion in patients with congenital heart disease and right-to-left shunts.

Cardiac dyspnea usually begins as breathlessness on strenuous exertion and, over the course of months or years, progresses until the patient is dyspneic at rest. Occasionally, a nonproductive cough developing in the recumbent position, particularly at night, may be the first complaint.

Orthopnea, i.e., dyspnea in the recumbent position, and *paroxysmal nocturnal dyspnea*, i.e., attacks of shortness of breath which usually occur at night and awaken the patient from sleep, are characteristic of more advanced forms of heart failure associated with elevations of pulmonary venous and capillary pressures and are discussed in Chap. 182. Orthopnea is the result of the alteration of gravitational forces when the recumbent position is assumed. This augmentation of intrathoracic blood volume elevates pulmonary venous and capillary pressures which increases the pulmonary closing volume (Chap. 201) and reduces the vital capacity. An additional factor associated with recumbency is the elevation of the diaphragm, which results in a lower end-expiratory lung volume. This combination of lower end-expiratory lung volume and increase in closing volume results in a significant alteration of alveolar-capillary gas exchange.

PAROXYSMAL (NOCTURNAL) DYSPNEA Also known as *cardiac asthma*, this condition is characterized by attacks of severe shortness of breath which generally occur at night and usually awaken the patient from sleep. The attack is precipitated by stimuli which aggravate the previously existing pulmonary congestion; frequently the total blood volume is augmented at night because of the reabsorption of edema from dependent portions of the body during recumbency; the redistribution of blood volume which takes place results in an increase in intrathoracic blood volume and therefore produces pulmonary congestion. A sleeping patient can tolerate relatively severe pulmonary engorgement and may awaken only when actual pulmonary edema and bronchospasm have developed, with the feeling of suffocation and with wheezing respirations.

CHEYNE-STOKES RESPIRATION See Chap. 182.

DIAGNOSIS The diagnosis of cardiac dyspnea depends on the recognition of heart disease on the basis of the history and physical examination. There may be a history of antecedent myocardial infarction, third and fourth heart sounds may be audible, and/or there may be evidence of left ventricular enlargement, jugular neck vein

distention, and/or peripheral edema. Often there are radiographic signs of heart failure, with evidence of interstitial edema, pulmonary vascular redistribution, and accumulation of liquid in the septal planes and pleural cavity. Cardiomegaly is often present, but the overall heart size may be normal, particularly in patients with dyspnea due to acute myocardial infarction or mitral stenosis; an enlarged left atrium is usually evident in the latter condition. The electrocardiogram (Chap. 176) is rarely specific for heart disease and cannot specifically indicate whether a patient's dyspnea is caused by heart disease; however, it is rarely normal in patients with cardiac dyspnea.

Differentiation between cardiac and pulmonary dyspnea In most patients with dyspnea there is obvious clinical evidence of disease of either heart or lungs. The dyspnea of chronic obstructive lung disease tends to develop more gradually than that of heart diseases; exceptions, of course, occur in patients with obstructive lung disease who develop an episode of infectious bronchitis, pneumonia, or pneumothorax, or an exacerbation of asthma. Like patients with cardiac dyspnea, patients with chronic obstructive lung disease may also waken at night with dyspnea, but this is usually associated with sputum production; the dyspnea is relieved after these patients rid themselves of secretions.

The difficulty in the distinction between cardiac and pulmonary dyspnea may be compounded by the coexistence of diseases involving both organ systems. Patients with a history of chronic bronchitis or asthma who develop left ventricular failure tend to develop recurrences of bronchoconstriction and wheezing in association with bouts of paroxysmal nocturnal dyspnea and pulmonary edema. This condition, i.e., cardiac asthma, usually occurs in patients with overt clinical evidence of heart disease. Acute cardiac asthma is further differentiated from acute attacks of bronchial asthma by the presence of diaphoresis, more bubbly airway sounds, and the more common occurrence of cyanosis.

It is desirable to carry out pulmonary function testing in patients in whom the etiology of dyspnea is not clear, for these tests should be helpful in determining whether dyspnea is produced by heart disease, lung disease, abnormalities of the chest wall, or anxiety. In addition to the usual means of assessing patients for heart disease (Chap. 174), determination of the ejection fraction at rest and during exercise by radionuclide ventriculography (Chap. 178) is helpful in the differential diagnosis of dyspnea; the left ventricular ejection fraction is depressed in left ventricular failure while the right ventricular ejection fraction may be low at rest or may decline during exercise in patients with severe lung disease; both ejection fractions are normal at rest and during exercise in dyspnea due to anxiety or malingering. Careful observation during the performance of an exercise treadmill test will often help in the identification of the patient who is malingering or whose dyspnea is secondary to anxiety. Under these circumstances the patient usually complains of severe shortness of breath but appears to be breathing either effortlessly or totally irregularly. In less than obvious cases, measurements of P_{O_2}, pH, and P_{CO_2} in arterial blood and CO_2 and O_2 levels in mixed expired gas may be helpful in establishing either that gas exchange is normal or that a significant abnormality that is not detectable at rest exists during exercise.

Anxiety neurosis Dyspnea experienced by someone with an anxiety neurosis is a difficult symptom to evaluate. The signs and symptoms of acute and chronic hyperventilation do not serve to distinguish between anxiety neurosis and other processes, such as recurrent pulmonary emboli. Another potentially confusing situation is seen when chest pain and electrocardiographic changes accompany the hyperventilation syndrome. When present and attributable to this condition, often referred to as *neurocirculatory asthenia* (Chap. 16), the chest pain is often sharp, fleeting, and in various loci, and the electrocardiographic changes are most often seen during repolarization; yet occasional ventricular ectopic activity can be seen as well. A rather extensive series of pulmonary and cardiac function tests, carried out both at rest and during exercise, may be needed to be certain that anxiety is, in fact, the cause of the dyspnea. Certain clues are helpful in leading one to suspect a psychogenic origin. Frequent sighing respirations and a bizarre, irregular breathing pattern are helpful. Often the breathing pattern returns to normal during sleep.

PULMONARY EDEMA

CARDIOGENIC PULMONARY EDEMA   An increase in pulmonary venous pressure, which results initially in the engorgement of the pulmonary vasculature, is common in most instances of dyspnea in association with congestive heart failure. The lungs become less compliant, the resistance of small airways increases, and there is an increase in lymphatic flow which apparently serves to maintain a constant pulmonary extravascular liquid volume. At this early stage there is usually mild tachypnea, and if arterial blood gases are measured, the arterial P_{O_2} and P_{CO_2} are both lowered with an increase in the alveolar-to-arterial oxygen difference. Tachypnea itself, which might result from stimulation of receptors in the pulmonary interstitium, apparently increases lymphatic flow by augmenting ventilatory pumping of lymphatic vessels. The changes described are seen well in advance of auscultatory findings or radiographic signs pointing to congestive heart failure. If sufficient both in magnitude and duration, the increase in intravascular pressure results in a net gain of liquid in the extravascular space despite further increases in lymphatic flow. It is at this point that symptoms worsen, tachypnea increases, gas exchange deteriorates further, and radiographic changes, such as Kerley B lines and loss of distinct vascular margins, are seen. Even at this intermediate stage, the capillary endothelial intercellular junctions have been shown to widen and allow passage of macromolecules into the interstices. Up to and including this stage, the edema is purely *interstitial*. Sufficient further elevations in intravascular pressure result in disruption of the tighter junctions between alveolar lining cells, and alveolar edema ensues with outpouring of liquid, which contains both red blood cells and macromolecules. At this point *alveolar edema* is present. Although at one time considered an early and subtle radiographic sign of interstitial edema, current evidence suggests that an antigravity redistribution of pulmonary blood flow occurs only after the onset of alveolar edema. With yet more severe disruption of the alveolar-capillary membrane, edematous liquid floods the alveoli and airways. At this point, full-blown clinical pulmonary edema with bilateral wet rales and rhonchi will occur, and the chest radiograph may show diffuse haziness of the lung fields with greater density in the more proximal hilar regions. Typically, the patient is anxious and perspires freely, and the sputum is frothy and blood-tinged. Gas exchange is more severely compromised with worsening hypoxia and possibly hypercapnia. Without effective treatment (Chap. 182), progressive acidemia, hypoxia, and respiratory arrest ensue.

The earlier sequence of liquid accumulation described above follows the Starling law of capillary–interstitial fluid exchange:

Liquid accumulation $= K[(P_c - P_{IF}) - \sigma(\pi_{pl} - \pi_{IF})] - Q_{lymph}$
where K = permeability coefficient
 P_c = mean intracapillary pressure
 π_{IF} = oncotic pressure of interstitial liquid
 σ = reflection coefficient of macromolecules
 P_{IF} = mean interstitial liquid pressure
 π_{pl} = oncotic pressure of the plasma
 Q_{lymph} = lymphatic flow

The pressures tending to move liquid out of the vessel are P_c and π_{IF}, which are normally more than offset by pressures tending to move liquid back into the vasculature, i.e., the algebraic sum of P_{IF} and π_{pl}. Implicit in the above equation is that lymphatic flow can increase in the case of imbalance of forces and result in no net accumulation of interstitial liquid. However, in later sequences, with opening of first the endothelial and then the alveolar intercellular junctions, the permeability and reflection coefficients change strikingly. Thus, the initial process of hemodynamic pulmonary edema is one of liquid filtration and clearance. With further increasing pressures, disruption of both the structure and the function of the alveolar-capillary membrane occurs.

NONCARDIOGENIC PULMONARY EDEMA   There are several clinical conditions which are associated with pulmonary edema based upon an imbalance of Starling forces other than through primary elevations of pulmonary capillary pressure. Although diminished plasma oncotic pressure in hypoalbuminemic states (e.g., severe liver disease, nephrotic syndrome, protein-losing enteropathy) might be expected to lead to pulmonary edema, the balance of forces normally so strongly favors resorption that even under these conditions some elevation of capillary pressure is necessary before interstitial edema develops. Increased negativity of interstitial pressure has been implicated in the genesis of unilateral pulmonary edema following rapid evacuation of a large pneumothorax. In this situation the findings may be apparent only by radiography, but occasionally the patient experiences dyspnea with physical findings localized to the edematous lung. It has been recently proposed that large negative intrapleural pressures during acute severe asthma may be associated with the development of interstitial edema. If this proposal can be supported by sufficient clinical data, then asthma would represent an additional example of edema due to increased negativity of interstitial pressure. Lymphatic blockade secondary to fibrotic and inflammatory diseases or lymphangitic carcinomatosis may lead to interstitial edema. In such instances both clinical and radiographic manifestations are dominated by the underlying disease process.

There are other conditions characterized by increases in the interstitial liquid content of the lungs which begin neither with an imbalance between intravascular and interstitial forces nor with alterations in lymphatics, but rather appear to be associated primarily with disruption of the alveolar-capillary membranes. Any number of spontaneously occurring or environmental toxic insults, including diffuse pulmonary infections, aspiration, shock (particularly due to gram-negative septicemia and hemorrhagic pancreatitis, and following cardiopulmonary bypass), are associated with diffuse pulmonary edema which clearly does not have a hemodynamic origin. These conditions, which may lead to the adult respiratory distress syndrome, are discussed in Chap. 218.

Other forms of pulmonary edema   There are three forms of pulmonary edema which have not been clearly related to increased permeability, inadequate lymphatic flow, or an imbalance of Starling forces; hence their precise mechanism remains unexplained. *Narcotic overdose* is a well-recognized antecedent to pulmonary edema. Although illicit use of parenteral heroin has been the most frequent cause, parenteral and oral overdoses of legitimate preparations of morphine, methadone, and dextropropoxyphene have also been associated with pulmonary edema. Thus the earlier idea that injected impurities lead to the disorder is untenable. Available evidence suggests that there are alterations in the permeability of alveolar and capillary membranes rather than elevation of pulmonary capillary pressure.

Exposure to high altitude in association with severe physical exertion is a well-recognized setting for pulmonary edema in unacclimatized, yet otherwise healthy, persons. Recent data show that acclimatized high-altitude natives also develop this syndrome upon return to high altitude after a relatively brief sojourn at low altitudes. The syndrome is far more common in persons under the age of 25 years. The mechanism for high-altitude pulmonary edema remains obscure, and studies have been conflicting, some suggesting pulmonary venous constriction and others indicating pulmonary arteriolar constriction as the prime mechanisms. A role for hypoxia at altitude is suggested by the fact that patients respond to the administration of oxygen and/or return to lower altitudes. Hypoxia per se does not alter permeability of the alveolar-capillary membrane. Hence, increased cardiac output and pulmonary arterial pressures with exercise combined with hypoxic pulmonary arteriolar constriction, which is more prominent in young persons, may combine to make this an example of prearteriolar, high-pressure pulmonary edema.

Neurogenic pulmonary edema has been suspected in patients with central nervous system disorders and without apparent preexisting left ventricular dysfunction. Although most experimental equivalents have implicated sympathetic nervous system activity, the mechanism whereby sympathetic efferent activity leads to pulmonary edema is a matter of speculation. It is known that a massive adrenergic discharge leads to peripheral vasoconstriction with elevation of blood pressure and shifts of blood to the central circulation. In addition, it is probable that a decrease in left ventricular compliance also occurs, and both factors serve to increase left atrial pressures sufficiently to induce pulmonary edema on a hemodynamic basis. Some experimental evidence suggests that stimulation of adrenergic receptors increases capillary permeability directly, but this effect is relatively minor as compared to the imbalance of Starling forces.

TREATMENT OF PULMONARY EDEMA   See Chap. 182.

REFERENCES

CHERNIACK NS, ALTOSE MD: Mechanisms of dyspnea. Clin Chest Med 8:207, 1987

INGRAM RH JR, BRAUNWALD E: Pulmonary edema: Cardiogenic and noncardiogenic, in *Heart Disease*, E. Braunwald (ed). Philadelphia, Saunders, 1988, p 544

MALIK AB: Mechanisms of neurogenic pulmonary edema. Circ Res 57:1, 1985

McFADDEN ER, INGRAM RH JR: Relationship between diseases of the heart and lungs, in *Heart Disease*, E Braunwald (ed). Philadelphia, Saunders, 1988, p 1870

RASANEN J et al: Continuous positive airway pressure by face mask in acute cardiogenic pulmonary edema. Am J Cardiol 55:296, 1985

ROUSSOS C, MACKLEM PT: Disorders of the respiratory muscle function, in *Update III: Harrison's Principles of Internal Medicine*, KJ Isselbacher et al (eds). New York, McGraw-Hill, 1982, p 83

SCHOENE RB et al: High altitude pulmonary edema: Characteristics of lung lavage fluid. JAMA 256:63, 1986

SPRUNG CL et al: The spectrum of pulmonary edema: Differentiation of cardiogenic, intermediate, and noncardiogenic forms of pulmonary edema. Am Rev Resp Dis 124:718, 1981

WASSERMAN K, CASABURI R: Dyspnea: Physiological and pathophysiological mechanisms. Ann Rev Med 39:503, 1988

37   HYPOXIA, POLYCYTHEMIA, AND CYANOSIS

EUGENE BRAUNWALD

HYPOXIA

The fundamental purpose of the cardiorespiratory system is to deliver oxygen (and substrates) to the cells and to remove carbon dioxide (and other metabolic products) from them. Proper maintenance of this function depends on intact cardiovascular and respiratory systems and a supply of inspired gas containing adequate oxygen. Changes in oxygen and in carbon dioxide tension as well as changes in the intraerythrocytic concentration of certain *organic phosphate compounds*, especially 2,3-diphosphoglyceric acid (2,3-DPG), cause shifts in the oxygen dissociation curve. These are discussed in detail in Chap. 290 and are illustrated in Fig. 290-4. When hypoxia results as a consequence of respiratory failure, Pa_{CO_2} usually rises (Chap. 210), and the oxygen dissociation curve tends to be displaced to the right. Under these conditions the percentage saturation of the hemoglobin in the arterial blood at a given level of alveolar oxygen (Pa_{O_2}) tension declines. Thus arterial hypoxia and cyanosis are likely to be more marked in proportion to the degree of depression of Pa_{O_2} when such depression results from pulmonary disease than when the depression occurs as the result of a decline in the partial pressure of oxygen in the inspired air, in which case Pa_{CO_2} falls and the oxygen dissociation curve is displaced to the left.

DIFFERENTIAL DIAGNOSIS   Anemic hypoxia   Any decrease in hemoglobin concentration is attended by a corresponding decline in the oxygen-carrying capacity. The Pa_{O_2} remains normal, but the absolute amount of oxygen transported per unit volume of blood is diminished. As the anemic blood passes through the capillaries, and the usual amount of oxygen is removed from it, the P_{O_2} in the venous blood declines to a greater degree than would normally be the case.

Circulatory hypoxia   As in anemic hypoxia, Pa_{O_2} is normal, but venous and tissue P_{O_2} are reduced as a consequence of reduced tissue perfusion in the face of normal tissue oxygen consumption. For this reason the term *stagnant hypoxia* may be used for this condition. Generalized circulatory hypoxia occurs in heart failure (Chap. 182) and in most forms of shock (Chap. 39).

Specific organ hypoxia   Decreased circulation to a specific organ resulting in localized stagnant hypoxia may be due to organic arterial or venous obstruction or may occur as a consequence of vasoconstriction. The latter may occur in the upper extremities in Raynaud's phenomenon. Reduced circulation may occur in all limbs in patients with heart failure or hypovolemic shock in an attempt to maintain adequate perfusion to more vital organs. Ischemic hypoxia with accompanying pallor occurs in organic arterial obliterative disease. Localized hypoxia may also result from venous obstruction and the resultant congestion. Edema, which increases the distance through which oxygen diffuses before it reaches the cells, can also cause localized hypoxia.

Increased oxygen requirements   Even if oxygen diffusion into blood perfusing the pulmonary capillary bed is unhampered and the hemoglobin is qualitatively and quantitatively normal, the P_{O_2} in venous blood (hence, capillary and tissue P_{O_2}) may be reduced if the oxygen consumption of the tissues is elevated without a corresponding increase in volume flow per unit of time. Such a situation may be encountered when fever or thyrotoxicosis occurs in patients in whom the cardiac output cannot rise normally. Under such conditions the circulation may be considered deficient relative to the metabolic requirements.

Ordinarily, the clinical picture of patients with hypoxia due to an elevated basal metabolic rate is quite different from that in other types of hypoxia; the skin is warm and flushed, owing to increased cutaneous blood flow which dissipates the excessive heat produced, and cyanosis is usually absent.

Exercise is a classic example of increased tissue oxygen requirements. The increased demands are normally met by several mechanisms: (1) increasing the cardiac output and ventilation and thus oxygen delivery to the tissues; (2) preferentially directing the blood to the exercising muscles and away from resting muscles and skin (by changing vascular resistances in various circulatory beds, directly and/or reflexly); (3) increasing oxygen extraction from the delivered blood and widening the arteriovenous oxygen differences; (4) reducing the pH of the tissues and capillary blood, thereby unloading more oxygen from hemoglobin. If the capacity of these mechanisms is exceeded, then hypoxia, especially of the exercising muscles, will result.

Carbon monoxide intoxication (Chap. 374)   This condition is analogous to anemic hypoxia in that the hemoglobin which is combined with the carbon monoxide (carboxyhemoglobin) is unavailable for oxygen transport. In addition, the presence of carboxyhemoglobin shifts the dissociation curve of hemoglobin to the left, so that the oxygen can be unloaded only at lower tensions. By such formation of carboxyhemoglobin a given degree of reduction in oxygen-carrying power produces a far greater degree of tissue hypoxia than the equivalent reduction in hemoglobin due to simple anemia.

Improper oxygen utilization   Cyanide (Chap. 374) and several other similarly acting poisons cause a paradoxic state in which the tissues are unable to utilize oxygen and as a consequence the venous blood tends to have a high oxygen tension. This condition has been termed *histotoxic hypoxia*. Cyanide produces cellular hypoxia by paralyzing the electron-transfer function of cytochrome oxidase so that it cannot pass electrons to oxygen, whereas diphtheria toxin is believed to inhibit the synthesis of one of the cytochromes and thus interfere with oxygen consumption and energy production by the cells involved.

EFFECTS OF HYPOXIA Changes in the central nervous system, particularly the higher centers, are especially important. Acute hypoxia produces impaired judgment, motor incoordination, and a clinical picture closely resembling that of acute alcoholism. When hypoxia is long-standing, fatigue, drowsiness, apathy, inattentiveness, delayed reaction time, and reduced work capacity occur. As hypoxia becomes more severe, the centers of the brainstem are affected, and death usually results from respiratory failure. With reduction of Pa_{O_2}, cerebrovascular resistance decreases and cerebral blood flow increases, which tends to reduce the cerebral hypoxia. On the other hand when the reduction of Pa_{O_2} is accompanied by hyperventilation and diminution of Pa_{CO_2}, cerebrovascular resistance rises, blood flow falls, and hypoxia is enhanced. Compared with the brain, the phylogenetically older spinal cord and peripheral nerves are relatively insensitive to hypoxia. Hypoxia also causes pulmonary arterial constriction, which serves the useful function of shunting blood away from poorly ventilated areas toward better-ventilated portions of the lung. However, it has the disadvantage of causing increased pulmonary vascular resistance and increased right ventricular afterload.

A complex disturbance of cellular functions results from the metabolic effects of severe acute hypoxia. In liver and muscles the breakdown of the primary foodstuff, carbohydrate, normally proceeds anaerobically (i.e., without oxidation) to the stage of formation of pyruvic acid. The breakdown of pyruvate requires oxygen, and when this is deficient, increasing proportions of pyruvate are reduced to lactic acid, which cannot be broken down further (Chap. 51). Hence, there is an increase in the blood lactate, with decrease in bicarbonate and a corresponding metabolic acidosis. Under these circumstances the total energy obtained from foodstuff breakdown is greatly reduced, and the amount of energy available for continuing resynthesis of energy-rich phosphate compounds becomes inadequate, leading to a complex disturbance of cellular function.

Most of the useful respiratory response to hypoxia originates in special chemosensitive cells in the carotid and aortic bodies, although the respiratory center is also stimulated directly by oxygen lack. The resultant increase in ventilation, with loss of carbon dioxide, leads to respiratory alkalosis. On the other hand, the diffusion of additional quantities of lactic acid from the tissues into the blood tends to produce metabolic acidosis. In either case the total amount of bicarbonate, and hence the carbon dioxide–combining power, tends to be diminished.

Diminished oxygen tension in any tissue results in local vasodilatation, and the diffuse vasodilatation which occurs in generalized hypoxia causes an elevation of total cardiac output (Fig. 290-5). In patients with preexisting heart disease, particularly coronary artery disease, the combination of hypoxia and the requirements of the peripheral tissues for an increase of cardiac output may precipitate congestive heart failure. Prolonged or severe hypoxia may also impair hepatic and renal function.

One of the important mechanisms of compensation for prolonged hypoxia is an increase in the quantity of hemoglobin in the blood (Fig. 290-5). This is due not to direct stimulation of the bone marrow but to the effect of erythropoietin, which originates primarily in the kidneys (Chap. 290). Assayable levels of erythropoietin are increased by hypoxia, and its production has been found to be regulated by the balance between tissue oxygen supply and demand.

POLYCYTHEMIA (See also Chap. 297)

The term *polycythemia* signifies an increase above the normal in the number of red blood cells in the circulating blood. This elevation is usually, though not always, accompanied by a corresponding increase in the quantity of hemoglobin and in the hematocrit. The increase may or may not be associated with an elevation in the total quantity of red blood cells in the body. It is important to distinguish between *absolute* polycythemia (an increase in the total red cell mass) and *relative* polycythemia, which occurs when, through loss of blood plasma, the *concentration* of the red cells becomes greater than normal in the circulating blood. This may be the consequence of abnormally lowered fluid intake, of the loss of plasma into the interstitial fluid, or of the marked loss of body fluids, such as occurs in persistent vomiting, severe diarrhea, copious sweating, or acidosis.

Because the term polycythemia is used loosely to refer to all varieties of increase in the number of red corpuscles, the terms *erythrocytosis* and *erythremia* are preferred in referring to two forms of *absolute* polycythemia. Erythrocytosis denotes absolute polycythemia which occurs in response to some known stimulus (secondary polycythemia); erythremia (polycythemia vera) refers to the disease of unknown etiology (Chap. 297). An approach to the differential diagnosis of erythrocytosis should begin with a consideration of its mechanisms (Table 37-1). Erythrocytosis develops as a consequence of a variety of factors and represents a physiologic response to conditions of hypoxia.

Sojourn at high altitudes leads to defective saturation of arterial blood with oxygen and stimulates the production of more red cells. The oxygen saturation, rather than oxygen tension, appears to be the more important determinant of the erythropoietic response to chronic hypoxia (Fig. 37-1). A disorder may set in insidiously after several years of continued residence at high altitudes, leading to the development of a condition known as *chronic mountain sickness* or *seroche* (Monge's disease), which appears to be caused by the development of alveolar hypoventilation superimposed on a lowered inspired O_2 concentration. Prominent manifestations are a florid color which turns to cyanosis on mild exertion, mental torpor, fatigue, and headache. Those affected are usually in the fourth to sixth decades. Return to sea level promptly relieves the symptoms. Living at high altitudes also evokes a number of compensatory reactions which act to increase oxygen delivery to the tissues. These include hyperventilation, which reduces the oxygen gradient between inspired and alveolar air, an augmentation of pulmonary capillary blood volume, an increase of diffusing capacity, and an increase in cardiac output.

Any pulmonary disease which produces chronic hypoxia may lead to erythrocytosis. The increased blood viscosity secondary to the polycythemia elevates pulmonary arterial pressure and, combined with the elevation of pulmonary vascular resistance resulting from

---

TABLE 37-1 Differential diagnosis of erythrocytosis

ABSOLUTE (↑ RED CELL MASS)

I Autonomous erythroid proliferation (↓ EP*); polycythemia vera
II Secondary erythroid proliferation
  A Autonomous or inappropriate increase in EP
    1 Neoplasm
    2 Renal lesions
    3 Familial erythrocytosis (autosomal recessive inheritance)
  B Secondary increase in EP
    1 Hypoxia (↓ arterial P_{O_2})
      a High altitude
      b Alveolar hypoventilation
      c Pulmonary disease
      d Cardiac right-to-left shunt
    2 Abnormal hemoglobin function (normal arterial P_{O_2})
      a High-affinity variants (autosomal dominant inheritance)
      b Congenital methemoglobinemia
      c Carboxyhemoglobin (smokers')
  C Hormonal stimulus to erythropoiesis
    1 Cushing's syndrome
    2 Androgen or corticosteroid administration

RELATIVE (REDUCED PLASMA VOLUME, NORMAL RED CELL MASS)

I Dehydration
II Stress erythrocytosis

* Erythropoietin.
SOURCE: Adapted from HF Bunn et al, *Human Hemoglobins*, Philadelphia, Saunders, 1988.

FIGURE 37-1   Relationship between mean arterial oxygen saturation (percent) and the mean hemoglobin content (grams per deciliter) in healthy male residents at various altitudes. *(From Hurtado, by permission of Annals of Internal Medicine.)*

hypoxia, further elevates right ventricular pressure, contributing to the development or intensification of cor pulmonale (Chap. 191). The *abnormal ventilatory conditions* present in very obese individuals may cause alveolar hypoventilation and result in arterial unsaturation, erythrocytosis, hypercapnia, and somnolence (the Pickwickian syndrome, Chap. 217). This syndrome is observed less commonly in nonobese persons (sleep-apnea syndrome) in whom decreased sensitivity of the respiratory center to CO_2 may play a role (Chap. 217).

The partial shunting of blood from the pulmonary circuit, such as occurs in *congenital heart disease,* causes the most striking erythrocytosis resulting from abnormalities in the heart or lungs (Chap. 186). Erythrocyte counts as high as 13 million per microliter, which are possible only when the red corpuscles are smaller than normal, have been observed in such patients, with volumes of packed red blood cells as high as 860 mL/L (86 mL/dL) of blood. As the polycythemia develops, there is a progressive elevation of blood viscosity, which begins to rise logarithmically when the volume of packed red blood cells exceeds 55 percent. The commonest defects producing such polycythemia in the adult are tetralogy of Fallot and Eisenmenger's complex. Other conditions include transposition of the great arteries, tricuspid atresia, and persistent truncus arteriosus. The polycythemia of cyanotic congenital heart disease may lead to spontaneous thrombosis at any site, including the central nervous system. The increase in hematocrit and the sharp increase in viscosity which occur when these patients become dehydrated are particularly hazardous. This condition may also be accompanied by a variety of blood coagulation defects, including reduced fibrinogen and prothrombin concentrations, as well as thrombocytopenia. Reduction in red blood cell volume (phlebotomy with reinfusion of the plasma) is sometimes performed in severely symptomatic patients with extremely high hematocrit levels, but it must be carried out slowly and with caution. It results in a reduction of the elevated blood viscosity which improves blood flow.

The excessive use of coal-tar derivatives and other forms of chronic poisoning, by producing abnormal hemoglobin pigments such as *methemoglobin* and *sulfhemoglobin* (Chap. 295), also may cause erythrocytosis. Patients with abnormal hemoglobins which displace the oxygen dissociation curve to the left and interfere with oxygen unloading in the tissues stimulate the production of erythropoietin and a secondary erythrocytosis *unassociated* with leukocytosis or thrombocytosis (Chap. 295).

Mild erythrocytosis is sometimes found in *Cushing's syndrome*

and can be produced by the administration of large amounts of adrenocortical steroids. Androgens also exert an erythropoietic effect and when administered to normal individuals can produce erythrocytosis. Especially intriguing are the instances of erythrocytosis observed in association with various *tumors* which produce erythropoietin or an erythropoietin-like substance. These have been chiefly of two varieties, *infratentorial* and *renal.* The tumors in the posterior fossa have usually been vascular (hemangioblastomas). The renal tumors have included renal cell carcinoma, adenoma, and sarcoma. Other tumors that have been associated with erythrocytosis include uterine myoma, hepatic carcinoma, and pheochromocytoma. Erythrocytosis also has been reported in association with solitary and polycystic disease of the kidneys, with hydronephrosis, and with renal artery stenosis. However, only a small proportion of the renal disorders mentioned above have been associated with polycythemia. Plasma erythropoietin levels have been found to be elevated in a number of these patients. Erythropoietin-like activity has been demonstrated in tumor extracts and in renal cyst fluid, and erythrocytosis has disappeared after the associated tumor was removed.

The term *stress erythrocytosis* has been applied to the polycythemia seen occasionally in very active, hard-working, middle-aged white males who are typically hypertensive and overweight and in a state of anxiety, who appear florid but who have none of the other characteristic signs of polycythemia vera—no splenomegaly or leukocytosis with immature cells in the blood. In such persons the total red blood cell mass is normal, and the plasma volume is below normal. Thus, they have an elevated hematocrit and *relative* polycythemia. *Smokers' polycythemia* is a closely related condition, but the high carboxyhemoglobin concentration may cause a small absolute increase in red cell mass which is often associated with a reduced plasma volume.

The *clinical features* of polycythemia include, in addition to the symptoms of the underlying condition (in the secondary forms), a characteristic "ruddy" cyanosis, dizziness, headache, epistaxes, and an increased incidence of thrombotic complications.

The *differential diagnosis* of absolute polycythemia is discussed in Chap. 297. In polycythemia vera, erythropoietin levels are usually absent, leukocyte alkaline phosphatase and vitamin B_{12} levels and platelet and total white blood cells are usually elevated, and splenomegaly is common; the bone marrow shows hyperplasia of all elements. In secondary polycythemia with hypoxia, Pa_{CO_2} is reduced, erythropoietin levels are elevated, while levels of leukocyte alkaline phosphatase, serum vitamin B_{12}, platelet, total white blood cell, and differential counts are all normal, and the liver and spleen are not enlarged; the bone marrow shows only erythroid hyperplasia. In the absence of features of either polycythemia vera or polycythemia secondary to hypoxia or to a tumor, a hemoglobin with a high affinity for oxygen should be sought for.

CYANOSIS

Cyanosis refers to a bluish color of the skin and mucous membranes resulting from an increased amount of reduced hemoglobin, or of hemoglobin derivatives, in the small blood vessels of those areas. It is usually most marked in the lips, nail beds, ears, and malar eminences. The "red cyanosis" of polycythemia vera (Chap. 297) must be distinguished from the true cyanosis discussed here. A cherry-colored flush, rather than cyanosis, is caused by carboxyhemoglobin (Chap. 374). The degree of cyanosis is modified by the quality of cutaneous pigment, the color of the blood plasma, and the thickness of the skin, as well as by the state of the cutaneous capillaries. The accurate clinical detection of the presence and degree of cyanosis is difficult, as proved by oximetric studies. In some instances central cyanosis can be reliably detected when the arterial saturation has fallen to 85 percent; in others, particularly dark-skinned persons, it may not be detected until the saturation has declined to 75 percent.

The increase in the quantity of reduced hemoglobin in the cutaneous vessels which produces cyanosis may be brought about either by an increase in the quantity of venous blood in the skin as the result of dilatation of the venules and venous ends of the capillaries, or by a reduction in the oxygen saturation in the capillary blood. In general, cyanosis becomes apparent when the mean capillary concentration of reduced hemoglobin exceeds 50 g/L (5 g/dL). It is the *absolute* rather than the *relative* quantity of reduced hemoglobin which is important in producing cyanosis. Thus, in a patient with severe anemia the relative amount of reduced hemoglobin in the venous blood may be very large when considered in relation to the total amount of hemoglobin. However, since the concentration of the latter is markedly reduced, the *absolute* quantity of reduced hemoglobin may still be small, and therefore patients with severe anemia and even *marked* arterial desaturation do not display cyanosis. Conversely, the higher the total hemoglobin content, the greater the tendency toward cyanosis; thus, patients with marked polycythemia tend to be cyanotic at higher levels of arterial oxygen saturation than patients with normal hematocrit values. Likewise, local passive congestion, which causes an increase in the total amount of reduced hemoglobin in the vessels in a given area, may cause cyanosis. Cyanosis also is observed when nonfunctional hemoglobin such as methemoglobin or sulfhemoglobin (Chap. 295) is present in blood.

Cyanosis may be subdivided into *central* and *peripheral* types. In the *central* type, there is arterial blood unsaturation or an abnormal hemoglobin derivative, and the mucous membranes and skin are both affected. *Peripheral* cyanosis is due to a slowing of blood flow to an area and abnormally great extraction of oxygen from normally saturated arterial blood. It results from vasoconstriction and diminished peripheral blood flow, such as occurs in cold exposure, shock, congestive failure, and peripheral vascular disease. Often, in these conditions the mucous membranes of the oral cavity or those beneath the tongue may be spared. Clinical differentiation between central and peripheral cyanosis may not always be simple, and in conditions such as cardiogenic shock with pulmonary edema there may be a mixture of both types.

DIFFERENTIAL DIAGNOSIS (See Table 37-2) **Central cyanosis** Decreased arterial oxygen saturation results from a marked reduction in the oxygen tension in the arterial blood. This may be brought about by a decline in the tension of oxygen in the inspired air without sufficient compensatory alveolar hyperventilation to maintain alveolar oxygen tension. Cyanosis does not occur in a significant degree in an ascent to an altitude of 2500 m (8000 ft) but is marked in a further ascent to 5000 m (16,000 ft). The reason for this becomes clear on studying the *S* shape of the oxygen dissociation curve (Fig. 290-4). At 2500 m (8000 ft) the tension of oxygen in the inspired air is about 120 mmHg, the alveolar tension is approximately 80 mmHg, and the hemoglobin is nearly completely saturated. However, at 5000 m (16,000 ft) the oxygen tensions in atmospheric air and alveolar air are about 85 and 50 mmHg, respectively, and the oxygen dissociation curve shows that the arterial blood is only about 75 percent saturated. This leaves 25 percent of the hemoglobin in the reduced form, an amount likely to be associated with cyanosis in the absence of anemia. Similarly, a mutant hemoglobin with a low affinity for oxygen (Hb Kansas) causes lowered arterial oxygen saturation and resultant central cyanosis (Chap. 295).

Seriously *impaired pulmonary function,* through alveolar hypoventilation or perfusion of unventilated or poorly ventilated areas of the lung, is a common cause of central cyanosis (Chap. 201). This may occur acutely, as in extensive pneumonia or pulmonary edema, or with chronic pulmonary diseases (e.g., emphysema). In the last situation polycythemia is generally present and clubbing of the fingers may occur. However, in many types of chronic pulmonary disease with fibrosis and obliteration of the capillary vascular bed, cyanosis does not occur because there is relatively little perfusion of underventilated areas.

Another cause of decreased arterial oxygen saturation is *shunting of systemic venous blood into the arterial circuit.* Certain forms of congenital heart disease are associated with cyanosis (Chap. 186). Since blood normally flows from a higher pressure to a lower pressure region, in order for a cardiac defect to result in a right-to-left shunt, it must ordinarily be combined with an obstructive lesion distal to the defect or with elevated pulmonary vascular resistance. The commonest congenital cardiac lesion associated with cyanosis in the adult is the combination of ventricular septal defect and pulmonary outflow tract obstruction (tetralogy of Fallot). The more severe the obstruction, the greater the degree of right-to-left shunting and resultant cyanosis. The mechanisms for the elevated pulmonary vascular resistance which may produce cyanosis in the presence of intra- and extracardiac communications without pulmonic stenosis are discussed elsewhere (Chap. 186). In patients with patent ductus arteriosus, pulmonary hypertension, and right-to-left shunt, *differential cyanosis* results; i.e., cyanosis occurs in the lower extremities but not in the upper extremities.

Pulmonary arteriovenous fistulas may be congenital or acquired, solitary or multiple, microscopic or massive. The degree of cyanosis produced by these fistulas depends upon their size and number. They occur with some frequency in hereditary hemorrhagic telangiectasia (Chap. 288). Arterial oxygen unsaturation also occurs in some patients with cirrhosis, presumably as a consequence of pulmonary arteriovenous fistulas or portal vein–pulmonary vein anastomoses.

In patients with cardiac or pulmonary right-to-left shunts, the presence and severity of cyanosis depend on the size of the shunt relative to the systemic flow as well as on the oxyhemoglobin saturation of the venous blood. In patients with central cyanosis due to arterial oxygen unsaturation, the severity of cyanosis increases with exercise. With increased extraction of oxygen from the blood by the exercising muscles, the venous blood returning to the right side of the heart is more unsaturated than at rest, and shunting of this blood or its passage through lungs incapable of normal oxygenation intensifies the cyanosis. Also, since the systemic vascular resistance normally decreases with exercise, the right-to-left shunt is augmented by exercise in patients with congenital heart disease and communications between the two sides of the heart. Secondary polycythemia occurs frequently in patients with arterial unsaturation and contributes to the cyanosis.

Cyanosis can be caused by small amounts of circulating methemoglobin and by even smaller amounts of sulfhemoglobin (Chap. 295). Although they are uncommon causes of cyanosis, these abnormal hemoglobin pigments should be sought by spectroscopy when cyanosis is not readily explained by malfunction of the circulatory or respiratory systems. Generally, clubbing does not occur with them. The diagnosis of methemoglobinemia can be suspected if, on mixing the patient's blood in a test tube and exposing it to air, it remains brown.

TABLE 37-2 Causes of cyanosis

I Central cyanosis
  A Decreased arterial oxygen saturation
    1 Decreased atmospheric pressure—high altitude
    2 Impaired pulmonary function
      a Alveolar hypoventilation
      b Uneven relationships between pulmonary ventilation and perfusion (perfusion of hypoventilated alveoli)
      c Impaired oxygen diffusion
    3 Anatomic shunts
      a Certain types of congenital heart disease
      b Pulmonary arteriovenous fistulas
      c Multiple small intrapulmonary shunts
    4 Hemoglobin with low affinity for oxygen
  B Hemoglobin abnormalities
    1 Methemoglobinemia—hereditary, acquired
    2 Sulfhemoglobinema—acquired
    3 Carboxyhemoglobinemia (not true cyanosis)
II Peripheral cyanosis
  A Reduced cardiac output
  B Cold exposure
  C Redistribution of blood flow from extremities
  D Arterial obstruction
  E Venous obstruction

Peripheral cyanosis   Probably the most common cause of peripheral cyanosis is generalized vasoconstriction resulting from exposure to cold air or water. This is a normal response. When cardiac output is low, as in severe congestive heart failure or shock, cutaneous vasoconstriction occurs as a compensatory mechanism, so that blood is diverted from the skin to more vital areas such as the central nervous system and heart (Chap. 182), and intense cyanosis associated with cool extremities may result. Even though the arterial blood is normally saturated, the reduced volume flow through the skin and the reduced oxygen tension at the venous end of the capillary result in cyanosis.

Arterial obstruction to an extremity, as with an embolus, or arteriolar constriction, as in cold-induced vasospasm (Raynaud's phenomenon, Chap. 198), generally results in pallor and coldness, but there may be associated cyanosis. If there is venous obstruction and the extremity is congested and with stagnation of blood flow, cyanosis is also present. Venous hypertension, which may be local (as in thrombophlebitis) or generalized (as in tricuspid valve disease or constrictive pericarditis), dilates the subpapillary venous plexuses and thereby intensifies cyanosis.

APPROACH TO THE PATIENT WITH CYANOSIS   Certain features are important in arriving at the proper cause of cyanosis:

1 The history, particularly the duration (cyanosis present since birth is usually due to congenital heart disease); possible exposure to drugs or chemicals which may produce abnormal types of hemoglobin.
2 Clinical differentiation of central as opposed to peripheral cyanosis. Objective evidence by physical or radiographic examination of disorders of the respiratory or cardiovascular systems. Massage or gentle warming of a cyanotic extremity will increase peripheral blood flow and abolish peripheral but not central cyanosis.
3 The presence or absence of clubbing of the fingers. Clubbing without cyanosis is frequent in patients with infective endocarditis and in association with ulcerative colitis, it may occasionally occur in healthy persons, and in some instances it may be occupational, e.g., in jackhammer operators. Slight cyanosis of the lips and cheeks, without clubbing of the fingers, is common in patients with mitral stenosis and is probably due to minimal arterial hypoxia resulting from fibrotic changes in the lungs secondary to longstanding congestion combined with reduction of cardiac output (Chap. 188). The combination of cyanosis and clubbing is frequent in many patients with certain types of congenital cardiac disease and is seen occasionally in persons with pulmonary disease such as lung abscess or pulmonary arteriovenous shunts. On the other hand, peripheral cyanosis or acutely developing central cyanosis is not associated with clubbed fingers.
4 Determination of arterial blood oxygen tension or oxygen saturation, spectroscopic and other examinations of the blood for abnormal types of hemoglobin.

CLUBBING   The selective bullous enlargement of the distal segment of a digit due to an increase in soft tissue is termed *clubbing*. It may be hereditary or idiopathic, or acquired and associated with a variety of disorders, including cyanotic heart disease, infective endocarditis, and a variety of pulmonary conditions (among them, primary and metastatic lung cancer, bronchiectasis, lung abscess, and mesothelioma), as well as with some gastrointestinal diseases (including regional enteritis, chronic ulcerative colitis, and hepatic cirrhosis). Primary lung cancer, mesothelioma, neurogenic diaphragmatic tumors, and rarely cyanotic congenital heart disease may be associated with hypertrophic osteoarthropathy, the subperiosteal formation of new bone in the distal diaphyses of the long bones of the extremities. Although the mechanism of clubbing is unclear, it appears to be secondary to a (presumably humoral) substance which causes dilation of the vessels of the fingertip.

REFERENCES

DOLL DC, GREENBERG BR: Cerebral thrombosis in smokers' polycythemia. Ann Intern Med 102:786, 1985

ERSLEV AJ: Erythrocytosis (sec 17, Chaps 73–75), in *Hematology*, 4th ed, WJ Williams et al (eds). New York, McGraw-Hill, 1990, p 705

HURTADO A: Some clinical aspects of life at high altitudes. Ann Intern Med 53:247, 1960

LUPINETTI FM et al: Pathophysiology of chronic cyanosis in a canine model. Functional and metabolic response to global ischemia. J Thorac Cardiovasc Surg 90:291, 1985

ROSENTHAL A, TYLER DC: Effect of red cell volume reduction or pulmonary blood flow in polycythemia of cyanotic congenital heart disease. Am J Cardiol 33:410, 1974

SCHOENE RB, HORNBEIN TF: High altitude adaptation, in *Textbook of Respiratory Medicine*, JF Murray, JA Nadel (eds). Philadelphia, Saunders, 1988

SMITH JR, LANDAW SA: Smokers' polycythemia. N Engl J Med 298:6, 1978

SZIDON JP, FISHMAN AP: Cyanosis and clubbing, in *Pulmonary Diseases and Disorders*, 2d ed, A Fishman (ed). Philadelphia, Saunders, 1988, 351

38   EDEMA

EUGENE BRAUNWALD

Edema is defined as an increase in the extravascular (interstitial) component of the extracellular fluid volume, which may expand by several liters before the abnormality is recognized. Therefore, a weight gain of several kilograms usually precedes overt manifestations of edema, and a similar weight loss from diuresis can be induced in a slightly edematous patient before "dry weight" is achieved. *Ascites* (Chap. 48) and *hydrothorax* refer to accumulation of excess fluid in the peritoneal and pleural cavities, respectively, and are considered to be special forms of edema. *Anasarca* refers to gross, generalized edema. Depending on its etiology and mechanism, edema may be localized or have a generalized distribution; it is recognized in its generalized form by puffiness of the face, which is most readily apparent in the periorbital areas, and by the persistence of an indentation of the skin following pressure; this is known as "pitting" edema. In its more subtle form, it may be detected by the fact that after the stethoscope is removed, the rim of the bell leaves an indentation on chest skin for a few minutes. An early symptom a patient may note is the ring on a finger fitting more snugly than in the past, or difficulty in putting on shoes, particularly in the evening.

PATHOGENESIS (See also Chap. 50)   About one-third of the total-body water is confined to the extracellular space. This compartment, in turn, is composed of the plasma volume and the interstitial space. Under ordinary circumstances the plasma volume represents about 25 percent of the extracellular space, and the remainder is interstitial fluid. The forces that regulate the disposition of fluid between these two components of the extracellular compartment are frequently referred to as the Starling forces (see p. 223). In general terms, the hydrostatic pressure within the vascular system and the colloid oncotic pressure in the interstitial fluid tend to promote movement of fluid from the vascular to the extravascular space. In contrast, the colloid oncotic pressure contributed by the plasma proteins and the hydrostatic pressure within the interstitial fluid, referred to as the *tissue tension*, promote the movement of fluid into the vascular compartment. As a consequence of these forces there is a movement of water and diffusible solutes from the vascular space at the arteriolar end of the capillaries. Fluid is returned from the interstitial space into the vascular system at the venous end of the capillary and by way of the lymphatics, and unless these channels are obstructed, lymph flow tends to increase if there is net movement of fluid from the vascular compartment to the interstitium. These forces are usually balanced so that a steady state exists in the size of the intravascular and interstitial compartments, and yet a large exchange between them is permitted. However, should any one of these forces be altered significantly, a net movement of fluid from one component of the extracellular space to the other will occur.

An increase in capillary pressure as a cause of edema may result from an increase in venous pressure due to local obstruction in venous drainage, to congestive heart failure, or rarely to the simple expansion of the vascular volume by the administration of large volumes of fluid at a rate in excess of the ability of the kidneys to excrete them. The colloid oncotic pressure of the plasma may be reduced, owing to any factor that may induce severe hypoalbuminemia, such as malnutrition, liver disease, loss of protein into the urine or into the gastrointestinal tract, or a severe catabolic state.

Edema may also result from damage to the capillary endothelium, which increases its permeability and permits the transfer to the interstitial compartment of fluid containing more protein than usual. Injury to the capillary wall can result from chemical, bacterial, thermal, or mechanical agents. Increased capillary permeability may also be a consequence of a hypersensitivity reaction and is characteristic of immune injury. Damage to the capillary endothelium is presumably responsible for inflammatory edema, which is usually nonpitting, localized, and accompanied by other signs of inflammation—redness, heat, and tenderness.

To formulate a hypothesis about the pathophysiology of an edematous state, it is important to discriminate between the *primary* events, such as venous or lymphatic obstruction, reduction of cardiac output, hypoalbuminemia, trapping of fluid in spaces such as the peritoneal cavity, or an increase in capillary permeability, and the predictable *secondary* consequences, which include the renal retention of salt and water in an attempt to restore the plasma volume. There are also instances in which an abnormal positive balance of salt and water may, in fact, be the primary disturbance. In these circumstances the edema is a secondary manifestation of the generalized increase in extracellular fluid volume. These special instances are usually related to conditions characterized by a reduction in renal function (either acute, as in acute tubular necrosis or acute glomerulonephritis, or chronic, as in chronic renal failure). Vasodilators such as minoxidil can also induce primary renal sodium retention.

The pathogenesis of edema depends on one or more alterations in the Starling forces so that there is a net movement of fluid from the vascular system into the interstitium or into a "third space" or from the arterial compartment of the vascular space into the chambers of the heart or into the venous circulation itself. The *effective arterial blood volume*, an as yet poorly defined parameter of the filling of the arterial tree, is reduced, and as a consequence a series of physiologic responses designed to restore it to normal are set into motion. A key element of these responses is the retention of an increment of salt and therefore of water, and in many instances this repairs the deficit of the effective arterial blood volume; often this occurs without the development of overt edema. If, however, the retention of salt and water is insufficient to restore and maintain the effective arterial blood volume, the stimuli are not dissipated, the retention of salt and water continues, and edema develops. This sequence of events is operative in dehydration and hemorrhage. Although in these conditions there is a reduction of effective arterial blood volume and activation of the entire sequence shown in the center of Fig. 38-1, including the diminished excretion of salt and water, edema does not occur because the net sodium and water balance is negative. In most conditions that lead to edema the mechanisms responsible for maintaining a normal effective osmolality in the body fluids operate efficiently so that sodium retention promotes thirst and secretion of the antidiuretic hormone, which, in turn, lead to the ingestion and retention of approximately 1 L of water for each 140 mmol sodium retained. In edematous states, isotonic expansion of the extracellular fluid space may be massive, while the intracellular fluid volume is changed little or not at all.

Reduced cardiac output A reduction of cardiac output, whatever the cause, is associated with a reduction of the effective arterial blood volume as well as of renal blood flow and an elevation of the filtration fraction, i.e., the ratio of glomerular filtration rate to renal plasma

FIGURE 38-1 Sequence of events leading to the formation and retention of salt and water and the development of edema. ANP, atrial natriuretic peptide; RPF, renal plasma flow. Inhibitory influences are shown by dashed lines.

flow. In severe heart failure the blood flow to the outer renal cortex, in particular, is reduced with less depression in the more central regions of the kidney, and there is a reduction in the glomerular filtration rate. This constriction of renal cortical vessels plays an important role in the retention of salt and water and in the formation of edema in heart failure. At different stages of heart failure, activation of the sympathetic nervous system or of the renin-angiotensin systems is responsible for renal vasoconstriction. Activation of the former can be counteracted by the administration of alpha-adrenergic blocking agents, a finding which indicates that the elevated renal vascular resistance in heart failure is mediated, at least in part, by sympathetic stimuli. The augmented renal blood flow and diuresis induced by treatment with angiotensin-converting enzyme inhibitors point to the involvement of the renin-angiotensin system in the retention of salt and water in heart failure.

Renal factors An increase in the tubular reabsorption of glomerular filtrate plays a principal role in the salt and water retention of heart failure. Although there is evidence for both proximal and distal increases in sodium reabsorption in heart failure, the precise role of each tubule segment, including the thick ascending limb of Henle and the collecting duct, requires further elucidation. Alterations in intrarenal hemodynamics appear to play a significant role. Heart failure, by augmenting renal arteriolar constriction, reduces the hydrostatic pressure and raises the colloid osmotic pressure in the peritubular capillaries, thus enhancing salt and water reabsorption in the proximal tubule. The reduction of renal perfusion pressure may be responsible for augmentation of sodium reabsorption in the ascending limb of the loop of Henle.

In addition, the diminished renal blood flow characteristic of states in which the effective arterial blood volume is reduced is translated by the renal juxtaglomerular cells into a signal for increased renin release (Chap. 317). The specific nature of the signal is complex. One factor involves a baroreceptor mechanism, in which reduced renal perfusion results in incomplete filling of the renal arterioles and diminished stretch of the juxtaglomerular cells, a signal that provides for the elaboration or release, or both, of renin. A second mechanism involves the macula densa; as a result of reduced glomerular filtration the sodium chloride load reaching the distal renal tubules is reduced. This is sensed by the macula densa, which in an undefined manner signals the neighboring juxtaglomerular cells to secrete renin. A third mechanism involves the sympathetic nervous system and circulating catecholamines. Activation of the beta-adrenergic receptors in the juxtaglomerular cells stimulates renin release. These three mechanisms generally act in concert.

The renin-angiotensin-aldosterone system Renin, an enzyme with a molecular weight of about 40,000, acts on its substrate, angiotensinogen, an alpha$_2$ globulin synthesized by the liver, to release angiotensin I, a decapeptide, which is broken down to angiotensin II, an octapeptide. This has vasoconstrictor properties and independently increases Na reabsorption in the proximal tubule. The intrarenal production of angiotensin II may also contribute to renal vasoconstriction and to the salt and water retention in heart failure. Angiotensin II also enters the circulation and stimulates the production of aldosterone by the zona glomerulosa of the adrenal cortex. In patients with heart failure, not only is aldosterone secretion elevated, but the biologic half-life of aldosterone is prolonged, which further increases the plasma level of the hormone. A depression of hepatic blood flow, particularly during exercise, secondary to a reduction in cardiac output, is responsible for the reduced hepatic catabolism of aldosterone.

Although increased quantities of aldosterone are secreted in heart failure and in other edematous states and although blockade of the action of aldosterone by spironolactone often induces a moderate diuresis in edematous states, persistent augmented levels of aldosterone (or other mineralocorticoids) do not always promote accumulation of edema, as witnessed by the lack of striking fluid retention in most instances of primary aldosteronism (Chap. 317). Furthermore, although normal subjects retain some salt and water under the influence

of a potent mineralocorticoid, such as deoxycorticosterone acetate or fludrocortisone, the accumulation is self-limiting, despite continued exposure to the steroid and to salt and water (mineralocorticoid escape). The failure of normal subjects to accumulate large quantities of fluid is probably a consequence of an increase in glomerular filtration rate, other hemodynamic influences, and most importantly the increase in volume which promotes an increased excretion of salt that is independent of the filtered load of sodium, i.e., through the action of natriuretic substance(s) or of pressure natriuresis. The role of aldosterone in the accumulation of fluid in edematous states may be more important because these patients are unable to repair the deficit in effective arterial blood volume.

Atrial natriuretic peptide Atrial distention and/or a sodium load cause release into the circulation of atrial natriuretic peptide (ANP), a polypeptide (Chap. 173); a high-molecular-weight precursor of ANP is stored in secretory granules within atrial myocytes. Release of ANP causes (1) excretion of sodium and water by augmenting glomerular filtration rate, inhibiting sodium reabsorption in the papillary collecting duct, and inhibiting release of renin and aldosterone; and (2) arteriolar and venous dilatation. Thus, ANP has the capacity to oppose sodium retention and arterial pressure elevation in states characterized by hypervolemia. There is also some evidence for the existence of a distinctly different natriuretic factor, a low-molecular-weight substance that is activated or released as a result of the expansion of the extracellular fluid and causes natriuresis by inhibiting renal sodium reabsorption through inhibiting ouabain-sensitive Na^+,K^+-ATPase. The role of this factor and of ANP in normal and pathophysiologic conditions requires clarification. For example, it is not yet clear why patients with heart failure and hepatic cirrhosis have low rates of sodium excretion despite often having high circulating levels of ANP.

Obstruction of venous (and lymphatic) drainage of a limb In this condition the hydrostatic pressure in the capillary bed upstream to the obstruction increases so that more fluid than normal is transferred from the vascular to the interstitial space; since the alternate route (i.e., the lymphatic channels) may also be obstructed, this event causes an increased volume of interstitial fluid in the limb, i.e., a trapping of fluid in the extremity, at the expense of the blood volume in the remainder of the body, thereby reducing effective arterial blood volume and leading to the consequences shown in Fig. 38-1.

As fluid accumulates in the interstitium of the limb in which venous and lymphatic drainage are obstructed, tissue tension rises until it counterbalances the primary alterations in the Starling forces, at which time no further fluid accumulates in that limb. At this point the additional accumulation of fluid repairs the deficit in plasma volume, and the stimuli to retain more salt and water are dissipated. The net effect is an increase in the volume of interstitial fluid in a local area, and the secondary responses repair the plasma volume deficit incurred by the primary event. This same sequence occurs in ascites and hydrothorax in which fluid is trapped or accumulates in the cavitary space, depleting the intravascular volume and leading to secondary salt and fluid retention as already described.

Congestive heart failure (See also Chap. 182) In this disorder the defective systolic emptying of the chambers of the heart and/or the impairment of ventricular relaxation promotes an accumulation of blood in the heart and venous circulation at the expense of the arterial volume, and the aforementioned sequence of events (Fig. 38-1) is initiated. In some instances of mild heart failure, a small increment of total blood volume may repair the deficit of arterial volume and establish a new steady state because, through the operation of Starling's law of the heart, up to a point, an increase in the volume of blood within the chambers of the heart promotes a more forceful contraction and may thereby increase the cardiac output (Fig. 182-1). However, if the cardiac disorder is more severe, retention of fluid cannot repair the deficit in effective arterial blood volume. The increment accumulates in the venous circulation, and the increase in hydrostatic pressure therein promotes the formation of edema. The formation of edema in the lungs (Chap. 36) impairs gas exchange and may induce hypoxia, which embarrasses cardiac function still further.

Incomplete ventricular emptying and/or inadequate ventricular relaxation leads to an elevation of ventricular diastolic pressure. If the impairment of cardiac function involves the right ventricle, pressures in the systemic veins and capillaries may rise, thereby augmenting transudation of fluid into the interstitial space and enhancing the likelihood of peripheral edema. The elevated systemic venous pressure is transmitted to the thoracic duct with consequent reduction of lymph drainage, further increasing the accumulation of edema.

If the impairment of cardiac function (incomplete ventricular emptying and/or inadequate relaxation) involves the left ventricle, then pulmonary venous and capillary pressures rise [leading in some instances to pulmonary edema (Chap. 36)], as does pulmonary artery pressure; this in turn interferes with the systolic emptying of the right ventricle, leading to an elevation of right ventricular diastolic and central and systemic venous pressures, enhancing the likelihood of formation of peripheral edema.

Nephrotic syndrome and other hypoalbuminic states (See also Chap. 227) The traditional view holds that the primary alteration in this disorder is a diminished colloid oncotic pressure due to massive losses of protein into the urine. This promotes a net movement of fluid into the interstitium, causes hypovolemia, and initiates the sequence of events described above, including activation of the renin-angiotensin-aldosterone system. As long as the hypoalbuminemia is severe, the salt and water retained cannot be restrained within the vascular compartment, and hence the stimuli to retain salt and water are not abated. A similar sequence of events occurs in other conditions which lead to *severe* hypoalbuminemia, including severe nutritional deficiency states, protein-losing enteropathy, congenital hypoalbuminemia, and severe, chronic liver disease. However, in the nephrotic syndrome, particularly when the serum albumin exceeds approximately 2 g/dL, edema is probably more related to primary renal sodium retention.

Cirrhosis (See also Chaps. 48 and 254) The *total* blood volume in cirrhosis of the liver is commonly increased when the disorder is accompanied by a system of dilated venous radicles and multiple small arteriovenous fistulas. On the other hand, effective systemic perfusion, the effective arterial blood volume, and the intrathoracic blood volume appear to be diminished, probably as a consequence of the passage of blood through these fistulas, as well as from the portal venous hypertension and the obstruction of the lymphatic drainage of the liver. These alterations are frequently complicated by reduced serum albumin, which reduces the effective arterial blood volume even further, leading to activation of the renin-angiotensin-aldosterone system and other salt- and water-retaining mechanisms. Initially, the excess interstitial fluid is localized preferentially behind the congested portal venous system and obstructed hepatic lymphatics, i.e., in the peritoneal cavity. In late stages of the disease, particularly when there is severe hypoalbuminemia, peripheral edema may also be noted.

Idiopathic edema This syndrome, which occurs almost exclusively in women, often with psychosocial difficulties, is characterized by periodic episodes of edema, frequently accompanied by abdominal distention. Fairly large, diurnal alterations in weight occur, so that the patient may weigh several pounds more after having been in the upright posture for several hours. Such large diurnal weight changes suggest an increase in capillary permeability which appears to fluctuate in severity and is aggravated by hot weather. The fact that it occurs most commonly in women, appears to be most prominent during the premenstrual period, and may be improved by progesterone administration suggests that there may be a hormonal effect on the permeability of the vessels that permits the loss of plasma volume into the interstitial space in the upright position and that leads in turn to a contraction in plasma volume and the subsequent retention of salt and water. There are also some cases in which the edema appears to be "diuretic-induced." It has been postulated that in these patients,

chronic diuretic administration leads to mild blood volume depletion which causes chronic hyperreninemia and juxtaglomerular hyperplasia. *Acute* withdrawal of diuretics can then leave the sodium-retaining forces unopposed, leading to fluid retention and edema.

The treatment of idiopathic cyclic edema includes a reduction in salt intake, rest in the supine position for several hours each day, the wearing of elastic stockings which are put on before arising in the morning, and an attempt to understand any underlying emotional problems. A variety of pharmacologic agents including angiotensin-converting enzyme inhibitors, progesterone, the dopamine receptor agonist bromocriptine, and the sympathomimetic amine dextroamphetamine have all been reported to be useful when administered to patients who do not respond to simpler measures. Diuretics are initially useful but may lose their effectiveness with continuous administration; accordingly, they should be employed sparingly, if at all. Persistent discontinuation of diuretics paradoxically leads to diuresis in "diuretic-induced" edema, described above.

DIFFERENTIAL DIAGNOSIS As a rule, localized edema can be readily differentiated from generalized edema. The great majority of patients with generalized edema of significant degree suffer from advanced cardiac, renal, hepatic, or nutritional disorders. Consequently, the differential diagnosis of generalized edema should be directed toward identifying or excluding these several conditions.

Localized edema Edema originating from inflammation or hypersensitivity is usually readily identified. Localized edema due to venous or lymphatic obstruction may be caused by thrombophlebitis, chronic lymphangitis, resection of regional lymph nodes, filariasis, etc. Lymphedema is particularly intractable because restriction of lymphatic flow results in increased protein concentration in the interstitial fluid, a circumstance which aggravates retention of fluid.

Edema of heart failure Evidence of heart disease, as manifested by cardiac enlargement and gallop rhythm together with evidence of cardiac failure, such as dyspnea, basilar rales, venous distention, and hepatomegaly, usually provides an indication on clinical examination that edema results from heart failure. Noninvasive tests such as echocardiography and radionuclide angiography may be helpful in establishing the diagnosis of heart failure (see also Chaps. 177 and 182).

Edema of the nephrotic syndrome Massive proteinuria (> 3.5 g/d), severe hypoalbuminemia, and in some instances hypercholesterolemia are present. This syndrome may occur during the course of a variety of kidney diseases, which include glomerulonephritis, diabetic glomerulosclerosis, and hypersensitivity reactions. A history of previous renal disease may or may not be elicited (see also Chap. 227).

Edema of acute glomerulonephritis and other forms of renal failure The edema occurring during the acute phases of glomerulonephritis is characteristically associated with hematuria, proteinuria, and hypertension. Although some evidence supports the view that the fluid retention is due to increased capillary permeability, in most instances the edema in this disease results from primary retention of sodium and water by the kidneys owing to renal insufficiency. This state differs from congestive heart failure in that it is characterized by a normal or increased cardiac output and a normal arterial–mixed venous oxygen difference. Patients commonly have evidence of pulmonary congestion on chest roentgenograms before cardiac enlargement is significant and do not usually develop orthopnea. Patients with chronic impairment of renal function (including some patients with the nephrotic syndrome *without* severe hypoalbuminemia) may also develop edema due to primary renal retention of sodium and water.

Edema of cirrhosis Ascites and evidence of hepatic disease (collateral venous channels, jaundice, and spider angiomas) characterize edema of hepatic origin. The ascites is frequently refractory to treatment because it collects as a result of a combination of obstruction of hepatic lymphatic drainage, portal hypertension, and hypoalbuminemia. Edema may also occur in other parts of the body in these patients as a result of hypoalbuminemia. Furthermore, the sizable accumulation of ascitic fluid may increase intraabdominal pressure and impede venous return from the lower extremities; hence, it tends to promote accumulation of edema in this region as well (see also Chap. 254).

Edema of nutritional origin   A grossly deficient diet over a prolonged period may produce hypoproteinemia and edema, which may be intensified by beriberi heart disease, in which multiple peripheral arteriovenous fistulas result in reduced effective systemic perfusion and effective arterial blood volume, thereby enhancing edema formation (Chap. 194). Edema may actually become intensified when these famished subjects are first provided with an adequate diet. The ingestion of more food may increase the quantity of salt ingested, which is then retained along with water. Refeeding edema may also be linked to increased release of insulin, which directly increases tubular sodium reabsorption. In addition to hypoalbuminemia, hypokalemia and caloric deficits may be involved in the edema of starvation.

Other causes of edema   These include hypothyroidism, in which myxedema may be located typically in the pretibial region and which may also be associated with periorbital puffiness. Exogenous hyperadrenocortism, pregnancy, and administration of estrogens and vasodilators, particularly the calcium antagonist nifedipine, may also all cause edema.

Distribution   The distribution of edema is an important guide to the cause. Thus, edema of one leg or of one or both arms is usually the result of venous and/or lymphatic obstruction. Edema resulting from hypoproteinemia characteristically is generalized, but it is especially evident in the very soft tissues of the eyelids and face and tends to be most pronounced in the morning because of the recumbent posture assumed during the night. Edema associated with heart failure, on the other hand, tends to be more extensive in the legs and to be accentuated in the evening, a feature also determined largely by posture. When patients with heart failure have been confined to bed, edema may be most prominent in the presacral region. In the rare types of cardiac disease, such as tricuspid stenosis and constrictive pericarditis, in which orthopnea is absent and the patient actually prefers the recumbent posture, the factor of gravity may be equalized and facial edema observed. Less common causes of facial edema include trichinosis, allergic reactions, and myxedema. Unilateral edema occasionally results from lesions in the central nervous system affecting the vasomotor fibers on one side of the body; paralysis also reduces lymphatic and venous drainage on the affected side.

Additional factors in diagnosis   The color, thickness, and sensitivity of the skin are significant. Local tenderness and increase in temperature suggest inflammation. Local cyanosis may signify a venous obstruction. In individuals who have had repeated episodes of prolonged edema, the skin over the involved areas may be thickened, indurated, and often red.

Measurement of the venous pressure is of importance in evaluating edema. Elevation in an isolated part of the body usually reflects localized venous obstruction. Generalized elevation of systemic venous pressure usually suggests the presence of congestive heart failure, although it may occur with the hypervolemia that accompanies acute renal insufficiency. Ordinarily, significant increase in venous pressure can be recognized by the level at which cervical veins collapse; in doubtful cases and for accurate recording, the central venous pressure should be measured manometrically. In patients with obstruction of the superior vena cava, edema is confined to the face, neck, and upper extremities, where the venous pressure is elevated compared with that in the lower extremities. Measurement of venous pressure in the upper extremities is also useful in patients with massive edema of the lower extremities and ascites; it is elevated when the edema is on a cardiac basis (e.g., constrictive pericarditis or tricuspid stenosis) but is normal when it is secondary to cirrhosis. Severe heart failure may cause ascites that may be distinguished from the ascites caused by hepatic cirrhosis by the jugular venous pressure, which is elevated in heart failure and low-normal in cirrhosis.

Determination of the concentration of serum albumin aids impor-

tantly in identifying those patients in whom edema is due, at least in part, to diminished intravascular colloid oncotic pressure. The presence of proteinuria affords useful clues. The total absence of protein in the urine is evidence against renal disease as a cause of edema. Slight to moderate proteinuria is the rule in patients with heart failure, whereas persistent massive proteinuria is usually due to the nephrotic syndrome.

APPROACH TO THE PATIENT WITH EDEMA   A significant question to ask is whether the edema is localized or generalized. If it is localized, those phenomena that may be responsible should be concentrated upon. In this context, *localized* edema may include hydrothorax, ascites, or both, in the absence of congestive heart failure or hypoalbuminemia. Either of these collections may be a consequence of local venous or lymphatic obstruction, as in inflammatory disease or carcinoma.

If the edema is generalized, it should be determined, first, if there is hypoalbuminemia of significant degree, e.g., serum albumin concentration less than 2.5 g/dL. If there is, the history, physical examination, urinalysis, and other laboratory data will help evaluate the question of cirrhosis, severe malnutrition, protein-losing gastroenteropathy, or the nephrotic syndrome as the underlying disorder. If hypoalbuminemia is not present, it should be determined if there is evidence of congestive heart failure of a severity to promote generalized edema. Finally, it should be ascertained whether the patient has an adequate urine output, or if there is significant oliguria or even anuria. These abnormalities are discussed in Chaps. 49, 223, and 224. The major differential diagnosis in patients with generalized edema and normal serum albumin is between primary renal retention of salt and water and congestive heart failure.

REFERENCES

BERNARD DB: Extrarenal complications of the nephrotic syndrome. Kidney Int 33:1184, 1988

GOLDEN MHN: Protein deficiency, energy deficiency, and the oedema of malnutrition. Lancet 1:1261, 1982

ROSE BD: Edematous states, in *Clinical Physiology of Acid-Base and Electrolyte Disorders.* New York, McGraw-Hill, 1989, pp 416–463

SEIFTER JL et al: Control of extracellular fluid volume and pathophysiology of edema formation, in *The Kidney,* 3d ed, BM Brenner, FC Rector (eds). Philadelphia, Saunders, 1986, p 343

STAUB NB, TAYLOR AE (eds): *Edema.* New York, Raven Press, 1984

STREETEN DHP: Idiopathic edema: Pathogenesis, clinical features, and treatment. Metabolism 27:353, 1978

SUZUKI H et al: Effect of the angiotensin converting enzyme inhibitor, captopril (SQ14, 225), on orthostatic sodium and water retention in patients with idiopathic edema. Nephron 39:244, 1985

---

39   SHOCK

JOSEPH E. PARRILLO

Shock may be defined as the state in which profound and widespread reduction of tissue perfusion leads first to reversible, and then, if prolonged, to irreversible, cellular injury. Since reduction of tissue perfusion is central to this definition, it is useful to consider the factors that control this vital function.

CONTROL OF ARTERIAL BLOOD PRESSURE   Maintenance of adequate perfusion of vital organs is critical for survival. Organ perfusion is dependent on an appropriate perfusion pressure, which, in turn, is determined by two variables, the cardiac output and the systemic vascular resistance. The latter is proportional to the vessel length and the viscosity of blood and inversely proportional to the fourth power of the vessel radius. Therefore, the cross-sectional area of a vessel is the overriding determinant of the resistance to blood flow. Since vascular smooth-muscle tone regulates the cross-sectional area of the arteriolar bed (the major site of systemic resistance in the vascular tree), any variable that affects vascular smooth-muscle tone has a profound effect on vascular resistance and, in turn, on perfusion pressure.

The second critical determinant of arterial pressure is the cardiac output, which itself is the product of stroke volume and heart rate. The stroke volume is a function of three major variables, as discussed in detail in Chap. 181: (1) preload, generally reflected in the ventricular end-diastolic volume; (2) impedance to blood flow (afterload), which is related to the systemic vascular resistance; and (3) myocardial contractility.

Physiologic mechanisms can affect the arterial pressure by acting on one or more of the variables mentioned above. These mechanisms include the local release of vasodilator metabolites such as adenosine; the activity of the autonomic (sympathetic and parasympathetic) nervous system and the modulation of this activity by baroreceptor reflexes and the vasomotor center in the brainstem, which, in turn, is acted on by higher centers in the nervous system; the release into the bloodstream of the catecholamines epinephrine or norepinephrine by the adrenal medulla and sympathetic nerve endings (Chap. 67); the activity of the renin-angiotensin system (Chap. 317); the release of vasopressin (Chap. 315); the release of vasodilators, including the kinins and prostaglandins; and alterations in intravascular volume via control of fluid and electrolyte balance (Chap. 38). All of these can affect the arterial pressure by altering the vascular resistance and/or cardiac output. Through the integrated operation of these several mechanisms the mean arterial pressure (the average pressure throughout the cardiac cycle) in young, healthy adults is maintained within a relatively narrow range of 90 to 100 mmHg.

CLASSIFICATION OF SHOCK A classification of shock based on etiology is shown in Table 39-1.

✓Oligemic or hypovolemic shock Hemorrhage or a large loss of fluid secondary to vomiting, diarrhea, burns, or dehydration leads to inadequate ventricular filling, i.e., to severely decreased preload, reflected in decreased left and right ventricular end-diastolic volumes and pressures. These changes lead to shock by causing an inadequate stroke volume and inadequate cardiac output. This is probably the most frequent cause of shock and also the best studied, because all gradations of oligemic shock can be produced in animal models.

✓Cardiogenic shock (See Chap. 189) This is due to a severe depression of systolic cardiac performance. Systolic arterial pressure is <80 mmHg. The cardiac index is reduced below 1.8 (L/min)/m^2, and the left ventricular filling pressure is elevated, generally above

---

TABLE 39-1   Classification of forms of shock

Cardiogenic shock
  Myopathic (reduced systolic function)
    Acute myocardial infarction
    Dilated cardiomyopathy
    Myocardial depression in septic shock
  Mechanical
    Mitral regurgitation
    Ventricular septal defect
    Ventricular aneurysm
    LV outflow obstruction (aortic stenosis, idiopathic hypertrophic subaortic stenosis)
  Arrhythmic
Extracardiac obstructive shock
  Pericardial tamponade
  Constrictive pericarditis
  Pulmonary embolism (massive)
  Severe pulmonary hypertension (primary or Eisenmenger)
  Coarctation of the aorta
Oligemic shock
  Hemorrhage
  Fluid depletion
Distributive shock
  Septic shock
  Toxic products, e.g., overdose
  Anaphylaxis
  Neurogenic shock
  Endocrinologic shock

SOURCE: Adapted with permission from Parker and Parrillo.

---

18 mmHg; pulmonary edema may or may not be evident. The patient is frequently obtunded, the urine output is less than 20 mL/h, and the extremities are cold and cyanotic. The most frequent cause is infarction involving 40 percent or more of the left ventricular myocardium, leading to a severe reduction in left ventricular contractility and failure of the left ventricular pump. Other causes include acute myocarditis and the depression of myocardial contractility following cardiac arrest and prolonged cardiac surgery.

Another form of cardiogenic shock is caused by mechanical abnormalities of the ventricle. Acute mitral or aortic regurgitation or acutely acquired ventricular septal defect or ventricular aneurysm, usually caused by acute myocardial infarction, can cause a severe reduction in *forward* cardiac output (blood flow through the aortic valve into the systemic arterial circulation) and thereby result in cardiogenic shock.

✓Extracardiac obstructive shock This form of shock is best exemplified by pericardial tamponade (Chap. 193). Physiologically, the major abnormality is the inability of the ventricle to fill during diastole, markedly limiting the stroke volume and ultimately the cardiac output. Another common cause of extracardiac obstructive shock is massive pulmonary embolism (Chap. 213). Although the mechanism responsible for the reduced cardiac output in extracardiac obstructive shock differs from that in cardiogenic shock, the actual cause of shock, i.e., the severe reduction in tissue perfusion, is similar.

✓Distributive shock Examples of this form of shock are septic shock (Chap. 89), neurogenic shock, and anaphylactic shock (Chap. 267), all of which usually cause a profound *decrease* in peripheral vascular resistance; the first is now the most common cause of death in intensive care units in the United States. The pathogenesis of septic shock probably involves abnormalities of both the peripheral vascular system and the heart. It is considered in detail below.

Patients may suffer from more than one form of shock simultaneously. Thus, septic and oligemic shock sometimes coexist. These two forms of shock may produce dissimilar, even opposing cardiovascular effects, and treatment of one form may unmask the presence of the other.

PATHOGENESIS Some characteristics of the pathogenesis of shock are the same regardless of the underlying cause. The final pathway of shock is cell death. Once large numbers of cells from vital organs have reached this stage, shock becomes irreversible, and death occurs despite correction of the underlying cause. This concept of irreversibility is useful because it emphasizes the need to prevent the progression of shock.

The pathogenetic mechanism leading to cell death is incompletely understood. One of the common denominators of the first three forms of shock listed in Table 39-1 is a low cardiac output (see Fig. 39-1). Patients with oligemic shock, cardiogenic shock, extracardiac obstructive shock, and a minority of patients with distributive shock develop a severe decrease in cardiac output and, hence, in perfusion of vital organs. Initially, compensatory mechanisms such as vasoconstriction may maintain arterial pressure at a near-normal level. However, if the process causing shock continues, these compensatory mechanisms ultimately fail, leading to the clinical manifestations of the shock syndrome. If shock persists, cell death will ensue and result in irreversible shock.

Of the forms of shock with low cardiac output, *oligemic shock* has been studied the most carefully, both in humans and in animal models, and it provides lessons applicable to other forms of low-output shock. A healthy adult can compensate for the loss of 10 percent of total blood volume using the mechanisms described previously, principally sympathetically mediated vasoconstriction. However, if 20 to 25 percent of the blood volume is lost, the compensatory mechanisms usually begin to fail, and the clinical shock syndrome ensues. The cardiac output declines, and there is hypotension despite generalized vasoconstriction. Regulation of local blood flow maintains perfusion of the heart and brain until late in the course, when these mechanisms also fail. Vasoconstriction, which

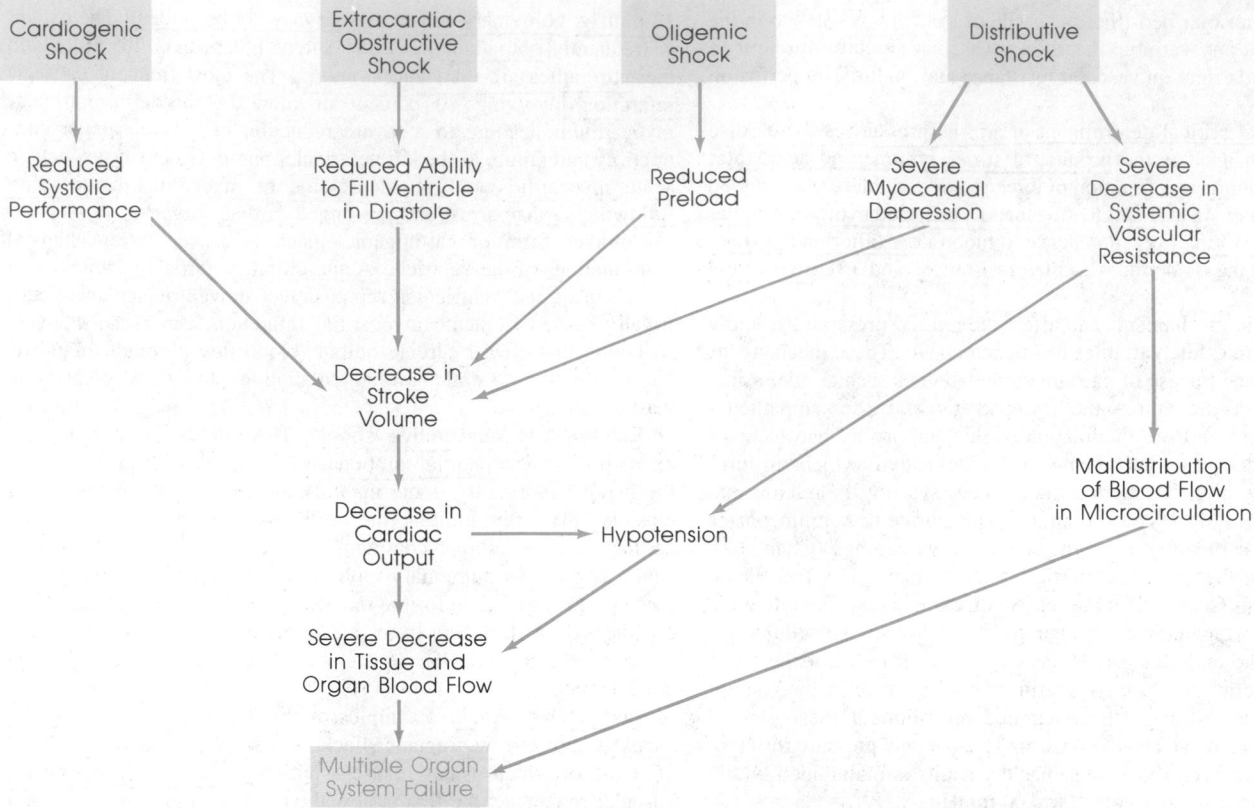

FIGURE 39-1 Pathogenesis of shock in humans. This schematic diagram depicts our present understanding of the pathogenetic relationships among the different types of shock and the cardiovascular abnormalities they usually produce.

begins as a compensatory mechanism in shock, may become excessive in some tissues and cause destructive lesions such as ischemic necrosis of the intestines or digits. A myocardial depressant factor has been characterized in the dog with hemorrhagic shock, but this factor has not been clearly related to clinical myocardial dysfunction. Ultimately, if shock continues, end organ damage occurs, precipitating the adult respiratory distress syndrome (Chap. 218), acute renal failure (Chap. 223), disseminated intravascular coagulation (Chap. 288), and multiorgan failure leading to death.

Distributive shock has a different and more complicated pathogenesis. Septic shock (Chap. 89) is characterized, at least initially, by a low systemic vascular resistance and an elevated cardiac output. As shown in Fig. 39-2, septic shock usually begins with a nidus of infection that releases microbes and/or one or more mediators into the bloodstream. Many mediators [e.g., histamine, kinins, most prostaglandins, lipid A (the toxic component of endotoxin), endorphins, tumor necrosis factor, interleukin 1, and interleukin 2] produce vascular dilatation, while others (some prostaglandins and leukotrienes) produce vasoconstriction. The peripheral vasodilatation results in a reduced systemic vascular resistance and a high cardiac output; the latter occurs in virtually all patients with septic shock, who are volume-loaded. The maldistribution of blood flow, evidenced by lactic acidemia despite a high cardiac output, probably results from circulating mediators with either dilating or constricting properties, causing inappropriate dilatation in some vascular beds and constriction in others.

It has been argued that the high cardiac output in humans with septic shock suggests good ventricular function. However, left and right ventricular ejection fractions are reduced and the ventricles dilate during the initial phase of septic shock. Both ventricles are usually dilated; the increase in preload maintains a normal stroke volume despite the depression of myocardial contractility. The normal stroke volume, combined with tachycardia, results in an elevated cardiac output. However, expansion of blood volume in such patients demonstrates depressed ventricular function curves (Chap. 181), i.e.,

the response of stroke work as a function of filling pressure is subnormal. The reduced ejection fraction, ventricular dilatation, and decreased ventricular stroke work response to volume infusion all demonstrate that myocardial depression occurs frequently in human septic shock. A similar pattern of cardiac dysfunction has been reported with anaphylactic shock. The mechanism of this depressed ventricular performance is unknown; a circulating myocardial depressant substance probably plays a role.

If septic shock persists, the combined peripheral vascular abnormalities and the myocardial depression result in a mortality of approximately 50 percent (Fig. 39-2). Death results from unrelenting hypotension and/or organ system failure. The hypotension is usually associated with a severe and irreversible reduction in systemic vascular resistance, though occasionally (in 10 to 20 percent of nonsurvivors) myocardial depression progresses and results in a low cardiac output that worsens the hypotension. Death from multiple organ failure usually results from insufficiency of kidney, liver, brain, or lung function.

Other pathogenetic mechanisms in septic shock appear to relate to neutrophil aggregation, which produces microthrombi and endothelial cell injury that contribute to alterations in microvascular perfusion. These are discussed in Chap. 89.

CLINICAL MANIFESTATIONS Some symptoms and signs are the same for all types of shock. This condition is almost always characterized by hypotension, which in adults generally refers to a mean arterial pressure of less than 60 mmHg. However, in interpreting any given level of arterial pressure the *chronic* level of pressure must be considered. Thus, patients with severe, chronic hypertension may be hypotensive when their mean arterial pressure declines by 40 mmHg, even if it still exceeds 60 mmHg. Conversely, patients with chronic hypotension may not exhibit acute relative hypotension until mean pressures decline below 50 mmHg. Other common manifestations of shock are tachycardia, oliguria, a clouded sensorium, and cool, mottled extremities indicative of reduced blood flow to the skin (the latter sign usually is not characteristic of distributive shock).

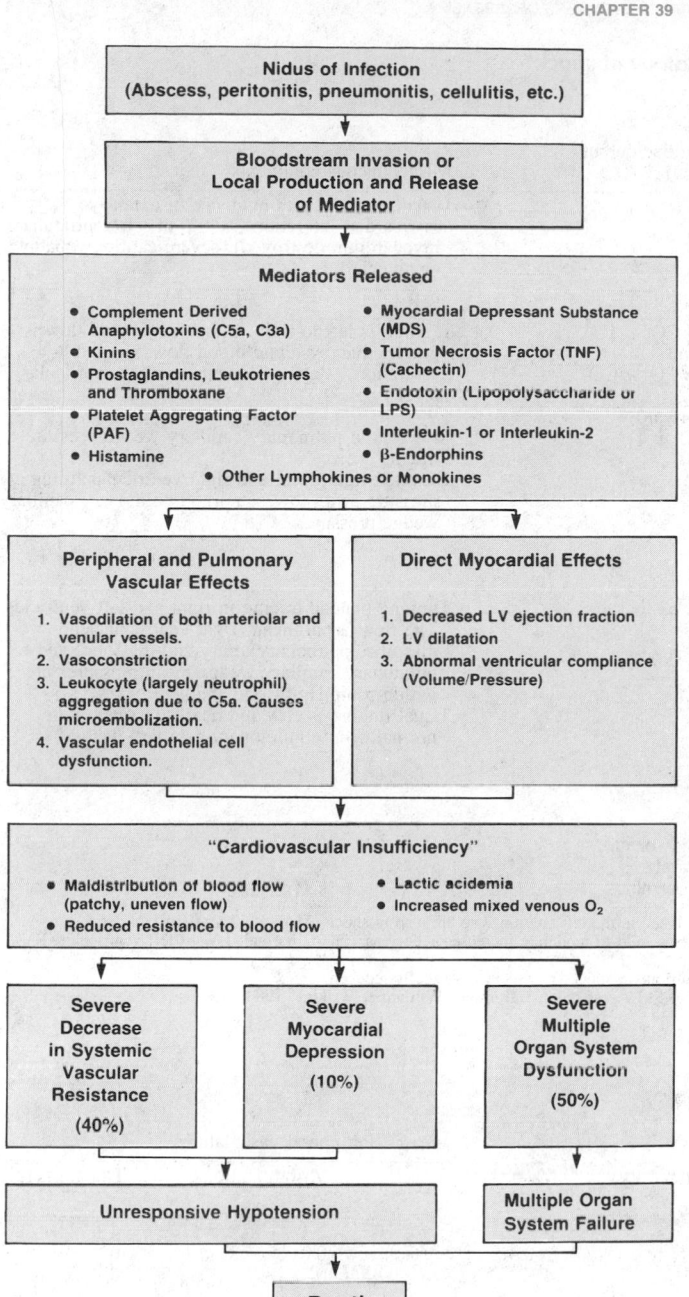

Nidus of Infection
(Abscess, peritonitis, pneumonitis, cellulitis, etc.)

↓

Bloodstream Invasion or
Local Production and Release
of Mediator

↓

Mediators Released

- Complement Derived Anaphylotoxins (C5a, C3a)
- Kinins
- Prostaglandins, Leukotrienes and Thromboxane
- Platelet Aggregating Factor (PAF)
- Histamine
- Myocardial Depressant Substance (MDS)
- Tumor Necrosis Factor (TNF) (Cachectin)
- Endotoxin (Lipopolysaccharide or LPS)
- Interleukin-1 or Interleukin-2
- β-Endorphins
- Other Lymphokines or Monokines

Peripheral and Pulmonary Vascular Effects

1. Vasodilation of both arteriolar and venular vessels.
2. Vasoconstriction
3. Leukocyte (largely neutrophil) aggregation due to C5a. Causes microembolization.
4. Vascular endothelial cell dysfunction.

Direct Myocardial Effects

1. Decreased LV ejection fraction
2. LV dilatation
3. Abnormal ventricular compliance (Volume/Pressure)

↓

"Cardiovascular Insufficiency"

- Maldistribution of blood flow (patchy, uneven flow)
- Reduced resistance to blood flow
- Lactic acidemia
- Increased mixed venous O₂

Severe Decrease in Systemic Vascular Resistance (40%) | **Severe Myocardial Depression (10%)** | **Severe Multiple Organ System Dysfunction (50%)**

↓

Unresponsive Hypotension | Multiple Organ System Failure

↓

Death

FIGURE 39-2 Pathogenesis of human septic shock. This schematic diagram represents our present understanding of the interrelationships in the pathogenesis of septic shock in humans. *(Adapted from JE Parrillo, in Major Issues in Critical Care Medicine, JE Parrillo, SM Ayres, eds, Baltimore, Williams & Wilkins, 1984.)*

Metabolic acidosis, often due to elevated blood lactic acid levels (Chap. 51), reflects prolonged inadequate blood flow to multiple tissues.

Other clinical manifestations are specific to the type of shock. Patients with cardiogenic shock usually have symptoms and signs of heart disease, including elevated filling pressures, a gallop rhythm, and other evidence of acute heart failure. Mechanical causes of cardiogenic shock frequently cause heart murmurs, such as those of acute mitral regurgitation or ventricular septal defect. Patients with pericardial tamponade may demonstrate evidence of pericardial effusion, e.g., pulsus paradoxus, distant heart sounds. Patients with oligemic shock frequently have a history of gastrointestinal bleeding or hemorrhage from another site or clear evidence of large volume losses via diarrhea and/or vomiting. In patients with distributive shock due to sepsis in the absence of severe neutropenia there may be

evidence of a localized infection (pneumonitis, pyelonephritis, or abdominal abscess) as well as fever and chills. Patients with septic shock and severe neutropenia are less likely to have a clinically evident nidus of infection and may be septic from their own skin or bowel flora.

CLINICAL EVALUATION OF THE SHOCK PATIENT   Shock is usually an emergency. Optimal management requires a balance of the need to institute therapy before shock causes irreversible damage to vital organs against the need to complete the clinical assessment required to ensure a comprehensive understanding of the cause. A practical approach is to make a rapid evaluation initially, based on a limited history, physical examination, and specific diagnostic procedures directed to determining the cause and severity of shock. Initial laboratory tests may include a chest x-ray, electrocardiogram, arterial blood P_{O_2}, P_{CO_2}, and pH; a right heart catheterization with a balloon-tipped flow-directed (Swan-Ganz) catheter; and other x-rays or tests directed at specific questions raised by the initial examination. Once this brief evaluation is completed and if the shock is severe or progressive, therapy should be initiated. After the condition has stabilized, a more comprehensive conventional diagnostic evaluation should be undertaken, and the response to the initial therapeutic interventions should be assessed.

Use of right heart catheterization to evaluate shock   The different categories of shock (Table 39-1) have different cardiovascular profiles (Table 39-2). Patients with mild hypovolemic shock may be treated successfully with fluid replacement, the nature of the fluid depending upon the cause of the shock. However, in patients with moderate or severe shock, the flow-directed balloon-tipped pulmonary artery (Swan-Ganz) catheter is often useful for providing hemodynamic assessment and following the response to therapy, because clinical evaluation is frequently incorrect in estimating filling pressure and cardiac output.

Table 39-2 summarizes the usual hemodynamic profiles of patients with the different forms of shock. When these profiles are combined with clinical findings and the calculation of systemic vascular resistance, the etiology of most bouts of shock can be categorized, allowing the physician to concentrate attention on management.

MANAGEMENT   Whenever possible, patients should be treated in an intensive care unit and should receive continuous electrocardiographic monitoring and an arterial line to provide a beat-to-beat measure of systolic, diastolic, and mean arterial pressures. In most cases of shock that cannot be rapidly reversed, serial measurement of left and right ventricular filling pressures and cardiac output should be performed. Frequent determinations of arterial blood gases (P_{O_2}, P_{CO_2}, and pH), electrolytes, complete blood count, and clotting parameters should be made. Serum calcium and phosphorus values should be followed, because substantial reductions in these ions can be associated with myocardial depression. The frequency of measurements should depend on the clinical course and the perceived need to assess the response to therapy.

In general, the goals of treating shock are threefold: (1) Maintain blood flow to those organs most frequently damaged by shock, i.e., kidney, liver, central nervous system, and lungs. It is useful to follow urine flow hourly as a rough guide to renal perfusion. (2) Maintain mean arterial pressure above 60 mmHg (in a normal adult) to ensure adequate perfusion of vital organs. (3) Maintain arterial blood lactate below 22 mmol/L. (Since lactate measurements are not usually available "on line," the last goal must often be assessed retrospectively.)

Specific forms of shock require therapy directed at the underlying process.

Oligemic shock usually presents with clinical evidence of blood or fluid loss and low pulmonary artery wedge and right atrial pressures. Rapid infusion of blood plasma or plasma expanders is the correct therapy while the source of blood or fluid loss is identified and corrected.

In *cardiogenic shock* (Chap. 189) therapy should be directed toward reducing ischemia and salvaging severely ischemic but re-

TABLE 39-2 Use of right heart catheterization to diagnose the etiology of shock*

Diagnosis	Pulmonary capillary wedge pressure†	Cardiac output (CO)	Miscellaneous comments
Cardiogenic shock 　Cardiogenic shock due to myocardial dysfunction	↑ ↑	↓ ↓	Usually occurs with evidence of extensive myocardial infarction (>40% of left ventricular myocardium destroyed), severe cardiomyopathy, or myocarditis
Cardiogenic shock due to a mechanical defect 　Acute ventricular septal defect	↑ or nl	LVCO ↓ ↓ and RVCO > CO	If shunt is left to right, pulmonary blood flow is greater than systemic blood flow: oxygen saturation "step-up" occurs at right ventricular level
Acute mitral regurgitation	↑ ↑	Forward CO ↓ ↓	V waves in pulmonary capillary wedge pressure tracing
Right ventricular infarction	nl or ↓	↓ ↓	Elevated right atrial and right ventricular filling pressures with low or normal pulmonary capillary wedge pressures
Extracardiac obstructive forms of shock 　Pericardial tamponade	↑ ↑	↓ or ↓ ↓	Dip and plateau tracing in right and left ventricles. The right atrial mean, right ventricular end-diastolic, pulmonary artery end-diastolic, and pulmonary capillary wedge mean pressures are within 5 mmHg of one another
Massive pulmonary emboli	nl or ↓	↓ ↓	Usual finding is elevated heart pressures with normal or low pulmonary capillary wedge
Oligemic shock (hypovolemia)	↓ ↓	↓ ↓	
Distributive forms of shock 　Septic shock	↓ or nl	↑ ↑ or nl, rarely ↓	
Anaphylactic shock	↓ or nl	↑ or nl	

* The hemodynamic profiles summarized in this table refer to patients with the diagnosis listed in the left column who are also in shock (MAP <60 mmHg).
† ↑ ↑ or ↓ ↓ designates a moderate-to-severe increase or decrease; ↑ or ↓ designates a mild-to-moderate increase or decrease; nl = normal; LV = left ventricular; RV = right ventricular.
NOTE: Systemic vascular resistance is increased, initially, in all forms of shock except distributive shock, in which it is usually reduced.
SOURCE: Modified from JE Parrillo, in *Major Issues in Critical Care Medicine*, JE Parrillo, SM Ayres (eds), Baltimore, William & Wilkins, 1984.

TABLE 39-3 Commonly used vasopressor agents (relative potency*)

Agent	Dose	Cardiac		Peripheral vasculature		
		Heart rate	Contractility	Vasoconstriction	Vasodilatation	Dopaminergic
Dopamine	1–4 (μg/kg)/min	2+	2+	0	2+	4+
	4–20 (μg/kg)/min	2+	2+	2–3+	0	0
Levarterenol (norepinephrine)	2–8 μg/min	2+	2+	4+	0	0
Dobutamine	1–10 (μg/kg)/min	1+	4+	1+	2+	0
Isoproterenol	1–4 μg/min	4+	4+	0	4+	0
Epinephrine	1–8 μg/min	4+	4+	4+	3+	0
Phenylephrine	20–200 μg/min	0	0	4+	0	0

* The 1 to 4+ scoring system represents an arbitrary quantitative scoring system to allow a judgment of comparative potency among these vasopressor agents.
SOURCE: Adapted from JE Parrillo, *Major Issues in Critical Care Medicine*, JE Parrillo, SM Ayres (eds), Baltimore, Williams & Wilkins, 1984.

versibly damaged myocardium at the infarct border. This may be accomplished by administration of oxygen and nitrates, institution of intraaortic balloon pumping to unload mechanically the ventricle and augment coronary perfusion, and, perhaps most importantly, by attempting to restore myocardial perfusion to salvage nonirreversibly damaged myocardium. Depending on the specific situation, the latter may include the administration of thrombolytic agents, cardiac catheterization and coronary arteriography to define coronary anatomy, and early coronary angioplasty or coronary bypass surgery in patients with appropriate anatomy. This aggressive approach may reduce the mortality of cardiogenic shock from approximately 90 to approximately 60 percent. Prospective, randomized studies are needed to document the true efficacy of this approach. Cardiogenic shock also occurs after a prolonged period of induced cardiac arrest, often during reparative cardiac surgery. The impaired (stunned) myocardium may require hours or days to recover sufficiently to support the circulation.

Treatment consists of the combination of intraaortic balloon counterpulsation and sympathomimetic amines such as dopamine or dobutamine (Table 39-3). In cardiogenic shock due to mechanical abnormalities, such as acute mitral regurgitation or ventricular septal defect, surgical correction is usually necessary.

Pericardial tamponade, the prototype of *extracardiac obstructive shock*, may be recognized by clinical manifestations (hypotension, pulsus paradoxus, distended neck veins) and characteristic findings on electrocardiography (Chap. 193) or by echocardiography (Chap. 177). Although expansion of intravascular volume and the administration of inotropic agents, particularly sympathomimetic amines such as norepinephrine and/or dopamine, may temporarily improve hemodynamics and act as a "holding maneuver," pericardiocentesis or surgical pericardial drainage is the only effective treatment.

The management of *septic shock* is discussed in Chap. 89.

REFERENCES

Bone RC et al and the Methylprednisolone Severe Sepsis Study Group: A controlled clinical trial of high-dose methylprednisolone in the treatment of severe sepsis and septic shock. N Engl J Med 317:653, 1987

Connors AF et al: Evaluation of right-heart catheterization in the critically ill patient without acute myocardial infarction. N Engl J Med 308:263, 1983

Ellrodt AG et al: Left ventricular performance in septic shock: Reversible segmental and global abnormalities. Am Heart J 110:402, 1985

Guyton AC: Local control of blood flow by the tissues; and nervous and humoral regulation, in Human Physiology and Mechanisms of Disease, 3d ed. Philadelphia, Saunders, 1982, pp 161–169

———: Cardiac output and circulatory shock, in Human Physiology and Mechanisms of Disease, 3d ed. Philadelphia, Saunders, 1982, pp 187–200

Natanson C et al: Gram negative bacteremia produces both severe systolic and diastolic cardiac dysfunction in a canine model that simulates human septic shock. J Clin Invest 77:259, 1986

Ognibene FP et al: Neutrophil aggregation activity and septic shock in humans: Neutrophil aggregation by a C5a-like material occurs more frequently than complement component depletion and correlates with depression of systemic vascular resistance. J Crit Care 3:103, 1988

——— et al: Depressed left ventricular performance in response to volume infusion in patients with sepsis and septic shock. Chest 93:903, 1988

Parker MM, Parrillo JE: Septic shock and other forms of distributive shock, in Current Therapy in Critical Care Medicine. Toronto, B.C. Decker, 1987, pp 44–55

Parrillo JE: Septic shock in humans: Clinical evaluation, pathogenesis, and therapeutic approach, in Textbook of Critical Care, 2d ed, W.C. Shoemaker et al (eds). Philadelphia, Saunders, 1989, pp 1006–1023

——— et al: A circulating myocardial depressant substance in humans with septic shock: Septic shock patients with a reduced ejection fraction have a circulating factor that depresses in vitro myocardial cell performance. J Clin Invest 76:1539, 1985

Rock P et al: Efficacy and safety of naloxone in septic shock. Crit Care Med 13:28, 1985

Schaer GL et al: Norepinephrine alone versus norepinephrine plus low-dose dopamine: Enhanced renal blood flow with combination pressor therapy. Crit Care Med 13:492, 1985

Ziegler EJ et al: Treatment of gram-negative bacteremia and shock with human antiserum to a mutant Escherichia coli. N Engl J Med 307:1225, 1982

40 CARDIOVASCULAR COLLAPSE, CARDIAC ARREST, AND SUDDEN DEATH

ROBERT J. MYERBURG / AGUSTIN CASTELLANOS

OVERVIEW AND DEFINITIONS

Cardiac disorders account for the vast majority of natural sudden deaths. The magnitude of the problem of *cardiac* causes is highlighted by estimates that more than 300,000 sudden cardiac deaths (SCD) occur each year in the United States, and that as many as 50 percent of all cardiac deaths are sudden and unexpected. Since techniques and systems are now available to save patients who have out-of-hospital cardiac arrest, which was uniformly fatal in the past, understanding the SCD problem has practical importance.

SCD must be defined carefully. In the context of time, "sudden" was previously defined as death within 24 h of the onset of the clinical event which led to a fatal cardiac arrest; this was subsequently shortened for most clinical and epidemiologic purposes to 1 h or less between the onset of the terminal illness and death. However, because of community-based interventions, victims may remain biologically alive for days or weeks after a cardiac arrest that has resulted in irreversible central nervous system damage. Confusion in terms can be avoided by adhering strictly to definitions of death, cardiac arrest, and cardiovascular collapse, as outlined in Table 40-1. Death is biologically, legally, and literally an absolute and irreversible event. Death may be delayed in a survivor of cardiac arrest, but "survival after sudden death" is contradictory. Currently, the accepted definition of SCD is *natural death* due to *cardiac* causes, heralded by abrupt loss of consciousness within *1 h* of the onset of acute symptoms, in an individual who may have known *preexisting* heart disease, but in

TABLE 40-1 Distinction between death, cardiac arrest, and cardiovascular collapse

Term	Definition	Qualifiers or exceptions
Death	Irreversible cessation of all biologic functions	None
Cardiac arrest	Abrupt cessation of cardiac pump function which may be reversible by a prompt intervention but will lead to death in its absence	Rare spontaneous reversions; likelihood of successful intervention relates to mechanism of arrest and clinical setting
Cardiovascular collapse	A sudden loss of effective blood flow due to cardiac and/or peripheral vascular factors which may reverse spontaneously (e.g., vasodepressor syncope) or only with interventions (e.g., cardiac arrest)	Nonspecific term which includes cardiac arrest and its consequences and also events which characteristically revert spontaneously

SOURCE: Myerburg and Castellanos, with permission.

whom the *time* and *mode* of death are *unexpected*. When biologic death of the cardiac arrest victim is delayed because of interventions, the relevant pathophysiologic event remains the sudden and unexpected cardiac arrest which leads ultimately to death, even though delayed by artificial methods. Thus, the terminology used should reflect the fact that the index event was a cardiac arrest, and that death was due to its delayed consequences.

CAUSES, CONTRIBUTING FACTORS, AND CLINICAL EPIDEMIOLOGY

Extensive epidemiologic studies have identified populations at high risk for SCD. In addition, a large body of pathologic data provide information on the underlying *structural abnormalities* in victims of SCD, and clinical/physiologic studies highlight the *contributing functional factors* which may convert a long-standing underlying structural abnormality from a stable to an unstable state (Table 40-2). This mass of information is developing into an understanding of the causes and mechanisms of SCD.

Cardiac disorders constitute the most common causes of sudden *natural* death. After an initial peak incidence of sudden death between birth and 6 months of age (the sudden infant death syndrome), the incidence of sudden death falls abruptly and then increases to a second peak in the age range of 45 to 75 years. Moreover, increasing age is a powerful risk factor for sudden *cardiac* death. It follows that the *proportion* of *cardiac* causes among all sudden *natural* deaths increases dramatically with advancing years. From 1 to 13 years of age, only one of five sudden natural deaths is due to cardiac causes. Between 14 and 21 years of age, the proportion increases to 30 percent, and then to 88 percent in the middle aged and elderly.

Men and women have very different susceptibilities to SCD, which tend to decrease with advancing age. The overall male/female ratio is approximately 4:1, but in the 55- to 64-year-old age group, the male SCD excess is nearly 7:1. It falls to approximately 2:1 in the 65- to 74-year-old age group. The difference in risk for SCD parallels the risks for other manifestations of coronary heart disease in men and women. As the gap for other manifestations of coronary heart disease closes in the seventh and eighth decades of life, the excess risk of SCD narrows. Despite the lower incidence in women, the classic coronary risk factors still operate in the proportionately smaller subgroup of women—cigarette smoking, diabetes, hyperlipidemia, hypertension.

Hereditary factors contribute to the risk of SCD, but largely in a nonspecific manner, merely as one expression of the hereditary predisposition to coronary heart disease. Except for a few very

TABLE 40-2   Cardiac arrest and sudden cardiac death

I Structural causes

   A Coronary heart disease
     1 Coronary atherosclerosis
       a Chronic obstructive lesions
       b Acute lesion
         (plaque fissuring, platelet aggregation, acute thrombosis)
     2 Myocardial infarction
       a Healed
       b Acute

   B Myocardial hypertrophy
     1 Secondary
     2 Hypertrophic cardiomyopathy
       a Obstructive
       b Nonobstructive

   C Cardiomyopathy, dilated

   D Myocarditis

   E Valvular heart disease

   F Electrophysiologic abnormalities, structural
     1 Anomalous pathways
     2 Conducting system disease

II Functional contributing factors

   A Transient ischemia and reperfusion
     1 Loss of substrates
     2 Generation of injurious substances
     3 Disturbed membrane electrical properties

   B Low cardiac output states
     1 Heart failure
       a Chronic
       b Acute decompensation
     2 Shock

   C Systemic metabolic abnormalities
     1 Electrolyte imbalance
     2 Hypoxemia, acidosis

   D Neurophysiologic disturbances
     1 Autonomic fluctuations
       a Central, neural, humoral
     2 Receptor function
     3 Long QT syndrome, congenital

   E Toxic responses
     1 Proarrhythmic drug effects
     2 Cardiac toxins

infrequent syndromes, such as the genetic hyperlipoproteinemias (Chap. 326), there are no *specific* hereditary risk factors for SCD. Higher levels of life stress, lower levels of education, social isolation, changes in lifestyle after myocardial infarction, cigarette use, alcohol consumption, obesity, absence of regular exercise, and type A–personality features, all have been *suggested* as contributors to risk of SCD. Among women, those who are unmarried, and those who have fewer children or have greater educational disparity with their spouses, appear to be at higher risk.

The major categories of structural causes of, and functional factors contributing to, the SCD syndrome are listed in Table 40-2. Worldwide, and especially in western cultures, coronary atherosclerotic heart disease is the most common structural abnormality associated with SCD. Up to 80 percent of all SCDs in the United States are due to the consequences of coronary atherosclerosis. The cardiomyopathies (dilated and hypertrophic, collectively, Chap. 192) account for another 10 to 15 percent of SCDs, and all of the remaining diverse etiologies cause only 5 to 10 percent of these events. The relative role of various factors contributing to the initiation of cardiac arrest has not been quantitated as well as the structural basis. Transient ischemia in the previously scarred or hypertrophied heart, electrolyte disturbances, fluctuations in autonomic nervous system activity, and transient changes in the electrophysiologic properties of the diseased heart have all been implicated as mechanisms responsible for transition from electrophysiologic stability to instability.

PATHOLOGY   Data from necropsies of SCD victims parallel the clinical observations on the prevalence of coronary heart disease as the major structural etiologic factor. More than 80 percent of SCD victims have pathologic findings of coronary heart disease which are commonly accompanied by ruptured atherosclerotic plaques and/or coronary thrombi. The most consistent *coronary artery* abnormality is extensive coronary atherosclerosis. Seventy-five percent of the victims have two or more major vessels with ≥75 percent stenosis. In one study, atherosclerotic plaque fissuring, platelet aggregates, and/or acute thrombosis were observed in 95 of 100 individuals who had pathologic studies after SCD. The majority of these acute changes were superimposed on preexisting chronic lesions. However, only 44 percent of the SCD victims had more than 50 percent luminal narrowing by recent coronary thrombi, raising issues about interactions between breakdown of preexisting noncritical lesions, local thrombus formation and spontaneous lysis, and acute coronary spasm with ischemia in the initiation of the terminal event.

The pathology of the *myocardium* in SCD also reflects the extensive coronary heart disease which usually precedes the fatal event. As many as 70 to 75 percent of males who die suddenly have prior myocardial infarctions (MIs), and 20 to 30 percent have recent acute

MIs. A high incidence of left ventricular (LV) hypertrophy coexists with prior MIs. Clinical and epidemiologic data suggest that LV hypertrophy itself predisposes to SCD, and it is likely that coexistence with prior MI adds a dimension of risk.

CLINICAL DEFINITION OF FORMS OF CARDIOVASCULAR COLLAPSE   The definitions of the terms listed in Table 40-1 have important clinical applications. Cardiovascular collapse is a general term connoting loss of effective blood flow due to acute dysfunction of the heart and/or peripheral vasculature. Cardiovascular collapse may be caused by vasodepressor syncope (vasovagal syncope, postural hypotension with syncope—see Chap. 21), a transient severe bradycardia, or by cardiac arrest. The latter is distinguished from the transient forms of cardiovascular collapse in that it requires an intervention to achieve resuscitation. In contrast, vasodepressor syncope and many primary bradyarrhythmic syncopal events are transient, and the patient will regain consciousness spontaneously.

The most common electrical mechanism for true cardiac arrest is ventricular fibrillation (VF), which is responsible for 65 to 80 percent of cardiac arrests. Severe persistent bradyarrhythmias and asystole cause another 20 to 30 percent. Sustained ventricular tachycardia (VT) with hypotension is a less common cause, as is electromechanical dissociation in which organized electrical activity is present but no mechanical response. Acute low cardiac output states, having precipitous onset, may also present clinically as a cardiac arrest. The causes include massive acute pulmonary emboli, internal blood loss from ruptured aortic aneurysm, intense anaphylaxis, cardiac rupture after myocardial infarction, and unexpected fatal arrhythmia due to electrolyte disturbances.

CLINICAL CHARACTERISTICS OF CARDIAC ARREST

PRODROME, ONSET, ARREST, DEATH   Long-term studies in both unselected and high-risk populations suggest that SCD may be presaged by days, weeks, or months of increasing angina, dyspnea, palpitations, easy fatigability, and other nonspecific complaints. However, these *prodromal complaints* are generally predictive of any major cardiac event; they are not specific for predicting SCD. In one study, nearly 50 percent of SCD victims saw a physician within the month prior to death, but the complaints generally appeared to be unrelated to the heart. Among survivors of out-of-hospital cardiac arrest, 28 percent retrospectively reported new onset of worsening angina pectoris or dyspnea prior to cardiac arrest. Prodromes are useful for identifying patients at risk for cardiovascular events, but not for identifying the subgroup of SCD victims.

The *onset of the terminal event*, leading to cardiac arrest, may be abrupt and instantaneous or may be heralded by up to 1 h of symptoms reflecting an acute change in cardiovascular status. Continuous ECG recordings, fortuitously obtained prior to a cardiac arrest, demonstrate changes in cardiac electrical activity in the minutes or hours before the event. There is a tendency for the heart rate to increase and for advanced grades of premature ventricular contractions to evolve. Most cardiac arrests that occur by the mechanism of VF begin with a run of sustained or nonsustained VT which then degenerates into VF.

In the clinical classification proposed by Hinkle and Thaler, sudden unexpected loss of effective circulation was separated into ''arrhythmic events'' and ''circulatory failure.'' Arrhythmic events are characterized by a high incidence of patients being awake and actively moving immediately prior to the event, are dominated by VF as the electrical mechanism, and have a short duration of terminal illness (<1 h). In contrast, circulatory failure deaths occur in patients who are inactive or comatose, have a higher incidence of asystole than VF, have a tendency to a longer duration of terminal illness, and are dominated by noncardiac events preceding the terminal illness.

The onset of cardiac arrest may be characterized by typical symptoms of an acute cardiac event, such as prolonged angina or the pain of myocardial infarction, acute dyspnea or orthopnea, or the sudden onset of palpitations, sustained tachycardia, or light-headedness. However, in many patients, the onset is precipitous, without forewarning.

Cardiac arrest is, by definition, abrupt. Mentation may be impaired in patients with sustained VT during the onset of the terminal event. However, complete loss of consciousness is a *sine qua non* in cardiac arrest. Although rare spontaneous reversions occur, it is generally accepted that cardiac arrest progresses to death within minutes (i.e., SCD has occurred) if active interventions are not undertaken promptly.

The ability to resuscitate the victim of cardiac arrest is related to the setting in which the event occurs, the mechanism (VF, VT, electromechanical dissociation, asystole), and the clinical status of the patient prior to the cardiac arrest. Those settings in which it is possible to institute prompt cardiopulmonary resuscitation (CPR) provide a better chance of a successful outcome. However, the outcome in intensive care units and other in-hospital environments is heavily influenced by the patient's preceding clinical status. The immediate outcome is good for cardiac arrest occurring in the intensive care unit in the presence of an acute cardiac event or transient metabolic disturbance, but the outcome for patients with advanced noncardiac disease (e.g., renal failure, pneumonia, sepsis, diabetes, cancer) is no more successful in hospital than in the out-of-hospital environment.

The success rate for initial resuscitation and ultimate survival from an out-of-hospital cardiac arrest depends in part upon the mechanism of the event. When the mechanism is VT, the outcome is best (67 percent); VF is the next most successful (30 percent), and asystole and electromechanical dissociation have dismal outcome statistics (Fig. 40-1). Age also influences the chances of successful resuscitation, with statistics for the elderly being poor.

Progression to biologic death is a function of the mechanism of cardiac arrest and the length of the delay before interventions. VF or asystole, without CPR within the first 4 to 6 min, has a poor outcome, and there are few survivors among patients who have had no life support activities for 8 min. Outcome statistics are dramatically improved by lay bystander intervention (basic life support—see below) prior to definitive interventions (advanced life support—defibrillation). The most common causes of death during hospitalization after resuscitated cardiac arrests are related to the severity of injury to the central nervous system. Anoxic encephalopathy and infections subsequent to prolonged respirator-dependence account for 60 percent of the deaths. Another 30 percent occur as a consequence of low cardiac output states which fail to respond to interventions. Paradoxically, recurrent arrhythmias are the least common cause of death, accounting for only 10 percent of in-hospital deaths.

FIGURE 40-1 Initial electrophysiologic mechanisms recorded during out-of-hospital cardiac arrest. The figures highlighted by the boxes indicate the number of patients in each of three mechanism categories (ventricular fibrillation, ventricular tachycardia, and bradyarrhythmia/asystole), plus totals. In each category, the data indicate the number of prehospital cardiac arrests (*top*), the number of patients successfully resuscitated in the field and transferred to the hospital alive (*middle*), and the number of patients who survived to be discharged from hospital (*bottom*). The percentages in parentheses indicate survivals between each level of care for each category. (*Modified from Myerburg RJ et al: Clinical, electrophysiologic, and hemodynamic profile of patients resuscitated from prehospital cardiac arrest. Am J Med 68: 568, 1980, with permission*).

Outcome during hospitalization, particularly in patients with acute MI, is very different for patients with primary and secondary cardiac arrests. *Primary* cardiac arrests refer to those which occur in the absence of hemodynamic instability, and *secondary* cardiac arrests are those which occur in patients in whom abnormal hemodynamics dominate the clinical picture before cardiac arrest. The success rate for immediate resuscitation in primary cardiac arrest during acute MI should approach 100 percent. In contrast, as many as 70 percent of patients with secondary cardiac arrest succumb immediately or during the same hospitalization.

IDENTIFICATION OF PATIENTS AT RISK FOR SUDDEN CARDIAC DEATH Primary prevention of cardiac arrest depends upon the ability to identify individual patients at high risk. One must view the problem in the context of the total number of events and the population pools from which they are derived. In Fig. 40-2, the inverted triangle demonstrates that the annual incidence of SCD among an unselected adult population is 1 to 2 per 1000 population, largely reflecting the prevalence of those coronary heart disease patients among whom SCD is the first clinical manifestation (20 to 25 percent of first coronary events). The incidence (percent per year) increases progressively with addition of coronary risk factors to populations free of prior coronary events. The most powerful factors are age, elevated blood pressure, cigarette smoking, elevated serum cholesterol level, obesity, and nonspecific electrocardiographic abnormalities. These coronary risk factors are not specific for SCD, but rather represent increasing risk for all coronary deaths. The proportion of coronary deaths that are sudden remains at approximately 50 percent in all risk categories. Despite the marked *relative* increase of risk of SCD with addition of multiple risk factors (from 1 to 2 per 1000 population per year in an unselected population to as much as 50 to 60 per 1000 in the highest risk subgroups), the *absolute* incidence remains relatively low when viewed in terms of the relationship between the number of individuals to have a preventive intervention versus the number of events which can be prevented. Specifically, a 50 percent reduction in annual SCD risk would be a huge *relative* decrease, but would require an intervention in up to 200 unselected individuals to prevent one sudden death. These figures highlight the importance of primary prevention of coronary heart disease. Control of coronary risk factors may be the only practical method to prevent SCD in major segments of the population, since the majority of events occur in the large unselected subgroups rather

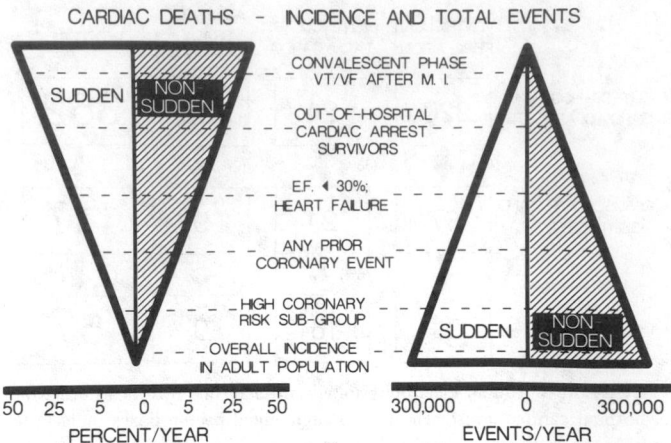

CARDIAC DEATHS - INCIDENCE AND TOTAL EVENTS

FIGURE 40-2 Incidence of sudden and nonsudden cardiac deaths in population subgroups, and the relation of total number of events per year to incidence figures. Approximations of subgroup incidence figures, and the related population pool from which they are derived, are presented. Approximately 50 percent of all cardiac deaths are sudden and unexpected. The incidence triangle on the left ("Percent/Year") indicates the approximate percentage of sudden and nonsudden deaths in each of the population subgroups indicated, ranging from the lowest percentage in unselected adult populations (0.1 to 2 percent/year), to the highest percentage in patients with VT or VF during convalescence after an MI (approximately 50 percent/year). The triangle on the right indicates the total number of events per year in each of these groups, to reflect incidence in context with the size of the population subgroups. The highest risk categories identify the smallest number of total annual events, and the lowest incidence category accounts for the largest number of events per year. (EF = ejection fraction; VT = ventricular tachycardia; VF = ventricular fibrillation; MI = myocardial infarction.)

than the specific high-risk subgroups (contrast "Events/Year" to "Percent/Year" in Fig. 40-2).

For patients with acute or prior clinical manifestations of coronary heart disease, high-risk subgroups having a much higher ratio of SCD risk to population base can be identified. The acute, convalescent, and chronic phases of MI provide large population subsets with more highly focused risk (Chap. 189). The potential risk of cardiac arrest from the onset through the first 72 h after acute MI (the acute phase) may be as high as 15 to 20 percent. The highest risk of SCD in relation to MI is found in the subgroup who have VT or VF during the convalescent phase (3 days to 8 weeks) after MI. A 50 to 80 percent mortality in 6 to 12 months has been observed among these patients, when managed with conventional therapy, and at least 50 percent of the deaths are sudden. Aggressive interventions appear to reduce the incidence dramatically to 15 to 20 percent in 18 months, or better.

Chronic premature ventricular complexes (PVCs) after the acute phase of MI identify a long-term risk for total cardiac mortality and SCD. Increasing *frequency* of PVCs, with a plateau above the range of 10 to 30 PVCs per h on 24-h ambulatory monitor recordings, indicates increased risk; but advanced *forms* (salvos, nonsustained VT) are probably the more powerful predictor. PVCs interact strongly with the size of MI, as reflected by decreased left ventricular ejection fraction (EF). The combination of frequent PVCs, salvos or nonsustained VT, and an EF ≤ 30 percent identifies patients who have an annual risk of 20 percent. The risk falls off sharply with decreasing PVC frequency and the absence of advanced forms, and with higher EF. Whether suppression of PVCs alters risk has not yet been determined.

Beyond the specific problem of coronary heart disease, the general factors of extent of underlying disease due to any cause and a prior clinical expression of risk of SCD (i.e., survival after out-of-hospital cardiac arrest, not associated with acute MI) identify very high risk patients. Survival after out-of-hospital cardiac arrest predicts a 30

percent 1-year recurrent cardiac arrest rate in the absence of specific interventions (see below) in this group of patients.

A general rule is that the risk of SCD is approximately one-half of the total cardiovascular mortality rate. Thus, the SCD risk is approximately 20 percent per year for patients with advanced coronary heart disease or dilated cardiomyopathy severe enough to result in a 40 percent 1-year total mortality rate. Figure 40-2 demonstrates a much more focused population fraction ("Percent/Year") for identifying high-risk patients for interventions in the high-risk subgroups, but the overall impact on the population, indicated by the absolute number of preventable events ("Events/Year"), is considerably smaller.

MANAGEMENT OF CARDIAC ARREST

The individual who collapses suddenly is managed in five stages: (1) the initial response; (2) basic life support; (3) advanced life support; (4) postresuscitation care; and (5) long-term management. The initial response and basic life support can be carried out by physicians, nurses, paramedical personnel, and trained lay persons. There is a requirement for increasing skills as the patient moves through the stages of advanced life support, postresuscitation care, and long-term management.

INITIAL RESPONSE The initial response will confirm whether a sudden collapse is indeed due to a cardiac arrest. Observations for respiratory movements, skin color, and the presence or absence of pulses in the carotid or femoral arteries will immediately determine whether a life-threatening cardiac arrest has occurred. Agonal respiratory movements may persist for a short time after cardiac arrest, but it is important to observe for severe stridor with a persistent pulse as a clue to aspiration of a foreign body or food. If this is suspected, a prompt Heimlich maneuver (see below) may dislodge the obstructing body. A precordial blow, or "thump," delivered firmly to the junction of the middle and lower third of the sternum may occasionally revert VT or VF, but there is concern about converting VT *to* VF. Therefore, it has been recommended to use precordial thumps only in monitored patients; this recommendation remains controversial. The third action during the initial response is to clear the airway. The head is tilted back and chin lifted so that the oropharynx can be explored to clear the airway. Dentures or foreign bodies are removed, and the Heimlich maneuver is performed if there is reason to suspect that a foreign body is lodged in the oropharynx. If respiratory arrest precipitating cardiac arrest is suspected, a second precordial thump is delivered after the airway is cleared.

BASIC LIFE SUPPORT More popularly known as cardiopulmonary resuscitation (CPR), basic life support is intended to maintain organ perfusion until definitive interventions can be accomplished. The elements of CPR are the establishment and maintenance of ventilation of the lungs and compression of the chest. Mouth-to-mouth respiration may be used if no specific rescue equipment is immediately available (e.g., plastic oropharyngeal airways, esophageal obturators, masked Ambu bag). Conventional ventilation techniques during CPR require the lungs to be inflated once every 5 s when two persons are performing the resuscitation, and twice in succession every 15 s when one person is carrying out both ventilation and chest wall compression. Chest compression is based on the assumption that cardiac compression allows the heart to maintain a pump function by sequential filling and emptying of its chambers, with competent valves maintaining forward direction of flow. The technique is illustrated in Fig. 40-3. The palm of one hand is placed over the lower sternum, with the heel of the other resting on the dorsum of the lower hand. The sternum is depressed, with the arms remaining straight, at a rate of approximately 80/min. Sufficient force is applied to depress the sternum 3 to 5 cm, and relaxation is abrupt. This conventional technique for CPR is currently being compared to a new technique based on simultaneous compression and ventilation. While measurable carotid artery flow can be achieved with conventional CPR, experimental data and theoretical considerations suggest

FIGURE 40-3 Major steps in cardiopulmonary resuscitation. *A.* Make certain the victim has an open airway. *B.* Start respiratory resuscitation immediately. *C.* Feel for the carotid pulse in the groove alongside the "Adam's apple" or thyroid cartilage. *D.* If pulse is absent, begin cardiac massage. Use 60 compressions a minute with one lung inflation after each group of 5 chest compressions. *(From J Henderson, Emergency Medical Guide, 4th ed, New York, McGraw-Hill, 1978.)*

that flow may be optimized by a pumping action produced by pressure changes in the entire thoracic cavity, as is achieved by simultaneous compression and ventilation. However, it is not yet clear whether this technique causes an unacceptable impedance of coronary blood flow, and whether the increased *carotid flow* produces equivalent increases in *cerebral perfusion*. Until these issues are clarified, conventional CPR remains the generally accepted technique.

ADVANCED LIFE SUPPORT   Advanced life support is intended to achieve adequate ventilation, control cardiac arrhythmias, stabilize the hemodynamic status (blood pressure and cardiac output), and to restore organ perfusion. The activities carried out to achieve these goals include: (1) intubation with an endotracheal tube; (2) defibrillation/cardioversion and/or pacing; and (3) insertion of an intravenous line. Ventilation with O_2 (room air if O_2 is not immediately available) may promptly reverse hypoxemia and acidosis. The speed with which defibrillation/cardioversion is carried out is an important element for successful resuscitation. When possible, immediate defibrillation should precede intubation and insertion of an intravenous line; CPR should be carried out while the defibrillator is being charged. As soon as a diagnosis of VT or VF is obtained a 200-J shock should be delivered. Additional shocks at higher energies, up to a maximum of 360 J, are tried if the initial shock does not successfully abolish VT or VF. If the patient is less than fully conscious upon reversion,

or if two or three attempts fail, prompt intubation, ventilation, and arterial blood gas analysis should be carried out. Intravenous $NaHCO_3$, which was formerly used in large quantities, is no longer considered routinely necessary and may be dangerous in larger quantities. However, the patient who is persistently acidotic after successful defibrillation and intubation should be given 1 mmol/kg of $NaHCO_3$ initially, and a 50 percent addition of the dose repeated every 10 to 15 min.

After initial defibrillation attempts, whether successful or not, a bolus of 1 mg/kg of lidocaine is given intravenously (Chap. 189) and the dose repeated in 2 min in those patients who have persistent ventricular arrhythmias or remain in VF. This is followed by a continuous infusion at a rate of 1 to 4 mg/min. If lidocaine fails to provide control, intravenous procainamide (loading infusion of 100 mg/5 min to a total dose of 500 to 800 mg, followed by continuous infusion at 2 to 5 mg/min) or bretylium tosylate (loading dose 5 to 10 mg/kg in 5 min; maintenance dose 0.5 to 2 mg/min) may be tried. For persistent VF, epinephrine (0.5 to 1.0 mg) may be given intravenously every 5 min during resuscitation with attempts to defibrillate between each dose. The drug may be given by an intracardiac route if intravenous access is not available. Intravenous calcium gluconate is no longer considered safe or necessary for routine administration. It is used only in patients in whom acute hyperkalemia is known to be the triggering event for resistant VF, in the presence of known hypocalcemia, or in patients who have received toxic doses of calcium channel antagonists.

Cardiac arrest secondary to bradyarrhythmias or asystole are managed differently. Once it is known that this type of rhythm is present, there is no role for external shock. The patient is promptly intubated, CPR is continued, and an attempt is made to control hypoxemia and acidosis. Epinephrine and/or atropine are given intravenously or by an intracardiac route. External pacing devices are now available to attempt to establish a regular rhythm, but the prognosis is generally very poor in this form of cardiac arrest. The one exception is bradyarrhythmic/asystolic cardiac arrest secondary to airway obstruction. This form of cardiac arrest may respond promptly to removal of foreign bodies by the Heimlich maneuver; or, more commonly in hospitalized patients, by intubation and suctioning of obstructing secretions in the airway.

POSTRESUSCITATION   This phase of care is determined by the clinical setting of the cardiac arrest. *Primary VF in acute MI* (Chap. 189) is generally very responsive to life support techniques and easily controlled after the initial event. Patients are maintained on a lidocaine infusion at the rate of 2 to 4 mg/min for 24 to 72 h after the event. In the in-hospital setting, respirator support is usually not necessary or needed for only a short time, and hemodynamics stabilize promptly after defibrillation or cardioversion. In *secondary VF in acute MI* (those events in which hemodynamic abnormalities predispose to an arrhythmic event), resuscitative efforts are less often successful; and in those patients who are successfully resuscitated, the recurrence rate is high. The clinical picture is dominated by hemodynamic instability. In fact, the outcome is determined more by the ability to control hemodynamic dysfunction than electrophysiologic abnormalities. Bradyarrhythmias, asystole, and electromechanical dissociation are commonly secondary events in hemodynamically unstable patients, and are less responsive to interventions.

The outcome after in-hospital cardiac arrest associated with *noncardiac* diseases is poor; and in the few successfully resuscitated patients, the postresuscitation course is dominated by the nature of the underlying disease. Patients with cancer, renal failure, acute central nervous system disease, and uncontrolled infections, as a group, have a survival rate of less than 10 percent after in-hospital cardiac arrest. Some major exceptions to the poor outcome of cardiac arrest due to noncardiac causes are patients with transient airway obstruction, electrolyte disturbances, proarrhythmic effects of drugs, and severe metabolic abnormalities, most of whom may have an excellent chance of survival if they can be promptly resuscitated and maintained while the transient abnormalities are being corrected.

POST-CARDIAC ARREST CARE AFTER SURVIVAL FROM OUT-OF-HOSPITAL CARDIAC ARREST This form of care has evolved into a major area of specialized clinical activities since the development of community-based emergency rescue systems. Patients who do not suffer irreversible injury of the central nervous system and who become hemodynamically stable should have extensive diagnostic and therapeutic testing to guide long-term management. This aggressive approach is driven by the fact that early statistics indicated survival after out-of-hospital cardiac arrest was followed by a 30 percent recurrent cardiac arrest rate at 1 year, 45 percent at 2 years, and a total mortality rate of almost 60 percent at 2 years. Historical comparisons suggests that these dismal statistics may be significantly improved by newer interventions.

Among those patients in whom a transmural, acute MI is the cause of out-of-hospital cardiac arrest, the management is the same as any other patient who suffers cardiac arrest during the acute phase of a documented MI (see Chap. 189). For almost all other categories of patients, however, extensive diagnostic studies are carried out to determine etiology, functional impairment, and electrophysiologic instability as guides to future management. In general, patients who have out-of-hospital cardiac arrest due to chronic ischemic heart disease, without an acute MI, are evaluated to determine whether transient ischemia or chronic electrophysiologic instability was the more likely cause of the event. If there is reason to suspect an ischemic mechanism, anti-ischemic surgery or medical interventions (angioplasty, drugs) are used to reduce the ischemic burden. Electrophysiologic instability is best identified by the use of programmed electrical stimulation to determine whether the patient is inducible into a sustained VT or VF (Chap. 184). If so, this information can be used as a baseline against which to evaluate drug efficacy for prevention of inducibility, which is considered a satisfactory endpoint for long-term management. Using this technique for patients with ejection fractions of 30 percent or more, the recurrent cardiac arrest rate is less than 10 percent during the first year of follow-up. The outcome is not as good for patients with ejection fractions under 30 percent, but is still better than the apparent natural history of survival after cardiac arrest. For patients for whom successful drug therapy cannot be identified by this technique, insertion of an automatic implantable cardioverter/defibrillator or antiarrhythmic surgery (coronary bypass surgery, aneurysmectomy, cryoablation), should be considered (Chap. 184). The array of interventions available for these patients, properly applied, is providing continuing improvement in long-term outcome.

REFERENCES

BEDELL SE et al: Survival after cardiopulmonary resuscitation in the hospital. N Engl J Med 309:569, 1983

BIGGER JT, FLEISS JL, KLEIGER R, MILLER JP, ROLNITZKY LM, AND THE MULTICENTER POST-INFARCTION RESEARCH GROUP: The relationships among ventricular arrhythmias, left ventricular dysfunction, and mortality in the two years after myocardial infarction. Circulation 69:250, 1984

COBB LA, HALLSTROM AP: Community-based cardiopulmonary resuscitation: What have we learned? Ann NY Acad Sci 382:330, 1982

HEIMLICH HJ: A life-saving maneuver to prevent food-choking. JAMA 234:398, 1975

HINKLE LA, THALER HT: Clinical classification of cardiac deaths. Circulation 65:457, 1982

KANNEL WB, SCHATZKIN A: Sudden death: Lessions from subsets in population studies. J Am Coll Cardiol 5 (Suppl 6): 141B, 1985

KULLER L et al: An epidemiological study of sudden and unexpected deaths in adults. Medicine 46:341, 1967

MYERBURG RJ, CASTELLANOS A: Cardiac arrest and sudden cardiac death, in Heart Disease, 3d ed, E Braunwald (ed). Philadelphia, Saunders, 1988, chap 24, pp 742–777

—— et al: Long-term survival after prehospital cardiac arrest: Analysis of outcome during an 8-year study. Circulation 70:538, 1984

—— et al: A biological approach to sudden cardiac death: Structure, function, and cause. Am J Cardiol, 63:1512, 1989

PACKER M: Sudden unexpected death in patients with congestive heart failure: A second frontier. Circulation 72:681, 1985

ROBERTS WC, JONES AA: Quantitation of coronary arterial narrowing at necropsy in sudden cardiac death. Analysis of 31 patients and comparison with 25 controls. Am J Cardiol 44:39, 1979

Standard and guidelines for cardiopulmonary resuscitation (CPR) and emergency cardiac care (ECC). JAMA 255:290, 1986

WILBER DJ et al: Out-of-hospital cardiac arrest: Use of electrophysiologic testing in the prediction of long-term outcome. N Engl J Med 318:19, 1988

section 5   Alterations in gastrointestinal function

41   ORAL MANIFESTATIONS OF DISEASE

JOHN S. GREENSPAN / PAUL GOLDHABER

A thorough oral examination, to include the oral and pharyngeal soft tissues as well as the teeth, is an important part of the physical examination. The common oral diseases are due to infection by bacteria, fungi, and viruses. The complex development of the orofacial structures leads to close interposition of a wide range of tissues, most of which are prone to developmental anomalies, growth disturbances, and neoplasia.

DISEASES OF THE TEETH

DENTAL CARIES, PULPAL AND PERIAPICAL DISEASE, AND COMPLICATIONS Dental caries is a destructive disease of the hard tissues of the teeth due to infection with *Streptococcus mutans* and other bacteria. Formerly one of the commonest human diseases, caries has shown marked changes in recent years. In the United States fewer than half of those 17 years and younger now have carious lesions, although in many segments of the population and in the third world this decrease has not occurred. Much of the decline is due to artificial fluoridation of drinking water to a level of 1 part per million, with additional effects due to fluoride-containing toothpastes and topical fluoride administration. Conversely, retention of teeth and the aging of the population have led to an increase in root caries. Increasing numbers of patients surviving with the consequences of cancer therapy and other special populations (diabetics and those with xerostomia due to Sjögren's syndrome or to medications) may experience severe caries unless appropriate topical fluoride prophylaxis is used. Treatment of caries involves removal of the softened and infected hard tissues, sealing of the exposed dentine, and restoration of the lost tooth structure with silver amalgam, composite plastic, gold, or porcelain.

If the carious lesion progresses, infection of the dental pulp may occur, causing *acute pulpitis*. The tooth may become sensitive to hot or cold and then severe continuous throbbing pain ensues. At this stage, pulp damage is irreversible and it becomes necessary to remove the contents of the pulp chamber and root canals, followed by thorough cleaning, antisepsis, and filling with an inert material (root canal therapy). Alternatively, extraction of the tooth may be indicated.

If the pulpitis is not successfully treated, infection may spread beyond the tooth apex into the periodontal ligament. If the infection causes acute inflammation, pain on chewing or percussion is present and a *periapical abscess* may form, while chronic inflammation can produce a *periapical granuloma* within the alveolar bone. This may cause slight pain and tenderness or may be asymptomatic. Proliferation of epithelial cell rests may convert the granuloma into a *periapical cyst*. Both the granuloma and the cyst produce periapical radiolucencies, whereas the periapical abscess does not do so unless it forms as a complication of one of the other two lesions. The pus in the periapical abscess may track through the alveolar bone into soft tissues, causing cellulitis and bacteremia, or may discharge into the oral cavity (*parulis* or *gumboil*), into the maxillary sinus, or through the skin of the face or submandibular area. A severe form of cellulitis, *Ludwig's angina*, originates from an infected mandibular molar, involves the submandibular space, and extends throughout the floor of the mouth, with elevation of the tongue, dysphagia, and difficulty in breathing. Glottal edema may occur, necessitating emergency tracheotomy.

EFFECT OF SYSTEMIC FACTORS ON TEETH   Systemic factors, occurring in utero or in infancy during the stages of crown formation, may influence the development and structure of the teeth. Enamel hypoplasia of the primary and/or permanent teeth, manifested by alterations ranging from white spots to gross defects in the surface structure of the crowns, may be caused by disturbances of calcium and phosphate metabolism such as are found in vitamin D–resistant rickets, hypoparathyroidism, gastroenteritis, and celiac disease. Premature birth or high fevers may also give rise to enamel hypoplasia. Tetracycline, given during the second half of pregnancy, in infancy, and in childhood up to 8 years of age, causes both a permanent discoloration of the teeth and enamel hypoplasia. Daily ingestion of more than 1.5 mg fluoride can result in enamel discoloration (*mottling*). Prenatal factors appear to influence crown size. Larger teeth are associated with maternal diabetes, maternal hypothyroidism, and large birth size. Tooth size is reduced in Down's syndrome. Premature loss of the deciduous dentition is frequently the first symptom in juvenile hypophosphatasia. Systemic disease may give rise to pain that simulates pulpal disease. Maxillary sinusitis is frequently manifested as pain in the maxillary teeth, including sensitivity to thermal changes and percussion. Cardiac disease with angina pectoris may result in pain referred to the lower jaw, probably through the vagus nerve.

PERIODONTAL DISEASES

In adults, chronic destructive periodontal disease becomes responsible for more loss of teeth than caries, particularly in the aged. However, the prevalence and incidence of periodontal disease also appears to be declining in the United States. The commonest form of periodontal disease starts as inflammation of the marginal gingiva (*gingivitis*) which is painless, although the gingiva may bleed on brushing. The disease spreads to involve the periodontal ligament and alveolar bone. As the latter is slowly resorbed, there is loss of periodontal ligament attachment between tooth and bone. The soft tissue separates from the tooth surface, causing "pocket" formation with bleeding on probing and during chewing. Acute inflammation may become superimposed on this chronic process, with the production of pus and the formation of a *periodontal abscess*. Ultimately, extreme bone loss, tooth mobility, and recurrent abscess formation leads to tooth exfoliation or may mandate tooth extraction.

Gingivitis and periodontitis are infections associated with the accumulation of *bacterial plaque* which may become mineralized (*calculus*) and which can be prevented by appropriate *oral hygiene* measures including tooth brushing, flossing, antibacterial mouth rinses, and the removal of impacted food debris. Poorly fabricated or deteriorated restorations may contribute through overextended or inadequate margins, while the role of occlusal trauma is unclear.

Therapy is directed at the causative microflora and consists of removal of plaque and calculus, debridement of the pocket lining and superficial infected cementum, combined with elimination of other contributing factors.

Periodontal disease appears to be a group of conditions, including *adult periodontitis*, associated with *Bacteroides gingivalis*, *B. intermedius*, and other gram-negative organisms. *Localized juvenile periodontitis* (LJP) causes rapid, severe pocketing and bone loss and is associated with *Actinobacillus actinomycetemcomitans* (*A.a*), *Capnocytophaga*, *Eikenella corrodens*, and other anaerobes. *Acute necrotizing ulcerative gingivitis* (ANUG) involves sudden inflammation of the gingivae with necrosis, tissue loss, pain, bleeding, and halitosis and is associated with *B. intermedius* and spirochetes. ANUG and an aggressive and rapid form of periodontitis (HIV-P) are seen in association with human immunodeficiency virus (HIV) infection. Some of these cases progress to a destructive gangrenelike lesion of oral soft tissues and bone (*necrotizing stomatitis*) resembling the *noma* formerly seen in severely malnourished populations. Therapy involves local antibacterial measures, debridement and, in severe cases, systemic antibiotics effective against gram-negative anaerobes.

Host factors may be involved in the pathogenesis of periodontal disease in other populations also. Thus, familial defects in neutrophil chemotaxis are found in LJP and these may predispose to tissue destruction caused by the toxins of *A.a.* including leucotoxin, collagenase, endotoxin, and a factor further inhibiting neutrophil chemotaxis. Patients with IgA deficiency and agammaglobulinemia probably have less periodontal disease than matched healthy individuals, whereas in *Down's syndrome* and *diabetes mellitus* severe periodontal disease may occur. During pregnancy there may be severe gingivitis and the formation of localized *pyogenic granulomas*. Certain drugs, notably the anticonvulsant *phenytoin* and the antiangina calcium channel blocker *nifedipine*, cause *fibrous hyperplasia* of the gingiva which may cover the teeth, interfere with eating, and be unsightly. Similar clinical appearances can be due to *idiopathic familial gingival fibromatosis*. Surgical management is used for both conditions, although a change in medication may be appropriate for the drug-induced form.

Periapical and periodontal bacterial infections can cause transient bacteremia after tooth extraction and even routine dental prophylaxis. These can lead to bacterial endocarditis in patients with a history of rheumatic fever, other valvular disease, valvular graft, or heart or joint prostheses. Antibiotic coverage is appropriate in such cases.

DISEASES OF THE ORAL MUCOSA

INFECTIONS   Most oral mucosal diseases involve microorganisms (see Table 41-1).

PIGMENTED LESIONS   (See Table 41-2)

DERMATOLOGIC DISEASES   (See Tables 41-1, -2, and -3 and Chaps. 55 to 60)

DISEASES OF THE TONGUE   (See Table 41-4)

HALITOSIS   (See Table 41-5)

HIV DISEASE AND AIDS   (See Table 41-6 and Chaps. 134 and 264)   Immunosuppression induced by HIV infection predisposes to numerous oral infections, neoplasms, and autoimmune and idiopathic lesions. Some of these, such as *oral candidiasis* and *hairy leukoplakia* (a benign epithelial hyperplasia associated with Epstein-Barr virus, or EBV), are common features of HIV disease and often precede or accompany full-blown AIDS. Some, such as oral Kaposi's sarcoma and lymphoma, are diagnostic of AIDS. While most oral lesions of HIV disease are also found in the general population, both hairy leukoplakia and HIV-P are strongly associated with HIV infection and are seen only very rarely in other circumstances. Only small and variable amounts of HIV can be found in saliva but blood, tissue fluid, and gingival crevicular exudate, found in the mouth as a result of lesions or of clinical manipulation, are certainly sources of other

TABLE 41-1   Vesicular, bullous, or ulcerative lesions of the oral mucosa

Condition	Usual location	Clinical features	Course
VIRAL DISEASES			
Primary acute herpetic gingivo-stomatitis (herpes simplex virus type 1, rarely type 2)	Lip and oral mucosa	Labial vesicles which rupture and crust, and intraoral vesicles which quickly ulcerate; extremely painful; acute gingivitis, fever, malaise, foul odor, and cervical lymphadenopathy; occurs primarily in infants, children, and young adults	Heals spontaneously in 10–14 days unless secondarily infected
Recurrent herpes labialis	Mucocutaneous junction of lip perioral skin	Eruption of groups of vesicles which may coalesce, then rupture and crust; painful to pressure or spicy foods	Lasts about 1 week, but condition may be prolonged if secondary infection occurs
Recurrent intraoral herpes simplex	Palate and gingiva	Small vesicles which rupture and coalesce; painful	Heal spontaneously in about 1 week
Chickenpox (varicella-zoster virus)	Gingiva and oral mucosa	Skin lesions may be accompanied by small vesicles on oral mucosa that rupture to form shallow ulcers; may coalesce to form large bullous lesions that ulcerate; mucosa may have generalized erythema	Lesions heal spontaneously within 2 weeks
Herpes zoster (reactivation of varicella-zoster virus)	Cheek, tongue, gingiva, or palate	Unilateral vesicular eruption and ulceration in linear pattern following sensory distribution of trigeminal nerve or one of its branches	Gradual healing without scarring; postherpetic neuralgia is common
Infectious mononucleosis (Epstein-Barr virus)	Oral mucosa	Fatigue, sore throat, malaise, low-grade fever, and enlarged cervical lymph nodes; numerous small ulcers usually appear several days before lymphadenopathy; gingival bleeding and multiple petechiae at junction of hard and soft palates	Oral lesions disappear during convalescence
Warts (papillomavirus)	Any place on skin and oral mucosa	Single or multiple papillary lesions, with thick, white keratinized surfaces containing many pointed projections; cauliflower lesions covered with normal colored mucosa or multiple pink or pale bumps (focal epithelial hyperplasia)	Lesions grow rapidly and spread
Herpangina (coxsackievirus A; also possibly coxsackievirus B and echovirus)	Oral mucosa, pharynx, tongue	Sudden onset of fever, sore throat, and oropharyngeal vesicles, usually in children under 4 years, during summer months; diffuse pharyngeal injection and vesicles (1–2 mm), grayish white surrounded by red areola; vesicles enlarge and ulcerate	Incubation period 2–9 days; fever for 1–4 days; recovery uneventful
Hand, foot, and mouth disease (type A coxsackieviruses)	Oral mucosa, pharynx, palms, and soles	Fever, malaise, headache with oropharyngeal vesicles which become painful, shallow ulcers	Incubation period 2–18 days; lesions heal spontaneously in 2–4 weeks
Primary HIV infection	Gingiva, palate, and pharynx	Acute gingivitis and oropharyngeal ulceration, associated with febrile illness resembling mononucleosis and including lymphadenopathy	Followed by HIV seroconversion; asymptomatic HIV infection and usually ultimately by HIV disease
BACTERIAL OR FUNGAL DISEASES			
Acute necrotizing ulcerative gingivitis ("trench mouth", Vincent's infection)	Gingiva	Painful, bleeding gingiva characterized by necrosis and ulceration of gingival papillae and margins plus lymphadenopathy and foul odor	Continued destruction of tissue followed by remission, but may recur
Prenatal (congenital) syphilis	Palate, jaws, tongue, and teeth	Gummatous involvement of palate, jaws, and facial bones; Hutchinson's incisors, mulberry molars, glossitis, mucous patches, and fissures of corners of mouth	Tooth deformities in permanent dentition irreversible
Primary syphilis (chancre)	Lesion appears where organism enters body; may occur on lips, tongue, or tonsillar area	Small papule developing rapidly into a large, painless ulcer with indurated border; unilateral lymphadenopathy; chancre and lymph nodes containing spirochetes; serologic tests positive by third to fourth weeks	Healing of chancre in 1–2 months, followed by secondary syphilis in 6–8 weeks
Secondary syphilis	Oral mucosa frequently involved with mucous patches, primarily on palate, also at commissures of mouth	Maculopapular lesions of oral mucosa, 5–10 mm in diameter with central ulceration covered by grayish membrane; eruptions occurring on various mucosal surfaces and skin accompanied by fever, malaise, and sore throat	Lesions may persist from several weeks to a year
Tertiary syphilis	Palate and tongue	Gummatous infiltration of palate or tongue followed by ulceration and fibrosis; atrophy of tongue papillae produce characteristic bald tongue and glossitis	Gumma may destroy palate, causing complete perforation

(continued)

TABLE 41-1   Vesicular, bullous, or ulcerative lesions of the oral mucosa (continued)

Condition	Usual location	Clinical features	Course
BACTERIAL OR FUNGAL DISEASES			
Gonorrhea	Lesions may occur in mouth at site of inoculation or secondarily by hematogenous spread from a primary focus elsewhere	Earliest symptoms are burning or itching sensation, dryness, or heat in mouth followed by acute pain on eating or speaking; tonsils and oropharynx most frequently involved; oral tissues may be diffusely inflamed or ulcerated; saliva develops increased viscosity and fetid odor; submaxillary lymphadenopathy with fever in severe cases	Lesions may resolve with appropriate antibiotic therapy
Tuberculosis	Tongue, tonsillar area, soft palate	A solitary, irregular ulcer covered by a persistent exudate; ulcer has an undermined, firm border	Lesions may persist
Cervicofacial actinomycosis	Swellings in region of face, neck, and floor of mouth	Infection may be associated with an extraction, jaw fracture, or eruption of molar tooth; in acute form resembles an acute pyogenic abscess, but contains yellow "sulfur granules" (gram-positive mycelia and their hyphae)	Acute form may last a few weeks; chronic form lasts months or years; prognosis excellent; actinomycetes respond to antibiotics (tetracyclines or penicillin) but not to antifungal drugs
Histoplasmosis	Any area in mouth, particularly tongue, gingiva, or palate	Numerous small nodules which may ulcerate; hoarseness and dysphagia may occur because of lesions in larynx, usually associated with fever and malaise	May be fatal
Candidiasis	Any area of oral mucosa	Pseudomembranous form with white patches which are easily wiped off leaving red, bleeding, sore surface; erythematous form is flat and red while rarely candida leukoplakia appears as white patch in tongue which does not rub off; angular cheilitis due to *Candida* involves sore cracks and redness at angle of mouth; *Candida* seen on KOH preparation in all forms	Responds to antifungals
DERMATOLOGIC DISEASES			
Mucous membrane pemphigoid	Primarily mucous membranes of the oral cavity, but may also involve the eyes, urethra vagina, and rectum	Painful, grayish white collapsed vesicles or bullae with peripheral erythematous zone; gingival lesions desquamate, leaving ulcerated area	Protracted course with remissions and exacerbations; involvement of different sites occurs slowly; glucocorticoids may temporarily reduce symptoms but do not control the disease
Erythema multiforme (Stevens-Johnson syndrome)	Primarily the oral mucosa and skin of hands and feet	Intraoral ruptured bullae surrounded by an inflammatory area; lips may show hemorrhagic crusts; the "iris," or "target" lesion, on the skin is pathognomonic; patient may have severe signs of toxicity	Onset very rapid; condition may last 1–2 weeks; may be fatal; acute episodes respond to steroids
Pemphigus vulgaris	Oral mucosa and skin	Ruptured bullae and ulcerated oral areas; mostly in older adults	With repeated recurrence of bullae, toxicity may lead to cachexia, infection, and death within 2 years; often controllable with steroids
Lichen planus	Oral mucosa and skin	White striae in mouth; purplish nodules on skin at sites of friction; occasionally causes oral mucosal ulcers and erosive gingivitis	Protracted course, may respond to topical steroids
NEOPLASTIC DISEASES			
Squamous cell carcinoma	Any areas in mouth, most commonly on lower lip, tongue, and floor of mouth	Ulcer with elevated, indurated border; failure to heal, pain not prominent; lesions tend to arise in areas of leukoplakia or in smooth or atrophic tongue	Invades and destroys underlying tissues and may metastasize to regional lymph nodes
Acute leukemia	Gingiva	Gingival swelling and superficial ulcerations followed by hyperplasia of gingiva with extensive necrosis and hemorrhage; deep ulcers may occur elsewhere on the mucosa complicated by secondary infection	Fatal if untreated
Lymphoma	Gingiva, palate, tongue, and tonsillar area	Elevated, ulcerated area which may proliferate rapidly, giving the appearance of a traumatic inflammatory lesion; swelling of regional lymph nodes	Fatal if untreated
Metastatic tumors	Deep in jaw bone, usually in premolar-molar area of mandible	May arise from carcinoma of distant organ such as breast, lung, or kidney; advanced lesion may expand and destroy bone, loosen and spread teeth, involve inferior alveolar nerve, cause pain and numbness of lower lip	Usually fatal

(continued)

TABLE 41-1   Vesicular, bullous, or ulcerative lesions of the oral mucosa (continued)

Condition	Usual location	Clinical features	Course
OTHER CONDITIONS			
Recurrent aphthous ulcers	Any place on nonkeratinized oral mucosa (lips, tongue, buccal mucosa, floor of mouth, soft palate, oropharynx)	Single or clusters of painful ulcers with surrounding erythematous border; lesions may be 1–2 mm in diameter in crops (herpetiform), 1–5 mm (minor), or 5–15 mm (major)	Lesions heal in 1–2 weeks but may recur monthly or several times a year; topical steroids give symptomatic relief; systemic glucocorticoids may be needed in severe cases; a tetracycline oral suspension may decrease severity of herpetiform ulcers
Behçet's syndrome	Oral mucosa, eyes, genitalia, gut, and CNS	Multiple aphthous ulcers in mouth; inflammatory ocular changes, ulcerative lesions on genitalia; inflammatory bowel disease and CNS disease	Ulcers may persist for several weeks and heal without scarring
Traumatic ulcers	Any place on oral mucosa; dentures frequently responsible for ulcers in vestibule	Localized, discrete ulcerated lesion with red border; produced by accidental biting of mucosa, penetration by a foreign object, or chronic irritation by a denture	Lesions usually heal in 7–10 days when irritant is removed, unless secondarily infected

viruses, such as herpes simplex virus (HSV) and EBV, and the same may be true for HIV.

HEMATOLOGIC AND NUTRITIONAL DISEASE   Gingival bleeding, necrotic ulcers, and enlargement due to malignant infiltrates are seen in all forms of leukemia, particularly *monocytic leukemia*. In agranulocytosis severe oral mucosal ulcers are seen, while in *thrombocytopenia* oral petechiae, ecchymoses, and gingival bleeding occur. In *Plummer-Vinson syndrome* (see Chaps. 290 and 291), atrophy of oral mucosa, particularly the tongue papillae, causes redness and soreness as well as dysphagia. This is associated with increased susceptibility to oral cancer. A smooth tongue can also be seen in *pernicious anemia* (Chap. 292). Severe oral mucositis with ulcers, candidiasis, bacterial infections, and xerostomia complicate local radiotherapy for head and neck malignancies as well as chemotherapy for both local and other malignancies. Although now rarely seen in the United States, oral features of vitamin deficiency include oral mucositis and ulcers, glossitis, and burning sensations in the tongue (*B group vitamins*) and petechiae, gingival swelling, bleeding, and ulceration as well as loosening of teeth (*scurvy* of vitamin C deficiency).

ORAL CANCER

Oral *squamous cell carcinoma* accounts for 2 to 4 percent of malignancies in the United States (excluding skin carcinomas) and

TABLE 41-2   Pigmented lesions of the oral mucosa

Condition	Usual location	Clinical features	Course
Oral melanotic macule	Any area of the mouth	Discrete or diffuse localized, brown to black macule	Remains indefinitely
Diffuse melanin pigmentation	Any area of the mouth	Diffuse pale to dark-brown pigmentation; may be physiologic ("racial") or due to smoking	Remains indefinitely
Nevi	Any area of the mouth	Discrete, localized, brown to black pigmentation	
Malignant melanoma	Any area of the mouth	Can be flat and diffuse, painless, brown to black, or can be raised and nodular	Expands and invades early; metastasis leads to death
Addison's disease	Any area in mouth but mostly on buccal mucosa	Blotches or spots of bluish-black to dark-brown pigmentation occurring early in the disease, accompanied by diffuse pigmentation of skin; other symptoms of adrenal insufficiency	Condition controlled by steroid therapy
Peutz-Jeghers syndrome	Any area in mouth	Dark-brown spots on lips, buccal mucosa, with characteristic distribution of pigment around lips, nose, eyes, and on hands; concomitant intestinal polyposis	Pigmented lesions remain indefinitely; polyps may become malignant
Drug ingestion (tranquilizers, oral contraceptives, antimalarials)	Any area in mouth	Brown, black, or gray areas of pigmentation	Disappears following cessation of drug
Amalgam tattoo	Gingiva and mucobuccal fold	Small blue-black pigmented areas associated with embedded amalgam particles in soft tissues; these may show up on radiographs as radiopaque particles in some cases	Remains indefinitely
Heavy metal pigmentation (bismuth, mercury, lead)	Gingival margin	Thin blue-black pigmented line along gingival margin; due to prior treatment for syphilis with bismuth or mercury or from accidental absorption of lead	Long-lasting
Black hairy tongue	Dorsum of tongue	Elongation of filiform papillae of tongue, which take on a brown to black coloration	Long-lasting but may disappear spontaneously
Fordyce's "disease"	Buccal and labial mucosa	Aggregation of numerous small yellowish spots just beneath mucosal surface; no symptoms; due to hyperplasia of sebaceous glands	Remains without apparent change indefinitely

TABLE 41-3   White lesions of oral mucosa

Condition	Usual location	Clinical features	Course
Lichen planus	Buccal mucosa, tongue, gingiva, and lips; skin	Striae, white plaques, red areas, ulcers in mouth; purplish papules on skin; may be asymptomatic, sore, or painful; lichenoid drug reactions may look similar	Protracted; responds to topical steroids
White sponge nevus	Oral mucosa, vagina, anal mucosa	Painless white thickening of epithelium; adolescent/early adult onset; familial	Benign and permanent
Smokers leukoplakia and smokeless tobacco lesions	Any area of oral mucosa, sometimes related to location	White patch that may become firm, rough, or red fissured and ulcerated; may become sore and painful but usually painless	Occasionally premalignant; may or may not resolve on cessation of habit
Nicotinic stomatitis	Palate in pipe smokers	White nodular elevations on hard palate with central red areas	Benign; usually resolves on cessation of pipe smoking
Frictional keratosis	Any area in mouth	Elevated white lesion due to hyperkeratosis and thickening of the oral epithelium secondary to chronic irritation	Removal of irritant leads to healing in 2–3 weeks
Candidiasis ("candidosis," "moniliasis")	Any area in mouth	*Pseudomembranous type* ("thrush"): creamy white curdlike patches that reveal a raw, bleeding surface when scraped; found in sick infants, debilitated elderly patients receiving high doses of glucocorticoids or broad spectrum antibiotics, or in patients with AIDS	Responds favorably to antifungal therapy and correction of predisposing causes where possible
		Erythematous type: flat, red, sometimes sore areas, same groups of patients	
		Candidal leukoplakia: nonremovable white thickening of epithelium due to *Candida*	Responds to prolonged antifungals
		Angular cheilitis: sore fissures at corner of mouth	Responds to topical antifungals
Hairy leukoplakia	Usually lateral tongue, rarely elsewhere on oral mucosa	White areas ranging from small and flat to extensive and "hairy"; found in HIV carriers in all risk groups for AIDS; rarely causes discomfort	Due to EBV; many patients develop AIDS; responds to high dose acyclovir but recurs
Chemical burns	Any area in mouth	White slough due to necrosis of epithelium and underlying connective tissue caused by contact with agents (e.g., aspirin) applied locally or the use of undiluted sodium perborate or hydrogen peroxide as a mouthwash; removal of slough leaves a raw, painful surface	Lesion heals in several weeks if not secondarily infected

in most western countries, but represents up to 50 percent of malignancies in India. Globally, oral cancer is fourth in incidence for men and sixth for women. The disease is age related, occurring in those over 40 years of age and increasing in incidence with age. The male/female ratio is 3:1 but the incidence of lip and mouth cancer is decreasing in white males and increasing in black males and in females. However, both the overall incidence and death rate are fairly static. *Lip cancer* has shown significant decreases in incidence in recent years, probably because of changes in pipe-smoking habits, while *tongue cancer* has become commoner. Lip cancer is still the commonest oral site followed by tongue, floor of mouth, and other intraoral locations. The etiology involves *tobacco* smoked in pipes, cigars, and cigarettes and chewed or "dipped." The role of pipe smoking in lip cancer may also include the effects of

TABLE 41-4   Alterations of the tongue

Type of change	Clinical features
SIZE OR MORPHOLOGY CHANGES	
Macroglossia	Enlarged tongue that may be part of a syndrome found in developmental conditions such as Down's syndrome; may be due to tumor (hemangioma or lymphangioma), metabolic disease (such as primary amyloidosis), or endocrine disturbance (such as acromegaly or cretinism)
Fissured ("scrotal") tongue	Dorsal surface and sides of tongue covered by painless shallow or deep fissures that may collect debris and become irritated
Median rhomboid glossitis	Congenital abnormality of tongue with ovoid, denuded area in median posterior portion of the tongue; may be associated with candidiasis and may respond to antifungals
COLOR CHANGES	
"Geographic" tongue (benign migratory glossitis)	Asymptomatic inflammatory condition of the tongue, with rapid loss and regrowth of filiform papillae, leading to appearance of denuded red patches "wandering" across the surface of the tongue
Hairy tongue	Elongation of filiform papillae of the medial dorsal surface area due to failure of keratin layer of the papillae to desquamate normally; brownish black coloration may be due to staining by tobacco, food, or chromogenic organisms
"Strawberry" and "raspberry" tongue	Appearance of tongue during scarlet fever due to the hypertrophy of fungiform papillae plus changes in the filiform papillae
"Bald" tongue	Atrophy may be associated with xerostomia, pernicious anemia, iron-deficiency anemia, pellagra, or syphilis; may be accompanied by painful burning sensation; may be an expression of erythematous candidiasis and respond to antifungals

TABLE 41-5 Causes of halitosis

I Upper respiratory infection
  A Bronchiectasis
  B Lung abscess
II Oral infection
  A Acute primary herpetic gingivostomatitis
  B Acute necrotizing ulcerative gingivitis
  C Periodontal disease
  D Caries
III Smoking
IV Hepatic failure (fishy odor)
V Azotemia (ammoniacal or urinary odor)
VI Diabetic ketoacidosis (sweet, fruity odor)

heat and other irritants. Other factors include *alcohol*, iron deficiency (Plummer-Vinson syndrome), and deficiencies of vitamins. Evidence linking oral *syphilitic* lesions and oral *candidiasis* with oral cancer is circumstantial, but a growing body of data indicates roles for *herpes simplex virus* and *human papillomavirus*. There are no data supporting the idea that irritation from sharp teeth or dental appliances cause oral cancer.

The most common precancerous lesion in the oral cavity presents as *leukoplakia*, a white patch on the mucosa that cannot be rubbed off. Histologically such lesions show hyperkeratosis, acanthosis, and *atypia* (*dysplasia*). Leukoplakias include homogeneous and nonhomogeneous types. The nonhomogeneous nodular leukoplakias (white nodules on a red background), have a much higher potential for malignant transformation than homogeneous leukoplakia. Recent evidence suggests that the asymptomatic, red velvety lesion (*erythroplasia*) of the floor of the mouth, ventrolateral aspect of the tongue, or soft palate–anterior pillar complex is more likely to be carcinoma in situ or invasive carcinoma than is the white lesion. All chronic ulcerative lesions that fail to heal within 1 to 2 weeks should be considered potentially malignant and must be biopsied in order to make a definitive diagnosis. It is noteworthy that in their early stages intraoral squamous cell carcinomas are rarely painful, in contrast to similar-appearing inflammatory lesions.

The prognosis for patients with carcinoma of the lip is usually good, since these malignant tumors are noted sooner and apparently metastasize later. Patients with carincoma of the tongue have a poorer prognosis, particularly if the tumor occurs more posteriorly on the tongue. Intraoral carcinomas may spread by direct invasion to the

TABLE 41-6 Oral lesions of HIV disease and AIDS

I Fungal
  A Candidiasis
    1 Pseudomembranous
    2 Erythematous
    3 Candidal leukoplakia
    4 Angular cheilitis
  B Histoplasmosis
  C Cryptococcosis
II Bacterial
  A Acute necrotizing ulcerative gingivitis
  B HIV-gingivitis
  C HIV-periodontitis
  D Necrotizing stomatitis
  E Mycobacterium avium intracellulare complex and tuberculosis
  F Stomatitis due to enteric organisms
III Viral
  A Herpes simplex
  B Herpes zoster
  C Hairy leukoplakia
  D Warts
IV Neoplastic
  A Kaposi's sarcoma
  B Lymphoma
V Other
  A Recurrent aphthous ulcers
  B Immune thrombocytopenic purpura
  C Xerostomia
  D Salivary gland enlargement

underlying bone. Depending on the site of origin of the intraoral carcinoma, metastases usually spread to the submaxillary or cervical lymph nodes. Death may result from recurrent or uncontrollable disease above the clavicles, metastatic disease beyond the neck, treatment complications, or a second primary cancer, usually in the oral cavity or the upper parts of the gastrointestinal or respiratory tract. Metastatic tumors to the jaw may occur from carcinomas of the lung, breast, kidney, or gastrointestinal tract.

DISEASES OF THE SALIVARY GLANDS

The major and minor salivary glands can be involved in mumps, sarcoidosis, tuberculosis, lymphoma, and Sjögren's syndrome (Chap. 273). The latter may cause dry eyes and dry mouth (*xerostomia*) and be associated with features of connective tissue diseases, including rheumatoid arthritis or systemic lupus erythematosus. Xerostomia may also be due to medications such as diuretics, antihistamines, or tricylic antidepressants as well as therapeutic irradiation for head and neck cancer. It may cause *cervical or incisal caries* and oral candidiasis. Management includes fluoride mouth rinses and topical applications, saliva substitutes, salivary stimulation with sugarless candies, and the avoidance of sugar-containing drinks or food. Candidiasis is treated with nystatin or other antifungals. Salivary stones (*sialolithiasis*), usually in the duct of a major salivary gland, cause *sialoadenitis* with pain and swelling, often on eating. Recurrent parotitis without apparent cause is seen in children.

The commonest neoplasm of the salivary glands is the *pleomorphic adenoma* which is benign but will recur unless fully enucleated; malignant tumors include *mucoepidermoid carcinoma*, *adenoid cystic carcinoma*, and *adenocarcinoma*. The pleomorphic adenoma causes a firm, slowly growing mass in the parotid, palate, or cheek while malignant tumors grow faster and can cause ulceration and invade nerves, producing numbness or facial paralysis.

NEUROLOGIC DISTURBANCES AND OROFACIAL PAIN

The mouth and face may be the site of pain from a number of vascular, neurologic, muscle/connective tissue, or joint conditions. Interdisciplinary diagnosis and management programs involving neurologists, restorative dentists, oral surgeons, otorhinolaryngologists, and other specialists, together with new imaging techniques to diagnose or exclude organic lesions, have begun to clarify this complex field. *Temporal arteritis* causes pain in the face, jaws, and tongue and may mimic temporomandibular joint disease. Glucocorticoids may provide relief. *Myofascial pain* is a dull, constant ache with local tenderness in the muscles of the jaws and difficulty in opening the mouth. This may be related to clenching and grinding habits (*bruxism*). *Arthralgia* of the temporomandibular joint causes local pain which may extend to the face and head. Both myofascial pain and arthralgia can be relieved with heat, rest, and anti-inflammatory agents. Displacement of the meniscus or condyle may cause pain, clenching, or locking of the mandible in the open position. The joint may become involved in *osteoarthritis* with minimal symptoms, while *rheumatoid arthritis* causes pain and swelling in the joint, limitation of movement and, in the *juvenile* form, severe malocclusion in children. *Ankylosis* may occur, necessitating condylectomy (see Chap. 270).

Trigeminal neuralgia (tic douloureux) causes sudden, severe, unilateral lancinating pain initiated by touching a "trigger zone" or occurring spontaneously. Confusion with pulpal or periapical pain is common, leading to inappropriate endodontic or surgical therapy. Many cases respond to carbamazepine and phenytoin although, for a few, surgical intervention to decompress the trigeminal nerve is indicated. Similar symptoms in the distribution of the ninth cranial nerve (tongue, pharynx, soft palate) are due to *glossopharyngeal neuralgia*, which may be triggered by swallowing and may produce referred pain in the temporomandibular joint. *Postherpetic neuralgia* may follow trigeminal herpes zoster (see Chap. 360) and cause burning, aching, and long-lasting pain. *Facial palsy* is usually unilateral and may be due to trauma, surgical intervention, tumor, or infection of the seventh cranial nerve. *Bell's palsy* is a form with acute onset and unknown cause, possibly viral infection such as herpes zoster. The corner of the mouth droops, there may be difficulty in speech, eating, and in closing the eye. The symptoms usually disappear spontaneously but residual facial immobility and lip drooping may persist. Abnormal or reduced *taste sensation* may be due to xerostomia, disturbances of the facial and glossopharyngeal nerves or their central connections, aging, or the wearing of dentures. Disease involving the hypoglossal nerve may cause atrophy of the tongue muscles with protrusion, if bilateral, or deviation towards the affected side, if unilateral.

REFERENCES

GENCO R et al: *Contemporary Periodontics*. St. Louis, Mosby, 1989
GREENSPAN D et al: *AIDS and the Dental Team*. Chicago, Yearbook, 1987
LYNCH MA et al: *Burket's Oral Medicine, Diagnosis and Treatment*, 8th ed. Philadelphia, Lippincott, 1984
NEWBRUN E: *Cariology*, 3d ed. Chicago, Quintessence, 1989
WRIGHT BA et al: *Oral Cancer: Clinical and Pathological Considerations*. Boca Raton, Fla. CRC Press, 1988

42 DYSPHAGIA

RAJ K. GOYAL

Dysphagia is defined as a sensation of "sticking" or obstruction of the passage of food through the mouth, pharynx, or the esophagus.

Dysphagia should be distinguished from other symptoms related to swallowing. *Aphagia* signifies complete esophageal obstruction, which is usually due to bolus impaction and represents a medical emergency. *Difficulty in initiating a swallow* occurs in disorders of the voluntary phase of swallowing. Once initiated, however, swallowing is completed normally. *Odynophagia* means painful swallowing. Frequently, odynophagia and dysphagia occur together. *Globus hystericus* is the sensation of a lump lodged in the throat. No difficulty, however, is encountered when actual swallowing is performed. *Phagophobia*, meaning fear of swallowing, and *refusal to swallow* may occur in hysteria, rabies, tetanus, and pharyngeal paralysis due to fear of aspiration. Painful inflammatory lesions that cause odynophagia may also cause refusal to swallow. Some patients may feel the food as it goes down the esophagus. This esophageal sensitivity is not associated with sticking of the food or obstruction, however. Similarly, the *feeling of fullness in the epigastrium* that occurs after a meal or after swallowing air should not be confused with dysphagia.

PHYSIOLOGY OF SWALLOWING The process of swallowing begins with a voluntary (oral) phase during which a bolus of food is pushed backward into the pharynx. The bolus activates oropharyngeal sensory receptors which initiate the involuntary (pharyngeal and esophageal) phase, or deglutition reflex. The deglutition reflex is a complex series of events which serves both to propel food through the pharynx and the esophagus and to prevent its entry into the airway. At the same time as the bolus is propelled backward by the tongue, the larynx moves forward and the upper esophageal sphincter opens. As the bolus moves into the pharynx, contraction of the superior pharyngeal constrictor against the contracted soft palate initiates a peristaltic contraction that proceeds rapidly downward to move the bolus through the pharynx and the esophagus. The lower

esophageal sphincter opens as the food enters the esophagus and remains open until the peristaltic contraction has swept the bolus into the stomach. Peristaltic contraction in response to a swallow involves inhibition followed by sequential contraction of muscles along the entire swallowing passage and is called *primary peristalsis*. The inhibition that precedes the peristaltic contraction is called *deglutitive inhibition*. Local distention of the esophagus due to food activates intramural reflexes in the smooth muscle and results in *secondary peristalsis*, limited to the thoracic esophagus. *Tertiary contractions* are nonperistaltic as they occur simultaneously over a long segment of the esophagus. Tertiary contractions may occur in response to a swallow or esophageal distention, or they may occur spontaneously.

PATHOPHYSIOLOGY OF DYSPHAGIA The normal transport of an ingested bolus through the swallowing passage depends on (1) the size of the ingested bolus, (2) the luminal diameter of the swallowing passage, (3) the peristaltic contraction, and (4) deglutitive inhibition, including normal relaxation of upper and lower esophageal sphincters during swallowing. Dysphagia caused by a large bolus or luminal narrowing is called *mechanical dysphagia*, while dysphagia due to incoordination or weakness of peristaltic contractions or to impaired deglutitive inhibition is called *motor dysphagia*.

Mechanical dysphagia Mechanical dysphagia could be caused by a very large food bolus, intrinsic narrowing, or extrinsic compression of the lumen. In an adult, the esophageal lumen can distend up to a diameter of 4 cm because of the elasticity of the esophageal wall. When the esophagus cannot dilate beyond 2.5 cm in diameter, dysphagia can occur, but it is always present when it cannot distend beyond 1.3 cm. Circumferential lesions produce dysphagia more consistently than do lesions that involve only a portion of circumferences of the esophageal wall, as uninvolved segments retain their distensibility. The causes of mechanical dysphagia are listed in Table 42-1. Common causes include: (1) carcinoma, (2) peptic and other benign strictures, and (3) lower esophageal ring.

Motor dysphagia Motor dysphagia may result from difficulty in initiating a swallow or abnormalities in peristalsis and deglutitive inhibition due to diseases of the esophageal striated or smooth muscle.

Diseases of the striated muscle involve the pharynx, upper esophageal sphincter, and the upper part of the esophagus. The striated muscle is innervated by a somatic component of the vagus with cell bodies of the lower motor neurons located in the nucleus ambiguus. These neurons are cholinergic and excitatory and are the sole determinant of the muscle activity. Peristalsis in the striated muscle segment is due to sequential central activation of neurons innervating muscles at different levels along the esophagus. Motor dysphagia of the pharynx results from neuromuscular disorders causing muscle paralysis, simultaneous nonperistaltic contraction, or loss of opening of the upper esophageal sphincter. Loss of opening of the upper sphincter is caused by paralysis of geniohyoid and other suprahyoid muscles or loss of deglutitive inhibition of the cricopharyngeus muscle. Because each side of the pharynx is innervated by ipsilateral nerves, a lesion of motor neurons occurring only on one side leads to unilateral pharyngeal paralysis. Although lesions of striated muscle also involve the cervical part of the esophagus, the clinical manifestations of pharyngeal dysfunction usually overshadow the manifestations due to esophageal involvement.

Diseases of the smooth muscle segment involve the thoracic part of the esophagus and the lower esophageal sphincter. The smooth muscle is innervated by the parasympathetic component of the vagal preganglionic fibers and postganglionic neurons in the myenteric ganglia. These nerves exert a predominantly inhibitory influence on the lower esophageal sphincter and cause inhibition followed by contraction in the esophageal body. Peristalsis in this segment is due to neuromuscular mechanisms in the wall of the esophagus itself. Dysphagia results when the peristaltic contractions are weak or nonperistaltic or when the lower sphincter fails to open normally. Loss of contractile power occurs due to muscle weakness, as in scleroderma, or to loss of myenteric neurons, as in achalasia. The cause of nonperistaltic contractions, typically seen in diffuse esoph-

TABLE 42-1   Causes of dysphagia

Mechanical dysphagia	Motor (neuromuscular) dysphagia

I Luminal
  A Large bolus
  B Foreign body
II Intrinsic narrowing
  A Inflammatory condition causing edema and swelling
    1 Stomatitis
    2 Pharyngitis, epiglottitis
    3 Esophagitis
      a Viral (herpes simplex, varicella-zoster, cytomegalovirus)
      b Bacterial
      c Fungal (candidal)
      d Mucocutaneous bullous diseases
  B Webs and rings
    1 Pharyngeal (Plummer-Vinson syndrome)
    2 Esophageal (congenital, inflammatory)
    3 Lower esophageal mucosal ring (Schatzki ring)
  C Benign strictures
    1 Peptic
    2 Caustic and pill-induced
    3 Inflammatory (Crohn's disease, candidal, mucocutaneous lesions)
    4 Ischemic
    5 Postoperative, postirradiation
    6 Congenital
  D Malignant tumors
    1 Primary carcinoma
      a Squamous cell carcinoma
      b Adenocarcinoma
      c Carcinosarcoma
      d Pseudosarcoma
      e Lymphoma
      f Melanoma
      g Kaposi's sarcoma
    2 Metastatic carcinoma
  E Benign tumors
    1 Leiomyoma
    2 Lipoma
    3 Angioma
    4 Inflammatory fibroid polyp
    5 Epithelial papilloma
III Extrinsic compression
  A Cervical spondylitis
  B Vertebral osteophytes
  C Retropharyngeal abscess and masses
  D Enlarged thyroid gland
  E Zenker's diverticulum
  F Vascular compression
    1 Aberrant right subclavian artery
    2 Right-sided aorta
    3 Left atrial enlargement
    4 Aortic aneurysm
  G Posterior mediastinal masses
  H Pancreatic tumor, pancreatitis
  I Postvagotomy hematoma and fibrosis
	I Difficulty in initiating swallowing reflex
	  A Oral lesions and paralysis of tongue
	  B Oropharyngeal anesthesia
	  C Lack of saliva (e.g., Sjögren's syndrome)
	  D Lesions of sensory components of vagus and glossopharyngeal nerves
	  E Lesions of swallowing center
	II Disorders of pharyngeal and esophageal striated muscle
	  A Muscle weakness
	    1 Lower motor neuron lesion (bulbar paralysis)
	      a Cerebrovascular accident
	      b Motor neuron disease
	      c Poliomyelitis
	      d Polyneuritis
	      e Amyotrophic lateral sclerosis
	      f Familial dysautonomia
	    2 Neuromuscular
	      a Myasthenia gravis
	    3 Muscle disorders
	      a Polymyositis
	      b Dermatomyositis
	      c Myopathies (myotonic dystrophy, oculopharyngeal myopathy)
	  B Simultaneous onset contractions or impaired deglutitive inhibition
	    1 Pharynx and upper esophagus
	      a Rabies
	      b Tetanus
	      c Extrapyramidal tract disease
	      d Upper motor neuron lesions (pseudobulbar paralysis)
	    2 Upper esophageal sphincter (UES)
	      a Paralysis of suprahyoid muscles (causes same as paralysis of pharyngeal musculature)
	      b Cricopharyngeal achalasia
	III Disorders of esophageal smooth muscle
	  A Paralysis of esophageal body causing weak contractions
	    1 Scleroderma and related collagen vascular diseases
	    2 Hollow visceral myopathy
	    3 Myotonic dystrophy
	    4 Metabolic neuromyopathy (amyloid, alcohol?, diabetes?)
	    5 Achalasia (classical)
	  B Simultaneous-onset contractions or impaired deglutitive inhibition
	    1 Esophageal body
	      a Diffuse esophageal spasm
	      b Achalasia (vigorous)
	      c Variants of diffuse esophageal spasm
	    2 Lower esophageal sphincter
	      a Disorders of achalasia
	        (1) Primary
	        (2) Secondary
	          (a) Chagas' disease
	          (b) Carcinoma
	          (c) Lymphoma
	          (d) Neuropathic intestinal pseudoobstruction syndrome
	          (e) Toxins and drugs
	      b Lower esophageal muscular (contractile) ring

ageal spasm, is not understood. Impairment of deglutitive inhibition of the lower esophageal sphincter is associated with a defect in inhibitory nerves to the sphincter and is the major cause of dysphagia in achalasia.

The causes of motor dysphagia are listed in Table 42-1. The important causes are pharyngeal paralysis, cricopharyngeal achalasia, scleroderma of the esophagus, achalasia, diffuse esophageal spasm and related motor disorders.

APPROACH TO THE PATIENT WITH DYSPHAGIA   History   The history can provide a correct presumptive diagnosis in over 80 percent of patients. The type of food causing dysphagia provides useful information. Difficulty only with solids implies mechanical dysphagia with a lumen that is not severely narrowed. The impacted bolus may be forced through the narrowed area by drinking liquids. In advanced obstruction dysphagia occurs with liquids as well as solids. In contrast, motor dysphagia due to achalasia and diffuse esophageal spasm is equally affected by solids and liquids from the very onset. Patients with scleroderma have dysphagia to solids that is unrelated to posture and to liquids in the recumbent but not in the upright posture. When peptic stricture develops in these patients dysphagia becomes more persistent.

The duration and course of dysphagia are helpful in diagnosis. Transient dysphagia of short duration may be due to an inflammatory process. Progressive dysphagia of a few weeks' to a few months' duration is suggestive of carcinoma of the esophagus. Episodic dysphagia to solids of several years' duration indicates a benign disease and is characteristic of a lower esophageal ring.

The localization of dysphagia is helpful when it is described in the chest, where the site of dysphagia generally correlates with the site of esophageal obstruction. However, localization of dysphagia to the neck is of no diagnostic value because lesions of even the lower esophagus may cause dysphagia to be perceived in the neck.

Associated symptoms provide important diagnostic clues. Nasal regurgitation and tracheobronchial aspiration with swallowing are hallmarks of pharyngeal paralysis or a tracheoesophageal fistula. Tracheobronchial aspiration unrelated to swallowing may be secondary to achalasia, a Zenker's diverticulum, or gastroesophageal reflux. Severe weight loss out of proportion to the degree of dysphagia is highly suggestive of carcinoma. When hoarseness precedes dysphagia, the primary lesion is usually in the larynx. Hoarseness following dysphagia may suggest involvement of the recurrent laryngeal nerve by extension of esophageal carcinoma beyond the walls of the esophagus. Sometimes hoarseness may be due to laryngitis secondary to gastroesophageal reflux. Association of laryngeal symptoms and dysphagia also occurs in various neuromuscular disorders. Hiccups suggest a lesion in the distal portion of the esophagus. Unilateral wheezing with dysphagia indicates a mediastinal mass involving the esophagus and a large bronchus. Chest pain with dysphagia occurs in diffuse esophageal spasm and in related motor disorders. Chest pain resembling diffuse esophageal spasms also may occur in acute aphagia due to a large bolus. A prolonged history of heartburn and reflux preceding dysphagia indicates peptic stricture. Similarly, a history of prolonged nasogastric intubation, ingestion of caustic agents, ingestion of pills without water, previous radiation therapy, or associated mucocutaneous diseases may provide the cause of esophageal stricture. If odynophagia is present, candidal or herpes esophagitis should be suspected. In patients with AIDS or other immunodeficiency states, esophagitis due to opportunistic infections such as *candida*, herpes simplex virus, cytomegalovirus, and tumors such as Kaposi's sarcoma and lymphoma should be suspected.

Physical examination Physical examination is important in motor dysphagia due to skeletal muscle, neurologic, and oropharyngeal diseases. Signs of bulbar or pseudobulbar palsy, including dysarthria, dysphonia, ptosis, tongue atrophy, and hyperactive jaw jerk, in addition to evidence of generalized neuromuscular disease, should be carefully searched for. The neck should be examined for thyromegaly or a spinal abnormality. A careful inspection of the mouth and pharynx should disclose lesions that may cause interference with passage of food from the mouth or esophagus because of pain or obstruction. Changes in the skin and extremities may suggest a diagnosis of scleroderma and other collagen vascular diseases, or mucocutaneous diseases such as pemphigoid or epidermolysis bullosa which may involve the esophagus. Metastatic diseases to lymph nodes and liver may be evident. Pulmonary complications of acute aspiration pneumonia or chronic aspiration may be present.

Diagnostic procedures Dysphagia is one of the major symptoms of esophageal disease, and a cause for this symptom can invariably be determined. Therefore, all patients with dysphagia must be thoroughly investigated until a specific cause is determined. This is particularly important because the treatment depends upon the underlying cause of dysphagia. Barium swallow with cineradiography, esophagogastroscopy with biopsy and exfoliative cytology, and esophageal motility study are the main diagnostic procedures (see Chap. 237). The treatment is dependent upon the cause of dysphagia.

REFERENCES

CASTELL DO, JOHNSON LF (eds): *Esophageal Function in Health and Disease.* New York, Elsevier Biomedical, 1983

DURANCEAU A et al: Oropharyngeal dysphagia and operations on the upper esophageal sphincter. Surg Annu 19:317, 1987

ENTERLINE H, THOMPSON, J: *Pathology of the Esophagus.* New York, Springer-Verlag, 1984

FRIEDMAN SL, OWEN RL: Gastrointestinal manifestations of AIDS and other sexually transmitted diseases, in *Gastrointestinal Diseases*, MH Sleisenger, JS Fordtran (eds). Philadelphia, Saunders, 1989, pp 1250–1251

GIDDA JS, GOYAL RK: Regional gradient of initial inhibition and refractoriness in esophageal smooth muscle. Gastroenterology 89:843, 1985

GOYAL RK, PATERSON WG: Esophageal motility, in *Handbook of Physiology: Gastrointestinal System I. American Physiological Society* 1989, pp 865–908

OTT DJ: Radiologic evaluation of esophageal dysphagia. Curr Probl Diag Radiol 17:1, 1975

SCHULZE-DELNIEU K, CHRISTENSEN J: The esophagus, in *The Gastroenterology Annual*, F Kern, A Blum (eds). New York, Elsevier Science, 1984, pp 1–28

43 ANOREXIA, NAUSEA, VOMITING, AND INDIGESTION

LAWRENCE S. FRIEDMAN / KURT J. ISSELBACHER

ANOREXIA

Anorexia is a loss of appetite or lack of desire to eat. It must be differentiated from specific food intolerances and early satiety, a sense of fullness after the ingestion of a small amount of food. Anorexia is a prominent symptom in a wide variety of intestinal and extraintestinal disorders but as an isolated symptom is of little specific diagnostic value.

The mechanisms whereby hunger and appetite are modified in various disease states are poorly understood. Food intake is regulated by two hypothalamic centers—a lateral "feeding center" and a ventromedial "satiety center." The latter inhibits the feeding center following a meal, leading to the sensation of satiety. The brain-gut peptide cholecystokinin (CCK) appears to have a satiety effect and may be involved in the regulation of feeding behavior.

Anorexia is commonly seen in *diseases of the gastrointestinal tract and liver*. For example, it may precede the appearance of jaundice in acute hepatitis, or it may be a prominent symptom in gastric carcinoma. In the setting of intestinal disease, anorexia should be clearly differentiated from *sitophobia* (fear of eating because of subsequent abdominal discomfort). In such circumstances, appetite may persist, but the ingestion of food is curtailed nonetheless. Sitophobia may occur, for example, in regional enteritis (especially with partial obstruction) or in chronic mesenteric vascular insufficiency ("abdominal angina").

Anorexia may also be a prominent feature of *extraintestinal diseases*. Chronic pain from any source may lead to loss of appetite. Anorexia may be profound in severe congestive heart failure and may be a major symptom in patients with uremia, respiratory failure, and various endocrinopathies (e.g., hyperparathyroidism, Addison's disease, and panhypopituitarism). In patients with cancer, anorexia may result from anxiety, depression, pain, a decreased sense of taste and smell, the effect of the tumor on the gastrointestinal tract (e.g., partial intestinal obstruction) or liver (metastases), chemotherapeutic agents, and, possibly, the release of an anorectic substance by the tumor (possibly tumor necrosis factor). Medications such as antihypertensives, diuretics, digitalis, and narcotic analgesics may cause anorexia. Finally, anorexia often accompanies psychogenic disturbances such as depression and may result from emotional upset, boredom, or exposure to unpleasant sights, odors, or thoughts. For a discussion of anorexia nervosa, see Chap. 73.

NAUSEA AND VOMITING

Nausea and vomiting may occur independently of each other but generally are closely allied and are presumed to be mediated by the same neural pathways, so that they may be considered together. *Nausea* denotes the feeling of an imminent desire to vomit, usually referred to the throat or epigastrium. *Vomiting* (or emesis) refers to the forceful oral expulsion of gastric contents. *Retching* denotes the labored rhythmic contraction of respiratory and abdominal musculature that frequently precedes or accompanies vomiting.

Nausea often precedes or accompanies vomiting. It is usually associated with diminished functional activity of the stomach (e.g., hypotonicity, hypoperistalsis, and hyposecretion) and altered small-intestinal motility (e.g., hypertonicity and reversed peristalsis of the duodenum). Often accompanying severe nausea is evidence of altered autonomic (especially parasympathetic) activity, such as skin pallor, increased perspiration, hypersalivation, defecation, and, occasionally, hypotension and bradycardia (vasovagal syndrome); anorexia is also usually present.

Nausea, retching, and hypersalivation frequently precede the act of vomiting, which is a highly integrated sequence of involuntary visceral and somatic motor events. The stomach plays a relatively passive role in the vomiting process, the major ejection force being provided by the abdominal musculature. With relaxation of the gastric fundus and gastroesophageal sphincter, a sharp increase in intraabdominal pressure is brought about by forceful contraction of the diaphragm and abdominal wall muscles. This, together with concomitant annular contraction of the gastric pylorus, results in the expulsion of gastric contents into the esophagus. Increased intrathoracic pressure results in the further movement of esophageal contents into the mouth. Reversal of the normal direction of esophageal peristalsis may play a role in this process. Reflex elevation of the soft palate during the vomiting act prevents the entry of the expelled material into the nasopharynx, whereas reflex closure of the glottis and inhibition of respiration help to prevent pulmonary aspiration.

Repeated emesis may have deleterious effects in a number of ways. The process of vomiting, if forceful, may lead to pressure rupture of the esophagus (Boerhaave's syndrome) or to linear mucosal (Mallory-Weiss) tears in the region of the cardioesophageal junction with resulting hematemesis. Prolonged vomiting may lead to dehydration, the loss of gastric secretions (especially hydrochloric acid) resulting in metabolic alkalosis with hypokalemia, malnutrition with various deficiency states, and dental caries. In states of central nervous system depression (e.g., coma), gastric contents may be aspirated into the lungs, with a resulting aspiration pneumonitis.

VOMITING MECHANISM   The act of vomiting is under the control of two functionally distinct medullary centers: the *vomiting center* in the dorsal portion of the lateral reticular formation and the *chemoreceptor trigger zone* in the area postrema of the floor of the fourth ventricle. The vomiting center controls and integrates the actual act of emesis. It receives afferent stimuli from the gastrointestinal tract and other parts of the body, from higher brainstem and cortical centers, especially the labyrinthine apparatus, and from the chemoreceptor trigger zone. Persons vary considerably in the threshold of their vomiting centers to different stimuli. The important efferent pathways in vomiting are the phrenic nerves (to the diaphragm), the spinal nerves (to the intercostal and abdominal musculature), and visceral efferent fibers in the vagus nerve (to the larynx, pharynx, esophagus, and stomach). The vomiting center is located near other medullary centers regulating respiratory, vasomotor, and autonomic functions that may be involved in the act of vomiting.

The chemoreceptor trigger zone by itself is incapable of mediating the act of vomiting; rather activation of this zone results in efferent impulses to the medullary vomiting center, which in turn initiates emesis. The chemoreceptor trigger zone is an emetic chemoreceptor that can be activated by a variety of stimuli or drugs, including apomorphine and other opiates, levodopa (after decarboxylation to dopamine), digitalis, bacterial toxins, radiation, and metabolic abnormalities as occur with uremia and hypoxia.

CLINICAL CLASSIFICATION   Nausea and vomiting are common manifestations of many organic and functional disorders. The precise mechanisms triggering vomiting in various clinical conditions are not well understood, making classification of mechanisms difficult.

Many *acute abdominal emergencies* which lead to the "surgical abdomen" are associated with nausea and vomiting. Vomiting may be seen with inflammation of a viscus, as in acute appendicitis or acute cholecystitis, intestinal obstruction, or acute peritonitis (see Chap. 246).

Other *disorders of the alimentary tract*, including those associated with chronic indigestion (see below), are frequently accompanied by nausea and vomiting. In peptic ulcer, emesis may be either spontaneous or self-induced and may lead to relief of symptoms, particularly if antral or pyloric edema has resulted in gastric outlet obstruction. Nausea and vomiting are also prominent in patients with disordered gastrointestinal motility, including postvagotomy, diabetic, or idio-

pathic gastroparesis (gastric atony), other gastric "dysrhythmias" resulting from abnormal myoelectric activity, and intestinal pseudo-obstruction due to abnormal intestinal myogenic or neurogenic function. Gastroparesis may be demonstrated by gastric scanning after a radiolabeled meal or by radiography after ingestion of indigestible radiopaque solid markers. Experimentally, some patients with otherwise unexplained nausea and vomiting have been demonstrated to have accelerated ("tachygastria") or irregular ("gastric tachyarrhythmia") gastric electrical activity as measured by electrodes implanted surgically on the serosa of the stomach or placed on the abdominal surface ("electrogastrogram"). Typically intestinal obstruction of any cause (e.g., adhesions, malignancy, hernia, volvulus) leads to vomiting, as do other disorders of the liver, pancreas, and biliary tract. Nausea and vomiting may accompany the distention and pain seen in the aerophagic syndromes (see below).

Viral, bacterial, and parasitic *infections of the intestinal tract* are typically associated with severe nausea and vomiting, often with diarrhea. *Acute systemic infections* with fever, especially in young children, are also frequently accompanied by vomiting and often by severe diarrhea. The mechanism whereby infections remote from the gastrointestinal tract produce these manifestations may relate to stimulation of the medullary chemoreceptor trigger zone by toxins or abnormal metabolites.

Central nervous system disorders which lead to increased intracranial pressure (e.g., neoplasms, encephalitis, hydrocephalus) may be accompanied by vomiting, which is often *projectile* (intensely forceful). Vertigo due to disorders of the labyrinthine apparatus, such as acute labyrinthitis and Ménière's disease, may be accompanied by vomiting with nausea and retching. Similarly, motion sickness is typically associated with anorexia, nausea, and vomiting as well as apathy, increased salivation, cold sweating, and headache. Additionally, migraine headaches, tabetic crises, acute meningitis, and the reactive phase of hypotension with syncope may be associated with nausea and vomiting.

Nausea and vomiting may be present in *acute myocardial infarction*, especially when posterior in location or transmural in extent, and in *congestive heart failure*, perhaps in relation to congestion of the liver. The possibility that these symptoms may also be due to drugs (e.g., opiates or digitalis) should always be borne in mind in patients with cardiac disease. Nausea and vomiting are common in cancer patients, especially those who are terminally ill.

Nausea and vomiting commonly accompany several *metabolic and endocrinologic disorders*, including uremia, diabetic ketoacidosis, hypo- and hyperparathyroidism, hyperthyroid crisis, and adrenal insufficiency, especially adrenal crisis. The morning sickness of early pregnancy is another instance of nausea and vomiting possibly related to hormonal changes; the term *hyperemesis gravidarum* is applied when fluid and electrolyte disturbances or nutritional deficiency results.

The *side effects of many drugs and chemicals* include nausea and vomiting. In some cases drugs have central emetic effects, as with digitalis, morphine, histamine, and some chemotherapeutic agents. In other cases drug-induced gastric irritation leads to stimulation of the medullary vomiting center, as with salicylates, aminophylline, and ipecac. The ingestion of a toxin (e.g., food poisoning) may also cause acute vomiting.

Psychogenic vomiting refers to chronic or recurrent vomiting which may result from an emotional or psychological disturbance. Often patients with emotional disorders and chronic vomiting maintain a relatively normal state of nutrition because only a relatively small amount of the ingested food is vomited. In some cases regurgitation rather than vomiting may predominate, and the degree of weight loss may be out of proportion to the patient's description of the frequency and severity of vomiting. As discussed in Chap. 73, anorexia nervosa and bulimia are emotional disturbances which may be associated with vomiting and weight loss.

DIFFERENTIAL DIAGNOSIS   Vomiting should be distinguished from *regurgitation*, which refers to the expulsion of food in the absence of nausea and without the abdominal diaphragmatic muscular contraction associated with vomiting. Regurgitation of esophageal contents may occur with esophageal strictures or diverticula. Regurgitation of gastric contents is generally seen with gastroesophageal sphincter incompetence, especially with hiatus hernia and gastroesophageal reflux, with pyloric spasm or obstruction due to peptic ulcer, or with gastroparesis. *Rumination* is the regurgitation, rechewing, and reswallowing of food from the stomach, one mouthful at a time; psychological factors are thought to play a role.

The temporal relationship of vomiting to eating may be of help diagnostically. Vomiting that occurs predominantly in the morning is often seen early in pregnancy and in uremia. Alcoholic gastritis is also commonly accompanied by early morning retching and emesis, the so-called dry heaves. Vomiting that occurs during or shortly after eating may suggest psychogenic vomiting or peptic ulcer with pylorospasm. Vomiting that occurs 4 to 6 h or longer after eating and involves the elimination of large quantities of undigested food often indicates gastric retention (e.g., pyloric obstruction, gastroparesis) or certain esophageal disorders (achalasia, Zenker's diverticulum). Vomiting that is projectile or without antecedent nausea suggests the possibility of a central nervous system lesion.

Associated symptoms may also provide diagnostic clues. For example, vertigo and tinnitus indicate the possibility of Ménière's disease. A long history of vomiting with little or no weight loss suggests psychogenic vomiting. Relief of abdominal pain with vomiting is typical of peptic ulcer. Early satiety is typical of gastroparesis.

The character of the vomitus also offers clues to the diagnosis. If the vomitus contains large amounts of free hydrochloric acid, gastric outlet obstruction due to an ulcer or a hypersecretory state such as Zollinger-Ellison syndrome should be considered. Absence of free hydrochloric acid is more compatible with gastric malignancy. A feculent or putrid odor reflects the results of bacterial action on the intestinal contents and may occur with distal intestinal obstruction, peritonitis, or gastrocolic fistula. Bile is commonly present in gastric contents whenever vomiting is prolonged; it has no significance unless constantly present in large quantities, when it may signify an obstructing lesion below the ampulla of Vater. The presence of blood in the gastric contents usually denotes bleeding from the esophagus, stomach, or duodenum.

TREATMENT Effective therapy of nausea and vomiting usually depends on correction of the underlying cause. *Antiemetic agents* vary in their usefulness depending on the cause of the symptoms, responsiveness of the patient, and occurrence of side effects. *Antihistamines* such as dimenhydrinate and promethazine hydrochloride are effective for the control of nausea and vomiting due to inner ear dysfunction; they do not act on the chemoreceptor trigger zone and are of little value in other causes of vomiting. *Anticholinergics* such as scopolamine are also effective in motion sickness. *Phenothiazine* derivatives such as prochlorperazine and the structurally related butyrophenone haloperidol inhibit cerebral dopamine receptors and act principally at the chemoreceptor trigger zone. They are often ineffective for severe nausea and vomiting and have the potential for causing sedation, hypotension, and Parkinson-like effects. *Metoclopramide* is the prototype of selective dopamine antagonists called *substituted benzamides*. In contrast to the phenothiazines, which have anticholinergic effects, metoclopramide has powerful peripheral cholinergic effects that enhance gastric emptying. Metoclopramide may be superior to phenothiazines in the treatment of severe nausea and vomiting and is particularly useful in the treatment of gastroparesis. The usual oral dosage is 5 to 20 mg four times daily, but intravenous doses up to 1 to 3 mg/kg may be effective as prophylaxis prior to potent chemotherapeutic agents (e.g., cisplatin). Unfortunately, neurologic side effects are frequent, including muscle spasm, tremor, parkinsonism, and confusion. Experimental agents (not yet licensed for use in the United States) such as *domperidone* and *cisapride* exert peripheral antiemetic effects without the central nervous system side effects of metoclopramide. *Tetrahydrocannabinol*, the active ingredient of marijuana, is marketed as dronabinal for the prevention of nausea and vomiting after cancer chemotherapy; the mechanism of action is unknown.

INDIGESTION

Indigestion is a term frequently used by patients to describe a variety of symptoms generally appreciated as distress associated with the intake of food. The term is nonspecific and may not have the same meaning for the patient and physician. Thus, in approaching the patient with indigestion, it is important for the physician first to elicit a precise description of this complaint. To some patients indigestion refers to actual abdominal pain, pressure, or heartburn. Others may use the term to describe either a vague feeling that digestion has not proceeded naturally or intolerances to specific foods. Still others may use it to describe belching, a feeling of excessive gas, or flatulence. The term *dyspepsia* has often been used interchangeably with indigestion but is increasingly used to refer specifically to upper abdominal pain or discomfort typical of (but not necessarily due to) peptic ulcer.

After having ascertained the patient's definition of indigestion, it is important to determine (1) the location and duration of the discomfort, (2) the temporal relation of the symptoms to the ingestion of food, and (3) the possible relation of the symptoms to the ingestion of specific types of food (e.g., milk, fatty foods) or drugs.

Indigestion may occur in association with diseases of the gastrointestinal tract or pathologic states in other organ systems. As a result of a systematic clinical and laboratory investigation, a definable pathophysiologic process sometimes can be shown to be responsible for the symptoms in a given case of indigestion. Frequently, however, a clear etiologic explanation for the patient's complaint of indigestion cannot be established. If the symptoms are typical of peptic ulcer, but an ulcer is not found, the designation *nonulcer dyspepsia* may be applied. Other cases may be designated as "functional indigestion," with the implication that psychosomatic factors underlie the complaint. Although it is evident that psychological factors may lead to symptoms of indigestion, the designation of "functional indigestion" is rarely a satisfactory explanation, serving only to rephrase the patient's description of the symptoms. Moreover, on the basis of electrophysiologic studies, some cases of functional indigestion, including some cases of nonulcer dyspepsia, appear to result from subtle disturbances of gastrointestinal motility. Indeed, some patients with functional indigestion also have features of the irritable bowel syndrome, suggesting a diffuse intestinal motility disturbance (see Chap. 242).

SYNDROMES COMMONLY DESCRIBED AS INDIGESTION Pain A careful elucidation of the pattern of pain may provide important diagnostic information. Visceral abdominal pain is mediated by visceral afferent nerves which accompany the abdominal sympathetic pathways (see Chap. 17). Visceral pain is described as dull and aching in nature, with a diffuse midline localization, or as fullness or pressure. The location of the discomfort generally corresponds to the segmental level of neural innervation of the affected organ. Abdominal visceral pain can be produced experimentally by artificially increasing pressure in a hollow viscus and results from distention or exaggerated muscular contraction of the viscus. Inflammation generally lowers the threshold for pain from such stimuli.

The visceral pain of indigestion should be distinguished from the sharp, localized pain patterns of many acute abdominal processes involving the peritoneum. In contrast to visceral pain, this somatic pain is mediated by cerebrospinal afferent nerves.

In view of the diffuse nature of visceral abdominal pain, the main clue to the cause comes from the *location* of the pain and the corresponding segmental level of neural innervation; however, in any given segmental region there is no way of determining which of several viscera is the source of the pain (Table 43-1). The following rules, already described in Chap. 17, are useful: *Substernal pain* of gastrointestinal origin usually arises from disorders of the esophagus

TABLE 43-1   Distribution of visceral pain and examples of disorders frequently involving the specific organ

Organ	Location of pain	Examples of disorders
Esophagus	Substernum, epigastrium	Peptic esophagitis, stricture, esophageal spasm, carcinoma
Stomach	Epigastrium	Gastritis, gastric ulcer, carcinoma
Duodenum (first and second portions)	Epigastrium	Duodenal ulcer
Small intestine (excluding first and second portions of duodenum)	Periumbilical region	Infectious gastroenteritis, regional enteritis, lymphoma, intestinal obstruction
Gallbladder	Epigastrium, right upper quadrant, right upper back	Cholelithiasis, cholecystitis
Pancreas	Epigastrium, left upper quadrant, left side of back	Pancreatitis, pancreatic carcinoma
Liver	Right upper quadrant	Hepatitis, cirrhosis, passive congestion
Colon	Below umbilicus	Infectious colitis, ulcerative colitis, carcinoma, partial obstruction

or cardia of the stomach. Because pain in this area can emanate from the heart, cardiac disease must be carefully considered and excluded. *Epigastric pain* is generally of gastric, duodenal, biliary, or pancreatic origin. (The epigastrium is also a frequent location for "functional" pain.) As pathologic processes in the biliary tract or pancreas become more intense, pain may lateralize and localize, e.g., biliary pain to the right upper quadrant and tip of the scapula and pancreatic pain to the left upper quadrant and back. *Periumbilical pain* is generally associated with disease involving the small intestine. *Pain below the umbilicus* is often of appendiceal, colonic, or pelvic origin.

The unraveling of the *temporal relationships* of the patient's symptoms often provides additional diagnostic clues. It is important to ascertain whether the symptoms are *constant* (continually present over extended periods of time), as may occur with an infiltrating gastric carcinoma, or *intermittent*, as in acute gastritis or biliary colic. The symptoms may have a *diurnal* pattern, as in reflux esophagitis in which pain often occurs nocturnally and with recumbency. Pain that awakens the patient from a sound sleep may occur with duodenal ulcer. Occasionally symptoms are *seasonal*, as in peptic ulcer disease, in which some patients experience more discomfort in the spring and autumn than at other times.

Another helpful diagnostic feature is the relation of pain to *food ingestion*. Early postprandial symptoms may reflect esophageal disease, acute gastritis, or gastric carcinoma. Late postprandial indigestion, i.e., occurring several hours after eating, may reflect failure of the stomach to empty adequately, as in gastric outlet obstruction, gastroparesis and other disorders of gastric motility, or duodenal ulcer, in which case pain results from exposure of ulcerated mucosa to acid secreted by the stomach and unbuffered by food. Conversely, the relief of pain following ingestion of food or antacids is characteristic of duodenal ulcer and is presumably due to the neutralization of acid. Late postprandial indigestion also may result from impaired digestive and absorptive processes, as in pancreatic insufficiency.

It is important to recognize that the pain patterns and relationships to the intake of food described above are generalizations, and many cases do not conform to classic "textbook" descriptions. For example, although pain limited to the right upper quadrant is often caused by gallbladder disease, about half of patients with this condition experience only epigastric pain. Similarly, there are some patients with peptic ulcer whose pain is not relieved by food or antacids; there are

other patients with functional indigestion and even gastric carcinoma whose pain improves with food or antacids.

Nonulcer dyspepsia   Nonulcer dyspepsia (also referred to as *idiopathic* or *essential dyspepsia*) refers to symptoms that suggest a diagnosis of peptic ulcer despite the absence of an ulcer by endoscopy or barium x-ray studies and the absence of any other demonstrable organic disorder (e.g., biliary tract disease) or evidence of the irritable bowel syndrome to account for the symptoms. Nonulcer dyspepsia is twice as common as peptic ulcer and may affect up to 20 to 30 percent of the population. The pathogenesis is poorly understood; most patients with nonulcer dyspepsia have normal gastric acid secretion, and a relation between nonulcer dyspepsia and duodenitis or duodenal ulcer has not been demonstrated. Similarly, the role of *Helicobacter pylori* and associated chronic gastritis in causing dyspeptic symptoms in persons without peptic ulcer is uncertain (see Chap. 238). A role for disordered gastroduodenal and small-intestinal motility in nonulcer dyspepsia has been suggested but requires further investigation. In contrast to peptic ulcer, nonulcer dyspepsia improves inconsistently following antacids and other standard ulcer therapy.

Heartburn   Heartburn, or pyrosis, is a sensation of warmth or burning located substernally or high in the epigastrium with radiation into the neck and occasionally to the arms. Occasional heartburn is common in normal persons, but frequent and severe heartburn is generally a manifestation of esophageal dysfunction. Heartburn may result from abnormal motor activity or distention of the esophagus, reflux of acid or bile into the esophagus, or direct esophageal mucosal irritation (esophagitis).

Heartburn is most often associated with gastroesophageal reflux (see Chap. 237). In this setting, heartburn typically occurs after a large meal, with stooping or bending, or when the patient is supine. It may be accompanied by the spontaneous appearance in the mouth of fluid which may be salty ("water brash"), sour (gastric contents), or bitter and green or yellow (bile). Heartburn may arise following the ingestion of certain foods (e.g., citrus fruit juices) or drugs (e.g., alcohol and aspirin). Characteristically heartburn is alleviated promptly, even if only temporarily, by antacids.

Heartburn may also occur in the absence of a demonstrable anatomic or physiologic condition. In this setting, it is frequently accompanied by aerophagia, which may represent an attempt by the patient to relieve discomfort, and is often attributed to psychological factors for lack of other explanations.

Food intolerance   In some persons specific foods or types of foods appear to be related to indigestion. Careful documentation of this relationship is sometimes of great help in arriving at an etiologic diagnosis.

Some foods may be poorly tolerated because of their consistency. Patients with esophageal stricture or carcinoma may tolerate liquids well but may experience discomfort, especially substernal distress, after ingesting solids (see Chaps. 42 and 237). Citrus fruits, with their relatively low pH, often provoke symptoms in patients with peptic ulcer disease or peptic esophagitis. Certain foods may be tolerated poorly because of impaired intestinal digestion or absorption, as with the ingestion of fatty foods in patients with pancreatic or biliary tract disease.

Patients may have a congenital or acquired *deficiency of a specific enzyme* required for intestinal absorption of a certain nutrient. One example is the deficiency of lactase, the intestinal mucosal enzyme which catalyzes the hydrolysis of lactose. In persons who are lactase-deficient, the ingestion of milk (which contains lactose) results in abdominal cramps, distention, diarrhea, and flatulence (Chap. 240). Certain nutrients may lead to profound systemic effects because of *biochemical defects* in the patient that render the substances particularly hazardous, as in galactose intolerance in persons with galactosemia (see Chap. 337).

Some foods may initiate *allergic reactions*, which should be suspected when symptoms occur immediately after ingestion of the food, recur on challenge testing, and are associated with other features of an allergic reaction, such as lip swelling, urticaria, angioedema, asthma, or, rarely, anaphylactic shock. Other foods may exert *toxic effects* on the intestine in susceptible persons (e.g., gluten in patients with celiac sprue).

In many instances we do not understand the mechanism by which indigestion is associated with the ingestion of specific foods. Thus, a history of fatty food intolerance or distress after eating spicy foods is commonly obtained from patients with indigestion; however, the mechanisms leading to these symptoms in these circumstances are often unclear.

Aerophagia Patients with a complaint of *chronic, repetitive eructation* (belching) can usually be observed to precede each belch with a swallow of air, most of which passes only partway down the esophagus and is then regurgitated. Thus, excessive eructation results from *aerophagia*, or air swallowing, not from excessive gas production in the stomach or the intestine. A degree of aerophagia occurs in normal persons, but some individuals gulp air excessively because of chronic anxiety, rapid eating, drinking carbonated beverages, gum chewing, postnasal drip, poorly fitting dentures, or esophageal speech. Because eructation which follows aerophagia may provide a temporary sense of relief to the patient, a vicious cycle of aerophagia and eructation may ensue.

About 20 to 60 percent of intestinal gas represents swallowed air. Because nitrogen and oxygen are the only gases present in the atmosphere in appreciable concentrations and because they are not produced in the gastrointestinal tract, their detection on chromatographic analysis of intestinal gas indicates that swallowed air is the source. Swallowed air that is not eructated passes into the stomach and intestine. Accumulation of swallowed air in the stomach may lead to postprandial fullness and pressure and the finding by x-ray of a large amount of air in the gastric fundus. This symptom complex, referred to as the *magenblase* (i.e., gastric bubble) *syndrome,* may occur when a patient lies supine after a large meal, thereby permitting gastric air to be "trapped" below the gastroesophageal junction by overlying fluid and unable to be eructated. Inability to eructate is also thought to underlie the "gas-bloat" syndrome observed after surgical repair of a hiatal hernia. Acute gastric distention by swallowed air can sometimes produce sharp pains which may mimic angina pectoris. Swallowed air which successfully passes the stomach may either produce diffuse abdominal distention or become trapped in the splenic flexure of the colon. The latter condition, or *splenic flexure syndrome,* is characterized by a sensation of left upper quadrant fullness and pressure with radiation to the left side of the chest. Relief of pain often follows defecation or the expulsion of flatus. The diagnosis is suggested by the finding of increased tympany in the extreme left lateral portion of the upper abdomen on physical examination or of large amounts of air in the splenic flexure of the colon on a plain abdominal radiograph.

Gaseousness, bloating, and flatulence Despite the widely held belief that feelings of *diffuse abdominal pain and bloating* are often caused by excessive quantities of intestinal gas, studies employing an intestinal gas wash-out technique suggest that patients complaining of excessive gas have normal volumes of intestinal gas. The primary abnormality causing functional bloating and pain in such persons appears to be a motility disturbance that causes the patient to perceive pain with an intestinal gas volume that is well tolerated by normal subjects. Alternatively, intestinal motility may be normal in such persons, but they may be excessively responsive to normal impulses arising from the intestinal tract.

A major source of intestinal gas is the fermentative action of intestinal bacteria on carbohydrates and proteins within the lumen. Normally such bacteria are limited to the colon, and the principal gases produced are carbon dioxide and hydrogen (in addition to minute quantities of odoriferous gases—indole, skatols, and sulfur-containing compounds—which give flatus its characteristic odor). In the upper small bowel carbon dioxide is also produced when hydrochloric acid from the stomach or ingested fatty acids are neutralized by bicarbonate. (This may explain, in part, indigestion associated with fatty foods.) About one-third of adults produce

appreciable quantities of methane in the colon; this appears to be a familial trait and unrelated to food ingestion.

An increase in intraluminal gas production resulting in *abdominal distention, bloating, and flatulence* occurs following the ingestion of certain foods, such as legumes and some grains, which contain significant quantities of nonabsorbable carbohydrates that pass into the colon where they supply gas-forming substrates for colonic bacteria. The best-studied example of this is beans, which contain oligosaccharides (stachyose and raffinose) that cannot be split by intestinal mucosal enzymes but are metabolized by colonic bacteria. Increased intraluminal gas production may also result from abnormal bacterial colonization of the small intestine (bacterial overgrowth syndrome) or infection with *Giardia lamblia*.

Indigestion due to extraintestinal disease A number of extraintestinal diseases may lead to indigestion. Thus, indigestion may be prominent in congestive heart failure, pulmonary tuberculosis, neoplastic disease, and uremia. Also, a variety of drugs such as aspirin, nonsteroidal anti-inflammatory agents, and glucocorticoids may cause indigestion because of their ulcerogenic properties.

DIAGNOSTIC APPROACH TO THE PATIENT WITH INDIGESTION Indigestion represents a challenging and difficult diagnostic problem because of its nonspecific nature. It is essential to obtain a clear and detailed description of the specific symptoms, particularly the patient's definition of the term indigestion. The nature of the distress, its frequency and time of occurrence, its relationship to meals, and the special circumstances which lead to its exacerbation or relief should be elicited. Associated intestinal symptoms such as nausea and vomiting, abnormal bowel habits, diarrhea, steatorrhea, and melena should be sought, and an assessment of nutritional status, appetite, and changes in weight should be made. A careful history should also include an assessment of the patient's general health, including the possible presence of extraintestinal disorders which may produce indigestion. A careful evaluation of psychological factors is crucial, because they often play an etiologic or contributory role; of particular importance are anxiety, depressive symptoms, and hysteria.

Physical examination rarely establishes the specific diagnosis but may be useful in detecting diseases in other organ systems which can affect intestinal function (e.g., congestive heart failure). Stools should be examined for appearance and occult blood.

Whether further diagnostic studies are indicated depends on the specific nature of the patient's complaints and the patient's age (concern about the possibility of gastrointestinal malignancy being greater in older patients). Abdominal pain may be evaluated with radiologic and imaging studies of the esophagus, stomach, small intestine, colon, pancreas, and biliary tract. Esophagogastroscopy, endoscopic cholangiopancreatography, sigmoidoscopy, or colonoscopy may also be helpful or necessary. On the other hand, in patients under age 40 with epigastric pain typical of peptic ulcer, routine diagnostic studies are unlikely to disclose serious diseases (such as gastric carcinoma) and are often in fact negative; thus, an empiric trial of antacids, H-2-receptor-blocking drugs, or sucralfate may be appropriate. Esophagogastroscopy may be reserved for patients with symptoms that persist despite therapy or that recur soon after therapy is discontinued. In patients with *C. pylori* on endoscopic antral biopsy, a trial of bismuth subsalicylate or an oral antibiotic active against *C. pylori* (or both) may be considered. In individuals complaining of excessive eructation, a simple demonstration that aerophagia reproduces the symptoms may suffice to confirm the diagnosis and hopefully break the habit. Patients complaining of excessive gas, bloating, distention, and flatulence must be questioned carefully about dietary preferences and the relation of symptoms to ingestion of specific foods. In some cases elimination of certain foods (e.g., milk, legumes) from the diet followed by rechallenge may be confirmatory. In other cases a more detailed assessment, including stool examination for fat and muscle fibers and for parasites such as *G. lamblia*, breath tests to detect carbohydrate malabsorption, and gastrointestinal motility studies, may be desirable. The therapeutic value of activated charcoal in reducing gaseousness associated with carbohydrate malabsorption is uncertain.

In many cases of indigestion no clear explanation is obtained, even after careful diagnostic studies and therapeutic trials. Some cases represent nonulcer dyspepsia or intestinal motility disturbances, perhaps due to subtle physiologic derangements not detectable by currently available methods. In some such instances, an empiric trial of dopamine antagonists (e.g., metoclopramide) which augment gastrointestinal motility may be beneficial. Other cases represent early stages of actual disease processes which may only be diagnosed by conventional methods at a later date. Still others are psychogenic and may respond to appropriate psychiatric measures. The ultimate evaluation of indigestion requires, therefore, the utmost in sensitivity, diligence, and concern on the part of the examining physician.

REFERENCES

FELDMAN M: Nausea and vomiting, in *Gastrointestinal Disease*, 4th ed, MH Sleisenger, JS Fordtran (eds). Philadelphia, Saunders, 1989, pp 222–238

HANSON JS, McCALLUM RW: The diagnosis and management of nausea and vomiting. Am J Gastroenterol 80:210, 1985

HEALTH AND PUBLIC POLICY COMMITTEE, AMERICAN COLLEGE OF PHYSICIANS: Endoscopy in the evaluation of dyspepsia. Ann Intern Med 102:266, 1985

HEATLEY RV, RATHBONE BJ: Dyspepsia: A dilemma for doctors? Lancet ii:779, 1987

LEVITT MD, BOND JH: Intestinal gas, in *Gastrointestinal Disease*, 4th ed, MH Sleisenger, JS Fordtran (eds). Philadelphia, Saunders, 1989, pp 257–263

MALAGELADA J-R, CAMILLERI M: Unexplained vomiting: A diagnostic challenge. Ann Intern Med 101:211, 1984

TALLEY NJ, PHILLIPS SF: Non-ulcer dyspepsia: Potential causes and pathophysiology. Ann Intern Med 108:865, 1988

VANTRAPPEN G et al: Gastrointestinal motility disorders. Dig Dis Sci 31:5S, 1986

44   CONSTIPATION AND DIARRHEA

STEPHEN E. GOLDFINGER

NORMAL COLONIC FUNCTION   Each day approximately 9 L of fluid enters the digestive tract; 2 L represents ingested fluids and the remainder comes from salivary, gastric, biliary, pancreatic, and intestinal secretions that are needed to provide an appropriate milieu for food digestion. Most of this fluid is absorbed in the upper bowel. Approximately 1 L containing undigested dietary residue and cellular debris passes across the ileocecal valve to the colon. Little of nutritional value remains following the extensive digestive processing and absorption that occurs in the small intestine. The colon's principal function is to convert this liquid ileal effluent to solid feces before it is advanced to the rectum and evacuated. Several important physiologic processes underlie normal colonic function; among these are *absorption* of fluid and electrolytes; *peristaltic contractions* that facilitate mixing, desiccation, and passage of feces to the rectum; and, finally, *defecation*.

Absorption of fluid and electrolytes (See also Chap. 240)   In western societies where dietary fiber content is relatively low, the average daily stool weight is less than 200 g, of which 60 to 80 percent is water. Thus, the colon normally absorbs approximately 80 to 90 percent of the fluid it receives, and this occurs well within its absorptive capacity of 6 L water and 800 mmol sodium per day. Fluid and electrolyte absorption occurs primarily in the ascending and transverse colon. Water absorption occurs passively, osmotically following the active transport of sodium and chloride ions. In addition, bicarbonate is secreted in exchange for chloride. The secreted bicarbonate is converted, in part, to carbon dioxide by reacting with acids produced by colonic bacteria.

The term *diarrhea* generally connotes *frequent* or *loose* stools. Based on physiologic events described above, diarrhea may be defined more quantitatively as a fecal output exceeding 200 g per day when dietary fiber content is low. Diarrhea can be further classified on the basis of underlying mechanisms (see Table 44-1). In *secretory diarrhea*, fecal fluid rich in sodium and potassium is lost as a consequence of impaired absorption and/or excessive secretion of electrolytes by the bowel. In *osmotic diarrhea*, absorption of water is decreased by the osmotic effect of nonabsorbable, intraluminal molecules. *Exudative diarrhea* is caused by an outpouring of necrotic mucosa, colloid, fluid, and electrolytes from an inflamed colon which, in addition, is less able to carry out its normal absorptive function. Increased amounts of arachidonic acid metabolites present in inflamed mucosa may also promote increased ion secretion. *Anatomic derangements* of the bowel and *motility disorders* cause diarrhea by reducing the surface area or the contact time necessary for adequate absorption to occur.

Colonic innervation and motility   The colon and rectum are innervated by fibers that release norepinephrine, acetylcholine, and a variety of other neurotransmitters. Signals transmitted by autonomic nervous system fibers originating centrally, local reflex arcs confined to the autonomous "enteric nervous system," and intrinsic contractile responses of smooth muscle all play a part in the coordination of colonic motility. Parasympathetic nerves, which stimulate peristaltic contraction as well as electrolyte secretion, dominate the neurogenic regulation of colonic motor activity; adrenergic tone inhibits cholinergic stimulation and also increases electrolyte absorption. The precise integration of all neural and nonneural mediators of colonic motility and ion transport remains poorly understood.

The basal motor activity of the colon corresponds to the function of its various segments. In the ascending colon, where most fluid absorption occurs, rhythmic, retrograde contractions occur to prolong fecal contact time. In the midcolon, segmental contractions continue the process of absorption while feces are gradually advanced to the left colon. The most distal portion of the colon, which is under the greatest neurogenic control, propels feces caudally in preparation for defecation. In addition, massive peristalsis occurs several times per day.

Since colonic motility plays an important role in both absorption and movement of contents to the rectum, alterations of bowel tone occurring as a result of disease, stress, or various drugs tend to have an important influence on bowel movements. In view of the number of pharmacologic agents that may influence smooth muscle contractility, it is essential to take a careful drug history when evaluating patients with constipation or diarrhea of recent onset.

TABLE 44-1   Classification of diarrhea

Type	Mechanism	Stool characteristics	Examples
Secretory	↑ Secretion of electrolytes ↓ Absorption of electrolytes	Clear Negative osmotic gap* No polymorphs	Cholera Diarrheogenic islet cell tumors Bile salt enteropathy
Exudative	Impaired colonic absorption; outpouring of cells and colloid	Purulent Polymorphs present Gross or occult blood	Ulcerative colitis Shigellosis Amebiasis
Decreased absorption			
Osmotic	Nonabsorbable intraluminal molecules	Clear High osmotic gap* No polymorphs	Lactase deficiency Mg^{2+}-containing cathartics
Anatomic derangement	Decreased absorption surface	Variable	Subtotal colectomy Gastrocolic fistula
Motility disorder	Decreased contact time	Variable	Hyperthyroidism Irritable bowel syndrome

* See Shiau et al.

Defecation The defecatory reflex is initiated by acute distention of the rectum. When it is allowed to progress by supraspinal centers, sigmoidal and rectal contractions heighten the pressure within the rectum and also obliterate the rectosigmoidal angle. Concomitant relaxation of the internal and external anal sphincters then permits the evacuation of feces. This can be augmented by an increase in intraabdominal pressure created by the Valsalva maneuver. Conversely, defecation may be consciously prevented by the voluntary contraction of the striated muscles of the pelvic diaphragm and external anal sphincter. The functional value of voluntary control of defecation requires little elaboration, but the opportunity for individuals to resist the defecatory urge, when abused, may lead to chronic rectal distention, reduced afferent signals, lax tone, and chronic constipation.

DIARRHEA AND CONSTIPATION The bowel habits of apparently healthy persons vary widely. For this reason, the complaint of *diarrhea* and *constipation* should be evaluated in terms of the degree of change from an individual's customary pattern. Reasonably detailed information is important in either abnormality. When patients complain of diarrhea, it is important to obtain an estimate of the volume as well as frequency of fecal output and, whenever possible, to examine directly a stool sample for consistency, blood, oiliness, and malodor. For example, the repeated elimination of small quantities of solid material admixed with gas, so typical in the irritable bowel syndrome, has a far different connotation than the same number of movements of liquid, blood-tinged feces. It is also useful to learn if fecal incontinence is present. Involuntary loss of feces may be an embarrassing symptom for a patient to verbalize, but such information may point to a potentially correctable anal sphincter abnormality. The term *constipation* may be used by the patient to refer to a variety of changes including reduction in frequency of defecation, a constant sensation of rectal fullness with incomplete evacuation of feces, and sometimes painful defecation due to hard stools or perianal pathology. Excessively hard stools are usually due to increased absorption of fluid as a result of prolonged contact of the luminal contents with the colonic mucosa consequent to delayed transit. In an assessment of complaints of diarrhea or constipation, it is important to consider the patient's emotional state since in many instances the recent onset of psychological stress is the major reason for altered bowel habits. However, it can be hazardous to assume this to be the case, even when the relationship seems convincing. For this reason, the judicious use of laboratory, proctoscopic, and radiologic procedures is recommended to make certain that organic disease will not be overlooked.

Acute diarrhea Diarrhea of abrupt onset occurring in otherwise healthy persons is usually due to an infectious cause. A variety of accompanying symptoms are often observed, including fever, headache, anorexia, vomiting, malaise, and myalgia, but they cannot be used to distinguish with certainty among viral, bacterial, and protozoal causes. When bacterial and protozoal pathogens are not recovered from the feces, so-called nonspecific diarrhea is usually considered to be of viral etiology. However, enterotoxin-producing strains of *Escherichia coli*, which are not distinguishable from "normal flora" on routine culture, may account for a number of cases that are usually ascribed to viral infection.

Acute diarrhea presumed to be of viral etiology typically lasts for a period of 1 to 3 days; death is extremely rare except in previously debilitated individuals who become severely dehydrated. When human volunteers have been infected with the Norwalk virus, which is believed to account for approximately one-third of epidemics of acute viral diarrhea in American adults, transient malabsorption of fat and xylose has been described. Changes in the small intestine include abnormalities of intestinal cell morphology such as villous shortening, an increase in the number of crypt cells, and increased cellularity of the lamina propria. The colonic mucosa is unaffected in viral diarrhea; this is consistent with the absence of polymorphonuclear leukocytes when fresh stool is examined microscopically after preparation with Loeffler's methylene blue.

Bacterial diarrhea is likely if there is a history of a similar and simultaneous illness in individuals who have shared contaminated food with the patient. Diarrhea developing within 12 h of the meal is most likely due to ingestion of a preformed toxin (e.g., staphylococcal exotoxin). A lag period of up to 3 days after consumption of contaminated food can occur with salmonellosis. The pathogenesis of bacterial diarrhea is due to two mechanisms, direct mucosal invasion by bacteria and the elaboration of toxins; the latter may cause direct tissue damage (cytotoxin) or promote intestinal secretion without causing any morphologic change (enterotoxin). Invasive bacteria (shigella, salmonella, *Campylobacter*, *Vibrio parahaemolyticus*) and cytotoxin-producing bacteria (*Clostridium difficile*, *Escherichia coli* 0157:H7) typically cause edema, leukocytic infiltration, and frank ulceration of colonic mucosa. Lower abdominal cramps and tenderness are prominent, as are tenesmus and rectal urgency. In severe cases the stool is grossly bloody. Microscopic examination of the stool will often reveal neutrophils along with erythrocytes. The prototypical example of enterotoxin-mediated bacterial diarrhea is *cholera*, in which the organism *Vibrio cholerae* adheres to, but does not invade, the surface epithelial cells and releases an enterotoxin which stimulates massive secretion of fluid and electrolytes by the small intestine. This may be produced experimentally in animals by placing the enterotoxin, free of the organism itself, into isolated intestinal loops. Hypersecretion reaches a peak at 4 to 6 h and is mediated by the stimulation of mucosal adenylate cyclase by the toxin. Because mucosal morphology is essentially normal and intestinal absorptive capacity is preserved, cholera is effectively treated by oral rehydration therapy with solutions containing simple sugars and sodium chloride, the former stimulating absorption of the latter. Other species of bacteria that produce enterotoxins include *E. coli*, *Clostridium*, *Staphylococcus aureus*, and *Aeromonas*.

Protozoal infections may also be responsible for acute diarrhea. *Entamoeba histolytica*, prevalent in some areas of the United States and in the homosexual male population, produces an inflammatory colitis which can closely mimic idiopathic ulcerative colitis. Giardiasis is a cause of nonexudative diarrhea that may last for weeks or even months; it is acquired by drinking contaminated water. *Cryptosporidial* infection, initially described as occurring in immunocompromised patients, has also been linked to diarrheal illness in otherwise normal persons. Careful microscopic examination of fresh stools by experienced personnel is required for the diagnosis of protozoal infection.

Travelers' diarrhea may result from any one or several of the pathogens described above. When no specific agent is identified, the etiology is usually assumed to be due to enterotoxin-producing coliform organisms or viruses; both Norwalk virus and rotavirus have been implicated. Prolonged bowel irregularity often occurs following the acute illness.

Ulcerative colitis and *Crohn's disease* may begin as acute diarrhea (Chap. 241). Bloody stools, abdominal cramping, tenderness, and fever are often observed. When Crohn's disease is limited to the small bowel (regional enteritis), the diarrhea tends to be milder, is often nonbloody, and is associated with right lower quadrant pain and tenderness. Diarrhea may be caused by a variety of *drugs*, including cholinergic agents, magnesium-containing antacids, antimetabolites used in cancer chemotherapy, and many antibiotics. A necrolytic toxin produced by *Clostridium difficile* is the cause of pseudomembranous colitis occurring during or after antibiotic use. Diarrhea due to *diverticulitis* is usually accompanied by fever, tenesmus, and rectal urgency, together with cramps and tenderness in the left lower quadrant (Chap. 243). When there is no evidence of acute inflammation, diarrhea in the presence of colonic diverticula is probably due to a spastic (irritable) colon, a disorder which may set the stage for the development of diverticula. In elderly and debilitated individuals with *fecal impaction*, the presenting symptom may be the frequent expulsion of small amounts of liquid stool overflowing from colonic distention behind the impaction. This is sometimes termed *paradoxical diarrhea*. Fecal incontinence due to anal sphincter impairment is a problem that may be encountered in certain neurologic disorders or following local surgical procedures (e.g., hemorrhoidectomy, episiotomy). Acute *psychological stress* can cause diarrhea at any age.

DIAGNOSTIC APPROACH   The appropriate tempo and approach in the evaluation of acute diarrhea depend so heavily on the clinical setting in which it occurs that only very general guidelines can be offered. It is entirely reasonable to withhold studies in mild, self-limited cases such as are seen as part of an epidemic viral illness. When dealing with sporadic severe diarrhea or when a suggestive epidemiologic history is obtained, bacterial cultures and microscopic examination of the stool for parasites and inflammatory cells are appropriate. Proctoscopy is generally reserved for patients with bloody diarrhea or those who show no improvement within 10 days. Likewise, radiologic studies should usually be deferred until the initial course of the illness has been observed. In cases of massive fluid loss, measurement of serum electrolytes is useful to aid in determining replacement therapy.

TREATMENT   General and nonspecific treatment of acute diarrhea includes rest and encouragement of fluid intake. Intravenous fluid and electrolyte replacement may be necessary in infants and the elderly. The use of opiate-containing drugs to control diarrhea is potentially dangerous if an enteroinvasive organism is suspected, but is a reasonable comfort measure in cases of mild, undifferentiated diarrhea. As a result of success achieved with cholera patients, the use of oral sugar-electrolyte solutions is being extended to the treatment of patients with acute diarrhea considered to be due to other enterotoxin-producing bacteria. The relative pros and cons of antimicrobial treatment of specific enteric infections are reviewed in their respective sections of this textbook. Biofeedback therapy has proved helpful for some patients who suffer from fecal incontinence due to anal sphincter impairment.

Chronic diarrhea   Diarrhea persisting for weeks or months, whether constant or intermittent, may be a functional symptom or a manifestation of serious illness. For this reason, it is incumbent upon the physician to search carefully for evidence of organic disease, such as fever, weight loss, malnutrition, or anemia. Abdominal tenderness and fever suggest the presence of inflammation. When there is involvement of the large bowel, the major diseases to be considered include ulcerative colitis, Crohn's disease of the colon, amebiasis, and diverticulitis. Crohn's disease of the small intestine may involve one or more of its segments. The ileum is most frequently affected. Other diarrheal conditions that may resemble Crohn's disease radiographically include tuberculous and fungal enteritis, lymphoma, amyloidosis, and argentaffin (carcinoid) tumors of the small bowel.

Prolonged diarrhea without evidence of inflammation may reflect a primary malabsorptive disorder. Selective derangements of absorption, such as those due to *bile salt enteropathy* and *lactase deficiency,* are usually not accompanied by weight loss or malnutrition. *Mucosal disorders,* best exemplified by sprue, are frequently associated with weight loss, malodorous stools, abdominal distention, and anemia, and, when more severe, with osteomalacia, bleeding due to hypoprothrombinemia, avitaminotic neuropathies, and tetany. Both osmotic and secretory mechanisms contribute to the diarrhea of sprue. *Pancreatic insufficiency* resulting from chronic pancreatitis, carcinoma, resection, or cystic fibrosis produces steatorrhea and weight loss of varying severity. A number of factors may be responsible for *postgastrectomy diarrhea* (see Chap. 238). These include the dumping syndrome, postvagotomy motility derangements, inadequate stimulation of pancreatic digestive enzymes, and incomplete mixing of these enzymes with food. On rare occasions severe postgastrectomy diarrhea and malnutrition are due to the inadvertent creation by the surgeon of a gastroileostomy instead of a gastrojejunostomy. *Bacterial overgrowth* in the small intestine, as may occur with extensive diverticulosis and prolonged bowel stasis secondary to disorders of peristalsis (e.g., scleroderma, diabetic visceral neuropathy), can also lead to chronic diarrhea and weight loss. This has been attributed to the secretory action of deconjugated bile salts and hydroxylated fatty acids that are produced by bacterial enzymes, to consumption of nutrients by the microorganisms, and to mucosal abnormalities

believed to be caused by bacteria or their metabolites (see Chap. 240). At times, diarrhea may accompany stasis in the absence of bacterial overgrowth.

Endocrine disorders that may be accompanied by chronic diarrhea include thyrotoxicosis, diabetes mellitus, adrenal insufficiency, and hypoparathyroidism. The release of potent secretagogues from neoplastic tissue in the Zollinger-Ellison syndrome (gastrin), medullary carcinoma of the thyroid (calcitonin, prostaglandins), the pancreatic cholera syndrome (vasoactive intestinal peptide), and the carcinoid syndrome (serotonin) makes diarrhea a prominent feature of these disorders. *Rectal villous adenomas* may secrete large quantities of fluid and electrolytes, which are promptly evacuated as a clear, odorless liquid. When marked fluid loss occurs, hypokalemia and dehydration may result.

Habitual *cathartic abuse* must be suspected when the cause of prolonged diarrhea remains perplexing. Even if this is denied by the patient, a stool sample should be alkalinized with sodium hydroxide; this will produce a lavender color if phenolphthalein-containing laxatives have been surreptitiously ingested. The observation of melanosis coli by sigmoidoscopy indicates chronic usage of anthraquinone laxatives.

Constipation   Constipation is a common complaint often resulting from the inordinate expectation of "regularity" in bowel-conscious individuals. Stools are described as infrequent, incomplete, or unduly hard; unusual straining may be required to achieve defecation. A review of the patient's habits often reveals contributory and correctable causes, such as insufficient dietary roughage, lack of exercise, suppression of defecatory urges arising at inconvenient moments, inadequate allotment of time for full defecation, and prolonged travel. Appropriate adjustments of these patterns and reassurance are preferable to the prescription of laxatives and may be all that is required for improvement. When the patient also has symptoms such as fatigue, malaise, headaches, or anorexia, the possibility should be considered that such symptoms reflect an underlying depression of which constipation is but one component. Decreased colonic motility is responsible for the constipation associated with the use of parasympatholytic drugs, spinal cord injury, scleroderma, and Hirschsprung's disease. A variety of derangements have been described in patients with severe idiopathic constipation. These include: histopathologic abnormalities of the myenteric plexi; functional outlet obstruction during defecation due to incomplete relaxation of the internal anal sphincter; excessive contraction of the external sphincter (anismus); a reduced anorectal angle as detected by defecatory radiography; and absence of rectosigmoid myoelectric and pressure responses to feeding. It is uncertain whether these abnormalities represent primary or secondary events and whether any of them will be responsive to specific therapeutic interventions.

Hemorrhoids, anal fissures, perineal abscesses, and rectal strictures often prevent easy and adequate stool evacuation. When constipation and tenesmus of recent onset are reported, the possibility of carcinoma of the rectum or sigmoid colon must be seriously considered. In such instances sigmoidoscopic and barium enema examinations should be obtained early and are virtually obligatory if fecal blood has been observed or if occult blood is detected on any of three successive stool specimens. Stools of abnormally thin caliber occur in patients with rectal or sigmoid colon carcinoma but are more commonly due to a spastic colon. Other mechanical causes of constipation include volvulus of the sigmoid colon, diverticulitis, intussusception, and hernias. A variety of metabolic abnormalities, such as hypothyroidism, hypercalcemia, hypokalemia, porphyria, lead poisoning, and dehydration are often associated with constipation. Prolonged fecal retention, leading to impaction, may occur in certain neurologic disorders (e.g., spinal cord injury, multiple sclerosis, cerebral palsy, senility), and in these instances, when autonomic regulation of evacuation is unachievable, vigorous and sustained enema programs are often necessary.

IRRITABLE BOWEL   The irritable bowel syndrome (also referred to as *spastic colon* and *mucous colitis*) is one of the most frequent gastrointestinal disorders (see Chap. 243). This condition is characterized by periodic or chronic bowel symptoms which include diarrhea, constipation, a sense of incomplete evacuation, and abdominal pain. These symptoms flare during periods of psychological stress, but the anxiety produced by the bowel disturbance is sometimes regarded by the patient as the fundamental cause of the emotional upset. During periods of discomfort, stools are apt to become thin, fragmented, or pelletlike, and are accompanied by excessive mucus and gas. It is estimated that 17 percent of adults have irritable bowel syndrome, but most do not seek medical evaluation; those who do are apt to have greater concern about personal health and fear of illness. Efforts to ameliorate symptoms with mild cathartics or various drugs may yield adverse and exaggerated responses. A number of therapeutic approaches, including the avoidance of foods which tend to upset the patient, addition of bulk-forming agents, judicious use of antispasmodics and tranquilizers, and psychotherapy may provide some degree of relief. If the patient's life goals can be shifted away from the quixotic search for the perfect stool, much can be accomplished. At the same time, it must be remembered that such individuals are not exempt from developing bowel cancer, and any worrisome deviation from their general pattern of derangement must be seriously evaluated.

FLATULENCE A significant amount of flatus is passed each day by normal persons, and the complaint of flatulence often reflects a heightened and embarrassing awareness of this natural occurrence. Excessive quantities of flatus may be caused by aerophagia or the formation of increased amounts of gas by intestinal bacteria. The latter process can be associated with malabsorption syndromes but is more frequently a consequence of eating foods such as beans, broccoli, and cabbage which have a high content of nondigestible polysaccharides. The oligosaccharides stachyose and raffinose, isolated from beans, are particularly effective substrates for fermentation to carbon dioxide, hydrogen, and methane by colonic flora. Chromatographic analysis of a sample of flatus will show these gases to predominate, in contrast to the high nitrogen levels that occur when excessive flatus is caused by aerophagia. The treatment of flatulence is generally undertaken to reduce embarrassment and consists of measures to decrease aerophagia along with avoidance of foods that cause excessive gas.

REFERENCES

ANTONY MA et al: Infectious diarrhea in patients with AIDS. Dig Dis Sci 33:1141, 1988

BLACKLOW NR, CUKOR GC: Viral gastroenteritis. N Engl J Med 304:397, 1981

CHRISTENSEN J: Motility of the colon, in *Physiology of the Gastrointestinal Tract*, LR Johnson et al (eds). New York, Raven Press, 1981, vol 1, chap 14

DROSSMAN DA et al: Psychosocial factors in the irritable bowel syndrome. Gastroenterology 95:701, 1988

FIELD M et al (eds): *Secretory Diarrhea*, Clinical Physiology Series. Bethesda, Md, American Physiological Society, 1980

GERSHON MD, ERDE SM: The nervous system of the gut. Gastroenterology 80:1571, 1981

KREJS GT, FORDTRAN JS: Diarrhea, in *Gastrointestinal Disease*, MH Sleisenger, JS Fordtran (eds). Philadelphia, Saunders, 1983, chap 16

LIEBERMAN DA: Common anorectal disorders. Ann Intern Med 101:837, 1984

READ NW et al: Chronic diarrhea of unknown origin. Gastroenterology 78:2644, 1980

REYNOLDS JC et al: Chronic severe constipation. Gastroenterology 92:414, 1987

SCHULTZ SG: Ion transport by mammalian large intestine, in *Physiology of the Gastrointestinal Tract*, LR Johnson et al (eds). New York, Raven Press, 1981, vol 2, chap 38

SHIAU YF et al: Stool electrolyte and osmolality measures in the evaluation of diarrheal disorders. Ann Intern Med 102:773, 1985

SHOULER P, KEIGHLEY MRB: Changes in colorectal function in severe idiopathic chronic constipation. Gastroenterology 90:414, 1986

SNOOKS SJ et al: Damage to the innervation of the pelvic floor musculature in chronic constipation. Gastroenterology 89:977, 1985

WALDRON D et al: Colonic and anorectal motility in young women with severe idiopathic constipation. Gastroenterology 95:1388, 1985

45 GAIN AND LOSS IN WEIGHT

DANIEL W. FOSTER

GENERAL PRINCIPLES In normal persons weight is stable because food intake is matched to energy expenditure by the coordinated activity of "feeding" and "satiety" centers in the hypothalamus. The signals that regulate the interactions of these centers are probably multifactorial, and both short- and long-term controls are thought to be operative. Whatever the mechanisms, the system is normally efficient over periods of months to years.

Gain or loss in tissue mass is determined by the net balance between food intake and energy expenditure. Food intake is determined by availability and attractiveness of food and by emotional and physical factors. The bulk of energy expenditure is due to basal metabolism and physical activity. The former is defined as the requirement when the body is in the supine position, motionless except for quiet respiration; it is the energy required to maintain structural and functional integrity of the body in the absence of physical activity. About half the total daily intake is normally consumed by basal processes. Nonsedentary persons spend about 40 percent of energy in physical activity; athletes may utilize 50 percent or more of ingested energy in exercise. Persons sedentary because of habit, illness, or obesity expend far less in activity. In nonobese, nonsedentary subjects 10 percent of ingested food is released as heat associated with the absorption of food, a process called *dietary thermogenesis*. This fraction, previously designated *specific dynamic action*, is usually considered a separate component of energy costs. Heat generated during and after exercise and heat released for maintenance of body temperature (*regulatory thermogenesis*) are included in the energy costs of physical activity and basal metabolism, respectively.

Change in body weight as a consequence of voluntary alteration in diet or exercise is never worrisome; change in weight that is not deliberately sought, on the other hand, is a frequent reason for consultation with the physician and often indicates the presence of disease. Changes in weight may reflect alteration in either tissue mass or body fluid content. Even when tissue mass is changing, fluid loss or gain plays a major role in the measured change in weight, particularly over the short run. This point is illustrated in Table 45-1, where the composition of weight loss was estimated during a 24-day period of semistarvation in 13 normal men [daily intake, 4200 kJ (1010 kcal)]. During the first 3 days 70 percent of the decrease in weight was due to water loss, while in subsequent stages a diminution of protein and fat accounted for essentially all the weight loss. This varying contribution of fluid explains why a fixed formula cannot be used for predicting weight loss or gain. It is frequently stated that a net change of 32,000 kJ (7700 kcal) will be accompanied by a 1-kg change in body mass. While this estimate is reasonable for long-term changes in food intake, the apparent cost per kilogram of weight lost or gained varies with the accompanying fluid shifts. In the experiment

TABLE 45-1 Percentage composition of mean daily weight loss in 13 young men during food restriction for 24 days

Days	Mean weight loss, kg/day	Water, %	Fat, %	Protein, %	Food equiv. of weight loss, kJ/kg (kcal/kg)
1–3	0.80	70	25	5	10,900 (2600)
11–13	0.23	19	69	12	29,500 (7000)
22–24	0.17	0	85	15	36,400 (8400)

SOURCE: After Brožek et al.

summarized in Table 45-1, for example, a negative balance of only 10,900 kJ (2600 kcal) resulted in the loss of 1 kg of weight between days 1 and 3, while between days 22 and 24, loss of 1 kg of weight required a deficit of 36,400 kJ (8700 kcal). In general if weight loss or gain has occurred over a period of weeks or months, it is safe to assume that change in tissue mass has occurred; weight loss or gain limited to a several-day period may be due to fluid shifts alone. Occasionally true loss of tissue mass is obscured by fluid retention as in the case of the patient with cirrhosis of the liver who develops ascites or the patient with anorexia nervosa who has significant edema.

WEIGHT GAIN

While obesity is a major public health concern (see Chap. 72), its diagnosis is usually uncomplicated. Obese subjects often deny overeating, but the true situation can be assessed either by tabulating actual food intake and determining its caloric content from standard tables, by interviewing the patient's family and friends, or by estimating metabolic rates from indirect calorimetry.

Regardless of history, excess caloric intake is the cause of obesity in the majority of cases. Pathologic causes are rare. In the adult, Cushing's syndrome can result in acquired obesity, but usually the diagnosis is suggested by the pattern of fat distribution and the clinical picture. Other endocrine diseases such as hypothyroidism, hypogonadism, and insulin-secreting tumors are frequently listed in the differential diagnosis of obesity but do not represent significant diagnostic problems. Congenital diseases that cause obesity such as the Prader-Willi, Laurence-Moon-Biedl, and Alström syndromes are readily recognizable and appear early in life. Rarely, a disease involving the hypothalamus, such as craniopharyngioma, may cause acquired obesity. Extensive workup of the central nervous system is not indicated in obesity, however, in the absence of suspicious symptoms (headache, visual difficulties, vomiting, or endocrine changes).

WEIGHT LOSS

Weight loss in the absence of deliberate dieting is a more serious problem than weight gain, because there is a high chance that organic disease is present. Mechanisms include decreased food intake, accelerated metabolism, and loss of calories in urine or stool, acting singly or in combination. Almost any serious illness can cause weight loss either through direct effects or by inducing malaise and depression. The signals that cause decreased appetite and accelerated tissue loss are not known. The negative nitrogen balance that occurs following trauma, surgery, or stressful illness is likely mediated at least partially by glucagon and other catabolic hormones. Additional candidate molecules for disease-induced weight loss are cytokines such as tumor necrosis factor (cachectin) and adipsin, but proof of their involvement is lacking.

The general categories of disease that need to be considered when weight loss is a prominent complaint are discussed next.

DIABETES MELLITUS Initial weight loss with the onset of diabetes is largely fluid and is due to the osmotic diuresis induced by hyperglycemia. Subsequently, loss of tissue mass occurs in the insulin-dependent form of the disease as a result of caloric wastage (the consequence of glycosuria) and of the hormonal abnormalities that characterize the illness. Insulin deficiency and glucagon excess result in impaired synthesis of protein and fat and simultaneously cause accelerated proteolysis and lipolysis such that the net energy state is catabolic. Weight loss in diabetes is frequently associated with increased food intake.

ENDOCRINE DISEASE Thyrotoxicosis is the most common endocrine disease producing weight loss. Increased appetite and food intake are the rule, and patients often consume a high-carbohydrate diet. Energy expenditure is enormous, primarily because of an increased metabolic rate, but increased motor activity also plays a

role. The molecular mechanism whereby thyrotoxicosis causes weight loss is not settled. In rodents thyroid hormone increases Na-K adenosine triphosphatase (ATPase) activity in many tissues resulting in a futile cycle of ATP synthesis and breakdown with energy lost as heat. This abnormality does not appear to operate in humans. Whatever the mechanism, metabolism is "uncoupled" in thyrotoxicosis, accounting for excess generation of heat and caloric wastage.

In "apathetic" hyperthyroidism weight loss and weakness may predominate with little evidence of nervousness or other symptoms. Another cause of weight loss due to hypermetabolism is pheochromocytoma, the inducing agent being catecholamine release. Panhypopituitarism and adrenal insufficiency are often associated with weight loss, largely as a consequence of diminished appetite secondary to cortisol deficiency.

GASTROINTESTINAL DISEASE Overt or occult steatorrhea due to sprue, chronic pancreatitis, or cystic fibrosis may produce wasting despite major increases in food intake. A variety of other diseases of the gastrointestinal tract cause weight loss: inflammatory bowel disease, parasites, esophageal strictures, obstruction secondary to chronic peptic ulcer, pernicious anemia, and cirrhosis of the liver. Mechanisms of weight loss include anorexia, obstruction with vomiting, malabsorption, and the effects of inflammation. Intraabdominal masses (e.g., massive splenomegaly) act by compressing the stomach, while weight loss in heart failure is due to visceral congestion.

INFECTION Hidden infection must always be sought in patients with unexplained weight loss. Tuberculosis, fungal disease, amebic abscess, and subacute bacterial endocarditis should be high on the list of suspects. Infection with human immunodeficiency virus must be considered, especially in high-risk groups (male homosexuals, intravenous drug users, recipients of multiple transfusions). Weight loss with infection is probably due to inflammatory cytokines.

MALIGNANCY Occult malignancy is probably the most common cause of weight loss in the absence of major signs and symptoms. In the search for malignancy particular emphasis must be placed on the gastrointestinal tract, pancreas, and liver. Lymphoma and leukemia should also be considered. While silent (except for weight loss) malignancy can occur in any organ, the gastrointestinal tract is the most common site. Mechanisms of weight loss in cancer vary, and more than one factor is often operative. Anorexia is usually present, but increased metabolism may also play a role, particularly in lymphomas and leukemias. Thus far, no increase in weight-loss-inducing cytokines has been documented.

PSYCHIATRIC DISEASE The classic psychiatric illness associated with profound weight loss is anorexia nervosa (Chap. 73). Conversion disorders, schizophrenia, and depression may also cause weight loss due to decreased food intake. While organic disease causing both anorexia and depression has to be ruled out, ordinarily the psychiatric nature of the problem will be clear.

RENAL DISEASE One of the earliest manifestations of uremia is anorexia. As a consequence all patients with unexplained weight loss should be given screening renal function tests.

SUMMARY

Weight loss is more often a diagnostic problem than weight gain and more often a sign of serious organic illness. If the weight loss is associated with increased food intake, the diagnosis is likely diabetes, thyrotoxicosis, or malabsorption; less frequently, leukemias or lymphomas cause weight loss in the presence of increased food intake. If food intake is normal or decreased, malignancy, infection, renal disease, psychiatric syndromes, or endocrine deficiency is more common.

REFERENCES

BEUTLER B, CERAMI A: Cachectin: More than a tumor necrosis factor. N Engl J Med 316:379, 1987

Brožek J et al: Changes in body weight and body dimensions in men performing work on a low calorie carbohydrate diet. J Appl Physiol 10:412, 1957

Flier JS et al: Severely impaired adipsin expression in genetic and acquired obesity. Science 237:405, 1987

Foster DW: Eating disorders: Obesity and anorexia nervosa, in *Williams Textbook of Endocrinology*, 7th ed, JD Wilson, DW Foster (eds). Philadelphia, Saunders, 1985, p 1081

Garfinkel PE et al: Differential diagnosis of emotional disorders that cause weight loss. Can Med Assoc J 129:939, 1983

Marton KI et al: Involuntary weight loss: Diagnostic and prognostic significance. Ann Intern Med 95:568, 1981

Morley JE: Neuropeptide regulation of appetite and weight. Endocrine Rev 8:256, 1987

Socher SH et al: Tumor necrosis factor not detectable in patients with clinical cancer cachexia. J Natl Cancer Inst 80:595, 1988

46 GASTROINTESTINAL BLEEDING

JAMES M. RICHTER / KURT J. ISSELBACHER

Hematemesis is defined as the vomiting of blood, and *melena* as the passage of stools rendered black and tarry by the presence of altered blood. These symptoms of gastrointestinal hemorrhage should bring the patient to medical attention and suggest the anatomic site of bleeding. The color of vomited blood will vary depending on the concentration of hydrochloric acid in the stomach and its mixture with the blood. Thus, if vomiting occurs shortly after the onset of bleeding, the vomitus appears red; and later the appearance will be dark red, brown, or black. Precipitated blood clots in the vomitus will produce a characteristic "coffee grounds" appearance. Hematemesis usually indicates bleeding proximal to the ligament of Treitz, since blood entering the gastrointestinal tract below the duodenum rarely enters the stomach.

While bleeding sufficient to produce hematemesis usually results in melena, less than half of patients with melena have hematemesis. *Melena* usually denotes bleeding from the esophagus, stomach, or duodenum, but lesions in the jejunum, ileum, and even ascending colon may cause melena provided the gastrointestinal transit time is sufficiently prolonged. Approximately 60 mL of blood is required to produce a single black stool; acute blood loss greater than this may produce melena for up to 3 days. After the stool color returns to normal, tests for occult blood may remain positive for up to a week or longer. The black color of stools secondary to intestinal bleeding results from contact of the blood with hydrochloric acid to produce hematin. Characteristically, such stools are tarry ("sticky"). This tarry consistency is in contrast to black or dark stools occurring after the ingestion of iron, bismuth, or licorice. Similarly, red stools may result from the ingestion of beets or intravenous administration of sulfobromophthalein. Gastrointestinal bleeding, even if detected only by positive tests for occult blood, indicates potentially serious disease and must be further investigated.

Hematochezia, the passage of red blood per rectum, generally signifies bleeding from a source distal to the ligament of Treitz. However, since blood must remain in the gut for approximately 8 h to produce melena, rapid hemorrhage into the esophagus, stomach, or duodenum may also result in hematochezia.

The clinical manifestations of gastrointestinal bleeding depend upon the extent and rate of hemorrhage and the presence of coincidental diseases. Blood loss of less than 500 mL is rarely associated with systemic signs; exceptions include bleeding in the elderly or in the anemic patient in whom smaller amounts of blood loss may produce hemodynamic alterations. Rapid hemorrhage of greater volume results in decreased venous return to the heart, decreased cardiac output, and increased peripheral resistance due to reflex vasoconstriction. Orthostatic hypotension greater than 10 mmHg usually indicates a 20 percent or greater reduction in blood volume. Concomitant symptoms include syncope, lightheadedness, nausea, sweating, and thirst. When blood loss approaches 40 percent of blood volume, shock frequently ensues with pronounced tachycardia and hypotension. Pallor is prominent, and the skin is cool.

In the setting of rapid hemorrhage the hematocrit may not accurately reflect magnitude of blood loss, since equilibration with extravascular fluid and hemodilution require several hours. Common laboratory findings include mild leukocytosis and thrombocytosis which develop within 6 h after the onset of bleeding. The blood urea nitrogen may be mildly elevated, particularly in upper gastrointestinal bleeding, due to breakdown of blood proteins to urea by intestinal bacteria as well as from a mild reduction in the glomerular filtration rate.

Occult bleeding, detected by the physician or patient with a simple card test for hemoglobin peroxidase, has been recognized as an important means of finding colorectal neoplasia at early stages, when it is more amenable to cure. Testing is advocated for patients over age 40 as a part of the periodic checkup, and test kits are available for purchase by patients. The interpretation of the test is complicated by the need for examining multiple stools (usually two samples from three stools) and multiple examinations for positive tests. A positive result can be due to physiologic blood loss, dietary peroxidases, vitamin C, or any cause of upper or lower gastrointestinal bleeding. In order to limit the confounding variables, patients should be tested on a high-fiber and low-meat diet with no ingestion of nonsteroidal anti-inflammatory agents or vitamin C.

ETIOLOGY OF UPPER GASTROINTESTINAL BLEEDING A careful history and physical examination of the oropharynx and nasal cavity should serve to exclude swallowed blood as a source of hematemesis or melena.

The four most common causes of upper gastrointestinal hemorrhage are (1) peptic ulceration, (2) erosive gastritis, (3) varices, and (4) esophagogastric mucosal tear. These entities account for up to 90 percent of all cases of upper gastrointestinal hemorrhage in which a definite lesion can be found.

Peptic ulcer Peptic ulcer is the most common cause of upper gastrointestinal bleeding; the majority of such ulcers are found in the duodenum. Because hemorrhage may be the initial manifestation of a peptic ulcer, this lesion should be seriously considered even when a history characteristic of ulcer disease is not obtained.

Gastritis Gastritis may be associated with recent alcohol ingestion, portal hypertension, or the use of anti-inflammatory drugs, such as aspirin or ibuprofen. Gastric erosions also frequently develop in patients with major trauma, surgery, and severe systemic disease, particularly burn victims and patients with increased intracranial pressure. Because there are no characteristic physical findings, the diagnosis of gastritis must be suspected when the appropriate clinical setting is encountered. When a specific diagnosis is required, endoscopy is usually needed to confirm the diagnosis since radiologic examination generally lacks sufficient sensitivity.

Varices Variceal bleeding is characteristically abrupt and massive; chronic gastrointestinal blood loss is unusual. Bleeding from esophageal or gastric varices is usually the result of portal hypertension, secondary to cirrhosis. Although alcoholic cirrhosis is the most prevalent cause of esophageal varices in the United States, any condition producing portal hypertension, even in the absence of hepatic disease (i.e., portal vein thrombosis or idiopathic portal hypertension), may result in variceal bleeding. Further, while the presence of varices usually connotes long-standing portal hypertension, acute hepatitis or severe fatty infiltration of the liver may occasionally produce varices which disappear once the hepatic abnormality resolves. Although upper gastrointestinal bleeding in a patient with cirrhosis suggests a variceal source, approximately half those patients will be bleeding from other lesions (e.g., gastritis, ulcers). Consequently, it is essential to exclude nonvariceal causes of bleeding so that the appropriate treatment can be instituted.

Esophagogastric mucosal tear (Mallory-Weiss syndrome) With the advent of esophagogastroduodenoscopy, the Mallory-Weiss syndrome has been demonstrated with increasing frequency as a cause of acute upper gastrointestinal hemorrhage (see also Chap. 43). Mucosal laceration occurs in the region of the esophagogastric junction and is often characterized historically by retching or non-bloody vomiting followed by hematemesis.

Other lesions Less common bleeding esophageal lesions include esophagitis and carcinoma; these generally cause chronic blood loss and rarely produce massive bleeding.

Gastric carcinoma may result in chronic gastrointestinal bleeding. Lymphoma, polyps, and other tumors of the stomach and small bowel are uncommon and are infrequent causes of hemorrhage. Leiomyoma and leiomyosarcoma are likewise rare, but they can lead to massive hemorrhage. Bleeding from duodenal and jejunal diverticula is relatively unusual. Vascular insufficiency of the mesenteric vessels, including occlusive and nonocclusive disease, may lead to bloody diarrhea.

Arteriosclerotic aortic aneurysms may rupture into the small intestine; such an event is almost always fatal. Rupture usually occurs following arterial reconstructive surgery with fistula formation between synthetic graft and bowel lumen. A small or herald bleed may precede a sudden massive hemorrhage from an aortoenteric fistula. Sudden bleeding may also occur after trauma resulting in hepatic laceration; this may result in blood loss into the bile ducts (i.e., hemobilia).

Primary blood dyscrasias, vasculitis, and connective tissue disorders may result in significant gastrointestinal bleeding. Uremia may produce gastrointestinal blood loss; the most common presentation is chronic, occult bleeding from diffuse involvement of the mucosa of the stomach and small bowel.

ETIOLOGY OF LOWER GASTROINTESTINAL BLEEDING   Anal and rectal lesions Small amounts of bright red blood on the surface of the stool and toilet tissue are often caused by hemorrhoids; such bleeding is generally precipitated by the strained passage of a hard stool. Anal fissures and fistulas may present in a similar fashion. Proctitis is another source of rectal bleeding. It is often an idiopathic, limited variant of ulcerative colitis. In others, particularly male homosexuals, proctitis may be due to gonorrheal or mycoplasma infections. Rectal trauma is a cause of hematochezia, and the placement of foreign objects in the rectal vault may precipitate perforation as well as acute rectal hemorrhage. It must be emphasized that anal pathology does not preclude other sources of blood loss, and these must be sought and excluded.

Colonic lesions Carcinoma of the colon, as well as colonic polyps, may produce chronic blood loss. Angiodysplasia, a mucosal telangiectasia usually involving the ascending colon, is a major source of acute or chronic bleeding in elderly patients. Frankly bloody diarrhea is common and may be the presenting symptom in patients with ulcerative colitis; it is less frequent in granulomatous colitis, but occult blood may be present in the stool. Bleeding may also accompany diarrhea due to infections such as shigellosis, amebiasis, campylobacterosis, and rarely, salmonellosis. In the elderly patient, ischemic colitis may be a cause of bloody diarrhea; this lesion may also be seen in younger women who use oral contraceptive agents.

Diverticula Colonic diverticula are most often located in the sigmoid colon; however, diverticular bleeding may originate anywhere in the colon. Bleeding from colonic diverticula is a cause of massive lower gastrointestinal hemorrhage. The usual presentation of a diverticular hemorrhage is that of painless passage of a maroon-colored stool. Meckel's diverticulum, a congenital anomaly of the distal ileum, is present in about 2 percent of the population and is an important cause of acute hemorrhage in children and young adults. Although only about 15 percent of these diverticula contain gastric mucosa, half of the lesions which cause acute bleeding contain gastric mucosa.

APPROACH TO THE PATIENT WITH GASTROINTESTINAL BLEEDING The approach to the bleeding patient depends upon the site, extent, and rate of bleeding. Patients with hematemesis have usually bled greater amounts (often greater than 1000 mL) than those who have melena alone (usually 500 mL or less), and mortality with the former is about twice that of the latter. When first seen, the patient may be in shock. Prior to taking a history and performing a

thorough physical examination, vital signs should be noted, blood sent for typing and cross-matching, and a large-bore intravenous line placed for infusion of saline or other plasma expanders. The primary consideration in the care of the bleeding patient is maintaining adequate intravascular volume and hemodynamic stability.

History A history or symptoms suggestive of ulcer disease may provide a useful clue. Similarly, recent heavy use of alcohol or anti-inflammatory drugs should make erosive gastritis suspect. If such alcohol use has been long-standing, esophageal varices may be a more likely source of hemorrhage. Aspirin use may also cause gastroduodenitis, peptic ulceration, and bleeding. Prior history of gastrointestinal bleeding may be helpful, as may a family history of intestinal disease or hemorrhagic diathesis. Recent retching followed by hematemesis should suggest the possibility of the Mallory-Weiss syndrome. The acute onset of bloody diarrhea may indicate the presence of inflammatory bowel disease or an infectious colitis. Associated systemic illnesses, burns, or recent trauma may lead to erosive gastritis.

Physical examination Following evaluation for orthostatic changes in pulse and blood pressure and institution of volume repletion, the patient should be examined for clues to the underlying illness. A nonintestinal bleeding source should be excluded by careful examination of the oral cavity and nasopharynx. Dermatologic examination may disclose the characteristic telangiectasia of Osler-Weber-Rendu disease (although these will not be visible if severe anemia is present), the perioral pigmentation of Peutz-Jeghers syndrome, the dermal fibromas of neurofibromatosis, the sebaceous cysts and bony tumors of Gardner's syndrome, the palpable purpura frequently seen with vasculitis, or the diffuse pigmentation seen in hemochromatosis. Stigmata of chronic liver disease such as spider angiomata, gynecomastia, testicular atrophy, jaundice, ascites, and hepatosplenomegaly suggest portal hypertension resulting in bleeding from esophageal or gastric varices. Significant lymph node enlargement or abdominal masses may reflect underlying intraabdominal malignancy. Careful rectal examination is important to exclude local pathology as well as to observe the color of the stool.

Laboratory studies Initial studies should include the hematocrit, hemoglobin, careful assessment of red blood cell morphologic features (hypochromic, microcytic red blood cells suggest that blood loss is chronic), white blood cell count, differential, and platelet count. Prothrombin time, partial thromboplastin time, and other coagulation studies are needed to exclude primary or secondary clotting defects. Radiography of the abdomen is rarely helpful in establishing a diagnosis unless a perforated or ischemic viscus is suspected. Though the initial studies are valuable and essential, repeated evaluation of the laboratory data is important as one follows the clinical course of the bleeding.

Diagnostic and therapeutic approach The diagnostic approach to the patient with gastrointestinal hemorrhage must be individualized. The management of gastrointestinal bleeding is often under the direction of the internist, but it is prudent to consult a surgeon in the event that surgery is required.

When there is a history of melena or hematemesis or the suspicion of bleeding from the upper part of the gastrointestinal tract, the patient should have a nasogastric tube passed to empty the stomach and to determine whether the bleeding is in the esophagus, stomach, or duodenum. If the initial nasogastric aspirate is clear, the tube should be left in place for several hours, since active duodenal bleeding may occur with an initially clear nasogastric aspirate. If the aspirate is negative for blood during a period of active bleeding, it is reasonable to conclude that active bleeding is not occurring in the gastroduodenal region, and the nasogastric tube can be removed. However, if there is no evidence of active bleeding at the time the nasogastric tube is placed, one cannot assume bleeding did not come from the stomach or duodenum and endoscopy may be required.

If red blood or "coffee grounds" material is aspirated from the nasogastric tube, saline irrigation of the stomach should be initiated. Irrigation serves two purposes: it provides the clinician with an assessment of the rapidity of the bleeding, and it clears the stomach of old blood prior to possible endoscopy. Subsequent diagnostic maneuvers will depend on whether bleeding continues; this can be assessed by vital signs, transfusion requirements, and the number and consistency of stools.

If the bleeding has stopped and the patient is stable, one may proceed with either esophagogastroduodenoscopy or upper gastrointestinal barium studies. Although *endoscopy* provides a higher diagnostic yield, it has not been proved conclusively that survival is increased by early endoscopy. *Barium examination* may identify a potential source of hemorrhage, but there are important limitations to such x-rays. First, lesions such as erosive gastritis and Mallory-Weiss lacerations are not visualized by x-ray. Second, if the patient rebleeds following a barium exam, the retained contrast material will make endoscopy difficult and angiography impossible. Clearly the approach in this setting must be individualized. The decision to employ esophagogastroduodenoscopy or barium studies will depend on several variables, including the availability of an experienced endoscopist and the condition of the patient. Although studies have shown that emergency endoscopy and a vigorous diagnostic approach do not generally decrease patient morbidity or mortality, emergency endoscopy may be important in planning therapy in certain patients with cirrhosis or previous gastric surgery. By identifying other patients with visible vessels and thus a high risk for recurrent bleeding, possible complications can be anticipated.

Persistent upper gastrointestinal hemorrhage must be viewed differently, and most clinicians would proceed immediately to esophagogastroduodenoscopy (Fig. 46-1). Determination of the site and cause of bleeding is essential to plan for appropriate therapy, particularly if varices are suspected. Thus, anticipation of surgery, angiography, or the suspicion of bleeding varices are strong indications for esophagogastroduodenoscopy in the evaluation of the patient with persistent upper gastrointestinal bleeding. Bleeding from an arteriole in a peptic ulcer may be controlled by endoscopic coagulation using Nd:YAG laser, heater probe, or electrocautery. However, esophagogastroduodenoscopy is more difficult in the evaluation of *massive* hemorrhage, since large amounts of blood obscure visualization of mucosal pathology, and angiography may be required in addition to endoscopy.

Should bleeding continue and endoscopy fail to reveal the bleeding source, the site of hemorrhage may be beyond the ligament of Treitz. In this situation angiography is frequently valuable in establishing a diagnosis. Angiographic demonstration of the bleeding site requires blood loss at a rate of at least 0.5 mL/min. Clinical correlates reflecting this degree of blood loss include postural hypotension and the necessity for blood transfusion to maintain stable vital signs. Emergency angiography may localize the site of bleeding; however,

the cause of the bleeding may not be determined unless varices, vascular malformations, or aneurysms are present.

Therapeutic angiography is a helpful approach to the control of persistent hemorrhage. Continuous intraarterial infusion of vasoconstrictor agents, such as vasopressin, is often successful in controlling hemorrhage due to gastric ulcer or Mallory-Weiss tear. Additionally, embolic material may be injected directly into the artery perfusing the bleeding site. However, intravenous infusions of vasopressin and endoscopic sclerosis for control of variceal bleeding are more valuable than angiographic techniques.

If bleeding esophageal varices are identified on upper endoscopy, peripheral infusions of vasopressin may control the bleeding. The response to such therapy depends upon the general condition of the patient as assessed by clinical and laboratory parameters. It has been shown that intraarterial vasopressin is no more effective than intravenous administration in the control of variceal bleeding. Endoscopic sclerosis of varices has emerged as an effective therapy for bleeding esophageal varices and when available should be attempted prior to surgery. Periodic endoscopic sclerotherapy also appears to limit further bleeding in patients who have bled from varices. Varices may also be controlled by balloon tamponade with a Sengstaken-Blakemore tube. Unlike vasopressin, this technique is generally used as a preoperative stabilizing measure which should be followed by definitive therapy within 48 h whenever possible.

In the evaluation of *lower gastrointestinal bleeding* the most important procedures are the digital examination, anoscopy, and sigmoidoscopy. The last of these may identify a bleeding site or document bleeding coming from above the range of the instrument. Colonoscopy is a valuable technique for the evaluation of patients with small to moderate lower gastrointestinal bleeds. Preparation of the colon with saline lavage solutions permits a colonoscopic evaluation of the bowel within hours. Many colonic abnormalities can be detected and treated with polypectomy or electrocoagulation. If bleeding is brisk, arteriography may serve to localize the bleeding site and allow local infusion of vasoconstrictor agents to control bleeding. Because arteriography detects actively bleeding lesions only when blood loss exceeds 0.5 mL/min and gastrointestinal bleeding tends to be intermittent, arteriography is often nondiagnostic. Radiolabeled erythrocyte scanning is more sensitive than arteriography in detecting blood loss of 0.1 mL/min and may be used to investigate less severe bleeding. However, bleeding scans are less specific than arteriography, generally localizing the lesion and seldom making a discrete diagnosis. Bleeding scans are most helpful in detecting active, low-grade, or intermittent bleeding in order to better time arteriography and obtain the maximal diagnostic yield. Finally, a barium enema has a limited role in the evaluation of acute rectal bleeding. Although it may localize potential bleeding sources, it will not define the

FIGURE 46-1 Endoscopic photographs from a patient with hematemesis. *A*. A gastric ulcer along the lesser curvature of the stomach is identified (*arrows*). *B*. The same ulcer is bleeding actively from a spurting artery (*arrows*).

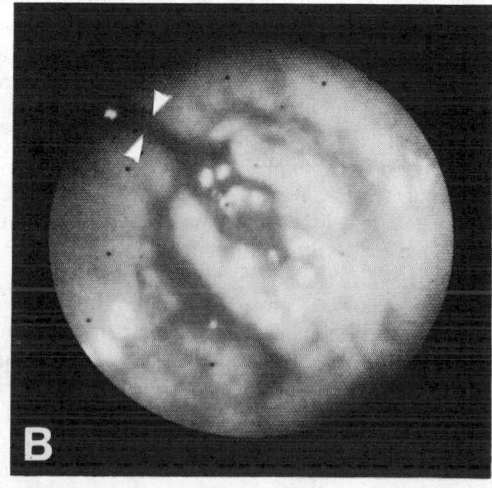

bleeding site. Furthermore, if brisk bleeding recurs, subsequent colonoscopy or angiography will be difficult to interpret due to retained contrast material. Therefore, it is advisable to withhold barium studies of both the upper and lower bowel for at least 48 h after the cessation of active bleeding.

Patients with occult bleeding are evaluated principally to exclude colorectal neoplasia. Any symptoms or history of disease should be investigated as well. If there are no symptoms, evaluation should focus on the colon with either a barium enema and sigmoidoscopy or colonoscopy. If there is no symptom or anemia, evaluation of the colon is sufficient. Patients with anemia are unlikely to have a physiologic or trivial basis for their test result, and the evaluation should be pursued until a full explanation is obtained.

REFERENCES

Cello JP et al: Endoscopic sclerotherapy versus portacaval shunt in patients with severe cirrhosis and acute variceal hemorrhage; Long-term follow-up. N Engl J Med 316:11, 1987

Chojkier M et al: A controlled comparison of continuous intra-arterial and intravenous infusions of vasopressin in hemorrhage from esophageal varices. Gastroenterology 77:540, 1979

Laine L: Multipolar electrocoagulation in the treatment of active upper gastrointestinal tract hemorrhage. N Engl J Med 316:1613, 1987

Levy M: et al: Major upper gastrointestinal tract bleeding; Relation to the use of aspirin and other nonnarcotic analgesics. Arch Intern Med 148:281, 1988

Lichtenstein JL: Accuracy and reliability of endoscopy and x-ray in upper gastrointestinal bleeding. Dig Dis Sci 26:70s, 1981

Peterson WL et al: Routine early endoscopy in upper gastrointestinal tract bleeding: A randomized, controlled trial. N Engl J Med 304:925, 1981

Priebe HJ et al: Antacid versus cimetidine in preventing acute gastrointestinal bleeding. A randomized trial in 75 critically ill patients. N Engl J Med 302:426, 1980

Richter JM et al: Angiodysplasia: Clinical presentation and colonoscopic diagnosis. Dig Dis Sci 29:481, 1984

Steer ML, Silen W: Diagnostic procedures in gastrointestinal hemorrhage. N Engl J Med 309:646, 1983

47   JAUNDICE AND HEPATOMEGALY

KURT J. ISSELBACHER

JAUNDICE

Jaundice, or *icterus*, refers to the yellow pigmentation of the skin or scleras by bilirubin. This in turn is a result of elevated levels of bilirubin in the bloodstream. Jaundice may be brought to clinical attention by a darkening of the urine or a yellow discoloration of the skin or sclera; the latter often is the site where clinical icterus may first be detected. Scleral pigmentation is attributed to richness of this tissue in elastin, which has a special affinity for bilirubin. Jaundice must be distinguished from other causes of yellow pigmentation such as carotenemia (see Chap. 76), which is due to carotenoid pigments in the bloodstream and is associated with a yellowish discoloration of the skin but not of the sclera.

Normal serum bilirubin concentrations range from 5 to 17 μmol/L (or 0.3 to 1.0 mg/dL), and normally most of this is unconjugated (see Fig. 47-1). The precise level at which jaundice becomes clinically evident varies, but it can usually be recognized when the total serum bilirubin exceeds 34 to 43 μmol/L (2 to 2.5 mg/dL). With pronounced jaundice the skin may take on a greenish hue because of the conversion of bilirubin to biliverdin, an oxidation product of bilirubin. Oxidation occurs more readily with conjugated bilirubin, and hence a greenish hue is seen more frequently in conditions with pronounced conjugated hyperbilirubinemia. When bilirubin is exposed to visible blue light (430 to 470 nm), metastable isomers are produced. These photoisomers are polar (because they permit no intramolecular hydrogen bonding) and can

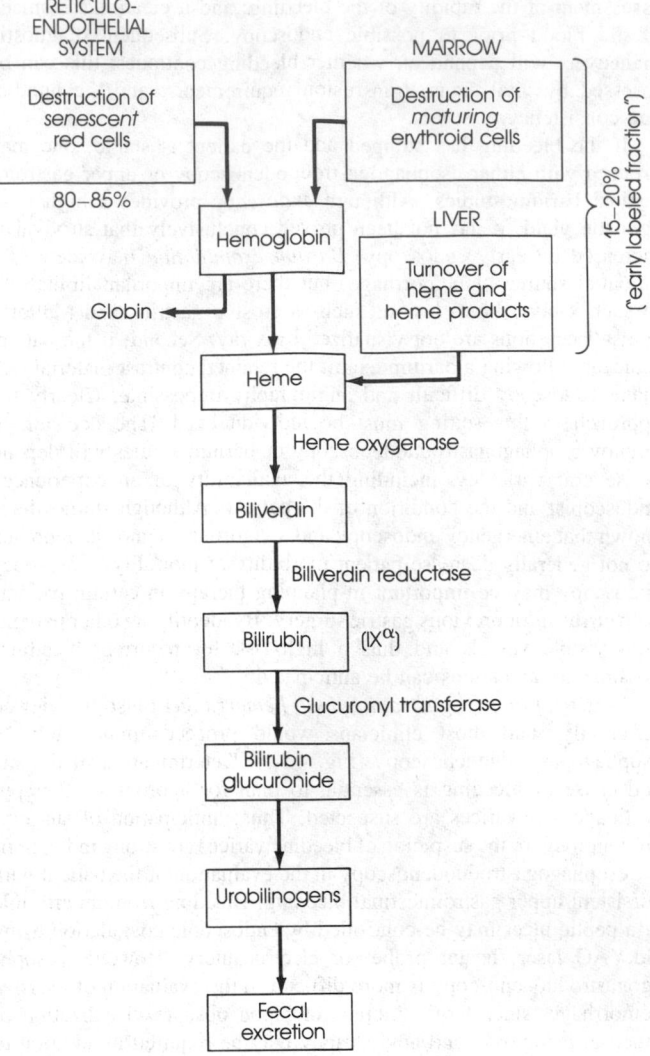

FIGURE 47-1 The sources and precursors of bilirubin and steps in its subsequent metabolism and excretion.

be excreted by the liver into bile without having to be conjugated (see below and Fig. 47-2).

PRODUCTION AND METABOLISM OF BILIRUBIN Normal sources of bilirubin (Fig. 47-2)   Most bilirubin is derived from the catabolism of hemoglobin present in senescent red blood cells. This normally accounts for about 80 to 85 percent of the daily bilirubin production. When a circulating red blood cell reaches the end of its normal life span of approximately 120 days, it is destroyed in the reticuloendothelial system. In the catabolism of hemoglobin, globin is first dissociated from heme, after which the heme moiety (ferroprotoporphyrin IX) is oxidatively cleaved and converted to biliverdin by a microsomal heme oxygenase (which is inhibited by protoporphyrins; see below). This enzyme system requires oxygen and a cofactor, reduced nicotinamide adenine dinucleotide phosphate (NADPH). Bilirubin (in the chemical form of bilirubin IXα) is then formed from biliverdin by biliverdin reductase.

About 15 to 20 percent of the bilirubin is derived from sources other than senescent erythrocytes. One source is the *destruction of maturing erythroid cells in the bone marrow,* or so-called ineffective erythropoiesis (see Chap. 294). The other is *nonerythroid components,* especially in the liver, and involves the turnover of heme and heme proteins (such as cytochrome, myoglobin, and heme-containing enzymes). These two sources of bilirubin are collectively referred to as the *early labeled fraction,* a term derived from experiments with labeled glycine and Δ-aminolevulinic acid (ALA). Thus when labeled glycine is administered to a normal subject, approximately 15 percent

FIGURE 47-2   Scheme showing the conversion of bilirubin IXα to water-soluble derivatives by photoisomerization or conjugation. In *A* the normal, unconjugated pigment Z-Z isomer is shown; the dashed line shows the upright position of the hydrogen at the methene bridges linking the pyrrole molecules. *B* shows the effect of light leading to the formation of the water-soluble E-E isomer; the dashed-line box serves to emphasize the inversion of the hydrogens at the methene bridges between the pyrrole molecules. *C* shows the formation of water-soluble bilirubin diglucuronide formation; the dashed-line box encloses one of the two glucuronic acid moieties.

of the label appears in stool urobilinogens in the first 3 to 5 days; 85 percent of the label appears over a broad range with the peak at about 120 days and reflects bilirubin produced from the normal destruction of senescent red blood cells.

Transport of bilirubin   Following liberation of unconjugated bilirubin into the plasma, virtually all the pigment is tightly *bound to albumin*. The maximum binding capacity is 2 mol bilirubin per mole of albumin in a reversible, noncovalent manner. Certain organic anions, such as sulfonamides and salicylates, compete with bilirubin for common binding sites on albumin and may displace bilirubin from albumin, permitting it to enter tissues such as the central nervous system. Most of the evidence for albumin binding has been obtained from studies using unconjugated bilirubin. Conjugated bilirubin is also bound to albumin, but in both a reversible and an irreversible manner. The reversible binding is similar to the noncovalent binding of unconjugated bilirubin, but the binding is much weaker. The second type involves a very tight, irreversible albumin-bilirubin complex that appears in the serum when hepatic excretion of bilirubin is impaired (i.e., with cholestasis). Due to the nature of the binding, the complex does *not* appear in urine. Also this bilirubin-albumin conjugate may remain detectable in the serum for several weeks after the relief of the obstruction or during recovery from hepatocellular jaundice.

Bilirubin is found in body fluids (cerebrospinal fluid, joint effusions, cysts, etc.) in proportion to the albumin content of the fluids and is absent from true secretions such as tears, saliva, and pancreatic juice. The appearance of jaundice is also influenced by blood flow and edema. Paralyzed extremities and edematous areas tend to remain uncolored, and "unilateral" jaundice in patients with hemiplegia and edema may be seen if jaundice develops.

Hepatic metabolism of bilirubin (Fig. 47-3)   The liver occupies a central role in the metabolism of the bile pigments. Three distinct phases are recognized: (1) *hepatic uptake*, (2) *conjugation*, and (3) *excretion* into bile. Of these three steps, excretion appears to be the rate-limiting step and the one most susceptible to impairment when the liver cell is damaged.

UPTAKE   Unconjugated bilirubin bound to albumin is presented to the liver cell, and upon entry the pigment and albumin become dissociated. The uptake phase and subsequent hepatocyte storage of bilirubin involves binding of bilirubin to certain cytoplasmic anionic binding proteins, especially ligandin. This binding may prevent efflux of bilirubin back into the plasma.

CONJUGATION   Unconjugated bilirubin is water-insoluble and must be converted to a *water-soluble derivative* in order to be excreted by the liver cell into bile. This is accomplished by conjugation whereby bilirubin is predominantly converted to bilirubin glucuronide. The reaction occurs in the endoplasmic reticulum of the hepatocytes

FIGURE 47-3   Scheme of bilirubin uptake, conjugation, and excretion by the liver cell. Although the conversion of BMG to BDG appears to be catalyzed by glucuronyl transferase, some have also postulated its formation by a plasma membrane transglucuronidase. B = bilirubin; BMG = bilirubin monoglucuronide; BDG = bilirubin diglucuronide; UDP = uridine diphosphate.

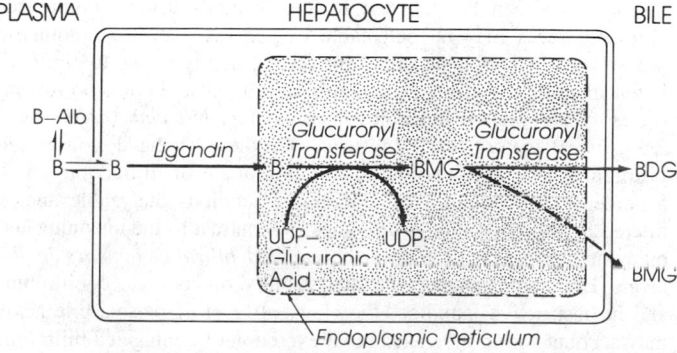

by action of bilirubin glucuronyl transferase. As shown in Fig. 47-3, this appears to be a two-step reaction, resulting first in the formation of the monoglucuronide followed by the production of the diglucuronide. Normally, bile contains 85 percent of bilirubin diconjugates and 15 percent monoconjugates. Unconjugated bilirubin usually is *not* excreted by the liver into the bile (except following photooxidation, see below).

EXCRETION OR SECRETION INTO BILE   Normally, for bilirubin to be excreted into bile, *the pigment must be in the conjugated form.* Although the overall process is not well understood, the excretion of conjugated bilirubin into bile appears to be an energy-dependent and *rate-limiting* step in the hepatic metabolism of bilirubin. When this step is compromised, two consequences occur: (1) decreased excretion of bilirubin into the bile and (2) "regurgitation," or reentry of conjugated bilirubin from the liver cells into the bloodstream.

As indicated above, bilirubin IXα can exist as four geometric isomers. The naturally occurring isomer is the Z-Z form (see Fig. 47-2), which permits intramolecular hydrogen bonding, making the molecule hydrophobic. The other isomers (Z-E, E-Z, and E-E, depending on the position of the hydrogens at the two bridge double bonds) can be formed upon exposure to blue light and are unstable. They are *water-soluble* because their geometric configuration prevents intramolecular hydrogen bonding. Thus, these isomers (photoisomers) can be *excreted* into bile *without having to be conjugated.* The natural Z-Z isomer is also rendered water-soluble by conjugation with glucuronic acid. Bilirubin glucuronide formation prevents intramolecular hydrogen bonding, makes the molecule polar, and permits excretion of the pigment into bile (Fig. 47-2).

Intestinal phase of bilirubin metabolism   After its appearance in the intestinal lumen, bilirubin glucuronide may be excreted in the stool or metabolized to urobilinogen and related products. Because of its polarity, *conjugated bilirubin is not reabsorbed* by the intestinal mucosa, a mechanism which may serve to rid the body of this pigment. The formation of urobilinogen from conjugated bilirubin requires the action of bacteria and occurs in the lower part of the small intestine and colon.

In contrast to conjugated bilirubin, *urobilinogen is reabsorbed* from the small intestine into the portal blood and is thus subject to the enterohepatic circulation. Some urobilinogen is reexcreted by the liver into the bile; the rest is excreted in the urine in an amount usually not exceeding 4 mg daily. When the hepatic excretory mechanism is impaired (e.g., in hepatocellular disease) or the production of bilirubin is greatly increased (e.g., in hemolytic anemia), the urinary urobilinogen may increase significantly.

The normal output of fecal urobilinogen ranges from 50 to 280 mg per day. Under conditions of decreased excretion of conjugated bilirubin into the intestine (e.g., liver disease, bile duct obstruction) or suppression of intestinal flora by antibiotics, fecal output will be diminished. In hemolytic anemia, urinary and fecal urobilinogen excretion is greatly increased.

In a normal person with a blood volume of 5 L and a hemoglobin concentration of 150 g/L (15 g/dL), the total circulating hemoglobin is 750 g. Because approximately 0.8 percent of the red blood cells are destroyed daily, 6.3 g hemoglobin is released for catabolism.

Renal excretion of bilirubin   Normally the urine contains no bilirubin that can be detected by the methods usually employed, although traces may be detectable by sensitive spectrophotometric procedures. Unconjugated bilirubin, being tightly bound to albumin, is not filtered by the renal glomeruli, and because there is no tubular secretory process for bilirubin, *unconjugated bilirubin (as the IXα, Z-Z isomer) is not excreted in urine.* On the other hand, conjugated bilirubin is less tightly bound to albumin, and a small fraction (about 5 percent) is unbound. The unbound fraction is dialyzable and is filtered by the renal glomeruli. Thus, in contrast to the unconjugated pigment, a fraction of plasma *conjugated bilirubin appears in the urine.* Bile salts enhance the dialyzability of conjugated bilirubin, and in obstructive jaundice, the elevated level of plasma bile acids may account for an increased renal excretion of conjugated bilirubin.

This may also explain why in biliary tract obstruction, serum conjugated bilirubin levels tend to plateau and not to exceed 510 to 680 μmol/L (30 to 40 mg/dL), while with severe hepatocellular injury bilirubin levels higher than this may occur.

CHEMICAL TESTS FOR BILE PIGMENTS   The most widely employed chemical test for the bile pigments in serum is the van den Bergh reaction. In this reaction the bilirubin pigments are diazotized with sulfanilic acid, and the chromogenic products are measured colorimetrically. The van den Bergh reaction can be used to distinguish between unconjugated and conjugated bilirubin because of the different solubility properties of the pigments. When the reaction is carried out in an *aqueous* medium, the water-soluble conjugated bilirubin reacts to give the so-called direct van den Bergh reaction. When the reaction is carried out in *methanol,* the intramolecular hydrogen bonds of unconjugated bilirubin are broken; thus, both conjugated and unconjugated pigments react, giving a measure of the *total* bilirubin level. The total minus the direct-reacting bilirubin give the *indirect* value, which is a measure of the unconjugated bilirubin level.

In the direct van den Bergh reaction, the most accurate measurements are those carried out at 1 min. If the reaction is allowed to proceed longer, a small amount of the unconjugated pigment may begin to react in the aqueous medium. As a result, if the reaction is carried out at 30 min in a patient with unconjugated hyperbilirubinemia, falsely low values for the indirect-reacting bilirubin may be obtained. This serves to emphasize that the direct and indirect van den Bergh reactions represent *approximations* (not absolute measurements) of the conjugated and unconjugated pigments.

The most accurate method for measuring bilirubin in biologic fluids involves the formation of bilirubin methyl esters (by alkaline methanolysis) and measuring the products by high-performance liquid chromatography (HPLC). Studies with this procedure show that *normal serum contains mostly unconjugated bilirubin* with less than 4 percent of the total bilirubin being conjugated. This confirms the long-held suspicion that the small amount of "direct-reacting" bilirubin measured by the van den Bergh method (2 to 5 μmol/L or 0.1 to 0.3 mg/dL) is not correct and is an overestimate of the amount of conjugated bilirubin actually present in normal serum. The HPLC method also shows that in patients with liver disease and conjugated hyperbilirubinemia, the serum contains significant amounts of *monoconjugates as well as diconjugates.* A summary of the key differences in the properties and reactions of the bilirubin pigments is presented in Table 47-1.

The qualitative measurement of bilirubin in the urine may be carried out with Ictotest tablets or the dipstick method. The foam test is also a simple and qualitatively valid procedure. When normal urine is vigorously shaken in a test tube, the foam is absolutely white. In urine containing bilirubin, the foam will be yellow. This difference may be subtle and may become evident only by comparing a normal urine specimen and one containing bilirubin side by side.

Except for concentrated urine, the most common cause of a deep-yellow-brown or dark urine is bilirubinuria. However, other mechanisms and diseases associated with a dark urine need to be considered. These include yellow urine due to drugs (e.g., sulfasalazine); red

TABLE 47-1   Comparison of the major differences between conjugated and unconjugated bilirubin

Properties and reactions	Unconjugated*	Conjugated
Water solubility	0	+
Affinity for lipids	+	0
Renal excretion	0	+
van den Bergh reaction	Indirect (total minus direct)	Direct
Binding to serum albumin (reversible)	+ + +	+
Formation of bilirubin-albumin complex (irreversible)	0	+ †

* These properties apply to the naturally occurring bilirubin IXα. Other geometric and photoisomers behave like conjugated bilirubin. See text for details.
† Detectable in plasma under conditions of cholestasis (see text).

urine due to porphyria, hemoglobinuria, myoglobinuria, or drugs (e.g., pyridium); and dark-brown or black urine due to homogentisic acid (in ochronosis) or melanin (with melanoma).

APPROACH TO THE PATIENT WITH JAUNDICE   Once jaundice is recognized clinically or chemically, it is important to determine whether it is predominantly due to unconjugated or to conjugated hyperbilirubinemia. *A simple clue in this regard is to determine whether bilirubin is present in the urine.* Its absence in the urine suggests unconjugated hyperbilirubinemia (since this pigment is not filtered by the glomerulus); its presence indicates conjugated hyperbilirubinemia. One can then proceed to the chemical measurement of the bilirubin pigments in the serum. In predominantly unconjugated hyperbilirubinemia, 80 to 85 percent of the total serum bilirubin is measured as unconjugated by the van den Bergh reaction, but more than 96 percent by the more accurate HPLC method. The patient is considered to have predominantly conjugated hyperbilirubinemia when more than 50 percent of the serum bilirubin is of the conjugated type. The serum of such patients will contain both mono- and diglucuronide conjugates.

An approach to the classification of jaundice based on this important distinction is presented in Table 47-2. Derangements of bilirubin metabolism may occur through any of four mechanisms: (1) overproduction, (2) decreased hepatic uptake, (3) decreased hepatic conjugation, and (4) decreased excretion of bilirubin into bile (due to both intrahepatic and extrahepatic factors). Jaundice may also be described on the basis of the pathogenetic mechanisms or disease processes leading to increased bilirubin levels. Thus, the terms *hemolytic jaundice, hepatocellular jaundice,* and *obstructive* (or *cholestatic*) *jaundice* are often used. Though these classifications and terms are helpful, in any one patient more than a single derangement or more than one "type" of jaundice may be present. For example, a patient with cirrhosis may have not only impaired liver cell function (and hence hepatocellular jaundice) but also hemolysis. Furthermore, obstructive jaundice may be due to either *mechanical* obstruction of the biliary radicles or *functional* factors causing impaired hepatic excretion of bilirubin into bile.

In the present chapter a brief description of the major types of

---

TABLE 47-2   Classification of jaundice based on underlying derangement of bilirubin metabolism

I Predominantly *unconjugated* hyperbilirubinemia
  A Overproduction
    1 Hemolysis (intra- and extravascular)
    2 Ineffective erythropoiesis
  B Decreased hepatic uptake
    1 Drugs (e.g., flavaspidic acid)
    2 Prolonged fasting [< 1255 kJ/d (< 300 kcal/d)]
    3 Sepsis
  C Decreased bilirubin conjugation (decreased glucuronyl transferase activity)
    1 Gilbert's syndrome (*mild* decrease in transferase)
    2 Crigler-Najjar type II (*moderate* decrease in transferase)
    3 Crigler-Najjar type I (*absent* transferase)
    4 Neonatal jaundice
    5 Acquired transferase deficiency
       a Drug inhibition (e.g., pregnanediol, chloramphenicol)
       b Hepatocellular disease (hepatitis, cirrhosis)*
    6 Sepsis
II Predominantly *conjugated* hyperbilirubinemia
  A Impaired hepatic excretion (intrahepatic defects)
    1 Familial or hereditary disorders
       a Dubin-Johnson syndrome; Rotor syndrome
       b Recurrent (benign) intrahepatic cholestasis
       c Cholestatic jaundice of pregnancy
    2 Acquired disorders
       a Hepatocellular disease* (e.g., viral or drug-induced hepatitis)
       b Drug-induced cholestasis (e.g., oral contraceptives, methyltestosterone)
       c Sepsis
  B Extrahepatic biliary obstruction (mechanical obstruction, e.g., stones, stricture, tumor of bile duct)

---

* In hepatocellular disease (hepatitis and cirrhosis) there is usually interference in the three major steps of bilirubin metabolism—uptake, conjugation, and excretion. However, excretion is the rate-limiting step and is usually impaired to the greatest extent. As a result, conjugated hyperbilirubinemia predominates.

---

jaundice is given. A more detailed discussion of the individual disease entities is found in Chap. 251.

Jaundice with predominantly unconjugated bilirubin in the serum   OVERPRODUCTION OF BILIRUBIN   When an increased amount of hemoglobin is released from red blood cells into either the bloodstream or tissues, increased bilirubin production occurs. This is reflected by an increase in unconjugated bilirubin levels in the serum, but with levels rarely exceeding 51 to 68 μmol/L (3 to 4 mg/dL). There may also be a slight increase in conjugated bilirubin, but on a percentage basis the amount is comparable to what is found in normal serum, i.e., 4 percent or less of total bilirubin. For a detailed description of the causes of increased bilirubin production, see Chap. 251.

IMPAIRED HEPATIC UPTAKE OF BILIRUBIN   As indicated previously, the uptake of bilirubin by the liver cell involves dissociation of the pigment from albumin, and then binding to ligandin. In some cases of drug-induced jaundice (e.g., due to flavaspidic acid) and possibly in some patients with Gilbert's syndrome, there may be a derangement in this phase of bilirubin metabolism (see Chap. 251).

IMPAIRED GLUCURONIDE CONJUGATION   Both acquired and genetic derangements in hepatic glucuronyl transferase occur. In the fetus and at birth, glucuronyl transferase activity is low and appears to account in part for the *neonatal jaundice* normally found between the second and the fifth days of life. *Mild* decreases in glucuronyl transferases occur in Gilbert's syndrome, *moderate* decreases are found in Crigler-Najjar syndrome type II, and the enzyme is totally *absent* in the rare Crigler-Najjar syndrome type I (see Chap. 251).

Acquired defects in bilirubin glucuronyl transferase activity may be produced by drugs (i.e., enzyme inhibition) or intrinsic liver disease. However, with liver cell damage, the excretory capacity of the liver is impaired to a greater extent than is the conjugating capacity. Therefore in most hepatocellular diseases, the hyperbilirubinemia is predominantly of the conjugated type (see Chap. 251).

Jaundice with predominantly conjugated bilirubin in the serum
IMPAIRED EXCRETION OF BILIRUBIN BY THE LIVER   The impaired excretion of bilirubin into the biliary canaliculi, whether due to functional or mechanical factors, results in predominantly conjugated hyperbilirubinemia and bilirubinuria. The presence of *bilirubin in the urine is evidence of conjugated hyperbilirubinemia* and is a most important point in the differential diagnosis of jaundice. Such findings are identical to those occurring in complete obstruction of the bile duct, emphasizing that *jaundice due to hepatocellular disease can seldom be differentiated from that due to extrahepatic obstruction solely on the basis of changes in bile pigment metabolism.* Indeed there are often instances when the two conditions are not distinguishable by any biochemical criteria, and liver biopsy or other diagnostic procedures (e.g., ultrasound) are needed for the definitive diagnosis.

When there is interference in the excretion of conjugated bilirubin into bile, by what mechanism does this pigment enter the systemic circulation? Several postulates have been proposed for this "reentry": (1) rupture of the bile canaliculi secondary to the necrosis of the hepatic cells that constitute their walls; (2) occlusion of the canaliculi by inspissated bile or their compression by swollen hepatic cells; (3) obstruction of the terminal intrahepatic bile ducts (cholangioles) by inflammatory cells; (4) altered hepatic cell permeability; and (5) impaired excretion, resulting in accumulation of conjugated bilirubin in the hepatocytes, and secondary diffusion into the plasma. Although some of these postulates are speculative, it is likely that several of these mechanisms occur. For example, occasionally in histologic sections, escape of bile through rents in the walls of canaliculi in areas of necrosis is apparent. Also, microscopic studies of the liver of rats injected with fluorescent dyes have shown reflux of bile from canaliculi into sinusoids. However, no anatomic damage needs to be invoked, because when unconjugated bilirubin is infused into normal subjects at high rates, conjugated hyperbilirubinemia occurs; this is explained most logically by passive diffusion.

EXTRAHEPATIC BILIARY OBSTRUCTION   Complete obstruction of the extrahepatic bile ducts leads to jaundice with predominantly conjugated hyperbilirubinemia, bilirubinuria, and clay-colored stools. Failure of bile to reach the intestine results in virtual disappearance of urobilinogen from the stool and urine. The concentration of bilirubin rises progressively but then usually plateaus at a level of 510 to 680 µmol/L (30 to 40 mg/dL). To some extent this plateau may be explained by a balance between renal excretion and diversion of bilirubin to other metabolites. In hepatocellular jaundice, such a plateau tends not to occur, and bilirubin levels in excess of 855 µmol/L (50 mg/dL) may be found, in part due to concomitant hemolysis and renal insufficiency.

Partial obstruction of the extrahepatic bile ducts can also give rise to jaundice but only if the intrabiliary pressure is increased, because the excretion of bilirubin does not diminish until the intraductile pressure approaches the maximal secretory pressure of approximately 250 mmHg bile. Jaundice may occur at much lower pressures if the obstruction is complicated by infection of the ducts or hepatocellular injury. Therefore, jaundice, bilirubinuria, and clay-colored stools are inconstant findings in partial biliary obstruction, and the amount of urobilinogen in urine and stool varies with the degree of occlusion.

The functional reserve of the liver is so great that *occlusion of the intrahepatic bile ducts* does not give rise to jaundice unless the drainage of bile from a large segment of the parenchyma is interrupted. Either of the two major hepatic ducts or a large number of secondary radicles may be occluded without production of jaundice. In experimental animals the ducts draining at least 75 percent of the parenchyma must be occluded before jaundice appears.

Additional points of terminology In clinical practice, a patient may be described as having *obstructive,* or *cholestatic,* jaundice. By this is meant that clinically, and especially biochemically, there is little to suggest hepatocellular damage and that the main features point to interference with, or obstruction in, the flow of bile. Typically one would expect such a patient to show (1) predominantly conjugated hyperbilirubinemia, (2) minimal biochemical changes of parenchymal liver damage, and (3) a moderate to a marked increase in the serum alkaline phosphatase level [usually three or four times normal (or greater than 250 IU/L)]. As emphasized in Chaps. 248 and 250, an *elevated alkaline phosphatase level* in a patient with jaundice or liver disease, in the absence of other disorders such as bone disease, is most suggestive of interference with bile secretion or an infiltrative process in the liver. However, *laboratory tests alone may not permit differentiation of intrahepatic from extrahepatic cholestasis.*

Some clinicians reserve the term *obstructive jaundice* for those cases in which anatomic obstruction can be demonstrated and use the term *cholestatic jaundice* for cases of parenchymal liver disease in which the obstructive phase is on a functional basis. Nevertheless, because these two entities frequently are indistinguishable by clinical and biochemical criteria, the terms obstructive jaundice and cholestatic jaundice are often used interchangeably.

Hepatocellular disorders in which jaundice associated with an obstructive, or cholestatic, phase occurs include (1) occasional cases of viral hepatitis, (2) drug reactions, especially those due to chlorpromazine and methyltestosterone, (3) some cases of alcoholic hepatitis or alcohol-induced fatty liver, (4) jaundice in the last trimester of pregnancy, (5) most cases of Dubin-Johnson or Rotor syndrome, (6) benign recurrent intrahepatic cholestasis, and (7) certain types of postoperative jaundice. These and other conditions are discussed in Chaps. 251 and 252.

In summary, all forms of conjugated hyperbilirubinemia have by definition an impairment in the excretion of bilirubin into bile. In most cases of parenchymal liver disease, a broad derangement is shown by the biochemical tests of liver function. However, when the major detectable alterations of liver function tests include (1) conjugated hyperbilirubinemia and (2) moderate to marked elevation of the serum alkaline phosphatase level, the terms obstructive or cholestatic jaundice may be appropriate. Additional procedures, including operation, are often needed to determine the cause of the cholestasis (see Chaps. 247 to 249).

HEPATOMEGALY

In the supine position, the major part of the liver lies beneath the right rib cage. In some normal persons the liver edge may be palpable 1 to 2 cm below the right costal margin, and a palpable liver edge by itself does not necessarily indicate hepatomegaly. In evaluating liver size by physical examination, two factors other than ability to palpate the liver edge need to be considered, namely, (1) the location of the upper border of liver dullness by percussion and (2) the body habitus.

Normally, the upper edge of liver dullness on the right side in the midclavicular line is at the level of the fifth rib, but in asthenic habitus it may be lower. The liver edge normally descends 1 to 3 cm with deep inspiration. In hypersthenic subjects, the liver may extend over to the left side of the abdominal wall, with the lower edge high and not palpable; in hyposthenic subjects with a very acute costal angle, the liver may lie in the right half of the abdomen, the edge being palpable by as much as 6 to 8 cm below the right costal margin lateral to the right rectus abdominis muscle. Thus, palpability does not necessarily imply hepatomegaly.

In determining liver enlargement by palpation, one should be certain that the liver is being palpated rather than other right upper quadrant masses such as gallbladder, colonic neoplasm, or fecal material in the colon. Liver enlargement is often confirmed by radiologic studies, including hepatic scintiscans, computed tomography, and ultrasonography.

In many cases of generalized liver enlargement, the left lobe will be felt in the epigastrium between the xiphoid and umbilicus. The liver should be carefully palpated during deep inspiration to determine whether the edge is tender, regular or irregular, firm or soft, rounded and thickened, or sharp. The edge is tender and often rounded with hepatic inflammation, as in hepatitis, or when the liver is acutely congested, as in cardiac decompensation. Pulsation of the liver may be found with tricuspid valvular incompetence. A carcinomatous liver may be rocklike in hardness; the cirrhotic liver is very firm in consistency. The largest livers are often found with carcinoma (primary or metastatic), marked fatty infiltration, congestive cardiac decompensation, Hodgkin's disease, and amyloidosis. Rapid decrease in liver size may occur with improvement of congestive failure, mobilization of fat from the liver, or massive hepatic necrosis.

In a patient with hepatomegaly, auscultation is sometimes helpful.

TABLE 47-3   Causes of a palpable liver and hepatomegaly

I Palpable liver without hepatomegaly
  A Right diaphragm displaced downward (e.g., emphysema, asthma)
  B Subdiaphragmatic lesion (e.g., abscess)
  C Aberrant lobe of liver (Riedel's lobe)
  D Extremely thin or relaxed abdominal muscles
  E Occasionally present in normal persons
II Hepatomegaly
  A Vascular congestion (e.g., congestive heart failure, hepatic vein thrombosis)
  B Bile duct obstruction (e.g., lesion in common duct leading to hepatomegaly and subsequently to biliary cirrhosis)
  C Infiltrative disorders
    1 Bone marrow and reticuloendothelial cells
      a Extramedullary hematopoiesis
      b Leukemia
      c Lymphoma
    2 Fat
      a Fatty liver (e.g., secondary to alcohol, diabetes, or toxins)
      b Gaucher's disease and some other lipidoses
    3 Glycogen (e.g., diabetes, especially after insulin excess)
    4 Amyloid
    5 Iron (hemochromatosis and hemosiderosis)
    6 Granuloma (tuberculosis, sarcoid)
  D Inflammatory disorders
    1 Hepatitis—due to drugs or infectious agents
    2 Cirrhosis—except in late stages when prolonged scarring may lead to a *small,* shrunken liver
  E Tumors—primary or metastatic
  F Cysts—polycystic disease, congenital hepatic fibrosis

A friction rub may be audible (and palpable) in the right upper quadrant; it is usually due to a recent biopsy, tumor, or perihepatitis. In portal hypertension a venous hum may be audible between the umbilicus and the xiphoid. An arterial murmur or bruit over the liver may indicate tumor, usually hepatocellular carcinoma.

Some of the causes of a palpable liver and hepatomegaly are given in Table 47-3.

REFERENCES

BERLIN N, BERK P: Quantitative aspects of bilirubin metabolism for hematologists. Blood 57:983, 1981

BLANKAERT N, SCHMID R. Physiology and pathophysiology of bilirubin metabolism, in *Hepatology: A Textbook of Liver Disease*, D Zakim, T Boyer (eds). Philadelphia, Saunders, 1982, pp 246–296

CHOWDHURY JR et al: Hereditary jaundice and disorders of bilirubin metabolism, in *The Metabolic Basis of Inherited Disease*, 6th ed, CR Scriver et al (eds). New York, McGraw-Hill, 1989, pp 1367–1408

KAPPAS A et al: Sn-Protoporphyrin use in the management of hyperbilirubinemia in term newborns with direct Coombs-positive ABO incompatibility. Pediatrics 81:485, 1988

MCDONAGH AF et al: Blue light and bilirubin excretion. Science 208:145, 1980

MURACA M et al: Relationship between serum bilirubins and production and conjugation of bilirubin. Studies in Gilbert's syndrome, Crigler-Najjar disease, hemolytic disorders and rat models. Gastroenterology 92:309, 1987

VAN HOOTEGEM P et al: Serum bilirubins in hepatobiliary disease: Comparison with other liver function tests. Hepatology 5:112, 1985

WEISS JS et al: The clinical importance of a protein-bound fraction of serum bilirubin in patients with hyperbilirubinemia. N Engl J Med 309:147, 1983

48 ABDOMINAL SWELLING AND ASCITES

ROBERT M. GLICKMAN / KURT J. ISSELBACHER

ABDOMINAL SWELLING Abdominal swelling or distention is a common problem in clinical medicine and may be the initial manifestation of a systemic disease or of otherwise unsuspected abdominal disease. *Subjective* abdominal enlargement, often described as a sensation of fullness or bloating, is usually transient and is often related to a functional gastrointestinal disorder when it is not accompanied by objective physical findings of increased abdominal girth or local swelling. *Obesity* and lumbar lordosis, which may be associated with prominence of the abdomen, may usually be distinguished from true increases in the volume of the peritoneal cavity by history and careful physical examination.

Clinical history Abdominal swelling may first be noticed by the patient because of a progressive increase in belt or clothing size, the appearance of abdominal or inguinal hernias, or the development of a localized swelling. Often, considerable abdominal enlargement has gone unnoticed for weeks or months, either because of coexistent obesity or because the ascites formation has been insidious, without pain or localizing symptoms. Progressive abdominal distention may be associated with a sensation of "pulling" or "stretching" of the flanks or groins and vague low back pain. Localized *pain* usually results from involvement of an abdominal organ (e.g., a passively congested liver, large spleen, or colonic tumor). Pain is uncommon in cirrhosis with ascites and when it is present, pancreatitis, hepatoma, or peritonitis should be considered. Tense ascites or abdominal tumors may produce increased intraabdominal pressure, resulting in *indigestion* and *heartburn* due to gastroesophageal reflux or *dyspnea*, *orthopnea*, and *tachypnea* from elevation of the diaphragm. A coexistent pleural effusion, more commonly on the right, presumably due to leakage of ascitic fluid through lymphatic channels in the diaphragm, may also contribute to respiratory embarrassment. The patient with diffuse abdominal swelling should be questioned about increased alcoholic intake, a prior episode of jaundice or hematuria,

a change in bowel habits, or a past history of rheumatic heart disease. Such historical information may provide the clues that will lead one to suspect an occult cirrhosis, a colonic tumor with peritoneal seeding, congestive heart failure, or nephrosis.

Physical examination A carefully executed *general physical examination* can yield valuable clues concerning the etiology of abdominal swelling. Thus palmar erythema and spider angiomas suggest an underlying cirrhosis, while supraclavicular adenopathy (Virchow's node) should raise the question of an underlying gastrointestinal malignancy. *Inspection* of the abdomen is an important but often cursorily performed aspect of the abdominal examination. By noting the abdominal contour, one may be able to distinguish localized from generalized swelling. The tensely distended abdomen with tightly stretched skin, bulging flanks, and everted umbilicus is characteristic of ascites. A prominent abdominal venous pattern with the direction of flow away from the umbilicus often is a reflection of portal hypertension; venous collaterals with flow from the lower part of the abdomen toward the umbilicus suggest obstruction of the inferior vena cava; flow downward toward the umbilicus suggests superior vena cava obstruction. "Doming" of the abdomen with visible ridges from underlying intestinal loops is usually due to intestinal obstruction or distention. An epigastric mass, with evident peristalsis proceeding from left to right, usually indicates underlying pyloric obstruction. A liver with metastatic deposits may be visible as a nodular right upper quadrant mass moving with respiration.

Auscultation may reveal the high-pitched, rushing sounds of early intestinal obstruction or a succussion sound due to increased fluid and gas in a dilated hollow viscus. Careful auscultation over an enlarged liver occasionally reveals the harsh bruit of a vascular tumor, especially a hepatoma, or the leathery friction rub of a surface nodule. A venous hum at the umbilicus may signify portal hypertension and an increased collateral blood flow around the liver. A fluid wave and flank dullness which shifts with change in position of the patient are important signs that indicate the presence of peritoneal fluid. In obese patients, small amounts of fluid may be difficult to demonstrate; on occasion the fluid may be detected by abdominal percussion with patients on their hands and knees. Doubt about the presence of peritoneal fluid may be resolved by careful paracentesis with a small-gauge (no. 19 or 20) needle. Careful percussion should serve to distinguish generalized abdominal enlargement from localized swelling due to an enlarged uterus, ovarian cyst, or distended bladder. Percussion can also outline an abnormally small or large liver. Loss of normal liver dullness may result from massive hepatic necrosis; it may also be a clue to free gas in the peritoneal cavity, as from perforation of a hollow viscus.

Palpation is often difficult with massive ascites, and ballottement of overlying fluid may be the only method of palpating the liver or spleen. A slightly enlarged spleen in association with ascites may be the only evidence of an occult cirrhosis. When there is evidence of portal hypertension, a soft liver suggests that obstruction to portal flow is extrahepatic; a firm liver suggests cirrhosis as the likely cause of the portal hypertension. A very hard or nodular liver is a clue that the liver is infiltrated with tumor, and when accompanied by ascites, it suggests that the latter is due to peritoneal seeding. The presence of a hard periumbilical lymph node (Sister Marie Joseph's nodule) suggests metastatic disease from a pelvic or gastrointestinal primary tumor. A pulsatile liver and ascites may be found in tricuspid insufficiency.

An attempt should be made to determine whether a mass is solid or cystic, smooth or irregular, and whether it moves with respiration. The liver, spleen, and gallbladder should descend with respiration unless they are fixed by adhesions or extension of tumor beyond the organ. A fixed mass not descending with respiration may indicate that it is retroperitoneal. Tenderness, especially if localized, may indicate an inflammatory process such as an abscess; it may also be due to stretching of the visceral peritoneum or tumor necrosis. Rectal and pelvic examinations are mandatory; they may reveal otherwise undetected masses due to tumor or infection.

Radiographic and laboratory examinations are essential for confirming or extending the impressions gained on physical examination. Upright and recumbent films of the abdomen may demonstrate the dilated loops of intestine with fluid levels characteristic of intestinal obstruction or the diffuse abdominal haziness and loss of psoas margins suggestive of ascites. Ultrasonography is often of value in detecting ascites, determining the presence of a mass, or evaluating the size of the liver and spleen. CT scanning provides similar information. A plain film of the abdomen may reveal the distended colon of otherwise unsuspected ulcerative colitis and give valuable information as to the size of the liver and spleen. An irregular and elevated right side of the diaphragm may be a clue to a liver abscess or hepatoma. Studies of the gastrointestinal tract with barium or other contrast media are usually necessary in the search for a primary tumor.

ASCITES The evaluation of a patient with ascites requires that the *cause* of the ascites be established. In most cases ascites will appear as a part of a well-recognized illness, i.e., cirrhosis, congestive heart failure, nephrosis, or disseminated carcinomatosis. In these situations, the physician should determine that the development of ascites is indeed a consequence of the basic underlying disease and not due to the presence of a separate or related disease process. This distinction is necessary even when the cause of ascites seems obvious. For example, when the patient with compensated cirrhosis and minimal ascites develops progressive ascites that is increasingly difficult to control with sodium restriction or diuretics, the obvious temptation is to attribute the worsening of the clinical picture to progressive liver disease. However, an occult hepatoma, portal vein thrombosis, spontaneous bacterial peritonitis, or even tuberculosis may be responsible for the decompensation. The disappointingly low success in diagnosing tuberculous peritonitis or hepatoma in the patient with cirrhosis and ascites reflects the too-low index of suspicion for the development of such superimposed conditions. Similarly, the patient with congestive heart failure may develop ascites from a disseminated carcinoma with peritoneal seeding. The thorough evaluation of each patient with ascites, even in the presence of an "obvious" cause, will help avoid these errors.

Diagnostic paracentesis (50 to 100 mL) should be part of the routine evaluation of the patient with ascites. The fluid should be examined for its gross appearance; and protein content, cell count, and differential cell count should be determined, and Gram's and acid-fast stains and culture performed. Cytologic and cell-block examination may disclose an otherwise unsuspected carcinoma. Table 48-1 presents some of the features of ascitic fluid typically found in various disease states. In some disorders, such as cirrhosis, the fluid has the characteristics of a transudate (less than 25 g protein per liter and a specific gravity less than 1.016); in others, such as peritonitis, the features are those of an exudate. Although there is variability of the ascitic fluid in any given disease state, some features are sufficiently characteristic to suggest certain diagnostic possibilities. For example, blood-stained fluid with more than 25 g protein per liter is unusual in uncomplicated cirrhosis but is consistent with tuberculous peritonitis or neoplasm. Cloudy fluid with a predominance of polymorphonuclear cells and a positive Gram stain are characteristic of bacterial peritonitis; if most cells are lymphocytes, tuberculosis should be suspected. The complete examination of each fluid is most important, for occasionally only *one* finding may be abnormal. For example, if the fluid is a typical transudate but contains more than 250 white blood cells per microliter, the finding should be recognized as atypical for cirrhosis, nephrosis, or congestive heart failure and should warrant a search for tumor or infection. This is especially true in the evaluation of cirrhotic ascites where occult peritoneal infection may be present with only minor elevations in the white blood cell count of the peritoneal fluid (300 to 500 cells per microliter). Since Gram's stain of the fluid may be negative in a high proportion of such cases, careful culture of the peritoneal fluid is mandatory. Direct visualization of the peritoneum (laparoscopy) may disclose peritoneal deposits of tumor, tuberculosis, or metastatic disease of the liver. Biopsies are taken under direct vision often adding to the diagnostic accuracy of the procedure.

Chylous ascites refers to a turbid, milky, or creamy peritoneal fluid due to the presence of thoracic or intestinal lymph. Such a fluid shows Sudan-staining fat globules microscopically and an increased triglyceride content by chemical examination. A turbid fluid due to leukocytes or tumor cells may be confused with chylous fluid (pseudochylous), and it is often helpful to carry out alkalinization and ether extraction of the specimen. Alkali will tend to dissolve cellular proteins and thereby reduce turbidity; ether extraction will lead to clearing if the turbidity of the fluid is due to lipid. Chylous

TABLE 48-1   Ascitic fluid characteristics in various disease states

Condition	Gross appearance	Specific gravity	Protein, g/dL	Cell count — Red blood cells, >10,000/μL	Cell count — White blood cells, per μL	Other tests
Cirrhosis	Straw-colored or bile-stained	<1.016 (95%)*	<25 (95%)	1%	<250 (90%);* predominantly mesothelial	
Neoplasm	Straw-colored, hemorrhagic, mucinous, or chylous	Variable, >1.016 (45%)	>25 (75%)	20%	>1000 (50%); variable cell types	Cytology, cell block, peritoneal biopsy
Tuberculous peritonitis	Clear, turbid, hemorrhagic, chylous	Variable, >1.016 (50%)	>25 (50%)	7%	>1000 (70%); usually >70% lymphocytes	Peritoneal biopsy, stain and culture for acid-fast bacilli
Pyogenic peritonitis	Turbid or purulent	If purulent, >1.016	If purulent, >2.5	Unusual	Predominantly polymorphonuclear leukocytes	+Gram's stain, culture
Congestive heart failure	Straw-colored	Variable, <1.016 (60%)	Variable, 15–53	10%	<1000 (90%); usually mesothelial, mononuclear	
Nephrosis	Straw-colored or chylous	<1.016	<25(100%)	Unusual	<250; mesothelial, mononuclear	If chylous, ether extraction, Sudan staining
Pancreatic ascites (pancreatitis, pseudocyst)	Turbid, hemorrhagic, or chylous	Variable, often >1.016	Variable, often >25	Variable, may be blood-stained	Variable	Increased amylase in ascitic fluid and serum

* Since the conditions of examining fluid and selecting patients were not identical in each series, the percentage figures (in the parentheses) should be taken as an indication of the order of magnitude rather than as the precise incidence of any abnormal finding.

ascites is most often the result of lymphatic obstruction from trauma, tumor, tuberculosis, filariasis (see Chap. 169), or congenital abnormalities. It may also be seen in the nephrotic syndrome.

Rarely, ascitic fluid may be *mucinous* in character, suggesting either pseudomyxoma peritonei (Chap. 246) or rarely a colloid carcinoma of the stomach or colon with peritoneal implants.

On occasion, ascites may develop as a seemingly isolated finding in the absence of a clinically evident underlying disease. It is then that a careful analysis of ascitic fluid may indicate the direction the evaluation should take. A useful framework for the workup starts with an analysis of whether the fluid is an exudate or transudate. *Transudative ascites* of unclear etiology is most often due to occult cirrhosis, right-sided venous hypertension raising hepatic sinusoidal pressure, or hypoalbuminemic states such as nephrosis or protein-losing enteropathy. Cirrhosis with well-preserved liver function (normal albumin) resulting in ascites invariably is associated with significant portal hypertension (see Chap. 254). Evaluation should include liver function tests, liver spleen scan or other hepatic imaging procedure (i.e., CT or ultrasound) to detect nodular changes in the liver, or a colloid shift of isotope to suggest portal hypertension. On occasion a wedged hepatic venous pressure can be useful to document portal hypertension. Finally, if clinically indicated, a liver biopsy will confirm the diagnosis of cirrhosis and perhaps suggest its etiology. Other etiologies may result in hepatic venous congestion and resultant ascites. Right-sided cardiac valvular disease and particularly constrictive pericarditis should raise a high index of suspicion and may require cardiac imaging and cardiac catheterization for definitive diagnosis. Hepatic vein thrombosis is evaluated by visualizing the hepatic veins using imaging techniques (angiography, CT scans, magnetic resonance imaging) to demonstrate obliteration, thrombosis, or obstruction by tumor. Uncommonly, transudative ascites may be associated with benign tumors of the ovary, particularly fibroma (Meigs's syndrome) with ascites and hydrothorax.

Exudative ascites should initiate an evaluation for primary peritoneal processes, most importantly infection and tumor. Routine bacteriologic culture of ascitic fluid often will yield a specific organism causing infectious peritonitis. Tuberculous peritonitis (Table 48-1) is best diagnosed by peritoneal biopsy, either percutaneously or via laparoscopy. Histologic examination invariably shows granulomata that may contain acid-fast bacilli. Since cultures of peritoneal fluid and biopsies for tuberculosis may require 6 weeks, characteristic histology with appropriate stains allows antituberculosis therapy to be started promptly. Similarly the diagnosis of peritoneal seeding by tumor can be made by cytologic analysis of peritoneal fluid or by peritoneal biopsy. Appropriate diagnostic studies can then be undertaken to determine the nature and site of the primary tumor. Pancreatic ascites (Table 48-1) is invariably associated with an extravasation of pancreatic fluid from the pancreatic ductal system, most commonly from a leaking pseudocyst. Ultrasound or CT examination of the pancreas followed by visualization of the pancreatic duct by direct cannulation (viz., endoscopic retrograde cholangiopancreatography, ERCP) will usually disclose the site of leakage and permit resective surgery to be carried out.

An analysis of the physiologic and metabolic factors involved in the production of ascites (see Chap. 254 for details), coupled with a complete evaluation of the nature of the ascitic fluid, will invariably disclose the etiology of the ascites and permit appropriate therapy to be instituted.

REFERENCES

CATTAN EL JR et al: The accuracy of the physical examination in the diagnosis of suspected ascites. JAMA 247:1146, 1982
EPSTEIN M: Treatment of refractory ascites. N Engl J Med 321:1675, 1989
GARCIA-TSAO G et al: The diagnosis of bacterial peritonitis. Hepatology 5:91, 1985
PINTO PC et al: Large volume paracentesis in nonedematous patients with tense ascites: Its effect on intravascular volume. Hepatology 8:207, 1988
RECTOR WG JR, REYNOLDS TB: Superiority of the serum: Ascites albumin difference over the ascites total protein concentration in separation of "transudative" and "exudative" ascites. Am J Med 77:83, 1984
RUNYON BA: Patients with deficient ascitic fluid opsonic activity are predisposed to spontaneous bacterial peritonitis. Hepatology 8:632, 1988

section 6 Alterations in urinary function and electrolytes

49 ALTERATIONS IN URINARY FUNCTION

FREDRIC L. COE

AZOTEMIA, OLIGURIA, AND ANURIA

AZOTEMIA   Measurements of urea and creatinine concentrations in serum are often obtained to assess the glomerular filtration rate (GFR). Both substances are produced at a reasonably constant rate, by the liver and muscles, respectively. As discussed in Chap. 222, they undergo complete glomerular filtration and are not reabsorbed extensively by the renal tubules; hence their clearances tend to reflect the GFR. An increase in their serum concentrations, termed *azotemia* (*azo*, "containing nitrogen"), occurs as the GFR falls. Creatinine is a more reliable index of GFR than urea because of the latter's lower back diffusion from tubule lumen to peritubular blood. The GFR may be reduced by a fall in the filtration rates of individual functioning nephrons or by a reduction in the total number of functioning nephrons. (See Table 49-1.)

Reduced single-nephron GFR   TUBULAR FUNCTION NORMAL   An important response of the normal kidney to a severe sodium-conserving stimulus, such as extracellular fluid volume depletion, is reduction of the single-nephron glomerular filtration rate (SNGFR) and subsequent reabsorption of an increased fraction of the reduced amounts of NaCl and water that enter the tubules. The resulting azotemia is called *prerenal azotemia*, in which urinary Na concentration falls below 20 (often below 1) mmol/L (see Table 49-1). The fractional excretion of Na can be calculated (see Chap. 223) and used as an additional index of prerenal azotemia. Secretion of vasopressin is stimulated by depletion of extracellular fluid volume, and as a consequence, the distal tubules and collecting ducts become fully permeable to water. The concentrating mechanisms in the inner medulla (Chap. 222) are very efficient when flow rates through the loops of Henle and the collecting ducts are low. As a result, the filtrate that escapes reabsorption in the proximal tubule undergoes maximal osmotic concentration, the urine volume becomes small, and it has a high osmolality, above 500 mosmol per kilogram of water. Most of the filtered creatinine escapes tubular reabsorption,

TABLE 49-1 Pathophysiologic mechanisms of azotemia

Mechanism of reduced GFR	Clinical examples	Laboratory findings					
		Oliguria	Urine osm, mosmol/kg	Urine [Na$^+$], mmol/L	$\left(\dfrac{U}{P}\right)_{creat}$	$\left(\dfrac{U}{P}\right)_{urea}$	BUN / Serum creat
REDUCED SNGFR							
Tubules normal (prerenal azotemia)	Severe dehydration, edema-forming states, diuretic agents, systemic hypotension, acute glomerular disease,* acute urinary obstruction, incomplete renal vascular obstruction	Nearly always present	>500	<20	>40	>8	>10
Tubules damaged (acute renal failure)	Acute tubular necrosis, nephrotoxic agents, glomerulonephritis with tubule injury	Common	<350	>40	<20	>2	10
REDUCED NEPHRON NUMBER							
Elevated SNGFR	Chronic tubulointerstitial-renal disease Surgical loss of renal tissue	Rare†	[290	>40	3–10	3–10]	10
Normal SNGFR	Diffuse chronic glomerulonephritis Diabetic nephropathy	Rare†	[100–350‡	10–100‡	>10	>3]	>10
Reduced SNGFR	Any of the factors that can reduce SNGFR (listed above) may lower SNGFR in a patient who has a reduced number of functioning nephrons	Common	290	>20	>10	<3	>10

* Acute obstruction causing reduced SNGFR is called postrenal azotemia.
† Occurs only when total GFR is below 5% normal; urine chemistry values are helpful only when oliguria is present and are therefore enclosed in brackets.
‡ Varies with diet and with the level of GFR. When GFR is below 20% normal, osmotic concentration of the urine is usually impossible.
NOTE: osm = osmolality; creat = creatinine concentration; U = urine; P = plasma.

and consequently the ratio of the urine-to-plasma (U/P) creatinine concentrations is very high, 40 or more. Because urea can back-diffuse more completely than creatinine, the blood urea nitrogen (BUN) level rises more than the serum creatinine concentration. Normally, the ratio of BUN to serum creatinine concentration is 10:1; with depletion of the extracellular fluid volume this ratio rises. An elevated ratio can also be produced by unrelated factors such as tetracycline administration, adrenocortical steroid therapy, the presence of blood in the gastrointestinal tract, and increased protein turnover due to trauma or burn.

Prerenal azotemia can occur in any edema-forming condition during the phase in which NaCl and water accumulate. Typical examples include the nephrotic syndrome and hepatic cirrhosis with ascites (Chaps. 38 and 227). When a diuretic is being administered to inhibit the tubular reabsorption of NaCl, urine volume and Na concentration may be normal or elevated, even though SNGFR falls in response to the combination of the underlying edema-forming stimulus and further extracellular fluid volume depletion from the drug. Oliguria may appear upon withdrawal of the drug as the renal tubules resume intense reabsorption of NaCl and water. Prerenal azotemia may also be seen when renal blood flow is reduced by systemic hypotension, incomplete renal arterial or venous occlusion, or other cause (Chap. 132). Acute incomplete obstruction of the ureter and acute glomerular injury may also reduce SNGFR and leave tubule function relatively intact; postrenal azotemia is a term often applied when acute obstruction lowers SNGFR and causes azotemia. Whenever chronic obstruction of any portion of the urinary tract or glomerulonephritis damages nephrons extensively, the high urinary osmolality, U/P ratios for creatinine or urea, and low urinary Na concentrations disappear, and the kidneys behave as they do when nephron number is reduced.

TUBULE FUNCTION IMPAIRED   Certain acute renal diseases which produce azotemia lower SNGFR and at the same time damage the tubules sufficiently to reduce or even abolish their reabsorptive function, producing *acute renal failure*. Acute tubular necrosis, nephrotoxic agents, and all forms of acute tubulointerstitial disease are excellent examples. Azotemia and oliguria appear, but the urinary Na concentration exceeds 20 mmol and usually 40 mmol/L; the U/P

ratios for urea and creatinine are below 2 and 20, respectively; and urine osmolality is below 350 mosmol per kilogram of water. The ratio of BUN to serum creatinine is not elevated (see Chap. 223).

Reduced nephron number INCREASED SNGFR If one kidney is removed, the other grows larger, its nephrons enlarge, and the SNGFR increases until the total GFR becomes nearly normal for two kidneys. The tubules are overperfused with filtrate, but they appear to cope well with their increased reabsorptive burdens, perhaps in part because they are longer and wider and possess more cells. If more kidney tissue is removed, the remnant nephrons enlarge further, and their SNGFR rises. Extreme overperfusion of the tubules interferes with Na conservation. At the same time, total GFR comes to depend more and more upon expansion of the extracellular fluid volume largely because the increase in SNGFR is due not only to anatomic growth of the glomeruli but also to a relatively high rate of blood flow per glomerulus. Nephron adaptations to reduced nephron number are detailed in Chap. 222.

Azotemia occurs because the total GFR, i.e., the product of the elevated SNGFR and the markedly reduced nephron number, is low. Tubular conservation of filtered H_2O and Na conservation are poor, so fluid and salt intake must be liberal. Clinical states that produce this picture include surgical loss of renal substance secondary to trauma, neoplasm, stone, and destruction of kidneys by bacterial infection or tuberculosis, polycystic and medullary cystic renal diseases, and all the chronic tubulointerstitial nephropathies (Chaps. 229 and 231). In each of these disorders, the nephrons that remain viable are either fully intact or behave as though the SNGFR is better preserved than tubule function.

SNGFR NORMAL   The SNGFR does not appear to increase despite a reduction of nephron number in diseases such as glomerulonephritis and diabetic glomerulosclerosis, where the glomerulus is the primary site of damage. In these diseases total GFR falls directly with nephron number and is not supported by elevated SNGFR. Since the tubules are not confronted with an excessive reabsorptive burden, sodium conservation is adequate. In these disorders, superimposed conditions that lower SNGFR, such as depletion of extracellular fluid volume, can cause oliguria with low urine sodium concentration and U/P ratios for creatinine and urea above 20 and 3, respectively. The serum urea to creatinine ratio will rise distinctly.

SNGFR REDUCED In patients with chronic renal disease in whom total GFR has been sufficient to support life only because of a very high SNGFR, inadvertent dehydration or any other factor (Table 49-1 and Chaps. 222 and 223) that lowers the SNGFR can provoke oliguria and severe azotemia. Under these circumstances, urine Na concentration falls, but not below 20 mmol/L., as in the normal person, because SNGFR, though reduced from a previously elevated level, may still be above normal. The U/P ratios for creatinine and urea will be low, usually below 10 and 3, respectively, despite oliguria, and urine osmolality will not rise above the plasma level. The serum urea to creatinine ratio may rise, but not above 20. In less extreme situations, reduction of SNGFR will worsen azotemia and alter urine chemistry in the same directions but to a lesser extent.

OLIGURIA AND ANURIA *Oliguria* refers to a urine volume insufficient to sustain life, usually less than 400 mL per day in an adult of average size. Daily urine volume is difficult to measure when flow rate is low, because small absolute errors of volume measurement, in the range of 50 to 100 mL of urine each day, or of timing of collection, may represent large percentage errors.

Anuria, which is the absence of urine flow, is caused mainly by urinary obstruction, which must be excluded as a first step (Chap. 233). Total renal arterial and venous occlusion is another important cause. Severe renal diseases such as cortical necrosis and rapidly progressive glomerulonephritis produce anuria in the adult, but so rarely that anuria should never be ascribed to a primary renal disease until patency of the urinary tract and major renal blood vessels has been established.

Approach to the patient with azotemia or oliguria A critical issue is whether azotemia has been stable and long-standing (chronic renal failure, Chap. 221) or is recent and increasing (acute renal failure, Chap. 223; pre- and postrenal azotemia). If azotemia is recent, and oliguria present, the most discriminating additional measurements include serum urea and creatinine concentrations, and the Na, urea, and creatinine concentrations and osmolality of a concurrent urine sample. Reduction of SNGFR with well-preserved tubule function is usually present when urine osmolality exceeds 500 mosmol per kilogram of water, Na < 20 mmol/L, the U/P ratios for urea and creatinine > 8 and 40, respectively, the urinalysis is normal, and the BUN is more than 10 times the serum creatinine concentration. The prognosis for recovery of adequate GFR is good, if the cause of reduced SNGFR can be reversed. When urine osmolality is below 350 mosmol per kilogram of water, Na > 40 mmol, the U/P values for urea and creatinine < 2 and 20, respectively, and the BUN exceeds the serum creatinine by only tenfold, tubule function has been lost, and some form of acute or chronic renal failure usually is present.

ABNORMAL URINARY CONSTITUENTS

PROTEINURIA Normal adults may excrete up to 150 mg protein daily. Of this, only 10 to 15 mg is albumin; the rest is composed of over 30 different plasma proteins and of glycoproteins that derive from the renal cells. Tamm-Horsfall mucoprotein, the most prevalent of the urine proteins that do not arise from plasma, is produced by the cells of the ascending limb of the loop of Henle and is excreted at the rate of 25 mg per day. Daily excretion of more than 150 mg protein is properly termed *pathologic proteinuria,* but in common usage the word *proteinuria* suffices. Protein excretion above 3.5 g per 24 h is termed *massive* proteinuria and usually occurs when glomeruli have been damaged enough to allow plasma proteins, especially albumin, to enter the urine. Urinary albumin loss lowers serum albumin concentration, and the consequent fall in intracapillary oncotic pressure fosters the accumulation of tissue edema (Chap. 38); serum lipids rise, for reasons detailed in Chap. 227. The combination of *massive proteinuria, hypoalbuminemia, edema,* and *hyperlipidemia*

is often called the *nephrotic syndrome;* but this term is becoming synonymous with massive urinary protein loss alone. Hypoalbuminemia, elevated blood lipids, and edema are pathophysiologic consequences of massive proteinuria and occur only when hepatic albumin synthesis, though normal or even increased, fails to compensate for urine albumin losses; these features are not a direct result of renal disease.

Detection of proteinuria Proteinuria is usually detected by urine "dipsticks" that register a trace result in response to as little as 50 mg protein per liter, and a distinct color change of the 1+ level at about 300 mg protein per liter. Since proteinuria can be missed if the urine is very dilute, fasting morning samples that tend to be concentrated are usually studied. Dipsticks respond best to albumin, so that a negative result can occur when large amounts of other protein, or protein fragments such as light chains, are being excreted. Dipstick proteinuria requires additional evaluation by the measurement of 24-h excretion rate. If total protein excretion is abnormal, it is helpful to characterize the proportions of albumin and globulins in the urine by cellulose acetate electrophoresis or other methods. Immunoelectrophoresis is required to identify immunoglobulin fragments, kappa or lambda light chains, when their presence is suggested by a monoclonal peak on routine urine electrophoresis.

Mechanisms of proteinuria TUBULAR PROTEINURIA Normal low-molecular-weight (<40,000) serum proteins, such as beta$_2$ microglobulin (11,600 mol wt), lysozyme (14,000 mol wt), or light chains (22,000 mol wt) are readily filtered by the glomeruli but are reabsorbed so efficiently that only trace amounts enter the urine. Diseases that selectively damage the tubules more than glomeruli (Chap. 229) cause excessive excretion of these small proteins with little or no increase in albumin excretion. The resulting proteinuria is usually between 1 and 3 g per 24 h, and edema and lipid disorders do not occur because albumin losses are small. Bence Jones protein, which is probably a dimer of two light chains, light chains themselves, and myoglobin are examples of proteins whose plasma concentrations may increase as a consequence of disease. If their filtered load rises enough to exceed tubular reabsorptive capacity, "overflow" proteinuria may occur.

GLOMERULAR PROTEINURIA Normal glomeruli filter very little albumin or globulin. Glomerular capillary endothelial cells form a barrier penetrated by pores of about 100 nm diameter that holds back cells and other particles but offers no impediment to most proteins. The glomerular basement membrane traps molecules about 5 nm in effective radius, above 100,000 daltons molecular mass. The *foot processes (podocytes)* of the visceral epithelial cells (Fig. 49-1) cover the urinary aspect of the glomerular basement membrane and produce a series of narrow channels through which molecules that traverse the basement membrane must pass. Anionic molecules, like albumin, are filtered less freely than are neutral or positively charged molecules of the same size, so little albumin enters the filtrate. This charge selectively appears to be due to anionic glycoproteins that cover the surfaces of the foot processes and contribute to the matrix structure of the basement membrane (Chap. 222). The glycoproteins are anionic because they contain the dicarboxylic amino acids, glutamic and aspartic acid, and sialic acid. At the pH of blood (7.4) or urine (4.5 to 7.5) carboxylic and sialic acid residues are dissociated and, therefore, have a negative charge; albumin also carries an overall negative charge. The negatively charged portions of the glycoproteins repel those of albumin and retard filtration.

Glomerular disease can disrupt any of these filtration barriers. Injury limited to the polyanion glycoproteins would tend to produce selective losses of anionic proteins, such as albumin, that would be filtered more completely by the normal glomerulus but for their charge. Extensive injury that involves the entire basement membrane, not only its polyanion components, may increase losses of very large proteins as well as albumin.

The selectivity of proteinuria varies with the extent of glomerular injury. However, the clinical value of measuring selectivity has not been fully defined. The basis of such measurements is to express the

FIGURE 49-1 Top. Diagram showing normal structures separating the capillary lumen and urinary space in the glomerulus. In the process of glomerular filtration, an ultrafiltrate of plasma traverses the glomerular capillary wall through endothelial fenestrae, basement membrane, and slit diaphragms. Macromolecules in the plasma are believed to be restricted from entry into glomerular urine by each of these wall structures. In addition, circulating polyanions (e.g., albumin) are thought to be retarded by negatively charged glycosialoproteins, which, as shown by the shaded area in the upper panel, are distributed throughout the glomerular wall. Bottom. A corresponding electron micrograph of the same structures. *(Drawing by NL Gahan from BM Brenner, R Beeuwkes, Hosp Prac, vol 13, no 7, 1978. Reproduced with permission.)*

excretion rate of a protein as a fraction of its theoretical maximal filtered load, which is the product of its serum concentration and the GFR. This fraction must reflect the relative filtration efficiency of the protein to that of a completely filtered GFR marker, usually inulin or creatinine, provided that tubular reabsorption and renal production or catabolism are negligible. The slope of a plot of such a clearance ratio against the molecular weight for a variety of serum proteins is one index of filtration selectivity. A more practical version of this test is based upon the ratio of the clearance fractions of two proteins of different molecular weight, such as IgG and transferrin (Chap. 227).

Approach to the patient with proteinuria Given dipstick proteinuria of the 1+ level or more, 24-h urine protein excretion should be measured. If it is above 150 mg, electrophoresis should be carried out to determine the proportions of albumin and other proteins. Excretion mainly of albumin signifies a glomerular lesion. When the total daily protein excretion exceeds 3.5 g, by definition the nephrotic syndrome is considered to be present; milder albuminuria is called an *asymptomatic urinary abnormality*. The initial steps in evaluating proteinuria are outlined in Chap. 221. Subsequent details of differential diagnosis are in Chaps. 227 and 228. Tubular proteinuria usually reflects a hereditary or acquired tubular disorder (Chap. 231) or tubulointerstitial nephropathy (Chap. 229). The presence of large amounts of Bence Jones protein suggests that multiple myeloma may be present (Chap. 265).

HEMATURIA AND CASTS   Isolated hematuria Bleeding in the urinary tract from the urethra to the renal pelvis produces isolated hematuria, without significant proteinuria, cells, or urinary casts.

Total hematuria, which occurs evenly throughout voiding, means that blood has had the opportunity to mix fully with the bladder urine. When bleeding occurs mainly at the beginning or end of micturition, a prostatic or urethral origin is more likely.

Common causes of *isolated* hematuria are urinary tract stones, benign and malignant neoplasms of the urinary tract, tuberculosis, trauma, and prostatitis; few primary renal diseases cause it. As discussed in Chaps. 221 and 227, *focal glomerulitis*, in the syndrome of benign recurrent hematuria or in Berger's disease, i.e., IgA nephropathy, is usually associated with red blood cell casts. Analgesic nephropathy and sickling states cause isolated hematuria, but modest proteinuria; papillary necrosis or azotemia often is present and suggests a renal origin. Hemoglobin electrophoresis is appropriate whenever a sickling disorder is suspected.

Examination of the prostate and external urethra is the basic first step in the evaluation of isolated hematuria. Intravenous pyelography and renal ultrasonography are the next. If no lesion is found and no obvious cause of bleeding such as renal stone passage is present, cystoscopy and retrograde pyelography may become necessary. At cystoscopy, blood may be found to issue from only one ureter, a helpful clue which indicates a localized lesion rather than a primary renal disease. Disorders of coagulation, and thrombocytopenia, as well as urinary infection, must be excluded. Because infection with tuberculosis and fungi may be difficult to detect, multiple urine samples must be cultured and examined by microscopy. Computed tomography of the kidney and sometimes renal arteriography may be needed to disclose anatomic lesions such as cysts or tumors. Urine cytology may give a clue to malignant neoplasms of the kidneys or urinary tract that otherwise escape detection.

Hematuria associated with urinary tract infection Bacterial infection of the lower urinary tract or of the kidneys frequently causes hematuria. The presence of associated pyuria suggests the diagnosis of infection, and the demonstration of pathogenic bacteria in concentrations above 10^5 colonies per milliliter of urine establishes it. Acute cystitis or urethritis in women is an especially common cause of gross hematuria; in such symptomatic patients infection is documented by colony counts above 10^2 colonies per milliliter. Urinary tuberculosis can produce isolated hematuria, but pyuria often is present as well.

Hematuria with evidence of renal disease NEPHRONAL HEMATURIA   Blood that enters the tubular fluid anywhere along the nephron can be trapped in a cylindrical mold of gelled Tamm-Horsfall protein to produce red blood cell casts. Tamm-Horsfall protein gels when concentrated at a low pH, as occurs during dehydration, or when exposed to myoglobin, hemoglobin, albumin, Bence Jones protein, and pyelographic contrast media. Degenerated red blood cells and clumps of hemoglobin can produce deeply pigmented casts that have the same significance—nephronal hematuria—as red blood cell casts.

Nephronal hematuria always connotes significant renal disease such as glomerulonephritis, tubulointerstitial injury, or a vasculitis that has damaged the circulation of the nephron. Glomerular or tubular proteinuria often accompanies renal bleeding, as a consequence of nephron injury. In general, nephronal hematuria, or proteinuria alone, arise from primary renal diseases that have a better prognosis than those in which proteinuria and hematuria occur in combination (Chap. 221).

Hematuria with proteinuria or casts Frequently, hematuria is accompanied by proteinuria, but red blood cell and deeply pigmented granular casts are absent. The presumption then is that bleeding is of nephronal origin, but a coincident independent lesion of the urinary tract must always be considered, because common renal diseases, such as diabetic glomerulosclerosis and arteriolar nephrosclerosis associated with hypertension, produce mainly proteinuria.

TYPES OF CASTS   Heavy albuminuria or dehydration can cause showers of transparent, refractile "hyaline" casts. During heavy proteinuria, tubule cells fill with cholesterol-rich lipid droplets that display a Maltese-cross appearance in polarized light. Casts that incorporate these cells are called *fatty casts* because the lipid droplets are prominent. The same lipid-rich cells free in urine are called *oval fat bodies*.

White blood cell and *epithelial cell casts* can occur in any inflammatory state that involves the nephrons. White blood cell casts are particularly common in pyelonephritis, in nephritis associated with systemic lupus erythematosus, and during transplant rejection. When white blood or epithelial cells degenerate, they form granular nonpigmented casts that contain cellular debris and aggregated proteins. So-called *waxy* casts, with few granules and very distinct margins, arise when cell debris has broken down to a fine dispersion so that granules are no longer visible and are most common in chronic and progressive renal diseases.

Broad casts, of unusual width, are thought to arise in the dilated tubules of enlarged nephrons that have undergone compensatory hypertrophy in response to a reduction of functioning renal mass. A urine sample that contains a combination of broad and waxy casts as well as cellular or granular casts or red blood cells indicates a chronic smoldering process and has been termed a *telescoped* urine. This abnormality, first described in polyarteritis nodosa and systemic lupus erythematosus, can also be found in many chronic forms of glomerulonephritis with active glomerulitis.

Approach to the patient with hematuria Many urinalyses should be performed to determine whether the hematuria is isolated or associated with other features of primary renal disease, i.e., cells, casts, or proteinuria. The magnitude and type of associated proteinuria should be determined. As a general rule intravenous pyelography should be performed, if it can be done safely, even when the hematuria is of definite nephronal origin. Not only lesions of the urinary tract, but renal tumors or cysts, discrete areas of papillary necrosis, or signs of renal venous obstruction may be present. The source of isolated hematuria must always be ascertained, and this means a detailed examination of the urinary tract by cystoscopy, retrograde pyelography, and arteriography to disclose tumor, stone, cysts, or other cause. Renal ultrasonography and computed tomography are particularly helpful in detecting and evaluating renal cysts and tumors and should precede cystoscopy and arteriography. If all the studies disclose normal structures, a nephronal origin of hematuria is likely even if no red blood cell casts are present. The role of renal biopsy in such cases is detailed in Chaps. 227, 228, and 229. Hematuria with infection or overt renal disease usually requires no steps beyond intravenous pyelography. Evaluation of hematuria is detailed further in Chap. 215.

POLYURIA AND NOCTURIA

POLYURIA A reasonable definition of polyuria is a urine volume above 3 liters per day, but this should be qualified to exclude normal individuals who desire a large fluid intake and therefore form large volumes of urine. Patients cannot always distinguish polyuria from urinary frequency, the frequent voiding of small volumes. Since voiding volumes may not be clear from the history, polyuria must be substantiated by 24-h urine collection before one begins an investigation of causes.

Causes Polyuria can arise from inadequate secretion of vasopressin, failure of the renal tubules to respond to vasopressin, solute diuresis, or natriuresis (Table 49-2). It may also occur as a physiologic adaptation to deliberate excessive water drinking. The normal physiology of urine formation and mechanisms responsible for renal water conservation are discussed in Chap. 222.

DIABETES INSIPIDUS (See also Chap. 315) The term *diabetes insipidus* is applied to situations in which inadequate renal water conservation causes polyuria and secondary thirst. Either vasopressin insufficiency (central diabetes insipidus) or renal unresponsiveness to vasopressin (nephrogenic diabetes insipidus) may be responsible. In both, water reabsorption is reduced all along the distal nephron, because passive water movement from tubules into the hypertonic outer and inner medullary interstitium is slow. But even though the

---

TABLE 49-2 Causes of polyuria

I Inadequate renal water conservation
  A Diabetes insipidus
    1 Vasopressin-sensitive (posthypophysectomy; posttrauma; postpituitary ablation; idiopathic; supra- or intrasellar tumors or cysts; histiocystosis or granuloma; encroachment by aneurysm; Sheehan's syndrome; meningoencephalitis; Guillain Barré syndrome; fat embolus; empty sella)
    2 Nephrogenic
      a Acquired tubulointerstitial renal disease (pyelonephritis, analgesic nephropathy, multiple myeloma, amyloidosis, obstructive uropathy, sarcoidosis, hypercalcemic or hypokalemic nephropathy, Sjögren's syndrome, sickle cell anemia, renal transplantation)
      b Drugs or toxins (lithium, demeclocycline, methoxyflurane, ethanol, diphenylhydantoin, propoxyphene, amphotericin)
      c Congenital (hereditary nephrogenic diabetes insipidus, polycystic or medullary cystic disease)
  B Solute diuresis (glucosuria, high-protein tube feedings, urea or mannitol infusion, radiographic contrast media, chronic renal failure)
  C Natriuretic syndromes (salt-losing nephritis, diuretic phase of acute tubular necrosis, diuretic agents)
II Primary polydipsia
  A Psychogenic
  B Hypothalamic disease
  C Drugs (thioridazine, chlorpromazine, anticholinergic agents)

---

rate of water movement out of the collecting ducts is low for a given osmotic difference between the tubule lumen and interstitial fluid, the fluid that enters the collecting ducts is so abnormally dilute and copious in volume that more water enters the inner medulla than under normal circumstances and medullary solutes are washed out into the vasa recta. Wash-out is incomplete and vasopressin administration can lead to formation of an osmotically concentrated urine, but the maximal urine osmolality that can be attained is below normal.

Vasopressin-sensitive (central) diabetes insipidus may be idiopathic or secondary to hypophysectomy or trauma or to neoplastic, inflammatory, vascular, or infectious causes (Table 49-2). Idiopathic diabetes insipidus can be inherited as an autosomal dominant trait; but more commonly it is sporadic and appears in childhood. In both forms there is selective destruction of the neurons that produce vasopressin in the supraoptic nucleus.

Rarely, nephrogenic diabetes insipidus is familial and congenital; but usually it is acquired from renal disease (Table 49-2). Hypercalcemia and hypokalemic nephropathy are important reversible causes of nephrogenic diabetes insipidus. Lithium carbonate, methoxyflurane anesthesia, and demeclocycline can also produce nephrogenic diabetes insipidus.

SOLUTE DIURESIS Excessive filtration of a poorly resorbed solute such as glucose, mannitol, or urea can depress reabsorption of NaCl and water in the proximal tubule and cause their loss in the urine, producing polyuria. Urine Na concentration is below that of blood, so that more water than salt is lost from the body and serum hypertonicity can be produced. Glucosuria in diabetes mellitus is a common cause of solute diuresis. Iatrogenic solute diuresis may arise from mannitol infusion, angiographic contrast media, and high-protein gavage feedings, which produce an excessive excretion of urea. Any degree of solute diuresis can cause polyuria, so further evaluation of renal concentrating ability should be postponed until the solute diuresis is corrected.

NATRIURETIC SYNDROMES Excessive chronic Na loss may occur during the course of tubulointerstitial or cystic renal diseases. Polyuria and polydipsia are accompanied by an unusually large daily Na requirement. Examples of this phenomenon include medullary cystic disease, Bartter's syndrome, and the diuretic phase of acute tubular necrosis, in which Na and water losses are very large.

PRIMARY POLYDIPSIA Whether because of habit, predilection, psychiatric disorder, a specific lesion in the brain, or medication (Table 49-2), some people drink enough water every day to produce polyuria. The body and the kidneys rarely if ever are injured by chronic polydipsia, but the condition can be confused with diabetes insipidus, which it resembles closely. During deliberate polydipsia, extracellular fluid volume is normal or high, and vasopressin secretion is reduced to a basal level because serum osmolality tends to be near the lower limits of normal. Reabsorption of water from the end distal convoluted tubule and collecting ducts is reduced so that all the surplus water can be excreted into the urine. The inner medulla loses its urea and NaCl gradients because of wash-out, as in diabetes insipidus. Wash-out may be more severe than in diabetes insipidus because primary polydipsia tends to cause expansion of the extracellular fluid volume, whereas primary renal water loss does the opposite. Volume expansion raises total delivery of NaCl and water to the thick ascending limb of Henle's loop and therefore to the inner medulla, all things being equal. It also raises renal blood flow, and increased flow through the vasa recta reduces their ability to trap solutes in the medulla.

Approach to the patient with polyuria Solute diuresis and natriuretic syndromes usually are apparent from the history, physical examination, urinalysis (glucosuria), clinical setting, blood count, blood glucose, and serum creatinine or the BUN. Diagnostic problems occur mainly when stable, chronic polyuria and polydipsia of uncertain origin are present. Here, one must try to distinguish between vasopressin-sensitive diabetes insipidus, nephrogenic diabetes insipidus, and primary polydipsia; the best-established way to do this is by measuring the response of urine osmolality to water deprivation and the administration of vasopressin.

The patient should have free access to water and receive a normal diet that provides approximately 100 mmol NaCl per day for 3 days; then a total fast is instituted. During the fast, pulse and blood pressure should be measured every 30 min and body weight every hour, using an accurate balance. When 3 percent of the initial body weight has been lost or 14 h have elapsed, urine and serum osmolality are measured. The normal subject will lower urine volume below 0.5 mL/min and raise urine osmolality to above 700 mosmol per kilogram of water. In complete diabetes insipidus, nephrogenic or vasopressin-sensitive, the urine osmolality will remain below 200 mosmol/kg water and urine flow above 0.5 mL/min, but some rise in osmolality and fall in flow will occur in incomplete diabetes insipidus. If urine osmolality is below 700 mosmol/kg water, by the end of the fasting period, 5 mU/min of aqueous vasopressin is administered by intravenous drip. Patients with complete or partial vasopressin-sensitive diabetes insipidus will raise their urine osmolality above the level achieved by fasting alone by more than 9 percent (see Chap. 315). No increase will occur given complete nephrogenic diabetes insipidus, although incomplete forms of nephrogenic diabetes insipidus will permit some response to vasopressin. Infusion of hypertonic saline (Chap. 315) is useful in defining defects of osmoregulator function.

The response of patients with primary polydipsia is quite different. During fluid restriction the secretion of vasopressin increases, and at the completion of the test the flow rate and osmolality of the urine will reflect a physiologic level of vasopressin acting upon normal tubules that traverse a medullary interstitium whose urea and NaCl concentrations have been reduced by chronic wash-out. In other words, the wash-out will set the upper limit on urine osmolality, and patients with primary polydipsia thus demonstrate a submaximal concentrating ability in spite of intact vasopressin secretion. Exogenous vasopressin can increase urine osmolality very little, < 9 percent, because medullary wash-out, not vasopressin insufficiency or insensitivity, is the main limiting factor. Usually the urine osmolality will be above 400 mosmol/kg water by the end of the fluid deprivation test, in contrast to the lower values of approximately 200 mosmol/kg water encountered in patients with diabetes insipidus; but it may be impossible to distinguish incomplete diabetes insipidus from primary polydipsia, in some cases, by using the fluid deprivation test alone. However, measurement of serum antidiuretic hormone levels by radioimmunoassay may increase diagnostic accuracy.

NOCTURIA Whether an individual sleeps through the night without urinating depends upon a diurnal rhythm in which the volume of urine formed during sleep does not exceed bladder capacity, because of reduced renal osmotic concentration, high sodium excretion, solute diuresis, or low bladder capacity.

All the polyuric states may cause nocturia. Urinary concentrating ability falls in most renal diseases (Chap. 222), often at an early stage. Even though overt polyuria may be absent, overnight urine volume frequently exceeds bladder capacity. Nocturia also occurs in edema-forming states. In congestive heart failure, nephrotic syndrome, and hepatic cirrhosis with ascites, fluid accumulates preferentially in dependent portions of the body during the day. At night, with recumbency, tissue capillary forces change and some edema fluid is mobilized, producing the effect of an intravenous saline infusion. Venous insufficiency may produce dependent edema of the legs that is often also mobilized at night, causing nocturia.

Reduced bladder capacity also causes nocturia. Infection, tumor, or stone can cause inflammation and increased irritability. Chronic partial bladder-outflow obstruction, from prostatic hypertrophy, urethral stricture, or benign or malignant neoplasm or stone, causes a frequent stimulus to void and also a thickening of the muscular wall that reduces its compliance. Frequent small voidings may be a clue to this lower urinary tract cause of nocturia, but in its earlier phases chronic obstruction may lead to only one nocturnal voiding of reasonable volume.

DYSURIA, FREQUENCY AND URGENCY, INCONTINENCE, AND ENURESIS

DYSURIA, FREQUENCY, AND URGENCY *Dysuria* refers to pain or a burning sensation during urination. *Urinary frequency* means voiding at abnormally brief intervals, due to a sense of bladder fullness that is due not to a full bladder but to a bladder that is irritable and feels full even when it is not. *Urgency* is an exaggerated sense of needing to urinate, due to an irritable or inflamed bladder.

Mechanisms of dysuria REDUCED BLADDER COMPLIANCE When the bladder has a decreased ability to expand, frequency, nocturia, and urgency usually result. When decreased expansion is due to inflammation of the mucosa (cystitis) from infection, radiation, chemicals, or foreign bodies (catheters, stones), a burning sensation usually is more prominent than when it is due to infiltration of the muscle by tumors of the bladder or from adjacent organs (prostate, rectum, uterus).

INFECTION   Acute bacterial cystitis, which occurs more frequently in women, usually causes great frequency day and night, a burning sensation on urination, and, not infrequently, gross hematuria. Prostatitis or prostatocystitis in men can cause a picture similar to acute cystitis in women. When only the prostate is involved, milder symptoms such as vague pain or discomfort in the lower abdomen, groin, perineum, rectum, testes, or penis occur. The symptoms may be associated with urination but more frequently are noticed at times other than during micturition or ejaculation.

PSYCHOSOMATIC CYSTITIS   The functional bladder syndrome and chronic glandular urethrotrigonitis are synonyms for a very common but poorly understood affliction of middle-aged and older women, in which pain is usually vague, aching in nature, and in the lower abdomen or vagina. There is daytime frequency without nocturia; pyuria is absent. A complete urologic evaluation usually becomes necessary because symptoms are chronic and hard to eradicate. The functional bladder syndrome must be distinguished from the effects of a cystocele, which can be repaired surgically.

Approach to the patient with dysuria The medical history should focus on past as well as present urinary problems. A pelvic examination in women and prostatic examination in men are necessary components of the physical examination. Microscopic examination of a two-glass urinary sediment in all patients and of the prostatic fluid in men, obtained by prostatic massage, is also necessary. The first 20 mL of a voiding, if collected separately, may contain a higher concentration of leukocytes and bacteria than the remainder of the voided urine, when the urethra is the principal site of inflammation or infection. Normal prostatic fluid, not subjected to centrifugation, contains less than 10 leukocytes per high-power field; excessive leukocytes in the prostatic fluid are an important clue to prostatitis and may, when prostatitis is chronic, be the only detectable abnormality. Further diagnostic studies will depend upon such positive findings as a history of chronic or recurrent episodes or associated fever, which are rare in lower urinary tract infections except in acute prostatitis, or an abnormality on physical examination such as a pelvic or rectal mass or tenderness, hematuria or pyuria, or excessive leukocytes and macrophages in the prostatic fluid. Serum acid phosphatase may be elevated when carcinoma of the prostate has extended beyond the boundary of the prostatic capsule.

Additional evaluation of dysuria, when the cause is not evident from clinical examination, may include cultures of urine and prostatic fluid for aerobic and anaerobic bacteria, tubercle bacilli, and myco-plasmas; excretory urography; and voiding cystourethrography. If these examinations do not reveal the diagnosis, but symptoms are troublesome, urologic evaluations, including cystoscopy and ureth-roscopy with endoscopic biopsies of visualized abnormalities, and dynamic urinary tract studies may be useful.

INCONTINENCE *Incontinence* refers to the inability to retain urine in the bladder. It results from neurologic or mechanical disorders of the complicated system that controls normal micturition.

Normal bladder function The detrusor muscle, which provides the propulsive force for emptying the bladder, consists of interlacing fibers of smooth muscle that are under parasympathetic autonomic control through the pelvic nerves from sacral spinal cord segments S2, S3, and S4. The smooth muscle of the trigonal portion of the bladder, between the ureteral orifices and the posterior area of the bladder outlet, is innervated by motor fibers from thoracolumbar segments (T11 to L2) of the sympathetic nervous system, in which alpha receptor sites predominate. This layer of muscle extends into the posterior urethra and acts as an involuntary internal sphincter that helps maintain urinary continence even in the absence of voluntary control. The external urethral sphincter and perineal muscles are under voluntary control via the pudendal nerves.

Sensory tracts of pain, temperature, and distention pass from the bladder via the pelvic nerves to sacral spinal levels S2, S3, and S4, creating a simple spinal voiding reflex between the bladder and the sacral spinal cord. The sensory tracts from the bladder further ascend through sacrobulbar pathways to the medulla of the brain and ultimately to cortical centers, from which impulses arise, pass back down the lateral and ventral reticulospinal tracts, and normally suppress the sacral spinal reflex arc controlling bladder emptying.

The normal adult bladder can accommodate as much as approxi-mately 400 mL fluid without a significant increase in intravesical pressure (< 20 cmH$_2$O). Above this point, sensations of fullness are transmitted to the sacral cord. If not suppressed by cortical control, the sacral cord reflexly discharges motor impulses that cause powerful sustained detrusor contraction. Urination can be prevented by cortical suppression of the reflex arc or by voluntary contraction of the external sphincter and perineal muscles. Infants, and adults with spinal cord damage above S2, urinate spontaneously when the bladder fills sufficiently.

Normal urination is initiated by voluntary suppression of cortical inhibition of the reflex arc and by relaxation of the muscles of the pelvic floor and the external sphincter. The base of the bladder falls; then the trigone contracts, an action that occludes the ureters as they pass through the bladder wall and helps to prevent vesicoureteral reflux of urine during voiding. Finally, the detrusor contracts and voiding occurs.

Causes of incontinence DETRUSOR INSTABILITY In this con-dition, the bladder becomes prone to uncontrollable contractions—that cause incontinence—because inhibitory neural pathways are damaged. Among the elderly, detrusor instability causes as much as 70 percent of urinary incontinence, and arises from diseases of the central nervous system such as cerebrovascular accidents, Alzheimer's dementia, neoplasm, and, possibly, normal pressure hydrocephalus. Any lesion that disrupts the lateral and ventral reticulospinal tracts can reduce or abolish descending inhibiting impulses to the sacral spinal reflex and can result in detrusor instability. If the descending

tracts are completely destroyed, the bladder will empty automatically. Bladder or pelvic infection or tumor, fecal impaction, uterine prolapse, and prostatic hypertrophy are other causes. Whatever the cause, the usual clinical picture is of unpredictable, involuntary voiding, usually >160 mL each time. Imipramine, 25 mg at bedtime, or calcium channel blockers (such as nifedipine) reduce detrusor contractions, and improve continence. Local infection, tumors, or fecal impaction are treated conventionally.

STRESS INCONTINENCE This condition is common in postmeno-pausal parous women. The structures of the female urethra atrophy when deprived of estrogen, and many become unable to resist the passage of urine under the stress of increased intraabdominal pressure during coughing, sneezing, climbing stairs, and other physical activity, so small amounts of urine escape. Parturition may damage the pelvic support of the bladder so that the bladder and urethra can slip downward from their normal position above the pelvic diaphragm. As they do, the urethra shortens, and the normal urethrovesical angle, important in closing the urethral sphincter, is lost. In men, stress incontinence usually is secondary to prostatic surgery for benign prostatic hypertrophy or prostatic carcinoma. If the external sphincter has also been damaged during operation, total incontinence may result. Surgical elevation of the urethrovesical angle is helpful in women. Estrogen replacement therapy may prevent atrophy of the urethral mucosa.

MECHANICAL INCONTINENCE Some congenital anomalies, extro-phy of the bladder, patent urachus, and ectopic ureteral openings distal to the vesical neck cause mechanical incontinence. They are correctable only by surgery. Mechanical incontinence can follow transurethral resection of the prostate that damages both the internal and external sphincter mechanisms. Pelvic surgery or irradiation of the uterus or rectum may cause incontinence because of vesicovaginal, ureterovaginal, vesicoperineal, or ureteroperineal fistulas.

OVERFLOW OR PARADOXICAL INCONTINENCE This form of in-continence arises from large residual volumes of urine secondary to obstruction at the bladder neck or along the urethra (urethral stricture) or from neurologic damage. Benign prostatic hypertrophy afflicts upward of 75 percent of older men. It is manifested by nocturia, reduced size and force of the urinary stream, straining to urinate, and terminal dribbling, all due to outflow obstruction. Functional outflow obstruction can occur because of spinal cord disease; the detrusor and external sphincter contract dyssynergistically, i.e., at the same time. Hypotonic neurogenic bladders may occur in diseases which produce autonomic peripheral neuropathy, such as diabetes mellitus, uremia, hypothyroidism, chronic alcoholism, Guillain-Barré syndrome, collagen vascular diseases, and toxic neuropathies asso-ciated with some carcinomas (especially lung and kidney). It also may occur because of prolonged overdistention of the bladder. Hydronephrosis and impaired renal function can occur in patients with chronic overflow incontinence. All causes produce a dilated, palpable bladder. Especially in diabetes, patients can control mictu-rition but lose their sensory awareness of bladder filling. Their incontinence can be avoided by scheduled reminders. Outlet obstruc-tion is treated surgically. If the bladder has become adynamic because of prolonged overfilling, bethanechol chloride, 50 to 100 mg per day, may improve emptying.

PSYCHOGENIC AND FUNCTIONAL INCONTINENCE Children, and even some young adults, draw attention to themselves by feigning incontinence and thereby derive some secondary emotional satisfac-tion. A complete diagnostic evaluation usually is necessary to rule out organic disease even when psychogenic incontinence is strongly suspected. In elderly people, especially those who have a limited ability to walk or who are confused because of central nervous system disease or drugs, incontinence may be *functional*, i.e., due simply to an inability to reach a toilet in time. Treatment depends upon correcting the individual problem in each case.

ENURESIS *Enuresis* refers to the involuntary passage of urine at night or during sleep—hence, the synonym bed-wetting. Some clinicians reserve the term enuresis for those bed wetters who have no gross urologic abnormalities, but it should be used for bed-wetting in general.

The sacral spinal reflex arc alone controls urination in the infant; therefore, enuretic incontinence is normal under the age of 2 years. As the nervous system matures, cortical control over the spinal reflex arc results in the voluntary control over urination and defecation by the age of 2½ years. Even so, enuresis beyond the age of 3 years occurs to some degree in approximately 10 percent of all otherwise normal children and probably is due to a delay in maturation of bladder control, which may be familial.

Although the majority of bed wetters will be dry by the age of puberty, organic diseases, especially infections of the urinary tract, obstructive lesions with overflow incontinence, neurovesical dysfunction, and polyuric conditions that overload the bladder must be suspected in any child who is enuretic beyond the age of 3 years. Patients with organic disease usually, but not always, are incontinent during the day as well as at night. For the majority, who have no overt lesions, imipramine (75 mg at bedtime) may be useful.

REFERENCES

Azotemia, oliguria, and anuria

ABUELO JG: Proteinuria: Diagnostic principles and procedures. Ann Intern Med 98:186, 1983

BRENNER BM et al: Molecular basis of proteinuria of glomerular origin. N Engl J Med 298:826, 1978

BRIDGES CR et al: Glomerular charge alterations in human minimal charge nephropathy. Kidney Int 22:677, 1982

GLASSOCK RJ et al: Primary glomerular diseases, in The Kidney, 3d ed, BM Brenner, FC Rector Jr (eds). Philadelphia, Saunders, 1986, p 929

KURTZMAN NA (ed): Seminars in Nephrology: Acute Renal Failure, JP Knochel (guest ed). New York, Grune & Stratton, 1981

——— (ed): Seminars in Nephrology: Chronic Renal Failure, G Eknoyan (guest ed). New York, Grune & Stratton, 1981

LEVEY AS et al: Idiopathic nephrotic syndrome. Ann Intern Med 107:697, 1987

OKEN DE: On the differential diagnosis of acute renal failure. Am J Med 71:916, 1981

PARDO V et al: Benign primary hematuria: Clinicopathologic study of 65 patients. Am J Med 67:817, 1979

Polyuria and nocturia

BERL T (ed): Disorders of water metabolism, in Seminars in Nephrology, vol 4. New York, Grune & Stratton, 1984, p 285

ROBERTSON GL, BERL W: Pathophysiology of water metabolism, in The Kidney, 3d ed, BM Brenner, FC Rector Jr (eds). Philadelphia, Saunders, 1986, p 385

SCHRIER RW, BICHET DG: Osmotic and nonosmotic control of vasopressin release and the pathogenesis of impaired water excretion in adrenal, thyroid, and edematous disorders. J Lab Clin Med 98:1, 1981

ZERBE RL, ROBERTSON GL: A comparison of plasma vasopressin measurements with a standard indirect test in the differential diagnosis of polyuria. N Engl J Med 305:1539, 1981

Dysuria, frequency and urgency, incontinence, and enuresis

BRADLEY WE: Diagnosis of urinary bladder dysfunction in diabetes mellitus. Ann Intern Med 92:323, 1980

———, SCOTT FB: Physiology of the urinary bladder, in Urology, 4th ed, JH Harrison et al (eds). Philadelphia, Saunders, 1978, vol 1, p 87

DEGROAT WC, BOOTH AM: Physiology of the urinary bladder and urethra. Ann Intern Med 92:312, 1980

HINDMARSH HR, BYRNE PO: Adult enuresis: A symptomatic and urodynamic assessment. Br J Urol 52:88, 1980

KELLOGG JA et al: Clinical relevance of culture versus screens for the detection of microbial pathogens in urine specimens. Am J Med 83:739, 1987

MEARES EM JR: Prostatitis syndromes: New perspectives about old woes. J Urol 123:141, 1980

MIKKELSEN EJ, RAPOPORT JL: Enuresis: Psychopathology, sleep stage, and drug response. Urol Clin North Am 7:361, 1980

PLATT R: Quantitative definition of bacteriuria. Infectious Diseases Symposium, July 28, 1983, p 44, Supplement to Am J Med

TURNER-WARWICK R, WHITESIDE CG (eds): Symposium on Clinical Urodynamics: The Urologic Clinics of North America, vol 6. Philadelphia, Saunders, 1979

WILLIAMS ME, PANNELL FC: Urinary incontinence in the elderly. Ann Intern Med 97:895, 1982

50   FLUIDS AND ELECTROLYTES

NORMAN G. LEVINSKY

SODIUM AND WATER

PHYSIOLOGIC CONSIDERATIONS (See also Chap. 222)   Both physiologically and clinically, sodium and water metabolism are closely interrelated. The sodium content of the body depends on the balance between dietary intake and renal excretion of sodium. In health, extrarenal losses of sodium are negligible. Renal sodium excretion is closely regulated to match dietary content. Within 2 to 4 days after sodium intake stops, urinary excretion decreases to 5 mmol/d or less. If dietary sodium is abruptly increased, sodium excretion promptly rises and equals intake within a few days. Thus, in normal persons the sodium content of the body remains quite constant despite wide variations in sodium intake; over the range of 0 to 400 mmol/d, total body sodium varies only by about 10 percent.

Renal sodium excretion   This is regulated by the interplay of multiple control mechanisms. Sodium loads or deficits tend to produce corresponding changes in the central blood volume. Receptors, apparently located in the atria and central arteries, respond to changes in local pressure or flow which signal the volume/capacity relation of the central circulation (*effective blood volume*). If the effective volume is depleted, salt retention is induced, while expansion triggers multiple factors that favor natriuresis. With volume (salt) depletion, renal blood flow falls, due to decreased cardiac output, increased renal sympathetic nerve activity, and activation of the renin-angiotensin system. Glomerular filtration also tends to fall, which reduces filtered sodium. Tubular reabsorption of sodium is enhanced. Proximal reabsorption is stimulated by changes in Starling forces (e.g., increased plasma protein concentration) in the peritubular circulation and by sympathetic nerves which innervate proximal segments directly. Distal tubular reabsorption is enhanced by aldosterone, which is secreted at an increased rate in response to stimulation of the adrenal gland by angiotensin. Volume expansion leads to the opposite changes in renal hemodynamics and in these various regulators of tubular transport. Moreover, one or more natriuretic hormones are released in response to increased extracellular volume. A natriuretic peptide secreted by the atria augments sodium excretion both by increasing glomerular filtration and by inhibiting tubular sodium reabsorption. Another natriuretic hormone may decrease tubular salt transport by inhibiting Na^+, K^+ adenosine triphosphatase (ATPase). Prostaglandins and kinins secreted within the kidney reduce sodium reabsorption in distal nephron segments. The exact role of these natriuretic factors in the regulation of sodium excretion is uncertain.

Undoubtedly, other regulatory mechanisms remain to be defined. The multiplicity of control mechanisms prevents abnormalities of any single mechanism from grossly distorting the regulation of sodium excretion. For example, increased aldosterone secretion leads only to limited and transient sodium retention, because the initial accumulation of sodium stimulates opposing natriuretic factors such as increased glomerular filtration and decreased proximal tubular sodium reabsorption.

Distribution of sodium   All but 2 to 5 percent of the sodium in the body is located in the extracellular fluids. (Approximately 40 percent of total body sodium is in bone, but this fraction does not participate significantly in most physiologic processes and will not be considered further.) Except for minor differences in concentration due to the Gibbs-Donnan effect of plasma proteins, the electrolyte compositions of plasma and interstitial fluid are essentially equal. Consequently, plasma composition can be considered representative of the entire extracellular compartment. Total extracellular volume approximates 20 percent of body weight. Of this, 5 percent represents plasma volume and 15 percent the volume of interstitial fluids. Thus, in a 70-kg individual with plasma sodium concentration of 140 mmol/

L, extracellular sodium content will approximate 2000 mmol. The volume of intracellular fluid is approximately twice as great as that of extracellular fluid, i.e., about 40 percent of body weight. However, since intracellular sodium concentration is less than 5 mmol/L, total intracellular sodium content is only about 100 to 150 mmol. The asymmetric distribution of sodium across cell membranes is maintained by expenditure of a large fraction of the energy derived from cell metabolism, which is required constantly to pump sodium out of cells against its electrochemical gradient. All the principal electrolytes are asymmetrically distributed across cell membranes. The principal electrolytes of the extracellular fluids are sodium, chloride, and bicarbonate. The major electrolytes of the intracellular fluids are potassium, magnesium, calcium, and organic anions, including proteins.

Since sodium salts account for more than 90 percent of the total osmolality of the extracellular fluid, variations in plasma sodium concentration are almost always reflected in equivalent changes in plasma osmolality. Exceptions due to accumulation of other solutes in plasma are discussed later. Although the electrolyte compositions of intracellular and extracellular fluids differ markedly, they are always in osmotic equilibrium, since water moves rapidly across cellular membranes to dissipate osmotic gradients. Therefore, although sodium is largely confined to extracellular fluids, plasma sodium concentration is an index of not only the relative proportions of sodium and water in those fluids but also the relation between total body solute and total body water. An example is the effect of shift of sodium from extracellular to intracellular fluid without a change in total body solute. Movement of sodium into cells would not cause hyponatremia, since water would shift into cells with the sodium. On the other hand, a primary decrease in the concentration of osmotically active solute within cells would decrease total body solute; although there would be no change in total body sodium or water, hyponatremia would result from the shift of intracellular water into the extracellular compartment.

Role of antidiuretic hormone A very effective mechanism involving the *hypothalamus,* the *neurohypophysis,* and the kidney regulates plasma osmolality. Changes of 2 percent or less in plasma osmolality can be detected by osmoreceptors in the hypothalamus. Small increases in osmolality stimulate the secretion of vasopressin (the antidiuretic hormone, ADH) from the neurohypophysis, while small decreases suppress secretion of the hormone. Normal plasma osmolality is approximately 280 to 300 mosmol per kilogram of water; the exact level is determined by the "set" of the hypothalamic osmoreceptors in a given individual. When ADH secretion is maximal, urine volume will be about 500 mL/d, and urine osmolality will be 800 to 1400 mosmol/kg. In the absence of ADH, minimal urine osmolality is 40 to 80 mosmol/kg, and maximum water diuresis can reach 15 to 20 L/d or more. The capacity of this receptor-effector system is sufficient to maintain plasma osmolality within narrow limits despite large variations in the volume and concentration of dietary fluids. ADH secretion is also regulated by changes in extracellular volume. A reduction of 10 percent or more may trigger ADH release even in the absence of changes in plasma osmolality. If volume contraction is sufficiently severe, volume-mediated stimulation of ADH may override osmotic signals and cause water retention despite progressive dilution of body fluids. Conversely, extracellular volume expansion tends to suppress ADH release even if the body fluids are hypertonic.

The total sodium *content* of the body is determined by the renal sodium regulatory mechanisms described earlier. However, the principal determinant of plasma sodium *concentration* is water metabolism rather than total body sodium content. If excess sodium were to be ingested and retained, hypernatremia would be only transient. Water intake would increase because of thirst, and the fluid ingested would be retained because hypernatremia (hyperosmolality) would stimulate ADH secretion. Expanded extracellular volume, not hypernatremia, would be the end result. Conversely, if the osmoregulatory system is functioning normally, loss of moderate amounts of sodium without

water would not result in permanent reduction of plasma sodium concentration. The initial reduction would shut off secretion of ADH, and a water diuresis would ensue. The final outcome would be contraction of extracellular volume, while plasma sodium concentration would be restored to normal. It follows that changes in total sodium content tend to cause changes in extracellular volume. In this sense, the sodium content of the extracellular fluid determines extracellular volume. On the other hand, changes in plasma sodium concentration reflect altered regulation of water excretion, not changes in total body sodium content alone. Clinically, plasma sodium concentration per se gives no information about the amount of sodium present in the body. Total body sodium content is determined by the volume of extracellular fluids as well as by the concentration of sodium in these fluids. Extracellular volume is usually the dominant factor since changes in volume tend to be proportionately greater than changes in sodium concentration. Plasma sodium concentration reflects the relative proportions of sodium and water (or, more exactly, of total body solute and water), not the absolute amount of sodium in the body. Either hyponatremia or hypernatremia may occur when total body sodium content is decreased, normal, or increased.

CLINICAL DISORDERS Deficits and excesses of sodium and water occur in a great variety of clinical circumstances. The manifestations of the underlying illness may overshadow the clinical features of the fluid and electrolyte disorder. Theoretically, disturbances of sodium and water metabolism can be classified into four categories, reflecting a primary excess or deficit of water or sodium. Practically, such isolated disturbances are uncommon. A primary excess of sodium leads to edema; it is not ordinarily considered as an electrolyte disorder but as a feature of underlying disease, such as congestive heart failure, hepatic cirrhosis, or nephrotic syndrome. Primary sodium deficits are nearly always accompanied by water depletion, leading to the clinical syndrome of extracellular volume depletion. Pure or disproportionate water excess leads to hyponatremia, relative or absolute water depletion to hypernatremia. A practical clinical classification of the principal disorders of sodium and water metabolism is given in Table 50-1.

VOLUME DEPLETION Combined sodium and water deficits are far more frequent than isolated deficits of either constituent. Although the term *dehydration* is often used for combined deficits, this usage is confusing. Dehydration should be used to describe relatively pure water depletion leading to hypernatremia; *volume depletion* or some similar term should be used for combined deficits.

Pathogenesis As noted earlier, elimination of sodium from the diet will not by itself lead to sodium depletion in the presence of normal renal function, since urinary sodium excretion will quickly fall to very low levels. Therefore, sodium depletion is always due either to extrarenal losses or to abnormal renal losses.

GASTROINTESTINAL The most common cause of volume depletion is loss of a significant fraction of the 8 to 10 L of gastrointestinal fluids secreted daily. As the sodium concentration of these fluids is high, their loss causes combined sodium and water deficits. Since the principal secretions contain potassium and hydrogen ion or bicarbonate in large amounts, volume depletion due to such losses is often combined with potassium depletion and acidosis or alkalosis.

Significant volume depletion may be caused by sequestration of secretions within an obstructed gastrointestinal tract or within the peritoneal cavity in peritonitis. Rapid reaccumulation of ascites after paracentesis may reduce the effective circulating blood volume.

SKIN The sodium concentration of sweat varies from 5 to 50 mmol/L; sodium concentration increases with higher rates of sweating and in adrenal insufficiency. Because sweat is always a hypotonic solution, sweating leads to water deficits out of proportion to sodium losses. In burns, capillary damage may lead to sequestration of large amounts of sodium and water in the injured skin.

RENAL Abnormal losses of sodium and water in the urine may occur in both acute and chronic renal diseases. Early in the recovery (diuretic) phase of *acute renal failure,* urinary sodium concentration tends to be high (50 to 100 mmol/L), and substantial deficits of both

TABLE 50-1 Disorders of sodium and water metabolism*

I Combined sodium and water depletion (volume depletion)
 A Extrarenal losses
  1 Gastrointestinal (vomiting, diarrhea, gastrointestinal suction, fistulas)
  2 Abdominal sequestration (peritonitis, rapid reaccumulation of ascites)
  3 Skin (sweating, burns)
 B Renal losses
  1 Renal disease (diuretic phase of acute renal failure, postobstructive diuresis, chronic renal failure, salt-wasting tubular disease)
  2 Diuretic excess
  3 Osmotic diuresis (diabetic glycosuria)
  4 Mineralocorticoid deficiency (Addison's disease, hypoaldosteronism)
II Hyponatremia
 A Associated with extracellular volume depletion (see list of causes above)
 B Associated with extracellular volume excess and edema
 C Associated with normal or modestly expanded extracellular volume (no edema)
  1 Acute and chronic renal failure
  2 Temporary impairment of water diuresis (pain, drugs, emotion)
  3 Syndrome of inappropriate secretion of antidiuretic hormone (SIADH)
  4 Endocrine (glucocorticoid deficiency, hypothyroidism)
  5 Severe polydipsia
  6 Essential ("sick cell syndrome")
 D Without plasma hypoosmolality
  1 Osmotic (hyperglycemia, mannitol)
  2 Artifactual (hyperlipemia, hyperproteinemia, laboratory error)
III Hypernatremia
 A Due solely to water loss
  1 Extrarenal
   a Skin (insensible losses)
   b Lungs
  2 Renal
   a Diabetes insipidus (central, nephrogenic)
  3 Hypothalamic dysfunction
 B Due to water loss associated with sodium loss
  1 Extrarenal
   a Sweat
  2 Renal
   a Osmotic diuresis (glycosuria, urea)
 C Due to sodium gain
   a Excessive sodium administration
   b Adrenal hyperfunction (hyperaldosteronism, Cushing's syndrome)

* For differential diagnosis, see Fig. 50-1, p. 283.

sodium and water may ensue. With rare exceptions, severe sodium and water wasting does not persist beyond the first few days. It is important to discriminate between increased excretion, which represents elimination of excess retained during the oliguric period, and true tubular sodium and water wasting, which depletes normal extracellular volume. Only the latter requires replacement. Acute salt and water wasting due to tubular damage may also occur immediately after relief of prolonged *obstruction* of the urinary tract. Although such a postobstructive diuresis may be severe, it rarely persists for more than several days as a clinically important phenomenon.

Patients with *chronic renal failure* have limited ability to decrease sodium and water excretion in response to decreased intake. They will become progressively volume-depleted if their intake is restricted by the anorexia, nausea, and vomiting characteristic of uremia or because of their physician's instructions. Large deficits may develop insidiously over many days or weeks. A "self-perpetuating cycle" may result, in that volume depletion will tend further to compromise renal function. Severe sodium-wasting renal disease, i.e., negative sodium balance when dietary sodium is normal, is rare. It occurs in occasional patients with tubulointerstitial diseases of the kidney, especially medullary cystic disease.

Renal sodium wasting in the presence of normal intrinsic renal function occurs in three clinical circumstances. Perhaps the most common is sodium depletion due to continued administration of potent *diuretics* to patients after edema has been relieved or to patients whose edema is sequestered and cannot be mobilized. For example, attempted treatment of cirrhotics with ascites may result in depletion of extracellular volume rather than mobilization of ascitic fluid. An obligatory *osmotic diuresis* may also cause renal sodium and water wasting despite normal renal function. Marked glycosuria in uncon-

trolled diabetes mellitus is the most frequent clinical example. Volume depletion in patients receiving high-protein enteral or parenteral alimentation may be due to an osmotic diuresis of urea formed by protein metabolism. Administration of solutes such as mannitol, which act as osmotic diuretics, may cause volume depletion. Finally, renal sodium wasting despite normal intrinsic function occurs in Addison's disease and hypoaldosteronism due to a *deficiency of mineralocorticoids.*

Clinical features and diagnosis The cause of volume depletion can usually be suspected from a history of inadequate salt and water intake together with vomiting, diarrhea, or excessive sweating; the symptoms of poorly controlled diabetes mellitus or of renal or adrenal disease may be elicited. The key findings on physical examination are those of interstitial and plasma volume depletion. Decreased interstitial volume may be recognized from reduced skin turgor, which is usually present in patients with significant volume contraction but may be difficult to evaluate in the elderly. It can be estimated clinically by noting the slow rate of return of skin to its original position when it is raised between the examiner's fingers. An area of skin normally free of wrinkles and not subject to wide variations in the thickness of subcutaneous tissue, such as that over the sternum, should be selected for this maneuver. Oral mucous membranes may be dry and axillary sweating decreased; these are less reliable diagnostic features than decreased skin turgor. Plasma volume depletion is indicated by changes in blood pressure. With moderate volume depletion, blood pressure is usually normal when the patient is recumbent, although resting tachycardia may be present. Postural hypotension, i.e., a drop of at least 5 to 10 mmHg in the sitting or standing position, is often present. With greater degrees of volume depletion, even recumbent blood pressure is reduced, and frank shock may occur. The patient with moderate or severe degrees of volume contraction is often lethargic, weak, confused, or obtunded. Such patients are usually oliguric, even when recumbent blood pressure is normal. However, an osmotic diuresis, as occurs in hyperglycemia, tends to prevent oliguria despite volume contraction.

LABORATORY FINDINGS The hematocrit and plasma protein concentration are increased, but increases within the normal range are interpretable only if prior values are known. Plasma sodium concentration may be decreased, normal, or increased, depending upon the proportion between deficits of sodium and of water. Plasma creatinine and urea nitrogen are usually increased, since the glomerular filtration rate is decreased ("prerenal azotemia"). Blood urea nitrogen (BUN) tends to rise proportionately more than plasma creatinine. Urinary sodium concentration may be of value in differentiating extrarenal and renal sources of sodium loss if the probable cause is not clear from the history. With extrarenal losses, urinary sodium concentration is less than 10 mmol/L; the concentration will usually exceed 20 mmol/L if renal or adrenal disorders are at fault. However, urinary sodium may ultimately fall below this level even in patients with renal salt wasting if sodium depletion becomes severe.

Treatment The principal clinical manifestations of extracellular volume depletion are due to reduction of plasma and interstitial fluid volume. Since there is no convenient clinical method for quantifying these volumes, the effect of treatment must be determined by following the changes in clinical features such as blood pressure, urine output, and skin turgor. Modest deficits of sodium and water can often be corrected by increased oral intake in patients not suffering from gastrointestinal disorders. Severe depletion requires therapy with intravenous solutions. Isotonic saline (0.85%) is the infusion of choice in patients whose serum sodium concentration is approximately normal. The amount to be infused can be estimated from the history of prior losses and from the severity of the physical findings of extracellular volume contraction. Patients with moderate volume contraction usually require replacement with 2 to 3 L of saline, while patients with severe depletion may require much larger volumes. The need for correction of other concurrent electrolyte abnormalities may alter the composition of the required infusion; e.g., some of the sodium may be given as bicarbonate to patients with volume contraction and metabolic acidosis, or potassium may be added in patients with concurrent potassium depletion. In estimating the total amount to be infused, allowance for ongoing losses must be included. Since the amount to be infused cannot be calculated precisely, patients should be monitored carefully to avoid fluid overload and congestive failure.

HYPONATREMIA Pathophysiology Hyponatremia indicates that the body fluids are diluted by an excess of water relative to total solute. Hyponatremia is not equivalent to sodium depletion, which is only one of the clinical states in which it may occur (see Table 50-1). Most types of hyponatremia result from defective urinary dilution. The normal response to dilution of body fluids is a water diuresis, which corrects the hypoosmotic state. Normal water diuresis requires three factors: (1) Secretion of ADH must be suppressed. (2) Sufficient sodium and water must reach the diluting sites of the nephron, in the ascending limb of Henle's loop and the distal convoluted tubule. (3) These nephron segments must function normally, reabsorbing sodium while remaining impermeable to water.

Correspondingly, three mechanisms may cause defective water diuresis in patients with hyponatremia. (1) Secretion of ADH may continue "inappropriately" despite hypotonicity of extracellular fluid, which normally shuts off secretion of the hormone. This may be due to unregulated release of ADH by neoplasms or to nonosmotic stimuli to ADH secretion. The latter include volume depletion, neural factors such as pain and emotion, and certain drugs. (2) Insufficient sodium may reach the diluting segments to permit the formation of an adequate amount of dilute urine. Inadequate delivery of tubular fluid to distal sites may be due to reduced glomerular filtration and/or enhanced proximal tubular reabsorption. Even in the absence of ADH, distal tubular segments are not absolutely impermeable to water; small amounts of water continue to leak from the hypotonic tubular fluid into the isotonic cortical and slightly hypertonic medullary interstitial fluid. The amount of water leaking back in this manner becomes an increasingly larger fraction of the volume of dilute urine formed, as the diluting process is progressively limited by decreasing delivery. Hence, urine osmolality rises progressively. In some instances, this mechanism may even result in excretion of a urine hypertonic to plasma, despite the absence of ADH. (3) Sodium transport in the diluting segments may be defective, or water permeability may be excessive at these sites even in the absence of ADH. One of these three factors can account for most types of hyponatremia, as described below.

Types of hyponatremia (Table 50-1) In patients with extracellular *volume depletion,* delivery of sodium and water to the diluting segments of the nephron is reduced because of decreased glomerular filtration, increased proximal tubular reabsorption, or both. ADH secretion is stimulated by the volume contraction. These changes in renal function and hormone secretion limit water diuresis during extracelluar volume depletion. Hyponatremia per se is usually of little clinical significance in sodium (volume) depletion. The major features are those of extracellular volume contraction, described above. Reduction of plasma sodium concentration by more than 10 to 15 mmol/L is rare in the absence of obvious decreases in skin turgor, postural or recumbent hypotension, and some degree of azotemia. Treatment is directed to correction of the volume deficits. In the occasional symptomatic patient with sodium depletion whose plasma sodium concentration is less than 125 mmol/L, some of the intravenous sodium replacement fluids should be administered as hypertonic saline.

Multiple factors contribute to hyponatremia caused by *diuretics.* Salt loss may cause volume depletion, which limits water diuresis by mechanisms already described. Furosemide, ethacrynic acid, and thiazides inhibit salt reabsorption in the diluting segments of the nephron and thereby directly limit water diuresis. Thiazides appear to be the diuretics most commonly associated with hyponatremia, probably because they interfere with elaboration of a hypotonic urine by inhibiting sodium reabsorption in the distal convoluted tubule but, unlike loop diuretics, do not limit urine concentration and water

retention by interfering with salt transport in the loop of Henle. In addition, potassium depletion caused by many diuretics contributes to hyponatremia through uncertain mechanisms. Hyponatremia due to diuretic therapy is frequent but usually minor in severity. However, moderate or severe hyponatremia may occur in patients who receive diuretics and who drink large quantities of water or other hypotonic fluids. Progressive hyponatremia is an important complication of diuretic therapy in edematous patients, in whom the underlying disease tends to cause hyponatremia (see below) and to whom large doses of diuretics may be given. The treatment of hyponatremia due to diuretics is water restriction and repletion of potassium deficits.

In *edematous states* such as congestive heart failure, cirrhosis, and the nephrotic syndrome, hyponatremia paradoxically appears to result from mechanisms similar to those that cause hyponatremia in patients with volume depletion. Although total extracellular volume is increased in edematous patients, it is believed that the "effective" volume is reduced by decreased cardiac output or sequestration of fluid outside the central circulation. The decrease in "effective" volume results in diminished delivery of sodium and water to nephron diluting segments, because of reduced glomerular filtration, increased proximal tubular reabsorption, or both. Volume-mediated secretion of ADH is also triggered in these conditions. In some edematous patients essential hyponatremia may be an additional mechanism (see below). In edematous states, the severity and frequency of hyponatremia correlate to some extent with the magnitude of the edema and the seriousness of the underlying condition. Hyponatremia is usually present in patients with advanced disease unless water intake is restricted. The hyponatremia itself is often of little clinical significance. The principal features are those of the underlying disease. However, symptomatic hyponatremia may occur, most often in connection with vigorous diuretic therapy or excessive oral or parenteral intake of dilute fluids.

Hyponatremia associated with edema responds to effective treatment of the underlying disease. Moderate nonprogressive hyponatremia in edematous patients usually does not cause symptoms. Attempts to correct such hyponatremia by restriction of fluid intake induce thirst and discomfort without improving the clinical picture or longevity. Patients with severe or progressive hyponatremia may require some restriction of water intake, especially during vigorous treatment with diuretics. However, moderate limitation to the range of 1 to 1.5 L/d will often suffice to avoid symptoms of progressive hyponatremia. More severe restriction should be instituted only if specific clinical or laboratory observations warrant. Since edematous subjects have excess total extracellular sodium, hypertonic saline should not be administered except in rare instances in which clinical manifestations of extreme hyponatremia, such as coma or convulsions, justify emergency measures. Furosemide should be given concurrently in such cases to avoid further expansion of the extracellular space. Dialysis can also be used to correct severe hyponatremia without increasing volume in edematous patients.

Hyponatremia may result from *impaired water excretion* not associated with a substantial deficit or excess of salt. In this case, extracellular volume is only modestly expanded. Since excess water is distributed throughout both intracellular and extracellular fluids in proportion to their volumes, only one-third of a water excess will be retained in the extracellular compartment. *Oliguric* patients develop dilutional hyponatremia if the volume of oral and intravenous fluids is not restricted appropriately. The ability to excrete a normal volume of dilute urine is progressively limited in advancing *chronic renal failure.* Regulation of water intake by thirst usually prevents dilutional hyponatremia. However, hyponatremia may be precipitated by increased fluid intake (for example, if the patient is instructed to force fluids). Since the ability to regulate salt excretion is also limited in chronic renal failure, in many patients hyponatremia is associated with edema or salt depletion. In patients with normal renal function, *water diuresis* may be *limited temporarily* by ADH secretion induced by various neural stimuli such as pain and narcotics. In the postoperative state, these factors, together with administration of large volumes of hypotonic fluids, may cause hyponatremia. The etiology of hyponatremia due to impaired water excretion is usually evident from the clinical setting and a careful review of fluid intake and output. This type of hyponatremia is treated by water restriction. Only if severe symptoms occur is hypertonic saline infusion required.

In the *syndrome of inappropriate antidiuretic hormone* (SIADH) secretion (see also Chap. 315), ADH is released "inappropriately" despite dilution of body fluids and increased extracellular volume. Hyponatremia in patients with SIADH is principally due to water retention, but urinary losses of sodium may also contribute to a mild negative sodium balance. Renal sodium wasting is due to water retention and consequent modest volume expansion, which increases sodium excretion by mechanisms discussed above. Clinically, SIADH is characterized by a number of features: (1) Urine osmolality is not maximally dilute even when marked hyponatremia is induced by water loading. In most cases, urine osmolality exceeds plasma osmolality. (2) Plasma creatinine and urea are normal or low, indicating that the glomerular filtration rate is normal or increased. (The elaboration of hypertonic urine is presumptive evidence of ADH secretion if the glomerular filtration rate is normal.) (3) During fluid loading (even if the fluid is saline), hyponatremia increases due to water retention and urinary sodium wasting. It should be noted that sodium wasting during volume expansion may be minimal or even absent in patients with extreme degrees of hyponatremia. (4) Since hyponatremia and salt wasting are not direct effects of vasopressin but are due to retention of ingested water, they are corrected by restriction of fluid intake. This response is helpful in occasional patients in whom it may be difficult to distinguish SIADH from mild volume depletion as the cause of hyponatremia. The plasma uric acid also may be of value in making this distinction. Since uric acid excretion tends to vary with "effective" extracellular volume, hyperuricemia is common in volume depletion while hypouricemia is usual in SIADH.

SIADH occurs commonly in patients with oat cell carcinoma of the lung but has also been described in patients with a variety of other *neoplasms*. In some of these patients the tumor secretes ADH or a substance with analogous biologic activity (see also Chap. 315). The syndrome has also been reported in patients with various disorders of the *central nervous system,* including meningitis, encephalitis, tumors, trauma, stroke, and in acute *porphyria*. It is assumed that ADH in these patients is secreted in response to direct stimulation of the hypothalamic osmoreceptors. *Pulmonary* diseases associated with SIADH, in addition to tumors, include a wide variety of infections, asthma, and chronic obstructive lung disease.

Pharmacologic agents that induce SIADH include (1) the oral hypoglycemic agents chlorpropamide and tolbutamide; (2) the antineoplastic and immunosuppressive agents vincristine and cyclophosphamide; (3) psychoactive drugs such as haloperidol, thioridazine, carbamazepine, and amitriptyline; and (4) clofibrate. These agents exert their antidiuretic effect either by potentiating the tubular action of small amounts of ADH or by stimulating inappropriate secretion of ADH.

Hyponatremia due to SIADH can be treated by limiting fluid intake; restriction to the range of 1 to 1.2 L/d is ordinarily adequate. Occasional patients who are symptomatic despite water restriction may be treated by enhancing water excretion. This can be accomplished either by increasing solute excretion (by taking a high-salt, high-protein diet or ingesting urea) or by antagonizing ADH with demeclocycline or lithium. Initial therapy with hypertonic saline infusions may be required in a few patients with marked hyponatremia. Concurrent administration of furosemide may facilitate correction of hyponatremia in those patients who do not respond promptly to hypertonic saline alone.

Hyponatremia may occur in certain *endocrine* disorders, notably adrenal insufficiency and hypothyroidism. Multiple factors appear to play a role in limiting water diuresis in patients with *adrenal insufficiency*. Deficient secretion of mineralocorticoid hormones may lead to sodium depletion, with consequent reduction of glomerular

filtration and enhancement of proximal tubular sodium reabsorption. Moreover, glucocorticoid deficiency directly reduces filtration. Therefore, adrenal insufficiency will tend to decrease delivery of sodium to diluting sites. In addition, glucocorticoid deficiency prevents the maintenance of normal water impermeability in distal diluting segments of the nephron. This appears to be due to inappropriate secretion of ADH, although glucocorticoid deficiency may have a direct effect on water permeability of distal tubular epithelium. Since patients with adrenal insufficiency may have the combination of defective dilution of the urine and sodium wasting, hyponatremia due to Addison's disease can occasionally be confused with SIADH. Usually, other clinical features of adrenal insufficiency such as hyperkalemia, pigmentation, and hypoglycemia suggest the correct diagnosis. However, specific tests of adrenal function are indicated whenever the diagnosis is in doubt. Hyponatremia due to adrenal insufficiency is corrected by appropriate hormonal therapy.

Hyponatremia may develop in moderate or severe *hypothyroidism*. Decreased delivery of tubular fluid to diluting segments and persistent release of ADH both limit water excretion in this condition. The diagnosis of this type of hyponatremia is made by recognizing the clinical features of hypothyroidism and from the response to treatment with thyroid hormone.

The normal kidney can excrete 15 to 20 L of dilute urine per day. Normal water intake, regulated by thirst and habit, is a small fraction of this maximum excretory capacity. Rarely, *psychogenic polydipsia* may be so severe that the rapid ingestion of huge quantities of fluids may overwhelm normal excretory capacity and produce symptomatic dilutional hyponatremia despite normal renal diluting mechanisms. Hyponatremia of this type is diagnosed from the history of massive fluid intake, most often in patients with other evidence of psychiatric illness. Since water excretory capacity is normal, the urine is maximally dilute in this condition. Hyponatremia due to psychogenic polydipsia responds to water restriction. Rare patients who are symptomatic due to extreme degrees of hyponatremia may require intravenous infusion of hypertonic saline.

Some patients may be hyponatremic in the absence of a defect in water diuresis. The terms *essential hyponatremia* and *sick cell syndrome* have been applied to this category. Osmoreceptor cells in the hypothalamus are thought to be "reset" to maintain a decreased level of body fluid osmolality as though it were normal. Urine becomes dilute or concentrated, respectively, if plasma sodium falls or increases slightly from the new "normal" level for the particular patient. The genesis of such a syndrome is speculative. Changes in cellular metabolism may lead to a primary reduction in cellular osmolality. Another possibility is that essential hyponatremia is a variant of SIADH in which there is a nonosmotic stimulus to ADH secretion. When plasma osmolality is reduced sufficiently, osmotic suppression of ADH secretion overcomes the nonosmotic stimulus.

Essential hyponatremia may occur in a variety of chronic illnesses, such as pulmonary tuberculosis, congestive heart failure, and hepatic cirrhosis. This type of hyponatremia is asymptomatic; skin turgor, blood pressure, and renal function are normal, unless altered by the primary disease. Definitive diagnosis of essential hyponatremia requires the demonstration of normal urinary dilution in response to water loading, normal urinary concentration during dehydration, and normal renal sodium excretory responses to sodium loading and restriction. This type of hyponatremia does not require treatment.

Hyponatremia due to *accumulation* of *osmotically active solutes* in the plasma is the sole exception to the rule that hyponatremia means decreased plasma osmolality. In this type of hyponatremia, plasma osmolality is increased. Plasma sodium is diluted by movement of water out of cells along the osmotic gradient created by the addition of a solute such as glucose or mannitol. (High plasma urea levels in patients with renal failure do not cause hyponatremia because urea concentration is equal across cell membranes.) The diagnosis of hyponatremia due to increased plasma concentrations of osmotically active solutes is usually apparent from the history and clinical features of uncontrolled diabetes. Plasma sodium concentration will decrease by about 1.6 mmol/L with every elevation of 1 g/L in plasma glucose above normal. This type of hyponatremia should also be considered whenever there is a history of recent administration of mannitol, especially to oliguric patients unable to excrete it promptly. Since plasma osmolality is increased, clinical manifestations of hypotonicity are absent in this type of hyponatremia.

In patients with severe hyperlipemia or, very rarely, with extreme hyperproteinemia, *artifactual* hyponatremia may be reported by the laboratory. In severe hyperlipemia part of any unit volume of plasma taken for analysis will be lipid, which is sodium-free. This type of hyponatremia rarely occurs unless the plasma is grossly milky. In patients with extreme hyperproteinemia, proteins occupy more than the normal 7 percent of plasma volume, thereby reducing the proportion of aqueous sodium-containing fluid per unit of plasma taken for analysis. In both cases, hyponatremia will be reported by the laboratory because the sodium concentration will be low in millimoles per liter of plasma. However, sodium concentration per liter of plasma water and plasma osmolality are normal; hence, this type of hyponatremia has no clinical significance. Laboratories increasingly have adopted the sodium-selective electrode as the method for measuring plasma sodium. This technique eliminates artifactual hyponatremia because it gives accurate values regardless of plasma lipid or protein concentration.

Differential diagnosis Although the type of hyponatremia can be defined easily in most patients, precise diagnosis may be difficult in some. Figure 50-1 is a flow chart that outlines the major steps in determining the cause of hyponatremia. First, assess extracellular fluid (ECF) volume. The history and physical examination are usually sufficient to determine whether the hyponatremia is associated with a decreased, increased, or normal extracellular volume. In occasional patients, moderate volume depletion may not readily be separable from normovolemia by clinical examination. In that event, measurement of BUN and plasma creatinine may be helpful. The plasma creatinine, and especially the BUN, tend to be increased when hyponatremia is associated with volume depletion and normal or decreased when it is associated with a normal or expanded extracellular volume, as in SIADH. The various types of normovolemic hyponatremia can frequently be recognized by a careful review of specific features of the history, such as associated diseases, drug therapy, and fluid intake. However, laboratory tests, such as measurement of serum cortisol, may be needed to confirm a diagnosis.

Measurements of urinary sodium concentration and osmolality are common in the workup. *Urinary sodium concentration* is low (under 10 mmol/L) if hyponatremia is associated with edema or with volume depletion due to extrarenal causes. Urine sodium concentration usually exceeds 20 mmol/L if hyponatremia is due to renal salt losses or to renal failure with water retention. In SIADH, urine sodium concentration usually exceeds 20 mmol/L unless fluid intake has been restricted. Since impaired water diuresis is the mechanism of most types of hyponatremia, measurement of *urinary osmolality* is not usually of value. A maximally dilute urine would be expected only in hyponatremia due to extreme polydipsia or during water loading in essential hyponatremia. With other causes, urinary osmolality exceeds 150 mosmol per kilogram of water; usually the urine is hypertonic to plasma.

Clinical manifestations Neurologic dysfunction is the principal clinical manifestation of hyponatremia. It is due to intracellular movement of water, leading to swelling of brain cells. The severity of symptoms is related both to the degree of hyponatremia and to the rapidity with which it develops. In chronic hyponatremia, the degree of brain swelling caused by any given reduction in body fluid osmolality is reduced because solute, largely potassium and sodium chloride, is lost from the cells. Patients may be lethargic, confused, stuporous, or comatose. If hyponatremia develops rapidly, signs of hyperexcitability such as muscular twitches, irritability, and convulsions may occur. Hyponatremia rarely causes clinical symptoms when plasma sodium is above 125 mmol/L, although symptoms may occur at higher levels if the decrease in concentration has been rapid.

Treatment Appropriate therapy for the various types of hyponatremia has been outlined. Hyponatremia itself is often of little significance and requires no specific treatment. If severe, symptomatic hyponatremia requires intravenous treatment; the amount of sodium given should be calculated by multiplying the deficit in plasma sodium concentration (millimoles per liter) by the total body water (approximately 50 to 60 percent of body weight). Although the administered sodium will remain in the extracellular compartment, the osmotic

FIGURE 50-1 Flow chart for differential diagnosis of causes of hyponatremia. Categories (A, B, C, D) and types (C1–6) are keyed to Table 50-1. Abbreviations: Nl = normal; ECF = extracellular fluid; creat = creatinine; CHF = congestive heart failure; BP = blood pressure; Uosm = urinary osmolality; U_{Na} = urinary Na, mmol/L; ↓ = decreased, ↑ = increased; Hx = history, PE = physical examination.

effect of hypertonic saline will cause water to shift out of cells. The appropriate rate and extent of initial correction of hyponatremia is controversial. Severe hyponatremia itself is potentially hazardous; on the other hand, some studies suggest that rapid correction of hyponatremia may cause neurologic damage (central pontine myelinolysis). Although the issue has not yet been resolved, the following regimen seems reasonable. The amount of hypertonic (5%) saline needed to raise plasma sodium to 125 mmol/L should be calculated and infused at a rate estimated to increase plasma sodium by 1 to 2 mmol/h. The symptoms and clinical status, especially with respect to circulatory congestion, should be carefully assessed throughout the infusion. Furosemide may be given if fluid overload is present initially or develops during the infusion. Complete correction of hyponatremia, if indicated, is usually best carried out more slowly by water restriction or oral sodium supplementation if possible.

HYPERNATREMIA **Pathophysiology** Hypernatremia is due to a deficit of body water relative to total body solute or sodium content. Without exception, hypernatremia indicates that the body fluids are hypertonic. Normally, minimal increases in tonicity stimulate both thirst and release of ADH. Although renal water retention induced by ADH helps to correct hypernatremia, thirst appears to be the principal defense mechanism. Hypernatremia is usually modest in patients with diabetes insipidus, who lack ADH and may excrete 15 L or more of urine per day. Thirst stimulates water intake enough to balance even such large water losses. Severe persistent hypernatremia occurs only in patients who cannot respond to thirst by voluntary ingestion of fluid, e.g., infants or mentally obtunded patients, or in rare patients with disorders of thirst mechanisms. In such individuals, loss of dilute body fluids progressively elevates body fluid osmolality. Initial losses of water are from the extracellular compartment, but water deficits are rapidly equilibrated throughout total body water. The rise in extracellular fluid tonicity causes intracellular water to shift into the extracellular compartment. In effect, approximately two-thirds of pure water deficits are derived from intracellular fluid. Hence, extracellular volume depletion is clinically significant in patients with relatively pure deficits of water only when such deficits are large. The principal clinical features are attributable to decreased intracellular volume, especially dehydration of cells in the central nervous system. Brain cells appear to adapt to chronic hyperosmolality by accumulating increased intracellular solute. When hyperosmolality is rapidly corrected, the increase in total intracellular solute may promote brain swelling even at normal or slightly elevated plasma osmolality. These mechanisms may account for the fact that rapid correction of hypertonicity sometimes causes deterioration of central nervous function. The identity of the excess brain solute is uncertain; electrolyte accumulation accounts for only part of the excess.

Pathogenesis (Table 50-1) For clinical purposes it is useful to classify hypernatremia as due to water loss alone; to water deficits associated with, but proportionately in excess of, sodium deficits; or to retention of sodium. *Pure water deficits* may be due to extrarenal or renal water losses that are not replaced. Insensible losses of water from the skin or lungs may reach several liters per day, especially in patients with fever, increased respirations, or extensive burns. Renal losses may lead to hypernatremia in diabetes insipidus. Alert patients with diabetes insipidus ordinarily maintain normal or only slightly hypertonic body fluids despite massive renal water wasting by increasing fluid intake appropriately. However, diabetes insipidus may develop acutely after cerebral trauma or neurosurgical procedures. In such patients, careful attention to replacement of urinary losses is mandatory to avoid severe hypernatremia. Defective thirst and ADH regulation occurs in rare patients with hypothalamic disorders, which may be idiopathic ("essential hypernatremia") or due to specific causes such as tumors, granulomas, and cerebrovascular accidents.

Water losses leading to hypernatremia are often *associated with sodium deficits*. In such cases, the clinical features of extracellular volume depletion and hypernatremia may both be present, and either may predominate. Extrarenal losses of salt and water due to profuse sweating and renal losses due to osmotic diuresis are the major causes of hypernatremia in this category. Since sweat is hypotonic, hypernatremia will develop if profusely sweating patients cannot drink. In an osmotic diuresis, urinary sodium concentration is less than plasma concentration; therefore, hypernatremia tends to occur. Hypernatremia due to urea diuresis may develop when patients unable to complain of thirst are placed on high-protein feeding. Examples include patients with severe cerebrovascular accidents who are unable to swallow and postoperative neurosurgical patients. In the syndrome of hyperosmolar nonketotic diabetic coma, severe hyperosmolality of the body fluids is due to a combination of hyperglycemia and relative or absolute hypernatremia. The hypernatremia is a consequence of an intense glucose osmotic diuresis in patients who are unable to ingest fluids. Since hyperglycemia itself causes hyponatremia by inducing a shift of water from cells, the presence of hypernatremia in the face of extreme hyperglycemia indicates that total body water is severely depleted.

Infrequently, hypernatremia may result from an absolute *excess of sodium* rather than from water depletion. Examples are hypernatremia caused by accidental substitution of salt for sugar in infant feeding formulas and administration of excessive amounts of hypertonic sodium chloride or bicarbonate infusions to comatose adults unable to drink. The cause of the common mild hypernatremia in patients with adrenal hyperfunction is uncertain. Presumably, stimulation of renal tubular sodium reabsorption by adrenal steroids initiates the hypernatremia, and the hypervolemia that results resets upward the threshold for ADH release. It is not known why the thirst mechanism fails to maintain normal body fluid osmolality.

Clinical features and diagnosis The principal manifestations of hypernatremia are observed in the central nervous system. Confusion and other evidence of altered mental state; increased neuromuscular irritability, such as twitching and seizures; and obtundation, stupor, or coma may all occur. The magnitude of symptoms depends on the severity of the hyperosmolality. The symptoms are similar whether hyperosmolality is due to hypernatremia or extreme hyperglycemia. The neurologic symptoms appear to be due to dehydration of brain cells. The clinical manifestations of acute hypernatremia are more marked than those of slowly developing hypernatremia. Severe hyperosmolality may cause irreversible neurologic sequelae, apparently due to vascular consequences such as venous sinus thrombosis and hemorrhage from vessels that rupture when the brain shrinks. High mortality rates are associated with extreme hyperosmolality, especially in children and in the elderly.

In patients with pure water deficits, manifestations of extracellular volume depletion are minimal because only one-third of the deficit is derived from extracellular fluid. As noted, combined deficits are common, especially in patients who sweat or experience an osmotic diuresis; in such individuals, the signs and symptoms of volume depletion may overshadow those of hypernatremia.

The cause of hypernatremia can usually be inferred from the history when it is due to extrarenal water loss, an osmotic diuresis, or sodium excess. In these cases, the urine is hypertonic to plasma. The differential diagnosis of pituitary and nephrogenic diabetes insipidus, in which urine concentrating ability is impaired, is discussed in Chap. 315.

Treatment Hypernatremia itself is corrected with water by mouth or by intravenous infusion of 5% dextrose in water. Calculation of water requirements must be based on total body water, since water deficits are drawn from both intracellular and extracellular fluid and both must be repleted. For example, suppose a 70-kg man has a plasma sodium of 160 mmol/L which is to be lowered to 140. Total body water is estimated as 60 percent of 70 kg, which is 42 L. To reduce plasma sodium, this volume must be increased to (160/140) × 42 L, which equals 48 L. Thus, a positive water balance of 6 L (48 − 42) is required. Hypernatremia should be corrected slowly; no more than half the water deficit should be replaced in the first 12 to 24 h. As stated above, rapid correction of hypertonicity may cause central nervous function to deteriorate.

In patients with associated sodium deficits, saline solutions should be infused. If the predominant clinical feature is extracellular volume depletion with circulatory insufficiency, treatment should begin with 0.9% saline to replete extracellular volume promptly. If the neurologic effects of hypertonicity predominate, therapy can start with 0.45% saline. In patients with hyperosmolar diabetic coma, sodium deficits are usually large, due to prior glucose osmotic diuresis. Plasma hypertonicity is due to both hyperglycemia and hypernatremia. Treatment consists of isotonic saline (0.9%) to replete extracellular volume and insulin to lower plasma glucose and thereby partly correct hypertonicity. Later, hypotonic saline (0.45%) can replace the remaining water and salt deficits and return plasma sodium to normal.

POTASSIUM

PHYSIOLOGIC CONSIDERATIONS Potassium is the principal intracellular cation. Active transport mediated by Na^+,K^+–stimulated ATPase in cell membranes maintains a cellular concentration of approximately 160 mmol/L, 40 times that in extracellular fluid. All but 2 percent of the 2500 to 3000 mmol potassium in the body is within cells. Since potassium is a large fraction of total cellular solute, it is a major determinant of the volume of the cell and the osmolality of the body fluids. Moreover, potassium is an important cofactor in a number of metabolic processes. Extracellular potassium, while a small fraction of the total, greatly influences neuromuscular function. The ratio of intracellular to extracellular potassium concentration is the principal determinant of membrane potential in excitable tissues. Since extracellular potassium concentration is low, small deviations in concentration produce large variations in this ratio; conversely, only large changes in intracellular potassium influence the ratio significantly. These relationships have practical consequences. For example, toxic effects of hyperkalemia can be mitigated by inducing movement of potassium from extracellular fluid into cells.

With the exception of changes in acid-base balance (see below), in most circumstances extracellular and intracellular potassium change in the same direction. Hence, alterations in plasma potassium are a useful index of alterations in total body potassium. During potassium depletion, plasma potassium initially decreases about 1 mmol/L for each 100 to 200 mmol lost. However, plasma potassium falls more slowly after it reaches 2 mmol/L. Thus, a plasma potassium in the range of 2 to 3.5 mmol/L is a reasonably accurate guide to the magnitude of depletion, but plasma potassium concentrations less than 2 mmol/L may reflect a wide range of deficits, from moderate to severe. Plasma concentration increases about 1 mmol/L after acute administration of 100 to 200 mmol potassium. Assuming an extracellular volume of 15 L, 150 mmol would be expected to raise plasma potassium by about 10 mmol/L. Thus, the largest fraction of administered potassium rapidly enters cells. Renal excretion also increases promptly. Chronic exposure to high-potassium diets enhances both tissue uptake and renal excretion of the ion; the mechanism of these adaptations is uncertain. Sustained hyperkalemia rarely is caused by excess intake, because these mechanisms normally function so efficiently. Impaired renal excretion and cellular transfer are the usual causes of hyperkalemia.

The relation between plasma and cellular potassium is influenced by acid-base balance and by hormones. Acidosis tends to shift potassium out of cells, and alkalosis favors movement from extracellular fluid into cells. The relation between blood pH and plasma potassium is complex and is influenced by several factors, including the type of acidosis, the duration of the altered acid-base state, and the change in plasma bicarbonate per se. In general, plasma potassium changes less with respiratory acidosis than with metabolic acidosis and less with alkalosis than with acidosis. While the magnitude of the change in plasma potassium cannot be predicted from changes in blood pH alone, a patient with normal total body potassium tends to be hyperkalemic if acidotic and hypokalemic if alkalotic. Hormones appear to be important parts of the mechanism for moving potassium

loads out of plasma. Insulin and beta-adrenergic catecholamines promote movement of potassium into cells. Conversely, alpha-adrenergic agonists impair potassium uptake into cells.

Of the usual potassium intake of 50 to 150 mmol/d, most is excreted in the urine. Normally, stool and sweat contain only about 5 mmol/d. As noted, the kidneys respond to acute and chronic changes in potassium intake by corresponding changes in excretion. Excess potassium is excreted promptly; about half of an acute load appears in the urine within 12 h. The renal response to potassium depletion is more sluggish. Excretion does not fall to minimal levels for 7 to 14 days. During this period, a deficit of 200 mmol or more may develop in an individual on a potassium-deficient diet. Renal excretory mechanisms for potassium are complex. Potassium in the urine is derived almost entirely from potassium secreted in the distal convoluted tubule and collecting duct; filtered potassium is nearly quantitatively reabsorbed in more proximal segments. Potassium secretion appears to be determined by the potassium concentration of tubular cells and by an electrochemical gradient favoring diffusion of the ion into tubular fluid. Among the key influences on potassium secretion are aldosterone, distal tubular fluid flow rate, acid-base balance, and factors that alter distal tubular electronegativity. Aldosterone stimulates potassium secretion. Thus, hyperkalemia increases potassium excretion by two mechanisms: it stimulates adrenal secretion of aldosterone, and it directly enhances renal secretion, presumably via increased tubular cell potassium. Potassium secretion in the distal tubule is flow-dependent; increased distal delivery of tubular fluid favors potassium excretion. For example, loop diuretics, which enhance distal volume delivery, increase potassium excretion, especially in patients with edema and secondary aldosteronism. Alkalosis enhances and acidosis depresses renal potassium secretion, probably by inducing corresponding changes in tubular cell potassium. If delivery to distal segments of sodium salts of unreabsorbable anions such as excess bicarbonate or carbenicillin is augmented, tubular electronegative potential will increase as sodium is reabsorbed. The enhanced electrical gradient will promote potassium excretion.

POTASSIUM DEPLETION AND HYPOKALEMIA Pathogenesis The principal causes of potassium depletion are listed in Table 50-2. As noted above, renal excretion of potassium falls slowly in persons on potassium-deficient diets. During the 10 to 14 days before balance is achieved, significant deficits may occur. Thus, in contrast to sodium, moderate potassium depletion may result from *poor intake* alone. Potassium deficiency is frequent in *gastrointestinal disorders* in which vomiting, diarrhea, or loss of gastrointestinal secretions is prominent. Diarrhea may cause large potassium deficits, since the potassium concentration of liquid stool is 40 to 60 mmol/L. *Loss of*

TABLE 50-2 Causes of potassium depletion and hypokalemia

I Gastrointestinal
  A Deficient dietary intake
  B Gastrointestinal disorders (vomiting, diarrhea, villous adenoma, fistulas, ureterosigmoidostomy)
II Renal
  A Metabolic alkalosis
  B Diuretics, osmotic diuresis
  C Excessive mineralocorticoid effects
    1 Primary aldosteronism
    2 Secondary aldosteronism (including malignant hypertension, Bartter's syndrome, juxtaglomerular cell tumor)
    3 Licorice ingestion
    4 Glucocorticoid excess (Cushing's syndrome, exogenous steroids, ectopic ACTH production)
  D Renal tubular diseases
    1 Renal tubular acidosis
    2 Leukemia
    3 Liddle's syndrome
    4 Antibiotics
  E Magnesium depletion
III Hypokalemia due to shift into cells (no depletion)
  A Hypokalemic periodic paralysis
  B Insulin effect
  C Alkalosis

gastric secretions through vomiting or nasogastric suction is also a common cause of potassium depletion. The potassium concentration of gastric fluid is only 5 to 10 mmol/L; direct losses contribute modestly to negative potassium balance. The potassium deficit is primarily due to increased renal excretion. Potassium excretion appears to be stimulated by three mechanisms. Loss of gastric acid leads to *metabolic alkalosis,* which increases tubular cell potassium concentration. The elevated plasma bicarbonate concentration also increases delivery of bicarbonate and fluid to the distal nephron. At that site, as noted above, excess bicarbonate acts as a nonreabsorbable anion to augment potassium excretion. Finally, secondary hyperaldosteronism due to associated extracellular volume contraction may play a role in maintaining potassium excretion at high levels despite potassium depletion.

Diuretics are among the most frequent causes of hypokalemia and potassium depletion. Thiazides, loop diuretics, and carbonic anhydrase inhibitors all increase potassium excretion. These agents augment sodium and fluid delivery to the distal potassium secretory site by inhibiting reabsorption in more proximal nephron segments. Carbonic anhydrase inhibitors such as acetazolamide, which inhibit proximal bicarbonate reabsorption, also enhance potassium excretion by increasing distal delivery of nonreabsorbable bicarbonate. Hypokalemia and potassium depletion are frequent when diuretics are used to treat edematous patients, in whom secondary aldosteronism is the rule. Although hypokalemia also occurs in patients receiving diuretics for treatment of hypertension, potassium depletion is modest if dietary potassium is normal. Surreptitious abuse of diuretics should be considered when hypokalemic patients have renal potassium wasting of uncertain cause.

Potassium excretion is increased during an *osmotic diuresis.* This mechanism leads to potassium depletion in patients with diabetic ketoacidosis, in whom the osmotic diuresis is due to glycosuria and to increased excretion of keto acid anions. However, plasma potassium may be normal or even high due to the shift of potassium out of tissues caused by the diabetic acidosis and insulin deficiency. Failure to recognize potassium depletion may lead to serious cardiotoxicity from sudden hypokalemia when the acidosis is corrected with insulin or alkali. A normal plasma potassium concentration in an acidotic patient strongly suggests potassium depletion.

Urinary potassium loss is often due to *excessive mineralocorticoid activity.* Hypokalemia is characteristic of *primary aldosteronism* (Chap. 317). It may be minimal in patients with restricted sodium intake because potassium excretion is limited by decreased distal salt and fluid delivery. *Secondary aldosteronism* causes renal potassium wasting and hypokalemia in patients with malignant hypertension, Bartter's syndrome, and renin-secreting renal tumors. However, patients with congestive heart failure, hepatic cirrhosis, and nephrotic syndrome usually are not hypokalemic despite secondary aldosteronism. The decrease in effective blood volume in such patients reduces distal delivery of salt and fluid, thereby limiting potassium excretion. As noted above, treatment with diuretics, which increase distal delivery, will often provoke hypokalemia in these patients. Some forms of *licorice* contain a compound with mineralocorticoid activity; patients who consume huge amounts may become hypokalemic. Excessive levels of *glucocorticoids* stimulate secretion of renal potassium (and hydrogen), leading to hypokalemia and alkalosis in patients with *Cushing's syndrome* (Chap. 317) and some receiving *therapeutic steroids.*

Renal tubular potassium wasting is a feature of *renal tubular acidosis* (Chap. 231). Some patients with monocytic or myelomonocytic *leukemia* develop hypokalemia. The mechanism is uncertain. Renal potassium wasting in some patients appears to correlate with lysozymuria, and the enzyme may interfere with tubular function. In *Liddle's syndrome,* a rare familial disorder (Chap. 231), renal potassium wasting is an intrinsic tubular abnormality. Certain *antibiotics* may cause hypokalemia by increasing potassium excretion. Carbenicillin in large amounts promotes distal tubular secretion by acting as an unreabsorbed anion; amphotericin B alters distal tubular permeability. Gentamicin has also been reported to cause hypokalemia by unknown mechanisms.

Magnesium depletion can cause potassium depletion, apparently due to increased renal and possibly gastrointestinal losses. Increased aldosterone secretion may play a role in stimulating potassium excretion. Hypokalemia in this condition is associated with hypocalcemia.

Clinical features and diagnosis   The most prominent features of hypokalemia and potassium depletion are neuromuscular. Moderate degrees of depletion may be asymptomatic, especially if they develop slowly. Some patients, however, complain of muscle weakness, especially in the lower extremities. With more severe or acute degrees of hypokalemia and potassium deficiency, marked and generalized weakness of skeletal muscles is prominent. Very severe or abrupt development of hypokalemia may lead to virtually total paralysis, including the respiratory muscles. Rhabdomyolysis may occur. On physical examination, in addition to decreased motor power, the patient may demonstrate decreased or absent tendon reflexes. The smooth muscle of the gastrointestinal tract may be affected, resulting in paralytic ileus.

Abnormalities in the electrocardiogram are common (Chap. 176). The characteristic changes include flattening and inversion of the T wave, increased prominence of the U wave, and sagging of the ST segment. These alterations are not well correlated with the severity of the disturbance in potassium metabolism and cannot be relied on as indexes of the clinical significance of a potassium deficit. Although moderate potassium depletion rarely affects cardiac action, severe or rapid reduction in serum potassium may cause cardiac arrest. Potassium deficiency enhances the cardiac toxicity of digitalis preparations. A variety of atrial and ventricular arrhythmias may occur in hypokalemia, especially in patients receiving digitalis.

Renal tubular function is markedly impaired by potassium depletion (Chap. 229). The most prominent abnormality is decreased concentrating ability, which may cause polyuria and polydipsia. Glomerular filtration rate is normal or slightly reduced; moderate reductions may occur with chronic potassium depletion nephropathy. Renal regulation of potassium excretion remains normal. The urinalysis is benign: protein excretion is normal or minimally increased, and the urinary sediment is normal or demonstrates only a slight increase in hyaline or granular casts.

DIAGNOSIS   The cause of hypokalemia and potassium depletion is usually evident from the history. However, patients whose potassium deficiency is caused by chronic abuse of laxatives; psychogenic, self-induced vomiting; or surreptitious use of diuretics rarely volunteer an accurate history. Patients with villous adenomas of the rectum sometimes report that their feces are formed; careful questioning will reveal the elimination of the characteristic mucous secretion of the tumor.

Figure 50-2 is a flow chart that outlines the steps in differential diagnosis of hypokalemia when the cause is not evident from the history. The presence of *hypertension,* which suggests hyperaldosteronism (except Bartter's syndrome) or glucocorticoid excess, may be a clue to diagnosis. Blood pressure is normal in patients whose potassium depletion is due to the other causes listed in Table 50-2. Evaluation of *urinary potassium excretion* may be helpful in determining the origin of the potassium deficit. If gastrointestinal losses have occurred, urinary excretion is usually less than 20 to 25 mmol/L or per day. Although renal conservation of potassium is slow, excretion falls to these levels by the time that clinically significant deficits of potassium have accumulated. On the other hand, when renal potassium wasting is the cause, urinary excretion usually exceeds 20 to 25 mmol/L or per day. However, lower concentrations and lower excretion rates may be found in severe depletion, in those patients with excessive mineralocorticoid activity while on low sodium intake, and in patients whose diuretics have been stopped at the time of examination. Evaluation of blood *acid-base status* may help in differential diagnosis. Hypokalemia is associated with metabolic acidosis in renal tubular acidosis, diarrhea, and diabetic ketoacidosis,

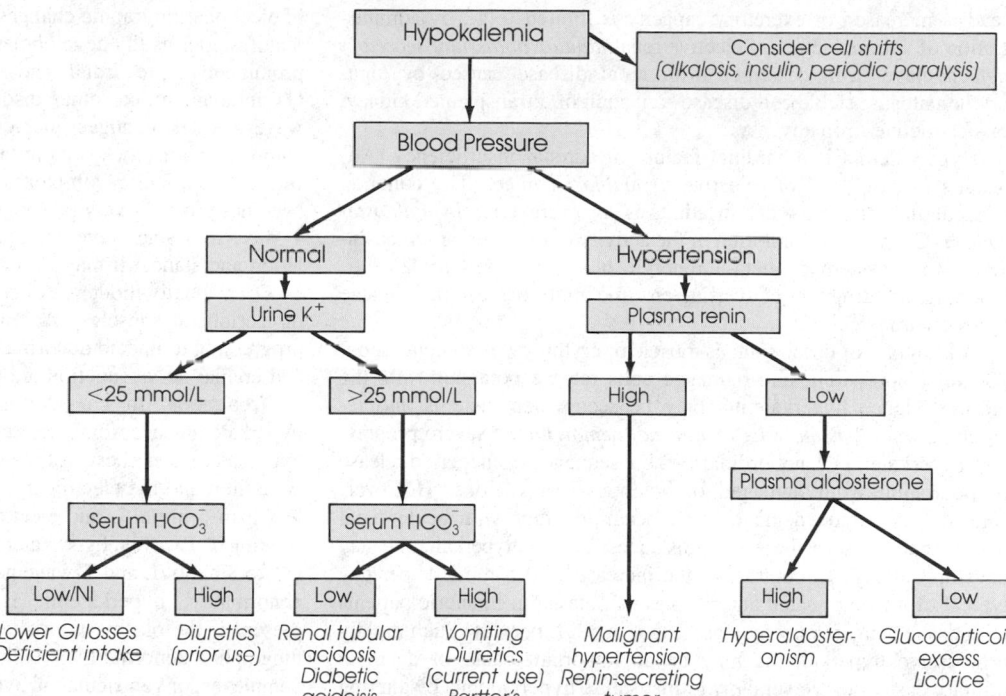

FIGURE 50-2 Flow chart for differential diagnosis of principal causes of hypokalemia. Nl = Normal.

and in patients treated with carbonic anhydrase inhibitors. With other causes of hypokalemia, blood bicarbonate is normal, or elevated due to associated metabolic alkalosis.

Treatment When possible, potassium depletion should be corrected by increased dietary intake or supplementation with potassium salts. Potassium chloride is the salt of choice, especially in alkalotic patients. It may be given in the form of an elixir or in tablets in which potassium chloride crystals are imbedded in a wax. Enteric-coated potassium chloride tablets have been responsible for ulceration of the small bowel, due to release of high concentrations of potassium salts, and should be avoided. Organic salts such as gluconate or citrate are adequate in patients who are not severely alkalotic and often are used to treat hypokalemia due to renal tubular acidosis. In edematous patients treated with diuretics that cause hypokalemia, potassium deficits should be prevented or treated by increased dietary potassium intake, supplementation with potassium chloride, or addition of ''potassium-sparing'' diuretics such as spironolactone. More controversial is the need for routine dietary supplements in patients receiving diuretics for treatment of hypertension. Patients with adequate dietary potassium intake usually do not develop significant hypokalemia and probably do not require routine supplements to prevent potassium depletion. However, those who do develop hypokalemia despite adequate diets should probably receive potassium salts, since hypokalemia may be associated with an increased frequency of arrhythmias.

Intravenous treatment is required for patients with gastrointestinal disorders or when the potassium deficiency is severe. It must be emphasized that the potassium *concentration* in commonly available intravenous solutions of potassium chloride is 2000 mmol/L. Concentrations in intravenous infusions should not exceed 40 or at the most 60 mmol/L. The rate of infusion should not exceed 20 mmol/h or approximately 200 to 250 mmol/d, unless the need for more rapid infusion has been demonstrated in the individual patient by evidence of continuing losses large enough to justify more intensive therapy. The results of treatment are best monitored by repeated determinations of plasma potassium and evaluation of clinical symptoms such as muscular weakness or paralysis. Disappearance of electrocardiographic abnormalities correlates only roughly with improvement in total body potassium content. However, during rapid intravenous administration of potassium, the electrocardiogram should be monitored to avoid cardiac toxicity from inadvertent hyperkalemia.

Hypokalemia and hypocalcemia may occur together, for example, in patients with malabsorption syndrome. The neuromuscular effect of each electrolyte abnormality is masked by the other. Treatment of either disorder alone may precipitate symptoms. Thus, treatment of hypokalemia alone may precipitate tetany, and conversely, treatment of hypocalcemia without correcting the hypokalemia may exacerbate the manifestations of potassium deficiency.

HYPERKALEMIA Pathogenesis The causes of hyperkalemia are shown in Table 50-3. *Inadequate renal excretion* is the most frequent cause (see also Chaps. 223 and 224). When oliguria or anuria is present, as in acute renal failure, progressive hyperkalemia is the rule. Plasma potassium rises by about 0.5 mmol/L per day if there are no abnormal loads. Chronic renal failure does not cause severe or progressive hyperkalemia unless oliguria supervenes. Adaptive changes of unknown etiology increase potassium excretion per residual nephron as chronic renal failure progresses. However, patients with chronic renal failure function at the limits of their excretory capacity. Hence, hyperkalemia may develop rapidly if the potassium

---

TABLE 50-3 Causes of hyperkalemia

I Inadequate excretion
  A Renal failure
    1 Acute renal failure
    2 Severe chronic renal failure
    3 Tubular disorders
  B Adrenal insufficiency
    1 Hypoaldosteronism
    2 Addison's disease
  C Diuretics which inhibit potassium secretion (spironolactone, triamterene, amiloride)
II Shift of potassium from tissues
  A Tissue damage (muscle crush, hemolysis, internal bleeding)
  B Drugs: succinylcholine, arginine, digitalis poisoning, beta-adrenergic antagonists
  C Acidosis
  D Hyperosmolality
  E Insulin deficiency
  F Hyperkalemic periodic paralysis
III Excessive intake
IV Pseudohyperkalemia
  A Thrombocytosis
  B Leukocytosis
  C Poor venipuncture technique
  D In vitro hemolysis

load is increased or excretory capacity is limited, e.g., by administration of spironolactone. Selective renal *tubular potassium secretory defects* have been described with renal disease caused by lupus erythematosus, sickle cell disease, rejection of a transplanted kidney, or obstructive uropathy.

Hyperkalemia is a cardinal feature of adrenal insufficiency (Addison's disease) and of selective *hypoaldosteronism*. The common form of the latter disorder in adults is *hyporeninemic hypoaldosteronism* (Chap. 317). Inhibition of the activity of the renin-angiotensin-aldosterone system by beta-adrenergic blockers, nonsteroidal antiinflammatory drugs, or converting enzyme inhibitors also may induce hyperkalemia.

A kilogram of tissue such as muscle or erythrocytes contains about 80 mmol potassium, and damaged cells release potassium into the plasma. Hence hyperkalemia may be seen when there is *muscle-crushing injury, hemolysis,* or *internal hemorrhage.* Severe progressive hyperkalemia is not ordinarily a consequence of increased release of potassium from damaged or acidotic tissues alone. However, acidosis and tissue damage often occur together with acute renal insufficiency; under these circumstances, severe hyperkalemia may develop quickly. In contrast to the increase of 0.5 mmol/L per day typical of uncomplicated anuria, plasma potassium in anuric patients with tissue damage may increase 2 to 4 mmol/L per day. Such rapidly progressive hyperkalemia may be an important cause of death in military casualties. Several *drugs* may cause hyperkalemia by altering tissue uptake of potassium. In patients with trauma, burns, or neuromuscular diseases such as paraplegia and multiple sclerosis, the muscle relaxant succinylcholine may cause dangerous hyperkalemia. This agent apparently releases potassium from muscle by depolarizing cell membranes. Arginine hydrochloride, used to treat metabolic alkalosis, drives potassium out of cells. If potassium excretion is impaired, clinically significant hyperkalemia may occur during arginine infusions. Extreme digitalis poisoning may cause severe hyperkalemia; potassium leaks out of cells because Na^+,K^+-ATPase is inhibited by the drug. Beta-adrenergic blockers may induce hyperkalemia by interfering with the action of endogenous beta-catecholamines to enhance movement of potassium into tissues. *Metabolic acidosis* causes hyperkalemia by shifting potassium out of cells. Respiratory acidosis has less striking effects. *Hyperosmolality* also enhances potassium movement from cells. *Insulin deficiency* is conducive to hyperkalemia because the action of insulin to promote potassium movement into cells is diminished. Hyperosmolality or metabolic acidosis may be additional mechanisms of hyperkalemia in insulin-deficient patients. In *hyperkalemic periodic paralysis*, the hyperkalemia is associated with repeated attacks of muscular paralysis. The mechanism of this syndrome is not understood. Ingestion of increased amounts of potassium may precipitate attacks.

The severity of hyperkalemia caused by large oral or intravenous *potassium loads* is influenced by factors that modulate tissue uptake and renal excretion of potassium. For example, insulin deficiency and treatment with beta-adrenergic blockers tend to augment hyperkalemia by limiting tissue uptake. Volume depletion enhances hyperkalemia by limiting the rate at which the kidney excretes such loads.

Patients with extreme thrombocytosis or, more rarely, extreme leukocytosis in leukemia may demonstrate the phenomenon of pseudohyperkalemia. Platelets or white blood cells release potassium during blood clotting in vitro. While serum potassium may be grossly abnormal, plasma potassium is not increased. Artifactual elevation of plasma potassium may occur if blood is drawn after repeated fist clenching to make veins more prominent during application of a tourniquet, due to leakage of potassium from exercising muscle. Improper technique during collection or processing of blood samples may cause hemolysis and hence hyperkalemia in vitro. Artifactual hyperkalemia may be suspected when electrocardiographic abnormalities are absent despite elevation of measured potassium levels.

Clinical features and diagnosis   The most important toxic effects of hyperkalemia are cardiac arrhythmias. The characteristic sequence of electrocardiographic changes is shown in Fig. 176-15. The earliest manifestation is the development of high-peaked T waves, especially prominent in precordial leads. Hyperkalemia does not prolong the QT interval, unlike other disorders which induce peaking of the T waves. Later changes include prolongation of the PR interval, complete heart block, and atrial asystole. As plasma potassium rises further, ventricular complexes may deteriorate. The QRS complex becomes progressively prolonged and finally tends to merge with the T wave in a sine wave configuration. Terminally, ventricular fibrillation and standstill may occur.

Occasionally moderate or severe hyperkalemia has striking effects on peripheral muscles. Ascending muscular weakness can occur, progressing to flaccid quadriplegia and respiratory paralysis. Cerebral and cranial nerve function are normal, as is sensation.

Treatment   In considering therapy, it is helpful to classify hyperkalemia according to degree of severity. The seriousness of hyperkalemia is best estimated by considering both the plasma potassium and the electrocardiogram. When the plasma potassium is less than 6 mmol/L and electrocardiographic changes are limited to peaking of T waves, hyperkalemia is mild. When the plasma potassium is 6 to 8 mmol/L and T-wave peaking is the only electrocardiographic abnormality, hyperkalemia is moderate. Severe hyperkalemia is present if the plasma potassium exceeds 8 mmol/L or if electrocardiographic abnormalities include absent P waves, widened QRS complexes, or ventricular arrhythmias. Mild hyperkalemia can usually be treated by elimination of a cause, such as potassium-sparing diuretics, or by treatment of accompanying acidosis.

More severe or progressive hyperkalemia requires vigorous therapy. Severe cardiac toxicity responds most rapidly to infusion of calcium; 10 to 30 mL of 10% calcium gluconate may be infused intravenously within a period of 1 to 5 min under constant electrocardiographic monitoring. While calcium infusions do not alter plasma potassium, they counteract the adverse effects of potassium on neuromuscular membranes. The effect of calcium infusions, while almost immediate, is transient if the hyperkalemia is not treated directly.

In moderate or severe hyperkalemia, infusion of hypertonic glucose solutions decreases toxicity by provoking insulin release and shifting potassium into cells. In the first 30 min, 200 to 500 mL of 10% glucose may be given. An additional 500 to 1000 mL may be infused over the next several hours. Ten units of regular insulin are given intravenously or subcutaneously, although this is probably necessary only in insulin-deficient diabetic patients. This treatment may reduce serum potassium by 1 to 2 mmol/L, and effects persist for a number of hours. The infusion of sodium bicarbonate also helps lower serum potassium rapidly by causing potassium to shift into cells; 50 to 150 mmol alkali (two to three ampuls) may be added to a liter of glucose. Although this agent is most valuable in acidotic patients, it also is effective in individuals with normal acid-base status. The effect occurs within 1 h and persists for a number of hours. The infusion of hypertonic sodium solutions may also be effective in reversing cardiac toxicity, especially in hyponatremic or volume-depleted patients. In part, the effect depends simply on dilution of plasma potassium, but there may be a direct effect of elevated plasma sodium to antagonize hyperkalemic neuromuscular toxicity as well. Glucose, bicarbonate, and sodium may be combined in a "therapeutic cocktail," formulated by adding an ampul or two of sodium bicarbonate to a liter of 5% dextrose in 0.9% saline.

None of the measures just described removes potassium from the body. Cation exchange resins such as sodium polystyrene sulfonate are useful to remove potassium in the treatment of moderate or severe hyperkalemia. Fifty grams of the resin is mixed with 50 mL of 70% sorbitol and 100 mL of tap water and given by retention enema. Enough potassium may be removed by a single enema to reduce potassium by 0.5 to 2 mmol/L within an hour, and repeated enemas can be given. These resins can also be given repeatedly by mouth to maintain low plasma potassium concentration. Twenty grams is given three or four times a day together with 20 mL of a 70% sorbitol solution, as required to ensure the passage of several loose stools daily. In patients with renal failure, hemodialysis and peritoneal dialysis effectively control hyperkalemia. However, they are relatively slow techniques, and patients with severe hyperkalemia should be treated first with one of the methods previously discussed.

REFERENCES

Sodium and water

Ayus JC et al: Treatment of symptomatic hyponatremia and its relation to brain damage. N Engl J Med 317:1190, 1987

Narins RG et al: Diagnostic strategies in disorders of fluid, electrolyte and acid-base homeostasis. Am J Med 72:496, 1982

Robertson GL: Thirst and vasopressin function in normal and disordered states of water balance. J Lab Clin Med 101:351, 1983

Sterns RH et al: Osmotic demyelination syndrome following correction of hyponatremia. N Engl J Med 314:1535, 1986

Weiner M, Epstein FH: Signs and symptoms of electrolyte disorders. Yale J Biol Med 43:76, 1970

Weisberg LS et al: Pseudohyponatremia: A reappraisal. Am J Med 86:315, 1989

Zerbe R et al: Vasopressin function in the syndrome of inappropriate diuresis. Ann Rev Med 31:315, 1980

Potassium

Bia MJ, DeFronzo RA: Extrarenal potassium homeostasis. Am J Physiol 240:F257, 1981

Hollenberg NK, Brown RS (eds): Electrolytes and cardiovascular disease. Am J Med 77(5A):1, 1984

Knochel JP: The syndrome of hyporeninemic hypoaldosteronism. Ann Rev Med 30:145, 1979

————: Neuromuscular manifestations of electrolyte disorders. Am J Med 72:521, 1982

————: Hypokalemia. Adv Int Med 30:317, 1984

Ponce SP et al: Drug-induced hyperkalemia. Medicine 64:357, 1985

Richardson RMA, Kunau RT Jr: Renal regulation of potassium: Abnormal, in The Kidney: Physiology and Pathophysiology, 2d ed, DW Seldin, G Giebisch (eds). New York, Raven, 1985, p 1251

Seldin DW, Giebisch G (eds): The Regulation of Sodium and Chloride Balance. New York, Raven, 1989, 350 pp

Sterns RH et al: Internal potassium balance and the control of the plasma potassium concentration. Medicine 60:339, 1981

Stokes JB: Potassium intoxication: Pathogenesis and Treatment, in The Regulation of Potassium Balance, DW Seldin, G Giebisch (eds). New York, Raven, 1989, p 269

Tanner RL: Diuretic-induced hypokalemia. Kidney Int 28:988, 1985

51 ACIDOSIS AND ALKALOSIS

NORMAN G. LEVINSKY

PHYSIOLOGIC CONSIDERATIONS Acids are produced continuously during normal metabolism. Despite the addition of some 20,000 mmol of carbonic acid and 80 mmol of nonvolatile acids to body fluids daily, the free hydrogen ion concentration of these fluids is fixed within a narrow range. The pH of extracellular fluid is normally between 7.35 and 7.45 (hydrogen ion, 45 to 35 nmol/L). The pH of intracellular fluids cannot be determined with precision, but most methods suggest a mean intracellular pH in the range of 6.9. Intracellular hydrogen ion concentration is not uniform; it varies among intracellular organelles within individual cells. Although the free hydrogen ion concentration of body fluids is low, protons are so reactive that even minute changes in concentration influence enzymatic reactions and physiologic processes. Immediate defense against untoward changes in pH is provided by buffers that can take up or release protons instantaneously in response to changes in acidity of body fluids. Regulation of pH ultimately depends on the lungs and the kidneys.

Role of the lungs The principal acid product of metabolism is carbon dioxide, equivalent to potential carbonic acid. The normal concentration of carbon dioxide in body fluids is fixed around 1.2 mmol/L [P_{CO_2} = 5.3 kPa (40 mmHg)] by the lungs; at this concen-

tration, pulmonary excretion equals metabolic production. Although carbon dioxide reacts with water and body buffers during transport from cells to pulmonary alveoli, no net change in body fluid composition results, since the CO_2 excreted by the lungs is equal to the CO_2 produced by cells.

Nonvolatile acids When a nonvolatile acid is produced by metabolism, the protons are removed instantaneously from body fluids by reaction with buffers. In extracellular fluid, bicarbonate is converted to water and carbon dioxide, which is excreted by the lungs. Although this mechanism minimizes changes in acidity, it destroys bicarbonate and uses up cell buffer capacity. The total buffer capacity of the body fluids is about 15 mmol per kilogram of body weight. Thus, the normal rate of production of nonvolatile acids would be sufficient to deplete the body buffers completely in 10 to 20 days, were it not for the ability of the kidney to eliminate protons from the body by secretion into the urine, thereby regenerating bicarbonate and cell buffer capacity.

The principal source of nonvolatile acid is metabolism of methionine and cystine in dietary proteins, which produces sulfuric acid. Additional sources include the incomplete combustion of carbohydrates and fats, which produces organic acids; the metabolism of nucleoproteins, which produces uric acid; and the metabolism of organic phosphorus compounds, which releases protons and inorganic phosphates. The diet does not normally contain significant amounts of preformed acid or alkali, but significant amounts of potential acid (e.g., an excess of cationic acids, such as lysine) or alkali (e.g., citrate) may be present.

Role of the kidneys The principal functions of the kidney in acid-base metabolism can be viewed as retention of existing bicarbonate and generation of new bicarbonate to replace that used to buffer nonvolatile acids. Bicarbonate is reabsorbed in both proximal and distal segments by secretion of protons into tubular fluid. New bicarbonate is generated by secretion of protons onto urinary buffers. Normally, one-third is titrated onto phosphate, converting HPO_4^{2-} to $H_2PO_4^-$, and the remainder onto ammonia. The amount of free acid which can be excreted in the urine is negligible, even at the minimum urine pH of 4.8. However, acidification of the urine is essential for titration of protons onto phosphate and ammonia. Changes in the pH of body fluids lead to regulatory responses by the kidney. Acidosis stimulates renal hydrogen ion secretion. Ammonia production increases, and more protons can be excreted as ammonium. In extreme acidosis, ammonia production may increase tenfold or more above the normal rate of 40 to 50 mmol/d. The bicarbonate concentration of extracellular fluid is, in effect, set by the renal rate of proton secretion (bicarbonate reabsorption and generation). If plasma bicarbonate rises without an increase in renal reabsorptive capacity, bicarbonate is excreted rapidly and normal plasma bicarbonate is restored promptly. For example, chronic ingestion of even large amounts of sodium bicarbonate normally produces only minimal sustained elevation of plasma bicarbonate.

The rate of proton secretion is influenced by a number of factors, important among them carbon dioxide tension of body fluids, extracellular volume, aldosterone, and body potassium stores. Bicarbonate reabsorption is directly related to carbon dioxide concentration; hypercapnia tends to stimulate, and hypocapnia tends to inhibit, renal bicarbonate retention. Contraction of extracellular volume enhances tubular bicarbonate reabsorption, while volume expansion has the opposite effect. Aldosterone stimulates renal proton secretion; by this effect, hyperaldosteronism promotes metabolic alkalosis, while hypoaldosteronism causes acidosis. In experimental animals, renal bicarbonate reabsorption is inversely related to body potassium stores. In humans, the relation is less clear, but severe potassium depletion has been associated with increased bicarbonate reabsorption and metabolic alkalosis.

The respiratory response to changes in blood pH is almost instantaneous. Acidosis stimulates and alkalosis depresses ventilation. The respiratory center in the medulla appears to respond to a pH intermediate between those of blood and cerebrospinal fluid.

EVALUATION OF ACID-BASE BALANCE   In practice, classification of acid-base disorders is based on measurements of changes in the bicarbonate–carbonic acid system, the principal buffer of extracellular fluid. Because intracellular and extracellular buffers are functionally linked, measurement of the plasma bicarbonate system provides useful information about total body buffers. The relationship among the elements of the bicarbonate system is usually described in terms of the Henderson-Hasselbalch equation:

$$pH = pK + \log \frac{[HCO_3^-]}{[H_2CO_3]}$$

Acidosis is defined as a disturbance which tends to add acid or remove alkali from body fluids, while *alkalosis* is any disturbance which tends to remove acid or add base. Since compensatory processes may minimize or prevent a change in the hydrogen ion concentration of the plasma, some authors prefer to use the terms *acidemia* and *alkalemia* to indicate those situations in which the pH of the plasma is measurably altered. *Metabolic* disorders are those in which the primary disturbance is in the concentration of bicarbonate. Since bicarbonate appears in the numerator of the buffer salt/acid ratio in the Henderson-Hasselbalch equation, increased bicarbonate concentration causes increased pH (alkalemia) while a decrease in bicarbonate causes decreased pH (acidemia). *Respiratory* disorders are those in which the primary change is in the concentration of carbon dioxide (carbonic acid). As can be seen from the Henderson-Hasselbalch equation, a fall in carbon dioxide concentration causes alkalemia, while an increase in carbon dioxide concentration causes acidemia.

A major problem in the assessment of acid-base disorders results from the compensatory responses of the lungs and the kidney. A primary change in carbon dioxide concentration induces a compensatory renal response which alters plasma bicarbonate in the same direction. Conversely, a primary alteration of plasma bicarbonate induces a compensatory respiratory response, which changes plasma carbon dioxide in the same direction. Consider a patient with chronic respiratory insufficiency who has the following set of acid-base parameters: P_{CO_2} = 9.3 kPa (70 mmHg), $[HCO_3^-]$ = 31 mmol/L, pH = 7.25. The clinician needs to know whether the elevation of plasma bicarbonate is merely the appropriate renal response to the primary hypercapnia or a metabolic acid-base disorder is superimposed. No calculations or a priori reasoning will provide the answer to this key question. Such information can be derived only from in vivo observations in which the usual compensatory response to a given degree of chronic hypercapnia is determined.

Clinical and experimental observations in humans (and animals) have been made in all common primary acid-base disturbances. They are most readily visualized and used for analysis of clinical acid-base disorders by the "confidence band" technique, as shown in Fig. 51-1. Each band represents the mean ± 2 SD, that is, 95 percent of observations, for the compensatory response to each primary disturbance. In the example under discussion, inspection of the confidence band marked *chronic respiratory acidosis* indicates that 95 percent of individuals with chronic elevation of P_{CO_2} to 9.3 kPa (70 mmHg) would have $[HCO_3^-]$ between 34 and 44 mmol/L, due to renal compensation. Thus, the $[HCO_3^-]$ of 31 mmol/L in the example cannot be interpreted as the sole result of an appropriate compensatory response to chronic hypercapnia. A second acid-base disorder, presumably metabolic acidosis, must be superimposed to account for the fact that plasma bicarbonate, although increased in response to hypercapnia, is not as high as usually observed when P_{CO_2} is 9.3 kPa (70 mmHg). Obviously, the use of this figure is no panacea, nor does it obviate the need for commonsense clinical evaluation of alternative possibilities. For example, if the patient under discussion had only recently developed hypercapnia, the $[HCO_3^-]$ of 31 mmol/L would be too high for a purely compensatory response to acute respiratory acidosis and would be interpreted as superimposed metabolic alkalosis. The difference between these two interpretations depends entirely on the clinical recognition of the chronicity of the primary respiratory disorder. The use of Fig. 51-1 in each type of

FIGURE 51-1 Nomogram, showing bands for uncomplicated respiratory or metabolic acid-base disturbances in intact subjects. Each "confidence" band represents the mean ± 2 SD for the compensatory response of normal subjects or patients to a given primary disorder. Ac = acute; chr = chronic, resp = respiratory; met = metabolic; acid = acidosis; alk = alkalosis. (*Modified from Arbus.*)

acid-base disturbance is described in the appropriate sections of this chapter.[1]

METABOLIC ACIDOSIS

PATHOPHYSIOLOGY   Metabolic acidosis is caused by one of three mechanisms (see Table 51-1): (1) increased production of nonvolatile acids, (2) decreased acid excretion by the kidney, (3) loss of alkali. In intracellular fluid excess protons replace potassium, which shifts out of cells, tending to elevate plasma levels. Extracellular bicarbonate is reduced by reaction with hydrogen ions or, in patients wasting alkali, by loss of bicarbonate in urine or stool. The decrease in pH stimulates respiration, and P_{CO_2} is lowered. Inspection of the confidence band for metabolic acidosis (Fig. 51-1) indicates that a decrease in P_{CO_2} of about 0.16 kPa (1.2 mmHg) can be expected for each decrement of 1 mmol/L in plasma bicarbonate. Complete respiratory compensation for primary metabolic acidosis does not occur. Respiratory compensation for acute acidosis tends to be somewhat greater than for chronic metabolic acidosis. The minimum level of P_{CO_2} that can be attained is approximately 1.3 kPa (10 mmHg); levels below 2 to 2.7 kPa (15 to 20 mmHg) are rarely maintained in chronic metabolic acidosis. When kidney function is normal, net acid excretion increases promptly in response to metabolic acidosis. Most of the initial rise is due to increased titration of urinary phosphate as urine pH falls below 5.2. Over several days, ammonia

[1] Although the confidence band method does not permit automatic identification of simple or complicated acid-base disorders, it is preferable to techniques such as "buffer base" or "base excess-deficit" for reasons discussed in detail by Schwartz and Relman, N Engl J Med 268:1382, 1963. These terms are not used in this chapter.

TABLE 51-1   Causes of metabolic acidosis

Increased anion gap
I Increased acid production
  A Ketoacidosis
    1 Diabetic
    2 Alcoholic
    3 Starvation
  B Lactic acidosis
    1 Secondary to circulatory or respiratory failure
    2 Associated with various disorders (see text)
    3 Drugs and toxins
    4 Enzyme defects
  C Poisoning (salicylates, ethylene glycol, methanol)
II Renal failure

Normal anion gap (hyperchloremic)
III Renal tubular dysfunction
  A Renal tubular acidosis
  B Hypoaldosteronism
  C "Potassium-sparing" diuretics
IV Loss of alkali
  A Diarrhea
  B Ureterosigmoidostomy
  C Carbonic anhydrase inhibitors
V Ammonium chloride, cationic amino acids (excess intake)

production by the kidney increases and becomes the most important mechanism for excreting excess protons. Net acid excretion may increase 5 to 10 times above normal, reaching a maximum of several hundred millimoles per day.

The most common cause of *acute* metabolic acidosis is increased production of nonvolatile acids. In *diabetic ketoacidosis*, acetoacetic and β-hydroxybutyric acids are produced more rapidly than they can be metabolized (Chap. 319). Severe ketoacidosis may occur in *association* with *acute* and *chronic alcoholism*. Typically patients give a history of prolonged abstention from food, protracted vomiting, and appreciable alcohol intake just before development of the ketoacidosis. β-Hydroxybutyrate, acetoacetate, and lactate accumulate in the plasma. The ketosis may be overlooked because the ratio of β-hydroxybutyrate to acetoacetate tends to be high; the nitroprusside test used for clinical detection of plasma ketones responds only to the latter. Blood sugar is usually normal or mildly elevated in these patients. The mechanism of the syndrome is uncertain. *Starvation* may cause mild ketoacidosis because of increased fat catabolism.

Lactic acidosis   This is one of the most common types of metabolic acidosis. Metabolic production and consumption of lactate are normally in balance. Under basal conditions the liver and kidney consume lactate produced by tissues such as erythrocytes, skin, intestine, and muscle. However, if oxygen delivery is inadequate to meet energy requirements, any tissue will generate lactate. Deficient oxygen impairs electron flow through the cytochrome transport chain; ATP formation is decreased and cell redox pairs, such as NADH/NAD, are shifted toward the reduced state. Decrease in ATP and reciprocal increases in ADP and AMP concentrations activate phosphofructokinase, the key enzyme regulating glycolysis. Accelerated glycolysis leads to increased production of pyruvate and the increase in NADH/NAD ratio decreases its oxidation. Pyruvate and lactate are in a near-equilibrium reaction catalyzed by lactic dehydrogenase, as follows:

$$\text{Pyruvate} + \text{NADH} + \text{H}^+ \rightleftharpoons \text{lactate} + \text{NAD}$$

Thus lactate will tend to increase when pyruvate concentration increases and when the ratio of NADH to NAD rises. Since both conditions occur when tissues are oxygen-deprived, lactate formation is increased. Lactate will accumulate because it can be consumed only by conversion back to pyruvate, which is blocked so long as pyruvate concentration and the NADH/NAD ratio are elevated. Since the overall process of glycolysis generates one H^+ for each lactate produced, acid production increases proportionately with lactate production.

These mechanisms, probably compounded by decreased uptake

or, even, production of lactate by the liver, account for the development of lactic acidosis in patients with *shock* due to any cause (e.g., sepsis, myocardial infarction, hemorrhage) or with respiratory arrest. Since severe acidosis depresses myocardial and arteriolar contractility, lactic acidosis may compound the underlying cause of shock. Less commonly, lactic acidosis may be caused by *pulmonary diseases* leading to extreme hypoxia or by diminished blood oxygen–carrying capacity in severe *anemia* and *carbon monoxide* poisoning. The mortality rate is high in patients with lactic acidosis secondary to shock and tissue hypoxia. During vigorous *exercise* or convulsions, local disproportion between oxygen supply and demand in contracting muscle may lead to transient, clinically benign lactic acidosis.

Lactic acidosis also is *associated* with disorders in which tissue hypoxia does not appear to be present. It has been reported in patients with leukemia, lymphoma, and solid tumors; with poorly controlled diabetes mellitus; and with severe hepatic failure. Mechanisms causing lactic acidosis in these disorders are poorly understood. Overproduction of lactate by neoplastic tissue probably is a factor in lactic acidosis associated with tumors. Insulin deficiency, which inhibits pyruvate oxidation, presumably is an important factor in patients with poorly controlled diabetes. Decreased hepatic lactate metabolism seems a likely mechanism in severe liver disease.

A variety of *drugs* and *toxins* have been associated with lactic acidosis. *Drugs* include fructose used in parenteral alimentation; sodium nitroprusside; epinephrine and norepinephrine infusions; and, before the drug was removed from general use, the biguanide hypoglycemic agent, phenformin. Lactic acidosis may contribute to the severe acidosis in *poisoning* by salicylates, ethylene glycol, or methanol. Ethanol elevates serum lactate but clinically significant lactic acidosis does not occur in alcohol intoxication unless there are associated disorders such as hepatic or circulatory failure.

In infants and children a number of congenital defects in enzymes of carbohydrate metabolism cause lactic acidosis. These include defects of glucose-6-phosphatase, fructose-1,6-biphosphatase, pyruvate carboxylase, and pyruvate dehydrogenase. *Primary* lactic acidosis in patients without an underlying disease has been reported, but the existence of such a spontaneous disorder is uncertain.

Acute metabolic acidosis   *Poisoning* and drug toxicity are causes of acute metabolic acidosis. Among the more common agents are salicylates, ethylene glycol, and methyl alcohol (Chap. 374). Salicylates create a metabolic block, which leads to production of a mixture of endogenous organic acids. Methanol and ethylene glycol are converted to acid metabolites, methanol to formic acid and ethylene glycol to glyoxylic and oxalic acids. In addition, these intoxicants create metabolic blocks, which may lead to increased production of endogenous organic acids. Salicylates have the additional effect of stimulating the respiratory center directly. Respiratory alkalosis is the earliest derangement in salicylate intoxication and may be the only acid-base disorder in some patients.

Chronic metabolic acidosis   Renal disease is the most common cause of *chronic* metabolic acidosis. In *chronic renal failure* (Chap. 224), the principal defect is decreased ability to excrete ammonium, but some patients also waste bicarbonate, especially at plasma levels of 18 mmol/L or above. Acidification of the urine and formation of titratable acidity are usually normal. Plasma bicarbonate tends to fall progressively as renal insufficiency becomes increasingly severe, but plasma bicarbonate usually stabilizes at levels of 12 to 18 mmol/L; it rarely falls below 10 mmol/L, even in advanced uremia. The mechanisms of stabilization are thought to be (1) stimulation of acid excretion by advancing acidosis, which occurs to some extent even in the diseased kidney; and (2) buffering of the daily metabolic acid load by carbonate and phosphate in bone. In *acute renal failure* (Chap. 223), plasma bicarbonate decreases by about 1 to 2 mmol/L per day if reduced renal acid excretion is the only cause of metabolic acidosis. Greater rates of fall suggest the presence, in addition, of some cause of increased acid production.

Chronic metabolic acidosis is the hallmark of *renal tubular acidosis* (Chap. 231), which may be an isolated disorder of tubular acid excretion; part of a Fanconi syndrome, in which other tubular functions are also abnormal; or associated with nonrenal primary disorders (Chap. 335). The acidosis is due to defective renal tubular acidification mechanisms, which limit renal conservation and regeneration of bicarbonate.

Aldosterone stimulates distal tubular acid and potassium secretion. In *hypoaldosteronism,* loss of this effect leads to metabolic acidosis and hyperkalemia. The acidosis is due not only to loss of the direct effect of aldosterone on acid excretion but also to the hyperkalemia, which decreases renal ammonia production. The same factors account for metabolic acidosis caused by the diuretic spironolactone, which blocks the action of aldosterone, and other "potassium-sparing" diuretics such as triamterene and amiloride, which directly inhibit distal tubular secretion of acid and potassium.

Loss of alkali may cause acute or chronic metabolic acidosis. Severe *diarrhea* or intestinal malabsorption usually causes mild to moderate acidosis due to the loss of bicarbonate in liquid stool, in which concentrations of 40 to 60 mmol/L may be present. Uretero-sigmoidostomy, i.e., transplantation of the ureters into the sigmoid colon, leads to metabolic acidosis both because of exchange of chloride for bicarbonate by intestinal epithelium and because renal disease (obstructive uropathy and pyelonephritis) often develops. However, acidosis is not a problem with the more modern technique for urinary diversion, in which a bladder is formed from a small isolated loop of ileum. Carbonic anhydrase inhibitors, such as acetazolamide, cause mild to moderate acidosis by increasing bicarbonate loss in the urine.

Acidosis can be caused by administration of ammonium chloride and lysine or arginine hydrochloride, which form HCl during metabolism. This type of acidosis also may occur during parenteral alimentation with amino acid infusates that contain an excess of the cationic amino acids arginine, lysine, and histidine.

CLINICAL FEATURES AND DIAGNOSIS   There are few specific symptoms or signs of metabolic acidosis; diagnosis depends on recognition of the clinical setting and appropriate laboratory studies. In acute metabolic acidosis, hyperventilation is usual and may be intense (Kussmaul respiration). However, it is ordinarily impossible to detect increased respiration by physical examination in patients with chronic metabolic acidosis, despite substantial reduction of P_{CO_2}. Acute, severe acidosis produces a variety of nonspecific symptoms ranging from fatigue through confusion, stupor, and coma. Cardiovascular effects include decreased cardiac contractility and vasodilatation, which may lead to heart failure or hypotension. Chronic metabolic acidosis may produce no symptoms or may be associated with fatigue and anorexia, although it is usually difficult to determine whether these symptoms reflect the acidosis per se or are related to the underlying disease.

The characteristic laboratory features are reduction of plasma bicarbonate and blood pH, together with a compensatory reduction in P_{CO_2} (see Fig. 51-1). Hyperkalemia is often present, due to shift of potassium out of cells. This phenomenon may mask significant potassium depletion (see Chap. 50). Hypokalemia is a clue to conditions in which concomitant potassium depletion is severe, for example, diarrhea or diabetic ketoacidosis, or in which renal potassium-regulating mechanisms are affected, such as renal tubular acidosis or administration of carbonic anhydrase inhibitors.

When the cause of metabolic acidosis is not evident from the history or clinical setting, calculation of unmeasured anions (anion gap) may help in differential diagnosis. Unmeasured anions are calculated by subtracting the sum of plasma bicarbonate and chloride from plasma sodium concentration; the normal value is 8 to 16 mmol/L. The negative charges on plasma proteins, principally albumin, make up most of the anion gap. Phosphate, sulfate, and organic acid anions normally contribute to unmeasured anions to a lesser degree. When metabolic acidosis is due to increased acid production or renal insufficiency (categories I and II, Table 51-1), the anion gap is usually increased. In acidosis resulting from increased acid production, the increased anion gap is due to accumulation in

plasma of the anions of the various acids such as acetoacetate or lactate, which are produced faster than they can be metabolized or excreted. In renal failure, the anion gap increases because sulfate, phosphate, and organic acid anions are not excreted efficiently.

The cause of acidosis with an increased anion gap usually is easily determined from the clinical setting and simple laboratory tests. *Ketoacidosis* should be considered when acidosis occurs in patients with uncontrolled diabetes mellitus (Chap. 319), alcoholism, or starvation. Ketonemia can be detected by testing serum dilutions with nitroprusside (Acetest) reagent. In occasional patients this test, which reacts to acetoacetate but not β-hydroxybutyrate, may be misleading. If the clinical diagnosis is uncertain, a specific assay for β-hydroxybutyrate is available. The diagnosis of *lactic acidosis* is suspected in patients with severe circulatory insufficiency when other causes of acidosis can be ruled out. A specific assay for plasma lactate is available if the diagnosis is uncertain. Plasma salicylate concentration in the toxic range [>2.9 mmol/L (>40 mg/dL)] will confirm suspected *salicylate intoxication* (Chap. 374). Acidosis due to *poisoning* with ethylene glycol or methanol (Chap. 374) may be suspected if measured plasma osmolality exceeds calculated plasma osmolality [(2 × plasma Na) + glucose/18 + BUN/2.8 (with plasma Na in mmol/L, glucose and BUN in mg/dL)]. This "osmolal gap" reflects the plasma level of methanol or ethylene glycol, small molecules that at toxic concentrations add significantly to plasma osmolality. (Since ethanol has a similar effect, it must be measured if alcohol intoxication is suspected.) Detection of an "osmolal gap" in a patient with severe acidosis may permit prompt treatment to be instituted while awaiting confirmation of the diagnosis with specific tests for the toxins.

In all other types of metabolic acidosis (categories III, IV, V, Table 51-1), the anion gap is normal since there is neither increased production nor decreased excretion of organic acids, sulfate, and phosphate. Plasma chloride concentration is increased approximately as much as plasma bicarbonate is decreased (hyperchloremic acidosis). In diabetic ketoacidosis a variety of plasma acid-base patterns may develop, depending on the balance between production and renal excretion of ketoacid anions. In most patients there is renal dysfunction, and the anions are retained, leading to an anion-gap acidosis in which the elevation in plasma unmeasured anion is about equal to the reduction in bicarbonate concentration. Patients whose renal function is not impaired may present with a component of hyperchloremic acidosis due to renal excretion of ketone anions and retention of chloride. After therapy that repairs volume depletion and hence renal dysfunction, most patients develop some degree of hyperchloremia, due to the same mechanisms.

TREATMENT   The treatment of metabolic acidosis depends on its cause and severity. In *chronic renal failure,* mild or moderate metabolic acidosis does not require treatment. When plasma bicarbonate falls below 15 mmol/L, it is reasonable to treat patients with oral alkali, such as sodium bicarbonate or sodium citrate. The dose is gradually increased until plasma bicarbonate concentration rises to about 18 to 20 mmol/L. Some patients appear to benefit symptomatically from elevation of bicarbonate to this level, and fatigue, anorexia, and malaise tend to be alleviated. Caution must be exerted to avoid excessively rapid alkalination of the plasma, which may precipitate tetany; excess sodium given with alkali may aggravate hypertension or edema. Acidosis should be corrected as completely as possible in patients with type 1 (distal) *renal tubular acidosis;* this will avoid hypercalciuria, osteomalacia, nephrocalcinosis, and lithiasis. In type 2 (proximal) renal tubular acidosis, therapy is usually not required (see Chap. 231). Patients with *acute renal failure* also do not ordinarily require specific therapy for acidosis. Dialysis instituted for management of the renal failure should maintain an adequate plasma bicarbonate.

Diabetic *ketoacidosis* responds to insulin, and most patients do not require treatment with alkali (see Chap. 319). However, when acidosis is extreme (pH less than 7.1 or [HCO_3^-] less than 6 to 8 mmol/L), intravenous bicarbonate therapy is justified. The ketoacidosis associated with alcoholism responds rapidly to infusions of glucose and saline. Insulin is not required, nor should alkali be given unless acidosis is extreme. The ketoacidosis of starvation is mild and requires no specific treatment.

In *lactic acidosis,* if the underlying disorder can be reversed, the acidosis will be corrected by metabolism of lactate, which generates bicarbonate. Since lactic acidosis is usually associated with severe circulatory or respiratory failure, the mortality rate is high. Because production of lactate and H+ in lactic acidosis can be very rapid, it is usually resistant to treatment with alkali. Large amounts of bicarbonate may be required to raise or even to stabilize plasma bicarbonate. Some studies have suggested that alkali therapy in lactic acidosis may be counterproductive because correction of acidosis appears to increase lactate production. However, extreme acidosis may contribute to circulatory collapse (see above), thereby perpetuating the underlying cause of the lactic acidosis. Hence, it seems reasonable to treat lactic acidosis with intravenous bicarbonate at a rate at least sufficient to maintain plasma bicarbonate at 8 to 10 mmol/L and pH above 7.10. If vigorous administration of sodium bicarbonate leads to circulatory overloading, diuretics should be given or dialysis with a bicarbonate-buffered fluid may be instituted. Dichloroacetate, an investigational agent that enhances pyruvate dehydrogenase activity, has shown promise for treating lactic acidosis in experimental and clinical studies.

The acidosis due to *diarrhea* or loss of alkaline upper intestinal secretions is usually associated with volume depletion and potassium deficiency. Treatment of such electrolyte disorders with intravenous infusions appropriate for the patient's specific abnormalities may be required.

Some general points about therapy with alkali are worth emphasis. Oral treatment with sodium bicarbonate should usually begin with 1 g three times daily and be increased to maintain the desired plasma bicarbonate level. Some patients find that sodium bicarbonate leads to upper gastrointestinal discomfort; a 10% sodium citrate solution may be more palatable. In the intravenous treatment of acute metabolic acidosis, sodium bicarbonate is the agent of choice. The amount of bicarbonate to be given depends upon the severity of the acidosis and any associated disorders of serum sodium concentration. Typically, concentrations of bicarbonate between 50 and 150 mmol/L are achieved by adding one to three vials of sodium bicarbonate to a liter of dextrose in water. The concentration of bicarbonate in these vials is 1000 mmol/L (50 mmol in 50 mL); these bicarbonate solutions should never be given undiluted in the treatment of acidosis, since rapid infusion may induce serious or even fatal cardiac arrhythmias, especially if given as a bolus through a central venous catheter.

The total amount of alkali needed to raise plasma bicarbonate can be estimated from the effects of administration of acid loads. Approximately equal amounts of acid appear to be buffered by extracellular bicarbonate and by intracellular buffers. (In severe acidosis, a greater fraction of the acid load may be buffered within cells.) Therefore, it is appropriate to calculate the amount of alkali needed by assuming that approximately half will accept protons from intracellular buffers and be destroyed; the other half will elevate plasma bicarbonate concentration. Thus, the calculation would be: millimoles of bicarbonate required equals desired increment in plasma concentration (millimoles per liter) times 40 percent of body weight. The 40 percent figure represents twice the extracellular volume. It is rarely desirable to infuse enough alkali to elevate plasma bicarbonate to normal. Possible untoward effects include hypokalemic cardiac toxicity in patients who are substantially potassium-depleted, tetany in patients with renal failure or hypocalcemia, and congestive failure due to excess sodium. Moreover, alkalosis may supervene. Cerebrospinal fluid bicarbonate does not equilibrate rapidly with plasma. Hence the respiratory center, which responds to acidity both of blood and cerebrospinal fluid, maintains some degree of hyperventilation as plasma bicarbonate is increasing. This type of respiratory alkalosis may sometimes persist for several days after correction of metabolic acidosis. In acute acidosis due to overproduction of metabolic acids, successful treatment of the primary disorder will cause rapid metabolic

conversion of lactate and ketone bodies to bicarbonate. Thus, excessive administration of bicarbonate early in therapy also may lead to metabolic alkalosis at a later stage of treatment, when endogenous bicarbonate has been reconstituted by improvement in metabolism.

METABOLIC ALKALOSIS

PATHOPHYSIOLOGY Metabolic alkalosis is usually initiated by increased loss of acid from the stomach or the kidney. However, excretion of bicarbonate at high plasma concentrations is normally so rapid that alkalosis will not be sustained unless bicarbonate reabsorption is enhanced or alkali is continuously generated at a great rate. Clinically, maintenance of metabolic alkalosis is most often due to stimulation of bicarbonate reabsorption by a volume (chloride) deficit. During volume depletion, renal conservation of sodium takes precedence over other homeostatic mechanisms, such as correction of alkalosis. Since in alkalosis a large fraction of plasma sodium is paired with bicarbonate, complete reabsorption of filtered sodium requires reabsorption of bicarbonate as well. Alkalosis is sustained until volume depletion is corrected by administration of sodium chloride. This diminishes tubular avidity for sodium and provides chloride as an alternative anion for reabsorption with sodium; excess bicarbonate can then be excreted with sodium.

The other major mechanism which can maintain metabolic alkalosis is hypermineralocorticoidism. Mineralocorticoids stimulate renal hydrogen ion secretion. In patients with excess mineralocorticoid activity, elevation of plasma bicarbonate is initiated by increased urinary loss of protons as ammonium and titratable acidity. Stimulation of tubular acid secretion also enhances bicarbonate reabsorption, thereby sustaining the metabolic alkalosis. Patients with excess mineralocorticoid activity are not volume- or chloride-deficient. Hence, this type of metabolic alkalosis does not respond to sodium chloride administration.

The relation between metabolic alkalosis and potassium is incompletely understood. Alkalosis and hypokalemia often occur together. Alkalosis may cause hypokalemia and potassium depletion through mechanisms discussed in Chap. 50. Conversely, potassium depletion may help to sustain metabolic alkalosis because tubular acid secretion, and hence bicarbonate reabsorption, is stimulated. Whether potassium depletion alone can generate metabolic alkalosis is uncertain; if so, severe potassium depletion is required.

Respiratory compensation for metabolic alkalosis is limited. Alveolar ventilation decreases, and P_{CO_2} is elevated. However, since this response is limited by hypoxia, P_{CO_2} rarely rises above 7.3 to 8 kPa (55 to 60 mmHg).

PATHOGENESIS The principal causes of metabolic alkalosis are outlined in Table 51-2. *Vomiting* and *gastric drainage* usually induce only minimal or moderate alkalosis, but occasional patients, especially those with increased gastric acid secretion, e.g., with acid-peptic disease or the Zollinger-Ellison syndrome, may develop very severe alkalosis. Loss of hydrochloric acid in the gastric fluid initiates the alkalosis. Water and sodium chloride are lost in the vomitus or gastric aspirate. Initially, sodium is lost in the urine as well, coupled

---

TABLE 51-2 Causes of metabolic alkalosis

I Associated with volume (chloride) depletion
   A Vomiting or gastric drainage
   B Diuretic therapy
   C Posthypercapnic alkalosis
II Associated with hyperadrenocorticism
   A Cushing's syndrome
   B Primary aldosteronism
   C Bartter's syndrome
III Severe potassium depletion
IV Excessive alkali intake
   A Acute
   B Milk-alkali syndrome

to increased bicarbonate excretion (which results from elevation of plasma bicarbonate above the tubular reabsorptive threshold). These losses cause a volume (chloride) deficit, which stimulates tubular reabsorption of bicarbonate and thus maintains the elevated plasma bicarbonate generated by gastric losses of hydrochloric acid.

Alkalosis may be present in patients treated with "loop" *diuretics* (furosemide, ethacrynic acid, bumetanide) or with thiazides. The diuretics cause extracellular volume contraction and inhibit sodium chloride reabsorption in the loop of Henle or distal convoluted tubule, which increases delivery of tubular fluid to more distal nephron segments. The volume deficit and consequent hyperaldosteronism stimulate proton secretion in these segments, generating and maintaining the alkalosis. Alkalosis due to treatment with oral diuretics is usually mild. Acute administration of potent intravenous diuretics such as furosemide or ethacrynic acid to patients on low-sodium diets may induce more severe alkalosis due to rapid loss of sodium chloride in the urine. Sudden contraction of extracellular volume elevates plasma bicarbonate; renal excretion of excess bicarbonate is prevented by the mechanism discussed above. Diuretics that specifically inhibit bicarbonate reabsorption, such as acetazolamide, or inhibit distal cation secretion, such as spironolactone, amiloride, and triamterene, cause acidosis rather than alkalosis (see above).

Patients with chronic hypercapnia due to respiratory insufficiency maintain high plasma bicarbonate concentrations (see "Respiratory Acidosis," below). If respiration improves, P_{CO_2} falls promptly. However, urinary excretion of excess bicarbonate previously generated by renal compensatory mechanisms takes a number of days. In patients on low-salt diets or diuretics who have a volume (chloride) deficiency, *posthypercapnic* alkalosis of this type may persist indefinitely unless sodium or potassium chloride is added to the diet. The mechanism in this condition is the same as that which causes persistent alkalosis in vomiting, described earlier.

Alkalosis is variable in patients with excess mineralocorticoid activity. Minimal or moderate alkalosis is usually present in patients with *Cushing's syndrome* or *primary aldosteronism*. More marked alkalosis may be seen in patients with extreme adrenal hyperfunction associated with ACTH-secreting tumors, such as bronchogenic carcinoma. Moderate alkalosis is typical of patients with *Bartter's syndrome*.

Although alkalosis and *potassium depletion* are often associated, mild or moderate potassium depletion does not cause sustained metabolic alkalosis. However, extreme degrees of potassium depletion (serum potassium usually 2 mmol/L or less) may cause metabolic alkalosis. This type of alkalosis is not corrected by administration of sodium chloride but does respond to administration of potassium.

For reasons noted earlier, alkalosis due to administration of alkali cannot be sustained unless large amounts are given. When renal function is compromised, alkalosis may be sustained by small exogenous loads. This is apparently the mechanism of alkalosis in the milk-alkali syndrome, in which hypercalcemic nephropathy and alkalosis develop in response to excessive intake of absorbable alkali. The nephropathy limits bicarbonate excretion, thus maintaining the alkalosis.

CLINICAL FEATURES AND DIAGNOSIS   There are no specific clinical signs or symptoms. Severe alkalosis may cause apathy, confusion, and stupor. If serum calcium is borderline or low, rapid development of alkalosis may lead to tetany. The diagnosis of metabolic alkalosis depends on recognition of the clinical setting and appropriate laboratory studies. Plasma bicarbonate is increased. P_{CO_2} increases by about 0.01 kPa (0.6 mmHg) for each mmol/L increase in bicarbonate. Elevation of P_{CO_2} is insufficient to prevent alkalemia (see Fig. 51-1). Plasma potassium concentration is often reduced, and the electrocardiogram may reveal changes in T and U waves typical of hypokalemia (Chap. 176). These changes may be due to alkalosis itself or to associated alterations in potassium metabolism. Despite elevation of plasma bicarbonate, the urine pH is usually less than 7 in patients with sustained metabolic alkalosis.

This "paradoxical aciduria" reflects the fact that bicarbonate reabsorption must be increased if metabolic alkalosis is to be sustained.

Differential diagnosis is usually made from clinical features, such as a history of vomiting or the manifestations of Cushing's syndrome. The urinary chloride concentration may be a helpful clue if the diagnosis is not evident. When the alkalosis is associated with volume contraction (category I, Table 51-2), urinary chloride is low, usually less than 10 mmol/L. When the alkalosis is caused by hyperadrenocorticism or severe potassium depletion (categories II and III), urinary chloride is higher, usually 20 mmol/L or more.

TREATMENT   Mild or moderate metabolic alkalosis rarely requires specific treatment. In patients with gastric alkalosis, infusion of saline solutions is usually sufficient to enhance renal bicarbonate excretion and to correct alkalosis by mechanisms discussed above. Administration of potassium chloride is also helpful in treating or preventing alkalosis in these patients and those with diuretic-induced alkalosis. In patients with adrenal hyperfunction, alkalosis is corrected by specific treatment of the underlying disease. In Bartter's syndrome hypokalemia, potassium wasting, and alkalosis may be partly corrected by treatment with prostaglandin synthetase inhibitors such as indomethacin. Whenever alkalosis and potassium depletion occur together, potassium depletion should be treated with potassium chloride, not with an organic salt of potassium.

Rarely, with prolonged gastric metabolic alkalosis losses may be severe enough to require intravenous therapy with acidifying agents. Dilute hydrochloric acid or acidifying salts such as ammonium chloride or arginine hydrochloride may be given slowly under such circumstances. In most patients the use of acidifying agents can be avoided by appropriate treatment with saline and potassium chloride. In patients who are volume-expanded or in whom volume loading is inadvisable, therapy with acetazolamide, which enhances renal bicarbonate excretion, may be helpful.

RESPIRATORY ACIDOSIS

PATHOPHYSIOLOGY   Failure of ventilation promptly increases P_{CO_2} (carbonic acid) because metabolic production of carbon dioxide is so rapid. Acute respiratory acidosis is modulated to a limited degree by tissue buffers. As can be seen from the curve labeled *acute respiratory acidosis* in Fig. 51-1, immediate tissue buffering elevates plasma bicarbonate only slightly, by about 1 mmol/L for each increase of 1.3 kPa (10 mmHg) in P_{CO_2}. If hypercapnia is sustained, renal acid excretion is enhanced, and bicarbonate reabsorption is stimulated. Over a period of several days, plasma bicarbonate rises approximately 3 mmol/L for each increase of 1.3 kPa (10 mmHg) in P_{CO_2}, thereby minimizing the degree of acidemia. The increment in plasma bicarbonate attributable to renal activity is represented by the difference between the curves marked *chronic respiratory acidosis* and *acute respiratory acidosis*.

PATHOGENESIS (See also Table 217-1)   *Acute* respiratory acidosis occurs whenever there is a sudden failure of ventilation. Common causes include depression of the respiratory center by cerebral disease or drugs, neuromuscular disorders, and cardiopulmonary arrest. *Chronic* respiratory acidosis occurs in pulmonary diseases such as chronic emphysema and bronchitis, in which ventilation and perfusion are mismatched and effective alveolar ventilation is decreased. Chronic hypercapnia may also result from primary alveolar hypoventilation or from alveolar hypoventilation related to extreme obesity (Pickwickian syndrome). Acute and chronic diseases characterized principally by interference with alveolar gas exchange, such as chronic pulmonary fibrosis, pneumonia, and pulmonary edema, usually cause hypocapnia rather than hypercapnia. In these conditions, hypoxia stimulates increased ventilation; since carbon dioxide is much more diffusible than oxygen, excretion of carbon dioxide is enhanced despite the barrier to gas exchange. Hypercapnia occurs only with respiratory fatigue or extremely severe disease.

CLINICAL FEATURES AND DIAGNOSIS It is often difficult to separate the manifestations of respiratory acidosis from those of associated hypoxia. Moderate hypercapnia, especially if it develops slowly, probably has no specific clinical features. When P_{CO_2} exceeds 9.3 kPa (70 mmHg), patients become progressively confused and obtunded. Asterixis may be present. Papilledema may occur, apparently because intracranial pressure is increased by the cerebral vasodilation characteristic of hypercapnia. Dilatation of conjunctival and superficial facial blood vessels may be noted.

The diagnosis of acute respiratory acidosis is usually evident from the clinical situation, especially if respiration is obviously depressed. Proof requires laboratory confirmation that P_{CO_2} is elevated. Acidemia is always present in patients with *acute* hypercapnia. Acidosis in acute cardiopulmonary arrest is usually a combination of a metabolic lactic acidosis and acute respiratory acidosis. Patients with *chronic* hypercapnia are usually acidemic. However, some individuals with minimal or moderate chronic hypercapnia may have normal or even slightly elevated plasma pH, as may be seen from Fig. 51-1. The mechanism of full compensation or of "overcompensation" in such instances is unknown. However, significant elevation of pH in patients with chronic hypercapnia is almost always due to complicating metabolic alkalosis. Diuretics, low-sodium diets, and posthypercapnic alkalosis are frequent causes of this type of superimposed acid-base disorder.

Because of the differences between plasma bicarbonate in acute hypercapnia and in chronic hypercapnia, proper interpretation of acid-base parameters in respiratory acidosis depends on clinical information.

TREATMENT The only worthwhile approach to treatment of respiratory acidosis is correction of the underlying disorder. Rapid infusion of alkali is justified in cardiopulmonary arrest. In other circumstances, infusions of alkali have no role in practical management of respiratory acidosis.

RESPIRATORY ALKALOSIS

PATHOPHYSIOLOGY Acute reduction in carbon dioxide concentration releases hydrogen ion from tissue buffers, which minimize alkalemia by reducing plasma bicarbonate. Acute alkalosis also enhances glycolysis; increased production of lactic and pyruvic acids lowers serum bicarbonate and raises plasma concentrations of the corresponding anions by a millimole or two. In chronic hypocapnia, plasma bicarbonate is further reduced because the decreased P_{CO_2} inhibits tubular reabsorption and generation of bicarbonate. As in respiratory acidosis, compensation for the chronic state is much more complete than for the acute (Fig. 51-1). In acute hypocapnia, plasma bicarbonate falls only about 2 mmol/L for each 1.3-kPa (10-mmHg) reduction in P_{CO_2}. In chronic hypocapnia, plasma bicarbonate is reduced by 4 to 5 mmol/L for each 1.3-kPa (10-mmHg) decrease in P_{CO_2}. The decrement in plasma bicarbonate attributable to renal compensatory activity is shown by the difference between the curves labeled acute and chronic respiratory alkalosis in Fig. 51-1.

PATHOGENESIS Respiratory alkalosis is due to acute or chronic hyperventilation, which lowers P_{CO_2}. The causes of respiratory alkalosis are shown in Table 51-3.

TABLE 51-3 Causes of respiratory alkalosis

I Hypoxia
   A Acute (e.g., pneumonia, asthma, pulmonary edema)
   B Chronic (e.g., pulmonary fibrosis, cyanotic heart disease, high altitudes)
II Respiratory center stimulation
   A Anxiety
   B Fever
   C Salicylate intoxication
   D Cerebral disease (tumor, encephalitis, etc.)
III Exercise
IV Gram-negative sepsis
V Hepatic cirrhosis
VI Pregnancy
VII Excessive mechanical ventilation

CLINICAL FEATURES AND DIAGNOSIS Depending on its severity and acuteness, hyperventilation may or may not be clinically apparent. In acute respiratory alkalosis, the clinical picture is rather characteristic: patients complain of paresthesias, numbness, and tingling; of light-headedness; and, if alkalosis is sufficiently severe, of manifestations of tetany. Alkalosis directly enhances neuromuscular excitability; this effect, rather than the modest decrease in ionized plasma calcium induced by alkalosis, is probably the major cause of tetany. Severe respiratory alkalosis may cause confusion or loss of consciousness, perhaps due to cerebral vasospasm induced by hypocapnia.

The diagnosis may be suspected from the clinical setting but must be confirmed by analysis of the plasma bicarbonate system. Hypocapnia together with a variable degree of alkalemia is found; plasma bicarbonate is decreased but is rarely below 15 mmol/L.

TREATMENT The only successful treatment for respiratory alkalosis is elimination of the underlying disorder. In the acute hyperventilation syndrome, sedation, reassurance, and, if symptoms are sufficiently severe, rebreathing into a bag will usually terminate the attack.

REFERENCES

ADROGUE HJ et al: Plasma acid-base patterns in diabetic ketoacidosis. N Engl J Med 307:1603, 1982

ARBUS GS: An in vivo acid-base nomogram for clinical use. Can Med Assoc J 109:291, 1973

BATTLE DC, KURTZMAN NA: Renal regulation of acid-base homeostasis: Integrated response, in *The Kidney: Physiology and Pathophysiology*, 2d ed, DW Seldin, G Giebisch (eds). New York, Raven, 1986, p 1539

EMMETT M, NARINS RG: Clinical use of the anion gap. Medicine 56:38, 1977

HARRINGTON JT: Metabolic alkalosis. Kidney Int 26:88, 1984

KASSIRER JP, MADIAS NE: Respiratory acid-base disorders. Hosp Practice 15:57, 1980

LEVY LH et al: Ketoacidosis associated with alcoholism in non-diabetic subjects. Ann Intern Med 78:213, 1973

MADIAS NE: Lactic acidosis. Kidney Int 29:752, 1986

NARINS RG, EMMETT M: Simple and mixed acid-base disorders: A practical approach. Medicine 59:161, 1980

ROCHER LL, TANNEN RL: The clinical spectrum of renal tubular acidosis. Ann Rev Med 37:319, 1986

SCHWARTZ WB, RELMAN AS: A critique of the parameters used in the evaluation of acid-base disorders. N Engl J Med 268:1382, 1963

SELDIN DW, GIEBISCH G (eds): *Regulation of Acid-Base Balance*. New York, Raven, 1989, 616 pp

STACPOOLE PW et al: Dichloroacetate in the treatment of lactic acidosis. Ann Int Med 108:58, 1988

52 IMPOTENCE

JOHN D. MCCONNELL / JEAN D. WILSON

A variety of endocrine, vascular, neurologic, and psychiatric diseases disrupt normal sexual and reproductive function in men. Furthermore, sexual dysfunction may be the presenting symptom of systemic disease.

NORMAL SEXUAL FUNCTION

Penile erection is initiated by neuropsychologic stimuli that ultimately produce vasodilation of the sinusoidal spaces and arteries within the paired corpora cavernosa. Erection is normally preceded by sexual desire (or libido), which is regulated in part by androgen-dependent psychic factors. Although nocturnal and diurnal spontaneous erections are suppressed in men with androgen deficiency, erections in response to erotic stimuli may continue. Thus, continuing action of testicular androgens appears to be required for normal libido but not for the erectile mechanism itself.

The penis receives innervation from sympathetic, parasympathetic, and somatic fibers. Somatic fibers in the dorsal nerve of the penis form the afferent limb of the erectile reflex by transmitting sensory impulses from the penile skin and glans to the S2-S4 dorsal root ganglia via the pudendal nerve. Unlike the corpuscular-type endings in the penile shaft skin, the majority of afferent terminations in the glans are free nerve endings. The efferent limb begins with parasympathetic preganglionic fibers from S2-S4 which pass in the pelvic nerves to the pelvic plexus. Sympathetic fibers emerging from the intermediolateral gray areas of T11-L2 travel through the paravertebral sympathetic chain ganglia, superior hypogastric plexus, and hypogastric nerves to enter the pelvic plexus along with parasympathetic fibers. Somatic efferent fibers from S3-S4 traveling in the pudendal nerve to the ischiocavernosus and bulbocavernosus muscles—as well as postganglionic sympathetic fibers innervating the smooth muscle of the epididymis, vas deferens, seminal vesicle, and internal sphincter of the bladder—mediate rhythmic contraction of these structures at the time of ejaculation.

Autonomic nerve impulses, integrated in the pelvic plexus, project to the penis through the cavernous nerves which course along the posterolateral aspect of the prostate before penetrating the pelvic floor muscles immediately lateral to the urethra. Distal to the membranous urethra, some fibers enter the corpus spongiosum, while the remainder enter the corpora cavernosa along with the terminal branches of the pudendal artery and exiting cavernous veins. If disruption of the cavernous nerves occurs following pelvic trauma or surgery, erectile impotence may ensue.

The brain exerts an important modulatory influence over spinal reflex pathways that control penile function. A variety of visual, auditory, olfactory, and imaginative stimuli elicit erectile responses that involve cortical, thalamic, rhinencephalic, and limbic input to the medial preoptic–anterior hypothalamic area, which is an important integrating center. Other areas of the brain, such as the amygdaloid complex, may inhibit sexual function.

Although the parasympathetic nervous system is the primary effector of erection, the transformation of the penis to an erect organ is a vascular phenomenon. In the flaccid state the arteries, arterioles, and sinusoidal spaces within the corpora cavernosa are constricted due to active contraction of smooth muscle in the walls of these structures. The venules between the sinusoids and the dense tunica albuginea surrounding the cavernosa open freely to the emissary veins. Erection begins when relaxation of the smooth muscles leads to dilatation of the sinusoids and a decrease in peripheral resistance, causing a rapid increase in arterial blood flow through internal pudendal and cavernosal arteries. Blood is trapped in the expanding sinusoidal system, which compresses the venules against the tunica albuginea, resulting in venous occlusion. The increase in intracorporeal pressure leads to tumescence and rigidity. Full rigidity, however, may in addition require stimulation of somatic fibers in the pudendal nerve and contraction of the ischiocavernosus muscle.

The neurotransmitter responsible for vasodilation in the penis has not been identified. Although the corpora cavernosa have cholinergic terminals, acetylcholine is unlikely to be the transmitter directly responsible for erection. Indeed, acetylcholine may produce vasodilation indirectly, either by acting on vascular endothelium to release a vasodilator substance, *endothelium-derived relaxing factor*, which then acts on the smooth muscle, or by decreasing adrenergic-induced tone. A variety of neuropeptides in corporal tissues, including vasoactive intestinal peptide (VIP) and substance P, produce tumescence when injected into the penis but have uncertain physiologic roles. Furthermore, high tissue levels of norepinephrine and the rich concentration of adrenergic receptors (predominantly alpha) suggest an important role of adrenergic mechanisms in both tumescence and detumescence, perhaps via synaptic "cross talk" with cholinergic nerves.

Seminal emission and ejaculation are under control of the sympathetic nervous system. Emission results from alpha-adrenergic-mediated contraction of the epididymis, vas deferens, seminal vesicles, and prostate, which causes seminal fluid to enter the prostatic urethra. Concomitant closure of the bladder neck prevents retrograde flow of semen into the bladder. Antegrade ejaculation results from contraction of the muscles of the pelvic floor, including the bulbocavernosus and ischiocavernosus muscles.

Orgasm is a psychosensory phenomenon in which the rhythmic contraction of the pelvic muscles is perceived as pleasurable. Orgasm can occur without either erection or ejaculation and in the presence of retrograde ejaculation.

Detumescence after orgasm and ejaculation is incompletely understood. Presumably, active tone in the vessels of the sinusoidal spaces is restored by active (probably adrenergic-mediated) contraction of smooth muscles, which decreases the inflow of blood to the penis and promotes emptying of the erectile tissue. Following orgasm, there is an refractory period that varies with age, physical condition, and psychic factors during which erection and ejaculation are inhibited.

IMPOTENCE

Simply defined, impotence is the failure to achieve erection, ejaculation, or both. Men with sexual dysfunction present with a variety of complaints, either singly, or in combination: loss of libido, inability to initiate or maintain an erection, ejaculatory failure, premature ejaculation, or inability to achieve orgasm. Sexual dysfunction can be secondary to systemic disease processes or their treatment, to specific disorders of the urogenital or endocrine systems, or to psychological disturbance. Previously, it was felt that the majority of men with erectile impotency had a psychogenic etiology for their dysfunction. It is now believed that the majority of impotent men have a component of underlying organic disease. Since the selection and success of subsequent therapy depends upon the specific etiology, it is essential to evaluate all aspects of the erectile mechanism.

LOSS OF DESIRE A decrease in sexual desire, or libido, may be due to androgen deficiency (arising from either pituitary or testicular disease), psychological disturbance, or to some types of prescribed or habitually abused drugs. The possibility of androgen deficiency can be tested by measurement of plasma testosterone and gonadotropins. The level of testosterone required for normal erectile function remains unknown. Hypogonadism may also result in the absence of emission, secondary to decreased secretion of ejaculate by the seminal vesicles and prostate.

FAILURE OF ERECTION The organic causes of erectile impotence can be grouped into endocrine, drug, local, neurologic, and vascular causes (Table 52-1).

Decreased plasma testosterone secondary to testicular failure is an uncommon but easily recognized and treated disorder. However, hyperprolactinemia may cause impotence in some men with pituitary tumors and may not be obvious on physical examination; hyperprolactinemia suppresses luteinizing hormone–releasing hormone (LHRH) production, resulting in plasma gonadotropins and testosterone values in the low normal range. Bromocriptine, a dopamine agonist, may lower prolactin levels and reverse impotence in such patients.

TABLE 52-1 Some organic causes of erectile impotence in men

I Endocrine causes
  A Testicular failure (primary or secondary)
  B Hyperprolactinemia
II Drugs
  A Antiandrogens
    1 H-2 blockers (e.g., cimetidine)
    2 Spironolactone
    3 Ketoconazole
  B Antihypertensives
    1 Central-acting sympatholytics (e.g., clonidine and methyldopa)
    2 Peripheral acting sympatholytics (e.g., guanadrel)
    3 Beta blockers
    4 Thiazides
  C Anticholinergics
  D Antidepressants
    1 Monoamine oxidase inhibitors
    2 Tricyclic antidepressants
  E Antipsychotics
  F Central nervous system depressants
    1 Sedatives (e.g., barbiturates)
    2 Antianxiety drugs (e.g., diazepam)
  G Drugs of habituation or addiction
    1 Alcohol
    2 Methadone
    3 Heroin
III Penile diseases
  A Peyronie's disease
  B Previous priapism
  C Penile trauma
IV Neurologic diseases
  A Anterior temporal lobe lesions
  B Diseases of the spinal cord
  C Loss of sensory input
    1 Tabes dorsalis
    2 Disease of dorsal root ganglia
  D Disease of nervi erigentes
    1 Radical prostatectomy and cystectomy
    2 Rectosigmoid operations
  E Diabetic autonomic neuropathy and various polyneuropathies
V Vascular disease
  A Aortic occlusion (Leriche syndrome)
  B Atherosclerotic occlusion or stenosis of the pudendal and/or cavernosal arteries
  C Venous leak
  D Disease of the sinusoidal spaces

Although many drugs are associated with impotence, antihypertensive agents, cimetidine, and monoamine oxidase (MAO) inhibitors are more likely to lead to erectile dysfunction. Antihypertensive drugs with peripheral and central sympatholytic action or beta-adrenergic-receptor blocking activity are the most frequently implicated. Angiotensin-converting enzyme inhibitors, calcium channel blockers, and peripheral vasodilators do not cause a significant incidence of sexual dysfunction. Histamine (H-2)-receptor antagonists, such as cimetidine, have antiandrogenic properties in addition to increasing prolactin secretion. MAO inhibitors, antipsychotic drugs, and tricyclic antidepressants may impair sexual function via anticholinergic and sympatholytic action.

Penile diseases including previous priapism, penile trauma, and Peyronie's disease can cause impotence due to fibrosis of the sinusoidal spaces of the corpora cavernosa, corporeal artery occlusion, or neurogenic mechanism. Peyronie's disease is not rare; patients present with a painful plaque on the dorsum of the penis and may progress to development of penile curvature and decreased rigidity.

Many types of neurologic disorders cause impotence, including lesions in the anterior temporal lobe, spinal cord disorders, insufficiency of sensory input such as can occur in tabes dorsalis, or damage to parasympathetic nerves, for example, following surgical procedures such as radical (total) prostatectomy or cystectomy. In contrast, transurethral prostatectomy does not cause organic impotence. Furthermore, the nerve supply to the penis (the nervi erigentes) runs on the posterolateral surface of the prostate, and if the nerves are preserved during radical prostate and bladder surgery, potency can be preserved in many men. If spinal cord injury is above the thoracolumbar region, reflex erections may occur, whereas diffuse injury of the spinal cord results in total impotence. As many as half of men with diabetes mellitus develop impotence within 6 years of the onset of diabetes, and impotency may be the first clinical manifestation of diabetic neuropathy. Several factors contribute to neuropathic impotence, including abnormalities in afferent sensory pathways, motor neuropathy in the cavernosal nerves (which carry the efferent pathways for vasodilation in the penis), and decreased level of cavernosal neurotransmitters. Although the autonomic pathways in the penis cannot be tested directly, most patients demonstrate other manifestations of autonomic neuropathy on careful examination. Many of the other polyneuropathies associated with impotence have similar effects.

Men with vasculogenic impotence may present with total erectile impotence, decreased penile rigidity, or loss of erection during intercourse. Vascular insufficiency may be due to aortic occlusion (Leriche syndrome) or to more distal atherosclerotic disease in the hypogastric, pudendal, and cavernosal arteries. Significant disease in the pudendal and cavernosal arteries can occur in the absence of other clinical manifestations of peripheral vascular disease. Together with neuropathy, vascular insufficiency contributes to the impotence in many men with diabetes mellitus.

PREMATURE EJACULATION This disorder seldom has an organic cause. It is usually related to anxiety in the sexual situation, unreasonable expectations about performance, or emotional disorder. A variety of successful therapeutic modalities have been described by Levine.

ABSENCE OF EMISSION This symptom may be produced by (1) retrograde ejaculation, (2) sympathetic denervation, (3) androgen deficiency, or (4) drugs. Retrograde ejaculation may occur following surgery on the bladder neck or develop spontaneously in diabetic men. Demonstration of sperm in a postcoital urine specimen establishes the diagnosis. Following sympathectomy or occasionally after extensive retroperitoneal surgery, the autonomic innervation of the prostate and seminal vesicles is lost, resulting in absence of smooth-muscle contraction at the time of ejaculation. Androgen deficiency results in a decrease in secretions of the prostate and seminal vesicles and in a diminution of the volume of ejaculate. Finally, drugs such as guanethidine, phenoxybenzamine, and phentolamine primarily impair ejaculation rather than erection or libido.

ABSENCE OF ORGASM If libido and erectile function are normal, the absence of orgasm is almost always due to a psychiatric disorder.

FAILURE OF DETUMESCENCE

Priapism is a persistent painful erection, often unrelated to sexual activity. Priapism can be distinguished from a normal erection by the absence of tumescence of the glans penis. Priapism may be idiopathic but can be associated with sickle cell anemia, chronic granulocytic leukemia, spinal cord injury, or injection of vasodilator agents (such as papaverine) into the penis. The disorder may be secondary to clotting of blood within the sinusoidal spaces of the penis or to abnormalities of the adrenergic-mediated mechanism for detumescence. Failure to treat priapism promptly usually results in fibrosis and subsequent loss of erectile function. In early phases, detumescence can sometimes be achieved by aspiration, irrigation of the corpora cavernosa, and injection of dilute vasoconstrictors. If this fails, surgical relief by shunting procedures may be necessary. In patients with priapism secondary to sickle cell anemia, conservation measures such as transfusion, oxygenation, and irrigation are generally preferred to shunting procedures.

EVALUATION OF IMPOTENCE

The relative frequency of organic as opposed to psychogenic causes of erectile impotence is still debated. Nevertheless, anxiety and depressive states are common causes of impotence (see Chap. 29). Other psychological factors such as disinterest in the sexual partner, fear of sexual incompetence, marital discord, guilt about deviant sexual attitudes, worry, fatigue, and ill health often operate in various combinations to reduce sexual impulse. The central issue in the evaluation of impotence is to separate those instances due to psychological factors from those due to organic causes (Table 52-1). Often, the separation can be made on the basis of history. With the exception of those with severe depression, men with psychogenic impotence usually have normal nocturnal and early morning erections. From early childhood through the eighth decade, erections occur during normal sleep. This phenomenon, termed *nocturnal penile tumescence* (NPT), occurs during rapid eye movement sleep, and the total time of NPT averages 100 min per night. Consequently, if the impotent man gives a history of rigid erections under any circumstances (often when awakening in the morning), the efferent neurologic and circulatory systems that mediate erection are intact, and dysfunction is probably due to a psychiatric disorder. In these patients the workup should be limited. (Occasional patients with early sensory neuropathy may have nocturnal erections.)

If the history of nocturnal erections is questionable, measurements of NPT can be made with the use of a strain gauge attached to a recorder or by snap gauge. Although false-negative and false-positive results are possible, this procedure helps to differentiate psychogenic and organic impotence. Patients with vasculogenic impotence may have some degree of penile tumescence without the development of adequate rigidity, which may result in a false-positive NPT test. Other features in favor of organic impotence include a similar degree of erectile dysfunction under all circumstances, onset not associated with any particular psychiatric symptomatology, a previous uninterrupted period of normal erectile function, and persistent sexual desire.

Having deduced an organic cause, the fundamental problem is the differential diagnosis of the etiology (Table 52-1). The history should be probed for diabetes mellitus, manifestations of peripheral neuropathy or bladder dysfunction, symptoms referable to the vascular system such as intermittent claudication, and symptoms of penile disease such as a history of priapism or penile curvature (Peyronie's). A thorough drug history should be obtained, and inquiry made concerning past surgery that may have produced neurologic damage.

Physical examination should include a detailed genital examination to identify abnormalities of the penis, especially Peyronie's disease which is usually easily felt as a fibrotic plaque on the dorsum of the penis. The testes should be palpated for size, symmetry, and abnormal masses; if the length is less than 3.5 cm, hypogonadism should be considered. Evidence of feminization such as gynecomastia and abnormal body hair distribution should be sought. All pulses should be palpated, and the presence of bruits should be sought. Often, the pulse in the dorsal penile artery can be felt. If there is an indication from either history or physical examination of a vascular etiology, direct measurement of penile blood flow may be indicated.

Pudendal arteriography provides the most accurate assessment of penile arterial disease, but it is expensive and invasive. Moreover, distal arterial lesions may not be identified unless the procedure is performed under conditions of chemical erection (papaverine injection). The penile/brachial index can be used to estimate penile blood flow, by dividing the penile systolic blood pressure, as determined by Doppler technique, by the simultaneously determined supine brachial systolic pressure. An index of less than 0.6 is suggestive of vasculogenic impotence. However, the test only evaluates flow through the dorsal penile artery, which is not directly involved in the erectile process. Significant disease may be present in the cavernosal arteries despite normal flow through the dorsal artery. Pulsed Doppler analysis and high-resolution ultrasonography can be used in conjunction with intracorporeal papaverine to assess blood flow in the cavernosal arteries. Abnormalities in the venous occlusive mechanism of the penis can cause impotence due to venous leak and can be diagnosed with the use of papaverine-induced erection in combination with ultrasonography. The incidence of venous leakage in men with normal erectile function is unknown. Moreover, venous leak may be secondary to arterial inflow and sinusoidal disease. Nevertheless, in carefully selected patients, surgical ligation or clinical obliteration of the incompetent veins can improve erectile function.

The neurologic examination should measure anal sphincter tone, perineal sensation, and the bulbocavernosus reflex. This reflex is elicited by squeezing the glans penis and noting the degree of anal sphincter constriction. An examination for peripheral neuropathy, including assessment of distal muscle function, the tendon reflexes in the legs, and vibratory, position, tactile, and pain sensation, should also be performed. In the presence of peripheral neuropathy, tests to evaluate penile neuropathy are seldom necessary. In cases with an uncertain neurogenic component, electromyographic sacral signal tracing of the bulbocavernosus reflex may be helpful. A specific test to document abnormalities in the penile autonomic efferent pathways is not available.

In the absence of hypogonadism or feminization, the serum testosterone is usually normal. Hyperprolactinemia, however, may not be suspected on the basis of history and physical examination. Although endocrine causes of erectile dysfunction are uncommon, measurement of serum prolactin and pooled serum testosterone and LH (see Chap. 321) is appropriate since abnormalities of these parameters are treatable.

TREATMENT OF IMPOTENCE

Medical therapy with androgens offers little more than placebo benefit except in hypogonadal men, and empirical therapy may actually delay identification of organic etiologies. If a prolactin-secreting pituitary tumor is present, however, either surgical removal or treatment with bromocriptine usually results in return of potency. Surgical therapy may be useful in the treatment of decreased potency related to aortic obstruction; however, potency can be lost rather than improved after aortic surgery if the autonomic nerve supply to the penis is damaged. The efficacy of penile revascularization and balloon embolization therapy for vasculogenic impotency remains uncertain. Men with primary venous leak impotence, without associated arterial or sinusoidal disease, may benefit from venous ligation.

A variety of vasoactive substances produce erection when injected into the corpora cavernosa. Self-injection with papaverine, with or without phentolamine, produces erection in patients with psychogenic, neurogenic, and mild vasculogenic impotency. Lack of FDA approval, pain on injection, and the possible complications of priapism and penile fibrosis limited the use of this therapy. Commercially available mechanical devices that utilize a vacuum to produce an erection and a rubber band to restrict venous return at the base of the penis, provide a successful nonsurgical alternative in many patients, including some with diabetes mellitus.

Penile prostheses are the most common therapeutic alternative in impotent patients refractory to other forms of therapy. Malleable silastic rode implanted into the penis provide the simplest system and the lowest complication rates, however, the cosmetic and functional performance of the device is not uniformly satisfactory. Multicomponent, hydraulically operated prostheses offer the advantage of more physiologic erection and greater increase in penile diameter. However, these devices are subject to mechanical failure.

Even in patients with organic impotence, psychotherapy is often beneficial in alleviating concomitant psychogenic factors that limit the success of medical and surgical therapy.

REFERENCES

ABRAMOWICZ M et al: Drugs that cause sexual dysfunction. Med Lett 29:65, 1987

DEGROAT WC, STEERS WD: Neuroanatomy and neurophysiology of penile erection, in *Contemporary Management of Impotence and Infertility*, EA Tanagho et al (eds). Baltimore, Williams & Wilkins, 1988, pp 3–27

FISHMAN JF et al: Experience with inflatable penile prosthesis. Urol 23:86, 1984

GOLDSTEIN I: Electromyography: Evoked-response evaluations, in *Controversies in Neuro-Urology*, DM Barret, AJ Wein (eds). New York, Churchill Livingstone, 1984

KAISER FE, KORENMAN SG: Impotence in diabetic men. Am J Med 85(Suppl 5A):147, 1988

KWAN M et al: The nature of androgen action on male sexuality: A combined laboratory–self-report study on hypogonadal men. J Clin Endocrinol Metab 57:557, 1983

LEVINE SB: Marital sexual dsyfunction: Ejaculation distubances. Ann Intern Med 84:575, 1976

LEWIS RW, PUYAU FA: Procedures for decreasing venous drainage. Semin Urol 4:263, 1986

LUE TF, TANAGHO EA: Functional anatomy and mechanism of penile erection, in *Contemporary Management of Impotency and Infertility*, EA Tanagho et al (eds). Baltimore, Williams & Wilkins, 1988, pp 39–50

——— et al: Functional evaluation of penile veins by cavernosography in papaverine-induced erection. J Urol 135:479, 1986

MEYER J: Disorders of sexual function, in *Textbook of Endocrinology*, JD Wilson, DM Foster (eds). Philadelphia, Saunders, 1985, vol 7, pp 476–491

NATH RL et al: The multidisciplinary approach to vasculogenic impotence. Surgery 89:124, 1981

SAYPOL DC et al: Impotence. Are the newer diagnostic methods a necessity? J Urol 130:260, 1983

WABEK AJ: Bulbocavernosus reflex testing in 100 consecutive cases of erectile dysfunction. Urology 25:495, 1985

WALSH PC et al: Impotency following radical prostatectomy: Insight into etiology and prevention. J Urol 128:492, 1982

WINTER CC: Priapism. Urol Surv 28:163, 1978

WITHERINGTON R: Vacuum constriction device for management of erectile impotence. J Urol 141:320, 1989

ZORGNIOTTI AW: Auto-injection of the corpus cavernosum with a vasoactive drug combination for vasculogenic impotence. J Urol 133:39, 1985

53 DISTURBANCES OF MENSTRUATION AND SEXUAL FUNCTION IN WOMEN

BRUCE R. CARR / JEAN D. WILSON

Complaints related to the female reproductive tract can usually be categorized as disturbances of menstruation, pelvic pain, disturbances in sexual function, or infertility. However, a single disorder, for example, leiomyoma of the uterus, can present with symptoms referable to any one or more of these categories. Furthermore, sexual dysfunction can interdigitate with other complaints in several ways. On the one hand, in women who present with complaints related to other reproductive tract functions, the underlying problem may actually be severe sexual dysfunction or marital conflict. Alternatively, women with severe organic disorders of the pelvis, for example, pelvic inflammatory disease, may present with sexual dysfunction such as dyspareunia which in fact is only a minor manifestation of the underlying disease.

Since normal reproductive function depends on the integrated action of the central nervous system, the endocrine glands, and the reproductive organs, menstrual cycle abnormalities, sexual dysfunction, and infertility may be the result of a variety of systemic and psychological disorders as well as of primary defects in the endocrine and reproductive organs. The endocrine and physiologic control—normal and abnormal—of puberty, reproductive life, and menopause are discussed in Chap. 322. The focus of this chapter is on the initial evaluation of women with disturbances of the reproductive tract.

DISTURBANCES IN MENSTRUATION Disorders of menstruation can be divided into abnormal uterine bleeding and amenorrhea.

Abnormal uterine bleeding The menstrual cycle is defined as the interval between the onset of one bleeding episode and the onset of the next. In normal women the cycle averages 28 ± 3 days, the mean duration of menstrual flow is 4 ± 2 days, and the average blood loss is 40 to 100 mL. Between menarche and the menopause most women experience one or more episodes of abnormal uterine bleeding, here defined as any bleeding pattern outside the normal ranges of frequency, duration, and/or amount of blood loss described above. The decision to evaluate a patient with an abnormal bleeding pattern depends on the severity and frequency of the abnormal bleeding episodes.

When uterine bleeding is suspected, it is essential to establish first that the blood observed by the patient is derived from the uterine endometrium. Rectal, bladder, cervical, and vaginal sources of bleeding must be excluded. Once the bleeding is documented to be uterine in origin, a pregnancy-related disorder (such as threatened or incomplete abortion or ectopic pregnancy) must be excluded by physical examination and appropriate laboratory tests. Abnormal uterine bleeding may also be the initial or principal manifestation of a generalized bleeding diathesis. The remaining causes of abnormal uterine bleeding can be divided into those associated with ovulatory cycles and those associated with anovulatory cycles.

OVULATORY CYCLES Menstrual bleeding with ovulatory cycles is spontaneous, regular in onset, predictable in duration and amount of flow, and frequently associated with discomfort. Uterine bleeding with ovulatory cycles is due to progesterone withdrawal at the end of the luteal (postovulatory) phase and requires prior estrogen priming of the endometrium during the follicular (preovulatory) phase of the cycle. When deviations from an established pattern of menstrual flow occur but the cycles are still regular, the usual cause is organic disease of the outflow tract. For example, regular, prolonged, excessive bleeding episodes unassociated with a bleeding diathesis are usually due to abnormalities of the uterus such as submucous leiomyomas, adenomyosis, or endometrial polyps. On the other hand, cyclic, predictable menstruation characterized by spotting or light bleeding is often due to obstruction of the outflow tract as with uterine synechiae or scarring of the cervix. Intermittent bleeding between cyclic ovulatory menses is often due to cervical or endometrial lesions.

ANOVULATORY CYCLES Uterine bleeding that is irregular in occurrence, unpredictable as to amount and duration of flow, and usually painless is called dysfunctional uterine bleeding. This type of bleeding is the result of a failure of normal follicular maturation with consequent anovulation and may be either transient or chronic. Transient disruption of the synchronous hypothalamic-pituitary-ovarian hormonal control necessary for ovulatory cycles occurs most often in the early menarcheal years, during the perimenopausal period, or as the secondary consequence of a variety of stresses and intercurrent illnesses. Persistent dysfunctional uterine bleeding during the reproductive years can occur in several organic diseases that affect ovarian function and is most often due to estrogen breakthrough bleeding. Estrogen breakthrough bleeding occurs when prolonged continuous estrogen stimulation of the endometrium is not interrupted by cyclic progesterone withdrawal. For example, chronic acyclic estrogen production not associated with ovulation can occur in polycystic ovarian disease.

Amenorrhea   Amenorrhea is defined as failure of menarche by age 16, regardless of the presence or absence of secondary sexual characteristics, or the absence of menstruation for 6 months in a woman with previous periodic menses. Amenorrhea in a woman who has never menstruated is termed primary; cessation of menses is termed secondary amenorrhea. Because some disorders can cause both primary and secondary amenorrhea, we prefer a functional classification based upon the nature of the underlying defect, namely anatomic defects of the outflow tract (uterus, cervix, or vagina), ovarian failure, and chronic anovulation.

Anatomic defects of the outflow tract include congenital defects of the vagina, imperforate hymen, transverse vaginal septa, cervical stenosis, intrauterine adhesions (synechiae), absence of the vagina or uterus, and uterine maldevelopment. The diagnosis of an anatomic defect is usually made by physical examination and confirmed by demonstrating failure of bleeding following administration of estrogen plus a progestogen for 21 days or by a hysterosalpingogram or hysteroscopy.

Causes of *ovarian failure* include gonadal dysgenesis, deficiency of 17α-hydroxylase or 17,20-desmolase, resistant ovary syndrome, and premature ovarian failure. Ovarian failure encompasses those disorders in which the ovary is deficient in germ cells and those in which the germ cells are resistant to FSH (follicle-stimulating hormone). The diagnosis of ovarian failure as the cause of amenorrhea is confirmed by a plasma FSH greater than 40 IU/L.

Women with *chronic anovulation* fail to ovulate spontaneously but have the capability of ovulating with appropriate therapy. In some women with chronic anovulation estrogen production is adequate, but estrogen is not secreted in a cyclic fashion. In others estrogen production is deficient.

Women who have adequate estrogen production and demonstrate withdrawal bleeding after progesterone challenge usually have polycystic ovarian disease (see Fig. 322-7). Unusual causes include hormone-secreting ovarian and adrenal tumors. Women with deficient or absent estrogen production, and therefore with absence of withdrawal bleeding after progestogen administration, usually have hypogonadotropic hypogonadism due either to organic or functional disorders of the pituitary or central nervous system such as brain tumors, pituitary tumors (especially prolactin-secreting adenomas), primary hypopituitarism, or Sheehan's syndrome.

PELVIC PAIN   Pelvic pain may originate in the pelvis or be referred from another region of the body. A pelvic source for such pain is often suggested by the history (for example, dysmenorrhea and dyspareunia) and physical findings, but a high index of suspicion must be entertained for extrapelvic disorders that refer to the pelvis, such as appendicitis, cholecystitis, intestinal obstruction, and urinary tract infections (see Chap. 17).

"Physiologic" pelvic pain   PAIN ASSOCIATED WITH OVULATION ("MITTELSCHMERZ") Many women experience low abdominal discomfort with ovulation, typically a dull aching pain at midcycle in one lower quadrant lasting from a few minutes to hours. It is rarely severe or incapacitating. The relationship of the pain to the mechanisms of ovulation is unknown. It may result from peritoneal irritation by follicular fluid released into the peritoneal cavity at the time of ovulation. The onset at midcycle and a short duration of pain are often diagnostic.

PREMENSTRUAL OR MENSTRUAL PAIN   In normal ovulatory women somatic symptoms during the few days prior to menses may be insignificant or disabling. Such symptoms include edema, breast engorgement, and abdominal bloating or discomfort. A symptom complex of cyclic irritability, depression, and lethargy is known as the *premenstrual syndrome* (PMS). The cause of PMS is unknown, and there is no consensus about therapy.

Severe or incapacitating uterine cramping in women with ovulatory menses but no demonstrable disorders of the pelvis is termed *primary dysmenorrhea*. Primary dysmenorrhea is caused by prostaglandin-induced uterine ischemia and is treated with prostaglandin synthetase inhibitors or oral contraceptive agents.

Pelvic pain due to organic causes   Severe dysmenorrhea associated with disease of the pelvis is termed *secondary dysmenorrhea*. Organic causes of pelvic pain can be classified as (1) uterine, (2) adnexal, (3) vulvar or vaginal, and (4) pregnancy-associated.

UTERINE PAIN   Pain of uterine etiology is often chronic and continuous and increases in intensity during menstruation and intercourse. Causes include leiomyomas of the uterus (particularly submucous and degenerating leiomyomas), adenomyosis, and cervical stenosis. Infections of the uterus associated with intrauterine manipulation following dilatation and curettage or with intrauterine devices can also cause significant pelvic pain (see Chap. 322). Pelvic pain due to endometrial or cervical cancer is usually a late manifestation of disseminated disease (see Chap. 322).

ADNEXAL PAIN   The most common cause of pain in the adnexae (fallopian tubes and ovaries) is infection (see Chap. 94). Acute salpingo-oophoritis presents as low abdominal pain, fever, and chills, begins a few days after a menstrual period, and is usually due to chlamydia or gonococcal disease with or without a superimposed pyogenic infection. Chronic pelvic inflammatory disease results from either a single episode or multiple episodes of infection and may present as infertility associated with chronic pelvic pain that increases in intensity with menses and intercourse. On physical examination the adnexae are tender, and adnexal thickening with or without masses may be present. Pelvic inflammatory disease may become a surgical emergency if peritonitis results from rupture of a tuboovarian abscess. Ovarian cysts or neoplasms may cause pelvic pain that becomes more severe with torsion or rupture of the mass, and ectopic pregnancy must be considered in the differential diagnosis (see below). Endometriosis involving fallopian tubes, ovaries, or peritoneum may cause both chronic low abdominal pain and infertility; the magnitude of tissue involvement does not always correlate with the severity of symptoms. Endometriosis pain typically increases with menstruation and, if the posterior ligaments of the uterus are involved, with intercourse.

VULVAR OR VAGINAL PAIN   Pain in these areas is most often due to infectious vaginitis caused by organisms such as *Monilia, Trichomonas,* or *Gardnerella* and is characteristically associated with vaginal discharge and pruritus. Herpetic vulvitis, condyloma acuminatum, and cysts or abscesses of Bartholin's glands may also cause vulvar pain.

PREGNANCY-ASSOCIATED DISORDERS   Pregnancy must be considered in the differential diagnosis of pelvic pain during the reproductive years. Threatened abortion or incomplete abortion often presents with uterine cramping, bleeding, or passage of tissue following a period of amenorrhea. Ectopic pregnancy may be insidious in presentation and result in severe intraperitoneal hemorrhage and maternal death.

Evaluation of pelvic pain   The evaluation of pelvic pain includes a careful history and pelvic examination. This often leads to the correct diagnosis and institution of appropriate treatment. If the pain is severe and the diagnosis is unclear, the workup should follow that outlined for the acute abdomen (Chap. 17). A culdocentesis is indicated if a ruptured ectopic pregnancy is suspected. If there is a question of an adnexal mass or if the patient is so obese as to preclude a thorough pelvic examination, sonography may be useful. Serial human chorionic gonadotropin (hCG) measurements may be helpful in establishing a diagnosis of tubal pregnancy. Finally, diagnostic laparoscopy and laparotomy may be indicated with severe or prolonged pain of undetermined etiology.

SEXUAL DYSFUNCTION   Some women with sexual dysfunction describe minor complaints related to the reproductive tract as a means of bringing sexual problems to the attention of the physician. Alternatively, sexual dysfunction may be thought to be the cause of low abdominal discomfort or dyspareunia when the actual etiology is organic. However, more and more women seek medical advice because of sexual problems that interface in provenance between medicine and sociology.

The normal sexual response begins with sexual arousal which causes genital vasocongestion that results in vaginal lubrication in preparation for intromission. The lubrication is due to the formation of a transudate in the vagina and in conjunction with genital congestion produces the so-called orgasmic platform prior to orgasm. Sexual stimuli (visual, tactile, auditory, and olfactory) as well as healthy vaginal tissue are prerequisites for genital vasocongestion and vaginal lubrication. During the second stage of the sexual response involuntary contractions of the muscles of the pelvis result in a pleasurable cortical sensory phenomenon known as orgasm. Direct or indirect stimulation of the clitoris is important in the production of the female orgasm. In simple terms, sexual dysfunction can be due to interference with the arousal or orgasmic phases of the sexual response. Either disorder can be due to an organic or functional cause or both.

Illnesses that impair neurologic function such as diabetes mellitus or multiple sclerosis may prevent normal sexual arousal. Local pelvic diseases such as vaginitis, endometriosis, and salpingo-oophoritis may preclude normal sexual response because of resulting dyspareunia. Debilitating systemic diseases such as cancer and cardiovascular diseases may impair normal sexual response indirectly.

More commonly, failure of a normal sexual response is due to psychological factors that impair sexual arousal. Such problems include misinformation, for example, the perception of sexual satisfaction as bad, or feelings of guilt about previous psychologically traumatic events such as incest, rape, or unwanted pregnancy. In addition, women who have had previous hysterectomy or mastectomy may perceive themselves as "incomplete." Stresses such as anxiety, depression, fatigue, and marital or interpersonal conflicts may lead to failure of the vasocongestive response and prevent normal vaginal lubrication. Women with such experiences may be unable to achieve normal sexual response unless they receive professional counseling by a family physician, psychiatrist, or sex therapist. Such problems are approached by attempting to identify and reduce the causative stresses.

Failure to achieve orgasm is a specific form of sexual dysfunction. In the absence of orgasm many women enjoy sexual encounters to variable degrees because of the pleasure derived from closeness in a cherished relationship, particularly with a loving partner. However, for other women sexual relations with rare or absent orgasms are frustrating and unsatisfying. In many instances, failure of orgasm is due to insufficient clitoral stimulation and may be rectified by appropriate counseling and patient education.

A specific entity, "vaginismus," painful, involuntary contractions of the musculature surrounding the entrance to the vagina, is a rare cause of dyspareunia. It is a conditioned response to a previous real or imagined frightening or traumatic sexual experience. Treatment is directed to elimination of the conditioned response by progressive vaginal dilation by the patient in conjunction with marital therapy.

REPRODUCTION Problems of infertility are discussed in detail in Chap. 322. The approach to infertile couples always involves evaluation of both the man and woman. The initial evaluation includes a thorough history and physical examination. The history should elicit information as to the frequency of intercourse, the sexual responses of both, the use of contraceptives or lubricants, previous or past medical illnesses, and all medications taken.

Male-associated factors account for a third of infertility problems. Therefore, one of the first procedures in the workup of infertile couples should be a semen analysis (see Chap. 321). The initial evaluation of the female includes documentation of normal ovulatory cycles. A history of regular, cyclic, predictable, spontaneous menses usually indicates ovulatory cycles, which may be confirmed by basal body temperature graphs, properly timed endometrial biopsies, or plasma progesterone measurements during the luteal phase of the cycle. Also, the diagnosis of luteal-phase dysfunction (low progesterone secretion during the luteal phase) can be established by these methods. If the woman is anovulatory, attempts to induce ovulation can be undertaken by a variety of methods including clomiphene, human menopausal gonadotropins, bromocriptine, luteinizing hormone–releasing hormone (LHRH) agonists, or wedge resection of the ovaries (Chap. 322).

The most common cause of infertility in women is tubal disease, usually due to infection (pelvic inflammatory disease) or endometriosis. Tubal disease can be evaluated by obtaining a hysterosalpingogram or by diagnostic laparoscopy. The treatment of tubal causes of infertility is primarily surgical.

A cervical factor as a cause of infertility is identified by a properly timed postcoital examination. During this examination the sperm motility in cervical mucus is observed. Also, immunologic etiologies for infertility can be tested for by a variety of laboratory tests. The cause of infertility is unknown in 10 percent of couples. In many instances of infertility reproductive technology now makes possible the successful use of in vitro fertilization and embryo transfer, gamete intrafallopian tube transfer, transfer of cryopreserved ova and embryos, and intrauterine insemination.

The desire for fertility control or contraception is also a frequent cause for women to seek medical treatment or evaluation. The most widely used methods for fertility control include (1) rhythm and withdrawal techniques, (2) barrier methods, (3) intrauterine devices, (4) oral steroid contraceptives, (5) sterilization, and (6) abortion. A discussion of these methods and the possible complications of each is found in Chap. 322.

REFERENCES

Cunningham FG et al: *Williams Obstetrics,* 18th ed. Norwalk, Appleton-Century-Crofts, 1989
Droegemuller W et al: *Comprehensive Gynecology.* St. Louis, Mosby, 1987
Fordney DS: Dyspareunia and vaginismus. Clin Obstet Gynecol 21:205, 1978
Hatcher RA et al: *Contraceptive Technology 1986–1987.* New York, Irvington, 1986
Masters W, Johnson V: *Human Sexual Response.* Boston, Little, Brown, 1966
——, ——: *Human Sexual Inadequacy.* Boston, Little, Brown, 1970
Speroff L et al: *Clinical Gynecologic Endocrinology and Infertility,* 4th ed. Baltimore, Williams & Wilkins, 1988

54 HIRSUTISM AND VIRILIZATION

WILLIAM J. KOVACS / JEAN D. WILSON

Hirsutism, male pattern hair growth in women, is a common and perplexing problem. The distribution and growth of hair in normal persons is under complex genetic and endocrine control so that there is considerable variability in hair growth in normal men and women. As a consequence, abnormal hair growth is sometimes difficult to define: Some patients may seek medical attention because of what the physician may consider an insignificant cosmetic defect. Others, because of personal or cultural differences, may be undisturbed by surprising degrees of hirsutism. The central issue in dealing with such patients is the separation of those infrequent instances in which hirsutism is a manifestation of a serious and remediable underlying disorder from the vast majority of hirsute women in whom excess hair is fundamentally a cosmetic problem.

CONTROL OF NORMAL HAIR GROWTH AND DISTRIBUTION
Endocrine control Androgens are the major determinants of hair distribution in both sexes. There are three principal circulating androgens in women—dehydroepiandrosterone, derived from the adrenal; androstenedione, which is derived equally from adrenal and ovary; and testosterone, which is both secreted by the ovary and

adrenal and formed in peripheral tissue from circulating dehydroepi-androsterone and androstenedione. The production of adrenal andro-gen is regulated primarily by ACTH, while ovarian androgen secretion is regulated by luteinizing hormone (LH). These various androgens must be converted to testosterone (or dihydrotestosterone) before they can bind to the androgen receptor of target cells and induce an androgenic response. Thus, adrenal androgens virilize only in so far as they serve as precursors for testosterone and dihydrotestosterone.

Several types of relationships can be defined between hair growth and androgens in normal individuals. Eyebrows, eyelashes, and lanugo (fine, downy hair) are not dependent on androgens, while axillary and lower pubic hair are sensitive to the small amounts of androgen secreted by the adrenal. Hair in these regions therefore grows to an approximately equal extent in men and women. Hair growth in areas typical of males appears to require the greater androgen levels normally produced by the testes; such areas include the face, upper pubic triangle, chest, and ears. Finally, scalp hair exhibits androgen-mediated regression. The reason different body regions respond differently to the same or similar androgen is unknown. Theoretically, the metabolism of androgens might differ in the various sites, or hormone receptors might vary. The hair follicle, like some other androgen targets, requires conversion of testosterone to dihydrotestosterone for expression of androgen action, and hair follicles from all regions of the body perform this conversion equally well. Moreover, the same receptor that is essential for androgen action in other cells (Chap. 321) mediates the effects of dihydrotestosterone in the hair follicle. Genetic disorders with normal testosterone production but absent androgen receptor have deficient or absent axillary, pubic, facial, truncal, and limb hair (Chap. 324). Regional differences in androgen responsiveness of hair in normal individuals may be the consequence of regional differences in the amount of androgen receptor in hair follicles.

Genetic factors   Despite similar hormone levels, there is con-siderable diversity in the distribution of hair between individuals and among different racial groups in regard to facial, truncal, and pubic hair. Dark-haired, darkly pigmented whites of either sex tend to be more hirsute than blond or fair-skinned persons. Orientals, American Indians, and blacks on average are less hirsute than whites. Orientals rarely have facial or body hair except in the pubic and axillary regions, and American Indians, in addition, rarely develop baldness in either sex. Heterogeneity of hair patterns also exists within families. The inheritance of hair patterns is complex and probably polygenic in nature.

Other factors   Aging is a prerequisite for the expression of some types of hair development. For example, in men hair on the trunk and extremities frequently increases for several years after maximal levels of plasma androgens have been reached. Conversely, loss of androgen may not result in diminution of normal hair growth in men or complete reversal of hirsutism in women. The appearance of pubic hair is frequently the heralding event of puberty in females. Women in the first trimester of pregnancy commonly observe increased hairiness of the face, extremities, and breasts. Menopause is often associated with the loss of hair in the pubic area, axillae, and extremities, whereas growth of hair on the face increases in post-menopausal women. The physiologic basis for these changes is unclear and cannot be explained entirely by changes in androgen levels.

PATHOLOGIC HAIR GROWTH AND DISTRIBUTION   A central consideration in the evaluation of women with hirsutism is whether evidence of virilization or defeminization is also present (Table 54-1) since such signs suggest a more significant degree of androgen excess. In patients with overproduction of androgen, defeminizing signs, such as disturbances of menstruation, are more frequently observed than are the signs of virilization. However, the presence or absence of overt virilization should be interpreted with caution for at least two reasons. First, signs of virilization (clitoromegaly, balding, coarsening of the hair, hirsutism) indicate androgen excess at some time in the patient's life but do not necessarily mean that active

TABLE 54-1   Clinical signs of defeminization and virilization

Signs of defeminization	Signs of virilization
Amenorrhea	Frontal balding
Decrease in breast size	Increase in size of shoulder girdle
Loss of female body contours	muscles
	Clitoromegaly
	Coarsening of the voice
	Acne

After Karp L, Herrmann WL: Diagnosis and treatment of hirsutism in women. Obstet Gynecol 41:283, 1973.

disease is present at the time of evaluation. It is necessary to measure plasma androgen levels and/or production rates to determine if androgen excess is ongoing. Second, severe overandrogenization may exist in the absence of marked virilization; i.e., at the same level of androgen production clitoromegaly may be present in one patient and not another.

Diagnostic considerations   DRUGS   Excessive hair growth can be caused by drugs that do not produce signs of defeminization or virilization. Such drugs include phenytoin, minoxidil, diazoxide, cyclosporin, and hexachlorobenzene. Androgens produce hirsutism as well as virilization. Some synthetic progestogens have androgenic activity.

TUMORS   The rapid onset of hair growth with or without accom-panying signs of frank virilization suggests a neoplastic source of androgen. Such tumors include androgen-secreting adenomas and carcinomas of the adrenal and ovarian tumors such as arrhenoblastoma, which secrete androgens directly, and Krukenberg tumors of the ovary, which stimulate the surrounding ovarian stromal tissue to produce excess androgen.

POLYCYSTIC OVARIAN DISEASE   The most common cause of ovar-ian hyperandrogenism is polycystic ovarian disease. This disorder has a broad clinical spectrum that ranges from mild hirsutism to complete amenorrhea and virilization. The salient feature for the diagnosis is the pubertal onset of chronic anovulation and hirsutism; enlarged cystic ovaries, obesity, and amenorrhea (i.e., the Stein-Leventhal syndrome) are present in only half or fewer of women with this disorder and need not be present for the diagnosis (see Chap. 322). The fundamental abnormality in polycystic ovarian disease is not fully understood. Elevation of plasma LH concentration causes enhanced androgen secretion by stromal and thecal cells of the ovary.

ATTENUATED FORMS OF ADRENAL HYPERPLASIA   The adrenal can also be the source of excess androgen in the absence of tumor. Heritable defects in adrenal steroidogenesis (congenital adrenal hy-perplasia) such as 21-hydroxylase deficiency, 11β-hydroxylase defi-ciency, and 3β-hydroxysteroid dehydrogenase deficiency can produce virilization, and each of these enzyme deficiencies can occur in a "late-onset" form in which hirsutism or virilization and menstrual irregularities appear at the time of expected puberty or in adulthood (see Chap. 324). The clinical presentation in these cases is usually indistinguishable from polycystic ovarian disease. Late-onset 21-hydroxylase deficiency is the most common of these attenuation forms of congenital adrenal hyperplasia and has been most extensively studied; its incidence in the general population of hirsute, oligomen-orrheic women is probably on the order of a few percent. The presence of elevated plasma levels of adrenal androgens (such as dehydroepiandrosterone sulfate) or of dexamethasone-suppressible hyperandrogenism does not necessarily imply that the overandrogen-ization is due to a specific adrenal steroidogenic defect, but these findings may be useful as a guide to therapy.

IDIOPATHIC HIRSUTISM   In many women with hirsutism a specific diagnosis cannot be made. The term *idiopathic hirsutism* applies to those women with evidence of androgen excess but with normal menses, normal-sized ovaries, no evidence of tumors of the adrenal or ovary, and normal adrenal function. Slight elevations of plasma androstenedione and testosterone are commonly present in such women, and testosterone production rates are increased above normal, although to a lesser degree than in patients with polycystic ovarian disease.

Experience outside the United States with the antiandrogen cyproterone acetate indicates that this form of hirsutism is androgen-mediated, since therapy results in improvement. Women with idiopathic hirsutism could constitute the extreme end of a normal continuum of androgen production or represent a true pathologic subset. Some women with the tentative diagnosis of idiopathic hirsutism actually have mild or early polycystic ovarian disease, but in most, hirsutism is not accompanied by or followed by signs of ovarian dysfunction. If such women are merely extremes of the normal range of androgen production, then their hirsutism is fundamentally a cosmetic defect.

DIAGNOSTIC EVALUATION The decision as to when to undertake a complex diagnostic evaluation depends on several factors. Such evaluation is appropriate in all women with hirsutism and virilization; whether it should be performed in women with isolated hirsutism depends upon the severity, distribution, and rate of hair growth. An approach to the diagnostic evaluation of hirsute patients is shown in Fig. 54-1. The clinical history is taken with particular attention to drug ingestion and to the details of pubertal development and menstrual history and their relation to the onset of excessive hair growth. The physical examination is directed to the assessment of sites of growth of androgen-dependent hair (pubic, axillary, facial, truncal, and extremity) and evaluation for signs of virilization, which correlate with higher levels of androgen overproduction and raise the concern of androgen-producing neoplasms. Such signs include laryngeal enlargement (deepening of the voice), temporal balding, clitoromegaly, and increased muscle mass in the limb girdles. Signs of cortisol excess (plethora, centripetal obesity, striae, and dorsocervical and supraclavicular fat pads) should also be sought. Pelvic examination should include a search for palpable ovarian masses. Appropriate laboratory tests include measurement of serum androgens and, when appropriate, radiologic imaging of ovaries and adrenal glands. Basal measurements of dehydroepiandrosterone sulfate greater than 22 nmol/L (8000 ng/mL) or of serum testosterone over 7 nmol/L (2ng/mL) suggest neoplastic sources of androgen excess; plasma testosterone levels in the normal range are more difficult to interpret because total levels in women do not necessarily reflect the free or unbound levels of hormone under conditions when testosterone binding globulin levels are either increased or decreased. Suspected Cushing's syndrome should be evaluated with standard dexamethasone suppression testing if a screening test (such as urinary free cortisol excretion or overnight dexamethasone suppression test) is abnormal. The diagnosis of polycystic ovarian disease is made from the history and clinical features in a woman with chronic anovulation. Women with severe hirsutism associated with cystic acne may be screened for delayed-onset adrenal hyperplasia by the short cosyntropin stimulation test and measurement of plasma 17-hydroxyprogesterone (see Chap. 317).

MANAGEMENT In the case of drug-induced hirsutism and neoplastic disease of the ovary or adrenals treatment is straightforward; administration of the drugs should be stopped, or the tumor should be removed. Adrenal steroidogenic defects are treated with glucocorticoids to suppress excess ACTH and hence inhibit adrenal androgen secretion. In most instances (polycystic ovarian disease as well as idiopathic hirsutism) both cosmetic treatment and suppression of androgen production or antagonism of its action at the receptor level need to be employed.

Cosmetic therapy is directed at the concealment or removal of hair from exposed skin areas. Small amounts of hair can be bleached with hydrogen peroxide. Methods for removal of hair are classified as depilatory (removal of hair from the surface of the skin) or epilatory (removal of the intact hair with the root). Depilatory techniques include shaving and chemical methods. Shaving does not have an adverse effect on hair growth rate or coarseness (although the blunt ends may feel coarse), but shaving of areas other than axillae or legs is unacceptable to most women. Chemical depilatories are effective for limited areas of hair removal and are generally safe if used properly. Most available depilatories are substituted mercaptans, such as thioglycollic acid, which reduce the disulfide bonds in the peptide chains of keratin. The hair fiber swells and softens to a consistency that can be washed from the skin. Care must be taken to avoid skin irritation because of the alkalinity of these preparations. Temporary epilation can be achieved by plucking (useful only for isolated hairs) or wax treatment. The waxes are melted and applied to the skin. When the wax cools and sets, it is stripped off, removing hair with it. The procedure is uncomfortable, and best results can be obtained by salon treatments. Permanent epilation can be achieved only by electrolysis. The treatments are expensive and time-consuming, and success depends on the skill of the electrologist.

While cosmetic treatment is undertaken, attempts to suppress androgen overproduction may also be appropriate. Treatment with combination oral contraceptives suppresses ovarian androgen secretion when restoration of fertility is not an objective. To minimize side effects the lowest effective dosage of estrogen should be used. Women over 35 years of age, smokers, and those with hypertension, a history

FIGURE 54-1 Diagnostic approach to the hirsute patient. T = testosterone; DHEA-S = dehydroepiandrosterone sulfate.

of thromboembolic disease, impaired liver function, or suspected estrogen-dependent neoplasm should not be treated with oral contraceptives. Suppression of adrenal androgen overproduction can be achieved with small doses of dexamethasone and is useful in the treatment of women with late-onset 21-hydroxylase deficiency.

Antagonism of the effects of androgens at the hair follicle is the basis for the other main treatment modality, the antiandrogens. Cyproterone acetate has been used with success but is unavailable in the United States. Spironolactone has a dual action of blocking the androgen receptor and of inhibiting androgen production and is a useful alternative therapy. Cimetidine also binds to the androgen receptor and acts as an androgen antagonist, but it is not of general benefit in the treatment of hirsutism.

If pharmacologic therapy is undertaken, the patient should be prepared to make a commitment of 6 months for an adequate trial of efficacy. Even when treatment is long-term, dramatic reversal of established hair growth is unlikely to be achieved by interference with androgen synthesis or action. Such hormonal manipulations can arrest or slow the rate of hair growth, but established hair must be dealt with by use of cosmetic treatment.

REFERENCES

BRODIE BL, WENTZ AC: Late onset congenital adrenal hyperplasia—a gynecologist's perspective. Fertil Steril 48:175, 1987

LESHIN M: Hirsutism. Am J Med Sci 294:369, 1987

LUCKY AW et al: Plasma androgens in women with acne vulgaris. J Invest Dermatol 81:70, 1983

RAJ SG et al: Normalization of testosterone levels using a low-estrogen-containing oral contraceptive in women with polycystic ovary syndrome. Obstet Gynecol 60:15, 1982

RICHARDS RN et al: Electroepilation (electrolysis) in hirsutism: 35,000 hours experience on the face and neck. J Am Acad Dermatol 15:693, 1986

RITTMASTER RS, LORIAUX DL: Hirsutism. Ann Intern Med 106:95, 1987

RUBENS R: Androgen levels during cyproterone acetate and ethinyl estradiol treatment of hirsutism. Clin Endocrinol 20:313, 1984

TREMBLAY RR: Treatment of hirsutism with spironolactone. Clin Endocrinol Metab 15:363, 1986

section 8   Alterations in the skin

55   EXAMINATION OF THE SKIN

THOMAS J. LAWLEY / KIM B. YANCEY

The challenge of examining the skin lies in distinguishing normal from abnormal and significant findings from trivial ones and in integrating pertinent signs and symptoms into an appropriate differential diagnosis. The fact that the largest organ in the body is visible is both an advantage and a disadvantage to those who examine it. It is advantageous because no special instrumentation, other than a magnifying glass, is necessary and because the skin can be biopsied with little morbidity. However, the casual observer can be overwhelmed by a variety of stimuli and overlook important, subtle signs of skin or systemic disease. For instance, the sometimes minor differences in color and shape that distinguish a malignant melanoma from a benign pigmented nevus can be difficult to recognize. To aid in the interpretation of skin lesions, a variety of descriptive terms have been developed to characterize cutaneous lesions (Tables 55-1 and 55-2; Fig. 55-1). Mastery of this terminology is important not only for categorizing the skin lesions of a particular case but also in formulating a differential diagnosis (Table 55-3). For instance, the finding of large numbers of scaling papules, usually indicative of a primary skin disease, places the patient in a different diagnostic category than would hemorrhagic papules, which may indicate vasculitis or sepsis. It is important to differentiate primary skin lesions from secondary skin changes. If the examiner focuses on linear erosions overlying an area of erythema and scaling, he or she may incorrectly assume that the erosion is the primary lesion and the redness and scale are secondary, while the correct interpretation would be that the patient has a pruritic eczematous dermatitis and the erosions have been caused by scratching.

AN APPROACH TO THE PATIENT   In examining the skin it is usually advisable to assess the patient before taking a history. This way, the entire cutaneous surface is sure to be evaluated and objective findings can be integrated with relevant historical data. Four basic features of any cutaneous lesion must be noted and considered in the examination of skin: the distribution of the eruption, the type(s) of primary lesion, the shape of individual lesions, and the arrangement of the lesions. In the initial examination it is important that the patient be disrobed as completely as possible. This will minimize chances of missing important individual skin lesions and make it possible to assess accurately the distribution of the eruption. The patient should first be viewed from a distance of about 1.5 to 2 m (4 to 6 ft), so that the general character of the skin and the distribution of lesions can be evaluated. Indeed, distribution of lesions often correlates highly with diagnosis (Fig. 55-2). For example, a hospitalized patient with a generalized erythematous exanthem is more likely to have a drug eruption than is a patient with a similar rash limited to the sun-exposed portions of the face. The presence or absence of lesions on mucosal surfaces should also be determined. Once the distribution of the lesions has been established, the nature of the primary lesion must be determined. Thus, when lesions are distributed on elbows, knees, and scalp, the most likely possibilities based solely on distribution are psoriasis or dermatitis herpetiformis. The primary

---

TABLE 55-1   Descriptions of primary skin lesions

1 Macule: A flat, colored lesion, <2 cm in diameter, not raised above the surface of the surrounding skin. A "freckle," or ephelid, is a prototype pigmented macule.

2 Patch: A large (>2 cm), flat lesion with a color different from the surrounding skin. This differs from a macule only in size.

3 Papule: A small, solid lesion, <1 cm in diameter, that is raised above the surface of the surrounding skin and hence palpable (e.g., a closed comedone, or whitehead, in acne).

4 Nodule: A larger (1–5 cm), firm lesion raised above the surface of the surrounding skin. This differs from a papule only in size (e.g., dermal nevus).

5 Tumor: A firm, solid, raised growth >5 cm in diameter.

6 Plaque: A large (>1 cm) flat-topped raised lesion; edges may either be distinct (e.g., in psoriasis) or gradually blend with surrounding skin (e.g., in eczematous dermatitis).

7 Vesicle: A small, fluid-filled lesion <1 cm in diameter that is raised above the plane of surrounding skin. Fluid is often visible, and the lesions are often translucent [e.g., vesicles in allergic contact dermatitis caused by *Rhus* (poison ivy)].

8 Pustule: A vesicle filled with leukocytes. Note: The presence of pustules does not necessarily signify the existence of an infection.

9 Bulla: A fluid-filled, raised, often translucent lesion >1 cm in diameter.

10 Cyst: A soft, raised, encapsulated lesion filled with semisolid or liquid contents.

11 Wheal: A raised, erythematous papule or plaque, usually representing short-lived dermal edema.

12 Telangiectasia: Dilated, superficial blood vessels.

TABLE 55-2 Common dermatologic terms

1 Lichenification: A distinctive thickening of the skin that is characterized by accentuated skin-fold markings and that feels thick and firm on palpation.
2 Crust: Dried exudate of body fluids that may be either yellow (serous exudate) or red (hemorrhagic exudate).
3 Milia: Small, firm, white papules that are filled with keratin (and may in part resemble pustules).
4 Erosion: Epithelial deficit resulting in a superficial disruption of skin integrity.
5 Ulcer: Epithelial deficit resulting in a deep surface disruption.
6 Excoriations: Linear, angular erosions that may be covered by crust and are caused by scratching.
7 Atrophy: An acquired loss of substance. In the skin, this may appear as a depression with intact epidermis (i.e., loss of dermal or subcutaneous tissue) or as sites of shiny, delicate, wrinkled lesions (i.e., epidermal atrophy).
8 Scar: A change in the skin secondary to trauma or inflammation. Sites may be erythematous, hypopigmented, or hypertrophic, depending on their age or character. Sites on hair-bearing areas may be characterized by destruction of hair follicles.

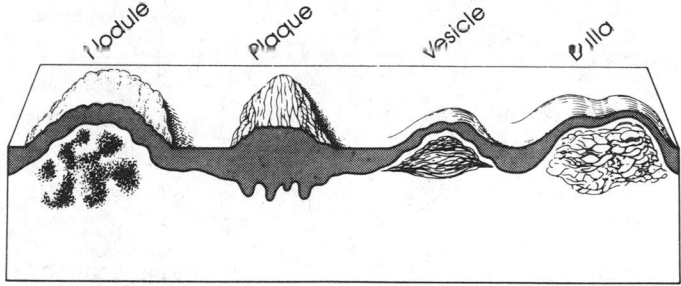

FIGURE 55-1 A schematic representation of several common primary skin lesions (see Table 55-1).

lesion in psoriasis is a scaly papule that soon forms erythematous plaques covered with a white scale, while that of dermatitis herpetiformis is an urticarial papule that quickly becomes a small vesicle. In this manner, identification of the primary lesion directs the examiner toward the proper diagnosis. Secondary changes in skin can also be

TABLE 55-3 Selected common dermatologic conditions

Diagnosis	Common distribution	Usual morphology	Diagnosis	Common distribution	Usual morphology
Acne vulgaris	Face, upper back	Open and closed comedones, erythematous papules, pustules, cysts	Folliculitis	Any hair-bearing area	Perifollicular pustules
Rosacea	Blush area of cheeks, nose, forehead, chin	Erythema, telangiectasias, papules, pustules	Impetigo	Anywhere	Papules, vesicles, pustules often with honey-colored crusts
Seborrheic dermatitis	Scalp, eyebrows, perinasal	Erythema with greasy yellow-brown scale	Herpes simplex	Lips, genitalia	Grouped vesicles progressing to crusted erosions
Atopic dermatitis	Antecubital and popliteal fossae; may be widespread	Patches and plaques of erythema, scaling, and lichenification	Herpes zoster	Dermatomal, usually trunk but may be anywhere	Vesicles limited to a dermatome (often painful)
Stasis dermatitis	Ankles, lower legs	Patches of erythema and scaling on background of hyperpigmentation associated with signs of venous insufficiency	Varicella	Face, trunk, relative sparing of extremities	Lesions arise in crops and quickly progress from erythematous macules to papules to vesicles to pustules to crusts
Dyshidrotic eczema	Palms, soles, sides of fingers and toes	Deep vesicles	Pityriasis rosea	Trunk (Christmas tree pattern) herald patch followed by multiple smaller lesions	Symmetric erythematous patches with a collarette of trailing scale
Plant dermatitis (poison ivy)	Anywhere	Linear patches of erythema and vesicles			
Allergic contact dermatitis	Anywhere	Localized erythema, vesicles, and scale, e.g., fingers, earlobes—nickel; dorsal aspect of foot—shoe dermatitis, etc.	Tinea versicolor	Chest, back, abdomen, proximal extremities	Scaly hyper- or hypopigmented macules
Psoriasis	Elbows, knees, scalp, lower back, fingernails (may be generalized)	Papules and plaques covered with silvery scale; nails have pits	Candidiasis	Groin, beneath breasts, vagina, oral cavity	Erythematous macerated areas with satellite pustules; white, friable patches on mucous membranes
Lichen planus	Wrists, ankles, mouth (may be widespread)	Violaceous flat-topped papules and plaques	Dermatophytosis	Feet, groin, beard, or scalp	Varies with site, e.g., tinea corporis—scaly annular patch
Keratosis pilaris	Extensor surfaces of arms and thighs, buttocks	Keratotic follicular papules with surrounding erythema	Scabies	Groin, axillae, between fingers and toes, beneath breasts	Excoriated papules, burrows
Melasma	Forehead, cheeks, temples, upper lip	Tan to brown patches	Insect bites	Anywhere	Erythematous papules with central puncta
Vitiligo	Periorificial, trunk, extensor surfaces of extremities, flexor wrists, axillae	Chalk-white macules	Cherry angioma	Trunk	Red, blood-filled papules
			Keloid	Anywhere (site of previous injury)	Firm tumor; pink, purple, or brown
Actinic keratosis	Sun-exposed areas	Skin-colored or red-brown macule or papule with dry adherent scale	Dermatofibroma	Anywhere	Firm red to brown nodule that shows dimpling of overlying skin with lateral compression
Basal cell carcinoma	Face	Papule with pearly border on sun-damaged skin	Acrochordons (skin tags)	Groin, axilla, neck	Fleshy papules
Seborrheic keratosis	Trunk, face	Brown plaques with adherent greasy scale; "stuck on" appearance	Urticaria	Anywhere	Wheals, sometimes with surrounding flare
			Transient acantholytic dermatosis	Trunk, especially anterior chest	Erythematous papules
			Xerosis	Extensor extremities, especially legs	Dry, erythematous, scaling patches

FIGURE 55-2*A–D.* The distribution of some common dermatologic diseases and lesions.

quite helpful. For example, scale represents excessive epidermis, while crust is the result of an inadequate or inconsistent epithelial cell layer. Palpation of skin lesions can also yield insight into the character of an eruption. Thus, red papules on the lower extremities that blanch with pressure can be a manifestation of many different diseases, but red papules that do not blanch with pressure indicate palpable purpura characteristic of necrotizing vasculitis.

The shape of lesions is also an important feature. Flat, round, erythematous macules are common in many cutaneous diseases. However, target-shaped lesions that consist in part of erythematous macules are specific for erythema multiforme. In the same way, the arrangement of individual lesions is important. Erythematous papules and vesicles can occur in many conditions, but their arrangement in a specific linear array suggests an external etiology such as allergic contact or primary irritant dermatitis. In contrast, lesions with an annular or arciform arrangement are common and suggest a systemic etiology.

As in other branches of medicine, a complete history should be obtained to emphasize the following features:

1 Evolution of lesions
  a Site of onset
  b Manner in which eruption progressed or spread
  c Duration
  d Periods of resolution or improvement in chronic eruptions
2 Symptoms associated with eruption
  a Itching, burning, pain, numbness
  b What, if anything, has relieved symptoms
  c Time of day when symptoms are most severe
3 Current or recent medications (prescribed, as well as over-the-counter)

4 Associated systemic symptoms (e.g., malaise, fever, arthralgias)
5 Ongoing or previous illnesses
6 History of allergies
7 Presence of photosensitivity
8 Review of systems

DIAGNOSTIC TECHNIQUES Many skin diseases can be diagnosed on gross clinical appearance, but sometimes relatively simple diagnostic procedures can yield valuable information. In most instances, they can be performed at the bedside with a minimum of equipment.

Skin biopsy A skin biopsy is a straightforward minor surgical procedure; however, it is important to biopsy the anatomic site most likely to yield diagnostic findings. This decision may require expertise in skin diseases and knowledge of superficial anatomic structures in selected areas of the body. In this procedure a small area of skin is anesthetized with 1% xylocaine with or without epinephrine. The skin lesion in question can be excised with a scalpel or removed by punch biopsy. In the latter technique, a punch is pressed against the surface of the skin and rotated with downward pressure until it penetrates to the subcutaneous tissue. The circular biopsy is then lifted with forceps, and the bottom is cut with iris scissors. Biopsy sites may or may not need suture closure, depending on size and location.

KOH preparation A potassium hydroxide (KOH) preparation is performed on scaling skin lesions when a fungal etiology is suspected. The edge of such a lesion is scraped gently with a scalpel blade, and the removed scale is collected on a glass microscope slide and treated with 1 to 2 drops of a solution of 10 to 20% KOH. KOH dissolves keratin and allows easier visualization of fungal elements. Brief heating of the slide accelerates dissolution of keratin. When the preparation is viewed under the microscope, the refractile hyphae will be seen more easily when the light intensity is reduced. This technique can be utilized to identify hyphae in dermatophyte infections, pseudohyphae and budding yeast in *Candida* infections, and fragmented hyphae and spores in tinea versicolor. The same sampling technique can be used to obtain scale for culture of selected pathogenic organisms.

Tzanck smear A Tzanck smear, named after Arnault Tzanck, is a cytologic technique most often used in the diagnosis of herpesvirus infections (simplex or varicella-zoster). An early vesicle, not a pustule or crusted lesion, is unroofed, and the base of the lesion is scraped gently with a scalpel blade. The material is then placed on a glass slide, air-dried, and stained with Giemsa or Wright's stain. Multinucleated giant cells suggest the presence of herpes, but culture must be performed to identify the specific virus.

Diascopy Diascopy is designed to assess whether a skin lesion will blanch with pressure as, for example, in determining whether a red lesion is hemorrhagic or simply blood-filled. For instance, a hemangioma will blanch with pressure, while a purpuric lesion caused by necrotizing vasculitis will not. Diascopy is performed by pressing a microscope slide or magnifying lens against a specified lesion and noting the amount of blanching which occurs. Granulomas often have an "apple jelly" appearance on diascopy.

Wood's light A Wood's lamp generates 360 nm ultraviolet (or "black") light and causes erythrasma to show a characteristic coral-red color and *Pseudomonas*, a pale blue. Tinea capitis caused by certain dermatophytes such as *Microsporum canis* or *M. audouini* exhibits a yellow fluorescence. Pigmented lesions of the epidermis such as freckles are accentuated, while dermal pigment such as postinflammatory hyperpigmentation fades under a Wood's light. Vitiligo appears totally white under a Wood's lamp, and previously unsuspected areas of involvement often become apparent. A Wood's lamp may also aid in the demonstration of tinea versicolor and in recognition of ash leaf spots in patients with tuberous sclerosis.

Patch tests Patch testing is designed to document sensitivity to a specific antigen. In this procedure a battery of suspected allergens is applied to the patient's back under occlusive dressings and allowed to remain in contact with the skin for 48 h. The dressings are then removed, and the area is examined for evidence of delayed hypersensitivity reactions. This test is best performed by physicians with special expertise in patch testing and is often helpful in the evaluation of patients with chronic dermatitis.

REFERENCES

FITZPATRICK TB et al (eds): *Dermatology in General Medicine,* 3d ed. New York, McGraw-Hill, 1987
LOOKINGBILL DP, MARKS JG: *Principles of Dermatology.* Philadelphia, Saunders, 1986
ROOK A et al (eds): *Textbook of Dermatology,* 4th ed. Oxford, Blackwell Scientific, 1986

56 ECZEMA, PSORIASIS, CUTANEOUS INFECTIONS, ACNE, AND OTHER COMMON SKIN DISORDERS

THOMAS J. LAWLEY / ROBERT A. SWERLICK

COMMON SKIN DISORDERS

ECZEMA Eczema, or dermatitis, is a reaction pattern manifested by variable clinical and histologic findings. Eczema is the final common expression for atopic dermatitis, allergic contact and irritant contact dermatitis, dyshidrotic eczema, nummular eczema, lichen simplex chronicus, asteatotic eczema, and seborrheic dermatitis. Primary lesions may include papules, erythematous macules, and vesicles, which can coalesce to form patches and plaques. In severe eczema, secondary lesions such as weeping and crusting may predominate. Long-standing dermatitis is often dry and is characterized by thickened, scaling skin (lichenification). The histologic changes correlate with the clinical findings. The histologic features of dermatitis have been divided into three patterns: acute, subacute, and chronic. Acute dermatitis shows a mixture of epidermal and dermal edema, epidermal vesiculation, and a mononuclear cell infiltrate. Chronic dermatitis demonstrates epidermal acanthosis, hyperkeratosis, upper dermal fibrosis, and a predominantly perivascular mononuclear cell infiltrate. Mixtures of these two histologic reaction patterns occur in subacute dermatitis. Any of these patterns may be associated with the various clinical forms of dermatitis, and the histopathologic findings are rarely diagnostic.

ATOPIC DERMATITIS Atopic dermatitis is the cutaneous expression of the atopic state, and up to 70 percent of patients have a family history of asthma, hay fever, or dermatitis. Atopic individuals often have dry, itchy skin, abnormal cutaneous vascular responses, and, in some instances, elevations in serum IgE. The clinical presentation falls into three patterns related to age: the infantile form (ages 2 months to 2 years), the childhood form (ages 4 to 10 years), and the adolescent and adult form. In severe cases, the infantile or childhood forms of the disease may persist into adult life.

The infantile form is characterized by inflammatory patches and weeping, crusted plaques on the face, neck, extensor surfaces, and groin. Pruritus is prominent, and many of the cutaneous findings are secondary to rubbing and scratching. Dermatitis of flexural areas is characteristic of the childhood form, particularly in the antecubital and popliteal fossae. Lesions on the wrists, neck, and face are common. Other cutaneous stigmata that may become apparent at this stage are perioral pallor, an extra fold of skin beneath the lower eyelid (Dennie's line), and increased palmar markings. Cutaneous infections, particularly with *Staphylococcus aureus,* occur frequently.

The adult form is usually more localized than the infantile or childhood forms of the disease. Atopic dermatitis often resolves spontaneously as children enter adulthood, but the persistent variant tends to localize to the hands (see "Hand Dermatitis"), neck, face, genitalia, or legs and may resemble nummular eczema or lichen simplex chronicus (see below).

Diagnosis is based upon a family history of atopy, presence of other forms of allergy (asthma or allergic rhinitis), history of infantile or childhood eczema, and the pattern of eruption. In severe disease, serum IgE should be measured to rule out the possibility of hyper-IgE syndrome (see Chap. 81). Patients who do not respond to conventional therapies should be considered for patch testing to exclude allergic contact dermatitis.

Therapy of atopic dermatitis should be based upon avoidance of cutaneous irritants, adequate cutaneous hydration, judicious use of low- or midpotency topical glucocorticoids (Table 56-1), and treatment of infected skin lesions. The most common irritants are soaps and hot water. Patients should bathe using warm, but not hot, water and should limit their use of soap, particularly on extremities. Immediately after bathing, the skin should be lubricated with a low- or midpotency topical glucocorticoid in a cream or ointment base. Crusted and weeping lesions should be treated with systemic antibiotics with activity against *S. aureus* and *Streptococcus pyogenes,* since secondary infection often exacerbates eczema. Antihistamines are useful to control the pruritus that accompanies eczema, but sedation may limit their usefulness.

The role of dietary allergens in atopic dermatitis is controversial, but there is little evidence that it plays any role except in infancy. A significant number of children under age 3 who do not respond to conventional therapy have food sensitivities. Unfortunately, parental histories of food intake do not correlate with actual food allergens, and identification of the offending agents is best done with double-blind food challenges.

Treatment with systemic glucocorticoids should be limited to severe exacerbations unresponsive to topical therapy. In the patient with chronic atopic eczema, therapy with systemic glucocorticoids will generally clear the skin only briefly, but cessation of the systemic therapy will invariably be accompanied by return, if not worsening, of the dermatitis. The side effects of daily doses of systemic glucocorticoids preclude chronic use in virtually all patients with atopic dermatitis, and the efficacy of alternate-day regimens in this disease is limited.

ALLERGIC CONTACT DERMATITIS The most commonly recognized form of allergic contact dermatitis (ACD) is phytodermatitis or plant dermatitis. Members of the *Rhus* family, including poison ivy, poison oak, and poison sumac, cause an allergic reaction marked by erythema, vesiculation, and severe pruritus. The eruption is often linear, corresponding to areas where plants have touched the skin. Other allergens are much more difficult to identify, especially if the exposure is chronic and the skin becomes thickened and scaly.

If ACD is suspected and an offending agent is identified and removed, the eruption resolves. Usually, treatment with high-potency fluorinated topical glucocorticoids is enough to relieve symptoms while the ACD runs its course. Patients with particularly widespread disease, or disease involving the face or genitalia, may require treatment with oral glucocorticoids. Since the natural course of ACD is 2 to 3 weeks, therapy should be continued for that length of time. Treatment of ACD with short, rapidly tapered courses of oral glucocorticoids is usually followed by recurrence of skin lesions.

Identification of a contact allergen can be a difficult and time-consuming task. Patients with a dermatitis unresponsive to conventional therapy or with an unusual and patterned distribution should be suspected of having ACD. They should be questioned carefully regarding occupational exposures, topical medications, and oral medications. Common sensitizers include preservatives in topical preparations, nickel sulfate, potassium dichromate, neomycin sulfate, fragrances, formaldehyde, and rubber curing agents. Standard patch test trays are helpful in identifying these agents, but should not be used in patients with widespread active dermatitis or in those on systemic glucocorticoids.

HAND ECZEMA Hand eczema, a common chronic skin disorder, may be associated with other cutaneous disorders such as atopic dermatitis or psoriasis or may occur by itself. Like other forms of dermatitis, both exogenous and endogenous factors play important roles in the expression of hand dermatitis. Chronic, excessive exposure to water and detergents may initiate or aggravate this disorder. It may present with dryness and cracking of the skin of the hands, as well as with variable amounts of erythema and edema. Often, the dermatitis begins under rings, where water and irritants are trapped. A variant of hand dermatitis, dyshidrotic eczema, presents with multiple, intensely pruritic, small papules and vesicles on the thenar and hypothenar eminences and the sides of the fingers. Lesions tend to occur in crops, slowly crust over, and are followed by another outbreak.

Therapy of hand dermatitis is directed toward avoidance of irritants, identification of possible contact allergens, treatment of coexistent infection, and application of topical glucocorticoids. The most common hand irritants are soap and water. Health care professionals, housewives, and food handlers are prone to hand eczema. Use of mild soap, avoidance of hot water, and compulsive use of emollients can alleviate some symptoms. Whenever possible, the hands should be protected by gloves, preferably vinyl gloves, since many patients with hand eczema may become sensitive to curing agents in rubber gloves. Predominant involvement of the dorsal surface of the hands with sparing of the palmar surface should suggest a possible contact dermatitis. Most patients can be treated by application of cool, moist compresses (dressings) to dry and debride acute inflammatory lesions and to decrease swelling, followed by a midpotency topical glucocorticoid in a cream or ointment base. If allergic contact dermatitis is suspected, ointments are preferable. Chronic use of very high potency topical glucocorticoids can lead to cutaneous atrophy and is often accompanied by loss of effectiveness. As with atopic dermatitis, treatment of secondary infection with *Staphylococcus* or *Streptococcus* is essential. All patients with hand dermatitis should be examined for dermatophyte infection by KOH preparation and culture (see "Dermatophyte Infections").

NUMMULAR ECZEMA Nummular eczema is characterized by circular or oval "coinlike" lesions. Initially, this eruption consists of small edematous papules that become crusted and scaly. The most common locations are on the trunk or the extensor surfaces of the extremities, particularly on the pretibial areas or dorsum of the hands. It occurs most frequently in middle-aged men. The etiology is unknown but appears to be related to dryness of the skin and exogenous irritants. Unlike other forms of dermatitis, nummular eczema does not respond well to hydration, topical glucocorticoids,

---

TABLE 56-1 Selected topical glucocorticoid preparations*

Group†	Generic name	Brand name
1	Clobetasol propionate	Temovate cream 0.05%
	Clobetasol propionate	Temovate ointment 0.05%
	Betamethasone dipropionate	Diprolene cream 0.05%
	Betamethasone dipropionate	Diprolene ointment 0.05%
	Diflorasone diacetate	Psorcon ointment 0.05%
2	Flucinonide	Lidex cream 0.05%
	Flucinonide	Lidex ointment 0.05%
	Betamethasone dipropionate	Diprosone ointment 0.05%
	Halcinonide	Halog cream 0.1%
3	Betamethasone dipropionate	Diprosone cream 0.05%
	Betamethasone valerate	Valisone ointment 0.1%
	Diflorasone diacetate	Maxiflor cream 0.05%
4	Triamcinolone acetonide	Kenalog ointment 0.1%
	Triamcinolone acetonide	Aristocort ointment 0.1%
	Flurandrenolide	Cordran ointment 0.05%
5	Triamcinolone acetonide	Kenalog cream 0.1%
	Fluocinolone acetonide	Synalar cream 0.025%
	Hydrocortisone valerate	Westcort cream 0.2%
6	Desonide	Tridesilon cream 0.05%
	Desonide	DesOwen cream 0.05%
	Alclometasone dipropionate	Alcovate cream 0.05%
7	Hydrocortisone	Many

* List not meant to be comprehensive.
† Preparations grouped according to potency: group 1 is most potent; group 7 is least potent.

or antihistamines. Overt infection should be treated appropriately with antibiotics; however, even in instances where infection is not apparent, treatment with oral antibiotics, such as tetracycline or erythromycin, may be useful.

LICHEN SIMPLEX CHRONICUS Lichen simplex chronicus may represent the end stage of a variety of eczematous disorders. It consists of a well-circumscribed plaque or plaques with lichenified or thickened skin due to chronic scratching or rubbing. Common areas involved include the posterior nuchal region, dorsum of the feet, or ankles. Treatment of lichen simplex chronicus centers around breaking the cycle of chronic itching and scratching. High-potency topical glucocorticoids may be helpful in alleviating pruritus, but in recalcitrant cases application of topical glucocorticoids under occlusion or intralesional injection of glucocorticoids may be required.

ASTEATOTIC ECZEMA Asteatotic eczema, also known as xerotic eczema or "winter itch," is a mildly inflammatory variant of eczematous dermatitis that develops most commonly on the lower legs of elderly individuals during dry times of year. Fine cracks, with or without erythema, resembling cracks seen in china or porcelain characteristically develop on the anterior surface of the lower extremities. Pruritus is variable. Asteatotic eczema responds well to avoidance of excessive dryness, rehydration of the skin, and application of topical emollients, particularly those containing urea or α-hydroxy acids (lactic acid or glycolic acid).

STASIS DERMATITIS AND STASIS ULCERATION Stasis dermatitis develops on the lower extremities secondary to chronic edema and venous incompetence. The disorder usually begins as mild erythema and scaling associated with pruritus over the medial aspect of the ankle, often over a varicose vein. The dermatitis progresses to become pigmented as the result of extravasation of blood and hemosiderin deposition. Stasis dermatitis may become acutely inflamed, with crusting and exudation. Chronic stasis dermatitis is often associated with dermal fibrosis which results in brawny edema and may be complicated by the development of stasis ulcers.

Elevation of the legs, compression stockings, and topical emollients are the cornerstone of therapy. Patients should be instructed to elevate the affected extremity when sitting. Support stockings are a useful adjunct, particularly in individuals who stand for long periods of time. A graded compression stocking is more desirable than an antiembolism hose, which is designed for individuals confined to bed. The dermatitic component can be treated with cool dressings and the application of midpotency topical glucocorticoids. Glucocorticoids should not be applied to ulcerations, since they may retard healing. Secondarily infected lesions should be treated with appropriate oral antibiotics.

Stasis ulcerations are difficult to treat, and resolution of these lesions is slow even under the best of circumstances. The affected limb should be elevated as much as possible. External compression dressings such as an Unna boot are also helpful in aiding healing. The ulcer should be kept clear of necrotic material, and debridement may be facilitated by frequent soaks. The use of semipermeable and hydrocolloid dressings may be helpful. Some ulcerations may take months to heal and require skin grafting. Healed areas are prone to recurrent ulceration.

SEBORRHEIC DERMATITIS Seborrheic dermatitis is a common, chronic disorder usually affecting the central face and scalp, and on occasion the groin, axilla, submammary folds, and gluteal clefts. Rarely, it may cause a widespread generalized dermatitis. Patients commonly complain of itching or burning. It is characterized by greasy scales overlying erythematous patches or plaques. In the scalp it may be recognized as severe dandruff. On the face it affects the eyebrows, eyelids, glabella, nasolabial fold, or ears. Scaling within the external ear is often mistaken for a chronic fungal infection (otomycosis), and postauricular dermatitis often becomes macerated and tender.

Seborrheic dermatitis may be evident in infancy in the scalp ("cradle cap"), face, or groin. It is not seen in children beyond infancy but becomes evident again during adult life. Although it is frequently seen in patients with Parkinson's disease, in those who have had cerebrovascular accidents, and in those with human immunodeficiency virus (HIV-1) infection, the overwhelming majority of individuals with seborrheic dermatitis have no underlying disorder.

Treatment with low- to midpotency topical glucocorticoids in conjunction with shampoos containing coal tar and/or salicylic acid is generally sufficient to control activity of this disorder. Selenium sulfide shampoos may also be effective. Fluorinated topical glucocorticoids should not be used on the face.

PAPULOSQUAMOUS DISORDERS

PSORIASIS Psoriasis is one of the most common dermatologic diseases, affecting 1 to 2 percent of people. It is a chronic inflammatory skin disorder characterized by erythematous, sharply demarcated papules and rounded plaques, covered by silvery micaceous scale. The lesions are variably pruritic. The most common areas of involvement are the elbows, knees, gluteal cleft, and the scalp. Lesions tend to be symmetric. Traumatized areas are often involved (Koebner or isomorphic phenomenon). Most patients will have stable, slowly growing infiltrated plaques, which remain unchanged for long periods. Eruptive psoriasis in children and young adults is notable for the development of many small lesions after upper respiratory tract infection with beta-hemolytic streptococci.

About half of patients have fingernail involvement, appearing as a punctate pitting, nail thickening, or subungual hyperkeratosis. About 5 to 10 percent of psoriatics have joint complaints, often when there is fingernail involvement. Although some have typical rheumatoid arthritis (see Chap. 270), many have joint disease specifically associated with psoriasis: (1) disease limited to a single or a few small joints (70 percent of cases); (2) a seronegative rheumatoid arthritis–like disease; (3) involvement of the distal interphalangeal joints; (4) severe destructive arthritis with the development of "arthritis mutilans"; and (5) disease limited to the spine (see Chap. 283).

The histologic picture can be variable but is usually diagnostic in early lesions or at the advancing edge of a well-established plaque. The epidermis demonstrates elongation of the rete ridges, suprapapillary thinning, loss of the granular layer, parakeratotic keratin, and intraepidermal collections of neutrophils. Dilated capillaries and mononuclear cell infiltrates are common in the dermal papillae.

Treatment depends on the type, location, and extent of disease. All patients should be instructed to avoid excess drying or irritation of the skin and to maintain adequate cutaneous hydration. Most patients with localized plaque-type psoriasis can be managed with midpotency topical glucocorticoids, although their long-term use is often accompanied by loss of effectiveness. The effectiveness of topical glucocorticoids may be increased if used in conjunction with a keratolytic agent, such as salicylic acid, which removes surface scale and allows greater penetration. Crude coal tar (1 to 5% in an ointment base) is an old but useful method of treatment in conjunction with ultraviolet light therapy.

Ultraviolet light is useful for widespread psoriasis. The ultraviolet B (UV-B) spectrum is effective alone or may be combined with coal tar (Goeckerman regimen) or anthralin (Ingram regimen). Natural sunlight or an artificial light source can be used. The combination of the ultraviolet A (UV-A) spectrum and either oral or topical psoralens is also extremely effective for the treatment of psoriasis, but the photosensitizing potential of psoralens and unknown long-term toxicity may limit the use of this therapy.

Other agents can be used for widespread disease. Methotrexate is useful in patients with associated psoriatic arthritis. Long-term liver toxicity limits its use to patients with widespread disease not responsive to standard agents. The synthetic retinoid etretinate is effective in some patients with severe psoriasis, but it is a potent teratogen with an extremely long tissue half-life, thus precluding its use in women of childbearing age.

LICHEN PLANUS Lichen planus is a papulosquamous disorder in which the primary lesions are pruritic, polygonal, flat-topped, violaceous papules. Close examination of the surface of these papules will often reveal a network of grayish lines (Wickham's striae). The skin lesions have a predilection for the wrists, shins, lower back, and genitalia. Involvement of the scalp may lead to hair loss. Lichen planus commonly involves mucous membranes, particularly the buccal mucosa, where it can present as a netlike, whitish eruption. The etiology is unknown, but cutaneous eruptions clinically resembling lichen planus can occur after administration of numerous drugs, including thiazide diuretics, gold, antimalarials, and phenothiazines, and in patients with skin lesions of chronic graft-versus-host disease. Histologic examination of lesions of lichen planus will demonstrate hyperkeratosis, irregular acanthosis, a bandlike dermal infiltrate of lymphocytes adjacent to the epidermis, and damage to the epidermal basal cells. The course is variable, but most patients have spontaneous remissions 6 months to 2 years after the onset of disease. Topical glucocorticoids are the mainstay of therapy.

PITYRIASIS ROSEA Pityriasis rosea is a papulosquamous eruption of unknown etiology that occurs more commonly in the spring and fall. Its first manifestation is the development of a 2- to 6-cm annular lesion (the herald patch). This is followed in a few days to a few weeks by many smaller annular or papular lesions with a truncal predilection. The lesions are generally oval with their long axis parallel to the skin-fold lines. The individual lesions may be red to brown in color with an erythematous border and trailing scale. Many clinical features resemble the eruption of secondary syphilis, but palm and sole lesions are rare in pityriasis rosea. The eruption tends to be moderately pruritic and lasts 3 to 8 weeks. The histologic picture is often not diagnostic, because it can resemble an acute or subacute dermatitis. Treatment is generally directed at alleviating pruritus and consists of oral antihistamines, midpotency topical glucocorticoids, and, in some cases, the use of ultraviolet B phototherapy.

CUTANEOUS INFECTIONS

IMPETIGO AND ECTHYMA *Impetigo* is a common superficial bacterial infection caused by group A beta-hemolytic streptococci or *S. aureus*. The primary lesion is a superficial pustule that ruptures and forms a characteristic yellow-brown "honey-colored" crust. Lesions caused by *Staphylococcus* may be tense, clear bullae, and this form of the disease is called *bullous impetigo*. Lesions may occur on normal skin or in areas already affected by another skin disease. Ecthyma is a variant of impetigo on the lower extremities and causes punched-out ulcerative lesions. In addition to improving hygiene, treatment of both ecthyma and impetigo involves gentle debridement of adherent crusts, which is facilitated by the use of soaks and topical antibiotics in conjunction with appropriate oral antibiotics.

ERYSIPELAS AND CELLULITIS See Chap. 101.

DERMATOPHYTOSIS Fungi that infect skin, hair, and nails include members of the species *Trichophyton*, *Microsporum*, and *Epidermophyton*. Infection of the foot is most common and is referred to as *tinea pedis* (athlete's foot). Tinea pedis is often chronic and is characterized by variable erythema and edema, scaling, pruritus, and occasionally vesiculation. Involvement may be widespread or localized, but almost invariably the web space between the fourth and fifth toes is affected. Infection of the nails (tinea unguium) is characterized by opacified, thickened nails and subungual debris. The groin is the next most commonly involved area, with men affected predominantly. It presents as a scaling erythematous eruption, which spares the scrotum. Microscopic examination of scale after digestion with potassium hydroxide (KOH preparation) of either untreated tinea pedis or tinea cruris usually demonstrates hyphae. However, even short courses of topical antifungal agents may make demonstration of hyphae difficult.

Dermatophyte infection of the scalp (tinea capitis) is quite common,

particularly in inner city clinics. The predominant organism, *Trichophyton tonsurans*, can produce a relatively noninflammatory infection that may present with either well-defined or irregular, diffuse areas of mild scaling and hair loss. Close examination of the scalp may reveal many broken off hairs appearing as small black dots. Unlike infections with *Microsporum* sp., which was previously the most common cause of tinea capitis, lesions caused by *Trichophyton tonsurans* are not fluorescent under a Wood's lamp. Tinea capitis caused by *Microsporum audouini* is characterized by a sharply delineated noninflammatory area in which hairs are broken off close to the surface. Hairs infected with *M. audouini* fluoresce bright bluish green when examined with a Wood's lamp. Tinea corporis, or widespread infection on non-hair-bearing skin, may have a variable appearance, depending on the extent of the associated inflammatory reaction. It may have the typical annular appearance of "ringworm" or appear as deep inflammatory nodules (on the scalp known as *kerions*) or granulomas. KOH examination of scale or hair from patients with tinea capitis or inflammatory tinea corporis often does not reveal hyphae, and diagnosis may require culture.

Both topical and systemic therapies may be used to treat dermatophyte infection. Topical imidazoles and triazoles, including miconazole, ketaconazole, and econazole, may be effective. Haloprogin, undecylic acid, ciclopirox olamine, and tolnaftate are also effective, but nystatin is not active against dermatophytes. Griseofulvin is the drug of choice for dermatophyte infections requiring systemic therapy. While older preparations of griseofulvin required the use of as much as 1 to 2 g of drug daily, newer microsized and ultramicrosized preparations are better absorbed and allow treatment with much lower doses of drug. Generally, a daily dose of 500 mg of microsized or 350 mg of ultramicrosized griseofulvin is adequate. Unresponsive infections may respond to doubling the dose. Griseofulvin is best absorbed if administered with a fatty meal. The most common side effects of griseofulvin are gastrointestinal distress and headache. It is also rarely associated with hematologic and liver function abnormalities, and patients on long-term therapy should be carefully monitored.

The choice of treatment depends on the site involved and the type of infection. For chronic noninflammatory tinea pedis, topical imidazoles or keratolytics are useful to limit pruritus and scaling but are rarely curative. Treatment with oral griseofulvin is effective but may require months of therapy for mycologic cure and, even then, is associated with a high relapse rate, particularly if the nails are involved. The therapy of tinea corporis depends on the extent of disease. Localized infection is best treated with topical imidazoles, but widespread disease, particularly in patients with decreased cellular immunity, requires systemic antifungal therapy.

Dermatophyte infection of hair-bearing areas (such as tinea capitis) requires systemic antifungal therapy, and treatment should be continued for 6 to 8 weeks. The adjunctive use of topical antifungals in addition to systemic therapy may be useful, but topical therapy alone is not adequate. Markedly inflammatory tinea capitis may result in scarring and hair loss, and systemic or topical glucocorticoids may prevent this sequela.

TINEA VERSICOLOR Tinea versicolor is caused by a nondermatophyte dimorphic fungus which is a normal inhabitant of the skin. As the yeast form (*Pityrosporum orbiculare*), it generally does not cause disease (except for folliculitis in certain individuals). However, in some individuals, it converts to the hyphal form and causes characteristic lesions. Infection is promoted by heat and humidity. The typical lesions consist of oval scaly macules, papules, and patches concentrated on the chest, shoulders, and back and rarely on the face or distal extremities. On dark skin they often appear as hypopigmented areas, while on light skin they are slightly hyperpigmented. In some darkly pigmented individuals, they may only appear as scaling patches. A KOH preparation from scaling lesions will demonstrate a confluence of short hyphae and round spores (so-called spaghetti and meatballs). There are many effective topical treatments for tinea versicolor. Solutions containing sulfur, salicylic acid, or selenium sulfide will clear the infection if used daily for a week and then intermittently thereafter. Topical imidazoles are also effective.

CANDIDIASIS Candidiasis is caused by a related group of yeasts, whose manifestations may be localized to the skin or may be systemic and life-threatening. The causative organism is usually *Candida albicans* but may also be *C. tropicalis*, *C. parapsilosis*, and *C. krusei*. These organisms are normal saprophytic inhabitants of the gastrointestinal tract but can overgrow (usually due to broad-spectrum antibiotic therapy) and cause disease at cutaneous sites. Other predisposing factors include diabetes mellitus, chronic intertrigo, and cellular immune deficiency. The oral cavity is commonly involved. Lesions may occur on the tongue or buccal mucosa (thrush) and appear as white plaques. Microscopic examination of scrapings demonstrates both pseudohyphae and yeast forms. Fissured, macerated lesions at the corners of the mouth (perleche) are often seen in individuals with poorly fitting dentures and may also be associated with candidal infection. Additionally, candidal infections have an affinity for sites that are chronically wet and macerated and may occur around nails (onycholysis and paronychia) and in intertriginous areas. Intertriginous lesions are characteristically edematous, erythematous, and scaly, with scattered "satellite pustules." In men there is often involvement of the penis and scrotum as well as the inner aspect of the thighs, and in women the introitus and vagina may be infected. Diagnosis is based upon the clinical pattern and demonstration of yeast on KOH preparation or on culture. Treatment involves removing any predisposing factors such as antibiotic therapy or chronic wetness, the careful control of diabetes mellitus if present, and the use of appropriate topical or systemic antifungal agents.

WARTS Warts are cutaneous neoplasms caused by papillomaviruses. Over 50 different human papillomaviruses (HPV) have been described. Types 1, 2, 4, and 7 cause typical verrucae vulgaris. These lesions are sessile, dome-shaped, usually about a centimeter in diameter, and have a surface made up of many small filamentous projections. These papillomaviruses also cause typical plantar warts and filiform warts in intertriginous areas. Plantar warts are endophytic and are covered by thick keratin. Paring of the wart will generally demonstrate a central core of keratinized debris and punctuate bleeding points. Filiform warts are most common on the face, neck, and skin folds and present as papillomatous lesions on a narrow base. HPV types 3 and 10 are associated with flat warts or verrucae plana. These lesions are only slightly elevated and have a velvety, nonverrucous surface. They have a propensity for the face, arms, and legs and often are spread by shaving.

HPV types 6, 11, 16, 18, 31–35, 39, 48, and 51–54 cause genital tract lesions. Types 6 and 11 are associated with typical lesions of condyloma acuminata, which generally begin as small papillomas and may grow to form large fungating lesions. In women, they may involve either the labia, perineum, or perianal skin. Additionally, the mucosa of the vagina, urethra, and anus can be involved, as well as the cervical epithelium. In men, the lesions often occur initially in the coronal sulcus, but may be seen on the shaft of the penis, the scrotum, perianal skin, or in the urethra. They initially appear as soft, pink filiform lesions, which may enlarge and coalesce to form large cauliflower-like aggregates. HPV types 6 and 11 can also cause juvenile laryngeal papillomas.

HPV also plays a role in the development of neoplasia of the uterine cervix and external genitalia. A high rate of coexistence of condyloma acuminata with cervical dysplasia or carcinoma was initially reported, and HPV DNA has been found in association both with cervical carcinoma and dyplasia and with cancerous and precancerous lesions of the external genitalia. HPV types 16 and 18 have been most intensely studied; other types are also implicated. In men these lesions may initially appear as small, flat, hyperpigmented papules on the penis or perianal skin. The surface of the lesions is generally smooth and velvety, but may be verrucous. The detection of subtle lesions may be improved by treatment with 5% acetic acid, which makes them appear white. In women, cutaneous lesions are generally multiple and often pigmented. They can be located on the

labia majora and minora of the vulva and in the perianal region. Histologic examination of biopsies from affected sites may reveal changes associated with typical warts (hyperkeratosis, papillomatosis, and vacuolated cells) and/or features typical of intraepidermal carcinoma (Bowen's disease). Features in the latter include a disordered maturational sequence of dyskeratotic keratinocytes with hyperchromatic nuclei.

Squamous cell carcinomas are also associated with papilloma virus infections in extragenital skin. This has been seen in patients immunosuppressed after renal transplantation and in patients with the disorder epidermodysplasia verruciformis. Patients in both groups tend to develop multiple cutaneous squamous cell carcinomas on sun-exposed sites associated with several HPV types, including types 5, 8, and 14.

There are many ways to treat warts, but none is universally effective. Perhaps the most useful and convenient method is cryotherapy with liquid nitrogen. Equally effective, but requiring much more patient compliance is the use of keratolytic agents such as salicylic acid plasters or combinations of lactic acid and salicylic acid in flexible collodion. Keratolytic agents are of limited use on mucous membranes and genital lesions. For genital warts, podophyllin solution is moderately effective but may be associated with marked local reactions. Other topical agents used include trichloracetic acid or cantharidin. Electrodesiccation and curettage or carbon dioxide laser are also effective but require local anesthesia. Some caution should be exercised with electrodesiccation or carbon dioxide laser ablation as infectious viral particles may be in the vaporized tissue. Recurrence of warts appears to be common to all these modalities because viral genomic material is present in normal-appearing skin adjacent to the clinical lesions. Treatment should be tempered by recognition that most warts in normal individuals resolve spontaneously within 1 to 2 years. Also, only a fraction of warts are associated with neoplasia, and those are almost exclusively located on the genitalia or perianal skin.

HERPES SIMPLEX See Chap. 135.
HERPES ZOSTER See Chap. 136.

ACNE

ACNE VULGARIS Acne vulgaris is usually a self-limited disorder of teenagers and young adults, although 10 to 20 percent of adults may experience some form of the disorder. The permissive factor for the expression of the disease is the increase in sebum release by sebaceous glands after puberty. Small cysts, called comedones, form in hair follicles due to blockage of the follicular orifice by retention of sebum and keratinous material. The action of lipophilic yeast (*Pityrosporum orbiculare*) and bacteria (*Proprionibacterium acnes*) within the comedones releases free fatty acids from sebum, causes inflammation within the cyst, and results in rupture of the cyst wall. An inflammatory reaction develops as a result of extrusion of oily and keratinous debris from the cyst.

The clinical hallmark of acne vulgaris is the comedo, which may be closed (whitehead) or open (blackhead). Closed comedones appear as 1- to 2-mm pebbly white papules that are accentuated when the skin is stretched. They are the precursors of inflammatory lesions, and the contents are not easily expressed. Open comedones, which rarely result in inflammatory acne lesions, have a large dilated follicular orifice and are filled with easily expressible oxidized, darkened oily debris. Closed comedones are usually accompanied by inflammatory lesions: papules, pustules, or nodules.

The earliest lesions in adolescence are generally mildly inflamed or noninflammatory comedones on the forehead followed by more typical inflammatory lesions on the cheeks, nose, and chin. The most common location for acne is the face, but the chest and back may be involved. Most diseases remain mild and do not lead to scarring; a subset of patients develop large inflammatory cysts and nodules, which may drain, and result in significant scarring.

Exogenous and endogenous factors can alter the expression of acne vulgaris. Friction and trauma may rupture preexisting microcomedones and elicit inflammatory acne. This is commonly seen with headbands or chin straps of athletic helmets. Agents that predispose to comedone formation include topical agents in cosmetics or hair preparations such as lanolin, petrolatum, butylstearate, lauryl alcohol, and oleic acid, and chronic topical exposure to certain industrial compounds that contain insoluble cutting oils (impure paraffin oil mixtures), halogenated hydrocarbons, and coal tar and its derivatives. Glucocorticoids, applied topically or administered systemically, may also elicit acne. Other systemic medications such as isoniazid, halogens, dilantin, and phenobarbital may produce acneiform eruptions or aggravate preexisting acne.

Treatment is directed toward elimination of comedones, decreasing the population of lipophilic bacteria and yeast, and decreasing inflammation. Although areas affected with acne should be kept clean, removal of surface oils does not play an important role in therapy. Indeed, overly vigorous scrubbing may aggravate acne due to mechanical rupture of comedones. Oral tetracycline or erythromycin in doses of 250 to 1000 mg daily will decrease follicular colonization with some lipophilic organisms and may have an anti-inflammatory effect independent of antibacterial effects. Topical agents such as retinoic acid, benzoyl peroxide, or salicylic acid may alter the pattern of epidermal desquamation, prevent the formation of comedones, and aid in the resolution of preexisting cysts. Topical antibacterial agents like benzoyl peroxide, topical erythromycin, clindamycin, or tetracycline are also useful adjuncts to therapy. Severe nodulocystic acne not responsive to oral antibiotics and topical therapy may be treated with the synthetic retinoid isotretinoin at doses of 0.5 to 1.0 mg/kg body weight per day for 15 to 20 weeks. The use of this drug is limited by its teratogenicity, and women must be screened for pregnancy prior to initiating therapy, maintain a fail-safe method of birth control during treatment, and be screened for pregnancy during treatment. Patients receiving this medication develop extremely dry skin and cheilitis and must be followed for development of hypertriglyceridemia. Patients treated with isotretinoin, particularly those on long-term therapy for disorders other than acne, are also at risk to develop calcifications of tendons and bony overgrowths of vertebrae.

ACNE ROSACEA Acne rosacea is an inflammatory disorder predominantly affecting the central face. It rarely affects patients under age 30. Rosacea is more common in women, but those most severely affected are men. It is characterized by erythema, telangiectasias, and superficial pustules and is not associated with comedones. Rosacea rarely involves the chest or back.

There is a relationship between the tendency for pronounced facial flushing and the subsequent development of acne rosacea. Initially, individuals with rosacea demonstrate a pronounced flushing reaction. This may be in response to heat, emotional stimuli, alcohol, hot drinks, or spicy foods. As the disease progresses, the flush persists longer and longer, eventually becoming permanent. Papules, pustules, and telangiectasias then become superimposed on the persistent flush.

Rosacea of long standing may lead to connective tissue overgrowth, particularly of the nose (rhinophyma), and may be complicated by inflammatory disorders of the eye, including keratitis, blepharitis, iritis, and recurrent chalazion. These ocular problems potentially threaten vision and warrant ophthalmologic evaluation.

Acne rosacea can generally be effectively treated with oral tetracycline in doses ranging from 250 to 1500 mg/d. Topical metronidazole is also effective, and low-potency, nonfluorinated topical glucocorticoids, particularly after cool soaks, may alleviate facial erythema. Fluorinated topical glucocorticoids should be avoided since chronic use of these preparations may actually elicit rosacea. Topical therapy is not effective for ocular disease.

REFERENCES

FITZPATRICK TB et al (eds): *Dermatology in General Medicine*, 3d ed. New York, McGraw-Hill, 1987

LEVER WP, LEVER GS: *Histopathology of the Skin*, 6th ed. Philadelphia, Lippincott, 1983

MOSCHELLA SL, HURLEY HH (eds): *Dermatology*, 2d ed. Philadelphia, Saunders, 1985

PETO R, ZUR HAUSEN H: *Viral Etiology of Cervical Cancer: Banbury Report*. Cold Spring Harbor, Cold Spring Harbor Laboratory, 1986

PLEWIG G, KLIGMAN AM: *Acne: Morphogenesis and Treatment*. New York, Springer-Verlag, 1975

57   CUTANEOUS DRUG REACTIONS

BRUCE U. WINTROUB / ROBERT S. STERN

Cutaneous reactions are among the most frequent adverse reactions to drugs. Early in drug-induced illness, prompt therapeutic intervention may limit toxicity. This chapter focuses on adverse cutaneous reactions to drugs other than topical agents and reviews the incidence, patterns, and pathogenesis of cutaneous reactions to drugs and therapeutic agents.

USE OF PRESCRIPTION DRUGS IN THE UNITED STATES As of 1981, about 54,000 drug products, comprising nearly 1900 different active agents, were available in the United States with more than 1000 new chemical entities introduced since 1940. Hospital inpatients alone annually receive about 120 million courses of drug therapy, and half of adult Americans receive prescription drugs on a regular outpatient basis. Approximately 1 in 7 hospital days is devoted to treatment for drug toxicity, at a cost exceeding $12 billion per year.

INCIDENCE OF CUTANEOUS REACTIONS Although adverse drug reactions are common, it is difficult to ascertain their incidence, seriousness, and ultimate health effects. The fact that comprehensive information on these reactions is inadequate in part reflects the difficulty in establishing a system for postmarketing surveillance that is both economically feasible and capable of generating clinically useful data. Available information comes from evaluation of hospitalized patients, epidemiologic surveys, premarketing studies, and voluntary reporting.

In one study about 2 percent of medical inpatients had skin reactions consisting of rash, urticaria, or pruritus during hospitalization, and the overall reaction rate per course of drug therapy was 3:1000. Penicillins, sulfonamides, and blood products accounted for two-thirds of cutaneous reactions. In another study of 491 case records, drug-specific reaction rates were estimated for 42 days. This study showed that most cutaneous reactions occur within 1 week of exposure to the drug; exceptions were semisynthetic penicillins and ampicillin; about half of the reactions to these drugs occurred more than 1 week after initial administration. The risk of allergic reactions was not related to age, diagnosis, or blood level of urea nitrogen on admission. Skin reactions were more frequent among women.

In one study of 464 patients with drug eruptions cared for within hospital dermatology departments over a multiyear period, the most common morphologic patterns were classified as exanthematous (46 percent), urticaria and/or angioedema (23 percent), fixed drug eruption (19 percent), erythema multiforme (5.4 percent), and Stevens-Johnson syndrome (4.0 percent). Four percent of cases had exfoliative dermatitis, 3 percent had photosensitivity reactions, 1.5 percent had anaphylaxis, and 1.5 percent had toxic epidermal necrolysis; two patients died. The eruptions were attributed to more than 50 drugs, the most common being sulfonamide- and penicillin-related antibiotics.

PATHOGENESIS OF DRUG REACTIONS

Untoward cutaneous responses to drugs can arise as the result of immunologic or nonimmunologic mechanisms. Immunologic reactions require activation of host immunologic pathways and are designated *drug allergy*. Drug reactions occurring through nonimmunologic mechanisms may be due to activation of effector pathways, overdosage, cumulative toxicity, side effects, ecologic disturbance, interactions between drugs, metabolic alterations, exacerbation of preexisting dermatologic conditions, or inherited protein or enzyme deficiencies. Nonimmunologic cutaneous reactions to drugs are more common, and immunologic reactions are unpredictable when they do occur. It is often not possible to specify the responsible drug or pathogenic mechanism because the skin responds to a variety of stimuli through a limited number of reaction patterns. The mechanism of many drug reactions is unknown.

IMMUNOLOGIC DRUG REACTIONS Drugs frequently elicit an immune response, but only a small number of individuals experience clinical hypersensitivity reactions. For example, most patients exposed to penicillin develop demonstrable antibodies to penicillin but do not manifest drug reactions when exposed to penicillin. Multiple factors determine the capacity of a drug to elicit an immune response, including the *molecular characteristics* of the drug and *host effects*.

Increases in *molecular* size and complexity are associated with increased immunogenicity, and macromolecular drugs such as protein or peptide hormones are highly antigenic. Most drugs are small organic molecules less than 1000 daltons in size, and the capacity of such small molecules to elicit an immune response depends upon their ability to act as haptens, that is, to form stable, usually covalent, bonds with tissue macromolecules. Fortunately, most drugs have little or no ability to form covalent bonds with tissue components, and clinical sensitization results from minor contaminants or conversion of the drugs themselves to reactive metabolic products.

Route of administration of a drug or simple chemical can influence the nature of the *host* immune response. For example, topical application of antigens tends to induce delayed hypersensitivity, and exposure to antigens via oral or nasal cavities stimulates production of secretory immunoglobins, IgA and IgE, and occasionally IgM. Some agents, such as pentadecacatechol, sensitize readily if applied to the skin but do so poorly if orally ingested or applied to a mucosal surface. Frequency of sensitization through intravenous administration of drugs varies, but anaphylaxis is a more likely clinical consequence with this route of exposure.

The degree of drug exposure and individual variability in absorption and metabolism of a given agent may alter immunogenic load. The variable degree of in vivo acetylation of hydralazine provides a clinical example of this phenomenon. Hydralazine produces a lupus-like syndrome associated with antinuclear antibody formation more frequently in patients who acetylate the drug slowly. Frequent high-dose and interrupted courses of therapy are also important risk factors for development of drug allergy.

Pathogenesis of allergic drug reactions IgE-dependent drug reactions are usually manifest in the skin and gastrointestinal, respiratory, and cardiovascular systems (see Chap. 267). Primary symptoms and signs include pruritus, urticaria, nausea, vomiting, cramps, bronchospasm, and laryngeal edema and, on occasion, anaphylactic shock with hypotension and death. Immediate reactions may occur within minutes of drug exposure, and accelerated reactions occur hours or days after drug administration. Accelerated reactions are usually urticarial and may include laryngeal edema. IgE-dependent reactions are usually due to penicillins, manifestations are caused by release from sensitized tissue mast cells or circulating basophilic leukocytes of chemical mediators such as histamine, adenosine, leukotrienes, prostaglandins, platelet activating factor, enzymes, and proteoglycans. Release is triggered when polyvalent drug protein conjugates cross-link IgE molecules fixed to sensitized cells. The clinical manifestations are determined by interaction of the released chemical mediator with its target organ, i.e., skin, respiratory, gastrointestinal, and/or cardiovascular systems. Certain routes of administration favor different clinical patterns (i.e., oral route: gastrointestinal effects; intravenous route: circulating effects).

Immune-complex-dependent reactions Serum sickness is produced by circulating immune complexes and is characterized by fever, arthritis, nephritis, neuritis, edema, and an urticarial, papular, or pruritic rash (see Chap. 268). The syndrome requires an antigen that remains in the circulation for prolonged periods so that when antibody is synthesized, circulating antigen-antibody complexes are formed. Serum sickness was first described following administration of foreign sera, but drugs are now the usual cause. Drugs that produce serum sickness include the penicillins, sulfonamides, thiouracils, cholecystographic dyes, phenytoin, aminosalicylic acid, streptomycin, and antilymphocyte globulin. Symptoms develop 6 days or more after exposure to a drug, the latent period representing the time needed to synthesize antibody. The antibodies responsible for immune-complex-dependent drug reactions are largely of the IgG or IgM class.

Cytotoxic drug-induced reactions Immunologic reactions to drugs may damage kidneys, heart, lungs, liver, muscle, peripheral nerves, or formed elements of the blood by at least three mechanisms. First, a drug may react with the tissue and introduce haptenic groups on a cell surface that renders the tissue susceptible to antibody- or lymphocyte-mediated cytotoxicity. Second, drug-antibody complexes formed in the fluid phase may bind to the cell surface and damage the cell as an "innocent bystander." Third, drugs may induce immune responses that involve formed blood elements such as platelets and erythrocytes but do not cause cutaneous allergic drug reactions.

Cell-mediated immune responses play a role in contact drug hypersensitivity and are suspected to participate in other allergic drug reactions (i.e., pulmonary infiltration).

NONIMMUNOLOGIC DRUG REACTIONS Nonimmunologic mechanisms are responsible for the majority of drug reactions.

Nonimmunologic activation of effector pathways Drug reactions may result from nonimmunologic activation of effector pathways by three mechanisms: First, drugs may directly release mediators from mast cells and basophils and present as anaphylaxis or as urticaria and/or angioedema. Urticarial anaphylactic reactions induced by opiates, polymyxin B, tubocurarine, radiocontrast media, and dextrans may occur by this mechanism. Second, drugs may activate complement in the absence of antibody. This is an additional mechanism through which radiocontrast media may act. Third, drugs such as aspirin and other nonsteroidal anti-inflammatory agents may alter pathways of arachidonic acid metabolism; such drugs inhibit the cyclooxygenase that catalyzes the generation of prostaglandins from arachidonic acid in vitro.

Overdosage The manifestations of overdosage are predictable for most drugs; symptoms are an exaggeration of the drug's pharmacologic action. Overdosage can, at times, be observed in patients given the usual doses of the drug because of differing rates of absorption, metabolism, or excretion. An example is easy bruisability caused by warfarin overdose.

Phototoxicity Phototoxic reactions may be drug-induced or may occur in metabolic disorders in which an appropriate photosensitizing chemical is overproduced. In each case, the phototoxic reaction occurs when enough chromophore (drug or metabolic product) absorbs sufficient radiation in reactive tissue. Drug-induced phototoxic reactions can occur on first exposure, and the incidence of phototoxicity is a direct function of the concentration of sensitizer and amount of light. At least three distinct photochemical mechanisms have been described: First, the reaction between the excited state of a phototoxic molecule and a biologic target may cause formation of a covalent photoaddition product. Second, the phototoxic molecule may absorb protons to form stable photoproducts that are toxic to biologic substrates. Third, radiation of a phototoxic molecule may result in transfer of energy to oxygen molecules and cause formation of toxic oxygen species, such as singlet oxygen, superoxide anion, or hydroxyl radical. Interaction of these species with biologic targets produces photooxidized molecules. Serum protein-dependent systems and circulating effector cells play a role in acute in vivo phototoxic tissue damage due to exogenous agents; normal numbers of polymorphonuclear leukocytes and an intact complement system are required for the full development of demeclocycline-induced phototoxic lesions.

Cumulative toxicity The cumulative effects of drug deposition in skin may cause disturbance in skin color. In some instances, the drug is deposited in phagocytic cells of skin or mucous membranes, as occurs after prolonged administration of silver, bismuth, mercury, or gold. In other instances, the drug or its metabolic derivatives may bind to a component of the skin (for instance, melanin) as in patients taking high doses of chlorpromazine.

Secondary or side effects Secondary effects occur uniformly as part of the normal pharmacologic action of a drug but are not the primary therapeutic objective. Examples include alopecia, gastrointestinal disturbances, or hematopoietic depression during use of chemotherapeutic agents.

Ecologic disturbances These reactions result from drug-dependent alterations of normal flora of the skin, gut, or mucous membranes, permitting overgrowth of an organism (e.g., anogenital and oral candidiasis during administration of a broad-spectrum antibiotic).

Drug interactions Drugs may interact to cause adverse reactions. First, drugs may compete for the same plasma protein binding sites. For example, warfarin may be displaced from its binding site by phenylbutazone or aspirin and result in hemorrhage. Second, a drug may inhibit or stimulate metabolic enzymes important to its degradation or to that of another agent. Third, one drug may interfere with the excretion of another; for example, probenecid reduces penicillin excretion by the kidney.

Metabolic changes Drugs may sufficiently alter nutritional or metabolic status to induce cutaneous changes. For example, drugs, such as phenytoin, that interfere with folate absorption or metabolism increase the risk of aphthous stomatitis. In addition, drugs that alter lipid metabolism, such as isotretinoin, cause xanthomas by elevation of very low-density lipoproteins.

Exacerbation of preexisting diseases A variety of agents can exacerbate preexisting diseases. For example, lithium can exacerbate acne and psoriasis in a dose-dependent manner. Beta-blocking agents may induce a psoriasiform dermatitis, and withdrawal of glucocorticoids can exacerbate psoriasis or atopic dermatitis. Exacerbations of cutaneous lupus have been noted in association with cimetidine use. Vasodilators may exacerbate rosacea.

Inherited enzyme or protein deficiencies Drug reactions may also occur as the result of inherited enzyme deficiencies. For example, patients may be deficient in an enzyme required for metabolism of the drug or clearance of a toxic drug metabolite. The phenytoin hypersensitivity syndrome occurs in patients deficient in epoxide hydrolase, an enzyme required for metabolism of a toxic epoxide derived from phenytoin. Second, patients may be deficient in an enzyme required for normal function of a biochemical pathway, and further drug-induced lowering of the factor may cause pathologic manifestations. An example is warfarin sodium (Coumadin) necrosis of skin in patients with heterozygote deficiency of protein C, a proenzyme required for normal thrombolytic function.

CHARACTERISTIC FEATURES OF CUTANEOUS DRUG REACTIONS

Cutaneous disorders induced by drugs by known mechanisms include: urticaria, photosensitivity, disturbances of pigmentation, vasculitis, phenytoin hypersensitivity syndrome, and warfarin necrosis of skin. Reactions of uncertain mechanism include: morbilliform reactions, erythema multiforme, fixed drug reactions, erythema nodosum, lichenoid reactions, bullous drug reaction, and toxic epidermal necrolysis.

REACTIONS OF KNOWN CAUSE **Urticaria** Urticaria is a skin reaction characterized by pruritic, red wheals. Lesions may vary from a small point to a large area. Individual lesions rarely last more than 24 h. When deep dermal and subcutaneous tissues are also swollen, this reaction is known as *angioedema*. Angioedema may involve mucous membranes and may be part of a life-threatening anaphylactic reaction. Urticarial lesions, along with pruritus and morbilliform (or maculopapular) eruptions, are among the most frequent types of cutaneous reactions to drugs.

Drug-induced urticaria may be caused by three mechanisms: an IgE-dependent mechanism, circulating immune complexes (serum sickness), and nonimmunologic activation of effector pathways. IgE-dependent urticarial reactions usually occur within 36 h but can occur within minutes. Reactions occurring within minutes to hours of drug exposure are termed *immediate reactions*, while those that occur 12 to 36 h after drug exposure are designated *accelerated reactions*. Immune-complex-induced urticaria associated with serum sickness may occur from 4 to 12 days after challenge. In this syndrome, the urticarial eruption may be accompanied by fever, hematuria, and arthralgias, hepatic dysfunction, and neurologic symptoms.

Certain drugs, such as nonsteroidal anti-inflammatory agents and radiographic dyes, may induce urticarial reactions whose time course resembles that of immediate IgE-dependent reactions. Drug-specific antibody does not play a role in such reactions, and they are thought to be induced by the action of drug on cutaneous mast cells, complement, or arachidonic acid–dependent pathways. Although aspirin, penicillin, and blood products are the most frequent causes of urticarial eruptions, urticaria has been observed in association with nearly all drugs.

Drugs may also cause chronic urticaria, which lasts more than 6 weeks. The mechanisms of chronic urticaria are unclear. Aspirin frequently exacerbates this problem.

Photosensitivity eruptions Photosensitivity eruptions are usually most marked in sun-exposed areas but may extend to sun-protected areas. Phototoxic reactions are more common than photoallergic reactions. Phototoxic reactions usually resemble sunburn, can occur with the first exposure to a drug, and are dose-related. The action spectrum for phototoxicity is similar to the ultraviolet absorption spectrum of the drug. No single test system seems to be a successful predictor of the photosensitivity potential for a given compound.

The mechanism for photoallergy to systemic medications is not well defined. Drug, immune response, and light are required to produce clinical photoallergy, and photoallergic reactions may be delayed hypersensitivity responses. Eruptions range from lichenoid papules to eczematous changes.

Orally administered drugs that cause photoallergic or phototoxic reactions include chlorpromazine, tetracycline, thiazides, nalidixic acid, and two nonsteroidal anti-inflammatory agents, benoxaprofen and piroxicam. Based on test systems, the majority of the common photosensitizers seem to have action spectrums in the long-wave ultraviolet (UV-A) range and are usually phototoxic. This is fortunate since phototoxic reactions will abate with removal of either the drug or ultraviolet radiation, but some photoallergic reactions may persist after the drug is withdrawn.

Drugs may also induce photosensitivity diseases. For example, procainamide may induce systemic lupus erythematosus.

Pigmentation changes Drugs may cause a variety of pigmentary changes in the skin. Some drugs stimulate melanocytic activity and increase pigmentation. Drug deposition can also lead to pigmentation; this phenomenon occurs with heavy metals. Phenothiazines may be deposited in the skin and cause a slate-gray color. Antimalarial drugs may cause a slate-gray or yellow pigmentation. Inorganic arsenic, once used to treat psoriasis, is associated with diffuse macular pigmentation. Other heavy metals that cause pigmentary changes include silver, gold, bismuth, and mercury. Long-term use of phenytoin can produce a chloasma-like pigmentation in women. Certain cytostatic agents can also cause pigmentary changes. Histologic examination is often diagnostic for drug deposition diseases.

Clofazimine, an aminophenazine dye used in the treatment of leprosy, causes a red skin color that is so marked that some patients discontinue therapy. Methysergide produces a red color in the skin and an orange-peel-like texture. Nicotinic acid in large doses may cause brown pigmentation. Oral contraceptives may produce chloasma, and adrenocorticotropin may cause a hypermelanosis similar to that of primary adrenal insufficiency. In addition, amiodarone may cause violaceous hyperpigmentation which is increased in sun-exposed skin. Drugs such as heavy metals, copper, antimalarial and arsenical agents, and ACTH may also discolor oral mucosa.

Vasculitis Cutaneous necrotizing vasculitis often presents as palpable purpuric lesions that may be generalized or limited to the lower extremities or other dependent areas (see Chap 276). Urticarial lesions, ulcers, or hemorrhagic blisters also occur. Vasculitis may involve other organs, including the liver, kidney, brain, and joints. Drugs are only one cause of vasculitis. Immune-complex-dependent mechanisms are probably responsible for drug-induced vasculitis and/ or serum sickness. Propylthiouracil induces a cutaneous vasculitis that is accompanied by leukopenia and splenomegaly. Direct immunofluorescent changes in these lesions suggest immune-complex deposition. Drugs implicated in vasculitic eruptions include allopurinol, thiazides, penicillin, and phenytoin.

Phenytoin hypersensitivity reaction The phenytoin hypersensitivity reaction, one of many phenytoin-induced cutaneous reactions, is an erythematous eruption that eventually becomes purpuric and is accompanied by fever, facial and periorbital edema, tender generalized lymphadenopathy, leukocytosis (often with atypical lymphocytes and eosinophils), hepatitis, and sometimes nephritis. The cutaneous reaction usually begins 1 to 3 weeks after phenytoin is begun and resolves rapidly with drug cessation and treatment with systemic glucocorticoids. The eruption recurs with rechallenge. This syndrome apparently results from an inherited deficiency of epoxide hydrolase, an enzyme required for metabolism of a toxic intermediate arene oxide that is formed during metabolism of phenytoin by the cytochrome P_{450} system.

Warfarin necrosis of the skin This rare reaction occurs usually between the third and tenth days of therapy with warfarin derivatives, usually in women. Lesions are sharply demarcated, erythematous, indurated, and purpuric and may resolve or progress to formation of large, irregular, hemorrhagic bullae with eventual necrosis and slow-healing eschar formation.

Development of the syndrome is unrelated to drug dose or underlying condition. Favored sites are breasts, thighs, and buttocks. The course is not altered by discontinuation of the drug after the onset of the eruption. Similar reactions have been associated with heparin. Warfarin reactions are associated with protein C deficiency. Protein C is a vitamin K–dependent protein with a shorter half-life than other clotting proteins and is in part responsible for control of fibrinolysis. Since warfarin inhibits synthesis of vitamin K–dependent coagulation factors, warfarin anticoagulation in heterozygotes for protein C deficiency causes a precipitous fall in circulating levels of protein C, permitting hypercoagulability and thrombosis in the cutaneous microvasculature, with consequent areas of necrosis.

REACTIONS OF UNCERTAIN CAUSE Morbilliform reactions Morbilliform or maculopapular eruptions may be the most common of all drug-induced reactions, often start on the trunk or areas of pressure or trauma, and consist of erythematous macules and papules that are frequently symmetric and may become confluent. Involvement of mucous membranes, palms, and soles is variable; the eruption may be associated with moderate to severe pruritus and fever.

The pathogenesis is unclear. A hypersensitivity mechanism has been suggested, although these reactions do not always recur following drug rechallenge. Diagnosis is rarely assisted by laboratory tests; differentiation from viral exanthem is the principal differential diagnostic consideration. While these reactions usually require discontinuation of drug (dechallenge), eruptions may occasionally decrease or fade with continued use of the responsible drug.

Morbilliform reactions usually develop within 1 week of initiation of therapy and last 1 to 2 weeks; however, reactions to some drugs, especially penicillin, may begin more than 2 weeks after therapy has begun, and last as long as 2 weeks after therapy has ceased. These eruptions are common in patients receiving ampicillin, amoxicillin, or allopurinol; trimethoprim-sulfamethoxazole causes frequent reactions in acquired immunodeficiency syndrome (AIDS) patients.

Erythema multiforme Erythema multiforme is an acute, self-limited inflammatory disorder of skin and mucous membranes characterized by distinctive iris or target lesions, often associated with sore throat and malaise. Many drugs, including sulfonamides, penicillin, phenytoin, and phenylbutazone, can cause erythema multiforme; long-acting sulfonamides are the best-studied. Erythema multiforme resulting from sulfonamides typically begins after 1 to 2 weeks of drug therapy and is accompanied by fever and mucous membrane reaction (Stevens-Johnson syndrome). An immune-complex-induced, lymphocyte-mediated mechanism may be responsible.

Fixed drug reactions These reactions are characterized by one or more sharply demarcated, erythematous lesions in which hyperpigmentation results after resolution of the acute inflammation; with rechallenge, the lesion recurs in the same (i.e., "fixed") location. Lesions often involve the face, genitalia, and oral mucosa and cause burning. Fixed drug eruptions have been associated with phenolphthalein, sulfonamides, tetracycline, phenylbutazone, and barbiturates. Although cross-sensitivity appears to occur between different tetracycline compounds, cross-sensitivity was not elicited when different sulfonamide compounds were administered to patients as part of provocation testing.

Documentation of a characteristic papillary-dermal mononuclear cell infiltrate in close approximation to the dermoepidermal junction may confirm the clinical diagnosis. Extensive basal cell degeneration can lead to formation of bullae and pigment dispersion. Even when lesions are completely healed, melanin-laden macrophages are present in the dermis.

Erythema nodosum Erythema nodosum is a panniculitis characterized by tender, subcutaneous, erythematous nodules, usually on the anterior portion of the legs. Drug hypersensitivity, frequently involving oral contraceptives, is one cause of this reaction. The mechanism is unknown.

Lichenoid drug eruptions A lichenoid cutaneous reaction, clinically and morphologically indistinguishable from lichen planus, is associated with a variety of drugs and chemicals. Eosinophils in lichen planus are more common when the reaction is drug-induced. Gold and antimalarials are most often associated with this eruption. Antihypertensive agents, including beta blockers and captopril, have also been reported to cause a lichenoid reaction.

Bullous eruptions Blisters accompany a wide variety of cutaneous reactions, especially the severe morbilliform eruptions, and may be an integral part of erythema multiforme, toxic epidermal necrolysis, and fixed drug eruptions. Nalidixic acid and furosemide cause blistering eruptions indistinguishable from the primary bullous diseases. Other examples are a pemphigus foliaceus–like eruption seen with penicillamine and cicatricial pemphigoid that has been seen with clonidine.

Toxic epidermal necrolysis Toxic epidermal necrolysis is the most serious cutaneous drug reaction and may be fatal. Drugs are the most frequent cause in adults. Onset is generally acute and is characterized by epidermal necrosis with a minimal dermal inflammatory process. This reaction is often associated with allopurinol and has been reported with measles vaccine, fumigants, phenytoin, sulfonamides, and nonsteroidal anti-inflammatory agents.

DRUGS OF SPECIAL INTEREST

PENICILLIN The incidence of reactions to penicillin is about 1 percent. Not all adverse reactions are immunologic, as illustrated by ampicillin-induced morbilliform eruptions and central nervous system reactions to procaine penicillin.

IgG, IgM, and IgE antibodies can be produced; IgG and IgM anti-penicillin antibodies play a role in the development of hemolytic anemia, whereas anaphylaxis and serum sickness appear to be due to IgE antibodies in serum.

Since penicillin reactions often occur in patients without a prior history of penicillin allergy, the utility of accurate and easily administered tests for sensitization is apparent. Current practice is to perform skin testing with a commercially available penicilloyl determinant preparation (Pre-pen, Kremers-Urban) and with fresh penicillin and if possible with another source of minor (nonpenicilloyl) determinants such as aged or base-treated penicillin. Antibodies to minor determinants are common in patients experiencing anaphylaxis. Testing with major determinants alone detects most patients at risk for anaphylaxis.

Twenty-seven percent (10 to 36 percent) of patients with a positive history of penicillin allergy also have a positive skin test, while 6 percent (3 to 10 percent) with a negative history demonstrate a positive skin response to penicillin. Administering penicillin to those patients with a positive skin test produces reactions in a high proportion (50 to 100 percent); conversely, only a few patients (about 0.5 percent) with negative skin tests react to the drug, and reactions tend to be mild and to occur late. Since a negative skin test may occur during or just after an acute reaction, testing should be performed either prospectively or several months after a suspected reaction. As many as 80 percent of patients lose anaphylactic sensitivity and IgE antibody after several years. Radioallergosorbent test (RAST) and other in vitro tests offer no advantage over properly performed skin testing.

Some cross-reactivity exists between penicillin and nonpenicillin β-lactam antibiotics (e.g., cephalosporins). About half of patients who react to penicillin skin testing also react to cephalosporin skin testing; anaphylaxis from cephalosporins has occurred in patients testing positive to penicillin. The benefit of skin testing with penicillin derivatives and cephalosporins in addition to penicillin is uncertain; in one study none of 120 patients with negative results to penicillin skin tests reacted to semisynthetic penicillinase-resistant agents.

In the face of a positive clinical history of penicillin reaction, another drug should be chosen. If this is not feasible or prudent (e.g., in a pregnant patient with syphilis; with enterococcal endocarditis), skin testing with penicillin is warranted. If skin tests are negative, cautious administration of penicillin is acceptable, although some recommend desensitization of such patients. In those with positive skin tests, desensitization is mandatory if therapeutic use of β-lactam antibiotics is to be undertaken. Various protocols are available, including oral and parenteral approaches. Oral desensitization appears to carry a lesser risk of serious anaphylactic reactions during desensitization. However, desensitization carries the risk of anaphylaxis regardless of how it is performed. After desensitization many patients experience non-life-threatening IgE-mediated untoward reactions to penicillin during their course of therapy. Desensitization is not effective in those with exfoliative dermatitis or morbilliform reactions due to penicillin.

NONSTEROIDAL ANTI-INFLAMMATORY DRUGS Nonsteroidal anti-inflammatory drugs (NSAIDs), including aspirin (but not salicylates in general) and indomethacin (indometacin), cause two broad categories of allergic-like symptoms in susceptible individuals: (1) approximately 1 percent of persons experience urticaria or angioedema; (2) about half as many (0.5 percent) experience rhinosinusitis and asthma; however, about 10 percent of adult asthmatics and one-third of individuals with nasal polyposis and sinusitis may respond adversely to aspirin.

Urticaria/angioedema may be delayed up to 24 h and may occur at any age. The rhinosinusitis-asthma syndrome generally develops within 1 h of drug administration. In young people, the reaction pattern often begins as watery rhinorrhea that can be complicated by nasal and sinus infection, and polyposis, bloody discharge and nasal eosinophilia. In many individuals with this syndrome, asthma eventually ensues that can be life-threatening whenever NSAIDs are subsequently ingested, and symptoms may persist despite avoidance of these drugs. Proof of the association of symptoms and NSAIDs use requires either clear-cut history of symptoms following drug ingestion or an oral challenge. For the latter to be performed with relative safety, (1) asthma must be under good control, (2) the procedure must be conducted in a hospital setting by experienced personnel capable of recognizing and treating acute respiratory responses, and (3) the challenge should begin with very low doses (i.e., <30 mg) of aspirin and increase every 1 to 2 h in doubling doses as tolerated to 650 mg. In a study of 50 consecutive patients with a positive history of aspirin-induced bronchospasm, 84 percent developed pulmonary or nasoocular symptoms with aspirin, but 16 percent did not react; moreover, when subjects who initially tested positive to a challenge were reexposed to aspirin, the clinical reaction pattern was identical in only 60 percent.

While cross-reactivity between NSAIDs is common, it is not immunologic, and patients who are sensitive to NSAIDs cannot be identified by assessment of IgE antibody to aspirin, lymphocyte sensitization, or in vitro immunologic testing. All cross-reacting drugs are cyclooxygenase inhibitors, although salicylates also inhibit cyclooxygenase but (except for aspirin) do not cause the response.

"Desensitization" to the adverse effects of NSAIDs can be accomplished by the challenge procedure above, although repeated challenge at the initial provocation dose may be required. Desensitization works by unknown mechanisms, renders the subject tolerant to all NSAIDs yet studied, persists for at least 24 and up to 96 h, and is probably universal but does not have a positive effect on the underlying disorder.

RADIOCONTRAST MEDIA Large numbers of patients are exposed to radiocontrast agents, and 5 to 10 percent of patients receiving them develop some reaction: urticaria in 1 percent, dyspnea in 0.25 percent, and death in 0.01 percent. Reactions consisting of urticaria and angioedema, asthma, and hypotension mimicking anaphylaxis occur in less than 1 percent of radiocontrast procedures. About one-third of those with mild reactions to previous exposure reeact upon reexposure.

There is no proof of an immunologic mechanism for radiocontrast media reactions. Elevations in plasma histamine occur in those with and without reaction, and may be due to the hypertonicity of these media. In addition, complement activation by both classical and alternative pathways occurs in normal and reactive individuals. In short, the mechanism for these reactions is not understood and no test identifies patients at risk for a radiocontrast medium reaction. Because repeat reactions are common, obtaining a thorough history is the best available technique for identifying those most likely to experience an adverse reaction. Several pretreatment regimens are claimed to decrease repeat reaction rate to about 10 percent. One such regimen consists of 50 mg prednisone at 13, 7, and 1 h before the procedure, and 50 mg diphenhydramine 1 h before the procedure.

HYDANTOINS Phenytoin and other hydantoins cause morbilliform eruptions, erythema multiforme, and toxic epidermal necrolysis, as well as a hypersensitivity reaction (described above) and the pseudolymphoma syndrome. In one study, 5 percent of children treated with phenytoin developed a mild dose-dependent, maculopapular eruption lasting 3 to 5 days and occurring within 2 weeks of starting treatment.

The pseudolymphoma syndrome, consisting of lymphadenopathy and histopathologic lymph node atypia, is a more chronic form of the phenytoin hypersensitivity syndrome, and the cutaneous changes are less marked in this syndrome.

Use of phenytoin is frequently associated with gingival hyperplasia and rarely with a syndrome similar to systemic lupus erythematosus, severe exfoliative dermatitis, and polyarteritis nodosa. Because many hydantoin side effects may be dose-related, drugs that interfere with its elimination (e.g., chloramphenicol) effectively prolong those effects.

Sulfasalazine and allopurinol cause reactions that are indistinguishable from the phenytoin hypersensitivity syndrome. Unlike the hydantoins, an immunologic mechanism seems the most likely explanation for hypersensitivity to these drugs.

THIAZIDES AND SULFONAMIDES Thiazides are among the most common causes of drug-induced urticaria and morbilliform eruptions; they also cause erythema multiforme, drug-induced cutaneous vasculitis, and lichenoid and photosensitivity eruptions. Because they are substituted sulfonamides, antibodies to these diuretics may cross-react with sulfonamide antibiotics and sulfonamide-based hypoglycemic agents. The combination of sulfamethoxazole and trimethoprim causes two distinct cutaneous reactions: (1) an urticarial eruption beginning in the first few days of treatment and (2) a morbilliform eruption often occurring more than 1 week after therapy has begun. The morbilliform reaction is frequent in patients with AIDS and is associated with pancytopenia in some patients. The eruption may have an intensely purpuric character, independent of the presence of vasculitis. One patient developed toxic epidermal necrolysis and pancytopenia following administration of sulfamethoxazole-trimethoprim.

AGENTS USED IN CANCER CHEMOTHERAPY Since many agents used in cancer chemotherapy inhibit cell division, rapidly proliferating elements of the skin, including hair, mucous membranes, and appendages, are sensitive to their effects; as a result, stomatitis and alopecia are among the most frequent dose-dependent side effects of chemotherapy. Onychodystrophy (dystrophic changes in nails) is also seen with bleomycin, hydroxyurea (hydroxycarbamide), and 5-fluorouracil. Sterile cellulitis and phlebitis and ulceration of pressure areas occur with many of these agents. Urticaria, angioedema, exfoliative dermatitis, and erythema of the palms and soles have also been seen, as has local and diffuse hyperpigmentation. Diagnosis and treatment of these reactions are especially difficult because of the underlying malignancy.

TETRACYCLINES While urticaria and morbilliform eruptions are unusual, tetracyclines sometimes cause other cutaneous side effects, including a photosensitivity reaction (as a result of drug-induced phototoxicity) and onycholysis (sometimes with no apparent cutaneous photosensitivity). These reactions occur with demeclocycline, doxycycline, minocycline, tetracycline, and oxytetracycline. Tetracyclines also cause fixed drug and lichenoid eruptions. An acnelike, gram-negative folliculitis with long-term use of tetracycline is due to overgrowth of resistant bacteria.

Several pigmentary abnormalities have been noted. If used during pregnancy or early childhood, tetracycline stains the teeth, sometimes permanently. Minocycline can cause hyperpigmentation in sun-exposed areas and in areas of previous inflammation. Histiocytes that contain iron are responsible for the pigmentary changes. Tetracycline has also been associated with a flulike syndrome (accompanied by headaches, malaise, and eosinophilia) that recurred with rechallenge. A serum sickness–like reaction to minocycline has also been reported.

GLUCOCORTICOIDS Both systemic and topical glucocorticoids cause a variety of skin changes, including acneiform eruptions, atrophy, striae, and other stigmata of Cushing's syndrome, and in sufficiently high doses can retard wound healing. Patients using glucocorticoids are at higher risk for bacterial, yeast, and fungal skin infections that may be misinterpreted as drug eruptions but are in fact drug side effects instead.

ANTIMALARIAL AGENTS Antimalarial agents are used as therapy for several skin diseases, including the skin manifestations of lupus and polymorphous light eruption, but they also can induce cutaneous reactions. In patients with asymptomatic porphyria cutanea tarda, chloroquine increases porphyrin levels and may exacerbate the disease.

Pigmentation disturbances, including black pigmentation of the face, mucous membranes, pretibial and subungual areas, occur with antimalarials, and quinacrine (mepacrine) causes generalized, cutaneous yellow discoloration. Antimalarial agents may exacerbate psoriasis, and exfoliative dermatitis, fixed drug eruptions, lichenoid dermatitis, and erythema annulare centrifugum have all been reported with their use.

GOLD Chrysotherapy has been associated with a variety of dose-related dermatologic reactions (including maculopapular eruptions) that can develop as long as 2 years after initiation of therapy and require months to resolve. Erythema nodosum, psoriasiform dermatitis, vaginal pruritus, eruptions similar to pityriasis rosea, hyperpigmentation, and lichenoid eruptions resembling those seen with antimalarial agents have been reported. After a cutaneous reaction, it is sometimes possible to reinstitute gold therapy at lower doses without recurrence of the dermatitis.

DIAGNOSIS OF DRUG REACTIONS

Possible causes of an adverse reaction can be assessed as definite, probable, possible, or unlikely, based on six variables: (1) previous experience with the drug in the general population, (2) alternative etiologic candidates, (3) timing of events, (4) drug levels or evidence of overdose, (5) patient reaction to dechallenge, and (6) patient reaction to rechallenge.

PREVIOUS EXPERIENCE Tables of relative reaction rates are available and are useful to assess the likelihood that a given drug is responsible for a given cutaneous reaction. The specific morphologic pattern of a drug reaction, however, may modify these reaction rates by increasing or decreasing the likelihood that a given drug is responsible for a given reaction. For example, since fixed eruptions due to drug are more often seen with barbiturates than with penicillin, a fixed drug reaction in a patient taking both types of agents is more likely to be due to the barbiturate even though penicillins have a higher overall drug reaction rate.

ALTERNATIVE ETIOLOGIC CANDIDATES A cutaneous eruption may be due to exacerbation of preexisting disease or to development of new disease unrelated to drugs. For example, a patient with psoriasis may have a flare-up of disease coincidental with administration of penicillin for streptococcal infection; in this case infection is a more likely cause for the flare-up than drug reaction.

TIMING OF EVENTS Since most drug reactions of the skin occur within 1 to 2 weeks of initiation of therapy, reactions beginning after 2 weeks are less likely to be due to drugs.

DRUG LEVELS Some cutaneous reactions are dependent on dosage or cumulative toxicity. For example, lichenoid dermatoses due to gold administration appear more often in patients taking high doses.

DECHALLENGE Most adverse cutaneous reactions to drugs remit with dechallenge (removal of the suspected agent). A reaction is unlikely to be drug-related if improvement occurs without dechallenge or if a patient fails to improve after dechallenge and appropriate therapy.

RECHALLENGE Rechallenge provides the most definitive information concerning adverse cutaneous reactions to drugs, since a reaction failing to recur on rechallenge with a drug is unlikely to be due to that agent. Rechallenge is frequently impractical, however, because the need to ensure patient safety and comfort outweighs the value of the possible information derived from rechallenge.

DIAGNOSIS OF DRUG ALLERGY

Tests for IgE responses include in vivo and in vitro methods, but such tests are available only for a limited number of drugs, including penicillins and cephalosporins, some peptide and protein drugs (insulin, xenogeneic sera), and some agents used for general anesthesia. In vivo testing is accomplished by prick puncture and/or by intradermal skin testing. A wheal-and-flare response 2 by 2 mm greater than that seen with a saline control within 20 min is considered indicative of IgE-mediated mast cell degranulation, provided (1) the patient is not dermographic, (2) the drug does not nonspecifically degranulate mast cells, (3) the drug concentration is not high enough to be irritating, and (4) the buffer itself does not cause wheal-and-flare responses.

Skin testing with major and minor determinants of penicillins or cephalosporins has proved useful for identifying patients at risk of anaphylactic reactions to these agents. However, skin tests themselves carry a small risk of anaphylaxis. Negative skin tests do not rule out IgE-mediated reactivity, and the risk of anaphylaxis in response to penicillin administration in patients with negative skin tests is about 1 percent; about two-thirds of patients with a positive skin test and history of a previous adverse reaction to penicillin experience an allergic response on rechallenge. Skin tests may be negative in allergic patients receiving antihistamines or in those whose allergy is to determinants not present in the test reagent. Although less well studied, similar techniques can identify patients who are sensitive to protein drugs and to agents such as gallamine and succinylcholine. Most other drugs are small molecules, and skin testing with them is unreliable.

In vitro testing for IgE may be done by assessing the ability of serum to bind to antigen and then to bind radiolabeled antibody to IgE (RAST test) or by assessing the ability of the drug to cause histamine release from basophils from drug-sensitive individuals. The RAST test is sensitive and specific but is not available for most drugs; even in the case of penicillin it is available for major determinants only. Similarly, basophil histamine release is a research technique that is not generally available.

There are no generally available and reliable tests for sensitivity to NSAIDs, to agents that directly degranulate mast cells, or to drugs that cause manifestations via immune-complex-mediated complement activation. Although it is possible to screen for the absence of IgA antibody, the utility of this maneuver in preventing transfusion-associated anaphylaxis in IgA-deficient individuals has not been documented.

REFERENCES

ARNDT KA, JICK H: Rates of cutaneous reactions to drugs. JAMA 235:918, 1976
GREENBERGER PA: Contrast media reaction. J Allergy Clin Immunol 74:600, 1984
———, PATTERSON R: Management of drug allergy in patients with acquired immunodeficiency syndrome. J Allergy Clin Immunol 79:484, 1989
PARKER CW: Drug allergy. N Engl J Med 292:511, 1975
PASRICHA JS: Drugs causing fixed eruptions. Br J Dermatol 100:183, 1979
PLESKOW W et al: Aspirin desensitization in aspirin sensitive asthmatics: Characterization of the refactory period. J Allergy Clin Immunol 69:11, 1982
REVUZ J et al: Toxic epidermal necrolysis: Clinical findings and prognosis factors in 87 patients. Arch Dermatol 123:160, 1987
SAXON A: Immediate hypersensitivity reactions to beta-lactam antibiotics. Rev Infect Dis 5:5368, 1983
SOGN DD: Penicillin allergy. J Allergy Clin Immunol 74:589, 1984
SPEILBERG SP et al: Predisposition to phenytoin hepatotoxicity assessed *in vitro.* N Engl J Med 307:722, 1981
STANLEY J, FALLON-PELLICCI V: Phenytoin hypersensitivity reaction. Arch Dermatol 14:1350, 1978
STERN RS, BIGBY M: An expanded profile of cutaneous reactions to non-steroidal antiinflammatory drugs. JAMA 252:1433, 1984

58   IMMUNOLOGICALLY MEDIATED SKIN DISEASES

KIM B. YANCEY / THOMAS J. LAWLEY

A number of immunologically mediated skin diseases and the cutaneous manifestations of immunologically mediated systemic disorders are now recognized as distinct entities with relatively consistent clinical, histologic, and immunopathologic findings. Many of these disorders are due to autoimmune mechanisms. Clinically, they are characterized by morbidity (pain, pruritus, disfigurement) and in some instances by mortality (largely due to loss of epidermal barrier function and/or secondary infection). The major features of the more common immunologically mediated skin diseases are summarized in this chapter. See Table 58-1.

PEMPHIGUS VULGARIS   Pemphigus vulgaris (PV) is a blistering skin disease seen predominantly in elderly patients. Jewish patients with PV have an increased incidence of the HLA-DR4 haplotype. This disorder is characterized by the loss of cohesion between epidermal cells (a process termed *acantholysis*) with the resultant formation of intraepidermal blisters. Clinical lesions of PV typically consist of flaccid blisters on either normal-appearing or erythematous skin. These blisters rupture easily, leaving denuded areas that may crust and enlarge peripherally. Substantial portions of the body surface may be denuded in severe cases. Manual pressure to the skin of these patients may elicit the separation of the epidermis from the dermis—Nikolsky's sign. This finding, while characteristic of PV, is not specific to this disorder and is also seen in toxic epidermal necrolysis, Stevens-Johnson syndrome, and a few other skin diseases. The skin lesions in PV typically present on the scalp, face, neck, axilla, trunk, and oral cavity. In half or more patients, lesions begin in the mouth; approximately 90 percent of patients have oromucosal involvement at some time during the course of their disease. Involvement of other mucosal surfaces (e.g., pharyngeal, laryngeal, esophageal, conjunctival, vulval, or rectal) can also occur in severe disease. Extensive denudation may be associated with pain of varying severity. Lesions usually heal without scarring except at sites complicated by secondary infection or mechanically induced dermal wounds. Nonetheless, postinflammatory hyperpigmentation is usually present at sites of healed lesions for some time. Although pemphigus occurs in several autoimmune diseases, its association with thymoma and/or myasthenia gravis is particularly significant. To date, more than 30 cases of thymoma and/or myasthenia gravis have been reported in association with pemphigus, usually with pemphigus foliaceus (see below).

Biopsies of early lesions demonstrate intraepidermal vesicle formation secondary to loss of cohesion between epidermal cells (i.e., acantholytic blisters). Blister cavities contain epidermal acantholytic cells which appear as round homogeneous cells containing hyperchromatic nuclei. Basal keratinocytes remain attached to the epidermal basement membrane so that blister formation is within the suprabasal portion of the epidermis. In addition, lesional skin may contain focal collections of intraepidermal eosinophils and granulocytes within blister cavities; dermal alterations are slight, usually limited to an eosinophil-predominant leukocytic infiltrate. Direct immunofluorescence microscopy of normal-appearing, perilesional skin shows IgG on the surface of keratinocytes; deposits of the third component of complement (C3) may occur in the same distribution. These deposits of IgG are derived from a circulating autoantibody directed against keratinocyte cell surface antigens. Circulating autoantibodies can be demonstrated in 80 to 90 percent of PV patients by indirect immunofluorescence microscopy; monkey esophagus is the optimal substrate for demonstration of these autoantibodies. These autoantibodies are responsible for dysadhesion of epidermal cells probably through the activation of endogenous proteases in keratinocytes. The titer of circulating autoantibody (determined by indirect immunofluorescence microscopy) correlates roughly with disease activity. These immunopathologic findings aid the diagnosis of PV and its differentiation from other blistering skin diseases.

PV can be life-threatening. Prior to the availability of glucocorticoids, the mortality ranged from 60 to 90 percent. The current mortality is approximately 5 to 15 percent. Common causes of morbidity and mortality are infection and complications of treatment with glucocorticoids. Bad prognostic factors include advanced age, widespread involvement, and the requirement for high doses of glucocorticoids (with or without other immunosuppressive agents) for control of disease. The course of PV in individual patients is variable and difficult to predict. Some patients achieve remission after variable periods of treatment (40 percent of patients in some series) but others may require long-term treatment or succumb to complications of their disease or its treatment. The mainstay of treatment is systemic glucocorticoids. Patients with moderate to severe disease are usually started on prednisone 60 to 80 mg/d. If new lesions continue to appear after 1 to 2 weeks of treatment, the dose should be increased. Many regimens have combined an immunosuppressive agent with systemic glucocorticoids for control of PV. The two most frequently used are either azathioprine (1 mg/kg per day) or cyclophosphamide (1 mg/kg per day). It is important to

TABLE 58-1 Immunologically mediated blistering skin diseases

Disease	Clinical	Histology	Immunopathology
Pemphigus vulgaris	Flaccid blisters, denuded skin, oromucosal lesions	Blister formed in suprabasal layer of epidermis	Cell surface deposits of IgG on keratinocytes
Pemphigus foliaceus	Crusts and shallow erosions on scalp, central face, neck, upper chest, and back	Blister formed in superficial layers of epidermis	Cell surface deposits of IgG on keratinocytes
Bullous pemphigoid	Large tense blisters on flexor surfaces	Blister formed in subepidermal region, usually eosinophil-rich	Linear band of IgG or C3 at BMZ*
Dermatitis herpetiformis	Extremely itchy small papules and vesicles on elbows, knees, buttocks, and posterior nuchal area	Subepidermal blister with neutrophils in dermal papillae	Granular deposits of IgA in dermal papillae
Linear IgA dermatosis	Extremely itchy small papules and vesicles on extensor surfaces, occasionally larger arciform blisters	Subepidermal blister with neutrophils in dermal papillae	Linear band of IgA at BMZ
Epidermolysis bullosa acquisita	Blisters and scarring on dorsum of hands, elbows, knees, oromucosal lesions	Blister is subepidermal and can be inflammatory or not	Linear band of IgG or C3 at BMZ

* BMZ = basement membrane zone.

bring severe or progressive disease under control quickly to lessen the severity and/or duration of this disorder.

PEMPHIGUS FOLIACEUS Pemphigus foliaceus (PF) is distinguished from PV by several features. In PF, acantholytic blisters are located high within the epidermis, usually just beneath the stratum corneum. Hence, PF is a more superficial blistering disease than PV. The distribution of lesions in the two disorders is much the same except that in the former, mucous membrane lesions are rare and usually limited to superficial erosions. Patients with PF rarely demonstrate intact blisters but rather exhibit shallow erosions associated with erythema, scale, and crust formation. Mild cases of PF resemble severe seborrheic dermatitis; severe PF may cause extensive exfoliation. Sun exposure (ultraviolet irradiation) may be an aggravating factor. A blistering skin disease endemic to south central Brazil known as fogo selvagem or Brazilian pemphigus is clinically, histologically, and immunopathologically indistinguishable from PF.

Patients with PF have immunopathologic features in common with PV. Specifically, direct immunofluorescence microscopy of apparently normal, perilesional skin demonstrates IgG and C3 on the surface of keratinocytes. As in PV, patients with PF frequently have circulating IgG autoantibodies against keratinocyte cell surface antigens. Guinea pig esophagus is the optimal substrate for indirect immunofluorescence microscopy studies of sera from patients with PF.

PF is generally a far less severe disease than PV and carries a better prognosis. Localized disease can be treated conservatively with topical or intralesional glucocorticoids; more active cases can usually be controlled with systemic glucocorticoids, such as prednisone 20 to 40 mg/d.

BULLOUS PEMPHIGOID Bullous pemphigoid (BP) is a subepidermal blistering skin disease usually seen in the elderly. Lesions typically consist of tense blisters on either normal-appearing or erythematous skin. The lesions are usually distributed over the lower abdomen, groin, and flexor surface of the extremities; oral mucosal lesions are found in 10 to 40 percent of patients. Pruritus may be nonexistent or severe. As lesions evolve, tense blisters tend to rupture and be replaced by flaccid lesions or erosions with or without surmounting crust. Nontraumatized blisters heal without scarring. There is no ethnic or HLA association. Patients with BP do not have an increased incidence of malignancy in comparison with appropriately age- and sex-matched controls.

While biopsies of early lesional skin demonstrate subepidermal blisters, the histologic features depend on the character of the particular lesion. Lesions on normal-appearing skin generally show a sparse perivascular leukocytic infiltrate with some eosinophils. Biopsies of inflammatory lesions typically show an eosinophil-rich, leukocytic infiltrate within the papillary dermis, at sites of vesicle formation, and in perivascular areas. In addition to eosinophils, these cell-rich lesions also contain mononuclear cells and neutrophils. It is not always possible to distinguish BP from other subepidermal blistering skin diseases by routine histologic techniques.

Immunopathologic studies have broadened our understanding of this disease and aided its diagnosis. Direct immunofluorescence microscopy of normal-appearing, perilesional skin shows linear deposits of IgG and/or C3 in the epidermal basement membrane. Other immunoreactants such as factor B or C4 may be found in the same location. The sera of approximately 70 percent of these patients contain circulating IgG autoantibodies that bind the epidermal basement membrane of normal human skin in indirect immunofluorescence microscopy. No correlation exists between the titer of these autoantibodies and disease activity. The autoantibodies recognize a 220,000-dalton glycoprotein constituent of the basement membranes of normal stratified squamous epithelial cells. Autoantibodies are believed to develop against this antigen, deposit in situ, activate complement, elicit the accumulation and activation of leukocytes, and prompt dermal mast cell degranulation. The net consequence is to cause blister formation and tissue damage.

BP is generally benign, but may persist for months to years, with exacerbations or remissions. Although extensive involvement may result in widespread erosions and compromise cutaneous integrity, the mortality rate is low even in the absence of treatment. Nonetheless, deaths may occur in elderly and/or debilitated patients. The mainstay of treatment is systemic glucocorticoids. Patients with local or minimal disease can sometimes be controlled with topical glucocorticoids alone; patients with more extensive lesions generally respond to systemic glucocorticoids either alone or in combination with immunosuppressive agents. Patients will usually respond to prednisone 40 to 60 mg/d. In some instances azathioprine (1 mg/kg per day) or cyclophosphamide (1 mg/kg per day) are necessary adjuncts.

DERMATITIS HERPETIFORMIS Dermatitis herpetiformis (DH) is an intensely pruritic, chronic papulovesicular skin disease. The lesions are usually symmetrically distributed over extensor surfaces, including elbows, knees, buttocks, back, scalp, and posterior neck. The primary lesion in this disorder is a papule, papulovesicle, or urticarial plaque. Because pruritus is prominent, patients may present with excoriations and crusted papules but no observable primary lesions. Patients also sometimes report that their pruritus may have a distinctive burning or stinging component, and the onset of these local symptoms reliably heralds the development of distinct clinical lesions 12 to 24 h later. Granular deposits of IgA (with or without C3) are present in the epidermal basement membrane zone in both normal and lesional skin. Thus, while cutaneous deposits of IgA are thought to be very important in the pathogenesis of DH, they are not sufficient to cause lesions. Exactly what else is necessary to induce clinical lesions is not known. Almost all of these patients have an associated, usually subclinical, gluten-sensitive enteropathy (also see Chap. 240) and more than 90 percent express the HLA-B8/DRw3 and HLA-DQw2 haplotypes. Patients with DH and granular deposits of IgA within their epidermal basement membrane zone are distinguished from those with linear deposits of IgA at this site in their skin (see "Linear IgA Dermatosis"). DH may present at any age, including childhood; onset in the second to fourth decades is most common. The disease is typically chronic.

Biopsy of early lesional skin reveals neutrophil-rich infiltrates within dermal papillae. Neutrophils, fibrin, edema, and microvesicle formation at these sites are characteristic of early disease. Older lesions may demonstrate nonspecific features of a subepidermal bulla or an excoriated papule. Because the clinical and histologic features of this disease can be variable and resemble other subepidermal blistering disorders, the diagnosis can be confirmed by direct immunofluorescence microscopy of normal-appearing, perilesional skin. Such studies demonstrate the previously described granular deposits of IgA in the sublamina densa region of the basement membrane zone. Circulating autoantibodies directed against this site in skin have not been demonstrated. Hence, the importance of studying tissue samples for the presence of immunoreactants in situ for evidence of circulating autoantibodies is apparent. IgA deposits in the skin are unaffected by control of disease with medication; however, these immunoreactants may diminish in intensity or disappear in patients maintained for long periods on a strict gluten-free diet (see below).

Although most DH patients do not report overt gastrointestinal symptoms or laboratory evidence of malabsorption, biopsies of small bowel usually reveal blunting of intestinal villi and a lymphocytic infiltrate in the lamina propria. As is true for patients with celiac disease, this gastrointestinal abnormality can be reversed by a gluten-free diet. Moreover, if maintained for a long enough period of time, this diet alone may control the skin disease, and eventually it may not be possible to demonstrate IgA in the epidermal basement membrane zone. Subsequent gluten exposure in the latter patients alters the morphology of their small bowel, elicits a flare of their skin disease, and is associated with the reappearance of IgA in their epidermal basement membrane zone. Patients with DH also have an increased incidence of thyroid abnormalities, achlorhydria, atrophic gastritis, and antigastric parietal cell antibodies. These associations likely relate to the high frequency of the HLA-B8/DRw3 haplotype in these patients since this phenotype is commonly linked to autoimmune disorders. The mainstay of treatment is dapsone. Patients respond rapidly (24 to 48 h) to dapsone but require careful pretreatment evaluation and close follow-up to ensure that complications are avoided or controlled. All patients on more than 100 mg/d dapsone will have some hemolysis and methemoglobinemia. These are expected pharmacologic side effects of dapsone. It is important to employ the lowest possible maintenance dose of dapsone to control symptoms and lesions. Gluten restriction can control DH and lessen dapsone requirements, but this diet must rigidly exclude gluten to be of benefit. Moreover, many months of dietary restriction may be necessary before a beneficial result is achieved. Good dietary counseling by a trained dietitian is essential.

LINEAR IgA DERMATOSIS Linear IgA dermatosis (or linear IgA disease) was formerly considered a variant form of dermatitis herpetiformis. However, this disorder is actually a separate and distinct entity. Clinically, these patients may resemble typical cases of DH, bullous pemphigoid, or other subepidermal blistering skin diseases. Lesions typically consist of papulovesicles, bullae, and/or urticarial plaques, predominantly on extensor (as seen in "classic" DH), central, or flexural sites. Oral mucosal involvement does occur in selected patients. Severe pruritus resembles that in patients with DH. Patients with linear IgA dermatosis do not have an increased frequency of the HLA-B8/DRw3 haplotype or an associated enteropathy and hence are not candidates for a gluten-free diet.

The histologic alterations in early lesions may be virtually indistinguishable from those in DH. However, direct immunofluorescence microscopy of normal-appearing, perilesional skin reveals linear deposits of IgA (and often C3) in the epidermal basement membrane. Selected patients with linear IgA dermatosis demonstrate circulating IgA autoantibodies against normal epidermal basement membrane. As in classic DH, patients respond promptly to treatment with dapsone, 50 to 200 mg/d.

EPIDERMOLYSIS BULLOSA ACQUISITA Epidermolysis bullosa acquisita (EBA) is a rare, noninherited, polymorphic, subepidermal blistering skin disease. Since lesions generally occur in sites prone to minor trauma (e.g., dorsum of the hands, elbows, knees, etc.), EBA is regarded as a mechanobullous disease. Patients with the classic or noninflammatory form of this disease have blisters on noninflamed skin as well as atrophic scarring, milia, nail dystrophy, and oral lesions. Other patients with EBA have widespread inflammatory, scarring, bullous lesions and oromucosal involvement. Cases of inflammatory EBA resemble severe BP. In fact, many cases of EBA were probably incorrectly classified in the past as some other inflammatory blistering skin disease. Some patients present with an inflammatory bullous skin disease that subsequently evolves into the classic noninflammatory form of this disease. In general, EBA is a chronic disorder. Association with multiple myeloma, amyloidosis, inflammatory bowel disease, and diabetes mellitus has been reported. The HLA-DR2 haplotype is found with increased frequency.

The histology of lesional skin varies depending on the type or character of the lesion being studied. Noninflammatory bullae show subepidermal blisters with a sparse leukocytic infiltrate, and resemble those in lesional skin from patients with porphyria cutanea tarda. Inflammatory vesiculobullous lesions consist of a subepidermal blister with a neutrophil-rich leukocytic infiltrate within the superficial dermis. EBA patients have continuous deposits of IgG (and frequently C3) in a linear pattern within the epidermal basement membrane. These immunoreactants are also found in the sublamina densa region in association with anchoring fibrils. Approximately 25 to 50 percent of patients have circulating autoantibodies against normal epidermal basement membrane. These autoantibodies can be distinguished from those in BP by mapping the pattern of binding in indirect immunofluorescence microscopy. In brief, EBA sera bind to the base of 1-M NaCl split-skin substrate, while BP sera bind the roof. The antigen recognized by EBA autoantibodies is the globular carboxyl terminal domain of type VII procollagen.

Treatment of EBA is generally unsatisfactory. Some patients with inflammatory EBA may respond to systemic glucocorticoids, either alone or in combination with immunosuppressive agents. Other patients (especially those with neutrophil-rich inflammatory lesions) may respond to dapsone. The chronic, noninflammatory form of this disease is largely resistant to treatment.

AUTOIMMUNE SYSTEMIC DISEASES WITH PROMINENT CUTANEOUS FEATURES

DERMATOMYOSITIS The cutaneous manifestations of dermatomyositis (see Chap. 364) are often distinctive but at times may resemble those of systemic lupus erythematosus (SLE), scleroderma, or other overlapping connective tissue diseases. The extent and severity of cutaneous disease may or may not correlate with the extent and severity of the myositis. Patients with severe muscle involvement may have relatively minor skin changes, while patients with marked skin involvement may have mild muscle disease. The cutaneous manifestations of dermatomyositis are similar whether the disease appears in childhood or old age, except that calcification of subcutaneous tissue is a common late sequela in childhood dermatomyositis.

The cutaneous signs of dermatomyositis may precede or follow the development of myositis by weeks to years. The most common manifestation is a purple/red discoloration of the upper eyelids, sometimes associated with scaling ("heliotrope" erythema) and with periorbital edema. Erythema on the cheeks and nose in a "butterfly" distribution may resemble the eruption in SLE. Erythematous or violaceous scaling patches are common on the upper, anterior chest and the extensor surfaces of the arms, legs, and hands. Erythema and scaling may be particularly prominent over the elbows, knees, and the dorsal interphalangeal joints. Approximately one-third of patients have violaceous, flat-topped papules over the dorsal interphalangeal joints that are pathognomonic of dermatomyositis (Gottron's sign or Gottron's papules). These lesions can be contrasted with the erythema and scaling on the dorsum of the fingers in some patients with SLE which spares the skin over the interphalangeal joints. Periungual telangiectasia may be prominent, and a lacy or reticulated erythema may be associated with fine scaling on the extensor surfaces of the thighs and upper arms. Other patients, particularly those with long-standing disease, develop areas of hypopigmentation, hyperpigmentation, mild atrophy, and telangiectasia, known as poikiloderma vasculare atrophicans. Poikiloderma is rare in both SLE and scleroderma and thus can serve as a clinical sign that distinguishes dermatomyositis from these two diseases. However, cutaneous changes may be similar in scleroderma and dermatomyositis and may include thickening and binding down of the skin of the hands, sclerodactyly, and Raynaud's phenomenon. However, the presence of severe muscle disease, Gottron's papules, heliotrope erythema, and poikiloderma serve to distinguish these patients as having dermatomyositis. Skin biopsy of erythematous, scaling lesions of dermatomyositis may reveal only mild nonspecific inflammation but sometimes may show changes indistinguishable from those found in SLE including epidermal atrophy, hydropic degeneration of basal keratinocytes, edema of the upper dermis, and a mild mononuclear cell infiltrate. Direct immunofluorescence of lesional skin is usually negative. Treatment should be directed at the systemic disease. In the few instances where adjunctive cutaneous therapy is desirable, topical glucocorticoids are sometimes useful. These patients should avoid exposure to ultraviolet irradiation and use photoprotective measures such as sunscreens.

LUPUS ERYTHEMATOSUS   The cutaneous manifestations of lupus erythematosus (LE) (see Chap. 269) can be divided into acute, subacute, and chronic (i.e., discoid LE) types. Acute cutaneous LE is characterized by erythema of the nose and malar eminences in a "butterfly" distribution. The erythema is often sudden in onset, accompanied by edema and fine scale, and correlated with systemic involvement. Patients may have widespread involvement of the face as well as erythema and scaling of the extensor surfaces of the extremities and upper chest. These acute lesions, while sometimes evanescent, usually last for days and are often associated with exacerbations of systemic disease. Skin biopsy of acute lesions may show only a sparse dermal infiltrate of mononuclear cells and dermal edema. In some instances cellular infiltrates around blood vessels and hair follicles are notable, as is hydropic degeneration of basal cells of the epidermis. Direct immunofluorescence of lesional skin frequently reveals deposits of immunoglobulin and complement in the epidermal basement membrane zone. Treatment is aimed at control of systemic disease; photoprotection in this, as well as other forms of LE, is very important.

Subacute cutaneous lupus erythematosus (SCLE) is characterized by a widespread photosensitive, nonscarring eruption that may take two forms. About one-half of these patients have SLE in which severe renal and CNS involvement is uncommon. The two forms of SCLE are a papulosquamous eruption that can resemble psoriasis and an annular form that may resemble erythema multiforme. In the papulosquamous form, discrete erythematous papules arise on the back, chest, shoulders, extensor surfaces of the arms, and the dorsum of the hands but are uncommon on the face, flexor surfaces of the arms, and below the waist. The slightly scaling papules tend to merge into large plaques, some with a reticulate appearance. The annular form involves the same areas and also begins as an erythematous papule but tends to develop oval, circular, or polycyclic lesions. The lesions of SCLE are more widespread but have less tendency for scarring than do lesions of discoid LE. Skin biopsy reveals a dense mononuclear cell infiltrate around hair follicles and blood vessels in the superficial dermis, combined with hydropic degeneration of basal cells in the epidermis. Direct immunofluorescence of lesional skin reveals deposits of immunoglobulin at the epidermal basement membrane zone in about half of cases. Most SCLE patients have anti-Ro antibodies. Local therapy is usually unsuccessful, and most patients require treatment with aminoquinoline antimalarials. Low-dose therapy with oral glucocorticoids is sometimes necessary; photoprotective measures are important.

Discoid lupus erythematosus (DLE) is characterized by discrete lesions, most often on the face, scalp, or external ears. The lesions are erythematous papules or plaques with a thick adherent scale that occludes hair follicles (follicular plugging). When the scale is removed, its underside will show small excrescences that correlate with the opening of hair follicles and is termed a "carpet tack" appearance. This finding is relatively specific for discoid LE. Long-standing lesions develop central atrophy, scarring, and hypopigmentation, but frequently have erythematous, sometimes raised, borders at the periphery. These lesions persist for years and tend to expand slowly. Only 5 to 10 percent of patients with DLE meet the American Rheumatism Association criteria for SLE. However, typical discoid lesions are frequently seen in patients with SLE. Biopsy of discoid LE shows hyperkeratosis, follicular plugging, and atrophy of the epidermis. The dermal-epidermal junction reveals hydropic degeneration of basal keratinocytes, and a mononuclear cell infiltrate surrounds hair follicles and blood vessels. Direct immunofluorescence demonstrates immunoglobulin and complement deposits at the basement membrane zone in about 90 percent of cases. Treatment is focused on control of local cutaneous disease and consists mainly of photoprotection and topical or intralesional glucocorticoids. If local therapy is ineffective, use of aminoquinoline antimalarials may be indicated.

SCLERODERMA AND MORPHEA   The skin changes of scleroderma (see Chap. 271) usually begin on the hands, feet, and face, with episodes of recurrent nonpitting edema. Sclerosis of the skin begins distally on the fingers (sclerodactyly) and spreads proximally, usually accompanied by resorption of bone of the fingertips, which may have punched out ulcers, stellate scars, or areas of hemorrhage. The fingers may actually shrink in size and become sausage-shaped, and since the fingernails are usually unaffected the nails may curve over the end of the fingertips. Periungual telangiectasias are usually present, but periungual erythema is rare. In advanced cases, the extremities show contractures and calcinosis cutis. Face involvement includes a smooth, unwrinkled brow, taut skin over the nose, shrinkage of tissue around the mouth, and perioral radial furrowing. Matlike telangiectasias are often present, particularly on the face and hands. Involved skin feels indurated, smooth, and bound to underlying structures; hyperpigmentation and hypopigmentation are often also present. Raynaud's phenomenon, that is, cold-induced blanching, cyanosis, and reactive hyperemia, is present in almost all patients with scleroderma and can precede development of scleroderma by many years. The combination of calcinosis cutis, Raynaud's phenomenon, esophageal dysmotility, sclerodactyly, and telangiectasia has been termed the CREST syndrome. Anticentromere antibodies have been reported in a very high percentage of patients with the CREST syndrome but in only a small minority of patients with scleroderma. Skin biopsy reveals thickening of the dermis and homogenization of collagen bundles. Direct immunofluorescence of lesional skin is usually negative.

Morphea, which has been called localized scleroderma, is characterized by localized thickening and sclerosis of skin, usually affecting young adults or children. Morphea begins as erythematous or flesh-colored plaques that become sclerotic, develop central hypopigmentation, and demonstrate an erythematous border. In most cases, patients have one or a few lesions, and the disease is termed *localized morphea*. In some patients, widespread cutaneous lesions may occur, without systemic involvement. This form is called *generalized morphea*. Most patients with morphea do not have autoantibodies. Skin biopsy of morphea is indistinguishable from that of scleroderma. Linear scleroderma is a limited form of disease which presents in a linear, bandlike distribution and tends to involve deep as well as superficial layers of skin. Scleroderma and morphea are usually quite resistant to therapy with medications. For this reason, physical therapy to prevent joint contractures and to maintain function is employed and is often helpful.

Eosinophilic fasciitis is a clinical entity that can sometimes be confused with scleroderma. There is usually the sudden onset of swelling, induration, and erythema of the extremities frequently following significant physical exertion. The proximal portions of extremities (arms, forearms, thighs, legs) are more often involved than are the hands and feet. While the skin is indurated, it is usually not bound down as in scleroderma. These skin findings are accompanied by peripheral blood eosinophilia, increased erythrocyte sedimentation rate, and sometimes hypergammaglobulinemia. Deep biopsy of affected areas of skin reveals inflammation and thickening of the deep fascia overlying muscle. An inflammatory infiltrate composed of eosinophils and mononuclear cells is usually found. Patients with eosinophilic fasciitis appear to be at increased risk to develop bone marrow failure or other hematologic abnormalities. While the ultimate course of eosinophilic fasciitis is uncertain, many patients respond favorably to treatment with prednisone in doses ranging from 40 to 60 mg/d.

REFERENCES

BRAVERMAN IM: Connective tissue diseases, in *Skin Signs of Systemic Disease*. Philadelphia, Saunders, 1981, pp 255–377

GAMMON WR et al: Epidermolysis bullosa acquisita—a pemphigoid-like disease. J Am Acad Dermatol 11:820, 1984

HALL RP: The pathogenesis of dermatitis herpetiformis: Recent advances. J Am Acad Dermatol 16:1129, 1987

KATZ SI et al: Dermatitis herpetiformis: The skin and the gut. Ann Intern Med 93:857, 1980

KORMAN N: Pemphigus. J Am Acad Dermatol 18:1219, 1988

SHULMAN LE: Diffuse fasciitis with eosinophilia: A new syndrome. Arthritis Rheum 20 (Suppl):205, 1977

STANLEY JR: Bullous pemphigoid, in *Symposium on Blistering Disease, Dermatologic Clinics*, BV Jegasothy, GS Lazarus (eds). Philadelphia, Saunders, 1983, pp 205–216

YANCEY KB, LAWLEY TJ: The immunology of the skin, in *Allergy: Principles and Practice*, 3d ed, E Middleton, CE Reed, EF Ellis (eds). St. Louis, Mosby, 1988, pp 206–223

59   SKIN MANIFESTATIONS OF INTERNAL DISEASE

JEAN BOLOGNIA / IRWIN M. BRAVERMAN

It is now a generally accepted concept in medicine that the skin can show signs of internal disease. Therefore in textbooks of medicine, one finds a chapter describing in detail the major systemic disorders that can be identified by cutaneous signs. The underlying assumption of such a chapter is that the clinician has been able to identify the disorder in the patient and needs only to read about it in the textbook. In reality, concise differential diagnoses and the identification of these disorders is actually difficult for the nondermatologist because he or she is not well versed in the recognition of cutaneous lesions or their spectrum of presentations. Therefore the authors of this chapter have decided to cover this particular topic of cutaneous medicine not by discussing individual disorders but by describing and discussing the various presenting clinical signs and symptoms that indicate the presence of these disorders. Concise differential diagnoses will be generated in which the significant diseases will be briefly discussed and distinguished from the more common disorders that have no significance for internal diseases. The latter disorders are reviewed in table form and always need to be excluded when considering the former. For a detailed description of individual diseases, the reader should consult a dermatologic text. The categories of skin lesions that are discussed include: papulosquamous, erythroderma, alopecia, figurate, acne, telangiectasias, hypopigmentation, hyperpigmentation, vesicles/bullae, exanthems, urticaria, papulonodular, purpura, and ulcers. In an attempt to determine the appropriate category for a particular lesion, it is important to carefully examine its surface qualities, shape, and color in addition to the location and distribution (see Chap. 55).

PAPULOSQUAMOUS SKIN LESIONS (Table 59-1) When an eruption is characterized by elevated lesions, papules (<1 cm), or plaques (>1 cm), in association with scale, it is referred to as papulosquamous. The most common papulosquamous diseases— *psoriasis, tinea, pityriasis rosea*, and *lichen planus*—are primary cutaneous disorders (Table 59-2). When psoriatic lesions are accompanied by arthritis, the possibility of psoriatic arthritis or *Reiter's disease* should be considered. A history of oral ulcers, conjunctivitis, uveitis, and/or urethritis point to the latter diagnosis. In *guttate psoriasis*, there is an acute onset of small, widely scattered, uniform lesions, often in association with a streptococcal infection. Lithium, beta blockers, human immunodeficiency virus (HIV) infection, and a rapid taper of systemic glucocorticoids are also known to exacerbate psoriasis. Epidermal hyperproliferation and incomplete maturation are responsible for the plaque formation and scale that is characteristic of psoriasis.

Whenever the diagnosis of pityriasis rosea or lichen planus is made, it is important to review the patient's medications because the eruption can be treated by simply discontinuing the offending agent. Pityriasis rosea-like drug eruptions are seen most commonly with beta blockers, captopril, clonidine, gold, griseofulvin, isotretinoin, metronidazole, penicillin, and tripelennamine, while the drugs which can produce a lichenoid eruption include gold, antimalarials, thiazides, quinidine, phenothiazines, sulfonylureas, furosemide, methyldopa, griseofulvin, beta blockers, and captopril. Lichen planus-like lesions are also observed in chronic graft-versus-host disease. *Bowen's disease* represents squamous cell carcinoma in situ and it usually presents as a single lesion. The plaque is well demarcated, pink to red in color, and the amount of scale varies. Bowen's disease is found in both sun-exposed and sun-protected areas of the body, and the possibility of arsenic exposure should be explored in these patients, and an examination of the palms and soles for arsenical keratoses should be included.

Parapsoriasis is an intermediate disease, for it can remain solely as a primary cutaneous disease or it can progress to cutaneous T-cell lymphoma (CTCL) after a latency period of as long as 40 years. There are several forms of *parapsoriasis*, including small plaque (0.5 to 5 cm), large plaque (>6 cm), and retiform. The lesions of both small plaque and large plaque parapsoriasis are thin and salmon-pink in color with fine white scale. In small plaque, they are commonly on the trunk, but can be widely scattered. In large plaque, the most common location is the "girdle" area, and fine wrinkling secondary to epidermal atrophy is often seen. Retiform parapsoriasis forms a netlike pattern and the individual papules are red-brown and flat-topped. The latter two forms of parapsoriasis, large plaque and retiform, can progress to CTCL.

TABLE 59-1   Causes of papulosquamous skin lesions

Primary cutaneous disorders
  A Psoriasis
  B Tinea
  C Pityriasis rosea
  D Lichen planus
  E Parapsoriasis
  F Bowen's disease
Drugs
Systemic diseases
  A Lupus erythematosus
  B Cutaneous T-cell lymphoma
  C Secondary syphilis
  D Reiter's disease
  E Bazex' syndrome

TABLE 59-2 Papulosquamous skin diseases (primary cutaneous disorders)

	Characteristic lesion	Location	Other findings	Diagnostic aids
Psoriasis	Pink-red, silvery scale, sharply demarcated	Elbows, knees, scalp, presacral area	Nail dystrophy: pitting, onycholysis, yellow discoloration Arthritis, primarily small joints (hands and feet)	Skin biopsy
Tinea	Pink-red, central clearing common, active, scaling border	Inner thigh (tinea cruris), palms, soles, any area of body	Invasion of stratum corneum by dermatophytes	KOH and/or fungal culture of scale
Pityriasis rosea	Salmon-pink, oval shape, long axis follows lines of cleavage in the skin, peripheral collarette of scale	Trunk, proximal, extremities	Herald patch: initial lesion and usually the largest in size Spontaneous resolution over 2–3 months	Skin biopsy, VDRL to exclude secondary syphilis
Lichen planus	Violet-colored, polygonal, flat-topped, traversed by thin white lines (Wickham's striae)	Flexor wrists, ankles, presacral area, glans penis	Oral mucosa: lacelike white plaques and/or erosions Pruritus	Skin biopsy

Cutaneous T-cell lymphoma (CTCL), *secondary syphilis, lupus* (see "Papulonodular Skin Lesions," below), and *Bazex' syndrome* are less common papulosquamous disorders that are associated with systemic disease. A clue to the development of *CTCL* within lesions of large plaque or retiform parapsoriasis is an increase in the palpable component of the plaque (increased infiltration). In its early stages, CTCL may be confused with eczema or psoriasis, but it often fails to respond to the appropriate therapy for those inflammatory diseases. The diagnosis of CTCL is established by skin biopsy in which collections of atypical T lymphocytes are found in the epidermis and dermis. As the disease progresses, cutaneous tumors and lymph node involvement may appear.

In *secondary syphilis,* there are scattered red-brown papules with thin scale. The eruption often involves the palms and soles and it can resemble pityriasis rosea. Associated findings are helpful in making the diagnosis and they include annular plaques on the face, nonscarring alopecia, condyloma lata (broad-based and moist), and mucous patches as well as lymphadenopathy, malaise, fever, headache, and myalgias. The interval between the primary chancre and the secondary stage is usually 4 to 8 weeks and spontaneous resolution without appropriate therapy is seen. When psoriasiform lesions are seen on the nose, ears, fingers, and toes, *Bazex' syndrome* should be considered. It is a distinctive paraneoplastic eruption associated with squamous cell carcinomas of the oropharynx, tracheobronchial tree, and esophagus.

ERYTHRODERMA (Table 59-3) Erythroderma is the term used when the majority of the skin surface is erythematous (red in color). There may be associated scale, erosions, or pustules as well as shedding of the hair and nails. Potential systemic manifestations include fever, chills, hypothermia, reactive lymphadenopathy, peripheral edema, hypoalbuminemia, increased transepidermal water loss and high-output cardiac failure. The major etiologies of erythroderma are: (1) *cutaneous diseases* such as psoriasis and dermatitis (Table 59-4); (2) *drugs;* (3) *systemic diseases,* most commonly CTCL; and (4) *idiopathic.* In the first three groups, the location and description of the initial lesions, prior to the development of the erythroderma, aid in the diagnosis. For example, a history of red scaly plaques on the elbows and knees would point to psoriasis. It is also important

to examine the skin carefully for a migration of the erythema and associated secondary changes such as pustules or erosions. Migratory waves of erythema studded with superficial pustules are seen in *pustular psoriasis,* whereas erosive migratory erythema of the face and girdle area is seen in *necrolytic migratory erythema* (glucagonoma syndrome).

An erythroderma secondary to an underlying cutaneous disease is most commonly due to *psoriasis* or one of the various forms of *dermatitis* (eczema). Each type of dermatitis has its own distinguishing features, but they may be limited to the initial lesions. Uncontrolled dermatitis can evolve into an erythroderma through a process known as "autosensitization" (conditioned hyperirritability), where initially uninvolved skin becomes pruritic and eventually dermatitic.

Drug-induced erythroderma (exfoliative dermatitis) may begin as a morbilliform eruption or it may arise as diffuse erythema. Fever and peripheral eosinophilia often accompany the eruption. There are a number of *drugs* that can produce an erythroderma, including penicillins, sulfonamides, barbiturates, phenytoin, gold, allopurinol, captopril, D-penicillamine, sulfonylureas, and furosemide. Reactions to allopurinol may also be accompanied by hepatitis and nephropathy, especially in patients with impaired renal function given full doses of allopurinol plus a diuretic.

The most common malignancy that is associated with erythroderma is *CTCL;* in some series, up to 25 percent of the cases of erythroderma were due to CTCL. The patient may progress from isolated plaques and tumors, or the erythroderma may be the initial manifestation (Sézary syndrome). In the Sézary syndrome, there are circulating atypical T lymphocytes, pruritus, and lymphadenopathy. Additional findings include keratoderma and leonine facies. In cases of erythroderma where there is no apparent cause (idiopathic), longitudinal follow-up is mandatory to monitor the possible development of CTCL. Other types of *lymphoma* can be associated with erythroderma, including Hodgkin's and non-Hodgkin's lymphoma, the former being more common. There have also been isolated case reports of erythroderma secondary to some solid tumors—lung, liver, prostate, thyroid, and colon—but it is usually in a late stage of the disease.

ALOPECIA (Table 59-5) The two major forms of alopecia are scarring and nonscarring. In scarring alopecia, there is associated fibrosis, inflammation, and loss of hair follicles. A smooth scalp with a decreased number of follicular openings is usually observed clinically, but in some cases, the changes are only seen in biopsy specimens from the affected areas. In nonscarring alopecia, the hair shafts are gone, but the hair follicles are preserved, explaining the reversible nature of nonscarring alopecia.

Primary cutaneous disorders are the most common causes of nonscarring alopecia and they include *telogen effluvium, androgenetic alopecia, alopecia areata, tinea capitis,* and *traumatic alopecia* (Table 59-6). In women with androgenetic alopecia, an elevation in circulating levels of androgens may be seen as a result of ovarian or adrenal gland dysfunction. When there are signs of virilization, such

TABLE 59-3 Causes of erythroderma

Primary cutaneous disorders
  A Psoriasis
  B Dermatitis (atopic, stasis, contact, seborrheic)
  C Pityriasis rubra pilaris
Drugs
Systemic diseases
  A Cutaneous T-cell lymphoma
  B Lymphoma
  C Necrolytic migratory erythema
Idiopathic

TABLE 59-4 Erythroderma (primary cutaneous disorders)

	Initial lesions	Location of initial lesions	Other findings	Diagnostic aids
Psoriasis	Pink-red, silvery scale, sharply demarcated	Elbows, knees, scalp, presacral area	Nail dystrophy, arthritis, pustules	Skin biopsy
Dermatitis:				
Atopic	Acute: Erythema, fine scale, crust, indistinct borders Chronic: Lichenification (increased skin markings)	Antecubital and popliteal fossae, neck, hands	Pruritus Family history of atopy, including asthma, allergic rhinitis or conjunctivitis, and atopic dermatitis Rule out secondary infection with *S. aureus* Rule out superimposed irritant contact dermatitis	Skin biopsy
Stasis	Erythema, crusting, excoriations	Lower extremities	Pruritus, lower extremity edema History of venous ulcers, thrombophlebitis, and/or cellulitis Rule out cellulitis Rule out superimposed contact dermatitis, e.g., topical neomycin	Skin biopsy
Contact (local)	Erythema, crusting, vesicles and bullae	Depends upon offending agent	Irritant—onset often within hours Allergic—delayed-type hypersensitivity; lag time of 48 h	Patch testing
Contact (systemic)	Erythema, fine scale, crust	Generalized	Patient has history of allergic contact dermatitis to topical agent then receives systemic medication that is structurally related, e.g., ethylenediamine (topical) aminophyline (IV)	Patch testing
Seborrheic	Pink-red, greasy scale	Scalp, nasolabial folds, eyebrows, intertriginous zones	Flares with stress HIV infection Associated with Parkinson's disease	None
Pityriasis rubra pilaris	Orange-red, perifollicular, papules	Generalized, but characteristic "skip" areas of normal skin	Wax-like keratoderma Rule out cutaneous T-cell lymphoma	Skin biopsy

TABLE 59-5 Causes of alopecia

Nonscarring alopecia
  A Primary cutaneous disorders
    1 Telogen effluvium
    2 Androgenetic alopecia
    3 Alopecia areata
    4 Tinea capitis
    5 Traumatic alopecia
  B Drugs
  C Systemic diseases
    1 Lupus erythematosus
    2 Secondary syphilis
    3 Hypothyroidism
    4 Hyperthyroidism
    5 Deficiencies of protein, iron, biotin, and zinc

Scarring alopecia
  A Primary cutaneous disorders
    1 Lichen planus
    2 Folliculitis decalvans
    3 Pseudopelade
    4 Linear scleroderma (morphea)
  B Systemic diseases
    1 Lupus erythematosus
    2 Sarcoidosis
    3 Cutaneous metastases

as a deepened voice and enlarged clitoris, the possibility of an ovarian or adrenal gland tumor should be considered.

Exposure to various *drugs* can also cause diffuse hair loss, usually by inducing a telogen effluvium. An exception is the anagen effluvium observed with antimitotic agents such as daunorubicin. Alopecia is a side effect of the following drugs: warfarin, heparin, propylthiouracil, carbimazole, vitamin A, isotretinoin, etretinate, lithium, beta blockers, levodopa, amphetamines, and thallium. Fortunately, spontaneous regrowth usually follows the discontinuation of the offending agent.

Less commonly, nonscarring alopecia is associated with *lupus erythematosus* and *secondary syphilis*. In systemic lupus, there are two forms of alopecia—one is scarring secondary to discoid lesions (see below) and the other is nonscarring. The latter form may be diffuse and involve the entire scalp or it may localized to the frontal

TABLE 59-6 Nonscarring alopecia (primary cutaneous disorders)

	Clinical characteristics	Pathogenesis
Telogen effluvium	Diffuse shedding of normal hairs Follows either major stress (high fever, severe infection) or change in hormones (post partum) Reversible without treatment	Stress causes the normally asynchronous growth cycles of individual hairs to become synchronous; therefore, large numbers of growing (anagen) hairs simultaneously enter the dying (telogen) phase
Androgenetic alopecia	Miniaturization of hairs along the midline of the scalp Recession of the anterior scalp line in men and some women	Increased sensitivity of affected hairs to the effects of testosterone Increased levels of circulating androgens (ovarian or adrenal source)
Alopecia areata	Well circumscribed, circular areas of hair loss, 2–5 cm in diameter In extensive cases, coalescence of lesions and/or involvement of other hair-bearing surfaces of the body	The germinative zones of the hair follicles are surrounded by T lymphocytes Occasional associated diseases: hyperthyroidism, hypothyroidism, vitiligo, Down's syndrome
Tinea	Varies from scaling with minimal hair loss, to discrete patches with "black dots" (broken hairs), to boggy plaque with pustules (kerion)	Invasion of hairs by dermatophytes, most commonly *Trichophyton tonsurans*
Traumatic alopecia	Broken hairs Irregular outline	Traction with curlers, rubber bands, braiding Exposure to heat or chemicals Mechanical pulling (trichotillomania)

TABLE 59-7 Causes of figurate skin lesions

Primary cutaneous disorders
  A Tinea
  B Urticaria
  C Erythema annulare centrifugum
  D Granuloma annulare
Systemic diseases
  A Migratory
    1 Erythema chronicum migrans
    2 Erythema gyratum repens
    3 Erythema marginatum
    4 Pustular psoriasis
    5 Necrolytic migratory erythema
  B Nonmigratory
    1 Sarcoidosis
    2 Subacute lupus erythematosus
    3 Secondary syphilis
    4 Cutaneous T-cell lymphoma
    5 Elastosis perforans serpiginosa

scalp in the form of multiple short hairs ("lupus hairs"). Scattered, poorly circumscribed patches of alopecia with a "moth-eaten" appearance are a manifestation of the secondary stage of syphilis (see "Papulosquamous Skin Lesions"). Diffuse thinning of the hair is also associated with hypothyroidism, hyperthyroidism, hypopituitarism, and deficiencies of protein, iron, biotin, and zinc.

Scarring alopecia is more frequently the result of a primary cutaneous disorder such as *lichen planus, folliculitis decalvans,* or *linear scleroderma (morphea)* than it is a sign of systemic disease. For example, the scarring lesions of *discoid lupus* are seen in patients with systemic lupus; however, in the majority of cases, the disease process is limited to the skin. Less common causes of scarring alopecia include *sarcoidosis* (see "Papulonodular Skin Lesions"), cutaneous *metastases,* and *pseudopelade.* The latter disease may be idiopathic and arise de novo or it can represent the inactive end-stage phase of a previous inflammatory process such as lichen planus, sarcoid, or discoid lupus. The irregularly shaped areas of alopecia lack inflammation and often arise at an acute angle from the midline.

In the early phases of discoid lupus, lichen planus, and folliculitis decalvans, there are circumscribed areas of alopecia. Fibrosis and subsequent loss of follicles are observed primarily in the center of the individual lesions while the inflammatory process is most prominent at the periphery. The areas of active inflammation in *discoid lupus* are erythematous with scale. The areas of previous inflammation are often hypopigmented with a rim of hyperpigmentation. In *lichen planus,* the peripheral perifollicular papules are violet-colored and postinflammatory hyperpigmentation is a characteristic finding. Complete examination of the skin and oral mucosa combined with a biopsy and direct immunofluorescence will aid in distinguishing these two entities. The peripheral active lesions in *folliculitis decalvans* are perifollicular pustules which routinely grow *Staphylococcus aureus* or normal flora. These patients often have other forms of acne and folliculitis and can develop a reactive arthritis.

FIGURATE SKIN LESIONS (Table 59-7) In figurate eruptions, the lesions form rings and arcs which are usually erythematous, but can be flesh-colored to brown. Most commonly, they are due to primary cutaneous diseases such as *tinea, urticaria, erythema annulare centrifugum,* and *granuloma annulare* (Table 59-8). An underlying systemic illness is found in a second, less common, group of migratory annular erythemas. It includes *erythema gyratum repens, erythema chronicum migrans* (ECM), and *erythema marginatum.*

In *erythema gyratum repens,* one sees hundreds of mobile concentric arcs and wavefronts which resemble the grain in wood. A search for an underlying malignancy is mandatory in a patient with this eruption. *ECM* is the cutaneous manifestation of Lyme disease, which is caused by the spirochete *Borrelia burgdorferi.* In the initial stage (3 to 30 days after tick bite), a single annular lesion is usually seen, which can expand to ≥10 cm in diameter. Within several days, approximately half of the patients develop multiple smaller erythematous lesions at sites distant from the bite. Associated symptoms include fever, headache, myalgias, photophobia, arthralgias, and malar rash. *Erythema marginatum* is seen in patients with rheumatic fever, primarily on the trunk. Lesions are pink-red in color, flat to mildly elevated, and transient. If pustules are noted within a figurate eruption, consider *pustular psoriasis,* and if erosions are seen, consider *necrolytic migratory erythema.*

There are additional cutaneous diseases that present as annular eruptions, but they lack an obvious migratory component. Examples include *CTCL,* annular cutaneous *lupus,* also referred to as subacute lupus (see "Papulonodular Skin Lesions"), secondary *syphilis,* and *sarcoidosis* (see "Papulonodular Skin Lesions"). The most common clinical setting for the annular form of secondary lues is the face of black patients; a clue to this diagnosis is the presence of central hyperpigmentation. If keratotic plugs are noted within the annular or arciform lesions, particularly if they are localized to the neck and antecubital fossae, consider *elastosis perforans serpiginosa* (EPS). EPS is seen as a side effect of D-penicillamine and in patients with Down's syndrome and disorders of elastin and collagen. The latter include Ehlers-Danlos type IV and Marfan's syndromes, pseudoxanthoma elasticum, and osteogenesis imperfecta.

ACNE (Table 59-9) *Acne vulgaris* and *acne rosacea* are the two major forms of acne (Table 59-10). Estrogens decrease sebaceous gland activity, whereas androgens enhance sebum production. Therefore, acne vulgaris in an adult, especially if it is of recent onset, may be a reflection of increased levels of circulating *androgens.* Dysfunction of the ovary or adrenal gland, e.g., polycystic ovary disease, Cushing's syndrome or partial deficiency of the enzyme 21-hydroxylase, can lead to the hormonal imbalance. Examination of the patient for signs such as hirsutism, androgenetic alopecia, hypertension, and redistribution of subcutaneous fat will aid in the diagnosis. In patients with acne conglobata, a more severe form of acne characterized by multiple cysts and bridging scars, an associated inflammatory arthritis has been described.

Exposure to chlorinated aromatic hydrocarbons such as dioxin (TCDD) leads to a particular form of acne known as chloracne, which is characterized by open comedones and straw-colored cysts. Patients exposed to dioxin can also develop the signs and symptoms of porphyria cutanea tarda (see "Vesicles"). Exacerbations of acne

TABLE 59-8 Figurate eruptions (primary cutaneous disorders)

	Clinical characteristics	Pathogenesis
Tinea	Active, scaling erythematous border with central clearing Expands slowly	Invasion of stratum corneum by dermatophytes
Urticaria	Central wheal with erythematous flare Transient and/or migratory Pruritic	Release of histamine from mast cells via immunologic (IgE, type 1 hypersensitivity) or nonimmunologic mechanisms
Erythema annulare centrifugum	Enlarges slowly Erythematous, flat or slightly raised "Trailing scale"—scale on inner aspect of expending ring Buttock, upper thighs	Not known Usually idiopathic Sometimes associated with tinea pedis, drug hypersensitivity Rarely, paraneoplastic
Granuloma annulare	Border composed of flesh-colored to red-brown papules Extremities	Granulomatous process is limited to the skin Unknown etiology Disseminated form is associated with diabetes mellitus

TABLE 59-9   Causes of acneiform eruptions

Primary cutaneous disorders
    A Acne vulgaris
    B Acne rosacea
Drugs
Systemic diseases
    A Increased androgen production
        1 Adrenal origin, e.g., Cushing's disease, 21-hydroxylase deficiency
        2 Ovarian origin, e.g., polycystic ovary disease
    B Cryptococcosis, disseminated

vulgaris follow the ingestion of several *drugs,* such as iodides, bromides, vitamin B_{12}, glucocorticoids, and lithium, as well as the application of oil-containing compounds. In addition, high dose oral glucocorticoids can cause a widespread eruption of perifollicular pustules (folliculitis) on the trunk, characterized by lesions in the same stage of development. In immunocompromised hosts, disseminated *cryptococcosis* may present as an acneiform eruption.

Patients with the carcinoid syndrome have episodes of flushing of the head, neck, and sometimes the trunk. Resultant skin changes of the face, in particular telangiectasias, mimic the clinical appearance of acne rosacea. Suffusion of the face, as is seen in polycythemia vera, can also be confused with acne rosacea.

TELANGIECTASIAS (Table 59-11) In order to distinguish the various types of telangiectasias, it is important to examine the shape and configuration of the dilated blood vessels. *Linear telangiectasias* are seen on the face of patients with *actinically damaged skin* and *acne rosacea* and are found on the legs of patients with *venous hypertension* and *essential telangiectasia* (Table 59-12). Patients with an unusual form of *mastocytosis* (telangiectasia macularis eruptiva perstans), the *carcinoid* syndrome (see "Acne"), and *ataxia-telangiectasia* also have linear telangiectasias. In ataxia-telangiectasia, linear telangiectasias appear on the bulbar conjunctiva during childhood. Eventually, there is involvement of the ears, eyelids, cheeks, and/or flexural areas such as the antecubital and popliteal fossae. Lastly, linear telangiectasias are found in areas of cutaneous inflammation. For example, lesions of discoid lupus frequently have telangiectasias within them.

Poikiloderma is a term used to describe a patch of skin with (1) reticulated hypo- and hyperpigmentation, (2) wrinkling secondary to epidermal atrophy, and (3) telangiectasias. Poikiloderma does not imply a single disease entity—it is seen in skin damaged by *ionizing radiation,* in the disorders *poikiloderma vasculare atrophicans* (PVA) and *xeroderma pigmentosum,* as well as in patients with connective tissue diseases, primarily *dermatomyositis.* PVA is a precursor lesion of CTCL, and the areas of poikiloderma usually begin in the flexural areas of the axillae and groin.

In *scleroderma,* the dilated blood vessels have a unique configuration and are known as *mat telangiectasias.* The lesions are broad macules that usually measure 2 to 7 mm in diameter; occasionally they are larger in size. Mats have a polygonal or oval shape and their erythematous color may be uniform or the result of delicate telangiectasias. The most common locations for mat telangiectasias are the face, oral mucosa, and hands—peripheral sites that are prone to intermittent ischemia. One theory is that the mats represent a form

of neovascularization in these areas. In the CREST variant of scleroderma (see Chap. 271), which is associated with a chronic course and anticentromere antibodies, the *T* stands for telangiectasias. Mat telangiectasias are an important clue to the diagnosis of the CREST syndrome as well as systemic scleroderma, for they may be the only cutaneous finding. A minority of the patients with scleroderma will have telangiectasias indistinguishable from those found in hereditary hemorrhagic telangiectasia (see below).

Periungual telangiectasias are pathognomonic signs of the three major connective tissue diseases—*lupus erythematosus, scleroderma,* and *dermatomyositis* (DM). They are easily visualized by the naked eye and they occur in at least two-thirds of these patients. In both DM and lupus, there is associated nailfold erythema and in DM, the erythema is often accompanied by "ragged" cuticles and fingertip tenderness. Under $10\times$ magnification, the blood vessels in the nailfolds of lupus patients are tortuous and resemble "glomeruli," whereas in scleroderma and DM, there is a loss of capillary loops and those that remain are markedly dilated.

In *hereditary hemorrhagic telangiectasia* (Osler-Rendu-Weber disease), the lesions usually appear during adulthood and are most commonly seen on the mucous membranes, face, and distal extremities, including under the nails. They represent arteriovenous (AV) malformations of the dermal microvasculature, are dark red in color, and are usually slightly elevated. When the skin is stretched over an individual lesion, an eccentric punctum with radiating legs is seen. Although the degree of systemic involvement varies in this autosomal dominant disease, the major symptoms are recurrent epistaxis and gastrointestinal bleeding. The fact that these mucosal telangiectasias are actually AV malformations helps to explain their tendency to bleed. Patients should also be screened for pulmonary AV fistulas because of the associated complications of hypoxia, bleeding, and paradoxic emboli.

HYPOPIGMENTATION (Table 59-13) Disorders of hypopigmentation are classified as either diffuse or localized. The classic example of *diffuse* hypopigmentation is *oculocutaneous albinism* (OCA). The two most common forms are tyrosinase-negative OCA and tyrosinase-positive OCA; the former is characterized by a lack of enzyme activity. At birth, both types of OCA appear similar—white hair, gray-blue eyes, and pink-white skin. The patients with tyrosinase-negative OCA maintain this phenotype, whereas those with tyrosinase-positive OCA will acquire some pigmentation of the eyes, hair, and skin as they age. The degree of pigment formation is a function of their racial background, but a pigmentary dilution is readily apparent when they are compared to their first-degree relatives.

The ocular findings in OCA correlate with the degree of hypopigmentation and they include decreased visual acuity, nystagmus, photophobia, and monocular vision. Patients with OCA, particularly those who reside in the tropics, develop cutaneous squamous cell carcinomas in association with severe actinic damage. The diagnosis of tyrosinase-positive OCA in a patient from Puerto Rico (Arecibo region) or southern Holland raises the possibility of the Hermansky-Pudlak syndrome. In addition to the signs and symptoms of OCA, these patients have a bleeding diathesis secondary to a platelet storage pool defect and restrictive lung disease secondary to deposits of

TABLE 59-10   Acne (primary cutaneous disorders)

	Clinical characteristics	Pathogenesis
Acne vulgaris	Erythematous papules, pustules, open comedones (blackheads), closed comedones (whiteheads), and cysts	Epithelial hyperproliferation within the infundibulum of the hair follicle leads to comedone formation
	Areas that contain sebaceous glands: face, neck, upper trunk	Additional factors: sebum-derived free fatty acids, *Propionibacterium acnes*
Acne rosacea	Papules, pustules; central face	Unknown
	Telangiectasias of nose and cheeks	No increased reactivity of cutaneous blood vessels to vasodilators
	Facial erythema	Sebum production normal
	Flushing reaction to hot foods and alcohol	
	Ocular involvement: conjunctivitis, blepharitis, keratitis	

TABLE 59-11   Causes of telangiectasias

Primary cutaneous disorders	Systemic diseases
A Linear	A Linear
1 Acne rosacea	1 Carcinoid
2 Actinically damaged skin	2 Ataxia-telangiectasia
3 Venous hypertension	3 Mastocytosis
4 Essential telangiectasia	B Poikiloderma
B Poikiloderma	1 Dermatomyositis
1 Ionizing radiation	2 Xeroderma pigmentosa
2 Poikiloderma vasculare atrophicans	C Mat
	1 Scleroderma
C Spider angioma	D Periungual
1 Idiopathic	1 Lupus erythematosus
2 Pregnancy	2 Scleroderma
	3 Dermatomyositis
	E Papular
	1 Hereditary hemorrhagic telangiectasia
	F Spider angioma
	1 Cirrhosis

ceroidlike material. Generalized vitiligo, phenylketonuria, and homocystinuria are other unusual causes of diffuse pigmentary dilution. In generalized vitiligo, melanocytes are not found in affected skin, whereas in OCA they are present but have decreased activity. Appropriate laboratory tests exclude the other disorders of metabolism.

The differential diagnosis of *localized* hypomelanosis includes the following primary cutaneous disorders: *vitiligo, chemical leukoderma, piebaldism, nevus depigmentosus* (see below), *postinflammatory hypomelanosis,* and *tinea versicolor* (Table 59-14). In this group of diseases, the areas of involvement are macules or patches with a decrease or absence of pigmentation, and in the first four disorders, secondary changes such as scale or crust are absent. Patients with vitiligo have an increased incidence of several autoimmune disorders, including hypothyroidism, Graves' disease, pernicious anemia, Addison's disease, uveitis, alopecia areata, chronic mucocutaneous candidiasis, and the polyglandular autoimmune syndromes (types I, II, and III). Diseases of the thyroid gland are the most frequently associated disorders, occurring in up to 30 percent of patients with vitiligo. Circulating autoantibodies are often found and the most common ones are antithyroglobulin and antimicrosomal and antiparietal cell antibodies.

There are three systemic diseases which should be considered in a patient with skin findings suggestive of vitiligo—*Vogt-Koyanagi-Harada syndrome, scleroderma,* and *melanoma-associated leukoderma.* A history of aseptic meningitis, nontraumatic uveitis, tinnitus, hearing loss, and/or dysacusis points to the diagnosis of the Vogt-Koyanagi-Harada syndrome. In these patients, the face and scalp are the most common locations of pigment loss. The vitiligo-like leukoderma seen in patients with scleroderma has a clinical resemblance to idiopathic vitiligo that has begun to repigment as a result of treatment; that is, there are perifollicular macules of normal pigmentation within areas of depigmentation. The basis of this leukoderma is unknown; there is no evidence of inflammation in areas of

involvement, but it can resolve if the underlying connective tissue disease becomes inactive. In contrast to idiopathic vitiligo, melanoma-associated leukoderma often begins on the trunk and its appearance should prompt a search for metastatic disease. The possibility exists that the destruction of normal melanocytes is the result of an immune response against malignant melanocytes.

There are two systemic disorders that have the cutaneous findings of piebaldism (partial albinism) (Table 59-14). They are Hirschsprung's disease and Waardenburg's syndrome. A possible explanation for both disorders is an abnormal embryonic migration or survival of two neural crest-derived elements, one of them being melanocytes and the other myenteric ganglion cells (Hirschsprung's disease) or auditory nerve cells (Waardenburg's syndrome). The latter syndrome is characterized by congenital sensorineural hearing loss, dystopia canthorum (lateral displacement of the inner canthi, but normal interpupillary distance), heterochromic irises, and a broad nasal root, in addition to the piebaldism.

In *tuberous sclerosis,* the earliest cutaneous sign is the ash leaf spot. These lesions are often present at birth; however, detection may require Wood's lamp examination, especially in fair-skinned individuals. The pigment within them is reduced but not absent. The average size is 1 to 3 cm and the common shapes are oval, polygonal, and lance-ovate, while the less common shapes are dermatomal and confettilike. The terms lance-ovate and ash leaf are used to describe lesions with a particular shape, that is, tapered at one end and round at the other. Examination of the patient for additional cutaneous signs such as adenoma sebaceum (multiple angiofibromas of the face), ungual and gingival fibromas, fibrous plaques of the forehead, and connective tissue nevi (shagreen patches) is recommended. It is important to remember that an ash leaf spot on the scalp will result in poliosis, which is a circumscribed patch of gray-white hair. Internal manifestations include seizures, mental retardation, central nervous system (CNS) and retinal hamartomas, renal angiomyolipomas, and cardiac rhabdomyomas.

Nevus depigmentosus is a stable, well-circumscribed hypomelanosis that is present at birth. There is usually a single circular or rectangular lesion, but occasionally the nevus has a dermatomal or whorled pattern. It is important to distinguish this lesion from ash leaf spots and hypomelanosis of Ito, for it is rarely associated with CNS findings. *Hypomelanosis of Ito* (incontinentia pigmenti achromians) is an autosomal dominant disorder in which swirls and streaks of hypopigmentation run parallel to one another. The pattern resembles that of a marble cake. Associated abnormalities are found in the musculoskeletal system (asymmetry), the CNS (seizures and mental retardation), and the eyes (strabismus and hypertelorism). Chromosomal mosaicism and diploid/triploid mixoploidy have been reported in these patients; this lends support to the hypothesis that the pattern is the result of the migration of two clones of primordial melanocytes, each with a different pigment potential.

Localized areas of decreased pigmentation are commonly seen as a result of cutaneous inflammation (Table 59-14) and have been observed in the skin overlying active lesions of *sarcoidosis* (see

TABLE 59-12   Telangiectasias (primary cutaneous disorders)

Type	Associated disorder	Clinical characteristics	Pathogenesis
Linear: Simple red or blue line that disappears with diascopy (pressure)	Acne rosacea	Face Associated with flushing, erythema, papulopustules, and rhinophyma	Vasodilatation
	Actinically damaged skin	Face, arms, upper trunk Associated with hypopigmentation, hyperpigmentation, and keratoses	Damage to supportive connective tissue
	Essential telangiectasia	Netlike sheets Begins on lower extremities May be widespread More common in women	Unknown
Spider angioma: Central pulsating punctum with radiating legs	Idiopathic	Upper half of the body	Proliferation of blood vessels in association with increased circulating estrogens
	Pregnancy	Halo of pallor secondary to local steal phenomenon	

TABLE 59-13 Causes of hypopigmentation

Primary cutaneous disorders	Systemic diseases
A Diffuse	A Diffuse
1 Generalized vitiligo	*1* Oculocutaneous albinism
B Localized	B Localized
1 Vitiligo	*1* Vogt-Koyanagi-Harada
2 Chemical leukoderma	*2* Scleroderma
3 Piebaldism	*3* Melanoma-associated leukoderma
4 Nevus depigmentosus	*4* Tuberous sclerosis
5 Postinflammatory	*5* Hypomelanosis of Ito
6 Tinea versicolor	*6* Sarcoidosis
	7 Tuberculoid leprosy
	8 Cutaneous T-cell lymphoma

''Papulonodular Skin Lesions'') as well as *CTLC*. Cutaneous infections also present as disorders of hypopigmentation and in *tuberculoid leprosy*, there are a few asymmetric patches of hypomelanosis that have associated anesthesia, anhidrosis, and alopecia. Biopsy specimens of the palpable border show dermal granulomas that lack *Mycobacterium leprae* organisms.

HYPERPIGMENTATION (Table 59-15) Disorders of hyperpigmentation are also divided into two groups—localized and diffuse. The *localized* forms are due to an epidermal alteration, a proliferation of melanocytes, or an increase in pigment production. Both *seborrheic keratoses* and *acanthosis nigricans* belong to the first group (Table 59-16). Seborrheic keratoses are common lesions, but in one clinical setting they are a sign of systemic disease, and that setting is the sudden appearance of multiple lesions, often in association with

acrocordons (skin tags) and acanthosis nigricans. This is termed the *sign of Leser-Trélat* and it signifies an internal malignancy. *Acanthosis nigricans* can also be a reflection of an internal malignancy, most commonly of the gastrointestinal tract, and it appears as velvety hyperpigmentation (Table 59-16). In the majority of patients, acanthosis nigricans is associated with obesity, but it may be a reflection of an endocrinopathy such as acromegaly, Cushing's syndrome, Addison's disease, the Stein-Leventhal syndrome, or insulin-resistant diabetes mellitus (type A, type B, and lipoatrophic forms).

A proliferation of melanocytes results in the following pigmented lesions: *lentigo*, nevocellular *nevus*, and *melanoma* (Table 59-16). In an adult, the majority of lentigines are related to sun exposure, which explains their distribution. However, in the Peutz-Jeghers and LEOPARD syndromes, lentigines do serve as a clue to systemic disease. The lentigines in patients with *Peutz-Jeghers* syndrome are located primarily around the nose and mouth, on the hands and feet, and within the oral cavity. While the pigmented macules on the face may fade with age, the oral lesions persist. However, similar intraoral lesions are also seen in Addison's disease and as a normal finding in darkly pigmented individuals. Patients with this autosomal dominant syndrome have multiple benign polyps of the gastrointestinal tract, ovarian tumors, and an approximately 6 percent risk of developing a gastrointestinal malignancy when the polyps arise in the stomach, duodenum, or colon.

In the multiple lentigines or *LEOPARD syndrome*, hundreds of lentigines develop during childhood and are scattered over the entire surface of the body. The syndrome consists of *L*, lentigines; *E*, ECG abnormalities, primarily conduction defects; *O*, ocular hypertelorism;

TABLE 59-14 Hypopigmentation (primary cutaneous disorders, localized)

	Clinical characteristics	Wood's lamp examination (UV-A: peak = 365 nm)	Skin biopsy	Pathogenesis
Vitiligo	Acquired; progressive Symmetric areas of complete pigment loss Periorifical—around mouth, nose, eyes, nipples, umbilicus, anus Other areas—flexor wrists, extensor distal extremities Segmental form is less common—unilateral, dermatomal-like	More apparent Chalk-white	Absence of melanocytes Occasional inflammation	Possible autoimmune phenomenon that results in destruction of melanocytes—humoral and/or cellular Alternative hypothesis is self-destruction of melanocytes and circulating antibodies against melanocytes as a secondary phenomenon
Chemical leukoderma	Similar appearance to vitiligo Often begins on hands Satellite lesions in areas not exposed to chemicals	More apparent Chalk-white	Decreased number or absence of melanocytes	Exposure to chemicals that selectively destroy melanocytes, in particular, phenols and catechols (germicides; rubber products) Release of cellular antigens and activation of circulating lymphocytes may explain satellite phenomenon
Piebaldism	Autosomal dominant Congenital, stable White forelock Areas of hypomelanosis contain normally pigmented and hyperpigmented macules of various sizes Symmetric involvement of central forehead, ventral trunk, and mid regions of upper and lower extremities	Enhancement of leukoderma and hyperpigmented macules	Hypomelanotic areas—few to no melanocytes	Defect in migration of melanoblasts from neural crest to ventral skin or failure of melanoblasts to survive or differentiate in these areas
Post-inflammatory	Hypopigmentation can develop within active lesions, as in subacute lupus, or after the lesion fades, as in dermatitis	Depends upon particular disease Usually less enhancement than in vitiligo	Type of inflammatory infiltrate depends upon specific disease	Block in transfer of melanin from melanocytes to keratinocytes could be secondary to edema or decrease in contact time Destruction of melanocytes if inflammatory cells attack basal layer
Tinea versicolor	Common disorder Upper trunk and neck Shawl-like distribution Young adults Macules have fine white scale when scratched	Golden fluorescence	Hyphae and spores in stratum corneum	Invasion of stratum corneum by the yeast *Pityrosporum* Yeast is lipophilic and produces C_9 and C_{11} dicarboxylic acids which in vitro inhibit tyrosinase

TABLE 59-15   Causes of hyperpigmentation

Primary cutaneous disorders
  A Localized
    1 Epidermal alteration
      a Seborrheic keratosis
      b Acanthosis nigricans (obesity)
    2 Proliferation of melanocytes
      a Lentigo
      b Nevus
      c Melanoma
    3 Increased pigment production
      a Ephelides (freckles)
      b Café au lait spots
  B Localized and diffuse
    1 Drugs
Systemic diseases
  A Localized
    1 Epidermal alteration
      a Seborrheic keratoses (sign of Leser-Trélat)
      b Acanthosis nigricans (endocrine disorders, paraneoplastic)
    2 Proliferation of melanocytes
      a Lentigos (Peutz-Jeghers, LEOPARD syndromes)
      b Nevi (LAMB and NAME syndromes)
    3 Increased pigment production
      a Café au lait spots (neurofibromatosis, Albright's syndrome)
    4 Dermal pigmentation
      a Incontinentia pigmenti
      b Dyskeratosis congenita
  B Diffuse
    1 Endocrinopathies
      a Addison's disease
      b Nelson's syndrome
      c Ectopic ACTH syndrome
    2 Metabolic
      a Porphyria cutanea tarda
      b Hemochromatosis
      c Vitamin B_{12}, folate deficiency
      d Pellagra
      e Malabsorption, Whipple's disease
    3 Melanosis secondary to metastatic melanoma
    4 Autoimmune
      a Biliary cirrhosis
      b Scleroderma
      c POEMS syndrome
    5 Drugs

P, pulmonary stenosis and subaortic valvular stenosis; A, abnormal genitalia (cryptorchidism, hypospadias); R, retardation of growth; and D, deafness (sensorineural). Lentigines are also seen in association with cardiac myxomas and have been described under the mnemonics LAMB syndrome and NAME syndrome. The findings in these two syndromes overlap and include L, lentigines; A, atrial myxomas; M, mucocutaneous myxomas; and B, blue nevi versus N, nevus; A, atrial myxoma; M, myxoid neurofibroma, and E, ephelides (freckles). These patients can also have evidence of endocrine overactivity in the form of Cushing's disease, acromegaly, or sexual precocity.

The third type of localized hyperpigmentation is due to a local increase in pigment production and it includes ephelides (Table 59-16) and café au lait spots. The latter are most commonly associated with two disorders—neurofibromatosis and Albright's syndrome. Café au lait (CAL) spots are flat, uniformly light brown in color, and can vary in size from 0.5 to 12 cm. Approximately 80 percent of the patients with neurofibromatosis will have six or more CAL spots measuring 1.5 cm or greater in diameter. Additional findings are discussed in the section on neurofibromas (see "Papulonodular Skin Lesions"). In comparison to neurofibromatosis, the CAL spots in patients with Albright's disease (polyostotic fibrous dysplasia with precocious puberty in females) are usually larger, more irregular in outline, respect the midline, and rarely contain macromelanosomes. CAL spots have also been associated with pulmonary stenosis, temporal dysrhythmia, tuberous sclerosis, the LEOPARD syndrome, and ataxia telangiectasia, but a few such lesions can be found in normal individuals.

In incontinentia pigmenti, dyskeratosis congenita, and bleomycin pigmentation, the areas of localized hyperpigmentation form a pattern—swirled in the first, reticulated in the second, and flagellate in the third. Patients with the X-linked dominant disorder incontinentia pigmenti can have linear blisters and verrucous papules during infancy. During childhood, parallel swirls and streaks of hyperpigmentation appear on the trunk, and occasionally streaks of hypopigmentation appear on the extremities. Associated findings include seizures, mental retardation, spastic paraplegia, strabismus, cataracts, and delayed or impaired dentition. Biopsy of the streaks will show pigment within dermal macrophages ("incontinent pigment"). In dyskeratosis congenita, atrophic reticulated hyperpigmentation is seen on the neck, thighs, and trunk and it is accompanied by nail dystrophy, pancytopenia, and leukoplakia of the oral and anal mucosa. The latter often develops into squamous cell carcinoma. In addition to the flagellate pigmentation (linear streaks) on the trunk, patients receiving bleomycin often have hyperpigmentation on the elbows, knees and small joints of the hand.

Localized hyperpigmentation is seen as a side effect of several other systemic medications, including those that produce fixed-drug reactions (phenolphthalein, tetracyclines, sulfonamides, barbiturates,

TABLE 59-16   Hyperpigmentation (primary cutaneous disorders, localized)

	Clinical characteristics	Histopathology
Seborrheic keratosis	Tan to black papule Warty and/or greasy surface "Stuck on" appearance Trunk	Epidermal hyperplasia
Acanthosis nigricans	Velvety surface Neck, axillae, groin Occasionally on dorsum of the hand, corners of mouth	Epidermal folds
Ephelides (freckles)	2–5-mm macule Tan color Sun-exposed surfaces Darkens following sun exposure	Increased pigment in epidermis
Lentigo	0.3–1.5-cm macule Tan to black Most commonly in sun-exposed areas Face, upper trunk, and extremities	Increased number of melanocytes in epidermis
Nevus		
Junctional	Brown to black macule 2–6 mm	Nests of melanocytes at dermoepidermal junction
Compound	Tan to brown papule 2–6 mm	Nests of melanocytes in epidermis and dermis
Dermal	Flesh-colored Papule	Nests of melanocytes in dermis
Melanoma	Variation in color—brown, black, blue, red, white Irregular outline and surface >5 mm in diameter Asymmetric	Malignant neoplasm of melanocytes

and analgesics) and those that can bind to melanin (antimalarials). Fixed-drug eruptions recur in the same location as circular areas of erythema that can become bullous and then resolve as brown macules. The eruption usually appears within hours of administration of the offending agent and common locations include the genitalia, extremities, and perioral region. Chloroquine, hydroxychloroquine, and quinacrine produce gray-brown to blue-black discoloration of the shins, hard palate, and face, while blue macules are seen on the lower extremities and in sites of inflammation with prolonged minocycline administration. Estrogen in oral contraceptives can induce melasma (chloasma)—symmetric brown patches on the face, especially the cheeks, upper lip, chin, and forehead. Similar changes are seen in pregnancy, in patients receiving hydantoin, and in the adult form of Gaucher's disease. In the latter group, there is also hyperpigmentation of the distal lower extremities.

In the *diffuse* forms of hyperpigmentation, the darkening of the skin may be of equal intensity over the entire body or it may be accentuated in sun-exposed areas. The causes of diffuse hyperpigmentation can be divided into four groups—endocrine, metabolic, autoimmune, and drugs. The endocrinopathies that frequently have associated hyperpigmentation include *Addison's disease, Nelson's syndrome,* and *ectopic ACTH syndrome.* In these diseases, the increased pigmentation is diffuse, but it is accentuated in the palmar and plantar creases, sites of friction, scars, and the oral mucosa. An overproduction of any or all of the pituitary hormones α-MSH (melanocyte stimulating hormone), ACTH, and β-lipotropin can lead to an increase in melanocyte activity. All of these peptides are products of the pro-opiomelanocortin gene and therefore they can exhibit homology, e.g., α-MSH and ACTH share 13 amino acids. A minority of the patients with Cushing's disease or hyperthyroidism have generalized hyperpigmentation.

The metabolic causes of hyperpigmentation include *porphyria cutanea tarda* (PCT), *hemochromatosis, vitamin B$_{12}$ deficiency, folic acid deficiency, pellagra, malabsorption,* and *Whipple's disease.* In patients with PCT (see "Vesicles/Bullae"), the skin darkening is seen in sun-exposed areas and is a reflection of the photoreactive properties of porphyrins. The increased level of iron in the skin of patients with hemochromatosis stimulates melanin pigment production and leads to the classic bronze color. Patients with pellagra have a brown discoloration of the skin, especially in sun-exposed areas, as a result of nicotinic acid (niacin) deficiency. In the areas of increased pigmentation, there is a thin varnishlike scale. These changes are also seen in patients who are vitamin B$_6$ deficient, have functioning carcinoid tumors (increased consumption of niacin), or take isoniazid. Approximately 50 percent of the patients with Whipple's disease have an associated generalized hyperpigmentation in association with diarrhea, weight loss, arthritis, and lymphadenopathy. A diffuse slate-blue color is seen in patients with melanosis secondary to *metastatic melanoma* and melanogenuria. There is a debate as to whether the color is due to single-cell metastases in the dermis or to a widespread deposition of melanin resulting from the high concentration of circulating melanin precursors.

Of the autoimmune diseases associated with diffuse hyperpigmentation, *biliary cirrhosis* and *scleroderma* are the most common and, occasionally, both disorders are seen in the same patient. The skin is dark brown in color, especially in sun-exposed areas. In biliary cirrhosis, the hyperpigmentation is accompanied by pruritus, jaundice, and xanthomas, while in scleroderma, it is accompanied by sclerosis of the extremities, face, and, less commonly, the trunk. Additional clues to the diagnosis of scleroderma are telangiectasias, calcinosis cutis, Raynaud's phenomenon, and distal ulcerations (see "Telangiectasias"). The differential diagnosis of cutaneous sclerosis with hyperpigmentation includes the *POEMS syndrome: P,* polyneuropathy; *O,* organomegaly (liver, spleen, lymph nodes); *E,* endocrinopathies (impotence, gynecomastia); *M,* M-protein; and *S,* skin changes. The skin changes include hyperpigmentation, skin thickening, hypertrichosis, hyperhidrosis, and angiomas.

Diffuse hyperpigmentation that is due to *drugs* or metals can result from one of several mechanisms—induction of melanin pigment formation, complexing of the drug or its metabolites to melanin, and deposits of the drug in the dermis. Busulfan; cyclophosphamide; long-term, high-dose ACTH; and inorganic arsenic induce pigment production. Complexes containing melanin or hemosiderin plus the drug or its metabolites are seen in patients receiving chlorpromazine and minocycline. The sun-exposed skin as well as the conjunctivae of patients on long-term, high-dose chlorpromazine can become blue-gray in color. Patients taking minocycline may develop a diffuse blue-gray, muddy appearance in sun-exposed areas in addition to pigmentation of the mucous membranes, teeth, nails, bones, and thyroid. Administration of amiodorone can result in both a phototoxic eruption (exaggerated sunburn) and/or a brown or blue-gray discoloration of sun-exposed skin. Biopsy specimens of the latter show yellow-brown granules in dermal macrophages, which represent intralysosomal accumulations of lipids, amiodarone, and its metabolites. Actual deposits of a particular drug or metal in the skin are seen with silver (argyria), where the skin appears blue-gray in color; gold (chrysiasis), where the skin has a brown to blue-gray color; and clofazimine, where the skin appears reddish-brown. The associated hyperpigmentation is accentuated in sun-exposed areas, and discoloration of the eye is seen with gold (sclerae) and clofazimine (conjunctivae).

VESICLES/BULLAE (Table 59-17) Depending upon their size, cutaneous blisters are referred to as vesicles (<0.5 cm) or bullae (>0.5 cm). The primary blistering disorders include *pemphigus vulgaris, pemphigus foliaceus, pemphigus erythematosus, bullous pemphigoid, herpes gestationis, cicatricial pemphigoid, epidermolysis bullosa acquisita,* and *dermatitis herpetiformis* (see Chap. 58).

Vesicles and bullae are also seen in *contact dermatitis,* both allergic and irritant forms (see "Erythroderma"). When there is a linear arrangement of vesicular lesions, an exogenous cause should be suspected. Bullous disease secondary to the ingestion of drugs can take one of several forms, including phototoxic eruptions, isolated bullae, toxic epidermal necrolysis, and erythema multiforme. Clinically, phototoxic eruptions resemble an exaggerated sunburn with diffuse erythema and bullae in sun-exposed areas. The most commonly associated drugs are chlorothiazides, tetracyclines, sulfonylureas, sulfonamides, phenothiazines, griseofulvin, and psoralens. The development of a phototoxic eruption is dependent upon the dose of both the drug and the UV-A irradiation.

There are several drugs, including penicillins, sulfonamides, D-penicillamine, phenobarbital, phenytoin, furosemide, and nonsteroidal anti-inflammatory agents, that cause isolated bland bullae to arise on normal skin. The characteristics of these blisters are such that they can not be assigned to a particular cutaneous disease. The most common location for these isolated bullae is the distal extremity. In contrast, *toxic epidermal necrolysis* (TEN) is characterized by bullae

---

TABLE 59-17   Causes of vesicles/bullae

Primary cutaneous diseases	Systemic diseases
A Primary blistering diseases	A Infections
1 Pemphigus	*1* Cutaneous emboli
2 Bullous pemphigoid	B Metabolic
3 Herpes gestationis	*1* Diabetic bullae
4 Cicatricial pemphigoid	*2* Porphyria cutanea tarda
5 Dermatitis herpetiformis	*3* Porphyria variegata
6 Epidermolysis bullosa	*4* Pseudoporphyria
acquisita	*5* Bullous dermatosis of
B Secondary blistering diseases	hemodialysis
1 Contact	
2 Erythema multiforme	
3 Toxic epidermal necrolysis	
C Infections	
1 Varicella/zoster*	
2 Herpes simplex*	
3 Staphylococcal scalded-skin	
syndrome	
4 Bullous impetigo	

* Also systemic.

that arise on widespread areas of erythema and then slough. This results in large areas of denuded skin. The associated morbidity, such as sepsis, and mortality are relatively high and they are a function of the extent of epidermal necrosis. In addition, these patients may also have involvement of the mucous membranes and the intestinal tract. Drugs are the primary cause of TEN, and the most common offenders are phenytoin, barbiturates, sulfonamides, penicillins, allopurinol, phenolphthalein, and phenylbutazone. Severe acute graft-versus-host disease (grade 4) can also resemble TEN.

In *erythema multiforme* (EM), the primary lesions are pink-red macules and edematous papules, the centers of which may become vesicular. The clue to the diagnosis of EM rather than of a drug-induced morbilliform exanthem is the development of a "dusky" violet color or petechiae in the center of the lesions. Target or iris lesions are also characteristic of EM and they arise as a result of active centers and borders in combination with centrifugal spread. However, iris lesions need not be present to make the diagnosis of EM. Preferred sites of involvement include the hands, extensor forearms, palms, soles, and mucous membranes (oral, nasal, ocular, and genital). Hemorrhagic crusts of the lips are characteristic of EM as well as two other blistering disorders—pemphigus vulgaris and TEN. Fever, malaise, myalgias, sore throat, and cough may precede or accompany the eruption. The lesions of EM usually resolve over 3 to 6 weeks, but they may be recurrent.

Drugs can induce EM, in particular sulfonamides, phenytoin, barbiturates, penicillins, phenolphthalein, and carbamazepine, but they do not cause the majority of cases, especially in young adults. Infections with herpes simplex are a common cause of EM in this age group and the lesions appear 7 to 12 days after the viral eruption. Other infectious agents associated with EM include *Mycoplasma pneumoniae, Histoplasma capsulatum, Coccidioides immitis, Yersinia enterocolitica, Francisella tularensis,* and several viruses (echo, coxsackie, Epstein-Barr, and influenza). EM can also follow vaccinations with BCG, poliomyelitis or vaccinia viruses; radiation therapy; and exposure to environmental toxins; and it has been observed in a few patients with lupus erythematosus, Wegener's granulomatosis, and internal malignancy.

In addition to primary blistering disorders and hypersensitivity reactions, bacterial and viral infections can lead to vesicles and bullae. The most common infectious agents are herpes simplex, herpes varicella-zoster, and staphylococci.

Staphylococcal scalded-skin syndrome (SSSS) and bullous impetigo are two blistering disorders associated with staphylococcal (phage group II) infection. In SSSS, the initial findings are redness and tenderness of the central face, neck, trunk, and intertriginous zones. This is followed by short-lived flaccid bullae and a slough or exfoliation of the superficial epidermis. Crusted areas then develop, characteristically around the mouth. SSSS is distinguished from TEN by the following features: younger age group, more superficial site of blister formation, no oral lesions, shorter course, less morbidity and mortality, and an association with staphylococcal exfoliative toxin ("exfoliatin"), not drugs. A rapid diagnosis of SSSS versus TEN can be made by a frozen section of the blister roof or exfoliative cytology of the blister contents. In SSSS, the site of staphylococcal infection is usually extracutaneous (conjunctivitis, rhinorrhea, otitis media, pharyngitis, tonsillitis), and the lesions are sterile, whereas in *bullous impetigo* the lesions are the site of infection. Impetigo is more localized than SSSS and it usually presents with honey-colored crusts. Occasionally, superficial purulent blisters also form. *Cutaneous emboli* from gram-negative infections may present as isolated bullae, but the base of the lesion is purpuric or necrotic and it may develop into an ulcer (see "Purpura").

There are several metabolic disorders that are associated with blister formation including diabetes mellitus, renal failure, and porphyria. Local hypoxia secondary to decreased cutaneous blood flow can also produce blisters, which explains the presence of bullae over pressure points in comatose patients (coma bullae). In *diabetes mellitus,* tense bullae with clear viscous fluid arise on normal skin.

TABLE 59-18 Causes of exanthems

Morbilliform
  A Drugs
  B Viral
    1 Rubeola
    2 Rubella
    3 Erythema infectiosum
    4 Epstein-Barr, echo, coxsackie, and adenovirus
    5 Early HIV
  C Bacterial
    1 Typhoid fever
    2 Early secondary syphilis
    3 Early Rickettsia
    4 Early meningococcus
  D Acute graft-versus-host disease
Scarlatiniform
  A Scarlet fever
  B Toxic shock syndrome
  C Kawasaki's disease

The lesions can be as large as 6 cm in diameter and they are located on the distal extremities. There are several types of porphyria, but the most common form with cutaneous findings is *porphyria cutanea tarda* (PCT). In sun-exposed areas (primarily the face and hands), the skin is very fragile and trauma leads to erosions and tense vesicles. These lesions then heal with scarring and formation of milia; the latter are firm 2 to 3 mm white or yellow papules that represent epidermoid inclusion cysts. Associated findings can include hypertrichosis of the lateral malar region (males) or face (females) and, in sun-exposed areas, hyperpigmentation and firm sclerotic plaques. An elevated level of urinary uroporphyrins confirms the diagnosis and is due to a decrease in uroporphyrinogen decarboxylase activity. Precipitating agents include alcohol, estrogen, iron, and chlorinated hydrocarbons.

The differential diagnosis of PCT includes: (1) *porphyria variegata*—the skin signs of PCT plus the systemic findings of acute intermittent porphyria; it has a diagnostic plasma porphyrin fluorescence emission at 626 nm; (2) *drug-induced bullous photosensitivity* (pseudoporphyria)—the clinical and histologic findings are similar to PCT, but porphyrins are normal; etiologic agents are furosemide, tetracycline, nalidixic acid, dapsone, naproxen, and pyridoxine; (3) *bullous dermatosis of hemodialysis*—the same appearance as PCT, but porphyrins are usually normal or occasionally borderline elevated; patients have chronic renal failure and are on hemodialysis; (4) PCT associated with hepatomas, hepatic carcinomas, and hemodialysis; and (5) *epidermolysis bullosa acquisita* (see Chap. 58).

EXANTHEMS (Table 59-18) Exanthems are characterized by an acute generalized eruption. The two most common presentations are erythematous macules and papules (morbilliform) and confluent blanching erythema (scarlatiniform). *Morbilliform* eruptions are usually due to either *drugs* or viral infections. For example, at least 5 percent of the patients receiving penicillins, sulfonamides, captopril, phenytoin, or gold will develop a maculopapular eruption. Accompanying signs may include pruritus, fever, eosinophilia, and transient lymphadenopathy. Similar maculopapular eruptions are seen in the classic childhood viral exanthems including: (1) *rubeola* (measles)—a prodrome of coryza, cough, conjunctivitis, and Koplik's spots on the buccal mucosa whose onset coincides with a second fever spike; the eruption begins behind the ears, at the hair line, and on the forehead then spreads down the body, often becoming confluent; (2) *rubella*—it begins on the forehead and face, then spreads down the body; it resolves in the same order and is associated with retroauricular and suboccipital lymphadenopathy; and (3) *erythema infectiosum* (fifth disease)—erythema of the cheeks is followed by a reticulated pattern on extremities; it is secondary to a parvovirus infection and in adults, an associated arthritis is seen.

Both measles and rubella are seen in unvaccinated young adults and an atypical form of measles is seen in adults immunized with either killed measles vaccine or killed vaccine followed in time by live vaccine. In contrast to classic measles, the eruption of atypical measles begins on the palms, soles, wrists, and knuckles, and the lesions may become purpuric. The patient with atypical measles can have pulmonary involvement and be quite ill. Rubelliform and roseoliform eruptions are also associated with *Epstein-Barr* (5 to 15 percent of patients), *echo, coxsackie,* and *adenovirus* infections. Detection of specific IgM antibodies allows the proper diagnosis. Occasionally, a maculopapular eruption is the result of a drug-viral interaction. For example, about 95 percent of the patients with infectious mononucleosis who are given ampicillin will develop a rash.

Of note, early in the course of infections with *Rickettsia* and *meningococcus,* prior to the development of purpura, the lesions may be erythematous macules and papules. This is also the case in chickenpox prior to the development of vesicles. Maculopapular eruptions are associated with early *HIV* infection, early secondary *syphilis, typhoid fever,* and *acute graft-versus-host* disease. In the last, lesions frequently begin on the palms and soles; the macular rose spots of typhoid fever involve primarily the anterior trunk.

The prototypic *scarlatiniform* eruption is seen in *scarlet fever* and is due to an erythrotoxin produced by group A beta-hemolytic streptococcal infections, most commonly pharyngitis. There are a diffuse erythema, which begins on the neck and upper trunk, and red perifollicular puncta. Additional findings include a white strawberry tongue (white coating with red papillae) followed by a red strawberry tongue (red tongue and red papillae); petechiae of the palate; a facial flush with circumoral pallor; linear petechiae in the antecubital fossae; and desquamation of the involved skin, palms, and soles 5 to 20 days after the onset of the eruption. A similar desquamation of the palms and soles is seen in toxic shock syndrome, Kawasaki's disease, and after severe febrile illnesses. Certain strains of staphylococci also produce an erythrotoxin that leads to the same clinical findings as in streptococcal scarlet fever, except that the antistreptolysin O titers are not elevated.

In *toxic shock syndrome* (TSS), staphylococcal (phage group I) infections produce an exotoxin, which causes the fever and rash, as well as an enterotoxin. Initially, the majority of cases were reported in menstruating women who were using tampons. However, other sites of infection, including wounds and vaginitis, may produce TSS. The diagnosis of TSS is based upon clinical criteria and three of these involve mucocutaneous sites. The clinical criteria are: (1) fever; (2) diffuse erythema of the skin; (3) desquamation of the palms and soles 1 to 2 weeks after onset of illness; (4) hypotension; and (5) involvement of three or more organ systems, including the gastrointestinal tract, muscles, kidney, liver, CNS, hematologic (thrombocytopenia), and mucous membranes. The latter is characterized as hyperemia of the vagina, oropharynx, or conjunctivae.

Although the cutaneous eruption in *Kawasaki's disease* (mucocutaneous lymph node syndrome) is polymorphous, the two common types are morbilliform and scarlatiniform. The majority of cases are seen in children less than 5 years of age, but adult cases have been reported. The diagnosis is based upon a fever lasting more than 5 days plus four of the five following criteria: (1) bilateral conjunctival injection; (2) exanthem; (3) cervical lymphadenopathy, usually unilateral; (4) erythema and edema of the hands and feet followed by desquamation; and (5) diffuse erythema of the oropharynx, red strawberry tongue, and erosions with crusting on the lips. This clinical picture can resemble TSS and scarlet fever, but clues to the diagnosis of Kawasaki's disease are the cervical lymphadenopathy, lip erosions, and increased platelets. The more serious associated systemic finding in this disease is coronary aneurysms secondary to arteritis. The latter may lead to sudden death, primarily within the first 30 days of the illness. Scarlatiniform eruptions are also seen in the early phase of SSSS (see "Vesicles/Bullae") and as reactions to drugs.

URICARIA (Table 59-19) *Urticaria* (hives) are transient lesions that are composed of a central wheal surrounded by an erythematous halo. Individual lesions are round, oval, or figurate and they are often pruritic. *Acute* and *chronic* urticaria have a wide variety of allergic etiologies. Less common systemic causes of urticaria are mastocytosis (urticaria pigmentosa), hyperthyroidism, malignancy,

TABLE 59-19   Causes of urticaria

Primary cutaneous disorders
  A   Acute and chronic urticaria
  B   Physical urticaria
     1   Dermatographism
     2   Solar urticaria
     3   Cold urticaria*
     4   Cholinergic urticaria*
  C   Angioedema (hereditary and acquired)
Systemic diseases
  A   Urticarial vasculitis
  B   Hepatitis B infection
  C   Serum sickness
  D   Angioedema (acquired)

* Also systemic.

and juvenile rheumatoid arthritis (JRA). In JRA, the lesions coincide with the fever spike and they are transient, but not migratory as in erythema marginatum.

The common *physical urticarias* include *dermatographism, solar urticaria, cold urticaria,* and *cholinergic urticaria.* Patients with dermatographism exhibit linear wheals following minor pressure or scratching of the skin. It is a common disorder, affecting approximately 5 percent of the population. Solar urticaria characteristically occurs within minutes of sun exposure and is a skin sign of one systemic disease—erythropoietic protoporphyria. In addition to the urticaria, these patients have subtle pitted scarring of the nose and hands. Cold urticaria is precipitated by exposure to the cold and therefore exposed areas are usually affected. In some cases, the disease is associated with abnormal circulating proteins—more commonly, cryoglobulins and cold hemolysins, and less commonly, cryofibrinogens and cold agglutinins. Additional systemic symptoms include wheezing and syncope, thus explaining the need for these patients to avoid swimming in cold water. Cholinergic urticaria is precipitated by heat, exercise, or emotion and is characterized by small wheals with relatively large flares. It is occasionally associated with wheezing.

Whereas urticaria is the result of dermal edema, subcutaneous edema leads to the clinical picture of *angioedema.* Sites of involvement include the eyelids, lips, tongue, larynx, and gastrointestinal tract as well as the subcutaneous tissue. Angioedema occurs alone or in combination with urticaria, including urticarial vasculitis and the physical urticarias. Both acquired and hereditary (autosomal dominant) forms of angioedema occur (see Chap. 267), and in the latter, urticaria is rarely seen.

Urticarial vasculitis is an immune complex disease that may be confused with simple urticaria. In contrast to simple urticaria, individual lesions tend to last longer than 24 h and they usually develop central petechiae that can be observed even after the urticarial phase has resolved. The patient may also complain of burning rather than pruritus. On biopsy, there is either a lymphocytic or leukocytoclastic vasculitis of the small blood vessels. Although many cases of urticarial vasculitis are idiopathic in origin, it can be a reflection of an underlying systemic illness such as lupus erythematosus, Sjögren's syndrome, or hereditary complement deficiency. There is a spectrum of urticarial vasculitis which ranges from purely cutaneous to multisystem involvement. The most common systemic signs and symptoms are arthralgias and/or arthritis, nephritis, crampy abdominal pain, asthma, and chronic obstructive lung disease. Hypocomplementemia is seen in one- to two-thirds of patients, even in the idiopathic cases. Similar cutaneous, joint, and renal findings can be seen in the prodrome of *hepatitis B* infection, *serum sickness,* and *serum sickness–like illnesses.*

PAPULONODULAR SKIN LESIONS (Table 59-20) In the papulonodular diseases, the lesions are elevated above the surface of the skin and they may coalesce to form plaques. The location, consistency, and color of the lesions are the keys to their diagnosis. This section is organized on the basis of color and the color groups are white, flesh, pink, yellow, red, red-brown, blue, violaceous, purple, and brown-black.

TABLE 59-20 Papulonodular skin lesions according to color groups

White
  A Calcinosis cutis
Flesh
  A Rheumatoid nodule
  B Neurofibromas
    (von Recklinghausen's disease)
  C Angiofibromas
    (tuberous sclerosis)
  D Neuromas
    (multiple endocrine neoplasia
    syndrome, type 2b)
  E Adnexal tumors
    1 Basal cell epitheliomas
      (basal cell nevus syndrome)
    2 Tricholemmomas
      (Cowden's disease)
  F Primary cutaneous disorders
    1 Epidermal inclusion cysts
    2 Lipomas
Pink/translucent
  A Amyloidosis
  B Papular mucinosis
Yellow
  A Xanthomas
  B Tophi
  C Necrobiosis lipoidica
  D Pseudoxanthoma elasticum
  E Sebaceous adenomas
    (Torre's syndrome)
Red
  A Papules
    1 Angiokeratomas
      (Fabry's disease)
    2 Hemangioma-like lesions
      (disseminated cat-scratch
      disease in AIDS)
  B Papules/plaques
    1 Cutaneous lupus
    2 Lymphoma cutis
    3 Leukemia cutis
	C Nodules
	    1 Panniculitis
	    2 Cutaneous polyarteritis
	      nodosa
	    3 Systemic vasculitis
	  D Primary cutaneous disorders
	    1 Arthropod bites
	    2 Cherry hemangiomas
	    3 Infections, e.g., erysipelas,
	      sporotrichosis
	    4 Polymorphous light eruption
	    5 Lymphocytoma cutis
	      (pseudolymphoma)
	Red-brown
	  A Sarcoidosis
	  B Sweet's syndrome
	  C Urticaria pigmentosa
	  D Erythema elevatum diutinum
	    (chronic leukocytoclastic
	    vasculitis)
	  E Lupus vulgaris
	Blue
	  A Cavernous hemangiomas
	    (blue rubber bleb syndrome)
	  B Primary cutaneous disorders
	    1 Venous lake
	    2 Blue nevus
	Violaceous
	  A Lupus pernio (sarcoidosis)
	  B Lymphoma cutis
	  C Cutaneous lupus
	Purple
	  A Kaposi's sarcoma
	  B Angiosarcoma
	  C Palpable purpura
	Brown-black
	  See "Hyperpigmentation"
	Any color
	  A Metastases

usually in combination with six or more café au lait spots measuring >1.5 cm (see "Hyperpigmentation") and multiple Lisch nodules, are seen in von Recklinghausen's disease. Lisch nodules are 1-mm yellow-brown spots within the iris that are best observed with 10× magnification. Additional manifestations include axillary freckling and peripheral and CNS tumors (see Chap. 358). In some patients, the neurofibromas are localized and unilateral while in others, they are limited to the CNS.

Angiofibromas are pink to flesh-colored firm papules that measure from 3 mm to several centimeters in diameter. When they are located on the central cheeks (adenoma sebaceum) or under and around the nails, the patient has tuberous sclerosis. It is an autosomal disorder and the associated findings are discussed in the section on ash leaf spots (see "Hypopigmentation").

Neuromas (benign proliferation of nerve fibers) are also flesh-colored firm papules. They are more commonly found at sites of amputation and as rudimentary supernumerary digits. However, when there are multiple neuromas on the eyelids, lips, distal tongue, and/or oral mucosa, the patient should be investigated for other signs of the multiple endocrine neoplasia syndrome, type 2b. Associated findings include marfanoid habitus, protuberant lips, intestinal ganglioneuromas, and medullary thyroid carcinoma (>75 percent of patients) (see Chap. 325).

Adnexal tumors are derived from pluripotential cells of the epidermis that can differentiate toward hair, sebaceous, apocrine, or eccrine glands or remain undifferentiated. *Basal cell epitheliomas* (BCEs) are examples of adnexal tumors that have little or no evidence of differentiation. Clinically, they are translucent papules with rolled borders, telangiectasias, and central erosion. BCEs commonly arise in sun-damaged skin of the head and neck. When a patient has multiple BCEs, especially prior to age 30, the possibility of the basal cell nevus syndrome should be raised. It is inherited as an autosomal dominant trait and is associated with jaw cysts, palmar and plantar pits, frontal bossing, rib anomalies, spina bifida occulta, and calcification of the falx cerebri and diaphragma sellae. *Tricholemmomas* are also flesh-colored adnexal tumors, but they differentiate towards hair follicles and can have a wartlike appearance. The presence of multiple tricholemmomas on the face and oral mucosa points to the diagnosis of Cowden's disease (multiple hamartoma syndrome). The oral tricholemmomas are found primarily on the tongue and gingiva and give these areas a cobblestone appearance. Internal organ involvement (in decreasing order of frequency) includes fibrocystic disease and carcinoma of the breast, adenomas and carcinomas of the thyroid, and gastrointestinal polyposis. Keratoses of the palms, soles, and dorsa of the hands are also seen.

Pink lesions The cutaneous lesions associated with primary systemic *amyloidosis* are pink in color and translucent. Common locations are the face, especially the periorbital and perioral regions, and intertriginous areas. On biopsy, homogeneous deposits of amyloid are seen in the dermis and in the walls of blood vessels; the latter leads to an increase in vessel wall fragility. As a result, petechiae and purpura develop in clinically normal skin as well as in lesional skin following minor trauma, hence the term "pinch purpura." Amyloid deposits are also seen in the striated muscle of the tongue and this results in macroglossia.

Even though specific mucocutaneous lesions are rarely seen in secondary amyloidosis and are present in only about 30 percent of the patients with primary amyloidosis, a rapid diagnosis of systemic amyloidosis can be made by an examination of abdominal subcutaneous fat. By special staining, deposits are seen around blood vessels or individual fat cells in 40 to 50 percent of patients. There are also three forms of amyloidosis that are limited to the skin and that should not be construed as cutaneous lesions of systemic amyloidosis. They are macular amyloid (upper back), lichenoid amyloidosis (usually lower extremities), and nodular amyloidosis. In macular and lichenoid amyloidosis, the deposits are composed of altered epidermal keratin.

Patients with multicentric reticulohistiocytosis also have pink-colored papules and nodules on the face and mucous membranes as

White lesions In *calcinosis cutis,* there are firm white to white-yellow papules with an irregular surface. When the contents are discharged, a chalky white material is seen. *Dystrophic* calcification is seen at sites of previous inflammation or damage to the skin. It develops in acne scars as well as on the distal extremities of patients with scleroderma and in areas of muscle necrosis in dermatomyositis. The latter is more extensive and is more commonly seen in children. An elevated calcium phosphate product, as in secondary hyperparathyroidism, can lead to nodules of *metastatic* calcinosis cutis, which tend to be subcutaneous and periarticular. This form is often accompanied by calcification of muscular arteries and subsequent ischemic necrosis.

Flesh-colored lesions There are several types of flesh-colored lesions including epidermoid inclusion cysts, lipomas, rheumatoid nodules, neurofibromas, angiofibromas, neuromas, and adnexal tumors such as tricholemmomas. Both *epidermoid inclusion cysts* and *lipomas* are very common mobile subcutaneous nodules—the former are rubbery and compressible and they drain cheeselike material (sebum and keratin) if incised. Lipomas are firm and somewhat lobulated on palpation. When extensive facial epidermoid inclusion cysts develop in childhood or there is a family history of such lesions, the patient should be examined for other signs of Gardner's syndrome, including desmoid tumors (see Chap. 242). *Rheumatoid nodules* are firm 0.5- to 4-cm nodules that tend to localize around pressure points, especially the elbows. They are seen in approximately 20 percent of patients with rheumatoid arthritis and 6 percent of patients with Still's disease. Biopsies of the nodules show palisading granulomas. Similar lesions that are smaller and shorter-lived are seen in rheumatic fever.

Neurofibromas (benign Schwann cell tumors) are soft papules or nodules that exhibit the "button-hole" sign, that is, they invaginate into the skin with pressure in a manner similar to a hernia. Single lesions are seen in normal individuals, but multiple neurofibromas, well as on the extensor surface of the hands and forearms. They have a polyarthritis that can mimic rheumatoid arthritis clinically. On histologic examination, the papules have characteristic giant cells which are not seen in biopsies of rheumatoid nodules. Pink to flesh-colored papules that are firm, 2 to 5 mm in diameter, and often in a linear arrangement are seen in patients with *papular mucinosis*. This disease is also referred to as lichen myxedematosus or scleromyxedema. The latter name comes from the brawny induration of the face and extremities that may accompany the papular eruption. Biopsy specimens of the papules show localized mucin deposition, and serum protein electrophoresis demonstrates a monoclonal spike of IgG, usually with a λ light chain.

Yellow lesions   Several systemic disorders are characterized by yellow-colored cutaneous papules or plaques—hyperlipidemia (xanthomas), gout (tophi), diabetes (necrobiosis lipoidica), pseudoxanthoma elasticum, and Torre's syndrome (sebaceous tumors). Eruptive xanthomas are the most common form of *xanthomas* and they are associated with hypertriglyceridemia (types I, III, IV, and V). Crops of yellow papules with erythematous halos occur primarily on the extensor surface of the extremities and the buttocks in association with elevations of the circulating triglycerides. They spontaneously involute with a fall in serum lipids. Increased β-lipoproteins (primarily types II and III) result in one or more of the following types of xanthoma: xanthelasma, tendon xanthomas, and plane xanthomas. Xanthelasma are found on the eyelids, while tendon xanthomas are frequently associated with the Achilles and extensor finger tendons; plane xanthoma are flat and favor the palmar creases, face, upper trunk, and scars. Tuberous xanthomas are frequently associated with hypertriglyceridemia, but they are also seen in patients with hypercholesterolemia (type II) and they are found most frequently over the large joints or hand. Biopsy specimens of xanthomas show collections of lipid-containing macrophages (foam cells).

Patients with several disorders, including biliary cirrhosis, can have a secondary form of hyperlipidemia with associated tuberous and planar xanthomas. However, patients with myeloma have *normolipemic* flat xanthomas. This latter form of xanthoma may be ≥12 cm in diameter and is most frequently seen on the upper trunk or side of the neck. It is also important to note that the most common setting for eruptive xanthomas is uncontrolled diabetes mellitus. The least specific sign for hyperlipidemia is xanthelasma because at least 50 percent of the patients with this finding have normal lipid profiles.

In tophaceous gout, there are deposits of monosodium urate in the skin around the joints, particularly those of the hands and feet. Additional sites of *tophi* formation include the helix of the ear and the olecranon and prepatellar bursae. The lesions are firm, yellow in color, and occasionally discharge a chalky material. Their size varies from 1 mm to 7 cm and the diagnosis can be established by polarization of the aspirated contents of a lesion. Lesions of *necrobiosis lipoidica* are found primarily on the shins (90 percent) and the majority of patients have diabetes mellitus or develop it subsequently. Characteristic findings include a central yellow color, atrophy (transparency), telangiectasias, and an erythematous border. Ulcerations can also develop within the plaques. Biopsy specimens show necrobiosis of collagen, granulomatous inflammation, and obliterative endarteritis.

In *pseudoxanthoma elasticum* (PXE), there is an abnormal deposition of calcium upon the elastic fibers of the skin, eye, and blood vessels. In the skin, the flexural areas such as the neck, axillae, antecubital fossae, and inguinal area are the primary sites of involvement. Yellow papules coalesce to form reticulated plaques that have an appearance similar to that of plucked chicken skin. In severely affected skin, hanging, redundant folds develop. Some patients have a more subtle macular form of the disease and careful inspection is required. Biopsy specimens of involved skin show swollen and irregularly clumped elastic fibers with deposits of calcium. In the eye, the calcium deposits in Bruch's membrane lead to angioid streaks and choroiditis; in the arteries of the heart, kidney, gastrointestinal tract and extremities, the deposits lead to angina, hypertension, gastrointestinal bleeding, and claudication, respectively. Four types

of PXE have been described—two with autosomal dominant and two with autosomal recessive inheritance. The extent of vessel and skin involvement varies depending upon the type.

Adnexal tumors that have differentiated toward sebaceous glands include sebaceous adenoma, sebaceous epithelioma, sebaceous carcinoma, and sebaceous hyperplasia. Except for sebaceous hyperplasia, which is commonly seen on the face, these tumors are solitary and uncommon. Patients with Torre's syndrome have *sebaceous adenomas*, and, in the majority of cases, there are multiple such tumors. These patients can also have sebaceous carcinomas and sebaceous hyperplasia as well as keratoacanthomas. The internal manifestations of Torre's syndrome include *multiple* carcinomas of the gastrointestinal tract (primarily colon) as well as cancers of the larynx, genitourinary tract, ovary, and endometrium. Some patients have a strong family history of cancer.

Red lesions   Cutaneous lesions that are red in color have a wide variety of etiologies and in an attempt to simplify their identification, they will be subdivided into papules, papules/plaques, and subcutaneous nodules. Common red papules include *arthropod bites* and *cherry hemangiomas;* the latter are small, bright-red, dome-shaped papules that represent benign proliferation of capillaries. In patients with AIDS, the development of multiple red hemangioma-like lesions points to disseminated *cat-scratch disease*, and biopsy specimens show collections of gram-negative rods. Multiple *angiokeratomas* are seen in Fabry's disease, an X-linked recessive lysosomal storage disease that is due to a deficiency of alpha galactosidase A. The lesions are red to red-blue in color and can be quite small in size (1 to 3 mm) with the most common location being the lower trunk. Associated findings include chronic renal failure, peripheral neuropathy, and corneal opacities (cornea verticillata). Electron photomicrographs of angiokeratomas and clinically normal skin demonstrate lamellar lipid deposits in fibroblasts, pericytes, and endothelial cells that are diagnostic of this disease. Widespread acute eruptions of erythematous papules are discussed in the section on exanthems.

There are several infectious diseases that present as erythematous papules or nodules in a sporotrichoid pattern, that is, in a linear arrangement along the lymphatic channels. The two most common etiologies are *Sporothrix schenckii* (*sporotrichosis*) and *Mycobacterium marinum* (atypical mycobacteria). The organisms are introduced as a result of trauma, and a primary inoculation site is often seen in addition to the lymphatic nodules. Additional causes include *Nocardia, Leishmania,* and other dimorphic fungi; culture of lesional tissue will aid in the diagnosis.

The diseases that are characterized by erythematous plaques with scale are reviewed in the papulosquamous section and the various forms of dermatitis are discussed in the section on erythroderma. Additional disorders in the differential diagnosis of red papules/plaques include *erysipelas, polymorphous light eruption, lymphocytoma cutis, cutaneous lupus, lymphoma cutis,* and *leukemia cutis.* The first three diseases represent primary cutaneous disorders. Polymorphous light eruption (PMLE) is characterized by erythematous papules and plaques in a primarily sun-exposed distribution—dorsum of the hand, extensor forearm, and face. Lesions follow exposure to both UV-B and UV-A, and in northern latitudes PMLE is most severe in the late spring and early summer. A process referred to as "hardening" occurs with continued UV exposure and the eruption fades, but in temperate climates it will recur in the spring. PMLE must be differentiated from cutaneous lupus and this is accomplished by histologic examination and direct immunofluorescence of the lesions. Lymphocytoma cutis (pseudolymphoma) is a *benign* proliferation of lymphocytes in the skin that presents as infiltrated pink-red to red-purple papules and plaques. It must be distinguished from cutaneous lupus and lymphoma cutis.

Several types of red plaques are seen in patients with systemic *lupus* including: (1) erythematous urticarial plaques across the cheeks and nose in the classic butterfly rash; (2) erythematous discoid lesions with fine or "carpet-tack" scale, telangiectasias, central hypopigmentation, peripheral hyperpigmentation, follicular plugging, and atrophy located on the face, scalp, external ears, arms, and upper trunk; and (3) psoriasiform or annular lesions of subacute lupus with hypopigmented centers located on the face, extensor arms, and upper trunk. Additional cutaneous findings include: (1) a violaceous flush on the face and vee of the neck; (2) urticarial vasculitis (see "Urticaria"); (3) lupus panniculitis (see below); (4) diffuse alopecia; (5) alopecia secondary to discoid lesions; (6) periungual telangiectasias and erythema; (7) erythema multiforme-like lesions which may become bullous; and (8) distal ulcerations secondary to Raynaud's phenomenon, vasculitis, or livedoid vasculitis. Patients with only discoid lesions usually have the form of lupus that is limited to the skin. However, 2 to 10 percent of these patients eventually develop systemic lupus. Direct immunofluorescence of involved skin shows deposits of IgG and C3 in a granular distribution along the dermal-epidermal junction.

In *lymphoma cutis,* there is a proliferation of malignant lymphocytes or histiocytes in the skin and the clinical appearance resembles that of lymphocytoma cutis—infiltrated pink-red to red-purple papules and plaques. Lymphoma cutis can occur anywhere on the surface of the skin, whereas the sites of predilection for lymphocytomas are the malar ridge, tip of the nose, earlobes, forearms, and scrotum. Patients with non-Hodgkin's lymphomas have specific cutaneous lesions more often than those with Hodgkin's disease and occasionally the skin nodules precede the development of extracutaneous non-Hodgkin's lymphoma. Arcuate lesions are sometimes seen in lymphoma and lymphocytoma cutis as well as in CTLC. *Leukemia cutis* has the same appearance as lymphoma cutis and specific lesions are seen more commonly in monocytic leukemias than in lymphocytic or granulocytic leukemias. Cutaneous chloromas (granulocytic sarcomas) may precede the appearance of circulating blasts in acute nonlymphocytic leukemia and as such represent a form of aleukemic leukemia cutis.

Common causes of erythematous subcutaneous nodules include inflamed epidermoid inclusion cysts, acne cysts, and furuncles. *Panniculitis,* an inflammation of the fat, also presents as subcutaneous nodules and is frequently a sign of systemic disease. There are several forms of panniculitis including erythema nodosum, erythema induratum, lupus profundus, Weber-Christian disease, α_1-antitrypsin deficiency, facticial, and fat necrosis secondary to pancreatic disease. In all of these disorders, except for erythema nodosum, the lesions may break down and ulcerate or heal with a scar. The shin is the most common location for the nodules of erythema nodosum while the calf is the most common location for lesions of erythema induratum. In erythema nodosum, the nodules are initially red, but then they develop a blue color as they resolve. Patients with erythema nodosum and no underlying systemic illness can still have fever, malaise, leukocytosis, arthralgias and/or arthritis, and unilateral or bilateral hilar adenopathy. However, the possibility of an underlying illness should be excluded and the most common associations are streptococcal infections, upper respiratory infections, sarcoidosis, and inflammatory bowel disease. The less common associations include tuberculosis, histoplasmosis, coccidioidomycosis, psittacosis, drugs (oral contraceptives, sulfonamides, aspartame, bromides, iodides), cat-scratch fever, and infections with *Yersinia, Salmonella,* and *Chlamydia.*

In most patients, erythema induratum/nodular vasculitis is an idiopathic disease, while in a few it may be a reflection of extracutaneous tuberculosis. The lesions of lupus profundus are found primarily on the face, upper arms, and buttocks (sites of abundant fat) and they are seen in both the cutaneous and systemic forms of lupus. The overlying skin may be normal, erythematous, or have the changes of discoid lupus. The subcutaneous fat necrosis that is associated with pancreatic disease is presumably secondary to circulating lipases and is seen in patients with pancreatic carcinoma as well as with acute and chronic pancreatitis. In this disorder and in Weber-Christian disease, there may be an associated arthritis, fever, and inflammation of visceral fat. Histologic examination of deep incisional biopsy specimens will aid in the diagnosis of the particular type of panniculitis.

Subcutaneous erythematous nodules are also seen in *cutaneous polyarteritis nodosa* (PAN) and as a manifestation of *systemic vasculitis,* e.g., systemic PAN, allergic granulomatosis, or Wegener's granulomatosis. Cutaneous PAN presents with painful subcutaneous nodules and ulcers within a red-purple, netlike pattern of livedo reticularis. The latter is due to slowed blood flow through the superficial horizontal venous plexus. The majority of lesions are found on the lower extremity, and while arthralgias and myalgias may accompany cutaneous PAN, there is no evidence of systemic involvement. In both the cutaneous and systemic forms of vasculitis, skin biopsy specimens of the associated nodules will show the changes characteristic of a vasculitis; the size of the vessel involved will depend upon the particular disease.

Red-brown lesions The cutaneous lesions in *sarcoidosis* are classically red to red-brown in color, and with diascopy (pressure with a glass slide) a yellow-brown residual color is observed that is secondary to the granulomatous infiltrate. The waxy papules and plaques may be found anywhere on the skin, but the face is the most common location. Usually there are no surface changes, but occasionally the lesions will have scale. Biopsy specimens of the papules show "naked" granulomas in the dermis, that is, granulomas surrounded by a minimal number of lymphocytes. Other cutaneous findings in sarcoidosis include annular lesions with an atrophic or scaly center, papules within scars, hypopigmented macules and papules, alopecia, acquired ichthyosis, erythema nodosum, and lupus pernio (see below). Additional physical findings are peripheral lymphadenopathy and parotid and lacrimal gland enlargement. When there is cutaneous involvement of the hands, radiographs will often show lytic leisons in the underlying bone.

The differential diagnosis of sarcoidosis includes foreign body granulomas produced by chemicals such as beryllium and zirconium, late secondary syphilis, and *lupus vulgaris.* Lupus vulgaris is a form of cutaneous tuberculosis that is seen in previously infected and sensitized individuals. There is often underlying active tuberculosis elsewhere, usually in the lungs or lymph nodes. At least 90 percent of the lesions occur in the head and neck area and they are red-brown plaques with a yellow-brown color on diascopy. Secondary scarring and squamous cell carcinomas can develop within the plaques. Cultures of the lesions should be done because it is rare for the acid-fast stain to show bacilli within the dermal granulomas.

Sweet's syndrome is characterized by red-brown plaques and nodules that are frequently painful and occur primarily on the head, neck, and upper extremities. The patients also have fever, neutrophilia, and a dense dermal infiltrate of neutrophils in the lesions. In approximately 10 percent of the patients, there is an associated malignancy, most commonly acute nonlymphocytic leukemia. Lymphoma, chronic leukemia, myeloma, myelodysplastic syndromes, and solid tumors (primarily of the genitourinary tract) have also been reported. Extracutaneous sites of involvement include joints, muscles, eye, kidney (proteinuria, occasionally glomerulonephritis), and lung (neutrophilic infiltrates). The idiopathic form of Sweet's syndrome is seen more often in women, following a respiratory tract infection.

A generalized distribution of red-brown macules and papules is seen in the form of mastocytosis known as *urticaria pigmentosa.* Each lesion represents a collection of mast cells in the dermis with hyperpigmentation of the overlying epidermis. Stimuli such as rubbing and heat cause these mast cells to degranulate and this leads to the formation of localized urticaria (Darier's sign). Additional symptoms can result from mast cell degranulation and these include headache, flushing, diarrhea, and pruritus. Mast cells also infiltrate various organs such as the liver, spleen, and gastrointestinal tract in up to 30 to 50 percent of patients with urticaria pigmentosa, and accumulations of mast cells in the bones may produce either osteosclerotic or osteolytic shadows on radiographs. In the majority of these patients, however, the internal involvement remains fairly static. A subtype of chronic leukocytoclastic vasculitis, *erythema elevatum diutinum* (EED), also presents with papules that are red-brown in color. The papules coalesce into plaques on the extensor surface of knees, elbows, and small joints of the hand. Flares of EED have been associated with streptococcal infections.

Blue lesions Lesions that are blue in color are the result of either vascular ectasias and tumors or melanin pigment in the dermis. *Venous lakes* (ectasias) are compressible dark blue lesions that are found commonly in the head and neck region. *Cavernous hemangiomas* are also compressible blue papules and nodules that can occur anywhere on the body, including the oral mucosa. When they are multiple rather than single congenital lesions, the patient may have the blue rubber bleb syndrome or Mafucci's syndrome. Patients with the blue rubber bleb syndrome also have hemangiomas of the gastrointestinal tract that may bleed, whereas patients with Mafucci's syndrome have associated dyschondroplasia and osteochondromas. In the case of single cavernous hemangiomas that are relatively large in size, there can be associated platelet consumption (Kasabach-Merritt syndrome) or musculoskeletal defects. *Blue nevi* (moles) are seen when there are collections of pigment-producing nevus cells in the dermis. These benign papular lesions are dome-shaped and they occur most commonly on the dorsum of the hand and arm.

Violaceous lesions Violaceous papules and plaques are seen in *lupus pernio, lymphoma cutis,* and *cutaneous lupus.* Lupus pernio is a particular type of sarcoidosis that involves the tip of the nose and the earlobes, with lesions that are violaceous in color rather than red-brown. This form of sarcoidosis is associated with involvement of the upper respiratory tract. The plaques of lymphoma cutis and cutaneous lupus may be red or violaceous in color and are discussed above.

Purple lesions Purple-colored papules and plaques are seen in vascular tumors, such as *Kaposi's sarcoma* (see Chap. 264) and *angiosarcoma,* and when there is extravasation of red blood cells into the skin in association with inflammation, as in *palpable purpura* (see purpura). Patients with congenital or acquired arteriovenous fistulas can develop purple papules on the lower extremities that can resemble Kaposi's sarcoma clinically and histologically, and this condition is referred to as pseudo-Kaposi sarcoma (acral angiodermatitis). *Angiosarcoma* is found most commonly on the scalp and face of elderly patients or within areas of chronic lymphedema and it presents as purple papules and plaques. In the head and neck region, the tumor often extends beyond the clinically defined borders and may be accompanied by facial edema.

Brown and black-colored papules are reviewed in the section on hyperpigmentation.

Cutaneous metastases are discussed last because they can have a wide range of colors. Most commonly they present as either firm flesh-colored subcutaneous nodules or red to red-brown firm papulonodules. The lesions of lymphoma cutis range from pink-red to plum in color while metastatic melanoma can be pink, blue, or black in color. Cutaneous metastases develop from hematogenous or lymphatic spread and are most often due to the following primary carcinomas: in men, lung, colon, melanoma, and oral cavity; and in women, breast, colon, and lung. These metastatic lesions may be the initial presentation of the carcinoma, especially when the primary site is the lung, kidney, or ovary.

PURPURA (Table 59-21) Purpura are seen when there is an extravasation of red blood cells into the dermis and, as a result, the lesions do not blanch with pressure. This is in contrast to those erythematous or violet-colored lesions that are due to localized vasodilatation—they do blanch with pressure. Purpura (≥3 mm) and petechiae (≤2 mm) are divided into two major groups, palpable and nonpalpable. The most frequent causes of *nonpalpable* petechiae and purpura are primary cutaneous disorders such as *trauma, solar purpura,* and *steroid purpura.* Less common causes are *capillaritis* and *livedoid vasculitis* (see "Ulcers"). Solar purpura are seen primarily on the dorsum of the hand and extensor forearm while glucocorticoid purpura, secondary to potent topical steroids, or endogenous or exogenous Cushing's syndrome can be more widespread. In both cases, there is alteration of the supporting connective tissue that surrounds the dermal blood vessels. In contrast, the

TABLE 59-21 Causes of purpura	
Primary cutaneous disorders	*d* Warfarin reaction
A Nonpalpable	4 Emboli
1 Trauma	*a* Cholesterol
2 Solar purpura	*b* Fat
3 Steroid purpura	5 Possible immune complex
4 Capillaritis	*a* Gardner-Diamond syn-
5 Livedoid vasculitis	drome (autoerythrocyte
Systemic diseases	sensitization)
A Nonpalpable	*b* Waldenström's hypergam-
1 Clotting disturbances	maglobulinemic purpura
a Thrombocytopenia	*B* Palpable
b Abnormal platelet	1 Vasculitis
function	*a* Leukocytoclastic vasculi-
c Clotting factor defects	tis (oval outline)
2 Vascular fragility	*b* Polyarteritis nodosa (ir-
a Amyloidosis	regular outline)
b Ehlers-Danlos syndrome	2 Emboli (irregular outline)
c Scurvy	*a* Acute meningococcemia
3 Thrombi	*b* Disseminated gonococcal
a Disseminated intravascu-	infection
lar coagulation	*c* Rocky mountain spotted
b Monoclonal cryoglobuli-	fever
nemia	*d* Ecthyma gangrenosum
c Thrombotic thrombocyto-	
penic purpura	

petechiae that result from capillaritis are found primarily on the lower extremities. In capillaritis, there is an extravasation of erythrocytes as a result of perivascular lymphocytic inflammation. The petechiae are bright red, 1 to 2 mm in size, and scattered within annular or coin-shaped yellow-brown macules. The yellow-brown color is caused by hemosiderin deposits within the dermis.

Systemic causes of nonpalpable purpura fall into several categories and those secondary to clotting disturbances and vascular fragility will be discussed first. The former group includes *thrombocytopenia, abnormal platelet function* as is seen in uremia, and *clotting factor defects.* The initial site of presentation for thrombocytopenia-induced petechiae is the distal lower extremity. Capillary fragility leads to nonpalpable purpura in patients with systemic *amyloidosis* (see "Papulonodular Skin Lesions") and disorders of collagen production such as *Ehlers-Danlos syndrome* and *scurvy.* In scurvy, there are flattened corkscrew hairs with surrounding hemorrhage on the lower extremities, in addition to gingivitis. Vitamin C is a cofactor for lysyl hydroxylase, an enzyme involved in the posttranslational modification of procollagen that is necessary for cross-link formation.

In contrast to the previous group of disorders in which either capillary fragility or a clotting abnormality is responsible for the nonpalpable purpura, the purpura seen in the following group of diseases are associated with thrombi formation within vessels. It is important to note that these thrombi are demonstrable in skin biopsy specimens. This group of disorders includes *disseminated intravascular coagulation, monoclonal cryoglobulinemia, thrombotic thrombocytopenic purpura* and *reactions to warfarin.* Disseminated intravascular coagulation (DIC) is triggered by several types of infection (gram-negative, gram-positive, viral, and rickettsial) as well as by tissue injury and neoplasms. Widespread purpura and hemorrhagic infarcts of the distal extremities are seen. Similar lesions are found in purpura fulminans, which is a form of DIC associated with fever and hypotension that occurs more commonly in children following an infectious illness such as varicella, scarlet fever, or an upper respiratory tract infection. In both disorders, hemorrhagic bullae can develop in involved skin.

Monoclonal cryoglobulinemia is associated with multiple myeloma, Waldenström's macroglobulinemia, lymphocytic leukemia, and lymphoma. Purpura, primarily of the lower extremities, and hemorrhagic infarcts of the fingers and toes are seen in these patients. Exacerbations of disease activity can follow cold exposure or an increase in serum viscosity. Biopsy specimens show precipitates of the cryoglobulin within dermal vessels. Similar deposits have been found in the lung, brain, and renal glomeruli. Patients with *thrombotic thrombocytopenic purpura* can also have hemorrhagic infarcts as a result of intravascular thromboses. Additional signs include thrombocytopenic purpura, fever, and microangiopathic hemolytic anemia (see Chap. 294).

Administration of *warfarin* can result in painful areas of erythema that become purpuric then necrotic with an adherent black eschar. This reaction is seen more often in women and in areas with abundant subcutaneous fat—breasts, abdomen, buttocks, thighs, and calves. The erythema and purpura develop between the third and tenth day of therapy, most likely as a result of a transient imbalance in the levels of anticoagulant and procoagulant vitamin K–dependent factors. Continued therapy does not exacerbate preexisting lesions, and patients with an inherited or acquired deficiency of protein C are at increased risk for this particular reaction as well as for purpura fulminans.

Purpura secondary to *cholesterol emboli* are usually seen on the lower extremities of patients with atherosclerotic vascular disease. They often follow anticoagulant therapy or an invasive vascular procedure such as an arteriogram, but they also occur spontaneously from disintegration of atheromatous plaques. Associated findings include livedo reticularis, gangrene, cyanosis, subcutaneous nodules, and ischemic ulcerations. Multiple step sections of the biopsy specimen may be necessary to demonstrate the cholesterol clefts with the vessels. Petechiae are also an important sign of *fat embolism* and they occur primarily on the upper body 2 to 3 days after a major injury. By using special fixatives, the emboli can be demonstrated in biopsy specimens of the petechiae. Emboli of tumor or thrombus are seen in patients with atrial myxomas and marantic endocarditis.

In the *Gardner-Diamond* syndrome (autoerythrocyte sensitivity), female patients develop large ecchymoses within areas of painful, warm erythema. An episode of significant trauma frequently precedes the onset of this syndrome. Intradermal injections of autologous erythrocytes or phosphatidyl serine derived from the red cell membrane can reproduce the lesions in most patients; however, there are instances where a reaction is seen at an injection site of the forearm, but not in the midback region. The latter has led some observers to view Gardner-Diamond syndrome as a cutaneous manifestation of severe emotional stress. *Waldenström's hypergammaglobulinemic purpura* is a chronic disorder characterized by petechiae on the lower extremities. There are circulating complexes of IgG; anti-IgG molecules and exacerbations are associated with prolonged standing or walking.

Palpable purpura are further subdivided into vasculitic and embolic. In the group of vasculitic disorders, *leukocytoclastic vasculitis* (LCV), also known as allergic vasculitis, is the one most commonly associated with palpable purpura (see Chap. 276). *Henoch-Schönlein purpura* is a subtype of acute LCV that is seen primarily in children and adolescents following an upper respiratory infection. The majority of lesions are found on the lower extremities and buttocks. Systemic manifestations include fever, arthralgias (primarily of the knees and ankles), abdominal pain, gastrointestinal bleeding, and nephritis. Direct immunofluorescence examination shows deposits of IgA within dermal blood vessel walls. In *polyarteritis nodosa,* specific cutaneous lesions result from a vasculitis of arterial vessels rather than from postcapillary venules as in LCV. The arteritis leads to ischemia of the skin and this explains the irregular outline of the purpura (see below).

Several types of emboli can give rise to palpable purpura. Infectious embolic lesions are usually *irregular* in outline as opposed to the lesions of leukocytoclastic vasculitis which are *circular* in outline. The irregular outline is indicative of a cutaneous infarct, and the size correponds to the area of skin that received its blood supply from that particular arteriole or artery. The palpable purpura in LCV are circular because the erythrocytes simply diffuse out evenly from the postcapillary venules as a result of inflammation. Infectious emboli are most commonly due to gram-negative cocci (meningococcus, gonococcus), gram-negative rods (Enterobacteriacae), and gram-positive cocci (staphylococcus). Additional causes include *Rickettsia* and, in immunocompromised patients, *Candida* and *Aspergillus.*

The embolic lesions in *acute meningococcemia* are found primarily on the trunk, lower extremities, and sites of pressure, and a gunmetal-gray color often develops within them. Their size varies from 1 mm to several centimeters, and the organisms can be cultured from the lesions. Associated findings include a preceding upper respiratory tract infection, fever, meningitis, disseminated intravascular coagulation, and, in some patients, a deficiency of the terminal components of complement. In *disseminated gonococcal infection* (arthritis-dermatitis syndrome), a small number of papules and vesicopustules with central purpura or hemorrhagic necrosis are found over the joints of the distal extremities. Additional symptoms include arthralgias, tenosynovitis, and fever. To establish the diagnosis, a Gram stain of these lesions should be performed. *Rocky mountain spotted fever* is a tick-borne disease that is caused by *Rickettsia rickettsii.* A several-day history of fever, chills, severe headache, and photophobia precedes the onset of the cutaneous eruption. The initial lesions are erythematous macules and papules on the wrists, ankles, palms, and soles. With time the lesions spread centripetally and become purpuric.

Lesions of *ecthyma gangrenosum* begin as edematous erythematous papules or plaques and then develop central purpura and necrosis. Bullae-formation also occurs in these lesions, and they are frequently found in the girdle region. The organism that is clasically associated with ecthyma gangrenosum is *Pseudomonas aeruginosa*, but other gram-negative rods such as *Klebsiella, E. coli,* and *Serratia* can produce similar lesions. In immunocompromised hosts, the list of potential pathogens is expanded to include *Candida* and *Aspergillus.*

ULCERS (Table 59-22) As an approach to the patient with a cutaneous ulcer, the etiologies are divided into two major groups: (1) primary cutaneous disorders and (2) underlying systemic diseases. Within the group of primary cutaneous disorders, there are three categories: vascular, tumor-associated, and infectious. The *peripheral vascular* group is the first to be discussed because it contains the most common cause of lower extremity ulcers in adults, *venous insufficiency.* Stasis ulcers are characteristically painless and contain adequate granulation tissue. They are often found on the medial malleoli against a background of varicosities, stasis dermatitis, edema, and hemosiderin deposition (yellow-brown discoloration of the skin).

In contrast, lower extremity ulcers due to *arteriosclerosis obliterans* are often painful and are associated with cool, hairless, atrophic skin and dystrophic nails—all a reflection of a decrease in blood flow. The majority of patients are men and they frequently have evidence of atherosclerosis in other large- and medium-sized arteries. *Thromboangiitis obliterans* (Buerger's disease) and *Mönckeberg's arteriosclerosis* are two less common arterial diseases that can lead to ulcers of the distal upper extremity as well as the lower extremity. The latter is found in patients with primary or secondary hyperparathyroidism, and the calcification of the tunica media of involved muscular arteries is seen radiographically as a diffuse pipe-stem

---

TABLE 59-22 Causes of cutaneous ulcers

Primary cutaneous disorders
  A Peripheral vascular disease
    1 Venous
    2 Arterial
  B Livedoid vasculitis
  C Squamous cell carcinoma, e.g., within scars
  D Infections, e.g., ecthyma
Systemic diseases
  A Legs
    1 Leukocytoclastic vasculitis
    2 Hemoglobinopathies
    3 Cryoglobulinemia
    4 Cholesterol emboli
    5 Necrobiosis lipoidica
  B Hands and feet
    1 Raynaud's phenomenon
  C Generalized
    1 Pyoderma gangrenosum
  D Mucosal
    1 Behçet's syndrome
    2 Erythema multiforme

calcification. Buerger's disease occurs primarily in young men (ages 25 to 40) who smoke or have been smokers.

Livedoid vasculitis (atrophie blanche) represents a combination of a vasculopathy with intravascular thrombosis. Purpuric lesions and livedo reticularis are found in association with painful ulcerations of the lower extremities. These ulcers are often slow to heal, but when they do, irregularly shaped white scars are formed. The majority of cases are idiopathic in origin, but possible underlying illnesses include systemic lupus, the antiphospholipid syndrome, scleroderma, and cryoglobulinemia. Patients with the antiphospholipid syndrome have anticardiolipin antibodies, biologic false-positive tests for syphilis, and prolonged activated partial thromboplastin times; the latter are due to a circulating lupus anticoagulant. These antiphospholipid antibodies are seen most commonly in patients with systemic lupus, but they are also associated with other connective tissue diseases. In addition to the lesions of livedoid vasculitis, patients with the antiphospholipid syndrome have recurrent venous thrombosis, arterial thrombosis (including cerebrovascular accidents), spontaneous abortions, and thrombocytopenia.

Several *carcinomas* can present as cutaneous ulcers, e.g., basal cell carcinoma, squamous cell carcinoma, and, less often, melanoma. When an ulcer on the lower extremity does not heal, despite correction of the presumed cause, it should be biopsied to rule out carcinoma, primarily squamous cell carcinoma. The same holds true for ulcers that develop with scars. Bacterial and viral *infections* also lead to cutaneous ulceration, and one of the more commonly isolated organisms is streptococcus. The term ecthyma is used to describe the often widespread ulcerative lesions that are caused by this bacteria. Ecthyma is a primary cutaneous disorder and should not be confused with ecthyma gangrenosum, which is secondary to blood-borne emboli (see ''Purpura''). In Meleney's ulcer, a gradually expanding ulcer begins at a site of trauma or surgery. The clinical appearance is similar to that of pyoderma gangrenosum, but it is due to a synergistic infection that usually includes anaerobic streptococci.

For one group of patients with cutaneous ulcers, the lower extremity is the primary location for those due to an underlying systemic disease. In a young patient, ischemic cutaneous ulcers on the leg should raise the possibility of a *hemoglobinopathy* or *hereditary spherocytosis*. Intravascular thrombosis is the presumed cause of these ulcers as well as for the ulcers seen in patients with *monoclonal cryoglobulinemia* (see ''Purpura''). Primary and secondary forms of *LCV* as well as *emboli of cholesterol* can result in cutaneous ulceration, again primarily on the lower extremities (see ''Purpura''). For example, lower extremity ulcers in patients with rheumatoid arthritis are often due to vasculitis. In addition, the yellow atrophic plaques of *necrobiosis lipoidica* can break down centrally into an ulcer (see ''Papulonodular Skin Lesions'').

Vasospasm occurs in patients with *Raynaud's phenomenon* and can lead to ulcerations of the hands as well as the feet. Raynaud's phenomenon is defined as a triphasic reaction of pallor, cyanosis, and hyperemia in response to cold or emotional stress. Vasospasm is also seen in patients who receive systemic noradrenaline, vasopressin, ergot, and bleomycin. The patient with Raynaud's phenomenon and ulcerations on the tips of the digits should be examined carefully for periungual and mat telangiectasias, the subtle signs of scleroderma. Raynaud's phenomenon is also seen in patients with dermatomyositis, systemic lupus, cryoglobulinemia, cervical rib and scalenus anticus syndromes, pneumatic hammer disease, and occupational acroosteolysis (associated with the manufacture of polyvinyl chloride).

In *pyoderma gangrenosum*, the border of the ulcers has a characteristic appearance of an undermined necrotic bluish edge and a peripheral erythematous halo. The ulcers often begin as pustules that then expand rather rapidly to a size as large as 20 cm. Although these lesions are most commonly found on the lower extremities, they can arise anywhere on the surface of the body, including sites of trauma (pathergy). An estimated 30 to 50 percent of cases are idiopathic, and the most common associated disorders are ulcerative

colitis and Crohn's disease. Less commonly, it is associated with chronic active hepatitis, seropositive rheumatoid arthritis, acute and chronic granulocytic leukemia, polycythemia vera, and myeloma. Additional findings in these patients, even those with idiopathic disease, are cutaneous anergy and a benign monoclonal gammopathy. Because the histology of pyoderma gangrenosum is nonspecific, the diagnosis is made clinically by excluding less common causes of similar-appearing ulcers such as necrotizing vasculitis, Meleney's ulcer (see above), dimorphic fungi, cutaneous amebiasis, spider bites, and factitial. In the myeloproliferative disorders, the ulcers may be more superficial with a pustulobullous border and these lesions provide a connection between classic pyoderma gangrenosum and acute febrile neutrophilic dermatosis (Sweet's syndrome).

The diagnosis of *Behçet's* disease requires the presence of three major clinical criteria, one of which must be recurrent aphthae. The major criteria include: (1) recurrent aphthous stomatitis; (2) recurrent genital ulcers, primarily of the scrotum and labia; (3) uveitis; (4) vasculitis of either cutaneous or large vessels—the skin lesions may be papules, pustules, or nodules; (5) synovitis; (6) meningoencephalitis; and (7) pathergy, which is defined as reproduction of cutaneous lesions by trauma. A test for pathergy is the injection of sterile saline into the dermis. The oral ulcers are painful and well-defined with an erythematous halo, whereas the genital ulcers tend to be deeper and heal with scarring. Patients can also have ulceration of the gastrointestinal tract, superficial and deep thrombophlebitis, pyoderma, and furunculosis. Disorders that must be excluded include recurrent *erythema multiforme* (see ''Vesicles/Bullae''), herpes simplex, inflammatory bowel disease, systemic lupus, and Reiter's disease.

REFERENCES

BORK K: *Cutaneous Side Effects of Drugs*. Philadelphia, Saunders, 1988

BRAVERMAN IM: *Skin Signs of Systemic Disease*, 2d ed. Philadelphia, Saunders, 1981

DEVITA VT JR et al: (eds): *Cancer—Principles and Practice of Oncology*, 2d ed. Philadelphia, Lippincott, 1985

JORRIZZO JL: *Dermatology Clinics*, vol 3: No 1: *Urticaria*. Philadelphia, Saunders, 198.

LEVER WF, SCHAUMBURG-LEVER G: *Histopathology of the Skin*, 6th ed. Philadelphia, Lippincott, 1983

ROOK A et al (eds): *Textbook of Dermatology*, 4th ed. Oxford, Blackwell Scientific, 1986.

60   PHOTOSENSITIVITY AND OTHER REACTIONS TO LIGHT

DAVID R. BICKERS

SOLAR RADIATION   Sunlight is the most visible and obvious source of comfort in the environment, and it is in the nature of humans to love light. This natural proclivity for the sun has the beneficial results of warmth and vitamin D synthesis but also can produce pathologic consequences of cutaneous sun exposure. Few effects due to exposure to the sun beyond those on the skin have been identified, but cutaneous exposure to sunlight can alter immunologic responses at sites distant from the skin.

The sun's energy encompasses a broad range from ultrashort ionizing radiation (10^{-2} µm) to ultralong radiowaves of very low photon energy (10^7 µm). Thus, the emission spectrum has a range of nine orders of magnitude, but the component that reaches the earth's surface is narrow and includes the components of the ultraviolet, visible light, and portions of the infrared. The cutoff at the short end of the ultraviolet is at approximately 290 nm, because stratospheric ozone is formed by ionizing radiation of wavelengths less than 100 nm and ozone absorbs incident energy between 120 and 310 nm. In effect, stratospheric ozone prevents the penetration to the earth's surface of the shorter, more energetic, potentially more harmful wavelengths of solar radiation. Indeed, concern about the destruction of ozone by chlorofluorocarbons released into the atmosphere has led to international agreements to reduce production of these chemicals.

Measurements of solar flux in various areas indicate that there is a twentyfold variation in the amount of ultraviolet B at 300 nm that reaches the surface of the earth. This variability is in part related to seasonal effects, the path of sunlight transmission through ozone and air, the altitude (4 percent increase for each 300 m of elevation), the latitude (increasing intensity with decreasing latitude), and the amount of cloud cover, fog, and pollution.

The major components of the photobiologic action spectrum include the ultraviolet and visible wavelengths between 290 and 700 nm. In addition, the wavelengths beyond 700 nm in the infrared primarily evoke heat, but warming of the skin may enhance the response to wavelengths in the ultraviolet and visible spectrum.

The ultraviolet (UV) spectrum is arbitrarily divided into three major segments: C, B, and A. This includes the wavelengths between 10 and 400 nm. UV-C consists of wavelengths between 10 and 290 nm and does not reach the earth because of its absorption by stratospheric ozone. These wavelengths are not a cause of photosensitivity except in occupational settings where artificial sources of this energy are employed, for example, for germicidal effects. UV-B consists of wavelengths between 290 and 320 nm. This portion of the photobiologic action spectrum is the most efficient in producing redness or erythema in human skin, and hence it is sometimes known as the sunburn spectrum. UV-A represents those wavelengths between 320 and 400 nm and is approximately a thousandfold less efficient in producing skin hyperemia than is UV-B.

The visible wavelengths between 400 and 700 nm include the familiar white light which when directed through a prism can be shown to consist of various colors including violet, indigo, blue, green, yellow, orange, and red. The energy possessed by photons in the visible spectrum usually is not capable of damaging human skin in the absence of a photosensitizing chemical. Photon energy levels are critical to photosensitivity since the absorption process requires that sufficient energy be present. The absorption of a photon is an all-or-none phenomenon, and when absorbed, the photon ceases to exist. The absorption of energy is critical to the development of photosensitivity. Thus, the *absorption spectrum* of a molecule is defined as the range of wavelengths absorbed by it, whereas the *action spectrum* for an effect of incident radiation is defined as the range of wavelengths that evoke the response.

Photosensitivity occurs when a photon-absorbing chemical (*chromophore*) present in the skin absorbs incident energy, becomes excited, and transfers the absorbed energy to various structures or to oxygen. The absorbed energy must subsequently be dissipated by processes including heat, fluorescence, and phosphorescence. It is important to emphasize that absorption spectra and action spectra need not be superimposable, but there must be overlap at some point to produce photosensitization.

STRUCTURE AND FUNCTION OF SKIN The skin is accessible to incident solar radiation and has a structural heterogeneity that permits the absorption of some wavelengths and the transmission of others. Essentially, human skin is a sandwich of two distinctive compartments, the epidermis and dermis. The outer epidermis is a stratified squamous epithelium comprising the surface stratum corneum (a protein- and lipid-rich compact acellular membrane), the stratum granulosum, stratum Malphigii, and the basal cell layer. The basal cell layer contains a heterogeneous population of dividing cells and resting cells, some of which begin an upward migratory process of terminal differentiation that results in keratinization to form the stratum corneum. The cells of the epidermis include resident keratinocytes and melanocytes and immigrant cells including the immunologically active Langerhans cells, lymphocytes, polymorphonuclear

leukocytes, monocytes, and macrophages. The epidermis is a major component of the immune system. Branches of sensory nerve endings also reach into this compartment.

The second major component of skin is the dermis, which is relatively large and less densely populated with cells that include fibroblasts, endothelial cells within dermal vessels, and mast cells. Tissue macrophages and sparsely distributed inflammatory cells are also present. All of these cells exist within an extracellular matrix of collagen, elastin, and glycosaminoglycans. In contrast to the epidermis, rich vascularization of the dermis allows it to play an important role in temperature regulation.

UV RADIATION AND SKIN The epidermis and the dermis contain several chromophores capable of interacting with incident solar energy. These interactions include reflection, refraction, absorption, and transmission. The stratum corneum is a major impediment to the transmission of UV-B, and less than 10 percent of incident wavelengths in this region penetrate the basement membrane. Approximately 3 percent of radiation below 300 nm, 20 percent of radiation below 360 nm, and 33 percent of short visible radiation reaches the basal cell layer in untanned human skin. Proteins and nucleic acids absorb intensely in the short UV-B. In contrast, the UV-A penetrates the epidermis efficiently to reach the dermis, where it likely produces changes in structural and matrix proteins that contribute to the appearance of chronically exposed skin, particularly in individuals of light complexion.

Proteins and nucleic acids in the epidermis are major absorbers of UV-B, and one of the consequences of this absorption process is the production in DNA of pyrimidine, particularly thymine dimers. These structural changes are produced primarily by UV-B, but also by UV-A, and can be repaired by mechanisms that result in their excision and the reestablishment of normal base sequences. The efficient repair of these structural aberrations is crucial since individuals with defective DNA repair are at high risk for the development of cutaneous cancer. For example, patients with xeroderma pigmentosum, an autosomal recessive disorder, are characterized by variably decreased repair of UV-induced pyrimidine dimers and may develop the xerotic appearance of photoaging as well as basal cell and squamous cell carcinomas and melanoma in the first two decades of life.

Cutaneous optics and chromophores Chromophores are endogenous or exogenous chemical components that can absorb physical energy. Endogenous chromophores of skin are of two types: (1) chemicals that are normally present in the biologic structure of the skin, including nucleic acids, proteins, lipids, and cholesterol derivatives such as the precursor of vitamin D, and (2) chemicals, such as porphyrins, synthesized elsewhere in the body that circulate in the bloodstream and diffuse into the skin where they can absorb incident radiation and evoke cutaneous photosensitivity. Normally, only trace amounts of porphyrins are present in the skin, but in the porphyrias increased amounts of porphyrins are released into the circulation and are transported to the skin, where they absorb incident energy both in the Soret band around 400 nm (short visible) and to a lesser extent in the red portion of the visible spectrum (580 to 660 nm). This results in structural damage to the skin that may be manifest as erythema, edema, urticaria, or blister formation (see Chap. 328).

Acute effects of sun exposure The immediate cutaneous consequences of sun exposure include sunburn and vitamin D synthesis.

SUNBURN This very common affliction of human skin is the result of sun exposure. Generally speaking, the ability of an individual to tolerate sunlight is inversely proportional to melanin pigmentation. Melanin is a complex polymer of tyrosine that functions as an efficient neutral-density filter with broad absorbance within the UV portion of the solar spectrum. Melanin is synthesized in specialized epidermal dendritic cells termed *melanocytes* and packaged into *melanosomes* that are transferred via dendritic processes into *keratinocytes*, where they provide photoprotection. A single melanocyte can provide melanin pigment for approximately 36 keratinocytes, and this group of cells is termed the *epidermal-melanin unit*. Tolerance of sun exposure is a function of the efficiency of the epidermal melanin unit and can usually be ascertained by asking an individual two questions: (1) Do you always, sometimes, or never burn after sun exposure on unprotected skin? and (2) Do you never, sometimes, or always tan? By the answers to these questions, it is usually possible to divide the population into six skin types varying from type I (always burn, never tan) to type VI (never burn, always tan) (see Table 60-1).

There are two general theories about the pathogenesis of the sunburn response. First, the lag phase in time between skin exposure and the development of visible redness (usually 4 to 12 h) may be due to an epidermal chromophore that causes a delayed production and/or release of vasoactive mediator(s) that diffuse to the dermal vasculature to evoke vasodilatation. Other evidence suggests that the small amount of incident UV-B radiation (10 percent or less) that penetrates to the dermis can be absorbed by endothelial cells in the vasculature, thereby directly resulting in vasodilatation. The issue remains unresolved.

The action spectrum for sunburn erythema includes the UV-B and the UV-A. Photons in the shorter UV-B are perhaps a thousandfold more efficient than photons in the longer UV-B and the UV-A in evoking the response. However, UV-A may contribute to sunburn erythema at midday when much more UV-A than UV-B is present.

The mechanism of injury remains pooly defined, but the action spectrum for UV-B erythema closely resembles the absorption spectrum for DNA after adjusting for the absorbance of incident energy by the stratum corneum. Damaged keratinocytes (so-called sunburn cells) are visible histologically within an hour and are maximal within 24 h of exposure. UV-A is less effective than UV-B in producing sunburn cells. Mast cells may release inflammatory mediators after exposure to UV-B and UV-A radiation. For example, erythema doses of both UV-B and UV-A increase histamine levels in suction blisters of human skin that return to normal by 24 h (before visible erythema has subsided). Prostaglandin E_2 (PGE_2) increases to approximately 150 percent of control levels by 24 h and then diminishes. Since prostaglandins evoke both pain and redness when injected intradermally, their presence in suction blisters after UV-B radiation suggests a role in UV-B erythema. There may be an age-related decline in the amount of inflammatory mediators detectable in human skin after UV-B irradiation. UV-A erythema results in few epidermal sunburn cells, but vascular endothelial injury is greater than with UV-B. In addition, there are increased levels of arachidonic acid and of prostaglandins D_2, E_2, and I_2 that peak within 5 to 9 h and then subside before peak redness occurs. Despite the evidence for elevated prostaglandins in both UV-B- and UV-A-irradiated skin, administration of nonsteroidal anti-inflammatory drugs is more effective in reducing erythema evoked by UV-B than by UV-A.

VITAMIN D PHOTOCHEMISTRY   Cutaneous exposure to UV-B causes photolysis of epidermal provitamin D_3 (7-dehydrocholesterol) to previtamin D_3, which then undergoes a temperature-dependent isomerization to form the stable hormone vitamin D_3. This compound then diffuses to the dermal vasculature and circulates to the liver and kidney, where it is converted to the functional hormone 1,25-dihydroxy vitamin D_3 [1,25(OH)$_2$D$_3$] (see also Chap. 399). There are age-related differences in the rates of conversion of provitamin D_3 to previtamin D_3. Aging substantially decreases the ability of human skin to produce vitamin D_3. This, coupled with the widespread recommended use of sunscreens that filter out UV-B, has led to

concern that vitamin D deficiency may become a significant clinical problem in the elderly. Indeed, studies have shown that the use of a sunscreen with a sun protection factor of 8 can prevent the production of vitamin D_3 in human skin.

Chronic effects of sun exposure: nonmalignant   The clinical features of photodamaged sun-exposed skin consist of wrinkling, blotchiness, telangiectasia, and a roughened irregular "weatherbeaten" appearance. Whether these changes, which some refer to as "photoaging" or dermatoheliosis, represent accelerated chronologic aging or a separate and distinct process is not clear.

Within chronically sun-exposed epidermis there is thickening (acanthosis) and morphologic heterogeneity within the basal cell layer. Higher but irregular melanosome content may be present in some keratinocytes, indicating prolonged residence of the cells in the basal cell layer. These structural changes may help to explain the leathery texture and the blotchy discoloration of sun-damaged skin.

The dermis is the major site for sun-associated chronic damage, manifest as a massive increase in thickened irregular masses of tangled elastic fibers containing uncharacterized electron-dense material. Collagen fibers are also abnormally clumped in the deeper dermis. Fibroblasts are increased in number and show morphologic signs suggesting enhanced metabolic activity. Degraded mast cells may be present in the dermis, the relevance of which remains unclear.

These morphologic changes, both gross and microscopic, are features of chronically sun-exposed skin. The chromophore(s), the action spectra, and the specific biochemical events that result in these changes are unknown. Although topical retinoids, particularly vitamin A acid, are being used for the treatment of these photoaging changes in human skin, neither the efficacy nor the long-term safety has been verified.

Chronic effects of sun exposure: malignant   One of the major known consequences of chronic skin exposure to sunlight is nonmelanoma skin cancer. The two types of skin cancer are basal cell and squamous cell carcinoma (see Chap. 307). There are three major steps for cancer induction: initiation, promotion, and progression. Chronic exposure of animal skin to artificial light sources that mimic solar UV radiation results in *initiation*, a step whereby structural (mutational) changes in DNA evoke an irreversible change in the target cell (keratinocyte) that begins the tumorigenic process. Exposure to a tumor initiator is believed to be a necessary but not sufficient step in the malignant process. Thus, initiated cells that are not exposed to tumor promoters do not generally develop into tumors. The second stage in tumor development is promotion, a multistep process whereby initiated cells are exposed to chemical and physical agents that evoke epigenetic changes that culminate in the clonal expansion of initiated cells and cause the development, over a period of weeks to months, of benign growths known as *papillomas*. UV-B radiation is a complete carcinogen, meaning that it can function as both an initiator and a promoter leading to tumor induction. Incomplete carcinogens can initiate tumorigenesis but require additional skin exposure to tumor promoters to cause the production of tumors. The prototype tumor promoter is the phorbol ester 12-0-tetradecanoyl phorbol-13-acetate (TPA). Tumor promotion usually requires multiple exposures over time to evoke a neoplasm.

The first tumors that develop in skin exposed to solar radiation are benign papillomas. The final step in the malignant process is the conversion of the benign papillomas into malignant squamous cell carcinomas, a process thought to require additional genetic alterations in already transformed cells.

Sun exposure is believed to promote the development of both nonmelanoma and melanoma cancers of the skin, although the evidence is far more direct for its role in nonmelanoma (basal cell and squamous cell carcinoma) than in melanoma cancers. Approximately 80 percent of nonmelanoma skin cancers develop on exposed body areas, including the face, the neck, and the hands. The nose and cheeks are the most commonly affected sites. Men of fair complexion who work outdoors are twice as likely as women to develop these types of cancers. Whites of darker complexions (e.g.,

TABLE 60-1   Skin type and sunburn sensitivity

Type	Description
I	Always burn, never tan
II	Always burn, sometimes tan
III	Sometimes burn, always tan
IV	Never burn, always tan
V	Darker pigment
VI	Darkest pigment

Hispanics) have one-tenth the risk of developing such cancers as do light-skinned individuals. Blacks are at lowest risk for all forms of skin cancer. Between 400,000 and 500,000 individuals in the United States annually develop nonmelanoma skin cancer, and the lifetime risk for a white individual to develop such a neoplasm is estimated at approximately 15 percent. A consensus exists that the incidence of nonmelanoma skin cancer is rising as a result of greater opportunities for sun exposure in the population.

The relationship of sun exposure to melanoma is less clear-cut, but suggestive evidence supports an association. Melanomas may develop by the teenage years, indicating that the latent period for tumor growth is less than that of nonmelanomas. Epidemiologic studies of immigrants of similar ethnic stock indicate that individuals born in one area or who migrated to the same locale before age 10 have higher age-specific melanoma rates than individuals arriving later. It is thus reasonable to conclude that life in a sunny climate from birth or early childhood increases the risk of melanoma. In general, risk does not correlate with cumulative sun exposure but may relate to sequelae of sun exposure in childhood. Thus, a blistering sunburn is associated with a doubling of melanoma risk at the site of the reaction.

Immunologic effects Exposure to solar radiation influences both local and systemic immune responses. UV-B appears to be most efficient in altering immune responses, likely related to the capacity of such energy to affect antigen presentation in skin by interacting with epidermal Langerhans cells. These bone marrow–derived dendritic cells possess surface markers characteristic of monocytes and macrophages. Following skin exposure to erythema doses of UV-B, Langerhans cells undergo both morphologic and functional changes that result in decreased contact allergic responses when haptens are applied to the radiated site. This diminished capacity for sensitization is due to the induction of antigen-specific suppressor T lymphocytes. Indeed, while the immunosuppressive effect of irradiation is limited to haptens applied to the irradiated site, the net result is systemic immune suppression to that antigen because of the induction of suppressor T cells that spread throughout the body.

Higher doses of radiation evoke diminished immunologic responses to antigens introduced either epicutaneously or intracutaneously at sites distant from the irradiated site. These suppressed responses are also associated with the induction of antigen-specific suppressor T lymphocytes and may be mediated by as yet undefined factors that are released from epidermal cells at the irradiated site. The implications of this generalized immune suppression in terms of altered susceptibility to infection remain to be defined.

The photoimmunologic effects of solar radiation may also play a role in carcinogenic responses to UV radiation in the skin. UV-induced-tumors in murine skin are antigenic and are rapidly rejected when transplanted into normal syngeneic animals. If the tumors are transplanted into animals previously exposed to subcarcinogenic doses of UV radiation, they are not rejected and instead grow progressively in the recipients. This failure of irradiated animals to reject the transplanted tumors is due to the development of T suppressor cells that prevent the rejection response. While the mechanism of suppression of tumor rejection is unknown, such a response might be a critical determinant of cancer risk in human skin. Namely, in human subjects cutaneous exposure to erythema doses of UV-B causes changes in T-helper- and -suppressor-cell ratios and diminishes the effectiveness of natural killer cell function.

PHOTOSENSITIVITY DISEASES The diagnosis of photosensitivity requires a careful history to define the duration of the signs and symptoms, the length of time between exposure to sunlight, and the development of subjective complaints and visible changes in the skin. The age of onset can also be a helpful clue; for example, the acute photosensitivity of erythropoietic protoporphyria almost always begins in childhood, whereas the chronic photosensitivity of porphyria cutanea tarda typically begins in the fourth and fifth decades. A history of exposure to topical and systemic drugs and chemicals may provide important information. Many classes of drugs can cause photosensitivity either on the basis of phototoxicity or photoallergy. Fragrances such as musk ambrette contained in numerous cosmetic products are also potent photosensitizers.

Examination of the skin may also offer important clues. Anatomic areas that are naturally protected from direct sunlight such as the hairy scalp, the upper eyelids, the retroauricular areas, the infranasal, and the submental regions may be spared when the exposed areas show characteristic features of the pathologic process. These anatomic localization patterns are often helpful but not infallible in making the diagnosis. For example, airborne contact sensitizers that are blown on to the skin may produce dermatitis that can be difficult to distinguish from photosensitivity, despite the fact that such material may trigger skin reactivity in areas shielded from direct sunlight.

Many dermatologic conditions may be caused or aggravated by light (Table 60-2). The role of light in evoking these responses may be dependent upon genetic abnormalities ranging from the well-described defect in DNA repair that occurs in xeroderma pigmentosum to the inherited abnormalities in heme synthesis that characterize the porphyrias. In certain photosensitivity diseases the chromophore has been identified, whereas in the majority, the energy-absorbing agent is unknown.

Polymorphous light eruption After sunburn, the most common type of photosensitivity disease is polymorphous light eruption, the mechanism of which is unknown. Many affected individuals never seek medical attention because the condition is often transient, becoming manifest each spring with initial sun exposure, but then subsiding spontaneously with continuing exposure, a phenomenon known as "hardening." The major manifestations of polymorphous light eruption include pruritic (often intensely so) erythematous

TABLE 60-2 Classification of photosensitivity diseases

Type	Disease
Genetic	Erythropoietic porphyria
	Erythropoietic protoporphyria
	Albinism
	Xeroderma pigmentosum
	Rothmund-Thompson disease
	Bloom's disease
	Cockayne's disease
	Familial porphyria cutanea tarda
	Phenylketonuria
	Hepatoerythropoietic porphyria
Metabolic	Sporadic porphyria cutanea tarda
	Variegate porphyria
	Hartnup disease
	Kwashiorkor
	Pellagra
	Carcinoid
	Pseudoporphyria
Phototoxic	
Internal	Drugs
External	Drugs, plants, food
Photoallergic	
Immediate	Solar urticaria
Delayed	Drug photoallergy
	Persistent light reaction
Neoplastic and degenerative	Photoaging
	Actinic keratoses
	Basal cell carcinoma
	Squamous cell carcinoma
	Melanoma
	Dysplastic nevus syndrome
	Bowen's disease
Idiopathic	Polymorphous light eruption
	Hydroa aestivale
	Actinic reticuloid
Photoaggravated	Lupus erythematosus
	Systemic
	Subacute cutaneous
	Dermatomyositis
	Pemphigus foliaceus
	Herpes simplex
	Lichen planus actinicus
	Acne vulgaris
	Atopic dermatitis
	Transient acantholytic dermatosis

TABLE 60-3   Phototoxic drugs and chemicals

	Topical	Systemic
Coal tar derivatives		
Acridine	+	
Anthracene	+	
Phenanthrene	+	
Drugs		
Amiodarone		+
Dacarbazine		+
5-Fluorouracil	+	+
Furosemide		+
Nalidixic acid		+
Phenothiazines		+
Psoralens	+	+
Retinoids	+	+
Sulfonamides		+
Sulfonylureas		+
Tetracyclines		+
Thiazides		+
Vinblastine		+
Dyes		
Anthraquinone		+
Eosin		+
Methylene blue		+
Rose bengal		+

TABLE 60-4   Photoallergenic drugs and chemicals

	Topical	Systemic
Antibiotics		
Sulfonamides		+
Antifungals		
Fenticlor	+	
Jadit	+	
Multifungin	+	
Diuretics		
Thiazides		+
Fragrances		
Musk ambrette	+	
6-Methylcoumarin	+	
Plant oleoresins	+	
Halogenated salicylanilides		
Bithionol	+	
Tetrachlorosalicylanilides	+	
Tribromosalicylanilide	+	
Nonsteroidal anti-inflammatory agents		
Piroxicam	+	
Phenothiazines		
Chlorpromazine	+	
Promethazine	+	
Sulfonylureas		+
Sunscreens		
p-Aminobenzoic acid and esters	+	
Whitening agents		
Stilbenes	+	

papules that may coalesce into plaques on exposed areas of the face and arms or other areas as well, making the distribution spotty and uneven.

The diagnosis can be confirmed by skin biopsy and by performing phototest procedures in which skin is exposed to multiple erythema doses of the UV-A and UV-B. The action spectrum for polymorphous light eruption is usually within these portions of the solar spectrum.

Treatment of this disease includes the induction of "hardening" by the cautious administration of light either alone or in combination with photosensitizers such as the psoralens (see below).

Phototoxicity and photoallergy Another photosensitivity disorder is related to the topical or systemic administration of drugs and other chemicals. Photosensitivity reactions are of two broad types, phototoxicity and photoallergy, both of which require the absorption of energy by a drug or chemical resulting in the production of an excited state photosensitizer that can transfer its absorbed energy to a bystander molecule or to molecular oxygen, thereby generating tissue-destructive chemical species.

Phototoxicity is a nonimmunologic reaction caused by drugs and chemicals, a few of which are listed in Table 60-3. The usual clinical manifestations include erythema resembling a sunburn that quickly desquamates or "peels" within several days. In addition, edema, vesicles, and bullae may occur.

Photoallergy is distinct in that the immune system participates in the pathologic process. The excited-state photosensitizer may create highly unstable haptenic free radicals that bind covalently to macromolecules to form a functional antigen capable of evoking a delayed hypersensitivity response. Some of the drugs and chemicals that produce photoallergy are listed in Table 60-4. The clinical manifestations typically differ from those of phototoxicity in that an intensely pruritic eczematous dermatitis tends to be predominant and evolves into lichenified, thickened, "leathery" changes in sun-exposed areas. A small subset (perhaps 5 to 10 percent) of patients with photoallergy may develop a persistent exquisite hypersensitivity to light even when the offending drug or chemical is identified and eliminated. This is known as persistent light reaction and may be incapacitating for many years.

Diagnostic confirmation of phototoxicity and photoallergy can often be obtained using phototest procedures. In patients with suspected phototoxicity, determination of the minimal erythema dose (MED) while the patient is exposed to a suspected agent and then repeating the MED after discontinuation of the agent may provide a clue to the causative drug or chemical. Photopatch testing can be performed to confirm the diagnosis of photoallergy. This is a simple variant of ordinary patch testing in which a series of known

photoallergens is applied to the skin in duplicate and one set irradiated with a suberythema dose of UV-A. Development of eczematous change at sites exposed to sensitizer and light is a positive result. The characteristic abnormality in patients with persistent light reaction is a diminished threshhold to erythema evoked by UV-B.

The management of drug photosensitivity is first and foremost to eliminate exposure to the chemical agents responsible for the reaction and to reduce sun exposure to the minimum possible. The acute symptoms of phototoxicity may be ameliorated by cool, moist compresses, topical glucocorticoids, and systemically administered nonsteroidal anti-inflammatory agents. In severely affected individuals, a rapidly tapered course of systemic glucocorticoids may be useful. Judicious use of analgesics may be necessary.

Photoallergic reactions require similar management techniques. Furthermore, individuals suffering from persistent light reactivity must be protected against light exposure. In selected patients in whom chronic systemic high-dose glucocorticoids pose unacceptable risks, it may be necessary to employ cytotoxic agents such as azathioprine or cyclophosphamide.

Porphyria The porphyrias (see Chap. 328) are a group of diseases that have in common various derangements in the synthesis of heme. Heme is a nonchelated tetrapyrrole or porphyrin, and the porphyrins are potent photosensitizers that absorb light intensely in both the short (400 to 410 nm) and the long (580 to 650 nm) portions of the visible spectrum.

Heme cannot be reutilized and must be continuously synthesized, and the two compartments with the largest requirement for its production are the bone marrow and the liver. Accordingly, the porphyrias originate in one or the other of these organs with the end result of excessive endogenous production of potent photosensitizers. The porphyrins circulate in the bloodstream and diffuse into the skin, where they absorb solar energy, become photoexcited, and evoke cutaneous photosensitivity. The mechanism of porphyrin photosensitization is known to be a photodynamic or oxygen-dependent reaction that can be mediated by reactive oxygen species such as superoxide anions.

Two forms of human porphyria, porphyria cutanea tarda and erythropoietic protoporphyria, will be discussed briefly. Porphyria cutanea tarda is the most common type of human porphyria and is associated with decreased activity of the enzyme uroporphyrinogen decarboxylase. There are two basic types of porphyria cutanea tarda: the sporadic or acquired type, generally seen in individuals ingesting ethanol or receiving estrogens and associated with increased hepatic iron stores, and the inherited type, in which there is autosomal dominant transmission of deficient enzyme activity.

In both types of porphyria cutanea tarda, the predominant feature is a chronic photosensitivity characterized by increased fragility of sun-exposed skin, particularly areas subject to repeated trauma such as the dorsa of the hands, the forearms, the face, and the ears. The predominant skin lesions are vesicles and bullae that rupture, producing moist erosions often with a hemorrhagic base that heal slowly with crusting and purplish discoloration of the affected skin. Hypertrichosis, mottled pigmentary change, and scleroderma-like induration are associated features. Biochemical confirmation of the diagnosis can be obtained by measurement of urinary porphyrin excretion and by assay of uroporphyrinogen decarboxylase.

Treatment consists of repeated phlebotomies to diminish the excessive hepatic iron stores and/or intermittent low doses of the antimalarial drugs chloroquine and hydroxychloroquine. Long-term remission of the disease can be achieved if the patient eliminates exposure to porphyrinogenic agents.

Erythropoietic protoporphyria originates in the bone marrow and is due to a decrease in the enzyme ferrochelatase. The major clinical features include an acute photosensitivity characterized by subjective burning and stinging of exposed skin that often develops during or just after exposure. There may be associated skin swelling and, after repeated episodes, a waxlike scarring.

The diagnosis is confirmed by demonstration of elevated measurement of free erythrocyte protoporphyrin. Detection of increased plasma protoporphyrin helps to differentiate lead poisoning and iron-deficiency anemia, in both of which elevated erythrocyte protoporphyrin occurs in the absence of cutaneous photosensitivity and of elevated plasma protoporphyrin.

Treatment consists of reducing sun exposure and the oral administration of the carotenoid β-carotene, which is an effective scavenger of free radicals. Many affected individuals are able to tolerate sun exposure while ingesting this drug, but it has no effect upon the metabolic defect in porphyrin-heme synthesis.

PHOTOPROTECTION Since photosensitivity of the skin results from exposure to sunlight, it follows that avoidance of the sun would eliminate these disorders. Unfortunately, social pressures make this an impractical alternative for most individuals, and this has led to a search for better approaches to photoprotection.

Natural photoprotection is provided by structural proteins in the epidermis, particularly keratin and melanin. The amount of melanin and its distribution in cells is genetically regulated, and individuals of darker complexion (skin types IV to VI) are at decreased risk for the development of cutaneous malignancy.

Other forms of photoprotection include clothing and sunscreens. Clothing constructed of tightly woven fabrics irrespective of color affords substantial protection. Wide-brimmed hats, long sleeves, and pants all reduce direct exposure. Sunscreens are of two major types—chemical and physical. Chemical sunscreening agents are chromophores that absorb energy in the UV-B and/or UV-A, thereby diminishing photon absorption by the skin (Table 60-5). Sunscreens are rated for their photoprotective effect by their *sun protective factor* (SPF). The SPF is simply a ratio of the time required to produce sunburn erythema with and without sunscreen application. SPF ratings of 15 or higher provide effective protection against UV-B and, to a lesser extent, UV-A. The major categories of chemical sunscreens include *p*-aminobenzoic acid and its esters, benzophenones, anthranilates, cinnamates, and salicylates. Physical sunscreens are light-opaque mixtures containing zinc oxide, talc, or titanium oxide that scatter light, thereby reducing absorption by the skin.

In addition to light absorption, a critical determinant of the photoprotective effect of sunscreens is their ability to remain on the skin, a property known as *substantivity*. In general, the PABA esters formulated in moisturizing vehicles provide the greatest substantivity.

Photoprotection can also be achieved by limiting the time of exposure during the day. Since as much as half of an individual's total lifetime sun exposure may occur by the age 18, it is important

TABLE 60-5 Properties of selected sunscreens

Ingredients	Trade names	SPF* (outdoors)	Substantivity†
p-Aminobenzoic acid (PABA) (5% in ethanol)	Pre-Sun-15	10–12	Excellent
p-Aminobenzoic acid esters (3.5% padimate A + 3.0% octyldimethyl PABA)	Original Eclipse	4–6	Fair
p-Aminobenzoic acid ester combinations (7.0% padimate 0 + 2.5% oxybenzone + 5.0% dioxybenzone)	Bain de Soleil	9	Excellent
Non-*p*-aminobenzoic acid (3% 2-hydroxy-4-methoxy benzophenone)	Ti-Screen-15	10–12	Excellent
Physical sunscreens (5% titanium Dioxide + 5% methyl anthranilate)	A-Fil	4–6	Good

*SPF = sun protective factor.
†Substantivity = ability to remain on the skin.

to educate parents and young children about the hazards of sunlight. Simply eliminating exposure at midday will achieve substantial reduction in UV-B exposure.

PHOTOTHERAPY AND PHOTOCHEMOTHERAPY While greatest attention has been paid to the damaging effects of sunlight in the skin, this same energy is employed in the management of selected dermatologic diseases. The administration of UV-B alone or in combination with topically applied compounds such as emollient ointments with or without crude coal tar induces remissions in psoriasis, an inflammatory disorder in which excessively rapid epidermal cell turnover is associated with thick scaling and redness of the skin.

Photochemotherapy in which UV-A radiation is administered in combination with topically applied or systemically administered psoralens (PUVA) is also effective in treating psoriasis and in the early stages of cutaneous T-cell lymphoma and vitiligo. Psoralens are tricyclic furocoumarins which when intercalated into DNA and exposed to UV-A produce monofunctional adducts to pyrimidine bases and eventually form DNA cross-links. These structural changes are thought to decrease DNA synthesis and effect the improvement that occurs in psoriasis. The reason that PUVA photochemotherapy is effective in cutaneous T-cell lymphoma is not clear.

In addition to its effects on DNA, PUVA photochemotherapy also stimulates melanin synthesis, and this provides the rationale for its use in the depigmenting disease vitiligo. Oral 8-methoxypsoralen and UV-A appear to be most effective in this regard, but as many as 100 treatments extending over 12 to 18 months may be required to promote satisfactory repigmentation.

The major side effects of phototherapy and PUVA photochemotherapy are due to the cumulative effects of photon absorption and include skin dryness, actinic keratoses, and an increased risk of nonmelanoma skin cancer. Despite these risks, the therapeutic index of these modalities is positive.

REFERENCES

FRAIN-BELL W: *Cutaneous Photobiology.* Oxford, Oxford University Press, 1985

HARBER LC, BICKERS DR: *Photosensitivity Diseases*, 2d ed. Toronto, Decker, 1989

MAGNUS IA: *Dermatological Photobiology.* Oxford, Blackwell, 1976

PATHAK MA et al: Preventive treatment of sunburn, dermatoheliosis and skin cancer with sun-protective agents, in *Dermatology in General Medicine*, 3d ed, TB Fitzpatrick et al (eds). New York, McGraw-Hill, 1987

URBACH F, GANGE RW: *The Biological Effects of UVA Radiation.* New York, Praeger, 1986

section 9 Hematologic alterations

---

61 ANEMIA

H. FRANKLIN BUNN

By definition patients with anemia have a significant reduction in red cell mass and a corresponding decrease in the oxygen-carrying capacity of the blood. Normally, blood volume is maintained at a nearly constant level. Therefore, anemia entails a decrease in the concentration of red cells or hemoglobin in peripheral blood.

Under unusual circumstances, the blood values do not accurately reflect alterations in the red cell mass. For example, hemoglobin level and hematocrit are falsely elevated in patients who have sustained an acute reduction in plasma volume owing to hemorrhage, extensive burns, vigorous diuresis, or other types of severe dehydration. In contrast, the blood values may be falsely low in patients who have an expanded blood volume, as in pregnancy or congestive heart failure.

Normal blood values for individuals of various ages are shown in the Appendix. In women in the childbearing age group the blood values are 10 percent lower than in men. At high altitudes, higher values are found, roughly in proportion to the elevation above sea level. Anemia may be defined as a reduction of more than 10 percent below the mean values for the sex. However, since the variations in normal hemoglobin values approach this limit, the documentation of mild anemia may be uncertain.

SIGNS AND SYMPTOMS OF ANEMIA The clinical presentation of the anemic patient depends on the underlying disease as well as on the severity and chronicity of the anemia. The manifestations of anemia per se can be explained by the pathophysiologic principles outlined in this chapter and in Chap. 290. Most of these signs and symptoms represent cardiovascular and ventilatory adjustments which compensate for the decrease in red blood cell mass.

The degree to which symptoms occur in an anemic patient depends on several contributing factors. If the anemia has developed rapidly, there may not be adequate time for compensatory adjustments to take place, and the patient may have more marked symptoms than if an anemia of equivalent severity had developed insidiously. Furthermore, the patient's complaints may depend on the presence of local vascular disease. For example, angina pectoris, intermittent claudication, or transient cerebral ischemia may be unmasked by the development of anemia.

Individuals with mild anemia are often asymptomatic. They may complain of fatigue as well as dyspnea and palpitation, particularly following exercise. Severely anemic patients will often be symptomatic at rest and unable to tolerate significant exertion. When the hemoglobin concentration falls below 75 g/L (7.5 g/dL), resting cardiac output rises significantly with an increase in both heart rate and stroke volume. The patient may be aware of this hyperdynamic state and complain of palpitation or a pounding pulse. Symptoms of cardiac failure may develop if the patient's myocardial reserve is reduced.

The symptoms of severe anemia extend to other organ systems. Patients often complain of dizziness and headache and may experience syncope, tinnitus, or vertigo. Many patients are irritable and have difficulty sleeping or concentrating. Because of decreased blood flow to the skin, patients may become hypersensitive to cold. Gastrointestinal symptoms such as anorexia, indigestion, and even nausea or bowel irregularity are attributable to shunting of blood away from the splanchnic bed. Females commonly develop abnormal menstruation, both amenorrhea and increased bleeding. Males may complain of impotence or loss of libido.

Physical findings *Pallor* is the physical finding most commonly associated with anemia. However, the usefulness of this sign is limited by other factors that affect the color of the skin. The thickness and texture of the skin vary widely among individuals. Furthermore, the blood flow to the skin can undergo wide fluctuations. Normal individuals will appear sallow when blood is shunted away from the skin, whereas anemic patients may appear flushed when overheated or during periods of excitement. The concentration of melanin in the epidermis is another important determinant of skin color. Individuals with a fair complexion may look pale even though they are not anemic. Conversely, pallor is difficult to detect in deeply pigmented individuals. Furthermore, acquired disorders of melanin pigmentation (e.g., Addison's disease, hemochromatosis) or jaundice may interfere with detection of pallor. Nevertheless, even in blacks, the presence of anemia may be suspected by the color of the palms or of noncutaneous tissues such as oral mucous membranes, nail beds, and palpebral conjunctivas. The color of the creases of the palm is a useful sign. When they are as pale as the surrounding skin, the patient usually has a hemoglobin of less than 70 g/L (7 g/dL).

Two factors contribute to the development of pallor in patients with anemia. There is, of course, a decrease in the hemoglobin concentration of blood perfusing the skin and mucous membranes. Also, blood is shunted away from the skin and other peripheral tissues, permitting enhanced blood flow to vital organs. Redistribution of blood flow is an important mode of compensation in anemia.

Other physical findings associated with anemia include tachycardia, wide pulse pressure, and a hyperdynamic precordium. A systolic ejection murmur is often heard over the precordium, particularly at the pulmonic area. In addition, a venous hum may be detected over the neck vessels. These cardiac findings disappear when the anemia is corrected. Patients with hemolytic anemia often have icterus and splenomegaly and occasionally develop superficial skin ulceration over the ankle bones.

APPROACH TO THE PATIENT WITH ANEMIA

In evaluating the anemic patient, the physician should proceed in an orderly fashion so that the correct diagnosis can be established with a minimum of laboratory tests and procedures. As in other clinical disciplines, a comprehensive history and meticulous physical examination are of paramount importance in the initial workup of the anemic patient. For example, a family history which reveals a dominant inheritance pattern provides strong support for the diagnosis of hereditary spherocytosis. The discovery of a heart murmur and splenomegaly raises the possibility that the anemic patient may have subacute bacterial endocarditis.

The evaluation of the anemic patient should be based on a firm understanding of the pathophysiologic principles outlined in Chap. 290. As shown in Table 61-1, the clinician must first ask whether the anemia is due to a decreased production of red cells or to enhanced destruction. Moreover, the possibility of blood loss either as the sole etiology or as a contributing factor must always be considered. The examination of the stool for occult blood is an indispensable part of the evaluation of all anemic patients.

TABLE 61-1 Initial evaluation of anemia

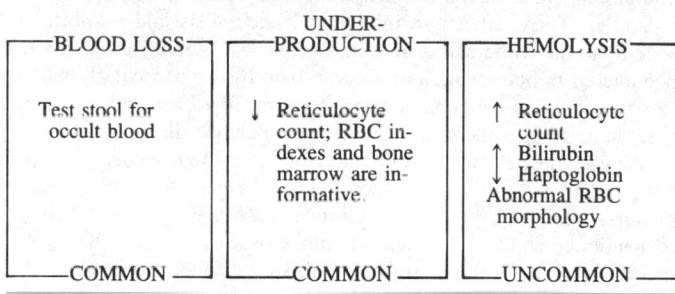

BLOOD LOSS	UNDER-PRODUCTION	HEMOLYSIS
Test stool for occult blood	↓ Reticulocyte count; RBC indexes and bone marrow are informative.	↑ Reticulocyte count ↑ Bilirubin ↓ Haptoglobin Abnormal RBC morphology
COMMON	COMMON	UNCOMMON

RETICULOCYTE COUNT This is the most useful laboratory test for distinguishing underproduction from hemolysis. When an appropriate supravital stain is applied to a sample of peripheral blood, the 1- to 2-day-old red cells exhibit a network of purple strands which are aggregates of ribosomes. Reticulocytosis is a reflection of the release of an increased number of young cells from the bone marrow. The degree of increased erythropoiesis can be assessed more quantitatively by determining the reticulocyte index, which uses the hematocrit or packed cell volume (PCV) and is calculated as follows:

$$\text{Reticulocyte index} = \text{reticulocyte \%} \times \frac{\text{patient's PCV}}{\text{normal PCV}}$$

This measure fails to consider the distribution of reticulocytes between the bone marrow and the peripheral blood. When the marrow is greatly stimulated, marrow reticulocytes enter the circulation prematurely. On a routinely prepared smear, these "shift reticulocytes" appear larger than average and have a lavender hue, so-called polychromatophilia. Since the circulation of "shift reticulocytes" in the peripheral blood is prolonged, the reticulocyte index should be divided by about 2. This factor varies from 1.5 to 3 depending upon the severity of the anemia and the degree of erythropoietin stimulation. This correction should always be made if normoblasts are encountered in the peripheral blood since this finding indicates the premature release of red cell precursors into the circulation.

A failure to produce red cells is reflected in an inappropriately low reticulocyte count. In contrast, a significant elevation of reticulocytes is suggestive of hemolysis. Exceptions include (1) the brisk reticulocyte response that is seen in a patient with hemorrhage, (2) reticulocytosis encountered in patients recovering from impaired erythropoiesis (e.g., an individual with pernicious anemia who received an injection of vitamin B_{12} 1 week earlier), and (3) mild to moderate elevations in reticulocytes (3 to 7 percent) encountered in myelophthisic anemia in which the orderly release of cells is affected by alterations of the marrow stroma owing to tumor, fibrosis, or granulomata. These exceptions are often readily appreciated in the initial evaluation of the patient. Furthermore, a number of ancillary laboratory tests described below are useful in determining to what extent hemolysis is occurring. The measurement of unconjugated bilirubin in the serum is a particularly useful guide to the presence of accelerated red blood cell breakdown. Once this information is obtained, the workup can be directed toward the establishment of a specific etiology.

Three additional baseline studies are of critical importance in the initial workup of the patient with anemia: *measurement of red cell indexes, examination of the peripheral blood smear,* and, in many patients, *bone marrow examination.*

RED CELL INDEXES Red cell indexes can be calculated from determinants of hematocrit, hemoglobin concentration, and red blood cell count. Measuring the hematocrit or PCV is the simplest and one of the most precise ways to ascertain the concentration of red cells in the blood. Generally, a small sample of anticoagulated blood is drawn into a capillary tube which is sealed at one end and centrifuged. The PCV is the ratio of the volume of packed red cells to the total

volume. Alternatively, the concentration of hemoglobin can be determined spectrophotometrically from the absorbance of the cyanmethemoglobin form at a specific wavelength. With the advent of automated red blood cell counting technology, very precise measurements of red blood cell indexes are now readily available in nearly all hospitals and clinical laboratories. The electronic counter makes a direct measurement of the red cell count (RBC/μL) and the mean red cell volume (MCV):

$$\text{MCV (fL)} = \frac{\text{PCV (L/L)}}{(\text{RBC/μL}) \times 10^{-9}}$$

This instrument calculates the PCV from the direct measurement of MCV and RBC/L. In addition, hemoglobin concentration is measured directly on a separate channel. The mean corpuscular hemoglobin concentration (MCHC) is then computed as follows:

$$\text{MCHC (g/dL)} = \frac{\text{Hb (g/dL)}}{\text{PCV (L/L)}}$$

A third red blood cell index, the mean corpuscular hemoglobin (MCH), is determined as follows:

$$\text{MCH (pg)} = \frac{\text{Hb (g/dL)}}{(\text{RBC/μL}) \times 10^{-7}}$$

Generally, an automated system provides a printout which includes hemoglobin concentration, red cell count, packed cell volume, and the three red cell indexes (MCV, MCHC, and MCH). The MCHC, when calculated by an electronic counter, is not reliable and is of little use to the clinician.

As Table 61-2 shows, the MCV is particularly useful in classifying the anemias due to decreased red cell production. Microcytic anemias have low MCV values. On microscopic examination, the red cells appear small and often pale. In contrast, in the macrocytic anemias the MCV is elevated and large oval cells (macroovalocytes) are seen on microscopic examination. Unlike the anemias of underproduction, nearly all the hemolytic anemias are normocytic or slightly macrocytic owing to the preponderance of young red cells. Exceptions include the severe forms of thalassemia in which microcytic red cells are accompanied by brisk hemolysis.

TABLE 61-2 Anemias due to decreased red cell production

RBC Indexes	Marrow	Additional lab tests	Diagnosis
Hypochromic, microcytic (↓ MCV)	0 Iron	↓ Fe, ↑ TIBC	Iron deficiency
	+ Iron	↑ Hb A_2, ↑ Hb F	β Thalassemia
	Ring sideroblasts	↓ Hb A_2	Sideroblastic anemia
Macrocytic (↑ MCV)	Megaloblastic	↓ Serum B_{12}, achlorhydria	Vitamin B_{12} deficiency, pernicious anemia
		↓ Serum folate	Folic acid deficiency
Normochromic, normocytic	Normal	↓ Fe, ↓ TIBC	Anemia of chronic inflammation
		↑ Creatinine	Anemia of uremia
		Abn LFT	Anemia of liver disease
		↓ T_4	Anemia of myxedema
Normoblasts, teardrops	Aplastic	Pancytopenia	Aplastic anemia
	Infiltrated: tumor, lymphoma, etc.		Myelophthisic
	Fibrosis	↑ LAP	Myeloid metaplasia

NOTE: Fe, iron; TIBC, total iron-binding capacity; Hb, hemoglobin; LAP, leukocyte alkaline phosphatase; LFT, liver function tests; Abn, abnormal; MCV, mean corpuscular volume.

EXAMINATION OF THE BLOOD SMEAR   In the evaluation of patients with anemia, the physician should take the time to examine a well-stained peripheral blood film. Figures A5-1 to A5-12 show examples of abnormalities in red cell morphology encountered in various types of anemia. Many subtleties escape the attention of the technologist whose primary purpose in examining the slide is to obtain a white cell differential count. Furthermore, the clinician can approach the specimen with a prepared mind and can scrutinize it for specific abnormalities. As suggested above, the examination can confirm the size and color of red cells as estimated by RBC indexes. Furthermore, while these indexes provide mean statistical values, the microscopic examination can reveal variation in red cell size (anisocytosis) or shape (poikilocytosis), changes which are helpful in the diagnosis of specific anemias. Examination of the blood smear is particularly important in evaluating a patient with hemolysis. Most hemolytic anemias have characteristic morphologic abnormalities. Finally, this practice may yield unexpected dividends. The finding of rouleaux suggests the presence of dysproteinemia as occurs in multiple myeloma. The examination may provide the initial clue that the patient has significant thrombocytopenia.

BONE MARROW EXAMINATION   A microscopic examination of the bone marrow is generally indicated in the workup of any *unexplained* anemia. Study of the bone marrow is particularly informative in the anemias of underproduction. The more severe the anemia, the more likely that the procedure will be informative. An assessment of the quantity and quality of red cell precursors may determine whether there is a primary defect in cell production. A marrow biopsy is particularly useful in estimating overall cellularity. The normal differential of nucleated cells in the marrow is shown in the Appendix. The ratio of myeloid (M) to erythroid (E) precursors is normally about 2:1 but may be artifactually increased by the inclusion of circulating leukocytes. The ratio is increased in patients with infection, a leukemoid reaction, or neoplastic proliferation of myeloid cells. Rarely, a high M/E ratio is due to selective aplasia of the red cell precursors. A decreased M/E ratio indicates erythroid hyperplasia (seen in hemolysis or hemorrhage) or ineffective erythropoiesis (e.g., megaloblastic and sideroblastic anemias). The morphology of the precursors may reveal a maturation deficit such as megaloblastic anemia. The bone marrow examination is also important in demonstrating the presence of cellular infiltrates such as those found in leukemia, lymphoma, or multiple myeloma. The demonstration of tumor, fibrosis, or granulomata usually requires a biopsy. A portion of the marrow specimen should be stained with Prussian blue. In addition to providing an assessment of iron stores, the iron stain is required for the identification of sideroblasts.

VARIOUS FORMS OF ANEMIA

ANEMIA DUE TO BLOOD LOSS   This form of anemia varies considerably in its clinical presentation depending upon the site, severity, and rapidity of the hemorrhage. At opposite extremes are acute fulminant bleeding producing hypovolemic shock and chronic occult blood loss leading to iron-deficiency anemia.

Patients who have sustained an acute hemorrhage generally present with signs and symptoms secondary to hypoxia and hypovolemia. Depending on the severity of the process, the patient will have weakness, fatigue, lightheadedness, stupor, or coma and will often appear pale, diaphoretic, and irritable. Vital signs are a reflection of cardiovascular compensation for the acute blood loss (Chap. 39). The patient will have hypotension and tachycardia in proportion to the degree of hemorrhage. Elicitation of postural signs is useful in the initial evaluation of patients with acute blood loss. If the pulse rises 25 percent or more, or the systolic blood pressure falls 20 mmHg or more upon going from a supine to sitting position, the patient is likely to have significant hypovolemia (blood loss >1000 mL) and requires prompt replacement. Acute blood loss in excess of 1500 mL usually leads to cardiovascular collapse.

If the blood loss has been acute and recent, the peripheral blood may not reveal a significant decrease in packed cell volume or hemoglobin, since the red cell mass and plasma volume are contracted in parallel. There often is a moderate leukocytosis and a "shift to the left" in the white cell differential count. Thrombocytosis may be encountered in both acute and chronic blood loss, particularly when the patient is iron-deficient. During the first few days following an acute hemorrhage there is usually an increase in reticulocytes. Occasionally nucleated red cells may appear in the peripheral blood. Since young red cells are larger than old ones, the patient may develop slightly macrocytic red cell indexes (MCV = 95 to 105 fL). As mentioned above, sustained reticulocytosis will be seen if significant blood loss continues, or until iron stores have been exhausted. Internal bleeding may be accompanied by an increase in unconjugated bilirubin. This abnormality is a reflection of an increase in catabolism of heme from extravasated red cells. Patients with acute gastrointestinal blood loss will often have an elevation of blood urea nitrogen owing to impaired renal blood flow and perhaps to the absorption of digested blood protein.

It is of critical importance to assess these patients promptly and institute treatment without delay. A large-bore intravenous line should be placed. While blood is being typed and cross matched, saline, Ringer's lactate, or, preferably, a colloid such as 5% albumin should be infused to correct hypovolemia. Whole blood is then administered as soon as it is available. Monitoring of vital signs and central venous pressure is useful in determining the appropriate amount of volume replacement. During and following these emergency measures, diagnostic studies may reveal the site or sites of bleeding. If the bleeding is unexplained an emergency coagulation profile should be obtained. Demonstration of bleeding from the gastrointestinal tract may require the insertion of a nasogastric tube. Appropriate radiologic studies may be indicated to determine sites of internal bleeding such as retroperitoneal hemorrhage.

Chronic blood loss is usually due to lesions in the gastrointestinal tract or the uterus. The testing of stool specimens for occult blood is an essential, though frequently overlooked, part of the evaluation of anemia. It may be necessary to examine serial specimens over a prolonged period of time since gastrointestinal bleeding is often intermittent. The hematologic manifestations of chronic blood loss are those of iron-deficiency anemia, discussed in detail in Chap. 291.

ANEMIAS DUE TO DECREASED RBC PRODUCTION   As shown in Table 61-2, red cell indexes are useful in classifying the anemias due to underproduction of red cells. They can be conveniently grouped into three major categories: microcytic, macrocytic, and normocytic.

The *microcytic* anemias include iron-deficiency anemia (Chap. 291), sideroblastic anemias (Chap. 291), and the thalassemias (Chap. 295). Collectively, they represent a decrease in the availability or synthesis of one of the three major constituents of the hemoglobin molecule: iron, porphyrin, and globin. Since hemoglobin makes up over 90 percent of the protein within the erythrocyte, it is not surprising that these defects in hemoglobin synthesis result in the formation of small, pale red cells. These disorders involve a variable degree of ineffective erythropoiesis (Chap. 290). In addition, the anemias of chronic inflammation and malignancy may be slightly microcytic (Chap. 293). This phenomenon is due to a defect in the availability of iron. However, these disorders are more often normocytic and have been so classified in Table 61-2. Measurement of serum iron and iron-binding capacity and evaluation of marrow iron stores are particularly useful in distinguishing between these anemias.

The *macrocytic* anemias generally are associated with megaloblastic morphology in the bone marrow. In most cases, a deficiency of either vitamin B_{12} or folic acid results in an impairment of the replication of DNA, particularly in cells having a high turnover rate. Because nuclear maturation lags behind cytoplasmic development, large red cells tend to be produced in the bone marrow. Megaloblastic anemias are discussed in detail in Chap. 292. Like the microcytic anemias, these disorders are maturation defects associated with ineffective erythropoiesis. Macrocytosis, generally of a lesser degree, may also be encountered in patients with liver disease, hypothyroidism, acute blood loss, hemolytic anemia, aplastic anemia, and alcoholism. However, in these conditions, the red cell precursors in the bone marrow do not appear megaloblastic. The macrocytes in liver disease and hypothyroidism may be related to an increased deposition of lipid in the red cell membrane.

The *normocytic* anemias of underproduction comprise a diverse group of disorders. As shown in Table 61-2, this group can be conveniently subdivided into two categories: those secondary to some other underlying disease and those due to intrinsic pathology within the bone marrow.

The primary disorders of the bone marrow are best approached by microscopic examination of a marrow aspirate and biopsy. This group of anemias is often accompanied by leukopenia and thrombocytopenia. Pancytopenia, usually to a lesser degree, can also be seen in hypersplenism and in the megaloblastic anemias. Aplastic anemia and the myelophthisic anemias are discussed in Chap. 298.

The diagnosis of anemia secondary to some underlying disease is usually quite straightforward. Conversely, the presence of an unexplained normocytic anemia should prompt the search for an underlying disorder such as chronic renal failure, infection, or myxedema. If the presence of such an illness is established, the physician is obliged to investigate whether other factors such as blood loss or a nutritional deficiency contribute to the patient's anemia. Generally, the anemias due to liver disease, chronic inflammation, or an endocrinopathy are of only moderate severity. Unlike the other "secondary" anemias, that due to chronic renal failure can be severe. All these anemias are discussed in more detail in Chap. 293.

HEMOLYTIC ANEMIAS Hemolytic anemias (Table 61-3) are encountered much less frequently than the anemias due to decreased red cell production. Although they are a diverse group, the hemolytic anemias have a number of clinical features in common. Signs and symptoms of patients with hemolysis are briefly mentioned above.

A number of laboratory tests are available to establish the presence of accelerated breakdown of red cells. The reticulocyte count is the single most useful test. Patients with hemolysis nearly always have an elevated reticulocyte count. A variety of serum and urine tests are useful in confirming the presence of hemolysis and assessing its magnitude. Serum unconjugated bilirubin and haptoglobin are particularly useful (Table 61-1). Others are described in detail in Chap. 294 and are summarized in Table 294-2.

Classification of hemolytic anemias Once the presence of hemolysis is established, a large battery of laboratory tests is available for determining the specific diagnosis. Some of these tests are listed in Table 61-3. No other area of internal medicine is better suited to

detailed and fruitful diagnostic probing. In the interest of time and money, the clinician should use the available tests in an orderly fashion. This complex group of disorders is easier to approach diagnostically if a concise and workable classification is used. The hemolytic anemias can be grouped in several ways: congenital versus acquired, intracorpuscular versus extracorpuscular, or by anatomic site of the erythrocyte defect. The various kinds of hemolytic anemia are discussed in Chap. 294.

TREATMENT OF ANEMIA

The effective treatment of anemia, like other disorders, is predicated upon a thorough diagnostic evaluation. There is no reason to administer hematinics such as iron, vitamin B_{12}, or folic acid unless a specific deficiency of these substances has been demonstrated or is anticipated. Although the indiscriminate administration of vitamin B_{12} is not deleterious per se, it lulls both the patient and the physician into false security. In contrast, the inappropriate use of iron preparations over a prolonged period of time can be directly harmful, leading to a state of iron overload. Pyridoxine is indicated only in the treatment of sideroblastic anemias.

Many kinds of anemias can be corrected if a precipitating cause can be uncovered and reversed. If a drug or toxin can be incriminated, its withdrawal may allow full recovery. The outcome of the "secondary" anemias is dependent on whether the underlying condition can be corrected. Anemias due to an endocrinopathy or infection should respond favorably to appropriate treatment. Occasionally, the anemia of malignancy is corrected by the removal of the primary tumor. One of the most dramatic sequelae of a successful renal transplant is the prompt correction of the "anemia of uremia." Moreover, the anemia associated with renal failure can be corrected by the administration of recombinant human erythropoietin. This agent may also prove to be effective in the treatment of anemia associated with other chronic disorders such as hepatic cirrhosis, rheumatoid arthritis, or AIDS.

Primary disorders of the bone marrow such as aplastic anemia or myelophthisic anemia are often irreversible and are treated with supportive measures such as transfusions of red cells and platelets. *Androgens* are sometimes employed in this group of anemias, but their efficacy is marginal. The recent availability of recombinant hematopoietic growth factors may provide more specific and effective treatment. Because prognosis is so bleak in these disorders, a radical approach to treatment seems justified. As described in Chaps. 298 and 299, bone marrow transplantation and immunosuppressive therapy are now reasonable therapeutic alternatives in selected cases of severe aplastic anemia and acute leukemia.

Several factors should be weighed in determining whether an anemic patient should be transfused. The risks and complications of the administration of blood products are discussed in Chap. 286. Patients with chronic or long-standing anemias are able to compensate in several ways, discussed earlier in this chapter. A considerable reduction in red cell mass can be surprisingly well tolerated, especially if the patient is young or sedentary. Transfusion is seldom indicated in a patient with a chronic anemia whose hemoglobin is 90 g/L (9 g/dL) or greater. Those who are expected to respond to the administration of a specific agent such as iron, folic acid, or vitamin B_{12} can usually be spared transfusions. If the anemia has precipitated an episode of congestive heart failure or myocardial ischemia, prompt but cautious administration of packed red cells is indicated. In general, whole blood should be given only if the patient is hypovolemic.

Glucocorticoids have only a limited role in the treatment of anemia. These agents are not effective in stimulating erythropoiesis. High doses of a glucocorticoid are indicated in the treatment of immunohemolytic anemia, thrombotic thrombocytopenic purpura, and pure red cell anemia. Otherwise, steroids should be prescribed sparingly unless some coexisting condition dictates their use.

Splenectomy is indicated in the treatment of certain hemolytic

TABLE 61-3 Hemolytic anemias

Blood smear	Additional lab tests	Diagnosis
Schistocytes, helmet cells		Traumatic hemolytic anemia
Spherocytes	+ Coombs' test	Immunohemolytic anemia
	↑ Osmotic fragility	Hereditary spherocytosis
Spur cells	Abnormal LFT	Spur cell anemia
	+ Sucrose lysis	Paroxysmal nocturnal hemoglobinuria
Sickle cells	+ Sickle prep	Sickle cell syndromes
Target cells	Abn Hb electrophoresis	Hb C, D, etc.
Heinz bodies	Abn Hb electrophoresis	Congenital Heinz body hemolytic anemia
	↓ G6PD	G6PD deficiency

NOTE: Hb, hemoglobin; G6PD, glucose-6-phosphate dehydrogenase; LFT, liver function tests; Abn, abnormal.

anemias. The efficacy of splenectomy correlates with the degree to which the abnormal or defective red cells are sequestered. Splenectomy is virtually curative in hereditary spherocytosis. The operation may be beneficial in selected patients with immunohemolytic anemia, congestive splenomegaly, spur cell anemia, and certain hemoglobinopathies and enzymopathies. The operative morbidity and mortality from elective splenectomy are very low. Occasional patients develop a left subphrenic abscess. Following splenectomy, young children are at risk of developing overwhelming septicemia. This complication is much rarer in adults. Thrombocytosis generally develops promptly following splenectomy. However, in most cases, it is transient. In patients with continued hemolysis or a myeloproliferative disorder (Chap. 297), the thrombocytosis usually persists and may occasionally be associated with thromboembolic phenomena.

REFERENCES

Babior BM, Stossel TP: *Hematology, A Pathophysiological Approach.* New York, Churchill Livingstone, 1984
Beck WS (ed): *Hematology.* 2nd ed. Boston, MIT Press, 1990
Crosby WH: Red cell mass: Its precursors and perturbations. Hosp Prac 15:2, 71, 1980
Erslev AJ, Gabuzda TG: *Pathophysiology of Blood.* Philadelphia, Saunders, 1985
Jandl JH: *Blood, Textbook of Hematology.* Boston, Little, Brown, 1987
Williams WJ et al (eds): *Hematology.* 4th ed. New York: McGraw-Hill, 1990.
Wintrobe MM (ed): *Blood, Pure and Eloquent.* New York, McGraw-Hill, 1980

62   BLEEDING AND THROMBOSIS

ROBERT I. HANDIN

Hemorrhage, intravascular thrombosis, and embolism are common clinical manifestations of many diseases. The normal hemostatic system limits blood loss by precisely regulated interactions between components of the vessel wall, circulating blood platelets, and plasma proteins. However, when disease or trauma damage large arteries and veins, excessive bleeding may occur, despite a normal hemostatic system. Less frequently, hemorrhage is caused by an inherited or acquired disorder of the hemostatic machinery itself. A large number of such bleeding disorders have now been identified.

In addition, unregulated activation of the hemostatic system may cause thrombosis and embolism, which can reduce blood flow to critical organs like the brain and myocardium. Although we understand less about the pathophysiology of thrombosis than of hemostatic failure, certain patient groups have been identified that are particularly prone to thrombosis and embolism. These include patients (1) immobilized after surgery, (2) with chronic congestive heart failure, (3) with atherosclerotic vascular disease, (4) with malignancy, or (5) who are pregnant. Most of these "thrombosis-prone" patients have no identifiable hemostatic disorder. However, there are certain patient groups who have inherited or acquired a "hypercoagulable" or "prethrombotic" state which predisposes them to recurrent thrombosis.

The cardinal manifestations of disordered hemostasis which cause bleeding or thrombosis are discussed below, along with the clinical approach to diagnosis and evaluation of these patients. Certain information in the patient's history, such as the mode of onset and sites of bleeding, a family bleeding tendency, and a record of drug ingestion help establish the correct diagnosis. Physical examination can identify bleeding in the skin or joint deformities due to previous hemarthroses. Ultimately, however, bleeding disorders are diagnosed by laboratory tests. General screening tests are utilized first, to document a systemic disorder, and are then supplemented by specific tests of coagulation protein or platelet function to arrive at an accurate diagnosis.

The hypercoagulable or prethrombotic patient can also be identified by a careful history. There are three important clues to this diagnosis: (1) repeated episodes of thromboembolism without an obvious predisposing condition; (2) a family history of thrombosis; and (3) well-documented thromboembolism in adolescents and young adults. There are, as yet, no clinically useful screening tests for the prethrombotic state. However, several of the prethrombotic disorders can be diagnosed with specific immunologic and functional assays.

NORMAL HEMOSTASIS

Accurate diagnosis and treatment of patients with either bleeding or thrombosis requires some knowledge of the pathophysiology of hemostasis. The process can be divided into primary and secondary components and is initiated when trauma, surgery, or disease disrupt the vascular endothelial lining and blood is exposed to subendothelial connective tissue. *Primary hemostasis* is the name given to the process of platelet plug formation at sites of injury. It occurs within seconds of injury and is of prime importance in stopping blood loss from capillaries, small arterioles, and venules (see Fig. 62-1). *Secondary hemostasis* describes the reactions of the plasma coagulation system which result in fibrin formation. It requires several minutes for completion. The fibrin strands which are produced strengthen the primary hemostatic plug. This reaction is particularly important in larger vessels and prevents recurrent bleeding hours or days after the initial injury. Although presented here as separate events, primary and secondary hemostasis are closely linked. For example, activated platelets accelerate plasma coagulation, and products of the plasma coagulation reaction, such as thrombin, stimulate platelet aggregation.

Effective primary hemostasis requires three critical events—platelet adhesion, granule release, and platelet aggregation. Within a few seconds of injury, platelets adhere to collagen fibrils in vascular subendothelium via a specific platelet collagen receptor made up of glycoprotein Ia and IIa. As shown in Fig. 62-2, this interaction is stabilized by the von Willebrand factor, an adhesive glycoprotein which allows platelets to remain attached to the vessel wall despite the high shear forces generated within the vascular lumen. The von Willebrand factor accomplishes this task by forming a link between a platelet receptor site on glycoprotein Ib and subendothelial collagen fibrils. The adherent platelets then release preformed granule con-

FIGURE 62-1 Schematic presentation of the major events in primary hemostasis. The first event is platelet adhesion, the interaction of platelets with a nonplatelet surface such as vascular subendothelium. This is followed by platelet activation and secretion. Some of the products secreted by platelets are depicted. Abbreviations—ADP, adenosine diphosphate; PDGF, platelet-derived growth factor, vWF, von Willebrand's factor. The final event is the binding of activated platelets to the adherent monolayer in the process of platelet aggregation.

Activation/Secretion

ADP   Factor Va   Thrombospondin

Thromboxane A$_2$ PDGF

Heparinase   vWF

Fibrinogen   Fibronectin

Adhesion   Aggregation

FIGURE 62-2 The molecular basis of platelet adhesion and aggregation. Adhesion of platelets to vascular subendothelium is facilitated by the von Willebrand's factor, which forms a bridge between collagen fibrils in the vessel wall and receptors on platelet glycoprotein Ib (GpIb). In a similar manner, platelet aggregation is mediated by fibrinogen which links adjacent platelets via receptors on the platelet glycoprotein IIb and IIIa complex (GpIIb–IIIa).

stituents and generate de novo mediators like those depicted in Fig. 62-1.

As in other cells, platelet activation and secretion are regulated by changes in the level of cyclic nucleotides, the influx of calcium, hydrolysis of membrane phospholipids, and phosphorylation of critical intracellular proteins. The relevant pathways are depicted in Figs. 62-3 and 62-4. The binding of agonists such as epinephrine, collagen, or thrombin to platelet surface receptors activates two membrane enzymes—phospholipase C and phospholipase A_2. These enzymes

FIGURE 62-3 Generation of thromboxane A_2 in platelets and prostacyclin (PGI_2) in endothelial cells.

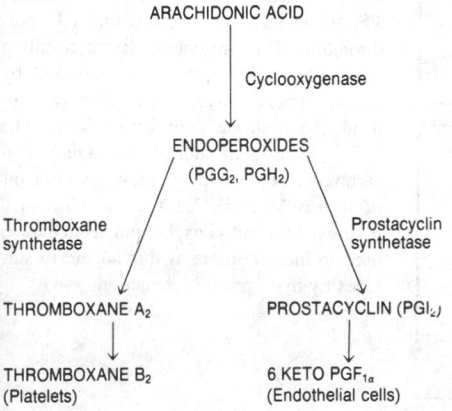

FIGURE 62-4 The biochemical basis of platelet activation and secretion. Binding of agonists such as thrombin, epinephrine, or collagen sets in motion a chain of events which hydrolyzes membrane phospholipids, inhibits adenylate cyclase, mobilizes intracellular calcium, and phosphorylates critical intracellular proteins. The net result is shape change, movement of granules to the canalicular system, generation of mediators like thromboxane A_2, and granule secretion. Abbreviations—A.C., adenylate cyclase; G, guanine nucleotide–binding protein; PIP_2, phosphatidylinositol-4,5-bisphosphate; PLC, phospholipase C; DAG, diacylglycerol; PLA_2, phospholipase A_2; PC, phosphatidylcholine; AA, arachidonic acid; CO, cyclooxygenase; O_2, oxygen; IP_3, inositol triphosphate; cAMP, cyclic AMP; Ca-CM, calcium calmodulin complex; MLCK, myosin light chain kinase.

catalyze the release of arachidonic acid from two of the major membrane phospholipids, phosphatidylinositol and phosphatidylcholine. Initially, a small quantity of the released arachidonic acid is converted to thromboxane A_2 (TXA_2), which, in turn, can activate phospholipase C. The formation of TXA_2 from arachidonic acid is mediated by the enzyme cyclooxygenase (see Fig. 62-3). This enzyme is inhibited by aspirin and nonsteroidal anti-inflammatory drugs. Inhibition of TXA_2 synthesis is a cause of mild bleeding in some patients, as well as the basis for the action of some antithrombotic drugs.

Hydrolysis of the membrane phospholipid, phosphatidylinositol 4,5-bisphosphate (PIP_2), produces diacylglycerol (DAG) and inositol triphosphate (IP_3), both of which play critical roles in platelet metabolism. IP_3 mediates the movement of calcium into the platelet cytosol and stimulates the phosphorylation of myosin light chains. The latter interact with actin to facilitate granule movement and platelet shape change. DAG activates protein kinase C which, in turn, phosphorylates a 47,000-dalton protein (plekstrin) that may regulate platelet granule secretion.

A finely balanced mechanism controls the rate and extent of platelet activation, which is illustrated in Fig. 62-3. TXA_2, a platelet product of arachidonic acid, increases phospholipase C activity, which stimulates platelet activation and secretion. In contrast, prostacyclin (PGI_2), an endothelial cell product of arachidonic acid, inhibits phospholipase C activity by raising the intraplatelet cyclic AMP levels, which in turn inhibits platelet activation. Similar pathways to regulate activation and secretion occur in other cells.

Following activation, platelets secrete their granule contents into plasma. Endoglycosidases and a heparin-cleaving enzyme are released from lysosomes; calcium, serotonin, and adenosine diphosphate (ADP) are released from the dense granules; and several proteins including the von Willebrand factor, fibronectin, thrombospondin, and a heparin-neutralizing protein (platelet factor 4) are released from

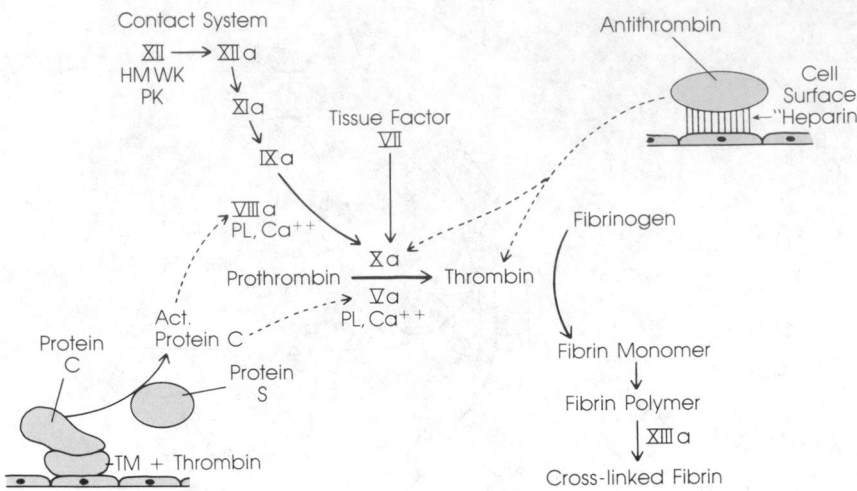

FIGURE 62-5 A schematic diagram of some of the clinically important coagulation reactions. The unactivated or precursor proteins are indicated by roman numerals, and the active form by the addition of a lowercase "a"—a standard convention. Other abbreviations are HMWK, high-molecular-weight kininogen; PK, prekallikrein; PL, phospholipid; TM, thrombomodulin; Ca^{2+}, calcium. There are two independent activation pathways, the contact system and the tissue factor–mediated or extrinsic system. They both merge at the point of factor X activation and lead to the generation of thrombin, which converts fibrinogen into fibrin. These reactions are regulated by antithrombin, which forms complexes with all of the coagulation protein serine proteases except factor VII, and the protein C–protein S system which inactivates factors V and VIII.

alpha granules. Released ADP modifies the platelet surface so that fibrinogen can attach to a complex formed between membrane glycoproteins IIb and IIIa, thereby linking adjacent platelets into a hemostatic plug (Fig. 62-2). Platelet-derived growth factor (PDGF), another alpha granule protein, stimulates the growth and migration of fibroblasts and smooth muscle cells within the vessel wall, which is an important part of the repair process.

As the primary hemostatic plug is being formed, plasma coagulation proteins are activated to initiate secondary hemostasis. An overall picture of the coagulation scheme, including the role of various inhibitors, is shown in Fig. 62-5. The coagulation pathway can be broken down into a series of reactions (outlined in Fig. 62-6) which culminate in the production of sufficient thrombin to convert a small portion of plasma fibrinogen to fibrin. Each of the reactions requires the formation of a surface-bound complex, the conversion of inactive precursor proteins into active proteases by limited proteolysis, and each is regulated by both plasma and cellular cofactors and calcium.

In *reaction 1*, the intrinsic or contact phase of coagulation, three plasma proteins, Hageman factor (factor XII), high-molecular-weight kininogen (HMWK), and prekallikrein (PK) are thought to form a complex on vascular subendothelial collagen. After binding to HMWK, factor XII is slowly converted to an active protease (XIIa), which then converts both PK to kallikrein and factor XI to its active form (XIa). Kallikrein (K) in turn accelerates XII conversion to XIIa, while XIa participates in subsequent coagulation reactions. Although

these interactions are well-characterized in vitro, an alternative mechanism for the activation of factor XI may exist, as patients who are deficient in factor XII, HMWK, or PK have apparently normal hemostasis and no clinical bleeding.

Reaction 2 provides a second pathway to initiate coagulation by converting factor VII to an active protease. In this extrinsic or tissue-factor-dependent pathway, a complex is formed between factor VII, calcium, and tissue factor, a ubiquitous lipoprotein present in cellular membranes which is exposed following cellular injury. Factor VII and three other coagulation proteins—factors II (prothrombin), IX, and X—require calcium and vitamin K for biologic activity. These proteins are synthesized in the liver, where a vitamin K–dependent carboxylase catalyzes a unique posttranslational modification which adds a second carboxyl group to certain glutamic acid residues. Pairs of these di-γ-carboxyglutamic acid (Gla) residues bind calcium, which anchors these proteins to negatively charged phospholipid surfaces and confers biological activity. Inhibition of this posttranslational modification by vitamin K antagonists (e.g., warfarin) is the basis of one of the most common forms of anticoagulant therapy.

In *reaction 3*, factor X is activated by the proteases generated in the two previous reactions. In one reaction, a calcium- and lipid-dependent complex is formed between factors VIII, IX, and X. Within this complex, factor IX is first converted to IXa by factor XIa that was generated within the intrinsic pathway (reaction 1). Factor X is then activated by factor IXa in concert with factor VIII. Alternatively, both factors IX and X can be activated more directly

FIGURE 62-6 The major coagulation reactions are subdivided and depicted in schematic form to emphasize their similarity. They all rely on the formation of surface bound enzyme-cofactor complexes. Abbreviations are PK, prekallikrein; K, kallikrein; HMWK, high-molecular-weight kininogen; TF, tissue factor; Ca^{2+}, calcium; PT, prothrombin; Thr, thrombin. By convention other coagulation factors are indicated by roman numerals, with a lowercase "a" appended to indicate their active form. The ∧∧∧ is used to indicate the Gla (di-γ-carboxyglutamic acid)–containing domains of factors VII, IX, X, Xa, and PT which bind calcium and phospholipid. Hatching is used to indicate proteins that adhere to surfaces by hydrophobic interaction.

by factor VIIa, which has been generated via the extrinsic pathway (reaction 2). Activation of factors IX and X provides an important link between the intrinsic and extrinsic coagulation pathways (see Fig. 62-5).

Reaction 4, the final step, converts prothrombin to thrombin in the presence of factor V, calcium, and phospholipid. Although prothrombin conversion can take place on various natural and artificial phospholipid-rich surfaces, it accelerates several-thousand-fold on the surface of activated platelets. Thrombin, the product of this reaction, has multiple functions in hemostasis. Although its principal role in hemostasis is the conversion of fibrinogen to fibrin, it also activates factors V, VIII, and XIII and stimulates platelet aggregation and secretion. Following the release of fibrinopeptides A and B from the alpha and beta chains of fibrinogen, the modified molecule, now called fibrin monomer, polymerizes into an insoluble gel. The fibrin polymer is then stabilized by the cross-linking of individual chains by factor XIIIa, a plasma transglutaminase (Fig. 62-5).

Clot lysis and vessel repair begin immediately after the formation of the definitive hemostatic plug. There are three major activators of the fibrinolytic system, Hageman factor fragments, urokinase (UK), and tissue plasminogen activator (t-PA). The principal physiologic activator, t-PA, diffuses from endothelial cells and converts plasminogen, adsorbed to the fibrin clot, into plasmin (see Fig. 62-7). Plasmin then degrades fibrin polymer into small fragments which are cleared by the monocyte-macrophage scavenger system. Although plasmin can also degrade fibrinogen, the reaction remains localized because (1) t-PA activates plasminogen more effectively when it is adsorbed to fibrin clots, and (2) any plasmin that enters the circulation is rapidly bound and neutralized by the alpha₂ plasmin inhibitor. The importance of this inhibitor is underscored by the fact that patients who lack it have unchecked fibrinolysis and bleed. In addition endothelial cells release a plasminogen activator inhibitor (PAI) which blocks the action of t-PA.

As noted above, the plasma coagulation system is tightly regulated so that only a small quantity of each coagulation enzyme is converted to its active form. As a consequence, the hemostatic plug does not propagate beyond the site of injury. Precise regulation is important, since there is enough clotting potential in a single milliliter of blood to clot all the fibrinogen in the body in 10 to 15 s. Blood fluidity is maintained by the flow of blood itself, which reduces the concentration of reactants, the adsorption of coagulation factors to surfaces, and

the presence of multiple inhibitors in plasma. Antithrombin and proteins C and S are the most important inhibitors which help maintain blood fluidity.

These inhibitors have distinct modes of action. Antithrombin forms complexes with all the serine protease coagulation factors except factor VII (see Fig. 62-5). Rates of complex formation are accelerated by heparin and heparin like molecules on the surface of the endothelial cells. This ability of heparin to accelerate the activity of antithrombin is the basis for heparin's action as a potent anticoagulant. Protein C is converted to an active protease by thrombin after it is bound to an endothelial cell protein called thrombomodulin. Activated protein C then inactivates the two plasma cofactors V and VIII to slow down two critical coagulation reactions. Protein C may also stimulate the release of tissue plasminogen activator from endothelial cells. The inhibitory function of protein C is enhanced by protein S. As one might predict, reduced levels of antithrombin or proteins C and S, or dysfunctional forms of the molecule, result in a hypercoagulable or prethrombotic state.

The preceding description of blood coagulation implies that the process is uniform throughout the body. In fact, the process is not uniform and composition of the blood clot varies with the site of injury. Hemostatic plugs or thrombi that form in veins where blood flow is slow are richly endowed with fibrin and trapped red blood cells and contain relatively few platelets. They are often called red thrombi due to their appearance in surgical and pathologic specimens. The friable ends of these red thrombi, which often form in leg veins, can break off and embolize to the pulmonary circulation. Conversely, clots that form in arteries under conditions of high flow are predominantly composed of platelets and have little fibrin. These white thrombi may readily dislodge from the arterial wall and embolize to distant sites to cause temporary or permanent ischemia. This is particularly common in the cerebral and retinal circulation and may lead to transient neurologic dysfunction (transient ischemic attacks) including temporary monocular blindness (amaurosis fugax) or strokes. In addition, there is increasing evidence that many episodes of myocardial infarction are due to thrombi which form within atherosclerotic coronary arteries. It is important to remember that there is little difference between hemostatic plugs, which are a physiologic response to injury, and pathologic thrombi. To underscore the similarity, thrombosis is often described as coagulation occurring in the wrong place or at the wrong time.

CLINICAL EVALUATION

HISTORY   Certain elements of the history are particularly useful in determining whether bleeding is caused by an underlying hemostatic disorder rather than a local anatomic defect. One clue is a history of bleeding following common hemostatic stresses such as dental extraction, childbirth, or minor surgery. Bleeding that is sufficiently severe to require a blood transfusion merits special attention. A family history of bleeding and bleeding from multiple sites that cannot be linked to trauma or surgery also suggest a systemic disorder. Since bleeding can be mild, lack of a family history of bleeding does not exclude an inherited hemostatic disorder.

It may be possible to localize the defect to the platelet or plasma coagulation system (Table 62-1). Bleeding from a platelet disorder is usually localized to superficial sites such as the skin and mucous membranes, comes on immediately after trauma or surgery, and is readily controlled by local measures. In contrast, bleeding from secondary hemostatic or plasma coagulation defects occurs hours or days after injury and is unaffected by local therapy. Such bleeding most often occurs in deep subcutaneous tissues, muscles, joints, or body cavities.

PHYSICAL EXAMINATION   In conjunction with a careful history, physical examination can also be of help in evaluating patients with hemostatic disorders. The most common site to observe bleeding is in the skin and mucous membranes. Collections of blood in the skin

FIGURE 62-7   A schematic diagram of the fibrinolytic pathway. t-PA (tissue plasminogen activator) is released from endothelial cells, enters the fibrin clot, and activates plasminogen to plasmin. Any free plasmin is complexed with α₂ PI (alpha₂ plasmin inhibitor). Fibrin is degraded to low-molecular-weight fragments, abbreviated as FDPs, fibrin degradation products.

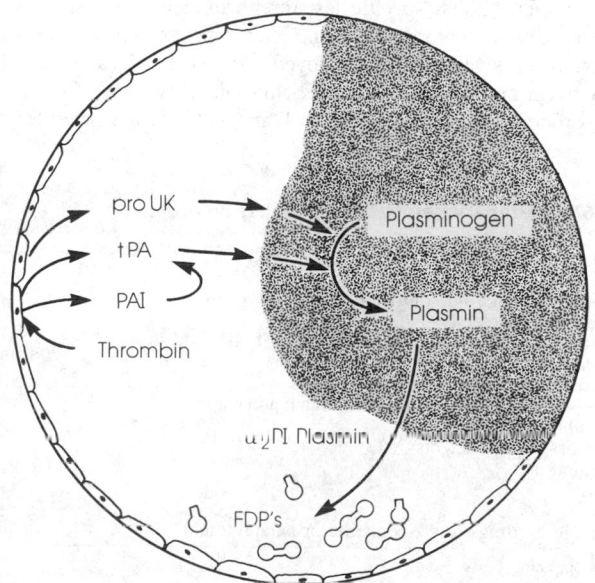

TABLE 62-1   Differences in the clinical manifestations of disorders of primary and secondary hemostasis

	Primary hemostasis (platelet defect)	Secondary hemostasis (plasma proteins)
Onset of bleeding after trauma	Immediate	Delayed—hours or days
Sites of bleeding	Superficial—skin; mucous membranes; nose; gastrointestinal, genitourinary tracts	Deep—joints, muscle, retroperitoneum
Physical findings	Petechiae, ecchymoses	Hematomas, hemarthroses
Family history	Autosomal dominant	Autosomal or X-linked recessive
Response to therapy	Immediate; local measures effective	Requires sustained systemic therapy

TABLE 62-2   Causes of thrombocytopenia

I Decreased marrow production of megakaryocytes
  A Marrow infiltration with tumor, fibrosis
  B Marrow failure—aplastic, hypoplastic anemias
II Splenic sequestration of circulating platelets
  A Splenic hypertrophy—tumor, portal hypertension
III Increased destruction of circulating platelets
  A Nonimmune destruction
    1 Vascular prostheses, cardiac valves
    2 Disseminated intravascular coagulation
    3 Sepsis
    4 Vasculitis
  B Immune destruction
    1 Autoantibodies to platelet antigens
    2 Drug-associated antibodies
    3 Circulating immune complexes—systemic lupus erythematosus, viral agents, bacterial sepsis

are called *purpura* and may be subdivided on the basis of the site of bleeding in the skin. Small pinpoint hemorrhages into the dermis due to the leakage of red cells through capillaries are called *petechiae* and are characteristic of platelet disorders—in particular, severe thrombocytopenia. Larger subcutaneous collections of blood due to leakage of blood from small arterioles and venules are *ecchymoses* (common bruises) or, if somewhat deeper and palpable, *hematomas*. They are also common in patients with platelet defects and result from minor trauma. There are other skin and mucous membrane lesions like dilated capillaries or *telangiectasia* that may cause bleeding without any hemostatic defect. In addition, the loss of connective tissue support for capillaries and small veins that accompanies aging increases the fragility of superficial vessels, such as those on the dorsum of the hand, leading to extravasation of blood into subcutaneous tissue—*senile purpura*. Menorrhagia is a serious problem in women with severe thrombocytopenia or platelet dysfunction. In addition, some patients with primary hemostatic defects, especially von Willebrand's disease, may have recurrent gastrointestinal hemorrhage.

As mentioned previously, bleeding into body cavities, retroperitoneum, or joints is a common manifestation of plasma coagulation defects. Repeated joint bleeding may cause synovial thickening, chronic inflammation, and fluid collections and may erode articular cartilage and lead to chronic joint deformity and limited mobility. Such deformities are particularly common in factor VIII and IX deficiency, the two sex-linked coagulation disorders referred to as the hemophilias. For unclear reasons, hemarthroses are much less common in other plasma coagulation defects. Blood collections in various body cavities or soft tissues can cause secondary necrosis of tissues or nerve compression. Retroperitoneal hematomas can cause femoral nerve compression, and large collections of poorly coagulated blood in soft tissues may occasionally mimic malignant growths—the pseudotumor syndrome. Two of the most life-threatening sites of bleeding are in the oropharynx, where bleeding can compromise the airway, and in the central nervous system. Intracerebral hemorrhage is one of the leading causes of death in patients with severe coagulation disorders.

LABORATORY TESTS The most important screening tests of the primary hemostatic system are (1) a *bleeding time* (a sensitive measure of platelet function) and (2) a *platelet count*. The latter is particularly useful as it is readily available and correlates well with the propensity to bleed. The normal platelet count is 150,000 to 450,000 platelets per cubic millimeter of blood. As long as the count is above 100,000 per cubic millimeter, patients are not symptomatic and the bleeding time remains normal. Platelet counts of 50,000 to 100,000 per cubic millimeter cause mild prolongation of the bleeding time and bleeding occurs only after severe trauma or other stress. Patients with platelet counts less than 50,000 per cubic millimeter have easy bruising, which is manifested by skin purpura with minor trauma and bleeding after mucous membrane surgery. Patients with a platelet count below 20,000 per cubic millimeter have an appreciable

incidence of spontaneous bleeding, usually have petechiae, and may have intracranial or other spontaneous internal bleeding. The major causes of thrombocytopenia are outlined in Table 62-2.

Patients with qualitative platelet abnormalities have a normal platelet count and a prolonged bleeding time (Table 62-3). The bleeding time is ascertained by making a small, superficial skin incision and timing the duration of blood flow from the wounded area. Although this is a rather crude "bioassay," by careful standardization it has become a reliable and sensitive test of platelet function. The most widely used technique uses a template or an automated scalpel to control the length and depth of the incision (usually 1 mm deep by 9 mm long), and a sphygmomanometer inflated to 40 mmHg to distend the capillary bed of the forearm uniformly. Although any patient with a bleeding time over 10 min has a slightly increased risk of bleeding, the risk does not become great until the bleeding time exceeds 15 or 20 min. When a defect in primary hemostasis is uncovered, specialized testing is needed to determine the cause of the platelet dysfunction (Table 62-3). A precise diagnosis is important since patients with bleeding due to a primary hemostatic disorder may need therapy with platelets, one of several hormones (desmopressin, estrogen, glucocorticoids), or plasma fractions, depending on the nature of the disorder.

Plasma coagulation function is readily assessed with a few simple laboratory tests—the partial thromboplastin time (PTT), prothrombin time (PT), thrombin time (TT), or a quantitative fibrinogen determination (Fig. 62-5, Table 62-4). The PTT screens the intrinsic limb of the coagulation system and tests for the adequacy of factors XII, HMWK, PK, XI, IX, and VIII. The PT screens the extrinsic or tissue factor-dependent pathway. Both tests also evaluate the common coagulation pathway involving all the reactions that occur after the activation of factor X. A specific test for fibrinogen conversion to fibrin is needed when both the PTT and PT are prolonged—either a TT or fibrinogen level can be employed. A test for factor XIII–dependent fibrin cross-linking, such as clot solubility in 5 *M* urea, should be ordered when the PT and PTT are both normal but there

TABLE 62-3   Primary hemostatic (platelet) disorders

Platelet adhesion defects:
  Von Willebrand's disease
  Bernard-Soulier syndrome (absence of platelet GpIb)*
Platelet aggregation defects:
  Glanzmann's thrombasthenia (absence of GpIIb–IIIa)
Platelet release defects:
  Decreased cyclooxygenase activity
    Drugs—aspirin, nonsteroidal anti-inflammatory agents
    Congenital
  Granule storage pool defects
    Congenital
    Acquired
  Uremia
Platelet coating by drugs (e.g., penicillin or paraproteins)

* Gp = glycoprotein.

TABLE 62-4 Relationship between secondary hemostatic disorders and coagulation test abnormalities

Prolonged partial thromboplastin time (PTT):
  No clinical bleeding—factors XII, HMWK, PK
  Mild or rare bleeding—factor XI
  Frequent, severe bleeding—factors VIII and IX
Prolonged prothrombin time (PT):
  Factor VII deficiency
  Vitamin K deficiency—early
  Warfarin anticoagulant ingestion
Prolonged PTT and PT:
  Factor II, V, or X deficiency
  Vitamin K deficiency—late
  Warfarin anticoagulant ingestion
Prolonged thrombin time (TT):
  Mild or rare bleeding—afibrinogenemia
  Frequent, severe bleeding—dysfibrinogenemia
  Heparin-like inhibitors or heparin administration
Clot solubility in 5 *M* urea:
  Factor XIII deficiency
  Inhibitors or defective cross-linking
Rapid clot lysis
  Alpha₂ plasmin inhibitor

NOTE: HMWK = high-molecular-weight kininogen; PK = prekallikrein.

is a strong history of bleeding. The fibrinolytic system can be assessed by measuring the rate of clot lysis with the euglobulin lysis or whole blood clot lysis tests and by measuring the level of alpha₂ plasmin inhibitor. When abnormalities are noted in any of the screening tests, more specific coagulation factor assays can be ordered to determine the nature of the defect.

There are no clinical tests to screen patients suspected of having hypercoagulable or prethrombotic disorders, although tests are being developed in research laboratories which measure small peptides or enzyme-inhibitor complexes generated during coagulation. For example, radioimmunoassays have been developed for fibrinopeptides A and B, for the thrombin-antithrombin complex, and for prothrombin cleavage fragments. Elevated levels of these products have been reported in patients with prethrombotic disorders and in patients with thromboembolism. At present, patients suspected of having a hypercoagulable state, on the basis of clinical information, should have specific assays to screen for the small number of known defects. Currently available tests can identify 10 to 20 percent of the cases of familial thrombosis and represent only a small fraction of the many patients who present to physicians with thromboembolism.

Inhibitor syndromes or circulating anticoagulants are usually due to antibodies which impair coagulation factor activity. They are an infrequent cause of bleeding which require specialized diagnostic testing. Inhibitors are likely when screening test abnormalities cannot be reversed by adding normal plasma to patient plasma. Antibodies against specific coagulation factors may develop in (1) postpartum females; (2) patients with autoimmune disorders such as systemic lupus erythematosus; (3) patients taking drugs like penicillin and streptomycin; and (4) otherwise healthy elderly individuals. In addition, between 10 and 20 percent of patients with severe hemophilia who have received multiple plasma infusions develop inhibitor antibodies. Some patients, especially those with systemic lupus erythematosus, may also have a nonspecific form of anticoagulant antibody which interferes with phospholipid binding of coagulation factors and prolongs the PT and PTT but does not cause clinical bleeding. The presence of the lupus anticoagulant may increase the risk of thromboembolism and may cause placental infarction and recurrent midtrimester abortion. Occasionally, patients develop inhibitors that are not antibodies. For example, several patients with circulating mucopolysaccharides that have heparin-like activity have been described with clinical bleeding.

REFERENCES

COLMAN RW et al (eds): *Hemostasis and Thrombosis: Basic Principles and Clinical Practice*, 2d ed. Philadelphia, Lippincott, 1986

HANDIN RI: Physiology of coagulation: The platelet, in *Hematology of Infancy and Childhood*, 3d ed, DG Nathan, FA Oski (eds). Philadelphia, Saunders, 1987, pp 1271–1292
ROSENBERG RD: Physiology of coagulation: The fluid phase, in *Hematology of Infancy and Childhood*, 3d ed, DG Nathan, FA Oski (eds). Philadelphia, Saunders, 1987
WILLIAMS WJ et al (eds): *Hematology*, 4th ed. New York, McGraw-Hill, 1990

63 ENLARGEMENT OF LYMPH NODES AND SPLEEN

BARTON F. HAYNES

Lymph nodes and spleen constitute a major portion of the peripheral immune system, and become enlarged in a wide spectrum of infectious, malignant, autoimmune, and metabolic diseases. Enlargement of lymph nodes (lymphadenopathy) and spleen (splenomegaly) are common clinical findings that can lead to a wide range of diagnostic and therapeutic procedures. The goal of this chapter is to serve as an introduction to these two components of the immune system and to highlight clinical features and diagnostic evaluation of some of the diseases in which lymphadenopathy and splenomegaly occur.

LYMPH NODES

LYMPH NODE STRUCTURE AND FUNCTION Lymph nodes are peripheral lymphoid organs that are connected to the circulation by afferent and efferent lymphatic vessels (Fig. 63-1) and by postcapillary high-endothelial venules. A number of cell types make up the lymph node supportive framework and stroma. Fibroblasts are the predominant cell type in the lymph node capsule and trabeculae. Fibroblast-derived reticular cells are supporting cells found frequently in the follicles and germinal centers, that is, the B-cell areas of lymph nodes. Tissue macrophages derived from circulating monocytes are present throughout the normal node. Within cortical areas are interdigitating reticular cells (also called dendritic cells) and Langerhans cells both of which are specialized nonphagocytic, Ia-bearing cells of bone marrow origin that along with macrophages participate in antigen presentation to thymus-derived (T) and B cells (Chap. 13). The outer lymph node cortex contains lymphoid follicles with germinal centers that are the B-cell areas of lymph node (Fig. 63-1). Primary lymphoid follicles are aggregates of IgM- and IgD-bearing B cells and CD4+ helper/inducer T cells prior to antigenic challenge. Secondary lymphoid follicles are the result of antigen stimulation, and contain an outer or mantle layer of IgM- and IgD-bearing B cells

FIGURE 63-1 Schematic lymph node structure. Lymph flows into nodes via afferent lymphatics (A) and leaves nodes via efferent lymphatics (E). B-cell areas are primary and secondary follicles in lymph node cortex while T cells are concentrated in paracortical areas.

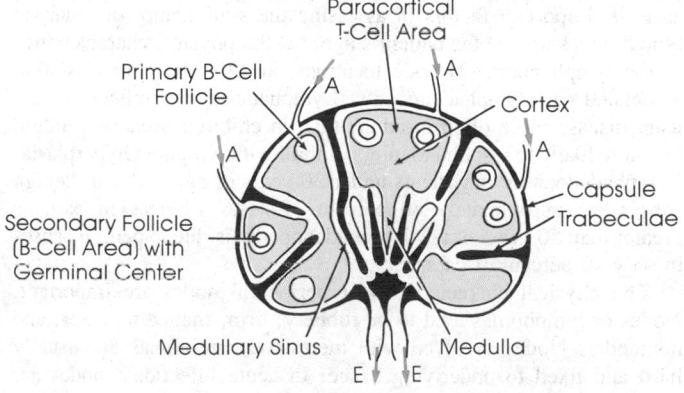

and an inner zone (germinal center) of activated B cells, macrophages, reticular cells, and scattered CD4 + helper T cells. Between primary and secondary follicle areas (interfollicular zones) and inner lymph node medullary regions are T-cell (paracortical) areas. The majority of T cells in lymph nodes are CD4 + helper T cells (approximately 80 percent) while the minority are CD8 + suppressor/cytotoxic T cells (approximately 20 percent).

The two most important factors contributing to the composition and distribution of lymphoid cells within lymph node are (1) generation of memory B and T cells de novo from proliferation of antigen-stimulated percursors within lymph nodes, and (2) selective recirculation to and homing of specific types of lymphoid cells to lymph nodes from the circulation. Traffic through lymph nodes is via two general routes (Fig. 63-1). Afferent lymph, containing lymphocytes, macrophages, and antigens, enters the lymph node via the subcapsular space, and drains through paracortical and medullary areas into medullary sinuses that converge to form efferent lymphatic vessels through which lymph exits. B cells from bone marrow and T cells from the thymus enter lymph nodes from the circulation by binding to specific receptors on cells of postcapillary high-endothelial venules. After activation by antigen and clonal expansion, sensitized T and B cells and antibody-secreting plasma cells leave the node in efferent lymph and rejoin the peripheral blood circulation via the thoracic duct.

Lymph nodes function as sites of macrophage, T-cell, and B-cell contact with antigen, with a specialized structure that gives rise to optimal T cell, B cell, and macrophage interactions. Under normal conditions such interactions result in efficient recognition of antigen, activation of the cellular and humoral arms of the immune response, and ultimate elimination of antigen (see Chap. 13).

Lymph node enlargement can be due to (1) an increase in the number of benign lymphocytes and macrophages during response to antigens, (2) infiltration by inflammatory cells in infections involving lymph nodes (lymphadenitis), (3) in situ proliferation of malignant lymphocytes or macrophages, (4) infiltration of nodes by metastatic malignant cells, or (5) infiltration of lymph nodes by metabolite-laden macrophages in lipid storage diseases.

In normal immune responses, antigen stimulation of macrophages and lymphocytes in lymph nodes exerts profound influences on lymphocyte traffic. One of the earliest effects of antigen is to increase blood flow through the affected node, which during antigen stimulation may reach 10 to 25 times normal levels. Lymphocytes accumulate in antigen-stimulated nodes by increase in traffic through the node, decreased egress of lymphocytes from antigen-stimulated nodes, and proliferation of responding T and B cells. A lymph node may thus reach 15 times its normal size 5 to 10 days after antigenic stimulation.

DISEASES ASSOCIATED WITH LYMPHADENOPATHY Under normal conditions in adults, the inguinal lymph nodes may be palpable, and are generally 0.5 cm to 2 cm in size. Elsewhere in the body, smaller lymph nodes due to past infections may be present normally. Enlargement of lymph nodes requires investigation when there are one or more new nodes present equal to or greater than 1 cm in diameter, and not known to arise from a previously recognized cause. However, this is not a rigid criterion and under certain circumstances new multiple or single smaller lymph nodes may warrant investigation as well. Important factors in assessing the significance of enlarged lymph nodes are (1) the patient's age, (2) the physical characteristics of the lymph node, (3) node locations, and (4) the clinical setting associated with lymphadenopathy. Lymphadenopathy reflects significant disease more often in adults than in children because children are more likely to respond to minor stimuli with lymphoid hyperplasia. Lymphadenopathy in patients under 30 years of age is due to benign causes in approximately 80 percent of cases whereas in patients greater than 50 years of age lymphadenopathy is due to benign causes in only 40 percent of cases.

The physical characteristics of peripheral nodes are important. Nodes of lymphomas tend to be rubbery, firm, matted together, and nontender. Nodes involved with metastatic carcinomas are usually hard and fixed to underlying tissue. In acute infections, nodes are tender, asymmetrically enlarged, matted together, and the overlying skin may be erythematous.

The clinical setting is important in assessing lymphadenopathy. In a young college student with fever and recent onset of lymph node enlargement, infectious mononucleosis syndromes are important to consider. In homosexuals, hemophiliacs, and intravenous drug users with systemic lymphadenopathy, the acquired immunodeficiency syndrome (AIDS) or an AIDS-related complex syndrome should be considered (see Chap. 264).

The location of enlarged lymph nodes may suggest important clues to the diagnosis. Enlarged posterior cervical nodes are frequently present in scalp infections, toxoplasmosis, and rubella, whereas anterior auricular nodes suggest infections of the eyelids and conjunctiva. Lymphomas commonly involve cervical lymph nodes and can occasionally involve posterior auricular and occipital nodes as well. Enlarged suppurative cervical nodes are seen in mycobacterial lymphadenitis (scrofula). Unilateral jugular or mandibular lymph node enlargement suggests lymphoma or nonlymphoid head-and-neck malignancy. Supraclavicular and scalene lymph node enlargement is always significant, and frequently results from metastasis from intrathoracic or gastrointestinal malignancies or from lymphomas. Virchow's node is an enlarged left supraclavicular lymph node infiltrated with metastatic tumor usually from the gastrointestinal tract. Unilateral epitrochlear node enlargement is usually due to hand infections; bilateral epitrochlear node enlargement is seen in sarcoidosis, tularemia, and secondary syphilis.

Unilateral axillary adenopathy can be seen with breast carcinoma, lymphomas, infections of the upper extremities, cat-scratch disease, and brucellosis.

Bilateral inguinal adenopathy can be seen in a variety of venereal infections; however, lymphogranuloma venereum and syphilis are associated with unilateral inguinal adenopathy. Progressive inguinal lymph node enlargement without obvious infection suggests malignant disease. Femoral node involvement has been reported to occur in *Pasteurella pestis* infections and lymphomas.

Symptoms that should raise the suspicion of hilar or mediastinal node enlargement are cough or wheezing due to airway compression, recurrent laryngeal nerve compression with hoarseness, paralysis of the diaphragm, dysphagia with esophageal compression, and swelling of the neck, face, or arms due to superior vena cava or subclavian vein compression. Bilateral mediastinal adenopathy is frequently seen in lymphomas, especially the nodular sclerosing type of Hodgkin's disease. Unilateral hilar adenopathy indicates a high likelihood of metastatic carcinoma (usually lung), while bilateral hilar adenopathy is more often benign and is seen in sarcoidosis, tuberculosis, and systemic fungal infections. Bilateral hilar adenopathy in asymptomatic patients or in association with erythema nodosum or uveitis is almost always due to sarcoidosis (Chap. 277). The association of bilateral hilar adenopathy with an anterior mediastinal mass, pleural effusion, or pulmonary mass suggests neoplastic disease.

Enlarged retroperitoneal and intraabdominal nodes are not usually inflammatory in origin, but are frequently due to lymphomas or other neoplastic diseases. Tuberculosis can cause mesenteric lymphadenitis with large matted and sometimes calcified nodes.

Some of the diseases associated with lymph node enlargement are listed in Table 63-1 and fall into six general categories: infectious diseases, immunologic diseases, malignant diseases, endocrine diseases, lipid storage diseases, and miscellaneous.

The manifestations of infectious diseases are protean and are best considered according to the type of infectious agent. The most common viral infection associated with systemic lymphadenopathy is Epstein-Barr (EB) virus–associated infectious mononucleosis (see Chap. 137). A variety of other viral diseases including viral hepatitis, cytomegalovirus, rubella, and influenza can cause clinical syndromes similar to those induced by the EB virus. AIDS is caused by a retrovirus, human immunodeficiency virus (HIV). In the HIV-associated lymphadenopathy syndrome, cervical, axillary, and occipital nodes are the most commonly involved (see Chap. 264).

TABLE 63-1 Diseases associated with lymph node enlargement

I Infectious diseases
  A Viral infections: infectious hepatitis, infectious mononucleosis syndromes (cytomegalovirus, EB virus), AIDS, rubella, varicella–herpes zoster, vaccinia
  B Bacterial infections: streptococci, staphylococci, salmonella, brucella, Francisella tularensis, *Listeria monocytogenes, Pasteurella pestis, Haemophilus ducreyi,* cat-scratch disease
  C Fungal infections: coccidioidomycosis, histoplasmosis
  D Chlamydial infections: Lymphogranuloma venereum, trachoma
  E Mycobacterial infections: tuberculosis, leprosy
  F Parasitic infections: trypanosomiasis, microfilariasis, toxoplasmosis
  G Spirochetal diseases: syphilis, yaws, endemic syphilis (bejel), leptospirosis
II Immunologic diseases
  A Rheumatoid arthritis
  B Systemic lupus erythematosus
  C Dermatomyositis
  D Serum sickness
  E Drug reactions: phenytoin, hydralazine, allopurinol
  F Angioimmunoblastic lymphadenopathy
III Malignant diseases
  A Hematologic: Hodgkin's lymphoma, acute and chronic T-, B-, myeloid, and monocytoid cell leukemias and lymphomas, malignant histiocytosis
  B Metastatic tumors to lymph nodes: melanoma, Kaposi's sarcoma, neuroblastoma, seminoma, tumors of lung, breast, prostate, kidney, head and neck, gastrointestinal tract
IV Endocrine diseases: hyperthyroidism
V Lipid storage diseases: Gaucher's and Niemann-Pick diseases
VI Miscellaneous diseases and diseases of unknown cause
  A Giant follicular lymph node hyperplasia
  B Sinus histiocytosis
  C Dermatopathic lymphadenitis
  D Sarcoidosis
  E Amyloidosis
  F Mucocutaneous lymph node syndrome
  G Lymphomatoid granulomatosis
  H Multifocal Langerhans cell (eosinophilic) granulomatosis

Chronic bacterial infections as well as fungal infections may produce considerable lymph node enlargement without signs of local inflammation. Cat-scratch disease is a regional lymphadenitis occurring approximately 2 weeks following a cat scratch or bite. The nodes involved relate to lymph drainage of the wound site with upper extremity adenopathy being the most common, occurring in 50 percent of cases. Fungi associated with primary pulmonary infections (coccidioidomycosis, histoplasmosis) can cause hilar adenopathy. Acute and chronic mycobacterial, parasitic, and spirochetal diseases against which there is a profound cellular and humoral immune response all can result in either systemic or regional enlarged lymph nodes depending on the clinical syndrome in question. Virtually any disease characterized by immune cell activation (systemic lupus erythematosus, rheumatoid arthritis, serum sickness, reactions due to drugs such as diphenylhydantoin, angioimmunoblastic lymphadenopathy) can be associated with regional or systemic adenopathy. Lymph node enlargement associated with malignant disease may be due to direct node involvement by tumor, lymphoid hyperplasia in response to tumor, or both. Generalized lymphoid hyperplasia may occur with hyperthroidism. Patients with lipid storage diseases such as Gaucher's and Niemann-Pick disease can have enlarged lymph nodes, particularly in the abdomen, due to accumulation of lipid-laden macrophages.

A number of diseases of unknown cause are associated with lymphadenopathy and in many of the diseases in this group, lymphadenopathy is a major manifestation of the disease. Sarcoidosis frequently presents with generalized lymph node enlargement, especially in cervical, inguinal, and epitrochlear areas (Chap. 277). Although giant follicular lymph node hyperplasia can occur in extrathoracic lymph nodes, mediastinal or hilar nodes are involved in 70 percent of cases. In sinus histiocytosis, massive cervical lymph node enlargement often associated with generalized lymphadenopathy occurs and is associated with fever and leukocytosis. Patients with exfoliative dermatitis or other dermatologic syndromes can develop enlarged superficial lymph nodes (called dermatopathic lymphadenitis)

which usually regress with resolution of the dermatitis. Lymph node involvement occurs in approximately 30 percent of cases of primary and secondary amyloidosis; only rarely is amyloid lymphadenopathy the major or the only organ involvement. The mechanism of node enlargement in amyloidosis is the accumulation of extracellular masses of amyloid fibrils that compress and eventually obliterate normal lymph node architecture (Chap. 266).

Mucocutaneous lymph node syndrome (Kawasaki's disease) is a systemic lymphadenopathy syndrome, the hallmarks of which are fever, conjunctivitis, erythema of the tongue with protrusion of papillae (strawberry tongue), a truncal exanthem with desquamation of palms and soles, and acute nonsuppurative enlargement of cervical lymph nodes (see Chap. 276).

Lymphomatoid granulomatosis is a disease characterized by infiltration of various organs (lungs, skin, central nervous system) with an angiocentric and angioinvasive polymorphic cellular infiltrate consisting of atypical lymphocytes and macrophages. The disease has characteristics of both an inflammatory granulomatous process and a lymphoproliferative disease, with progression to frank lymphoma in up to 50 percent of cases. Lymphadenopathy in the prelymphoma state of lymphomatoid granulomatosis occurs in 40 percent of cases affecting primarily intrathoracic nodes while peripheral adenopathy occurs only rarely (10 percent) (see Chap. 276).

Angioimmunoblastic lymphadenopathy is a disease characterized by fever, generalized lymphadenopathy, hepatosplenomegaly, polyclonal hypergammaglobulinemia, and Coombs-positive hemolytic anemia. Although it is not thought to be a malignant disease, it evolves into B-cell lymphoma in 35 percent of patients (see Chap. 302).

Diseases characterized by benign and malignant proliferation of tissue macrophages (histiocytes) or of specialized bone marrow–derived cells called Langerhans cells have been termed *histiocytoses* or *histiocytosis X.* In the past, these terms encompassed a number of diseases including unifocal and multifocal eosinophilic granuloma, Hand-Schüller-Christian syndrome, Letterer-Siwe disease, and frank neoplasms of undifferentiated histiocytes. Recently, the identification of the Langerhans cell as the predominant cell in forms of eosinophilic granuloma has prompted reevaluation of these syndromes.

One term currently in use for eosinophilic granuloma syndromes is *Langerhans cell (eosinophilic) granulomatosis,* and this term will be used here. The term histiocytosis X is an outmoded term that refers to a spectrum of diseases encompassing both the benign disorder of Langerhans cell (eosinophilic) granulomatosis and malignant lymphomatous disease.

The classic triad of the *Hand-Schüller-Christian syndrome* (exophthalmus, diabetes insipidus, and destructive bone lesions) occurs with 25 percent of cases of multifocal eosinophilic granuloma but also may occur in malignant lymphoma and carcinoma. *Letterer-Siwe disease* is an acute clinical syndrome of unknown etiology in infants that consists of hepatosplenomegaly, lymphadenopathy, hemorrhagic diathesis, anemia, no familial occurrence, and generalized hyperplasia of tissue macrophages in a variety of organs. It is currently felt that Letterer-Siwe disease represents an unusual form of malignant lymphoma, and is distinct from forms of eosinophilic granuloma.

Histologically, Langerhans cell granulomatosis consists of aggregates of mature eosinophils and Langerhans cells. Langerhans cells are bone marrow–derived cells normally found among epidermal cells of skin and rarely in B-cell areas of lymph node and the medulla of thymus. Langerhans cells contain distinct cytoplasmic granules (Birbeck granules) and contain adenosine triphosphatase and alpha naphthyl acetate esterase. Surface markers of Langerhans cells include class II major histocompatibility complex antigens (Ia-like) and the T6 antigen that is also expressed by the cortical (immature) thymocytes (see Chap. 13).

Unifocal Langerhans cell (eosinophilic) granulomatosis is a benign disease of children and young adults, predominantly in males. Occasionally, it occurs as late as 60 to 70 years of age, and presents as a solitary osteolytic lesion in the femur, skull, vertebrae, ribs, or occasionally the pelvis. Since there are no consistent accompanying laboratory abnormalities, the diagnosis of unifocal Langerhans cell granulomatosis requires biopsy of the lytic bone lesion. Treatment of choice of this condition is excision or curettage of the lesion. Rarely, lesions in inaccessible sites such as cervical vertebrae require moderate doses of irradiation [3 to 6 Gy (300 to 600 rad)]. After initial bone scan and radiographic survey to assess extent of disease, follow-up studies should be performed at 6-month intervals for 3 years. If no additional lesions are present 12 months after diagnosis, development of subsequent lesions is unlikely.

Multifocal Langerhans cell (eosinophilic) granulomatosis also usually presents in childhood, and is characterized by the development of multiple bony lesions at virtually any site—though less commonly in the feet and hands.

Transient or permanent diabetes insipidus due to granulomatous involvement of the hypothalamus occurs in one-third of patients; 20 percent develop hepatomegaly, 30 percent splenomegaly, and one-half of the patients have focal or generalized lymph node involvement. Lesions may also involve the skin, vulva, gingiva, lung, and thymus. Laboratory studies are rarely helpful in the diagnosis of multifocal Langerhans cell granulomatosis, necessitating biopsy of lesions. While generally a benign disease, multifocal Langerhans cell granulomatosis is best treated with low to moderate doses of methotrexate, prednisone, or vinblastine, usually with regression of lesions.

EVALUATION OF THE PATIENT WITH LYMPHADENOPATHY

Good physical examination techniques for palpation and assessment of lymph nodes are essential for providing useful information on which diagnostic and therapeutic decisions can be based. For serial evaluation of nodes, the documentation of each node with regard to size, location, consistency, and mobility at each examination is critical. For cervical nodes the examiner may stand behind or in front of the seated patient to palpate the neck and to examine in sequence the sites of various groups of nodes. Submental nodes are under the chin in the midline and on either side; submandibular nodes are under the jaw near its angle; jugular nodes are along the anterior border of the sternocleidomastoid muscle; supraclavicular nodes are found behind the mid portion of the clavicle. Suboccipital nodes are found in the apex of the posterior cervical triangle, and pre- and postauricular nodes are found in front of and behind the ear pinnae, respectively. Central axillary nodes occur near the middle of the thoracic wall of the axilla; lateral axillary nodes are located near the upper part of the humerus along the axillary vein and are best felt by having the patient's arm elevated. Subscapular nodes can be felt under the anterior edge of the latissimus dorsi muscle, and pectoral nodes are beneath the lateral edge of the pectoralis major muscle. Infraclavicular nodes can be felt under the distal end of the clavicle. Epitrochlear nodes are located approximately 3 cm proximal to the medial humeral epicondyle. Palpation of epitrochlear nodes is best accomplished by palpation across the epitrochlear node area in an anterior to posterior direction. Enlarged abdominal lymph nodes can be difficult to palpate and may only be felt if the patient has a shallow abdominal cavity. Pelvic nodes are best evaluated with deep palpation of the lower abdomen by rolling the extended fingers over the pelvic brim.

The investigation of lymphadenopathy can be organized according to where nodes occur and the type of clinical symptoms present. Enlarged supraclavicular nodes most often result from lymphoma, gastrointestinal, or intrathoracic tumors and should be biopsied. Acute onset of cervical adenopathy in young adults in the absence of head-and-neck infections suggests the diagnosis of infectious mononucleosis syndromes. If localized cervical node enlargement persists and serologic evaluation for EB virus, cytomegalovirus, and toxoplasmosis infections as well as chest x-ray and intermediate-strength PPD skin test are negative, then lymph node biopsy is indicated to seek lymphoma, sarcoidosis, carcinoma, and other diseases listed in Table 63-1.

Unilateral cervical adenopathy warrants a careful ear, nose, and throat examination for malignancy. In the asymptomatic patient with persistent new axillary and/or inguinal adenopathy, a biopsy specimen

should be obtained. If fever and constitutional symptoms are present, the cause of infectious mononucleosis–like syndromes should be sought prior to node biopsy.

Generalized lymph node enlargement can be caused by systemic infections, drug reactions, malignancy, or one of the systemic lymphadenopathy syndromes (Table 63-1). History and physical examination can yield clues regarding the possibility of these diagnoses and direct further evaluation (e.g., complete blood count, blood cultures, chest x-ray, serologies, skin tests). If systemic adenopathy persists without an obvious cause being identified, lymph node biopsy is warranted. Once the decision to perform lymph node biopsy has been made, tissue should be processed for culture of appropriate organisms, frozen in liquid nitrogen for lymphocyte typing or other special diagnostic studies for malignant cell types, and processed for routine pathologic evaluation. One can expect information that will lead to a diagnosis in 50 to 60 percent of lymph node biopsies. About 25 percent of patients with nondiagnostic lymph node biopsies will subsequently develop within a year a disease (usually a lymphoma) related to the indication for biopsy. Therefore there should be little hesitation to repeat a nondiagnostic biopsy, especially if enlarged lymph nodes and symptoms persist.

The term *atypical hyperplasia of lymph nodes* refers to neither a clinical nor a pathologic entity, but designates cases in which the pathologist expresses concern about neoplasia and is unable to unequivocally diagnose lymphoma. Since 30 percent of patients whose lymph node biopsies are read as atypical hyperplasia subsequently develop lymphoma, a repeat biopsy is recommended at a later date if node enlargement persists. Needle aspiration biopsy is a safe technique for initial evaluation of superficial adenopathy. While lymph node aspiration can aid in the diagnosis of metastatic tumor and infections, it is rarely helpful in the diagnosis of lymphomas and other hematologic malignancies.

SPLEEN

SPLEEN STRUCTURE AND FUNCTION The spleen is a lymphoreticular organ that serves at least four major physiologic functions. First, it is an organ of the immune system and a major site of clearance of microorganisms and particulate antigens from the bloodstream and of generation of humoral or cellular responses to foreign antigens. Second, the spleen is instrumental in sequestration and removal of normal and abnormal blood cells. Third, the vasculature of the spleen plays a role in regulation of portal blood flow. Fourth, while hematopoiesis in the normal adult takes place primarily in the bone marrow, under pathologic conditions when the marrow is replaced or overstimulated to respond, the spleen may become a major site of extramedullary hematopoiesis.

The spleen is arranged into units of areas called red and white pulp (Fig. 63-2). Red pulp contains blood-filled sinuses and pulp cords lined by reticuloendothelial cells. White pulp contains centrally located arterioles, surrounded by densely packed small lymphocytes, which are primarily CD4+ helper T lymphocytes. Adjacent to the T-cell periarteriolar lymphocyte sheath is the follicular zone of B lymphocytes which also contains germinal centers made up of B cells and macrophages. The outermost portion of white pulp is another B-cell layer called the marginal zone which blends into red pulp areas.

The blood supply and the route of blood flow are unique in the spleen, and splenic anatomy can best be defined in terms of route of blood flow (Fig. 63-2). Blood enters the spleen by the splenic artery. The splenic artery divides into branches which penetrate into the spleen via connective tissue projections called trabeculae and from the trabeculae branch into smaller arteries called central arteries. From central arteries the bloodstream reaches the arterial capillaries. The periarteriolar lymphoid sheaths of T cells surrounding B-cell follicles persist around the arterial vessels until they become small arterioles. Blood in central arterioles empties partly through arterial capillaries directly into splenic venules and then into splenic veins.

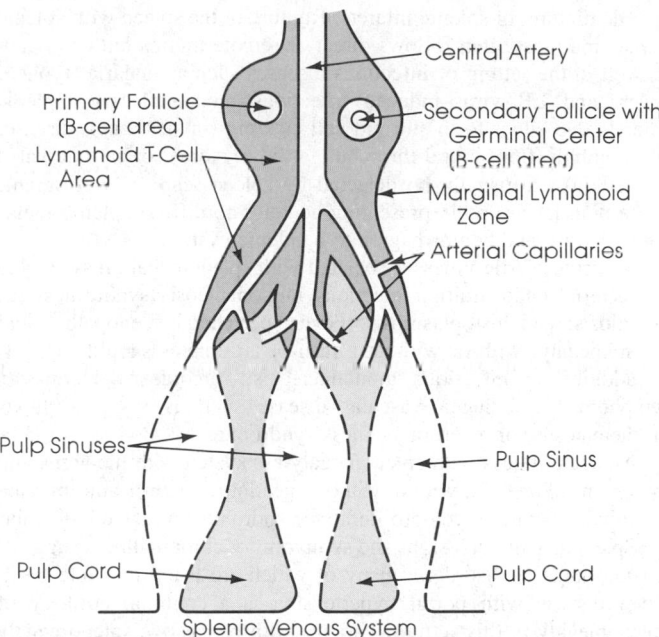

FIGURE 63-2 Schematic spleen structure. The spleen is made up of multiple units of red and white pulp centered around small branches of the splenic artery called central arteries. White pulp areas of spleen are lymphoid areas while red pulp areas include pulp sinuses and pulp cords. In white pulp, B-cell areas are primary and secondary follicles and the marginal lymphoid zone, while T-cell areas are lymphoid cells around follicles and arterial capillaries. (*Redrawn with permission from Videbaek et al.*)

The central arterioles also empty into macrophage-lined sinuses of red pulp and into the fibrous network of reticuloendothelial cells and tissue macrophages called pulp cords. Blood in red pulp sinuses and pulp cords empties directly into the splenic venous system. During red blood cell passage from central arteries to pulp cords, and finally to spleen sinuses, red cells are concentrated in the macrophage-rich pulp cords. Normally circulating red cells accumulate in pulp cords with subsequent passage through critical small openings of sinus endothelium into red pulp sinuses and on to the splenic venous system. Packing of red cells in pulp cords with subsequent passage through small slits into sinuses is termed *erythrocyte conditioning*. Upon senescence, red cells become less deformable and are unable to pass into sinuses; they are retained in pulp cords and phagocytosed by macrophages—a process termed *culling*. Erythrocyte particulate matter such as nuclear material (Howell-Jolly bodies), denatured hemoglobulin (Heinz bodies), or malaria parasites can be pinched off during passage of red cells from pulp cords into sinuses and retained in the spleen while the rest of the red cell passes back into the circulation—a process termed *pitting*.

Many of the mechanisms of spleen enlargement are exaggerated forms of normal spleen function. While there is a wide variety of diseases associated with enlargement of the spleen, there are six basic pathophysiologic mechanisms of splenic enlargement. (1) Splenic enlargement occurs from reticuloendothelial or immune system hyperplasia in infectious diseases such as bacterial endocarditis or in immune diseases such as Felty's syndrome. Reticuloendothelial hyperplasia also occurs in diseases associated with destruction of abnormal red blood cells such as hereditary spherocytosis, thalassemia, or early in the course of sickle cell disease. (2) Splenic enlargement occurs due to altered splenic blood flow in hepatic cirrhosis or splenic, hepatic, or portal vein thrombosis. (3) Malignant neoplasms can involve the spleen either primarily as with lymphomas or angiosarcomas, or secondarily with leukemias or metastatic solid tumors. (4) Splenic enlargement can occur in situations leading to extramedullary hematopoiesis in the spleen such as in myeloid metaplasia or other myelophthisic syndromes. (5) Infiltration of the spleen with abnormal material in amyloidosis and Gaucher's disease can result in splenomegaly. (6) Splenomegaly can also result from space-occupying lesions such as hemangiomas and cysts.

DISEASES ASSOCIATED WITH SPLENIC ENLARGEMENT A wide variety of diseases lead to an increase in cellularity and vascularity of the spleen (Table 63-2). Increase in cellularity in infections is due to lymphocyte and macrophage proliferation in both red and white pulp areas. Splenomegaly is often present in acute systemic bacterial infections. Infectious granulomas due to mycobacterial and fungal infections occur in both red and white pulp. In diseases associated with disordered immunoregulation such as rheumatoid arthritis and systemic lupus erythematosus, splenic enlargement is often due to lymphoid hyperplasia with enlarged lymphoid follicles present in white pulp areas and increased number of plasma cells and macrophages around red pulp arterioles and pulp cords. Splenic enlargement associated with abnormal splenic blood flow is most commonly due to chronic passive congestion from increased portal vein pressure, or from portal vein obstruction. *Banti's syndrome* is *congestive splenomegaly* with hypersplenism associated with cirrhosis and portal hypertension and is manifested histologically by red pulp congestion with accumulation and concentration of erythrocytes in widened pulp cords and sinuses. In congestive splenomegaly, reticuloendothelial hyperplasia occurs with proliferation of cells lining red pulp cords and sinuses. In splenic enlargement in conditions associated with abnormal erythrocytes such as hereditary spherocytosis, there is pooling of abnormal red cells in sinuses and pulp cords because of

TABLE 63-2 Diseases associated with enlargement of the spleen

I Infections
  A Infectious mononucleosis
  B Bacterial septicemias
  C Bacterial endocarditis
  D Tuberculosis
  E Malaria
  F Leishmaniasis
  G Trypanosomiasis
  H Acquired immunodeficiency syndrome
  I Viral hepatitis
  J Congenital syphilis
  K Splenic abscess
  L Disseminated histoplasmosis
II Diseases of disordered immunoregulation
  A Rheumatoid arthritis (Felty's syndrome)
  B Systemic lupus erythematosus
  C Immune hemolytic anemias
  D Angioimmunoblastic lymphadenopathy
  E Drug reactions with serum sickness syndromes
  F Immune thrombocytopenias and neutropenias
III Diseases of disordered splenic blood flow
  A Laennec's and postnecrotic cirrhosis
  B Hepatic vein obstruction
  C Hepatic schistosomiasis
  D Portal vein obstruction or cavernous sinus transformation
  E Splenic vein obstruction
  F Chronic congestive heart failure
  G Splenic artery aneurysm
IV Diseases associated with abnormal erythrocytes
  A Spherocytosis
  B Sickle cell disease
  C Ovalocytosis
  D Thalassemia
V Infiltrative diseases of the spleen
  A *Benign*—amyloidosis, Gaucher's disease, Niemann-Pick disease, Hurler's syndrome, Tangier disease, multifocal Langerhans cell (eosinophilic) granulomatosis, extramedullary hematopoiesis, hamartomas, fibromas, hemangiomas, lymphangiomas, splenic cysts
  B *Malignant*—leukemias, lymphomas, Hodgkin's lymphoma, primary splenic tumors, angiosarcomas, metastatic tumors, myeloproliferative syndromes
VI Miscellaneous diseases or diseases of unknown cause
  A Idiopathic splenomegaly
  B Thyrotoxicosis
  C Iron-deficiency anemia
  D Sarcoidosis
  E Berylliosis

increased red cell rigidity and therefore decreased ability to traverse the red pulp sinusoidal endothelium.

Myelosclerosis with myeloid metaplasia is characterized by splenic intrasinusoidal extramedullary hematopoiesis involving all three myeloid cell lines associated with dilated and distended pulp sinuses. In cases of secondary extramedullary hematopoiesis such as in myelophthisic syndromes, extramedullary hematopoiesis may only involve one or two cell lineages, particularly red cells. Infiltrative malignant disease can cause focal or generalized increases in white pulp lymphoid cells as in the case of Hodgkin's disease and lymphocytic lymphoma, or infiltration of red pulp areas with malignant cells as in chronic granulocytic leukemia, acute leukemia syndromes, systemic mast cell disease, and metastatic carcinoma. Infiltrative diseases of the spleen such as Gaucher's and Niemann-Pick disease produce splenic enlargement by increase in number of splenic red pulp histiocytes. Thyrotoxicosis can be associated with splenomegaly and is due to thyroid hormone–induced lymphoid hyperplasia. Sarcoidosis causes splenic enlargement by the development of areas of granulomatous inflammation in white pulp lymphoid tissue. A splenic artery aneurysm may cause unexplained splenomegaly, cramping, and left upper abdominal pain; a calcified ring in the splenic area may be seen on x-ray.

The degree of splenomegaly varies with the disease entity. Slight or mild enlargement occurs in chronic passive congestion of the liver due to congestive heart failure, acute malaria, typhoid fever, bacterial endocarditis, systemic lupus erythematosus, rheumatoid arthritis, and thalassemia minor. Moderate splenic enlargement occurs in hepatitis, cirrhosis, lymphomas, infectious mononucleosis, hemolytic anemias, splenic abscesses and infarcts, and amyloidosis. Massive enlargement of the spleen occurs in chronic myelocytic leukemia, agnogenic myeloid metaplasia with myelofibrosis, hairy cell leukemia, Gaucher's and Niemann-Pick diseases, sarcoidosis, thalassemia major, chronic malaria, congenital syphilis, leishmaniasis, and in some cases of portal vein obstruction.

DIAGNOSTIC EVALUATION OF THE PATIENT WITH SPLENIC ENLARGEMENT   When normal in size and position, the spleen is generally inaccessible to abdominal palpation. A normal-sized spleen is about 12 cm long and 7 cm wide. Because of the oblique orientation of the spleen to the abdominal cavity, its long axis lies behind and parallel to the tenth rib in the midaxillary line, with splenic width located between the ninth and eleventh ribs. Therefore, to percuss for splenic dullness the patient is placed on the right side and the ninth intercostal space is located by finding the tip of the scapula lying in the seventh intercostal space and counting down to the ninth intercostal space. Dullness outside the ninth and eleventh intercostal spaces suggests splenomegaly, although fluid in the stomach and feces in the colon can cause splenic area dullness as well. Palpation of the left upper quadrant is performed with the patient supine or on the right side by the examiner's right hand; the examiner's left hand is placed under the lower thorax grasping the lower ribs posteriorly. Palpation for spleen enlargement is performed with the patient taking deep breaths to permit the examiner to feel the inferior tip of an enlarged spleen. To avoid missing a massively enlarged spleen, palpation of the left upper quadrant should begin in the lower abdominal cavity with gradual movement up to the left upper quadrant.

Demonstration of mild to moderate splenic enlargement by physical examination may be difficult, particularly in obese patients. Other techniques for assessment of spleen size include ^{99}Tc-colloid liver-spleen scan, computed tomography, and ultrasound scanning of the left upper quadrant. These three techniques can be useful in defining splenic defects such as cysts, infarct, or tumors, or in defining accessory splenic tissue that may be due to congenital accessory spleens or residual foci of splenic tissue following splenic rupture (splenosis).

In the evaluation of the patient with splenomegaly, it is helpful to consider splenomegaly with acute or subacute illnesses separately from splenomegaly with chronic illness. Acute left upper quadrant pain with an enlarged tender spleen suggests subcapsular hematoma,

splenic rupture, or splenic infarcts. Rupture of the spleen with splenic hematoma most often follows direct or remote trauma but can occur as well in the setting of infectious diseases such as malaria, typhoid fever, and EB virus–induced infectious mononucleosis. Splenic infarcts due either to in situ red cell sickling (in sickle cell disease) or to emboli (from mural thrombus, atrial myxoma, or cardiac valve vegetation) can usually be detected by spleen scan or arteriogram. More unusual disorders presenting acutely are diffuse splenic metastatic disease and hemorrhage into a splenic cyst.

An acute febrile illness associated with splenomegaly may be due to bacterial endocarditis, infectious mononucleosis syndromes, tuberculosis, and histoplasmosis. Fever, peripheral adenopathy, and splenomegaly, with or without a rash or arthralgias should suggest, in addition to infectious mononucleosis, sarcoidosis, Hodgkin's lymphoma, a collagen vascular disease such as systemic lupus erythematosus, or a serum sickness syndrome.

An acute illness with splenomegaly associated with the signs and symptoms of anemia, with or without bleeding, suggests autoimmune hemolytic anemia, myeloproliferative syndromes, or acute leukemia.

Splenomegaly with signs and symptoms of chronic illness suggests a wide range of disorders, many of which are listed in Table 63-2. Liver disease with portal hypertension is a common etiology of splenomegaly in this setting. Patients with congestive splenomegaly from liver disease or portal or splenic vein thrombosis are often asymptomatic. With clinical features of rheumatoid arthritis and leukopenia, Felty's syndrome should be considered. The presence of lymphadenopathy should suggest chronic lymphocytic leukemia or lymphoma. Plethora and an elevated hematocrit suggest polycythemia vera or chronic lung disease, with right heart failure and congestive splenomegaly. Weight loss or other signs of chronic illness suggest leukemia or other myeloproliferative syndromes as well as a variety of hemoglobinopathies. Bone marrow aspiration and biopsy can aid in the diagnosis of leukemia and lymphoma, lipid storage diseases, disseminated fungal or mycobacterial diseases, metastatic malignant diseases, and amyloidosis.

Occasionally laparotomy and splenectomy are indicated in the evaluation of splenomegaly. The decision to perform diagnostic laparotomy in a patient with unexplained splenomegaly is difficult and must take into account the patient's age and clinical signs, symptoms, and laboratory abnormalities present. One study has documented palpable spleens in 3 percent of entering college freshmen and no increased risk of any disease during the ensuing 6 years. In another study of older subjects (average age 49) who had undergone splenectomy for undiagnosed splenomegaly and had signs and symptoms of chronic illness, a diagnosis of an underlying disorder was obtained in the majority of patients by splenectomy.

HYPERSPLENISM   The term hypersplenism applies to any clinical situation in which the spleen removes excessive quantities of erythrocytes, granulocytes, or platelets from the circulation. General mechanisms of removal of formed blood elements include increased sequestration of cells due to hemodynamic abnormalities of splenic blood flow, or by production of anti-red cell, granulocyte, or platelet antibodies, making the cells vulnerable to clearance by splenic macrophages. Situations in which passive congestion of the spleen occurs produce abnormal sludging of blood in sinuses and red pulp cords. Under these conditions there is plasma pooling, producing marked intrasplenic hemoconcentration and hypoxia, making blood cells more vulnerable to the phagocytic action of pulp cord macrophages. Criteria for diagnosis of hypersplenism include (1) splenomegaly, (2) splenic destruction of one or more cell lines in the peripheral blood, (3) normal or hyperplastic cellularity of bone marrow with normal representation of the cell line deficient in the circulation, and (4) variably, evidence of increased cell turnover in the cell lines affected, i.e., reticulocytosis, increased band forms of neutrophils, or circulating immature platelet forms.

Therapy for hypersplenism relates in large part to the underlying disease or the underlying pathophysiologic process. If the underlying disorder responsible for hypersplenism cannot be corrected, splenectomy is an option for cases in which a severe deficit is present (see below for indications for splenectomy).

HYPOSPLENISM The terms hyposplenia or asplenia are used to indicate diminished or absent splenic function. The usual causes of hyposplenism are splenectomy, congenital absence of the spleen, sickle cell anemia in patients older than 5 years (with autosplenectomy due to repeated infarcts), and splenic irradiation. In sickle cell anemia, persistence of a palpable spleen after age 5 suggests coexisting α thalassemia. Findings in the peripheral blood that indicate diminished splenic function include the presence of nucleated red cells, erythrocyte Howell-Jolly bodies, erythrocyte Heinz bodies, as well as target and burr forms of red cells.

Splenectomized patients or patients with functional asplenia (such as in sickle cell disease) are prone to bacterial infections, which are frequently overwhelming and life-threatening, particularly with encapsulated organisms such as *Streptococcus pneumoniae*, *Neisseria meningitidis*, *Escherichia coli*, and *Haemophilus influenzae*. This is due to a reduction or absence of the filtration function of the spleen for clearance of antibody-coated bacteria as well as to decreased production of IgG and IgM antibodies (opsonins) needed to bind bacteria. Immunization with pneumococcal vaccine is recommended in patients older than 2 years with hyposplenism and prior to elective splenectomy. The presence of peripheral blood manifestations of hyposplenism (Howell-Jolly bodies) in the presence of a normal-sized or enlarged spleen suggests the presence of splenic infiltrative disease such as a primary splenic angiosarcoma.

INDICATIONS FOR SPLENECTOMY Splenic trauma, whether accidental blunt trauma or intraoperative iatrogenic injury, is the most common indication for splenectomy. En bloc removal of the spleen may be indicated either because of tumor involvement or for a splenorectal shunt. Staging laparotomy with splenectomy remains a major diagnostic procedure for many early stage Hodgkin's disease patients being considered for radiation therapy alone. Splenectomy for selected patients with idiopathic splenomegaly is often necessary when other investigations fail to produce a diagnosis; however, the spleen should not be removed simply because it is palpable. Hypersplenism in lymphomas can cause persistent cytopenias and in select cases responds to splenectomy. B-cell hairy cell leukemia frequently presents with hypersplenism, and splenectomy is often beneficial, producing remission in the majority of cases with a 5-year survival of 50 percent.

Felty's syndrome (rheumatoid arthritis and hypersplenism) and Gaucher's disease both require splenectomy when splenomegaly leads to symptomatic neutropenia or other complications of hypersplenism. Immune thrombocytopenic purpura which persists after trials of medical therapy may benefit from splenectomy (see Chap. 287). Of the hemolytic anemias, hereditary spherocytosis, hereditary elliptocytosis, immune hemolytic anemia with warm-reacting IgG antibody, and pyruvate-kinase deficiency have been improved by splenectomy. Splenectomy is usually necessary late in the course of thalassemia major when neutropenia or thrombocytopenia develops, or when transfusion requirements double. Chronic lymphocytic leukemia (CLL), chronic granulocytic leukemia, and agnogenic myeloid metaplasia may be complicated by symptomatic hypersplenism or, in the case of CLL, immune hemolytic anemia and thrombocytopenia, often necessitating splenectomy. (Chaps. 297 and 296.)

REFERENCES

Lymph node enlargement

BUTCHER E, WEISSMAN I: Lymphoid tissues and organs in *Fundamental Immunology*, WE Paul (ed). New York, Raven, 1984, pp 109–127

GREENFIELD S, JORDAN MC: The clinical investigation of lymphadenopathy, in primary care practice. JAMA 240:1388, 1978

IOACHIM HL: *Lymph Node Biopsy*. Philadelphia, Lippincott, 1982

LENNERT K, STEIN H: The germinal center, in *Morphology, Histochemistry, and Immunohistology in Lymphoproliferative Diseases of Skin*, M Goos, E Christopher (eds). Berlin, Heidelberg, New York, Springer-Verlag, 1982

LIEBERMAN PH et al: A reappraisal of eosinophilic granuloma of bone, Hand-Schüller-Christian syndrome, and Letterer-Siwe syndrome. Medicine 48:375, 1969

NATHWANI BN et al: Malignant lymphoma arising in angioimmunoblastic lymphadenopathy. Cancer 41:578, 1978

POPPEMA S et al: Distribution of T cell subsets in human lymph nodes. J Exp Med 153:30, 1981

SCHROER KR, FRANSSILA KO: Atypical hyperplasia of lymph nodes: A follow-up study. Cancer 44:1155, 1979

SINCLAIR S et al: Biopsy of enlarged, superficial lymph nodes. JAMA 228:602, 1974

THOMAS JA et al: Combined immunological and histochemical analysis of skin and lymph node lesions in histiocytosis X. J Clin Pathol 35:327, 1982

WINTERBAUER RH et al: A clinical interpretation of bilateral hilar adenopathy. Ann Intern Med 78:65, 1973

YEN-TSU N et al: Lymph node biopsy for diagnosis: A statistical study. J Surg Oncol 14:53, 1980

Splenic enlargement

BUTLER JJ: Pathology of the spleen in benign and malignant conditions. Histopathology 7:453, 1983

EICHNER ER, WHITFIELD CL: Splenomegaly: An algorithmic approach to diagnosis. JAMA 246:2858, 1981

ENRIQUEZ E, NEIMAN RS (eds): *The Pathology of the Spleen: A Functional Approach*. Chicago, American Society of Clinical Pathologists, 1976

HERMANN RE et al: Splenectomy for the diagnosis of splenomegaly. Ann Surg 168:896, 1964

LEWIS SM (ed): *Clinics in Haematology*, vol 12: *The Spleen*. London, Saunders, 1983, pp 361–608

McINTYRE OR, EBAUGH FG: Palpable spleens in college freshmen. Ann Intern Med 66:301, 1967

STEINBERG MH et al: Evidence of hyposplenism in the presence of splenomegaly. Scand J Haematol 31:437, 1983

VIDEBAEK A et al: *The Spleen in Health and Disease*. Chicago, Yearbook, 1982

64 LEUKOCYTOSIS, LEUKOPENIA, AND EOSINOPHILIA

DAVID C. DALE

Alterations of leukocytes occur in many hematologic, infectious, inflammatory, and neoplastic diseases. For this reason, the laboratory evaluation of many patients begins with measurement of leukocyte count and examination of a stained blood smear. Five types of leukocytes usually are seen: neutrophils, lymphocytes, monocytes, eosinophils, and basophils. It is generally accepted that they all derive from a common hematopoietic stem cell. Beyond this common origin, different mechanisms govern their production, distribution, and function. For simplicity, clinical inferences often are made from the total leukocyte count and the differential count expressed as a percentage. It is more precise to express the counts for each type of leukocyte in terms of the concentration or absolute count per microliter. This is determined by multiplying the total count by the percent value or by direct counting on automated systems (Table 64-1).

Several terms are used to describe alteration of leukocyte counts. *Leukocytosis* and *leukopenia* indicate increases or decreases in the total number of leukocytes. *Granulocytosis* and *granulocytopenia* describe increases or decreases of granulocytes, i.e., neutrophils,

TABLE 64-1 Normal values for concentration of blood leukocytes*

Cell type	Mean, cells per microliter	95% Confidence limits, cells per microliter
Neutrophil	3650	1830–7250
Lymphocyte	2500	1500–4000
Monocyte	430	200–950
Eosinophil	150	0–700
Basophil	30	0–150

* Total leukocyte counts from venous blood samples were done in a Coulter counter, and 200 leukocytes were differentiated on Wright-stained blood smears made on coverglass.

eosinophils, and basophils. *Neutrophilia* and *neutropenia, lymphocytosis* and *lymphopenia, monocytosis* and *monocytopenia, eosinophilia* and *eosinopenia* are used for increases or decreases in the absolute counts of neutrophils, lymphocytes, monocytes, and eosinophils, respectively. It is best to use these terms to describe changes to levels above or below the 95 percent confidence limits of normal values (Table 64-1).

LEUKOCYTOSIS

Leukocytosis occurs by several mechanisms. Normally about half of the blood leukocytes are in a *marginal pool,* i.e., loosely adherent to the vascular endothelium or trapped in the microcirculation. With exercise or epinephrine administration, these cells are released into the *circulating pool* and the leukocyte count rises, a process called *demargination.* For neutrophils, but not for other leukocytes, there is a storage pool of mature cells in the marrow, the *marrow neutrophil reserves.* Normally neutrophils are released from the storage pool into the blood in response to stress, with infections, and after corticosteroid administration. With a strong stimulus, e.g., a severe bacterial infection, immature neutrophils, i.e., bands and metamyelocytes, are released, a response sometimes called a *left shift.* Leukocytosis also occurs due to increased cell production. If production is stimulated intensely, the leukocyte counts can rise to 25,000 to 50,000 per microliter, a response called a *leukemoid reaction.* The rates for these processes differ substantially. A shift of cells from the marginal to the circulatory pool can occur within a few minutes, whereas the release of neutrophils from the marrow usually occurs over several hours. Increases in production take several days.

The mechanisms maintaining normal leukocyte production and blood counts are not well understood. It is presumed that under basal conditions, factors made in the marrow, thymus, lymph nodes, and spleen provide local control (see Chaps. 81 and 297). Two groups of factors, the interleukins and colony stimulating factors, may be involved in normal regulation and play important roles in causing leukocytosis. Interleukin 2 (IL-2) and IL-4 are known to expand T- and B-lymphocyte populations, respectively (see Chap. 13). Granulocyte colony stimulating factor (G-CSF), granulocyte-macrophage colony stimulating factor (GM-CSF), macrophage colony stimulating

factor (M-CSF), and four interleukins, IL-1, IL-3, IL-5, and IL-6, are involved in neutrophil, monocyte, and eosinophil production (Fig. 64-1).

Leukocytosis usually is due to neutrophilia (Table 64-2). Leukocytosis due to lymphocytosis occurs in acute and chronic lymphatic leukemia and some infectious diseases, e.g., infectious mononucleosis, infectious hepatitis, infectious lymphocytosis, pertussis, tuberculosis, brucellosis, and syphilis. A moderate increase in the absolute lymphocyte count is seen with thyrotoxicosis and Addison's disease.

Increases in blood monocytes are observed with chronic inflammation, e.g., tuberculosis, bacterial endocarditis, brucellosis, Rocky Mountain spotted fever, malaria and kala azar, sarcoidosis, Crohn's disease, and some collagen vascular diseases. Monocytosis occurs in pre-leukemia. It may be a prominent feature of histiocytic leukemia and the myeloproliferative syndromes.

LEUKOPENIA

NEUTROPENIA   Neutropenia is the most frequent cause of leukopenia. It is usually defined as "severe" if the neutrophil count is less than 500 cells per microliter, "moderate" with 500 to 1000 cells per microliter, and "mild" with 1000 to 2000 cells per microliter. Neutropenia is an important risk factor for infections; as the counts decline below about 1000 cells per microliter, the risk of infection increases (see Chap. 82). This risk also relates to the duration of

TABLE 64-2   Causes of neutrophilia

Physiologic: Exercise, excitement, stress, epinephrine

Infections: Chiefly bacterial, also fungal, parasitic, and some viral

Inflammation: Burns, tissue necrosis, as in myocardial and pulmonary infarction, collagen vascular diseases, hypersensitivity states, other inflammatory diseases

Metabolic disorders: Ketoacidosis, acute renal failure, eclampsia, acute poisoning

Myeloproliferative diseases: Myelocytic leukemia, myeloid metaplasia, polycythemia vera

Other: Metastatic carcinoma, acute hemorrhage or hemolysis, glucocorticoids, lithium therapy, idiopathic

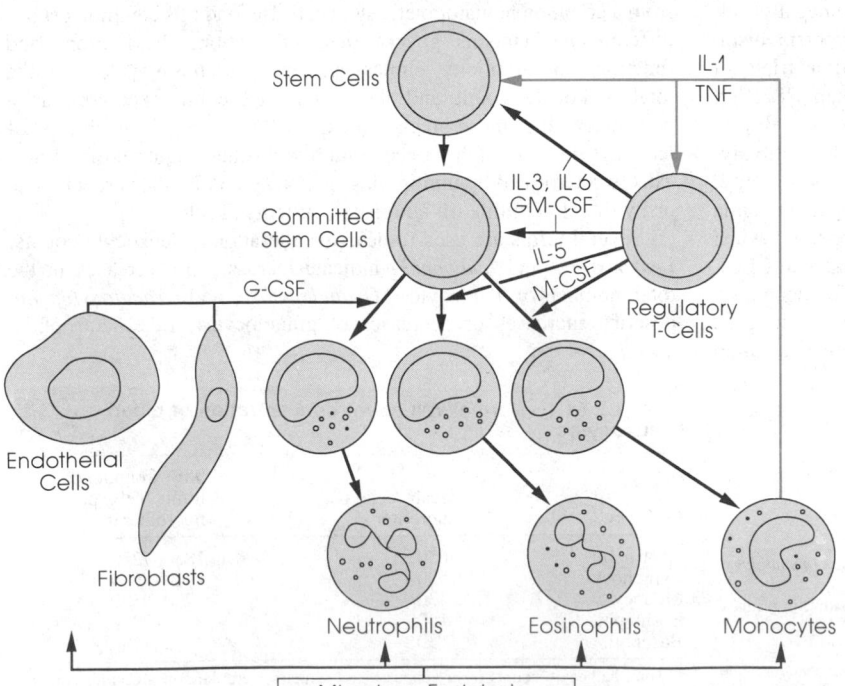

FIGURE 64-1 A simplified schema for the stimulation of neutrophil, eosinophil, and monocyte production by microbial infection or endotoxin. At tissue sites of inflammation, monocytes produce interleukin 1 (IL-1) and tumor necrosis factor (TNF). The IL-1 and TNF directly activate stem cells and stimulate regulatory T lymphocytes to produce additional factors: IL-3, IL-6, and granulocyte-macrophage colony stimulating factor (GM-CSF) from endothelial cells and fibroblasts, and IL-5 and macrophage colony stimulating factor (M-CSF). These factors stimulate production of neutrophils, eosinophils, and monocytes, respectively. All of the colony stimulating factors and interleukins can be produced by other types of cells.

TABLE 64-3 Causes of neutropenia

DECREASED PRODUCTION

Hematologic diseases: Aplastic anemia, leukemia, myelodysplastic syndromes, infantile genetic disorders, cyclic neutropenia, chronic idiopathic neutropenia, neutropenia with clonal expression of T8 cells, Chédiak-Higashi syndrome

Drug-induced: Alkylating agents (nitrogen mustard, busulfan, chlorambucil, cyclophosphamide); antimetabolites (methotrexate, 5-fluorocytosine); non-cytotoxic agents [antibiotics (chloramphenicol, penicillins, sulfonamides), phenothiazines, tranquilizers (meprobamate), certain diuretics, anti-inflammatory agents, antithyroid drugs, many others]

Tumor invasion: Myelofibrosis

Nutritional deficiency: Vitamin B_{12}, folate (especially in alcoholics)

Infection: Tuberculosis, typhoid fever, brucellosis, tularemia, measles, infectious mononucleosis, viral hepatitis, malaria, histoplasmosis, leishmaniasis

PERIPHERAL DESTRUCTION

Antineutrophil antibodies and/or splenic trapping

Autoimmune disorders: Felty's syndrome, systemic lupus erythematosus

Drugs: Aminopyrine α-methyldopa, phenylbutazone, mercurial diuretics, some phenothiazines

PERIPHERAL MARGINATION

Overwhelming bacterial infection

Hemodialysis

Cardiopulmonary bypass

---

neutropenia, the intactness of other host defense mechanisms, and the nature of the primary disease process.

Neutropenia occurs by several mechanisms: reduced or ineffective production, increased margination, accelerated utilization, or a combination of these mechanisms (Table 64-3). Most patients fit into one of the following general categories:

Disorders of production Probably the most frequent cause of severe neutropenia in the United States is marrow suppression from cytotoxic drugs given for cancer or immunosuppressive therapy. Neutropenia is a prominent effect of these drugs because of the high proliferative rate of the neutrophil precursors and the rapid turnover of neutrophils in the blood and tissues. Suppression of neutrophil formation can occur as an idiosyncratic reaction to many other drugs (see below). Neutropenia due to impaired production is a feature of several diseases affecting hematopoietic stem cells, e.g., leukemia and the myelodysplastic syndromes (see Chap. 296) or aplastic anemia (see Chap. 61). With vitamin B_{12} and folic acid deficiency (see Chap. 76), neutropenia is attributed to ineffective production, i.e., defective neutrophils being destroyed in the marrow before they can enter the blood. Most other disorders of production are rare.

GENETIC NEUTROPENIAS *Congenital hypoplastic neutropenia,* Kostmann's syndrome, is a autosomal recessive disease causing severe neutropenia and infections from birth. Some early neutrophil precursors may be present in the marrow, but numbers of more mature cells are severely reduced. With antibiotic therapy and good supportive care, survival to adulthood is not uncommon. Neutropenia with immunodeficiency is a stem cell disorder involving both neutrophils and lymphocytes. It is associated with markedly enhanced susceptibility to infection. Both congenital neutropenia and the immunodeficiency syndromes have been treated successfully with bone marrow transplantation; colony stimulating factors are a promising experimental therapy.

Cyclic neutropenia is an unusual disorder, characterized by fever, malaise, mouth ulcers, cervical adenopathy, and the absence of blood neutrophils, usually at 21-day intervals. Between episodes, the patients are generally well. Cyclic fluctuations of other blood leukocytes, platelets, and reticulocytes also occur. Usually this disease is detected in early childhood, but cases with adult onset are occasionally seen.

This disorder is attributed to a regulatory defect of stem cells. It has been shown that G-CSF will stimulate neutrophil production, shorten the duration of neutropenia, and reduce symptoms and infections in these patients.

The Chédiak-Higashi syndrome is discussed in Chap. 81.

NEUTROPENIAS OF UNKNOWN CAUSE In *chronic idiopathic neutropenia,* neutrophils are selectively decreased, and monocytes often are increased. The marrow is normocellular and shows decreased mature neutrophils. In some, but not all cases, antineutrophil antibodies can be detected; but their significance is often unclear. Only individuals with severe neutropenia tend to have recurrent fever and frequent infections.

Spontaneous remissions have occurred, and evolution of idiopathic neutropenia to leukemia has been reported very rarely. Alternate-day glucocorticoids may be helpful. G-CSF recently has been found to elevate the neutrophil counts and reduce infections in severely affected patients.

Syndromes have been described where clonal expansion of T8 cells is associated with neutropenia. T8 cells are granulated T lymphocytes, and patients with T8 cell lymphocytosis have moderate blood and bone marrow lymphocytosis, neutropenia, polyclonal hypergammaglobulinemia, splenomegaly, and absence of lymphadenopathy. They have a chronic and relatively stable course. Recurrent bacterial infections are frequent. It is not clear whether this is a benign or malignant disease. In some patients a spontaneous regression has occurred even after 11 years, suggesting an immunoregulatory defect as the basis for the disorder. It is likely patients with T8 cell lymphocytosis and neutropenia will ultimately be shown to represent a biologically heterogeneous group of patients.

DRUG-INDUCED NEUTROPENIA Idiosyncratic drug reactions are an important cause of neutropenia (see Chap. 66). In most instances, the patient presents acutely ill with fever and a sore throat or perianal ulcerations several weeks or months after beginning a new drug. The total leukocyte count is often 1000 to 2000 per microliter. Mature neutrophils are absent from the blood, and marrow aplasia is rare. If administration of the offending drug is discontinued, recovery is the rule, provided good supportive care is available. The mechanisms responsible for these reactions are poorly understood but probably involve both immunologic and toxic injury to the neutrophils and their precursors. With some drugs, e.g., chloramphenicol, phenothiazines, and propylthiouracil, neutropenia may occur gradually. As a rule, a presumed offending drug should always be discontinued whenever the neutrophil count falls to less than 2000 per microliter.

Neutropenia affecting margination and utilization IMMUNE-MEDIATED NEUTROPENIA Isoimmune neonatal neutropenia is a transient disorder due to the transplacental passage of maternal antibodies directed toward neutrophil specific antigens which were inherited from the patient's father. Ordinarily it resolves spontaneously in the first few months of life and does not recur. Autoimmune neutropenia must be diagnosed by the finding of antineutrophil antibodies in the plasma and on the cells of affected individuals. It is usually a benign condition causing a selective reduction in blood neutrophils. Careful observation and prompt antibiotic therapy for suspected episodes of infection are cornerstones for care of these individuals.

In systemic lupus erythematosus, mild neutropenia is common. Some patients with rheumatoid arthritis have severe neutropenia associated with splenomegaly and very high rheumatoid factor titers, i.e., Felty's syndrome. Usually the marrow is hypercellular. In many patients infections are surprisingly infrequent given the level of the neutrophil counts. Splenectomy usually increases blood neutrophils but should be reserved for patients with well-documented problems with infections. In other autoimmune syndromes, e.g., Sjögren's syndrome and autoimmune hepatitis, autoantibodies and enlargement of the spleen may play a role in the development of neutropenia: splenic trapping of neutrophils may occur.

NEUTROPENIA WITH INFECTIONS Neutropenia can result from bacterial, viral, parasitic, or rickettsial diseases. Depending upon the infection the mechanisms can involve abnormal production, increased margination or utilization, or varying combinations of all. In certain viral infections, e.g., infectious mononucleosis, infectious hepatitis, and human immunodeficiency virus (HIV) infections, severe and protracted neutropenia may be due to infection of the hematopoietic stem cells; neutrophil production is impaired. In addition, antineutrophil antibodies have been described in some HIV-infected patients, and therapy with cytotoxic agents such as azidothymidine may complicate the picture (see Chap. 264). In other infections, neutropenia may be attributed to increased neutrophil adherence to endothelial cells, e.g., measles, influenza, malaria, rickettsial, and *Babesia* infections. With severe bacteremic gram-negative or rarely grampositive infections, neutropenia is probably due to increased margination and increased utilization at sites of infection. Other bacteremic infections such as typhoid and brucellosis are often associated with a relative but not an absolute neutropenia (< 1500 per microliter) and a left shift with bands seen in the peripheral blood. In tuberculosis, histoplasmosis, and leishmaniasis neutropenia can be associated with marrow invasion by these organisms and decreased myeloid precursors; the mechanism of suppression of myelopoiesis is unknown. With splenomegaly increased trapping of neutrophils may be an additional mechanism for neutropenia.

Miscellaneous causes of neutropenia   Conditions which cause splenomegaly (e.g., cirrhosis, sarcoidosis) may have associated neutropenia due to splenic trapping of neutrophils. Neutropenia followed by a neutrophilic leukocytosis is commonly seen in patients undergoing hemodialysis. Increased adhesion of neutrophils to vascular endothelium appears to be responsible for the neutropenia with C5a-mediated increased expression of neutrophil adhesion proteins (see Chap. 87).

LYMPHOCYTOPENIA,   MONOCYTOPENIA,   EOSINOPENIA
Lymphocytopenia, i.e., less than 1500 cells per microliter in adults or less than 3000 cells per microliter in young children, is a feature of the congenital immunodeficiency syndromes; it also occurs acutely following stress, radiation injury, or cytotoxic drug and corticosteroid therapy. Other etiologies include lymphoma, aplastic anemia, renal failure, impaired intestinal lymph drainage, severe right-sided heart failure, and cachexia of any cause. Monocytopenia occurs with acute infections, stress, and following administration of glucocorticoids. Monocytopenia also occurs in aplastic anemia, acute myelogenous leukemia, and as a direct result of myelotoxic and immunosuppressive drugs. Eosinopenia occurs with stress, infections, and after steroid administration.

EOSINOPHILIA

Eosinophilia can be defined as a blood eosinophil count of more than 500 per microliter. The blood eosinophil pool is relatively small compared to the tissue pool; however, significant tissue eosinophilia can occur without an elevated blood count.

TABLE 64-4   Causes of blood eosinophilia

Drug reactions: Iodides, aspirin, sulfonamides, nitrofurantoin, penicillins, cephalosporins

Parasitic infections: Hookworm disease, strongyloidiasis, toxocariasis, trichuriasis, trichinosis, filariasis, schistosomiasis, echinococcosis, cysticercosis

Allergic diseases: Hay fever, asthma, angioedema, serum sickness, allergic vasculitis, eczema, pemphigus

Collagen vascular diseases: Rheumatoid arthritis, dermatomyositis, periarteritis nodosa

Malignancy: Hodgkin's disease, mycosis fungoides, chronic myelogenous leukemia, cancer of lung, stomach, pancreas, ovary, or uterus

Hypereosinophilic syndromes: Loeffler's syndrome, Loeffler's endocarditis, eosinophilic leukemia

---

There are many causes for eosinophilia (Table 64-4). A useful diagnostic approach is to begin by reexamining the blood smear to be sure the cells are not peculiarly stained neutrophils, i.e., pseudoeosinophilia, and to consider the possibility of chronic myelogenous leukemia, which may present with eosinophilia. Rarely, filarial parasites will be seen on the blood smear. The next step is to review carefully the patient's history with close attention to drugs, diet, and travel. Many drugs can cause eosinophilia (see Chap. 66). The travel and diet history may suggest a specific parasitic infection. The physical examination initially may reveal evidence for a chronic inflammatory disease or a malignancy as the cause of eosinophilia (Table 64-4). Stools should be collected and examined for ova and parasites, in particular looking for evidence of worms (see Chap. 157). If the diagnosis is not obvious, examination of serum for antibodies may reveal infestation with *Dirofilaria immitis* (see Chap. 169) or cysticercosis (see Chap. 171). In most patients, eosinophilia will remit when the primary disease is treated effectively. When other diagnoses are excluded, the *idiopathic hypereosinophilic syndrome* should be considered. This syndrome is characterized by a wasting illness with hepatosplenomegaly, peripheral neuropathy, cardiac murmurs, and congestive heart failure (see Chap. 81).

REFERENCES

CANNISTRA SA, GRIFFIN JD: Regulation of the production and function of granulocyte and monocytes. Semin Hematol 25:173, 1988

DALE DC: "Neutropenia" and "Neutrophilia," in *Hematology*, 4th ed, WJ Williams et al (eds). New York, McGraw-Hill, 1990, pp 807–820

GALLIN JI et al: *Inflammation: Basic Principles and Clinical Correlates.* New York, Raven Press, 1988

GLEICH GJ, LOEGERING DA: Immunobiology of eosinophils. Ann Rev Immunol 2:429, 1984

JOHNSTON RB JR: Monocytes and macrophages. N Engl J Med 318:747, 1988

SHURIN SB: Pathologic states associated with activation of eosinophils and with eosinophilia. Hematol Oncol Clin North Am 2:171, 1988

65 PRINCIPLES OF DRUG THERAPY

JOHN A. OATES / GRANT R. WILKINSON

QUANTITATIVE DETERMINANTS OF DRUG ACTION

Safe and effective therapy with drugs requires their delivery to target tissues in concentrations within the narrow range that yields efficacy without toxicity. Optimal precision in achieving concentrations of drug within this therapeutic "window" can be achieved with regimens that are based on the kinetics of the drug's availability to target sites. This chapter deals with the principles of drug elimination and distribution that form the basis for loading and maintenance regimens for the average patient and considers instances in which elimination of the drug is impaired (e.g., renal failure). The basis for optimal utilization of plasma level data is also discussed.

PLASMA LEVELS AFTER A SINGLE DOSE The levels of lidocaine in plasma following intravenous administration decline in two phases as illustrated in Fig. 65-1; such a biphasic decline is typical for many drugs. Immediately following rapid injection, essentially all of the drug is in the plasma compartment, and the high initial plasma level reflects its confinement to this small volume. Subsequently, the drug is transferred into the extravascular compartment, and the period of time during which this occurs is referred to as the *distribution phase*. For lidocaine the distribution phase is virtually complete within 30 min; then a slower rate of fall ensues, referred to as the *equilibrium phase* or *elimination phase*. During this latter phase, the drug levels in plasma and those in the tissues change in parallel.

Distribution phase Pharmacologic events during the distribution phase depend on whether the level of drug at the receptor site is similar to that in the plasma. If this is the case, the pharmacologic effects, whether favorable or adverse, may be inordinately great during this period because of the high initial levels in plasma. For example, following a small bolus dose (50 mg) of lidocaine, antiarrhythmic effects may be evident during the early distribution phase but disappear as levels fall below those that are minimally effective and even before equilibrium between plasma and tissue is reached. Thus, larger single doses or multiple small doses must be administered to achieve an effect that is sustained into the equilibrium phase. Toxicity resulting from high levels of some drugs during the distribution phase precludes administration of a single intravenous loading dose that will achieve therapeutic levels during the equilibrium phase. For example, the administration of a loading dose of phenytoin as a single intravenous bolus can cause cardiovascular collapse due to the high levels during the distribution phase. If a loading dose of phenytoin is administered intravenously, it must be given in fractions at intervals sufficient to permit substantial distribution of the prior dose before the next is given (for example, 100 mg every 3 to 5 min). For similar reasons, the loading dose of many potent drugs that rapidly equilibrate with their receptors is divided into fractional doses for intravenous administration.

After an oral dose that delivers an equivalent amount of drug into the systemic circulation, plasma levels during the initial period after administration are not as high as after an intravenous bolus dose.

Because the drug is not absorbed instantly after oral administration and is delivered into the systemic circulation more slowly, much of the drug is distributed by the time absorption is complete. Thus, procainamide, which is almost totally absorbed after oral administration, can be given as a single 750-mg loading dose with little risk of hypotension; in contrast, loading of the drug by the intravenous route is more safely accomplished by giving the dose in fractions of about 100 mg at 5-min intervals to avoid the hypotension that might ensue during the distribution phase if the entire loading dose were given as a single bolus.

In contrast, other drugs are distributed slowly to their sites of action during the distribution phase. For example, levels of digoxin at the receptor site (and its pharmacologic effect) do not reflect plasma levels during the distribution phase. Digoxin is transported (or bound) to its cardiac receptors more slowly by a process that proceeds throughout distribution. Thus, plasma levels fall during a distribution phase of several hours, while levels at the site of action and pharmacologic effect increase. Only at the end of the distribution phase, when the drug has reached equilibrium with the receptor, does the concentration of digoxin in plasma reflect pharmacologic effect. For this reason, there should be a 6- to 8-h wait after administration before plasma levels of digoxin are obtained for a guide to therapy.

Equilibrium phase After distribution has proceeded to the point where the concentration of drug in plasma is in dynamic equilibrium with that in the tissues outside the vascular compartment, the levels in plasma and tissues fall in parallel as the drug is eliminated from the body. Thus, the *equilibrium phase* is sometimes also referred to as the *elimination phase*. Measurement of drug concentration in plasma provides the best reflection of drug level in tissues during this phase.

Most drugs are eliminated as a first-order process. During the equilibrium phase, a characteristic of the first-order process is that the time required for the level of drug in plasma to fall to one-half the original value (the half-life, $t_{1/2}$) is the same regardless of which point on the plasma level curve is chosen as a starting point for the measurement. Another characteristic of the first-order process is that

FIGURE 65-1 Concentrations of lidocaine in plasma following the administration of 50 mg intravenously. The half-life of 108 min is computed as the time required for levels to fall from any given value during the equilibrium phase ($Cp_{initial}$) to one-half that level. Cp_0 is the hypothetical concentration of lidocaine in plasma at time zero if equilibrium had been achieved instantly.

a semilogarithmic plot of the concentrations in plasma versus time during the equilibrium phase is linear. From such a plot (Fig. 65-1) it can be seen that the half-life of lidocaine is 108 min.

One can calculate what amount of the administered dose remains in the body at any multiple of the half-life interval following administration:

Number of half-lives	Amount of dose remaining in the body, %	Amount of dose eliminated, %
1	50	50
2	25	75
3	12.5	87.5
4	6.25	93.75
5	3.125	96.875

In theory, the elimination process never reaches completion. From a clinical standpoint, however, elimination is essentially complete when it has reached 90 percent. Therefore, for practical purposes, *a first-order elimination process reaches completion after 3 to 4 half-lives.*

DRUG ACCUMULATION—LOADING AND MAINTENANCE DOSES

With repeated administration of a drug, the amount in the body accumulates if the elimination of the first dose is incomplete when the second dose is given, and both the amount of drug in the body and its pharmacologic effect increase with continuing administration until they reach a plateau. The accumulation of digoxin administered in repeated maintenance doses (without a loading dose) is illustrated in Fig. 65-2. As digoxin's half-life is about 1.6 days in a patient with normal renal function, 65 percent of digoxin remains in the body at the end of 1 day. Thus, the second dose will raise the amount of digoxin in the body (and average plasma level) to 165 percent of that following the first dose. Each subsequent dose will result in greater amounts in the body until a *steady state* is achieved. At this point drug intake per unit of time is the same as the rate of elimination, with the fluctuation between peak and trough plasma levels remaining constant. If the rate of drug delivery is subsequently altered, a different and new steady state will be attained. Continuing infusion of a drug at constant rate will also result in progressive accumulation to a predictable steady state (Fig. 65-3). In this case a constant plasma level (Cp_{ss}) is achieved which is between the peak and trough values attained when the same rate of drug delivery is administered in an intermittent fashion. For *all* drugs with first-order kinetics, the time required to achieve steady state levels can be predicted from the half-life because accumulation also is a first-order process with a half-life identical to that for elimination. Hence, accumulation reaches 90 percent of steady state levels at the end of 3 to 4 half-lives. For digoxin, with a half-life of 1.6 days (with normal renal function), accumulation will be practically complete in 5 days. Continuing

FIGURE 65-2 The time course of digoxin accumulation when a single daily maintenance dose is given without a loading dose. Note that accumulation is more than 90 percent complete by the end of 4 half-lives.

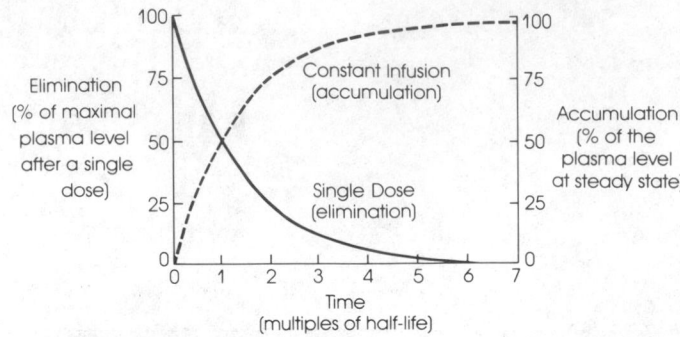

FIGURE 65-3 The time course of plasma levels of a drug following a single intravenous dose (——) compared with those during a constant intravenous infusion (----). This relationship applies to all drugs that rapidly achieve equilibrium between plasma and tissues.

infusion of a drug at a constant rate also will result in progressive accumulation to a steady state with a time course predictable from the elimination curve for that drug (Fig. 65-3).

When the time required to reach steady state levels is longer than one wishes to wait, plasma levels may be achieved more rapidly by the administration of a *loading dose.* Loading entails the administration of an amount that will bring the concentration in plasma (at equilibrium) to the level present during steady state. If the desired plasma level (Cp_{ss}) is known, the loading dose can be estimated with knowledge of the extent of the drug's extravascular distribution at equilibrium; the apparent volume of distribution, or V_d:

$$\text{Loading dose} = \frac{\text{desired plasma level}}{\text{at steady state}} \times \frac{\text{volume of}}{\text{distribution}}$$

$$= Cp_{ss} \times V_d$$

Loading may be accomplished by the administration of the loading amount as a single dose, or in the case of drugs for which there is risk of toxicity if all of the drug is introduced into the plasma compartment rapidly, the loading amount is administered in a series of fractions of the total loading amount. As the accumulation of procainamide to 90 percent of steady state by infusion would require approximately 10 h (the $t_{1/2}$ is 3 h), a loading regimen is almost always desirable. The load required to suppress an arrhythmia, however, varies among individuals from 300 to 1000 mg, and rapid intravenous administration of the *average loading dose* causes hypotension during the distribution phase in some patients. Therefore, the intravenous loading dose of procainamide is given in fractions (e.g., 100 mg every 5 min) until the arrhythmia is controlled or adverse effects such as hypotension indicate that no further drug should be given. Dividing the loading dose into fractions is appropriate for most drugs that have a low therapeutic index. (the therapeutic index is the ratio of toxic dose to the therapeutic dose). This permits better individualization of the loading amount and minimizes adverse effects.

The size of the loading dose required to achieve the plasma levels at steady state also can be determined from the fraction of drug eliminated during the dosage interval and the maintenance dose (in the case of intermittent drug administration). For example, if the fraction of digoxin eliminated daily is 35 percent and the planned maintenance dose is to be 0.25 mg daily, then the loading dose to achieve steady state levels should be 100/35 times the maintenance dose, or approximately 0.75 mg. Thus,

$$\frac{\text{Loading}}{\text{dose}} = \frac{100}{\substack{\text{\% of drug eliminated} \\ \text{per dosage interval}}} \times \text{maintenance dose}$$

The fraction of drug eliminated during any dosage interval can be determined from a semilogarithmic graph, in which the total amount in the body at time zero is set at 100 percent and the fraction remaining at the end of 1 half-life is 50 percent.[1] Conversely, if the loading dose is known, the maintenance dose can be similarly calculated.

To calculate a loading dose designed to achieve the plasma concentration of a known infusion rate at steady state

$$\text{Loading dose} = \frac{\text{infusion rate}}{k}$$

where k is the fractional elimination constant that describes the rate of drug elimination.[1]

Regardless of the size of the loading dose, *after maintenance therapy has been given for 3 to 4 half-lives, the amount of drug in the body is determined by the maintenance dose.* The independence of the plasma levels at steady state from the load is illustrated in Fig. 65-3, which indicates that the elimination of any drug would be practically complete after 3 to 4 half-lives.

DETERMINANTS OF PLASMA LEVELS DURING THE EQUILIBRIUM PHASE An important determinant of the level of drug in plasma during the equilibrium phase after a single dose is the extent to which the drug is distributed outside the plasma compartment. For example, if the distribution of a 3-mg dose of a large macromolecule is confined to a plasma volume of 3 L, then the concentration in plasma will be 1 mg/L. However, if a different drug is distributed so that 90 percent of it leaves the plasma compartment, then only 0.3 mg will remain in the 3-L plasma volume and the concentration in plasma will be only 0.1 mg/L. The *apparent volume of distribution,* or V_d, expresses the relationship between the amount of drug in the body and the plasma concentration at equilibrium:

$$V_d = \frac{\text{amount of drug in body}}{\text{plasma concentration}}$$

The amount of drug in the body is expressed as mass (e.g., milligrams), and the plasma concentration is expressed as mass per volume (e.g., milligrams per liter). Thus V_d is a hypothetical volume into which a quantity of drug would distribute if its concentration in the entire volume were the same as that in plasma. Although it is not a real volume, it is an important concept because it determines the fraction of total drug in the plasma and therefore the fraction available to the organs of elimination. An approximation of V_d in the equilibrium phase can be obtained by estimating the concentration of drug in plasma at time zero (Cp_0) by back-extrapolation of the equilibrium phase plot to zero time as illustrated in Fig. 65-1. Then, after intravenous administration when the amount in the body at time zero is the dose, we have

$$V_d = \frac{\text{dose}}{Cp_0}$$

For the administration of the large macromolecule mentioned above, the measured Cp_0 of 1 mg/L after a 3-mg dose indicates a V_d that is a real volume, the plasma volume. This is the exception, however, for the V_d of most drugs is larger than plasma volume; many drugs are so extensively taken up by cells that cellular levels exceed those in plasma. For such drugs, the hypothetical V_d is large, even greater than the volume of body water. For example, Fig. 65-1 indicates that the Cp_0 obtained by extrapolation after administration of 50 mg lidocaine is 0.42 mg/L, yielding a V_d of 119 L.

As elimination is performed largely by the kidney and liver, it is useful to consider the elimination of drugs according to the *clearance* concept. For example, in the kidney, regardless of the extent to which removal of drug is determined by filtration, secretion, or reabsorption, the net result is a reduction of the concentration of drug in plasma as it passes through the organ. The extent to which the

concentration is reduced is expressed as the *extraction ratio,* or E, which is constant as long as first-order elimination occurs.

$$E = \frac{C_a - C_v}{C_a}$$

where C_a = arterial plasma concentration
  C_v = venous plasma concentration

If the extraction is complete, $E = 1$. If the total plasma flow to the kidneys is Q (mL/min), the total volume of plasma from which drug is completely removed in a unit time (clearance from the body, Cl) is determined as

$$Cl_{renal} = QE$$

If the renal extraction ratio of penicillin is 0.5 and renal plasma flow is 680 mL/min, then penicillin's renal clearance is 340 mL/min. If the extraction ratio is high, as is the case for renal extraction of aminohippurate or hepatic extraction of propranolol, then clearance is a function of organ blood flow.[2]

Clearance from the body is the sum of clearance from all organs of elimination and is the best measure of the efficiency of the elimination processes. If a drug is removed by both the kidney and liver, then

$$Cl = Cl_{renal} + Cl_{hepatic}$$

Thus, if penicillin is eliminated by both renal clearance (340 mL/min) and hepatic clearance (36 mL/min) in a normal individual, total clearance is 376 mL/min. If renal clearance is reduced to half, total clearance is 170 + 36 or 206 mL/min. In anuria, total clearance equals hepatic clearance.

Only the drug in the vascular compartment can be cleared during each passage through an organ. To ascertain the effect of a given plasma clearance by one or more organs on the rate of removal of drug from the body, the clearance must be related to the volume of "plasma equivalents" to be cleared, that is, the volume of distribution. If the volume of distribution is 10 L and clearance is 1 L/min, then one-tenth of the drug in the body is eliminated per minute. This fraction, Cl/V_d, is known as a *fractional elimination constant* and is designated as k:

$$k = \frac{Cl}{V_d}$$

If the fraction k is multiplied by the total amount of drug in the body, the actual rate of elimination at any given time can be determined:

$$\text{Rate of elimination} = k \times \text{amount in body} = ClCp$$

This is the general equation for all first-order processes and expresses the fact that rate is proportional to the declining quantity in a first-order process.

As half-life is a temporal expression of the exponential first-order process, half-life ($t_{1/2}$) can be related to k as follows:

$$t_{1/2} = \frac{0.693}{k}$$

Because $$k = \frac{Cl}{V_d}$$

then $$t_{1/2} = \frac{0.693 V_d}{Cl}$$

As shown in the section on drug dosage in renal failure, the linear relationship of k to creatinine clearance makes k a useful parameter upon which to estimate changes in drug elimination with reduction in creatinine clearance in renal insufficiency. Half-life is not linearly related to clearance.

---

[1] Alternatively, the fraction of drug lost from the body during a dosage interval can be determined nongraphically from this equation:

$$\text{Fraction of drug lost from body} = 1 - e^{-kt}$$

Values for e^{-kt} can be obtained from a table of natural exponential functions or by a calculator, where k ($= 0.693/t_{1/2}$) is the fractional elimination constant (described in the next section) and t is the time interval after drug administration.

[2] When drug is present in the formed elements of blood, then calculation of extraction and clearance from blood is more physiologically meaningful than from the plasma.

The important relationship

$$t_{1/2} = \frac{0.693 V_d}{Cl}$$

indicates clearly the dependency of half-life, a measure of rate of elimination, on the two physiologically independent variables of volume of distribution and clearance, which expresses the efficiency of elimination. Thus, half-life is shortened when phenobarbital induces the enzymes responsible for hepatic clearance of a drug, and half-life is lengthened when a drug's renal clearance is attenuated in renal failure. Also, the half-life of some drugs is shortened when their volume of distribution is reduced. If, as in the case of cardiac failure, the volume of distribution is reduced at the same time that clearance is reduced, there may be little change in drug half-life to reflect the impaired clearance, but steady state plasma levels will be increased, as is the case with lidocaine. In treating patients after an overdose, the effects of hemodialysis on a drug's elimination are dependent on its volume of distribution. When the volume of distribution is large, as with tricyclic antidepressants (V_d of desipramine equals more than 2000 L), the removal of drug, even with a high-clearance dialyzer, proceeds slowly.

The extent to which a drug is bound to plasma protein also determines the fraction extracted by the organ(s) of elimination. Altered binding changes the extraction ratio significantly, however, only when elimination is limited to the unbound (free) drug in plasma. The extent to which binding influences elimination depends on the relative affinity of the plasma binding versus the affinity of the drug for the extraction process. The high affinity of the renal tubular anion transport system for many drugs leads to extraction of bound and unbound drug, and the efficient process by which the liver removes propranolol extracts most of this highly bound drug from blood. However, in the case of drugs with low organ extraction ratios, only unbound drug is available for elimination.

STEADY STATE   With a constant infusion of drug, the infusion rate equals elimination rate at steady state. Therefore,

$$\begin{array}{ccc} \text{Infusion rate} & = & Cp_{ss} & \times & Cl \\ \text{(amt/unit time)} & & \text{(amt/vol)} & & \text{(vol/unit time)} \end{array}$$

when the units for amount, volume, and time are consistent.

Thus, if clearance (Cl) is known, the infusion rate to achieve a given steady state plasma level can be calculated. Estimation of drug clearance is discussed in the section on renal disease.

When the dose is given intermittently instead of by infusion, the above relationship between plasma concentration and the dose administered at each dosage interval can be expressed as

$$\text{Dose} = Cp_{av} \times Cl \times \text{dosage interval}$$

The average plasma concentration (Cp_{av}) implies, as seen in Fig. 65-2, that levels can be higher and lower than the average during the dosage interval.

When a drug is given orally, the fraction (F) of the administered dose that reaches the systemic circulation is an expression of the drug's *bioavailability*. A reduction in bioavailability may reflect a poorly formulated dosage form that fails to disintegrate or dissolve in the gastrointestinal fluids. Regulatory standards have reduced the extent of this problem. Drug interactions also can impair absorption after oral dosing. Bioavailability may also be reduced due to drug metabolism in the gastrointestinal tract and/or the liver during the absorption process, the *first-pass effect*. This is a particular problem for drugs that are extensively extracted by these organs, and considerable interpatient variability often exists in bioavailability. Lidocaine for the control of arrhythmias is not administered orally because of the first-pass effect. Drugs that are injected intramuscularly may also have low bioavailability, e.g., phenytoin. An unexpected drug response should lead to consideration of bioavailability as a possible factor. Calculation of a dosage regimen should be corrected for bioavailability:

$$\begin{array}{c} \text{Oral} \\ \text{dose} \end{array} = \frac{Cp_{av} \times Cl \times \text{dosage interval}}{F}$$

DRUG ELIMINATION THAT IS NOT FIRST-ORDER   The elimination of some drugs such as phenytoin, salicylate, and theophylline does not follow first-order kinetics when amounts of drug in the body are in the therapeutic range. For these drugs, the clearance changes as levels in the body fall during elimination or after alterations in dose. This pattern of elimination is said to be *dose-dependent*. Accordingly, the time for the concentration to fall to one-half becomes less as plasma levels fall; this halving time is not truly a half-life, because the term *half-life* applies to first-order kinetics and is a constant. The elimination of phenytoin is dose-dependent, and when very high levels are present (in the toxic range), the halving time may be longer than 72 h, whereas as the concentration in plasma declines, the clearance increases and the concentration in plasma will halve in 20 to 30 h. When a drug is eliminated by first-order kinetics, the plasma level at steady state is directly related to the amount of the maintenance dose, and a doubling of the dose should lead to doubling of the steady state plasma level. However, for drugs with dose-dependent kinetics, increases in the dose may be accompanied by disproportionate increases in plasma level. Thus, if the daily dose of phenytoin is increased from 300 to 400 mg, plasma levels rise by more than 33 percent. The extent of increase is not predictable because of the interpatient variability in the extent to which clearance deviates from first order. Salicylates are also eliminated by dose-dependent kinetics at high plasma levels, and in children particular caution must be taken with the administration of high doses. Ethanol metabolism also is dose-dependent, with obvious implications. The mechanisms involved in dose-dependent kinetics may include the saturation of the rate-limiting step in metabolism or a feedback inhibition of the rate-limiting enzyme by a product of the reaction.

INDIVIDUALIZATION OF DRUG THERAPY

Recognition of factors modifying drug action is essential for therapy that provides optimal benefit and minimal risk to each patient.

ALTERATION OF DRUG DOSAGE IN RENAL DISEASE   Where urinary excretion is an important route of elimination, renal failure results in decreased drug clearance and therefore slower removal of the drug from the body, so that administration of the usual dosage leads to greater accumulation and an increased likelihood of toxicity. The goal in such cases is to modify the dosage schedule so that a similar drug concentration–time profile is achieved in the plasma of the patient with renal insufficiency and the steady state is reached after a similar time interval as in the patient with normal renal function. This is particularly appropriate for drugs with long half-lives and narrow therapeutic indexes (e.g., digoxin). Since,

$$\begin{aligned} Cp_{av} &= \frac{\text{dose}}{\text{dose interval}} \times \frac{1}{Cl} \\ &= \frac{\text{dose}}{\text{dose interval}} \times \frac{1}{k V_d} \end{aligned}$$

the Cp_{av} achieved with normal renal function can be obtained in patients with renal impairment, i.e., decreased Cl, by either decreasing the dose while maintaining the normal dosing interval, administering the usual dose but less frequently, or a combination of the two. Moreover, the modification factor for the dosage regimen is dependent on the ratio of the drug's clearance or rate of elimination in renal failure to that in uncompromised patients. Although such pharmacokinetic strategies in renal failure result in the same Cp_{av} during the dosage interval, the peak-to-trough fluctuations differ considerably from those seen in patients with normal renal function. Selection of the most appropriate modifications, therefore, depends on the levels associated with efficacy or toxicity, e.g., peak, Cp_{av}, or trough, and the drug's therapeutic index.

One approach is to calculate the *fraction of the normal dose* that is to be given at the usual dosage interval. This fraction can be determined from either drug clearance (Cl) or the fractional rate constant (k), based on the fact that both renal clearance and k are proportional to creatinine clearance (Cl_{cr}). Creatinine clearance is best determined directly. However, serum creatinine (C_{cr}) may be used to estimate the value by the following equation which is applicable to men:

$$Cl_{cr} = \frac{(140 - age) \times weight\,(kg)}{72 \times C_{cr}\,(mg/dL)}\,(mL/min)$$

For women, the value should be reduced to 85 percent of that estimated by this equation. This approach to estimation of Cl_{cr} is invalid in severe renal insufficiency ($C_{cr} > 5$ mg/dL) or with rapidly changing renal function.

The clearance approach   Calculation of drug dosage is most accurately based on the clearance of a drug. From data on the clearance of a drug, the dose in renal insufficiency ($Dose_{ri}$) may be calculated as follows:

$$Dose_{ri} = dose \times \frac{Cl_{ri}}{Cl}$$

where ri = renal insufficiency
Cl = clearance from the whole body with normal renal function
Cl_{ri} = clearance from the whole body with renal insufficiency
Dose = maintenance dose with normal renal function ($Cl_{cr} \sim$ 100 mL/min)

The normal clearance and that in renal impairment can be obtained by employing the data in Table 65-1 in the following equations:

$$Cl = Cl_{renal} + Cl_{nonrenal}$$

$$Cl_{ri} = Cl_{renal} \times \frac{measured\,Cl_{cr}}{100\,mL/min} + Cl_{nonrenal}$$

The Cl_{renal} values in Table 65-1 are those found with $Cl_{cr} = 100$ mL/min, and the renal clearance of drug in renal insufficiency is obtained by multiplying Cl_{renal} by the ratio of measured Cl_{cr} (in milliliters per minute) to 100 mL/min.

For gentamicin, with a normal Cl_{renal} of 78 mL/min and $Cl_{nonrenal}$ of 3 mL/min, Cl = 81 mL/min. Therefore, with a Cl_{cr} of 12 mL/min, $Cl_{ri} = 78 \times (12/100) + 3 = 12.4$ mL/min. If the dose of gentamicin for a given infection should be 1.5 mg/kg per 8 h in the presence of normal renal function, then

$$Dose_n \quad \frac{1.5\,mg/kg}{8\,h} \times \frac{12.4\,mL/min}{81\,mL/min} = \frac{0.23\,mg/kg}{8\,h}$$

In the patient with renal insufficiency, this computation provides an average plasma level during a dosage interval that is the same as the average plasma level during the dosage interval with normal renal function; the fluctuations between peaks and troughs, however, will be less pronounced, but the peak value could be below the therapeutic level. Alternatively, the normal (1.5 mg/kg) dose of gentamicin could be administered but the dosage interval prolonged by the modification factor based on the change in clearance

$$8\,h \times \frac{81\,mL/min}{12.4\,mL/min} = 52\,h$$

In this case, the plasma levels may be subtherapeutic for a deleterious length of time during the dosage interval.

In some instances it may be desirable to calculate a dose that will yield a certain plasma level at steady state. This approach is most appropriate for constant intravenous infusions where 100 percent of the dose is delivered to the systemic circulation. When clearance of a drug in a patient with renal insufficiency is calculated as above, then

$$\underset{(amt/unit\,time)}{Dose_{ri}} = \underset{(vol/unit\,time)}{Cl_{ri}} \times \underset{(amt/vol)}{Cp}$$

where the time, amount, and volume terms are uniform.

If a plasma concentration of carbenicillin of 100 μg/mL is the therapeutic objective in a patient with a creatinine clearance of 25 mL/min, the infusion rate is calculated as follows. Carbenicillin clearance is

$$Cl_{ri} = \left(68 \times \frac{25}{100}\right) + 10 = 27\,mL/min$$

Therefore, carbenicillin should be infused at a rate of 2700 μg/min.

Should the method of calculating dose based on the desired plasma level be applied to intermittent-dose therapy, particular attention should be given to the fact that the calculation is based on an *average* plasma level and that peak plasma levels will be higher. In addition, if an oral drug is not completely absorbed, the computed dose must be divided by the fraction (*F*) that reaches the systemic circulation (see "Steady State" above).

The fractional rate constant (*k*) approach   For many drugs, clearance data in renal failure are not available. In these cases, the fraction of the normal dose that is required in a patient with renal failure can be approximated from the ratio of the fractional rate constant for elimination from the body in renal failure (k_{ri}) to that with normal renal function (*k*). This approach requires the assumption that the distribution of the drug (V_d) is not affected by renal disease. The approach is the same as that employed with clearance data:

$$Dose_{ri} = Dose \times \frac{k_{ri}}{k}$$

As the ratio k_{ri}/k is the fraction of the usual dose employed in a given degree of renal insufficiency, it is termed the *dose fraction* and may be estimated from the information in Table 65-2 and the nomogram (Fig. 65-4). Table 65-2 gives the fraction of the usual dose of a drug

FIGURE 65-4 Nomogram for estimation of the dose fraction (k_{ri}/k) in patients with renal insufficiency. The application of the nomogram is described in the text.

TABLE 65-1   Clearance of drugs

Drug	Renal clearance,* mL/min	Nonrenal clearance, mL/min
Ampicillin†	340	12
Carbenicillin	68	10
Digoxin†	110	36
Gentamicin	78	3
Kanamycin	60	0
Penicillin G‡	340	36

* The "normal" renal clearances are those associated with a clearance of creatinine of 100 mL/min.
† The fraction of digoxin absorbed after an oral dose (*F*) is approximately 0.75, and *F* for ampicillin is 0.5.
‡ One microgram of penicillin G = 1.6 units.

TABLE 65-2 Estimated fraction of usual dose of drug required for a patient with a creatinine clearance of zero (dose fraction$_0$) and average overall fractional elimination rate constant for a patient with normal renal function (k)

Drug	Dose fraction$_0$	k (per hour)
ANTIBIOTICS		
Amikacin	0.05	0.4
Amoxicillin	0.15	0.7
Ampicillin	0.1	0.6
Aztreonam	0.25	0.4
Carbenicillin	0.1	0.6
Cefazolin	0.06	0.35
Cefotaxime*	0.3	0.7
Cefoxitin	0.1	0.8
Ceftazidime	0.1	0.4
Ceftriaxone†	0.5	0.09
Cephalexin	0.04	0.7
Cephalothin	0.02	1.4
Chloramphenicol	0.8	0.3
Ciprofloxacin	0.33	0.2
Clindamycin	0.8	0.2
Cloxacillin	0.25	1.2
Dicloxacillin	0.5	1.2
Doxycycline	0.8	0.03
Erythromycin	0.7	0.5
Gentamicin	0.05	0.3
Imipenem	0.25	0.7
Isoniazid:		
Fast inactivators	0.8	0.5
Slow inactivators	0.5	0.25
Methicillin	0.12	1.4
Minocycline	0.9	0.06
Nafcillin	0.4	1.2
Norfloxacin	0.5	0.2
Oxacillin	0.25	1.4
Penicillin G	0.1	1.4
Piperacillin	0.33	0.5
Rifampin	1.0	0.25
Streptomycin	0.05	0.25
Sulfadiazine	0.45	0.7
Sulfamethoxazole	0.85	0.07
Tetracycline	0.12	0.08
Ticarcillin	0.1	0.6
Tobramycin	0.05	0.35
Trimethoprim	0.45	0.06
Vancomycin	0.03	0.12
MISCELLANEOUS DRUGS		
Chlorpropamide	0.4	0.02
Lidocaine	0.9	0.4
Sulfinpyrazone	0.55	0.3

CARDIAC GLYCOSIDES		k (per day)
Digitoxin	0.7	0.1
Digoxin	0.3	0.45

* See text on dosage in renal disease.
† Extrarenal clearance also may be reduced in patients with renal failure who are uremic and/or ill.

required at a creatinine clearance of zero (dose fraction$_0$). The nomogram presents the dose fraction as a linear function of creatinine clearance.

To calculate the dose fraction$_{ri}$, the dose fraction$_0$ is obtained from Table 65-2, plotted on the left ordinate of the nomogram, and connected by a straight line to the upper-right-hand corner of the nomogram. This line describes the dose fraction over a range of creatinine clearances from 0 to 100 mL/min. The point of intersection between the measured creatinine clearance (on the lower abscissa) and this dose fraction line is a coordinate with the dose fraction (on the left ordinate) corresponding with that particular creatinine clearance. For example, if a patient with a creatinine clearance of 20 mL/min requires penicillin G for an infection that would be treated with 10 million units daily in patients with normal renal function, then an appropriate dose would be 2.8 million units daily. This dose is estimated by plotting the dose fraction$_0$ for penicillin G (0.1) on the

left-hand ordinate and connecting it to the top right-hand corner of the nomogram (Fig. 65-4). On this dose fraction line for penicillin G, the coordinate for a creatinine clearance of 20 mL/min corresponds on the left ordinate with a dose fraction of 0.28. Hence, the dose is 0.28×10 million units daily.

The loading dose In addition to adjusting the maintenance dose in renal failure, consideration must also be given to the loading dose. Since this dose is designed to bring the plasma concentration, or more particularly the amount of drug in the body, rapidly to the level at steady state, there is no need to modify the usual loading dose, if one is normally used. The elimination of many drugs is sufficiently rapid in patients with normal renal function that the time required to reach steady state is not significant, and no loading dose is usually used. On the other hand, in renal failure where the half-life may be significantly prolonged, this accumulation period may become unacceptably long. In such a case, a loading dose may be indicated; it would be the same amount of drug administered with normal renal function as described in "Drug Accumulation" above.

General considerations for determining dosage in renal insufficiency Because of the differences in volumes of distribution and rates of metabolism, calculations of drug dose in renal failure must be viewed as valuable approximations which prevent the use of doses that are grossly excessive or inadequate for most patients. However, *maintenance dosages are most accurate when plasma level data are employed to enable adjustment of the dose where necessary.*

In all the above calculations, it is assumed that the nonrenal clearance and nonrenal k are constant in renal failure. In fact, when cardiac failure accompanies renal failure, metabolic clearance for many drugs is reduced. Accordingly, when a drug with a narrow therapeutic index, such as digoxin, is used in cardiac failure, an appropriate precaution would be to reduce the value for nonrenal clearance (or k) to about one-half.

Active or toxic metabolites of drugs also may accumulate in renal failure. Meperidine, for example, is cleared largely by metabolism, and its concentration in plasma is little altered by renal insufficiency. However, the plasma concentration of one of its metabolites, normeperidine, is increased when its renal elimination is impaired. As normeperidine has more convulsant activity than meperidine, its accumulation in patients with renal failure probably accounts for the signs of central nervous system excitation such as irritability, twitching, and seizures that result from the administration of multiple doses of meperidine to patients in renal insufficiency.

The metabolite of procainamide, N-acetylprocainamide, also has cardiac effects. As N-acetylprocainamide is eliminated almost entirely by the kidney, its concentration in plasma is increased by renal failure. Thus, the potential of procainamide to produce toxicity in renal insufficiency cannot be assessed by measuring the plasma concentration of procainamide alone. Cefotaxime is metabolized predominately to desacetylcefotaxime, which also has antimicrobial activity. Desacetylcefotaxime accumulates in renal failure to an even greater degree than does the parent drug, but no adverse effects are known to accrue to the accumulation of this metabolite.

LIVER DISEASE In contrast to the predictable decline in renal clearance of drugs when glomerular filtration is reduced, it is not possible to make a general prediction of the effect of liver disease on hepatic biotransformation of drugs (Chap. 247). Rather, in hepatitis and cirrhosis changes may range from impaired to increased drug clearance. Even in advanced hepatocellular disease, the magnitude of impairment in drug clearance usually is only about two- to fivefold. The extent of such changes, however, cannot be predicted by the common tests of liver function. Consequently, even when it is suspected that drug elimination is altered in liver disease, there is no quantitative base upon which to adjust the dosage regimen other than assessment of clinical response and concentration of drug in plasma.

Portacaval shunting creates a special situation because the effective hepatic blood flow is reduced. This situation has its greatest effect on drugs that normally have a high hepatic extraction ratio so that their clearance is largely a function of blood flow; thus the clearance of such drugs (e.g., propranolol and lidocaine) is remarkably reduced by portacaval shunting. In addition, the fraction of an administered oral dose reaching the systemic circulation is increased, because drug that is shunted around the liver during the absorption process escapes the first-pass metabolism by this organ (e.g., meperidine, pentazocine).

CIRCULATORY INSUFFICIENCY—CARDIAC FAILURE AND SHOCK Under conditions of decreased tissue perfusion, redistribution of the cardiac output occurs to preserve blood flow to the heart and brain at the expense of other tissues (Chap. 39). As a result, the drug is distributed into a smaller volume of distribution, higher drug concentrations are present in the plasma, and the tissues that are best perfused are exposed to these higher concentrations. If either the brain or heart is sensitive to the drug, an alteration in response will occur.

Furthermore, the decreased perfusion of the kidney and liver may impair drug clearance by these organs directly or indirectly. Thus, in severe congestive heart failure, in hemorrhagic shock, and in cardiogenic shock, the response to the usual dose of drug may be excessive, and dosage modification may be necessary. For example, the clearance of lidocaine is reduced by about 50 percent in cardiac failure, and therapeutic plasma levels are achieved at infusion rates of only about half of those usually required. In cardiac failure there also is a significant reduction in lidocaine's volume of distribution which results in the requirement of a smaller loading dose. Similar situations are thought to exist for procainamide, theophylline, and possibly quinidine. Unfortunately, predictors of these types of pharmacokinetic alterations are unavailable. Therefore, loading doses should be conservative, and continued therapy should be monitored closely, following clinical indicators of toxicity and plasma levels.

DISEASE-INDUCED CHANGES IN PLASMA BINDING Many drugs circulate in the plasma partly bound to the plasma proteins. Since only the unbound or free drug can distribute to the site of pharmacologic action, the therapeutic response should be related to the free rather than the total circulating plasma drug concentration. In most cases the degree of binding is fairly constant across the therapeutic concentration range so that significant error is not caused by individualizing therapy on the basis of total drug levels in plasma. However, states such as hypoalbuminemia, liver disease, and renal disease can decrease the extent of drug binding, particularly of acidic and neutral drugs, so that at any total plasma level there is a greater concentration of free drug and a risk of increased response and toxicity. Other conditions, e.g., myocardial infarction, surgery, neoplastic disease, rheumatoid arthritis, and burns, that lead to an increased plasma concentration of the acute-phase reactant alpha$_1$-acid glycoprotein have the opposite effect on the basic drugs that are bound to this macromolecule. The drugs for which changes in binding are important are those that are normally highly bound in the plasma (>90 percent) because a small alteration in the extent of binding produces a large change in the amount of drug in the unbound form.

The consequences of these binding changes, particularly with respect to total drug levels, depend on whether the clearance and distribution are dependent on the unbound or total drug. For many drugs, elimination and distribution are largely restricted to the unbound fraction, and therefore a decrease in binding leads to an increase in the clearance and distribution of the drug. The relative magnitudes of these changes are such that the net effect is to shorten the half-life. The appropriate modification of the dosage regimen in conditions with reduced drug binding, as is the case of phenytoin in renal failure, is simply to administer the usual daily dose of the drug but in divided doses at more frequent intervals. Individualization of therapy can then be based on either the clinical response or the plasma concentration of unbound drug. It is critical that the patient not be titrated into the usual therapeutic range for concentration of *total* drug in plasma since this will lead to excessive response and toxicity.

In the case of drugs bound to alpha$_1$-acid glycoprotein, the disease-induced increase in binding has the opposite effects of reducing the clearance and distribution of total drug. Accordingly, constant rate infusion of lidocaine to control arrhythmias after myocardial infarction leads to an accumulation of total drug. However, the clearance of unbound and pharmacologically active drug remains essentially unchanged. Again, it is critical that the patient not be dosed on the basis of total drug concentrations in the plasma since this will be associated with subtherapeutic levels of unbound drug.

INTERACTIONS BETWEEN DRUGS

The effect of some drugs can be altered markedly by the administration of other agents. Such interactions can sabotage therapeutic intent by producing excessive drug action (with adverse effects) or decreasing the action of a drug, rendering it ineffective. Drug interactions must be considered in the differential diagnosis of unexpected responses to drugs, recognizing that patients often come to the physician with a legacy of drugs acquired during previous medical experiences. A meticulous drug history will minimize the unknown elements in the therapeutic milieu; it should include examination of the patient's medications and calls to the pharmacist to identify prescriptions, if necessary.

There are two principal types of interactions between drugs. *Pharmacokinetic interactions* result from alteration in the delivery of drugs to their sites of action. *Pharmacodynamic interactions* are those in which the responsiveness of the target organ or system is modified by other agents.

An index of the drug interactions discussed in this chapter is provided in Table 65-3. Included are interactions which have verified significance in patients and a few of such potential danger that cognizance should be taken of experimental data or case reports suggesting their likely occurrence.

I PHARMACOKINETIC INTERACTIONS CAUSING DIMINISHED DRUG DELIVERY

A Impaired gastrointestinal absorption Cholestyramine, an ionic exchange resin, binds thyroxine, triiodothyronine, and the cardiac glycosides with sufficiently high affinity to impair their absorption from the gastrointestinal tract. This resin probably also interferes with the absorption of other drugs, and it is safest not to give it within 2 h of their administration. Aluminum ions, present in antacids, form insoluble chelates with the tetracyclines, thereby preventing absorption of these drugs. Ferrous ions similarly block tetracycline absorption. Kaolin-pectin suspensions bind digoxin, and when the drugs are administered together, digoxin absorption is reduced by about one-half. However, when kaolin-pectin is administered 2 h after digoxin, there is no effect on absorption of digoxin.

Ketoconazole is a weak base that dissolves well only at acidic pH. Thus, histamine-2 antagonists such as cimetidine, by neutralizing gastric pH, impair the dissolution and subsequent absorption of ketoconazole. Oral administration of aminosalicylate interferes with the absorption of rifampin by an unknown mechanism.

Impaired absorption results in reduction in the total amount of drug absorbed, with reduced area under the plasma level curve, reduced peak plasma levels, and lower steady state concentrations of the drug involved.

B Induction of hepatic drug-metabolizing enzymes When the elimination of the drug is largely by metabolism, an increase in the rate of metabolism reduces its availability to sites of action. The metabolism of most drugs occurs largely in the liver, because of its mass, high blood flow, and concentration of enzymes that metabolize drugs. The initial step in metabolism of many drugs is executed by a group of mixed-function oxidase isoenzymes in the endoplasmic reticulum. These enzyme systems containing cytochrome P$_{450}$ oxidize the molecule by a variety of reactions including aromatic hydroxylations, N-demethylations, O-demethylations, and sulfoxidations. The products of these reactions are usually more polar (and more readily excreted by the kidney).

TABLE 65-3 Drug interaction index

Drug	Section of chapter describing interaction
Acetohexamide	IIB
Allopurinol	IIA
p-Aminosalicylate	IA
Amiodarone	IIC
Amphetamine	IC
Antidepressants, tricyclic (desipramine, nortriptyline, imipramine, doxepin, protriptyline, amitriptyline)	IC
Aspirin	IIB, III
Azathioprine	IIA
Barbiturates (class)	IB
Bethanidine	IC
Carbamazepine	IB, IIA
Chlorpromazine	IC
Cholestyramine	IA
Cimetidine	IA, IIA, IIB
Clofibrate	IIA
Clonidine	IC
Cyclosporine	IB, IIA
Dexamethasone	IB
Digitoxin	IA, IB, IIC
Digoxin	IA, IIC
Diuretics	III
Erythromycin	IIA
Ephedrine	IC
Ethanol	IIA
Famotidine	IIA
Guanadrel	IC
Guanethidine	IC
Indomethacin	III
Isoniazid	IIA
Kaolin-pectin	IA
Ketoconazole	IA, IB, IIA
Lidocaine	IIA
6-Mercaptopurine	IIA
Methadone	IB
Methotrexate	IIB
Metronidazole	IB, IIA
Metyrapone	IB
Mexiletine	IB
Nifedipine	IIA
Nonsteroidal anti-inflammatory drugs	III
Oral contraceptive steroids	IB
Phenobarbital	IB
Phenylbutazone	IIA, IIB
Phenytoin (diphenylhydantoin)	IB, IIA
Piroxicam	III
Potassium	III
Prednisone	IB
Probenicid	IIB
Procainamide	IIB
Propranolol	III
Quinidine	IB, IIA, IIC, III
Ranitidine	IA, IIA
Rifampin	IA, IB
Salicylate	IIB
Spironolactone	III
Tetracycline	IA
Theophylline	IIA
Thiazide diuretics	III
Tolbutamide	IIA
Triamterene	III
Triazolam	IIA
Verapamil	IIC
Warfarin	IB, IIA, III

The biosynthesis of some of the mixed-function oxidase isoenzymes is under regulatory control at the transcriptional level, and their content in the liver can be induced by a number of drugs. Phenobarbital is the prototype of these inducers, and all barbiturates in clinical use increase mixed-function oxidase isoenzymes. Induction with phenobarbital can occur with doses of as little as 60 mg daily. Mixed-function oxidases also are induced by rifampin, carbamazepine, phenytoin, and glutethimide, by occupational exposure to chlorinated insecticides such as DDT, and by chronic alcohol ingestion.

Phenobarbital and other inducers lower plasma levels of many drugs, including warfarin, digitoxin, quinidine, mexiletine, ketocon-

azole, cyclosporine, dexamethasone, prednisolone (the active metabolite of prednisone), oral contraceptive steroids, methadone, metronidazole, and metyrapone. These interactions all have obvious clinical significance. With the coumarin anticoagulants, the patient is placed at major risk when an appropriate level of anticoagulation is achieved while the coumarin drug is coadministered with an inducing agent. Should the inducer then be discontinued, e.g., following discharge from the hospital, plasma levels of the coumarin anticoagulant will rise as the induction effect wears off, leading to excessive anticoagulation. Barbiturates have been shown to lower the plasma levels of phenytoin in some patients, but the clinical effect of reduced phenytoin levels is probably counterbalanced by the anticonvulsant effects of phenobarbital.

There is considerable variation among individuals in the extent to which drug metabolism can be induced. In some patients phenobarbital leads to marked acceleration in the rate of drug metabolism, whereas little induction is seen in others.

In addition to inducing certain of the mixed-function oxidase isoenzymes, phenobarbital has other effects on hepatic function. It increases liver blood flow, bile flow, and the hepatocellular transport of organic anions. The conjugation of drugs and bilirubin may also be enhanced by inducing agents.

C Inhibition of cellular uptake or binding The guanidinium antihypertensives, guanethidine, guanadrel, and bethanidine, are transported to their site of action in adrenergic neurons by an energy-requiring membrane transport system for biogenic monoamines. Although the physiologic function of the transport system is reuptake of the adrenergic neurotransmitter, it also transports a variety of ring-substituted bases, including guanethidine and related guanidiniums, into the adrenergic neuron against a concentration gradient. Inhibitors of norepinephrine uptake prevent the uptake of the guanidinium antihypertensives into adrenergic neurons and thereby block their pharmacologic effects. The tricyclic antidepressants are potent inhibitors of norepinephrine uptake. Consequently, concomitant administration of clinical doses of tricyclic antidepressants including desipramine, protriptyline, nortriptyline, and amitriptyline almost totally abolishes the antihypertensive effects of guanethidine, guanadrel, and bethanidine. Although they are less potent inhibitors of norepinephrine uptake, doxepin and chlorpromazine, when given in doses of greater than 100 mg daily, produce dose-related antagonism of the action of the guanidinium antihypertensives. In patients with severe hypertension, the loss of control of blood pressure from these drug interactions can lead to stroke and malignant hypertension.

Ephedrine, a component of many drug combinations used in asthma, also antagonizes the effect of guanethidine, probably by both inhibition of uptake and displacement from the neuron.

The antihypertensive effect of clonidine is partially antagonized by tricyclic antidepressants. Clonidine lowers arterial pressure by reducing sympathetic outflow from the blood-pressure-regulating centers in the hindbrain (Chap. 196). This central hypotensive action is antagonized by the tricyclic antidepressants.

II PHARMACOKINETIC INTERACTIONS CAUSING INCREASED DRUG DELIVERY

A Inhibition of drug metabolism If the active form of a drug is cleared largely by biotransformation, inhibition of its metabolism leads to a reduced clearance, prolonged half-life, and accumulation of the drug during maintenance therapy. Excessive accumulation due to inhibited metabolism can lead to adverse effects.

Cimetidine is a potent inhibitor of the oxidative metabolism of warfarin, quinidine, nifedipine, lidocaine, theophylline and phenytoin. Adverse reactions, many of them severe, have resulted from the administration of these drugs in conjunction with cimetidine. Cimetidine is a more potent inhibitor of mixed-function oxidases than ranitidine, whereas ranitidine is more potent as a histamine-2 antagonist. Thus, ranitidine, when administered in doses of 150 mg twice daily, does not inhibit the oxidative metabolism of most drugs; where reduced drug elimination has been observed, the effects of ranitidine have been less than those of cimetidine and devoid of appreciable pharmacodynamic consequence. Doses of ranitidine higher than 150 mg, however, may produce greater inhibition of drug oxidation. Famotidine, like ranitidine, is not known to produce clinically appreciable inhibition of drug metabolism.

Erythromycin inhibits the metabolism of several drugs, including cyclosporine, warfarin, carbamazepine, triazolam, and theophylline. Adverse effects, some severe, have been the consequence of these drug interactions. The extent to which disposition of these drugs is impaired by erythromycin is a function of erythromycin concentration in plasma (and its dose) and probably also of the duration of erythromycin administration. Erythromycin is metabolized by an isozyme of cytochrome P_{450} to a nitroso metabolite that binds to and inhibits the P_{450} isozyme.

Other drugs that inhibit biotransformation of pharmacologic compounds include (with examples of drugs that have their metabolism blocked by the inhibitor listed in parenthesis):

Clofibrate (phenytoin, tolbutamide)
Excessive ingestion of ethanol (warfarin)
Isoniazid (phenytoin)
Ketoconazole (cyclosporine)
Metronidazole (warfarin)
Phenylbutazone (warfarin, phenytoin, tolbutamide)

Cyclosporine inhibits the disposition of some other drugs. Cyclosporine lowers the clearance of prednisolone. The administration of lovastatin to cardiac transplant patients receiving cyclosporine has been associated with a high prevalence of rhabdomyolysis that can be severe. As the concentration of lovastatin was noted to be elevated when measured in these patients with rhabdomyolysis, impairment of its clearance by cyclosporine has been inferred but not proved as a cause of this severe drug interaction.

Azathioprine is readily converted in the body to an active metabolite, 6-mercaptopurine, which in turn is oxidized by xanthine oxidase to 6-thiouric acid. When allopurinol, a potent inhibitor of xanthine oxidase, is administered concurrently with standard doses of azathioprine or 6-mercaptopurine, life-threatening toxicity (bone marrow suppression) can result.

B **Inhibition of renal elimination** A number of drugs are secreted by the renal tubular transport systems for organic anions. Inhibition of this tubular transport system can cause excessive accumulation of a drug. Phenylbutazone, probenecid, and salicylates competitively inhibit this transport system. Salicylate, for example, reduces the renal clearance of methotrexate, an interaction that may lead to methotrexate toxicity. Renal tubular secretion contributes substantially to the elimination of penicillin, which can be inhibited by probenecid.

Inhibition of the tubular cation transport system by cimetidine impedes the renal clearance of procainamide and its active metabolite *N*-acetylprocainamide.

C **Inhibition of clearance by multiple mechanisms** The concentrations of digoxin and digitoxin in plasma are elevated by quinidine, due largely to inhibition of renal elimination and in part from inhibition of nonrenal clearance as well. An increase in cardiac arrhythmia may occur when quinidine is given in conjunction with a cardiac glycoside.

Amiodarone, cyclosporine, and verapamil also inhibit the clearance of digoxin and increase the concentration of digoxin in plasma.

III **PHARMACODYNAMIC AND OTHER INTERACTIONS BETWEEN DRUGS** Therapeutically useful interactions occur in which the combined effect of two drugs is greater than that of either drug alone. These favorable drug combinations are described in specific therapeutic sections in this text, and the following is directed toward those interactions that create unwanted effects. Two drugs may act on separate components of a common process and yield effects greater than either alone. For example, small doses of aspirin (less than 1 g daily) do not alter the prothrombin time appreciably in patients who are on warfarin therapy. However, the addition of aspirin to patients

anticoagulated with warfarin increases the risk of bleeding because aspirin inhibits platelet aggregation. Thus the combination of impaired functions of platelets and the clotting system increases the potential for hemorrhagic complications in patients receiving warfarin therapy.

Indomethacin, piroxicam, and probably other nonsteroidal antiinflammatory drugs antagonize the antihypertensive effects of beta-adrenergic receptor blockers, diuretics, converting enzyme inhibitors, and other drugs. The resultant elevation in blood pressure ranges from trivial to severe. Aspirin and sulindac, however, do not elevate the blood pressure in treated hypertensive patients.

Polymorphic ventricular tachycardia (torsades de pointes) during quinidine administration occurs much more frequently in patients receiving diuretics, probably as a consequence of potassium and/or magnesium depletion.

The administration of supplemental potassium leads to more frequent and more severe hyperkalemia when potassium elimination is reduced by concurrent treatment with spironolactone or triamterene.

VARIABLE ACTIONS OF DRUGS CAUSED BY GENETIC DIFFERENCES IN THEIR METABOLISM

ACETYLATION Isoniazid, hydralazine, procainamide, and a number of other drugs are metabolized by acetylation of a hydrazino or amino group. This reaction is catalyzed by *N*-acetyl transferase, an enzyme in the liver cytosol that transfers an acetyl group from acetyl coenzyme A to the drug. Individuals differ markedly in the rate at which drugs are acetylated, and there is a bimodal distribution of the population into ''rapid acetylators'' and ''slow acetylators.'' The rate of acetylation is under genetic control; slow acetylation is an autosomal recessive trait.

Responses to hydralazine therapy are dependent upon the acetylation phenotype. The hypotensive effect of hydralazine is greater in patients who acetylate the drug slowly, and the lupus erythematosus-like syndrome produced by hydralazine occurs almost exclusively in those with slow acetylation. Thus it may be of value to know the acetylation phenotype as a predictor of which patients with hypertension might benefit from an increase in the dose of hydralazine above the 200 mg daily that can be safely employed in the population at large.

Acetylation phenotype can be determined by measuring the ratio of acetylated to nonacetylated dapsone or sulfamethazine in plasma or urine following administration of a test dose of these acetylation substrates. The ratio of monoacetyldapsone to dapsone in plasma at 6 h after dapsone administration is less than 0.35 for slow acetylators and greater than 0.35 for rapid acetylators. At 6 h following the administration of sulfamethazine, less than 25 percent of the drug in the plasma is in the acetylated form in slow acetylators (rapid acetylators, more than 25 percent); in the urine collected in the 5- to 6-h interval after administration, less than 70 percent of the drug is in the acetylated form in slow acetylators (rapid acetylators, more than 70 percent).

METABOLISM BY MIXED-FUNCTION OXIDASES In healthy individuals taking no other medications, the major determinant of the rate of metabolism of drugs by the hepatic mixed-function oxidases is genetic. Hepatic endoplasmic reticulum contains a family of cytochrome P_{450} isoenzymes with different substrate specificities. Many drugs undergo oxidative metabolism by more than one isoenzyme, and the steady state concentrations of such drugs in the plasma is a function of the sum of the activities of these and other metabolizing enzymes. When a drug is metabolized by multiple pathways, the catalytic activities of the participating enzymes are regulated by a number of genes so that the frequency of clearance rates and steady state concentrations of the drug tend to distribute unimodally within the population. The range of activity may differ markedly (tenfold or more) between different individuals, as is the case for chlorpromazine, and there is no way to make a prior prediction of the rate.

For certain metabolic pathways bimodally distributed activity suggests control by a single gene, and several polymorphisms have been identified. As a result, two phenotypic populations are usually present analogous to the situation with N-acetylation (see above). A majority of the population are extensive metabolizers (EM), and a smaller group of individuals of the poor metabolizer phenotype (PM) have an impaired, if not an absent, ability to metabolize the drug. For example, about 8 to 10 percent of whites are unable to form the 4-hydroxy metabolite of the test drug debrisoquin, and this trait is inherited in an autosomal recessive fashion. Importantly, the putatively involved cytochrome P_{450} isoenzyme is also involved in the biotransformation of other drugs whose metabolic fate, therefore, cosegregates with the debrisoquin trait. A similar situation occurs with other oxidative polymorphisms that characterize the metabolism of mephenytoin and possibly tolbutamide. The situation is further complicated by interethnic differences in the frequency of the polymorphisms. For example, impaired hydroxylation of mephenytoin is present in only 3 to 5 percent of whites, but the incidence is about 20 percent in individuals of Japanese descent; likewise, the frequency of the PM phenotype for debrisoquin hydroxylation appears to decrease as one moves from western (8 to 10 percent) to eastern (0 to 1 percent) population groups.

Polymorphisms in drug metabolizing ability may be associated with large differences in the disposition of the drug among individuals, especially when the involved pathway is a major contribution to the overall elimination of the drug. For example, the oral clearance of mephenytoin differs 100- to 200-fold between individuals of the EM and PM phenotypes. As a result, peak plasma concentrations and bioavailability after oral administration may be profoundly increased and the rate of drug elimination decreased in PM individuals. This in turn results in drug accumulation and exaggerated pharmacologic responses, including toxicity, when usual drug dosages are administered to patients with the PM phenotype. Effective individualization of drug therapy is even more critical when using drugs exhibiting polymorphic drug metabolism.

CONCENTRATION OF DRUGS IN PLASMA AS A GUIDE TO THERAPY

Optimal individualization of therapy is assisted by measuring the concentration of certain drugs in plasma. Genetic variation in elimination rates, interactions with other drugs, disease-induced alterations in elimination and distribution, and other factors combine to yield a wide range of plasma levels in patients given the same dose. Furthermore, the problem of noncompliance with prescribed regimens during continuing therapy is an endemic and elusive cause of therapeutic failure (see below). Clinical indicators assist the titration of some drugs into the desired range, and no chemical determination is a substitute for careful observations of the response to treatment. However, the therapeutic and adverse effects are not precisely quantifiable for all drugs, and in complex clinical situations estimates of the action of a drug may be misleading. For example, previously existing neurologic disease may obscure the neurologic consequences of intoxication with phenytoin. Because clearance, half-life, accumulation, and steady state plasma levels are difficult to predict, the measurement of plasma levels is often useful as a guide to the optimal dose. This is particularly so when there is a narrow range between the plasma levels yielding therapeutic and adverse effects. For drugs having such characteristics, e.g., digoxin, theophylline, lidocaine, aminoglycosides, and anticonvulsants, numerous dosing methods have been developed in an attempt to improve the relationship between dosing, plasma drug concentration, and response. Some of these methods are accurate and useful, for example, the Bayesian feedback approach, but others are not accurate or have not been sufficiently validated. Further examination of their cost effectiveness is necessary to establish their place in routine patient care.

The variability among individual responses to given plasma levels must be recognized. This is illustrated by a hypothetical population

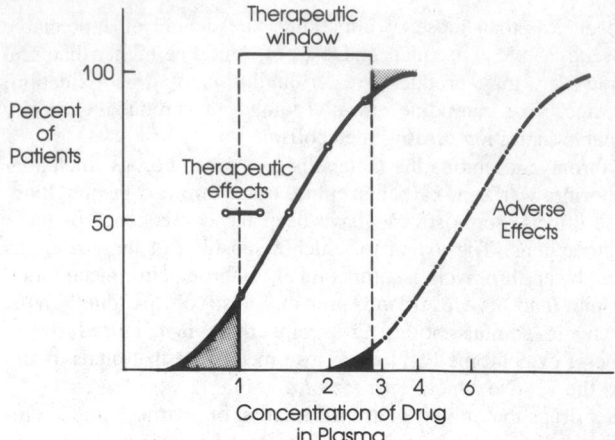

FIGURE 65-5 The cumulative percentage of patients responding to increasing levels of drug in plasma with both therapeutic and adverse effects. The therapeutic "window" defines the range of concentrations of drug that will achieve therapeutic effects in most patients with adverse effects in only a small percentage.

dose-response curve (Fig. 65-5) and its relationship to the therapeutic range or therapeutic "window" of desired plasma levels. The defined therapeutic window should include the levels at which the majority of patients achieve the intended pharmacologic effect. However, a few people are sensitive to the therapeutic effects of most drugs, responding to lower levels, whereas others are sufficiently refractory as to require levels that impose the likelihood of adverse effects as a price for therapeutic benefit. For example, a few patients with strong seizure foci require plasma levels of phenytoin exceeding 20 μg/mL to control seizures. Dosages to achieve this effect may be appropriate.

As also illustrated in Fig. 65-5, some patients are prone to adverse effects at levels that are tolerated by most of the population, and therefore elevation of levels to those with a high probability of therapeutic effect may bring on unwanted actions in the exceptional patient. Table 65-4 presents the concentrations of a number of drugs in plasma that are associated with adverse and therapeutic effects in most patients. Its use within the guidelines discussed should permit more effective and safer therapy for those patients who are not "average."

TABLE 65-4 Concentrations of drugs in plasma: Relation to efficacy and adverse effects

Drug	Efficacy*	Adverse effects†
Amikacin (peak)	20 μg/mL	40 μg/mL
Carbenicillin	100 μg/mL‡	300 μg/mL
Carbamazepine	3 μg/mL	10 μg/mL
Digitoxin	12 ng/mL	25–30 ng/mL
Digoxin	0.8 ng/mL	2.0 ng/mL
Ethosuximide	40 μg/mL	100 μg/mL
Gentamicin (peak)	5 μg/mL	10 μg/mL
Gentamicin (predose)		2.5 μg/mL
Lidocaine	1.5 μg/mL	5 μg/mL
Lithium	0.5 meq/liter	1.3 meq/liter
Penicillin G	1–25 μg/mL¶	
Phenytoin (diphenylhydantoin)	10 μg/mL	20 μg/mL
Procainamide	4 μg/mL	10 μg/mL
Quinidine	2.5 μg/mL	6 μg/mL
Theophylline	8 μg/mL	20 μg/mL

* The therapeutic effect is infrequent or slight at levels below these.
† The frequency of adverse effects increases sharply when these levels are exceeded.
‡ Minimal inhibitory concentration (MIC) for most strains of Pseudomonas aeruginosa. MIC for other, more sensitive, organisms is less.
§ Dependent on the MIC. Higher levels may be desired when host defenses are impaired.
¶ There is a wide range of MIC of penicillin for various organisms, and the MIC of all those for which penicillin is used is < 20. "Massive" penicillin therapy with 20 million units daily achieves levels of 20 to 25 μg/mL in patients with clearance of creatinine of 100 mL/min.

EFFECTIVE PARTICIPATION OF THE PATIENT IN THERAPEUTIC PROGRAMS Measurement of the concentration of a drug in plasma is the most effective approach to determining when patients have failed to take the drug. Such "noncompliance" is a frequent problem in the long-term treatment of diseases such as hypertension and epilepsy, occurring in 25 percent or more of patients in therapeutic environments that lack special efforts to involve patients in the responsibility for their own health. Occasionally, noncompliance can be uncovered by sympathetic, nonincriminating questioning, but more often it is recognized only after determining that the concentration of drug in plasma is nil or is recurrently low. Because other factors can cause plasma levels to be lower than expected, comparison with levels obtained during inpatient treatment may be required to confirm that noncompliance did, in fact, occur. Once the physician is certain of noncompliance, a nonaccusatory discussion of the problem with the patient may elucidate a reason for the noncompliance and serve as a basis for more effective participation of the patient in the care subsequently. Many approaches have been tried to enhance the patients' exercise of responsibility for their own treatment, most based on improved communication regarding the nature of the disease and the expectations of treatment success and treatment failure. This communication includes an opportunity for the patient to relate problems associated with treatment, and it may be improved by involving nurses and other paramedical personnel in the process. Minimizing the complexity of the regimen is helpful, both in terms of the number of drugs and the frequency of administration. Educating patients to assume the principal role in their own health care requires a blend of the art and science of medicine.

REFERENCES

BENET LZ, SHEINER LB: Design and optimization of dosage regimens: Pharmacokinetic data, in *Goodman and Gilman's The Pharmacological Basis of Therapeutics*, 7th ed. AG Gilman et al (eds). New York, Macmillan, 1985, p 1663, Appendix II.

BENNETT WM et al: *Drug Prescribing in Renal Failure. Dosing Guidelines for Adults*. Philadelphia, American College of Physicians, 1987

BURTON ME et al: Comparison of drug dosing methods. Clin Pharmacokinet 10:1, 1985

CHENNAVASIN P, BRATER DC: Nomograms for drug use in renal disease. Clin Pharmacokinet 6:193, 1981

ROWLAND M, TOZER TN: *Clinical Pharmacokinetics—Concepts and Applications*, 2d ed. Philadelphia, Lea & Febiger, 1988

SHAND DG et al: Pharmacokinetic drug interactions, in *Handbook of Experimental Pharmacology*, vol 28: *Concepts in Biochemical Pharmacology*, JR Gillette, JR Mitchell (eds). New York, Springer Verlag, 1975, p 272

SHEINER LB, TOZER TN: Clinical pharmacokinetics: The use of plasma concentrations of drugs, in *Clinical Pharmacology: Basic Principles in Therapeutics*, 2d ed, KL Melmon, HF Morrelli (eds). New York, Macmillan, 1978, p 71

66 ADVERSE REACTIONS TO DRUGS

ALASTAIR J. J. WOOD / JOHN A. OATES

The beneficial effects of drugs are coupled with the inescapable risk of untoward effects. The morbidity and mortality from these untoward effects often present diagnostic problems because they can involve every organ and system of the body.

Major advances in the investigation, development, and regulation of drugs ensure in most instances their uniformity, effectiveness, and relative safety, as well as identify their recognized hazards. However, the large number and variety of drugs available over the counter (OTC) or by prescription make it impossible for patient or physician to obtain or retain the knowledge necessary to use all drugs well. It is understandable, therefore, that many OTC drugs are used unwisely by the public and that restricted drugs may be prescribed incorrectly by physicians.

Most physicians use no more than 50 drug products in their practice, gaining familiarity with their effectiveness and safety. Most patients probably use only a limited number of OTC drugs. Nevertheless, many patients receive care and drug prescriptions from more than one physician, and in any 30-day period patients consume more than three different OTC drug products containing nine or more different chemical agents.

Twenty-five to fifty percent of patients may make errors in self-administration of prescribed medicines, and this can be responsible for adverse drug effects. Elderly patients are most likely to commit such errors. One-third or more of patients also may not take their prescribed medications. Similarly, patients commit errors in taking OTC drugs by not reading or following the directions for use of the medicines on the containers. Physicians must recognize that providing directions with prescriptions does not always guarantee compliance.

Every drug can produce untoward consequences, even when used according to standard or recommended methods of administration. When used incorrectly, the effectiveness may be reduced, and adverse reactions can be expected to occur more frequently. The administration of several drugs during the same period of time also may result in adverse interactions between drugs (see Chap. 65).

In the hospital all drugs a patient is given should be under the control of a physician, and patient compliance is, in general, ensured. Errors may occur nevertheless, in that the wrong drug or dose may be given, or the drug may be given to the wrong patient, although improved drug distribution and administration systems have reduced this problem. On the other hand, there are no means for controlling how ambulatory patients take prescription or OTC drugs.

EPIDEMIOLOGY Epidemiologic studies of adverse drug reactions have been helpful in evaluating the magnitude of the overall problem, in calculating the rate of reactions to individual drugs, and in characterizing some of the determinants of adverse drug effects.

Patients receive on the average 10 different drugs during each hospitalization. The sicker the patient, the more drugs are given, and there is a corresponding increase in the likelihood of adverse drug reactions. When fewer than 6 different drugs are given to hospitalized patients, the probability of an adverse reaction is about 5 percent, but if more than 15 drugs are given, the probability is over 40 percent. Retrospective analyses of ambulatory patients have revealed adverse drug effects in 20 percent.

Thus, the magnitude of drug-induced disease is large. Two to five percent of patients are admitted to the medical and pediatric services of general hospitals because of illnesses attributed to drugs. The case/fatality ratio from drug-induced disease in hospitalized patients varies from 2 to 12 percent. Furthermore, some fetal or neonatal abnormalities are due to medicines taken by the mother during pregnancy or parturition.

A small group of widely used drugs account for a disproportionate number of reactions; aspirin, digoxin, anticoagulants, diuretics, antimicrobials, steroids, and hypoglycemic agents account for 90 percent of reactions.

ETIOLOGY Most adverse reactions can be classified into two groups. The most frequent result from the exaggerated but predicted pharmacologic action of the drug. Other adverse reactions ensue from toxic effects unrelated to the intended pharmacologic actions. These therefore are often unpredictable, are frequently severe, and result from recognized as well as undiscovered mechanisms. Some mechanisms of extrapharmacologic toxicity include direct cytotoxicity, initiation of abnormal immune responses, and perturbation of metabolic processes in individuals with genetic enzymatic defects.

EXAGGERATION OF THE INTENDED PHARMACOLOGIC EFFECT By prior consideration of the known factors that modify drug action, these adverse reactions often are preventable.

Abnormally high drug concentration at the receptor site (site of action) due to the pharmacokinetic variability is the usual cause (see Chap. 65). For example, reduction in the volume of distribution, in the rate of metabolism, or in the rate of excretion all result in higher than expected concentration of drug at the receptor site with consequent increase in pharmacologic effect.

Alteration in the dose-response curve due to increased receptor sensitivity results in an increase in drug effect at the same concentration. An example of this is seen in the excessive response to the anticoagulant warfarin at normal or lower than normal blood levels in the elderly.

The shape of the dose-response curve itself also determines the likelihood of the development of adverse drug reactions. Drugs with a steep dose-response curve are more likely to be associated with dose-related toxicity because of the small increase in dose required to produce a large change in pharmacologic effect. An increase in the dose of drugs which exhibit nonlinear kinetics, such as phenytoin (see previous chapter), may produce a proportionately greater increase in the blood level, resulting in toxicity.

Concomitant drug therapy may affect the pharmacokinetics or pharmacodynamics of other drugs. Pharmacokinetics may be affected by alterations in bioavailability, protein binding, or the rate of metabolism or excretion. Pharmacodynamics may be altered by competition for receptor sites, by prevention of the drug's reaching its site of action, or by antagonism or enhancement of the drug's pharmacologic effect. These subjects are discussed in detail in the previous chapter.

TOXICITY UNRELATED TO A DRUG'S PRIMARY PHARMACO-LOGIC ACTIVITY   Cytotoxic reactions   The understanding of so-called idiosyncratic reactions has greatly improved with the recognition that many of these reactions are due to irreversible binding of drug or metabolites to tissue macromolecules by shared electron (covalent) bonds. Some chemical carcinogens such as the alkylating agents combine directly with DNA. Usually, it is only after metabolic activation to reactive metabolites that covalent binding occurs. This activation usually occurs in the microsomal mixed-function oxidase system, the hepatic enzyme system responsible for the metabolism of many drugs (Chap. 65). During the course of drug metabolism, reactive metabolites may covalently bind to tissue macromolecules, causing tissue damage. Because of the reactive nature of these metabolites, covalent binding often occurs close to the site of production, such as the liver, but the mixed-function oxidase system is found in other tissues as well.

An example of this type of adverse drug reaction is the hepato-toxicity associated with isoniazid, which is metabolized principally by acetylation to acetylisoniazid, which is then hydrolyzed to ace-tylhydrazine. The further metabolism of acetylhydrazine by the mixed-function oxidase system liberates reactive metabolites that covalently bind to hepatic macromolecules, causing hepatic necrosis. The administration of drugs known to increase the activity of the mixed-function oxidase system, such as phenobarbital or rifampin, together with isoniazid, is associated with the production of increased amounts of reactive metabolites, increased covalent binding, and hepatic damage.

The hepatic necrosis produced by overdosage of acetaminophen is also caused by reactive metabolites. Normally these metabolites are detoxified by combining with hepatic glutathione. When gluta-thione becomes exhausted, the metabolites bind instead to hepatic protein with resultant hepatocyte damage. The hepatic necrosis produced by the ingestion of acetaminophen can be prevented, or at least attenuated, by the administration of substances such as *N*-acetylcysteine, which reduce the binding of electrophilic metabolites to hepatic proteins. The risks of hepatic necrosis are increased in patients receiving drugs such as phenobarbital that increase the rate of drug metabolism and rate of production of toxic metabolite(s).

It is likely, though as yet unproved, that other idiosyncratic reactions are caused by the covalent binding of reactive metabolites to tissue macromolecules, with either direct cytotoxicity or via the initiation of an immunologic response.

Immunologic mechanisms   Most pharmacologic agents are poor immunogens since they consist of small molecules with molecular weights less than 2000. Stimulation of antibody synthesis or sensitization of lymphocytes by a drug or one of its metabolites usually requires in vivo activation and covalent linkage to protein, carbohydrate, or nucleic acid.

Drug stimulation of antibody production may mediate tissue injury by one of several mechanisms. The antibody may attack the drug affixed to a cell by covalent linkage and thereby destroy the cell, as occurs in penicillin-induced hemolytic anemia. Complexes of antibody-drug-antigen may be passively adsorbed by a bystander cell which is destroyed by activation of complement; this occurs in quinine- and quinidine-induced thrombocytopenia. Drugs or their reactive metabolites may alter host tissue, rendering it antigenic, and stimulate autoantibodies; for example, hydralazine and procainamide can chemically alter nuclear material, stimulate formation of anti-nuclear antibodies, and occasionally cause lupus erythematosus. Autoantibodies may be stimulated by drugs which neither interact with the host antigen nor have any chemical similarity to the host tissue; for example, alpha methyldopa frequently stimulates formation of antibodies to host erythrocytes, yet the drug does not itself attach to the erythrocyte or share any chemical similarities with the antigenic determinants on the erythrocyte.

Drug-induced *pure red cell aplasia* (Chap. 298) is due to an immunologic-based drug reaction. Red cell formation in bone marrow cultures can be inhibited by phenytoin and purified IgG obtained from a patient with pure red cell aplasia associated with phenytoin.

Serum sickness (Chap. 267) results from deposition of circulating drug-antibody complexes on endothelial surfaces. Complement activation occurs, chemotactic factors are generated locally, and an inflammatory response appears at the site of complex entrapment. Arthralgias, urticaria, lymphadenopathy, glomerulonephritis, or cerebritis may result. Penicillin is the most common cause of serum sickness today. Many drugs, particularly the antimicrobial agents, induce production of IgE, which affixes to mast cell membranes. Contact with a drug antigen initiates a series of biochemical events within the mast cell and results in the release of mediators that may produce urticaria, wheezing, flushing, rhinorrhea, and occasionally hypotension characteristic of anaphylaxis.

Drugs may also excite cell-mediated immune responses. Topically administered substances may interact with sulfhydryl or amino groups in the skin and react with sensitized lymphocytes to produce the rash characteristic of contact dermatitis. Other types of rashes may also appear from the interaction of serum factors, drugs, and sensitized lymphocytes. The role of drug-activated lymphocytes in the immune mechanisms governing destruction of visceral tissue is unknown.

Toxicity associated with genetically determined enzymatic defects   In the porphyrias, drugs that increase the activity of enzymes proximal to the deficient enzyme in the biosynthetic pathway of porphyrins can increase the quantity of porphyrin precursors that accumulate proximal to the deficient enzyme (Chap. 328). These drugs are listed in Table 66-1.

Patients with a deficiency of glucose-6-phosphate dehydrogenase (G6PD) develop hemolytic anemia on primaquine and a number of other drugs (Table 66-1) that do not cause hemolysis in patients with adequate quantities of this enzyme (Chap. 294).

Diagnosis   The manifestations of drug-induced diseases frequently resemble those of other diseases and may be produced by different and dissimilar drugs. Recognition of the role of a drug or drugs responsible for illness is dependent upon appreciation of the possible adverse reactions to drugs in any disease, identification of a temporal relationship between drug administration and development of illness, and familiarity with the manifestations most often caused by particular drugs. Although specific reactions have been described as resulting from the use of particular drugs, there is always a ''first,'' and any drug should be suspected of causing an adverse effect if the clinical setting is appropriate.

Illness related to a drug's pharmacologic action may be more easily recognized than illness attributable to immunologic or other mechanisms. For example, side effects such as cardiac arrhythmias in patients receiving digitalis, hypoglycemia in patients given insulin, and bleeding in patients receiving anticoagulants are more easily related to the drug than are symptoms like fever or rash, which may be caused by many drugs or by other factors.

TABLE 66-1 Clinical manifestations of adverse reactions to drugs

I MULTISYSTEM MANIFESTATIONS

Anaphylaxis	Angioedema	Drug-induced lupus	Fever
Cephalosporins	Captopril	erythematosus	Aminosalicylic acid
Demeclocycline	Enalapril	Acebutolol	Amphotericin B
Dextran	Lisinopril	Asparaginase	Antihistamines
Insulin		Barbiturates	Novobiocin
Iodinated drugs or contrast		Bleomycin	Penicillins
media		Cephalosporins	Hyperpyrexia
Iron dextran		Hydralazine	Antipsychotics
Lidocaine		Iodides	Serum sickness
Penicillins		Isoniazid	Aspirin
Procaine		Methyldopa	Penicillins
Streptomycin		Phenolphthalein	Propylthiouracil
Sulfobromophthalein		Phenytoin	Streptomycin
		Procainamide	Sulfonamides
		Quinidine	
		Sulfonamides	
		Thiouracil	

II ENDOCRINE MANIFESTATIONS

Addisonian-like syndrome	Sexual dysfunction	Thyroid function tests,	Vaginal carcinoma
Busulfan	*1* Impaired ejaculation:	disorders of	Diethylstilbestrol (given to
Ketoconazole	Bethanidine	Acetazolamide	mother)
Galactorrhea (may also	Debrisoquin	Amiodarone	
cause amenorrhea)	Guanethidine	Bromsulfophthalein	
Methyldopa	Thioridazine	Chlorpropamide	
Phenothiazines	*2* Decreased libido and	Clofibrate	
Reserpine	impotence:	Colestipol and	
Tricyclic antidepressants	Beta blockers	nicotinic acid	
Gynecomastia	Clonidine	Dimercaprol	
Calcium channel	Diuretics	Gold salts	
antagonists	Lithium	Iodides	
Digitalis	Major tranquilizers	Lithium	
Estrogens	Methyldopa	Oral contraceptives	
Ethionamide	Oral contraceptives	Phenindione	
Griseofulvin	Sedatives	Phenothiazines (long-term)	
Isoniazid	*3* Impairment of	Phenylbutazone	
Methyldopa	spermatogenesis or	Phenytoin	
Phenytoin	oogenesis:	Sulfonamides	
Reserpine	Cytotoxics	Tolbutamide	
Spironolactone	*4* Priapism:		
Testosterone	Trazodone		

III METABOLIC MANIFESTATIONS

Hyperbilirubinemia	Hyperkalemia	Hyperuricemia	Metabolic acidosis
Novobiocin	Angiotensin-converting	Aspirin	Acetazolamide
Rifampin	enzyme inhibitors	Chlorthalidone	Paraldehyde (degraded)
Hypercalcemia	Amiloride	Cytotoxics	Phenformin
Antacids with absorbable	Cytotoxics	Ethacrynic acid	Salicylates
alkali	Digitalis overdose	Fructose (IV)	Spironolactone
Thiazides	Heparin	Furosemide	Porphyria exacerbation
Vitamin D	Lithium	Hyperalimentation	Barbiturates
Hyperglycemia	Potassium preparations	Thiazides	Chlordiazepoxide
Chlorthalidone	including salt substitute	Hyponatremia	Chlorpropamide
Diazoxide	Potassium salts of drugs	*1* Dilutional:	Estrogens
Encainide	Spironolactone	Carbamazepine	Glutethimide
Ethacrynic acid	Succinylcholine	Chlorpropamide	Griseofulvin
Furosemide	Triamterene	Cyclophosphamide	Meprobamate
Glucocorticoids	Hypokalemia	Diuretics	Oral contraceptives
Growth hormone	Alkali-induced alkalosis	Octreotide	Phenytoin
Oral contraceptives	Amphotericin B	Vincristine	Rifampin
Thiazides	Carbenoxolone	*2* Salt wasting:	Sulfonamides
Hypoglycemia	Corticosteroids	Diuretics	
Insulin	Diuretics	Enemas	
Oral hypoglycemics	Gentamicin	Mannitol	
Quinine	Insulin		
	Laxative abuse		
	Mineralocorticoids,		
	some glucocorticoids		
	Osmotic diuretics		
	Sympathomimetics		
	Tetracycline (degraded)		
	Theophylline		
	Vitamin B_{12}		

(continued)

TABLE 66-1   Clinical manifestations of adverse reactions to drugs (continued)

IV DERMATOLOGIC MANIFESTATIONS

Acne
  Anabolic and androgenic
    steroids
  Bromides
  Glucocorticoids
  Iodides
  Isoniazid
  Oral contraceptives
  Troxidone
Alopecia
  Cytotoxics
  Ethionamide
  Heparin
  Oral contraceptives
    (withdrawal)
Eczema
  Captopril
  Cream and lotion
    preservatives
  Lanolin
  Topical antihistamines
  Topical antimicrobials
  Topical local anesthetics

Erythema multiforme or
  Steven-Johnson
  syndrome
  Barbiturates
  Chlorpropamide
  Codeine
  Ethosuximide
  Penicillins
  Phenylbutazone
  Phenytoin
  Salicylates
  Sulfonamides
  Sulfones
  Tetracyclines
  Thiazides
Erythema nodosum
  Oral contraceptives
  Penicillins
  Sulfonamides
Exfoliative dermatitis
  Barbiturates
  Gold salts
  Penicillins
  Phenylbutazone
  Phenytoin
  Quinidine
  Sulfonamides
Fixed drug eruptions
  Barbiturates
  Captopril
  Phenolphthalein
  Phenylbutazone
  Quinine
  Salicylates
  Sulfonamides

Hyperpigmentation
  Bleomycin
  Busulfan
  Chloroquine and other
    antimalarials
  Corticotropin
  Cyclophosphamide
  Gold salts
  Hypervitaminosis A
  Oral contraceptives
  Phenothiazines
Lichenoid eruptions
  Aminosalicylic acid
  Antimalarials
  Chlorpropamide
  Gold salts
  Methyldopa
  Phenothiazines
Photodermatitis
  Captopril
  Chlordiazepoxide
  Furosemide
  Griseofulvin
  Nalidixic acid
  Oral contraceptives
  Phenothiazines
  Sulfonamides
  Sulfonylureas
  Tetracyclines, particularly
    demeclocycline
  Thiazides
Purpura (see also
    thrombocytopenia)
  Aspirin
  Glucocorticoids

Rashes (nonspecific)
  Allopurinol
  Ampicillin
  Barbiturates
  Indapamide
  Methyldopa
  Phenytoin
Skin necrosis
  Warfarin
Toxic epidermal necrolysis
    (bullous)
  Allopurinol
  Barbiturates
  Bromides
  Iodides
  Nalidixic acid
  Penicillins
  Phenolphthalein
  Phenylbutazone
  Phenytoin
  Sulfonamides
Urticaria
  Aspirin
  Barbiturates
  Captopril
  Enalapril
  Penicillins
  Sulfonamides

V HEMATOLOGIC MANIFESTATIONS

Agranulocytosis (see also
    pancytopenia)
  Aprindine
  Captopril
  Carbimazole
  Chloramphenicol
  Cotrimoxazole
  Cytotoxics
  Gold salts
  Indomethacin
  Methimazole
  Oxyphenbutazone
  Phenothiazines
  Phenylbutazone
  Propylthiouracil
  Sulfonamides
  Tolbutamide
  Tricyclic antidepressants
Clotting abnormalities/
    Hypothrombinemia
  Cefamandole
  Cefoperazone
  Moxalactam
Eosinophilia
  Aminosalicylic acid
  Chlorpropamide
  Erythromycin estolate
  Imipramine
  l-Tryptophan
  Methotrexate
  Nitrofurantoin
  Procarbazine
  Sulfonamides

Hemolytic anemia
  Aminosalicylic acid
  Cephalosporins
  Chlorpromazine
  Dapsone
  Insulin
  Isoniazid
  Levodopa
  Mefenamic acid
  Melphalan
  Methyldopa
  Penicillins
  Phenacetin
  Procainamide
  Quinidine
  Rifampin
  Sulfonamides
Hemolytic anemia (in G6PD
    deficiency)
  Aminosalicylic acid
  Antimalarials, e.g.,
    primaquine
  Aspirin
  Chloramphenicol
  Cotrimoxazole
  Dapsone
  Nalidixic acid
  Nitrofurantoin
  Phenacetin
  Probenecid
  Procainamide
  Quinidine
  Sulfonamides
  Vitamin C
  Vitamin K

Leukocytosis
  Glucocorticoids
  Lithium
Lymphadenopathy
  Phenytoin
  Primidone
Megaloblastic anemia
  Cotrimoxazole
  Folate antagonists
  Nitrous oxide (repeated or
    prolonged exposure)
  Oral contraceptives
  Phenobarbital
  Phenytoin
  Primidone
  Triamterene
  Trimethoprim
Pancytopenia (aplastic
    anemia)
  Carbamazepine
  Chloramphenicol
  Cytotoxics
  Gold salts
  Mepacrine
  Mephenytoin
  Oxyphenbutazone
  Phenylbutazone
  Phenytoin
  Potassium perchlorate
  Quinacrine
  Sulfonamides
  Trimethadione
  Zidovudine (AZT)

Pure red cell aplasia
  Azathioprine
  Chlorpropamide
  Isoniazid
  Phenytoin
Thrombocytopenia
    (see also pancytopenia)
  Acetazolamine
  Aspirin
  Carbamazepine
  Carbenacillin
  Carbenicillin
  Chlorpropamide
  Chlorthalidone
  Cotrimoxazole
  Digitoxin
  Furosemide
  Gold salts
  Heparin
  Indomethacin
  Isoniazid
  Methyldopa
  Moxalactam
  Novobiocin
  Oxyphenbutazone
  Phenylbutazone
  Phenytoin and other
    hydantoins
  Quinidine
  Quinine
  Thiazides
  Ticarcillin

(continued)

Once an adverse reaction is suspected, discontinuance of the suspected drug followed by disappearance of the reaction is presumptive evidence of a drug-induced illness. Reappearance of the reaction upon cautious readministration of the drug may provide confirmatory evidence of the relationship if such confirmation adds useful information to the future management of the patient without entailing undue risk. With concentration-dependent adverse reactions, lowering the dosage may also be followed by disappearance of the reaction, and increasing the dose may cause it to reappear. When the reaction is thought to be allergic, however, readministration

TABLE 66-1 Clinical manifestations of adverse reactions to drugs (continued)

VI CARDIOVASCULAR MANIFESTATIONS

Acute chest pain (nonischemic)	Arrhythmias	Fluid retention or congestive heart failure	Hypertension
Bleomycin	Adriamycin	Carbenoxolone	Clonidine withdrawal
Angina exacerbation	Antiarrhythmic drugs	Diazoxide	Corticotropin
Alpha blockers	Atropine	Estrogens	Cyclosporinc
Ergotamine	Anticholinesterases	Indomethacin	Glucocorticoids
Excessive thyroxine	Beta blockers	Mannitol	Monoamine oxidase inhibitors with sympathomimetics
Hydralazine	Daunomycin	Minoxidil	
Methysergide	Digitalis	Phenylbutazone	NSAIDs (some)
Minoxidil	Emetine	Propranolol	Oral contraceptives
Nifedipine	Guanethidine	Steroids	Sympathomimetics
Oxytocin	Lithium	Verapamil	Tricyclic antidepressants with sympathomimetics
Propranolol withdrawal	Papaverine	Hypotension (see also arrhythmias)	
Vasopressin	Phenothiazines, particularly thioridazine	Calcium channel blockers, e.g., nifedipine	Pericarditis
	Sympathomimetics	Citrated blood	Emetine
	Thyroid hormone	Diuretics	Hydralazine
	Tricyclic antidepressants	Levodopa	Methysergide
	Verapamil	Morphine	Procainamide
	AV block	Nitroglycerin	Thromboembolism
	Clonidine	Phenothiazines	Oral contraceptives
	Methylclopa	Protamine	
	Verapamil	Quinidine	
	Cardiomyopathy		
	Adriamycin		
	Daunorubicin		
	Emetine		
	Lithium		
	Phenothiazines		
	Sulfonamides		
	Sympathomimetics		

VII RESPIRATORY MANIFESTATIONS

Airway obstruction (bronchospasm, asthma; see also anaphylaxis)	Cough	Pulmonary infiltrates	Respiratory depression
Beta blockers	Angiotensin-converting enzyme inhibitors	Amiodarone	Aminoglycosides
Cephalosporins	Nasal congestion	Azothioprine	Hypnotics
Cholinergic drugs	Decongestant abuse	Bleomycin	Opiates
Nonsteroidal anti-inflammatory drugs, e.g., aspirin, indomethacin	Guanethidine	Busulfan	Polymyxins
	Isoproterenol	Carmustine (BCNU)	Sedatives
	Oral contraceptives	Chlorambucil	Trimethaphan
Penicillins	Reserpine	Cyclophosphamide	
Pentazocine	Pulmonary edema	Melphalan	
Streptomycin	Contrast media	Methotrexate	
Tartrazine (drugs with yellow dye)	Heroin	Methysergide	
	Hydrochlorthiazide	Mitomycin C	
	Methadone	Nitrofurantoin	
	Propoxyphene	Procarbazine	
		Sulfonamides	*(continued)*

of the drug may be hazardous, since anaphylactic shock may develop. Readministration is unwise under these conditions unless alternative drugs are not available and treatment is mandatory.

If the patient is receiving many different drugs when an adverse reaction is suspected, the drugs most likely to be incriminated can usually be identified. All drugs may be discontinued at once, or if this is not practical, then drugs should be discontinued one at a time, starting with the drug under greatest suspicion, and the patient observed for signs of improvement. The time taken for the disappearance of a concentration-dependent adverse effect depends on the time for the concentration to fall below the range associated with the adverse effect, and this in turn depends on the initial blood level and on the rate of elimination or metabolism of the drug. Adverse effects of drugs with long half-lives, such as phenobarbital, take a considerable time to disappear.

Drugs recognized as producing a number of reactions are listed in Table 66-1. This table includes well-documented and some less well-documented reactions that are sufficiently devastating as to require consideration. It should be used to suggest the likely causative drug, but the absence of a drug from the table does not mean that it is not responsible for the reaction.

Serum antibody has been demonstrated in some persons with drug allergy involving cellular blood elements, as in agranulocytosis, hemolytic anemia, and thrombocytopenia. For example, both quinine and quinidine can produce platelet agglutination in vitro in the presence of complement and the serum from a patient who has developed thrombocytopenia following this drug.

Eliciting a drug history from patients is important for diagnosis. Attention must be directed to nonprescription, or OTC, as well as to prescription drugs. Each type can be responsible for adverse drug effects, and adverse interactions may occur between OTC drugs and prescribed drugs. In addition, it is common for patients to be cared for by several physicians, and duplicative, additive, counteractive, or synergistic drugs may therefore be taken if the physicians are not aware of the patients' drug histories. Every physician should determine what drugs a patient has been taking, at least during the preceding 30 days, before prescribing any medications. A history of previous adverse drug effects in patients is common. Since these patients have a predisposition to other drug-induced illnesses, eliciting such a history should dictate added caution in prescribing drugs.

Patients with biochemical abnormalities such as erythrocyte G6PD deficiency can be identified; patients with the defect are usually blacks or of Mediterranean descent. Drug-induced hemolytic crisis can be avoided by testing for the enzyme defect before administering these

TABLE 66-1   Clinical manifestations of adverse reactions to drugs *(continued)*

VIII GASTROINTESTINAL MANIFESTATIONS

Cholestatic jaundice
  Acetohexamide
  Anabolic steroids
  Androgens
  Chlorpropamide
  Erythromycin estolate
  Gold salts
  Methimazole
  Nitrofurantoin
  Oral contraceptives
  Phenothiazines
Constipation or ileus
  Aluminum hydroxide
  Barium sulfate
  Calcium carbonate
  Ferrous sulfate
  Ganglionic blockers
  Ion exchange resins
  Opiates
  Phenothiazines
  Tricyclic antidepressants
  Verapamil
Diarrhea or colitis
  Antibiotics (broad-
    spectrum)
  Clindamycin
  Colchicine
  Digitalis
  Guanethidine
  Lactose excipients
  Lincomycin
  Magnesium in antacids
  Methyldopa
  Purgatives
  Reserpine

Diffuse hepatocellular
  damage
  Acetaminophen
    (paracetamol)
  Allopurinol
  Aminosalicylic acid
  Aprindine
  Dapsone
  Erythromycin estolate
  Ethionamide
  Glyburide
  Halothane
  Isoniazid
  Ketoconazole
  Methimazole
  Methotrexate
  Methoxyflurane
  Methyldopa
  Monoamine oxidase
    inhibitors
  Niacin
  Nifedipine
  Nitrofurantoin
  Oxyphenisatin
  Phenytoin and other
    hydantoins
  Propoxyphene
  Propylthiouracil
  Pyridium
  Rifampin
  Salicylates
  Sodium valproate
  Sulfonamides
  Tetracyclines
  Verapamil
  Zidovudine (AZT)

Intestinal ulceration
  Solid KCl preparations
Malabsorption
  Aminosalicylic acid
  Antibiotics (broad-
    spectrum)
  Cholestyramine
  Colchicine
  Colestipol
  Cytotoxics
  Neomycin
  Phenobarbital
  Phenytoin
  Primidone
Nausea or vomiting
  Digitalis
  Estrogens
  Ferrous sulfate
  Levodopa
  Opiates
  Potassium chloride
  Tetracyclines
  Theophylline
Oral conditions
  1 Dental discoloration:
    Tetracycline
  2 Drymouth:
    Anticholinergics
    Clonidine
    Levodopa
    Methyldopa
    Tricyclic antidepressants
  3 Gingival hyperplasia:
    Calcium antagonists
    Cyclosporine
    Phenytoin

4 Salivary gland swelling:
    Bethanidine
    Bretylium
    Clonidine
    Guanethidine
    Iodides
    Phenylbutazone
5 Taste disturbances:
    Biguanides
    Captopril
    Griseofulvin
    Lithium
    Metronidazole
    Penicillamine
    Rifampin
6 Ulceration:
    Aspirin
    Cytotoxics
    Gentian violet
    Isoproterenol (sublingual)
    Pancreatin
Pancreatitis
  Azathioprine
  Ethacrynic acid
  Furosemide
  Glucocorticoids
  Opiates
  Oral contraceptives
  Sulfonamides
  Thiazides
Peptic ulceration or
    hemorrhage
  Aspirin
  Ethacrynic acid
  Glucocorticoids
  NSAIDs
  Reserpine (large doses)

IX RENAL MANIFESTATIONS

Bladder dysfunction
  Anticholinergics
  Disopyramide
  Monoamine oxidase
    inhibitors
  Tricyclic antidepressants
Calculi
  Acetazolamide
  Vitamin D
Concentrating defect with
    polyuria (or
    nephrogenic diabetes
    insipidus)
  Demeclocycline
  Lithium
  Methoxyflurane
  Vitamin D

Hemorrhage cystitis
  Cyclophosphamide
Interstitial nephritis
  Allopurinol
  Furosemide
  Penicillins, esp.
    methicillin
  Phenindione
  Sulfonamides
  Thiazides
Nephropathies
  Due to analgesics
    (e.g., phenacetin)

Nephrotic syndrome
  Captopril
  Gold salts
  Penicillamine
  Phenindione
  Probenecid
Obstructive uropathy
  Extrarenal: methysergide
  Intrarenal: cytotoxics
Renal dysfunction
  Cyclosporine
  NSAIDs
  Triamterene
Renal tubular acidosis
  Acetazolamide
  Amphotericin B
  Degraded tetracycline

Tubular necrosis
  Aminoglycosides
  Amphotericin B
  Cephaloridine
  Colistin
  Cyclosporin
  Methoxyflurane
  Polymyxins
  Radioiodinated contrast
    medium
  Sulfonamides
  Tetracyclines

X NEUROLOGIC MANIFESTATIONS

Exacerbation of myasthenia
  Aminoglycosides
  Polymyxins
Extrapyramidal effects
  Butyrophenones,
    e.g., haloperidol
  Levodopa
  Methyldopa
  Metoclopramide
  Oral contraceptives
  Phenothiazines
  Reserpine
  Tricyclic antidepressants
Headache
  Bromides
  Ergotamine (withdrawal)
  Glyceryl trinitrate
  Hydralazine
  Indomethacin

Peripheral neuropathy
  Amiodarone
  Chloramphenicol
  Chloroquine
  Chlorpropamide
  Clioquinol
  Clofibrate
  Demeclocycline
  Disopyramide
  Ethambutol
  Ethionamide
  Glutethimide
  Hydralazine
  Isoniazid
  Methysergide
  Metronidazole
  Mustine
  Nalidixic acid
  Nitrofurantoin

Peripheral neuropathy *(cont.)*
  Perhexiline
  Phenelzine
  Phenytoin
  Polymyxin, colistin
  Procarbazine
  Streptomycin
  Tolbutamide
  Tricyclic antidepressants
  Vincristine
Pseudotumor cerebri (or
    intracranial
    hypertension)
  Amiodarone
  Glucocorticoids,
    mineralocorticoids
  Hypervitaminosis A
  Oral contraceptives
  Tetracyclines

Seizures
  Amphetamines
  Analeptics
  Imipenem
  Isoniazid
  Lidocaine
  Lithium
  Nalidixic acid
  Penicillins
  Phenothiazines
  Physostigmine
  Theophylline
  Tricyclic antidepressants
  Vincristine
Stroke
  Oral contraceptives

(continued)

TABLE 66-1 Clinical manifestations of adverse reactions to drugs (continued)

XI OCULAR MANIFESTATIONS

Cataracts	Corneal edema	Optic neuritis	Retinopathy
Busulfan	Oral contraceptives	Aminosalicylic acid	Chloroquine
Chlorambucil	Corneal opacities	Chloramphenicol	Phenothiazines
Glucocorticoids	Chloroquine	Clioquinol	
Phenothiazines	Indomethacin	Ethambutol	
Color vision alteration	Mepacrine	Isoniazid	
Barbiturates	Vitamin D	Penicillamine	
Digitalis	Glaucoma	Phenothiazines	
Methaqualone	Mydriatics	Phenylbutazone	
Streptomycin	Sympathomimetics	Quinine	
Sulfonamides		Streptomycin	
Thiazides			
Troxidone			

XII EAR MANIFESTATIONS

Deafness	Vestibular disorders
Aminoglycosides	Aminoglycosides
Aspirin	Mustine
Bleomycin	Quinine
Chloroquine	
Erythromycin	
Ethacrynic acid	
Furosemide	
Mustine	
Nortriptyline	
Quinine	

XIII MUSCULOSKELETAL MANIFESTATIONS

Bone disorders	Myopathy or myalgia
1 Osteoporosis:	Amphotericin B
Glucocorticoids	Carbenoxolone
Heparin	Chloroquine
2 Osteomalacia:	Clofibrate
Aluminum hydroxide	Glucocorticoids
Anticonvulsants	Oral contraceptives
Glutethimide	Myositis
	Lovastatin

XIV PSYCHIATRIC MANIFESTATIONS

Delirious or confusional	Depression	Hallucinatory states	Schizophrenic-like or
states	Amphetamine withdrawal	Amantadine	paranoid reactions
Amantadine	Beta blockers	Beta blockers	Amphetamines
Aminophylline	Centrally acting	Levodopa	Bromides
Anticholinergics	antihypertensives	Meperidine	Corticosteroids
Antidepressants	(reserpine, methyldopa,	Narcotics	Levodopa
Bromides	clonidine)	Pentazocine	Lysergic acid
Cimetidine	Glucocorticoids	Tricyclic antidepressants	Monoamine oxidase
Digitalis	Levodopa	Hypomania, mania, or	inhibitors
Glucocorticoids	Drowsiness	excited reactions	Tricyclic antidepressants
Isoniazid	Antihistamines	Glucocorticoids	Sleep disturbances
Levodopa	Anxiolytic drugs	Levodopa	Anorexiants
Methyldopa	Clonidine	MAO inhibitors	Levodopa
Penicillins	Major tranquilizers	Sympathomimetics	Monoamine oxidase
Phenothiazines	Methyldopa	Tricyclic antidepressants	inhibitors
Sedatives and hypnotics	Reserpine		Sympathomimetics
	Tricyclic antidepressants		

drugs. Similarly, persons with an abnormal serum pseudocholines-terase may have abnormally prolonged apnea when given succinyl-choline.

General comments No drug is completely without side effects, and a side effect in one patient may be the desired pharmacologic effect in another. Current drug regulations allow physicians to prescribe drugs with considerable confidence in their purity, bio-availability, and effectiveness. However, physicians have to weigh the potential toxicity against the possible benefits. Thus toxicity that would be acceptable for an effective antineoplastic agent would not be permitted in an oral contraceptive. Because of the necessarily small number of patients treated in premarketing studies, rare adverse reactions cannot be identified, so that the first responsibility for identifying and reporting these effects must rest with the practicing clinician through the use of the various national adverse reaction reporting systems, such as those operated by the Food and Drug Administration in the United States and the Committee on Safety of Medicines in Great Britain. The publication of a newly recognized adverse reaction can in a short time stimulate many similar such reports of reactions that previously had gone unrecognized.

The prevention of adverse drug reactions first involves a high index of suspicion that the development of a new symptom or sign may be drug-related. Reduction of the dose or discontinuation of the suspected agent usually clarifies the position in concentration-de-pendent toxic reactions. Physicians should be familiar with the common adverse effects of the drugs they use and, if they are in doubt, should consult the literature.

REFERENCES

DAVIES DM: *Textbook of Adverse Drug Reactions*, 3d ed. New York, Oxford University Press, 1985

DESSYPRIS EN et al: Diphenylhydantoin-induced pure red cell aplasia. Blood 65:789, 1985

GOLDSTEIN RA: Drug allergy: Prevention, diagnosis, and treatment. Ann Intern Med 100:302, 1984

ROSSI AC, KNATT D: Discovery of new adverse drug reactions. JAMA 252:1030, 1984

STEEL K et al: Iatrogenic illness on a general medical service at a university hospital N Engl J Med 304:398, 1981

TIMBRELL JA: Drug hepatotoxicity. Br J Clin Pharmacol 15:3, 1983

67   PHYSIOLOGY AND PHARMACOLOGY OF THE AUTONOMIC NERVOUS SYSTEM

LEWIS LANDSBERG / JAMES B. YOUNG

FUNCTIONAL ORGANIZATION OF THE AUTONOMIC NERVOUS SYSTEM

The autonomic nervous system innervates vascular and visceral smooth muscle, exocrine and endocrine glands, and parenchymal cells throughout the various organ systems. Functioning below the conscious level, the autonomic nervous system responds rapidly and continuously to perturbations that threaten the constancy of the internal environment. The many functions governed by this system include the distribution of blood flow and the maintenance of tissue perfusion, the regulation of blood pressure, the regulation of the volume and composition of the extracellular fluid, the expenditure of metabolic energy and supply of substrate, and the control of visceral smooth muscle and glands.

Autonomic responses, like those of the somatic nervous system, are induced promptly and dissipated quickly, in contrast to the slower, more prolonged effects of circulating hormones. The autonomic nervous system, like the endocrine system, regulates the rate of processes that have intrinsic activities of their own, while the somatic nervous system initiates responses de novo. Although certain autonomic responses are discriminating, many are generalized and influence a variety of effectors in different organs. The interface between the autonomic nervous system and the endocrine system is exemplified by the adrenal medulla. This gland, homologous in many respects with the postganglionic sympathetic neuron, secretes a hormone (epinephrine) into the circulation to interact with adrenergic receptors throughout the body.

ANATOMIC ORGANIZATION   The autonomic neurons, located in ganglia outside the central nervous system, give rise to the postganglionic autonomic nerves that innervate organs and tissues throughout the body. The activity of autonomic nerves is regulated by central neurons responsive to diverse afferent inputs. After central integration of afferent information, autonomic outflow is adjusted to permit the functioning of the major organ systems in accordance with the needs of the organism as a whole. Connections between the cerebral cortex and the autonomic centers in the brainstem coordinate autonomic outflow with higher mental functions.

The sympathetic and parasympathetic divisions   The preganglionic neurons of the parasympathetic nervous system leave the central nervous system in the third, seventh, ninth, and tenth cranial nerves and in the second and third sacral nerves, while the preganglionic neurons of the sympathetic nervous system exit the spinal cord between the first thoracic and the second lumbar segments. Responses to sympathetic and parasympathetic stimulation are frequently antagonistic, as exemplified by their opposing effects on heart rate and gut motility. This antagonism reflects highly coordinated interactions within the central nervous system; the resultant changes in parasympathetic and sympathetic activity, often reciprocal, provide more precise control of autonomic responses than could be achieved by the modulation of a single system.

Neurotransmitters   *Acetylcholine* (ACh) is the preganglionic neurotransmitter for both divisions of the autonomic nervous system, as well as the postganglionic neurotransmitter of the parasympathetic neurons. Nerves that release ACh are said to be cholinergic. *Norepinephrine* (NE) is the neurotransmitter of the postganglionic sympathetic neurons; these nerves are said to be adrenergic. Within the sympathetic outflow postganglionic neurons innervating the eccrine sweat glands (and perhaps some blood vessels supplying skeletal muscle) are of the cholinergic type.

THE SYMPATHETIC NERVOUS SYSTEM AND THE ADRENAL MEDULLA

CATECHOLAMINES   All three of the naturally occurring catecholamines, NE, *epinephrine* (E), and *dopamine,* function as neurotransmitters within the central nervous system. NE, the neurotransmitter of postganglionic sympathetic nerve endings, exerts its effects locally, in the immediate vicinity of its release. E, the circulating hormone of the adrenal medulla, influences processes throughout the body. A peripheral dopaminergic system also exists but has not been characterized in detail.

Biosynthesis (Fig. 67-1)   Catecholamines are synthesized from the amino acid tyrosine, which is sequentially hydroxylated to form dihydroxyphenylalanine (dopa), decarboxylated to form dopamine, and hydroxylated on the beta position of the side chain to form NE. The initial step, the hydroxylation of tyrosine, is rate-limiting and is regulated so that synthesis of dopa is coupled to norepinephrine release. This regulation is achieved by alterations in both the activity and the amount of tyrosine hydroxylase. In the adrenal medulla and in those central neurons utilizing E as neurotransmitter, NE is N-methylated to E by the enzyme phenylethanolamine-N-methyltransferase (PNMT). A major portion of the blood perfusing the adrenal medulla is enriched with glucocorticoids from the adrenal cortex, and since adrenal PNMT is inducible by glucocorticoids, the capacity of the adrenal medulla to form E may be related to its strategic location within the adrenal cortex.

Catecholamine metabolism (Fig. 67-1)   The major metabolic transformations of catecholamines involve O-methylation at the meta-hydroxyl group and oxidative deamination. O-methylation is catalyzed by the enzyme catechol-O-methyltransferase (COMT), and oxidative deamination is promoted by monoamine oxidase (MAO). COMT in liver and kidney is important in the metabolism of circulating catecholamines. MAO, a mitochondrial enzyme present in most tissues including nerve endings, has a lesser role in the metabolism of circulating catecholamines but is important in regulating the catecholamine stores within the peripheral sympathetic nerve endings. The metanephrines and 4-hydroxy-3-methoxymandelic acid (VMA) are the major end products of N and NE metabolism. Homovanillic acid (HVA) is the end product of dopamine metabolism.

STORAGE AND RELEASE OF CATECHOLAMINES   Both in the adrenal medulla and sympathetic nerve endings catecholamines are stored in subcellular granules and released by exocytosis. The large stores of catecholamines in these tissues provide an important physiologic reserve that maintains an adequate supply of catecholamines in the face of intense stimulation.

Adrenal medulla   The adrenal medullary chromaffin tissue in a pair of normal human adrenal glands weighs about 1 g and contains approximately 6 mg of catecholamines, 85 percent of which is E. Catecholamines are maintained in high concentration within the storage (chromaffin) granule by an active uptake process involving the granule membrane and by an intragranular storage complex that appears to involve ATP, calcium, and a specific granule protein, chromagranin A. The latter, isolated originally from chromaffin granules, has been found to be a common constituent of secretory granules in a number of different endocrine cells, including those of the anterior pituitary, pancreatic islets, and parathyroids. Its role in hormone storage and secretion is still unknown. Catecholamine secretion, stimulated by ACh from the preganglionic sympathetic nerves, occurs after calcium influx triggers fusion of the chromaffin granule membrane and cell membrane; obliteration of the cell membrane at the point of fusion and extrusion of the entire soluble contents of the granule into the extracellular space complete the process of exocytosis (Fig. 67-1). Approximately 2 to 10 percent of the total adrenal medullary catecholamine store is turned over each day.

Peripheral sympathetic nerve endings   The peripheral sympathetic nerve endings form a reticulum or ground plexus that brings the terminal fibers into close contact with effector cells. All the NE in peripheral tissues is in the sympathetic nerve endings, and heavily

FIGURE 67-1 Catecholamine biosynthesis, release, and metabolism. Schematic representation of a peripheral sympathetic nerve ending is shown at the top; the bulbous areas on the terminal fiber represent varicosities identified by histochemical fluorescence techniques as areas of high neurotransmitter concentration. The processes of biosynthesis, release, modulation, and reuptake are shown sequentially for demonstration purposes only; in vivo they proceed concurrently. Adrenal medullary chromaffin cells are shown at the bottom of the diagram. (TH = tyrosine hydroxylase, AAD = aromatic-L-amino acid decarboxylase, DA = dopamine, DBH = dopamine-β-hydroxylase, NE = norepinephrine, PNMT = phenylethanolamine-N-methyltransferase, E = epinephrine, COMT = catechol-O-methyltransferase, NMN = normetanephrine, MAO = monoamine oxidase, DHMA = 3,4-dihydroxymandelic acid, VMA = 3-methoxy-4-hydroxymandelic acid.)

innervated tissues contain as much as 1 to 2 μg per gram of tissue. NE stored in the nerve endings is in discrete subcellular particles analogous to the adrenal medullary chromaffin granules. MAO in the mitochondria of the nerve endings plays an important role in regulating the local concentration of NE (Fig. 67-1). Amines in storage vesicles are protected from oxidative deamination; amines within the cytoplasm, however, are deaminated to inactive metabolites. Release from the nerve ending occurs in response to action potentials propagated in terminal sympathetic fibers (Fig. 67-1).

THE PERIPHERAL ADRENERGIC NEUROEFFECTOR JUNCTION Neuronal uptake The peripheral sympathetic nerve endings possess an amine transport system that actively takes up amines from the extracellular fluid. A variety of synthetic and naturally occurring amines are substrates for this process. Neuronal uptake or recapture of locally released NE terminates the action of the transmitter and contributes to the constancy of the NE stores (Fig. 67-1).

Prejunctional modulation A variety of factors alter the relationship between neuronal impulse traffic and NE release. Diminished temperature and acidosis, for example, both decrease the amount of NE released in response to sympathetic impulses. Several chemical mediators operate at the peripheral sympathetic nerve ending (referred to as prejunctional or presynaptic sites) to modify sympathetic neurotransmission by influencing the amount of NE released in response to nerve impulses. Prejunctional modulation may be either inhibitory or facilitatory. Certain modulators, such as catecholamines and ACh, may either inhibit or facilitate NE release, antagonistic effects that are mediated by different adrenergic or cholinergic receptors, respectively. Those compounds exerting an *inhibitory* effect on NE release at the prejunctional nerve ending include the following: catecholamines (alpha$_2$ receptor), ACh (muscarinic receptor), dopamine (D-2 receptor), histamine (H-2 receptor), serotonin, adenosine, enkephalins, and prostaglandins. *Facilitatory* prejunctional modulators include catecholamines (beta$_2$ receptor), ACh (nicotinic receptor),

and angiotensin II. The overall significance of prejunctional modulation, as well as the relative importance of the various mediators, has yet to be established.

PREJUNCTIONAL ADRENERGIC RECEPTORS Catecholamines reduce NE release via prejunctional alpha receptors in a classic negative feedback system. Feedback regulation is complicated by the fact that beta-receptor activation facilitates NE release. Two hypotheses have been advanced to explain how the antagonistic alpha and beta effects on NE release may be integrated physiologically. One hypothesis is based on the observation that beta-mediated effects occur at lower agonist concentrations than those mediated by the alpha receptor, whereas alpha-mediated responses predominate at higher concentrations of agonist. During low levels of sympathetic stimulation, therefore, when NE concentrations in the synaptic cleft are low, beta-mediated positive feedback may predominate with facilitation of NE release. Conversely, at higher levels of sympathetic stimulation with increased NE concentration in the synaptic cleft, alpha-mediated negative feedback predominates and NE release is inhibited. The other hypothesis is that prejunctional beta receptors (beta$_2$, see below) are more sensitive to E than NE; circulating levels of E, therefore, might stimulate the prejunctional beta receptors, thereby augmenting NE release and enhancing sympathetic neurotransmission.

PREJUNCTIONAL CHOLINERGIC RECEPTORS Though both inhibitory and facilitatory effects of ACh on NE release have been described, the inhibitory effect of ACh, mediated by the muscarinic cholinergic receptor, occurs at lower ACh concentrations and is probably of greater physiologic significance. This peripheral inhibitory effect of ACh on adrenergic neurotransmission may reinforce the reciprocal changes in central parasympathetic and sympathetic outflow that occur in the regulation of numerous physiologic responses.

CENTRAL REGULATION OF SYMPATHOADRENAL OUTFLOW
Brainstem sympathetic centers Sympathetic outflow is initiated from the reticular formation of the medulla oblongata and pons and

from centers in the hypothalamus. Descending fibers originating from these centers synapse in the intermediolateral cell column of the spinal cord with the preganglionic sympathetic neurons. The brainstem sympathetic centers, which have an intrinsic activity of their own, are regulated by many stimuli, including impulses from more rostral areas of the central nervous system (cortex, limbic lobe, hypothalamus); neural afferents that interact at the level of the brainstem centers and at the higher centers; and changes in the physical and chemical properties of the extracellular fluid, including the circulating levels of hormones and substrates. The higher centers, which have connections with the brainstem, coordinate sympathetic outflow with higher mental functions, emotional reactions, and the homeostatic needs of the internal environment. Although the hallmark of intense sympathoadrenal stimulation is a global response (the fight-or-flight reaction of Cannon), discrete changes in sympathetic outflow to different organ systems influence many autonomic functions.

RELATIONSHIP BETWEEN THE SYMPATHETIC NERVOUS SYSTEM AND THE ADRENAL MEDULLA   Sympathetic nervous system activity and adrenal medullary secretion are coordinated but not always congruent. During periods of intense sympathetic stimulation, such as cold exposure and exhaustive exercise, the adrenal medulla is progressively recruited, and circulating E reinforces the physiologic effects of sympathetic stimulation. In other situations the sympathetic nervous system and the adrenal medulla are stimulated independently. The response to upright posture, for example, involves predominantly the sympathetic nervous system while hypoglycemia stimulates only the adrenal medulla. An important role for the adrenal medulla may be to provide circulating catecholamines to support vital functions when the sympathetic nervous system is suppressed.

Sympathetic regulation of the cardiovascular system   The sympathetic nervous system plays a major role in the regulation of the circulation. Stretch receptors in the systemic and pulmonary arteries and veins continuously monitor intravascular pressures; the resulting afferent impulses, after relay and integration in the brainstem, alter sympathetic activity in defense of blood pressure and blood flow to critical areas (Fig. 67-2).

ARTERIAL BARORECEPTORS   An increase in blood pressure stimulates receptors in the carotid sinus and aortic arch. The ensuing afferent impulses, after relay within the nucleus of the solitary tract (NTS) in the brainstem, suppress the brainstem sympathetic centers (Fig. 67-2). This baroreceptor reflex arc forms a negative feedback loop in which a rise in arterial pressure results in the inhibition of central sympathetic outflow. A brainstem noradrenergic pathway interacts with the NTS to participate in suppression of sympathetic outflow. This noradrenergic inhibitory pathway is stimulated by centrally acting alpha-adrenergic agonists and may be involved in the action of certain antihypertensive drugs, such as clonidine, that potentiate the baroreceptor-mediated vasodepressor response (Chap. 196). In the opposite manner, when the blood pressure falls, decreased afferent impulses diminish central inhibition, resulting in an increase in sympathetic outflow and a rise in arterial pressure.

CENTRAL VENOUS PRESSURE   Receptors in the walls of the great veins and within the atria are also involved in the regulation of sympathetic outflow. Stimulation of these receptors by high venous pressure suppresses the brainstem sympathetic centers; when central venous pressure is low, sympathetic outflow increases. The central connections are poorly understood, but the afferent impulses are carried in the vagus (Fig. 67-2).

ASSESSMENT OF SYMPATHOADRENAL ACTIVITY   The clinical assessment of sympathoadrenal activity involves the measurement of catecholamines in plasma and of catecholamines and catecholamine metabolites in urine. Quantitation of urinary catecholamines and metabolites is useful in the diagnosis of pheochromocytoma (Chap. 318).

Plasma catecholamines   Catecholamines in human plasma may be measured by radioenzymatic isotope derivative techniques or by high performance liquid chromatography in conjunction with electrochemical detection. Plasma catecholamine measurements provide an index of sympathetic nervous system and adrenal medullary activity and have been widely used to assess sympathoadrenal activity in clinical investigation in human subjects. The usefulness of plasma catecholamine measurements is, however, compromised by factors that alter the relationship between the plasma concentration of catecholamines and the functional state of the sympathoadrenal system. The clinical usefulness of plasma catecholamine levels is limited to the evaluation of patients with autonomic insufficiency and, on occasion, patients with suspected pheochromocytoma (Chap. 318).

Basal plasma NE concentrations are in the range of 0.09 to 1.8 nmol/L (150 to 350 pg/mL; basal E levels are about 135 to 270 pmol/L (25 to 50 pg/mL). The half-time of disappearance of NE from the circulation is approximately 2 min. The plasma NE level is markedly affected by a variety of factors, including posture; accordingly, the conditions under which blood is obtained for assay must be controlled. By convention, basal plasma NE levels are those obtained through an indwelling intravenous line after the patient has rested supine in a relaxed environment for 30 min.

PLASMA NE RESPONSE TO UPRIGHT POSTURE   The predictable increase in circulating NE concentration during upright posture provides a convenient test of sympathetic nervous system function. Five minutes of quiet standing results in a two- to threefold increase in plasma NE level. A normal response requires an intact afferent system, appropriate central nervous system relays, and an intact peripheral sympathetic nervous system; a defect of any of these components reduces the increment in circulating NE.

Plasma E levels are also dependent on the physical and mental state of the subject. Change in plasma E with upright posture is usually small. Hypoglycemia and various types of mental stress, however, can cause large increments in the plasma E level.

PERIPHERAL DOPAMINERGIC SYSTEM

In addition to its role as neurotransmitter in the central nervous system, dopamine functions as an inhibitory transmitter in the carotid body and the sympathetic ganglia. A distinct peripheral dopaminergic system is also believed to exist. Dopamine elicits a variety of responses not attributable to stimulation of classic adrenergic receptors; it relaxes the lower esophageal sphincter, delays gastric emptying,

FIGURE 67-2 Sympathetic regulation of the circulation. Receptors in the venous and arterial circulations are stimulated by stretch, caused by an increase in pressure; afferent impulses from these receptors are carried to the central nervous system by the ninth and tenth cranial nerves. The net result of these afferent impulses, after relay in the brainstem, is to inhibit central sympathetic outflow. The arterial baroreceptor reflex involves a relay in the nucleus of the tractus solitarius (NTS). (+ = stimulation; − = inhibition.)

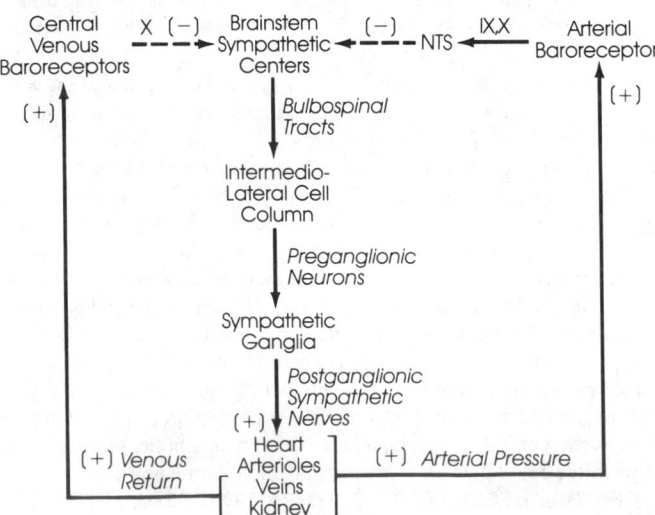

causes vasodilation in the renal and mesenteric arterial circulation, suppresses aldosterone secretion, directly stimulates renal sodium excretion, and suppresses NE release at sympathetic nerve terminals by a presynaptic inhibitory mechanism. The mediation of these dopaminergic effects in vivo is poorly understood. Dopamine does not appear to be a circulating hormone. Unequivocal evidence of peripheral autonomic dopaminergic nerves has not been produced, although such nerves may be present in the kidney. The kidney, furthermore, produces much of the dopamine in the urine since the amount excreted each day (approximately 200 μg per 24 h) cannot be accounted for by clearance of plasma dopamine. Decarboxylation of circulating dopa, which is present in high concentration in the plasma [9 nmol/L (1500 pg/mL)] may contribute to urinary dopamine production. Dopamine generated from the decarboxylation of circulating dopa might also be involved in the mediation of dopaminergic effects in the kidney and other sites. Thus, the nature of the peripheral dopaminergic system is obscure, but the existence of a dopaminergic system in those tissues that respond uniquely to dopamine seems likely.

ADRENERGIC RECEPTORS

Catecholamines influence effector cells by interacting with specific *receptors* on the cell surface. When stimulated by catecholamines, the adrenergic receptor initiates a series of membrane changes followed by a cascade of intracellular events that culminates in a measurable response. Compounds that elicit the response are referred to as *agonists;* those that block the interaction of the agonist with the receptor are referred to as adrenergic *receptor blocking agents* or *antagonists.*

Two major categories of response to catecholamines reflect the activation of two populations of adrenergic receptors, designated *alpha* and *beta*. Selective agonists and antagonists are available, enabling pharmacologic stimulation or blockade of the physiologic effects mediated by one receptor without influencing those mediated by the other. Both alpha and beta receptors have been further divided into subtypes that serve different functions and are susceptible to differential stimulation and blockade.

ALPHA-ADRENERGIC RECEPTORS The alpha-adrenergic receptor mediates vasoconstriction, intestinal relaxation, and pupillary dilatation. E and NE are approximately equipotent as alpha-receptor agonists. Distinct alpha$_1$- and alpha$_2$-receptor subtypes are also recognized. Originally the postsynaptic or postjunctional alpha-adrenergic receptors on effector cells were designated alpha$_1$, while the prejunctional alpha-adrenergic receptors on the sympathetic nerve endings were designated alpha$_2$. Several additional nonneuronal (postsynaptic) processes appear to be mediated by the alpha$_2$ receptor. The alpha$_1$ receptor mediates the classic alpha effects including vasoconstriction; phenylephrine and methoxamine are selective alpha$_1$ agonists, and prazosin is a selective alpha$_1$ antagonist. The alpha$_2$ receptor mediates presynaptic inhibition of NE release from adrenergic nerves and other responses including inhibition of ACh release from cholinergic nerves, inhibition of lipolysis in adipocytes, inhibition of insulin secretion, stimulation of platelet aggregation, and vasoconstriction in some vascular beds. Specific alpha$_2$ agonists include clonidine and α-methylnorepinephrine; these agents, the latter derived from α-methyldopa in vivo, exert an antihypertensive effect by interacting with alpha$_2$ receptors within the brainstem sympathetic centers that regulate blood pressure. Yohimbine is a specific alpha$_2$ antagonist.

BETA-ADRENERGIC RECEPTORS Physiologic events associated with beta-adrenergic receptor responses include stimulation of heart rate and contractility, vasodilation, bronchodilation, and lipolysis. Beta-receptor responses can also be divided into two types. The beta$_1$ receptor responds equally to E and NE and mediates cardiac stimulation and lipolysis. The beta$_2$ receptor is more responsive to E than to NE and mediates responses such as vasodilation and bron-

chodilation. Isoproterenol stimulates and propranolol blocks both beta$_1$ and beta$_2$ receptors. Other agonists and antagonists that have partial selectivity for the beta$_1$ or beta$_2$ receptors have been used therapeutically where the desired response involves predominantly one of the two subtypes.

DOPAMINERGIC RECEPTORS Specific dopaminergic receptors, distinct from the classic alpha- and beta-adrenergic receptors, are present in the central and peripheral nervous system and in several nonneural tissues. Two types of dopaminergic receptor serve different functions and have different second messengers. Dopamine is a potent agonist of both types of receptor; the action of dopamine is antagonized by phenothiazines and thioxanthenes. The dopamine 1 receptor mediates vasodilation in the renal, mesenteric, coronary, and cerebral vascular beds. Fenoldopam is an investigational agonist selective for the dopamine 1 receptor. The dopamine 2 receptor inhibits transmission in the sympathetic ganglia, inhibits NE release from sympathetic nerve endings by an effect on the presynaptic membrane (Fig. 67-1), inhibits prolactin release from the pituitary, and causes vomiting. Selective agonists of the dopamine 2 receptor include bromocriptine, lergotrile, and apomorphine, while butyrophenones such as haloperidol (active within the central nervous system) and domperidone (does not cross blood-brain barrier readily) and the benzamide sulpiride are relatively selective dopamine 2 antagonists.

STRUCTURE AND FUNCTION OF ADRENERGIC RECEPTORS The utilization of recombinant DNA technology has substantially increased current understanding of the structure and function of adrenergic receptors. cDNAs of the four major adrenergic receptor subtypes have been cloned and their primary amino acid sequences deduced. It is clear from these studies that the adrenergic receptors belong to a family of related membrane proteins that includes the visual protein rhodopsin and the muscarinic acetylcholine receptors. These proteins share significant sequence homologies and, as deduced from the properties of the constituent amino acids, a similar topographic structure in the cell membrane (Chap. 173). The postulated structure of this family of receptor proteins is shown schematically in Fig. 67-3. The characteristic features include seven membrane-spanning hydrophobic domains containing 20 to 28 amino acids each (possibly arranged as alpha helices), a hydrophilic extracellular *N*

FIGURE 67-3 Proposed structure of adrenergic receptors as deduced from primary amino acid sequences. The single protein chain contains a hydrophilic *N* terminus (extracellular) and *C* terminus (intracellular) connected by seven lipophilic membrane-spanning regions (M-I to M-7) which are interconnected by three extracellular loops (E-I to E-III) and three cytoplasmic loops (C-I to C-III). The beta$_1$, beta$_2$, alpha$_1$, and alpha$_2$ adrenergic receptors have appreciable sequence homologies and are believed to fit the general structural model represented. Specificity of agonist binding may be conferred by the tertiary structure of several of the membrane-spanning domains while specificity of intracellular response may be related to the length and tertiary structure of the cytoplasmic loops and *C* terminus. (*Modified from RJ Lefkowitz and MG Caron.*)

FIGURE 67-4 Interaction of autonomic agonists with membrane-bound regulatory proteins and cellular effectors systems. The designations α and β refer to adrenergic receptors, DA refers to dopaminergic receptors, and M, to muscarinic receptors. G designates the GTP-associated regulatory protein which may have a stimulatory (s) or inhibitory (i) effect on adenylyl cyclase or may stimulate phospholipase C (p). (+) designates stimulation; (−) designates inhibition. PIP_2 = phosphatidylinositol-4,5-bisphosphate; DAG = 1,2-diacylglycerol; IP_3 = inositol-1,4,5-trisphosphate. See text for details.

terminus and three extracellular connecting loops, and a hydrophilic intracellular *C* terminus with three cytoplasmic connecting loops.

Specificity for agonist binding and effector response is apparently conferred by differences in the tertiary structure of the various domains. Beta receptors, for example, have short third cytoplasmic loops (C-III) and long *C*-terminal chains, while the alpha$_2$ receptor has a long C-III and a short *C* terminus. The C-III loop appears to influence binding to the appropriate regulatory protein within the cell membrane (see below). The membrane-spanning domains, particularly M-VII (Fig. 67-3), appear to be important in determining the characteristic agonist binding.

Coupling of receptor occupancy with cellular response The major mediators of adrenergic (as well as many other) cellular responses are a family of regulatory proteins termed G (or N) proteins that, when activated, bind the nucleotide guanosine triphosphate (GTP). The best-characterized G proteins are those that stimulate or inhibit adenylyl cyclase, designated G_s or G_i, respectively (Fig. 67-4) (see Chap 68). The beta$_1$, beta$_2$, and dopamine 1 receptors are coupled to G_s; receptor occupancy is therefore associated with stimulation of adenylyl cyclase and results in an increase in intracellular cyclic adenosine monophosphate (AMP), which in turn results in activation of protein kinase A and other cAMP-dependent protein kinases. The resultant protein phosphorylation alters the activity of enzymes and the function of other proteins, culminating in a cellular response that is characteristic of the tissue being stimulated. The alpha$_2$, M-2 subtype of the muscarinic acetylcholine receptor and the dopamine 2 receptor are coupled to G_i, resulting in diminished adenylyl cyclase activity and a fall in cAMP. The subsequent alterations in enzyme activity and function of other proteins produce an alternate, frequently opposite, series of cellular responses. Not all alpha$_2$ responses can be explained by inhibition of adenylyl cyclase; independent changes in ion fluxes are involved as well.

The alpha$_1$ adrenergic receptor (as well as the M-1 subtype of the acetylcholine receptor) appears to be coupled to a different G protein that activates phospholipase C; this G protein has not been well characterized but is sometimes tentatively designated G_p. Receptor occupancy in this system stimulates phospholipase C, which catalyzes the breakdown of membrane-bound phospholipids, particularly phosphatidylinositol-4,5-bisphosphate (PIP_2) with the production of inositol-1,4,5-trisphosphate (IP_3) and 1,2-diacylglycerol (DAG), both of which act as second messengers (Fig. 67-4). IP_3 rapidly mobilizes calcium from intracellular stores within the endoplasmic reticulum producing an increase in free cytoplasmic calcium which by itself and via calcium-calmodulin–dependent protein kinases influences cellular processes appropriate to the stimulated cell. The transient rise in calcium induced by IP_3 from the intracellular stores is reinforced in the presence of continued agonist stimulation by alterations in membrane calcium flux that result eventually in net calcium uptake from the extracellular fluid by mechanisms that have been incompletely defined.

DAG, the other second messenger produced by the action of phospholipase C on PIP_2 (as well as other membrane phospholipids), remains associated with the cell membrane and activates protein kinase C, which has different substrates than the calcium-calmodulin kinases stimulated by IP_3. Protein phosphorylation stimulated by protein kinase C contributes to the tissue-specific response in ways that remain poorly understood.

REGULATION OF ADRENERGIC RECEPTORS Radiolabeled adrenergic-receptor agonists and antagonists have been utilized as ligands to study adrenergic receptors. In combination with studies of peripheral tissue sensitivity these studies demonstrated that changes in adrenergic receptors occur under a variety of physiologic conditions. Prolonged exposure to alpha- or beta-adrenergic agonists decreases the number of corresponding adrenergic receptors on effector cells. Although the biochemical mechanisms involved are obscure, internalization of the beta-adrenergic receptor within the cell occurs during agonist exposure in some systems, suggesting that internal translocation causes the decrease in receptor number. Alteration in agonist concentration may also affect the affinity of the receptor for the agonist. Adrenergic receptors that utilize adenylate cyclase for the second messenger (beta receptors, alpha$_2$ receptors) exist in high and low affinity states; exposure to agonist diminishes the proportion of receptors in the high affinity state. Such alterations in adrenergic receptors induced by adrenergic agonists are termed *homologous regulation*. Agonist-induced alterations in adrenergic-receptor density and affinity are believed to contribute to the diminished physiologic response that occurs after prolonged exposure of an effector tissue to adrenergic agonist, a phenomenon known as *tachyphylaxis* or *desensitization*. Recent evidence suggests that phosphorylation of the beta receptor by a specific beta-receptor kinase is involved in the desensitization phenomenon.

Adrenergic receptors are also influenced by factors other than adrenergic agonists, so-called heterologous regulation. Enhanced alpha-adrenergic-receptor affinity, for example, may underlie the potentiation of alpha-adrenergic responses that occur in response to lowered environmental temperatures. Thyroid hormones potentiate beta-receptor responses by alterations in beta-receptor number and in the efficiency of coupling receptor occupancy with physiologic response. Estrogen and progesterone alter the sensitivity of the myometrium to catecholamines by effects on alpha-adrenergic receptors. Glucocorticoids may influence adrenergic function by antagonizing agonist-induced decreases in adrenergic receptors, thereby counteracting tachyphylaxis in response to intense adrenergic stimulation. Some forms of heterologous desensitization may involve modifications in the membrane regulatory proteins or in adenylyl cyclase itself.

Alterations in sensitivity to catecholamines also occur as a consequence of postreceptor changes, although the latter remain poorly characterized.

PHYSIOLOGY OF THE SYMPATHOADRENAL SYSTEM

Catecholamines influence all the major organ systems. The effects take place in seconds as compared with the minutes, hours, or days that characterize the actions of the endocrine system and most other control systems that regulate bodily processes. The sympathoadrenal system, moreover, may respond in anticipation of physiologic requirement. An increase in sympathoadrenal activity prior to strenuous exercise, for example, lessens the impact of exercise on the internal environment.

DIRECT EFFECTS OF CATECHOLAMINES Cardiovascular system Catecholamines stimulate vasoconstriction in the subcutaneous, mucosal, splanchnic, and renal vascular beds by an alpha-receptor-mediated mechanism. Since vasoconstriction in the coronary and cerebral circulations is minimal, flow to these areas is maintained. The adaptive significance of this priority given the heart and brain is clear; in both of these organs the metabolic requirements relative to blood flow are high, and continuous perfusion is essential for life. Skeletal muscle vasculature contains beta receptors sensitive to low circulating levels of E so that skeletal muscle blood flow is augmented during adrenal medullary activation.

The effects of catecholamines on the heart are mediated by beta$_1$ receptors and include increase in heart rate, enhancement of cardiac contractility, and increase in conduction velocity. The increase in myocardial contractility is illustrated by a leftward and upward shift of the ventricular function curve (Fig. 181-6) that relates cardiac work to ventricular diastolic fiber length; at any initial fiber length catecholamines increase cardiac work. Catecholamines also enhance cardiac output by stimulating venoconstriction, enhancing venous return, and by increasing the force of atrial contraction, thereby augmenting diastolic volume and hence fiber length. The acceleration of conduction in the junctional tissues results in a more synchronous, and hence more effective, ventricular contraction. Cardiac stimulation increases myocardial oxygen consumption, a major factor in the pathogenesis and treatment of myocardial ischemia.

Metabolism Catecholamines increase metabolic rate. In small mammals mitochondrial respiration in brown adipose tissue is functionally uncoupled by NE. In a reaction unique to brown adipose tissue, NE activates a specific mitochondrial uncoupling protein that dissipates the proton gradient between the inner mitochondrial matrix and the cytoplasm, thereby uncoupling substrate utilization and ATP synthesis. In humans a functional role for brown adipose tissue has not been established with certainty, but increasing evidence suggests a potential role for this tissue in catecholamine-stimulated heat production in human beings.

SUBSTRATE MOBILIZATION In a variety of tissues catecholamines stimulate the breakdown of stored fuel with the production of substrate for local consumption; glycogenolysis in the heart, for example, provides substrate for immediate metabolism by the myocardium. Catecholamines also accelerate fuel mobilization in liver, adipose tissue, and skeletal muscle, liberating substrates (glucose, free fatty acids, lactate) into the circulation for use throughout the body. Activation of enzymes involved in fuel breakdown occurs by a beta-receptor (beta$_1$) mechanism for adipose tissue lipolysis and by alpha- and beta-receptor (beta$_2$) mechanisms for hepatic glycogenolysis and gluconeogenesis. In skeletal muscle catecholamines stimulate glycogenolysis (beta receptor), thereby increasing lactate efflux.

Fluids and electrolytes Catecholamines contribute to the regulation of the volume and composition of extracellular fluid. By a direct action on the renal tubule, NE stimulates sodium reabsorption, thereby defending extracellular fluid volume. Dopamine, in contrast, promotes sodium excretion. NE and E also promote cellular uptake of potassium, thereby defending against the development of hyperkalemia. Effects of catecholamines on calcium, magnesium, and phosphate metabolism are complex and depend on a variety of factors.

Viscera Catecholamines affect visceral function by actions on smooth muscle and glandular epithelium. Urinary bladder and intestinal smooth muscle are relaxed while the corresponding sphincters are stimulated. Gallbladder emptying also involves sympathetic mechanisms. Catecholamine-mediated smooth-muscle contraction in the female aids ovulation and ovum transport along the fallopian tubes, and in the male provides propulsive force for the seminal fluid during ejaculation. Inhibitory alpha$_2$ receptors on cholinergic neurons within the gut contribute to intestinal relaxation. Catecholamines induce bronchodilation by a beta$_2$-receptor mechanism.

INDIRECT EFFECTS OF CATECHOLAMINES The ultimate physiologic response induced by catecholamines involves changes in hormone secretion and in blood flow distribution, both of which support and amplify the direct effects of catecholamines.

Endocrine system Catecholamines influence the secretion of renin, insulin, glucagon, calcitonin, parathormone, thyroxine, gastrin, erythropoietin, progesterone, and, possibly, testosterone. Secretion of each of these hormones is governed by complex feedback loops. With the exception of thyroxine and the gonadal steroids, each is a polypeptide not under the direct control of the pituitary gland. Sympathoadrenal input into the secretion of these hormones provides a mechanism for regulation by the central nervous system and ensures a coordinated hormonal response in accord with the homeostatic needs of the organism.

RENIN The juxtaglomerular apparatus of the kidney is heavily innervated. Sympathetic stimulation increases renin release by a direct beta-receptor effect independent of vascular changes within the kidney. The renin response to volume depletion is sympathetically mediated and is initiated by a fall in central venous pressure. Since renin secretion activates the angiotensin-aldosterone system, angiotensin-induced vasoconstriction supports the direct effects of catecholamines on blood vessels, while aldosterone-mediated sodium reabsorption complements the direct increase in sodium reabsorption induced by sympathetic stimulation. Beta-receptor blocking agents suppress renin secretion.

INSULIN AND GLUCAGON The pancreatic islets also receive an extensive sympathetic innervation. Stimulation of pancreatic sympathetic nerves or an elevation in circulating catecholamines suppresses insulin and increases glucagon release. Inhibition of insulin secretion is mediated by the alpha$_2$ receptor, and stimulation of glucagon is mediated by the beta receptor. This combination of effects supports substrate mobilization, reinforcing the direct effects of catecholamines on hepatic glucose output and lipolysis. Although alpha-receptor-mediated suppression of insulin release usually predominates, a beta-receptor mechanism may augment insulin secretion under some circumstances.

SYMPATHOADRENAL FUNCTION IN SELECTED PHYSIOLOGIC AND PATHOPHYSIOLOGIC STATES Support of the circulation The sympathetic nervous system functions to maintain an adequate circulation. During upright posture and volume depletion, reduction of afferent venous and arterial baroreceptor impulse traffic diminishes an inhibitory input to the vasomotor center, thereby increasing sympathetic activity (Fig. 67-2) and reducing efferent vagal tone. As a result, heart rate is increased, and cardiac output is diverted from the skin, subcutaneous tissues, mucosa, and viscera. Sympathetic stimulation of the kidney increases sodium reabsorption, and sympathetically mediated venoconstriction enhances venous return. With pronounced hypotension, the adrenal medulla is recruited and E reinforces the effects of the sympathetic nervous system. A similar pattern of sympathetic activation occurs in the postprandial state when blood and extracellular fluid are sequestered in the splanchnic circulation and in the lumen of the gut, respectively.

CONGESTIVE HEART FAILURE   The sympathetic nervous system also provides circulatory support during congestive heart failure (Chap. 182). Venoconstriction and sympathetic stimulation of the heart increase cardiac output while peripheral vasoconstriction directs blood flow to the heart and brain. The afferent signals are less clear than in simple volume depletion since the venous pressure is usually elevated. In severe heart failure depletion of cardiac NE may impair the effectiveness of sympathetic circulatory support.

TRAUMA AND SHOCK   In acute traumatic injury or shock, adrenal catecholamines support the circulation and mobilize substrates. It is presumed, but unproved, that the sympathetic nervous system is activated as well. In the chronic, reparative phase following injury catecholamines contribute to substrate mobilization and to the elevation in metabolic rate.

EXERCISE   Sympathetic activation during exercise increases cardiac output, maintains blood flow, and ensures sufficient substrate to meet the increased needs. Central neural factors, such as anticipation, and circulatory factors, such as fall in venous pressure, trigger the sympathetic response. Mild degrees of exercise stimulate the sympathetic nervous system alone; during more severe exertion the adrenal medulla is activated as well. Conditioning is associated with a decrease in sympathetic nervous system activity both at rest and during exercise.

Hypoglycemia   Hypoglycemia causes a marked increase in adrenal medullary E secretion. When glucose concentrations fall below overnight fasting levels, regulatory glucose-sensitive neurons in the central nervous system initiate a prompt increase in adrenal medullary secretion. The increase is especially intense when plasma glucose levels drop below 2.8 mmol/L (50 mg/dL) when plasma E levels increase 25 to 50 times above baseline, thereby increasing hepatic glucose output, providing alternative substrate in the form of free fatty acids, suppressing endogenous insulin release, and inhibiting insulin-mediated glucose utilization in muscle. Many clinical manifestations of hypoglycemia, such as tachycardia, palpitations, nervousness, tremor, and widened pulse pressure, are secondary to increased E secretion. These manifestations of epinephrine secretion constitute an "early warning" system in insulin-requiring diabetics. In patients with long-standing diabetes mellitus, however, the epinephrine response to hypoglycemia may be diminished or absent, leaving affected patients at greater risk to develop severe hypoglycemia.

Cold exposure   The sympathetic nervous system plays a critical role in the maintenance of normal body temperature during exposure to a cold environment. Receptors in the skin and central nervous system respond to a fall in temperature by activating hypothalamic and brainstem centers that increase sympathetic activity. Sympathetic stimulation leads to vasoconstriction in the superficial vascular beds, thereby diminishing heat loss. Heat production is simultaneously increased by shivering, generation of metabolic heat, and substrate mobilization. Acclimatization during chronic cold exposure increases the capacity for metabolic heat production in response to sympathetic stimulation.

Dietary intake   Fasting suppresses and overfeeding stimulates the sympathetic nervous system. The reduction in sympathetic activity during fasting or starvation may contribute to the decrease in metabolic rate, bradycardia, and hypotension in these states. Enhanced sympathetic activity during periods of increased caloric intake may contribute to the elevation in metabolic rate associated with a chronic increase in dietary intake.

Hypoxia   Chronic hypoxia is associated with stimulation of the sympathoadrenal system, and some of the cardiovascular changes in hypoxia may be dependent upon catecholamines.

THE SYMPATHETIC NERVOUS SYSTEM IN PATHOGENESIS OF SELECTED DISEASE STATES

HYPERTENSION (See also Chap. 196)   As shown in Fig. 67-5, regulation of arterial pressure by the sympathetic nervous system involves blood vessels, the heart, and the kidneys. The sympathetic nervous system increases peripheral resistance by direct stimulation of the resistance vessels and by activation of the renin-angiotensin system. Increased cardiac output is the result of enhanced cardiac contractility and augmented venous return, the latter a result of venoconstriction and increased renal sodium reabsorption. Stimulation of sodium retention diminishes the capacity of the kidney to compensate for the increase in blood pressure. Antiadrenergic agents lower blood pressure by interacting at many of the sites shown in Fig. 67-5.

Whether sympathetic overactivity plays a role in the pathogenesis of primary hypertension is uncertain due to the insensitivity of currently available methods of assessing sympathetic activity in humans. It is well established, however, that the sympathetic nervous system plays at least a permissive role in hypertension (Chap. 39). Despite the elevated blood pressure, sympathetic nervous system activity is not suppressed in hypertensive patients, and reflex control of the circulation is retained, due in part to upward resetting of the baroreceptors. In addition, peripheral sensitivity of the vasculature to NE is either normal or enhanced. The maintenance of sympathetic nervous system activity in patients with hypertension accounts for the hypotensive effects of antiadrenergic agents.

During antihypertensive treatment with vasodilators or diuretics, the sympathetic nervous system may be activated in response to decreased pressure in either the venous or arterial circulation (Fig. 67-2). The heightened sympathetic activity that results, in addition to causing tachycardia, may oppose the antihypertensive therapy by activating the various effector systems shown in Fig. 67-5. Antiadrenergic agents, therefore, have a fundamental role in the therapy of most hypertensive patients.

ANGINA PECTORIS (Chap. 190)   Sympathetic stimulation of the cardiovascular system increases myocardial oxygen consumption as a consequence of elevated heart rate, enhanced myocardial contractility, and increased myocardial wall tension. Attacks of angina,

FIGURE 67-5 Sympathetic nervous system effects on blood pressure. Sympathetic stimulation (+) increases blood pressure by effects on the heart, the veins, the kidneys, and the arterioles. The net result of sympathetic stimulation is an increase in both cardiac output and peripheral resistance. *[From JB Young, L Landsberg, in P Sleight et al (eds), Scientific Foundations of Cardiology, London, Heinemann, 1981.]*

therefore, are often precipitated by situations associated with sympathetic activation such as exercise, eating, and cold exposure. Beta blockade is beneficial in the treatment of angina because of reduction in sympathetic stimulation of the heart. Alpha-adrenergically mediated coronary vasoconstriction may also contribute to coronary spasm.

HYPERTHYROIDISM (Chap. 316)   Many of the peripheral manifestations of hyperthyroidism suggest a hyperadrenergic state. Enhancement of beta-receptor responses in hyperthyroidism is due in part to effects on the beta receptor. Thyroid hormone, in some tissues and in some species, increases receptor number; in other tissues, even when beta-receptor number is not increased, coupling of receptor occupancy to the adenylate cyclase cyclic-AMP system is augmented to amplify catecholamine-induced responses. Since thyroid hormone excess does not suppress sympathetic nervous system activity (plasma NE levels are normal in thyrotoxic patients), a "normal" level of sympathetic activity may evoke an exaggerated physiologic response. Many of the adrenergic manifestations of hyperthyroidism are diminished by treatment with beta-receptor blocking agents.

ORTHOSTATIC HYPOTENSION (Chap. 39)   The maintenance of arterial pressure during upright posture depends upon an adequate blood volume, an unimpaired venous return, and an intact sympathetic nervous system. Significant postural hypotension, therefore, often reflects extracellular fluid volume depletion or dysfunction of the circulatory reflexes. Diseases of the nervous system, such as tabes dorsalis, syringomyelia, or diabetes mellitus, may disrupt these sympathetic reflexes with resultant orthostatic hypotension. Although any antiadrenergic agent may impair the postural sympathetic response, orthostatic hypotension is most prominent with drugs that block neurotransmission within the ganglia or adrenergic neurons.

The term *idiopathic orthostatic hypotension* refers to a group of degenerative diseases involving either the pre- or postganglionic sympathetic neurons. Involvement of the peripheral sympathetic nervous system is characterized by low basal NE levels, while involvement at the level of the central nervous system or preganglionic sympathetic neurons is associated with normal basal plasma NE levels. In both cases the plasma NE response to upright posture is deficient. Orthostatic hypotension caused by disruption of the preganglionic autonomic neurons within the intermediolateral cell column of the spinal cord often occurs in association with degenerative changes of basal ganglia and other portions of the central nervous system. In the latter situation, known as *multiple systems atrophy*, or the *Shy-Drager* syndrome, orthostatic hypotension occurs along with a variety of neurologic disturbances including Parkinson's disease.

Treatment of orthostatic hypotension is usually unsatisfactory except in the mildest cases. There is no way of reestablishing the normal relationship between fall in venous return and sympathetic neuronal activation. Volume expansion with fludrocortisone and a liberal salt diet in conjunction with fitted stockings to the waist, and elevation of the head of the bed to avoid recumbency, will maintain plasma volume and venous return and frequently provide symptomatic improvement. Rarely a beneficial response may be obtained from treatment with sympathomimetic amines (including clonidine).

PHARMACOLOGY OF THE SYMPATHOADRENAL SYSTEM

A variety of therapeutic agents affect sympathetic nervous system function or interact with adrenergic receptors, making it possible to stimulate or suppress effects mediated by catecholamines with some degree of specificity (Table 67-1).

SYMPATHOMIMETIC AMINES   Sympathomimetic amines may directly activate adrenergic receptors (direct acting) or release NE from the sympathetic nerve endings (indirect acting). Many agents have both direct and indirect effects.

Epinephrine and norepinephrine   The naturally occurring catecholamines act predominantly by the direct stimulation of adrenergic receptors. NE is employed to support the circulation and elevate the blood pressure in hypotensive states (Chap. 39). Peripheral vasoconstriction is the major effect although cardiac stimulation occurs as well. E, also employed as a pressor, has special usefulness in the treatment of allergic reactions, especially those associated with anaphylaxis. E antagonizes the effects of histamine and other mediators on vascular and visceral smooth muscle and is useful in the treatment of bronchospasm.

Dopamine   *Dopamine* is used in treating hypotension, shock (Chap. 39), and certain forms of heart failure (Chap. 182). At low infusion rates it exerts a positive inotropic effect both by a direct action on the cardiac beta$_1$ receptors and by the indirect release of NE from sympathetic nerve endings in the heart. At low doses direct stimulation of dopaminergic receptors in the renal and mesenteric vasculature also results in vasodilation in the gut and kidney and facilitates sodium excretion. At higher infusion rates interaction with alpha-adrenergic receptors results in vasoconstriction, an increase in peripheral resistance, and an elevation of blood pressure.

Beta-receptor agonists   *Isoproterenol*, a direct-acting beta-receptor agonist, stimulates the heart, decreases peripheral resistance, and relaxes bronchial smooth muscle. It raises the cardiac output and accelerates atrioventricular conduction while increasing the automaticity of ventricular pacemakers. Isoproterenol is used in the treatment of heart block and bronchoconstriction. *Dobutamine*, a congener of dopamine with relative selectivity for the beta$_1$ receptor and with a greater effect on myocardial contractility than on heart rate, is also used in the treatment of congestive heart failure, often in combination with vasodilators (Chap. 182).

SELECTIVE BETA$_2$-RECEPTOR AGONISTS   The cardiac stimulation caused by nonselective beta agonists, such as isoproterenol or epinephrine, is occasionally dangerous when these agents are used in the treatment of bronchoconstriction. Selective beta$_2$ agonists (*metaproterenol, albuterol, terbutaline*, and *isoetharine*) improve the therapeutic ratio by achieving bronchial dilatation with less activation of the cardiovascular system (Chaps. 204 and 210); selectivity is relative, and cardiac stimulation does occur with these agents, particularly at the higher dose levels. *Ritodrine*, another selective beta$_2$ agonist, is used as a tocolytic agent (as is *terbutaline*) to relax the uterus and antagonize premature labor.

Alpha-adrenergic agonists   *Phenylephrine* and *methoxamine* are direct-acting alpha agonists that elevate blood pressure by increasing peripheral vasoconstriction. They are used primarily in the treatment of hypotension and paroxysmal supraventricular tachycardia (Chap. 185), in the latter case by increasing cardiac vagal tone through reflex baroreceptor stimulation. Phenylephrine and a related proprietary compound, *phenylpropanolamine*, are common constituents of decongestant medications (often combined with antihistamines) for the treatment of allergic rhinitis and upper respiratory infections.

Miscellaneous sympathomimetic amines with mixed actions   *Ephedrine* has both direct beta-receptor agonist properties and an indirect effect on sympathetic nerve endings, from which it releases NE, and is used primarily as a bronchodilator. *Sudephedrine*, a congener of ephedrine, is less potent at dilating bronchi and serves as a nasal decongestant. *Metaraminol* has both direct and indirect effects on sympathetic nerve endings and is employed in the treatment of hypotensive states.

Dopaminergic agonists   The dopamine 2–receptor agonist *bromocriptine* is used to suppress prolactin secretion (Chap. 313). *Apomorphine*, another dopamine 2–receptor agonist, is used to induce emesis.

ANTIADRENERGIC OR SYMPATHOLYTIC AGENTS (See also Chap. 196)   **Agents inhibiting central sympathetic outflow**   The antihypertensive agents *methyldopa, clonidine, guanabenz*, and *guanfacine* diminish central sympathetic outflow by stimulating a central alpha-adrenergic pathway (alpha$_2$ receptor) that diminishes vasomotor outflow. Central nervous system side effects such as sedation are common. When administration of clonidine is stopped abruptly, a withdrawal syndrome characterized by rebound hyperactivity of the

TABLE 67-1   Some commonly used autonomic drugs[a,b,c]

Agent	Indication	Dose and Route	Comment
ADRENERGIC AGONISTS[d]			
Epinephrine	Anaphylaxis	100–500 μg SC or IM (0.1–0.5 mL of 1/1000 solution of hydrochloride salt); 25–50 μg IV (slowly) every 5–15 min; titrate as needed	Nonselective alpha and beta agonist; increases BP, heart rate Bronchodilation
Norepinephrine	Shock Hypotension	2–4 μg of NE base/min IV; titrate as needed	Alpha and beta$_1$ agonist Vasoconstriction predominates Extravasation causes tissue necrosis; infuse through IV cannula
Isoproterenol	Cardiogenic shock Bradyarrhythmias AV block Asthma	0.5–5.0 μg/min IV; titrate as needed Inhalation	Nonselective beta agonist Increases cardiac rate and contractility (beta$_1$) Tachycardia limits usefulness Dilates bronchi (beta$_2$); cardiac stimulation also occurs
Dobutamine	Refractory CHF Cardiogenic shock	2.5–25 (μg/kg)/min IV	Selective beta$_1$ agonist with greater effect on contractility than heart rate; a congener of dopamine but not a dopaminergic agonist
Phenylephrine	Hypotension	40–180 μg/min IV	Selective alpha$_1$ agonist; useful in antagonizing hypotension of spinal anesthesia
	Supraventricular tachycardia	150–800 μg slow IV push	Pressor effect induces vagotonic response; do not exceed 21 kPa (160 mmHg) systolic BP
Terbutaline	Asthma	2.5–5.0 mg PO tid; 0.25–0.5 mg SC; inhalation every 4–5 h	Selective beta$_2$ agonist; beta$_1$ (cardiac) effects at higher doses
Albuterol	Asthma	2.0–4.0 mg PO tid or qid; inhalation every 4–6 h	Selective beta$_2$ agonist; beta$_1$ effects (cardiac) at higher doses
Isoetharine	Asthma	Inhalation every 2–4 h	Selective beta$_2$ agonist; some beta$_1$ effects
Metaproterenol	Asthma	10–20 mg PO tid or qid; inhalation every 3–4 h	Selective beta$_2$ agonist; some beta$_1$ effects
Ritodrine	Premature labor	100–350 μg/min IV; 10–20 mg every 4–6 h PO	Selective beta$_2$ agonist; hypokalemia. hyperglycemia, hypotension, cardiac stimulation may occur Neonatal hypoglycemia, hypocalcemia reported
DOPAMINERGIC AGONISTS			
Dopamine	Shock	2–5 (μg/kg)/min IV (dopaminergic range) 5–10 (μg/kg)/min IV (dopaminergic and beta range) 10–20 (μg/kg)/min IV (beta range) 20–50 (μg/kg)/min IV (alpha range)	Pharmacologic effects are dose dependent: renal and mesenteric vasodilation predominate at lower doses; cardiac stimulation and vasoconstriction develop as the dose is increased
Bromocriptine	Amenorrhea-galactorrhea	2.5 mg PO bid or tid	Selective agonist of dopamine-2 receptor; inhibits prolactin secretion
	Acromegaly	5–15 mg PO tid or qid	Lowers growth hormone in a minority of patients with acromegaly
INHIBITORS OF CENTRAL SYMPATHETIC OUTFLOW			
Clonidine	Hypertension	0.1–0.6 mg PO bid	Selective alpha$_2$ agonist; potentiates central baroreceptor depressor reflex Abrupt discontinuation may result in withdrawal syndrome with rebound hypertension
Methyldopa	Hypertension	250–500 mg PO every 6–8 h	Metabolized by decarboxylation and beta hydroxylation to α-methyl-norepinephrine, a centrally active selective alpha$_2$ agonist
ADRENERGIC NEURON BLOCKING AGENTS			
Guanethidine	Hypertension	10–100 mg PO qd	Concentrated in sympathetic nerve endings; blocks release of NE in response to nerve impulses and depletes NE stores; prominent orthostatic hypotension
Bretylium	Ventricular fibrillation and tachycardia	5 mg/kg IV	In addition to blocking NE release, has direct effect on electrical properties of cardiac muscle
BETA BLOCKING AGENTS[e]			
Propranolol	Hypertension	40–160 mg PO bid (or higher)	Lipophilic, nonselective Dosage highly variable
	Angina	10–40 mg PO tid or qid	
	Myocardial infarction	60–80 mg PO tid	Prolongs survival post MI
	Arrhythmias	10–30 mg PO tid or qid; 1–3 mg IV	
	Hypertrophic cardiomyopathy	20–40 mg PO tid or qid	
	Pheochromocytoma	10–20 mg PO tid or qid; 0.5–2.0 mg IV	After alpha blockade initiated
	Essential tremor	20–80 mg PO tid	
	Migraine	20–80 mg PO bid or tid	
	Hyperthyroidism	10–60 mg PO tid or qid	

TABLE 67-1 Some commonly used autonomic drugs[a,b,c] *(continued)*

Agent	Indication	Dose and Route	Comment
BETA BLOCKING AGENTS[e] *(continued)*			
Metoprolol	Hypertension	50–200 mg PO bid	Selective beta$_1$ (cardiac), lipophilic
	Myocardial infarction	100 mg PO bid	Prolongs survival post MI
Nadolol	Hypertension	80–320 mg PO qd	Hydrophilic, nonselective; lengthen dosage interval
	Angina	80–240 mg PO qd	with renal failure
Timolol	Hypertension	10–30 mg PO bid	Lipophilic, nonselective
	Myocardial infarction	10 mg PO bid	Prolongs survival post MI
Atenolol	Hypertension	50–100 mg PO qd	Selective beta$_1$, hydrophilic; lengthen dosage interval with renal failure
Pindolol	Hypertension	5–30 mg PO bid	Nonselective, lipophilic with partial agonist activity
	Angina	10 mg PO qid	
Acebutolol	Hypertension	200–800 mg qid	Selective beta$_1$, hydrophilic, partial agonist activity
	Arrhythmias	200–600 mg bid	
Esmolol	Supraventricular tachycardia	50–200 (μg/kg)/min after loading dose of 500 (μg/kg)/min for 1 min	Selective beta$_1$, very short duration of action
ALPHA BLOCKING AGENTS			
Phenoxybenzamine	Pheochromocytoma	10–60 mg PO bid; titrate as needed	Noncompetitive, nonselective alpha blockade
Phentolamine	Pheochromocytoma	5 mg IV (after test dose of 0.5 mg)	Competitive, nonselective alpha blockade
Prazosin	Hypertension	1–5 mg PO bid or tid	Competitive, selective alpha$_1$ blockade
	CHF	2–7 mg PO qid	
Terazosin	Hypertension	1–5 mg PO qid	Competitive, selective alpha$_1$ blockade, long duration of action
COMBINED ALPHA-BETA BLOCKING AGENT			
Labetalol	Hypertension	100–1200 mg PO bid; titrate slowly as needed; 20–80 mg IV (by increments up to 300 mg); 2 mg/min by IV infusion	Competitive alpha and beta antagonist with relatively more activity against beta receptors
DOPAMINERGIC ANTAGONIST[f]			
Metoclopramide	Diabetic gastroparesis	10 mg PO qid	Competitive dopaminergic antagonist with prominent cholinergic agonist activity
	Gastroesophageal reflex	10–15 mg PO qid	
	Antiemetic (cancer chemotherapy)	10 mg IV	
GANGLIONIC BLOCKING AGENT			
Trimethaphan	Hypertensive crisis (aortic dissection)	1–3 mg/min IV	Competitive ganglionic blocker; some direct vasodilating effects; inhibits parasympathetic as well as sympathetic nervous system
CHOLINERGIC AGONIST			
Bethanechol	Urinary retention (nonobstructive)	10–100 mg PO tid or qid; 5 mg SC	M-2 receptor agonist
ANTICHOLINESTERASE AGENTS[g]			
Physostigmine	Central cholinergic blockade	1–2 mg IV (slow)	Tertiary amine; penetrates CNS well; may cause seizures; used to reverse central anticholinergic effects produced by overdose of atropine or tricyclic antidepressants
Edrophonium	Paroxysmal supraventricular tachycardia	5 mg IV (after 1.0-mg test dose)	Induces vagotonic response; rapid onset, short duration of action; effects reversed by atropine
CHOLINERGIC BLOCKING AGENTS[h]			
Atropine	Bradycardia and hypotension	0.4–1.0 mg IV every 1–2 h	Competitive inhibition of M-1 and M-2 receptor; blocks hemodynamic changes associated with increased vagal tone

[a] Consult complete prescribing information.
[b] Doses for children are not given.
[c] Only the more common indications and routes of administration are listed.
[d] Dopaminergic agonists are listed separately although dopamine, at high doses, is an adrenergic agonist as well.
[e] Clinical efficacy of most beta blockers appears similar for major indications. Not all beta blockers are FDA approved for all indications listed in the table. When beta blocking agents are discontinued, gradual dosage reduction is recommended.
[f] Neuroleptic and antipsychotic agents are also dopaminergic antagonists; these are not included in the table.
[g] A major use of cholinesterase inhibitors is in the treatment of myasthenia gravis (Chap 368). These agents, quaternary amines that do not penetrate the CNS, are not included in the table.
[h] A wide variety of synthetic atropine derivatives are available for the purpose of (1) diminishing GI tract motility and secretion and (2) increasing urinary bladder capacity. Their usefulness is limited by anticholinergic side effects. Some may be useful as adjuncts in the treatment of peptic ulcer disease.

sympathetic nervous system can produce a syndrome resembling the crises of patients with pheochromocytoma. *Opiates* may also exert a central sympatholytic effect; the sympathetic excitation of morphine withdrawal responds to clonidine and vice versa. *Propranolol* and *reserpine* may exert some sympatholytic effects at the level of the central nervous system.

Ganglionic blocking agents Ganglionic transmission may be antagonized by drugs that block the (nicotinic) cholinergic synapse between the preganglionic and postganglionic autonomic nerves. These agents inhibit the parasympathetic as well as the sympathetic nervous system. Only *trimethaphan* is in general clinical use; its major application is in the treatment of hypertensive crises, particularly aortic dissection, when controlled hypotension and decreased myocardial contractility are desirable (Chap. 197).

Agents acting at the peripheral sympathetic nerve endings Adrenergic neuron-blocking agents depress the function of the peripheral sympathetic nerves by decreasing the amount of neurotransmitter released. *Guanethidine*, the prototype of this class of drugs, is concentrated in the sympathetic nerve endings by the amine-uptake mechanism. Within the terminal it blocks the release of NE in response to nerve impulses and eventually depletes the nerve of NE by displacing it from the intraneuronal storage granules. The drug is occasionally useful in the management of severe hypertension, although orthostatic hypotension is a limiting side effect. *Bretylium*, an agent whose effects are similar to those of guanethidine, is employed in the treatment of ventricular fibrillation (Chap. 185). Both guanethidine and bretylium are antagonized by agents that affect the amine-uptake transport process such as sympathomimetic amines, tricyclic antidepressants, phenoxybenzamine, and phenothiazines. The antihypertensive action of guanethidine may be rapidly reversed by these drugs.

Reserpine depletes catecholamines from the peripheral sympathetic nerve endings, the brain, and the adrenal medulla. Its antihypertensive effect in humans is usually attributed to depletion of peripheral NE stores within sympathetic nerve endings. The sedation and occasionally morbid depression attending its use result from NE depletion within the central nervous system.

Adrenergic-receptor blocking agents Adrenergic blocking agents antagonize the effects of catecholamines at the level of the peripheral tissue.

ALPHA-ADRENERGIC-RECEPTOR BLOCKING AGENTS *Phenoxybenzamine* and *phentolamine* are utilized principally in treating pheochromocytoma (Chap. 318). Phenoxybenzamine produces prolonged, noncompetitive alpha blockade, while phentolamine leads to reversible, competitive blockade. Because of its rapid action and short duration, phentolamine is commonly used in the treatment of acute hypertensive paroxysms secondary to catecholamine excess, such as occur with pheochromocytoma, with pressor reactions in patients receiving monoamine oxidase inhibitors, and in clonidine withdrawal. Both phentolamine and phenoxybenzamine antagonize alpha$_1$ and alpha$_2$ receptors, although phenoxybenzamine is more potent at the alpha$_1$ receptor site. *Prazosin*, an alpha-adrenergic blocking agent with selectivity for the alpha$_1$ receptor, possesses properties that resemble those of primary vasodilators and is used in the treatment of essential hypertension and as an afterload reducing agent in congestive heart failure. Terazosin, a long-acting selective alpha$_1$ blocker, is used in the treatment of essential hypertension. Since none of these agents have much effect on the beta-adrenergic receptor, unopposed beta stimulation may result in tachycardia.

BETA-ADRENERGIC-RECEPTOR BLOCKING AGENTS Beta blocking agents antagonize the cardiovascular effects of catecholamines in angina pectoris, hypertension, and cardiac arrhythmias. The benefit of beta blockade in angina derives from the decrease in myocardial oxygen consumption following reduction in heart rate and myocardial contractility (Chap. 190). The hypotensive effect of beta blockade is not clearly understood (Chap. 196). Diminished cardiac output, decreased NE release at postganglionic sympathetic nerve endings, reduced renin secretion, and suppressed central sympathetic outflow

are possible mechanisms. The efficacy of beta blocking agents in the treatment of arrhythmias depends upon reduction of the rate of spontaneous depolarization of pacemaker cells in the sinus node and junctional pacemakers and upon slowing conduction within the atria and atrioventricular node. Beta blockade is also effective in the symptomatic management of hyperthyroidism and the control of tachycardia and arrhythmias in patients with pheochromocytoma. Beta-adrenergic blocking agents are also useful in the treatment of migraine, essential tremor, idiopathic hypertrophic subaortic stenosis, aortic dissection, and possibly in the period following myocardial infarction. Several trials have suggested that beta blocking agents, administered long-term, diminish mortality following acute myocardial infarction. The mechanism may involve antiarrhythmic action, prevention of reinfarction, and reduction in infarct size (Chap. 189).

PHARMACOLOGIC PROPERTIES OF BETA-RECEPTOR BLOCKING AGENTS
Eight beta blocking agents (atenolol, acebutolol, esmolol, metoprolol, nadolol, pindolol, propranolol, and timolol) are available for use in the United States. Other agents (alprenolol, bevantolol, oxprenolol, sotalol, etc.) are in use in other countries and investigational within the United States. The utility of these agents is derived predominantly from blockade of beta-adrenergic receptors. In general, the various agents have similar clinical efficacy.

Although much has been written about other pharmacologic properties including cardioselectivity, membrane stabilizing (local anesthetic) effects, intrinsic sympathomimetic (partial-agonist) activity, and lipid solubility, the clinical significance of these additional properties is small. Local anesthetic properties are most prominent with propranolol; however, membrane stabilization probably does not contribute substantially to the clinical utility. The various beta blockers do differ in their water and lipid solubility. The lipophilic agents (propranolol, metoprolol, oxprenolol) are readily absorbed from the gastrointestinal tract, metabolized by the liver, have large volumes of distribution, and penetrate the central nervous system well; the hydrophilic agents (acebutolol, atenolol, nadolol, sotalol) are less readily absorbed, not extensively metabolized, and have relatively long plasma half-lives. As a consequence, the hydrophilic agents may be administered once per day. Hepatic failure may prolong the plasma half-life of the lipophilic agents, and renal failure prolongs the action of the hydrophilic group. The degree of lipid solubility, therefore, may provide a basis for choice of a particular agent in patients with hepatic or renal insufficiency. Although the hydrophilic agents penetrate the central nervous system less well, central nervous system side effects (sedation, depression, hallucinations) probably occur as frequently with the hydrophilic as with the lipophilic agents.

Some beta-adrenergic blocking agents possess beta-agonist activity. This has been referred to as "intrinsic sympathomimetic activity" or "ISA." Agents with partial agonist activity (pindolol, alprenolol, acebutolol, oxprenolol) cause little or no depression of resting heart rate (partial agonist effect) while blocking the increase in heart rate that occurs in response to exercise or the administration of a beta agonist such as isoproterenol. The presence of partial agonist activity may be useful when bradycardia limits treatment in patients with slow resting heart rates. Although intrinsic sympathomimetic activity may also be useful in patients with depressed left ventricular function and reactive airways, no clear advantage of these agents over beta blockers without partial agonist activity has been demonstrated. Pindolol also produces mild vasodilation, perhaps in part related to peripheral beta$_2$ stimulation. On theoretical grounds intrinsic sympathomimetic activity would be undesirable in the treatment of thyrotoxicosis, idiopathic hypertrophic subaortic stenosis, and aortic dissection.

CARDIOSELECTIVE (BETA$_1$)-ADRENERGIC-RECEPTOR BLOCKING AGENTS
Propranolol, the prototype of the nonselective beta-adrenergic blocking agent, induces a competitive blockade of both beta$_1$ and beta$_2$ receptors. Other nonselective beta blocking agents include alprenolol, nadolol, oxprenolol, pindolol, sotalol, and timolol. Metoprolol, acebutolol, and atenolol possess relative selectivity for the beta$_1$ receptor. Although beta$_1$ selective agents have the theoretical advan-

tage of producing less bronchoconstriction and less peripheral vaso-constriction, a clear-cut clinical advantage of the cardioselective agents has not been demonstrated, since the beta$_1$ selectivity is only relative. Bronchoconstriction may occur when beta$_1$ selective agents are administered in full therapeutic doses.

ADVERSE EFFECTS OF BETA BLOCKING AGENTS   Aside from the effects on the central nervous system, most adverse reactions to beta blocking agents are consequences of beta-adrenergic blockade. These include the precipitation of heart failure in patients in whom cardiac compensation depends upon enhanced sympathetic drive; the aggravation of bronchospasm in patients with asthma; predisposition to the development of hypoglycemia in insulin-requiring diabetics (blockade of catecholamine-mediated counterregulation and antagonism of the adrenergic warning signs of hypoglycemia); the development of hyperkalemia in diabetic or uremic patients with impaired potassium tolerance; and the enhancement of coronary or peripheral arterial vasospasm.

MISCELLANEOUS ADRENERGIC BLOCKING AGENTS   *Labetalol,* approved for use in the United States as an antihypertensive agent, is a competitive antagonist of both alpha- and beta-adrenergic receptors. Although labetalol induces relatively more beta- than alpha-receptor blockade, fall in peripheral resistance may be marked following acute administration of the drug. Vasodilation may be mediated in part by a partial agonist effect on the beta$_2$-adrenergic receptor; labetalol does not possess partial agonist activity for the beta$_1$ (cardiac) receptor.

Metoclopramide is a dopaminergic antagonist with cholinergic agonist properties. It enhances gastric emptying, increases the tone of the lower esophageal sphincter, increases prolactin and aldosterone secretion, and antagonizes emesis induced by apomorphine. It is useful clinically in enhancing gastric emptying (in the absence of organic obstruction such as in diabetic gastroparesis), in antagonizing gastroesophageal reflux, and as an antiemetic during cancer chemotherapy.

THE PARASYMPATHETIC NERVOUS SYSTEM

ACETYLCHOLINE   Acetylcholine (ACh) serves as the neurotransmitter at all autonomic ganglia, at the postganglionic parasympathetic nerve endings, and at the postganglionic sympathetic nerve endings innervating the eccrine sweat glands. The enzyme choline acetyltransferase catalyzes the synthesis of ACh from acetyl CoA produced within the nerve ending and from choline, actively taken up from the extracellular fluid. Within the cholinergic nerve endings ACh is stored in discrete synaptic vesicles and released in response to nerve impulses that depolarize the nerve terminals and increase calcium influx.

Cholinergic receptors   Different receptors for ACh exist on the postganglionic neurons within the autonomic ganglia and at the postjunctional autonomic effector sites. Those within the autonomic ganglia and adrenal medulla are stimulated predominantly by nicotine (*nicotinic receptors*) and those on autonomic effector cells by the alkaloid muscarine (*muscarinic receptors*). Ganglionic blocking agents antagonize the nicotinic receptors while atropine blocks the muscarinic receptors. The muscarinic (M) receptor, furthermore, has been recently subdivided into two types. The M-1 receptor is localized to the central nervous system and perhaps parasympathetic ganglia; the M-2 receptor is the nonneuronal muscarinic receptor on smooth muscle, cardiac muscle, and glandular epithelium. Bethanechol is a selective agonist of the M-2 receptor; pirenzepine, an investigational agent, is a selective antagonist of the M-1 receptor. This agent markedly reduces gastric acid secretion. The M-2 receptor inhibits adenylyl cyclase and utilizes the regulatory G$_i$ protein; the M-1 receptor interacts with G$_p$ and stimulates phospholipase C (Fig. 67-4).

Acetylcholinesterase   Hydrolysis of ACh by acetylcholinesterase inactivates the neurotransmitter at cholinergic synapses. This enzyme (also known as specific or true cholinesterase) is present within neurons and is distinct from butyrocholinesterase (serum

cholinesterase or pseudocholinesterase). The latter enzyme is present in plasma and nonneuronal tissues and is not primarily involved in the termination of the effects of ACh at autonomic effector sites. The pharmacologic effects of anticholinesterase agents are due to inhibition of neuronal (true) acetylcholinesterase.

PHYSIOLOGY OF THE PARASYMPATHETIC NERVOUS SYSTEM   The parasympathetic nervous system participates in the regulation of the cardiovascular system, the gastrointestinal tract, and the genitourinary system. Tissues such as liver, kidney, pancreas, and thyroid also receive parasympathetic innervation, suggesting a role for the parasympathetic nervous system in metabolic regulation as well, although cholinergic effects on metabolism are not well characterized.

Cardiovascular system   Parasympathetic effects on the heart are mediated by the vagus nerve. ACh reduces the rate of spontaneous depolarization of the sinoatrial node and decreases heart rate. The heart rate in different physiologic states is the result of coordinated interaction between sympathetic stimulation, parasympathetic inhibition, and the intrinsic activity of the sinoatrial pacemaker. ACh also delays impulse conduction within the atrial musculature while shortening the effective refractory period, a combination of factors which may initiate or perpetuate atrial arrhythmias. At the atrioventricular node ACh reduces conduction velocity, increases the effective refractory period, and thus diminishes the ventricular response during atrial flutter or fibrillation (Chap. 185). The decrease in inotropy induced by ACh is related to a prejunctional inhibitory effect on sympathetic nerve endings as well as to a direct inhibitory effect on the atrial myocardium. The ventricular myocardium is not much affected since innervation by cholinergic fibers is minimal. A direct cholinergic contribution to the regulation of peripheral resistance appears unlikely since parasympathetic innervation of the vasculature is not extensive. The parasympathetic nervous system, however, may influence peripheral resistance indirectly by inhibiting NE release from sympathetic nerves.

Gastrointestinal tract   Parasympathetic innervation of the gut is via the vagus nerve and the pelvic sacral nerves. The parasympathetic nervous system increases the tone of gastrointestinal smooth muscle, enhances peristaltic activity, and relaxes the gastrointestinal sphincters. ACh stimulates exocrine secretion from the glandular epithelium and enhances the secretion of gastrin, secretin, and insulin.

Genitourinary and respiratory systems   Sacral parasympathetic nerves supply the urinary bladder and genitalia. ACh increases ureteral peristalsis, contracts the urinary detrusor muscle, and relaxes the trigone and sphincter, thereby playing a critical role in the coordination of urination. The respiratory tract is innervated with parasympathetic fibers derived from the vagus nerve. ACh increases tracheobronchial secretions and stimulates bronchial constriction.

PHARMACOLOGY OF THE PARASYMPATHETIC NERVOUS SYSTEM   Cholinergic agonists   ACh itself has no therapeutic role because of its widespread effects and short duration of action. Congeners of ACh are less susceptible to hydrolysis by cholinesterase and have a narrower range of physiologic effects. Bethanechol, the only systemic cholinergic agonist in general use, stimulates gastrointestinal and genitourinary smooth muscle with minimal effect on the cardiovascular system. It is used in the treatment of urinary retention in the absence of outflow tract obstruction and, less commonly, in gastrointestinal disorders such as postvagotomy gastric atony. Pilocarpine and carbachol are topical cholinergic agonists used in the treatment of glaucoma.

Acetylcholinesterase inhibitors   Cholinesterase inhibitors enhance the effects of parasympathetic stimulation by diminishing the inactivation of ACh. The therapeutic application of reversible cholinesterase inhibitors depends upon the role of ACh as neurotransmitter at the skeletal muscle neuroeffector junction and within the central nervous system and includes the treatment of myasthenia gravis (Chap. 366), the termination of neuromuscular blockade following general anesthesia, and the reversal of intoxication by agents with a central anticholinergic action. Physostigmine, a tertiary amine, penetrates the central nervous system well, while related quaternary amines (neostigmine, pyridostigmine, ambenonium, and edrophonium) do not. Organophosphorous cholinesterase inhibitors produce irreversible cholinesterase blockade; these agents are used principally as insecticides and are primarily of toxicologic interest. With regard to the autonomic nervous system, cholinesterase inhibitors are of limited use in the treatment of intestinal and bladder smooth-muscle dysfunction such as occurs in paralytic ileus and atonic urinary bladder. Cholinesterase inhibitors induce a vagotonic response in the heart and may be useful in terminating attacks of paroxysmal supraventricular tachycardia (Chap. 185).

Cholinergic-receptor blocking agents *Atropine* blocks muscarinic cholinergic receptors, with little effect on cholinergic transmission at the autonomic ganglia and the neuromuscular junctions. Many of the central nervous system actions of atropine and atropine-like drugs are attributable to blockade of central muscarinic synapses. The related alkaloid, *scopolamine,* is similar to atropine but causes drowsiness, euphoria, and amnesia, effects that make it suitable as a preanesthetic medication.

Atropine increases heart rate and enhances atrioventricular conduction, actions that may be useful in combating the bradycardia or heart block associated with heightened vagal tone. In addition, atropine reverses cholinergically mediated bronchoconstriction and diminishes respiratory tract secretions. These effects contribute to its utility as a preanesthetic medication.

Atropine also decreases gastrointestinal tract motility and secretion. Although various derivatives and congeners of atropine (such as *propantheline, isopropamide,* and *glycopyrrolate*) have been advocated in patients with peptic ulcer or with diarrheal syndromes, the chronic use of such agents is limited by other manifestations of parasympathetic inhibition such as dry mouth and urinary retention. The investigational selective M-1 inhibitor pirenzepine inhibits gastric secretion at doses that have minimal anticholinergic effects at other sites; this agent may be useful in the treatment of peptic ulcer. Atropine and its congener *ipratropium,* when given by inhalation, cause bronchodilation and have been used experimentally in the treatment of asthma.

REFERENCES

BERRIDGE MJ: Inositol trisphosphate and diacylglycerol: Two interacting second messengers. Ann Rev Biochem 56:159, 1987

EXTON JH: Mechanisms of action of calcium-mobilizing agonists: Some variations on a young theme. FASEB J 2:2670, 1988

———: Mechanisms involved in alpha-adrenergic phenomena. Am J Physiol 248:E633, 1985

FRISHMAN WH: Clinical significance of beta₁ selectivity and intrinsic sympathomimetic activity in a beta-adrenergic blocking drug. Am J Cardiol 59:33F, 1987

FRISHMAN WH: Beta-adrenoceptor antagonists: New drugs and new indications. N Engl J Med 305:500, 1981

INSEL PA: Identification and regulation of adrenergic receptors in target cells. Am J Physiol 247:E53, 1984

LANDSBERG L, YOUNG JB: Catecholamines and the adrenal medulla, in *Williams Textbook of Endocrinology,* 7th ed, JD Wilson, DW Foster (eds). Philadelphia, Saunders, 1985, p 891

———, ———: The influence of diet on the sympathetic nervous system, in *Neuroendocrine Perspective,* vol 4, EE Muller et al (eds). Amsterdam, Elsevier, 1985, p 191

LEFKOWITZ RJ, CARON MG: Adrenergic receptors: Models for the study of receptors coupled to guanine nucleotide regulatory proteins. J Biol Chem 263:4993, 1988

LIMBIRD LE: Receptors linked to inhibition of adenylate cyclase: Additional signaling mechanisms. FASEB J 2:2686, 1988

WILLIAMSON JR: Role of inositol lipid breakdown in the generation of intracellular signals: State of the art lecture. Hypertension 8(Suppl II):II-140, 1986

68 G PROTEINS AND THE REGULATION OF SECOND MESSENGER SYSTEMS

MICHAEL FREISSMUTH / ALFRED G. GILMAN

For expression of their biological effects, hormones, neurotransmitters, growth factors, and autacoids (local transmitters such as histamine and serotonin) need interaction with specific receptors. These receptors are classified into distinct categories, based on structural homologies and on similarities in their mechanism of action. For example, the receptors for insulin and certain growth factors (e.g., platelet-derived growth factor) are membrane-bound tyrosine protein kinases, and this enzymatic activity is essential for their function (see Chap. 319). The binding site for ANF (atrial natriuretic factor; see Chap. 38) is in the extracellular domain of a guanylate cyclase that spans the plasma membrane; the intracellular portion of this protein synthesizes a second messenger, guanosine-3′,5′-monophosphate (cyclic GMP). Steroid hormones and triiodothyronine form hormone-receptor complexes that act as regulators of gene transcription (see Chap. 311). Yet another class of receptors, exemplified by the nicotinic cholinergic receptor, incorporate ion channels. Lastly, a large family of plasma membrane–bound receptors (the known number approximates 100) activate guanosine triphosphate–binding (GTP-binding) regulatory proteins, or *G proteins,* in the plasma membranes of cells. Each G protein in turn controls the activity of one or more membrane-bound effectors, such as adenylate cyclase, ion channels, and phospholipases (Table 68-1).

G PROTEIN–LINKED RECEPTORS A diverse group of ligands interact with G protein–linked receptors. These include peptide hormones (e.g., glucagon, ACTH), lipids (prostaglandins), nucleosides and nucleotides (adenosine, ATP), and amines (epinephrine, histamine). Nevertheless, all such receptors possess some structural features in common—including the topology of the proteins with respect to the plasma membrane (Fig. 68-1). The amino terminus of each receptor is outside the cell and is attached to *N*-linked oligosaccharides. The carboxyl terminus is intracellular and contains sites that can be phosphorylated and that play a crucial role in desensitization to hormone actions. The central portion of the receptor molecule is believed to fold into seven α helices that span the membrane bilayer and form the hydrophobic core of the receptor. The ligand-binding site lies within this hydrophobic core and is formed by reactive side chains that are contributed by more than one transmembrane helix. Portions of the intracellular loops that connect the individual membrane-spanning α helices form the site of interaction between the ligand-bound receptor and the appropriate G protein.

G PROTEINS AND THEIR EFFECTORS G proteins are composed of three different subunits designated α, β, and γ in order of decreasing mass. A few of the distinctive properties of individual G protein subunits are summarized in Table 68-2.

G Protein α subunit G proteins are classified on the basis of the α subunit. The hormone-sensitive adenylate cyclase system and the retinal cyclic GMP phosphodiesterase that participates in vision have served as models for the elucidation of the mechanisms of G protein–mediated transmembrane signaling. In both cases, the α subunit of the G protein interacts with and regulates the effector. The α subunits bind Mg^{2+} and guanine nucleotide (GTP or GDP) with high affinity and also possess GTPase activity that is essential for deactivation of the pathway. In addition, many G protein α subunits are substrates for bacterial toxins that catalyze the incorporation of an ADP-ribosyl moiety into the polypeptide at specific amino acid residues. G_s (the G protein that activates adenylate cyclase) and G_t (the major retinal G protein that activates the cyclic GMP phosphodiesterase) are substrates for cholera toxin; G_s in intestinal cells is the natural target for the toxin since cholera is an intraluminal infection. The incorporation of ADP-ribose into G_s causes its persistent activation, and

TABLE 68-1 Hormones, neurotransmitters, and autacoids that control G protein–linked second messenger systems

Agonist	Adenylate cyclase Stimulation	Adenylate cyclase Inhibition	Phospholipase C (IP$_3$, diacylglycerol) Stimulation	Arachidonic acid release Stimulation
Acetylcholine		+(M$_2$, M$_4$)*	+(M$_1$, M$_3$, M$_5$)	+
Adenosine	+(A$_2$)	+(A$_1$)		
ADP			+	+
Adrenocorticotropin	+			
Angiotensin		+	+	+
ATP		+(P$_2$)	+(P$_2$)	+
Bombesin			+	
Bradykinin			+	
Calcitonin	+			
Chemotactic peptides (e.g., FMLP)			+	+
Cholecystokinin			+	
Dopamine	+(D$_1$)	+(D$_2$)		
Enkephalin/endorphin		+(δ, μ?)		
Epinephrine/norepinephrine	+(β$_1$, β$_2$)	+(α$_2$)	+(α$_1$)	+(α$_1$)
Follicle stimulating hormone	+			
Glucagon	+(G$_2$)		+(G$_1$)	
Histamine	+(H$_2$)		+(H$_1$)	+(H$_1$)
5-Hydroxytryptamine	+(5HT$_{1A}$)	+(5HT$_{1A}$)	+(5HT$_2$, $_{1B,1C,1D}$)	
Leukotrienes			+	+
Luteinizing hormone (LH)	+			
Luteinizing hormone releasing hormone (LHRH)	+		+	
Parathyroid hormone	+			
Platelet activating factor			+	
Prostacyclin	+			
Prostaglandins (e.g., PGE$_2$)	+	+		
Somatostatin		+		
Tachykinins (substance P,K)			+	
Thromboxane A$_2$			+	
Thyrotropin releasing hormone (TRH)	+		+	
Vasoactive intestinal peptide (VIP)	+			
Vasopressin	+(V$_2$)	+(V$_1$)	+	

*Receptor subtypes, where known, are indicated in parentheses. M = muscarinic; P = purinergic.

FIGURE 68-1 Schematic representation of the topology of a G protein–coupled receptor. The barrels represent membrane-spanning α helices. The ligand-binding site of the receptor is located within the core formed by these membrane-spanning segments.

three closely related α subunits, designated G$_{i\alpha 1}$, G$_{i\alpha 2}$, and G$_{i\alpha 3}$. G$_{o\alpha}$ is an abundant brain G protein that is structurally similar to the G$_{i\alpha}$ family. While none of the G$_{i\alpha}$ subunits by itself is probably of great relevance in the inhibition of adenylate cyclase (see "Mechanism," below), each of these proteins can activate a K$^+$ channel in atrial myocardial cells. Stimulation of this pathway by muscarinic cholinergic agonists hyperpolarizes the cell and results in both negative chronotropic and inotropic responses. In the central nervous system, G$_o$ and the G$_i$ family apparently couple a variety of receptors to Ca^{2+} channels; G$_o$ can also modulate K$^+$ currents in brain cells. The resulting ion fluxes mediate the actions of myriad neurotransmitters. Two or three of the G$_{i\alpha}$ polypeptides and, in some cases, G$_{o\alpha}$ as well control the same effector. The precise role of each α subunit is thus difficult to assess, particularly since single cell types can contain several of these polypeptides. G$_{o\alpha}$- or G$_{i\alpha}$-like polypeptides may also

TABLE 68-2 Properties of G protein subunits

Subunit	M$_r$($\times 10^{-3}$)	Toxin	Role
α$_s$ (× 4)	44.5–46	Cholera toxin	Activates adenylate cyclase and voltage-sensitive calcium channels
α$_{s,olf}$	44.7	Cholera toxin	Presumed to activate olfactory adenylate cyclase
α$_i$ (× 3)	40.4–40.5	Pertussis toxin	Inhibits adenylate cyclase (weak); stimulates K$^+$ channels; implicated in pertussis toxin–sensitive activation of phospholipase C
α$_o$	39.9	Pertussis toxin	Regulates neuronal Ca^{2+} and K$^+$ channels; implicated in pertussis toxin–sensitive activation of phospholipase C
α$_{t,r}$	40.5	Pertussis toxin, cholera toxin	Activates cyclic GMP phosphodiesterase in retinal rods
α$_{t,c}$	40.9	Pertussis toxin, cholera toxin	Activates cyclic GMP phosphodiesterase in retinal cones
α$_z$	40.9	Unknown	Pertussis toxin–insensitive events
β (× 2)	37.4	—	βγ required for interaction of α with receptor; deactivates α subunit; direct regulation of effectors(?)
γ (× 3?)	8–10	—	

this is the crucial reaction in the pathogenesis of cholera. G$_o$, G$_t$ family, and the G$_i$'s are ADP-ribosylated by pertussis toxin, and this modification blocks the ability of the G protein to interact with receptors. The precise role of ADP-ribosylation in the pathogenesis of whooping cough is not clear.

G$_S$ ALPHA SUBUNIT All molecular species of G$_{s\alpha}$ can activate adenylate cyclase and in addition activate Ca^{2+} channels in skeletal and cardiac muscle. The fact that a single G protein α subunit can interact with more than one effector is an important general point. Not only can G proteins integrate the input from several receptors, they also represent a branch point for regulation of multiple effectors in response to a single signal.

G$_I$ AND G$_O$ ALPHA SUBUNITS G$_i$ mediates hormonal inhibition of adenylate cyclase. The G$_i$ family consists of oligomers with at least be involved in the regulation of phospholipase C, since GTP-dependent activation of this enzyme by hormones can be blocked by pertussis toxin in some tissues.

G_T ALPHA SUBUNIT   Retinal G protein, G_t or *transducin*, plays a pivotal role in vision. The photon receptor, *rhodopsin*, is localized in membranous disks in the outer segments of retinal rod cells; analogous color receptors are present in the cones. These molecules resemble the other G protein–linked receptors. Upon activation by light, rhodopsin interacts with and activates G_t; G_t in turn activates a cyclic GMP–specific phosphodiesterase. Intracellular concentrations of cyclic GMP fall rapidly, resulting in the closing of Na^+ channels and hyperpolarization of the rod cells. This represents the initial electrical signal that is eventually transmitted to the visual cortex. Retinal rods and cones differ not only in their individual photon receptors; they also have distinct G_t molecules ($G_{t,r}$ and $G_{t,c}$) and distinct cyclic GMP phosphodiesterases.

G_Z ALPHA SUBUNIT G_z is a G protein α subunit that lacks a site for ADP-ribosylation by pertussis toxin and is thus a candidate for regulation of transmembrane signaling pathways that cannot be disrupted by this toxin (e.g., stimulation of phospholipase C in many cells; regulation of certain ion channels).

G protein $\beta\gamma$-subunit complex   Two separate genes encode closely related but distinct β subunits (termed β_1 and β_2). Different forms of the γ polypeptide probably exist as well. The functional implication of this heterogeneity is unclear, since the β and γ subunits form a tightly associated complex and have not been resolved in active forms. In addition, the properties of $\beta\gamma$ complexes isolated from G_s, G_i, or G_o oligomers are indistinguishable. The $\beta\gamma$ complex contributes to the formation of the receptor recognition site on the G protein oligomer and facilitates the attachment of α subunits to the inner face of the plasma membrane. The $\beta\gamma$ complex is believed to deactivate the α subunit by formation of the intact G protein. In addition, the free $\beta\gamma$ subunit may also regulate effectors, possibly inhibiting adenylate cyclase and activating phospholipase A_2 directly.

MECHANISM OF G PROTEIN–MEDIATED SIGNAL TRANSDUCTION   A widely accepted model of the mechanism of G protein–mediated signal transduction is shown schematically in Fig. 68-2. The central thesis is that the G protein α subunit cycles between an inactive, GDP-liganded oligomeric form and an active, GTP-liganded monomeric state. *These two forms of the α subunit represent the "off" and "on" positions of a molecular switch.* The dissociation of GDP from α is the rate-limiting step. That is, the slow rate of spontaneous dissociation of GDP from α holds the switch in the off position. Interaction of the G protein with an agonist-receptor complex (H·R) facilitates dissociation of GDP. Binding of GTP to this ternary complex of hormone, receptor, and G protein has two consequences. First, the affinity of the receptor for the agonist is lowered, resulting in dissociation of the ternary complex. The receptor is thus free to recycle and activate additional G protein molecules, as long as agonist is present. As a result, considerable amplification occurs at this step. Second, the α subunit is activated by its dissociation from the $\beta\gamma$ complex. The switch is now on, and the activated α subunit interacts with the appropriate effector and modulates its activity. The G protein switch is programmed to turn itself off automatically, since deactivation results from hydrolysis of bound GTP by the α subunit.

FIGURE 68-2   Model of the regulatory cycles involved in G protein–mediated signal transduction. H = hormone or agonist; R = receptor; E = effector; G = G protein; α and $\beta\gamma$ = G protein subunits. Starred complexes are activated species. For further explanation, see text.

However, the lifetime of the activated α subunit is relatively long (several seconds), since the intrinsic rate of hydrolysis of GTP is slow; this kinetic feature permits additional signal amplification. To complete the cycle, the GDP-bound α subunit associates with $\beta\gamma$, and the system relaxes to its basal state. As mentioned above, the free $\beta\gamma$ subunit may itself regulate effectors directly.

Inhibition of adenylate cyclase is attributed at least in part to the capacity of the $\beta\gamma$ subunit, released upon activation of G_i, to interact with and deactivate G_s; $\beta\gamma$ can thus inhibit adenylate cyclase indirectly. This subunit exchange hypothesis predicts that the activation of one pathway can cause inhibition of effectors that are controlled by other G protein α subunits if the concentration of $\beta\gamma$ in the membrane is raised sufficiently.

SECOND MESSENGER SYSTEMS UNDER THE CONTROL OF G PROTEINS (Fig. 68-3)   Cyclic AMP   The conversion of ATP to cyclic AMP is accomplished by the catalytic subunit of the adenylate cyclase complex. This membrane-bound enzyme is believed to span the plasma membrane several times; the topology of the protein resembles that usually found in transporters and channels.

Cyclic AMP acts as a second messenger for a number of hormones (Table 68-1). The primary mechanism of action of the cyclic nucleotide is to cause dissociation of a dimer of cyclic AMP–binding regulatory subunits from the catalytic subunits of a protein kinase. The free catalytic subunits of the protein kinase are enzymatically active, and they transfer the γ phosphate from ATP to serine and threonine residues in target proteins. Such phosphorylation can either increase the activity (e.g., glycogen phosphorylase kinase, triacylglycerol lipase, protein phosphatase inhibitor 1) or decrease the activity (e.g., glycogen synthase, myosin light chain kinase) of the various substrates.

Termination of cyclic AMP action is accomplished by several mechanisms that are themselves subject to regulation by cyclic AMP and Ca^{2+}-calmodulin, a molecule with related second messenger functions (see below). Cyclic AMP is degraded to 5'-AMP by cyclic nucleotide phosphodiesterases. Some of these isoenzymes are activated by Ca^{2+}-calmodulin; they are inhibited by several drugs, including the methylxanthines (caffeine and theophylline) and milrinone. In addition, most cells possess a mechanism for the facilitated extrusion of cyclic AMP.

The regulatory effects of protein kinases are reversed by phosphoprotein phosphatases, which hydrolytically cleave the phosphate ester bond. These enzymes differ in their substrate specificities and in their regulation. For example, in the presence of elevated concentrations of cyclic AMP, protein phosphatase inhibitor 1 is phosphorylated by the cyclic AMP–dependent protein kinases; in this phosphorylated form, the inhibitor suppresses the activity of protein phosphatase 1. By contrast, protein phosphatase 2B is activated by Ca^{2+}-calmodulin. This network of stimulatory and inhibitory mechanisms integrates input from additional second messenger systems, which is necessary for efficient fine-tuning of cellular activities. All intracellular effects of cyclic AMP were initially believed to result from activation of protein phosphorylation, but ionic (Na^+) channels in olfactory neuroepithelial cells can be regulated (gated) directly by cyclic AMP.

Inositol trisphosphate, diacylglycerol, and calcium   Inositol-1,4,5-trisphosphate (IP_3) and diacylglycerol are second messengers generated by activation of a family of phosphoinositidases, commonly termed *phospholipase C*. These enzymes use phosphatidylinositol-4,5-bisphosphate, a phospholipid component of the plasma membrane, as substrate. Inositol trisphosphate can be phosphorylated to inositol-1,3,4,5-tetrakisphosphate, which may also serve as a second messenger. A large number of hormones and related molecules are known to activate phospholipase C (Table 68-1). This pathway is dependent on GTP, and it can be blocked by pertussis toxin in certain cells (e.g., granulocytes and mast cells). By contrast, the toxin has no effect on this response in certain other cells (e.g., cardiac myocytes and hepatocytes). More than one G protein may be involved in the regulation of phospholipase C.

FIGURE 68-3   The role of G proteins in transmembrane signaling. The top panel shows pathways that are regulated by identified G proteins. The bottom panel depicts pathways in which the participation of G proteins is probable, but the specific proteins have not yet been identified.

AA = arachidonic acid
AC = adenylate cyclase
Ca^{2+}/Cam PKC = calcium-calmodulin-dependent protein kinase
Cam = calmodulin
CH = channel
DG = diacylglycerol
E.R./S.R. = endoplasmic/sarcoplasmic reticulum
G = G protein
12-HETE = 12-hydroxyeicosatetraenoic acid
15-HETE = 15-hydroxyeicosatetraenoic acid
IP_3 = inositol trisphosphate
LL = lysophospholipid
LT = leukotriene
PDE = cyclic nucleotide phosphodiesterase
PG = prostaglandin
PIP_2 = phosphatidylinositol trisphosphate
PLC = phospholipase C
PKA = cyclic AMP–dependent protein kinase
PKC = protein kinase C
R = receptor for hormone or agonist

Inositol trisphosphate releases Ca^{2+} from intracellular stores (endoplasmic/sarcoplasmic reticulum) and promotes Ca^{2+} influx from the extracellular fluid. Additional mechanisms for entry of Ca^{2+} into the cytosolic compartment include voltage-gated Ca^{2+} channels and exchange mechanisms activated by other ions. G proteins regulate the activity of some of these channels and exchangers.

Ca^{2+} both regulates the activity of target enzymes directly and, more importantly, exerts its second messenger functions by interactions with Ca^{2+}-binding proteins such as troponin C and calmodulin. Calmodulin is a ubiquitous intracellular protein that binds four molecules of Ca^{2+}. This Ca^{2+}-calmodulin complex regulates several enzymes of the cyclic AMP system, including one type of adenylate cyclase, certain cyclic nucleotide phosphodiesterases, and protein phosphatase 2B (calcineurin). Several protein kinases are also activated by Ca^{2+}-calmodulin; the resulting effect can be either synergistic with (e.g., activation of phosphorylase kinase) or antagonistic to (e.g., activation of myosin light chain kinase) the cyclic AMP–mediated action. The effects of Ca^{2+}-calmodulin on its target enzymes can be blocked by certain phenothiazine drugs. The relationship

between this effect and the therapeutic efficacy or toxicity of these drugs is unknown.

Deactivation of the pathway is achieved by active transport of Ca^{2+} into intracellular compartments and extrusion of the ion by plasma membrane–bound, Ca^{2+}-pumping ATPases. Inositol trisphosphate is degraded by sequential dephosphorylation. The phosphatase that catalyzes the removal of phosphate from inositol-1-phosphate is inhibited by Li^+. It is not known whether this effect of Li^+ is related to its efficacy in psychiatric disorders.

The second product of the phospholipase C reaction is diacylglycerol, which acts as a second messenger by activating a family of isoenzymes referred to as *protein kinase C*. Upon binding of diacylglycerol, the requirement of these enzymes for Ca^{2+} decreases into the range of free Ca^{2+} concentrations found in cytosol. Activated protein kinase C phosphorylates many intracellular proteins, including some substrates of cyclic AMP–dependent protein kinase. The phorbol esters, which act as tumor promoters, are structurally related to diacylglycerol and also bind to and activate protein kinase C. This action is believed to explain their carcinogenicity.

The effect of diacylglycerol is terminated by enzymatic recycling to form phosphatidylinositol. Alternatively, diacylglycerol is broken down by a diacylglycerol lipase. Of interest, one of the fatty acids in the diacylglycerol molecule is usually arachidonate, the precursor of prostaglandins, leukotrienes, and other eicosanoids.

STIMULATION OF PHOSPHOLIPASE A$_2$ AND RELEASE OF ARACHIDONIC ACID Release of arachidonate from membrane phospholipids is the rate-limiting step in the biosynthesis of prostaglandins, leukotrienes, and other eicosanoids (see Chap. 69). Free arachidonate can arise by two distinct mechanisms. First, a family of enzymes, termed *phospholipase A$_2$*, cleaves the ester bond at the 2 position of the glycerol moiety of membrane phospholipids, giving rise to equimolar amounts of arachidonate and lysophospholipids. The enzymes require Ca^{2+} for activity. Second, as mentioned above, free arachidonate can be produced by the sequential action of phospholipase C and diacylglycerol lipase. Thus, hormones that stimulate the hydrolysis of phosphatidylinositol-4,5-bisphosphate also cause the release of arachidonate and the subsequent synthesis of eicosanoids (Table 68-1). In addition, these hormones increase intracellular concentrations of free Ca^{2+} and stimulate protein kinase C through inositol trisphosphate and diacylglycerol, respectively. Both of these effects may also contribute to the generation of free arachidonate via activation of phospholipase A$_2$. Phospholipase A$_2$ is activated by Ca^{2+}, and direct stimulation of protein kinase C by phorbol esters promotes release of arachidonate.

In view of the interdigitation of the regulatory mechanisms that control these pathways, it is not surprising that the regulation of phospholipase A$_2$ by G proteins is poorly understood. However, phospholipase A$_2$ can be activated independently of concomitant stimulation of phospholipase C. Moreover, purified G protein $\beta\gamma$ subunit complex may stimulate phospholipase A$_2$ activity in cell membranes.

Most eicosanoids are not second messengers as defined originally, since they produce their biologic effects by interacting with specific cell surface receptors coupled to G proteins. However, some metabolites of the 12-lipoxygenase pathway, in particular HEPETE (8-hydroxy-11,12-epoxy-5,9,14-icosotrienoic acid), may affect neuronal K^+ channels through a direct intracellular mechanism and thus act as typical second messengers.

REGULATION OF RECEPTOR-EFFECTOR COUPLING Desensitization Prolonged exposure of cells to a hormonal stimulus leads to a gradual attenuation of the biologic response, despite the continuing presence of the stimulus, a process usually termed desensitization, refractoriness, or tolerance. This type of adaptation is a general biologic mechanism, as exemplified by pharmacodynamic tolerance to massive concentrations of opioids. Desensitization is traditionally divided into two categories. *Homologous* or *receptor-specific desensitization* refers to the refractoriness that develops only to agonists that act on the same receptor as the desensitizing stimulus. In addition, stimulation of a particular receptor by an agonist can lead to the subsequent attenuation of the response to multiple hormones that influence the same pathway through distinct receptors. This phenomenon is termed *heterologous desensitization.*

Beta-adrenergic receptor-mediated stimulation of adenylate cyclase has served as a model system for elucidation of the molecular events that underlie desensitization, and both homologous and heterologous desensitization appear to result from phosphorylation of the receptor on its carboxyl-terminal domain.

Homologous desensitization is a multistep process. Initially (within minutes) receptors are uncoupled from G$_s$, as judged in part by their inability to stimulate adenylate cyclase. This process is reversible upon removal of agonist. However, the continued presence of agonist eventually leads to a decline in the concentration of receptors in the plasma membrane. This "down regulation" occurs over several hours and is not readily reversible, since protein synthesis is required to replenish the receptors on the cell surface. A novel protein kinase termed βARK (beta-adrenergic receptor kinase) specifically phosphorylates the agonist-bound receptor, whereas unliganded or antagonist-bound receptor will not serve as substrate. However, βARK

also phosphorylates other agonist-bound receptors that stimulate adenylate cyclase, such as the receptor for prostaglandin E$_1$. Phosphorylation of the beta-adrenergic receptor uncouples it from G$_s$ and is presumed to initiate sequestration of the receptor into an ill-defined subcellular compartment. The sequestered receptor may recycle to the functionally active pool upon hydrolytic cleavage of the incorporated phosphate by a phosphatase, or it may undergo degradation. Long-term exposure of cells to agonists apparently also reduces the number of receptors by decreasing the steady-state concentration of the mRNA that encodes the protein.

Heterologous desensitization of receptors that stimulate adenylate cyclase is probably mediated predominantly by a classic negative feedback loop. Activation of cyclic AMP–dependent protein kinase leads to phosphorylation of the receptors in a largely agonist-independent manner, and this modification also interferes with their ability to interact with G$_s$.

An analogous mechanism of desensitization is observed with receptors that mediate stimulation of phospholipase C (e.g., the alpha-adrenergic receptor). As a result of release of diacylglycerol, protein kinase C phosphorylates the receptors near the carboxyl terminus and is thereby presumed to interfere with the receptor–G protein interaction.

Additional forms of regulation The steady-state concentration of receptors in the plasma membrane represents the balance between synthesis and insertion into the bilayer versus internalization and degradation. As mentioned, the continuous presence of agonist tilts this balance in favor of degradation. Conversely, removal of agonist by pharmacologic blockade of the receptor, denervation of tissue, or extirpation of the source of the agonist favors accumulation of receptors on the cell surface and sensitization of target tissues to the appropriate agonist. Such sensitization may underlie the clinical syndrome associated with abrupt withdrawal of beta-adrenergic blocking agents.

Several other regulatory mechanisms influence signal transduction and, thus, the sensitivity of target cells to agonists. Since these events are not promoted by the receptor agonist, they are referred to as heterologous regulation. The most remarkable examples of heterologous regulation at the clinical level are the alterations in adrenergic receptor-effector coupling produced by thyroid and steroid hormones. Both triiodothyronine and glucocorticoids appear to be necessary to maintain normal coupling between beta-adrenergic receptors and G$_s$. In addition, thyroid hormones and glucocorticoids can increase transcription of mRNA for beta-adrenergic receptors. As one example, symptoms of increased sympathetic activity in the absence of elevated concentrations of plasma catecholamines is characteristic of hyperthyroidism. Similarly, heterologous regulation may underlie the permissive role of glucocorticoids in neurohormonal control of blood pressure.

ROLE OF G PROTEIN SYSTEMS IN DISEASE The pivotal role of G proteins in regulatory biology is understood in considerable detail. Comparatively little is known about the degree to which perturbations of these pathways participate in pathophysiology. However, a link to alterations in a G protein–regulated second messenger system has been established in several entities.

Cholera (See also Chap. 122) Pathogenic strains of *Vibrio cholerae* produce an exotoxin that transfers an ADP-ribosyl moiety to the α subunit of G$_s$, using intracellular nicotinamide adenine dinucleotide (NAD) as the donor. This reaction can occur in virtually all cells. However, the bacteria remain confined to the intestinal lumen, and the toxin binds to the intestinal epithelium but is not absorbed into the systemic circulation. Cell-surface binding of cholera toxin is dependent on the interaction between the B subunits of the toxin and gangliosides (GM$_1$) on the cell surface. Following such binding, the catalytically active A subunit of the toxin penetrates the cell. The ensuing modification of G$_{s\alpha}$ leads to its persistent activation, and the resultant high intracellular concentrations of cyclic AMP trigger the secretion of water and electrolytes into the intestinal lumen. The resulting watery diarrhea is the hallmark of cholera. Enteropathogenic strains of *Escherichia coli* produce a heat-labile toxin that is quite similar to cholera toxin and causes diarrhea by an identical mechanism (see Chap. 92). By contrast, other strains of *E. coli* cause diarrhea by elaboration of a low-molecular-weight, heat-stable toxin that activates guanylate cyclase. Enzymes capable of removing mono ADP-ribosyl moieties from cellular proteins have not been detected. Upon removal of the toxin, its effects fade slowly as ADP-ribosylated $G_{s\alpha}$ is gradually replaced by newly synthesized protein. This explains why the symptoms of cholera persist after eradication of the bacteria.

Pertussis (See also Chap. 116) The molecular pathogenesis of whooping cough and cholera are similar. *Bordetella pertussis* remains confined to the bronchi and produces two exotoxins. The first is commonly referred to as pertussis toxin or islet-activating protein. Like cholera toxin, this protein is an enzyme that catalyzes the NAD-dependent ADP-ribosylation of proteins; the targets for pertussis toxin are receptors of the $G_{i\alpha}$ family and $G_{o\alpha}$ (see above). This modification interferes with the ability of these G proteins to interact with receptors; cyclic AMP concentrations are thus elevated. Again, restoration of normal G protein function depends on de novo synthesis of the α subunits, explaining in part why the symptoms of pertussis can persist for weeks after eradication of the microorganisms. In contrast to cholera, the sequence of events that links ADP-ribosylation of G protein α subunits to clinical symptoms is not understood. However, *B. pertussis* also interferes with cellular regulation of cyclic AMP concentrations by another mechanism, since the second exotoxin is itself an invasive calmodulin-dependent adenylate cyclase. Elevated concentrations of cyclic AMP in neutrophils impair their ability to kill ingested bacteria. In addition, ADP-ribosylation of a neutrophil G protein α subunit (presumably $G_{i\alpha 2}$) uncouples the neutrophil chemotactic receptor from the pathway that controls superoxide generation and bactericidal activity. This may contribute to the increased susceptibility to pulmonary infection by other pathogens—a frequent complication of whooping cough.

Anthrax (See also Chap. 104) Cutaneous infection with *Bacillus anthracis* produces a lesion characterized by central necrosis and prominent subcutaneous edema. The edema is due to the presence of a bacterial exotoxin, referred to as *edema factor*. Edema factor is an adenylate cyclase that shares many characteristics with the *B. pertussis* enzyme, including host cell penetration and dependence on calmodulin. Rare patients who ingest *Bacillus* organisms can develop a watery diarrhea indistinguishable from cholera. This syndrome may result from penetration of edema factor into cells of the intestinal mucosa.

Pseudohypoparathyroidism (See also Chap. 340) Pseudohypoparathyroidism type I is an inherited disorder characterized by target organ resistance to parathyroid hormone. In addition, many patients exhibit partial resistance to other hormones that act by stimulation of adenylate cyclase (e.g., thyroid stimulating hormone, vasopressin, glucagon). In one variation of the disorder (termed pseudohypoparathyroidism type Ia), the molecular defect results in reduced cellular concentrations of $G_{s\alpha}$, and this partial deficiency is apparently due to lower cellular levels of the mRNAs that encode the polypeptide. These observations point to a mutation that impairs transcription of the $G_{s\alpha}$ gene or that decreases the stability of the mRNA. Pseudohypoparathyroidism Ib is a similar syndrome in which cellular concentrations of $G_{s\alpha}$ are normal.

Other disorders Alterations of G proteins are postulated to occur in diabetes mellitus and hypertrophic congestive cardiomyopathy. The relationship between these alterations and the pathogenesis of the disease remain to be established.

Certain point mutations within the genes that encode G protein α subunits interfere with the GTPase activity, and in vivo such mutations would be expected to cause constitutive activation of the pathways that they regulate. Analogous mutations also occur in the related guanine nucleotide–binding p21^{ras} proteins of human cancer cells (see Chap. 10). Expression of these mutated p21^{ras} proteins causes transformation of the cells, thus proving a cause-and-effect relationship. Similar mutations in G protein α subunits could also cause human tumors, since the growth rate of some cells (in particular

pituitary, adrenal, thyroid, gonads) depends in part on the intracellular concentration of cyclic AMP. Membranes of pituitary adenomas have been reported to contain a constitutively activated $G_{s\alpha}$ subunit. Tumor-promoting phorbol esters are believed to act by persistent activation of protein kinase C, and constitutive activation of this pathway via a mutated G protein α subunit that regulates phospholipase C would conceivably also promote tumor development.

REFERENCES

BERRIDGE MJ: Inositol trisphosphate and diacylglycerol: Two interacting second messengers. Ann Rev Biochem 56:159, 1987

BROWN AM, BIRNBAUMER L: Direct G protein gating of ion channels. Am J Physiol 254:H401, 1988

CARTER A et al: Reduced expression of multiple forms of the α subunit of the stimulatory GTP-binding protein in pseudohypoparathyroidism type Ia. Proc Natl Acad Sci USA 84:7266, 1987

GILMAN AG: G proteins: Transducers of receptor-generated signals. Ann Rev Biochem 56:615, 1987

SIBLEY DR et al: Regulation of transmembrane signaling by receptor phosphorylation. Cell 48:913, 1987

VALLAR L et al: Altered G_s and adenylate cyclase activity in human GH-secreting pituitary adenomas. Nature 330:566, 1987

69 EICOSANOIDS AND HUMAN DISEASE

R. PAUL ROBERTSON

This chapter focuses on the formation and mechanism of action of the physiologically active metabolites of arachidonic acid and on the biologic phenomena in which these compounds may be involved.

FORMATION OF THE EICOSANOIDS Prostaglandins, the first arachidonic acid metabolites to be recognized, were so named because they were originally identified in seminal fluid and thought to be secreted by the prostate. As other active metabolites were characterized, two major pathways—the cyclooxygenase and the lipoxygenase pathways—became apparent. These synthetic pathways are summarized schematically in Fig. 69-1, and structures of representative metabolites are shown in Fig. 69-2. All products of both the cyclooxygenase and the lipoxygenase pathways are called *eicosanoids*. The products of the cyclooxygenase pathway—the prostaglandins and the thromboxanes—are termed *prostanoids*.

The initial synthetic step for both pathways involves the cleavage of arachidonic acid from phospholipid in the plasma membrane of cells. Phospholipase A_2 cleaves arachidonic acid from phospholipid. Free arachidonic acid can also be derived by phospholipase C cleavage of diacylglycerol from phosphoinositides and subsequent cleavage of arachidonic acid from diacylglycerol by diacylglycerol lipase. Free arachidonic acid can then be oxygenated by the cyclooxygenase or lipoxygenase pathway. The first product of the cyclooxygenase pathway is the cyclic endoperoxide prostaglandin G_2 (PGG$_2$), which is converted to prostaglandin H_2 (PGH$_2$). PGG$_2$ and PGH$_2$ are the key intermediates in the formation of physiologically active prostaglandins (PGD$_2$, PGE$_2$, PGF$_{2\alpha}$, and PGI$_2$) and thromboxane A_2 (TXA$_2$). The first product of the 5-lipoxygenase pathway is 5-hydroperoxyeicosatetraenoic acid (5-HPETE) which is an intermediate in the formation of 5-hydroxyeicosatetraenoic acid (5-HETE) and the leukotrienes (LTA$_4$, LTB$_4$, LTC$_4$, LTD$_4$, and LTE$_4$). Two fatty acids other than arachidonic acid [3,11,14-eicosatrienoic acid (dihomo-γ-linolenic acid) and 5,8,11,14,17-eicosapentaenoic acid] can be converted to metabolites closely related to these eicosanoids. Prostanoid products of the former substrate carry the subscript 1; the leukotriene subscript is 3. Prostanoid products of the latter substrate have the subscript 3 while leukotrienes have the subscript 5. Arachidonic acid forms prostaglandin products with subscripts 2 and leukotrienes with

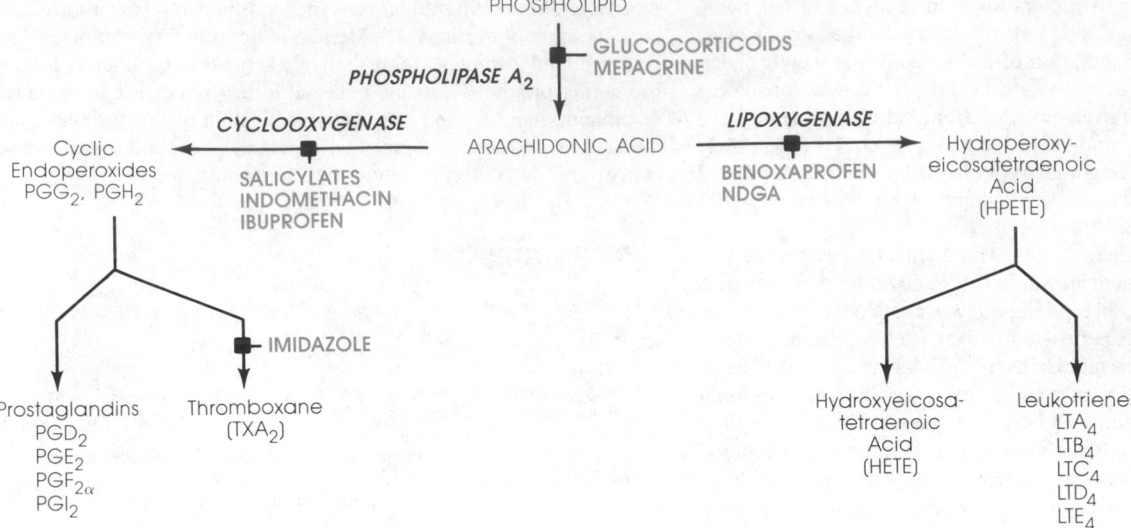

FIGURE 69-1 The overall scheme of arachidonic acid metabolism. The various drugs act at the various enzymatic steps to inhibit the reactions. The major pathways are the cyclooxygenase and the lipoxygenase pathways. Phospholipase A_2 is inhibited by glucocorticoids and mepacrine; cyclooxy- genase is inhibited by certain salicylates, indomethacin, and ibuprofen; and lipoxygenase is inhibited by benoxaprofen and nordihydroguaiaretic acid (NDGA). Imidazole prevents TXA_2 synthesis.

the subscript 4. (The subscripts designate the number of double bonds between carbon atoms in the side chains.)

Virtually all cells have the necessary substrates and enzymes to form some of the metabolites of arachidonic acid, but tissues differ in the enzymes they possess and consequently in the products they form. Eicosanoids are synthesized according to immediate need and are not stored in significant amounts for later release.

The cyclooxygenase products   Prostaglandins D_2, E_2, $F_{2\alpha}$, and I_2 are formed from the cyclic endoperoxides PGG_2 and PGH_2. Of these, PGE_2 and PGI_2 exert the broadest physiologic effects. PGE_2 has notable effects in, and is synthesized by, many tissues. PGI_2 (also called prostacyclin) is a dominant product of arachidonic acid in the endothelial and smooth muscle cells of vessel walls and in some nonvascular tissues. PGI_2 is a vasodilator and an inhibitor of platelet aggregation. PGD_2 is also believed to play a role in platelet aggregation and brain function. $PGF_{2\alpha}$ plays a role in uterine and ovarian function.

Thromboxane synthetase catalyzes the incorporation of an oxygen atom into the ring of the endoperoxide PGH_2 to form the thromboxanes. TXA_2 is synthesized by platelets and enhances platelet aggregation.

FIGURE 69-2   Structures of representative biologically active eicosanoids.

Prostaglandin	5-HETE
COOH OH OH PGE_2	OH COOH 5-HETE
Prostacyclin	Leukotriene
HOOC PGI_2 OH OH	NH_2 S-CH$_2$-CHCONHCH$_2$COOH COOH OH LTD_4 (SRS-A)
Thromboxane	
COOH OH TXA_2	

The lipoxygenase products   The leukotrienes and HETE are the end products of the lipoxygenase pathway. The leukotrienes have histamine-like actions, including induction of increased vascular permeability and of bronchospasm, and appear to have mediator activities for leukocytes. LTC_4, LTD_4, and LTE_4 together have been identified as slow-reacting substance of anaphylaxis (SRS-A). (The pathophysiology of the leukotrienes is discussed in detail in Chap. 204.)

EFFECTS OF DRUGS ON THE SYNTHESIS OF EICOSANOIDS
Many drugs block the synthesis of eicosanoids by inhibiting one or more enzymes in their biosynthetic pathways. Glucocorticoids and antimalarial drugs such as mepacrine interfere with the cleavage of arachidonic acid from phospholipids (Fig. 69-1). Cyclooxygenase is directly inhibited by nonsteroidal anti-inflammatory drugs including salicylates, indomethacin, and ibuprofen. Benoxaprofen, another nonsteroidal anti-inflammatory drug, inhibits the lipoxygenase-me-diated conversion of arachidonic acid to HPETE. Tranylcypromine, an antidepressant drug, inhibits the conversion of cyclic endoperoxides to PGI_2, and imidazole inhibits thromboxane synthesis. The fact that a drug inhibits the synthesis of a certain eicosanoid does not mean that a given drug effect is the direct result of a deficiency of that eicosanoid. Most of these drugs inhibit early reactions in the synthetic pathways and therefore block the formation of more than one product. Additionally, some of these drugs have other effects. For example, indomethacin not only inhibits formation of cyclic endoperoxides by cyclooxygenase but may also disrupt calcium flux across membranes, inhibit cyclic adenosine monophosphate (cyclic AMP)–dependent protein kinase and phosphodiesterase, and inhibit one of the enzymes responsible for degradation of PGE_2.

No truly specific synthesis inhibitors nor specific receptor antag-onists for individual arachidonic acid metabolites are suitable for human use. The lack of such drugs is a major barrier to elucidating the role of these metabolites in physiologic and pathophysiologic processes.

METABOLISM AND ASSAY OF EICOSANOIDS   Arachidonic acid metabolites are catabolized rapidly in vivo. Prostaglandins of the E and F series, although chemically stable, are almost completely degraded during a single passage through the liver or the lung. Thus, essentially all nonmetabolized PGE_2 measurable in urine is derived from renal and seminal vesicle secretion, whereas PGE_2 metabolites in urine represent total-body PGE_2 synthesis. PGI_2 and TXA_2 are both chemically unstable and also rapidly catabolized. Because PGE_2,

PGI_2, and TXA_2 are short-lived in vivo, measurement of their inactive metabolites is commonly used as an index of the rates of their formation. PGE_2 is converted to 15-keto-13,14,-dihydro-PGE_2, PGI_2 is converted to 6-keto-$PGF_{1\alpha}$, and TXA_2 is converted to TXB_2. Five methods are generally available to measure arachidonic acid metabolites in physiologic fluids: bioassay, radioimmunoassay, chromatography, receptor assay, and mass spectrometry. Bioassay provides direct physiologic data but is not very sensitive. Radioimmunoassay is the most convenient and sensitive but, as with bioassay and receptor assay, should be preceded by extraction and chromatography of samples to ensure specificity. Mass spectrometry preceded by chromatography is accurate but laborious. With each method precautions must be taken in handling samples because prostaglandin synthesis may be enhanced during the collection of biologic samples. For example, if blood is allowed to clot or if platelets are not carefully separated from plasma, the generation of large amounts of PGE_2 and TXA_2 during processing can lead to erroneous results. Use of an inhibitor of prostaglandin synthesis in the collection tube minimizes this problem.

PHYSIOLOGY Prostaglandins and leukotrienes have specific receptor sites on the plasma membranes of cells such as liver, corpus luteum, adrenal gland, adipocytes, thymocytes, uterus, pancreatic islets, platelets, and red blood cells. Most of the binding sites exhibit specificity for eicosanoids of a given type. For example, the liver plasma membrane PGE receptor binds PGE_1 and PGE_2 with high affinity but not prostaglandins of the A, F, and I configurations. The postreceptor mechanisms by which the binding of the prostaglandins alters cell function are poorly understood. Some of these mechanisms involve modulation of cyclic AMP production through interactions with two G-proteins, the stimulatory (G_s) and inhibitory (G_i) subunits of adenylate cyclase (see Chap. 68). The normal physiologic actions of eicosanoids are not mediated via the plasma. Instead, eicosanoids act as local, intercellular, and/or intracellular modulators of biochemical activity in the tissues in which they are formed (e.g., a paracrine function). They are autacoids, not hormones. Most are short-lived in the circulation because of chemical instability and/or rapid degradation.

Lipolysis PGE_2 is synthesized by adipocytes, has specific receptors in adipocytes, and is a potent endogenous inhibitor of lipolysis. Since the formation of cyclic AMP is necessary in the action of hormones that stimulate lipolysis, the interactions between PGE and adenylate cyclase have been examined in considerable detail. PGE inhibits lipolysis by decreasing the formation of cyclic AMP in response to epinephrine, adrenocorticotropic hormone (ACTH), glucagon, and thyroid-stimulating hormone (TSH). Thus, PGE may act as an endogenous antilipolytic substance by interfering with the stimulation of cyclic AMP formation by hormones.

Insulin and PGE may act independently during their antilipolytic actions on the adipocyte. For example, insulin but not PGE inhibits the stimulation of lipolysis by exogenous cyclic AMP in isolated adipocytes, but both agents inhibit hormone-stimulated generation of cyclic AMP. This suggests a site of action of insulin distal to the stimulation of adenylate cyclase. In some animals PGE inhibits glucagon-induced lipolysis whereas insulin does not.

Sodium and water balance The renin-angiotensin-aldosterone system is a major regulator of sodium homeostasis, and vasopressin exerts the principal control over water balance. Arachidonic acid metabolites influence both systems. PGE_2 and PGI_2 stimulate renin secretion, and inhibitors of prostaglandin synthesis have the opposite effect. PGI_2 and PGE_2 decrease renal vascular resistance and increase blood flow; this results in redistribution of blood flow from the outer renal cortex to the juxtamedullary region of the kidney. Conversely, inhibitors of prostaglandin synthesis, such as indomethacin and meclofenamate, decrease total renal blood flow and shunt the remaining flow to the outer cortex, which can lead to acute renal venoconstriction and acute renal failure in circumstances such as volume depletion and edematous states. PGE_2 is natriuretic whereas cyclooxygenase inhibitors cause sodium and water retention.

Indomethacin also increases sensitivity to exogenous vasopressin in dogs. Conversely, PGE_2 decreases vasopressin-stimulated water transport. Since this effect of PGE_2 is circumvented by the administration of dibutyryl–cyclic AMP, PGE_2 most likely interferes with the stimulation of adenylate cyclase by vasopressin.

Platelet aggregation Platelets synthesize PGE_2, PGD_2, and TXA_2. Although a physiologic role has not been established for PGE_2 and PGD_2 in platelet function, TXA_2 is a potent stimulator of platelet aggregation; in contrast PGI_2, formed by the endothelial cells of blood vessel walls, is a potent antagonist of platelet aggregation. TXA_2 and PGI_2 may exert their opposing effects by decreasing and increasing, respectively, platelet generation of cyclic AMP.

Inhibitors of endogenous prostaglandin synthesis interfere with platelet aggregation. For example, a single dose of aspirin can suppress normal platelet aggregation for 48 h and longer, presumably by suppressing cyclooxygenase-mediated TXA_2 synthesis. Cyclooxygenase inhibition by a single dose of aspirin is of longer duration in platelets than in other tissues, because the platelet, in contrast to nucleated cells that can synthesize new proteins, does not have the machinery to form new enzyme. Consequently, the effect of aspirin persists until newly formed platelets have been released. Endothelial cells, on the other hand, rapidly recover cyclooxygenase activity following discontinuation of treatment with aspirin, and PGI_2 production is thus restored. This is one reason that patients taking aspirin are not predisposed to excessive formation of platelet thrombi. In addition, the platelet is more sensitive than the endothelial cell to aspirin.

Endothelial damage may lead to platelet aggregation along the blood vessel wall by causing a local decrease in PGI_2 synthesis, thereby allowing unbridled platelet aggregation at the site of vessel wall damage.

Vascular effects The vasoactive properties of arachidonic acid metabolites are among their most impressive actions. PGE_2 and PGI_2 are vasodilators where $PGF_{2\alpha}$, TXA_2, and LTC_4-LTD_4-LTE_4 are vasoconstrictors in most vascular beds. These effects appear to be the result of direct action on the smooth muscle of the vessel wall. Provided that systemic blood pressure is maintained, the vasodilatory arachidonic acid metabolites act to increase blood flow. If blood pressure falls, however, blood flow decreases because with systemic hypotension catecholamine induced vasoconstriction offsets the vasodilatory effect of the prostaglandins. Thus, significant alterations in systemic blood pressure must be excluded when evaluating the effects of arachidonic acid metabolites on organ blood flow.

Gastrointestinal effects Prostaglandins of the E series influence gastrointestinal function. Infusion of either PGI_2 or PGE_2 into the gastric artery of dogs causes increases in blood flow and inhibition of acid output, and several PGE analogues both inhibit gastric acid output and directly protect the gastrointestinal mucosa when taken orally. In in vitro experiments prostaglandins stimulate gastrointestinal smooth muscle and thereby increase motility, but it is not clear whether these actions are physiologically important.

Neurotransmission PGE inhibits egress of norepinephrine from sympathetic nerve terminals. The effect of PGE on norepinephrine secretion appears to be prejunctional, i.e., at a site on the nerve terminal proximal to the synaptic cleft, and can be reversed by increases in calcium concentration in the perfusing medium. Therefore, PGE_2 may inhibit norepinephrine release by blocking calcium influx. Inhibitors of PGE_2 synthesis can augment norepinephrine release in response to stimulation of adrenergic nerves.

Catecholamines can release PGE_2 from a variety of tissues, probably by an alpha-adrenergic–mediated mechanism. For example, in innervated tissues such as the spleen, nerve stimulation or injection of norepinephrine causes release of PGE_2. This release is blocked after denervation or administration of alpha-adrenergic blockers. Thus, a stimulus that activates the nerve causes release of norepinephrine, which in turn stimulates synthesis and release of PGE_2; PGE_2 then feeds back at the prejunctional level of the nerve terminal to decrease the amount of norepinephrine released.

Pancreatic endocrine function PGE$_2$ has primarily inhibitory effects on insulin secretion by the pancreatic beta cell in vitro and on insulin response to intravenous glucose. This effect is at least partially mediated by G$_i$, the inhibitory regulatory subunit of adenylate cyclase, since it is associated with decreased production of cyclic AMP and is preventable by pertussis toxin, an agent that inhibits G$_i$ activity. This inhibitory effect appears to be specific for glucose because the insulin responses to other secretagogues are not influenced by PGE$_2$. Studies with inhibitors of prostaglandin synthesis support the concept that endogenous PGE$_2$ acts in vivo to inhibit insulin secretion. In general, such drugs augment insulin secretion and improve carbohydrate tolerance. An exception is indomethacin, which inhibits glucose-induced insulin secretion and can cause hyperglycemia. The discordant results with indomethacin are likely due to some action other than inhibition of cyclooxygenase. The lipoxygenase pathway appears to play a role in potentiating insulin secretion by participating in stimulus-secretion coupling. In this case a likely active arachidonic acid product may be 12-HPETE.

Luteolysis In the sheep hysterectomy during the luteal phase of the ovarian cycle results in maintenance of the corpus luteum, suggesting that the uterus normally produces a luteolytic substance. A candidate for this substance is PGF$_{2\alpha}$ since it can cause luteal regression.

PATHOPHYSIOLOGY Most postulated roles for arachidonic acid metabolites in disease involve excessive production, but a few disorders may be the result of decreased production. The latter could result from dietary deficiency of arachidonic acid (an essential fatty acid), from damage to a tissue required for prostaglandin synthesis, or from therapy with drugs that inhibit enzymes in the synthetic pathway.

Bone resorption: Hypercalcemia of malignancy (Also see Chaps. 309 and 340) Hypercalcemia occurs in association with nonparathyroid malignancies of many different types. Parathyroid hormone excess, as the result either of autonomous production by parathyroid tissue or ectopic formation by the tumor itself, causes a portion of these cases. However, most patients with hypercalcemia of malignancy do not have elevated plasma levels of parathyroid hormone, and the etiology of the hypercalcemia has been the subject of considerable interest.

Prostaglandin E$_2$ is a potent inducer of bone resorption and of calcium release from bone, and PGE$_2$ production is elevated in certain hypercalcemic animals with transplantable tumors. Treatment of these animals with inhibitors of PGE$_2$ synthesis causes reduction of PGE$_2$ levels and a concomitant decrease in hypercalcemia. Likewise, occasional patients with hypercalcemia and malignancy have excessive amounts of PGE$_2$ metabolites in urine, whereas equally elevated levels do not occur in normocalcemic patients with otherwise similar malignancies. Drugs that inhibit prostaglandin synthesis decrease circulating calcium levels in some patients with hypercalcemia of malignancy. Thus, a subset of approximately 5 to 10 percent of patients with hypercalcemia and malignancy have elevated PGE production and can be treated with drugs that inhibit prostaglandin synthesis.

The source of the excess PGE$_2$ in these patients has not been identified. Increased liver and lung degradation of PGE would be expected to compensate if large amounts of PGE were present in the circulation. It is possible, of course, that such large amounts of PGE$_2$ are released by a tumor into the circulation that liver and lung degradation cannot handle the load. Alternatively, if lung metastases are present, the venous drainage from the tumors could be delivered into the systemic circulation without passing through lung tissue. A third possible mechanism involves metastatic seeding of bone. Tumor cells synthesize PGE in culture, and metastatic tumor cells in bone could synthesize PGE that acts locally to cause bone resorption. Part of this hypothetical mechanism may involve PGE$_2$ production by circulating white cells which congregate at metastatic sites. Hypercalcemia of malignancy can occur in the absence of demonstrable bone metastases, but the clinical tools for excluding such metastases,

such as radioisotope scans, may not be sensitive enough to detect many small lesions.

Bone resorption: Rheumatoid arthritis and dental cysts (See Chap. 270) Overproduction of PGE$_2$ has been postulated as a cause of the juxtaarticular osteoporosis and bony erosions in some patients with rheumatoid arthritis. Rheumatoid synovia synthesize PGE$_2$ in tissue culture, and media from these cultures promote bone resorption; moreover, the inclusion of indomethacin in the culture medium blocks this resorptive capacity. Since indomethacin does not prevent bone resorption due to preformed PGE$_2$, the PGE$_2$ produced by the synovia is presumed to be responsible for the resorptive activity.

Cells from benign dental cysts also cause bone resorption and synthesize PGE$_2$ in tissue culture. Again, bone resorption caused by the culture medium from such cells is decreased if indomethacin is added prior to the incubation. A related problem is that of alveolar bone resorption in patients with periodontal disease, a common inflammatory disease of the gums. PGE$_2$ levels in inflamed gingiva are greater than in healthy gingival tissue. Thus, it is possible that alveolar resorption might be due, in part at least, to local overproduction of these metabolites.

Bartter's syndrome (See Chap. 231) Bartter's syndrome is characterized by elevated levels of plasma renin, aldosterone, and bradykinin; resistance to the pressor effect of angiotensin; hypokalemic alkalosis; and renal potassium wasting in the presence of normal blood pressure. The basis for the postulated role of prostaglandins in the disorder is that PGE$_2$ and PGI$_2$ stimulate the release of renin and that the pressor response to infused angiotensin is blunted by the vasodilator effects of PGE$_2$ and PGI$_2$. The increase in renin release leads to increased aldosterone secretion, which in turn can increase urinary kallikrein activity.

In keeping with this postulate, elevated levels of PGE$_2$ and 6-keto-PGF$_{1\alpha}$ are present in urine of patients with the syndrome. Hyperplasia of renal medullary interstitial cells (which synthesize PGE in culture) has also been demonstrated. These findings led to therapeutic trials of inhibitors of prostaglandin synthesis in the disorder. Indomethacin (and other inhibitors) reverse virtually all the abnormalities except hypokalemia. Thus, a prostaglandin, probably PGE$_2$ and/or PGI$_2$, probably mediates some of the manifestations of Bartter's syndrome.

Diabetes mellitus (See Chap. 319) Intravenous administration of large amounts of glucose to normal individuals causes a sudden (first-phase) increase in secretion of insulin into plasma followed by a slower, more prolonged response termed second-phase insulin secretion. Patients with type II (non-insulin-dependent, adult-onset) diabetes mellitus have absent first-phase insulin release in response to glucose and a variable decrease in second-phase insulin secretion. Insulin response to other secretagogues, such as arginine, isoproterenol, glucagon, and secretin, is preserved. Thus, diabetics appear to have a specific defect that interferes with normal perception of glucose signals. Since PGE inhibits glucose-induced insulin secretion in normal individuals, inhibitors of endogenous prostaglandin synthesis have been given to patients with type II diabetes mellitus to ascertain whether insulin secretion can be improved. Both sodium salicylate and aspirin elevate basal plasma insulin levels, partially restore the first-phase insulin response, increase second-phase insulin secretion, and improve glucose tolerance. This suggests that the defect in glucose-induced insulin secretion in patients with type II diabetes mellitus may be associated with excessive local production of, or hypersensitivity to, endogenous PGE$_2$.

Patent ductus arteriosus (See Chap. 186) The ductus arteriosus in sheep is sensitive to the vasodilatory properties of PGE$_2$, and PGE-like material is present in the ductal wall. Thus, enhanced endogenous PGE$_2$ might maintain prenatal patency of the ductus. Since inhibitors of prostaglandin synthesis cause constriction of the ductus of fetal lambs, trials with indomethacin were undertaken in premature human infants with isolated patent ductus arteriosus. Such treatment for several days is followed by closure of the vessel in the majority, although some require a second course of therapy, and a minority require surgical ligation. Infants under 35 weeks of gestational age are most likely to respond.

Patients with certain types of congenital heart disease require a patent ductus arteriosus to survive. Ductus-dependent pulmonary blood flow is essential under circumstances in which the ductus is the major channel by which nonoxygenated blood reaches the lungs from the aortic arch, for example, in pulmonary atresia and tricuspid atresia. Since PGE relaxes the smooth muscle in the lamb ductus arteriosus, clinical trials of intravenous PGE were undertaken to attempt to maintain patency of the ductus in such patients as an alternative to emergency surgery. Such PGE infusions for a short time cause a temporary increase in blood flow to the lungs and improve arterial oxygen saturation until the necessary corrective heart surgery can be performed. The large right-to-left shunt in these cardiac malformations allows the intravenously infused PGE_2 to escape pulmonary degradation before arriving at the ductus. In this instance, the disease process itself facilitates delivery of the therapeutic agent.

Peptic ulcer disease (See Chap. 238) Excessive gastric acid secretion in patients with peptic ulcer disease is involved in damaging the mucosa. Various analogues of PGE_2 inhibit gastric acid secretion and are also inherently cytoprotective. These agents are more effective than placebo in relieving pain and decreasing gastric acid secretion in patients with ulcer disease. Moreover, acceleration of the healing of ulcer craters as assessed by endoscopic criteria has been reported in patients receiving PGE analogues as compared with placebo-treated groups.

Dysmenorrhea (See Chap. 322) Dysmenorrhea is usually associated with increased uterine contractions. The fact that some analgesics used to treat this disorder also inhibit prostaglandin synthesis suggests that arachidonic acid metabolites may play a role in the pathogenesis of dysmenorrhea. Prostaglandins of the E and F series are present in human endometrium. Intravenous infusion of either produces uterine contractions, and PGF and PGE levels in menstrual blood are decreased by administration of prostaglandin synthesis inhibitors. Controlled trials comparing prostaglandin synthesis inhibitors with placebo in women with dysmenorrhea suggest that symptomatic improvement is greater following drug therapy.

Asthma (See Chap. 204)

Inflammatory response and immune response (See Chaps. 13 and 267) Drugs such as aspirin have antipyretic, anti-inflammatory, and analgesic effects. Several arguments support a relation between inflammation and the arachidonic acid metabolites: (1) Inflammatory stimuli such as histamine and bradykinin release endogenous prostaglandins in parallel. (2) Leukotriene C_4-D_4-E_4 is more potent than histamine in causing bronchoconstriction. (3) Several arachidonic acid metabolites cause vasodilatation and hyperalgesia. (4) PGE_2 and LTB_4 are present in areas of inflammation. Polymorphonuclear cells release these products during phagocytosis, and they are chemotactic

for leukocytes. (5) Some prostaglandins cause increased vascular permeability, a feature of the inflammatory response that gives rise to local edema. (6) Vasodilation induced by PGE is not abolished by atropine, propranolol, methysergide, or antihistamines, known antagonists of other possible mediators of the inflammatory response. Thus, PGE may have a direct inflammatory effect, and some mediators of inflammation may act by influencing PGE release. (7) Some arachidonic acid metabolites can cause pain in animal models and hyperalgesia or an increased sensitivity to pain in humans. (8) PGE can cause fever after injection into the cerebral ventricles or into the hypothalamus of animals. (9) Pyrogens cause increased concentrations of prostaglandins in cerebrospinal fluid, whereas prostaglandin synthesis inhibitors decrease fever and decrease release of prostaglandins into cerebrospinal fluid.

Arachidonic acid metabolites may also play a role in the immune response. Small amounts of PGE_2 can suppress stimulation of human lymphocytes by mitogens such as phytohemagglutinin, and the inflammatory response is associated with the local release of arachidonic acid metabolites; thus, these substances may act as negative modulators of lymphocyte function. The release of PGE by mitogen-stimulated lymphocytes may constitute a portion of a negative feedback control mechanism by which lymphocyte activity is regulated. Sensitivity of lymphocytes to the inhibiting effects of PGE_2 increases with age, and indomethacin augments lymphocyte responsiveness to mitogens to a greater degree in the elderly. Lymphocytes cultured from patients with Hodgkin's disease release more PGE_2 after the addition of phytohemagglutinin, and lymphocyte responsiveness is enhanced by indomethacin. When suppressor T cells are removed from the cultures, the amount of PGE_2 synthesized is diminished, and the responsiveness of the lymphocytes from the Hodgkin's patients and controls is no longer different. Depressed cellular immunity in patients with Hodgkin's disease may be the result of PGE inhibition of lymphocyte function.

REFERENCES

Advances in prostaglandins and gastroenterology. Symposium. Am J Med 83 (1A): 1, 1987

ALESSANDRINI P et al: Thromboxane biosynthesis and platelet function in type I diabetes mellitus. N Engl J Med 319:208, 1988

HEYMAN MA: Prostaglandins and leukotrienes in the perinatal period. Clin Perinatol 14:857, 1987

METZ SA et al: Prostaglandins as mediators of paraneoplastic syndromes: Review and update. Metabolism 30:299, 1981

NEEDLEMAN P et al: Arachidonic acid metabolism. Ann Rev Biochem 55:69, 1986

ROBERTSON RP (ed): Symposium on prostaglandins in health and disease. Med Clin North Am 65:711, 1981

———: Arachidonic acid metabolite regulation of insulin secretion. Diab Metab Rev 2:261, 1986

SCHARSCHMIDT L et al: Glomerular prostaglandins, angiotensin II, and nonsteroidal anti-inflammatory drugs. Am J Med 81(2B):30, 1986

A1-12 **Perlèche** consists of painful small fissures at the angles of the mouth, often covered with yellow crusts. Perlèche most often occurs with poorly fitting dentures and in moniliasis and secondary syphilis.

A1-13 **Rosacea,** usually limited to the face, consists of tiny, erythematous papules and pustules 1 to 5 mm in size. The pustules, often tiny and sometimes hardly visible, sit on the dome of the papules. The diffuse redness of the face is due to vasodilatation, as well as to myriad telangiectases. In men, rhinophyma, a disfiguring enlargement of the nose, may occur.

A1-14 **Seborrheic dermatitis,** a common disorder found in all age groups, occurs most frequently on the scalp, eyebrows, and nasolabial folds and behind the ears. Scaling is the prominent feature and is loose and branny; it may be yellow and oily or dry and white. The lesion may become exudative and crusted or eczematous.

A1-15 **Seborrheic keratosis** appears in middle life and may occur on exposed or unexposed areas but is especially common on the trunk. The lesions are irregularly round or oval flat-topped papules or plaques that seem "stuck" on the skin. The margins are distinct, and the surface is often warty or consists of multiple tiny projections (vegetation). In fair-skinned persons, the lesions are light brown at first but, enlarging, become more heavily pigmented and may be confused with malignant melanoma.

A1-16 **Senile angioma ("cherry red spot")** appears in the third decade. On the lip, the lesion is usually singular and consists of a bluish red round nodule. On the trunk, the lesions are small (2 to 3 mm), bright red, globular papules.

A1-17 **Senile lentigo** occurs as a single macule or as a group of isolated, sharply circumscribed macules on the exposed areas, especially on the dorsal surfaces of the hands and arms and on the forehead and cheeks. The macules are usually light yellowish brown, but may be dark brown; the color is somewhat variegated, rather than uniform as it is in a café au lait macule. Rarely, dark brown *papules* develop in these lesions, and then the condition is called *lentigo maligna,* which may slowly develop, over a period of years, into a melanoma (lentigo maligna melanoma).

Al-6 **Dermatophytosis** is identified by the striking polycyclic, annular shape of the scaling, especially on the feet and hands, where there is often a scalloped pattern. A positive diagnosis of dermatophytosis is quickly established by direct examination of scales from the advancing border; the mycelia are revealed when the scales are immersed in 10% potassium hydroxide or Swartz stain.

Al-7 **Eczematous dermatitis** is a very common cutaneous reaction that is localized to the hands of housewives, to the legs in patients with chronic venous insufficiency, and behind the ears in patients with seborrheic dermatitis. In subacute eczematous dermatitis, there are mild erythema, dry scales, and often small red papules, many of which are excoriated. In chronic eczematous dermatitis, lichenification is the most prominent feature.

Al-8 **Localized lichenification** results from repeated rubbing of the skin and consists of isolated, circumscribed plaques. These single lesions vary in size from 2 to 10 cm and occur most often on the extensor aspect of the forearm and in the scrotal, nuchal, inguinal, and anogenital areas. The perianal and vulvar areas may become diffusely lichenified. Lichenification is thought to be more frequent in persons with an atopic background.

Al-9 **Melasma (chloasma)** is the so-called "mask" of pregnancy, but it also occurs in men and in women taking progestational agents. The pigmentation is uniform and is limited to the exposed areas of the face. There is no scaling or epidermal change. In fair-skinned persons, the pigment may be any shade from light tan to a very dark brown. It is most often seen on the cheek and upper lip, as here, and on the forehead.

Al-10 **Milia** are a collection of lesions, occurring most commonly on the face, and consist of tiny (1 to 2 mm), white, hard, rounded, superficial papules. There is no orifice, and the keratinous contents are easily expressed by lateral compression after the making of a tiny incision in the dome of the lesion.

Al-11 **Psoriasis,** affecting more than 2 percent of the population, consists of isolated scaling papules or plaques and is quite commonly observed in the routine physical examination. The lesions occur most frequently on the scalp, elbows, and knees. The color and type of scales are the identifying features of the lesions. The scales are either dense and lamellated with peripherally detached edges or loose and branny. The plaques are pink to deep red, and the borders are distinct.

A1-18 **Senile sebaceous adenoma** occurs on the face in patients over 40 and is often diagnosed as basal-cell carcinoma. The lesions are soft, small, flat-topped papules, varying in size from 1 to 8 mm, and are characterized by a minute central depression from which sebaceous material can be exuded by lateral compression.

A1-19 **Solar keratosis** (1) occurs usually in persons with light skin prone to sunburn or with darker skin after chronic excessive exposure; (2) is strictly limited to exposed skin, especially on the face and dorsal surfaces of the hands; (3) is more easily felt than seen (gritty and sandpaperish); (4) in fair-skinned persons, consists of skin-colored or light brown macules or slightly raised papules with superficial adherent scales not easily removed; and (5) is associated with marked wrinkling, telangiectasia, and often diffuse, tiny, pale yellow papules indicating solar degeneration of connective tissue ("turkey skin").

A1-20 **Spider nevus** consists of a central, punctate, bright red macule or papule (the body) from which fine red lines radiate like spider legs. There is often a red flare between the radiating vessels. On diascopy, the central body pulsates.

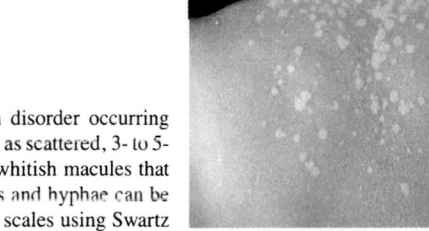

A1-21 **Tinea versicolor** is a relatively common disorder occurring primarily on the trunk and appearing in two forms: as scattered, 3- to 5-mm, very slightly scaling brown macules or as whitish macules that may be confused with vitiligo. The fungal spores and hyphae can be easily demonstrated on direct examination of the scales using Swartz stain.

A1-22 **Verruca vulgaris** may occur at any age, but it is most common in children. The lesions, which vary in size from 0.5 to 2.0 cm, are round or oval, firm, skin colored papules with multiple tiny keratotic, rounded or filiform projections covering the surface (vegetation). They occur most frequently on the hands and soles.

A1-23 **Xanthelasma** consists of one or more bright yellow, sharply marginated plaques with no epidermal change, usually occurring on the eyelids. All patients with xanthelasma should be investigated for evidence of plasma lipid abnormalities.

A1-24 **Systemic lupus erythematosus.** Erythematous, confluent, butterfly-like eruption with fine scaling.

A1-25 **Necrotizing vasculitis syndrome.** Scattered discrete, purpuric eruption on the legs. The purpura is "palpable."

A

A1-26 **Glucagonoma** (*A*) and **acquired zinc deficiency** (*B*). Circinate and gyrate areas of blistering, erosion, and maceration. The eruption is often mistaken for psoriasis or mucocutaneous moniliasis.

B

A1-27 **Porphyria cutanea tarda.** Violaceous suffusion in the periorbital skin is evident. There are erosions and pink atrophic scars at sites of previous bullae on the dorsa of the hands.

A1-28 **Necrobiosis lipoidica.** The lesion often begins as a small, dusky red, elevated nodule with a sharp border. It slowly enlarges, becomes flattened and eventually depressed as the dermis becomes atrophic. The color becomes brownish yellow except for the border, which may remain reddened. Delicate vessels can be seen through the atrophic epidermis.

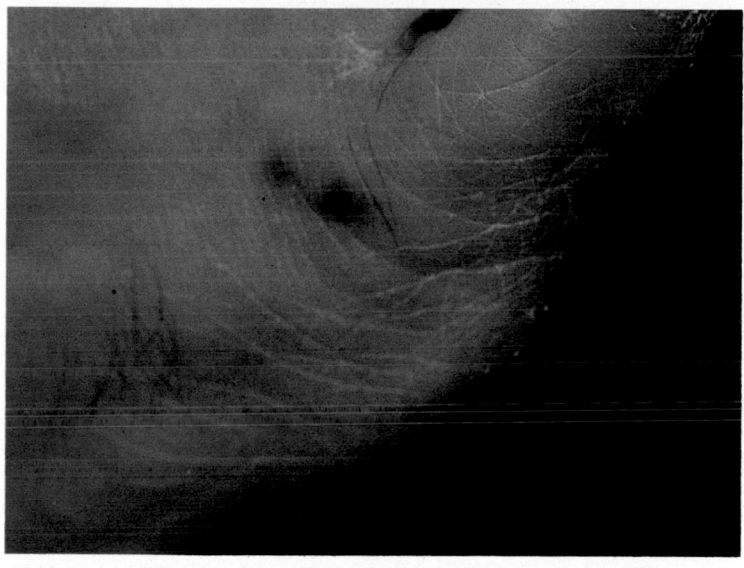

A1-29 Two purplish red nodules of **Kaposi's sarcoma** in a patient with AIDS.

A1-30 **Carcinoid** showing the effect of stroking. In contrast to the flushing that occurs in other disorders, the flush in carcinoid is typically a panorama of colors, ranging from bizarre pinkish orange to bright red to violaceous to blanching white. The flush (which lasts only a few minutes) spreads from the face to the neck, shoulders, chest, and arms.

A

B

C

D

E

A1-31 **Malignant melanoma.** On close inspection melanomas shown are characterized by irregular surface (*A*), irregular border and notching (*B*), and nodularity (*C*). Also shown are a reniform melanoma (*D*), an extensive lentigo maligna on face of patient (*E*) and a regressive melanoma characterized by grayish color infiltrated with pink areas (*F*). (From Hospital Practice, January 1982, with permission.)

F

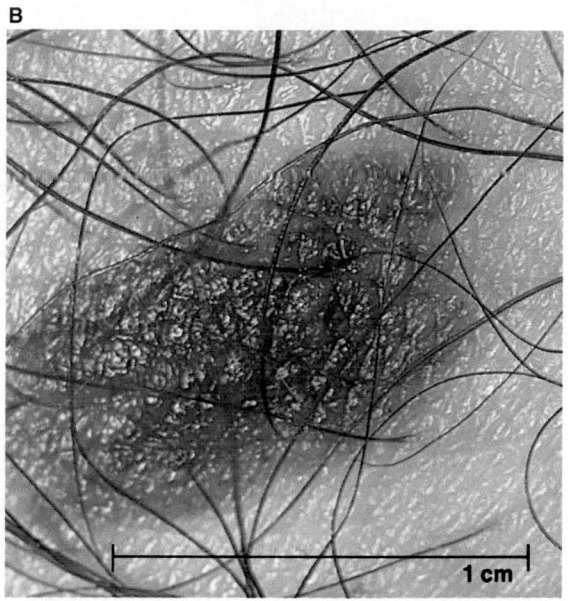

A1-32 **Dysplastic melanocytic nevi.** (*A*) Round, essentially macular lesions in which the slightly elevated area is present at 12:00 o'clock. The elevation is detectable only by oblique lighting. Note striking variegation of color with tan, brown, and pink areas. (*B*) This lesion is more obviously elevated in the central portion. Note "pebbly" surface. Both lesions have indistinct and irregular borders. (From Dermatologic Capsule & Comment 7(4):4, 1985, with permission.)

A1-33 **Malignant melanoma — dysplastic nevus syndrome.** This 28-year-old woman gave a history of a rapidly growing (3 to 6 months), asymptomatic lesion on her right scapular area. Her mother had melanoma and both mother and siblings had many dark "moles." Diagnosis: (1) Superficial spreading melanoma, level IV, 4.75 mm. (2) Regional nodes — of 32 removed, 1 was positive. (3) Dysplastic nevus syndrome with family history of melanoma. Note primary lesion and many dark "moles" on back (*A*) and dysplastic nevi on untanned areas under the bathing suit straps (*B*). (From Dermatologic Capsule & Comment 6(4):3, 1984, with permission.)

A2-1 **Varicella** (chickenpox).[3]

A2-2 **Measles** (rubeola).[3]

A2-3 **Rocky Mountain spotted fever** — early rash.[2]

A2-4 **Rocky Mountain spotted fever** — late rash.[2]

A2-7 **Pseudomonas septicemia**.[3]

A2-8 **Facial erysipelas**.[3]

A2-5 **Meningococcemia**.[3]

A2-6 **Disseminated gonococcal infection** — skin lesion.[4]

A2-9 **Lyme disease: erythema chronicum migrans** — secondary lesion.[5]

A2-10 **Lyme disease: erythema chronicum migrams** — primary lesion.[5]

A2-11 Mucous patches involving the tongue in **secondary syphilis.**[4]

A2-12 **Papulosquamous lesions of secondary syphilis** on the sole of the foot.[4]

A2-13 **Macular syphilids** in early secondary syphilis.[4]

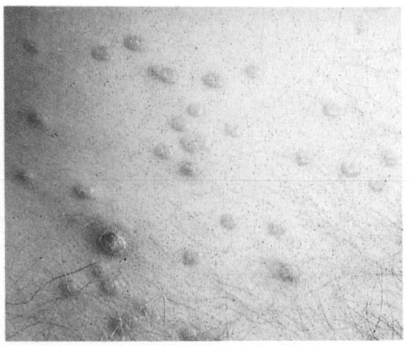

A2-14 **Molluscum contagiosum** of the lower abdomen in a patient with coexisting genital molluscum lesions. Note central umbilication and pale-salmon color.[4]

A2-15 **Esthiomene** due to lymphogranuloma venereum.[4]

A2-16 **Severe primary HSV* infection** with extensive vesicles, ulcerations, and penile edema.[4]

A2-17 **Primary HSV* pharyngitis** showing ulcerative lesions on the uvula and palate together with exudative tonsillitis. HSV-2 was recovered from pharyngeal and genital lesions.[4]

A2-18 **Neonatal HSV* infection.** Ulcers and crusting lesions on the buttocks.[4]

*Herpes Simplex Virus

A2-19 **Herpetic whitlow.**[1]

A2-20 **Keratodermia blenorrhagica** in Reiter's syndrome.[4]

A2-21 Grouped excoriations due to **scabies** on the lower buttocks, simulating dermatitis herpetiformis.[4]

A2-22 **Cervicofacial actinomycosis.**[3]

A2-23 Lesions of **Kaposi's sarcoma** on the cheek of a homosexually active man.[4]

A2-24 **Kaposi's sarcoma** involving the palate of a homosexually active man.[4]

Sources

1 Courtesy of Lawrence Corey, M.D.
2 Courtesy of Theodore E. Woodward, M.D.
3 Fitzpatrick TB et al: *Dermatology in General Medicine,* 2nd ed. New York, McGraw-Hill, 1984
4 Holmes KK et al: *Sexually Transmitted Diseases.* New York, McGraw-Hill, 1984
5 Steere AC et al: Ann Intern Med 86:685, 1977 (reprinted with permission)

A3-1 **Normal esophagus;** normal fine vasculature can be seen.

A3-2 **Peptic regurgitant esophagitis;** linear red streaks with a central white streak are noted extending up the esophagus.

A3-3 **Ulcerated squamous cell carcinoma,** with a depressed center, involving one wall of the esophagus.

A3-4 **Moniliasis of the esophagus.** A white exudate is seen with underlying erythematous mucosa.

A3-5 **Barrett's metaplasia of the esophagus with an adenocarcinoma.** The squamo-columnar junction is noted in the proximal esophagus. A mucosal irregularity in the center of the photograph was an adenocarcinoma.

A3-6 **Normal body of the stomach with rugal folds.**

A3-7 **Large, benign, lesser curve, gastric ulcer.** The folds end at the ulcer margin.

A3-8 **Gastric polyp.** The histologic type must be determined by excision and pathologic examination.

A3-9 **Arteriovenous malformation of the gastric mucosa.**

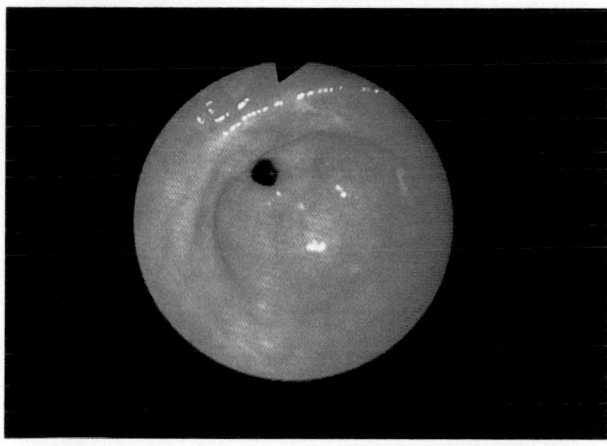

A3-10 **Normal pylorus.** Note the absence of gastric rugal folds in the antrum proximal to the pylorus.

A3-11 **Normal duodenal bulb.**

A3-12 **Normal papilla of Vater.** The fold pattern surrounding the papilla is normal; bile is seen adjacent to the papilla.

A3-13 **Periampullary carcinoma.** The mass at the papilla of Vater has been catheterized during ERCP.

A3-14 **Endoscopic papillotomy.** A papillotome has been passed into the papilla, the wire bowed, and an incision made, with electrosurgical current, in the superior aspect of the papilla.

A3-15 **Normal colon;** typical haustral folds and a normal vascular pattern can be seen.

A3-16 **Colonic adenomatous polyp.** The polyp is erythematous; a stalk is seen covered with normal mucosa.

A3-17 **Multiple, small, colonic adenomatous polyps** in a case of familial polyposis coli. This colon must be removed to prevent the development of cancer.

A3-18 **Colon adenocarcinoma.** The cancer is multilobed and growing into the lumen.

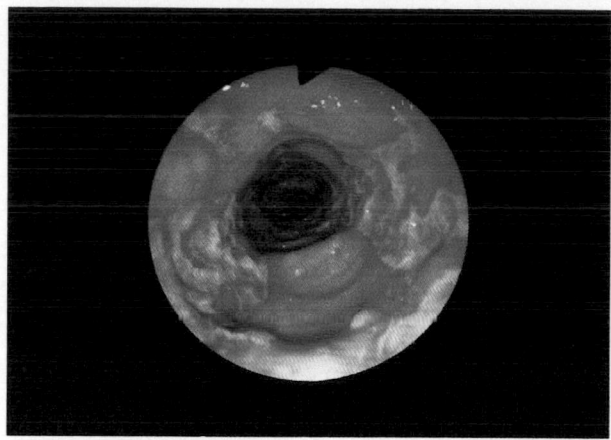

A3-19 **Crohn's colitis** with linear, serpiginous, white-based ulcers surrounded by colonic mucosa which is relatively normal.

A3-20 **Severe ulcerative colitis** with diffuse ulceration, bleeding, and exudation.

A3-21 **Kaposi's sarcoma involving the colon** in a patient with AIDS. The erythematous lesions involve most of the colonic mucosa in the photograph.

Source: Courtesy of FE Silverstein and GN Tytgat: *Atlas of Gastrointestinal Endoscopy.* Gower Medical Publishing, New York, 1987.

A4-1 **Normal optic nerve and retina.**

A4-2 **Central retinal artery occlusion.**

A4-3 **Central retinal vein occlusion.**

A4-4 **Early papilledema.**

A4-5 **Drusen of the optic nerve head.**

A4-6 **Anterior ischemic optic neuropathy.**

A4-7 **Primary optic atrophy.**

A4-8 **Angioid streaks.**

A4-9 **Retinitis pigmentosa.**

A4-10 **Band keratopathy.**

A4-11 **Glaucomatous optic disk with secondary atrophy.**

A4-12 **Diabetic retinopathy with microaneurysms.**

A4-13 **Proliferative diabetic retinopathy.**

A4-14 **Cytomegalovirus retinitis in AIDS.**
(Courtesy of Donald J. D'Amico, M.D.)

A4-15 **Retinal arteriovenous malformation in the Wyburn-Mason syndrome.**

A4-16 **Kayser-Fleischer ring in Wilson's disease.**
(Note: The ring is the golden brown pigment at the periphery of the cornea and is characteristically broader superiorly and inferiorly than it is medially and laterally.)

A5-1 **Normal blood smear.** Normal red blood cells are round, possess an area of central pallor, appear slightly smaller than the nucleus of a mature lymphocyte, and vary little in size (anisocytosis) or in shape (poikilocytosis).

A5-2 **Megaloblastic anemia.** Oval macrocytes, well filled with hemoglobin, are admixed with lesser numbers of small teardrop-shaped red blood cells. Note also hypersegmented granulocyte.

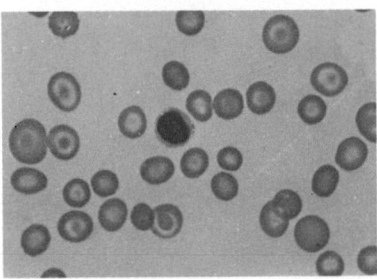

A5-3 **Liver disease.** Round macrocytes of rather uniform size are seen. Many of the macrocytes are also target cells.

A5-4 **Iron-deficiency anemia.** In severe iron deficiency, the red blood cells are smaller than normal (microcytosis), and their central area of pallor is expanded (hypochromia) so that the cells appear to have only a thin rim of hemoglobin.

A5-5 **β thalassemia intermedia.** Microcytic and hypochromic red blood cells are seen that resemble the red blood cells of severe iron deficiency anemia shown in Fig. A5-4. Many elliptical and teardrop-shaped red blood cells are noted.

A5-6 **Sickle cell anemia.** The elongated and crescent-shaped red blood cells seen on this smear represent circulating irreversible sickled cells. Target cells and a nucleated red blood cell are also seen.

A5-7 **Traumatic hemolysis.** The helmet-shaped red blood cell and the small triangular shaped red blood cells seen on this smear represent morphologic evidence of mechanical damage to red blood cells within the circulatory tree.

A5-8 **Spur cell anemia.** Spur cells are recognized as distorted red blood cells containing several irregularly distributed thornlike projections. Cells with this morphologic abnormality are also called acanthocytes.

A5-9 **Uremia.** The red blood cells in uremia may acquire numerous, regularly spaced, small spiny projections. Such cells, called burr cells or echinocytes, are readily distinguishable from the irregularly spiculated acanthocytes shown in Fig. A5-8.

A5-10 **Hereditary spherocytosis.** Small, densely staining red blood cells are seen that have lost their central area of pallor (microspherocytes). Microspherocytes may also be found in other hemolytic disorders (Fig. A5-11).

A5-11 **Immunohemolytic anemia.** Microspherocytes are seen on this blood smear along with several macrocytes with a slight purple tinge (polychromasia). The latter represent new red blood cells released early from the bone marrow. The microspherocytes seen in immunohemolytic anemia may be indistinguishable from the microspherocytes seen in hereditary spherocytosis (Fig. A5-10).

A5-12 **Myeloid metaplasia.** Teardrop-shaped red blood cells, a nucleated red blood cell, and immature myeloid cells are seen on this blood smear.

A   **B**

A5-13 A. **Normal granulocyte.** The normal granulocyte has a segmented nucleus with heavy, clumped chromatin; fine neutrophilic granules are dispersed throughout its cytoplasm. *B.* **Normal monocyte and lymphocyte.** The normal monocyte is a large cell with an indented or folded nucleus containing loose, strandlike chromatin; the cytoplasm is a blue-gray color and usually contains fine azurophilic granules. The normal lymphocyte is a smaller cell. Its nucleus is usually round but may be indented, as in the cell shown in this plate. The nuclear chromatin has a smudgy appearance; the cytoplasm is a blue color.

A   **B**

A5-14 A. **Normal eosinophil.** The eosinophil contains large, bright-orange granules; the nucleus is bilobed. *B.* **Basophil.** The basophil contains large purple-black granules which fill the cell and obscure the nucleus.

A5-15 **Normal granulocyte precursors in marrow.** The earliest granulocytic precursor (myeloblast) possesses a round nucleus with fine, punctate chromatin and one or more nucleoli; the cytoplasm is blue. As nuclear differentiation proceeds, the nucleoli disappear, the chromatin coarsens, and the nucleus becomes increasingly indented and finally segmented. As cytoplasmic differentiation proceeds, azurophilic granules appear and the cytoplasm changes color from blue to the yellow-pink-gray hue of the mature granulocyte, and as this occurs the azurophilic granules become obscured by fine neutrophilic granules.

A5-16 **Neutrophils with toxic granulation.** In infection and other toxic states, azurophilic granules may become visible in mature granulocytes as coarse, dark-staining cytoplasmic granules.

A5-17 **Band with Döhle body** (center). Döhle bodies are discrete, blue-staining, nongranular areas found in the periphery of the cytoplasm of the neutrophil in infections and other toxic states. They represent aggregates of rough endoplasmic reticulum.

A5-18 **Hypersegmentation.** Frequent five-lobed granulocytes on a blood smear or granulocytes with more than five lobes are evidence of hypersegmentation, an important clue to the diagnosis of megaloblastic anemia.

A **B**

A5-19 A. **Chédiak-Higashi anomaly.** In this ultimately fatal disorder, the granulocytes contain huge cytoplasmic granules, formed from aggregation and fusion of azurophilic and specific granules. Large, abnormal granules are found in other granule-containing cells throughout the body. *B.* **Pelger-Hüet anomaly.** In this benign disorder, the majority of granulocytes are bilobed. The nucleus frequently has a spectacle-like or "pince-nez" configuration.

A5-20 **Reactive lymphocytes** (infectious mononucleosis). Reactive lymphocytes are usually large, cytoplasmic lymphocytes. The nucleus may be eccentrically placed and may have irregular borders and indentations (not seen on this plate). The cytoplasm contains areas that stain a darker blue due to their increased content of RNA. The cytoplasm may be indented where it abuts against a red blood cell.

A5-21 **Chronic granulocytic leukemia.** The peripheral blood WBC count is high due to increased numbers of granulocytes and their precursors. The majority of the WBCs are segmented granulocytes or band forms, but as seen on this plate, myelocytes and promyeloblasts (not seen on this plate) may also be found on review of the blood smear.

A5-22 **Leukemic cell in acute promyelocytic leukemia.** Note multiple Auer rods.

A5-23 **Chronic lymphocytic leukemia.** The peripheral blood WBC count is high due to increased numbers of small, well-differentiated lymphocytes. However, the leukemic lymphocytes are fragile, and substantial numbers of broken, smudged cells are usually also present on the blood smear.

A5-24 **Leukemic cells in acute lympho-blastic leukemia** characterized by round or convoluted nuclei, high nuclear/cytoplasmic ratio and absence of cytoplasmic granules.

A5-25 **Hodgkin's disease:** Reed-Sternberg cell in marrow (center). The Reed-Sternberg cell is recognized by its bilobed, mirror-image nucleus, which contains in each lobe a giant, inclusion body–like nucleolus. The cytoplasmic borders of the cell cannot be identified on this plate.

A5-26 **Non-Hodgkin's nodular lymphoma** (lymph node). This low-power view illustrates that a proliferative process has caused the normal architecture of the lymph node to be replaced by multiple nodules of varying size that extend throughout the entire lymph node.

A5-27 **Multiple myeloma** (marrow). The cells bear the characteristic morphologic features of plasma cells, round or oval cells with an eccentric nucleus composed of coarsely clumped chromatin, a densely basophilic cytoplasm, and a perinuclear clear zone (hof) containing the Golgi apparatus. Binucleate and multinucleate malignant plasma cells can also be seen.

70 NUTRITION AND NUTRITIONAL REQUIREMENTS

IRWIN H. ROSENBERG

Maintenance of good nutrition is essential for both the comprehensive management and the prevention of disease. Many debilitating complications can be prevented or modified by attention to nutritional status and prevention of nutritional deficits. The effective management of the sick patient, therefore, requires detailed evaluation of diet and nutritional status and a projection of the interaction of diet and nutritional status on the clinical course. Only then can proper goals and techniques of nutritional management be selected and nutritional guidance be provided for disease prevention and health promotion.

The purpose of the chapters in this section is to summarize some of the basic considerations for the estimation of nutritional needs and the setting of goals for treatment. Determination of the nutritional needs of the individual patient must take into account both the physiologic responses to normal dietary intake and the nutritional impairments induced by disease.

EATING BEHAVIOR AND NUTRITIONAL NEEDS Eating behavior is by nature intermittent, yet energy needs are continuous. This basic feature of mammalian biology has resulted in the evolution of an elaborate set of metabolic controls that promote the ebb and flow of nutrients after feeding and during the postabsorptive period and, in addition, provide for the maintenance of near-normal function during periods of fasting.

In a nutritional perspective, the mechanisms that control appetite and eating behavior are directed to maintain energy intake adequate for the needs of the healthy adult, for the extra needs of growth in the child, and for the requirements of pregnancy and lactation. Under conditions of disease or trauma, the increased requirements must be met through appropriate modifications in eating behavior or caloric supplementation if energy balance is to be maintained.

The usual remarkable stability of body weight and body composition requires that energy intake and expenditure must be balanced over time. The precise nature of the internal signals that relay the information that caloric intake is appropriate for energy needs during the preceding days is not known. Such signals do not adjust eating behavior on a meal-to-meal time scale. At the time of an individual meal, volume and chemoreceptors in the stomach and small bowel initiate neural and hormonal responses that contribute to satiety. The nutrient density of the food eaten, in terms of the protein or calorie content per unit volume, is not sensitively perceived, and therefore total energy or protein intake can fluctuate substantially over the short run. The neurophysiologic mechanisms that control eating behavior recognize calorie deficiencies on roughly a 24- to 48-h time scale and make compensatory changes in the volume of food eaten over periods of 1 to 2 days. That these controls work remarkably well is attested to by the stability of body weight and general nutritional health of most people who have access to adequate food intake. Aberrations in these control factors can produce serious and even life-threatening imbalance, as evidenced by obesity and syndromes of anorexia and depletion related to manifest disease.

METABOLIC RESPONSES TO CALORIC INTAKE When dietary or energy intake is adequate, several metabolic controls act to maintain essential body functions. One essential function is the maintenance of a steady fuel supply to the brain. Under the usual conditions the brain uses glucose for energy at a rate of about 5 g/h, and such a supply must be available in both the fasted and fed states. The brain is also capable of utilizing ketones as an energy source and will do so in preference to glucose if the ketones are present in sufficiently high concentration. In contrast to tissues such as skeletal muscle, the brain uses energy at a fairly constant rate, whether awake, sleeping, thinking, or dreaming.

During the influx of nutrients into blood after feeding and absorption, the energy and amino acid needs of the body are readily met by the supply entering from the gastrointestinal tract. When this flow of nutrients subsides, however, the body's needs are met by release of energy from stores. In the period immediately after feeding, these stores are generated and maintained under hormonal control, particularly insulin. The excess amino acids, fatty acids, and glucose not required immediately for energy are stored in the form of proteins, triglycerides, and glycogen. This storage process also serves to modulate the large extracellular osmotic shifts that might occur between the fed and the fasting states by depositing excess nutrients in intracellular depots.

NUTRITIONAL REQUIREMENTS To formulate an overall plan for nutritional management, one must consider the nutritional requirements of the patient and the impact of disease on these requirements. Energy balance in simplest terms means energy intake that maintains a steady body weight. Energy insufficiency is reflected in weight loss, and energy overabundance causes weight gain. Conditions that can substantially modify nutritional requirements include infection, trauma (including surgery), alcohol abuse, and malabsorption.

ESTIMATION OF ENERGY REQUIREMENT Malnutrition occurs when nutrient intake is below nutrient needs. Although the disorder can result from excessive nutritional intake, in general the term commonly refers to undernutrition. Undernutrition can be due to inadequate intake or absorption or to increased metabolic requirements imposed by disease, including loss and secretion of nutrients and drug-nutrient antagonisms.

The components of energy requirements in humans are summarized in Table 70-1. Total daily energy requirement consists of basal

TABLE 70-1 Example of estimation of daily energy requirement

The information presented above can be utilized as in the following example: A 45-year old, 70-kg male office worker presents with rheumatoid arthritis of mild severity. Calorie intake is good, but recent activity has been limited.

Resting energy expenditure (based on weight and sex)	7500 kJ (1800 kcal)
Activity-related expenditure	1700 kJ (400 kcal)
Illness-related expenditure (10 percent of 1800 kcal)	750 kJ (180 kcal)
Diet-induced thermogenesis (10 percent of 2380 kcal)	955 kJ (238 kcal)
Total	10,945 kJ (2618 kcal)

TABLE 70-2   Estimation of resting metabolic rate (RMR)

Age (years)	Male kJ†	Male kcal†	Female kJ†	Female kcal†
3–10	Wt* × 95 + 2110	Wt* × 22.7 + 505	Wt* × 85 + 2033	Wt* × 20.3 + 486
10–18	Wt × 74 + 2754	Wt × 17.7 + 659	Wt × 56 + 2898	Wt × 13.4 + 693
18–30	Wt × 63 + 2896	Wt × 15.1 + 693	Wt × 62 + 2036	Wt × 14.8 + 487
30–60	Wt × 48 + 4653	Wt × 11.5 + 1113	Wt × 34 + 3538	Wt × 8.1 + 846
>60	Wt × 59 + 2459	Wt × 11.7 + 588	Wt × 38 + 2755	Wt × 9.1 + 659

*Body weight in kilograms
†To convert the RMR from kJ to kcal multiply kJ by 0.239.
  To convert the RMR from kcal to kJ multiply the kcal by 4.186.
SOURCE: Modified from WN Schofield.

metabolic rate (BMR) plus energy of activity and the thermic effect of food. Basal metabolic rate (BMR) or, more appropriately, resting metabolic rate (RMR) is a measure of the amount of energy expended at rest and without food; energy of activity is a measure of the energy expended to support a variety of physical activities; thermic effect of food (TEF) [also called diet-induced thermogenesis (DIT) and previously called specific dynamic action] is an estimate of the number of calories produced as heat during the digestion, absorption, and metabolism of food. RMR accounts for about two-thirds of the total energy requirements and is affected by body size (height and weight), age, sex, and habitus (Table 70-2). Several clinical methods are available for estimating energy expenditure.

Estimation of resting metabolic rate (RMR)   Most methods are based on calorimetry, a measurement of oxygen consumption under carefully controlled conditions, e.g., during fasting, in the morning, and for one hour. A more meaningful metabolic rate would reflect the rate at which energy is consumed in a normal life situation at rest throughout the day, including the period of food assimilation. The usual clinical estimates of RMR discussed below are based on indirect assessments rather than true measurements. Nonetheless, such estimates are frequently very useful.

The method of estimation devised by Harris and Benedict is used most commonly to estimate BMR. The formulas for calculating BMR (in kcal per day) using the four variables of age, height, weight, and sex are as follows:

$$BMR_{women} = 655 + (9.5 \times W) + (1.8 \times H) - (4.7 \times A)$$
$$BMR_{men} = 66 + (13.7 \times W) + (5 \times H) - (6.8 \times A)$$

where W is actual or usual weight (kg), H is height (cm), and A is age (years).

The equations for RMR are simpler than those of Harris and Benedict and are based on more comprehensive data. Because people of the same weight but of different heights have similar RMRs, the formulas are based only on weight, age, and sex (Table 70-2). The values differ from earlier formulas mostly for women, in whom there was an overestimation for weight above 40 kg, reaching an error of nearly 18 percent by a weight of 80 kg. It should be remembered that predicted RMR (or BMR) may over- or underestimate the measured values by 20 or even 30 percent for any individual.

Diet-induced thermogenesis (DIT)   The ingestion of nutrients in food causes heat or energy production in excess of basal metabolic rates. A mixed diet causes approximately a 6 to 10 percent increase above basal in calories expended as heat. Thermogenic effect of protein is greatest, that of carbohydrate is next, and fat is least effective. The calorigenic effect of food seems to be closely related to the energy required for ATP formation, in which protein (via amino acid breakdown and urea synthesis) is the oxidative substrate. Most of the effect is generated in the muscle and liver and occurs whether intake is enteral or parenteral. In hypermetabolic patients, diet-induced thermogenesis is less marked because heat production is already elevated. In calculating additional energy requirements for hypermetabolic patients, the DIT should be estimated at no more than 5 percent of total energy requirements.

Estimates of energy for activity   The energy expenditure of physical activity accounts for about one-third of total energy expend-

itures under most conditions and can vary from 6 to 36 kJ (1.5 to 8.5 kcal) per kilogram body weight per hour (Table 70-3). This factor is obviously more important in calculating energy requirements for active, ambulatory patients. Some types of work (e.g., gardening) can fatigue certain muscle groups without using a large number of calories. Usually, any exercise that results in lifting the body from the ground (e.g., running) uses the most calories. Although precise measurements by calorimetry are available for a wide range of activities, it is easiest to use an approximation when estimating energy needs.

Additional energy requirements of illness   Heat production increases with fever and inflammation. However, as oxygen consumption increases, DIT decreases, and the energy of activity declines owing to immobility. For these reasons, the daily energy requirement in ill persons is usually only slightly greater than the requirement when well. Indeed, the energy requirement for most patients, even during severe illness, rarely exceeds 12,500 kJ (3000 kcal) per day. (The earlier estimates of massively increased calorie requirements in patients with sepsis have not been substantiated.) Approximately 20 percent should be added to resting energy estimates for a patient confined to bed, and 30 percent should be added for ambulatory patients. Severe illness requires additional caloric supplementation, namely, addition of 10 percent of estimated RMR for mild illness, 25 percent for moderate illness, and 50 percent for severe illness.

Malabsorption is a special cause of increased energy requirement. The most accurate but impractical way to assess calorie loss would be calorimetry of the feces. However, fat excretion in grams per day (as determined in a 72-h fecal fat assay) × 38 kJ (9 kcal) per gram equals the daily energy loss due to fat malabsorption. To estimate total fecal energy loss from all sources, the fecal energy loss from fat (in kJ or kcal) is multiplied by 2.5. This estimate assumes an average dietary composition and equivalent malabsorption of fat, carbohydrate, and protein.

ESTIMATION OF PROTEIN REQUIREMENT   Protein balance, like energy balance, is a function of intake relative to utilization and loss. Normally, nitrogen derived from amino acids is excreted in urine and feces and lost from the skin. Unlike the energy stored in triglycerides and glycogen, no proteins (or amino acids) are stored in the body solely for subsequent utilization. Every protein serves either a structural or metabolic function; when excess protein is ingested the amino acids are transaminated, and the nonnitrogenous portion of the molecule serves as a source of calories for storage as glycogen and/or fat.

TABLE 70-3   Estimation of additional energy expenditure by activity

Type of work	Calories added to BMR kJ/d	Calories added to BMR kcal/d
Sedentary	1670–3350	400–800
Light: office, professional and clerical	3350–5000	800–1200
Moderate: walking, lifting	5000–7500	1200–1800
Heavy: construction, athletic	7500–19,000	1800–4500

SOURCE: Modified from DW Wilmore, *The Metabolic Management of the Critically Ill.* New York, Plenum Press, 1977.

Obligatory nitrogen losses Urea accounts for over 80 percent of urinary nitrogen. The remaining nitrogen is excreted as creatinine, porphyrins, and other nitrogen-containing compounds. Thus, total urine loss of nitrogen = urea nitrogen (mg/dL) × daily volume (dL) ÷ 0.8. Urinary nitrogen is related to the RMR. The larger the body muscle mass, the more transamination of amino acids occurs to fulfill energy needs. Each kilocalorie needed for basal metabolism leads to the excretion of 1 to 1.3 mg of urinary nitrogen. For the same reason, nitrogen excretion increases during exercise and heavy work.

Fecal and skin losses account for a large proportion of nitrogen loss from the body (about 40 percent) in normal circumstances, but the magnitude of these losses varies in disease states. Thus, measurement of urinary nitrogen often provides a useful index of daily nitrogen requirement.

Minimal nitrogen loss (in grams per day) from a 70-kg person on a diet that is nitrogen free but energy adequate approximates 1.9 to 3.1 in urine, 0.7 to 2.5 in stool, and 0.3 from skin for a mean total loss of 4.4 g per day. Equivalent protein loss can be calculated by multiplying nitrogen loss by 6.25 so that total loss by metabolism of protein is 4.4 × 6.25 or 27.5 g/d or about 0.4 g/kg body weight for a 70-kg person. The recommended protein allowance for adults varies from 0.6 to 0.9 g/kg to allow for a margin of safety. Vigorous exercise may increase protein requirements to 1 g/kg body weight or higher.

Protein requirements are highest during the growth spurts of infancy and adolescence. During infancy, total body protein reserve is lowest, and obligatory losses are greatest. Thus, protein deficiency is most common in infancy. Protein requirements decline slightly during childhood and again increase during adolescence. Minimal requirements for these stages of life are about 1.5 g/kg body weight per day. The recommended allowance (2 g/kg body weight per day) exceeds this figure to allow a margin of safety for children who have increased needs or who ingest proteins of low biologic value. Low quality proteins include certain vegetable proteins that do not support growth as well as protein from milk, eggs, or meat. The differences in the nutritional value of protein are largely due to the higher content of essential amino acids in animal proteins and to differences in digestibility. Protein (and energy) requirements also increase during pregnancy and lactation.

CALORIC REQUIREMENTS FOR PROTEIN UTILIZATION
Amino acids ingested without other energy sources are not efficiently incorporated into protein partly because of the energy lost during amino acid metabolism. Moreover, incorporation of each amino acid molecule into peptides requires three high-energy phosphate bonds. Consequently, excess of dietary energy over basal needs improves the efficiency of nitrogen utilization. During the period of intense growth in children, about 300 kJ (76 kcal) of nonprotein energy are required for each gram of protein. In ambulatory adults about 200 kJ (50 kcal) from nonprotein sources are needed per gram of protein. This high ratio usually cannot be achieved with parenteral feeding, since energy intake is limited by the volume needed to be infused. Acceptable figures for parenteral nutrition are about 100 to 125 kJ (25 to 30 kcal) from nonprotein sources per gram of protein or 600 to 750 kJ (150 to 180 kcal) per gram of nitrogen.

RECOMMENDED DIETARY ALLOWANCES OF PROTEIN AND MICRONUTRIENTS
Guidelines of nutritional requirements in health have been formulated in the reports, updated periodically, of the Food and Nutrition Board of the National Research Council of the United States. These Recommended Dietary Allowances, expressed for age and sex and modified for such conditions as pregnancy and lactation, are designed to cover the requirements of virtually all healthy individuals. With the exception of energy, the allowances are not average requirements but rather a recommended intake sufficient to meet the needs of all healthy individuals.

The recommended dietary allowances for protein (nitrogen), iron, and calcium are based upon experiments in which normal requirement is defined as the intake necessary to achieve zero balance between intake versus output. For most vitamins the recommended allowance is the daily intake required to maintain full function and safe levels

TABLE 70-4 Recommended dietary allowances for healthy adults

	Range of allowance	
	Men	Women
Protein, g	45–63	44–50
Vitamin A, μg retinol equivalents	1000	800
Vitamin D, μg	5–10	5–10
Vitamin E, mg α-tocopherol equivalents	10	8
Vitamin K, μg	45–80	45–65
Vitamin C, mg	50–60	50–60
Thiamine, mg	1.2–1.5	1–1.1
Riboflavin, mg	1.4–1.8	1.2–1.3
Niacin, mg niacin equivalents	15–20	13–15
Vitamin B_6, mg	1.4–2.0	1.4–1.6
Folate, μg	150–200	150–180
Vitamin B_{12}, μg	2.0	2.0
Biotin, μg*	30–100	50–100
Pantothenic Acid, mg*	4–10	4–7
Calcium, mg	800–1200	800–1200
Phosphorus, mg	800–1200	800–1200
Magnesium, mg	270–400	280–300
Iron, mg	10–12	10–15
Zinc, mg	15	12
Iodine, μg	150	150
Selenium, μg	40 70	45 55
Copper, mg*	1.5–3	1.5–3
Manganese, mg*	2–5	2–5
Fluoride, mg*	1.5–4	1.5–4
Chromium, μg*	50–200	50–200
Molybdenum, μg*	75–250	75–250

*Estimated safe and adequate daily dietary intakes. From the National Research Council: *Recommended Dietary Allowances*, 10th ed. Washington, D.C., National Academy of Sciences, 1989.

of body stores. Most estimates assume normal digestion and absorption and normal metabolism. In some cases, estimates of daily turnover by radioisotope or stable isotope tracer techniques are used to determine the amount of nutrient required to maintain body stores. It follows, therefore, that diseases that influence efficiency of absorption or that change the metabolism or nutritional requirements will change the safe allowance for that individual. It further follows that the recommended dietary allowances are at best a rough guide for requirements for enteral nutrient intake by any individual. Such allowances may be an overestimation of parenteral requirements, particularly in the case of micronutrients, since in that case no allowance need be made for the inefficiency of extraction from food and absorption. A listing of these essential nutrients and an estimation of the ranges of required intake for healthy adults are presented in Table 70-4.

The recommended dietary allowances make little provision for changes in nutrient requirements for the elderly. Energy requirements decline progressively beyond age 50 or 60 as the lean (muscle) mass declines and resting metabolic energy expenditure decreases. Energy needs for activity also decline as aging often leads to more sedentary lifestyle. There are few studies in the elderly that define specific differences in nutrient requirements. At present, it is prudent to recommend full adult levels of protein, vitamins, and minerals even in the face of declining energy intake. For small elderly people, especially small women, this may require heightened dietary planning and vigilance. Increased physical activity at all ages promotes the retention of lean muscle mass and also increases appetite and food intake.

REFERENCES

ALPERS DH et al: *Manual of Nutritional Therapeutics.* Boston, Little, Brown, 1987, chap 3

HAVEL RJ: Caloric homeostasis and disorders of fuel transport. N Engl J Med 1987:1186, 1972

KISSILEFF HR, VAN ITALLIE TB: Physiology of the control of food intake. Ann Rev Nutr 2:271, 1982

SCHOFIELD WN: Predicting basal metabolic rate, new standards and review of previous work. Human Nutr Clin Nutr 39C(Suppl 1), 1985

THE NATIONAL RESEARCH COUNCIL: *Recommended Dietary Allowances*, 10th ed. Washington, DC, National Academy of Sciences, 1989

71   PROTEIN-ENERGY MALNUTRITION

JOEL B. MASON / IRWIN H. ROSENBERG

Protein-energy malnutrition (PEM), or protein-calorie malnutrition (PCM), is present when there is insufficient energy or protein available to meet metabolic demands. Inadequate dietary intake is only one of several mechanisms by which this may occur: Increased metabolic demands due to disease and increased nutrient losses can also result in PEM. Protein deficiency may also arise in the face of adequate protein intake if the dietary protein is of poor quality (i.e., the content of one or more essential amino acids is inadequate and thus becomes the limiting factor in protein utilization); such is the case when the entire protein intake is derived from a single vegetable source. Protein nutrition is also influenced by the intake of energy relative to the intake of protein because the efficient utilization of dietary protein requires energy from nonprotein calories.

Adaptive responses function over the short term when protein and energy sources are limited. As a consequence, the pathologic consequences of undernutrition require a sustained inadequacy of protein or energy sources. The adaptive mechanisms that respond to protein and calorie deprivation are finite, particularly because protein has no storage form in the body.

The rapidity with which an individual develops PEM and the severity of the resulting syndrome depend on a number of factors, including the nutritional state when the nutritional deprivation begins, the underlying illness, and the developmental stage. Some of these factors are outlined in Table 71-1.

PROTEIN-ENERGY MALNUTRITION AS A GLOBAL PROBLEM Recognition of PEM emerged from studies in the tropics that were focused primarily on the problem in children. Preschool children, particularly infants, are more susceptible to PEM. They are dependent on others for determining the quantity and quality of food intake; protein and energy requirements of children are substantially higher per unit weight; and unhygienic habits and immaturity of the immune system heighten susceptibility to infections. Gastrointestinal infections, in particular, constitute a major precipitant of PEM in infants and children because such illnesses result in altered feeding habits, vomiting, decreased intestinal absorption, increased metabolic needs, and increased metabolic losses. The magnitude of the problem is immense; the World Health Organization estimated in 1983 that 300 million children have growth retardation secondary to malnutrition. Increased mortality and impaired cognitive, social, and economic development are additional features of this condition.

PEM is confined neither to infants and children nor to the less-developed countries. Although the overall prevalence of PEM is low, specific sectors of the U.S. population, such as the institutionalized elderly and children of the poor, have a significant prevalence. For example, the Ten State Survey, which focused on low income areas

in the United States, found that 22 to 35 percent of the children aged 2, 4, and 6 were below the 15th percentile for weight. In this survey income level and minority status were predictors of growth retardation among children. Moreover, in large urban teaching hospitals and smaller community hospitals 30 to 70 percent of general medical and surgical patients have anthropometric and/or biochemical evidence of PEM. Similar statistics have been noted in surveys of pediatric inpatients. It is perhaps more disturbing that the nutritional status of the majority of hospitalized patients *declines* during the course of hospitalization. Positive associations between the degree of PEM and the incidence of postoperative infections, impaired healing of surgical wounds, and prolongation of hospitalization indicate that more attention needs to be paid to the maintenance of adequate nutrition in individual patients. There are tangible benefits from such nutritional diligence because aggressive preoperative nutritional restitution of malnourished patients can decrease perioperative morbidity such as infection.

Most modern-day hospital malnutrition is compounded by insufficient attention by medical personnel to nutrition (Table 71-2). Indeed, most factors contributing to the high prevalence of malnutrition in hospitalized patients are reversible or preventable.

PROTEIN-ENERGY METABOLISM DURING STRESS Physiological adaptation to starvation During periods of protein and/or energy deficit, compensatory mechanisms serve to lessen the pathologic impact of these deficiencies. To understand how malnutrition develops, it is therefore important to understand the responses to such inadequate intake. During the first 24 h of fasting, circulating glucose, fatty acids, and triglycerides and liver and muscle glycogen are used as fuel sources. However, the sum of these stores in a 70-kg man is only about 5000 kJ (1200 kcal) and provides less fuel than is needed for basal metabolism for a single day. Triglycerides, derived primarily from adipose tissue, can be catabolized to fatty acids and ketone bodies by most tissues. However, over the short run tissues such as the brain can only use glycolytic pathways to obtain energy. Since the conversion of fatty acids to carbohydrate is inefficient in animals, these glycolytic tissues must utilize either glucose or substrates that can be converted to glucose. Amino acids derived primarily from skeletal muscle constitute the major endogenous substrate for glucose production for this purpose. Since there is no storage form of protein in the body, a fasting individual sustains a daily loss of functionally significant protein.

The provision of adequate fuel substrate to critical tissues, particularly the brain, has homeostatic priority during protein/energy deprivation. Brief starvation leads to acute adaptive responses that sustain the supply of glucose to tissues that require it and minimize the amount of protein breakdown to meet this need. To accomplish this end, certain tissues, such as the heart, kidney, and skeletal muscle, change their primary fuel substrate from glucose to fatty acids and ketone bodies. Other tissues, such as the bone marrow, renal medulla, and peripheral nerves, switch from the full oxidation of glucose to anaerobic glycolysis, resulting in the production of

---

TABLE 71-1   Factors that influence the response to inadequate nutrient intake

I Nutritional factors
  A Underlying adequacy of reserves/depot of that nutrient
  B Severity and duration of the inadequate intake
  C Concurrent deficiencies of other nutrients
II Underlying illnesses
  A Fever, infection, trauma, and other conditions associated with increased requirements and catabolic losses
  B Malabsorptive and maldigestive states
  C Disorders associated with excessive loss of nutrients (e.g., protein-losing enteropathy, nephrotic syndrome, enteric fistulas)
  D Conditions associated with altered metabolism of nutrients (e.g., diabetes mellitus, hyperthyroidism)
III Physiologic states in which increased requirements are present
  A Pregnancy, lactation
  B Growth and development during infancy, childhood, and adolescence

---

TABLE 71-2   Undesirable practices affecting the nutritional assessment and/or status of hospitalized patients

Failure to record height and weight in the hospital chart
Diffusion of responsibility for patient care
Prolonged use of glucose and saline intravenous feedings
Failure to observe and record dietary intake
Withholding meals because of diagnostic tests
Use of enteral or parenteral feedings of uncertain composition and in inadequate amounts
Ignorance of the composition of nutritional products
Failure to recognize increased nutritional needs due to injury or illness
Lack of communication between physician, nurse, and dietician
Delay of nutritional support until severe depletion has developed
Limited availability of laboratory tests to assess nutritional status; failure to use those that are available
Limited emphasis on nutrition education in medical education

SOURCE: After CE Butterworth, in Nutr Today 9:4, 1974

lactate and pyruvate. These compounds can be converted to glucose in the liver with energy derived from fat oxidation and then released for systemic consumption. This shuttle, the Cori cycle, enables energy stored as fat to be utilized for glucose synthesis and thus conserves protein energy that would otherwise be necessary for the de novo synthesis of glucose.

With more extended starvation other adaptations appear. A decrease in physical exertion decreases energy consumption, and the resting metabolic rate generally declines by about 10 percent. The brain, which ordinarily obtains energy only by glucose oxidation, acquires the ability to use keto acids for its fuel requirements, and this contributes further to protein conservation. Animal studies and, less definitively, human studies suggest that protein that is consumed during relative protein starvation is utilized more efficiently. Moreover, chronic protein deprivation leads to a reduced rate of protein turnover, and amino acids are reutilized more efficiently for the synthesis of new proteins, contributing to savings in both energy and amino acid requirements.

During relative or total caloric starvation, such adaptations allow the body to provide the energy necessary for metabolism and to minimize the obligatory loss of protein, which appears primarily as nitrogen-containing compounds in the urine. After several weeks of starvation, nitrogen loss in the urine may decrease by more than 65 percent. However, these homeostatic mechanisms do not compensate entirely for the imposed deficits, and eventually the negative caloric and/or protein balance lead to pathologic consequences.

Effects of physical stress Infection, trauma, and other physical stress cause inflammatory responses. In such situations, protein and energy metabolism change in ways that increase both energy demands and nitrogen losses and thereby predispose to the development of PEM.

Resting metabolic rate (RMR) increases dramatically during critical illness. Patients with burns over more than 40 percent of the body have a RMR approximately twice normal, and patients with sepsis have a RMR that is about one and a half times normal. Factors that contribute to the increased energy consumption include increases in circulating catecholamines and increase in energy expenditure required for gluconeogenesis.

Nitrogen loss during critical illness is also increased. A healthy adult loses approximately 12 g of nitrogen in urine per day in the fasting state; sepsis and trauma commonly increase that value by 50 to 100 percent. Since 1 g of urinary nitrogen represents approximately 30 g of lean body mass, critical illness induces a daily loss of 0.6 kg of lean body mass. Most of this loss comes from the skeletal muscle, and the efflux of amino acids from skeletal muscle increases two- to sixfold in critically ill patients. Increased efflux from skeletal muscle is probably due to increased protein catabolism rather than decreased protein synthesis.

The amino acids mobilized from skeletal muscle are in part used as fuel and in part taken up by the liver and other visceral organs. The proteolysis of muscle under physical stress thus enables the body to shift protein substrate from the somatic compartment to visceral organs whose function is more critical for immediate survival. Hormonal factors play a significant role in this shift; circulating levels of cortisol, glucagon, epinephrine, and growth hormone are increased in physically stressed individuals. Increased circulating levels of interleukin 1 and tumor necrosis factor in septic and traumatized patients may participate in the sparing of the visceral protein compartment at the expense of the skeletal muscle. Eventually, continued deficits in protein and energy, particularly when superimposed on sustained physical stress, lead to a constriction of the visceral protein compartment and its associated functions.

DIAGNOSIS, ASSESSMENT, AND CLASSIFICATION OF PROTEIN-ENERGY MALNUTRITION Protein-energy malnutrition may be primary, due to an inadequate intake of protein and/or energy source, or secondary, due to illness that impairs intake or utilization of nutrients or that increases nutrient requirements or metabolic losses. Malignancy, intestinal malabsorption, inflammatory bowel disease,

acquired immunodeficiency syndrome, and chronic renal failure are a few of the illnesses commonly associated with secondary PEM.

There are no universally accepted criteria for defining the severity of PEM although it is often categorized as mild, moderate, or severe. An effective nutritional assessment requires the synthesis of information provided by a dietary history, physical examination, and anthropometric and biochemical assessment. No single piece of evidence is sufficient to indicate the nutritional status. A corollary is that each parameter used to assess nutritional status can be, and often is, influenced by factors that have little to do with the nutritional state.

In adults, the most commonly used indicator of caloric status is body weight. Standard tables of desirable or ideal body weight are available, but individual variation is such that comparison with the premorbid weight may be most useful in the identification of PEM. An obese individual with ongoing deficits in protein or energy balance, although considerably above ideal body weight, can develop PEM with its pathologic consequences. A decrease of more than 10 percent of the usual body weight, particularly when the rate of loss is greater than 3 to 6 percent per month, is a good predictor of PEM.

Fat stores are the major energy reserve in the body and, as such, can also be used to assess energy status. Reduction in subcutaneous fat together with weight loss constitute the most obvious and constant physical features of PEM in adults. Children with PEM have retarded physical development such as stunted (low height for age) or wasted (low weight for height) body habitus and delayed puberty. Cognitive and psychosocial development is commonly retarded.

Reduction in subcutaneous fat is usually evident by inspection of the extremities or face, although a significant reduction in fat mass can be overlooked unless quantitative criteria are assessed, such as skin-fold measurements or assessment of body composition. The triceps fat fold, when compared to standard values, provides an indication of the adequacy of body fat since more than half of total body fat is subcutaneous (Table 71-3).

Protein nutrition can be assessed in several ways. Separate assessments of the somatic and visceral protein compartments are useful since the two protein depots are handled differently. Decreased muscle mass can frequently be recognized on physical examination, although mild malnutrition is usually underestimated. The somatic compartment (primarily skeletal muscle) can be assessed by comparing the midarm muscle area to normative values (Table 71-4). The creatinine-height index performs a similar function (Table 71-5). The visceral compartment can be assessed by estimation of the total lymphocyte count in peripheral blood and by measuring the delayed cutaneous hypersensitivity response. Levels of serum proteins such as albumin are also useful. However, the validity of serum albumin as a reflection of the status of the visceral protein compartment is poor in the setting of acute or critical illness; the long half-life of albumin (20 days), the fact that it is distributed extensively in the extravascular as well as intravascular compartment, and the fact that its synthesis is influenced by the presence of circulating inflammatory mediators and by liver function all limit its value as a measure of nutrition. Serum proteins with shorter half-lives, such as transferrin, thyroxine-binding prealbumin, and retinol-binding protein, are better than albumin in this regard (Table 71-6).

The reduction in lean body mass in mild to moderate PEM is usually not as great as the reduction in fat mass. Nevertheless, the midarm muscle area or the creatinine-height index may be below the standard values. The decrease in urinary urea nitrogen, in contrast, reflects physiologic adjustments to inadequate intake of protein and/or energy rather than loss in skeletal mass. Functionally, work capacity decreases, particularly in very active individuals. Pregnant women with mild to moderate PEM are at risk of delivering infants with low weight or length for gestational age. The volume and fat and energy content of breast milk in such women are decreased.

More severe forms of PEM cause more marked alterations in body habitus and laboratory parameters. Deficiency states of specific micronutrients (see Chap. 76) may be present although PEM itself

TABLE 71-3　Normative values for triceps skin-fold thickness

Age group, years	Sample size	Estimated population, millions	Mean, mm	Percentile 5	10	25	50	75	90	95
MEN										
18–74	5261	61.18	12.0	4.5	6.0	8.0	11.0	15.0	20.0	23.0
18–24	773	11.78	11.2	4.0	5.0	7.0	9.5	14.0	20.0	23.0
25–34	804	13.00	12.6	4.5	5.5	8.0	12.0	16.0	21.5	24.0
35–44	664	10.68	12.4	5.0	6.0	8.5	12.0	15.5	20.0	23.0
45–54	765	11.15	12.4	5.0	6.0	8.0	11.0	15.0	20.0	25.0
55–64	598	9.07	11.6	5.0	6.0	8.0	11.0	14.0	18.0	21.5
65–74	1657	5.50	11.8	4.5	5.5	8.0	11.0	15.0	19.0	22.0
WOMEN										
18–74	8410	67.84	23.0	11.0	13.0	17.0	22.0	28.0	34.0	37.5
18–24	1523	12.89	19.4	9.4	11.0	14.0	18.0	24.0	30.0	34.0
25–34	1896	13.93	21.9	10.5	12.0	16.0	21.0	26.5	33.5	37.0
35–44	1664	11.59	24.0	12.0	14.0	18.0	23.0	29.5	35.5	39.0
45–54	836	12.16	25.4	13.0	15.0	20.0	25.0	30.0	36.0	40.0
55–65	669	9.98	24.9	11.0	14.0	19.0	25.0	30.5	35.0	39.0
65–74	1822	7.28	23.3	11.5	14.0	18.0	23.0	28.0	33.0	36.0

SOURCE: Heymsfield and Williams.

usually has the most impact on health. There is further loss of subcutaneous fat and worsening of muscle wasting in the extremities; this disorder in children is termed *marasmus*. The decrease in muscle mass can sometimes be recognized in the interosseous muscles in the hand and the temporalis muscles of the head, and confirmation is obtained by determining the midarm muscle area. The loss of subcutaneous fat and muscle mass, in conjunction with a loss of the normal elasticity of the skin, commonly results in loose fitting, wrinkled skin with reduplicated folds. Skin lesions in advanced PEM may be shiny, erythematous, atrophic areas or hyperkeratotic, hyperpigmented regions ("flaky paint" dermatitis). Decubitus ulcers are also common in severe disease. The hair may become sparse and dry; it loses its usual sheen and can be pulled out with little effort. The color of the hair may change to reddish or dull brown, and alternating periods of nutritional depletion and repletion may give rise to bands of such color changes in the hair.

Lethargy is a common feature. Alterations in gastrointestinal function include constipation and difficulty ingesting normal-sized meals due to early satiety and vomiting. The heart rate, blood pressure, and core body temperature are frequently subnormal. Infections may not be accompanied by fever and appropriate tachycardia.

Severe PEM due to an inadequate intake of both protein and energy (*combined PEM*) is characterized by a diminution in somatic protein out of proportion to the reduction in the visceral protein compartment. Individuals with combined PEM have muscle wasting in the extremities and trunk but maintain a relatively normal visceral compartment. Weakness can be profound. Loss of subcutaneous fat combined with the loss in muscle mass results in a "skin and bones" appearance. The fact that edema is absent constitutes the major clinical feature separating combined PEM from pure protein malnutrition.

When inadequate availability of protein outweighs the extent of energy deprivation, the subcutaneous fat and somatic protein compartment tend to be spared in comparison to the reduction in the visceral protein compartment. Interpretation of the anthropometric measurements of the somatic protein and fat compartments may be complicated by the presence of edema, but serum protein levels are consistently low in so-called hypoproteinemic PEM. (In children this disorder is termed *kwashiorkor*.) Pure protein malnutrition is unusual

TABLE 71-4　Normative values for midarm muscle area*

Age group	Arm muscle area percentiles, mm² 5	10	25	50	75	90	95
MEN							
16–16.9	3625	4044	4352	4951	5753	6576	6980
17–17.9	3998	4252	4777	5286	5950	6886	7726
18–18.9	4070	4481	5066	5552	6374	7067	8355
19–24.9	4508	4777	5274	5913	6660	7606	8200
25–34.9	4694	4963	5541	6214	7067	7847	8436
35–44.9	4844	5181	5740	6490	7265	8034	8488
45–54.9	4546	4946	5589	6297	7142	7918	8458
55–64.9	4422	4783	5381	6144	6919	7670	8149
65–74.9	3973	4411	5031	5716	6432	7074	7453
WOMEN							
16–16.9	2308	2567	2865	3248	3718	4353	4946
17–17.9	2442	2674	2996	3336	3883	4552	5251
18–18.9	2398	2538	2917	3243	3694	4461	4767
19–24.9	2538	2728	3026	3406	3877	4439	4940
25–34.9	2661	2826	3148	3573	4138	4806	5541
35–44.9	2750	2948	3359	3783	4428	5240	5877
45–54.9	2784	2956	3378	3858	4520	5375	5964
55–64.9	2784	3063	3477	4045	4750	5632	6247
65–74.9	2737	3018	3444	4019	4739	5566	6214

* Estimates based on data from the U.S. Health and Nutrition Examination Survey, 1971–1974 (HANES I).
SOURCE: AJ Frisancho, Am J Clin Nutr 34:2540, 1981.

TABLE 71-5　Normative values for creatinine excretion based on height

Men* Height, cm	Ideal creatinine, mg	Women† Height, cm	Ideal creatinine, mg
157.5	1288	147.3	830
160.0	1325	149.9	851
162.6	1359	152.4	875
165.1	1386	154.9	900
167.6	1426	157.5	925
170.2	1467	160.0	949
172.7	1513	162.6	977
175.3	1555	165.1	1006
177.8	1596	167.6	1044
180.3	1642	170.2	1076
182.9	1691	172.7	1109
185.4	1739	175.3	1141
188.0	1785	177.8	1174
190.5	1831	180.3	1206
193.0	1891	182.9	1240

* Creatinine coefficient (men) = 23 mg/kg of ideal body weight.
† Creatinine coefficient (women) = 18 mg/kg of ideal body weight.
SOURCE: GL Blackburn et al., J Parent Ent Nutr 1:11, 1977.

TABLE 71-6 Serum proteins used in nutritional assessment

Serum protein	Approximate molecular mass, Da	Biosynthetic site	Normal value $\overline{X} \pm$ SD or (range)*	Half-life, days	Function	Comment†
Albumin	66,000	Hepatocyte	45 (35–50)	14–20	Maintain plasma oncotic pressure; carrier for small molecules	Serum levels are determined by many different processes
Transferrin	77,000	Hepatocyte	2.3 (2.0–3.2)	8–9	Binds Fe^{2+} in plasma and transports to bone	Iron nutriture influences plasma level; increased during pregnancy, estrogen therapy, and acute hepatitis; reduced in protein-losing enteropathy and nephropathy, chronic infections, uremia, and acute catabolic states; often measured indirectly as total iron-binding capacity
Prealbumin	61,000	Hepatocyte	0.30 (0.2–0.5)	2–3	Binds T_3 and to a lesser extent T_4. Carrier for retinol-binding protein	Increased in patients with chronic renal failure on dialysis; reduced in acute catabolic states, after surgery, in hyperthyroidism; serum level determined by overall energy and nitrogen balance
Retinol-binding protein (RBP)	21,000	Hepatocyte	0.0372 ± 0.0073‡	0.5	Transports vitamin A in plasma; binds noncovalently to prealbumin	Catabolized in renal proximal tubular cell; with renal disease RBP increases and $t_{1/2}$ is prolonged; low in vitamin A deficiency, acute catabolic states, after surgery, and in hyperthyroidism

* Units are g/L. Normal range varies between centers; check local values.
† All of the listed proteins are influenced by hydration and the presence of hepatocellular dysfunction.
‡ Normal values are age- and sex-dependent. Table value is for pooled subjects.
SOURCE: Heymsfield and Williams.

in malnourished hospitalized patients, but a mixed form with features of both hypoproteinemic and combined PEM is more common. Such individuals have subnormal fat and somatic protein compartments, as indicated by anthropometric measurements, as well as depressed levels of the serum proteins and accompanying edema. The edema in hypoproteinemic PEM is usually dependent but may be generalized in severe cases. Pure hypoproteinemic PEM is often not recognized because fat and muscle wasting is less marked than that with combined PEM. This does not imply that this type of PEM is associated with less morbidity. Indeed, hospitalized patients with hypoproteinemic PEM may have a worse prognosis and a greater propensity for development of infections than those with combined PEM.

The liver in hypoproteinemic PEM may be enlarged and tender to palpation. Histologic examination reveals fatty infiltration; fat droplets initially appear in the periportal hepatocytes and, with increasing severity, spread to the pericentral regions of the hepatic lobule. The fatty liver is thought to be due to the inadequate movement of lipids out of the hepatic parenchyma caused by the decreased availability of lipoproteins for lipid transport (see Chap. 326). Serum concentrations of very low density lipoproteins (VLDL) and low density lipoproteins (LDL) are subnormal in hypoproteinemic PEM, and the severity of fatty infiltration of the liver correlates with the degree of depression of these lipoproteins.

Several factors influence whether a malnourished child develops a combined, hypoproteinemic, or mixed form of PEM. For example, infection in an undernourished child is more likely to precipitate hypoproteinemic than combined PEM. Individual host responses to the same type of nutritional deprivation may also play a role. Children with combined PEM have a more responsive adrenocortical axis than those with hypoproteinemic PEM, and this difference may maintain the visceral protein compartment at the expense of skeletal muscle.

PHYSIOLOGIC IMPAIRMENTS ASSOCIATED WITH PROTEIN-ENERGY MALNUTRITION Gastrointestinal tract The alterations in gastrointestinal structure and function arise partially from under-

nutrition itself and partially from decreased stimulation of the gut by ingested nutrients. Sustained absence of nutrients in the intestine of a nutritionally-replete, parenterally fed individual causes structural and functional atrophy of the intestine as described below. The changes have been best characterized in malnourished children in the less-developed countries, and similar alterations are presumed to occur in adult PEM. Blunting or absence of the intestinal villi is associated with decreased levels of disaccharidases and aminopeptidases in the mucosa. Gastric and pancreatic secretions are reduced in volume and contain decreased amounts of acid and digestive enzymes. The volume of bile and the concentration of conjugated bile acids in bile are reduced. Substantial populations of facultative and strict anaerobic bacteria in the upper small bowel convert conjugated bile acids to free bile acids. The impairments in pancreatic and biliary function, in conjunction with the structural alterations in the small intestine, result in malabsorption of carbohydrates, vitamins, and fat; the degree of steatorrhea is proportional to the severity of PEM. These alterations in absorption further exacerbate the inability to assimilate nutrients.

Immunologic function PEM impairs both cell-mediated and humoral immune systems. In vitro responses that assess the functional integrity of T lymphocytes, polymorphonuclear leukocytes, and the complement system are uniformly blunted. There is some disagreement as to whether B-lymphocyte function is impaired. A cycle is established in which malnutrition impairs host defenses and thereby enhances the susceptibility to infection, which, in turn, worsens the malnourished state. Additional PEM-associated phenomena, such as impaired epithelial integrity and decreased gastric acid and lysozyme secretion, may accelerate the propensity to infection and promote malnutrition by several mechanisms. These mechanisms include anorexia, which decreases the intake of nutrients; a shift in the balance of protein metabolism, which assumes a catabolic character and thereby promotes the loss of lean body mass; and enhancement of the metabolic rate, which increases about 13 percent for every 1°C elevation of body temperature. The macrophage-derived peptide interleukin 1 (IL-1) may play a role in these secondary effects. Proteolysis-inducing factor (PIF), a cleavage product of IL-1, is present in the blood of infected individuals and causes a marked increase in muscle proteolysis as indicated by increases in the rate of amino acid release from muscle. Cachectin (or tumor necrosis factor) also participates in mediating the effects of infection on host metabolism; it inhibits lipid metabolism and therefore inhibits the utilization of fat stores as an energy source.

Total lymphocyte count and measurements of delayed skin hypersensitivity, as well as some of the nutritional indexes that incorporate these items (see below), serve as reasonable predictors for susceptibility to postoperative infections and, in some cases, to postoperative mortality. Nevertheless, factors other than nutritional status also influence the assessment of lymphocytes (see Chap. 13).

Endocrine function   Most hormonal alterations in PEM appear to be the consequence of physiologic adaptations to the undernourished state. Inadequate food intake leads to a decrease in the availability of circulating glucose and amino acids, resulting in low circulating levels of insulin and increased levels of growth hormone and glucagon (see Chap. 320). These alterations, in conjunction with decreased levels of somatomedins and increased levels of glucocorticoids, promote muscle protein catabolism and enhance the incorporation of the liberated amino acids into visceral organs. Urea synthesis is inhibited, decreasing nitrogen loss and enhancing the reutilization of amino acids. Enhancement of lipolysis and gluconeogenesis provides more energy substrate.

The serum levels of triiodothyronine (T_3) and thyroxine (T_4) are commonly decreased in association with increased concentrations of 3,5,5'-triiodothyronine (reverse T_3), resembling the pattern observed in the "euthyroid sick syndrome" (see Chap. 316). The decrease in T_3 levels may play a role in the decrease in metabolic rate and decrease in protein catabolism in PEM. Primary gonadal dysfunction is accompanied by decreased concentrations of circulating testosterone and estrogen and impairment in reproductive potential. Amenorrhea is common. Impaired secretion of luteinizing hormone–releasing hormone (LHRH) may play a role in the hypogonadism. Fertility in women is further reduced by an increased rate of resorption of implanted embryos. In prepubertal children with PEM the basal level of follicle-stimulating hormone and the response of the gonadotropin to LHRH are variously reported to be low or normal. Delay of puberty appears to be related to failure to achieve a critical lean body mass rather than to a decrease in absolute weight.

Cardiovascular system   Moderate to severe PEM produces both quantitative and qualitative alterations in the myocardium. Myocardial mass is decreased, although proportionally less than the loss in body weight. Microscopic analysis reveals myofibrillar atrophy, edema, and, less commonly, patchy necrosis and infiltration with chronic inflammatory cells. Involvement of the myocardial conduction system may explain the conduction abnormalities associated with anorexia nervosa and total starvation. The structural changes in the myocardium are also associated with alterations in myocardial performance, most evident under conditions of increased demand as a decrease in cardiac output, stroke volume, and maximal work capacity. The alterations in cardiac structure and function are not irreversible: both left ventricular mass and maximal cardiac output increase after nutritional repletion.

Respiratory system   The mass of the diaphragm decreases in proportion to the loss in body weight. This atrophy results in decreases in the maximal inspiratory pressure. Energy deprivation, regardless of nitrogen balance, also blunts the ventilatory drive in response to hypoxia, although the clinical significance of this phenomenon is unclear. In tracheostomy patients, bacterial adherence to tracheal epithelial cells is enhanced. Nutritional repletion leads to reversal of impaired pulmonary function. Repletion associated with weight gain or an improved serum albumin level results in improved respiratory muscle function and a greater likelihood of weaning patients from ventilators.

Wound healing   Even mild malnutrition impairs the capacity to deposit collagen in wounds during the early stages of healing, and the provision of adequate nutrition after surgery enhances the deposition of collagen at the wound. Likewise, intestinal anastomoses in well-nourished animals have a higher tensile strength than those in malnourished animals. Nevertheless, those malnourished animals surviving for 8 weeks ultimately develop wounds with equivalent integrity to those of their well-nourished counterparts.

INFLUENCE OF MALNUTRITION ON HOSPITAL COURSE

The correlation between those parameters used to assess nutritional status and the outcome of hospitalization is clear-cut. For example, in hospitalized patients a depressed serum albumin or transferrin level, a recent unintentional weight loss of >10 percent of body weight, a decreased total lymphocyte count (<1200/μL) and an anergic skin response to foreign antigens are all predictive of an increased in-hospital incidence of morbid events such as infection. Moreover, some of these parameters are predictors of the duration of postoperative hospitalization as well as of mortality.

Several nutritional indexes, each of which incorporates various combinations of these measurements, have been developed to assess the nutritional status of hospitalized patients, as outlined in Table 71-7. However, every index for the clinical assessment of nutritional status and all indexes that integrate several of them into a single "nutritional score" are also influenced by nonnutritional factors. Consequently, such an index is more properly considered to be an assessment of the severity of illness and of the likelihood of malnutrition rather than to be an indicator of nutritional status alone. It therefore remains unclear whether the ability of these indexes to

TABLE 71-7   Prognostic indices in hospitalized patients

	Incorporated parameters	Correlates with	Reference
Likelihood of malnutrition	Serum folate Serum vitamin C Serum albumin Lymphocyte count Hematocrit Triceps skin fold Arm muscle circumference Weight	Duration of hospitalization	Am J Clin Nutr 32:418, 1979
Prognostic nutritional index	Serum albumin Serum transferrin Delayed hypersensitivity Triceps skin fold	Incidence of postoperative complications and mortality	Cancer 47:2375, 1981
Instant nutritional index	Serum albumin Lymphocyte count	Incidence of postoperative infection	J Parent Ent Nutr 12:195, 1988
Hospital prognostic index	Serum albumin Delayed hypersensitivity Presence of sepsis or cancer	Hospital mortality	Am J Clin Nutr 34:2013, 1981

predict morbidity and mortality is determined solely by nutritional state.

REFERENCES

ARONA NS, ROCHESTER DF: Effect of body weight and muscularity on human diaphragm muscle mass, thickness and area. J Appl Physiol 52:64, 1982

BARACOS V et al: Stimulation of degradation of muscle proteins during fever. A mechanism for the increased degradation of muscle proteins during fever. N Engl J Med 308:553, 1983

BECKER DJ: The endocrine responses to protein calorie malnutrition. Ann Rev Nutr 3:187, 1983

BEUTLER B, CERAMI A: Cachectin: More than a tumor necrosis factor. N Engl J Med 316:379, 1987

BISTRIAN BR et al: Protein status of general surgical patients. JAMA 230:858, 1974

BISTRIAN BR et al: Prevalence of malnutrition in general medical patients. JAMA 235:1567, 1976

CAHILL GF: Starvation in man. N Engl J Med 282:668, 1970

DINARELLO CA: Interleukin 1. Rev Infect Dis 6:51, 1984

HEYMSFIELD SB, WILLIAMS PJ: Nutritional assessment by clinical and biochemical methods, in Modern Nutrition in Health and Disease, 7th ed, ME Shils, VR Young (eds). Philadelphia, Lea & Febiger, 1988

HEYMSFIELD SB et al: Cardiac abnormalities in cachectic patients before and during nutritional repletion. Am Heart J 95:584, 1978

KEUSCH GT, FARTHING MJG: Nutrition and infection. Ann Rev Nutr 6:131, 1986

ROSENBLATT S et al: Exchange of amino acids by muscle and liver in sepsis. Arch Surg 118:167, 1983

TEN-STATE NUTRITION SURVEY, 1968-70. US Department of Health, Education, and Welfare Publication (HSM) 72, 1972

WEINSIER RL et al: A prospective evaluation of general medical patients during the course of hospitalization. Am J Clin Nutr 32:418, 1979

WORLD HEALTH ORGANIZATION: Infant and Young Child Nutrition. Report by the Director General to the World Health Assembly. Document WHA 36/1983/70, March, 1983

72 OBESITY

JERROLD M. OLEFSKY

The ability to store food energy as fat provides survival value when the food supply is scarce or sporadic. Unlike glycogen or protein, triglyceride does not require water or electrolytes for storage purposes and can be retained essentially as pure fat; 1 g adipose tissue yields close to the full theoretical equivalent of 38 kJ (9 kcal). Because of the efficient storage of energy in adipose tissue, an individual of normal weight can survive up to 2 months of total starvation. However, western society is generally not characterized by periodic or insufficient food supply but rather by constant and abundant food. As a consequence, the ability to store fat all too frequently is of negative survival value because of overconsumption and the resulting obesity.

DEFINITION AND INCIDENCE Obesity can most easily be assessed in terms of height and weight. One way is to relate weight to an average range for height and age. This measure of relative weight can lead to an underestimation of the incidence of obesity, since in the United States the "average" individual is somewhat obese. Tables of ideal and desirable weight are based on actuarial estimates of what is consistent with longest life expectancy. Such tables are more useful if adjusted for differences in body build. An alternative method of estimating obesity is the body mass index or BMI [body weight (in kilograms) divided by height (in meters)²]. For adults ages 20 to 29, the 85th percentile for BMI is 27.8 for males and 27.3 for females. Although relative weight and BMI correlate with the degree of adiposity, excess poundage can be either lean or fat tissue. For example, heavily muscled individuals would be considered obese using these measurements. Nevertheless, such assessments correlate fairly well with the risk of adverse effects on health and longevity. More precise assessment of obesity can be made with measurements of body density or with isotopic dilution methods, but these are unsuitable for routine use. Alternatively anthropometry can be utilized for assessing the degree of adiposity. Assessment of skin-fold thickness over various areas of the body together with height, weight, and age can be used to assess the degree of adiposity. Triceps and subscapular skin folds are most commonly employed (see Chap. 71). From a health standpoint, certain patterns of obesity may be less desirable than others. Fat deposition about the waist and flank, as evidenced by a high ratio of waist to hip circumference, is associated with a greater health risk than fat deposition at the hips.

The term obesity implies an excess of adipose tissue, but the meaning of excess is hard to define. Aesthetic considerations aside, obesity can best be viewed as any degree of excess adiposity that imparts a health risk. This cutoff between normal and obese can only be approximated, and the health risk imparted by obesity is probably a continuum with increasing adiposity. The Framingham Study demonstrated that a 20 percent excess over desirable weight clearly imparted a health risk. A National Institutes of Health consensus panel on obesity agreed with this definition and concluded that a 20 percent increase in relative weight or a BMI above the 85th percentile for young adults constitutes a health risk; by use of these criteria 20 to 30 percent of adult men and 30 to 40 percent of adult women are obese, with the highest rates among the poor and minority groups. Significant health risks at lower levels of obesity can occur in the presence of diabetes, hypertension, heart disease, or other associated risk factors.

The Surgeon General's 1988 Report on obesity notes that even mild obesity increases the risk for premature death, diabetes, hypertension, atherosclerosis, gallbladder disease, and certain types of cancer. In the United States the prevalence of obesity has increased in the past few decades. Because of the high prevalence of obesity and its health consequences, its prevention and treatment should be a high public health priority.

ETIOLOGY When energy intake exceeds expenditure, the excess calories are stored in adipose tissue, and if this net positive balance is prolonged, obesity results, i.e., there are two components to weight balance, and an abnormality on either side (intake or expenditure) can lead to obesity.

The regulation of eating behavior is incompletely understood. To some extent, appetite is controlled by discrete areas in the hypothalamus: a feeding center in the ventrolateral nucleus of the hypothalamus (VLH) and a satiety center in the ventromedial hypothalamus (VMH). The cerebral cortex receives positive signals from the feeding center that stimulate eating (Fig. 72-1), and the satiety center modulates this process by sending inhibitory impulses to the feeding center. In animals destruction of the feeding center results in decreased food intake, and destruction of the satiety center leads to overeating and obesity. Several regulatory processes may influence these hypothalamic centers. The satiety center may be activated by the increases in plasma glucose and/or insulin that follow a meal. It is of interest in this regard that the VMH contains insulin receptors and is insulin-sensitive. Meal-induced gastric distention is another possible inhibitory factor. The total adipose tissue mass may also influence the activity of the hypothalamic centers; i.e., there is a relatively fixed "set point" for body adiposity. An elevated set point may account for the frequent recidivism in obese patients who have lost weight. How the "set point" is established and how the hypothalamus senses total fat stores are unknown. Glycerol release from fat cells, ascending neural impulses, and/or circulation of adipocyte-derived peptides such as adipsin may be signals of adipose tissue size. Additionally, the hypothalamic centers are sensitive to catecholamines, and beta-adrenergic stimulation inhibits eating behavior. This provides at least one rationale for the anorexiant effects of amphetamines.

Ultimately, the cerebral cortex controls eating behavior, and impulses from the feeding center to the cerebral cortex are only one input. Psychological, social, and genetic factors also influence food intake. In many obese subjects these influences are overriding; indeed, obese subjects usually respond to external signals such as time of day, social setting, and smell or taste of food to a greater extent than do persons of normal weight.

Eating Behavior

Cortex ← Social, Cultural, Genetic Influence

(+)

Feeding Center VLH ← "Set Point" or Adipostat Based On Body Fat Mass

(−)

Satiety Center VMH

↑ Gastric Distention   ↑ Plasma Glucose and Insulin   ↑ Adrenergic Influences

FIGURE 72-1 The regulation of eating. The ventromedial satiety center is considered to be inhibitory, and the ventrolateral feeding center stimulatory. See text for discussion.

Although overeating is the usual cause of obesity, other factors may participate. Daily caloric needs normally range between 110 to 130 kJ (27 to 32 kcal) per kilogram of body weight; this figure is higher in active and lower in sedentary individuals. Physical activity clearly modulates overall caloric balance, and obese individuals tend to be less active. This can be a contributory factor in the maintenance of excess weight, but decreased physical activity is unlikely to be an important cause of major weight gain in most obese subjects. Rather, obesity leads to inactivity. The modest increase in weight that often accompanies the middle years may be related more directly to diminished physical activity. Injury or illness may lead to chronic restricted activity and predispose to weight gain unless caloric intake is appropriately curtailed. Perhaps the greatest factor tending to diminish the output side of the equation is simply a sedentary lifestyle.

Decreased caloric expenditure and a metabolic abnormality associated with overefficient caloric utilization have also been postulated as involved in the pathogenesis of obesity. With rare exceptions major metabolic abnormalities have not been detected in obese individuals, although subtle defects may be undetected. There are three major components to overall energy expenditure: resting metabolic rate, exercise-induced thermogenesis, and the thermic response to food.

The resting metabolic rate accounts for 60 to 75 percent of daily energy expenditure and is measured in a thermoneutral environment while the subject is at rest following an overnight fast and several hours after any significant physical activity. An average resting metabolic rate in a 70-kg man is 6300 kJ (1500 kcal)/d. The resting metabolic rate should be expressed as a function of fat-free body weight (by subtracting the subject's total adipose mass from body weight), since triglyceride mass is metabolically inert in that negligible energy is expended to maintain triglyceride depots. When expressed in this way, the resting metabolic rate is normal in most obese subjects. However, a distinction must be made between static obesity and the actual process of gaining weight. When normal subjects consume hypercaloric diets, less weight is gained than would be predicted on the basis of the excess calories ingested. This effect is most marked when carbohydrate is consumed and disappears when the excess calories consist of fat. Thus, humans can apparently partially adapt to chronic excessive carbohydrate and protein intake,

and this protective effect attenuates the weight gain. Part of this adaptive response is related to an increase in thermogenesis manifested as an increase in the resting metabolic rate. The mechanism of adaptive thermogenesis is unknown, but overeating of carbohydrate or mixed nutrients leads to increased plasma levels of triiodothyronine (T_3) and decreased levels of reverse T_3 (rT_3). A converse effect is seen in starvation with decreased T_3 and increased rT_3 levels. The conversion of thyroxine to T_3 occurs largely in the liver; excess food may induce adaptive thermogenesis by increasing the concentration of T_3 relative to that of T_4 and rT_3. Increased central or peripheral sympathetic outflow leading to increased catecholamine-induced caloric utilization and increased heat production may also play a role in the thermogenic response to overnutrition. Adaptive thermogenesis can lead to a 10- to 15-percent increase in resting metabolic rate, and this effect is seen after a 2- to 3-week period of hypercaloric intake. The rate of onset and the degree of adaptive thermogenesis is the same in obese and nonobese individuals when expressed on the basis of fat-free body mass. Specifically, the increase in resting metabolic rate, changes in thyroid hormone metabolism, and thermic responses to infused catecholamines are similar in normal and obese subjects during periods of overnutrition.

Work performance, or energy expenditure per standard physical work load, can be normal or increased in obesity depending on the kind of work performed. The energy expenditure of exercise is increased in obese compared to lean subjects due to the extra effort involved in moving or supporting an increased body mass. When this effect of increased body mass is taken into account, work performance is normal in obesity. Clearly, normal or increased energy expenditure during physical work cannot contribute to the development of obesity. On the other hand, the total daily energy expenditure due to exercise is less in many sedentary obese subjects simply because they engage in less daily physical activity than their lean counterparts.

The third important aspect of caloric balance is the thermic response to food, so-called dietary thermogenesis. This consists of the heat, or energy, expended above the resting metabolic rate for several hours after the ingestion of a meal. About 75 percent of the thermic response to food is due to the energy cost of digestion, absorption, metabolism, and storage of foodstuffs; the remainder is probably due to activation of the sympathetic nervous system. The heat produced following nutrient ingestion is a form of caloric expenditure and is greater for protein and less for carbohydrate and fat. The thermic response to mixed meals can equal 10 to 15 percent of the calories ingested, and decreased thermic responses have been described in some studies of human obesity. This difference may be due to altered flux rates through different pathways of intermediary metabolism, with more energy-efficient pathways being favored in obesity. As an example, the higher the rate of glucose utilization, the greater the thermic response to carbohydrate-containing meals, and small decreases in the thermic response to food may be due to insulin resistance and decreased glucose disposal in obese subjects. It is clear that small differences in caloric utilization maintained over years can lead to a significant net positive caloric balance. However, while it is tempting to postulate that this decreased thermic response may contribute to obesity, most of the published comparisons have been made between normal persons and subjects who are already obese. Thus, the obesity-associated changes in thermic response to food may be secondary to the obese state rather than a primary abnormality. More importantly, differences in the thermic response to meals between the obese and nonobese are at most in the range of 125 to 210 kJ (30 to 50 kcal)/d. Such minor differences can easily be counterbalanced by minor decreases in food intake and/or increases in exercise-induced thermogenesis. Since such compensation does not occur, it seems more probable that obesity is the result of impaired coupling between caloric intake and expenditure.

Another potential regulatory process in the control of adipose tissue mass involves adipose tissue lipoprotein lipase (ATLPL). This enzyme is synthesized within adipocytes, secreted into the extracellular space, and attached to the luminal surface of nearby endothelial cells.

At this location ATLPL hydrolyzes fatty acids from the triglycerides of circulating triglyceride-rich lipoproteins. The released fatty acids are taken up by adipocytes, converted to triglycerides, and stored. Thus, ATLPL participates in the storage of excess fat calories in adipose tissue. The *lipoprotein lipase hypothesis* holds that in some obese states excessive levels of this enzyme induce obesity by causing preferential deposition of fat calories in adipose tissue. In support of this hypothesis, ATLPL levels are increased in obese rodents and humans. More importantly, levels of this enzyme do not return to normal following weight reduction. This latter finding is of particular interest since it is one of the few characteristics of the obese state that is not corrected by weight reduction and could explain the propensity of obese patients to regain lost weight.

Environmental, cultural, and genetic influences all contribute to obesity, and in population studies it is impossible to quantitate the separate impact of these factors. Nevertheless, the importance of genetics has been demonstrated in studies of twins and adopted siblings. The BMI of adopted individuals correlates better with that of the biologic rather than the adoptive parents. Among biologic and adoptive siblings, the amount and distribution of fat is associated with a genetic relationship, and similarities are not as close among adopted siblings. Most likely, both nature and nurture contribute to the etiology of obesity.

SECONDARY OBESITY Hypothyroidism Obesity can result from hypothyroidism because of decreased caloric needs. However, only a minority of hypothyroid patients are truly obese, and an even smaller proportion of obese patients are hypothyroid. Indiscriminate use of thyroid hormone in the treatment of obesity is to be deplored and should never be instituted in the absence of documentation of decreased thyroid function.

Cushing's disease Cushing's disease is a rare cause of obesity. Hyperadrenocorticism elicits a typical pattern of obesity with predominantly centripetal fat stores, characteristic rounded or moon facies, and cervical or supraclavicular fat deposits.

Insulinoma Hyperinsulinemia, secondary to an insulinoma, can occasionally cause obesity, presumably because of increased caloric intake secondary to recurrent hypoglycemia. Most patients with islet cell tumors and hypoglycemia are not obese.

Hypothalamic disorders Froehlich's syndrome in boys is characterized by obesity and hypogonadotrophic hypogonadism with other variable features such as diabetes insipidus, visual impairment, and mental retardation. The anterior pituitary is usually normal, and the syndrome is thought to be the result of hypothalamic dysfunction. This syndrome likely includes a number of overlapping disorders having in common a hypothalamic lesion that leads to overeating and to hypogonadotrophism. Occasionally pituitary tumors are present (as in Froehlich's original case) that may physically impair the hypothalamus.

Other rare causes of obesity include the Laurence-Moon-Biedl syndrome, characterized by retinitis pigmentosa, mental retardation, skull deformities, polydactyly and syndactyly, and the Prader-Willi syndrome, which is associated with hypotonia, mental retardation, and a predilection for diabetes mellitus. Both of these disorders also feature obesity and hypogonadism that are thought to be hypothalamic in origin.

PATHOLOGIC SEQUELAE Increased adipose tissue stores are deposited subcutaneously, around all internal organs, throughout the omentum, and in the intramuscular spaces. Obese individuals also have an expansion of lean body mass as evidenced by increased size of the kidneys, heart, liver, and skeletal muscle mass. Fatty livers are common in extreme obesity.

Adipocyte size and number Attempts have been made to classify obese individuals on the basis of the relative degree of adipocyte hypertrophy versus hyperplasia. This classification scheme was generated as the result of experimental data indicating that in several rodent species and in humans the capacity to increase adipocyte number exists for only a limited period in early life and perhaps at the time of puberty. Thus, prior to reaching adulthood the ability to increase the number of adipocytes declines, and after this time expansion of adipose tissue mass is accompanied primarily by an increase in fat-cell size. Individuals with severe obesity have both increased adipocyte size and number, and those with the greatest degree of adipocyte hyperplasia have a strong tendency toward onset of obesity early in life. Patients having mild to moderate obesity show predominantly adipocyte hypertrophy, and the onset is usually during adult life. Weight reduction leads to a decrease in adipocyte size with no change in cell number. The above observations led to the concept of the existence of a "critical period" in early life when final adipocyte number is determined and after which cell number cannot be changed. This formulation implies that alterations in adipocyte number can only be induced during this critical period. However, the concept of a strictly defined critical period for hyperplasia of the adipocytes is only partially correct. When severe obesity is induced in adult rats, both adipocyte number and cell size increase. Adipocyte hypercellularity also occurs in some patients with adult-onset obesity.

Thus while substantial overnutrition at any stage of life can lead to hypertrophy of individual existing adipocytes, there are periods during childhood and adolescence when overnutrition has an enhanced ability to induce the development of new adipocytes. Furthermore, even in adult life, if the degree of overnutrition is sufficient to induce existing adipocytes to enlarge to some limiting size, then new adipocytes will form. Whether this latter population of cells represents new cell formation or simply the filling with lipid of previously undetectable preadipocytes formed earlier in life is not known. Regardless of the cause or time of development of increased adiposity (adipocyte hypertrophy with or without hyperplasia), subsequent weight reduction only leads to a decrease in the size of existing adipocytes and not a decrease in adipocyte number. Thus, once a given complement of adipocytes is attained, this number is fixed and cannot be reduced.

METABOLIC SEQUELAE Obesity has a profound impact on diabetes mellitus and on various hyperlipoproteinemic states primarily through its influences on insulin secretion and insulin sensitivity.

Hyperinsulinemia: Insulin resistance Increased insulin secretion is a common feature of obesity. It occurs in the basal state and in response to a wide variety of insulinogenic agents. A correlation exists between the degree of obesity and the magnitude of the hyperinsulinemia—particularly the basal insulin levels. Some obese patients exhibit hyperglycemia or frank diabetes in the face of hyperinsulinemia. The combination of hyper- or euglycemia and hyperinsulinemia indicates an insulin-resistant state, and decreased hypoglycemic responses to insulin are common in obese humans and animals. Insulin resistance could be due to an abnormal beta-cell product, circulating insulin antagonists, or tissue insulin insensitivity. Since abnormal islet secretory products or circulating antagonists have not been identified, it is thought that the insulin resistance of obesity is primarily due to tissue insensitivity. The initial step in the cellular action of insulin involves binding to cell surface receptors in target tissues. Cells from obese animals and humans contain decreased numbers of insulin receptors, and this decrease doubtless plays a role in the insulin resistance. However, other factors participate. The enlarged adipocytes of obese rats have both a decrease in insulin receptors and an even greater defect in the capacity to metabolize glucose, suggesting a major biochemical abnormality distal to the receptor mechanism. A similar postreceptor defect presumably exists in other insulin target tissues such as muscle and liver. In the obese human insulin resistance is due to a combination of receptor and postreceptor defects in insulin action. In those obese patients with the mildest degree of hyperinsulinemia and insulin resistance, the decrease in insulin action is predominantly due to a decreased number of insulin receptors. As the insulin-resistant state worsens, a postreceptor defect emerges, and in obese subjects with the most severe degree of insulin resistance, the postreceptor defect is the predominant abnormality.

Diabetes mellitus (See also Chap. 319)   Although only a minority of obese patients are diabetic, the converse is not the case. Non-insulin-dependent, or type II, diabetes comprises about 90 percent of the diabetic population in the United States, and 80 to 90 percent of type II diabetics are obese. Obesity is an important contributory factor to the diabetes in these patients, predominantly through its influences on insulin resistance. Obesity exacerbates the diabetic state, and in many cases diabetes can be ameliorated by weight reduction.

Hyperlipoproteinemia (See also Chap. 326)   Most plasma cholesterol circulates in the low-density lipoprotein (LDL) fraction, and, in the fasting state, very low density lipoproteins (VLDL) contain most of the circulating triglyceride. The association between obesity and elevated LDL levels is modest at best, especially when the relationship is corrected for factors such as age. Total-body cholesterol is increased in obesity, but this is mainly accounted for by adipose tissue cholesterol stores. Cholesterol turnover may be increased, leading to increased biliary excretion of cholesterol. This may contribute to the increased incidence of gallstone formation. Obesity has a more pronounced effect on VLDL metabolism. Hypertriglyceridemia is frequent, and the degree of obesity correlates with the level of hypertriglyceridemia. The increased triglyceride levels are due to increased hepatic VLDL production with no defect in the removal of VLDL from plasma. As discussed above, plasma insulin levels are elevated, particularly in the portal venous blood. Hyperinsulinemia can promote increased hepatic VLDL synthesis and secretion. In addition, increased plasma free fatty acid (FFA) turnover exists in obesity, and FFA extraction by the liver provides an important precursor for hepatic triglyceride synthesis. Thus, the hypertriglyceridemia in obesity may be secondary to increased hepatic VLDL secretion due to hyperinsulinemia and augmented FFA availability.

MANIFESTATIONS AND COMPLICATIONS   Gross obesity produces mechanical and physical stresses that aggravate or cause a number of disorders including osteoarthritis (especially of the hips) and sciatica. Varicose veins, thromboembolism, ventral and hiatal hernias, and cholelithiasis are also more common.

Hypertension   In significantly obese persons, use of the standard size blood pressure cuff leads to erroneously high readings; an oversize cuff should always be used. A strong association between hypertension and obesity is observed even when accurate measurements are obtained. The mechanism by which obesity causes hypertension is uncertain, but peripheral vascular resistance is usually normal while blood volume is increased. Weight loss leads to reductions in systemic blood pressure independent of changes in sodium balance.

Hypoventilation syndrome (Pickwickian syndrome)   The obesity-hypoventilation syndrome is a heterogeneous group of disorders with differing clinical manifestations. The hypersomnolence that can occur in obesity is a manifestation of nighttime sleep apnea. In these individuals, once sleep begins, upper airway obstruction leads to hypoxemia and hypercapnia, causing arousal with return of normal respiration. Many such episodes occur each night, leading to chronic sleep deprivation and daytime somnolence. The combination of the obese habitus plus sleep-induced relaxation of the pharyngeal musculature is believed to be the cause of the intermittent upper airway obstruction. Occasionally such episodes are life-threatening (causing serious cardiac arrhythmias) and require long-term tracheostomy therapy. Chronic daytime hypoventilation is usually not as severe as that occurring during sleep and may be due to abnormalities of the respiratory control centers. Patients with hypoventilation display blunted ventilatory responses to hypercapnia and hypoxia and often develop hypercapnia and hypoxemia due to decreased basal ventilation; in addition, ventilation-perfusion mismatch may result from mechanical factors. In severe cases polycythemia, pulmonary hypertension, and cor pulmonale can result. Weight reduction will reverse these abnormalities if instituted before permanent cardiac damage develops. Some obese patients with sleep apnea and hypersomnolence

do not have daytime hypoventilation and have normal ventilatory responses to hypoxia and hypercapnia. Progestational agents have been used therapeutically in the obesity-hypoventilation syndrome since they stimulate the ventilatory response to hypercapnia and hypoxia in normal subjects. Medroxyprogesterone increases ventilation and improves heart failure and erythrocytosis in these patients, although obstructive sleep apnea continues.

Adrenal function   Although Cushing's disease can usually be distinguished from simple obesity on clinical grounds, laboratory testing is occasionally necessary. This can lead to confusion since 24-h urinary 17-hydroxycorticoid excretion is often elevated in obesity. Less commonly, plasma cortisol levels are also increased. Corticosteroid levels are usually suppressible with dexamethasone in obesity, but occasionally suppression is incomplete, rendering the diagnosis difficult (also see Chap. 317).

Growth hormone   Secretory responses of growth hormone to a variety of stimuli such as hypoglycemia, exercise, and arginine infusion are reduced, and the starvation-induced rise in plasma growth hormone levels is attenuated.

Atherosclerosis   Obesity is a risk factor for the development of coronary artery disease and stroke. Most of the risk is mediated through the associated hypertension, hyperlipoproteinemia, and diabetes. Nevertheless, even when these abnormalities are factored out, an additional, smaller risk can be ascribed to obesity per se.

TREATMENT   Amelioration of hyperinsulinemia, insulin resistance, diabetes, hypertension, and hyperlipidemia can occur following weight loss. These changes are significant and enduring provided the weight loss is maintained. During weight loss all adipose tissue depots diminish proportionately. Sometimes generalized loss does not produce the attractive cosmetic effects desired. Many techniques have been proposed to effect selective adipose tissue reduction over particular regions of the body, but none is effective.

Methods of weight reduction   In instances where obesity is secondary, the appropriate therapy is to treat the underlying disease. Most of the time the difficult problem of primary weight reduction must be undertaken.

Diet   Caloric restriction is the cornerstone of weight reduction. From the standpoint of patient and physician this is a frustrating and demanding undertaking. The basic principles are simple. If food intake is less than energy expenditure, stored calories, predominantly in the form of fat, will be consumed. In general, a deficit of 32,000 kJ (7700 kcal) leads to loss of about 1 kg fat. By estimating the patient's daily caloric needs [approximately 125 to 150 kJ (30 to 35 kcal) per kilogram of body weight], one can calculate the daily deficit necessary to achieve a given rate of weight loss.

Dietary restriction can range from total starvation to mild caloric deprivation, and these approaches will be discussed separately. Dietary recommendations are most effective when they are specific and geared to the patient's life-style. A dietitian or a similarly trained health professional should interview each patient and estimate average daily caloric intake, identify food preferences, and characterize the eating patterns. The amount of calories to be consumed on the restricted diet should be carefully explained in terms of quantities of specific foodstuffs. Frequently, the therapist must balance the degree of restriction against potential noncompliance. The more restrictive the diet, the more rapid the weight loss, but this often leads to a greater rate of nonadherence. It is preferable to design a diet with which the patient is comfortable and that produces a modest but steady weight loss.

Schemes for weight reduction have become a profitable business in the United States, and there are almost as many diets as there are therapists. Each proponent claims that the presence or absence of certain foodstuffs is desirable for more effective weight loss. However, little evidence exists to support the claim that calorie for calorie one hypocaloric diet will lead to a greater weight loss than another. The relationship between the patient and the therapist, plus patient education and encouragement, are more important to success than are the specific dietary constituents. The major virtue of "fad" diets is that patients are usually motivated to try them, at least initially, and patient cooperation is often better. Provided a particular diet is not harmful, probably the best course for the therapist is to maintain flexibility in the treatment program. Nevertheless, diets markedly deficient in any major class of foodstuff are to be avoided. For example, whole-food diets that are exceedingly low in carbohydrate are by nature high in fat and, depending on the type and quantity of fat ingested, may lead to hypercholesterolemia. The major virtue of a low-carbohydrate diet is the attendant ketosis (ketone bodies have a central anorexiant effect). This provided part of the rationale for the widely touted liquid or powdered protein diets that were previously popular. These diets have been dubbed "protein-sparing modified fasts," and claims were made that they allowed drastic long-term caloric restriction without inducing negative nitrogen balance. These claims have not been substantiated, nor has it been shown that the diets lead to a greater degree of fat tissue weight loss than mixed diets of equal caloric value. Basically a calorie is a calorie whether it comes from protein, carbohydrate, or fat. Furthermore, deaths have been reported in otherwise healthy individuals participating in such long-term dietary programs, even under medical supervision. This has been attributed to the fact that some of these diets contain mostly collagen-derived protein of low biologic value. Other very low calorie diets involve formula preparations containing 500 to 800 kcal/d, with 50 to 80 g of high-quality protein. The remaining calories consist of carbohydrate and fat. Vitamin and micronutrient supplements are incorporated in the formula or provided as an added supplement. Such high-quality low-calorie diet formulas lead to relatively rapid weight loss but should not be taken continuously as the sole caloric source for more than 6 weeks. In the absence of coexisting diseases such as gout, renal insufficiency, cardiac arrhythmias, etc., such diets are safe when taken under medical supervision. Such very low calorie diets are contraindicated in pregnant women and growing children.

Prior to therapy it is wise to warn patients that when caloric restriction is started, there is usually a marked initial weight loss, in large part due to fluid loss, but such rapid rates of loss will not persist. Likewise, positive shifts in fluid balance can sometimes mask loss of adipose mass, a fact that can sometimes be demonstrated to the patient's satisfaction by recording skin-fold thickness at periodic intervals.

Total-starvation diets have been advocated for the treatment of obesity; provided gout, renal insufficiency, and ketosis-prone diabetes are not present, short-term (2- to 3-day) fasts are usually well tolerated. Ketonemia and hyperuricemia regularly develop during starvation but rarely lead to acidosis or gout. Because of these potential complications, total fasting should be carried out only under medical supervision. Probably the major usefulness of total fasting is as a motivational aid at the beginning of a dietary program or when weight loss has stopped. Even though much of the weight loss during short-term fasting represents fluid, this weight loss can be encouraging to frustrated patients and motivate them to improve compliance with the long-term weight reduction program.

The major problem in the treatment of obesity is not weight reduction but maintenance of the reduced weight. Provided the therapist works hard and long enough, most motivated patients can eventually lose weight. Unfortunately, only the rare patient maintains the weight loss permanently. Obesity is an eating disorder, and the underlying mechanisms are not reversed by limiting food intake.

Behavior modification In recognition of the problems involved, the techniques of behavior modification have been devised to treat abnormal patterns of eating behavior. Many studies demonstrate that obese individuals respond less well than normal individuals to internal cues that regulate eating behavior such as gastric contractions, fear, and previous food ingestion. Conversely, obese subjects overrespond to external cues such as taste, smell, food attractiveness, food abundance, and the ease of obtaining food. Given the fact that the obese individual is unusually susceptible to external stimuli, food intake may be altered by changing the pattern and nature of these external cues, and this is the major premise underlying the behavior modification approach to weight reduction.

Behavior modification begins with a detailed individual history of the patient's eating patterns with respect to time of day, length of eating period, place of ingestion (restaurant, dining table, standing in front of open refrigerator), simultaneous activities (watching television, reading, idleness), emotional state, companions (relatives, friends, or alone), and finally the kinds and quantities of foods ingested. Once this detailed record is obtained, the therapist and patient can design specific behavioral changes aimed at disrupting or aborting recurring behavior patterns which initiate or prolong abnormal eating activity. As examples: if a patient eats in response to certain emotional states, then other activities can be substituted when the patient perceives such a state; if the patient snacks frequently from readily available food storage areas (refrigerators, cookie jars, etc.), then he or she is encouraged to eat only while sitting down at a table with a fixed place setting; if eating frequently occurs while watching television alone, then efforts to avoid this activity can be initiated. Many other examples of specific and general interventions could be given. Results with behavior modification techniques indicate that many patients can maintain long-term weight reduction providing the new behavior patterns are truly "learned."

Exercise Exercise has a place in any weight reduction program. However, the importance of exercise in terms of caloric balance must be clearly understood. Even moderate daily exercise would not lead to a large enough increase in energy expenditure to alter significantly the initial rate of weight reduction (Table 72-1). This does not mean exercise is unimportant in weight reduction, since even modest increases in caloric expenditure can lead to large long-term differences in caloric balance, provided exercise is performed on a regular basis. For example, a daily increase in caloric expenditure of 1250 kJ (300 kcal) over a period of 4 months could lead to a 4.5-kg weight loss. More importantly, incorporation of regular exercise into the overall weight reduction program improves the chances that the patient will maintain the weight loss.

Drugs Two classes of drugs are frequently used in the treatment of obesity: anorexiants and thyroid hormone supplements. The addition of levothyroxine or triiodothyronine to a weight reduction program is ineffective in promoting adipose tissue loss and, if anything, accentuates lean tissue loss and causes negative nitrogen balance. In susceptible individuals, cardiotoxicity may occur. Thus, unless clear-cut hypothyroidism is present, thyroid supplementation has no role in the treatment of obesity.

The major anorexiants are amphetamine-like agents that presumably exert their effect at the level of the hypothalamus. They probably have a modest effect in promoting short-term weight loss in some individuals. However, they are effective only for short periods, and problems of habituation, addiction, and drug abuse limit their usefulness. Two anorexiants, diethylpropion and fenfluramine, may be less addictive and, therefore, somewhat more useful. However, none of these agents treats the underlying eating disorder, and they are of little use in maintenance of weight reduction.

Injections of human chorionic gonadotropin (hCG) have been tried as an adjunct to weight reduction, but no evidence exists to indicate a beneficial effect. The primary effectiveness of the hCG-diet program is due to the calorically restricted diet, frequent physician contact, and placebo effects. Comparable weight loss is achieved if saline injections are substituted for hCG, suggesting a placebo or physiologic effect of the act of parenteral injection.

Jejunoileal shunt Small-bowel bypass is an effective means of achieving weight reduction in morbidly obese patients. However, it is an experimental procedure and should be attempted only in institutions where a trained team is committed to regular, systematic, and long-term follow-up. Because of accompanying morbidity and mortality most such institutions have abandoned this form of surgery in favor of the more benign and effective gastric plication or bypass approach described below.

The most common operative procedures for the jejunoileal shunt

TABLE 72-1   Energy equivalents of food calories expressed in minutes of activity

Food	Energy value, kJ (kcal)	Activity Walking*	Riding bicycle†	Swimming‡	Running§	Reclining¶
Apple, large	422 (101)	19	12	9	5	78
Bacon, 2 strips	401 (96)	18	12	9	5	74
Beer, 1 glass	477 (114)	22	14	10	6	88
Bread and butter	326 (78)	15	10	7	4	60
Carbonated beverage, 1 glass	444 (106)	20	13	9	5	82
Carrot, raw	176 (42)	8	5	4	2	32
Cheese, cottage, 1 tbsp	113 (27)	5	3	2	1	21
Chicken, fried, ½ breast	971 (232)	45	28	21	12	178
Cookie, chocolate chip	213 (51)	10	6	5	3	39
Egg, fried	460 (110)	21	13	10	6	85
Ham, 2 slices	699 (167)	32	20	15	9	128
Ice cream, ⅙ qt	808 (193)	37	24	17	10	148
Mayonnaise, 1 tbsp	385 (92)	18	11	8	5	71
Milk, skim, 1 glass	339 (81)	16	10	7	4	62
Milk shake	1762 (421)	81	51	38	22	324
Orange, medium	285 (68)	13	8	6	4	52
Pancake with syrup	519 (124)	24	15	11	6	95
Peas, green, ½ cup	234 (56)	11	7	5	3	43
Pizza, cheese, ¼	753 (180)	35	22	16	9	138
Potato chips, 1 serving	462 (108)	21	13	10	6	83
Sandwiches:						
Hamburger	1456 (350)	67	43	31	18	269
Tuna fish salad	1163 (278)	53	34	25	14	214
Sherbet, ⅙ qt	741 (177)	34	22	16	9	136

* Energy cost of walking for 70-kg individual = 22 kJ (5.2 kcal)/min.
† Energy cost of riding bicycle = 34 kJ (8.2 kcal)/min.
‡ Energy cost of swimming = 47 kJ (11.2 kcal)/min.
§ Energy cost of running = 81 kJ (19.4 kcal)/min.
¶ Energy cost of reclining = 5 kJ (1.3 kcal)/min.

involve end-to-end or end-to-side anastomosis of about 38 cm of proximal jejunum to 10 cm of terminal ileum. Weight loss is initially rapid, reaching a plateau at 18 to 24 months. While all patients lose weight, few return to ideal weight. The mean weight loss is about 30 to 50 percent of initial excess weight, leaving patients still about 50 percent overweight once a steady state is reached. Although some degree of malabsorption occurs, the major portion of the weight loss is due to decreased food intake.

Teams still performing this surgery select patients who are at least 50 kg overweight and in whom adequate attempts at medical management have failed repeatedly. Because of postoperative morbidity, older patients (>50 years) and psychologically unstable individuals are usually excluded.

The overall surgical mortality ranges from 0.5 to 7.8 percent with an average of around 4 percent. Mortality is inversely related to the experience of the surgical team. The major postoperative morbidity is related to wound infection and thromboembolism. The common serious medical complications are cirrhosis and hepatic failure, nephrolithiasis, electrolyte imbalances, cholelithiasis, and arthritis (Table 72-2). Severe liver disease probably occurs in 5 percent of patients, and milder degrees of hepatic dysfunction are more common. The long-range implications of mild hepatic abnormalities are unknown. Possible causes of liver damage following small-bowel bypass include (1) protein and particularly essential amino acid deficiency, (2) accumulation of hepatotoxic, secondary bile salts, and (3) release of unknown toxic substances from the excluded bowel. Hypokalemia is most likely secondary to diarrhea. Persistent deficiency of calcium and magnesium can result from malabsorption and must be treated with appropriate replacement. Transient depression of plasma 25-hydroxyvitamin D levels may also contribute to abnormal mineral metabolism. Nephrolithiasis occurs in up to 30 percent of patients and is due to hyperoxaluria secondary to calcium malabsorption. It can be treated by calcium supplements and a low oxalate intake. Migratory polyarthritis occurs in up to 6 percent of patients and may be due to circulating immune complexes. This operation is now rarely performed, in part due to the decision of many insurance companies not to render compensation for this procedure.

Gastric surgery   Gastroplasty establishes a small upper gastric remnant connected to a larger lower gastric pouch by a narrow 1- to 1.5-cm channel. Gastric bypass excludes the lower 90 percent of the stomach pouch and maintains intestinal continuity of the upper 10 percent via a retrocolic gastrojejunostomy. Both of these procedures

TABLE 72-2   Complications of bypass surgery

Complication	Percentage
EARLY	
Perioperative mortality	2–6
Thromboembolic disease	1–5
Wound infection	2–5
Renal failure	3
Severe nausea, vomiting	3
Wound dehiscence	1–3
LATE	
Urinary calculi	3–10
Severe electrolyte imbalance	5–8
Acute cholecystitis	0–5
Progressive liver disease	2–4
Intestinal obstruction	2
Peptic ulcer	1–2
Osteoporosis	?
Tuberculosis	1
MINOR	
Diarrhea	100
Weakness	80
Hypokalemia	80
Hypoproteinemia	50
Vomiting	50
Thirst	50
Hypocalcemia	30
Arthralgias	15
Incisional hernias	3
Hyperuricemia	<10
Anemias	<10

cause patients to limit food intake by delaying gastric emptying and providing a small gastric reservoir so that fullness is experienced after a small meal. Weight loss with these procedures is comparable with that achieved with small-bowel bypass operations but without the complications related to malabsorption, diarrhea, and hepatic dysfunction. The procedure can be reversed if a decision to restore normal anatomy is made at a later time. For these reasons, gastroplasty is frequently performed for the surgical treatment of morbid obesity in patients who have failed standard weight loss regimens.

SUMMARY For most patients obesity is an eating disorder, and a major hope for effective long-term treatment of this disease lies in understanding the causes of overeating. No single etiology explains all cases, and different causes exist for different individuals. At present a variety of techniques are available to effect initial weight loss. Unfortunately, initial weight loss is not the real therapeutic goal. Rather, the problem is that most obese patients eventually regain their weight. An effective means to sustain weight loss is the major challenge in the treatment of obesity today. The technique of behavioral modification, when professionally and rigorously applied, is the best tool for this task. As information develops concerning the hypothalamic "set point," or *adipostat*, and the factors that regulate it, other therapies may emerge that will effect long-term correction of abnormal eating patterns.

REFERENCES

Bray GA: Current status of intestinal bypass surgery in the treatment of obesity. Diabetes 26:1072, 1977

———, Gray IS: Treatment of obesity: Overview. Diabetes/Metabolism Rev 4:653, 1988

Foster DW: Eating disorders: Obesity and anorexia nervosa, in *Williams Textbook of Endocrinology,* 7th ed, JD Wilson, DW Foster (eds). Philadelphia, Saunders, 1985, p 1081

Hashim SA, Porikos K: Food intake behavior in man: Implications for treatment of obesity. Clin Endocrinol Metab 5:503, 1976

Henry RR et al: Metabolic consequences of very low calorie diet therapy in obese non-insulin dependent diabetic and non-diabetic subjects. Diabetes 35:155, 1986

Horton ES, Danforth E Jr: Energy metabolism and obesity, in *Diabetes Mellitus and Obesity,* SJ Bleicher, BN Brodoff (eds). Baltimore, Williams & Wilkins, 1981, p 261

Kolterman OG et al: Mechanisms of insulin resistance in human obesity. Evidence for receptor and postreceptor defects. J Clin Invest 65:1272, 1980

Mann GV: The influence of obesity on health. N Engl J Med 291:226, 1974

National Institutes of Health Consensus Development Panel on the Health Implications of Obesity: Health implications of obesity. Ann Intern Med 103:147, 1985

Olefsky JM et al: Insulin action and insulin resistance in obesity and non-insulin dependent, type II diabetes mellitus. Am J Physiol 243:E15, 1982

Salans L: The obesities, in *Endocrinology and Metabolism,* 2d ed, P Felig et al (eds). New York, McGraw-Hill, 1987, chap 21, p 1203

Stunkard AJ et al: An adoption study of human obesity. N Engl J Med 314:193, 1984

The Surgeon General's Report on Nutrition and Health. US Department of Health and Human Services Public Health Service (DHHS PHS) Publication 88-50210, 1988

Woo R et al: Regulation of energy balance, in *Annual Review of Nutrition,* vol 5. Palo Alto, Annual Reviews Inc, 1985, pp 411–433

73 ANOREXIA NERVOSA AND BULIMIA

DANIEL W. FOSTER

Anorexia nervosa and bulimia are eating disorders in young, previously healthy women who develop a paralyzing fear of becoming fat. The population at risk consists largely of white women from middle- and upper-class backgrounds. The disorders rarely occur in black or oriental women, are unusual in the poor, and are almost never seen in men. The driving force is the pursuit of thinness, all other aspects of life being secondary. In the anorexia nervosa syndrome this aim is achieved primarily by radical restriction of caloric intake, the end result being emaciation. In bulimia massive binge eating is followed by vomiting and excessive use of laxatives. Weight loss in bulimic

subjects is not great despite the obsession with food. Some authors consider anorexia nervosa and bulimia to be distinct illnesses, while others classify bulimia as a variant of anorexia nervosa. Overlap syndromes exist since emaciated patients fulfilling the criteria of true anorexia nervosa may exhibit bulimic behavior, while subjects with bulimia often pass through a phase of anorexia. In this chapter it is assumed that the two disorders are different clinical expressions of a primary psychologic obsession with body weight.

PREVALENCE Estimates of prevalence for anorexia nervosa range from 0.4 to 1.5 per 100,000 population. In adolescent white girls from middle- or upper-class families rates as high as 1 per 100 have been reported. Prevalence is believed to be increasing. Subclinical variants may occur in up to 5 percent of the socioeconomic group at highest risk. The incidence of bulimia is less certain. Vomiting after eating may occur in as many as 18 percent of women college students. The frequency of self-induced vomiting is probably 1 to 2 percent, but the full-blown bulimic syndrome is less frequent.

DIAGNOSIS The diagnosis of both anorexia nervosa and bulimia is made on clinical grounds. No specific diagnostic tests exist. For many years the criteria of Feighner et al. (Table 73-1) were the basis for diagnosis in research studies. Less strict requirements were formulated for the American Psychiatric Association's *Diagnostic and Statistical Manual of Mental Disorders* (revised, third edition; DSM-IIIR.)

In the revised criteria the weight loss required for diagnosis was decreased from 25 to 15 percent of expected or ideal weight. Three other requirements were listed: intense fear of gaining weight or becoming fat even when underweight; disturbance in the way body weight, size, or shape is experienced such that the individual "feels fat"; and, in women, either primary amenorrhea or secondary amenorrhea for at least three consecutive periods. The Feighner criteria remain useful, although it seems reasonable to substitute the 15 percent figure for weight loss. In actuality the spectrum of restricted eating ranges from a mild disorder of little consequence to life-threatening starvation. For this reason neither set of criteria is definitive.

The uniqueness of the disturbance in body image in patients with eating disorders has been questioned, and some authorities have recommended its omission on the grounds that many normal young women demonstrate the same perceptual distortion. In practice a presumptive diagnosis of anorexia nervosa is justified if the following elements are elicited: (1) a history of major weight loss; (2) absence of organic disease sufficient to account for weight loss; (3) absence of severe primary psychiatric illness that might account for failure to eat; (4) extreme restriction of food intake with or without intermittent induction of vomiting; (4) ritualized exercise; and (5) denial of hunger, fatigue, or emaciation.

The criteria for the diagnosis of bulimia in DSM-IIIR appear to be less useful. The picture is that of a normal- or near-normal-weight subject whose life is dominated by gorging and regurgitation in the absence of profound weight loss.

ETIOLOGY The cause of anorexia nervosa and bulimia is unknown. Although primary dysfunction of the hypothalamus has been

---

TABLE 73-1 Criteria for the diagnosis of anorexia nervosa

1 Onset prior to age 25
2 Anorexia with weight loss of at least 25 percent of original body weight
3 Distorted attitude toward eating, food, or weight that overrides hunger, admonitions, reassurances, and threats
4 No known medical illness that could account for the weight loss
5 No other known psychiatric disorder
6 At least two of the following manifestations:
  a Amenorrhea
  b Lanugo hair
  c Bradycardia (persistent resting pulse of 60 beats per minute or less)
  d Periods of overactivity
  e Episodes of bulimia
  f Vomiting (may be self-induced)

SOURCE: After Feighner et al.

postulated, the associated hypothalamic abnormalities revert to normal with weight gain and thus are secondary rather than causal.

Most investigators favor a psychiatric etiology, but there is disagreement about its nature. One view holds that the disorders begin in response to inadequate or destructive interpersonal relationships in upper middle class families that are goal-oriented and highly achieving. Despite an outward appearance of normality, interpersonal communication among family members tends to be inadequate, frequently following a pattern in which the father seeks success in his work while the mother turns to her children for fulfillment and in the process becomes overdirective. It is often stated that the families are "enmeshed," meaning that generational boundaries are blurred and that parents and children are constantly involved in each other's problems. Psychoanalytic interpretation tends to focus on anorexia as a mechanism whereby the patient reestablishes control of her own life in a way that is independent of parental direction. It is not clear how this sequence might cause the intense fear of being fat that is the central feature of both anorexia and bulimia.

Although the absence of psychiatric disease is a common criterion for diagnosis (Table 73-1), it is now widely held that depression plays a significant role in the eating disorders. Abnormalities of neurotransmitter concentrations have been reported in blood and cerebrospinal fluid, but such changes are inconsistent and are likely secondary rather than primary.

Cultural issues are also important in anorexia nervosa. The quest for health and slimness is a powerful force in modern western society and may reinforce the fear of fatness in patients with established anorexia or tip the borderline case into full-blown disease. Occupation may play a role; dancers, for example, have a prevalence of anorexia nervosa 10 times that of the general population. Likewise athletes, particularly runners, often seek to decrease body fat to very low levels (5 to 7 percent).

Whatever the mechanism(s) involved, the behavioral response is obsessive and is difficult to treat.

CLINICAL PICTURE   While anorexia nervosa and bulimia may coexist in the same patient, the clinical pictures are ordinarily distinct (Table 73-2).

Anorexia nervosa   The anorexia nervosa syndrome usually begins before or shortly after puberty but may appear later (rarely later than the middle twenties). Many patients have been overweight in childhood. Emaciation is equivalent to that seen in the concentration camp victims of World War II. Despite profound weight loss the patients deny hunger, thinness, or fatigue. They are often physically active, and ritualized exercise programs are common. Frenzied calisthenics or running may follow food intake. There is a preoccupation with food, and elaborate meals may be prepared for others. If social circumstances require them to eat more than usual, vomiting is induced as soon as possible, often in a public restroom. As noted, episodic binge eating may occur and is also followed by emesis. Amenorrhea usually accompanies or follows weight loss but in a sixth of patients may appear prior to any physical change. Constipation and cold intolerance are common. The latter is presumably due to a defect in regulatory thermogenesis secondary to hypothalamic dysfunction.

In advanced cases bradycardia, hypothermia, and hypotension are present. Body fat is undetectable, and the bones protrude through the skin. Interestingly, breast tissue is often preserved. The skin may be dry and scaly and is often yellow due to carotenemia, (particularly visible in the palms). Body hair is often increased; it is usually of fine, lanugo quality, but frank hirsutism may occur. Parotid glands may be enlarged as in other forms of starvation. Mitral valve prolapse is common and is due to valve-ventricular volume mismatch secondary to starvation-induced decrease in left ventricular volume. Edema in the absence of hypoalbuminemia is thought to be due to failure of extracellular fluid volume to diminish proportionally with body mass during weight loss. Because of edema in the legs and parotid enlargement, which gives a fullness to the face, the true state of emaciation may be masked when the patient is fully dressed.

Laboratory abnormalities include anemia and leukopenia (with hypocellularity of the bone marrow), hypokalemia, and hypoalbuminemia. Serum β-carotene levels tend to be elevated. Prerenal azotemia may occur if vomiting or laxative use are prominent. The blood urea nitrogen may be as high as 21 to 25 mmol/L (60 to 70 mg/dL). Renal concentrating ability is impaired, possibly due to blunted responsiveness to antidiuretic hormone. Release of vasopressin in response to an osmotic stimulus is also abnormal. Plasma cholesterol is occasionally high, but triglyceride levels are not increased despite low activities of hepatic and lipoprotein lipases. Glucose tolerance is abnormal as in other forms of starvation.

Miscellaneous abnormalities include low levels of IgG, IgM, and a variety of proteins in the complement pathways. Despite these findings immune function is generally preserved, and serious infections are rare. Plasma iron and ceruloplasmin are normal, but iron binding capacity is decreased. Serum zinc and copper are decreased, but concentrations of these metals are normal in hair. Serum amylase may be increased in the absence of signs or symptoms of pancreatitis.

A variety of endocrine abnormalities are seen. Basal levels of luteinizing hormone (LH) and follicle-stimulating hormone (FSH) are low when weight loss is severe, and the LH response to luteinizing hormone–releasing hormone (LHRH) is impaired. FSH response to LHRH is normal, although time to peak increase may be delayed. Studies of the 24-h circadian pattern of LH secretion show regression of the maturational stage to the pattern characteristic of prepubertal or early pubertal girls; i.e., episodic LH release is missing or occurs only during sleep. These findings presumably account, at least in part, for the amenorrhea. Menses return with weight gain, although the weight required for reinitiation of menstruation may be somewhat higher (~ 10 percent) than that needed for the original induction of menarche. Ovulatory menses may be induced in subjects with anorexia nervosa by prolonged treatment with LHRH agonists, suggesting that pituitary gonadotropin release is impaired because of hypothalamic dysfunction. Prolactin levels are normal. Plasma estradiol levels are low, but plasma testosterone is in the normal female range. Testosterone levels are low in men with anorexia nervosa.

Growth hormone (GH) in the basal state may be normal or elevated. A rise in GH occurs after injection of thyrotropin-releasing hormone (TRH), as in other states with elevated basal levels of GH such as acromegaly, uremia, and protein-calorie malnutrition. Insulin-like growth factor I (somatomedin C) concentrations are low and may contribute to growth hormone elevation via diminished negative feedback. Plasma cortisol levels are high due to increased secretion of corticotropin-releasing hormone from the hypothalamus. The

TABLE 73-2   The eating disorders

	Anorexia nervosa	Bulimia
Predominant sex	Female	Female
Method of weight control	Restriction of intake	Vomiting
Binge eating	Uncommon	Invariant
Weight at diagnosis	Markedly decreased	Near normal
Ritualized exercise	Usual	Rare
Amenorrhea	~100%	~50%
Antisocial behavior	Rare	Frequent
Cardiovascular changes (bradycardia, hypotension)	Common	Uncommon
Skin changes (hirsutism, dryness, carotenemia)	Usual	Rare
Hypothermia	Usual	Rare
Edema	+/−	+/−
Medical complications	Hypokalemia, cardiac arrhythmias	Hypokalemia, cardiac arrhythmias, aspiration of gastric contents, esophageal or gastric rupture

NOTE: These features are characteristic of pure anorexia nervosa and pure bulimia. Overlap syndromes occur, and anorexia may evolve to bulimia (the bulimia → anorexia transformation is rare).

cortisol negative feedback mechanism in the hypothalamus is believed to be impaired. Dexamethasone suppression tests may be abnormal. Norepinephrine concentrations in plasma are depressed.

Thyroxine (T_4) levels are in the low-normal range; free T_4 is normal. Triiodothyronine (T_3) concentrations are reduced, while reverse T_3 (rT_3) levels are increased. Basal levels of thyroid-stimulating hormone (TSH) are usually normal, and TSH response to TRH is intact. The primary defect in thyroid hormone metabolism is decreased activity of the $5'$-deiodinase that converts T_4 to T_3 and rT_3 to diiodothyronine in nonthyroidal tissues. These changes are characteristic of starvation and wasting diseases and are not specific for anorexia nervosa.

Bone density is decreased in women with anorexia nervosa. The mechanism is thought to be estrogen deficiency rather than an abnormality in vitamin D metabolism. Cortisol excess may contribute.

Bulimia Bulimia, which means "ox-hunger," refers to the episodic ingestion of large amounts of food in a compulsive fashion, coupled with awareness that the eating pattern is abnormal, a fear that eating cannot be stopped voluntarily, and feelings of depression at completion of the act. Bulimics have a morbid fear of becoming fat. While binge eating may occur in several types of emotional disorders, a high percentage of patients give a history of overt or cryptic anorexia nervosa, suggesting that bulimia is a variant of anorexia nervosa. Episodes of binge eating are followed by induced vomiting, with or without the subsequent ingestion of laxatives. Initially vomiting is induced by placing a toothbrush or fingers in the throat, but eventually most patients learn to vomit reflexly.

Binge eating generally occurs daily in the active phase; in a series of 40 patients the mean number of episodes per week was 12, ranging from 1 to 46. The duration of the eating period averaged 1.2 h but could last as long as 8 h. The amount of food ingested can be enormous, up to 200,000 kJ (50,000 kcal). High-carbohydrate foods are favored, and more than one food is usually eaten. The order of frequency in one report was: ice cream→bread→candy→doughnuts→soft drinks. The term "dietary chaos" describes the eating pattern. Because of the high sugar content of the diet, dental caries are frequent.

Other behavioral abnormalities are common. Secrecy about the eating-vomiting sequence is characteristic so that family and friends are often unaware. Stealing is common, and food is the item most often taken. There is a high rate of alcohol and drug abuse. Depression tends to be more severe than in anorexia nervosa, making suicide a definite risk. Hysterical behavior may occur. Families of patients with bulimia have a higher incidence of affective disorders, alcoholism, and illicit drug use than is seen in families of patients with anorexia nervosa.

Despite the close relationship with anorexia nervosa, a number of differences are noted. While many patients with bulimia are thin, emaciation is not seen; generally weight is within 15 percent of the normal range as defined by life insurance tables of ideal weight. Fluctuating weight is common, with cyclical gains and losses. Some patients are modestly overweight. In contrast to anorexia nervosa, about half of the patients continue to menstruate, and a number have become pregnant. Persistent menstruation probably reflects the absence of extreme weight loss. Sexual activity is greater in bulimic subjects than in those with anorexia.

The physical findings associated with bulimia are usually minimal, although subjects with more extensive weight loss may manifest some of the changes seen with anorexia nervosa.

The most common laboratory abnormality is hypokalemia with metabolic alkalosis secondary to vomiting and laxative use. Endocrine abnormalities are similar to those in anorexia nervosa. One study suggested that LH response to LHRH is exaggerated in bulimic patients, but this has not been confirmed. Dexamethasone suppression is frequently abnormal. Unlike patients with anorexia nervosa, some women with bulimia have low basal prolactin levels and an exaggerated prolactin response to TRH.

COMPLICATIONS Patients with anorexia nervosa are vulnerable to sudden death from ventricular tachyarrhythmias. Electrocardiograms show prolonged QT intervals. The risk of death becomes high when weight loss reaches 35 percent below ideal, probably because of protein deficiency. (Since there is no reserve store of protein, critical enzymes and cellular structures are affected by starvation-induced decreases in lean body mass; see Chap. 71.) Major complications of bulimia include aspiration, esophageal or gastric rupture, pneumomediastinum, hypokalemia with cardiac arrhythmias, pancreatitis, and ipecac-induced myopathy and/or cardiomyopathy.

PROGNOSIS The course of anorexia nervosa is variable. In long-term follow-up about half of patients achieve normal weight, 20 percent improve but remain underweight, 20 percent continue anorexic, 5 percent become obese, and 6 percent die. Even when weight gain occurs, signs of persistent illness remain since intermittent dieting, binge eating, vomiting, and laxative use persist in up to two-thirds of patients. Death is usually due to starvation (cardiac arrhythmias primarily) or suicide. Poor prognostic signs include older age of onset, longer duration of illness, history of bulimia or vomiting, extreme weight loss, and presence of significant depression. Fewer reports of long-term follow-up are available for bulimia than for anorexia nervosa. Because the psychiatric disturbance tends to be more severe (suicide occurs at higher rates) and because the medical dangers of gorging are greater, prognosis is believed to be even worse in bulimia than in anorexia. One report indicates that 40 percent of treated patients remained bulimic after 18 months of treatment and that relapse occurred in 65 percent after 1 year of recovery.

TREATMENT There is no specific treatment for anorexia nervosa or bulimia. The intense fear of becoming fat coupled with a perceptual disturbance that causes overestimation of body size results in powerful resistance to therapy. The benefits of psychiatric intervention are marginal. The same can be said of behavior modification techniques and for group and family therapy. Supportive care by an understanding physician may accomplish as much as formal psychotherapy. The patient should be seen regularly for a review of weight change, diet, and exercise patterns. It is often useful to establish a mutually agreeable explicit contract; e.g., if the patient weighs 65 pounds and ideal body weight determined from life insurance tables is 115 pounds, a goal of 90 pounds might be set as a first stage. At every visit the patient should be reassured by the physician that "we will not let you get fat." A calm but realistic review of the dangers of starvation, including sudden death, should be given, coupled with statements like "my job is to help you deal with this illness so that you can have a normal life expectancy with reasonable happiness." The physician must be perceived not as an enemy or a parental surrogate but an advisor and partner in the struggle.

A similar approach should also be used with bulimic patients. Even if the gorging-regurgitation cycle cannot be stopped, the lesser goal of limiting the load of food ingested (to minimize the chance of aspiration or gastric rupture) and decreasing the frequency of events may be achieved. Because depression and antisocial behavior are more common in bulimia, psychiatric therapy is usually required. It is now common to use antidepressants in both anorexia nervosa and bulimia. Imipramine and phenelzine may be the best choices. Potassium supplementation may be required for vomiters.

Hospitalization may be a lifesaving measure with severe anorexia nervosa. Sudden death may occur at weights more than 35 percent below ideal, particularly if weight loss has been rapid. Hypokalemia, hypotension, and prerenal azotemia due to volume depletion are other indications for hospitalization. If the patient refuses to eat, a nasogastric tube will be required, but it is better to persuade the patient to eat. Supervision of every meal is initially required, ideally by the same person. During the hospitalization the patient should never be allowed to eat alone. Total parenteral nutrition is rarely indicated. Instruction about nutrition, occupational therapy, group work with the family, and individual psychotherapy should be included in the treatment plan. The "safety" of eating and assurances that obesity will not result should be emphasized repetitively. Some specialists feel that all seriously affected anorexia patients benefit from initial hospitalization, but this is not a universal view. Hospitalization for bulimic subjects is normally only required for medical complications (e.g., aspiration).

Treatment of patients with the anorexia-bulimia syndrome is a long-term proposition, rife with failure, and requires perseverance by the subject, family, and physician.

REFERENCES

FEIGHNER JP et al: Diagnostic criteria for use in psychiatric research. Arch Gen Psychiatry 26:57, 1972

FOSTER DW: Eating disorders: Obesity and anorexia nervosa, in *Williams Textbook of Endocrinology*, 7th ed, JD Wilson, DW Foster (eds). Philadelphia, Saunders, 1985, pp 1081–1107

HERZOG DB, COPELAND PM: Eating disorders. N Engl J Med 313:295, 1985

———, ———: Bulimia nervosa—psyche and satiety. N Engl J Med 319:716, 1988

ISNER JM et al: Anorexia nervosa and sudden death. Ann Intern Med 102:49, 1985

LEVY AB: Neuroendocrine profile in bulimia nervosa. Biol Psychiatry 25:98, 1989

——— et al: How are depression and bulimia related? Am J Psychiatry 146:162, 1989

LUCAS AR: Anorexia nervosa in Rochester, Minnesota: A 45-year study. Mayo Clin Proc 63:433, 1988

MITCHELL JE et al: Medical complications and medical management of bulimia. Ann Intern Med 107:71, 1987

NEWMAN MM, HALMI KA: The endocrinology of anorexia nervosa and bulimia nervosa. Endocrin Metab Clin North Am 17:195, 1988

74   DIET THERAPY

JOHANNA T. DWYER / JODI ROY

The primary role of diet therapy is to prevent or treat malnutrition, to control diet-related signs and symptoms of disease, to delay the progression of chronic degenerative diseases, and to provide adjunctive support for other medical or surgical treatments. Diet therapy also plays an important role in rehabilitation and in palliation. For example, it may aid in maintaining or enhancing the quality of life in the terminally ill. Nutrition therapy may involve feeding by parenteral and enteral routes and/or use of special purpose oral supplements. Dietary advice may also be useful for health promotion, disease prevention, nutritional support, and rehabilitation.

There are four essential principles for sound diet therapy. First, a nutrition-related problem must be present for which an accepted dietary therapy exists. Second, the diet therapy should be based on a solid scientific rationale. Evidence on the effectiveness of therapeutic diets in ameliorating symptoms, slowing progression, lessening secondary problems or otherwise positively affecting function must be available from sound clinical trials. Anecdotal evidence of improvement alone is insufficient to warrant diet therapy. Third, the patient must be able to eat and must have a functional gastrointestinal tract. (For patients who require enteral nutrition therapy, see Chap. 75.) Finally, the patient must adhere to the diet. Little motivation may be required for a patient to consume a therapeutic diet in the hospital since no other food choice may be available, but a great deal of motivation is needed to buy, prepare, and eat therapeutic diets after discharge.

PLANNING DIET THERAPY

ASSESSMENT   Dietary assessment attempts to discover what is eaten, whereas assessment of nutrition status (Chap. 71) is aimed at measuring the interaction of diet, disease, and requirements. Both types of information are needed to identify nutrition-related problems and plan therapeutic diets. Dietary assessment requires cataloging what an individual usually eats and the nutritional quality and adequacy of that diet; it also helps determine nutritional status, establishes or refines differential diagnoses, and furnishes the background infor-

mation on food intakes and preferences that are needed for implementing dietary therapy.

There are qualitative and quantitative levels of dietary assessment. Qualitative assessment involves determining (1) if the patient is currently eating, following a specific diet, and/or has had recent weight loss or gain; (2) the number of meals per day, any use of nutritional supplements (e.g., amounts and types of vitamin or mineral supplements), special dietary preferences or dietary practices (e.g., consumption of only one or a few foods); and (3) assessment of the physical state (e.g., chewing problems, dysphagia, diarrhea). If the qualitative assessment suggests that nutritional problems may exist, more quantitation should be obtained. For example, the current dietary intake (e.g., the past day) is catalogued using 24-h recalls. The patient is asked to describe, starting with the meal last eaten, what has been consumed over the past 24 h. The intake is then assessed by calculating intakes of nutrients or by comparing intakes to a food grouping system that assumes dietary adequacy. This method is easy to administer, places little burden on the patient, and provides some estimate of intakes. However, 24 h may not be a long enough period to provide a representative intake, and habitual diet may not be assessed. Dietary intake data must reflect a sufficient period of time (weeks or months) for its effects on nutritional status to be meaningful. If changes in intake have occurred, it may also be helpful to recall previous intakes before illness or other events caused dietary alteration.

The patient's habitual diet is assessed using either semiquantitative food-frequency questionnaires, which permit a standardized dietary history to be taken using a list of foods and portion sizes, or the periodic collection of food records for several days at a time. Semiquantitative food-frequency questionnaires make it possible to estimate habitual diet and can be analyzed on a computer. Food records are better for identifying the intake of unusual foods not included on food-frequency questionnaires, but such records are more difficult to obtain and to analyze. Other methods for dietary assessment include the dietary history, in which the patient provides information on usual intakes in an interview with a dietitian. In skilled hands this can reveal usual dietary patterns quickly and is less burdensome to the patient than keeping food records, but training and time are needed to interview in a reproducible manner.

PRESCRIPTION   A diet prescription specifies the dietary modifications needed for nutritional therapy. It is usually brief, stated in terms of further assessment needed, the disease to be treated, and the modifications to deal with the disease. The physician is also responsible for making timely changes in diet orders. Failure to make changes can result in such unfortunate events as keeping patients indefinitely on nutritionally inadequate "clear liquid" diets, with resulting debilitation and/or delayed healing.

The rendering of nutrition care requires knowledge about food composition, dietary assessment, diet planning, and diet-counseling techniques. In acute care and inpatient settings the diet order is translated by dietitians to actual foods, menus, or eating plans acceptable to the patient. In outpatient settings, the physician may counsel patients directly, or they may be referred to dietitians.

CARE PLAN   The diet order is the first step in the implementation of nutritional intervention. A nutrition care plan is then formulated for the implementation of the diet. The individual who takes responsibility for diet therapy needs to record the nutritional care plan in the medical record and supervise its implementation. The care plan should include a summary of the needs discovered during patient assessment and an implementation plan describing how nutritional objectives are to be reached in terms of food behaviors and any additional resources needed, such as assistance in purchasing food, counseling, education, and help with eating (if necessary). Plans for review, follow-up, and evaluation of progress should also be specified.

IMPLEMENTING DIET THERAPY

USUAL INTAKE   The starting point for planning therapeutic diets is the patient's usual intake. The fewer the changes from usual intake, the greater the likelihood that individual preferences will be met and that the new eating plan will be followed. If the usual intake is not nutritionally adequate, the therapeutic plan includes modifications to ensure nutritional sufficiency.

MODIFICATIONS Therapeutic diets involve up to three basic alterations: modifications in route of feeding (see Chap. 75), in consistency, and in food constituents. The appropriate diet for a given condition depends on the stage or severity of disease, characteristics of the patient (age, sex, educational level, ethnicity), the treatment environment (e.g., inpatient, outpatient), and the social situation. For example, there is no single diabetic diet; there are many diets for diabetics, depending upon individual requirements such as whether the patient is on insulin, whether there is a need for weight reduction, and whether coexisting medical complications (such as hyperlipidemia, hypertension or renal disease) are present. Individual planning may be necessary to meet medical demands while ensuring that the planned diet is palatable.

Additional considerations must be taken into account in planning therapeutic diets. The first is meeting the recommended dietary allowances (RDAs) for nutrients (see Table 70-4), and the second is to deal with relevant medical concerns (such as ease of swallowing in a stroke patient, or the timing of feeding in insulin-dependent diabetes mellitus), patient food preferences, and drug-nutrient interactions. Individual hospital manuals specify the diets available in the institution.

Consistency (See Table 74-1) Variations in consistency usually involve two factors. The first is liquidity; major modifications are *clear liquid, full liquid,* and *soft.* The form in which the food constituents are prepared and the type of ingredients constitute the second factor. Options include common foods that have been chopped and blenderized, commercial nutritional supplements formulated with ingredients not usually available in the home, and "elemental diets" using nutrients in simple forms such as protein hydrolysates or amino acids. In general, the commercial products are more appetizing because they use stabilizers and other means to keep particles in suspension and because the mixtures are more palatable.

Nutritional adequacy and palatability must be considered in plans that alter consistency. *Clear liquid* diets are nutritionally inadequate and include only a few foods that most people eat regularly, but they

may be all that is tolerated immediately after surgery or during severe medical emergencies. *Full liquid* diets include more foods and may be nutritionally adequate, but they are limited in choice compared to normal diets. *Soft* diets are also limited in terms of palatability and deviation from usual diets. For these reasons, modifications in consistency should only be used when absolutely necessary and for as limited a time as feasible.

Composition (See Table 74-2) Modifications in the composition of diets may include energy level, type and amount of nutrients (e.g., lactose-free; low-fat, low saturated fat), or type and amount of other constituents in the diet (e.g., 30 gm soluble fiber, 300 mg cholesterol; low oxalate). Other therapeutic regimens are described in various standard texts.

Several points need emphasis in planning alterations in dietary composition: First, the supporting evidence and documentation of benefits for therapeutic diets vary in their completeness (Table 74-2). For some diseases, such as the hyperlipidemias, the role of diet modification in decreasing serum cholesterol and risk of coronary artery disease is well-documented. For other diseases, such as diabetes mellitus, diet can control acute and short-term symptoms, but its efficacy in altering the long-term sequelae, such as retinopathy and kidney disease, is not established. Patients need to be informed as to what can be expected from the diet therapy instituted.

Second, changes both in consistency and in constituents may be required. For example, simultaneous modifications in a number of constituents are mandatory in diabetes mellitus and renal failure. Such a patient may require an eating plan that controls energy intake, type and amount of carbohydrate, timing of carbohydrate intake, amount of dietary fiber, and the content of fat, protein, and sodium. In some cases there are so many constraints that priority ranking must be given to the most important alteration. With other modifications, less precision is acceptable. Otherwise, it may be impractical to implement the diet therapy.

Third, additional modifications in nutrient composition may be necessary to meet normal physiologic needs (infancy, puberty, pregnancy, lactation). Factors that may need to be considered include inadequacies in recent intake, the timing of nutrient intake (as in insulin-dependent diabetes mellitus), and the presence of specific food allergies or intolerances (e.g., patients on monoamine oxidase

TABLE 74-1 Modifications in diet consistency

Consistency	Purpose	Use	Nutritional adequacy	Comments
Clear liquid: clear broth, gelatin, popsicles, ices; sugar, honey, hard candy; clear fruit juices; clear coffee, tea, and carbonated beverages (as tolerated); low-residue, high-protein, high-calorie clear oral supplements	Short term (1–2 days preferably): to supply fluid and some energy [~2500 kJ/d (~600 kcal/d)] in a form that requires minimal digestion after surgery, trauma, or in acute illness.	Initial feeding after surgery or IV feeding to relieve thirst and hydrate, while minimizing the need to chew and GI-tract stimulation.	Falls seriously short of nutrient needs in energy, protein, vitamins, and minerals; if this diet is to continue beyond 3–5 days, nutritional support is necessary.	Produces few or no feces; greatly different from usual diets.
Full liquid: clear liquids plus: all milk and milk drinks, yogurt; vegetable and fruit juices; refined cooked cereals; butter, margarine; custard, ice cream, pudding; high-protein, high-calorie oral supplements	Supply fluid and meet energy and other nutrient needs more completely with foods that are liquid at body temperature; usually higher in calories than clear liquid diet.	Transition between clear liquid and solid foods after surgery and in acute illness; in esophageal or stomach disorders with strictures or anatomical irregularity; and for inability to chew or swallow solid foods.	May be inadequate in niacin, folacin, and iron due to lack of meat, whole grain, and vegetable intake; adequacy may be improved using high-protein, high-calorie supplements or the addition of a multivitamin supplement.	More complete diet than clear liquid; beneficial as a transitional feeding for weak patients who cannot adequately chew food; greatly different from usual diets.
Soft	Provide foods that can be swallowed with little or no chewing.	For patients who are alert or acutely ill with difficulty in chewing/swallowing, or who are too ill or weak to tolerate a usual diet; for head and neck surgical patients; those with esophageal strictures or poor dentition.	Can be adequate in all nutrients based on menu selection.	Textures can range from pureed (blenderized, strained or smooth foods) to ground, chopped, or soft solids.

TABLE 74-2 Dietary modifications in various diseases

Therapeutic diet modification	Disease	Known benefit(s)	Possible benefit(s)
ENERGY			
Energy controlled	Diabetes mellitus	Increased glucose tolerance, decreased acute side effects	Decreased long-term complications (large vessel atherosclerosis, nephropathy, hypertension)
Low energy	Obesity	Weight loss	
	Hypertension	Decreased systolic and diastolic blood pressure	
	Non-insulin dependent diabetes mellitus	Increased glucose tolerance, decreased short-term symptoms	Decreased long-term complications
High energy	Anorexia	Increased weight, lean body mass, and fat; promotes normal fat and lean tissue	
	Emaciation		
Small feedings	Gastroesophageal reflux	Decreased gastric volume, decreased likelihood of reflux (small feedings in an upright position)	
ENERGY-YIELDING NUTRIENTS			
Protein			
Low protein	Chronic renal failure (end stage renal disease)	Control of blood urea nitrogen, electrolytes, and phosphorus levels (amino acid supplements are used)	
	Hepatic encephalopathy	Prevention of hepatic encephalopathy	
	Early chronic progressive renal disease		Decreased decline in glomerular filtration rate
	Nephrotic syndrome		Decreased protein wasting
Fat			
Low fat	Steatorrhea	Decreased malabsorption	
	Gastroesophageal reflux	Increased lower esophageal sphincter pressure	
	Acute hepatic, pancreatic, and gall bladder disease	Decreased need for bile salts	
	Crohn's disease	Decreased malabsorption in patients with functional lactase deficiency	
	Postgastrectomy dumping	Decreased malabsorption in patients with functional lactase deficiency	
Minerals			
Low sodium	Hypertension	Decreased blood pressure in salt-sensitive individuals	
	Congestive heart failure	Decreased sodium retention, reducing hypertension	
	Chronic renal failure	Decreased sodium retention, reducing hypertension	
	Ascites	Decreased sodium retention	
Low potassium	Hyperkalemia	Decreased serum potassium	
	Chronic renal failure	Decreased serum potassium	
High potassium	Hypokalemia	Increased serum potassium	
High calcium	Osteoporosis		Risk reduction in premenopausal women
Low phosphorus	Hyperphosphatemia	Decreased serum phosphorus	
	Renal failure	Decreased serum phosphorus	
Oxalate			
Low oxalate	Oxalate kidney stones	Decreased concentration of oxalate in the urine	
	Crohn's disease	Decreased malabsorption in patients with steatorrhea	
	Radiation enteritis	Decreased malabsorption	
	Colon, prostate, and breast cancers		Reduced risks in promotional stage via hormonal actions
Low fat, low saturated fat, low cholesterol	Hyperlipidemia	Reduced serum lipids	
	Coronary heart disease	Reduced serum lipids	Fosters regression of some arterial plaques (if diet is extreme and long-continued)

(continued)

inhibitors). Other problems, such as the inability to feed oneself, vegetarianism, religious beliefs that prohibit certain foods, alcoholism, and specific likes and dislikes also need to be taken into account.

Fourth, elaborate diet prescriptions place a burden on patients. Complicated diets may cause only minor problems in the hospitalized patient but create major compliance problems for outpatients. When the continuation of such diets is necessary, diet counseling prior to discharge should be supplemented by frequent outpatient visits.

Even within a given disease category the role of dietary therapy may vary, and there may be no single "therapeutic diet" for a given disease.

Modifications for hypercholesterolemia The associations between dietary modifications and lowering of serum cholesterol are well-described and, at least in men, predictable, and the association between lowering of serum cholesterol and decreases in the complications of coronary artery disease is clear-cut. Hence, diet therapy is the first step in the treatment of most hyperlipidemic states. Table 74-3 summarizes the current recommendations for diet therapy of

TABLE 74-2 Dietary modifications in various diseases *(continued)*

Therapeutic diet modification	Disease	Known benefit(s)	Possible benefit(s)
OTHER CONSTITUENTS			
Fiber			
High fiber	Atonic constipation	Increased stool bulk and decreased transit time	
	Diverticulosis	Increased stool bulk and decreased colonic pressure, preventing the production of diverticula	
	Irritable bowel syndrome	Decreased constipation	
	Colon cancer		Risk reduction
	Crohn's disease (inactive)		Symptom control
	Diabetes mellitus	Improved glycemic control, reduced insulin requirements	
	Hyperlipidemia		Decreased serum cholesterol (high water-soluble fiber)
Low fiber	Crohn's disease/ulcerative colitis (active phase)	Reduced diarrhea and pain	
	Crohn's disease (inactive phase)		Symptom control
Gluten			
Gluten-free	Celiac disease	Decreased malabsorption and gut damage due to gluten enteropathy	
Lactose			
Lactose-free	Lactose intolerance	Decreased malabsorption	

TABLE 74-3 Recommendations of American Heart Association/National Cholesterol Education Program: step 1 and step 2 diets for hypercholesterolemia

Indications
  LDL cholesterol >4.1 mmol/L (>160 mg/dL)
  LDL cholesterol >3.4 mmol/L (>130 mg/dL) with definite coronary disease or two other risk factors*
Minimal goals
  Without coronary disease or two risk factors: Lower LDL cholesterol below 4.1 mmol/L (160 mg/dL)
  With coronary disease or two risk factors: Lower LDL cholesterol below 3.4 mmol/L (130 mg/dL)

	% of total calories	
Recommended intake	Step 1 diet	Step 2 diet (if serum lipid goal not reached)
Total fat	<30%	<30%
Saturated fatty acids	<10%	< 7%
Polyunsaturated fatty acids	<10%	<10%
Monounsaturated fatty acids	10–15%	10–15%
Carbohydrates	50–60%	50–60%
Protein	10–20%	10–20%
Cholesterol	<300 mg/d	<200 mg/d
Total energy intake	To achieve and maintain desirable weight	To achieve and maintain desirable weight

* Risk factors include male sex, family history of premature coronary distress, cigarette smoking, hypertension, low HDL cholesterol level, diabetes mellitus, history of definite cerebrovascular or occlusive peripheral vascular disease, severe obesity.
NOTE: LDL = low-density lipoprotein; HDL = high-density lipoprotein.
SOURCE: Adapted from National Cholesterol Education Program: Arch Intern Med 148:36, 1988.

TABLE 74-4 Nutritional recommendations for patients with diabetes mellitus

Energy intake: Achieve and maintain a desirable body weight.
Carbohydrate: (1) Up to 55–60% of the total calories; (2) Substitute unrefined complex carbohydrates with fiber for highly refined carbohydrates; (3) Modest amounts of sucrose and other refined sugars acceptable.
Protein: Consistent with the RDA of 0.8 g/kg of ideal body weight.
Total fat and cholesterol: Restrict to <30% total calories from fat, and cholesterol <300 mg/d.
Alternative sweeteners: Nutritive and non-nutritive sweeteners both acceptable in moderation.
Salt intake: <3000 mg/d.
Alcohol: If at all, in moderation.
Vitamins and minerals: Meet the RDA.

SOURCE: Adapted from Franz MJ et al: J Am Diet Assoc 87:28, 1987.

those adults at high risk [(e.g., total serum cholesterol >6.2 mmol/L (<240 mg/dL)] jointly endorsed by the National Cholesterol Education Program (NCEP) and the American Heart Association (AHA) and includes the indications for diet therapy in terms of the individual's serum lipid values (also see Chaps. 195 and 326).

The NCEP recommends a "step-care" approach in dealing with hyperlipidemia. Patients at risk are first placed on the step 1 diet (unless they are at very high risk), which is modified in total fat, saturated fat, cholesterol, and energy intake. After a period of 2 months the serum cholesterol is evaluated. Those who, despite adherence, do not achieve the goals of therapy on the step 1 diet are asked to continue the diet trial and are provided with additional assistance. Patients who still fail to lower their serum cholesterol to acceptable levels with diet are moved to the step 2 diet, which is even lower in saturated fat and cholesterol. If serum cholesterol levels are still not reduced sufficiently, drug therapy is added, and, if dietary efforts fail completely, drug therapy alone may be used.

Hyperlipidemic patients may also have hypertension, diabetes mellitus, chronic renal insufficiency, or other diseases that require additional dietary modifications.

Modifications for diabetes mellitus Table 74-4 outlines the nutritional recommendations for individuals with diabetes mellitus, and Table 74-5 summarizes a widely used tool—the exchange list. Exchange lists describe the serving size of various foods in groups that are similar in nutrient value. Exchange lists vary depending on the disease and the desired dietary modifications. Such lists provide an overall meal plan that allows selection of different foods and menus. However, the type and amount of dietary carbohydrate and fat and the energy intake ingested throughout the day need to be considered in planning the diet, drug schedule, and physical activity patterns. Diet therapy in diabetes is helpful in controlling the acute manifestations (excessive thirst, frequent urination, blurred vision, etc.) of hyperglycemia. Diet may also reduce the risk of accelerated atherosclerosis.

Alterations in dietary fiber Modifications in the type and amount of dietary fiber can sometimes ameliorate functional constipation or diarrhea. Increased dietary fiber intakes, particularly of water-insoluble fibers like wheat bran, also provide symptomatic relief in diverticulosis of the colon. Some water-soluble fibers in large doses may decrease serum cholesterol levels; these include fiber derived from oat bran, beans, and psyllium seeds.

Lactose-free diets Many adults, especially Orientals and blacks, have hereditary intestinal lactase deficiency. Lactose intolerance may

TABLE 74-5　Exchange list for meal planning for diabetics

Exchange list food group	Carbohydrate, grams	Protein, grams	Fat, grams	Energy intake, kilojoules (kilocalories)
Starch/bread ½ cup (120 mL) cereal, grain, or pasta 1 ounce (30 g) of a bread product	15	3	Trace	335 (80)
Meat 1 ounce (30 g) cooked				
Lean	—	7	3	230 (55)
Medium-fat	—	7	5	315 (75)
High-fat	—	7	8	415 (100)
Vegetable ½ cup (120 mL) cooked or juice 1 cup (240 mL) raw	5	2	—	105 (25)
Fruit ½ cup (120 mL) fresh or juice ¼ cup (60 mL) dried	15	—	—	250 (60)
Milk 1 cup (240 mL)				375 (90)
Skim	12	8	Trace	500 (120)
Low-fat	12	8	5	625 (150)
Whole	12	8	8	
Fat 1 tsp. butter, margarine, oil, mayonnaise (5 mL) 1 Tbsp. salad dressing (15 mL)	—	—	5	190 (45)

NOTE: Saturated fat, fiber and sodium intakes are controlled by choices within food groups
SOURCE: American Diabetes Association and the American Dietetic Association: *Exchange Lists for Meal Planning*, 1986.

also be secondary, either acquired or as the result of gastrointestinal disease. Elimination of lactose from the diet reduces the diarrhea due to the osmotic action of unabsorbed lactose in the gut lumen (see Chap. 240).

Gluten-free diets Gluten, a protein found primarily in wheat products, produces a toxic reaction causing villous atrophy in patients with sprue or celiac disease. Elimination of gluten from the diet is essential and requires substitution of foods from sources such as rice or potato (see Chap. 240).

Caffeine Caffeine can cause untoward behavioral effects in large doses (e.g., 1000 mg or more—the equivalent of 10 cups of coffee a day). Some patients with reflux esophagitis, hypermotility syndrome,

and peptic ulcer disease may also benefit from reducing or eliminating caffeine from the diet.

Unproven dietary remedies Many legitimate therapeutic diets exist in addition to those mentioned in Table 74-2. However, not all popular dietary remedies are well-documented and useful. For example, there is no evidence that special diets have any role in alleviating or treating premenstrual syndrome, migraine headaches, hyperactivity, fibrocystic disease of the breast, or acne; that a polyunsaturated fat diet is beneficial for multiple sclerosis; or that a macrobiotic diet is useful in patients with cancer.

HOW DIETARY CHANGES ARE ACHIEVED Dietary change is achieved by altering the amounts and the frequency of food con-

TABLE 74-6　Rich food sources of vitamins

Vitamin	Alternative names	Richest sources	Vitamin	Alternative names	Richest sources
Vitamin A (plus carotenoids)	Retinol (vitamin A alcohol)	Liver, egg yolk, chicken meat; whole milk, butter; breakfast cereals; margarines fortified with vitamin A	Niacin	Nicotinic Acid	Meats, poultry, fish; yeast; whole- and enriched-grain products; legumes; nuts; in addition, some of the tryptophan present in meats, poultry, fish, cheese, legumes, and seeds can be converted in the body to niacin
Carotenoids	β-Carotene (most plentiful)	Dark-green leafy vegetables like spinach, chard; yellow vegetables like carrots, squash; yellow fruits like mango, cantaloupe			
			Vitamin B₆	Pyridoxine Pyridoxal Pyridoxamine	Meat, poultry, fish; bananas; yeast; bran; and nuts
Vitamin D	D₃ (cholecalciferol) D₂ (ergocalciferol)	Fatty fish like salmon and fish oils; eggs; butter; liver; milk fortified with vitamin D	Vitamin B₁₂	Cobalamin	Only in foods of animal origin: liver, muscle meats, fish, eggs, and milk and milk products
Vitamin E	Alpha tocopherol	Oils from soybean, sunflower, corn, and cottonseed; germ of whole grains; fish liver oils; nuts	Folacin	Folic Acid Folate	Liver; dark-green leafy vegetables like spinach, romaine lettuce; dry beans, peanuts, wheat germ, whole grains; yeast
Thiamin	Vitamin B₁	Whole grains, dried legumes; pork muscle, liver; products made with enriched flour			
Riboflavin	Vitamin B₂	Milk and milk products; eggs; whole- and enriched-grain products; lean meat, liver, poultry, fish; dark-green vegetables like spinach, asparagus	Vitamin C	Ascorbic Acid	Citrus fruits like oranges, lemons, grapefruit; dark-green leafy vegetables like broccoli, asparagus

SOURCE: National Academy of Sciences Committee on Diet and Health: *Diet and Health Report*, 1989.

sumption. Nutrients are not equally distributed throughout all foods, and Tables 74-6 and 74-7 list food sources rich in selected vitamins and minerals.

Substitutions within food groups can alter diet composition. For example, using skim milk instead of whole milk lowers the amount of fat but does not alter its contribution of other nutrients (protein, calcium, and phosphorus). Lean cuts of meat, skinned chicken, and lean fish contain less fat than fried meats, but have the same content of protein, vitamins, and minerals.

When many simultaneous reductions must be made in nutrient intakes, development of a reasonable eating plan can be time-consuming and difficult. Computerized menu planning systems or use of simplified exchange systems and menu-planning guides may be helpful in some circumstances.

ORAL NUTRITIONAL SUPPLEMENTS WITH SPECIAL CHARACTERISTICS Diets to meet therapeutic needs may utilize readily available foods, but flexibility is enhanced by the inclusion of specially formulated dietary products (Table 74-8). These products can be of great help in planning menus that are palatable and that permit some latitude on the part of the patient. Some of the products are particularly useful for complex therapeutic diets.

SPECIAL PROBLEMS IN DIET THERAPY

TRANSITIONS FROM ONE ROUTE OF FEEDING TO ANOTHER
Transitional feeding refers to the return to the usual feeding pattern

TABLE 74-7 Rich food sources of minerals

Mineral	Sources
Calcium	Milk, cheese, broccoli, dark-green leafy vegetables such as collard, turnip, and mustard greens
Phosphorus	Meats, milk products, grains, phosphate, food additives
Magnesium	Green vegetables, nuts, seeds, dried beans, whole grains, and meats
Iron	Liver, red meat, whole-grain and enriched-grain products, beans, nuts, and dark-green leafy vegetables
Zinc	Shellfish, meat, poultry, cheese, whole grains, dry beans, nuts
Copper	Crab meat, fresh vegetables and fruits, nuts, seeds, legumes
Sodium	Salt (sodium chloride); cured meats (ham, bacon, sausage, frankfurters, luncheon meats); cheeses, olives; pickles; condiment sauces; frozen and canned meat and fish entrees and dinners; canned and dried soups; commercial pasta, noodle, and potato dishes; salted snacks; commercial mixes for waffles, muffins, and cakes; canned vegetables with sauces; baking powder; baking soda; certain emulsifiers and other food additives; drinking water; drugs such as some antacids.
Potassium	Milk, fruits (especially oranges, prunes, apples, pears, peaches, bananas, and grapefruit), vegetables (especially fresh broccoli, carrots, tomatoes, and potatoes), fish, shellfish, turkey, chicken, and cooked oatmeal.

SOURCE: National Academy of Sciences Committee on Diet and Health: *Diet and Health Report*, 1989.

TABLE 74-8 Nutrient composition of oral nutritional supplements

	Manufacturer	kJ/mL	kcal/mL	Percent of energy			Comments
				Protein	Fat	Carbohydrate	
CLEAR LIQUID FORMULAS							
Citrotein	Sandoz Nutrition	2.8	0.66	25	2	73	
Ross SLD (surgical liquid diet)	Ross	2.9	0.70	21	1	78	
FULL LIQUID FORMULAS							
Milk-based formulas							
Carnation Instant Breakfast	Carnation Company	4.4	1.06	21	27	52	
Meritene Liquid	Sandoz Nutrition	4.0	0.96	24	30	46	
Meritene Powder	Sandoz Nutrition	4.4	1.06	26	29	45	
Sustacal Nutritional Powder	Mead Johnson	5.4	1.30	23	23	54	
Sustagen	Mead Johnson	7.7	1.85	24	8	68	
Blenderized formulas							
Compleat Modified Formula	Sandoz Nutrition	4.5	1.07	16	31	53	Lactose-free; gluten-free
Compleat Regular Formula	Sandoz Nutrition	4.5	1.07	16	36	48	
Vitaneed	Sherwood Medical	4.2	1.00	16	35	49	Lactose-free
Formulas with fiber							
Enrich	Ross	4.6	1.10	14	29	57	Lactose-free; 14 g fiber per L
Sustacal with Fiber	Mead Johnson	4.4	1.06	17	29	54	Lactose-free; 5 g fiber per L
Jevity	Ross	4.4	1.06	16	30	54	Isotonic,* lactose-free; 14 g fiber per L
Lactose-free formulas							
Ensure	Ross	4.4	1.06	14	31	55	Low-residue*
Resource Plus Liquid	Sandoz Nutrition	6.2	1.50	15	32	53	Gluten-free; low-residue
Sustacal Liquid	Mead Johnson	4.2	1.01	24	20	56	Low-residue
Travasorb MCT Diet	Clinitec Nutrition Co.	6.7	1.60	20	30	50	
Resource Instant Crystals	Sandoz Nutrition	4.4	1.06	14	31	55	Low-residue
Resource Liquid	Sandoz Nutrition	4.4	1.06	14	31	55	Gluten-free; low-residue
Comply	Sherwood Medical	6.2	1.50	16	36	48	
Ensure Plus	Ross	6.2	1.50	15	32	53	Low-residue
Sustacal HC	Mead Johnson	6.4	1.52	16	34	50	Low-residue
Ensure Plus HN	Ross	6.2	1.50	17	30	53	Low-residue
Isocal HCN	Mead Johnson	8.4	2.00	15	45	40	
Magnacal	Sherwood Medical	8.4	2.00	14	36	50	Low-residue
Two Cal HN	Ross	8.4	2.00	17	40	43	
Isotonic formulas*							
Attain	Sherwood Medical	4.2	1.00	16	36	48	Lactose-free; low-residue
Osmolite	Ross	4.4	1.06	14	32	54	Lactose-free; low-residue
Precision Isotonic Diet	Sandoz Nutrition	4.0	0.96	12	28	60	Lactose-free; gluten-free; purine-free

(continued)

TABLE 74-8   Nutrient composition of oral nutritional supplements (continued)

	Manufacturer	kJ/mL	kcal/mL	Percent of energy Protein	Fat	Carbohydrate	Comments
FULL LIQUID FORMULAS (continued)							
Isotonic formulas* (continued)							
Isocal	Mead Johnson	4.4	1.06	13	37	50	Lactose-free; low-residue
Isosource	Ross	5.2	1.25	14	30	56	Lactose-free; low-residue; gluten-free
Isotein HN	Sandoz Nutrition	5.0	1.20	23	25	52	Lactose-free; low-residue; gluten-free
Isosource HN	Sandoz Nutrition	5.4	1.28	17	30	53	High-nitrogen; isotonic; lactose-free; gluten-free; low-residue
Osmolite HN	Ross	4.4	1.06	17	31	52	Lactose-free; low-residue
Specialized use formulas							
Amin-Aid Instant Drink	Kendall McGraw	8.2	1.96	4	21	75	Requires vitamin, mineral, and electrolyte supplementation
Attain L.S.	Sherwood Medical	4.2	1.00	16	36	48	Lactose-free; low-residue
Pre-Attain	Sherwood Medical	2.1	0.50	16	36	48	Lactose-free
Hepatic Aid II Instant Drink	Kendall McGraw	4.9	1.18	15	28	57	Requires vitamin, mineral, and electrolyte supplementation
Lonalac	Mead Johnson	4.2	1.00	21	49	30	
Portagen	Mead Johnson	4.2	1.01	14	41	45	Lactose-free
Precision High Nitrogen Diet	Sandoz Nutrition	4.4	1.05	17	1	82	Lactose-free; low-residue; gluten-free
Precision LR Diet	Sandoz Nutrition	4.2	1.10	9	1	90	Lactose-free; low-residue; gluten-free
Pulmocare	Ross	6.3	1.50	17	55	28	Lactose-free
Stresstein	Sandoz Nutrition	5.0	1.20	23	21	56	Lactose-free; no residue
Traum-Aid HBC	Kendall McGraw	4.2	1.00	24	6	70	Lactose-free; low-residue
TraumaCal	Mead Johnson	6.3	1.50	22	40	38	Lactose-free
Travasorb Hepatic	Clinitec Nutrition Co.	4.6	1.10	11	12	77	Low aromatic amino acids
Travasorb Renal	Clinitec Nutrition Co.	5.7	1.35	7	12	81	Requires vitamin, mineral, and electrolyte supplementation
Hydrolyzed protein-elemental formulas*							
Carnation Peptamen Liquid, Isotonic, Complete, Elemental Diet	Clinitec Nutrition Co.	4.2	1.00	16	34	50	Lactose-free
Criticare HN	Mead Johnson	4.4	1.06	14	3	83	Lactose-free; low-residue
Pepti 2000	Sherwood Medical	4.2	1.00	16	9	75	Lactose-free; low-residue
Travasorb HN	Clinitec Nutrition Co.	4.2	1.00	18	12	70	Lactose-free; low-residue
Travasorb STD	Clinitec Nutrition Co.	4.2	1.00	12	12	76	Lactose-free; low-residue
Vital High Nitrogen	Ross	4.2	1.00	17	10	73	Lactose-free; low-residue
Vivonex HN	Norwich Eaton	4.2	1.00	18	1	81	Lactose-free; no residue
Vivonex Standard	Norwich Eaton	4.2	1.00	9	1	90	Lactose-free; no residue
Vivonex T.E.N.	Norwich Eaton	4.2	1.00	15	3	82	Lactose-free; low-residue
HIGH CALORIE SOFT SUPPLEMENTS		kJ/g	kcal/g				
Puddings							
Ensure Pudding	Ross	7.5	1.8	11	35	54	Gluten-free
Sustacal Pudding	Mead Johnson	7.5	1.7	11	36	53	
Forta Pudding	Ross	7.5	1.8	14	32	54	Lactose free

(continued)

after total parenteral nutrition, peripheral hyperalimentation, or enteral feeding by gastrostomy, jejunostomy, esophagostomy, or nasogastric tube. After extended periods of disuse, the gut may not function normally, and unless the transition process is carefully monitored, ad libitum oral intakes and/or food absorption may be inadequate.

ADHERENCE TO DIET Compliance with therapeutic dietary recommendations is relatively easy to monitor if the patient is hospitalized. A menu that conforms to the diet orders is offered and choices are made in line with the therapeutic prescription (and if the choices are not appropriate, substitutes are made). However, the

TABLE 74-8 Nutrient composition of oral nutritional supplements (continued)

	Manufacturer	kJ/g or /mL	kcal/g or /mL	Protein	Fat	Carbohydrate	Comments
					Percent of energy		
MODULAR SYSTEMS (SINGLE NUTRIENT SOURCES)							
Protein nodules							
Casec	Mead Johnson	15.5	3.7	96	4	<1	Powder
Nutrisource Amino Acids	Sandoz Nutrition	16.3	3.9	100	0	0	Powder
Nutrisource Amino Acids -High BCAA	Sandoz Nutrition	15.9	3.8	100	0	0	Powder
Nutrisource Protein	Sandoz Nutrition	16.7	4.0	75	19	6	Powder
Pro Mod	Ross	17.6	4.2	72	19	9	Powder
Propac	Sherwood Medical	16.7	4.0	77	18	5	Powder
RDP	Corpak, Inc.	15.1	3.6	84	10	6	Powder
Fat nodules							
High Fat Supplement	Corpak, Inc.	25.5	6.12	3	70	27	Powder
MCT Oil	Mead Johnson	32.3	7.7	0	100	0	Liquid
Nutrisource Lipid-Long-Chain Triglycerides	Sandoz Nutrition	9.2	2.2	0	100	0	Liquid
Nutrisource Lipid-Medium Chain Triglycerides	Sandoz Nutrition	8.4	2.0	0	100	0	Liquid
Microlipid	Sherwood Medical	18.8	4.5	0	100	0	Liquid
Carbohydrate nodules							
Liquid Carbohydrate Supplement	Corpak, Inc.	10.5	2.5	0	0	100	Liquid
Moducal	Mead Johnson	15.9	3.8	0	0	100	Powder
Nutrisource Carbohydrate	Sandoz Nutrition	13.4	3.2	0	0	100	Liquid
Polycose Powder	Ross	15.9	3.8	0	0	100	Powder
Polycose Liquid	Ross	8.4	2.0	0	0	100	Liquid
Pure Carbohydrate Supplement	Corpak, Inc.	16.7	4.0	0	0	100	Powder
Sumacal	Sherwood Medical	15.9	3.8	0	0	100	Powder
LOW-PROTEIN PRODUCTS		kJ/50 g	kcal/50 g				
Low-protein noodles	Aproten	322	77	1	2	97	
Low-protein cookies	Kingsmill	1046	250	<1	41	59	
Low-protein bread	Dietary Specialties	527	126	2	20	78	
FIBER SUPPLEMENTS		kJ/20 g	kcal/20 g				
Fiber Med	Purdue Frederick Co.	243	70	11	26	63	
Fiberall	Ciba-Geigy Corp.	331	79	5	46	49	

* Definitions: Low-residue = producing little or no stool; isotonic = having the tonicity of plasma (308 mosmol/L); hydrolyzed protein-elemental formula = nutrients partially or completely digested.

SOURCE: Modified from the American Dietetic Association: *Manual of Clinical Dietetics*, 1988.

patient may refuse to eat or may miss meals because of diagnostic tests. Therefore, nutritional status and patient adherence should be monitored carefully even in the hospital.

To implement outpatient therapeutic diets, the patient must be motivated and must understand the diet instructions and the changes in what is to be eaten. New habits of food buying, food preparation, cooking, and eating may be required. Selections when dining out are also altered. These changes are difficult to make and even more difficult to sustain.

Psychological support; assistance in learning new food preparation, buying, and management skills; help with eating (in disabilities such as stroke); help in obtaining financial assistance to buy special foods; and general education about the importance of diet are as important as nutritional advice.

ASSURING THE CONTINUITY OF NUTRITIONAL CARE: THE TEAM CONCEPT Nutrition is too important to be the sole responsibility of a single member of the health team. Nutritional counseling can and does change dietary habits, and each health-care provider has a critical role in assuring that nutrition is adequate. However, physicians rarely obtain thorough diet histories, address potential barriers to change in eating habits, or offer special guidance on food selection. The major role of physicians is to expand the content of the nutritional information they provide, to emphasize the health benefits of good nutrition, and to refer those requiring help to specialized providers when available.

REFERENCES

NATIONAL RESEARCH COUNCIL: *Recommended Dietary Allowances*, 10th ed. Washington, DC, National Academy of Sciences, 1989

OLSON RE et al: *Present Knowledge in Nutrition.* Washington, DC, The Nutrition Foundation, 1984

PAIGE DM: *Clinical Nutrition.* St Louis, 1988

SHILS ME, YOUNG VR: *Modern Nutrition in Health and Disease.* Philadelphia, Lea & Febiger, 1988

SLEISENGER MH, FORDTRAN JS: *Gastrointestinal Disease: Pathophysiology, Diagnosis and Management*, 4th ed. Philadelphia, Saunders, 1988, pp 1971–2023

75 PARENTERAL AND ENTERAL NUTRITION THERAPY

LYN J. HOWARD

Parenteral and enteral nutrition provide life-sustaining therapy for patients who cannot take adequate nutrition by mouth and who consequently are at risk for the debilitating complications of malnutrition. These complications include greater susceptibility to infection and to the consequences of hypomotility (aspiration, pulmonary embolism), delayed recovery from illness and surgery, and an increased likelihood of death.

Although the term *enteral* refers to feeding via the gut and hence includes normal eating, in the present context it refers to the infusion of chemically defined formulas via a tube into the upper gastrointestinal tract. *Parenteral*, which means outside the gut, refers to the infusion of nutrient solutions into the bloodstream. While these approaches to nutritional support are technically different, the goals of therapy are by and large the same, and the techniques are best discussed concurrently. Wherever feasible, enteral nutrition is the preferred therapy because it better preserves immunologic defense mechanisms and is less expensive than parenteral nutrition.

Enteral tube feeding initially involved large-bore rubber tubes placed via the nose or through an ostomy into the stomach or jejunum, but these large tubes have been replaced by small-bore pliable tubes that remain soft with continued exposure to digestive juices. Endoscopic techniques have also been developed for placement of gastrostomy feeding tubes without the need for a surgical laparotomy. For many years, long-term tube feeding was used principally in hospitalized patients with chronic swallowing dysfunction or upper intestinal obstruction, but enteral feeding is now also used in the home setting.

Parenteral nutrition therapy has younger roots. After the life raft studies in the 1940s by Gamble demonstrated that small amounts of glucose (100 g/d) spared protein in fasting subjects, hypocaloric intravenous glucose infusions became routine therapy for hospitalized patients unable to eat. In the 1960s Dudrick and his colleagues demonstrated that it is possible to provide energy, amino acids, minerals, and vitamins via long-term infusion into a central vein catheter adequate to produce positive nitrogen balance and promote wound healing in adults and to support growth and development in infants. Subsequently, total parenteral nutrition became practical in hospitalized patients and in outpatients.

Isotonic amino acid solutions are more effective than isotonic glucose in counteracting negative nitrogen balance in fasting subjects, and the development of high-energy, isotonic intravenous fat solutions made it possible to deliver adequate amino acids and calories via a peripheral vein. However, peripheral veins usually do not withstand these nutrient infusions indefinitely, and long-term support usually requires access to a central vein.

INDICATIONS FOR ASSISTED THERAPY

The principles of nutritional assessment are discussed in Chap. 71. Some criteria used to define moderate and severe malnutrition in hospitalized patients are summarized in Table 75-1. Since none of these measurements is entirely specific for malnutrition, a weighted combination of the individual measurements has been developed, the so-called prognostic nutritional index. This index predicts, with reasonable sensitivity (0.88) and specificity (0.45), patients at risk

for malnutrition-associated complications. Clinical assessment provides a somewhat better combination of sensitivity (0.82) and specificity (0.72). For this purpose the medical history must address recent weight change and the effects of the primary disease on nutritional and functional status, and the physical examination must assess muscle mass and fat, edema, glossitis, and other signs indicative of micronutrient deficiencies. On the basis of this information, the physician categorizes patients as well-nourished, mildly malnourished, or severely malnourished. The inter-observer agreement is high.

In some clinical situations (e.g., the early phase of the extreme short-bowel syndrome, severe hemorrhagic pancreatitis, pseudomembranous colitis, necrotizing enterocolitis, and clinical conditions causing prolonged ileus) parenteral nutrition and bowel rest improve survival (Table 75-2). In other situations, where the need for total bowel rest may not be essential, enteral nutrition or a combination of enteral and limited parenteral nutrition can be successful and perhaps preferable. Disorders in this category include enterocutaneous fistulas, intractable diarrhea of infancy, and the later stages of the extreme short-bowel syndrome.

It is important to demonstrate that nutrition support leads to improved clinical outcome and not just to better nitrogen balance or increased serum albumin. Valid clinical end points include improved survival, fewer complications, or shorter hospital stays.

PERIOPERATIVE PERIOD Perioperative nutrition has a beneficial effect on complications and survival of surgical patients. Studley pointed out in 1936 that mortality rates after surgery for peptic ulcer are greater in patients with severe preoperative weight loss, and subsequent studies have confirmed the association between poor nutrition and poor surgical outcome. In a review of 18 controlled trials, 14 of which involved patient randomization, perioperative parenteral nutrition reduced the relative risk[1] of a major surgical complication, such as wound dehiscence, abscess, prolonged ileus, and sepsis, by a fifth and the relative risk of death by a third. A major complication of parenteral nutrition, including pneumothorax, central vein thrombosis, or sepsis, occurred in 7 percent of this pooled patient sample. In addition preliminary results of a large cooperative Veterans Administration trial indicate that perioperative nutrition also reduces noninfectious complications that relate both to prolonged immobility (pulmonary embolus) and to delayed wound healing in patients with moderate and severe malnutrition. Unfortunately, perioperative parenteral nutrition increased infectious complications, even infections not directly related to the central line. Because of these iatrogenic complications, perioperative nutrition provides medical benefit only to severely malnourished surgical patients.

CANCER Although early nonrandomized studies suggested that significant benefit ensues from parenteral nutritional support of cancer patients, randomized trials have largely shown no clinical benefit,

---

[1]Relative risk is the absolute difference in rate of events in the control group and represents the proportionate reduction in events attributable to perioperative parenteral nutrition.

TABLE 75-1 Quantitative values commonly used to stratify nutritional status

Method of assessment	Moderately malnourished	Severely malnourished
Ideal weight, %	60–80	<60
Creatinine-height index: (24-h urine creatinine) $\dfrac{\text{Actual}}{\text{Ideal for height and sex}} \times 100$ (see Table 71-5)	60–80	<60
Serum albumin, g/L (g/dL)	21–30 (2.1–3.0)	<21 (<2.1)
Serum transferrin, g/L (mg/dL)	1–1.5 (100–150)	<1 (<100)
Total lymphocyte count, 10^6/L (per mm^3)	0.8–1.2 (800–1200)	<0.8 (<800)
Delayed hypersensitivity index*	1	0
Prognostic nutritional index, %†	40–50	>50

* Delayed hypersensitivity index quantitates the amount of induration elicited by skin testing with a common antigen such as *Candida*, trichophyton, or mumps. Induration grade: 0 = <0.5 cm, 1 = 0.5 cm, 2 = 1.0 cm.
† Prognostic nutritional index (PNI) is a weighted combination of four individual measurements: PNI (%) = 158 − 1.66 × albumin (g/L) − 0.78 × triceps skinfold (mm) − 2.0 × transferrin (g/L) − 5.8 × delayed hypersensitivity index (0–2).

TABLE 75-2 Indications for nutritional support

HOSPITALIZED PATIENT	Enteral nutrition (EN)	Parenteral nutrition (PN)
Part of routine care	Protein-energy malnutrition [>10% acute weight loss, serum albumin <35 g/L (<3.5 g/dL)], no intake for >5 days Normal nutritional status but no intake for >10 days Severe dysphagia or anorexia Major full-thickness burns Massive small-bowel resection in combination with PN Low output enterocutaneous fistulas	Massive small bowel resection (>70%) Moderate to severe acute pancreatitis Established or clinically predictable malnutrition when the gastrointestinal tract is not usable for >7 days Necrotizing enterocolitis
Usually helpful	Major trauma Radiation therapy Mild chemotherapy Severe hepatic, renal and chronic pulmonary failure	Severe preoperative malnutrition Major surgery, trauma, including burns, where enteral absorption inadequate High output enterocutaneous fistulas Severe Crohn's disease requiring bowel rest or involving marked growth failure Inflammatory adhesions leading to small-bowel obstruction Hyperemesis gravidarum Intensive chemotherapy resulting in severe diarrhea
Benefit not established	Intensive chemotherapy Immediate postoperative period or poststress period Massive small-bowel resection (>90%) Severe diarrhea Severe bowel hypomotility	Minimal stress and trauma, where well-nourished and gastrointestinal tract expected to recover within 10 days Suspected untreatable disease state
Contraindicated	Complete mechanical or functional bowel obstruction High-output fistulas Severe acute pancreatitis Shock and bowel ischemia Necrotizing enterocolitis Prognosis not warranting nutritional support	Patients who have a functional and usable gastrointestinal tract When dependence on PN is anticipated to be <5 days Urgent operation should not be delayed for PN buildup Proven untreatable disease
HOME PATIENT*		
Usually helpful	Chronic severe dysfunction of swallowing Chronic upper gastrointestinal obstruction Gastrointestinal function insufficient to sustain growth or weight Period of gastrointestinal recovery and adaptation after major resection or severe enteritis	Extreme short-bowel syndrome Severe radiation enteritis Chronic obstruction due to adhesions or dysmotility Severe Crohn's disease Enterocutaneous fistula Congenital bowel dysfunction Hyperemesis gravidarum
Benefit not established	Chronic severe brain damage (vegetative state) Malnutrition of systemic illness such as chronic renal, hepatic, pulmonary disease or AIDS	Disorders of multiple systems including GI tract Neoplasms with bowel obstruction AIDS
Contraindicated	Prognosis not warranting aggressive nutritional support Patient refusing treatment Legal surrogate refusing treatment for an incompetent, terminal patient	Patient without adequate social support to deal with risks of therapy Proven untreatable disease where some meaningful quality of life cannot be sustained

* Includes patients in nursing homes.
SOURCE: Adapted from guidelines published by the American Society for Parenteral Enteral Nutrition, J Parent Enteral Nutr 10:441, 1986, 11:342, 439, 1987.

except in severely malnourished cancer patients undergoing surgery. Parenteral nutrition may enable patients to survive toxic chemotherapy and bone marrow transplantation. In patients undergoing bone marrow transplantation, parenteral and enteral nutrition support are equally effective.

LIVER DISEASE Patients with alcoholic liver disease tend to be chronically malnourished, both because of anorexia and because of the substitution of alcohol for food. Patients with both acute and chronic liver disease also may have decreased branched chain amino acids (BCAA) and elevated aromatic amino acids (AAA) in plasma and brain. In randomized prospective trials in patients with borderline hepatic encephalopathy, BCAA-enriched formulas improve nitrogen balance without precipitating encephalopathy, but only one study was large enough to show improved patient survival. Since the BCAA-enriched formula is expensive, it can only be justified in patients with hepatic failure who cannot tolerate adequate protein from standard enteral or parenteral formulas without developing encephalopathy.

RENAL DISEASE One controlled trial reported improved survival of patients with acute renal failure who received parenteral solutions of essential amino acids and glucose. Subsequent studies have suggested similar benefit from solutions that supply equal amounts of essential and nonessential amino acids.

PULMONARY DISEASE Weight loss in patients with advanced pulmonary disease is usually the consequence of increased work of breathing and of poor food intake. In cystic fibrosis, malnutrition may worsen pulmonary deterioration, and enteral feeding via gastrostomy tubes accelerates growth and stabilizes or improves pulmonary function. The greatest benefit is seen in the younger patients. The criteria for patient selection and the psychological costs of such invasive treatment have not been established. Clinical outcome studies of nutrition support are not available for other types of pulmonary disease.

THE DESIGN OF INDIVIDUAL REGIMENS

FLUID REQUIREMENTS These can be estimated by adding the normal daily requirement (120 mL/kg body weight for infants, 40 mL/kg body weight for adults) to any abnormal loss. If the patient is on parenteral therapy, any enteral intake should be subtracted from

TABLE 75-3 Estimation of daily fluid requirements

NORMAL 70-KG MAN

Intake	Output
Normal: 40 × 70 = 2800 mL/d [derived from oral liquids of 1500 mL, or 7 glasses/cups per day, and solid food providing 1300 mL (1000 mL from water in food, 300 mL from water generated by metabolism of foods)]	Urine: 1900 mL/d Insensible loss: 800 mL/d Stool: 100 mL/d (sweat loss can be up to 2 L/d; for each °C of fever add 200 mL/d)

TUBE ENTERAL PATIENT

55 kg-woman recovering from total gastrectomy for gastric cancer and supported by jejunostomy feedings, taking nothing by mouth or intravenously but experiencing 600 mL of diarrheal losses per day.

Normal requirement, 40 × 55	= 2200 mL/d
Abnormal loss, 600 − 100	= 500 mL/d
Total requirement	= 2700 mL/d

PARENTERAL PATIENT

65 kg-man with a high jejunostomy following massive bowel resection for Crohn's disease with oral intake of 2000 mL/d and jejunostomy loss of 4000 mL/d.

Normal requirement 40 × 65	= 2600 mL/d
Abnormal loss (4000 − 100) minus oral intake (2000)	= 1900 mL/d
Total requirement	= 4500 mL/d

the abnormal loss. For clinical examples see Table 75-3. Since abnormal loss of enteric fluid implies significant mineral losses, extra amounts of these nutrients (Table 75-4) must also be added to any standard parenteral or enteral formula.

ENERGY REQUIREMENTS These may be calculated by indirect calorimetry using a bedside metabolic cart and simultaneously measuring urine urea nitrogen and calculating energy expenditure, the respiratory quotient (RQ), and hence the mixture of fuels the patient is burning (fat, carbohydrate, protein). An RQ of greater than 1 suggests the patient is synthesizing fat and is at risk for hepatic dysfunction due to steatosis. If indirect calorimetry is not available, the patient's basal energy expenditure (BEE) can be calculated using the Harris-Benedict equation.

For women:

$$BEE(kcal/d) = 655.10 + 9.56 \times wt(kg) + 1.85 \times ht(cm) - 4.68 \times age(years)$$

For men:

$$BEE(kcal/d) = 66.47 + 13.75 \times wt(kg) + 5.00 \times ht(cm) - 6.76 \times age(years)$$

TABLE 75-4 Enteric fluid volumes and their sodium, potassium, chloride and bicarbonate content*

	L/d†	Na, mmol/L	K‡, mmol/L	Cl, mmol/L	HCO₃§ mmol/L
Oral intake	2–3				
Enteric secretions					
Saliva	1–2	10	30	10	30
Gastric juice	2	60	9	90	0
Bile	2–3	150	10	90	70
Small bowel	1	100	5	100	20
Colon	Variable	40	100	15	60

* Enteric secretions are also rich in divalent cations (Ca, Mg, Zn, Cu) and their loss is increased by steatorrhea, a high bowel fistula, or prolonged suction.
† Of the 9 L/d of oral and enteric fluid presented to the upper small bowel, normally 50% is absorbed in the jejunum, 40% in the ileum, and 10% in the colon. In short-bowel patients, the colon can absorb greater amounts, up to 3 L/d.
‡ Potassium losses are small except in secretions distal to the ileocecal valve. The colon ion exchange is partly controlled by aldosterone, and Na⁺ depletion increases K⁺ loss in the stool.
§ Bicarbonate losses must be replaced in parenteral solutions as acetate or lactate because of potential precipitation of bicarbonate with ingredients such as calcium.

To the BEE should be added a value of 20 percent of the BEE for patients without significant metabolic stress, 50 percent for patients with marked stress such as sepsis and trauma, and 100 percent for patients with severe stress such as a 40 percent surface burn. A simpler method of estimating energy requirements is to provide 105 kJ/kg (25 kcal/kg) body weight per day for unstressed patients and 126, 146, and 167 kJ/kg (30, 35, and 40 kcal/kg) body weight per day for patients who are mildly, moderately, and severely stressed or malnourished, respectively.

The most desirable balance of carbohydrate to fat in parenteral and enteral solutions is unsettled. There is a relative dependence of wound tissue, white blood cells, and the cerebral and renal cortex on glucose metabolism. The majority of energy is usually supplied as glucose in parenteral solutions and as oligosaccharides and disaccharides in enteral solutions. Parenteral lipid solutions are available as 10% or 20% emulsions of vegetable oils (soybean or safflower oils emulsified into artificial lipoproteins with egg phospholipid and made isotonic with glycerin). Polyunsaturated vegetable oils are used in most enteral formulas since they are better absorbed by the compromised gastrointestinal tract. The fat in parenteral and enteral formulas must supply the essential fatty acid requirement (1 to 2 percent of energy from linoleic and linolenic acid), and the provision of 30 percent of energy as fat may reduce the problems that arise from providing excess carbohydrate (e.g., hepatic steatosis and excess carbon dioxide production). Substitution of ω6 polyunsaturated vegetable fat by ω3 polyunsaturated fish oils may reduce the inflammatory response to burn injury, trauma, and radiation by reducing the synthesis of prostaglandins that may alter the gut mucosal barrier.

PROTEIN OR AMINO ACID REQUIREMENTS The recommended dietary protein allowance of 0.8 g/kg body weight per day is adequate for nonstressed patients (e.g., a patient with a high-grade esophageal stricture or anorexia nervosa). More catabolic patients require 1.2 or 1.5 g/kg body weight per day of protein to induce positive nitrogen balance and reconstitute the normal body mass. In a stable patient the adequacy of protein and energy support can be assessed by a balance study:

$$\text{Protein balance} = \text{protein intake} - \text{protein loss}$$

where protein loss = [24-h urine urea nitrogen (g) + 4] × 6.25, and by documenting healing, restoration of normal body composition, or resumption of longitudinal growth.

In states of disturbed protein utilization, such as renal and hepatic failure, azotemia and abnormal plasma amino acid patterns develop. The use of enteral and parenteral solutions to correct these aberrations is justified only in specific clinical circumstances. (See section on medical effectiveness of nutrition support, above.)

Glutamine is an important fuel for the gastrointestinal tract. The oxidation of one molecule of glutamine produces 30 mmol of ATP, which makes this amino acid almost as rich an energy source as one molecule of glucose. The free amino acid pool of the enterocyte is glutamine rich. Although this amino acid can be synthesized endogenously, it appears to be a relatively essential nutrient in stressed patients. Glutamine is fairly insoluble, and it is present in low concentrations in most enteral solutions. Arginine, carnitine, and certain nucleotides may promote optimal gut repair and function in stressed patients. Enteral nutrition provides the best vehicle for supplying nutrients with special trophic and immune benefit for the gut and also stimulates the secretion of gut hormones such as epidermal growth factor and gastrin.

MINERAL AND VITAMIN REQUIREMENTS (See Table 75-5) The parenteral requirements of some vitamins may be higher than the enteral requirements for several reasons: First, the micronutrients are delivered into the systemic rather than the portal circulation, thereby potentially bypassing the liver and being rapidly excreted by the kidneys. Second, many patients requiring parenteral support have large enteric losses that can result in sodium, potassium, chloride, and bicarbonate wasting (Table 75-4) and also in loss of divalent

TABLE 75-5 Daily enteral (EN) and parenteral (PN) requirements of essential fatty acids, minerals, and vitamins

Nutrient	Daily requirement, adult range	
	EN	PN
Essential fatty acids, % kcal	1–2	± 2–4
Calcium, g	0.8–1.2	0.4
Phosphorus, g	0.8 1.2	0.4
Potassium, g	2–5	4
Sodium, g	1–3	1–2
Chloride, g	2–5	2
Magnesium, g	0.3	0.3
Iron, mg	10	1–2
Zinc, mg	15	3–12
Copper, mg	2–3	0.3–0.5
Iodine, mg	0.15	0.15
Manganese, mg	2–5	2–5
Chromium, mg	0.05–0.2	0.015
Molybdenum, mg	0.15–0.3	0.01–0.5
Selenium, mg	0.05–0.2	.05–0.1
Ascorbic acid, mg	60	100
Thiamine, mg	1.4	3.0
Riboflavin, mg	1–6	3.6
Niacin, mg	18	40
Biotin, μg	60	60
Pantothenic acid, mg	5	15
Pyridoxine, mg	2.0	4.0
Folic acid, μg	400	400
Cobalamin, μg	3.0	5
Vitamin A, μg	1000	1300
Vitamin D, μg	10	5
Vitamin E, mg	8–10	10–15
Vitamin K, μg	70–140	200

cations and vitamins that normally have an enterohepatic circulation such as folate, cobalamin, vitamin D, and perhaps other fat-soluble vitamins. The tubing and delivery bags themselves and exposure to oxygen and light can also absorb and destroy vitamins (particularly vitamin A) before they reach the patient.

PARENTERAL NUTRITION

INFUSION TECHNIQUE AND PATIENT MONITORING Partial and short-term parenteral nutrition can be provided via a peripheral vein if the majority of the energy intake is supplied by isotonic fat solutions, but long-term total parenteral support should be administered via a central vein catheter because hypertonic glucose must be rapidly diluted in a high-flow system. The preferred sites for central vein access and the catheter choices available are summarized in Table 75-6, and typical nutrient contents for a standard daily parenteral formula are given in Table 75-7. The glucose content is increased gradually as the patient demonstrates tolerance of the high glucose load. Appropriate clinical and laboratory monitoring for patients on parenteral nutrition is summarized in Table 75-8.

COMPLICATIONS (See Table 75-9) **Mechanical** The insertion of a central venous catheter should only be done by trained personnel using stringently aseptic techniques. Major mechanical complications include pneumothorax, hemothorax from laceration of the subclavian artery or vein, brachial plexus injury, and malpositioning of the catheter in a cerebral vein, the azygos vein, or in the right ventricle. The correct catheter position must be confirmed by x-ray before the hypertonic nutrient solution is infused. Catheters can subsequently back out of the vein, develop leaks, or become detached from the hub and embolize into the heart or pulmonary artery. Catheter thrombosis may occur, especially if the catheter is used for withdrawing blood samples. Thrombosis of the catheter extending to the central vein is frequently coincident with infection. Thrombosed catheters may be unblocked by urokinase treatment.

Metabolic Early problems, especially in elderly and debilitated patients, include fluid overload producing congestive heart failure

TABLE 75-6 Central vein parenteral nutrition catheters

I Sites of venous access
  A Distal tip of catheter best placed in mid-portion of superior vena cava.
  B Enters venous system via:
    1 Percutaneous stick into the subclavian, external or internal jugular, or anterior cubital vein.
    2 Cutdown site on external jugular (via common facial vein), femoral, axillary, or intercostal vein.
  C All catheters can be tunneled superficially to a distal site, which:
    1 May provide a barrier to skin organisms infecting the line.
    2 Places exit site at convenient place for self care in patients going home.
II Types of catheters
  A Externalized
    1 Single, double, or triple lumen.
      a 2d and 3d channels used for IV medications or drawing of blood.
      b Higher incidence of infectious complications with multiple-lumen catheters.
    2 In home patients, avoids the need to do a nightly needle stick but requires constant aseptic dressing.
    3 Repair kits available if a leak or tear develops in the externalized portion.
  B Subcutaneous port
    1 Involves a small reservoir with an overlying rubber diaphragm that is self-sealing.
    2 Port must be entered by a J-shaped needle.
    3 Not all patients like the daily needle stick.
    4 If line is not in use, the buried port makes taking showers and swimming less hazardous.
III Catheter material
  A Polyvinylchloride, polyethylene, polyurethane, or polytetrafluoroethylene
    1 Advantage:
      a Inherent stiffness allows easy threading into the vein.
    2 Disadvantages:
      a Stiffness allows catheter to be in direct contact with vessel wall, causing thrombosis.
      b Stiffness increases over time, causing kinks or fractures.
  B Silicone rubber
    1 Advantages:
      a Very pliable; less kinking.
      b Less traumatic to vessel wall.
      c Inert, inducing little reaction or adherence.
    2 Disadvantages:
      a Difficult to thread into vein.
      b Falls out more easily owing to nonadherence.
      c Potential for tearing.

and glucose overload leading to osmotic diuresis and, as a result of stimulation of insulin secretion, massive extracellular to intracellular shifts of phosphorus and potassium. Such shifts are most likely in cachectic patients with total body phosphorus and potassium depletion and can result in arrhythmias, cardiopulmonary dysfunction, and neurologic symptoms. To avoid these complications, parenteral nutrition should be begun slowly and monitored carefully. Late metabolic complications include cholestatic liver disease with bile sludging and gallstone formation. The exact cause of the liver disease is not understood but appears to be linked to the lack of enteral stimulation; the disease is less likely if some enteral feeding is maintained. Parenteral nutrition induces hypercalcuria, which can result in negative calcium balance and osteopenia. The hypercalcuria appears to reflect several factors, including the calcuric effect of amino acid infusion and the high fixed acid load. Prior to the advent of synthetic amino acid solutions, many protein hydrolysates were contaminated with aluminum, which blocked bone mineralization. Once patients on long-term parenteral nutrition move from catabolic breakdown to sustained anabolism, deficiencies of micronutrients, such as essential fatty acids, trace minerals, and vitamins, may develop unless they are adequate in the parenteral nutrient solution (see Table 75-5).

Infectious Infection of the access line rarely occurs in the first 72 h, and early fever usually points to some alternative infectious site or other cause of hyperpyrexia. Infection of the access line is likely if the patient defervesces when the infusion rate of the parenteral nutrient is tapered. Positive central line cultures suggest catheter

TABLE 75-7   Standard total parenteral nutrition solution (24 h) for a 70-kg adult

Fluid	3L
Protein (amino acids)	0.2–0.3 g nitrogen per kg
Energy value*	105–165 kJ/kg (25–40 kcal/kg)
Essential fatty acids (lipids)	2% of total energy
Electrolytes	
Sodium	100 mmol
Potassium	100 mmol
Chloride	130 mmol
Acetate/gluconate	90 mmol
Calcium	30 mmol
Magnesium	40 mmol
Phosphorus	300 mg
Trace Elements	
Zinc	5 mg
Copper	1.5 mg
Iodine	120 μg
Selenium	100 μg
Chromium	15 μg
Manganese	2 mg
Vitamins	
Ascorbic acid	100 mg
Thiamine	3 mg
Riboflavin	3.6 mg
Niacin	40 mg
Pantothenic acid	15 mg
Pyridoxine	4 mg
Biotin	60 μg
Folid acid	400 μg
Cobalamin	5 μg
Vitamin A	1300 RE
Vitamin D	10 μg
Vitamin E	15 mg
Vitamin K	200 μg

* Provided principally as dextrose.

sepsis, especially if no other infectious source is identified and if the organism is staphylococcus or a *Candida* species. While removal of the central catheter may allow the patient to clear fungemia spontaneously, antibiotic therapy is usually necessary for bacterial infections. Catheter sepsis is less likely if central vein parenteral nutrition is provided via a single-lumen catheter; triple-lumen catheters, even if frequently replaced over a guidewire, are associated with a two or three times greater incidence of sepsis.

ENTERAL NUTRITION

TUBE PLACEMENT AND PATIENT MONITORING   The different types of enteral tubes, the techniques for inserting them, their clinical uses, and potential problems are outlined in Table 75-10. Available enteral formulas and their nutrient compositions are listed in Table 74-8. Patients on enteral feeding are at risk for some of the same metabolic complications as parenterally fed patients and should receive

TABLE 75-8   Monitoring the patient on total parenteral nutrition

Clinical data checked daily
  Patient's sense of well being, symptoms suggesting fluid overload, high or low blood glucose, electrolyte imbalance, etc.
  Patient's strength as judged by graded activity, getting out of bed, walking, stair climbing.
  Vital signs: temperature, blood pressure, pulse rate, and respiratory rate.
  Fluid balance: weight; fluid input (intravenous +/− enteral) versus fluid output (urine, stool, gastric suction, etc.).
  Delivery equipment for parenteral nutrition: composition of nutrient solution, tubing, pump, filter catheter, dressing (skin checked for local infection at time of dressing change).

Laboratory data	
Urine quantitative glucose	Four times daily
Blood glucose Na^+, K^+, Cl^-, HCO_3^- Blood urea nitrogen	Daily until glucose infusion load and patient stable, then twice weekly
Serum albumin, transferrin Liver function studies Serum creatinine Ca^{2+}, PO_4^{2-}, Mg^{2+} Hb/Ht, WBC	Baseline, then twice weekly
Prothrombin time	Baseline, then weekly
Micronutrient tests as indicated	

the same clinical and laboratory monitoring (Table 75-8). Since small-bore tubes are easily displaced, tube position should be tested by aspirating and measuring the pH of the gut fluid (<4 in stomach, >6 in jejunum). A generic description of the types of tubes required for different enteral formulas is given in Table 75-11.

COMPLICATIONS   Aspiration   The debilitated patient with poor gastric emptying and an impaired swallow and cough mechanism is at risk for aspiration. In patients on respirators, effective tracheal suctioning induces coughing and provokes gastric regurgitation, and the cuff on the endotracheal tube or tracheostomy seldom provides adequate protection against aspiration. Under these circumstances, it may be safer to use a large-bore rubber feeding tube, rather than a fine-bore soft collapsible tube, to allow for an accurate check of residual gastric contents and, if necessary, temporary removal of gastric contents prior to tracheal suction.

Although normal gastric motility provides a churning and fragmenting activity with intermittent propulsion of liquid and small food fragments into the duodenum, constant gastric infusion of an enteral formula is better tolerated in sick patients than is intermittent bolus feeding. A continuous infusion is best achieved with an enteral feeding pump, especially when using fine-bore feeding tubes that have a greater potential to clog. If long-term gastric feeding is anticipated, endoscopic, radiologic, or surgical placement of a gastric tube is preferable.

A nasojejunal tube reduces the risk of aspiration, but placement

TABLE 75-9   Complications of total parenteral nutrition (PN)

	First 48 h	First 2 weeks	After 3 months

Mechanical	Complications from catheter insertion:
	  Cephalad displacement
	  Pneumothorax
	  Hemothorax
	Detachment of line at catheter hub with blood loss or air embolism
		Catheter coming out vein more common if Silastic
		Detachment of line at catheter hub with blood loss or air embolism
			Detachment of line at catheter hub with blood loss or air embolism
			Fractures or tears in catheter

Metabolic	Fluid overload Hyperglycemia Hypophosphatemia Hypokalemia	Cardiopulmonary failure Hyperosmolar nonketotic hyperglycemic coma Acid-base imbalance Electrolyte imbalance	Essential fatty acid deficiency Zinc, copper, chromium, selenium, molybdenum deficiency Iron deficiency Vitamin deficiencies Refeeding edema PN metabolic bone disease PN liver disease
Infectious		Catheter-induced sepsis	Catheter-induced sepsis Tunnel infections

TABLE 75-10   Enteral feeding tubes

Type of tube	Placement technique	Clinical uses	Potential problems
Nasogastric	External measurement: nostril, ear to xiphisternum. Placed by professional or, with instruction, by family member or patient. Tube stiffened by ice water or a stylet. Position tested by injecting air and auscultating air bubble passing through fluid, or by aspirating acid gastric contents.	Short-term clinical situations (a few weeks). Placement can be intermittent. Normal gastric emptying required. Bolus feeds or continuous drip.	Aspiration pneumonia from regurgitated stomach contents. Irritation of nasopharynx or esophagogastric junction with bleeding and/or stricture.
Nasoduodenal or nasojejunal	External measurement: nostril, ear to anterior superior iliac spine in adults; to the medial malleolus in infants. Weighted tube may pass spontaneously through pylorus if patient lies on right side; or tube is placed with stiffening stylet under fluoroscopy. Position tested by aspirating alkaline duodenal contents or checking by x-ray.	Short-term clinical situations. Used if gastric emptying is impaired or to infuse beyond a high bowel fistula such as an esophageal tear or gastric or duodenal fistula.	Passing tube through pylorus. Preventing the spontaneous pulling back into stomach. Continuous drip required and tends to cause diarrhea. Tubes stiffen with time, can lacerate pylorus or gastroesophageal junction if pulled out rapidly.
Pharyngostomy/esophagostomy	Tube placed surgically through side of neck into pharynx.	Long-term access. No nasopharyngeal irritation. Once tract is established, tubes can be replaced.	Aspiration if tube in stomach. Pharyngeal scarring causes distortion of normal anatomy.
Gastrostomy	Tube placed through the abdominal wall into the stomach, either by a percutaneous endoscopic technique using local anesthetic or surgically via an abdominal incision using a spinal or general anesthetic.	Long-term access. Once tract is established, tubes can be replaced. Used when swallowing is impaired because of either mechanical obstruction or neurologic discoordination.	Irritation around tube site. Aspiration of stomach contents. Displacement of tube into peritoneal cavity or, if held in situ by balloon, obstruction of the pylorus.
Jejunostomy	Tube placed surgically through abdominal wall into proximal loop of jejunum and tethered to anterior wall by suture. Fine-bore tube inserted by diagonal tract into bowel lumen or large bore secured with an anchoring suture.	Long-term access. Used for defective gastric emptying. Fine-bore tube recommended as postoperative backup when prolonged gastric atony might occur.	Irritation at tube exit site, especially with large-bore tube. Clogging or displacement of tube. Continuous drip usually required. Diarrhea common.
Combined gastrojejunostomy	Tube placed surgically with jejunal arm threaded beyond the pylorus.	Allows for simultaneous gastric suction and jejunal infusion. Used in patient particularly at risk for aspiration of gastric contents.	Not yet widely available.

TABLE 75-11   Types of enteral feeding formulas

Formula category	Description	Clinical indications	Tube of choice	Comments
Blenderized	Mixture of pureed meat, fruit, vegetables, sometimes added nonfat milk, fiber, vitamins, and minerals; highly viscous	Normal digestion and absorption required; used with pharyngostomy, cervical esophagostomy, or gastrostomy tubes	Large-bore (12–18 French)	Lowest cost; 2 or more liters daily; bolus feed
Polymeric	Mixture of whole proteins, polysaccharides, and triglycerides; contains no fiber; lower viscosity than blenderized formulas	Normal digestion and absorption required; can be fed into esophagus, stomach, duodenum or jejunum	Small-bore (8–10 French)	2 or more liters needed daily; bolus, gravity, or pump feed
Monomeric	Mixture of predigested protein, carbohydrate (CHO), and a small amount of triglyceride; contains no fiber; has lowest viscosity of all formulas	Used for inflammatory bowel disease, chronic pancreatitis, GI fistula, enteritis from radiation or chemotherapy, panmalabsorption, or as a transition feeding from parenteral to enteral therapy	Small-bore (5–6 French)	Higher cost than polymeric formulas; 1.5–3 liters needed daily; pump feed
Disease-related	Devised to meet the nutritional needs of specific disease states; varying amounts of protein, amino acid ratios, CHO, and electrolytes; low viscosity.	Used for renal failure, hepatic encephalopathy, stress, trauma, and respiratory failure	Small-bore (5–6 French)	Highest cost; 2 liters or more needed daily; gravity or pump feed
Modular	Made-to-order feedings of individual constituents; viscosity depends on quantities of protein, CHO, and fat	Used for specific metabolic abnormalities, such as glycogen storage disease	Varies, depending on viscosity	Higher cost than monomeric formula; 1.5 or more liters needed daily; bolus, gravity, or pump feed

of such tubes through the pylorus is time-consuming, and such tubes frequently pull back into the stomach. If a debilitated patient with poor gastric emptying goes to surgery, it is appropriate to ask the surgeon to place a jejunostomy tube for feeding. This can involve a traditional rubber tube (12 to 14 French) or a fine-bore (5 to 8 French) tube inserted through an oblique needle track that seals rapidly when the jejunostomy tube is removed.

Diarrhea Enteral feeding often causes diarrhea, especially if absorption is compromised by bowel disease or drugs such as antibiotics. The diarrhea may be controlled by the use of continuous drip or administration of enteral bulking agents, such as psyllium hydrophilic mucilogs or an anticholinergic medication, in the formula. Diarrhea, stimulated by enteral feeding, does not necessarily imply inadequate absorption. Furthermore, since luminal nutrients induce trophic effects on the gut mucosa and stimulate the enteric immunologic barrier, it may be appropriate to persist despite the diarrhea, even when this necessitates temporary supplemental parenteral support.

OVERALL IMPACT OF NUTRITION SUPPORT

In 1986 about 1.5 million patients in the United States received parenteral and enteral nutrition at a cost of about 5 billion dollars, thus accounting for about 1 percent of health-care costs.

HOSPITAL SETTING Most nutrition support is for hospitalized patients, predominantly for patients whose length of stay is four times the average hospital stay and who are high users of other life-sustaining therapies (ventilators, kidney dialysis, intensive care units, cardiac monitoring). Such patients are typically referred from smaller hospitals to tertiary care centers. Perioperative parenteral nutrition is cost-effective for surgical patients who are severely malnourished preoperatively and for well-nourished patients in whom surgery results in ileus of 10 days duration or more. The costs and complications of parenteral nutrition can be reduced if patient management is supervised by a nutrition support service. In one study, catheter sepsis decreased from 28.6 percent to 4.7 percent after such a service was instituted, and in another study routine consultations with a nutrition support service resulted in a 20 percent reduction in average hospital stay and a 26 percent average reduction in costs per patient receiving parenteral nutrition.

NON-HOSPITAL SETTING In patients with benign causes of extreme short-bowel syndrome, home parenteral nutrition therapy is associated with low morbidity and high rates of good rehabilitation. For example, in patients with Crohn's disease on home parenteral nutrition, complete or partial rehabilitation was achieved in 97 percent, the mortality was only 3 percent per year, and the rehospitalization rate was only 1 percent per year. Home parenteral nutrition costs about half as much as similar treatment in hospital.

ETHICAL ASPECTS OF NUTRITIONAL SUPPORT As with all other forms of therapy, nutrition support is contraindicated if the risks exceed the potential benefit, and the consent of the patient or the legal surrogate is required. Because artificially supplied nutrition can protract the terminal phase of many illnesses, withholding or withdrawing nutrition support can be a major ethical and legal problem, especially in incompetent and institutionalized patients.

REFERENCES

ABEL RM et al: Improved survival from acute renal failure after treatment with intravenous essential L. amino acids and glucose. N Engl J Med 288:695, 1973

ALEXANDER WJ et al: The importance of lipid type in the diet after burn injury. Ann Surg 240:1, 1986

ANDERSON GF, STEINBERG EP: DRG's and specialized nutritional support: The need for reform. J Parent Enteral Nutr 10:3, 1986

BLACKBURN GL et al: Peripheral intravenous feeding with isotonic aminoacid solutions. Am J Surg 125:447, 1973

CERRA FB et al: Disease-specific amino acid infusion (F080) in hepatic encephalopathy. A prospective randomized, double blind controlled trial. J Parent Enteral Nutr 9:288, 1985

DETSKY AS et al: Evaluating the accuracy of nutritional assessment techniques applied to hospitalized patients: Methodology and comparisons. J Parent Enteral Nutr 8:153, 1984

———: A cost-effective analysis of the home parenteral nutrition program at Toronto General: 1970–1982. J Parent Enteral Nutr 10:49, 1986

———: Perioperative parenteral nutrition: A Meta analysis. Ann Intern Med 107:195, 1987

DUDRICK SJ et al: Long-term total parenteral nutrition with growth, development and positive nitrogen balance. Surgery 64:134, 1968

FOX AD et al: Effect of glutamine-supplemented enteral diet on methotrexate-induced enterocolitis. J Parent Enteral Nutr 12:325, 1988

HOWARD L et al: Vitamin A deficiency: A complication of long-term parenteral nutrition. Ann Intern Med 93:576, 1980

ISSELL BF et al: Protection against chemotherapy by IV hyperalimentation. Cancer Treat Rep 62:1139, 1978

OASIS Home Nutrition Support Patient Registry, Annual Report, 1986 Data. Oley Foundation, Albany Medical College, Albany, NY, 1986

SHILS ME et al: Long-term parenteral nutrition through an external arteriovenous shunt. N Engl J Med 283:341, 1970

STUDLEY HO: Percentage of weight loss. JAMA 106:458, 1936

SZELUGA DJ et al: Nutritional support of bone marrow transplant recipients: A prospective randomized clinical trial comparing total parenteral nutrition to an enteral feeding program. Cancer Res 47:3309, 1987

WEINSIER RL et al: Cost containment: A contribution of aggressive nutritional support in burn patients. J Burn Care Rehabil 6:436, 1985

WEISDORF S et al: Influence of prophylactic total parenteral nutrition on long-term outcome of bone marrow transplantation. Transplantation 43:833, 1987

76   VITAMIN DEFICIENCY AND EXCESS[1]

JEAN D. WILSON

Vitamins play several roles in human disease. Deficiencies of single vitamins are now rarely endemic, even in developing nations, and are more likely to occur either as a portion of states of general malnutrition, as a result of food faddism, as a complication of more widespread disease such as malabsorption, as a complication of complex therapy such as hemodialysis or total parenteral nutrition, or as the result of an inborn error of metabolism. Indeed, disorders of vitamin excess may now be more common than vitamin deficiency.

In considering the pathophysiology of vitamins several points are worth emphasis. (1) The fact that organic compounds cannot be synthesized within the body and are required constituents of the diet is the result of mutations, and the provision of vitamins in the diet is a form of therapy for an inborn error of metabolism. In some instances, such as the limited ability to synthesize thiamine, the requirement is common to many if not all animals, and the mutation must have occurred early in evolution; in others, such as the single-gene defect that prevents ascorbic acid synthesis, humans share the defect with only a few other species, such as the guinea pig. (2) The feature that separates vitamins from other necessary organic constituents in the diet is that small amounts of them are required, in contrast to the relatively large amounts of essential amino acids and essential fatty acids. This is a consequence of the fact that vitamins function not as building blocks of tissue mass or as substrates for energy production but rather as prosthetic groups for quantitatively minor tissue constituents or as catalytic cofactors for biologic reactions; like most catalysts they are required only in small amounts. (3) Deficiency of some vitamins has never been described in humans (e.g., pantothenic acid) implying that these vitamins are either so ubiquitous in food sources or are conserved so efficiently by the body that deficiency can become manifest, if at all, only in the context of a mixed nutritional and vitamin deficiency. (4) Alcoholism is the background upon which many vitamin deficiencies develop in the United States. This is the consequence of several interlocking factors including diminished intake, impairment of absorption and storage of vitamins, and, in some cases, predisposing genetic factors. (5) Biochemical means of proving vitamin deficiency, once suspected,

---

[1] For vitamin D, see Chap. 341 and for the hematologic vitamins, see Chap. 292.

are limited, and the role of vitamin deficiency in disease states is frequently not recognized because nonspecific vitamin therapy is a common part of standard supportive care. As a consequence, recognition of the manifestations of vitamin deficiency and a high index of suspicion in the appropriate clinical setting are essential for considering the diagnosis, and demonstration of a response to replacement therapy may be the most accurate way to confirm a diagnosis. (6) The consumption of excessive amounts of vitamins can occur either as the indirect consequence of dietary practice or, more commonly, as the result of deliberate ingestion. Syndromes of excess for the fat-soluble vitamins A and D are well characterized, whereas the toxicity syndromes produced by the water-soluble vitamins are inconsistent and less well understood.

DEFICIENCY STATES

NIACIN (PELLAGRA) **Biochemistry** *Niacin* is the generic term for nicotinic acid (3-pyridinecarboxylic acid) and derivatives that exhibit the nutritional activity of nicotinic acid (Fig. 76-1). In one sense niacin is not a vitamin since it can be formed from the essential amino acid tryptophan. In the human an average of about 1 mg of niacin is formed from 60 mg of dietary tryptophan. Accordingly, estimates of the adequacy of dietary intake must take into account the tryptophan content of the diet as well as the content of niacin. Many foodstuffs, especially cereals, contain bound forms of niacin from which the vitamin is not nutritionally available.

The absorption, tissue distribution, and metabolism of the vitamin are poorly understood. Approximately one-fifth of the vitamin is decarboxylated to nicotinuric acid, and the remainder is excreted in the urine as methylated products, largely *N*-methylnicotinamide and *N*-methyl-2-pyridone-5-carboxamide.

Mechanism of action Niacin is an essential component of nicotinamide adenine dinucleotide (NAD) and nicotinamide adenine dinucleotide phosphate (NADP), coenzymes for many oxidation-reduction reactions.

Requirements The requirements and recommended daily allowances for niacin and tryptophan are listed in Table 70-1. In contrast to most vitamins, the requirement for niacin does not appear to be increased during pregnancy. Requirement is primarily determined by the amino acid composition of the diet.

FIGURE 76-1 The structure and principal functions of some of the vitamins associated with human disorders.

Vitamin	Active Derivative or Cofactor Form	Principal Function
Niacin	Nicotinamide Adenine Dinucleotide Phosphate (NADP) and Nicotine Adenine Dinucleotide (NAD)	Coenzymes for Oxidations and Reductions
Thiamine	Thiamine Diphosphate	Coenzyme for Cleavage of Carbon-Carbon Bonds
Pyridoxine	Pyridoxal Phosphate	Cofactor for Enzymes of Amino Acid Metabolism
Riboflavin	Flavin Mononucleotide (FMN) and Flavin Adenine Dinucleotide (FAD)	Cofactor for Oxidation-Reduction Reactions and Covalently Attached Prosthetic Groups for Some Enzymes
Ascorbic Acid	Ascorbic Acid and Dehydroascorbic Acid	Participation as a Redox Ion in Many Biological Oxidation Reactions
Vitamin A	Retinol, Retinal, and Retinoic Acid	Formation of Carotenoid Proteins (Vision) and Glycoproteins (Epithelial Cell Function)
Vitamin E	Tocopherol	Antioxidant
Vitamin K	Menaquinone	Cofactor for Post-Translational Carboxylation of Many Proteins Including Essential Clotting Factors

Experimental depletion   After the institution of a diet deficient in niacin and tryptophan, the urinary excretion of niacin metabolites reaches minimal values (<1.5 mg/d) after 1 to 2 months and remains constant thereafter. Clinical deficiency develops shortly after excretion becomes stable at a low level and consists of dermatitis, glossitis, stomatitis, diarrhea, proctitis, mental depression, abdominal pain, vaginitis, dysphagia, and amenorrhea, findings similar to those in pellagra.

Clinical deficiency   Pellagra was previously an endemic disease in the American south and in many other parts of the world. The endemic disease is usually associated with a high intake of maize (American corn) or of millet (sorghum; jowar) and can be cured by the administration of niacin; nevertheless, the fact that large populations of people exist on a diet in which maize is the major source of protein but nevertheless are free of endemic pellagra implies that the relation between maize intake and the development of the disease is not straightforward. As a consequence, the concept of the pathogenesis of pellagra has evolved from that of a pure vitamin deficiency or a mixed deficiency of tryptophan and available niacin in the diet to a more complicated etiology. The disorder may be due to an imbalance in dietary amino acids or to a complex vitamin deficiency; the niacin equivalent (available niacin and tryptophan) of maize, although low, is no lower than that of some cereals that are unassociated with endemic pellagra. An alternative possibility is that the milling of maize influences the bioavailability of the niacin in the cereal. Treatment of maize with alkali in the preparation of foods in Latin America may serve to hydrolyze bound nicotinic acid and to inactivate toxins that may accumulate in stored grain contaminated with molds. Alternatively, degermination of the cereal during the common milling process in the United States may inhibit the liberation of bound niacin. The effect of these treatments, respectively, would be to prevent or to predispose to the development of pellagra when maize is a major element of the diet.

Whatever the cause, endemic pellagra disappeared coincident with the improvement of nutritional education and with the widespread supplementation of grain cereals with niacin. At present, pellagra is an occasional secondary manifestation of two disorders that profoundly affect tryptophan metabolism, the carcinoid syndrome, in which up to 60 percent of tryptophan is catabolized by what is ordinarily a minor pathway of metabolism (see Chap. 262), and Hartnup disease (see Chap. 335), an inherited disorder in which several amino acids including tryptophan are absorbed poorly from the diet. In both conditions pellagra is due to diminished availability of effective niacin equivalents and can be cured by the administration of large amounts of the vitamin.

Pellagra is a chronic wasting disease typically associated with dermatitis, dementia, and diarrhea. The dermatitis is bilateral, symmetric, and present in sites exposed to sunlight, and is due to photosensitivity. The mental changes are less discrete; fatigue, insomnia, and apathy may precede the development of an encephalopathy characterized by confusion, disorientation, hallucination, loss of memory, and eventually, frank organic psychosis. Paresthesias and polyneuritis may be the result of coexisting deficiencies of other vitamins. Diarrhea, when present, results from widespread inflammation of the mucous surfaces; other mucosal abnormalities include achlorhydria, glossitis, stomatitis, and vaginitis. The course is progressive over a several-year period, and death is usually due to secondary complications.

The relation between the known coenzyme function of NAD and NADP and these various symptoms has not been defined. Levels of NAD and NADP in erythrocytes are lower in patients with pellagra than in normal individuals, but the coenzymes are essential to so many reactions in intermediary metabolism that profound deficiency of the coenzymes is incompatible with life. The mental changes in pellagra may be associated with diminished conversion of tryptophan to serotonin.

No biochemical test is of diagnostic value, and diagnosis must be based upon suspicion and response to replacement therapy. As predicted, excretion in the urine of the metabolites of nicotinic acid and tryptophan is lower than average but not lower than in patients with generalized malnutrition. Plasma tryptophan and erythrocyte NAD and NADP levels are also low. The skin lesions are characterized by hyperkeratosis, hyperpigmentation, and desquamation.

The administration of small amounts of niacin (10 mg/d) in the face of adequate amounts of dietary tryptophan is sufficient to cure endemic pellagra. Large amounts of niacin (40 to 200 mg/d) may be required in Hartnup disease and in the carcinoid syndrome.

THIAMINE (BERIBERI)   Biochemistry   Thiamine contains pyrimidine and thiazole moieties linked by a methylene bridge (Fig. 76-1). The vitamin is synthesized by a variety of plants and microorganisms but not ordinarily by animals. However, rats and pigeons fed a thiamine-free diet can be protected from deficiency by large quantities of the pyrimidine and thiazole moieties, suggesting a small capacity to couple the subunits together. Small amounts of the vitamin may be synthesized by microorganisms in the gastrointestinal tract. Thiamine is absorbed both by an active-transport process and by passive diffusion. The capacity to absorb the vitamin in the human intestine is about 5 mg/d. Approximately 25 to 30 mg is stored in the body, 80 percent as thiamine diphosphate (pyrophosphate), 10 percent as thiamine triphosphate, and the remainder as thiamine monophosphate. Large amounts are present in skeletal muscles (about one-half of body stores), heart, liver, kidneys, and brain. A number of thiaminase enzymes inactivate thiamine by splitting the vitamin into its two component parts. Several metabolites are excreted in the urine, principally thiamine itself (which is secreted by the renal tubules), an acetylated derivative, and end products of thiamine catabolism, mainly derivatives of thiazole acetate and pyrimidine carboxylate.

Mechanism of action   Thiamine diphosphate acts as a coenzyme for several reactions that cleave carbon-carbon bonds—the oxidative decarboxylation of α-keto acids (pyruvate and α-ketoglutarate) and keto analogues of leucine, isoleucine, and valine, and the transketolase reaction in the pentose phosphate pathway. Many features of thiamine deficiency are the result of inhibition of these enzymatic reactions and/or the accumulation of the proximal metabolites. Thiamine may also have a specific role in neurons independent of its coenzymatic function in general metabolism; thiamine and its esters are present in axonal membranes, and electrical stimulation of nerves effects the hydrolysis and release of thiamine diphosphate and triphosphate.

Requirements   The recommended daily allowances for thiamine are given in Table 70-1. The vitamin has a widespread distribution in food and is absent only from oils, fats, cassava, and refined sugar. In vegetable products the vitamin is largely in the form of thiamine. The outer layers of cereal grains are especially rich in the vitamin; hence, machine-milled rice is a poor source. In animal tissues thiamine is present largely in the form of phosphate esters. The esters are dephosphorylated by phosphatases in the intestine, and only the free vitamin is absorbed. A substantial loss of the vitamin takes place during cooking above 100°C.

Several factors influence the absorption and metabolism of the vitamin (and hence alter daily requirements). One is the presence of thiaminases in foods such as fresh fish, clams, shrimp, mussels, and some raw animal tissues and in microorganisms in the colon. Two, daily needs decrease when fat forms a large part of the diet and increase as carbohydrate intake increases. Requirements are increased in pregnancy, during lactation, in thyrotoxicosis, and by fever. Accelerated loss of thiamine from the body may occur with diuretic therapy, hemodialysis, peritoneal dialysis, and diarrhea. Defective intestinal absorption can occur in malabsorption states, alcoholism, chronic malnutrition, and folate deficiency.

Experimental depletion   Following the institution of a thiamine-free diet in control subjects, thiamine excretion in the urine decreases to 5 percent of the control value after a week and becomes undetectable after 2 weeks. However, the excretion of the pyrimidine and thiazole catabolites of thiamine remains unchanged for as long as a month, indicating that the body pool is slowly utilized during a period of deficient intake.

Within a week after the institution of a deficient diet, subjects develop a resting tachycardia, followed by the onset of weakness, decreased deep tendon reflexes, and (in some) a sensory neuropathy. Subjective symptoms include generalized malaise, headache, nausea, and aching of the muscles. Appearance of these symptoms is paralleled by a fall in red blood cell transketolase activity. Within a week of thiamine repletion (2 mg/d) all abnormal physical findings disappear, and the subjective symptoms clear after 2 weeks. (Experimental depletion in humans has not been carried to the point of development of severe cerebral or cardiovascular symptoms.)

Clinical deficiency In developed nations thiamine deficiency occurs in alcoholics or food faddists or in the context of special clinical situations, such as chronic peritoneal dialysis, hemodialysis, refeeding after starvation, or after the administration of glucose to asymptomatic but thiamine-depleted patients. In developing countries the disorder is commonly due to the consumption of milled rice or foods containing thiaminases or (possibly) other antithiamine factors.

Development of thiamine deficiency in chronic alcoholics is due to low thiamine intake, impaired thiamine absorption and storage, accelerated destruction of thiamine diphosphate, and varying degrees of energy expenditure. However, clinical manifestations develop in only a fraction of alcoholics and other chronically malnourished persons. Genetic factors may be involved in susceptibility.

The two major manifestations of thiamine deficiency involve the cardiovascular (wet beriberi) and nervous systems (dry beriberi and the Wernicke-Korsakoff syndrome). The typical patient has mixed symptoms involving both the cardiovascular and nervous systems, but pure cardiovascular, pure neuropathic, and pure cerebral forms also occur. The factors that determine the relative preponderance of these manifestations are related in part to the duration and severity of the deficiency, the degree of physical exertion, and the caloric intake. Severe physical exertion, high carbohydrate intake, and a moderate degree of chronic deficiency favor wet beriberi with little or no peripheral neuritis, whereas an equal deficiency with caloric restriction and relative inactivity favors the development of dry beriberi.

Beriberi heart disease comprises three major physiologic derangements: (1) peripheral vasodilatation leading to a high-output state, (2) biventricular myocardial failure, and (3) retention of sodium and water leading to edema. In the chronic form peripheral vasodilatation leads to increased arteriovenous shunting of blood, rapid circulation time, tachycardia, increased cardiac output, and a venous congestive state characterized by elevated peripheral venous pressure, elevated right ventricular end-diastolic pressure, decreased arteriovenous extraction of oxygen, sodium retention, and edema. Disordered blood flow (decreased cerebral and renal blood flow and increased flow to muscles) is common. Cardiac output increases so that notwithstanding the lowered peripheral vascular resistance ventricular work, arterial blood pressure, and pulmonary wedge pressure tend to be elevated. Temporary appearance or worsening of hypertension may occur during thiamine repletion, presumably due to closing of arteriovenous shunts and temporary volume overload.

In acute fulminant cardiovascular (shoshin) beriberi, the myocardial lesion is the central feature of a course in which severe dyspnea, restlessness, and anxiety eventuate in acute cardiovascular collapse and death within hours to days. Physical findings include stocking-glove cyanosis, extreme tachycardia, marked cardiomegaly, hepatomegaly, arterial bruits, and neck vein distention. The venous pressure is high, and the circulation time is rapid. Because of the fulminant course edema may be minimal or absent. Administration of thiamine rapidly restores peripheral vascular resistance, but improvement in the myocardial abnormality may be delayed so that low-output failure supervenes during treatment.

Three types of nervous system involvement occur: peripheral neuropathy, Wernicke's encephalopathy (cerebral beriberi), and the Korsakoff syndrome. The neuropathy may or may not be painful and

is characterized by a symmetric impairment of sensory, motor, and reflex function that affects the distal segments of limbs more severely than the proximal ones. The histologic lesion is a noninflammatory degeneration of myelin sheaths. No meaningful distinction can be made between this disorder and so-called alcoholic neuropathy on the basis of either clinical or neurologic criteria.

Wernicke's encephalopathy ordinarily develops in an orderly sequence and consists of vomiting, nystagmus (horizontal more commonly than vertical), palsies of the rectus muscles leading to unilateral or bilateral ophthalmoplegia (and decrease in the nystagmus), fever, ataxia, and progressive mental deterioration that eventuates in a global confusional state and may progress to coma and death. Improvement occurs after thiamine replacement, although Korsakoff's syndrome may supervene. Thus, the eye palsies are corrected, the nystagmus improves in one-half, the ataxia improves or disappears in two-thirds, and the global confusional state disappears to be replaced by Korsakoff's syndrome. The latter consists of retrograde amnesia, impaired ability to learn, and (usually) confabulation. The patient is typically alert and responsive and exhibits no serious defect in behavior. Recovery (complete or partial) from Korsakoff's syndrome can be expected only in one-half.

In summary, Wernicke's encephalopathy and the amnesic psychosis of Korsakoff's syndrome are not separate clinical events; instead, the changing ocular and ataxic signs, the transformation of the global confusional state into the amnesic-confabulatory syndrome, and the development of a nonconfabulatory amnesic state are successive stages in the recovery from a single process. The clinical features, differential diagnosis, course, and pathology of cerebral beriberi are discussed in detail in Chap. 357.

Various biochemical tests to detect thiamine deficiency include the measurement of blood thiamine, pyruvate, α-ketoglutarate, lactate, and glyoxylate; measurement of the urinary excretion of thiamine and thiamine metabolites; a thiamine-loading test; and measurement of urinary methylglyoxal. The most reliable is the measurement of whole-blood or erythrocyte transketolase activity. Any enhancement in enzymatic activity resulting from added thiamine diphosphate (TPP) is referred to as the TPP effect (expressed in percent). If the activity of the enzyme is increased more than 15 percent by the added thiamine diphosphate, then a deficiency state is probably present. Due to variability in activity, measurement of isolated transketolase levels is not useful, but demonstration of an increase in activity after treatment coupled with a significant stimulation in vitro by added thiamine diphosphate prior to treatment suggests the presence of thiamine deficiency.

Another criterion for the diagnosis is the assessment of clinical response to thiamine administration. Clinical improvement may be dramatic in cardiovascular beriberi, and an increase in blood pressure and decrease in heart rate may be seen within 12 h after start of therapy. Diuresis and reduction in heart size may be apparent within 1 to 2 days.

Prompt administration of thiamine is indicated when beriberi is diagnosed or suspected. Fifty milligrams per day should be given intramuscularly for several days after which 2.5 to 5 mg/d can be administered by mouth. Larger amounts are usually not absorbed. All patients should also receive other water-soluble vitamins in therapeutic quantities.

Thiamine-responsive inborn errors of metabolism A number of thiamine-responsive inborn errors of metabolism have been described in which patients respond to pharmacologic doses of thiamine. These include thiamine-responsive megaloblastic anemia, for which the mechanism is unknown; thiamine-responsive lactic acidosis, which is due to low activity of pyruvate carboxylase in liver; thiamine-responsive branched-chain ketoaciduria, which is due to low activity of a ketoacid dehydrogenase; and intermittent cerebellar ataxia which may result from an abnormal pyruvate dehydrogenase. In addition, the autosomal recessive disorder subacute necrotizing encephalomyelopathy (Leigh's disease) may be related to a diminished amount of thiamine triphosphate in neural tissue; a factor has been isolated from the urine of such patients that inhibits the enzyme that synthesizes thiamine triphosphate. The clinical response of patients with Leigh's disease to pharmacologic doses of the vitamin appears to be minor, however.

PYRIDOXINE (VITAMIN B₆) **Biochemistry** The biologic activity of the vitamin B_6 group is displayed by pyridoxine, pyridoxal, and pyridoxamine and their 5-phosphate esters (Fig. 76-1). The coenzyme form is pyridoxal-5-phosphate, and the other compounds owe their activity to conversion to pyridoxal-5-phosphate. The vitamin is widely and uniformly distributed in all foods; muscle meats, liver, vegetables, and whole-grain cereals are among the best sources.

Mechanism of action Pyridoxal phosphate acts as a cofactor for many enzymes involved in amino acid metabolism, including transaminases, synthetases, and hydroxylases. In humans the vitamin is of particular importance in the metabolism of tryptophan, glycine, serine, glutamate, and the sulfur-containing amino acids. Pyridoxal phosphate is also required for the synthesis of the heme precursor δ-aminolevulinic acid. A large portion of body stores of pyridoxine is in muscle phosphorylase, where it functions to stabilize the enzyme rather than as a catalyst. It also plays a poorly understood role in neuronal excitability, possibly as a result of its function in transsulfuration reactions or in γ-aminobutyric acid metabolism.

Requirements The recommended daily allowances are given in Table 70-1. Even more than for most vitamins, the requirement is increased in pregnancy and by the administration of estrogens. In both conditions the pattern of excretion of tryptophan metabolites in urine changes, and this can be prevented by supplementation with pyridoxine. Estrogens appear to inhibit the role of pyridoxal phosphate in tryptophan metabolism. Pyridoxine requirement may also be increased by high protein intake. The ethanol metabolite acetaldehyde displaces pyridoxal phosphate from proteins and thus enhances its degradation.

Experimental depletion The feeding of pyridoxine-deficient diets leads to chemical evidence of deficiency (increased xanthurenic acid and decreased pyridoxine in urine) within a week. Electroencephalographic abnormalities are demonstrable within 3 weeks, and some subjects have grand mal seizures. Deficiency induced with the pyridoxine antagonist deoxypyridoxine causes, in addition, seborrheic dermatitis, cheilosis, glossitis, nausea, vomiting, weakness, and dizziness.

Clinical deficiency The widespread occurrence of the vitamin in food is probably the reason that pure pyridoxine deficiency does not occur except when the pyridoxine content of food is either destroyed or converted to less available protein-bound forms during processing, as has happened in some infant formulas. It is a paradox, therefore, that pyridoxine deficiency is now frequent because many commonly used drugs act as pyridoxine antagonists. Hydrazines such as *isoniazid* combine with pyridoxal and pyridoxal phosphate to form hydrazones. The hydrazones inhibit enzymes such as pyridoxal kinase, induce convulsions directly, and accelerate pyridoxine loss in the urine and thus induce a vitamin deficiency. *Cycloserine* also causes an increase in the excretion of the vitamin in the urine and produces profound neurologic effects, presumably by forming a complex with pyridoxal phosphate that competes with the cofactor for apoenzymes. *Penicillamine* acts as an antagonist by forming a thiazolidine derivative with pyridoxal phosphate. In each of these instances abnormal tryptophan metabolism and convulsions can be prevented by supplementation with the vitamin.

Estimates of vitamin deficiency have been based upon the correction of clinical signs of deficiency following administration of the vitamin, measurement of the excretion of tryptophan metabolites after tryptophan-loading tests, measurement of various amino acid transferase activities in blood, and measurement of the excretion of pyridoxine or its metabolites or of oxalate in urine. The most commonly used index is the measurement of urinary tryptophan metabolites, particularly xanthurenic acid, following tryptophan loading. Alternatively, cystathionine can be assayed after administration of a methionine load. In vitro measurement of red blood cell glutamic

pyruvic transaminase in the presence and absence of pyridoxal phosphate may be a better indicator of pyridoxine status than either loading test.

The appropriate management is prevention of deficiency. Supplementation of the diet with 30 mg of pyridoxine returns tryptophan metabolism to normal in pregnancy, in users of oral contraceptives, and in patients taking isoniazid. Doses as high as 100 mg/d may be required in subjects taking penicillamine.

Pyridoxine-responsive diseases Several genetic disorders cause abnormalities in vitamin B_6 metabolism. In one group, infants develop convulsions and brain damage and die if not provided with large daily supplements of pyridoxine; these children have an apoenzyme for glutamic acid decarboxylase that has a decreased binding affinity for pyridoxal phosphate. Consequently they do not form normal amounts of γ-aminobutyric acid, a physiologic inhibitor of neurotransmission. Another group of patients has pyridoxine-responsive chronic anemia; pyridoxine supplementation results in prompt hematologic improvement but does not correct the morphologic abnormality in the erythrocytes.

The synthesis of cystathionine from homocystine and serine and its cleavage to cysteine and homoserine are catalyzed by two pyridoxal phosphate enzymes. The changes that occur in deficiency of these two enzymes and in xanthurenic aciduria due to kynureninase deficiency have been reviewed by Mudd. Some patients with vitamin B_6–responsive xanthurenic aciduria or cystathioninuria have a mutant apoenzyme that interacts abnormally with pyridoxal phosphate, a defect that can be largely corrected by elevated concentrations of the cofactor. In contrast, the vitamin B_6 response in patients with homocystinuria due to cystathionine synthetase deficiency is due to an enhancement of the activity of the residual amount of normal enzyme present rather than a restoration of the affected enzyme levels to normal.

RIBOFLAVIN Riboflavin in the form of the coenzymes flavin mononucleotide (FMN) and flavin adenine dinucleotide (FAD) (Fig. 76-1) participates in a variety of oxidation-reduction reactions. In addition, covalently attached flavins are essential to the structure of such enzymes as succinate dehydrogenase and monoamine oxidase. The vitamin is absorbed from the gastrointestinal tract either as free riboflavin or the 5′-phosphate by a specific transport process. The recommended daily allowance is listed in Table 70-1. Covalently linked vitamin accounts for less than one-tenth of the tissue pool. The vitamin is excreted in urine predominantly in the free form although a small fraction of the daily turnover is the result of catabolism by microorganisms in the gastrointestinal tract.

Riboflavin deficiency can be induced in humans by feeding a riboflavin-deficient diet or by the administration of riboflavin antagonists such as galactoflavin. The deficiency syndrome is characterized by sore throat, hyperemia and edema of the pharyngeal and oral mucous membranes, cheilosis, angular stomatitis, glossitis, seborrheic dermatitis, and normochromic, normocytic anemia due to red cell hypoplasia of the bone marrow. These features can be reversed by riboflavin administration. Thyroid hormones and adrenal steroids enhance FMN and FAD synthesis; certain psychotropic agents (phenothiazines and tricyclic antidepressants) competitively inhibit flavin coenzyme biosynthesis, but these agents alone do not induce deficiency. Instead, riboflavin deficiency almost invariably occurs in combination with other vitamin deficiencies.

VITAMIN C (SCURVY) **Biochemistry** In most animals ascorbic acid (vitamin C) can be synthesized from glucose. However, humans, other primates, and the guinea pig are unable to synthesize L-ascorbic acid and require vitamin C in the diet. These species can perform the various reactions required for the biosynthesis of the vitamin from D-glucose except for one step, the conversion of L-gluconogamma-lactone to L-abscorbic acid. The enzyme that catalyzes this reaction (L-gluconolactone oxidase) is missing because of a mutation; thus the need for vitamin C in the diet is the result of an inborn error in carbohydrate metabolism.

Mechanism of action L-Ascorbic acid readily undergoes reversible oxidation and reduction as follows:

$$\text{L-ascorbic acid} \rightleftharpoons \text{dehydro-L-ascorbic acid} + 2H^+ + 2e$$

This property of the vitamin is the key to understanding its role as a redox agent for biologic oxidation. However, ascorbic acid does not act as a conventional cofactor since its requirement can usually be replaced by other compounds with similar redox properties. The best understood function is in the synthesis of collagen; absence of the vitamin leads to impairment of peptidyl hydroxylation of procollagen and a reduction in collagen formation and secretion by connective tissue. Nonhydroxylated collagen is unstable and cannot form the triple helix required for normal tissue structure. Many features of scurvy result from this defect in collagen synthesis, including the capillary fragility that underlies the hemorrhagic features, the poor healing of wounds, and (in part) the bony abnormalities of children. Collagens that normally have the highest content of hydroxyproline are most severely affected, accounting for the early disruption of the adventitia, media, and basal laminae of blood vessels. Ascorbic acid also functions to prevent oxidation of tetrahydrofolate and thus protect the active folic acid pool and to regulate iron distribution and storage, probably by influencing the valence of stored iron and maintaining a normal ratio of ferritin to hemosiderin. Scorbutic patients excrete incompletely oxidized products of tyrosine metabolism, but the significance is not clear.

Requirements The recommended daily allowance for vitamin C is described in Table 70-1. The vitamin is present in milk and some meats (kidney, liver, fish) and is widely distributed in fruits and vegetables. A portion is lost after prolonged storage of unprocessed fruits and vegetables (for example, potatoes), but it is partially preserved (half or greater) by most means of food processing (boiling, steaming, pressure cooking, preserving jams and jellies, freezing, dehydration, and canning). As a consequence the recommended daily allowances can be met with even a modest intake of fruits and vegetables. The utilization of the vitamin is increased during pregnancy and lactation and in thyrotoxicosis, and absorption is decreased in diarrheal states and in achlorhydria.

Experimental depletion The total-body pool of vitamin C varies from 1.5 to 3 g. When a deficient diet is instituted, the pool is depleted at a constant rate that may be as high as 4 percent per day. In monkeys the major catabolic pathway involves oxidation of the alcohol at carbon 6 to an aldehyde and then to an acid. Because of differences in initial pool size and rates of turnover, differences in the completeness of deficiency in various experimental diets, and variation among normal subjects at the cellular or enzymatic level, the time required for development of symptoms ranges from 1 to 3 months in different studies. Manifestations of deficiency correlate better with the total pool size than with plasma or blood levels. The first symptoms (petechial hemorrhages and ecchymoses) develop when the pool size is less than 0.5 g; with further depletion (pool size 0.1 to 0.5 g) manifestations include gum involvement, hyperkeratosis, congested hair follicles, arthralgias, Sjögren's syndrome, coiled hairs, and joint effusions. When depletion is extreme (pool size <0.1 g), dyspnea, edema, oliguria, and neuropathy supervene. Progress of the disease may then be rapid.

Symptoms do not improve until the normal pool is repleted, and the larger the therapeutic dose, the more rapid the repletion. However, with doses as small as 6.5 mg/d the body pool eventually returns to normal, and amelioration of symptoms follows.

Clinical deficiency Clinical scurvy now occurs for the most part in areas of urban poverty. An increased incidence occurs at 6 to 12 months of age in infants whose processed milk formulas are unsupplemented with citrus fruit or vegetables as a result of maternal error or neglect. Another peak occurs in middle and old age; edentulous men who live alone and cook for themselves are particularly prone to develop scurvy. Clinical scurvy is more severe than the experimental disease, doubtlessly because affected individuals usually have defi-

ciencies of other dietary constituents as well and because the groups at risk (infants and the elderly) are especially vulnerable.

In adults the features include perifollicular hyperkeratotic papules in which hairs become fragmented and buried; perifollicular hemorrhages; purpura beginning on the backs of the lower extremities coalescing to become ecchymoses (Fig. 76-2); hemorrhage into the muscles of the arms and legs with secondary phlebothromboses; hemorrhages into joints; splinter hemorrhages in the nail beds; gum involvement (only in people with teeth) that includes swelling, friability, bleeding, secondary infection, and loosening of the teeth; poor healing of wounds and breakdown of recently healed wounds; petechial hemorrhages in the viscera; and emotional changes. Symptoms resembling those of Sjögren's syndrome may occur. Terminally, icterus, edema, and fever are common, and convulsions, shock, and death may occur abruptly.

In infancy and childhood hemorrhage into the periosteum of long bones causes painful swellings and may result in epiphyseal separation. The sternum may sink inward, leaving a sharp elevation at the rib margins (scorbutic rosary). Purpura and ecchymoses may develop in the skin, and gum lesions occur if the teeth have erupted. Retrobulbar, subarachnoid, and intracerebral hemorrhages rapidly culminate in death if treatment is delayed.

Severe to moderate anemia is common in children and in adults, is usually normochromic and normocytic, and is due to bleeding into tissues. The anemia may be macrocytic and/or megaloblastic (one-fifth of patients in one series). Many foods that contain vitamin C also contain folate, and diets that cause scurvy may also cause folate deficiency. However, ascorbic acid deficiency also results in an increased oxidation of formyl tetrahydrofolic acid to inactive folate

FIGURE 76-2 Hemorrhages and ecchymoses in a patient with scurvy. *(Photograph courtesy of Leonard L. Madison.)*

metabolites and may cause a decrease in the active folate pool. Whether changes in iron distribution and storage are involved in the pathogenesis of the anemia is unclear. The anemia is corrected with refeeding and replenishment of vitamin C and the institution of a balanced diet.

In some hospitals platelet ascorbic acid levels are useful in diagnosing scurvy and are usually less than one-fourth of the normal value. Plasma levels of the vitamin correlate less well with the clinical state. In infants x-ray changes of the bones may be diagnostic. Indirect bilirubin is frequently elevated. Capillary fragility is abnormal. The remainder of the laboratory tests are nondiagnostic.

Scurvy is potentially fatal; if the diagnosis is suspected, blood should be obtained, and ascorbic acid therapy should be instituted promptly. The usual dose in adults is 100 mg three to five times a day by mouth until 4 g has been administered, then 100 mg/d. In infants and children administration of 10 to 25 mg three times a day is adequate. A diet rich in vitamin C should be initiated simultaneously. Spontaneous bleeding usually ceases within 24 h, muscle and bone pains subside quickly, and the gums begin to heal within 2 to 3 days. Even large ecchymoses and hematomas resolve in 10 to 12 days, although pigmentary changes in areas of extensive hemorrhage may persist for months. Serum bilirubin becomes normal within 3 to 5 days, and the anemia is ordinarily corrected within 2 to 4 weeks.

VITAMIN A   Biochemistry   Vitamin A (retinol) can either be ingested or synthesized within the body from plant carotenoids (Fig. 76-1). Preformed vitamin A is present in animal tissues, and the best sources are liver, milk, and kidney, where it occurs largely in the form of fatty acid esters. The esters are hydrolyzed during digestion, absorbed in the free form, reesterified with fatty acids within the intestinal mucosa, and enter the circulation in association with lymph chylomicrons. The carotenoid substrates for synthesis of vitamin A, mainly β-carotenes, are widely distributed in plants. β-Carotene can either be absorbed intact or cleaved in the intestinal tract to form two molecules of retinaldehyde. Retinaldehyde is subsequently reduced by an aldehyde reductase to retinol. Retinol from whatever source is stored as retinyl esters in the parenchymal cells of the liver. The normal body retinol pool varies from 300 to 900 mg.

Prior to release from the liver retinyl esters are hydrolyzed, and the free alcohol is mobilized bound to a specific transport protein, retinol-binding protein (RBP), for transport to peripheral tissues. In vitamin A deficiency the release of RBP from the liver is inhibited, and the protein accumulates in liver; with repletion RBP is rapidly released from preformed stores. Approximately equal amounts of retinol are excreted in the bile and urine.

Mechanism of action   The best-defined function of vitamin A is its role in vision; in the retina vitamin A constitutes the prosthetic group of a series of carotenoid proteins that provide the molecular basis for visual excitation. In addition, vitamin A is required for growth, reproduction, and the maintenance of life. Retinol-phosphate-mannose glycolipid is present in a variety of cell membranes, and the vitamin plays a primary role in the synthesis of glycoproteins. The importance of glycoprotein to every cell implies that this is an equally important function of the vitamin.

Requirements   The recommended daily allowance for vitamin A is listed in Table 70-1. The assumed utilization efficiency for the conversion of β-carotene to vitamin A in the human is one-sixth (0.167). Other carotenoids with provitamin A activity have, on the average, about half the activity of β-carotene. Pregnancy and disease states in which there is impaired absorption or storage, excessive utilization, or increased excretion of vitamin A may lead to increased requirements.

Experimental depletion   When experimental subjects are fed a diet deficient in both retinol and carotene, plasma levels fall, and the body pool shrinks to less than half the control value. Deficiency is manifested by follicular hyperkeratosis, impaired dark adaptation, and abnormalities of the electroretinogram. These changes are corrected after supplementation with 150 μg of retinol or 300 μg of β-carotene per day.

Clinical deficiency   Endemic deficiency results from inadequate amounts of the vitamin and of the carotene provitamins in the diet and probably always occurs in conjunction with deficiency of other nutrients or complicating diseases. In some developing countries vitamin A deficiency is a major cause of blindness in the young as a consequence of failure to incorporate green leafy vegetables or other sources of the provitamin or vitamin into the diet. Such children appear to be particularly susceptible to the complications of measles. Vitamin A deficiency may also accompany protein-calorie malnutrition, and here the deficiency is due in part to a defective release mechanism from the liver secondary to inadequate retinol-binding protein. In developed nations vitamin A deficiency is usually due either to intestinal malabsorption (as in sprue or after intestinal bypass surgery), abnormal storage (liver disease), or enhanced destruction or excretion of the vitamin (proteinuria). Vitamin A deficiency has also occurred in patients receiving total parenteral nutrition because of loss of vitamin A after prolonged storage of intravenous fluid.

Night blindness is the earliest symptom of deficiency, followed by degenerative changes in the retina. The bulbar conjunctiva becomes dry (xerosis), and small gray plaques with foamy surfaces develop (Bitôt's spots). These early lesions are reversible with vitamin A. The more serious effects of vitamin A deficiency are ulceration and necrosis of the cornea (keratomalacia), leading to perforation, endophthalmitis, and blindness. Such patients may also exhibit dryness and hyperkeratosis of the skin.

Vitamin A levels in plasma are not reliable for the assessment of stores in individual cases. Measurements of dark adaptation, rod scotometry, and electroretinography are useful indicators of vitamin A stores but require trained personnel and expensive equipment; consequently, the diagnosis is usually based upon a high index of suspicion in malnourished children or in patients with known predisposing factors for its development.

Night blindness and the milder conjunctival changes respond well to 30,000 IU of vitamin A daily for a week. Corneal damage constitutes a therapeutic emergency, and the usual treatment is 20,000 IU/kg body weight per day for 5 days. Children who are at risk for vitamin A deficiency and who develop measles should be given 200,000 IU orally each day for 2 days.

VITAMIN E   Biochemistry   Eight naturally occurring tocopherols possess vitamin E activity. The structure of alpha tocopherol, the most widely distributed and most active of the tocopherols, is shown in Fig. 76-1. The vitamin is absorbed from the gastrointestinal tract by a mechanism similar to that for other fat-soluble vitamins and enters the bloodstream via the lymph, associated first with chylomicrons and then with plasma betalipoproteins. Indeed, plasma levels correlate closely with plasma lipid levels. The vitamin is stored in all tissues, and the tissue stores can protect against vitamin deficiency for long periods. Approximately three-fourths of the vitamin is excreted in bile, and the balance is excreted as glucuronides in urine. Metabolites with quinone structures (including one similar to ubiquinone) are present in tissues.

Mechanism of action   The vitamin probably acts as an antioxidant rather than as a specific cofactor. In so acting it presumably inhibits oxidation of essential cellular constituents and prevents the formation of toxic oxidation products. Other antioxidants such as selenium, sulfur-containing amino acids, and the ubiquinone group can reverse the symptoms of vitamin E deficiency in animals.

Requirements   The recommended daily requirement is 10 to 30 mg/d (Table 70-1). Diets containing large amounts of polyunsaturated fatty acids increase and diets containing antioxidants decrease the requirement. The vitamin is widely distributed in food, so that a primary deficiency state has never been recognized in otherwise healthy children or adults. Newborn infants have plasma concentrations about one-fifth that of maternal levels, implying poor placental transfer, but human milk (in contrast to cow's milk) has sufficient levels to meet the requirements in infants.

Experimental depletion   In long-term studies vitamin E concentrations in plasma declined significantly only after months on a deficient diet. No manifestations of the depletion were detected in normal volunteers, making it difficult to establish that tocopherol is a human vitamin.

Clinical deficiency In the appropriate clinical setting vitamin E deficiency is associated with a discrete syndrome. Rarely, deficiency is due to a selective malabsorption of the vitamin. More commonly intestinal fat malabsorption can cause deficiency of all fat-soluble vitamins including vitamin E, and children with chronic cholestatic liver disease appear to be particularly susceptible, due to a combination of malabsorption of vitamin E and trapping of the vitamin in plasma by the associated hyperlipoproteinemia, so that tissue stores may be depleted despite a normal tocopherol level in serum. Indeed, the ratio of serum vitamin E to total serum lipid is the preferred index for assessing vitamin E status. The manifestations of deficiency include areflexia, gait disturbance, decreased proprioceptive and vibratory sensation, and paresis of gaze and are associated with degeneration of the posterior columns of the spinal cord, selective loss of large-caliber, myelinated axons in peripheral nerves, and appearance of spheroids in the gracile and cuneate nuclei of the brain. Treatment (50 to 100 IU/d by mouth) is most effective when initiated early in the course of the disease.

VITAMIN K Vitamin K consists of a quinone ring attached to a side chain (labeled *R* in Fig. 76-1) that varies depending on the source of the vitamin. Vitamin K_1 (phylloquinone) is present in most edible vegetables, particularly in green leaves, and vitamin K_2 is produced by intestinal bacteria. The many compounds with vitamin K activity are structurally related to the simpler compound, 2-methyl-1,4-naphthoquinone (menadione). Menadione is formed in the gut by the removal of the side chain from the vitamin by intestinal bacteria. After absorption, menadione is converted in the body to the active menaquinone. The vitamin is a component of a specialized microsomal enzyme system that effects the posttranslational γ carboxylation of glutamic acid in proteins of the plasma, bone, kidney, and urine, including the precursor proteins for the clotting factors VII, IX, X, and possibly V. Death from hemorrhage in deficiency states ensues before deficiency of the other carboxylated proteins becomes manifest.

Under ordinary circumstances about 80 percent of vitamin K is absorbed from the small bowel into the intestinal lymph. Because the naturally occurring forms of vitamin K are fat-soluble and are poorly stored in the body, deficiency can occur in association with diseases that interfere with fat absorption. In addition, long term treatment with oral antibiotics may temporarily eliminate intestinal bacteria as a source for vitamin K and promote deficiency when the diet is marginal or deficient. The warfarin anticoagulant drugs induce hypoprothrombinemia by inhibiting the γ carboxylation of the precursor protein.

Newborn infants tend to be deficient in vitamin K and have low plasma levels of several coagulation factors in the prothrombin complex. Such deficiencies result from minimal stores of vitamin K at birth, lack of an established intestinal flora, and a limited dietary intake of the vitamin.

Routine determination of prothrombin should be performed prior to surgical procedures or delivery. Subjects with levels below 70 percent of normal should receive therapy with vitamin K. Vitamin K deficiency can be separated from hypoprothrombinemia of liver disease by measurement of the noncarboxylated prothrombin precursor that accumulates in plasma in the vitamin deficiency.

VITAMIN EXCESS

Fat-soluble vitamins are stored to a variable extent in the body and hence are more likely to cause adverse effects when taken in excess; excess states for vitamins D (see Chap. 341) and A are particularly well characterized. Water-soluble vitamins are readily excreted in the urine and stored only to a limited extent. Consequently, toxicity states for these vitamins only occur when large amounts are taken for prolonged periods.

VITAMIN A AND CAROTENES Carotenemia Carotenemia results from excessive intake of vitamin A precursors in foods, principally carrots. Excess carotene is not injurious apart from the cosmetic effect; the fact that carotenemia does not cause hypervitaminosis A indicates that the conversion of carotene to vitamin A must be regulated. Carotenemia is manifested by yellowing of the skin with greatest intensity on the palms and soles and by a corresponding yellowness of serum. The yellowing of the skin can be distinguished from jaundice in that the scleras remain white. Hypothyroid patients are particularly susceptible. The omission of carrots from the diet leads to the rapid disappearance of the pigmentation. Discoloration of the skin can also result from the consumption of excessive amounts of other colored fruits and vegetables.

Vitamin A toxicity Hypervitaminosis A can result from accidental overingestion by hunters or explorers (polar bear liver), as the result of food faddism (usually caused by overly solicitous parents), or as a side effect of inappropriate therapy. Acute toxicity from a single massive dose consists of abdominal pain, nausea, vomiting, headache, dizziness, sluggishness, papilledema, and in infants a bulging fontanel followed within a few days by generalized desquamation of the skin and recovery. Chronic toxicity occurs following ingestion of 25,000 units or more daily for protracted periods and is characterized by bone and joint pain, hyperostoses, hair loss, dryness and fissures of the lips, anorexia, benign intracranial hypertension, low-grade fever, pruritus, weight loss, and hepatosplenomegaly. The only diagnostic laboratory finding is elevation of the vitamin in serum, chiefly in the form of retinyl esters. The concentration of retinol-binding protein is normal, and the excess vitamin A circulates in association with lipoprotein. Relief is prompt on withdrawal of the vitamin from the diet.

VITAMIN E Relatively large doses of vitamin E have been taken by some for extended periods without causing apparent harm. In others, a variety of nonspecific complaints have been reported including malaise, gastrointestinal complaint, headaches, and possibly hypertension. However, true toxicity appears to occur in two situations—in subjects receiving oral anticoagulants and in premature infants. In large amounts, vitamin E can apparently antagonize vitamin K and inhibit prothrombin time; this phenomenon results in a marked potentiation of oral anticoagulants. Premature infants given parenteral vitamin E are reported to have developed ascites associated with hepatosplenomegaly, cholestatic jaundice, azotemia, and thrombocytopenia.

VITAMIN K Large amounts of vitamin K can block the effects of oral anticoagulants and when given to pregnant women can cause jaundice in the newborn.

PYRIDOXINE Most adults can consume up to 10 times the recommended daily allowance of 2 mg pyridoxine per day without adverse effects. However, severe peripheral neuropathies have developed after ingestion of several grams per day for prolonged periods; symptoms include ataxia, perioral numbness, and clumsiness of the hands and feet, and the findings include loss of position and vibration sense without impairment of reflexes or sensory function. Recovery is slow after ingestion ceases. Lower doses (25 mg/d) can antagonize the effects of levodopa in Parkinson's disease and decrease the anticonvulsant effects of phenytoin barbiturates.

VITAMIN C Vitamin C is widely used in megavitamin therapy because of the claim that large amounts of the vitamin (a gram or greater per day) are effective in preventing or minimizing the symptoms of the common cold. However, in controlled studies, no significant differences in occurrence, severity, or duration of colds have been demonstrated in subjects treated with a placebo compared with the vitamin. Use of the vitamin in this way is unwarranted and probably unwise. The long-term use of ascorbic acid in these doses can interfere with the absorption of vitamin B_{12}, enhance blood levels of estrogens in women on exogenous estrogens, cause uricosuria, and predispose to formation of oxalate kidney stones. In addition, large doses enhance the development of metabolizing enzymes in the fetus and may cause rebound scurvy in the offspring of mothers who have ingested large amounts of the vitamin during pregnancy. However, pharmacologic doses (200 mg daily) may correct leukocyte abnormalities in patients with the Chédiak-Higashi syndrome (see Chap. 64).

NIACIN Large doses of niacin are used for treatment of hypercholesterolemia and occasionally for other purposes. The vitamin causes release of histamine, which in turn can cause severe flushing, pruritus, and gastrointestinal disturbances and may aggravate asthma. Acanthosis nigricans may occur. In doses of 3 g/d niacin has been reported to cause elevation of serum uric acid and of fasting glucose. Large doses can also cause hepatic toxicity including cholestatic jaundice.

REFERENCES

General

ELSAS LJ, McCORMICK DB: Genetic defects in vitamin utilization. Part I: General aspects and fat-soluble vitamins. Vitam Horm 43:103, 1986

GOODHART RS, SHILS ME (eds): *Modern Nutrition in Health and Disease*, 6th ed. Philadelphia, Lea & Febiger, 1980

HOYUMPA AM: Mechanisms of vitamin deficiencies in alcoholism. Alcoholism (NY) 10:573, 1986

MACHLIN LJ (ed): *Handbook of Vitamins. Nutritional, Biochemical, and Clinical Aspects.* New York, Dekker, 1984

MUDD SH: Inborn errors of metabolism. Vitamin-responsive genetic disease. J Clin Pathol 27(Suppl) 8:38, 1974

RUDMAN D, WILLIAMS PJ: Nutrient deficiencies during total parenteral nutrition. Nutr Rev 43:1, 1984

Niacin deficiency

CARPENTER KJ: The relationship of pellagra to corn and the low availability of niacin in cereals. Experientia(Suppl) 44:197, 1983

———, LEWIN WJ: A reexamination of the composition of diets associated with pellagra. J Nutr 115:543, 1985

CASTIELLO RJ, LYNCH PJ: Pellagra and the carcinoid syndrome. Arch Dermatol 105:574, 1972

DE LANGE DJ, JOUBERT CP: Assessment of nicotinic acid status of population groups. Am J Clin Nutr 15:169, 1964

GOLDSMITH GA: Experimental niacin deficiency. J Am Dietetic Assoc 32:312, 1956

HENDERSON LM: Niacin. Ann Rev Nutr 3:289, 1983

LEVY HL: Hartnup disorder, in *The Metabolic Basis of Inherited Disease*, 6th ed, CR Scriver et al (eds). New York, McGraw-Hill, 1989, p 2515

JUKES TH et al: The conquest of pellagra. Fed Proc 40:1519, 1980

Thiamine deficiency

BROWN GM: Biogenesis and metabolism of thiamine, in *Metabolic Pathways*, 3d ed, DM Greenberg (ed). New York, Academic, 1970, p 369

DURAN M, WADMAN SK: Thiamine-responsive inborn errors of metabolism. J Inherited Metab Dis 8(Suppl 1):70, 1985

DYCKNER T et al: Aggravation of thiamine deficiency by magnesium depletion. Acta Med Scand 218:129, 1985

HARPER CG et al: Clinical signs in the Wernicke-Korsakoff complex: A retrospective analysis of 131 cases diagnosed at necropsy. J Neurol Neurosurg Psychiatry 49:341, 1986

HOYUMPA AM: Mechanisms of thiamine deficiency in chronic alcoholism. Am J Clin Nutr 33:2750, 1980

KAWAI C et al: Reappearance of beriberi heart disease in Japan. Am J Med 69:383, 1980

KOZAM RL et al: Cardiovascular beriberi. Am J Cardiol 30:418, 1972

KURIYAMA M et al: Blood vitamin B_1, transketolase, and thiamine pyrophosphate (TPP) effect in beriberi patients. Clin Chim Acta 108:159, 1980

PINCUS JH et al: Thiamine derivatives in subacute necrotizing encephalomyelopathy. Pediatrics 51:716, 1973

VICTOR M et al: *The Wernicke-Korsakoff Syndrome*. Philadelphia, Davis, 1971

ZIPORIN ZZ et al: Excretion of thiamine and its metabolites in the urine of young adult males receiving restricted intakes of the vitamin. J Nutr 85:287, 1965

Pyridoxine deficiency

BHAGAVAN HN, BRIN M: Drug–vitamin B_6 interaction. Curr Concepts Nutr 12:1, 1983

FRIMPTER GW et al: Vitamin B_6–dependency syndromes: New horizons in nutrition. Am J Clin Nutr 22:794, 1969

GERSHOFF SN: Vitamin B_6, in *Nutrition Reviews' Present Knowledge in Nutrition*, 4th ed, DM Hegsted et al (eds). Washington, DC, The Nutrition Foundation, 1976, p 149

HARRIS JW, HORRIGAN DL: Pyridoxine-responsive anemia-prototype and variations on the theme, in *Vitamins and Hormones*, RS Harris et al (eds). New York, Academic, 1964, vol 22, p 721

JAFFE IA: The antivitamin B_6 effect of penicillamine: Clinical and immunological implications, in *Advances in Biochemical Psychopharmacology*, MS Ebodi et al (eds). New York, Raven Press, 1972, vol 4

LUHBY AL et al: Vitamin B_6 metabolism in users of oral contraceptive agents: I.

Abnormal urinary xanthurenic acid excretion and its correction by pyridoxine. Am J Clin Nutr 24:684, 1971

MUDD SH: Pyridoxine-responsive genetic disease. Fed Proc 30:970, 1971

SAUBERLICH HE et al: Biochemical assessment of the nutritional status of vitamin B_6 in the human. Am J Clin Nutr 25:629, 1972

Riboflavin deficiency

BATES CJ: Human riboflavin requirements, and metabolic consequences of deficiency in man and animals. World Rev Nutr Diet 50:215, 1987

MERRILL AH JR et al: Formation and mode of action of flavoproteins. Ann Rev Nutr 1:281, 1981

PINTO JT, RIVLIN RS: Drugs that promote renal excretion of riboflavin. Drug Nutr Interact 5:143, 1987

——— et al: Mechanisms underlying the differential effects of ethanol on the bioavailability of riboflavin and flavin adenine dinucleotide. J Clin Invest 79:1343, 1987

Ascorbic acid deficiency

BARNES MJ, KODICEK E: Biological hydroxylations and ascorbic acid, in *Vitamins and Hormones*, P Munson et al (eds). New York, Academic, 1972, vol 30, p 1

BARNESS LA: Nutritional aspects of vegetarianism, health foods, and fad diets. Nutr Rev 59:153, 1977

BOXER LA et al: Correction of leucocyte function in Chédiak-Higashi syndrome by ascorbate. N Engl J Med 295:1041, 1971

BURNS JJ et al: Third conference on vitamin C. Ann NY Acad Sci 498, 1987

ENGLAND S, SEIFTER S: The biochemical functions of ascorbic acid. Ann Rev Nutr 6:365, 1986

HODGES RE et al: Clinical manifestations of ascorbic acid deficiency in man. Am J Clin Nutr 24:432, 1971

LEVINE M: New concepts in the biology and biochemistry of ascorbic acid. N Engl J Med 314:892, 1986

REID GM: Scurvy: Old disease—New insight. Med Hypotheses 12:167, 1983

REULER JB et al: Adult scurvy. JAMA 253:805, 1985

SATO P, UNDENFRIEND S: Studies on ascorbic acid related to the genetic basis of scurvy, in *Vitamins and Hormones*, P Munson et al (eds). New York, Academic, 1978, vol 36, p 33

TOLBERT BM et al: New information on synthesis and metabolism of ascorbic acid. Nutr Rev 35:22, 1977

VILTER RW: Effects of ascorbic acid deficiency in man, in *The Vitamins*, WH Sebrell Jr et al (eds). New York, Academic, 1967, vol 1, p 457

WALLERSTEIN RO, WALLERSTEIN RO JR: Scurvy. Sem Hematol 13:211, 1976

Vitamin A deficiency

BARCLAY AJG et al: Vitamin A supplements and mortality related to measles: A randomised clinical trial. Br Med J 294:294, 1987

DeLUCA LM: The direct involvement of vitamin A in glycosyl transfer reactions of mammalian membranes, in *Vitamins and Hormones*, PL Munson et al (eds). New York, Academic, 1977, vol 35, p 1

GOODMAN DS: Vitamin A and retinoids in health and disease. N Engl J Med 310:1023, 1984

HOWARD L et al: Vitamin A deficiency from long-term parenteral nutrition. Ann Intern Med 93:576, 1980

SAUBERLICH HE et al: Vitamin A metabolism and requirements in the human studied with the use of labeled retinol, in *Vitamins and Hormones*, RS Harris et al (eds). New York, Academic, 1974, vol 32

SMITH FR, GOODMAN DS: Vitamin A transport in human vitamin A toxicity. N Engl J Med 294:805, 1976

SOMMER A et al: Clinical characteristics of vitamin A responsive and nonresponsive Bitôt's spots. Am J Ophthalmol 90:160, 1980

TIELSCH JM, SOMMER A: The epidemiology of vitamin A deficiency and xerophthalmia. Ann Rev Nutr 4:183, 1974

VAHLQUIST A: Clinical use of vitamin A and its derivatives—physiological and pharmacological aspects. Clin Exp Dermatol 10:133, 1985

Vitamin A for measles. Lancet 1:1067, 1987

WALD G: Molecular basis of visual excitation. Science 162:230, 1968

Vitamin E deficiency

BIERI JG et al: Medical uses of vitamin E. N Engl J Med 308:1063, 1983

HORWITT MK: Interrelations between vitamin E and polyunsaturated fatty acids in adult men, in *Vitamins and Hormones*, GF Marrian, KV Thimann (eds). New York, Academic, 1962, vol 20, p 541

———: The promotion of vitamin E. J Nutr 116:1371, 1986

PERLMUTTER DH et al: Intramuscular vitamin E repletion in children with chronic cholestasis. Am J Dis Child 141:170, 1987

ROSENBLUM JL et al: A progressive neurologic syndrome in children with chronic liver disease. N Engl J Med 304:503, 1981

SITRIN MD et al: Vitamin E deficiency and neurologic disease in adults with cystic fibrosis. Ann Intern Med 107:51, 1987

SOKOL RJ et al: Vitamin E deficiency with normal serum vitamin E concentrations in children with chronic cholestasis. N Engl J Med 310:1209, 1984

——— et al: Isolated vitamin E deficiency in the absence of fat malabsorption—familial and sporadic cases: Characterization and investigation of causes. J Lab Clin Med 111:548, 1988

TRABER MG et al: Lack of tocopherol in peripheral nerves of vitamin E–deficient patients with peripheral neuropathy. N Engl J Med 317:262, 1987

Vitamin K deficiency

ALLISON PM et al: Effects of a vitamin K-deficient diet and antibiotics in normal human volunteers. J Lab Clin Med 110:180, 1987

BERTINA RM et al: New method for the rapid detection of vitamin K deficiency. Clin Chim Acta 105:93, 1980

DOISY EA JR, MATSCHINER JT: Biochemistry of vitamin K, in *Fat-Soluble Vitamins*, RA Morton (ed). Elmsford, NY, Pergamon, 1970, vol 9, p 293

IBER FL et al: Vitamin K deficiency in chronic alcoholic males. Alcoholism (NY) 10:679, 1986

OLSON RE, SUTTIE JW: Vitamin K and α-carboxyglutamate biosynthesis, in *Vitamins and Hormones*, PL Munson et al (eds). New York, Academic, 1977, vol 35, p 59

SHEARER MJ et al: Studies on the absorption and metabolism of phylloquinone (vitamin K) in man, in *Vitamins and Hormones*, RS Harris et al (eds). New York, Academic, 1974, vol 32, p 513

SUTTIE JW: *Vitamin K Metabolism and Vitamin K-Dependent Proteins*. Baltimore, University Park Press, 1980

Vitamin excess

ALHADEFF L: Toxic effects of water-soluble vitamins. Nutr Rev 42:33, 1984

CHALMERS TC: Effects of ascorbic acid on the common cold. Am J Med 58:532, 1975

CORRIGAN JJ JR: The effect of vitamin E on warfarin-induced vitamin K deficiency. Ann NY Acad Sci 82:361, 1982

HERBERT V: The vitamin craze. Arch Intern Med 140:173, 1980

LEMONS JA, MAISELS MJ: Vitamin E—How much is too much? Pediatrics 76:625, 1985

LOMBAERT A, CARTON H: Benign intracranial hypertension due to A-hypervitaminosis in adults and adolescents. Eur Neurol 14:340, 1976

LORCH V et al: Unusual syndrome with fatalities among premature infants: Association with a new intravenous vitamin E product. Morb Mort Week Rep 33:198, 1984

Megavitamin E supplementation and vitamin K–dependent carboxylation. Nutr Rev 41:268, 1986

SCHAUMBURG H et al: Sensory neuropathy from pyridoxine abuse: A new megavitamin syndrome. N Engl J Med 309:445, 1983

SHIN HB et al: Ascorbic acid–induced uricosuria: A consequence of megavitamin therapy. Ann Intern Med 84:385, 1976

Toxic effects of vitamin overdosage. Med Lett Drugs Ther 26:73, 1984

WOOLLISCROFT JO: Megavitamins: Fact and fancy. Dis-A-Month 24:1, 1983

77 DISTURBANCES IN TRACE ELEMENT METABOLISM

KENNETH H. FALCHUK

CLASSIFICATION AND FUNCTIONS The "trace elements" comprise metals in biologic fluids at concentrations below one microgram per gram of wet weight. Most are essential nutrients for human beings (Table 77-1). Others (As, Ni, Sn, V, Si) are essential for some plants and/or vertebrates including mammals and may be required by humans. The functions of trace elements and of other, more abundant metals (Na, K, Ca, Mg) are determined, in part, by their charges, mobilities, and binding constants to biologic ligands. Elements in one group (Na, K) bind weakly to negatively charged ligands and can cross cellular membranes without major impediment. They are used by living systems as charge carriers to conduct electric impulses along nerves, etc. Those in a second group (Mg, Ca) form moderately stable but not tight complexes with enzymes, nucleic acids, and other ligands. They act as biochemical "triggers," altering and/or controlling the functions of these molecules, e.g., Ca affects muscle contraction and relaxation (Chap. 365). Those in a third group (Fe, Zn, Cu, and others) form strong, static complexes with and become integral functional components of enzymes (Table 77-1).

METAL DEFICIENCY OR TOXICITY Metals can cause disease through deficiency, imbalance, or toxicity. Deficiency usually results when dietary intake is inadequate or when intake is adequate but other conditioning factors come into play. Deficiencies can be caused by metal malabsorption in chronic diarrheal diseases, surgical resection of the small intestine, or formation of metal complexes with dietary components that are not readily absorbed, e.g., between phytates and Zn. Deficiency states can also result from increased losses through urine, pancreatic juice, or other exocrine secretions or from metabolic imbalances produced by antagonistic or synergistic interactions between metals. Large amounts of Ca, for example, decrease the absorption of and induce deficiency of Zn. Similarly, Mo and Cu compete with each other; excessive Mo in cattle leads to Cu deficiency characterized by diarrhea and wasting. Proven manifestations of trace element deficiencies in humans, except for iron, were previously rare but have been recognized more frequently with the use of total parenteral nutrition (TPN) (Chap. 75). Clinical criteria for the recognition of deficiency states include decreases in metal content of whole blood, serum, hair and/or other accessible fluids and tissues, changes in the activities of metalloenzymes, and characteristic signs and symptoms (Table 77-2).

Toxic effects are dependent on the chemical form, the amount ingested, the route of entry into the body, the biologic ligands associated with the metal, the tissue distribution, the concentration

TABLE 77-1 Requirements and functions of trace elements in humans

Element	Requirements, mg/day*	Amount† Total, g per 70 kg body weight	Serum µmol/L	Serum µg/dL	Selected biochemical functions	Enzymes Class	Enzymes Example
Fe	10–20	4.0	18	100	Oxygen transport	Oxidoreductases	Cytochrome oxidase
Zn	15–20	3.0	15	100	Nucleic acid and protein synthesis and degradation, alcohol metabolism	Transferases, hydrolases, lyases, isomerases, ligases, oxidoreductases	RNA polymerases, alcohol dehydrogenases, transcription factors
Cu	2–6	0.25	16	100	Hemoglobin synthesis, connective tissue metabolism, bone development	Oxidoreductases	Superoxide dismutase, ferroxidase (ceruloplasmin)
Co	0.0001	1.1	0.0001	0.0007	Methionine metabolism	Transferases	Homocysteine methyltransferase
Mn	2–5	0.02	0.001	0.06	Oxidative phosphorylation; fatty acid, mucopolysaccharide, and cholesterol metabolism	Oxidoreductases, hydrolases, ligases	Diamine oxidase, pyruvate carboxylase
Mo	0.15–0.5	0.07	0.007	0.07	Xanthine metabolism	Oxidoreductases	Xanthine oxidase
Se	0.05–0.2	(−)	1.6	13	Antioxidant	Oxidoreductases, transferases	Glutathione peroxidase
Ni	(−)	(−)	0.02	0.1	?Stabilizing RNA structure	Oxidoreductases, hydrolases	Urease
Cr	0.005–0.2	0.0006	0.004	0.02	?Binding of insulin to cells, glucose metabolism		

* Requirements may differ for different age groups and physiologic states, e.g., pregnancy.
† Reported normal values vary owing to differences in sample preparation, analytical instruments, and small quantities present in biologic materials.
(−), Reported values variable or not available.

TABLE 77-2 Disorders of metal metabolism in humans

Element	Deficiency	Toxicity*
Fe	Anemia	Hepatic failure, diabetes, testicular atrophy, arthritis, cardiomyopathy, peripheral neuropathy, hyperpigmentation
Zn	Growth retardation, alopecia, dermatitis, diarrhea, immunologic dysfunction, failure to thrive, psychological disturbances, gonadal atrophy, impaired spermatogenesis, congenital malformations.	Gastric ulcer, pancreatitis lethargy, anemia, fever, nausea, vomiting, respiratory distress, pulmonary fibrosis
Cu	Anemia, growth retardation, defective keratinization and pigmentation of hair, hypothermia, degenerative changes in aortic elastin, mental deterioration, scurvy-like changes in skeleton	Hepatitis, cirrhosis, tremor, mental deterioration, Kayser-Fleischer rings, hemolytic anemia, renal dysfunction (Fanconi-like syndrome)
Mn	Bleeding disorder (increased prothrombin time)	Encephalitis-like syndrome, Parkinson-like syndrome, psychosis, pneumoconiosis
Co	Anemia (B_{12} deficiency)	Cardiomyopathy, goiter
Mo	? Esophageal cancer	? Hyperuricemia
Cr	? Impairment of glucose tolerance	Renal failure, dermatitis (occupational), pulmonary cancer
Se	Cardiomyopathy, congestive heart failure, striated muscle degeneration	Alopecia, abnormal nails, emotional lability, lassitude, garlic odor to breath
Ni	?	Dermatitis (occupational), lung and nasal carcinomas, liver necrosis, pulmonary inflammation
Si	? Impaired early bone development	Pulmonary inflammation, granuloma, fibrosis
F	? Impaired bone and dental structure	Motted dental enamel, nausea, abdominal pain, vomiting, diarrhea, tetany, cardiovascular collapse

* Symptoms are dependent on route of entry and tissue distribution (see text).

achieved, and the excretion rate. Mechanisms of toxicity include inhibition of enzyme activity by binding to essential amino acid residues, alterations in nucleic acid function and structure, alteration in protein synthesis, effects on membrane permeability, and inhibition of phosphorylation, among others. Metal toxicity in patients undergoing chronic renal dialysis is important because of the frequency and severity of the resulting problems and because of the number of metals involved, e.g., Al, Zn, Cu, Ni, and Sn (Chap. 225). For example, even when it is present only in trace amounts in dialysis fluids, Al is readily absorbed into blood and accumulates in brain, bone, and erythroid tissues, causing disabling neurologic, skeletal, and hematologic disorders. These include malaise, memory loss, asterixis, dementia, twitches, and other manifestations of metabolic encephalopathy including seizures and death. Osteomalacia unresponsive to vitamin D, fractures, muscular pain, weakness, and anemia may occur. Documentation of increase in plasma Al concentration following deferoxamine administration is diagnostic.

DISORDERS OF METABOLISM OF SPECIFIC METALS Zinc
Absorption of Zn in the small intestine is decreased by fibers, phytate, phosphate, Ca, and Cu. In contrast, amino acids, peptides, iodoquinol and other chelating agents increase Zn absorption. Excretion of Zn occurs principally through secretions of the pancreas and intestine. Nearly 99 percent of total-body Zn is inside cells, the remainder is in plasma and extracellular fluids. Serum Zn, approximately 70

percent of which is loosely bound to albumin and other proteins, is the source of metal for cellular needs. Serum Zn content does not normally vary, but it decreases when intake or absorption is reduced (e.g., in regional enteritis) or when urinary losses are increased (e.g., in nephrotic syndrome; in cirrhosis of the liver or other hypoalbuminemic states; during the administration of penicillamine or other chelating agents; in high catabolic states as after trauma, burns, or surgery; and in hemolytic anemias and sickle cell disease). Plasma Zn also decreases in the acute phase of myocardial infarction, infections, malignancies, hepatitis, and other diseases. The decreases may be due to redistribution from plasma to tissues and are probably mediated by ACTH, cortisol, and/or a leukocyte protein (leukocyte endogenous mediator). Clinical deficiency may follow these decreases in serum content. The Zn requirement of the developing fetus, pregnant woman, and growing child or adolescent is higher than that of adult men or nonpregnant women. Therefore, the former groups are more susceptible to Zn depletion. Zn deficiency in pregnant animals can lead to fetal Zn deficiency, which results in high mortality rates or congenital malformations of nearly all organ systems. Zinc deficiency has not been described in pregnant women, but has been reported in adolescents who eat dirt, in patients who receive TPN without supplemental Zn (see Chap. 75), and in patients with the autosomal recessive defect acrodermatitis enteropathica. In the latter disease, deficiency in plasma Zn may be the consequence of a defect in Zn absorption. The onset of symptoms often occurs when an affected infant is weaned from human to cow's milk. Zn may also play a role in the maintenance of normal taste and in wound healing.

Tissues with a high cellular turnover, including skin, gastrointestinal mucosa, chondrocytes, spermatogonia, and thymocytes are characteristically affected (Table 77-2). The dermatologic abnormalities (hyperkeratosis, parakeratosis, acrodermatitis, and alopecia) call attention to the possibility of Zn deficiency. The usual distribution of the keratotic lesions is in areas that are readily traumatized (elbows, knees), but the lesions can develop in other areas as well. The keratotic lesions can become pustular or crusting, red, scaly plaques. Superinfections are common with either fungi or bacteria.

Toxicity follows inhalation of Zn fumes (by welders), oral ingestion, or intravenous administration. Inhalation of high concentrations of zinc oxide fumes leads to an acute illness called metal-fume fever or brass chills, manifested by fever, chills, excessive salivation, headaches, cough, and leukocytosis. Dialysis fluids can be contaminated with Zn from the adhesive plaster used on the dialysis coils or from galvanized pipes. The toxic syndrome associated with hemodialysis is characterized by anemia, fever, and central nervous system disturbances (Table 77-2). Toxic amounts of Zn decrease chemotaxis, phagocytosis, pinocytosis, and platelet aggregation.

Copper The liver, kidney, heart, and brain contain the highest amounts of Cu. Over 90 percent of plasma Cu is associated with ceruloplasmin, while 60 percent of that in red blood cells is bound to superoxide dismutase. The major excretory pathway is through the bile. The serum Cu concentration is normally constant. Increases occur in patients with acute myocardial infarction, leukemia, solid tumors, infections, portal and biliary cirrhosis, hemochromatosis, thyrotoxicosis, and connective tissue disorders. The consequences of the increases are unknown. Decreases occur in the nephrotic syndrome, kwashiorkor, the hepatolenticular degeneration of Wilson's disease (see Chap. 330), severe diarrheal diseases with malabsorption, and other conditions associated with increased excretion or decreased synthesis of ceruloplasmin. Premature infants who are fed diets deficient in Cu develop decreased serum ceruloplasmin and Cu levels, anemia, osteopenia, skin and hair depigmentation, and psychomotor retardation. Cu deficiency in subjects receiving TPN causes anemia and neutropenia.

A more complex disorder of Cu metabolism occurs in Menkes' disease, an X-linked recessive disorder (see also Chap. 336). Intestinal Cu uptake is normal, and tissue Cu content varies; that of intestinal, kidney, and skin (fibroblast) cells is normal or high, while that of serum, liver, brain, and (likely) vascular cells is low. Ceruloplasmin content and the activities of some Cu enzymes (e.g., connective tissue amine oxidases) also are decreased. The clinical picture is similar to that of nutritional Cu deficiency in animals except that anemia does not occur (Table 77-2). The patients have kinky hair, and decreased amounts of mature collagen and elastin cause dissecting aneurysms, sudden cardiac rupture, emphysema, and osteoporosis. Death usually occurs in the first 5 years of life.

Excessive oral intake of Cu or hemodialysis with water contaminated with Cu is toxic. The acute symptoms include hemolytic anemia, nausea, vomiting, and diarrhea. The renal and hepatic failure and the central nervous system disorders that eventually develop (Table 77-2) are typical of the Cu toxicity syndrome in hepatolenticular degeneration (Wilson's disease). (See Chap. 330.)

Cobalt Co is a component of vitamin B_{12}, and deficiency syndromes are those associated with deficiency of the vitamin (see Chap. 292). Pharmacologic doses of Co induce erythropoiesis. Chronic administration blocks iodine uptake by the thyroid, resulting in development of goiter.

Cardiomyopathy, congestive heart failure with pericardial effusions, polycythemia, thyroid enlargement, and neurologic abnormalities have been reported as manifestations of Co toxicity in drinkers of beer to which the metal had been added as a foam stabilizer. Co accumulates in the heart, forms a complex with lipoic acid, and interferes with decarboxylation reactions critical to both pyruvate and fatty acid metabolism.

Manganese Mn acts both as an activator of enzymes and as a component of metalloenzymes (Table 77-1). Defects of the skeletal, central nervous, and gonadal systems occur in Mn deficiency in animals. Humans obtain sufficient Mn from normal dietary intake so that a deficiency syndrome is rare. In one reported instance an increase in prothrombin time, unresponsive to Vitamin K, was noted. In serum, Mn is bound to transmanganin. Mn is excreted primarily in bile and pancreatic secretions.

Serum Mn increases following myocardial infarction and decreases for unknown reasons in children with convulsive disorders. Miners who inhale large quantities of Mn dust over long periods of time develop asthenia, anorexia, apathy, headache, impotence, leg cramps, speech disturbances, and occasionally even more severe toxic symptoms (Table 77-2).

Selenium Se is a component of glutathione peroxidase and plays a critical role in the control of oxygen metabolism, particularly in catalyzing the breakdown of H_2O_2. The metal is required for the growth of human fibroblasts and other cells in tissue culture. Furthermore, Se cures or prevents Keshan disease, a syndrome that is endemic to Keshan Province in China where the soil may be deficient in the metal. Keshan disease is characterized by multifocal myocardial necrosis and reduced blood and serum Se content. The clinical severity varies from severe arrhythmias and cardiogenic shock to a mild form with cardiac enlargement as the only significant finding. Peripheral myopathies may develop as a consequence of muscle degeneration (Table 77-2). Children and women of childbearing age are particularly susceptible. Se protects animals from a number of carcinogenic chemicals and viral agents; a role in human cancer prevention is not established. Se binds Cd, Hg, and other metals and mitigates their toxic effects, even though the measurable levels of the metals remain elevated.

Se toxicity occurs in animals, but humans who have consumed vegetables grown in soil containing high selenium content have not become ill. Se poisoning has been reported due to ingestion of water containing large amounts of the metal.

Other trace elements *Silicon* is present in bone and skin and may play a role in the cross-linkage of collagen. Deficiency in animals results in decreased growth, abnormal early bone development, and decreased hexosamine content of epiphyses and epiphyseal plates. No instance of deficiency in humans has been described. Inhalation of fine particles of SiO_2 causes granuloma formation and chronic fibrosis (silicosis) of the lungs (see Chap. 206).

Fluoride is a constituent of teeth and bone. It prevents dental caries, and its use in patients with osteoporosis has resulted in increased mineralized bone (see Chap. 345). Complications of longterm ingestion by such patients include calcification of bony ligaments and tendons. Chronic intake of fluorides also causes fluorosis, a syndrome characterized by weakness, weight loss, anemia, brittle bones, and mottling of teeth (if taken during stages of enamel formation). Acute ingestion of toxic amounts, as found in some insect poisons, causes severe abdominal pain, nausea, vomiting, diarrhea, and hypocalcemia. Eventually, tetany and cardiorespiratory arrest occur.

A deficiency of any one of *arsenic, nickel, tin,* and *vanadium* causes pathologic manifestations in plants and some vertebrates. Their roles in human health are undefined.

REFERENCES

Falchuk KH: Effect of acute disease and ACTH on serum zinc proteins. N Engl J Med 296:1129, 1977

Karcioulu ZA, Sarper RM: *Zinc and Copper in Medicine*, Springfield, Ill., Charles C Thomas, 1980

Metabolic and physiological consequences of trace element deficiency in animals and man. Philos Trans R Soc Lond [Biol] 294:1, 1981

Millner DS et al: Use of the deferoxamine infusion test in the diagnosis of aluminum-related osteodystrophy. Ann Intern Med 101:775, 1984

Prasad AS: *Trace Elements in Human Health and Disease*. New York, Academic, 1976, vol II

Reinhold JG: Trace elements—A selective survey. Clin Chem 21:476, 1975

Ting-Kai L, Vallee BL: The biochemical and nutritional roles of other trace elements, in *Modern Nutrition in Health and Disease*, 6th ed, RS Goodhart and ME Shils (eds). Philadelphia, Lea and Febiger, 1980

Underwood EJ: *Trace Elements in Human and Animal Nutrition*, 3d ed. New York, Academic, 1971

Williams RJP: The Tilden lecture. Q Rev Chem Soc (Lond) 24:331, 1970

section 1 Basic considerations in infectious disease

78 INTRODUCTION TO INFECTIOUS DISEASES: PATHOGENIC MECHANISMS AND HOST RESPONSES

FREDERICK P. HEINZEL / RICHARD K. ROOT

THE SCOPE OF INFECTIOUS DISEASES Infectious diseases pervade human existence. Great plagues have shaped our history, literature, plumbing, personal hygiene, and societal mores. Just centuries ago, cities were devastated by bubonic plague, populations scarred by smallpox, and whole armies defeated by vibrio and spirochetes. Fortunately, a century of advance in medicine and public health has markedly attenuated the risk of most infectious diseases. As a result, modern day children no longer fear diphtheria, tetanus, polio, or pertussis. Smallpox has been completely eradicated. Mosquito control has removed malaria and yellow fever as endemic threats in the United States, while improved disposal of human waste has decreased the frequency of bacterial and helminthic enteric infections. Unfortunately, many old enemies are with us still; malaria, typhoid, tuberculosis, and other infections remain prevalent in developing nations, where they continue to impede agricultural and economic development. Sexually transmitted diseases, such as chlamydia and gonorrhea, are rampant in most modern cities. Pneumococcus is still occasionally "the old man's friend."

Some technologic advances have created their own problems; the foremost of these has been the development of antibiotic resistance in microbes. In this regard, hospitals have bred strains of staphylococcus and pseudomonas that are increasingly unresponsive to available antibiotics. Poultry and cattle fed antimicrobials to improve their commercial yield now harbor multiply resistant salmonella that have caused outbreaks of disease among humans. Both falciparum malaria and its mosquito vector have become refractory to formerly effective drugs and insecticides.

Similarly, our advanced medical science has inadvertently provided niches in which less pathogenic microorganisms can produce mischief. Transplant and cancer patients are treated with cytotoxic drugs that attenuate host defenses while receiving antibiotics that remove normal pathogens. These patients become a fertile field for formerly unusual species of pathogenic bacteria and fungus. The use of indwelling metal and plastic prosthetic devices has produced access and microecologies favorable for infection with previously "nonpathogenic" coagulase-negative staphylococci and diphtheroids.

If new tricks learned by old microbes were not trouble enough, novel pathogens have been discovered in the last decade. Most prominent among these is the human immunodeficiency virus (HIV), the cause of acquired immunodeficiency syndrome. The immune devastation produced by this virus has in turn given clinical and research prominence to opportunistic pathogens that were previously mere curiosities. Similarly, the clinical entity of Lyme disease has been described and its causative agent, *Borrelia burgdorferi*, characterized. Human parvovirus and human herpesvirus 6 have been implicated in the etiology of erythema infectiosum and erythema subitum, respectively, both previously idiopathic febrile exanthems of infancy. Even peptic ulcers may prove to be of microbial origin, as evidence accumulates linking *Campylobacter pylori* with that disease.

The need for all health care practitioners to study the pathogenesis, diagnosis, and treatment of infectious diseases has not changed in this century of medical progress. It is still true that the study of medicine is greatly involved with the study of infectious disease. It is also true that to understand infection, we must first know how microbes interact with their human hosts.

MICROBIAL FACTORS Infectious disease occurs when a pathogenic organism causes signs and symptoms of inflammation or organ dysfunction. This may be caused by infection, when the etiologic agent multiplies in the host, or from intoxication of the host by cellular poisons generated by a noninfecting organism. Many infections are subclinical, not producing the usual manifestations of ill health. Whether infection is clinically evident or not, the outcome is (1) eradication of the infecting agent (resolution), (2) chronic infection, (3) prolonged excretion of agent (carrier state), or (4) latency of the agent within host tissues.

A wide variety of viruses, bacteria, protozoa, fungi, helminths, and arthropods have been demonstrated to infect humans. The ability of a specific pathogen to cause disease depends on the interaction between its intrinsic pathogenic potential, or virulence, and the defensive measures used by the host to contain and neutralize the infectious threat (Fig. 78-1). The virulence of a pathogen is a relative term; many organisms with normally low virulence can cause severe disease in hosts with compromised immunity. These are called *opportunistic pathogens*. Virulence factors are characteristics of the organism that allow it to colonize, proliferate, invade, and destroy host tissues. In some cases, tissue damage is caused by mass effect from parasitic accumulations or by exuberant host responses.

A relatively uniform series of events must occur before a particular microbe produces clinical disease in humans. At the most basic level, pathogen and host must meet. All etiologic agents have some normal habitat, or reservoir, where they reside and multiply. The most proximate place that the pathogen exists before transmittal to host is termed the source and may be distinct from the reservoir. An infecting agent can be from endogenous or exogenous sources. Endogenously acquired organisms are typically those residing on mucosal surfaces or resting latent in various tissues. Exogenous pathogens are transmitted from source to host by direct or indirect contact, by common vehicle, by airborne particles, or by arthropod or animal vectors. Transmittal by contact occurs when the host encounters the source directly, as in person-to-person spread, or indirectly through secretions, excretions, or objects contaminated by the source. A common

FIGURE 78-1 Schematized interplay between microorganisms and host factors that lead to infection, infectious disease, and resolution. The circled numbers indicate sites at which the designated host responses may interrupt or modify the pathogenesis of disease. *(Modified and used with permission from RK Root, WL Heirholzer, in Clinical Pharmacology: Basic Principles in Therapeutics, 2d ed, KL Melmon, HF Morelli, (eds), Macmillan, New York, 1978.)*

vehicle is a shared item, such as food, water, or blood, that transmits a pathogen to multiple hosts. Airborne transmittal occurs when infectious agents travel through the air on small water or dust particles, often for great distances. Animal or arthropod vectors may transmit disease agents from source to host; in some cases the vector may serve double duty as reservoir and host. Knowledge of the route of transmission of an infectious agent not only will help the physician to understand how disease develops but will provide important diagnostic clues in the case of pet-, travel-, and food-related outbreaks. Additionally, such information is critical to the public health official or hospital epidemiologist who must prevent further illness by disrupting routes of transmission or by removing sources of infection.

Disease does not immediately or inevitably occur once a prospective pathogen is transmitted to its host. Many infections are preceded by colonization of body surfaces, wounds, or hollow viscera with

the infecting agent. The agent typically first colonizes at the site to which it is transmitted (the portal of entry). Success there is supported when the infecting dose is sufficiently large and adherence to epithelium or other tissue is possible. Epithelial attachment is promoted by microbial adhesins, molecules that bind to distinct tissue receptors. In bacteria, these molecules are usually located on filamentous structures (pili, fimbriae) and demonstrate affinity for specific epithelial receptors, such as surface glycoproteins and gangliosides. Pili increase the virulence of pathogenic strains of *Escherichia coli* and *Neisseria gonorrheae*, allowing these organisms to attach to uroepithelium, persist against the opposing flow of urine, and thus better cause disease. Surface polysaccharides of other pathogens may serve similar functions. Dextran produced by certain viridans streptococci glues bacteria to tooth surfaces, where they participate in causing gingival disease. Similarly, complex carbohydrate slime secreted by

Staphylococcus epidermidis promotes adherence to prosthetic devices, a common site for infection with that bacterium.

Pathogens that colonize a site in the body may subsequently proliferate there, greatly increasing the opportunity for tissue invasion or toxin production. Growth of the infecting agent at the portal of entry is determined by the prevailing moisture, oxygen content, pH, and availability of nutrients. Additionally, the agent must be able to surmount competition from the normal flora for required nutrients and epithelial attachment sites. When the protective normal flora is diminished by antibiotics or ill health, pathogenic organisms, such as *Clostridium difficile*, may proliferate inappropriately and cause disease. Alternatively, the proliferative phase may not result in invasive disease, but instead continue and cause prolonged excretion of infectious organisms (carrier state).

Infectious disease becomes evident when microbes invade and disseminate in host tissue. Most infections will present as a primary lesion, usually at the site of initial entry, colonization, and proliferation. If proliferation results in spread along mucosal surfaces, lymphatic channels, or fascial planes, lesions may appear at sites distant from the point of entry. Bloodborne infection can result either in symptoms and signs of overwhelming, multisystem sepsis or in distant metastatic infection. Bacteria often localize to specific organs during dissemination, depending on local factors, such as blood flow, oxygen content, and tissue receptors for microbial adherence factors. For instance, the dextran used by viridans streptococci to promote adherence to teeth also may mediate adherence to heart valve lesions, which could explain the propensity of such bacteria to cause infective endocarditis.

Specific virulence factors that allow pathogens to invade tissue in a predictable fashion have been characterized. Entry may be facilitated by digestive enzymes secreted from the invading organism. Schistosomula and hookworm larvae generate proteases that digest a passage as the worm enters through the skin of the host. Similarly, pyogenic bacteria, such as *Staphylococcus aureus*, *Streptococcus pyogenes*, *Pseudomonas aeruginosa*, and *Clostridium perfringens*, secrete complex cocktails of collagenases, hyaluronidases, lecithinases, and streptokinases that destroy connective tissue and permit invasion and dissemination of infection.

For viral, bacterial, and protozoan agents which are obligate intracellular pathogens, invasion necessarily precedes proliferation. Most of these organisms possess surface molecules that mediate binding and entry into their cellular targets. Influenza viruses adhere to *N*-acetylneuraminic acid residues on respiratory epithelia via hemagglutinating (H) protein expressed on the viral coat. A viral neuraminidase (N) then allows penetration of the cell membrane and uncoating of the virus. Chlamydia and rickettsia have evolved surface proteins that induce phagocytosis by their normally nonphagocytic host cells. *Leishmania* spp., also obligate intramacrophage parasites, use at least three distinct ligand interactions to ensure that they are efficiently phagocytosed by the cells they infect.

Outside of factors that promote colonization, proliferation, and tissue invasion, important virulence factors include bacterial toxins. These are either secreted proteins (exotoxins) or structural portions of the organism, such as endotoxins. Exotoxins can cause disease without antecedent infection. Toxin preformed in food by *S. aureus* or *Bacillus cereus* will cause food poisoning without any further participation of the bacteria following ingestion. Other exotoxins are produced during local proliferation, causing disease without evidence of invasion. Examples include the diarrhea caused by colonization and proliferation within the intestine of *Vibrio cholerae*, which produces a locally active enterotoxin. Toxins formed during bacterial proliferation at one site may be carried considerable distances in the body to produce dysfunction systemically or in other organ systems, as occurs during staphylococcal toxic shock syndrome, scarlet fever, diphtheria, and tetanus.

In contrast to these protein exotoxins, endotoxins from gram-negative bacteria are highly heterogeneous lipopolysaccharides that are part of the bacterial cell wall. Release of this substance during infection, or during infusion of contaminated parenteral fluids, results in an intense host response. Endotoxin potently activates coagulation, complement, and kallikrein pathways, as well as stimulating production of cytokines that can cause fever, widespread circulatory disturbances, and organ dysfunction. The resulting clinical picture of septic shock is discussed in Chap. 89.

HOST IMMUNE FACTORS   Life in such a hostile microbial environment is possible because mammalian hosts possess efficient physical, cellular, and molecular host defenses. The first level of protection is provided by epithelial and epidermal barriers. Would-be pathogens may colonize, but may be unable to penetrate these surfaces. The normally acidic conditions that prevail in the stomach, urine, and vagina additionally limit proliferation of microbes at these sites. Other local secretions contain antimicrobial substances, such as lysozyme and fatty acids, or contain antibodies that block microbial adherence. Surface flow of fluids in the hollow viscera and mucociliary flow of secretions in the respiratory passages further act to prevent internal spread of microbes colonizing the external orifices. Unfortunately, these mechanisms are only as good as their physical integrity, which is often violated by environmental trauma or by the well-meant insertion of urinary and intravenous catheters.

When these external surfaces are penetrated by infectious agents, additional immune mechanisms can be recruited to contain infection (see Chap. 13). The defenses provided by phagocytes, complement, antibodies, and cellular immunity are traditionally described separately, but are in fact tightly interrelated systems that rarely operate in isolation. These responses may occur in either a nonspecific or a specific fashion. Nonspecific responses, although indiscriminate and inefficient, have the advantage of being rapidly available during acute infection and may permit survival of the host until specific responses focus subsequent defenses. Phagocytes and the alternative pathway of complement account for the bulk of nonspecific immune responses, most occurring within hours of the stimulus. In contrast, antibody- and cell-mediated immunities take days to weeks to develop following primary exposure but are often required for complete resolution of disease. Because they have intrinsic memory functions, antibodies and T lymphocytes provide the basis for long-term immunity to reinfection. Their immune specificity is determined by the enormous repertoire of recognition sites available in normal populations of antibodies and T-cell receptors. The importance of these various systems is demonstrated by the markedly increased infectious morbidity and mortality that accompanies genetic or acquired defects of the immune system, which are specifically discussed in Chap. 82.

Polymorphonuclear cells (PMNs) and macrophages are the host's "professional" phagocytes; eosinophils have comparatively minor roles in host defense (see Chap. 64). Polymorphonuclear cells are highly mobile, short-lived blood cells that rapidly enter sites of infection to ingest and destroy microbial invaders. When infection occurs, PMNs can be provided in large numbers from marrow precursors or from preformed pools. Under the guidance of substances diffusing from infection sites, including both microbial products and elicited host factors, PMNs adhere to and cross the endothelium. These same factors then elicit directed migration (chemotaxis) of PMNs to the inflammatory site. Pathogens are bound by PMN surface adhesins, ingested, and subsequently exposed during phagolysosomal fusion to an acidic internal environment rich in hydrolytic enzymes and antibacterial proteins. In addition, the polymorphonuclear cell consumes oxygen during microbial ingestion and generates toxic oxidants such as superoxide anion and hydrogen peroxide. The lysosomal enzyme myeloperoxidase augments the already considerable microbicidal activity of these oxidants by producing hypochlorous acid from chloride ion and hydrogen peroxide. Disorders of phagocytes are discussed in Chap. 81.

In contrast, macrophages circulate transiently and then establish long-lived residency in tissue, particularly the spleen, liver, and lung. They are favorably situated to remove infectious threats in transit through the lungs or bloodstream. Macrophages share many of the phagocytic and microbicidal activities of PMNs. However they can markedly increase these functions when activated by factors, notably γ-interferon, produced by stimulated T lymphocytes. In addition, macrophages have accessory cell functions, such as antigen presentation and interleukin 1 production, that are critical for initiating cellular and humoral immunity.

Complement and antibodies are the major soluble mediators of immunity in serum and provide important specific and nonspecific protection against extracellular and viral pathogens. The complement system is a collection of some 25 proteins that enzymatically generates membrane-associated opsonizing and microbicidal protein complexes. Specific activation of complement, by the classical pathway, is triggered when antibodies bind to microbe. Nonspecific activation (alternative pathway) is stimulated upon exposure to certain types of microbial surface components and does not require the presence of antibody.

Antibodies are complex glycoproteins, produced by B lymphocytes, that bind to microbial antigens and that subsequently activate microbicidal responses. The antigen-binding site of antibody exhibits any of approximately 10^8 variable protein sequences capable of specifically binding to macromolecules, such as microbial antigens, by means of complementary charge and molecular topography. Other portions of the antibody are invariant in structure and are responsible for initiating complement activation, antibody-dependent cellular cytotoxicity (ADCC), or phagocytosis when antibody is bound to a microbial target. Antibodies may, in addition, neutralize viruses, bacteria, and toxins by blocking adhesins or functional sites.

The constant regions of the antibody define the five classes of immunoglobulin: IgM, IgG, IgA, IgD, and IgE. Each class of immunoglobulin has a distinct distribution within host tissues. IgM antibodies are largely found within the intravascular compartment, whereas IgG antibodies are distributed widely throughout the extracellular space. Both may appear on mucosal surfaces during inflammation. Otherwise, mucosal immunity is largely due to IgA secretory antibodies that inhibit colonization, multiplication, and invasion by bacteria and viruses.

Cellular immunity is the host response mediated by macrophages, T lymphocytes, and their soluble products. Whereas PMNs and humoral immunity are most effective against extracellular pathogens, cellular immunity is best suited for the control of intracellular parasites. T lymphocytes are activated by antigen presented in conjunction with major histocompatibility antigen (MHC) on the surfaces of macrophages and B lymphocytes. Following activation, T lymphocytes may assume a variety of functional roles. They may differentiate into T cells that stimulate B-cell growth and synthesis of immunoglobulin. Alternatively, they may secrete proteins that activate the microbicidal or cytotoxic functions of macrophages and cytotoxic T cells. Both macrophages and T lymphocytes secrete other proinflammatory cytokines that cause fever, increase serum levels of acute phase reactants, or stimulate bone marrow production of leukocytes. Other T lymphocytes are capable of lysing host cells infected with virus or that have become neoplastic. Similar cytotoxic functions are provided by large granular lymphocytes that lack T-cell receptors and that do not require MHC for recognition of their target; these lymphocytes are called natural killer (NK) cells.

Each step in the pathogenesis of infectious disease is a complex interplay of microbial action and host reaction. These battle lines are far from static, as many infectious agents have evolved strategies to evade host immunity. Certainly colonizing organisms that elude local host defenses are better able to proliferate and cause eventual disease. Not surprisingly, a wide variety of such stratagems are recognized. One such mechanism is the avoidance of early nonspecific immune responses. For example, antiphagocytic surfaces of encapsulated bacteria protect against ingestion by leukocytes; other bacteria are intrinsically resistant to complement activation when in the bloodstream. Similarly, microbes may evade phagocytes and antibodies by dwelling within host cells, a technique used to great advantage by chlamydia, rickettsia, toxoplasma, and leishmania. Antigenic variation may foil recognition by antibodies and is used by some

species of borrelia and trypanosoma, accounting for the chronic, relapsing course of those diseases. Influenza viruses regularly undergo antigenic change; epidemics result when the neoantigen is unrecognized by the human population. Pathogens may generate molecules that inactivate host immune responses. Lumen-dwelling bacteria, such as *N. gonorrhea*, produce IgA proteases that degrade mucosal antibodies, whereas some strains of *S. aureus* and streptococci possess surface proteins that bind immunoglobulin in nonfunctional conformations. Other bacteria, such as clostridia and bordetella, produce toxins that kill or inactivate leukocytes.

The balance of microbial virulence and host immunity determines the outcome of disease. When host responses eradicate the offending agent, resolution occurs—often with complete immunity to reinfection. When host responses are evenly balanced against microbial factors, chronic disease may result. Alternatively, the immune response may simply drive the pathogen into a latent state in some protected site, such as a nerve ganglion cell following infection with herpes simplex or varicella-zoster viruses. Any waning of host surveillance then results in reactivation of infection, as often happens with herpes viruses, toxoplasma, and mycobacteria following immunosuppression. When host defenses eliminate invasive infection but allow continued proliferation of the microbe at mucosal sites, a carrier state may develop.

HOST RESPONSES TO INFECTION Infectious diseases have long been known by the host responses they provoke: fever, chills, local inflammation, leukocytosis, protein catabolism, and the serum acute phase reaction. Fever and chills, often accompanied by increased pulse rate, are the usual herald signs of severe infection. Although the pattern and duration of fever may give useful diagnostic clues, body temperature is better used to assess the course of infection and the response to therapy (see Chap. 20). Signs of inflammation (heat, erythema, pain, and swelling) are the characteristic features of localized infection. Infected viscera become recognizable by tenderness upon palpation, by the inflammatory changes (usually polymorphonuclear leukocytes) present in adjacent body fluids, by their radiographic appearance, or by altered organ function. Like fever, an increased neutrophil count in the peripheral blood gives information about the presence and intensity of infection. However, as the severity of infection increases, neutropenia may develop and is a poor prognostic sign during sepsis or pneumonia. Other blood constituents are affected; thrombocytopenia, anemia, and coagulopathy may accompany subacute or chronic infection.

The profile of serum proteins changes during infection. Collectively referred to as the acute phase reaction, it reflects altered hepatic synthesis of protein. Typically, serum albumin concentration is reduced while serum amyloid A protein, C-reactive protein, and various proteinase inhibitors increase, sometimes up to 1000-fold. Serum levels of zinc and iron decrease in the serum at the same time, probably due to chelation with lactoferrin and similar acute phase products. A catabolic state is further augmented by simultaneous increases in levels of circulating cortisol, glucagon, catecholamines, and other hormones.

Although discrete inflammatory roles have been described for prostanoids, complement products, and monamines, the most dramatic effects are mediated by a few proinflammatory cytokines: interleukin 1, tumor necrosis factor, interleukin 6, and γ-interferon. These factors, singly or in combination, promote fever, stimulate hepatic acute phase responses, produce local inflammatory signs, and trigger catabolic responses. Responding lymphocytes and macrophages similarly elaborate a variety of colony-stimulating factors which promote bone marrow production of leukocytes.

When mild to moderate in intensity, inflammatory responses probably serve important host defense functions. For instance, increased body temperatures accentuate lymphocyte responses and may inhibit viral replication. Inflammatory hyperemia and systemic neutrophilia optimize phagocyte delivery to sites of infection. The decreased availability of iron "starves" certain microbes of a necessary nutrient. However, when these responses become extreme, extensive tissue damage can result, as typified in the extreme by fulminant septic shock (see Chap. 89).

Other infections may be similarly accompanied by deleterious side effects as a result of prolonged or inappropriate immune reactivity. The wasting of body fat and muscle during lengthy infections probably reflects the strong catabolic and anorexic effects of circulating interleukin 1 and tumor necrosis factor. In certain circumstances, antigen and antibody may form immune complexes that will independently initiate inflammatory reactions at sites of deposition, causing vasculitis and glomerulonephritis syndromes. When microbe and host by chance share common immunologic epitopes, autoimmune disease may be triggered. The classic example is provided by rheumatic cardiomyopathy, thought to arise from molecular mimicry of cardiac muscle antigen by streptococcal M protein. Celiac disease, Reiter's syndrome, and juvenile-onset diabetes mellitus may be initiated by similar events.

DIAGNOSIS AND TREATMENT OF INFECTIOUS DISEASES
The basic goals of diagnosis in infectious disease are to determine which organ system is affected and which agent is responsible for the disease. This evaluation requires a careful history, complete physical examination, and intelligent use of laboratory tests. The clinician is usually first presented with certain clinical symptoms and signs highly suggestive of infection, including abrupt onset, fever, chills, myalgia, photophobia, pharyngitis, acute lymphadenopathy and splenomegaly, gastrointestinal upset, and leukocytosis or leukopenia. When infectious disease is likely, three important items should be addressed by the history, physical examination, and initial laboratory tests: the organ system involved, the tempo of the illness, and the presence of unusual risk factors. The affected organ system is usually obvious from complaints such as dysuria, productive cough, localized pain, swelling, or erythema. Occasionally symptoms are diffuse and may represent systemic infection. Because certain organs are infected by relatively predictable agents, the classification of the patient's disorder as pneumonia, meningitis, urinary tract infection, septic shock, cellulitis, etc., will help direct diagnostic and therapeutic strategies. This syndromic approach to infectious disease is illustrated in the following chapters. The tempo of onset may incriminate certain types of pathogen as possible causes of infectious disease. For example, viruses and pyogenic bacteria tend to have acute or subacute courses; fungal or mycobacterial infections are indolent and often cause chronic diseases. Relapsing or recurrent symptoms may be critical diagnostic clues during infection with borrelia, plasmodia, or brucella.

Most infectious agents have sharply defined reservoirs and routes of communication, so that unusual exposures should be sought in the patient's history. An extensive review of occupational, travel, sexual, and social information may be required. This is exemplified by the workup for atypical pneumonia, which necessitates a detailed inquiry about travel- and animal-related exposures that might implicate psittacosis, coccidioidomycosis, tularemia, or Q fever. Similarly, sexual histories are essential when genital lesions are present, and information about sexual practices, intravenous drug abuse, or transfusions is required to assess a patient's risk for HIV infection. Many unusual risks are iatrogenic or nosocomially acquired, the most obvious being previous antibiotic use, irradiation, or cytotoxic therapy for neoplasm and organ transplantation (see Chaps. 82 and 83).

Once a list of suspect pathogens has been generated, laboratory tests are used to identify the offender. Direct methods of identification typically include stains and culture of body fluids, secretions, and tissue. The type of stain and culture to use in atypical scenarios is best decided after consultation with the microbiology laboratory (see Chap. 80). Another direct means of microbial diagnosis is to assay for microbial antigen in fluid or tissue using immunofluorescence, ELISA, or RIA techniques. Indirect methods measure the host response to infecting agent by assaying titers of specific antibody or by measuring skin test reactivity. These give less satisfactory diagnostic information because the measured responses often are delayed in onset, persist for years, and may not occur at all in immunocom-

promised patients. Because no microbiologic or serologic assay is perfect, very few diagnoses are made from these data alone; the clinician must interpret the facts supplied by the laboratory examination in the context of a patient's history and examination.

When infection does occur, numerous therapeutic options are available. Many simple viral infections will, of course, resolve without specific treatment. Minor cutaneous or mucosal infections may respond to topical therapy. With increasing severity of disease, systemic antibiotics become necessary. The choice of agent should be based on the efficacy, toxicity, cost, and ease of administration (see Chaps. 85 to 88). Although sometimes therapy can be initiated on minimal microbiologic data, such as penicillin for streptococcal pharyngitis, nosocomial infections may require a careful review of susceptibility data to uncover acquired antibiotic resistances.

In infectious diseases, prevention is preferable to cure. Immunization has become a cornerstone of modern medicine, and it is essential that it be a part of primary care (see Chap. 84). Most active vaccines contain an immunizing agent that is either inactivated or attenuated and are typically used before infectious exposure can occur. However, administration of vaccine in conjunction with specialized immune globulins may be effective even after exposure to certain infectious agents such as hepatitis B, rabies, and *Clostridium tetani*. Passive immunization alone, such as provided by pooled human serum globulin, is still used to protect travelers against the acquisition of hepatitis A. Other practices to avoid infection have become standard procedure, such as the use of asepsis during surgery and the aggressive debridement and cleaning of traumatic wounds. In appropriate circumstances, antibacterial prophylaxis may additionally decrease the risk of infection inherent in some surgical procedures or from exposure to communicable agents (see Chap. 85).

REFERENCES

BURNET FM, WHITE DO: *Natural History of Infectious Disease*, 4th ed. Cambridge University Press, 1972
MANDELL GL et al (eds): *Principles and Practice of Infectious Diseases*, 3d ed. New York, Wiley, 1990
MIMS CA: *The Pathogenesis of Infectious Disease*, 3d ed. London, Academic, 1987
ROOT RK: Infectious diseases: Pathogenetic mechanisms and host responses, in *Pathophysiology—The Biological Principles of Diseases*, 2d ed, LH Smith Jr, SO Thier (eds). Philadelphia, Saunders, 1985

79 INFECTIOUS DISEASES AND THE NEW BIOLOGY

DON GANEM

Fundamental recent developments in molecular biology have revolutionized our understanding of the basic chemistry of living things. These developments have enormous potential for the study and treatment of human diseases in general and infectious diseases in particular. In this chapter we review selected advances in the study of microbial pathogens that illustrate the nature and scope of progress in this area.

The conceptual cornerstone of molecular biology is the marriage of genetic reasoning and biochemical methodology. In this approach, biochemical phenomena are characterized by the isolation and study of mutant organisms with genetic lesions affecting these phenomena. Initially this was done with simple organisms, most commonly *Escherichia coli* and its bacteriophages. It has since become possible to extend these studies to higher organisms and to the parasites and viruses that infect them. Thus, virtually from its inception, molecular biology has had a disproportionate impact on the study of microorganisms. A major watershed was crossed in the mid-1970s when the technology was developed to clone and characterize segments of DNA from any organism in *E. coli*. (For a discussion of the details of this methodology, see Chap. 6.) This *recombinant DNA (rDNA)* technology has further facilitated the study of microbial pathogens and also made possible new approaches to diagnostics and therapeutics. The impact of these developments for our understanding of the origins, pathogenesis, and treatment of human infectious diseases are considered below.

MOLECULAR GENETICS AND PATHOGENESIS

BACTERIAL DISEASES   Recent progress in understanding the nature of phase and antigenic variation in gonococci provides a beautiful example of the power of genetic reasoning to understand microbial pathogenesis. Early studies of pathogenic gonococci indicated that piliated strains (i.e., those with the protein *pilin* organized as surface projections called *pili*) are substantially more pathogenic than nonpiliated ones, perhaps because they show increased adherence to mucosal cells or resistance to phagocytosis (see Chap. 110). However, when cultured apart from the host, strains often lose their surface pili; with further passage the same organism can regain surface pili. This is referred to as pilin *phase variation*. It is even more important that the antigenic structure of these pili often changes radically as the organisms grow; such *antigenic variation* is believed to contribute greatly to the organism's ability to evade the host's immune response.

Cloning and characterization of pilin revealed that the gonococcal genome contains many incomplete genes harboring fragmentary coding information for pilin polypeptides in a silent, unexpressed form and only one (or, rarely, two) locus at which pilin genes can be actively expressed as RNA and protein. Variant pilins arise when stretches of coding sequences originating from the silent pilin loci recombine into the expression site. As a result of this genetic exchange, new pilin coding sequences are created. If these sequences are untranslatable, the organism loses its pili altogether (phase variation); if translatable, they often give rise to antigenic variation. These studies indicate that phase and antigenic variation proceed from a single recombinational mechanism and have important potential implications for the design of vaccination strategies.

Another important example of the use of genetics to define virulence pathways has been the study of plasmid-associated virulence factors. For example, both *Yersinia enterocolitica* and *Shigella sonnei* produce an invasive intestinal infection, and both harbor large extrachromosomal DNA molecules (plasmids) that replicate apart from the bacterial genome. In both cases, derivative strains lacking the plasmid have been isolated. When compared with their parental strains, each plasmidless variant was virtually avirulent when inoculated into animal hosts, indicating that important virulence factors are either encoded or regulated by the plasmid sequences. This finding set the stage for the identification of these factors by isolating and characterizing mutants of the plasmid that would not restore virulence upon transfer to plasmidless strains. In this way, multiple plasmid gene products that contribute to virulence have been identified in both organisms. The availability of each of these genes in cloned form now makes possible rigorous study of the biosynthesis and function of their products.

Genetic analysis of bacterial virulence factors is not limited to those mediated by plasmids. In *Yersinia*, for instance, important chromosomal loci exist that mediate additional functions in pathogenesis. It has long been known that *Yersinia* of several species can invade and replicate within eukaryotic host cells, even including cells not overtly specialized for phagocytosis. Two genetic loci governing such invasion have now been identified by cloning *Yersinia* DNA in *E. coli* and screening the recombinant bacteria (carrying cloned sequences) for the ability to invade cells in culture. Two distinct genes of *Yersinia* have emerged from this selection, each of which

can mediate entry into host cells, albeit at different efficiencies. At least one of these genes encodes a surface protein involved in cell attachment and invasion. Neither gene, however, allows intracellular growth of *E. coli*, suggesting that additional loci mediate these functions.

This brief survey of genetically identified bacterial virulence factors is intended to be illustrative. Over the years many other equally important virulence determinants have been identified using these approaches. These include enterotoxins (in *Vibrio cholerae* and enterotoxigenic *E. coli*), cytotoxins (in *Pseudomonas aeruginosa*, *Shigella*, and enterohemorrhagic *E. coli*), adhesins (in uropathogenic and enterotoxigenic *E. coli*), and IgA proteases (in pathogenic *Neisseriae*), to name but a few.

VIRAL REPLICATION   Viruses have proven invaluable as tools for the study of gene expression in higher eukaryotic cells. Much of what is currently known about transcription, RNA processing, and translation in mammalian cells was learned through the study of animal viruses. Conversely, in the course of these studies the basics of virus structure and replication were elucidated in great detail, setting the stage for further progress in the understanding of virus-host biology and pathogenesis. In no other area of infectious disease research has the impact of molecular biology been as profound as in virology (see Chap. 133).

The course of research into the acquired immunodeficiency syndrome (AIDS) bears eloquent testimony to this fact (see Chap. 264). In the space of only a few years from the first isolation of human immune virus (HIV), the viral genome was cloned and its complete nucleotide sequence determined. This led to the recognition of a number of new viral genes not previously encountered among standard animal retroviruses, including genes involved in the regulation of viral transcription (*tat*) and RNA processing (*rev*), as well as others affecting viral infectivity and morphogenesis. The molecular basis of the antigenic variation of the viral surface glycoproteins has been determined, and highly conserved sites on this protein involved in receptor binding and membrane fusion identified. Such regions are of obvious importance in the design of potential strategies for immunoprophylaxis. The viral receptor has been identified as the cell surface protein CD4, and the regions of the receptor involved in virus binding have been mapped. Cloning of the receptor itself also has been achieved, and mutant variants of the protein secreted from cultured cells have been shown to block viral infectivity. These recombinant CD4 preparations have been used in clinical trials as candidate antiviral agents.

These advances in the understanding of HIV are particularly striking because they illustrate how rapidly such information can be obtained with contemporary approaches. Most of these technologies were developed through the study of other viruses prior to the advent of the AIDS epidemic. Using these methods, for instance, the receptors for many viruses, including Epstein-Barr virus, poliovirus, and rhinoviruses have been identified and cloned. For some viruses, including poliovirus and influenza, the details of the virion surface structure and receptor-binding site are known at atomic resolution.

Recombinant DNA technology has also made possible the detailed study of many aspects of viral replication and gene expression without the requirement for virus growth in culture. This can be done by transfection of cloned viral genes into cultured cell lines, as well as by the analysis of viral DNA and RNA in infected human or animal tissues. This has allowed characterization of many medically important viruses whose study was impossible by classic virologic means. The hepatitis viruses provide an important case in point. The involvement of reverse transcription in the replication of hepatitis B virus (HBV) was discovered, and its mechanism defined, entirely in the absence of cell culture. The replicative program of the virus of delta hepatitis, a satellite of HBV, was similarly elucidated. More recently a candidate viral genome has been cloned from the serum of a recipient of blood products implicated in the transmission of non-A, non-B hepatitis. Even though this agent (tentatively termed hepatitis C virus) also has not been grown in culture, serodiagnostic tests based on recombinant antigens can now be developed and should have a major positive impact on the safety of the blood supply.

The human papilloma viruses (HPV) also cannot be grown in culture, but analysis of infected tissues with cloned HPV DNA probes has revealed that there is a strong association between cervical and genital carcinoma and infection with specific biotypes of HPV. Tumors arising in the context of infection by these viruses harbor viral DNA sequences integrated into the host genome; analysis of the host DNA invariably reveals the retention of certain regions of the viral genome, while others are typically deleted. These studies have provided powerful clues to the viral genes involved in malignant transformation.

No discussion of contemporary molecular virology would be complete without mention of the use of animal viruses as genetic vectors for the delivery of foreign DNA to somatic cells. Viruses are attractive vehicles for such gene transfer because they have evolved efficient mechanisms for entry into and persistence within host cells. In most strategies for viral vectoring, genes are first removed from the virus genome and replaced with the exogenous DNA of interest. The resulting recombinant genome, once packaged inside the virus particle, is then used to infect the appropriate host cell. Assuming the genes excised from the virus are not required for its replication, the recombinant genome will be capable of replication and spread within the recipient. If the deleted sequences are required for viral growth, the recombinant will be defective (nonviable) and will not spread beyond the original infected cell unless complemented by a helper virus.

Many types of virus has been employed as genetic vectors, including polyomavirus, parvovirus, adenovirus, papillomavirus, retrovirus, poxvirus, and even herpesvirus. As yet only retrovirus, adenovirus, and poxvirus show promise as clinically useful vectors. Defective murine retrovirus is the most likely vector to be used in initial efforts at somatic gene therapy, particularly for disorders involving cells of the blood or bone marrow (e.g., adenosine deaminase deficiency; see Chap. 263). The principal advantages of this virus include its efficient infection of hematopoietic cells and the ability to prepare helper-free stocks of replication-incompetent vectors, which ensures that there will be no spread of the virus in the recipient of the treated marrow.

By contrast, there are situations in which a limited amount of viral replication in the host is desirable—for example, in the design of live-virus vaccines—where this serves to mimic natural infection and provoke both humoral and cell-mediated immunity. For these applications, a nondefective poxvirus (e.g., vaccinia) or adenovirus has found favor. Attenuated live-virus strains with long records of human use as vaccines are available for both virus families; these serve as starting material for recombinant design. Foreign genes encoding antigens of interest are then cloned into nonessential regions of the viral genome and the recombinants isolated in pure culture for use. This practice is most highly developed for vaccinia, where recombinants have been constructed bearing antigens from HBV, HIV, influenza, and even *Plasmodium falciparum*. Like all live-virus vaccines, these recombinant viruses carry with them the risk of disease induction in the immunodeficient host (as well as other potential risks) and will require careful experimental and clinical scrutiny before they can be contemplated for widespread use.

PARASITOLOGY The same features that have allowed molecular biologists to study noncultivatable viruses have also proven useful in the study of difficult-to-grow protozoan and metazoan parasites. Spectacular progress has been made, for example, in the study of the biology of the African trypanosomes, the causative agents of sleeping sickness (see Chap. 161). These organisms undergo a remarkable program of antigenic variation to evade host immune responses during their protracted bloodstream infection. It consists of sequential expression of variants of a major surface glycoprotein, brought about, as in gonococci, by movement of coding information from silent chromosomal reservoirs into active expression sites.

Equally remarkable progress is being made in the study of malarial

parasites. Genes governing the production of the major surface protein of the sporozoite have been cloned and extensively characterized, and the protein products of the recombinants have been tested as candidate vaccine components. Similar work is underway to express important antigens from the merozoite (bloodstream) and even the gametocyte stages (see Chaps. 156 and 159). While an effective vaccine has not been developed, there is renewed hope that a combination of such antigens affecting a number of steps in the parasite's complex life cycle may yet prove effective in attenuating disease and preventing transmission.

Perhaps the most surprising and provocative result yet to emerge from the application of molecular biology to parasites concerns the characterization of *Pneumocystis carinii* (see Chap. 163). Examination of the sequence of ribosomal RNA from this organism yields the unexpected finding that this agent, widely classified as a protozoan, is taxonomically closer to yeasts!

DIAGNOSTIC AND THERAPEUTIC APPLICATIONS

Although the aforementioned advances will form the bases of the diagnostic and therapeutic approaches of the future, many more direct applications of rDNA technology are having immediate impact on present-day clinical practice. Some of these are summarized below.

DIAGNOSTICS Once any organism is available in reasonable quantity and purity, molecular clones of its genome can be prepared, irrespective of its ability to be readily grown in culture. These DNA clones can then be used as hybridization probes to detect the organism's genome in clinical specimens. A variety of formats are available for such DNA:DNA hybridization tests, both in solid phase (*filter hybridization*) and in solution. Methods even exist for the detection of microbial genomes or transcripts in histologic specimens (*in situ hybridization*). While detailed consideration of the methodologic aspects of such testing is beyond the scope of this chapter (see Chap. 81), the advantages of these tests can be simply summarized as follows: (1) they can be performed on noncultivatable as well as cultivatable organisms; (2) they can be much more rapid than culture-based tests for organisms that are difficult to grow; and (3) they can display extraordinary specificity. However, such testing is not a diagnostic panacea. Widespread use of these tests has been limited by several features. Optimal sensitivity often requires the use of radiolabeled probes with isotopes with a short half-life; particularly where radiolabeled probes are required, a high level of technical expertise is necessary to maintain quality in the environment of mass testing in clinical laboratories. Finally, like most biochemical tests, the sensitivity of filter hybridization tests is generally less than that of culture, where replication of the organism affords rapid and enormous amplification of the signal. These considerations suggest that such tests will not replace cultures for most conventional bacteria but will be of greatest use in the diagnosis of organisms (e.g., viruses, *Chlamydia,* and parasites) where culture is either impossible, difficult, or inefficient.

An even more powerful DNA-based diagnostic technology has recently been developed that promises to mitigate the problem of sensitivity mentioned above. This is the enzymatic amplification of DNA in vitro also known by its technical name, the polymerase chain reaction (see Chap. 6). Basically, this method uses DNA polymerases to amplify the signal from the microbial genome in the test tube, in a fashion analogous to what authentic replication would do during culture. As a result, each copy of the microbial genome in the specimen undergoes replication many thousandfold in vitro during the brief period (hours) of the reaction. The amplified DNA segment can then be specifically identified by filter hybridization or other means. The method has the advantage of enormous sensitivity, rivaling that of culture for some organisms. Its disadvantages are the expense and high level of technical expertise needed to perform the test. Its exquisite sensitivity may also impose some limits on its clinical utility. False-positive results from degrees of laboratory contamination too trivial to be detected by conventional tests have already occurred.

The other area in which rDNA technology is already having an impact is in the development of improved reagents for serologic testing. The expression of foreign antigens in *E. coli* is now routine and is increasingly being used to generate pure antigens for use in diagnostic serology. This has been particularly valuable for agents that are difficult to grow in quantity or hard to purify. For example, recombinant core and surface antigens of HBV and *gag* and envelope antigens of HIV are now commonly used in commercial testing kits (see Chaps. 252 and 264).

THERAPEUTICS The other major area in which rDNA technology is already affecting clinical practice is in the production of therapeutic agents and vaccines. This area is still in its infancy but will certainly undergo rapid expansion in the future. The development of live virus vaccines based on viral vectors has already been discussed. More conventional vaccines composed of recombinant antigens produced in bacteria, yeast, or cultured cells can be anticipated with certainty. Already one such product has been licensed, recombinant hepatitis B surface antigen (produced in yeast cells). Similar strategies are underway for vaccine development against HIV, herpes simplex, rabies, and other agents.

A wide variety of biologically active polypeptides with therapeutic potential have also been produced using this technology, including a number of growth factors, hormones, and cytokines. Some of these, e.g., hematopoietic growth factors like GM-CSF, may be useful in shortening periods of neutropenia induced by cytotoxic cancer chemotherapy. Other polypeptides with immunoregulatory or antiviral activity, such as interferons or other lymphokines, may also have therapeutic value.

Finally, the expression of microbial products by rDNA technology in large quantities facilitates x-ray crystallographic structure determination. For those proteins (e.g., metabolic enzymes or adhesins) that are good targets for antimicrobial drugs, knowledge of the protein's fine structure may one day make possible the rational design of inhibitors targeted to the relevant active site.

REFERENCES

GANEM D, VARMUS H: The molecular biology of the hepatitis B viruses. Ann Rev Biochem 56:651, 1987

MILLER V, FALKOW S: Evidence for two genetic loci in *Yersinia enterocolitica* that can promote invasion of epithelial cells. Infect Immun 56:1242, 1988

NOTKINS A, OLDSTONE MB (eds): *Concepts in Viral Pathogenesis.* New York, Springer-Verlag, 1984

SCAIFE J et al (eds): *The Genetics of Bacteria.* London, Academic, 1985

SPARLING PF et al: Phase and antigenic variation of pili and outer membrane protein II in *Neisseria gonorrheae.* J Infect Dis 153:196, 1986

TURNER M, ARNOT D (eds): *Molecular Genetics of Parasitic Protozooa.* New York, Cold Spring Harbor Press, 1988

80   THE DIAGNOSIS OF INFECTIOUS DISEASES

JAMES J. PLORDE

The diagnosis of an infectious disease requires the direct or indirect demonstration of a pathogenic microbe on or within the tissues of the afflicted host. The major ways in which this is accomplished are described in this chapter.

DIRECT MICROSCOPIC EXAMINATION

The direct microscopic examination of body fluids, exudates, and tissues is both the simplest and one of the most helpful laboratory procedures available for the diagnosis of infectious diseases. In many situations the examination allows an accurate, highly specific identification of the causative agent. Examples include the recognition of *Borrelia* or *Plasmodium* species in blood smears taken from patients with relapsing fever or malaria. More commonly, only a tentative identification can be made on the basis of microbial morphology. Nevertheless, this is often sufficiently precise to allow the selection of an appropriate chemotherapeutic agent pending the results of more definitive investigations.

WET MOUNTS Dark-field examination of fluid from genital lesions for the spirochete of syphilis is a well-known, but neglected, procedure. More often, wet mounts are used for the diagnosis of fungal and parasitic infections. The examination of hair fragments, skin scrapings, or nail clippings in a drop of 10% KOH or KOH-calcofluor is useful in establishing the presence of superficial mycoses. Occasionally a presumptive diagnosis of a systemic fungus infection can also be established with this procedure. Two examples are cryptococcal meningitis diagnosed by demonstrating the encapsulated organism in an india ink preparation of cerebrospinal fluid, and coccidioidomycosis identified by finding characteristic spherules in expectorated sputum.

Examination of wet mounts of stool or duodenal drainage is also the initial step in establishing the diagnosis of intestinal protozoal infections such as amebiasis, giardiasis, and cryptosporidiosis. Moreover, it is the definitive procedure diagnosing intestinal helminthic infections including ascariasis, trichuriasis, strongyloidiasis, and hookworm. Filariasis and sleeping sickness can be recognized by demonstrating the characteristic motility of microfilariae and trypanosomes in blood or other body fluids.

STAIN-ENHANCED MICROSCOPY Despite many technical advances in the field of microbiology, the Gram stain remains, after 100 years of use, the best single technique available for the rapid diagnosis of bacterial infections. It is of particular value in the examination of exudates, aspirates, and body fluids, including cerebrospinal fluid and urine. Stains are examined first under the lower-power objective to demonstrate the presence of pink-staining inflammatory cells. The paucity of such cells in the presence of many squamous epithelial cells suggests that the specimen was contaminated during the process of collection and may not be representative of the inflammatory process. The smear is then examined for the presence of bacteria using the oil immersion lens; bacteria appear either as dark blue (gram-positive) or pink (gram-negative) bodies. Their color and morphologic appearance often make possible a presumptive identification of the genus and occasionally the species of the organism. The demonstration of pneumococci in the sputum, Enterobacteriaceae in the urine, staphylococci in localized abscesses, gonococci in urethral exudates, clostridia in foul-smelling discharge, and pneumococci, meningococci, or *Haemophilus influenzae* in stained smears of the cerebrospinal fluid permits the initiation of specific chemotherapy with the assurance that the regimen is the proper one.

Mycobacteria have the unique capacity to resist the decolorization by strong mineral acid alcohol solutions once they have been stained with basic carbol-fuchsin (Ziehl-Neelsen, Kinyoun stains) or one of the newer fluorochromes. This allows their immediate recognition in body tissues and fluids. The presence of a large number of acid-fast bacilli in the expectorated sputum establishes the presumptive diagnosis of respiratory tuberculosis and is sufficient evidence for initiating isolation procedures and antituberculosis therapy once additional specimens are collected for culture.

Acid-fast smears can also be used to identify *Cryptosporidium* and *Isospora* spp. in the stool of patients with diarrhea. If mineral acid rather than acid alcohol is used for decolorization, pathogenic strains of *Nocardia* may be visualized in body fluids or exudates.

A number of stains are available for the definitive identification of parasites. *Pneumocystis carinii* can be recognized in induced sputum, bronchial lavage fluid, and transbronchial brush biopsies using a modified Wright's stain, toluidine blue, or methenamine silver. Blood and tissue protozoa such as plasmodia and *Leishmania* can be demonstrated best with Romanowsky-type mixtures containing methylene blue and eosin. These render the nuclei red to violet and the cytoplasm blue. The identification of intestinal protozoa, on the other hand, requires the use of stains such as iron hematoxylin or trichrome to demonstrate the taxonomically important nuclear detail.

IMMUNE MICROSCOPY This method combines the specificity of immunologic procedures with the speed of direct microscopy. In the immunofluorescent technique, smears thought to contain viral, bacterial, fungal, or parasitic organisms are stained with specific antibody preparations labeled with fluorescent compounds and examined with a fluorescent microscope. The most useful application of this technique is the examination of brain tissue for herpes simplex or rabies virus; respiratory specimens for cytomegalovirus, *Legionella* spp., and *P. carinii;* cervical, urethral, conjunctival, and nasopharyngeal specimens for *Chlamydia trachomatis;* and genital lesions for herpes simplex virus. Direct fluorescent antibody staining of nasopharyngeal cells may also be used for the rapid diagnosis of pertussis, influenza, parainfluenza, and respiratory syncytial virus infections.

The accuracy and reliability of immunofluorescent techniques continues to improve as older polyclonal antisera are replaced with more specific monoclonal reagents. The need for expensive fluorescent microscopes and well-trained technologists restricts the routine use of these procedures to larger laboratories.

Enzyme-linked immunosorbent assay (ELISA) tests are similar to the immunofluorescence test except that the antiserum is reacted with an enzyme-labeled antispecies conjugate. After treatment with an appropriate substrate, a color change can be visualized with the ordinary light microscope, obviating expensive equipment.

HYBRIDIZATION MICROSCOPY It has been shown that microbes fixed on glass slides can be hybridized with small, fluorescently labeled, oligonucleotide probes complementary to 16 S ribosomal RNA and visualized by fluorescent microscopy. Identification is accomplished by utilizing probes complementary to group- or species-specific 16 S rRNA sequences. A variety of microbes can be identified on the same microscopic slide with the simultaneous use of multiple probes labeled with different fluors.

DETECTION OF MICROBIAL ANTIGENS, BY-PRODUCTS, AND GENOMES

The relative nonspecificity of many direct microscopic methods and the delay inherent in culture procedures have resulted in the introduction of a variety of techniques aimed at the rapid detection of microbial antigens, by-products, or genomes. Such procedures are particularly useful when prior antibiotic therapy has rendered microscopic and culture tests negative.

PARTICLE AGGLUTINATION Particle (e.g., latex, erythrocytes) agglutination tests are the most commonly employed antigen detection procedures. They are technically simpler and frequently more sensitive than the counterimmunoelectrophoresis (CIE) method which they have supplanted. Agglutination tests have been plagued by false-positive reactions from heat-labile serum and urine components and from rheumatoid factor. Like CIE, latex and coagglutination tests have proved most useful for the rapid detection of pneumococcal, meningococcal, group B streptococcal, or *H. influenzae* antigens in the urine and spinal fluid of children with acute meningitis and cryptococcal antigen in the blood and spinal fluid of patients with chronic meningoencephalitis. Agglutination tests have been introduced for the detection of pneumococci in the sputum, group A streptococci (*Streptococcus pyogenes*) in throat swabs, *Candida* antigen in serum, and rotavirus, as well as a product of *C. difficile,* in stool.

Of these, tests for the detection of *S. pyogenes* in throat swabs have attracted the most clinical attention. Over 30 such assays are commercially available; in each the group A carbohydrate is extracted from the swab with acid or enzyme treatment and then tested in a latex agglutination, coagglutination, or enzyme-linked immunosorbent assay (see below). Results are generally available within minutes.

The speed and ease with which these tests can be performed have resulted in their widespread utilization in primary and emergency care settings. Although antigen detection tests have generally demonstrated high specificity ($\geq$90 percent) vis-à-vis culture results, their sensitivities have varied (62 to 100 percent) from study to study. The adequacy of quality control and culture procedures, the skill of the tester, the patient's age, and the number of organisms present on the swab all appear to influence outcome. Of primary concern is the relative insensitivity of these procedures in patients whose simultaneous throat cultures yield fewer than 100 streptococcal colonies. Because a significant proportion of such patients demonstrate fourfold serum streptococcal antibody rises, true infections may be missed by the current generation of antigen tests. While their ultimate role in the diagnosis of streptococcal pharyngitis remains to be determined, they are now widely used as a culture substitute in outpatient settings lacking adequate laboratory services and in patient populations unable or unlikely to return for culture results. In clinical settings where throat cultures are practical, the simultaneous use of both tests may facilitate patient management. Patients with positive antigen test results could then be treated immediately, and therapeutic decisions on the antigen-negative patients postponed pending the availability of culture results.

ENZYME-LINKED IMMUNOSORBENT ASSAYS The method, as described above under "Direct Microscopic Examination," can be adapted for the visual or spectrophotometric detection of microbial antigens. It has largely replaced radioimmunoassay techniques in the diagnosis of hepatitis A and B infections and is extensively utilized to ascertain the presence of rotavirus and enteric adenovirus in the diarrheal stool of infants and immunosuppressed adults. It has been successfully used to detect circulating antigens in candidiasis, aspergillosis, and toxoplasmosis as well as urinary antigens in legionellosis. Enzyme immunoassays are also beginning to play an important role in the diagnosis of *C. trachomatis* and gonococcal cervicitis and urethritis, genital herpes, and viral respiratory tract infections.

URINE SCREENING TESTS A number of nonmicroscopic bacteriuria screening tests are commercially available. Each is designed to decrease the time and cost involved in the diagnosis of urinary tract infections. Bioluminescence, filtration-colorimetry, or chemical procedures are employed to determine the presence or absence of bacterial and/or leukocytic enzymes in the urine specimen. The tests can be performed reliably by individuals with minimal technical training and require only minutes to complete. Generally, specimens demonstrating a positive screening test are cultured; a negative result is reported as such, and the specimen is discarded. The sensitivity, specificity, and reproducibility of these tests do not differ significantly from those obtained with a microscopic examination of a stained urine smear conducted by a competent microbiologist; all reliably detect specimens containing 10^5 or more colony-forming units (CFU) per milliliter of urine, but are insufficiently sensitive at lower colony counts. The considerably higher cost of the screening tests vis-à-vis microscopic examination is partially offset by their technical simplicity. The ultimate role of these screening tests may be in the selection of specimens requiring culture techniques capable of detecting low colony count bacteriuria.

DNA PROBES The utilization of recombinant DNA techniques has made it possible to isolate, reproduce, and label single-stranded nucleotide sequences from the genome of specific microorganisms that are unique to that particular strain, species, genus, or group. These labeled DNA fragments, or probes, can be added to microbial cultures, body fluids, exudates, or tissues thought to contain the pathogen in question and the mixture treated with heat or chemicals to separate the microbial DNA into single strands. Following treatment, the DNA strands reanneal. This reassociation, or hybridization, is highly specific, occurring only between strands bearing complementary nucleotide sequences. If the specimen contains nucleotide sequences complementary to those of the probe, they will be hybridized and labeled.

The potential advantages of such probes are in their unique

specificity, their capacity to detect a single pathogen among a plethora of others, and the capacity to identify microorganisms that are either difficult or impossible to recover by cultural methods. Their most immediate impact will be on the diagnosis of viral, chlamydial, mycobacterial, enteric bacterial, and parasitic infections. Probes have already been developed for a wide variety of agents, including herpes simplex virus I and II, cytomegalovirus, enteroviruses, Epstein-Barr virus, hepatitis B virus, adenovirus, varicella-zoster virus, rotavirus, human papillomavirus, human immunodeficiency and T-cell leukemia viruses, *Mycoplasma pneumoniae*, *C. trachomatis*, enterotoxigenic and enteroadherent *Escherichia coli*, *Yersinia enterocolitica*, *Salmonella* spp., *Shigella* spp., *Campylobacter* spp., *Legionella* spp., *Mycobacteria* spp., *Leishmania mexicana*, *L. braziliensis*, and *Plasmodium falciparum*. Only a few of these, including mycoplasmal, mycobacterial, legionella, gonococcal, and human papillomavirus probes, are commercially available.

Ultimately, the utility of DNA probes in clinical medicine will rest on the simplification and commercialization of the hybridization procedure and the development of practical, highly sensitive labels. To date, most probes have utilized radioisotopic markers (usually ^{32}P). These demonstrate a high level of sensitivity but require prolonged processing for autoradiographic detection, have an extremely limited shelf life, and require the storage and disposal of radioactive materials, making them impractical for the clinical laboratory. Colorimetrically detected or fluorescent enzymatic labels have been developed which circumvent these drawbacks; however, all appear to be somewhat less sensitive than the radiometric labels and decidedly less sensitive than most cultural procedures. A gene amplification method known as the polymerase chain reaction (PCR) is capable of synthesizing millions of copies of a single nucleotide sequence within a few hours. Application of the PCR methodology to clinical specimens make it possible, in combination with DNA probes, to detect the presence of microbes present in extremely small numbers (see Chap. 6). This technique has already proved useful in the research laboratory for the detection of human immunodeficiency virus (HIV) in the peripheral blood cells of infected patients. With the anticipated development of more satisfactory, nonradiometric labels, the DNA probe may well alter the diagnosis and management of infectious diseases in a dramatic way. They are unlikely, however, to displace culture methods for infections in which the recovery, characterization, and susceptibility testing of the pathogenic agent is critical to the management of a sick patient.

CULTURE TECHNIQUES

Despite the time and complexity, the isolation of the etiologic agent by cultivation in artificial media, tissue cultures, or animals is generally the most definitive procedure available.

The diagnostic value of a culture specimen, however, depends to a large extent on the likelihood that it has been collected free of contamination with the resident microbial flora and transported to the laboratory in a fashion that ensures survival of fastidious organisms.

SPECIMEN COLLECTION When specimens from deep closed lesions are collected, the site of percutaneous needle aspiration should be cleansed first by using 70% isopropyl or ethyl alcohol and then disinfected with a 2% tincture of iodine or an appropriate iodophor. If the specimen for culture is drawn through an indwelling cannula, the site of withdrawal must be disinfected in the same fashion.

When specimens are to be collected from the uterus or a draining wound or sinus tract, the orifice must be thoroughly cleansed and disinfected as described above, a sterile intravenous catheter or multilumen tube is introduced as deeply as possible through the orifice, and the specimen aspirated into a sterile syringe. Culture from an open lesion may be collected by biopsy, aspiration from the margin, or by swabbing the surface. In the first two situations the wound is prepared as for a deep closed lesion. For swab cultures, the wound surface is cleansed only with sterile saline to remove debris and saprophytic flora.

TRANSPORTATION All specimens submitted for microbial culture should be transported to the laboratory as rapidly as possible, preferably within 1 h. Delay beyond this time may result in death of fastidious organisms, overgrowth of contaminants, and/or change in the number of bacteria unless special procedures are employed to overcome these problems. Respiratory secretions, urine, large pieces of tissue, and large volumes of fluid can be safely transmitted in plastic containers with leakproof lids. Aspirates are conveniently and safely transported in the same syringe used in the collection procedure, providing all air is expressed from the syringe. Alternatively, such fluid may be injected into a sealed gassed-out vial suitable for transport of anaerobic specimens. Small pieces of tissue (less than 1 cm^2) are transported best in sterile rubber-stoppered gassed-out tubes. Swabs should be submitted in one of several commercially available transport media. These prevent both the desiccation of organisms implanted on the swab and the overgrowth of hardy organisms at the expense of more fastidious ones. Although special anaerobic transport materials are available, use of swab specimens for the recovery of such organisms is not encouraged.

UPPER RESPIRATORY TRACT SPECIMENS Because the throat and nasopharynx are normally heavily colonized by both saprophytic and potentially pathogenic bacteria, culture of this area is seldom useful except when a particular bacterial pathogen is being sought, e.g., *S. pyogenes*, *Bordetella pertussis*, *Corynebacterium diphtheriae*, meningococci, or gonococci.

When *throat cultures* are submitted to the laboratory without specifying the pathogen being sought, the laboratory will generally report only the presence or absence of *S. pyogenes*. Since a single properly obtained throat swab will detect at least 90 percent of patients with streptococcal pharyngitis, a negative culture is very helpful in excluding the possibility of this disease. Similarly, a heavy or predominant growth of group A beta-hemolytic streptococci in patients presenting with the signs and symptoms of streptococcal pharyngitis is highly predictive of an antibody response to streptococcal antigens and, therefore, presumably disease. It is far more difficult to interpret cultures with a light or nonpredominant growth of *S. pyogenes*. At least half of these patients do not mount an appreciable immunologic response, suggesting that bacterial growth often represents a carrier state.

LOWER RESPIRATORY TRACT SPECIMENS Although culture of expectorated sputum is the most frequently employed technique for the diagnosis of lower respiratory tract infections, both its sensitivity and specificity have been questioned. Studies of patients with bacteremic pneumococcal pneumonia have shown the etiologic agent to be present in the sputum in only 50 to 94 percent of cases. Moreover, expectorated sputum is almost always contaminated with oropharyngeal flora including, in many cases, bacterial species commonly associated with pulmonary infections. Some confusion can be avoided if the specimen is collected appropriately and screened carefully for both gross and microscopic characteristics prior to inoculation of the culture.

Specimens demonstrating a Gram-stain smear with fewer than 10 squamous epithelial cells (SEC) and greater than 25 leukocytes per low-power field are likely to contain lower tract flora. This is particularly true if a single or clearly predominant bacterial type grows, or, in the case of chronic obstructive pulmonary disease, if both pneumococci and *H. influenzae* are isolated. If SEC number more than 10 per low-power field, the specimen can be considered heavily contaminated with oropharyngeal flora and should be discarded. In most cases a second carefully collected expectorated sputum will yield a satisfactory specimen. If the patient is unable to produce sputum, coughing may be stimulated by lowering the head of the patient's bed for a few minutes or exposing the patient to an aerosol of warm hypertonic saline.

Direct endotracheal or endobronchial aspiration may be employed when a satisfactory expectorated or induced sputum cannot be produced. However, such specimens are subject to contamination by oropharyngeal flora which is introduced during the passage of the aspiration instrument. Fiberoptic bronchoscopy, which allows the direct visualization and aspiration of bronchial secretions, may result in a somewhat better specimen. When it is accompanied by a brush biopsy performed through an occluded double-lumen tube, the material obtained is unlikely to be diluted with saliva or topical anesthetics and may be utilized for anaerobic cultures. Alternatively, the specimen may be collected by a technique that totally bypasses the oropharynx. The most widely used is transtracheal aspiration. This method entails a definite risk of hemoptysis, subcutaneous and mediastinal emphysema, vagal discharge, or respiratory embarrassment and is contraindicated in the presence of a bleeding diathesis. It should be used only when results from expectorated sputum are unsatisfactory and the infection is severe enough to merit the attendant risks (see Chap. 207).

Needle aspiration of a pulmonary infiltrate under fluoroscopic control also produces specimens of excellent quality. The percutaneous method gives both a high yield and accurate results but has at least a 5 percent chance of complications, particularly pneumothorax. The morbidity risk is greater than with transtracheal aspiration biopsy, but the diagnostic yield may be superior.

Whatever technique is used to sample the lower respiratory tract, a concomitant blood culture should always be obtained. If a pleural effusion is present, it should also be aspirated and cultured.

In addition to bacterial pathogens, pneumonia can be caused by viruses, *Rickettsia*, *Chlamydia*, *M. pneumoniae*, *Legionella*, and *Pneumocystis* and related agents. Techniques for the recovery of these agents from the sputum are generally not available in a routine clinical microbiology laboratory, and the diagnosis is most frequently made by clinical, immunologic, and/or serologic methods. *P. carinii* and cytomegalovirus can be recovered by bronchoalveolar lavage. *L. pneumophila* can be cultured from expectorated sputum, lung tissue, or empyema fluid. In addition, the organism can be demonstrated by direct fluorescent antibody staining and DNA probing of respiratory specimens, and its antigens may be detected in urine with ELISA procedures. These methods permit early diagnosis and rapid institution of appropriate therapy.

URINE SPECIMENS   Voided urine, like expectorated sputum, is usually contaminated with the normal microbial flora, in this case from the urethra and external genitalia. Urine cultures, however, are more reliable than those of expectorated sputum, because the periurethral area can be disinfected and the urethra itself flushed with the first portion of the urine stream before a sample is taken by the clean-voided, midstream collection technique. In addition, quantitation of the bacterial growth is helpful in separating contaminated specimens from true infection. When this procedure is followed conscientiously, a single specimen from a male which yields a colony count in excess of 100,000 organisms per milliliter is highly indicative of bacteriuria. In women, the colony count must exceed 100,000 organisms per milliliter in two consecutive urine specimens before infection can be considered to be present. Because urine is a good culture medium, contaminating organisms will multiply to large numbers if the urine is allowed to stand at room temperature for prolonged periods of time. For this reason, specimens which cannot be dispatched to the laboratory within an hour should be refrigerated. They can be held at 4°C for 4 to 6 h without an appreciable change in the bacterial colony count. In most instances, urinary tract infections are caused by a single bacterial species. The isolation of three or more species in a urine culture usually reflects contamination even when the colony count is high. True polymicrobial bacteriuria does occur but is generally restricted to patients with chronic indwelling urethral catheters. In contrast, colony counts of less than 100,000 organisms per milliliter may represent true bacteriuria. For example, $\geq 10^2$ CFU per milliliter in symptomatic dysuric women and $\geq 10^3$ in symptomatic men are significant counts. In fact, up to one-third of urinary tract infections are associated with counts less than 100,000 organisms per milliliter. Patients receiving antimicrobial therapy and specimens obtained by ureteral or urethral catheterization and by suprapubic aspiration also are likely to contain a low number of organisms.

When an adequate clean-voided urine specimen cannot be obtained,

or when anaerobic cultures are desired, suprapubic aspiration may be employed. Specimens obtained in this manner are unlikely to be contaminated, and even slight growth may be significant. When an indwelling catheter is in place, a specimen should be collected directly from the catheter by means of a sterile needle and syringe after careful disinfection of the exterior surface or sampling port. Urine should not be taken from the drainage tube or bag, because these are frequently contaminated.

BLOOD SPECIMENS   Cultures should be obtained from all febrile patients who have rigors, are seriously ill, are thought to have endocarditis or intravascular infection, or are immunosuppressed. If viremia, fungemia, brucellosis, tularemia, leptospirosis, or an infection with cell wall–deficient bacteria is suspected, the laboratory should be contacted for special instructions. The sensitivity of most culture techniques is volume-dependent, with yields increasing approximately 2 percent for each milliliter of blood drawn over 5 mL. In general, three blood cultures of 10 to 30 mL taken at intervals of no less than 60 min are adequate to document the presence of bacteremia in an adult. In emergent situations, two cultures taken simultaneously from different anatomic sites will usually suffice. In patients who have received antimicrobial agents within the previous 2 weeks or in whom endocarditis is suspected, a total of six cultures taken over a 2-day period may be useful. If the patient is receiving antimicrobial agents, the cultures should be taken immediately prior to the next dose, and the laboratory should be notified to allow use of an antibiotic removal device, or extensive dilution of the blood specimen. The collection of specimens over and above the number listed above is seldom helpful in detecting occult bacteremia unless the culture procedures, media, or conditions of incubation are altered to allow detection of fastidious organisms.

Specimens are best collected by percutaneous venipuncture. If possible, aspirations from the femoral vein should be avoided since disinfecting the skin of the groin is often difficult and the concentration of organisms in the venous drainage of the lower extremity is generally less than that found in the venous blood of the arms. The increasingly common practice of drawing blood for culture through an indwelling intravascular cannula often results in a higher level of contamination without substantially improving the detection of bacteremia. Similarly there is no evidence that arterial blood cultures possess any advantage over venous cultures. Bone marrow cultures may reveal the etiologic agent when it cannot be obtained by other means in occasional patients with disseminated salmonellosis, tuberculosis, and deep mycoses.

To minimize the chance of contamination with skin flora, the site of aspiration should be carefully disinfected as described above. Following aspiration, the blood should be inoculated into both aerobic and anaerobic broths immediately. The dilution ratio of blood to broth should be at least 1:5 to minimize the normal bactericidal activity of serum and the activity of any antimicrobial agents that may be present. If direct inoculation into broth is not feasible, the blood may be drawn into a sterile Vacutainer tube containing sodium polyethanol sulfanate (SPS). This anticoagulant is anticomplementary and inactivates leukocytes and certain aminoglycoside and polypeptide antibiotics. Nevertheless, it will not delay bacterial death indefinitely, and Vacutainer specimens should be sent to the laboratory for dilution in broth within 30 min of the time the blood is drawn. If fungemia is suspected, the laboratory should be notified since some of the standard techniques described above are less satisfactory for the isolation of fungi.

Approximately two-thirds of blood cultures from bacteremic patients are found to be positive within 24 h and 90 percent within 3 days. Despite strict adherence to disinfectant procedures on the ward and sterile technique in the laboratory, contamination occasionally occurs. The following are characteristics of "false-positive" blood cultures: (1) repeat cultures are seldom positive for the same organism, (2) bacterial growth in broth generally occurs after 2 days of incubation, and (3) the organisms are often identified as diphtheroids, *Bacillus*, or *Staphylococcus epidermidis*. However, any of these species, particularly coagulase-negative staphylococci, can occasionally be responsible for true bacteremia, particularly in immunosuppressed patients.

CEREBROSPINAL FLUID SPECIMENS Bacterial meningitis can be rapidly fatal if treatment is delayed or inadequate, and appropriate therapy often requires specific identification of the etiologic agent. Because of the clinical urgency, CSF specimens should be collected as soon as the diagnosis is considered, and the specimen promptly transported to the laboratory. The laboratory should be notified if the specimen has been collected from an abscess within the central nervous system to ensure that it is cultured both aerobically and anaerobically. If possible, at least 2 mL CSF should be obtained and the specimen sent for glucose, quantitative protein level, and cell count in addition to microbiologic studies. A simultaneous blood sugar also should be drawn for correlation with the CSF glucose level. Fastidious organisms, particularly *Neisseria meningitidis,* may not survive prolonged storage at temperatures below that of the body. If a delay in CSF examination cannot be avoided, specimens should be held at 37°C.

After receipt, the specimen is concentrated by centrifugation or filtration, Gram stained, and cultured. The inflammatory response in the CSF is helpful in distinguishing acute bacterial meningitis from nonbacterial forms of the disease. In bacterial meningitis, polymorphonuclear leukocytes predominate, while in tuberculous, fungal, or protozoal meningitis, the inflammatory cells usually consist of lymphocytes, and the response is less intense. Although polymorphonuclear leukocytes may dominate early in the course of aseptic meningitis, there is usually a clear shift to mononuclear cells within 8 h. Cytologic changes in the CSF may also be seen in patients with brain abscess. However, smears and cultures are generally negative in these cases unless the abscess ruptures into the subarachnoid space or into the ventricles (see Chap. 354). The Gram's stain smear of the CSF should be examined carefully for stainable organisms, particularly meningococci, pneumococci, *Enterobacteriaceae, Listeria,* and staphylococci in patients with atrioventricular shunts. Stainable, but nonviable, organisms occasionally contaminate sterile plastic containers and may result in a "false-positive" Gram's stain. In addition, in cases of partially treated bacterial meningitis there is a tendency for gram-positive organisms to stain gram-negative.

When a large number of organisms are present and specific antiserums are available, the etiologic agent can often be rapidly identified by the particle agglutination tests described above. Moreover, detection of microbial antigens in the CSF is often the only method of identification of an infectious agent from a patient with partially treated meningitis. In the presence of a significant number of mononuclear cells without stainable bacteria cryptococcal antigen can be identified by latex agglutination tests.

Regardless of the results of these studies, the CSF must be cultured and any resulting growth identified to the species level. In patients presenting with an acute mononuclear meningitis, the viral cultures should be submitted simultaneously with bacterial cultures. Coxsackie B, mumps, herpes simplex virus, and HIV may be recovered in appropriate clinical settings. Mycobacterial and fungal cultures should be set up on patients who present with chronic meningitis and a mononuclear inflammatory response in the CSF.

Naegleria fowleri, the cause of amebic meningoencephalitis, can often be recognized by its ameboid movements in wet-mount preparations of cerebrospinal fluid. This organism should be looked for in patients who develop hemorrhagic meningoencephalitis during the summer months (see Chap. 158).

GASTROINTESTINAL TRACT SPECIMENS Cultures of the mouth, periodontal lesions, or saliva usually yield a mixed flora of aerobic and anaerobic organisms including *Actinomyces* spp. and *Candida* spp. The isolation of these organisms is without significance unless the specimen was collected in a way which avoided contamination with indigenous flora. If actinomycosis is suspected, the laboratory should be contacted for special instructions. The diagnosis of oral thrush and Vincent's infection can be made with stained smears from scrapings of the suspected lesion.

Cultures of ileostomy or colostomy stomas, gastrointestinal fistulas, and rectal fissures invariably grow both aerobic and anaerobic intestinal flora. They are seldom helpful, therefore, unless a search is made for specific intestinal pathogens.

Fecal cultures are helpful in determining the etiology of diarrhea and in detecting carrier states. Such specimens are routinely cultured for species of *Salmonella, Shigella,* and *Arizona.* Many laboratories are now also looking for *Vibrio parahaemolyticus, Yersinia enterocolitica, Campylobacter jejuni, E. coli* 0157:H7, and *Clostridium difficile.* Cell culture and particle agglutination techniques can be used for the direct detection of *C. difficile* toxin and other diarrhea-associated products of this organism in the stool of diarrheal patients. There is at present no convenient and reliable cultural method of identifying enterotoxogenic strains of *E. coli* or the Norwalk-like viruses in the clinical laboratory. The laboratory should be alerted as to whether any of these, or any other unusual infection such as candidiasis, clostridial food poisoning, or cholera, is suspected.

Although rectal swabs are adequate for the diagnosis of bacterial diarrhea, they are less satisfactory for the detection of carrier states. If swabs are used, they should show obvious soiling and be sent to the laboratory in appropriate transport media. Whole stool should be collected free of urine, placed in clean, waxed cardboard cartons, and promptly dispatched to the laboratory. If delivery cannot be made within 1 h, the stool should be preserved in phosphate-buffered glycerol to prevent death of fastidious organisms such as *Shigella* spp. It is seldom necessary to submit more than three consecutive daily specimens.

GENITAL TRACT SPECIMENS Genital specimens are submitted primarily for the diagnosis of venereal disease including gonorrhea, syphilis, herpes, chancroid, trichomoniasis, chlamydial, CMV, and HIV infections. Instructions for the collection of specimens should be sought in the sections of the text dealing with these specific diseases. In addition to the venereal pathogens, a number of organisms may infect the endometrium, tuboovarian tissues, and vagina. Endometrial cultures must be collected through a double- or triple-lumen tube inserted through a decontaminated cervical os if contamination with vaginal and cervical flora is to be avoided. The specimens should be delivered to the laboratory in either a gassed-out vial or a sealed syringe to ensure recovery of anaerobic organisms. When a patient presents with vaginitis, a specimen is collected by swabbing the vaginal fornix under direct visualization. Candidiasis and bacterial vaginosis are best diagnosed by examination of a Gram-stained smear.

EXUDATES AND BODY FLUIDS Pus from undrained abscesses as well as pericardial, pleural, peritoneal, and synovial fluids is best collected by syringe and needle aspiration through disinfected skin. Prior rinsing of the syringe with a sterile anticoagulant such as heparin or SPS will help prevent formation of clots. Because anaerobic organisms are commonly involved in infection of these areas, the syringe should be sealed and sent immediately to the microbiology laboratory. Alternatively, the aspirate may be injected into a gassed-out anaerobic transport vial. The use of swabs is not encouraged since the sample size is small and fastidious organisms including anaerobes are unusually susceptible to desiccation and oxidation. Deep suppurative lesions which communicate with the surface of the body through fistulas or sinus tracts present a difficult problem in specimen collection. The communicating pathway is generally colonized by a wide variety of bacterial flora which contaminate drainage being ejected through the fistula opening. The degree of contamination can be lessened in many instances by carefully disinfecting the orifice and aspirating material via a sterile plastic catheter inserted deep into the sinus. Even when these precautions are taken, however, sinus tract cultures often fail to correlate well with pathogens isolated from operative specimens. For this reason, a bacteriologic diagnosis of draining suppurative lesions should be based on a culture of currettings or biopsy rather than sinus drainage. If actinomycosis is suspected, the draining sinus tract may be covered with gauze which is left in place until it is thoroughly saturated. The gauze is then submitted to the laboratory where it is carefully examined for the presence of granules which can be picked out and then identified.

SKIN, SOFT TISSUE, AND SUPERFICIAL WOUNDS Specimens collected from these areas are usually heavily contaminated with the normal flora of their respective sites. Swab cultures should be obtained only if gross pus is present or if there is need to confirm the presence or absence of only a single bacterial pathogen, such as *C. diphtheriae;* in this case, the wound should first be cleansed mechanically with saline to remove as much exudate as possible. Material from bullae and areas of cellulitis is best obtained with a syringe. Successful aspiration of an area of cellulitis may require several thrusts and withdrawals, care being taken to maintain the tip of the needle beneath the surface of the skin and a significant vacuum in the barrel of the syringe. If sterile saline is injected prior to aspiration, this solution should not contain a preservative which may affect the viability of some bacteria. Alternatively, a punch biopsy may be obtained of the area after appropriate disinfection. Similarly, cultures from open lesions may be obtained by biopsy or by aspirating from the margins of these lesions using a syringe and needle. Semiquantitative cultures of burn eschars are useful in identifying patients at risk of bacteremia.

Intravenous and intraarterial catheter segments are best collected by disinfecting the area of the skin penetrated by the catheter, carefully withdrawing the catheter, and aseptically cutting off the 5-cm section that had been located just under the skin into a sterile container. This is then delivered to the microbiology laboratory where semiquantitative cultures are done. In general, catheters which are contaminated during removal will have only a few colonies on agar plates, while infected catheters will show heavy growth.

IMMUNOLOGIC METHODS

These diagnostic methods are intended to supply evidence of past or present infection by demonstrating antibodies in serum or other body fluids, or indicating changed reactivity of the host (hypersensitivity, allergy) to products of the organism.

SEROLOGIC TESTS The finding on a single occasion that a patient's serum contains antibody which reacts with a certain antigen merely indicates that the patient has had previous contact with the antigen or a closely related substance. For this reason, with rare exceptions, the clinical interpretation of serologic tests depends on serial determinations. If the antibody titer is found to *rise or fall significantly,* or, alternatively, if specific IgM antibody is detected, the response likely is a result of recent contact with the antigen. With infections caused by herpes family or other latent viruses, caution must be exercised in interpreting serologic data. Reactivation may occur with or without changes in antibody titer. Cytomegalovirus IgM may persist for months after primary infection in transplant patients. *In any patient with a puzzling illness, a sterile specimen of serum should be preserved in a frozen state so that it can, if necessary, be studied and compared with serum collected at a later date.*

Prior contact with an antigen may be the result of past immunization with vaccines; interpretation of serum agglutinin titers for typhoid bacilli is often made difficult by prior immunization. The so-called anamnestic reaction, a nonspecific stimulation of antibody formation by an acute illness (e.g., a rise in *Brucella* agglutinins in a patient with acute tularemia), occurs only when the two organisms are antigenically related, and rarely presents a serious problem.

Some mention of "nonspecific" serologic changes may serve to emphasize again that clinical laboratory tests have come into use *only because they have been found to correlate reasonably well with clinical findings.* In several diseases it has been found, often accidentally, that serum antibody develops which will react with antigens derived from sources other than the etiologic agent (which may actually be unknown). Common examples are heterophil agglutinins in infectious mononucleosis, cold agglutinins in mycoplasma pneumonia, and the agglutination of certain strains of *Proteus* bacilli by

serum of patients with rickettsial diseases. The VDRL test for syphilis and related flocculation tests are performed with antigens derived from sources completely unrelated to *Treponema pallidum.*

The results of serologic tests must be interpreted in the light of other information about the patient, including such factors as previous immunizations and illnesses, the possibility of exposure to chemically but etiologically unrelated antigens, and the importance of a changing titer in serial tests as opposed to a single isolated observation.

VIROLOGIC SPECIMENS

The selection of specimens for the diagnosis of viral illness depends on both the stage of the disease and its clinical presentation. If the patient is seen early in the course of illness, frequently it is possible to demonstrate viral antigen in body tissue or fluids and/or to recover the virus by appropriate culture techniques. If the patient is seen later, during the recovery or convalescent stages, the diagnosis is often best established by serologic means. The type of specimen submitted for culture and the method of specimen transport depend to some extent on the nature of the illness. Throat swabs are helpful in the diagnosis of most viral infections. Because respiratory viruses are extremely labile, the swabs are placed in a buffered, high-protein transport medium containing antibiotic agents. If the specimen is to be transported to another institution, the specimen should be transported on ice (4°C). If delays of more than 24 h are anticipated, specimens should be stored at $-60°C$ and shipped on dry ice.

Cerebrospinal fluid from patients presenting with meningitis or encephalitis can also be submitted for culture. As with throat swabs, these specimens should be stored at low temperatures and shipped on dry ice. Stool should be collected in patients with respiratory illnesses, meningitis, or encephalitis, if either adenoviruses or enteroviruses are thought to be involved. Although these organisms are hardy, the feces should be collected in any sterile screw-top bottle and dispatched promptly to avoid bacterial overgrowth. Urine cultures are helpful in the diagnosis of congenital cytomegalovirus and rubella infections and in the late diagnosis of mumps. Vesicular fluid is a rich source of virus and viral antigen in patients presenting with exanthems. Pericardial fluid may be of help in patients with myocarditis or pericarditis. Viral blood cultures are seldom useful except in the diagnosis of arboviral infections. Isolation techniques for these viruses are highly specialized and are not available in most virus laboratories. Buffy coat cultures for cytomegalovirus and herpesvirus are often helpful in AIDS, transplant, and other immunosuppressed patients. Brain biopsy is the best single method for diagnosing herpes simplex encephalitis (see Chap. 135). The biopsy specimen should be placed in viral transport and dispatched, at 4°C, as quickly as possible.

REFERENCES

CENTOR RM et al: Throat cultures and rapid tests for diagnosis of Group A streptococcal pharyngitis. Ann Intern Med 105:892, 1986

EISENBERG HD et al: Collection, handling and processing of specimens, in *Manual of Clinical Microbiology,* 4th ed, EH Lennette et al (eds). Washington, DC, American Society for Microbiology, 1985

MINNICH LL et al: Cumitech 24, Rapid detection of viruses by immunofluorescence, S Specter (coordinating ed). Washington, DC, American Society for Microbiology, 1988

PEZZLO M: Detection of urinary tract infections by rapid methods. Clin Microbiol Rev 1:268, 1988

SIMOR AE et al: Cumitech 23, Infections of the skin and subcutaneous tissues, JS Smith (coordinating ed). Washington, DC, American Society for Microbiology, 1988

WASHINGTON JA II: Bacterial, fungi and parasites, the clinician and microbiology laboratory, in *Principles and Practice of Infectious Diseases,* 3d ed, GL Mandell et al (eds). New York, Wiley, 1990

81 DISORDERS OF PHAGOCYTIC CELLS

JOHN I. GALLIN

Leukocytes are the major cellular components of inflammatory and immune responses and include neutrophils, lymphocytes, monocytes, eosinophils, and basophils. The blood is the most readily obtainable source of leukocytes and serves as the vehicle for their delivery to the various tissues from the bone marrow, where they are produced. Normal blood leukocyte counts for adults are given in Chap. 64 and those for different ages in the Appendix. The various leukocytes are thought to derive from a common stem cell in the bone marrow. Three-fourths of the nucleated cells of bone marrow are committed to the production of leukocytes. Leukocyte maturation in the marrow is generally thought to be under the regulatory control of a number of different factors, which are incompletely defined (see Chap. 64). Because an alteration in the number and type of leukocytes is a frequent association with disease processes, a total white blood count (WBC) (cells per microliter) and differential counts are obtained frequently. The lymphocytes and basophils are discussed elsewhere. This chapter focuses on the neutrophils, monocytes, and eosinophils.

NEUTROPHILS

MATURATION Important events in the neutrophil life are summarized in Fig. 81-1. In normal humans neutrophils are only produced in the bone marrow. Best estimates indicate that the appropriate number of stem cells necessary to support hematopoiesis is between 400 and 500. There is convincing evidence that human blood monocytes and tissue macrophages produce colony stimulating factors, hormone(s) required for the growth of monocytes and neutrophils in the bone marrow. The hematopoietic system not only produces enough neutrophils (approximately 1.3×10^{11} cells per 80-kg person per day) to carry out physiologic functions but also has a large reserve stored in the marrow which can be mobilized in response to inflammation or infection. An increase in the number of blood neutrophils is called *neutrophilia*, and the presence of immature cells is termed a "shift to the left." A diminution in the number of blood neutrophils is referred to as *neutropenia* (see Chap. 64).

Neutrophils evolve from pluripotent stem cells. The final stages of hematopoiesis are characterized by the appearance of cells with distinct morphologic features. The myeloblast is the first recognizable precursor cell and is followed by the *promyelocyte* (see Fig. A5-15). The promyelocyte evolves when the classic lysosomal granules, called the *primary* or *azurophil granules*, are produced. The primary granules contain hydrolases, elastase, myeloperoxidase,

and cationic proteins. The promyelocyte divides to produce the *myelocyte*, a cell responsible for the synthesis of the *specific* or *secondary granules* which contain unique (specific) constituents such as lactoferrin, vitamin B_{12}–binding proteins, and probably cytochrome b, histaminase, and receptors for certain chemoattractants and adherence promoting factors. The secondary granules do not contain acid hydrolases and therefore are not classic lysosomes. They are readily released extracellularly, and their mobilization is probably important in modulating inflammation. During the final stages of maturation there is no cell division and the cell passes through the *metamyelocyte* stage and then to the *band* neutrophil with a sausage-shaped nucleus. As the band cell matures, the nucleus assumes a lobulated configuration.

In settings of severe acute bacterial infection, prominent neutrophil cytoplasmic granules called *toxic granulations* are occasionally seen. Toxic granulations are thought to be immature or abnormally staining azurophil granules. Cytoplasmic inclusions, also called *Doehle bodies*, (see Fig. A5-17) can also be seen during infection and probably represent fragments of endoplasmic reticulum. Large neutrophil vacuoles are often present in acute bacterial infection and probably represent pinocytosed (internalized) membrane.

Neutrophils have long been thought to be a homogeneous population of cells. However, studies of neutrophil function have suggested they are heterogeneous. Recently monoclonal antibodies have been developed that recognize only a subset of mature neutrophils. The meaning of neutrophil heterogeneity is not known.

MARROW RELEASE AND CIRCULATING COMPARTMENTS
Specific signals, including interleukin 1, tumor necrosis factor-α, the colony stimulating factors (see Chap. 64), or the complement fragment C3e, mobilize leukocytes from the bone marrow and deliver them to the blood in an unstimulated state. Under normal conditions about 90 percent of the neutrophil pool is in the bone marrow, 2 to 3 percent in the circulation, and the remainder in the tissues. The blood pool exists as two compartments: the marginated pool adherent to endothelial cells and the freely flowing circulating pool. In response to chemotactic stimuli from tissues (e.g., the complement product C5a, the arachidonic acid derivative leukotriene B_4, or the bacterial product *N*-formylmethionylleucylphenylalanine), neutrophil adhesiveness increases and the circulating cells aggregate to each other and adhere to the endothelium. An increased expression of a glycoprotein receptor for C3bi (also called CR3) appears to be intimately involved with the increased adhesion. Receptors for chemoattractants and opsonins are probably also mobilized; the cells orient toward the chemoattractant source in the extravascular space, increase their motile activity (chemokinesis), and migrate with direction (chemotaxis) into tissues. The process of migration into tissues is called *diapedesis* and involves the crawling of neutrophils between postcapillary endothelial cells which open junctions between adjacent cells to permit leukocyte passage. The endothelial responses (increased blood flow secondary to increased vasodilation and permeability) are mediated by anaphylatoxins (e.g., complement products

FIGURE 81-1 Schematic diagram of the life cycle of the neutrophil. MPO, myeloperoxidase.

C3a and C5a) as well as vasodilators such as bradykinin and prostaglandins E and I. In the healthy adult most neutrophils leave the body by migration through the mucous membrane of the gastrointestinal tract. Normally neutrophils spend a relatively short time in the circulation with a half-life of 6 to 7 h. Once in the tissues neutrophils release enzymes such as collagenase and elastase, which may help establish abscess cavities. Neutrophils ingest (phagocytose) pathogenic materials that have been properly altered (opsonized) by substances such as immunoglobulin G (IgG) and the complement product C3b. Fibronectin and the tetrapeptide tuftsin facilitate the phagocytic process.

Concomitant with phagocytosis there is a burst of oxygen consumption and activation of the hexose-monophosphate shunt. Nicotinamide-adenine dinucleotide phosphate (NADPH) oxidase is activated, and through a complex enzyme system consisting of membrane and cytosolic components, toxic oxygen products (e.g., hydrogen peroxide and hydroxyl radical) are generated. Hydrogen peroxide + chloride + neutrophil myeloperoxidase provide a particularly toxic system that generates hypochlorous acid, hypochlorite, and chlorine. These products oxidize and halogenate microorganisms and tumor cells and when uncontrolled, can damage host tissue. Strongly cationic proteins and small peptides known as "defensins" also participate in microbial killing. Other enzymes, such as lysozyme and acid proteases, help digest microbial debris. After 1 to 4 days in tissues neutrophils die. Under certain conditions, such as following delayed-type hypersensitivity immunity, a second wave of inflammation, associated with monocyte accumulation, occurs within 6 to 12 h of initiation of inflammation. Neutrophils, monocytes, microorganisms in various states of digestion, and altered local tissue cells make up pus, which derives its characteristic green color from myeloperoxidase. Myeloperoxidase and other factors may be important in turning off the inflammatory process by inactivating chemoattractants and immobilizing phagocytic cells.

NEUTROPHIL DYSFUNCTION A defect anywhere in the neutrophil life cycle summarized in Fig. 81-1 can lead to dysfunction and compromised host defenses. Inflammation is often depressed and the clinical result is often recurrent and severe bacterial and fungal infections creating novel and often difficult management problems. Diagnosis of phagocytic cell disorders is suggested by clinical evaluation. Neutropenia or impaired neutrophil function are frequently associated with depressed inflammation. Aphthous ulcers of mucous membranes (gray ulcers without pus) are common. Gingivitis and periodontal disease are common. Characteristically, patients with phagocyte defects have recurrent and often severe bacterial or fungal infections which often present as difficult management problems. Patients with congenital phagocyte defects can have infections within the first few days of life. Skin, ear, upper and lower respiratory tract, and bone infections are common. Sepsis and meningitis are rare. In some disorders the frequency of infection is variable, and patients can go for months or even years without major infection. Adults over 30 years of age with congenital defects are unusual, suggesting that patients with such defects die at an early age. However, with aggressive management, adults with these diseases are being seen with increasing frequency.

Neutropenia The consequences of absent neutrophils represent a dramatic demonstration of their importance in host defense. When the neutrophil count is below 1000 per microliter, there is an increased risk for infection (Chap. 82); when there are fewer than 200 cells per microliter, the inflammatory process is absent. The causes of neutropenia are multiple and are related to depressed production, peripheral destruction, and peripheral pooling. They are discussed in Chap. 64.

Neutrophilia Neutrophilia results from increased neutrophil production, marrow release, or defective margination. These are discussed in Chap. 64.

ABNORMAL NEUTROPHIL FUNCTION Congenital deficiencies and acquired abnormalities of phagocyte function are described in Table 81-1. The resulting diseases are best considered in terms of the functional defects of adherence, chemotaxis, and microbicidal activity. The distinguishing features of the important congenital lesions are shown in Table 81-2, several of which are discussed below.

Patients with congenitally (autosomal recessive) abnormal phagocyte adherence, *C3bi (CR3) deficiency*, lack the plasma membrane receptor for the fragment of the third complement component called C3bi (CR3 by other terminology). Patients with this syndrome have recurrent bacterial and fungal infections, severe periodontal disease, persistent leukocytosis (15,000 to 20,000 neutrophils per microliter), and usually a history of delayed separation of the umbilical stump. Neutrophils (and monocytes) from these patients have defective adherence, spreading, aggregation, and chemotaxis.

Abnormal neutrophil and monocyte chemotaxis occurs in the *hyperimmunoglobulin E–recurrent infection (Job's) syndrome*. For many years the cold abscesses were thought to be a reflection of impaired chemotaxis with too few phagocytes arriving too late, perhaps secondary to a lymphocyte factor inhibiting chemotaxis. However, it is now clear that the chemotactic defect in these patients is variable and the fundamental basis for the impaired defenses is complex and inadequately delineated.

The most common neutrophil defect is *myeloperoxidase deficiency*, which is inherited as an autosomal recessive trait and may have an incidence as high as about 1 in 2000 persons. Isolated myeloperoxidase

TABLE 81-1 Types of neutrophil dysfunction

Function	Drug-induced	Acquired disease	Congenital disorder
Adherence-aggregation	Aspirin; colchicine; alcohol; glucocorticoids; ibuprofen; piroxicam	Neonates, hemodialysis	C3bi (CR3) receptor deficiency
Deformability		Leukemia, neonates, diabetes mellitus, immature neutrophils	
Chemokinesis-chemotaxis	Glucocorticoids (high-dose); auranofin; colchicine (weak effect); phenylbutazone; naproxen; indomethacin	Thermal injury; malignancy; malnutrition; periodontal disease; neonates; systemic lupus erythematosus; rheumatoid arthritis; diabetes mellitus; sepsis; influenza virus infection; herpes simplex virus infection; acrodermatitis enteropathica; Down's syndrome; α-mannosidase deficiency; severe combined immunodeficiency; Wiskott-Aldrich syndrome	Hyper IgE–recurrent infection (Job's) syndrome; Chédiak-Higashi syndrome; specific granule deficiency
Microbicidal activity	Colchicine; cyclophosphamide; glucocorticoids (high-dose)	Leukemia; aplastic anemia; certain neutropenias; tuftsin deficiency; thermal injury; sepsis; neonates; diabetes mellitus; malnutrition	Chédiak-Higashi syndrome, specific granule deficiency; chronic granulomatous disease

TABLE 81-2 Distinguishing features of congenital phagocyte dysfunction syndromes

Disease/inheritance*	Defect	Clinical manifestations
C3bi (CR3) receptor deficiency/AR	Adherence, aggregation, spreading, chemotaxis, leukemoid reaction	Delayed separation of umbilical stump, depressed inflammation, bacterial infections, gingivitis, periodontal disease
Hyperimmunoglobulin E–recurrent infection (Job's) syndrome/Non X-linked	Variable chemotactic defects, very high IgE with anti-*S. aureus* IgE; low anti-*S. aureus* IgA	"Coarse" facies in most patients, "cold" cutaneous abscesses; recurrent pulmonary, bone, upper airway infections with *S. aureus* or *Haemophilus influenzae;* mild eosinophilia; mucocutaneous candidiasis
Myeloperoxidase deficiency/AR	Absent myeloperoxidase	Minimal unless another defect present, then *Candida albicans* or other fungal infections
Chédiak-Higashi syndrome/AR	Giant lysosomal granules; neutropenia, chemotaxis, degranulation, microbicidal activity, excess O_2 consumption and H_2O_2 production	Recurrent pyogenic infections, especially with *S. aureus;* many patients get lymphomatous-like illness during adolescence; periodontal disease; partial oculocutaneous albinism, nystagmus, progressive peripheral neuropathy
Specific granule deficiency/AR (?)	Absent specific granules; chemotaxis, O_2^- production, bactericidal activity decreased	Recurrent cutaneous, ear, and pulmonary bacterial infections; diminished inflammation
Chronic granulomatous disease/X, AR, AD (rare)	H_2O_2 production absent in neutrophils and monocytes; defective "turn-off" of inflammation	Severe infections of skin, ears, lungs, liver, bone with catalase-positive microorganisms such as *S. aureus, Pseudomonas cepacia, Aspergillus* sp., *Chromobacterium violaceum;* often hard to culture organism; excessive inflammation with granulomas; frequent lymph node suppuration; granulomas can obstruct gastrointestinal or genitourinary tracts; gingivitis, aphthous ulcers

* X = x-linked; AR = autosomal recessive; AD = autosomal dominant.

deficiency is not associated with severely compromised defenses, because other defense systems such as hydrogen peroxide generation are accelerated. However, if another underlying defect in host defense, such as poorly controlled diabetes mellitus, accompanies myeloperoxidase deficiency, then host defenses are likely to be significantly compromised. An acquired form of myeloperoxidase deficiency occurs in myelomonocytic leukemia and acute myeloblastic leukemia (also referred to as myelogenous leukemia).

Chédiak-Higashi syndrome (CHS) is a rare disease with autosomal recessive inheritance. Neutrophils and all cells containing lysosomes from patients with CHS characteristically have large granules (see Fig. A5-19). CHS neutrophils and monocytes have impaired chemotaxis and abnormal rates of microbial killing due to slow rates of fusion of the lysosomal granules with phagosomes.

Chronic granulomatous disease (CGD) represents a group of patients with disorders of neutrophil and monocyte oxidative metabolism. Although CGD is rare, occurring in about 1 in 1 million individuals, it is an important model of defective neutrophil oxidative metabolism. Most often CGD is inherited as an X-linked recessive pattern, although in 35 percent of patients the disease is inherited with an autosomal recessive pattern and an autosomal dominant pattern has been reported in one family. Leukocytes from patients with CGD have severely diminished hydrogen peroxide production. Defects anywhere in the leukocyte's hexose-monophosphate shunt or the NADPH oxidase enzyme system can lead to clinical disease, and specific defects of cell membrane and cytosolic components have been identified. The genes involved in several of the defects have been cloned. Patients with CGD characteristically have increased infection with catalase-positive microorganisms (organisms which destroy their own hydrogen peroxide). When patients with CGD become infected, they often have extensive inflammatory reactions, and lymph node suppuration is common despite the administration of appropriate antibiotics. Aphthous ulcers and chronic inflammation of the nares are usually present. Granulomas are frequent and can obstruct the gastrointestinal or genitourinary tracts. The excessive inflammatory reactions probably reflect abnormal turnoff of inflammation by failure to degrade chemoattractants and antigens which cause persistent neutrophil accumulation. Impaired killing of intracellular microorganisms by macrophages may lead to persistent cell-mediated immunity and granuloma formation.

MONONUCLEAR PHAGOCYTES

The mononuclear phagocyte system is defined as a continuum linking monoblasts, promonocytes, and monocytes with the structurally diverse tissue macrophages which make up what was previously referred to as the reticuloendothelial system. Macrophages are long-lived phagocytic cells capable of many of the functions of neutrophils. In addition, they are important secretory cells that, through their receptors and secretory products, participate in many complex immunologic and inflammatory processes not attributed to neutrophils. Monocytes leave the circulation by diapedesis more slowly than neutrophils and have a half-life in the blood of 12 to 24 h.

After blood monocytes arrive in the tissues, they differentiate into macrophages ("big eaters") with specialized functions suited for specific anatomic locations. Macrophages are particularly abundant in capillary walls of the lung, spleen, liver, and bone marrow, where they function to remove microorganisms and other noxious elements from the blood. Alveolar macrophages, liver Kupffer cells, splenic macrophages, peritoneal macrophages, bone marrow macrophages, lymphatic macrophages, brain microglial cells, and dendritic macrophages all have specialized functions. Macrophage secreted products include lysozyme, neutral proteases, acid hydrolases, arginase, numerous complement components, enzyme inhibitors (plasmin, α_2-macroglobulin), binding proteins (transferrin, fibronectin, transcobalamin II), nucleosides, cachectin, and interleukin 1 (pyrogen). Interleukin 1 (see Chaps. 13 and 20) has many important functions, including stimulating the hypothalamus to initiate fever, mobilizing leukocytes from the bone marrow, as well as activating lymphocytes and neutrophils. Cachectin (also called tumor necrosis factor) is a pyrogen that duplicates many of the actions of interleukin 1 and plays an important role in the pathogenesis of gram-negative shock (see Chap. 89). It can stimulate vigorous production of hydrogen peroxide and related toxic oxygen species by macrophages and neutrophils. In addition, cachectin induces catabolic responses of chronic inflammation which contribute to the profound wasting (cachexia) associated with many chronic diseases.

Other macrophage secreted products include reactive oxygen metabolites, bioactive lipids (arachidonate metabolites and platelet activating factors), a neutrophil chemoattractant, factors regulating synthesis of proteins by other cells, bone marrow colony stimulating factors, factors stimulating fibroblast and microvasculature proliferation, as well as factors inhibiting replication of lymphocytes, tumors, viruses, and certain bacteria (*Listeria monocytogenes*). Macrophages are key effector cells in the elimination of intracellular microorganisms. Their ability to fuse to form giant cells which coalesce into granulomas in response to some inflammatory stimuli is important in the elimination of intracellular microbes and may be under the control of γ-interferon.

Macrophages play an important role in the immune response (see Chap. 13). They process antigen for presentation to lymphocytes, their secreted products modulate lymphocyte function, and macrophages participate in autoimmune phenomena by removing immune complexes and other immunologically active substances from the circulation. Furthermore, they play a role in wound healing, in the disposal of senescent cells, and in the development of atheromas.

DISORDERS OF THE MONONUCLEAR PHAGOCYTE SYSTEM
Many disorders of neutrophils extend to mononuclear phagocytes. Thus, drugs which suppress neutrophil production in the bone marrow usually lead to monocytopenia. Transient monocytopenia can also be seen after stress or glucocorticoid administration. Monocytosis is associated with certain infections such as tuberculosis, brucellosis, subacute bacterial endocarditis, Rocky Mountain spotted fever, and malaria. Monocytosis is also seen in kala azar, malignancies, leukemias, myeloproliferative syndromes, hemolytic anemias, chronic idiopathic neutropenias, granulomatous diseases such as sarcoidosis, regional enteritis, and some collagen vascular diseases. Patients with neutrophil C3bi receptor deficiency, the hyperimmunoglobulin E–recurrent infection (Job's) syndrome, Chédiak-Higashi syndrome, and chronic granulomatous diseases all have defects in the mononuclear phagocyte system.

Certain viral infections impair mononuclear phagocyte function. For example, influenza virus infection is associated with abnormal monocyte chemotaxis. Mononuclear phagocytes can be infected by the human immunodeficiency virus (HIV), and abnormal monocyte chemotaxis and abnormal clearance of IgG-coated erythrocytes (discussed below) by macrophages is also seen in the acquired immunodeficiency syndrome (AIDS) (see Chap. 264). It is likely that these defects of the monocyte-macrophage system in AIDS contribute to the disordered immunoregulation and increased susceptibility to opportunistic infection due to intracellular microorganisms such as *Pneumocystis carinii* and *Mycobacterium avium-intracellulare*. T lymphocytes produce γ-interferon, which induces Fc-receptor expression and phagocytosis as well as stimulates hydrogen peroxide production by mononuclear phagocytes. In certain diseases, such as AIDS, γ-interferon production may be deficient, while in other diseases, such as T-cell lymphomas, excessive release of γ-interferon is thought to cause erythrophagocytosis by splenic macrophages.

Specific defects of the mononuclear phagocytes have been described in certain autoimmune diseases. Removal of IgG-coated radiolabeled autologous erythrocytes, presumably via the Fc receptor of splenic macrophages, is profoundly abnormal in patients with active systemic lupus erythematosus. Patients with other autoimmune diseases characterized by tissue deposition of immune complexes, as seen in Sjögren's syndrome, mixed cryoglobulinemia, dermatitis herpetiformis, and chronic progressive multiple sclerosis, also have defects in Fc-receptor function as judged by clearance of IgG-coated erythrocytes (see Chap. 268). Clinically, normal subjects with genetic haplotypes commonly associated with autoimmune disease (i.e., HLA-B8/DRw3) also have an increased incidence of defective Fc receptor–specific functional activity, suggesting that this defect may predispose individuals with this genetic profile to immune-complex disease.

EOSINOPHILS

Eosinophils and neutrophils share similar morphology, many lysosomal constituents, most chemotactic responses, phagocytic capacity, and oxidative metabolism. However, there are major differences between the two cell types, and little is known about the natural function of eosinophils. Eosinophils are much longer lived than neutrophils, and unlike neutrophils, tissue eosinophils can recirculate. During most infections eosinophils do not appear to have any important function. However, in invasive parasite infections, such as hookworm, schistosomiasis, strongyloidiasis, toxocariasis, trichinosis, filariasis, echinococcosis, and cysticercosis, the eosinophil likely plays a central role in host defense. Eosinophils are also associated with bronchial asthma, cutaneous allergic reactions, and other hypersensitivity states.

The characteristic red-staining eosinophil granules (Wright's stain) contain a number of unique constituents. The distinctive feature of the eosinophil granule is its crystalline core consisting of an arginine-rich protein (major basic protein) with histaminase activity, which is probably important in host defense against parasites. Eosinophil granules also contain a unique eosinophil peroxidase which catalyzes the oxidation of many substances by hydrogen peroxide and may facilitate killing of microorganisms.

Eosinophil peroxidase, in the presence of hydrogen peroxide and halide, initiates mast cell secretion in vitro and thereby may contribute to inflammation. Other substances found in eosinophils include cationic proteins, some of which bind to heparin and reduce its anticoagulant activity. Eosinophil cytoplasm contains Charcot-Leyden crystal protein, a hexagonal bipyramidal crystal first described in leukemia and then in sputum from asthma patients, which is lysophospholipase and may function to restrict the toxicity of certain lysophospholipids. Eosinophils also contain a powerful neurotoxin. Because patients with hypereosinophilic syndrome and cerebral spinal fluid eosinophilia exhibit varied neurologic abnormalities, eosinophil-derived neurotoxin may play an important role in central nervous system disease.

Several factors enhance the eosinophil's function in host defense. For example, T-cell-derived eosinophil stimulation promoter enhances the ability of eosinophils to kill parasites. Mast cell–derived eosinophil chemotactic factor of anaphylaxis (ECFa) increases the number of eosinophil complement receptors and enhances eosinophil killing of parasites. In addition, eosinophil colony stimulating factors produced by macrophages may not only increase eosinophil production in the bone marrow but may also activate eosinophils to kill parasites.

EOSINOPHILIA   The presence of more than 500 eosinophils per microliter of blood is common in many settings besides parasite infection (see Chap. 64). The most common cause of eosinophilia is probably allergic reactions to drugs such as iodides, aspirin, and sulfonamides. Allergies such as hay fever, asthma, and eczema commonly are associated with eosinophilia. Eosinophilia is also seen in collagen vascular diseases (e.g., rheumatoid arthritis, eosinophilic fasciitis, allergic angiitis, and granulomatosis) and malignancies (e.g., Hodgkin's disease, mycosis fungoides) as well as the hyperimmunoglobulin E–recurrent infection (Job's) syndrome and the chronic granulomatous diseases; the mechanisms for the eosinophilia in these diseases are not known. The most dramatic increases in eosinophils occur in hypereosinophilic syndromes, including Loeffler's syndrome, eosinophilic leukemia, and idiopathic hypereosinophilic syndrome (with counts as high as 50,000 to 100,000 eosinophils per microliter).

The idiopathic hypereosinophilic syndrome represents a heterogeneous group of disorders with the common feature of prolonged eosinophilia of unknown cause and associated organ system dysfunction, including the heart, central nervous system, kidneys, lungs, gastrointestinal tract, and skin. The bone marrow is involved in all subjects, but the most severe complications involve the heart and central nervous system. Eosinophils are found in the involved tissues and are thought to cause tissue damage by local deposition of toxic eosinophil proteins such as eosinophil cationic protein and eosinophil major basic protein. In the heart the pathologic changes lead to thrombosis which may result in endocardial fibrosis and restrictive endomyocardiopathy. Similar pathologic changes are thought to contribute to the damage of tissues in other organ systems. Although the mechanism for the hypereosinophilia is not known, it has been shown that chemotherapy with glucocorticoids usually induces remission. In patients unresponsive to glucocorticoids, a cytotoxic agent such as hydroxyurea has been used successfully to lower the peripheral blood eosinophil counts and to improve markedly the prognosis. Aggressive medical and surgical approaches are also employed when managing patients with cardiovascular complications.

EOSINOPENIA This occurs with stress, such as acute bacterial infection, and following administration of glucocorticoids. The mechanism of eosinopenia of acute bacterial infection is unknown but is independent of endogenous glucocorticoids since it occurs in animals following total adrenalectomy. There is no known adverse effect of eosinopenia.

LABORATORY DIAGNOSIS AND MANAGEMENT OF PHAGOCYTE DYSFUNCTION

Initial studies of white blood count and differential and often a bone marrow examination are followed by assessment of bone marrow reserves (steroid challenge test), marginated circulating pool of cells (epinephrine challenge test), and marginating ability (endotoxin challenge test). In vivo assessment of inflammation is possible with a Rebuck skin window test, in which the ability of leukocytes to accumulate at a superficial abrasion and adhere to a glass coverslip is tested. In vivo clearance of IgG-coated erythrocytes provides a useful way to monitor the mononuclear-phagocytic (reticuloendothelial) system. In vitro tests of phagocyte aggregation, adherence, chemotaxis, phagocytosis, degranulation, and microbicidal activity (for *Staphylococcus aureus*) help pinpoint cellular or humoral lesions which can then be further characterized at the molecular level. Deficiencies of oxidative metabolism are screened with the nitroblue tetrazolium dye (NBT) test, which is based on the ability of products of oxidative metabolism to reduce yellow, soluble NBT to blue-black formazan, an insoluble material which precipitates intracellularly and can be seen microscopically. Further aspects of neutrophil oxidative metabolism are defined by studies of superoxide and hydrogen peroxide production.

The most important aspect of patient management is to appreciate that patients often have delayed inflammatory responses. Therefore, clinical manifestations may be minimal despite overwhelming infection, and unusual infections must always be suspected in some patients. Early signs of infection demand prompt, aggressive use of antibiotics and surgical drainage of abscesses. Prolonged antibiotics are often required, and in life-threatening infections daily white blood cell transfusions (enriched for neutrophils) are probably beneficial, although their use is still controversial. In patients with the chronic granulomatous diseases, prophylactic antibiotics (trimethoprim-sulfamethoxazole) probably diminish the frequency of life-threatening infections. Surgery is required for thorough drainage of abscesses in lung, liver, and bones. Short courses of glucocorticoids have been of benefit in the management of the granulomas of CGD. Recent studies indicate that γ-interferon may correct the biochemical and functional defects in certain patients with CGD. Rigorous oral hygiene reduces but does not eliminate the discomfort of gingivitis, periodontal disease, and aphthous ulcers; tooth brushing with a hydrogen peroxide–sodium bicarbonate paste helps some patients. Ketoconazole has caused dramatic improvement of mucocutaneous candidiasis in patients with the hyperimmunoglobulin E–recurrent infection (Job's) syndrome. Treatment to restore myelopoiesis in patients with neutropenia due to impaired production has included use of androgens, glucocorticoids, lithium, and immunosuppressive therapy. Studies with granulocyte and macrophage colony stimulating factors suggest these agents will be useful in the management of certain forms of neutropenia. Cure of some congenital phagocyte defects is theoretically possible by bone marrow transplantation (see Chap. 299). However, complications of bone marrow transplantation are still great, and with rigorous medical care many patients with phagocytic disorders can go for years without a life-threatening infection. The identification of specific gene defects in certain patients with phagocyte abnormalities makes gene therapy an exciting future possibility.

REFERENCES

ANDERSON DC, SPRINGER TA: Leukocyte adhesion deficiency: An inherited defect in the Mac-1, LFA-1, and p150,95 glycoproteins. Ann Rev Med 38:175, 1987
CLARK RA et al: Genetic variants of chronic granulomatous disease: Prevalence of deficiencies of two discrete cytosolic components of the NADPH oxidase system. N Engl J Med 321:647, 1989
CURNUTTE JT (ed): Phagocyte defects: Abnormalities outside of the respiratory burst. Hematol Clin North Am 2:1988
DONABEDIAN H, BALLIN JI: The hyperimmunoglobulin E–recurrent infection (Job's) syndrome. A review of the NIH experience and the literature. Medicine 62:185, 1983
GALLIN JI: Phagocytic cells: Disorders of function, in: *Inflammation: Basic Principles and Clinical Correlates*, JI Gallin et al (eds). New York, Raven Press, 1988, pp 493–511
———: Neutrophil specific granule deficiency. Ann Rev Med 36:263, 1985
GLEICH GJ, LOEGEUNG DA: Immunobiology of eosinophils. Ann Rev Immunol 2:429, 1984
JOHNSTON RB: Monocytes and macrophages. N Engl J Med 318:747, 1988
LEUNG DYM, GEHA R: Clinical and immunologic aspects of the hyperimmunoglobulin E syndrome. Hematol Oncol Clin North Am 2:81, 1988
LOMAX KJ et al: Recombinant 47-kD cytosol factor restores NADPH oxidase in chronic granulomatous disease. Science 245:409, 1989
——— et al: The molecular biology of selected phagocyte defects. Blood Rev 3:94, 1989
MALECH HL, GALLIN JI: Neutrophils in human disease. N Engl J Med 317:687, 1987
NUNOI H et al: Two forms of autosomal chronic granulomatous disease lack distinct neutrophil cytosol factors. Science 242:1298, 1988
SAMTER M (ed): *Immunological Diseases*, 4th ed. Boston, Little, Brown, 1988
SECHLER JMG et al: Recombinant human interferon-γ reconstitutes defective phagocyte function in patients with chronic granulomatous disease of childhood. Proc Natl Acad Sci USA 85:4874, 1988
SHERRY B, CERAMI A: Cachectin/tumor necrosis factor exerts endocrine, paracrine, and autocrine control of inflammatory responses. J Cell Biol 107:1269, 1988

82   INFECTIONS IN THE COMPROMISED HOST

HENRY MASUR / ANTHONY S. FAUCI

DEFINITION Patients who lack resistance to infection because of a deficiency in any of their multifaceted host defenses are referred to as "compromised hosts." Other terms such as "abnormal host," "immunosuppressed host," or "immunocompromised patient" are often used, but they have different connotations. The latter two refer specifically to a subpopulation of compromised hosts whose major deficiency in antimicrobial activity is related to their defective immune response.

Deficient host defense can be caused by many different factors including inherited disorders, coexisting disease, trauma, alcoholism, malnutrition, or drug therapies. The drugs that most often cause deficient host defense are cytotoxic agents and glucocorticoids, which are administered to treat malignant neoplasms, collagen vascular disorders, and organ transplants. An expanding spectrum of diseases can now be controlled or cured by complex and aggressive surgery, implantation of foreign bodies, or powerful cytotoxic or anti-inflammatory drugs. As noninfectious complications such as hemorrhage or uremia or graft rejection are being managed with increasing success, infection is becoming the major threat to the quality and duration of survival in many different patient populations.

HOST DEFENSE MECHANISMS

Antimicrobial defense mechanisms (Table 82-1) consist of complex, interacting systems that protect the host from endogenous and exogenous microbes (Chap. 78). The degree to which a patient becomes abnormally susceptible to infection by this microbial envi-

TABLE 82-1 Mechanisms of host defense

Physical and chemical barriers
   Morphologic integrity of skin, mucous membranes
   Sphincters
   Epiglottis
   Normal secretory and excretory flow
   Endogenous microbial flora
   Gastric acidity
Inflammatory response
   Circulating phagocytes
   Complement
   Other humoral mediators (bradykinins, fibrinolytic systems, arachidonic
     acid cascade)
Reticuloendothelial system
   Tissue phagocytes
Immune response
   T lymphocytes and their soluble products
   B lymphocytes and immunoglobulins

ronment depends on the mechanism compromised, the severity of the derangements, and their interactions. For instance, as isolated abnormalities, total absence of serum IgA or complement component C9 would probably have minor, if any, impact on host susceptibility to infection. In contrast, isolated abnormalities such as total absence of circulating neutrophils, serum IgG, or complement component C3 would lead to recurrent and life-threatening infections. Similarly, partial deficiencies in host defense mechanisms can have variable impact on susceptibility to infection depending on the specific mechanism, the degree of deficiency, and the presence of concomitant abnormalities. A modest decrease in circulating neutrophil count to 25 percent of the lower limit of normal or a decrease in serum IgG concentration to 50 percent of the lower limit of normal are usually tolerated with little or no difficulty if either is an isolated and transient abnormality. If such a neutrophil count were present concurrently with a major defect in the skin or mucous membranes for a prolonged period of time, complicating infection is more likely to occur.

Recognition of which specific and nonspecific host defenses are compromised is important in order to develop effective clinical strategies for predicting the probable onset of infection and the most likely causative organisms; for formulating the appropriate diagnostic approach; and for developing the optimal therapeutic and preventive plan. However, based on an understanding of the mechanisms of host defenses, such an approach must be supplemented by clinical experience with specific patient populations. Because there are complexities of various host defense mechanisms that are not fully understood, it cannot be assumed that all patient populations with the same measured deficiency in antimicrobial defense (as assessed by current laboratory techniques) will behave identically. For example, patients with cytomegalovirus infection (Chap. 138) have immunologic profiles that are similar in certain respects to those of patients in the early phases of the acquired immunodeficiency syndrome (AIDS) (Chap. 264). However, the susceptibility of these two populations to life-threatening opportunistic infection is vastly different, with AIDS patients being far more susceptible.

PHYSICAL AND CHEMICAL BARRIERS Physical and chemical barriers (Table 82-1) are part of a complex and interacting system of nonspecific host defense mechanisms that are essential for preventing the introduction and spread of microbial pathogens. These barriers utilize a wide variety of properties to protect the host, including the morphologic and functional integrity of skin or mucous membranes, the epiglottis, or sphincters; chemical processes (e.g., gastric acidity, pancreatic enzymes, cutaneous fatty acids or lysozyme); physical removal of organisms (e.g., peristalsis, sloughing of squamous cells, urine flow); and competition from less virulent flora. Interference with any of these mechanisms can increase the host's susceptibility to infection.

INFLAMMATORY RESPONSES Circulating phagocytes (neutrophils, monocytes, eosinophils, and basophils) arise from the bone marrow and upon appropriate signals enter the peripheral circulation and are distributed to local tissues, where they form the cornerstone of the inflammatory response. Recruitment of phagocytes from the bloodstream is a complicated process which involves the phagocytes' aggregation, adherence to the vascular endothelium, passage through endothelial spaces, and migration to local tissue sites (Chap. 81). An effective inflammatory response depends on the ability of the phagocyte to adhere, deform, have random locomotion, and respond to a chemical signal with directed movement. Humoral mediators influence local structures in ways that affect the phagocyte's ability to reach various loci: an example is the influence the complement cascade (especially C3a and C5a) has on the potential spaces between endothelial cells. Humoral mediators including the complement system, the arachidonic acid cascade, kinin-generating systems, and cellular products such as interleukin 1 and tumor necrosis factor, microbial peptides, or endotoxins also promote directed locomotion of the phagocytes. Once the phagocyte arrives at a focus of infection, it can adhere to the microorganism, ingest it, and digest it, particularly if the organism has been opsonized by antibodies or complement products. A wide variety of bacteria as well as fungi are killed by neutrophils in this manner.

RETICULOENDOTHELIAL SYSTEM Circulating microorganisms are cleared from the bloodstream by tissue phagocytes that are derived from circulating monocytes. These phagocytes include macrophages in the liver (Kupffer cells), spleen, lymph nodes, lung (alveolar macrophages), kidney (mesangial cells), and brain (microglial cells). The antimicrobial activities of these monocytes and macrophages are strongly influenced by opsonins such as IgG or C3b, which enhance the rate of particle ingestion, and by a large variety of soluble mediators produced primarily by mononuclear leukocytes (see Chap. 81). The efficacy of the reticuloendothelial system is also influenced by characteristics of specific organisms which allow the microbes to resist phagocytosis, lysosome-phagosome fusion (toxoplasma), or intraphagosomal inactivation (leishmania).

Immune response The major cellular components of the immune response are T lymphocytes and B lymphocytes (Chap. 13). These cells are distributed throughout the body in the bloodstream and at tissue sites. They interact in a highly complex fashion among themselves and with monocytes, macrophages, immunoglobulins, and the complement cascade. T lymphocytes are major components of the cell-mediated immune system. They secrete a multitude of cytokines which influence the functional status of other T lymphocytes, B lymphocytes, monocytes, and macrophages to eradicate infection, and participate directly in cytotoxic reactions against tumor cells, HLA-incompatible cells, and certain virus-infected host cells. B lymphocytes and plasma cells secrete specific antibodies which have important roles in eradicating certain infections. The ability of the monocytes and macrophages to ingest and kill a wide variety of bacteria, fungi, and protozoa is augmented by lymphokines released by T lymphocytes, in particular, γ-interferon. Production of opsonizing, neutralizing, or microbicidal antibodies can also be profoundly influenced by the regulatory effect of T lymphocytes on B lymphocytes (Chap. 13).

ETIOLOGY AND PATHOGENESIS OF INFECTION

In compromised hosts the development of infections reflects the interaction of impaired immunologic and nonimmunologic host defense mechanisms with the host's endogenous and exogenous microbial environment. Factors which change the microbial flora have an important impact on the organisms that are likely to cause disease. Such factors include antimicrobial therapy, invasive procedures or trauma, ingestion or inhalation of infected material, and hospitalization itself. The type of infections which develop are usually the consequence of specific alterations in host defenses, however. Numerous processes can predispose to serious infection by compromising the anatomic and physical barriers of host defense. For example, the skin and mucous membranes can be breached by tumor invasion, tumor necrosis, or vascular insufficiency induced by arteritis or atherosclerosis; by injury such as burns, pressure, or trauma; by radiation or cytotoxic chemotherapy; by a drug-induced cutaneous slough; and by procedures such as venipuncture or surgery. The respiratory tract can become the site of infection when its anatomic barriers are disrupted: the epiglottis may fail to protect the lower tract when the patient's consciousness is impaired or during intubation or bronchoscopy. The patient's ability to expel organisms may be adversely affected by infection, tumor, or drugs that alter the state of consciousness or prevent coughing; by disruption of mucociliary transport by a congenital disorder of ciliary subunits (such as Kartagener's syndrome) or by smoke or other inhaled toxins, anesthetic agents, or cytotoxic therapy; or by airway obstruction as a result of tumor, a foreign body, or lymph node enlargement. The gastrointestinal tract can become a less effective barrier against entry of organisms if gastric acidity is abolished by a surgical procedure or antacid therapy (infections with *Salmonella* and other gram-negative rods are a particular consequence); or if its mucosa is eroded by tumor or cytotoxic therapy, especially in neutropenic patients. Obstruction of the intestinal or biliary tract by tumor, a stricture, or a stone allows endogenous or introduced flora to gain access to the involved tissues and often the bloodstream. The genitourinary tract can become a portal of entry for infections if its mucosa is eroded by tumor,

irradiation, or cytotoxic therapy or there is urinary obstruction. Renal failure associated with oliguria or anuria deprives the genitourinary system of the ability to flush out microorganisms and obviates the antimicrobial effects of urine itself. The insertion of foreign bodies into the urethra during catheterization or cystoscopy allows exogenous organisms to be introduced into the urinary tract. Any locus in the body can become the site of infection if devitalized tissue or foreign bodies are seeded by bacteria or become infected by direct penetration. Hematomas, necrotic tissue, infarcts, calcified heart valves, and prosthetic devices (joints, heart valves, or central nervous system appliances) are particularly prone to bacterial infection.

Defects in inflammatory and immune function may permit infections that would normally be promptly eradicated to progress and cause clinically important disease. These quantitative or qualitative defects may be due to a congenital disorder, an underlying acquired disease, or drug therapy. Several specific types of defects are associated with particularly frequent or severe infectious complications.

LEUKOCYTE DISORDERS The clinical consequences of leukocyte disorders depend on which subpopulations of leukocytes are numerically or functionally affected and the duration of the dysfunction (Table 82-2) (Chap. 81). Neutropenia (less than 1800 neutrophils per

TABLE 82-2 Infections associated with common defects in inflammatory or immunologic response

Host defect	Examples of diseases or therapies associated with defects	Common etiologic agents of infections
INFLAMMATORY RESPONSE		
Neutropenia	Hematologic malignancies, cytotoxic chemotherapy, aplastic anemia	Gram-negative bacilli, *Staphylococcus aureus*, *Candida* species, *Aspergillus* species
Chemotaxis	Chédiak-Higashi syndrome	*Staphylococcus aureus*, *Streptococcus pyogenes*
	Job's syndrome	*Staphylococcus aureus*, *Haemophilus influenzae*, gram-negative bacilli
	Protein-calorie malnutrition	
Phagocytosis (cellular)	Systemic lupus erythematosus, chronic myelogenous leukemia, megaloblastic anemia	*Streptococcus pneumoniae*, *Haemophilus influenzae*
Splenectomy		*Haemophilus influenzae*, *Streptococcus pneumoniae*, other streptococci, DF-2, *Babesia microti*
Microbicidal defect	Chronic granulomatous disease	Catalase-positive bacteria and fungi: Staphylococci, *Escherichia coli*, *Klebsiella* species, *Pseudomonas aeruginosa*, *Candida* species, *Aspergillus* species, *Nocardia* species
	Chédiak-Higashi syndrome	*Staphylococcus aureus*, *Streptococcus pyogenes*
COMPLEMENT SYSTEM		
C3	Congenital liver disease	*Staphylococcus aureus*, *Streptococcus pneumoniae*
	Systemic lupus erythematosus	*Pseudomonas* species, *Proteus* species
C5	Congenital	*Neisseria* species, Gram-negative rods
C6, C7, C8	Congenital, systemic lupus erythematosus	*Neisseria meningitidis*, *Neisseria gonorrhoeae*
Alternate pathway	Sickle cell disease	*Streptococcus pneumoniae*, *Salmonella* species
IMMUNE RESPONSE		
T-lymphocyte deficiency/dysfunction	Thymic aplasia, thymic hypoplasia, Hodgkin's disease, sarcoid, lepromatous leprosy	*Listeria monocytogenes*, *Mycobacterium* species, *Candida* species, *Aspergillus* species, *Cryptococcus neoformans*, *Herpes simplex*, *Herpes zoster*
	Acquired immunodeficiency syndrome	*Pneumocystis carinii*, cytomegalovirus, *Herpes simplex*, *Mycobacterium avium-intracellulare*, *Cryptococcus neoformans*, *Candida* species
	Mucocutaneous candidiasis	*Candida* species
	Purine nucleoside phosphorylase deficiency	Fungi, viruses
B-cell deficiency/dysfunction	Bruton's X-linked agammaglobulinemia, agammaglobulinemia, chronic lymphocytic leukemia, multiple myeloma, dysglobulinemia	*Streptococcus pneumoniae*, other streptococci, *Haemophilus influenzae*, *Neisseria meningitidis*, *Staphylococcus aureus*, *Klebsiella pneumoniae*, *Escherichia coli*, *Giardia lamblia*, *Pneumocystis carinii*, enteroviruses
	Selective IgM deficiency	*Streptococcus pneumoniae*, *Haemophilus influenzae*, *Escherichia coli*
	Selective IgA deficiency	*Giardia lamblia*, Viral hepatitis, *Streptococcus pneumoniae*, *Haemophilus influenzae*
Mixed T- and B-cell deficiency/dysfunction	Common variable hypogammaglobulinemia	*Pneumocystis carinii*, cytomegalovirus, *Streptococcus pneumoniae*, *Haemophilus influenzae*, various other bacteria
	Ataxia-telangiectasia	*Streptococcus pneumoniae*, *Haemophilus influenzae*, *Staphylococcus aureus*, rubella, *Giardia lamblia*
	Severe combined immunodeficiency	*Candida albicans*, *Pneumocystis carinii*, varicella, rubella, cytomegalovirus
	Wiskott-Aldrich	Infections seen in T- and B-cell abnormalities

microliter) is the most commonly encountered defect in inflammatory host defense mechanisms (Chap. 64). When the neutrophil count falls below 1000 cells per microliter, there is a progressive increase in susceptibility to bacterial and fungal infections and a progressive decrease in the localizing signs and symptoms of inflammation. Susceptibility to infection increases dramatically when the peripheral neutrophil count falls below 500 cells per microliter, particularly when the count falls below 100 cells per microliter. The rate of decline and the duration of neutropenia are also important parameters which influence the development of infection. Neutropenia can occur because of bone marrow failure, peripheral destruction, or pooling or sequestration of cells. The most common causes of neutropenia are cytotoxic chemotherapy, neoplastic invasion of the bone marrow, aplastic anemia, and idiosyncratic drug reactions.

Neutrophil dysfunction can also result in a substantial predisposition to serious infection. Dysfunction may be a manifestation of a congenital disorder such as chronic granulomatous disease or Chédiak-Higashi syndrome (Chap. 81). Glucocorticoids and some multiple drug chemotherapeutic regimens may alter both the number and the function of circulating neutrophils.

Lymphopenia in adults is defined as less than 1000 lymphocytes per microliter. The clinical consequences of lymphopenia depend on which subset(s) is affected. Regardless of the total lymphocyte count, severe infections may occur if profound deficiencies of either B lymphocytes or T lymphocytes are present. Substantial reductions in helper T lymphocytes (<200 per microliter) have particularly important infectious consequences. The most common causes of lymphopenia are hematologic malignancies, glucocorticoid therapy, antilymphocyte globulins, cytotoxic drugs, and infection with certain viruses such as cytomegalovirus (Chap. 138) and HIV (Chap. 264). Congenital lymphopenias can also have severe consequences (Chap. 263).

Lymphocyte dysfunction can predispose to life-threatening infection even if the lymphocyte number is normal. Lymphocyte dysfunction is most often a consequence of therapy with glucocorticoids or cytotoxic drugs.

IMMUNOGLOBULIN DISORDERS Decreased production of functional immunoglobulins, particularly IgG, can cause a marked increase in susceptibility to microbial disease (Chap. 263). Patients with significant reductions in IgG (usually less than 200 to 300 mg/dL) characteristically have recurrent infections due to encapsulated bacteria, particularly *Streptococcus pneumoniae*, *Haemophilus influenzae*, and *Neisseria meningitidis*, and to certain protozoa (*Pneumocystis carinii* and *Giardia lamblia*). Selective IgA deficiency can lead to respiratory or systemic bacterial infections (particularly when accompanied by IgG_2 deficiency) as well as intestinal giardiasis or severe viral hepatitis. The few documented cases of selective IgM deficiency have also been associated with severe infections, in particular, with gram-negative organisms such as *Neisseria meningitidis*. Clinically important causes of immunoglobulin deficiency or dysfunction include congenital and acquired disorders, such as malignancies (multiple myeloma, chronic lymphocytic leukemia), sickle cell disease, and splenectomy (Table 82-2) (Chap. 263).

COMPLEMENT DISORDERS The consequences of total absence of functional complement proteins depend on which of the specific components are deficient (Table 82-2) (Chap. 13). Deficiencies of C1 or C3 have been associated with pneumococcal infections while deficiencies of C5, C6, C7, or C8 may lead to relapsing *Neisseria meningitidis* or *Neisseria gonorrhoeae* infections. Most severe deficiencies are due to inherited disorders, although there are reports of significant deficiencies in patients with systemic lupus erythematosus, cirrhosis, or splenectomy.

SPLENECTOMY The spleen contains large numbers of B lymphocytes, monocytes, and macrophages and is a major site for T cell–independent immune responses such as the production of antibodies to polysaccharide antigens. The spleen has an important role in the phagocytosis of circulating opsonized organisms. Following splenectomy young children are at high risk for fulminant infections due to *Streptococcus pneumoniae*, *Haemophilus influenzae*, *Neisseria*

meningitidis, and the fastidious gram-negative bacterium DF-2. Adults who undergo splenectomy are also at increased risk for these infections, especially during the first 3 years after surgery. Splenectomized patients may develop fulminant infection with intraerythrocytic protozoa such as *Plasmodium malariae* and *Babesia*.

DIAGNOSIS

Clinicians managing compromised patients must recognize that the diagnosis of infectious processes requires special attention, persistence, and expertise. Compromised patients often present initially with manifestations that may be subtle or atypical. All infections can become life-threatening in extremely short time periods in many of these patients, so that the diagnostic evaluation needs to begin promptly when the first signs or symptoms or laboratory abnormalities become apparent. These evaluations should proceed in rapid sequence using tests that have the shortest feasible processing times. A thorough approach is necessary to make certain that the true etiologic agent is being treated and to minimize the likelihood that unnecessary drugs with unneeded toxicities will be employed. The spectrum of potential etiologic agents is usually wide, so that the diagnostic tests must often be broad-gauged as well. Based on knowledge of the factors that render the patient compromised, the organisms associated with particular defects in host defense, and the patient's individual history and presentation, the clinician in concert with the laboratory must consider whether special testing should be done for unusual bacteria, fungi, viruses, helminths, protozoa, or other microorganisms. It is usually desirable to have a standard protocol for evaluating common clinical syndromes (e.g., pneumonia, fevers, meningitis) in compromised patients, with modifications being made in the protocol as warranted by the individual patient's circumstances. For instance, when an HIV-infected patient has a helper-T-lymphocyte (T4-positive or CD4-positive) count below 200 to 300 per microliter, and especially when the count falls below 100 per microliter, mild cough with fever must be evaluated promptly and aggressively since pneumocystis or cytomegalovirus pneumonia are much more likely than in HIV-positive patients with normal T4 counts. Kidney transplant recipients are known to be at very high risk for bacterial wound and urinary tract infections during the first postoperative month, while opportunistic viral, fungal, and protozoan diseases are more common during the second through sixth months. The development of fever during the first postoperative month should prompt an evaluation that focuses initially on the wound and urinary tract, while similar symptoms occurring several months after surgery should direct studies for protozoan, fungal, or viral infections.

Patients with leukemias and lymphomas need particular scrutiny for complicating bacterial or fungal infections when their neutrophil counts fall below 100 cells per microliter (a time that is usually predictable from the pharmacokinetics of the chemotherapeutic regimen).

THERAPY

In compromised patients the therapy of infectious complications should include drainage of localized collections of infected material, specific antimicrobials, and, if possible, reconstitution of deficient antimicrobial defenses. Examples include the infusion of fresh frozen plasma to augment complement components, the administration of immune serum globulin to restore IgG levels, and the tapering of immunosuppressive drugs (such as glucocorticoids or cytotoxic agents) to restore cell-mediated immune mechanisms or neutrophil production. In certain neutropenic patients augmentation or restoration of neutrophils can be achieved temporarily by the use of colony stimulating factors (see Chap. 64) or white blood cell transfusions, or permanently by bone marrow transplantation. Patients must be carefully selected for which of these procedures is likely to be effective.

Empiric antimicrobial therapy is clearly appropriate for some patient populations. For example, newly developing fever in severely neutropenic patients is frequently due to infection with bacteria, and therapy using a broad-spectrum regimen directed against potential major gram-positive and gram-negative pathogens before culture results are available can be lifesaving. The use of antibiotic combinations that are synergistic against infecting bacteria has been more successful in reducing morbidity and mortality from bacterial infection in neutropenic patients than single agents or nonsynergistic combinations. Examples of such combinations are vancomycin, ticarcillin, and amikacin or ceftazidime and amikacin (for dosages see Chap. 85). Empiric use of amphotericin B in the febrile neutropenic patient unresponsive after several days of antibacterial treatment is a common practice and may reduce mortality from fungal superinfection.

PREVENTION OF INFECTION

In compromised patients certain types of infections can be prevented by avoiding damage to physical barriers, bolstering host defenses, reducing acquisition of new potential pathogens, and suppressing colonizing flora. The use of invasive procedures including repeated venipuncture, indwelling peripheral venous catheters, and urinary catheterization should be minimized or avoided completely. Surgical procedures should be chosen only when absolutely essential and performed with meticulous care. Bolstering host defenses can be accomplished directly in some patient groups. For example, immune serum globulin can be given prophylactically to hypogammaglobulinemic patients (see Chap. 263); hyperimmune varicella-zoster immunoglobulin can prevent or reduce the severity of varicella-zoster virus disease after acute exposure; immunization with vaccines against pneumococci, *Haemophilus,* and meningococci may be helpful for patients with conditions of particular susceptibility such as following splenectomy (see Chap. 81).

Maintaining an optimal nutritional status will improve cellular immune mechanisms and aid wound repair. Most other methods to enhance depressed cell-mediated immunity have been clinically ineffective. Colony stimulating factors offer promise in restoring neutrophil numbers and preventing infection in neutropenic subjects but requires further investigation (see Chap. 64). Reducing the acquisition of potential pathogens can be facilitated by simple techniques such as having hospital personnel wash their hands before patient contact and by appropriate isolation from specific potentially contagious organisms such as *Herpes zoster, Mycobacterium tuberculosis,* or multiply antibiotic-resistant gram-negative bacilli (see Chap. 83). More stringent measures such as laminar flow isolation or control of sterility of food and water have not proved to be useful or cost-effective for ultimate survival, although these measures will decrease the rate of infection for patients with prolonged and profound granulocytopenia. Suppression of endogenous bacteria or fungi is an important concept, since they cause more than 80 percent of infections in neutropenic cancer patients. Gut sterilization or prophylactic systemic antibiotics have proved useful as temporary measures in neutropenic patients but cannot be practically sustained for more than a few weeks. Prolonged antimicrobial prophylaxis of certain specific infections that have exceedingly high attack rates in certain defined populations can be quite effective. The impressive protection provided by trimethoprim-sulfamethoxazole or aerosolized pentamidine against *Pneumocystis carinii* pneumonia in patients with AIDS or acute lymphocytic leukemia is a striking example.

REFERENCES

THE EORTC INTERNATIONAL ANTIMICROBIAL THERAPY COOPERATIVE GROUP: Ceftazidime combined with a short or long course of amikacin for empirical therapy of gram-negative bacteremia in cancer patients with granulocytopenia. N Engl J Med 317:1692, 1987

GALLIN JI, FAUCI AS: *Advances in Host Defense Mechanisms,* vol 2, *Lymphoid Cells.* New York, Raven Press, 1983

HUGHES WT et al: Successful chemoprophylaxis for *Pneumocystis carinii* pneumonitis. N Engl J Med 297:1419, 1977

MASUR H et al: CD4 counts as predictors of pneumonias in human immunodeficiency virus infected individuals. Ann Intern Med 111:223, 1989

NOSSAL GJV: Current concepts: Immunology: The basic components of the immune system. N Engl J Med 316:1320, 1987

PIZZO PA, MEYERS J: Infections in the cancer patient, in *Cancer Medicine: Principles and Practice of Oncology,* V DeVita et al (eds). Philadelphia, Lippincott, 1989

——— et al: Fever in the pediatric and young adult patient with cancer: A prospective study of 1001 episodes. Medicine 61:153, 1982

ROSEN FS, YOUNG LS: The primary immunodeficiencies. N Engl J Med 311Z:235, 1984

ROSS SC, DENSEN P: Complement deficiency states and infection. Epidemiology, pathogenesis, and consequences of neisserial and other infections in an immune deficiency. Medicine 63:243, 1984

RUBIN LS, YOUNG LS: *The Clinical Approach to Infection in the Immunocompromised Host,* 2d ed. New York, Plenum, 1988

SANDE MA, VOLBERDING PA: *The Medical Management of AIDS.* Philadelphia, Saunders, 1988

SHENEP JL et al: Vancomycin, ticarcillin, and amikacin compared with ticarcillin-clavulanate and amikacin in the empirical treatment of febrile, neutropenic children with cancer. N Engl J Med 319:1053, 1988

83　HOSPITAL-ACQUIRED INFECTIONS

PIERCE GARDNER / JOSEPH J. KLIMEK

DEFINITIONS Hospital-acquired infections (also called nosocomial infections) are defined as infections occurring in patients after admission to the hospital that were neither present nor incubating at the time of admission. Infections acquired in the hospital but not manifest until after the patient is discharged are also included in this definition. Although many of these infections can be prevented, some cannot, and the term *hospital-acquired infection* should not be equated with *iatrogenic infection,* which indicates an infection caused by a diagnostic or therapeutic intervention such as the insertion of a urethral or intravenous catheter. *Opportunistic infections* occur in patients with impaired host defenses and are commonly caused by infectious agents that do not ordinarily produce disease in healthy individuals. Many opportunistic infections are caused by organisms in the patient's own flora (*autochthonous infections*) and are often unavoidable because they are related to defects in mucosal barriers or other host defenses rather than preventable environmental risks.

ETIOLOGY AND EPIDEMIOLOGY　Incidence and cost Hospital-acquired infections occur in from 2 to 10 percent (average, 5 percent) of patients admitted to general hospitals. The highest infection rates are reported from municipal hospitals and tertiary-care centers, while the prevalence of these infections is much lower in community hospitals. These differences in rates appear to be due to the greater severity of underlying disease in patients in municipal and tertiary-care hospitals and may also reflect greater utilization of invasive procedures and diagnostic tests in the management of these patients. On the average, hospital-acquired infections have a mortality rate of 1 percent and contribute to the death of at least an additional 3 percent. Therefore the estimated 2 million hospital-acquired infections which occur annually in the United States result in approximately 20,000 deaths and contribute to the mortality of an additional 60,000 patients. Nosocomial infections add over 7.5 million hospital days and over 1 billion dollars to national health care costs.

Causative pathogens Gram-negative bacilli lead the list of nosocomial pathogens. Their statistical importance is due in large part to their role in urinary tract infections, but gram-negative bacilli also are important pathogens at other sites. Many of these organisms, especially pseudomonads and *Klebsiella,* require minimal nutrients and are able to establish reservoirs in the inanimate hospital environment, as well as in patients. In large part, antimicrobial resistance among gram-negative bacilli is due to the acquisition of plasmids called *resistance factors* (R factors). R-factor plasmids consist of extrachromosomal circular DNA, which mediates antibiotic resistance by coding for enzymes that inactivate the drug or by modifying systems involved in antibiotic uptake. Several properties of plasmids are of major public health concern: (1) Resistance to several antibiotics is often linked on the same R factor; (2) R-factor transfer can occur across species and even genera of gram-negative bacilli; (3) small gene fragments encoding for a single antibiotic-inactivating enzyme have been incorporated into diverse plasmids which are spread among many genera of gram-negative bacilli. Certain gram-negative bacilli (most often *Enterobacter, Pseudomonas,* and *Serratia*) have developed an additional chromosomal mechanism of resistance to penicillin and cephalosporin drugs, i.e., the induction of β-lactamase enzymes. Because production of these enzymes is enhanced by exposure to β-lactam antibiotics (especially the newer cephalosporins), widespread use of these antibiotics in hospitals exerts selective pressure for the emergence of these difficult-to-treat gram-negative bacilli.

Among gram-positive cocci, *Staphylococcus aureus,* the scourge of the 1950s and early 1960s, remains the most important pathogen. During the past decade an alarming increase in methicillin-resistant *S. aureus* (MRSA) has been noted, especially in debilitated immunocompromised patients in intensive care units (see Chap. 101). These strains are generally resistant to all β-lactam agents and often to erythromycin, clindamycin, and the aminoglycosides as well. For serious infections caused by these strains, vancomycin is the drug of choice. Other antimicrobials with activity against MRSA include rifampin, ciprofloxacin, and trimethoprim-sulfamethoxazole (see Chap. 85). Bacterial tolerance (organisms are inhibited but not killed by bactericidal drugs) is common among currently isolated strains of *S. aureus* and may dictate the use of bactericidal antibiotic combinations in serious infections, such as endocarditis (see Chap. 90). The enterococcus (group D streptococcus), long recognized as an important pathogen in nosocomial urinary tract infections, is emerging as a significant wound pathogen particularly in patients who have received broad-spectrum cephalosporins (to which enterococci are uniformly resistant).

The spectrum of microorganisms recognized to be important nosocomial pathogens has expanded considerably. Opportunistic infections caused by low-virulence bacteria (*Staphylococcus epidermidis,* JK diphtheroid) and fungi (*Aspergillus, Candida,* and agents causing mucormycosis) have become commonplace. Respiratory viruses, especially respiratory syncytial virus and influenza, have gained increased recognition as causes of significant morbidity when acquired during hospitalization. Other viruses transmissible in blood (hepatitis viruses, human immunodeficiency virus, cytomegalovirus) are of concern to hospital personnel as well as patients.

Transmission of nosocomial pathogens Contact with hospital personnel remains the principal means of transmission of nosocomial pathogens and hand-washing by hospital personnel remains the principal control measure. Other less important modes of transmission include the airborne route, by which infections such as chickenpox and tuberculosis are spread, and contact with environmental sources. The inanimate hospital environment usually is not the source of infecting pathogens. However, environmental reservoirs have proved to be of primary importance in clusters of cases of aspergillosis caused by inhalation of spores from dust or fireproofing material, and in epidemics of Legionnaires' disease.

Host factors The age and underlying disease of patients, the integrity of their mucosal and integumentary surfaces, and the status of their immunologic defenses are among the major determinants of both the incidence and outcome of hospital-acquired infections (see Chap. 82).

COMMON HOSPITAL-ACQUIRED INFECTIONS Urinary tract infections Approximately 40 percent of hospital-acquired infections occur in the urinary tract and are usually a consequence of instrumentation of the urethra, bladder, or kidneys. The most common predisposing factor is the insertion of an indwelling urethral catheter which bypasses the normal anatomic barriers to ascending infection. Hospital surveys show that 10 to 15 percent of all adult patients have indwelling urinary catheters, many of which are unnecessary. Because

the urinary tract is the most common site of infection resulting in gram-negative bacteremia, steps to prevent catheter-related infections merit special emphasis and include the following:

1 Restrict the use of indwelling catheters except when required for management of bladder outlet obstruction or for close monitoring of urine output.
2 Rigorously adhere to sterile technique during insertion of the catheter.
3 Maintain a system of closed drainage. Good technique can usually keep the urine sterile for 5 to 7 days.
4 Keep the collecting tubing and bag unobstructed and in a dependent position.
5 When urine specimens are required, aspirate the specimen from the sampling port in the collecting tubing by use of a sterile needle and syringe rather than by breaking the closed drainage system.
6 Consider intermittent straight catheterization for patients with anticipated short-term needs for bladder drainage.

Wound infections Most surgical wound infections are caused by organisms introduced directly into the tissues at the time of operative procedures. Most infecting organisms originate from the resident flora of the patient, although personnel in the operating theater may occasionally be the source of infection, especially with group A streptococci or *S. aureus.* The major factors affecting the incidence of wound infection include the type of operation, its duration, the skill of the surgeon, and the basic health of the patient. Operations involving contaminated sites, such as the bowel or vagina, are more likely to be complicated by infection than operations on sites which are sterile prior to surgery. Operations of long duration, or ones in which devitalized tissue, foreign bodies, or hematomas are left behind, are associated with increased rates of wound infection. Adverse host factors include advanced age, poor nutritional status, the presence of distant foci of infection, diabetes mellitus, renal failure, and glucocorticoid therapy.

Most wound infections become apparent from 3 to 7 days following surgery. Early postoperative wound infections (those occurring within 24 to 48 h of surgery) are commonly caused by group A *Streptococcus* or *Clostridium* spp. Staphylococcal wound infections characteristically become evident 4 to 6 days after surgery, and those caused by gram-negative bacilli and anaerobic bacteria may not appear for a week or more. If perioperative antibiotics are used, the manifestations of infection may be delayed. Gram-stained smears of wound exudate, together with culture, often provide valuable early clues to the bacterial cause of wound infections.

In addition to emphasis on maintaining sterility in the operating room and insistence on operative techniques that minimize tissue trauma and blood loss, short prophylactic courses of antibiotics during the perioperative period may be beneficial in certain operations (see Chap. 85). The principles that should govern the use of antibiotics in this situation include (1) beginning the drug during the immediate preoperative period but not earlier, (2) ensuring adequate tissue levels throughout the surgery, giving intraoperative doses of antibiotics if necessary, and (3) discontinuing antibiotic prophylaxis within 24 to 48 h following surgery. These brief courses of antibiotics do not appear to alter the patient's flora or promote colonization with resistant strains. Prolonged pre- and postoperative courses are unnecessary, expensive, and potentially harmful because of the increased risk of drug toxicity and superinfection. Antibiotic prophylaxis administered according to these principles has reduced infectious morbidity in a wide variety of operative procedures that are traditionally associated with major risk of infection including colon surgery and vaginal hysterectomy.

Nonsurgical wounds that are common sites of nosocomial infection include burns, decubitus ulcers, and cutaneous ulcers resulting from venous or arterial occlusive disease. In general, the offending pathogens are similar to those found in surgical wound infections, except that burn wound infections are frequently caused by *Pseudo-*

monas aeruginosa, and ulcers of the pelvis and lower extremities usually contain fecal flora.

Pneumonia Lower respiratory tract infections are the leading cause of mortality among hospital-acquired infections, although they rank third in incidence behind urinary tract infections and wound infections. The major pathogens are the gram-negative bacilli and *S. aureus*, all of which characteristically cause a necrotizing bronchopneumonia. These organisms usually reach the lower respiratory tract by aspiration from the pharynx rather than by hematogenous spread. This is consistent with the observation that the pharyngeal flora of seriously ill patients contains an increased number of gram-negative bacilli. The three settings in which nosocomial pneumonias occur most commonly are in (1) obtunded patients whose gag reflex and cough are ineffective, (2) patients with underlying pulmonary disease or congestive heart failure whose pulmonary clearance mechanisms are impaired, and (3) patients who require respiratory tract instrumentation or ventilatory assistance.

Because antibiotic treatment of nosocomial pneumonia is often ineffective, preventive measures assume special importance. Positioning the patient in a swimmer's or Gatch position is the cornerstone for preventing aspiration in obtunded patients. Treatment of congestive heart failure will improve the effectiveness of the lung's defenses and will reduce lung edema fluid that serves as an excellent culture medium. Emphasis should be placed on sterile technique when performing tracheal toilet, and the breathing circuits on ventilatory assistance equipment must be properly maintained. Nosocomial spread of the tubercle bacillus is uncommon; however, recognition of active cases of pulmonary tuberculosis and prompt institution of respiratory isolation and appropriate chemotherapy are the principal means by which in-hospital spread of the disease can be limited.

Hospital transmission of viral respiratory pathogens is common, but except for influenza and respiratory syncytial virus, rarely results in severe disease. Epidemiologic studies indicate that direct and indirect contact spread of viruses on the hands of personnel is a more important route of transmission than airborne spread. When influenza A is widespread in the community, amantadine prophylaxis should be considered for unimmunized hospital patients identified as being at high risk for complications of influenza. Increasing the immunization levels among hospital personnel is likely to reduce nosocomial transmission of influenza viruses.

Bacteremia Although invasion of the bloodstream can occur in any nosocomial infection, the infected vascular cannula is the most common and also most preventable cause of hospital-acquired primary bacteremia and fungemia. Annually in the United States more than 10 million persons (more than one in four hospitalized patients) receive intravenous therapy, and therefore even a low rate of infection assumes major clinical significance. Infections related to intravenous therapy account for about 5 percent of all nosocomial infections and 10 percent of all positive blood cultures. The most common causative organisms are *S. epidermidis*, *S. aureus*, gram-negative bacilli, and enterococci; when hyperalimentation fluid is administered through the catheter, *Candida* also is an important pathogen. Although microorganisms can enter a fluid delivery system at any point, contamination most commonly occurs at the site of entry into the skin during cannula insertion or subsequent manipulation and may be followed by migration of organisms along the cannula into the bloodstream. Occasionally hematogenous seeding of the cannula may occur. Intravenous fluids may become contaminated as a result of adding medications, or, rarely, in the process of manufacture. A clue to the possible presence of infusate contamination is unexpected bacteremia caused by one of the few pathogens (*Enterobacter, Klebsiella, Serratia, Pseudomonas cepacia*, or *Citrobacter freundii*) capable of sustained growth in intravenous solutions containing 5% dextrose.

The type of cannula, the choice of insertion site, the adequacy of skin preparation, and the duration of cannula use influence the risk of cannula-related sepsis. Suppurative phlebitis, one of the most feared complications of cannula-related infections, is virtually unknown with steel needles. Arms are better insertion sites than legs owing to lower rates of phlebitis and sepsis. When cannula infection is suspected, semiquantitative microbiologic evaluation of the removed cannula tip by culture or by direct examination of a Gram-stained catheter segment is useful in identifying patients with heavily colonized cannulas who are at high risk of developing bacteremia or fungemia. With meticulous care, central venous catheters used for parenteral hyperalimentation can be maintained free of infection for prolonged periods. However, infectious complications, particularly *Candida* sepsis, are not uncommon in this setting. Intravascular catheters used for pressure monitoring pose many of the same risks as those used for infusion therapy; in addition, the presence of an indwelling pulmonary artery catheter during a period of bacteremia may increase the risk of developing endocarditis.

Transient bacteremia following diagnostic or therapeutic manipulations of the mouth or respiratory, gastrointestinal, or genitourinary tract are usually well-tolerated by the normal host. However, the patient with valvular or congenital heart disease or a prosthetic valve may be at risk of developing endocarditis during such episodes and should receive antibiotic prophylaxis when undergoing procedures associated with significant risk of bacteremia. These procedures include dental manipulations, urinary tract instrumentation, abdominal surgery, and other surgery involving infected tissue. For patients with prosthetic heart valves, these recommendations have been extended. Detailed programs of prophylaxis are given in the chapter on infectious endocarditis (see Chap. 90).

NOSOCOMIAL PATHOGENS OF SPECIAL INTEREST Human immunodeficiency virus (HIV) Nosocomial transmission of HIV has been a major problem for patients with hemophilia and others who have received HIV-infected blood products, but has been reassuringly rare in other health care settings. The incidence of *acquired immunodeficiency syndrome* (AIDS) among health care workers does not exceed the rate in the general public, and the risk of HIV transmission following a needle-stick accident from an infected patient is less than 1 percent. Nevertheless, the recognition of a large reservoir of infected asymptomatic people and the potential risk to health care workers exposed to blood and certain other body fluids (cerebrospinal fluid, pleural fluids, peritoneal fluid, pericardial fluid, and amniotic fluid) has led the Centers for Disease Control to recommend blood and body fluid precautions in the handling of all such specimens. These "universal precautions" might also be expected to reduce health worker risks of nosocomial hepatitis B virus and other bloodborne viruses. Universal precautions represent a significant departure from traditional disease-focused infection control methods. The impact of this approach on HIV and HBV transmission to health care workers and the effects on rates of bacterial nosocomial infections have not been determined (see Chap. 264).

Hepatitis B virus (HBV) The risk of hospital-acquired HBV is significant not only for patients but also for hospital personnel who work with infected patients or handle their blood specimens. Patients at special risk of HBV infection include those who receive blood products or undergo hemodialysis. Screening of blood products for hepatitis B surface antigen (HBsAg) has markedly reduced the incidence of posttransfusion HBV and most posttransfusion hepatitis is now caused by other hepatitis viruses (non-A, non-B hepatitis). However, transmission of HBV remains an endemic problem on many hemodialysis units and oncology services.

Measures to prevent nosocomial HBV infection of health care workers should include: (1) HBV immunization for all hospital personnel whose work places them at risk; (2) meticulous attention to precautions to limit spread of pathogens by needle accidents or body fluid contact (see "Universal Precautions" in Chap. 264); and (3) prompt passive-active immunization with hepatitis B immune globulin and HBV vaccine for susceptible personnel who have been subjected to a specific hepatitis risk (i.e., needle stick from an infectious patient) (see Chap. 252).

Legionnaires' disease Nosocomial Legionnaires' disease usually affects immunocompromised patients. Although contamination of hospital cooling tower water accounts for some cases, sustained epidemic or hyperendemic problems have almost always been traced to heavy contamination of hot tap water by *Legionella* species. Infectious aerosols of tap water can be produced by showers and during operation of some humidifiers and respiratory devices filled with tap water. A causative role of contaminated hospital tap water has been substantiated by the efficacy of hyperchlorination or super-heating of hospital tap water in curtailing epidemics.

Clostridium difficile colitis Bacterial superinfection with *C. difficile* is a consequence of alteration of bowel flora by antimicrobial therapy. Patients with *C. difficile* colitis excrete large numbers of organisms and represent a risk to other patients. Therefore, enteric precautions and thorough cleaning of bathroom areas of patients with *C. difficile* disease should be implemented.

CONTROL MEASURES Infection control team The goals of those concerned with infection control are (1) to reduce the risk of patients acquiring infections in the hospital, (2) to provide adequate care for patients with a potentially communicable infection, and (3) to minimize the infectious risks of employees, visitors, and community contacts. The functions of the infection control team include (1) development of enforceable policies necessary for appropriate management of patients with communicable infections; (2) development of a surveillance system which identifies patients with communicable infections, quantitates the incidence and prevalence of hospital-acquired infection, and focuses on problems requiring further investigation; (3) feedback to physicians and other staff regarding identified problems and surveillance findings, including surgical wound infection rates; (4) liaison with personnel from nursing, central supply, housekeeping, maintenance, pharmacy, and other hospital services to ensure that an appropriate infection control environment is maintained; (5) education of employees in appropriate techniques to prevent the spread of infectious agents; (6) communication with employee health services to ensure adequate immunization of hospital employees and to provide care when personnel are exposed to a potentially communicable disease; and (7) monitoring of antibiotic utilization and susceptibility patterns of common nosocomial pathogens. Generally an effective infection control program can reduce nosocomial infection rates by one-third.

Prevention The basic principles of hand-washing between patient contacts, appropriate isolation of patients harboring communicable microorganisms, and application of epidemiologic methods to identify and correct potential sources of infection remain the cornerstones of prevention of nosocomial infections.

EMPLOYEE HEALTH SERVICE   Preventive medicine also applies to hospital personnel. The employee health service should maintain an employee surveillance program for communicable diseases such as tuberculosis and routinely offer indicated adult immunizations (see Chap. 84). Personnel of both sexes who are likely to come into contact with pregnant women should be tested for rubella antibodies, and, if susceptible, immunized before being allowed to work in areas where contact with pregnant women is likely. HBV immunization is strongly indicated for all personnel whose work involves frequent handling of blood or direct contact with patients. Annual influenza immunization should be encouraged both to reduce the risk of nosocomial influenza transmission to patients and to minimize winter absenteeism.

Hospital personnel with highly communicable infections should be removed from patient contact during the period of communicability. The dangers of pustular lesions are often underestimated and it is commonly forgotten that susceptible contacts may develop chickenpox following exposure to persons with herpes zoster.

Approximately 1 percent of physicians and dentists are asymptomatic carriers of HBV. Although several instances of transmission from health care workers to patients have been identified, the great majority of HBV-infected personnel do not appear to present a hazard to patients. They should be encouraged to pay particular attention to personal hygiene and hand-washing and should wear gloves during invasive procedures or contact with mucous membranes. If these precautions are observed, their patient-related activities need not be restricted. There is no evidence to suggest that HIV infected health personnel present an infectious risk to patients.

ADMISSION SCREENING   A patient scheduled for elective admission who has, or is thought to be incubating, an acute communicable disease should not be admitted until the period of communicability has passed. Screening on admission for communicable infections is particularly important for pediatric patients and for patients being admitted to oncology and transplant services where there may be a concentration of immunocompromised patients. Infections usually considered to be of minor importance, such as chickenpox or measles, can be devastating in such patients.

CONTAINMENT   Isolation procedures are time-consuming and expensive and can hinder essential patient care activities if applied too rigidly. They should be used only when necessary and for the shortest period consistent with good medical practice. Several alternative isolation systems are presently in common use: (1) A "category" system of seven unique isolation and precaution practices each designed to protect against one kind of disease transmission such as "respiratory," "enteric," or "wound and skin"; (2) a system listing each disease or pathogen separately along with specific individual isolation practices; (3) a system treating all body substances as potentially infectious (universal precautions).

Differences in patient population and hospital size and function may be important determinants of which system (or combination) is most appropriate for any given institution.

If preventive measures fail and a communicable infection develops in an inpatient, the following principles of containment should be observed:

1 Prevent further transmission of disease by the index case by either isolating the patient or, if the patient's condition allows, arranging for discharge from the hospital.
2 Identify all contacts of the index case and determine their susceptibility and degree of exposure.
3 If prophylactic measures are available, administer them appropriately to exposed susceptible individuals.
4 Design a plan to prevent the spread of the infectious agent from the exposed susceptibles to other patients and personnel. This plan must recognize the epidemiology of the communicable disease in question, the effectiveness and feasibility of various control measures, and the potential consequences of further disease transmission.

Methods commonly employed to limit the tertiary spread of communicable diseases by exposed susceptibles are (1) early discharge of patients when feasible, (2) arranging assignments of exposed personnel to avoid patient contact during the period of communicability, and (3) cohorting exposed susceptible patients and personnel together and treating them as an epidemiologic unit. Although cohorting is cumbersome, it remains a major measure for control of hospital outbreaks of chickenpox and epidemic diarrhea.

PROGNOSIS Most nosocomial infections are diseases of medical progress, and the ever-increasing orientation of modern medicine to technologically sophisticated procedures, both diagnostic and therapeutic, makes it likely that the risk of patients acquiring infections in the hospital will continue to increase. On the other hand, many of the factors that promote infections in the hospital have been identified, and measures for their control have been developed. Influencing hospital personnel to carry out these control measures, such as hand-washing, catheter care, and restraint in the use of antibiotics, remains a major challenge.

REFERENCES

BENNETT JV, BRACHMAN PS (eds): *Hospital Infections*. Boston, Little, Brown, 1985
CENTERS FOR DISEASE CONTROL: Recommendations for prevention of HIV transmission in health care settings. Morb Mort Week Rep Supp 2S, 1987
CHAMBERS HF: Methicillin resistant staphylococci. Clin Microbial Rev 1:173, 1988
MAKI DG et al: Prospective study of replacing administration set for intravenous therapy at 48- vs 72-hour intervals. JAMA 258:1777, 1987
WILLIAMS WW et al: Immunization policies and vaccine coverage among adults. Ann Intern Med 108:616, 1988
YU VL: Nosocomial legionellosis: Current epidemiological issues, in *Current Clinical Topics in Infectious Diseases*, JS Remington, MN Swartz (eds). New York, McGraw-Hill, 1986.

section 2 Prevention and therapy of infectious disease

---

84 IMMUNIZATION

ADAM FINN / STANLEY A. PLOTKIN

"Prevention is better than cure" is an old and familiar saying that remains valid for the modern physician, nowhere more so than in the field of infectious diseases. Figure 84-1 depicts the three main approaches to the prevention of infection. Of these, removal of the infecting microorganism from the general environment of the host and enhancement of the host immune response to invasion have had by far the greatest impact on disease. Active immunization works through both these strategies. A single vaccine, appropriately administered, can have effects on morbidity and mortality in a population which far outweigh the benefits a single doctor practicing curative medicine could hope to have in an entire lifetime. For example, it has been estimated that during the first 20 years since its licensure, measles vaccine has prevented 52 million cases, 5210 deaths, and 17,370 cases of mental retardation in the United States alone.

PRINCIPLES OF IMMUNIZATION

ACTIVE IMMUNIZATION Active immunization is highly effective because it works through the adaptive immune system, which is specific for an infecting agent and has long-lasting memory (see Chap. 13). Vaccination provides the stimulus to activate this system and arms the vaccinee with protection which may be lifelong. Important factors that affect the development of useful active vaccines include: (1) the number and stability of critical antigens involved in the virulence of microorganisms; (2) the role of local as opposed to systemic immunity in protection against infection by parenteral or orally administered vaccines; (3) the ability of vaccine antigens to stimulate a lasting host response that mimics natural immunity; (4) the safety of the vaccine; and (5) the existence of effective mechanisms

FIGURE 84-1 Ways of preventing infection. Examples of infectious diseases significantly influenced are shown in brackets; i.m.o., infecting microorganism.

ENVIRONMENT   HUMAN HOST

Invasion by | Microorganism

1

Remove i.m.o. From
General Environment
of Host:

1. Improve sanitation
and living conditions
(cholera, plague)

2. Active immunization
of human (or animal)
host (smallpox,
rabies)

2

Give Agent(s) to Kill or
Inhibit i.m.o. on
Contact with/Invasion
of Host:

1. Passive immunization
(hepatitis A)

2. Antimicrobial
chemoprophylaxis
(malaria)

3

Enhance Host Immune
Response

1. Active immunization
(measles, diphtheria)

2. Improve nutrition
and general health
(tuberculosis)

to ensure vaccine delivery and compliance with vaccination strategies in populations at risk.

Antigenic diversity has limited development of effective vaccines against rhinoviruses and is a major problem in the design of a vaccine against the human immunodeficiency virus (HIV). Other factors have limited development of highly effective vaccines against cholera and salmonellae (see Chaps. 107 and 122). Despite the challenges the dramatic successes of active vaccines against smallpox, polio, measles, mumps, rubella, pertussis, diphtheria, tetanus, and, most recently, against hepatitis B virus testify to the value and utility of this approach in the prevention of disease worldwide.

HERD IMMUNITY AND VACCINATION RATES Active immunization has two points of impact on the prevention of disease (see Fig. 84-1). First, it may provide the individual vaccinee with immune protection, and, second, it may reduce the circulation of the infecting agent in the population, thereby protecting unvaccinated individuals as well. This phenomenon is known as *herd immunity* and is of relevance in many immunization programs directed against infections that are transferred from person to person. Once adequate rates of vaccination are achieved, herd immunity will operate and the incidence of the disease will fall rapidly. Highly contagious infections such as measles require higher vaccination rates for effective herd immunity. If vaccination rates fall and the pathogen is still circulating, the incidence of new infections will rise as herd immunity is lost. For example, large outbreaks of pertussis occurred in the mid-1970s in the United Kingdom following a dramatic fall in vaccination rates after reports of possible adverse neurologic effects were publicized in the mass media. The very success of a vaccine mitigates against its continued use because, as the memory of the specific infection fades within the population, so does the will to ensure adequate immunization. All this underlines the need for good education of physicians, other health professionals, and the public about the use and continuing benefits of immunization.

IMMUNIZATION STRATEGIES Vaccine efficacy is determined by its ability to induce a detectable immune response, the documentation of substantially reduced or abolished infection rates under experimental and natural conditions, the production of lasting immunity, proper application of the vaccine to key target populations, and acceptance of vaccination by these populations and their health care providers.

Extensive development and testing must be carried out with documentation of safety and efficacy in well-designed field trials before vaccines are licensed for routine use. When effective vaccines are developed against a particular disease, there are many factors that influence the strategy chosen for subsequent use. A simplified scheme is depicted in Fig. 84-2. The epidemiologic characteristics of the disease will be the primary influence on all the elements of strategy. For example, the severity and widespread endemicity of smallpox, together with its lack of carrier state and lack of nonhuman reservoir, enabled a worldwide strategy to be adopted which led to its complete elimination.

Target population In some cases universal immunization of the population (usually as children) will be appropriate (e.g., for diphtheria-pertussis-tetanus and polio), whereas in others only selected high-risk groups should be vaccinated (e.g., for hepatitis B, influenza). With some vaccines, the target group for vaccination may not be the group which the program is principally designed to protect. Rubella vaccination of all children and females of child-bearing age aims to

Strategy:

Target Population:
Universal/high risk groups

Vaccine and Regimen:
Choice of vaccine if > 1 available
Dose, interval, boosters, etc.

Factors Influencing Strategy:

Disease Epidemiology:
1. End-epidemic incidence prevalence
2. Mode of transmission
3. Associated morbidity/mortality
4. Infectious reservoirs (zoonotic/environmental)
5. Existence of asymptomatic carrier state
6. Antigenic heterogeneity and change
7. Groups at high risk of infection or severe illness
8. Need for immune maturation for adequate vaccine response
9. Other pathogens interfering with vaccine response

Vaccine Characteristics:
1. Size and duration of vaccine-induced immune response and protection
2. Vaccine adverse effects

Factors Affecting Vaccine Delivery:
1. Funds available and prioritization of spending
2. Cost of vaccine and administration to patient
3. Health services structure and ways to reach the target population
4. Surveillance of vaccine quality and disease epidemiology
5. Vaccine stability and need for special handling
6. Acceptibility and ease of administration

Strategy:

Age at Immunization

Delivery System:
eg. Continuous program
Seasonal use
Epidemic control
Mass campaigns

FIGURE 84-2   Genesis of an immunization strategy.

prevent infection of the fetus by reducing the likelihood of primary infection in women during pregnancy.

Vaccine and regimen   The choice of vaccine and appropriate dosage regimen can vary with the disease, specific target populations, health systems, and even climates. For example, debate continues concerning the relative efficacies of live and inactivated polio vaccines in both temperate and tropical climates.

Age at immunization   Regional differences in infection rates and severity may influence the age at which vaccine is routinely administered. Measles vaccine is administered to children at 15 months of age in the United States; in developing countries it is often given to younger infants, aged 6 to 9 months, since measles infection and mortality rates in infants are high. The aim of this approach is to prevent infection at an earlier age even though seroconversion rates may be somewhat lower because of the persistence of maternal antibody.

Delivery system   The delivery system can vary with different diseases, vaccine efficacy, and local practical issues. In countries where health service facilities are not available for a continuing policy of universal vaccination of infants against polio, mass campaigns are often used to vaccinate large numbers in a single day.

SURVEILLANCE AND RECORDS   Vaccine programs require continuous and rigorous monitoring. First, the quality and purity of vaccine must be subject to close surveillance in order to avoid the occurrence of mishaps such as the notorious "Cutter incident" in 1955 in which 192 vaccinees and their contacts developed paralytic polio as a result of incomplete inactivation of live virus in the Salk-type vaccine. Second, the balance of risks and benefits must be constantly reevaluated in the context of vaccine efficacy and risks of vaccination and the current epidemiology of the disease. In response

to data from the United States demonstrating more effective prevention of the congenital rubella syndrome, the strategy of rubella vaccination in the United Kingdom was changed in 1988 from one of selective vaccination of prepubertal females to include universal vaccination of children at 15 months of age. Accurate records of immunizations should be kept by both physicians and vaccinees; such records are often required for travel from one country to another and, in the United States, for entry into school.

LIVE AND "KILLED" VACCINES   Live vaccines utilize an attenuated strain of the original pathogen which can replicate and induce an immune response in the host but fails to cause significant illness. These vaccines mimic true infection and tend to induce long-lasting immunity. They may also cause significant illness in a small minority of vaccinees either because of reversion to virulence during replication in the host or because of immune defects in the host. Other intercurrent infection may interfere with live vaccines and prevent an adequate response. "Killed" vaccines, really a misnomer as not all of this group are prepared from inactivated organisms, challenge the vaccinee's immune system with antigens common to the original pathogen that do not replicate. In general effective immune responses require relatively large vaccine dosages and protection may be less persistent, but there is no risk of serious vaccine-induced infection. The term "subunit" vaccines refers to vaccines that are constructed of key antigenic components of microorganisms essential for infection and/or virulence.

HYPERSENSITIVITY   Vaccines occasionally induce allergic reactions ranging from mild to anaphylactic responses that contraindicate further administration of that vaccine. Sometimes these responses are due to materials other than the vaccine itself. For example, measles vaccine contains small quantities of neomycin and traces of protein from the chick fibroblasts in which the virus is propagated. Individuals who have had anaphylaxis following neomycin should not be given the vaccine, and those who have had anaphylactic reactions to eggs should be vaccinated with special precautions. A vague history of allergic symptoms is inadequate grounds for denying an individual the benefit of immunization, and specific recommendations for each vaccine should always be consulted.

TABLE 84-1   Recommended schedule for active immunization of healthy infants and children in the United States

Recommended age	Immunization(s)	Comments
2 Months	DTP,[1] OPV[2]	Can be initiated as early as 2 weeks of age in areas of high endemicity or during epidemics.
4 Months	DTP, OPV	2-month interval desired for OPV to avoid interference from previous dose.
6 Months	DTP	A 3d dose of OPV is not indicated in the US, but is desirable in geographic areas where polio is endemic.
15 Months	Measles, mumps, rubella (MMR)[3]	MMR preferred to individual vaccines.
18 Months	DTP,[4,5] OPV[6] PRP-D[7]	
4–6 Years	DTP,[8] OPV	At or before school entry.
12 Years	MMR or measles	At entrance to middle school. However, may be given instead at entry to kindergarten.
14–16 Years	Td[9]	Repeat every 10 years throughout life.

[1] DTP, diphtheria and tetanus toxoids with pertussis vaccine. Given IM.
[2] OPV, oral poliovirus vaccine containing attenuated poliovirus types 1, 2, and 3.
[3] MMR, live measles, mumps, and rubella viruses in a combined vaccine. Given SC.
[4] Should be given 6 to 12 months after the third dose.
[5] May be given simultaneously with MMR at 15 months of age.
[6] May be given simultaneously with MMR at 15 months of age or at any time between 12 and 24 months of age.
[7] PRP-D, *Haemophilus* b diphtheria toxoid conjugate vaccine. Given IM.
[8] Up to the seventh birthday.
[9] Td, adult tetanus toxoid (full dose) and diphtheria toxoid (reduced dose) for adult use. Given IM.
SOURCE: American Academy of Pediatrics, *Report of the Committee on Infectious Diseases*, 1988.

IMMUNIZATION PROGRAMS

VACCINATION OF CHILDREN   Most general immunization programs have been directed primarily at the pediatric population. In the United States, it is currently recommended that all children receive vaccines against eight common diseases (Table 84-1). The practice of vaccination of children is well-established, generally well-accepted by pediatricians and the public, and is reinforced by regulations requiring records of immunization for school entry. Consequently immunization rates in many areas are high. Special indications for extra vaccines are similar to those in adults (Tables 84-3 and 84-4). Infants born to hepatitis B surface-antigen-positive mothers should be immunized with both hepatitis B immune globulin (one dose) and hepatitis B vaccine (three doses).

VACCINATION OF ADULTS   In contrast to pediatric practice, immunization of adults is often neglected. It lacks established tradition, and legal requirements are not broad, so that despite the availability of a large number of effective vaccines, utilization rates are often low.

There are three target groups for adult immunization. First, all normal individuals should receive vaccines as part of universal programs. Some require additional vaccines because the lack of previous immunization or infection renders them susceptible. Visitors, students, immigrants, and refugees from countries with poor general immunization programs are particularly likely to be unimmunized, so such individuals should make vaccination a high priority. Table 84-2 lists vaccines documented to be effective in producing an immune response and reducing disease in normal adults and indicates appropriate target groups.

Second, certain conditions or occupations, such as health care work, can place normal adults at significant risk of vaccine-preventable infection and illness. Table 84-3 lists vaccines that fall into this category. In some cases the objective is to prevent illness of key personnel likely to have high exposure rates to influenza, hepatitis B, and rabies. In others, the vaccines are to be employed in outbreaks of disease (e.g., meningococcal vaccine) or immediately upon potential exposure to a lethal infectious agent (e.g., postexposure prophylaxis for rabies). Because of the relatively low frequency of tuberculosis, the lack of proven efficacy in large population studies in the country, and the availability of effective prophylaxis (isoniazid),

---

TABLE 84-2   Vaccines for active immunization of normal civilian adults in the United States

Vaccine	Schedule and target group	Delivery	Comments
Combined diphtheria and tetanus toxoids (Td)	Each 10 years. All adults (e.g., age 25, 35, 45, etc.). Also, after potentially tetanus-contaminated wound if no immunization in previous 5 years. Primary course: 3 doses at 0, 1–2, 6–12 months.	Primary care offices and clinical emergency rooms.	Td has reduced dose of diphtheria toxin relative to combined vaccine used in primary immunization of children. Td should always be used in preference to tetanus toxoid alone. Previously unimmunized adults seen at time of injury should also receive passive immunization.
Inactivated influenza vaccine for current year	Yearly in autumn. All adults, from age 65 (see also Tables 84-3 and 84-4).	Hospital wards (at discharge). Hospital clinics. Primary care offices and clinics. Residential homes for elderly.	Both this vaccine and 23-valent pneumococcal vaccine can be given simultaneously at separate sites.
23-Valent pneumococcal vaccine	One dose. All adults at age 65 (or over). See also Table 84-4.	See above.	See above.
Live measles vaccine	One dose. All adults (particularly males) without history of previous infection or immunization born after 1956.	College clinics. Primary care offices and clinics.	Serologic testing for immunity is not considered necessary as previous infection or immunization does not contraindicate revaccination. A combined measles-mumps vaccine is available
Live mumps vaccine	One dose. All adults (particularly males) without history of previous infection or immunization.	See above.	See above.
Live rubella vaccine	One dose. All females shown to be seronegative (e.g., on antenatal or hospital employee screening).	Postnatal wards, obstetric and gynecologic clinics. Primary care.	Immunization of the many women of childbearing age who are seronegative is needed so long as rubella continues to circulate in the community.

TABLE 84-3 Vaccines for additional active immunization of normal individuals with high-risk circumstances in the United States

Vaccine	Schedule/target group	Notes
Bacille Calmette-Guérin (BCG) (against tuberculosis)	One dose. 1. Tuberculin-negative individuals in populations and groups with high frequency of TB transmission and inadequate health provision for normal methods of case detection and isoniazid prophylaxis (e.g., ghettos, alcoholics, and migrants). 2. Tuberculin-negative health care personnel caring for such populations.	BCG should not be given to immunodeficient individuals (e.g., with HIV infection).
Inactivated influenza vaccine for current year	Yearly, in fall. IM (preferred) or SC. 1. Health care personnel caring for high-risk patients (see Table 84-4). 2. Residents of institutions housing patients with chronic medical conditions (see also Tables 84-2 and 84-4).	Acute febrile illness is a contraindication. Most individuals with egg allergy can be immunized with special precautions.
Hepatitis B vaccine	3 Doses at 0, 1, and 6 months. IM in deltoid muscle. Susceptible or probably susceptible individuals in the following groups: 1. Health care personnel (ideally in training) who will be at risk of exposure to blood, blood products, and needles. 2. Household and sexual contacts of known hepatitis B carriers. 3. Clients and staff of institutions for the mentally handicapped. 4. Hemodialysis patients and recipients of clotting factor concentrates. 5. Homosexual men and heterosexual persons with multiple sexual partners. 6. Users of illicit injectable drugs. 7. Prison inmates. 8. Groups with highly endemic disease (e.g., Alaskan Eskimos, Pacific Islanders, immigrants from east Asia and sub-Saharan Africa). 9. Infants born to hepatitis B surface-antigen-positive mothers (see Table 84-5).	Pregnancy is not a contraindication for women at risk of contracting hepatitis B.
Rabies vaccine [human diploid cell vaccine (HDCV) or other licensed vaccine]	1. Preexposure prophylaxis: 3 doses at 0, 7, and 28 days IM (boosters may be necessary). Individuals at high risk of exposure (e.g., veterinarians, laboratory workers). 2. Postexposure prophylaxis: (see Table 84-5).	
Inactivated polio vaccine (enhanced potency)	3 Doses at 0, 1–2, and 6–12 months, SC. Unimmunized adults likely to be exposed to wild poliovirus (health care workers). For immediate risk of exposure [e.g., contact with known polio case, household contact of child receiving oral polio vaccine (OPV)] unimmunized adults should receive OPV 4 doses at 0, 1–2, 3–4, 9–16 months (see also Table 84-4). Previously partially immunized adults should complete course of vaccine.	Routine immunization against polio of adults resident in United States is not recommended.
Meningococcal polysaccharide vaccine	Bivalent (groups A, C) or quadrivalent (gps. A, C, Y, W135) vaccine. One dose, SC. 1. Household contact of patient with type A, C, Y, or W135 meningococcal infection. 2. Local control of outbreak of type A, C, Y, or W135 meningococcal disease (see also Table 84-4).	Type B infection against which there is no vaccine is most common. Contacts are given rifampin also.

BCG (bacille Calmette-Guérin) is not routinely employed in the United States.

Third, because of underlying medical conditions some individuals are likely to develop particularly severe illness from infections which may be prevented by appropriate vaccination. Table 84-4 lists indications for use of influenza, pneumococcal, meningococcal, and polio vaccines in different patient groups in this category.

IMMUNE DEFICIENCY Patients with reduced immunity present a particular problem. On the one hand, they are particularly at risk for severe infections, but on the other, they are often unable to mount a good immune response. Furthermore, live-virus vaccines are as a rule contraindicated, so these patients are usually given less immunogenic toxoids and other inactivated vaccines. When patients will be medically immunosuppressed, for example, as part of cancer chemotherapy or following splenectomy, appropriate vaccination should, whenever possible, be undertaken before initiation of treatment. If this is not feasible, vaccination should be delayed for at least a month after chemotherapy has been completed to allow for immune recovery.

Persons infected with HIV are a group for whom vaccination recommendations are under constant review (see Chap. 264). In the United States it is recommended that symptomatic HIV infection contraindicate the use of some live vaccines [e.g., oral polio vaccine (OPV) and BCG]. Asymptomatic HIV-seropositive individuals with preserved CD4-positive lymphocyte numbers can be given live vaccines except BCG, unless they have household contacts with

TABLE 84-4 Vaccines for additional active immunization of individuals who have an inherently increased risk of severe vaccine-preventable infections

Vaccine	Schedule and target group	Notes
Inactivated influenza vaccine for current year	Yearly, in autumn (children should only be given "split" vaccine). Individuals with chronic cardiovascular, pulmonary, renal, and metabolic (e.g., diabetes mellitus) diseases, severe anemia, and immune deficiency or suppression (including symptomatic HIV infection). See also Tables 84-2 and 84-3.	Acute febrile illness is a contraindication. Most individuals with egg allergy can be immunized with special precautions.
23-Valent pneumococcal vaccine	One dose. Individuals with chronic cardiovascular, pulmonary disease, cirrhosis, renal failure, alcoholism, anatomic or functional asplenia (including sickle cell anemia), Hodgkin's lymphoma, myeloma, cerebrospinal fluid leaks, and immune deficiency or suppression (including symptomatic HIV infection). See Table 84-2.	
Quadrivalent meningococcal vaccine (groups A, C, Y, W135)	One dose. Individuals with anatomic or functional asplenia (including sickle cell anemia). Individuals with terminal complement component defects. See also Table 84-3.	
Inactivated polio vaccine (IPV) (enhanced potency)	3 Doses at 0, 1–2, and 6–12 months. Individuals with immune deficiency or suppression and their household contacts should be given IPV, not oral polio vaccine. See also Table 84-3.	Although immune response may be reduced, some protection may be achieved.

symptomatic HIV infection, in which case inactivated polio vaccine should be used instead of OPV. Measles vaccine, either monovalent or as measles, mumps, and rubella combined vaccine, is advocated for all HIV-infected children because of reports of severe or fatal natural measles in this group and no reports of vaccine complications. Pneumococcal vaccine, preferably administered at a time before depression of CD4-positive lymphocytes occurs, is also recommended.

PREGNANCY In general, the administration of vaccines, like drugs, should be avoided in pregnancy or delayed until the second or third trimester. The theoretical risks include teratogenic effects of vaccines on the fetus and, in the case of live vaccines, of congenital infection. However, diphtheria and tetanus toxoids are considered to be safe, and where there is genuine, substantial, and unavoidable risk of exposure, a nonimmune pregnant woman may be given live oral polio and yellow fever vaccines. Hepatitis B vaccine may also be given to susceptible pregnant women who are at high risk because the risk of infection to the infant outweighs theoretical concerns about the vaccine. Rubella vaccine is of special interest in this context because of the congenital rubella syndrome (CRS). Although the vaccine is contraindicated in pregnancy and transplacental infection of the fetus with the vaccine virus has been observed, CRS has not been reported in infants born to women inadvertently vaccinated in pregnancy. Therefore, such vaccination is not a priori an indication for abortion. In the case of influenza, the risk of severe disease, particularly in the third trimester, is greater than the theoretical risk to the fetus of inactivated vaccine.

PASSIVE IMMUNIZATION Passive immunization involves providing exogenous antibody in an attempt to prevent or to attenuate an anticipated infection. Although this method lacks many of the advantages of active immunization and protection may be short-lived, it has the advantage that the effect is immediate. This is important in the use of antibody preparations in prophylaxis against tetanus and rabies and in the protection of contacts with measles, varicella, and hepatitis A and B (see Table 84-5). Passive immunization is also used to protect travelers against hepatitis A, where no vaccine is yet commercially available. Pooled human serum immune globulins contain a wide variety of IgG antibodies against different agents. The increasing availability of intravenous preparations which can be safely administered in high dosages has broadened the use of this treatment. Individuals with congenital deficiency of immunoglobulins treated with regular infusions of immune globulin have a reduced number of infections due to a wide variety of pathogens (see Chap. 263). There is also limited evidence to suggest that similar therapy reduces the frequency of serious infections in children with symptomatic HIV infection (see Chap. 264). Studies are being conducted to evaluate intravenous gamma globulin treatment in other individuals at high risk for sepsis (e.g., burn and intensive care patients).

Passive immunization may interfere with immune responses to some antigens, as with measles vaccine. However, combined active and passive immunization is used effectively against both rabies and hepatitis B.

IMMUNIZATION OF TRAVELERS The presentation of an individual for immunization advice prior to travel is an opportunity to ensure that routine vaccinations have been performed (Table 84-2). Often the risks of measles and diphtheria will be much greater outside the United States, in underdeveloped countries. The need for supplementary protection will vary not only with the travel destinations but also with the activities planned. For example, immunization against hepatitis B would routinely be undertaken only if the individual were susceptible and expected to have prolonged close contact with the local population in an area of endemic infection (e.g., health care workers). Finally, many countries have regulations governing the immunization status of visitors. Table 84-6 lists some of the immunizations commonly advised for use in travelers. As specific recommendations vary from one area to another and are subject to change, up-to-date information can be obtained in the United States

---

TABLE 84-5　Preparations currently recommended for passive immunization of exposed or infected patients

Disease	Preparation of choice	Target group and schedule	Comment
POSTEXPOSURE PROPHYLAXIS OF CONTACTS			
Hepatitis A	Immune globulin (human) (IG)	Contacts in day care centers, households, and custodial institutions. 0.02 mL/kg IM.	See Table 84-6 for preexposure prophylaxis for foreign travel.
Hepatitis B	Hepatitis B immune globulin (HBIG)	1. Infants of hepatitis B surface antigen positive mothers. 0.5 mL IM. 2. Possible percutaneous or sexual contact with hepatitis B. 0.06 mL/kg IM.	HBIG is usually given with appropriate doses of hepatitis B vaccine (see Table 84-3).
Varicella	Varicella-zoster immune globulin (VZIG)	1. Exposed infants and children at high risk of severe infection. 2. Exposed susceptible adults. 125 units (1 vial)/10 kg IM (minimum 125, maximum 625).	
Tetanus	Tetanus immune globulin (TIG)	Patients with wounds (other than clean minor wounds) without a clear history of full, up-to-date tetanus immunization 500–3000 units IM, part of dose infiltrated around wound.	Tetanus with diphtheria toxoids (Td) normally given as well.
Rabies	Human rabies immune globulin (HRIG)	Individuals thought to have had significant exposure to a rabid or potentially rabid animal. Patients known to be immune and/or fully immunized against rabies do not require HBIG but only 2 doses of rabies vaccine on days 0 and 3 (see Table 84-3). 20 IU/kg, half infiltrated around wound, half IM.	Give early and follow with a 5-dose course of rabies vaccine on days 0, 3, 7, 14, and 28.
Measles	Immune globulin (human) (IG)	Susceptible household and close contacts, within 6 days of exposure, particularly immunosuppressed individuals (including those with HIV infection) and infants. 0.25 mL/kg IM.	Routine measles vaccination should be postponed until 3 months after IG administration.
Rubella	Immune globulin (human) (IG)	Pregnant women exposed in early pregnancy, where termination is not an option. 0.55 mL/kg IM.	Passive immunization does not ensure protection of the fetus.
TREATMENT OF ESTABLISHED DISEASE			
Botulism	Equine trivalent antitoxin*	Patients with food-borne or wound botulism.	Not used to treat infant botulism.
Diphtheria	Equine diphtheria antitoxin*	Patients with clinical diagnosis of diphtheria.	Probably of no value in cutaneous diphtheria.
Tetanus	Tetanus immune globulin (TIG)	Patients with clinical diagnosis of tetanus.	

* Tests for sensitivity and if necessary desensitization should be undertaken for these products.

TABLE 84-6 Immunizations and chemoprophylaxis commonly required by travelers abroad in addition to routine requirements*

Disease	Schedule	Notes
ACTIVE IMMUNIZATION		
Polio	Where time allows, previously unimmunized adults should receive inactivated polio vaccine (regimen as in Table 84-3). For rapid immunization: killed polio vaccine, 2 doses at least 4 weeks apart. For immediate protection, oral polio vaccine should be given.	If a pregnant woman requires rapid protection against polio, because of significant risk of exposure, oral polio vaccine may be given.
Yellow fever	Single dose of live-virus vaccine must be administered at registered vaccination center, which will issue certificate of vaccination, which may be required for travel in certain areas.	Certificate is valid for 10 years. Vaccination is contraindicated in immune-suppressed persons. Pregnant women and infants less than 6 months old should not be vaccinated unless risk of exposure is unavoidable.
Typhoid	Killed whole-cell vaccine may be used to protect travelers to areas where typhoid is endemic.	These vaccines have relatively high rates of local and systemic adverse effects.
Cholera	Vaccination is not recommended unless it is a requirement for entry into the country of destination.	Infection is more effectively prevented by taking precautions in handling food and drink.
Japanese B encephalitis	Killed-virus vaccine; recommended for travelers to rural areas of the Far East, including China and Korea.	Routinely given to children in endemic areas.
PASSIVE IMMUNIZATION		
Hepatitis A	Up to 0.06 mL/kg immune serum globulin is given by IM injection, affording protection against hepatitis A (HAV) infection for 3–4 months.	Individuals who are seropositive for anti-HAV need not be immunized.
CHEMOPROPHYLAXIS		
Malaria	Chemoprophylaxis should be started prior to departure and continued after return. Regimens change with changing plasmodial resistance.	Chemoprophylaxis does not provide absolute protection.

* Indications and further details should be sought from *Health Information for International Travel*.

from the latest edition of the Centers for Disease Control booklet entitled *Health Information for International Travel*. For recommendations regarding chemoprophylaxis against malaria see Chap. 159.

ASSESSMENT OF IMMUNIZATION PROGRAMS Vaccine efficacy The ultimate test of a vaccine is in its ability to reduce or prevent widespread disease. The dramatic fall in the reported cases of the seven diseases that have been the object of sustained immunization programs in the United States is shown in Table 84-7. Information of this type is much more important than specific measurements of an immune response in vaccinated subjects and testifies to effective application of highly immunogenic vaccines to large populations. The latter involves a well-coordinated and -supported public and private health effort.

Cost-benefit The rising cost of health care in wealthy nations and the limited resources available in many poorer countries mandate the rigorous assessment of cost-benefit for all medical interventions (see Chap. 3). In all analyses to date effective immunization programs have been shown to be less costly than most other preventive health strategies and far less expensive than the cost of treating established disease.

TABLE 84-7 Comparison of maximum and current morbidity of vaccine-preventable diseases

Disease	Maximum cases (year)	1986	% Change
Diphtheria	206,939 (1921)	0	100.00
Measles	894,134 (1941)	6282	99.30
Mumps*	152,209 (1968)	7790	94.88
Pertussis	265,269 (1934)	4195	98.42
Polio (paralytic)	21,269 (1952)	3	99.99
Rubella†	57,686 (1969)	551	99.05
Congenital rubella syndrome	20,000 (1964–5)	14	99.93
Tetanus‡	608 (1948)	64	89.35

* First reportable in 1968.
† First reportable in 1966.
‡ First reportable in 1947.
SOURCE: AR Hinman, in Plotkin and Mortimer.

Legal considerations Successful vaccination programs can militate against their own continued use. This phenomenon is compounded by the growing number of lawsuits filed on behalf of individuals claiming compensation for alleged vaccine-induced damage. Because pediatric vaccination is a legal requirement, persons or the families of persons thought to have been damaged by a vaccine will often consider that they are entitled to compensation, particularly if they were not informed of the inherent risks involved. No vaccines are perfect, although serious adverse effects are extremely rare. Furthermore, it is often impossible to define whether there is a causal connection between a coincidental acute illness and immunization. The costs and uncertainties that accompany such legal proceedings act as disincentives to health professionals to administer vaccines and to pharmaceutical firms to manufacture them. Some programs of immunization, most notably that against pertussis, are under threat as a result, with possibly disastrous consequences. The best solution to this problem may prove to be the institution of an effective no-fault compensation scheme for vaccine-related injury. Several European countries have used such programs successfully, and the United States has recently instituted one.

LICENSED VACCINES IN CURRENT ROUTINE USE

DIPHTHERIA AND TETANUS TOXOIDS These are two of the most successful vaccines ever made. Both are based on the use of an inactivated toxin to produce antitoxin antibodies. The vaccines are protective because the diseases are mediated through the action of extracellular toxins, which are neutralized by the antitoxin.

PERTUSSIS Widespread use of the conventional whole cell pertussis vaccine has greatly reduced the frequency of the infection. Mono- and combined-component acellular pertussis vaccines were developed and used initially in Japan in children over 2 years of age. Field trials of such vaccines in younger infants in Scandinavia and the United States are in progress and suggest that they may be efficacious and have fewer side effects.

POLIO Two types of vaccine are available. One is a live attenuated vaccine administered orally, the other is a formalin-inactivated vaccine administered parenterally. Both are mixtures of the three poliovirus serotypes. While both are effective in individual vaccinees, their relative efficacy in different populations may vary with the local epidemiology of polio. The oral vaccine is preferred for routine use in the United States. The antigenicity of the inactivated vaccine has been enhanced, and this more potent product may eventually receive greater use in the United States.

MEASLES Use of the live attenuated vaccine has brought measles to a low ebb in the United States, but earlier hopes of eradicating the disease have not been borne out. There have been persistent epidemics in unvaccinated infants in poor areas of large cities, and occasional outbreaks in older vaccinated children. Proposed new strategies include strenuous efforts to vaccinate young infants whenever possible, and mass revaccination of students in schools where an outbreak occurs without attempting to confirm old records or to identify seronegative individuals. Live attenuated measles vaccine should be given to previous recipients of the older inactivated vaccine to prevent attacks of atypically presenting measles (see Chap. 141).

MUMPS Epidemic mumps is now virtually gone from the United States through immunization with mumps vaccine, although not every state mandates its use.

RUBELLA Congenital rubella syndrome is now rare, and the high immunity due to vaccination may make eradication of the virus from the United States a possibility.

HAEMOPHILUS TYPE B A particular problem of polysaccharide vaccines, which contain the polymers that constitute the bacterial cell wall, is their poor immunogenicity in children under 2 years. Since much of the most serious illness caused by *Haemophilus influenzae* type b occurs in this age group, a newly licensed vaccine contains the polysaccharide bound to diphtheria toxoid, a protein antigen. This T-cell-dependent antigen enhances immunogenicity and gives added protection to younger children (see Chap. 115).

HEPATITIS B The licensure of recombinant hepatitis B vaccine made in yeast has sharply diminished fears concerning the widespread use of this vaccine for high-risk populations, including medical personnel.

PNEUMOCOCCUS This vaccine has recently been improved to contain 23 capsular serotypes which together cause over 90 percent of bacteremic pneumococcal infections in children and adults. However, this polysaccharide vaccine is poorly immunogenic in infants and some other high-risk groups. Debate persists regarding its efficacy in adult populations at high risk of developing serious pneumococcal infections (e.g., splenectomized and elderly patients). It is generally well-tolerated, and there are few contraindications to its use (see Chap. 99).

INFLUENZA This is a trivalent vaccine, containing two prevalent type A strains with different hemagglutinins, and a type B strain. Each autumn the composition of the vaccine is changed to reflect a prediction of the important strains of the coming winter's epidemic.

NEW DEVELOPMENTS Much work in vaccine development is in progress. Attempts are being made both to improve the quality of vaccines already in use and to develop vaccines against other infectious diseases not hitherto preventable by immunization. In addition, a number of newly developed molecular genetic techniques may enhance vaccine research.

Rabies The main impediment to the use of the highly effective human diploid cell vaccine against rabies in the poorer countries of the world where rabies is common is its high cost. A number of vaccines are becoming available which use animal cell lines to propagate the virus. These may prove to be substantially cheaper.

Adenovirus Live attenuated adenovirus vaccines have been used extensively in military recruits and have been effective in preventing outbreaks of acute respiratory diseases (see Chap. 140). They have not been used in civilians.

Cytomegalovirus (CMV) Congenital CMV infection of the fetus and disseminated CMV infection in transplant recipients are important causes of morbidity and mortality. Both live attenuated and subunit CMV vaccines are under development and may contribute to prevention of these infections (see Chap. 138).

Rotavirus Multiple serotype viruses of this group are a major cause of infantile gastroenteritis throughout the world. A number of live vaccines have been developed from viruses of animal origin. Further work may include genetic manipulation of human rotaviruses to produce a safe and immunogenic multivalent vaccine (see Chap. 145).

Varicella A live attenuated varicella vaccine was developed in Japan in 1974. It has been shown to be safe and immunogenic in several field trials conducted in normal children or children with malignancies. It has been licensed in Japan and Europe, and it may be licensed either for restricted or general use in the United States in the near future (see Chap. 136).

Hepatitis A Several vaccines against hepatitis A are under development. In areas where the disease is prevalent, the induction of lasting immunity by active immunization, perhaps as part of the routine childhood immunization program, would be an important step forward.

Measles The availability of the Edmonston-Zagreb strain of measles virus that is more immunogenic in 7- to 9-month-old children holds promise for future use in areas of the world with high endemic rates in young children.

REFERENCES

AMERICAN ACADEMY OF PEDIATRICS: Report of the Committee of Infectious Diseases 1986 ("Red Book"), 20th ed., 1986

BLOCH AB et al: The health impact of measles vaccination in the United States. Pediatrics 76:524, 1985

CENTERS FOR DISEASE CONTROL: Rubella vaccination during pregnancy-United States 1971–1986. Morb Mort Week Rep 36:457, 1987

———: *Health Information for International Travel.* Atlanta, GA, Centers for Disease Control, United States Department of Health and Human Services, Public Health Service (published annually)

Communicable Disease Statistics 1986: England and Wales. Her Majesty's Stationery Office, ser MB2, no 13, 1986

FENNER F et al: Smallpox and its eradication. Geneva, World Health Organization, 1988

Guide for Adult Immunization. Philadelphia, American College of Physicians, 1985

HERMAN JJ et al: Allergic reactions to measles (rubeola) vaccine in patients hypersensitive to egg protein. Pediatrics 102:196, 1983

——— et al: Live-inactivated poliovirus vaccine. Pediatr Infect Dis J 6:881, 1987

PLOTKIN SA, MORTIMER EA: *Vaccines.* Philadelphia, Saunders, 1988

WALKER D et al: Measles, mumps, and rubella: The need for a change in immunization policy. Br Med J 292:1501, 1986

WORLD HEALTH ORGANIZATION EXPANDED PROGRAMME ON IMMUNIZATION: Conclusions and recommendations of the Global Advisory Group. Wkly Epidemiol Rec 60:13, 1985

85 THERAPY AND PROPHYLAXIS OF BACTERIAL INFECTIONS

HAROLD C. NEU

INTRODUCTION Changes in the host, the appearance of new pathogens, and the resistance of new and old pathogens to previously available antimicrobial agents explain the large number of antimicrobial agents. Changes in the host include prolonged survival of critically ill patients due to use of cancer chemotherapy, transplantation, and prosthetic devices. The problem of resistance has been severe due to the worldwide dissemination of plasmids that convey resistance to multiple antimicrobial agents. Considerations of efficacy and toxicity have a major impact on the selection of antimicrobial agents, but cost is increasingly important. This chapter deals with general observations on antimicrobial therapy, and a description of most antibacterial agents. Recommendations for therapy of infections are made in the chapters dealing with individual diseases. Tables 85-1 and 85-2 summarize important information concerning the drugs discussed in this chapter.

FACTORS INFLUENCING SELECTION OF ANTIMICROBIALS Several factors bear directly on the selection of an antimicrobial agent. Knowledge of the infecting microorganism may not be available

TABLE 85-1 Serum and body fluid levels after oral administration of various antibiotics

| Drug | Unit dose* (oral) | Average peak level, μg/mL | | | | Half-life, h | | Dose adjustment renal failure |
		Blood†	Urine‡	Bile§	CSF¶	$C_{cl} > 80$ mL	$C_{cl} < 10$ mL	
Amoxicillin	0.5 g	10	1000	10	NA	1	6	Minor
Ampicillin	0.25 g	1.5	50	5	NA	1	6	Minor
Cefaclor	0.5 g	15	200	5	NA	1	2	No
Cephalexin	0.25 g	8	500	3	NA	1	8–20	Major
Cephradine	0.25 g	8	500	5	NA	1	8	Major
Chloramphenicol	1 g	13	100	3	6	2	5	Minor
Ciprofloxacin	0.75 g	4	300	8	1	3.5	5–10	Major
Clindamycin	0.15 g	2	30	20	NA	2	6–10	Minor
Cloxacillin	0.5 g	8	200	—	NA	1	4	Minor
Dicloxacillin	0.5 g	15	200	—	NA	1	2	Minor
Doxycycline	100 mg	2.5	100	15	NA	15–20	15–20	No
Erythromycin estolate	0.25 g	1.4	200	800	NA	1.5–2	4–6	No
Indanyl carbenicillin	1 g	15	600	NA	NA	1–2	15	Major
Metronidazole	0.25 g	5	50	5	2	8	8	Minor
Minocycline	100 mg	2.5	100	15	NA	15	15–25	Minor
Norfloxacin	500 mg	4	200	2	NA	3	8–20	Major
Ofloxacin	400 mg	6	500	5	NA	6	10–20	Major
Penicillin V	0.25 g	2	300	4	NA	1	2	No
Rifampin	8 mg/kg	10	50	100	0.5	1.5–5	1.5–5	No
Sulfadiazine	1.0 g	25	100	25	15	10	12–25	Major
Tetracycline	0.25 g	2.2	100	15	NA	6–8	30–50	Major
TMP/SMX	0.16 g TMP + 0.8 g SMX	1 + 30	10 + 100	3 + 30	0.5 + 15	10	25	Major

* Doses listed are the lowest doses that would normally be employed for adults or children over 32 kg with normal renal function in the treatment of systemic infections.
† Blood levels are at 1–2 h after IM or at the end of 20–30 min IV infusion. In most instances considerably higher serum levels are attainable with higher dosages. For example, 2 g of ampicillin would yield a peak blood level of 70–90 μg/mL, 2 g of cefoxitin a peak blood level of 120–140 μg/mL.
‡ Drug concentrations may be significantly lower if the patient is producing a very dilute urine or if creatinine clearance is below 10 mL/min. Concentration based on mean levels for the first 4 h after drug is administered.
§ Assuming normal liver function.
¶ Meningeal inflammation; in meningitis higher doses than those listed would normally be employed resulting in higher CSF levels.
NOTE: NA = not appropriate therapy for meningitis; — = data not available; TMP/SMX = trimethoprim-sulfamethoxazole.

TABLE 85-2 Serum and body fluid levels after parenteral administration of various antibiotics

| Drug | Unit dose[a] (parenteral) | Average peak level, μg/mL | | | | Half-life, h | | Dose adjustment renal failure | Effect of hemodialysis |
		Blood[b]	Urine[c]	Bile[d]	CSF[e]	$C_{cl} > 80$ mL	$C_{cl} < 10$ mL		
Amdinocillin	1.0 g IV	70	>1000	20	1–5[f]	1	4	Minor	Yes
Amikacin	5 mg/kg IM or IV	25	200	5	5	2	30	Major	Yes
Ampicillin	1.0 g IV	35	500	10	3[f]	1	4	Minor	Yes
Azlocillin	3.0 g IV	190	>2000	100	16	1	4	Minor	Yes
Aztreonam	1.0 g IV	160	>1000	20	1–5[f]	1.5–2	6	Minor	Yes
Carbenicillin	4.0 g IV	250	>1000	50	20	1	15	Major	Yes
Cefamandole	1.0 g IV	70	1000	100	NA	0.7	8	Minor	Yes
Cefazolin	1.0 g IV	110	>1000	50	NA	2	25	Major	Yes
Cefoperazone	2.0 g IV	250	>1000	>100	1–5	2	2–4	No	No
Cefotaxime	1.0 g IV	80	>1000	15	10[f]	1	4	Minor	Yes
Cefoxitin	1.0 g IV	70	1000	100	1–5	0.8	10	Major	Yes
Ceftazidime	1.0 g IV	80	>1000	5–10	1–20[f]	1.8	1.5	Major	Yes
Ceftizoxime	1.0 g IV	80	>1000	30	1–10[f]	1.6	19	Major	Yes
Ceftriaxone	1.0 g IV	150	>1000	200	1–20[f]	8	16	No	Yes
Cefuroxime	0.75 g IV	40	>1000	10–30	1–20[f]	1.5	20	Major	Yes
Cephalothin	1.0 g IV	70	500	10	0.7	0.5	8	Minor	Yes
Cephapirin	1.0 g IV	70	500	10	NA	0.5	8	Minor	Yes
Chloramphenicol	1.0 g IV	15	100	3	10	1–2	3–5	No	Yes
Ciprofloxacin	300 mg IV	3	100	10	1	3–4	5–10	Yes	Yes
Clindamycin	0.6 g IV	15	30	40	NA	2	6–10	No	No
Erythromycin	1.0 g IV	10	20	80	1	1–2	4–6	No	No
Gentamicin	1.5 mg/kg IM or IV	6	50	2	1	1–2	4–6	Major	Yes
Imipenem	0.5 g IV	30	100	10	1	1	6	Major	Yes
Kanamycin	5.0 mg/kg IM or IV	20	200	5	NA	2	35	Major	Yes
Methicillin	2.0 g IV	80	1000	30	5	0.5	4	Minor	Yes
Metronidazole	8.0 mg/kg IV	25	100	20	10	8	8	Minor	Yes
Mezlocillin	3.0 g IV	190	>2000	100	16	1	4	Minor	Yes
Moxalactam	1.0 g IV	100	>1000	60	1–30[f]	2	19	Major	Yes
Nafcillin	1.0 g IV	70	150	40	2	1	2	Minor	No
Oxacillin	1.0 g IV	70	500	2.5	1	1	2	Minor	No
Penicillin G	3 million units IV	115	300	15	6	1	4	Minor	Yes
Piperacillin	3.0 g IV	190	>2000	50	20	1	4	Minor	Yes
Ticarcillin	3.0 g IV	190	>2000	50	20	1	15	Major	Yes
Tobramycin	1.5 mg/kg IM or IV	6	50	2	1	2	35	Major	Yes
Vancomycin	0.5 g IV	30	100	3	3	6	120	Major	No

[a] Doses listed are the lowest doses that would normally be employed for adults or children over 32 kg with normal renal function in the treatment of systemic infections.
[b] Blood levels are at 1–2 h after IM or at the end of 20–30 min IV infusion. In most instances considerably higher serum levels are attainable with higher dosages. For example, 2 g of ampicillin would yield a peak blood level of 70–90 μg/mL, 2 g of cefoxitin a peak blood level of 120–140 μg/mL.
[c] Drug concentrations may be significantly lower if the patient is producing a very dilute urine or if creatinine clearance is below 10 mL/min. Concentration based on mean levels for the first 4 h after drug is administered.
[d] Assuming no biliary obstruction.
[e] Meningeal inflammation; in meningitis higher doses than those listed would normally be employed resulting in higher CSF levels. For example, 2 g of cefotaxime is usually used.
[f] Value at higher dose.
NOTE: NA = not appropriate therapy for meningitis; — = data not available.

at the time therapy is initiated. Antimicrobial therapy is started empirically in many situations. Empiric selection of an antimicrobial agent should be based on a knowledge of the likely pathogens and their antimicrobial susceptibility. For example, the most common cause of urinary tract infections is *Escherichia coli*. When dealing with outpatient urinary tract infections, therapy should be selected to inhibit this microorganism; therapy for treatment of a nosocomial urinary tract infection might be quite different. Bacteria other than *E. coli* are likely to produce urinary infection, particularly in the presence of an indwelling urethral catheter, and nosocomial pathogens are likely to be resistant to many antibiotics.

The host plays an extremely important role in the selection of an antimicrobial. The antibiotics chosen to treat a febrile, neutropenic patient will be different than those for a healthy individual with a minor infection. Host factors also have an important impact on the route of administration of antimicrobial agents and upon the duration of therapy.

IDENTIFICATION OF THE INFECTING ORGANISMS   There are a number of techniques for the rapid identification of the infecting microorganism. A Gram stain is a simple, inexpensive, and rapid method to identify many bacteria and fungi. This technique should be applied to all available body fluids such as urine, wound exudate, synovial fluid, pleural fluid, peritoneal fluid, and cerebrospinal fluid. In situations in which material for diagnosis is not available, knowledge of the most likely pathogens will be beneficial in directing the selection of an antimicrobial agent. For example, following an animal bite an organism such as *Pasteurella multocida* should be suspected. Cellulitis in the foot of a diabetic patient should suggest hemolytic streptococci, *Staphylococcus aureus,* as well as anaerobes.

SUSCEPTIBILITY OF INFECTING MICROORGANISMS   There are a number of different methods for determining the susceptibility of bacteria to antimicrobial agents. Susceptibility tests for viruses and fungi are less well developed, and very few laboratories have the ability to determine susceptibility of parasites to antiparasitic drugs.

A commonly used method to determine bacterial susceptibility to antibiotics is a disk diffusion method, which provides data within 24 h. It is semiquantitative, not useful for many slow-growing or fastidious organisms, and has not been adequately standardized for anaerobic bacteria. With the disk method, results are usually given as susceptible, resistant, and intermediate. A *susceptible* zone of inhibition correlates with serum and urine levels that are readily achievable with standard doses of the agent being tested. A *resistant* reading indicates that the zone of inhibition, using regression analysis, is less than that which would correspond to a concentration that could be achieved in blood under normal circumstances. *Intermediate* susceptibility means that the organism falls into a category that is necessary because of the splay in data correlating zone size with minimum inhibitory concentrations (MIC). This is particularly true if the infecting organism is found in a urine specimen in which the concentration of antimicrobial agent would be much higher than in blood or tissues.

Quantitative data on the susceptibility of particular organisms can be determined by micro or macro broth-dilution techniques. These methods detect the lowest concentration of antimicrobial agent that prevents visible growth after an 18- to 24-h incubation period (MIC). To understand MIC values it is essential to understand the pharmacokinetics of an antimicrobial agent. In general, an organism is considered susceptible when the MIC is no more than one-fourth of the readily obtainable peak serum level of the antimicrobial agent. It is also possible to determine the minimal bactericidal concentration (MBC) or minimal lethal concentration (MLC). This is defined as the concentration of drug that reduces the original inoculum by 99.9 percent as judged by subculture on antibiotic-free medium. MBC determinations are necessary in only a few situations that will be discussed below.

The large number of antimicrobial agents has made it difficult to test all antimicrobial agents against an isolate, and a particular compound is used as the class representative for a group of compounds. For example, among the first-generation cephalosporins, cephalothin is the representative drug that, either in a disk or in a broth-dilution system, is used to represent susceptibility to cephapirin, cefazolin, cephalexin, cephradine, and cefaclor. Occasionally, susceptibility tests provide incorrect information. For example, methicillin-resistant *S. aureus* appear susceptible to cephalosporin antibiotics, but are not. Most susceptibility tests do not readily identify a resistant subpopulation.

Some microorganisms have remained susceptible to the same drugs since antibiotics were discovered, and in them development of resistance is exceedingly rare. Examples are group A streptococci which are susceptible to penicillins and cephalosporins. Hence most laboratories do not report susceptibilities of group A streptococci. However, group A streptococci may be resistant to erythromycin, and if the use of this drug is contemplated, susceptibility tests may be necessary. Most strains of *Streptococcus pneumoniae* remain susceptible to penicillin. However, some isolates have intermediate susceptibility; that is, the MICs are between 0.1 and 1.0 μg/mL. Although such a penicillin concentration can readily be achieved in the blood and lung, it may be difficult to achieve cerebrospinal fluid concentrations that are tenfold this level. For this reason, pneumococci isolated from the CSF should be tested for penicillin susceptibility.

CLINICAL PHARMACOLOGY   Knowledge of the clinical pharmacology of antimicrobial agents is important in selecting therapeutic programs that are both effective and safe. Antimicrobial agents can be administered by the oral, intramuscular, intravenous, intraperitoneal, or topical routes. After absorption they dissolve in the plasma and are variably bound to plasma proteins. From the plasma they are distributed to various extracellular tissues and fluids in which they may be free or bound. As an antibiotic is distributed into extravascular compartments, there is an initial fall in plasma concentration. Peak concentrations of antimicrobial agents after intravenous infusion occur at the end of the infusion. In contrast, after intramuscular injection, and after oral ingestion, there is an initial slow distribution phase, that is, a combination of absorption and simultaneous excretion or metabolism. Peak serum levels following oral ingestion of antimicrobial agents usually occur in 1 to 2 h. Continued decrease in serum levels of antimicrobial agents is related to renal and biliary excretion and to the hepatic metabolism of some drugs. The amount of drug that reaches the extravascular tissues in which the infection is present depends not only on the concentration gradient from serum to tissue, but also on protein binding in serum and in tissues and the diffusibility of the agent. The diffusibility of antimicrobial agents is a function of their molecular size, dissociation constant, and lipid solubility.

Several pharmacokinetic indexes are useful in adjusting the dosage of antimicrobial agents. The half-life of a drug is the time required for the plasma concentration to fall by one-half as it is being eliminated from the body. Half-life refers to the drug elimination phase after the absorption of the drug has been completed and the drug has been distributed throughout its entire volume of distribution. The assumption is that the fall in plasma concentration parallels the fall in the total amount of drug in the body. Direct extrapolation of the frequency of dosing from half-life considerations is not completely appropriate. The MIC of the infecting organism, site of infection, and host defense mechanisms must be considered in determining dose frequency.

Another pharmacokinetic index that may be useful for guiding therapy is the volume of distribution (V_d). This is the volume in which the total amount of drug in the body would have to be uniformly distributed in order to give the observed plasma concentration. Simplistically it is calculated by the formula $V_d = A/C_p$, where A is amount of drug administered and C_p is plasma concentration. The volume of distribution does not correspond to an actual anatomic or physiologic space. It is useful for determining initial or loading doses and in calculating subsequent or maintenance doses to achieve safe, therapeutic plasma concentrations. When a drug dose is given repetitively at regular intervals, the peak concentration and the minimal concentration eventually reach a constant state if there is no change in the rate of drug elimination. With most antimicrobial agents it is not necessary to use an initial loading dose. However, when agents such as the aminoglycosides are used to treat serious infections such as suspected bacteremia or pneumonia, a loading dose which will provide an initial plasma and tissue concentration well above the MIC of the suspected infecting microorganisms is used.

The half-lives of many antibiotics have been determined in healthy young males. Prolongation of a drug half-life often may result from renal or hepatic dysfunction. Half-life may also be influenced by age and may be shortened in certain disease states. Other drugs administered concomitantly can also either prolong or shorten a drug's half-life.

HOST FACTORS   A number of different host factors have a significant influence on the efficacy and toxicity of antimicrobial agents.

Allergic history   It is critical to obtain a history of previous adverse reactions to antimicrobial agents since similar reactions may occur to drugs within the same class.

Age   Certain antimicrobial agents should not be given to individuals in some age groups. Sulfonamides should not be administered to pregnant females or to newborns because they bind to serum albumin, displacing bilirubin, which may result in kernicterus. Premature and newborn babies produce an inadequate amount of glucuronyltransferase, the enzyme that inactivates chloramphenicol, and some newborns treated with this drug may develop the "gray baby syndrome," which is characterized by progressive pallor, cyanosis, vasomotor collapse, and death. Tetracyclines should not be administered to pregnant females, newborn infants, or to children below 8 years of age because the drugs bind to developing bone and tooth structure, which may cause permanent brownish discoloration of the teeth.

Renal function   Many antimicrobial agents are removed from the body by renal excretion. Glomerular and some tubular functions do not develop to adult levels until at least 2 months of age, and drugs administered to premature or newborn infants must be given at different dosage schedules than those used for older children or adults. With advancing age, renal function decreases, and approximately 1 percent of glomerular clearance is lost per year over the age of 30. Antimicrobial agents removed from the body purely by glomerular filtration will accumulate as glomerular filtration declines, resulting in toxicity to other organs or to the kidney itself. Even compounds removed from the body by tubular secretion will accumulate as renal function falls below creatinine clearance of 20 mL/min. Toxic levels of certain penicillins, aminoglycosides, tetracyclines, and quinolones may develop in the presence of markedly reduced renal function. Serum creatinine or blood urea nitrogen may not reflect the true state of renal function in an elderly individual with a small body mass. Hence in calculating the dose of antimicrobial agent it is necessary to consider age, sex, and body weight.

Hepatic function   Some antimicrobial agents are metabolized and removed from the body primarily by hepatic mechanisms. These include some of the macrolides, rifamycins, imidazoles, chloramphenicol, quinolones, and linconoid drugs. Reductions in dose may be necessary to avoid toxic concentrations of these agents. Chloramphenicol, clindamycin, and tetracyclines accumulate in patients with severe liver disease. The half-lives of both rifampin and isoniazid are prolonged in patients with extensive hepatic disease. Some drugs which are excreted by biliary mechanisms are excreted by the kidney in the presence of hepatic failure. Conversely, some compounds that are normally excreted by the kidney are excreted in the bile in the presence of renal failure. In the presence of combined biliary and hepatic disease, toxic levels may be reached. Examples are cefoperazone, which is primarily excreted by biliary mechanisms, and carbenicillin and ticarcillin, which are primarily renally excreted but in the presence of combined hepatic and renal failure accumulate in the plasma.

Pregnancy   Antimicrobial agents cross the placenta to varying degrees. Most penicillins, cephalosporins, and erythromycins are not teratogenic and are safe in pregnant women. Tetracyclines should not be used in pregnancy not only because of their effect upon fetal dentition but also because they have a propensity to cause fatty necrosis of the liver, pancreatitis, and possible renal damage in pregnant females. If streptomycin is used to treat tuberculosis in pregnancy, it can cause abnormalities of vestibular function and hearing in the child.

Genetic factors   A number of different antimicrobial agents will produce hemolysis in patients with glucose-6-phosphate dehydrogenase deficiency. These include sulfonamides, nitrofurantoin, furazoline, chloramphenicol, pyrimethamine, and various sulfones.

The rate at which isoniazid is inactivated by acetylation in the liver is genetically determined. In the United States and North European populations, 50 to 60 percent of individuals are slow inactivators of this drug. Polyneuritis is seen more frequently as a complication of isoniazid therapy in individuals who are slow acetylators.

Site of infection   The site of infection is one of the most important factors in determining the choice of a dose and route by which the antimicrobial is administered. Adequate concentrations of a drug must be delivered to the site of the infection. In many situations, if the local concentration of an antimicrobial equals or exceeds the minimum inhibitory concentration of the infecting microorganism, cure will result, but only in those areas of the body in which there are adequate host defenses such as polymorphonuclear cells, complement, and antibody. Where these factors are inadequate or absent, such as in the spinal fluid or on the heart valves, concentrations at least fourfold and preferably five- to tenfold above the MIC, or even MBC, are needed to achieve a cure. Even when concentrations above the MICs are not achieved, there will be an effect on the microorganisms that will aid the host's counterattack. Subinhibitory concentrations of antimicrobial agents alter the adherence properties of microorganisms, thereby decreasing further invasion. Subinhibitory concentrations also alter surface structures, enhancing phagocytosis. Subinhibitory concentrations of antibiotics, by binding to the surface of microorganisms, enhance the intracellular killing of bacteria ingested by phagocytic cells. These factors may explain the unusual circumstances in which antimicrobial agents in seemingly inadequate doses result in clinical cure. Nonetheless, the major goal of therapy should be to achieve concentrations above the MIC in all tissues.

In general, antimicrobial agents are widely distributed and reach adequate concentrations in many infected sites, including pleural, pericardial, and infected joint fluids and infections in muscles or skin structures. An exception are vegetations on the heart valves in endocarditis. Although the valves are exposed to the circulation, the bacteria often are trapped deep within the fibrin vegetation. The organisms are growing less rapidly, making them less susceptible to many antibiotics, and there is inadequate phagocytic function in the focal valvular infection. Because of these factors, therapy of bacterial endocarditis requires bactericidal agents that are administered for long periods of time and that achieve such high concentration in the blood that diffusion of the antibiotic into the vegetation occurs (see Chap. 90).

Meningitis is another disease in which the concentration of antimicrobial agent in the infected site is critical. Many antimicrobial agents cross the blood-brain barrier poorly and do not produce adequate cerebrospinal fluid levels, for example, parenteral aminoglycosides. Lipid-soluble agents can cross the spinal fluid barrier easily, accounting for the utility of chloramphenicol. This agent has proved highly effective in the therapy of meningitis due to *Streptococcus pneumoniae*, *Haemophilus influenzae*, and *Neisseria meningitidis* because of the bactericidal concentrations it produces in the cerebrospinal fluid. Chloramphenicol is not useful in treating meningitis due to *E. coli* or *Klebsiella pneumoniae*, even if the organisms are susceptible in vitro, because it is not bactericidal for these organisms, and concentrations eightfold above the MBC cannot be achieved within the cerebrospinal fluid. Fortunately, antimicrobials such as cefotaxime, ceftizoxime, ceftriaxone, ceftazidime, and moxalactam all enter the cerebrospinal fluid in concentrations adequate to treat both the common causes of meningitis and the less frequently encountered gram-negative organisms.

An infectious site that may be particularly refractory to treatment involves bones in areas of devitalized tissue, as occurs in diabetics and other patients with inadequate blood supply due to vascular insufficiency. Penetration of the antimicrobial agents to the site of the infection may be only borderline or inadequate. Antimicrobial agents must be administered in high concentrations for prolonged periods to yield adequate concentration within bone. Even with extended therapy, many cases of chronic osteomyelitis are never completely cured since some of the bacteria are in a resting state and do not come into contact with the antimicrobial agent.

In some instances the surgeon's knife is the only mechanism by which an abscess can be cured. Others, like lung abscess, can be treated without surgical intervention in most situations since the abscess can drain via the bronchi, and the antimicrobial agents kill bacteria in the surrounding inflammatory tissue (see Chap. 207). Lung abscesses 8 to 10 cm in diameter frequently do not respond to antimicrobial therapy alone since there is inadequate diffusion of the antimicrobial agent into the cavity and organisms persist. Other abscesses which may respond to antimicrobial therapy alone are those of the ovary, brain, and liver. Ultrasound, computed tomography (CT) scanning, and magnetic resonance imaging (MRI) have demonstrated detectable decreases in abscess size with antimicrobial treatment alone. In general, abscesses in other parts of the abdomen require external drainage, since antimicrobial agents by themselves fail to sterilize the majority of them. Exceptions have been noted with some anaerobic microorganisms; compounds such as metronidazole diffuse into the abscess and destroy the anaerobic organisms.

Local factors within an abscess can have an important impact upon the activity of certain antimicrobial agents. For example, in the case of a mixed aerobic and anaerobic abscess, the anaerobic organisms may produce β-lactamases that will destroy the β-lactam compound that is being used to inhibit the aerobic gram-negative bacilli. Aminoglycoside antibiotics are significantly less active in an anaerobic abscess since they require an aerobic environment for antimicrobial activity. They are less effective at an acid pH than at pH 7.4. Gentamicin or tobramycin might inhibit a *Klebsiella* at 0.1 μg/mL at pH 7.4, but in the infected lung the pH is 6.4 to 6.5. Aminoglycosides are ten- to thirtyfold less active at this pH than they are at pH 7.4. Cellular debris from decaying white cells will complex with aminoglycosides and reduce their activity. In a hyperosmolar environment some β-lactam antimicrobial agents may be less effective because they will not produce death of the microorganism. Agents such as methenamine, nitrofurantoin, and chlortetracycline are more active at an acid pH; the activities of erythromycin, clindamycin, and aminoglycosides are greater in an alkaline milieu.

Foreign bodies have an extremely important effect on the response to antimicrobial agents. Infections of prosthetic heart valves or joint implants usually are not cured by antimicrobial agents even though the organisms infecting the foreign body are highly susceptible to antibiotics. It is thought that a glycocalyx develops that adheres to the foreign material and provides a cover for the microorganisms. Organisms such as *Staphylococcus epidermidis* send projections into small defects in the polypropylene material used in catheters and other foreign devices. The methylmethacrylate used in artificial joints provides a large number of interstices in which microorganisms avoid exposure to antimicrobial agents. Indwelling urethral catheters are another example of a foreign body which makes it virtually impossible to eradicate infecting microorganisms. Unless the catheter is removed, the organisms will not be eradicated. Calculi, whether in the urinary or biliary tracts, provide a haven for microorganisms.

ANTIMICROBIAL COMBINATIONS Although the majority of infections can be treated with a single antimicrobial agent, there are definite situations in which the combination of antimicrobial agents is indicated. However, combination antimicrobial therapy is used much more frequently than necessary and may have deleterious results.

The combination of two or three antimicrobial agents may have one of three different effects. Drugs are *additive* when their activity in combination equals the sum of their separate, independent activities. *Synergistic* activity implies that the activity of two or three antimicrobials is greater than the sum of their independent activities. Drugs are *antagonistic* when the activity of the combination is less than the sum of the independent effects.

Preventing the emergence of resistant organisms is one of the most common indications for combination therapy. For example, the mycobacteria causing tuberculosis consist of a population of organisms of varying susceptibility to antituberculous drugs. The large number of bacilli in a tuberculous lung cavity contain organisms that are intrinsically resistant to the antituberculous agent. Mutants resistant to antituberculosis agents occur at a rate of 1 in 10^{-6} organisms. For this reason, two or three drugs are utilized in the treatment of this disease. The concept of the use of multiple drugs in the treatment of tuberculosis is particularly important for isoniazid-resistant organisms.

Use of rifampin as a single agent to treat staphylococcal infections rapidly results in the emergence of strains resistant to the antibiotic. However, the combination of a β-lactam antibiotic with rifampin reduces the chance for the emergence of such resistant strains. Combination of an aminoglycoside with a cephalosporin has not been shown to prevent the emergence of resistance in *Enterobacter* or *Citrobacter* species.

A second major reason for combination therapy is to treat polymicrobial infections. Intraperitoneal and pelvic infections are usually due to an aerobic and anaerobic flora. Although some antimicrobial agents inhibit both aerobic and anaerobic species, it may not always be feasible to use these drugs clinically. Combination therapy might include an agent effective against the anaerobic organism and an agent effective against the aerobic gram-negative rod. Brain abscesses are frequently caused by *Bacteroides* and anaerobic or microaerophilic streptococci. Metronidazole penetrates extremely well into the abscess and has excellent activity against the *Bacteroides* species. However, it has poor activity against streptococcal species. Penicillin will penetrate into the brain adequately to kill the streptococcal species but cannot be used singly since it would be destroyed in the brain abscess by the β-lactamases frequently elaborated by the *Bacteroides* strains.

A theoretical reason for the use of drug combinations is to lower concentrations of compounds that have toxic potential. However, there is no clinical evidence to substantiate the use of two drugs at lower concentrations than that at which they would normally be utilized.

One of the major indications for combined antimicrobial therapy is to provide a broad spectrum of coverage for the patient who is neutropenic and has significantly compromised host defenses. It has been the practice to use a broad-spectrum antipseudomonas penicillin or cephalosporin combined with an aminoglycoside as initial therapy for the febrile neutropenic patient. The increasing number of infections due to β-lactam-resistant gram-positive species has led to the use of vancomycin in combination with β-lactams.

Although synergism can be demonstrated in the laboratory with many antimicrobial combinations, in only a few clinical settings has combination therapy proved more effective than single agents. The most widely accepted combination therapy is penicillin G or ampicillin with an aminoglycoside, streptomycin or gentamicin, for the treatment of enterococcal endocarditis. The drugs enhance the uptake of each other, and the enterococci are killed. Similar synergism can be demonstrated between semisynthetic penicillinase-resistant penicillins, such as nafcillin or oxacillin, and gentamicin against *S. aureus*. However, clinical data do not show that this combination has advantages over use of a single drug. Combinations of antipseudomonas penicillins with aminoglycosides are synergistic against many strains of *Pseudomonas aeruginosa*. Clinical trials have demonstrated the superiority of these combinations in neutropenic patients.

The combination of trimethoprim with sulfamethoxazole inhibits two critical points in the folic acid cycle, which is part of the production pathway of DNA. In vitro and animal experiments demonstrate that the two drugs are more effective than either drug alone. The major situation in which the combination is necessary is in treatment of *Pneumocystis carinii* infection. In urinary tract infections trimethoprim alone is as effective as the combination.

Examples of drug synergism are combinations of a β-lactam drug with a β-lactamase inhibitor: an amoxicillin and clavulanate (augmentin), ticarcillin and clavulanate (timentin), and sulbactam with ampicillin. Combination of a β-lactamase-susceptible β-lactam with a β-lactamase inhibitor enhances the antibacterial spectrum of a drug that would normally be destroyed by β-lactamase. Amoxicillin-clavulanate and sulbactam-ampicillin inhibit *Haemophilus, Branhamella, E. coli, Salmonella, S. aureus, Fusobacterium, Bacteroides, Neisseria,* and *Klebsiella,* which are resistant to amoxicillin or ampicillin.

Another form of synergy is that shown by amdinocillin, which binds to a specific penicillin-binding protein different from the proteins to which other penicillins and cephalosporins bind. When combined with various β-lactams, amdinocillin synergistically inhibits some gram-negative bacteria.

Disadvantages of antimicrobial combinations There are a few examples of antagonism of antimicrobial agents. In the 1950s it was demonstrated that penicillin alone was more effective than a combination of penicillin and chlortetracycline for the treatment of pneumococcal meningitis.

Combination therapy may result in superinfection with other organisms, particularly fungi, since the combination obliterates the normal protective flora of the oropharynx and the intestine. This problem can be avoided by discontinuing unnecessary empiric combination therapy once the diagnosis has been established. Another adverse effect of combination therapy may be increased drug reactions or other metabolic side effects.

ROUTE OF ADMINISTRATION OF ANTIMICROBIAL AGENTS Having determined the most appropriate agent to treat a given infection, the most appropriate route of administration should be determined. The choice usually lies between the oral and the parenteral route. Oral administration of antimicrobial agents has generally been for infections that are mild and are treated on an outpatient basis. As hospital costs have risen, reevaluation of this concept is necessary. Some serious infections initially may be treated parenterally; then therapy can be completed with an oral antibiotic. Examples would be osteomyelitis, pneumonitis, or severe skin infections that have begun to respond to parenteral therapy. When drugs are administered by the oral route, it is important to be certain that the patient takes the drug in a manner that will result in the best blood and tissue levels. The absorption of many antimicrobial agents is markedly decreased by food. Tetracyclines form a soluble chelate with magnesium, calcium, aluminum, or iron. Quinolone absorption is reduced by aluminum and magnesium but not by calcium. In a number of infections it may be possible to administer an oral antimicrobial agent twice a day rather than four times a day. This may be important for patient compliance.

The parenteral route is used for agents that are not absorbed from the gastrointestinal tract, and for serious infections in which a high concentration of the antimicrobial agent is needed immediately. Examples are suspected bacteremia, meningitis, and gram-negative pneumonia. Intravenous administration of most drugs is preferred since it provides for high serum concentration. There are no definitive data that show whether bolus, 3- to 5-min injection, infusion over 15 to 30 min, or continuous administration of a drug by the intravenous route is more effective in curing bacterial infection. Serum concentrations adequate to treat many infections are achieved after intramuscular administration. With some agents with extremely long half-lives it may be possible to complete therapy of serious infections by administration of the drug intramuscularly once a day. It is rarely necessary to instill antimicrobial agents into infected cavities. Peritonitis in patients receiving peritoneal dialysis may respond better to administration of the antimicrobial agent in the dialysis solution. Meningitis due to *Coccidioides immitis* and some gram-negative species may require intraventricular or intrathecal therapy.

MONITORING PATIENT RESPONSE With some antimicrobial agents it is essential that serum levels of the agent be monitored. For the aminoglycoside antibiotics, peak levels should be obtained to determine that effective concentrations are being achieved and trough levels should be measured to determine that the drugs are not accumulating and producing nephrotoxicity or ototoxicity. Except for renal failure, it is not necessary to monitor serum concentrations of β-lactam antibiotics.

Serum bactericidal titers, defined as the dilution of serum which will kill the infecting pathogen in vitro, have been used extensively to monitor therapy of bacterial endocarditis. There has been wide variation in the performance of serum bactericidal titers, but guidelines for their use have been developed. If a standardized inoculum of organisms is used and standard media and techniques employed, the tests are useful in certain clinical situations. For example, a peak serum bactericidal titer $>1:64$ correlates with a 98 percent bacteriologic cure of endocarditis. However, clinical cure cannot be predicted since damage to the valve as a result of the endocarditis may result in valvular insufficiency requiring surgery. A peak serum bactericidal titer greater than 1:8 correlates with a successful outcome in osteomyelitis, bacteremia, septic arthritis, and empyema.

PROPHYLAXIS WITH ANTIMICROBIAL AGENTS Antibiotic prophylaxis should be directed at preventing specific bacterial infection. This means that a particular species or several species of microorganisms have been shown to produce the infection, that an effective antibiotic is available, and that the risk of the infection outweighs the hazard of the antibiotic. The antibiotic must achieve adequate concentrations at the site at which infection would occur, and it must prevent colonization or eliminate organisms that could potentially cause infection. In the case of surgical prophylaxis, the antibiotic must be delivered to the site of probable infection in time to inhibit bacteria that would colonize the area and produce subsequent infection, and the agent must be present for 3 to 4 h after the incision. In some situations it is sufficient to decrease the number of pathogens but not eradicate them. The duration of prophylaxis must be short to avoid toxicity and prevent selection of a resistant bacterial flora by eliminating the normal flora.

Prophylaxis can be divided into medical and surgical situations. Medical situations in which it has been successful include meningococcal meningitis, *Haemophilus influenzae* meningitis, recurrence of rheumatic fever, postsplenectomy, pneumococcal or *Haemophilus* infection, cellulitis complicating lymphedema, recurrent cystitis, tuberculosis, and bacterial endocarditis. A special medical problem is the prevention of infection in the neutropenic patient. Many of the bacteremias in neutropenic patients are of gastrointestinal origin, and use of agents that eliminate the aerobic gram-negative flora reduces the incidence of gram-negative sepsis (see Chap. 82).

Numerous surgical situations qualify for prophylaxis—upper gastrointestinal surgery, cholecystectomy, colon surgery, appendectomy, head and neck surgery, cardiac surgery, prosthetic hip and other joint surgery, hysterectomy, and cesarean section. The optimum agent for each clinical situation has not been established.

Prophylaxis can be effective without eradicating all of the bacteria in an area. Topical application of silver sulfadiazine or mafenide to burn eschars will reduce the number of bacteria in the burn eschar to less than 10^5 per gram of tissue. This prevents sepsis in the burn and allows healing.

Antibiotics do not alter an underlying pathophysiologic state. Trimethoprim-sulfamethoxazole (TMP/SMX) will prevent recurrent urinary tract infections in women with recurrent cystitis. However, even if an individual uses TMP/SMX for 6 months, reinfection can recur when the antimicrobial agent is discontinued if the patient's perineal area is recolonized with *E. coli* that have fimbriae with receptors for the urethra and bladder of the patient (see Chap. 95).

SPECIFIC ANTIMICROBIAL AGENTS

β-LACTAM ANTIBIOTICS β-Lactam antibiotics interfere with bacterial cell wall biosynthesis by binding to proteins, referred to as penicillin-binding proteins (PBPs), which by transpeptidation produce crosslinking of peptidoglycan chains that form the bacterial cell wall. The most common form of resistance is that due to β-lactamases. In staphylococci, β-lactamases are plasmid-mediated exoenzymes with affinity primarily for penicillins. In gram-negative aerobic and anaerobic species, β-lactamase synthesis is either plasmid- or chromosomally mediated and the enzymes are in the periplasmic space. β-Lactamases of gram-negatives can have affinity primarily for penicillins or for cephalosporins, or they may be capable of destroying both classes of compounds.

Resistance to β-lactams can be due to failure to bind to PBPs, as occurs with methicillin-resistant staphylococci and penicillin-resistant pneumococci. Resistance can be due to failure of the β-lactam to reach a receptor, i.e., cross the bacterial cell wall. Rarely, resistance of gram-positive bacteria to β-lactams is due to failure to activate autolysins.

PENICILLINS   Penicillins can be divided into several classes on the basis of antibacterial activity.

Natural penicillins   Penicillin G and penicillin V are the two natural penicillins. Penicillin G is available as an orally, intramuscularly, and intravenously administered compound. Penicillin G is combined with procaine as a 1:1 molar salt which extends the half-life of the drug, and it is combined with benzathine to produce a long-acting repository form. Penicillin V is available only for oral use. The antibacterial activity of penicillin G and penicillin V includes *S. pneumoniae*, beta-hemolytic streptococci, viridans group streptococci, and microaerophilic and anaerobic streptococci. Most *S. aureus* and *S. epidermidis* produce β-lactamases which destroy both penicillin G and V. *Neisseria meningitidis* are susceptible to penicillin G. In many parts of the world penicillinase-producing *N. gonorrhoeae* are a significant problem. Penicillin G has excellent activity against clostridial species and also inhibits many oral *Bacteroides* species and *Fusobacterium* species. Penicillin V does not have good activity against species such as *Haemophilus* or *Branhamella*, which are important pathogens causing sinusitis, otitis, and other upper respiratory infections. Infrequently encountered organisms for which penicillin G remains an excellent drug are *Erysipelothrix, Listeria monocytogenes, Pasteurella multocida, Streptobacillus, Spirillum, Fusospirochetes, Treponema pallidum*, and *Actinomyces israelii*, as well as the *Borrelia* which causes Lyme disease.

Penicillin G is not stable in gastric acid and should not be used as an oral preparation. In contrast, penicillin V is 60 percent absorbed when given orally, and food causes only a minor decrease in absorption. Penicillin V is an effective agent in treatment of streptococcal infections and less serious forms of pneumococcal pneumonia. It should not be used to treat syphilis, gonorrhea, or *Haemophilus* infections. Penicillin G remains the treatment of choice for viridans group streptococcal endocarditis and for most cases of pneumococcal and meningococcal meningitis. Since penicillin G has a short half-life due to rapid tubular secretion, it must be administered on a 4- or 6-hourly basis. Only minor dosage adjustments are necessary until the creatinine clearance falls below 30 mL/min. Even in the presence of renal failure, doses of 4,000,000 to 6,000,000 units per day can be administered safely. Benzathine penicillin, which has a half-life of a week, can be used in the treatment of streptococcal pharyngitis, in the therapy of primary and early syphilis, and in the prevention of recurrences of rheumatic fever when administered once monthly.

Aminopenicillins   Aminopenicillins have an amino group on the β-acyl side chain of the penicillin nucleus. A number of different compounds are available. They differ microbiologically to a minor degree. Ampicillin was the first aminopenicillin. Subsequently, amoxicillin was produced, and other agents such as bacampicillin, cyclacillin, epicillin, hetacillin, and pivampicillin have been synthesized. Aminopenicillins retain the in vitro activity of penicillin G. In addition, they inhibit many *H. influenzae* and are more active against *Enterococcus faecalis*. Many *E. coli* are inhibited by aminopenicillins, as are *Proteus mirabilis*. In the United States, many *Salmonella*

species and *Shigella* species are inhibited by ampicillin, but in developing countries most strains are resistant to aminopenicillins. Aminopenicillins inhibit most mouth organisms, but do not inhibit *Pseudomonas* species, *Klebsiella, Enterobacter*, and the majority of *Bacteroides fragilis* species. In some parts of the United States, 35 percent of *H. influenzae* contain a β-lactamase, making them resistant to the aminopenicillins.

Amoxicillin and bacampicillin are absorbed approximately twice as well as ampicillin. Bacampicillin is an ester of ampicillin that is converted in the intestinal mucosa and in plasma to free ampicillin. Administered parenterally, ampicillin is well distributed to most body compartments and therapeutic concentrations are achieved in the cerebrospinal, pleural, joint, and peritoneal fluids in the presence of inflammation. Urinary levels are high. Although ampicillin can be administered intramuscularly, orally administered amoxicillin will produce serum levels comparable to those achieved by intramuscular injection of similar amounts of ampicillin. Ampicillin currently is used in the treatment of outpatient urinary tract infections, upper respiratory infections, otitis media, sinusitis, bacterial exacerbations of bronchitis, and community-acquired pneumonia. It is effective therapy for pneumococcal and meningococcal meningitis, and is used in the therapy of enterococcal endocarditis, always in combination with an aminoglycoside. For oral therapy, amoxicillin should replace ampicillin due to its better absorption. The one clinical setting in which amoxicillin is inferior to ampicillin is in the treatment of shigellosis. Amoxicillin and bacampicillin can be administered three times a day and still attain adequate blood, tissue, and urinary levels for treatment of susceptible organisms.

Although allergic reactions of the hypersensitivity type to the aminopenicillins occur with the same frequency as with penicillin G or V, there is an increased risk of skin rash with oral ampicillin. It is estimated that 8 to 10 percent of patients receiving oral ampicillin develop a skin rash. As many as 90 percent of patients with infectious mononucleosis receiving ampicillin develop a maculopapular rash beginning approximately 4 days after therapy is instituted. This rash does not represent true penicillin allergy and does not mean that the patient can never receive a penicillin again.

Penicillinase-resistant penicillins   A number of different penicillinase-resistant penicillins were developed for the treatment of staphylococcal infections. These agents inhibit *S. aureus* and coagulase-negative staphylococci, as well as *S. pyogenes* and *S. pneumoniae*. None of them has activity against *E. faecalis* or against aerobic or anaerobic gram-negative bacilli. Methicillin was the first antistaphylococcal β-lactamase-stable penicillin.

S. aureus resistant to all β-lactams are referred to as methicillin-resistant. These isolates have an altered penicillin-binding protein as the basis of their resistance, and hence these *S. aureus* and similar strains of coagulase-negative staphylococci are resistant to all penicillins and to cephalosporins as well. In vitro tests of methicillin-resistant staphylococci against cephalosporins tend to be unreliable, and may show false-positive susceptibility. The drug of choice for methicillin-resistant staphylococci is vancomycin.

Methicillin can only be used parenterally since it is not acid-stable, and it has a short half-life, necessitating intravenous administration every 4 h. Since interstitial nephritis is a relatively common side effect, methicillin is rarely used today.

Nafcillin has more intrinsic activity than methicillin against both staphylococci and streptococci. It is excreted primarily by the liver, and to a lesser extent by the kidney. Nafcillin should not be used orally since absorption by this route is erratic. The usual dosage of nafcillin is 4 to 12 g/d, depending upon the severity of the infection, and 100 to 200 mg/kg per day for children. Intravenous nafcillin may result in more severe phlebitis than other antistaphylococcal penicillins, and in high doses may result in more neutropenia.

The isoxazolyl penicillins consist of oxacillin, which should be used only parenterally due to poor oral absorption, and the oral preparations cloxacillin and dicloxacillin. In many countries, flucloxacillin is also available as an oral drug, and in some countries cloxacillin is available for parenteral use. Although dicloxacillin produces higher blood levels than cloxacillin, it is slightly more protein-bound, 96 vs. 94 percent, than cloxacillin. The active antibiotic levels of the two drugs are quite similar. In general, cloxacillin or dicloxacillin are administered in doses of 0.5 or 0.25 g four times a day, respectively.

Although the primary indication for the use of antistaphylococcal penicillins is infection due to penicillinase-producing staphylococci, they are often administered before the etiologic agent is known. Blood levels with the penicillinase-resistant penicillins are adequate to inhibit S. pneumoniae, except in the CSF, and most hemolytic streptococci; therefore, it is not necessary to give both a penicillinase-resistant penicillin and penicillin G simultaneously. However, infections caused by E. faecalis and Neisseria do not respond to penicillinase-resistant penicillins, and ampicillin should also be used if these organisms are suspected.

Carboxy penicillins Carbenicillin was the first penicillin with activity against P. aeruginosa and certain indole-positive Proteus species. Ticarcillin is also a carboxy penicillin, but it is fourfold more active than carbenicillin against P. aeruginosa and has replaced carbenicillin. These compounds are destroyed by β-lactamases of gram-positive and some gram-negative organisms but are less readily destroyed by the β-lactamases of species such as Pseudomonas, Enterobacter, Morganella, and Proteus-Providencia. Carbenicillin and ticarcillin are less active than ampicillin against S. pyogenes, S. pneumoniae, and E. faecalis. They have excellent activity against non-β-lactamase-producing Haemophilus, N. meningitidis, and N. gonorrhoeae. In general, the antibacterial activity of the carboxy penicillins against E. coli, Proteus, Salmonella, and Shigella species is similar to ampicillin. They are inactive against Klebsiella since they are destroyed by the β-lactamase of these organisms. Ticarcillin has activity against oral and intestinal Bacteroides species, although higher concentrations are required than are needed to inhibit the Enterobacteriaceae. Ticarcillin acts synergistically with aminoglycosides to inhibit P. aeruginosa. This group of compounds is rarely used intramuscularly since peak serum levels are inadequate for tissue Pseudomonas infections, but they provide adequate concentrations in the urine. Ticarcillin is administered in dosage of 200 to 300 mg/kg per day, divided into 4- or 6-hourly doses for 24 h. Ticarcillin is excreted by the renal tubules and accumulates in the presence of renal dysfunction. Since the drug contains 4.7 mmol of sodium, full doses of 12 to 30 g/d may precipitate congestive heart failure. Hypokalemia may also result since the nonreabsorbable portion of the anion is delivered to the distal tubule where it triggers a hydrogen ion exchange, resulting in potassium loss. Ticarcillin and other penicillins bind to ADP receptor sites on platelets and prevent normal platelet aggregation. Bleeding times are prolonged and clinical bleeding may occur in the presence of high serum levels. Ticarcillin cannot be administered in the same solution as aminoglycosides since it complexes with the aminoglycoside, rendering the aminoglycoside inactive. This does not normally occur in the body, except in the presence of renal failure, when very high concentrations of the antipseudomonas penicillins result in complexing with aminoglycosides. Ticarcillin has proved useful in the therapy of aspiration pneumonia in the hospital setting, in the therapy of the febrile neutropenic patient, in treatment of intraabdominal infection, and in treatment of gynecologic infections.

In the United States, there is only one oral antipseudomonas penicillin, indanyl carbenicillin. This is an alpha-carboxy ester of carbenicillin that has no intrinsic activity of its own, but is acid-stable and moderately well absorbed in the gastrointestinal tract, where it is hydrolyzed to yield free carbenicillin. Indanyl carbenicillin does not provide adequate serum or tissue levels for systemic infection and is useful only for the treatment of urinary tract infections or prostatitis. In the presence of decreased renal function, urine levels may be lower and may be inadequate to treat Pseudomonas urinary tract infections. This drug should be replaced by the quinolones.

Ureido penicillins Ureido penicillins, azlocillin, mezlocillin, and piperacillin, in contrast to the carboxy penicillins, are derivatives of ampicillin in which the presence of a side chain linked to the amino group on the alpha carbon provides increased binding to penicillin-binding proteins and more rapid passage through porin channels of gram-negative bacteria. Ureido penicillins are destroyed by β-lactamases of S. aureus, E. coli, Klebsiella, and Bacteroides. Azlocillin is 4 times more active than ticarcillin against P. aeruginosa and is less active against indole-positive Proteus species. It has the same activity as ampicillin against streptococcal species. It is not absorbed orally and must be given by the intravenous route to provide adequate serum levels to treat Pseudomonas infections. Since ureido penicillins show nonlinear pharmacokinetics, these drugs should be used in a larger dose administered at intervals of 6 h, rather than the 4-h interval used for ticarcillin. Azlocillin does not accumulate in the blood in renal failure to the same degree as ticarcillin. Its half-life increases to a maximum of only 4 h, even when renal insufficiency is present, necessitating less adjustment in dosage. Azlocillin enters the cerebrospinal fluid in the presence of meningeal inflammation, but levels are only 10 percent of serum levels. The drug is used primarily to treat Pseudomonas infections; the usual dose is 12 to 18 g/d.

Mezlocillin is a ureido penicillin that differs from ticarcillin by being more active against streptococci, particularly enterococci, and it inhibits approximately 60 percent of Klebsiella pneumoniae in a concentration of 16 μg/mL; virtually no Klebsiella are inhibited by ticarcillin. It is also more active against B. fragilis and H. influenzae. Mezlocillin has activity against P. aeruginosa similar to that of ticarcillin. Mezlocillin can be given at 6-hourly intervals, and the dose needs to be reduced only moderately as renal function declines. It is the least likely of the broad-spectrum penicillins to alter bleeding times, but the clinical significance of this is unknown. The drug has been effective in the treatment of respiratory, urinary, gynecologic, and surgical infections. Usual doses are 12 to 18 g/d for adults.

Piperacillin has excellent activity against streptococcal species, Neisseria, and Haemophilus, and it is the most active penicillin against P. aeruginosa. Like the other acyl ureido penicillins, it is destroyed by β-lactamases. It inhibits some community-acquired Klebsiella and Bacteroides species but will not inhibit Enterobacteriaceae which contain the plasmid β-lactamase. The human pharmacology of piperacillin is similar to the other ureido penicillins. It should be administered in a dose of 12 to 18 g/d, at 6-hourly intervals.

Other penicillins Amdinocillin is a penicillin active only against gram-negative species since it does not bind to the penicillin-binding proteins of gram-positive organisms. It has poor activity against Haemophilus and Neisseria, but is extremely active against E. coli, many Klebsiella, Enterobacter, and Citrobacter species. It has variable activity against Proteus species and does not inhibit Pseudomonas or Bacteroides fragilis. Amdinocillin acts synergistically with other penicillins and has been used in this way. Amdinocillin is not acid-stable and cannot be used orally except as the pivolyl ester which is well absorbed and immediately hydrolyzed, yielding the free compound.

Untoward reactions to penicillins The major adverse effects of penicillins are hypersensitivity reactions which range from minor rashes to immediate anaphylaxis. Anaphylactic reactions and accelerated urticarial reactions are due to IgE antibody. Patients who have had such reactions should not receive penicillins. Drug fever is common with all penicillins. Intestinal side effects produced by penicillins are diarrhea or bouts of enterocolitis, some of which are due to overgrowth of Clostridium difficile. Neutropenia, platelet dysfunction, and hemolytic anemia have followed the use of all the penicillins. Minor elevations in serum glutamic oxaloacetic transaminase (SGOT) occur most often with oxacillin, nafcillin, or carbenicillin. Neurologic adverse effects in the form of seizures will occur if penicillin G is administered in high doses to patients with decreased renal function. Renal toxicity has varied from allergic angiitis to interstitial nephritis most commonly with methicillin, but this complication can occur with all penicillins.

CEPHALOSPORINS Cephalosporins differ from penicillins by the presence of a dihydrothiazine ring rather than the five-membered thiazolidine ring fused to the four-membered β-lactam ring. Because of their structural configuration, cephalosporins have been modified chemically to produce compounds with different microbiologic and pharmacologic properties. It is useful to divide cephalosporins into so-called generations. In a particular group of cephalosporins, there may be marked differences in microbiologic activity and pharmacologic properties. Like the penicillins, cephalosporins inhibit cell wall biosynthesis and are bactericidal.

First-generation cephalosporins First-generation cephalosporins include some compounds that can be used only parenterally and some that can be used orally. The parenteral agents are cephalothin, cephapirin, cefazolin, and cephradine. Oral compounds are cephalexin, cephradine, cefadroxil, and cefaclor. First-generation cephalosporins inhibit group A, B, C, and G streptococci and most viridans group streptococci. They are active against *S. pneumoniae*, *S. aureus*, and *S. epidermidis*. Among the Enterobacteriaceae, *E. coli*, *P. mirabilis*, and *Klebsiella* species are inhibited. None of these first-generation drugs inhibit *Serratia*, *Enterobacter*, indole-positive *Proteus*, *P. aeruginosa*, or *B. fragilis* species. Only cefaclor can be considered therapeutically useful against *Haemophilus*. None of these agents is therapeutic for *Neisseria* species, although all of them have some inhibitory activity against these organisms in vitro.

In some hospitals, 20 to 30 percent of *E. coli* and *Klebsiella* are resistant to first-generation cephalosporins. Nonetheless, one of these agents, cefazolin, has continued to be useful. Cefazolin has a half-life of approximately 2 h and can be administered either by the intramuscular or intravenous routes. It accumulates in the body in the presence of decreased renal function, in which event dosage adjustments must be made. It is normally administered in doses of 0.5 to 1 g every 8 h. Cefazolin has proved useful as therapy of respiratory, skin, and urinary tract infections, and as therapy of endocarditis due to viridans streptococci in penicillin-allergic patients. It is also appropriate therapy for osteomyelitis due to staphylococcal species. Cefazolin is useful as a prophylactic antimicrobial agent at the time of orthopedic surgery, prosthetic valve surgery, and upper gastrointestinal operations. Cephalothin and cephapirin have half-lives of 4 h and are converted in the body to less active desacetyl derivatives. These drugs should be administered every 4 h.

Both cephalexin and cephradine are well absorbed after oral ingestion, yielding peak blood levels in the range of 15 to 20 μg/mL after a 0.5-g dose. Although these cephalosporins are less active against *S. aureus* than the parenteral first-generation cephalosporins, serum and tissue concentrations are adequate to treat many minor staphylococcal infections in penicillin-allergic patients. Both drugs have a half-life of approximately 1 h and are usually administered three or four times daily. The drugs are totally excreted in the urine, yielding high concentrations inhibitory to common urinary pathogens.

Cefadroxil is a parahydroxy derivative of cephalexin which has a longer half-life, allowing it to be administered twice daily. Otherwise, its antimicrobial activity is identical to that of cephalexin.

Cefaclor has found utility primarily as a therapeutic agent for respiratory infections in children caused by *H. influenzae* or other susceptible organisms. It is partially β-lactamase-stable, but the concentrations in ear fluid are adequate to eradicate β-lactamase-producing *H. influenzae*. It should not be used for serious infections caused by β-lactamase-producing strains and is ineffective in urinary tract infections due to β-lactamase-producing *E. coli* and *Klebsiella*.

Second-generation cephalosporins Second-generation cephalosporins probably should not be grouped as a class since the compounds within this class have markedly different antibacterial and pharmacologic properties. They are most frequently used by the intravenous route; only cefuroxime axetil can be used orally. Cefamandole has excellent activity against streptococcal and staphylococcal species with the exception of *E. faecalis*. It is more active than

first-generation cephalosporins against *E. coli* and *Klebsiella* and has increased activity against *H. influenzae*. It is destroyed by β-lactamases of some gram-negative species, and is not active against *Bacteroides* or *Pseudomonas* species. Cefamandole has a relatively short half-life, 0.7 h, and is administered every 4 to 6 h in doses of 1 to 2 g. The drug does not produce adequate concentrations in the cerebrospinal fluid, and should not be used in patients in whom meningitis is suspected. Because of potential nephrotoxicity, this drug is used rarely and has been replaced by other cephalosporins.

Cefuroxime is a β-lactamase-stable cephalosporin that inhibits most streptococcal and staphylococcal species, *H. influenzae*, penicillinase-producing *N. gonorrhoeae*, and β-lactamase-producing Enterobacteriaceae. It is not active against *E. faecalis*, *Bacteroides fragilis*, or *P. aeruginosa*. Cefuroxime has a half-life of approximately 1.5 h, permitting administration at 8-hourly intervals. It enters the cerebrospinal fluid in concentrations adequate to treat meningitis due to *H. influenzae*, *S. pneumoniae*, and *N. meningitidis*. CSF concentrations are inadequate to treat meningitis due to *E. coli* or *Klebsiella* species. Cefuroxime has been used in the therapy of respiratory infections, biliary tract infections, soft tissue infections, osteomyelitis, and urinary tract infections. It can also be used for therapy of meningitis in children and young adults. Cefuroxime axetil is an oral form for use in respiratory infections, particularly those in which β-lactamase-producing *H. influenzae* are suspected, and for cutaneous infections.

Cefonicid is a cephalosporin structurally related to cefamandole. However, substitution of a different moiety at position 3 of the dihydrothiazine ring has provided the compound with a long half-life of approximately 4 to 5 h. Cefonicid activity is similar to that of cefamandole and cefuroxime, with the exception of lower activity against *S. aureus*. Cefonicid has been used in a single daily dose administered either intravenously or intramuscularly to treat respiratory, skin, and urinary tract infections due to susceptible organisms. It should not be used to treat meningeal infections.

Cefoxitin is a cephalosporin which possesses a methoxy group affixed to the β-lactam that provides excellent β-lactamase resistance but decreases activity against gram-positive organisms such as staphylococci. Cefoxitin inhibits most staphylococci at concentrations of 2 to 4 μg/mL, and *S. pneumoniae* are inhibited at similar concentrations. It possesses no activity against *E. faecalis*. Cefoxitin inhibits *E. coli* and *Klebsiella* species resistant to first-generation cephalosporins. It lacks activity against *Enterobacter* and *Citrobacter* species, and does not inhibit *Pseudomonas*. Cefoxitin has good activity against *B. fragilis*, inhibiting 85 percent of clinical isolates at a concentration between 16 to 32 μg/mL, which is readily achieved in humans. Cefoxitin has a half-life of approximately 0.8 h. It does not yield adequate concentrations within the CSF. The drug accumulates in the presence of decreased renal function, so that dose adjustments must be made. Cefoxitin has been widely used as therapy of mixed aerobic and anaerobic intraabdominal infections and in the treatment of gynecologic infections. Cefoxitin combined with doxycycline is effective therapy for pelvic inflammatory disease. Cefoxitin has also been used as a parenteral prophylactic agent for colon surgery, particularly in patients in whom oral prophylactic programs are not feasible.

Third-generation cephalosporins Third-generation cephalosporins can be grouped into several convenient classes. The first of these are the aminothiazolyl iminomethoxy cephalosporins which consist of cefotaxime, ceftizoxime, cefmenoxime, and ceftriaxone. These agents possess excellent activity against hemolytic streptococci and *S. pneumoniae*, inhibiting these species at concentrations <0.1 μg/mL. They do not inhibit *E. faecalis*. The compounds are highly active against *H. influenzae*, *N. meningitidis*, and *N. gonorrhoeae*, including β-lactamase-producing strains. Because of their high affinity for penicillin-binding proteins, these compounds inhibit the majority of the Enterobacteriaceae at concentrations below 4.0 μg/mL, although some *Enterobacter* and *Citrobacter* are resistant. These four agents do not show adequate activity against *P. aeruginosa* and *Acinetobacter*.

Cefotaxime has a half-life of approximately 1 h, and it is converted to a desacetyl derivative which has a half-life of approximately 1.6 h. Although the desacetyl derivative is less active than the parent compound, it is more active than most second-generation cephalosporins and acts synergistically with the parent compound to inhibit some microorganisms. Cefotaxime produces concentrations in the CSF ranging from 1 to 30 μg/mL, depending upon the degree of inflammation and the dose used. It has proved effective as therapy of meningitis due to group B streptococci, E. coli, H. influenzae, N. meningitidis, S. pneumoniae, and Klebsiella. Although cefotaxime has a relatively short half-life, its high activity and the presence of an active metabolite indicate that it can be administered 8-hourly in most infections, except in febrile neutropenic patients.

Ceftizoxime has a slightly longer half-life than cefotaxime at 1.6 h, and can be administered every 8 to 12 h in the majority of infections.

Ceftriaxone differs from the aforementioned compounds because it has a half-life of approximately 7 h in normal individuals. Sixty percent of ceftriaxone is cleared by the kidney, and the remainder of the drug is cleared through the biliary system. Although ceftriaxone is 95 percent bound to serum proteins, it produces such high serum levels that adequate free drug is available to inhibit the majority of gram-positive and gram-negative bacteria with the exception of E. faecalis, Pseudomonas, and Bacteroides. Ceftriaxone enters the CSF and is removed from the CSF extremely slowly. Levels well above the minimum inhibitory concentration for most meningeal pathogens are present 24 h after the administration of a single dose. Ceftriaxone has been administered once and twice daily to treat a variety of infections and offers the possibility of once-daily intramuscular therapy in the home setting to complete treatment initially instituted within the hospital.

Moxalactam is an oxacephalosporin with oxygen replacing the sulfur in the bicyclic ring structure. The drug possesses an N-methylthiotetrazole group at position 3 of the bicyclic structure. This structure has been associated with two adverse reactions. The first is a disulfiram reaction when alcohol is ingested. This is caused by interference with alcohol dehydrogenase and the accumulation of acetaldehyde. The second is hypoprothrombinemia which appears related to dimer formation of the N-methylthiotetrazole which interferes with the production of vitamin K. Moxalactam administered in doses above 4 g/d also will cause platelet dysfunction due to its effect on ADP receptors on the platelets. Because of these factors, patients receiving moxalactam should receive vitamin K at least twice weekly, and platelet function should be assessed by bleeding times. Concern over bleeding problems associated with moxalactam has limited its use in the United States.

Cefotetan is a 7-alpha-methoxy cephalosporin that has in vitro activity similar to cefoxitin against anaerobic microorganisms and activity slightly less than that of the aminothiazolyl cephalosporins against gram-positive cocci and the Enterobacteriaceae. It does not inhibit Pseudomonas species. Cefotetan has a half-life of approximately 4 h, and can be administered twice or three times daily.

Cephalosporins with activity against Pseudomonas aeruginosa
Cefoperazone inhibits Enterobacteriaceae and the majority of gram-positive microorganisms, and will inhibit most P. aeruginosa at concentrations below 32 μg/mL. It is destroyed by some β-lactamase-producing E. coli, Klebsiella, and B. fragilis strains. Cefoperazone is approximately 85 percent protein bound. Following a 2-g dose, peak blood levels of 250 μg/mL are achieved. The half-life of the drug is approximately 2 h. Only 25 percent of cefoperazone is removed from the body by the kidney; the remainder is removed by biliary mechanisms. Cefoperazone is used in a dose of 2 g twice daily to treat gram-positive and gram-negative infections. Higher doses are usually needed to treat serious Pseudomonas infections. Since cefoperazone contains an N-methylthiotetrazole group, it can produce disulfiram reactions and prolongation of the prothrombin time. Therefore vitamin K should be administered once a week to patients treated with this agent. It does not alter platelet function.

Ceftazidime is an aminothiazolyl cephalosporin that contains a propyliminocarboxy group which has excellent activity against P. aeruginosa and many strains of P. cepacia and Acinetobacter. It is slightly less active than cefotaxime against streptococcal species and fourfold to eightfold less active against S. aureus, but has similar activity against the Enterobacteriaceae. Ceftazidime has no activity against B. fragilis and is inactive against many clostridial species. Ceftazidime is cleared primarily by glomerular filtration and has a half-life of approximately 1.8 h. It enters the CSF in concentrations adequate to inhibit the majority of organisms producing meningitis and has been used successfully to treat a number of patients with meningitis caused by Haemophilus, Neisseria, and even P. aeruginosa. Ceftazidime accumulates in the presence of decreased renal function, and dosage adjustments must be made in patients with markedly decreased renal function. Ceftazidime has proved to be a successful drug in various serious infections, including pneumonia, bacteremia, urosepsis, osteomyelitis, and deep skin structure infections due to Enterobacteriaceae and P. aeruginosa. It is widely used to treat suspected infection in the febrile neutropenic patient singly or in combination with vancomycin.

OTHER β-LACTAM ANTIBIOTICS A number of novel compounds belonging to the β-lactam class have been developed. These agents differ widely in their antibacterial and pharmacologic properties.

Imipenem Imipenem is a carbapenem which has excellent in vitro activity against aerobic gram-positive species such as the hemolytic streptococci and S. pneumoniae; it inhibits E. faecalis, S. aureus, and S. epidermidis, including β-lactamase-producing strains, and Listeria monocytogenes. The majority of the Enterobacteriaceae are inhibited by concentrations <1 μg/mL, as are H. influenzae and N. gonorrhoeae. P. aeruginosa, including strains resistant to penicillins and to aminoglycosides, are inhibited by concentrations of 1 to 8 μg/mL. P. cepacia and Acinetobacter are inhibited, but P. maltophilia are resistant. Imipenem inhibits the majority of anaerobic species including B. fragilis. Imipenem is not absorbed after oral ingestion due to its instability in gastric acid. It is hydrolyzed in the kidney by a peptidase, dehydropeptidase-1, which is located on the brush border of the proximal renal tubular cells. To overcome the problem of destruction of imipenem, a dehydropeptidase inhibitor, cilastatin, is administered with imipenem.

Imipenem has a relatively short half-life of approximately 1 h; doses of 500 mg to 1 g provide plasma, tissue, and urine concentrations sufficient to inhibit the majority of bacteria. Imipenem has been used to treat bacteremia, respiratory infections, intraabdominal infections, bone and joint infections, endocarditis, and urinary tract infections due to organisms that are susceptible to it and that are resistant to other β-lactams and to aminoglycosides. Nausea occurs in some patients following too rapid infusion. The most important toxic effect is seizures, which occur in less than 5 percent of patients.

Monobactams Aztreonam is a monocyclic β-lactam which inhibits only aerobic gram-negative bacteria and does not inhibit gram-positive or anaerobic organisms. Most Enterobacteriaceae, Haemophilus, and Neisseria species, including β-lactamase-producing strains, are inhibited by <1 μg/mL. Most P. aeruginosa are inhibited by 16 μg/mL. Aztreonam is not absorbed following oral ingestion. It has a half-life between 1.5 and 2 h, and following doses of 1 g, serum and urine concentrations above the MICs of most Enterobacteriaceae and Pseudomonas are readily achieved. Aztreonam accumulates in the presence of renal failure with an increase in half-life to 6 h. The drug has been used to treat a variety of serious infections due to aerobic gram-negative species including E. coli, Klebsiella, Serratia, and Pseudomonas. It has been used in combination with clindamycin, antistaphylococcal penicillins, or vancomycin in mixed infections where it has been utilized as a replacement for the aminoglycosides. Aztreonam enters the CSF, but only a small number of patients with meningitis have been treated. The drug does not cross-react with penicillins and cephalosporins and is safe to administer to patients allergic to these agents.

β-LACTAMASE INHIBITORS Clavulanate is a β-lactamase inhibitor that has minimal antibacterial activity of its own but inhibits the β-lactamases of *S. aureus*, many Enterobacteriaceae, *Bacteroides*, *Klebsiella*, and *Branhamella* species. Clavulanate is a suicide inhibitor of β-lactamases. Potassium clavulanate is moderately well absorbed from the gastrointestinal tract and peak serum levels occur approximately at the same time as with amoxicillin, with which it is combined. The combination of clavulanate and amoxicillin (augmentin) does not alter the pharmacologic properties of either drug. Augmentin can be administered every 8 h and has been used to treat skin and bite wound infections due to β-lactamase-producing bacteria, otitis due to *H. influenzae*, and urinary tract infections due to β-lactamase-producing *E. coli* and *Klebsiella*. It has also been used in deep cutaneous infections due to anaerobic microorganisms and in upper respiratory infections in which *Branhamella* has been shown to be an important component.

Timentin is a combination of 3 g ticarcillin and 100 or 200 mg of clavulanate. Timentin increases the activity of ticarcillin to include *S. aureus*, β-lactamase-producing *Haemophilus*, *Branhamella*, *Bacteroides* species, *Klebsiella*, and many of the β-lactamase-producing *E. coli* strains. Timentin has been used to treat respiratory, cutaneous, gynecologic, and intraabdominal infections, osteomyelitis, and urinary tract infections, and as combination therapy in the febrile neutropenic patient.

Sulbactam is a penicillanic acid sulfone that inhibits the plasmid and chromosomally mediated β-lactamases inhibited by clavulanate. It has been combined with ampicillin, and in the presence of concentrations of 8 μg/mL of sulbactam and 16 μg/mL of ampicillin, most species of staphylococci, *Klebsiella*, *Haemophilus*, *Branhamella*, *E. coli*, and *Bacteroides* are inhibited. Sulbactam has pharmacokinetics in humans similar to ampicillin. It is administered intravenously. The ampicillin-sulbactam combination has been used successfully to treat urinary tract, intraabdominal, skin, gynecologic, and respiratory infections due to β-lactamase-producing microorganisms.

VANCOMYCIN Vancomycin is a glycopeptide that is active only against gram-positive species. It has assumed increasing importance because of the widespread appearance of methicillin-resistant staphylococci and the recognition of antibiotic-associated colitis caused by *C. difficile*. Vancomycin inhibits cell wall synthesis and is bactericidal. It is active against all hemolytic streptococcal species, *viridans* group streptococci, *S. pneumoniae*, *L. monocytogenes*, and the *Corynebacterium* species resistant to other β-lactam drugs. For most infections vancomycin is administered by the intravenous route. It is eliminated from the body by glomerular filtration and has a half-life of approximately 6 h in individuals with normal renal function. In the presence of anuria, its half-life may be prolonged to between 5 to 9 days, and it may be detected in serum for as long as 21 days after a single 1-g dose. Vancomycin is not absorbed from the gastrointestinal tract. It can be used orally, but not parenterally, to treat enterocolitis, since it is not secreted into the intestine. Following intravenous administration of a 1-g dose, peak levels of 20 to 125 μg/mL are found in serum, and when given orally, concentrations between 100 to 800 μg/mL are found in the stool. Vancomycin enters the CSF poorly. It may be administered once weekly to patients in renal failure as therapy for serious staphylococcal or streptococcal infections. Hemodialysis does not remove vancomycin. Rapid infusion of vancomycin will produce a "red man" syndrome due to histamine release, with fever, chills, and generalized erythema. This reaction can be mitigated by antihistamine drugs, e.g., diphenhydramine. Vancomycin also produces ototoxicity. It is probably minimally nephrotoxic, but when used with an aminoglycoside, nephrotoxicity and ototoxicity may be increased. Vancomycin is the therapy of choice for methicillin-resistant staphylococcal infections and for therapy of *E. faecalis* endocarditis in penicillin-allergic patients. Vancomycin is also useful in the prevention of bacterial endocarditis in patients allergic to penicillin, particularly those who have a prosthetic heart valve (see Chap. 90).

AMINOGLYCOSIDES AND SPECTINOMYCIN Aminoglycoside antibiotics are defined by the presence of amino sugars linked by a glycoside bound to an aminocyclitol ring. All aminoglycosides contain amino groups and hydroxyl groups which are important in the antibacterial activity of the compounds, as well as being the sites of enzymatic inactivation by bacterial enzymes. The drugs' ototoxicity and nephrotoxicity is also determined by their structure. Aminoglycosides are bactericidal since they bind irreversibly to proteins in the ribosomes and cause the interruption of the flow of genetic information. Enzymatic modification of the aminoglycosides by enzymes in plasmid-carrying bacteria results in their inactivation since compounds that have been adenylated, phosphorylated, or acetylated do not bind well to ribosomes and fail to induce a protein which facilitates their uptake by bacteria.

Their antibacterial activity is to inhibit members of the Enterobacteriaceae, that is, *E. coli*, *Klebsiella*, *Serratia*, *Enterobacter*, etc. Gentamicin, tobramycin, amikacin, sisomicin, and netilmicin all inhibit *P. aeruginosa*, but kanamycin does not. None of the agents are active against anaerobic species such as *Clostridium* or *Bacteroides*. They are not active against a number of gram-positive cocci, including *S. pneumoniae* or hemolytic streptococci. Aminoglycosides act synergistically with penicillins to inhibit *E. faecalis* and with antipseudomonas penicillins (aztreonam, imipenem, and ceftazidime) to inhibit *Pseudomonas*. They also act synergistically with nafcillin or oxacillin against *S. aureus*.

Aminoglycosides are highly water soluble and stable over a wide pH range but are markedly less active at acid pH, and their activity is decreased in the presence of divalent cations such as calcium and magnesium. An anaerobic environment decreases their effectiveness against both Enterobacteriaceae and staphylococci. They are inactivated by nucleic acid debris from decaying cells.

Aminoglycosides are not normally absorbed from the intestine. However, the small amounts absorbed can be sufficient to produce toxicity in the patient with markedly decreased renal function. This is particularly true when neomycin is administered orally in large amounts. The drugs can be absorbed when applied to burns or after irrigation of ulcers or wounds if excessive amounts are used, and they will produce oto- and nephrotoxicity following such topical application. Aminoglycosides are well absorbed after intramuscular use. Peak serum levels occur 30 to 90 min after an intramuscular injection, and in normal individuals with creatinine clearances >100 mL, their half-life is approximately 2 h. Aminoglycosides are distributed in the extracellular fluid and enter pleural, peritoneal, and synovial fluids. They do not penetrate the CSF or the eye. Extremely high concentrations are present in renal cortical tissue and persist there for up to several weeks after a course of therapy. All aminoglycosides are removed from the body by glomerular filtration. The drugs are not metabolized, and biliary excretion is minimal. With all the aminoglycosides, there is marked accumulation in the presence of decreased renal function. The half-life of the drugs in the presence of anuria is 35 to 50 h. Urinary concentrations in normal individuals are 25 to 100 times the plasma concentrations. However, in the presence of decreased renal function, only a small amount of drug is present in the urine.

The pharmacokinetics of aminoglycosides in children and the elderly are markedly different than those in young healthy adults. Although the volume of distribution in the elderly is similar to that in young adults, half-lives are considerably longer due to decreased glomerular function. Glomerular function in the elderly may not necessarily be reflected by a higher serum creatinine because of decreased creatinine production in this group. It is therefore important always to use a calculated creatinine clearance in order to estimate the half-life of an aminoglycoside in the elderly. The equation of Cockroft and Gault by which aminoglycoside concentrations may be calculated is

$$C_{cr}(\text{min}) = \frac{(140 - \text{age}) \times \text{wt (kg)}}{\text{Cr (mg/dL)} \times 72}$$

In obese patients, the volume of distribution of aminoglycosides is approximately 75 percent of that in normal patients. In calculating doses, this must be taken into consideration. Conversely, in a markedly protein-malnourished individual, there will be a larger volume of distribution so that the total body weight should be multiplied by 120 percent compared to that of the normal patient.

In initiating therapy with aminoglycosides, a loading dose should be administered in order to achieve a therapeutic serum level as quickly as possible. Reasonable serum levels, 30 to 60 min after the initial dose, are between 5 and 10 μg/mL for gentamicin, tobramycin, netilmicin, and sisomicin, and between 20 and 40 μg/mL for kanamycin and amikacin. A loading dose of 2 mg/kg for gentamicin, tobramycin, and netilmicin and a loading dose of 8 mg/kg for amikacin are satisfactory. The loading dose is the same whether or not elimination is impaired by renal dysfunction. Since loading doses are sizable, they should be given intravenously over 20 to 30 min to avoid the risk of neuromuscular toxicity. In individuals with creatinine clearances >80 mL/min, a dose of 1.5 to 2 mg/kg of gentamicin, tobramycin, or netilmicin every 8 h, or 5 mg/kg of amikacin every 8 h, provides adequate peak and trough levels. The daily dose of aminoglycosides must be reduced in patients whose renal function is impaired. A simple way of calculating the total daily dose is to calculate the patient's creatinine clearance based on age, sex, weight, and serum creatinine. The clearance of aminoglycosides is linearly related to creatinine clearance. Therefore, the ratio of the patient's creatinine clearance to a normal creatinine clearance approximates the aminoglycoside clearance. An individual with a creatinine clearance of 30 mL/min or 30 percent should receive 30 percent of the usual daily dose. Instead of 4.5 to 6 mg/kg per day, the dose should be reduced to 1.5 to 2 mg/kg per day. This dose can be administered either as a reduced dose at the regular time interval of 8 h, or the total dose can be divided and administered at less frequent intervals. Calculated predictions of aminoglycoside levels provide reasonable approximations, but blood levels should be measured, both at the peak and trough, and dose adjustments should be made accordingly.

Toxicity of aminoglycosides All aminoglycosides share similar toxicity. Hypersensitivity is exceedingly rare, but all of these drugs will produce some degree of nephrotoxicity. The initial renal toxicity is nonoliguric renal failure. There is a loss of concentrating ability, proteinuria, casts in the urine, and renal enzymuria. Subsequently, the serum creatinine and blood urea nitrogen (BUN) will rise. Nephrotoxicity involves the proximal tubular cells. Risk factors for development of toxicity are old age, concomitant hypotension at the onset of aminoglycoside therapy, use of other nephrotoxic agents simultaneously, and, perhaps, concomitant liver disease. Aminoglycoside nephrotoxicity is usually mild and reversible. However, it can result in renal failure and may even require dialysis. For this reason, it is critical to follow aminoglycoside blood levels in patients receiving these drugs. Ototoxicity can be aimed at either the cochlea or the vestibular apparatus. The mechanism of the toxicity is the destruction of hair cells within the organ of Corti or those in the ampullar cristae. Once these cells have been damaged, they cannot regenerate. Detectable toxicity occurs in 3 to 5 percent of patients receiving aminoglycosides. Although tinnitus and a feeling of fullness in the ears may precede hearing loss, it is not a useful guide to hearing damage. Since the high tones outside the conversation range are affected first, ototoxicity may not be recognized initially. Less frequent forms of toxicity seen with these drugs are neuromuscular blockade and malabsorption. There is evidence that administration of the total daily dose to nonneutropenic patients as a single dose provides a similar response with less toxicity.

Individual aminoglycosides Streptomycin is used for treatment of selected cases of tuberculosis (for which it is administered twice weekly), tularemia, plague, and brucellosis. It is used in the treatment of endocarditis due to *E. faecalis* or viridans streptococci, provided that the strains are susceptible to less than 2000 μg/mL. Neomycin's sole use today is in bowel preparation for intestinal surgery, combined with erythromycin or metronidazole. Kanamycin has been superseded

by other aminoglycosides. Gentamicin remains useful as a first-line agent in the treatment of gram-negative infections, particularly because of its relatively low cost. Tobramycin is more active than gentamicin against *P. aeruginosa* and less active against *Serratia* species. Its clinical efficacy is equivalent to that of gentamicin, but there is some evidence that tobramycin is somewhat less nephrotoxic than gentamicin. Amikacin is less likely to be inactivated by plasmid-mediated resistance enzymes and should be used particularly in those situations in which it is likely that there is aminoglycoside resistance. Netilmicin is a derivative of gentamicin which is less nephrotoxic and ototoxic. It is less active against *Pseudomonas* than is gentamicin or tobramycin, but it inhibits a number of strains of *E. coli*, *Klebsiella*, and *Serratia* resistant to gentamicin and tobramycin.

Spectinomycin is an amino cyclitol antibiotic that has been used in a single 2-g intramuscular dose to treat gonorrhea due to penicillinase-producing strains. Its use has been superseded by compounds such as ceftriaxone, which can be administered in 125- to 250-mg intramuscular doses to treat penicillinase-producing gonococcal strains.

TETRACYCLINES Tetracyclines are bacteriostatic agents that inhibit protein biosynthesis. By binding to the 30 S ribosome they inhibit binding of aminoacyl tRNA. Resistance to tetracyclines is due to plasmid-mediated synthesis of a protein which results in a drug efflux. Tetracycline-resistant bacteria bind less drug; what does enter is pumped out by an energy-dependent process. They inhibit many gram-positive and gram-negative species and are active against other important organisms, including Rickettsiae, *Chlamydia*, and *Mycoplasma*. They also inhibit *Actinomyces*, but do not inhibit *Nocardia*. Resistance to the tetracyclines has appeared in many species. Some strains of *S. pneumoniae* and *S. pyogenes* are resistant. Many staphylococci are resistant to the tetracyclines as well as many enteric organisms such as *Shigella*. In general, organisms resistant to one tetracycline are resistant to all members of the group. Tetracyclines can be divided into three groups based on pharmacology. The short-acting group consists of tetracycline, chlortetracycline, and oxytetracycline. The intermediate group consists of demeclocycline and methacycline, and the long-acting compounds are doxycycline and minocycline. Tetracyclines are incompletely absorbed from the gastrointestinal tract, and their absorption is increased if they are taken in the fasting state. Their absorption is decreased by milk, milk products, and magnesium-containing antacids and iron. The binding of tetracyclines to plasma proteins varies with the type of drug. They enter the CSF, but concentrations are inadequate for treatment of meningitis. Since the agents cross the placenta, they cannot be given to pregnant women since they will be sequestered into bone and tooth structures causing abnormalities. High concentrations of the drugs are found in the bile, and there is a significant enterohepatic circulation. Minocycline is excreted in saliva and lacrimal secretions producing antibacterial concentrations in the oropharynx; for this reason it has been used as prophylaxis for meningococcal disease. However, since minocycline can cause vestibular toxicity, it has been supplanted by rifampin. With the exception of doxycycline and chlortetracycline, the tetracyclines are eliminated from the body primarily by glomerular filtration. In the presence of renal failure, the half-life of all tetracyclines, except these two drugs, increases markedly.

The tetracyclines may cause skin rashes, particularly with solar exposure. Gastrointestinal effects include nausea, vomiting, and diarrhea. The diarrhea may be either a direct toxic effect, or due to pseudomembranous colitis. Severe hepatotoxicity has occurred during prolonged therapy with high doses, particularly in pregnant women. In some, often debilitated, patients there may be catabolic effects with protein breakdown, weight loss, and nitrogen retention. Tetracycline's effect on the gut flora may cause prolongation of prothrombin time.

Tetracyclines are rarely the drugs of choice in most common bacterial infections because of the large number of other drugs available. There are specific indications for use of these compounds. In rickettsial infections such as Rocky Mountain spotted fever, typhus, or scrub typhus, tetracycline remains the drug of choice. They are drugs of choice in the treatment of sexually transmitted chlamydial infections and are useful in the treatment of *Mycoplasma* infections. Tetracyclines have proved useful in the therapy of Lyme disease in adults, brucellosis, relapsing fever due to *Borrelia*, and, combined with streptomycin, for treatment of complicated plague. They have also proved useful in therapy of infections due to *Actinomyces* and in *Pasteurella multocida* infections in penicillin-allergic patients. Tetracyclines have been used in a number of syndromes such as acne, bacterial exacerbations of bronchitis, malabsorption syndrome, and sinusitis. They are not the drugs of choice for streptococcal or pneumococcal infections or for anaerobic infections in the abdomen.

CHLORAMPHENICOL   Chloramphenicol binds to 50 S ribosomes inhibiting peptide bond formation. It is bacteriostatic. Resistance is due to acetylation of the drug by the plasmid-mediated enzyme chloramphenicol transacetylase. Acetylation of the OH of the C-1 carbon prevents binding to ribosomes. Chloramphenicol is extremely active against aerobic and anaerobic bacteria, *Rickettsia*, *Chlamydia*, *Mycoplasma*, and *Spirochaeta*. The organisms most commonly causing meningitis in childhood, *H. influenzae*, *S. pneumoniae*, and *N. meningitidis*, are highly susceptible to this agent and most *Bacteroides* species are inhibited by it.

Chloramphenicol is well-absorbed from the gastrointestinal tract. Blood levels following oral ingestion are superior to those achieved after intravenous injection since the inactive chloramphenicol succinate ester which is used in the intravenous preparation is incompletely hydrolyzed within the body. Chloramphenicol is metabolized in the liver where it is conjugated with glucuronic acid and is excreted in an inactive form by the kidneys. It diffuses well into many tissues and body fluids and produces excellent concentrations in the cerebrospinal fluid and brain tissue. In the presence of renal disease, the half-life of the drug is not significantly increased. In contrast, in patients with hepatic disease, serum levels may increase yielding levels capable of producing bone marrow suppression.

The most important toxic effect of chloramphenicol is on bone marrow. Approximately 1 in 25,000 patients who receive the drug develop aplastic anemia. This is an unpredictable, idiosyncratic response. There is also a dose-related anemia and leukopenia which is predictable when blood levels are above 25 μg/mL. This toxicity is reversible when the antibiotic is discontinued. Chloramphenicol cannot be given to newborns since they are unable to conjugate the drug and develop toxicity due to excessive levels of free compound.

In the United States, chloramphenicol is now rarely used. The new cephalosporins enter the CSF and provide concentrations that are effective against many pathogens. Metronidazole, clindamycin, cefoxitin, and imipenem are available to treat severe *B. fragilis* infections. Many strains of *S. typhi* are resistant to chloramphenicol, and other drugs such as trimethoprim-sulfamethoxazole or ciprofloxacin should be used.

Chloramphenicol undergoes a number of significant drug interactions. It prolongs the half-life of tolbutamide, chlorpropamide, phenytoin, and warfarin by inhibiting hepatic microsomal enzymes.

ERYTHROMYCIN   Erythromycin is a macrolide antibiotic that acts primarily in a bacteriostatic fashion by binding to 50 S ribosomes and preventing peptidyl transfer and translocation. Resistance is due to methylation of two adenine nucleotides in the 23 S component of the 50 S RNA. The resistance is normally repressed in nonresistant bacteria and is induced in the presence of a plasmid. The drug inhibits *S. pyogenes*, *S. pneumoniae*, many strains of *Neisseria*, some strains of *H. influenzae*, *C. diphtheriae*, *Clostridium*, *Listeria*, *Treponema*, and a number of anaerobic cocci and oral *Bacteroides* species. It is effective against *Mycoplasma pneumoniae* and *Legionella pneumophila*.

Erythromycin is used by either the oral or intravenous route. There are a number of different erythromycin preparations available. Esters and salts of erythromycin are more acid-stable. The erythromycin base and ethyl succinate forms are better absorbed when taken in the fasting state. The stearate form is better absorbed when taken with meals. The estolate salt is associated with more cholestatic

hepatitis in adults than are the other forms. The normal half-life of erythromycin is 1.5 h, and appreciable serum levels are maintained for at least 6 h. Therefore, in a number of infections such as streptococcal pharyngitis, the drug can be administered on a twice-daily basis. In anuric patients, reduction in dosage is generally not necessary.

Erythromycin is one of the safest antibiotics, and untoward reactions are extremely uncommon except for cholestatic hepatitis. The main side effect has been epigastric distress and nausea. Hearing loss does occur in association with large doses administered to elderly patients with renal insufficiency. Erythromycin used concomitantly with oral theophylline preparations may cause increased blood levels of theophylline and potential theophylline toxicity. Erythromycin also causes elevation in urinary catecholamines and in 17-hydroxycorticosteroids. The major use of erythromycin is to treat streptococcal pharyngitis in the penicillin-allergic patient, or in the treatment of otitis media in combination with sulfonamides. Erythromycin can also be used during pregnancy to treat skin infections or, in high doses, to treat syphilis in pregnancy. Erythromycin in a dose of 0.5 to 1 g every 6 h is the therapy of choice for *Legionella* pneumonia, and it is the drug of choice for *M. pneumoniae* and some *Ureaplasma* infections.

LINCOMYCIN AND CLINDAMYCIN   Lincosamide antibiotics inhibit many of the same organisms as do the erythromycins. Their mechanism of action is inhibition of protein synthesis. Clindamycin is a less effective inducer of the methylating enzyme. The clinical significance becomes evident in the development of resistance of erythromycin-resistant, clindamycin-susceptible *S. aureus* infections. Lincomycin is rarely used today and clindamycin is the primary agent in this class. Clindamycin inhibits *S. pneumoniae*, *S. pyogenes*, and viridans group streptococci. It lacks activity against *E. faecalis*. Many strains of *S. aureus* and *S. epidermidis* are inhibited by clindamycin, and it has excellent activity against most anaerobic species, including *Clostridium* and *Bacteroides*. It also inhibits *Chlamydia*.

Clindamycin is well-absorbed following oral ingestion and can also be administered intramuscularly or intravenously. The serum half-life is approximately 2.5 h, and the drug is metabolized primarily in the liver. Dosage adjustments are minor except in the presence of hepatic failure. Clindamycin produces high concentrations in bone, and has been found to enter white blood cells. Its most significant toxic effect is diarrhea, which has often been associated with pseudomembranous colitis caused by *C. difficile*. If diarrhea develops during clindamycin therapy, the drug should be discontinued. If diarrhea persists, proctoscopy or assay for *C. difficile* toxin should be performed and therapy with oral vancomycin or metronidazole instituted.

The major therapeutic use of clindamycin is for anaerobic infections or as a combination with an aminoglycoside or aztreonam. Clindamycin provides coverage against streptococcal, staphylococcal, and anaerobic species while the aerobic gram-negative organism is attacked by the other agent. Clindamycin has proved to be an excellent agent for the therapy of anaerobic pulmonary disease, particularly in patients who have failed to respond to penicillin. Topical solutions of clindamycin are useful in the treatment of severe acne. Clindamycin should not be used for serious staphylococcal infections due to erythromycin-resistant bacteria because resistance to clindamycin will develop. Furthermore, its bacteriostatic activity against *S. aureus* makes it a less desirable choice against this organism than active β-lactams or vancomycin.

RIFAMPIN   Rifampin is a macrocyclic antibiotic produced by a *Streptomyces*. It inhibits DNA-directed RNA polymerase. Resistance is due to change of one amino acid on the beta subunit of the polymerase altering the binding of rifampin to the enzyme. The degree of resistance is related to the degree that the enzyme is changed. Resistance can develop during therapy due to selection of a subpopulation of microorganisms that contain altered polymerase. Rifampin is available in the United States only for oral use. The drug has been used primarily in the treatment of tuberculosis. However, rifampin inhibits many microorganisms: coagulase-positive and -negative staphylococci, as well as *N. meningitidis*, *N. gonorrhoeae*, and *H. influenzae*. It is the most active agent known against *L. pneumophila* and is also effective against *L. micdadei* and *L. dumoffei*. It inhibits *C. difficile* at concentrations less than 1 μg/mL and inhibits the majority of streptococci and *S. pneumoniae* at concentrations of less than 0.1 μg/mL. Although rifampin inhibits many of the Enterobacteriaceae and some strains of *Pseudomonas*, resistance develops rapidly. The drug inhibits *Chlamydia*, but *Ureaplasma urealyticum* and *Treponema pallidum* usually are resistant.

Rifampin is well-absorbed from the gastrointestinal tract and, following ingestion of 600 mg in an adult or 10 mg/kg in children, peak serum concentrations of approximately 8 μg/mL are reached. With repeated doses, drug levels decrease slightly because the drug stimulates the hepatic enzymes responsible for its metabolism. The drug is approximately 75 percent protein-bound. Rifampin is both metabolized and excreted by the liver. The desacetyl derivative is not reabsorbed and is excreted via the stool; only 5 to 30 percent of the dose is excreted in the urine. In general, dosage adjustment is unnecessary in renal failure, but a lower dose should be used in patients with severe hepatic dysfunction. Food will interfere with the absorption of rifampin, lowering and delaying peak blood levels. Rifampin penetrates into all body tissues and enters white cells. High concentrations are found in lacrimal and salivary secretions; the drug penetrates well into bone. Cerebrospinal fluid levels as high as 1.3 μg/mL have been observed during treatment of meningitis.

The adverse effects of rifampin are few. On occasion, it will produce a flulike syndrome in individuals who take the drug intermittently. There have also been reports of interstitial nephritis, thrombocytopenia, and hemolytic anemia. Rifampin alters the metabolism of a number of drugs; it decreases the effect of exogenous steroids and interferes with birth control pills. It artificially lowers the serum concentration of thyroxine; tri-iodothyronine remains normal. Patients should be warned that rifampin will cause red discoloration of urine and can cause permanent staining of soft contact lenses. Rifampin crosses the placenta and has produced teratogenic effects in rodents, but such effects have not been observed in humans. However, during pregnancy the drug should be used only for severe tuberculosis. The major use of rifampin is in short-term (6 to 9 months) treatment of tuberculosis, combined with isoniazid (see Chap. 125). It is also used as prophylaxis for contacts of patients with meningococcal meningitis in a dose of 600 mg for 2 days in adults and 20 mg/kg for 2 days in children. It has also been recommended for prophylaxis of children under 4 years of age who have had close contact with a child with *H. influenzae* type B meningitis. Rifampin, combined with cloxacillin, has proved effective in eradicating nasal carriage in individuals with recurrent furunculosis. It may also be used to eradicate methicillin-resistant staphylococci when used in combination with vancomycin or trimethoprim-sulfamethoxazole. Rifampin has been used in the therapy of endocarditis due to tolerant *S. aureus* and for treatment of *Corynebacterium* species endocarditis. It is useful in treating patients with *L. pneumophila* infection who have failed to respond to erythromycin. Rifampin also may be useful combined with nafcillin or vancomycin in the treatment of chronic staphylococcal osteomyelitis.

METRONIDAZOLE   Metronidazole is a nitroimidazole which, following reduction of the nitro group of the nitrosohydroxyl amino group, causes breaks in strands of DNA. Plasmids that prevent reduction of imidazoles have been found. The drug kills organisms within a twofold dilution of the inhibitory concentration: 99 percent of *B. fragilis* are inhibited by 8 μg/mL and 100 percent of *Fusobacterium* by 4 μg/mL. Most clostridial species are inhibited by 4 μg/mL. However, anaerobic gram-positive cocci may be less susceptible, as are *Actinomyces* and *Arachnida*. It is highly active against *C. difficile*. *Propionibacterium acnes* are resistant, but *Gardnerella vaginalis*, *Campylobacter fetus*, and oral *Spirochaeta* are inhibited by metronidazole.

Metronidazole is rapidly and almost completely absorbed when given orally. It can also be absorbed by rectal instillation and is available as an intravenous solution. There is minimal protein binding; the drug has a long half-life of 8 h. Absorption of metronidazole is not affected by food although peak levels are markedly delayed. Metronidazole is metabolized in the liver to a variety of hydroxy and glucuronide derivatives. Both metronidazole and its metabolites are eliminated in the urine and in the feces. Metronidazole dosage does not need to be adjusted in renal failure, but the drug is rapidly removed by hemodialysis. Therefore, additional doses should be given after dialysis. Given its long half-life, dosage of 500 mg every 8 h is adequate.

There are a number of adverse effects related to metronidazole. Rare but important reactions are seizures and encephalopathy, peripheral neuropathy, disulfiram-like reaction with alcohol, potentiation of the effects of warfarin, and, extremely rarely, pseudomembranous colitis. Minor problems that are associated with the drug are development of gastrointestinal disturbance, metallic taste, maculopapular rashes, or vaginal burning. Metronidazole is tumorigenic in rats, but there is no evidence that this occurs in humans. Nevertheless, the drug should probably not be used in pregnancy unless no other drug is feasible.

Metronidazole is effective in treatment of serious anaerobic infections, with some exceptions. It is not useful in actinomycosis, and it has not been very effective in aspiration pneumonia, probably because of the large number of streptococci found in this infection. It is particularly useful in intraabdominal infections since it is able to penetrate abscesses and kill *Bacteroides* within the abscess. It has also been used in other anaerobic infections including bacteremia, endocarditis, osteomyelitis, and head-and-neck infections. Metronidazole can be used in the management of pseudomembranous colitis due to *C. difficile* either orally or parenterally. Metronidazole is useful in the treatment of amebic liver abscess, intestinal amebiasis, and vaginitis due to *Trichomonas*. It may be useful in *Blastocystis hominis* infections. Metronidazole has been used as prophylaxis for elective colonic and gynecologic surgery or at the time of emergency appendectomy. However, it has no activity against gram-positive or gram-negative aerobic organisms.

POLYMYXINS   Polymyxins are cyclic basic polypeptides. There are two compounds available, polymyxin B sulfate and polymyxin E, or colistin. Polymyxins are active only against aerobic gram-negative bacteria such as *Pseudomonas* and members of the Enterobacteriaceae. The compounds are not absorbed when given orally and must be administered parenterally. They are rapidly sequestered within the kidney and liver, reducing their clinical value. Both drugs produce very serious neuro- and nephrotoxicity. In view of the large number of other compounds available, there is no reason to use them.

SULFONAMIDES AND TRIMETHOPRIM   Sulfonamides are bacteriostatic and act by interfering with folic acid metabolism in bacteria. Resistance is due to the presence of an altered or new dihydropteroic synthetase enzyme that binds para-aminobenzoic acid (PABA) better than sulfonamides. They are generally classified as short-, medium-, or long-acting sulfonamides, sulfonamides limited to the gastrointestinal tract, and topical sulfonamides. Sulfonamides inhibit some gram-positive bacteria and members of the Enterobacteriaceae, including *E. coli*, *Klebsiella*, and *Proteus*. They are also active against *Haemophilus*, but do not have activity against *P. aeruginosa*. The major problem with sulfonamides is that bacteria have become resistant on the basis of plasmid-mediated production of altered enzymes. Most sulfonamides are administered orally, although sulfamethoxazole is available for intravenous use. Sulfonamides are absorbed rapidly from the small intestine and stomach. The compounds are distributed throughout the body and enter the CSF, synovial, pleural, and peritoneal fluids in concentrations that approximate 80 percent of serum levels. Sulfonamides are metabolized in the liver by acetylation and glucuronidation. They are excreted via glomerular filtration with partial reabsorption and tubular secretion. Sulfonamides differ widely in their protein binding, plasma half-life, metabolism, and solubility.

Sulfonamides produce a number of serious side effects. These include a rash that appears in 3 to 5 percent of individuals (more frequently in AIDS patients), fever, jaundice, serum sickness–like syndrome, and acute hemolysis in the G6PD-deficient patient. They also may cause agranulocytosis, thrombocytopenia, and leukopenia. Sulfonamides cannot be administered during the last month of pregnancy since they cross the placenta and displace bilirubin from albumin and increase the risk of kernicterus. Long-acting sulfonamides have been associated with fatal hypersensitivity reactions; this has been noted particularly with the longer-acting sulfonamides used in malarial preparations. By binding to albumin sites, sulfonamides may displace drugs such as warfarin, methotrexate, and hypoglycemic agents such as chlorpropamide. Sulfonamide concentrations are increased by indomethacin, salicylates, and probenecid. Tubular necrosis due to deposition of sulfa crystals within the kidney rarely occurs today.

Sulfadiazine is the most active sulfonamide attaining the highest blood and cerebrospinal fluid levels. However, it tends more often to produce crystalluria; hence sulfisoxazole and sulfamethoxazole are used more frequently. Mixtures of three sulfonamides are also available and can be used in the treatment of toxoplasmosis. Long-acting sulfonamides should be avoided because of the risk of severe erythema multiforme. Topical sulfonamide preparations such as silver-sulfadiazine or mafenide inhibit Enterobacteriaceae, *P. aeruginosa*, staphylococci, and streptococci and are extremely useful to reduce the number of bacteria in burn eschars.

Trimethoprim is a 2,4-diaminopyrimidine that inhibits dihydrofolate reductase. Resistance is plasmid- and transposon-mediated due to production of altered dihydrofolate reductase enzyme which has markedly reduced affinity for trimethoprim. Trimethoprim is active against most gram-positive cocci and gram-negative rods with the exception of *P. aeruginosa* and *Bacteroides*. It also has relatively poor activity against *Neisseria* species, and against *Chlamydia* and *Nocardia*. Resistance to trimethoprim has been fairly slow to develop. However, in the far east, strains of *Salmonella* and *Shigella* have become resistant, and toxigenic *E. coli* have been isolated in Central America that are resistant to trimethoprim and the combination of trimethoprim and sulfamethoxazole.

Trimethoprim is available as a single agent or a combined agent in a fixed combination of one part trimethoprim to five parts sulfamethoxazole. It is also available as an intravenous combination which contains one part trimethoprim and five parts sulfamethoxazole. Like the sulfonamides, trimethoprim is well-absorbed from the gastrointestinal tract. Most of the drug is excreted in the urine via tubular secretion; it has a serum half-life of 9 to 11 h in normal individuals. Trimethoprim-sulfamethoxazole can usually be given to patients with creatinine clearances greater than 30 mL/min in the usual doses and given in half doses to patients whose creatinine clearances are in the range of 15 to 30 mL/min. Trimethoprim itself may cause fever and rash and depression of white cells and platelets. This problem often can be avoided by the simultaneous administration of folinic acid. Pseudomembranous enterocolitis also can occur following use of trimethoprim-sulfamethoxazole.

Trimethoprim-sulfamethoxazole has been useful in the treatment of urinary tract infections, acute bacterial exacerbations of chronic bronchitis, otitis media, and gastrointestinal infections due to *Salmonella*, *Shigella*, and toxigenic *E. coli*. Trimethoprim also is useful in the treatment of gonorrhea and chancroid. It can be used to treat *Listeria* meningitis in patients allergic to penicillins. It has had some success in therapy of methicillin-resistant *S. aureus*. Trimethoprim-sulfamethoxazole is used in high-dose oral or intravenous therapy of *Pneumocystis carinii* infections. Trimethoprim-sulfamethoxazole has also proved useful as prophylaxis in neutropenic children and in chronic granulomatous disease of childhood. The combination has been of particular value in the prevention of recurrent bacteriuria in women with recurrent urinary tract infections.

QUINOLONES Quinolones are synthesized chemically. Nalidixic acid which inhibits gram-negative bacteria has been used only for the treatment of urinary tract infections. Quinolones bind to an enzyme, DNA gyrase, which is involved in the production of new DNA molecules. Resistance is due to an altered DNA gyrase A subunit and to failure of uptake of the drugs due to loss of outer membrane proteins.

The compounds can be considered in groups; nalidixic acid, oxolinic acid, and cinoxacin are one group. They inhibit the majority of strains of *E. coli*, *P. mirabilis*, *Klebsiella*, and *Enterobacter* at concentrations that can be achieved in urine. *Pseudomonas* species are resistant as are gram-positive organisms, *S. aureus*, *S. pneumoniae*, and *E. faecalis*. Cross-resistance occurs between all three of the compounds. These agents are given by the oral route and are almost completely absorbed from the gastrointestinal tract. They are metabolized in the liver to biologically active and inactive compounds that are excreted by the kidney. The major difficulty with these agents has been the rapid development of resistance to them; hence they have not proved very effective for urinary tract infections.

The carboxyfluoroquinolones norfloxacin, enoxacin, pefloxacin, ofloxacin, and ciprofloxacin differ from the previously mentioned drugs because they have an extended antibacterial spectrum. All of these agents inhibit virtually all of the Enterobacteriaceae at concentrations below 1 μg/mL. They have varying activity against *Pseudomonas*, depending upon the particular compound. Ciprofloxacin is extremely active against *P. aeruginosa*, inhibiting isolates resistant to β-lactam and aminoglycoside antibiotics at ≤ 0.5 μg/mL. The agents also inhibit *Haemophilus*, *Branhamella*, and methicillin-resistant staphylococci. They tend to have less activity against *S. pneumoniae* and hemolytic streptococci and generally do not inhibit *Bacteroides* and many clostridial species except at high concentrations. Ciprofloxacin inhibits most *S. pneumoniae* and *S. pyogenes* at ≤ 2.0 μg/mL.

These agents differ in their oral absorption. Ofloxacin and enoxacin are more readily absorbed than are norfloxacin and ciprofloxacin. Absorption is markedly reduced in the presence of aluminum and magnesium antacids, but not by H-2-blocking agents. The compounds are widely distributed in the body and are metabolized to both active and inactive products within the liver. The majority of excretion products leave the body via the urinary tract or biliary tract. Ciprofloxacin enters the CSF at therapeutic concentrations against *H. influenzae*, *N. meningitidis*, and Enterobacteriaceae, but not *S. pneumoniae*. High concentrations are achieved in bone. Ciprofloxacin and norfloxacin are available for use in the United States. Ciprofloxacin has been used in the treatment of urinary tract infections, respiratory tract infections, gastrointestinal disease due to *Salmonella* and *Shigella*, and pathogenic *E. coli* and *Campylobacter*. Ciprofloxacin and ofloxacin have been successfully used in the treatment of osteomyelitis and skin infections. Ciprofloxacin has been extremely effective in therapy of *Pseudomonas* infections, including those occurring in cystic fibrosis patients. Norfloxacin has been restricted to use in urinary tract infections.

Toxic and adverse reactions to these agents have been infrequent. Gastrointestinal side effects have included nausea, vomiting, and occasionally diarrhea. Nonspecific rashes and urticaria have occurred. Ophthalmologic side effects are rare. Central nervous system symptoms noted with nalidixic acid include headache, vertigo, seizures, and psychosis, but such reactions are extremely uncommon with ciprofloxacin, norfloxacin, and ofloxacin. Ciprofloxacin prolongs the half-life of theophylline; all the agents increase caffeine's half-life.

ANTITUBERCULOSIS DRUGS See Chap. 125.

ANTIFUNGAL AGENTS See Chap. 87.

ANTIVIRAL AGENTS See Chap. 86.

ANTIPARASITIC AGENTS See Chap. 88.

REASONS FOR FAILURE OF CHEMOTHERAPY

There are few microorganisms with the exception of fungi and viruses that are not susceptible to some antimicrobial agents. Nonetheless, a large number of patients who develop infections continue to die. In these patients, antimicrobial agents appear to have failed. The failure of chemotherapy often is more apparent than real, and may be attributed to a number of different causes.

First, the infection being treated may not be due to a treatable microorganism but to a viral infection that will not respond to the chemotherapeutic agents that are being used. Antibiotics do not prevent bacterial complications of most viral infections.

A second common reason for failure of antimicrobial therapy is that purulent material has not been drained, or that a focus of obstruction or a foreign body has not been removed. Antimicrobial agents do not work well in these situations.

Third, fever may continue, not due to the infection, but as the result of development of hypersensitivity to one of the agents being used to treat the patient. Drug fever is particularly common with antimicrobial agents of the β-lactam and sulfonamide classes.

Occasionally, chemotherapy fails because the incorrect drug has been chosen or the culture results have been misinterpreted. This may be particularly true in respiratory infections. One of the most common errors when such a patient is not responding is to add more antimicrobial agents indiscriminately, when the correct course would be to discontinue therapy and observe the patient.

With many of the new antimicrobial agents, failure to provide an adequate dose of antibiotic is less frequently a problem than it was formerly. However, this still may be true in certain infections in which penetration of the antimicrobial agent to the particular area of the body is inadequate unless large doses are utilized.

More and more, today's patients lack host defenses, and include elderly patients with degenerative and debilitating diseases, or patients who have received multiple antimicrobial agents, antineoplastic or immunosuppressive drugs, or who have undergone major surgical procedures. These individuals will have much more difficulty in responding to antimicrobial therapy than normal uncompromised hosts, most of whom remain free of life-threatening infections.

REFERENCES

Acar JF, Neu HC (eds): Gram-negative aerobic bacterial infections: A focus on directed therapy, with special reference to aztreonam. Rev Infect Dis 7(Suppl 4):537, 1985
Andriole VT (ed): *The Quinolones*. London, Academic, 1988
Antimicrobial prophylaxis in surgery. Med Lett Drugs Ther 31:105, 1989
Bruchat MA, Dajani AS (eds): Sulbactam/ampicillin in clinical practice. Drugs 35(Suppl 7):1, 1988
Donowitz GR, Mandell GL. Beta-lactam antibiotics. N Engl J Med 319:419, 1988
Drusano GL et al: The acylampicillins: Mezlocillin, piperacillin, and azlocillin. Rev Infect Dis 6:13, 1984
Geddes AM, Stille W (eds): Imipenem, the first thienamycin antibiotic. Rev Infect Dis 7(Suppl 3), 1985
Levy SB et al: Antibiotic use and antibiotic resistance worldwide. Rev Infect Dis 9(Suppl 3):231, 1987
Neu HC (ed): Beta-lactamase inhibition: Therapeutic advances. Am J Med 79(Suppl 5B):1, 1985
—— (ed): Update on antibiotics I. Med Clin North Am 71(6):1051, 1987
—— (ed): Update on antibiotics II. Med Clin North Am 72(3):555, 1988
—— et al (eds): Ciprofloxacin: A major advance in quinolone chemotherapy. Am J Med 82(4A):1, 1987
Norrby SR et al (eds): Evaluation of new beta-lactam antibiotics. Rev Infect Dis 8(Suppl 3):235, 1986
Platt R et al: Perioperative antibiotic prophylaxis for herniorrhaphy and breast surgery. N Engl J Med 322:153, 1990

86 ANTIVIRAL CHEMOTHERAPY

RAPHAEL DOLIN

INTRODUCTION The use of antiviral compounds for chemotherapy and chemoprophylaxis of viral diseases is a relatively new development in the field of infectious diseases, particularly when compared to the more than 40 years of experience with antibacterial antibiotics. The principles which underlie the use of antiviral com-

pounds have been modeled after those successfully employed in the treatment of bacterial infections, as outlined in Chap. 85. However, application of these principles to antiviral chemotherapy and chemoprophylaxis presents a number of unique problems.

First, antiviral compounds must possess a high degree of selectivity because of the biologic properties of viruses. Bacteria can replicate extracellularly and have evolved metabolic and structural features which differ considerably from those of mammalian cells. However, viruses must replicate intracellularly and often employ host cell enzymes, macromolecules, and organelles for the synthesis of virus particles. Therefore, safe and effective antiviral compounds must be able to discriminate with a high degree of efficiency between cellular and virus-specific functions. Inhibitors of virus replication which lack this selectivity are likely to be too toxic for clinical use.

Second, because of the nature of virus replication, evaluation of the in vitro sensitivity of virus isolates to antiviral compounds must be carried out in a complex culture system consisting of living cells (e.g., tissue culture). The results from such assay systems vary widely according to the type of tissue culture cells which are employed and the conditions of assay. Furthermore, the precise relationship between the in vitro sensitivity of an isolate and the outcome of antiviral therapy is not well worked out.

Third, information regarding the pharmacokinetics of antiviral compounds, particularly in diverse clinical settings, is limited, particularly when compared to that available for antibacterial antibiotics. For compounds such as acyclovir, considerable detailed pharmacokinetic data are available, while for others such as rimantadine, relatively little information exists. Assays to determine concentrations of antivirals, particularly of active moieties within cells, are not widely available. There are few guidelines with which to adjust dosage levels to maximize antiviral activity and to minimize toxicity. Therefore, clinical use of antiviral compounds must be accompanied by particular vigilance for unanticipated side effects or toxicities.

Fourth, it is clear that highly complex host defense systems play critical roles in the course of viral infections. The presence or absence of preexisting immunity, and the ability to mount humoral and/or cell-mediated immune responses, are especially important determinants in the outcome of viral infections. For example, profound "immunosuppression" may result in infections in which prolonged viral replication is present, and inhibition of such replication by antiviral compounds may be particularly useful. On the other hand, if host defenses are severely depressed, as in bone marrow transplants, antiviral therapy may be relatively ineffective. The state of host defenses and their interactions with antiviral compounds need to be considered when antivirals are utilized or evaluated.

Finally, as with antibacterial antibiotics, the optimal use of antiviral compounds requires that a specific and timely diagnosis be made. For some viral infections, such as herpes zoster, the clinical manifestations are so characteristic that a diagnosis can be made on clinical grounds alone. For other viral infections, such as influenza A, epidemiologic information (i.e., community-wide outbreaks) can be utilized to make a presumptive diagnosis with a high degree of accuracy. However, for most other viral infections, including herpes simplex encephalitis, cytomegalovirus infections, and acute viral gastroenteritis, diagnosis on clinical grounds alone cannot be accomplished with certainty. For such infections, rapid, noninvasive viral diagnostic techniques are sorely needed, and considerable effort is being expended to develop such tests.

Despite the above complexities, the efficacy of several antiviral compounds has been clearly established in rigorously conducted and controlled studies. The compounds which are currently available or likely to be made available in the immediate future for clinical use are discussed below and summarized in Table 86-1.

AMANTADINE AND RIMANTADINE Amantadine (1-adamantanamine hydrochloride) and the closely related compound rimantadine (α-methyl-1-adamantanemethylamine hydrochloride) are primary symmetric amines with antiviral activity limited to influenza A viruses.

TABLE 86-1   Antiviral chemotherapy and chemoprophylaxis

Infection	Antiviral drug	Administration	Dosage	Comment
Influenza A (prophylaxis)	Amandatine or rimantadine	Oral Oral	Adults: 200 mg/d for period at risk Children ≤9 yrs: 4.4–8.8 mg/kg per day not to exceed 150 mg/d As above	Needs to be administered for the duration of the outbreak. Dosage should be reduced in renal failure and in the elderly. Can be administered along with vaccine. Not yet licensed by FDA. May be better tolerated than amantadine.
Influenza A (therapy)	Amandatine or rimantadine	Oral Oral	As above for 5–7 days As above for 5–7 days	Both amantadine and rimantadine are effective in uncomplicated influenza. Neither drug has been demonstrated to be effective in complicated influenza (e.g., pneumonia). Under study for treatment of complicated influenza in placebo-controlled trials.
Respiratory syncytial virus	Ribavirin	Aerosol	Administered continuously by small-particle aerosol from a reservoir containing 20 mg/mL for 3–6 days	Utilized for treatment of infants and young children hospitalized with RSV pneumonia and bronchiolitis.
Herpes simplex encephalitis	Acyclovir or vidarabine	IV IV	10 mg/kg every 8 h for 10 days 15 mg/kg per day as a continous infusion for 12 h for 10 days	Acyclovir is the drug of choice for this infection on the basis of comparative trials vs. vidarabine. Optimal results are obtained when therapy is initiated early in illness.
Neonatal herpes simplex	Vidarabine or acyclovir	IV IV	30 mg/kg per day given as a continuous infusion over 12 h per day for 10 days 10 mg/kg every 8 h for 10 days	Vidarabine reduces mortality, but severe morbidity is frequent. Currently being compared with acyclovir in a clinical trial.
Genital herpes simplex: primary infection	Acyclovir	IV Oral Topical	5 mg/kg every 8 h for 5–10 days 200 mg 5 times per day for 10 days 5% ointment; 4–6 applications per day for 7–10 days	IV route is preferred if infection is of sufficient severity to warrant hospitalization, or if neurologic complications are present. Preferred route of administration for patients who do not warrant hospitalization. Adequate hydration should be maintained. Largely supplanted by oral therapy. May be of use in pregnant women in order to avoid systemic therapy. Systemic symptoms and untreated areas are not affected.
Genital herpes simplex: recurrent infections (therapy)	Acyclovir	Oral	200 mg 5 times per day for 5 days	Clinical effect is modest and is enhanced if therapy is initiated early. No effect on subsequent recurrence rates.
Genital herpes simplex: recurrent infections (suppression)	Acyclovir	Oral	200 mg 3 times per day for up to 6 months	Suppressive therapy is recommended only for patients with frequent recurrences, at least 6 to 10 per year. Occasional "breakthrough" may occur, and asymptomatic shedding of virus occurs.
Mucocutaneous herpes simplex in immunocompromised patients (treatment)	Acyclovir or vidarabine	IV Oral Topical IV	250 mg/m² every 8 h for 7 days 200 mg PO 5 times per day for 10 days 5% ointment; 4–6 applications per day for 7 days or until healed 10 mg/kg per day for 7 days given as a 12-h infusion	Choice of intravenous or oral route will depend on severity of infection and whether patient can take oral medication. Oral or IV administration has supplanted topical therapy except for small, easily accessible lesions. Efficacy has been demonstrated in HSV-1 infections and in patients who were older than 40. Appears to be less useful than acyclovir in this setting.
Mucocutaneous herpes simplex in immunocompromised patients (prevention of recurrences during periods of intense immunosuppression)	Acyclovir	Oral IV	200 mg 4 times per day 5 mg/kg every 12 h	Acyclovir is administered during periods when intense immunosuppression is expected, e.g., antitumor chemotherapy, after transplantation. After therapy is discontinued, lesions recur.
Herpes simplex keratitis	Trifluorothymidine or vidarabine	Topical Topical	One drop of 0.1% ophthalmic solution every 2 h while awake (maximum 9 drops per day) 0.5-in ribbon of 0.5% ophthalmic ointment 5 times per day	Therapy should be undertaken in consultation with an ophthalmologist. As above.
Varicella in immunocompromised patients	Acyclovir or vidarabine	IV IV	500 mg/m² every 8 h for 7 days 10 mg/kg per day in a 12-h infusion for 5 days	Studies comparing acyclovir with vidarabine in the treatment of varicella have not been performed. Limited placebo-controlled studies suggest the effects of both drugs on varicella are similar.

TABLE 86-1 Antiviral chemotherapy and chemoprophylaxis *(continued)*

Infection	Antiviral drug	Administration	Dosage	Comment
Herpes zoster in immunocompromised patients	Acyclovir or	IV	500 mg/m^2 every 8 h for 7 days	Efficacy of acyclovir and vidarabine are established for localized zoster, particularly when treated early and acyclovir appears to be more effective. Studies of the effect on disseminated zoster of the two drugs are under way. Oral acyclovir (4 g/d) is under study in herpes zoster in immunosuppressed patients and in ''normal'' hosts.
	vidarabine	IV	10 mg/kg per day in a 12-h infusion for 5 days	
Herpes zoster ophthalmicus	Acyclovir	Oral	600 mg PO 5 times a day for 10 days	Reduces ocular complications including keratitis and uveitis
Cytomegalovirus infections	Ganciclovir	IV	5 mg/kg twice a day for 14–21 days, then 5 mg/kg per day as maintenance	Investigational drug used to treat CMV infections, particularly in AIDS patients. May be effective in retinitis, colitis, ''wasting syndromes'' associated with CMV—probably less so in CMV pneumonitis.
Human immunodeficiency virus infection	Zidovudine	Oral	200 mg PO every 4 h	Licensed for treatment of AIDS and ARC patients with CD4 counts less than 200/μL. Beneficial effects on mortality and morbidity wane after 1 year of therapy. Efficacy of lower doses and efficacy in patients with early ARC or with asymptomatic HIV infections are under study.

They inhibit influenza A virus replication at an as yet unspecified step after virus attachment to the cell, possibly through interaction with the influenza A M2 matrix protein. In several experimental systems, rimantadine is two to four times more active than amantadine against isolates of influenza A.

Amantadine and rimantadine have been demonstrated to be effective in the prophylaxis of influenza A in large-scale studies in young adults, and to a lesser extent in children and in elderly subjects. In such studies, efficacy rates of 55 to 80 percent in prevention of influenza-like illness were noted, and even higher rates were reported when virus-specific attack rates were calculated. Amantadine and rimantadine have also been demonstrated to be effective in the treatment of influenza A infection, in studies carried out predominantly in young adults and, to a lesser extent, in children. Administration of these compounds within 24 to 72 h after the onset of illness has resulted in a reduction of duration of signs and symptoms by approximately 50 percent when compared to a placebo-treated group. The effect on signs and symptoms of illness has been demonstrated to be superior to that of commonly used antipyretic-analgesics. Only anecdotal reports are available concerning the efficacy of amantadine or rimantadine in the prevention or treatment of complications of influenza (e.g., pneumonia).

Amantadine and rimantadine are available only in oral formulations and are ordinarily administered in a dose of 200 mg/d for adults, given once or twice daily. Despite their structural similarities, the pharmacokinetics of the two compounds are different. Amantadine is not metabolized and is excreted almost entirely by the kidney, with a half-life of 12 to 17 h and peak plasma concentrations of 0.4 μg/mL. Rimantadine is extensively metabolized to hydroxylated derivatives and has a half-life of 30 h. Only 30 percent of an orally administered dose is recovered in the urine. The peak plasma levels of rimantadine are approximately one-half those of amantadine, but rimantadine is concentrated in respiratory secretions to a greater extent than amantadine. For prophylaxis, the compounds must be administered daily for the period at risk (i.e., the duration of the outbreak). For therapy, amantadine or rimantadine is generally administered for 5 to 7 days.

Although these compounds are generally well tolerated, 5 to 10 percent of amantadine recipients experience mild central nervous system side effects, consisting primarily of dizziness, anxiety, insomnia, and difficulty in concentrating. These side effects are rapidly reversible upon cessation of the drug. In a dose of 200 mg/d, rimantadine is better tolerated than amantadine, and in a large-scale study in young adults, side effects were no more frequent in rimantadine recipients than in placebo recipients. Seizures and worsening of congestive heart failure have also been reported in patients treated with amantadine, although a causal relationship has not been established.

Amantadine is licensed for the prophylaxis and therapy of influenza A in the United States, while rimantadine remains experimental. Because of its effectiveness and lack of toxicity, rimantadine may be particularly advantageous for long-term prophylaxis, or for therapy of influenza in subjects at particular risk for development of CNS toxicity, such as elderly individuals. When amantadine is employed in the latter group, the recommended dose is 100 mg/d.

RIBAVIRIN Ribavirin is a synthetic nucleoside analogue that inhibits a wide range of RNA and DNA viruses. The mechanism of action of ribavirin is not completely defined and may be different for different groups of viruses. Ribavirin-5'-monophosphate blocks the conversion of inosine-5'-monophosphate to xanthosine-5'-monophosphate, and interferes with the synthesis of guanine nucleotides and both RNA and DNA synthesis. Ribavirin-5'-monophosphate also inhibits capping of virus-specific RNA in certain viral systems. In studies demonstrating the effectiveness of ribavirin, the compound has been administered as a small-particle aerosol. It has been utilized to treat respiratory syncytial virus (RSV) infection in infants, and to a lesser extent, parainfluenza infections in children and influenza A and B infection in young adults. In RSV infection in infants, ribavirin administered by continuous aerosol for 3 to 6 days resulted in more rapid resolution of illness, lower respiratory tract signs, and arterial oxygen desaturation when compared to placebo-treated groups. Its use for severe RSV infections in adults has not resulted in any clear benefit. Orally administered ribavirin has not been effective in the treatment of influenza A infections. Ribavirin is under evaluation for adenovirus and arenavirus infections, including Lassa fever, and for patients with acquired immunodeficiency syndrome (AIDS).

Large doses of ribavirin administered orally (800 to 1000 mg/d) have been associated with reversible hematopoietic toxicity, but this has not been observed with aerosolized ribavirin, apparently because little drug is absorbed systemically. Aerosolized administration of ribavirin has been approved for treatment of respiratory syncytial virus infection in infants. Because of the need for aerosolized administration, the drug can only be given for this indication under close supervision. Health care workers exposed to the drug have experienced minor toxicity including eye and respiratory tract irritation.

ACYCLOVIR Acyclovir, 9-[(2-hydroxyethoxy)methyl]guanine, is a highly potent and selective inhibitor of replication of certain herpesviruses, including herpes simplex 1 (HSV-1), herpes simplex 2 (HSV-2), varicella-zoster virus (VZV), and Epstein-Barr virus (EBV). It is relatively ineffective in human cytomegalovirus (CMV) infections.

The high degree of selectivity of acyclovir is related to its mechanism of action, which requires that the compound first be phosphorylated to acyclovir monophosphate. This phosphorylation occurs efficiently in herpesvirus-infected cells by means of a virus-coded thymidine kinase. In uninfected mammalian cells, little phosphorylation of acyclovir occurs, and therefore, the drug is concentrated in herpesvirus-infected cells. Acyclovir monophosphate is subsequently converted by host cell kinases to a triphosphate which is a potent inhibitor of virus-induced DNA polymerase but has relatively little effect on host cell DNA polymerase. Acyclovir triphosphate can also be incorporated into viral DNA, with early chain termination.

Acyclovir is available in intravenous, oral, and topically administered forms. Intravenous acyclovir has been demonstrated to be markedly effective in the therapy of mucocutaneous HSV infections in immunocompromised hosts, reducing time to healing, duration of pain, and virus shedding. When administered prophylactically during periods of intense immunosuppression such as chemotherapy for leukemia or transplantation, but before lesions are present, intravenous acyclovir has also reduced the frequency of HSV-associated disease. After prophylaxis was discontinued, recurrent HSV lesions developed. Intravenous acyclovir has also been demonstrated to be effective in the treatment of HSV encephalitis, and two comparative trials have indicated that acyclovir is more effective than vidarabine for treatment of the latter infection (see below). Varicella-zoster virus is generally less sensitive to acyclovir than is herpes simplex virus, so that higher doses of acyclovir must be used to treat varicella-zoster virus infections. In immunocompromised patients with herpes zoster, intravenous acyclovir reduced the frequency of cutaneous dissemination and visceral complications and was more effective than vidarabine in one comparative trial. Acyclovir administered orally at doses of 800 mg five times a day had a modest beneficial effect on localized herpes zoster lesions in both immunocompromised and immunocompetent patients and is being evaluated in large-scale collaborative trials. Orally administered acyclovir (600 mg five times a day) reduced complications of herpes zoster ophthalmicus in a placebo-controlled trial.

The most widespread use of acyclovir is in the therapy of genital herpes simplex virus infections. Both intravenous and oral formulations have shortened the duration of symptoms, reduced virus shedding, and accelerated healing when employed for the treatment of primary genital HSV infections. Oral acyclovir also had a modest effect in the therapy of recurrent genital HSV infections. However, treatment of either primary or recurrent disease did not reduce the frequency of subsequent recurrences, indicating that acyclovir was ineffective in elimination of latent infection. Chronically administered oral acyclovir for periods ranging from 1 to 6 years has been shown to reduce the frequency of recurrences markedly while on therapy, although once the drug was discontinued, lesions recurred. In AIDS patients chronic administration of acyclovir has been associated with the development of strains resistant to the action of the drug and with clinical failures.

With the availability of the oral and intravenous forms, there are few indications for topical acyclovir, although treatment with this formulation has shown modest beneficial effects in the therapy of primary genital herpes infections and of mucocutaneous HSV infections in immunocompromised hosts.

Overall, acyclovir is remarkably well tolerated and generally free of toxicity. The most frequently encountered toxicity has been occasional renal dysfunction, particularly after rapid intravenous administration or when patients have been inadequately hydrated. Central nervous system changes, including lethargy and tremors, occasionally have been reported, primarily in immunosuppressed patients. However, whether these changes are related to acyclovir, to concurrent administration of other therapy, or to underlying infection remains unclear. Acyclovir is excreted primarily unmetabolized by the kidney, both by glomerular filtration and tubular secretion. Approximately 15 percent of a dose of acyclovir is metabolized to 9-[(carboxymethoxy)methyl]guanine or other minor metabolites. Reduction in dosage is indicated in patients with creatinine clearances less than 50 mL/min per 1.73 m². The half-life of acyclovir is approximately 3 h in normal adults, and peak plasma concentrations after a 1-h infusion employing a 5 mg/kg dose are 9.8 μg/mL. Approximately 22 percent of acyclovir administered orally is absorbed, and peak plasma concentrations of 0.3 to 0.9 μg/mL are attained after administration of a 200-mg dose. Acyclovir penetrates relatively well into the cerebrospinal fluid, with CSF concentrations approaching one-half of those found in plasma.

GANCICLOVIR An analogue of acyclovir, ganciclovir, 9-[(1,3-dihydroxy-2-propoxy)methyl]guanine, has markedly increased activity against CMV. Ganciclovir triphosphate inhibits CMV DNA polymerases and can be incorporated into CMV DNA but, in contrast to acyclovir, does not function as a chain terminator. CMV, unlike HSV, does not code for its own thymidine kinase, and the mechanism by which phosphorylation of ganciclovir takes place in host cells is not defined. Ganciclovir has been utilized most extensively in the treatment of CMV infection in AIDS and otherwise immunosuppressed patients, and the drug has been used in neonatal CMV infections as well. Much of the clinical experience with ganciclovir has been uncontrolled, but available evidence indicates that it is effective in treatment of CMV retinitis for which it is approved by the Federal Drug Administration (FDA). Its efficacy in CMV colitis, CMV-associated "wasting," and, perhaps less so, in CMV pneumonitis remains to be established. It is currently investigational for the latter conditions, and is available only as an intravenous preparation. The most commonly employed dosage for initial therapy is 5 mg/kg twice a day for 14 to 21 days, followed by a maintenance dose of 5 mg/kg per day, possibly for as long as the immunosuppression persists. Administration of ganciclovir has been associated with profound bone marrow suppression, particularly neutropenia, which represents a major limitation of its use in many patients. Bone marrow toxicity is potentiated when other bone marrow suppressants such as zidovudine are used concomitantly. Clinical trials to determine optimal dosage and to evaluate oral formulations of ganciclovir are under way.

Foscarnet is another inhibitor of CMV DNA polymerase which has shown antiviral activity in vitro and in vivo. The major toxicity appears to be renal, with little bone marrow suppression, which makes the drug an attractive alternative in patients who cannot tolerate ganciclovir. It also has activity against human immunodeficiency virus (HIV) in vitro. Clinical trials to determine the efficacy and toxicity of foscarnet are currently being carried out.

ZIDOVUDINE Zidovudine (ZDV), also known as azidothymidine (AZT), inhibits the replication of HIV-1 through a competitive inhibition of HIV reverse transcriptase by AZT triphosphate, and possibly through chain termination of viral DNA synthesis as well. A large-scale placebo-controlled trial carried out in patients with AIDS or with advanced AIDS-related complex (ARC) demonstrated that administration of ZDV was associated with prolonged survival and with a decreased frequency and severity of opportunistic infections. On this basis, ZDV was licensed for treatment of patients with AIDS or patients with ARC who have less than 200 CD4 lymphocytes per microliter in peripheral blood. Median survival for the patients in the study who received ZDV was 85 percent at the end of the first year, but fell markedly during the second year. The reasons for this decline in efficacy are unclear but may be related to the progressive bone marrow toxicity associated with ZDV. Anemia or granulocytopenia sufficient to require blood transfusion and/or interruption or discontinuation of ZDV occurred in 70 percent of subjects during 21 months of study. In addition, relative resistance of HIV-1 to ZDV has been described after more than 6 months of administration of the drug. Trials are underway to define the role of myelopoietic growth factors (G-CSF and GM-CSF) and erythropoietin in reversing ZDV bone marrow toxicity.

The recommended dose of ZDV is 200 mg by mouth every 4 h, but because of drug toxicity, reduced doses, usually to 200 mg by mouth every 8 h, are frequently employed. The efficacy of reduced doses is under study as is the efficacy of ZDV in the prevention of disease progression in patients who are infected with HIV but are asymptomatic or who have early stages of ARC.

Other inhibitors of HIV replication are also being evaluated in laboratory and clinical studies. Among the most promising are dideoxycytidine and dideoxyinosine, which are nucleoside analogues that are active in vitro and have shown anti-HIV-1 activity in phase one studies in humans. Comparative studies of these drugs with ZDV are in progress.

VIDARABINE Vidarabine (9-β-D-arabinofuranosyladenine) is a purine nucleoside analogue with activity against HSV-1, HSV-2, VZV, and EBV. Vidarabine inhibits viral DNA synthesis through its 5'-triphosphorylated metabolite, although the precise molecular mechanisms of action are not completely understood. In the therapy of herpes zoster in immunosuppressed patients, vidarabine, administered in a dose of 10 mg/kg per day for 5 days, resulted in reduction of rates of cutaneous and visceral dissemination, and of postherpetic neuralgia but was less effective than acyclovir in a comparative trial. Beneficial effects have also been observed in the treatment of varicella in immunosuppressed patients. Vidarabine administered in a higher dose (15 mg/kg per day for 10 days) was demonstrated to be effective in the therapy of herpes simplex encephalitis in a placebo-controlled study in which mortality was reduced from 70 to 40 percent in vidarabine recipients at 6 months after therapy. However, comparative studies indicate that acyclovir (30 mg/kg per day) is more effective than vidarabine in the therapy of herpes simplex encephalitis, and acyclovir has supplanted vidarabine as the treatment of choice for that infection. The above studies also indicated that the success of therapy was closely related to administration of the drug early in the illness.

Vidarabine treatment has also reduced the mortality of neonatal herpes simplex infection from 74 percent in placebo recipients to 38 percent, although the majority of survivors have severely impaired central nervous system function. Vidarabine has also been effective in the treatment of HSV mucocutaneous infections in immunosuppressed patients, although the effects observed were limited to patients who had HSV-1 infections and were older than 40. Topically administered vidarabine has been generally ineffective in the treatment of mucocutaneous genital or orofacial HSV infections, but is effective in the treatment of HSV keratitis.

For systemic administration, vidarabine is available only as an intravenous preparation with poor solubility and is administered as a constant 12-h infusion, so that a substantial fluid load can result which may be a significant problem in central nervous system infections. In humans, vidarabine is rapidly deaminated by a serum adenosine deaminase to its hypoxanthine derivative, ara-Hx, which has tenfold less antiviral activity than the parent compound, but is the major antiviral moiety in the plasma.

Large-scale controlled trials of vidarabine at doses of 10 to 15 mg/kg per day have not been attended by significant toxicity. At somewhat higher doses (20 mg/kg per day), vidarabine has been associated with hematopoietic side effects, including anemia, leukopenia, and thrombocytopenia. Neurotoxicity has also been reported, particularly with high dosages, in patients with hepatic or renal insufficiency, and possibly with concurrent interferon or allopurinol administration. The neurotoxic effects have included tremor, alterations in mentation, rarely coma or seizures, and unusual pain syndromes in the extremities, which have lasted up to 6 months after cessation of therapy.

TOPICAL ANTIVIRALS IUdR (5'-iodo-2'-deoxyuridine) is an inhibitor of DNA virus replication, including herpesviruses and poxviruses. It was formerly used systemically to treat herpesvirus infections, including HSV encephalitis, but because of associated toxicity and lack of demonstrated efficacy, its systemic use has largely been abandoned. Topical IUdR has been effective in the treatment of HSV keratitis, particularly in superficial epithelial infections, but has been largely supplanted by topically applied trifluorothymidine or vidarabine.

Trifluorothymidine (TFT) is an analogue of deoxythymidine, which is also effective against herpesvirus infections. Because of bone marrow suppression, its use is restricted to topical application in the eye, where it appears to be somewhat more effective and better tolerated than IUdR, and at least as effective as vidarabine. TFT has also been effective in some patients who had not responded clinically to topical IUdR or vidarabine.

INTERFERONS From its earliest descriptions, considerable interest has existed in the application of interferon to the prophylaxis and/or therapy of viral infections. Early studies with human leukocyte interferon demonstrated an effect in the prophylaxis of experimentally induced rhinovirus infections in humans, and in the treatment of varicella-zoster infections in immunosuppressed patients. DNA recombinant technology has made available highly purified α-, β-, and γ-interferons, which have been evaluated in a variety of viral infections. Results available from such trials have confirmed the effectiveness of intranasally administered interferon in the prophylaxis of rhinovirus infections, although its use has been associated with nasal mucosal irritation. Administration of either intralesional or intramuscular interferons has resulted in beneficial effects on genital warts, and trials of interferon therapy in papilloma virus infection are under way. Interferon therapy is undergoing evaluation in chronic hepatitis B infections, and as an additive treatment to ZDV in therapy of AIDS. α-Interferon has been demonstrated to be effective in reducing the manifestations of Kaposi's sarcoma in AIDS patients.

REFERENCES

DOLIN R: Antiviral chemotherapy and chemoprophylaxis (review). Science 227:1296, 1985

——— et al: A controlled trial of amantadine and rimantadine in the prophylaxis of influenza A infection. N Engl J Med 307:580, 1982

FISCHL M et al: The efficacy of azidothymidine (AZT) in the treatment of patients with AIDS and AIDS-related complex; a double blind placebo-controlled trial. N Engl J Med 317:185, 1987

HALL CB et al: Aerosolized ribavirin treatment of infants with respiratory syncytial viral infection: A randomized double blind study. N Engl J Med 308:1443, 1983

NEYERS JD: Management of cytomegalovirus infection. Am J Med 85(Suppl 2A):102, 1988

REICHMAN RC et al: Treatment of recurrent genital herpes simplex with acyclovir. A controlled trial. JAMA 251:2103, 1984

WHITLEY RJ et al and the NIAID Collaborative Antiviral Study Group: Herpes simplex encephalitis: Adenine arabinoside versus acyclovir therapies. N Engl J Med 314:144, 1986

87 ANTIFUNGAL THERAPY

JOHN E. BENNETT

TOPICAL AGENTS **Imidazoles and triazoles** These synthetic compounds act by inhibiting ergosterol synthesis in the fungal cell wall and when given topically may cause direct damage to the cytoplasmic membrane. Drug resistance rarely arises in the previously sensitive strains. Imidazoles available for cutaneous application include clotrimazole, econazole, and miconazole. Vaginal formulations include three imidazoles: miconazole, clotrimazole, and butoconazole; and one triazole: terconazole. Miconazole lotion is available without prescription. As yet, no substantial difference in efficacy or local intolerance between these agents has appeared. All are effective in treatment of cutaneous candidiasis, tinea versicolor, and mild to moderately severe ringworm of the glabrous skin. Vaginal formulations are effective in vulvovaginal candidiasis. Clotrimazole is poorly absorbed from the gastrointestinal tract, but the oral troche is useful as a topical treatment for oral and esophageal candidiasis.

Polyene macrolide antibiotics   These broad-spectrum antifungal agents combine with sterol in the fungal cytoplasmic membrane, increasing membrane permeability. Topically they are not active against ringworm but are effective against candidiasis of the skin and mucous membranes. Nystatin suspension is effective in oral thrush, and vaginal troches are effective in vulvovaginal candidiasis. Both nystatin and amphotericin B are available in topical preparations for cutaneous candidiasis. Natamycin ophthalmic suspension is marketed in some countries (but not in the United States) for mycotic keratitis and conjunctivitis.

Other topical antifungals   Ciclopirox olamine, haloprogin, and naftifine have the same clinical spectrum among the cutaneous mycoses as the imidazoles. Tolnaftate and undecylenic acid are effective against ringworm but not candidiasis. Keratolytic agents, such as salicylic acid, are helpful as accessory drugs for some hyperkeratotic skin lesions.

SYSTEMIC ANTIFUNGALS   Griseofulvin   Griseofulvin is a useful drug in treating certain kinds of ringworm; however, it is ineffective in treating candidiasis. The microcrystalline and ultramicrocrystalline preparations differ in dose but not in efficacy. Absorption of both is enhanced when ingested with fat-containing foods. Griseofulvin interacts with phenobarbital and coumarin-type anticoagulants.

Imidazoles and triazoles   Ketoconazole is the only systemically absorbed oral drug of this class that is currently available, though similar drugs are undergoing clinical trial. Absorption of ketoconazole is variable between individuals, is not affected by food, and is poor in patients taking cimetidine or other H-2 blocking agents. Simultaneous administration of antacids can also impair absorption. Metabolism is chiefly hepatic, but substantial liver disease has minimal effect on plasma ketoconazole concentrations. Ketoconazole plasma levels are decreased in patients taking rifampin and also in some taking isoniazid. Ketoconazole administration can elevate cyclosporin blood levels and, occasionally, can enhance the anticoagulant effect of warfarin. The drug is contraindicated during pregnancy and, because it appears in breast milk, during breast feeding. Neither renal disease nor hemodialysis affects the metabolism of ketoconazole. The most common toxicity of ketoconazole is dose-related nausea, anorexia and, occasionally, vomiting. Hepatotoxicity is idiosyncratic and usually mild but rarely can be serious and fatal. Several dose-related, temporary endocrine effects have been observed: decreased adrenal cortical reserve; gynecomastia; decreased serum testosterone, libido, and potency in males; and menstrual irregularity in females. Pruritus or rash may also occur. Ketoconazole is effective in blastomycosis, histoplasmosis, paracoccidioidomycosis, chronic mucocutaneous candidiasis, esophageal candidiasis, and some forms of disseminated coccidioidomycosis and pseudallescheriasis. The usual adult dose is 400 mg, taken once daily. Partial improvement may be seen in cutaneous sporotrichosis and chromomycosis. Although vulvovaginal candidiasis, ringworm, and tinea versicolor are responsive to the drug, the toxicity of oral ketoconazole makes topical imidazoles or other drugs preferable for these indications. Miconazole is available as both a topical and an intravenous preparation. The latter is rarely indicated.

Itraconazole and fluconazole are systemic triazoles under clinical investigation. Toxicity and hormonal suppression are less than with ketoconazole. There is preliminary evidence that fluconazole may be useful in cryptococcosis and in coccidioidal meningitis. Itraconazole has compared favorably with ketoconazole for most indications. Therapeutic indications, significant drug interactions, and dosage remain to be defined for both agents.

Amphotericin B   A colloidal preparation of this drug is available for intravenous or intrathecal administration. The drug cannot be given intramuscularly and is not absorbed orally. Sodium or potassium salts must not be added to the infusion solutions because the colloidal drug will precipitate out of solution. In-line filters with 0.22-μm pore

diameter may trap some of the colloid. Catabolism is extremely slow and is not influenced by renal failure, hepatic failure, or hemodialysis. Penetration into cerebrospinal fluid and vitreous humor is poor; however, concentrations in pleural, peritoneal, and articular exudates are adequate for many mycoses. Histoplasmosis, blastomycosis, paracoccidioidomycosis, candidiasis, and cryptococcosis are the most responsive mycoses. Coccidioidomycosis, extraarticular sporotrichosis, aspergillosis, and mucormycosis are less responsive; chromomycosis, mycetoma, and pseudallescheriasis show little if any response. The usual course is 8 to 10 weeks of 0.4 to 0.6 mg/kg daily. Infusions are generally given in 5% dextrose over 2 to 4 h. Severe febrile reactions to initial doses generally prompt use of an initial test dose with 1 mg, followed by escalating doses based upon the gravity of the patient's infection and tolerance of the drug. Virtually all patients show toxic reactions that are related to the dose and duration of therapy. These side effects include azotemia, anemia, hypokalemia, nausea, anorexia, weight loss, phlebitis and, occasionally, hypomagnesemia. Intrathecal amphotericin B is indicated in coccidioidal meningitis and refractory cryptococcal meningitis, though this therapy is associated with considerable toxicity. Doses of 0.1 to 0.5 mg are given three times per week initially, then with decreasing frequency.

Flucytosine   Flucytosine (5-fluorocytosine) is a synthetic oral drug useful in cryptococcosis, candidiasis, and chromomycosis. Within the fungal cell, flucytosine is converted to the antimetabolite 5-fluorouracil. Drug resistance appears rather rapidly when flucytosine is used alone. For this reason the drug is generally used in combination with amphotericin B, permitting a lower dose of the latter. The usual regimen is amphotericin B 0.3 mg/kg daily and flucytosine 37.5 mg/kg every 6 h. Flucytosine is well absorbed from the gastrointestinal tract, even in the presence of food. The drug penetrates well into the cerebrospinal fluid and is excreted unchanged in the urine. Hemodialysis results in significant drug removal. Even modest reductions in renal function may elevate flucytosine blood levels into the toxic range, ≥ 100 to 125 μg/mL. Elevated levels are associated with a significant incidence of neutropenia and thrombocytopenia. Elevated flucytosine blood levels also seem to predispose to colitis, the other major toxicity of this drug. Hepatotoxicity is idiosyncratic and uncommon. An allergic rash may also occur.

REFERENCES (See Chap. 151)

88   THERAPY OF PARASITIC INFECTIONS

JAMES J. PLORDE

INTRODUCTION   Despite some gains, treatment of parasitic diseases remains unsatisfactory. The total number of available agents remains small, and for some infections, including cryptosporidiosis, satisfactory drugs have yet to be developed. Few of the newer chemotherapeutics are at once inexpensive, effective in single oral dose, and safely dispensed with limited medical supervision, essential attributes if they are to be fully useful in developing countries, where the burden of parasitism is greatest. Drug resistance, a phenomenon so common to bacterial pathogens, now threatens the usefulness of several antiparasitic chemicals. This is particularly serious among the antimalarials. Chloroquine-resistant *Plasmodium falciparum*, long present in southeast Asia and Latin America, has spread to most parts of tropical Africa, the area most devastated by this disease. Some Asian strains of this organism have developed resistance to the

TABLE 88-1 Agents available through the parasitic diseases division, CDC*	
Infection	Therapeutic agent
Amebiasis	Dehydroemetine
	Diloxanide furoate
Chagas' disease	Nifurtimox
(*Trypanosoma cruzi*)	
Fascioliasis	Bithionol
Leishmaniasis	Sodium antimony gluconate (stibo-
	gluconate sodium)
Malaria	Parenteral quinine dihydrochloride
Onchocerciasis	Ivermectin
	Suramin
Paragonimiasis	Bithionol
Sleeping sickness	Melarsoprol
(*Trypanosoma brucei*)	Suramin

* Parasitic Diseases Division, Centers for Disease Control, Atlanta, Ga 30333. Telephone: (404)639-3670 (day); (404)639-2888 (evenings, weekends, or holidays).

pyrimethamine-sulfadoxine drug combination and to newly introduced agents such as mefloquine, sharply limiting the armamentarium available for the management of this lethal disease. The availability of many antiparasitic drugs is sharply limited, both in the United States and around the world. In fact, many of the drugs recommended in the following chapters have not been approved by the U.S. Food and Drug Administration either for use in this country or for the particular disease indicated. Those available as investigational agents through the Centers for Disease Control are listed in Table 88-1. Others, such as albendazole, DL-α-difluoromethylornithine (DFMO), and ivermectin, must be obtained directly from the manufacturer. When a clinician prescribes such an agent, the patient should be informed of the drug's investigational status and potential side effects.

STRUCTURE AND MODE OF ACTION   Characteristically, antiparasitic agents have been synthesized de novo rather than derived from naturally occurring antibiotics. Most are relatively simple, often containing benzene or other ring structures. Nitrocompounds are common, despite studies documenting that chemicals of this class may be teratogenic and carcinogenic in experimental animals. A few of the currently used drugs resemble the original chemotherapeutics in their possession of heavy metal moieties, specifically arsenic or antimony.

It has been difficult to determine the precise mechanisms by which chemotherapeutic agents kill or injure parasites, given the metabolic complexity of these organisms and the difficulties involved in maintaining them in vitro. Nevertheless, there is both direct and indirect evidence that most antiprotozoan agents act by interfering with nucleic acid synthesis. Anthelmintics, in contrast, are thought to compromise glycolytic pathways or interfere with neuromuscular function. As both parasite and host share similar, and in some cases identical, target sites, differential toxicity is achieved by differences in the susceptibility of functionally equivalent sites, metabolic alteration of the drug within the parasite, or preferential uptake by the parasite. The development of parasite resistance usually results from mutation and selection in the face of intensive drug use. The responsible mechanisms most commonly appear to be related to altered uptake of drug.

DRUG CATEGORIES   Heavy metals   Although nearly a century has passed since the introduction of the first organic heavy metal chemotherapeutic agents, a few such agents survive for want of adequate substitutes. Such drugs are thought to inhibit cellular enzyme systems necessary for metabolism by binding to sulfhydryl groups; arsenate ion may block ATP generation through the inhibition of pyruvate kinase. The drugs have their greatest impact on cells that are the most metabolically active, and their differential toxicity for parasites probably results from the intense metabolic activity of these pathogens. Pentavalent compounds, which appear to penetrate mammalian cells less effectively than their trivalent analogues, are generally preferred for human use. They appear, however, to be less effective parasitologic agents than the trivalent compounds and may require

intracellular conversion to the trivalent form for full activity. Side chain substitutions of the organic structure alter drug solubility and other pharmacologic properties.

Melarsoprol (Mel B), a trivalent compound capable of penetrating the blood-brain barrier, is the only arsenical still widely used for the treatment of human disease. It is administered for sleeping sickness when less toxic agents have failed or the central nervous system is involved. It must be given intravenously, and tissue extravasation produces an intense inflammatory reaction. Arsenic-induced enteropathy, hepatitis, nephritis, or dermatitis may occur. The most serious side effect is an often fatal encephalopathy, which occurs in up to 20 percent of patients with central nervous system involvement.

Antimonial agents are now restricted to the management of leishmanial infections. In the United States, the pentavalent compound sodium stibogluconate (Pentostam) is the drug of choice. It may be given intravenously, intramuscularly, or, in the case of cutaneous leishmaniasis, by local infiltration. In disseminated disease, prolonged therapy is often required and relapse occurs with some frequency. In localized cutaneous leishmaniasis, cure is usually achieved with a single, relatively brief course. Toxic side effects are similar to that produced by the arsenicals. Anaphylaxis, hemolytic anemia, arthropathies, bradycardia, electrocardiogram abnormalities, and vascular collapse have also been reported.

Antimalarial quinolines   Following the isolation of quinine from cinchona bark in 1820, this alkaloid rapidly became the most widely used antimalarial agent in the world. Synthesis of new antimalarials, which share a double-ring quinoline structure with quinine, was stimulated by the interruption of quinine supplies during two world wars and the subsequent development and spread of resistant strains of *P. falciparum*. The synthetic analogues fall into three major groups, the 4-aminoquinolines, 8-aminoquinolines, and 4-quinolinemethanols. The first two appear to block nucleic acid synthesis by intercalation into double-stranded DNA; the failure of the 4-quinolinemethanols to intercalate indicates that other mechanisms, possibly interference with hemoglobin digestion by the malaria parasite, may also be involved. Quinine, 4-aminoquinolines, and 4-quinolinemethanols concentrate in parasitized erythrocytes and rapidly destroy the intracellular schizonts. As these parasite forms are responsible for the clinical manifestations of malaria, blood schizonticides rapidly terminate the acute malarial paroxysm; administered prophylactically, they prevent clinical manifestations should infection occur. As they are not selectively concentrated in tissue cells, hepatic schizonts survive administration of these agents and may later invade the bloodstream and reestablish erythrocytic infection, producing a clinical relapse. The 8-aminoquinolines accumulate in tissue cells and, by damaging parasite mitochondria, destroy hepatic hypnozoites. This prevents subsequent relapse and effects a radical cure. While active against mature gametocytes of all four malaria species, the 8-aminoquinolines are minimally effective against erythrocytic schizonts; accordingly, they are not used in the treatment of acute disease. The discrepancy between the high level of activity demonstrated by these drugs against hepatic hypnozoites and mature gametocytes and their minimal activity against erythrocytic schizonts is not fully understood. As the two former parasitic stages are metabolically dormant, it is possible they lack the capacity for mitochondrial repair, making them more sensitive to the damaging effects of the 8-aminoquinolines.

Quinine is the most toxic of the quinolines. Normal doses produce tinnitus and reversible alterations in auditory and visual acuity (cinchonism). Rapid intravenous administration may induce cardiac arrythmia and/or hypotension. Its use is currently restricted to the treatment of multiresistant strains of *P. falciparum*. Chloroquine phosphate, a 4-aminoquinoline, is the most widely used of the blood schizonticidal drugs. In the doses recommended for long-term malaria prophylaxis, it has proved remarkably free of untoward effects, even in pregnant women. Although irreversible retinopathy has occurred in patients receiving high daily doses over prolonged periods for conditions such as rheumatoid arthritis, this phenomenon has been seen rarely among those taking the lower doses recommended for malaria prophylaxis, even after decades of use. Its use in acute malaria is occasionally accompanied by transient gastrointestinal or visual disturbances. Chloroquine overdose can produce convulsions and cardiorespiratory arrest. The major toxic effect of primaquine phosphate, the 8-aminoquinoline used to eradicate persistent hepatic parasites, relates to its oxidant activity. Methemoglobinemia and hemolytic anemia are particularly frequent in patients with glucose-6-phosphate dehydrogenase deficiency, because they are unable to generate sufficient quantities of NADPH to respond to this oxidant stress. Typically, anemia is severe in patients of Mediterranean and Oriental ancestry and mild in blacks.

Strains of *P. falciparum* resistant to several of the blood schizonticidal agents are spreading rapidly through Asia, Latin America, and Africa. Chloroquine resistance is the most frequent and worrisome because there are few suitable alternatives to this safe and highly effective agent. The mechanism of resistance is not clearly understood. Mefloquine, a newly developed oral 4-quinolinemethanol, displays high level of activity against most chloroquine-resistant parasites. However, its structural similarity to chloroquine, the ready in vitro induction of mefloquine resistance in *P. falciparum,* and reports of mefloquine-resistant falciparum malaria from the field raise the specter that cross-resistance to this new agent may develop quickly.

Folate antagonists In protozoa, as in bacteria, the active form of folic acid is produced in vivo by a simple two-step process. The first, the conversion of para-aminobenzoic acid (PABA) to dihydrofolic acid, is blocked by sulfonamides. The second, the transformation of dihydro- to tetrahydrofolic acid, is suppressed by folic acid analogues (folate antagonists), which competitively inhibit the enzyme dihydrofolate reductase. Used together with sulfonamides, these antagonists are very effective inhibitors of protozoan growth.

The trimethoprim and sulfamethoxazole combination so widely used as an antibacterial agent is also effective in the management of some parasitic diseases, most notably *Pneumocystis carinii* pneumonia. Because of its high affinity for sporozoan dihydrofolate reductase, pyrimethamine has been particularly effective, when used in combination with a sulfonamide, in the management of malaria and toxoplasmosis. Proguanil also demonstrates antimalarial activity. Because this folate antagonist is slow-acting, it is used as a prophylactic rather than a therapeutic agent. Although unavailable in this country, it is used in many endemic areas of Africa and Asia. Acquired protozoan resistance is mutational in origin and generally has been limited to species of plasmodia; the mechanism is presumed to be identical to that described for bacteria. Cross-resistance among drugs of this class is common.

Manifestations of folate deficiency may be seen when these agents are used in individuals with limited folate stores, such as newborns, pregnant women, and the malnourished. It is particularly frequent when large doses are used for a prolonged period of time, as in the treatment of acute toxoplasmosis. When administered with sulfonamides, the entire range of toxicities associated with this class of antimicrobials may be seen. Of particular concern are the serious cutaneous reactions such as erythema multiforme, toxic epidermal necrolysis, and the highly lethal Stevens-Johnson syndrome reported in individuals receiving long-term malaria prophylaxis with the pyrimethamine-sulfadoxine combination. Patients with acquired immunodeficiency syndrome (AIDS) appear to suffer an unusually high incidence of toxic side effects to trimethoprim-sulfamethoxazole given for the treatment of *P. carinii* pneumonia. In approximately half, the reactions are severe enough to require discontinuation of the drugs.

Nitroimidazoles Metronidazole, one of the first of the new generation of antiparasitic agents, was introduced in 1959 for the treatment of trichomoniasis. Subsequently, it was found to be effective in the management of giardiasis and amebiasis as well. In all three of these protozoan agents, generation of energy is dependent upon the presence of low redox potential compounds such as ferredoxin to serve as electron carriers. They reduce the 5-nitro group of the imidazoles to intermediate products responsible for the death of protozoal cells, possibly by alkylation of DNA. Resistance, although uncommon, has been noted in strains of *Trichomonas vaginalis* lacking nitroreductase activity. Since low redox potential compounds are unique to obligate anaerobes, the nitroimidazoles are ineffective against aerobic or facultatively anaerobic pathogens. Metronidazole is rapidly absorbed after oral administration, reaching peak levels in 2 h; it diffuses well into all tissues, including the brain and cerebrospinal fluid. Side effects are uncommon and generally mild, including a metallic taste, epigastric discomfort, urethral and vaginal burning, overgrowth of *Candida,* and reversible neutropenia. Excreted metabolites often impart a reddish-brown color to the urine. Although an Antabuse-like reaction has been reported with metronidazole, this is not common. Rarely, central nervous system toxicity including vertigo, ataxia, sensory neuropathy, and convulsions has been observed. Of greater concern is metronidazole's mutagenicity for a variety of bacteria, an indication of its potential carcinogenicity in mammals. This appears to be mediated by the nitro group's reduction metabolites. Although tumorigenic activity has been demonstrated in chronically dosed rodents, it has not been noted in two retrospective human studies. Longer observation periods will be required before a definitive judgment about human carcinogenicity can be made. Although there is no evidence of teratogenicity in either animals or humans, it is probably unwise to use this agent during the first trimester of pregnancy. Metronidazole is the drug of choice for trichomoniasis and invasive amebiasis. Although not yet approved for treatment of giardiasis, the drug is effective in this infection as well. Tinidazole, a newer nitroimidazole not yet available in the United States, appears to be both more effective and less mutagenic.

Benzimidazoles As the name implies, the basic structure of these broad-spectrum anthelmintic agents consists of linked imidazole and benzene rings. The prototype drug, thiabendazole, acts against both adult and larval nematodes and was shown to be useful in the management of cutaneous larva migrans, trichinosis, and most intestinal nematode infections. It remains the drug of choice of cutanea larva migrans, strongyloidiasis, toxocariasis, and trichinosis. The mechanism by which it exerts its anthelmintic action is uncertain; it is known to inhibit fumarate reductase, an important mitochondrial enzyme of helminths. Thiabendazole is rapidly absorbed from the intestinal tract, reaches peak levels within 1 h of dosing, and, after hydroxylation in the liver, is almost totally eliminated in the urine within 24 h. Most side effects are mild, related to the gastrointestinal tract or liver, and rapidly disappear with the discontinuation of the drug. Occasionally dizziness, paresthesias, and drowsiness are noted. Hypersensitivity reactions, induced either by the drug or by antigens released from the damaged parasite, may occur.

Mebendazole, a carbamate benzimidazole, has a spectrum similar to that of thiabendazole. It also has been found to be effective against a number of cestodes including *Taenia, Hymenolepsis,* and *Echinococcus.* It is the drug of choice for pinworm infections, trichuriasis, ascariasis, and hookworm disease. Although not yet approved for use in tapeworm infections, mebendazole has proved to be useful in the management of the cestode infections mentioned above, particularly as an adjunct to the surgical removal of echinococcal cysts. It irreversibly blocks glucose uptake of both adult and larvae worms resulting in glycogen depletion, cessation of ATP formation, and paralysis or death. It does not appear to affect glucose metabolism in humans and is thought to exert its effect in worms by binding to tubulin and interfering with the assembly of cytoplasmic microtubules, structures essential to glucose uptake. Unlike thiabendazole, the drug is not well absorbed from the gastrointestinal tract, and it may owe part of its effectiveness against intestinal-dwelling adult worms to its high concentrations in the gut. Because of its poor absorption, systemic toxicity is uncommon. Nevertheless teratogenic effects have been observed in experimental animals. Accordingly its use in infants and pregnant women is contraindicated.

Albendazole, a benzimidazole carbamate not yet approved for use in the United States (available from manufacturer), has a spectrum similar to that of its close relative, mebendazole. It may be more effective than mebendazole in the management of echinococciasis, and is effective in the management of many intestinal nematode infections when administered as a single-dose treatment.

Avermectins   Avermectins are macrocyclic lactones produced as fermentation products of *Streptomyces avermitilis*. They are effective at extremely low concentrations against a wide variety of nematodes and arthropods, possibly by mimicking the action of the parasites' inhibitory neurotransmitter, γ-aminobutyric acid (GABA), thereby producing neuromuscular paralysis; host immune mechanisms may synergize and prolong drug activity. GABA receptors also are found in the mammalian brain, but because avermectins penetrate the blood-brain barrier poorly, significant untoward effects in humans appear to be uncommon. As might be suspected by their unique mode of action, these antibiotics have not demonstrated cross resistance with other antiparasitic agents.

Ivermectin, a 22,23-dihydro derivative of avermectin B_1 widely used in veterinary medicine, has become the drug of choice for the treatment of onchocerciasis. Peak blood levels are achieved within 3 h of oral administration, but little is known about subsequent distribution or metabolism of the drug in humans. While pharmacokinetic studies have demonstrated a half-life of only 22 h, microfilaricidal activity appears to persist for months. Dose-dependent, mild to moderate hypotension occurs in approximately 5 percent of drug recipients, but only rarely requires therapy. Rash, tenderness, and lymph node enlargement have also been reported. Ocular reactions are minimal, even in patients with severe corneal involvement. Its usefulness in other nematode infections of humans remains to be established. Not yet approved for use in the United States, the drug may be obtained from the manufacturer for investigational purposes.

Praziquantel   As an extremely safe, single-dose oral agent effective against a broad range of cestodes and trematodes, praziquantel more closely approaches the definition of an ideal antiparasitic than any other currently used anthelmintic. This heterocyclic pyrazine-isoquinoline is rapidly absorbed from the gastrointestinal tract and metabolized in the liver; it diffuses well into most tissues, including the central nervous system. Activity appears dependent on the agent's ability to penetrate the helminthic cuticle; the thick outer membrane of the nematodes protects this class of worms from the action of the drug. In the susceptible platyhelminths, praziquantel induces the loss of intracellular calcium with tetanic muscular contraction, paralysis, and tegmental damage. The latter results in the loss of attachment organs and the exposure of surface antigens to the host's immune mechanisms. Differential toxicity appears related to the inability of susceptible worms to metabolize the drug. Aside from the transient, mild gastrointestinal symptoms, the drug is remarkably free of side effects; it is well tolerated by patients with glucose-6-phosphate dehydrogenase deficiency and hemoglobinopathies, and does not appear to be mutagenic or carcinogenic. It is currently the drug of choice for the treatment of schistosomiasis, neurocysticercosis, *Hymenolepsis nana* infections, and all infections produced by hermaphroditic flukes, *Fasciola hepatica* excepted. Good activity has been demonstrated against other common trematode and cestode infections, and it may displace currently used agents for these diseases as well. Its effectiveness as a single dose and its high level of safety make it likely that this agent will play a significant role in worldwide mass therapy campaigns.

Ornithine decarboxylase inhibitors   Elfornithine (DL-α-difluoromethylornithine, DFMO) is a potent inhibitor of *Trypanosoma*

TABLE 88-2   Miscellaneous antiparasitic medications

Compound	Drug class	Route	Mechanism of action	Clinical use	Side effects and comments
Bithionol	Phenol	Oral	Uncouples phosphorylation	Paragonimiasis	Rare leukopenia, toxic hepatitis Availability: CDC
Dehydroemetine	Synthetic alkaloid	SQ	Blocks movement of ribosome along messenger RNA	Tissue amebiasis	Occasional GI disturbances, neuropathy, heart failure; use only in severe disease Availability: CDC
Diethylcarbamazine	Piperazine	Oral	Neuromuscular paralysis	Filarial infections	Allergic reactions to filarial antigens Rare loss of vision in onchocerciasis Availability: Lederle
Diloxanide furoate	Acetanilide	Oral	Unknown	Intestinal amebiasis	Flatulence, urticaria Indications: asymptomatic carriers Availability: CDC
Iodoquinol (diiodohydroxyquin)	Halogenated quinoline	Oral	Unknown	Intestinal amebiasis, *Dientamoeba* infections	Rare optic atrophy with prolonged use
Niclosamide	Phenol	Oral	Uncouples phosphorylation	Intestinal tapeworms	Occasional nausea, abdominal pain Does not kill eggs
Nifurtimox	Nitrofuran	Oral	Alkylates DNA	Acute Chagas' disease	Rare convulsions, pulmonary infiltrates Therapy prolonged, effectiveness marginal Availability: CDC
Pentamidine	Diamidine	IV	Binds DNA	Pneumocystosis, leishmaniasis, trypanosomiasis	Extremely toxic
Pyrantel pamoate	Tetrahydropyrimidine	Oral	Neuromuscular blockade Inhibits fumarate reductase	Pinworm infection, hookworm infection, ascariasis	Occasional GI disturbance, fever Single-dose therapy
Suramin	Sulfated naphthylamine	IV	Inhibits a glycerophosphate oxidase and dehydrogenase	African trypanosomiasis, onchocerciasis	Occasional renal toxicity, blood dyscrasia, optic atrophy, shock Not effective in CNS disease

SOURCE: After JJ Plorde.

TABLE 88-3 Fecal egg counts associated with illness

Worm	Approximate egg output per female worm per day	Minimum egg output usually associated with illness
Necator americanus	25,000	>2000/mL
Trichuris trichiura	7500	>3000/g
Schistosoma mansoni	60–300	>200/g

SOURCE: After DP Stevens, Clin Gastroenterol 7:236, 1978.

brucei, the protozoan agent of African trypanosomiasis (sleeping sickness). It acts by specifically and irreversibly inhibiting ornithine decarboxylase (ODC), an enzyme required in the biosynthesis of polyamines such as putrescine, spermidine, and spermine—substances thought to play an important role in cell division and differentiation. In *T. brucei,* DFMO slows nucleic acid synthesis and alters parasite morphology. Its effect appears to be cytostatic; an intact immune system is required for optimal effect. Although ornithine decarboxylase is present in mammalian as well as protozoan cells, *T. brucei* is 100 times more sensitive to the effects of elfornithine than are mammalian cells, possibly related to its high affinity for the trypanosomal enzyme or its active uptake by trypanosomes. Diarrhea, a common side effect, can be controlled with symptomatic therapy and dose reduction. Reversible anemia occurs in one-third of patients. Seizures have occurred in 10 percent of patients with late-stage trypanosomiasis. The drug may be given orally or intravenously and readily penetrates the blood-brain barrier. Early clinical trials in *T.b. gambiense* infections have shown the drug to be highly effective, even in patients failing arsenical therapy. It seems likely that this agent will supplant melarsoprol in the treatment of central nervous system trypanosomal infections. Not yet approved for use in the United States, the drug may be obtained from the manufacturer for investigational purposes.

Miscellaneous agents The names of a number of other important antiparasitic agents, the diseases for which they are used, their mode of action, and other comments are provided in Table 88-2.

THERAPEUTIC GOALS The principles governing the treatment of helminthic infections differ significantly from those employed for the management of prokaryotic or protozoan disease. Unlike the latter pathogens, worms, with few exceptions, do not multiply within the human host. Although they produce prodigious numbers of offspring, these mature to their infectious state outside the body. Subsequent contact of a human with an infectious egg or larva results in the development of a single adult worm within the host's body. Multiple worm infections require the repeated acquisition of infectious stage parasites. Because there is a direct correlation between the total number of worms harbored by the human host and the disability incurred, clinical disease is manifest only in those who have accumulated large worm burdens through repeated infections. Worm burdens do not follow a normal distribution in human populations. Most infected patients harbor fewer than a dozen adult worms; only a small minority harbor the large numbers required to produce clinical illness. In endemic areas, focusing treatment on the clinically ill will alleviate the medical impact of a helminthic disease on a community at a cost dramatically lower than that required for treatment of all who are infected. Short, subcurative doses will often produce sufficient decrease in the worm burden to alleviate clinical symptoms. This approach reduces cost, minimizes the likelihood of drug toxicity, and decreases the transmission of disease by targeting the major reservoir of the helminths. In general, light infections need to be treated only when (1) a small number of worms may be dangerous, as in the case of strongyloidiasis, (2) the chance of reinfection is slight, and/or (3) the anthelmintic agent in question is without serious side effects. The intensity of many infections can be determined by enumerating the eggs found in stool (Table 88-3). Multiplying the total seen on direct smear by 750 provides a rough estimate of the number present per gram of feces. The Stoll dilution and the various modifications of the Kato thick-smear technique provide more precise results.

REFERENCES

CAMPBELL WC, REW RS (eds): *Chemotherapy of Parasitic Diseases.* New York, Plenum, 1986

Drugs for parasitic infections. Med Lett 30:15, 1988

Health Information for International Travel 1988. US Department of Health and Human Services Publication (CDC) 88-8280, 1988

PLORDE JJ: Pathogenesis and chemotherapy of parasitic diseases, in *Medical Microbiology: An Introduction to Infectious Diseases,* 2d ed, JC Sherris (ed). New York, Elsevier–North Holland, 1989

section 3 Clinical syndromes

89 SEPTICEMIA AND SEPTIC SHOCK

RICHARD K. ROOT / RICHARD JACOBS

DEFINITION Septicemia and septic shock are dramatic clinical syndromes which result from acute invasion of the bloodstream by certain microorganisms or their toxic products. Fever, chills, tachycardia, tachypnea, and altered mentation are common acute manifestations of septicemia. When hypotension and signs of inadequate organ perfusion develop, the condition is termed *septic shock.* The circulatory insufficiency is characterized by a lowered systemic vascular resistance, decreased myocardial contractile function, and pooling and altered distribution of blood in the microcirculation. Diffuse cell and tissue injury and, ultimately, widespread organ failure develop. Even with appropriate antimicrobial and supportive care many patients die of septic shock, making strategies for prevention and more effective treatment of critical importance.

ETIOLOGY Manifestations of septicemia can be seen with severe systemic infection with all classes of organisms; however, frank septic shock is most commonly caused by gram-negative bacteria (60 to 70 percent of cases). Staphylococci, pneumococci, streptococci, and other gram-positive organisms are less frequent causes (20 to 40 percent of cases), as are opportunistic fungi (2 to 3 percent), and, rarely, mycobacteria or certain viruses (e.g., dengue–hemorrhagic fever and herpesviruses) or protozoans (e.g., *Falciparum malaria*). In septic shock, *Escherichia coli, Klebsiella-Enterobacter, Proteus, Pseudomonas,* and *Serratia* are the most frequent blood culture isolates, followed by staphylococci and pneumococci. Gram-negative bacteremia is complicated by shock in about 40 percent of patients; shock is seen in 5 to 15 percent of patients with acute bacteremias caused by pneumococci or staphylococci. In the setting of systemic purpura and meningitis, *Neisseria meningitidis* is the most frequent isolate. Patients may develop manifestations of sepsis and frank septic shock with severe localized infection but without detectable organisms on blood culture. The sepsis syndrome and shock are triggered by the interactions of various microbial products in the blood, in particular, gram-negative endotoxins, with host mediator systems.

EPIDEMIOLOGY In the 1970s the incidence of gram-negative rod bacteremia in the United States was estimated at between 100,000 and 300,000 cases per year; the incidence now may approach 300,000 to 500,000 cases per year. About two-thirds of cases are seen in already hospitalized patients, most of whom have underlying diseases or procedures which render their bloodstreams susceptible to invasion. Despite the introduction of new antimicrobial agents, the overall mortality from gram-negative bacteremia has averaged about 25 percent over the past two decades and is highest in patients who have major associated diseases or shock. Predisposing factors include diabetes mellitus; cirrhosis; alcoholism; leukemia; lymphoma or disseminated carcinoma; cytotoxic chemotherapy and immunosuppressive drugs which cause neutropenia; total parenteral nutrition; a variety of surgical procedures; and infections arising from the urinary, biliary, or gastrointestinal tracts. Neonates and elderly patients with urinary tract obstruction or dysfunction are particularly at risk. Gram-positive bacteremias are more often community-acquired except staphylococcal sepsis from indwelling intravenous catheters. In the 1970s gram-positive organisms accounted for less than 10 percent of cases of septic shock in most hospitals, but their relative incidence appears to be increasing and now approximates 30 percent in prospective studies. Opportunistic fungal sepsis is seen most often in immunosuppressed patients with severe neutropenia or in postoperative patients with intravenous catheters and usually follows prolonged antibiotic therapy. The widespread use of antibiotics, glucocorticoids, mechanical ventilation, and urinary and intravenous catheters and drainage tubes in other sites, as well as the increased longevity of patients with chronic diseases, contributes to the changing incidence and profile of this serious clinical problem.

PATHOGENESIS AND PATHOLOGY Most of the bacteria causing gram-negative sepsis are normal commensals in the gastrointestinal tract. From there they may spread to contiguous structures, as in peritonitis after appendiceal perforation, or they may migrate from the perineum into the urethra or bladder. Gram-negative bacteremia follows infection in a primary focus, usually the genitourinary tract, biliary tree, gastrointestinal tract, or lungs and, less commonly, the skin, bones, and joints. In burn patients and in patients with leukemia, the skin or the lungs are often portals of entry. In about 30 percent of cases, notably in patients with debilitating diseases, cirrhosis, and cancer, no primary focus is apparent. Gram-positive bacteremias usually arise from the skin or respiratory tract. Metastatic abscess formation may complicate bacteremia, particularly that caused by gram-positive or anaerobic organisms. More often, however, the autopsy findings in gram-negative sepsis reflect primarily the infection

at the primary locus and show involvement of target organs: pulmonary edema, hemorrhage, and hyaline membrane formation in the lungs; tubular or cortical necrosis in the kidney; patchy necrosis in the myocardium; superficial ulceration or even hemorrhagic necrosis in the gastrointestinal tract; and leukocyte-platelet or, less commonly, fibrin thrombi in the capillaries in many tissues.

PATHOPHYSIOLOGY The clinical manifestations of septicemia and septic shock are the result of an interplay between microbial products and host mediator systems. From the standpoint of vascular perfusion and organ function a vicious circle is established that results in altered blood flow in the microcirculation and progressive injury to the capillary endothelium and tissues. Unless this circle is interrupted by control of the infection and correction of the hemodynamic and metabolic alterations, death usually results.

Microbial factors Microbial factors that are most important include gram-negative lipopolysaccharides (LPS), in particular, the lipid A component, peptidoglycans from gram-positive organisms or mannan from fungal cell walls, certain polysaccharides, and extracellular enzymes (e.g., streptokinase) or toxins (e.g., toxic shock enterotoxins of staphylococci) (see Chap. 100). The mechanisms of action of LPS and lipid A have been studied most extensively. LPS can directly activate humoral or cellular systems, which, in turn, promote the development of the septicemic and shock syndromes. Although not as well defined, other microbial products affect the same systems to varying degrees.

Host mediators A variety of host mediators have been implicated in the pathogenesis of septic shock including active metabolites of the complement, kinin, and coagulation systems as well as factors released from stimulated cells, in particular, the cytokines, tumor necrosis factor-α (TNF) and interleukin 1 (IL-1), enzymes and oxidants from polymorphonuclear leukocytes (PMNs), vasoactive peptides (e.g., histamine), and products of the metabolism of arachidonic acid. The precise sequence of events and the critical initiating steps need further clarification. Furthermore, the secretion and action of counterregulatory vasoactive catecholamines, angiotensin, pituitary hormones, insulin, and glucagon all contribute to the clinical and laboratory events in sepsis.

HUMORAL SYSTEMS LPS can directly activate both the *coagulation* and *kinin systems* through its effect on Hageman factor (Fig. 89-1). The intrinsic coagulation cascade is triggered (see Chap. 62); and increased turnover of factors XII, VIII, and V and fibrinogen is measurable in sepsis. Plasmin is also generated by activated Hageman factor. Bradykinin and related kinins are potent vasodilators, increase capillary permeability, and increase gastrointestinal motility. They are produced when activated Hageman factor cleaves prekallikrein to kallikrein. Reduction of these precursors and increases in plasma kinins have both been documented in septic shock.

LPS and other microbial products can activate the *complement system* (see Chap. 13); reduction of C3 levels in septic shock has

FIGURE 89-1 Schematized interactions between gram-negative lipopolysaccharides (LPS) and host humoral and cellular mediator systems in sepsis. PMNs = polymorphonuclear leukocytes; IL-1 = interleukin 1; TNF = tumor necrosis factor-α.

been correlated with a fatal outcome. Generation of the anaphylatoxins C3a and C5a can contribute to vasodilation and increased capillary permeability; free C5a and C3a have been detected in the plasma of septic patients. Effects on PMNs include aggregation, increased adhesion to endothelial cells, promotion of lysosomal enzyme release, and activation of the superoxide-generating system (see Chap. 81).

CYTOKINES   A primary mechanism for the multiple actions of LPS and other microbial products in sepsis appears to reside in their ability to induce formation and release of both IL-1 and TNF (or "cachetin") by macrophages, endothelial cells, and perhaps other cells (see Chap. 20). Cardinal manifestations of sepsis—fever, somnolence, myalgias, and leukocytosis—follow administration of small amounts of recombinant TNF or IL-1 to human beings. Large doses of TNF in experimental animals produce all the systemic and pathologic features of LPS- or bacteria-induced septic shock, including hypotension, pulmonary injury with platelet and leukocyte thrombi, hemorrhagic necrosis of the intestine, acute renal failure, severe metabolic acidosis, and death. Anti-TNF antibodies block the manifestations of experimental LPS- and bacteria-induced sepsis, as does pretreatment with glucocorticoids, which inhibit TNF and IL-1 production, or cyclooxygenase inhibitors, which block their actions.

TNF appears in the plasma of human beings following LPS administration. During naturally occurring sepsis the levels of TNF in some studies correlate with severity and mortality, although more investigation of this is needed. Less precise correlations have been observed with measurements of circulating IL-1; however, it acts synergistically with TNF when administered in vivo to animals. Furthermore, many of the effects of IL-1 may be exerted at a local cellular level by the nonsecreted IL-1α form. The mechanisms by which TNF and IL-1 are produced and act and their relevance to the acute inflammatory responses characteristic of sepsis are discussed in detail in Chap. 20.

In experimental animals TNF and IL-1 can act synergistically to mobilize amino acids from muscles by proteolysis and lipids from adipose tissue, producing hyperlipidemia, and they also promote hepatic glycogenolysis and gluconeogenesis. Albumin synthesis is inhibited and may lead to hypoalbuminemia; formation of acute phase reaction proteins is enhanced. Finally, both TNF and IL-1 can release insulin and glucagon from pancreatic cells, and adrenocorticotropic hormone (ACTH), β-endorphins, growth hormone, and arginine vasopressin (AVP) from the pituitary. These studies suggest that both cytokines contribute to characteristic hormonal and metabolic alterations seen in sepsis in human beings.

Other cytokines found in high levels in the plasma of patients with sepsis include interleukin 6 (IL-6) and interferon γ (IFN-γ). These cytokines may act synergistically with IL-1 and TNF (IL-6) or augment cellular responses to TNF (IFN-γ).

ARACHIDONATE METABOLITES   In experimental animals inhibition of cyclooxygenase or thromboxane synthetase has been protective against lethal endotoxin shock. Elevated levels of thromboxane B_2 (TBX_2) and the end product of prostacyclin metabolism, 6-keto-prostaglandin $F_{1\alpha}$, are present in patients with sepsis. Thromboxanes, produced by activated platelets and PMNs, are platelet aggregating agents and induce pulmonary arteriolar constriction. Prostacyclins formed by endothelial cells oppose the action of thromboxanes (see Chap. 69), are potent vasodilators, and increase capillary permeability. Production of these products, as well as of the classic prostaglandins of the E series, by a variety of cells may be induced by IL-1 and TNF as well as LPS. For example, induction of prostaglandin E_2 synthesis in the brain is a key step in fever production by IL-1 and TNF (see Chap. 20); IL-1- or TNF-induced PGE_2 production in muscles promotes proteolysis. Circulating PGE_2 is a systemic vasodilator and promotes gastrointestinal motility. By direct effects on PMNs, endothelial cells, platelets, macrophages, and mast cells, LPS can promote the formation of leukotrienes and platelet activating factor (PAF) (see Chap. 69). Leukotrienes can induce asthma and pulmonary edema, and leukotriene B_4, specifically, has potent effects on PMNs which reproduce the actions of C5a and TNF. PAF

aggregates platelets, is a vasodilator, increases capillary permeability, and also has effects on PMNs that duplicate those of the leukotrienes.

Once triggered, the interactions become very complex, with recruitment of a wide array of inflammatory mediators. Endothelial cells and the microcirculation appear to be major targets of this intravascular inflammatory response. There is evidence of cytotoxicity, precapillary shunting, the plugging of postcapillary venules with PMN and platelet thrombi, and fibrin deposition. A generalized capillary leak syndrome manifested in the lungs as pulmonary edema is a common event. Kinins, C3a, C5a, histamine released by mast cells, arachidonate metabolites, proteases, and oxygen products released by activated neutrophils, monocytes, and macrophages can all contribute to the vasomotor alterations characteristic of sepsis and can participate in capillary damage. Widespread tissue hypoxia and eventual cell death result from the disordered microcirculation.

CARDIOPULMONARY MANIFESTATIONS   The cardiovascular features of septicemia and septic shock can be distinguished from cardiogenic or hypovolemic shock in that the systemic vascular resistance (SVR) is low and the cardiac output is increased. A maldistribution of blood flow in the microcirculation occurs, presumably through the actions of various vasodilators and constrictors. Leakage of plasma constituents from capillaries contributes to functional hypovolemia. These findings appear to be universal and independent of the type of organism causing the infection. The cardiovascular abnormalities in sepsis with shock are discussed in detail in Chap. 39. In brief, in addition to a low SVR and early functional hypovolemia, which contribute to hypotension, about half the patients exhibit depression of myocardial contractile function. With successful treatment both the SVR and myocardial function return to normal over a several-day period. Death is associated with refractory hypotension and persistently low SVR, progressive lactic acidosis, and evidence of multiple organ failure despite administration of fluids, pressors, and antibiotics.

Hyperventilation is a characteristic early response to sepsis leading to varying degrees of respiratory alkalosis. The precise mechanisms for the initial hyperventilation remain to be defined, but at later stages, increased lung water, decreased compliance, stimulation of lung stretch receptors, and incipient or manifest pulmonary edema all play a role. Hypoxemia and increased blood lactate concentrations also cause hyperventilation through central mechanisms in the brain. Ventilation-perfusion mismatching early in sepsis causes a fall in arterial P_{O_2}. With progression of sepsis a widening alveolar-arterial oxygen gradient often signals lung injury, which becomes fully expressed as the adult respiratory distress syndrome (ARDS).

METABOLIC RESPONSES   Blood lactate concentrations rise early in sepsis, and in the late stages marked metabolic acidosis usually predominates. While increased lactate production by poorly perfused tissues may be a factor, reduced removal of lactate by the liver and kidneys appears to play the major role. In the late stages of septic shock generalized hypoperfusion and the use of vasoconstricting pressors also aggravate the acidosis.

Elevations in plasma ACTH, growth hormone, AVP, cortisol, catecholamines, glucagon and insulin, lipids, and amino acids occur in sepsis. Some hormonal responses can exacerbate hyperglycemia in diabetic patients by antagonizing the action of insulin and promoting ketosis (see Chap. 319). Conversely, some patients with sepsis develop hypoglycemia. The mechanisms are not fully understood, but diminished hepatic glycogen stores (in neonates, with starvation, and with preexisting liver disease) and excessive insulin release may both contribute.

COMPLICATIONS   Respiratory failure   Sepsis is the leading cause of ARDS (see Chap. 218). A progressively widening alveolar-arterial oxygen gradient and the appearance of diffuse pulmonary infiltrates on chest x-ray are characteristic features. Histopathologically the lungs show pulmonary edema, hemorrhage, atelectasis, hyaline membrane formation, and platelet-PMN-fibrin capillary thrombi. ARDS develops in 20 to 45 percent of patients with severe sepsis. Infection with gram-negative organisms and the development of clinical shock are the major risk factors. Overly vigorous intravenous fluid administration may also contribute. When ARDS results from sepsis, the mortality rates are 80 to 90 percent in most studies, with complicating secondary pneumonias responsible for many of the deaths which occur late (>48 h) in the course.

Coagulation defects Thrombocytopenia of modest (<150,000 platelets per microliter) to moderate (<50,000 to 100,000 platelets per microliter) degree is seen in up to 70 percent of patients with septicemia. Direct effects of LPS as well as activation of platelet aggregation by multiple mechanisms are responsible. Platelet counts below 50,000 per microliter (in the absence of antecedent marrow failure) are usually associated with evidence of disseminated intravascular coagulation (DIC) (see Chap. 62). Activation of Hageman factor also contributes to this syndrome, as does release of plasminogen activator from macrophages and endothelial cells. The development of overt DIC in septic shock is an ominous prognostic sign.

Renal failure Most patients will have evidence of renal hypoperfusion or renal injury including oliguria, azotemia, variable degrees of proteinuria, and the appearance of tubular and epithelial cells and coarse granular casts in the urine. Late complications include acute tubular necrosis (ATN) (see Chap. 223) or, rarely, renal cortical necrosis as part of a generalized Shwartzman reaction.

Other organs Patchy myocardial necrosis with heart failure, hemorrhagic necrosis of the intestine, and hepatic necrosis may occur terminally in sepsis as in other shock syndromes.

CLINICAL MANIFESTATIONS The abrupt onset of the full-blown picture of sepsis, with fever, chills, tachycardia, tachypnea, mental status changes, and hypotension, is easily recognized. However, during the early stages of sepsis and depending upon various host factors (e.g., age extremes, underlying disease, treatment with glucocorticoids), the clinical manifestations may be subtle and the diagnosis difficult. Fever and chills occur commonly, but up to 13 percent of patients may be hypothermic, with rectal temperature of <36.5°C (97.6°F), at the onset of sepsis, and an additional 5 percent of patients who are not initially hypothermic may fail to mount a febrile response above 37.5°C (99.6°F). The absence of fever is seen primarily in the elderly and in those with underlying diseases such as alcoholism and uremia and has been associated with a poor prognosis. Up to 40 percent of patients who present with hypothermia may have severe infection or bacteremia as the cause, and the mortality rate is higher in those with infection than in those with hypothermia of other causes.

Hyperventilation with respiratory alkalosis and changes in mental status are extremely important signs, because they occur early, often before the onset of fever, chills, and hypotension. In the initial stages of sepsis, alterations in mental status may be subtle, with disorientation or personality change as the only manifestation; later in the disease more obvious changes of obtundation and coma may be present. Focal neurologic signs are absent, and the findings are usually more pronounced in neonates, the elderly, or those with preexisting central nervous system disease, but they may be seen in any patient.

Cutaneous manifestations occur with variable frequency, are diverse in presentation, and are not usually specific for the sepsis syndrome. They are extremely important, however, because a Gram stain of a scraping may confirm the presence of sepsis and indicate a preliminary microbiologic diagnosis. When bacteria or fungi invade the skin, pustules or vesiculopustular lesions are usually seen. In some gram-negative infections, particularly those caused by *Pseudomonas aeruginosa*, necrotizing or bullous skin lesions may occur and have been termed *ecthyma gangrenosum*. Sepsis associated with DIC is often accompanied by acrocyanosis with eventual necrosis of peripheral tissues (tip of the nose, fingertips, toes, and ears).

Gastrointestinal manifestations are seen in approximately one-third of patients. They include nausea, vomiting, diarrhea, or ileus and may obfuscate the diagnosis of septicemia by suggesting the possibility of acute gastroenteritis. Upper gastrointestinal bleeding may occur; on endoscopy small ulcers of the stomach and duodenum are seen. The appearance and prevalence of ulceration is similar to that seen in other conditions of extreme systemic stress (e.g., severe head trauma). Rarely hemorrhagic necrosis of the bowel occurs and may be exacerbated by preexisting atherosclerotic disease. Mild to moderate jaundice may be present, related to a sepsis-induced defect in bile secretion. Less frequently shock-induced hepatic necrosis occurs.

LABORATORY FINDINGS The laboratory data in sepsis are variable and depend primarily upon whether shock with end organ damage and other complications have occurred. There is usually a leukocytosis with a left shift, but normal white blood cell counts and even leukopenia can occur. Toxic granulations, Döhle bodies, and intracytoplasmic vacuolization may been seen within neutrophils. Thrombocytopenia is often present; when severe (<50,000 per microliter), it is usually a manifestation of concomitant DIC and is associated with a prolonged thrombin time, decreased fibrinogen level, and elevated fibrin degradation products. In the absence of DIC with a microangiopathic hemolytic anemia, red blood cell morphology and numbers are usually normal.

Many patients will demonstrate mild abnormalities on urinalysis, such as proteinuria. With shock, acute tubular necrosis (ATN) may develop with oliguria, azotemia, and cellular or granular casts. In patients with normal renal function, the urinary sodium is low (<20 meq/L) in the initial phases of shock but rises in the presence of ATN or with the use of diuretics.

During the early phases of sepsis there is respiratory alkalosis and arterial blood gases reveal an elevated pH and decreased P_{CO_2}. With shock a metabolic acidosis develops with elevated lactate levels. Hypoxemia is present in varying degrees and is most severe when ARDS develops. Abnormalities in the chest x-ray may include an underlying pneumonia as the source of sepsis, congestive heart failure as a result of myocardial depression and volume resuscitation, or the diffuse infiltrates of ARDS. The ECG often shows nonspecific ST-T wave abnormalities; as with any hypotensive patient an initial and follow-up ECGs are indicated to exclude myocardial infarction.

Hypoglycemia is an uncommon manifestation of overwhelming sepsis. Most diabetics will have hyperglycemia, and severe infection is a leading cause of diabetic ketoacidosis which may contribute to the development of shock (see Chap. 314). Abnormalities in serum electrolytes can include an elevated anion gap with reduction of the bicarbonate concentration and metabolic acidosis. Liver function test abnormalities include modest hyperbilirubinemia and elevations of the transaminases that may be more pronounced in severe shock. Hypoalbuminemia, mild at first, may progress as sepsis continues and malnutrition supervenes. Serum lipids are often elevated. Rarely, changes in serum calcium and phosphorus levels are seen.

DIAGNOSIS Because many of the signs and symptoms of sepsis are nonspecific, the bedside diagnosis may be difficult. Once shock with end organ dysfunction has supervened in the febrile patient with a primary focus, the diagnosis is usually obvious. The presence of hyperventilation with a normal chest x-ray and unexplained confusion or disorientation should raise the possibility of sepsis. Other entities often confused with septic shock include myocardial infarction, pulmonary embolus, drug overdose, occult hemorrhage, cardiac tamponade, rupture of an aortic aneurysm, and aortic dissection.

The diagnosis and etiology of sepsis is confirmed by finding pathogenic organisms in the blood or at other sites of infection. Because bacteremia is intermittent and low grade (usually less than 10 organisms per milliliter of blood), obtaining a single small volume of blood (5 to 10 mL) prior to initiating antibiotic therapy may only result in positive cultures 50 to 60 percent of the time. Obtaining a single large volume of blood (30 mL) and dividing it equally into three culture bottles will increase the yield. Blood cultures usually become positive within 3 days of incubation; the failure to do so may be due to the intermittent nature of the bacteremia, prior administration of antibiotics, or the presence of slow-growing, fastidious organisms. In several large prospective studies of septic shock blood cultures were positive in only 50 to 60 percent of patients; the diagnosis was established by documenting infection at a local site. A Gram stain and culture of the primary site of infection or skin lesions, if present, are essential to establish the diagnosis, determine the etiology, and assist in immediate management.

In some patients a rapid diagnosis of bacteremia can be made by doing a Gram stain of the buffy coat. Although results are conflicting, this simple technique has been reported to give positive results in up to 10 to 50 percent of patients with bacteremia. The presence of intracytoplasmic vacuoles in neutrophils may also correlate with the presence of bacteremia.

TREATMENT Reversal of sepsis and septic shock depends upon aggressive treatment of the underlying infection as well as careful monitoring of hemodynamic and respiratory function in order to ensure adequate perfusion and oxygenation of vital organs. In the severely ill patient, clinical assessment of hemodynamic function does not correlate well with values measured more precisely. Even though pulmonary artery catheterization has not been shown to improve survival, its use allows for accurate measurement of volume status, cardiac output, and peripheral resistance, and it is an invaluable aid in monitoring the administration of fluids and pressors. Although not absolutely required, a peripheral arterial line is helpful in monitoring pressure and obtaining arterial samples to assess oxygenation. Management of the patient with sepsis and septic shock requires attention to the following:

Reversal of the underlying disease The outcome of sepsis depends in large part upon the severity of the underlying disease of the patient. Patients who are immunosuppressed by virtue of drugs or a disease will have an improved outcome if the immunosuppressive medication can be decreased or discontinued or if the underlying disease can be effectively treated. In patients with neutropenia or neutrophil dysfunction who have persistent bacteremia despite appropriate antibiotic therapy, granulocyte transfusions should be considered, but their benefit is controversial.

Removal of the source of infection A careful search for the site of origin of a bacteremia is always indicated since, if possible, removal or drainage of the source can turn a potentially fatal disease into an easily treatable one. Intravenous catheters should be removed and replaced. Foley and drainage catheters should be checked for patency and replaced if necessary.

Support of respiration Arterial oxygen should be monitored by pulse oximetry or by direct measurement. Oxygen should be provided nasally or by mask sufficient to maintain arterial oxygen saturations in excess of 95 percent. If respiratory failure develops, intubation with mechanical ventilation should be employed. The use of positive end-expiratory pressure (PEEP) does not prevent ARDS from developing but is useful to improve oxygenation at the lowest possible fraction of inspired oxygen (see Chap. 218).

Hemodynamic support Many patients have a relative depletion of intravascular volume, and the initial response to a falling blood pressure should be the administration of fluid. Whether colloids or crystalloids are superior has not been established. Anemia severe enough to compromise peripheral oxygen delivery (e.g., hematocrit acutely <30 percent) requires red blood cell transfusions. The pulmonary capillary wedge pressure should be maintained between 15 and 20 mmHg or the central venous pressure between 10 and 12 cmH$_2$O. Adequate fluid usually requires initial administration of 1 to 1.5 L over 1 to 2 h although on occasion much larger volumes are needed. Once volume has been repleted, a diuretic such as furosemide can be given to maintain hourly urine output above 20 mL/h and to prevent the occurrence of pulmonary edema. If the mean arterial pressure is sufficient to maintain adequate mentation and urine output and to prevent chest pain, it is not necessary to raise blood pressure to normal levels. In previously normotensive patients this can usually be accomplished at mean arterial pressures of >60 mmHg. About a third of patients will respond to fluid administration alone with reversal of the hypotension; if volume resuscitation fails to increase blood pressure, pressor drugs should be given. Dopamine is the agent most frequently used. When given in doses of 5 to 10 (μg/kg)/min, it primarily has a beta$_1$ effect, augmenting cardiac output and dilating splanchnic, renal, and cerebral arterioles through stimulation of dopaminergic receptors (see Chap. 39). Higher doses stimulate alpha receptors and can result in peripheral vasoconstriction severe enough to cause ischemia and gangrene. Dobutamine, 2 to 20 (μg/kg)/min, acts primarily on beta$_1$- and beta$_2$-adrenergic receptors and may be particularly useful in the rare patients with low cardiac output states. Because of its alpha$_1$ effect, norepinephrine, 10 to 15 μg/min, should be reserved for situations in which blood pressure cannot be maintained by other means; it can be used in combination with dopamine.

Therapy of acidosis and DIC Acidosis often resolves with therapy of the underlying infection and correction of hypoperfusion. If the pH falls below 7.20, sodium bicarbonate should be given (see Chap. 51).

Treatment of the underlying infection is of critical importance in the management of DIC. Asymptomatic DIC (laboratory abnormalities only) or mild manifestations, such as ecchymoses or oozing at venipuncture sites, do not require specific therapy. If major bleeding is encountered, replacement of clotting factors and platelets is prudent. Use of heparin and fibrinolytic agents is controversial (see Chap. 62).

Antibiotics Antibiotics should be initiated as soon as the diagnosis of sepsis is seriously entertained. Prior to the institution of antibiotics, blood cultures as well as cultures of relevant body fluids and exudates should be obtained, but administration of antibiotics should not be unduly delayed just to obtain cultures. Identification of a portal of entry or localized site of infection can guide initial antibiotic therapy. In the absence of this information, it is important to note that the signs and symptoms of sepsis due to gram-positive and gram-negative organisms are identical and indistinguishable at the bedside. When considering the choice of antibiotics prior to the availability of culture results, an antibiotic or combination of antibiotics should be chosen with activity against both gram-positive and gram-negative organisms. Once the results of culture are known, therapy can be more specific. Drugs should be given intravenously, and, generally, bactericidal drugs are preferred over bacteriostatic agents. The dosage of drug used should be the maximum recommended in order to ensure adequate serum and tissue levels. Knowledge of local bacteriologic patterns is very important in choosing initial therapy. Many nosocomial pathogens may only be susceptible to drugs that may be potentially toxic, such as aminoglycosides. In such cases, even if the patient has renal insufficiency, it is usually necessary to give aminoglycosides to ensure adequate therapy, taking into account that nephrotoxicity from these agents usually requires 3 to 5 days to develop. Ideally, during that period the causative organism will be identified and less toxic drugs can be substituted. In most situations a single agent is adequate to treat sepsis with a known pathogen. Combination therapy is indicated in the following circumstances:

1 As initial therapy to cover all likely pathogens until culture results are available
2 To treat certain pathogens for which antibiotic synergy has been demonstrated, such as *Pseudomonas aeruginosa* and enterococcus
3 For therapy in immunosuppressed patients, particularly those with neutropenia

The following are examples of initial therapy for various infections by site until culture results and antimicrobial susceptibilities are known. The precise antimicrobial dosages are provided in Chap. 85.

Urosepsis is usually caused by gram-negative rods or enterococci, and initial therapy with ampicillin plus gentamicin (vancomycin for the penicillin-allergic patient) is appropriate. If only gram-negative rods are seen in the urine, then gentamicin alone should suffice unless there is reason to suspect resistance to this drug (see Chap. 95).

Intraabdominal infections are usually polymicrobial and caused by anaerobes and enteric gram-negative organisms. They can be treated with metronidazole and gentamicin (ampicillin can be added to cover the possibility of enterococcus). Ticarcillin plus gentamicin or cefoxitin plus gentamicin are equally effective as initial treatment.

Imipenem may be used as a single drug or in combination with an aminoglycoside (see Chap. 108).

Outpatient *pneumonia* in an otherwise healthy adult is usually caused by *Streptococcus pneumoniae*, and penicillin can be used. In alcoholics or smokers, *Klebsiella pneumoniae* and *Haemophilus influenzae* become important pathogens, and a second- or third-generation cephalosporin (e.g., cefuroxime, cefotaxime, or ceftizoxime) can be given (see Chap. 207).

Nosocomial pneumonias frequently are caused by resistant gram-negative rods, and an aminoglycoside (gentamicin or tobramycin), usually in combination with an antipseudomonal penicillin (ticarcillin, mezlocillin, azlocillin, or piperacillin) or ceftazidime, is indicated (see Chap. 207).

Cellulitis is usually caused by streptococci and staphylococci, and a first-generation cephalosporin (e.g., cefazolin) or oxacillin is adequate coverage.

Sepsis from an *intravenous catheter* is usually caused by *Staphylococcus aureus*, *S. epidermidis*, or gram-negative rods. The catheter should be removed, and therapy with vancomycin and gentamicin is indicated.

Meningitis in adults can be treated with high-dose penicillin to cover *S. pneumoniae* and *Neisseria meningitidis;* if a gram-negative organism is suspected (posttraumatic or nosocomial meningitis) or the Gram stain is negative, a third-generation cephalosporin, such as cefotaxime or ceftriaxone, should be given (see Chap. 354).

In 30 percent of cases no source will be evident, and broad-spectrum coverage for gram-negative and gram-positive bacteria is important. A choice of vancomycin, metronidazole and gentamicin, or cefotaxime and gentamicin is reasonable.

Other agents Studies in animals have suggested that under highly controlled conditions administration of glucocorticoids may reduce mortality in sepsis. The clinical use of these drugs has been controversial due to the lack of well-designed studies evaluating large numbers of septic patients. Two prospective, randomized, placebo-controlled, and blinded studies have assessed the effect of early administration of large doses of glucocorticoids (30 mg/kg methylprednisolone every 6 h for four doses or 30 mg/kg of methylprednisolone followed by a constant infusion of 5 mg/kg per hour for 9 h) on the outcome of patients with severe sepsis and shock. In both studies the addition of glucocorticoids did *not* improve survival, prevent the development of shock, or reverse shock in those who presented with it. Furthermore, superinfection was more likely to occur in patients treated with glucocorticoids, and the mortality rate was higher in steroid-treated patients with azotemia. Based on these data, there is little support for the use of glucocorticoids in the therapy of acute sepsis.

Naloxone, an opiate antagonist, has been demonstrated in animal studies to prevent endotoxin-induced shock. Although uncontrolled studies have suggested that naloxone can reverse septic shock in humans, most controlled studies involving small numbers of patients have not confirmed this finding. Thus, the use of naloxone remains of unproven benefit.

Administration of polyclonal antibodies directed at common core LPS antigens of the J5 mutants of *E. coli* has been shown to decrease mortality in patients with gram-negative bacteremia and septic shock and to prevent the development of shock when given prophylactically to high-risk patients. Immunotherapy for gram-negative sepsis is under investigation using monoclonal antibodies to core components of LPS and to TNF. Results are not yet available, but both techniques hold promise as a possible novel approach to therapy.

PROGNOSIS The outcome of gram-negative sepsis depends more upon host factors than virulence factors of organisms. A major determinant of mortality is the presence of underlying diseases: patients with rapidly fatal diseases (e.g., acute leukemia) have higher mortality rates than do patients with ultimately fatal (likely to be fatal in 5 years) or nonfatal diseases. With the exception of *Pseudomonas aeruginosa*, which has been associated with an increased mortality, the specific organism causing infection is not a major

determinant of outcome. The development of complications such as shock, lactic acidosis, DIC, and ARDS all contribute to a poor prognosis. Other less important factors associated with increased mortality include azotemia, failure to mount a febrile response, polymicrobial infections, and high-grade bacteremia (>10 organisms per milliliter of blood). Conversely, early and appropriate antibiotic therapy is associated with improved survival.

The overall mortality in gram-negative sepsis is about 25 percent; most deaths occur in the first 48 h. These early deaths are usually due to acute events such as irreversible shock. Deaths occurring after 48 h are usually due to persistent poorly controlled infection or to other complications of intensive care.

PREVENTION Despite the availability of new broad spectrum antibiotics with increased activity, the incidence and outcome of sepsis and septic shock have not decreased significantly in the last two decades. This is due in part to the failure of early recognition and therapy of underlying infection, a problem particularly common in the elderly, who may not manifest classic signs of infection. Even more important, though, is the increased longevity of patients with chronic diseases. Up to 75 percent of all episodes of gram-negative sepsis are nosocomial in nature. This fact emphasizes the need to limit invasive procedures, limit the use of intravenous lines, avoid Foley catheterization, and practice good infection control at all times in an attempt to prevent the occurrence of these infections (see Chap. 83). Finally, the use of active and passive immunization against cell wall components of gram-negative organisms holds promise as a preventive measure in the future.

REFERENCES

BALL HA et al: Role of thromboxane, prostaglandins, and leukotrienes in endotoxic and septic shock. Intensive Care Med 12:116, 1986

BEUTLER B, CERAMI A: Cachectin: More than a tumor necrosis factor. N Engl J Med 316:379, 1987

BONE RC et al: A controlled clinical trial of high dose methylprednisolone in the treatment of severe sepsis and septic shock. N Engl J Med 317:653, 1987

DEGROOTE MA et al: Plasma tumor necrosis factor levels in patients with presumed sepsis. Results in those treated with antilipid A antibody vs. placebo. JAMA 26:2, 1989

DINARELLO CA: Interleukin 1. Amino acid sequences, multiple biologic activities, and comparison with tumor necrosis factor. Year Immunol 2:68, 1986

THE EORTC INTERNATIONAL ANTIMICROBIAL THERAPY COOPERATIVE GROUP: Ceftazidime combined with a short or long course of amikacin for empirical therapy of gram-negative bacteremia in cancer patients with granulocytopenia. N Engl J Med 317:1692, 1987

GIRARDIN E et al: Tumor necrosis factor and interleukin 1 in the serum of children with severe infectious purpura. N Engl J Med 319:397, 1988

HACK CE et al: Increased plasma levels of interleukin-6 in sepsis. Blood 74:1704, 1989

HARRIS RL et al: Manifestations of sepsis. Arch Intern Med 147:1895, 1987

HIGGINS TL, CHENOW B: Pharmacotherapy of circulatory shock. Dis-a-Month 33:309, 1987

JACOBS ER, BONE RC: Clinical indicators in sepsis and septic adult respiratory distress syndrome. Medical emergencies I. Med Clin North Am 70:921, 1986

KREGER BE et al: Gram-negative rod bacteremia III: Reassessment of etiology, epidemiology, and ecology in 612 patients. Am J Med 68:332, 1980

——— et al: Gram-negative rod bacteremia IV: Re-evaluation of clinical features and treatment in 612 patients. Am J Med 68:344, 1980

MICHIE HR et al: Detection of circulating tumor necrosis factor after endotoxin administration. N Engl J Med 318:1481, 1988

PARKER MM et al: Profound but reversible myocardial depression in patients with septic shock. Ann Intern Med 100:483, 1984

ROBERTS DE et al: Effects of prolonged naloxone infusion in septic shock. Lancet 2:699, 1988

ROOT RK, SANDE MS (eds): *Contemporary Issues in Infectious Diseases*, vol 4, *Septic Shock*. New York, Churchill Livingstone, 1985

THE VETERANS ADMINISTRATION STUDY GROUP: Effects of high-dose glucocorticoid therapy in patients with clinical signs of systemic sepsis. N Engl J Med 317:659, 1987

WILSON JJ et al: Infection induced thrombocytopenia. Semin Thrombos Hemostas 8:217, 1982

YOUNG LS: Gram negative sepsis, in *Principles and Practices of Infectious Diseases*, 3d ed, G Mandell et al (eds). New York, Wiley, 1990, pp 611–635

ZIEGLER EJ et al: Treatment of gram negative bacteremia and shock with antiserum to a mutant *E. coli*. N Engl J Med 303:1225, 1982

90 INFECTIVE ENDOCARDITIS

DONALD KAYE

DEFINITION Infective endocarditis is an infection which produces vegetations on the endocardium. It is virtually always fatal if untreated. A heart valve is usually involved, but infection may be on a septal defect or mural endocardium. Infection of an arteriovenous shunt or coarctation of the aorta is more properly called endarteritis and produces a similar clinical syndrome. The subsequent discussion of endocarditis also applies to endarteritis.

CLASSIFICATION

Endocarditis can be divided into native valve endocarditis, endocarditis in intravenous drug abusers, and prosthetic valve endocarditis, each with different infecting microorganisms and courses. Endocarditis can also be classified as acute or subacute. Acute endocarditis most frequently is caused by *Staphylococcus aureus*, occurs on a normal heart valve, is rapidly destructive, produces metastatic foci, and untreated, is fatal in less than 6 weeks. Subacute endocarditis usually is caused by viridans streptococci, occurs on damaged valves, does not produce metastatic foci, and untreated, takes more than 6 weeks and even a year to be fatal. Correlations between organism and course are not perfect. Viridans streptococci can be associated with an acute course and *S. aureus* with a subacute course. Most important is classification by infecting organisms (e.g., *S. aureus* endocarditis), because the organism has implications for therapy as well as course.

NATIVE VALVE ENDOCARDITIS Etiology Although almost any bacteria can produce endocarditis, streptococci and staphylococci account for the vast majority of cases.

STREPTOCOCCI Streptococci cause 60 to 80 percent of cases of native valve endocarditis in patients who do not abuse intravenous drugs. Viridans streptococci (most commonly *S. sanguis*, *S. mutans*, or *S. mitior*) account for over half of these; *S. bovis*, enterococci,[1] and other streptococci cause 25, 15, and 5 percent respectively. Viridans streptococci are normal inhabitants of the oropharynx and generally are highly susceptible to penicillin.

Enterococci and group A beta-hemolytic streptococci attack normal or damaged heart valves and may cause their rapid destruction. Other streptococci are much more likely to infect damaged valves and rarely cause rapid valve destruction. Enterococci and *S. mitior* can cause metastatic abscesses, which are uncommon with other streptococci.

Enterococci are alpha-, beta-, or gamma-hemolytic and are normal inhabitants of the gastrointestinal tract, the anterior urethra, and occasionally the mouth. All enterococci are in Lancefield's group D and may be distinguished from other streptococci by biochemical tests. They are relatively resistant to penicillin G, and an aminoglycoside must be added to achieve a bactericidal effect. Enterococcal endocarditis is most common in males, who develop infection at an average age of 60, while the average age of women with enterococcal endocarditis is under 40. Many patients give a recent history of genitourinary tract manipulation, trauma, or disease (e.g., cystoscopy, urethral catheterization, prostatectomy, abortion, pregnancy, or cesarean section) which occur mainly in older men and younger women.

Two other group D streptococci, *S. bovis* and *S. equinus*, differ from enterococci biochemically and are highly susceptible to penicillin G. Endocarditis caused by these organisms can be treated like viridans streptococcal endocarditis. *S. bovis* endocarditis occurs in elderly individuals (80 percent over 60 years of age), over one-third of whom have a malignant or premalignant gastrointestinal lesion (most often colonic cancer or a villous adenoma or polyp of the colon).

STAPHYLOCOCCI Staphylococci cause about 25 percent of cases of native valve endocarditis (with *S. aureus* 5 to 10 times more frequent than *S. epidermidis*). *S. aureus* attacks normal or damaged heart valves, often causing rapid destruction. The course is often fulminant, with death from bacteremia within days or heart failure within weeks. Abscesses are common at multiple sites (e.g., kidneys, lungs, and brain). *S. epidermidis* infects abnormal valves without causing rapid destruction.

OTHER BACTERIA Almost all species of bacteria are occasional causes of endocarditis, including *Strep. pneumoniae*, *Neisseria gonorrhoeae*, enteric gram-negative bacilli, *Pseudomonas*, *Salmonella*, *Streptobacillus*, *Serratia marcescens*, *Bacteroides*, *Haemophilus*, *Brucella*, *Mycobacterium*, *N. meningitidis*, *Listeria*, *Legionella*, and diphtheroids, and can result in an acute or chronic course.

FUNGI Fungi rarely cause native valve endocarditis in nonintravenous drug abusers. However, *Candida* and *Aspergillus* endocarditis can occur in patients with intravascular catheters who frequently have received glucocorticoids, broad spectrum antimicrobial drugs, or cytotoxic agents. The course is usually subacute. Large friable vegetations are common and give rise to large emboli, often to the lower extremities. The prognosis is grave, partly because of the relatively poor activity of available antifungal agents.

OTHER MICROORGANISMS Spirochetes (e.g., *Spirillum minor*), cell wall–deficient bacteria, rickettsiae (*Coxiella burnetti*), and chlamydiae (*C. psittaci* and *C. trachomatis*) are rare causes of endocarditis.

Epidemiology In native valve endocarditis, the proportion of males is higher than females, and most patients are over age 50. Endocarditis is uncommon in children.

Between 60 and 80 percent of patients have an identifiable predisposing cardiac lesion. *Rheumatic valvular disease* accounts for about 30 percent of cases. The mitral valve is most commonly involved, followed by the aortic. Right-sided endocarditis usually affects the tricuspid valve but is rare on rheumatic valves.

Congenital heart disease other than mitral valve prolapse is the underlying lesion in about 10 to 20 percent of patients with endocarditis. Predisposing lesions include patent ductus arteriosus, ventricular septal defect, tetralogy of Fallot, coarctation of the aorta, pulmonary stenosis, and bicuspid aortic valve but not uncomplicated atrial septal defect. *Mitral valve prolapse* is the underlying lesion in about 10 to 33 percent of cases.

Degenerative heart disease predisposes to endocarditis. *Calcific aortic stenosis* (from degenerative disease or bicuspid valve) is an important lesion in the elderly. Other predisposing but unusual lesions are *asymmetric septal hypertrophy*, *Marfan's syndrome*, and *syphilitic aortic valve*. Arterioarterial or arteriovenous fistulas can also be underlying lesions. In 20 to 40 percent of patients with infective endocarditis, *no underlying heart disease* can be recognized.

ENDOCARDITIS IN INTRAVENOUS DRUG ABUSERS Drug abusers with endocarditis are frequently young males. The skin is the most frequent source of microorganisms responsible for endocarditis; contamination of drugs is less common. *S. aureus* causes over 50 percent of cases, streptococci about 15 percent and fungi (mainly *Candida*) and gram-negative bacilli (usually *Pseudomonas* species) about 10 to 15 percent each. Infection with multiple organisms is common. The onset is usually acute. Only about 20 percent of addicts with their first episode of endocarditis have previously damaged heart valves. The tricuspid valve is infected in over 50 percent of cases, the aortic in 25 percent, and the mitral in about 20 percent. Over 75 percent with *S. aureus* infection and a much lower percent with other organisms have tricuspid valve endocarditis. Pulmonary emboli or pneumonia consequent to septic pulmonary emboli are common in tricuspid valve endocarditis, and murmurs are frequently absent.

PROSTHETIC VALVE ENDOCARDITIS Any intravascular prosthesis predisposes to endocarditis and makes cure difficult. Infections of prosthetic valves now account for 10 to 20 percent of cases of endocarditis. Intravascular sutures, pacemaker wires, and Teflon-Silastic tubes can also be foci of infection. Patients with prosthetic valve endocarditis are mainly males over age 60. Endocarditis occurs

---

[1] Although enterococci have been classified as a separate genus, in this chapter they are considered with the streptococci.

in 1 to 2 percent of these patients during the first year after operation and 1 percent per year thereafter. Aortic valve prostheses are much more likely to be involved than mitral valve prostheses. The infection is usually on the suture line.

Early-onset endocarditis (onset of symptoms within 60 days of surgery) is a consequence of valve contamination during the procedure or bacteremia perioperatively. *Late-onset endocarditis* (onset of symptoms after 60 days) may have the same pathogenesis as early endocarditis (especially during the first year) but with a long incubation period, or may result from transient bacteremia.

About half the episodes of early and one-third of late endocarditis are caused by staphylococci, and *S. epidermidis* is more frequent than *S. aureus*. Gram-negative bacilli cause up to 15 percent and fungi (most commonly *Candida*) up to 10 percent of early cases and are less common in late endocarditis. A prosthetic valve may malfunction because of large fungal vegetations. Streptococci are the most frequent single cause of late endocarditis (about 40 percent of cases) but are uncommon in early endocarditis.

Early prosthetic valve endocarditis is often associated with valve dysfunction or dehiscence and a fulminant course. Although late endocarditis may be similarly fulminant, the course is commonly indistinguishable from that of patients without prosthetic valves, especially when the organism is a streptococcus.

PATHOGENESIS AND PATHOLOGY

The characteristic lesions of infective endocarditis are vegetations on valves or elsewhere on endocardium. The disease usually arises secondary to localization of microorganisms on sterile vegetations composed of platelets and fibrin. Sterile vegetations, termed nonbacterial thrombotic endocarditis, form over areas of trauma to the endothelium (e.g., from intracardiac foreign bodies), in areas of turbulence (as on deformed valves), over scars, or in patients with wasting disease, particularly malignancy (marantic endocarditis).

Infection of a sterile vegetation is most likely when bacteremia occurs with bacteria that adhere well to platelets, fibrin, and fibronectin. The vegetation of infective endocarditis then results from deposition of platelets and fibrin over the bacteria, forming a "protected site" into which phagocytic cells penetrate poorly.

Endocarditis tends to occur in high-pressure areas (left side of heart) and downstream from where blood flows through a narrow orifice at a high velocity from a high- to low-pressure chamber (e.g., distal to the constriction in coarctation of the aorta). Endocarditis is unusual in sites with a small pressure gradient, as in atrial septal defects. Endocarditis occurs more frequently in valvular incompetence than pure stenosis and is characteristically on the atrial side of the regurgitant mitral valve and the ventricular surface of the regurgitant aortic valve. A high-velocity stream of blood can produce satellite-infected lesions at distant points of impact.

Microorganisms that possess little pathogenicity in other situations, e.g., viridans streptococci, usually implant only on deformed heart valves with nonbacterial thrombotic endocarditis, but more virulent microorganisms, e.g., *S. aureus* and *Strep. pneumoniae*, can infect apparently normal valves.

Transient bacteremia is common in various infections and during traumatic procedures involving epithelial surfaces that are colonized by a bacterial flora (oropharynx, genitourinary and gastrointestinal tracts, and skin). For example, after trauma to tissues of the mouth, viridans streptococci are the most common bacteria isolated from blood, alone or more often mixed with other bacteria. The frequency and magnitude of bacteremia are related to the severity of periodontal disease and the severity of trauma. The portal of entry for the initiating episode of bacteremia is usually not apparent in viridans streptococcal endocarditis. Dental procedures, the most common apparent portals of entry, precede viridans streptococcal endocarditis in only 15 to 20 percent of cases.

Bacteremia also is common with prostatic surgery, cystoscopy,

urethral dilation or catheterization, and procedures on the female reproductive tract. The organisms are usually enterococci and gram-negative bacilli. About 50 percent of patients with enterococcal endocarditis have had a recent operation or instrumentation on the genitourinary or gastrointestinal tracts. About 35 percent with staphylococcal endocarditis have had a preceding staphylococcal infection at a remote site.

The clinical features of endocarditis result from the vegetations and an immune reaction to the infection. Extensive vegetations, especially in fungal endocarditis, may occlude the valve orifice. Rapid destruction with consequent valvular regurgitation may occur, especially with *S. aureus*. Healing may cause scar formation with subsequent valvular stenosis or regurgitation. Infection may extend into the myocardium producing burrowing abscesses. Conduction abnormalities, fistulas (between chambers of the heart and the pericardium or major vessels), or rupture of the chordae, a papillary muscle, or the ventricular septum may result.

Pieces of vegetation break off and embolize to the heart, brain, kidney, spleen, liver, extremities, and lung (in right-sided endocarditis). Infarcts and occasionally abscesses result. Septic embolization to the vasa vasorum or direct bacterial invasion of the arterial wall may result in formation of mycotic aneurysms which may rupture. Mycotic aneurysms most often develop in the cerebral arteries, aorta, sinuses of Valsalva, ligated ductus arteriosus, and the superior mesenteric, splenic, coronary, and pulmonary arteries.

Patients with endocarditis usually have high antibody titers against the infecting microorganism. This contributes to formation of circulating immune complexes that may result in glomerulonephritis (focal, membranoproliferative, or diffuse), arthritis, or various mucocutaneous manifestations of vasculitis.

Myocarditis may be due to small coronary artery emboli, myocardial abscesses, or immune complex vasculitis.

MANIFESTATIONS

Symptoms of endocarditis generally start within two weeks of the precipitating event. The *onset* is usually gradual, with mild fever and malaise, with organisms of low pathogenicity (e.g., viridans streptococci). With organisms of high pathogenicity (e.g., *S. aureus*), the onset is often acute with high fever. *Fever* is present in almost all patients with endocarditis (except occasionally in the elderly or those with renal failure, congestive heart failure, or severe debility). The fever is usually low grade (less than 39.4°C) except with acute disease. Arthralgias are common, and arthritis occurs occasionally.

Cardiac murmurs are almost always present except early in acute endocarditis or in intravenous drug abusers with tricuspid valve infection. True changes in murmurs or the appearance of a new murmur are uncommon except in acute endocarditis where a new murmur (particularly aortic regurgitation) is frequent. Changes in intensities of murmurs are often due to changes in heart rate and/or cardiac output (e.g., from anemia) and not necessarily from progressive valvular damage.

Splenomegaly and *petechiae* each tend to occur in about 30 percent of cases in disease of long duration. Petechiae are most frequently found on the conjunctivae, palate, buccal mucosa, and upper extremities. *Splinter hemorrhages* are subungual, linear, dark-red streaks that may appear in endocarditis but also commonly result from trauma. *Roth spots* (oval, retinal hemorrhages with a clear pale center) are seen in less than 5 percent of patients and may also occur in connective tissue disease and severe anemia. *Osler nodes* (small tender nodules usually on the finger or toe pads which persist for hours to days) occur in 10 to 25 percent of patients but also in other diseases. *Janeway lesions* are small hemorrhages with a slightly nodular character on the palms and soles and are most commonly seen in acute endocarditis. *Clubbing* of the fingers is present in some patients with longstanding disease. *Embolic episodes* are recognized in about one-third of patients and may occur during or after therapy. Emboli to large arteries (e.g., femoral arteries) are often the result of fungal endocarditis with its large friable vegetations. Pulmonary emboli are common in drug abusers with right-sided endocarditis and may be seen in left-sided endocarditis with left-to-right cardiac shunts.

Mycotic aneurysms occur in about 10 percent of patients. Symptoms are usually lacking but may be those of an expanding mass. They can rupture during or even years after therapy. *Neurologic manifestations* are present in about one-third of patients with endocarditis. Major cerebral emboli as well as mycotic aneurysms usually involve the middle cerebral artery system. Brain abscess and purulent meningitis are most common with *S. aureus* endocarditis. *Heart failure* may occur during the course of the disease or long after cure. Contributing factors are valve destruction, myocarditis, coronary artery emboli with infarction, and myocardial abscesses. *Renal disease* is present in most patients with endocarditis and is due to renal emboli or glomerulonephritis. Renal insufficiency may result.

LABORATORY FEATURES

A normocytic normochromic anemia is usual in infective endocarditis. The white blood cell and differential counts are often normal. However, in acute disease, leukocytosis without anemia may be present. Proteinuria and/or microscopic hematuria are found in most patients, and the serum creatinine may be elevated. The erythrocyte sedimentation rate is almost always elevated except when heart failure is present.

About 50 percent of patients with endocarditis for at least six weeks have a positive serum test for rheumatoid factor, and virtually all have circulating immune complexes. These tend to disappear with cure. The serum complement may be decreased, especially with diffuse glomerulonephritis. Large mononuclear cells in the first drop of blood obtained after massage of the ear lobe ("ear lobe histiocytes") occur in about 25 percent of patients with endocarditis as well as in some with other chronic infections. Serum antibodies to teichoic acid (a cell wall antigen in *S. aureus*) suggest endocarditis or other deep infection in patients with staphylococcal bacteremia. Bacteria can be seen inside leukocytes in buffy coat preparations of blood in about 50 percent of patients with endocarditis.

The critical diagnostic finding in endocarditis is bacteremia or fungemia. Blood cultures are positive in over 95 percent of patients. The bacteremia is continuous; if any cultures are positive, all are likely to be positive. There is no advantage to obtaining cultures at any particular time or body temperature. Arterial blood or bone marrow offers no advantage over antecubital vein blood.

In subacute disease, in the absence of previous therapy, three cultures should be obtained over 3 to 6 h and therapy initiated. With previous therapy, treatment may be expeditiously delayed in an attempt to obtain positive blood cultures. In general, in acute disease, therapy should not be delayed for more than 2 to 3 h while obtaining cultures. Only one culture should be obtained from each venipuncture, using anaerobic as well as aerobic techniques. The yield of positive cultures is increased by observing them over three weeks and making periodic blind Gram stains and subcultures. Addition of pyridoxal hydrochloride to the media will improve the chances of isolating nutritionally deficient variant streptococci.

Blood cultures may be negative in infections with fastidious organisms such as *Haemophilus parainfluenzae*. Fifty percent of patients with *Candida* endocarditis and almost all with *Aspergillus*, *Histoplasma*, and *Coxiella burnetii* endocarditis have negative blood cultures. With fungi, large peripheral emboli are common, necessitating embolectomy. Histologic examination and culture of the embolus may be diagnostic. Serologic tests for *C. burnetii* and *C. psittaci* are positive in endocarditis caused by these organisms.

Although not diagnostic, echocardiograms will demonstrate the vegetation in up to 80 percent of patients with native valve endocarditis. Serial phonocardiography and cineradiography are useful in evaluating infection on prosthetic valves. Disappearance of an opening click or sound produced by a closing valve suggests presence of a vegetation. With dehiscence, cineradiography of the valve will show abnormal motion.

DIAGNOSIS

Endocarditis should be suspected either when a heart murmur and unexplained fever are present for at least 1 week or in febrile intravenous drug abusers even in the absence of a murmur. However, a definitive clinical diagnosis requires positive blood cultures.

Atrial myxoma, nonbacterial thrombotic endocarditis, acute rheumatic fever, lupus erythematosus, and sickle cell disease can duplicate the syndrome of infective endocarditis. Any patient with an existing heart murmur can develop fever related to another occult illness or to drugs. Therefore, in the absence of positive blood cultures, a search must be made for other causes of fever.

Following cardiac surgery, fever may be related to infection at other sites, to the post-cardiotomy syndrome, or to a "postpump syndrome" (e.g., cytomegalovirus infection).

TREATMENT

PRINCIPLES OF THERAPY   Cure of endocarditis requires eradication of all microorganisms from the vegetation. Therefore, microbicidal drug regimens must be used in high enough concentrations and for a long enough duration to sterilize the vegetation. Regimens including penicillins, cephalosporins, and vancomycin give far better results than when these drugs cannot be used because of resistant organisms or drug reactions.

The minimal inhibitory and bactericidal concentrations (MIC and MBC) should be determined. Evidence suggests that peak serum concentrations of a regimen that are bactericidal at a 1:8 dilution generally indicate adequate therapy. While this determination is not necessary in most cases, it may be useful when infection is caused by organisms other than gram-positive cocci, treatment has failed, or regimens do not include penicillins, cephalosporins, or vancomycin. Except for unusual circumstances, antibiotic administration should be parenteral to guarantee adequate absorption of drugs. The infecting microorganism should be saved for future testing (e.g., serum antibacterial activity, evaluation of different antibiotics, or comparison with a relapse strain).

SPECIFIC ANTIMICROBIAL REGIMENS   Therapy before culture results are known   The treatment of subacute infective endocarditis on a native valve while awaiting culture results should be for streptococci, and such "expectant" therapy should be directed against the most antibiotic-resistant streptococci, enterococci.

With an acute course, therapy should be directed against *S. aureus*. In intravenous drug abusers, therapy should be directed against *S. aureus* and gentamicin should be included for gram-negative bacilli. In many cities, most *S. aureus* isolated from drug abusers are methicillin-resistant and vancomycin must be used. With prosthetic valves, vancomycin plus gentamicin should be used because of the high incidence of methicillin-resistant *S. epidermidis* as well as to cover enterococci.

Once the organism is isolated, the regimen should be altered appropriately. If cultures remain sterile and culture-negative endocarditis is likely, treatment is continued provided that the response is adequate.

Streptococci   Most streptococci are inhibited by serum concentrations of 0.1 μg/mL penicillin G. Three regimens including penicillin G (Table 90-1) can be used for these highly penicillin-susceptible strains. Penicillin G alone for 4 weeks (regimen A) gives cure rates of 99 percent. Addition of gentamicin or streptomycin (regimen B) results in a more rapid bactericidal effect and gives equivalent cure rates in 2 weeks. Regimen B should be standard for uncomplicated infection, but regimen A is preferred in patients likely to have side

TABLE 90-1 Therapy of infective endocarditis caused by gram-positive cocci*

STREPTOCOCCI† WITH MIC ≤ 0.1 μg/mL PENICILLIN G

Regimen A	Penicillin G, 10–20 million units/d IV in divided doses every 4 h × 4 weeks *or*
Regimen B	Penicillin as in regimen A plus streptomycin, 7.5 mg/kg IM every 12 h or gentamicin, 1 mg/kg IV every 8 h, both × 2 weeks *or*
Regimen C	Penicillin plus streptomycin or gentamicin × 2 weeks as in regimen B with penicillin continued 2 weeks longer *or*
Regimen D	Cefazolin 1–2 g IV or IM every 6–8 h × 4 weeks *or*
Regimen E	Vancomycin, 15 mg/kg IV every 12 h × 4 weeks

ENTEROCOCCI OR OTHER STREPTOCOCCI WITH MIC > 0.5 μg/mL PENICILLIN G

Regimen F	Penicillin G, 20–30 million units/d or ampicillin, 12 g/d IV in divided doses every 4 h plus gentamicin, 1 mg/kg IV every 8 h or streptomycin 7.5 mg/kg IM every 12 h, both × 4–6 weeks *or*
Regimen G	Vancomycin, 15 mg/kg IV every 12 h plus gentamicin or streptomycin as in regimen F, both × 4–6 weeks

STREPTOCOCCI OTHER THAN ENTEROCOCCI WITH MIC > 0.1 BUT < 0.5 μg/mL PENICILLIN G

Regimen H	Use regimen C *or* regimen E if penicillin allergic

METHICILLIN-SUSCEPTIBLE *S. AUREUS* OR *S. EPIDERMIDIS*

Regimen I	Nafcillin, 2 g IV every 4 h × 4–6 weeks with or without gentamicin, 1 mg/kg IV every 8 h × the first 3–5 d *or*
Regimen J	Cefazolin, 2 g IV every 6 h × 4–6 weeks with or without gentamicin as in regimen I *or*
Regimen K	Vancomycin 15 mg/kg IV every 12 h × 4–6 weeks with or without gentamicin as in regimen I

METHICILLIN-RESISTANT STAPHYLOCOCCI OR *CORYNEBACTERIUM SP.*

Regimen L	Vancomycin with or without gentamicin as in regimen K

ENDOCARDITIS ON A PROSTHETIC VALVE

Regimen C but with 20 million units of penicillin each day and a longer duration of penicillin (a total of 6 weeks)
Regimen D × 6 weeks with gentamicin or streptomycin × the first 2 weeks
Regimen E × 6 weeks with gentamicin or streptomycin × the first 2 weeks
Regimen F or G × 6 weeks
Regimen H, but continue penicillin × 6 weeks
Regimen I, J, or K × 6–8 weeks with gentamicin × the first 2 weeks
Regimen L × 6–8 weeks with gentamicin × the first 2 weeks
In the presence of *S. epidermidis* also add rifampin, 300 mg orally every 8 h × 6–8 weeks. The use of rifampin with *S. aureus* is controversial.

* Peak serum concentrations of gentamicin should be about 3 μg/mL. Streptomycin peaks should be about 20 μg/mL. The maximum dose of vancomycin is 1 g every 12 h.
† For Group A streptococci or *S. pneumoniae* use regimen A.
NOTE: MIC = minimal inhibitory concentration.

effects with aminoglycosides (i.e., those with renal insufficiency or eighth nerve disease, or older than 65 years). Penicillin for 4 weeks with an aminoglycoside for the first 2 weeks (regimen C) is used for nutritionally deficient variant strains, a relapse, or complications (e.g., metastatic abscesses or shock). Regimen D can be substituted with a history of a delayed rash to penicillin. Regimen E should be used with a history of anaphylaxis to penicillin.

Penicillin, ampicillin, and vancomycin are not bactericidal for most enterococci. With the addition of an aminoglycoside a synergistic bactericidal effect occurs. Enterococcal endocarditis requires penicillin, ampicillin, or vancomycin plus an aminoglycoside for cure of most patients (regimens F and G, with G used for hypersensitivity to penicillin G). An alternative to regimen G consists of skin testing with major and minor determinants of penicillin, followed by attempts at desensitization to penicillin. This involves a scratch test through a drop of penicillin G (100 units per mL). This is followed in 30 min by graded amounts of penicillin intradermally, begun at 0.01 units in 0.1 mL of saline solution and continued in tenfold increments every 30 min; with increasing amounts, administration is changed to the subcutaneous, intramuscular, and finally intravenous route. Epinephrine and diphenhydramine should be on hand for emergency use during the procedure in case of anaphylaxis, and preferably the procedure should be carried out in an intensive care unit. If a reaction occurs, alternative therapy should be initiated.

Therapy is usually given for 4 weeks but is prolonged to 6 weeks when symptoms have been present for longer than 3 months or the course is complicated. Cephalosporins cannot be used in enterococcal endocarditis because the organisms are highly resistant.

A synergistic bactericidal effect against enterococci occurs with aminoglycosides only when growth is inhibited by 2000 μg/mL. Synergism is most likely with gentamicin. However, enterococci resistant to 2000 μg/mL of gentamicin are more common than in the past. Some of these gentamicin-resistant strains are inhibited by 2000 μg/mL of streptomycin, but most are resistant to 2000 μg/mL of all aminoglycosides. With aminoglycoside-resistant strains, it may be best to exclude aminoglycosides from the regimen and treat for 6 to 8 weeks. However, relapses may occur.

Endocarditis caused by non-enterococcal streptococci with a MIC > 0.1 but < 0.5 μg/mL penicillin G is managed with regimen H, a compromise between the regimens for highly susceptible (MIC ≤ 0.1 μg/mL) and relatively resistant (MIC ≥ 0.5 μg/mL) streptococci.

Staphylococci Methicillin-susceptible *S. aureus* and *S. epidermidis* are treated with regimens I or J. Methicillin-resistant staphylococci are resistant to all penicillins and cephalosporins. In these cases, or in patients who cannot tolerate penicillins or cephalosporins, vancomycin as in regimens K and L must be used. Some experts advocate addition of gentamicin for the first 3 to 5 days because of an increase in the rate of bactericidal activity. However, clinical evidence of improved outcome is lacking and routine administration of gentamicin is not recommended. Therapy for 4 weeks is standard, but with metastatic or intracardiac abscess formation or an otherwise complicated course, therapy should be prolonged to 6 weeks or even longer.

As indicated in Table 90-1, in prosthetic valve endocarditis, therapy should be prolonged and combinations containing an aminoglycoside are usually used. When a methicillin-resistant *S. epidermidis* infects a prosthetic valve, results have been improved with addition of rifampin.

Other organisms In endocarditis caused by other organisms, bactericidal antibiotics, preferably a penicillin, cephalosporin, or vancomycin with or without an aminoglycoside, should be given, and therapy continued for 4 to 6 weeks. With gram-negative bacilli, the penicillin or cephalosporin which has the greatest potency against the infecting bacteria in vitro should be administered in large doses intravenously along with an aminoglycoside to which the bacterium is susceptible (e.g., ampicillin, 2 g every 4 h; piperacillin, 3 g every 4 h; cefotaxime, 2 g every 4 to 6 h; or ceftazidime, 2 g every 8 h plus gentamicin 1.7 mg/kg every 8 h). Ciprofloxacin alone, which is bactericidal for gram-negative bacilli, should also be useful.

When the organisms are resistant to penicillins, cephalosporins, ciprofloxacin, and vancomycin, therapy will probably be unsuccessful. Under these circumstances, treatment should be with the bactericidal drug grouping that demonstrates the best activity in vitro. If the response is poor or relapse occurs, antimicrobial therapy plus valve replacement will probably be necessary.

SURGERY IN THE MANAGEMENT OF ENDOCARDITIS   When appropriate microbicidal therapy is not available (as in fungal endocarditis) and positive blood cultures persist on therapy or relapse occurs after therapy, the valve should be replaced. Ideally, surgery should be performed after several days of the best available anti-microbial therapy. With organisms that tend to produce metastatic foci, therapy should then be continued long enough to eradicate these foci. Persistence of infection with the same organism following valve replacement has been uncommon. Immediate replacement (even after only hours of therapy) is essential in patients developing heart failure secondary to severe valvular regurgitation. Surgery is necessary to drain myocardial or valve ring abscesses and should be considered with recurrent emboli despite adequate antimicrobial therapy. It should also be considered in patients with aortic valve endocarditis who develop first and second degree atrioventricular block. In some centers, the presence of a large vegetation on echocardiography is also an indication for surgery.

Replacement of a prosthesis is often necessary for infections with organisms other than streptococci, for valve dysfunction or dehiscence, or for myocardial invasion. Myocardial invasion is common with prosthetic valves and is suggested by continued fever after 10 days of therapy, a new regurgitant murmur, and/or atrioventricular conduction disturbance.

COURSE

Defervescence usually occurs after 3 to 7 days of antimicrobial therapy. Blood cultures should be obtained periodically during treatment and generally become negative after several days of therapy. Lack of response of fever and bacteremia may be associated with myocardial or metastatic abscess formation (especially associated with *S. aureus*).

The most common cause of persistent or recurrent fever during therapy is a drug reaction and, less commonly, emboli. If a rash develops, therapy can be continued and antihistamines or even glucocorticoids given to suppress the reaction. If the rash is severe, therapy should be altered.

Weight gain and a rise in hemoglobin may not be seen until weeks after therapy has been completed. Petechiae, Osler nodes, and emboli may occur during and for weeks after successful antimicrobial therapy. Mycotic aneurysms may regress on drug therapy or may rupture weeks to years later. Heart failure may occuring during or after therapy and is the principal cause of death.

Anticoagulants should be used only with a pressing indication (such as certain prosthetic valves, but not including infected emboli) because of increased risk of hemorrhage (especially intracranial). Coumadin is preferable to heparin. Blood cultures 2 and 4 weeks after discontinuation of the therapy detect the vast majority of relapses.

PROGNOSIS

Factors that predispose to a poor prognosis are (1) non-streptococcal disease, (2) development of heart failure, (3) aortic valve involvement, (4) infection on a prosthetic valve, (5) older age, and (6) valve ring or myocardial abscess. The cure rate in streptococcal endocarditis is

about 90 percent. Failures are not due to uncontrolled infection but to death from heart failure, embolus, rupture of mycotic aneurysm, or renal failure. The mortality rate in nonaddicts with *S. aureus* endocarditis is at least 40 percent, and most deaths are due to overwhelming infection or heart failure. In drug addicts with *S. aureus* infection on the tricuspid valve, cure rates are over 90 percent and treatment may be shortened in the absence of infected emboli to 2 weeks of nafcillin plus an aminoglycoside. Results are poor in endocarditis caused by fungi and gram-negative bacilli resistant to penicillins and cephalosporins. The presence of large vegetations on echocardiogram may indicate a poorer prognosis than small or absent vegetations. About 10 percent of patients will have additional episodes of endocarditis, months or years later. The prognosis in early prosthetic valve endocarditis is much worse than in late disease, with mortality rates of 40 to 80 percent versus 20 to 40 percent.

ANTIMICROBIAL PROPHYLAXIS OF ENDOCARDITIS

Although the risk of endocarditis is small and there is no proof of efficacy, prophylaxis is recommended for patients with predisposing cardiac lesions undergoing procedures known to cause bacteremia. The conditions for which prophylaxis is recommended are valvular or congenital heart disease (except uncomplicated atrial septal defect), intracardiac prostheses, asymmetric septal hypertrophy, and previous episode of endocarditis. Mitral valve prolapse increases the risk of endocarditis to a low to moderate extent. However, it is so common, that it is neither risk- nor cost-effective to give prophylaxis to all patients with prolapse for all procedures. It is, however, reasonable to use prophylaxis in individuals with mitral valve prolapse who have holosystolic murmurs and who presumably are at greatest risk.

Oral hygiene should be optimal in patients with cardiac lesions that predispose to endocarditis, especially those who are to have prosthetic cardiac valves implanted.

For dental and other procedures in the mouth, nose, or throat likely to cause bleeding or significant trauma, prophylaxis is aimed at viridans streptococci. The regimen recommended by the American Heart Association is penicillin V, 2 g orally, 1 h before the procedure followed by 1 g 6 h later. An effective alternative regimen is a single oral dose of 3 g of amoxicillin 1 h before the procedure. With penicillin allergy, erythromycin is recommended, 1 g orally 1 h before, followed by 0.5 g 6 h later. In high-risk patients (e.g., those with prosthetic valves), the regimen is ampicillin, 2 g intramuscularly or intravenously plus gentamicin, 1.5 mg/kg intramuscularly or intravenously both 30 min before and 1 g penicillin V orally 6 h later or, with penicillin allergy, vancomycin, 1 g intravenously over 1 h starting 1 h before.

For genitourinary and gastrointestinal tract procedures likely to cause significant trauma (e.g., urethral catheterization, prostatic surgery, and colonic or gallbladder surgery), prophylaxis is directed against enterococci. The regimen is ampicillin plus gentamicin as above. With penicillin allergy, the vancomycin regimen above is given, but 1.5 mg/kg gentamicin intravenously or intramuscularly is added 1 h before the procedure. For low-risk patients with minor procedures, amoxicillin may be used, 3g orally 1 h before the procedure followed by 1.5 g 6 h later. Fiberoptic endoscopy without biopsy and barium enema are at such low risk for endocarditis that prophylaxis is difficult to justify. If used, it should be only in high-risk patients.

Prophylaxis for cardiac surgery with placement of intracardiac prostheses, patches, or sutures is directed against staphylococci and has usually consisted of 2 g of cefazolin intravenously plus 1.5 mg/kg gentamicin intravenously starting immediately preoperatively, fol-lowed by repeated doses 8 and 16 h later. However, as strains of *S. epidermidis* may be methicillin-resistant, substitution of vancomycin for cefazolin in a dose of 15 mg/kg intravenously over 1 h, starting 1 h before the procedure, 10 mg/kg after completion of by-pass, and then 7.5 mg/kg every 6 h for 3 doses is reasonable. Vancomycin can also be used when patients have hypersensitivity to penicillins and cephalosporins.

Patients with coronary artery bypass grafts or transvenous pacemakers in place do not require prophylaxis for endocarditis nor is it indicated for patients undergoing cardiac catheterization.

REFERENCES

Bisno AL et al: Antimicrobial treatment of infective endocarditis due to viridans streptococci, enterococci and staphylococci. JAMA 261(10):1471, 1989

Buda AJ et al: Prognostic significance of vegetations detected by two-dimensional echocardiography in infective endocarditis. Am Heart J 112(6):1291, 1986

Chambers HF et al: Right-sided *Staphylococcus aureus* endocarditis in intravenous drug abusers: Two-week combination therapy. Ann Intern Med 109:619, 1988

Durack D: Prophylaxis of infective endocarditis, in *Principles and Practice of Infectious Diseases*, 3d ed, GL Mandell et al (eds). New York, Churchill Livingstone, 1990

Hoffman SA, Moellering RC: The enterococcus: "Putting the bug in our ears." Ann Intern Med 106:757, 1987

MacMahon SW et al: Risk of infective endocarditis in mitral valve prolapse with and without precordial systolic murmurs. Am J Cardiol 59:105, 1987

McKinsey DS et al: Underlying cardiac lesions in adults with infective endocarditis. Am J Med 82:681, 1987

Prevention of bacterial endocarditis. Med Lett Drugs Ther 31:112, 1989

Sande MA et al (eds): *Contemporary Issues in Infectious Diseases*, vol 2: *Endocarditis*. New York, Churchill Livingstone, 1984

Scheld M, Sande M: Endocarditis and intravascular infections, in *Principles and Practice of Infectious Diseases*, 3d ed, GL Mandell et al (eds). New York, Churchill Livingstone, 1990

Shulman ST et al: Prevention of bacterial endocarditis. Circulation 70:1123A, 1984

Sussman JI et al: Viridans streptococcal endocarditis: Clinical, microbiological and echocardiographic correlations. J Infect Dis 154(4):597, 1986

Threlkeld M, Cobbs G: Infections of prosthetic valves and intravascular devices, in *Principles and Practice of Infectious Diseases*, 3d ed, GL Mandell et al (eds). New York, Churchill-Livingstone, 1990

91 LOCALIZED INFECTIONS AND ABSCESSES

JAN V. HIRSCHMANN

GENERAL CONSIDERATIONS

While many pathogens produce a characteristic clinical syndrome, in some infections the location of the process rather than the identity of the responsible organisms determines the clinical manifestations. Examples include abscesses, soft tissue infections, bacterial endocarditis (see Chap. 90), pyogenic infections of the central nervous system (see Chap. 354), urinary tract infections (see Chap. 95), lung abscess (see Chap. 207), mediastinitis (see Chap. 216), appendicitis and appendiceal abscess (see Chap. 245), diverticulitis (see Chap. 243), osteomyelitis (see Chap. 97), and infections of the pericardium (see Chap. 193). Many pathogens can cause infections in these sites; but knowledge of the usual flora causing them should permit appropriate therapy before the results of cultures are available.

ETIOLOGY Localized pyogenic infection can develop in any region or organ of the body, and may be initiated by *trauma* and secondary bacterial contamination, by some *alteration in local conditions* that renders a tissue susceptible to infection with organisms already present as part of the "normal flora" to which it is ordinarily resistant, by *contiguous spread* from a nearby lesion, or by *metastatic implantation* of microorganisms carried in blood or lymph.

Infection in some areas is more likely to be caused by certain organisms, such as staphylococci in the skin and coliform bacteria in the urinary tract, and special features of the tissue reaction produced by some bacterial species make it possible to recognize infection by them with considerable accuracy. The *staphylococci* produce rapid necrosis and early suppuration with large amounts of creamy yellow pus (see Chap. 100). Group A beta-hemolytic streptococcal infections (see Chap. 101) tend to spread rapidly through tissues, causing intense edema and erythema but relatively little necrosis and thin, serumlike exudate; anaerobic bacteria (see Chap. 108) may produce necrosis and profuse, foul-smelling pus.

The identification of infecting organisms is important in the choice of antimicrobial chemotherapy. However, when infection occurs in certain areas, as in paranasal sinuses or cutaneous ulcers, or shows up in sputum, it is unlikely that treatment will render cultured specimens sterile. In these locations, serial cultures during antimicrobial administration are typically unhelpful, and therapy should be guided largely by the clinical response.

PATHOGENESIS Factors predisposing to the initiation and persistence of infection in a tissue include trauma, obstruction of normal drainage (sweat glands, biliary tract, bronchial tree, urinary tract), ischemia (infarction, gangrene), chemical irritation (by gastric contents, bile, or intramuscularly injected drugs), hematoma formation, accumulation of fluid (lymphatic obstruction, cardiac edema), foreign bodies (bullets, splinters, sutures), and others such as the occurrence of stasis or turbulence in the vascular system. When these conditions severely compromise local host defenses almost any common bacteria can initiate an infection, and the organisms responsible are often part of the normal flora of an adjacent cutaneous or mucosal surface.

Infection in soft tissue usually begins as a *cellulitis*, a diffuse acute inflammation with hyperemia, edema, and leukocytic infiltration but little or no necrosis and suppuration. With some organisms, this is followed by necrosis, liquefaction, accumulation of leukocytes and debris, suppuration, loculation of the pus, and formation of one or more *abscesses*.

Infection may spread locally via the path of least resistance along fascial planes or by the lymphatic system, which may lead to lymphangitis or regional lymphadenitis, sometimes with suppuration. Involvement of local venules or large veins may cause infective thrombophlebitis with resulting bacteremia, septic embolization, and systemic dissemination of infection.

Depending upon the infecting organism and the anatomy of the affected region, a small abscess may subside completely; there may be gradual encapsulation of the accumulated pus and persistence of the focus in a quiescent state; or the lesion may "point" and rupture into adjacent tissues or to the outside surface of the body, as usually happens with furuncles. Spontaneous drainage ordinarily leads to resolution of a superficial abscess. However, if it is deeply situated and well encapsulated, persistence of a fistulous tract and the formation of a chronic, draining sinus may occur. *The development of persistent sinuses over an area of suppuration produced by ordinary pyogenic bacteria should always suggest involvement of underlying bone or the presence of a foreign body.* Fistulas that open onto the skin are, of course, soon colonized by microorganisms from the external environment. Routine bacterial cultures of drainage fluid almost invariably show a mixed flora and are unreliable for the etiologic diagnosis of the underlying disease, particularly in disorders that characteristically lead to persistent sinus formation, such as tuberculosis and actinomycosis.

MANIFESTATIONS Infections of the skin and subcutaneous tissues almost invariably produce the classic manifestations: *redness, tenderness, heat,* and *swelling*. Reddish streaks extending proximally and associated with tender enlargement of regional lymph nodes indicate lymphangitis. Systemic symptoms may be absent or mild, or there may be fever, malaise, prostration, and leukocytosis.

Infection and suppuration in deeper tissues or in body cavities often cause pain and tenderness, but locating and determining the exact nature of the lesion may be difficult. Palpating a tender mass is helpful and fluctuation indicates that it contains fluid, usually pus, but muscle spasm and intervening structures often interfere with identifying the site. Auscultation may reveal a friction rub over an abdominal viscus, the pleura, or the pericardium. The rapid development of an effusion in the pericardium, pleura, abdomen, or a joint should suggest infection. Similarly, fluid detected by transillumination of paranasal sinuses or inspection of the tympanic membrane may be the first sign of infection.

An abscess may produce symptoms and signs by encroaching upon adjacent structures. Respiratory obstruction may be the first sign of mediastinal abscess; dysphagia often first calls attention to peritonsillar or retropharyngeal abscesses; and tamponade is sometimes the initial clue to pericardial infection. Localizing signs of dysfunction are especially striking and important with brain and spinal cord abscesses, although brain abscesses may be clinically silent (see Chap. 354). In some patients local pain and tenderness or signs of dysfunction are absent, mild, or equivocal, and fever, prostration, fatigue, and weight loss predominate. The fever may be low-grade but is often hectic, with repeated rigors and drenching night sweats. Fatigue and anemia are frequent, and weight loss may be so rapid that emaciation occurs within a few weeks. A patient with these symptoms and signs may have a chronic intraabdominal abscess without any detectable physical sign to indicate its location.

LABORATORY FINDINGS Peripheral polymorphonuclear leukocytosis is frequent with abscesses, and significant unexplained elevation of the white blood cell count in any patient may indicate localized suppuration. An elevated sedimentation rate is common in infections of all durations, but the "anemia of chronic disease" may occur with a protracted course. Mild albuminuria, occasionally noted in febrile patients, has no diagnostic import.

Pus or fluid obtained by needle aspiration or incision of a suspected lesion should *always* be stained and examined directly in addition to being cultured aerobically and anaerobically. *Failure to examine exudates with Gram's stain is the single greatest deterrent to appropriate antimicrobial therapy.*

Blood cultures are usually positive in intravascular infections such as septic thrombophlebitis and endocarditis and may be positive in localized abscesses, especially when metastatic, as in staphylococcal, streptococcal, and *Salmonella* bacteremias. Moreover, manipulation, including surgical incision, of any localized infection may cause transient bacteremia.

Noninvasive techniques are often helpful in the diagnosis of abscess. Radiographic examinations may indicate localized collections of pus when they show atypical collections of gas, displacement of organs, and tissue densities in abnormal locations. Diagnostic ultrasound is not only useful in localizing abscess but also may provide clues to the size of the abscess and to the presence of multiple abscesses or loculation. Computed tomography (CT) scan is usually the most accurate technique in demonstrating abscesses, especially in the brain and abdominal cavity, including the retroperitoneum. Radionuclide scans using labeled leukocytes may be helpful when other imaging technologies are negative or equivocal, but they also may be misleading. Magnetic resonance imaging (MRI) scans may be preferred when metal causes artifacts or in further defining brain abscesses or those invading soft tissues and contiguous bone (e.g., vertebral body abscesses with spinal cord compression).

THERAPEUTIC CONSIDERATIONS Striking symptomatic improvement usually follows adequate drainage of pus, but incision of infected tissue before the stage of liquefaction is often deleterious, fails to relieve discomfort, and may even at times facilitate spread of infection. For this reason, it is sometimes necessary to wait until an abscess "ripens," i.e., localizes and "comes to a head." The *application of heat* to an area of superficial inflammation may relieve pain and speed the subsidence of cellulitis without suppuration. If necrosis of tissue is already under way, hot applications appear to facilitate localization of the process and accumulation of pus, making incision and drainage feasible at an earlier time. Another procedure that helps reduce swelling and relieve pain is *elevation of the affected part*.

Antimicrobial therapy is used in many types of abscesses. Some agents, notably the penicillins, retain their antibacterial activity in the presence of pus, while others, exemplified by the aminoglycosides, are partially inactivated. The inability of the drug to penetrate into an area of suppuration, however, is rarely the reason for therapeutic

failure. Although this possibility exists in some infections, such as osteomyelitis, it is usually overcome by increasing dosage.

An established inflammatory exudate is a relatively poor environment for rapid bacterial multiplication. Because some antibiotics are bactericidal only against multiplying organisms, failure of these agents to eradicate infection in an abscess may be related to the organisms' inactive metabolic state. Because bacteriostatic drugs inhibit, but do not kill, bacteria, the death of organisms in any infection treated with these agents depends on other mechanisms, especially phagocytosis. In fluid-filled cavities, particularly in the metabolically unfavorable milieu of an abscess, phagocytosis may occur, but intracellular killing is reduced. Consequently, despite inhibition of bacterial multiplication, organisms can remain dormant and survive for long periods of time. It is probably a combination of these two circumstances, decreased multiplication of bacteria and decreased phagocytosis, that makes infection in the heart valves, for example, so relatively resistant to antimicrobial therapy. Large doses of bactericidal drugs for long periods are needed to achieve cure.

Antimicrobial drugs may obviate suppuration if given early or prevent spread of an existing abscess, but usually are no substitute for drainage of purulent material. Indeed, their use in the face of a lesion requiring evacuation of pus is one of the most common serious errors in treating pyogenic infections.

In thoracic empyema, suppurative pericarditis, or pyarthrosis, excellent therapeutic results are sometimes achieved by aspiration of pus and systemic antimicrobial therapy. Success, however, depends as fully on the adequacy of drainage as it does upon the administration of the antibiotic, and if loculation occurs or the exudate becomes too viscid to remove, surgical or catheter drainage may be necessary. An exception to the general rule of the essential role of surgical drainage for cure may be seen in the treatment of brain abscesses; if small or inaccessible, good therapeutic responses have been obtained with prolonged (>6 weeks) administration of antimicrobials (see Chap. 354).

In infective thrombophlebitis, surgical interruption of the veins by ligation or, in some cases, by total excision of an infected segment is sometimes indicated to prevent seeding of other organs by infected emboli.

CLINICAL FEATURES OF INFECTIONS IN VARIOUS REGIONS

SUPERFICIAL ABSCESSES Skin and subcutaneous tissues *Impetigo* is a superficial infection caused by group A hemolytic streptococci, sometimes combined with *Staphylococcus aureus*. Primarily a disease of children and common in warm weather, it is characterized by multiple, pruritic, erythematous lesions, which become vesicles and pustules that rupture to form a crust. In adults impetigo is most commonly an infectious complication of a chronic dermatitis. Local spread occurs through scratching and release of infected vesicle fluid. Serious complications are metastatic abscesses and acute glomerulonephritis. Treatment consists of local and general cleansing of the skin, appropriate systemic antibiotics, and therapy of any underlying dermatologic condition.

About one-fourth of cutaneous abscesses, especially on the extremities, are due to *S. aureus*. The rest yield other organisms, usually anaerobes alone or a combination of aerobes and anaerobes. The bacteria isolated are usually part of the normal flora on that region of the skin where the abscess developed. These organisms ordinarily possess little cutaneous virulence, but when inoculated into the dermis or subcutaneous tissue by trauma or other mechanisms, they can produce suppuration. In most patients with normal host defenses the appropriate treatment is incision and drainage of the abscess and packing of the wound. Gram stain, culture, and antibiotic therapy are unnecessary unless the patient is immunocompromised or the lesion is complicated by extensive cellulitis, cutaneous gangrene, or systemic manifestations of infection.

Lymphadenitis with or without suppuration may complicate any pyogenic skin lesion and is often striking with superficial streptococcal infections. Specific diseases characterized by suppurative regional lymphadenitis include lymphogranuloma venereum (see Chap. 155), cat-scratch disease (see Chap. 98), tularemia (see Chap. 120), and bubonic plague (see Chap. 121).

Infections of the hand These are almost invariably secondary to trauma. Because of the rapidity with which infection can spread through the complex fascial spaces of the hand, wrist, and forearm, and produce irreparable functional damage, *any deep infection in this area should receive expert surgical attention immediately.* The availability of antibiotics has in no way lessened the importance of such care.

The ordinary *paronychia,* or "run-around," is a superficial infection of the epithelium lateral to a nail, usually a result of tearing a hangnail and most frequently caused by staphylococcus. Hot applications will lead to subsidence of paronychial cellulitis, but often a superficial blister of pus appears. A small incision or simply separation of the nail fold from the nail will promote adequate drainage. If the infection burrows beneath the nail to form a painful *subungual abscess,* incision and drainage with partial or complete removal of the nail are necessary. Recurrence is common, especially in nail biters, and this seemingly trivial infection can cause painful disability. Chronic paronychial inflammation, usually from *Candida,* occurs in those with prolonged or frequent immersion of hands in water.

What appears to be a small furuncle of the webs of the fingers sometimes produces a *collar-button abscess,* consisting of a superficial and deep compartment connected by a narrow tract. Evacuation of the shallow pocket without emptying the deeper abscess can lead to puzzling persistence of infection. Sometimes a foreign-body granuloma forms in the skin of the digital webs. This is most common in barbers, in whom a hair is the core of the foreign-body granuloma, the "barber's interdigital pilonidal sinus."

Infection of the distal phalanx of a finger, usually acquired by pinprick, thorn prick, burn, or sliver, may lead to the formation of a *felon,* or *whitlow.* This is a suppurative infection in the tightly enclosed fibrous compartments of the finger pulp, that can compromise the distal blood supply by compressing the digital arteries, cause skin necrosis, and produce osteomyelitis of the phalanx. The manifestations are swelling, extreme pain, and tenderness of the palmar surface of the fingertip. The treatment is immediate incision directly over the lesion to drain the locus of purulence.

Suppurative tenosynovitis, usually a complication of a puncture wound, is a very serious hand infection in which early diagnosis and treatment are mandatory to prevent permanent disability from destruction of the tendon or its sheath. The cardinal manifestations of tenosynovitis are (1) generalized swelling of the digit, (2) exquisite tenderness over the flexor tendon sheath, (3) flexion of the fingers, and (4) excruciating pain, most marked at the base of the digit, on extension of the involved finger. *Immediate incision* of the sheath is indicated, to prevent not only tendon damage but also proximal extension of the process into the major fascial spaces of the hand or forearm. Vigorous antibiotic treatment should accompany surgery.

Human bites may lead to hand infections that, if neglected, almost invariably produce a highly destructive, necrotizing lesion contaminated by a mixture of aerobic and anaerobic organisms (see Chap. 98). A deliberately inflicted bite on the hand or elsewhere is usually recognized as dangerously contaminated, but wounds on the knuckles produced by striking an opponent's teeth with the fists may not be recognized as potentially dangerous. In general, bite wounds should be cleaned thoroughly and not sutured. Patients should be given prophylaxis for tetanus and antibiotics, a good choice being amoxicillin-clavulanic acid.

Chronic cutaneous ulcers Chronic cutaneous ulcers from a variety of causes, including vascular disease, burns, bedsores, or neurologic disease, usually become colonized with bacteria, commonly a complex flora of aerobic and anaerobic organisms, often including streptococci, staphylococci, and anaerobic gram-negative bacilli. These organisms ordinarily do not retard healing and tend to persist until the wound becomes covered with epithelium, even in those patients treated with topical or systemic antibiotics. Chronic cutaneous ulcers do not require routine cultures or antimicrobial therapy, which should be reserved for substantial surrounding cellulitis, osteomyelitis, signs of systemic infection, or formation of abscesses, which should be drained.

INFECTIONS OF THE HEAD AND NECK Pustules of the nose and upper lip may be particularly dangerous, because they can extend intracranially through the angular vein to the cavernous sinus. These lesions should be treated conservatively, manipulation or incision should be avoided if possible, and systemic antibiotics should be used if local swelling or redness appears.

Suppurative parotitis Typically, suppurative parotitis occurs in elderly and chronically ill patients who have a dry mouth from decreased oral intake, following general anesthesia and surgery, or from medications with atropine-like effects, such as antihistamines or phenothiazines. In most patients, it is an ascending infection due to *S. aureus,* which can colonize the opening to Stensen's duct. Occasionally, there is an obstructing calculus. Its onset, usually sudden, is heralded by unilateral local pain and swelling, frequently with fever and chills. Frank pus can often be expressed from the duct and may show gram-positive cocci in clumps. The gland itself is firm and tender, often with redness and edema of the overlying skin. Treatment consists of systemic antimicrobial therapy with a penicillinase-resistant penicillin or some other agent effective against *S. aureus,* unless another organism is isolated, combined with improved hydration and oral hygiene. Massage of the gland and sialagogues, like lemon drops, help promote drainage through the duct. Surgery is usually unnecessary and should be reserved for patients failing to improve after several days of medical management.

Miscellaneous Infections Antibiotics have reduced the incidence of many suppurative complications of streptococcal pharyngitis. However, as a result of streptococcal sore throat, *Bacteroides* infections of the pharynx, or introduction of infection by trauma to the floor of the mouth or the pharyngeal wall, abscesses of the deep cervical structures still occur. *Suppurative cervical adenitis,* once an all-too-common sequel to streptococcal pharyngitis in children, is now rare. *Peritonsillar abscess (quinsy)* is manifested by fever, sore throat, cervical lymphadenopathy, unilateral pain radiating to the ear on swallowing, and enlargement of the tonsil with redness and swelling of the adjacent soft palate. Treatment with penicillin and irrigations of warm saline solution sometimes suffices, but if digital palpation reveals fluctuation, needle aspiration is indicated. Tonsillectomy is usually reserved for patients with recurrent tonsillar infections. Organisms associated with peritonsillar abscess include *Streptococcus pyogenes* and oral anaerobic bacteria.

The course of *deep cervical infections* depends upon the anatomic arrangement of fascial planes. Infection in this area is serious and is attended by fever, prostration, and leukocytosis. It is usually caused by a mixture of aerobes, predominantly streptococci, and anaerobes, particularly *Peptostreptococcus, Fusobacterium,* and *Bacteroides* (mostly *melaninogenicus*) (see Chap. 108).

Infection of the *sublingual* and submandibular spaces, so-called Ludwig's angina, causes brawny induration of the submaxillary region, edema of the floor of the mouth, and elevation of the tongue. It usually originates from apical abscesses of the second and third mandibular molars and causes severe pain, dysphagia, drooling, stiff neck, and, within hours, dyspnea from respiratory obstruction. *Treatment* consists of large doses of penicillin and careful observation. With significant airway obstruction, tracheostomy, tracheal intubation, or cricothyroidotomy is necessary. Since the infection is largely a cellulitis, incision and drainage are reserved for evidence of abscess formation detected by physical or radiographic (especially CT) examination.

The retropharyngeal space lies between the muscles anterior to the cervical vertebrae and the pharyngeal mucosa. *Retropharyngeal abscess*, formerly common in children, is manifested by dysphagia, progressive stridor, pain, and fever. The bulging mass is easily seen and can completely occlude the airway within hours. Incision and drainage are mandatory; spontaneous rupture may lead to death by aspiration. Another complication is extension of infection into the mediastinum, causing posterior mediastinitis, mediastinal abscess that may rupture into the pleura, or pericarditis, frequently with tamponade. Esophageal perforation during endoscopy may result in abscess as a late complication. Tuberculous abscess, secondary to spinal disease, occasionally appears in the retropharyngeal space; it is painless, and relief of obstruction follows surgical incision.

Lateral pharyngeal space infections, occurring in the lateral portion of the neck between the hyoid bone inferiorly and the sphenoid bone superiorly, can develop from infections throughout the neck, including those involving the teeth, lymph nodes, pharynx, and parotids. Patients usually have fever and leukocytosis. When the anterior portion of this space is involved, trismus, indurated edema of the mandibular angle, and medial bulging of the pharyngeal wall are typically present. Infection of the posterior compartment causes fewer signs, and many patients have only fever. A very serious complication of lateral space infections is involvement of the contiguous vessels. Suppurative jugular venous thrombophlebitis can cause bacteremia, septic pulmonary emboli, and thrombosis of the intracranial venous sinuses. Infection adjacent to the carotid artery may result in an aneurysm that may compress nearby structures to produce a Horner's syndrome, or palsies of the ninth to twelfth cranial nerves. These aneurysms may rupture, causing fatal bleeding.

Therapy of head and neck abscesses includes surgical incision and drainage, open treatment of infected wounds, and systemic antibiotics, which should include agents active against anaerobic organisms. Penicillin is usually the drug of choice; clindamycin or chloramphenicol can be used in penicillin-allergic patients.

INTRAABDOMINAL ABSCESSES

A useful classification divides intraabdominal abscesses, according to location, into three major types, each with several subdivisions: (1) intraperitoneal, (2) retroperitoneal, and (3) visceral. The clinical features vary but usually include fever, with no characteristic pattern (ranging from mild to hectic), leukocytosis, and an elevated erythrocyte sedimentation rate. Common, but not universal, are pain near the abscess, anorexia, weight loss, nausea, vomiting, and altered bowel habits. A tender mass may be palpable. Plain abdominal films may suggest an abscess by showing a soft tissue density, displacement of adjacent organs, or extraintestinal gas from a perforated viscus or produced by the infecting organisms within the abscess cavity.

The most useful noninvasive diagnostic techniques are ultrasound and CT examinations. Ultrasound has a diagnostic accuracy of about 80 percent and is most effective in detecting abscesses in the right upper quadrant, retroperitoneum, and pelvis. It shows a sonolucent mass that may have internal echoes when debris and septations are present. The appearance is usually indistinguishable from other fluid-filled masses, but clinical features and, if necessary, needle aspiration of the mass should discriminate among the possible causes. Since gas blocks the beam, ultrasound is not useful when large amounts of gas are present, as occurs in the stomach and splenic flexure, which makes the left upper quadrant a difficult area to examine. Similarly, loops of gas-filled bowel impair evaluation of the midabdomen. Since the transducer must have good skin contact, wounds, fistulas, stomata, and surgical dressings may make ultrasound examination impossible.

These factors do not affect CT scans, which are therefore especially useful in the postoperative patient, when there are no focal signs or symptoms, or when the area of concern is the left upper quadrant, pancreas, or midabdomen. CT scans are positive in over 90 percent of patients with abscesses, characteristically demonstrating fluid collections with well-defined walls that enhance following intravenous administration of contrast material. MRI is preferred to CT scanning

if steel clips obscure visualization by artifact; it may also be better for detecting pelvic abscesses. Unless gas lies within the mass, however, these findings do not distinguish abscesses from simple cysts, old hematomas, or mucinous metastases. Clinical features or needle aspiration should determine the correct diagnosis.

Effective treatment must include antimicrobial agents active against the responsible organisms. While the infecting flora varies, it commonly comprises bowel organisms, a complex mixture of aerobic and anaerobic bacteria, including *Bacteroides fragilis*. An appropriate initial therapeutic choice is a combination of an aminoglycoside, such as gentamicin, and an antianaerobic agent such as clindamycin, chloramphenicol, or metronidazole. Cefoxitin, cefotetan, or cefotaxime are effective alternatives, but an aminoglycoside should be added if the infection is hospital-acquired or the patient has received previous antimicrobial therapy.

Antimicrobial therapy alone is often sufficient for some abscesses—appendiceal, renal, and some hepatic—but cure usually also requires drainage of pus, either by surgery or percutaneous catheters, inserted with ultrasonic or CT guidance. Criteria for percutaneous drainage include (1) pus thin enough to be evacuated through the catheter; (2) few abscess cavities or loculations; (3) a drainage route that does not traverse bowel, uncontaminated organs, or sterile pleural or peritoneal spaces. The absence of a safe drainage route prevents catheter drainage in most pelvic and interloop abscesses, and this technique is not very successful in pancreatic abscesses because of its inability to remove thick necrotic debris. When used appropriately, however, its success rate is about 70 percent, with the catheters typically remaining in place for about 10 to 20 days.

INTRAPERITONEAL ABSCESS   These infections usually arise from a generalized peritonitis caused by perforated abdominal viscera, penetrating trauma, or postoperative infections. Some derive from localized peritonitis when infection extends from a contiguous site. With generalized peritonitis, the effects of gravity, intraabdominal pressure, and respiratory movements favor localization to the subphrenic spaces, the pelvis, and paracolic gutters lateral to the ascending and descending colon.

Subphrenic abscess   These abscesses occur in the subphrenic space, arbitrarily defined as lying between the diaphragm and the transverse colon and possessing four subdivisions. The *suprahepatic* and *subhepatic* spaces are located on the right side; on the left there is a single *subphrenic* space plus the *lesser sac*, a space posterior to the stomach and anterior to the pancreas. About 55 percent of subphrenic abscesses are right-sided, 25 percent left-sided, and 20 percent multiple. Over 90 percent are complications of abdominal surgery, especially on the biliary tract, stomach, and duodenum. The contamination causing infection can occur during surgery or afterward, especially from anastomotic leaks. Symptoms typically begin 3 to 6 weeks after surgery, but occasionally develop only months later. Fever, nearly universal, is often mild, rather than dramatic. Abdominal pain is usual, but localized tenderness less common, and a palpable mass rare. By causing diaphragmatic irritation, inflammation that spreads to the pleural cavity, and abdominal distention, subphrenic abscesses often produce thoracic symptoms such as cough, dyspnea, and chest pain. Shoulder discomfort, referred pain from an irritated diaphragm, and hiccups sometimes occur. On chest examination there may be dullness to percussion, diminished breath sounds, basilar crackles, and rarely, a pleural friction rub. Chest roentgenograms, usually abnormal, may demonstrate ipsilateral atelectasis, pleural effusion, elevated hemidiaphragm, and basilar pneumonia.

Midabdominal abscess   These abscesses include those in the right and left lower quadrants and between loops of bowel (interloop abscesses). *Right lower quadrant abscesses* usually arise as a complication of acute appendicitis, but occasionally from colonic diverticulitis, Crohn's disease, or upper alimentary tract perforations that drain down into the right paracolic gutter. Most commonly, fever, right lower quadrant pain, and a palpable mass occur following symptoms suggesting acute appendicitis. Occasionally, the abscess causes partial or complete small bowel obstruction. Appendiceal abscesses are usually treatable with antibiotics alone. *Left lower quadrant abscesses* complicate left colonic perforations, usually from diverticulitis, carcinoma, or Crohn's disease, and cause fever, left lower quadrant pain, and a palpable mass. *Interloop abscesses* are collections of pus between the folded surfaces of the small and large intestines and their mesenteries, generally arising from anastomotic disruptions, bowel perforations, or Crohn's disease. The clinical features, which are often very subtle, include mild fever, with or without vague abdominal discomfort. Abdominal tenderness, mechanical bowel obstruction, or a palpable mass occasionally occurs. Plain abdominal roentgenograms may show bowel wall edema, separation of bowel loops, localized ileus, and air-fluid levels on upright films.

Pelvic abscess These are complications of acute appendicitis, colonic diverticulitis, or acute salpingitis. The major symptoms are fever and lower abdominal discomfort. Those adjacent to the colon may cause diarrhea; those next to the bladder may cause urinary frequency and urgency. On abdominal examination tenderness is common, but peritoneal signs, guarding, or a palpable mass are unusual. Rectal or vaginal examination may reveal a mass anterior to the rectum or in the cul-de-sac. Pelvic abscesses usually require surgical drainage, but those arising from acute salpingitis typically resolve with antibiotic therapy alone.

RETROPERITONEAL ABSCESS The retroperitoneum is the space between the posterior peritoneum and the transversalis fascia lining the posterior portion of the abdominal cavity. The *anterior retroperitoneal* space, lying between the posterior peritoneum and the anterior renal fascia, contains the extraperitoneal portion of the alimentary tract: the ascending and descending colon, the duodenal loop, and the pancreas. Abscesses in this space usually develop from pancreatitis or perforations in these extraperitoneal parts of the intestines. The major clinical features are fever, abdominal or flank pain and tenderness, and a palpable mass.

The *perinephric* space, situated between the anterior and posterior layers of the renal (Gerota's) fascia on each side of the body, contains the kidney, adrenal, and ureter. Perinephric abscesses usually occur from rupture of a renal parenchymal abscess through the renal capsule. Such an abscess may be staphylococcal following hematogenous dissemination from another site, usually the skin, but more commonly it arises from pyelonephritis, often associated with urinary tract obstruction by stones, malignancies, or other causes. Perinephric abscesses may also follow urologic surgery or, occasionally, suppuration may extend from contiguous infections of the intestinal tract, liver, gallbladder, or bone. The causative organisms, therefore, are usually aerobic gram-negative bacilli or staphylococci; a minority are polymicrobial. The major symptoms are fever, chills, and unilateral flank pain. Dysuria is frequent, and most patients have unilateral flank or abdominal tenderness, often with a palpable mass. Leukocytosis is typical; pyuria, and a positive urine culture occur in about 60 percent. Blood cultures are positive in 20 to 40 percent of patients. Perinephric abscess usually differs clinically from uncomplicated acute pyelonephritis by the longer duration of symptoms before hospitalization (usually more then 5 days) and the failure of patients to become afebrile within 5 days after receiving antimicrobial therapy. Chest roentgenograms often show ipsilateral pneumonia, atelectasis, pleural effusion, or elevated hemidiaphragm. Suggestive findings on excretory urogram occur in about 60 percent of cases and include a nonvisualizing or poorly visualizing kidney, distorted calyces, anterior renal displacement, and unilateral fixation of the kidney, best demonstrated by fluoroscopy or inspiration-expiration films. Ultrasound usually demonstrates the abscess, but is less reliable than CT, which is almost always positive. Treatment includes appropriate systemic antibiotics, drainage of pus by percutaneous catheters or surgery, and relief of any urinary obstruction; occasionally, nephrectomy is necessary.

VISCERAL ABSCESS Hepatic abscess These abscesses are usually amebic (see Chap. 158) or bacterial (pyogenic). Bacterial liver abscesses usually develop by one of five mechanisms: (1) portal

vein bacteremia arising from an infected intraabdominal site, such as appendicitis, diverticulitis, or perforated bowel; (2) systemic bacteremia originating from a distant site, causing bacteria to reach the liver via the hepatic artery; (3) ascending cholangitis in a biliary tract completely or partially obstructed by stone, malignancy, or stricture; (4) direct extension from a contiguous focus of infection outside the biliary tract, such as a subphrenic abscess; or (5) trauma, either penetrating, with direct introduction of organisms into the liver, or blunt, causing a hematoma that becomes secondarily infected. In most cases the cause is apparent, but in some the pathogenesis of the abscess is unexplained ("cryptogenic"). Most abscesses are single; multiple abscesses are typically microscopic and are associated with systemic bacteremia or complete biliary tract obstruction. In these cases, the onset is acute, and the clinical features of the predisposing disease usually predominate.

Most other cases of hepatic abscess have a subacute onset, and an illness lasting several weeks is the rule. Fever is nearly always present and is accompanied by such nonspecific symptoms as chills, nausea, vomiting, anorexia, weight loss, and weakness. Right upper quadrant abdominal pain or tenderness is present in about one-half of patients, as is hepatomegaly. Some complain of right pleuritic chest pain. Jaundice is usually evident only when there is biliary tract obstruction.

Laboratory findings in most patients include one or more of the following: anemia, leukocytosis, increased erythrocyte sedimentation rate, increased alkaline phosphatase, decreased serum albumin, and usually mildly increased serum bilirubin. The chest roentgenogram is abnormal in about one-half of patients, showing right-sided basilar atelectasis, pneumonia, pleural effusion, or an elevated hemidiaphragm.

Ultrasound scans are usually positive and can distinguish fluid-filled from solid masses, helping to discriminate between infectious and neoplastic lesions. CT scan is the most accurate method of demonstrating multiple abscesses.

The bacteriology of liver abscesses depends upon the cause. With systemic bacteremia staphylococci or streptococci are common. Abscesses originating from an intraabdominal infection, however, usually contain aerobic gram-negative rods, especially *Escherichia coli* and *Klebsiella-Enterobacter;* anaerobic bacteria, especially anaerobic gram-positive cocci, *F. nucleatum,* and *B. fragilis;* or a mixture of aerobes and anaerobes. Blood cultures are positive in about half of patients but may not grow all the organisms present in the abscess.

Although some patients respond to antibiotic therapy alone, most also require evacuation of pus. Percutaneous catheter drainage, if technically feasible, is generally preferable to surgery, provided that no other indication for laparotomy exists. When the bacteriology is unknown, chloramphenicol or a combination of clindamycin and an aminoglycoside should be effective. Antibiotics are usually continued for several weeks following drainage.

In correctly diagnosed and treated patients, the mortality rate is about 20 to 40 percent and is higher in those with multiple rather than single abscesses.

In patients with clinical and roentgenographic findings suggesting a liver abscess who may have had previous exposure to *Entamoeba histolytica*, it is important to distinguish between a bacterial and an amebic etiology, since the latter rarely requires drainage. Features suggesting an amebic abscess are age under 50; single rather than multiple lesions; an acute presentation (<2 weeks of symptoms); male sex; the presence of *E. histolytica* in the stool; and the absence of a condition predisposing to bacterial liver abscess. The most helpful differential point is that nearly all patients with amebic liver abscesses have a positive serology for *E. histolytica*.

Splenic abscess Most splenic abscesses are multiple, small, and clinically silent lesions found incidentally at autopsy and occurring as a terminal manifestation of uncontrolled infection elsewhere. Clinically important splenic abscesses are generally solitary and arise from (1) systemic bacteremia originating in another site, such as endocarditis or salmonellosis; (2) infection, probably by the hematogenous route, of a spleen damaged by bland infarction (as occurs in hemoglobinopathies, especially sickle cell trait or sickle cell disease), trauma, penetrating or blunt (with superinfection of a subcapsular hematoma), or other diseases (malaria, hydatid cysts); or (3) extension from a contiguous focus of infection, such as a subphrenic abscess. The most common organisms are staphylococci, streptococci, anaerobes, and aerobic gram-negative rods, including *Salmonella*. In neutropenic hosts fungi, predominantly *Candida* species, may cause splenic abscesses.

The onset is typically subacute, and the major features are fever and leukocytosis. Left-sided pain, often pleuritic, may occur in the upper abdomen, lower chest, or flank, sometimes radiating to the left shoulder. Left upper quadrant abdominal tenderness and splenomegaly are common, but an audible splenic friction rub is rare.

Radiographic findings may include (1) a left upper quadrant soft tissue abdominal mass, (2) extraintestinal gas from gas-forming organisms in the abscess, (3) displacement of other organs, including the colon, kidney, and stomach, (4) elevation of the left hemidiaphragm, and (5) left pleural effusion. An ultrasound scan may be positive for macroscopic splenic abscesses, but CT scan is the most reliable diagnostic test.

Treatment consists of appropriate systemic antibiotics and removal of pus by percutaneous catheter, splenotomy, or splenectomy. Splenic abscesses should be considered a possible, although rare, cause of continued bacteremia in acute endocarditis despite appropriate chemotherapy, and splenectomy may be necessary to achieve final eradication of the infection. Successful treatment of fungal splenic abscesses in immunodeficient patients has usually included splenectomy and prolonged administration of amphotericin B, but some patients have been cured with antifungal drugs alone.

Pancreatic abscess These abscesses usually occur in a site of pancreatic necrosis following acute pancreatitis. Typically, the patient improves after the attack of pancreatitis, but about 10 to 21 days later fever, abdominal pain and tenderness, nausea, vomiting, and sometimes persistent ileus occur. Less commonly, the abscess develops shortly after the attack begins. In those cases, persistent fever, leukocytosis, and abdominal findings beyond 7 to 10 days should suggest an abscess. A mass is sometimes palpable. The serum amylase is irregularly elevated, but leukocytosis is usually present. The serum alkaline phosphatase may be increased and the albumin decreased.

Chest roentgenograms often show a left pleural effusion, basilar atelectasis or pneumonia, or a raised hemidiaphragm. Ultrasound is very useful in revealing fluid-filled pancreatic masses but may be unable to distinguish infected from uninfected fluid. CT is the most accurate test for abscesses and may show pancreatic gas, peripancreatic fluid collections, or masses, but only pancreatic gas is diagnostic of infection.

Treatment is appropriate antibiotic therapy and drainage of pus by percutaneous catheters or surgery. Catheter drainage often fails because of inability to remove thick, necrotic debris. Since the usual organisms are coliforms, staphylococci, streptococci, and anaerobes in varying combinations, clindamycin and an aminoglycoside are a reasonable choice until culture results return. Even with appropriate treatment the mortality rate is about 20 to 40 percent, and recurrent abscesses requiring multiple drainage procedures are common.

Renal abscess Single or multiple abscesses of the renal *cortex* may be the result of metastatic implantation of staphylococci from another focus. There is no relationship to previous renal disease; the infection occurs in younger individuals, is usually unilateral, and occurs on the right side oftener than on the left. Many patients give a history of recent skin infection such as furuncle. Medullary abscesses usually develop from acute pyelonephritis when foci of cellular infiltrates in the interstitium coalesce to form single or multiple distinct cavities.

The onset of renal abscess is abrupt, with chills and fever, followed by costovertebral pain and tenderness. If the abscess is cortical, the urine contains *no white blood cells;* medullary abscesses are usually accompanied by pyuria. The stained urinary sediment may show myriads of gram-positive cocci in cortical abscesses and gram-negative organisms in medullary abscesses. Transient gross or microscopic hematuria may occur at the onset. The white blood cell count is usually elevated and may exceed 30,000 cells per cubic millimeter. Physical signs are usually localized to the region of the kidney, but abdominal spasm may lead to confusion with appendicitis, cholecystitis, or pancreatitis. Early in the disease, ureteral calculus or acute hydronephrosis may be considered as possible diagnoses. Sudden onset of *fever, leukocytosis, and renal pain in the absence of pyuria* should suggest the diagnosis of a renal cortical abscess, especially in a patient with infection elsewhere. Obstruction of the ureter by pus or cellular debris may also yield a urine sediment sparse in white blood cells and bacteria. Excretory urograms typically reveal an intrarenal mass, and ultrasound and CT scans usually demonstrate the abscess as a fluid-filled defect. *Treatment* consists of appropriate antibiotics, adequate fluids, and relief of pain. An abscess may suddenly discharge into the renal pelvis, with relief of pain and the passage of cloudy urine containing enormous numbers of leukocytes and bacteria. Recovery is ordinarily prompt, and chronic sequelae are rare. Failure to achieve prompt defervescence following treatment suggests an incorrect diagnosis or the necessity of drainage, by needle aspiration, percutaneous catheter, or surgery.

MISCELLANEOUS ABSCESSES

RETROFASCIAL ABSCESS The retrofascial space, lying between the transversalis and psoas fascias, contains the psoas and quadratus lumborum muscles. Abscesses in this area usually derive from infections in the vertebrae, ilium, and sacroiliac joints. Less frequently, they represent extensions from abscesses in the anterior retroperitoneal space. Sometimes no adjacent source of infection is apparent; these "primary" infections are usually staphylococcal and almost surely have a hematogenous origin. The symptoms of retrofascial abscesses are abdominal pain in the iliac or inguinal region and, particularly with psoas muscle involvement, hip pain and posterior thigh pain and paresthesias. Careful palpation of the lower abdomen or groin often reveals a mass, and rectal or vaginal examination may disclose fullness and tenderness. Pain on hip motion is common, the hip is flexed, and extension or internal rotation of the hip is very painful. Plain abdominal films may demonstrate a mass or loss of the psoas shadow; excretory urograms may show displacement of the kidney or ureter and scoliosis with concavity on the side of infection. Ultrasound usually reveals a soft tissue mass, but CT and MRI scans typically provide more precise information, including evaluation of the adjacent bones. Appropriate antimicrobial therapy alone may sometimes be curative, but drainage by percutaneous catheter or open surgery is often necessary.

PROSTATIC ABSCESS These abscesses, typically occurring in middle age, are complications of acute prostatitis, cystitis, urethritis, or epididymitis. Most patients are *afebrile* and have urinary frequency, retention, or dysuria. Less common features are hematuria, perineal pain, and a purulent urethral discharge. Some patients have persistent or recurrent urinary infections despite apparently adequate antimicrobial therapy. Rectal examination may reveal prostatic tenderness or fluctuance, but sometimes there is only prostatic enlargement or even no abnormality at all. Pyuria and positive urine cultures are usual, but not invariably so. Many of these abscesses are unexpected discoveries at prostatic surgery or endoscopy performed for apparent benign prostatic hypertrophy. Treatment is appropriate antibiotics and surgical drainage by transurethral or perineal incision. The usual pathogens are aerobic gram-negative rods and, less frequently, *S. aureus.*

RECTAL ABSCESS Most of these infections are superficial and involve the perirectal region, and many are associated with fistulas. Infection in the apocrine glands (hidradenitis) or folliculitis in the perianal region, extension of cryptitis or obstructions in the "anal glands" which open into the crypts of Morgagni, and contamination of submucosal hematomas, sclerosed hemorrhoids, or anal fissures may lead to abscess formation. In most patients, the cause of infection is not apparent. These are usually painful, easily palpable, often visible on inspection. Treatment is incision and drainage, even when no fluctuance is present or the patient is neutropenic. Antibiotics are rarely necessary unless there is extensive perineal cellulitis.

Difficulties in diagnosis are likely to arise with infections higher in the rectum. Most are in the ischiorectal area, but those above the pelvic diaphragm, the so-called supralevator abscess, are particularly elusive. Patients with this type of infection often have fever, malaise, and leukocytosis for several days or even weeks before any symptoms referable to the rectum develop. There is vague pelvic discomfort, relieved by defecation, and constipation punctuated by short episodes of diarrhea is common. In males, the inflammation often involves the base of the bladder, and urinary urgency or retention may occur, falsely centering attention on the urinary tract as the source of fever and malaise. Eventually, the abscess produces severe pain, chills, and fever; palpation and instrumentation will reveal the swelling in the rectal ampulla. Such an abscess may surround the rectum and produce narrowing that is differentiated from neoplasm by the fact that the mucosa remains intact. A useful sign of deep rectal abscess is severe pain with pressure in the region between the anus and the coccyx. The supralevator space is continuous with the ischiorectal space, with both the gluteal and obturator regions, and with the retroperitoneal space. In neglected cases, the abscess may drain through the skin of the perineum, the groin, or the buttock or may extend as high as the perirenal areas. Rectal abscesses often occur in patients with preexisting anorectal disease, diabetes, alcoholism, and neurologic disease; infections in this area are also peculiarly frequent in patients with acute leukemia, especially when neutropenia is present. Because the clinical picture may be that of "fever of unknown origin" for a long period, it is important that thorough digital and endoscopic examination of the rectum be carried out in patients with unexplained fever. Identification and localization of the abscess are best achieved by CT or MRI scan. Patients with diabetic ketoacidosis should receive a careful rectal examination because a rectal abscess may be the infection responsible for precipitating the ketoacidosis.

A rectal abscess may be a forerunner of both ulcerative colitis and regional enteritis, and may occur months and even years before other overt manifestations of these diseases. For this reason, proctosigmoidoscopy, colonoscopy, barium enema, and, often, upper gastrointestinal roentgenograms are indicated in nonhealing or recurrent rectal lesions.

Treatment of high rectal abscesses consists of incision and drainage, analgesics, and antibiotics directed at *E. coli, Klebsiella-Enterobacter, Bacteroides,* and a variety of streptococci, which constitute the polymicrobial flora of these lesions.

REFERENCES

BARNES PF et al: A comparison of amebic and pyogenic abscess of the liver. Medicine 66:472, 1987

BLOMQUIST IK et al: Life-threatening deep fascial space infections of the head and neck. Infect Dis Clin North Am 2:237, 1988

EDELSTEIN H et al: Perinephric abscess. Modern diagnosis and treatment in 47 cases. Medicine 67:118, 1988

GOLIGHER JC: *Surgery of the Anus, Rectum, and Colon,* 5th ed. New York, Macmillan, 1984

GYORFFY EJ et al: Pyogenic liver abscess. Diagnostic and therapeutic strategies. Ann Surg 206:699, 1987

LINSCHEID RL et al: Common and uncommon infections of the hand. Orthop Clin North Am 6:1063, 1975

NELKEN N et al: Changing clinical spectrum of splenic abscess. A multicenter study and review of the literature. Am J Surg 154:27, 1987

PRUETT TL et al: Status of percutaneous catheter drainage of abscesses. Surg Clin North Am 68:89, 1988

STEINER E et al: Complicated pancreatic abscesses: Problems in interventional management. Radiology 167:443, 1988

92 ACUTE INFECTIOUS DIARRHEAL DISEASES AND BACTERIAL FOOD POISONING

CHARLES C. J. CARPENTER

Acute diarrheal illnesses caused by bacterial, viral, or protozoal pathogens vary from slightly annoying bowel dysfunction to fulminant, life-threatening diseases. Largely because of the recognition of enterotoxigenic *Escherichia coli* as a major cause of acute diarrheal disease in adults and the identification of rotavirus as a frequent cause in young children, specific etiologic agents have been isolated from 80 to 85 percent of patients with acute diarrheal illnesses. Those illnesses caused by bacterial pathogens are more often life-threatening, at least among adults, and for that reason they will be addressed first. This chapter is aimed at presenting an overview of these diseases; in most instances, the entities are discussed in more detail in the chapters dealing with the specific etiologic agent.

In considering the bacterial diarrheas, it is useful to divide them into two groups, those caused by invasive and those caused by noninvasive microorganisms. The invasive pathogens, of which *Shigella* (see Chap. 114) may be considered the prototype, generally cause abdominal pain, fever, and other systemic symptoms, often including headache and myalgia. Illness caused by the noninvasive pathogens, of which cholera (see Chap. 122) is the prototype, is generally characterized by the absence of fever and few systemic symptoms (except those directly related to intestinal fluid loss). The invasive pathogens characteristically destroy gut mucosal cells, typically involving the terminal ileum and colon, and both leukocytes and erythrocytes are present, to a variable degree, in the stool. Inflammatory cells are generally absent from the stool in acute diarrheal disease caused by noninvasive bacterial pathogens.

NONINVASIVE BACTERIAL PATHOGENS

ENTEROTOXIGENIC *ESCHERICHIA COLI* Etiology and epidemiology Enterotoxin-producing *E. coli* (ETEC), which have the dual capacity to adhere to small-bowel epithelial cells and to produce one or more diarrheagenic toxins, are recognized as a major cause of acute diarrheal disease throughout most of the world and are the most common cause of "traveler's diarrhea." Largely because current techniques for demonstrating toxigenicity remain cumbersome, the epidemiology of ETEC diarrhea is poorly understood. ETEC are responsible for the majority of cases of traveler's diarrhea in visitors to the developing nations in South America, Africa, and Asia. ETEC are also one of the two (with rotavirus) leading causes of acute diarrheal illnesses in children throughout the developing world. ETEC have been implicated as a major cause of fulminant, cholera-like diarrheal disease in adult patients in south and southeast Asia but generally cause milder, self-limited diarrhea in adults in other parts of the developing world. There is no satisfactory explanation for the difference in severity in diarrhea caused by ETEC in different geographic areas. ETEC are occasionally incriminated in episodic diarrheal illness in children and adults in the United States.

Pathogenesis The ability to cause diarrheal disease is not restricted to any one *E. coli* serotype but appears to be dependent upon the presence of both a plasmid-mediated colonization factor, which allows the *E. coli* to adhere to small-bowel mucosal cells, and one or more plasmids which code for the production of one or both of the two distinct classes of diarrheagenic toxins that may be produced by *E. coli.* The kinetics and mode of action of one class, which is heat labile (LT) and of relatively high molecular mass (~83,000 daltons), are similar to those of cholera enterotoxin (see Chap. 122); the diarrheagenic effect results from stimulation of adenylate cyclase in the gut epithelial cells. The other class, which is heat stable (ST) and of a lower molecular mass (<2000 daltons), has a more rapid onset of action and probably exerts its effect through stimulation of guanylate cyclase in the gut mucosal cells. Either or both classes of toxins may be produced by ETEC. Most isolates from patients with severe diarrheal disease in Bangladesh produce both LT and ST, whereas isolates from patients in other developing nations have shown widely varying capacities for the production of LT, ST, or both. The wide clinical spectrum may be, in part, related to the predominant production of either LT or ST by the culpable microorganisms. The nutritional status of the host may also be a factor in determining the clinical response to ETEC.

Manifestations Both clinical observations and volunteer studies indicate that the incubation period is generally between 24 and 72 h. The illness which follows is quite variable, ranging from the fulminant, cholera-like disease often seen on the Indian subcontinent to the much milder Mexican "turista," in which the symptoms of mild, watery diarrhea, abdominal cramps, and occasional low-grade fever are more troublesome than life-threatening. Vomiting occurs in fewer than half the adults with *E. coli* diarrhea and is seldom responsible for major fluid losses.

In fulminant cases, the severe diarrhea seldom lasts longer than 24 to 36 h, and the response to either oral or intravenous electrolyte repletion is predictable and dramatic. With milder disease, the symptoms may subside more gradually, occasionally persisting for a week or longer.

Laboratory findings As with cholera, no erythrocytes and few, if any, polymorphonuclear leukocytes are seen in a stool preparation stained with Loeffler's methylene blue. Because *E. coli* occurs normally among stool flora and its ability to produce enterotoxin is not restricted to any specific serotype, there is no rapid and simple means to make the laboratory diagnosis of enterotoxigenic *E. coli*. Bioassays for LT, based on the ability of *E. coli* isolates to produce fluid in isolated intestinal loops of experimental animals or to stimulate adenylate cyclase in cells in tissue culture, as well as the suckling mouse bioassay for ST, are reliable but of little value in patient management. Newer technology, utilizing DNA probes for rapid identification of the genes responsible for ST and LT production, appears promising and may be adapted for widespread use for epidemiologic purposes in the future.

Treatment The intestinal fluid losses are qualitatively identical to those in cholera. Therefore, in those patients who develop clinically significant saline depletion, the principles of fluid administration are identical to those described for cholera (see Chap. 122). Oral solutions containing electrolytes plus glucose or sucrose are consistently effective in correcting the saline depletion. Antibiotics (tetracycline, 30 mg/kg per day, given orally at 6-h intervals for 48 h; trimethoprim, 200 mg twice daily for 5 days; or trimethoprim, 160 mg, with sulfamethoxazole, 800 mg, twice daily for 5 days) are effective in decreasing the duration of illness but are not essential. One of the quinolone drugs (norfloxacin or ciprofloxacin) is also effective (see Chap. 85). Bismuth subsalicylate, 60 mL hourly for four doses, provides symptomatic relief (less frequent stools, less severe abdominal cramps). Both diphenoxylate and loperamide may provide rapid relief of abdominal cramps, but neither drug has been shown to alter the volume of intestinal fluid loss.

Prognosis Even in the more fulminant cases of disease caused by ETEC, with adequate peroral or intravenous fluid replacement, the prognosis is excellent.

Prevention Careful hygienic practices, with special attention to ingestion of clean water (boiled for 2 min if its source is uncertain) and adequately cooked foods, provide the most certain protection against enterotoxigenic *E. coli*. Doxycycline, 100 mg/d, is 60 to 90 percent effective as a prophylactic agent, the effectiveness varying with the tetracycline sensitivity of the ETEC in the geographic area. Trimethoprim, 160 mg, with sulfamethoxazole, 800 mg, taken once daily, is also effective in prophylaxis against traveler's diarrhea caused by ETEC.

NONTOXIGENIC ENTEROPATHOGENIC *E. COLI* The classically recognized enteropathogenic *E. coli* (EPEC) strains neither invade gut mucosa nor produce an identifiable toxin, yet produce occasional outbreaks of acute, sometimes severe, diarrheal disease in infants and are associated with sporadic cases of mild diarrhea in adults, in both industrialized and developing countries. Most such EPEC strains demonstrate plasmid-encoded adherence to small-gut mucosal cells, which is associated with dissolution of the glycocalyx and effacement of the microvilli. The exact mechanism by which diarrhea is produced is not known. Infants may require oral, or occasionally intravenous, fluid repletion therapy. Since the illness is self-limited, antimicrobial agents are of no demonstrable benefit.

CHOLERA See Chap. 122.

OTHER ENTEROTOXIGENIC ENTEROBACTERIACEAE Noninvasive strains of *Klebsiella* and *Enterobacter* occasionally have been implicated in acute diarrheal disease in developing areas of the world. The clinical illness produced is indistinguishable from the milder cases of diarrhea caused by enterotoxigenic *E. coli*, and treatment is the same.

CLOSTRIDIUM PERFRINGENS (See Chap. 107) This organism remains a significant cause of diarrheal disease and is implicated in many cases of acute food poisoning in the United States. Both the epidemiologic background and the clinical picture of *C. perfringens* diarrhea differ strikingly from those of *E. coli*. *Clostridium perfringens* diarrhea tends to occur in a microepidemic pattern following ingestion of contaminated meat, poultry products, or legumes. The relatively short incubation period of 6 to 12 h is an important diagnostic clue. Typically, two or more patients who have ingested the same meat dish become ill at roughly the same time. The production of a specific enterotoxin by the actively sporulating microorganisms in the intestinal tract appears to be responsible for all the symptoms. The clinical picture of diarrhea caused by *C. perfringens* is different from that caused by enterotoxigenic *E. coli* in one important respect, because moderately severe cramping abdominal pain, which is usually less prominent with *E. coli*, is a major presenting symptom. Treatment consists of symptomatic therapy to alleviate the cramping abdominal pain and intravenous fluid therapy in the small proportion of patients in whom there is clinical evidence of saline depletion. The illness is self-limited and rarely lasts for more than 24 h. Because of the relatively short natural course of the illness, antimicrobial therapy is of no value. Because *C. perfringens* normally inhabits mammalian and avian intestinal tracts, prevention is dependent upon adequate cooking and handling of meat and poultry products. The practice of allowing cooked meat products to cool slowly toward room temperature over 12 to 24 h permits germination of contaminating clostridial spores and this practice must be avoided.

STAPHYLOCOCCUS AUREUS (See Chap. 100) Acute staphylococcal diarrhea, classic "food poisoning," is due entirely to ingestion of preformed enterotoxin, and the causative organisms are often absent from the stool during the acute illness. This form of diarrhea often occurs in institutional outbreaks and is characterized by a short incubation period (2 to 6 h), relatively short duration (usually less than 10 h), and very high attack rates (often greater than 75 percent of the population at risk). In addition to its distinctive epidemiologic features, acute staphylococcal diarrhea differs from other noninvasive bacterial diarrheas by the prominence of vomiting, which is an almost constant feature and is apparently mediated by a direct effect of the absorbed toxin on the central nervous system. Treatment is directed toward correction of the saline depletion (intravenous fluids are required in 10 to 20 percent of patients) and, when necessary, toward symptomatic relief of vomiting. Because staphylococcal food poisoning is caused by preformed enterotoxin and is not perpetuated by viable microorganisms, antimicrobials are of no value.

A good example of the explosive nature of staphylococcal food poisoning was provided by an outbreak on a jet liner flying from Anchorage to Copenhagen. In this episode, 57 percent of 343 passengers developed an acute illness characterized by vomiting, diarrhea, and cramping abdominal pain. Of the 200 affected individuals, 30 required intravenous fluids, but none had serious sequelae. The food, contaminated by a pustule on the hand of a food handler, had not been adequately refrigerated aboard the plane, allowing abundant growth of the staphylococcus, with production of enterotoxin. Since staphylococci are ubiquitous, the prevention of massive contamination is dependent largely on control of growth conditions, primarily temperature. *Staphylococcus aureus* can multiply at temperatures from 4 to 46°C, and if contaminated food is allowed to remain at ambient temperatures after cooking, these organisms have ample opportunity to multiply, especially in such items as cream pastries, potato salad, and mayonnaise.

BACILLUS CEREUS *Bacillus cereus* is a cause of acute diarrheal disease which, although uncommon, has been identified with increasing frequency in Europe. The illness results from gross contamination of food with this gram-positive rod, which is capable of producing at least two discrete enterotoxins, one having characteristics similar to those of the labile enterotoxin of *E. coli* and the other having effects similar to that of staphylococcal enterotoxin. *Bacillus cereus* may, therefore, cause two distinct clinical syndromes, a diarrheal form resulting from the *E. coli* LT type of enterotoxin and an emetic form caused by the staphylococcal type of enterotoxin. The diarrheal syndrome caused by *B. cereus* is generally similar to that caused by enterotoxin-producing *E. coli,* with the exceptions that abdominal cramps are more common (75 percent of cases) and both the incubation period (6 to 14 h) and median duration of illness (20 h) are shorter. The emetic syndrome is clinically indistinguishable from that caused by staphylococcal enterotoxin, with a short incubation period (median 2 h), short duration (median 9 h), and prominent vomiting (100 percent compared with less than 25 percent in the diarrheal syndrome). Because both syndromes are self-limited and generally mild, no specific therapy is indicated. When *B. cereus* food poisoning is suspected clinically, the diagnosis can be confirmed by demonstration of 10^5 or more *B. cereus* organisms per gram in epidemiologically incriminated food. *Bacillus cereus* grows readily on simple laboratory media, including blood agar, but will not generally be identified as a pathogen unless such identification is specifically requested. Isolation of *B. cereus* from stool alone does not establish it as the etiologic agent because the organism is frequently found in the fecal flora of normal individuals. Since *B. cereus* is ubiquitous in soil, as well as in many raw, dried, and processed foods, proper food handling is the only practical means of preventing this form of food poisoning. The emetic form of *B. cereus* food poisoning almost invariably has been associated with ingestion of contaminated fried rice. *Bacillus cereus* is commonly present in uncooked rice, and its spores survive boiling and germinate, with production of the enterotoxin, when boiled rice is left unrefrigerated. Brief rewarming before serving is not adequate to destroy the relatively heat-stable toxin. Prompt refrigeration of boiled rice will prevent this disease.

INVASIVE AND/OR DESTRUCTIVE ENTERIC PATHOGENS

INTRODUCTION Shigellae characteristically invade the colon and terminal ileum, destroy segments of intestinal mucosa, cause extensive inflammatory changes in the lamina propria, and are the prototype of the invasive and/or destructive enteric bacterial pathogens. Other important invasive bacterial enteric pathogens include *Salmonella, Yersinia enterocolitica, Campylobacter jejuni, Vibrio parahemolyticus,* and enteroinvasive *E. coli* (EIEC). As opposed to the noninvasive pathogens, the invasive enteric organisms frequently cause systemic symptoms, including headache, myalgias, chills, and fever. As a general rule, antiperistaltic agents such as opiates, diphenoxylate, loperamide, and atropine are contraindicated in diarrheal disease caused by invasive enteric pathogens because they clearly worsen the clinical course in shigellosis.

The major therapeutic challenge in invasive bacterial diarrheas is that of distinguishing between (1) shigellosis and yersiniosis, in which antimicrobial therapy decreases the duration and severity of illness and shortens the period of fecal shedding of the pathogen, and (2) infections caused by *Salmonella* in which antimicrobial therapy does not alter the duration of illness and may cause prolonged excretion of the pathogen.

SHIGELLOSIS See Chap. 114.

SALMONELLOSIS See Chap. 113.

YERSINIA ENTEROCOLITICA See Chap. 121.

CAMPYLOBACTER JEJUNI **Etiology and epidemiology** *Campylobacter jejuni* is second only to *Giardia lamblia* among recognized causes of waterborne diarrheal disease outbreaks in the United States. Attack rates have been highest in adolescents and young adults. *C. jejuni* occurs in the intestinal flora of many wild and domestic animals and poultry and can be transmitted to humans by milk and water polluted by such animal carriers. The distribution of *C. jejuni* is worldwide, and *C. jejuni* appears to cause from 5 to 10 percent of acute diarrheal illnesses in adults in both the industrialized and the developing areas of the world. Ingestion of raw milk and of water from contaminated mountain streams has been implicated in *Campylobacter* enteritis in North America; in outbreaks associated with ingestion of raw milk, attack rates have reached 60 percent.

Pathogenesis *C. jejuni* causes patchy destruction of mucosa of both the small intestine, especially the distal ileum, and the colon; the stools, therefore, regularly contain pus cells and occasionally are grossly bloody. *C. jejuni* rarely produces transient bacteremia; when it does, it is likely to occur in an immunocompromised host.

Manifestations An incubation period of 2 to 6 days, longer than that of most bacterial enteric pathogens, is followed by fever, cramping abdominal pain, and diarrhea that is initially watery but later contains blood and mucus. The diarrhea, generally mild but occasionally voluminous, usually ceases within 2 to 5 days without specific antimicrobial therapy; on rare occasions the diarrhea may persist for 3 to 4 weeks. In some cases, the abdominal pain may be more prominent than the diarrhea, and the clinical picture may simulate acute appendicitis or, rarely, pancreatitis. (This may also be true in *Yersinia* enterocolitis; see Chap. 121.) In such cases, laparotomy has revealed acutely inflamed mesenteric lymph nodes as well as patchy inflammation of the small bowel. Acute reactive arthritis, similar to that associated with other invasive bacterial diarrheas (*Shigella, Salmonella, Yersinia*) may follow *C. jejuni* enteritis and is often associated wtih the HLA-B27 antigen.

Laboratory findings Diagnosis depends upon isolating *C. jejuni* from stool. Since this curved, motile bacillus does not compete well with other enteric flora on standard enteric media, it will rarely be isolated from stool unless special techniques are utilized. These include incubation at 42°C in a microaerobic atmosphere on blood agar to which a number of antimicrobials have been added. Serologic diagnosis is rarely helpful, as there are many serotypes of *C. jejuni,* and agglutination tests require use of the homologous organism.

Treatment Since *C. jejuni* usually produces a short, self-limited illness, antimicrobial therapy is not essential to management. Erythromycin, 30 mg/kg per day, does, however, significantly decrease the duration of fecal shedding of *C. jejuni* and may shorten the mean duration of illness. In the occasional patient who develops clinical signs of saline depletion, oral and/or intravenous fluids of the same sort used in cholera are uniformly effective (see Chap. 122).

OTHER *CAMPYLOBACTER* INFECTIONS The observation of small, curved, gram-negative rods with characteristic corkscrew-like motility in many stool specimens from which *C. jejuni* cannot be isolated has led to the identification of several additional species of *Campylobacter* which are associated with human disease. The *Campylobacter* genus causes a broad range of human illness, including gastritis and systemic infection as well as enteritis. All such species, like *C. jejuni,* appear to be epizootic, but precisely which animals are the most common vectors for specific *Campylobacter* species is not known. This discussion will be limited to four species of *Campylobacter,* which represent the spectrum of illness caused by these microorganisms.

Campylobacter coli, although slightly different in biochemical characteristics, is identical to *C. jejuni* in morphology, growth characteristics and epidemiology, as well as in the illness it produces.

Campylobacter fetus is similar to *C. jejuni* in morphology and growth characteristics but has a marked predilection for patients with chronic renal, hepatic, and neoplastic disease, alcoholism, and compromised immune function. Although the intestinal tract of the compromised host is the presumed site of entry, the intestinal infection may be mild or subclinical, and overshadowed by a bacteremic illness, associated with high fever, which often follows a prolonged or relapsing course and may be complicated by endocarditis, infection of preexisting aortic aneurysms, and/or septic phlebitis. Persistent bacteremia may be enhanced by the relative resistance of *C. fetus* to the bactericidal activity of normal serum. Although occasional patients have had self-limited *C. fetus* sepsis, *C. fetus* bacteremia is usually fatal unless treated with antimicrobials. Gentamicin is thought to be the drug of choice, although no controlled observations are available. At least 4 weeks of antimicrobial treatment is recommended because of the tropism of *C. fetus* for intravascular sites.

Campylobacter cinaedi sp. n. has been the most frequently isolated of four *Campylobacter*-like organisms (CLOs) which have been associated with proctitis, proctocolitis, and enteritis in homosexual males. Although morphologically similar to *C. jejuni*, the CLOs grow poorly at 42° (and are therefore missed by the standard technique used to isolate *C. jejuni* and *C. fetus*), and prototype CLO strains show little (< 2 percent) DNA homology with *C. jejuni* and *C. fetus*. The CLO organisms grow slowly in a microaerophilic environment on modified brucella agar supplemented with 10% sheep blood.

A distinct species, *Campylobacter pylori* (formerly *C. pyloridis*), has been strongly associated with antral gastritis and with peptic ulcer disease. *C. pylori* has been isolated from over 50 percent of both adults and children with primary antral gastritis, and from an even higher proportion of patients with demonstrable duodenal ulcers, but rarely from normal gastric mucosa. *C. pylori*–associated antral gastritis has been shown to heal after administration of appropriate antimicrobials. *C. pyloris* is therefore thought to be an etiologic factor in primary antral gastritis and associated peptic ulcer disease. Data are not adequate to determine what proportion of cases of antral gastritis may be associated with *C. pyloris*. *C. pyloris* is readily grown in a microaerobic atmosphere on blood agar to which several antimicrobials have been added; like the CLOs, *C. pyloris* grows well at 37°C but poorly at 42°C.

Despite the differing growth characteristics, the CLOs produce changes which are indistinguishable from those caused by *C. jejuni* on sigmoidoscopic and histologic examination. Although the CLOs are sensitive to erythromycin, no controlled studies of antimicrobial therapy are available.

VIBRIO PARAHEMOLYTICUS   Etiology and epidemiology *Vibrio parahemolyticus* is a curved, aerobic, nonmotile, gram-negative bacillus. Although present in coastal waters throughout the temperate zone, it has most commonly been associated with acute diarrheal illness in Japan, presumably in relation to ingestion of raw seafood. It is regarded as the prototype of the halophilic vibrios because it grows more rapidly in 6% NaCl solutions than in the isotonic or hypotonic media used to culture most bacterial pathogens. *V. para-hemolyticus* is responsible for a relatively small (<10 percent) proportion of acute diarrheal illnesses in both adults and children in rural Bangladesh, where an association with seafood is less clearly established. It has been implicated in several outbreaks of acute diarrheal disease in the coastal United States, always as a common-source outbreak related to ingestion of inadequately cooked seafood, usually shrimp. Secondary cases caused by person-to-person transmission occur rarely. Several outbreaks of *V. parahemolyticus* infections on cruise ships have occurred.

Pathogenesis   Although *V. parahemolyticus* produces a toxin capable of causing intestinal fluid accumulation in experimental animals, the role of this toxin in human disease is not certain. *V. parahemolyticus* causes patchy mucosal damage in both distal ileum and colon; stools usually contain numerous polymorphonuclear leukocytes and are occasionally grossly bloody. The volume of fluid lost with *V. parahemolyticus* infection is relatively small, and intravenous fluids are seldom required. The illness is self-limited, with a median duration of just under 24 h.

Manifestations   Within 6 to 48 h after ingestion of raw or inadequately cooked seafood, the patient develops an acute diarrheal illness. The volume of fluid lost is not great, moderately severe abdominal cramps may be a prominent feature, and chills and fever are observed in roughly half the cases. Vomiting is generally not prominent and occurs in no more than one-third of patients. The illness is self-limited, and no deaths have been reported in outbreaks in the United States.

Laboratory findings   When a common-source outbreak of acute diarrheal disease occurs in a group exposed to fresh or frozen seafood, the index of suspicion should be high and the diagnosis should be confirmed by plating a rectal swab on thiosulfate–citrate–bile salt–sucrose (TCBS) agar, on which typical colonies of *V. parahemolyticus* appear in 24 h. (This organism grows poorly and is therefore easily overlooked on deoxycholate culture plates.) The stool generally has numerous polymorphonuclear leukocytes and a smaller number of erythrocytes, but these findings are less prominent than in shigellosis.

Treatment   No therapy is required for the majority of patients. Antimicrobial therapy shortens neither the course nor the duration of pathogen excretion. Antiperistaltic agents are not of clear-cut benefit. An occasional patient may lose sufficient quantities of intestinal fluid to require oral or intravenous fluid therapy.

Prognosis   The outcome is almost always good. Fatal cases, occasionally reported from Japan, have occurred in rare instances in patients with serious underlying disease.

VIBRIO MIMICUS   *Vibrio mimicus* has been identified as a pathogen in sporadic cases of acute diarrheal disease, occurring in previously healthy individuals of all age groups who have ingested raw seafood (especially oysters) along the Gulf Coast. The epidemiology of *V. mimicus* infections differs from that caused by *V. parahemolyticus* in that, with the exception of one small outbreak, all isolates have represented single, sporadic cases. Although *V. mimicus*, like *V. cholerae*, is not a halophilic vibrio (it grows more rapidly in 1% NaCl than in higher salt solutions), it does not produce cholera enterotoxin, and it causes an illness in which the presenting features are clinically indistinguishable from those caused by *V. parahemolyticus*.

Fever occurs in at least 40 percent of cases and bloody diarrhea in roughly 15 percent. Since the illness is self-limited, treatment is symptomatic. Antibiotic therapy is of no value.

VIBRIO VULNIFICUS   *Vibrio vulnificus*, like *V. parahemolyticus*, is a true halophilic vibrio that is common in shellfish along the Gulf of Mexico and less frequent along the Atlantic and Pacific coasts. It has been recognized as the cause of serious illness in at least 60 individuals in the last decade. *V. vulnificus* produces two clinical syndromes distinct from those caused by other vibrio species. In the compromised host, most frequently in individuals with liver disease, *V. vulnificus* may cause fulminant septicemia, usually associated with the early (within 36 h) development of cutaneous bullae and/or ulcers. In the noncompromised host, after contamination of a superficial wound by seawater, *V. vulnificus* may cause rapid development of intense cellulitis and local ulceration, often associated with bacteremia.

V. vulnificus should be suspected, and therapy with intravenous tetracycline should be initiated immediately in any individual with chronic liver disease who develops signs of septicemia (especially if associated with cutaneous lesions) within 1 to 3 days of ingestion of shellfish.

INVASIVE ESCHERICHIA COLI   Enteroinvasive *E. coli*, which are far less common pathogens than enterotoxigenic *E. coli*, may cause a clinical syndrome quite similar to shigellosis with the exceptions that vomiting seldom occurs with EIEC and the illness is of shorter duration. Diarrhea caused by EIEC is rare in the United States but has been a significant cause of short-term disability in eastern Europe and southeast Asia. Since the illness is relatively short-lived, antimicrobial therapy has not been shown to be helpful.

ENTEROHEMORRHAGIC ESCHERICHIA COLI (EHEC)   A small number of *E. coli* strains, most commonly 0157:H7, have been responsible for widely distributed sporadic cases of hemorrhagic colitis in the United States. Undercooked meat, especially hamburger, has been the most frequently identified mode of transmission. All age groups have been affected. The clinical illness is most commonly heralded by crampy abdominal pain and watery diarrhea, followed within 24 h by frankly bloody stools, which may simulate lower gastrointestinal bleeding. Unlike those with other bacteria associated with bloody diarrhea (e.g., *Shigella, Campylobacter*), patients are usually afebrile, and inflammatory cells are seldom present in the stool. Colonoscopy demonstrates inflammation, edema, and hemorrhage, primarily in the ascending and proximal transverse colon. The mean duration of illness has been 8 days.

All isolates tested have been noninvasive (Sereny test negative) but EHEC consistently produce verocytotoxin that is immunologically indistinguishable from the Shiga toxin of *Shigella dysenteriae* type I. Verocytotoxin can be isolated from the stool of virtually all patients with EHEC enteritis. Available data indicate that the hemolytic-uremic syndrome (HUS) is at least as frequent following EHEC colitis as it is following enteritis caused by *S. dysenteriae* type I. Despite the production of a toxin immunologically identical to the Shiga toxin, EHEC are not invasive, appear to cause disease by a direct effect of the verocytotoxin on colonic mucosal cells, and generally cause few systemic symptoms.

With the exception of the individuals who develop HUS, the illness is generally self-limited. HUS may, however, develop in any age group, and the mortality rate has been especially high in elderly individuals who develop this complication. Treatment with appropriate antimicrobials has not been shown to alter the duration or severity of the illness, but the sporadic occurrence of cases has prevented controlled studies of antibiotic therapy.

ACUTE VIRAL DIARRHEAS

Acute viral gastroenteritis is discussed in detail in Chap. 145. These illnesses are both more common and more life-threatening in small children than adults. In the United States, rotaviruses account for a large proportion of diarrheal illnesses during the first 2 years of life and usually occur during the winter. They have seldom been implicated in adult illness. In rural Bangladesh, infection with rotavirus accounts for roughly 60 percent of episodes of diarrhea in children from 6 to 24 months of age and for about 5 percent in the 2- to 5-year-old age group; it seldom occurs in adolescents and adults. The illness usually presents with vomiting followed by watery diarrhea and low-grade fever, with little or no associated abdominal pain. Vomiting is a prominent and almost constant early manifestation of rotavirus enteritis but rarely persists beyond the first 24 h. Diarrhea often persists for 4 to 8 days. Although the illness is generally not life-threatening, many patients require fluid and electrolyte repletion. Since the vomiting is usually short-lived, fluid repletion can generally be achieved by the oral route, using the same fluids that are effective in the treatment of cholera (see Chap. 122).

The diagnosis can be confirmed by a variety of tests including demonstration of the virus in stool by electron microscopy, a rise in complement-fixing antibody titers, and radioimmunoassay. The most useful and reliable test for rapid diagnosis under field conditions consists of direct demonstration of the antigen in stool by the enzyme-linked immunosorbent assay (ELISA).

Norwalk and Norwalk-like viruses, now implicated in roughly a third of episodes of epidemic gastroenteritis involving adults in the United States, usually cause relatively mild, short (<36 h), and self-limited disease, for which neither fluid nor drug therapy is necessary (see Chap. 145).

ACUTE PROTOZOAL DIARRHEAS

Giardia lamblia has emerged as a major cause of acute diarrheal disease (see Chap. 165). Although formerly thought to be a pathogen only in children and later considered to be a significant cause of diarrheal disease only in developing nations, this organism is the pathogen most commonly incriminated in outbreaks of waterborne diarrheal disease in the United States. It occurs most commonly in the Rocky Mountain states and more frequently causes disease in visitors than in the indigenous population. The illness characteristically presents with the sudden onset of watery diarrhea and malabsorption, accompanied by mild to moderate abdominal discomfort, bloating, and flatulence. Symptoms may occasionally persist for weeks unless appropriate antimicrobials are administered. Prolonged disease with malabsorption occurs from time to time in previously normal individuals but is particularly common in patients with IgA deficiency, who tend to have the most severe form of giardiasis.

The attack rate may be quite high (>50 percent) in individuals exposed to contaminated water sources. In North American travelers returning from Leningrad, where the water supply has been heavily contaminated with *Giardia* cysts, up to 60 percent of individuals have developed clinical giardiasis. The usual incubation period is 10 to 20 days. The illness, therefore, frequently develops after a traveler returns home, and the travel history is critical in suspecting the diagnosis. Occasionally the disease occurs endemically in individuals who have not traveled. The diagnosis can be confirmed in approximately half the cases by examining the stool for cysts; if the stool examination is negative in a patient with characteristic clinical features, duodenal aspirates or biopsies will usually yield the characteristic trophozoites. Treatment with quinacrine, 100 mg tid for 5 to 7 days, is generally curative; metronidazole, 250 mg tid for 7 days, is an equally effective alternative.

TRAVELER'S DIARRHEA

Diarrhea is by far the most common health problem of travelers to developing countries. Of more than 16 million travelers annually from industrialized nations to developing countries, approximately one-third will develop diarrhea. The incidence of traveler's diarrhea (TD) varies markedly by destination.

Etiology and epidemiology   Virtually all cases of TD are caused by infectious agents, acquired through ingestion of fecally contaminated food and/or water. Especially risky foods include raw vegetables, raw meats, and raw seafood. Foods sold by street vendors are a common source of enteropathogens. Bacterial pathogens account for the great majority of episodes. Overall, the most common etiologic agents in TD are enterotoxigenic *E. coli* (ETEC), which are responsible for 50 to 75 percent of episodes. The culpable ETEC may produce LT, ST, or both enterotoxins, with considerable geographic variation. Other recognized enteropathogens can be isolated from most of the remainder of cases, but with great regional differences in prevalence. For example, *Shigella* causes up to 10 percent of TD in Mexico but is an unusual etiologic agent in North Africa. *Vibrio parahemolyticus* is a relatively common cause of TD in Japanese travelers in Asia but has not been associated with TD in South America. Viruses (rotavirus, Norwalk-like virus) and protozoa (amebas, *Giardia*) are collectively responsible for fewer than 10 percent of cases of TD.

Pathogenesis   The pathogenesis varies with the culpable etiologic organism, but most cases of TD, even when caused by *Shigella*, are self-limited and have not been associated with serious sequelae in previously healthy individuals.

Manifestations   Episodes of TD usually begin abruptly, with urgent diarrhea, abdominal cramps, nausea, and often low-grade fever. In the great majority of cases, the fluid loss is not voluminous, and symptoms subside within 3 to 5 days.

Treatment   For the great majority of patients, fluid losses do not demand specific replacement fluids. Patients want relief from the two specific problems of abdominal cramps and diarrhea. Bismuth subsalicylate, taken as Pepto-Bismol liquid, in a dose of 60 mL qid, can decrease the severity of symptoms. Diphenoxylate and loperamide both provide symptomatic relief, but should not be used in the rare patient with high fever or blood in the stool; the antimotility agents should be discontinued if symptoms persist beyond 48 h. Patients with more severe symptoms (e.g., more than three loose stools within

8 h) may benefit from antimicrobial treatment. Trimethoprim, 160 mg, with sulfamethoxazole, 800 mg, twice daily, or trimethoprim alone, 200 mg twice daily for 3 days, has proved effective in shortening the mean duration of symptoms from 4 to 1.5 days. It is not certain that these antimicrobials will prove equally effective in all parts of the developing world.

Prevention The only sure prevention is to avoid ingestion of contaminated water and food, a goal that is not practical for most travelers. Carefully controlled studies have demonstrated that three antimicrobials, doxycycline, trimethoprim-sulfamethoxazole, and norfloxacin, when taken prophylactically, are consistently effective in reducing the incidence of TD by 50 to 86 percent in various parts of the developing world. Because of the calculable risks of administration of prophylactic antimicrobials to several million travelers annually, balanced against the generally self-limited course of TD, prophylactic antimicrobials are not routinely recommended for prevention of TD. Travelers are advised, however, to obtain therapeutic doses of effective antimicrobial agents prior to travel to high-risk areas, so that the more severe episodes of TD can be treated early, without recourse to potentially dangerous over-the-counter drugs.

REFERENCES

BARKER WH JR et al: *Vibrio parahemolyticus* outbreak in Covington, Louisiana, in August, 1972. Am J Epidemiol 100:316, 1974

BLACKLOW NR, CUKOR G: Viral gastroenteritis. N Engl J Med 304:397, 1981

BLASER MJ et al: *Campylobacter* enteritis in the United States: A multicenter study. Ann Intern Med 98:360, 1983

CARTER AO et al: A severe outbreak of *Escherichia coli* 0157:H7-associated hemorrhagic colitis in a nursing home. N Engl J Med 317:1496, 1987

CLOVER TL, ABER RD: *Yersinia enterocolitica.* N Engl J Med 321:16, 1989

DUPONT HL et al: Pathogenesis of *Escherichia coli* diarrhea. N Engl J Med 285:1, 1971

——— et al: Symptomatic treatment of diarrhea with bismuth subsalicylate among students attending a Mexican university. Gastroenterology 73:715, 1977

——— et al: Treatment of traveler's diarrhea with trimethoprim/sulfamethoxazole and with trimethoprim alone. N Engl J Med 307:841, 1982

GORBACH SL et al: Traveler's diarrhea and toxigenic *Escherichia coli.* N Engl J Med 292:933, 1975

GRIFFIN PM et al: Illnesses associated with *Escherichia coli* 0157:H7 infections. A broad clinical spectrum. Ann Intern Med 109:705, 1988

GUERRANT RL et al: Prospective study of diarrheal illnesses in northeastern Brazil: Patterns of disease, nutritional impact, etiologies and risk factors. J Infect Dis 148:986, 1983

LEVINE MM: *E. coli* that cause diarrhea. J Infect Dis 155:377, 1987

MARSHALL BJ: *Campylobacter pyloridis* and gastritis. J Infect Dis 153:650, 1986

NATIONAL INSTITUTES OF HEALTH: Consensus development conference on traveler's diarrhea. JAMA 253:2700, 1985

NEILL MA et al: Hemorrhagic colitis with *Escherichia coli* 0157:H7 preceding adult hemolytic uremic syndrome. Arch Intern Med 145:2215, 1985

QUINN TC et al: Infections with *Campylobacter jejuni* and Campylobacter-like organisms in homosexual men. Ann Intern Med 101:187, 1984

SACK DA et al: Oral rehydration in rotavirus diarrhea: A double blind comparison of sucrose with glucose electrolyte solution. Lancet 2:280, 1978

TERRANOVA W et al: Current concepts: *Bacillus cereus* food poisoning. N Engl J Med 298:143, 1978

WALKER RI et al: Physiology of *Campylobacter* enteritis. Microbiol Rev 50:81, 1986

93 SEXUALLY TRANSMITTED DISEASES

KING K. HOLMES / H. HUNTER HANDSFIELD

Venereology encompasses not only the five "venerable" venereal diseases (syphilis, gonorrhea, chancroid, lymphogranuloma venereum, and granuloma inguinale) but also a growing number of other diseases which might be considered the "new generation" of sexually transmitted diseases (STDs). The most recently recognized STD, and in certain populations the most important, is infection with human immunodeficiency virus (HIV) (see Chap. 264). Like gonorrhea, many of these newer STDs became epidemic in nearly all countries of the world during the past quarter-century. With increasing interest in these diseases and improved methods for diagnosis has come awareness of the growing consequences of STD to health and society, which extend far beyond the traditional sphere of venereology, encompassing such diverse problems as acquired immunodeficiency syndrome (AIDS), neoplasia, infertility, and serious congenital and perinatal morbidity.

CLASSIFICATION OF SEXUALLY TRANSMITTED DISEASES These diseases can be classified on the basis either of their etiologies or their clinical manifestations. Table 93-1 summarizes the etiologic classification of STD.

APPROACH TO SEXUALLY TRANSMITTED DISEASE No single STD can be regarded as an isolated problem, because multiple coinfections are common and because the presence of an STD denotes the occurrence of high-risk sexual behavior that is often associated with the risk of other, more serious infections. STDs are not endogenous, nor are they transmitted by fomites, food, flies, or casual contact. *At least one infected partner always exists.* The sexual history and management of sexual partners are therefore of paramount importance. Failure to identify and examine or refer the infected partner(s) represents a failure in management, both at the community level (since sources of spread of infection are not identified) and at the patient level (since reinfection is not prevented).

Most persons with genital discharges, lesions, or pain cease sexual activity and seek medical care. Accordingly, those who transmit infection usually are among the minority who are infected but asymptomatic, or who do not understand the implications of their symptoms. Therefore, they do not seek medical attention spontaneously, and physicians must see that they are examined and treated, or referred. In the United States, local health departments will usually identify and treat contacts of some diseases (e.g., syphilis, gonococcal pelvic inflammatory disease), but for most STDs this responsibility is shared by the patient and the physician. With the increasing importance of potentially incurable viral STDs (HIV infection, genital herpes, human papillomaviruses, chronic hepatitis B virus infections), the role of counseling to reduce transmission is growing.

STDs are propagated most efficiently in core populations with high levels of sexual activity and frequent changes of sexual partners. In most of the United States, these core groups consist of predominantly young urbanites of low socioeconomic level, who are disproportionately black and Hispanic. They often reside within circumscribed high-prevalence neighborhoods. The treatable bacterial STDs, such as syphilis, gonorrhea, and chancroid, are heavily concentrated in core populations and increasingly involve prostitutes and their sex partners and others involved in illicit drug use. These individuals are difficult to reach for educational programs and contact tracing and may continue sexual activity despite STD symptoms. Other STDs are more evenly distributed in society, chlamydial infections, for example. For these, available control measures (e.g., widespread screening, contact tracing) have not been widely applied, even in noncore populations. Chlamydial infection and the incurable viral STDs persist, often asymptomatically, and they are propagated widely in populations which do not share the above characteristics of STD core groups. Table 93-2 lists some of the most common clinical syndromes and their complications associated with sexually transmitted pathogens. Strategies for the management of some of the common syndromes are outlined below. AIDS is discussed in Chap. 264.

URETHRITIS IN MEN Urethritis in men is classified as gonococcal or nongonococcal. During the past decade the incidence of gonococcal urethritis has fallen in many western countries, while that of nongonococcal urethritis (NGU) remains at high levels, suggesting that current measures for control of NGU are relatively ineffective. In general, gonorrhea and NGU have similar frequencies among men seen in STD clinics in the United States, whereas NGU is approximately three times as common as gonorrhea among men seen by physicians in private practice and 10 times as common as gonorrhea among college students.

TABLE 93-1 Sexually transmitted pathogens

Bacteria	Virus	Other*
TRANSMITTED IN ADULTS PREDOMINANTLY BY SEXUAL INTERCOURSE		
Neisseria gonorrhoeae	Human immunodeficiency viruses (HIV-1 and -2)	Trichomonas vaginalis
Chlamydia trachomatis	Herpes simplex virus, type 2 (HSV-2)	Phthirus pubis
Treponema pallidum	Human papilloma virus (genital types HPV 6, 11, 16, 18, 31, 33, 35, 39, 42, 43, 44, 45, 51–56)	Sarcoptes scabiei
Calymmatobacterium granulomatis	Cytomegalovirus	
Ureaplasma urealyticum	Molluscum contagiosum virus	
SEXUAL TRANSMISSION REPEATEDLY DESCRIBED BUT NOT WELL DEFINED OR NOT THE PREDOMINANT MODE OF TRANSMISSION		
Mycoplasma hominis	Human T-lymphotrophic virus (HTLV I)	Candida albicans
Gardnerella vaginalis and other vaginal bacteria	(?) Hepatitis C, D viruses	
Group B streptococcus	Herpes simplex virus type 1 (HSV-1)	
	(?) Epstein-Barr virus (EBV)	
TRANSMITTED BY SEXUAL CONTACT INVOLVING ORAL-FECAL EXPOSURE; OF DECLINING IMPORTANCE IN HOMOSEXUAL MEN		
Shigella spp.	Hepatitis A virus†	Giardia lamblia
Campylobacter spp.		Entamoeba histolytica

* Other includes protozoa, ectoparasites, fungi.
† Among U.S. patients for whom a risk factor can be ascertained, most hepatitis B virus infections are sexually transmitted.

About 40 percent of NGU is caused by *Chlamydia trachomatis.* Herpes simplex virus and, perhaps, *Trichomonas vaginalis* each cause a small additional proportion of NGU cases in the United States, but over half of the cases cannot be attributed to any of these three pathogens. *Ureaplasma urealyticum* has been implicated in case-control studies as a probable cause of many of the *Chlamydia*-negative cases. Two other organisms, *Mycoplasma genitalium* and *Bacteroides urealyticum,* are also under investigation as possible causes of this syndrome. Since facilities for detection of these agents are not widely available and their role is not certain, the diagnosis

TABLE 93-2 Common STD syndromes and etiologic agents

Syndrome	Primary sexually transmitted (ST) agent
Urethritis: males	N. gonorrhoeae, C. trachomatis, U. urealyticum, HSV
Epididymitis	C. trachomatis, N. gonorrhoeae; non-ST agent: urinary tract pathogens
Lower genital tract infections: females	
Cystitis/urethritis	C. trachomatis, N. gonorrhoeae, HSV; non-ST agent: urinary tract pathogens
Mucopurulent cervicitis	Same as cystitis/urethritis
Vulvovaginitis	C. albicans, T. vaginalis; non-ST agent: urinary tract pathogens
Bacterial vaginosis (BV)	BV-associated flora (see text)
Acute pelvic inflammatory disease	N. gonorrhoeae, C. trachomatis, BV-associated flora; non-ST agent: coliform bacteria
Ulcerative lesions of the genitalia	HSV-1, HSV-2, T. pallidum, H. ducreyi, C. trachomatis (LGV strains), C. granulomatis; non-ST agent: pyogenic bacteria (e.g., S. pyogenes, C. albicans)
Proctitis	Same as urethritis, cervicitis; T. pallidum
Acute arthritis	N. gonorrhoeae (e.g., DGI), C. trachomatis (e.g., Reiter's syndrome), HBV, HIV
Genital and anal warts	Human papillomavirus (genital types)
AIDS	HIV-1, HIV-2; also many opportunistic pathogens
Glandular fever (acute fever, lymphadenopathy, atypical lymphocytosis)	Cytomegalovirus, HIV; non-ST agent: EBV
Neoplasias	
Squamous cell cancer of the cervix, anus, vulva, or penis	Human papillomavirus (?)
Kaposi's sarcoma	HIV, other (?); non-ST agent: EBV
Lymphoid neoplasia	HIV, HTLV-I
Hepatocellular carcinoma	
Scabies	S. scabiei
Pubic lice	P. pubis

NOTE: HSV, herpes simplex virus; EBV, Epstein-Barr virus

of male urethritis usually does not include cultures for these organisms. However, diagnostic testing for *C. trachomatis* is now widely available, by isolation of the agent in tissue cell culture or by immunochemical detection of chlamydial antigens. The following steps should be taken in evaluating sexually active men with symptoms of urethral discharge and/or dysuria:

1 *Establish the presence of urethritis.* Commonly in NGU, and less often in gonorrhea, discharge can be demonstrated only by milking the urethra after the patient has not voided for several hours, preferably overnight. If no overt discharge is demonstrable, urethral inflammation can be documented by inserting a small urethrogenital swab 2 to 3 cm into the urethra and examining the Gram-stained direct smear prepared from this swab for leukocytes. Five or more leukocytes per $1000\times$ field in areas containing cells suggests urethritis. Patients with symptoms who lack objective confirmatory evidence of urethritis on two occasions 1 week apart may have functional problems and generally do not benefit from repeated courses of antibiotics.

2 *Evaluate for complications or alternative diagnoses.* Epididymitis and systemic complications, such as the gonococcal arthritis-dermatitis syndrome and Reiter's syndrome, should be excluded by brief history and examination. Bacterial prostatitis and cystitis should be excluded by appropriate tests in men with dysuria who lack evidence of urethritis or in sexually inactive men with urethritis. Digital examination of the prostate gland is seldom informative in patients with urethritis.

3 *Evaluate for gonococcal and chlamydial infection.* The diagnosis of gonorrhea is confirmed by demonstrating typical gram-negative diplococci within neutrophils. The diagnosis of NGU is warranted if gram-negative diplococci are not found. Isolation of *N. gonorrhoeae* by culture should be attempted to document antimicrobial susceptibility, and also because the predictive value of Gram-stained urethral smears is dependent on the experience of the laboratory. Diagnostic testing for *C. trachomatis* should also be performed if resources are available, regardless of the presence or absence of gonorrhea, since coinfection with *N. gonorrhoeae* and *C. trachomatis* is common in men with urethritis. An approach to the diagnosis of urethritis is illustrated in Fig. 93-1. The treatment of gonorrhea and chlamydial infections is discussed in Chaps. 110 and 155, respectively.

EPIDIDYMITIS Acute epididymitis is almost always unilateral and must be differentiated from testicular torsion, tumor, and trauma. Torsion, a surgical emergency, usually occurs in the second or third

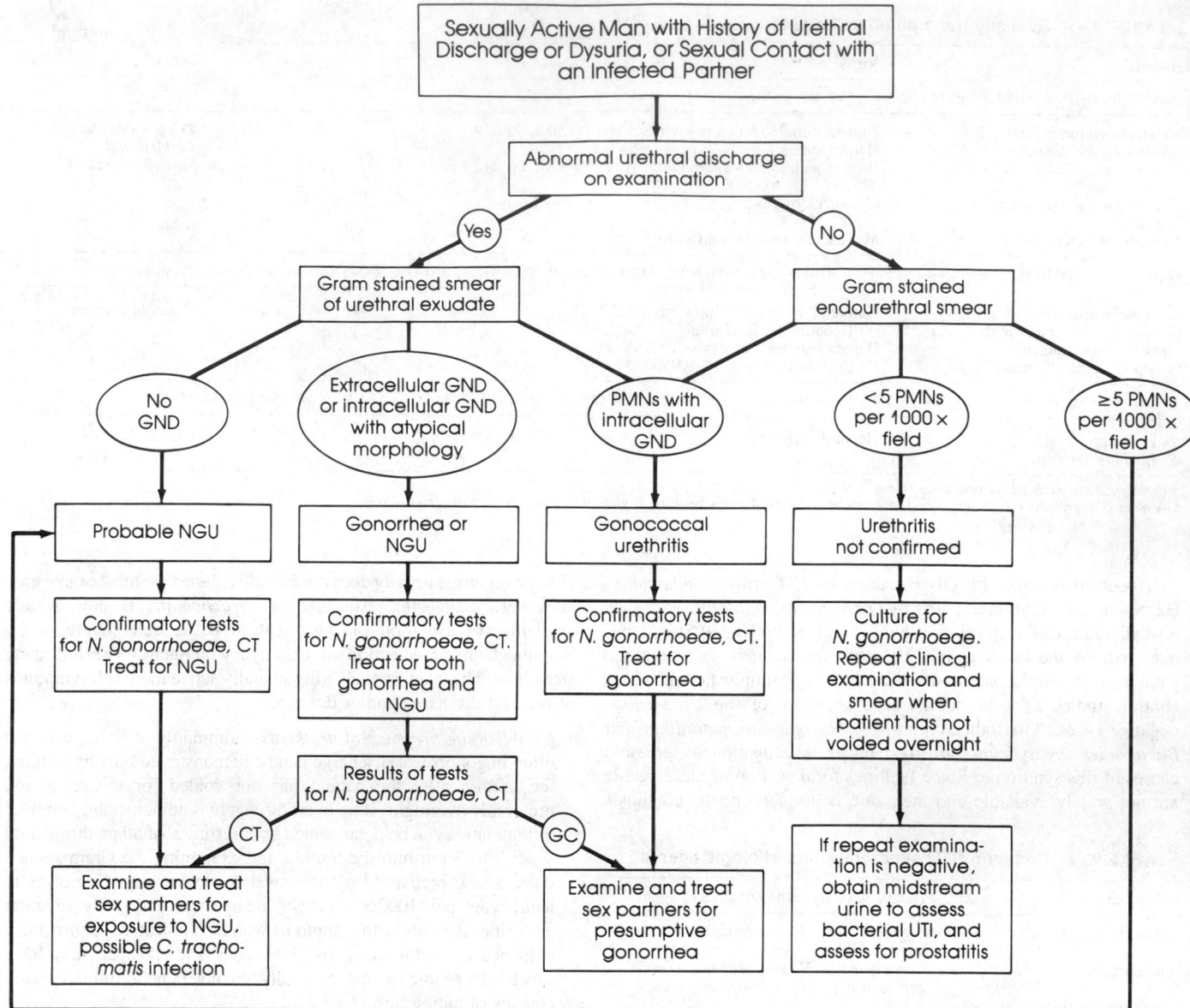

FIGURE 93-1 Evaluation of sexually active men with suspected urethritis. PMN = polymorphonuclear leukocyte; GND = gram-negative diplococci; NGU = nongonococcal urethritis; UTI = urinary tract infection; GC = *Neisseriae gonorrhoeae;* CT = *chlamydia trachomatis.*

decade and is suggested by sudden onset of pain, elevation of the testicle within the scrotal sac, and absence of blood flow on Doppler examination or 99Tc scan. In sexually active men under age 35, acute epididymitis is usually caused by *C. trachomatis,* or less commonly by *Neisseria gonorrhoeae,* and is usually associated with overt or subclinical urethritis. Antimicrobial agents are the mainstay of therapy; optimal treatment for epididymitis due to *C. trachomatis* is doxycycline, 100 mg twice daily for 10 days. For gonococcal epididymitis, the recommended treatment is ceftriaxone, 250 mg intramuscularly, followed by the same doxycycline regimen. Bed rest and scrotal elevation may hasten symptomatic relief.

Acute epididymitis in older men or following urinary tract instrumentation is usually caused by gram-negative bacilli or other urinary pathogens. Urethritis is usually absent, but bacteriuria is present.

LOWER GENITOURINARY TRACT INFECTION IN WOMEN Infections of the female urinary tract, cervix, vulva, and vagina produce dysuria, vulvar irritation, dyspareunia, and increased or altered vaginal discharge. Diagnostic confusion may be attributable not only to the symptomatology, which is nonspecific, but also to the lack of consistent application of available laboratory tests, and to the difficulty

in differentiating true inflammatory conditions from functional genitourinary complaints. Two steps are required in the evaluation of lower genitourinary symptoms in women: (1) differentiation among cystitis, urethritis, vaginitis, cervicitis, and cervical ectopy, and (2) exclusion of associated upper tract disease (e.g., pyelonephritis, salpingitis).

Cystitis and urethritis Although dysuria is more common in bacterial urinary tract infection (UTI) than in vaginitis, dysuria is often attributable to vaginitis in young women because vaginitis is substantially more common than UTI. Localization of dysuria as "internal" is suggestive of UTI or urethritis, while "external dysuria" (caused by painful contact of urine with the labia) is associated with vulvovaginitis. Among sexually active young women with internal dysuria, up to 25 percent have fewer than 100 urinary pathogens per milliliter of urine and are considered to have the *urethral syndrome.* About half of these have pyuria, and most of them are infected with *C. trachomatis* or *N. gonorrhoeae.* Sexually active women with urethral syndrome who lack pyuria have no apparent infection, and their symptoms usually resolve spontaneously. In a study of female college students with dysuria, urgency, or frequency without vaginal infection, about half had bacterial cystitis with 10^5 bacteria or more per milliliter of urine, and one-quarter had bacterial cystitis with less than 10^5 bacteria per milliliter (usually between 10^2 and 10^5 per milliliter). About one-quarter had urethral symptoms without bacteriuria. In the latter group, about half had pyuria, and most of these were infected with *C. trachomatis*, while most of those without pyuria had no demonstrable infection and improved with placebo therapy. In populations whose risk of gonorrhea is higher than that of college students, *N. gonorrhoeae* is also a common cause of the urethral syndrome.

DIAGNOSIS AND THERAPY Among women with acute dysuria and frequency, the first step is to exclude evidence of acute pyelonephritis (e.g., costovertebral pain and tenderness, and fever). As outlined in Fig. 93-2, the next step in sexually active women is the differentiation of cystitis or urethritis from vaginal infection. Among women without vaginal infection, bacterial UTI must then be differentiated from the urethral syndrome. The finding of a single conventional urinary pathogen, such as *Escherichia coli* or *Staphylococcus saprophyticus*, in a concentration of $\geq 10^2$ per milliliter in a properly collected midstream urine specimen from a symptomatic woman with pyuria indicates probable bacterial UTI, whereas pyuria with $<10^2$ conventional uropathogens per milliliter of urine ("sterile pyuria") suggests the diagnosis of acute urethral syndrome due to *C. trachomatis* or *N. gonorrhoeae*. Gonorrhea should be evaluated by Gram stain and culture of the cervix and urethra. Chlamydial infection should be evaluated by culture or specific immunologic tests for chlamydial antigen in urethral and cervical specimens. Treatment with a tetracycline (e.g., doxycycline, 100 mg twice daily for 7 days) has been shown to alleviate dysuria in women with "sterile" pyuria, but not in women without pyuria or isolation of a pathogen. The sexual partners of such patients should also be examined and considered for treatment.

VULVOVAGINAL INFECTIONS In self-referred women attending STD clinics, vaginal infection is the most common diagnosis. Bacterial vaginosis is the most common cause of vulvovaginal symptoms, followed by candidiasis and then trichomoniasis. Vaginal infection may be characterized by one or more of the following: increased volume of discharge; abnormal yellow color of discharge caused by increased concentration of polymorphonuclear leukocytes; vulvar itching, irritation, or burning, often with external dysuria; vulvar dyspareunia; and vaginal malodor. An important component of the clinical evaluation of vaginal discharge is ascertaining by speculum examination whether the discharge emanates from the vagina or the cervix, and whether the discharge is, in fact, abnormal. Occasionally, symptoms of increased discharge or other vaginal symptoms are not associated with objective signs of vaginitis or cervicitis. Although psychological testing is normal in most such cases, possible causes of functional symptoms should be explored. The diagnosis and therapy of the three major types of vaginal infection are summarized in Table 93-3.

***Trichomonas vaginalis* vaginitis** (See Chap. 167) Sexual transmission of *T. vaginalis* is well established. Routine culture testing indicates that many women and most men with infection are asymptomatic. However, treatment of asymptomatic as well as symptomatic cases is recommended to reduce the reservoir of infection and the risk of transmission and to prevent the future development of symptoms.

DIAGNOSIS AND THERAPY Trichomoniasis characteristically produces a profuse, yellow, purulent, homogeneous vaginal discharge. The vaginal epithelium is inflamed, and petechial lesions can be seen by colposcopy on the cervix ("strawberry cervix") in about 50 percent of cases. In women with typical symptoms and signs of trichomoniasis, the diagnosis can usually be confirmed by demonstration of motile trichomonads and polymorphonuclear leukocytes in vaginal secretions mixed with normal saline and promptly examined microscopically. In such patients, wet-mount examination is at least 80 percent as sensitive as culture. However, in women without symptoms or signs, culture is often required to detect the organism. The pH of vaginal secretions is usually ≥ 5.0. The diagnosis of *T.*

vaginalis infection in men is more difficult and requires culture of early morning first-voided urine sediment or of a urethral swab specimen obtained before voiding.

Nitroimidazoles are the only consistently effective drugs for treating trichomoniasis. Several studies show that a single 2.0-g oral dose of metronidazole is at least 90 percent as effective as more prolonged dosage schedules. Other nitroimidazoles such as tinidazole and ornidazole have longer half-lives than metronidazole, but have not been clearly shown to give better results in trichomoniasis. Routine treatment of sex partners is recommended to reduce both the risk of reinfection and the reservoir of infection. Metronidazole should not be given to women during the first trimester of pregnancy. Alcohol must be avoided for 24 h after treatment because of a disulfiram-like effect of the drug. The partners of patients with trichomoniasis (and all sexually transmitted infections) should be examined; they should not be treated without examination and counseling.

Bacterial vaginosis Vaginal discharge not associated with *T. vaginalis*, yeast, or cervical infection is usually due to bacterial vaginosis. This syndrome (formerly termed *nonspecific vaginitis* or *Gardnerella-associated vaginal discharge*) is characterized by vaginal malodor and increased white discharge that is homogeneous, low in viscosity, and uniformly coats the vaginal walls. It is unclear whether bacterial vaginosis is a sexually transmitted infection. The syndrome is associated with STD risk factors, such as number of sexual partners and recent intercourse with a new partner, but no single sexually transmitted pathogen has been clearly identified as a cause. Antibiotic treatment of the male sexual partners has not conclusively been shown to influence the recurrence rate in affected women. It is likely that poorly understood factors associated with sexual activity somehow alter the vaginal milieu, resulting in the characteristic alterations of the vaginal flora. Formerly considered a benign condition, bacterial vaginosis has been implicated as a risk factor for acute salpingitis, premature labor, and related neonatal and perinatal complications.

The concentration of *Gardnerella vaginalis* (formerly *Haemophilus vaginalis*), *Mycoplasma hominis*, *U. urealyticum*, and certain anaerobic bacteria is increased in vaginal washings from women with this syndrome. Two closely related species of curved, motile, gram-negative anaerobic rods (*Mobiluncus curtisii*, *Mobiluncus mulieris*) are particularly closely associated with this syndrome. The prevalence and concentration of other anaerobic bacteria, such as vaginal *Bacteroides* spp. and *Peptostreptococcus* spp., also are increased and probably contribute to the pathogenesis of bacterial vaginosis. However, many of these are common among women without this syndrome; e.g., *G. vaginalis* has been isolated from the vagina of up to 50 percent of normal women. The aerotolerant *Lactobacillus* species, which constitute most of the normal vaginal flora (e.g., *L. acidophilus*, *L. jenseni*), are absent or present only in reduced concentration in the vagina in bacterial vaginosis. These species produce lactic acid, hydrogen peroxide, and other factors thought to be important in regulating the vaginal flora.

DIAGNOSIS AND TREATMENT In a patient with symptoms of abnormal vaginal discharge and malodor or objective signs of increased white homogeneous vaginal discharge, the diagnosis of bacterial vaginosis can be made with reasonable certainty by the following:

1 Exclusion of candidal and trichomonal vaginitis and mucopurulent cervicitis, including collection of endocervical specimens to test for *C. trachomatis* and *N. gonorrhoeae*.
2 Microscopic demonstration of "clue cells" and characteristic alterations of the vaginal microflora. Clue cells are vaginal epithelial cells coated with coccobacillary organisms. On wet mount, prepared by mixing vaginal secretions 1:1 with normal saline, clue cells have a granular appearance and their borders are obscured (Fig. 93-3). Clue cells also can be detected on a Gram-stained smear, which permits assessment of the vaginal flora; the normally predominant lactobacilli are largely or completely replaced by a profusion of bacterial morphotypes consistent with *G. vaginalis*

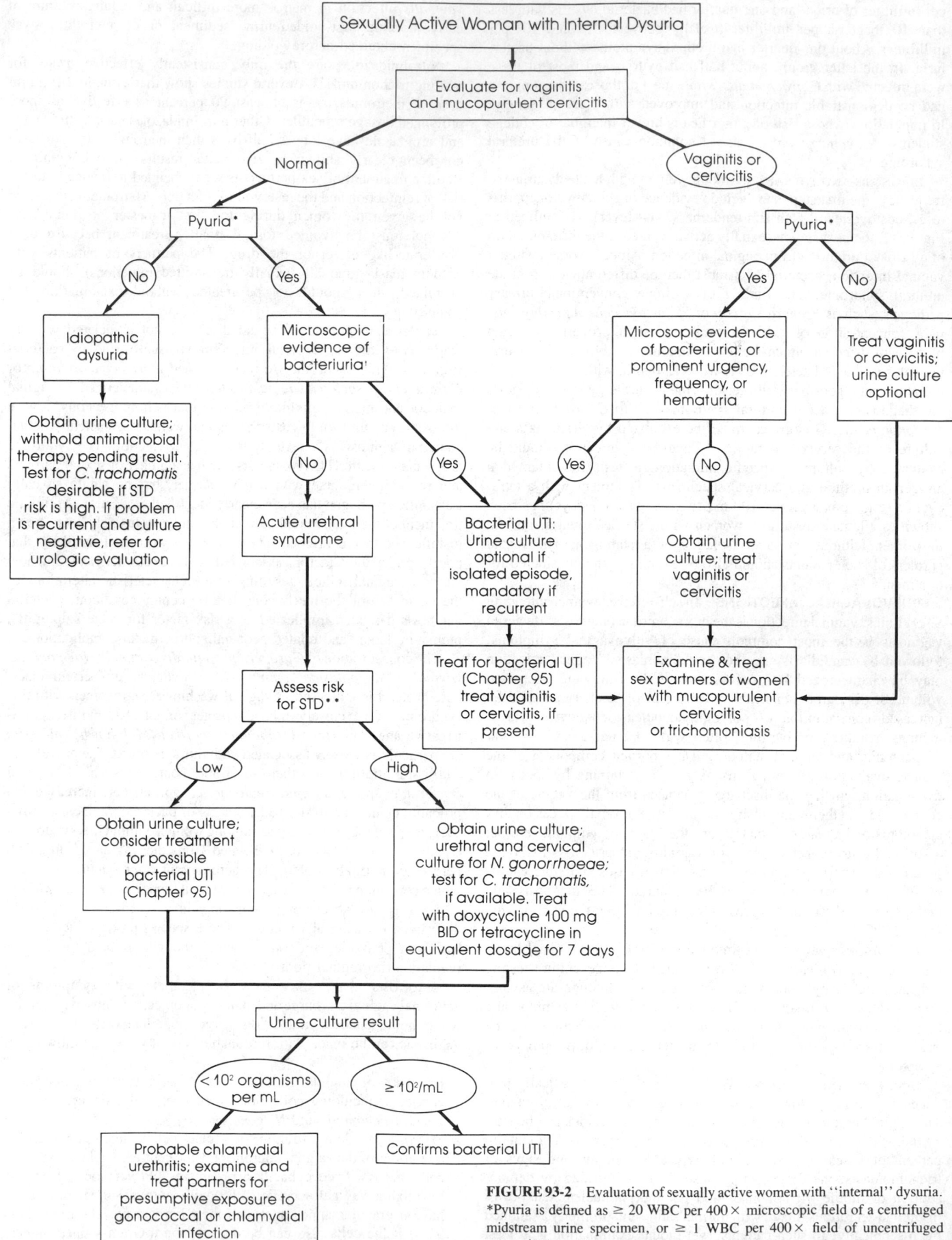

FIGURE 93-2 Evaluation of sexually active women with ''internal'' dysuria. *Pyuria is defined as ≥ 20 WBC per 400× microscopic field of a centrifuged midstream urine specimen, or ≥ 1 WBC per 400× field of uncentrifuged urine. †Microscopic evidence of bacteriuria is the presence of ≥ 1 bacillus per 400× field of an uncentrifuged midstream specimen of urine. **Evaluation of STD risk is based on number and nature of sexual partner(s), recent change in partner, marital status, past history of STD, etc.

TABLE 93-3   Diagnostic features and management of vaginal infection

	Normal vaginal exam	Yeast vaginitis	Trichomonal vaginitis	Bacterial vaginosis (BV)
Etiology	Uninfected; *Lactobacillus* predominant	*Candida albicans* and yeasts	*Trichomonas vaginalis*	Associated with *G. vaginalis*, various anaerobic bacteria, and mycoplasma
Typical symptoms	None	Vulvar itching and/or irritation, increased discharge	Profuse purulent discharge; vulvar itching	Malodorous, slightly increased discharge

Discharge:
  Amount
  Color*
  Consistency
	Variable; usually scant
	Clear or white
	Nonhomogeneous, floccular
		Scant to moderate
		White
		Clumped; adherent plaques
			Profuse
			Yellow
			Homogeneous
				Moderate
				Usually white or gray
				Homogeneous, low viscosity; uniformly coating vaginal walls

Inflammation of vulvar or vaginal epithelium	None	Erythema of vaginal epithelium, introitus; vulvar dermatitis common	Erythema of vaginal and vulvar epithelium; colpitis macularis	None
pH of vaginal fluid†	Usually ≤4.5	Usually ≤4.5	Usually ≥5.0	Usually ≥4.7
Amine ("fishy") odor with % KOH	None	None	May be present	Present
Microscopy‡	Normal epithelial cells; lactobacilli predominant	Leukocytes, epithelial cells; yeast, mycelia, or pseudomycelia in up to 80%	Leukocytes; motile trichomonads seen in 80–90% of symptomatic patients, less often in the absence of symptoms	Clue cells; few leukocytes; lactobacilli outnumbered by profuse mixed flora, nearly always including *G. vaginalis* plus anaerobic species on Gram stain
Usual treatment	None	Miconazole or clotrimazole, intravaginally each 100 mg daily for 7 days. Nystatin, 100,000 units intravaginally twice daily for 7–14 days	Metronidazole or tinidazole, 2 g orally (single dose). Metronidazole, 500 mg orally twice daily for 7 days	Metronidazole, 500 mg orally twice daily for 7 days
Usual management of sex partner	None	None; topical treatment if candidal dermatitis of penis is present	Examine for STD; treat with metronidazole, 2 g, orally (single dose)	Examine for STD; no treatment if normal

* Color of discharge is determined by examining vaginal discharge against the white background of a swab.
† pH determination is not useful if blood is present.
‡ To detect fungal elements, vaginal fluid is digested with 10% KOH prior to microscopic examination; to examine for other features, fluid is mixed (1:1) with physiologic saline. Gram's stain also is excellent for detecting yeasts and pseudomycelia and for distinguishing normal flora from the mixed flora seen in bacterial vaginosis, but it is less sensitive than the saline preparation for detection of *T. vaginalis*.
SOURCE: From KK Holmes et al.

and anaerobic organisms. The demonstrations of clue cells by wet-mount microscopy and of characteristically altered vaginal flora by Gram stain represent the most sensitive, specific, and objective criteria for the diagnosis of bacterial vaginosis in women with symptoms and/or signs of this condition.

3 Liberation of a distinct fishy odor immediately after mixing vaginal secretions with a 10% solution of KOH. This odor is attributable to volatile amines (e.g., putrescine, cadaverine) present in the vaginal fluid, presumably the result of anaerobic bacterial metabolism.

4 Demonstration of pH of vaginal secretions greater than 4.5. The elevated pH may be partly due to the presence of amines as well as to decreased production of lactate by lactobacilli.

The most consistently effective therapy for bacterial vaginosis is metronidazole, 500 mg twice daily for 7 days, perhaps because of the role of the anaerobes, most of which are highly susceptible to metronidazole in this infection. Amoxicillin, 500 mg three times daily for 7 days, has been effective in about 40 to 50 percent of cases of bacterial vaginosis, and is the primary alternative to metronidazole. Systemic or vaginal therapy with clindamycin is also effective. Sulfonamide-containing vaginal creams are usually ineffective, probably because sulfonamides are inactive against both *G. vaginalis* and many vaginal anaerobes, and there is no rationale for their use. Tetracycline therapy also is ineffective. Treatment of male partners of women with this syndrome is not routinely indicated. However, because bacterial vaginosis is associated with sexual

behavioral risks, it is not unreasonable to examine partners for evidence of other STDs.

Vulvovaginal candidiasis The predominant symptom in vulvovaginal candidiasis is vulvar pruritus. There is usually no distinct odor. Vulvar erythema commonly is present. The vaginal discharge typically is white, scanty, and often takes the form of thrush-like plaques or cottage cheese-like curds adhering to the vaginal mucosa. *Candida albicans* accounts for about 80 percent of yeasts isolated from the vagina, while *Torulopsis glabrata* and other less commonly encountered *Candida* species are found in the remainder. Overt vulvovaginitis is more common among women colonized by *C. albicans* than among those colonized with *T. glabrata* or other species. Most cases of vulvovaginal candidiasis probably result from increased growth of yeasts that previously colonized the vagina or the intestinal tract. Some cases of recurrent vulvovaginal candidiasis may be due to sexual transmission from a colonized male.

DIAGNOSIS AND THERAPY   The diagnosis of vulvovaginal candidiasis involves demonstration of fungi by microscopic examination of vaginal secretions in saline or 10% KOH, or by Gram's stain. Demonstration of pseudohyphae strengthens the diagnosis of vaginitis due to *C. albicans*. Polymorphonuclear leukocytes usually are present. Microscopic examination is less sensitive than culture, but culture detects asymptomatic carriage in women who may not require therapy. The pH of vaginal secretions is usually less than 4.5, and an amine odor is not produced when vaginal secretions are mixed with 10% KOH. Vulvitis often accompanies vaginitis and may result in superficial erosions that must be differentiated from genital herpes. In most

A

B

FIGURE 93-3 *A.* Vaginal epithelial "clue cells." Note granular appearance due to adherent *G. vaginalis* and indistinct cell margins. 400×. *B.* Normal vaginal epithelial cells. The cell margins are distinct and lack granularity.

circumstances, therapy for candidal vaginal infection is indicated only if the patient is symptomatic, has signs of vulvovaginitis, or if inflammatory cells or pseudohyphae are present. The usual treatment is intravaginal miconazole, clotrimazole, or butoconazole for 3 to 7 days; intravaginal nystatin is less effective. Oral treatment with ketoconazole may be indicated for especially severe or frequently recurrent cases or for cases that do not respond to vaginal therapy. Such patients should be evaluated for HIV infection. Treatment of the sex partner is not routinely indicated, although this has not been studied rigorously.

MUCOPURULENT CERVICITIS Mucopurulent cervicitis refers to inflammation of the columnar epithelium and subepithelium of the endocervix, and of any contiguous columnar epithelium that lies exposed in an ectopic position on the exocervix. Mucopurulent cervicitis in the female can be regarded as the "silent" partner of urethritis in the male, being equally common and caused by the same agents but more difficult to recognize. It is the most common major STD syndrome in women and can lead to pelvic inflammatory disease, and in pregnant women may lead to obstetrical complications. Improved recognition and treatment of this syndrome would greatly improve the control of STD. Mucopurulent cervicitis most commonly is caused by *C. trachomatis* and sometimes by *N. gonorrhoeae*, but about one-third to one-half of cases are associated with neither of these organisms. The syndrome can usually be differentiated clinically from cervicitis caused by primary or recurrent herpes simplex virus infection, which produces lesions on the stratified squamous epithelium of the exocervix, as well as on the columnar epithelium; and from vaginitis caused by *C. albicans* or *T. vaginalis*.

DIAGNOSIS AND THERAPY   The diagnosis is made by demonstrating mucopurulent discharge from the cervical os or by demonstrating

increased numbers of polymorphonuclear leukocytes in Gram-stained or Papanicolaou smears of endocervical discharge. Cervical ectopy (see below) that is edematous and endocervical bleeding induced by gentle swabbing are common signs of mucopurulent cervicitis due to *C. trachomatis*. The color of cervical mucus on a white swab removed from the endocervix should be noted; a yellow color indicates the presence of mucopus. The cervical mucus should be rolled *thinly* on a slide for Gram staining. An area of the slide should be identified which contains strands of cervical mucus which are not contaminated by vaginal squamous epithelial cells or bacteria. The presence of ≥30 polymorphonuclear cells per 1000× microscopic field within strands of cervical mucus suggests cervicitis. The prevalence of *C. trachomatis* infection or gonorrhea has been significantly greater among women with mucopurulent cervicitis by the above criteria than among women without it. The presence of a characteristic pattern of inflammatory cells on endocervical Papanicolaou smears has been used by cytopathologists to suggest the possibility of chlamydial infection and the need for specific confirmatory testing.

Mucopurulent cervicitis requires antimicrobial therapy. An etiologic diagnosis should always be established to guide management of sexual partners, but therapy should usually be initiated against the most likely causes of this syndrome, while results of diagnostic tests are pending. The diagnosis of gonococcal cervicitis is made by culture of an endocervical specimen. When carefully collected endocervical specimens are examined by experienced personnel, Gram's stain is an insensitive but highly specific test, and observation of intracellular gram-negative diplococci indicates gonococcal infection, even if the culture is negative. The sensitivity of a single endocervical culture for *N. gonorrhoeae* is 80 to 90 percent. Chlamydial infection of the cervix can be confirmed by culture or antigen detection (see Chap. 155).

While diagnostic test results are pending, therapy for mucopurulent cervicitis should be initiated with a single-dose regimen effective for gonorrhea (ceftriaxone, 250 mg intramuscularly), followed by doxycycline, 100 mg twice daily, orally for 1 week. For pregnant women, erythromycin base or stearate, in a dose of 500 mg four times daily for 7 to 14 days, can be substituted for doxycycline. The male sex partners of women with nongonococcal mucopurulent cervicitis should be examined and treated as described for gonococcal and nongonococcal urethritis.

Cervical ectopy Cervicitis must be differentiated from cervical ectopy, which is often mislabeled "cervical erosion." Ectopy represents the presence of the one-cell-thick columnar endocervical epithelium in an exposed visible "ectopic" position on the cervix, where it appears redder than the several-cells-thick stratified squamous vaginal epithelium. When ectopy is present, the cervical os may contain clear or slightly cloudy mucus, but usually not mucopus. Colposcopy shows that the epithelium is intact and not ulcerated. Ectopy is normally present during early adolescence and gradually recedes as squamous metaplasia replaces the ectopic columnar epithelium. Oral contraceptive usage or pregnancy favors persistence or reappearance of ectopy. The use of cauterizing procedures to eliminate simple ectopy is not warranted. The presence of ectopy may make the cervix more susceptible to infection with *N. gonorrhoeae* or *C. trachomatis* by exposing a larger surface area of susceptible columnar epithelium. If mucopurulent cervicitis supervenes, the area of ectopy may become edematous and fragile, with bleeding induced by gentle swabbing. In addition, edema of the cervix may result in eversion of the os, enlarging the apparent area of ectopy.

ULCERATIVE LESIONS OF THE GENITALIA The incidence and etiology of ulcerative lesions of the genitalia vary greatly in different areas of the world. In Asia and Africa, genital ulcers are seen as frequently as gonorrhea in some STD clinics, and chancroid is the commonest cause, while genital herpes is relatively uncommon. In the industrialized western countries, genital ulcers are considerably less common than urethritis, mucopurulent cervicitis, and vaginitis. Genital herpes is the commonest cause, and chancroid is relatively uncommon. Syphilis is the second most common form of genital ulcer in almost all areas of the world and must always be excluded. Lymphogranuloma venereum (LGV) and donovanosis (granuloma inguinale) are very rare in North America and Europe. Other causes include candidiasis and traumatized genital warts, both of which usually are readily recognized; and various nonsexually transmitted dermatoses. Chancroid, syphilis, genital herpes, and probably all causes of genital ulcer enhance the efficiency of sexual transmission and acquisition of HIV. Moreover, genital ulcers, especially chancroid and syphilis, are most common in inner city populations with low socioeconomic status and high rates of prostitution and illicit drug use, independent risk factors for HIV infection. From 1985 through 1988, chancroid and syphilis have been spreading at epidemic rates in such populations,

DIAGNOSIS AND THERAPY   In industrialized countries, the differential diagnosis of genital ulceration, when nonsexually transmitted lesions are excluded, usually involves genital herpes simplex virus (HSV) infection, syphilis, and chancroid. The clinical findings are occasionally definitive (e.g., presence of herpetic vesicles), and clinical findings plus epidemiologic considerations usually help to guide initial therapy pending further studies. Nevertheless, most genital ulcerations cannot be diagnosed confidently on clinical grounds. It is axiomatic to exclude syphilis by appropriate serology in all cases. Dark-field examination should also be performed, by experienced technicians when possible, on lesions consistent with primary or secondary syphilis. Direct immunofluorescence using antibodies to *T. pallidum* is at least as sensitive and specific as dark-field microscopy for detection of *T. pallidum* in lesion exudate and can be performed on specimens sent to a central laboratory. This procedure should be used more widely. Selective enrichment media are available for isolation of *Haemophilus ducreyi*.

The following general guidelines are recommended for management of ulcerative genital lesions (Fig. 93-4):

1 If typical painful herpetic vesicles or pustules are present: In this case the clinical diagnosis of herpes is warranted, although a serologic test for syphilis should be performed. If desired, the diagnosis can be confirmed by isolation of HSV or by immunochemical detection with specific antibody. Cytologic methods to detect HSV-infected cells (Tzanck preparation or Papanicolaou stain) are insensitive.

2 If painful nonvesicular ulcer(s) raise the suspicion of herpes or chancroid: If there are painful lesion(s) or enlarged, tender inguinal lymph nodes or if other features suggest herpes or chancroid, attempts to demonstrate HSV or *H. ducreyi* are indicated. All methods of HSV detection are less sensitive in the ulcerative stage than in the vesicular stage. Syphilis should be excluded by dark-field examination and serologic testing, both of which should be repeated 1 to 2 weeks later if negative initially and if another diagnosis cannot be confirmed.

3 If painless ulcerative lesions suggest the diagnosis of syphilis: If lesions are at all suggestive of syphilis, or there are epidemiologic reasons to suspect syphilis, such as recent exposure, then dark-field examination and a rapid serologic test for syphilis should be performed for prompt diagnosis. If these are negative, two more dark-field examinations on successive days are recommended, and the serologic test should be repeated 1, 2, and 6 weeks later. Direct immunofluorescent detection of *T. pallidum* should be used if dark-field examination by experienced examiners is not available.

4 If genital ulceration is chronic and painless: In addition to the tests for syphilis and chancroid, biopsy is indicated to exclude donovanosis and carcinoma.

Antibacterial therapy is not indicated for undiagnosed ulcerative genital lesions. Oral acyclovir speeds resolution of systemic and local manifestations of initial episodes of genital and anorectal herpes if started early; therefore, acyclovir should be started promptly if the diagnosis of these forms of herpes seems likely (see Chap. 135). Treatment for syphilis should not be instituted until the diagnosis is established. The value of antimicrobial therapy for idiopathic ulcer-

ative lesions of the genitalia is uncertain, but treatment for presumptive chancroid with ceftriaxone or erythromycin (see Chap. 117) sometimes may be reasonable for lesions of recent onset that persist or progress during several days of observation and that cannot be attributed to herpes or syphilis. Antimicrobial therapy should be given promptly when chancroid is probable, especially if regional lymph node suppuration is present or appears imminent. If patients worsen or do not improve during 1 or 2 weeks of observation and the diagnosis remains obscure, attempts to isolate *H. ducreyi* should be made or repeated, and other noninfectious and infectious etiologies (e.g., donovanosis) should be considered.

PROCTITIS, PROCTOCOLITIS OR ENTEROCOLITIS, AND ENTERITIS   Sexually acquired proctitis, or inflammation limited to the rectum, results from direct rectal inoculation of typical STD pathogens. In contrast, inflammation which extends from the rectum to the colon (proctocolitis) and involves the small and large bowel (enterocolitis) or the small bowel alone (enteritis) can result from ingestion of typical intestinal pathogens through sexual contact involving oral-fecal exposure. Anorectal pain and mucopurulent or bloody rectal discharge suggest proctitis or proctocolitis. Proctitis is commonly associated with tenesmus and constipation, whereas proctocolitis and enterocolitis are more often associated with diarrhea. In both, anoscopy usually shows the presence of mucosal inflammation with exudate and easily induced mucosal bleeding (i.e., positive "wipe test"). Petechial or mucosal ulcers also may be observed. Exudate should be sampled for microbiologic studies and Gram stain. Sigmoidoscopy or colonoscopy, performed if possible without an enema, shows inflammation limited to the rectum in proctitis, or disease extending at least into the sigmoid colon in proctocolitis.

Most cases of sexually transmitted intestinal infection have in the past involved homosexual men. During the AIDS era, there has been an extraordinary shift in the clinical and etiologic spectrum of intestinal infections in homosexual men. The number of opportunistic intestinal infections—not described in this chapter—has risen rapidly in homosexual men with AIDS. At the same time, the number of sexually transmitted intestinal infections, described below, has fallen rapidly as high-risk sexual behaviors have become less common in this group.

Most cases of infectious proctitis are due to *N. gonorrhoeae*, HSV, or *C. trachomatis;* these are acquired via receptive rectal intercourse. Primary and secondary syphilis can also produce anal or rectal lesions, with or without symptoms. Gonococcal proctitis and proctitis due to non-LGV strains of *C. trachomatis* typically involve the most distal rectal mucosa and the anal crypts and are clinically mild, without systemic manifestations. In contrast, primary HSV proctitis and LGV proctocolitis usually produce severe anorectal pain and fever. Perianal ulcers and inguinal lymphadenopathy may occur with either, but most commonly are due to herpes. Sacral nerve root radiculopathies, usually with urinary retention, are common in primary herpetic proctitis. Sigmoidoscopy most commonly shows ulcerative proctitis with either herpes or LGV, but may reveal intact vesicopustular lesions with anorectal herpes. In herpes, biopsy of the rectal mucosa shows microulcerations and may show intranuclear inclusions or perivascular lymphocytic cuffing. In LGV, biopsy typically shows crypt abscesses, granulomas, and giant cells, findings that may be indistinguishable from those of Crohn's disease. Syphilis can also produce rectal granulomas, usually associated with infiltration by plasma cells or other mononuclear cells.

The occurrence of diarrhea and abdominal bloating or cramping pain, without anorectal symptoms, in association with normal anoscopy and sigmoidoscopy, is consistent with inflammation of the small intestine or more proximal colon. In homosexual men, without HIV infection, enteritis limited to the small intestine is often attributable to *Giardia lamblia*, while *Campylobacter* spp., *Shigella* spp., and *Entamoeba histolytica* can produce enterocolitis with or without lesions involving the distal colon or rectum. Sexually acquired proctocolitis, enterocolitis, and enteritis due to *Campylobacter* spp., *Shigella* spp., *E. histolytica*, and *G. lamblia* are clinically indistin-

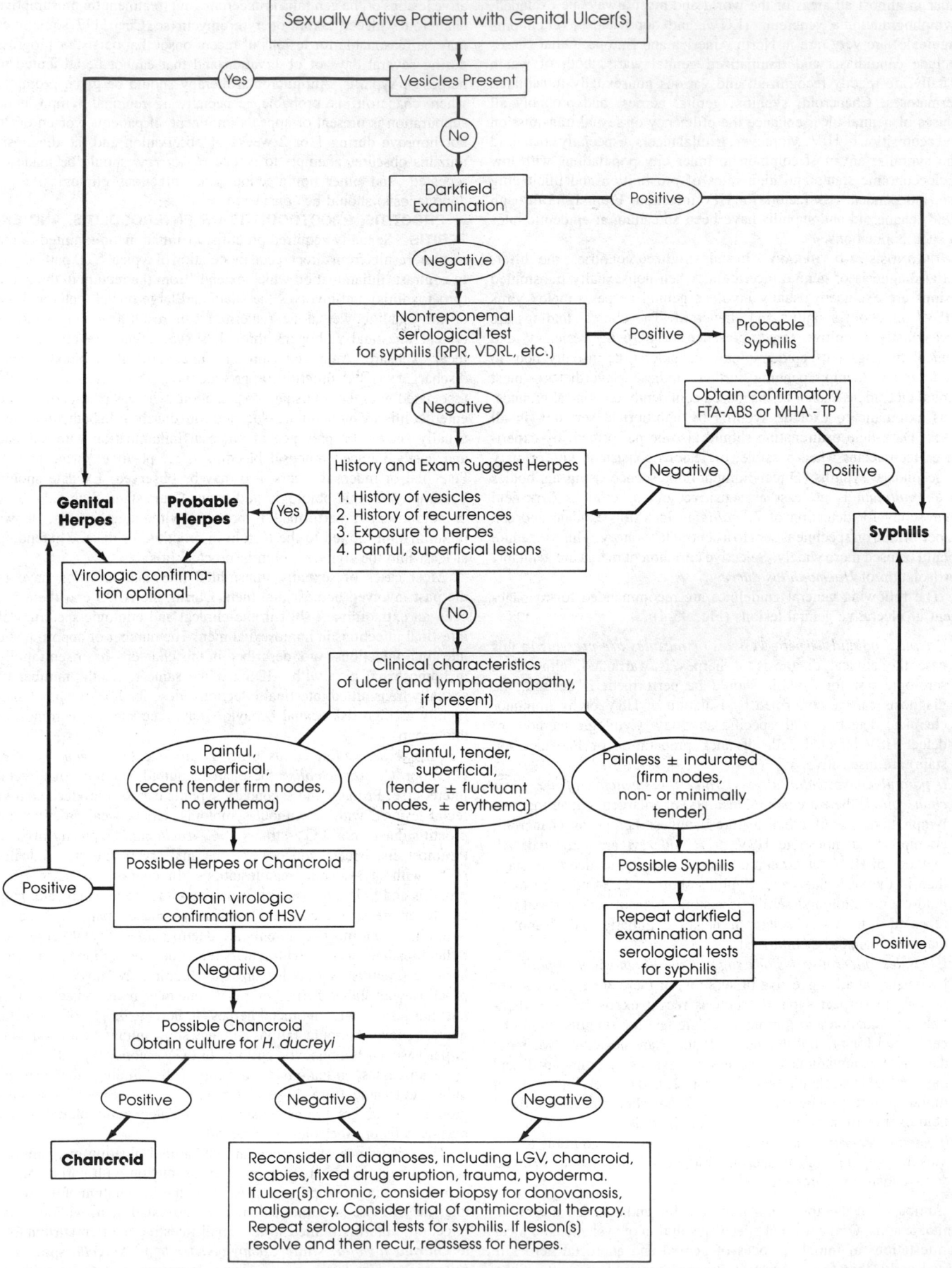

FIGURE 93-4 Evaluation of sexually active persons with genital ulcer-inguinal lymphadenopathy syndromes.

guishable from nonsexually transmitted infections with the same symptoms.

ACUTE ARTHRITIS The gonococcal arthritis-dermatitis syndrome probably is the most common form of acute arthritis in sexually active young adults, and Reiter's syndrome is the second commonest. These must be differentiated from each other and from other forms of infective arthritis, various diseases associated with immune-complex deposition, crystal-induced arthritis, acute rheumatoid arthritis, and other less common rheumatic disorders such as systemic lupus erythematosus. Meningococcemia, *Yersinia* infection, sarcoidosis, and syphilis are other occasional causes of acute arthritis.

Demonstration of *N. gonorrhoeae* by culture or a specific immunochemical method in synovial fluid, blood, skin lesions, or cerebrospinal fluid is diagnostic of DGI. Failing this, gonococcal arthritis is highly probable if *N. gonorrhoeae* is recovered from a mucosal site of infection or from the patient's sex partner, typical pustular or hemorrhagic skin lesions are distributed primarily on the extremities, and a therapeutic antibiotic trial produces prompt improvement. Suspected and confirmed cases of DGI should be treated promptly with an antibiotic effective against antibiotic-sensitive and -resistant gonococci, such as ceftriaxone (see Chap. 110). Some patients with septic gonococcal arthritis may require repeated closed-joint irrigations with saline before improvement occurs.

Reiter's syndrome occurs in a sporadic (apparently sexually transmitted) form and a postdysenteric form, which sometimes occurs in discrete epidemics. It is described in detail in Chap. 274.

VIRAL WARTS See Chap. 150.

PREVENTION AND CONTROL OF SEXUALLY TRANSMITTED DISEASES The control of bacterial STD has traditionally depended on secondary prevention of spread by early diagnosis and treatment. The emergence of the incurable viral STDs has required increasing emphasis on health education and health promotion as primary prevention strategies. Medical students and physicians require training to develop skills in eliciting a sexual history, in determining the extent to which their patients, especially adolescents and young adults, are at risk for STD, and in counseling them appropriately. Public education and personal counseling should begin in early adolescence and should emphasize responsible sexual behavior (abstinence, maintenance of monogamous relationships); the use of condoms for nonmonogamous sexual encounters; avoidance of traumatic sexual practices, such as anal intercourse; the recognition of early symptoms and signs of STD; and early health care for such symptoms and signs. Genital self-examination, analogous to breast self-examination, is a practice to prevent sequelae and improve control of STD.

Maintenance of clinical skills in the recognition, diagnosis, and treatment of STDs is essential for secondary prevention of STD by early treatment. Screening tests for gonorrhea, chlamydial infection, syphilis, and HIV infection should be widely available and used by physicians serving populations at risk. Similarly, health departments should provide high-quality STD clinical services and screening for high-risk populations. Health departments also are responsible for STD surveillance and for coordinating targeted control measures; this requires the cooperation of physicians in reporting cases. Notification of the sexual partners of infected persons is the joint responsibility of the patient and physician. In most communities, the local health department will assist in this effort for cases of syphilis, some cases of gonorrhea, and, increasingly, for cases of HIV infection.

REFERENCES

General

CENTERS FOR DISEASE CONTROL: 1989 sexually transmitted diseases treatment guidelines. Morb Mort Week Rep 38(Suppl 8):1–43, 1989

HANDSFIELD HH (ed): Sexually transmitted diseases. Infect Dis Clin North Am 1:1, 1987

HOLMES KK et al (eds): *Sexually Transmitted Diseases*, 2d ed. New York, McGraw-Hill, 1989

Urethritis in males

BOWIE WR et al: Etiology of nongonococcal urethritis: Evidence for *Chlamydia trachomatis* and *Ureaplasma urealyticum*. J Clin Invest 59:735, 1977

JACOBS NF, KRAUS SF: Gonococcal and nongonococcal urethritis in men: Clinical and laboratory differentiation. Ann Intern Med 82:7, 1975

Epididymitis

BERGER RE et al: Etiology, manifestations, and therapy of acute epididymitis: Prospective study of 50 cases. J Urol 121:750, 1979

Urethral syndrome

STAMM WE et al: Urinary tract infections: From pathogenesis to treatment. J Infect Dis 159:400, 1989

Vaginitis

ESCHENBACH DA et al: Diagnosis and clinical manifestations of bacterial vaginosis. Am J Obstet Gynecol 158:819, 1988

HOLMES KK: Lower genital tract infections in women, in *Sexually Transmitted Diseases*, 2d ed, KK Holmes et al (eds). New York, McGraw-Hill, 1989

SOBEL J: Genital candidiasis, in *Sexually Transmitted Diseases*, 2d ed, KK Holmes et al (eds). New York, McGraw-Hill, 1989

WOLNER-HANSSEN P et al: Clinical manifestations of vaginal trichomoniasis. JAMA 261:571, 1989

Cervicitis

BRUNHAM RC et al: Mucopurulent cervicitis—the ignored counterpart in women of urethritis in men. N Engl J Med 311:1, 1984

Genital ulcers

KROCKTA WP, BARNES RC: Genital ulceration with regional adenopathy. Infect Dis Clin North Am 1:217, 1987

SIMONSEN JN et al: Human immunodeficiency virus infection among men with sexually transmitted diseases. N Engl J Med 319:274, 1988

Proctitis, proctocolitis, enterocolitis, and enteritis

QUINN TC et al: The polymicrobial etiology of intestinal infections in homosexual men. N Engl J Med 309:576, 1983

Arthritis

HANDSFIELD HH, POLLOCK PS: Arthropathies associated with sexually transmitted diseases, in *Sexually Transmitted Diseases*, 2d ed, KK Holmes et al (eds). New York, McGraw-Hill, 1989

94 PELVIC INFLAMMATORY DISEASE

KING K. HOLMES

DEFINITION The term *pelvic inflammatory disease (PID)* usually refers to ascending infection of the uterus, fallopian tubes, and broad ligaments. Intrauterine infection can be primary (spontaneously occurring and usually sexually transmitted) or secondary to invasive intrauterine surgical procedures (e.g., dilatation and curettage, termination of pregnancy, insertion of an intrauterine device, or hysterosalpingography), or to parturition. Endometritis or endomyometritis is particularly common following delivery by cesarean section.

PID is uncommon during pregnancy itself. The uterotubal junction is closed as early as the seventh week of pregnancy, and the chorioamnion becomes approximated to the endocervical os, sealing off the intrauterine cavity, at the twelfth to fifteenth week of gestation. As a consequence, ascending intrauterine infection prior to the twelfth week of gestation may be associated (either as cause or effect) with endometritis and spontaneous abortion, while ascending infection after the twelfth week may be associated with chorioamnionitis. Rarely, infection may extend secondarily to the pelvic organs from adjacent foci of inflammation, such as appendicitis, regional ileitis, or diverticulitis; as a result of hematogenous dissemination, such as tuberculosis; or as a rare complication of certain tropical diseases, such as schistosomiasis.

Spontaneously occurring PID can be divided into chronic and acute types. Chronic PID due to tuberculosis has become uncommon;

other forms of chronic PID, due to chronic infection with *Chlamydia trachomatis* or secondary to IUD usage, have been described but have not been adequately studied.

PID is most often used today to refer to cases of acute spontaneously occurring infection ascending from the cervix or vagina. The clinical diagnosis of PID is imprecise. Use of endometrial biopsy together with laparoscopy provides evidence of a continuum, progressing from cervicitis alone to endometritis, to salpingitis, to pelvic peritonitis, to generalized peritonitis, to perihepatitis, or to pelvic abscess. In this chapter, PID is used to refer to the clinical syndrome which includes each of these conditions, and the term *salpingitis* is restricted to patients with visually or histopathologically confirmed inflammation of the fallopian tubes. The distinction between endometritis and salpingitis may be important, because long-term sequelae are common after salpingitis. These sequelae include infertility due to bilateral tubal occlusion, peritubal adhesions, ectopic pregnancy due to tubal damage without occlusion, chronic pelvic pain, and recurrent PID.

ETIOLOGY The etiology of PID has seemed to vary greatly in several studies for reasons related to patient selection as well as methodology. As is summarized in Table 94-1, the agents most often implicated in acute PID include those which are primary causes of cervicitis (*Neisseria gonorrhoeae* and *C. trachomatis*) and those which can be regarded as abnormal components of the vaginal flora.

In the United States, gonococci were isolated from 44 percent of women with acute PID in a multicity cooperative study during the 1970s. From 1980 through 1989 in Seattle, *N. gonorrhoeae* or *C. trachomatis* have been found in over three-fourths of patients with proven salpingitis and endometritis; about one-fourth had gonorrhea alone, one-fourth had chlamydial infection alone, and one-fourth had both. However, in Scandinavian countries, where gonococcal infection is under much better control, endocervical gonococcal infection has been found in less than one-fourth of women with PID during the past decade, while chlamydial infection has remained common in this group. For example, in Sweden the proportion of women with acute PID who had gonorrhea fell from 50 percent in 1970 to 5 percent in 1985. In general, PID is most often associated with gonorrhea where there is a high incidence of gonorrhea, for example, in developing countries and in indigent, inner city populations in developed countries. In several studies of women with PID, up to two-thirds with positive endocervical cultures for *N. gonorrhoeae* have had positive endometrial, peritoneal, or tubal cultures for this organism. Similarly, studies of women with proven PID have shown that *C. trachomatis* can be demonstrated by culture or immunofluorescent staining in the endometrium or tubes of the majority of those who have endocervical chlamydial infection.

Anaerobic and facultative anaerobic organisms (especially *Bacteroides* species, peptostreptococci, *Escherichia coli*, and groups B and D streptococci) and genital mycoplasmas have been isolated from specimens obtained at laparoscopy from the peritoneal fluid or fallopian tubes in a varying proportion—typically one-fourth to one-third—of women with PID studied in the United States. These vaginal organisms can be found in association with chlamydial or gonococcal infection, as well as in women without them. The importance of vaginal organisms in salpingitis has probably been overestimated in studies based on culture of specimens obtained by culdocentesis or endometrial aspiration, procedures in which contamination of the aspirated specimen by vaginal flora could occur. However, specimens obtained by laparoscopy have also contained anaerobic and facultative species in some patients with PID. It is extremely difficult to determine the exact microbial etiology in the individual patient with PID because of the frequency of mixed infection, the difficulty in sampling the fallopian tube itself, and the complexity of microbiologic techniques required to detect the various fastidious pathogens involved.

In general, first episodes of acute PID are particularly likely to be caused by *N. gonorrhoeae* and/or *C. trachomatis*. These sexually transmitted pathogens are somewhat less often implicated in recurrent bouts of acute PID, episodes occurring in IUD users, and episodes precipitated by invasive intrauterine diagnostic or therapeutic procedures, which are often associated with ascending infection caused by the more virulent components of the endogenous vaginal flora.

EPIDEMIOLOGY It has been estimated that the annual incidence of PID in the United States during the mid-1970s was about 850,000 cases per year. PID is not a reportable disease in the United States; surveillance of physicians in private practice and of hospital discharges suggests that the incidence of PID increased from the mid-1960s through the mid-1970s and may then have decreased. The incidence of a major sequela of salpingitis, ectopic pregnancy, progressively rose each year from 13,200 cases in 1967 to 78,400 cases in 1985. Similar trends in ectopic pregnancies have been seen in Canada and England. Some of this increase may be due to improved tests for ectopic pregnancy. There is some evidence that involuntary infertility also increased in the United States during the 1970s.

Acute PID is almost exclusively a disease of sexually active women. The risk appears to be greater in sexually active teenagers than among older women. Important risk factors other than young age include a history of gonorrhea or of salpingitis, and use of an intrauterine device, particularly the Dalkon shield. In most studies, the relative risk of PID among IUD users was higher in nulliparous women than in parous women. On the other hand, women using oral contraceptives appear to be at decreased risk of PID. Barrier methods of contraception also prevent PID by reducing the risk of chlamydial and gonococcal infection. Tubal sterilization reduces (but does not completely eliminate) the risk of salpingitis by preventing intraluminal spread of infection into the tubes.

PATHOGENESIS Factors cited as possibly contributing to intracanalicular upward spread of gonococci and *Chlamydia* from the endocervix to the endometrium and endosalpinx include estrogen-dominated (thin) cervical mucus, attachment to sperm which migrate upward into the tubes, use of an intrauterine device, vaginal douching, and menstruation. The onset of symptoms of gonorrhea-associated PID and of *Chlamydia*-associated PID often occurs during or soon after the menstrual period. In fallopian tube organ cultures in vitro, gonococci attach to the surface of the secretory columnar cells (but not the ciliated cells) of the endosalpinx. Gonococcal pili and perhaps other surface proteins are important in this attachment. Gonococci then are taken into the secretory cells by endocytosis. They pass through the cells, and perhaps between cells, and are extruded through the base of the cell into the submucosal connective tissue. Ciliary motion ceases, and then ciliated cells, although not directly invaded by gonococci, are sloughed from the mucosa during this process—a factor which may render the tubes more susceptible to superinfection by other organisms. It is uncertain whether this loss of ciliated cells is irreversible in vivo. Gonococcal endotoxin and peptidoglycan are at least partly responsible for these cytotoxic effects. Gonococci associated with PID have been significantly more resistant to penicillin and less likely to belong to the Arg-Hyx-Ura auxotype than are strains causing uncomplicated gonorrhea.

C. trachomatis also infects the columnar cells of the fallopian tube, but produces little damage in tubal organ cultures, perhaps

---

TABLE 94-1   Cervical and vaginal organisms most often implicated in acute PID

Cervical pathogens	Vaginal flora
N. gonorrhoeae	Anaerobic bacteria
C. trachomatis	*Bacteroides* spp.
	Peptostreptococci
	Mobiluncus spp.
	Actinomyces spp.
	Facultative bacteria
	Enterobacteriaceae
	H. influenzae
	G. vaginalis
	Streptococcus, groups B, D
	Mycoplasma
	M. hominis
	U. urealyticum

because the host response is more important in the pathogenesis of chlamydial salpingitis. In chlamydial mucopurulent cervicitis (MPC), cervical biopsies show inclusions containing *Chlamydia* within columnar cells; columnar epithelial infiltration by neutrophils; submucosal and stromal infiltration by plasma cells, lymphocytes, histiocytes, and neutrophils; and lymphoid aggregates containing transformed lymphocytes. Routine endometrial biopsies from consecutive women with chlamydial MPC show endometritis in approximately one-half. Although endometritis detected in this way is sometimes associated with uterine tenderness, abnormal menstrual bleeding, and leukocytosis, symptoms of abdominal pain and fever are usually lacking, underscoring the subclinical nature of many cases of upper genital tract chlamydial infection. It is not known what proportion of those with endometritis also have salpingitis, since laparoscopy has not been performed in the absence of more suggestive symptoms and signs of salpingitis. However, among women with chlamydial MPC who lack such symptoms and signs, the great majority who undergo endometrial biopsy and laparoscopy have both endometritis and salpingitis. Chlamydial inclusions are demonstrable by direct immunofluorescence in columnar epithelial cells of the endometrium and endosalpinx. The endometrial biopsies usually show neutrophils infiltrating the epithelium and plasma cells infiltrating the stroma, findings also seen in gonococcal endometritis, but not in the uninfected endometrium. Other inflammatory changes analogous to those seen in the cervix are also found in the endometrium with chlamydial infection. Experimental inoculation of the fallopian tubes of lower primates produces mild acute salpingitis and ciliary sloughing, which is completely reversible. However, if experimental tubal inoculation is preceded by repeated inoculation of the fallopian tubes or cervix, a more intense salpingitis results and progresses to peritubular scarring. This suggests that in the female genital tract, as in the eye, repeated exposure to *C. trachomatis* leads to the greatest degree of tissue inflammation and damage.

The pathogenesis of PID attributable to mycoplasmas or other vaginal anaerobic or facultative organisms is less well studied. It is possible that other vaginal organisms implicated in PID cause tubal infection in women whose tubes have already been damaged by a primary sexually transmitted pathogen (i.e., *N. gonorrhoeae* or *C. trachomatis*). Since the anaerobic organisms and mycoplasmas implicated in PID are found in the vagina most often and in greatest concentration in bacterial vaginosis (nonspecific vaginitis), it is possible that bacterial vaginosis itself is a predisposing factor for PID (just as poor oral hygiene is a risk factor in aspiration pneumonia).

Certain other iatrogenic factors, such as dilatation and curettage or cesarean section, are known to pose a greater risk of causing PID in women with endocervical gonococcal or chlamydial infection. It remains to be determined whether such procedures are also a greater risk in women with bacterial vaginosis.

CLINICAL MANIFESTATIONS **Tuberculous salpingitis** Unlike nontuberculous salpingitis, genital tuberculosis often occurs in older women, and about half are postmenopausal. In a large review of cases in Sweden, 38 percent had had previously diagnosed tuberculosis. The commonest presenting symptoms were abnormal vaginal bleeding, pain, including dysmenorrhea, and infertility. Most had normal bimanual pelvic examinations, though about one-quarter had adnexal masses. The most common method of diagnosis was endometrial biopsy, showing tuberculous granulomas, often associated with a positive culture.

Nontuberculous salpingitis The evolution of symptoms classically proceeds from a mucopurulent vaginal discharge caused by cervicitis—possibly associated with dysuria and frequency due to urethritis, or with anorectal pain, tenesmus, rectal discharge, and bleeding due to proctitis—to midline abdominal pain and abnormal vaginal bleeding caused by endometritis, followed by bilateral lower abdominal and pelvic pain caused by salpingitis, with nausea and vomiting and increased abdominal tenderness caused by peritonitis. Some patients have diffuse abdominal pain caused by generalized peritonitis, or pleuritic right upper quadrant pain caused by perihep-

atitis. The pattern in which symptoms evolve varies from patient to patient and is also related to the etiology of the PID.

The onset of IUD-associated PID is typically gradual, and may be preceded by typical malodorous vaginal discharge characteristic of bacterial vaginosis. The onset of gonococcal PID has been more acute than that of chlamydial PID in some, but not all studies, and both are often associated with menses.

The abdominal pain is usually described as dull or aching. In some cases, pain is lacking or is atypical, and active inflammatory changes can be found in the course of an unrelated evaluation or procedure such as a tubal ligation or laparoscopic evaluation for infertility. Abnormal uterine bleeding precedes or coincides with the onset of pain in about 40 percent of women with PID, symptoms of urethritis occur in 20 percent, and symptoms of proctitis in 7 percent of patients.

Speculum examination shows evidence of mucopurulent cervicitis in the majority of women with gonococcal or chlamydial PID. Cervical motion tenderness is produced by stretching of the adnexal attachments on the side toward which the cervix is pushed. Bimanual examination reveals uterine fundal tenderness due to endometritis, and abnormal adnexal tenderness due to salpingitis which is usually, but not necessarily, bilateral. Adnexal swelling is palpable in about one-half of women with acute salpingitis, but evaluation of the adnexae in a patient with marked tenderness is not reliable, even by an experienced examiner. An initial temperature >38°C is found in only about one-third of patients with acute salpingitis, and fever is not required for the diagnosis.

Laboratory findings include elevation of the erythrocyte sedimentation rate (ESR) in 75 percent and elevation of the peripheral white blood cell count in up to 60 percent of patients with acute salpingitis. Microscopic examination of a saline wet-mount preparation of vaginal fluid has revealed more than one polymorphonuclear leukocyte per vaginal epithelial cell in nearly all patients with laparoscopically confirmed salpingitis in Swedish studies. However, exceptions have not been uncommon in U.S. studies of the same population.

Certain clinical manifestations of acute PID have been correlated with etiologic findings. For example, the onset of salpingitis is related to menses in women with gonorrhea or chlamydial infection. Women with gonorrhea or chlamydia associated salpingitis are significantly younger than women with other forms of salpingitis. Women with chlamydia-associated salpingitis reportedly tend to have an indolent disease with mild symptoms of significantly longer duration and with less fever compared to women who have gonorrhea-associated salpingitis, but paradoxically, those with chlamydia-associated salpingitis have had significantly higher ESR and more severe inflammatory reactions seen at laparoscopy. It is suspected that for all recognized cases of symptomatic *Chlamydia* salpingitis, there is a comparable number of unrecognized cases of indolent subclinical *Chlamydia* salpingitis, and that subclinical chronic or recurrent *Chlamydia* salpingitis may be a major cause of infertility in women.

IUD-associated PID has been much less common since withdrawal of the Dalkon shield from the market. It tends to be indolent and is less often associated with fever, but more often with adnexal masses, than is PID not associated with IUD use.

Perihepatitis and periappendicitis Symptoms of perihepatitis, including pleuritic upper abdominal pain and tenderness, usually localized to the right upper quadrant, occur in 3 to 10 percent of women with acute PID. The onset of symptoms of perihepatitis occurs during or after onset of symptoms of PID and may overshadow the lower abdominal symptoms, leading to a mistaken diagnosis of cholecystitis. In perhaps 5 percent of cases of acute salpingitis, laparoscopy performed early reveals inflammation ranging from edema and erythema of the liver capsule to exudate with fibrinous adhesions between the visceral and parietal peritoneum. When treatment is delayed, and laparoscopy is performed late, dense "violin-string" adhesions are seen over the liver; these cause chronic exertional or positional right upper quadrant pain when traction is placed on the adhesions. Although perihepatitis, also known as the Fitz-Hugh–

Curtis syndrome, was for many years attributed to gonococcal PID, it has been recognized that most cases of perihepatitis have been associated with chlamydial salpingitis. In patients with chlamydial salpingitis, serum microimmunofluorescent antibody titers against *C. trachomatis* are typically much higher when perihepatitis is present than when it is absent, and it has been suggested that repeated chlamydial infections are responsible for perihepatitis.

Physical findings include right upper quadrant tenderness and usually include adnexal tenderness and cervicitis, even in patients whose symptoms are not suggestive of salpingitis.

Liver function tests are nearly always normal, since inflammation is largely limited to the liver capsule, usually sparing the parenchyma. Oral cholecystogram may show nonfunction of the gallbladder, but ultrasonography of the right upper quadrant is normal. The presence of mucopurulent cervicitis and pelvic tenderness in a young woman with subacute pleuritic right upper quadrant pain with normal ultrasonography of the gallbladder points to a diagnosis of perihepatitis.

Periappendicitis (appendiceal serositis without involvement of the intestinal mucosa) has been found in approximately 5 percent of patients undergoing appendectomy for suspected appendicitis, and can occur as a complication of gonococcal or chlamydial salpingitis.

DIAGNOSIS Early diagnosis and initiation of therapy are essential to minimize tubal scarring. Appropriate treatment must not be withheld from patients who have an equivocal diagnosis. Since delay in therapy may lead to progression of tubal scarring, it is better to err on the side of overdiagnosis and overtreatment. On the other hand, it is essential to differentiate between salpingitis and other pelvic pathology, particularly surgical emergencies such as appendicitis and ectopic pregnancy.

No clinical or laboratory finding short of laparoscopy is pathognomonic for salpingitis, and there is reluctance to perform laparoscopy in all cases of suspected salpingitis. Most patients with acute PID have lower abdominal pain of <3 weeks' duration, pelvic tenderness on bimanual pelvic examination, and evidence of lower genital tract infection (e.g., white blood cells outnumber all other cells in the vaginal fluid). Approximately 60 percent of such patients had salpingitis at laparoscopy. Among the patients with these findings, a rectal temperature above 38°C, a palpable adnexal mass, and elevation of the ESR over 15 mm/h also raise the probability of salpingitis, which was found at laparoscopy in 68 percent of patients with one of these additional findings, 90 percent of patients with two or more, and 96 percent of patients with three or more additional findings. However, only 17 percent of all patients with laparoscopy-confirmed salpingitis had three additional findings.

Mucopurulent cervicitis is probably responsible for the presence of neutrophils in vaginal fluid in PID. In a woman with pelvic pain and tenderness, demonstration of an increased number of neutrophils (≥30 per 1000× microscopic field in strands of cervical mucus) increases the predictive value of a clinical diagnosis of acute PID.

Several clinical features other than the presence of cervicitis also favor the diagnosis of acute PID. These include onset with menses, history of recent abnormal menstrual bleeding, presence of an IUD, history of previous salpingitis, and exposure to a male with urethritis. Detection of polymorphonuclear leukocytes in fluid aspirated by culdocentesis supports a diagnosis of suspected salpingitis. Urethritis or proctitis may occur in chlamydial or gonococcal infection but may also represent a urinary tract infection or an intestinal source for the patient's symptoms. Early onset of nausea and vomiting favors appendicitis or other disorders of the gut. A missed menstrual period dictates evaluation for ectopic pregnancy. The more sensitive assays for human beta-chorionic gonadotropin are usually positive. Ultrasonography is sometimes useful to differentiate pelvic abscess from an inflammatory mass involving tubes, ovary, bowel, and omentum, but is not sufficiently sensitive to detect salpingitis.

Laparoscopy is the most specific method for diagnosis of acute salpingitis. Although it may be normal if inflammation is limited to the endosalpinx or endometrium, patients with suspected PID who have normal laparoscopy have a better prognosis, with few if any

TABLE 94-2 Laparoscopic findings in patients with false-positive or false-negative clinical diagnoses of acute PID

False-positive clinical diagnosis		False-negative clinical diagnosis, unexpected PID at laparoscopy	
Laparoscopic diagnosis	Percent	Clinical diagnosis	Percent
Acute appendicitis	24	Ovarian tumor	20
Endometriosis	16	Acute appendicitis	18
Corpus luteum bleeding	12	Ectopic pregnancy	16
Ectopic pregnancy	11	Chronic salpingitis	6
Pelvic adhesions only	7	Acute peritonitis	6
Benign ovarian tumor	7	Endometriosis	5
Chronic salpingitis	6	Uterine myoma	5
Miscellaneous	15	Atypical pelvic pain	6
		Miscellaneous	6

SOURCE: L Jacobsen and L Weström, Am J Obstet Gynecol 105:1088, 1969.

sequelae, when compared with patients who have abnormal laparoscopic findings. The primary and uncontested value of laparoscopy in women with lower abdominal pain is exclusion of other surgical problems. Table 94-2 clearly shows that the most common and serious problems that may be confused with salpingitis are usually unilateral. Unilateral pain or pelvic mass, though not incompatible with PID, is a strong indication for laparoscopy unless the clinical picture warrants laparotomy instead. Atypical clinical findings such as the absence of lower genital tract infection, a missed menstrual period, or failure to respond to appropriate therapy are other frequent indications for laparoscopy.

Laparoscopic criteria used for the diagnosis of salpingitis include (1) erythema of the fallopian tube; (2) edema of the fallopian tube; and (3) seropurulent exudate or fresh, easily lysed adhesions at the fimbriated end or on the serosal surface of a fallopian tube. Laparoscopic findings are further scored as mild, where the above manifestations are mild and the tubes are freely movable and patent; moderate, when the above manifestations are more marked, tubes are not freely movable, and patency is uncertain; and severe, when findings consist of an inflammatory mass.

Endometrial biopsy is relatively sensitive and specific for the diagnosis of endometritis when the changes described above are present and are found in at least three-fourths of women with laparoscopically confirmed salpingitis, and absent in women without PID.

The etiologic diagnosis of PID can be further studied by cultures or specimens obtained by endocervical swab, endometrial aspiration, or culdocentesis, or by laparoscopy or laparotomy. Endocervical swab specimens should be examined by Gram stain for neutrophils and gram-negative diplococci and by culture for *N. gonorrhoeae*. The sensitivity of Gram stain is about 60 percent and specificity >95 percent, compared with culture. The endocervical swab specimen should also be tested for *C. trachomatis* by culture, immunofluorescence, or antigen-capture assay. Although isolation of either *N. gonorrhoeae* or *C. trachomatis* from the cervix does not prove that either agent is also present in the upper genital tract, this finding strongly supports the diagnosis of PID. The clinical diagnosis of PID made by expert gynecologists is confirmed by laparoscopy or endometrial biopsy in only about 60 percent of all consecutive patients, but in about 90 percent of those who also have positive cultures for *N. gonorrhoeae* or *C. trachomatis*. There is no evidence that isolation of anaerobes or facultative anaerobes from the cervix or vagina correlates with the presence of these organisms in the upper genital tract in acute PID, but this has not been well studied. The value of culture of culdocentesis and endometrial aspirate specimens is disputed because of the risk of contamination of the specimen with vaginal flora. When laparoscopy is performed, material can be obtained directly from the cul-de-sac or the fimbriated opening of the tube, or by tubal aspiration if pyosalpinx is present. Such specimens should be cultured for anaerobic and facultative pathogens, as well as for *N. gonorrhoeae* and *C. trachomatis*.

TABLE 94-3 Relative activities of the antimicrobial agents most commonly used to treat PID

	N. gonorrhoeae	C. trachomatis	Vaginal anaerobes GPC*	GNR†	Facultative GNR	M. hominis
Ampicillin/amoxicillin	3+	2+	4+	2+	2+	0
Tetracycline HCl	3+	4+	4+	2+	2+	2+
Doxycycline	3+	4+	4+	3+	2+	2+
Cefoxitin, cefotetan	3+	0	4+	3+	4+	0
Ceftriaxone	4+	0	3+	2+	4+	0
Gentamicin/tobramycin	2+	0	1+	0	4+	2+?
Fluoroquinolones	3 to 4+	Variable	1+	1+	4+	Variable
Clindamycin	1+	2+	4+	4+	0	3+
Metronidazole	0	0	4+	4+	0	0

* GPC = Gram-positive cocci (peptostreptococci).
† GNR = Gram-negative rods (anaerobic GNR include Bacteroides, facultative GNR include Enterobacteriaceae, H. influenzae).
NOTE: No single antimicrobial agent offers optimal activity against all of these pathogens, but certain combinations (e.g., cefoxitin plus doxycycline, gentamicin plus clindamycin) have complementary activity.

TREATMENT Hospitalization should be considered in all women with PID. Hospitalization is strongly recommended when (1) the diagnosis is uncertain, (2) surgical emergencies such as appendicitis and ectopic pregnancy must be excluded, (3) a pelvic abscess is suspected, (4) severe illness precludes outpatient management, (5) the patient is pregnant, (6) the patient is an adolescent, (7) the patient is assessed as unable to follow or tolerate an outpatient regimen, (8) the patient has failed to respond to outpatient therapy, or (9) clinical follow-up after 48 to 72 h of instituting antibiotic treatment cannot be arranged. The treatment of choice is not established. No single agent is active against the entire spectrum of pathogens (Table 94-3). Several antimicrobial combinations do provide a broad spectrum of activity against the major pathogens in vitro, but many have not been adequately evaluated for clinical efficacy in PID.

Examples of combination regimens with broad activity against major pathogens in PID

1 Doxycycline 100 mg, twice a day, IV, plus cefoxitin 2.0 g, four times a day, IV, or cefotetan 2.0 g, every 12 h, IV. These drugs should be continued IV for at least 48 h after the patient improves. Doxycycline should be continued in a dose of 100 mg by mouth, twice a day, after discharge from the hospital to complete 14 days of therapy. This regimen provides excellent coverage for N. gonorrhoeae, including penicillinase-producing N. gonorrhoeae (PPNG), and C. trachomatis.

2 Clindamycin 900 mg, every 8 h, IV, plus gentamicin 2.0 mg/kg, IV, followed by 1.5 mg/kg, every 8 h, IV, in patients with normal renal function. These drugs should be continued for at least 48 h after the patient improves. After discharge from the hospital doxycycline 100 mg orally, twice a day, should be given to complete 14 days of therapy. This regimen provides good activity against anaerobes and facultative gram-negative rods, and is active against C. trachomatis and N. gonorrhoeae. Doxycycline provides definitive therapy for chlamydial infection.

Patients who are not hospitalized should also receive a combined regimen with broad activity, such as ceftriaxone 250 mg, IM, followed by doxycycline 100 mg, by mouth, twice a day for 14 days. Cefoxitin, 2.0 g, IM, given concurrently with probenecid 1.0 g, orally, could be used in place of ceftriaxone. Tetracycline could also be used in a dose of 500 mg, four times a day, in place of doxycycline, but requires more frequent dosing which is a major drawback in the treatment of PID.

Management of sexual partners All persons who are sexual partners of patients with PID should be examined for STD and promptly treated with a regimen effective against uncomplicated gonococcal and chlamydial infection.

Follow-up All patients who are treated as outpatients should be clinically reevaluated in 48 to 72 h. Those not responding favorably should be hospitalized. A culture to test whether cure has been achieved should be performed as needed.

Removal of an intrauterine device Although possible benefit of IUD removal on the response of acute salpingitis to antimicrobial therapy and on the risk of recurrent salpingitis has not been proven, removal of the IUD soon after antimicrobial therapy has been initiated seems reasonable. When an IUD is removed, contraceptive counseling is necessary.

Surgery Surgery is necessary only rarely for treatment of salpingitis, except in the face of life-threatening infection such as rupture or threatened rupture of a tuboovarian abscess, or for drainage of an abscess. Ultrasonography is useful for diagnosing and following pelvic abscesses. When surgery is performed, conservative procedures are usually sufficient. Pelvic abscesses can often be drained by posterior colpotomy, and peritoneal lavage can be used if there is generalized peritonitis.

PROGNOSIS In a cooperative trial in the United States, nearly 20 percent of women treated for PID on an ambulatory basis with IM penicillin followed by a 10-day course of ampicillin, or with a 10-day course of tetracycline alone, were judged to be clinical failures.

Among 900 women who underwent long-term follow-up for a mean period of 8 years after successful treatment of the acute episode with various regimens in Sweden, late sequelae included infertility due to bilateral tubal occlusion, ectopic pregnancy due to tubal scarring without occlusion, chronic pelvic pain, and recurrent salpingitis. Chronic pain lasting longer than 6 months was seen in 18 percent of patients and infertility due to tubal occlusion in 17 percent; 4 percent of pregnancies that did occur were ectopic, representing approximately a sixfold increase over the expected rate of ectopic pregnancies. The rate of infertility after salpingitis was found to be related to age of the patient, duration of symptoms when treatment was started, severity of salpingitis by laparoscopy at the time of diagnosis, and number of episodes of salpingitis. The rate of infertility due to tubal occlusion among women exposed to a chance of pregnancy was 14 percent for women 15 to 24 years of age and 26 percent for women 25 to 34 years of age; the risk for women of all ages combined was 11 percent after one episode of salpingitis, 23 percent after two episodes, and 54 percent after three or more episodes. The risk of infertility after gonococcal salpingitis was comparable to the risk after chlamydial salpingitis in one small prospective study.

A striking relationship has also been shown in several countries between infertility due to tubal occlusion and the prevalence and titer of antibody to C. trachomatis. Recurrent salpingitis has been seen in approximately 15 to 25 percent of women treated for salpingitis in various studies.

PREVENTION Prevention of PID depends first on the effective control of gonococcal and chlamydial infection. Effective methods include promotion of changes in sexual behavior and use of barrier contraceptives while providing ready access to modern methods of diagnosis and effective treatment, and treatment of sex partners to control further spread. The decline in popularity of the intrauterine device, particularly in nulliparous women, has undoubtedly helped to reduce the incidence of PID. It is also possible, but not proven, that use of oral contraceptives and avoidance of vaginal douching might reduce the risk of PID.

The complications of salpingitis can be minimized by early diagnosis and prompt treatment. It seems logical, but is unproven, that broad-spectrum therapy effective against all of the common causes of PID would offer the best outcome. Similarly, hospitalization to ensure rest and adequate compliance may improve the rather dismal long-term prognosis for tubal function. One placebo-controlled study showed that concurrent anti-inflammatory therapy with prednisolone hastened the reduction of acute inflammatory changes but did not improve the end results as measured by fertility, hysterosalpingo-graphic findings, or chronic pain. However, the potential value of anti-inflammatory therapy remains to be evaluated adequately.

REFERENCES

CATES WJ et al: Worldwide patterns of infertility: Is Africa different? Lancet 2:596, 1985

CENTERS FOR DISEASE CONTROL: 1989 sexually transmitted diseases treatment guidelines. Morb Mort Week Rep 38 (Suppl 8):1, 1989

ESCHENBACH DA et al: Polymicrobial etiology of acute pelvic inflammatory disease. N Engl J Med 293:166, 1975

FALK V et al: Genital tuberculosis in women. Am J Obstet Gynecol 138:974, 1980

HADGU A et al: Predicting acute PID: A multivariate analysis. Am J Obstet Gynecol 155:954, 1986

KIVIAT N et al: Endometrial histopathology in patients with culture-proven upper genital tract infection and laparoscopically diagnosed acute salpingitis. Am J Clin Pathol 1990 (in press)

MÅRDH PA et al: *Chlamydia trachomatis* infection in patients with acute salpingitis. N Engl J Med 296:1377, 1977

MØLLER BR et al: Pelvic infection after elective abortion associated with *Chlamydia trachomatis*. Obstet Gynecol 59:210, 1982

PAAVONEN J et al: Microbiological and histological findings in acute pelvic inflammatory disease. Br J Obstet Gynaecol 94:454, 1987

PLUMMER FA et al: Postpartum upper genital tract infections in Nairobi, Kenya: Epidemiology, etiology, and risk factors. J Infect Dis 156:92, 1987

ST JOHN RK, BROWN ST (eds): International symposium on pelvic inflammatory disease. Am J Obstet Gynecol 138:845, 1980

SVENSSON L et al: Differences in some clinical and laboratory parameters in acute salpingitis related to culture and serologic findings. Am J Obstet Gynecol 138:1017, 1980

——— et al: Infertility after acute salpingitis—with special reference to *Chlamydia trachomatis*–associated infections. Fertil Steril 40:322, 1983

WASSERHEIT JN et al: Microbial causes of proven pelvic inflammatory disease and efficacy of clindamycin with tobramycin. Ann Intern Med 104:187, 1986

WESTRÖM L, MÅRDH PA: Acute pelvic inflammatory disease, in *Sexually Transmitted Diseases*, KK Holmes et al (eds). New York, McGraw-Hill, 1989, pp 593–613

WØLNER-HANSSEN P et al: Outpatient treatment of pelvic inflammatory disease with cefoxitin and doxycycline. Obstet Gynecol 71:595, 1988

——— et al: Atypical pelvic inflammatory disease: Subacute, chronic, or subclinical upper genital tract infections in women, in *Sexually Transmitted Diseases*, KK Holmes et al (eds). New York, McGraw-Hill 1990, pp 615–620

95   URINARY TRACT INFECTIONS AND PYELONEPHRITIS

WALTER E. STAMM / MARVIN TURCK

DEFINITIONS   Acute infections of the urinary tract can be subdivided into two general anatomic categories: lower tract infection (urethritis, cystitis, and prostatitis) and upper tract infection (acute pyelonephritis). Infections at these various sites may occur together or independently, and may be asymptomatic or present as the clinical syndromes outlined below.

Microbiologically, urinary tract infection exists when pathogenic microorganisms are detected in the urine, urethra, kidney, or prostate. In most instances, growth of more than 10^5 organisms per milliliter from a properly collected midstream "clean catch" urine sample

indicates infection. However, significant bacteriuria may be absent in some circumstances when true urinary infection exists. Especially in symptomatic patients, a smaller number of bacteria (10^2 to 10^4 per milliliter of midstream urine) may accompany infection. In urine specimens obtained by suprapubic aspiration or "in and out" catheterization, or from a patient with an indwelling catheter, colony counts of 10^2 to 10^4 per milliliter generally indicate infection. Conversely, colony counts in excess of 10^5 per milliliter of midstream urine are occasionally due to specimen contamination.

Recurrent infections after antibiotic therapy can be due to the originally infecting strain, as judged by species identification, serotype, and antibiogram, or to reinfection with a new strain. "Same strain" recurrent infections that occur within 2 weeks of cessation of therapy can result from unresolved renal or prostatic infection or from unresolved vaginal colonization that leads to rapid reinfection of the bladder.

Symptoms of dysuria, urgency, and frequency unaccompanied by significant bacteriuria have been termed the acute urethral syndrome. Although widely used, this term lacks anatomic precision because many cases of urethral syndrome are in actuality bladder infections. Moreover, since the causative agent can usually be identified in these patients, the term *syndrome*, implying unknown causation, is inappropriate.

Chronic pyelonephritis refers to chronic interstitial nephritis believed to result from bacterial infection of the kidney (see Chap. 229). Many noninfectious diseases also cause an interstitial nephritis indistinguishable pathologically from chronic pyelonephritis.

ACUTE INFECTIONS OF THE URINARY TRACT: URETHRITIS, CYSTITIS, AND PYELONEPHRITIS

EPIDEMIOLOGY   Epidemiologically, urinary tract infections should be subdivided into catheter-associated (or nosocomial) infections and non-catheter-associated (or community-acquired) infections. In either category, infections may be symptomatic or asymptomatic. Acute infections in noncatheterized patients occur very commonly, especially in women, and account for over 6 million office visits annually in the United States. These infections occur in 1 to 3 percent of schoolgirls, and then increase markedly in incidence with the onset of sexual activity in adolescence. The vast majority of acute symptomatic infections occur in young women. Acute symptomatic urinary infections are rare in men under the age of 50. The occurrence of asymptomatic bacteriuria parallels that of symptomatic infection and is rare in men under 50, but is common in women between the ages of 20 and 50. Asymptomatic bacteriuria is most common in elderly men and women.

ETIOLOGY   Many different microorganisms can infect the urinary tract, but by far the most common agents are the gram-negative bacilli. *Escherichia coli* causes approximately 80 percent of acute infections in patients without urologic abnormalities or calculi. Other gram-negative rods, especially *Proteus* and *Klebsiella* and occasionally *Enterobacter*, *Serratia*, and *Pseudomonas*, account for a smaller proportion of uncomplicated infections. These organisms assume increasing importance in recurrent infections and infections associated with urologic manipulation, calculi, or obstruction. They play a major role in nosocomial, catheter-associated infections (see below). *Proteus* species, by virtue of urease production, and *Klebsiella* species, through production of extracellular slime and polysaccharides, predispose to stone formation and are isolated more frequently from patients with calculi.

Gram-positive cocci play a lesser role in urinary tract infections. However, *Staphylococcus saprophyticus,* a novobiocin-resistant, coagulase-negative staphylococcus, accounts for 10 to 15 percent of acute symptomatic urinary tract infections in young females. Enterococci and *Staphylococcus aureus* cause infections in patients with renal stones or previous instrumentation. Isolation of *S. aureus* from the urine should arouse suspicion of bacteremic infection of the kidney.

About one-third of women with dysuria and frequency have either a nonsignificant number of bacteria in midstream urine cultures or completely sterile cultures, and have been previously defined as having the urethral syndrome. About three-quarters of these women have pyuria, while one-quarter have no pyuria and little objective evidence of infection. In the women with pyuria, two groups of pathogens account for the majority of infections. Low quantities (10^2 to 10^4 bacteria per milliliter) of typical bacterial uropathogens such as *E. coli, S. saprophyticus, Klebsiella,* or *Proteus* in midstream urine specimens are found in the majority of these women. They are probably the causative agents in these women because they can usually be isolated from a suprapubic aspirate, are associated with pyuria, and respond to appropriate antimicrobial therapy. In other women with acute urinary symptoms, pyuria, and sterile urine (even on suprapubic aspiration), sexually transmitted urethritis-producing agents such as *Chlamydia trachomatis, Neisseria gonorrhoeae,* and herpes simplex virus are important etiologic agents. These sexually transmitted agents are more frequently found in young, sexually active women with new sexual partners.

Viruses may increase the kidney's susceptibility to infection with gram-negative bacteria. In humans, viruses (cytomegalovirus, for example) are most commonly recovered from the urine without evidence of acute urinary disease, although some adenoviruses cause acute hemorrhagic cystitis. *Candida* and other fungi may colonize the urine of catheterized patients or diabetics, and in some patients cause acute symptomatic infection.

PATHOGENESIS AND SOURCES OF INFECTION The urinary tract should be viewed as a single anatomic unit connected by a continuous column of urine that extends from the urethra to the kidney. In the vast majority of infections, bacteria gain access to the bladder via the urethra. Ascent of bacteria from the bladder may then follow and is probably the usual pathway for most renal parenchymal infections.

The vaginal introitus and distal urethra are normally colonized with diphtheroids, streptococcal species, lactobacilli, and staphylococcal species, but not with the enteric gram-negative bacilli that commonly cause urinary tract infections. In females prone to development of cystitis, however, enteric gram-negative organisms residing in the bowel colonize the introitus, the periurethral skin, and the distal urethra prior to and during episodes of bacteriuria. Factors predisposing to periurethral colonization with gram-negative bacilli remain poorly understood but probably involve alteration of the normal perineal flora by antibiotics or by contraceptives, especially diaphragm and spermicide. Small numbers of periurethral bacteria probably gain entry to the bladder frequently, facilitated in some women by urethral massage during intercourse. Whether bladder infection ensues then depends upon interaction between the pathogenicity of the strain, the inoculum size, and local and systemic host defense mechanisms.

Under normal circumstances, bacteria placed in the bladder are rapidly cleared. This results partly from the flushing and dilutional effects of voiding, but also from direct antibacterial properties of urine and the bladder mucosa. Due mostly to high urea concentration and high osmolarity, the bladder urine of many normal persons inhibits or kills bacteria. Prostatic secretions possess antibacterial properties as well. Polymorphonuclear leukocytes in the bladder wall also appear to play a role in clearing bacteriuria. The role of locally produced antibody remains unclear. Hematogenous pyelonephritis occurs most often in debilitated patients who either have chronic illnesses or who are receiving immunosuppressive therapy. Staphylococcal pyelonephritis may follow bacteremia from distant foci of infection in the bone, skin, endothelium, or elsewhere.

CONDITIONS AFFECTING PATHOGENESIS   Gender and sexual activity The female urethra appears particularly prone to colonization with colonic gram-negative bacilli, owing to its proximity to the anus, its short length (about 4 cm), and its termination beneath the labia. Urethral massage, as occurs during sexual intercourse, causes introduction of bacteria into the bladder, and appears to be important in the pathogenesis of urinary infections in younger women. (Voiding after intercourse has been shown to reduce the risk of cystitis, probably because it promotes eradication of bacteria introduced during intercourse.) In addition, diaphragm and spermicide use dramatically alter the normal introital bacterial flora and have been associated with a marked increase in vaginal colonization with *E. coli* and risk of urinary infection. In males, prostatitis or urethral obstruction due to prostatic hypertrophy are important factors predisposing to bacteriuria. Homosexuality also predisposes to an increased risk of cystitis, probably associated with rectal intercourse.

Pregnancy Depending on socioeconomic status, urinary infections are detected in 2 to 8 percent of pregnant women. In particular, symptomatic upper tract infections occur more commonly during pregnancy; fully 20 to 30 percent of pregnant women with asymptomatic bacteriuria subsequently develop pyelonephritis. This predisposition to upper tract infection during pregnancy results from the decreased ureteral tone, decreased ureteral peristalsis, and temporary incompetence of the vesicoureteral valves seen in pregnancy. Bladder catheterization during or after delivery causes additional infections. Cystitis and pyelonephritis are no more common in women with toxemia of pregnancy than in other pregnant women. An increased prevalence of prematurity and newborn mortality may result from urinary infections during pregnancy, particularly those involving the upper urinary tract.

Obstruction Any impediment to the free flow of urine—tumor, stricture, stone, or prostatic hypertrophy—results in hydronephrosis and greatly increased frequency of urinary tract infection. Infection superimposed on urinary tract obstruction may lead to rapid destruction of renal tissue. It is of utmost importance, therefore, when infection is present, to repair obstructive lesions. On the other hand, with minor degrees of obstruction that are not progressive or associated with infection, great caution should be exercised in attempting surgical correction. The introduction of infection in such patients may be more damaging than uncorrected minor obstructions that do not significantly impair renal function.

Neurogenic bladder dysfunction Interference with the nerve supply to the bladder, as in spinal cord injury, tabes dorsalis, multiple sclerosis, diabetes, or other diseases, may be associated with urinary tract infection. The infection may be initiated by the use of catheters for bladder drainage and is favored by the prolonged stasis of urine in the bladder. An additional factor often present in these patients is bone demineralization due to immobilization, which causes hypercalciuria, calculus formation, and obstructive uropathy.

Vesicoureteral reflux This condition is defined as reflux of urine from the bladder cavity up into the ureters and sometimes into the renal pelvis. It occurs during voiding or with elevation of pressure in the bladder. In practice, vesicoureteral reflux exists when retrograde movement of radiopaque or radioactive material can be demonstrated. However, since a fluid connection between the bladder and kidney always exists in the patent urinary system, during infections some retrograde movement of bacteria probably occurs normally but is not detected by radiologic techniques. An anatomically impaired vesicoureteral junction facilitates reflux of bacteria.

Vesicoureteral reflux is common in children with anatomic abnormalities of the urinary tract and in children with anatomically normal but infected urinary tracts. In the latter group, reflux disappears with advancing age and probably results from causes other than urinary infection. Follow-up of children with urinary tract infection who were found to have reflux establishes that renal damage correlates with marked reflux, not with infection.

The routine search for reflux would be aided by development of noninvasive tests applicable to young children, where the need is greatest. In the meantime, it appears reasonable to search for reflux in anyone with unexplained failure of renal growth or renal scarring, because urinary tract infection per se is an insufficient explanation for these abnormalities. On the other hand, it is doubtful that all children with recurrent urinary tract infections but normal urinary tracts on pyelography should be subjected to voiding cystoureterography merely to detect the rare patient with marked reflux that did not reveal itself on the intravenous pyelogram.

Bacterial virulence factors Bacterial virulence factors influence the likelihood that a given strain, once introduced into the bladder, will cause urinary tract infection. Not all *E. coli* are equally able to infect the intact urinary tract. The majority of strains that cause symptomatic urinary tract infections in noncatheterized patients belong to a small number of serogroups (O, K, and H), produce hemolysin, and share certain other "uropathogenic" properties. Adherence of bacteria to uroepithelial cells is a critical first step in the initiation of infection. For both *E. coli* and *Proteus*, fimbriae (hairlike surface appendages) mediate bacterial attachment to specific receptors on epithelial cells. Nearly all *E. coli* strains that cause pyelonephritis in patients with anatomically normal urinary tracts possess a particular pilus (the P pilus or gal-gal pilus) that mediates attachment to the digalactoside portion of glycosphingolipids present on uroepithelium. Strains that produce pyelonephritis are also usually hemolysin producers, have aerobactin (a siderophore for scavenging iron), and are resistant to the bactericidal action of human serum. Since most strains that produce acute pyelonephritis in the intact host possess all or nearly all of these virulence factors, the concept has arisen that a small number of uropathogenic clones cause most such cases of infection. In patients with structural or functional abnormalities of the urinary tract, infections are frequently caused by bacterial strains that lack these uropathogenic properties, implying that these properties are not needed for infection of the compromised urinary tract.

Genetic factors Increasing evidence suggests that genetic factors influence susceptibility to urinary infection. The number and type of receptors on uroepithelial cells to which bacteria may attach is at least in part genetically determined. Many of these antigens are found on both erythrocytes and uroepithelial cells. For example, P fimbriae mediate attachment of *E. coli* to P-positive erythrocytes and are present on nearly all strains causing acute uncomplicated pyelonephritis. Conversely, P-negative individuals, who lack these receptors, have a decreased likelihood of pyelonephritis. It has also been demonstrated that nonsecretors of blood group antigens may have an increased risk of recurrent urinary infection.

LOCALIZATION OF INFECTION Infections involving the upper urinary tract usually cause a significant rise in serum antibodies directed against the O antigen of the infecting strain. They also produce a temporary defect in renal concentrating ability in many patients, and may be associated with formation of leukocyte casts. Lower tract infections rarely result in increased antibody titers, concentrating defects, or white cell casts. Unfortunately, these methods of distinguishing renal parenchymal infection from cystitis are neither reliable nor convenient enough for routine clinical use. More sensitive tests for distinguishing pyelonephritis from cystitis (bilateral ureteral catheterization and the bladder wash-out technique originated by Fairley) are inherently invasive and too complex for routine clinical practice. The development of a simpler and clinically applicable test to separate upper and lower tract infections based upon antibody coating of bacteria in the urine has been studied. In this test, urinary bacteria from patients with pyelonephritis demonstrate antibody coating on their surface when they have been exposed to a fluorescein-labeled antihuman globulin and are viewed under a fluorescence microscope. No surface antibodies can be seen on bacteria from patients with cystitis. This antibody response consists mainly of IgG. The antibody-coated bacteria test does not have sufficient sensitivity and specificity to be of value in the routine clinical management of patients. An elevated C-reactive protein often accompanies acute pyelonephritis and rarely is seen in cystitis, but this acute phase reactant is nonspecific and occurs in infections other than pyelonephritis as well.

CLINICAL PRESENTATION Clinical signs and symptoms cannot be relied upon to diagnose urinary tract infection accurately or to localize the site of infection. Many patients with significant bacteriuria (including some with upper tract infection) have no symptoms at all. Of those with significant bacteriuria and symptoms of cystitis, about one-half have lower tract infection and about one-half have clinically silent upper tract infection that is evident only upon performing localization studies. Clinical symptoms and signs of pyelonephritis, though usually suggestive, do not always indicate upper tract infection. Finally, among women presenting with acute dysuria and frequency, only 60 to 70 percent have significant bacteriuria, but the majority of those without significant bacteriuria also have urinary tract or urethral infections.

Enumeration of the number of bacteria in the urine is an extremely important diagnostic procedure. In symptomatic infections of the urinary tract, bacteria are usually demonstrable in the urine in large numbers. Quantitative estimation of the number of bacteria in voided urine specimens as a rule makes it possible to distinguish contaminants from true bacteriuria, and 10^5 or more bacteria per milliliter has been the criterion traditionally used for this purpose. However, in symptomatic women with pyuria, counts of 10^2 to 10^4 *E. coli*, *Klebsiella*, *Proteus*, or *S. saprophyticus* per milliliter of midstream urine usually indicate infection, not contamination, and should not be disregarded. In asymptomatic patients, two or three consecutive urine specimens should be examined bacteriologically before instituting therapy, and 10^5 or more per milliliter of a single species should be demonstrable in the repeated specimens. Since the large number of bacteria in the bladder urine is due in part to bacterial multiplication during residence in the bladder cavity, samples of urine from the ureters or renal pelvis may contain fewer than 10^5 bacteria per milliliter and yet indicate infection. Similarly, the presence of bacteriuria of any degree in suprapubic aspirates or of 10^2 or more bacteria per milliliter of urine obtained by catheterization usually indicates infection. In some circumstances (antibiotics, high urea concentration, high osmolarity, low pH), urine will inhibit bacterial multiplication, resulting in a lower number of bacteria in the presence of infection. For this reason, antiseptic solutions should not be used in washing the periurethral area prior to collection of the urine specimen. Water diuresis or recent voiding also reduces the bacterial counts in urine. Rapid methods of detection of bacteriuria have been developed as alternatives to standard culture methods. They detect bacterial growth using photometry, bioluminescence, or other means and provide results rapidly, usually in 1 to 2 h. These methods generally achieve a sensitivity of 95 to 98 percent and >99 percent negative predictive value as compared with urine cultures when bacteriuria is defined as 10^5 cfu/mL. However, the sensitivity of these tests falls to 60 to 80 percent when bacteriuria of 10^2 to 10^4 colony forming units per milliliter is the standard of comparison.

Microscopy of urine from symptomatic patients can be of great diagnostic value. Microscopic bacteriuria, which is best assessed using Gram-stained, uncentrifuged urine, is found in over 90 percent of specimens from patients whose infections have colony counts of 10^5 per milliliter, and is a very specific finding. However, bacteria cannot usually be detected microscopically in lower colony count infections (10^2 to 10^4 per milliliter). The presence of bacteria on urinary microscopy is firm evidence of infection, but its absence does not exclude the diagnosis. When carefully sought using a chamber count microscopy method, pyuria is a highly sensitive indicator of urinary tract infection in symptomatic patients. Its absence should cause the diagnosis to be questioned. The leukocyte esterase "dipstick" method is less sensitive than microscopy in identifying pyuria, but is a useful alternative where microscopy is not available.

Cystitis Patients with dysuria, frequency, urgency, and suprapubic pain usually have cystitis. The urine often becomes grossly cloudy, malodorous, and, in about 30 percent of cases, bloody. White cells and bacteria should be present on examination of the unspun urine in most patients. However, some women with cystitis have only 10^2 to 10^4 bacteria per milliliter of urine, which cannot be seen on Gram's stain of unspun urine. Physical examination generally reveals only a tender urethra or suprapubic tenderness. If a genital lesion or a vaginal discharge is present, especially with fewer than 10^5 bacteria per milliliter on culture, causes of urethritis, vaginitis, or cervicitis such as *C. trachomatis*, gonorrhea, *Trichomonas*, *Can-*

dida, and *Herpesvirus hominis* should be considered. Prominent systemic manifestations like fever over 38.3°C (101°F), nausea, vomiting, and costovertebral angle tenderness usually indicate concomitant renal infection. However, the absence of these findings does not ensure that infection is limited to the bladder and urethra.

Acute pyelonephritis Symptoms generally develop rapidly over a few hours or a day and include fever which is often 39.4°C (103°F) or greater, shaking chills, nausea, vomiting, and diarrhea. Symptoms of cystitis may or may not be present. Besides fever, tachycardia, and generalized muscle tenderness, physical examination reveals marked tenderness on deep pressure in one or both costovertebral areas or on deep abdominal palpation. In some patients, signs and symptoms of gram-negative sepsis predominate. Most patients have significant leukocytosis, pyuria with leukocyte casts in the urine, and bacteria on a Gram's stain of unspun urine. Hematuria may be present during the acute phase of the disease, but if it persists after acute manifestations of infection have subsided, a stone, tumor, or tuberculosis should be considered.

Except in individuals with papillary necrosis or urinary obstruction, the manifestations of acute pyelonephritis usually subside within a few days, even without specific antibacterial therapy. However, despite the absence of symptoms, bacteriuria or pyuria may persist. With severe pyelonephritis, fever subsides more slowly and may not disappear for several days, even after appropriate antibiotic treatment has been instituted.

Urethritis Approximately 30 percent of women with acute dysuria, frequency, and pyuria have midstream urine cultures that show either no growth or nonsignificant bacterial growth. Clinically, these women cannot be readily distinguished from those with cystitis. In these women distinction should be made between those having sexually transmitted pathogens such as *C. trachomatis, Neisseria gonorrhoeae,* or herpes simplex virus, and those having low-count *E. coli* or staphylococcal infection of the urethra and bladder. Women with a gradual onset of illness, no hematuria, no suprapubic pain, and a history of more than 7 days of symptoms should be suspected of having chlamydial infection. The additional history of a recent sex partner change, especially if the patient's partner has recently had chlamydial or gonococcal urethritis, should heighten the suspicion of a sexually transmitted infection, as would the finding of mucopurulent cervicitis. Gross hematuria, suprapubic pain, abrupt onset of illness, a duration of illness of less than 3 days, and a history of previous urinary tract infections favor *E. coli* or staphylococcal infection.

Catheter-associated urinary tract infections Bacteriuria occurs in at least 10 to 20 percent of hospitalized patients with indwelling urethral catheters. The risk of infection is about 3 to 5 percent per day of catheterization. *Proteus, Pseudomonas, Klebsiella,* and *Serratia,* in addition to *E. coli,* usually cause these infections. Many infecting strains show marked antimicrobial resistance compared with organisms that cause community-acquired urinary infections. Factors associated with an increased risk of infection include female sex, lengthy period of catheterization, severe underlying illness, faulty catheter care, and poorly trained nursing personnel.

Infection occurs when bacteria reach the bladder by one of two routes: by migrating through the column of urine in the catheter lumen (intraluminal route); or by moving up the mucous sheath outside the catheter (periurethral route). Hospital-acquired pathogens reach the patient's catheter or urine-collecting system on the hands of hospital personnel, in contaminated solutions or irrigants, and via contaminated instruments or disinfectants. Entry of bacteria into the catheter system usually occurs at the catheter–collecting tube junction or at the drainage bag portal. Bacteria then ascend intraluminally into the bladder. More often, the patient's own bowel flora migrate to the perineal skin and periurethral area and reach the bladder via the external surface of the catheter. This route is particularly common in women.

Most catheter-associated infections appear to be benign. They cause minimal symptoms, no fever, and often resolve after withdrawal of the catheter. The frequency of upper tract infection associated with catheter-induced bacteriuria is unknown. Gram-negative bacteremia, which follows 1 to 2 percent of cases of catheter-associated bacteriuria, is the most significantly recognized complication of catheter-induced urinary infections. The catheterized urinary tract has repeatedly been demonstrated to be the most common source of gram-negative bacteremia in hospitalized patients. It has also been suggested that bacteriuria in hospitalized catheterized patients is associated with an adjusted increased relative risk of death of approximately threefold compared with similar patients without bacteriuria.

Catheter-associated urinary tract infections can be partially prevented in patients catheterized less than 2 weeks by use of a sterile closed collecting system, attention to aseptic technique during insertion and care of the catheter, use of meatal antiseptic ointments, and by measures to minimize cross infection. Despite these precautions, the majority of patients catheterized longer than 2 weeks develop bacteriuria. The optimal treatment for such patients has not been established. Removal of the catheter and a short course of antibiotics to which the organism is susceptible is probably the best course of action and nearly always eradicates the bacteriuria. If the catheter cannot be removed, antibiotic therapy usually proves to be unsuccessful and may result in infection with a more resistant strain. In this situation, the bacteriuria should be ignored unless the patient develops symptoms or is at high risk of developing bacteremia. In these cases, systemic antibiotics or urinary bladder antiseptics may reduce the degree of bacteriuria and the likelihood of bacteremia. In patients who require long-term catheterization, sterile intermittent in-and-out catheterization performed by a nurse or by the patient results in fewer infections than does continuous indwelling catheterization.

DIAGNOSTIC TESTING Although many authorities have recommended that urine culture and antimicrobial susceptibility testing be performed in any patient with a suspected urinary tract infection, it may be more cost-effective to manage patients who have symptoms and urinalysis findings characteristic of acute uncomplicated cystitis without an initial urine culture. We recommend that patients with symptoms and signs of acute cystitis in whom no complicating factors are present should have urinary microscopy (or alternatively, a leukocyte esterase test or rapid filtration-stain test) performed. If positive for pyuria, hematuria, and/or bacteriuria, these tests provide sufficient documentation of infection that a urine culture and susceptibility testing can be omitted and the patient treated empirically. Urine culture should be obtained, however, in patients in whom symptoms and urine examination findings leave the diagnosis of cystitis in question. Pretherapy cultures and susceptibility testing are also essential in the management of patients with suspected upper tract infections and those in whom complicating factors are present, since in these situations a variety of pathogens may be present and antibiotic therapy is best tailored to the individual organism.

TREATMENT Several therapeutic principles should underlie treatment of urinary tract infections:

1 In most circumstances a quantitative urine culture, a positive Gram stain, or an alternative rapid diagnostic test should be obtained to confirm infection before starting treatment. When cultures are obtained, antimicrobial sensitivity testing should be used to direct therapy.
2 Factors predisposing to infection, such as obstruction, neurogenic bladder, calculi, etc., should be identified and corrected if possible.
3 Relief of clinical symptoms does not always indicate bacteriologic cure.
4 After completion of therapy, each treatment episode should be classified as a failure (bacteriuria not eradicated during therapy or upon the immediate posttreatment culture) or a cure (resolution of symptoms and elimination of bacteriuria). Recurrent infections should be classified as same strain or different strain and early or late.
5 In general, uncomplicated infections confined to the lower urinary tract respond to low doses and short courses of therapy, while upper tract infections require longer periods of treatment. After

therapy, early recurrences with the same strain may result from an unresolved upper tract focus of infection but often (especially after short-course therapy) result from persistent vaginal colonization rather than from recurrent bladder infection. Recurrences that occur more than 2 weeks after the cessation of therapy are nearly always reinfections, even though some may be with the same strain.

6 Community-acquired infections, especially initial infections, are nearly always due to antibiotic-sensitive strains.

7 Patients with repeated infections, instrumentation, or recent hospitalization should be suspected of harboring resistant strains.

The anatomic location of a urinary tract infection greatly influences success or failure of a therapeutic agent. Bladder bacteriuria (cystitis) can usually be eliminated with nearly any antimicrobial to which the infecting strain is sensitive; as little as a single dose of 500-mg intramuscular kanamycin eliminates bladder bacteriuria in most patients. A 7-day course of therapy with oral drugs appears more than adequate. With upper tract infections, however, single-dose therapy fails in the majority of cases and even a 7-day course will be unsuccessful in many patients. Longer periods of treatment (2 to 6 weeks) aimed at eradicating a persistent focus of infection may be necessary in some cases.

In *acute uncomplicated cystitis,* more than 90 percent of infections are due to *E. coli,* and although resistance patterns vary geographically, most strains are sensitive to many antibiotics. Single-dose trimethoprim-sulfamethoxazole (4 to 6 single-strength tablets), trimethoprim (400 mg), and sulfa alone (2.0 g) have been used successfully to treat acute uncomplicated episodes of cystitis. A single 3-g dose of amoxicillin (amoxicilline) appears to result in lower cure rates than the other three agents, especially in women infected with amoxicillin-resistant strains. In most areas, about one-third of *E. coli* strains causing acute cystitis are amoxicillin-resistant. The advantages of single-dose therapy include less expense, ensured compliance, fewer side effects, and perhaps less intense selective pressure for emergence of resistant organisms in the gut or vaginal or perineal flora. However, two studies suggest that more recurrences with the same strain occur shortly after single-dose therapy than after longer treatment and that single-dose therapy does not effectively eradicate vaginal colonization with *E. coli.* Nevertheless, single-dose therapy does appear safe and efficacious for women presenting with *acute uncomplicated cystitis.* Single-dose therapy should be used only in reliable patients, in whom posttreatment follow-up can be ensured, and in patients in whom symptoms have been present for less than 10 days. Three days of therapy may preserve the lower side effects rate of single-dose therapy but may improve efficacy. Single-dose therapy should not be used in women with symptoms or signs of pyelonephritis and in women with urologic abnormalities or stones, or in women with previous infections due to antibiotic-resistant organisms. In these populations, 7 days of therapy with the antimicrobials listed above should be given. Alternatively, broader spectrum agents such as an oral cephalosporin, norfloxacin, or ciprofloxacin can be used. Males with urinary tract infection often have urologic abnormalities or prostatic involvement and positive antibody-coated-bacterial bacteriuria, and hence are not candidates for single-dose or 3-day therapy.

Treatment of the acute urethritis in women depends upon the etiologic agent involved. In chlamydial infection, doxycycline (100 mg orally bid for 7 days) should be used. Women with acute dysuria and frequency, negative urine cultures, and no pyuria do not usually respond to antimicrobial agents.

Acute pyelonephritis without accompanying clinical evidence of calculi or urologic disease is due to *E. coli* in most cases. Although the optimal route and duration of therapy have not been established, a 10- to 14-day course of trimethoprim-sulfamethoxazole, trimethoprim alone, an aminoglycoside, or a cephalosporin usually provides adequate therapy. Ampicillin or amoxicillin should not be used as initial therapy since 20 to 30 percent of *E. coli* are now resistant in vitro. Intravenous antibiotics, at least for the first several days of treatment, should probably be given to most patients, but minimally

symptomatic patients can be treated with 2 weeks of oral antibiotics. Some patients relapse following therapy and should be investigated to determine whether unrecognized suppurative foci, calculi, or urologic disease is present. If not, treatment should be extended to 2 to 6 weeks to eliminate a presumed upper tract focus causing recurrent bacteriuria.

When suspected *gram-negative sepsis* complicates acute pyelonephritis, hospitalization, prompt parenteral therapy with an aminoglycoside, and ancillary measures to treat sepsis should be provided (see Chap. 89). When the antibiotic sensitivities of the infecting strain are available, therapy can be changed to a less toxic agent. Similar therapy should be used for infected patients with calculi or urologic abnormalities who have suspected sepsis.

In *pregnancy,* acute cystitis can be managed with 7 days of amoxicillin, nitrofurantoin, or a cephalosporin. After treatment, a culture should be obtained to ensure cure and repeated monthly thereafter. Acute pyelonephritis in pregnancy should be managed by hospitalization and parenteral antibiotics, generally a cephalosporin or an extended-spectrum penicillin. Continuous low-dose prophylaxis with nitrofurantoin should be given to women who have recurrent infections during pregnancy.

Asymptomatic bacteriuria should be documented with at least two positive cultures before treatment is given. Seven days of an oral agent to which the organism is sensitive should be given initially. If bacteriuria persists, it can be followed without further treatment in most patients. In patients who may be at high risk because of neutropenia, compromised host defenses, renal transplant, or previous development of pyelonephritis or bacteremia, further treatment with either 6 weeks of oral therapy or 4 to 6 weeks of combined parenteral and oral therapy should be given.

Optimal treatment regimens for patients with *catheter-associated urinary tract infections* have not been well established. These infections often remit spontaneously or with short-term antibiotic therapy if the catheter can be removed. If the catheter cannot be removed, systemic antibiotics or urinary antiseptics may reduce bacteriuria, but do not usually eliminate it. Asymptomatic bacteriuria in catheterized patients can probably be left untreated in most patients who are not immunosuppressed or who are not at high risk for sepsis because of old age, severe underlying disease, diabetes, or pregnancy.

UROLOGIC EVALUATION   Very few women with recurrent urinary tract infections have correctable lesions discovered at cystoscopy or upon intravenous pyelography, and these procedures should not be routinely performed in such patients. In selected women, namely those with relapsing infection, those with a history of childhood infections, those with stones or painless hematuria, and those with recurrent pyelonephritis, urologic evaluation should be performed. All males with urinary infection should be evaluated urologically. Men or women presenting with acute infection and signs or symptoms suggestive of an obstruction or stones should undergo urologic evaluation, generally by means of ultrasound.

PROGNOSIS   In patients with uncomplicated cystitis or pyelonephritis, treatment ordinarily results in complete resolution of symptoms. In fact, symptoms usually remit even without specific therapy. Lower tract infections in adult women are of concern mainly because they cause discomfort, minor morbidity, and time lost from work. Cystitis may also result in upper tract infection or in bacteremia (especially during instrumentation), but there is little evidence to suggest that renal impairment follows. When repeated episodes of cystitis occur, they are nearly always reinfections, not relapses. Why a significant subpopulation of adult women develops a predisposition to multiple recurrent infections remains poorly understood. In some cases, residual urine, urethral stenosis, or other anatomic explanations exist, but most women with recurrent infections have no such demonstrable abnormality. Their uroepithelial cells appear highly prone to persistent colonization with *E. coli;* the explanation for this phenomenon is not clear.

Uncomplicated acute pyelonephritis in adults rarely progresses to functional impairment and chronic renal disease. Repeated upper tract infections often indicate relapse rather than reinfection, and a vigorous search for renal calculi or an underlying urologic abnormality should be undertaken. If neither is found, 6 weeks of chemotherapy may be useful in eradicating an unresolved focus of infection.

Repeated symptomatic urinary tract infections in children, and in adults with obstructive uropathy, neurogenic bladder, structural renal disease, or diabetes more often progress to chronic renal disease. Asymptomatic bacteriuria in these groups, as well as in adults without urologic disease or obstruction, predisposes to increased episodes of symptomatic infection but does not result in renal impairment in most instances.

PREVENTION Patients with frequent symptomatic infections may benefit from long-term low-dose antibiotics directed at preventing recurrences. A single dose of trimethoprim-sulfamethoxazole (80 mg trimethoprim and 400 mg sulfamethoxazole daily), trimethoprim alone (100 mg daily), or nitrofurantoin (50 mg daily) have been particularly effective. Prophylaxis should be initiated only after bacteriuria has been eradicated with a full-dose treatment regimen. Women having more than two infections every 6 months should be considered for preventive antibiotics. Low-dose antibiotics (nitrofurantoin 50 to 100 mg) after sexual intercourse may also be of benefit in preventing episodes of symptomatic infections. Other patients for whom prophylaxis appears to have some merit include men with chronic prostatitis; patients undergoing prostatectomy, both during the operation and in the postoperative period; and pregnant women with asymptomatic bacteriuria. All pregnant women should be screened for bacteriuria in the first trimester, and should be treated if bacteriuria is found.

CHRONIC PYELONEPHRITIS

Chronic interstitial nephritis thought to result from bacterial infection of the kidney has been termed *chronic pyelonephritis*. It may occur in patients with predisposing urologic abnormalities (obstruction, vesicoureteral reflux, or neurogenic bladder) or in patients with apparently normal urinary tracts. Unlike acute urinary tract infections, for which simple diagnostic criteria and characteristic clinical syndromes exist, no pathognomonic clinical, laboratory, or pathologic criteria can be used to identify cases of chronic pyelonephritis, and few reliable data on the incidence or prevalence of this condition have been collected. Many patients with renal lesions that fulfill the pathologic criteria for chronic pyelonephritis at autopsy have sterile urine cultures and were not known to have had clinical episodes of bacterial urinary tract infection or urinary obstruction during life. Such cases suggest that other forms of renal injury result in morphologic changes indistinguishable from those produced by bacterial infection. Conversely, relatively few individuals with acute urinary infection develop chronic infection or progressive renal impairment. Most often, this occurs in patients with anatomic obstruction, neurogenic bladder, or vesicoureteral reflux.

Patients with many episodes of urinary tract infection; impaired renal function; pyuria with white cell casts; bacteriuria; an intravenous pyelogram showing an irregularly outlined renal pelvis with caliectasis and cortical scars; and typical pathologic changes can be diagnosed as having chronic pyelonephritis. In less typical patients, the relationship of infection to renal damage is uncertain and the diagnosis often remains unclear.

PAPILLARY NECROSIS

The renal papilla is of major importance in the pathogenesis of chronic interstitial nephritis and, when complicated by bacterial infection, pyelonephritis. It has become evident that a variety of underlying conditions cause primary renal papillary damage, resulting eventually in the renal lesions of chronic interstitial nephritis. When urinary infection does not supervene, the resulting renal disease may progress slowly and silently to the point of renal insufficiency. The pathology of this renal injury may be indistinguishable from that of pyelonephritis. In addition to common diseases such as gout and diabetes mellitus, which cause renal papillary damage, many medications, which achieve enormous concentrations in the urine traversing the renal papilla, may be toxic for that zone of the kidney. The best known of these are phenacetin-containing analgesic mixtures. This problem is much more common than generally recognized, and diagnosis requires a careful history.

It is not known how many other substances may be important in the pathogenesis of primary renal papillary disease. However, in view of the benignity of urinary infection in persons without underlying renal papillary damage, it is reasonable to assume the presence of primary underlying renal papillary damage in any patient with urinary infection who shows the development of or progression to renal damage.

When severe infection of the renal pyramids is present in association with vascular diseases of the kidney or with urinary tract obstruction, renal papillary necrosis is likely to result. Patients with diabetes, sickle cell disease, chronic alcoholism, and vascular disease seem peculiarly susceptible to this complication. Hematuria, pain in the flank or abdomen, and chills and fever are the most common presenting symptoms. Acute renal failure with oliguria or anuria sometimes occurs. Rarely, sloughing of a pyramid may take place without symptoms in a patient with chronic urinary infection, and the diagnosis is made when the necrotic tissue is passed in the urine or identified as a "ring shadow" on pyelography. If renal function deteriorates suddenly in a diabetic or a patient with chronic obstruction, the diagnosis of renal papillary necrosis should be entertained, even in the absence of fever or pain. Although renal papillary necrosis is often bilateral, when it is unilateral, nephrectomy may be lifesaving in the management of overwhelming infection.

RENAL AND PERINEPHRIC ABSCESS

See Chap. 91.

PROSTATITIS

The term *prostatitis* has been used for various inflammatory conditions affecting the prostate, including acute and chronic infections with specific bacteria and, more commonly, instances in which signs and symptoms of prostatic inflammation are present but no specific organisms can be detected. To classify patients with suspected prostatitis correctly, each patient should be evaluated using first-void and midstream urine specimens, a prostatic expressate, and a post-massage urine specimen. All specimens should be quantitatively cultured and evaluated for numbers of leukocytes. Based on the results of these studies, patients can be classified as having acute or chronic bacterial prostatitis, nonbacterial prostatitis, or prostatodynia. Patients with suspected prostatitis usually have low back pain, perineal or testicular discomfort, mild dysuria, and lower urinary obstructive symptoms. Microscopic pyuria may be the only objective manifestation of prostatic disease.

ACUTE BACTERIAL PROSTATITIS This disease generally affects young male adults when it occurs spontaneously, but it may also be associated with an indwelling urethral catheter. It is characterized by fever, chills, dysuria, and a tense or boggy, extremely tender prostate on examination. Although prostatic massage usually produces purulent secretions with a large number of bacteria on culture, bacteremia may result from manipulation of the inflamed gland. For this reason, and because the etiologic agent can usually be identified on urine Gram stain and culture, vigorous prostatic massage should be avoided. In non-catheter-associated cases, the infection is generally due to one of the common gram-negative urinary tract pathogens or *Staphylococcus aureus*. Initially, intravenous trimethoprim-sulfamethoxazole, a cephalosporin, or an aminoglycoside can be utilized if gram-negative rods are seen in the urine Gram stain, and a cephalosporin or nafcillin if gram-positive cocci are seen. Although these drugs do not readily diffuse into the noninflamed prostate gland, the response to antibiotics is usually prompt, perhaps because drugs penetrate more readily into the acutely inflamed prostate. In catheter-associated cases, a broader spectrum of etiologic agents is seen, including hospital-acquired gram-negative rods and enterococci. In such cases, an aminoglycoside or a third-generation cephalosporin should be used for initial therapy until the organism has been isolated and susceptibilities determined. The long-term prognosis is good, although in some instances acute infection may result in abscess formation, epididymoorchitis, seminal vesiculitis, septicemia, and residual chronic bacterial prostatitis. Since the advent of antibiotics, the frequency of acute bacterial prostatitis has diminished markedly. Many so-called cases of acute prostatitis are probably posterior urethritis.

CHRONIC BACTERIAL PROSTATITIS This entity is a major cause of recurrent bacteriuria in males but may be difficult to diagnose. Symptoms are usually absent, the prostate feels normal on palpation, and although many white blood cells may be seen in the urinary sediment, results of conventional bacteriologic studies are often negative. Bacteria may be cultured from the expressed prostatic secretion or postmassage urine. The presence of these bacteria can be determined only by careful quantitative bacteriologic techniques when the bladder urine is sterile. Intermittently, symptoms of frequency, urgency, and dysuria occur when infection spreads to the bladder urine. The pattern of recurrent bladder infection in the male with chronic bacterial prostatitis is clinically not very different from that seen in the recurrent cystourethritis of the female. Antibiotics promptly relieve the symptoms associated with acute exacerbations, but have been less effective in eradicating the focus of chronic infection in the prostate. The relative ineffectiveness of antimicrobials, in terms of long-term cure, in part results from the poor penetration of most antibiotics into the prostate because the low pH which prevails in this organ precludes solubility of most drugs. Macrolides (erythromycin) do enter the prostatic secretions, but these agents are generally ineffective against gram-negative organisms. Sulfonamide-trimethoprim and the fluoroquinolines have been employed successfully in some cases, but they must be given for at least 12 weeks to be effective. Patients with frequent episodes of acute cystitis should be treated with prolonged courses of antimicrobials (usually sulfonamide, trimethoprim, or nitrofurantoin), with a view toward suppressing symptoms and keeping the bladder urine sterile. Total prostatectomy produces cure of chronic prostatitis but is associated with considerable morbidity. Transurethral prostatectomy is safer but cures only one-third of patients.

NONBACTERIAL PROSTATITIS Patients who present with symptoms and signs of prostatitis, increased leukocytes in their expressed prostatic secretions and postmassage urine, and no bacterial growth in cultures are classified as having nonbacterial prostatitis. Prostatic inflammation can be considered present when the expressed prostatic secretion and postmassage urine contain at least tenfold more leukocytes than the first-void and midstream specimens, or when the expressed prostatic secretion contains ≥1000 leukocytes per microliter. The presumed infectious etiology of this condition remains unidentified. Evidence for the causative role of both *Ureaplasma urealyticum* and *Chlamydia trachomatis* has been presented, but is not conclusive. Since most cases of nonbacterial prostatitis occur in young, sexually active men, and since many cases arise following an episode of nonspecific urethritis, the causative agent may well be sexually transmitted. The effectiveness of antimicrobial agents in this condition remains uncertain. Some patients benefit from a 4- to 6-week course of erythromycin, doxycycline, or trimethoprim-sulfamethoxazole, but controlled trials are lacking.

PROSTATODYNIA Patients who have symptoms and signs of prostatitis but no evidence of prostatic inflammation (normal leukocyte counts) and negative urine cultures are classified as having prostatodynia. Despite their symptoms, these patients most likely do not have prostatic infection and should not be given antimicrobial agents.

REFERENCES

BAILEY RR: Single-dose therapy for uncomplicated urinary tract infections. NZ Med J 98:327, 1985

JOHNSON JR, STAMM WE: Diagnosis and treatment of acute urinary tract infections. Infect Dis Clin North Am 1:773, 1987

KOMAROFF AL: Acute dysuria in women. N Engl J Med 310:368, 1984

———: Urinalysis and urine culture in women with dysuria. Ann Intern Med 104:212, 1986

KRIEGER JN: Complications and treatment of urinary tract infections during pregnancy. Urol Clin North Am 13:685, 1986

KUNIN CM: Use of antimicrobial agents in treating urinary tract infection. Adv Nephrol 14:39, 1985

———: *Detection, Prevention and Management of Urinary Tract Infections*, 4th ed. Philadelphia, Lea & Febiger, 1987

LIPSKY BA: Urinary tract infections in men. Ann Intern Med 110:138, 1989

MEARES EM JR: Acute and chronic prostatitis: Diagnosis and treatment. Infect Dis Clin North Am 1:855, 1987

PEZZLO M: Detection of urinary tract infections by rapid methods. Clin Microbiol Rev 1:268, 1988

RONALD AR: Current concepts in the management of urinary tract infections in adults. Med Clin North Am 68:335, 1984

STAMM WE et al: Causes of the acute urethral syndrome in women. N Engl J Med 303:409, 1980

——— et al: Diagnosis of coliform infection in acutely dysuric women. N Engl J Med 307:463, 1982

——— et al: Urinary tract infections: From pathogenesis to treatment. J Infect Dis 159:400, 1989

SVANBORG-EDEN C et al: Host-parasite relationship in urinary tract infection. J Infect Dis 157:421, 1988

WARREN JW: Catheter-associated urinary tract infections. Infect Dis Clin North Am 1:823, 1987

96   INFECTIOUS ARTHRITIS

DANIEL ROTROSEN

NONGONOCOCCAL SEPTIC ARTHRITIS Acute bacterial arthritis is a common medical problem affecting individuals of all ages. Prompt recognition and treatment are important to avoid permanent articular disability.

Etiology, pathogenesis, and predisposing factors Approximately 75 percent of nongonococcal pyoarthroses are due to gram-positive cocci, particularly *Staphylococcus aureus*. Pneumococci and group A beta-hemolytic and viridans streptococci collectively account for less than half of these. Among immunocompromised individuals, group G streptococci are an infrequent cause of septic arthritis, and group B streptococci are an important cause of arthritis in neonates. *Staphylococcus epidermidis* is the leading cause of prosthetic joint infection.

Gram-negative bacilli account for approximately 20 percent of cases, typically in patients with obvious risk factors for gram-negative bacteremia. *Pseudomonas aeruginosa* is an important cause of septic arthritis in intravenous drug addicts and neonates. *Haemophilus influenzae* type B is a prominent cause of pyoarthrosis among children under age 5.

Septic arthritis usually results from direct hematogenous seeding of the synovium. Conditions which predispose to septic arthritis include infancy, immunosuppressive therapy, alcoholism, drug abuse, some chronic systemic illnesses, hemoglobinopathies, complement and immunoglobulin deficiencies, phagocytic cell dysfunction, chronic arthritis, and previous joint damage. Infection may occur as a complication of arthroscopy, intraarticular glucocorticoid injection, or prosthetic joint surgery. A history of minor joint trauma is a common but often overlooked feature in patients with suppurative arthritis. An extraarticular focus of infection (e.g., cutaneous abscesses) can be identified in about 25 percent of patients and can be useful in both establishing a cause and choosing antibiotics before joint fluid culture results are available.

The synovium is well vascularized and lacks a limiting basement membrane, allowing relatively free access of bloodborne microorganisms to the joint space once extravasation has occurred. In experimentally induced arthritis, microorganisms are found scattered throughout the synovium 1 to 2 h after inoculation. Within 1 to 2 days vascular congestion, leukocyte infiltration, and hyperplasia of the synovial lining cells are prominent. The host response may be sufficient to eradicate infection in some cases, but early changes usually progress to purulent effusion accompanied by microabscess formation within the synovium and subchondral bone. Increased intraarticular pressure causes ischemia and impairs cartilage biomechanics and nutrition; chondrolytic enzymes released from neutrophils contribute to the destruction of articular cartilage, subchondral bone, and joint capsule. Irreversible changes may ensue as a consequence of synovial lining cell proliferation, mononuclear cell infiltration, and the appearance of granulation tissue; such changes may appear as early as 1 week after infection begins.

Clinical and experimental observations suggest that host immune mechanisms play a critical role in the development and maintenance of synovial inflammation. Sterile bacterial products, including endotoxins, exotoxins, and cell wall peptidoglycan induce acute and chronic arthritis in laboratory animals. Deposition of immune complexes in synovium and periarticular tissues may be followed by a sterile synovitis during the convalescent phase of certain bacterial and viral infections. Individuals who develop postinfectious arthritis or Reiter's syndrome following *Shigella*, *Salmonella*, *Yersinia*, and *Campylobacter* infection of the gastrointestinal tract are more likely than matched controls to have the specific histocompatibility antigen HLA-B27.

Manifestations Nongonococcal septic arthritis presents as a monarticular synovitis with a predilection for large weight-bearing joints. The knee is the most frequently involved joint in children and adults, followed by the hip. The ankle, wrist, elbow, shoulder, sternoclavicular, and sacroiliac joints are involved less often. The interphalangeal joints are rarely affected in bacterial arthritis, except in patients with gonococcal synovitis or mycobacterial infection. Gram-positive coccal arthritis usually presents as an acute illness with severe constitutional symptoms accompanied by swelling, pain, warmth, and restricted motion of the involved joint. In septic arthritis of the hip, effusion may not be readily appreciated, and pain may be minimal or referred to the groin, buttock, lateral thigh, or anterior knee. Patients with suppurative arthritis usually seek medical attention within 3 to 4 days of the onset of symptoms. Signs of inflammation may be masked in patients taking glucocorticoids or other immunosuppressive medications and in those with chronic debilitating illnesses. Individuals with coexistent rheumatoid or gouty arthritis often attribute their symptoms to a flare-up of the underlying disease and consequently delay medical evaluation. In this setting a high degree of suspicion is warranted, and studies to exclude infection are important when articular symptoms fail to respond to anti-inflammatory agents.

If medical attention is sought early in the illness, a source of bacteremia is usually identified, and the responsible pathogen can be isolated from the blood in about 50 percent of cases. In contrast, gram-negative bacillary arthritis follows a more indolent course with moderate constitutional symptoms and less prominent articular complaints. These differences contribute to the more prolonged time to diagnosis in gram-negative bacillary arthritis (typically 3 weeks from the onset of symptoms) and to the high incidence of coexistent osteomyelitis at the time of diagnosis. Rarely, *S. aureus* may have a less acute presentation when it causes arthritis (see Chap. 100).

Prosthetic joint infection is associated with mild symptoms and an indolent course resulting in a mean diagnostic delay of 2 to 8 months. *S. epidermidis* and *S. aureus* account for most of these infections, but multiple organisms, gram-negative bacilli, and anaerobes are not uncommon. Infection occurs in 1 to 4 percent of

prostheses followed for 10 years and is more frequent after revision of a previous total joint replacement. It invariably is accompanied by osteomyelitis at the site of implantation. Eradication of the infection usually requires removal of the prosthesis.

Certain pathogens are likely to cause infection at unusual sites. Spinal arthritis is most often associated with osteomyelitis of adjacent vertebral bodies. It is usually due to *S. aureus*, but *Brucella*, *Salmonella*, and *Mycobacterium tuberculosis* also preferentially involve the spine. Among intravenous drug addicts, *P. aeruginosa* infection can occur in the sternoclavicular and sacroiliac joints.

Laboratory findings and diagnosis Analysis of synovial fluid is essential in the evaluation of suspected bacterial arthritis. Fluid sufficient for complete analysis can usually be obtained by percutaneous arthrocentesis. Care should be taken not to contaminate the joint space by inserting the needle through an area of overlying cellulitis or through an infected bursa. Fluoroscopic guidance may facilitate aspiration of the hip, shoulder, spinal, or sacroiliac joints. When joints are difficult to aspirate, arthrotomy may be required to obtain fluid or synovial tissue. Synovial fluid in septic arthritis is usually turbid or grossly purulent. The synovial fluid leukocyte count is greater than 100,000 per microliter (range < 10,000 to > 300,000 per microliter, usually > 90 percent polymorphonuclear neutrophils) in one-third to one-half of patients. In patients with unexpectedly low leukocyte counts on initial evaluation, repeat joint aspiration 12 to 24 h later almost always demonstrates leukocytosis. The synovial fluid leukocyte count and differential are of limited diagnostic utility due to considerable overlap with values in other acute inflammatory arthritides. However, serial counts are important in monitoring response to therapy.

Gram's stain of synovial fluid is important in establishing an etiologic diagnosis of septic arthritis. Stains are positive in 75 to 95 percent of gram-positive coccal and in approximately 50 percent of gram-negative bacillary infections. Regardless of the results of Gram's stain, synovial fluid should be cultured aerobically and anaerobically to identify the specific pathogen and provide data on antimicrobial sensitivity. Joint fluid cultures are positive in most patients with nongonococcal bacterial arthritis. If the patient has taken oral antibiotics prior to arthrocentesis, the microbiology laboratory should be notified, because growth of the organism may be delayed and cultures may require special handling. Blood cultures should be obtained, and a diligent search should be made for occult sources of bacteremia. Bacterial antigen detection by counterimmunoelectrophoresis has been advocated as a rapid diagnostic test for certain etiologic agents (e.g., *Streptococcus pneumoniae* and *H. influenzae*), but is not widely used.

In septic arthritis the synovial fluid glucose level may be low and lactate elevated, compared to the corresponding levels in serum, but neither test is sufficiently sensitive or specific to be of general diagnostic utility. Elevated synovial fluid protein and poor mucin clot are diagnostically nonspecific.

Unless arthritis arises by extension of adjacent osteomyelitis, distention of the joint capsule and periarticular soft tissue swelling are the only radiographic findings expected on initial evaluation. Nonetheless, early films are useful to establish a baseline for subsequent evaluation. Destructive changes are rarely noted radiologically before the second to third week of untreated infection. At that time, periosteal elevation, juxtaarticular osteoporosis, bony erosions on the articular surface, and joint space narrowing due to cartilage destruction may be apparent. In prosthetic joint infection radiographic evidences of implant loosening and ostemyelitis are usually seen.

In the setting of staphylococcal or gram-negative bacillary arthritis, computed tomography (CT) or magnetic resonance imaging (MRI) of involved joints is helpful, particularly when the sternoclavicular joint or the hip is involved. These joints are poorly visualized by conventional techniques, and CT or MRI may reveal extensive bony involvement and parasynovial abscesses when conventional x-ray films are negative. Such findings have important implications for surgical intervention and for the duration of antimicrobial therapy.

Radioisotope scans lack diagnostic specificity and may be positive in noninfectious inflammatory joint disease. However, scans are useful to identify inapparent foci of osteomyelitis and to bolster suspicions of low-grade infection in the hip, shoulder, spine, and sacroiliac joints.

Other conditions to be considered in the differential diagnosis of oligoarticular arthritis include septic bursitis (usually olecranon or prepatellar), juvenile rheumatoid arthritis, psoriatic arthritis, acute rheumatic fever, Reiter's syndrome, sarcoid arthropathy, trauma, villonodular synovitis, aseptic necrosis, and intermittent hydroarthrosis. Infection that can present as oligoarticular arthritis include Lyme disease and infections caused by mycobacteria and fungi.

Management and outcome Optimal management of suppurative arthritis includes parenteral antimicrobial therapy, joint drainage, and articular rest. Most antibiotics achieve therapeutic levels in the infected joint following parenteral administration. There is accordingly no rationale for intraarticular administration of antibiotics, and in fact, direct injection of certain antibiotics can induce chemical synovitis. The initial choice of antibiotics should be guided by Gram's stain of synovial fluid and revised as dictated by culture results. Antibiotic regimens for specific organisms are provided in the chapters dealing with these organisms and in Chap. 85, which details the properties of each antibiotic. When no organisms are seen on Gram's stain, the antimicrobial regimen should be tailored to cover the likely pathogens based on the patient's age and the clinical setting. Infants under 1 month of age should be treated with a semisynthetic penicillin and an aminoglycoside to provide coverage against *S. aureus,* gram-negative bacilli, and group B streptococci. In children under 5 years of age therapy should be targeted against *S. aureus* and ampicillin-resistant *H. influenza.* Children over 5 years and adults should receive a semisynthetic penicillin and an aminoglycoside until culture results are available. Vancomycin is the drug of choice in patients with serious penicillin allergy and may be required in prosthetic joint infection due to methicillin-resistant *S. epidermidis.* The results of single-drug therapy of gram-negative bacillary arthritis have been disappointing, despite in vitro sensitivity to the agents used. Because of the high rates of failure and relapse in this setting combination chemotherapy is generally advised. After an initial clinical response (and if in vitro sensitivities permit) substitution of a newer β-lactam or quinolone antibiotic may be advisable to avoid the toxicities of prolonged aminoglycoside therapy.

Most cases of streptococcal arthritis are cured by a 10- to 14-day course of antibiotics, whereas staphylococcal and gram-negative bacillary infections require longer treatment, usually 3 to 6 weeks, particularly with complicating osteomyelitis. Drainage of purulent joint fluid is essential to relieve pain, diminish the risk of loculation and pressure necrosis, and remove chondrolytic products that promote destructive changes within the joint. As with other closed space infections, drainage of acidic, purulent fluid improves the bactericidal activity of neutrophils, cell-wall-active antibiotics, and aminoglycosides. Percutaneous needle aspiration and joint irrigation can be performed daily or twice daily for the first 5 to 7 days of therapy. The development of loculations, continued culture positivity, or persistence of a purulent effusion beyond that time are indications that arthroscopy or open drainage may be required. When the hip joint is involved, surgical intervention is usually warranted from the outset, especially in children, due to the technical difficulty of repeated percutaneous aspiration and the risk of vascular compromise from elevated intracapsular pressure. Early exploratory arthrotomy and open drainage have been beneficial in septic arthritis of the shoulder and sternoclavicular joints. Persistently positive cultures despite adequate drainage are an indication for reculture of the fluid to exclude emergence of antibiotic-resistant strains.

During the acute phase the joint should be immobilized in a position that minimizes capsular tension, usually midway between full extension and flexion. Passive range-of-motion exercises should be started as the synovitis improves, but weight bearing should be avoided until pain and signs of inflammation are gone.

Most cases of streptococcal arthritis resolve without sequelae, whereas in staphylococcal and gram-negative bacillary arthritis the response is generally less salutary. In this setting healing may be delayed by a sterile, postinfectious synovitis. Despite microbiologic cure such patients may be left with limitation of motion and persistence of pain. Other major determinants of a poor outcome are failure to recognize and treat the infection within 7 days of onset and involvement of the hip joint. In children with hip or ankle arthritis impaired ambulation and shortening of the extremity are not uncommon.

GONOCCOCAL ARTHRITIS (See Chap. 110) Gonoccocal infection is the leading cause of bacterial arthritis in young adults and the most common form of infectious arthritis seen at urban medical centers. It may be a complication of sexual abuse in young children. In disseminated gonococcal infection an early arthritis-dermatitis syndrome is typically followed by a joint-localization stage. The early phase is characterized by constitutional symptoms, migratory tenosynovitis and arthralgias, vesiculopustular skin lesions, and minimal joint effusion. The knee, shoulder, wrist, and interphalangeal joints of the hands are commonly involved. Cultures of blood and skin lesions may be positive at this stage of the illness, whereas culture and Gram's stain of synovial fluid are usually negative. A presumptive diagnosis can be made if the gonococcus is isolated from a silent primary focus (e.g., urogenital tract, pharynx, or rectum). Without treatment, constitutional symptoms and dermatitis usually abate, but joint involvement progresses to a purulent mon- or pauciarticular arthritis. Synovial fluid cultures may be positive at this stage whereas blood cultures are almost always negative. In 30 to 40 percent of patients a biphasic pattern of illness is not observed, and some patients present with a monarticular purulent arthritis and few systemic manifestations. Terminal complement component deficiencies, menstruation, and pregnancy predispose to gonococcal dissemination.

The differential diagnosis of disseminated gonoccocal infection includes acute rheumatic fever, Reiter's syndrome, chronic meningococcemia, and *Streptobacillus moniliformis* infection. In Reiter's syndrome constitutional toxicity is usually less pronounced, there is often a history of symptomatic urethritis and conjunctivitis, and distinct, but subtle mucocutaneous lesions are usually present. Sacroiliitis and Achilles tendonitis are more common in Reiter's syndrome, but involvement of the upper extremity, especially the wrist, is unusual. A clinical response to antibiotics (in gonoccocal disease) or to salicylates (in rheumatic fever) may help to differentiate among these syndromes.

In the United States most gonococcal isolates causing disseminated infection are penicillin-sensitive, enabling treatment with oral antibiotics on an outpatient basis. Hospitalization and administration of parenteral antibiotics are warranted for unreliable patients and for those with purulent monarticular arthritis or uncertain diagnoses. In documented penicillin resistance ceftriaxone or spectinomycin is effective. Penicillin-resistant species are more common in the Philippines, southeast Asia, and Africa (see Chap. 110).

CHRONIC MONARTICULAR ARTHRITIS Certain mycobacteria and fungi cause chronic oligoarticular arthritis that is clinically and histologically distinct from other forms of septic arthritis.

Tuberculous arthritis (See Chap. 125) *Mycobacterium tuberculosis* causes a slowly progressive arthritis that is monarticular in up to 90 percent of cases. With the decline in primary tuberculosis in developed countries, spinal arthritis is rare, and involvement of the knee, hip, wrist, ankle, or small joints of the hand is more common. These sites become infected by reactivation of long-dormant lymphohematogenous foci. Rupture of such a focus (often in the epiphyseal region of long bones) into the joint space causes effusion and a progressive granulomatous reaction of synovial membranes, articular cartilage, and tendons. Localized pain may precede other signs of inflammation or x-ray changes by weeks or even months. The insidious nature of the infection usually delays diagnosis by weeks or months (the average time elapsed was 19 weeks from onset in one series). The granulomatous process eventually imparts a boggy, doughy feeling to the joint and periarticular structures. Cold abscesses and draining sinuses may develop. Constitutional symptoms are not prominent, and active pulmonary tuberculosis is unusual. Most patients are tuberculin-positive. Radiographs initially show subchondral osteoporosis and periarticular bone destruction with overlying periosteal thickening. Eventually, destructive changes are noted within the joint. The synovial fluid leukocyte count ranges from about 1000 to >100,000 per microliter (average about 15,000 per microliter) with a preponderance of polymorphonuclear neutrophils when counts are high, but frankly purulent fluid is uncommon. Acid-fast bacilli are not often seen on smears of synovial fluid (approximately 20 percent yield), but cultures of synovial fluid or tissue are positive in 80 to 90 percent of cases. Demonstration of characteristic granulomatous changes with or without caseation on synovial biopsy is sufficient evidence to initiate antituberculous therapy while awaiting culture and sensitivity results. Infection due to atypical mycobacteria (e.g., *M. kansasii, M. marinum, M. avium-intracellulare*) may produce a chronic granulomatous arthritis with similar clinical and histopathologic features. The correct diagnosis and choice of an appropriate antimicrobial regimen depend on isolation of the organism from synovial fluid or tissues. For treatment of tuberculosis and nontuberculous mycobacterial infection see Chaps. 125 and 127. In spinal tuberculosis surgery is usually reserved for drainage of abscesses or stabilization of the spine and is rarely required for treatment of other joints. Arthritis due to *Brucella* sp., *Nocardia asteroides,* and fungi may resemble mycobacterial infection.

Fungal arthritis Any of the invasive mycoses may infect bone and articular structures (see Chap. 151). With the exception of acute arthritis due to *Candida* sp. or blastomycosis, the fungal arthritides tend to be slowly progressive and may elude accurate diagnosis for months or years. All show a predilection for involvement of large weight-bearing joints, especially the knee. While common in blastomycotic arthritis, a history of serious underlying illness in other fungal arthritides is often absent, and joint infection usually occurs without obvious evidence of extraarticular dissemination.

In acute pulmonary *coccidioidomycosis,* benign, self-limited, sterile synovitis occurs as a component of the acute hypersensitivity syndrome known as "desert fever." Persistent coccidioidal synovitis may arise via direct hematogenous seeding of the synovium or via extension from an adjacent osteomyelitic focus. In the former case the disease tends to follow an indolent course with recurrent effusion, maintenance of joint space integrity, no evidence of osteomyelitis, and only late progression to a destructive villonodular arthritis with pannus formation. With extension from an adjacent bony focus effusion is less prominent, and destructive changes tend to occur earlier. Diagnosis depends on culture and histology of synovial tissue; joint fluid cultures are positive in <5 percent of cases.

Sporotrichotic arthritis usually occurs in the complete absence of the more familiar lymphocutaneous syndrome. There is a predilection for involvement of the small joints of the hand and wrist in addition to the knee. Articular disability is uncommon until late in the disease. The etiologic agent, *Sporothrix schenckii* is easily cultured from synovial fluid. As opposed to cutaneous sporotrichosis, articular disease is relatively refractory to iodide therapy, and response to amphotericin B may be slow.

Isolated articular involvement is unusual in *blastomycosis,* and patients usually present with a rapidly progressive "pulmonary-cutaneous-arthritic" syndrome. Involvement of multiple joints is the rule. In contrast to other granulomatous arthritides, joint fluid is frankly purulent in articular blastomycosis, and the organism is easily visualized on wet-mount microscopy of synovial aspirates.

Candida arthritis usually follows direct hematogenous seeding of synovium in patients with risk factors for disseminated candidiasis. The acute articular infection may spread to involved adjacent bone.

In *histoplasmosis* a migratory polyarthritis accompanied by erythema nodosum may be analogous to the acute hypersensitivity syndrome of coccidioidomycosis; osseous and articular involvement is exceedingly rare.

In *cryptococcosis* bone involvement is common with dissemination, but synovitis is unusual.

Successful management of fungal arthritis usually requires prolonged administration of amphotericin B; surgical debridement is helpful in cases with extensive pannus formation.

VIRAL ARTHRITIS Self-limited polyarthritis is a common manifestation of rubella, type B hepatitis, and arboviral diseases not found in the western hemisphere (chikungunya and o'nyong-nyong in Africa and Ross River arthritis in Australia). Synovitis is less common in mumps, varicella, adenovirus, and parvovirus infection. Destructive joint changes are uncommon in viral arthritis even with recurrent disease.

Arthritis occurs in natural *rubella* infection and following immunization with live, attenuated rubella virus. Approximately 15 percent of postpubertal women develop frank arthritis in the course of natural rubella infection. Large and small joints may be involved; the small joints of the hand and wrist are most severely affected. Occasional involvement of the distal interphalangeal joints helps to differentiate this syndrome from the onset of rheumatoid arthritis. The onset of arthritis in rubella usually occurs at the same time or within a few days of the rash and within 2 to 10 weeks after immunization. Rubella arthritis usually abates spontaneously within 1 to 2 weeks; recalcitrant cases respond to salicylates. Joint symptoms may recur for a year or more in natural rubella, but rarely after rubella immunization.

The synovitis that accompanies *type B hepatitis* resembles serum sickness with abrupt onset of fever and articular symptoms. Symmetric polyarthritis of the small joints of the hand may be associated with rheumatoid arthritis-like morning stiffness. The knee, shoulder, ankle, elbow, and wrist are also involved, but the joints of the feet are typically spared. Synovitis is usually accompanied by an urticarial rash, but the rash may be erythematous, maculopapular, or petechial. The possibility of hepatitis-associated arthritis is rarely entertained at the onset of the illness because synovitis usually occurs in the anicteric/prodromal phase. Over a third of patients never become jaundiced, but liver function tests invariably show evidence of hepatitis. In overt hepatitis the arthritis usually resolves. Immune complexes containing hepatitis B antigens are present in serum and synovium during the prodromal stage of hepatitis, lending support to the concept that this form of synovitis is immunologically mediated.

In contrast to rubella, the arthritis of *mumps* has a predilection for men. It generally follows complete subsidence of parotitis, may be accompanied by high fever, and is resistant to salicylates. In children and adults, *coxsackie* and *adenoviral* infection have been associated with recurrent fever, polyarthritis, and polyserositis resembling Still's variety of juvenile rheumatoid arthritis. *Parvoviruses* can also cause a self-limited acute polyarthritis, predominately in women.

SPIROCHETAL ARTHRITIS Articular disease occurs in congenital, secondary, and tertiary *syphilis* (see Chap. 128). Congenital syphilis is associated with metaphyseal osteochondritis of the long bones that abates spontaneously after 6 months of age and ongoing periostitis that continues after that age. At puberty, a typically painless bilateral synovitis of the knees and elbows (Clutton's joints) may develop. Synovial fluid shows a lymphocytic pleocytosis. Arthralgias, arthritis, and tenosynovitis may accompany the classic signs of secondary syphilis. Gummatous synovitis of the large joints occurs in tertiary syphilis. Neurogenic joint degeneration (Charcot's joint) occurs in neurosyphilis. Articular manifestations may also occur in the nonvenereal treponematoses.

Lyme disease (see also Chap. 132) is a multisystem disorder caused by a spirochete, *Borrelia burgdorferi,* that is transmitted by the bite of *Ixodes dammini* or related ticks. The hallmark of the disease is a characteristic rash, erythema chronicum migrans, during the early phase of infection. Weeks to months later, neurologic and cardiac abnormalities occur, accompanied by polyarthralgias and tenosynovitis. Joint manifestations may evolve to frank arthritis, particularly of the large joints, and recur for years. Prompt oral therapy with penicillin or tetracycline eradicates the rash, and generally prevents late manifestations. Diagnosis is usually made by serologic studies. Less than 5 percent of patients are seronegative but develop late manifestations, possibly related to a spirochetal "persister" state induced by early oral antibiotic therapy. Established late manifestations are cured by parenteral penicillin or ceftriaxone; response to therapy may take several months, and repeated treatment may be necessary.

REFERENCES

Bayer AS, Guze LB: Fungal arthritis. II. Coccidioidal synovitis: Clinical, diagnostic, therapeutic, and prognostic considerations. Semin Arthritis Rheum 8:200, 1979

Goldenberg DL, Reed JI: Bacterial arthritis. N Engl J Med 312:764, 1985

Steigbigel NH: Diagnosis and management of septic arthritis, in *Current Clinical Topics in Infectious Diseases*, JS Remington, MN Swartz (eds). New York, McGraw-Hill, 1983, vol 4, pp 1–29

97 OSTEOMYELITIS

JON T. MADER

DEFINITION Osteomyelitis refers to an infection of the bone, generally of the cortical and/or medullary portions. While many types of microorganisms may cause osteomyelitis, it is usually bacterial in origin.

PATHOGENESIS Long bone infections are either hematogenous or secondary to a contiguous focus of infection. Contiguous focus osteomyelitis can be subdivided into bone infections occurring in (1) patients who have relatively normal vascularity and in (2) patients with generalized vascular insufficiency. Both hematogenous and contiguous focus osteomyelitis may be acute or chronic processes.

Hematogenous osteomyelitis occurs mainly in infants and children. The metaphyses of the long bones (tibia, femur) are the most frequently involved. The terminal vessels of the growth plates form large sinusoids that are easy targets for infection. Initially, the acute infection is usually focal, resulting in a breakdown of leukocytes, increased bone pressure, decreased pH, and decreased oxygen tension. The cumulative effects of these physiologic factors compromise the medullary circulation and predispose to extension of the infection. Eventually, the infection may extend laterally through the Haversian and Volkmann canal systems, perforate the bony cortex, and lift the periosteum from the surface of the bone. When this occurs, both periosteal and endosteal circulation are lost and large segments of dead cortical and cancellous bone result. A single pathogen is almost always recovered from the bone in hematogenous osteomyelitis, with *Staphylococcus aureus* being the most commonly isolated organism.

Hematogenous osteomyelitis also occurs in adults. Typically, the long bone infection begins in the diaphysis and spreads to involve the entire medullary canal. Adult hematogenous osteomyelitis most commonly occurs in the vertebrae. The infection is usually monomicrobic with *S. aureus* and aerobic gram-negative rods having the highest incidence. There is often a history of urinary tract infection or intravenous drug abuse. The lumbar vertebral bodies are most often involved, followed in frequency by the thoracic and cervical vertebrae. Spread of the infection to adjacent vertebral bodies may occur rapidly via the rich venous networks in the spine.

When bacteria are introduced into bone by direct trauma or by extension of adjacent soft tissue infections, contiguous focus osteomyelitis results. Open fractures, joint infections, and chronic soft tissue infections are common causes. Osteomyelitis can also occur from contamination at surgery. Most infections of hardware and joint prostheses arise in this way. Unlike hematogenous osteomyelitis, multiple bacterial organisms are usually isolated from the infected bone. The bacteriology is diverse, but *S. aureus* and *S. epidermidis*

are the most commonly isolated pathogens. In addition, aerobic gram-negative bacilli and anaerobic organisms are frequently isolated.

The small bones of the feet are common sites of contiguous focus osteomyelitis in patients with generalized vascular disease. Inadequate tissue perfusion predisposes these patients to infection by blunting the local inflammatory response. The infection commonly develops following minor trauma, infected nail beds, cellulitis, or trophic skin ulceration. Multiple aerobic and anaerobic bacteria are usually isolated from the infected bone.

PATHOLOGY Osteomyelitis may be acute or chronic. The acute disease is characteristically suppurative and is accompanied by edema, vascular congestion, and small vessel thrombosis. The vascular supply to the bone is compromised as the infection extends into the surrounding soft tissue. Large areas of dead bone (sequestra) may be formed when both the medullary and periosteal blood supplies are compromised. Despite an intense host response and/or antibiotic therapy, viable colonies of bacteria may be harbored within the necrotic and ischemic tissues. Once the antibiotics are discontinued or the host response declines, the organisms may again proliferate, which leads to a recurrence of the infection. The hallmarks of chronic osteomyelitis are a nidus of infected dead bone or scar tissue, an ischemic soft tissue envelope, and a refractory clinical course.

MANIFESTATIONS Some patients (particularly children) with hematogenous osteomyelitis present with abrupt fever, irritability, lethargy, and local signs of inflammation 3 weeks or less in duration. However, 50 percent of patients present with vague complaints including pain in the involved limb of 1 to 3 months' duration and minimal, if any, temperature elevation. The clinical signs of soft tissue extension often dominate the presenting findings and may lead to inappropriate diagnostic and therapeutic measures unless the clinical suspicion of osteomyelitis is considered.

The patient with hematogenous vertebral osteomyelitis presents with vague symptoms and signs: dull, constant back pain, spasms of the paravertebral muscles, point tenderness over the involved vertebral body, and low-grade or absent fever.

The clinical features of contiguous focus osteomyelitis include local pain, draining sinuses, tenderness, and erythema over the involved bone. The patient is often afebrile. In patients with vascular disease the clinical features are more subtle and are usually associated with foot ulcers.

Infection of a joint prosthesis may become evident shortly after surgery, especially if the infecting organism is virulent. Erythema and drainage at the operative site are common. More frequently, the onset is delayed, with persistent pain and loosening of the prosthesis developing 3 to 12 months after surgery. Local signs of infection are typically absent. Differentiating infections from noninfectious mechanical loosening of the prosthesis can be very difficult and can be substantiated only by the isolation of a pathogen by arthrocentesis or surgical culture.

DIAGNOSIS Bacterial osteomyelitis is confirmed by the identification of causative bacteria from bone or blood. However, chronic osteomyelitis is rarely accompanied by a bacteremia except in response to an acute extension of the infection into the soft tissues. Since sinus tract cultures are not reliable in identifying which organisms(s) will be isolated from the infected bone, antibiotic treatment of osteomyelitis should be based only on deep bone biopsy cultures.

Radiographic changes in acute hematogenous osteomyelitis are often nebulous. Initial radiographic changes include soft tissue swelling, periosteal thickening and/or elevation, and focal osteopenia. These subtle observations may be overlooked and occur at least 2 weeks following onset of the infection. Diagnostic lytic changes are more protracted and often accompany an indolent infection of several months' duration. In contiguous focus and chronic osteomyelitis the radiographic changes are even more vague, are often found in association with other nonspecific radiographic findings, and require a careful clinical correlation to achieve diagnostic significance.

An earlier diagnosis of osteomyelitis may be achieved with radionuclide imaging, such as technetium-99m diphosphonate, gallium-67 citrate, or indium-111 chloride scans. Although these studies may be definitive as early as 48 h after onset of infection, they may also be negative due to decreased blood flow. Positive scans may be difficult to interpret and require clinical correlation.

Computed tomography and magnetic resonance imaging (MRI) can be more useful than conventional radiographic approaches to define the extent of bone damage due to osteomyelitis. MRI is particularly helpful in defining abscesses and spinal cord impingement in vertebral osteomyelitis.

TREATMENT Acute hematogenous osteomyelitis In children, acute hematogenous osteomyelitis is primarily a medical disease which can be treated nonsurgically. In adults, debridement surgery is often required. Identification of the causative pathogen is essential. The infection will usually respond to specific antimicrobial therapy. Mismanagement with inappropriate antibiotic(s) or dosages results in disease extension, sequestra formation, and the development of a refractory infection. Surgical intervention is indicated in those patients in whom the infection has not responded to specific antimicrobial therapy within 48 h, or in those with evidence of a soft tissue abscess or a confirmed or suspected joint infection. The initial approach is to obtain appropriate culture material. A bone biopsy is essential unless blood cultures are positive and are accompanied by radiographic or bone scan findings consistent with osteomyelitis. Following cultures, a parenteral antimicrobial regimen is chosen which covers the clinically suspected pathogens. Gram's stains can direct the choice of initial antibiotic until culture results are known. In the event of a negative Gram's stain, initial treatment usually includes an anti-staphylococcal penicillin or a cephalosporin with good antistaphylo-coccal activity (e.g., cefazolin). Once the organism is isolated, the antibacterial activity of different antibiotic classes can be determined by appropriate sensitivity methods (see Chap. 85). Appropriate parenteral antimicrobial therapy should be administered for 4 to 6 weeks dated from the initiation of therapy or following the last major debridement surgery. Occasionally oral antibiotic therapy can be utilized for treatment of childhood osteomyelitis. However, 2 weeks of parenteral antibiotic therapy are recommended prior to changing to an oral agent.

Osteomyelitis secondary to contiguous focus infection, chronic osteomyelitis Common denominators of these types of osteomyelitis are infected necrotic bone and poorly perfused soft tissue enveloping the bone. Adequate drainage, thorough debridement, obliteration of dead space, wound coverage with viable soft tissue, and specific antimicrobial coverage are essential to successful therapy. Following diagnostic evaluation, a bone biopsy should be performed to obtain aerobic and anaerobic cultures. However, if immediate debridement surgery is required, antibiotics that cover clinically suspected pathogens are mandated until the bacteriologic tissue data are reported. These antibiotics may be modified, if necessary, after results of the debridement cultures and sensitivities are known.

Surgical exposure should be direct and designed to avoid unnecessary devitalization of bone and soft tissue. The cortical and cancellous bone remaining in the wound after debridement surgery must bleed uniformly to ensure antibiotic perfusion and avoid continued sequestration. Repeat debridements may be necessary.

Appropriate management of the dead space created by debridement surgery is mandatory to arrest the disease and maintain the integrity of the skeletal part involved. The goal of dead space management is to replace dead bone and scar with durable vascularized tissue. Complete wound closure should be attained whenever possible. Local tissue flaps, free tissue flaps, vascularized bone grafts, bone transfers, and antibiotic beads may be used to fill dead space. Cancellous bone grafts may be placed beneath local or transferred tissues when structural augmentation is necessary. Careful preoperative planning is crucial to making efficient use of the patient's limited cancellous bone reserves. Finally, if motion is present, stability of the skeletal unit must be achieved. This is usually managed with external fixators (Hoffmann, Orthofix), which allow soft tissue access, or fixators (Ilizarov) that allow segmental resection and bone transfer.

Since the soft tissue envelope enclosing the debrided bone requires 3 to 4 weeks to become revascularized after debridement surgery, antibiotics are used to treat live infected bone and to safeguard soft tissue and bone undergoing revascularization. Parenteral antimicrobial therapy is administered for 4 to 6 weeks after the last major debridement surgery. However, the duration of antibiotic administration for osteomyelitis remains controversial. Long-term intravenous access catheters make outpatient intravenous treatment possible and decrease hospitalization time. Oral therapy with the quinolone class of antibiotics is currently being evaluated in adult patients.

If bony stability is present, treatment of osteomyelitis associated with hardware requires removal, thorough debridement, and antimicrobial therapy. If bony stability is not present, rigid bony stability must be established. Debridement of infected material plus antimicrobial agents are essential to permit union to occur. Once stability is reestablished, the hardware can be removed, the bone debrided, and another course of antimicrobials begun. Osteomyelitis associated with a joint prosthesis generally requires removal of the appliance, thorough debridement, and appropriate antimicrobial therapy.

Osteomyelitis secondary to contiguous focus infection with vascular disease Osteomyelitis associated with vascular insufficiency is difficult to treat because of the reduced ability of the host to participate in the eradication of the infection. Most of these infections occur in the feet of diabetic individuals. They are insidious and are often beyond simple salvage by the time the patient seeks medical therapy. Polymicrobial infection is common, and the presence of a foul odor or gas in the surrounding soft tissues is indicative of anaerobic bacteria (see Chap. 108).

Assessment of the vascular status of the tissue at the infection site is essential. Several methods may be used to determine perfusion adequacy. Doppler flow, thermograms, arteriograms, and pulse pressures (ischemic index) have been used. Cutaneous oxygen tensions plus pulse pressures are most commonly employed. Cutaneous oxygen tensions are obtained by a modified Clark electrode applied to the skin surface. Cutaneous oxygen tension values provide rough guidelines for determining the location of adequate tissue perfusion. The values are also helpful in assessing whether local debridement surgery can be performed and in selecting surgical margins where wound healing can be expected to occur in cases requiring amputations. Hyperbaric oxygen therapy may facilitate healing in areas having marginally satisfactory tensions.

Suppressive antibiotic therapy, local debridement surgery, or ablative surgery may be indicated in selected patients. Management decisions must consider tissue oxygen perfusion at the infection site, extent of the osteomyelitis, and patient preference. If definitive surgical intervention would result in unacceptable patient morbidity or disability, long suppressive therapy may be preferable. This is also an option when the patient refuses local debridement or ablative surgery. Despite suppressive antibiotic therapy, most patients will eventually require ablative surgery. For localized osteomyelitis with good perfusion, debridement surgery and a 4-week course of antibiotics may be sufficient. Extensive osteomyelitis with poor tissue oxygen perfusion usually requires ablative surgery with the amputation level being dictated by the vascular status of the tissues proximal to the site of infection.

REFERENCES

CALHOUN JH et al: Treatment of diabetic foot infections: Wagner classification, therapy, and outcome. Foot Ankle J, 9:101, 1988

CIERNY G, MADER JT: Adult chronic osteomyelitis. Orthop 7:1557, 1984

MACKOWIAK PA et al: Diagnostic value of sinus tract cultures in chronic osteomyelitis. JAMA 239:2772, 1978

RUTTLE PE et al: Chronic osteomyelitis treated with a muscle flap. Orthop Clin North Am 15:451, 1984

SAPICO FL, MONTGOMERIE JZ: Pyogenic vertebral osteomyelitis: Report of nine cases and review of the literature. Rev Infect Dis 1:754, 1979

WALDVOGEL FA et al: Osteomyelitis: A review of clinical features, therapeutic considerations, and unusual aspects. N Engl J Med 282:198, 260, 316, 1970

98 INFECTIONS CAUSED BY ANIMAL BITES AND SCRATCHES

ROB ROY MACGREGOR

Millions of humans suffer scratches and bites from domestic and wild animals every year. Fortunately, few result in significant infections. Rabies, the most severe complication, is discussed elsewhere (see Chap. 147). This section will review three syndromes: animal bite–related infections in general, rat-bite fever, and cat-scratch disease.

ANIMAL BITE INFECTIONS

DEFINITION These infections result from the inoculation of an animal's oral flora into tissue traumatized by a bite.

EPIDEMIOLOGY AND ETIOLOGY The more than 100 million dogs and cats in the United States inflict between 1 and 2 million bites each year. Over 1 percent of all pediatric emergency room visits are for treatment of animal bites and their complications, and approximately 10,000 require hospitalization. Dogs account for 75 to 90 percent of reported bites, cats account for 8 to 15 percent, and the remainder are due to rodents, monkeys, and other animals.

Most animal bites are by pets known to their victims. Children and young adults are affected most commonly. In children 60 to 80 percent of reported bites are to the head and neck; in adults 75 percent are on the extremities. Infection rates are highest in bites to the hand; rates also vary by animal (5 to 15 percent for dog bites and 40 to 60 percent for cat bites). The difference is thought to result from the character of the bites: dog bites tend to cause laceration and tissue crush injury and as such are likely to receive careful debridement and cleansing; cat bites may appear more trivial initially, and cat tooth punctures are more difficult to clean. Rat and monkey bites appear to cause a low frequency of infection when given proper wound care. The most common organisms causing infection are *Pasteurella multocida*, *Staphylococcus aureus*, streptococcal species, and obligate anaerobes, all normal mouth flora in cats and dogs. In addition, a slow-growing gram-negative bacillus designated DF-2 (dysgonic fermenter type 2, CDC classification) can cause life-threatening septicemia following dog bites and licks.

P. multocida is a small, nonsporulating, nonmotile gram-negative coccobacillus found in 25 to 50 percent of dog bites and in up to 80 percent of cat-bite infections. The organism produces small, gray, nonhemolytic colonies on blood agar and will not grow on Mac-Conkey's agar. It ferments most sugars with the exception of lactose and is urease- and catalase-positive. It can be serotyped on the basis of capsular and somatic antigens. It can be cultured as a single pathogen from rapidly progressing cellulitis that develops within 12 to 24 h after a cat or dog bite (see below).

DF-2 is a gram-negative rod that grows slowly (4 to 10 days) in most blood culture systems and on chocolate agar or heart infusion agar supplemented with 5% rabbit blood in an increased CO_2 environment. On the latter medium organisms are 1 to 4 μm long and can be curved or filamentous in morphology. Owing to the difficulty in culturing, the 10 percent frequency of isolation from the canine oral cavity is probably an underestimate, as is the number of reported human infections. It has been recognized almost exclusively as a cause of septicemia and meningitis occurring usually 4 to 8 days after patients have sustained dog or cat bites and scratches. In the normal host it appears to be of low virulence, because 90 percent of reported cases are in patients at increased risk secondary to splenectomy, alcoholic liver disease, chronic lung disease, or other conditions known to compromise host resistance.

Other organisms have occasionally been identified as the cause of infection following animal bites and scratches: *Herpesvirus simile*

(B-virus) is inoculated by the bite of clinically healthy monkeys and causes an acute, usually lethal encephalomyelitis. Two animal pox viruses are pathogenic in human beings: *bovine papular stomatitis virus*, which produces stomatitis and skin lesions in young cattle and causes small painless papules or verrucous nodules in humans, and *Orf virus*, which causes watery, papillomatous lesions on the mucous membranes of goats and sheep and a papulovesicular lesion, which occasionally may become generalized or progress to a hyperplastic nodular mass, at sites of inoculation in humans. *Lymphocytic choriomeningitis* can be contracted from handling mice and hamsters (see Chap. 149). *Brucella* (see Chap. 119) can be inoculated by handling infected animal tissue, and *tularemia* (see Chap. 120) has occurred following bites and scratches from infected animals. *Leptospirosis* (see Chap. 130) may occur after bites of dogs, mice, and rats (even though organisms normally are not found in saliva). *Erysipeloid*, or "fish-handler's disease," is an acute cellulitis resulting from inoculation of *Erysipelothrix rhusiopathiae* through skin scratches while dressing fish; occasionally it can progress to septicemia and endocarditis (see Chap. 103).

CLINICAL MANIFESTATIONS Patients sustaining animal bites generally present at two distinct times after injury; clinical and management concerns are different at each. One group comes for care within several hours of the bite, before infection has had time to develop; management issues involve hemostasis, cleansing, repair, and prophylaxis (see below). Other patients seek medical aid 8 h to a week or more following injury and present with obvious evidence of infection. In most cases signs and symptoms of infection (swelling, pain, dysfunction) are restricted to the injured part. Fever and leukocytosis are seen in only a third of patients. Blood cultures are usually sterile. Infections caused by *P. multocida*, either alone or in concert with other mouth flora, can produce rapid onset of swelling, pain, and loss of function, often with attendant lymphangitis. Particularly in the hand, infection can spread quickly along tendon sheaths and fascial planes, leading to tissue destruction and long-term disability. Tenosynovitis, septic arthritis, and osteomyelitis are associated complications. In patients with chronic liver disease, *P. multocida* can also cause bacteremia and spontaneous bacterial peritonitis following animal bites and scratches. The striking exception to the pattern of localized bite-induced cellulitis is the systemic presentation of DF-2 infections, in which high fever, prostration, shock, purpura, and meningitis can rapidly lead to death from disseminated intravascular coagulation and bacteremia, often with little or no evidence of local wound infection.

DIAGNOSIS AND TREATMENT In most cases, the diagnosis of wound infection is obvious, although the small puncture wounds inflicted by cats may be masked by marked cellulitis and tenosynovitis. Specific microbiologic diagnosis requires culturing pus and tissue from debridement. In contrast, DF-2 infections often occur sufficiently long after animal exposure to obscure the association. Therefore, DF-2 bacteremia should be considered in any patient presenting with fulminant bacteremic shock and disseminated intravascular coagulation who has a history of splenectomy, liver disease, chronic lung disease, or immunosuppression. Often, the organism can be seen on Gram stain of buffy coat smears but takes 4 to 10 days to grow in blood cultures.

Treatment of bites and scratches depends upon the time elapsed since the bite: the fresh wound (with no signs of infection) requires careful and copious saline irrigation (puncture wounds should be entered with a 20-gauge needle) followed by exploration, debridement of devitalized tissue, and removal of foreign material. Some authorities recommend against suturing bite wounds, because of the risk of infection. However, many surgeons prefer primary closure of wounds of the face, neck, and hands because of their potential for disfiguring, and the risk of infection is small if suturing is performed in association with careful wound cleansing and prophylactic antibiotic administration. Internal fixation of fractures is contraindicated, and lacerations of tendons and nerves are usually repaired in a second procedure. Tetanus prophylaxis should be given if immunization has lapsed or if immune status is unknown. If the patient is seen later, when infection is present or suspected, incision and drainage are necessary, with exploration of tendon sheaths and other locations of possible deeper loculated infection (see Chap. 91). These wounds are usually not closed until several days later. Elevation of the extremity will reduce swelling and promote healing.

Antibiotics must often be chosen on the basis of presumptive evidence: procaine penicillin G, 600,000 units intramuscularly every 12 h, or penicillin V, 500 mg orally every 6 h, is recommended initial treatment for *P. multocida,* streptococci, and most anaerobic mouth organisms. If the Gram stain suggests presence of staphylococci, a penicillinase-resistant penicillin should be added; however, because many *P. multocida* are resistant to penicillinase-resistant penicillins, they should not be used as monotherapy. Alternatively, the fixed combination of amoxicillin plus clavulinic acid, which has a spectrum of activity that includes all organisms commonly encountered in bite wounds, has been used successfully as a single agent. Cefoxitin may be used when empiric intravenous therapy is required. The recommended treatment in penicillin-allergic patients is a tetracycline, although these drugs should not be used in pregnant women or in children with developing teeth; in such patients erythromycin (even though up to 50 percent of *P. multocida* are not susceptible) and cotrimoxazole appear to be effective alternatives. The required duration of therapy is not established, and recommendations vary from 1 to 4 weeks. In vitro testing shows DF-2 to be susceptible to penicillins, cephalosporins, tetracyclines, erythromycin, and clindamycin and to be resistant to aminoglycosides. Intravenously administered penicillin G, in doses up to 20 million units daily, is recommended for suspected and proven septicemia with this organism.

PREVENTION No studies of the efficacy of prophylactic antibiotics have been decisive, owing to the small number of infections encountered. Nonetheless, because of the potential severe consequences, most authorities recommend treatment of all but trivial lacerations and abrasions of the hands and face with a penicillinase-resistant penicillin (with or without addition of penicillin itself), ampicillin-clavulinic acid, or tetracycline for several days.

RAT-BITE FEVER

DEFINITION Rat-bite fever (RBF) is a syndrome characterized by relapsing fever, rash, and arthralgias occurring days to weeks after a rat bite.

ETIOLOGY AND EPIDEMIOLOGY The syndrome has two causes: *Streptobacillus moniliformis* and *Spirillum minus;* the former is a pleomorphic gram-negative bacillus that grows slowly in liquid medium, causing typical ''puffball'' colonies over 2 to 7 days. Growth on trypticase soy agar requires enrichment with 20% serum and incubation in 8% CO_2. Its pleomorphic morphology is best demonstrated by Giemsa stain and includes short rods, filaments, coccobacillary chains, and yeast-like swellings, which give it its name. In anaerobic cultures, it can be mistaken for bacteroides or fusospirochetal species. *Spirillum minus* is a short, thick, and tightly coiled gram-negative spiral organism with polar flagella that create rapid, darting motility under dark-field examination. It has not been grown in culture and is best isolated by intraperitoneal inoculation of infected tissues and blood into mice or guinea pigs. Both organisms are normal flora in wild and laboratory rats; infections have been reported following contact with rodents, pigs, squirrels, cats, and dogs and as a result of ingestion of contaminated milk. Infection is an occupational hazard to laboratory workers. Risk of infection from an individual bite appears to be low: in one series of 50 consecutive rat bites treated with local cleansing alone, only 1 became infected, and none developed RBF. The true incidence of the disease is unknown, but it appears to be uncommon in the United States, where *Streptobacillus moniliformis* is the more common documented cause (which may simply indicate the relative ease of finding the two organisms in tissue and blood). In Japan, where RBF is known as *sodoku,* *Spirillum minus* is more common.

CLINICAL MANIFESTATIONS With both organisms the infection begins with a rat bite, usually to the face or upper extremity. In the streptobacillary form, the wound heals uneventfully, usually without regional adenopathy, but is followed 2 to 10 days later by the abrupt onset of rigors, high fever, headache, myalgias, and prostration. Several days later patients develop a morbilliform or petechial rash, either on the extremities (including palms and soles) or generalized. At the same time, over two-thirds of patients experience severe arthralgias or frank arthritis, usually affecting large joints, which can be either monarticular or migratory and polyarthralgic. Untreated, the acute symptoms remit after several days and can be followed by an irregular pattern of relapsing fevers and other constitutional symptoms lasting for weeks to months. Complications include septic arthritis, endocarditis, pericarditis, pneumonia, and metastatic abscess. In spirillary RBF, the incubation period is longer, usually between 7 and 21 days. The healed bite wound often suppurates at the time of generalized symptoms and is associated with lymphangitis and regional adenopathy. The rash consists of large, reddish-brown macules, and arthritis is uncommon. Untreated, a relapsing fever course ensues similar to that in the streptobacillary form. A mortality of 10 percent has been reported, usually from endocarditis, but prognosis in antibiotic-treated patients is excellent. When the streptobacillary form occurs in the absence of documented animal exposure or in epidemic form, it has been called Haverhill fever or *erythema arthriticum epidemicum,* named for an epidemic in 1926 caused by ingestion of unpasteurized, contaminated milk.

DIAGNOSIS Symptoms of acute fever and prostration several days to weeks after a rat bite should cause consideration of RBF. If the incubation period is less than a week and if the syndrome includes prominent joint manifestations, the streptobacillary form is likely; a longer incubation period, particularly if associated with suppuration at the healed bite site, lymphangitis, and adenopathy, favors the spirillary form. *Streptobacillus moniliformis* can be grown from joint fluid, blood, and other body fluids when cultured in serum-enriched broth. Blood culture medium should be inoculated with twice the normal volume of patient's blood (for serum enrichment), and the commonly used anticoagulant sodium polyanethol sulfonate (SPS; Liquoid) should be omitted, as it is inhibitory to the organism. Gram stain of joint effusions may show pleomorphic gram-negative rods. Isolation of *Spirillum minus* requires intraperitoneal inoculation of blood or other infected material into mice or guinea pigs followed by dark-field examination of the animal's blood and peritoneal fluid 1 to 3 weeks later; occasionally, the organisms can be observed in direct dark-field examination of material from the patient's bite site, regional node, or blood. In both forms the white blood count may be normal or elevated, and a biologic false-positive test for syphilis occurs in up to 25 percent of streptobacillary cases and in more than 50 percent of spirillary cases. Differential diagnosis of a syndrome of fever, rash, and arthritis can be broad, especially when the history of rat bite is not elicited, as in Haverhill fever. Infectious causes include Rocky Mountain spotted fever (especially when the rash is limited to the extremities), viral exanthems, Lyme disease, gonococcal arthritis, and secondary syphilis; immune disorders include rheumatoid arthritis, systemic lupus erythematosus, and drug reactions.

TREATMENT Both organisms are susceptible to penicillin, and a dose of 600,000 units of procaine penicillin given every 12 h for 7 to 10 days should be curative. When endocarditis is present, most experts advise a dose of 15 to 20 million units per day for 4 weeks. When penicillin cannot be used, tetracycline and streptomycin are effective alternatives. Although the risk of infection from an individual rat bite appears to be low, prophylactic administration of oral penicillin V for 1 to 2 days may abort incipient infection.

CAT-SCRATCH DISEASE

DEFINITION Cat-scratch disease (CSD) is an indolent, self-limited disease characterized by a local infection at the site of the scratch followed by regional adenopathy and variable systemic symptoms lasting for weeks to months. The pathogen is a gram-negative cell-wall-defective rod, strongly associated with cats.

ETIOLOGY Over the years a number of agents were proposed as causing CSD, including viruses, chlamydiae, mycobacteria, and other bacteria. Since 1983 attention has focused on a small, pleomorphic, gram-negative bacillus that has been seen in lymph nodes, skin, and conjunctivae of patients with CSD. Margileth and colleagues have summarized the evidence supporting the etiologic role of this organism: (1) The organism has been grown on biphasic brain-heart infusion media from lymph nodes taken from 10 of 19 patients with clinical CSD and not from patients with other diseases. (2) Organisms of similar appearance have been demonstrated by Warthin-Starry stain in nodes and skin lesions from infected patients. (3) Patients have a rise in the antibody titers to the organism. (4) Antibody raised against the organism in a rabbit reacted with CSD bacilli in human tissue sections. (5) The organism causes dermal lesions in armadillos similar to those of early CSD. Several immunologically distinct subtypes may exist. In culture, the organism is thin (0.2 to 0.5 μm in diameter), short (0.2 to 2.5 μm long), and slightly curved with bulbous ends, connected in aggregates by delicate filaments. Transmission electron micrography shows that organisms in culture and tissue sections lack portions of their cell walls, which may contribute to the difficulty in culturing them. Nonetheless, the failure to grow or stain the organism in a higher percentage of patients warrants caution as to whether it is the true pathogen of CSD.

EPIDEMIOLOGY CSD is primarily a disease of childhood, the majority of cases occurring in children under age 10 and more than 90 percent of cases under age 18. The range is worldwide; all races are affected; a late summer-autumn seasonality is discernible in temperate climates. Ninty percent or more of patients report contact with a cat, although anecdotal cases suggest transmission through other mammals or by puncture wounds from inanimate objects. Cats that transmit the infection are not ill, and the duration of infectiousness is unknown. This stems partially from the fact that the disease is not very communicable: less than 5 percent of affected families have more than one case.

Subclinical disease may be common; reaction to the CSD skin test is around 20 percent in cat owners versus 1.5 percent in people who have minimal contact with cats.

PATHOLOGY The microscopic appearance of infected lymph nodes shows characteristic suppurative granulomatous inflammation but is nonspecific; other diseases causing similar pathologic appearance include lymphogranuloma venereum, tularemia, brucellosis, sarcoid, mycobacterial infection, and even some lymphomas. The characteristic delicate pleomorphic organisms can be demonstrated by Warthin-Starry silver stain in the majority of infected lymph nodes.

DIAGNOSIS The diagnosis is suggested when, with or without systemic symptoms, tender regional adenopathy and a lesion compatible with an inoculation site develop within several weeks after exposure to a cat, particularly in children. The diagnosis is confirmed when criteria in Table 98-1 are met. The CSD skin test, although unstandardized and not available commercially, is reliable, with false-positive and false-negative rates in the 5 percent range. Antigen is prepared by diluting pus aspirated from a suppurative CSD node, heating it to 60°C for 8 h, and testing for sterility and viral antigens such as hepatitis B and human immunodeficiency virus. Failure to develop at least 5 mm of induration 48 to 72 h after intracutaneous inoculation of 0.1 mL of this material on two occasions at least 4

TABLE 98-1   Criteria for the diagnosis of cat-scratch disease

Diagnosis confirmed if three of the first four or one of the first four plus number five are present:

1 History of cat contact and presence of a scratch or primary dermal or eye lesion
2 Positive cat-scratch disease skin test
3 Negative studies for other causes of lymphadenopathy
4 Characteristic histopathology of a biopsied lymph node
5 Presence of typical silver-staining bacteria in histopathologic sections of lymph nodes or primary skin or eye lesions

SOURCE: BL Hainer, Cat-scratch disease, J Fam Pract 25:497, 1987.

weeks apart makes the diagnosis very unlikely. Despite the crude nature of the test material, no serious side effects have been described.

It appears that the responsible organism has been identified, and it is likely that specific CSD antigen will provide for standardized skin testing and measurement of antibody response, thereby simplifying diagnosis. Diagnostic biopsy of involved lymph nodes or skin lesions should be restricted to the occasional case with atypical aspects such as protracted symptoms or lack of exposure to cats. Silver stain techniques should demonstrate the organism. The differential diagnosis includes infectious causes of localized adenopathy such as infectious mononucleosis, mycobacterial infection, streptococcal and staphylococcal infection, syphilis, tularemia, toxoplasmosis, sporotrichosis, and other fungi and noninfectious disorders such as lymphoma, sarcoid, congenital cysts, and Kawasaki disease.

TREATMENT Antibiotic therapy has not been studied systematically, but anecdotal evidence suggests that it has not been effective. However, the presumed causative bacillus appears to be susceptible to cefoxitin, cefotaxime, and aminoglycoside antibiotics in vitro, agents largely untried to date in CSD. Because of the benign and self-limited nature of the disease, treatment is largely supportive. Limitation of activity should be dictated by the level of constitutional symptoms, and sequential monitoring will help determine when needle aspiration of suppurative lymph nodes is warranted. A second aspiration is necessary in about half of cases. Incision and drainage or excisional biopsy of affected nodes is not recommended routinely. Isolation of affected patients is not appropriate because person-to-person spread has not been shown.

REFERENCES

CARITHERS HA: Cat-scratch disease; an overview based on a study of 1,200 patients. Am J Dis Child 139:1124, 1985

ELLIOT DL et al: Pet-associated illness. N Engl J Med 313:985, 1985

ENGLISH CK et al: Cat-scratch disease. Isolation and culture of the bacterial agent. Am J Dis Child 139:1124, 1985

FEDER HM et al: Review of 59 patients hospitalized with animal bites. Pediatr Infect Dis 6:24, 1987

HICKLIN H et al: Dysgonic fermenter 2 septicemia. Rev Infect Dis 9:884, 1987

HOLROYD KJ et al: *Streptobacillus moniliformis* polyarthritis mimicking rheumatoid arthritis: An urban case of rat bite fever. Am J Med 85:711, 1988

KOEHLER JE et al: Cutaneous vascular lesions and disseminated cat-scratch disease in patients with the acquired immunodeficiency syndrome and AIDS-related complex. Ann Intern Med 109:449, 1988

MARGILETH AM et al: Systemic cat scratch disease: Report of 23 patients with prolonged or recurrent severe bacterial infection. J Infect Dis 155:390, 1987

MCDONOUGH JJ et al: Management of animal and human bites and resulting human infections, in *Current Clinical Topics in Infectious Diseases,* JS Remington, MN Swartz (eds). New York, McGraw-Hill, 1987, vol 8, pp 11–36

SHANSON DC et al: *Streptobacillus moniliformis* isolated from blood in four cases of Haverhill fever. Lancet 2:92, 1983

Diseases caused by gram-positive organisms

99 PNEUMOCOCCAL INFECTIONS

ROBERT AUSTRIAN

ETIOLOGY The pneumococcus *(Streptococcus pneumoniae)* is a gram-positive encapsulated coccus that usually grows in pairs or short chains. In the diplococcal form, the adjacent margins are rounded and the opposite ends slightly pointed, giving the organisms a lancet shape. In stained preparations of exudate, gram-negative forms are sometimes present. Pneumococcal colonies are surrounded by greenish discoloration on or in blood agar and are confused at times with other alpha-hemolytic streptococci to which they are closely related. Their isolation from respiratory secretions may be facilitated by inclusion of 5 μg gentamicin per milliliter in the medium. Pneumococci can be distinguished by their bile solubility and mouse virulence or by serologic typing. Another method with approximately 90 percent specificity, utilizing inhibition of pneumococci by Optochin-impregnated paper disks, is less cumbersome.

The capsular substances are complex polysaccharides and are the basis for dividing pneumococci into serotypes. Organisms exposed to type-specific antiserum show a positive capsular precipitin reaction, the Neufeld quellung reaction; by this means, 84 serotypes have been identified. All are pathogenic for human beings, but types or groups 1, 3, 4, 7, 8, 9, and 12 are encountered most frequently in clinical practice. Types or groups 6, 14, 19, and 23 often cause pneumonia and otitis media in children but are less common in adults.

Specific typing of pneumococci remains of great clinical importance if pneumococcus is to be identified with regularity, and recognition of pneumococcus has decreased significantly since the abandonment of capsular typing by most clinical laboratories. The detection of pneumococcal capsular polysaccharides in sputum and in other body fluids by immunologic methods such as counter-immunoelectrophoresis (CIE) or latex agglutination provides an alternative to bacteriologic techniques for the presumptive diagnosis of pneumococcal infection. Because of cross reactions between the polysaccharides of pneumococci and of other bacterial species, immunologic diagnosis is less specific than bacteriologic diagnosis.

PATHOGENESIS The mechanism by which pneumococci damage the mammalian host is obscure, and no toxin elaborated by the organism has been shown to play a major pathogenic role in pneumococcal infection, although components of the cell wall may cause inflammation. The capsular polysaccharides, though nontoxic, are known to be necessary factors in virulence and to offer some protection of the organism from phagocytosis.

Although ''pneumococcal pharyngitis'' is a doubtful clinical entity, invasion of nasopharyngeal tissue may occur in the infant and occasionally in the nonimmune adult and be followed by spread to the circulation via the cervical lymphatics. At times, secondary infection of serous cavities in the absence of demonstrable focal infection of the upper or lower respiratory tract may occur. The organisms multiply readily in vivo and may produce acute inflammation of the lungs, serous cavities, and endocardium.

The normal human respiratory tract is provided with a variety of mechanisms which guard the lungs from infection. The lower respiratory tract is protected by the glottis and larynx, and material passing these barriers stimulates the expulsive cough reflex. Removal of small particles impinging on the walls of the trachea and bronchi is facilitated by their mucociliary lining (see Chap. 207); and growth of bacteria reaching normal alveoli is inhibited by their relative dryness and by the phagocytic activity of alveolar macrophages. Any anatomic or physiologic derangement of these coordinated defenses tends to augment the susceptibility of the lungs to infection. Anesthesia, alcoholic intoxication, convulsions, and disturbed innervation of the larynx depress the cough reflex and may permit aspiration of infected material. Alterations in the tracheobronchial tree leading to anatomic changes in the epithelial lining or to localized obstruction increase the vulnerability of the lungs to infection. Pulmonary edema, local or generalized, resulting from viral infection, inhalation of irritant gases, cardiac failure, or contusion of the chest wall, provides a fluid menstruum in the alveoli for the growth of bacteria and their spread to adjacent areas of the lung. Viral infection of the respiratory epithelium with concomitant disruption of its component cells interferes significantly with the clearance of bacteria from the lungs, an observation in accord with the high incidence of pneumococcal pneumonia during epidemics of viral influenza and its frequent clinical association with sporadic viral respiratory infections.

Pneumonia usually begins in the right lower, right middle, or left lower lobe, those areas to which gravity is most likely to carry upper respiratory secretions aspirated during sleep. Bronchial embolization with infected mucinous secretions during the course of an upper respiratory infection appears to be the initiating factor in many cases of pneumococcal pneumonia. Protected initially from phagocytosis by mucinous material, the bacteria multiply and, in infected alveoli, evoke the outpouring of proteinaceous fluid which serves both as a nutrient and as a vehicle for spread to adjacent alveoli. Soon thereafter, polymorphonuclear leukocytes migrate from the pulmonary capillaries to phagocytize a part of the pneumococcal population before the appearance of detectable antibody. Delay in the polymorphonuclear leukocytic response occurs during alcoholic intoxication and certain forms of anesthesia, permitting spread of infection. Glucocorticoids may also interfere with leukocyte migration. Later, as the pneumonic lesion evolves, macrophages appear in the exudate and remove the debris of fibrin and cells. It is probable that antibody to the capsular polysaccharide of the invading pneumococcus makes its appearance locally in the lung before being detectable in the circulation. Such antibody increases the efficiency of phagocytosis approximately twofold and causes agglutination of the organisms and their adherence to alveolar walls, thereby slowing their dissemination in the lung. The outcome of infection depends, therefore, on the rate at which bacteria can multiply in the edema fluid and spread, and on the host's ability to immobilize and destroy them by phagocytosis. Individuals with hypogammaglobulinemia and patients with multiple myeloma (see Chap. 265) incapable of producing anticapsular antibody are prone to recurrent attacks of pneumococcal pneumonia. Repeated infection with the same pneumococcal type should always prompt a search for dysgammaglobulinemia.

Failure of local defense mechanisms in the lung results in lymphatic spread of pneumococci to the hilar lymph nodes. In the sinusoids of these organs, a sequence of events not unlike that in the lung ensues. If infection is not checked in this secondary line of defense, organisms find their way into the thoracic duct and then into the circulation. Although transient bacteremia may occur at the onset of many cases of pneumococcal pneumonia, it is detectable in only 20 to 30 percent of cases. Bacteremia, which reflects the body's inability to localize the pulmonary infection, is a poor prognostic sign and carries with it the danger of metastatic infection. The mortality of treated or untreated bacteremic pneumococcal pneumonia is four times that resulting from comparably managed nonbacteremic infections. Metastatic infection secondary to bacteremia may occur in the meninges, joints, or peritoneum or on the endocardium. Direct spread from the infected lung may give rise to empyema or to pericarditis.

Natural recovery from pneumococcal infection coincides usually, but not invariably, with the appearance of detectable type-specific antibody in the circulation and is often accompanied by a dramatic and abrupt fall in temperature, the so-called crisis. Antibody aids recovery by increasing the efficiency of phagocytosis and by limiting dissemination of the organisms. Bacteriostatic drugs, such as sulfonamides, facilitate control of the infection by limiting the size of the pneumococcal population, but the host's defense mechanisms are still required for the elimination of the bacteria. Bactericidal agents, such as penicillin, cause the death of pneumococci in the lung and are effective when some of the host's defense mechanisms are compromised. With the arrest of infection, the alveolar exudate undergoes liquefaction, the inflammatory debris is removed by expectoration and via the lymphatic channels, and the lung is restored to its normal state. Necrosis of pulmonary tissue as a result of pneumococcal infection is distinctly uncommon. Primary pneumococcal lung abscess is a rare clinical entity, although the diagnosis is mistakenly made at times when pneumococcal infection complicates lung abscess of other origins.

In addition to causing pneumonia and its metastatic sequelae, pneumococcus can extend from the nasopharynx to its adjacent structures, giving rise to otitis media, mastoiditis, paranasal sinusitis, or conjunctivitis. Soft tissue abscesses are rare but may occur.

PNEUMOCOCCAL PNEUMONIA

Pneumococcal pneumonia is a disease of considerable uniformity, in contrast to other infections such as typhoid fever and tuberculosis. The diseases produced by different pneumococcal serotypes show little variation in severity or in clinical manifestations. The prognosis in type 3 pneumococcal pneumonia is usually regarded as poor, probably because type 3 infections occur frequently in the aged and in patients with other debilitating diseases, such as diabetes and congestive heart failure. The usual lesion in adults is segmental or lobar in distribution, but in children and the aged, bronchopneumonia, characterized by patchy involvement, is frequent.

MANIFESTATIONS Pneumonia is often preceded for a few days by coryza or some other form of common respiratory disease. The onset is frequently so abrupt that the patient can state the exact hour that illness began. There is a sudden *shaking chill* in more than 80 percent of the cases and a rapid rise in temperature, with corresponding tachycardia and an increase in respiratory rate (tachypnea). Most patients with pneumococcal pneumonia have a single rigor unless antipyretic drugs are administered, and repeated chills should suggest another etiologic agent.

About 75 percent of patients develop severe *pleuritic pain* and *cough,* productive of pinkish or "rusty" mucoid sputum within a few hours. The chest pain is agonizing, and respirations become rapid, shallow, and grunting as the patient tries to splint the affected side. Many patients are mildly cyanotic as a result of hypoxia caused by $\dot{V}/\dot{Q}$ (ventilation-perfusion ratio) abnormality or shunt, which accompanies altered respiration, and show dilatation of the alae nasi when first seen. Patients appear acutely ill; but nausea, headache, and malaise are not prominent, and most individuals are alert. Pleuritic pain and dyspnea are the dominant complaints.

In the untreated disease, there are sustained fever of 39.2 to 40.5°C (103 to 105°F), continued pleuritic pain, cough, and expectoration; and *abdominal distention* is frequent. *Herpes labialis* is a

common complication. After 7 to 10 days, there are diaphoresis, abrupt defervescence, and dramatic improvement in well-being, the "crisis."

In cases which terminate fatally, there is usually extensive pulmonary involvement, and dyspnea, cyanosis, and tachycardia are prominent. Circulatory collapse or a picture resembling adult respiratory distress syndrome has been observed. Death in a few patients is associated with empyema or some other suppurative complication such as meningitis or endocarditis.

Physical examination reveals restricted motion of the affected hemithorax. Tactile fremitus may be decreased during the initial day of illness but is usually increased when consolidation is fully established. Deviation of the trachea away from the affected lung suggests pleural effusion or empyema. The percussion note is dull, and if the lesion is in an upper lobe, impaired motion of the diaphragm can be detected on the affected side. Very early in the course of infection, breath sounds are diminished, but as the lesion evolves, they become tubular or bronchial in quality, and bronchophony and whispered pectoriloquy can be elicited. These findings are accompanied by fine crepitant rales.

EFFECT OF SPECIFIC CHEMOTHERAPY Pneumococcal pneumonia usually improves promptly when an appropriate antimicrobial drug is given. Within 12 to 36 h after initiation of treatment with penicillin, temperature, pulse, and respiration begin to fall and may reach normal values, pleuritic pain subsides, and the spread of the inflammatory process is halted. The temperature of approximately half the patients, however, requires 4 days or longer to become normal, and failure of the patient's temperature to reach normal in 24 to 48 h should not prompt a change in antibacterial therapy in the absence of other indications.

COMPLICATIONS The typical course of pneumococcal pneumonia can be modified by the development of one or more local or distant complications:

In the lung ATELECTASIS Atelectasis of all or part of a lobe may occur during the active stage of pneumonia or after treatment has been instituted. The patient may complain of sudden recurrence of pleuritic pain and show rapid respirations. Small areas of atelectasis are often detected by x-ray in the absence of symptoms. These areas usually clear with coughing and deep breathing, but bronchoscopic aspiration is occasionally necessary. If atelectasis is allowed to persist, the affected area becomes fibrotic and functionless.

DELAYED RESOLUTION Return of physical findings in the lung to normal after pneumococcal pneumonia is usually complete within 2 to 4 weeks. X-ray evidence of residual pulmonary consolidation, however, may persist as long as 8 weeks, and other radiologic manifestations of the infection (volume loss, stranding, and pleural disease) may persist for up to 18 weeks. The process of resolution may require a longer time in those over 50 years of age and in those with chronic obstructive airway disease or alcoholism.

ABSCESS Lung abscess is a rare sequel to pneumococcal infection, although pneumococcal pneumonia is a not uncommon complication of lung abscess of other origins. It is manifested by continued fever and profuse expectoration of purulent sputum. X-ray shows one or more cavities. This complication is exceedingly rare in patients who receive penicillin therapy and is most likely to follow infection with pneumococcus type 3.

In adjacent structures PLEURAL EFFUSION Pleural effusion detectable in lateral decubitus x-rays of the chest occurs in approximately half of patients with pneumococcal pneumonia and is associated with delay in the initiation of therapy and with bacteremia. Usually the effusion is sterile and is absorbed spontaneously within a week or two. At times, however, the effusion is large and requires aspiration or drainage.

EMPYEMA Before the introduction of effective chemotherapy, empyema occurred in 5 to 8 percent of patients with pneumococcal pneumonia; it is now observed in less than 1 percent of treated cases. It is manifested by persistent fever or pleuritic pain, together with signs of pleural effusion. In the early stages, the gross appearance of infected fluid may not differ from that of a sterile pleural effusion; later, there is a profuse outpouring of polymorphonuclear leukocytes and fibrin, resulting in an exudate of thick greenish pus containing large clots of fibrin. The quantity of exudate may become large enough to displace mediastinal structures. In neglected cases, this process leads to extensive pleural scarring, with limitation of thoracic movement. Rupture and drainage through the chest wall (*empyema necessitatis*) occur, but are rare. Metastatic *brain abscess* is an occasional complication of chronic empyema.

PERICARDITIS A particularly serious complication is spread of infection to the pericardial sac. This lesion is characterized by pain in the precordial region, a friction rub synchronous with the heartbeat, and distention of cervical veins, although one or all of these findings may be absent. The possibility of coexisting purulent pericarditis should be considered whenever a very ill patient with pneumonia develops empyema.

Metastatic infections *Arthritis* occurs more often in children than in adults. The affected joint is swollen, red, and painful, with a purulent effusion. It usually subsides promptly with systemic administration of penicillin, although aspiration and intraarticular injection of penicillin may be necessary in adults.

Acute bacterial endocarditis and *meningitis*, complications of pneumococcal pneumonia, are discussed subsequently.

Paralytic ileus Gaseous abdominal distention is commonly present and in severely ill patients may assume such serious proportions that the term *paralytic ileus* is justified. This complication further impairs respiratory movement by elevation of the diaphragm and constitutes a difficult problem in management. A rarer and more serious gastrointestinal complication is acute gastric dilatation.

Impaired liver function Alterations in hepatic function are common during the course of pneumococcal pneumonia, and mild jaundice is not at all rare. The pathogenesis of the jaundice is not entirely clear, although in some patients it appears to be related to glucose-6-phosphate dehydrogenase deficiency.

LABORATORY FINDINGS *Sputum* should be obtained in the physician's presence before the administration of antimicrobial drugs to ensure its quality. Although resort to transtracheal aspiration or lung puncture may be necessary on occasion to establish the cause of pneumonia, routine use of these invasive techniques is not recommended because of their attendant, albeit infrequent, complications. When stained by Gram's method, the sputum shows polymorphonuclear leukocytes and variable numbers of gram-positive cocci, singly and in pairs. These can be typed directly by the Neufeld quellung technique, and this procedure should be used to facilitate diagnosis whenever possible. The *blood culture* is positive for pneumococci during the first days of untreated illness in 20 to 30 percent of cases. The white blood cell count usually shows a polymorphonuclear *leukocytosis* ranging from 12×10^9/L to 25×10^9/L (12,000 to 25,000 cells per microliter). A normal white count or leukopenia is sometimes observed in patients with overwhelming infection and bacteremia. Occasionally, pneumococci may be seen directly in granulocytes of patients with bacteremia by examining the buffy coat after staining with Wright's stain. These patients often have asplenia. *X-ray of the chest* usually reveals a homogenous density in the affected area of the lung. In well-established cases, the density may occupy one or more entire lobes. Atypical patterns of consolidation may be seen in patients with underlying chronic pulmonary disease.

EXTRAPULMONARY PNEUMOCOCCAL INFECTION

PNEUMOCOCCAL MENINGITIS The pneumococcus is second only to the meningococcus as a cause of purulent meningitis in adults; in children, meningitis caused by *Haemophilus influenzae* is also more frequent than pneumococcal infection.

Pneumococcal meningitis can develop as a "primary" disease without preceding signs of infection elsewhere; as a complication of pneumococcal pneumonia; by extension from otitis, mastoiditis, or sinusitis; or following a skull fracture which creates an opening between the subarachnoid space and the nasal cavity or paranasal sinuses. Patients with pneumococcal endocarditis frequently develop meningeal infection. Patients with multiple myeloma and with sickle cell disease seem to be prone to pneumococcal infection of the meninges, just as they are to pneumonia.

The *manifestations* are of those of any acute pyogenic meningitis (see Chap. 354) and include chills, fever, headache, nuchal rigidity, Kernig's and Brudzinski's signs, delirium, and cranial nerve palsies. Evidence of otitis, sinusitis, or pneumonia should be carefully sought by physical and roentgenographic examination in all patients.

The *spinal fluid* is under increased pressure, appears cloudy, often with a greenish tint, and shows a high protein and low glucose content. Stained smears usually reveal gram-positive diplococci and polymorphonuclear leukocytes; in some patients, the number of cells in the spinal fluid is surprisingly small, and much of the cloudiness is produced by the bacterial content. The diagnosis can be established rapidly by identification of pneumococci in the spinal fluid by Gram's stain. Immunologic tests (CIE or latex agglutination) are positive in approximately 80 percent of culture-positive cases and may provide a presumptive bacterial cause of infection in some patients from whose spinal fluid no organism is recovered.

With appropriate chemotherapy, recovery can be expected in 70 percent of cases; the prognosis is better in children than in infants or in adults. Relapse may occur but is unusual if adequate treatment is carried out. Subarachnoid block, the result of accumulation of large amounts of thick exudate in the meningeal space and at the base of the brain, is an infrequent complication.

PNEUMOCOCCAL ENDOCARDITIS Endocarditis is a rare complication of pneumonia or meningitis. The clinical picture is that of acute bacterial endocarditis (see Chap. 90), with remittent fever, splenomegaly, and metastatic infection of the lungs, meninges, joints, eye, and other tissues. Petechiae are uncommon. The infection can attack normal valves and is particularly likely to occur on the aortic valve. The valvular infection is destructive, and loud murmurs and heart failure develop rapidly. Rupture or perforation of cusps or even rupture of the aorta may occur. The blood culture is consistently positive for the pneumococcus in the absence of treatment with antimicrobial drugs; yet at the same time antibodies to the infecting organism may be demonstrable in the blood, a combination of findings seldom observed except in endocarditis or brucellosis. Although the infection is relatively easy to cure with penicillin, damage to valve leaflets, especially to the cusps of the aortic valve, may be followed by rapidly progressive heart failure. Surgical repair or replacement of damaged valvular structures should be carried out early, before heart failure becomes intractable.

PNEUMOCOCCAL PERITONITIS Pneumococcal peritonitis is a rare disease and is probably the sequel to transient pneumococcal bacteremia, although, because of its somewhat greater frequency in young girls, it has been hypothesized that the organism may gain entry to the peritoneum via the vagina and fallopian tubes. Peritonitis was formerly a common complication of the nephrotic syndrome, particularly in children, but it occurs now with a frequency of less than 2 percent. In adults, the disease is seen in association with cirrhosis or with carcinoma of the liver. The diagnosis is made by examination of the ascitic fluid; blood cultures are often positive, and a polymorphonuclear leukocytosis is the rule.

TREATMENT

SPECIFIC ANTIMICROBIAL THERAPY Although resistance of pneumococci to antimicrobial drugs has not been regarded as a significant problem in the past, a small but increasing number of strains have been found to be resistant to one or all of the following agents: penicillins, cephalosporins, tetracyclines, chloramphenicol, erythromycin, clindamycin, co-trimoxazole, and aminoglycosides.

For this reason sensitivity of the infecting organism to the drug(s) to be used should be determined, particularly in treating extrapulmonary infection. In the absence of resistance or of hypersensitivity to it, penicillin G (benzylpenicillin) is the drug of choice for all manifestations of pneumococcal infection. Strains of pneumococcus manifesting increased resistance to penicillin have been recovered infrequently from humans; and although the level of such resistance does not often preclude treatment with this antibiotic, awareness of the phenomenon is necessary. A dose of 600,000 units daily provides a good margin of safety in treating adults with bacteremic or nonbacteremic infection in the absence of an extrapulmonary focus, but the occurrence of pneumococci showing increased resistance to penicillin makes the initiation of therapy with larger amounts desirable. Treatment may be started with doses of 600,000 units of aqueous crystalline penicillin G or procaine penicillin administered at 12-h intervals to be continued until the patient has been afebrile for 48 to 72 h. Pneumococcal pneumonia can be treated with an oral penicillin, preferably one resistant to gastric acid (see Chap. 85), in dosage equivalent to 2.4 to 4.8 million units of penicillin G. *Peritonitis* caused by sensitive strains responds usually within 36 to 48 h to 2 to 4 million units of penicillin daily.

Pneumococcal meningitis in adults should be treated with 18 to 24 million units of penicillin G daily intravenously. Larger amounts should not be used, to avoid neurotoxicity from excessive dosage. Intrathecal administration of penicillin is unnecessary, and supplementation of penicillin with broad-spectrum bacteriostatic drugs such as tetracyclines may exert a deleterious effect. All pneumococcal isolates from cerebrospinal fluid should be tested promptly for their sensitivity to antibacterial drugs. Vancomycin is the drug of choice for treatment of meningitis caused by pneumococci resistant to multiple antimicrobial agents.

Moderate doses of penicillin G are used to treat pneumococcal endocarditis—8 to 12 million units daily by intravenous infusion. Rapidly developing heart failure as a result of valvular injury and a tendency to form myocardial abscess, however, often lead to a fatal outcome despite the use of antibiotics. Prompt surgical repair or replacement of damaged heart valves should be considered when cardiac failure develops.

Cephalosporins in parenteral doses of 1 to 2 g daily are effective in pneumococcal pneumonia but must be administered with caution to those hypersensitive to penicillin. Many members of this class of β-lactam drugs cannot be used to treat meningitis because of their poor ability to penetrate the blood–cerebrospinal fluid barrier. Several of the newer cephalosporins, including cefotaxime and ceftriaxone, show promise of efficacy in treating pneumococcal meningitis although experience with each is limited. The tetracyclines in doses of 1 to 2 g daily, erythromycin in doses of 1.6 g daily, or clindamycin in doses of 1.2 g daily are effective treatment for pneumococcal pneumonia if it is caused by a sensitive strain, but they are recommended only for patients who have had untoward reactions to penicillins or cephalosporins. Despite its efficacy, chloramphenicol should not be used to treat pneumococcal infections other than meningitis in patients hypersensitive to penicillin who are infected with a drug-sensitive strain. For patients with illness caused by multiply drug-resistant pneumococci, vancomycin in doses of 2 g daily is the drug of choice. Sulfonamides have little place in the present-day treatment of pneumococcal pneumonia and are useless in endocarditis and meningitis. Aminoglycosides, such as gentamicin, tobramycin, and amikacin, should not be employed to treat pneumococcal infection.

Pneumococcal arthritis responds to systemic penicillin, but aspiration and intraarticular instillation of the drug may be necessary.

Empyema should be detected and treated as early as possible. When an effusion is found, fluid should be removed and examined for bacteria, leukocytes, glucose concentration, and pH. The presence of bacteria, pus, a pH below 7.0, and/or a pleural fluid glucose below 2.2 mmol/L (40 mg/dL) are indications for institution of closed-chest tube drainage. Failure to cure empyema early may be followed by pleural fibrosis and may necessitate subsequent surgical decortication of the lung to restore pulmonary function.

OTHER MEASURES   Oxygen administered through a face mask should be used to treat significant cyanosis, cardiac failure, and delirium. In the presence of adult respiratory distress syndrome, positive end-expiratory pressure may be indicated. Codeine, 32 to 64 mg every 4 h, will usually control pleuritic pain. When pain is severe, it may require intercostal nerve block with 1 to 2% procaine for relief.

PROGNOSIS AND PREVENTION

Although the mortality from pneumococcal pneumonia has diminished significantly since the advent of antimicrobial drugs, available evidence indicates that the incidence of the disease has changed little, if at all. The fatality rate in patients over the age of 12 years with bacteremic pneumococcal pneumonia treated with an antibiotic is 18 percent, and in patients over the age of 50 and in those with underlying systemic illness, it is significantly higher.

Signs of poor prognosis in pneumonia include leukopenia, bacteremia, multilobar involvement, any extrapulmonary focus of pneumococcal infection, presence of preexisting systemic disease, circulatory collapse, and occurrence of the infection in the first year of life or after the age of 55. Infection with pneumococcus type 3 has a higher mortality rate than that caused by other pneumococcal types. Death is most likely to occur in individuals sustaining irreversible physiologic damage early in the course which is unaltered by antimicrobial therapy. Until the nature of the injury produced by pneumococcus is understood and ways are devised to repair it, vaccination will remain the principal means of protecting those at high risk of a fatal outcome.

A 23-valent vaccine containing the capsular polysaccharides of pneumococcal types 1, 2, 3, 4, 5, 6B, 7F, 8, 9N, 9V, 10A, 11A, 12F, 14, 15B, 17F, 18C, 19F, 19A, 20, 22F, 23F, and 33F, which include the serotypes or groups responsible for 90 percent of bacteremic infections in the United States, is recommended for prevention of pneumococcal infection caused by these serotypes in individuals at high risk of a fatal outcome. Those at higher-than-average risk are individuals over the age of 55 and patients with a variety of chronic systemic illnesses including heart disease, chronic bronchopulmonary disease, hepatic disease, renal insufficiency, diabetes, and a variety of malignancies. Persons of all ages with sickle cell disease have an increased risk of developing pneumococcal infection, and the vaccine is recommended for those with this disorder over the age of 2 years. Since anatomic or functional asplenia is associated with fulminant overwhelming pneumococcal septicemia with disseminated intravascular coagulation, giving rise to a clinical picture resembling that of the Waterhouse-Friderichsen syndrome, such individuals should also be immunized. However, the vaccine does not contain the antigens of all pneumococcal types, and infection caused by nonincluded types may occur occasionally in immunized subjects. Reactions to the vaccine are usually absent or mild, although in the occasional individual they may resemble those following immunization with typhoid vaccine: local pain, erythema, and elevation of temperature. Because of the persistence of pneumococcal antibodies after a single injection of vaccine, reimmunization is not necessary. The aggregate efficacy of the vaccine in preventing bacteremic infection is 65 to 70 percent in immunocompetent adults. It may afford little, if any, protection, however, to those with agamma- or dysgammaglobulinemia or to patients who have been subjected recently to intensive antitumor chemotherapy and radiation. In children, immunologic responsiveness to different capsular antigens develops at different times prior to puberty as a result of maturational characteristics of the human immune system and, in infancy, may be manifested only by antibodies of the IgM class. Currently, vaccines of capsular polysaccharide conjugated to proteins such as diphtheria toxoid, which are antigenic in infancy, are under development for pediatric populations. If circumstances dictate, pneumococcal vaccine may be administered concomitantly with influenza viral vaccine, provided each vaccine is injected from a separate syringe at a separate site.

REFERENCES

APPLEBAUM PC: World-wide development of antibiotic resistance in pneumococci. Eur J Clin Microbiol 6.367, 1987

AUSTRIAN R: *Life with the Pneumococcus*. Philadelphia, University of Pennsylvania Press, 1985

————: Untreated pneumococcal bacteraemia of cryptic origin in the human adult with spontaneous recovery. S Afr Med J 70(Suppl):46, 1986

BOLAN N et al: Pneumococcal vaccine efficacy in selected populations in the United States. Ann Intern Med 104:1, 1986

FRUCHTMAN SM et al: Adult respiratory distress syndrome as a cause of death in pneumococcal pneumonia. Chest 83:598, 1983

HEFFRON R: *Pneumonia with Special Reference to Pneumococcus Lobar Pneumonia*. Cambridge, Harvard, 1979

KAPLAN SL: Antigen detection in cerebrospinal fluid—pros and cons. Am J Med 75:109, 1983

KLUGMAN KP, KOORNHOF HJ: Drug resistance patterns and serogroups or serotypes of pneumococcal isolates from cerebrospinal fluid or blood, 1979–1986. J Inf Dis 158:956, 1988

PATON JC et al: Antibody response to pneumococcal vaccine in children aged 5 to 15 years. Am J Dis Child 140:135, 1986

RESEARCH COMMITTEE, BRITISH THORACIC SOCIETY: Community-acquired pneumonia in adults in British hospitals in 1982–83: A study of aetiology, mortality, prognostic factors and outcome. Quart J Med 62:195, 1987

SHAPIRO ED, CLEMENS JD: A controlled evaluation of pneumococcal vaccine for patients at high risk of serious pneumococcal infections. Ann Intern Med 101:325, 1984

STEPHEN JJ et al: The radiographic resolution of *Streptococcus pneumoniae* pneumonia. N Engl J Med 293:798, 1975

TUOMANEN E et al: Induction of pulmonary inflammation by components of the pneumococcal cell surface. Am Rev Resp Dis 135:869, 1987

VILADRICH PF et al: Characteristics and antibiotic therapy of adult meningitis due to penicillin-resistant pneumococci. Am J Med 84:839, 1988

100 STAPHYLOCOCCAL INFECTIONS

RICHARD M. LOCKSLEY

The staphylococci, of which *Staphylococcus aureus* is the most important human pathogen, are hardy, gram-positive bacteria that colonize the skin of most human beings. If the skin or mucous membranes are disrupted by surgery or trauma, staphylococci may gain access to and proliferate in the underlying tissues, giving rise to a typically localized, superficial abscess. Although these cutaneous infections are most commonly harmless and self-limited, the multiplying organisms may invade the lymphatics and the blood, leading to the potentially serious complications of staphylococcal bacteremia. These complications include septic shock, which may be indistinguishable from that caused by gram-negative bacteria, and serious metastatic infections, including endocarditis (see Chap. 90), arthritis (see Chap. 96), osteomyelitis (see Chap. 97), pneumonia (see Chap. 207), and abscesses (see Chap. 91) in virtually any organ. Certain strains of *S. aureus* produce toxins that cause skin rashes or that mediate multisystem dysfunction, as in toxic shock syndrome. Coagulase-negative staphylococci, particularly *S. epidermidis*, are important nosocomial pathogens, with a particular predilection for infecting vascular catheters and prosthetic devices. *S. saprophyticus* is a common cause of urinary tract infection.

ETIOLOGY AND MICROBIOLOGY Staphylococci are gram-positive, nonmotile, aerobic or facultatively anaerobic, catalase-positive cocci within the family Micrococcaceae. The name derives from the typical clustering of organisms (the Greek *staphyle*, "bunch of grapes") observed microscopically in stained specimens taken from colonies grown on solid media. Pathogenic staphylococci are distinguished from nonpathogenic micrococci by the ability of staphylococci to ferment glucose anaerobically and by their sensitivity to lysostaphin

endopeptidase. *S. aureus*, the most important human pathogen in the genus, is named for the golden color of colonies grown aerobically on solid media. All staphylococcal strains producing coagulase are designated *S. aureus*. In contrast to coagulase-negative staphylococci, *S. aureus* ferments mannitol, produces DNase, and displays greater susceptibility to lysostaphin. *S. aureus* strains are generally hemolytic when cultured on blood agar and exhibit greater expression of biochemical activity (production of coagulase, toxins, hemolysis) than coagulase negative staphylococci.

There are 21 recognized species of coagulase-negative staphylococci. Twelve are part of the normal human flora, of which *S. epidermidis* and *S. saprophyticus* are the most important clinically.

Differentiation among strains of *S. aureus* or *S. epidermidis* has been used to identify a common source during epidemics or intrahospital outbreaks of staphylococcal disease. Strains may be distinguished by antimicrobial susceptibility profiles, patterns of lysis by staphylococcal bacteriophages (phage typing), and biochemical testing (biotyping) and molecular analysis of plasmids or of plasmid or chromosomal DNA. Of these three tests, antibiotic susceptibility testing has the least, and molecular analysis the most, discriminatory ability.

EPIDEMIOLOGY The coagulase-negative staphylococci are part of the normal flora of the skin, mucous membranes, and lower bowel; *S. epidermidis* is the commonest species isolated. *S. aureus* transiently colonizes the anterior nares in 70 to 90 percent of persons and may be recovered for relatively prolonged periods of time in 20 to 30 percent of them. Nasal carriage is often accompanied by secondary colonization of the skin. Independent colonization of the perineal area occurs in 5 to 20 percent of persons, and vaginal carriage has been demonstrated in 10 percent of menstruating females. Higher carriage rates of *S. aureus* have been documented in hospital employees (including physicians and nurses), hospitalized patients, persons with atopic dermatitis, and patients whose care requires frequent puncture of the skin, e.g., with insulin-dependent diabetes, dialysis-dependent renal failure, or frequent desensitization injections for allergies. Drug abusers who use needles also have enhanced *S. aureus* carriage rates. Presumably, disturbances in the local cutaneous barrier allow *S. aureus* to establish and maintain colonization successfully.

S. saprophyticus demonstrates enhanced adherence to urothelial cells compared to *S. epidermidis*. Approximately 5 percent of healthy males and females have low colony counts of *S. saprophyticus* in the urethral or periurethral areas (see Chap. 95).

Although staphylococci can survive in the environment for prolonged periods of time and airborne spread of organisms can be demonstrated, person-to-person transfer via contaminated hands is the most important mechanism for transmission of these organisms. Hospitalized patients with active staphylococcal infection or those who become heavily colonized, particularly at cutaneous sites (surgical wounds, burns, decubitus ulcers), constitute the greatest reservoir for nosocomially acquired infection. Such patients shed an enormous number of organisms, and the hands of hospital personnel caring for these patients are readily colonized. Failure to use aseptic technique and neglect of hand washing allows transmission of the organisms to the skin of other patients. Strains of both *S. aureus* and *S. epidermidis* may become endemic in areas of the hospital housing patients with large integumental defects, particularly when widespread antimicrobial use favors the acquisition of multiply resistant strains (burn units, intensive care units, bone marrow transplant units). Less frequently, otherwise healthy hospital employees who are nasal carriers have been implicated in nosocomial outbreaks. Upon careful examination, most of these carriers will have active dermatologic infections during the time that effective transmission of staphylococci is documented.

If infections arising from the urinary tract are excluded, *S. aureus* and *S. epidermidis* together have become the most common cause of nosocomial infection in United States hospitals. They are the most frequently isolated pathogens in both primary and secondary bacteremias and in cutaneous and surgical wound infections.

PATHOGENESIS Infection by staphylococci usually results from a combination of bacterial virulence factors and diminution in host defense. Important microbial factors include the ability of the staphylococcus to survive under harsh conditions, its cell wall constituents, the production of enzymes and toxins that promote tissue invasion, its capacity to persist intracellularly in certain phagocytes, and its potential to acquire resistance to antimicrobials. Important host factors include an intact mucocutaneous barrier, an adequate number of functional neutrophils, and removal of foreign bodies or devitalized tissues.

Microbial factors Cell wall components of *S. aureus* include a large peptidoglycan complex that confers rigidity on the organism and enables it to survive under unfavorable osmotic conditions, a unique teichoic acid linked to peptidoglycan, and protein A, found both attached to peptidoglycan over the outermost parts of the cell and released in soluble form. Both peptidoglycan and teichoic acid are capable of activating the complement cascade via the alternative pathway. Although important for opsonization of organisms for ingestion by phagocytes, complement activation may also play a role in the pathogenesis of shock and disseminated intravascular coagulation. Protein A binds in the Fc portion of certain classes of IgG as well as to the Fc receptor on phagocytes and may serve as a blocking factor preventing neutrophil ingestion of the organism. Specific receptors for laminin, the major glycoprotein of the vascular basement membrane, may mediate the widespread metastatic potential of *S. aureus*. Activation of tissue factor (procoagulant activity) occurs when endothelial cells and monocytes are incubated with *S. aureus*. Some strains of *S. aureus* may be coated by an antiphagocytic capsule that requires specific antibodies for ingestion. The cell wall of certain strains of *S. epidermidis* is also capable of activating complement; shock and disseminated intravascular coagulation during infections by these organisms have been described, although less frequently than with *S. aureus*. The capacity of *S. epidermidis* to adhere to intravascular cannulas and prosthetic devices may explain the propensity of these organisms to cause foreign body infections. These organisms bind fibronectin and other matrix proteins that coat catheters and secrete an exopolysaccharide slime that forms a protective biofilm over the colonizing organisms.

Certain enzymes produced by *S. aureus* may play a role in virulence. Catalase degrades hydrogen peroxide and may protect the organism during phagocytosis when it must withstand the phagocyte's respiratory burst. Coagulase is present in both soluble and cell-bound forms, and causes plasma to clot by formation of thrombinlike material. The high correlation between coagulase production and virulence suggests that this substance is important in the pathogenesis of staphylococcal infections, but its precise role as a determinant of pathogenicity has not been determined. Many strains also produce hyaluronidase, an enzyme that degrades hyaluronic acid in the connective tissue matrix and that may promote spreading of infection. A trypsinlike protease from some strains enhances influenza virus infection by proteolytic cleavage of the viral precursor hemagglutinin into its active fragments, and may contribute to the morbidity of such coinfections. *S. saprophyticus* produces urease, an enzyme capable of breaking down urea to ammonium, alkalinizing the urine and favoring the formation of struvite stones.

S. aureus may produce numerous extracellular toxins. The expression of multiple toxins, as in gram-negative bacilli, is coordinately regulated by an accessory gene regulator protein, presumably in response to physicochemical environmental stimuli. Toxins may be encoded by chromosomal or plasmid DNA. Four different red cell hemolysins—designated alpha, beta, gamma, and delta toxins—have been identified. Alpha toxin is also dermonecrotic when injected subcutaneously into animals. Delta toxin inhibits water absorption by elevating cyclic AMP in guinea pig ileum and may play a role in the acute watery diarrhea seen in some cases of staphylococcal infection. Leukocidin lyses granulocyte and macrophage membranes by producing membrane pores permeable to cations.

While the role of the above factors in virulence is incompletely understood, the exfoliatin toxins A and B, the staphylococcal enterotoxins, and the toxic shock syndrome toxin—TSST-1—have been implicated in disease. The exfoliatin toxins mediate the dermatologic manifestations of the staphylococcal scalded skin syndrome. The chromosomally mediated toxins cause intraepidermal cleavage of the skin at the stratum granulosum, leading to bullae formation and denudation. Antibodies to the toxins are protective in both humans and animals. Five serologically distinct enterotoxins (A through E) have been implicated in food poisoning due to *S. aureus*. The toxins enhance intestinal peristalsis and seem to induce vomiting by a direct effect on the central nervous system. Enterotoxins B and C may also mediate toxic shock syndrome (TSS), although this is more frequently due to TSST-1. TSST-1 is produced by over 90 percent of *S. aureus* recovered from women with menstrual TSS and over 60 percent of nonmenstrual cases. Most TSST-1 negative strains produce enterotoxin B and, rarely, enterotoxin C. TSST-1 is a 22-kDa protein that causes hypotension, conjunctival and cutaneous hyperemia, and fever when injected into rabbits; death may result from multisystem failure and mimics human TSS. TSST-1 is a potent stimulus for cytokine release by mononuclear cells: tumor necrosis factor (TNF) and interleukin 1 (IL-1) are released by monocytes, and lymphotoxin, IL-2, colony-stimulating factors, and interferon-γ are released by lymphocytes. Host cytokines presumably mediate most of the symptoms of TSS (see Chaps. 20 and 89). The *tst* gene encoding TSST-1 is present in 5 to 25 percent of clinical isolates of *S. aureus* as part of a large, mobile transposon-like element. Similar elements encode the enterotoxin B and C genes. Like TSST-1, enterotoxins B and C cause a TSS-like syndrome in animals, are pyrogenic, and are potent inducers of cytokine production by human T cells and macrophages.

Antimicrobial resistance by staphylococci favors their persistence in the hospital environment. Over 90 percent of both hospital and community strains of *S. aureus* causing infection are resistant to penicillin. Resistance is due to the production of β-lactamases, usually by plasmids. A subgroup of *S. aureus* hyperproduce β-lactamase in vitro and show borderline susceptibility to oxacillin that disappears when clavulanic acid (β-lactamase inhibitor) is added. Infections due to these organisms with "acquired resistance to oxacillin" can be treated safely with penicillinase-resistant β-lactam antimicrobial agents. The true penicillinase-resistant *S. aureus,* called methicillin-resistant *S. aureus* (MRSA), are resistant to all the β-lactam antimicrobics, as well as to the cephalosporins, despite the fact that standard disk susceptibility testing may indicate sensitivity to cephalosporin drugs. Resistance of MRSA is chromosomally mediated and involves production of an altered penicillin-binding protein (PBP 2a or PBP 2′) with a low binding affinity for β-lactams. Not uncommonly, MRSA has acquired R plasmids mediating some combination of resistance to erythromycin, tetracycline, chloramphenicol, clindamycin, and aminoglycosides. MRSA has become increasingly common worldwide, particularly in tertiary care referral hospitals. In the United States, approximately 5 percent of hospital isolates of *S. aureus* are MRSA; one-third of hospitals surveyed have experienced bacteremias due to MRSA. The isolation of these organisms has remained relatively constant since 1980. Outbreaks continue to occur periodically in the form of intrahospital epidemics. The community carriage rate of MRSA is low, although selected patient populations, like parenteral drug abusers, may have MRSA at the time of admission to the hospital. These isolates remain susceptible to vancomycin.

Tolerance of staphylococci to β-lactams is an in vitro phenomenon characterized by resistance to the lethal action of normally cidal antimicrobials. It is characterized by a marked discrepancy between the minimal inhibitory and the minimal bactericidal concentrations of the drug. The mechanism may relate to a defect in the normal activation of autolytic enzymes of the bacteria by cell wall-active antimicrobials. Demonstration of the trait is influenced markedly by physicochemical conditions. Although tolerance has been reported to influence the outcome of severe staphylococcal infection adversely, it has been difficult to incriminate tolerance to β-lactams as a significant cause of antibiotic failure. This may reflect the in vitro observation that continued treatment with β-lactams will kill tolerant *S. aureus*, although killing proceeds more slowly.

Most instances of *S. epidermidis* infection are nosocomially acquired and typically express greater variability and degrees of antimicrobial resistance than those of *S. aureus*. Virtually all isolates contain R plasmids that produce β-lactamase and are resistant to penicillin. Approximately one-third are resistant to aminoglycosides and two-thirds are resistant to tetracycline, erythromycin, clindamycin, and chloramphenicol. Hospital isolates of *S. epidermidis* containing multiple antimicrobial-resistant plasmids can serve as important reservoirs for the acquisition of resistance by *S. aureus* and *Enterococcus* species.

Methicillin resistance is common among *S. epidermidis* strains; over 80 percent of isolates from cases with prosthetic valve endocarditis in one study were methicillin-resistant. Conditions of temperature, pH, osmolality, and the presence of chelating agents and heavy metals all may influence the demonstration of resistance. Methicillin-resistant isolates may appear susceptible by routine susceptibility testing. The most reliable identification of these organisms is by their growth from a large inoculum (10^7 cells) spread on agar containing 6 µg/mL oxacillin. Cross-resistance to the other β-lactam antimicrobials and to the cephalosporins is always present, although as with MRSA, these bacteria may appear susceptible to cephalosporins using conventional disk testing. As with *S. aureus*, *S. epidermidis* strains remain susceptible to vancomycin, although resistance has occurred in strains of *S. haemolyticus*. Although the quinolone antibiotics are active against methicillin-resistant staphylococci, resistance has occurred when these drugs are used alone.

HOST FACTORS The importance of host factors in resisting staphylococcal infections is demonstrated by the observation that enormous numbers of bacteria are required to establish experimental infections in humans and animals. Areas where skin or mucosal continuity is broken provide portals of entry for staphylococci. More than 50 percent of serious staphylococcal infections of deep tissues arise from cutaneous foci; a smaller number originate from respiratory, gastrointestinal, or less frequently, the genitourinary tract. Direct inoculation of organisms into the blood is an important route of infection in hospitalized patients with intravenous catheters and in drug abusers.

Staphylococci often invade the integument via plugged hair follicles and sebaceous glands, or areas involved by burns, wounds, abrasions, insect bites, or dermatitis. Colonization and invasion of the lungs may occur when the normal mucociliary clearance mechanisms are either bypassed, as occurs with endotracheal intubation, or depressed, as occurs following viral infections of the lung (influenza) or in patients with cystic fibrosis. Mucosal damage to the gastrointestinal tract following cytotoxic chemotherapy or radiotherapy predisposes to invasion from that site.

Once the integument has been breached, local bacterial multiplication is accompanied by inflammation and tissue necrosis at the site of infection. Neutrophils rapidly enter the area and ingest large numbers of staphylococci. Thrombosis of surrounding capillaries occurs; fibrin is deposited about the periphery; later, fibroblasts create a relatively avascular wall about the area. The fully developed staphylococcal abscess consists of a central core of dead and dying leukocytes and bacteria which gradually liquefies to form characteristic thick, creamy pus, surrounded by a fibroblastic wall. When host mechanisms fail to contain the cutaneous or submucosal infection, staphylococci may enter the lymphatics and the bloodstream. Common sites of metastatic seeding include the diaphyseal ends of long bones in children, and the lungs, kidneys, cardiac valves, myocardium, liver, spleen, and brain.

Polymorphonuclear leukocytes appear to be the major protective mechanism against staphylococcal disease. Persons with neutropenia or inherited or acquired defects of neutrophil chemotaxis, ingestion, or killing are particularly susceptible to staphylococcal infections. A low number of staphylococci are capable of surviving within phagocytes, which may account for the relatively slow response of

staphylococcal infections to antimicrobials and the potential for relapse.

Although infections may occur in all age groups, serious staphylococcal infections most commonly afflict the young and old—particularly those with underlying debilitating disease. Primary staphylococcal pneumonia is common in infants but rare in adults. Acute staphylococcal osteomyelitis is almost exclusively a disease of children. Superficial staphylococcal pyoderma is more frequent in infants, whereas actual abscess formation occurs more often in adults. While these examples suggest some role for immunity in resistance against staphylococci, there has been no satisfactory demonstration that human staphylococcal disease is followed by effective immunity or that infection can be modified significantly by vaccination. Virtually 100 percent of adults possess antistaphylococcal antibodies in their serum. Except for the efficacy of neutralizing antibodies to toxins in staphylococcal toxin–mediated diseases, the role of humoral immunity in modifying or protecting against staphylococcal infection is unclear.

The presence of a foreign body such as a suture or a prosthetic device markedly decreases the inoculum of staphylococci required to produce experimental infection. Once established, such infections are very difficult to cure without removal of the foreign body. Strains of *S. epidermidis* are capable of adhering firmly to and invading plastic catheters and of secreting a protective glycocalyx covering the adherent colonies. Neutrophil function is also altered in the presence of a foreign body; phagocytosis and killing of *S. aureus* are diminished.

DIAGNOSIS The diagnosis of all staphylococcal infections is made by Gram's stain and culture of purulent material, either aspirated pus or involved tissue, or by culture of normally sterile body fluids. Typical clustering of organisms may not be seen in clinical specimens; individual cocci and even short chains of three or four organisms may be present. Bacteria in the static phase or within leukocytes may appear gram-negative. Abundant neutrophils, many containing intracellular organisms, are usually present, except in severely neutropenic patients.

SPECIFIC DISEASES **Superficial infections** Infection of hair follicles manifested as a collection of minute erythematous papules without involvement of the surrounding skin or deeper tissues is termed *folliculitis*. A more extensive and invasive follicular or sebaceous gland infection with some involvement of subcutaneous tissues is termed a *furuncle*, or *boil*. Itching and mild pain are followed by progressive local swelling and erythema, and the overlying skin becomes exquisitely painful on pressure or motion. Relief of pain occurs promptly after spontaneous or surgical drainage.

Furuncles occur most commonly in areas subjected to maceration or friction, poor personal hygiene, or involved by acne or dermatitis. The face, neck, axillae, buttocks, and thighs are common sites. Staphylococcal infection may involve the apocrine sweat glands in the axilla or groin (hidradenitis suppurativa). These infections may be deep-seated, slow to localize and drain, and are prone to recurrence and scarring.

Staphylococcal infections within the thick, fibrous, inelastic skin of the back of the neck and upper part of the back lead to formation of a *carbuncle*. The relative thickness and impermeability of the overlying skin lead to lateral extension and loculation, and a large, indurated, painful lesion with multiple ineffective drainage sites results. Carbuncles produce fever, leukocytosis, extreme pain, and prostration. Bacteremia is common.

Staphylococci frequently colonize impetiginous lesions, but most impetigo is due to group A streptococci. However, staphylococcal impetigo does occur, and while it cannot be clearly differentiated on the basis of its clinical features from streptococcal impetigo, it tends to produce multiple superficial, localized lesions at different stages of development, has a grayish rather than golden-yellow crust, and less often produces high fever.

Treatment of most superficial infections does not require the use of antibiotics. Local moist heat, attention to personal hygiene, and washing with germicidal soaps that leave an inhibitory residue on the skin (hexachlorophene, chlorhexidine, triclosan) are usually sufficient.

For more severe or recurrent disease, oral antibiotic therapy with dicloxacillin or cloxacillin (2 g/d in four divided doses) for 7 to 10 days may be effective. Incision and drainage should be utilized selectively. Disease presenting with prominent constitutional symptoms or facial or periorbital infection should be treated with intravenous doses of appropriate antimicrobials as outlined in the section on bacteremic disease.

Toxin-mediated staphylococcal diseases STAPHYLOCOCCAL SCALDED SKIN SYNDROME (SSSS) SSSS is a generalized exfoliative dermatitis complicating infection by toxin (exfoliatin)-producing strains of *S. aureus*. The disease typically occurs in newborns (Ritter's disease) and in children under the age of 5; it is rare in adults. Strains of *S. aureus* causing SSSS in the United States are frequently phage group II. The disease begins with a localized cutaneous infection often accompanied by a nonspecific viral-like prodrome. Fever and leukocytosis are mild. A scarlatiniform rash begins in the perioral area, becomes generalized over the trunk and extremities, and finally desquamates. The disease may consist of rash alone (staphylococcal scarlet fever), or large, flaccid bullae develop that may be localized (more common in adults) or generalized. The bullae burst, resulting in red, denuded skin resembling a burn. Friction applied to healthy areas of skin causes the epidermis to wrinkle and separate (Nikolsky's sign). *S. aureus* can usually be recovered from the skin and nasopharynx. Most adults with SSSS are immunosuppressed or have renal insufficiency. Blood cultures are frequently positive, and mortality is significant. Therapy includes antistaphylococcal antibiotics and local skin care. Recovery usually occurs in infants and children.

In adults, SSSS has been grouped with other severe scalding syndromes such as toxic epidermal necrolysis (Lyell's disease). Drug reactions are the most frequent cause of toxic epidermal necrolysis in adults, and the syndrome may be differentiated from SSSS by skin biopsy. Cleavage of the skin in drug-induced toxic epidermal necrolysis occurs at the basal cell layer resulting in full-thickness denudation, with a greater potential for superinfection and significant fluid and electrolyte loss. In SSSS, cleavage occurs within the epidermis. Kawasaki's disease and toxic shock syndrome should also be considered in the differential diagnosis of SSSS.

TOXIC SHOCK SYNDROME Toxic shock syndrome (TSS) was described in 1978 as a multisystem disease presenting with high fever, a "sunburn" rash that subsequently desquamated, and hypotension in children who had group I *S. aureus* isolated from mucosal or sequestered sites. In 1980 TSS became epidemic among young, primarily white, women, with onset during menstruation. A strong correlation was found between TSS and recovery of *S. aureus* from vaginal or cervical cultures of affected patients. The occurrence of a rash, the infrequency of bacteremia, and the association with *S. aureus* suggested a toxin-associated illness. Subsequently a marker toxin, TSST-1, that mediates most cases of this syndrome was identified. Staphylococcal enterotoxins B or C may also mediate TSS. The pathogenesis involves establishment of a toxin-producing strain in a nonimmune individual under conditions favoring toxin formation; i.e., an aerobic, nutrient environment favoring late-log to stationary phase growth of the organism. The attack rate of TSS among the 10 percent of persons lacking sufficient levels of antitoxin antibodies approaches 25 percent when infected with toxin-positive strains.

Epidemiologically, TSS was associated with the introduction of certain brands of hyperabsorbent tampons. Their prolonged intravaginal use enhances the aerobic surface area in the vagina favoring the growth of intravaginal *S. aureus* and TSST-1 production. Public education and removal of hyperabsorbent tampons from the market have resulted in a marked decrease in the number of reported cases of TSS. Although the majority of cases continue to occur among menstruating females, nonmenstrual TSS now accounts for up to 45 percent of TSS cases in the United States.

The diagnosis of TSS is based on clinical criteria that include high fever, a diffuse rash that desquamates on the palms and soles

over the subsequent 1 to 2 weeks, hypotension that may be orthostatic, plus evidence of involvement in three or more organ systems. These commonly include gastrointestinal dysfunction (vomiting or diarrhea), renal or hepatic insufficiency, mucous membrane hyperemia, thrombocytopenia, myalgias with elevated creatine phosphokinase (CK) levels, and disorientation with a normal cerebrospinal fluid examination. Milder forms of the syndrome have been reported.

The onset is acute and typically occurs around the start of menses in a young woman using tampons or barrier contraception methods. The vaginal mucosa is hyperemic, and *S. aureus* can be cultured from the vaginal discharge. Blood cultures are usually negative. Clinical findings are the same in nonmenstrual-associated TSS. Cutaneous infections, postpartum vaginal and cesarean section wound infections, focal tissue infections (abscesses, empyema, osteomyelitis), postinfluenza pneumonia, and rarely primary staphylococcal bacteremia have been associated with TSS. Signs of infection may be minimal among patients with postoperative wound infections where the onset typically occurs on the second day after surgery. Nosocomial transmission has been described. The mortality rate of TSS is 3 percent and is most often due to refractory hypotension and the development of the adult respiratory distress syndrome (ARDS) with or without disseminated intravascular coagulation.

Treatment is directed at correcting shock and treating renal failure, pulmonary insufficiency, and disseminated intravascular coagulation when present. Antistaphylococcal antibiotics should be administered parenterally. Focal collections of *S. aureus* must be drained. Because neutralizing antibodies are widespread, the use of intravenous pooled gamma globulin is being investigated. Up to 30 percent of menstruating women with TSS may have recurrences with subsequent menses, although these are generally milder. The use of antistaphylococcal antibiotics to treat TSS and discontinuation of tampon use significantly decrease the likelihood of recurrences.

The differential diagnosis of TSS includes Rocky Mountain spotted fever, meningococcemia, streptococcal scarlet fever, toxic epidermal necrolysis, and Kawasaki's syndrome. A similar syndrome has been described following group A streptococcal infection.

Staphylococcal food poisoning See Chap. 92.

Invasive staphylococcal infections BACTEREMIA AND ENDOCARDITIS Bacteremia due to *S. aureus* may arise from any local infection, either at extravascular (cutaneous infections, burns, cellulitis, osteomyelitis, arthritis) or intravascular foci (intravenous catheters, dialysis access sites, intravenous drug abuse). Up to one-third of patients do not have an identifiable focus.

Rarely, patients with bacteremia die within 12 to 24 h with high fever, tachycardia, cyanosis, and vascular collapse. Disseminated intravascular coagulation may produce a disease mimicking meningococcemia. Commonly, the disease progresses more slowly, with hectic fever and metastatic abscess formation in the bones, kidneys, lungs, myocardium, spleen, brain, or other tissues.

A major complication of *S. aureus* bacteremia is endocarditis (see Chap. 90). *S. aureus* is the second most common cause of endocarditis and the commonest cause among drug addicts. Among nonaddicts, normal valves are involved in 30 to 60 percent of cases, and older, frequently hospitalized, patients with underlying medical disease are most often infected. The mitral, aortic, or both valves may be involved. The disease typically pursues an acute course with high fever, progressive anemia, and frequent embolic and extracardiac septic complications. Progressive valvular insufficiency leads to significant murmurs in 90 percent of patients. Valve ring and myocardial abscesses are common. The mortality rate is 20 to 30 percent. Infection of the aortic valve, the development of uncontrolled congestive heart failure, or evidence of central nervous system involvement are poor prognostic signs; these patients frequently require surgical intervention.

Among addicts, *S. aureus* frequently involves the tricuspid valve. Evidence for septic pulmonary emboli (chest pain, hemoptysis, nodular infiltrates) is common. Audible murmurs and peripheral stigmata of endocarditis are less common than in nonaddicts. Myalgias and back pain may be the major presenting symptoms and obfuscate the diagnosis. The mortality rate is 2 to 10 percent.

Differentiation of bacteremia from endocarditis may be difficult. Patients with normal heart valves with an identifiable, easily managed or removable primary focus of infection, who receive and respond promptly to appropriate antibiotic therapy, and who do not develop evidence of metastatic complications during the subsequent 2 weeks on therapy usually can be treated for bacteremia alone. Patients with underlying valvular disorders, with murmurs of valvular regurgitation, with community-acquired disease and no obvious focus, with infection secondary to drug abuse, with evidence for embolic events, or with echocardiographic evidence for vegetations should be treated for endocarditis. The presence of antibodies to the teichoic acid cell-wall component of S. aureus after 2 weeks of illness does not distinguish reliably between endocarditis or bacteremia with metastatic foci and uncomplicated bacteremia.

Three carefully collected blood cultures are adequate for the diagnosis in most instances; usually all are positive for S. aureus. More cultures may be required if the patient has previously received antibiotics. Purulent skin lesions and urine should also be cultured before instituting antibiotic therapy. The urine may be positive in up to a third of cases of staphylococcal bacteremia (with colony counts typically lower than 10^5 per milliliter); staphylococcal bacteriuria in this setting does not indicate metastatic renal infection.

Intravenous therapy should be initiated with a penicillinase-resistant agent. Nafcillin (1.5 g every 4 h) and oxacillin (2.0 g every 4 h) are preferred to methicillin because of the high incidence of interstitial nephritis with methicillin. Gentamicin (1 mg/kg every 8 h, adjusted for renal function) is frequently added for the first 48 to 72 h because of evidence for synergy with β-lactam antimicrobials against S. aureus and the tendency for patients treated with both drugs to defervesce more rapidly and to achieve earlier sterilization of the bloodstream. Rare isolates that do not produce β-lactamase should be treated with intravenous penicillin G (4×10^6 units every 4 h). First-generation cephalosporins (cephalothin, cefazolin) have also been used successfully in infections with both penicillinase-positive and -negative strains of S. aureus. Patients with serious penicillin allergy or with infections due to methicillin-resistant S. aureus should be treated with vancomycin 30 mg/kg per day in two or three divided doses, adjusted for renal function.

Cases of uncomplicated S. aureus bacteremia can be treated for 2 weeks. These patients should be followed carefully; relapses should be treated as endocarditis. Uncomplicated right-sided endocarditis in drug addicts has been successfully treated with 2 weeks of intravenous nafcillin plus tobramycin or gentamicin. All other cases of endocarditis should receive 4 to 6 weeks of parenteral antimicrobials. Prosthetic valve endocarditis should be treated with an appropriate penicillin or vancomycin, plus gentamicin, with or without rifampin, for 6 weeks. Most cases will require surgery as well.

The response to antimicrobials in staphylococcal endocarditis may be slow. The fever may not disappear until the second week of therapy. Persistent fever or signs of sepsis should prompt a search for metastatic abscesses that require drainage.

S. epidermidis is the most common isolate in primary nosocomial bacteremias and the most frequent organism infecting intravenous access devices. It has been recognized as a major cause of bacteremia among neutropenic cancer patients, arising either from long-term, indwelling central catheters or from the gastrointestinal tract. Continued fever, progressive sepsis, multiple pulmonary abscesses, and death may result if this complication is left untreated.

Although an uncommon cause of native valve endocarditis, S. epidermidis is the commonest cause of prosthetic valve endocarditis (40 percent of cases). Most cases are due to inoculation of organisms at the time of surgery but may not become clinically apparent until 1 year later. Infections frequently involve the valve ring and require surgical intervention. Over 50 percent of patients die.

Because coagulase-negative staphylococci are frequent blood culture contaminants, distinguishing infection from contamination can be difficult. Positive blood cultures demand careful inspection of catheter sites and repeat blood cultures, even in the absence of symptoms, in patients with indwelling catheters, or with prosthetic heart valves or vascular grafts. Speciation of multiple isolates may be useful if isolates can be demonstrated to be the same; plasmid analysis may be required. Catheters should be removed and cultured, although antibiotic therapy alone has been successful for treatment of bacteremic catheter-related infections.

Hospital-acquired S. epidermidis infections are usually multiply antibiotic resistant. Methicillin resistance is heterotypic and difficult to exclude. For these reasons, all serious S. epidermidis infections should be treated with vancomycin in doses used for S. aureus. Prosthetic valve endocarditis should be treated for 6 weeks with vancomycin plus gentamicin, with or without rifampin. Monitoring of renal function and ototoxicity is required.

OSTEOMYELITIS   S. aureus is responsible for the majority of cases of acute osteomyelitis (see Chap. 97). This infection occurs most commonly in children under the age of 12, but adults are also susceptible to acute osteomyelitis, especially of the spine. Approximately 50 percent of patients give a history of a furuncle or superficial staphylococcal infection preceding osteomyelitis. In children, the frequent localization in the diaphyseal end of the long bones is thought to be due to the endarterial circulation of the diaphysis. Many patients give a history of preceding trauma to the involved area. Clavicular osteomyelitis has complicated septic thrombosis of a catheterized subclavian vein.

Once established, infection spreads through the newly formed juxtaepiphyseal bone to the periosteum or along the marrow cavity. If the infection reaches the subperiosteal space, the periosteum is lifted, a subperiosteal abscess forms, and rupture with infection of the subcutaneous tissues may occur. Rarely, the joint capsule is penetrated, producing pyogenic arthritis. There is death of bone, producing a sequestrum, followed by new bone formation, the involucrum. Occasionally indolent staphylococcal infections of bone may persist for years within dense granulation tissue about a central necrotic cavity, a so-called Brodie's abscess.

Osteomyelitis in children may present as an acute process beginning abruptly with chills, high fever, nausea, vomiting, and progressive pain at the site of bony involvement. Muscle spasm about the affected bone is a common early sign, and the child may refuse to move the affected limb. Leukocytosis is common. Blood cultures are positive for S. aureus in 50 to 60 percent of cases early in disease. The tissues overlying the involved bone become edematous and warm, and the skin becomes erythematous. Anemia develops during the course of untreated disease.

Staphylococcal vertebral osteomyelitis in the adult differs considerably from acute osteomyelitis in the child. The onset is less abrupt, and there is a greater tendency for bony fusion with obliteration of the disk space. The lumbar spine is most frequently affected.

Osteomyelitis should be suspected in any child with fever, limb pain, and leukocytosis. Similarly, back or neck pain in an adult, when accompanied by fever, should raise the possibility of vertebral osteomyelitis. A history of a preceding cutaneous infection, local tenderness over the bone, and culture of S. aureus from the blood are confirmatory. Roentgenograms are usually normal during the first week, but radionuclide scans may be abnormal. Bony rarefaction, local periosteal elevation, and new bone formation can frequently be seen during the second week. Needle aspiration or bone biopsy should be performed if necessary to obtain a specific etiologic diagnosis prior to institution of chemotherapy. In chronic osteomyelitis, sinus tracts are often present, but cultures of the sinus tracts are not reliable in the diagnosis.

Therapy should be initiated parenterally using a penicillinase-resistant semisynthetic penicillin as outlined for bacteremia and endocarditis and continued for 4 to 6 weeks. Cephalosporins and clindamycin have also been used. Uncomplicated osteomyelitis in children has been managed with 2 weeks of intravenous therapy followed by 2 to 4 weeks of oral therapy. Vancomycin can be used in penicillin-allergic patients and in infections due to methicillin-resistant organisms. Surgery may be required to remove devitalized bone and to drain soft tissue and periosteal abscesses. Neurologic findings due to epidural abscess and cord compression complicating vertebral osteomyelitis demand early surgical intervention. Aggressive treatment of acute osteomyelitis has decreased the incidence of chronic osteomyelitis, with its penchant for recurrent flare-ups and sinus formation. The cure rate for acute staphylococcal osteomyelitis is approximately 90 percent, and death is rare.

PNEUMONIA (See Chap. 207)   S. aureus causes approximately 1 percent of community-acquired bacterial pneumonias. This disease occurs sporadically except during influenza outbreaks, when staphylococcal pneumonia is relatively more common, although still less frequent than pneumococcal pneumonia.

Primary staphylococcal pneumonia in infants and children frequently presents with high fever and cough. Multiple thin-walled abscesses, or pneumatoceles, are present on the chest roentgenogram. Empyema formation is common. Cough may be nonproductive, and blood cultures are usually negative, frequently necessitating empiric antistaphylococcal therapy. In older children and healthy adults staphylococcal pneumonia is generally preceded by an influenza-like respiratory infection (influenza, measles, or other viruses). Onset of staphylococcal involvement is abrupt, with chills, high fever, progressive dyspnea, cyanosis, cough, and pleural pain. The sputum may be bloody or frankly purulent.

Staphylococci frequently colonize the bronchiectatic airways in children with cystic fibrosis and may cause recurrent episodes of bronchopneumonia. Nosocomial staphylococcal pneumonia typically occurs in intubated patients in intensive care units and in debilitated patients who are prone to aspiration. Residents of nursing homes may have an increased incidence of staphylococcal pneumonia. Infections distal to an obstructing bronchogenic carcinoma may also be caused by S. aureus. These infections can begin insidiously, with increasing fever, tachycardia, and tachypnea the only indications of infection. The disease may also be less abrupt when pulmonary involvement occurs during the course of staphylococcal bacteremia, as in patients with right-sided endocarditis or septic thrombophlebitis. Cavitation and pleural effusions are common, but empyema is unusual.

The course of staphylococcal pneumonia may be stormy despite adequate antimicrobial therapy. Gradual defervescence starting 48 to 72 h after the initiation of therapy is typical.

Staphylococcal pneumonia must be differentiated from other pneumonias. The preceding influenza-like illness, rapid onset of pleural pain, cyanosis, and prostration out of proportion to physical findings should suggest primary staphylococcal pneumonia. Sputum Gram's stain showing masses of neutrophils and gram-positive intraleukocytic cocci provides supportive evidence. Leukocytosis is generally present. Blood cultures are positive in 20 to 30 percent of cases. When pneumonia develops suddenly or insidiously in debilitated hospital patients, staphylococci should be considered.

Parenteral therapy should be initiated with antistaphylococcal antimicrobials as outlined for serious bacteremia and endocarditis. Two weeks of intravenous therapy is usually adequate if complications do not develop. Empyema usually necessitates chest tube drainage and may be complicated by the formation of loculations or bronchopleural fistulas. Ultrasound or computed tomography scan may be required to identify loculated collections of pus for drainage.

URINARY TRACT INFECTION   S. saprophyticus is, after Escherichia coli, the most common cause of primary, nonobstructive urinary tract infection in sexually active young women (see Chap. 95). It is responsible for 10 to 20 percent of infections in healthy outpatients. Symptoms of urgency, frequency, and burning are indistinguishable from urinary infections due to other agents. Fever is absent or low-grade. Although lower tract infection is most common, pyelonephritis has been reported.

The diagnosis is established by examination of the urinary sediment, which characteristically reveals pyuria, microscopic hematuria, and cocci in clumps. The organism may be identified by its resistance to novobiocin and nalidixic acid. S. saprophyticus grows readily on blood agar, but less well on MacConkey agar and may be missed by currently available rapid diagnostic methods that depend on nitrate reduction or glucose utilization. The criterion for greater than 10^5 bacteria per milliliter developed for gram-negative urinary tract infection is unreliable.

The organism is susceptible to most antimicrobials used for urinary tract infection, including ampicillin, trimethoprim, sulfonamides, and nitrofurantoin. Relapses after appropriate therapy should raise the consideration of infected renal calculi, which may be formed because of the organism's capacity to produce urease.

Isolation of S. aureus from a well-collected urine specimen should prompt consideration of staphylococcal bacteremia, which may have been complicated by renal, perinephric, or prostatic abscesses.

Other infections   Infection of the vascular-access site with S. aureus is a major cause of morbidity and death among patients on hemodialysis. Chronic nasal carriage is the source of most infections. The use of 5-day courses of oral rifampin and topical bacitracin every 3 months significantly decreases the incidence of infection, and should be considered in hemodialysis centers where such infections are endemic. S. epidermidis and S. aureus rank first and second among pathogens infecting prosthetic devices and intravascular grafts. S. epidermidis infections tend to be more insidious and frequently pursue a prolonged course with high morbidity due in part to the temptation to regard positive cultures as contaminants. Subtle clinical findings are common—prosthetic hip infections may present with pain and loosening of the prosthesis, and cerebrospinal fluid shunt infections may present as hypocomplementemic glomerulonephritis due to circulating immune complexes. S. epidermidis is a common cause of endophthalmitis complicating ocular surgery. S. aureus is a frequent cause of mastitis among nursing mothers.

CONTROL OF HOSPITAL OUTBREAKS (See Chap. 85)   Hospital outbreaks of staphylococcal disease may develop rapidly in burn units, intensive care units, or neonatal care units—areas housing debilitated patients under continuous antibiotic pressure. The index case is frequently a patient recently discharged or transferred from another hospital where the organism is endemic. The implicated strains of S. aureus are frequently methicillin-resistant (MRSA).

Control demands the rapid identification of the patient reservoir in the affected care units by cultures of wounds, nares, and perineum; urine cultures should be obtained from patients with indwelling urinary catheters. Isolation of culture-positive patients together with reinforcement of the need for proper aseptic technique and hand washing by hospital personnel decreases transmission. Housekeeping antisepsis using phenolic cleaning agents should be carried out in the rooms of colonized patients. Early discharge of colonized patients should be encouraged. Charts should be labeled and the patient returned to strict isolation upon readmission to the hospital until shown to be culture-negative.

Although nasal carriers among hospital personnel may transmit the organism, efficient dissemination is by cutaneous diseases (eczema, atopic dermatitis) that have become colonized with S. aureus. Such personnel should be removed from clinical duties until they become culture-negative either spontaneously or following therapy.

Decolonization of the skin and nares in patients and personnel has been accomplished by whole-body washing with antiseptic soaps that leave an inhibitory residue on the skin—hexachlorophene, chlorhexidine, or triclosan. Topical antibiotics are ineffective. Oral antibiotics may be required to abolish the carrier state. Rifampin (600 mg every day for 5 days) has been used successfully alone or, depending on the sensitivity of the staphylococcal isolate, combined with trimethoprim-sulfamethoxazole, doxycycline, or dicloxacillin to prevent the emergence of rifampin resistance.

REFERENCES

ARBUTHNOT J et al (eds): International Symposium on Toxic Shock Syndrome. Rev Infect Disease 11 (Suppl 1):S1, 1989

BRUMFITT W, HAMILTON-MILLER J: Methicillin-resistant *Staphylococcus aureus*. N Engl J Med 320:1188, 1989

CHAMBERS HF et al: Right-sided *Staphylococcus aureus* endocarditis in intravenous drug abusers: Two-week combination therapy. Ann Intern Med 109:619, 1988

MARTIN MA et al: Coagulase-negative staphylococcal bacteremia. Mortality and hospital stay. Ann Intern Med 110:9, 1989

PFALLER MA, HERWALDT LA: Laboratory, clinical and epidemiological aspects of coagulase-negative staphylococci. Clin Microbiol Rev 1:281, 1988

TODD JK: Staphylococcal toxin syndromes. Annu Rev Med 36:337, 1986

YU VL et al: *Staphylococcus aureus* nasal carriage and infection in patients on hemodialysis. Efficacy of antibiotic prophylaxis. N Engl J Med 315:91, 1986

101 STREPTOCOCCAL INFECTIONS

ALAN BISNO

Streptococci are among the commonest bacterial pathogens of humans. They are responsible for a diverse spectrum of diseases including pharyngitis and tonsillitis, scarlet fever, erysipelas, impetigo, lymphangitis, and perinatal infections of mother and child. Certain representatives of this genus are prominent causes of endocarditis and urinary tract infections. In addition to their role in causing acute pyogenic infections, strains of *Streptococcus pyogenes* are capable of giving rise to the delayed nonsuppurative sequels of acute rheumatic fever and acute glomerulonephritis.

ETIOLOGY AND CLASSIFICATION Streptococci are spherical or ovoid bacterial cells which grow in pairs or chains of varying lengths. Most are facultative anaerobes. The organisms are grampositive, usually nonmotile, non-spore-forming, and catalasenegative. No single system of classification suffices to differentiate this heterogeneous group of organisms. Instead, classification depends upon a combination of features, including patterns of hemolysis observed on blood agar plates, antigenic composition, growth characteristics, biochemical reactions, and genetic studies.

When cultivated on sheep blood agar plates, colonies of streptococci may exhibit complete (beta), partial (alpha), or no (gamma) hemolysis. The term *hemolytic streptococci* is currently applied to beta-hemolytic strains. Colonies of such strains are surrounded by clear colorless zones within which the red cells have been completely lysed. This pattern of hemolysis is characteristic of *S. pyogenes* and many other streptococci pathogenic for humans. Alpha-hemolytic colonies are surrounded by a zone of greenish discoloration, whence the often-used designation "viridans streptococci." Strains of *S. pneumoniae* are alpha hemolytic, as are many other streptococci which normally inhabit the upper respiratory and gastrointestinal tracts.

Although classification of streptococci on the basis of hemolytic reactions is quite useful in certain clinical situations, more precise identification of streptococci is accomplished by differentiation into serogroups, as originally described by Lancefield, on the basis of antigenic differences in cell wall carbohydrates or teichoic acids. The majority of beta-hemolytic streptococci isolated from human infections belong to groups A to D and G. Certain alpha-hemolytic and nonhemolytic strains also contain group-specific antigens. The most important of these are the group D streptococci, including the so-called enterococci, among which many strains fail to show beta hemolysis.

Species designation is based upon growth characteristics under varying conditions of temperature, pH, and media composition. Some species do not possess group antigens, and a number of serogroups do not encompass any of the recognized species.

Anaerobic streptococci include members of the family Peptococcaceae, genus *Peptostreptococcus;* four species are recognized. Hemolytic reactions of these organisms are variable, and no satisfactory method of classifying them has been devised.

GROUP A STREPTOCOCCAL INFECTIONS

Streptococci of Lancefield's group A (*S. pyogenes*) are uniquely important because of the frequency with which they cause human infections and their role as precursors of rheumatic fever and glomerulonephritis.

ETIOLOGY The *group-specific carbohydrate* of group A streptococci is a polymer of rhamnose and *N*-acetylglucosamine. There are approximately 80 recognized and provisional group A serotypes. The typing system is based upon antigenic differences in a cell wall constituent known as *M protein,* which is the principal virulence factor of group A organisms. Strains rich in M protein are highly resistant to phagocytosis by polymorphonuclear leukocytes in vitro and are capable of initiating disease in humans and experimental animals. Strains lacking M protein are avirulent. The antiphagocytic effect of M protein is due, at least in part, to its ability to prevent opsonization of the organism by the complement system. This effect is enhanced by the ability of M protein to precipitate fibrinogen directly onto the bacterial surface. Acquired human immunity to streptococcal infection is based upon development of opsonic antibodies directed against the antiphagocytic moiety of M protein. Immunity is type-specific and lasts for many years, perhaps indefinitely. M proteins of certain types share antigenic determinants with certain constituents of the human heart, including sarcolemmal membrane and cardiac myosin.

T protein serves as the basis of a subsidiary typing system which has been useful in classifying strains not typable by the M system; unlike M protein, the T antigen plays no role in virulence. *Lipoteichoic acid,* a substance which has a marked affinity for biological membranes, has been found to play a crucial role in colonization by binding group A streptococci to fibronectin sites on the surface of human epithelial cells. The streptococcal *cell membrane* contains a number of antigenic structures, certain of which have been reported to share determinants with constituents of human heart and with basement membrane of the renal glomerulus. During the early logarithmic phase of replication, streptococci are enveloped in a *hyaluronic acid capsule* which serves to retard phagocytosis and, therefore, represents an accessory virulence factor. Highly encapsulated group A streptococcal strains produce mucoid colonies on sheep blood agar plates. Such strains have been observed in association with epidemics of acute rheumatic fever.

As streptococci grow in vitro or in vivo, they elaborate a number of extracellular products. Streptococcal pyrogenic exotoxins (erythrogenic toxins) which are induced by lysogeny with temperate bacteriophages are responsible for the rash of scarlet fever. There are three serologically distinct toxins, the effects of which may be neutralized by antibody. Two distinct hemolysins are elaborated. *Streptolysin O* is reversibly inhibited by oxygen (hence exerting its effect primarily on subsurface colonies) and irreversibly inhibited by cholesterol. It is produced by almost all group A strains as well as by many group C and G organisms. In clinical practice, titration of antistreptolysin O (ASO) antibodies in human serums is the most widely used serologic procedure to detect group A streptococcal infection. Streptolysin S differs from streptolysin O in being oxygenstable and nonantigenic, but both hemolysins possess the capacity to damage membranes of polymorphonuclear leukocytes, platelets, and subcellular organelles. A number of other extracellular products exert effects which might serve to facilitate the organisms' survival in vivo by liquefying pus (streptokinase and deoxyribonucleases A to D) or by allowing spread through tissue planes (hyaluronidase and proteinase). Their role in streptococcal virulence remains unproved.

The two most frequent types of group A streptococcal infection are pharyngitis and pyoderma. They differ markedly in their epidemiologic, clinical, and bacteriologic characteristics.

STREPTOCOCCAL PHARYNGITIS Epidemiology The incidence of this ubiquitous infection is highest in children aged 5 to 15 years; males and females are affected equally. The great majority of such infections are due to group A streptococci, but strains of other serogroups, particularly group C or G, are involved occasionally. The organism is ordinarily transmitted directly from person to person, most likely by droplet spread, and crowding markedly facilitates interpersonal transmission. This may account for the increased incidence of streptococcal pharyngitis in northern latitudes during the colder months of the year, as well as for the explosive outbreaks which occur in military recruit camps and other crowded institutional settings. Common-source epidemics of streptococcal sore throat with high attack rates occasionally occur following contamination of a food item with beta-hemolytic streptococci.

Patients with acute streptococcal pharyngitis harbor large numbers of organisms in the anterior nares and throat. If antibiotics are not administered, the organisms may persist in the upper respiratory tract for weeks to months after symptoms have subsided. However, as the length of the carrier state increases, the organisms decrease in number, disappear from the anterior nasal secretions, and lose detectable M protein. Therefore, convalescent carriers are less likely than acutely ill patients to transmit group A streptococci to exposed individuals. Group A pharyngeal carriage rates vary with geographic location, season of the year, and age group. Among school-age children, rates of 15 to 20 percent have been reported; the carriage rate among adults is considerably lower.

Symptoms The usual incubation period of streptococcal pharyngitis is between 2 and 4 days. The classic syndrome, in older children and adults, is ushered in by the rather abrupt onset of sore throat, particularly by pain on swallowing. Associated symptoms include headache, malaise, feverishness, and anorexia. Chilliness is a frequent symptom, but true rigors are rare. Nausea, vomiting, and abdominal pain are common in children.

Physical signs The patient appears moderately ill with tachycardia and fever which frequently exceeds 38.3°C (101°F). There is diffuse erythema, edema, and lymphoid hyperplasia of the posterior pharynx. The uvula is edematous. The tonsils, if present, are enlarged, reddened, and covered by a punctate or coalescent exudate which may be yellow, gray, or white. Discrete areas of pinhead-size exudate may be present on the hypertrophied lymphoid follicles of the posterior pharynx. On the soft palate, small, red, raised follicular lesions with yellowish centers ("doughnut lesions") are occasionally seen. The anterior cervical lymph nodes at the angles of the jaw are enlarged and tender. Cough and hoarseness, if present, are mild and, in the absence of the signs and symptoms indicated above, do not suggest the diagnosis of streptococcal pharyngitis. Laryngeal involvement with hoarseness or loss of voice is not a feature.

The full-blown clinical syndrome of acute exudative tonsillopharyngitis is seen frequently during explosive epidemics of streptococcal disease, particularly those occurring in institutional settings. In endemically occurring infections among civilians, however, the illness is frequently much milder and only about half the children with sore throats and positive cultures for group A streptococci will have tonsillar exudate, and a third or less may have fever greater than 38.3°C (101°F) or marked leukocytosis. Patients who have undergone tonsillectomy tend to experience a milder clinical syndrome. In infants, streptococcal upper respiratory infections tend to be less sharply localized to the lymphoid tissue of the faucial and posterior pharyngeal areas. Infections at this age are characterized by rhinorrhea with excoriation of the nares, low-grade fever, anorexia, and a protracted clinical course. Exudative pharyngitis in children under 3 is rarely streptococcal in etiology.

Course The course of streptococcal pharyngitis is usually brief and self-limited. Fever abates within a week, usually within 3 to 5 days. Constitutional symptoms and sore throat disappear with defervescence or shortly thereafter. Several weeks may be required, however, for the tonsils and lymph nodes to return to normal size.

SCARLET FEVER When streptococcal pharyngitis is due to a lysogenic strain producing pyrogenic (erythrogenic) toxin, and when the host does not possess neutralizing antibody to the toxin, scarlet fever may ensue. A preexisting state of hypersensitivity to streptococcal products may predispose to the development of scarlet fever.

The rash usually appears within 2 days after onset of sore throat, involves first the neck, upper chest, and back, then spreads over the remainder of the trunk and the extremities, and spares the palms and soles. The rash may be difficult to appreciate in black patients. It consists of a diffuse erythema, which blanches on pressure, with numerous 1- to 2-mm punctate elevations that impart a "sandpaper" texture to the skin. Discrete lesions are absent from the face, but there is a generalized facial flush which contrasts with the prominent circumoral pallor. The rash is more intense along skin folds, such as those of the antecubital fossae and axillary folds, and in these locations often produces linear striations of confluent petechiae known as *Pastia's lines*, which are due to increased capillary fragility.

The exanthem of scarlet fever is accompanied by an enanthem, consisting of punctate erythema and petechiae on the soft palate. Early in the disease, the tongue is covered with a white coat through which hypertrophied papillae protrude as islands of red (white strawberry tongue). By the fourth or fifth day the coating is gone and the entire tongue appears beefy red (red strawberry or raspberry tongue). In rare cases, scarlet fever may be complicated by jaundice, hydrops of the gallbladder, pleural effusion, and arthralgia.

The rash usually lasts 4 to 5 days and is followed by extensive desquamation which begins as early as a few days or as late as 3 to 4 weeks after onset of the disease and is often a striking feature of the convalescent phase of scarlet fever.

Although scarlet fever usually follows upper respiratory infection due to group A streptococci, rarely pyrogenic toxins are produced by streptococci of other groups and by certain strains of staphylococci. Moreover, scarlet fever may follow streptococcal impetigo or secondary streptococcal infection of superficial wounds or surgical incisions. The disease must be differentiated from various of the childhood exanthems (e.g., rubeola, rubella, exanthem subitum), toxic shock syndrome, Kawasaki disease, infectious mononucleosis (when the latter is associated with rash), miliaria, and drug eruptions. Management consists of adequate treatment of the infection.

Streptococcal pyrogenic exotoxin A has been reported to have an amino acid homology of nearly 50 percent with staphylococcal enterotoxin B, a putative mediator of non-menstrual toxic shock syndrome. This fact may explain the existence of a toxic shock–like syndrome due to *S. pyogenes*. The cases have occurred in adults, in several instances with a localized cellulitis or soft tissue infection. Clinical manifestations include diffuse erythroderma, hypotension, and dysfunction of multiple organs.

Complications Streptococcal pharyngitis may give rise to suppurative complications, among which acute otitis media and acute sinusitis are the most frequent. Suppurative cervical lymphadenitis, peritonsillar cellulitis, peritonsillar abscess, or retropharyngeal abscess may also occur. The abscesses themselves, however, usually contain a variety of oropharyngeal flora, including anaerobic bacteria, with or without group A streptococci. Certain other complications, common in the past, are almost never seen in the antibiotic era: (1) extension up the cribriform plate of the ethmoid or via the mastoid, giving rise to meningitis, brain abscess, or thrombosis of cerebral venous sinuses; and (2) bacteremia with metastatic foci of infection such as suppurative arthritis, endocarditis, osteomyelitis, or liver abscess. Streptococcal pharyngitis is associated with two delayed nonsuppurative sequels: acute rheumatic fever (ARF) and acute glomerulonephritis (AGN). These are discussed in Chaps. 187 and 227, respectively.

Diagnosis Sore throat due to group A streptococci must be differentiated from that caused by a number of other agents. *Diphtheria* is rare in immunized populations. It is characterized by the presence of an extensive diphtheritic membrane, and in severe cases by respiratory embarrassment due to laryngeal involvement, as well as by myocarditis and cranial nerve palsies. Cultures on Loeffler's medium will be positive for *Corynebacterium diphtheriae*. *C. hemolyticum* may cause exudative pharyngitis and a scarlatiniform rash which is clinically indistinguishable from that due to *S. pyogenes*. Most such infections occur in teenagers and young adults. The organism is difficult to recognize on sheep blood agar plates.

Gonococcal tonsillopharyngitis is suggested by a history of homosexuality or fellatio and confirmed by appropriate cultures. *Yersinia enterocolitica* is a rare but life-threatening cause of pharyngitis in adults. Some, but not all, patients have associated gastrointestinal symptoms. *Vincent's angina* (*fusobacterial membranous tonsillitis*) is characterized by sore throat and tonsillopharyngeal exudate. Unlike streptococcal sore throat, however, there is an insidious onset without constitutional symptoms, pharyngeal ulcerations are frequent, and the disease is usually unilateral.

The major differential diagnostic confusion is with viral upper respiratory infections, which occur more frequently than streptococcal infections. In many cases, the viral etiology may be suspected because of the more prominent catarrhal, "common cold–like" symptoms. *Adenoviruses* may cause an exudative pharyngitis which is indistinguishable clinically from that due to group A streptococci. *Infectious mononucleosis* also produces severe exudative pharyngitis with fever and at times is accompanied by a rash which may be confused with scarlet fever. The generalized lymphadenopathy, splenomegaly, prolonged fever, and presence of abnormal lymphocytes and heterophile antibodies in the peripheral blood serve to differentiate this entity. Pharyngitis due to group A coxsackieviruses (*herpangina*) or to primary infection with *herpes simplex* is characterized by formation of vesicles, which rupture and leave shallow ulcers. *Influenza* virus infections frequently occur in epidemics; they are accompanied by severe myalgias, bronchitis is a frequent clinical feature, and all age groups are affected. *Mycoplasma pneumoniae* infections may cause pharyngitis that at times may be exudative. Bullous myringitis, if present, should suggest this diagnosis.

Although use of algorithms incorporating combinations of epidemiologic data, symptoms, and signs may enhance diagnostic accuracy, in many instances it is impossible to differentiate streptococcal from nonstreptococcal sore throat on clinical grounds alone. For this reason, precise diagnosis requires identification of the infecting organism in the pharynx. This is achieved most reliably by a throat culture. In obtaining the culture, it is important to rub the swab over both tonsils or tonsillar fossae, the oropharynx, and the nasopharynx posterior to the uvula. The swab should be inoculated onto a sheep blood agar plate to allow evaluation of patterns of hemolysis after overnight incubation. If beta-hemolytic streptococci are isolated, they may be identified presumptively as group A if growth is inhibited around a low-potency (0.04-unit) bacitracin disk. Definitive identification may be accomplished by fluorescent antibody, agglutination, or precipitin techniques. A number of the positive cultures obtained, particularly those with relatively few organisms on the culture plate, will emanate from streptococcal carriers rather than cases of acute infection. It is not possible to differentiate cases from carriers on the basis of culture results, but culture does serve to exclude from antimicrobial therapy the bulk of patients with sore throat (approximately 70 percent) who have negative cultures for beta-hemolytic streptococci. A number of commercial kits are available which allow detection of group A antigen directly from throat swabs by immunologic means. These kits provide results within an hour or less. The direct antigen tests are highly specific, and the physician may proceed confidently on the basis of a positive result. Although the immunologic tests are in general quite sensitive, they fail to identify reliably patients with weakly positive cultures. It is likely, however, that many such patients are asymptomatic carriers. Nevertheless, it is advisable to confirm negative direct antigen tests with throat cultures. This is especially important in epidemiologic settings in which there is an appreciable risk of acute rheumatic fever.

In selecting patients for throat culture or antigen testing, it should be borne in mind that group A streptococcal pharyngitis and acute rheumatic fever are extremely rare in children under 3 in the United States. Likewise, first attacks of rheumatic fever are rare in older adults. Routine use of streptococcal diagnostic procedures is less cost-effective in these groups.

Assays of serum antibodies to streptococcal extracellular products (e.g., ASO, anti-DNase B) provide confirmatory evidence of recent streptococcal infection in patients suspected of having ARF or AGN, but such tests are of no value in the diagnosis of acute infection.

Treatment Therapy of streptococcal pharyngitis is directed primarily toward prevention of ARF and of suppurative sequelae. It is unclear whether treatment of the antecedent streptococcal infection will prevent development of AGN. Prevention of ARF correlates with eradication of the infecting organism from the pharynx, which requires prolonged antibiotic treatment. Penicillin is the drug of choice. It is inexpensive and nontoxic, and all group A streptococci have remained exquisitely sensitive to it. A single intramuscular injection of benzathine penicillin G, 600,000 units for children weighing 27 kg (60 lb) or less and 1.2 million units for all others, ensures a prolonged penicillinemia and is a highly effective form of therapy. Many physicians now elect oral therapy for compliant patients. This is an attractive alternative because the risk of severe allergic reactions is presumed to be less with oral than with intramuscular penicillin. A full 10 days of therapy is required, however, but is often difficult to achieve, because patients are usually asymptomatic well before the 10 days have elapsed. If oral therapy is utilized, penicillin V, 250 mg, three times daily, is the treatment of choice.

Penicillin-allergic individuals may be treated with oral erythromycin estolate, 20 to 40 mg per kilogram of body weight per day, or erythromycin ethyl succinate, 40 mg/kg per day, which should be administered in two to four equally divided portions. The total dose should not exceed 1 g/d. Treatment should be continued for 7 to 10 days.

Nearly all group A streptococci in the United States have remained susceptible to erythromycin, but extensive resistance has been reported in Japan. On the other hand, tetracycline-resistant strains are encountered with some frequency in the United States, and this drug should not be used. Sulfonamides are ineffective in eradication of established streptococcal infection, although they are useful prophylactically in preventing new pharyngeal acquisitions of group A streptococci and in preventing recurrences of ARF (see Chap. 187).

A variable percentage of patients, ranging from 5 to 30 percent, continue to harbor group A streptococci in the pharynx following a course of antimicrobial therapy. This may be due to noncompliance, reinfection, or true treatment failure. Because patients in this category are frequently streptococcal carriers rather than acutely infected individuals, and because the risk of rheumatic fever remains low in most U.S. populations, routine follow-up cultures are not currently recommended in asymptomatic individuals. Exceptions should be made, however, if there is a history of ARF in the family or in family contacts, and in those areas of the United States wherein marked increases in rheumatic fever incidence have recently been reported.

Appropriate antibiotic therapy is effective in preventing ARF, even when initiated as long as 9 days after the onset of acute pharyngitis. Therefore, in the patient seen early in the course of illness, the delay in initiating therapy occasioned by processing a throat culture is not ordinarily a matter of concern. Although treatment also speeds resolution of fever, sore throat, and systemic symptoms associated with streptococcal pharyngitis, the effect of antibiotics is in most cases not dramatic. Indeed, given the self-limited course of the illness, it is difficult to demonstrate clinical improvement in antibiotic-treated vs. placebo-treated patients if therapy is initiated more than 24 h after onset of symptoms. Unless patients have high fever, severe systemic toxicity, or evidence of suppurative complications, initiation of antimicrobial therapy can await the results of throat culture.

In patients judged to be more severely ill, therapy may be initiated at the time of the initial visit after a throat culture has been obtained. If oral antibiotic therapy is elected, the throat culture serves as a guide to the necessity of completing a full 10-day course or, alternatively, of recalling the patient for definitive therapy with an injection of benzathine penicillin G. If signs or symptoms are present, a positive direct antigen test warrants therapy at the time of initial evaluation.

Patients with more severe suppurative complications, such as mastoiditis or ethmoiditis, require larger doses of penicillin than those used for treatment of uncomplicated sore throat. When streptococcal upper respiratory infection is complicated by the development of abscesses associated with suppurative cervical adenitis or in the peritonsillar or retropharyngeal soft tissues, incision and drainage are usually required.

The role of tonsillectomy, if any, in the management of patients with frequent recurrences of acute pharyngitis or in the prevention of ARF remains undefined. Clinical episodes of pharyngitis occur less frequently and tend to be milder following tonsillectomy, but this may make detection and appropriate treatment of immunologically significant streptococcal infections more difficult.

Family contacts of patients with streptococcal sore throat frequently develop symptomatic infections or become asymptomatic pharyngeal carriers. Symptomatic secondary cases in families should be treated appropriately. Asymptomatic family contacts should be cultured in high-risk circumstances. These include the presence of a rheumatic subject in the family or of known cases of ARF occurring in the general area. In situations where the risk is lower, cultures of asymptomatic family contacts need not be performed routinely.

STREPTOCOCCAL SKIN INFECTIONS Erysipelas Also known as Saint Anthony's fire, erysipelas is an acute infection of the skin, with marked involvement of cutaneous lymphatic vessels. It is caused by group A streptococci, and, rarely, other streptococci and *Staphylococcus aureus*. The disease most frequently affects infants, young children, and elderly individuals. The commonest site of involvement is the face, where cutaneous infection originates from an upper respiratory source, presumably by way of small or inapparent breaks in the skin. Erysipelas may also result from streptococcal infection of wounds, surgical incisions, or even areas of dermatophytosis, in which case any portion of the body may be involved.

The onset is usually abrupt; initial symptoms include malaise, chilliness, feverishness, headache, and vomiting. The skin lesion may begin with itching and mild discomfort at the site of infection and is followed shortly thereafter by a small area of erythema which enlarges during the ensuing hours. The lesion spreads rapidly, reaching its maximum extent in 3 to 6 days. It is warm, pink to deep red, and has an advancing elevated margin which protrudes irregularly into the surrounding areas of normal skin. Vesicles and bullae may appear; these rupture leaving crusts on the surface. While the advancing margin remains inflamed, central clearing may be evident with a return of the skin to normal appearance or with residual pigmentation. The eruption may be less well demarcated in areas where the skin is loose, but edema and erythema are constant features. Facial erysipelas commonly involves the bridge of the nose and one or more cheeks in a "butterfly" distribution.

The disease process may be accompanied by high fever and bacteremia. Recovery is usually apparent by the end of a week, but this varies with the severity of the infection. The substantial mortality attending bacteremic cases of erysipelas in the preantibiotic era has been markedly reduced by penicillin. Fatalities still occur among children within the first few months of life and in elderly, debilitated, immunosuppressed individuals. The disease tends to recur, especially in areas of chronic lymphatic obstruction. The diagnosis of erysipelas is primarily clinical. Group A streptococci may at times be isolated from the respiratory tract, the bloodstream, or the lesion itself.

Pyoderma This term is used collectively to denote localized purulent streptococcal skin infections. Some pyoderma lesions represent obvious secondary infections of wounds or burns. For the most part, however, the term is used synonymously with streptococcal impetigo or impetigo contagiosa and refers to discrete purulent lesions which appear to be primary infections of the skin. Streptococcal impetigo differs from streptococcal pharyngitis in a number of particulars (Table 101-1). Epidemiologically, impetigo is more prevalent among underprivileged children residing in warm, humid

TABLE 101-1 Comparative features of pharyngitis and pyoderma due to group A streptococci

	Pharyngitis	Pyoderma
Predominant geographic distribution	Ubiquitous	Subtropic-tropic
Season (temperate zone)	Winter-spring	Summer-fall
Peak age group	5–15 years	2–5 years
Mode of spread	Direct contact (droplet)	Unknown (?insects)
Clinical illness	Acute	Indolent
Streptococcal types	Generally lower-numbered M types	Generally higher-numbered M types
ASO responses	Good	Weak
Type-specific antibody responses	Generally good	Variable, often poor
Nonsuppurative sequelae	Acute rheumatic fever, acute glomerulonephritis	Acute glomerulonephritis

SOURCE: Modified from Wannamaker LW, N Engl J Med 282:23, 1970

climates such as the southeastern United States or the tropics. However, the disease may also occur during the summer in northern settings, such as the American Indian reservations of Minnesota. The peak incidence is in young children (2 to 6 years), and there is no definite sex or racial predisposition.

The mode of spread of streptococcal pyoderma is unknown, but personal contact and insect vectors such as *Hippelates* flies are probably both important. "Skin strains" of group A streptococci (i.e., strains of M and T types usually associated with pyoderma) are capable of contaminating unbroken skin, from where they may be inoculated intradermally by local scratches, abrasions, or insect bites. Nasal and pharyngeal carriage of skin strains is frequent in children with impetigo, but such carriage does not ordinarily occur until after establishment of cutaneous carriage or overt infection.

The pattern of immunologic responses to streptococcal impetigo differs from that associated with upper respiratory infection. In particular, the ASO response to impetigo is weak, perhaps because streptolysin O is inactivated by lipids present in the skin. However, antibody responses to anti-DNase B and anti-hyaluronidase, as well as to the Streptozyme slide hemagglutination reagent, are brisk. Type-specific anti-M responses are variable, depending in part upon the antigenicity of the infecting strain, but in general such responses are weaker than in pharyngeal infections. The role of type-specific antibodies in protection against reinfection in pyoderma has not been adequately studied.

Streptococcal impetigo occurs on exposed areas of the body, most frequently on the lower extremities. The lesions remain well-localized but are frequently multiple. They begin as papules but rapidly evolve into vesicles surrounded by an area of erythema. The vesicular lesions are rarely recognized clinically; they give rise to pustules which gradually enlarge, then break down over 4 to 6 days to form characteristic thick crusts. The lesions heal slowly, leaving depigmented areas. A deeply ulcerated form of impetigo is known as *ecthyma*. Although regional lymphadenitis often occurs, systemic symptoms are not ordinarily present.

In addition to the indolent, impetiginous skin infections of young children, a more severe and extensive form of pyoderma has been observed in combat troops serving in hot, wet environments such as the jungles of southeast Asia. In their most common form, they consist of multiple ecthymatous ulcers located on the ankle or dorsum of the foot. The ulcers are usually circular, punched-out lesions 0.5 to 3.0 cm in diameter, have borders, and are surrounded by a zone of erythema. They are filled with purulent material and covered with grayish-yellow adherent crusts. Secondary cellulitis or lymphadenitis may be present.

The diagnosis of streptococcal pyoderma is made by culture. Adequate cultures require removal of the surface crusts in order to obtain specimens from the base of the lesions. Although both *S. pyogenes* and *Staphylococcus aureus* may be isolated from the lesions, the former is the major pathogen. Morphologically characteristic lesions respond well to penicillin, even when penicillinase-resistant staphylococci are recovered. These lesions contrast with bullous impetigo, which is ordinarily due to *S. aureus* and not to streptococci. Antibiotic regimens are the same as those for pharyngitis, and benzathine penicillin G, oral penicillin V, or oral erythromycin all result in cure rates in excess of 95 percent. Topical antiseptics and antibiotics are of limited value. Prevention of pyoderma depends primarily upon adherence to good personal hygiene, with special attention to frequent scrubbing with soap and water.

Streptococcal pyoderma does not give rise to ARF. This observation remains unexplained, but may indicate a requirement for infection at the pharyngeal site, with its rich endowment of lymphoid tissue, in order to initiate the immunologic events leading to ARF. On the other hand, studies of populations in which ARF and AGN occur simultaneously indicate that the streptococcal strains responsible for each sequelum are distinct and suggest that "pyoderma strains" of group A streptococci may be nonrheumatogenic. When pyoderma is due to a nephritogenic strain of group A streptococcus, AGN may ensue. Indeed, pyoderma is by far the commonest antecedent of poststreptococcal glomerulonephritis in subtropical and tropical regions of the world. Strains of a number of M types (49, 55, 57, and others) have been associated with both sporadic cases and large epidemics of pyoderma-associated nephritis in diverse geographic areas. There are no conclusive data to indicate that treatment of an individual case of pyoderma will prevent the subsequent occurrence of AGN in that patient. Such treatment is important, however, in eradicating nephritogenic streptococci from the environment in epidemiologic settings in which these strains are prevalent.

Cellulitis Streptococcal cellulitis may occur in areas of tissue damage due to trauma, operative wounds, or stasis ulceration. Although such infections are frequently due to group A organisms, beta-hemolytic streptococci of groups G, B, or C may be responsible. Cellulitis is an acute inflammation of the skin and subcutaneous tissues marked by pain, tenderness, erythema, fever, and often regional lymphadenopathy. In contrast to erysipelas, the margins of the lesions are neither elevated nor sharply demarcated from the surrounding uninvolved tissue. Rarely such lesions may progress to frank gangrene. Certain patients who have undergone saphenous venectomy for coronary bypass surgery experience recurrent bouts of acute streptococcal cellulitis for months or years after surgery. The cellulitis always involves the saphenous donor extremity. Frequently the patients suffer from tinea pedis, and eradication of the superficial fungal infection, which may serve as a nidus for streptococcal colonization, may result in abolition of the recurrent attacks.

Cellulitis of the perianal area may be manifested by painful defecation or by pruritus; asymptomatic anal colonization has been the source of several outbreaks of hospital-acquired streptococcal infection. Vaginal colonization by group A streptococci has a number of features in common with perianal involvement. In both instances there is a close epidemiologic association with streptococcal upper respiratory infection. Anal and vaginal streptococcal infection may be either symptomatic or asymptomatic. Outbreaks of nosocomial streptococcal infection have been attributed to asymptomatic vaginal carriers.

LYMPHANGITIS, BACTEREMIA, AND PUERPERAL SEPSIS Local trauma, whether or not complicated by frank cellulitis, may give rise to *acute lymphangitis*. This entity is characterized by the appearance of red linear streaks extending from the portal of entry to the draining regional lymph nodes, which are enlarged and tender. Systemic symptoms, including chills, fever, malaise, and headache, are prominent, and the process may be accompanied by demonstrable bacteremia.

Streptococcal bacteremia, from whatever cause, may give rise to metastatic foci of infection, such as suppurative arthritis, osteomyelitis, peritonitis, endocarditis, meningitis, or visceral abscesses.

Streptococcal bacteremia may complicate parenteral drug abuse; such infections are often associated with local abscesses at the injection site and/or infective endocarditis (see Chap. 90). The clinical course of streptococcal bacteremia may be fulminant and lead rapidly to prostration, shock, purpura fulminans, disseminated intravascular coagulation, and death.

Puerperal sepsis follows abortion or childbirth when streptococci invade the endometrium and surrounding structures and then the lymphatics and bloodstream. The process may be further complicated by pelvic cellulitis, septic pelvic thrombophlebitis, peritonitis, or pelvic abscess. The causative organism may be transmitted to the pregnant woman directly by medical personnel or attendants. Group B streptococci have supplanted other organisms as the most frequent cause of perinatal streptococcal infections of mother and child (see below). Anaerobic streptococci, along with other anaerobic organisms, have also been implicated (see Chap. 108).

PNEUMONIA AND EMPYEMA Pneumonia due to group A streptococci is uncommon and usually occurs following influenza, measles, pertussis, or varicella. The illness occurs in epidemic form in military recruit camps and is characterized by abrupt onset of fever, chills, myalgia, dyspnea, cough, pleuritic chest pain, and hemoptysis. Patients are severely ill and often cyanotic. Pathologically and radiologically, this is usually a bronchopneumonia, and lobar consolidation is uncommon. A characteristic feature of streptococcal pneumonia is the early and rapid accumulation of copious amounts of thin, serosanguinous empyema fluid. Bacteremia occurs in 10 to 15 percent of cases. Extension of the pneumonic process to the pericardium may give rise to a purulent pericarditis. Other potential complications include mediastinitis, pneumothorax, and bronchiectasis. Therapy consists of at least 4 to 6 million units of parenteral penicillin daily in the form of aqueous procaine penicillin G, given every 6 to 12 h intramuscularly, or intravenous aqueous crystalline penicillin G, and adequate drainage of empyema fluid, which usually requires insertion of a chest tube.

MYOSITIS, GANGRENE, AND SEPTIC BURSITIS Myositis due to group A streptococci is a rare disorder characterized by severe pain and marked signs of local inflammation in the infected area. The patients are usually bacteremic, and the clinical course is frequently rapid and fulminant. The mortality rate is extremely high. Aggressive surgical debridement and penicillin therapy are required. *Hemolytic streptococcal gangrene* may occur after trauma or surgery or without an obvious portal of entry. It is characterized by necrosis of subcutaneous and dermal tissues which spreads along fascial planes. This entity is a form of necrotizing fasciitis, and a similar clinical picture can result from infection due to a variety of anaerobic and facultatively aerobic bacteria, often in combination. *Septic bursitis* of the olecranon bursa, although usually caused by *Staphylococcus aureus*, may also be due to *S. pyogenes*.

GROUP B STREPTOCOCCAL INFECTIONS

Streptococci belonging to serogroup B have been of interest to veterinarians because of their association with bovine mastitis, an association which led to their species designation as *S. agalactiae*. The organisms are usually, but not uniformly, beta-hemolytic and are resistant to bacitracin. In addition to the presence of group B carbohydrate in their cell walls, *S. agalactiae* may be identified by biochemical means, including production of hippuricase and so-called CAMP factor and failure to hydrolyze bile esculin agar. Group B streptococci may be subdivided into serotypes by means of surface polysaccharides and protein antigens. The capsular antigens are virulence factors and immunity to them is type-specific.

Human strains of group B streptococci, which appear to be biologically distinct from bovine strains, frequently colonize the female genital tract as well as the throat and rectum. Asymptomatic vaginal carriage rates in postpubertal women generally have ranged between 6 and 25 percent, depending on the bacteriologic methods employed and on the socioeconomic status and geographic residence of the women sampled. The majority of serious group B infections occur as perinatal events. Maternal infections include chorioamnionitis, septic abortion, and puerperal sepsis. *Streptococcus agalactiae* now ranks with *Escherichia coli* as one of the two most frequent causes of neonatal sepsis and meningitis. Neonatal disease takes one of two forms. Early-onset disease, occurring within the first 10 days of life, is usually due to organisms acquired from the maternal genital tract. It involves primarily the lungs, probably as a result of aspiration of infected amniotic fluid, but the organism can be cultured from the blood, nasopharynx, skin, and myocardium. Early-onset group B streptococcal infection occurs in approximately two of every thousand live births (the incidence is higher following prolonged or complicated delivery) and is attended by a high mortality rate. Late-onset disease occurs in infants over 10 days old, may be due to nosocomial transmission of group B streptococci, is manifested primarily by meningitis and bacteremia, and has a lower mortality rate than early-onset disease. Although the serotypes involved in early-onset illness are variable, type III organisms predominate as the cause of late-onset meningeal infection. Transplacentally acquired antibodies to type III organisms may protect against late-onset disease: they are present in serums of most women delivering healthy babies but are usually lacking in serums of mothers whose offspring develop late-onset meningitis due to type III group B streptococci.

Group B streptococci also cause adult infections not associated with the puerperium. These are often opportunistic and involve debilitated patients with diabetes mellitus, malignancy, or other severe illnessses. Adult infections due to group B organisms include urinary tract infections, suppurative soft tissue infections, bacteremia, endocarditis, pyogenic arthritis, pneumonia, empyema, meningitis, and peritonitis. Although recovered from a small proportion of throat cultures, group B streptococci are rarely the cause of clinically significant pharyngitis. All strains are susceptible to penicillin, which is the drug of choice, although group B organisms have higher minimal inhibitory concentrations for penicillin than do group A strains. Life-threatening group B infections in neonates are often treated initially with aminoglycosides in addition to high doses of penicillin because this combination is synergistic in vitro and avoids the occasional occurrence of penicillin tolerance in group B strains. Most strains are sensitive to erythromycin, but tetracyclines should not be used without prior susceptibility testing because resistance to them is common.

OTHER STREPTOCOCCAL INFECTIONS

Although streptococci of groups C and G are human commensals, both are capable of causing pharyngitis, and epidemics of upper respiratory disease due to these organisms have been reported, particularly following ingestion of contaminated foods. Strains of both serogroups produce streptolysin O, and pharyngeal infections with groups C and G elicit rises in ASO titer. Streptococci of groups C and G are highly susceptible to penicillin.

There have been several outbreaks of human disease due to group C in which the vehicle was unpasteurized or inadequately pasteurized milk or cheese. Clinical manifestations have included pharyngitis, cervical adenitis, and disseminated deep tissue infections. In two outbreaks, cases of poststreptococcal glomerulonephritis ensued.

Group G streptococcal bacteremia often arises from cutaneous foci such as localized cellulitis or decubitus ulcers, and chronic lymphatic obstruction and venous insufficiency are important predisposing factors. The patients involved frequently have underlying conditions such as malignancy, alcoholism, or parenteral drug abuse. Bacteremia may lead to severe, life-threatening complications such as endocarditis, meningitis, or septic arthritis.

Lancefield's group D include both enterococcal and nonenterococcal species. The former have recently been recognized as a distinct genus, of which the major human pathogens are *Enterococcus faecalis*

and *E. faecium*. Enterococci are frequent causes of urinary tract infection in patients with structural abnormalities of the urinary tract and are responsible for 10 percent or more of cases of bacterial endocarditis. They are isolated from infected decubitus ulcers and intraabdominal abscesses, usually in combination with other bacteria. These microorganisms are ordinarily alpha-hemolytic or nonhemolytic but may be beta-hemolytic. The treatment of severe enterococcal infections, particularly bacterial endocarditis, is complicated; the organisms are resistant to many antibiotics and are relatively resistant to the penicillins. In the therapy of enterococcal endocarditis, a combination of intravenous penicillin G or ampicillin in high doses plus an aminoglycoside should be used, because this combination exerts a synergistic effect in the killing of enterococci (see Chap. 90). Formerly, streptomycin was the aminoglycoside of choice, but high-level resistance (>2000 μg/mL) to streptomycin and kanamycin has been found in a significant number of enterococcal isolates and synergy is not observed in the presence of such high-level resistance. Gentamicin is the drug of choice along with penicillin or ampicillin in treatment of serious enterococcal infections due to organisms which are highly resistant to streptomycin. The combination of penicillin and tobramycin is not lethal in vitro for strains of *E. faecium*.

Fortunately, gentamicin remains an effective synergistic agent for treatment of most deep tissue enterococcal infections encountered in the United States. In treatment of individual cases, however, it is advisable to rule out the presence of high-level gentamicin resistance by in vitro testing. Treatment of life-threatening enterococcal infections in patients who cannot tolerate penicillin is difficult. The cephalosporins and clindamycin are of no value, but vancomycin, in combination with gentamicin, is likely to be effective. Strains of *E. faecalis* that produce beta lactamase have been described but are rare.

Nonenterococcal group D streptococci, of which *S. bovis* is the major pathogen, remain extremely sensitive to penicillin and are amenable to therapy with this agent alone. Bacteremia or endocarditis due to *S. bovis* has been associated with carcinoma of the colon. Enterococci can be differentiated from nonenterococcal group D streptococci by their ability to grow in 6.5% NaCl and by a positive PYR (pyroglutamyl aminopeptidase) test.

Streptococci of most groups have been isolated at least occasionally from infected heart valves, soft tissues, or visceral abscesses. Such infections may occur as "opportunists" following surgical manipulation or in patients with malignant disease. Group F streptococci occasionally are associated with abscess formation and bacteremia, and a number of instances of meningitis and bacteremia in humans due to streptococci of serogroup R, a group of organisms well-known as pathogens of swine, have been reported. In nearly all human cases there had been a history of contact with pigs.

Viridans streptococci are normal inhabitants of the oropharynx and gastrointestinal tract. They remain the most frequent causative agents of subacute bacterial endocarditis occurring on native heart valves (see Chap. 90). The taxonomy of these organisms is confused, but one classification scheme recognizes five species (in addition to *S. pneumoniae*): *salivarius, mitior, milleri, sanguis*, and *mutans*. Although viridans streptococci are not usually highly invasive, *S. milleri* is capable of causing serious pyogenic infections such as liver and brain abscesses, peritonitis, and empyema. Endocarditis due to *S. milleri* is more likely to be complicated by abscess formation in peripheral tissues than are similar infections due to other species of viridans streptococci. All the viridans species, including *S. milleri*, are susceptible to penicillin. Modest increases in the minimal inhibitory concentrations of oral streptococci to penicillin occur following prolonged oral or high-dose intravenous therapy.

Anaerobic streptococci (see Chap. 108) abound in the mouth, intestinal tract, and vagina. They may be found, often in combination with other anaerobic and aerobic microorganisms, in abscess cavities throughout the body. In the head and neck, anaerobic streptococci occur in infected paranasal sinuses, brain abscesses, dental abscesses, infections of the retropharyngeal or lateral pharyngeal spaces, and as Ludwig's angina. In the chest, these organisms occur in lung abscesses and empyema fluids. Abscesses of the liver and other intraabdominal viscera, as well as perirectal abscesses and pelvic abscesses in women, may be due in part to peptostreptococci. These organisms may also thrive in dead or devitalized muscle, skin, or subcutaneous tissue. *Anaerobic streptococcal myositis* is characterized by marked edema, crepitant myositis, pain, and the presence of chains of gram-positive cocci in a seropurulent exudate. *Progressive synergistic gangrene* usually develops about a surgical incision and consists of an ulcerated lesion surrounded by gangrenous skin. The infection is associated particularly with the use of through-and-through sutures after abdominal surgery and is thought most often to be due to the synergistic action of *Staph. aureus* and microaerophilic streptococci. *Chronic burrowing ulcer* is a deep soft tissue infection, caused by microaerophilic streptococci, which erodes through subcutaneous tissue to emerge as an ulcer at a distant site. Management of infections due to anaerobic and microaerophilic streptococci consists of drainage of abscesses, debridement of devitalized tissues, and high-dose intravenous penicillin therapy.

REFERENCES

ADAMS EM et al: Streptococcal myositis. Arch Intern Med 145:1020, 1985

AMERICAN HEART ASSOCIATION, COMMITTEE ON RHEUMATIC FEVER ENDOCARDITIS AND KAWASAKI DISEASE: Prevention of rheumatic fever. Circulation 70:1082, 1988

AUCKENTHALER R et al: Group G streptococcal bacteremia: Clinical study and review of the literature. Rev Infect Dis 5:196, 1983

BADDOUR LM, BISNO AL: Recurrent cellulitis after coronary bypass surgery: Association with superficial fungal infection in saphenous venectomy limbs. JAMA 251:1049, 1984

BARG NL et al: Group A streptococcal bacteremia in intravenous drug abusers. Am J Med 78:569, 1985

BRENNAN RO, DURACK DT: The viridans streptococci in perspective, in *Current Clinical Topics in Infectious Diseases*, JS Remington, MN Swartz (eds). New York, McGraw-Hill, 1984

CONE LA et al: Clinical and bacteriologic observations of a toxic-shock like syndrome due to *Streptococcus pyogenes*. New Engl J Med 317:146, 1987

EDWARDS MS, BAKER CJ: *Streptococcus agalactiae* (group B streptococci), in *Principles and Practice of Infectious Diseases*, 2d ed, GL Mandell et al (eds). New York, Wiley, 1985, p 1155

HOFFMAN S, MOELLERING RC JR: The enterococcus: "Putting the bug in our ears." Ann Intern Med 106:757, 1987

KELLOGG JA, MANZELLA JP: Detection of group A streptococci in the laboratory or physician's office. JAMA 255:2638, 1988

MILLER RA et al: *Corynebacterium hemolyticum* as a cause of pharyngitis and scarlatiniform rash in young adults. Ann Intern Med 105:867, 1986

STEVENS DL et al: Severe group A streptococcal infections associated with a toxic shock-like syndrome and scarlet fever toxin A. N Engl J Med 321:1, 1989

STOLLERMAN GH: *Rheumatic Fever and Streptococcal Infection*. New York, Grune & Stratton, 1975

102 DIPHTHERIA

RANDALL K. HOLMES[1]

DEFINITION Diphtheria is a localized infection of mucous membranes or skin caused by *Corynebacterium diphtheriae*. A characteristic pseudomembrane may be present at the site of infection. Some strains of *C. diphtheriae* produce diphtheria toxin, a protein that can cause myocarditis, polyneuritis, and other systemic toxic effects. Respiratory diphtheria is usually caused by toxinogenic (tox$^+$) *C. diphtheriae*, but cutaneous diphtheria is frequently caused by nontoxinogenic (tox$^-$) strains.

ETIOLOGY *C. diphtheriae* is an aerobic, nonmotile, nonsporulating, irregularly staining, gram-positive rod. The bacteria are 2 to 6 μm long, 0.5 to 1 μm wide, club-shaped, and often arranged in clusters (Chinese letters) or parallel arrays (palisades). *C. diphtheriae*

forms gray to black colonies on selective media containing potassium tellurite. Three biotypes, designated gravis, mitis, and intermedius, are distinguished on the basis of colonial morphology, hemolytic activity, sugar fermentation reactions, and other biochemical tests. Some strains of *C. diphtheriae* produce diphtheria toxin. Both tox$^+$ and tox$^-$ strains cause infections, and tox$^+$ strains of all three biotypes can cause severe disease. Individual strains of *C. diphtheriae* within a biotype can be identified by phage typing, analyzing bacterial polypeptides or bacterial DNA restriction patterns, or performing hybridization tests with specific DNA probes.

The gene for diphtheria toxin is present in specific corynephages. Nontoxinogenic *C. diphtheriae* acquire the ability to produce diphtheria toxin by infection with tox$^+$ phages, a process termed *phage conversion*. Growth of *C. diphtheriae* under low-iron conditions, which mimic the environment of host tissues, induces diphtheria toxin synthesis.

IMMUNOLOGY Treatment of diphtheria toxin with formaldehyde converts it to a nontoxic product called diphtheria toxoid. Immunization with toxoid elicits antibodies (antitoxin) that neutralize the toxin and prevent respiratory diphtheria. Antitoxin does not prevent colonization by *C. diphtheriae* or eradicate the carrier state. If most individuals in a population have antitoxic immunity, the carrier rate for tox$^+$ strains of *C. diphtheriae* usually decreases to a low level. Thus, herd immunity reduces the risk that nonimmune individuals in the population will be exposed to tox$^+$ *C. diphtheriae*. Nonimmune individuals may contract diphtheria if they travel to regions where the disease is prevalent or if tox$^+$ strains of *C. diphtheriae* are introduced into their community.

No specific amount of antitoxin provides absolute protection against diphtheria. Both the attack rate and the mortality rate for diphtheria are much lower in individuals with >0.01 units of antitoxin per milliliter, so that level is often used for epidemiologic studies as an index of immunity. Antitoxic immunity can also be determined by the Schick test, in which standardized doses of diphtheria toxin and toxoid are injected intracutaneously at separate sites on the volar surface of the forearm. A tender, swollen, erythematous lesion reaching maximal intensity at 4 to 5 days at the site of the toxin injection only (a positive reaction) is a direct toxic effect of diphtheria toxin; the individual is not immune. No lesion at either site (a negative reaction) indicates that the toxin was neutralized by circulating antitoxin; the individual has antitoxic immunity. Tuberculin-like reactions at both sites that reach a maximum at 2 to 3 days and then fade (a pseudoreaction) indicates delayed hypersensitivity to toxin/toxoid in an individual with antitoxin. Delayed hypersensitivity reactions at both sites combined with a subsequent positive reaction at the site of toxin administration only (a combined reaction) indicates delayed hypersensitivity in an individual without a protective level of antitoxin.

EPIDEMIOLOGY Humans are the reservoir for *C. diphtheriae*. Transmission occurs primarily by close contact of diphtheria patients or carriers with susceptible individuals, but the risk of transmission from patients appears to be substantially greater than from asymptomatic carriers. Transmission involving fomites and indirect routes is less common, although *C. diphtheriae* can survive for weeks to months in the environment. The incubation period for respiratory diphtheria is typically 2 to 5 days and, rarely, up to 8 days. Cutaneous diphtheria is usually a secondary infection, and the signs of infection develop an average of 7 days (range 1 to >21 days) after the appearance of primary skin lesions.

In unimmunized populations in temperate climates diphtheria primarily involves the respiratory tract, occurs year round with peak incidence in the colder months, and is usually caused by tox$^+$ *C. diphtheriae*. Most infants are immune because of transplacental transfer of maternal IgG antitoxin, but they become susceptible by 6 to 12 months of age. Diphtheria is primarily a disease of children that affects up to 10 percent of individuals and sometimes occurs in devastating epidemics. Approximately 75 percent of individuals become immune by age 10 from clinical or subclinical

[1]The opinions expressed herein are those of the author and do not necessarily represent the views of the Department of Defense or the Uniformed Services University of the Health Sciences.

infection with *C. diphtheriae*. Mortality rates of 30 to 40 percent are common in untreated disease and sometimes exceed 50 percent in epidemics.

Treatment with antitoxin can reduce the case mortality rate to 5 to 10 percent.

In the United States routine immunization with toxoid introduced in the 1920s has resulted in a progressive decrease in disease and shift of cases to older age groups. More than 206,000 cases of diphtheria occurred in 1921; only 22 cases were reported from 1980 to 1987. Forty-eight percent of cases in 1971 to 1981 were in persons over 15 years of age. Despite high rates of immunization in children by school entry (96 percent) 25 to 50 percent of older adults are susceptible to diphtheria. In the United States large local outbreaks of diphtheria occurred in San Antonio, Texas (1969 to 1970, 201 cases) and Seattle, Washington (1972 to 1982, 1100 cases). Alcoholism, low socioeconomic status, crowded living conditions, and Native American ethnic background were significant risk factors in these and other recent diphtheria outbreaks.

In the tropics cutaneous diphtheria is more common than respiratory diphtheria, occurs throughout the year, and often occurs as a secondary infection complicating other dermatoses. Isolates of *C. diphtheriae* from skin lesions are more often tox⁻ than tox⁺. A study in Rangoon, Burma, demonstrated *C. diphtheriae* (18.5 percent tox⁺ strains) in more than 60 percent of bacterially infected skin lesions in patients under 12 years of age. Eighty percent of isolates were from impetiginous scabies, with most other isolates from impetiginous eczema or impetigo. Cutaneous diphtheria has also been increasingly recognized in temperate climates during the past two decades and accounted for 86 percent of the 1100 cases in Seattle.

Molecular epidemiologic studies demonstrated that the Seattle epidemic actually consisted of three discrete but overlapping outbreaks involving intermedius, gravis, and mitis strains. The intermedius and gravis strains were shown to be distinct clones of *C. diphtheriae* with loss of toxigenicity occuring in the gravis clone late in the epidemic (1978–1982). The mitis strains isolated throughout the epidemic were predominantly tox⁻ and represented multiple clones. A recent outbreak in Sweden (1984–1986) with high mortality (>20 percent) was found to be caused by a single tox⁺ mitis strain that differed from *C. diphtheriae* strains isolated concurrently from carriers. These observations suggest that traits other than toxigenicity can contribute to virulence of *C. diphtheriae*. Evidence for initiation of an epidemic by phage conversion of tox⁻ to tox⁺ strains in vivo in one individual with subsequent dissemination to other susceptible subjects was found in an outbreak in England.

PATHOLOGY AND PATHOGENESIS   *C. diphtheriae* infects mucous membranes, most commonly in the respiratory tract, and also invades open skin lesions from insect bites or trauma. In infections caused by tox⁺ *C. diphtheriae*, initial edema and hyperemia are often followed by epithelial necrosis and acute inflammation. Coagulation of the dense fibrinopurulent exudate produces a pseudomembrane, and the inflammatory reaction accompanied by vascular congestion extends into the underlying tissues, accompanied by vascular congestion. The pseudomembrane contains large numbers of *C. diphtheriae*, but the bacterium is rarely isolated from the blood or internal organs.

Diphtheria toxin acts both locally and systemically. Very small amounts cause dermonecrosis, as in the Schick test, and toxin presumably contributes to pseudomembrane formation. The lethal dose of diphtheria toxin for nonimmune humans and highly susceptible animals is about 0.1 μg/kg body weight. Absorbed toxin can cause myocarditis, neuritis, and focal necrosis in other organs including the kidneys, liver, and adrenal glands. Early changes in diphtheritic myocarditis include cloudy swelling of muscle fibers and interstitial edema. These are followed in succeeding weeks by hyaline and granular degeneration of muscle fibers, sometimes with fatty degeneration of the myocardium, progressing to myolysis and, finally, replacement of lost muscle by fibrosis. Thus, diphtheria can cause permanent cardiac damage. In diphtheritic polyneuritis pathologic changes include patchy breakdown of myelin sheaths in peripheral

and autonomic nerves, but recovery of nerve damage is the rule if the patient survives.

Diphtheria toxin is produced by *C. diphtheriae* as an extracellular polypeptide. It is cleaved by proteases to form nicked toxin, consisting of fragments A and B which remain linked by a disulfide bond. Fragment B binds to specific receptors on plasma membranes of cells from humans or susceptible animals, and the bound toxin is internalized by receptor-mediated endocytosis. Fragment A is translocated across the endosomal membrane and released into the cytoplasm where it catalyzes the transfer of the adenosine diphosphate ribose moiety from nicotinamide adenine dinucleotide (NAD) to a modified histidine residue (diphthamide) on elongation factor 2 (EF-2), thereby inactivating EF-2 and inhibiting protein synthesis. One molecule of fragment A in the cytoplasm can kill a cell. Other metabolic alterations in intoxicated cells are secondary to inhibition of protein synthesis. In the intoxicated heart, depletion of carnitine occurs and may contribute to the pathogenesis of diphtheritic myocarditis. Diphtheria toxin and exotoxin A of *Pseudomonas aeruginosa* have the same enzymatic activity and their catalytic domains have homologous amino acid sequences. Nevertheless, their biologic effects differ because they bind to different cell surface receptors and exhibit different cellular tropisms.

CLINICAL MANIFESTATIONS   Patients with *C. diphtheriae* in the respiratory tract are classified as diphtheria cases if they have symptoms consistent with local infection and as diphtheria carriers if they are asymptomatic. Signs and symptoms vary depending on the site and severity of the local infection, patient's age, preexisting nasopharyngeal disease, and concomitant systemic disease. Onset is often gradual, but most patients seek medical care within a few days of becoming ill. Sore throat is the most common symptom, but children are less likely than adults to complain of sore throat and more likely to have nausea and vomiting. Fever of 37.8 to 38.9°C (100 to 102°F) and dysphagia occur in about half the patients, but cough, hoarseness, chills, and rhinorrhea are less common. Systemic manifestations are primarily due to toxic effects of diphtheria toxin. Patients without toxicity feel well except for discomfort associated with the local infection, whereas severely toxic patients may have listlessness, pallor, and tachycardia that can progress rapidly to vascular collapse.

Primary infection in the respiratory tract is most often tonsillopharyngeal (one-half to two-thirds of cases), followed in decreasing order of frequency by laryngeal, nasal, and tracheobronchial infection. Multiple sites are frequently involved, and secondary spread of pharyngeal infection upward to the nasal mucosa or downward to the larynx and tracheobronchial tree is much more common than primary infection at those sites. Systemic toxicity is usually less severe in nasal diphtheria than in tonsillopharyngeal diphtheria and most severe when extensive pseudomembrane extends from the tonsils and pharynx into contiguous regions. A small percentage of patients present with malignant or ''bull-neck'' diphtheria with abrupt onset, extensive pseudomembrane formation, foul breath, massive swelling of the tonsils and uvula, thick speech, cervical lymphadenopathy, striking edematous swelling of the submandibular region and anterior neck, and severe toxicity.

In tonsillopharyngeal diphtheria, only erythema may be noted initially, but isolated spots of grey or white exudate are common. These often extend and coalesce within a day to form a confluent, sharply demarcated pseudomembrane which becomes progressively thicker, more tightly adherent to the underlying tissue, and darker gray in color. Unlike the exudate in streptococcal pharyngitis, the diphtheritic pseudomembrane often extends beyond the margin of the tonsils onto the tonsillar pillars, palate, or uvula. Dislodging the membrane is likely to cause bleeding. Estimates of the proportion of patients with pharyngeal diphtheria who develop typical pseudomembranes vary widely, from as few as one-third to almost all. The higher estimates may be biased by failure to consider and confirm the diagnosis of diphtheria in patients who do not develop pseudomembranes. Patients with nasal diphtheria often present with serosanguinous nasal discharge, which may be unilateral or bilateral and cause irritation of the nares or lip. Laryngeal diphtheria often presents with hoarseness and cough. Demonstration of laryngeal pseudomembrane by laryngoscopy is helpful for distinguishing diphtheria from other infectious forms of laryngitis. Primary or secondary diphtheritic infection occasionally involves other mucous membranes, including conjunctiva, genitourinary tract, and gastrointestinal tract.

Cutaneous diphtheria usually presents as an infection by *C. diphtheriae* of preexisting dermatoses involving, in decreasing order of frequency, the lower extremities, upper extremities, head, or trunk. The clinical features are similar to other secondary cutaneous bacterial infections. In the tropics cutaneous diphtheria occasionally presents with morphologically distinct "punched-out" ulcers that are covered by necrotic slough or membrane and have well demarcated edges.

COMPLICATIONS Obstruction of the respiratory tract, presenting as tachypnea, dyspnea, stridor, cyanosis, and use of accessory muscles of respiration, can be caused by extensive pseudomembrane formation and swelling during the first few days of the disease or by sloughed pseudomembrane that becomes lodged in the airway at a later stage in the disease. The risk of respiratory obstruction is greater when infection involves the larynx or tracheobronchial tree and is higher in children because of the small size of the airways.

Myocarditis and polyneuritis are the most prominent toxic manifestations of diphtheria. Their risk is proportional to the severity of local disease, and both can occur in individual patients. Myocarditis may present during the acute phase of illness, develop as the local disease is improving, or begin insidiously after several weeks. One-half to two-thirds of patients with typical diphtheria have subtle evidence of cardiac dysfunction, including electrocardiographic abnormalities, but clinically apparent myocarditis develops in 10 to 25 percent of patients and is usually more severe when the onset is early. Electrocardiographic abnormalities include ST-T wave changes, varying degrees of heart block, and arrhythymias, including atrial fibrillation, ventricular premature beats, ventricular tachycardia, or ventricular fibrillation. Clinical signs include diminished heart sounds, gallop rhythm, systolic murmurs, and, less commonly, acute or insidiously progressive congestive heart failure. Serum aspartate aminotransferase levels reflect the intensity of myocardial damage and can be used to monitor its course.

Polyneuritis is uncommon in mild diphtheria but occurs in approximately 10 percent of cases of average severity and in up to 75 percent of severe cases. Bulbar dysfunction typically develops during the first 2 weeks. Palatal and pharyngeal paralysis usually develop first. Swallowing is difficult; the voice is nasal; and ingested fluids may be regurgitated through the nose. With unilateral pharyngeal infection, ipsilateral palatal paralysis is more common than contralateral or bilateral paralysis. Additional bulbar signs may develop over several weeks, with oculomotor and ciliary paralysis occurring more often than facial or laryngeal paralysis. Peripheral polyneuritis typically begins from 1 to 3 months after the onset of diphtheria with proximal weakness of the extremities that spreads distally. Severity varies from mild weakness of the pelvic muscles with unsteady gait to total paralysis including failure of respiration. Paresthesias may occur, most often in a "glove-and-stocking" distribution. Polyneuritis usually resolves completely, with the time needed for improvement approximately equal to that taken for development of symptoms. Severe muscular weakness may develop 1 to 2 weeks before maximal abnormalities in peripheral nerve conduction velocity can be demonstrated, resulting in a striking dissociation between clinical and electrophysiologic findings. Cerebrospinal fluid most often shows moderately increased albumin, occasionally with pleocytosis, but the abnormalities in CSF do not determine the prognosis.

Pneumonia occurs in more than half of fatal cases of diphtheria. Less common complications include renal failure, encephalitis, cerebral infarction, pulmonary embolism, and bacteremia or endocarditis due to invasive infection by *C. diphtheriae*. Serum sickness may result from antitoxin therapy.

COURSE AND PROGNOSIS Most cases of diphtheria occur in nonimmunized patients. The attack rate, severity of disease, and risk of complications are much lower when diphtheria occurs in immunized patients. The pseudomembrane may continue to increase in size during the first day after administration of antitoxin. During the next several days to a week it becomes softer, less adherent, and nonconfluent and it eventually disappears as the normal mucosa is regenerated. In the preantibiotic era, *C. diphtheriae* persisted in the throat for about 2 weeks in half of patients and for 1 month or more in about one-fifth. Mortality increases with increasing severity of local disease, extent of pseudomembrane formation, and delay between onset of local disease and administration of antitoxin. Mortality is highest during the first week of illness; in patients with "bull-neck" diphtheria; in patients with myocarditis who develop ventricular tachycardia, atrial fibrillation, or complete heart block; in patients with laryngeal or tracheobronchial involvement; in infants and those over 60 years of age; and in alcoholics. In cutaneous diphtheria both the mortality rate and the risk of developing myocarditis or peripheral neuropathy are significantly lower than in respiratory diphtheria.

DIAGNOSIS A characteristic pseudomembrane on the mucosa of the oropharynx, palate, nasopharynx, nose, or larynx suggests diphtheria, but pseudomembrane is not uniformly present. Diphtheritic pseudomembrane must be distinguished from other pharyngeal exudates, including those of group A beta-hemolytic streptococcal infections, infectious mononucleosis, viral pharyngitides, fusospirochetal infection, and candidiasis. Diphtheria should be considered in patients with sore throat, cervical adenopathy or swelling, and low-grade fever, especially when accompanied by systemic toxicity, hoarseness, stridor, palatal paralysis, or serosanguinous nasal discharge, with or without demonstrable pseudomembrane. Treatment with diphtheria antitoxin should be initiated as soon as the clinical diagnosis of diphtheria is made. Definitive diagnosis of diphtheria depends on isolation of *C. diphtheriae* from local lesions. The laboratory should be notified that diphtheria is suspected to ensure use of media appropriate for isolation of *C. diphtheriae*, such as Tinsdale's tellurite agar or Loeffler's coagulated serum medium. Rapid presumptive diagnosis of *C. diphtheriae* can sometimes be made by methylene blue or fluorescent antibody staining of bacteria from direct swabs, or preferably after several hours of selective cultivation, but confirmation of biochemical reactions to differentiate *C. diphtheriae* from corynebacteria of the normal flora (diphtheroids) requires days. Toxigenicity tests should be performed on all isolates of *C. diphtheriae*. Group A beta-hemolytic streptococci and *Staphylococcus aureus* are also isolated frequently from patients with diphtheria.

Cutaneous diphtheria may present with a characteristic "punched-out" ulcer with a membrane, but it is more often indistinguishable from other inflammatory dermatoses. Diagnosis depends on a high degree of suspicion and on the use of laboratory media appropriate for isolation of *C. diphtheriae* from culture of specimens from cutaneous lesions. Throat cultures for *C. diphtheriae* should be obtained from all patients with cutaneous diphtheria.

TREATMENT The decision to treat with diphtheria antitoxin is based on the clinical diagnosis of diphtheria, without definitive laboratory confirmation, since each day of delay is associated with increased mortality. Because diphtheria antitoxin is produced in horses, it is necessary to obtain a history of possible allergy to horse serum and to perform a conjunctival or intracutaneous test with diluted antitoxin for immediate hypersensitivity. Epinephrine must be available to treat any severe allergic reactions immediately. Patients with immediate hypersensitivity should be desensitized before a full therapeutic dose of antitoxin is given. The dose of diphtheria antitoxin currently recommended by the Committee on Infectious Diseases of the American Academy of Pediatrics is based on the site of the primary infection and the duration and severity of disease: 20,000 to 40,000 units for disease involving the pharynx or larynx and of ≤48 h duration; 40,000 to 60,000 units for nasopharyngeal infections; and

80,000 to 100,000 units if the disease is extensive, has been present for 3 or more days, or is accompanied by brawny anterior cervical edema. Antitoxin is administered intravenously by infusion in saline over 60 min to neutralize unbound toxin rapidly. The approximately 10 percent risk of developing serum sickness is acceptable because of the established therapeutic value of antitoxin in decreasing mortality from respiratory diphtheria. During the early phase of the Seattle epidemic, all patients with cutaneous diphtheria were treated with 20,000 units of antitoxin. Later, when most isolates were known to be tox⁻, antitoxin was withheld initially and administered only to patients from whom tox⁺ strains of *C. diphtheriae* were isolated. The potential systemic complications from cutaneous diphtheria must be weighed against the potential adverse effects from antitoxin treatment, and authorities are not unanimous in recommending antitoxin therapy for cutaneous diphtheria.

Antibiotics have little demonstrated effect on healing of the local infection in diphtheria patients treated with antitoxin. The primary goal of antibiotic therapy for patients or carriers is, therefore, to eradicate *C. diphtheriae* and prevent its transmission from the patient to susceptible contacts. Commonly recommended regimens for treatment of adults with respiratory diphtheria are erythromycin (500 mg four times daily, parenterally or orally) or intramuscular procaine penicillin G (600,000 units at 12-h intervals) for 14 days. Patients with cutaneous diphtheria and carriers can be treated orally with erythromycin (500 mg four times daily) or rifampin (600 mg once daily) for 7 days. If compliance is in question, a single dose of benzathine penicillin G (1.2 to 2.4 million units intramuscularly) can be substituted. Eradication of *C. diphtheriae* should be documented by negative cultures taken at least 24 h after completion of antibiotic therapy on two or three successive days, and some authorities also recommend a repeat throat culture 2 weeks later. The small percentage of patients who continue to be infected with *C. diphtheriae* after treatment should receive an additional 10-day course of oral erythromycin or rifampin. Plasmid-mediated resistance to erythromycin of the MLS type in *C. diphtheriae* emerged temporarily during the Seattle epidemic but declined dramatically in prevalence after routine use of erythromycin was discontinued.

Patients with respiratory diphtheria or cutaneous diphtheria caused by tox⁺ *C. diphtheriae* or strains of unknown toxinogenicity should be hospitalized, kept initially at bed rest, handled with respiratory and contact isolation procedures appropriate for the site of infection, and given supportive care as needed. Respiratory and cardiac function must be monitored closely. Early intubation or tracheostomy is recommended when the larynx is involved or signs of impending airway obstruction are present. Mechanical removal of a tracheobronchial membrane can sometimes be accomplished via the endotracheal tube or tracheostomy. Primary or secondary pneumonia should be diagnosed and treated promptly. Sedative or hypnotic drugs that may mask respiratory symptoms are contraindicated. Close electrocardiographic monitoring, treatment of arrhythmias, and electrical pacing for heart block are essential. Congestive heart failure should be treated as described in Chap. 182. Glucocorticoids do not reduce the risk of diphtheritic myocarditis or polyneuritis. Oral Therapy with DL-carnitine (100 mg/kg per day given in twice-daily doses for four days) may have a beneficial effect in diphtheritic myocarditis, but such therapy should be considered experimental until additional data are available. Ulcerative or ecthymatous cutaneous lesions should be treated with Burow solution as wet compresses after debridement of necrotic areas, and treatment for associated conditions such as pediculosis, scabies, or underlying dermatoses should be instituted.

PREVENTION Vaccines available in the United States for immunization against diphtheria include diphtheria and tetanus toxoids and pertussis vaccine adsorbed (DTP); diphtheria and tetanus toxoids adsorbed (DT) (for pediatric use); and tetanus and diphtheria toxoids adsorbed (Td) (for adult use). Each vaccine contains one dose in 0.5 mL and is administered intramuscularly. The adsorbent is alum, which functions as an adjuvant and enhances immunogenicity of the vaccines. Td contains less diphtheria toxoid than DPT or DT and causes fewer adverse reactions in adults.

Initial immunization against diphtheria requires completion of a primary series, and periodic booster doses throughout life are required to maintain immunity. The recommended primary series for immunization of children up to the seventh birthday is four doses of DTP: the first at 6 weeks to 2 months of age, two additional doses after successive intervals of 4 to 8 weeks, and a fourth dose at 6 to 12 months after the third. DT is substituted for DPT if pertussis vaccine is contraindicated. If primary immunization is delayed until after the seventh birthday, the primary series is three doses of Td: the second dose at 4 to 8 weeks after the first, and the third at 6 to 12 months after the second. If primary immunization is interrupted, the series should be completed, but there is no need to start a new series. Children who complete a primary series should receive one dose of DPT before entering kindergarten, unless the final dose of the primary series was given after the fourth birthday. Adults with an uncertain history of immunization should receive a primary series. Patients with diphtheria should be actively immunized after recovery. Booster doses of Td should be given at intervals of 10 years throughout life, preferably at the mid-decade ages of 15 years, 25 years, etc.

Close contacts of diphtheria patients should be cultured for *C. diphtheriae,* kept under surveillance for 1 week, and treated with appropriate antibiotics if cultures are positive. Previously immunized close contacts should receive an appropriate booster containing diphtheria toxoid if their last booster was given >5 years previously. If immunization status is uncertain, close contacts should receive an antibiotic regimen appropriate for carriers and primary immunization against diphtheria appropriate for their age.

REFERENCES

BJORKHOLM B et al: An outbreak of diphtheria among Swedish alcoholics. Infection 15:354, 1987

CENTERS FOR DISEASE CONTROL: Diphtheria, tetanus, and pertussis: Guidelines for vaccine prophylaxis and other preventive measures. Ann Intern Med 103:896, 1985

CHEN RT et al: Diphtheria in the United States, 1971–1981. Am J Public Health 75:1393, 1985

COYLE MB et al: The molecular epidemiology of three biotypes of *Corynebacterium diphtheriae* in the Seattle outbreak from 1972–1982. J Infect Dis 159:670, 1989

GORE I: Myocardial changes in fatal diphtheria. A summary of observations in 221 cases. Am J Med Sci 219:257, 1948

HARNISH JP et al: Diphtheria among alcoholic urban adults. A decade of experience in Seattle. Ann Intern Med 111:71, 1989

KJELDSEN K et al: Immunity against diphtheria and tetanus in the age group 30–70 years. Scand J Infect Dis 20:177, 1988

MACGREGOR RR: Other corynebacteria, in *Principles and Practice of Infectious Diseases,* G Mandell et al (eds), 3d ed. New York, Churchill Livingstone, 1990

MORTIMER EA Jr: Diphtheria toxoid, in *Vaccines,* SA Plotkin, EA Mortimer, Jr (eds). Philadelphia, Saunders, 1988, p 31

OLSNES S et al: Diphtheria toxin entry: Protein translocation in the reverse direction. Trends Biochem Sci 13:348, 1988

RAMOS ACMF et al: The protective effect of carnitine in human diphtheric myocarditis. Pediatr Res 18:815, 1984

RAPPUOLI R et al: Molecular epidemiology of the 1984–1986 outbreak of diphtheria in Sweden. N Engl J Med 318:12, 1988

COMMITTEE ON INFECTIOUS DISEASES: Diphtheria, in *Report of the Committee on Infectious Diseases,* 21st ed. Elk Grove Village, IL. American Academy of Pediatrics, 1988, p 174

SINGH M et al: Diphtheria in Afganistan—a review of 155 cases. J Trop Med Hyg 88:373, 1985

WARD, WHJ: Diphtheria toxin: A novel cytocidal enzyme. Trends Biochem Sci 12:28, 1987

INFECTIONS CAUSED BY *LISTERIA MONOCYTOGENES* AND *ERYSIPELOTHRIX RHUSIOPATHIAE*

PAUL D. HOEPRICH

LISTERIA MONOCYTOGENES INFECTIONS

DEFINITION Listeriosis, a disease caused by *L. monocytogenes*, consists of many clinical syndromes. Perinatal infection, acquired either transplacentally or during parturition, is the most nearly unique form of listeriosis, while meningitis is the most frequent clinical manifestation.

ETIOLOGY *Listeria monocytogenes* are gram-positive, non-acid-fast, microaerophilic, motile bacilli that form smooth colonies but do not produce either capsules or spores. Several serotypes have been defined on the basis of O and H antigens. The epidemiologically essential aid of typing is available from the Centers for Disease Control. Of the 17 types, 1/2a, 1/2b, and 4b account for more than 70 percent of the cases worldwide. Weakly hemolytic gram-positive bacilli are presumed to be *L. monocytogenes* if they are motile (when grown at 20 to 25°C), reduce 2,3,5-triphenyltetrazolium chloride, hydrolyze esculin, and display characteristic animal pathogenicity: (1) The Anton test—3 to 5 days after inoculation into the conjunctival sac of a rabbit or a guinea pig, *L. monocytogenes* cause a keratoconjunctivitis; (2) general listeriosis (intravenous or intraperitoneal inoculation) typically provokes a monocytosis in rabbits, and focal hepatic necrosis in mice.

EPIDEMIOLOGY AND PATHOGENESIS Found on every continent save the Antarctic, *L. monocytogenes* are distinct from the nonhemolytic, nonpathogenic, bacilli (found mainly in soil, decaying matter, and feces) that are designated *L. innocua* or assigned to the new genus *Murraya*. *Listeria ivanovii* and *L. seeligeri* have rarely been associated with disease in humans, whereas *L. welshimeri* has not; all three are differentiable from *L. monocytogenes* by biochemical and augmentation hemolysis (CAMP) tests. Although typical *L. monocytogenes* have been isolated from silage, other vegetative sources, and 1 to 5 percent of specimens of human feces, listeriosis is uncommon and occurs sporadically with a frequency of 3.6 cases per million population per year in the United States. Listeriosis is more common in urban than rural dwellers, occurring most frequently in July and August (northern hemisphere). Ingestion of food or drink contaminated with *L. monocytogenes* is the usual mode of infection in adults, as exemplified by outbreaks associated with coleslaw, pasteurized milk, ice cream, and fresh Mexican-style cheese.

Infection by direct transfer of *L. monocytogenes* occurs in two circumstances: (1) as an occupational hazard in butchers, abattoir workers, and veterinarians; and (2) from the infected pregnant woman to her offspring either transplacentally or intrapartum. Transplacental perinatal infection results in disseminated fetal listeriosis. The fetus is usually stillborn or is prematurely ejected, virtually always with lethal listeriosis. Fetal listeriosis acquired during delivery is typically not clinically evident for 1 or 2 weeks post partum and usually presents as meningitis.

Listeriosis is preponderantly a disease of persons under 1 year and over 55 years of age. Persons in apparent good health may develop listeriosis. However, other diseases, particularly those with diminished cell-mediated immunity (listerias can survive intracellularly), facilitate the occurrence of listeriosis: for example, neoplasms (especially of the lymphoreticular system) and any conditions requiring treatment with pharmacologic doses of glucocorticoids, irradiation, or cytotoxic agents; alcoholism; cardiovascular disease; diabetes mellitus; and tuberculosis.

MANIFESTATIONS *Listeriosis of the newborn* ranges from meningitis that is clinically apparent within 1 month post partum to diffuse disseminated disease in aborted, premature, stillborn infants, and neonates, who die within minutes to days after birth. If clinical disease is delayed to 1 to 4 weeks post partum, it is generally localized to the central nervous system, as is the rule when children 1 month to 6 years of age are afflicted.

Infants born alive with listeriosis may or may not have fever; yet these babies are critically ill, with cardiorespiratory distress, vomiting, and diarrhea. Dark-red skin papules are frequent, particularly on the lower extremities. Hepatosplenomegaly may be present. This form of listeriosis is also known as septic or miliary granulomatosis. The findings at necropsy are characteristic and mimic those seen in listeriosis of rodents: widely disseminated abscesses varying in size from grossly visible to microscopic, involving, in order of decreasing frequency, liver, spleen, adrenal glands, lungs, pharynx, gastrointestinal tract, central nervous system, and skin. Typically, the lesions are abscesses, but classic granulomas may be seen, depending principally on the duration of infection before death. Microscopic examination of a Gram-stained smear of meconium from the normal newborn infant does not disclose bacteria; fetal listeriosis results in meconium laden with gram-positive bacilli. For this reason, examination of meconium by Gram's stain and by culture should be carried out whenever there is gross soiling of the amniotic liquid with meconium, prematurity, or unexplained fever in the mother before or at the onset of labor. This is particularly important because listeriosis in the pregnant woman may be asymptomatic or may cause a mild, nonspecific illness. A week to a month ante partum, there may have been malaise, a chill, diarrhea, pain in the back or flanks, and itching. Even when symptomatic, the disease is benign and self-limited in the mother; however, as symptoms subside, a decrease or cessation of fetal movement may be noted. Infection of the fetus may occur as early as the fifth month of gestation but occurs most often in the third trimester. Following delivery of infants with proved fetal listeriosis, cervical cultures are, or soon become, negative for *L. monocytogenes*; subsequent conception, gestation, and delivery are normal.

Meningitis accounts for about three-fourths of the cases verified by culture and is the predominant clinical form of listeriosis. Meningitis caused by *L. monocytogenes* cannot be distinguished on clinical grounds from meningitis caused by other bacteria.

Nonmeningeal listeriosis of the central nervous system is associated with fever, nausea and vomiting, headache, and listeremia; the cerebrospinal fluid is normal. Localizing neurologic signs may develop (especially if abscess forms), or the picture may be that of an encephalitis.

Typhoidal listeriosis, i.e., listeremia that has no identifiable source and is associated with high fever and severe prostrating illness, occurs most often in patients with cancers and immunosuppression. However, primary listeremia may also develop in patients with cirrhosis, alcoholism, pregnancy, and no discernible underlying disease.

Listerial endocarditis is generally a chronic process without singular manifestations. About half of the patients have no known predisposing cardiac disease.

Other rare forms of listeriosis include ocular infections, dermatitis, infections of serous cavities, and abscesses in various organs.

LABORATORY FINDINGS Although *L. monocytogenes* grow well on the usual culture media, etiologic diagnosis by isolation and identification may be hampered by failure of differentiation from *Corynebacterium* spp., *Erysipelothrix rhusiopathiae*, and *Streptococcus* spp. Recognition of listerial colonies in a mixed culture, as may result with vaginal or cervical specimens, is difficult and may be aided by using selective media and/or enrichment procedures.

Serodiagnosis by assay for agglutinins has not been useful because of the common finding of so-called natural antibodies. Such nonspecific reactions may reflect the known antigenic relationship between *Staphylococcus aureus* and several listerial serotypes, or contact with nonpathogenic *Listeria* spp. or *Murraya* spp. The humoral antibody response to listeriosis in humans is almost exclusively IgM throughout the disease, whereas staphylococci elicit IgG as well as IgM; i.e., treatment of sera with 2-mercaptoethanol may not eliminate nonspecific reactivity.

Monocytosis is not common in human listeriosis. Leukocytosis with neutrophilia, as in any acute bacterial infection, is seen in listerial meningitis, nonmeningeal infection of the central nervous system, primary listeremia, listerial endocarditis, and abscesses in hosts capable of mounting a granulocytic response. In most patients with listerial meningitis, the findings in the cerebrospinal fluid do not differ from those found in other bacterial meningitides; however, a relative increase in mononuclear cells may be seen in patients with underlying malignancies.

DIFFERENTIAL DIAGNOSIS   Abortion, premature delivery, stillbirth, and neonatal death are more often due to causes other than listeriosis: Rh incompatibility, syphilis, or toxoplasmosis.

In patients with leptomeningitis, conjunctivitis, endocarditis, bacteremia, or polyserositis, reports of isolation of "diphtheroids" or "nonpathogens" must always be challenged. A statement that *L. monocytogenes* has been excluded is required.

TREATMENT   *Listeria monocytogenes* are susceptible to several antimicrobials in vitro, including penicillin G, ampicillin, erythromycin, rifampin, streptomycin, gentamicin, tobramycin, amikacin, trimethoprim-sulfamethoxazole, and the tetracyclines. *Listeria* are resistant to all classes of cephalosporins. Tolerance, i.e., inhibition at low concentrations with much higher concentrations needed for killing, is characteristic with the penicillins, erythromycin, rifampin, trimethoprim-sulfamethoxazole, and streptomycin. Accordingly, combination therapy is necessary for maximally listericidal therapy, e.g., penicillin G [150 to 200 mg (240,000 to 320,000 units) per kilogram of body weight per day, intravenously, as six equal portions every 4 h] plus tobramycin (5 to 6 mg/kg per day, intravenously, as three equal portions every 8 h). Ampicillin and gentamicin (same dosages) may be substituted but offer no advantage. Such treatment is appropriate for listeriosis of the newborn (2 weeks), listeremia in pregnancy (2 weeks), primary listeremia (4 weeks), listerial endocarditis (4 to 6 weeks), and any form of listeriosis outside the central nervous system in immunosuppressed patients (4 to 6 weeks).

As gentamicin and tobramycin do not enter the central nervous system reliably, high-dosage therapy with penicillin G [200 to 300 mg (320,000 to 480,000 units) per kilogram of body weight per day, intravenously, as six equal portions every 4 h] is the primary treatment. Ampicillin may be substituted in the same dose, but the cephalosporins, including the newer derivatives, should not be used. Optimal treatment of patients who are allergic to the penicillins is uncertain; candidate antimicrobials include erythromycin (40 to 50 mg/kg per day, intravenously, as four equal portions every 6 h); doxycycline (3 mg/kg, intravenously as a loading dose, and 1.5 mg/kg per day, intravenously, as two equal portions every 12 h for maintenance); trimethoprim/sulfamethoxazole (15/75 mg/kg per day, intravenously, as 3 equal portions every 8 h). Treatment should be continued in full dosage by intravenous injection for 14 to 21 days after defervescence.

PROGNOSIS   Prompt, vigorous antimicrobial treatment of the acute forms of listeriosis, excepting fetal listeriosis, is usually curative. On the basis of agglutinin titers, specific antibody disappears during the months following cure. However, reinfection has not been reported.

ERYSIPELOTHRIX RHUSIOPATHIAE INFECTIONS

DEFINITION   Erysipeloid is the commonest and most nearly unique form of infection in humans caused by *Erysipelothrix rhusiopathiae*. Infective endocarditis and arthritis are rare forms of erysipelothricosis in humans.

ETIOLOGY   As gram-positive, nonmotile, nonencapsulated, nonsporulating, microaerophilic bacilli, *E. rhusiopathiae* may be confused with nontoxinogenic *Corynebacterium* spp. and *Listeria monocytogenes*. However, *E. rhusiopathiae* is nonmotile and fails to grow on media selective for *Corynebacterium* spp. Also, unlike *L. monocytogenes*, *E. rhusiopathiae* only rarely causes conjunctivitis, following conjunctival inoculation, or monocytosis, after intravenous inocula-

tion, in the rabbit. Because alpha hemolysis is commonly evident after 48 h of incubation of *E. rhusiopathiae*, confusion with streptococci may also occur. Isolates of *E. rhusiopathiae* appear to be serologically homogeneous. Although serodifferentiation from other gram-positive bacilli is possible, few laboratories are capable of definitive serodiagnosis.

EPIDEMIOLOGY AND PATHOGENESIS   Primarily a saprobe, *E. rhusiopathiae* is worldwide in distribution. Humans are virtually always infected by traumatic dermal inoculation; erysipeloid is the usual result. The disease is almost wholly restricted to persons who in their occupations handle edible or nonedible dead animal products. If the bacilli are not successfully confined to the skin, bacteremia may result and may lead to infective endocarditis; in about two-thirds of the reported cases, there was no evidence of preexisting valvular heart disease and the aortic valve was involved in about 60 percent of the cases. Septic arthritis, usually in previously damaged joints, may also complicate bacteremia.

The seasonal incidence of erysipeloid parallels that of swine erysipelas, being highest in summer and early fall. Yet persons who tend pigs, even pigs ill with porcine erysipelas, do not commonly develop erysipeloid.

MANIFESTATIONS   Erysipeloid begins 2 to 7 days after injury, often after the initial lesion has healed. An itching, burning, painful irritation may precede and always accompanies the appearance of the maculopapular, nonvesiculated, sharply defined, raised, purplish-red zone surrounding the site of entry. There is local swelling, and when, as is usual, a finger or the hand is involved, nearby joints may become stiff and painful. Centrifugal spread from the site of inoculation is apparent in a day or two. Movement is slow, 1 to 2 cm per 24 h maximally, and more rapid proximally than distally; involvement of the terminal phalanx of a finger is rare, while spread to other fingers and the hand distal to the wrist is common. With extension, the original center subsides without desquamation or suppuration. There are usually no systemic signs or symptoms; regional lymphangitis and lymphadenitis are rare. Untreated, the disease heals within 3 weeks in most patients, although relapse has been observed.

The manifestations of erysipelothrical endocarditis may be either acute or chronic, depending on the virulence of the infecting strain and on the state of resistance of the host. Usually, there are no classic erysipeloid skin lesions to suggest the disease at the time that endocarditis is clinically evident. However, a history of recent erysipeloid may be helpful.

Erysipelothrical arthritis is not clinically characteristic but usually can be related to erysipeloid or erysipelothrical bacteremia. Isolation of *E. rhusiopathiae* from synovial fluid has not been reported.

LABORATORY FINDINGS   The usual culture media are adequate for the growth of *E. rhusiopathiae*. However, differentiation from diphtheroids, listerias, and streptococci depends primarily on the clinician's alerting the laboratory to the possibility of erysipelothricosis. In erysipeloid, *E. rhusiopathiae* are best recovered by incubating, in broth containing glucose, a full-thickness biopsy of skin removed from the advancing edge of a lesion. Culture of an aspirate obtained after injection of sterile, bacteriostat-free 0.9% NaCl solution into the periphery of a lesion is less likely to yield *E. rhusiopathiae*. With endocarditis and arthritis, the findings are in keeping with the respective clinical syndromes and are in no way characteristic for *E. rhusiopathiae*, whereas abrasion of a florid lesion with culture of the resultant exudate may be rewarding.

DIFFERENTIAL DIAGNOSIS   The appearance and location of erysipeloid, its slow and limited spread, the lack of constitutional reaction, the history of occupation and injury, all serve to identify this disease. The afflicted skin in *erysipelas* is very erythematous, and the face and scalp are affected; there are regional lymphangitis and lymphadenitis, leukocytosis, fever, and malaise. Eczematous lesions may itch, but they display vesicles and little abnormal color. The various erythemas have a different location and do not usually itch or burn; they are more apt to be chronic and nonmigratory.

TREATMENT The penicillins, the cephalosporins, erythromycin, clindamycin, the tetracyclines, and chloramphenicol inhibit *E. rhusiopathiae* in vitro at concentrations practical in therapy. Penicillin G is the agent of choice. Erysipeloid is adequately treated by injection of 1.2 million units of benzathine penicillin G. Erythromycin (15 mg/kg per day in four equal portions taken orally for 5 to 7 days) is an alternative. Cure of erysipelothrical endocarditis has been effected by the daily injection of 2 to 20 million units of penicillin per day or cefazolin (65 to 75 mg/kg per day, intravenously, as four equal portions every 6 h) for 4 to 6 weeks; the dose can be monitored by determination of the bactericidal activity of serum from the patient against the infecting strain. Intractable cardiac failure may oblige surgical excision of an infected valve and insertion of a prosthesis. Erysipelothrical arthritis usually responds to repeated needle aspiration drainage plus penicillin or cefazolin in the dosage given for endocarditis. Antimicrobial therapy should be continued for at least one week after the effusion clears.

PROGNOSIS Penicillin therapy is highly effective in curing erysipelothrical infections. As with infective endocarditis from any cause, the prognosis is primarily a function of the severity of the valvular damage. Despite appropriate antimicrobial therapy, the mortality remains 30 to 40 percent; earlier diagnosis, and, perhaps, earlier resort to surgical excision and replacement of infected valves, may improve the outcome.

REFERENCES

CHERUBIN CE et al: Listeria and gram-negative bacillary meningitis in New York City, 1972–1979. Am J Med 71:199, 1981

CIESIELSKI CA et al: Listeriosis in the United States: 1980–1982. Arch Intern Med 148:1416, 1988

FLEMING DW et al: Pasteurized milk as a vehicle of infection in an outbreak of listeriosis. N Engl J Med 312:404, 1985

GORBY GL et al: *Erysipelothrix rhusiopathiae* endocarditis: Microbiologic, epidemiologic, and clinical features of an occupational disease. Rev Infect Dis 10:317, 1988

HOEPRICH PD: Listeriosis, in *Infectious Diseases*, 4th ed, PD Hoeprich (ed). Philadelphia, Lippincott-Harper, 1989, chap 56

———: Erysipeloid, in *Infectious Diseases*, 4th ed, PD Hoeprich (ed). Philadelphia, Lippincott-Harper, 1989, chap 112

LINNAN MD et al: Epidemic listeriosis associated with Mexican-style cheese. N Engl J Med 319:823, 1988

NELSON E: Five hundred cases of erysipeloid. Rocky Mount Med J 52:40, 1955

ROCOURT J, GRIMONT PAD: *Listeria welshimeri* sp. nov. and *Listeria seeligeri* sp. nov. Int J Syst Bacteriol 33:866, 1983

SCHLECH WF III et al: Epidemic listeriosis—evidence for transmission by food. N Engl J Med 308:203, 1983

SEELIGER HPR: *Listeriosis*. Basel, Karger, 1961

104 ANTHRAX

RANDALL K. HOLMES

DEFINITION Anthrax is an acute bacterial infection caused by *Bacillus anthracis* that occurs most frequently in herbivorous animals. Humans become infected when spores of *B. anthracis* are introduced into the body by contact with infected animals or contaminated animal products, insect bites, inhalation, or ingestion. In humans the most common form is cutaneous anthrax, characterized by development of a localized skin lesion with a central eschar surrounded by marked nonpitting edema. Inhalation anthrax (woolsorter's disease) typically produces hemorrhagic mediastinitis, rapidly progressive systemic infection, and a very high mortality rate. Gastrointestinal anthrax is rare and has a high mortality rate.

ETIOLOGY *B. anthracis* is a large (1 to 1.5 μm by 4 to 10 μm), nonmotile, encapsulated, chain-forming, aerobic gram-positive rod that forms centrally located, oval spores. Oxygen is required for sporulation but not for germination of spores, and sporulation does not occur in living animals. The individual bacteria in the chains are rectangular, giving them a boxcar-shaped appearance. On blood agar virulent *B. anthracis* usually forms nonhemolytic or weakly hemolytic, gray-white, rough colonies with irregular, comma-shaped projections, said to resemble a Medusa's head; but if the medium contains bicarbonate and incubation is carried out in the presence of excess CO_2 the colonies are smooth and mucoid. Virulent strains of *B. anthracis* are pathogenic for animals, including mice and guinea pigs. Known virulence factors include three proteins collectively called *anthrax toxin* (see below) and an antiphagocytic capsular polypeptide, composed of D-glutamic acid residues linked by peptide bonds involving the gamma carboxyl group. The genes that determine production of anthrax toxin and of capsular polypeptide are present on separate plasmids of *B. anthracis*. Determination of susceptibility to bacillus phage gamma and demonstration of species specific antigens by direct fluorescent antibody tests or by hemagglutination tests are helpful in laboratory identification of *B. anthracis*. Spores of *B. anthracis* can survive for years in dry earth but are destroyed by boiling for about 10 min, by treatment with oxidizing agents such as potassium permanganate or hydrogen peroxide, or by dilute formaldehyde. Most strains of *B. anthracis* are susceptible to penicillin.

EPIDEMIOLOGY The distribution of anthrax is worldwide. All animals are susceptible to varying degrees, but the disease is most prevalent among domestic herbivores, including cattle, sheep, horses, and goats, and wild herbivores.

Grazing animals become infected when they are foraging for food in areas contaminated with spores of *B. anthracis* under appropriate climatic conditions. Anthrax in herbivores tends to be severe, with high mortality. Terminally ill animals have overwhelming bacteremic infections and often bleed from the nose, mouth, and bowel, thereby contaminating soil or watering places with vegetative *B. anthracis* that can subsequently sporulate and persist in the environment. The carcasses of infected animals provide additional potential foci of contamination. Whether or not *B. anthracis* multiplies to any significant extent in the soil is controversial, and environmental factors which affect the probability that animals grazing in infected areas will become infected are not fully defined. Epidemics among animals may spread from an initial focus to contiguous geographic areas, consistent with the movement of infected animals. Biting flies have also been implicated as vectors for the spread of anthrax, and vultures that feed on infected carcasses are believed to be involved in the occasional spread of anthrax from an infected area to noncontiguous areas, probably by contaminating surface water pools.

The natural resistance of humans to anthrax is greater than that of herbivorous animals. It is difficult to determine the annual worldwide incidence of human anthrax because many cases do not receive medical attention and are not reported; estimates of 20,000 to 100,000 cases per year have been made. Human cases are classified as agricultural or industrial based on the epidemiologic setting in which they occur. Agricultural cases result most often from contact with animals that have anthrax (skinning, butchering, dissecting, etc.), from bites of contaminated or infected flies, and rarely from consumption of contaminated meat. Industrial cases are associated with exposure to contaminated hides, goat hair, wool, or bones that are used for commercial purposes. Anthrax in animals has been a longstanding problem in Iran, Turkey, Pakistan, and Sudan, and probability is high that animal products, especially goat hair, originating from these areas will be contaminated with anthrax spores.

Only four cases of anthrax occurred in the United States from 1984 through 1988, and gastrointestinal anthrax has never been documented in the United States. Large epidemics of anthrax occurred in Sverdlovsk in the Soviet Union in April, 1979, and in Zimbabwe between 1978 and the early 1980s. The outbreak in Zimbabwe involved more than 9700 cases of agricultural anthrax in 1979 and 1980. The massive outbreak in Zimbabwe occurred during wartime and was associated with disruption of the veterinary and medical infrastructure and cessation of anthrax vaccination programs (see below).

PATHOGENESIS B. anthracis is an extracellular pathogen that can evade phagocytosis, invade the bloodstream, multiply rapidly to a high population density in vivo, and kill rapidly. Capsular polypeptide and anthrax toxin are recognized as virulence factors of B. anthracis.

Anthrax toxin was discovered by demonstrating that transfer of sterile blood from guinea pigs dying of anthrax to uninfected guinea pigs kills the recipient animals and that death is prevented by specific immune serum.

Anthrax toxin consists of three separate soluble proteins called protective antigen (PA), edema factor (EF), and lethal factor (LF). Antibodies against PA protect experimental animals and man against anthrax. PA is the major component of the vaccine against anthrax used for humans in the United States. Loss of the plasmid that encodes anthrax toxin is the probable basis for attenuation of the strain of B. anthracis developed by Pasteur for his original experiments on immunization of animals against anthrax. Capsular polypeptide of B. anthracis is antiphagocytic. Loss of ability to produce capsule is the primary basis for attenuation of the live spore vaccine (Sterne strain) used for animals in the United States. These nonencapsulated strains produce anthrax toxin and elicit antitoxic antibodies but are less invasive than wild-type strains.

PA, EF, and LF have been purified and characterized and their structural genes cloned and sequenced. PA binds to receptors on the plasma membrane of target cells and is then cleaved by trypsin or a protease with similar specificity to produce two fragments. The smaller fragment is released, but the larger fragment remains on the cell surface and displays a binding site for EF or LF. The large fragment of PA on the cell surface serves, therefore, as a specific receptor for EF or LF; and it mediates entry of EF or LF into target cells by receptor-mediated endocytosis. EF is a calmodulin-dependent adenylate cyclase. The enzymatic activity of EF is only expressed within target cells, which provide the required calmodulin activator as well as the ATP substrate that is converted into cyclic AMP. The actions of cyclic AMP in the intoxicated cells are presumed to be responsible for the biological effects of EF, which include formation of the edema characteristic of anthrax lesions as well as inhibition of phagocytosis by polymorphonuclear leukocytes. PA-mediated entry of LF into susceptible target cells leads to cell death, but the mechanism of action of LF has not yet been determined.

Cutaneous anthrax is initiated by introducing spores of B. anthracis into the skin through cuts or abrasions or by biting flies. The spores germinate within hours, and the vegetative cells begin to multiply and produce the components of anthrax toxin. Histologically the lesion in cutaneous anthrax is characterized by necrosis, vascular congestion, hemorrhage, and gelatinous edema. The number of leukocytes is disproportionately small in comparison with the amount of tissue damage. The clinical description of this lesion as a "malignant pustule" is not in concordance with the pathologic findings.

In inhalation anthrax B. anthracis spores in airborne particles of less that 5 μm diameter are deposited directly into the alveoli or alveolar ducts. The spores are phagocytized by alveolar macrophages and some are carried to and germinate in mediastinal nodes. Hemorrhagic necrosis of the nodes, associated with hemorrhagic mediastinitis and development of overwhelming B. anthracis bacteremia, may develop rapidly. Secondary pneumonia sometimes occurs.

Gastrointestinal anthrax usually results from ingestion of inadequately cooked meat from animals with anthrax. Primary infection can be initiated in the intestine by germination of spores that survive passage through the stomach, but an oropharyngeal form of the disease has also been described. Lesions in the throat or intestine are usually accompanied by hemorrhagic lymphadenitis.

B. anthracis bacteremia can develop in any form of anthrax and occurs in almost all fatal cases. Autopsies reveal large numbers of bacteria in blood vessels, lymph nodes, and many organs.

CLINICAL MANIFESTATIONS Approximately 95 percent of human cases are cutaneous anthrax, and about 5 percent are inhalation anthrax. Gastrointestinal anthrax occurs rarely. Anthrax meningitis

occurs in a small percentage of all cases but is a frequent complication of overwhelming B. anthracis bacteremia.

Cutaneous anthrax The cutaneous lesion in anthrax is most often found on exposed areas of skin. In Zimbabwe, lesions in children under 5 years old were significantly more likely to be on the head, neck, or face and less likely to be on the upper limbs than in adults. This correlated with the fact that children had less contact with carcasses of infected animals and were more likely to acquire infection by fly bites.

Within days after inoculation of B. anthracis spores into skin, a small, red macule appears. During the next week the lesion typically progresses through papular and vesicular or pustular stages, leading to formation of an ulcer with a blackened, necrotic eschar surrounded by a highly characteristic, expanding zone of brawny edema. The early lesion may be pruritic, and the fully developed lesion is painless. Small satellite vesicles may surround the original lesion, and painful nonspecific regional lymphadenitis is common. Most patients are afebrile, with mild or no constitutional symptoms, but in severe cases edema may be extensive and associated with septic shock. Spontaneous healing occurs in 80 to 90 percent of untreated cases, but edema may persist for weeks. In the 10 to 20 percent of untreated patients who develop progressive infection, bacteremia develops and is often associated with high fever and a rapidly fatal outcome. The differential diagnosis includes staphylococcal skin infections, tularemia, plague, and orf. Cutaneous anthrax should be considered in all patients who have painless ulcers associated with vesicles and edema as well as contact with animal products or animals.

Inhalation anthrax The presenting symptoms of inhalation anthrax (woolsorter's disease) are often similar to those of severe viral respiratory diseases, making early diagnosis difficult. After 1 to 3 days an acute phase supervenes, with increasing fever, dyspnea, stridor, hypoxia, and hypotension usually leading to death within 24 h. Occasionally patients present with the fulminant disease. A characteristic x-ray finding associated with the hemorrhagic mediastinitis is symmetrical mediastinal widening.

Gastrointestinal anthrax Symptoms of gastrointestinal anthrax are variable and include fever, nausea and vomiting, abdominal pain, bloody diarrhea, and sometimes rapidly developing ascites. Diarrhea is occasionally massive, causing hemoconcentration and severe contraction of intravascular volume. The major features of oropharyngeal anthrax are fever, sore throat, dysphagia, painful regional lymphadenopathy, and toxemia; respiratory distress may be present. The primary lesion is most often on the tonsils and features necrosis, hemorrhage and exudate formation.

LABORATORY DIAGNOSIS B. anthracis is present in large numbers in cutaneous lesions of anthrax and can be demonstrated by Gram's stain, direct fluorescent antibody staining, or culture unless the patient has been treated with antibiotics. A small proportion of patients with anthrax have bacteremia, but the disease may progress to a fatal outcome before cultures become positive. Patients with anthrax meningitis have bloody spinal fluid containing a large number of B. anthracis demonstrable by staining or culture. Virulence of suspected isolates of B. anthracis can be demonstrated by inoculating guinea pigs; death occurs within 24 h with positive cultures from heart blood. Patients with mild disease usually have normal leukocyte counts, but patients with disseminated disease typically have polymorphonuclear leukocytosis. Tests for antibody to B. anthracis are useful in confirming the diagnosis of anthrax.

TREATMENT Viable B. anthracis disappears from the lesions of cutaneous anthrax within 5 h in patients treated with parenteral penicillin G. Recommended therapy for adults is 2 million units of penicillin G at intervals of 6 h until edema subsides, followed by oral penicillin to complete a 7- to 10-d course of treatment. For penicillin-sensitive adults erythromycin or tetracycline (500 mg every 6 h) can be substituted. Chloramphenicol has also been used successfully. Antibiotics decrease local edema and systemic toxicity in patients with cutaneous anthrax but do not prevent eschar formation. Cutaneous lesions should be cleaned and covered, and used dressings should be decontaminated. For inhalation anthrax high-dose penicillin therapy (2 million units at 2-hourly intervals) is recommended, and a similar regimen is recommended for gastrointestinal anthrax or anthrax meningitis. A rational case can be made for passive immunization with anthrax antitoxin in addition to antibiotic therapy in severely ill patients with anthrax, but appropriate antitoxin is not commercially available.

PREVENTION Inhalation anthrax was virtually eliminated in England before 1940 by developing methods to decontaminate wool and goat hair and by improving working conditions for handlers of animal products. Nonliving vaccines consisting of alum precipitated or aluminum hydroxide adsorbed extracellular components of unencapsulated *B. anthracis* are available in the UK and USA for use in humans who are at risk for exposure to anthrax. The major active component of these vaccines is PA. Molecular engineering was recently used to produce a mutant form of PA that lacks the trypsin-sensitive sequence and cannot interact with EF or LF to mediate toxicity. The mutant PA is being tested as a potential new vaccine against anthrax. Immunization of domestic herbivores with spores of nonencapsulated strains of *B. anthracis* has a major role in decreasing the prevalence of anthrax in livestock both in developed and in developing countries. Living attenuated spore vaccines are not used for humans in the United States but are used both for humans and animals in the Soviet Union. Carcasses of animals that succumb to anthrax should be buried intact or cremated. Necropsies or butchering of infected animals should be avoided because sporulation of *B. anthracis* occurs only in the presence of oxygen.

PROGNOSIS The mortality rate is 10 to 20 percent for untreated cutaneous anthrax and is very low with appropriate antibiotic therapy. In contrast, the mortality rate of inhalation anthrax approaches 100 percent, and therapy is usually unsuccessful. The mortality rate in treated gastrointestinal anthrax is approximately 50 percent. Anthrax meningitis is usually fatal.

The opinions expressed herein are those of the author and do not necessarily represent the views of the Department of Defense or the Uniformed Services University of the Health Sciences.

REFERENCES

BRACHMAN PS: Inhalation anthrax. Ann NY Acad Sci 353:83, 1980

BRAGG TS, ROBERTSON UL: Nucleotide sequence and analysis of the lethal factor gene (lef) from *Bacillus anthracis*. Gene 81:45, 1989

DAVIES JCA: A major epidemic of anthrax in Zimbabwe, Part II. Distribution of cutaneous lesions. Central African J Med 28:291, 1982

————: A major epidemic of anthrax in Zimbabwe. The experience of the Beatrice Road Infectious Diseases Hospital, Harare. Central African J Med 31:176, 1985

DOGANAY M et al: Primary throat anthrax. A report of six cases. Scand J Infect Dis 18:415, 1986

————: A case of cutaneous anthrax with toxemic shock. Brit J Dermatol 117:659, 1987

GORDON VH et al: Adenylate cyclase toxins from *Bacillus anthracis* and *Bordetella pertussis*. Different processes for interaction with and entry into target cells. J Biol Chem 264:14792, 1989

HAMBLETON P et al: Anthrax: The disease in relation to vaccines. Vaccine 2:125, 1984

KNUDSON GB: Treatment of anthrax in man: History and current concepts. Military Medicine 151:71, 1986

LAFORCE FM: *Bacillus anthracis* (anthrax), in *Principles and Practice of Infectious Diseases*, 3d ed, GL Mandell et al (eds). New York, Churchill Livingstone, 1990, p 1593

MARSHALL L: Sverdlovsk: Anthrax capital? Science 240:383, 1988

O'BRIEN J et al: Effects of anthrax toxin components on human neutrophils. Infect Immun 45:306, 1986

SINGH Y et al: A deleted variant of *Bacillus anthracis* protective antigen is non-toxic and blocks anthrax toxin action in vivo. J Biol Chem 264:19103, 1989

105   TETANUS

ELIAS ABRUTYN

DEFINITION Tetanus is a neurologic disorder, characterized by increased muscle tone and spasms, that is caused by tetanospasmin, a powerful protein toxin elaborated by *Clostridium tetani*. Tetanus occurs in several clinical forms including generalized, neonatal, and localized disease.

MICROBIOLOGY The organism is an anaerobic, motile gram-positive rod that forms an oval, colorless, terminal spore creating a shape that resembles a tennis racket or drumstick. It is found worldwide in soil, in the inanimate environment, in animal feces, and occasionally in human feces. Spores may survive for years in some environments and are resistant to various disinfectants and boiling for 20 min. Vegetative cells, however, are easily inactivated and are susceptible to several antibiotics (penicillin, erythromycin, and others).

Tetanospasmin is formed in vegetative cells under plasmid control. It is a single polypeptide chain. With autolysis, the single-chain toxin is released and cleaved to form a heterodimer consisting of a heavy chain (93,000 mol wt) and a light chain (52,000 mol wt) joined by a disulfide bond. The amino acid structures of the two most powerful toxins known, botulinum and tetanus toxin, are partially homologous.

EPIDEMIOLOGY Tetanus occurs sporadically and almost always affects nonimmunized or partially immunized persons, or fully immunized individuals who fail to maintain adequate immunity with booster doses of vaccine. Although entirely preventable by immunization, worldwide the burden of disease is large. The disease is common where soil is cultivated, in rural areas, in warm climates, during summer months, and in males. In countries without a major immunization program, neonatal tetanus and tetanus in the young predominate; worldwide an estimated 800,000 neonates die each year. In the United States and other nations with successful immunization programs, neonatal tetanus rarely occurs and the disease affects other age groups and those in groups inadequately reached by immunization such as nonwhites. The elderly, in particular, are prominently involved. Under 100 cases have been reported to the Centers for Disease Control annually. 95 percent of cases occurred in persons over 20 years of age and 71 percent in individuals over 50.

In the United States, most tetanus occurs after an acute injury, such as a puncture wound or laceration, and is often acquired at home, either indoors or outdoors, frequently in a garden. The injury may be major, but often is trivial so medical attention is not sought. The disease may complicate chronic conditions such as skin ulcers, abscesses, and gangrene. Tetanus is also associated with burns, frostbite, ear infection, surgery, abortion, childbirth, and drug abuse, notably skin "popping." In some patients no portal of entry can be identified.

PATHOGENESIS Contamination of wounds with spores is probably frequent. Germination and toxin production, however, only occur in wounds with low oxidation-reduction potential such as those containing devitalized tissue, foreign bodies, or active infection. *Clostridium tetani* does not itself evoke inflammation.

Toxin released in the wound binds to peripheral motor neuron terminals, enters the axon, and is transported to the nerve cell body in the central nervous system by retrograde intraneuronal transport. It then crosses the synapse to enter the inhibitory interneurons where it acts to block neurotransmitter release, resulting in heightened motor activity. By a similar process the toxin causes increased sympathetic activity. Animal studies suggest that the toxin is disseminated via the bloodstream to other peripheral neurons; toxin in the blood does not cross the blood-brain barrier.

CLINICAL MANIFESTATIONS Generalized tetanus, the most common form, is characterized by increased muscle tone and generalized spasms. The median onset after injury is 7 days; 10 percent of cases occur within 3 days and 10 percent after 14 days.

Typically, the patient first notices increased tone in the masseter muscles (trismus or lockjaw). Dysphagia or stiffness or pain in the neck, shoulder, and back muscles may also be present. Soon other muscles are involved, producing a rigid abdomen and stiff proximal limb muscles; the hands and feet are relatively spared. Sustained contraction of the facial muscles produces a grimace or sneer (risus sardonicus), and contraction of the back muscles an arched back (opisthotonos). Some patients develop paroxysmal, violent, painful, generalized muscle spasms that may cause cyanosis and threaten ventilation. They occur repetitively and may be spontaneous or provoked by even the slightest stimulation. A constant threat during generalized spasms is reduced ventilation or apnea or laryngospasm. The severity of illness may be mild (muscle rigidity and few or no spasms), moderate (trismus, dysphagia, rigidity, and spasms), or severe (frequent explosive paroxysms). The patient may be febrile, although many have no fever; mentation is unimpaired. Deep tendon reflexes may be increased. Dysphagia or ileus may preclude oral feeding.

Sympathetic overactivity commonly complicates severe cases and is characterized by labile or sustained hypertension, tachycardia, hyperpyrexia, profuse sweating, arrhythmias, and increased plasma and urinary catecholamine levels. Late cardiovascular complications include hypotension and bradycardia which are easily reversed by physical stimulation such as suctioning. Hypotension, tachycardia, and hyperpyrexia are ominous signs.

Complications include pneumonia, fractures, muscle rupture, asphyxia, and unexplained cardiac arrest.

Neonatal tetanus usually occurs as generalized tetanus and usually is fatal. It develops in children born to inadequately immunized mothers, frequently after unsterile treatment of the umbilical cord or its stump. The onset generally occurs during the first 2 weeks of life. Poor feeding, rigidity, and spasms occur.

Local tetanus is an uncommon form in which manifestations are restricted to muscles near the wound; however, it may evolve to the generalized illness. The prognosis is excellent.

Cephalic tetanus, a rare form of local tetanus, follows head injury or ear infection. Trismus and dysfunction of one or more cranial nerves, often the seventh nerve, are found. The incubation period is a few days and the mortality is high.

DIAGNOSIS   The diagnosis of tetanus is made entirely on the basis of clinical findings. Wound cultures should be done. However, *C. tetani* can be isolated from wounds of patients without tetanus, and frequently the organism cannot be recovered from the wounds of those with tetanus. The leukocyte count may be elevated. The cerebrospinal fluid examination is normal. Electromyograms may show continuous discharge of motor units and shortening or absence of the silent interval normally seen after an action potential. Nonspecific changes may be seen on the electrocardiogram. Muscle enzyme levels may be raised.

The differential diagnosis includes local conditions also producing trismus such as alveolar abscess, strychnine poisoning, dystonic drug reactions (such as phenothiazines and metoclopramide), and hypocalcemic tetany. Other conditions possibly confused with tetanus include meningitis/encephalitis, rabies, and an acute intraabdominal process (because of the rigid abdomen). The marked increased tone in central muscles (face, neck, chest, back, and abdomen) with superimposed generalized spasms and relative sparing of the hands and feet strongly suggest tetanus.

TREATMENT   General measures   The goals of therapy are to eliminate the source of toxin, neutralize unbound toxin, prevent muscle spasms, and provide support, especially respiratory support, until recovery. Patients should be admitted to a quiet room in an intensive care unit where observation and cardiopulmonary monitoring can be maintained continuously, but stimulation can be minimized. Protection of the airway is vital. Wounds should be explored, carefully cleansed, and thoroughly debrided.

Antibiotic therapy   Although it is of questionable benefit, parenteral penicillin (10 to 12 million units daily for 10 days) is administered to eradicate vegetative cells, the source of the toxin. Clindamycin (150 to 300 mg every 6 h) or erythromycin (500 mg every 6 h) may be given as substitutes to patients with penicillin allergy. Specific therapy should be given for active infection caused by other organisms.

Antitoxin   Given to neutralize circulating toxin and unbound toxin in the wound, antitoxin effectively lowers mortality; toxin already bound to neural tissue is unaffected. Tetanus immune globulin (human) (TIG) is the preparation of choice and should be given promptly. The dose is 3000 to 6000 units intramuscularly, usually in divided doses, because the volume is large. It may be best to administer antitoxin before manipulating the wound and perhaps to inject a dose proximal to the wound; the value of infiltrating the wound is unclear. Additional doses are unnecessary because the half-life of the antitoxin is long. Antibody does not penetrate the blood-brain barrier. Intrathecal administration has been attempted, but should be considered experimental. Equine tetanus antitoxin (TAT) is also available. It is cheaper, but the half-life is shorter and hypersensitivity and serum sickness are common; doses up to 100,000 units are given, part intramuscularly and part intravenously, but 10,000 units may suffice.

Control of muscle spasms   Many agents, alone and in combination, have been used to treat the muscle spasms, which are painful and can threaten ventilation by causing laryngospasm or sustained contraction of ventilatory muscles. Ideal therapy would abolish spasmodic activity without causing oversedation and hypoventilation. Diazepam, a muscle relaxant that enhances presynaptic inhibition, is in wide use. The dose is titrated to as much as 120 mg/d or higher. Barbiturates and chlorpromazine are also used. Neuromuscular blockage (using pancuronium bromide or an equivalent agent) together with mechanical ventilation are highly effective for severe spasms, spasms that reduce ventilation, spasms unresponsive to medication, or hypoventilation from oversedation. Dantrolene and baclofen are being investigated as treatment to shorten the period of therapeutic paralysis.

Respiratory care   Intubation or tracheostomy, with or without mechanical ventilation, may be required to avert aspiration in patients with trismus, disordered swallowing, dysphagia, or laryngospasm. The need should be anticipated, and the procedure performed electively and early.

Sympathetic overactivity   The optimal therapy for sympathetic overactivity has not been defined. Beta blockers with alpha-blocking activity are used, although there are a few reports of associated profound hypotension and death. A simple alternative is morphine. Parenteral magnesium sulfate and epidural anesthesia have been used also. The relative efficacy of these four therapeutic modalities is unclear.

Vaccine   Active immunization should be initiated because immunity is not induced by the small amount of toxin that produces disease.

ADDITIONAL MEASURES   These include hydration to control insensible and other fluid losses which may be high, increased nutritional requirements which can be met by enteral or parenteral means, physiotherapy to prevent contractures, and heparin to prevent pulmonary emboli. Bowel, bladder, and renal function must be monitored. Gastrointestinal bleeding and decubitus ulcers must be prevented and intercurrent infection treated.

PREVENTION   Active immunization   All partially immunized and unimmunized adults should receive vaccine as should those recovering from tetanus. The primary series for adults consists of three doses: the first and second doses are given 4 to 8 weeks apart, and the third dose is given 6 to 12 months after the second. A booster dose is required every 10 years, and may be given at mid-decade ages, 35, 45, and so on. Combined tetanus and diphtheria toxoid adsorbed (for adult use) (Td) rather than single-antigen tetanus toxoid is preferred for persons over 7 years of age.

Wound management   Proper wound management requires consideration of the need for (1) passive immunization with TIG and (2) active immunization with vaccine, preferably Td in those over age

7. For clean, minor wounds, Td is administered to persons who have (1) unknown tetanus immunization histories, (2) received less than three doses of adsorbed tetanus toxoid, (3) received three or more doses of adsorbed vaccine, but more than 10 years have elapsed since the last dose, and (4) received three doses of *fluid* (nonadsorbed) vaccine. The recommendations for contaminated or severe wounds are identical, except that vaccine should be given to those who received three or more doses of adsorbed tetanus toxoid, if more than 5 years have elapsed since the last dose. TIG is not recommended for clean, minor wounds, but is given for all other wounds if the vaccination history indicates unknown or partial immunization. The dose of TIG for passive immunization of wounds of average severity is 250 units intramuscularly, which produces a protective antibody level (0.01 antitoxin unit per ml) in the serum for at least 4 to 6 weeks; the dose of equine antitoxin is 3000 to 6000 units. Vaccine and tetanus antitoxin should be administered at separate sites in separate syringes.

Neonatal tetanus Preventive efforts include vaccine, even during pregnancy, and measures to increase the number of in-hospital births and training for nonmedical birth attendants.

PROGNOSIS The application of methods to support respiration has markedly improved the prognosis in tetanus; mortality rates as low as 10 percent have been reported from units accustomed to handling such cases. In the United States, the overall mortality for the years 1985 to 1986 was 31 percent; it was 42 percent in those over 50 years of age, but only 5 percent for those under 50 (no neonatal disease); untreated neonatal disease, however, also has a poor prognosis. The outcome is poor in those with a short incubation period, a short interval from the onset of symptoms to admission, or a short period from onset of symptoms to the first spasm (period of onset).

The course of tetanus extends over 4 to 6 weeks, and patients may require ventilatory support for 3 weeks during this period. Increased tone and minor spasms can last for months, but recovery is usually complete.

REFERENCES

Bleck TP: Pharmacology of tetanus. Clin Neuropharmacol 9:103, 1986

Hinman AR et al: Neonatal tetanus: Potential for elimination in the world. Pediatr Infect Dis 6:813, 1987

Muller H et al: Intrathecal baclofen in tetanus. Ann NY Acad Sci 531:167, 1988

Rocke DA et al: Morphine in tetanus—The management of sympathetic nervous system overactivity. S Afr Med J 70:66, 1986

Trujillo MH et al: Impact of intensive care management on the prognosis of tetanus. Analysis of 641 cases. Chest 92:63, 1987

Vieira BI: Cephalic tetanus in an immunized patient: Clinical and electromyographic findings. Med J Austral 145:156, 1986

Wesley AG, Pather M: Tetanus in children: An 11-year review. Ann Trop Pediatr 7:32, 1987

106 BOTULISM

ELIAS ABRUTYN

DEFINITION Botulism is a paralytic disease that begins with cranial nerve involvement and progresses caudally to involve the extremities. It is caused by potent protein neurotoxins elaborated by *Clostridium botulinum*. The Centers for Disease Control (CDC) currently classifies cases as: (1) *food-borne botulism*, from ingestion of preformed toxin in food contaminated with *C. botulinum;* (2) *infant botulism*, from ingestion of spores and production of toxin in the intestine of infants; (3) *wound botulism*, from toxin produced in wounds contaminated with the organism; and (4) *indeterminate*, for patients over 1 year old with no recognized source for disease.

ETIOLOGY *C. botulinum*, a heterogeneous group of anaerobic gram-positive organisms that form subterminal spores, is found in soil and marine environments throughout the world and elaborates the most potent bacterial toxin known. Types A through G have been distinguished by the antigenic specificities of their toxins. Types with proteolytic activity can digest food and produce a spoiled appearance; nonproteolytic types leave the appearance of food unchanged.

Eight distinct toxin types (A, B, C_1, C_2, D, E, F, and G) have been described. All are neurotoxins, except for C_2, which is a cytotoxin of unknown significance. Toxicity is due to inhibition of acetylcholine release from cholinergic terminals at the motor end plate. The toxin resists degradation by acid and proteolytic enzymes but is inactivated by heat at 100°C for 10 min, as during routine home cooking. Spores, in contrast, are highly heat resistant, requiring exposure to 120°C for inactivation, as in steam sterilizers or pressure cookers.

Toxin types A, B, E, and rarely F cause human disease; type G has been associated with sudden death in a few patients in Switzerland; and types C and D cause animal disease.

EPIDEMIOLOGY Human botulism occurs worldwide. In the United States, the geographic distribution of cases by toxin type parallels the distribution of organism types found in the environment. Type A predominates west of the Rocky Mountains; type B is generally distributed, but is more common in the east; and type E is found in the Pacific northwest, Alaska, and the Great Lakes area. In the United States food-borne botulism has been associated primarily with home canned food, particularly vegetables, fruit, and condiments, and less commonly, with meat and fish. Type E outbreaks are frequently associated with fish products. Commercial products occasionally cause outbreaks, but some of these have resulted from improper handling after purchase. Outbreaks in restaurants, schools, and private homes have been traced to uncommon sources (commercial pot pies, beef stew, turkey loaf, sauteed onions, baked potatoes, and chopped garlic in oil). Food-borne botulism can occur when (1) a food to be preserved is contaminated with spores; (2) preservation does not inactivate the spores but kills other putrefactive bacteria that might inhibit growth of *C. botulinum* and also provides anaerobic conditions at a pH and temperature that allow germination and toxin production; and when (3) food is not heated before eating to a temperature that destroys toxin.

CLINICAL MANIFESTATIONS **Food-borne botulism** Following ingestion of food containing toxin, illness varies from a mild one for which no medical advice is sought to very severe disease which may result in death in 24 h. The incubation period is usually 18 to 36 h but depending upon toxin dose ranges from a few hours to several days. A symmetric descending paralysis is characteristic and can lead to respiratory failure and death. Cranial nerve involvement which almost always marks the onset of symptoms usually produces diplopia, dysarthria, and/or dysphagia; weakness progresses, often rapidly, from the head to involve the neck, arms, thorax, and legs. Nausea, vomiting, and abdominal pain may occur before or after onset of paralysis. Dizziness, blurred vision, dry mouth, and very dry, occasionally sore throat are common. Occasionally the weakness is asymmetric. Patients are generally alert and oriented, but may be drowsy, agitated, and anxious. Typically, fever is absent. Ptosis is frequent; the pupillary reflexes may be depressed, and fixed or dilated pupils are seen in half the patients. The gag reflex may be suppressed, and deep tendon reflexes may be normal or decreased. Paralytic ileus, severe constipation, and urinary retention are common.

Wound botulism When wounds are contaminated with *C. botulinum* spores, the spores may germinate to vegetative organisms that produce toxin. This rare condition resembles food-borne illness except that the incubation period is longer, averaging about 10 days, and gastrointestinal symptoms are absent. Wound botulism has been noted after traumatic wounds contaminated with soil, in chronic drug abusers, and after cesarean delivery. The illness has occurred even when antibiotics were given to prevent wound infection. When present, fever is probably from concurrent infection with other bacteria. The wound may appear benign.

Infant botulism   In infant botulism, the most common form of disease, toxin is produced in and absorbed from the intestine following germination of ingested spores. The severity ranges from mild illness with failure to thrive to fulminant, severe paralysis with respiratory failure and may be one cause of sudden infant death. Ingestion of contaminated honey has been defined as one source of spores, leading to the recommendation that honey not be fed to children less than 12 months of age. Most cases cannot be attributed to a particular food source, and the mechanism of intestinal colonization with *C. botulinum* is undefined. It is not clear why disease develops in some infants and not others and why it is so age-dependent, with over 90 percent of cases occurring in infants under 6 months of age.

DIAGNOSIS   Botulism must be considered in afebrile, mentally intact patients who have a symmetric descending paralysis without sensory findings. Conditions often confused with botulism include myasthenia gravis, which may be excluded by electromyography and appropriate antibody studies, and the Guillain-Barré syndrome, which is characterized by ascending paralysis, sensory abnormalities, and elevation in cerebrospinal fluid protein. The Miller-Fisher variant of Guillain-Barré—a descending paralysis—can be difficult to differentiate. Other conditions that may mimic botulism include poliomyelitis, tick paralysis, acute abdomen, pharyngitis, cerebrovascular accidents, and intoxications from drugs, mushrooms, or medications with anticholinesterase activities.

The demonstration of toxin in serum by bioassay in mice is definitive, but the test may be negative, particularly in wound and infant botulism. It is only performed by specific laboratories which can be identified by contacting regional public health authorities. The demonstration of toxin or the organism in vomitus, gastric fluid, or stool is strongly suggestive, because intestinal carriage is rare. Isolation of the organism from food without toxin is insufficient for diagnosis. Wound cultures showing the organism are suggestive. The edrophonium chloride (Tensilon) test for myasthenia gravis may be falsely positive in botulism but is usually less dramatic. Nerve conduction velocity is normal, but on electromyography, action potentials are decreased with a supramaximal stimulus and facilitation is found after repetitive stimulation at high frequency. The white blood cell count and sedimentation rate are normal.

TREATMENT   Patients should be hospitalized and monitored closely both clinically and by spirometry, pulse oximetry, and measurement of arterial blood gases for incipient respiratory failure. Intubation and mechanical ventilation should be strongly considered when the vital capacity is less than 30 percent of predicted, especially when paralysis is progressing rapidly and hypoxemia with absolute or relative hypercarbia is present (see Chap. 219).

In food-borne illness trivalent (types A, B, and E) equine antitoxin should be administered as soon as possible after obtaining specimens for laboratory analysis. Laboratory confirmation, which may take days, is unnecessary before initiating treatment. After testing for hypersensitivity to horse serum, two vials are given, either both intravenously or one intravenously and one intramuscularly; the dose may be repeated in 2 to 4 h. Anaphylaxis and serum sickness are risks inherent in using the equine product, and in allergic patients desensitization may be necessary. If there is no ileus, cathartics and enemas may be given to purge the gut of toxin; emetics or gastric lavage are used also if the time since ingestion is brief, e.g., only a few hours. Antibiotics to eliminate an intestinal source for possible continued toxin production and guanidine hydrochloride to reverse paralysis are of unproven value. In the United States antitoxin and help in clinical management and laboratory confirmation are available at *any* time by calling the state health department or the Centers for Disease Control.

Treatment of infant botulism requires supportive care; neither antitoxin nor antibiotics have been shown to be beneficial. In wound botulism antitoxin is administered. The wound should be thoroughly explored and debrided and an antibiotic such as penicillin given to eradicate *C. botulinum* from the wound, although the benefit of this therapy is unproven; results of wound cultures should guide the use of other antibiotics.

PROGNOSIS   Type A disease is generally more severe than type B, and mortality is higher above age 60. With improved respiratory and intensive care, the case-fatality rate in food-borne illness has fallen to about 7.5 percent and is low in infant botulism as well. Artificial respiratory support may be required for months in severe cases. Some patients experience residual weakness and autonomic dysfunction for as long as a year after disease onset.

REFERENCES

MacDonald K et al: The changing epidemiology of adult botulism in the United States. Am J Epidemol 124:794, 1986
McCroskey LM, Hatheway CL: Laboratory findings in four cases of adult botulism suggest colonization of the intestinal tract. J Clin Microbiol 26:1052, 1988
Mills DC, Arnon SS: The large intestine as the site of *Clostridium botulinum* colonization in human infant botulism. J Infect Dis 156:997, 1987
Smith LDS, Sugiyama H: *Botulism: The Organism, Its Toxins, the Disease*, 2d ed. Springfield, Charles C Thomas, 1988
Spika JS et al.: Risk factors for infant botulism in the United States. Am J Dis Child 143:828, 1989
St. Louis ME et al: Botulism from chopped garlic: Delayed recognition of a major outbreak. Ann Intern Med 108:363, 1988
Wainwright RB et al: Food-borne botulism in Alaska, 1947–1985: Epidemiology and clinical findings. J Infect Dis 157:1158, 1988
Wilcox P et al: Long-term follow-up of symptoms, pulmonary function, respiratory strength, and exercise performance after botulism. Am Rev Resp Dis 139:157, 1989

107   GAS GANGRENE AND OTHER CLOSTRIDIAL INFECTIONS

DENNIS L. KASPER

DEFINITION   Bacteria of the genus *Clostridium* are gram-positive, spore-forming, obligate anaerobes that are ubiquitous in nature. There are over 60 recognized species of clostridia, many of which generally are considered saprophytic. Some of these species are pathogenic for humans and animals, particularly under conditions of lowered oxidation-reduction potential. Infections associated with these organisms range from localized wound contamination to overwhelming systemic disease. The four major disease categories for which clostridia are responsible include intestinal disorders, deep tissue suppurative infections, skin and soft tissue infections, and bacteremias (see Table 107-1). Toxins play a major role in some of these syndromes.

ETIOLOGY   In humans, clostridia normally reside in the gastrointestinal tract and in the female genital tract, although they

TABLE 107-1   Classification of diseases caused by other clostridia

I Intestinal syndromes
  A Food poisoning
  B Enteritis necroticans
  C Antibiotic-associated colitis

II Suppurative deep tissue infections
  A Mixed bacterial infections
  B Only microorganism isolated

III Skin and soft tissue infections
  A Simple contamination
  B Local infection without systemic signs
  C Spreading cellulitis and fasciitis
  D Myonecrosis

IV Bacteremia
  A Transient bacteremia
  B Sepsis

occasionally can be isolated from the skin or the mouth. As with other pathogenic anaerobic bacteria, clostridia are quite aerotolerant. Of the known species of the genus *Clostridium,* at least 30 have been isolated from human infections. Clostridia characteristically produce abundant gas in artificial media and form subterminal endospores. *C. perfringens,* one of the most important of the species, is encapsulated, nonmotile, and rarely sporulates in artificial media; the spores usually can be destroyed by boiling. *C. tetani* and *C. botulinum* are discussed in Chaps. 105 and 106, respectively.

Clostridia are present in the normal colonic flora in concentrations of 10^9 to 10^{10} per gram. Of the 30 or more species that normally colonize humans, *C. ramosum* is the most common, followed by *C. perfringens.* These organisms are universally present in soil in concentrations of up to 10^4 per gram. Although clostridia morphologically are typical gram-positive organisms, many species appear to be gram-negative in clinical material or in stationary phase cultures. Therefore, Gram stains of cultures or clinical material should be interpreted with great care.

C. perfringens is the most common of the clostridial species isolated from tissue infections and bacteremias, followed in frequency by *C. novyi* and *C. septicum.* In the category of enteric infections, *C. difficile* is an important cause of antibiotic-associated colitis, and *C. perfringens* is associated with food poisoning and enteritis necroticans.

PATHOGENESIS   Severe infections due to clostridial species are relatively uncommon despite the fact that clostridia can be cultured from most severe, traumatic wounds. Essential to the development of severe disease appears to be the presence of tissue necrosis and a low oxidation-reduction potential. *C. perfringens* requires about 14 amino acids and 6 or 7 additional growth factors for optimum growth. These nutrients are not found in appreciable concentrations in normal body fluids but are present in necrotic tissue. When *C. perfringens* grows in necrotic tissue, a zone of tissue damage due to the toxins elaborated by the organism allows for progressive growth. In contrast, when only a few bacteria leak into the bloodstream from a small defect in the intestinal wall, the organisms do not have the opportunity to multiply rapidly because blood as medium for growth is relatively deficient in certain amino acids and growth factors. Therefore, in a patient without tissue necrosis, bacteremia is usually benign.

C. perfringens possesses 17 possible virulence factors, including 12 active tissue toxins and enterotoxins. *C. perfringens* has been divided into five types (A through E) on the basis of four major toxins: alpha, beta, epsilon, and iota. The alpha toxin is a phospholipase C (lecithinase) that splits lecithin into phosphorylcholine and diglyceride. This alpha toxin has been associated with gas gangrene and is known to be hemolytic, destroy platelets and polymorphonuclear leukocytes, and cause widespread capillary damage. When injected intravenously, it causes massive intravascular hemolysis and damages liver mitochondria. Alpha toxin may be important in the initiation of muscle infections that may progress to gas gangrene. Experimentally, the higher the concentration of alpha toxin present in the culture fluid, the smaller the infecting dose of *C. perfringens* required to produce infection. The protective effect of antiserum is directly proportional to its content of alpha antitoxin. Beta, epsilon, and iota toxins are also known to increase capillary permeability.

C. difficile produces a cytotoxin and an enterotoxin. Toxigenic strains are more resistant to phagocytosis than nontoxigenic strains. The cytotoxin is potent in tissue culture assays and is a relatively sensitive and specific marker for *C. difficile*–induced enteric disease. The enterotoxin, designated toxin A, appears to be substantially more potent in biologic assays using animal models. Therefore, this toxin may play an important role in the expression of clinical disease. Toxin A binds to a carbohydrate receptor (Galα1–3Galβ1–4GlcNAc) on brush border membranes. Most cases of antibiotic-associated colitis are caused by antibiotic-mediated suppression of the endogenous flora and overgrowth of *C. difficile.* The bowel flora may also produce β-lactamases which destroy some antibiotics, like ampicillin, and allow the overgrowth of *C. difficile.*

CLINICAL MANIFESTATIONS   Intestinal disorders   FOOD POISONING   *C. perfringens* is the second or third most common cause of food poisoning in the United States (see Chap. 92). Outbreaks generally have resulted from problems in the cooling and storage of foods cooked in bulk. The food sources primarily involved are meat, meat products, and poultry. Generally, the implicated meats have been cooked, allowed to cool, and then recooked the following day, often in a stew or hash. Strains of *C. perfringens* that contaminate meat manage to survive initial cooking. During reheating, the organisms sporulate and germinate. The disease is associated with an attack rate often as high as 70 percent. Symptoms of food poisoning from type A strains develop 8 to 24 h after ingestion of foods heavily contaminated with the organism. The primary symptoms include epigastric pain, nausea, and watery diarrhea lasting 12 to 24 h. Fever and vomiting are uncommon. Symptoms usually last less than 24 h. Diarrhea appears to be caused by a heat-labile protein enterotoxin. The enterotoxin inhibits glucose transport, damages the intestinal epithelium, and causes protein loss into the intestinal lumen.

ENTERITIS NECROTICANS   Enteritis necroticans (*pigbel*), caused by type C strains of *C. perfringens,* has been the cause of necrotizing enteritis and death, occurring after a feast, in children and adults in New Guinea. A similar disease, *darmbrand,* was epidemic in Germany after World War II and was also reported from an evacuation site on the Thai-Kampuchean border. Clinical features include acute abdominal pain, bloody diarrhea, vomiting, shock, and peritonitis; death occurs in 40 percent of patients. Pathologically, there is an acute ulcerative process of the bowel restricted to the small intestine. The mucosa is lifted off the submucosa, forming large denuded areas. Pseudomembranes composed of sloughed epithelium are common, and gas may dissect into the submucosa. The source of the organisms may be the patient's own intestinal flora, because cultures of ingested pig have failed to yield the organism. Antitoxin against the beta toxin of *C. perfringens* has been of considerable benefit in changing the course of established disease and in a large-scale trial, children immunized with *C. perfringens* beta toxoid were protected.

ANTIBIOTIC-ASSOCIATED COLITIS   Strains of *C. difficile* that produce toxins detectable in the stool have been identified as the major cause of colitis in patients with antibiotic-associated diarrhea. In order to diagnose this type of colitis, there should be no other identifiable cause of diarrhea and the onset of symptoms must occur either during antimicrobial administration or within 4 weeks after the implicated agent has been discontinued. The drugs implicated most commonly in *C. difficile* enterocolitis are clindamycin, ampicillin, and the cephalosporins. With the possible exceptions of vancomycin and parenterally administered aminoglycosides, nearly all antibiotics have been associated with this syndrome. Antibiotic-associated diarrhea is associated with up to 6 percent of clindamycin usage, and with 5 to 9 percent of ampicillin usage.

Antimicrobial-associated diarrhea can be divided into four anatomic categories: (1) normal colonic mucosa, (2) mild erythema with some edema, (3) granular, friable, or hemorrhagic mucosa, and (4) pseudomembrane formation. Most commonly, patients with antibiotic-associated diarrhea have a normal, minimally erythematous colonic mucosa with some edema. Occasionally colitis is more severe and is characterized by granular, friable, or hemorrhagic mucosa. Stool examination in these patients may reveal large numbers of red blood cells and some leukocytes. Biopsy shows subepithelial edema with round cell infiltration of the lamina propria and focal extravasation of erythrocytes. *C. difficile* toxin has been found in 15 to 46 percent of stools from patients in these first three categories, suggesting that other factors exist in the pathogenesis of antibiotic-associated diarrhea. The most characteristic form of antibiotic-associated colitis caused by *C. difficile* is pseudomembranous colitis (PMC). More than 95 percent of patients with documented PMC have positive stool toxin assays. Close inspection of pseudomembranes reveals exudative punctate raised plaques with skip areas or edematous hyperemic mucosa. These plaques can enlarge and coalesce over large segments of intestine in the later stages of disease. The clinical spectrum of antibiotic-associated PMC is diverse. Diarrhea is the common feature and is usually watery, voluminous, and without gross blood or mucus. Most patients have abdominal cramps and tenderness, fever, and leukocytosis. However, the symptoms may vary considerably. At one end of the spectrum are patients with annoying diarrhea but no systemic signs or symptoms, while at the other end there is severe systemic toxicity, fever to 40 or 40.6°C (104 or 105°F), and peripheral white blood cell counts of up to 50,000 per microliter. Fecal examination frequently reveals leukocytes. Without specific therapy, the course is highly variable. Some patients have prompt resolution of symptoms with discontinuation of the drug, while others have protracted diarrhea with large stool volumes for up to 8 weeks, with resultant hypoalbuminemia and electrolyte imbalance. Severely ill patients with toxic megacolon and colonic perforation have been reported. In those who are severely ill, mortality rates may be as high as 30 percent, while most patients with minimal symptoms have resolution of disease with discontinuation of antibiotics alone. In the majority of patients, symptoms begin 4 to 10 days after antibiotic therapy is initiated. However, about 25 percent of patients do not have symptoms until the implicated antimicrobial has been discontinued, in some cases as long as 4 weeks afterward. A few cases have been reported within hours after initiation of antibiotic therapy.

Diagnostic evaluation of patients with PMC should include examination of the stool for the presence of *C. difficile* cytotoxin. Although several assays are available, the tissue culture assay is the most practical and sensitive. The assay is performed by incubating stool filtrates with tissue culture cells and monitoring for a cytopathic effect which can be neutralized by antitoxin to either *C. sordellii* (which is cross-reactive with *C. difficile,* but does not cause PMC) or *C. difficile.* Endoscopy, although useful in establishing the presence of PMC, does not establish the etiology and should be reserved for more serious disease manifestations to exclude alternative diagnoses. Isolation of *C. difficile* from stool cultures is difficult, and *C. difficile* may be present as part of the "normal" flora in asymptomatic patients, particularly infants.

Suppurative deep tissue infection   Clostridia are recovered frequently from various suppurative conditions in conjunction with other anaerobic and aerobic bacteria, but can also be the only organisms isolated. These conditions exist with severe local inflammation, but usually without systemic signs induced by clostridial toxins. These infections include intraabdominal sepsis, empyema, pelvic abscess, subcutaneous abscess, frostbite with gas gangrene, infected stumps in amputees, brain abscess, prostatic abscess, perianal abscess, conjunctivitis, infection of a renal cell carcinoma, and infected aortic grafts.

Clostridia are isolated in approximately two-thirds of patients with intraabdominal infections resulting from intestinal perforation. *C. ramosum, C. perfringens,* and *C. bifermentans* are the most commonly isolated species. The clinical presentation does not differ from that of other patients with similar infections in which clostridia are not cultured and there is no adverse effect on outcome (see Chap. 108).

An association has been made between malignancy and the isolation of *C. septicum* in the absence of grossly contaminated deep traumatic wounds. A major site for these malignancies is the gastrointestinal tract, particularly the colon. An association with leukemia or with other solid tumors also has been noted. Some of these patients present with *C. septicum* bacteremia and have a fulminant clinical course (discussed below). Others develop localized suppurative infection in the abdomen or the abdominal wall, without bacteremia. Presumably this infection arises from a silent perforation that leads to intraabdominal abscess formation.

Clostridia have been isolated from suppurative infections of the female genital tract, particularly tuboovarian and pelvic abscess. The major species involved has been *C. perfringens.* Most of these are mild suppurative infections without evidence of uterine gangrene. Isolation of *C. perfringens* has been reported in as many as 20 percent of diseased gallbladders at surgery. One clinical syndrome, emphysematous cholecystitis, is caused by clostridial species at least 50 percent of the time. In this syndrome there is gas formation in the biliary radicles and the wall of the gallbladder. It is seen most often in diabetic patients. Although the mortality rate in this entity is higher than in more common forms of cholecystitis, there is no evidence of myonecrosis.

Clostridia are among the many organisms found in empyema fluid or isolated by transtracheal aspiration from patients with lung abscesses. There is no clinical clue to the presence of clostridia (as opposed to other organisms) in these infections. *C. perfringens* has been reported as a cause of empyema arising from aspiration pneumonia, pulmonary emboli, and infarction. However, the majority of cases of clostridial empyema are secondary to trauma.

Skin and soft tissue infections   Various categories of traumatic wound infections due to clostridia have been described: simple contamination, anaerobic cellulitis, fasciitis with or without systemic manifestations, and anaerobic myonecrosis.

SIMPLE CONTAMINATION   Clostridia are cultured most often from wounds in the absence of clinical signs of sepsis. As many as 30 percent of battle wounds can be contaminated by clostridia without signs of suppuration, and 16 percent of penetrating abdominal wounds yield clostridia on culture despite treatment with cephalothin and kanamycin. In cases of trauma, clostridia are isolated with equal frequency from suppurative and well-healing wounds. Based on these findings, the diagnosis of clostridial infection should be clinical rather than bacteriologic.

LOCALIZED INFECTION OF THE SKIN AND SOFT TISSUE WITHOUT SYSTEMIC SIGNS   This condition was originally referred to as anaerobic cellulitis. It is a localized infection involving the skin and soft tissue due to clostridia in pure or mixed culture. There are no systemic signs of toxicity, although the infection may invade locally, producing necrosis. These infections tend to be relatively indolent, spreading slowly to contiguous areas. Localized infections tend to be relatively free of pain and edema. Perhaps because of the lack of edema, gas that is limited to the wound and the immediately surrounding tissue may be more evident than in gas gangrene. In these localized infections gas is never found intramuscularly. Cellulitis, perirectal abscesses, and diabetic foot ulcers are typical infections from which clostridial species can be isolated. If inadequately treated, these localized infections advance by extension through subcutaneous tissue and fascial planes into muscle and may produce severe systemic disease with signs of toxemia.

A localized form of suppurative myositis has been described in heroin addicts. These patients develop local pain and tenderness in discrete areas (particularly the thigh and forearm) with the subsequent appearance of fluctuance and crepitance that require surgical drainage. The unusual aspect of these infections is that they remain localized without systemic signs of toxicity. Moreover these local areas are not necessarily sites of trauma or heroin injection. Pathologically there are subcutaneous abscesses, purulent myositis, and fasciitis, from which clostridia are recovered in pure culture; on occasion mixed infections involving aerobes and anaerobes are found.

SPREADING CELLULITIS AND FASCIITIS WITH SYSTEMIC TOXICITY   This is diffuse spreading cellulitis and fasciitis, but myonecrosis is absent, and only mild inflammation is seen in muscle. These patients present with the abrupt onset of a syndrome which progresses rapidly through the fascial planes within hours. When suppuration and gas in soft tissues as well as overwhelming toxemia are present, the infection is rapidly fatal. On physical examination there is subcutaneous crepitance, but little localized pain. Surgery is of no proven value because there are no discretely involved tissues amenable to resection, as may be the case in myonecrosis. However, incision of the affected area should be performed, because in rapidly advancing fasciitis, it is still the cornerstone of therapy. The initial local lesion may be quite innocuous and arises from an area involved by tumor or other infection and not from injury. The systemic toxic effects include hemolysis and injury of capillary membranes. Usually, this infection is uniformly fatal within 48 h, despite intensive therapy involving antitoxin and exchange transfusion. This syndrome is seen most commonly in patients with carcinoma, especially of the sigmoid or the cecum. Presumably, the tumor invades the fascia, and tumoral contents leak into the abdominal wall. These patients present with extreme toxicity and occasionally with total-body crepitance. The syndrome differs from necrotizing fasciitis caused by other organisms in three respects: (1) rapid mortality, (2) rapid tissue invasion, and (3) the systemic effects of the toxin typified by massive hemolysis.

CLOSTRIDIAL MYONECROSIS (GAS GANGRENE) Clostridial myonecrosis occurs when bacteria invade healthy muscle from adjacent traumatized muscle or soft tissue. The infection originates in a wound contaminated with clostridia. Despite the fact that more than 30 percent of deep wounds are infected with clostridia, the incidence of clostridial myonecrosis is quite low. These infections occur in military or civilian settings. An essential factor in the genesis of gas gangrene appears to be trauma, particularly involving deep lacerated muscle wounds. The entity of clostridial myonecrosis is relatively uncommon after simple, through-and-through bullet wounds without shattering of bone, and relatively common following shrapnel fragmentation wounds, particularly when deep muscle is involved. In civilian cases, gas gangrene can occur after trauma, surgery, or intramuscular injection. The trauma need not be severe; however, the wound must be deep, necrotic, and without communication to the surface.

The incubation period of gas gangrene is usually short: almost always less than 3 days, and frequently less than 24 h. Eighty percent of cases are caused by *C. perfringens*, while *C. novyi*, *C. septicum*, and *C. histolyticum* cause most of the other cases. Typically, gas gangrene begins with the sudden appearance of pain in the region of the wound, which helps to differentiate it from spreading cellulitis. Once established, the pain steadily increases in severity, but remains localized to the infected area and only spreads if the infection spreads. Soon after pain develops, local swelling and edema, accompanied by a thin, often hemorrhagic exudate, appear. These patients frequently develop marked tachycardia, but elevation in temperature may be only minimal. Gas usually is not obvious at this early stage and may be completely absent. Frothiness of the wound exudate may be noted. The skin is tense, white, often marbled with blue, and cooler than normal. The symptoms progress rapidly; swelling, edema, and toxemia increase and a profuse serous discharge, which may have a peculiar sweetish smell, appears. Gram stain of the wound exudate shows many gram-positive rods with relatively few inflammatory cells.

At surgery, the muscle is characteristically pale, edematous, and does not contract when probed with the scalpel. The muscle appears beefy red and nonviable and can progress to become black, friable, and gangrenous. It is important to establish a diagnosis early, preferably by frozen section biopsy of muscle.

Despite hypotension, renal failure, and often body crepitance, patients with myonecrosis often have a heightened awareness of their surroundings until just before death, when they lapse into toxic delirium and coma. In untreated cases, as the local wounds progress, the skin becomes bronzed; bullae appear, become filled with dark red fluid, and are accompanied by dark patches of cutaneous gangrene. Gas appears in later phases but may not be as obvious as in anaerobic cellulitis. Jaundice is rarely seen in wound gas gangrene (in contrast to uterine infections) and when it does appear, is almost invariably associated with hemoglobinuria, hemoglobinemia, and septicemia. There have been reports of cases of clostridial myonecrosis without a history of trauma. These patients have bullous lesions and crepitance of the skin; they present with a rapidly worsening course which includes myonecrosis, especially of the extremities.

Bacteremia and clostridial septicemia The relatively common entity of transient bacteremia due to clostridia can arise in any hospitalized patient but is most common with a predisposing focus in the gastrointestinal tract, biliary tract, or uterus. Fever frequently resolves within 24 to 48 h without therapy. Despite the finding of clostridial bacteremia following septic abortions and the frequent isolation of clostridia from the lochia, most of these patients do not have evidence of septicemia. In one series of 60 patients with clostridial bacteremia, half of the cases could be associated with an infected site, while the other half had a totally unrelated illness, such as tuberculous pneumonia, meningitis, or benign gastroenteritis. Frequently, by the time the blood culture reports return, the patients are completely well and sometimes have been discharged. Therefore, when a blood culture report is positive for clostridia, the patient must be assessed clinically rather than simply treated for the positive blood culture.

Clostridial septicemia is an uncommon but almost invariably fatal illness occurring after clostridial infection primarily of the uterus, colon, or biliary tract. This entity must be differentiated from transient clostridial bacteremia, which is much more common than septicemia. *C. perfringens* causes the majority of septicemic infections, as well as the majority of cases of transient bacteremia. *C. septicum*, *C. sordellii*, and *C. novyi* account for most of the remainder of cases. Clostridia account for 1 to 2.5 percent of all positive blood cultures in major hospital centers.

The majority of cases of clostridial septicemia originate from the female genital tract following septic abortion. Introduction of a foreign body is a common antecedent event. In the uterus there may be residual necrotic fetal and placental tissues and traumatized endometrium that allow the growth of clostridia. Only a small fraction of cases of septic abortion (1 percent) are followed by serious septicemic illness.

In these patients, sepsis, fever, and chills begin from 1 to 3 days after the attempted abortion. The initial signs are malaise, headache, severe myalgias, abdominal pain, nausea, vomiting, and occasionally diarrhea. Frequently a bloody or brown vaginal discharge is noted. Patients may rapidly develop oliguria, hypotension, jaundice, and hemoglobinuria. The hemolysis, which is secondary to *C. perfringens* alpha toxin, causes a characteristic bronzing of the skin. As in myonecrosis, the mental status of severely ill patients is characterized by increased alertness and apprehension. Local examination of the pelvis reveals foul cervical discharge, occasionally with gas. Frequently laceration marks around the cervix or perforation of the cervical segment are evident. If the infection involves the myometrium or has spread to the adnexa, extreme tenderness, guarding, and an adnexal mass may be found.

Laboratory studies in septicemic patients reveal an elevated white count and may show pink, hemoglobin-tinged plasma. Anemia is proportional to the degree of hemolysis, and the hematocrit may be extremely low. Platelets may be reduced, and there is often evidence of disseminated intravascular coagulation. Oliguria or anuria, increasingly refractory hypotension, and hemorrhage and bruising may develop.

Clostridia may enter the bloodstream from the gastrointestinal or biliary tract. This occurrence is associated with ulcerative lesions or obstruction of the small or large intestine, necrotic or infiltrating malignancy, bowel surgery, or various abdominal catastrophes. The patient may present with an acute febrile illness with chills and fever, but no other signs of localized infection. Intravascular hemolysis occurs in as many as half the cases. Biliary or gastrointestinal symptoms, if present, may be the only clue to the etiology. Positive blood cultures provide the definitive clue for the diagnosis.

Patients with malignant disease also can develop rapidly fatal clostridial sepsis, particularly from a gastrointestinal focus. The most common species in this setting is *C. septicum*. Characteristic signs and symptoms include fever, tachycardia, hypotension, abdominal pain or tenderness, nausea, vomiting, and, preterminally, coma. The tachycardia may be out of proportion to the fever. Only about 20 to 30 percent of patients develop hemolysis. A striking feature of this syndrome is the rapidity of death, which frequently occurs in less than 12 h.

DIAGNOSIS The diagnosis of clostridial disease must be based primarily on clinical findings. Because of the presence of clostridia in many wounds, their mere isolation from any site, including the blood, does not necessarily indicate severe disease. Smears of wound exudates, uterine scrapings, or cervical discharge may show abundant large gram-positive rods as well as other organisms. Cultures should be placed in selective media and incubated anaerobically for identification of clostridia.

The urine of patients with severe clostridial sepsis may contain protein and casts, and some patients may develop severe uremia. Profound alterations of circulating erythrocytes are seen in severely toxemic patients. Patients have a hemolytic anemia, which develops extremely rapidly, along with hemoglobinemia, hemoglobinuria, and elevated levels of serum bilirubin. Spherocytosis, increased osmotic and mechanical red blood cell fragility, erythrophagocytosis, and methemoglobinemia have been described. Disseminated intravascular coagulation may be seen in patients with severe infection. In patients with severe septicemia, a Wright or Gram stain smear of peripheral blood or buffy coat may demonstrate clostridia.

X-ray examination sometimes provides an important clue to the diagnosis by revealing gas in muscles, subcutaneous tissue, or the uterus. However, the finding of gas is not pathognomonic for clostridial infection. Other bacteria, particularly anaerobes, mixed with aerobic organisms may produce gas.

The diagnosis of clostridial myonecrosis can be established by frozen section biopsy of muscle. The diagnosis of *C. difficile*–associated colitis is made by the identification of *C. difficile* toxin in stool.

TREATMENT   The treatment of choice for clostridial infection is penicillin G, 20,000,000 units a day in adults. In cases of penicillin sensitivity or allergy, other antibiotics should be considered, but all should be tested for in vitro efficacy because of the occasional isolation of resistant strains. Chloramphenicol, 4 g/d, usually is an effective alternative. Clostridia are frequently, but not universally, susceptible in vitro to cefoxitin, carbenicillin, clindamycin, metronidazole, doxycycline, minocycline, tetracycline, third-generation cephalosporins, and vancomycin. For severe clostridial infections, sensitivity testing should be done before using an antimicrobial with unpredictable susceptibility. Simple contamination of a wound with clostridia should not be treated with antibiotics. Localized skin and soft tissue infection can be managed by debridement rather than with systemic antibiotics. Drugs are required when the process extends into adjacent tissue, or when fever and systemic signs of sepsis are present.

Suppurative infections should be treated with antibiotics. Frequently, broad-spectrum antibiotics must be used because of mixed flora in these infections. Aminoglycosides can be used for the aerobic gram-negative bacteria in mixed infections.

The use of a polyvalent gas gangrene antitoxin is still recommended by some authorities. At present the antitoxin is not produced in the United States, and most centers have discontinued its use in management of patients with suspected gas gangrene or clostridial postabortion sepsis because of questionable efficacy and the substantial risk of hypersentitivity to horse serum.

The use of hyperbaric oxygen in the treatment of gas gangrene is also controversial. Studies in humans are not well designed to answer questions on efficacy, but several knowledgeable authors believe that hyperbaric oxygen therapy has contributed to dramatic clinical improvement. It may, however, be associated with untoward effects due to oxygen toxicity and high atmospheric pressure. Some centers without hyperbaric chambers have reported acceptable mortality rates, indicating that expert surgical and medical management and control of complications are probably the most important factors in treating gas gangrene.

Treatment of *C. difficile* enterocolitis   The treatment of *C. difficile*–associated colitis requires discontinuation of the offending antimicrobial agent. In some patients symptoms will resolve over a period of 2 weeks. However, specific therapy has been beneficial. The most widely used agent in the treatment of antibiotic-associated diarrhea ascribed to *C. difficile* is oral vancomycin. Most strains of *C. difficile* are susceptible to achievable concentrations of oral vancomycin. This antibiotic is poorly absorbed after oral administration and high levels appear in the stool. Dosing should begin with 125 mg orally four times a day for 7 to 10 days, but the dose may

be increased to 500 mg orally four times a day. Oral metronidazole at a dose of 500 mg three times a day for 7 to 10 days is also effective. However, a few cases of *C. difficile* colitis have developed after oral metronidazole therapy for other infections. Because response to the two treatment regimens is comparable and metronidazole is less costly, it is reasonable to initiate treatment with metronidazole. If diarrhea persists, then therapy should be changed to oral vancomycin. Therapy with oral cholestyramine was initially reported to provide dramatic improvement in patients with pseudomembranous colitis (PMC). Subsequent studies have shown that cholestyramine, as well as other anionic resins, bind the cytotoxin produced by *C. difficile*. However, comparative trials in animals have shown that cholestyramine is distinctly inferior to oral vancomycin. Combination therapy with oral vancomycin and cholestyramine in refractory cases has been successful. Toxin production in PMC persists in 5 to 10 percent of treated patients. Relapses are reported in up to 20 percent of patients, but patients usually respond to a second course of oral vancomycin.

REFERENCES

BARTLETT JG et al: Antibiotic-associated pseudomembranous colitis due to toxin-producing clostridia. N Engl J Med 298:531, 1978

———, TAYLOR NS: Antibiotic-associated colitis, in *Medical Microbiology,* CSF Easman, J Jeljaszewicz (eds). London, Academic, 1982, pp 1–48

BORNSTEIN DL: Clostridial myonecrosis, in *Medical Microbiology and Infectious Diseases,* A Braude (ed). Philadelphia, Saunders, 1981, chap 239

DAILEY DC et al: Factors influencing the phagocytosis of *Clostridium difficile* by human polymorphonuclear leukocytes. Infect Immun 55:1541, 1987

FINEGOLD SM: *Anaerobic Bacteria in Human Disease.* New York, Academic, 1977

———: Anaerobic infections and *Clostridium difficile* colitis emerging during antibacterial therapy. Scand J Infect Dis (Suppl)49:160, 1986

GORBACH SL: Other *Clostridium* species (including gas gangrene), in *Principles and Practice of Infectious Diseases,* GL Mandell et al (eds). New York, Wiley, 1985

———, THADEPALLI H: Isolation of *Clostridium* in human infections: Evaluation of 114 cases. J Infect Dis 131:S81, 1975

JENDRZEJEWSKI JW et al: Nontraumatic clostridial myonecrosis. Am J Med 65:542, 1978

JOHNSON S et al: Enteritis necroticans among Khmer children at an evacuation site in Thailand. Lancet 2:496, 1987

KORANSKY JR et al: *Clostridium septicum* bacteremia. Am J Med 66:63, 1979

KRIVAN HC et al: Cell surface binding site for *Clostridium difficile* enterotoxin: Evidence for a glycoconjugate containing the sequence Gal alpha 1–3 Gal beta 1–4 Glc NAc. Infect Immun 53:573, 1986

PRITCHARD JA, WHALLEY PJ: Abortion complicated by *Clostridium perfringens* infection. Am J Gynecol 111:484, 1971

SMITH LDS: Virulence factors of *Clostridium perfringens.* Rev Infect Dis 1:254, 1979

TEASLEY DG et al: Prospective randomized trial of metronidazole versus vancomycin for *Clostridium difficile*–associated diarrhea and colitis. Lancet 2:1043, 1983

108   INFECTIONS DUE TO MIXED ANAEROBIC ORGANISMS

DENNIS L. KASPER

DEFINITIONS   Anaerobic bacteria are organisms that require reduced oxygen tension for growth, failing to grow on the surface of solid media in 10% CO_2 in air. Microaerophilic bacteria can grow in 10% CO_2 in air or under anaerobic or aerobic conditions. Facultative bacteria can grow in the presence or absence of air. This chapter addresses infections caused by nonsporulating anaerobic bacteria. In general, anaerobes associated with human infections are relatively aerotolerant. They can survive for as long as 72 h in the presence of oxygen, although generally they will not multiply in this environment. Less pathogenic anaerobic bacteria, which are also part of the normal flora, die after brief contact with oxygen, even in low concentrations.

The nonsporulating anaerobic bacteria exist as normal flora on the mucosal surfaces of humans and animals. The major reservoirs of these bacteria are the mouth, gastrointestinal tract, skin, and the female genital tract. Of the oral flora, anaerobes are the predominant commensal organisms, ranging in concentrations from 10^9 per milliliter in saliva to 10^{12} in gingival scrapings. In the oral cavity the relative concentration of anaerobic to aerobic bacteria ranges from 1:1 on the surface of the tooth to 100 to 1000:1 in the gingival crevice. Anaerobic bacteria are not found in appreciable numbers in the normal intestine until the distal ileum. In the colon, the proportion of anaerobes increases significantly, as does the overall bacterial count. For example, in the colon there are 10^{11} to 10^{12} organisms per gram of stool, with a ratio of anaerobes to aerobes of approximately 1000:1. In the female genital tract there are approximately 10^9 organisms per milliliter of secretions, with a ratio of anaerobes to aerobes of approximately 10:1. Hundreds of species of anaerobic bacteria have been identified as part of the normal flora of humans. Identification of as many as 500 different anaerobic species in fecal specimens reflects the diversity of the anaerobic flora. Despite the complex array of bacteria which exist in the normal flora, relatively few species are isolated commonly from human infection.

Anaerobic infections occur when the harmonious relationship between the host and bacteria is disrupted. Any site in the body is susceptible to infection with these indigenous organisms when the mucosal barriers or skin are compromised by surgery, trauma, tumor, or ischemia or necrosis, which reduce local tissue redox potentials. Because the sites that are colonized by anaerobic bacteria contain many species of bacteria, disruption of anatomic barriers allows penetration of many organisms, resulting in mixed infections involving multiple species of anaerobes combined with facultative or microaerophilic organisms. Such mixed infections are seen in the head and neck (chronic sinusitis, chronic otitis media, Ludwig's angina, and periodontal abscesses). Brain abscesses and subdural empyema are the most frequent anaerobic infections of the central nervous system. Anaerobes are responsible for pleuropulmonary diseases such as aspiration pneumonia, necrotizing pneumonia, lung abscesses, or empyema. Anaerobes play an important role in various intraabdominal infections such as peritonitis and intraabdominal and liver abscesses. They are isolated frequently in female genital tract infections such as salpingitis, pelvic peritonitis, tuboovarian abscess, vulvovaginal abscesses, septic abortions, and endometritis. Anaerobic bacteria also are frequently found in infections of the skin, soft tissue, bones, and in bacteremia.

ETIOLOGY The major anaerobic gram-positive cocci producing disease are *Peptostreptococcus* species. The major species involved in infections are *P. magnus, P. asaccharolyticus, P. anaerobius,* and *P. prevotii.* Clostridia are gram-positive rods which are isolated from wounds, abscesses, abdominal infections, and bacteremias; they are discussed in Chap. 107. The principal anaerobic gram-negative bacilli are the *Bacteroides* family, which includes the *Bacteroides fragilis* group, fusobacteria, and the pigmented *Bacteroides.* The *B. fragilis* group contains the anaerobic pathogens most frequently isolated from clinical infections. Members of this group are part of the normal bowel flora. Several distinct species comprise the group, including *B. fragilis, B. thetaiotaomicron, B. distasonis, B. vulgatis,* and *B. ovatis.* Of this group *B. fragilis* is the most important clinical isolate. However, in the normal fecal flora, the frequency with which *B. fragilis* is isolated is low compared to other *Bacteroides* species. A second major group of *Bacteroides* are part of the indigenous oral flora. These are primarily pigment-producing bacteria which were previously classified under the species *B. melaninogenicus.* The terminology of this group has changed so that several distinct species are recognized, including *B. gingivalis, B. asaccharolyticus,* as well as *B. melaninogenicus.* In female genital tract infections, *B. bivius* and *B. disiens* are the most frequent isolates, although *B. fragilis* is common. Fusobacteria are also isolated from clinical infections, including necrotizing pneumonia and abscesses.

Infections due to anaerobic bacteria most frequently are mixed infections with more than one organism. They may be due to one or several anaerobic species, or a combination of anaerobic organisms and aerobic bacteria acting synergistically.

APPROACH TO THE PATIENT WITH ANAEROBIC BACTERIAL INFECTIONS There are several features to remember when approaching the patient with presumptive infection due to anaerobic bacteria. (1) Most of these organisms are harmless commensals, and very few cause disease. (2) In order for these organisms to cause infection, they must spread beyond the normal mucosal barriers. (3) Conditions favoring the propagation of these bacteria, particularly a lowered oxidation-reduction potential, are necessary. These include sites of trauma, tissue destruction, compromised vascular supply, or complication of preexisting infection that produces necrosis. (4) There is a complex array of infecting flora. For example, as many as 12 different types of organisms can be isolated from a suppurative site. (5) Anaerobic organisms tend to be found in abscess cavities or in necrotic tissue. The detection of an abscess in a patient which fails to yield organisms on routine culture is the clue that the abscess is likely to contain anaerobic bacteria. However, often smears of this "sterile pus" are teeming with bacteria on Gram stain. The malodorous nature of the pus should suggest anaerobe infections. Although some facultative organisms, such as *Staphylococcus aureus,* also are capable of causing abscesses, abscesses in organs or within deeper body tissues should call to mind anaerobic infection. (6) Treatment need not be directed at all of the organisms in the infectious site. However, some species in particular require specific therapy. The best example of this principle is the need to treat the *B. fragilis* group. Many of these synergistic infections can be cured with antibiotics directed at some, but not all, of the organisms. Antibiotic therapy, combined with drainage, disrupts the interdependent relationship among the bacteria and species which are resistant to the antibiotic do not survive without the co-infective organisms. (7) Manifestations of disseminated intravascular coagulation are unusual in patients with anaerobic infection.

EPIDEMIOLOGY Difficulties in obtaining appropriate cultures, contamination of cultures by aerobic bacteria or normal flora, and the lack of readily available reliable culture techniques have made accurate incidence or prevalence data on anaerobic infections unavailable. However, these infections are encountered frequently in hospitals with active surgical, trauma, and obstetric and gynecologic services. In some centers anaerobic bacteria, particularly *B. fragilis,* account for approximately 8 to 10 percent of positive blood cultures.

PATHOGENESIS Anaerobic bacterial infections usually occur when an anatomic barrier becomes disrupted and the local flora enter a site which was previously sterile. The bacteria which are isolated from infected sites have survived changes in Eh and exposure to host defenses. Because of the specific growth requirements of anaerobic organisms and their presence as commensals on mucosal surfaces, conditions must arise which allow these organisms to penetrate mucosal barriers and enter tissue with a lowered oxidation-reduction potential. Therefore, tissue ischemia, trauma, surgery, perforated viscus, shock, or aspiration provide environments conducive to the proliferation of anaerobes. Highly fastidious anaerobes lack the enzyme superoxide dismutase (SOD) that in other organisms reduces toxic superoxide radicals, thereby lessening the potentially lethal effects of superoxide. A general correlation exists between the intracellular concentration of SOD and the oxygen tolerance of anaerobic bacteria; organisms that contain SOD have a selective advantage after exposure to aerobic environments. For example, in the case of a perforated viscus, hundreds of species of anaerobic bacteria are spilled into the peritoneal cavity, but many of these organisms are unable to survive because the highly vascularized tissue provides an adequate oxygen supply. The entry of oxygen into the environment results in selection of aerotolerant organisms.

The ability of an organism to adhere to host tissues is important to the establishment of infection. Some oral *Bacteroides* species adhere to crevicular epithelium in the oral cavity. *B. melaninogenicus* actually attach to other microorganisms. *B. gingivalis* is a common isolate in periodontal disease. These organisms have been shown to have fimbriae which facilitate attachment. Some unencapsulated

Bacteroides strains appear to be piliated which may account for their ability to adhere.

Anaerobic bacteria produce a number of exoenzymes which are capable of enhancing their virulence. These enzymes include a heparinase elaborated by *B. fragilis* which may contribute to intravascular clotting and lead to a requirement for increased doses of heparin in patients on heparin therapy. Collagenase, produced by *B. gingivalis*, may enhance tissue destruction. Both *B. fragilis* and *B. melaninogenicus* possess lipopolysaccharides (endotoxins) which lack the biologic potency characteristic of endotoxins associated with aerobic gram-negative bacteria. The biologic inactivity of the endotoxin may account for the rarity of disseminated intravascular coagulation and purpura in *Bacteroides* bacteremia compared to facultative and aerobic gram-negative rod bacteremia.

CLINICAL MANIFESTATIONS **Anaerobic infections of the mouth, head, and neck** Infections of the mouth can be divided into those infections that arise from the supragingival or subgingival dental plaque. Supragingival plaque formation begins with the adherence of gram-positive bacteria to the tooth surface. This form of plaque is influenced by salivary and dietary components, oral hygiene, and local host factors. Once established, the acquisition of pathogenic bacteria as well as an increase in the amount of plaque is responsible for the ultimate development of gingivitis. Early bacteriologic changes in the supragingival plaque initiate an inflammatory response in the gingiva, including edema, swelling, and increase in gingival fluid and are responsible for the development of caries and endodontic (pulp) infections. Also, these changes contribute to the subsequent pathogenic alteration in the subgingival plaque which arise from poor or inadequate oral hygiene. Subgingival plaque is associated with periodontal disease and disseminated infection arising from the oral cavity. Bacteria that colonize the subgingival area are primarily anaerobic. The black-pigmented gram-negative anaerobic bacilli belonging to the *Bacteroides* group, principally *B. gingivalis* and *B. melaninogenicus*, are the most important. Infections in this area are frequently mixed and involve both anaerobic and aerobic bacteria. After establishment of local infection either in root canals or in the periodontal area, infection may extend into the mandible, causing osteomyelitis; to the maxillary sinuses; or to local tissues in the submandibular or submental spaces, depending upon which teeth are involved. Periodontitis also may result in spreading infection that can involve adjacent bone or soft tissues. This form of infection may be due either to oral *Bacteroides* or to *Fusobacterium*.

GINGIVITIS Gingivitis may become a necrotizing infection (trench mouth, Vincent's stomatitis). The onset of disease is usually sudden and is associated with tender bleeding gums, foul breath, and a bad taste. The gingival mucosa, especially the papillae between the teeth, become ulcerated and may be covered by a gray exudate which is removable with gentle pressure. These patients may become systemically ill, developing fever, cervical lymphadenopathy, and leukocytosis. Occasionally, ulcerative gingivitis can spread to the buccal mucosa, the teeth, and the mandible or maxilla, resulting in widespread destruction of bone and soft tissue. This infection is termed *acute necrotizing ulcerative mucositis* (cancrum oris, noma). It destroys tissue rapidly, causing the teeth to fall out and large areas of bone, even the whole mandible, to be sloughed. A strong putrid odor frequently is present, although the lesions are not painful. The gangrenous lesions eventually heal, leaving large disfiguring defects. This infection is seen most commonly following a debilitating illness, or in severely malnourished children in underdeveloped areas. It has been known to complicate leukemia or to develop in individuals with a genetic deficiency of catalase.

ACUTE NECROTIZING INFECTIONS OF THE PHARYNX These usually occur in association with ulcerative gingivitis. There are an extremely sore throat, foul breath, and a bad taste in the mouth, accompanied by a sensation of choking and fever. Examination of the pharynx demonstrates that the tonsillar pillars are swollen, red, and ulcerated and covered with a grayish membrane that peels easily. Lymphadenopathy and leukocytosis are common. The disease may last for only

a few days or may persist for weeks if not treated. Lesions begin unilaterally but may spread to the other side of the pharynx or the larynx. Aspiration of the infected material by the patient can result in lung abscesses. Soft tissue infection of the oral-facial area may or may not be odontogenic in origin. *Ludwig's angina*, a periodontal infection usually arising from the third molar, may produce submandibular cellulitis that results in marked local swelling of tissues with pain, trismus, and superior and posterior displacement of the tongue. Submandibular swelling of the neck develops, which can impair swallowing and cause respiratory obstruction. In some cases tracheotomy may be life-saving.

FASCIAL INFECTIONS These arise from the spread of organisms originating in the upper airways to potential spaces formed by the fascial planes of the head and neck. Although there are few well-documented reports on the microbiology of these syndromes, anaerobes from the oral flora have been implicated in many cases. *Staph. aureus* and *Streptococcus pyogenes* infections may arise from boils or impetigo, whereas anaerobes are associated with space infections arising from diseases of the mucous membranes, dental manipulations, or occurring spontaneously.

SINUSITIS AND OTITIS The role of anaerobic bacteria in acute sinusitis may be underestimated because of improper collection of specimens. In chronic sinusitis anaerobic bacteria were found in 52 percent of specimens collected during external frontoethmoidotomy or radical antrotomy. Anaerobic bacteria are much more easily implicated in chronic suppurative otitis media than in acute otitis media. Purulent exudate from chronically draining ears has been found to contain anaerobes, particularly *Bacteroides* species, in up to 50 percent of patients. In contrast to other infections of the head and neck, *B. fragilis* has been isolated from up to 28 percent of patients with chronic otitis media.

COMPLICATIONS OF ANAEROBIC HEAD AND NECK INFECTIONS Contiguous spread of these infections craniad may result in osteomyelitis of the skull or mandible, or in intracranial infections such as brain abscesses or subdural empyema. Caudad spread can produce mediastinitis or pleuropulmonary infections. Hematogenous complications also may result from anaerobic infections of the head and neck. Bacteremia, which can occasionally be polymicrobial, can lead to endocarditis or other distant infections. When infections spread to produce suppurative thrombophlebitis of the internal jugular vein, a destructive syndrome with prolonged fever, bacteremia, septic emboli to both the lung and brain, and multiple metastatic foci of suppurative infection may develop. This syndrome has been reported with septicemia from species of *Fusobacterium* following exudative pharyngitis but is uncommon in this era of antimicrobial agents.

Central nervous system infections Brain abscesses are frequently associated with anaerobic bacteria (see Chap. 354). If optimal bacteriologic techniques are employed, as many as 85 percent of brain abscesses yield anaerobic bacteria. The anaerobic bacteria found most often in these infections are anaerobic gram-positive cocci, followed in frequency by fusobacteria and *Bacteroides* species. Frequently, facultative or microaerophilic streptococci and coliforms are involved in brain abscesses as mixed infections.

Pleuropulmonary infections Anaerobic pleuropulmonary infections result from the aspiration of oropharyngeal contents, which is often associated with an altered state of consciousness or absent gag reflex. There are four clinical syndromes associated with anaerobic pleuropulmonary infection produced by aspiration: simple aspiration pneumonia, necrotizing pneumonia, lung abscess, and empyema.

ANAEROBIC ASPIRATION PNEUMONITIS Anaerobic aspiration pneumonitis must be distinguished from two other types of aspiration pneumonitis, neither of which is bacterial. One aspiration syndrome results from aspiration of solids, usually food. Obstruction of major airways with resulting atelectasis is typical. Moderate nonspecific inflammation occurs. Therapy consists of removal of the foreign body.

A second aspiration syndrome is more easily confused with bacterial aspiration. This is the so-called Mendelson's syndrome, resulting from regurgitation of stomach contents and aspiration of chemical material, usually gastric juices. Pulmonary inflammation including destruction of alveolar lining with transudation of fluid into the alveolar space occurs with remarkable rapidity. Typically this syndrome develops within hours, often following anesthesia when the gag reflex is depressed. The patient becomes tachypneic, hypoxic, and febrile. The leukocyte count may rise, and the chest x-ray may evolve suddenly from normal to a complete whiteout bilaterally within 8 to 24 h. Minimal sputum production occurs. The pulmonary signs and symptoms can resolve quickly with symptomatic therapy or result in respiratory failure with subsequent development of bacterial superinfection over a period of days. Antibiotic therapy is not indicated unless bacterial infection supervenes. The signs of bacterial infection include sputum, persistent fever, leukocytosis, and clinical evidence of sepsis.

In contrast to these syndromes, bacterial aspiration pneumonia develops more slowly. It is seen in patients who are hospitalized and have a depressed gag reflex, elderly patients, or those with transient impaired consciousness in the wake of seizures or alcoholic blackouts. Patients who enter the hospital with this syndrome typically have been ill for several days, generally complain of low-grade fever, malaise, and sputum production. Usually the history reveals a predisposition for aspiration, such as alcohol overdose or residence in a nursing home. Sputum characteristically is not malodorous unless the process has been present for at least a week. Mixed bacterial flora with many polymorphonuclear leukocytes are present on Gram stain; reliable cultures can be obtained only by avoiding contamination with normal oral flora, i.e., by transtracheal aspiration. Chest x-rays show consolidation in dependent pulmonary segments. These are the basilar segments of the lower lobes if the patient aspirated while upright or sitting, or in the posterior segment of the upper lobe, usually on the right side, or in the superior segment of the lower lobe if aspiration has occurred in the supine position. Organisms isolated reflect the pharyngeal flora; *B. melaninogenicus*, *Fusobacterium* species, and anaerobic cocci are the most frequent isolates. The patient who aspirates in a hospital setting also may have mixed infection involving enteric gram-negative rods.

NECROTIZING PNEUMONITIS This is a form of anaerobic pneumonitis characterized by numerous small abscesses which spread to involve several pulmonary segments. The process can be indolent or fulminating. This syndrome is less common than either aspiration pneumonia or lung abscess, and includes features of both types of infection.

ANAEROBIC LUNG ABSCESSES These result from subacute anaerobic pulmonary infection. The clinical syndrome typically involves a history of constitutional symptoms including malaise, weight loss, fever, chills, and foul-smelling sputum which may occur over a period of weeks (see Chap. 207). Patients who develop lung abscesses characteristically have dental infection and periodontitis, but there are reports of lung abscesses in patients who are edentulous. Abscess cavities may be single or multiple, and generally occur in dependent pulmonary segments. Anaerobic abscesses must be distinguished from tuberculosis, neoplasia, and other causes of lung abscess, despite the fact that the clinical syndrome is usually typical. Oral anaerobes predominate, although *B. fragilis* is isolated in up to 10 percent of cases. *Staph. aureus* may be found as well. While in vitro resistance by *B. fragilis* to penicillin is common, this antibiotic generally is successful in treatment when combined with vigorous pulmonary toilet. Bronchoscopy is indicated only to rule out the presence of airway obstruction but should be delayed until the antimicrobial has begun to affect the disease process so that it does not spread the infection. Bronchoscopy has no role in enhancing drainage. Surgery is almost never indicated because of the danger of spilling the abscess contents into the lungs.

Empyema Empyema is a manifestation of long-standing anaerobic pulmonary infection. The clinical presentation resembles other anaerobic pulmonary infections including the presence of foul-smelling sputum. Patients may complain of pleuritic chest pain and marked chest wall tenderness.

Empyema may be masked by overlying pneumonitis and should be considered especially in cases of persistent fever in a patient receiving antibiotic therapy. Diligent physical examination and the use of ultrasound to localize a loculated empyema are important diagnostic tools. The presence of a foul-smelling exudate obtained by thoracentesis is typical. Drainage is required. Defervescence, a return to a feeling of well-being, and resolution of the process may require several months.

Extension from a subdiaphragmatic infection also may result in an anaerobic empyema. Septic pulmonary emboli may originate from intraabdominal or female genital tract infections and can produce anaerobic pneumonia.

Intraabdominal infections Because anaerobic bacteria outnumber aerobic bacteria in normal bowel flora by 100 to 1000:1, it is not surprising that disruption of the bowel wall will result in peritonitis with a preponderance of anaerobic bacteria. Colonic perforation releases large numbers of these bacteria and therefore entails a high risk of intraabdominal sepsis. Following peritonitis, abscesses may develop in any part of the peritoneal cavity and retroperitoneal spaces. The peritoneum reacts with a marked inflammatory response and effectively walls off the infection in a very short time. If an intraperitoneal abscess is localized, typical signs and symptoms appear (see Chap. 91). For example, *subphrenic abscess* may cause an ipsilateral sympathetic pleural effusion, and the patient may have pleuritic-type pain and splinting of the hemidiaphragm on the affected side. Constitutional symptoms include fever, chills, and malaise. There may be a history of abdominal surgery, trauma, or other conditions that predispose to disruption of the bowel wall. In contrast, more subtle clinical signs must be sought when an intraabdominal abscess is not readily localized. Peritonitis and abscess formation are closely related processes. Often following surgery to repair a bowel perforation, a patient may be febrile without localizing abdominal signs or general clinical deterioration. Persistent leukocytosis may be related to the operative procedure and/or resolving peritonitis. Profuse, cloudy, or foul-smelling wound drainage suggests the possibility of purulent anaerobic infection. Gram stain revealing a mixed fecal flora is frequently helpful. *B. fragilis* is isolated from approximately 70 percent of surgical wounds after trauma involving perforation of the lower gut, and a similar percentage of isolates follows elective colonic surgery. Antibiotics effective against *B. fragilis*, as well as facultative bacteria, are important in therapy, although they are not a replacement for surgical or percutaneous drainage. Appendicitis with perforation and abscess formation is the most common intraabdominal anaerobic infection. Diverticulitis involves nonsporulating anaerobes and can result in perforation followed by generalized peritonitis, but generally results in small walled-off infections that do not require surgical drainage. Abdominal ultrasound, gallium- or indium-labeled neutrophil scans, computed tomography (CT) scans, or magnetic resonance imaging may be helpful in localizing intraabdominal abscesses. Surgical exploration, however, may be necessary to establish the site of such an infection.

Among visceral abdominal infections involving nonsporulating anaerobes, the most common is *liver abscess;* nonsporulating anaerobes are isolated from approximately 50 percent of liver abscesses. Liver abscess results from both bacteremic spread (sometimes following blunt trauma with localized infarction of hepatic tissue) and from contiguous infection, especially within the peritoneal cavity. Infection may spread from the biliary tract or from the portal venous system (suppurative pyelophlebitis) which results from direct extension of pelvic or intraabdominal sepsis. Symptoms and signs often suggest infection that can be readily localized, but nonspecific symptoms of fever, chills, weight loss, nausea, and vomiting are also seen. Only half the patients have hepatomegaly, right upper quadrant abdominal tenderness, and jaundice. The diagnosis can be confirmed by ultrasound, CT scan, or radioisotopic scanning. Occasionally more than one diagnostic procedure may have to be utilized. More than 90 percent of patients with liver abscesses have a leukocytosis and elevation of the serum alkaline phosphatase and aspartyl transaminase.

Fifty percent have associated anemia, hypoalbuminemia, and elevated serum bilirubin. A basilar pulmonary infiltrate, pleural effusion, or elevated hemidiaphragm can be seen on chest x-ray. One-third of these patients have bacteremia. Open surgical drainage is indicated when an abscess is associated with other lesions requiring surgical drainage. Otherwise, percutaneous drainage using ultrasonography or CT scan to guide the catheter may be combined with antimicrobial therapy. If a liver abscess arises from contiguous gallbladder infection, cholecystectomy is essential.

Pelvic infections The vagina of a healthy woman is one of the major reservoirs of anaerobic and aerobic bacteria. In the normal flora of the female genital tract, anaerobes outnumber aerobes by a ratio of approximately 10:1. These anaerobes include anaerobic gram-positive cocci and *Bacteroides* species. Serious infections of the upper female tract contain organisms found in the normal vaginal flora. Anaerobes are isolated from the majority of such patients. The major pathogens consist of *B. fragilis, B. bivius, B. disiens, B. melaninogenicus,* anaerobic cocci, and clostridial species. Anaerobes frequently are encountered in tuboovarian abscess, septic abortion, pelvic abscess, endometritis, and postoperative wound infection, particularly following hysterectomy. Although these infections are frequently mixed, involving both anaerobes and coliforms, pure anaerobic infections without coliform or other facultative bacterial species occur more often in pelvic infections than intraabdominal infections. These infections are characterized by drainage of foul-smelling pus or blood from the uterus, generalized uterine or local pelvic tenderness, and continued fever and chills. Suppurative thrombophlebitis of the pelvic veins may complicate the infections and lead to repeated episodes of septic pulmonary emboli.

Skin and soft tissue infections Injury to skin, bone, or soft tissue by trauma, ischemia, or surgery creates a suitable environment for anaerobic infections. These infections are most frequently found when the site is prone to contamination with feces or upper airway secretions. Examples include wounds associated with intestinal surgery, decubitus ulcers, or human bites. Anaerobic bacteria can be isolated in cases of crepitant cellulitis, synergistic cellulitis, or gangrene and necrotizing fasciitis. These organisms have been isolated from cutaneous abscesses, rectal abscesses, and axillary sweat gland infections (hydradenitis suppurativa). Anaerobes frequently have been cultured from foot ulcers in diabetic patients.

These types of soft tissue or skin infections are usually polymicrobial. A mean of 4.8 bacterial species can be isolated with a roughly 3:2 ratio of anaerobes to aerobes. The most frequently isolated organisms include *Bacteroides* species, anaerobic streptococci, enterococci, clostridial species, and *Proteus* species. The presence of anaerobes in these types of infections is associated with a higher frequency of fever, foul-smelling lesions, or a visible foot ulcer.

Anaerobic bacterial *synergistic gangrene* (Meleney's) is exquisitely painful, red, and swollen, followed by induration. Erythema surrounds a central zone of necrosis. A granulating ulcer which may heal forms at the original center as necrosis and erythema extend outward. Symptoms are limited to pain. Fever is not typical. These infections most usually involve a combination of anaerobic cocci and *Staph. aureus.* Treatment includes surgical removal of necrotic tissue and antimicrobial therapy.

NECROTIZING FASCIITIS This is a rapidly spreading destructive disease of the fascia, usually attributed to group A streptococci, but it can be caused by anaerobic bacteria including *Peptostreptococcus* and *Bacteroides* species. Similarly, myonecrosis can be associated with mixed anaerobic infection. Fournier's gangrene is an anaerobic cellulitis involving the scrotum, perineum, and anterior abdominal wall in which mixed anaerobic organisms spread along deep external fascial planes and cause extensive loss of skin.

Bone and joint infections Although *actinomycosis* (see Chap. 152) accounts on a worldwide basis for the majority of anaerobic infections in bone, other organisms, including anaerobic or microaerophilic cocci, *Bacteroides* species, *Fusobacterium,* and *Clostridium* species, can be found. These infections frequently arise in the setting of adjacent soft tissue infections. Hematogenous seeding of bone is uncommon. Oral *Bacteroides* are seen in infections involving the maxilla and mandible, whereas *Clostridium* species have been reported as anaerobic pathogens in cases of osteomyelitis of the long bones, following fracture or trauma. Fusobacteria have been isolated in pure culture from osteomyelitis adjacent to the perinasal sinuses. Anaerobic and microaerophilic cocci have been reported as significant pathogens in infections involving the skull or mastoid.

In cases of anaerobic septic arthritis, the most common isolates are *Fusobacterium* species. Most of these patients have uncontrolled peritonsillar infections progressing to septic cervical venous thrombophlebitis and resulting in hematogenous dissemination which shows a predilection for the joints. Following the introduction of antibiotics, the isolation of *Fusobacterium* species from joints has been less common. Unlike anaerobic osteomyelitis, most cases of pyoarthritis caused by anaerobes are not polymicrobial and may be acquired hematogenously. Anaerobes are important pathogens in infections involving prosthetic joints; in these infections the causative organisms are part of the normal skin flora, such as anaerobic gram-positive cocci and *P. acnes.*

In patients with osteomyelitis (see Chap. 97), the most reliable source of culture is a bone biopsy obtained free from normal uninfected skin and subcutaneous tissue. If mixed flora is isolated from a bone biopsy, all isolates should be treated. When an anaerobic isolate is recognized as a major or sole pathogen involving a joint, the treatment regimen should be similar to treatment of arthritis caused by aerobic bacteria. Therapy includes management of underlying disease states, appropriate antimicrobial therapy, temporary joint immobilization, percutaneous drainage of effusions, and usually removal of infected prostheses or internal fixation devices. Surgical drainage and debridement such as sequestrectomy are essential for removal of necrotic tissue that would sustain anaerobic infections.

Bacteremia Transient bacteremia is a well-known event that occurs in healthy people when the anatomic mucosal barriers are injured (e.g., toothbrushing). These bacteremic episodes, which are often due to anaerobes, have no pathologic consequences. However, anaerobic bacteria compose nearly 10 to 15 percent of bacterial blood isolates from clinically ill patients when proper culture techniques are used. *B. fragilis* is the single most frequent anaerobic isolate. The portal of entry can usually be deduced along with the likely underlying problem that led to seeding of the bloodstream, by identification of the organism and understanding its place of normal residence. For example, mixed anaerobic bacteremia including *B. fragilis* implies colonic pathology with mucosal disruption from neoplasia, diverticulitis, or some other inflammatory lesion. The initial manifestations are determined by the portal of entry and reflect the localized condition. However, when bloodstream invasion occurs, patients can become extremely ill with rigors and hectic fevers ranging up to 40.6°C (105°F). The clinical picture may be quite similar to that seen in sepsis with aerobic gram-negative bacilli. Although other complications of anaerobic bacteremia such as septic thrombophlebitis and septic shock have been reported, the incidence of these complications in association with anaerobic bacteremia is low. Anaerobic bacteremia is potentially fatal and requires rapid diagnosis and appropriate therapy.

ENDOCARDITIS (See Chap. 90) Endocarditis due to anaerobes is uncommon. However, anaerobic streptococci, which are often classified incorrectly, are responsible for this disease more frequently than is appreciated. Gram-negative anaerobes are unusual causes of endocarditis.

DIAGNOSIS Because of the time and difficulty involved in the isolation of anaerobic bacteria, diagnosis of these infections must frequently be made on presumptive evidence. Certain clinical settings such as avascular, necrotic tissues with lowered oxidation-reduction potential favor the diagnosis of an anaerobic infection. When infections occur in proximity to mucosal surfaces normally harboring anaerobic flora, such as the gastrointestinal tract, female genital tract, or oropharynx, anaerobes should be considered as potential etiologic agents. A foul odor often is present since anaerobes produce certain organic acids as they proliferate in necrotic tissue. Although the presence of these odors is nearly pathognomonic for anaerobic infection, the absence of odor does not exclude these organisms as potential etiologic agents. Because anaerobes often coexist with other bacteria to form a mixed or synergistic infection, Gram-stained exudate frequently reveals numerous pleomorphic cocci and bacilli suggestive of anaerobes. Sometimes these organisms will have morphologic characteristics associated with specific species.

The presence of gas in tissues is highly suggestive, but not diagnostic, of anaerobes. Culture reports from obviously infected sites which yield no growth or only streptococci or a single aerobic species such as E. coli, when a Gram stain reveals mixed flora, imply that the anaerobic microorganisms failed to grow because of inadequate transport and/or culture techniques. Failure of a patient to respond to antibiotics that are not active against anaerobes, for example, aminoglycosides, and, in some circumstances, penicillin, cephalosporins, or tetracyclines, suggests the possibility of anaerobic infection.

There are three critical steps to diagnose anaerobic infection: (1) proper specimen collection, (2) rapid transportation of these specimens to the microbiology laboratory, preferably in anaerobic transport media, and (3) proper handling of these specimens by the laboratory. Collection of specimens must be performed by meticulously sampling infected sites avoiding contamination with normal flora. When there is a likely contamination of a specimen with normal flora, the specimen is unacceptable for processing by the bacteriology laboratory. Examples of unacceptable specimens for anaerobic culture include: (1) sputum collected by expectoration, or nasal tracheal suction, (2) bronchoscopy specimens, (3) direct collections through the vaginal vault, (4) collections of urine by voided specimen, and (5) feces. Specimens which can be cultured for anaerobes include blood, pleural fluid, transtracheal aspirates, pus obtained by direct aspiration from an abscess cavity, fluid obtained by culdocentesis, suprapubic bladder aspirates, cerebrospinal fluid, and lung puncture specimens.

Because even brief exposure to oxygen may kill some anaerobic organisms and result in failure to isolate them in the laboratory, abscess cavities which are aspirated with a syringe should have the air expelled and the needle capped with a sterile rubber stopper. Proper precautions should be utilized when handling contaminated needles. Specimens can be injected into transport bottles containing a reduced medium or brought immediately in syringes to the laboratory for direct culture on anaerobic media. In general, swabs should not be used. If a swab must be used, it should be placed in a reduced semisolid carrying medium before transport to the laboratory. Delays in transportation may lead to failure to isolate anaerobes due to exposure to oxygen, or overgrowth of facultative organisms which may eliminate or obscure the anaerobes that are present. All clinical specimens from suspected anaerobic infections should be Gram-stained and examined for organisms with characteristic morphology. It is not unusual for organisms to be observed on Gram stain but not isolated in culture. If purulent materials are found to be sterile, or organisms are seen on Gram stain, but do not grow in the culture, suspicion should be raised that anaerobes are involved.

TREATMENT   Successful therapy of anaerobic infections involves a combination of appropriate antibiotics, surgical resection, and drainage. Perforations must be closed promptly, devitalized tissues removed, closed spaces drained, tissue compartments decompressed, and adequate blood supply established. Drainage of abscess cavities should be carried out as soon as fluctuation or localization occurs. While surgery was formerly required to establish drainage, with the advent of CT scans and ultrasound, diagnostic radiologists now are able to perform percutaneous drainage of a number of abscess sites.

Patients with infections due to anaerobic bacteria require appropriate antibiotics. Most laboratories lack facilities to do antimicrobial susceptibility testing on anaerobic bacteria. In these instances presumptive therapy must be given and the patient's response followed closely. The selection of initial antibiotic therapy should be based on

TABLE 108-1 Antimicrobial therapy for anaerobic bacterial infection

	Bacteroides fragilis group or other penicillin-resistant anaerobes (usual source below diaphragm)	Other anaerobes in mixed infection (usual source above diaphragm)
Proven first-line therapy	Metronidazole* Clindamycin* Cefoxitin	Penicillin† Metronidazole‡ Clindamycin Cefoxitin
Alternatives	Chloramphenicol	Chloramphenicol
New drugs with good in vitro activity, but limited clinical experience	Imipenem Ampicillin-sulbactam Ticarcillin-clavulanic acid	Imipenem Ampicillin-sulbactam Ticarcillin-clavulanic acid

* Usually need to be given along with aerobic gram-negative bacterial coverage.
† The drug of choice for serious systemic clostridial infections
‡ Usually need to be given with aerobic gram-positive coverage in infections originating above diaphragm.

knowledge of the pathogens likely to be present in a specific clinical setting, in combination with the Gram-stain findings which should suggest the likelihood of certain species of organisms. Because many anaerobic infections tend to be mixed with coliforms and other facultative organisms, it is advisable, in general, to use drugs active against both aerobic and anaerobic components. If anaerobes are suspected, the choices of antibiotics can be made reliably since patterns of antimicrobial susceptibility are usually predictable (see Chap. 85 and Table 108-1).

Organisms belonging to the B. fragilis group or the species B. bivius are resistant to penicillin. In general they do not play a significant role in infections originating above the diaphragm, such as head and neck infections, pleuropulmonary infections, and central nervous system infections. However, septic processes originating below the diaphragm, including in the pelvic and abdominal cavity, frequently contain these bacteria and specific microbial therapy directed at penicillin-resistant anaerobic organisms should be employed. Treatment of infections arising from sources above the diaphragm with penicillin is accepted. Depending on the site of infection and the severity, the dose of penicillin recommended is variable. For the treatment of lung abscesses a dose of 6 to 12 million units of penicillin G per day for at least 4 weeks is recommended. Infrequently, infections arising from oral organisms will fail to respond to penicillin. In such cases these patients should be treated with drugs such as metronidazole or clindamycin which are effective against penicillin-resistant anaerobes. Occasional resistance of oral Bacteroides such as B. melaninogenicus to penicillin may account for some of these treatment failures.

Infections arising from a colonic source are likely to contain B. fragilis. Many therapeutic failures have been noted in patients with documented B. fragilis infection who are treated with penicillin or first-generation cephalosporins. In intraabdominal sepsis the use of antibiotics effective against anaerobes has clearly reduced the incidence of postoperative infection and serious infectious complications. The number of antimicrobial agents effective against B. fragilis has expanded and there are currently several choices which are useful (Table 108-1). In general, greater than 80 percent cure rates can be achieved in patients with B. fragilis infection when treated with appropriate antimicrobial therapy and drainage.

Several classes of antibiotics are active in the treatment of Bacteroides infection: (1) metronidazole; (2) clindamycin; (3) cefoxitin and selected other cephalosporins; (4) chloramphenicol; (5) broader spectrum penicillins when used in combination with β-lactamase inhibitors, such as ticarcillin-clavulanic acid, or ampicillin-sulbactam; and (6) imipenem. Of the newer types of antibiotics, the quinolines are notable for absence of activity against B. fragilis. In vitro metronidazole and clindamycin are the most active against B.

fragilis group organisms of any current classes of antibiotics. Resistance rates are high to tetracycline, cefoperazone, and cefotaxime and these drugs should not be used. Resistance to cefoxitin varies from 8 to 30 percent. In contrast, clindamycin resistance is encountered in approximately 5 percent of anaerobic isolates, and metronidazole resistance is uncommon. Cefotetan may be potentially useful for treatment of *B. fragilis* infection but is less active against non-*fragilis* *Bacteroides* species. In general, *B. fragilis* species are more sensitive to the third generation cephalosporins than other organisms of the *B. fragilis* group. In some patients treated with cefoxitin alone, treatment failures occur because of emergence of facultative gram-negative bacilli resistant to cefoxitin.

Resistance of *B. fragilis* has rarely been reported with metronidazole. This well-tolerated drug achieves significant serum levels and also can be found in high levels within abscess cavities. It should be considered first-line therapy against *B. fragilis* infection. The two other widely used drugs, clindamycin and cefoxitin, also could be considered as first-line therapy because despite the reports of in vitro resistance of *B. fragilis* to these agents, there are only scattered case reports of clinical failure. If a patient fails to respond to one of these drugs, consideration should be given to alternative therapy and to determining the resistance patterns among *B. fragilis* group isolates. Although in vitro resistance to chloramphenicol has not been reported, this drug does not appear to be as effective as others. Among new drugs, ampicillin-sulbactam, ticarcillin-clavulanic acid, and imipenem hold great promise in the treatment of *B. fragilis* infection.

Specific regimens must be tailored to the initial infecting site in clinical situations. Intraabdominal sepsis should be treated with an aminoglycoside plus either metronidazole, 7.5 mg/kg every 8 h, or clindamycin, 600 mg intravenously every 8 h. This regimen is the "gold standard" because it treats both facultative aerobic and strictly anaerobic gram-negative bacilli which are responsible for morbidity and mortality. If gram-positive bacteria are suspected, an appropriate penicillin should be added. Chloramphenicol can be used successfully in patients with anaerobic central nervous system infections at a dose of 30 to 60 mg/kg per day depending on the severity of illness. However, penicillin G and metronidazole also cross the blood-brain barrier and are bactericidal for many anaerobic organisms (see Chap. 354).

Nearly all the drugs mentioned have toxic side effects. These are described in detail in Chap. 85.

Anaerobic infections that have failed to respond to treatment or that relapse should be reassessed. Consideration should be given to additional surgical drainage or debridement. Superinfections with resistant gram-negative facultative or aerobic bacteria should be ruled out. Drug resistance must also be entertained particularly if chloramphenicol was the antibiotic used; repeated cultures should then yield the pathogenic organism.

Other supportive measures in the management of anaerobic infections include: careful attention to fluid and electrolyte balance since extensive local edema formation may lead to hypoalbuminemia; hemodynamic support for septic shock; immobilization of infected extremities; maintenance of adequate nutrition during chronic infections by parenteral hyperalimentation; relief of pain and anticoagulation with heparin for thrombophlebitis. Hyperbaric oxygen therapy is of no proven value.

REFERENCES

BARTLETT JG, FINEGOLD SM: Anaerobic infections of the lung and pleural space. Am Rev Resp Dis 110:56, 1974

BIELUCH VM et al: Clinical importance of cefoxitin-resistant *Bacteroides fragilis* isolates. Diagn Microbiol Infect Dis 2:119, 1987

FINEGOLD SM: *Anaerobic Bacteria in Human Disease.* New York, Academic, 1977

GIBBS RS: Microbiology of the female genital tract. Am J Obstet Gynecol 156:491, 1987

GORBACH SC: Anaerobic bacteria, in *Principles and Practices of Infectious Diseases,* 3d ed, GL Mandell et al (eds). New York, Wiley, 1990

———, BARTLETT JG: Anaerobic infections. N Engl J Med 290:1177, 1974

HARDING GKM et al: Prospective randomized comparative study of clindamycin, chloramphenicol and ticarcillin, each in combination with gentamicin in therapy for intraabdominal and female tract sepsis. J Infect Dis 142:384, 1980

KASPER DL et al: Virulence factors of anaerobic bacteria. Rev Infect Dis 1:246, 1979

——— et al: Capsular polysaccharides and lipopolysaccharides from two strains of *Bacteroides fragilis.* Rev Infect Dis 6:525, 1984

LEVIN S, GOODMAN LJ: Selected overview of nongynecologic surgical intraabdominal infections. Prophylaxis and therapy. Am J Med 79(5B):146, 1985

MATHISEN GE et al: Brain abscess and cerebritis. Rev Infect Dis 6:S101, 1984

NAKATA MN, LEWIS RP: Anaerobic bacteria in bone and joint infections. Rev Infect Dis 6:S165, 1984

NEWMAN MG: Anaerobic oral and dental infections. Rev Infect Dis 6:S107, 1984

ONDERDONK A et al: Use of a model of intraabdominal sepsis for studies of the pathogenicity of *Bacteroides fragilis.* Rev Infect Dis 6:S191, 1984

SUTTER VL et al: *Wadsworth Anaerobic Bacteriology Manual,* 3d ed. St Louis, Mosby, 1980

WEXLER HM, FINEGOLD SM: In vitro activity of imipenem against anaerobic bacteria. Rev Infect Dis 7:S417, 1985

ZALEZNIK DF, KASPER DL: *Bacteroides* species, in *Principles and Practice of Infectious Diseases,* 3d ed, GL Mandell et al (eds). New York, Wiley, 1990

———: Role of bacterial virulence factors in pathogenesis of anaerobic infections, in *Anaerobic Infections in Humans,* S. Finegold (ed). Orlando, FL, Academic, 1989

section 5   Diseases caused by gram-negative organisms

109   MENINGOCOCCAL INFECTIONS

J. McLEOD GRIFFISS

DEFINITION *Neisseria meningitidis* is an ordinary commensal of the human oropharynx that can cause a variety of diseases, most notably bacteremia and meningitis. Its pathogenic potential can be expressed as epidemic disease or as sporadic endemic cases and focal outbreaks.

ETIOLOGY Meningococci are gram-negative single cocci or diplococci with flattened adjacent sides. They grow well on media containing blood or serum at temperatures between 35 and 37°C in a moist atmosphere reduced in oxygen and containing 5 to 10 percent CO_2. The organism is recovered readily when fresh specimens are inoculated on warm chocolate agar and incubated 18 to 24 h in a candle jar or other apparatus that provides a suitable environment.

Neisseria make cytochrome oxidase, which is responsible for the positive "oxidase" test; species usually are differentiated by their ability to use simple and compound sugars as sources of energy. Typically, meningococci use both glucose and maltose. Meningococci differ from other *Neisseria* in that they are surrounded by a polysaccharide "capsule."

Meningococci are divided into serologic groups on the basis of antigenic differences among their capsular polysaccharides. Groups A, B, C, W, and Y cause most serious disease; other groups frequently colonize the oropharynx but only very rarely disseminate. The serogroups are further divided into serotypes and subtypes based on independent antigenic differences among outer membrane protein and glycolipid constituents.

EPIDEMIOLOGY The natural habitat of meningococci is the human throat. Transmission from person to person is through inhalation of droplets of infected oropharyngeal secretions. Colonization only rarely proceeds to disease, because specific antibodies and complement lyse the organisms as they enter the bloodstream and thereby provide an effective barrier to dissemination. The incidence of disseminated infection varies cyclically, with peaks of increased frequency occurring every 10 to 15 years and lasting 4 to 6 years. Each cycle spreads slowly and is called a "hyperendemic wave" to distinguish it from the truly endemic disease that occurs between waves. Hyperendemic waves are often punctuated by focal outbreaks. Widespread epidemics have been absent from temperate areas of the world since the end of World War II; hyperendemic waves continue to occur; the last was in 1981. The between-waves endemic incidence in temperate climates is a fairly constant 1 reported case per 100,000 population per year. The prevalence of meningococcal infection is also subject to seasonal influences; the lowest attack rate occurs in midsummer and the highest in winter and early spring.

Epidemic disease receives the greatest public attention. An epidemic begins as a focal outbreak in a demographically discrete population in which a strain of a single serotype, the "epidemic strain," emerges from among the endemic strains. In less developed areas the outbreak quickly spreads, develops high attack rates, and involves large segments of the community. It remains either multicentric or evolves in the same pattern as a hyperendemic wave. Each focal outbreak in multicentric epidemics lasts 1 to 3 years, while the epidemic as a whole may last 5 or more years. In developed areas foci usually involve economically deprived segments of the population and do not spread or develop into generalized epidemics.

Group A strains caused most epidemics in the United States in the first half of this century; since World War II, group B and C meningococci have caused outbreaks in both military and civilian populations. Hyperendemic waves are caused by group B, C, or W organisms that share a limited set of serotypes. Group A strains do not share serotypes with other groups and do not cause hyperendemic waves. Group W strains have been associated with endemic and hyperendemic disease only. Group Y organisms only cause sporadic disease in older children and teenagers. Endemic disease predominantly is caused by group B organisms of diverse serotypes.

The attack rate of endemic meningococcal disease is highest for children between 6 and 36 months of age. The age distribution of epidemic cases is always shifted to proportionately older individuals, and those of any age may be involved. The attack rate in household contacts of sporadic cases is up to 1000 times the overall endemic rate and may be as much as 15,000 times that of the general population in epidemic periods.

Carriers Between epidemics, 2 to 30 percent of individuals, depending on age, carry meningococci in their throats. When sporadic disease occurs, the carrier rate in close contacts may rise to 40 percent, and in closed populations or during epidemics, it may approach 100 percent. Despite this high carrier rate, the prevalence of meningococcal disease cannot be attributed to the prevailing carrier rate, because only a small proportion of the meningococci carried on the throats of those who share a patient's environment are of the same clonotype as the patient's and are able to cause disease. Case-to-case transmission of infection is rare; carriers, not patients, are the foci from which disease is spread. Although some individuals harbor meningococci for years, oropharyngeal infection is usually transient, and in 75 percent of carriers the organism disappears within a few weeks to a few months.

Immunity The occurrence of clinical disease is most dependent on the immunologic status of the host. Natural immunity is usually type-specific and develops in most individuals within the first two decades of life. Natural immunization may result from pharyngeal colonization during the first few years of life by a closely related bacterium, *Neisseria lactamica*. *N. lactamica* strains are genetically diverse but many share important outer membrane protein and lipooligosaccharide antigens with virulent strains of *N. meningitidis*. They are not encapsulated and therefore do not survive in the bloodstream to cause disseminated disease. *N. lactamica* colonizes the throat earlier in life than does *N. meningitidis*; colonized infants develop bactericidal antibodies that initiate complement-mediated lysis of a broad range of potentially pathogenic meningococci.

Colonization with *N. meningitidis* gradually replaces that with *N. lactamica* as the child grows older, and lactamica carriage is only rarely encountered in teenagers, in whom meningococcal carrier rates of 15 to 25 percent are the rule, regardless of season. Meningococcal carriage induces antibodies to the infecting strain as well as to other strains, thereby reinforcing and broadening naturally acquired immunity. Many enteric bacteria make capsules that are chemically similar to those of meningococci. Asymptomatic colonization with them can induce group-specific antibody. Second episodes of meningococcal disease are encountered. Deficiency of one of the terminal complement components, C6, C7, C8, or C9, is a risk factor for repeated episodes of bacteremia with pathogenic *Neisseria* and should always be sought in patients with second episodes.

PATHOGENESIS Meningococcal infection begins in the oropharynx. In most instances, this infection is subclinical, but occasionally mild symptoms develop. Dissemination from the pharynx is via the bloodstream, and generally is followed by clinical manifestations. Purulent meningitis, the most common manifestation, may predominate, or it may be associated with signs and symptoms of meningococcemia. Rarely, extensive inflammation may cause an acute diffuse encephalitis.

There is a correlation between susceptibility to meningococcal disease and the absence of complement-mediated bactericidal activity in serum. The pathogenetic mechanisms that account for the different epidemiologic forms of meningococcal disease all interfere with the generation of bactericidal activity by the membrane attack complex of complement (C5–9) (see Chap. 13). Hypogammaglobulinemia, deficiencies of complement components, and interference by the organisms' capsular polysaccharides with the effective deposition of the attack complex into its outer membrane account for endemic disease. Primary isolated IgM deficiency is a rare cause of susceptibility that is easy to detect and therefore disproportionately reported. Deficiencies of complement components are seen more frequently in patients than in the general population. They may be either primary or secondary. Approximately 1 in 1000 people are deficient in one or another of the five terminal components. Disseminated meningococcal and gonococcal infections occur with increased frequency in these patients. Inheritance of properdin deficiency and ineffective alternative pathway complement activity is sex-linked. Males in these pedigrees are at extremely high risk of fulminant meningococcal disease. Several systemic diseases can result in secondary deficiencies of complement components, primarily the early components of the classical pathway, and sporadic meningococcal disease. People with functional asplenia are also at increased risk of sporadic meningococcal disease, although pneumococcal disease is a much more common complication.

The generation of hyperendemic waves remains incompletely understood. An "out-of-phase" response to fluctuations in antibody levels in the population is a possible mechanism. Focal outbreaks during hyperendemic waves can be correlated with the presence of elevated levels of circulating, strain-specific IgA which blocks initiation of complement-mediated lysis by IgM or IgG, but the precise contribution of IgA-mediated susceptibility to hyperendemic waves remains unclear. When a sufficiently large part of the population has developed blocking serum IgA, conditions are established for an epidemic to occur. The environmental events that cause IgA levels to be elevated within the epidemic focus are not known with certainty, but epidemic disease has been correlated with prevalent enteric colonization with cross-reacting organisms. The extent of induction of blocking IgA in the epidemic focus may explain the extent and intensity of the epidemic as well as the failure of focal outbreaks to develop into generalized ones. Asplenia and coincidental diseases that interfere with the normal hepatic clearance of IgA, such as alcoholism, biliary tract disease, hemoglobinopathies, and hemosiderosis, increase susceptibility within the epidemic focus.

The meningococcal outer membrane contains lipooligosaccharides that are chemically and biologically similar to the lipopolysaccharide endotoxins of enteric bacilli. They induce tumor necrosis factor (TNF) and interleukin 1 (IL-1), which may be responsible for the hypotension and vascular collapse observed in fulminant meningococcemia and for the purpura and visceral hemorrhages associated with meningococcal bacteremia (see Chap. 89). Thrombosis of dermal venules, adrenal sinusoids, and renal glomerular capillaries is most commonly seen in patients who die of fulminant meningococcemia. The ability to form pili and release endotoxin from the outer membrane have been correlated with "virulence" and a poor prognosis, respectively.

CLINICAL MANIFESTATIONS   Of patients with meningococcal disease 90 to 95 percent have meningococcemia and/or meningitis.

Meningococcemia   Thirty to fifty percent of patients who develop overt disease have meningococcemia without meningitis. The onset of clinical illness may be abrupt, but patients usually have nonspecific prodromal symptoms of cough, headache, and sore throat followed by the sudden development of spiking fever, chills, arthralgias, and myalgias. Patients usually appear acutely ill with an inordinate degree of prostration. In addition to high fever, tachycardia, and tachypnea, mild hypotension may be present. However, clinical shock does not occur unless fulminant meningococcemia supervenes. In the course of meningococcal bacteremia, about three-fourths of the patients develop a characteristic petechial rash. Lesions are frequently sparse, and the axillae, flanks, wrists, and ankles are most commonly involved. Often petechiae are located in the center of lighter-colored macules, and they may become nodular as the disease progresses. The diagnosis of meningococcemia occasionally can be established by demonstrating gram-negative diplococci in scrapings from these nodular lesions. In severe cases, purpuric spots or large ecchymoses develop, and a widespread petechial or purpuric eruption suggests fulminating disease. However, the absence of rash does not necessarily indicate that the illness will be mild. The levels of circulating endotoxin, or of the cytokines it induces, are sensitive markers for the development of fulminant disease and a poor prognosis.

Fulminant meningococcemia, or the Waterhouse-Friderichsen syndrome, is meningococcemia associated with vasomotor collapse and shock. It occurs in the 10 to 20 percent of patients in whom high levels of endotoxin circulate. The onset is abrupt, and profound prostration frequently occurs within a few hours. Petechiae and purpuric lesions enlarge rapidly, and hemorrhage into the skin may be extensive. Early in the preshock stage, there is generalized vasoconstriction; patients are alert and pale, with circumoral cyanosis and cold extremities. Upon entering the shock stage, however, the cardiac output decreases, and the blood pressure falls; mentation decreases and coma may develop. Despite appropriate therapy, 40 to 60 percent of patients die from cardiac and/or respiratory failure. Patients who recover may have extensive sloughing of skin lesions or loss of digits because of gangrene.

Occult meningococcemia is an uncommon form of meningococcal infection that affects children between the ages of 3 and 24 months. It is characterized by fever and bacteremia without an obvious source. Infection usually resolves without treatment but may lead to the development of meningitis or other metastatic infection.

Chronic meningococcemia is a very rare form of meningococcal infection that lasts for weeks or months and is characterized by fever, rash, and arthritis or arthralgia. Typically, the fever is intermittent, and during afebrile periods, which may last several days, patients appear remarkably well. The usual maculopapular or polymorphous rash waxes and wanes with the fever. Petechial and nodular lesions are occasionally seen. Joint involvement is present in two-thirds of the patients, and splenomegaly is detected in about 20 percent. If treatment is delayed, meningitis, carditis, or nephritis may occur.

Meningitis   Meningitis is a common form of meningococcal disease that occurs primarily in children from 6 months to 10 years. Fever, vomiting, headache, and confusion or lethargy are the most common symptoms; in about one-fourth of the patients, symptoms begin abruptly and rapidly increase in severity. The more typical patient, however, has symptoms of an upper respiratory tract infection followed by an illness that progresses over several days. Twenty to forty percent of patients have meningitis without clinical evidence of meningococcemia, and the diagnosis depends upon bacteriologic examination of the cerebrospinal fluid. However, when meningitis occurs in association with a petechial or purpuric rash, a presumptive diagnosis of meningococcal disease is warranted because this pattern of illness is seen only rarely in other infections.

Rarer manifestations   The meningococcus may cause purulent conjunctivitis or sinusitis. Primary pneumonia occurs rarely, but secondary pneumonia not infrequently follows viral respiratory infections, particularly influenza. Bacterial endocarditis, primary pericarditis, arthritis, and osteomyelitis have also been reported. Meningococci can also produce genital infections clinically indistinguishable from gonococcal disease, including urethritis and endometritis.

LABORATORY FINDINGS   Aside from bacteriologic data, laboratory studies are of little value in establishing a specific diagnosis of meningococcal infection. Polymorphonuclear leukocyte counts usually are elevated but may be normal or low in meningococcemia; a left shift usually is present. Patients with hemorrhagic manifestations may have low platelet counts and decreased levels of circulating clotting factors as a result of disseminated intravascular coagulation (see Chap. 62). In meningitis, the cerebrospinal fluid (CSF) pressure is increased; the fluid usually contains from 10,000 to 40,000 polymorphonuclear leukocytes per microliter; the protein content is increased, and the concentration of glucose is low (see Chap. 354).

Meningococci usually can be recovered from cultures of blood or spinal fluid and, on occasion, of material aspirated from skin lesions or joints. In addition, gram-negative diplococci may be seen in stains of nodular petechiae or the buffy coat of blood from patients with meningococcemia. In meningococcal meningitis, a smear of the spinal fluid is diagnostic in about half the patients but often shows only a few intracellular bacteria, which are located with difficulty, particularly early in the course of the infection, when organisms may be present in the absence of CSF abnormalities. The infecting organisms shed their capsular polysaccharide, which usually can be detected in CSF, joint fluid, serum, or urine with use of highly specific antibodies in counterimmunoelectrophoresis (CIE) or latex agglutination (LA) assays. The sensitivity of these assays is dependent on the antibodies used and is least for group B; LA is somewhat more sensitive and easier to perform. In general, the immunoassays are more sensitive than culture alone and in combination with the Gram stain will provide a diagnosis in over 98 percent of cases. They are particularly helpful early in infection and when the patient has been treated with antibiotics, causing negative cultures.

COMPLICATIONS   Herpes labialis occurs in 5 to 20 percent of patients with meningococcal disease. Other complications, which result from neurologic damage or secondary foci of infection, are uncommon following appropriate treatment and are often transient. Seizures or deafness occur in 10 to 20 percent of patients during the acute stages of meningitis, but postmeningitic epilepsy is rare, and the frequency of permanent nerve damage is probably less than 5 percent. A number of patients complain of recurrent headache, emotional lability, insomnia, backache, memory loss, and difficulty in concentrating for months after an episode of meningitis. These symptoms usually disappear a year or two after the infection.

Septic arthritis is a not uncommon complication of meningococcemia that may accompany meningitis or occur as the only metastatic manifestation. The joint fluid usually contains many granulocytes (see Chap. 96), but meningococci are recovered infrequently. It can be diagnosed by Gram stain, CIE, or LA, or by recovery of the organism on culture. It is treated in the same way as meningitis; recovery without sequelae is to be expected.

Immune-complex arthritis occurs in about 10 percent of patients during convalescence. As a rule, multiple joints are involved, primarily the larger ones. Inflammation appears between days 7 and 15 of treatment when newly produced antibodies form insoluble complexes with the infecting organism's capsular polysaccharide. No specific therapy is indicated; permanent joint changes are rare.

Other pyogenic complications have become extremely uncommon since antibiotics have been used routinely. Bacterial endocarditis is quite rare, but a high proportion of patients who die of meningococcal infection have myocarditis. A pericardial friction rub or electrocardiographic changes of pericarditis are seen in about 5 percent of patients; rarely, purulent pericarditis may develop.

DIAGNOSIS The diagnosis of meningococcal disease depends upon recovering *N meningitidis* or detecting antigens in blood, spinal fluid, joint fluid, urine, or petechial scrapings from patients with a typical clinical picture. Capsular polysaccharides of serogroups A, B, C, Y, and W can be detected in fluids by LA or CIE. Recovery of meningococci from the pharynx does not establish the diagnosis of meningococcal disease; throat cultures are not indicated.

Few diseases need to be considered seriously in the differential diagnosis of meningococcal disease. If meningococcal meningitis is not accompanied by rash or other manifestations of bacteremia, it is indistinguishable from meningitis caused by other common pathogens (see Chap. 354). Occasionally, the common viral exanthems, mycoplasma infection, Rocky Mountain spotted fever (see Chap. 153), and vascular purpuras (see Chaps. 58 and 276) may be confused with meningococcemia.

TREATMENT In the absence of fulminant meningococcemia the treatment of meningococcal disease is not difficult, and the mortality rate should not exceed 5 percent. Therapy should be instituted as early as possible. Penicillin G is the drug of choice, and should be administered intravenously. The usual dosage for treatment of meningitis in adults with normal renal function is 12 to 24 million units per day (2 to 4 million units intravenously every 4 h), and in the pediatric age group, 300,000 to 400,000 units per kilogram per day, intravenously every 4 h in divided doses. When treatment is continued for a minimum of 7 days, or 4 to 5 days after the patient becomes afebrile, relapse is extremely rare. Chloramphenicol is just as effective as penicillin and may be the drug of choice in less-developed countries. It should be used when a patient is allergic to penicillin in a dosage of 50 mg/kg or, in adults, 2.0 to 4.0 g/d in divided doses every 4 h given intravenously until the patient is able to take oral medication. Some of the third-generation cephalosporins, such as cefotaxime, ceftriaxone, or cefuroxime (see Chaps. 85 and 354), are also effective and are often used to initiate therapy when the etiology of meningitis is uncertain. A significant proportion of meningococci are resistant to sulfonamides, so these should not be used routinely unless the infecting organism is shown to be susceptible. Sulfadiazine (2 to 3 g initially followed by 1 g 6-hourly thereafter given intravenously until the patient can take oral medication) or trimethoprim/sulfamethoxazole (160/800 mg intravenously every 6 h) is effective treatment for susceptible strains. The dosages must be reduced in renal failure and in children, depending on age (see Chap. 85).

Patients with meningococcal infections require supportive treatment as well as antimicrobial therapy. Maintenance of fluid and electrolyte balance and prevention of respiratory complications in comatose patients are of primary concern. When shock occurs, visceral perfusion must be improved. Vasoactive drugs should be employed according to the pathophysiologic derangement (see Chaps. 39 and 89). When disseminated intravascular coagulation is recognized, treatment with heparin, whole blood, or fibrinogen can be tried, but these are not certain to be effective.

PROGNOSIS Before the introduction of antibiotics, meningococcal meningitis and meningococcemia were almost invariably fatal. With prompt and appropriate chemotherapy, the mortality rate of meningitis without fulminant meningococcemia has dropped to less than 10 percent in the United States, and neurologic sequelae are rare. The mortality of fulminant infection remains high primarily

because patients are often in irreversible shock when treatment is instituted. Most deaths occur within 24 to 48 h of admission, and the capacity of the meningococcus to kill a previously healthy individual within a few hours remains one of the most awesome characteristics of this disease.

PREVENTION The capsular polysaccharides from organisms of serogroups A, C, Y, and W induce group specific bactericidal antibody responses after subcutaneous injection. A tetravalent vaccine containing these antigens is available for use to prevent or control outbreaks. Routine immunization of recruits has eliminated nearly all disease among military personnel, but in the United States immunization is recommended routinely only for travelers to areas where epidemic disease is occurring and for individuals with complement deficiencies or splenic dysfunction. An effective group B vaccine has not been developed. Chemoprophylaxis should be administered to intimate (usually household) contacts of sporadic cases. If the organism isolated from the patient is sensitive to sulfonamides, 2 days of prophylaxis with one of these drugs is recommended. When sensitivities are not known or the organism is resistant to sulfonamides, rifampin in a dosage of 600 mg every 12 h for 2 days for adults and 5 to 10 mg/kg every 12 h for children can be expected to eradicate the carrier state temporarily and minimize spread of meningococci. Vaccination is over 99 percent effective in preventing secondary cases (as compared with approximately 89 percent effectiveness for rifampin chemoprophylaxis), and vaccination of household or other intimate contacts should be encouraged.

REFERENCES

BRANDTZAEG P et al: Plasma endotoxin as a predictor of multiple organ failure and death in systemic meningococcal disease. J Infect Dis 159:195, 1989

COUNTS GW et al: Group A meningococcal disease in the U.S. Pacific Northwest: Epidemiology, clinical features, and effect of a vaccination control program. Rev Infect Dis 6:640, 1984

CROWE BA et al: Clonal and variable properties of *Neisseria meningitidis* isolated from cases and carriers during and after an epidemic in The Gambia, West Africa. J Infect Dis 159:686, 1989

DENSEN P et al: Familial properdin deficiency and fatal meningococcemia: Correction of the bactericidal defect by vaccination. N Engl J Med 316:922, 1987

ELLISON RT et al: Prevalence of congenital or acquired complement deficiency in patients with sporadic meningococcal disease. N Engl J Med 308:913, 1983

GRIFFISS J McL: Epidemic meningococcal disease: Synthesis of a hypothetical immunoepidemiologic model. Rev Infect Dis 4:159, 1982

JARVIS GA et al: Sialic acid of group B *Neisseria meningitidis* regulates alternative complement pathway activation. Infect Immun 55:174, 1987

KIM JJ et al: *Neisseria lactamica* and *Neisseria meningitidis* share lipooligosaccharide epitopes but lack common capsular and class 1, 2, and 3 protein epitopes. Infect Immun 57:602, 1989

WOLF RE, BIRBARA CA: Meningococcal infections at an army training center. Am J Med 44:243, 1968

110 GONOCOCCAL INFECTIONS

KING K. HOLMES / STEPHEN A. MORSE

DEFINITION Gonorrhea, an infection of columnar and transitional epithelium caused by *Neisseria gonorrhoeae*, is the most common reportable communicable disease in the United States. Anatomic sites which can be infected directly by the gonococcus include the urethra, rectum, conjunctivas, pharynx, and endocervix. Local complications include endometritis, salpingitis, peritonitis, and bartholinitis in the female, and periurethral abscess and epididymitis in the male. Systemic manifestations of gonococcemia include arthritis, dermatitis, endocarditis, and meningitis as well as myopericarditis and hepatitis.

ETIOLOGY *Neisseria gonorrhoeae* is a gram-negative coccus usually found in pairs with flattened adjacent sides. It forms oxidase-positive colonies and is differentiated from other *Neisseria* by its

FIGURE 110-1 Diagram of the envelope of *N. gonorrhoeae*, showing structures thought to influence pathogenesis, antimicrobial susceptibility, and antigenicity.

ability to utilize glucose but not maltose, sucrose, or lactose, and by specific immunologic reactions.

Colonies examined within 20 h of inoculation from clinical specimens contain organisms covered by fimbriae (pili). As the colonies grow older, their appearance changes, reflecting the loss of pili. Piliated organisms cause infection and urethritis after inoculation into the urethras of male volunteers, whereas nonpiliated organisms do not. Pili mediate attachment to various epithelial cells and interfere with neutrophil phagocytosis. Each pilus is composed of repeating peptide subunits (pilin) which have a molecular weight of about 20,000. The pilin subunits consist of conserved and variable regions. Pili undergo both *antigenic* and *phase variation*. Chromosomal rearrangements, leading to expression of any one of a large number of incomplete (silent) pilin genes, lead to antigenic variation in pili (pil α, pil β, etc.). If the rearrangement involves a defective pilin gene, piliated gonococci (pil⁺) produce nonpiliated variants (pil⁻), a process known as *phase variation*. Antigenic variation of pilin may allow gonococci to adapt rapidly to attachment onto different types of epithelial surfaces and to evade the host's antibody response to pilin. Phase variation from pil⁺ to pil⁻ may permit attachment and then persistence and spread.

The trilaminar outer membrane of the gonococcus contains several classes of proteins, including proteins I, II, and III, and lipopolysaccharide (Fig. 110-1). Like pili, protein II (now referred to as opacity-associated outer membrane proteins, or OPAs) also is thought to function as a ligand, mediating the attachment of gonococci to various types of human cells. As in the case with pili, individual strains of gonococci may or may not express OPAs. The serologic diversity of OPAs are relatively limited; up to seven or eight different OPAs may be expressed at different times by the same strain, and from zero to three may be expressed in the same gonococcal cell. The presence or absence of OPAs also influences colony opacity, and certain OPAs may be responsible for the clumping of gonococci that is so evident on Gram-stained smears of urethral exudate.

Opaque colonies contain organisms that express OPAs and predominate in isolates from the male urethra and in cervical isolates obtained from women in midcycle. Transparent colonies often lack OPAs and predominate in isolates from women during menses, and in isolates from blood, synovial fluid, or fallopian tubes.

Protein I (~32,000 mol wt) is quantitatively the major outer membrane protein. It appears to associate as a trimeric molecule, forming transmembrane channels (porins) that permit exchange of hydrophilic molecules through the outer membrane. Protein I also interacts with other outer membrane components, such as protein III and lipopolysaccharide (LPS), to form complex outer membrane structures. Protein molecules have been shown to move rapidly from gonococcal outer membranes to the more fluid cytoplasmic membrane of human cells. This process may initiate endocytosis of the gonococcus, the first step in gonococcal invasion of the epithelium.

The LPS of the gonococcus contains lipid A and an oligosaccharide. Gonococci have the ability to vary the composition of the oligosaccharide component of the LPS by a mechanism that is not well understood. One of the oligosaccharides is associated with serum resistance in *N. gonorrhoeae*. No capsular polysaccharide has been isolated, but high-molecular-weight surface polyphosphates have been demonstrated that may have functions similar to those of capsular polysaccharides in other organisms.

Gonococcal typing Gonococcal strains can be typed on the basis of nutritional requirements (auxotyping) or surface antigenic variation of protein I. Unlike pili and protein II, the protein I expressed by any single strain of gonococcus is antigenically stable, although there is considerable antigenic heterogeneity of protein I between strains. There are two structurally related forms of protein I, known as IA and IB, and individual strains contain either but not both. Protein IA and IB genes are alleles of the same gene. Monoclonal antibodies against different epitopes of protein IA and protein IB can be used to classify gonococci into a large number of serovariants, known as serovars IA1 to IA24, and IB1 to IB32.

EPIDEMIOLOGY The only natural hosts for *N. gonorrhoeae* are humans. In the United States the annual age-specific incidence rates tripled from 1963 to 1975, when over 1 million cases were reported and an equal number probably went unreported. During this period of epidemic gonorrhea, the incidence increased fastest in young white females. The incidence of gonorrhea has decreased from a peak of 473 cases per 100,000 in 1975 to about 300 per 100,000 in 1988.

Gonorrhea incidence and prevalence rates are known to be related to age, sex, sex preference, race, socioeconomic status, marital status, urban residence, and level of education—risk factors which influence sexual behavior, illness behavior, and accessibility of health care. Among sexually active individuals, the highest rates occur in teenagers, in nonwhites, in the poor and poorly educated, in large cities, and in unmarried persons—particularly those who live alone. Such individuals comprise a "core group" of "efficient transmitters" who play a disproportionate role in the spread of gonorrhea. Since 1985, the incidence of gonorrhea has continued to fall among white men and women, but has levelled off or increased among black men and women. There is some evidence that the spread of gonorrhea, like that of syphilis and chancroid, is associated with the crack cocaine epidemic and with exchange of sex by women for illegal drugs such as cocaine. The incidence of gonorrhea is highest in men, while the prevalence is highest in women. The prevalence rate is so high among women in the United States that routine endocervical cultures have been advocated for gonorrhea case detection in asymptomatic women age 30 or under who are considered to be at high risk because of sexual behavior or demographic factors cited above. However, greater reliance should be placed upon partner notification (contact tracing), which is far more efficient for control of gonorrhea, than upon routine endocervical culturing, which is expensive and does not focus on those most likely to transmit the infection. The single most important axiom about the epidemiology of this disease is that *gonorrhea is usually spread by carriers who have no symptoms or have ignored symptoms.* Symptomatic patients, male or female, have usually been recently infected by such carriers, who must in turn be traced and treated to prevent reinfection. *Men and women with symptomatic gonorrhea should always be interviewed to identify their recent sex contacts, who should be examined and treated if infected.* The growing association of gonorrhea, syphilis, and chancroid with the exchange of sex for drugs such as crack cocaine presents a new and unique challenge for sexually transmitted disease (STD) control and calls for intensified and innovative control efforts.

There are interesting regional differences in the antibiotic resistance of *N. gonorrhoeae*. In 1976, penicillinase-producing strains of *N. gonorrhoeae* (PPNG), completely resistant to penicillin and ampicillin, appeared almost simultaneously in two areas of the world: in England, where they had probably been imported from west Africa, and in the United States, where they had been imported from the Philippines. PPNG first became established and then spread in areas of the world where prostitution is exceptionally common and where access to subcurative antimicrobial therapy is unrestricted. PPNG now comprise 50 percent or more of all gonococci in many areas of Africa and Asia, and have by now become well established in many regions of the United States (e.g., Miami, New York, Los Angeles) and Europe. Plasmid-borne penicillin resistance results from the presence of a TEM-type β-lactamase gene on one of five small R factors which make up a very closely related family of plasmids. Plasmid-borne, tetracycline resistant *N. gonorrhoeae* (TRNG) is a highly resistant strain that results from the introduction of the streptococcal resistance determinant *tetM* into *N. gonorrhoeae*, where it resides on a plasmid derived in part from a conjugative plasmid. This new plasmid is self-transmissible and retains the capacity to mobilize some of the β-lactamase plasmids. TRNG are clinically resistant to tetracycline, minocycline, and doxycycline. Of equal importance has been the spread of gonococci with chromosomally mediated resistance to penicillin and tetracycline. These strains are referred to as chromosomally mediated resistant *Neisseria gonorrhoeae* (CMRNG). Auxotyping and monoclonal antibody serotyping have shown that in a midsized metropolitan city, as many as 60 to 100 different gonococcal strains are circulating, and new strains are being continuously introduced. Against this background, local outbreaks of PPNG, TRNG, or CMRNG belonging to a single auxotype-serovar class have been identified, and public health efforts have at times been successfully focused on the control of such strains.

IMMUNOLOGY AND PATHOGENESIS Epidemiologic data suggest that only about one-third of men become infected after a single exposure to gonorrhea, and under experimental conditions an inoculum of 10^3 organisms appears necessary to establish urethral infection in 50 percent of male volunteers. Factors that may confer resistance to infection are undefined. Components of the urethral or vaginal flora, such as *Candida albicans, Staphylococcus epidermidis,* and certain types of lactobacilli, can inhibit *N. gonorrhoeae* in vitro and may provide some natural resistance in vivo. Lactoferrin is present at mucosal surfaces, where it presumably competes with gonococci for iron, which is required for growth of the organism. However, when low environmental concentrations of iron are growth-limiting, gonococci produce iron repressible proteins, or FeRPs, that function in the removal of iron from lactoferrin or transferrin. Strains of gonococci requiring arginine, hypoxanthine, and uracil (AHU) for growth are generally unable to remove iron from lactoferrin, which could explain the tendency of such strains to cause asymptomatic mucosal infections. Gonococci infect mucus-secreting epithelial surfaces, and mucus could be a physical barrier or competitive inhibitor.

Attachment of gonococci to mucosal cells is mediated in part by pili and by protein II. Local antibody to pili or protein II can partially block attachment. Pili also impede phagocytosis of gonococci by neutrophils, and antibody to pili (as well as antibody to protein II) is opsonic. An enzyme produced by the pathogenic *Neisseria* IgA1 protease, which inactivates sIgA1, may interfere with IgA-mediated antiadherence activity, resulting in increased attachment.

Following attachment to columnar or transitional epithelium, gonococci penetrate through or between cells to reach the subepithelial connective tissue. Transfer of gonococcal protein I into the host cell may initiate endocytosis by the epithelial cell. Gonococcal LPS and peptidoglycan are toxic for fallopian tube organ cultures. Gonococci also produce several proteases, peptidases, phospholipases, and elastases which may play a role in pathogenesis. In subepithelial tissue, and in blood, gonococci presumably interact with serum antibody, including natural IgM antibody directed against LPS antigens, with generation of the chemotactic factor C5a and formation of the bactericidal C5b-C9 attack complex. Insertion of the attack complex into the outer membrane of serum-sensitive gonococci results in gonococcal cell lysis making antibody to LPS (like antibody to protein I) bactericidal. Although an attack complex is also formed when serum interacts with gonococci characterized by stable serum resistance, the insertion of the complex into the outer membrane of the organism has an abnormal configuration which does not result in rapid cell lysis. Furthermore, human serum also appears to contain non-complement-fixing IgG antibody directed against protein III which blocks the bactericidal action of IgM antibody for strains of gonococci with stable serum resistance.

Following phagocytosis by neutrophils, the susceptibility of gonococci to intracellular killing is controversial. During in vivo growth, gonococci apparently develop phenotypic serum resistance and resistance to neutrophil-mediated killing. The mechanisms responsible for these phenotypic changes are largely undefined but appear to involve the binding of host-derived CMP-*N*-acetyl neuraminic acid.

Spread of gonococci from the cervix to the endometrium and salpinges may be enhanced in women using an intrauterine device. Menstruation further increases the risk of intraluminal ascent from the cervix and also predisposes to gonococcal bacteremia.

CLINICAL MANIFESTATIONS The clinical spectrum of gonococcal infections depends upon the site of inoculation, the duration of infection, the virulence of the infecting strain, and the presence or absence of local or systemic spread of the organism. The influence of inoculum size, variations in host susceptibility, and of coinfection with *C. trachomatis* or other genital pathogens on clinical manifestations has not been well-defined.

Gonorrhea in the male The usual incubation period of gonococcal urethritis ("clap") in the male is 2 to 7 days following exposure, although longer intervals are not infrequent, and some men never develop symptoms. In one study, one auxotype with distinctive nutritional requirements was associated with 96 percent of asymptomatic infections and only 40 percent of symptomatic infections. Symptoms of urethritis include a purulent urethral discharge, usually associated with dysuria, frequent urination, and meatal erythema.

Although approximately 90 to 95 percent of men who acquire urethral gonococcal infection develop urethral discharge, most symptomatic men seek treatment and are removed from the infectious pool. The remaining men who never develop symptoms or who ignore their symptoms constitute about two-thirds of the infected men at any point in time, and they serve as the main source of spread of infection to women. Before antibiotic treatment became available, symptoms of urethritis persisted for an average of 8 weeks, and unilateral epididymitis occurred in 5 to 10 percent of untreated men. Epididymitis is now an uncommon complication (see below), and gonococcal prostatitis occurs rarely, if at all. Other local complications of gonococcal urethritis which are now unusual include inguinal lymphadenitis, edema of the penis due to dorsal lymphangitis or thrombophlebitis, submucous inflammatory "soft" infiltration of the urethral wall, periurethral abscess or fistula, unilateral inflammation or abscess of Cowper's gland (which lies between the thumb and forefinger when the forefinger is in the anal canal and the thumb is positioned anteriorly on the perineum), and, rarely, seminal vesiculitis.

In homosexual men, the frequency of gonococcal infection has fallen by 90 percent in many parts of the United States during the AIDS era of the 1980s. Gonococcal isolates from homosexual men tend to be more resistant to antimicrobials than are isolates from heterosexuals. This may be due to the fact that certain highly susceptible strains are rapidly killed by bile salts and fatty acids in feces and rarely occur in homosexual men, while gonococci possessing a gene for multidrug resistance (*mtr*) are resistant to bile salts and fatty acids and occur with increased frequency in homosexual men. Rectal infection may be asymptomatic from the outset or may produce anorectal pain, pruritus, tenesmus, and a bloody, mucopurulent rectal discharge. Proctoscopy and appropriate laboratory studies are essential to exclude several other conditions which cause similar symptoms (see Chap. 93). These symptoms may subside without treatment, leaving a chronic asymptomatic carrier state. Pharyngeal gonococcal infection occurs in approximately 20 percent of homosexual men or heterosexual women who engage in fellatio with men who have urethral infection, and in a smaller proportion of heterosexual men who engage in cunnilingus. Pharyngeal infection may produce exudative tonsillitis but frequently is asymptomatic; asymptomatic pharyngeal gonococcal infection usually clears spontaneously over several weeks, even without therapy.

Gonorrhea in the female Acute uncomplicated gonorrhea in the female often causes dysuria, frequent urination, increased vaginal discharge due to exudative endocervicitis, abnormal menstrual bleeding, and anorectal discomfort. While dysuria and frequency in young men arouse the suspicion of gonococcal urethritis, the same symptoms in a young woman are often automatically attributed to "cystitis." Actually, some of those without bacteriuria have gonococcal or chlamydial infection of the urethra. Young women with dysuria should have a thorough pelvic examination. Compression of the urethra through the anterior vaginal wall against the symphysis pubis may express urethral exudate which can be examined by Gram's stain and culture. Symptomatic young women with "sterile pyuria" (i.e., ≥10 neutrophils per 100× microscopic field in the centrifuged sediment of clean-catch midstream urine; no uropathogens isolated from the urine) should be evaluated for gonococcal and chlamydial infection. Acute symptoms of gonococcal urethritis in the female may subside spontaneously or following subcurative therapy with sulfonamides or urinary antiseptics. The proportion of women with gonorrhea who never develop symptoms is undefined.

Asymptomatic gonococcal infection in the female involves the endocervix, urethra, anal canal, and pharynx, in decreasing order of frequency. Extension of infection from the endocervix to the fallopian tubes occurs in at least 15 percent of women with gonorrhea. This tends to occur soon after acquisition of infection or during menstruation and results in acute endometritis, with abnormal menstrual bleeding and midline low abdominal pain and tenderness, followed by *acute salpingitis*, the major complication of gonorrhea. Coexisting *C. trachomatis* infection may increase the rate of pelvic inflammatory disease (PID). Extension of infection to the pelvis may produce signs of pelvic peritonitis, accompanied by nausea and vomiting, and may lead to pelvic abscess. Early antibiotic treatment, before development of adnexal masses, restores normal tubal function and fertility in nearly all cases of gonococcal salpingitis. However, if prominent adnexal swelling has occurred before treatment is begun, bilateral tubal damage occurs in 15 to 25 percent.

Spread of gonococci or chlamydia into the upper abdomen may cause *perihepatitis* (Fitz-Hugh–Curtis syndrome) manifested by right upper quadrant or bilateral upper abdominal pain and tenderness, and occasionally by a hepatic friction rub.

Acute inflammation of Bartholin's gland is usually unilateral and frequently is due to gonococcal infection. The acutely infected duct is surrounded by a red halo and exudes pus at the posterior third of the labium majus. Occlusion of the duct results in formation of a Bartholin's abscess. Chronic Bartholin cysts are rarely caused by active gonococcal infection.

There is suggestive evidence that peripartum endocervical gonococcal infection is associated with premature rupture of membranes, preterm delivery, and postpartum endometritis.

Gonorrhea in children During childbirth, the gonococcus may infect the conjunctivas, pharynx, respiratory tract, or anal canal of the newborn. The risk of contamination increases with prolonged rupture of membranes. Prevention of gonococcal ophthalmia by prophylactic use of 1% silver nitrate eyedrops or ophthalmic preparations containing erythromycin or tetracycline is a cost-effective measure in most areas of the world, including the United States. Since neonates and young infants lack bactericidal IgM antibody against *N. gonorrhoeae*, they may be at increased risk for gonococcal bacteremia. During the first year of life, infection of the infant usually results from accidental contamination of the eye or vagina by an adult. Between 1 year of age and puberty, many cases of gonorrhea involve vulvovaginitis in females who have been molested, and medicolegal considerations necessitate a complete bacteriologic diagnosis and child welfare consultation. Auxotyping and serotyping of isolates from the sexual assault victim and accused assailant have been used as evidence in court.

Disseminated gonococcal infection The incidence of disseminated gonococcal infection (DGI) varies with time and place, in relation to the local incidence of infection with strains of gonococci that have a propensity to produce bacteremia. Approximately two-thirds of patients with DGI are women, and symptoms of bacteremia often begin during menses. The majority of men and women with gonococcemia do not have symptoms of urogenital, anorectal, or pharyngeal gonococcal infection.

Patients typically present either with symptoms and signs of gonococcemia, or with purulent arthritis affecting one or two joints. The onset of gonococcemia is characterized by fever, polyarthralgias, and papular, petechial, pustular, hemorrhagic, or necrotic skin lesions. Approximately 3 to 20 such lesions appear, usually on the distal extremities. Gonococci are demonstrable by immunofluorescent staining in about two-thirds of gonococcal skin lesions. The initial joint involvement is characteristically limited to tenosynovitis involving several joints asymmetrically. The wrists, fingers, knees, and ankles are most often involved. Circulating immune complexes have been demonstrated at this stage of infection in some studies. Serum complement levels are normal (except in those with complement deficiency), and the role of immune complexes, if any, is uncertain. Without treatment, the duration of gonococcemia is variable; the systemic manifestations of bacteremia may subside spontaneously within a week. Alternatively, septic arthritis ensues, often without prior symptoms of fever, polyarthralgias, or skin lesions. Pain and swelling then increase in one or, very occasionally, more joints, with accumulation of purulent synovial fluid, leading to progressive destruction of the joint if treatment is delayed.

IgM antibody to gonococcal lipopolysaccharide, present in normal human serum, is bactericidal for most strains of gonococci in the presence of complement. Gonococci isolated from patients with DGI have stable resistance to normal human serum. These strains usually contain outer membrane protein IA, and are highly susceptible to penicillin. They often require arginine, hypoxanthine, and uracil for growth, and belong to the AHU auxotype. Patients deficient in complement components C5, C6, C7, and C8 are uniquely susceptible to gonococcemia and meningococcemia because they cannot mount a serum bactericidal response to gonococci or meningococci. Strains isolated from these patients may not be resistant to normal human serum. However, gonococci isolated from DGI patients without complement deficiency are resistant to pooled normal human serum. Isolates from patients with tenosynovitis and skin lesions are even more serum resistant than are isolates from patients with purulent arthritis, suggesting that the two different DGI syndromes may be determined by characteristics of the causative organism.

The probability of positive blood cultures decreases after 48 h of illness, and the probability of recovery of gonococci from synovial fluid increases with increasing duration of illness. Gonococci are infrequently recovered from early effusions containing less than 20,000 leukocytes per microliter, but are usually recovered from effusions containing more than 80,000 leukocytes per microliter. In the individual patient, gonococci are seldom recovered from blood and synovial fluid simultaneously.

Other common manifestations of disseminated gonococcal infection include mild myopericarditis and "toxic" hepatitis. Endocarditis and meningitis are infrequent but severe complications. Endocarditis is suggested by pathologic or changing heart murmurs, major embolic phenomena, severe myocarditis, deterioration of renal function, or an unusually large number of skin lesions.

DIFFERENTIAL DIAGNOSIS Gonococcal infection produces several common clinical syndromes which have multiple etiologies or which mimic other conditions. In particular, the epidemiology and clinical manifestations of *Chlamydia trachomatis* infections closely resemble those of gonococcal infections. The differential diagnosis of urethritis, epididymitis, and proctitis in men, vaginitis and cervicitis in women, and of acute arthritis in young adults is discussed in Chap. 93. The differential diagnosis of pelvic inflammatory disease is discussed in Chap. 94.

LABORATORY DIAGNOSIS A presumptive diagnosis of gonorrhea may be made if intracellular gram-negative diplococci are observed in leukocytes on Gram-stained smears of urethral or endocervical exudate. A diagnosis is equivocal if only extracellular or atypical gram-negative diplococci are seen, and is negative if no gram-negative diplococci are seen. When these criteria are employed by experienced microbiologists, the sensitivity and specificity of Gram's stain of the urethral exudate approach 100 percent. Presumptive diagnosis of gonorrhea cannot be made on the basis of gram-negative diplococci in pharyngeal smears because other *Neisseria* spp. are normal flora at this site. In areas where resistant gonococci are seen, culture should be performed to allow testing of isolates for antimicrobial resistance. The specificity of Gram's stain of purulent cervical exudate also is high, but the sensitivity is only about 50 percent. Selective media, i.e., Thayer-Martin (TM) medium, modified Thayer-Martin medium, and Martin-Lewis medium, which contain antibiotics to selectively inhibit most other organisms, are most useful for recovering the gonococcus from the urethra, endocervix, and pharynx. Rectal specimens are plated on modified Thayer-Martin medium or equivalent media containing trimethoprim lactate, which suppresses swarming organisms such as *Proteus* spp. The concentration of vancomycin in the selective medium should not exceed 3 µg/mL, and even this concentration may inhibit a small proportion of gonococci. After inoculation, the medium should be placed in a chamber with 70% humidity and an atmosphere containing 3 to 10% carbon dioxide to permit growth of the gonococcus. This can be accomplished in a candle jar, by generation of carbon dioxide chemically within packets that are sealed after inoculation, or within special CO_2 incubators. Inoculated media should be incubated at 35 to 37°C for 48 h, and putative gonococcal colonies should be confirmed by oxidase reaction, Gram's stain, sugar utilization tests, rapid

enzyme tests, or agglutination reactions using antibodies that are specific for *N. gonorrhoeae*. The latter three tests are especially important for isolates from the pharynx and rectum and for cultures obtained from populations which have a low prevalence of gonorrhea, such as prenatal patients. DNA probes have been introduced for the confirmatory identification of *N. gonorrhoeae*. Limited comparisons indicate that they are at least equivalent in effectiveness to other confirmatory tests.

In men with incubating or chronic asymptomatic urethral infection without exudate, or as a test of cure following treatment, a very thin swab should be inserted 2 cm into the anterior urethra and used to inoculate TM or other selective medium. Cultures of the pharynx and rectum should be obtained from homosexual men with suspected gonorrhea.

The most efficient test for gonorrhea in women is the endocervical culture, which is positive on a single examination in approximately 80 to 90 percent of those with gonorrhea. This diagnostic yield can be increased by performing a second endocervical culture and by performing cultures of the rectum, urethra, and pharynx.

Standard blood culture broth medium (tryptic soy, Columbia, brain-heart infusion) should be used in culturing blood and is also recommended for culturing synovial fluid. The broth should be vented and incubated under increased CO_2 tension. Synovial fluid can also be plated onto chocolate agar rather than a selective medium because it is not likely to be contaminated with commensal bacteria. In pus from skin lesions, *N. gonorrhoeae* is demonstrable by immunofluorescent staining, but this test is seldom performed. Techniques designed to detect gonococcal infection by testing of a single serum for antibody to *N. gonorrhoeae* have been limited by inability to differentiate antibody due to past gonorrhea from antibody due to current infection, and by false-positive tests caused by cross-reactive antibody to *N. meningitidis*. For these reasons, serologic tests for gonorrhea have had a very low predictive value and are not used in clinical practice.

Another diagnostic approach is the detection of gonococcal antigen in urethral or cervical secretion by enzyme-linked immunosorbent assay (ELISA). In men with urethritis, the Gram stain is just as accurate, quicker, and cheaper. In women, such tests may be an acceptable alternative to culture for diagnosis of endocervical gonococcal infection in settings where culture is not feasible. However, the positive predictive value of antigen detection tests requires careful study, particularly in populations with a low prevalence of gonorrhea. The medical-legal and psychosocial implications of a false-positive diagnosis of gonorrhea can be troublesome.

TREATMENT Until 1989 the preferred drugs for gonococcal infection have been penicillin G, ampicillin or amoxicillin, tetracycline hydrochloride, and spectinomycin. Although long-acting forms of penicillin (such as benzathine penicillin G) are effective in syphilotherapy, they have *no place* in the treatment of gonorrhea. Penicillin V and the isoxazolyl penicillins are not recommended for the treatment of gonococcal infection. Similarly, first-generation cephalosporins are not used for gonorrhea. In 1989, the Centers for Disease Control published new guidelines for treatment of gonorrhea. These guidelines, which are presented in this chapter, are based upon several observations: the importance of single-dose efficacy; the increasing proportion of infections due to antibiotic-resistant strains of *N. gonorrhoeae*, including PPNG, TRNG, and strains with chromosomally mediated resistance to multiple antimicrobials; the high frequency of coexisting chlamydial infections in persons with gonorrhea; the absence of a cheap, rapid test for chlamydial infection; and the severity of complications of gonococcal and chlamydial infections. The guidelines do not represent a comprehensive list of all possible treatment regimens. As is shown in Table 110-1, a regimen combining a single intramuscular dose of ceftriaxone, together with a 7-day course of tetracycline or doxycycline, is recommended for uncomplicated urethral, endocervical, rectal, or pharyngeal gonococcal infections in heterosexual adults. This combination regimen can be expected to provide adequate therapy for gonorrhea at any site and

TABLE 110-1　Recommended treatment for gonococcal infection

Diagnosis	Treatment of choice
Uncomplicated urethral, endocervical, rectal, or pharyngeal infection	Ceftriaxone 250 mg single IM dose plus Doxycycline 100 mg PO twice daily for 7 days.
Treatment failure	True treatment failure with the above regimen has so far occurred rarely, if ever. Evaluate for reinfection, alternative diagnosis.
Alternative regimen	For patients unable to take ceftriaxone, use spectinomycin, 2-g single IM dose, plus doxycycline.
Gonorrhea in pregnancy	Ceftriaxone 250 mg single IM dose plus Erythromycin base 500 mg PO four times daily for 7 days. Equivalent dose of erythromycin stearate (500 mg) or ethyl-succinate (800 mg) can be used.
Disseminated gonococcal infection (DGI)	Hospitalization is recommended. Ceftriaxone 1 g IM or IV every 24 h or Ceftizoxime 1 g IV every 8 h or Cefotaxime 1 g IV every 8 h (see text for duration of inpatient and subsequent ambulatory therapy).
Gonococcal PID	Hospitalization is recommended. See Chap. 94 for recommended therapy.
Gonococcal epididymitis	See Chap. 93.
Pediatric gonococcal infections　Infants	Ceftriaxone 25–50 mg/kg once daily or Cefotaxime 25 mg/kg twice daily. Usual duration of therapy is 7 days (longer for meningitis or endocarditis).
Children	Children who weigh 100 lb (45 kg) should receive adult doses; for those weighing less, see text.

will eliminate coexisting *C. trachomatis* infections. Tetracycline hydrochloride, 500 mg orally four times daily, can be substituted for doxycycline. Pregnant women and those unable to tolerate doxycycline or tetracycline can instead be given erythromycin base or stearate, 500 mg by mouth four times daily for 7 days, or erythromycin ethylsuccinate, 800 mg by mouth four times daily for 7 days, to accompany the ceftriaxone. All tetracyclines are ineffective as single-dose therapy for gonorrhea, and even a 7-day course of tetracycline has been ineffective in a growing proportion of patients, due to the spread of TRNG and the high proportion of strains with chromosomal resistance to tetracycline. Ceftriaxone can be prepared in 1% lidocaine as diluent (for intramuscular injection only) to reduce discomfort due to the injection. Other β-lactam antibiotics (cefotaxime, cefuroxime, ceftizoxime) and certain oxyquinolones (e.g., ciprofloxacin) are also very effective for resistant gonorrhea, but the long half-life of ceftriaxone, together with its in vitro activity, make it the optimal drug for single-dose therapy of gonorrhea. For patients who cannot take ceftriaxone, the preferred alternative is spectinomycin, 2 g intramuscularly as a single dose. Although spectinomycin resistance has emerged where that drug was used commonly for gonorrhea (e.g., in England and Korea), it has been rare in the United States. Other alternatives to ceftriaxone for uncomplicated urethral, endocervical, or rectal gonorrhea include ciprofloxacin, 500-mg single oral dose; cefuroxime axetil, 1-g single oral dose given simultaneously with probenecid, 1 g orally; cefotaxime, 1-g single intramuscular dose; or ceftizoxime, 500-mg single intramuscular dose.

All patients with gonorrhea should have a serologic test for syphilis at the time of diagnosis, and should be offered confidential testing for human immunodeficiency virus (HIV). Patients with incubating seronegative syphilis, without clinical signs of syphilis, are likely to be cured of syphilis by the recommended ceftriaxone-doxycycline regimen. However, patients with gonorrhea who also have syphilis or who are established contacts of someone with syphilis should be given additional treatment appropriate to the stage of syphilis (see Chap. 128).

Follow-up and treatment failure　Treatment failure following combined ceftriaxone-doxycycline therapy is exceedingly rare; therefore, a follow-up culture is not essential. Patients should be advised to return for reexamination if any symptoms persist or recur after completion of treatment. Persistent or recurrent symptoms or signs after treatment for gonorrhea should be evaluated by culture for *N. gonorrhoeae* and a specific test for chlamydial infection. Any gonococcal isolate should be tested for antibiotic susceptibility. Additional treatment for gonorrhea should be with ceftriaxone, 250 mg intramuscularly, or with 2.0 g spectinomycin intramuscularly (except in areas where spectinomycin resistance is a problem). Recurrent gonococcal infections after treatment with the recommended schedule are almost certainly due to reinfection or indicate a need for improved sex partner referral and patient education.

Postgonococcal urethritis (PGU) usually becomes apparent about 2 to 3 weeks after treatment of gonorrhea with a penicillin or a cephalosporin. PGU often is caused by *C. trachomatis* which may have been acquired at the same time as gonorrhea but did not become clinically apparent until later because of the longer incubation period of chlamydial infection. When PGU occurs, it can be managed, like nongonococcal urethritis, with doxycycline, 100 mg orally twice daily, or tetracycline, 0.5 g four times a day, for at least 7 days. Similarly, mucopurulent cervicitis in women often persists or appears after treatment of gonorrhea with cephalosporin, penicillin, or spectinomycin, is often caused by *C. trachomatis,* and can be treated like PGU. Men and women exposed to gonorrhea should be examined, cultured, and treated with one of the recommended treatment schedules.

All pregnant women should be cultured for *N. gonorrhoeae* (and tested for *C. trachomatis* infection and syphilis) at the time of the first visit as an integral part of the prenatal care. A second culture late in the third trimester (as well as tests for chlamydial infection and syphilis) should be obtained from women at high risk of sexually transmitted disease.

The regimen of choice for gonorrhea in pregnancy is ceftriaxone, in a 250-mg single intramuscular dose, plus erythromycin for a possible coexisting chlamydial infection. Pregnant women allergic to β-lactams can be treated with a single dose of spectinomycin, 2.0 g intramuscularly, plus erythromycin. Doxycycline and tetracycline should not be used in pregnant women because of potential toxic effects for mother and fetus.

The management of pelvic inflammatory disease is discussed in Chap. 94.

Treatment of gonococcal arthritis can be accomplished satisfactorily with several regimens. Gonococci recovered from patients with gonococcal arthritis have been significantly less resistant to penicillin or tetracycline than isolates from patients with uncomplicated gonorrhea. However, several cases of DGI caused by PPNG have been reported. Because of the threat of endocarditis, meningitis, and joint sepsis, all patients with disseminated infection should be hospitalized and treated with ceftriaxone intravenously, 1 g once a day, or with the alternatives listed in Table 110-1. Reliable patients without endocarditis or meningitis can be discharged 24 to 48 h after symptoms resolve, to complete a total of 7 to 10 days' therapy with an oral regimen of cefuroxime axetil, 500 mg twice a day; amoxicillin, 500 mg, with clavulanic acid, 125 mg, three times a day; or (if not pregnant) ciprofloxacin, 500 mg twice a day. If the infecting gonococcus is shown to be penicillin-sensitive, treatment can be completed with oral amoxicillin, 500 mg three times a day, without clavulanic acid. Failure to improve with appropriate antimicrobial regimens as listed above strongly suggests a diagnosis other than disseminated gonococcal infection. Repeated joint aspiration or closed irrigation of the joint with sterile saline may be required to reduce inflammation in patients with high synovial fluid leukocyte counts. Open drainage is seldom, if ever, required for gonococcal arthritis, except in infants with hip infection. Temporary immobilization of the joint may reduce discomfort and may be useful during initial ambulation in patients with persistent effusions of the knee or ankle. Antibiotics should not be injected directly into the joint. Once the diagnosis of gonococcal arthritis is proven, then occasional patients may benefit from use of anti-inflammatory agents along with anti-microbial therapy. However, if the diagnosis is suspected, but not proven, then early use of anti-inflammatory drugs will prevent monitoring the response to antimicrobial therapy, which is usually rapid and often of diagnostic importance in gonococcal arthritis.

Meningitis and endocarditis caused by the gonococcus require high-dose intravenous therapy with an agent effective against the strain causing the disease: ceftriaxone, 1 g intravenously every 12 h, for 10 to 14 days for meningitis and for 1 month for endocarditis. Patients with gonococcal endocarditis or meningitis, and perhaps all patients with DGI, should be evaluated for complement deficiency.

Gonococcal conjunctivitis in the adult or in children over 20 kg should be managed as a medical emergency by irrigation of the conjunctiva with saline, together with ceftriaxone, 1 g in a single intramuscular dose. All patients must have careful ophthalmologic evaluation, including slit-lamp examination.

Pediatric gonococcal infection The infant born to a mother with gonorrhea is at high risk of infection and requires prophylactic treatment with a single injection of ceftriaxone, 50 mg/kg intravenously or intramuscularly, not to exceed 125 mg. Ceftriaxone should be given with caution to hyperbilirubinemic infants, especially premature babies. Topical prophylaxis for neonatal ophthalmia is not adequate treatment for infections at other sites. Infants with gonococcal infection at any site (e.g., eye) should be evaluated for DGI by examination and culture of blood and CSF. They should be treated for 7 days with ceftriaxone, 25 to 50 mg/kg in a single daily intravenous or intramuscular dose. Alternatively, cefotaxime can be used in a dose of 25 mg/kg twice daily intravenously. Limited data suggest that uncomplicated gonococcal ophthalmia in the infant can be cured with a single injection of ceftriaxone, 50 mg/kg, up to a dose of 125 mg. Irrigation of the eyes with saline or buffered ophthalmic solutions should be performed immediately and then repeated as often as necessary to eliminate discharge. Topical antibiotic preparations alone are not sufficient or required when appropriate systemic antibiotic therapy is given. Both of the parents of a newborn with gonococcal ophthalmia must be treated for gonorrhea. The parents and infant should also be tested for chlamydial infection.

Children who weigh 45 kg or more should be treated with adult regimens. Children who weigh less than 45 kg should be treated as follows: For uncomplicated vulvovaginitis, cervicitis, urethritis, proctitis, and pharyngitis, the recommended treatment is ceftriaxone, a 125-mg single intramuscular dose. The alternative regimen is spectinomycin, a 40 mg/kg single intramuscular dose. Children 8 years of age or older can also be given doxycycline, 100 mg twice a day for 7 days. Children with gonorrhea should be evaluated for coexisting syphilis and chlamydial infection.

Topical and/or systemic estrogen therapy is of no benefit in gonococcal vulvovaginitis. All children should have follow-up cultures, and the source of infection should be identified, examined, and treated. Child abuse should be carefully considered and evaluated. For treatment of complicated disease, the alternative regimens recommended for adults may be used in appropriate pediatric dosages.

Treatment of gonorrhea in developing countries The proportion of gonococcal infections caused by PPNG or CMRNG is highest in developing countries, which can least afford ceftriaxone, spectinomycin, or other new antimicrobials effective against these strains. Inexpensive alternatives to penicillin G and tetracycline, the traditional mainstays of gonorrhea therapy, have been disappointing. For example, a sulfonamide-trimethoprim combination which initially cured over 95 percent of cases of gonorrhea in African countries, fell to less than 75 percent efficacy within 2 years after it became a popular regimen in Kenya. One approach has been the use of 4.8 million units of procaine penicillin G intramuscularly plus 1.0 g probenecid orally (a standard regimen for non-PPNG infections) together with 125 mg of clavulanic acid (in the form of one capsule of amoxicillin-clavulanate) to inhibit gonococcal β-lactamase. This inexpensive regimen has been effective in small trials in Kenya, even against PPNG infections. Gentamicin, in a 280-mg single intramuscular dose, has also been used effectively in this setting. Newer cephalosporins in lower than recommended doses, to reduce cost, should be discouraged. There is a growing need for clinical trials with less expensive regimens, and for ongoing surveillance of in vitro sensitivity of N. gonorrhoeae.

PREVENTION AND CONTROL There is probably no more striking illustration than gonorrhea of the failure of a specific treatment alone to eradicate a communicable disease. Vaccination is not available. A field trial of a purified gonococcal pili vaccine in U.S. soldiers in Korea showed that the vaccine was not effective. Use of the condom can prevent transmission, and the extensive use of condoms for contraception may be responsible for the low rates of gonorrhea in some countries (e.g., Japan). Spermicidal preparations used with a diaphragm or impregnated with nonoxynol-9 cervical sponges probably offer some protection against gonorrhea and chlamydial infection. Prophylactic antibiotics (e.g., 200 mg minocycline or doxycycline taken soon after sexual exposure) reduce the risk of infection, but are not recommended for general use or for individuals with known exposure to gonorrhea, who should receive one of the regimens recommended for established gonorrhea.

To contain the increasing spread of antimicrobial-resistant gonococci, several measures are important: (1) routine use of diagnosis by cultures and testing of isolates for antimicrobial resistance or β-lactamase production; (2) routine use of ceftriaxone to prevent gonorrhea treatment failures; and (3) rapid identification and treatment of sexual partners of patients with gonorrhea, particularly partners of those with recurrent infection and those known to be infected with resistant gonococci. The most effective public health measure now available for control of gonorrhea is treatment of sexual partners of infected patients.

REFERENCES

BOSLEGO JW et al: Effect of spectinomycin use on the prevalence of spectinomycin resistant and of penicillinase-producing Neisseria gonorrhoeae. N Engl J Med 317:272, 1987

BRITIGAN BE, SPARLING PF: Gonococcal infection: A model of molecular pathogenesis. N Engl J Med 312:1683, 1985

CENTERS FOR DISEASE CONTROL: 1989 Sexually transmitted diseases treatment guidelines. Morb Mort Week Rep 38(Suppl 8):1, 1989

———: Policy guidelines for the detection, management, and control of antibiotic resistant strains of Neisseria gonorrhoeae. Morb Mort Week Rep 36(5S):1, 1987

HANDSFIELD HH et al: Localized outbreak of penicillinase-producing Neisseria gonorrhoeae: Paradigm for introduction and spread of gonorrhea in a community. JAMA 261:2357, 1989

HOOK EH III, HOLMES KK: Gonococcal infections. Ann Intern Med 102:229, 1985

KNAPP JS et al: Serologic classification of Neisseria gonorrhoeae using monoclonal antibodies directed against outer membrane protein I. J Infect Dis 150:44, 1985

MORSE SA et al: High-level tetracycline resistance in Neisseria gonorrhoeae is result of acquisition of streptococcal tetM determinant. Antimicrob Agents Chemother 30:664, 1986

——— (eds): Perspectives on pathogenic Neisseria spp. Clin Microb Rev 2:1S, 1989

PLUMMER FA et al: Epidemiologic evidence for the development of serovar-specific immunity after gonococcal infection. J Clin Invest 83:1472, 1989

RICE PA et al: Immunoglobulin G antibodies directed against L protein III block killing of serum-resistant Neisseria gonorrhoeae by immune serum. J Exp Med 164:1735, 1986

SPARLING PF: Biology of Neisseria gonorrhoeae, in Sexually Transmitted Diseases, 2d ed, KK Holmes et al (eds). New York, McGraw-Hill, 1990, pp 131–147

111 DISEASES CAUSED BY GRAM-NEGATIVE ENTERIC BACILLI

DENNIS R. SCHABERG / MARVIN TURCK

The Enterobacteriaceae are a group of gram-negative nonsporing rods which are aerobic but can grow under anaerobic conditions, and which are commonly found in the gastrointestinal tract. They are characterized biochemically by their ability to ferment glucose, their ability to reduce nitrates to nitrites, and the fact that they are oxidase-negative. The diverse genera in this family, including *Escherichia, Salmonella, Shigella, Klebsiella, Serratia, Enterobacter, Proteus, Morganella, Yersinia, Providencia,* and other less common genera, are differentiated by serologic tests and computerized analysis of biochemical reactions. It is important to make this differentiation, not only taxonomically but also because of epidemiologic and therapeutic implications.

Other gram-negative bacilli which are not members of the family Enterobacteriaceae may also be causes of infection. Important genera include *Pseudomonas, Acinetobacter,* and *Eikenella.*

ESCHERICHIA COLI INFECTIONS

ETIOLOGY *Escherichia coli* is a commensal in the gastrointestinal tract. It may spread from there to infect contiguous structures if normal anatomic barriers are interrupted, as occurs in appendiceal perforation. It is believed that the urinary tract is infected via urethral contamination, but direct hematogenous spread may also account for renal infection. Once infection has occurred in a primary focus, further spread to distant organs may occur via the bloodstream. A consequence of bacteremia that occurs potentially with all gram-negative bacilli is septic shock (Chap. 89). In more than 50 percent of *E. coli* infections, the urinary tract is the portal of entry; infections emanating from the hepatobiliary tree, peritoneal cavity, skin, and lung are also common. Some patients with *E. coli* bacteremia have no demonstrable portal of entry; they often are leukopenic. There may be other defects in host resistance, including diabetes mellitus, cirrhosis, and sickle cell anemia or recent administration of irradiation, cytotoxic drugs, glucocorticoids, or antibiotics. There is also epidemiologic evidence that *E. coli* and other Enterobacteriaceae tend to colonize the skin and mucous membranes of debilitated patients, possibly accounting for the increased frequency of these infections in patients with advanced illness.

EPIDEMIOLOGY Strains of *E. coli* are characterized by their somatic (O), flagellar (H), and capsular (K) antigens, and there are hundreds of different serologic varieties. Any of the strains is capable of causing disease. Clinical and epidemiologic studies have demonstrated that certain specific *E. coli* serotypes are more frequently incriminated in diarrheal disease of the infant and newborn as well as in outbreaks of enteric disease in adults. Strains incriminated in infantile diarrhea probably are disseminated within nurseries by symptomatic or asymptomatic infant carriers, mothers, and staff. Although fecal contamination is the usual mode of spread, airborne contamination and fomite spread may also occur.

Some epidemiologic studies have suggested that *E. coli* O4, O6, and O75 are responsible for most *E. coli* infections other than infantile diarrhea. It is unclear whether these strains actually are more virulent or merely are more prevalent than other somatic types.

Strains of *E. coli* with K1 antigen are recovered from an inordinate number of neonates with meningitis. These K antigens have been implicated in promoting adherence to host cells and in resisting phagocytosis.

MANIFESTATIONS Urinary tract infections *Escherichia coli* accounts for over 75 percent of urinary tract infections, including cystitis, pyelitis, pyelonephritis, and asymptomatic bacteriuria (Chap. 95). Strains cultured from patients with acute uncomplicated urinary tract infections are almost invariably *E. coli,* whereas other Enterobacteriaceae and strains of *Pseudomonas* become prevalent among patients with chronic infection.

Peritoneal and biliary infections *Escherichia coli* can usually be cultured from a perforated or inflamed appendix or from abscesses secondary to perforated diverticula, peptic ulcers, subphrenic or lesser sac abscesses, or mesenteric infarction. Often, other organisms, including anaerobic streptococci, clostridia, and *Bacteroides,* are found along with *E. coli.* Acute cholecystitis with gangrene and perforation is often associated with *E. coli* infection. An air-fluid level associated with stones or a circumferential layer of gas in the wall of the gallbladder may be detectable by x-ray and is characteristic of acute emphysematous cholecystitis. From the gallbladder, infection may ascend via the biliary tree to produce cholangitis and multiple liver abscesses. More rarely, *E. coli* infection in the peritoneal cavity may produce a septic thrombophlebitis of the portal vein (pylephlebitis), which in turn is followed by liver abscesses.

Bacteremia Invasion of the bloodstream is the most serious manifestation of *E. coli* infection; it is characterized usually by the sudden onset of fever and chills but sometimes only by mental confusion, dyspnea, or unexplained hypotension. It is most common in patients with urinary tract infection and biliary or intraperitoneal sepsis. In some patients no portal of entry is evident. Most cases occur in elderly males, presumably because of the high incidence of urethral instrumentation and catheterization in this group. Hyperventilation may be an early sign. Hypotension may be present from the onset but usually occurs within 12 to 16 h after bacteremia; if it is persistent, it is accompanied by oliguria and often by mental confusion, stupor, and coma, a syndrome known as *gram-negative* or *septic shock* (Chap. 89). Occasionally, *E. coli* bacteremia develops in patients with cirrhosis without an overt portal of entry. This has been attributed to portosystemic shunts both in and around the liver, impaired reticuloendothelial function, and diminution in humoral and cellular defense mechanisms. Persistence or reappearance of bacteremia with *E. coli* or other members of the Enterobacteriaceae on therapy, so-called breakthrough bacteremia, has a poor prognosis and suggests an intraabdominal focus for infection or undrained pus.

Other manifestations *Escherichia coli* may produce abscesses anywhere in the body. Subcutaneous infections are found at the site of insulin administration in diabetics, in ischemic extremities, and in surgical wounds. Perirectal phlegmons are not uncommon in patients with leukemia. Subcutaneous abscesses, especially among diabetics, are often characterized by formation of gas in tissue, which may be detected by crepitation or by x-ray and which must be differentiated from clostridial infection. This is most rapidly accomplished by Gram's stain. *Escherichia coli* may cause pneumonia de novo; also, *E. coli* are often cultured from sputum in pulmonary superinfections.

Neonatal infection Neonates, particularly premature infants, often develop *E. coli* bacteremia associated with meningitis and bloodborne pyelonephritis. Fecal soiling and absence of maternal gamma-globulin (IgM) antibody are two of the factors which render this group particularly susceptible to *E. coli* infections.

Gastroenteritis Some strains of *E. coli* can interact with intestinal mucosa by a variety of pathogenic mechanisms to produce gastroenteritis. Some strains are enterotoxigenic (ETEC) and can produce one of two toxins, one heat labile (LT) and similar to the toxin elaborated by *Vibrio cholerae* and the other heat stable (ST) (see also Chaps. 92 and 122). As a toxin-mediated process the diarrhea from ETEC generally is large in volume and watery. Other *E. coli* produce bloody diarrhea and are referred to as enterohemorrhagic (EHEC). These strains were first recognized in patrons of fast-food restaurants; *E. coli* O157:H7 was isolated from hamburger in one outbreak. These strains produce Shiga's toxin, also called verotoxin, because of the cytotoxicity it produces with vero cells in tissue culture. A third clinical picture that can be due to *E. coli* is a dysenteric type of stools with low volume but with abdominal cramps, blood, and mucus. These strains are enteroinvasive (EIEC) and carry a large plasmid also found in invasive *Shigella* strains. Finally, some patients, especially children under 2 years of age, develop gastroenteritis typified by nausea, vomiting, and watery diarrhea. Most outbreaks of this disease have occurred in nurseries and have been due to specific serotypes of enteropathogenic *E. coli* (EPEC). These strains appear to have special adherence for mucosal cells, a property that correlates with ability to cause diarrhea. The rapid dehydration, with its attendant high mortality, demands prompt recognition of this condition, isolation of the infants, and treatment of both patients and contacts.

LABORATORY FINDINGS There are no characteristic laboratory abnormalities. The white blood cell count is usually elevated, and there is a preponderance of granulocytes. At times, however, the white count is normal or low. When *E. coli* infection occurs in previously healthy individuals, anemia is absent, but more commonly there is anemia which is usually related to underlying disease. *Escherichia coli* grows readily in a variety of bacteriologic media and should be cultured from appropriate secretions and blood. In the presence of bacteremia there can be metabolic derangements, including azotemia, metabolic acidosis, hypokalemia, and hyperkalemia as well as a variety of coagulation defects.

DIAGNOSIS *E. coli* cannot be differentiated from most other gram-negative bacteria on Gram's stain, and culture followed by appropriate biochemical characterization is necessary to identify the organism precisely. Serologic typing of *E. coli* may be useful in individual patients with recurrent urinary tract infections in order to help differentiate between relapse and reinfection.

TREATMENT As with other infections, drainage of pus and removal of foreign bodies are essential. If *E. coli* is suspected as the etiologic agent in a particular infection, choice of an appropriate antimicrobial will depend upon the site and type of infection as well as upon its severity; outcome is often related to underlying disease. For example, in acute, uncomplicated urinary tract infection in females, the disease is frequently self-limited even without antimicrobial therapy, and there is no evidence that antibiotics are superior to sulfonamides. Conversely, sustained *E. coli* bacteremia is associated with a high incidence of shock, and the response and survival are highly dependent on the choice of the correct antimicrobial.

In most situations, antibiotics should be selected on the basis of in vitro susceptibility tests. Although no drug is uniformly active against all strains of *E. coli*, a number of agents are effective against the majority of clinical isolates. Resistance to ampicillin is close to 30 percent in most hospitals, and for severe infections, cephalosporins are recommended as the initial treatment. Third-generation cephalosporins have lower minimal inhibitory concentrations (MICs) for *E. coli*; this increased activity coupled with slightly enhanced CNS penetration make them useful for the therapy of meningitis due to *E. coli* (Chap. 354). Gentamicin and tobramycin have been employed effectively in the initial treatment of severe *E. coli* infections in doses of 5 mg/kg per day in divided doses every 8 h. Amikacin is very active against isolates which are resistant to the other aminoglycosides in doses of 15 mg/kg per day, divided to be administered every 8 to 12 h. Tetracyclines and chloramphenicol are still used in the treatment of *E. coli* infection, but better drugs are now available. Although combinations of antimicrobials have been recommended, there is little need to employ more than one agent in most situations. Nitrofurantoin (400 mg) and nalidixic acid (2 to 4 g) are reserved for treating patients with *E. coli* bacteriuria, and should not be employed when infection is suspected outside the urinary tract. Trimethoprim-sulfamethoxazole and the fluoroquinolones are also useful, especially in urinary tract infections (Chap. 85). Intravenous trimethoprim-sulfamethoxazole is effective for treating severe *E. coli* infections and can be substituted for aminoglycosides, cephalosporins, or ampicillin.

PREVENTION Isolation and antimicrobial therapy of infants and contacts are essential to abort epidemic infantile diarrhea. In adults, many *E. coli* infections are hospital-associated, and their incidence can be reduced by limiting use of indwelling urinary and intravenous catheters, by careful surgical aseptic technique, by appropriate isolation of infection-prone patients, and by judicious use of antibiotics, glucocorticoids, and cytotoxic agents.

KLEBSIELLA-ENTEROBACTER-SERRATIA INFECTIONS

ETIOLOGY Next to *E. coli*, strains of *Klebsiella*, *Enterobacter*, and *Serratia* are the most important enteric organisms infecting humans. These are also of the family Enterobacteriaceae. In many laboratories *Klebsiella* are more resistant to antibiotics than are *E. coli*, and their isolation from blood, purulent exudates, and urine is of more serious epidemiologic and prognostic significance. The Friedlander bacilli (*K. pneumoniae*) are encapsulated gram-negative bacilli found among the normal flora of the mouth and intestinal tracts. *Klebsiella* are closely related to the genera *Enterobacter* and *Serratia* and may be differentiated only by certain amino acid decarboxylase tests. In addition to differentiation by these biochemical tests, which identify the *Klebsiella*, *Enterobacter*, and *Serratia* groups, strains of *Klebsiella* usually are nonmotile and form large mucoid colonies on solid media, whereas the other species are typically motile. Strains of *Klebsiella* can be further distinguished on the basis of type-specific capsular antigens; more than 75 known capsular types have been identified. There is little evidence that certain types are more virulent than others, and the main role of capsular typing of *Klebsiella* is as an epidemiologic tool in nosocomial outbreaks of infection.

Klebsiella rhinoscleromatis is probably the causative agent of rhinoscleroma, and *K. ozenae* has been isolated occasionally from the noses of patients with ozena, a chronic severe rhinitis associated with turbinate atrophy and progressive anosmia. *Klebsiella oxytoca* is the new designation for indole-positive strains of *K. pneumoniae*.

PATHOGENESIS *Klebsiella*, *Enterobacter*, and *Serratia* are all capable of causing disease in diverse anatomic sites. However, results of clinical and epidemiologic studies suggest that differences in pathogenicity may exist among these genera and that precise taxonomic identification is of value. Although infections of the respiratory tract with *K. pneumoniae* have been emphasized most in the past, the urinary tract presently accounts for the majority of clinical isolates. In this site clinical manifestations and pathogenesis are similar to those of infections produced by *E. coli*, but *Klebsiella* is more frequently found in patients with complicated and obstructive urinary tract disease. Infections of the biliary tract, peritoneal cavity, middle ear, mastoids, paranasal sinuses, and meninges also are not uncommon. In these locations, *Klebsiella* is more frequent than either *Enterobacter* or *Serratia* and is more likely to produce an illness of greater severity. The apparent increased frequency of infection by *Serratia* represents an increase primarily due to nosocomial spread of this organism. *Enterobacter* species have been incriminated frequently in outbreaks of in-hospital bacteremia attributed to contaminated intravenous solutions.

MANIFESTATIONS Symptoms and signs of common infections caused by *Klebsiella*—namely, those involving the urinary tract, biliary tree, and peritoneal cavity—are indistinguishable from those caused by *E. coli*. These infections commonly occur in diabetics and in the form of superinfections in patients who have received antimicrobials to which these organisms are resistant. *Klebsiella* infection is also an important etiologic agent in septic shock. *Serratia* and *Enterobacter* are almost exclusively nosocomial pathogens. These organisms have been implicated as pathogens in a wide variety of infections, most frequently pneumonia, urinary tract infections, and bacteremia.

Pneumonia *Klebsiella* is well recognized as a pulmonary pathogen but probably accounts for less than 1 percent of all cases of community-acquired bacterial pneumonia. The disease is most common in men over 40 years of age and is most frequently found in alcoholics. Other factors associated with increased susceptibility include diabetes mellitus and chronic bronchopulmonary disease. Aspiration of oropharyngeal secretions containing *Klebsiella* organisms is the likely inciting factor among alcoholic patients. The clinical manifestations are indistinguishable from those of pneumococcal pneumonia (Chap. 99), with sudden onset of chills, fever, productive cough, and severe pleuritic chest pain. Patients are frequently delirious and prostrated, but this may also occur with pneumococcal infection. The pulmonary lesion is most frequent in the right upper lobe but often rapidly progresses and, if untreated, may spread from lobe to lobe. Cyanosis and dyspnea develop rapidly, and jaundice, vomiting, and diarrhea may be present. Physical findings consist primarily of consolidation, unless pleural effusion or necrotizing pneumonitis with rapid cavitation has intervened. The blood leukocyte count may be elevated but is often low, which probably is a reflection of severe infection in an alcoholic patient with poor bone marrow reserve and folate deficiency. Lung abscess and empyema are much more frequent than they are in pneumococcal pneumonia; they are related to the destructive capabilities of this organism. So-called characteristic radiographic features such as bulging fissures and loss of lung volume occur only occasionally; they also may be found in pneumococcal infection as well as in necrotizing pneumonia caused by other gram-negative species.

Klebsiella, *Serratia*, and *Enterobacter* are frequently seen in nosocomial pneumonia. Older patients become colonized with gram-negative bacilli in the oropharynx, and these organisms can then gain access to the respiratory tract and cause pneumonia or purulent bronchitis. Common-source outbreaks, with contamination of a variety of respiratory therapy devices, have been implicated in infections with these pathogens, especially *Serratia*. As a general rule, the most drug-resistant strains of *Serratia* are nonpigmented and account for the majority of nosocomial isolates. However, pigmented and multiply sensitive *Serratia* isolates are also seen in device-related infections. Rarely, infection with *Klebsiella* may progress, often in indolent fashion, to a chronic necrotizing pneumonitis resembling tuberculosis. The principal symptoms are productive cough, weakness, and anemia.

DIAGNOSIS   Diagnosis of community-acquired pneumonia is established by an awareness of the clinical setting in which *Klebsiella* infections occur and by isolation of the organism. A presumptive diagnosis of *Klebsiella* pneumonia should be made on the basis of a Gram's stain of the sputum which shows a predominance of short, plump, gram-negative bacilli, frequently surrounded by a clear space because of the capsule. Often these gram-negative organisms occur together with gram-positive cocci, and because the gram-positives are easier to see, the gram-negative bacteria may be ignored and the diagnosis may be missed. This, in turn, may lead to potentially serious delays in instituting therapy. Additional proof of *Klebsiella* infection in the lung is the isolation of the organisms from blood and pleural exudate. In extrapulmonary infections, the organisms are readily seen in, or cultured from, pus or secretions of involved organs.

The diagnosis of nosocomial respiratory infection with these organisms may be more difficult, mainly because colonization has to be distinguished from infection. Careful evaluation of the clinical course is necessary in establishing a diagnosis. Transtracheal aspiration of sputum for culture and Gram's stain or bronchoscopy may be useful in difficult cases.

TREATMENT   *Klebsiella*, *Enterobacter*, and *Serratia* have variable susceptibility to antimicrobial drugs, and cultures of these organisms need to be tested in vitro. Frequently, antimicrobial therapy needs to be begun before results of antibiotic susceptibility tests are available. In general, most strains of *Klebsiella* are susceptible to the aminoglycosides and the third-generation cephalosporins. *Klebsiella* isolates do not respond to most penicillin analogues, although many isolates are inhibited by ureidopenicillins, e.g., mezlocillin. *Serratia* isolates are frequently resistant to many antimicrobials, and resistance to gentamicin and tobramycin is being encountered with increasing frequency. Amikacin has been used effectively in these drug-resistant infections. The antimicrobial regimen of choice in the treatment of *Klebsiella*, *Enterobacter*, and *Serratia* infection will vary from one institution to another depending on the resistance patterns as well as upon the degree of clinical severity of infection. In severely ill patients, the combination of an aminoglycoside such as tobramycin or gentamicin (3 to 5 mg/kg per day) or amikacin (15 mg/kg per day) with cephalothin, cephapirin, or cefazolin (4 to 12 g/d) is usually preferred. Cefoxitin, third-generation cephalosporins, aztreonam, or imipenem-cilastatin also may be active against *Klebsiella*, *Enterobacter*, and *Serratia*. Occasionally, one or all of these compounds may be more active than the older cephalosporins, and in vitro susceptibility tests will be required to select the most appropriate agent. Trimethoprim-sulfamethoxazole is often an effective agent against *Klebsiella*, *Serratia*, and *Enterobacter* species resistant to other antimicrobials. Aztreonam can be used to treat these and other serious gram-negative infections in patients who have experienced IgE-based β-lactam hypersensitivity in the past (Chap. 85). Regardless of the antimicrobial regimen employed, treatment should be continued for a minimum of 10 to 14 days and prolonged if there is extensive cavitation. Pleural effusions must be drained; antibiotic therapy alone is not sufficient treatment for closed-space infections of the pleural cavity. At times, rib resection with open drainage may be necessary and should be considered if effusions recur.

PROGNOSIS   Before the introduction of antimicrobials, the fatality rate from these infections varied from 50 to 80 percent, and death within 48 h was not infrequent. Even with antimicrobial treatment the course of these infections is quite variable and the prognosis must be guarded. For the most part, the prognosis reflects the age group involved and the frequent association of *Klebsiella* infections with alcoholism, malnutrition, and severe underlying disease.

PROTEUS, MORGANELLA, AND PROVIDENCIA INFECTIONS

ETIOLOGY   The genus *Proteus* of the family Enterobacteriaceae consists of gram-negative bacilli which do not ferment lactose and are characterized by their active motility and spreading growth on solid media. Organisms once thought to be related and once classified as *Proteus* have been renamed based on detailed DNA studies. *Proteus morganii* has been reclassified as *Morganella morganii*, while some biogroups of *Proteus rettgeri* have been reclassified as *Providencia stuartii* and *Providencia rettgeri*. *Proteus mirabilis* and *Proteus vulgaris* retain their nomenclature; *Proteus mirabilis* causes 75 to 90 percent of human infections. It is distinguishable from the other organisms mentioned by its inability to form indole. All four split urea, with production of ammonia. Some strains of *Proteus vulgaris* share a common antigen with certain rickettsia, which accounts for the appearance of antibodies against *Proteus* organisms (Weil-Felix reaction) in typhus, scrub typhus, and Rocky Mountain spotted fever. The *Providencia* group of organisms resembles those of the genus *Proteus* closely except for some differences in biochemical tests.

EPIDEMIOLOGY AND PATHOGENESIS   These organisms are normally found in soil, water, and sewage and are part of the normal fecal flora. Occasionally, they have been implicated as a cause of epidemic diarrhea in infants, but the evidence for this is inconclusive. They are frequently cultured from superficial wounds, draining ears, and sputum, particularly in patients who have received antibiotics; they replace the more susceptible flora eradicated by these drugs.

MANIFESTATIONS   These organisms are rarely primary invaders but produce disease in locations previously infected by other pathogens. These locations include skin, ears and mastoid, sinuses, eyes, peritoneal cavity, bone, urinary tract, meninges, lung, and bloodstream.

Cutaneous infections   These organisms can be isolated from surgical wounds, particularly after antimicrobial therapy, but they do not interfere with normal wound healing provided that the tissues are viable and foreign bodies are not present. Burns, varicose ulcers, and decubitus ulcers may become contaminated with these organisms, often in company with other gram-negative bacilli or staphylococci.

Infections of the ears and mastoid sinuses Otitis media and mastoiditis, especially with *Proteus mirabilis*, can result in extensive destruction of the middle ear and mastoid sinuses. Fetid otorrhea, cholesteatoma, and granulation tissue constitute a chronic focus of infection in the middle and inner ears and mastoid, and deafness ensues. Paralysis of the facial nerve is an occasional complication. The great danger of these infections lies in intracranial extension, leading to thrombosis of the lateral sinus, meningitis, brain abscess, and bacteremia.

Ocular infections These pathogens may cause corneal ulcers, usually following trauma to the eye, which occasionally terminate in panophthalmitis and destruction of the eyeball.

Peritonitis Because they are part of the normal intestinal flora, these organisms may be isolated from the peritoneal cavity following perforation of viscera or mesenteric infarction.

Urinary tract infections These organisms are a common cause of urinary tract infections, usually in patients with chronic bacteriuria, many of whom have had obstructive uropathy, a history of bladder instrumentation, and repeated courses of chemotherapy. They are often recovered from bacteriuric patients with renal or bladder calculi. This may be related to the urease activity which renders the urine alkaline and provides a fertile medium for formation of ammonium-magnesium-phosphate stones.

Bacteremia Bloodstream invasion is the most serious manifestation of infection with this organism. In 75 percent of cases, the urinary tract serves as the portal of entry; in the remainder, the biliary tree, gastrointestinal tract, ears and sinuses, and skin are the primary foci. Bacteremia is frequently preceded by cystoscopy, urethral catheterization, transurethral prostatic resection, or other operative procedures. Clinically, the signs, symptoms, and laboratory findings of sepsis—high fever, chills, shock, metastatic abscess, leukocytosis, and thrombocytopenia—are indistinguishable from those of bloodstream infections with *E. coli*, *Klebsiella*, or other gram-negative bacteria.

DIAGNOSIS The diagnosis of *Proteus*, *Morganella*, or *Providencia* infection depends on culture of the organism from blood, urine, or exudate and its identification by appropriate biochemical tests. It is especially important to separate *Proteus mirabilis*, the indole-negative species, from organisms that are indole-positive, because only *P. mirabilis* is susceptible to the action of penicillin and many other antibiotics. *Proteus* organisms are often present in mixed infections with other pathogens. Particular care should be exercised in the isolation of other organisms growing in the same medium with *Proteus mirabilis* or *Proteus vulgaris* lest they be masked by spreading growth. The spreading character of these bacteria also may make antibiotic sensitivity tests difficult to interpret.

TREATMENT Most strains of *Proteus mirabilis* are sensitive to penicillin in high concentration (10 units per milliliter or greater), ampicillin, carbenicillin, gentamicin, tobramycin, or amikacin, and the cephalosporin antibiotics. *Proteus mirabilis* bacteriuria can be readily eradicated with any of these drugs during treatment; ampicillin in dosage of 0.5 g every 4 to 6 h is highly effective. In severe infection, therapy should be parenteral: 6 to 12 g ampicillin or 20 million units of penicillin G plus tobramycin or gentamicin in divided doses of 5 mg/kg per day, if renal function is adequate. There is some evidence that an aminoglycoside is synergistic with ampicillin and penicillin G in *P. mirabilis* infections. In general, all strains of *P. mirabilis* are resistant to tetracycline. Most strains other than *P. mirabilis* are predictably sensitive only to aminoglycosides and the third-generation cephalosporins. Carbenicillin, ticarcillin, and the ureidopenicillins, imipenem-cilastatin, and aztreonam are effective against many isolates. Ideally, therapy should be based on in vitro susceptibility, or lacking this, an awareness of local resistance patterns. As with all other gram-negative infections, appropriate attention must be given to drainage of pus, maintenance of fluid and electrolyte status, and, if septic shock is present, treatment of circulatory collapse.

PSEUDOMONAS INFECTIONS

ETIOLOGY *Pseudomonas aeruginosa* is a motile gram-negative rod which generally is not encapsulated and forms no spores. It grows readily in all ordinary culture media, and on agar it forms irregular, soft, iridescent colonies which usually have a fluorescent yellow-green color because of diffusion into the medium of two pigments, pyocyanin and fluorescein. *Pseudomonas* produces acid but no gas in glucose, and it is proteolytic. It is oxidase-positive and produces ammonia from arginine. A number of different strains have been identified by immunofluorescent techniques or bacteriophage typing. There is no evidence that these strains vary in their virulence for humans. Other *Pseudomonas* species (*P. maltophilia*, *P. cepacia*, *P. fluorescens*, *P. testosteroni*, and *P. putida*) also may cause infection in human beings. For the most part, these organisms have been associated with common-source nosocomial outbreaks; in addition, they have been incriminated in bacteremia, endocarditis, and osteomyelitis in narcotic addicts.

EPIDEMIOLOGY *Pseudomonas* organisms are present on the skin of some normal persons, particularly in the axilla and anogenital regions. They are uncommon in the stools of adults not receiving antibiotics. In the majority of instances, *Pseudomonas* organisms are cultured as avirulent secondary contaminants in superficial wounds or from the sputum of patients treated with antibiotics. Ordinarily this is of little consequence because the organisms merely fill the bacteriologic vacuum left by the elimination of more sensitive bacteria. Occasionally, however, infections with *Pseudomonas* organisms occur in the ear, lung, skin, or urinary tract of patients, often after the primary pathogen has been eradicated by antibiotics. Serious infections are almost invariably associated with damage to local tissue or with diminished host resistance. Despite the many potential virulence factors shared by strains of *Pseudomonas*, the organism rarely causes disease in healthy persons. Patients compromised by cystic fibrosis and those with neutropenia appear at particular risk to severe infection with *P. aeruginosa*. Premature infants; children with congenital anomalies and patients with leukemia (who are usually receiving antibiotics, adrenal glucocorticoids or antineoplastic drugs); patients with burns; and geriatric patients with debilitating diseases are likely to develop *Pseudomonas* infections. Most often these infections occur in the hospital environment, and they generally are exogenous infections with the organism acquired from sources other than the patient's normal flora. In hospitals, the organisms have been cultured from a variety of sources that have in common an aqueous environment, including such items as sinks, antiseptic solutions, and aqueous medications. The organism is prevalent in urine receptacles and on catheters, and on the hands of hospital staff. In several outbreaks, *Pseudomonas* urinary tract infections appear to have been transmitted from patient to patient by human carriers. Similar epidemics have been reported in nurseries among premature infants, and cross-infection on burn wards is common. Although *P. aeruginosa* is found in the gastrointestinal tract of only approximately 5 percent of normal adults, carriage rates increase in hospitalized patients.

PATHOGENESIS The portal of entry of *Pseudomonas* organisms varies with the patient's age and underlying disease. In infancy and childhood, the skin, umbilical cord, and gastrointestinal tract predominate; in old age, the urinary tract is more often the primary focus. Often the infections remain localized to the skin or subcutaneous tissues. In burns, the region below the eschar may become massively infiltrated with bacteria and inflammatory cells and usually serves as the focus for bacteremia, the single most lethal complication. Hematogenous dissemination is characterized by hemorrhagic nodules in many areas, including the skin, heart, lungs, kidneys, and meninges. The histologic picture is one of necrosis and hemorrhage. Typically the walls of arterioles are heavily infiltrated with bacteria, and the vessels are partially or wholly thrombosed.

Most strains of *P. aeruginosa* produce a layer of slime which is rich in carbohydrate and shares heat-stable somatic antigenicity with the cell wall. Antibody against the specific serologic type of slime antigen affords protection to experimental challenge. Most isolates also produce a number of exotoxins. Exotoxin A, which shares many properties with diphtheria toxin, is the most potent toxin produced by *P. aeruginosa*. In life-threatening infection with *P. aeruginosa*, high antibody titers against exotoxin A correlate with increased survival.

MANIFESTATIONS   *Pseudomonas* infections occur in many locations, including the skin, subcutaneous tissues, bone and joints, eyes, ears, mastoid and paranasal sinuses, meninges, and heart valves. Bacteremia without a detectable primary focus may also occur and should raise the question of contaminated intravenous medications, intravenous solutions, or antiseptics used for preparing an intravenous site, especially when *Pseudomonas* species other than *P. aeruginosa* are isolated.

Infections of the skin and subcutaneous tissues   *Pseudomonas* organisms are frequently cultured from surgical wounds, varicose and decubitus ulcers, and burns, particularly following antibiotic therapy. Draining tuberculous or osteomyelitic sinuses may become secondarily infected. The mere presence of *Pseudomonas* in these sites is of little significance provided that bacterial multiplication deep in subcutaneous tissues does not occur and bacteremia does not ensue. Cutaneous infections usually heal after removal or slough of devitalized tissue. *Pseudomonas* organisms may be responsible for green nails in persons whose hands are excessively exposed to water, soap, and detergents, who have onychomycosis, or whose hands are subject to mechanical trauma. The organism can usually be cultured from the nail plate. It has been incriminated in whirlpool-associated dermatitis. The disease is benign and resolves spontaneously.

Osteomyelitis   Osteomyelitis is unusual with *Pseudomonas* except as a complication of bacteremia, intravenous drug abuse, or puncture wounds. If a puncture wound, especially a nail puncture of the foot in a child, fails to respond to standard therapy within 3 to 4 days, complicating *Pseudomonas* osteomyelitis must be considered.

Infections of the ear, mastoid, and paranasal sinuses   Otitis externa is the most common form of *Pseudomonas* infection which involves the ear. It is particularly troublesome in tropical climates and is characterized by chronic serosanguineous and purulent drainage from the external auditory canal. A rapidly progressive, severe infection due to *Pseudomonas* involving the ear, referred to as malignant otitis externa, can develop, especially in diabetics. In contrast to the usual otitis externa, this infection requires aggressive management including surgical debridement and parenteral antimicrobial therapy. Otitis media or mastoiditis usually occurs as a superinfection following eradication of gram-positive organisms by antimicrobial agents.

Infections of the eye   Corneal ulceration is the most severe form of ocular *Pseudomonas* infection. It usually follows a traumatic abrasion and may terminate in panophthalmitis and destruction of the globe. Purulent conjunctivitis occurs as a manifestation of *Pseudomonas* infection in premature infants. Contamination of contact lenses or lens fluid may be an important means of infecting the eyes with *Pseudomonas*.

Urinary tract infections   *Pseudomonas* organisms are common pathogens in the urinary tract and are usually found in patients with obstructive uropathy who have been subjected to repeated urethral manipulations or to urologic surgery. *Pseudomonas* bacteriuria is in no way unique and cannot be distinguished from infection with other organisms on clinical grounds.

Gastrointestinal tract   *Pseudomonas* organisms have been implicated as a cause of epidemic diarrhea of infancy. In addition, a number of infants dying from neonatal sepsis have the classic necrotic, avascular ulcers of *Pseudomonas* bacteremia in the bowel at autopsy. A "typhoidal" form of *Pseudomonas* infection characterized by fever, myalgia, and diarrhea occurs predominantly in the tropics. This illness, also called 13-day fever or Shanghai fever, is self-limited, and the prognosis is good.

Respiratory tract   Primary *Pseudomonas* pneumonia is infrequent, and culture of this organism from the sputum usually is indicative of aspiration of oropharyngeal contents with secondary infection following eradication of a more sensitive flora with antibiotics. The normal oropharyngeal flora of hospitalized patients is frequently replaced by gram-negative rods, including *Pseudomonas*, early in hospitalization. A variety of nosocomial events, most notably administration of sedative medications, endotracheal intubation, and intermittent positive pressure breathing treatments, can predispose to respiratory infection with *Pseudomonas*. Pulmonary infection is often associated with microabscesses. The organism is often isolated from the sputum of patients with bronchiectasis, chronic bronchitis, or cystic fibrosis who have lingering infections punctuated by multiple courses of chemotherapy, or from the stomata of tracheostomy sites. *Pseudomonas* bronchitis and bronchiolitis may be the terminal event in cystic fibrosis, and sputum isolates often have a characteristic mucoid colonial morphology when cultured on agar.

Meningitis   Spontaneous *Pseudomonas* meningitis is unusual, but the bacilli may be introduced into the subarachnoid space by lumbar puncture, spinal anesthesia, intrathecal medication, or head trauma. Shunts performed for hydrocephalus may become contaminated with *Pseudomonas*, and revision or removal of the shunt offers the best hope of cure.

Bacteremia   Bloodstream invasion tends to occur in debilitated patients, premature infants, children with congenital defects, patients with lymphomas, leukemias, or other malignant tumors, and elderly patients who have undergone surgery or instrumentation of the biliary or urinary tract. *Pseudomonas* bacteremia is an important cause of death in patients with severe burns. In adults, *Pseudomonas* bacteremia is indistinguishable from bloodstream infection with other bacterial species except for two findings: (1) ecthyma gangrenosum, the classic skin lesion, often located in the anogenital or axillary region as a round, indurated, purple-black area about 1 cm in diameter with an ulcerated center and a surrounding zone of erythema; and (2) rarely, the passage of green urine, presumably due to the hemoglobin pigment verdoglobin. Organisms usually can be cultured from cutaneous lesions and may provide an early clue to the diagnosis.

Bacterial endocarditis   A number of cases of *Pseudomonas* subacute bacterial endocarditis have followed open-heart surgery. Usually the organisms become implanted on a silk suture or a synthetic patch employed for closure of septal defects. Reoperation with removal of the vegetation and foreign bodies offers the best hope of cure. *Pseudomonas* endocarditis has been found on normal heart valves in patients with burns and in drug addicts. Metastatic abscesses in bone, joint, brain, adrenal glands, and lungs are frequent consequences of *Pseudomonas* endocarditis (see Chap. 90).

TREATMENT   Localized *Pseudomonas* infection can be treated by irrigation with 1% acetic acid or topical therapy with colistin or polymyxin B. Debridement and drainage of purulent material is essential when deeper tissues are involved. For deep-seated tissue infections and life-threatening infection, such as pneumonia or bacteremia, parenteral therapy must be employed. The aminoglycoside antibiotics tobramycin and gentamicin inhibit most strains of *Pseudomonas*. In patients with normal renal function, 5 mg/kg per day in divided doses will provide inhibitory levels. Amikacin is also active against *Pseudomonas* and is especially useful against strains which have developed enzyme-mediated drug resistance to tobramycin and gentamicin. It should be given in doses of 15 mg/kg per day in divided doses. Replacement of amikacin-sensitive by amikacin-resistant *Pseudomonas* has been reported in a few instances. Ticarcillin and mezlocillin are active against most strains of *Pseudomonas* in doses of 16 to 20 g/d. Piperacillin and azlocillin are active in vitro against some isolates not inhibited by ticarcillin. These isolates are usually nosocomial in origin. The combination of an aminoglycoside active against *Pseudomonas* plus an antipseudomonal penicillin is frequently employed to delay emergence of resistance during therapy and provides enhanced activity, especially in granulocytopenic patients with *Pseudomonas* infection. Ceftazidime plus an aminoglycoside makes for the most effective treatment for serious *Pseudomonas* infection. Asymptomatic bacteriuria, particularly when confined to the bladder, should be treated with the least toxic agent, which at times may be a sulfonamide or tetracycline. The fluoroquinolone antimicrobics such as norfloxacin or ciprofloxacin are very active against *P. aeruginosa* at urinary concentrations. Ciprofloxacin is also useful in prolonged oral treatment of osteomyelitis or pulmonary infections with *P. aeruginosa*. The antimicrobial susceptibility of *Pseudomonas*, except for *P. aeruginosa*, is variable, and some of these isolates may be resistant to aminoglycoside antibiotics. Some of the newer cephalosporins like cefoperazone and ceftazidime are also active in vitro against many isolates of *Pseudomonas*. Selective pressure of intense antimicrobial use in closed settings such as burn units or intensive care units has resulted sometimes in strains of *Pseudomonas* resistant to the usual β-lactams. Imipenem-cilastatin often remains active against such isolates, but should be combined with an effective aminoglycoside to avoid emergence of resistance.

PROPHYLAXIS *Pseudomonas* cross-infections in hospitals can be reduced by careful attention to aseptic techniques and good infection control practices (see Chap. 83). Systemic antibiotic prophylaxis aimed at preventing colonization and infection with *Pseudomonas* organisms has been notoriously unsuccessful and should be interdicted. A polyvalent vaccine for *Pseudomonas* has been developed, as well as hyperimmune gamma globulin. The latter is undergoing intensive evaluation in prophylaxis and therapy of serious *Pseudomonas* infections.

PROGNOSIS The mortality rate in *Pseudomonas* bacteremia is 75 percent and is highest in patients with shock or severe associated disease such as massive third-degree burns, leukemia, or prematurity. When bacteremia originates in the urinary tract and is not accompanied by shock, the prognosis is considerably better. Localized *Pseudomonas* infections do not present a threat to life unless hematogenous dissemination occurs.

ACINETOBACTER INFECTIONS

DEFINITION Organisms of the genus *Acinetobacter* are pleomorphic, gram-negative bacilli which are easily confused with members of the genus *Neisseria*. Severe infections with these organisms, including meningitis, bacterial endocarditis, pneumonia, and bacteremia, have been described with increasing frequency.

ETIOLOGY *Acinetobacter calcoaceticus* var. *lwoffi* was described by DeBord as *Mima polymorpha* in 1939. It is one of two well-characterized varieties of *Acinetobacter*, the other being *Acinetobacter calcoaceticus* var. *anitratus*, formerly called *Herellea vaginicola*. These organisms are pleomorphic, gram-negative, encapsulated, and nonmotile. They grow well on ordinary media, forming white, convex, smooth colonies. Diplococcal forms predominate in colonies grown on solid media; rods and filamentous forms are more common in liquid media. The species can be differentiated from the Enterobacteriaceae by their negative nitrate reaction and from members of the genus *Neisseria*, which they may resemble morphologically, by their simple growth requirements, their bacillary form in liquid media, and their usually negative oxidase reaction.

EPIDEMIOLOGY AND PATHOGENESIS *Acinetobacter* organisms are ubiquitous. Twenty-five percent of normal subjects are skin carriers of *Acinetobacter*. The striking association of *Acinetobacter* bacteremia with cutdowns or indwelling intravenous catheters favors the skin as a major portal of entry in human beings. *Acinetobacter* pneumonia, both as a primary infection and as a superinfection, also points to the respiratory tract as an important portal of entry. It appears that *Acinetobacter* organisms are normal human commensals of relatively low virulence which produce colonization much more frequently than infection. Infections seem to occur in patients subjected to the same epidemiologic pressures encountered with nosocomial, gram-negative bacilli; serious infections are produced under conditions of decreased host resistance, or in the presence of instrumentation, or with prior broad-spectrum antimicrobial therapy. An unexplained predominance of *Acinetobacter* pulmonary infections occurring in late summer has been noted. The role of these organisms as a cause of conjunctivitis, vaginitis, and urethritis requires further documentation.

MANIFESTATIONS Serious infections caused by *Acinetobacter* include (1) meningitis, (2) subacute and acute bacterial endocarditis, (3) pneumonia, (4) urinary tract infections, and (5) bacteremia. Usually, the signs and symptoms associated with infections in these sites are no different from those produced by other pathogens. Occasionally, *Acinetobacter* may be the cause of a fulminating bacteremia, with high fever, vascular collapse, petechiae, and ecchymoses, which is indistinguishable from fulminant meningococcemia. More often, however, bacteremia is associated with an overt portal of entry, such as infected cutdowns or indwelling intravenous catheters, surgical wounds, or burns; it may follow urethral or other surgical instrumentation. The clinical picture presented by these patients is dominated by endotoxemia, and the prognosis is poor.

DIAGNOSIS The diagnosis of *Acinetobacter* infection can be missed, either because the clinical bacteriology laboratory is unfamiliar with these organisms and reports them incorrectly or because they are considered contaminants. The confusion attending the taxonomic classification of these organisms has not simplified matters. For practical purposes, isolation of *Acinetobacter* from blood, spinal fluid, sputum, urine, or pus should be considered significant unless there is no evidence of infection on clinical grounds. Since *Acinetobacter* isolates are resistant to penicillin and members of the genus *Neisseria* are sensitive, differentiation of these organisms is of obvious importance.

TREATMENT Antibiotic sensitivities of *Acinetobacter* strains vary, but most strains are inhibited by gentamicin, tobramycin, amikacin, imipenem-cilastatin, the ureidopenicillins such as piperacillin, and aztreonam. Sensitivity to the tetracyclines is unpredictable, and most strains are resistant to penicillin, ampicillin, the cephalosporins, erythromycin, and chloramphenicol. For serious systemic infections, the appropriate antibiotic, generally an aminoglycoside, should be administered, and since these organisms may produce localized abscesses, surgical drainage may be necessary.

EIKENELLA INFECTIONS

ETIOLOGY *Eikenella corrodens* is a facultatively anaerobic or capnophilic gram-negative rod which is oxidase-positive. As colonies develop on blood agar, characteristic "pitting" or "corroding" of the agar is seen with many strains and generally requires 48 to 72 h of growth to develop.

EPIDEMIOLOGY *Eikenella corrodens* is an inhabitant of the mouth, upper respiratory tract, and gastrointestinal tract of mammals. Infections frequently involve bowel or oral contamination. A striking association between *Eikenella* infections and methylphenidate abuse has been noted, perhaps related to the low redox potential created by "skin popping" of this agent as well as a tendency for needles to become contaminated with oral secretions through needle licking.

MANIFESTATIONS The most common infection caused by *Eikenella* is that of skin or soft tissue. Endocarditis, pneumonia, osteomyelitis, and meningitis are reported but are rare. *Eikenella* infections frequently mimic infections caused by strict anaerobes such as *Bacteroides fragilis* or *Peptostreptococcus*. The infections are indolent and frequently mixed with aerobic gram-positive cocci, and drainage is often foul-smelling. Abscess formation is common.

TREATMENT *Eikenella corrodens* is susceptible to penicillin, ampicillin, carbenicillin, and tetracycline. Adequate drainage of purulent material is essential in the management of these infections. Ampicillin or penicillin coupled with surgical drainage generally provides a good response. Of note is the marked resistance of *Eikenella* to clindamycin, making the differentiation between *Eikenella* infections and those caused by mixed anaerobes even more important.

REFERENCES

Enterobacteriaceae: General

Boscia JA et al: Epidemiology of bacteriuria in an elderly ambulatory population. Am J Med 80:208, 1986

Karnad A et al: Pneumonia caused by gram-negative bacilli. Am J Med 79:61, 1985

Kreger BE et al: Gram-negative bacteremia. Am J Med 68:332, 1980

Maki DG: Nosocomial bacteremia: An epidemiologic overview. Am J Med 70:719, 1981

Moore RD et al: Association of aminoglycoside plasma levels with therapeutic outcome in gram-negative pneumonia. Am J Med 77:657, 1984

Tancrede CH, Andremont AO: Bacterial translocation and gram-negative bacteremia in patients with hematological malignancies. J Infect Dis 152:99, 1985

Escherichia coli infections

Geraci JE et al: Endocarditis due to gram-negative bacteria. Mayo Clin Proc 57:145, 1982

Levine MM: Escherichia coli that cause diarrhea: Enterotoxigenic, enteropathogenic, enteroinvasive, enterohemorrhagic, and enteroadherent. J Infect Dis 155:377, 1987

Ostroff SM et al: Infections with Escherichia coli 0157:H7 in Washington State. JAMA 262:355, 1989

Rahal JJ, Simberkoff MS: Host defense and antimicrobial therapy in adult gram-negative bacillary meningitis. Ann Intern Med 96:468, 1982

Klebsiella-Enterobacter-Serratia infections

Cooper R, Millis J: Serratia endocarditis. Arch Intern Med 140:199, 1980

Meltz DJ, Grieco MH: Characteristics of Serratia marcescens pneumonia. Arch Intern Med 132:359, 1973

Rennie RP, Duncan IBR: Emergence of gentamicin-resistant Klebsiella in a general hospital. Antimicrob Agents Chemother 11:179, 1978

Proteus infections

Berger SA: Proteus bacteremia in a general hospital. J Hosp Infect 6:293, 1985

Iannini PB et al: Multidrug-resistant P. rettgeri. Ann Intern Med 55:161, 1976

Senior BW et al: The ureases of Proteus strains in relation to virulence for the urinary tract. J Med Microbiol 13:468, 1982

Pseudomonas infections

Bagel J, Grossman ME: Subcutaneous nodules in Pseudomonas sepsis. Am J Med 80:528, 1986

Bodey GP et al: Infections caused by Pseudomonas aeruginosa. Rev Infect Dis 5:279, 1983

Gould IM, Rise R: Pseudomonas aeruginosa: Clinical manifestations and management. Lancet 2:1224, 1985

Hilf M et al: Antibiotic Therapy for Pseudomonas aeruginosa bacteremia: Outcome correlations in a prospective study of 200 patients. Am J Med 87:540, 1989

Maloney J et al: Analysis of amikacin-resistant Pseudomonas aeruginosa developing in patients receiving amikacin. Arch Intern Med 149:630, 1989

Morrison AJ, Wenzel RP: Epidemiology of infection due to Pseudomonas aeruginosa. Rev Infect Dis 6(Suppl):S627, 1984

Pollack M: The virulence of Pseudomonas aeruginosa. Rev Infect Dis 6(Suppl):S617, 1984

Acinetobacter infections

Bergogne-Berezin E et al: Epidemiology of nosocomial infections due to Acinetobacter calcoaceticus. J Hosp Infect 10:105, 1987

Harstein AI et al: Multiple intensive care unit outbreak of Acinetobacter calcoaceticus subspecies antitratus respiratory infection and colonization associated with contaminated, reusable ventilator circuits and resuscitation bags. Am J Med 85:624, 1988

Eikenella infections

Survangool SL et al: Pathogenicity of Eikenella corrodens in humans. Arch Intern Med 143:2265, 1983

112 MELIOIDOSIS AND GLANDERS

JAY P. SANFORD

MELIOIDOSIS

DEFINITION Melioidosis is an infection of humans and animals with a protean clinical spectrum. Melioidosis, which means "a resemblance to distemper of asses," bears a striking resemblance to glanders both clinically and pathologically, but is epidemiologically dissimilar.

ETIOLOGY Melioidosis is caused by a gram-negative motile bacillus, *Pseudomonas pseudomallei,* which can be differentiated from *P. mallei* by bacteriologic and serologic means. *P. pseudomallei* (also known as Whitmore's bacillus) is a small, gram-negative, motile, aerobic bacillus. When it is stained with methylene blue, Wayson's, or Wright's stain, marked irregularities with a bipolar "safety pin" pattern are observed. It grows well on standard bacteriologic media, with a characteristic wrinkling of colony surfaces after 48 to 72 h of incubation. Two antigenic types have been distinguished, type I (Asian), found widely, including in Australia, and type II (Australian), found mainly in Australia. The two types are equally pathogenic.

EPIDEMIOLOGY The disease is endemic in southeast Asia where human and animal cases occur commonly. Disease in humans has been reported from adjacent areas including India, Borneo, the Philippines, Guam, Indonesia, Sri Lanka, New Guinea, and Australia (north Queensland, Northern Territory). Cases in humans or animals have been reported from Madagascar, Chad, Kenya, Central West Africa (Niger, Upper Volta), Iran, and Turkey. In 1976, *P. pseudomallei* was isolated from animals in the Paris zoo. Human melioidosis has been described only rarely in the western hemisphere (Panama, Ecuador, Mexico)—a neonatal case in Hawaii, a case in Georgia, and a possible case in Oklahoma. With these exceptions, confirmed melioidosis has occurred in United States or European residents only when they have traveled in endemic areas. As of January 1973, when all American forces had been withdrawn from Vietnam, there had been 343 cases with 36 deaths reported in United States Army personnel who were or had been in Vietnam.

Pseudomonas pseudomallei is a saprophyte which can be isolated from soil, ponds, rice paddies, and market produce in endemic areas. Its ubiquitous nature is illustrated by its isolation as a laboratory contaminant or following an intraarticular injection. *Pseudomonas pseudomallei* is capable of causing disease in epizootic form among sheep, goats, swine, and horses. Occasional isolates have also been reported from cows, rodents, dogs, cats, wallabies, and birds. Although animals are susceptible to the disease, they apparently do not represent a reservoir for human disease. Attempts to culture *P. pseudomallei* from the urine and feces of a large variety of healthy animals have been unsuccessful. Arthropod-borne infection does not occur naturally. Humans contract melioidosis by soil contamination of skin abrasions. Ingestion, nasal instillation, and inhalation are other probable methods of spread. In contrast to glanders, infections have been uncommon, but can occur, in laboratory workers. *P. pseudomallei* has been recovered from urine specimens of patients who had urethral catheters, while hospitalized in an endemic area. Person-to-person transmission of melioidosis is rare. Venereal transmission is extremely rare. Also, the development of melioidosis in a 2-day-old newborn in Hawaii and demonstration of a significant antibody titer in a nurse who had never been in an endemic area but who had worked on wards with melioidosis patients raises the question of spread from person-to-person within a hospital.

PATHOLOGY In acute infections, the majority of lesions occur in the lungs, with occasional abscesses in other organs. In subacute infections, lung abscesses tend to be more extensive, and lesions are found throughout the body, in the skin, subcutaneous tissue, meninges, brain, eye, heart, liver, kidney, spleen, bone, prostate, synovial membranes, and lymph nodes. The acute abscesses are characterized by an outer border of hemorrhage, a medial zone heavily infiltrated with polymorphonuclear leukocytes, and an inner core of necrotic debris containing large histiocytes with two or three nuclei that have been termed giant cells. A striking histologic feature has been the marked karyorrhexis. In chronic infections, the lesion consists of a central area of caseation necrosis, mononuclear and plasma cells, and granulation tissue. Calcification does not occur.

Melioidosis is associated with impaired cellular immunity; total lymphocyte counts are usually less than 1000 per microliter; the percentage of total T cells is less than 50 percent due to a decrease in T helper cells; and skin tests with dinitrochlorobenzene are negative.

The number of T suppressor cells is normal, as is the number of B cells.

CLINICAL MANIFESTATIONS The clinical manifestations of melioidosis are variable. The illness can present as an acute, subacute, or chronic process. The incubation period has not been defined; however, judging by the lapse of time between injury and the development of infection, it may be as short as 2 days. Following a laboratory accident, an incubation period of 3 days ensued. Clinically inapparent infections may remain latent for a number of years after an individual leaves an endemic area, with an interval of 26 years reported in one patient. Men are more often affected than women, a finding which is thought to represent occupational exposure. Melioidosis may be recognized as inapparent infection, asymptomatic pulmonary infiltration, acute localized suppurative infection, acute pulmonary infection, acute septicemic infection, or chronic suppurative infection.

Inapparent infection In Thailand, Vietnam, and Malaysia, 6 to 8 percent of healthy adult men have significant antibody titers against *P. pseudomallei*, with the prevalence reaching 20 percent in a group of Army recruits from the rice-growing states of western Malaysia. Only 1 percent of Thai women had positive reactions. None of the sera from a control group from the United States was positive. The prevalence of significant antibody titers has been reported as 2 percent for Europeans living in Vietnam and 1 to 9 percent in unselected patients in United States Army hospitals and in a group of normal uninjured soldiers who had served in Vietnam. Occasionally, asymptomatic infections have been discovered by routine chest x-ray. In a serologic survey of 275 Chinese patients in a Hong Kong tuberculosis sanatorium, 14 percent had hemagglutinin titers of $\geq 1:80$.

Acute localized suppurative infection Infection by inoculation of a break in the skin usually results in a nodule with an area of acute lymphangitis and regional lymphadenitis. There are usually fever and generalized malaise. This form of infection may rapidly progress to the acute septicemic form.

Acute pulmonary infection The most common form of the disease has been pulmonary infection, which may represent a primary pneumonitis or hematogenous spread. The acute pulmonary infection can vary in severity from a mild bronchitis to overwhelming necrotizing pneumonia. The onset may be abrupt without prodromal symptoms or more gradual, with headache, anorexia, and generalized myalgia. Fever occurs in almost all patients, is often in excess of $38.9°C$ ($102°F$), and may be associated with rigors. Dull or pleuritic chest pain is common. Cough, with or without sputum, occurs. There may be mild pharyngitis. Tachypnea may be out of proportion to the fever and findings on physical or x-ray examination. Chest findings may be minimal but usually consist of rales in the area of pneumonitis. In the absence of dissemination, the spleen and liver are not palpable. Laboratory findings include total leukocyte counts ranging from normal to 20,000 cells per microliter. Mild normochromic, normocytic anemia may appear during the illness. The pneumonia usually involves the upper lobes with the radiographic appearance of consolidation. Thin-walled cavities, usually 2 to 7 cm in diameter, frequently occur. Without specific therapy, the temperature may become normal within a few days; however, the upper lobe cavitation persists, resulting in a radiographic appearance of tuberculosis. While uncommon, pleural effusions, a pleural mass, and bilateral hilar adenopathy have been reported. Progressive pulmonary spread or hematogenous dissemination with the development of septicemic manifestations may ensue.

Acute septicemic infection This is the form originally described primarily among narcotic addicts. Subsequent reports, however, have shown a predilection for debilitated patients with diabetes mellitus and alcoholism. The onset may be abrupt, with the dominant symptoms depending upon site of major involvement. In individuals with bacteremia complicating pneumonitis, symptoms may include disorientation, extreme dyspnea, severe headache, pharyngitis, watery diarrhea, and development of cutaneous pustular lesions on the head, trunk, or extremities. There is high fever, extreme tachypnea, a flushed skin, and cyanosis. Muscle tenderness may be striking. On

examination of the chest, signs may be absent, or rales, rhonchi, and pleural rubs may be heard. The liver and spleen may be palpable. Signs of arthritis or meningitis may appear. Patients with the septicemic form usually have a rapidly progressive fatal course, which in many instances may be too fulminant to be altered by therapy. The leukocyte count may be normal or slightly increased. Chest radiographs most commonly show irregular nodular densities 4 to 10 mm in diameter disseminated throughout the lungs. These enlarge, coalesce, and often undergo cavitation as the disease progresses. Pleural effusion is rare. Other radiographic patterns include unilateral irregular mottled densities which become confluent.

Chronic suppurative infection Acute or chronic abscesses dominate the clinical picture. Individuals have been misdiagnosed as having tropical pyomyositis which is caused by staphylococci. Organs involved include skin, brain, lung, myocardium, liver, spleen, prostate, bones, joints, lymph nodes, and even the eye. These patients may be afebrile.

Recrudescent infection Activation of inapparent or quiescent infection may present as acute localized suppurative, acute pulmonary, acute septicemic, or chronic suppurative disease remote from the probable time of exposure (up to 26 years having been reported). Surgery, trauma, intercurrent illness such as severe influenza pneumonia, diabetic ketoacidosis, alcoholic debauches, or radiation therapy appeared to act as triggering events. Since *P. pseudomallei* is an intracellular parasite and is associated with suppression of T helper lymphocytes, it seems only a matter of time before melioidosis will be added to the list of infections which occur in individuals with HIV infections, especially in areas where *P. pseudomallei* is endemic.

DIAGNOSIS Melioidosis should be considered in the differential diagnosis of any febrile illness in an individual who has been in an endemic area, especially if the presenting features are those of fulminant respiratory failure, if multiple pustular or necrotic skin or subcutaneous lesions develop, or if there is a radiographic pattern of tuberculosis in a patient from whom tubercle bacilli cannot be isolated.

Microscopic examination of exudates shows poorly staining, small, gram-negative bacilli with characteristic staining irregularities and "safety pin" bipolar staining with methylene blue. *Pseudomonas pseudomallei* will grow on most laboratory media, including eosin methylene blue agar (EMB) or MacConkey's agar, in 24 to 48 h. The organisms can be differentiated from *P. mallei* and *P. aeruginosa* by standard bacteriologic procedures, although isolates may pose problems in identification with some commercial medium kits. The hemagglutination, direct agglutination test, and complement fixation test are aids in diagnosis if a fourfold or greater rise in titer is demonstrated in paired sera. Single low titers are difficult to interpret because of nonspecific responses. The complement fixation test is said to be specific with titers above 1:8 during the acute illness, but may cross-react with *P. mallei*. A negative complement fixation test does not exclude disease. The hemagglutination and agglutination tests show more cross reactions. Titers of 1:40 or more suggest infection. In one-third of patients, with both fulminating and subacute disease, the serology has been negative at the time the culture became positive.

TREATMENT Virtually all strains of *P. pseudomallei* produce β-lactamase. In the past, most isolates have been sensitive in vitro to the tetracyclines, chloramphenicol, novobiocin, kanamycin, amikacin, and trimethoprim-sulfamethoxazole. In vitro studies with newer antimicrobial agents have shown over 90 percent of strains susceptible to ceftazidime, cefotaxime, cefoperazone, piperacillin, imipenem, amoxicillin-clavulanate, ampicillin-sulbactam, ticarcillin-clavulanate, and coumermycin (coumamycin). The fluorinated 4-quinolones such as ciprofloxacin and the monobacteram aztreonam have poor activity against *P. pseudomallei*. In Thailand, multiple resistant strains (resistant to chloramphenicol, tetracycline, trimethoprim-sulfamethoxazole), presumably permeability mutants, have been isolated from patients on admission and have emerged during treatment. In patients with pneumonitis who are not severely ill, currently recommended therapy is trimethoprim-sulfamethoxazole (4 mg/kg trimethoprim, 20 mg/kg sulfamethoxazole) for 60 to 150 days. In patients who are allergic to sulfonamides or in areas of trimethoprim-sulfamethoxazole resistance, alternatives include ceftazidime, 3 g daily (50 mg/kg), or cefotaxime, 3 g daily (30 mg/kg). Following clinical response to a third-generation cephalosporin, completion of a course with amoxicillin-clavulanate, 500 mg orally every 8 h, appears rational based on in vitro data; however, clinical experience is lacking. If the patient is severely ill, two antimicrobials in combination should be given for 30 days followed by another 30 to 120 days of trimethoprim-sulfamethoxazole. Although experience with the third-generation antipseudomonal cephalosporins is limited, a combination of ceftazidime (100 mg/kg per day) and trimethoprim (20 mg/kg per day)-sulfamethoxazole (100 mg/kg per day) is appropriate unless resistance is demonstrated. Individuals with low-titer positive serologic tests but with no clinical evidence of infection do not require therapy. The mean interval for sputum cultures to become negative has been 6 weeks. If sputum cultures remain positive for 6 months, surgery with lobectomy should be considered. In patients with extrapulmonary suppurative lesions, therapy should be continued for 6 months to 1 year and the usual principles of surgical drainage should be followed. In desperately ill patients with severe pneumonitis or the septicemic form, multiple antibiotics should be administered by the parenteral route. Levamisole[1] (150 mg twice per week) has been used as an adjunct to antibiotic therapy in several patients with results that suggest it may be beneficial in the treatment of relapses.

PROGNOSIS   Prior to antimicrobials, the mortality rate of apparent infection was 95 percent. With better diagnosis and more prolonged appropriate therapy, the mortality rate in all except the septicemic form is low. Even with vigorous appropriate antibiotics and supportive therapy, the mortality rate in patients with melioidosis septicemia is greater than 50 percent. Very few patients have had long-term follow-up, and the incidence of late relapses is approximately 20 percent.

PREVENTION   There is no means of active immunization. In endemic areas, vigorous cleansing of abrasions and lacerations is recommended.

GLANDERS

DEFINITION   Glanders is a serious infection of equine animals caused by *P. mallei*, which is transmitted occasionally to other domestic animals and to human beings.

ETIOLOGY   *Pseudomonas mallei* is a small, slender, nonmotile, gram-negative bacillus. When it is stained with methylene blue, marked irregularities in staining are observed. Organisms grow on most common meat infusion media but require glycerol for optimum growth.

EPIDEMIOLOGY   Glanders was at one time widespread throughout Europe, but owing to the introduction of control measures, its incidence has decreased steadily in most countries. The disease still occurs in Asia, Africa, and South America, but not in the United States and western Europe. Glanders has never been common in humans; the occasional infection, however, may be very serious. There have been no naturally acquired infections in the United States since 1938.

Glanders is primarily a disease of horses, mules, and donkeys, although goats, sheep, cats, and dogs sometimes naturally contract the disease. Pigs and cattle are resistant. In horses, the disease may be systemic, with prominent pulmonary involvement (*glanders*) or may be characterized by subcutaneous ulcerative lesions and lymphatic thickening with nodules (*farcy*). Inhalation, ingestion, and inoculation through breaks in the skin have been suggested as routes of infection in animals. In humans, the disease occurs primarily in individuals with close contact with horses, mules, or donkeys through inoculation of or a break in the skin or by exposing the nasal mucosa to contaminated discharges. A number of instances of airborne infection have been reported in laboratory workers.

CLINICAL MANIFESTATIONS   The manifestations, which frequently overlap, may be categorized as (1) acute localized suppurative infection, (2) acute pulmonary infection, (3) acute septicemic infection, and (4) chronic suppurative infection. Nearly 60 percent of patients have been between the ages of 20 and 40 years. The disease has been rare in women, probably because there is little opportunity for contact.

Infection acquired by inoculation through an abrasion in the skin usually results in a nodule with an area of acute lymphangitis. The incubation period is probably 1 to 5 days. In all types of acute glanders, there are usually fever, generalized malaise, and prostration.

Infection of the mucous membranes may result in a mucopurulent discharge involving the eye, nose, or lips followed by extensive ulcerating granulomatous lesions which may or may not be associated with systemic reactions. With systemic invasion, a generalized papular eruption which may become pustular is frequent. This septicemic form of disease is usually fatal in 7 to 10 days.

Infection by inhalation is followed by an incubation period of 10 to 14 days. The more common symptoms include fever, occasionally associated with rigors, generalized myalgia, fatigue, headache, and pleuritic chest pain. Other symptoms consist of photophobia, lacrimation, and diarrhea. Findings on physical examination are usually normal except for fever and occasional lymphadenopathy, especially in the cervical chain, and splenomegaly. Laboratory findings include mild leukocytosis with 60 to 80 percent neutrophilic leukocytes, but leukopenia with relative lymphocytosis has been recorded. In the acute pulmonary form, chest radiographs characteristically reveal circumscribed densities which suggest early lung abscesses. Other findings may include lobar or bronchopneumonia. In the chronic suppurative form of the disease, the most frequent finding consists of multiple subcutaneous and intramuscular abscesses which most often involve the arms or legs. Approximately one-half the patients will have associated fever, lymphadenopathy, and nasal discharge or ulceration. Visceral involvement including pulmonary or pleural, ocular, skeletal, hepatic, splenic, and meningeal or intracranial involvement occurs in some patients.

DIAGNOSIS   Microscopic examination of exudates may reveal small gram-negative bacilli which stain irregularly with methylene blue; however, organisms generally are very scanty. *Pseudomonas mallei* and *P. pseudomallei* cannot be distinguished morphologically. Growth occurs on most meat infusion nutrient media. Blood cultures are usually negative except in the terminal stages of disease. Serologic tests show a rapidly rising agglutination titer, which reaches levels of 1:640 within 2 weeks. Serum from normal persons has been reported to show agglutination titers in dilutions up to 1:320. The complement fixation test is less sensitive but more specific and usually becomes positive during the third week; it is considered positive in dilutions of 1:20 or greater.

TREATMENT   The limited number of recent infections in human beings has precluded evaluation of most of the antibiotic agents. Sulfadiazine has been found to be an effective agent in experimental animals and in humans. The dosage utilized has been approximately 100 mg/kg administered in divided doses. Treatment should be given for at least 30 days. Penicillin is ineffective. Tetracycline, chloramphenicol, the antipseudomonal aminoglycosides, carbenicillin, the third-generation antipseudomonal cephalosporins, and trimethoprim-sulfamethoxazole have not been evaluated. In the absence of clinical experience and pending in vitro susceptibility studies, it would seem most reasonable to utilize the regimens appropriate for patients with melioidosis. In the acute infections, appropriate supportive measures are essential, and in chronic suppurative infections, the usual principles of surgical drainage should be followed.

PROGNOSIS   The prognosis depends upon the type of infection. The acute septicemic form has been uniformly fatal. The localized or chronic forms have a much better prognosis.

---

[1] This drug has not been approved for this purpose by the Food and Drug Administration at the time of publication.

PREVENTION Next to acquisition from diseased horses, the commonest source of natural disease in human beings has been contact with human glanders. Isolation is indicated.

REFERENCES

BARNES PF et al: A case of melioidosis originating in North America. Am Rev Respir Dis 134:170, 1986

CHAOWAGUL W et al: Melioidosis: A major cause of community-acquired septicemia in Northeastern Thailand. J Infect Dis 159:890, 1989

DANCE DAB et al: Antibiotic resistance in *Pseudomonas pseudomallei*. Lancet 1:994, 1988

DODIN A, GALIMAND M: Whitmore's bacillus. Rec Med Vet 152:323, 1976

EVERETT ED, NELSON, R. Pulmonary melioidosis, observations in 39 cases. Am Rev Respir Dis 112:331, 1975

GILLESPIE SH et al: In vitro susceptibility of *Pseudomonas pseudomallei* to DNA gyrase inhibitors. J Antimicrob Chemother 20:612, 1987

GUARD LR et al: Melioidosis in far north Queensland. Am J Trop Med Hyg 33:467, 1984

JACKSON AE et al: Recrudescent melioidosis associated with diabetic ketoacidosis. Arch Intern Med 130:268, 1972

LUMBIGANON P et al: Neonatal melioidosis report of 5 cases. Pediatr Infect Dis J 7:634, 1988

McCORMICK JB et al: Human-to-human transmission of *Pseudomonas pseudomallei.* Ann Intern Med 83:512, 1975

McENIRY DW et al: Susceptibility of *Pseudomonas pseudomallei* to new beta-lactam and aminoglycoside antibiotics. J Antimicrob Chemother 21:171, 1988

MORRISON RE et al: Melioidosis: A reminder. Am J Med 84:965, 1988

SCHLECH WF III et al: Laboratory-acquired infection with *Pseudomonas pseudomallei* (melioidosis). N Engl J Med 305:1133, 1981

SO SY et al: Melioidosis: A serological survey in a tuberculosis sanatorium in Hong Kong. Trans Roy Soc Trop Med Hyg 81:1017, 1987

TANPHAICHITRA D, SRIMUANG S: Cellular immunity in tuberculosis, melioidosis, pasteurellosis, penicilliosis and role of levamisole and isoprinosine. Dev Biol Stand 57:117, 1984

WANVARIE S: Melioidosis: Certain interesting presentations and treatment. Trop Geo Med 36:165, 1984

WALL RA et al: A case of melioidosis in West Africa. J Infect Dis 152:424, 1985

WILKINSON L: Glanders: Medicine and veterinary medicine in common pursuit of a contagious disease. Med Hist 25:363, 1981

113 SALMONELLOSIS

GERALD T. KEUSCH

Organisms of the genus *Salmonella* are capable of causing a large variety of infections in humans, including typhoid (or enteric) fevers, focal systemic infections, septicemias, and gastroenteritis varying clinically from watery diarrhea to dysentery. Nontyphoidal salmonellosis usually refers to enteric disease caused by many members of the genus except *S. typhi*. Convalescent carriage of gastroenteritis strains is usually transient. A few subjects, generally young children under 5 years, may become long-term (longer than 1 year) asymptomatic carriers although they are not important in the spread of infection. Patients with *S. typhi* are more likely to become long-term carriers, for years or possibly for life, and they serve as reservoirs for the spread of infection.

ETIOLOGY The salmonellae are nonencapsulated gram-negative bacilli, almost always motile by means of peritrichous flagellae, expressing two or more forms of H antigens. They are generally lactose nonfermenters, and this property is used for initial selection in the clinical microbiology laboratory. The salmonellae ferment glucose, resulting in a typical acid butt and alkaline slant on triple sugar iron agar (TSI). They generally produce H_2S, which is detectable as a black reaction product and serves initially to distinguish isolates from *Shigella,* which also give an alkaline/acid TSI reaction. There are a very large number of *Salmonella* O and H antigens, allowing the separation of over 2200 different organisms on the basis of the patterns of the O and H antigens. As these isolates have often been named after the place they were first detected, *Salmonella* classification more closely resembles geography. On the basis of major somatic

antigens, a limited number of serogroups have been defined, and most human pathogens are members of groups A to D.

More rational classification schemes have been introduced that divide the genus into three species. One scheme includes *S. cholerasuis*, the prototype species; *S. typhi*, the major cause of typhoid (enteric) fever; and *S. enteritidis*, a catchall designation for all of the remaining serotypes only some of which are pathogenic for humans. These serotypes do not have the taxonomic rank of species and should not be italicized, but for clinical and epidemiologic ease the convention is to use only the serotype name. Thus, *S. enteritidis* serotype typhimurium becomes *S. typhimurium*, and *S. enteritidis* serotype enteritidis becomes *S. enteritidis*.

Some salmonellae are highly host-adapted to humans (e.g., *S. typhi, S. paratyphi A,* and *S. paratyphi B*) while most animal-adapted species cause no human disease. Others infect both man and lower animals causing gastroenteritis or less commonly, localized or septicemic infections.

TYPHOID FEVER

Typhoid fever is a distinctive acute systemic febrile infection of the mononuclear phagocytes and deserves separate consideration. Since it may be caused by several *species* (*S. typhi, S. paratyphi A* and *paratyphi B,* and occasionally *S. typhimurium*), many clinicians prefer the term *enteric fever*. But because typhoid is fundamentally not an enteric disease, this term is also inappropriate. On balance, *typhoid fever* is still the best term, for it is understood by nearly all clinicians to describe a particular syndrome that is, in fact, due primarily to *S. typhi*.

EPIDEMIOLOGY Because the cause of clinical typhoid fever is almost always a human-adapted *Salmonella*, most cases can be traced to a human carrier. The proximate cause may be water (the most common route) or food contaminated by a human carrier. Chronic carriers are generally over 50 years old, are more commonly women, and often have gallstones. *S. typhi* reside in the bile, even within the interiors of stones, and intermittently reach the lumen of the bowel, when they are excreted in the stool, thereby contaminating water or food.

With improvements in environmental sanitation in the United States, the incidence of typhoid has gradually dropped. Compared with 1920 when almost 36,000 cases were detected, the annual number now is approximately 500. Over 80 percent of these are active typhoid cases, and the others are convalescent carriers. The median age of a case is around 24 years, while the median age of carriers is over 60 years. Data gathered by the Centers for Disease Control (CDC) show that the incidence in the United States dropped fivefold from 1955 to 1966, from 1 per 100,000 to 0.2 per 100,000 population, and has remained steady since then. At the same time, the proportion of infections acquired abroad has increased, from 33 percent in the 1960s to over 60 percent in the 1980s. Mexico is the leading source for Americans, accounting for 39 percent of cases from 1975 to 1984; almost 60 percent were acquired somewhere in the Americas. The next most common location (17 percent) is the Indian subcontinent. Students are most at risk. In England, the majority of cases are also acquired abroad, usually in India or Pakistan. Known hot-spots for typhoid include Alexandria, Egypt; Jakarta, Indonesia; and Santiago, Chile.

Typhoid contracted in the United States is primarily due to association with known or newly diagnosed carriers (30 percent) or from food-borne outbreaks (28 percent). The highest rates occur in states bordering Mexico. The groups most likely to be at risk are bacteriology laboratory workers, other medical personnel, and sewage workers, but they actually have relatively low rates and account for less than 5 percent of identified cases. However, the number of patients is clearly underestimated, and an unknown proportion of patients escape detection because appropriate cultures are not done or the patients have already taken antibiotics.

PATHOGENESIS   Following ingestion of a suitable inoculum, *S. typhi* pass the gastric barrier to reach the small bowel. Experimental human infections with the Quailes strain have revealed that 10^3 organisms will not cause symptomatic disease but that 10^5 bacteria cause symptoms in 27 percent of volunteers. Higher doses result in more frequent illness, unless the organisms lack the ability to produce the Vi antigen. Animal studies suggest that *S. typhi* invade the host in the upper small bowel, resulting in a transient and asymptomatic bacteremia. The organisms are ingested by mononuclear phagocytes and must survive and multiply intracellularly to cause illness.

Persistent bacteremia initiates the clinical phase of infection. The ability of the inoculum to invade mononuclear cells and multiply intracellularly determines whether or not this secondary bacteremia occurs. The absence of bactericidal antibodies allows organisms to be phagocytized in a viable state. Intracellular survival is dependent upon microbial factors that promote resistance to killing and the state of specific T-lymphocyte–activated host cell–mediated immunity. Dose dependence of clinical disease appears to be governed by the balance between bacterial multiplication and acquired host extracellular and intracellular defenses. When the number of intracellular bacteria surpasses a critical threshold, secondary bacteremia occurs and results in the invasion of the gallbladder and Peyer's patches of the intestine. The sustained bacteremia is responsible for the persistent fever of clinical typhoid, while inflammatory responses to tissue invasion determine the pattern of clinical expression (cholecystitis, intestinal hemorrhage, or perforation). With invasion of the gallbladder and Peyer's patches, bacteria regain entry to the bowel lumen, and by the second week of clinical disease the prevalence of positive stool cultures increases. Seeding of the kidney leads to positive urine cultures but in a much lower percentage of patients. The lipopolysaccharide endotoxin of *S. typhi* may contribute to causing fever, leukopenia, and other systemic symptoms, but the occurrence of such symptoms in subjects made tolerant to endotoxin supports a role for other factors, such as cytokines released from infected mononuclear phagocytes, that can mediate inflammation (see Chap 20).

CLINICAL MANIFESTATIONS   The incubation period is variable and depends on both the inoculum size and the state of host defenses. A range of 3 to 60 days has been reported. The disease usually presents with a steplike daily increase in temperature to 40 to 41°C, associated with headache, malaise, and chills. The hallmark of typhoid fever is prolonged, persistent fever (4 to 8 weeks in untreated patients). Mild and brief illness may occur, but in some patients acute, severe infection with disseminated intravascular coagulation and central nervous system involvement may result in death. In other patients, necrotizing cholecystitis or intestinal bleeding and perforation can occur in the third or fourth week of illness, when the patient is otherwise improving. In most, the onset of these complications is dramatic and clinically obvious. Intestinal perforation appears to be less common in children under 5 years of age.

Early intestinal manifestations include constipation, especially in adults, or mild diarrhea in children, associated with abdominal tenderness. Mild hepatosplenomegaly is detectable in the majority of patients. Bradycardia relative to the height of the fever may be a clinical clue to typhoid, but is present in a minority of patients. Epistaxis may occur in the early stages of illness. "Rose spots," appearing as small, pale red, blanching, slightly raised macules, may be seen on the chest and abdomen during the first week. They can also evolve into nonblanching small hemorrhages that are difficult to see in dark skinned patients. While the major characteristics of untreated typhoid and persistent high fever, severe anorexia, weight loss, and changes in sensorium, a variety of other complications may be seen, including hepatitis, meningitis, nephritis, myocarditis, bronchitis, pneumonia, arthritis, osteomyelitis, parotitis and orchitis. The frequency of all of these complications, including hemorrhage and perforation, is reduced by prompt use of appropriate antibiotics.

Around 3 to 5 percent of patients become long-term asymptomatic carriers, some for life unless treated. Many carriers give no history of typhoid fever and probably had an undiagnosed mild infection.

LABORATORY FINDINGS   In the early phases of typhoid fever the white blood cell count is usually in the range of 4000 to 5000 cells per microliter, and a left shift is present. This relative leukopenia in relation to the degree of fever may be a clue to the diagnosis. Rarely, severe leukopenia (<2000 cells per microliter) can occur. In the event of intestinal perforation or pyogenic complications, secondary leukocytosis develops. The anemia of blood loss may be superimposed on the anemia of chronic infection.

Definitive diagnosis depends on isolation of the organism or a serologic response. The recovery of organisms from blood is highest in the first week of illness, when it approaches 90 percent. Bacteremia is detectable in 50 percent in the third week and at a progressively lower frequency later on. Early in the illness culture of bone marrow aspirates will yield the organism in the majority of patients, even after brief prior antimicrobial treatment. Stool cultures are frequently negative in the first week but usually become positive in 75 percent of patients during the third week. By the eighth week, stools are positive in only 10 percent of patients, but in approximately 3 to 5 percent of patients will remain so for at least 1 year. The frequency of positive urine cultures parallels the yield from stools and may represent, in some patients, contamination with feces.

Serologic diagnosis is less reliable than culture. Most, but not all, patients will develop agglutinating antibodies to O, H, and Vi antigens (the Widal test). In the absence of recent immunization, a high titer of antibody to O antigen (>1:640) is useful but not specific. Other serogroup D salmonellae share the antigen used in the Widal test, as do some organisms in groups A and B. H antibodies may be found in even higher titer, but because of their broad cross reactivity are difficult to interpret. A fourfold rise in antibody in paired samples is a good criterion but is of little use in the acutely ill patients and may be blunted by early effective antimicrobial therapy. The earlier the baseline sample is obtained, the more likely a significant rise will be detected. Vi antibodies typically rise later, after three to four weeks of illness, and are of less use in the early diagnosis of infection.

DIFFERENTIAL DIAGNOSIS   When all the classic clinical manifestations are present, including rose spots, prolonged fever, relative bradycardia, and leukopenia, the diagnosis of typhoid will be strongly suggested. However, most cases do not fit this "typical" profile. Differential diagnosis includes infections associated with prolonged fever such as the rickettsioses, brucellosis, tularemia, leptospirosis, miliary tuberculosis, viral hepatitis, infectious mononucleosis, cytomegalovirus infections, and malaria, as well as noninfectious causes such as lymphoma (see Chap. 20). In the United States, typhoid should be considered in any patient with prolonged, unexplained fever, especially after recent travel to places with endemic typhoid fever.

TREATMENT   Since its introduction, chloramphenicol has been the antimicrobial gold standard for treatment. No drug has been better in promoting a favorable clinical response, and this usually becomes apparent within 24 to 48 h of the start of treatment in the appropriate dosages (3 to 4 g/d in adults or 50 mg/kg body weight per day in young children). The drug is given orally for 2 weeks, and the dose may be reduced to 2 g/d or 30 mg/kg per day when the patient becomes afebrile, which usually is not before day five of treatment. Other effective oral regimens include amoxicillin (4 to 6 g/d in four divided doses in adults or 100 mg/kg per day in children); trimethoprim-sulfamethoxazole (640 and 3200 mg, respectively, in two divided doses daily in adults or 185 mg/m² body surface area per day of the trimethoprim component for children); or in those over 17 years, a 4-fluoroquinolone such as ciprofloxacin or ofloxacin. Parenteral ampicillin (8 g/d in adults or 200 mg/kg per day in four divided doses in children) is also effective. Chloramphenicol or trimethoprim-sulfamethoxazole may be given intravenously if patients are unable to tolerate oral therapy. Initial studies with ceftriaxone (75 mg/kg per day) administered for 5 days indicate that it is effective treatment.

Chloramphenicol-resistant *S. typhi* first appeared in 1972 and were responsible for an epidemic in Mexico. Resistant strains are still encountered sporadically in Mexico, the Indian subcontinent, and in Southeast Asia and Indonesia. Resistance is plasmid-mediated and usually carries multiple common antibiotic resistances to sulfonamides, streptomycin, and tetracycline. Occasional isolates are doubly resistant to chloramphenicol and trimethoprim-sulfamethoxazole or ampicillin. The availability of 4-fluoroquinolones for adults simplifies the problem of treating nonresponders or those in whom single or double resistance to one of the more generally used antimicrobials is encountered.

Patients with severe typhoid who present with central nervous system manifestations and/or evidence of disseminated intravenous coagulation should be given intravenous glucocorticoids such as dexamethasone, 3 mg/kg as a loading dose over 30 min followed by 1 mg/kg every 6 h for 24 h, in addition to parenteral antimicrobials. Salicylates should be avoided to reduce the danger of intestinal hemorrhage. It is often recommended that the late complications of hemorrhage and perforations be managed conservatively with antibiotics and general support. This is largely because these occur most commonly in developing countries where patients frequently present late in the course of illness, are usually malnourished, and are poor surgical risks, and where there are limitations in surgical and postoperative care. Bowel perforations occurring in patients in countries with sophisticated medical facilities should be treated surgically as indicated by the clinical state and not by the microbiologic diagnosis. Selective angiography or radioisotopic scanning methods (see Chap. 46) to localize the bleeding site can facilitate operative repair. Small perforations may localize with supportive care and antibiotics alone. In developing countries, limited surgery to close the site of perforation, without bowel resection, may be the wisest choice.

The early use of effective antimicrobials is associated with a relatively high rate of relapse; relapse rates of 20 percent can be expected, compared with 5 to 10 percent in untreated patients. This is presumably because prompt therapy inhibits the development of an adequate immune response. Relapses are usually milder than the initial attack and will respond to the same antimicrobial used initially.

Successful treatment of chronic carriers can be difficult. Administration of 100 mg/kg per day of ampicillin or amoxicillin plus probenecid (30 mg/kg per day) or trimethoprim/sulfamethoxazole (160/800 mg) twice daily plus rifampin 600 mg once daily for at least 6 weeks is usually successful if there are no gallstones. Prolongation of antimicrobial therapy for 3 months can cure some carriers with gallstones; however, the most reliable treatment is cholecystectomy plus antimicrobials. Regimens using 4 weeks of treatment with the quinolones may be equally effective; however, experience with this approach is still limited.

PREVENTION AND CONTROL Worldwide experience has shown that improvement of environmental sanitation, including sewage disposal and water supplies, will sharply reduce the incidence of typhoid fever. Where this approach is not yet possible, and for travelers, immunization has been used. Killed, whole typhoid bacillus vaccine provides limited protection for several months, presumably by inducing bactericidal antibodies. The vaccine produces fever and pain and will induce O and H antibodies that give a positive Widal test and impeded diagnostic interpretation of serologic data.

Other vaccines have been used in an attempt to improve efficacy and reduce toxicity. A purified Vi vaccine given intramuscularly has been shown to provide equal efficacy to whole killed vaccines with minimal side effects. Studies are also proceeding with live oral vaccines. Two approaches have achieved some success, but not sufficient for routine use. These are a galactose epimerase mutant *S. typhi*, Ty 21a, and auxotrophic mutants selected for aromatic metabolites not available inside cells. Both vaccine prototypes invade mononuclear cells and stimulate immunity, but neither survive within cells and, therefore, are avirulent. Because of these properties, there are many attempts to use these strains as "piggyback" vectors to carry unrelated antigens for immunization purposes.

Typhoid is a reportable disease in the United States. Patients should be monitored for prolonged carriage and treated for this if necessary. Precautions in food handling by carriers and in disposal of their stools are obvious and important (see Chap. 83).

PROGNOSIS Appropriate therapy of typhoid fever, especially if patients present for medical care in the early stage of disease, is highly successful. The mortality rate should be under 1 percent and few complications should occur.

NONTYPHOIDAL SALMONELLOSIS

Infections caused by any *Salmonella* other than *S. typhi* are termed nontyphoidal salmonellosis. These infections can present as acute diarrhea, a septicemic syndrome, focal abscesses, meningitis, osteomyelitis, endocarditis, or mycotic aneurysm or can be asymptomatic.

EPIDEMIOLOGY The species *S. cholerasuis* and *S. enteritidis* include a diverse group of organisms with both host-adapted and nonhost-adapted serotypes. Two human-adapted serotypes, *S. paratyphi A* and *S. schottmuelleri* (more often called *S. paratyphi B*), have been discussed under typhoid fever. Of the more than 2200 known *S. enteritidis*, just ten account for 75 percent of all human disease isolates in the United States, and four serotypes (*S. typhimurium, enteritidis, heidelberg,* and *newport*) cause about two-thirds of all disease. *S. typhimurium* is the most frequent isolate, representing around 35 percent of all strains reported to the CDC. In past surveillance studies, periodic increases in recovery of certain serotypes have represented either introduction of a new transmission source or the occurrence of a large outbreak. For example, the number of *S. typhimurium* isolates increased from an average of 12,000 per year to over 28,000 in 1985 due to a massive outbreak related to consumption of contaminated milk in the Chicago area. A fivefold increase in *S. enteritidis* isolates between 1976 and 1986 was due to ingestion of contaminated grade A eggs primarily in the northeastern United States.

Careful analysis of surveillance data in the United States has shown that not only is the number of nontyphoidal *Salmonella* isolates increasing, but the incidence appears to be increasing as well, from 8 per 100,000 of the general population in 1965, to 12 per 100,000 in 1975, to around 18 per 100,000 by 1985. These data are biased in part by excess reporting of investigated outbreaks, and because infants, the elderly, and severely ill patients are the most likely to have cultures performed. While the incidence of disease in young children is five times higher than in older subjects, the rate is also somewhat higher in adults over 70 years. Between 1970 and 1986 the median age of infected individuals rose from 6 years to 20 years. The greatest increase has been in the 20- to 39-year-old population, suggesting that foods consumed by young adults are becoming important vehicles or that they are traveling more to endemic areas. A reasonable estimate of the total incidence of symptomatic *Salmonella* infection in the United States is 1 to 2 million cases per year. This degree of morbidity implies a significant economic impact in lost productivity and medical costs and, by extension, a serious and underestimated cause of mortality.

Because nontyphoidal *Salmonella* are so often nonhost-adapted, many kinds of domestic animals can harbor the organism and serve as the source for human infection. Conditions of raising, shipping, slaughtering, and marketing contribute to the spread of *Salmonella* in the food supply. Introduction of the organism into processed foods can result in widespread dissemination, and contamination of such common foods as eggs or milk leads to large-scale outbreaks. Dried or frozen foods preserve viable salmonellae. For these reasons, salmonellosis is more a disease of the industrialized world than of the developing world. Additional sources of human infection are animals sold as pets, including baby chicks or ducks and turtles, and medical products of animal origin, such as carmine dye (from insects); pancreatin; bile salts; or tissue extracts from thyroids, adrenals, stomachs, or rattlesnakes.

A potentially serious problem is the selection of antibiotic-resistant strains of salmonellae by unregulated drug use in animal husbandry. There are a number of instances where transmission to humans has occurred. Persistent and severe salmonellosis has also been recognized as a problem among patients with acquired immunodeficiency syndrome (AIDS) (see Chap. 264).

PATHOGENESIS As with *S. typhi*, the events following ingestion of the organism are determined by environmental factors (dose), microbial factors (serotype, invasion, and other virulence properties), and host factors (resistance). As few as 10^3 virulent organisms may cause disease, especially in patients with achlorhydria or having recent antimicrobial therapy. Systemic invasion is more likely in patients with "reticuloendothelial blockade" due to hemolysis (malaria, bartonellosis, leptospirosis, sickle cell anemia) or intracellular infections (histoplasmosis). The incidence of documented bacteremia varies from 5 to 45 percent, but is assumed to occur early in the course of many, and possibly all, *Salmonella* infections and is quickly cleared in most patients infected with *S. enteritidis* serotypes. Certain serotypes, such as *dublin*, *infantis*, *virchow*, *panama*, and *newport*, may be more invasive and more commonly isolated from blood. *S. typhimurium* is the most frequent blood isolate, but the rate of isolation is no more than the average for all nontyphoidal *Salmonella*. Systemic and focal tissue infections are secondary to bacteremia. *S. cholerasuis* is a highly invasive serotype that usually causes a septicemia syndrome and is most commonly isolated from blood but not from stool. Microbial factors, which determine the invasiveness of salmonellae, include motility and the presence of plasmid genes needed to establish progressive infection of mononuclear phagocytes. Such genes have been identified on a small common Eco R1 restriction fragment in plasmids of varying size in *S. dublin*, *S. enteritidis*, and *S. cholerasuis*.

The pathogenesis of *Salmonella* enteritis is not clear. Virulent strains appear to be invasive and able to induce inflammatory responses in the gut mucosa, but these properties are not sufficient to cause intestinal fluid secretion. This may depend on a heat-labile enterotoxin which is structurally, functionally, and immunologically related to the cholera and *E. coli* LT toxins. This toxin has now been cloned and expressed in *E. coli*. Heat-labile cytotoxins that act like Shiga toxins to inhibit intestinal protein synthesis may also be involved.

CLINICAL MANIFESTATIONS Gastroenteritis The incubation period of *Salmonella* gastroenteritis is generally short, 24 to 48 h. Sporadic illness is likely to go undiagnosed because cultures are not taken. Large outbreaks, often considered as "food poisoning" and characterized by self-limited fever and diarrhea, are more likely to be investigated and diagnosed. Diarrhea may be associated with nausea, vomiting, and abdominal cramps and occasionally becomes bloody or even dysenteric when the colon becomes involved. The stool contains many leukocytes when examined by direct microscopy, a clue to the invasive nature of the infection. The illness is generally mild and resolves without use of specific therapy, but may cause severe dehydration or disseminate and lead to death in debilitated elderly patients or neonates. Blood cultures often become positive as the patient is improving. Treatment may be discontinued after identification of the organism unless there is an underlying immunosuppressive disease (e.g., sickle cell disease, AIDS, malignancy such as a lymphoma or the patient is receiving glucocorticoid or immunosuppressive drug therapy). In these conditions treatment with an appropriate antibiotic should be administered for 7 to 10 days. Carriage in the stool of salmonellae that can cause gastroenteritis lasts several weeks after symptomatic disease and rarely exceeds 2 months.

Localized systemic infections Blood-borne salmonellae can invade any tissue or organ. The most common isolates are *S. typhimurium*, *S. enteritidis*, and *S. cholerasuis*. Localized infections usually follow intestinal infection, although there may be no prior diarrhea. Endocarditis is rare, but when it occurs there may be destructive cardiac lesions including valve perforations or ring or septal abscesses. Therapy requires both appropriate antimicrobials and surgery when necessary (see Chap. 90).

Arterial infection generally occurs in preexisting arteriosclerotic infrarenal aortic aneurysms, especially in men older than 50. *S. cholerasuis* accounts for about 20 percent of the isolates, in contrast to being found in <1 percent of patients with diarrhea due to salmonella infection, reflecting its capacity to cause systemic invasive disease. *S. typhimurium* accounts for ~25 percent of isolates in arterial infections, consistent with its high incidence in causing gastrointestinal salmonellosis (about 35 percent of all cases). In addition to treatment with antimicrobials, eradication usually requires prompt excision and drainage with bypass through uninvolved tissue. The disease should be suspected when elderly men develop prolonged fever following gastroenteritis, accompanied by back, abdomen, or chest pain; when bacteremia is present or recurrent after therapy for the initial illness; or when it occurs in patients with vertebral osteomyelitis or in those with prosthetic valves.

Cholecystitis, other *hepatobiliary infection*, or *splenic abscess* are the most common intraabdominal localized infections due to salmonellae. In addition to *S. typhimurium* and *S. enteritidis*, *S. typhi* is an important cause.

Urinary tract infections sometimes occur, especially in patients with urolithiasis, structural abnormalities, or immunosuppressive diseases or therapy. Salmonella urinary tract infection sometimes coexists with renal tuberculosis or *Schistosoma haematobium* infection.

Pneumonia or *empyema* caused by salmonella is rare and usually seen in patients with preexisting abnormalities of the lungs or pleura or with conditions that predispose to infection, including malignancy, diabetes, glucocorticoid use, sickle cell disease, or alcohol abuse.

Meningitis caused by salmonella is also rare and is most prevalent in young infants and children. Gram stains of cerebrospinal fluid are usually positive. Mortality rates of 40 to 60 percent are reported in children and adults, respectively. In survivors, residua include seizures, hydrocephalus, subdural empyemas, and permanent disabilities such as retardation, paresis, athetosis, or visual disturbances.

Septic arthritis due to salmonella is associated with positive joint-fluid cultures and should not be confused with reactive arthritis (a culture-negative inflammatory joint disease occurring after invasive diarrheas, especially in HLA-B27 or -B7 positive patients). Underlying conditions that are often present include glucocorticoid or immunosuppressive drug therapy, sickle cell disease, prosthetic joints, or aseptic necrosis. Drainage may be needed in addition to appropriate antibiotics.

Salmonella *osteomyelitis* is predictably associated with sickle cell disease, sickle-C disease, or sickle thalassemia. It generally affects long bones and occurs primarily in young patients; blood cultures are often positive (the most common isolate is *S. typhimurium*).

Bacteremia Sepsis, with prolonged fever and positive blood cultures but generally without prior diarrhea, occurs most commonly with *S. cholerasuis* infection. While this presentation is "typhoidal," typical manifestations of typhoid (rose spots, relative bradycardia, leukopenia) are absent, and the disease is more acute in onset and duration. *S. cholerasuis* sepsis is a severe disease, associated with high mortality.

Intermittent symptomatic *Salmonella* bacteremia is seen in patients with hepatosplenic or urinary schistosomiasis. Clinically severe *Salmonella* sepsis due to *S. typhimurium* also occurs in AIDS patients (see Chap. 264), is often recurrent, and may develop before the diagnosis of AIDS is made. The infection may be refractory to treatment or recurrent in spite of appropriate therapy. The incidence of salmonellosis in AIDS patients in the United States is now estimated to be between 46 and 384 per 100,000, which is 100 to 1000-fold greater than the incidence in the general population (0.3 per 100,000).

DIAGNOSIS Specific diagnosis depends on the isolation of the organisms from stool, blood, or tissue fluids. All clinical laboratories should be able to make the initial isolation and identify common serotypes. Uncommon serotypes usually must be sent to reference laboratories for identification.

TREATMENT Treatment for focal systemic infections requires selection of the most appropriate antibiotic and, at times, drainage or resection of infected tissue. Bactericidal antibiotics by the parenteral route are the usual choice and may include ampicillin in a dose of 6 to 12 g/d in adults or 100 mg/kg in young children in divided doses; chloramphenicol in a dose of 2 to 4 g/d in adults or 50 mg/kg in children in divided doses; or appropriate doses of third-generation cephalosporins such as ceftriaxone or cefotaxime when the organism is ampicillin-resistant (see Chap. 85). Because the experience with these latter drugs is not great, they cannot be recommended for routine use. The results with 4-fluoroquinolones suggest that these agents will become increasingly valuable because they are effective by the oral route.

The proper treatment of *Salmonella* gastroenteritis is not clear; antibiotics do not shorten illness but do increase the duration of convalescent carriage. For this reason it is generally recommended that no treatment other than supportive care and fluid replacement be administered. Early results suggest that 4-fluoroquinolones reduce the duration of illness and eradicate the organism from stool. However, until these drugs are shown to be safe this approach should not be routinely employed in children. When blood cultures are positive in the setting of otherwise uncomplicated gastroenteritis, prolonged treatment is usually reserved only for patients with underlying immunosuppressive disease. In an infant under 3 months of age with diarrhea, the stool should be cultured, a workup to localize the septic process initiated, and presumptive treatment begun with a third-generation cephalosporin until culture results are available. Fever is often absent in very young infants and is not a reliable indicator of systemic infection. Asymptomatic patients with salmonellae other than *S. typhi* in the stool should *not* receive antimicrobial treatment, since active disease may be produced and the carriage state prolonged.

PREVENTION AND CONTROL It is probably not possible to eradicate nontyphoidal salmonellosis since the organisms are so widespread in nature. Reduction in the use in animal feed of antimicrobials employed for human infection and improved animal rearing and marketing practices would be useful. Vigilance in food preparation and in quality testing of the known and commonly contaminated foods should help as well. It is recommended that eggs be fully cooked and not eaten raw or partially cooked. If universal body substance precautions are not routinely utilized, hospital staff caring for patients with salmonellosis should be placed on "enteric precautions," with gowning and gloving when handling stool and urine, and careful hand washing after patient contact (see Chap. 83).

During outbreaks, food handlers may be responsible for transmission. Much effort is given to the identification by stool culture of asymptomatic food handlers who are carriers during food-borne outbreaks, and they are usually kept from work until they become culture-negative. However, it is more important to determine what standards of practice are maintained to ensure proper environmental and personal hygiene of food handlers to prevent the problem from occurring. This is because carriage may be intermittant and is often not uniform within a single stool sample, and because any food contaminated with the organism would require improper handling to permit the growth of a sufficient inoculum to cause disease. Perhaps the only situation where it may be truly justifiable to restrict carriers from the workplace is in the course of a hospital outbreak or when there are workers who refuse to improve their personal hygiene.

The development of effective vaccines may be difficult because of the great number of serotypes involved in infection. Some progress has been made with galactose epimerase or aroA vaccine mutants of *S. typhimurium* for use in animals, and these may ultimately be tested in humans. Of all of the nontyphoidal salmonellae, it would be most useful to have vaccines for *S. cholerasuis* serotypes typhimurium and enteritidis.

REFERENCES

ACHARYA IL et al: Prevention of typhoid fever in Nepal with the Vi capsular polysaccharide vaccine of *Salmonella typhi*. N Engl J Med 317:1101, 1987

CHOPRA AK et al: Cloning and expression of the salmonella enterotoxin gene. J Bacteriol 169:5095, 1987

COHEN JI et al: Extra-intestinal manifestations of *Salmonella* infections. Medicine 66:349, 1987

FERRECCIO C et al: Efficacy of ciprofloxacin in the treatment of chronic typhoid carriers. J Infect Dis 157:1235, 1988

HARGRETT-BEAN NT et al: *Salmonella* isolates from humans in the United States, 1984–1986. Morbidity and Mortality Annual Surveillance Reports 37 No. SS-2:25, 1988

HOFFMAN SL et al: Reduction of mortality in chloramphenicol-treated severe typhoid fever by high-dose dexamethasone. N Engl J Med 310:82, 1984

RYAN CA et al: *Salmonella typhi* infections in the United States, 1975–1984: Increasing role of foreign travel. Rev Infect Dis 11:1, 1989

SPIKA JS et al: Chloramphenicol-resistant *Salmonella newport* traced through hamburger to dairy farms: A major persisting source of human salmonellosis in California. N Engl J Med 316:565, 1987

ST LOUIS ME et al: The emergence of grade-A eggs as a major source of *Salmonella enteriditis* infections: New implication for the control of salmonellosis. JAMA 259:2103, 1988

TOPLEY JM: Mild typhoid fever. Arch Dis Child 61:164, 1986

114 SHIGELLOSIS

GERALD T. KEUSCH

DEFINITION Shigellosis is an acute infectious inflammatory colitis due to one of the members of the genus *Shigella*. Although the disease is often referred to as "bacillary dysentery," many patients have only mild watery diarrhea and never develop dysenteric symptoms. The less severe illness predominates in industrialized countries such as the United States, whereas more severe, often fatal dysentery occurs in patients in developing countries.

ETIOLOGY The *Shigellae* are slender, gram-negative, nonmotile bacilli and are members of the family Enterobacteriaceae and tribe *Escherichae*. They are so closely related to *Escherichia coli* that the two genera cannot be distinguished by DNA hybridization methods. There are four *Shigella* species (*dysenteriae*, *flexneri*, *boydii* and *sonnei*) defined on the basis of surface somatic O antigens and carbohydrate fermentation patterns. Most are lactose-negative (*S. sonnei* are late lactose fermenters) and produce acid but not gas from glucose, resulting in a typical acid butt and alkaline slant in triple sugar iron agar (TSI), without H_2S production, in contrast to *Salmonella*. The genus is characterized by its ability to invade intestinal epithelial cells and to produce highly potent protein toxins that irreversibly inhibit eukaryotic cell protein synthesis by a specific enzymatic action.

EPIDEMIOLOGY It is estimated that at least 140 million cases and almost 600,000 deaths occur annually due to shigellosis in young children under the age of 5 years. The organism is found everywhere in the world, but is most common in developing countries where poor environmental sanitation and crowding facilitate transmission from person to person. The incidence in the United States is much lower, and less than 15,000 cases each year are reported to the Centers for Disease Control (CDC). This is no doubt a gross underestimate, as organisms from many patients are neither cultured nor identified. In industrialized countries and developing countries alike, most patients are young children. In the United States from 1974 to 1980, 93,516 cases were identified by means of a nationwide passive surveillance system. While the overall isolation rate was 4.7 per 100,000 population per year, among children aged 1 to 4 the rate was 22.3 per 100,000 children per year. In the United States, the disease is most common in the urban poor, in infants in day-care centers, and in retarded children institutionalized for custodial care. One high-risk group has also been identified: male homosexuals, who transmit infection by anal-oral sexual practices.

Since the description of the genus, major global shifts in prevalence of the four species have been noted. Until World War I, *S. dysenteriae* type 1 was the predominant isolate, frequently occurring in devastating epidemics with high mortality until it was replaced by *S. flexneri*. Since World War II, however, *S. flexneri* has been steadily replaced by *S. sonnei* in the industrialized countries. The reasons for these shifts are not clear. In Bangkok, Thailand, *S. sonnei* is now overtaking *S. flexneri*, whereas in the countryside *S. flexneri* strains still predominate. *S. boydii*, the fourth species, has remained largely confined to the Indian subcontinent and is uncommon elsewhere.

The genus is highly host-adapted and is a natural pathogen of only humans and a few subhuman primates. Transmission is fecal-oral from person to person and is generally via direct contact, although contaminated food, water, and fomites may serve as vectors. Direct contact is efficient and only a few hundred organisms suffice to transmit disease. For this reason, rapid spread can occur among confined populations kept in close contact, as, for example, in day-care centers, in institutions for the mentally retarded, on cruise ships, or among military personnel. Shigella is also one of several pathogens associated with "gay bowel syndrome." These cases are almost always due to *S. flexneri*, and homosexual young men may be a major reservoir for these organisms in the United States.

Shigellosis is associated with a high secondary household transmission rate. As many as 40 percent of children and 20 percent of adult household contacts of a case (generally a preschool child) will develop *Shigella* infection, which is usually symptomatic in children but asymptomatic in adults, who seem to have an acquired immunity. In contrast, epidemic disease affects all ages, with a clustering of severe and fatal cases in the very young and very old. Since 1969, epidemic *S. dysenteriae* type 1 has reappeared first in Latin America, then in the Indian subcontinent and elsewhere in Asia, and in central Africa. In each place, the disease has been accompanied by relatively high mortality rates until the cause was recognized and effective therapy initiated. Prolonged asymptomatic carriage is uncommon, and unless there is underlying malnutrition which is associated with prolonged fecal excretion, organisms are cleared in a few weeks.

PATHOGENESIS AND PATHOLOGY *Shigellae* are orally ingested and, though they are acid labile in the laboratory, they seem to have little difficulty in passing the gastric acid barrier. An essential step in pathogenesis is invasion of colonic epithelial cells and cell-to-cell spread of infection. Both invasion and cell-to-cell spread involve the initial attachment of the organism to colonic cells and then entry by an endocytic mechanism in which organisms are initially encased in and then escape from plasma-membrane enclosed vesicles. This not only provides the organism with a means to evade host defenses, but also allows effective local spread. Although invasion is initially innocuous, with subsequent intracellular multiplication, cell damage and death occur, resulting in characteristic mucosal ulcerations.

These virulence properties of the organism are determined by both chromosomal and plasmid genes. Studies with *Shigella*–*E. coli* hybrids, produced by introducing *E. coli* genes into *Shigella*, have demonstrated at least three chromosomal regions to be necessary—one bounded by the *xyl* and *rhl* loci, the *his* locus, and the *purE* locus. The *xyl-rhl* region is known to code for aerobactin and iron-regulated outer membrane proteins (OMPs), while the *his* region controls specific side chains of lipopolysaccharide, which respectively may help the organism compete for iron with the host and protect it from host defenses. However, if these regions are transferred from *S. flexneri* to a recipient *E. coli* K12, the resulting recombinant hybrid is still avirulent until other genes present on the large 120- to 140-MDa plasmids in all virulent *Shigella* are transferred as well. These plasmids contain at least two loci within a 22-MDa region, the *ipa* (invasion plasmid antigen) region, which controls production of several OMPs, and the *inv* region, which is thought to control insertion of these OMPs into the outer membrane of the organism.

The large plasmids also carry other virulence-associated genes, such as *virF*, which regulates surface charge (affecting forces of attraction between the gut cell and the bacterium), and *virG*, which controls the production of a hemolysin that probably is involved in rapid escape of the organism from intracellular vesicles after invasion. Another gene, *ics*, codes for a 120-kDa OMP that polymerizes epithelial cell actin, allowing organisms to migrate along the actin network to the plasma membrane. From this location organisms can invade adjacent cells and spread locally. The multiple genes needed to induce the nonphagocytic colonic cell to mimic a phagocyte indicate the complexity of the process and the high degree of specialization of the organism.

A second property of apparent importance in virulence is the ability of *Shigellae* to produce protein toxins that cause cytotoxicity in susceptible cells. These toxins are composed of two distinct peptide subunits and seem to be related members of a family of Shiga toxins. The toxins have two highly conserved active regions. The first, located on the larger A subunit, is an *N*-glycosidase enzyme, which hydrolyzes adenine from specific sites of ribosomal RNA of the mammalian 60-S ribosomal subunit, resulting in the irreversible inhibition of protein synthesis. The second common region is a binding site on the B subunit that recognizes glycolipids terminating in a galactose $\alpha1{\rightarrow}4$-galactose disaccharide. The glycolipid Gb3, containing a "gal-gal" trisaccharide, is a specific receptor present on toxin-sensitive rabbit intestinal epithelial cells. In this species, Gb3 is only expressed on villus cells, and toxin action is specific for these cells, sparing the crypts. It is assumed that Gb3 is the toxin receptor on human intestinal epithelial cells as well. Following binding to the rabbit intestinal cell surface, toxin is transported from the coated pits on the cell surface by receptor-mediated endocytosis. Inhibition of protein synthesis in villus cells leads to functional impairment in neutral sodium absorption, with no effect on crypt cell chloride secretion. Unopposed chloride secretion results in accumulation of electrolytes and water in the gut lumen. If the same process occurs in the human gut, the modest fluid loss of shigellosis can be accounted for. In contrast, the prodigious fluid losses due to cholera toxin are caused by the combined effects of inhibition of villus sodium absorption and increased crypt cell chloride secretion.

In shigellosis, the epithelial surface of the human colon shows extensive ulcerations, with an exudate consisting of desquamated colonic cells, polymorphonuclear leukocytes, and erythrocytes; the ulcerations may resemble a pseudomembrane in severely affected areas. Marked mucus depletion and increased mitotic activity is seen in the crypt regions, presumably as a response to the loss of surface colonic cells. The lamina propria is edematous and hemorrhagic and infiltrated with neutrophils and plasma cells. There is also swelling of capillary and venular endothelial cells, with margination of neutrophils. At the ultrastructural level, bacteria can be seen within vesicles as well as free in the cytoplasm.

Epidemiologic evidence indicates that immunity develops and is serotype specific. The nature of this immunity, however, is not known. Common surface OMPs involved in invasion are known to elicit serum antibodies; however, these are cross-reactive for many *Shigella* species and serotypes. The serotype-specific determinants are likely to be somatic antigens, and there is evidence of IgA-mediated mucosal anti-O antigen responses during convalescence from shigellosis. Cellular mechanisms have also been proposed that involve antibody-dependent cellular cytotoxicity responses by Fc receptor–positive lymphocytes and phagocytic cells.

CLINICAL MANIFESTATIONS The spectrum of clinical shigellosis was expressed in a study in which human volunteers ingested 10,000 *S. flexneri* type 2a. While approximately one-quarter of the volunteers never became ill, over the first 24 to 48 h approximately 25 percent of volunteers developed a transient fever, another 25 percent had fever and a self-limited watery diarrhea, and the remaining 25 percent had fever and watery diarrhea that progressed to bloody diarrhea and dysentery. In young children, in particular, the temperature can rapidly rise to 40 to 41°C, and sometimes result in typical febrile seizures. Dysentery is characterized by small-volume stools consisting of blood, mucus, and pus, abdominal cramps, and tenesmus, with 40 or more bowel movements each day. Painful straining often leads to rectal prolapse, especially in young children. The likelihood of severe dysentery is greatest in *S. dysenteriae* type 1 and *S. flexneri* infection and least likely in *S. sonnei*. With mild disease, patients generally recover without specific therapy in a few days to a week. Severe shigellosis can progress to toxic dilatation and colonic perforation, which may be fatal.

Endoscopy shows the mucosa to be hemorrhagic with mucous discharge and focal ulcerations, sometimes with overlying exudate. The majority of the lesions are in the distal colon and progressively diminish in the more proximal segments of large bowel. Mild dehydration is common in patients with watery diarrhea; severe dehydration is very rare. With extensive colonic involvement, protein-losing enteropathy occurs and can have very important adverse nutritional consequences for the already poorly nourished child.

A variety of *extraintestinal complications* of shigellosis have been described. The majority of these occur in patients in developing countries and are related to both the prevalence of *S. dysenteriae* type 1 and *S. flexneri* infection as well as the poor nutritional state of the patients. For example, bacteremia, thought to be relatively infrequent in the United States, occurs in up to 8 percent of patients hospitalized for shigellosis in Dacca, Bangladesh. The causative *Shigella* species is isolated in half the patients; other Enterobacteriaceae are found in the remainder. Bacteremia is associated with higher than usual mortality and is more common in infants under 1 year of age and in those with protein-energy malnutrition. Persistent and clinically severe *Shigella* bacteremia has been encountered in the United States in patients with the acquired immunodeficiency syndrome (AIDS) (see Chap. 264).

Hemolytic-uremic syndrome (HUS) may occur with *S. dysenteriae* type 1 infection. In the United States, the more likely cause of HUS is a hemorrhagic colitis–causing strain of *E. coli* producing high levels of Shiga-family toxins, such as *E. coli* 0157:H7. HUS usually develops toward the end of the first week of shigellosis, when the dysentery is already resolving. Oliguria and a marked drop in hematocrit (as much as a 10 percent decrease within 24 h) are the first signs and may progress to anuria and renal failure or severe anemia with congestive heart failure, respectively. With HUS, leukemoid reactions with leukocyte counts over 50,000 per microliter may occur; thrombocytopenia (30,000 to 100,000 platelets per microliter) is common. Profound hyponatremia and severe hypoglycemia may be present. Central nervous system abnormalities include encephalopathic symptoms, seizures, altered consciousness, and bizarre posturing.

Other less common extraintestinal manifestations include seizures in some patients and in others reactive arthritis, both usually due to infection with *S. flexneri* strains. In patients expressing histocompatibility antigen HLA-B270, the full triad of Reiter's syndrome sometimes develops (see Chap. 274). Pneumonia, meningitis, vaginitis in prepubertal girls, keratoconjunctivitis, and "rose spot" rashes are rare events.

DIAGNOSIS AND LABORATORY FINDINGS Shigellosis is the principal bacterial cause of dysentery and should be considered in every patient presenting with bloody diarrhea. However, in the United States, because *S. sonnei* is the most common species, most patients will present with fever and a nonbloody watery diarrhea, while many patients with bloody diarrhea will have enterohemorrhagic *E. coli* as the cause. The specific diagnosis is made by culturing *Shigella* from the stool; most laboratories do not process *E. coli* found in stool cultures. The yield of *Shigella* is increased by culturing organisms from only those patients with fecal leukocytes or bloody diarrhea. The organism is very labile and must be quickly transferred to plates or holding media (such as buffered glycerol saline) or it will not survive. Stool samples are preferable to swabs; when the latter are used, a rectal sample should be obtained. For culturing, more than one selective medium should be used, including MacConkey and one other, such as Hektoen Enteric, Tergitol-7-tetrazolium, xylose-lysine-deoxycholate, or SS agars.

Serology can be performed as antibodies to somatic antigens develop early in the acute phase of disease; however, serum tests are not generally available and are usually used only for epidemiologic studies.

The differential diagnosis includes other microbial causes of inflammatory colitis: enterohemorrhagic and enteroinvasive *E. coli*, *Campylobacter jejuni*, *Salmonella enteriditis* serotypes, *Yersinia enterocolitica*, *Clostridium difficile*, and the protozoan *Entamoeba histolytica*. Ulcerative colitis or Crohn's colitis are among the "noninfectious" causes (see Chap. 241). All except *E. histolytica* are associated with the presence of large numbers of fecal leukocytes. Amebiasis can be diagnosed by finding erythrophagocytic trophozoites in the stool (see Chap. 158).

Other laboratory studies usually disclose a moderate neutrophilic leukocytosis, anemia due to blood loss with hemorrhagic diarrhea, prerenal azotemia, and a hyperchloremic acidosis if watery diarrhea has been pronounced. Laboratory findings in shigellosis complicated by the HUS are discussed above.

TREATMENT The mild dehydration in shigellosis can usually be easily corrected. Depending upon the severity of illness and the patient's ability to tolerate oral fluids, replacement therapy can be administered intravenously or orally. The oral replacement therapy recommended is similar to that for cholera (see Chap. 122).

The role of antibiotic therapy is variable and dependent upon the organism and severity of disease. Since *S. sonnei* infection is usually self-limited, culture results generally do not become available until the patient is better and there is little clinical need for further therapy. The use of antibiotics in more severe cases with bloody diarrhea or dysentery will reduce the duration of illness and can shorten the duration of the carriage state. Resistance to sulfonamides, streptomycin, chloramphenicol, and tetracyclines is almost universal, and many *Shigella* are now also resistant to ampicillin and trimethoprim-sulfamethoxazole. Knowledge of the pattern of resistance in a given population, which can change with time, is useful. In the United States, either ampicillin, 50 to 100 mg/kg per day in children or 2 g/d in adults in divided doses, or trimethoprim/sulfamethoxazole, 8/40 mg/kg per day in children or 2 regular strength tablets twice a day in adults, given for 5 days is generally recommended. Amoxicillin should *not* be substituted for ampicillin since it is not effective treatment for shigellosis. In developing countries, where resistance to both of these drugs is commonplace, the drug of choice for the treatment of multiresistant *S. dysenteriae* type 1 infections has been nalidixic acid, 55 mg/kg per day for 5 days. The 4-fluoroquinolones (e.g., ciprofloxacin) are highly effective for all strains (see Chap. 85), but are currently too costly for the third world and in the United States are not yet approved for use in children under 17 because of the concern for cartilage toxicity. Alternative drugs shown to be effective include pivamdinocillin (not yet approved by the Food and Drug Administration in the United States) and cefoperazone. In small clinical trials, cephalexin has had no effect in limiting symptoms; single doses of ceftriaxone may be effective, but more information is needed. No antibiotic treatment is recommended for the convalescent carriage state since this is usually limited to only several weeks' duration. Patients with AIDS may develop chronic carriage of shigella and be subject to relapsing infection with bacteremia (see Chap. 264). This cycle may be interrupted by prolonged (several weeks) treatment with a quinolone.

The role of antimotility agents such as atropine sulfate and diphenoxylate (Lomotil) and loperamide (Imodium) remains unclear in the early phases of shigellosis. They have had a limited effect in relieving diarrhea; conversely, they have not provoked more severe disease through retention of organisms. There is no indication for their use in the dysenteric phase of disease, and they are not recommended.

Treatment of complications of shigellosis often differs in developed and developing countries. For example, antibiotic-unresponsive toxic megacolon, with or without perforation, is often managed by colectomy in the United States. Surgery is less often employed in developing countries because of lack of availability or difficulties in ileostomy management. Hemolytic-uremic syndrome often requires dialysis. In developing countries this is less commonly used because azotemia is slow to develop; also the risk of significant hyperkalemia is often diminished because of the preexisting deficiency in total body potassium with malnutrition and wasting of lean body mass. The management of hyponatremia is governed by its severity and the symptomatic state of the patient as outlined in Chap. 50. Infusion of glucose can reverse clinical manifestations due to hypoglycemia and responses can be monitored by finger-stick blood glucose tests if no biochemistry laboratory is available. Optimal nutritional management is needed to correct the deficiencies due to underlying malnutrition and the superimposed catabolic stress and protein-losing enteropathy of shigellosis. This should begin during the acute illness and may require months of nutritional support afterwards (see Chap. 75).

PREVENTION Direct contact transmission of shigellosis can be prevented by appropriate environmental and personal hygiene. Hand washing with soap and water, decontamination of water supplies, use of sanitary latrines or toilets, protection of food preparation and its storage can all reduce the primary and secondary transmission of *Shigella* infection. In the highly endemic developing countries, infants are protected during the period of exclusive breast feeding, and this should be encouraged. Any measures that also reduce the burden of malnutrition will have a favorable effect on the population as well. Hospitalized patients should be put on stool precautions to ensure safe disposal of infected excreta and linens, and hospital personnel must wash their hands and medical instruments such as stethoscopes after each contact with an infected patient. Children in day-care must be kept at home while clinically ill and ideally should have a negative stool culture before returning to the group. Food handlers who develop shigellosis should also be required to be culture-negative before being allowed to return to work. Antibiotic treatment is not indicated for the asymptomatic carriage state. No effective vaccine is available.

REFERENCES

ASKENAZI S et al: Convulsions in shigellosis: Evaluation of possible risk factors. Am J Dis Child 141:208, 1987

BASKIN DH et al: Shigella bacteremia in patients with the acquired immune deficiency syndrome. Am J Gastroenterol 82:338, 1987

BENNISH ML et al: Death in shigellosis. Incidence and risk factors in hospitalized patients. J Infect Dis 161:507, 1990

CLEMENS JD et al: Breast feeding as a determinant of severity in shigellosis. Am J Epidemiol 123:710, 1986

CLERC PL, SANSONETTI PJ: Entry of *Shigella flexneri* into HeLa cells: Evidence of directed phagocytosis involving actin polymerization and myosin accumulation. Infect Immun 55:1681, 1987

HALE LH, FORMAL SB: Pathogenesis of Shigella infections. Pathol Immunopathol Res 6:117, 1987

KEUSCH GT, BENNISH ML: Shigella, in *Enteric Infection: Mechanisms, Manifestations, and Management.* MJG Farthing, GT Keusch (eds). London, Chapman & Hall, 1988, pp 265–282

115 HAEMOPHILUS INFECTIONS

DAVID C. WAAGNER / GEORGE H. McCRACKEN, JR.

INTRODUCTION Bacteria of the genus *Haemophilus* were first observed by Robert Koch in conjunctival exudates. The genus name, *Haemophilus*, reflects the growth requirements of these organisms for accessory factors found in erythrocytes. Many *Haemophilus* species are part of the normal respiratory tract flora, while others are identified only in the presence of disease. Of the 16 species within the genus, *H. influenzae* is encountered most frequently as a human pathogen. *H. parainfluenzae*, *H. ducreyi*, *H. aegyptius*, *H. aphrophilus*, and *H. paraphrophilus* are also associated with disease in humans.

Members of the genus are small, nonmotile, non-spore-forming, gram-negative bacilli. *Haemophilus* species are aerobic or facultatively anaerobic, reduce nitrates, and produce variable carbohydrate fermentation. Marked pleomorphism is characteristic of all *Haemophilus* species and is most prominent in those requiring only the V factor for growth. In cultures of pathologic materials, the organisms are primarily coccobacillary. The pleomorphic appearance and inconsistent uptake of safranin dye may promote confusion with other pathogens, most notably pneumococci and meningococci. *Haemophilus* species require at least one or both of two preformed growth factors present in erythrocytes: a heat-stable X factor (protoporphyrin X) and/or a heat-labile V factor [nicotinamide adenine dinucleotide (NAD) or NAD phosphate].

HAEMOPHILUS INFLUENZAE

BACTERIOLOGY *H. influenzae* strains are subdivided into eight distinct biotypes on the basis of indole production and urease and ornithine decarboxylase activity. Biotype I is isolated most frequently from patients with meningitis. Healthy children can harbor simultaneously several biotypes of *H. influenzae*, while usually only one biotype is recovered from healthy adults. *H. influenzae* strains are further subdivided by the presence or absence of an antigenically distinct polysaccharide capsule, demonstrable by quellung reaction with specific antisera. Six distinct antigenic capsule serotypes, a to f, have been described. Encapsulated strains of serotype b frequently produce invasive disease. Type b strains are further subdivided by differences in outer membrane proteins (OMPs). Antibodies to designated OMPs P1, P2, and P6 are partially protective in animal models. Encapsulated serotypes other than type b and nonencapsulated strains are more commonly associated with colonization of mucosal surfaces and disease of contiguous sites such as the middle ear (otitis media) and sinuses.

The virulence of *H. influenzae* is enhanced by several features. The polyribose ribitol phosphate (PRP) capsule of type b strain is protective against phagocytosis and serum complement activity. Outer membrane vesicles composed of lipooligosaccharide (LOS) and other membrane constituents are present on the cell wall surface and are excreted in vitro as membrane blebs. Antibodies to *H. influenzae* type b PRP capsule cross-react with antigens of certain pneumococcal and enterobacterial capsular polysaccharides. Utilizing monoclonal antibodies directed against epitopes present in the oligosaccharide portion of *Haemophilus* endotoxin, four distinct antigenic groups have been identified among *H. influenzae* type b strains. These LOS epitopes appear to be highly conserved among different strains. *H. influenzae* LOS produces a paralytic effect on ciliary motility in respiratory epithelial cells and induces meningeal inflammation when inoculated intracisternally in rabbits. *H. influenzae* produce three distinct IgA proteases capable of disrupting peptide bonds within IgA molecules, thereby enhancing infection of mucosal surfaces.

Growth of *H. influenzae* in culture media requires the presence of both X and V factors under aerobic conditions. *H. influenzae* grows poorly on ordinary blood agar, which contains heat-labile V factor inhibitors. Peptic digestion of blood (Fildes medium) or mild heating (Levinthal's medium or chocolate agar) liberates sufficient quantities of both factors for growth. Growth is maximally enhanced at 37°C and, in some strains, by the addition of 10% CO_2. On Levinthal's medium, encapsulated strains demonstrate a characteristic iridescence with obliquely transmitted light. When cultured under anaerobic conditions, *H. influenzae* does not require X factor for growth.

EPIDEMIOLOGY *H. influenzae* is indigenous to humans, residing primarily in the upper respiratory tract. *H. influenzae* infections have a worldwide distribution and are considered endemic. Nonencapsulated strains of *H. influenzae* colonize the oropharynx shortly after birth. Up to 90 percent of preschool children are currently or have been colonized with nonencapsulated *H. influenzae;* colonization and frequency of disease decrease with age. In contrast, asymptomatic colonization with *H. influenzae* type b occurs in less than 5 percent of children and adults. Rates of carriage can be markedly higher in closed crowded communities, such as day care centers and in close contacts, such as family members of an infant with disease. Carriage of *H. influenzae* type b can persist for months, despite orally or parenterally administered antibiotics or the presence of circulating antibody. In approximately 80 percent of patients with systemic *H. influenzae* type b infections, the organism can be recovered from pharyngeal culture.

Invasive *H. influenzae* is primarily a disease of infants and young children. *H. influenzae* type b meningitis, the most common invasive form, has a peak incidence between 6 and 7 months of age. The Centers for Disease Control estimate that the attack rate for *H. influenzae* type b meningitis in the United States is 1.45 per 100,000 population. Approximately two-thirds of *H. influenzae* type b infections occur in children under 2 years of age: specifically 90 percent of cellulitis and septic arthritis cases, 80 percent of cases of meningitis, and 75 percent of pneumonias. The peak incidence for epiglottitis occurs between ages 2 to 4 years. This age-related epidemiologic pattern is different in other countries such as Finland. A seasonal incidence for *H. influenzae* infections with peaks in both fall and early spring has been documented. A fourfold increase in the reported incidence of *H. influenzae* type b infections has occurred in the past four decades; it is not clear whether this is due to better diagnostic methods or represents a true increase in disease rates.

Certain host factors contribute to an increased risk for invasive *H. influenzae* disease. These include low socioeconomic status, large family size, neutropenia, immunoglobulin deficiency, sickle cell anemia, asplenia, low birth weight, and CSF shunt placement. Transplant recipients and patients with malignancies undergoing immunosuppression have an increased susceptibility to *H. influenzae*. Patients undergoing therapy for Hodgkin's lymphoma are notably at risk and often fail to produce protective anti-PRP antibody titers following infection. Alcoholism in adults is associated with an increased risk of *H. influenzae* pneumonia. Native Americans have a higher incidence of *H. influenzae* infections with younger peak attack rates and higher rates of recurrence than do other populations in the United States. Household contacts under 4 years of age of patients with *H. influenzae* type b meningitis have an approximately 500-fold greater likelihood of developing *H. influenzae* disease than does the general population.

PATHOGENICITY *H. influenzae* is transmitted through contact or inhalation of infected respiratory secretions. After nasopharyngeal colonization, organisms may infect the entire respiratory tract, spread contiguously to adjacent structures, or invade the bloodstream and seed distant foci. At least 95 percent of systemic diseases caused by *H. influenzae* are caused by type b strains.

Organisms are thought to reach the intravascular space from the nasopharynx as a result of transport within phagocytes from the mucosa into lymphatic channels. In experimental models, antecedent viral infection potentiates nasopharyngeal colonization of *H. influenzae* type b and enhances adherence to tissue culture cells. Within the bloodstream, the PRP capsule of type b organisms resists phagocytosis and complement activity. During bacteremia organisms can spread to all serous structures, most notably the meninges, pleura, joint spaces, and pericardium. The site of entry into the CSF from bloodborne organisms is the highly vascularized choroid plexus. The occurrence of meningitis correlates directly with the duration and magnitude ($>10^3$ colony forming units) of the bacteremia.

IMMUNITY The increased susceptibility of infants and young children to *H. influenzae* infections has been directly attributed to lack of sufficient anti-PRP antibody. Serum anti-PRP titers in relation to age correlate directly with the age-dependent susceptibility to *H. influenzae*. Newborns transiently acquire anti-PRP IgG antibody transplacentally, which diminishes after the first months of life. Acquisition of natural immunity generally does not occur until 2 to 4 years of age, leaving children between the ages of 2 months to 2 years at greatest risk for invasive disease.

Acquisition of anti-PRP antibody does not solely result from colonization of *H. influenzae* on mucosal surfaces. Many children naturally develop anti-PRP antibodies despite a lack of exposure to type b strains. This can result from colonization with organisms containing cross-reacting capsular antigens such as intestinal infection with *Escherichia coli* K100 strains. Children under 2 years of age produce low or undetectable concentrations of anti-PRP antibodies in response to *H. influenzae* infection or to PRP capsular vaccine. Antisomatic antibodies to noncapsular protein antigens from exposure to nonencapsulated strains can be cross-reactive with encapsulated *H. influenzae* strains as well. Passive immunization with antibodies to epitopes on the oligosaccharide portion of *Haemophilus* LOS has conferred protection in experimental disease, but their presence in acute phase sera of some infants with *H. influenzae* infection suggests that they are not protective in the clinical setting.

CLINICAL ILLNESSES *H. influenzae* is the most common cause of bacteremic illness in the pediatric population. Meningitis accounts for greater than 50 percent of invasive *H. influenzae* diseases, followed by pneumonia (12 to 15 percent), epiglottitis (5 to 17 percent), cellulitis (6 to 15 percent), and isolated bacteremia (2 to 11 percent). Osteomyelitis, pyogenic arthritis, and pericarditis occur less commonly. Healthy adults seldom develop invasive *H. influenzae* illness, but nonencapsulated strains of *H. influenzae* appear to play an important role in exacerbations of chronic bronchitis.

Meningitis *H. influenzae* type b is the most common cause of bacterial meningitis in children between 3 months and 5 years of age and is associated with a case fatality rate of approximately 5 percent and a long-term morbidity rate of 15 to 30 percent. Meningitis can develop insidiously over several days, usually associated with an upper respiratory infection, or abruptly, progressing in a few hours. The signs and symptoms of *H. influenzae* meningitis are identical to those seen in bacterial meningitis caused by other pathogens. Nonspecific findings include fever, lethargy, irritability, anorexia, emesis, respiratory distress, and altered mental status. Older children and adults often have headache, stiff neck, and photophobia. The characteristic stiff neck with Kernig's and Brudzinski's signs are seen infrequently in children younger than 15 months of age. Focal neurologic findings can appear early, with up to one third of patients having seizures before admission. Purpuric lesions identical to those seen in *Neisseria meningitidis* infection occur uncommonly and are usually associated with disseminated intravascular coagulation.

Epiglottitis Epiglottitis is characterized by the abrupt onset of epiglottic edema, which may progress rapidly to complete obstruction of the airway, representing a true medical emergency. *H. influenzae* type b is the principal cause of epiglottitis. The peak incidence occurs between 2 to 4 years of age. A genetic predisposition is suggested by a marked predominance in Caucasians, its unusual rarity in Native American and Eskimo populations, and the frequent association with certain HLA groups. *H. influenzae* bacteremia occurs in greater than 90 percent of patients with epiglottitis, yet extraepiglottic foci are uncommon.

Patients typically present with an abrupt onset of fever, sore throat, stridor, dyspnea, pooling of oral secretions, and drooling. They appear anxious, sitting in a prone position with their mouths open and their necks fully extended. Indirect visualization of the oropharynx with a tongue blade is contraindicated, as this maneuver can potentiate epiglottic edema resulting in acute respiratory obstruction. Adults can have a more insidious onset with sore throat and progressive dysphagia. Direct laryngoscopy should be performed in all patients only in a setting where immediate endotracheal intubation can be performed or an emergency tracheostomy placed if intubation is unsuccessful. The epiglottis is usually edematous with a cherry-red appearance, and the aryepiglottal folds and surrounding tissues are swollen and inflamed. Placement of an artificial airway (endotracheal tube or tracheostomy) is advocated because of the high mortality (up to 80 percent) when obstruction occurs. Radiographs of the lateral neck can demonstrate an enlarged epiglottis (the "thumb" sign).

Pneumonia Type b strains cause up to one-third of bacterial pneumonias in children between 4 months and 4 years of age. Many of the children with *H. influenzae* pneumonia have positive blood cultures, and almost half have evidence of additional foci of infection. *H. influenzae* pneumonia is clinically indistinguishable from *Streptococcus pneumoniae* infection. Radiographic appearance is more often segmented or lobar, although bronchopneumonia and interstitial patterns have been described. Pleural reaction with effusion or frank empyema is more common than with other pathogens. Pneumatocele formation occurs infrequently.

The exact incidence of pneumonia due to nonencapsulated strains of *H. influenzae* is unknown, as they are frequently found as part of the upper respiratory flora. Alcohol abuse significantly increases the risk of *H. influenzae* in adults. Some estimates place nonencapsulated *H. influenzae* strains as the second commonest cause of community acquired bacterial pneumonias in adults.

Cellulitis Cellulitis caused by *H. influenzae* primarily occurs in children under age 2 and predominantly in the buccal and periorbital areas. *H. influenzae* cellulitis has a rapid onset, develops within hours, and is associated with bacteremia in almost three-fourths of patients. Additional foci of infection are found in 10 percent of cases. The involved area often has a characteristic violaceous or reddish-blue appearance.

Septic arthritis *H. influenzae* type b strains are the most common cause of suppurative arthritis in young children. Cultures of joint fluid or blood will yield the pathogen in approximately 70 percent of cases. The presence of capsular antigen in joint fluid is usually diagnostic. Needle aspiration or open drainage of purulent material with antimicrobial therapy are the mainstays of management (see Chap. 96). Significant joint dysfunction has been described despite adequate antibiotic therapy.

Bacteremia without focal disease After *S. pneumoniae*, *H. influenzae* is the leading cause of bacteremia without localized disease in children less than 2 years of age. Older children and adults with asplenia, sickle cell disease, or immunodeficiency, or who are undergoing cancer chemotherapy are also at risk.

Pericarditis Purulent pericarditis caused by *H. influenzae* infrequently accompanies systemic *H. influenzae* disease. Pericarditis complicates *H. influenzae* pneumonia in approximately 5 percent of cases. Echocardiographic studies can identify the presence of excess fluid in the pericardial space which must be confirmed and managed by open drainage and antibiotic treatment (see Chap. 193).

Additional respiratory tract disease Nonencapsulated *H. influenzae* strains are a common cause of acute sinusitis and otitis media in all age groups and of chronic bronchial disease in adults. Greater than 90 percent of *H. influenzae* strains obtained from middle ear fluid in acute otitis media are nonencapsulated. Exacerbations of chronic bronchitis have been attributed to nonencapsulated *H. influenzae* strains, although their exact role is uncertain.

Other infections *H. influenzae* has been identified as a rare cause of osteomyelitis, endocarditis, endophthalmitis, pyelonephritis, mediastinitis, peritonitis, epididymitis, and tenosynovitis. Abscess formation is rare, but has been described in brain, lung, muscle, and peritonsillar tissue.

DIAGNOSIS A definitive diagnosis is made by recovery of *H. influenzae* from cultures of infected body tissues and fluids. Cultures of the nasopharynx are not useful. Examination and culture of the CSF must be considered in all infants and young children with evidence of systemic *H. influenzae* disease. Needle aspirations in areas of cellulitis should be performed at the site of maximal induration for highest yield.

Identification of organisms on Gram-stained smears of CSF correlates directly with bacterial density; 96 percent positive at a concentration $>10^5$ CFU/mL, 78 percent positive between 10^3 to 10^5 CFU/mL, and 0 at $\leq 10^3$ CFU/mL. The pleomorphic appearance of *H. influenzae* and its Gram stain variability can produce frequent misinterpretation, estimated at 15 percent in one series. Acridine orange stains can be useful in detecting intracellular bacteria and

small numbers of organisms in body fluids. Approximately one-third of patients with bacterial meningitis receive antimicrobial therapy before hospital admission, substantially reducing the diagnostic reliability of the Gram-stained smear and the culture.

The detection of PRP antigen in body fluids can be used to diagnose *H. influenzae* infection before culture results are available, or when prior antibiotic therapy has sterilized cultures. The most frequently used techniques in order of decreasing sensitivity are latex particle agglutination (LPA), coagulation, and countercurrent immunoelectrophoresis. LPA is capable of detecting PRP antigen at bacterial concentrations of approximately 100 CFU/mL or greater. Despite the occurrence of cross-reacting antigens among other organisms, false-positive results are uncommon. Enzyme-linked immunosorbent assays for PRP have been developed but are more difficult and time-consuming, offering few benefits over LPA identification.

THERAPY Antibacterial agents that are bactericidal in vitro and achieve adequate bactericidal activity in body fluids should be used for systemic *H. influenzae* infections. Regional differences in antimicrobial susceptibilities must be considered in selecting appropriate therapy. The high prevalence of β-lactamase-producing strains of *H. influenzae* type b (15 to 50 percent in the United States) dictates that an assay for β-lactamase and disk susceptibilities be performed on all isolates. Organisms should also be tested for chloramphenicol resistance (prevalence <10 percent in United States) as a result of plasmid-mediated acetyltransferase.

Empiric therapy with ampicillin (200 to 300 mg/kg per day for children, 4 to 6 g/d for adults, intravenously in four or six divided doses), in combination with chloramphenicol (75 to 100 mg/kg per day for children, 4 g/d for adults, intravenously in four divided doses) until results of susceptibility studies are available, has been used effectively for more than a decade. Chloramphenicol is bactericidal against *Haemophilus* strains. The unpredictable metabolism of chloramphenicol in patients with hepatic dysfunction or hypotension, in young infants, and in those receiving anticonvulsant therapy requires monitoring of serum chloramphenicol concentrations to maintain safe and therapeutic levels.

The emergence of multiply resistant strains of *H. influenzae* has promoted the development of newer antimicrobials which provide alternatives to conventional therapy with ampicillin and chloramphenicol. Cefotaxime and ceftriaxone are β-lactamase-stable and achieve high bactericidal titers in all body fluids, including CSF, providing effective single-drug therapy for *H. influenzae* infections. Ceftriaxone has a long serum half-life (6 to 8 h), permitting the option of single daily doses (see Chap. 85). Other, newer cephalosporins shown to be effective in systemic *H. influenzae* disease include ceftazidime, cefuroxime, and ceftizoxime. In comparative trials cefotaxime or ceftriaxone are as effective as ampicillin and chloramphenicol for the therapy of meningitis and in many centers in the United States are used as primary treatment.

Outpatient therapy of less severe *H. influenzae* infections may be accomplished with a variety of oral antimicrobials. Amoxicillin is the therapy of choice for susceptible isolates. Alternative oral antibiotic selections for resistant organisms or in penicillin-sensitive patients include trimethoprim-sulfamethoxazole, erythromycin-sulfasoxazole, cefaclor, cefuroxime axetil, and chloramphenicol (for dosages see Chap. 85). The routine use of oral chloramphenicol is discouraged due to emergence of resistance and hematologic toxicity. Pharmacologic combinations of amoxicillin and ampicillin with β-lactamase inhibitors such as potassium clavulanate and sulbactam permit these agents to be used for therapy of β-lactamase-producing strains of *H. influenzae*. Although not approved yet for use in children, the oral quinolones, such as ciprofloxacin, have excellent activity against *H. influenzae*.

Duration of antimicrobial therapy is dependent on the disease process and the patient's response to treatment. Invasive *H. influenzae* disease requires intravenous antimicrobial therapy until all infectious foci are sterilized and the patient is afebrile and without clinical or laboratory evidence of infection. Patients with meningitis traditionally receive 10 to 14 days of therapy; however, recent studies indicate that uncomplicated *H. influenzae* meningitis can be treated for only 7 to 10 days.

In addition to antimicrobial therapy, supportive care of systemic *H. influenzae* infection is of critical importance. Immediate attention must be directed at airway maintenance, reduction of increased intracranial pressure and cerebral edema, and support of the respiratory and cardiovascular systems. Establishment of a secure airway is of the utmost urgency in epiglottitis. Dexamethasone given intravenously in a dose of 0.15 mg/kg every 6 h for the first 4 days of therapy significantly diminishes meningeal inflammation and the incidence of moderate or severe hearing loss of *H. influenzae* meningitis. Patients with systemic *H. influenzae* infection should be kept in respiratory isolation for 24 h following initiation of appropriate antibiotic therapy.

PREVENTION Large epidemiologic studies have demonstrated significantly increased attack rates in young household contacts of patients with systemic *H. influenzae* infection. Age-specific attack rates range from 6 percent in those under 1 year of age to 0.5 percent for those between ages 4 and 6. Only rifampin (rifampicin) has proved effective in eliminating nasopharyngeal carriage and in preventing secondary cases among household contacts.

Currently, the American Academy of Pediatrics recommends rifampin (20 mg/kg per day for children, 600 mg/d for adults, in a single daily dose for 4 days) be given to all household contacts (including adults and the index case) of an index case when at least one sibling is under 4 years of age. Rifampin prophylaxis of day care contacts is recommended only if two or more cases of invasive disease occur within a 60-day period.

The low immunogenicity of PRP in infants and young children has hampered development of an effective vaccine. Vaccines composed of purified *H. influenzae* PRP are immunogenic for older children and adults, but have little immunogenicity in those under 24 months of age. A more immunogenic vaccine composed of PRP covalently linked to diphtheria toxoid (PRP-D) was licensed for use in the United States in December 1987, based on evidence from Finland indicating protective efficacy in young infants and children. It is likely that other *Haemophilus* PRP conjugated vaccines will be approved for use. The American Academy of Pediatrics recommends immunization of all children at 18 months of age with one injection of the conjugate vaccine.

HAEMOPHILUS AEGYPTIUS

H. aegyptius, also known as the *Koch-Weeks* bacillus, closely resembles nonencapsulated *H. influenzae* and demonstrates a 78 percent DNA homology. *H. aegyptius* can be distinguished by hemagglutination activity, lack of indole production, and triacetyloleandomycin (troleandomycin) susceptibility.

This organism is associated with a purulent conjunctivitis of worldwide distribution. The conjunctivitis responds to local irrigation, and therapy with topical aminoglycoside, polymyxin, or sulfonamide ophthalmic preparations. *H. aegyptius* also has been identified as the etiologic agent of Brazilian purpuric fever (BPF). BPF is a fulminant disease of infants and children characterized by the acute onset of conjunctivitis, fever, emesis, and abdominal pain, with rapid progression to purpura, vascular collapse, peripheral necrosis, and death within 48 h of onset. First recognized in 1984, BPF is endemic in South America, and has a case fatality rate approaching 70 percent.

HAEMOPHILUS DUCREYI

H. ducreyi grows poorly on most media, requiring X but not V factor. Isolation of organisms from clinical specimens occurs in only 60 to 70 percent of cases, even with selective media. Gram-stained

smears show gram-negative coccobacilli in chains or a "school of fish" pattern.

This organism causes chancroid, a sexually transmitted disease that occurs worldwide (see Chap. 93), most commonly in nonwhite uncircumcised men in poor socioeconomic conditions. Chancroid is manifested by painful, sharply demarcated ulcerations usually confined to the genitalia and perineal area. Suppurative inguinal lymphadenopathy develops in more than one-half of patients. Approximately 10 percent of patients with chancroid have concomitant primary syphilis. Clinical diagnosis can be confirmed by Gram stain and cultures of ulcers or lymph node aspirates. Most strains are resistant to ampicillin and many are resistant to sulfonamides and tetracycline. Erythromycin (2 g/d given orally in four divided doses) or trimethoprim/sulfamethoxasole (320 mg/1.6 g per day given orally in two divided doses) for a total of 10 days is the regimen of choice.

HAEMOPHILUS PARAINFLUENZAE

H. parainfluenzae is usually isolated as part of the microflora of the human nasopharynx and mouth. *H. parainfluenzae* requires V but not X factor, prompting confusion with *H. influenzae* when *H. influenzae* is incubated anaerobically as in stabbed cultures. A small percentage of isolates produce β-lactamase.

Infection with *H. parainfluenzae* may follow bloodstream invasion from dental manipulation. Risk factors include immune deficiency, alcoholism, and congenital or rheumatic valvular heart disease. Otitis media, pharyngitis, pneumonia, empyema, liver abscess, meningitis, endocarditis, and urinary tract infections have been described. Endocarditis is the most frequent manifestation of *H. parainfluenzae* infection, usually occurring in young or middle-aged adults with underlying valvular disease. Arterial embolization is more prominent than in endocarditis caused by other pathogens. Antimicrobial therapy consists of ampicillin or a third-generation cephalosporin often combined with an aminoglycoside.

HAEMOPHILUS APHROPHILUS

H. aphrophilus is part of normal human oral microflora. Optimal growth requirements include high CO_2 concentration and X factor (but not V factor)–enriched media. Most infections with *H. aphrophilus* follow oropharyngeal infection or trauma, resulting in bacteremia. *H. aphrophilus* causes endocarditis and brain abscess in patients with underlying heart disease. Sinusitis, pneumonia, emphysema, dental abscess, peritonitis, meningitis, osteomyelitis, and pyarthrosis caused by *H. aphrophilus* have been described. Most isolates are susceptible to ampicillin, third-generation cephalosporins, tetracycline, aminoglycosides, and chloramphenicol.

HAEMOPHILUS PARAPHROPHILUS

H. paraphrophilus is part of human oropharyngeal flora, requiring V factor (but not X) for growth. Reported disorders include endocarditis, osteomyelitis, and urinary tract infections.

REFERENCES

Haemophilus influenzae

American Academy of Pediatrics Committee on Infectious Diseases: *Haemophilus influenzae* infections, in *1988 Red Book*, G Peter et al (eds). Elk Grove Village, IL, American Academic of Pediatrics, 1988, pp 204–210

Borenstein DG, Simon GL: *Haemophilus influenzae* septic arthritis in adults. A report of four cases and a review of the literature. Medicine 65:191, 1986

Crowe HM, Levitz RE: Invasive *Haemophilus influenzae* disease in adults. Arch Intern Med 147:241, 1987

Ginsburg CM et al: Report of 65 cases of *Haemophilus influenzae* type b pneumoniae. Pediatrics 64:283, 1979

KATZ SL, MORTIMER EA: Proceedings of a round table. *Haemophilus influenzae* type b: The disease and its prevention. Pediatr Infec Dis J 6:773, 1987

LEBEL MH et al: Dexamethasone therapy for bacterial meningitis: Results of two double-blind placebo controlled trials. N Engl J Med 319:964, 1988

MAYOSMITH MF et al: Acute epiglottitis in adults. An eight-year experience in the state of Rhode Island. N Engl J Med 314:1133, 1986

MURPHY TF, APICELLA MA: Nontypable *Haemophilus influenzae:* A review of clinical aspects, surface antigens, and the human immune response. Rev Infect Dis 9:1, 1987

MURPHY TO et al: Risk of subsequent disease among day care contacts of patients with systemic *Haemophilus influenzae* type b disease. N Engl J Med 316:1, 1987

WEINBERG GA, GRANOFF DA: Polysaccharide-protein conjugate vaccines for the prevention of *Haemophilus influenzae* type b disease. J Pediatr 113:621, 1988

Haemophilus aegyptius

BRAZILIAN PURPURIC FEVER STUDY GROUP: Brazilian purpuric fever; epidemic purpura fulminans associated with antecedent purulent conjunctivitis. Lancet 2:757, 1987

————: Biochemical, genetic, and epidemiologic characterization of *Haemophilus influenzae* biogroup aegyptius (*Haemophilus aegyptius*) strains associated with Brazilian purpuric fever. J Clin Microbiol 26:1524, 1988

Haemophilus ducreyi

FAST MV: Antimicrobial therapy of chancroid: An evaluation of five treatment regimens correlated with *in vitro* sensitivity. Sex Trans Dis 8:192, 1981

Haemophilus parainfluenzae

BLACK CT et al: *Haemophilus parainfluenzae:* Haemophilus parainfluenzae infections in children with report of a unique case. Rev Infect Dis 10:342, 1988

Haemophilus aphrophilus

BIEGER RC et al: *Haemophilus aphrophilus:* A microbiologic and clinical review of 42 cases. Medicine 57:345, 1978

Haemophilus paraphrophilus

KILIAN M, BIBERSTEIN EL: Genus II, *Haemophilus,* in *Bergey's Manual of Systemic Bacteriology,* NR Kreig, JG Holt (eds). Baltimore, Williams & Wilkins, 1984, vol 1, p 567

116 WHOOPING COUGH

BISHARA J. FREIJ / GEORGE H. McCRACKEN, JR.

DEFINITION Pertussis, or whooping cough, is an acute infection of the respiratory tract caused by *Bordetella pertussis*. This illness occurs worldwide and is most severe when it afflicts unimmunized infants. The term *pertussis* (meaning intensive cough) is generally preferred to whooping cough because many patients, especially infants, with this infection do not manifest the characteristic whoop. Despite the availability of protective vaccines, worldwide control of pertussis has yet to be achieved because of large populations of unimmunized infants and children in developing countries and, in industrialized countries, because of the intense controversy surrounding the use of pertussis vaccines as a result of their purported severe reactions.

MICROBIOLOGY Of the three *Bordetella* species known to infect humans, *B. pertussis* is by far the most common cause of whooping cough. *B. parapertussis*, *B. bronchiseptica,* and adenovirus types 1, 2, 3, 5, 12, and 19 are infrequent causes of the pertussis syndrome.

B. pertussis is a small, encapsulated, nonmotile, gram-negative coccobacillus. Special strains are required to demonstrate the capsule because capsular swelling in the presence of antiserum does not occur. When grown on Bordet-Gengou medium, *B. pertussis* colonies are smooth, convex, glistening, and translucent with a zone of surrounding hemolysis. *B. pertussis* can be distinguished from *B. parapertussis* and *B. bronchiseptica* by biochemical reactions such as nitrate reduction, citrate utilization, and urease production and by the presence of species-specific heat-labile capsular K antigens (K1 for *B. pertussis*, K12 for *B. bronchiseptica,* and K14 for *B. parapertussis*). *B. bronchiseptica* possesses lateral flagella and is the only motile *Bordetella* species. There is extensive DNA homology between the three *Bordetella* species, suggesting that they may represent different biotypes of the same organism.

B. pertussis produces many biologically active substances that may function as virulence factors, including lymphocytosis-promoting factor (LPF, also known as leukocytosis-promoting factor), histamine-sensitizing factor, islet-activating factor, pertussis toxin, and pertussigen. Other potential virulence factors include filamentous hemagglutinin (FHA), adenylate cyclase (AC), lipopolysaccharide (LPS), tracheal cytotoxin (TCT), hemolysin, heat-labile toxin, and agglutinogens.

PATHOGENESIS *B. pertussis* is typically transmitted to a new host by inhalation of airborne respiratory secretions from an infected individual. The organisms colonize the respiratory tract by adhering to ciliated epithelial cells. FHA, LPF, and agglutinogens appear to be important for the attachment process because specific antibodies against these factors protect experimental animals from respiratory infection by *B. pertussis*. Persistence of infection may be accomplished through impairment of host immune effector cell function by both AC (inhibition of phagocyte function) and LPF (altered lymphocyte production), as well as by disruption of normal clearance mechanisms by tracheal cytotoxin. Local respiratory tract tissue damage can be mediated by TCT, AC, hemolysin, and heat-labile toxin. The leukocytosis and lymphocytosis observed in this disease are systemic effects of LPF. The pathogenesis of pertussis encephalopathy is unclear. Other systemic manifestations may be due to pertussis LPS, but its role in pathogenicity is not well-defined.

EPIDEMIOLOGY It is difficult to estimate the true worldwide impact of pertussis because of problems in accurately diagnosing the illness and of underreporting of cases. Approximately 600,000 pertussis-related deaths are believed to occur each year; most of these involve unimmunized infants. The total number of reported pertussis cases in the United States has declined annually over the past 10 years from about 115,000 to 270,000 (with 5000 to 10,000 deaths) per year in the prevaccine era to about 1200 to 4200 (with 4 to 11 deaths per year). The number of reported cases per 100,000 population in the United States, however, has recently increased from a range of 0.54 to 0.95 during the years 1978 to 1982 to 0.96 to 1.74 for the years 1983 to 1987. Reported cases are thought to represent only 15 to 25 percent of actual cases.

Pertussis is a highly communicable infection. Secondary attack rates of 70 to 100 percent have been reported for susceptible household contacts and of 25 to 50 percent in schools. Humans are the only known natural host of *B. pertussis*. Although asymptomatic transient carriage of this organism has been noted in some household contacts of index patients, a chronic carrier state does not exist.

Pertussis is endemic in the United States. Localized geographic outbreaks of this disease continue to occur largely because of failure to immunize large numbers of susceptible individuals. Seasonal variations in the incidence of pertussis have been noted; autumn appears to be the season of lowest incidence.

The attack rates for females are greater than those for males, and these differences become more prominent with increasing age. No racial differences in attack rates have been noted. About half of all reported cases in the United States are in infants under 1 year of age; an estimated 15 percent are in individuals 15 years of age or older. Clinical disease in adolescents or adults may be atypical and is frequently misdiagnosed as bronchitis. Pertussis can occur in adults who received vaccine in infancy and childhood. Such individuals can potentially serve as important reservoirs for transmitting the infection to susceptible infants and children.

CLINICAL MANIFESTATIONS The incubation period for pertussis ranges from 5 to 21 days with a mean of 7 to 10 days. In infants and young children the disease can be divided into three symptomatic stages. The initial *catarrhal* stage is characterized by nonspecific upper respiratory symptoms such as sneezing, rhinorrhea, conjunctival injection, tearing, mild cough, and low-grade fever. This stage lasts 1 to 2 weeks and represents the most infectious period of this disease.

In the second or *paroxysmal* stage, there is progression to increasing bouts of severe coughing. Each paroxysm is characterized by 5 to 20 forceful coughs within a span of a few seconds. The characteristic whoop is produced when air is forcefully inhaled through a narrowed glottis. At the peak of disease activity, patients may experience 15 to more than 25 such paroxysms over a 24-h period, usually more often at night. The attacks may be prolonged to such an extent that patients become hypoxic. Ventilatory support is sometimes required, especially in young infants. Other physical findings during an attack may include cyanosis, neck vein congestion, bulging eyes, and protrusion of the tongue. The paroxysms may be provoked by yawning, sneezing, or eating. Vomiting frequently follows paroxysms. Fever is generally absent unless secondary suppurative complications develop. Patients usually appear normal between attacks. This stage lasts from 2 to 4 weeks or longer.

During the third or *convalescent* stage, the paroxysms become less frequent and less intense. This stage can last several months although a 3- to 4-week course is more usual. Patients are not usually infectious during this period despite continued coughing. After recovery, noxious stimuli or a viral respiratory infection can provoke recrudescence of the paroxysmal cough.

The disease in older children and adults is much milder and usually consists only of a prolonged bronchitis, which lasts several weeks or, rarely, months.

COMPLICATIONS Approximately 40 percent of infants and young children with pertussis require hospitalization; the frequency is highest for infants younger than 6 months of age (75 percent) and decreases with advancing age. The mortality rate is highest in infancy and an estimated 1.0 percent of all infants under 6 months die from complications of this disease.

Pneumonia is the most frequent complication of pertussis. It occurs in 12 percent of all young patients and in about 20 percent of those under 1 year of age. The pneumonia may be caused by *B. pertussis* itself but is more commonly caused by secondary bacterial pathogens such as *Haemophilus influenzae*, *Streptococcus pneumoniae*, *S. pyogenes*, or *Staphylococcus aureus*. The development of significant temperature elevation should prompt evaluation for superinfection by any of these bacteria. Other pulmonary complications of pertussis include interstitial or subcutaneous emphysema, pneumothorax, atelectasis, and bronchiectasis.

Central nervous system complications are serious but uncommon. They are most likely to occur during the paroxysmal stage, and infants appear to be the most susceptible. Seizures occur in about 1.7 percent of all reported pertussis cases, while encephalopathy is noted in approximately 0.5 percent. Seizures are usually generalized but focal convulsions can occur. Other acute neurologic abnormalities include hemiplegia, paraplegia, deafness, blindness, ataxia, and aphasia. The cerebrospinal fluid of these patients is typically normal, although a mild lymphocytic pleocytosis of 100 cells or less per microliter and/or a protein concentration of 1.0 g/L (100 mg/dL) can be found. The prognosis for patients with pertussis who develop neurologic complications is poor. Of those who develop pertussis encephalopathy, approximately a third die, a third survive with permanent sequelae, and a third survive with no apparent deficits. Long-term residua can include focal or generalized convulsions, focal paralysis, mental retardation, or behavioral abnormalities.

Otitis media is common. Hemorrhagic complications are rare and include epistaxis, petechiae, melena, subdural or epidural hematomas, subarachnoid or intraventricular bleeding, subconjunctival and scleral hemorrhages, as well as hemorrhagic bullous myringitis. Other infrequent complications include activation of latent tuberculosis, diaphragmatic rupture, umbilical hernia, rectal prolapse, ulceration of the frenulum of the tongue, and weight loss, with or without dehydration, from poor nutritional intake.

DIAGNOSIS A clinical diagnosis of pertussis in infants and young children is usually first suggested during the paroxysmal stage of the disease. The nonspecific respiratory signs and symptoms encountered during the catarrhal stage are not suggestive of pertussis unless a history of contact with a known case is elicited or they occur in the setting of an outbreak of this disease. Spasmodic cough is, however, not pathognomonic of pertussis and can be associated with other diseases such as bronchiolitis; chlamydial, viral, or mycoplasmal pneumonia; cystic fibrosis; tuberculosis; and such noninfectious entities as foreign bodies or extrinsic airway compression caused by lymphadenopathy or malignancies. These conditions can generally be differentiated from pertussis by clinical and laboratory findings, by the chest x-ray, and by the course of the disease. In older children and adults the disease may mimic prolonged bronchitis from other causes; however, it can be distinguished from chronic bronchitis (see Chap. 210) by its acute onset and self-limited course.

The white blood cell count can be helpful in establishing the diagnosis. Characteristically, marked elevations of the white blood cell count (20,000 to 50,000 or more cells per microliter) with a lymphocytosis of 60 percent or more are seen at the end of the catarrhal and during the paroxysmal stages of pertussis; the degree of the lymphocytosis may correlate with disease severity. Both T and B lymphocytes are increased in number. Lymphocytosis is seen in older children and adults with the disease and helps to differentiate pertussis from other cases of prolonged bronchitis.

The definitive diagnosis of pertussis is made by recovering *B. pertussis*, *B. parapertussis*, or *B. bronchiseptica* from nasopharyngeal swabs. Dacron or calcium alginate swabs are preferred to cotton swabs because the latter contain fatty acids that may inhibit the growth of *B. pertussis*. Specimens should be directly plated on selective media to maximize the chance of obtaining a positive culture. The best selective media for isolation of *B. pertussis* are Regan-Lowe, Bordet-Gengou, and modified Stainer-Scholte agar.

Bacterial isolation rates are highest when cultures are obtained within the first 3 to 4 weeks of the illness. Factors that contribute to low recovery rates of *B. pertussis* include a delay in specimen collection (e.g., only 15 to 20 percent of cases are culture-positive at 6 weeks), antimicrobial therapy (especially with erythromycin, tetracycline, or trimethoprim-sulfamethoxazole), previous pertussis immunization, incorrect collection procedures or delays in specimen transport, overgrowth of contaminating bacteria, and inexperienced laboratory personnel who may fail to recognize the organism in culture. *B. pertussis* can be isolated from as many as 80 to 90 percent of patients during the catarrhal stage and from 50 percent or less of those in the paroxysmal stage of the disease.

A direct fluorescent antibody (DFA) test utilizes a polyclonal fluorescein-labeled antibody against *B. pertussis* to stain and directly identify the organism in nasopharyngeal specimens; however, its sensitivity is variable, with both high rates of false-negative or false-positive results reported in different laboratories.

Enzyme-linked immunosorbent assay (ELISA), complement fixation, immunodiffusion, and other antibody assays are not helpful in the diagnosis of pertussis. The detection of antipertussis antibodies may indicate natural infection with this organism or prior immunization. The demonstration of fourfold or greater rises in IgG titers against *B. pertussis* antigens is infrequent even in culture-positive cases, because the acute phase serum is usually not obtained early enough in the disease. Serum IgA responses to pertussis are found only after natural infection; however, many infants with this disease fail to produce detectable pertussis-specific IgA antibodies. These antibodies may also persist in normal populations because of subclinical infection, making it difficult to differentiate a recent acute infection from past disease.

B. pertussis–specific secretory IgA antibodies can be detected by ELISA in nasopharyngeal secretions after natural infection with this organism, but not after immunization. These secretory IgA antibodies usually appear during the second or third week of the disease and can persist for 3 months or longer. This test may ultimately prove to be useful in the diagnosis of pertussis in culture-negative cases.

TREATMENT Supportive care is of paramount importance in the management of patients with pertussis. Those with potentially severe disease, especially infants under 6 months, should be hospitalized. Strict respiratory isolation for 5 days after initiation of appropriate antibiotics is recommended before patients can be considered noninfectious. Close nursing observation, gentle suctioning to remove respiratory secretions, avoidance of stimuli that can provoke paroxysms such as invasive procedures or tobacco smoke, provision of adequate nutritional intake, attention to fluid and electrolyte balance, oxygen administration to avoid hypoxia, and management of apnea episodes all contribute to a satisfactory outcome. Neither cough suppressants nor antihistamines are helpful in reducing the intensity or frequency of paroxysms. The use of glucocorticoids and beta$_2$-adrenergic agonists to reduce coughing paroxysms remains controversial.

Antimicrobial therapy provided in the incubation period or catarrhal stage may prevent or ameliorate the disease. Antibiotics are generally considered ineffective in modifying the clinical course of the disease once it reaches the paroxysmal stage, but are administered to these patients to reduce their infectivity and to prevent spread of the organisms. Erythromycin in a dosage of 40 to 50 mg/kg per day in four equally divided doses (maximum, 2 g/d) given orally is preferred for treatment and is continued for 14 days. Erythromycin will eliminate *B. pertussis* from the nasopharynx in 4 or fewer days. Bacteriologic relapse occurs, however, in 10 percent of patients treated for periods shorter than 2 weeks. Trimethoprim/sulfamethoxazole (8/40 mg/kg per day in two divided doses) can be used in patients who cannot tolerate erythromycin, but its efficacy has not been established.

PREVENTION Management of contacts Household and other close contacts, whether children or adults, should be prophylactically treated with erythromycin in a dosage of 40 to 50 mg/kg per day (maximum, 2 g/d) in four equally divided doses given orally for 14 days. Even fully immunized individuals should receive chemoprophylaxis. In addition, close contacts younger than 7 years of age who have received at least four doses of pertussis vaccine (usually in the form of the triple diphtheria-tetanus-pertussis, DTP, vaccine) should be given a booster dose of DTP unless one has been given within the preceding 3 years. Those under age 7 who have not yet been completely immunized should continue with the recommended vaccine schedule and receive erythromycin prophylaxis.

Day-care center attendees should be treated as close contacts and managed accordingly. Children with pertussis may be allowed to return to day care after 5 days of erythromycin therapy, assuming their general condition permits unrestricted activity. All close contacts should be observed for the development of respiratory symptoms for 14 days after exposure to the index case. Those developing symptoms should be evaluated by a physician and excluded from day care until the cause of their symptoms is identified and appropriately managed.

Vaccines Currently available pertussis vaccines are generally prepared from either whole-cell suspensions or partially purified cell products. Only the adsorbed whole-cell vaccines are used in the United States; by contrast, Japan uses only the acellular type of pertussis vaccines. The efficacy of whole-cell vaccines is believed to be 80 to 90 percent. The duration of protection is uncertain, but limited data suggest that the efficacy declines to 50 percent 4 to 7 years after the last dose and is almost absent after 12 years. The efficacy of the acellular vaccines also appears to be approximately 85 to 90 percent based on studies conducted in Japan principally in children 2 years of age and older. The duration of protection with the acellular product is unknown.

Completely immunized individuals can still develop pertussis, but disease is typically milder. Although improvements in housing as well as in the general health of the population have been suggested as the cause for the decline in incidence of pertussis, industrialized countries such as the United Kingdom, Japan, and Sweden experienced major pertussis epidemics shortly after routine pertussis immunization was stopped because of concerns regarding vaccine safety.

A number of adverse reactions have been associated with pertussis immunization. Transient local and systemic reactions are common and include redness (7 percent), swelling (9 percent), and pain (51 percent) at the injection site; fever to 38°C or greater (47 percent); and vomiting (6 percent). These reactions occur within a few hours of vaccination, are transient, and tend to increase in frequency with subsequent doses of vaccine. These reactions do not constitute a contraindication to future pertussis immunization. The administration of acetaminophen in a dose of 15 mg/kg at the time of vaccination and 4 and 8 h later will reduce the incidence of these reactions. Sterile abscesses at the site of injection are rare. Similar reactions have been reported for the acellular vaccines but they are usually less frequent and milder in nature.

A number of other uncommon but more severe adverse reactions have been associated with pertussis immunization. These include fever of 40.5°C or greater (0.3 percent), seizures (0.06 percent), persistent or unusual crying for 3 h or longer (1 percent), shock-like hyporesponsive state (0.06 percent), encephalopathy, and severe allergic reactions. Several other serious problems have been blamed on the pertussis vaccine, but careful evaluation indicates that they are merely temporal associations and do not represent a cause-and-effect relationship. Among these unsubstantiated events are infantile spasms and sudden infant death syndrome.

Absolute contraindications to further administration of pertussis vaccines include:

1 Encephalopathy within 7 days of vaccination
2 Seizures within 3 days
3 Persistent or unconsolable crying for 3 h or longer or a high-pitched cry that is unusual for that infant within 2 days
4 Collapse or a shock-like hyporesponsive episode within 48 h of vaccination
5 Fever of 40.5°C or greater within 48 h
6 An immediate severe allergic reaction or anaphylaxis

In addition to these contraindications, the pertussis vaccine may be omitted or delayed in patients with infantile spasms, uncontrolled epilepsy, or progressive encephalopathy of unknown etiology.

Routine pertussis vaccination is not recommended after the age of 7 because the risk of severe disease is extremely low and reactions to vaccination may be higher. Vaccine has been employed in adults during outbreaks within hospitals with a prominent incidence of local reactions (>50 percent) and rarely occurring skin rashes.

The pertussis vaccine is almost always given in conjunction with other immunizing agents such as diphtheria and tetanus toxoids. Five 0.5-mL intramuscular doses of DTP are recommended for primary immunization; the first is given at about 2 months of age, the second and third doses are given 2 and 4 months later. A fourth dose is given 6 to 12 months after the third dose, and a fifth booster dose is given at about 4 to 6 years of age at the time of school entry. In outbreaks, pertussis immunization can be started as early as 2 weeks of age and the 2 subsequent doses given 4 weeks apart. Children in whom the recommended schedule for pertussis immunization has been interrupted or deferred and who need to resume vaccination can receive the next dose on schedule, regardless of the interval from the previous dose. No modifications in the immunization schedule are needed for premature infants.

REFERENCES

BLENNOW M et al: Primary immunization of infants with an acellular pertussis vaccine in a double-blind randomized clinical trial. Pediatrics 82:293, 1988

CHERRY JD et al: Report of the Task Force on Pertussis and Pertussis Immunization—1988. Pediatrics 81:939, 1988

FRIEDMAN RL: Pertussis: The disease and new diagnostic methods. Clin Microbiol Rev 1:365, 1988

GILLIS J et al: Artificial ventilation in severe pertussis. Arch Dis Child 63:364, 1988

HOFFMAN HJ et al: Diphtheria-tetanus-pertussis immunization and sudden infant death: Results of the National Institute of Child Health and Human Development Cooperative Epidemiological Study of Sudden Infant Death Syndrome risk factors. Pediatrics 79:598, 1987

LINNEMANN CC JR et al: Use of pertussis vaccine in an epidemic involving hospital staff. Lancet 2:540, 1975

ONORATO IM, WASSILAK SGF: Laboratory diagnosis of pertussis: The state of the art. Pediatr Infect Dis J 6:145, 1987

ROBERTSON PW et al: *Bordetella pertussis* infection: A cause of persistent cough in adults. Med J Aust 146:522, 1987

SHIELDS WD et al: Relationship of pertussis immunization to the onset of neurologic disorders: A retrospective epidemiologic study. J Pediatr 113:801, 1988

117 CHANCROID

ALLAN R. RONALD / FRANCIS A. PLUMMER

DEFINITION Chancroid, or soft chancre (ulcer molle), is an acute sexually transmitted infection characterized by painful genital ulcerations often associated with inflammatory inguinal adenopathy which may progress to suppuration. The diagnosis is established by isolation of *Haemophilus ducreyi* from the lesion or a suppurative node and by exclusion of syphilis, genital herpes, and other specific causes of genital ulceration.

ETIOLOGY The isolation of *H. ducreyi* from ulcers proves the microbial etiology of chancroid. Other organisms are often present, but there is no evidence that these are independent pathogens or require specific therapy. The clinical response to antimicrobial therapy parallels the susceptibility of *H. ducreyi*. In areas where chancroid is common, *H. ducreyi* can be isolated from up to 90 percent of ulcers that clinically appear to be chancroid. The organism is a gram-negative facultative aerobe which requires hemin (X factor) but not nicotinamide adenine dinucleotide (V factor) for growth. Although no unique biochemical or immunologic features are known, the colonial morphology of *H. ducreyi* is distinct in that the yellow gray colonies can be moved intact across the agar surface. Some strains demonstrate a typical streptobacillary "chaining" appearance on Gram stain.

EPIDEMIOLOGY The incidence of chancroid is unknown, owing to inaccurate diagnosis and incomplete reporting. It is common in southeast Asia and Africa, and is more prevalent than syphilis in many countries. A resurgence of chancroid is occurring in many U.S. urban centers, and endemic foci have been identified in Florida, New York City, and Dallas. The annual incidence has increased sixfold during the past decade and is continuing to rise. Over 5000 cases were reported in 1987. Uncircumcised males are more susceptible to the disease. Prostitution plays a major role in transmission, and among merchant seamen and military troops whose sexual contacts are prostitutes, chancroid is more common than syphilis. The role of asymptomatic female carriers, without ulcers, in the transmission of *H. ducreyi* is uncertain. Over one-half of the secondary sex partners of men with chancroid develop clinical chancroid.

Studies from Africa provide substantial evidence that chancroid is a major cofactor that facilitates the heterosexual spread of human immunodeficiency virus (HIV-1). Prostitutes with chancroid are more susceptible to HIV-1 infection following heterosexual intercourse and they also transmit HIV-1 much more frequently to their clients in the presence of genital ulcers. Almost one-half of bidirectional heterosexual transmission of HIV-1 may be attributed to chancroid in some African communities. Control and eradication of chancroid is now recognized as an urgent priority to curtail heterosexual transmission of HIV-1.

CLINICAL MANIFESTATIONS After an incubation period of 3 to 10 days, a small tender papule appears which rapidly ulcerates. The classic chancroidal ulcer is superficial, ranging in diameter from a few millimeters to several centimeters. The edge is ragged and undermined. The ulcer base is covered by a necrotic exudate. The ulcers are often multiple and may merge to form giant or serpiginous ulcers. Occasionally, the lesions remain pustular and resemble folliculitis or pyogenic infection. In contrast to syphilis, the chancroidal ulcer in males is painful and not indurated. The most frequent areas of localization are the preputial orifice, the internal surface of the prepuce, and the frenulum in men, and the labia, fourchette, and perianal region in women. The lesions in females tend to be more superficial and less painful. Extragenital ulcers are rare.

Acute, painful, tender inflammatory inguinal adenopathy occurs in almost 50 percent of patients and is frequently unilateral. If the patient is untreated, the involved nodes become matted, forming a unilocular suppurative bubo. The overlying skin becomes erythematous and tense and finally ruptures, forming a deep single ulcer.

DIAGNOSIS The morphologic diagnosis of genital lesions is fraught with error, and many lesions diagnosed as chancroid are actually genital herpes or syphilis. In the United States, one study of 100 consecutive men with penile ulceration disclosed genital herpes in 22, syphilis in 17, and traumatic lesions in 8. Classic chancroidal ulcers were noted in 12, only 2 of whom had ulcers that yielded *H. ducreyi*. In Kenya, of 97 consecutive men with penile ulceration, 60 were infected with *H. ducreyi*, 11 had syphilis, and only 4 had genital herpes.

Primary genital infection with herpes simplex virus produces tender inguinal adenopathy, but can be distinguished by the history of onset with vesicular lesions or of recent exposure to herpes and the presence of systemic symptoms such as fever and myalgia. Chancroid rarely causes systemic symptoms.

The chancre of primary syphilis is indurated, and the associated adenopathy is bilateral, nontender, and nonsuppurative. To exclude syphilis, all patients with genital ulcers should have two dark-field examinations performed on separate days, together with monthly serologic tests for syphilis for 3 months.

Lymphogranuloma venereum (LGV) differs from chancroid in that the adenopathy develops after the ulcer is healed. It is indolent, often bilateral and nontender, and develops multilocular suppuration and fistulas.

The diagnosis of chancroid is confirmed by the isolation of *H. ducreyi* from an ulcer. Exudate should be directly plated onto chocolate agar enriched with 1% Isovitalex and 5% sheep serum, plus 3 mg/L of vancomycin. Colonies usually appear within 48 h of incubation in 5% CO_2 with 100% humidity but may require 4 to 5 days. No serologic tests are available for the diagnosis of chancroid.

TREATMENT Untreated chancroid can persist for months. Small lesions may heal within 2 to 4 weeks. Although sulfonamides and tetracyclines were effective treatment, the emergence of multiresistant strains ended their usefulness. Many isolates of *H. ducreyi* possess plasmids which mediate resistance to sulfonamides, tetracyclines, chloramphenicol, ampicillin, and kanamycin. Trimethoprim/sulfamethoxazole, 320/1600 mg daily, or erythromycin, 2 g daily, each for 1 week are the regimens recommended by the Centers for Disease Control. Trimethoprim/sulfamethoxazole will not interfere with the dark-field examination for *Treponema pallidum* or with the development of a positive serologic test for syphilis. Ciprofloxacin, 500 mg orally, twice daily for three days is also effective. The usual time to healing after onset of therapy is about 9 days. Several single-dose regimens including trimethoprim/sulfamethoxazole, 640/3200 mg, spectinomycin, 2 g intramuscularly, and ceftriaxone, 250 mg intramuscularly have proved effective for chancroid in Kenya. HIV-infected patients appear to respond less well to therapy; the efficacy of regimens for chancroid treatment in patients concomitantly infected with HIV requires further study. Fluctuant buboes should be aspirated to prevent rupture. Lymph node suppuration may progress despite otherwise effective therapy. Buboes larger than 5 cm in diameter almost always require aspiration.

Sexual contacts of patients with chancroid should be examined for ulcers, and treatment of contacts is recommended. Although the epidemiology of chancroid suggests that effective control measures, specifically designed for limited target populations such as prostitutes and known sexual contacts, could halt the spread of this disease, further prospective epidemiologic studies to demonstrate this are required.

REFERENCES

BOWMER MI et al: Single dose ceftriaxone for chancroid. Antimicrob Agents Chemother 31:67, 1988

GREENBLATT RM et al: Genital ulceration as a risk factor for human immunodeficiency virus infection. AIDS 2:47, 1988

McNicol PJ et al: The plasmids of *Haemophilus ducreyi*. Antimicrob Agents Chemother 14:561, 1984

Salzman RS et al: Chancroid ulcers that are not chancroid: Cause and epidemiology. Arch Dermatol 120:636, 1984

Schmid GP et al: Chancroid in the United States. Reestablishment of an old disease. JAMA 258:3265, 1987

Simonsen JN et al: Human immunodeficiency virus infection among men with sexually transmitted diseases: Experience from a centre in Africa. New Engl J Med 319:274, 1988

118 DONOVANOSIS (GRANULOMA INGUINALE)

KING K. HOLMES

DEFINITION Donovanosis (granuloma inguinale) is a mildly contagious, chronic, indolent, progressive, autoinoculable, ulcerative disease involving the skin and lymphatics of the genital or perianal areas. The disease may be sexually transmitted and is associated with the presence in affected tissues of an intracellular microorganism, identified morphologically as the Donovan body.

ETIOLOGY Donovanosis was described by McLeod in India in 1882, and in 1905 Donovan described the intracellular bodies which are thought to cause the disease. Encapsulated bacteria resembling Donovan bodies have been recovered from lesions and pseudobuboes of granuloma inguinale by inoculation of chick embryo yolk sacs or yolk-agar medium. These bacteria, which are known as *Calymmatobacterium granulomatis*, measure 1.5 by 0.7 μm. They are antigenically related to *Klebsiella* species but do not reproduce the disease when inoculated intradermally in humans. It is uncertain whether these isolates are responsible for the disease. Electron microscopic studies of Donovan bodies confirm their morphologic resemblance to gram-negative bacteria.

EPIDEMIOLOGY Donovanosis is endemic in the tropics, particularly in New Guinea and among Hindus in India, and in parts of central Australia, the Caribbean, and Africa. In the United States the disease is rare. Most cases occur in the southeastern states and involve homosexual men. In reported cases the sex ratio of males to females is nearly 10:1. The disease is uncommon in Caucasians. The reported frequency of donovanosis in conjugal partners of chronically infected patients ranges from 1 to 64 percent. Evidence for sexual transmission includes the age-specific incidence, which corresponds to that of other sexually transmitted diseases, the frequent concomitant presence of syphilis, and the predilection for genital involvement in heterosexuals and for anorectal infection in homosexually active men.

CLINICAL MANIFESTATIONS The incubation period ranges from 8 days to 12 weeks, but most lesions appear within 30 days after sexual exposure.

Donovanosis begins as a papule that ulcerates and develops into a painless elevated zone of clean, beefy-red, friable granulation tissue. The edges are irregular and spread by continuity or by autoinoculation of approximated skin surfaces. Secondary anaerobic infection may produce pain and a foul-smelling exudate. Less common complications of the disease include deep ulcerations, chronic cicatricial lesions, phimosis, lymphedema, and exuberant epithelial proliferation which grossly resembles carcinoma. In men, the lesions are usually located on the glans, prepuce, or shaft of the penis or the perianal area, while infection of the labia is most common in women. Lesions in women often arise at the fourchette and progress anteriorly in a V shape along the vulva. Extragenital lesions may occur, involving the face, neck, mouth, and other sites. The chronicity of the disease is of diagnostic importance, since several months often elapse before patients seek treatment. Extension to the inguinal region by autoinoculation, by continuity, or via the lymphatics results in diffuse intradermal and subcutaneous swelling or suppuration, known as "pseudobubo," because involvement of the underlying lymph nodes is minimal. Locally destructive lesions and secondary infection may produce severe morbidity or death. Fatal disseminated disease, involving the bones, joints, or liver, has been reported after several years of chronic local infection. The relationship of donovanosis to subsequent carcinoma of the genitalia is uncertain.

DIAGNOSIS Early donovanosis may be mistaken for the primary chancre or condyloma latum of syphilis. Epithelial proliferation resembling carcinoma in the genital or perianal region in a young individual should always raise the suspicion of donovanosis if unnecessary destructive surgery is to be avoided. Chronic ulcerative or cicatricial changes may resemble lymphogranuloma venereum.

Amebiasis can produce penile lesions resembling donovanosis. In the United States, *Haemophilus ducreyi* has frequently been isolated from lesions resembling donovanosis; this has been termed *pseudogranuloma inguinale–chancroid*. Histologic studies in donovanosis reveal marked acanthosis and pseudoepitheliomatous hyperplasia. The dermis contains an inflammatory infiltrate consisting mainly of plasma cells and histiocytes. Because Donovan bodies are seldom detectable in sections stained with hematoxylin and eosin, these changes may lead to an erroneous diagnosis of carcinoma and to unnecessary destructive surgery. Although silver impregnation techniques are useful for demonstration of Donovan bodies in sections, the diagnosis is best made by examination of impression smears prepared from specimens obtained by punch biopsy of granulation tissue from the periphery of a lesion; the deep portion of the specimen is removed, crushed between two slides which are air-dried and fixed in methanol, and stained with Wright-Giemsa stain. With this method, Donovan bodies appear as very rounded coccobacilli, 1 by 2 μm in size, which lie within cystic spaces in the cytoplasm of large mononuclear cells. The capsule stains as a dense acidophilic zone surrounding the bacterium, which resembles a closed safety pin because of bipolar condensation of chromatin. The pathognomonic mononuclear cell is 25 to 90 μm in diameter and has many cystic areas containing Donovan bodies. Donovan bodies have also been identified in histiocytes in cervical Papanicolaou smears.

Perianal donovanosis may resemble condylomata lata of secondary syphilis. Other venereal diseases, particularly syphilis, very frequently coexist with donovanosis. Repeated dark-field examinations of lesions before treatment and a serologic test for syphilis should therefore be performed. In countries where donovanosis is endemic, the persistence of suspected condylomata lata after appropriate penicillin therapy for syphilis is highly suggestive of donovanosis. Other forms of genital ulcers (chancroid, syphilis, genital herpes) have been associated with increased risk of acquisition or transmission of human immunodeficiency virus. These diseases appear to be less responsive to therapy in HIV-seropositive individuals. Anecdotal cases of severe donovanosis associated with HIV infection have been reported, but the association has not been well studied.

TREATMENT The treatment of choice is tetracycline, 2 g daily, for at least 3 weeks, preferably continued until healing is complete. Healing is usually apparent within 3 weeks, as the lesions become pale and flatter and develop peripheral reepithelialization. Lack of objective clinical response within 7 days should lead to reassessment of the diagnosis and therapy. Donovan bodies disappear from lesions within a few days after onset of therapy. If tetracycline cannot be given, streptomycin may be used in a dose of 1 g intramuscularly every 12 h for 10 to 15 days. Chloramphenicol, 500 mg every 8 h orally, or gentamicin, 1 mg/kg twice daily, is used for cases which appear resistant to tetracycline. Co-trimoxazole (trimethoprim 160 mg, sulfamethoxazole 800 mg) twice daily for 10 days is also reported to be effective. In pregnant women, erythromycin, 500 mg every 6 h, may be effective.

REFERENCES

Hart G: Donovanosis, in *Sexually Transmitted Diseases*, 2d ed, KK Holmes et al (eds). New York, McGraw-Hill, 1990, chap 25, pp 273–277

Kraus SJ et al: Pseudogranuloma inguinale caused by *Haemophilus ducreyi*. Arch Dermatol 118:494, 1982

Kuberski T: Granuloma inguinale (donovanosis). Sex Transm Dis 7:29, 1980

Rosen T et al: Granuloma inguinale. J Am Acad Dermatol 11:433, 1984

Schneider J et al: Extragenital donovanosis: Three cases from Western Australia. Genitourinary Med 62:196, 1966

119 BRUCELLOSIS

DONALD KAYE

DEFINITION Brucellosis is an infection caused by bacteria of the genus *Brucella*. Human infection results from occupational contact with an infected animal or by ingestion of infected milk, milk products, or tissues. The symptoms of brucellosis are often nonspecific and include fever, malaise, and weight loss, often without physical findings.

ETIOLOGY There are four species of *Brucella* that cause infection in humans. The most pathogenic is *B. melitensis,* followed by *B. suis, B. abortus,* and *B. canis*. While each of these tends to produce infection in a specific animal host (*B. melitensis* in sheep and goats, *B. suis* in swine, *B. abortus* in cattle, and *B. canis* in dogs), cross-species infection occurs (e.g., *B. abortus* in sheep) and other animals may become infected.

Brucella are small, nonmotile, nonencapsulated, gram negative coccobacilli which do not form spores. *Brucella* grow best at 37°C under increased CO_2 tension and are separated from each other by biochemical and serologic techniques.

EPIDEMIOLOGY Animals acquire brucellosis either sexually or by ingesting contaminated milk or other animal products. Humans develop disease following ingestion of contaminated animal food products, by contact of *Brucella* with abraded skin, through the conjunctivae, or by inhalation. Person-to-person transmission rarely, if ever, occurs.

While there are 500,000 new cases of brucellosis reported annually worldwide, it has become a rare disease in the United States with fewer than 200 cases each year. However, it is estimated that only about 4 percent of cases are recognized and reported. *B. abortus* and *B. suis* cause most cases in the United States; *B. melitensis* and *B. canis* are rare. In the United States brucellosis is mainly an occupational disease with most cases occurring in working-age males who are abattoir workers, butchers, or farmers. Veterinarians may become infected by accidental inoculation of live attenuated *B. abortus* vaccine which causes mild disease. In most instances of brucellosis acquired in the United States from ingestion of contaminated milk products, the foods came from other parts of the world (Mexico, Mediterranean countries, the Far East, and South America).

Worldwide, *B. melitensis* is the most frequent cause of brucellosis. There are tremendous differences in the yearly incidence of human brucellosis in different countries, mainly depending on the extent of animal brucellosis. The areas with the highest prevalence are the Mediterranean countries, Asia, and Central and South America.

PATHOGENESIS AND PATHOLOGY After invading the body, *Brucella* are phagocytized by polymorphonuclear leukocytes and macrophages. Some *Brucella* are killed but others multiply within these cells and destroy them. Organisms spread via lymphatics to regional lymph nodes and, if not contained, to the bloodstream. Bacteremia may result in foci in cells of the reticuloendothelial system in the liver, spleen, and bone marrow and in other organs such as the kidneys. *Brucella* inside of phagocytic cells (as in the reticuloendothelial system and tissue macrophages) are protected against antibody and many antibiotics.

The reaction of tissues to *Brucella* is the formation of granulomas with epithelioid cells, giant cells, lymphocytes, and plasma cells. *B. abortus* usually causes mild disease with noncaseating granulomas in the liver and other reticuloendothelial organs. *B. suis* causes more severe disease with local suppurative complications and granulomas that may caseate. *B. melitensis* produces the most severe acute disease with symptoms that may be disabling. *B. canis* results in mild disease similar to that seen with *B. abortus*. Activated macrophages can kill *Brucella,* and this is the probable mechanism by which spontaneous cure and immunity occur. Granulomas in brucellosis eventually heal with fibrosis and often calcification.

Although brucellosis is a common cause of abortion in animals, there is no evidence that human abortions occur any more frequently with this disease than with other bacteremias.

MANIFESTATIONS Brucellosis may be asymptomatic with only serologic evidence of infection. Children are particularly prone to subclinical infection. The manifestations of symptomatic brucellosis may be divided into acute brucellosis, localized disease, and chronic brucellosis.

Acute brucellosis The incubation period of acute brucellosis usually varies between 7 and 21 days, but may be months. The onset is often insidious with a low-grade fever and no localizing complaints. Malaise, weakness, fatigue, headache, backache, myalgias, sweats, and chills are often prominent. Most patients are anorectic and lose weight. With *B. melitensis* infection the onset may be acute with high fever.

Typically, there are a multitude of complaints but a paucity of physical findings. When physical findings occur, the major manifestations are splenomegaly (which occurs in 10 to 20 percent of patients), lymphadenopathy (15 percent of patients), and hepatomegaly (less than 10 percent).

Localized brucellosis Localized disease may occur at almost any anatomic location, but osteomyelitis, splenic abscess, genitourinary tract infection, pulmonary disease, and endocarditis are among the more common. Osteomyelitis usually occurs in the vertebrae, with the lumbosacral area the most frequent site. There is a disc space infection with involvement of both adjacent vertebrae. Bone scans are positive early, followed by roentgenographic evidence of osteoporosis, anterior vertebral plate erosion, and formation of "parrot-beaked" osteophytes. Arthritis, which is much less common than osteomyelitis, most often involves the knee. Splenic abscesses may occur and result in areas of calcification. Epididymoorchitis and less often clinically apparent prostatic or renal infection may be observed. Neurologic complications are uncommon and include meningoencephalitis, myelitis, radiculitis, and peripheral neuropathy. Pleural effusion and pneumonia are occasional manifestations.

Endocarditis is the most common cause of mortality among patients with brucellosis. It has been reported predominantly in males, most often involves the aortic valve, has an indolent onset, results in bulky and ulcerative vegetations, is accompanied by a high rate of congestive heart failure and arterial embolization, and has usually required both valve replacement and antibiotic therapy to achieve cure.

Chronic brucellosis Chronic brucellosis is defined as ill health for more than 1 year following onset of brucellosis. It has mixed manifestations and includes patients with relapsing illness, with or without localized infection, as well as those who have no objective signs of infection (e.g., no fever) and no evidence of active brucellosis (by serology or culture). While the former clearly have brucellosis, it is doubtful that the latter have active brucellosis. Their complaints, fatigue and weakness, are more likely functional.

An unusual complication that occurs in veterinarians removing placentas from infected animals consists of an erythematous macular, papular, or postular rash on the hands and arms, which is presumed to be a hypersensitivity reaction to *Brucella* antigens.

DIAGNOSIS Brucellosis is a relatively rare disease, and there are many common illnesses that may mimic the most frequent presentation (i.e., fever without localizing symptoms or physical findings). Among them are infectious mononucleosis, toxoplasmosis, tuberculosis, hepatitis, systemic lupus erythematosus, typhoid fever, and many others. The clinical suspicion that the patient has brucellosis should be higher in farmers, abattoir workers, veterinarians, and others exposed to infected tissues or animal products. Most routine laboratory tests are not helpful. The white blood cell count is usually normal or low, and the erythrocyte sedimentation rate may be normal.

Cultures The definitive evidence of *Brucella* infection consists of isolating *Brucella* from the patient. However, culturing *Brucella* organisms may be dangerous to laboratory personnel. Therefore, specimens should be labelled as "suspected brucellosis" and should be processed only in laboratories that have Biosafety level 3 facilities. Up to half the untreated patients studied early in the course of infection will have *Brucella* in the blood when a culture is grown in trypticase soy broth for 1 to 3 weeks in the presence of 5 to 10% CO_2. Optimally, Casteñeda's medium (a biphasic trypticase soy broth and agar medium) should be used and incubated for 4 weeks. Bone marrow cultures are often positive in acute brucellosis when blood cultures are not. They are also more likely to remain positive later in the course of the disease and in spite of administration of antimicrobial agents. As the illness progresses, bacteremia is less frequent and organisms may then be isolated from infected lymph nodes or granulomas involving the spleen, liver, and bone. Altogether, only 15 to 20 percent of cases of brucellosis are confirmed by culture. In localized brucellosis, biopsy and isolation of *Brucella* may be necessary for diagnosis. In the majority of cases of brucellosis, the diagnosis is made serologically.

Serology The standard tube *Brucella* agglutination test (STA) has been used most in the diagnosis of brucellosis. It measures antibodies directed primarily at *Brucella* lipopolysaccharide antigens. A titer of $\geq$ 1:160 is considered positive and indicates past or present exposure to *Brucella* organisms or antigens that cross-react with *Brucella* species (*Brucella* skin tests, cholera vaccination, and infection with *Vibrio cholerae*, *Francisella tularensis*, or *Yersinia enterocolitica*). A fourfold or greater rise in titer of antibody in serum specimens drawn 1 to 4 weeks apart is indicative of recent exposure to *Brucella* or *Brucella*-like antigens. Paired specimens should be tested on the same day in the same laboratory. As measured by the STA, most patients develop a rise in titer within 1 to 2 weeks of illness, and by 3 weeks virtually all patients will show seroconversion. If there is strong clinical suspicion of brucellosis, dilutions as high as 1:1280 should be made, because false-negative tests due to blocking antibodies have been reported with blocking antibody titers as high as 1:640. True STA titers below 1:160 are strong evidence against active brucellosis.

The methods for serologic diagnosis of brucellosis use *B. abortus* antigens, because antibodies to *B. melitensis* and *B. suis* cross-react with *B. abortus*. However, antibodies to *B. canis* will not react with *B. abortus* antigen, and specialized serologic studies are necessary to detect these antibodies.

IgM antibody titers rise early in brucellosis (usually in the first week of infection), peak at about 3 months, and then fall gradually. However, high titers may persist for years. IgG antibodies appear 2 to 3 weeks after onset of illness, peak in about 8 weeks and persist as long as the infection is active. With cure, IgG antibody titers decrease rapidly and usually disappear within 1 year. The persistence of IgG antibody indicates continuing active infection. With relapse, both IgM and IgG titers increase. Use of 2-mercaptoethanol (2-ME) in the STA destroys the agglutinating activity of IgM antibodies and allows measurement of only the IgG-agglutinating antibody. In contrast to elevated IgM antibodies, a single titer of $\geq$ 1:160 in the 2-ME STA is good evidence of either current or very recent infection.

The *Brucella* skin test is only a measure of past infection. Because it may cause a rise in antibody titers, confusing the interpretation of the STA, it should not be performed.

TREATMENT The combination of tetracycline 30 mg/kg per day in four equally divided doses, orally, for 3 to 6 weeks plus streptomycin 15 mg/kg every 12 h intramuscularly for the first 2 weeks is considered the treatment of choice for brucellosis. The longer duration of tetracycline is recommended for patients with localized brucellosis. Patients who relapse are usually cured with retreatment. Tetracycline

should not be used in pregnant women or children below the age of 8 because of the danger of staining developing teeth. Streptomycin may cause eighth-nerve toxicity, and the dose must be decreased in patients with renal insufficiency.

A variety of other regimens, including tetracycline plus gentamicin or rifampin in lieu of streptomycin, doxycycline instead of tetracycline, or trimethoprim-sulfamethoxazole alone, have been tried in an attempt to decrease relapses and toxicity but none have been superior to the tetracycline-streptomycin combination. When tetracycline plus streptomycin cannot be used, trimethoprim/sulfamethoxazole (480/2400 mg/d) for 4 weeks is a reasonable substitute, although relapses are common. Addition of rifampin (900 mg/d) to the basic tetracycline-streptomycin or trimethoprim-sulfamethoxazole regimen may improve results when response is poor or when meningitis or endocarditis is present. Successful therapy of endocarditis has usually required valve replacement in addition to one of the above antimicrobial regimens. Despite apparent in vitro activity against strains of *Brucella*, the role of the third-generation cephalosporins in brucellosis remains to be determined.

Abscesses should be drained when indicated. Splenectomy has been performed in some patients with splenomegaly and multiple relapses and has apparently been successful in preventing further relapses.

Prednisone in an oral dose of 60 mg/d tapered rapidly over a 5- to 7-day period may be helpful in patients with brucellosis characterized by severe debility, but is rarely necessary. Headache, backache, and generalized aches and pains should be treated with analgesics.

PROGNOSIS Even before the advent of antimicrobial treatment, the mortality rate of brucellosis was less than 5 percent and only 15 percent of patients had an illness exceeding 3 months in duration. With chemotherapy, the mortality rate is less than 2 percent and long illnesses and complications are rare. When the morbidity exceeds 1 to 2 months, other causes, previously unsuspected underlying disease, or a complication of brucellosis should be considered.

PREVENTION The key to elimination of brucellosis in humans is the eradication of animal brucellosis. This can be accomplished by immunization of animals with a live attenuated *Brucella* vaccine which produces immunity. No vaccine is available for human immunization in the United States. The risk of acquiring brucellosis can be decreased by use of pasteurized milk and pasteurized milk products, by guarding against exposure to tissue from infected animals, and by protecting potential portals of entry in high risk individuals (veterinarians, meat inspectors, slaughterhouse workers) with protective bandages over cuts and by the use of protective clothing, gloves, and goggles.

REFERENCES

ARIZA J et al: Comparative trial of rifampin-doxycycline versus tetracycline-streptomycin in the therapy of human brucellosis. Antimicrob Agents Chemother 28(4):548, 1985
———— :Comparative trial of co-trimoxazole versus tetracycline-streptomycin in treating human brucellosis. J Infect Dis 152(6):1358, 1985
FERNANDEZ-GUERRERO ML et al: Prosthetic valve endocarditis caused by *Brucella melitensis*. Arch Intern Med 147:1141, 1987
GOTUZZO E et al: An evaluation of diagnostic methods for brucellosis—the value of bone marrow culture. J Infect Dis 153(1):122, 1986
HEWITT WG, PAYNE D: Estimation of IgG and IgM *Brucella* antibodies in infected and non-infected persons by a radioimmune technique. J Clin Pathol 37:692, 1984
JEROUDI M et al: Brucella endocarditis. Br Heart J 58:279, 1987
POLT SS et al: Human brucellosis caused by *Brucella canis:* Clinical features and immune response. Ann Intern Med 97:717, 1982
SHARDA DC, LUBANI M: A study of brucellosis in childhood. Clin Pediatr 25(10):492, 1986
YOUNG EJ: Human brucellosis. Rev Infect Dis 5:821, 1983
———— et al: Phagocytosis and killing of *Brucella* by human polymorphonuclear neutrophils. J Infect Dis 151:682, 1985

120   TULAREMIA

DONALD KAYE

DEFINITION   Tularemia (rabbit fever, deer fly fever) is an infection caused by *Francisella tularensis*. *F. tularensis* is found in many animals and is transmitted to human beings by direct contact or via an insect vector. The illness is characterized by an ulcerative lesion at the site of inoculation with regional lymphadenopathy, by pneumonia, or by fever without localizing findings.

ETIOLOGY   *F. tularensis* is a small, nonmotile, pleomorphic, gram-negative aerobic coccobacillus. It grows poorly in many media but will grow well in glucose-cysteine blood agar, thioglycolate broth, and other media supplemented with cysteine. *F. tularensis* is found only in the northern hemisphere. There are two types of *F. tularensis*. Type A is distributed solely in North America, is virulent for humans and rabbits, produces citrulline ureidase, and ferments glycerol. Type B is found in North America, Europe, and Asia, causes no or mild disease in humans and rabbits, does not produce citrulline ureidase, and does not ferment glycerol. *F. tularensis* cross-reacts serologically with *Brucella* species and *Yersinia pestis*.

EPIDEMIOLOGY   *F. tularensis* has been found in many mammals including rabbits, squirrels, muskrats, beavers, deer, cattle, and sheep, in birds, in amphibians, and in fish. Tularemia can result from skin contact with any of these species. Tularemia has also been caused by cat bite. Ticks and deer flies can transmit the bacterium. Ticks pass *F. tularensis* to their offspring via a transovarian route. The organism is found in tick feces but not in salivary glands. In the United States the disease can be carried by *Dermacentor andersoni* (Rocky Mountain wood tick), *Dermacentor variabilis* (American dog tick), *Dermacentor occidentalis* (Pacific Coast dog tick), and *Amblyomma americanum* (Lone Star tick). *F. tularensis* has also been recovered from streams.

In the United States most cases of tularemia result from skin contact with infected wild rabbits (especially cottontail rabbits) or tick feces. Infection occasionally results from ingestion or inhalation of infected material. Hunters and trappers are at greatest risk. Tularemia is most likely to occur in adult males, and person-to-person transmission rarely, if ever, occurs.

Tularemia has been reported from all parts of the United States, but mostly from Arkansas, Illinois, Missouri, Texas, Virginia, and Tennessee. Fewer than 200 cases are reported annually in the United States. Arthropod-borne disease occurs mainly in the spring and summer, and rabbit-produced infection mainly in the winter.

PATHOGENESIS AND PATHOLOGY   In human infection, the most common portal of entry is through the skin or mucous membranes either directly through inapparent abrasions or via the bite of a tick or other arthropod. Inhalation or ingestion of *F. tularensis* can also result in infection. Fewer than 50 organisms will result in infection when injected into the skin or inhaled, whereas more than 10^8 are usually required to produce infection via the oral route.

Following inoculation into the skin, the bacteria multiply locally and after 2 to 5 days (occasionally 1 to 10 days) produce an erythematous, tender, or pruritic papule. The papule rapidly enlarges and forms an ulcer with a black base. The bacteria spread to regional lymph nodes producing lymphadenopathy, and further spread with bacteremia may occur. With bacteremia, organisms are cleared from the blood by phagocytic cells of the reticuloendothelial system (mainly in the liver and spleen) and may survive intracellularly for long periods of time.

Affected organs (liver, spleen, lymph nodes) demonstrate areas of focal necrosis initially surrounded mainly by polymorphonuclear leukocytes. Subsequently granulomas form with epithelioid cells and lymphocytes and sometimes multinucleated giant cells surrounding the areas of necrosis which may resemble caseation necrosis. Coalescence of granulomas can lead to formation of abscesses. Nodes may occasionally become fluctuant and even rupture. Healing occurs with fibrosis and calcification of the granulomas.

Contamination of the conjunctiva can result in infection of the eye with regional lymph node enlargement. Aerosolization and inhalation of *F. tularensis* can result in pneumonia. Pneumonia can also occur via the hematogenous route. There is an inflammatory reaction with foci of alveolar necrosis and initially polymorphonuclear leukocytic and later mononuclear cell infiltration with granuloma formation. Chest roentgenograms usually reveal bilateral patchy infiltrates rather than large areas of consolidation. Mediastinal or other regional lymphadenopathy may occur.

Pharyngitis with cervical lymphadenopathy or gastrointestinal tularemia with mesenteric lymphadenopathy may follow ingestion of large numbers of *F. tularensis*. Typhoidal tularemia, which is characterized by fever and no localizing signs, is uncommon; the portal of entry is unknown.

CLINICAL MANIFESTATIONS   Tularemia usually has an incubation period of 2 to 5 days after which there is onset of one of a number of syndromes (listed below), all of which are usually associated with fever and chills and often with headache, myalgias, and malaise. Tender hepatosplenomegaly is common. About 20 percent of patients develop a generalized maculopapular rash which may occasionally become pustular, and some report erythema nodosum.

Ulceroglandular tularemia   Most patients with tularemia (75 to 85 percent) develop infection secondary to inoculation of the skin. In cases related to rabbits the portal of entry is usually on the finger or hand. In tick-related cases, the site of inoculation is usually on the lower extremities, inguinal or axillary areas, scalp, abdomen, or chest.

At time of onset of illness the patient usually has an erythematous papule that may be tender or pruritic, or an ulcer is already present at the portal of entry of the organism. If there is a papule, it evolves over a period of several days to form a punched out ulcer with sharply demarcated edges and a yellow exudate. The ulcer gradually develops a black base. The patient has very tender, large regional lymphadenopathy (usually axillary or epitrochlear with tularemia from rabbits, and inguinal or femoral lymphadenopathy with tick-borne disease). The nodes may become fluctuant and drain spontaneously. In 5 to 10 percent of patients, the skin lesion may be inapparent and the lymphadenopathy the only physical finding. This has been called "glandular tularemia."

Oculoglandular tularemia   In about 1 percent of patients, the conjunctiva serves as the portal of entry for the organism. Purulent conjunctivitis with regional lymphadenopathy (preauricular, submandibular, or cervical) is present. Corneal perforation may occur.

Oropharyngeal and gastrointestinal tularemia   Rarely tularemia occurs after ingestion of *F. tularensis* (usually in undercooked meat), resulting in acute exudative or membranous pharyngitis associated with cervical lymphadenopathy or ulcerative intestinal lesions with associated mesenteric lymphadenopathy, diarrhea, abdominal pain, nausea, vomiting, and gastrointestinal bleeding.

Pulmonary tularemia   Involvement of the lung can result from inhalation of *F. tularensis* or as a part of the bacteremia caused by tularemia at another site. Inhalation pulmonary disease occurs most often in laboratory workers and is a serious infection with high mortality. Pulmonary involvement occurs in 10 to 15 percent of patients with ulceroglandular tularemia and in about half of the patients with typhoidal tularemia. The patient has cough, which is usually nonproductive, and may have dyspnea or pleuritic chest pain. Most often the physical examination is normal. Roentgenograms of the chest usually reveal bilateral patchy infiltrates which have been described as "ovoid densities." Lobar pneumonia may occur, and pleural effusion(s) with a polymorphonuclear leukocytic (rarely mononuclear) exudate may be present.

Typhoidal tularemia   In about 10 percent of cases of tularemia fever develops without apparent skin lesion or lymphadenopathy. In the absence of a history of possible contact with a vector of the disease, diagnosis is extremely difficult.

Other manifestations Meningitis, pericarditis, peritonitis, endocarditis, and osteomyelitis have been reported. The meningitis causes a lymphocytic response in the spinal fluid.

DIAGNOSIS Differential diagnosis In patients with fever and large, tender lymphadenopathy the possibility of tularemia should be strongly considered, and an attempt should be made to determine if there was an appropriate animal or arthropod vector contact. The suspicion of tularemia should be especially high in hunters, trappers, game wardens, veterinarians, and laboratory workers. However, in up to 40 percent of patients with tularemia, no history of epidemiologic contact with an animal or arthropod vector can be elicited.

Ulceroglandular tularemia is often so characteristic that it does not present a problem in differential diagnosis, but on occasion it must be differentiated from other diseases. The skin lesion may resemble those seen in sporotrichosis, skin infection with coagulase-positive staphylococci or group A streptococci, syphilis, anthrax, rat bite fever (caused by *Spirillum minus*), rickettsial infections (such as scrub typhus), and *Mycobacterium marinum* infection. However, the regional lymphadenopathy in these diseases is usually not as impressive as in tularemia.

The lymphadenopathy of tularemia must be differentiated from that of plague (see Chap. 121), lymphogranuloma venereum (see Chap. 155), and cat-scratch fever (see Chap. 98). However, in these infections there is usually no local lesion resembling the ulcer of tularemia.

Typhoidal tularemia may resemble typhoid fever, other *Salmonella* bacteremias, rickettsial infections (such as Rocky Mountain spotted fever), brucellosis, infectious mononucleosis, toxoplasmosis, miliary tuberculosis, sarcoid, or hematologic malignancies. Tularemia pneumonia may resemble pneumonias caused by other bacteria as well as viral or *Mycoplasma* pneumonia.

Laboratory diagnosis Blood cultures are usually negative and the diagnosis is most frequently made serologically by agglutination methods. A significant rise in titer (i.e., fourfold or greater) in paired serum specimens over a 2- to 3-week period is diagnostic. Agglutinating antibody appears after 1 to 2 weeks of illness. Fifty percent of patients have antibody in the second week, and the rest develop antibody later in the course. Titers peak at 4 to 8 weeks and may remain elevated for years. A single agglutinating titer of $\geq$ 1:160 in a patient who has been ill for at least 2 weeks is highly suggestive of tularemia but may only indicate old infection. Antibodies to *F. tularensis* may cross-react with *Brucella*, but the titers to *Brucella* are usually much lower than the titers to *F. tularensis*. In the future enzyme-linked immunosorbent assay (ELISA) tests may offer an advantage because they tend to turn positive earlier than agglutinating antibody tests.

F. tularensis is rarely observed on Gram stains of skin lesions, sputum, or aspirates of nodes. However, the organisms can often be demonstrated by staining with a modified Dieterle stain or by fluorescent antibody staining techniques. Cultures of these materials or blood may be positive if processed on appropriate media, but there is a major risk of infection in laboratory personnel. Cultivation of *F. tularensis* should only be attempted in laboratories with adequate isolation techniques and experienced personnel.

Isolation of *F. tularensis* can be achieved by inoculation intraperitoneally into guinea pigs, which will die within 10 days, and by direct plating onto glucose-cysteine blood agar. Agents such as cycloheximide, polymyxin B, and penicillin are frequently added to media to suppress other organisms in specimens that may overgrow *F. tularensis*.

A delayed-type skin test (similar to the tuberculin test) with *F. tularensis* antigen or killed whole bacilli turns positive during the first week of illness, prior to the appearance of agglutinating antibody, and persists for years. However, the skin test antigen is not available commercially, and can boost titers of agglutinating antibodies.

The white blood cell count is usually normal, and the erythrocyte sedimentation rate may be normal as well. Pyuria is common.

TREATMENT Streptomycin, in a dose of 7.5 to 10 mg/kg every 12 h intramuscularly, is considered the drug of choice. In severe infections, 15 mg/kg every 12 h may be used for the first 48 to 72 h. Therapy is continued for 7 to 10 days. Gentamicin, in a dose of 1.7 mg/kg, intramuscularly or intravenously, every 8 h, is also effective. Virtually all strains are susceptible to streptomycin and gentamicin. Temperature response occurs within 2 days, but skin lesions and lymph nodes may take 1 to 2 weeks to heal. When therapy is not initiated until several weeks of illness have elapsed, the temperature response may be delayed. Relapses are very uncommon with streptomycin therapy.

Tetracycline or chloramphenicol, 30 mg/kg per day in four divided doses for 14 days, has also been used to treat tularemia. While response to these agents is good, the relapse rate is unacceptably high, occurring in up to 20 percent of patients.

If fluctuant nodes require aspiration or drainage, at least several days of antibiotic therapy should be given first to avoid exposure of medical personnel to aerosolization of infected material.

PREVENTION Prevention of tularemia is based on avoidance of exposure and vaccination of high-risk populations. Avoidance of skinning wild mammals, especially rabbits, and wearing gloves while handling rabbit carcasses will decrease the risk of transmission. Use of insect repellents and prompt removal of ticks will help prevent transmission by ticks in tick-infested areas.

A multiple-puncture intradermal vaccine (used in a fashion similar to vaccinia) made from live attenuated *F. tularensis* and available from the Centers for Disease Control, is effective in decreasing the frequency and severity of disease, but will not totally prevent tularemia. Protection is long-lasting. Veterinarians, hunters, trappers, game wardens, and others who are likely to come in contact with infected wild mammals are candidates for immunization. Laboratory workers who handle specimens containing *F. tularensis* should be immunized. Prophylactic treatment with streptomycin will prevent development of clinical disease in patients who are incubating *F. tularensis*.

PROGNOSIS If untreated, symptoms of tularemia usually last 1 to 4 weeks but may continue for months. The mortality of severe untreated infection (which includes all untreated tularemia pneumonia) can be as high as 30 percent. However, the overall mortality rate for untreated tularemia is less than 8 percent. Mortality is about 1 percent with appropriate therapy and is often associated with long delays in diagnosis and treatment. Following tularemia there is usually lifelong immunity.

REFERENCES

Evans ME et al: Tularemia: A 30-year experience with 88 cases. Medicine 64:251, 1985

Harper JL et al: Tularemic meningitis in a child with mononuclear pleocytosis. Pediatr Infect Dis 5:595, 1986

Kaiser AB et al: Tularemia and rhabdomyolysis. JAMA 253:241, 1985

Koskela P, Salminen A: Humoral immunity against *Francisella tularensis* after natural infection. J Clin Microbiol 22:973, 1985

Penn RL, Kinasewitz GT: Factors associated with a poor outcome in tularemia. Arch Intern Med 147:265, 1987

Sandstrom G et al: Antigen from *Francisella tularensis:* Nonidentity between determinants participating in cell-mediated and humoral reactions. Infect Immun 45:101, 1984

Sanford JP: Landmark perspective: Tularemia. JAMA 250:3225, 1983

121 PLAGUE AND OTHER *YERSINIA* INFECTIONS

DARWIN L. PALMER

PLAGUE

Plague is an acute infectious illness of humans, wild rodents, and their ectoparasites which is caused by the gram-negative bacillus *Yersinia pestis*. The disease persists because of its firm entrenchment in sylvatic rodent-flea ecosystems throughout the world. Wild rodent contact leads to sporadic human disease; the historically explosive urban epidemics resulted from transmission of disease into rats. Human bubonic plague follows bites by rodent fleas; after several days painful local adenopathy (the bubo) and sepsis spread to other organs, and death occurs. Primary plague pneumonia is transmitted between humans by cough-generated aerosols, has a fulminant course, and is almost universally fatal if untreated.

EPIDEMIOLOGY Sylvatic plague involves more than 200 species of wild rodents and is concentrated in the southwestern United States, the southern Soviet Union, India, Indochina, and South Africa. In the United States, ground squirrels, mice, voles, marmots, wood rats, prairie dogs, and chipmunks are potential carriers. Rodent disease is characterized by occurrence in the spring and summer, year-to-year variations in disease activity, chronicity in the populations involved, slow regional spread, and rare geographic regression. The disease dies off in some populations in cyclical fashion, leaving both resistant survivors and infected fleas seeking another host. Disease also persists in natural foci because of latent infection during animal hibernation, by prolonged viability of *Y. pestis* in soil of rodent burrows, by survival of infected fleas, and by persistent infection in relatively resistant rodents. Rodent predators may also spread plague; felines, such as domestic cats, generally die when infected with *Y. pestis*, while canines, such as foxes, coyotes, and dogs, often recover and may serve as serologic sentinels of wild rodent disease. Human disease can be readily acquired from domestic pets when the pets become infected or catch and return plague-infected rodents or their fleas to rural homes. Hares and rabbits are occasional nonrodent sources of the disease in humans, especially during the winter hunting season.

Rodent fleas are critical to the natural plague cycle and are implicated in about 85 percent of human cases. After infection, fleas develop obstruction of the foregut, causing regurgitation of plague bacilli during the next blood meal. The rat flea, *Xenopsylla cheopsis*, is an especially efficient plague vector both between rats and between rodents and humans. Transmission without fleas may occur by ingestion of infected carcasses by predators, possibly by contact with infected tissue through an open wound, or by inhalation of infected aerosols. Human body lice as well as ticks are also capable of interhuman or person-to-person transmission.

In the past three and one-half decades there has been a rising incidence of sporadic human plague originating in the western United States, with a death rate of 16 percent. This rate, double that seen in large outbreaks, reflects delay in the diagnosis or incorrect therapy due to travel during the incubation period out of plague endemic areas, or failure to elicit a history of animal exposure. Sporadic human plague occurs most frequently in the spring and summer, especially in males and children or youths under 20, reflecting their increased risk of wild rodent contact. While urban rat–related human outbreaks are now rare, they represent a continued threat; spread from sylvatic rodents into urban rats was documented as recently as 1983 in Los Angeles. Primary plague pneumonia arises as a secondary infection during bubonic/septicemic disease, with subsequent person-to-person spread via infectious aerosols. In closed quarters it is rapidly transmitted. A primary pneumonic plague outbreak in the United States last occurred in 1919, when 13 cases with 12 deaths (including two physicians and one nurse) developed before the disease was recognized and halted by case isolation. Cases of primary human pneumonic plague have also been acquired from domestic cats dying of plague pneumonia.

ETIOLOGY *Yersinia pestis* is a member of the family Enterobacteriaceae. It is a pleomorphic, gram-negative, nonmotile, aerobic bacillus which grows optimally at 28°C. The organism grows readily but slowly on routine media, and cultures should not be discarded before 72 h. Although weakly gram-negative, *Y. pestis* stains best with Giemsa's or Wayson's stain, with which it shows prominent bipolar "safety pin" microscopic morphology. The organism is a facultative intracellular parasite which maintains its virulence by the production of V and W antigens, enabling the organism to resist phagocytic intracellular killing, while production of capsular fraction 1 antigen partially protects the organism from phagocytosis by polymorphonuclear leukocytes. Other virulence factors include pesticin, fibrinolysin, coagulase, and a lipopolysaccharide endotoxin. The production of V and W antigens is plasmid-mediated, dependent on calcium, and may reflect the response of *Y. pestis* to its frequent intracellular location. No separate serotypes are recognized, but biotypes *antigua*, *orientalis*, and *mediaevalis* have geographic distributions which presumably mark previous epidemic spread. The organism is relatively resistant to drying and may maintain its viability in cool, moist conditions, such as the soil of an animal burrow, for many months. Antibiotic resistance can be developed in the laboratory, and both streptomycin- and tetracycline-resistant strains have been isolated from clinical specimens.

PATHOGENESIS After *Y. pestis* is inoculated into the skin by a flea bite, bacteria migrate to local lymph nodes, where they are taken up but not killed by mononuclear cells. Intracellular multiplication results in development of capsular envelopes containing fraction 1 protein; other toxins are elaborated. An acute inflammatory response is provoked in the lymph node in 2 to 6 days. At this stage the organisms are relatively resistant to phagocytosis by polymorphonuclear leukocytes because of the protection by capsules containing fraction 1 antigen and the lack of specific opsonic antibody. Characteristically, hemorrhagic necrosis of lymph nodes next occurs from which large numbers of bacteria gain access to the bloodstream and other organs. Extension along lymphatics involves both superficial nodes at the site of inoculation, the spleen, and nodes in the abdomen, mediastinum, or perihilar areas. The lung is secondarily infected in 10 to 20 percent, generally as a rapidly progressive, multilobar pneumonia, often with pleural exudate. The early acute inflammatory reaction is followed by lobar consolidation and hemorrhagic necrosis, and if death does not intervene, may progress to abscess formation. Fibrin thrombi may be extensive in the pulmonary vessels as well as in glomeruli and vessels of skin and other organs. Secondarily, the adult respiratory distress syndrome or a rise in pulmonary artery pressure may be seen. Pericarditis with a small amount of seropurulent exudate is frequent, and meningitis may occur late in untreated bacteremic plague. In 5 to 15 percent, the skin, predominantly of the extremities, is involved early on with petechiae and hemorrhages due to thrombocytopenia and vasculitis. Late in the disease, buboes may become fluctuant and occasionally may become superinfected with other bacteria. Endotoxemia may result in both endotoxin shock and disseminated intravascular coagulation.

MANIFESTATIONS Bubonic plague has an incubation period of 2 to 7 days from flea bite to onset of illness. Although many patients do not remember an insect contact, a small eschar may be found at the bite site. Patients present with a painful bubo and fever accompanied by headache, prostration, and abdominal distress. The bubo, a tender enlarged lymph node or nodes, ranges in size from 1 to 10 cm and is found in the groin in 70 percent; alternatively, buboes may develop in axillary or cervical nodes or in several lymphatic chains simultaneously. Buboes are extremely tender, not fixed to skin or underlying structures, and the overlying skin is often erythematous.

Fever and rigors are prominent and occasionally precede appearance of a bubo by 1 to 3 days. Gastrointestinal symptoms are present in more than half the patients, with abdominal pain often extending from the groin bubo and accompanied by anorexia, nausea, vomiting, and diarrhea, which may be bloody. Cutaneous petechiae and hemorrhages occur in 5 to 50 percent, and may be extensive late in the disease. Disseminated intravascular coagulation occurs in subclinical form in as many as 86 percent of patients, 5 to 10 percent of whom have clinical manifestations, including gangrene of the skin, fingers, toes, and penis. If untreated, bubonic disease may proceed without other organ system involvement to generalized sepsis, prostration, hypotension, and death within the next 2 to 10 days. Some patients have very prominent signs of sepsis with no demonstrable bubo. This represents a form of bubonic plague in which lymphatic involvement is limited to deep structures or where the buboes are so small as to be overlooked in the presence of overwhelming signs of infection. Septicemic disease may progress rapidly with chills, fever, rapid pulse, severe headache, nausea, vomiting, delirium, and death within 48 h. In such fulminant sepsis, bacteremia is so prominent that blood buffy coat may readily show *Y. pestis* on Gram stain.

Other than the lymphatics, the lung is the organ most commonly involved, with development of secondary pneumonia in 10 to 20 percent of all patients. Cough, fever, and tachypnea appear on days 2 to 3 of illness, accompanied by minimal pulmonary infiltrates. Later, or less commonly from the start, symptoms worsen rapidly with marked dyspnea, bloody sputum, and evidence of respiratory failure. There may be multilobar involvement, with variable degrees of consolidation, and the sputum may teem with *Y. pestis* and is highly contagious when disseminated by cough-generated aerosols. Primary plague pneumonia is a fulminant illness; time from the initial contact to death ranges from 2 to 6 days. The adult respiratory distress syndrome (ARDS), characterized by noncardiac pulmonary edema, anoxia, and respiratory failure, also occurs as a manifestation of plague sepsis and may be indistinguishable from plague pneumonia except for the absence of bacteria in respiratory secretions. Both *Y. pestis* pneumonia and the ARDS form of illness have a mortality in excess of 75 percent, despite appropriate antimicrobial and supportive therapy. Less commonly, marked perihilar adenopathy may present alone or accompany pneumonia.

Plague meningitis, as a late complication that occurs in 6 percent of untreated patients, is characterized by nuchal rigidity, headache, confusion, and coma, and is often preceded or accompanied by bacteremia. Most meningitis cases have been described in patients treated with antibiotics that do not readily cross the blood-brain barrier, such as tetracycline and streptomycin. Other contributory factors seem to be late or inadequate therapy. Meningitis due to plague is indistinguishable from that caused by other bacteria.

Rarely, patients with plague have a very mild illness manifested chiefly by low-grade fever and adenopathy. In this group are patients with tonsillar plague, who have positive throat cultures, serologic conversion, and minimal illness. Other less common late complications include persistent hectic fever despite appropriate therapy; fluctuance and spontaneous drainage from buboes; and pulmonary cavitation with abscess formation.

LABORATORY FINDINGS With the exception of definitive microbiologic studies, laboratory tests are of little diagnostic help. A polymorphonuclear leukocytosis of 15,000 to 20,000 cells per cubic millimeter is common, and the white cells may show toxic changes. Rarely, a marked leukemoid reaction with more than 100,000 white cells is seen. Modest elevations of serum glutamic oxaloacetic transaminase are common, but otherwise liver function studies are normal. Evidence of disseminated intravascular coagulation with low platelet counts, prolonged partial thromboplastin times, and positive fibrin degradation products is common. The electrocardiogram is usually normal but may show right axis deviation and peaked P waves indicative of acute cor pulmonale. The chest x-ray shows infiltrates, often with pleural effusion, in secondary or primary plague pneumonia or shows evidence of pulmonary edema in patients with

ARDS. In meningitis, examination of cerebrospinal fluid demonstrates polymorphonuclear pleocytosis, low sugar, elevated protein, and gram-negative coccobacillary organisms, although culture may demonstrate *Y. pestis* more reliably.

Confirmation of the clinical suspicion of bubonic plague may be obtained by needle-aspiration of a bubo with direct staining of the aspirated material. With either Wayson's or Giemsa's stain, the characteristic bipolar-staining "safety pin" forms are seen. By fluorescent antibody staining, a presumptive diagnosis may be specifically confirmed in about 80 percent of cases. Cultures of aspirated material, as well as sputum, pleural fluid, and blood, will be positive in a high percentage of patients. Microscopic examination of buffy coat smear may show *Y. pestis* in septicemic cases. A serologic response with a fourfold or greater rise in titer is detected in the second week of illness by complement fixation, hemagglutination or indirect immunofluorescent antibody.

DIAGNOSIS Bubonic plague must be suspected in any febrile patient with painful adenopathy who has a history of wild animal exposure in a plague endemic area, but may be confused with other illnesses. Presentation with fever and a painful groin bubo can mimic granuloma venereum or syphilis or, when more severe, an acute abdominal crisis such as incarcerated inguinal hernia, appendicitis, or a ruptured viscus. Abdominal pain and bloody diarrhea can be mistaken for shigellosis or other acute diarrheal processes. With an axillary or cervical bubo, acute streptococcal or staphylococcal lymphadenitis, tularemia, cat-scratch fever, granuloma venereum, or syphilis need to be considered. Bubonic/septicemic disease with an absent or minimal bubo, suggests typhoid fever or bacteremia due to other causes. Primary or secondary pneumonic plague may mimic bacterial pneumonia from any cause.

When plague is suspected, diagnostic maneuvers must include aspiration of buboes with appropriate stains and cultures, as well as blood cultures and cultures from other sources. Cultures should not be discarded early because the organism grows slowly and may only appear in 48 to 72 h. A serologic rise by passive hemagglutination is evident by day 5 and peaks by day 14. Newer serologic methods such as enzyme-linked immunosorbent assay compare well in sensitivity to standard passive hemagglutination tests and are more rapid.

TREATMENT If plague is strongly suspected on clinical and/or epidemiologic grounds, therapy must be started immediately, prior to completion of diagnostic studies. Antibiotic and supportive treatment should reduce the 40 to 100 percent mortality of untreated bubonic or pneumonic plague to 5 to 10 percent. Effective antibiotics include streptomycin, tetracycline, and chloramphenicol. Streptomycin should be given initially in a dosage of 7.5 to 15 mg/kg every 12 h intramuscularly; tetracycline, intravenously in a dosage of 5 to 10 mg/kg every 6 h, may be started concurrently and streptomycin discontinued when the patient becomes afebrile. Larger doses, even in those with severe illness, offer no benefit. Tetracycline should be continued for a total of 3 to 4 days after the fever has disappeared. In less severely ill patients, tetracycline alone at 5 to 10 mg/kg every 6 h may be given either by mouth or intravenously. Chloramphenicol in a dose of 12.5 to 25 mg/kg given intravenously every 6 h should be substituted for tetracycline in patients with meningitis because of its better central nervous system penetration. While antibiotic-resistant organisms have appeared only rarely, gentamicin is as effective as streptomycin. Tetracycline or trimethoprim-sulfamethoxazole are effective for the prophylaxis of case contacts and should be given orally for 5 days. Local treatment of the bubo is not indicated unless fluctuance or spontaneous drainage occurs, when cultures should be obtained to detect staphylococci. Ventilatory support for patients with plague pneumonia or ARDS may be necessary and lifesaving.

PREVENTION AND CONTROL Individuals working in high-risk occupations in plague endemic areas or conducting laboratory work with *Y. pestis* should consider use of the formalin-killed wholebacteria vaccine; however, the vaccine must be readministered every 6 months due to rapidly waning immunity. Alternatively, individuals briefly visiting a plague endemic area may take tetracycline or trimethoprim-sulfamethoxazole prophylaxis. Following the presumptive diagnosis of pneumonic plague, patients should be placed in respiratory isolation; simple hand-washing precautions suffice for bubonic cases. Contacts of a patient with plague pneumonia should be given oral tetracycline prophylaxis, 250 mg four times daily by mouth, and should be advised to seek medical attention if respiratory symptoms or fever develop. Possibly due to such precautions, transmission of primary plague pneumonia has not occurred in this country for many years.

The potential for spread of plague into urban rat populations from sylvatic rodent sources is an ever-present risk. Prevention depends on control of urban rat populations and their exclusion from dwellings as well as surveillance of sylvatic rodents and of their local predators. Picnickers, hikers, and others traveling into plague endemic regions during the spring-summer season should be warned that plague is a potential danger. They should avoid touching carcasses or sick rodents and should restrain and treat pets with flea-repellent powders. No practical measures exist for eliminating plague from wild rodent sources. Reducing rodent harborage around rural homes in endemic regions is important. Killing rodents around rural dwellings with rodenticides should be preceded by insect control to prevent displaced rodent fleas from seeking humans or domestic pets.

OTHER *YERSINIA* INFECTIONS (*Y. PSEUDOTUBERCULOSIS* AND *Y. ENTEROCOLITICA*)

ETIOLOGY *Y. enterocolitica* and *Y. pseudotuberculosis* are both non-lactose-fermenting, gram-negative, aerobic bacilli related to one another and to *Y. pestis* and are members of the Enterobacteriaceae. Both organisms grow slowly on media used for the detection of other enteric bacteria, and their detection can be enhanced by cold enrichment incubation at 20 to 25°C. Strains can be distinguished from one another and from *Y. pestis* on the basis of serologic and biochemical reactions as well as by antibiotic sensitivities. As in *Y. pestis*, both organisms elaborate W and V virulence factors and, with *Y. pseudotuberculosis*, virulence is also related to its ability to survive intracellularly. Both organisms produce an endotoxin and *Y. enterocolitica* elaborates a heat-stable enterotoxin which may be of significance in food-borne illness. A large number of serotypes of both organisms exist causing disease in many animal species, but most human infections are caused by a limited number of strains.

MANIFESTATIONS Although recognized most commonly in northern Europe and North America, *Y. enterocolitica* causes enteric infection worldwide and accounts for approximately 1 to 3 percent of all cases of acute bacterial enteritis. The origin of the disease is often unclear and outbreaks traced to both food and water have been reported; person-to-person as well as animal-to-person transmission is common. Manifestations of the disease vary with age. In infants and young children the predominant symptom is acute watery diarrhea lasting 3 to 14 days; 5 percent of children have blood in the stool. In older children and young adults, a syndrome of right lower quadrant pain accompanied by fever and moderate leukocytosis indistinguishable from acute appendicitis occurs. In adults, especially in women over age 40, erythema nodosum often follows enteritis by 1 to 2 weeks. Adults may develop a monarticular arthritis of the knee, foot, or hand with or without preceding enteritis. Rarely, a severe, disabling suppurative arthritis is seen. Among patients with arthritis, 65 percent have histocompatibility group HLA-B27. *Y. enterocolitica* also causes bacteremia, mostly in individuals with underlying illness such as diabetes mellitus, severe anemia, cirrhosis, or malignancy. Septicemic patients complain of headache, fever, and abdominal pain with or without diarrhea and frequently develop abscesses in multiple organs. Exudative pharyngitis with *Y. enterocolitica* was found in adult patients during the course of an outbreak of milk-borne yersiniosis.

Pseudotuberculosis is a rare illness acquired from humans or domestic and wild animals, presumably by fecal-oral contact. Most cases are sporadic and occur in the young, with males more commonly affected than females and with a peak in the winter months corresponding to the peak occurrence in animals. After ingestion, the organisms apparently penetrate the ileal mucosa, localize in the ileocecal lymph nodes, and produce an acute mesenteric adenitis, which is generally accompanied by vomiting, abdominal pain, and diarrhea. Fever is usually high and leukocytosis is common. At laparotomy the appendix appears normal, but enlarged mesenteric lymph nodes and inflammation of the terminal ileum may be seen. Complications appear in adults less commonly than with *Y. enterocolitica* but include arthritis, erythema nodosum, and septicemia.

DIAGNOSIS *Y. enterocolitica* and *Y. pseudotuberculosis* cause similar signs and symptoms but may have different reservoirs; the first is characterized primarily by diarrhea and the second by mesenteric adenitis. Therefore *Y. enterocolitica* causes disease similar to other bacterial diarrheas and must be distinguished from them by microbiologic means. Laboratory detection of the organism depends on special cultural techniques. The diagnosis is made best by isolation of the organism from stool in patients with enteritis, or atypical cases of appendicitis, erythema nodosum, or reactive arthritis. Cultures of the pharyngeal exudate, blood, peritoneal fluid, and other body fluids should be obtained where clinically indicated. Hemagglutination titers peak in 8 to 10 days and remain elevated for 18 months after infection. Cross-reactivity with some *Brucella*, *Salmonella*, and *Vibrio cholerae* antigens occurs. The diagnosis of *Y. pseudotuberculosis* is also made by culture of stool and mesenteric lymph nodes.

THERAPY AND PREVENTION *Y. enterocolitica* organisms are susceptible in vitro to aminoglycosides, chloramphenicol, tetracycline, trimethoprim-sulfamethoxazole, and the third-generation cephalosporins but are generally resistant to the penicillins and first-generation cephalosporins. However, the value of antimicrobial therapy is unclear, because most cases of enteritis are self-limited. Patients with very severe illness or septicemia should be treated, because treatment may shorten both the duration of disease and the shedding of organisms. *Y. pseudotuberculosis* is usually sensitive to ampicillin, tetracycline, choramphenicol, and cephalosporins. No controlled clinical trials demonstrate efficacy of treatment, although patients with septicemic disease should receive ampicillin or tetracycline, because severe infection has a high mortality. Prevention depends on hygienic measures such as careful food handling, availability of clean drinking water, and hand washing to prevent spread within families or other human contacts.

PASTEURELLA MULTOCIDA INFECTION (See Chap. 98)

REFERENCES

Plague

BARNES AM, POLAND JD: Plague in the United States, 1983, Centers for Disease Control Surveillance Summaries, Publication 33 (no 1SS), 1984

BECKER TB et al: Plague meningitis. A retrospective analysis of cases reported in the US, 1970–1979. West J Med 147(5):554, 1987

BUTLER T: A clinical study of bubonic plague: Observations on the 1970 Vietnam epidemic with emphasis on coagulation studies, skin histology, and electrocardiograms. Am J Med 53:268, 1972

KAUFMAN AF et al: Public health implications of plague in domestic cats. Am J Vet Assoc 179:875, 1981

REED WP et al: Bubonic plague in the Southwestern United States—A review of recent experience. Medicine 49:465, 1970

TOMICH PQ et al: Evidence for the extinction of plague in Hawaii. Am J Epidemiol 119: 261, 1984

Other *Yersinia* Infections

BOYCE JM: *Yersinia* species, in *Principles and Practice of Infectious Diseases*, 2d ed, GL Mandell et al (eds). New York, Wiley, 1985, pp 1296–1301

COVER TL, ABER RC: *Yersinia enterocolitica*. N Engl J Med 321:16, 1989

GRANFORS K et al: Yersinia antigens in synovial-fluid cells from patients with reactive arthritis. N Engl J Med 320:216, 1989

TACKET CO et al: *Yersinia enterocolitica* pharyngitis. Ann Intern Med 99:40, 1983

TERTTI R et al: An outbreak of *Yersinia pseudotuberculosis* infection. J Infect Dis 149:245, 1984

122   CHOLERA

GERALD T. KEUSCH

DEFINITION   Cholera is an acute diarrheal disease due to a highly motile, curved gram-negative rod, *Vibrio cholerae,* and it can result in severe and rapidly progressive dehydration and death in a matter of hours unless quickly treated. As a result, "cholera gravis" is a much feared disease, especially when it occurs in epidemics or in worldwide pandemics associated with high mortality rates.

ETIOLOGY AND EPIDEMIOLOGY   *V. cholerae* is a family of organisms, classified on the basis of their somatic O antigen. The major cause of clinical cholera belongs to O group 1 (O-1), which distinguishes it from the more than 70 other members of *V. cholerae* collectively known as non-O1 vibrios. While some of the latter cause diarrhea, only rarely is this cholera gravis. Eight other *Vibrio* species have been defined, of which *V. parahemolyticus, V. fluvialis, V. hollisae,* and *V. mimicus* also cause human diarrhea (see Chap. 92). *V. cholerae* exists in two biotypes, classical and El tor, that are distinguished on the basis of a number of diverse characteristics, such as phage susceptibility and hemolysin production. Both biotypes may be separated into serotypes known as Inaba and Ogawa, which are useful serologic markers for field epidemiologic studies.

Cholera is native to the Ganges delta in the Indian subcontinent, but since 1817, seven world pandemics have occurred. The last to reach the United States was in 1911, when the sixth pandemic made brief entry into New York and Massachusetts. In the past decade, sporadic endemic infection has been recognized along the Gulf coast of Louisiana and Texas, due to eating shellfish contaminated with free-living cholera vibrios. Small outbreaks on offshore oil rigs due to contaminated drinking water have occurred as well. In southern Asia, where the majority of cases in the world occur, fecal contamination of water from an infected human is the most common means of transmission, but contamination of food can contribute to intrafamilial spread. The infectious dose is relatively high, but is markedly reduced in hypochlorhydric subjects or when the gastric pH is buffered by a meal. In endemic areas, cholera is predominantly a pediatric disease, but it affects children and adults equally when the organism is newly introduced into a population. The seasonality of cholera in endemic areas is not fully explained, but may relate to environmental conditions that influence multiplication of vibrios and/or seasonal alterations in human behavior that affect their contact with water. Asymptomatic infections are frequent and are more common with El tor cholera. Young children under 2 years are less likely to develop severe cholera in endemic regions, which may be due in part to passive immunity from breast milk. For unexplained reasons, blood group status is significantly associated with cholera susceptibility; those with group O are at greater risk and those with group AB are at lesser risk.

PATHOGENESIS   Once the organism is ingested and safely passes through the stomach, it colonizes the upper small bowel. There are a number of bacterial adhesins that may mediate this phenomenon. Once established, the organism produces the protein, cholera toxin (CT), the principal cause of the watery diarrhea of cholera. CT binds to glycolipid receptors on jejunal epithelial cells, specifically to G_{M1} ganglioside, by a sugar-specific recognition mechanism. CT is an enzyme that transfers ADP-ribose from nicotine adenine dinucleotide (NAD) to a target protein in the adenylate cyclase enzyme system of intestinal epithelial cells. This G protein, the GTP-binding regulatory component of adenylate cyclase, permanently upregulates the cyclase catalytic unit when ADP-ribosylated, resulting in production of high levels of cyclic AMP. In turn, this alters transport of Na and Cl in both the Na-absorbing villus cell and the Cl-secreting crypt cells, leading to accumulation of NaCl in the intestinal lumen. Because water will move passively to maintain osmolality, isotonic fluid accumulates in the lumen, and when the volume exceeds the capacity of the rest of the gut to reabsorb the fluid, watery diarrhea occurs. Dehydration, leading to shock, and loss of base, leading to acidosis, then develop unless these fluids and electrolytes are replaced adequately.

The nature of immunity to cholera is poorly understood but seems to be primarily antibacterial at the level of the mucosa itself and, to a lesser extent, related to antitoxin antibody of the secretory IgA class. Serum antibody is more a marker of prior exposure than an indication of protection.

CLINICAL MANIFESTATIONS   After a 24 to 48 h incubation, the disease begins with the sudden onset of painless watery diarrhea that quickly becomes voluminous and is often quickly followed by vomiting. In severe cholera, adults can lose as much as 1 L/h and children 10 mL/kg per hour in the first 24 h. Without replacement, this fluid loss can cause lethal volume depletion. There is usually no fever, but muscle cramps may occur later due to potassium depletion. The stool has a characteristic appearance, a nonbilious, gray, slightly cloudy fluid with flecks of mucus and a somewhat sweet, inoffensive odor. Clinical symptoms parallel volume contraction, with thirst observed at 3 to 5 percent loss; postural hypotension, weakness, tachycardia, and decreased skin turgor at 5 to 8 percent; and oliguria, weak to absent pulses, sunken eyes and (in infants) sunken fontanelles, wrinkled ("washerwoman") skin, and somnolence progressing to coma with fluid losses in excess of 10 percent of normal body weight. When clinical manifestations of volume depletion are treated with fluid and salt, the process is self-limited to a few days at most, and complications such as renal failure due to acute tubular necrosis can be averted.

Laboratory data usually reveal elevation of the hematocrit in nonanemic patients; mild neutrophilic leukocytosis; elevations of BUN and creatinine consistent with prerenal azotemia; normal sodium, potassium, and chloride; a markedly reduced bicarbonate (<15 mmol/L); and elevation of the anion gap due to coexistent increases in serum lactate, protein, and phosphates. When measured, arterial pH is usually low (about 7.2).

DIAGNOSIS   Clinical suspicion of cholera can be proven by identification of the organism in stool. Dark-field microscopy by an experienced technician can directly detect the organism in a wet mount of fresh stool and even reveal serotype by immobilization with Inaba- or Ogawa-specific antisera. The best selective culture medium is thiosulfate–citrate–bile salt–sucrose (TCBS) agar, on which the organism grows as a flat yellow colony. In endemic areas there is little need for biochemical characterization, but this may be worthwhile where *V. cholerae* is an uncommon isolate. Standard biochemical testing for enterobacteriaceae will suffice. All vibrios are oxidase-positive, and *V. cholerae* can be distinguished from the otherwise similar *V. mimicus* by its ability to ferment sucrose. If a delay in processing samples is expected, it is recommended that Carey-Blair transport medium and/or alkaline-peptone water enrichment medium be inoculated as well.

TREATMENT   Cholera is simple to treat, needing only the rapid and adequate replacement of fluids, electrolytes, and base. Mortality rates are usually less than 1 percent. It has been conclusively proven that fluid may be given by the oral route, using the glucose-Na cotransport mechanism to move Na across the gut mucosa together with an actively transported molecule such as glucose. Since Na losses in the stool are high, fluid containing 90 mmol/L Na has been recommended by the World Health Organization (WHO) (Table 122-1). This amount of Na is higher than is needed in other diarrheas, but the solution is safe if alternated with Na-free fluid such as breast milk or water. For the sake of simplicity, WHO advises use of this single solution instead of multiple different formulae tailored for different etiologies. Because severe acidosis is common in severely dehydrated patients (pH <7.2), 50% *N* saline with added bicarbonate (44 mmoL/L) is the preferred solution for intravenous administration. For severely dehydrated patients the total fluid deficit (usually

TABLE 122-1 Oral rehydration fluids recommended by the World Health Organization

Component	Concentration, mmol/L		
	Bicarbonate based	Citrate based	Super-ORS*
Sodium	90	90	90
Potassium	20	20	20
Chloride	80	80	80
Citrate	—	10	—
Bicarbonate	30	—	30
Glucose	111	111	111
Glycine	—	—	111†

* Super-ORS refers to the use of solutions containing two substrates that are actively cotransported across the intestinal mucosa together with sodium, such as glucose and glycine.
† In the developing world, 30–50 g of rice powder is being substituted for glucose, as it is an inexpensive source of small-chain oligosaccharides that provide substrate for facilitated cotransport with sodium but do not increase osmolarity. In addition, rice-based ORS seems to provide more nutritional benefits than standard ORS and may reduce the net fluid output of diarrheal stool, an effect not seen with ordinary ORS.

REFERENCES

CLEMENS JD et al: Field trial of oral cholera vaccines in Bangladesh: Results of one year of follow-up. J Infect Dis 158:60, 1988
GLASS RI: Cholera and non-cholera vibrios, in *Enteric Infections: Mechanisms, Manifestations, Management*, MJG Farthing, GT Keusch (eds). London, Chapman & Hall, 1989, pp 317–325
LEVINE MM et al: Volunteer studies of deletion mutants of *Vibrio cholerae* O1 prepared by recombinant techniques. Infect Immun 56:262, 1988
MILLER CJ et al: Cholera epidemiology in developed and developing countries: New thoughts on transmission, seasonality, and control. Lancet 2:261, 1985
MORRIS JG JR, BLACK RE: Cholera and other vibrioses in the United States. N Engl J Med 312:343, 1985
WANG F et al: The acidosis of cholera. Contributions of hyperproteinemia, lactic acidemia and hyperphosphatemia to an increased serum anion gap. N Engl J Med 315:1591, 1986
WORLD HEALTH ORGANIZATION: *World Health Organization Guidelines for Cholera Control.* WHO/CDD/Ser/80.4 Revl, Geneva, 1986

estimated as 10 percent of body weight) can be safely replaced intravenously within the first 4 h following admission. Half of this may be given within the first hour. After this, oral therapy can usually be initiated to maintain fluid balance and intake equal to output. However, patients with continued large volume diarrhea may require prolonged administration of intravenous fluids to maintain adequate volume status until the diarrhea stops. Severe hypokalemia may be present, but will respond to potassium given by either the intravenous or oral route. Without adequate staff to monitor patient progress, the oral route is safer and is physiologically regulated by thirst and urine output.

The use of antibiotics to which the organism is susceptible will diminish the duration and the amount of fluid loss and more rapidly clear the organism from the stool, but is not necessary to achieve complete cure. Tetracycline is efficacious, but is not recommended for children under 8 years of age because of side effects on bone and developing teeth. Other antibiotics, including chloramphenicol, trimethoprim-sulfamethoxazole, and ampicillin are also effective.

CONTROL In outbreaks, attention should first be given to identification of case contacts and treatment of incubating carriers. Next, epidemiologic study is needed to establish the modes of transmission to help define the best control strategy. At the same time establishment of rehydration centers is essential to reduce mortality. The role of killed whole cholera vaccine is less clear.

PREVENTION Provision of safe water, facilities for sanitary disposal of feces, improved nutrition, and attention to food preparation and storage in the household could significantly reduce the incidence of cholera. Much attention has been given to the development of a cholera vaccine in the past two decades, focusing particularly on use of a live oral vaccine strain. The traditional killed cholera vaccine, consisting of three injections of 5 billion dead *Vibrios,* provides little protection to nonimmune subjects while predictably causing side effects, including local pain, malaise, and fever. A new approach consisting of oral administration of killed whole bacterial cells together with the toxin B-subunit has provided promising results. In trials in Bangladesh, the combined vaccine conferred 85 percent protection, compared to 58 percent for killed whole cells vaccine, 4 months after administration. However, the benefit of adding the B-subunit toxin was no longer detectable by 8 months, and by the end of 1 year protection was equivalent for the two vaccines (around 60 percent). Increasing the number of killed bacteria given by mouth may also increase its protective efficacy. Until this or another vaccine is available, parenteral cholera vaccine is not recommended for Americans traveling in cholera-endemic areas unless required by the country to be visited. Careful hygiene and attention to eating and drinking habits to reduce the likelihood of encountering the organism are recommended.

123 BARTONELLOSIS

JAMES J. PLORDE

DEFINITION Bartonellosis (Carrión's disease) is an infection with *Bartonella bacilliformis.* Two well-defined clinical stages occur: an acute febrile anemia of rapid onset and high mortality, designated *Oroya fever,* and a benign eruptive form with chronic cutaneous lesions, called *verruga peruana.* Either of these types may be mild, and asymptomatic cases constitute the greatest epidemiologic hazard.

ETIOLOGY *Bartonella bacilliformis* is a small, motile, aerobic, pleomorphic, gram-negative coccobacillus which stains reddish violet with Giemsa's stain. It can be cultured on enriched media and does not produce a hemolysin. The organisms are sensitive to several antibiotics in vitro.

EPIDEMIOLOGY The disease is limited to certain valleys in the Andes Mountains comprising parts of Peru, Ecuador, and Colombia. It occurs in regions between the altitudes of 750 and 2500 m (2400 and 8000 ft) where the phlebotamine sandfly vector, *Lutzomyia,* propagates. Although *L. verrucarum* is the principal vector of the disease, other species are involved in Colombia as well. Asymptomatic cases and convalescent carriers are the only known reservoir of infection. A low-grade bacteremia may persist for years following resolution of symptoms, and *B. bacilliformis* can be recovered from the blood of 5 to 10 percent of the apparently normal population in an endemic area. Epidemics often coincide with immigration of workers from uninfected areas.

PATHOLOGY AND PATHOGENESIS The manifestations of the disease are thought to reflect the immune status of the host. In nonimmune individuals Oroya fever develops. Large numbers of the *Bartonella* bacteria enter the bloodstream, adhere to erythrocytes, and invade the endothelial cells of the capillaries and lymphatics where they multiply. Subsequent invasion and multiplication within erythrocytes result in their phagocytosis and destruction by the liver and spleen. The red blood cell life span is greatly shortened, and anemia develops. This is accentuated by a defective erythropoietic response early in the course of infection. The pathogenesis of the hemolytic anemia remains unknown. Agglutinins and hemolysins have not been found, and tests for mechanical fragility of red blood cells have given variable results. Invasion and swelling of capillary endothelial cells may lead to vascular occlusion and tissue infarcts. It is thought that an impairment of reticuloendothelial function secondary to massive phagocytosis of red blood cells and immune suppression are responsible for the frequency with which *Salmonella* and other coliform bacteremias, staphylococcal infections, tuberculosis, malaria, and amebiasis are seen in Oroya fever.

With developing immunity, the bacteria nearly disappear from the peripheral blood and capillary endothelium. After a latent period they reappear in the skin and subcutaneous tissue where they are apparently responsible for the development of the hemangioid lesions of verruga peruana. Second attacks of Carrión's disease are unusual. When they occur, they almost invariably present as verruga.

CLINICAL MANIFESTATIONS The incubation period is approximately 3 weeks but may be longer. The initial symptoms are fever and pains in the bones, joints, and muscles. At this point the disease often resembles influenza or malaria, but blood cultures are positive. After these prodromes, the patient usually develops one of the two classic forms of the infection.

Oroya fever This form is characterized by sudden onset of high fever, extreme pallor, weakness, and a precipitous drop in the number of red blood cells. The count may fall from normal to 1 million per microliter within 4 or 5 days. The anemia is characterized by normochromic macrocytes in the peripheral blood, striking polychromasia and polychromatophilia, nucleated red blood cells, Howell-Jolly bodies, Cabot rings, and basophilic stippling. There may also be a mild leukocytosis with a shift to the left. Organisms are numerous in the blood, and stained smears may show 90 percent of the erythrocytes heavily invaded. Salmonellosis, malaria, amebiasis, tuberculosis, and other intercurrent infections may occur and are an important factor in fatal cases.

Muscle and joint pain and headache are severe, and insomnia, delirium, and coma are the terminal manifestations. In untreated patients, the mortality rate may exceed 50 percent; death occurs within 10 days to 4 weeks. With treatment, or sometimes spontaneously, recovery results if the organisms decrease and fever abates. The red blood cell count stabilizes and approaches normal values in about 6 weeks, when convalescence begins.

Verruga peruana This form of the disease, characterized by a profuse skin eruption, may follow the anemic form or may occur in patients without previous symptoms. The verrugas vary in color from red to purple. They may be miliary, nodular, or eroding, and they range in size from 2 to 10 mm up to 3 or 4 cm in diameter. They may resemble the lesions of Kaposi's sarcoma. The three types of verruga may occur together; since eruption takes place in successive crops, verrugas of all types and in all stages of development may be found on the same patient. The chief sites involved are the limbs and face, and less frequently the genitalia, scalp, and mucosa of the mouth and pharynx. They may persist for 1 month to 2 years. The eruption is accompanied by pain, fever, and moderate anemia. Bartonellas may be demonstrated in the lesions and cultured from the blood.

DIAGNOSIS A clinical diagnosis of verruga peruana can be made with accuracy in endemic areas. It is confirmed by demonstrating the Giemsa-stained organism in biopsy specimens from representative lesions. During Oroya fever the organism is easily seen on peripheral blood smears. It may be recovered from blood cultures in all stages of the disease.

TREATMENT Oroya fever responds dramatically to a number of antibiotics including tetracycline and chloramphenicol. The latter in a dose of 2 g per day for 7 days is often preferred because of the frequency with which *Salmonella* infections complicate this disease. Fever disappears within 48 h, and the patient recovers rapidly. Transfusions may be required when the anemia is severe. Antibiotic therapy [rifampin (rifampicin) 600 mg/d for 6 days] of the verrugal stage may hasten the involution of these lesions. The use of DDT in both the interior and exterior of human dwellings is highly effective in controlling the night-biting sandflies. Insect repellents and bed netting afford personal protection.

REFERENCES

Arias-Stella J et al: Verruga peruana, mimicking malignant neoplasms. Am J Dermatopathol 9:279, 1987

Caudra MC: Salmonellosis complication in human bartonellosis. Tex Rep Biol Med 14:97, 1956

Dooley JR: Haemotropic bacteria in man. Lancet 2:1237, 1980

Garcia FU: Tissue reaction in Bartonellosis may suggest Kaposi's sarcoma. Arch Pathol Lab Med 109:703, 1985

Schultz MG: Daniel Carrión's experiment. N Engl J Med 278:1323, 1968

124 *LEGIONELLA* INFECTIONS

MICHAEL S. BERNSTEIN / RICHARD M. LOCKSLEY

DEFINITION The family Legionellaceae consists of over 25 species of fastidious gram-negative, aerobic bacilli. The organisms are ubiquitous in the environment and cause disease when a sufficient environmental inoculum is aerosolized and inhaled by a human host. The course of the subsequent disease is determined both by virulence factors of the bacterium and by the immune competence of the host. The organism in humans behaves as a facultative intracellular bacterium. Legionnaire's disease, a fulminant pneumonia caused by *Legionella pneumophila*, is the prototypic illness caused by these organisms. Pontiac fever is a self-limited, flulike syndrome that occurs in immunocompetent individuals. The spectrum of disease caused by these organisms is designated legionellosis.

HISTORY Legionnaire's disease refers to an epidemic of pneumonia that affected 221 people and caused 34 deaths during the American Legion Convention at the Bellevue-Stratford Hotel in Philadelphia during July and August 1976. Initially referred to as the Legionnaire's disease agent, the organism was shown to be a new species of bacterium and subsequently designated *L. pneumophila*. Serotyping revealed that this organism had been responsible for previous epidemics of pneumonia, including 20 cases of severe pneumonia among attendees at a convention in Philadelphia at the same hotel in 1974. Furthermore, in July 1968, 144 employees and visitors in a health department building in Pontiac, Michigan, developed a self-limited illness consisting of fever, myalgias, headache, and malaise, subsequently termed Pontiac fever. Exposure of guinea pigs to aerosols of water from the building's air conditioning system led to isolation of the organism, eventually identified as *L. pneumophila*.

The discovery of *L. pneumophila* led rapidly to the isolation of related organisms within the family Legionellaceae (Table 124-1). There are more than 34 species (29 named) and over 50 distinct serogroups (46 named). Many isolates cause pneumonia indistinguishable from that caused by the initial strain, designated *Legionella pneumophila* serotype 1. This isolate accounts for 50 percent of human infection, followed in frequency by serotype 6 (10 percent). *L. micdadei* (Pittsburgh pneumonia agent) accounts for 7 percent of cases. The serologically unrelated, unnamed legionellae are designated *Legionella*-like organisms (LLOs).

ETIOLOGY The legionellae are classified in a single genus, *Legionella*, within the family Legionellaceae. The legionellae are gram-negative, aerobic, nonencapsulated bacilli measuring 0.3 to 0.9 μm in width and 2 to 5 μm in length. They are non-spore-forming, and most are motile due to polar or subpolar flagellae. Electron microscopy reveals multiple fimbriae (pili) extending from the surface. Legionellae have complex growth requirements and do not grow on standard bacteriologic media. All species require supplementation of growth media with L-cysteine and ferric salts and grow best at pH 6.8 to 7.0. Legionellae display an unusual dependence on amino acids, as opposed to carbohydrates, for energy and carbon sources. The fatty acids of legionellae contain an unusually high proportion of branched-chain acids, permitting identification by gas-liquid chromatography.

In most clinical laboratories legionellae are recognized by their growth on selective media. Identification is confirmed by serologic reactivity with defined antisera. A commercially available slide

TABLE 124-1 Identified *Legionella*

Species (serogroups)	Pneumonia	Pontiac fever	DFA*
L. pneumophila (14)	X	1,6†	1–10
L. micdadei	X		X
L. bozemanii (2)	X		1
L. dumoffii	X	?	X
L. gormanii	X		X
L. longbeachae (2)	X		1,2
L. jordanis	X		X
L. oakridgensis	X		
L. wadsworthii	X		
L. feeleii (2)	X	X	
L. sainthelensi	X	?	
L. anisa	X	X	
L. maceachernii	X		
L. jamestownensis			
L. rubrilucens			
L. erythra			
L. hackeliae (2)	X		
L. spiritensis		?	
L. parisiensis			
L. cherrii	X		
L. steigerwaltii			
L. santicrucis			
L. israelensis			
L. cincinnatiensis	X		
L. quinlivanii			
L. birminghamensis	X		
L. moravica			
L. brunensis			
L. tucsonensis	X		

* Direct fluorescent antibody reagents available.
† Numbers refer to serogroups.

agglutination test identifies 22 *Legionella* species and 33 serogroups. Further identification of a *Legionella* isolate may require analysis in a reference laboratory. Biochemical analysis, autofluorescence, immunofluorescence staining, and gas-liquid chromatography are used to characterize different species and strains. Less widely available techniques include restriction endonuclease analysis, alloenzyme typing, and plasmid DNA profiling.

ECOLOGY AND TRANSMISSION Legionellae are ubiquitous in aquatic environments. Diverse natural *reservoirs* harbor these organisms, including mud, frozen streams, hot springs, and stagnant lakes. Certain algae provide all of the nutritional and growth requirements for *L. pneumophila*. Some amebas and ciliated protozoa ingest legionellae and support their intracellular multiplication, protecting the bacteria from disinfectants and other adverse conditions. Legionellaceae have no animal or human reservoir.

Amplifiers are man-made water supplies that favor the growth of legionellae. Growth is enhanced by elevated temperatures (36 to 70°C), a source of iron and simple nutrients, and low levels of other competing bacteria. Hot water systems and heat exchange units are frequently contaminated due to stagnation, infrequent decontamination, and the presence of sediment or decayed plumbing, all of which contribute to suboptimal levels of chlorine. Decomposing rubber gaskets and sealing washers are capable of supporting the growth of these organisms. Legionellae have been isolated from such diverse man-made aqueous environments as potable water, ice machines, hot tubs, and humidifiers.

Disseminators facilitate transmission to the human respiratory tract by generating infectious aerosols. Airborne transmission by environmentally generated aerosols was suggested by epidemiologic evidence and has been reproduced in experimental animals. Aerosolized *L. pneumophila* can survive for more than 2 h and have been isolated nearly 1 mile downwind of cooling towers. Infectious aerosol particles are less than 5 μm in diameter and can be inhaled directly into the alveoli. A variety of sources have been identified in outbreaks of Legionnaire's disease, including cooling towers, air conditioning systems, humidifiers, whirlpool baths, respiratory nebulizers, and showers. Aerosolized legionellae have been traced to contaminated soil disturbed by excavation and to industrial lubricants used to cool machinery.

Other routes of transmission may exist. Microaspiration of contaminated water has been suggested by epidemiologic studies. Wound infection by *L. pneumophila* has been reported from a contaminated whirlpool bath. There is no evidence of person-to-person transmission.

EPIDEMIOLOGY *Legionella* infections account for 1 to 3 percent of community-acquired pneumonias and, in some studies, up to one-fourth of "atypical" community-acquired pneumonias. *L. pneumophila* may be responsible for 10 percent of nosocomial pneumonias and as much as 30 percent during endemic hospital outbreaks. About half of adults show evidence of prior exposure to at least one *Legionella* species.

Legionella infections occur in epidemic outbreaks, sporadic cases, or highly endemic clusters related to sustained nosocomial outbreaks. Both pneumonic and nonpneumonic legionellosis exist in epidemic form but differ in their attack rates and incubation periods. *Legionella* pneumonia has an attack rate of 1 to 7 percent, whereas Pontiac fever affects 95 to 100 percent of those exposed. The incubation period for pneumonia is 2 to 12 days, while that for nonpneumonic outbreaks is 24 to 48 h. There is a higher incidence of legionellosis during summer, presumably due to warmer water temperatures and increased use of water cooling systems that transmit the organism.

Pneumonic legionellosis affects men three times as often as women and is uncommon in children. Other risk factors for pneumonic disease include cigarette smoking, heavy alcohol use, advanced age, chronic illness, and use of immunosuppressive medication. Renal transplant patients appear to be at particular risk. Nonpneumonic legionellosis has no demonstrable risk factors.

PATHOGENESIS AND PATHOLOGY Direct alveolar deposition of infectious aerosols containing legionellae is the predominant form of inoculation in *Legionella* infections. The short incubation period and the association with environmental aerosols are consistent with this mechanism. The inoculum of aerosolized bacteria and poorly defined variability in virulence among strains may be important in determining the outcome of infection. Common-source exposures can result in nonpneumonic illness or severe pneumonia in different individuals, depending on the extent of exposure to infectious aerosols.

Legionellae appear to be susceptible to clearance by the mucociliary apparatus. Asymptomatic colonization does not occur, and, during disease, pathologic findings are limited to the lower respiratory tract. Alveolar deposition via aerosol and factors, such as smoking, that impair mucociliary clearance permit the organism to establish infection within resident alveolar macrophages. In the human host, legionellae are facultative intracellular pathogens of monocytes and macrophages. The organisms activate complement by the classic pathway but are resistant to lysis. Mononuclear phagocytes ingest *L. pneumophila* by a mechanism termed *coiling phagocytosis* that is mediated by complement receptors CR1 and CR3. Ingested organisms inhibit fusion of the phagosome to primary and secondary lysosomes, blocking the transfer of microbicidal substances into the phagosome and interfering with acidification of the vacuole. The sequestered organisms divide by binary fission within unusual vacuoles studded by host ribosomes and surrounded by glycogen granules and mitochondria. Continued replication results in lysis of the mononuclear cell and spread to adjacent cells. Both neutrophils and monocytes are recruited to the developing inflammatory lesion but are unable to inhibit bacterial growth efficiently. Specific antibody is produced, but the organisms remain resistant to antibody-mediated complement lysis. Phagocytosis is enhanced by specific antibody, thus further targeting the bacteria to the intracellular environment.

From the initial site, infection spreads by endobronchial, hematogenous, or lymphatic routes or by contiguous invasion. Bacteremia occurs in as many as one-third of patients with legionellosis and is the most common source of extrapulmonary infection.

Infection is controlled coincident with the appearance of cell-mediated immunity, similar to that with other intracellular pathogens. Sensitized T lymphocytes secrete macrophage activating factors, primarily interferon-γ, that enable the cell to inhibit intracellular replication. Interleukin 2–activated natural killer cells are also capable of destroying *Legionella*-infected monocytes in vitro. Immunization using aerosolized avirulent *L. pneumophila* or subcutaneous injection of a secreted bacterial protein protects guinea pigs against otherwise lethal aerosol challenge. The importance of cell-mediated immunity is supported by the increased incidence and severity of legionellosis among immunosuppressed patients, including transplant recipients.

Macroscopically, bronchopneumonia ranges from a patchy lobular process to more extensive multilobar consolidation. Round, nodular lesions are sometimes present. Abscesses with central necrosis occur in 25 percent of fatal cases. Pleuritis and small serosanguinous pleural effusions are common, but empyema is rare. Microscopically, infection is characterized by intense alveolitis and bronchiolitis. Alveolar spaces are filled with polymorphonuclear leukocytes, macrophages, fibrin, and proteinaceous exudate. Many inflammatory cells have undergone leukocytoclasis leaving only nuclear debris and fibrin. Organisms can be visualized using the Gimenez stain, Dieterle silver impregnation stain, or direct fluorescent antibody and are predominantly located within phagocytes. Alveolar septae and interstitial spaces are thickened by edema and inflammatory cells. More severe disease occurs in immunocompromised patients, including diffuse alveolar damage with hyaline membrane formation. Pathologic changes do not extend proximal to terminal bronchioles, a finding consistent with inoculation by aerosol. Pathologic changes are usually limited to the lungs. Brain tissue is normal even in cases with neurologic abnormalities.

CLINICAL MANIFESTATIONS Legionnaire's disease and Pontiac fever are the two well-described syndromes. The complete spectrum of infection by Legionellaceae remains undefined, however, and probably includes asymptomatic seroconversion, mild self-resolving illness, and isolated extrapulmonary manifestations.

Pneumonic illness typically begins with an abrupt prodrome of malaise, headache, myalgia, and weakness. Fever and intermittent rigors appear 24 h later, with temperatures exceeding 40°C in more than half of patients. Nonproductive cough is common. About half of patients eventually produce thin or minimally purulent sputum, and one-third may have scant hemoptysis. Pleuritic chest pain and dyspnea can raise the suspicion of pulmonary embolism. Gastrointestinal symptoms include diarrhea, nausea, vomiting, and abdominal pain. Altered mental status suggesting toxic encephalopathy may include confusion, disorientation, lethargy, hallucinations, depression, delirium, obtundation, or coma. Seizures are rare, but cranial or peripheral neuropathy and cerebellar dysfunction are not uncommon. Physical examination usually shows a toxic appearance and high fever. Relative bradycardia is common. Lung examination reveals rales and consolidation, but the physical findings are mild when compared to radiographic findings. Complications and systemic manifestations include lung abscess, empyema, respiratory failure, hypotension, shock, rhabdomyolysis, disseminated intravascular coagulation (DIC), thrombotic thrombocytopenic purpura (TTP), and renal failure.

Pontiac fever is an acute, self-limited illness lasting 2 to 5 days. A prodrome of malaise, myalgia, and headache is followed rapidly by fever, chills, and, variably, cough, coryza, and sore throat. Diarrhea, nausea, and mild neurologic symptoms such as dizziness or photophobia may be present.

Legionellae may also cause extrapulmonary infections related to bacteremia at the time of pneumonia or local exposure to contaminated water. Pericarditis, myocarditis, pyelonephritis, pancreatitis, sinusitis, and hemodialysis fistula infections; abscesses in liver, skin, and the perirectal area; and postoperative wound infections have been reported. *L. pneumophila* and *L. dumoffii* can cause subacute and chronic prosthetic valve endocarditis with annular and myocardial abscesses. The organisms are nosocomially acquired during the perioperative period when the primary infection may cause a postpericardiotomy–like syndrome. Emboli are rare.

LABORATORY FINDINGS *Legionella* pneumonia is usually accompanied by leukocytosis with an increase in early granulocyte forms; the total leukocyte count exceeds 20,000 cells per microliter

in 10 to 20 percent of cases. None of the laboratory abnormalities associated with pneumonic legionellosis is specific although hyponatremia occurs in 50 to 70 percent, more commonly than in other forms of pneumonia. Other laboratory findings may include hypophosphatemia, azotemia, microhematuria, proteinuria, and abnormal tests of liver function. Hematologic findings are typically normal unless the illness is complicated by DIC or TTP. Cerebrospinal fluid examination is usually normal although pleocytosis and elevated protein have been reported. Gram stain of the sputum may show inflammatory cells, but legionellae stain poorly or not at all in clinical specimens. *L. micdadei* is acid-fast by Kinyoun and modified Ziehl-Neelsen stains.

Early roentgenographic patterns include diffuse patchy infiltrates or ill-defined nodular densities. Pneumonia progresses to bilateral infiltrates in 50 percent of patients; a lobar-segmental pattern predominates. Small pleural effusions are present in 20 to 50 percent. Cavitation is uncommon but may occasionally be seen, particularly in immunosuppressed patients.

Leukocytosis is frequently the only laboratory abnormality in Pontiac fever.

DIAGNOSIS The diagnosis of *Legionella* infection may be made by culturing the organism, identifying its antigens or nucleic acids in tissue or secretions, or demonstrating a serologic response in the host (Table 124-2). A positive culture is diagnostic since no carrier state occurs. Cultures are performed on buffered charcoal yeast extract agar with α-ketoglutarate (BCYE-α agar), but 2 to 5 days may be required to identify the organism. BCYE-α agar is not selective, and supplementation with antibiotics or acidification is required for sputum samples to inhibit the growth of other bacteria. Typical results of the culture of clinical specimens are listed in Table 124-2. Blood cultures must be subcultured on BCYE-α agar after 24 h of aerobic incubation.

Legionellae may be visualized in clinical specimens by direct fluorescent antibody (DFA) staining. Clinical specimens are treated with fluorescein-conjugated rabbit antibody and examined by fluorescence microscopy. The test requires only 2 to 4 h. Commercially available DFA reagents detect over 90 percent of strains responsible for clinical disease (Table 124-1). However, the relatively low sensitivity (50 percent) and the need for an experienced technician are disadvantages. DFA may be less sensitive after a patient has received appropriate antibiotics.

Available tests for *Legionella* antigens in urine include an enzyme-linked immunosorbent assay, radioimmunoassay, and latex agglutination. The relative ease of specimen collection and assay performance may make this an attractive rapid test. However, antigenuria may persist for months, obscuring the distinction between acute and past infection. A radiolabeled nucleic acid hybridization kit is promising because it allows the detection of all *Legionella* species, although false-positive results have been reported. The radioactive isotope limits the shelf life of the assay.

Serum antibody is most commonly measured using the indirect fluorescent antibody (IFA) assay. Routinely available reagents detect antibody directed only against *L. pneumophila* serogroup 1, believed to account for half of human disease. A diagnosis of legionellosis is made by a fourfold rise in titer between acute and convalescent sera

TABLE 124-2 Laboratory tests in Legionnaire's disease

Test	Sensitivity, %	Specificity, %
Culture		
Sputum	60	100
Transtracheal	80	100
Lung biopsy	90	100
Blood	38	100
DFA	50	95
Urine antigen*	80	99
DNA probe	70	99
Serology (IFA)*	80	99

* *L. pneumophila* serogroup 1 only; indirect fluorescent antibody.

to at least 1:128, or a single titer of 1:256 or greater. Serum samples should be obtained acutely and after 3 weeks, although as many as one-fourth of patients may seroconvert within the first week of illness. Seroconversion develops in 80 percent of patients by 10 weeks.

While no clinical features of *Legionella* pneumonia are unique, the diagnosis should be suspected in a patient with severe pneumonia, high fever, nonproductive cough, hyponatremia, and altered mental status, particularly in the setting of immunosuppression. Each of the tests employed to diagnose legionellosis has its limitations. Combined approaches are recommended. No diagnostic test may be used to exclude the disease absolutely. Thus, clinical judgment must often prevail in decisions regarding therapy.

The diagnosis of Pontiac fever requires a compatible clinical illness, evidence of serologic conversion and, preferably, isolation of the organism from the environment. Viable legionellae have never been isolated from a case of Pontiac fever, raising the possibility that the pathogenesis involves hypersensitivity to bacterial antigens rather than true infection.

TREATMENT Erythromycin is the antibiotic of choice for pneumonic legionellosis. For serious infection, patients should receive 4 g/d intravenously. Dosage reduction may be necessary in renal failure to avoid ototoxicity. Immunocompromised patients and those with severe disease should receive rifampin (rifampicin) concurrently in a dose of 600 mg/d. Immunosuppressive medications should be tapered when possible. Response to therapy occurs in 24 to 48 h, although fever may persist for up to a week. With improvement, erythromycin may be reduced to 2 g/d orally. Therapy should continue for 3 weeks; shorter courses have been associated with relapse. Doxycycline or trimethoprim-sulfamethoxazole are potential alternatives when erythromycin is not tolerated, or in the rare patients failing to respond to erythromycin. Ciprofloxacin and other quinolones appear to be effective, but clinical experience with these agents is small. Effective antibiotics are those that diffuse readily into phagocytic cells, suggesting that their role may be to arrest intracellular multiplication until the development of cellular immunity.

Legionella prosthetic valve endocarditis usually requires valve replacement and prolonged antibiotic therapy (3 to 12 months). Pontiac fever is a self-limited illness requiring no therapy.

PROGNOSIS AND IMMUNITY Overall case fatality rates for *Legionella* pneumonia are approximately 15 percent. Mortality is 80 percent among untreated immunosuppressed patients and is reduced to 25 percent with appropriate antibiotic treatment. Untreated immunocompetent hosts have a 25 percent mortality rate; with proper therapy only 7 percent succumb.

Patients who survive usually have no permanent sequelae. Full recovery of pulmonary function is usual, although pulmonary fibrosis

with respiratory disability has been reported. Immunocompetent individuals who recover from infection are immune to reinfection with the same strain. Reinfection with an identical serotype has been reported in an immunocompromised patient.

PREVENTION AND CONTROL Understanding the chain of transmission of legionellae from natural reservoirs to man-made amplifiers and disseminators is important in devising control strategies. Surveillance efforts should concentrate on documenting human infection, rather than routinely screening the environment. During epidemic or endemic outbreaks, sentinel cases occur among immunosuppressed patients. Once detected, a careful search for the environmental source should be conducted. Multiple legionellae may be recovered from environmental cultures, many of which are not associated with human disease. Therefore, clinical isolates should be characterized so that control measures can focus on the source of pathogenic strains. Legionellosis is a reportable infection, and local health departments can provide assistance in the isolation and characterization of environmental strains.

Sources of environmental aerosols (disseminators), such as shower heads and air conditioning systems, must be identified so that transmission can be interrupted. Contaminated water systems (amplifiers) can be sterilized. Legionellae may be present in low titer in potable water systems, requiring culture of large volumes on selective media or following pretreatment with heat or acid to enhance recovery. Rusted plumbing and decayed rubber gaskets should be replaced. Sites of stagnation and sediment in water tanks may require elimination. Decontamination of potable water systems is accomplished by hyperchlorination (2 to 3 ppm) and/or intermittent heating to 60°C with flushing of distal outlets. During nosocomial outbreaks, prophylactic treatment of high-risk patients using oral erythromycin has been effective. Periodic monitoring of hospital water may be necessary to detect reemergence of the organism.

REFERENCES

CUNHA BA (ed): Legionnaire's disease. Semin Respir Infect 2:189, 1987

FANG GD et al: Disease due to the Legionellaceae (other than *Legionella pneumophila*). Historical, microbiological, clinical, and epidemiologic review. Medicine (Baltimore) 68:116, 1989

FRASER DW et al: Legionnaire's disease. Description of an epidemic of pneumonia. N Engl J Med 297:1189, 1977

MUDER RR et al: Mode of transmission of *Legionella pneumophila*. A critical review. Arch Intern Med 146:1607, 1986

TOMPKINS LS et al: Legionella prosthetic-valve endocarditis. N Engl J Med 318:530, 1988

WINN WC JR: Legionnaire's disease: Historical perspective. Clin Microbiol Rev 1:60, 1988

section 6 Mycobacterial diseases

125 TUBERCULOSIS

THOMAS M. DANIEL

DEFINITION Tuberculosis is a chronic bacterial infection caused by *Mycobacterium tuberculosis* that is characterized by the formation of granulomas in infected tissues and by cell-mediated hypersensitivity. The usual site of disease is the lungs, but other organs may be involved. In the absence of effective treatment for active disease, a

chronic wasting course is usual and death ultimately supervenes. Most cases of tuberculous infection are asymptomatic.

ETIOLOGY *Mycobacterium tuberculosis*, the tubercle bacillus, is one of more than 30 well-characterized and many unclassified members of the genus *Mycobacterium*. Along with the closely related *M. bovis*, it causes tuberculosis. *M. leprae* is the etiologic agent of leprosy (see Chap. 126), and a number of other mycobacterial species produce less common human diseases (see Chap. 127). Most mycobacteria are not pathogenic for humans, and many are readily isolated from environmental sources.

Mycobacteria are distinguished by their surface lipids which render them acid-fast so that they cannot be decolorized with acid alcohol after staining. Because of this lipid, heat or detergents are usually necessary to accomplish primary staining.

Important to understanding the pathogenesis of tuberculosis is recognition that *M. tuberculosis* contains many immunoreactive substances. Surface lipids of mycobacteria and water-soluble components of cell wall peptidoglycan are important adjuvants that may exert their effects through their primary actions on host macrophages. *M. tuberculosis* survives the intracellular milieu of macrophages, and this intracellular persistence may be facilitated by cell wall lipids which inhibit phagosome-lysosome fusion. Mycobacteria contain an array of protein and polysaccharide antigens, some probably species-specific but others clearly sharing epitopes broadly throughout the genus. Cell-mediated hypersensitivity is characteristic of tuberculosis and is an important determinant of the disease's pathogenesis.

EPIDEMIOLOGY Tuberculosis has been disappearing rapidly from Europe and North America, but in the rest of the world it continues as an important cause of death. In 1986, a total of 22,768 cases of tuberculosis were reported in the United States, a case rate of 9.4 per 100,000 per year. The case rate had been falling at a rate of 5 to 6 percent per year, but since 1985 this trend has been interrupted by AIDS. It is estimated that 10,000,000 Americans have a positive tuberculin test but that fewer than 1 percent of American children are tuberculin reactors. Tuberculosis in North America tends to be a disease of the elderly, the urban poor, of minority groups, and of patients with AIDS. At all ages case rates among nonwhites tend to be twice those in whites. Hispanic, Haitian, and southeast Asian immigrants may have case rates as high as those of the countries from which they come, and in these individuals the frequency of disease among younger persons reflects its occurrence in those countries. Increasingly, tuberculosis in the United States is being seen in microepidemics, often centered in families.

Because in the United States tuberculosis has become a disease of the elderly, it is frequently seen in nursing homes. Although transmission of infection can occur at any age, most disease in older persons represents a legacy of previous times. The elderly of today were children when transmission of tubercle bacilli occurred much more frequently. Of those who were infected, many developed disease in young adulthood. Some, especially males, did not and are only now developing reactivation disease in their late years. However, an increasing portion of elderly persons has never been infected, and have acquired nosocomial new infections in nursing homes.

In much of the world transmission of tuberculous infection is declining, but in many impoverished nations this is not true. In some countries estimated new case rates are as high as 400 per 100,000 per year. As in North America and Europe, poverty and tuberculosis go hand in hand. In high-prevalence areas, tuberculosis is seen with equal prevalence in rural and urban settings, and afflicts chiefly young adults. In countries where human immunodeficiency virus (HIV) infection is endemic, tuberculosis is a frequent cause of morbidity in AIDS patients. A reasonable estimate of the magnitude of tuberculosis in the world is that half of the population of the world is infected with *M. tuberculosis,* that there are 30 million cases of active tuberculosis in the world, that 10 million new cases occur annually, and that 3 million die of tuberculosis each year. Tuberculosis probably causes 6 percent of all deaths worldwide.

TRANSMISSION *M. tuberculosis* is transmitted from person to person via the respiratory route. Although other routes of transmission are possible and have been documented on occasion, none is of major importance. Tubercle bacilli in respiratory secretions form nuclei for water droplets expelled during coughing, sneezing, and vocalizing. Small droplets evaporate within a short distance from the mouth, and thereafter desiccated bacilli remain airborne for long periods. Infection of a susceptible host occurs when a few of these bacilli are inhaled. The number of bacilli excreted by most infected persons is not large; typically, household contact of many months is required for transmission. However, laryngeal tuberculosis, endobronchial disease, recent transbronchial spread of tuberculosis, and extensive cavitary pulmonary disease are often highly contagious. Infectiousness correlates with the number of organisms in the expectorated sputum, extent of pulmonary disease, and frequency of cough. Mycobacteria are susceptible to ultraviolet irradiation, and outdoor transmission of infection rarely occurs in daylight. Adequate ventilation is the most important measure to reduce the infectiousness of the environment. Fomites are not important in the transmission of tuberculosis. Most patients become noninfectious within 2 weeks after the institution of appropriate chemotherapy because of a decrease in the number of organisms excreted and a decrease in cough.

Transmission of infection with *M. bovis* has long been associated with the consumption of contaminated cow's milk. This organism is no longer a major cause of human disease in most of the world.

PATHOGENESIS The initial entry of tubercle bacilli into the lungs or other site of a previously uninfected individual elicits a nonspecific acute inflammatory response which is rarely noted and is usually accompanied by few or no symptoms. Bacilli are then ingested by macrophages and transported to the regional lymph nodes. If spread of the organism is not contained at the level of regional lymph nodes, then tubercle bacilli reach the bloodstream and widespread dissemination ensues. Most lesions of disseminated tuberculosis heal, as do most primary pulmonary lesions, although they remain potential foci of later reactivation. Dissemination may result in miliary or meningeal tuberculosis—illnesses with potential for major morbidity and mortality, especially in infants and young children.

During the 2 to 8 weeks after primary infection, while bacilli continue to multiply in their intracellular environment, cell-mediated hypersensitivity develops in the infected host. Immunologically competent lymphocytes enter areas of infection, where they elaborate chemotactic factors, interleukins, and lymphokines. In response, monocytes enter the area and undergo transformation into macrophages and subsequently into specialized histiocytic cells which are organized into granulomas. Mycobacteria may persist within macrophages for many years despite increased lysozyme production within these cells, but their further multiplication and spread are usually confined. Healing then occurs, often with late calcification of the granulomas, sometimes leaving a residual lesion visible on chest radiograph. The combination of a calcified peripheral lung lesion and calcified hilar lymph node is known as a Ghon complex.

In the United States, 95 percent of individuals undergo complete healing of primary tuberculous lesions with no subsequent evidence of disease. In other populations, where infective inocula may be higher and where nutritional status and other host factors may be less propitious, failure of complete healing may occur in more than 5 percent of individuals. Famine and many intercurrent diseases adversely affect healing and threaten the stability of healed tuberculous lesions.

Tuberculosis—the clinical disease—develops in the minority who do not successfully contain their primary infections. In some individuals tuberculosis develops within weeks after primary infection; in most, organisms lie dormant for many years before entering a phase of exponential multiplication leading to disease. Among many, age can be identified as a significant factor determining the course of tuberculosis. In infants tuberculous infection frequently progresses rapidly to disease, and the risk of disseminated disease including meningitis and miliary tuberculosis is high. In children older than 1 or 2 years up to about the age of puberty, primary tuberculous lesions almost always heal; most of those destined to develop tuberculosis do so during adolescence or young adulthood. Individuals infected in adulthood are at greatest risk of developing tuberculosis within approximately 3 years following infection. Tuberculous disease is more common in young adult women, whereas it is more common in men later in life.

IMMUNOLOGY **Immunity** Humans display native immunity to tuberculosis, with substantial individual variation. Twin studies have demonstrated that tuberculosis is more likely to occur in both members of monozygotic sibships than in dizygotic sibships or other family relationships. Attempts to link susceptibility to tuberculosis to HLA phenotype have produced conflicting data. Although susceptibility to tuberculosis has been associated with race, the evidence is largely anecdotal and is not convincing. As noted, age is an important determinant of native immunity to tuberculosis. Although specific data on nutrition and tuberculosis immunity are lacking, the association of tuberculosis with famine is clear.

Acquired immunity follows primary tuberculous infection. Disease due to exogenous reinfection is probably rare in North America and Europe; it may be more frequent in populations of high prevalence where risk of repeated exposure is great. It is useful to recall that *immunity* in the classic use of the word refers to resistance to infection, whereas *hypersensitivity* describes a state of altered host reactivity. In this sense, immunity may also result from vaccination with bacillus Calmette-Guérin (BCG) or from infection with other species of mycobacteria.

Antigen-specific immunity is T-lymphocyte-dependent and can be transferred adoptively with lymphocytes. It closely parallels cutaneous-type delayed hypersensitivity in its development.

Tuberculin hypersensitivity Tuberculin hypersensitivity is antigen-specific in nature and follows primary infection. It is chiefly or perhaps entirely directed against protein antigens. It is mediated by T lymphocytes through secretion of lymphokines which act upon effector monocytes.

Mycobacterial antigens have been subjected to extensive immunochemical study. It is clear that there is no single dominant antigen, and that infected and artificially sensitized hosts develop hypersensitivity to an array of mycobacterial proteins. Tuberculin purified protein derivative (PPD), the antigen preparation most frequently employed clinically and epidemiologically to demonstrate tuberculin hypersensitivity, is a crude mixture of largely denatured antigens and is a poor representative of native antigens. Nevertheless, its use has yielded much information.

Antigen recognition by the sensitized host follows processing by macrophages and depends upon expression by the macrophage at its surface of antigen-specific epitopes in association with Ia antigen, a gene product of the major histocompatibility locus. This complex is recognized by specific T lymphocytes. Macrophage synthesis and secretion of interleukin 1 is also necessary for T-lymphocyte response to the presented antigen. Following antigen presentation, T-lymphocyte clonal expansion occurs. Specific subsets of T lymphocytes develop which have antigen-specific immunoregulatory functions and which modulate the immune response (see Chap. 13).

Immunoreactive lymphocytes secrete mediators, and in response macrophages become activated and serve as the principal effector cells of tuberculin hypersensitivity. Peripheral blood monocytes from tuberculous patients have been shown to have several features characteristic of activated macrophages, including increased hexose monophosphate shunt activity, augmented surface adhesiveness, expression of characteristic membrane structures, and increased bactericidal activity. Animal studies have demonstrated that these features are T-lymphocyte-dependent. Activated monocytes/macrophages are important immunoregulatory cells possessing suppressor functions.

In tuberculosis, aberrations of this carefully modulated state of hypersensitivity occur with some frequency and are recognizable in 15 percent of acutely ill patients. This has given rise to the suggestion that tuberculosis may present with an immunologic spectrum similar to that seen in leprosy but more subtly expressed. At one pole are patients with chronic cavitary disease, relatively chronic courses, and florid expression of tuberculin hypersensitivity. At the other pole are the less frequently seen patients with cutaneous anergy, a few of whom have absence of granuloma formation and all other manifestations of cellular hypersensitivity and have pancytopenia, widely disseminated disease, and a progressive downhill course. Although the delayed tuberculin skin reaction is the best known manifestation of tuberculin hypersensitivity (see below), granuloma formation is probably its central and most important expression because it is important in containing the spread of infection.

Production of antibodies to protein and polysaccharide antigens of mycobacteria is readily demonstrated in tuberculosis. There is no evidence that these antibodies play a role in immunity, hypersensitivity, or pathogenesis of tuberculosis.

CLINICAL MANIFESTATIONS **Primary tuberculosis** Primary tuberculous infection is usually asymptomatic. A nonspecific pneumonitis typically occurs in the lower or midlung zones. Hilar lymph node enlargement is usual and in children is sometimes sufficient to produce bronchial obstruction. In low-prevalence areas primary infection may not occur until adulthood. It may progress directly to clinical disease which has the pathologic features of reactivation disease. In these persons such perplexing presentations as subapical pneumonias are common.

Reactivation tuberculosis Reactivation tuberculosis is a chronic wasting disease, and in pulmonary tuberculosis constitutional manifestations are often more prominent than respiratory symptoms. Weight loss and low-grade fever are common. Many patients present with typical drenching night sweats over the upper half of the body several times a week.

Pulmonary tuberculosis Pulmonary tuberculosis has a predilection for the apical posterior segments of the upper lobes and the superior segments of the lower lobes of the lungs. The location has been attributed both to posture and to higher intraalveolar oxygen concentration in the uppermost portions of the lung. The extent of disease varies from minimal infiltrates that produce no clinical illness and that are barely discernible on chest radiographs to massive involvement with extensive cavitation and debilitating constitutional and respiratory symptoms. In the absence of effective therapy, pulmonary tuberculosis pursues a chronic and progressive course. There are often long periods of stability and relative well-being, but in most patients these give way to episodes of disease progression with involvement of increasing lung parenchyma.

The onset of pulmonary tuberculosis is usually insidious, and illness may not be noted by the patient for some time. However, it is incorrect to view this onset as one of slow progression. In fact, pulmonary tuberculosis usually reaches its full extent within a few weeks. About one-third of patients will live long lives with chronic illness interspersed with periods of relative well-being. However, the overall death rate of untreated pulmonary tuberculosis probably approaches 60 percent, and the median course to death is about $2\frac{1}{2}$ years.

As pulmonary lesions progress, central necrosis occurs with development of caseation, so named because of the cheesy nature of necrotic material which only partly liquifies. Satellite lesions grow concomitantly. They can usually be recognized on chest x-ray films and are often helpful in distinguishing tuberculosis from pulmonary neoplasms. Necrotic material may empty into bronchi resulting in cavitation of the nodular disease. Other parts of the lung may be seeded transbronchially with the development of exudative lesions. In some patients tuberculous pneumonia develops in a lobar or segmental pulmonary distribution. Occasionally transbronchial spread following rupture of a tuberculous peribronchial lymph node into a bronchus leads to tuberculous pneumonia in the absence of other obvious disease. With the progression of pulmonary tuberculosis, the normal pulmonary architecture is lost. Fibrosis, volume loss, and upward contraction are typical. However, recently diseased areas may heal with relatively little destruction when effective chemotherapy is administered.

Pulmonary cavities may persist even though effective chemotherapy has resulted in apparent cure. In the absence of therapy, persistence of cavities is to be expected. Cavities may be a source of major hemoptysis, especially in the presence of continued active disease. Persistent terminal pulmonary arteries within cavities may be a source of profound bleeding (Rasmussen's aneurysm). Another cause of bleeding is an aspergilloma in a chronic tuberculous cavity, and bleeding in this instance may occur without persisting tuberculous disease. Rupture of a tuberculous cavity into the pleural space may lead to tuberculous empyema and bronchopleural fistula.

Chronic cough is the principal respiratory symptom. Sputum is usually scant and nonpurulent. Hemoptysis is frequent and is usually limited to blood streaking of the sputum. Massive, life-threatening hemoptysis is rare.

Findings on physical examination of the lung in patients with pulmonary tuberculosis are typically few and generally can be appreciated only in the presence of extensive disease. Rales which are accentuated or heard only posttussively are characteristic of apical disease. With extensive cavitation, amphoric breath sounds may be present. Dullness to percussion may sometimes be recognized in Krönig's isthmus and at the clavicles, reflecting extensive apical disease.

Extrapulmonary tuberculosis PLEURISY WITH EFFUSION Pleurisy with effusion results when the pleural space is seeded with *M. tuberculosis*. Following a peripheral primary infection, the pleural space may be contaminated by organisms that are transported lymphogenously to the pleura and hence across the surface of the lung to the hilum. Pleural effusion occurs, sometimes massively, usually with substantial pleuritic pain. The onset of symptoms is often abrupt. The effusion is most frequently, but not invariably, unilateral. Classically, tuberculous pleurisy with effusion occurs in younger individuals in the absence of pulmonary tuberculosis. However, in the United States this disease presents in many individuals past the age of 35 and simultaneous pulmonary tuberculosis is present in about one-third of patients. The effusion is exudative in nature, and a protein concentration greater than 3.0 g/dL is the most characteristic feature of the pleural fluid. Lymphocytes usually, but not invariably, predominate among the pleural fluid cells. Mesothelial cells are rare. Needle biopsy of the parietal pleura may reveal granulomas, confirming the diagnosis of tuberculous pleurisy. The tuberculin skin test is negative in one-third of patients, either because the disease presents early before tuberculin reactivity develops, or because this form of tuberculosis is particularly prone to aberrations of immunoregulation. Untreated, tuberculous pleurisy usually remits, but active pulmonary tuberculosis develops within 5 years in two-thirds of cases. Response to chemotherapy is good. Complete removal of pleural fluid is not necessary. There is rarely a need for surgical decortication.

Bronchopleural fistula and tuberculous empyema are catastrophic complications of untreated tuberculosis resulting from rupture of a pulmonary lesion into the pleural space. The diagnosis is usually not difficult, and acid-fast bacilli are usually readily demonstrated in the pleural exudate. Treatment consists of adequate surgical drainage and chemotherapy.

TUBERCULOUS PERICARDITIS AND PERITONITIS The pericardium and peritoneum may be the sites of tuberculosis. Pericarditis sometimes occurs in association with pleurisy and may represent an extension of that process. More commonly the pericardium is seeded by drainage from an infected lymph node. Exudative effusion occurs and patients present with fever and pericardial pain. A friction rub may be present. Cardiac tamponade occasionally occurs. Chronic constrictive pericarditis is a late sequel. The diagnosis of tuberculous pericarditis is often difficult and sometimes requires thoracotomy for pericardial biopsy.

Tuberculous peritonitis results from hematogenous seeding of the peritoneum or entry of bacilli from an abdominal lymphatic or genitourinary organ source. As with other serositis, an exudative effusion occurs. The onset is usually insidious, and the disease is often mistaken for hepatic cirrhosis in alcoholic patients. As with tuberculous pericarditis, the diagnosis is often difficult, and recovery of the organism from paracentesis fluid is possible only in a minority of cases. Surgical biopsy may be necessary for diagnosis.

LARYNGEAL AND ENDOBRONCHIAL TUBERCULOSIS Tuberculosis of the larynx is usually seen in association with far-advanced pulmonary disease. Occasionally it occurs with only minimal pulmonary involvement. It results from seeding of the mucosal surface during expectoration. The disease progresses from a superficial laryngitis to ulceration and granuloma formation. The epiglottis and hypopharynx are occasionally involved. Hoarseness is the principal symptom of tuberculous laryngitis. In a similar fashion the bronchial mucosa may be seeded, causing tuberculous bronchitis. Indeed, localized bronchitis in segmental bronchi leading to diseased portions of lung is common. Cough and minor hemoptysis are the chief clinical manifestations. Patients with tuberculous laryngitis and extensive bronchitis are usually highly infectious. These forms of disease respond rapidly to chemotherapy and have a favorable prognosis with treatment.

TUBERCULOUS ADENITIS Scrofula is chronic tuberculous lymphadenitis of the cervical lymph nodes. Any of the cervical nodes may be involved, but those high in the neck just below the mandible are the most frequent site of disease. Tuberculous nodes are usually rubbery and not tender. With progression, they become harder and matted. Chronic draining fistulas may develop, but these are rare, and the course of this form of tuberculosis is usually indolent. The diagnosis is commonly established by surgical biopsy. Lymph node biopsy specimens obtained for this purpose should always be submitted for culture as well as histologic examination, and chemotherapy should be instituted at or before the time of surgery to avoid postoperative fistulas in the surgical wound site. Lymph nodes other than those in the cervical regions are less commonly involved in tuberculosis and account for about 35 percent of tuberculous adenitis.

In children, *M. scrofulaceum* and *M. intracellulare* are frequently the cause of scrofula. The onset of this disease is usually before 5 years of age. As with tuberculosis, lymph nodes high in the neck are most frequently involved. A single enlarged node is commonly the presenting manifestation. Constitutional symptoms are absent, and the adenitis usually is not tender. Progression is common, with necrosis of the node and the development of fistulous sinus tracts. The organisms involved are usually not susceptible to drugs, and treatment, if necessary, is surgical excision. Spontaneous resolution is usual after puberty.

SKELETAL TUBERCULOSIS Bone and joint disease is a not infrequent manifestation of tuberculosis. Pott's disease, tuberculosis of the spine, usually involves the midthoracic spine. Tubercle bacilli reach the spine hematogenously or through lymphatic channels from the pleural space to paravertebral lymph nodes. Anterior erosion of vertebral bodies leads to collapse. The result is a sharply angulated kyphosis without scoliosis (gibbus deformity). Paraplegia may result. If there is no neurologic compromise, Pott's disease can be treated with chemotherapy. If the spine is unstable, surgical stabilization may be necessary. In the face of new paraparesis, immediate orthopedic consultation should be obtained. Paravertebral "cold abcesses" are a frequent concomitant of tuberculous spondylitis. They usually do not need to be drained, if adequate chemotherapy is given, unless they are very large. They may extend along fascial planes and point in the inguinal region or in other remote sites.

Tuberculosis of joints most frequently affects large weight-bearing joints such as the hips and knees. It responds well to immobilization and chemotherapy. Tuberculous synovitis may occur alone or in association with tuberculous arthritis.

GENITOURINARY TUBERCULOSIS Genitourinary tuberculosis may involve any part of either the male or female genitourinary system. Renal tuberculosis usually presents initially as microscopic pyuria and hematuria with a sterile urine culture. The diagnosis may be established by finding tubercle bacilli on culture of the urine. As the disease progresses, cavitation of the renal parenchyma occurs. In the past, nephrectomy was often performed for renal tuberculosis. However, with adequate chemotherapy surgical removal of a kidney is almost never necessary. The ureters and bladder may be infected by tubular spread of the organism, and ureteral stricture may result.

Tuberculous salpingitis often results in female sterility. Genital tuberculosis in the male most commonly involves the prostate, seminal vesicles, and epididymis. Prostatic and epididymal tuberculosis are characterized by nontender nodular induration detectable by physical examination. The presentation of genital tuberculosis in both males and females is insidious, with chronic or subacute symptoms. The diagnosis is usually made by culture of acid-fast bacilli.

MENINGEAL TUBERCULOSIS The leptomeninges are relatively frequently seeded by organisms which disseminate during primary infection. In young children, tuberculous meningitis may develop at this time. This chronic infection is manifested not only by meningeal signs but also frequently by cranial nerve signs, reflecting a tendency for basilar distribution of the infection. High protein content, low glucose, and lymphocytosis are characteristic of the cerebrospinal fluid. Prior to the advent of effective chemotherapy, this disease was almost always fatal. Chemotherapy with isoniazid, rifampin, and ethambutol is effective. Intrathecal drug administration is not necessary. Late reactivation of meningeal tuberculous foci may produce disease in adults who have no evidence of pulmonary tuberculosis. Tuberculomas of the meninges or brain may become evident in adult life many years after primary infection, and seizures are often their major clinical manifestation.

OCULAR TUBERCULOSIS Tuberculosis may involve almost any part of the eye. Chorioretinitis and uveitis are the most common manifestations. The diagnosis of tuberculosis of the eye is extremely difficult to establish, and most diagnoses are presumptive. The manifestations cannot be distinguished clinically from sarcoidosis or systemic mycoses, but phlyctenular keratitis strongly suggests tuberculosis. Phlyctenular lesions are thought to represent manifestations of tuberculin hypersensitivity rather than bacterial infection. Choroid tubercles are often present in patients with miliary tuberculosis, and their recognition may be helpful in the diagnosis of miliary tuberculosis. Ocular tuberculosis responds well to standard chemotherapeutic agents.

GASTROINTESTINAL TUBERCULOSIS The stomach is extremely resistant to tuberculous infection, and a large number of virulent tubercle bacilli can be swallowed without establishing an infection. Rarely, usually concomitantly with extensive cavitary pulmonary disease and severe debility, swallowed organisms reach the terminal ileum and cecum and tuberculous ileitis develops. Chronic diarrhea and fistula development are the principal manifestations, and the disease is difficult to distinguish from Crohn's disease. Tuberculosis of the liver can occur as an isolated event, but it is usually a manifestation of miliary tuberculosis.

ADRENAL TUBERCULOSIS Hematogenous seeding of the adrenal gland is probably fairly common, but disease due to this infection is rare and usually seen only in association with long-standing and extensive pulmonary tuberculosis. The cortex is most frequently involved and adrenal insufficiency may result. In contrast, carcinomatous involvement of the adrenal cortex, even though very extensive, rarely produces clinical adrenal insufficiency.

CUTANEOUS TUBERCULOSIS Tuberculous infection of the skin is rare in the absence of long-standing, untreated disease elsewhere. Lupus vulgaris is a granulomatous disease of the skin, and it responds well to treatment. Diagnosis is made by skin biopsy. Tuberculin hypersensitivity manifestations are common. Erythema nodosum may be present, although it much more commonly results from other granulomatous diseases including sarcoidosis and systemic mycoses. Tuberculids are poorly understood papular lesions of tuberculin hypersensitivity.

MILIARY TUBERCULOSIS Miliary tuberculosis results from widespread hematogenous dissemination. It often presents as a perplexing fever, sometimes with a double quotidian curve, often accompanied by anemia and splenomegaly. Miliary tuberculosis is apt to be more fulminating in children than in adults.

Classically, miliary tuberculosis develops following hematogenous dissemination at the time of primary infection, and patients present no antecedent history of tuberculosis. Lesions develop synchronously throughout the body. Patients become ill before radiographic changes, which take 4 to 6 weeks to become recognizable, appear. The typical radiologic findings are soft, uniformly distributed, fine nodules throughout both lung fields. They often can be recognized first on a lateral chest film or an underpenetrated anteroposterior radiograph. The diagnosis is difficult, and expectorated sputum rarely contains organisms. Transbronchial biopsy and liver biopsy are usually but

not invariably positive. Bone marrow biopsy is positive in approximately two-thirds of patients.

When hematogenous dissemination occurs in a previously diseased individual, a much more fulminant course results. Prostration is common. Diffuse but ragged nodular infiltrates develop within a few weeks, and the sputum is often positive. The diagnosis is rarely difficult.

The subacute form and the rare chronic form of miliary tuberculosis often present major problems in diagnosis. This type of disease is usually attributed to repeated seeding of the blood stream from a tuberculous focus. A very rare form of disseminated tuberculosis occurs with widespread dissemination of disease, a massive number of bacteria in tissues, complete absence of granuloma formation, and pancytopenia. It is termed disseminated nonreactive tuberculosis and has a poor prognosis, even with chemotherapy.

Tuberculin anergy is common in miliary tuberculosis, and a negative skin test should not be a deterrent to considering this diagnosis. Anergy may or may not extend to other delayed hypersensitivity antigens. In vitro cultured leukocyte studies also demonstrate hyporesponsiveness, suggesting that this anergy is mediated by monocytes with suppressor function. With treatment and stabilization of patients with miliary tuberculosis, tuberculin hypersensitivity is restored.

Without treatment, the prognosis for miliary tuberculosis is grave. This disease responds well to chemotherapy, however, and can be treated with the same drug regimens employed for other forms of tuberculosis.

SILICOTUBERCULOSIS Tuberculosis occurs with increased frequency in patients with silicosis and possibly in patients with some other pneumoconioses. The diagnosis is often difficult because of confounding radiographic changes due to the underlying pneumoconiosis. Even with therapy, the prognosis is less favorable than in other patients. Patients with silicotuberculosis should be treated for longer than customary periods. Patients with silicosis who are tuberculin-positive should be considered for isoniazid prophylaxis even when they do not meet other criteria for this form of therapy. Isoniazid prophylaxis may be less effective in persons with silicosis.

TUBERCULOSIS IN AIDS Tuberculosis occurs in more than 50 percent of individuals previously infected with M. tuberculosis who subsequently become infected with HIV. It usually precedes the development of other opportunistic infections associated with AIDS by about 3 months. In central Africa and Haiti, 30 to 50 percent of tuberculosis patients are HIV seropositive; only about one-third of these patients have other opportunistic infections associated with AIDS. In the United States, tuberculosis is most frequently seen in AIDS patients who are intravenous drug users or who are immigrants from Haiti or central Africa. Nearly half of AIDS patients with tuberculosis have extrapulmonary forms of the disease, with tuberculous lymphadenitis predominating. Among AIDS patients with pulmonary tuberculosis, nearly half have atypical roentgenographic findings, with diffuse infiltration. Mycobacterial infections other than tuberculosis are frequently seen in patients with AIDS. In the United States approximately half of AIDS patients develop disseminated disease due to M. avium-intracellulare, usually late in the course of AIDS (see Chap. 127).

DIAGNOSIS Bacteriology The diagnosis of tuberculosis is established when tubercle bacilli are identified in the sputum, urine, body fluids, or tissues of the patient. For the majority of patients who have pulmonary tuberculosis, the diagnosis can be most readily established by sputum examination. The staining characteristics of M. tuberculosis allow its ready identification in clinical specimens, although it is usually present in small numbers so that prolonged study of stained slides is necessary. A slender (less than 0.5 μm diameter), curved, often polychromatically beaded rod, it frequently presents in clinical specimens as pairs or clumps of a few organisms lying side by side. When stained with fluorescent auramine-rhodamine, tubercle bacilli can be seen under usual high-dry (100×) magnification. A more definitive stain consists of carbol fuchsin; this stain requires meticulous scanning with oil immersion (1000×) microscopy. Sputum culture adds to the diagnostic yield and also permits the specific identification of acid-fast bacilli and the determination of drug susceptibility. Primary isolation from clinical specimens usually requires 4 to 8 weeks on classical media. Radiometric techniques using highly selective media allow cultivation in 1 or 2 weeks, but confirmation of the identity of an isolated organism may require additional time. Mycobacteria are aerobes. Modern culture techniques are excellent, and there is no longer reason to inoculate guinea pigs for primary isolation. Niacin production characterizes *M. tuberculosis* and helps to distinguish it from other species. Nucleic acid hybridization probes have been developed for the rapid identification of mycobacteria in cultures. Probes for direct use with clinical specimens are under investigation.

If expectorated sputum is not readily available for examination, expectoration may be induced or samples obtained by nasotracheal aspiration. Early morning gastric aspiration provides excellent material for culture and for smear examination. Although nonpathogenic mycobacteria are occasionally found in gastric aspirates, their number is so small as to preclude their appearance in smears of gastric aspirates. Bronchoscopy has a high yield in the diagnosis of tuberculosis, but in the absence of other considerations it should not be undertaken unless multiple attempts by simpler means have failed and the diagnosis remains obscure.

The diagnostic yield of sputum smear and culture is directly related to the extent of pulmonary disease. About one-third of patients in whom a positive sputum culture can be obtained will have acid-fast bacilli identified on an initial sputum smear. With repeated examinations on separate days, this figure rises to about two-thirds. There is rarely an indication for obtaining more than five sputum examinations. However, only about one-third of patients with minimal pulmonary tuberculosis will have a positive sputum smear, even after multiple examinations. If there is no lesion visible on the chest radiograph, then there is usually little reason to obtain sputum examinations for tubercle bacilli. Conversely, if a patient with extensive cavitary disease or an exudative pneumonic process has a negative sputum smear, diagnoses other than tuberculosis should be sought.

Serology   Serologic tests for the diagnosis of tuberculosis remain experimental and are not routinely available. The most specific serologic tests have used highly purified antigens. Enzyme-linked immunosorbent assay (ELISA) techniques offer the potential for readily applied serologic tests for tuberculosis, and should have great value in the diagnosis of tuberculosis in children and in extrapulmonary disease where sputum is not available.

Radiology   The chest x-ray is an important tool for both the diagnosis and evaluation of tuberculosis. Healed primary lesions may leave a small peripheral nodule which may calcify with the passing of years. The Ghon complex comprises a calcified peripheral nodule together with a calcified hilar lymph node. Similar lesions result from histoplasmosis, and it is not possible to distinguish between healed primary lesions of these two diseases radiologically. Calcification of right paratracheal lymph nodes is more commonly seen in histoplasmosis.

Multinodular infiltration in the apical posterior segments of the upper lobes and superior segments of the lower lobes is the most typical lesion of pulmonary tuberculosis. Cavitation is frequently present and is usually accompanied by substantial amounts of infiltration in the same pulmonary segments. Laminagrams are often helpful in recognizing satellite nodular lesions, which are characteristic of tuberculosis and not usually seen in carcinoma. Lordotic views may be of help in evaluating disease obscured by the intersection of the third or fourth posterior rib, second anterior rib, and clavicle. They are of little use in evaluating disease located elsewhere. As tuberculosis becomes inactive or heals, fibrotic scarring becomes apparent on the chest radiograph. There is frequently volume loss in the involved upper lobes, and upward and medial retraction of hilar markings is common. Fibrotic lesions may develop calcifications.

The activity of tuberculosis may be judged from serial films. It is never wise to judge tuberculosis to be inactive on the basis of a single chest film.

Clinical pathology   Other than bacteriologic examinations, clinical laboratory tests contribute relatively little to the diagnosis of tuberculosis. Peripheral blood monocytosis in the range of 8 to 12 percent is common. The erythrocyte sedimentation rate is usually elevated, and modest anemia may be present.

Tuberculin test   The intracutaneous tuberculin skin test is a reliable means of recognizing prior mycobacterial infection. The preferred antigen is tuberculin purified protein derivative (PPD) and the intermediate-strength dose should be used. In North America this is 5 tuberculin units of material which is standardized by bioassay (bioequivalent) against reference antigen designated PPD-S. In other parts of the world, PPD lot RT-23, prepared in Denmark and widely distributed by the World Health Organization, is available. A gravimetric unit has been assigned to this material, and 2 units of this PPD are equivalent to 5 units of PPD-S. Diluents for PPD should contain polysorbate 80, which decreases loss of potency due to adsorption onto glass and plastic surfaces. Multiple puncture devices offer much convenience, but do so at the cost of decreased specificity. They can be recommended only as screening tests, and positive tests should be repeated using intracutaneous PPD.

The tuberculin test is usually applied on the forearm. Reactions should be read by measuring the transverse diameter of induration as detected by gentle palpation at 48 to 72 h. Patients with tuberculosis have normally distributed reaction sizes with the mean and mode at 17 mm. Infected but healthy, nondiseased individuals have similarly distributed reactions. Hence, a reaction to PPD is presumptive evidence of prior mycobacterial infection.

Tuberculin hypersensitivity may result from contact with nonpathogenic, environmental mycobacteria, and this nonspecific reactivity may confound the interpretation of tuberculin tests. Nonspecific tuberculin reactivity is rarely found in northern climates, and in such areas all reactivity to PPD can be considered to reflect infection with *M. tuberculosis*. In many warm and humid climatic zones, including all of the coastal areas of the southeastern United States, nonspecific tuberculin reactivity is common. In such regions it is customary to consider reactions smaller than 10 mm as not significant and attribute them to cross reactivity with environmental mycobacterial antigens. However, considering smaller reactions as not significant always incurs the risk of missing some reactions which bespeak infection with *M. tuberculosis*.

Repeated skin testing may boost reaction size, whether the primary reactivity was directed to *M. tuberculosis* or was nonspecific. Caution must be used in attributing a small increase in reactivity to new infection. It is well-established, however, that repeated skin testing with PPD does not lead to positive reactions in uninfected persons. Positive reactions do not occur as a result of allergy to components of the diluent. Tuberculin reactivity wanes with advancing age, and the booster phenomenon may be useful in this situation. For example, if an older person fails to react to initial testing, repeat testing with intermediate strength PPD may be done after 7 to 10 days. A reaction at this time should be accepted as significant.

PPD is also available in a second strength which contains 50 times the amount of PPD in intermediate-strength material. Except as a test for anergy, this product has little use. Because PPD at this strength so readily elicits nonspecific reactivity, a positive reaction to second-strength PPD is much more apt to give misinformation than to contribute to the correct diagnosis. A first-strength PPD is also available. It contains one-fifth the amount of PPD of intermediate PPD but is not useful clinically.

Anergy is the paradoxical absence of dermal tuberculin reactivity in infected persons. It occurs in association with a number of disease states and in immunosuppressed individuals. It also occurs in as many as 15 percent of tuberculous patients with newly active pulmonary disease. In these persons tuberculin reactivity reappears with stabilization of the disease process. One-half of patients with miliary tuberculosis and one-third of patients with newly diagnosed tuberculous pleurisy have negative tuberculin tests. It has become common practice in many medical centers to use a battery of delayed hypersensitivity antigens to serve as controls for tuberculin tests in demonstrating anergy. However, antigens standardized for this purpose are not available, and tuberculin anergy may be antigen-specific. False-negative tuberculin tests may result from technical errors including subcutaneous injection, use of outdated PPD, and permitting PPD to remain in syringes before use. Such errors should not be mistaken for anergy.

TREATMENT The modern treatment of tuberculosis is based on the administration of effective drugs. In the presence of adequate chemotherapy, hospitalization, rest, and improved diet do not contribute to achieving cures. In order to prevent the emergence of drug-resistant mutants which are present initially in very small numbers, two effective drugs are always required. Because of the slow generation time of mycobacteria and their long periods of metabolic inactivity, prolonged courses of drug therapy are always necessary. Treatment regimens do not differ for pulmonary and extrapulmonary tuberculosis.

Table 125-1 presents dosage and toxicity information on drugs currently in use for the treatment of tuberculosis. Table 125-2 describes several effective treatment regimens. Daily therapy with isoniazid and rifampin for 9 to 12 months represents the most effective regimen available and is capable of achieving a favorable outcome in 99 percent of patients. Many experts add ethambutol initially until the results of sensitivity tests become available. Daily therapy with isoniazid and ethambutol for 18 months is 90 to 95 percent effective, and is probably equal to isoniazid and rifampin in patients with minimal disease. In developing countries where drug costs are a limiting factor, the extremely low-cost combination of isoniazid and thioacetazone for 12 to 18 months provides a regimen which can achieve 80 to 90 percent cure rates.

An accepted hypothesis states that tubercle bacilli exist in tuberculous patients in three pools—a metabolically active extracellular pool and relatively metabolically inactive intracellular and necrotic caseum pools. Only rifampin is bactericidal for all of these pools, and it may not be necessary to continue rifampin-containing regimens for as long as other regimens which rely upon organisms entering the metabolically active pool to achieve sterilization. Isoniazid and streptomycin are both bactericidal against extracellular, metabolically

TABLE 125-2 Effective drug regimens for the treatment of tuberculosis

Regimen (adult drug dose)	Comment
Isoniazid (300 mg) and rifampin (600 mg) daily for 9–12 months	The usual regimen for initial treatment of all patients unless drug resistance is suspected, in which case ethambutol 15 mg/kg should be added.
Isoniazid (300 mg) and ethambutol (15 mg/kg) daily for 12–18 months	The least toxic effective regimen. Suitable for patients with minimal disease. The regimen of choice in pregnant women.
Isoniazid (300 mg) and thioacetazone (150 mg) daily for 12–18 months	The least expensive effective regimen. Streptomycin (0.75–1 g) may be added daily for the first 8 weeks to increase effectiveness, but this doubles both cost and toxicity.
Isoniazid (300 mg), rifampin (600 mg), pyrazinamide (2 g), and streptomycin (1 g) or ethambutol (15 mg/kg) daily for 2 months followed by one of the following:	Initial intensive phase for short course regimens. Short course regimens have only been demonstrated to be effective under conditions of close patient supervision.
a Isoniazid (300 mg) and rifampin (600 gm) daily for 4 months	
b Isoniazid (300 mg) and thioacetazone (150 mg) daily for 6 months	Inexpensive.
c Isoniazid (300 mg), rifampin (600 mg), and streptomycin (1 g) twice weekly for 6 months	Suitable for fully supervised therapy.
Isoniazid (300 mg) and rifampin (600 mg) daily for 1 month followed by isoniazid (900 mg) and rifampin (600 mg) twice weekly for 8 months	Effectiveness demonstrated in ambulatory treatment programs in Arkansas. Has not been compared with other regimens in clinical trials.

active organisms. Against intracellular organisms, isoniazid and pyrazinamide are bactericidal and streptomycin is inactive. In clinical trials, pyrazinamide has been found to be particularly useful during the first 2 months of treatment. Ethambutol is only bacteriostatic.

The major problem in tuberculosis treatment programs is patient default. It is unusual for a tuberculosis clinic to achieve a default rate of less than 15 percent, and default rates of 40 to 60 percent are common. Unfortunately, these rates tend to be highest in those parts of the world where high tuberculosis prevalence is coupled with limited resources. Default not only leads to treatment failure but also to the emergence and transmission of drug-resistant organisms. Since most patient defaults occur within the first 6 months of the treatment program, short-course therapy has been employed to mitigate the consequences of default. This strategy will be successful only if the resources conserved by shortening treatment are used to maintain patient compliance. Completely supervised regimens are successful for noncompliant patients, but their widespread use is costly. Twice weekly drug administration is effective and facilitates patient supervision.

Short-course treatment programs are best considered as consisting of two phases. An initial 2-month intensive phase of daily therapy should include isoniazid, rifampin, pyrazinamide, and either streptomycin or ethambutol. A consolidation phase of daily therapy with isoniazid and one other drug should be given for at least 4 months, and preferably 6 months. In the United States, a regimen of isoniazid 300 mg and rifampin 600 mg daily for 1 month, followed by isoniazid 900 mg and rifampin 600 mg twice weekly for 8 months has been highly effective. Patients with AIDS should be treated in the same manner as immunocompetent individuals with tuberculosis. Response to therapy is favorable in these patients, although they have more frequent drug reactions, particularly skin rashes. The optimum duration of therapy for these patients is not known, although it is

TABLE 125-1 Drugs used in the treatment of tuberculosis

Drug	Usual daily adult dose	Major toxicity
Isoniazid	300 mg	Hepatitis, peripheral neuropathy, drug fever
Rifampin	600 mg	Hepatitis, influenza-like syndrome, thrombocytopenia (rare)
Streptomycin	0.75–1 g	Deafness, loss of vestibular function, loss of renal function
Pyrazinamide	1.5–2 g	Hepatitis, hyperuricemia
Ethambutol	15 mg/kg	Optic neuritis (extremely rare at this dose)
p-Aminosalicylic acid	12 g	Diarrhea, hepatitis, hypersensitivity reactions
Ethionamide	1 g	Hepatitis
Cycloserine	1 g	Depression, personality changes, psychosis, convulsions
Thioacetazone	150 mg	Exfoliative dermatitis, hepatitis
Kanamycin	1 g	Deafness, loss of renal function, loss of vestibular function (rare)
Capreomycin	1 g	Deafness, loss of vestibular function, loss of renal function
Viomycin	1 g	Deafness, loss of vestibular function, loss of renal function

probably wise to avoid short-course regimens. AIDS patients should be followed for relapse after therapy for the rest of their lives.

Relapses after successful therapy should be less than 1 percent. Since these few relapses usually present with symptoms and are almost never found by routine x-rays, patients may be discharged from follow-up at the completion of therapy. Relapses are more frequent after short-course therapy, usually occurring within the first year, and follow-up for such patients for 1 or 2 years is justified.

Symptomatic improvement occurs within the first 2 to 3 weeks in most patients. Clearing of infiltrates on the chest radiograph may not occur within the first month but usually is readily recognized between the second and fourth months. Most patients reach a point of radiologic stability between 3 and 6 months. Therapy should be continued for 6 months after this point of stability is reached, even if this means prolonging the planned period of treatment. Sputum conversion occurs in most patients within the first 2 months. The fact that an individual patient responds more slowly than the norm should not necessarily be a cause for concern, provided the patient is taking effective drugs.

Since there are alternative effective drug regimens, toxicity becomes a factor in choice of therapy. Major individual drug toxicities are listed in Table 125-1; the toxicity of greatest concern is hepatitis. Toxicity sufficient to require change in regimen occurs in 3 to 5 percent of patients taking isoniazid and rifampin and in about 1.5 percent of patients taking isoniazid and ethambutol. The toxicity of isoniazid and thioacetazone appears to vary with the racial characteristics of the patient population. It reaches about 30 percent in oriental groups but is only 2 to 5 percent in other populations. Routine monitoring of serum enzymes or other blood tests reflecting liver disease is of little use and is not recommended. Normal values do not predict absence of toxicity, and serum enzymes in patients taking isoniazid may rise transiently to three times normal values without the subsequent development of hepatitis. A well-educated patient and an alert treatment supervisor are the principal safeguards against drug hepatitis. If medication is discontinued during the prodromal phase or promptly with the onset of jaundice, drug hepatitis can be expected to resolve without untoward incident. Isoniazid toxicity is probably due to toxic metabolites of acetyl isoniazid. Induction of cytochrome P_{450} enzymes by alcohol or long-acting barbiturates predisposes to isoniazid hepatitis. Isoniazid also causes a peripheral neuropathy which is preventable and reversible by the administration of pyridoxine. Patients with such predisposing factors as old age, diabetes, alcoholism, and malnutrition should be given pyridoxine concomitantly with isoniazid; the usual dose is 50 mg/d.

Isoniazid is safe in pregnant patients. Data are less complete for other drugs but suggest that ethambutol is the companion drug of choice. Rifampin should be used if the tuberculosis is disseminated or very extensive. Streptomycin should not be used in pregnancy because of the risk of fetal ototoxicity. Tuberculosis often pursues an unfavorable course during and just after pregnancy, and treatment of a pregnant woman should never be deferred. It is reasonable, however, to postpone isoniazid prophylaxis until just after delivery.

Patients with chronic renal failure also present special treatment problems, and these patients have tuberculosis case rates approximately 10 times those of the general population. Isoniazid is acetylated to an inactive form by the liver and then excreted by the kidney. Acetyl isoniazid is the precursor of hydrazines, which are probably hepatotoxic. Both isoniazid and acetyl isoniazid are not bound by plasma proteins and are dialyzable. In patients with renal failure isoniazid should be reduced to 5 mg/kg body weight (300 mg in adults) two or three times weekly. Patients on dialysis should receive the drug following each dialysis. Ethambutol behaves like isoniazid, except that it is excreted by the kidney as the active drug. As with isoniazid, the usual daily dose should be given at longer intervals, and administration should follow dialysis. Optic nerve toxicity of ethambutol appears to be related not to intermittent high drug levels but to sustained high drug levels. Patients with renal failure who are receiving ethambutol should have their color vision and visual acuity monitored regularly. Rifampin is protein-bound, nondialyzable, and

excreted in the bile by the liver. No change in dose or interval is necessary in the presence of renal failure. Caution should be exercised in using rifampin in patients with hepatic failure.

Faced with relapse in a previously treated patient, a major concern should be the possibility of drug resistance, and resistance studies of the organism should be obtained in a competent reference laboratory. In one-third of patients who relapse after adequate regular drug therapy, the relapse is caused by drug-resistant organisms. If, however, the patient took the drug sporadically or the previous regimen was inadequate, then the likelihood of drug resistance is about two chances in three. Therapy for presumed drug-resistant tuberculosis should be instituted with two drugs which the patient has not taken previously, provided that one of these two new drugs is isoniazid or rifampin. Otherwise, four drugs should be used, including as many new drugs as possible. When resistance studies become available, the regimen should be modified appropriately. It is beneficial to continue isoniazid even when laboratory studies indicate drug resistance. In general, all re-treatment regimens should be closely supervised and directed by physicians with special experience with this problem.

Primary drug resistance should be suspected in patients who appear to have contracted their infection from patients with known drug resistance or with known noncompliance and in patients who come from areas where drug resistance is common. In the United States, this group includes immigrants from Haiti, southeast Asia, and many areas of Latin America. While laboratory resistance studies are pending, drug therapy should be dictated by the prior treatment of the suspected index case. In immigrant populations, most of the drug resistance of concern is to isoniazid. In this circumstance, therapy should be initiated with isoniazid, rifampin, and ethambutol. One of these drugs may be discontinued when resistance studies become available.

PREVENTION Chemoprophylaxis In one of the largest controlled clinical trials ever conducted, 1 year of isoniazid has been shown to be effective in reducing the incidence of tuberculosis in tuberculin-positive individuals presumed to have been infected with *M. tuberculosis*. The benefit of isoniazid prophylaxis has been demonstrated so clearly that the question of its use now hinges primarily on the risk of drug toxicity, chiefly hepatitis.

In administering isoniazid prophylaxis, highest priority should be assigned to treating household contacts of persons with active tuberculosis and to persons known to have become infected within the preceding year. The risks of developing tuberculosis in these two groups are, respectively, 0.5 percent per year and 3 percent during the first year. Particular attention should be given to treating children in these categories. Prophylaxis of childhood household contacts with isoniazid should be started immediately. After 3 months of therapy, the child should be skin-tested with intermediate-strength PPD. If the skin test is negative at that time, isoniazid may be discontinued. If it is positive, 12 months of prophylaxis should be completed.

Younger individuals benefit most from isoniazid prophylaxis because the drug is most effective when the infection is recent and because older individuals have often already outlived a substantial part of their risk. The risk of hepatitis rises with age, reaching approximately 2 percent by the seventh decade. Cost-benefit analyses with large data bases have shown that there is a 1:1 ratio of cases of tuberculosis prevented and hepatitis caused at age 45 when individuals without added risks are considered. Based on this calculation, there is a general consensus that all persons younger than age 35 with a positive tuberculin reaction should receive isoniazid 300 mg/d for 1 year.

It is also possible to develop criteria for the prophylactic use of isoniazid in older persons with remote tuberculosis, either known historically or evident radiographically, who have never received adequate chemotherapy. The annual risk of tuberculosis in such persons is at least 0.5 percent. Isoniazid 300 mg/d should be given for 1 year to all persons in this category who have a life expectancy greater than 10 years. In compliant adults with fibrotic residuals of untreated tuberculosis visible on roentgenograms, 1 year of isoniazid prophylaxis reduced disease during the subsequent 5 years by 93 percent, and 6 months of isoniazid reduced disease by 69 percent. Others at high risk for the development of tuberculosis include tuberculin-positive individuals with AIDS or Hodgkin's disease (both of which alter T-lymphocyte-mediated immunity), patients with silicosis (which affects macrophage function), and persons who are (1) receiving immunosuppressive agents or glucocorticoids chronically or (2) who suffer from renal failure. As with therapy for active tuberculosis, monitoring serum enzymes is not useful in patients receiving isoniazid prophylaxis.

BCG vaccination Bacillus Calmette-Guérin (BCG) is an attenuated strain of *M. bovis* which has been given to more than 2 billion persons as a vaccine against tuberculosis. It is clearly safe, but its efficacy is in some dispute. In some controlled studies it offered little or no protection. However, even then, the disseminated forms of tuberculosis which have such high mortalities among children were virtually eliminated. While final judgment on the efficacy of BCG must be reserved, its continued use in high-prevalence areas appears justified.

BCG vaccination induces tuberculin hypersensitivity. However, the dermal reaction to PPD is usually not as large as that which follows natural infection, usually does not persist as long, and varies from strain to strain of vaccine. Individuals with large PPD reactions persisting for many years after vaccination should be viewed as infected and considered for isoniazid prophylaxis.

CONTROL PROGRAMS In most low-prevalence areas, such as North America, resources are relatively abundant and disease occurrence is mostly sporadic. Increasingly, tuberculosis is being seen in microepidemics, often centered in family groups. Immigrant groups and residents and employees of nursing homes are at highest risk. Central to any program is an efficient case-reporting and registry system. Contact investigation must be carried out effectively and is especially important when index cases occur in children. The major modality for decreasing the spread of infection is chemotherapy for all infectious patients. Chemoprophylaxis is necessary for contacts.

At the other end of the spectrum are high-prevalence areas with few or no resources for tuberculosis control. The single, most effective measure in this setting is a network of ambulatory tuberculosis treatment centers that provide diagnosis by direct sputum smear and standardized drug therapy. Successful treatment must entail no cost to the patient. Tuberculosis diagnostic and treatment programs should be integrated into national health programs, under expert supervision. Treatment records should be maintained, but complex registries are of little value.

In high-prevalence areas, BCG vaccine should be offered to every individual under 15 or 20 without prior tuberculin testing. Older individuals can be assumed to have been infected already. Before a mass BCG campaign is initiated, planning should begin for continuing vaccination of newborns or young schoolchildren. Community-wide isoniazid prophylaxis programs have not been successful.

REFERENCES

AMERICAN THORACIC SOCIETY: Diagnostic standards and classification of tuberculosis and other mycobacterial diseases (14th ed). Am Rev Respir Dis 123:343, 1981

————: Treatment of tuberculosis and other mycobacterial diseases. Am Rev Respir Dis 128:336, 1983

CHAISSON RE et al: Tuberculosis in patients with the acquired immunodeficiency syndrome. Am Rev Respir Dis 136:570, 1987

COMSTOCK GW, EDWARDS PQ: The competing risks of tuberculosis and hepatitis for adult tuberculin reactors. Am Rev Respir Dis 111:573, 1975

———— et al: The tuberculin skin test. Am Rev Respir Dis 124:356, 1981

————: Epidemiology of tuberculosis. Am Rev Respir Dis 125(suppl):8, 1982

DUTT AK et al: Short-course chemotherapy for extrapulmonary tuberculosis. Ann Intern Med 104:7, 1986

EDWARDS LB et al: An atlas of sensitivity to tuberculin, PPD-B, and histoplasmin in the United States. Am Rev Respir Dis 99(suppl):1, 1969

FOX W: The chemotherapy of pulmonary tuberculosis: A review. Chest 76(suppl):785, 1979

GLASSROTH J et al: Tuberculosis in the 1980s. N Engl J Med 302:1441, 1980

GROSSET J: Bacteriologic basis of short-course chemotherapy for tuberculosis. Clin Chest Med 1:231, 1980

GRZYBOWSKI S, ENARSON DA: The fate of cases of pulmonary tuberculosis under various treatment programmes. Bull Int Union Tuberc 53:70, 1978

PITCHENIK AE et al: Human T-cell lymphotrophic virus-III (HTLV-III) seropositivity and related disease among 71 consecutive patients in whom tuberculosis was diagnosed. A prospective study. Am Rev Respir Dis 135:875, 1987

SELWYN PA et al: A prospective study of the risk of tuberculosis among intravenous users with human immunodeficiency virus infection. N Engl J Med 320:545, 1989

SNIDER DE, JR: The tuberculin skin test. Am Rev Respir Dis 125(suppl):108, 1982

STEAD WW et al: Tuberculosis as an endemic and nosocomial infection among the elderly in nursing homes. N Engl J Med 312:1483, 1985

TENDAM HG et al: Present knowledge of immunization against tuberculosis. Bull WHO 54:255, 1976

126 LEPROSY (HANSEN'S DISEASE)

RICHARD A. MILLER

DEFINITION Leprosy (Hansen's disease) is a chronic granulomatous infection of humans which attacks superficial tissues, especially the skin and peripheral nerves. The clinical and immunologic manifestations of disease form a continuum extending from polar *tuberculoid* leprosy to polar *lepromatous* leprosy. The borderline portion of the spectrum lies between these two extremes, and is usually subdivided into *borderline tuberculoid, borderline,* and *borderline lepromatous* classes. In addition, an early indeterminate form is seen, which may spontaneously remit or develop into overt leprosy.

ETIOLOGY *Mycobacterium leprae,* or Hansen's bacillus, is the causal agent of leprosy. It is an acid-fast rod assigned to the family Mycobacteriaceae on the basis of morphologic, biochemical, antigenic, and genetic similarities to other mycobacteria. Although it has not been cultivated in artificial media or tissue culture, it can be consistently propagated in the foot pads of mice. The bacillus multiplies exceedingly slowly, with an estimated optimal doubling time of 11 to 13 days during logarithmic growth in mouse foot pads. The mouse model has been used extensively for the study of antileprosy drugs, and the high bacterial yield from armadillos has been crucial for immunologic studies.

Lepromin is a suspension of killed *M. leprae* prepared from heavily infected human or armadillo tissue. Intradermal injection elicits, somewhat variably, a tuberculin-like reaction at 48 h (Fernandez's reaction) and more consistently, a papular reaction at 3 to 4 weeks (Mitsuda's reaction). The Mitsuda reaction is usually positive in tuberculoid patients and is always negative in lepromatous patients. However, because it is also positive in nearly all normal adults, even those residing in areas free of endemic leprosy, it has no diagnostic value. Lepromin is not commercially available.

EPIDEMIOLOGY There are probably 10 to 20 million persons affected with leprosy in the world. The disease is more common in tropical countries, in many of which the prevalence rate is 1 to 2 percent of the population. A warm environment is not critical for transmission, and leprosy also occurs in certain regions with cooler climates, such as Korea and central Mexico. Distribution of infected individuals within countries is very nonhomogeneous, and districts in which 20 percent of the population is affected can be found. The distribution of cases across the spectrum of leprosy also varies between countries, with lepromatous disease predominating in some countries, such as Mexico, and tuberculoid disease in others, such as India. Ninety percent of the cases diagnosed in the United States in the past two decades have occurred in immigrants from leprosy-endemic countries. Indigenous transmission occurs primarily in Hawaii, the Pacific Island territories, and sporadically along the Gulf coast. The incidence of leprosy in the United States has fallen from a peak of 360 cases in 1985.

Leprosy can present at any age, although cases in infants less than 1 year of age are extremely rare. The age-specific incidence peaks during childhood in most developing countries; up to 20 percent of cases occur in children under 10. Since leprosy is most prevalent in poorer socioeconomic groups, this may simply reflect the age distribution of the high-risk population. The sex ratio of leprosy presenting during childhood is 1:1, but males predominate by a 2:1 ratio in adults.

Direct human-to-human transmission is believed responsible for most cases of leprosy. Animal reservoirs exist among feral armadillos and possibly among nonhuman primates, but there is little evidence that they have an important role in the epidemiology of human disease. Familial spread is facilitated by the indolence of the clinical illness and the potential for transmission prior to the development of symptoms. Among close family contacts (spouse-spouse or spouse-child) of untreated lepromatous patients the risk of disease is increased approximately eightfold, and the attack rate can be as high as 10 percent. Development of clinical disease in contacts of tuberculoid patients is less common, although immunologic tests suggest that most of these contacts have been sensitized to *M. leprae*. The site of entry remains a matter of conjecture, but is probably either the skin or the mucosa of the upper respiratory tract. The chief portal of exit is thought to be the nasal mucosa of untreated lepromatous patients.

The incubation period is frequently 3 to 5 years, but has been reported to range from 6 months to several decades.

PATHOGENESIS The early events following the entry of *M. leprae* into the body have not been described in humans. The bacilli are surrounded by a dense, nearly inert lipid capsule, produce no exotoxins, and engender little inflammatory response. Immunologic and epidemiologic studies suggest that only a small fraction, possibly 10 to 20 percent, of those exposed to viable bacilli will develop signs of indeterminate leprosy and that only about 50 percent of those with indeterminate disease will progress to full-blown clinical leprosy.

The intensity of the specific cell-mediated immune response to *M. leprae* correlates with the clinical and histologic disease class. Individuals with polar tuberculoid disease have an intense cellular response to *M. leprae* and a low bacillary load, whereas patients with lepromatous leprosy have no detectable cellular immunity to the leprosy bacillus. There is evidence from family studies that specific HLA-associated genes may be linked to different classes of disease. HLA-DR2 is inherited preferentially by children with polar tuberculoid disease, whereas HLA-MT1 is associated with polar lepromatous disease. The effect of the HLA-associated genes is limited to influencing the type of leprosy, and there is no association between HLA haplotypes and overall susceptibility to leprosy.

The defect in cell-mediated immunity in lepromatous patients is extremely specific. They do not suffer increased morbidity following infection by pathogens such as viruses or parasites for which cellular immunity is important, and they do not have an increased risk of neoplasia. Tuberculin reactivity may be suppressed in untreated lepromatous disease, but usually returns with treatment, unlike the lepromin response, which remains negative. Patients with lepromatous leprosy have been shown to have an increased number of circulating CD8+ ("suppressor") lymphocytes which can be specifically activated by *M. leprae* antigens, and the lymphocytes present in their cutaneous granulomas are almost exclusively CD8+. In contrast, CD4+4B4+ ("helper") cells predominate among the T cells in the cutaneous lesions of tuberculoid patients. In lepromatous leprosy, cells of the monocyte-macrophage family become engorged with *M. leprae* and are unable to kill or digest the organisms. Intracellular accumulation of large amounts of the *M. leprae*–specific surface lipid, phenolic glycolipid I, may contribute to the macrophage dysfunction. However, when studied in vitro, monocytes from these patients respond normally to lymphokines and display normal phagocytic and microbicidal activity. These results suggest that an underlying defect in regulation of T-lymphocyte subpopulations is responsible for the immunologic tolerance characteristic of lepromatous leprosy.

Intense bacillemia is very common in lepromatous leprosy, and organisms can often be seen in stained smears of peripheral blood or buffy coats, but high fever and signs of systemic toxicity are absent. Even in the most advanced cases, destructive lesions are limited to the skin, peripheral nerves, anterior portions of the eyes, upper respiratory passages above the larynx, testes, and structures of the hands and feet. The trophism of *M. leprae* for these tissues may be due to the fact that they are all usually several degrees cooler than 37°C. Two sites of preferential involvement are the ulnar nerves near the elbow and the peroneal nerves where they pass around the head of the fibula; above and below these areas where these nerves take deeper courses, they are less severely involved. In patients with lepromatous leprosy, collections of bacilli are also found in the liver, spleen, and bone marrow. No visceral organ system dysfunction has been associated with the presence of these bacilli, and it is unclear whether they are capable of reproduction at core body temperatures.

CLINICOPATHOLOGIC CLASSIFICATION The manifestations of leprosy are many and variable. The classification in general use is based on clinical and histopathologic findings.

Lepromatous leprosy is one of the polar forms. The cutaneous involvement is extensive, diffuse, and bilaterally symmetric. Even apparently normal skin will usually contain bacilli demonstrable by staining. Peripheral nerves are heavily infected but often better preserved than in the tuberculoid form. Histologically, there is a diffuse granulomatous reaction with macrophages, large foam (Virchow's) cells, and many intracellular bacilli, frequently in spheroidal masses (globi). Epithelioid cells and giant cells are not found.

Tuberculoid leprosy is the other polar type. Skin lesions are single or few and are sharply demarcated. Neurologic involvement is relatively pronounced and may occur in the absence of cutaneous lesions (pure neural leprosy). The histologic picture consists of lymphocytes, epithelioid cells, and perhaps giant cells; bacilli are frequently absent or difficult to demonstrate.

Classification within the borderline region of the spectrum is less precise. Lesions tend to increase in number and heterogeneity, but decrease in individual size as the lepromatous pole is approached. The histopathology of the granulomas also changes from an epithelioid cell to a macrophage predominance. The presence and number of lymphocytes are variable and correlate poorly with the disease class. Bacilli are present in large numbers in the skin granulomas of borderline and borderline lepromatous patients. For this reason, these groups, together with polar lepromatous leprosy, are referred to as "multibacillary leprosy." Borderline tuberculoid, polar tuberculoid, and indeterminate classes are grouped together as "paucibacillary leprosy." The borderline disease states are unstable and may shift toward the lepromatous form in the untreated patient or toward the tuberculoid pole during treatment. Change of either polar type to the other is exceedingly rare. In all forms of leprosy peripheral nerve involvement is a constant feature. In any histologic section involvement of nerves will tend to be more severe than involvement of other tissues. Much of the neural destruction appears to result from the granulomatous reaction of the host, rather than from an innate neurotoxic property of the bacillus.

CLINICAL MANIFESTATIONS **Early leprosy** The first signs of leprosy are usually cutaneous. One or more hypopigmented or hyperpigmented macules or plaques may be seen. Often an anesthetic or paresthetic patch is the first symptom noted by the patient, but on careful examination skin involvement can also be found. When contacts are examined, a single skin lesion is often noted, especially in children; usually, this is a hypesthetic macule that may clear spontaneously in a year or two, but specific treatment is usually recommended. Sensation is often preserved in early lesions, particularly those on the face.

Tuberculoid leprosy Early tuberculoid leprosy is frequently manifested by a hypopigmented macule which is sharply demarcated and hypesthetic. Later the lesions are larger, and the margins are elevated and circinate or gyrate. There is peripheral spread and central healing. Fully developed lesions are densely anesthetic and have lost the normal skin organs (sweat glands and hair follicles). The lesions appear singly or are few in number and are not symmetric. Nerve involvement occurs early, and the superficial nerves leading from the lesions may be enlarged. The larger peripheral nerves (especially the ulnar, peroneal, and greater auricular nerves) may be palpably and visibly enlarged, particularly those closest to the skin lesion. There may be severe neuritic pain. Neural involvement leads to muscle atrophy, especially of the small muscles of the hand. Contractures of the hand and foot are frequent. Trauma, especially from burns and splinters and from excessive pressure, leads to secondary infection of the hands and to plantar ulcers. Later, resorption and loss of phalanges may supervene. When the facial nerves are involved, there may be lagophthalmos, exposure keratitis, and corneal ulceration leading to blindness.

Lepromatous leprosy The skin lesions are macules, nodules, plaques, or papules. The macules are often hypopigmented. The borders of the lesions are ill defined and the centers of raised lesions are indurated and convex (rather than concave as in tuberculoid disease). There is also diffuse infiltration between the lesions. The sites of predilection are the face (cheeks, nose, brows), ears, wrists, elbows, buttocks, and knees. Involvement with infiltration and little or no nodulation may progress so subtly that the disease goes unnoticed. Loss of the lateral portions of the eyebrows is common. Much later the skin of the face and forehead becomes thickened and corrugated (leonine facies), and the earlobes become pendulous.

Nasal "stuffiness," epistaxis, and obstructed breathing are common early symptoms. Complete nasal obstruction, laryngitis, and hoarseness are also frequent. Septal perforation and nasal collapse lead to saddlenose. Invasion of the anterior portion of the eye leads to keratitis and iridocyclitis. Painless inguinal and axillary lymphadenopathy occurs. In adult males infiltration and scarring of the testes lead to sterility. Gynecomastia is common.

Involvement of major nerve trunks is less prominent in the lepromatous form, but diffuse hypesthesia involving the peripheral portions of the extremities is common in advanced disease.

Borderline leprosy The skin lesions of borderline tuberculoid leprosy generally resemble those of tuberculoid disease, but are greater in number and have more poorly defined borders. Involvement of multiple peripheral nerve trunks is more common than in polar tuberculoid disease. Increasing variability in the appearance of the skin lesions is characteristic of borderline leprosy (sometimes referred to as "dimorphic" leprosy). Papules and plaques may coexist with macular lesions. Anesthesia is less prominent than in tuberculoid disease. The earlobes may be slightly thickened, but the eyebrows and nasal regions are spared.

REACTIONAL STATES The general course of leprosy is indolent, but it may be interrupted by two types of reaction. Both forms of reactions can occur in untreated patients, but more often emerge as complications of chemotherapy.

Erythema nodosum leprosum Erythema nodosum leprosum (ENL), or type 2 lepra reaction, occurs in lepromatous and borderline lepromatous patients, most frequently in the latter half of the initial year of treatment. Tender, inflamed subcutaneous nodules develop, usually in crops. Each nodule lasts a week or two, but new crops may appear. ENL may last only a week or two, or it may continue for long periods. Low-grade fever, lymphadenopathy, and arthralgias can accompany severe ENL. Histologically, ENL is characterized by polymorphonuclear infiltration and deposits of IgG and complement, resembling an Arthus reaction.

Reversal reaction Reversal reaction, or type 1 lepra reaction, can complicate all three borderline categories. Existing skin lesions develop erythema and swelling, and new lesions may appear. An early influx of lymphocytes into existing lesions is followed by edema and a shift toward tuberculoid histology. Cellular immunity increases. Reversal reactions can be differentiated from disease progression or relapse by mouse inoculations to test bacillary viability and by histologic studies. Downgrading reactions, which clinically mimic reversal reactions, are most common in untreated patients and in women during the third trimester of pregnancy. Skin biopsies reveal a shift toward lepromatous histology and reflect a decrease in cellular immunity.

COMPLICATIONS Leprosy is probably the most frequent cause of crippling of the hand in the world. Trauma and secondary chronic infections can lead to loss of digits or distal extremities. Blindness is also common.

The *Lucio phenomenon*, characterized by arteritis, is limited to patients with diffuse, infiltrative, nonnodular lepromatous disease. Severe cases clinically resemble other forms of necrotizing vasculitis and are associated with a high mortality rate.

Secondary amyloidosis is a complication of severe lepromatous disease, especially in chronic ENL.

DIAGNOSIS The demonstration of acid-fast bacilli in skin smears made by the scraped-incision method is strong evidence for leprosy, but in tuberculoid disease bacilli may not be demonstrable. Wherever possible, a skin biopsy specimen from the affected area should be sent to a pathologist knowledgeable in leprosy. The histologic involvement of peripheral nerves is pathognomonic, even in the absence of bacilli.

Hematologic and blood chemistry tests are of little help in establishing the diagnosis. Lepromatous patients frequently have mild anemia, elevated erythrocyte sedimentation rate, and hyperglobulinemia. Between 10 and 20 percent of lepromatous patients have low titer false-positive serologic tests for syphilis or autoantibodies directed against nuclear or cellular antigens.

A specific serodiagnostic test for leprosy has been developed. Based on the detection of antibody to the *M. leprae*–specific surface antigen, phenolic glycolipid I, this assay has a sensitivity of over 95 percent in polar lepromatous disease and about 30 percent in tuberculoid disease. The level of antibody appears to correlate with the bacillary load which explains both the high false-negative rate in polar tuberculoid disease and the persistence of seropositivity in lepromatous patients, in whom bacterial remnant forms can persist for many years. Despite these limitations, the near 100 percent specificity of this assay makes it potentially useful for confirming the diagnosis of leprosy and monitoring the response to therapy, and as an epidemiologic tool for studying disease incubation and transmission.

The differential diagnosis includes lupus erythematosus, lupus vulgaris, sarcoidosis, yaws, dermal leishmaniasis, and a host of banal skin diseases. The skin lesions of leprosy, especially of tuberculoid disease, are characterized by hypesthesia, and peripheral nerve involvement can always be demonstrated. Peripheral neuropathy from other causes and syringomyelia may be confused with leprosy, although skin involvement is not a feature of other diseases causing peripheral neuropathy. The combination of a chronic skin disease and peripheral nerve involvement should always lead to the consideration of leprosy.

TREATMENT The management of leprosy involves a broad, multidisciplinary approach, including consultative services such as orthopedic surgery, ophthalmology, and physical therapy in addition to antimicrobial chemotherapy.

Specific chemotherapy Dapsone (4,4'-diaminodiphenylsulfone, DDS, diphenylsulfone), a folate antagonist, is the mainstay of therapy. The daily dosage is 50 to 100 mg in adults. Dapsone is very inexpensive, safe in pregnancy, and has a long serum half-life of about 24 h, allowing once daily administration. Major side effects are relatively uncommon, but include hemolysis, agranulocytosis, hepatitis, and potentially fatal exfoliative dermatitis. In lepromatous disease enough bacilli are killed during the first 10 to 12 weeks of dapsone monotherapy to render mouse foot pad inoculations negative. However, in this form of the disease nonviable bacilli disappear slowly and may be found in the tissues for 5 to 10 years. Moreover, a few viable bacilli (persisters) may survive in the tissues for many years and cause a relapse if treatment is discontinued.

Dapsone resistance is a problem of increasing concern. Secondary resistance is most common in lepromatous patients and presents as a clinical and bacteriologic relapse after several years of apparently successful, regular therapy. Sulfone resistance can be demonstrated by mouse foot pad inoculation. The frequency of this secondary resistance has been 2 to 30 percent in different countries, depending on the sulfone preparation used and the regularity of its administration. Primary dapsone resistance in as many as 30 percent of previously untreated patients has complicated empiric therapy in many parts of the world, but has remained uncommon in newly diagnosed patients in the United States. Because of the problems of dapsone-resistant bacilli and of persister bacilli, multiple drug therapy is now recommended for all multibacillary disease.

Rifampin is the most rapidly mycobactericidal drug known for *M. leprae*. The viability of skin bacilli falls to undetectable levels within 5 days following a single 1500-mg dose of oral rifampin. The usual dosage is 600 mg/d. The high cost of rifampin has limited its use in the developing world, and has led to regimens in which it is given at a dosage of 600 or 900 mg once per month. Until more clinical experience has been accumulated, however, many leprologists prefer to treat with daily or twice weekly rifampin. Rare cases of rifampin-resistant *M. leprae* have been reported. Rifampin has not been approved for the intermittent treatment of leprosy by the Food and Drug Administration.

Clofazimine is a compound derived from a phenazine dye. It is highly lipophilic and accumulates in the skin, the gastrointestinal tract, and in macrophages and monocytes. It is usually given in a dosage of 50 to 200 mg/d and has an apparent half-life of over 70 days. Major toxicity is restricted to the skin and the intestinal tract. The reddish skin pigmentation, often accompanied by ichthyosis, is unacceptable to many light-skinned patients and can lead to poor compliance. The intestinal toxicity is also dose-related and is reflected in diarrhea and cramping abdominal pain. Clofazimine is not safe for use during pregnancy.

Several other agents, including ethionamide, prothionamide, thiambutosine, and amithiozone, have limited activity against *M. leprae* and may be of value in multiple drug regimens. None of these drugs have been approved for this purpose by the Food and Drug Administration. Based on promising results in animal studies, clinical trials are underway with the quinolones, ofloxacin and pefloxacin, as well as with minocycline.

Therapy for multibacillary disease should consist of three drugs, usually dapsone, rifampin, and clofazimine. If the organism is known to be dapsone-sensitive, the combination of dapsone and rifampin may be adequate for borderline and borderline lepromatous cases, but the likelihood of secondary dapsone resistance makes the addition of a third drug advisable in lepromatous disease. Objective measures of response to therapy, including skin scrapings and biopsies, should be monitored and therapy continued at least until morphologically intact bacilli are consistently absent and the inflammatory cell infiltrate has resolved. The optimal duration of therapy is unknown, but a minimum of 2 years is recommended. Indefinite therapy may be required for lepromatous disease.

Therapeutic regimens containing two drugs, usually dapsone and rifampin, are adequate for paucibacillary leprosy. The World Health Organization recommends a 6-month course, which can be repeated if relapse occurs. Standard practice in the United States is to treat with dapsone and rifampin for the first 6 to 12 months (depending on the clinical response), followed by dapsone alone to complete a total of 24 months of therapy.

Evidence of clinical improvement should be visible by the second or third month of treatment. The clinical response to adequate therapy may be confused by intercurrent reactional states, but the disease stops progressing and the skin lesions gradually improve. Recovery from neurologic impairment is limited.

Treatment of reactional states Mild ENL is managed with antipyretics and analgesics. Severe cases can be rapidly controlled with high dosages of prednisone (60 to 120 mg/d). Antimicrobial therapy should be continued as glucocorticoid therapy promotes the viability of *M. leprae* in mice not given antileprosy drugs. Rifampin enhances the metabolism of glucocorticoids by the liver, necessitating administration of larger doses to achieve a given therapeutic effect. Thalidomide is the most effective drug for ENL. The usual initial dosage is 200 mg twice a day, which can be gradually tapered to a maintenance dosage of 50 to 100 mg/d for patients with chronic ENL. Thalidomide is absolutely contraindicated in women of child-bearing age because of its teratogenicity, but has proved relatively free of major side effects in other leprosy patients. This drug has not been approved by the Food and Drug Administration but is available through the Hansen's Disease Center, Carville, Louisiana, as an investigational agent. Clofazimine has anti-inflammatory properties as well as antimycobacterial activity and can be valuable in the treatment of chronic ENL, but requires at least 3 to 4 weeks to reach effective levels, making it of little use in acute attacks. Other classes of anti-inflammatory agents including antimalarials such as chloroquine and cytotoxic drugs have been used in difficult cases; in general these unusual situations should be managed in consultation with a leprosy specialist.

Reversal reactions are often acute and can lead to rapid and irreversible neurologic damage. Glucocorticoids are indicated for severe reversal reactions. Clofazimine is of some use in chronic situations, but it is generally necessary to continue glucocorticoids as well. Reversal reactions do not respond to thalidomide.

Other measures Many of the deformities and disabilities of leprosy are preventable. Plantar ulcers, which are very common, may be prevented by rigid-soled footwear or walking plaster casts, and contractures of the hand may be prevented by physical therapy and application of casts. Reconstructive surgery is sometimes helpful. Nerve and tendon transplants and release of contractures can give patients more functional ability. Vocational retraining is often necessary for those with permanent disability. Plastic repair of facial deformities assists acceptance of patients in society. The psychological trauma which resulted from prolonged segregation is now minimized by home therapy in virtually all cases.

Control Case finding and chemotherapy form the present basis of control. Infectiousness can be quickly suppressed with chemotherapy. Early detection of cases is especially important. In endemic countries this means establishing clinics or traveling teams. Family and other close contacts need regular examinations for leprosy. In the United States patients are eligible for treatment by the Public Health Service, and special clinics are located in several major cities, as well as an inpatient facility at the Hansen's Disease Center in Carville. Risk of transmission is very low, even in untreated patients, and no unusual infection control precautions are required when patients are hospitalized. Chemoprophylaxis with lowered doses of dapsone is effective, but contact screening by yearly physical examinations is preferred to empiric therapy in most situations. Vaccine trials with bacillus Calmette-Guérin in endemic areas continue despite conflicting results and modest efficacy. Two new experimental vaccines, one containing viable BCG and heat-killed *M. leprae*, and the second consisting of a cultivable mycobacterium (ICRC bacillus) are currently in field trials.

REFERENCES

BLOOM BR, GODAL T: Selective primary health care: Strategies for control of disease in the developing world. V. Leprosy. Rev Infect Dis 5:765, V, 1983
BULLOCK WE: Rifampin in the treatment of leprosy. Rev Infect Dis 5:S606, 1983
——: *Mycobacterium leprae* (leprosy), in *Principles and Practice of Infectious Diseases*, 2 ed, GL Mandell et al (eds). New York, Wiley, 1985, pp 1406–1413
HASTINGS RC (ed): *Leprosy*. New York, Churchill Livingstone, 1985
MODLIN RL et al: Learning from lesions: Patterns of tissue inflammation in leprosy. Proc Natl Acad Sci USA 85:1213, 1988
NEILL MA et al: Leprosy in the United States, 1971–1981. J Infect Dis 152:1064, 1985
RIDLEY DS, JOPLING WH: Classification of leprosy according to immunity: A five-group system. Int J Lepr 34:255, 1966
Serological tests for leprosy, editorial. Lancet 1:533, 1986
SHIELDS ED et al: Genetic epidemiology of the susceptibility to leprosy. J Clin Invest 79:1139, 1987
THOMAS DA et al: Armadillo exposure among Mexican-born patients with lepromatous leprosy. J Infect Dis 156:990, 1987
Vaccines against leprosy, editorial. Lancet 1:1183, 1987

127 OTHER MYCOBACTERIAL INFECTIONS

STANLEY D. FREEDMAN

INTRODUCTION Mycobacteria other than the tubercle bacilli were shown to be agents of human disease in the 1950s. A classification of these organisms based upon colonial morphology and growth characteristics was provided by Runyon. These bacteria are widely distributed in nature as saprophytes, primarily in soil and water. Animals can be infected and serve as reservoirs for infection of humans. Person-to-person transmission has not been documented. Epidemiologic studies using tuberculins from the various species demonstrated the extent of infection in the United States and other countries, as well as notable geographic differences. These organisms have been referred to as atypical mycobacteria or anonymous mycobacteria. Although the organisms are not always anonymous, the frequency with which they are found in the environment demands repeated isolation from a diseased area or isolation from blood or bone marrow before they can be accepted as the etiologic agent. With the steady improvement of laboratory techniques including radiometric cultures, species designations are now increasingly familiar and preferred in the study of these pathogens (Table 127-1). With increasing sophistication of medical practice and the emergence of newly recognized diseases, additional syndromes associated with different species have emerged and have assumed major importance.

MYCOBACTERIUM ULCERANS M. ulcerans is the etiologic agent of the Buruli or Bairnsdale ulcer. It grows only at 30 to 33°C. Colonies require 7 weeks to appear; isolation is enhanced by inoculation of mouse footpads. A disease of the tropics, it is concentrated in Australia and Africa. The first sign of infection with M. ulcerans is a small painless nodule developing into an extensive granulomatous ulceration usually affecting the extensor surfaces of the extremities. Characteristically, the ulcer is deep with a necrotic base and undermined edges. Tissue destruction may be due to a soluble bacterial toxin that may mute the host response. Wide surgical excision with skin grafting is curative; there are no clear data regarding chemotherapy.

MYCOBACTERIUM MARINUM This organism, previously called M. balnei, is a psychrophilic (30°C) photochromogen which inhabits fresh and salt water and causes disease in fish. Human infections are usually associated with some aquatic activity, like working in aquaria and swimming. The organism enters abraded skin and either forms a nodule, which can spread along lymphatics suggesting sporotrichosis, causes verrucous lesions, or, less commonly, ulcerates. The pathology consists of a granulomatous lesion usually without caseation—the so-called swimming pool or fishtank granuloma. Infection is frequently associated with a positive tuberculin test reflecting shared antigens with M. tuberculosis. Because the differential diagnosis includes sporotrichosis as well as other mycobacterial infections,

appropriate cultures (30 to 32°C incubation) are critical. Infections of tendon sheaths and synovia have been described in association with penetrating injuries. Ulcerations similar to those caused by M. ulcerans, as well as disseminated skin lesions, have been reported in immunocompromised patients. Minor lesions can resolve spontaneously. The organism is often sensitive in vitro to rifampin and ethambutol, and these drugs have been curative. Tetracycline, especially minocycline, and trimethoprim-sulfamethoxazole have also been used with favorable results. Surgical debridement is sometimes required.

MYCOBACTERIUM KANSASII M. kansasii produces pigment upon exposure to light, grows at 37°C, and is a long, thick, acid-fast organism with prominent transverse banding. Infections are more common in the central United States, Texas, England, and Wales. The reasons for these geographic variations are unknown, but likely relate to subtle ecologic properties of these organisms. Person-to-person spread is not recognized. Reported cases reflect a preponderance of white adult men.

Pulmonary disease is the commonest expression of this organism, and the clinical picture closely resembles pulmonary tuberculosis although signs and symptoms are milder. Pneumoconiosis and chronic obstructive pulmonary disease (COPD) are considered predisposing conditions. Thin-walled cavities with minimal inflammatory reaction are characteristic. The usual situation, without treatment, is slow progression.

Disseminated disease is now recognized as an important manifestation of M. kansasii infections. Such hematogenous spread is associated with pancytopenia, hairy cell leukemia, malignancies, acquired immunodeficiency syndrome (AIDS), and bone marrow and renal transplantations. Fever, anemia, and signs and symptoms of multiple organ system involvement occur. The diagnosis is confirmed by appropriate cultures of involved tissues. Skin and soft tissue involvement is seen and may mimic M. marinum infections. Tenosynovitis, osteomyelitis, lymphadenitis, pericarditis, and genitourinary tract infections have been reported.

Diseases due to M. kansasii respond well to treatment. Rifampin appears to be the most effective drug and should be used in all initial regimens. Ethambutol and isoniazid are usually the other drugs administered. Over 95 percent of patients respond to this combined regimen. Retreatment programs should be guided by in vitro sensitivity testing, and rifampin used if the organism is sensitive.

MYCOBACTERIUM SCROFULACEUM This bacillus, which forms pigment even in the dark (scotochromogenic), is a major cause of lymphadenitis in children. Cervical nodes are usually involved, and associated systemic symptoms are rare. Definitive diagnosis requires culture, and definitive therapy requires total excision of the node and sinus tract, if present. There are a few reports of pulmonary disease and osseous and soft tissue infections; dissemination usually is associated with serious underlying conditions. Sensitivity patterns vary, and multiple-drug regimens have been used.

MYCOBACTERIUM SZULGAI At 37°C this organism is scotochromogenic and can be confused with more common tap water contam-

---

TABLE 127-1 Human mycobacterial pathogens other than M. tuberculosis and M. leprae

Mycobacterium	Pigmentation of culture*	Usual site of disease	Usual source of infection	Response to drugs
M. marinum	P	Skin	Swimming pools, aquaria, fish	Good
M. ulcerans	N	Skin	Tropical environment	Variable
M. avium-intracellulare	N	Lungs	Environment, animals?	Poor
M. kansasii	P	Lungs	Environment?	Good
M. xenopi	S	Lungs	Water, animals?	Variable
M. szulgai	S†	Lungs	?	Good
M. scrofulaceum	S	Lungs, lymph nodes	Water, soil	Poor
M. fortuitum	N	Skin (abscesses), lungs	Soil, dirt, water	Poor
M. chelonei	N	Skin (abscesses), lungs	Soil, dirt, water	Poor

* P = photochromogenic (develops yellow-orange pigment only when exposed to light); N = nonpigmented; S = scotochromogenic (develops yellow-orange pigment in the dark).
† Scotochromogenic at 37°C, photochromogenic at 25°C.

inants. It was initially recognized as an uncommon pulmonary pathogen producing disease similar to *M. tuberculosis*. Bursitis, lymphadenitis, tenosynovitis, and disseminated disease have also been reported. Most isolates are sensitive to rifampin and ethambutol.

MYCOBACTERIUM XENOPI   *M. xenopi* is a slow-growing scotochromogen which infrequently causes tuberculosis-like pulmonary disease in humans usually with underlying diseases. Extrapulmonary disease is rare. However, reports of disseminated disease are becoming more common and include an association with AIDS (see below). Unlike a number of nontuberculous mycobacteria it is sensitive to most of the antituberculous drugs but combination therapy is required.

MYCOBACTERIUM AVIUM-INTRACELLULARE   Although seroagglutination, thin-layer chromatography, and enzyme-linked immunosorbent assays can distinguish *M. avium* from *M. intracellulare*, distinction is difficult and they are considered as a complex (MAC). These ubiquitous organisms are particularly prevalent in the southeastern United States and, overall, are the most commonly isolated mycobacteria other than *M. tuberculosis*. Colonization and inapparent infection are common; knowledge of transmission is limited. The lungs are most commonly involved, and the clinical picture is similar to pulmonary tuberculosis. Underlying pulmonary disease, a possible genetic predilection, and age are risk factors. Solitary pulmonary nodules are not uncommon. It is important to be certain of the etiology and the pathogenic role of the organism isolated, because chemotherapy is often associated with morbidity.

Skin involvement and musculoskeletal infections including vertebral osteomyelitis resembling Pott's disease have been described. MAC is a major cause of lymphadenitis in children. Disseminated disease is also recognized in children, and in adults in association with severe underlying diseases. Fever, anemia, leukocytosis, hypergammaglobulinemia, and hepatosplenomegaly are prominent features.

There is a striking association between organisms of the *Mycobacterium avium* complex and AIDS (see Chap. 264). The manifestations are unique and reflect overwhelming infection in these patients with impaired immunity. There is mycobacteremia, and organisms abound in most organs and body secretions. There is a minimal cellular response, granulomatous or otherwise. Profound diarrhea with intestinal pathology that resembles Whipple's disease, due to macrophages packed with MAC, is present. In other organs these macrophages resemble lepra cells. Blood cultures using the lysis centrifugation system combined with the radiometric systems and using DNA probes for identification can quickly confirm the diagnosis in many patients. The organisms are readily seen and cultured from other involved sites using standard techniques.

Treatment is difficult and unsatisfactory. The organisms are usually resistant to most of the antimycobacterial agents. Yet multiple-drug therapy is recommended with some demonstrable benefit possibly reflecting synergy which is difficult to prove in vitro. Drugs chosen should include those antimicrobials to which the organism is sensitive. Three to six drugs are used concurrently, chosen from among isoniazid, ethambutol, rifampin, ethionamide, pyrazinamide, cycloserine, streptomycin, kanamycin, amikacin, and capreomycin. Of these, ethambutol, rifampin, ethionamide, cycloserine, and amikacin appear more effective. Clofazamine may be useful in immunocompetent patients. Surgical excision is the treatment of choice for lymphadenitis and is a reasonable alternative for a few other localized infections. Treatment of patients with AIDS is problematic and controversial; combinations including rifampin, ethambutol, clofazamine, amikacin, one of the quinolones, along with immunomodulators, may be beneficial for some patients.

MYCOBACTERIUM FORTUITUM AND CHELONEI   The unique feature of these acid-fast bacteria is their rapid growth; initial growth may take 1 to 5 weeks, but subsequent subcultures grow within 5 days. Reflecting their meager nutritional requirements, they are readily cultured on most media. These two species account for virtually all the reported infections due to rapid growers. *M. fortuitum* is more frequently associated with posttraumatic and postsurgical skin and soft tissue infection. *M. chelonei* is a more common cause of pulmonary infections and disseminated disease. It has also been reported as a cause of chronic otitis media. Subspeciation is not necessary for clinical purposes. Widespread in nature and in hospital environments, and highly resistant to drugs, antiseptics, and disinfectants, rapid growers are important nosocomial pathogens.

Most human infections are associated with interruption of the integument and injury or alteration of the soft tissues. Inhalational pulmonary disease complicates underlying lung disease. Although a chronic granulomatous reaction with caseation may occur, the distinguishing feature is a suppurative process with microabscesses, and diphtheroid-like organisms on Gram stain. Infections have followed cardiothoracic surgery, augmentation mammoplasty, arthroplasty, injections, ocular surgery, and dialysis. Clinical manifestations include lymphadenitis, keratitis, osteomyelitis, meningitis, and endocarditis involving porcine, prosthetic, and natural valves. Hematogenous dissemination is uncommon, and affects primarily those with impaired host defenses.

Nodular erythematous skin lesions on the legs of renal transplant recipients are often due to *M. chelonei*.

Adequate debridement and drainage with removal of foreign bodies is indicated whenever possible. Many of these organisms are highly resistant to all antimicrobial agents. However, reflecting their growth characteristics, antimicrobial sensitivity testing is more reliable in determining appropriate chemotherapy than is the case with other atypical mycobacteria. Amikacin is most effective; other drugs reported to be of value include gentamicin, cefoxitin, doxycycline, minocycline, erythromycin, sulfonamides, rifampin, ethambutol, ciprofloxacin, imipenem, and clofazamine. Sulfonamides are more active against *M. fortuitum*, and erythromycin inhibits some *M. chelonei*. Because of the emergence of resistant organisms, two or three drugs may be preferable to one.

OTHER MYCOBACTERIA   *M. haemophilum* is a skin pathogen. It is psychrophilic, but requires iron supplements for growth. Virtually all reported cases have occurred in immunosuppressed patients, including some with AIDS. *M. malmoense* causes chronic pulmonary disease usually in the setting of pneumoconiosis. With increasing laboratory and clinical sophistication, the list of diseases caused by nontuberculous mycobacteria continues to expand.

REFERENCES

ALBERTS WM, CHANDLER KW: Pulmonary disease caused by *Mycobacterium malmoense*. Am Rev Respir Dis 135:1375, 1987

BENNETT C, VARDIMAN J: Disseminated atypical mycobacterial infection in patients with hairy cell leukemia. Am J Med 80:891, 1986

CHOW SP, IP FK: *Mycobacterium marinum* infection of the hand and wrist. Results of conservative treatment in twenty-four cases. J Bone Joint Surg [AM] 69:1161, 1987

COOPER JF et al: *Mycobacterium chelonei*: A cause of nodular skin lesions with a proclivity for renal transplant recipients. Am J Med 86:173, 1989

HAMPSON SJ, PORTAELS F: DNA probes demonstrate a single highly conserved strain of *Mycobacterium avium* infecting AIDS patients. Lancet 1:65, 1989

MALONEY JM, GREGG CR: Infections caused by *Mycobacterium szulgai* in humans. Rev Infect Dis 9:1120, 1987

PARROT RG, GROSSET JH: Post-surgical outcome of 57 patients with *Mycobacterium xenopi* pulmonary infection. Tubercle 69:47, 1988

PIMSLER M, SPONSLER TA: Immunosuppressive properties of the soluble toxin from *Mycobacterium ulcerans*. J Infect Dis 157:577, 1988

ROTH RI, OWEN RL: Intestinal infection with *Mycobacterium avium* in acquired immune deficiency syndrome (AIDS). Dig Dis Sci 30:497, 1985

WALLACE RJ: Treatment of nonpulmonary infections due to *Mycobacterium fortuitum* and *Mycobacterium chelonei* on the basis of in vitro susceptibilities. J Infect Dis 152:500, 1985

———, SWENSON JM: Spectrum of disease due to rapidly growing mycobacteria. Rev Infect Dis 5:657, 1983

WONG B, EDWARDS FF: Continuous high-grade *Mycobacterium avium-intracellulare* bacteremia in patients with the acquired immune deficiency syndrome. Am J Med 78:35, 1985

WOODS GL, WASHINGTON JA: Mycobacteria other than *Mycobacterium tuberculosis*: Review of microbiologic and clinical aspects. Rev Infect Dis 9:275, 1987

section 7 Spirochetal diseases

128 SYPHILIS

SHEILA A. LUKEHART / KING K. HOLMES

DEFINITION Syphilis is a chronic systemic infection caused by *Treponema pallidum* subspecies *pallidum*, is usually sexually transmitted, and is characterized by episodes of active disease interrupted by periods of latency. Following an incubation period averaging 3 weeks, a primary lesion appears and is often associated with regional lymphadenopathy; a secondary bacteremic stage is associated with generalized mucocutaneous lesions and generalized lymphadenopathy, followed by a latent period of subclinical infection lasting many years. In about one-third of untreated cases, the tertiary stage is characterized by progressive destructive mucocutaneous musculo-skeletal or parenchymal lesions, aortitis, or symptomatic central nervous system disease.

ETIOLOGY The discovery of *Treponema pallidum* in syphilitic material was made by Schaudinn and Hoffman in 1905. *Treponema pallidum* is one of the many spiral-shaped microorganisms which propel themselves by spinning around their longitudinal axis. The Spirochaetales include three genera which are pathogenic for humans and for a variety of other animals: the *Leptospira*, which cause human leptospirosis; the *Borrelia*, including *B. recurrentis* and *B. vincentii*, which cause relapsing fever and Vincent's angina, respectively, as well as *B. burgdorferi*, the causative agent of Lyme disease; and the *Treponema*, responsible for the diseases known as treponematoses. The *Treponema* include *T. pallidum* subspecies *pallidum* (hereafter called *T. pallidum*) which causes venereal syphilis, *T. pallidum* subspecies *pertenue* which causes yaws, *T. pallidum* subspecies *endemicum* which causes endemic syphilis or bejel, *T. carateum* which causes pinta (see Chap. 129), and *T. paraluiscuniculi*, the cause of rabbit syphilis. Other *Treponema* species are found in the human mouth, genital mucosa, and gastrointestinal tract but have no proven pathogenic role. These can be confused with *T. pallidum* on dark-field examination.

Treponema pallidum is a thin, delicate organism with 6 to 14 spirals and tapered ends, measuring 6 to 15 μm in total length and 0.2 μm in width. The cytoplasm is surrounded by a trilaminar cytoplasmic membrane, which in turn is surrounded by a delicate peptidoglycan layer providing some structural rigidity. The outer membrane is rich in lipid and contains relatively few integral membrane proteins. Six endoflagella wind around the cell body in a space between the inner cell wall and the outer membrane and may be the contractile elements responsible for motility. None of the four pathogenic treponemes has yet been cultured in vitro in quantity, and no convincing morphologic, serologic, or metabolic differences between them have been discerned. They are distinguished primarily according to the clinical syndrome they produce. The only known natural host for *T. pallidum* is the human. Many mammals can be infected with *T. pallidum*, but only humans, higher apes, and a few laboratory animals regularly develop syphilitic lesions. Virulent strains of *T. pallidum* are maintained in rabbits.

EPIDEMIOLOGY Nearly all cases of syphilis are acquired by sexual contact with infectious lesions (i.e., the chancre, mucous patch, skin rash, or condyloma latum). Less common modes of transmission include nonsexual personal contact and infection in utero or following blood transfusions.

The total reported number of cases of syphilis fell steadily from 575,593 in 1943 to a low of 64,621 in 1977, an 88 percent decrease, but has increased 60 percent in the past 11 years to 103,437 in 1988, with a 50 percent increase from 1986 through 1988. The number of new cases of infectious syphilis reached a peak in 1947, then fell to approximately 6000 in 1956; since then, there has been a rather steady increase in infectious syphilis punctuated by three periods of rapid growth: 10,000 more new cases by 1960 compared to 1956; 13,000 more new cases by 1982 compared to 1979; and from 1986 through 1988, an increase of 12,608 new infectious cases within only 2 years. In 1988, there were 40,117 reported cases of primary and secondary syphilis and 35,600 cases of early latent syphilis; the number of undiagnosed cases is estimated to be much greater.

The populations at highest risk for acquiring syphilis have changed. Between 1977 and 1982, approximately half of all patients with early syphilis in the United States were homosexual or bisexual men. Largely because of changing sexual practices in this population due to the AIDS epidemic, the proportion of early syphilis cases involving homosexual and bisexual men has decreased. The current epidemic of syphilis is occurring predominantly in black and Hispanic heterosexual men and women, largely in urban areas. In some cities, infectious syphilis is significantly correlated with exchange of sex for crack cocaine. The peak incidence of syphilis occurs in the age group 15 to 34. Although the reported incidence of syphilis is much higher in blacks and Hispanics than in whites and is higher in urban than in rural areas, these differences may reflect the fact that many members of urban minority groups are treated at public clinics, where case reporting is more complete. The case rates of early syphilis are highest in large urban population centers, including New York City, parts of Florida and Texas, Los Angeles, and the District of Columbia.

The incidence of congenital syphilis roughly parallels that of infectious syphilis in females. The number of reported cases of congenital syphilis in infants ≤1 year of age was lowest (107 cases) in 1978, when infectious syphilis was most prevalent in homosexual and bisexual men. The dramatic increase in primary and secondary syphilis in women from 1986 to 1988 has resulted in a proportional increase in the number of infants born with congenital syphilis, to 691 infants in 1988. Approximately one of two individuals named as contacts of infectious syphilis becomes infected. Many contacts will have already developed manifestations of syphilis when they are first seen, and about 30 percent of apparently uninfected contacts of infectious syphilis who are examined within 30 days of exposure will actually be in the incubation stage and will themselves develop infectious syphilis if not treated. Because of this, the identification and "epidemiologic" treatment of all recently exposed contacts has become an important aspect of syphilis control. Also important is the identification of syphilitics by serologic testing of pregnant women, hospital admissions, military inductees, and persons undergoing examination in physicians' offices. Of 45 million blood specimens examined during 1980 in the United States, 1.4 million tests were reactive, representing untreated syphilis, previously treated syphilis, or false-positive tests. Of all reported early syphilis cases of less than 1 year's duration in 1983, 47 percent were detected as a direct result of either contact tracing or serologic testing. More controversial are laws and regulations requiring routine premarital serologic testing for syphilis. Of 3.8 million premarital serologies performed in 1978, only 1 in 8461 was positive for infectious syphilis; the number positive for latent syphilis requiring treatment is probably larger, though national data are not available.

NATURAL COURSE AND PATHOGENESIS OF UNTREATED SYPHILIS *Treponema pallidum* rapidly penetrates intact mucous membranes or abraded skin and within a few hours enters the lymphatics and blood to produce systemic infection and metastatic foci long before the appearance of a primary lesion. Blood from a patient with incubating or early syphilis is infectious. The generation time of *T. pallidum* in vivo is estimated to be 30 to 33 h, and the incubation period of syphilis is inversely proportional to the number of organisms inoculated. The concentration of treponemes generally reaches at least 10^7 per gram of tissue before the appearance of a clinical lesion. In experimental infection in rabbits or humans, very low numbers of treponemes can initiate infection which leads to a discernible lesion only after several weeks, although histopathologic changes are evident earlier; intradermal injection of 10^6 organisms usually produces a lesion within 72 h. The number of organisms required for production of symptomatic infection in humans was determined by intradermal injection of three graded doses of *T. pallidum* simultaneously at separate inoculation sites into each of eight volunteers; based upon these results, the infectious dose 50 (ID_{50}) was calculated to be 57 organisms. The median incubation period in humans is about 21 days, suggesting an average inoculum of 500 to 1000 infectious organisms for naturally acquired disease. Experimental inoculations of humans and rabbits show that the period from inoculation until the primary lesion is discernible rarely exceeds 6 weeks. Subcurative therapy during the incubation period may delay the onset of the primary lesion, but it is not certain that this reduces the probability of ultimate development of symptomatic disease.

The primary lesion appears at the site of inoculation, usually persists for 2 to 6 weeks, and then heals spontaneously. Histopathology of primary lesions shows perivascular infiltration, chiefly by lymphocytes (including CD8 + and CD4 + cells), plasma cells, and histiocytes, with capillary endothelial proliferation, and subsequent obliteration of small blood vessels. At this time *T. pallidum* is demonstrable in the chancre in spaces between epithelial cells as well as within invaginations or phagosomes of epithelial cells, fibroblasts, plasma cells, and the endothelial cells of small capillaries, within lymphatic channels, and in the regional lymph nodes. Phagocytosis of organisms by macrophages ultimately causes their destruction.

The generalized parenchymal, constitutional, and mucocutaneous manifestations of secondary syphilis usually appear about 6 to 8 weeks after healing of the chancre, although 15 percent of patients with secondary syphilis have persisting or healing chancres. In other patients, secondary lesions may appear several months after the chancre has healed, and some patients may enter the latent stage without ever developing secondary lesions. Secondary maculopapular skin lesions show histopathologic features of hyperkeratosis of the epidermis, capillary proliferation with endothelial swelling in the superficial corium, and dermal papillae with transmigration of polymorphonuclear leukocytes, and in the deeper corium, perivascular infiltration by monocytes, plasma cells, and lymphocytes. Treponemes are found in many tissues including the aqueous humor of the eye and the cerebrospinal fluid. Cerebrospinal fluid abnormalities are detected in as many as 40 percent of patients during the secondary stage. Clinical hepatitis and immune complex–induced membranous glomerulonephritis are relatively rare but recognized manifestations of secondary syphilis; abnormal liver function tests may be demonstrated in up to 50 percent of patients with early syphilis. Generalized lymphadenopathy is present in 85 percent of patients with secondary syphilis and is characterized by marked follicular hyperplasia, with histiocytic infiltration and lymphocyte depletion of the paracortical areas, where treponema are present in greatest numbers. The reason for the paradoxical appearance of secondary manifestations in the face of high antibody titers (including immobilizing antibody) to *T. pallidum* is unknown. The secondary lesions subside within 2 to 6

weeks, and the patient enters the latent stage, which is detectable only by serologic testing. In the preantibiotic era, up to 25 percent of untreated patients experienced one or more subsequent generalized or localized mucocutaneous relapses at some time during the first 2 to 4 years after infection. Since 90 percent of such infectious relapses occur during the first year, identification and examination of sexual contacts are most important for patients with syphilis of less than 1 year's duration. Recurrent generalized rash is now rare.

In the preantibiotic era, about one-third of patients with untreated latent syphilis developed clinically apparent tertiary disease; today specific and coincidental therapy of early and latent syphilis have greatly reduced the incidence of apparent tertiary disease. In the past, the most common type of tertiary disease was the gumma, a usually benign granulomatous lesion. Today, gummas are very uncommon. The tertiary lesions are caused by obliterative small vessel endarteritis which usually involves the vasa vasorum of the ascending aorta and, less often, the central nervous system. Asymptomatic CNS involvement is demonstrable in up to 25 percent of patients with late latent syphilis. Factors which determine development and progression of tertiary disease are unknown.

The course of untreated syphilis has been studied retrospectively in a group of nearly 2000 patients with primary or secondary syphilis diagnosed clinically, before the dark-field and Wassermann tests came into use (the Oslo Study, 1891–1951); prospectively in 431 black men with seropositive latent syphilis of 3 or more years' duration (the Tuskegee Study, 1932–1972); and retrospectively in a review of 198 autopsies of patients with untreated syphilis (the Rosahn study).

In the Oslo Study, 24 percent of the patients developed relapsing secondary lesions within 4 years, and 28 percent eventually developed one or more manifestations of late syphilis. Cardiovascular syphilis, including aortitis, was detected in 10 percent, with no cases occurring in those infected before age 15; symptomatic neurosyphilis occurred in 7 percent, and 16 percent developed benign tertiary syphilis (gumma of the skin, mucous membranes, and skeleton). Syphilis was the primary cause of death in 15 percent of males and 8 percent of the females. Cardiovascular syphilis was found in 35 percent of men and 22 percent of women who eventually came to autopsy. In general, serious late complications were nearly twice as common in men as in women.

The Tuskegee Study showed that the death rate of untreated syphilitic black men, 25 to 50 years of age, was 17 percent greater than in nonsyphilitics, and 30 percent of all deaths were attributable to cardiovascular or central nervous system syphilis. The ethical issues raised by this study, begun in the preantibiotic era but continuing into the early 1970s, had a major influence on development of current guidelines for human medical experimentation. By far the most important factor in increased mortality was cardiovascular syphilis. Anatomic evidence of aortitis was found in 40 to 60 percent of autopsied syphilitics (versus 15 percent of controls), while CNS syphilis was found in only 4 percent. Hypertension was also increased in the syphilitics. These studies each show that about one-third of patients with untreated syphilis develop clinical or pathologic evidence of tertiary syphilis; about one-fourth die as a direct result of tertiary syphilis; and additional excess mortality not directly attributable to tertiary syphilis is also seen.

MANIFESTATIONS Primary syphilis The typical primary chancre usually begins as a single painless papule which rapidly becomes eroded and usually, but not always, is indurated, with a characteristic cartilagenous consistency on palpation of the edge and base of the ulcer (Fig. 128-1). Histologic examination of the ulcer shows lymphocytic and histiocytic infiltrates with obliterative endarteritis and periarteritis of small vessels. *Treponema pallidum* is seen by electron microscopy to lie in interstitial perivascular spaces and within invaginations or phagosomes of macrophages, neutrophils, endothelial cells, and plasma cells.

The chancre is usually located on the penis in heterosexual men while in homosexual men, it is often found in the anal canal or

FIGURE 128-1 Primary chancre on the penis. (*Reprinted, with permission, from Sexually Transmitted Diseases, Prof. Dr. E. Stolz, Rotterdam, ©Boehringer Ingelheim International, 1977.*)

rectum, within the mouth, or on the external genitalia. In women, common primary sites are the cervix and labia. Consequently primary syphilis may go unrecognized in women or in homosexual men.

Atypical primary lesions are common. The clinical appearance depends upon the number of treponemes inoculated and upon the immunological status of the patient. A large inoculum produces a dark-field–positive ulcerative lesion in nonimmune human volunteers, but in individuals with a previous history of syphilis may produce either a small dark-field–negative papule, an asymptomatic but seropositive latent infection, or no response at all. A small inoculum usually produces only a papular lesion, even in nonimmune humans. Therefore, syphilis should be considered even in the evaluation of trivial or atypical, dark-field–negative, genital lesions. The most common genital lesions which must be differentiated from primary syphilis include traumatic superinfected lesions, genital herpes simplex virus infection (see Chap. 135), and chancroid (see Chap. 117). *Primary genital herpes* may produce inguinal adenopathy, but the nodes are tender and associated with multiple painful vesicles which later ulcerate, and which are often accompanied by systemic symptoms including fever; *recurrent genital herpes* typically begins with a cluster of painful vesicles, usually without associated adenopathy. *Chancroid* produces painful, superficial exudative, nonindurated, more often multiple ulcers; adenopathy is either unilateral or bilateral, is tender, and may suppurate.

Regional lymphadenopathy usually accompanies the primary syphilitic lesion, appearing within 1 week of the onset of the lesion. The nodes are firm, nonsuppurative, and painless. Inguinal lymphadenopathy is bilateral and may occur with anal as well as with external genital chancres, since lymphatic drainage of the anus involves inguinal nodes. Rectal chancres result in perirectal lymphadenopathy, while chancres of the cervix and vagina result in iliac or perirectal adenopathy. The chancre generally heals within 4 to 6 weeks (range 2 to 12 weeks), but the lymphadenopathy may persist for months.

Secondary syphilis The manifestations of the secondary stage are protean but usually include localized or diffuse symmetric mucocutaneous lesions and generalized nontender lymphadenopathy. The healing primary chancre is still present in 15 percent of cases. The skin rash consists of macular, papular, papulosquamous, and occasionally pustular syphilides, often with one or more forms present simultaneously. The eruption may be very subtle, and approximately 25 percent of patients with a discernible rash of secondary syphilis may be unaware that they have dermatologic manifestations. Initial lesions are bilaterally symmetric, pale red or pink, nonpruritic, discrete, round macules, 5 to 10 mm in diameter, distributed on the trunk and proximal extremities (Fig. 128-2). After several days or weeks red, papular lesions 3 to 10 mm in diameter also appear. These

FIGURE 128-2 Maculopapular rash of secondary syphilis. (*Reprinted, with permission, from Sexually Transmitted Diseases, Prof. Dr. E. Stolz, Rotterdam, ©Boehringer Ingelheim International, 1977.*)

may progress to necrotic lesions (resembling pustules) in association with increasing endarteritis and perivascular mononuclear infiltration. These lesions are distributed widely, frequently involve the palms and soles (Fig 128-3), and may occur on the face and scalp. Tiny papular *follicular syphilides* involving hair follicles may result in patchy alopecia (alopecia areata) and loss of scalp hair, eyebrows, or beard in up to 5 percent of patients. Nonpatchy hair loss also occurs in secondary syphilis. Progressive endarteritis obliterans and ischemia result in superficial scaling of papules (*papulosquamous syphilides*) and eventually may lead to central necrosis (*pustular syphilides*). In warm, moist, intertriginous areas, including the perianal area, vulva, scrotum, and inner thighs, axillae, and the skin under

FIGURE 128-3 Secondary rash on palms and soles. [*From Ronald Roddy; reprinted, with permission, from Gynecology and Obstetrics, JW Sciarra (ed), New York, Harper & Row, 1985.*]

pendulous breasts, papules enlarge and become eroded, to produce broad, moist, pink or gray-white highly infectious lesions called *condylomata lata,* which are seen in 10 percent of patients with secondary syphilis. Superficial mucosal erosions, called *mucous patches,* occur in 10 to 15 percent of patients and may involve lips, oral mucosa, tongue (Fig. 128-4), palate, pharynx, vulva and vagina, glans penis, or inner prepuce. The typical mucous patch is a silver-gray erosion surrounded by a red periphery and is usually painless.

During relapses of secondary syphilis, condylomata lata are particularly common, and skin lesions tend to be asymmetrically distributed and more infiltrated, resembling skin lesions of late syphilis, perhaps reflecting increasing cellular immunity.

Constitutional symptoms which may accompany or precede secondary syphilis include sore throat (15 to 30 percent), fever (5 to 8 percent), weight loss (2 to 20 percent), malaise (25 percent), anorexia, headache (10 percent), and meningismus (5 percent). *Acute meningitis* occurs in only 1 to 2 percent of patients, but increased cells and protein have been found in the cerebrospinal fluid in 30 percent or more. *Treponema pallidum* has also been recovered from cerebrospinal fluid during primary and secondary syphilis in 30 percent of patients; this is often correlated with other CSF abnormalities, but may be seen in patients with normal CSF.

Other less common complications of secondary syphilis include hepatitis, nephropathy, gastrointestinal involvement (hypertrophic gastritis, patchy proctitis, ulcerative colitis, or a rectosigmoid mass), arthritis and periostitis, and iridocyclitis. Ocular findings which suggest secondary syphilis include otherwise unexplained pupillary abnormalities, optic neuritis, and a retinitis pigmentosa syndrome, as well as the classic iritis (especially granulomatous iritis) or uveitis. The diagnosis of secondary syphilis is often considered only after failure to respond to steroid therapy. Anterior uveitis has been reported in 5 to 10 percent of patients with secondary syphilis, and *T. pallidum* has been demonstrated in the aqueous humor from these cases. *Syphilitic hepatitis* is distinguished by an unusually high serum alkaline phosphatase and by a nonspecific histologic appearance which is unlike viral hepatitis and includes moderate inflammation with polymorphonuclear leukocytes and lymphocytes, some hepatocellular damage, and no cholestasis. The *renal involvement* is associated with proteinuria, an acute nephrotic syndrome, or rarely with hemorrhagic glomerulonephritis and is characterized by subepithelial electron-dense deposits and glomerular immune complexes, suggesting that this complication is a form of immune complex glomerulonephritis.

Latent syphilis A diagnosis of latent syphilis is established by the finding of a positive specific treponemal antibody test for syphilis, together with a normal cerebrospinal fluid examination and the absence of clinical manifestations of syphilis on physical examination and

chest films. The diagnosis is often suspected on the basis of a history of primary or secondary lesions, history of exposure to syphilis, or delivery of an infant with congenital syphilis. A previous negative serologic test and a history of lesions or exposure may help establish the duration of latent infection. *Early latent* syphilis encompasses the first year after infection, while *late latent* syphilis, beginning 1 year after infection, in the untreated patient, is associated with relative immunity to infectious relapse and with increasing resistance to reinfection. *Treponema pallidum* may still intermittently seed the bloodstream during this stage; pregnant women with latent syphilis may infect the fetus in utero; and transfusion syphilis has been transmitted from patients with latent syphilis of many years' duration. It was thought that untreated late latent syphilis had three possible outcomes: (1) it could persist throughout the life of the infected individual; (2) it could end in development of late syphilis; or (3) it could end with spontaneous cure of infection, with reversion of serologic tests to negative. It is now apparent, however, that the more sensitive treponemal antibody tests rarely if ever become negative. About seventy percent of untreated patients with latent syphilis never develop clinically evident late syphilis, but the occurrence of spontaneous cure is in doubt.

Late syphilis The onset of slowly progressive inflammatory disease leading to the tertiary stage begins early during the pathogenesis of syphilis, although it may not be clinically apparent for years. Evidence of early syphilitic aortitis is present soon after the secondary lesions subside, and it is patients who develop CSF abnormalities during the early stages of syphilis who appear to be at highest risk of late neurologic complications.

ASYMPTOMATIC NEUROSYPHILIS Central nervous system syphilis represents a continuum of early invasion, usually within the first weeks or months of infection, and asymptomatic involvement, which may or may not result in neurologic manifestations. Traditionally, the diagnosis of asymptomatic neurosyphilis has been made in patients who no longer have manifestations of primary or secondary syphilis, who lack neurologic symptoms and signs, and who have certain CSF abnormalities. Such abnormalities are found in up to one-quarter of patients with untreated late latent syphilis, and it is these patients who are known to be at risk for neurologic complications. However, evidence of CNS involvement can include isolation of *T. pallidum* from CSF even in the absence of other CSF abnormalities, and approximately 40 percent of patients with primary and secondary syphilis have had *T. pallidum* isolated from the CSF, abnormalities of the CSF consistent with asymptomatic neurosyphilis, or both. Although the therapeutic implications of these findings in early syphilis are uncertain, it seems appropriate to conclude that patients with early syphilis who have such findings do indeed have asymptomatic neurosyphilis. The risk of progression to symptomatic neurosyphilis is two or three times greater in whites than in blacks and is twice as common in men as in women. The risk of parenchymal neurosyphilis (tabes dorsalis or general paresis) is five times greater in men than in women. In patients with untreated asymptomatic neurosyphilis, the overall cumulative probability of progression to clinical neurosyphilis is about 20 percent in the first 10 years, but increases with passing time, and is highest in those who show the greatest degree of pleocytosis or protein elevation. Patients with untreated latent syphilis and normal CSF probably have no future risk of subsequently developing neurosyphilis.

SYMPTOMATIC NEUROSYPHILIS Although mixed features are common, the major clinical categories of symptomatic neurosyphilis include meningovascular and parenchymatous syphilis. The latter category includes general paresis and tabes dorsalis. The interval from infection to onset of symptoms is a few months to 12 years (average 7 years) for meningovascular syphilis, 20 years for general paresis, and 25 to 30 years for tabes dorsalis. However, many patients with symptomatic neurosyphilis, particularly in the antibiotic era, do not present a classic picture, but have mixed and subtle or incomplete syndromes. *Meningovascular syphilis* is associated with diffuse inflammation of the pia and arachnoid, together with evidence of

FIGURE 128-4 Mucous patches on the tongue. [*From Ronald Roddy; reprinted, with permission, from Sexually Transmitted Diseases, 2d ed, KK Holmes et al (eds), New York, McGraw-Hill, 1990.*]

focal or widespread arterial involvement of small, medium, or large vessels. The most common presentation is a stroke syndrome in a relatively young adult, involving the middle cerebral artery; however, unlike the usual thrombotic or embolic stroke syndrome of sudden onset, meningovascular syphilis often presents after a subacute encephalitic prodrome with headaches, vertigo, insomnia, and psychologic abnormalitics followcd by a gradually progrcssivc vascular syndrome. The manifestations of *general paresis* reflect widespread parenchymal damage and include abnormalities corresponding to the mnemonic *paresis* [*p*ersonality, *a*ffect, *r*eflexes (hyperactive), *e*ye (e.g., Argyll Robertson pupils), *s*ensorium (illusions, delusions, hallucinations), *i*ntellect (decreased recent memory, orientation, calculations, judgment, insight), and *s*peech]. *Tabes dorsalis* presents symptoms and signs of demyelinization of the posterior columns, dorsal roots, and dorsal root ganglia. Symptoms include ataxic, wide-based gait and footslap, paresthesias, bladder disturbances, impotence, areflexia, and loss of position, deep pain, and temperature sensation. Trophic joint degeneration (Charcot's joints) and perforating ulceration of the feet can result from loss of pain sensation. The Argyll Robertson pupil, seen in both tabes dorsalis and paresis, is a small, irregular pupil which reacts to accommodation but not to light. *Optic atrophy* also occurs frequently in association with tabes.

CARDIOVASCULAR SYPHILIS Cardiovascular manifestations are limited to the large vessels in which the blood supply is provided by vasa vasorum. Endarteritis obliterans of the vasa vasorum produces medial necrosis with destruction of elastic tissue, particularly in the ascending and transverse segments of the aortic arch, resulting in uncomplicated aortitis, aortic regurgitation, saccular aneurysm, or coronary ostial stenosis. The onset of symptoms occurs from 10 to 40 years after infection. Cardiovascular complications are more common and occur at an earlier age in men than in women, and in blacks than in whites. The incidence of symptomatic cardiovascular complications in late untreated syphilis is approximately 10 percent, with aortic regurgitation being two to four times as common as aneurysm. However, syphilitic aortitis was demonstrated at autopsy in about one-half of black men with untreated syphilis.

Asymptomatic syphilitic aortitis may be suspected if linear calcification of the ascending aorta is demonstrated on chest x-ray films, since arteriosclerotic disease seldom produces this sign. Aortic dilatation and a tambour quality of thc sound of aortic closurc arc unreliable signs of aortitis. Syphilitic aneurysms are usually saccular, occasionally fusiform, and do not lead to dissection. Approximately 1 in 10 aortic aneurysms of syphilitic origin may involve the abdominal aorta, but tend to occur above the renal arteries, whereas arteriosclerotic abdominal aneurysms usually are found below the renal arteries. With increasing age, the nervous system is also affected in up to 40 percent of patients with cardiovascular syphilis.

LATE LESIONS OF THE EYES Iritis associated with pain, photophobia, and dimness of vision or chorioretinitis occurs not only during secondary syphilis, but also as a relatively common manifestation of late syphilis. Adhesions of the iris to the anterior lens may produce a fixed pupil, not to be confused with Argyll Robertson pupil.

LATE BENIGN SYPHILIS (GUMMA) Gummas may be multiple or diffuse, but are usually solitary lesions which range from microscopic size to several centimeters in diameter, and histologically consist of granulomatous inflammation with central necrosis surrounded by mononuclear, epithelioid, and fibroblastic cells, occasional giant cells, and perivasculitis. Although *T. pallidum* is rarely demonstrated microscopically, it has reportedly been recovered from the lesions. The most commonly involved sites are the skin and skeletal systems, mouth and upper respiratory tract, larynx, liver, and stomach, although any organ may be involved. Gummas of skin produce painless nodular, papulosquamous, or ulcerative lesions, which are indurated, and form characteristic circles or arcs, with peripheral hyperpigmentation. The lesions are usually indolent, and may heal spontaneously with scarring, but may also bc cxplosivc in onset and are often destructive. These lesions may resemble many other chronic granulomatous conditions, including tuberculosis and sarcoidosis, leprosy,

and deep fungal infections. Skeletal gummas involve long bones of the legs with greatest frequency, although any bone may be affected. Trauma may predispose to involvement of a specific site. Presenting symptoms usually include focal pain and tenderness. When sufficiently advanced to produce radiographic abnormalities, the findings may include periostitis or destructive or sclerosing osteitis. Gummas of the upper respiratory tract can lead to perforation of the nasal septum or palate. Gummatous hepatitis may produce epigastric pain and tenderness and low-grade fever, and may be associated with splenomegaly and anemia.

The histopathology and extensive tissue necrosis associated with gummas suggest that delayed hypersensitivity to *T. pallidum* produces these lesions. Certain individuals appear to develop an exaggerated delayed hypersensitivity response to *T. pallidum*, presumably mediated by sensitized T lymphocytes and macrophages. Since the histologic changes may be suggestive but are nonspecific, the diagnosis of late benign syphilis is confirmed by serologic testing and by therapeutic trial. Treatment with penicillin results in rapid healing of active gummatous lesions.

Congenital syphilis Transmission of *T. pallidum* from a syphilitic woman to her fetus across the placenta may occur at any stage of pregnancy, but the lesions of congenital syphilis develop generally after the fourth month of gestation, when immunologic competence begins to develop. This suggests that the pathogenesis of congenital syphilis may depend upon the immune response of the host rather than upon a direct toxic effect of *T. pallidum*. The risk of infection of the fetus during untreated early maternal syphilis is estimated to be 75 to 95 percent, decreasing to about 35 percent for maternal syphilis of longer than 2 years' duration, with the risk of fetal infection apparently continuing throughout late latent maternal syphilis. Adequate treatment of the mother before the sixteenth week of pregnancy should prevent fetal damage. Untreated maternal infection may result in up to 40 percent fetal loss (stillbirth is more common than abortion, because of the late onset of fetal pathology), prematurity, neonatal death, or nonfatal congenital syphilis. Of mothers with untreated syphilis of <2 years' duration, 21 percent aborted or had a stillbirth, 13 percent had infants who died within 2 months, 43 percent had infants with syphilis alive at 2 months, and 23 percent had nonsyphilitic infants. Only fulminant cases of congenital syphilis arc clinically apparcnt in livc infants at birth, and thcse babies have a very poor prognosis. The most common clinical problem is the healthy-appearing baby born to a mother who has a positive serologic test. Routine serologic testing in early pregnancy is considered cost effective in virtually all populations, even in areas of low prenatal prevalence of syphilis. In noncompliant individuals, rapid plasma reagin (RPR) screening should be performed when pregnancy is detected to ensure prompt treatment. Where the prevalence of syphilis is high, and in high-risk patients, syphilis serology should be repeated in the third trimester and at delivery.

The recent dramatic rise in incidence of primary and secondary syphilis in women in the United States, particularly in indigent urban black women, has been accompanied by more than a sixfold increase in congenital syphilis in infants ≤1 year of age from 107 cases in 1978 to 691 in 1988.

The manifestations of congenital syphilis can be divided into (1) early manifestations, which appear within the first 2 years of life, often between 2 and 10 weeks of age, are infectious, and resemble severe secondary syphilis in the adult; (2) late manifestations, which appear after 2 years and are noninfectious; and (3) the residual stigmata of congenital syphilis. During 1988, 92 percent of reported cases of congenital syphilis were diagnosed during the first year of life.

The earliest sign of congenital syphilis is usually rhinitis ("snuffles") soon followed by other mucocutaneous lesions. These may include bullae (syphilitic pemphigus), vesicles, superficial desquamation, pctcchiae, and later, papulosquamous lesions, mucous patches, and condylomata lata. The most common early manifestations are osteochondritis and osteitis, particularly involving the metaphyses of long bones, progressing in severity during the first 6 months of life, then spontaneously subsiding; and periostitis, which continues to progress after the first 6 months. Hepatosplenomegaly, lymphadenopathy, anemia, jaundice, thrombocytopenia, and leukocytosis are common. The anemia is usually hypoproliferative but may be hemolytic (paroxysmal cold hemoglobinuria due to Donath-Landsteiner antibody, an IgG antibody that binds to the P antigen of red cells at low temperatures). The nephrotic syndrome in early congenital syphilis, as in adult secondary syphilis, represents an immune complex–induced glomerulonephritis. A compilation of clinical presentations of congenital syphilis in 9 studies involving a total of 212 infants included abnormal bone x-rays (61 percent), hepatomegaly (51 percent), splenomegaly (49 percent), petechiae (41 percent), other skin rash (35 percent), anemia (34 percent), lymphadenopathy (32 percent), jaundice (30 percent), pseudoparalysis (28 percent), and snuffles (23 percent).

Neonatal congenital syphilis must be differentiated from other generalized congenital infections, including rubella, cytomegalovirus or herpes simplex virus infection, and toxoplasmosis, and also from erythroblastosis fetalis. Neonatal death is usually due to pulmonary hemorrhage, secondary bacterial infection, or severe hepatitis. Pathologic findings include interstitial and perivascular inflammation followed by variable fibroblastic proliferation, involving skin, bones, liver, kidneys, pancreas, spleen, lungs, and intestines, and by extramedullary hematopoiesis.

Late congenital syphilis is defined as congenital syphilis which remains untreated after 2 years of age. In perhaps 60 percent of cases, the infection remains subclinical, while the clinical spectrum in the remainder differs in certain respects from that of acquired late syphilis in the adult. For example, cardiovascular syphilis rarely develops in late congenital syphilis, whereas interstitial keratitis is much more common and occurs between ages 5 and 25. The onset is acute with photophobia, pain, and circumcorneal injection, followed by superficial and deep vascularization of the cornea, which progresses despite antibiotic therapy, and eventually becomes bilateral. The symptoms and signs may be suppressed with glucocorticoid therapy. Although treponemes have occasionally been demonstrated in aqueous humor in interstitial keratitis, the pathogenesis is obscure and is ascribed to "hypersensitivity." Other manifestations associated with interstitial keratitis are eighth-nerve deafness and recurrent arthropathy. Bilateral knee effusions are known as *Clutton's joints*. Examination of CSF discloses asymptomatic neurosyphilis in about one-third of untreated patients without other late clinical manifestations, and clinical neurosyphilis occurs in a quarter of untreated individuals with congenital syphilis over 6 years of age. The clinical manifestations of congenital neurosyphilis correspond to those seen in adult neurosyphilis. Gummatous periostitis occurs between ages 5 and 20 and, as in nonvenereal endemic childhood syphilis, tends to cause destructive lesions of the palate and nasal septum.

Characteristic stigmata include *Hutchinson's teeth*, the centrally notched, widely spaced, peg-shaped upper central incisors, and "mulberry" molars, sixth-year molars which have multiple, poorly developed cusps, numbering more than the usual four. The abnormal facies of congenital syphilis, which includes frontal bossing, saddlenose, and poorly developed maxilla, may also be seen in congenital ectodermal dysplasia. Saber shins, or anterior tibial bowing, are rare but were probably more common in the past when syphilitic periostitis of the anterior tibia was accompanied by vitamin D deficiency. *Rhagades* are linear scars at the angles of the mouth and nose caused by secondary bacterial infection of the early facial eruption. Other stigmata include unexplained nerve deafness, old chorioretinitis, optic atrophy, and corneal opacities due to past interstitial keratitis.

LABORATORY EXAMINATIONS   Dark-field examination technique   Dark-field examination is essential in evaluating cutaneous lesions, such as the chancre of primary syphilis, or condylomata lata of secondary syphilis. Although it is often difficult to demonstrate *T. pallidum* in dry maculopapular lesions in secondary syphilis by dark-field examination, the organism may be demonstrated by saline

aspiration of lymph nodes during this stage. The surface of the suspected ulcerated lesion should be cleaned with saline and gauze, then gently abraded further with dry gauze, without production of bleeding. The lesion is then squeezed to express a serous transudate, and a drop of the transudate is picked up on the surface of a glass slide. A drop of saline (without bacteriostatic additives) may be mixed with the transudate if necessary, and this is then covered with a coverslip and examined immediately for *T. pallidum* with a dark-field or phase contrast microscope by an experienced individual. The identification of a single characteristic motile organism by a trained observer is sufficient for diagnosis. Examination of oral lesions by this method is not recommended, and it is also difficult to differentiate *T. pallidum* from other spirochetes that may be present in anal ulcers. A single negative examination does not exclude syphilis, since at least 10^4 treponemes per microliter of transudate must be present to be seen, and prior use of topical antiseptic or cleansing by the patient may obfuscate the results. Cleansing or use of topical medication should, therefore, be avoided, and ideally the dark-field examination should be repeated on three successive days before being considered negative.

Direct immunofluorescence   Most syphilis is diagnosed in private physicians' offices where dark-field microscopy is not available; alternative methods for the identification of *T. pallidum* in exudate are needed. The direct fluorescent antibody *T. pallidum* (DFA-TP) test, available at central laboratories, uses fluorescein-conjugated polyclonal antitreponemal antibody for detection of *T. pallidum* in fixed smears prepared from suspect lesions. Because of cross-reactive antibodies which will also stain commensal nonpathogenic spirochetes, the antiserum is extensively absorbed with cultured treponemes in an effort to produce a specific reagent.

A refinement of this technique using a monoclonal antibody which is specific for only the pathogenic treponemes has been developed, but is not yet commercially available. It has been shown in clinical trials to be as sensitive and specific as dark-field microscopy for examination of suspicious lesions.

Demonstration of *T. pallidum* in tissue   It is often necessary to demonstrate *T. pallidum* in tissue when clinical or histopathologic features suggest the diagnosis of syphilis. Although the organism can be found in tissue by appropriate silver stains, these should be interpreted with caution, because artifacts resembling *T. pallidum* are often seen. Treponemes can be demonstrated more reliably in tissue by immunofluorescence, using specific monoclonal or polyclonal antibodies against *T. pallidum*.

Serologic tests for syphilis   The profusion of serologic tests for syphilis causes much unnecessary confusion. Syphilitic infection produces two types of antibodies, the nonspecific *reaginic* antibody and specific antitreponemal antibody, which are measured by the nontreponemal and treponemal tests, respectively (Table 128-1). The treponemal tests, as well as the nontreponemal tests, are reactive in persons with any treponemal infection, including yaws, pinta, and endemic syphilis.

The nontreponemal antibodies produced in syphilis contain both IgG and IgM immunoglobulins directed against a lipoidal antigen that results from the interaction of *T. pallidum* with host tissues, and possibly against a lipoidal antigen of *T. pallidum* itself. The term *reagin* is unfortunate, since the unrelated IgE antibody involved in

---

TABLE 128-1   Common serologic tests for syphilis

Nontreponemal (reagin) tests
  Microscopic flocculation: Venereal Disease Research Laboratory (VDRL)
  Macroscopic flocculation: rapid plasma reagin (RPR)

Treponemal tests
  Immunofluorescence: fluorescent treponemal antibody-absorption (FTA-ABS)
  Hemagglutination: *T. pallidum* hemagglutination assay (MHA-TP, HATTS, TPHA)
  Immobilization: *Treponema pallidum* immobilization (TPI)

certain allergic phenomena is also known as reagin. The most widely used nontreponemal or reagin antibody tests for syphilis are the RPR test, which can be automated (ART), and the Venereal Disease Research Laboratory (VDRL) slide test. Other less frequently used nontreponemal tests include the unheated serum reagin (USR) and the reagin screen test (RST). In these tests, antibody is detected by the microscopic (VDRL, USR) or macroscopic (RPR, RST) flocculation of the antigen suspension (Table 128-1).

The RPR is often more expensive than the VDRL test but is easier to perform and uses unheated serum; it is the test of choice for rapid serologic diagnosis in a clinic or office setting. The VDRL reagents are less expensive, but must be prepared fresh daily. Although the development of the simpler macroscopic tests has resulted in the replacement of the VDRL by the RPR for examination of serum in many laboratories, the VDRL test remains the standard test for use with cerebrospinal fluid.

RPR and VDRL tests are equally sensitive and may be used for initial screening or for quantitation of serum reagin antibody titer. The reagin titer reflects the activity of the disease: a fourfold or greater rise in titer may be seen during the evolution of primary syphilis; VDRL titers usually reach 1:32 or higher in secondary syphilis; a persistent fall in titer following treatment of early syphilis provides essential evidence of an adequate response to therapy. VDRL titers do not correspond directly to RPR titers, and sequential quantitative testing (as for response to therapy) must employ a single test.

There are three standard treponemal tests: the fluorescent treponemal antibody-absorption (FTA-ABS), the microhemagglutination assay for antibodies to *T. pallidum* (MHA-TP), and the hemagglutination treponemal test for syphilis (HATTS). A third hemagglutination test, the TPHA is not available in the United States.

For the FTA-ABS test, the patient's serum is first diluted with a substance containing nonpathogenic treponemal antigens (sorbent) to bind group-specific antibodies which may be produced against saprophytic oral and genital treponemes. The patient's absorbed serum is then placed on a slide which contains fixed *T. pallidum*. If specific antibody to *T. pallidum* is present in the patient's serum, it is bound to the dried treponemes and is then detected by the addition of fluorescein-labeled antihuman gamma globulin and subsequent examination of the slide by fluorescence microscopy. The *T. pallidum* hemagglutination tests (MHA-TP, HATTS, and TPHA) also use a sorbent-like diluent for binding treponemal group antibodies. *T. pallidum*-specific antibody is detected by agglutination of *T. pallidum*-coated sheep or turkey erythrocytes. These hemagglutination tests are more commonly used than the FTA-ABS test. The *T. pallidum* immobilization (TPI) test, in which immobilization of live *T. pallidum* is produced by immune serum plus complement, is the most specific treponemal test, but is more laborious, and in the United States is available only in research laboratories. Both the hemagglutination and FTA-ABS tests are very specific and, when used for confirmation of positive reaginic antibody tests, have a very high positive predictive value for the diagnosis of syphilis. However, even these tests give false-positive rates as high as 1 to 2 percent when used for screening normal populations.

The relative sensitivities of the VDRL, FTA-ABS, and MHA-TP tests in the various stages of syphilis are shown in Table 128-2. The nontreponemal tests are nonreactive in nearly one-third of patients with primary or late syphilis. In early primary syphilis, the detection of antibody can be maximized either by performing an FTA-ABS test or simply by repeating a VDRL test after 1 to 2 weeks if the initial VDRL was negative. However, obtaining a reagin antibody test alone is not sufficient in evaluating late symptomatic syphilis; the more sensitive FTA-ABS test should be obtained routinely in suspected late syphilis. The hemagglutination tests are even less sensitive than the reagin tests in primary syphilis, but are as sensitive as the FTA-ABS in other stages. All treponemal and nontreponemal tests are reactive during secondary syphilis, and a nonreactive result virtually excludes syphilis in a patient with otherwise compatible

TABLE 128-2 Reactivity of serodiagnostic tests in untreated syphilis

| Test | Stage of disease, % positive* | | | |
	Primary	Secondary	Latent	Tertiary
VDRL	59–87	100	73–91	37–94
FTA-ABS	86–100	99–100	96–99	96–100
MHA-TP	64–87	96–100	96–100	94–100

* Percentage figures provided should not be interpreted as absolute values because there are small numbers in certain categories and test results vary from study to study.
SOURCE: Modified (with permission) from H Jaffe, D Musher, Management of the reactive syphilis serology, in *Sexually Transmitted Diseases*, KK Holmes et al (eds) 2d ed. New York, McGraw-Hill, 1990, p 935.

mucocutaneous lesions. (Less than 1 percent of patients with secondary syphilis have a nonreactive or weakly reactive VDRL test with undiluted serum which becomes positive in higher dilutions—the *prozone* phenomenon.) While the nontreponemal tests will become negative or decline in titer following therapy for early syphilis, the treponemal tests will usually remain reactive after therapy and are not helpful in determining the infection status in persons with past syphilis.

The presence of specific IgM antibody has been proposed as a marker for active syphilis, with the claim that IgM disappears following adequate therapy. The rate at which IgM declines after therapy is quite variable from patient to patient, and the use of this criterion for cure is not universally accepted. No IgM test for syphilis has been approved for use by the Centers for Disease Control.

False-positive serologic tests for syphilis Because the antigen used in the nontreponemal tests is found in other tissues, the tests may be reactive in persons without treponemal infection, although rarely in titers exceeding 1:8. In a population which has been selected for screening because of clinical suspicion, history of exposure, or increased risk for sexually transmitted infections, the percentage of reactive tests which are falsely positive is less than 2 percent. False-positive reagin tests are classified as acute if they become negative within 6 months and may occur during a variety of acute infections, such as viral diseases, mycoplasma pneumonia, and malaria, and following certain immunizations. Chronic reactions, which persist 6 months or longer, occur in intravenous drug addiction, autoimmune diseases, and aging. False-positive reagin tests occur in 25 percent of narcotic addicts, and in 10 to 20 percent of patients with active systemic lupus erythematosus. The autoimmune nature of the false-positive reagin test is suggested by the occurrence of systemic lupus erythematosus or other connective tissue diseases in 15 to 45 percent of chronic false-positive reactors. Other antibodies which have been found with great frequency in sera from chronic false-positive reactors include antinuclear, antithyroid, and antimitochondrial antibodies, as well as rheumatoid factor and cryoglobulins. The Donath-Landsteiner antibody responsible for paroxysmal cold hemoglobinuria is an autoimmune hemolysin which appears in syphilis. The prevalence of false-positive reagin tests increases with advancing age, and 10 percent of people over 70 years of age have false-positive reactions. Other diseases associated with hyperglobulinemia, such as leprosy, may also produce chronic false-positive reactions.

In the patient with a false-positive reagin test, syphilis is excluded by obtaining a nonreactive treponemal test. A typical *reactive* FTA-ABS occurs infrequently in conditions other than syphilis. Although false-positive FTA-ABS tests have been reported in 15 percent of patients with active systemic lupus erythematosus, the fluorescent staining is often weak or has an atypical "beaded" appearance. For practical purposes, most clinicians need to be familiar with the three uses of serologic tests for syphilis: (1) for testing large numbers of sera for screening or diagnostic purposes (e.g., RPR or VDRL); (2) for quantitative measurement of reaginic antibody titer in order to assess the clinical activity of syphilis, or to follow the reagin titer in response to therapy (e.g., VDRL or RPR); and (3) for confirmation of the diagnosis of syphilis in a patient with a positive reagin antibody test or with a suspected clinical diagnosis of syphilis (e.g., FTA-ABS, MHA-TP, HATTS).

Evaluation for asymptomatic neurosyphilis   Asymptomatic involvement of the central nervous system is detected by examination of cerebrospinal fluid. CSF abnormalities are very infrequent in the primary stage, but pleocytosis or elevated protein can be demonstrated in CSF from up to 40 percent of patients with secondary or latent syphilis. *T. pallidum* has been recovered by rabbit inoculation from up to 40 percent of those with secondary syphilis, but rarely from those with latent syphilis. The demonstration of *T. pallidum* in CSF is often associated with other CSF abnormalities; however, organisms can be recovered from patients without pleocytosis or elevated protein. In the prepenicillin era, the risk of developing clinical neurosyphilis was roughly proportional to the intensity of spinal fluid changes in early syphilis. CSF examination is essential in any seropositive patient with neurologic signs and symptoms and is recommended in all patients with untreated syphilis of unknown duration or of greater than 1 year's duration. The possibility that asymptomatic neurosyphilis is present in some patients with secondary and early latent disease is not addressed by these recommendations. Because standard penicillin G benzathine (benzathine benzylpenicillin) therapy for early syphilis fails to achieve treponemicidal levels in the CSF, some experts advise lumbar puncture in secondary and early latent syphilis, with follow-up examinations for patients with abnormalities.

CSF is examined for pleocytosis, increased protein concentration, and VDRL reactivity. The CSF-VDRL is very specific if the fluid is not contaminated with blood. The CSF-VDRL is relatively insensitive, however, and may be nonreactive even in progressive symptomatic neurosyphilis. Highest sensitivities are seen in meningovascular syphilis and paresis; lower sensitivities are seen in asymptomatic neurosyphilis and tabes dorsalis. The unabsorbed FTA test on cerebrospinal fluid is reactive far more often than the CSF-VDRL test in all stages of syphilis, but may reflect passive transfer of serum antibody into the CSF. Most specialists do not recommend performing an FTA test on spinal fluid. Similarly, the finding of a reactive CSF-FTA-ABS test without other cerebrospinal fluid abnormalities in a patient with nonspecific neurologic findings does not prove a diagnosis of neurosyphilis. Even in the absence of confirmatory CSF examination, a therapeutic trial of penicillin in doses adequate for neurosyphilis is warranted in any patient with a positive serum treponemal antibody test who also has neurologic findings consistent with neurosyphilis.

Attempts to identify a more sensitive and specific marker for neurosyphilis have included CSF oligoclonal banding and measurement of intrathecal production of antitreponemal IgM and IgG. CSF from 80 percent of patients with multiple sclerosis and approximately 40 percent of patients with other inflammatory CNS diseases (including neurosyphilis, bacterial meningitis, viral encephalitis, subacute sclerosing panencephalitis) have discrete oligoclonal immunoglobulin bands in the gamma globulin region following agarose gel electrophoresis of CSF. These antibodies are thought to be intrathecally produced and have specificity for the etiologic agent (e.g., *T. pallidum* in syphilis and measles virus in subacute sclerosing panencephalitis); however, an oligoclonal banding pattern per se is not specific for neurosyphilis in a seropositive patient.

Evaluation for syphilis in patients concurrently infected with human immunodeficiency virus (HIV)   Because persons at highest risk for acquiring syphilis (inner city populations and homosexually active men) are also at high risk for acquisition of HIV, these infections are frequently found in the same patient. There is evidence that syphilis and other genital ulcer diseases may be important risk factors for acquisition and transmission of HIV infection. Several studies propose that the manifestations of syphilis may be altered in patients with concurrent HIV infection; and multiple cases of neurologic relapse following standard therapy have been reported in HIV-infected patients. *T. pallidum* has been isolated from the CSF of patients following therapy for early syphilis with penicillin G benzathine. One case of VDRL and FTA-ABS seronegative secondary syphilis has been reported in a patient with AIDS; this patient finally seroconverted prior to therapy after weeks of secondary manifestations. HIV-infected patients with unusually high VDRL or RPR titers have also been described. The implications of these studies are numerous and alarming, but the nature and extent of the interaction between HIV infection and syphilis has not been well defined. The frequency of unusual clinical and laboratory manifestations of syphilis in patients coinfected with HIV is unknown, and such changes may be dependent upon the stage of HIV infection and degree of immunosuppression.

The evaluation of all syphilis patients should include serologic testing for HIV, with the patient's consent. Conversely, persons with newly diagnosed HIV infection should be tested for syphilis. Examination of CSF for evidence of neurosyphilis is recommended by some authorities for all coinfected patients, regardless of the clinical stage of syphilis. If CSF abnormalities are found, or if CSF examination is not performed, therapy adequate for neurosyphilis should be administered regardless of the apparent stage of infection. Serologic testing following treatment is important for all patients with syphilis, and particularly for those also infected with HIV.

TREATMENT OF ACQUIRED SYPHILIS   Penicillin G is the drug of choice for all stages of syphilis. *Treponema pallidum* is killed by very low concentrations of penicillin G, although a long period of exposure to penicillin is required for treatment because of the unusually slow rate of multiplication of the organism. The efficacy of penicillin for syphilis remains undiminished after nearly 50 years of use. Other antibiotics which are effective in syphilis include the tetracyclines, erythromycin, and the cephalosporins. Aminoglycosides and spectinomycin inhibit *T. pallidum* only in very large doses, and the sulfonamides and the quinolones are inactive. The optimal dose and duration of therapy have not been definitively established for any antimicrobial for any stage of syphilis.

It is necessary to achieve serum levels of penicillin G of 0.03 μg/mL or more for at least 7 days to cure early syphilis. Recurrence rates for a given regimen increase as infection progresses from incubating syphilis to seronegative primary to seropositive primary to secondary to late syphilis. Therefore it is probable, but unproved, that a longer duration of therapy is required to effect cure as the infection progresses. For these reasons some authorities use more prolonged penicillin therapy than that recommended by the U.S. Public Health Service when treating secondary, latent, or late syphilis.

The treatment regimens recommended for syphilis are summarized in Table 128-3 and described below.

Early syphilis   Preventive (abortive, "epidemiologic") treatment is recommended for seronegative individuals without signs of syphilis who were exposed to infectious syphilis within the previous 6 weeks. Before treatment is given, every effort should be made to establish a diagnosis by examination and serologic testing. *The regimens recommended for preventive treatment are the same as those recommended for early syphilis.*

For patients without known exposure to syphilis but who are undergoing treatment for other STDs, most currently recommended STD regimens involving beta lactam or tetracycline antibiotics are probably also effective for very early incubating syphilis. It is likely that the regimen currently recommended for treating gonorrhea [ceftriaxone 250 mg intramuscularly followed by doxycycline or tetracycline orally for 1 week (see Chap. 110)] is effective against incubating syphilis.

Penicillin G benzathine is the most widely used form of treatment for early syphilis, including primary, secondary, and early latent syphilis, although it is more painful on injection than penicillin G procaine. A single dose of 2.4 million units cures over 95 percent of cases of primary syphilis. Because efficacy for secondary syphilis may be slightly lower, some physicians administer a second dose of 2.4 million units 1 week after the initial dose for secondary syphilis. There are reports of treatment failure following penicillin G benzathine in patients coinfected with HIV and early syphilis. Therapeutic recommendations should be guided by knowledge of CSF abnormal-

TABLE 128-3 Recommendations for therapy of syphilis*

Stage of syphilis	Patients without penicillin allergy	Patients with confirmed penicillin allergy
Primary, secondary, or early latent	Benzathine penicillin G, 2.4 million units single dose IM (1.2 million units in each buttock).	Tetracycline hydrochloride, 500 mg PO 4 times daily; or doxycycline, 100 mg PO twice daily, for two weeks.
Late latent (or latent of uncertain duration), cardiovascular, or benign tertiary	Lumbar puncture CSF normal: Benzathine penicillin G, 2.4 million units IM weekly for 3 weeks. CSF abnormal: Treat as neurosyphilis.	Lumbar puncture CSF normal: Tetracycline hydrochloride, 500 mg PO 4 times daily, or doxycycline, 100 mg PO twice daily, for 4 weeks. CSF abnormal: Treat as neurosyphilis.
Neurosyphilis† (asymptomatic or symptomatic)	Aqueous penicillin G, 12–24 million units per day IV for 10–14 days. *Or* Aqueous procaine penicillin G, 2.4 million units IM daily plus oral probenecid 500 mg 4 times each day, both for 10–14 days.	Confirm penicillin allergy by skin-testing. If confirmed, desensitize and treat with penicillin.
Syphilis in pregnancy	According to stage.	Confirm penicillin allergy by skin-testing. If confirmed, desensitize and treat with penicillin.

* See test for discussion of syphilis therapy in HIV-infected individuals.
† Some authorities recommend following these regimens with three doses of 2.4 million units of benazathine penicillin G, given IM one week apart. Benzathine penicillin G alone has given inferior results for treatment of neurosyphilis. Drugs other than penicillin are not recommended. Many patients who give a history of penicillin allergy prove negative when skin-tested for immediate hypersensitivity to penicillin and could be given aqueous crystalline penicillin G for CNS syphilis under close supervision in the hospital. Certain third generation cephalosporins (e.g., ceftriaxone, cefotaxime) have some promise for certain penicillin-allergic patients with CNS syphilis but require further evaluation.
SOURCE: These recommendations are modified from Centers for Disease Control, 1989.

ities in such patients. CSF examination in HIV-seropositive individuals with syphilis of any stage is recommended. Patients without HIV infection may also benefit from CSF examination. Some experts recommend treatment with regimens effective against neurosyphilis for all HIV-seropositive individuals with syphilis of any stage.

Late latent and late syphilis Recommended treatment for late latent syphilis with normal CSF, for cardiovascular syphilis, and for late benign syphilis (gumma) is penicillin G benzathine, 2.4 million units intramuscularly once a week for 3 successive weeks (7.2 million units total). Lumbar puncture should be performed in the evaluation of latent syphilis of more than 1 year's duration, in suspected neurosyphilis, and also in late complications other than symptomatic neurosyphilis, since asymptomatic neurosyphilis may coexist with other late complications. Abnormal cerebrospinal fluid findings can then be followed serially as a guide to therapy.

In older asymptomatic individuals, the yield of lumbar puncture is relatively low. CSF examination is most clearly indicated in the following situations: neurologic signs or symptoms; treatment failure; serum reagin titer $\geq$ 1:32; HIV antibody–positive; other evidence of active syphilis (e.g., aortitis, gumma, visual or hearing changes); or nonpenicillin therapy planned.

No studies of penicillin G benzathine for cardiovascular syphilis have been reported, and the efficacy of penicillin therapy in any form for cardiovascular syphilis has not been proved. The response of cardiovascular syphilis to penicillin is seldom dramatic because aortic aneurysm and aortic regurgitation cannot be reversed by antibiotic treatment, although further progression of these lesions may be arrested. In contrast, the response of benign tertiary syphilis and of meningovascular syphilis to penicillin G is usually impressive. The response of parenchymal neurosyphilis has been variable. In a cooperative study of the treatment of 1086 general paretics with penicillin, the frequency of clinical improvement or termination of progression ranged from 38 percent of those with severe involvement to 81 percent of those with mild involvement. Tabes dorsalis or optic atrophy responds less often. In general, treatment of inactive neurosyphilis in which neurologic damage has already occurred may not produce any clinical change, and retreatment of such cases is not warranted. However, persistence of cerebrospinal fluid pleocytosis, or recurrence of pleocytosis following initial response to treatment, indicates continuing active infection, which should respond to additional treatment. The 1989 Centers for Disease Control treatment guidelines for neurosyphilis are presented in Table 128-3. Because penicillin G benzathine given in doses of up to 7.2 million units to adults or 50,000 units per kilogram to infants does not produce

detectable concentrations of penicillin G in cerebrospinal fluid, this form of penicillin is unreliable for the treatment of neurosyphilis in the adult or infant, and asymptomatic neurosyphilis has been found to relapse in up to one-quarter of patients treated with 2.4 million units of penicillin G benzathine. Therefore use of penicillin G benzathine alone for treatment of neurosyphilis is not recommended. On the other hand, administration of intravenous penicillin G in doses of 12 million units or more per day for 10 days or longer ensures treponemicidal concentrations of penicillin G in cerebrospinal fluid, and occasionally cures patients who failed to respond to conventional therapy. There are no data to support the use of antibiotics other than penicillin G for the treatment of neurosyphilis; however, some of the third-generation cephalosporins (e.g., ceftriaxone, cefotaxime) may deserve further evaluation. In patients with penicillin allergy documented by skin testing, desensitization may be the best course (see Chap. 90).

Management of syphilis in pregnancy Every pregnant woman should be tested with a nontreponemal test at her first prenatal visit, and women who are at high risk for acquiring sexually transmitted diseases should have a repeat test in the third trimester and at delivery. In the pregnant patient with presumed syphilis, evidenced by a reactive serology, with or without clinical manifestations, and with no history of treatment for syphilis, expeditious evaluation and initiation of treatment is essential. Therapy should be administered according to stage of the disease, as for nonpregnant patients. Patients should be warned of the risk of a Jarisch-Herxheimer reaction, which is often associated with mild premature contractions but rarely results in premature delivery.

Penicillin is the only recommended therapy for syphilis in pregnancy. If the patient has well-documented penicillin allergy, and this is confirmed by demonstration of an immediate wheal-and-flare response to skin testing with penicilloyl polylysine or penicillin G minor determinant mixture, desensitization should be carried out in a hospital using the 1989 STD guidelines issued by the Centers for Disease Control. After treatment, a quantitative reagin test should be repeated monthly throughout pregnancy, and if a fourfold rise in titer occurs, treatment should be repeated. Treated women who do not show a fourfold decrease in titer in a 3-month period should also be retreated.

Evaluation and management of congenital syphilis Newborn infants of mothers with reactive VDRL or FTA-ABS tests may themselves have reactive tests, whether or not they have become infected, because of transplacental transfer of maternal IgG antibody. Rising or persistent titers indicate infection, and the infant should be treated. If the seropositive mother received inadequate penicillin treatment or treatment other than penicillin, or her treatment status is unknown, or if the infant may be difficult to follow, the infant should be treated at birth. It is unwise to require proof of diagnosis before treatment in such cases. The CSF should be examined as a baseline before treatment of such infants. Penicillin is the only recommended drug for syphilis in infants. The calculation of penicillin dosage for treatment of late congenital syphilis is the same as that used in the infant, until dosage based upon weight reaches that used for adult neurosyphilis. Specific recommendations for treatment of infants can be found in the 1989 Centers for Disease Control treatment guidelines. Neonatal IgM antibody can be detected in cord or neonatal serums in a modified FTA-ABS test, employing fluorescein-labeled antihuman IgM to detect antitreponemal IgM antibody. However, the specificity of this test is questionable because of evidence that infants with a variety of congenital infections may produce IgM antibody to maternal allotypes of IgG (rheumatoid factor). IgM antibody detected in the IgM-FTA-ABS test may then be directed against maternal IgG antibody bound specifically to *T. pallidum*, rather than against *T. pallidum* itself. Because of the questionable sensitivity and specificity of this test, the IgM-FTA-ABS is not currently recommended. Instead, monthly quantitative reagin tests are performed on asymptomatic infants born to women who were treated adequately with penicillin during pregnancy.

Jarisch-Herxheimer reaction A dramatic reaction consisting of fever (average temperature elevation, 1.5°C), chills, myalgias, headache, tachycardia, increased respiratory rate, increased circulating neutrophil count (average total white blood cell count, 12,500 per microliter), and vasodilatation with mild hypotension, may occur following initiation of treatment for syphilis. This reaction occurs in approximately 50 percent of patients with primary syphilis, 90 percent with secondary, and 25 percent with early latent syphilis. The onset occurs within 2 h of treatment, the peak temperature occurs at about 7 h, and defervescence takes place within 12 to 24 h. The reaction is more delayed in neurosyphilis, with peak fever occurring after 12 to 14 h. In patients with secondary syphilis, an increase in erythema and edema of the mucocutaneous lesions occurs; occasionally subclinical or early mucocutaneous lesions may first become apparent during the reaction. The pathogenesis of this reaction is controversial. Patients should be warned to expect such symptoms, which can be managed by bed rest and aspirin. The Jarisch-Herxheimer reaction in neurosyphilis or cardiovascular syphilis has, on very rare occasions, been associated with acute progression of irreversible organ damage.

Follow-up evaluation of responses to therapy for all stages of syphilis The response of early syphilis to treatment should be determined by following the quantitative VDRL titer 1, 3, 6, and 12 months after treatment. More frequent serologic examination (1, 2, 3, 6, 9, and 12 months) is recommended for patients concurrently infected with HIV. Because the FTA-ABS and hemagglutination tests remain positive in nearly all patients treated for seropositive early syphilis, these tests are not useful in following the response to therapy. After successful treatment of seropositive primary or secondary syphilis, the VDRL titer progressively declines, becoming negative within 3 to 12 months in about 75 percent of seropositive primary cases and 40 percent of secondary cases. Two years after treatment for primary syphilis, nearly all patients have a negative VDRL, although 25 percent of secondary cases and a higher proportion of those treated for early latent syphilis maintain low reagin titers. If the VDRL becomes negative or reaches a fixed low titer within 1 or 2 years, performing a lumbar puncture is unnecessary at that time, since the spinal fluid examination is almost invariably normal and there is little risk of subsequent neurosyphilis. However, if a VDRL titer of 1:8 or more fails to fall at least fourfold within 12 months, if the VDRL titer rises fourfold, or if clinical symptoms persist or recur, retreatment is indicated. Every effort should be made to differentiate treatment failure from reinfection, and the CSF should be examined. Suspected treatment failures, especially those with abnormal CSF, should be treated as described for neurosyphilis. If

the patient remains seropositive but asymptomatic after such retreatment, no further therapy is necessary. Patients treated for late latent syphilis frequently have a low-titered VDRL prior to therapy and may not demonstrate a fourfold drop following therapy with penicillin; about half of these patients remain seropositive in low titer for years following therapy. Retreatment is not warranted unless the titer rises or signs and symptoms of syphilis recur.

The activity of neurosyphilis correlates best with the degree of cerebrospinal fluid pleocytosis. Changes in the cerebrospinal fluid cell count, and to a lesser extent, in cerebrospinal fluid protein concentration, provide the most sensitive index of response to treatment. Spinal fluid examination should be performed every 3 to 6 months for 3 years after treatment of asymptomatic or symptomatic neurosyphilis. An elevated cerebrospinal fluid cell count falls to 10 or less per microliter within 3 to 12 months in 95 percent of adequately treated cases, and becomes normal in all cases within 2 to 4 years. Elevated levels of cerebrospinal fluid protein fall more slowly, and the CSF reagin titer declines slowly over a period of several years.

Persistence of treponemal forms The persistence of *T. pallidum* in the aqueous humor, CSF, lymph nodes, brain, inflamed temporal arteries, and other tissues following "adequate" penicillin treatment of latent or late syphilis has been suggested by dark-field microscopy, immunofluorescent antibody and silver staining techniques, and rabbit inoculation. Because the data on persisting treponemes are scanty, no modification of the treatment recommendations for latent or late syphilis seems warranted. Adherence to recommendations regarding CSF examination prior to selection of therapy should minimize the possibility of *T. pallidum* persistence.

IMMUNITY AND PREVENTION OF SYPHILIS Only about 50 percent of the named contacts of primary and secondary syphilis become infected, but the actual risk of infection from a single exposure is probably much lower. The rate of development of acquired resistance to *T. pallidum* following natural or experimental infection is quantitatively related to the amount of the antigenic stimulus, which depends upon both the size of the infecting inoculum and the duration of infection prior to treatment. The role of serum antibody in conferring immunity to syphilis remains controversial. Reagin antibody is not protective. Passively administered antibody from rabbits recovering from experimental syphilis prevents or delays appearance of clinical manifestations of syphilis; it does not prevent infection. Cellular immunity is considered to be of major importance in the healing of early lesions and control of syphilis infection. The cellular infiltration of early lesions is predominantly composed of T lymphocytes and macrophages, and specifically sensitized T lymphocytes develop early in the course of infection in humans and experimentally infected rabbits.

Inability to cultivate pathogenic treponemes in vitro has hindered analysis, purification, and concentration of treponemal antigens. Attempts to induce immunity to syphilis by vaccination have shown limited promise, although several specific antigens have been identified and characterized. The outer membrane of *T. pallidum* contains few integral membrane proteins, although many of the major antigens appear to be proteolipins, which may be associated via their lipid tail with the outer membrane. Repeated injection of rabbits with gamma-irradiated motile strains has conferred immunity to a rechallenge. The prevention of syphilis depends upon use of condoms, antiseptic prophylactic agents, and detection and treatment of infectious cases.

REFERENCES

BERRY CD et al: Neurologic relapse after benzathine penicillin therapy for secondary syphilis in a patient with HIV infection. N Engl J Med 316:1587, 1987

BRYCESON ADM: Clinical pathology of the Jarisch-Herxheimer reaction. J Infect Dis 133:696, 1976

CENTERS FOR DISEASE CONTROL: Guidelines for the prevention and control of congenital syphilis. Morb Mort Week Rep (Suppl) 37(S-1):1, 1988

————: Recommendations for diagnosing and treating syphilis in HIV-infected individuals. Morb Mort Week Rep 37:600, 1988

————: 1989 Sexually transmitted diseases treatment guidelines. Morb Mort Week Rep 38(Suppl 8):1, 1989

Chapel T: The signs and symptoms of secondary syphilis. Sex Trans Dis 7:161, 1980

Fiumara NJ: Treatment of primary and secondary syphilis: Serologic response. JAMA 243:2500, 1980

Greene BM et al: Failure of penicillin G benzathine in the treatment of neurosyphilis. Arch Intern Med 140:1117, 1980

Hook EW III et al: Detection of *Treponema pallidum* in lesion exudate with a pathogen-specific monoclonal antibody. J Clin Microbiol 22:241, 1985

Hotson JR: Modern neurosyphilis: A partially treated chronic meningitis. West J Med 135:191, 1981

Luger A et al: Diagnosis of neurosyphilis by examination of the cerebrospinal fluid. Br J Vener Dis 57:232, 1981

Lukehart SA et al: Characterization of lymphocyte responsiveness in early experimental syphilis: II. Nature of cellular infiltration and *Treponema pallidum* distribution in testicular infection. J Immunol 124:461, 1980

———— et al: Invasion of the central nervous system by *Treponema pallidum*: Implications for diagnosis and treatment. Ann Intern Med 109:855, 1988

Mascola L et al: Congenital syphilis. Why is it still occurring? JAMA 252:17, 1984

Mohr JA et al: Neurosyphilis and penicillin in cerebrospinal fluid. JAMA 236:2208, 1976

Muller F, Moskophidis M: Estimation of the local production of antibodies to *Treponema pallidum* in the central nervous system of patients with neurosyphilis. Br J Vener Dis 59:80, 1983

Radolf JD et al: Outer membrane ultrastructure explains the limited antigenicity of virulent *Treponema pallidum*. Proc Natl Acad Sci 86:2051, 1989

Reimer CB et al: The specificity of fetal IgM: Antibody or anti-antibody? NY Acad Sci 254:77, 1975

Ross WH, Sutton HFS: Acquired syphilitic uveitis. Arch Ophthalmol 98:496, 1980

Simon RP: Neurosyphilis. Arch Neurol 42:606, 1985

Wendel GD et al: Penicillin allergy and desensitization in serious infections during pregnancy. N Engl J Med 312:1229, 1985

129 NONVENEREAL TREPONEMATOSES: YAWS, PINTA, AND ENDEMIC SYPHILIS

PETER L. PERINE

GENERAL CONSIDERATIONS Nonvenereal treponematoses occur in remote, impoverished areas of the world. Yaws, pinta, and endemic syphilis are distinguished from venereal syphilis solely by clinical and epidemiologic features. Yaws and pinta are caused by treponemes which are conventionally designated as unique species (*Treponema pertenue* causes yaws, and *T. carateum* pinta), but no significant morphologic or genetic differences have been demonstrated among *T. pertenue*, *T. carateum*, and *T. pallidum*. The etiologic agents of endemic syphilis and yaws are generally held to be identical with *T. pallidum* and have been designated as *T. pallidum* ssp. *endemicum* and ssp. *pertenue*, respectively. Pinta involves the skin alone; yaws affects skin and bones; and endemic syphilis involves the skin, bone, and mucous membranes. Each disease tends to progress by stages, but these are neither as distinct nor as predictable as in syphilis. Congenital infections and cardiovascular and central nervous system involvement occur rarely, if ever, in the nonvenereal treponematoses but are common in syphilis. It is unclear whether the clinical and epidemiologic differences among yaws, pinta, endemic syphilis, and venereal syphilis are solely determined by environmental and host factors or are attributable to undefined biologic differences among the causal treponemes. The relationship of the treponematoses is summarized in Table 129-1.

EPIDEMIOLOGY Treponemal antibodies are demonstrable in some proportion of nonhuman primates in regions of Africa where human yaws and endemic syphilis are common, and pathogenic treponemes have been found in skin lesions and lymph nodes of seropositive animals. These treponemes have produced yaws-like lesions in susceptible monkeys and hamsters.

Yaws and endemic syphilis are diseases of young children. Yaws occurs throughout the world between the tropics of Cancer and Capricorn, in humid, warm environments. Transmission of yaws among children is favored by scanty clothing, poor hygiene, and frequent skin trauma. Spread occurs by direct contact with infected lesions and perhaps by passive transfer of treponemes by insects. Endemic syphilis occurs in arid subtropical or temperate climates in Africa, the eastern Mediterranean, the Arabian peninsula, and central Asia. It is not observed in the western hemisphere. Skin-to-skin transmission is less important than in yaws; instead, infection of mucous membranes results from direct mouth-to-mouth contact or from contaminated fomites, such as shared drinking or eating utensils. Venereal syphilis can spread by nonvenereal contact among children and cause household outbreaks in modern cities when crowding and poverty favor transmission of *T. pallidum*.

Although cutaneous pigmentary changes resembling late stages of pinta occur in yaws or endemic syphilis, pinta is a separate, more benign disease which occurs only in the western hemisphere. The onset is typically later than in yaws or endemic syphilis, usually when the person is between 10 and 20 years of age. Pinta is not very contagious, and its mode of transmission is not well defined.

The WHO/UNICEF-assisted mass campaign for eradication of endemic nonvenereal treponematosis from 1948 to 1969 was an unusually successful public health campaign. Over 160 million people were examined in 46 countries, and approximately 50 million cases, contacts, and latent infections were treated. The impact of this program was remarkable. The prevalence of active yaws lesions was reduced from over 20 percent to less than 1 percent in many rural areas. In Bosnia, Yugoslavia, endemic syphilis was eradicated—the only example of eradication of an endemic treponematosis.

Relaxation of active surveillance activities after the mass campaigns has led to a resurgence of yaws, particularly in Africa. Yaws has not been eradicated in any large area. The Ivory Coast, Ghana, Togo,

TABLE 129-1 Etiology, epidemiology, and clinical manifestations of the treponematoses

	Venereal syphilis	Endemic syphilis	Yaws	Pinta
Organism	*T. pallidum* ssp. *pallidum*	*T. pallidum* ssp. *endemicum*	*T. pallidum* ssp. *pertenue*	*T. carateum*
Transmission	Sexual, transplacental*	Household contacts: mouth-to-mouth or via drinking, eating utensils	Skin-to-skin ? Insect vector	Skin-to-skin ? Insect vector
Usual age	Adult	Early childhood	Early childhood	Adolescent
Primary lesion	Cutaneous ulcer (chancre)	Rarely seen	Framboise (raspberry), or "mother yaw"	Nonulcerating papule with satellites
Secondary lesion	Mucocutaneous; occasional periostitis	Florid mucocutaneous lesions (mucous patch, split papule, condyloma latum); osteoperiostitis	Cutaneous papulosquamous lesions; osteoperiostitis	Pintides
Tertiary	Gumma, cardiovascular, and CNS lues	Destructive cutaneous osteoarticular gummas	Destructive cutaneous osteoarticular gummas	Dyschromic, achromic macules

* Since the nonvenereal treponematoses are usually acquired in childhood and treponemal bacteremia ceases with time, only in adult-onset venereal syphilis is there any likelihood of a mother giving birth to an infected child.

and Benin have large reservoirs of yaws and account for over 90 percent of cases reported to WHO since 1982. North of these countries, the Sahelian nations of Mali, Niger, Burkina Faso, and Senegal have prevalence rates in some areas of 10 to 15 percent for endemic syphilis. These rates exceed those reported before the mass treatment campaigns. Seroactivity and late manifestations of endemic syphilis continue to occur among nomads in Saudi Arabia. The resurgence of yaws and endemic syphilis led to a new yaws campaign in Ghana in 1980, and other national campaigns are planned to control resurgent yaws and endemic syphilis in Africa.

Antitreponemal and reaginic seroreactivity has been detected in a small percentage of children without clinical disease born after the mass campaigns in some areas (e.g., Nigeria, New Guinea, and Bosnia). This may represent attenuated or asymptomatic infection, or may simply reflect the decreased predictive value of serologic tests (probability that disease is present if the test is positive) when the prevalence of disease is sharply reduced.

In the Americas, foci of yaws persist in Haiti; Dominica, St. Lucia, and St. Vincent; Peru, Colombia, and Ecuador; a few areas of Brazil; and Guyana and Surinam. Pinta is confined to Central America and northern South America, where it appears to have regressed to remote Indian villages. Its prevalence today is probably less than 1 percent of that found 20 years ago.

BIOLOGIC RELATIONSHIPS Specific humoral antibodies to *T. pallidum* are produced in individuals with yaws, pinta, or endemic syphilis, but the time of appearance of antibodies after onset of infections is variable. The fluorescent treponemal antibody absorption (FTA-ABS) test, the *T. pallidum* hemagglutination test (TPHA), and the *T. pallidum* immobilization (TPI) test cannot differentiate among the treponematoses.

In addition to the clinical and epidemiologic differences among the treponematoses in humans, the range of susceptible animal hosts and some manifestations of experimental infection are also different. In particular, *T. carateum* has produced an infection in chimpanzees which resembles pinta, but attempts to infect other experimental animals have been unsuccessful. Individuals who have had yaws or pinta are considered relatively immune to syphilis, and persons with active pinta or syphilis cannot be superinfected with *T. pallidum* ssp. *pertenue* by experimental inoculation.

CLINICAL MANIFESTATIONS Yaws Also known as pian, framboesia, or bubas, yaws is a chronic infectious disease of childhood caused by *T. pallidum* ssp. *pertenue*. The disease is characterized by an initial skin lesion(s) followed by relapsing, nondestructive, secondary lesions of skin and bone. In the late stages, destructive lesions of skin, bone, and joints occur.

The incubation period following experimental inoculation of susceptible human beings is 3 to 4 weeks. Disruption of the skin by insect bites, abrasions, or injuries promotes acquisition of natural infection from infected contacts, most likely by fingers contaminated directly or indirectly with material from early yaws lesions. The initial early lesion is a single papule which is usually located on a leg. The lesion enlarges and becomes papillomatous (Fig. 129-1). This lesion also is known as a framboesioma (raspberry) or "mother yaw." It becomes superficially eroded and covered by a thin yellow crust of serous exudate containing *T. pertenue*. Erythema and induration do not occur. The lesion is mildly pruritic, and regional lymphadenopathy occurs. The initial lesion usually heals in 6 months. As a result of treponemal bacteremia and autoinoculation, a generalized secondary eruption of similar lesions appears either before or after the initial lesion has healed and is most extensive on the exposed surfaces of the body. These early cutaneous lesions of yaws have a variety of forms, including desquamative macular and papular as well as papillomatous types. Painful papillomata on the soles of the feet result in a crablike gait referred to as "crab yaws." Early lesions are infectious and heal slowly; they may result in scarring, hyperpigmentation, or depigmentation, resembling the pigmentary changes seen in pinta. Histologic findings are mononuclear-cell infiltration, acanthosis, hyperkeratosis, and the presence of many treponemes.

FIGURE 129-1 Young man with squamous micropapules of early yaws with papillomas in the left axilla and scapular area.

Other manifestations of early yaws include lymphadenopathy and nocturnal bone pain and polydactylitis due to periostitis. Fever and other constitutional symptoms are rare, however, unless lesions become secondarily infected. Infectious cutaneous relapses are characteristic during the first 5 years after infection. Late yaws lesions occur in about 10 percent of cases, starting 5 years or more after infection, and differ histologically from early lesions in showing endarteritis. Late lesions include gummas of the skin and long bones, particularly of the legs, hyperkeratoses of the soles and palms, osteitis, periostitis, juxtaarticular fibromatous nodes, and hydrarthrosis.

Late lesions of yaws are characteristically extensive and usually destructive. Destruction of the nose, maxilla, palate, and pharynx, termed *gangosa,* or *rhinopharyngitis mutilans,* occurs in late yaws, as well as in leprosy and leishmaniasis. Hypertrophic paranasal maxillary osteitis produces distinctive facies known as *goundou.*

The clinical features of yaws have become less reliable for diagnosis as the prevalence of yaws has decreased, necessitating the use of easily performed serologic tests, such as the rapid plasma reagin (RPR) card test. *T. pertenue* can be demonstrated by dark-field examination in early cutaneous lesions but should not be confused with other spirochetes found in tropical ulcers. The serum reagin antibody tests become positive after 1 month, and the FTA-ABS test is also positive.

Endemic syphilis Synonyms for endemic syphilis are Bejel, Siti, Dichuchwa, Njovera, and Skerljevo. It is a chronic nonvenereal, treponemal infection of childhood, characterized by early mucous membrane or mucocutaneous lesions, a latent period of indeterminate duration, and late complications including gummas of bone and skin. The causative organism is indistinguishable from *T. pallidum.* Endemic syphilis differs from congenital syphilis in that dental changes, interstitial keratitis, and neurosyphilis rarely, if ever, occur. Cardiovascular complications are considered rare in both endemic and congenital syphilis.

Primary cutaneous lesions are infrequent and when present are extragenital. The earliest manifestation of endemic syphilis is usually an intraoral mucous patch or mucocutaneous lesion resembling the split papules or condylomata of secondary syphilis. Periostitis is common. Regional lymphadenopathy occurs, but generalized lymphadenopathy is unusual. Treponemes are abundant in the moist early lesions and in aspirates from regional lymph nodes. After a variable latent period, late lesions may develop and are the most frequent clinical manifestations. These resemble the lesions of late benign syphilis and include osseous or cutaneous gummas. Destructive gummas, osteitis, and gangosa are more common than in late yaws. Gummas occur on the nipples of mothers who have themselves previously had endemic syphilis and who breastfeed infants with oral lesions. Both early and late forms of endemic syphilis thus may coexist in the same family. The tertiary lesions of endemic syphilis sometimes may be a consequence of repeated exposure of a previously sensitized host to reinfection.

Pinta Also known as mal del pinto, carate, azul, or purupuru, pinta is an infectious disease of the skin caused by *T. carateum*. This disease has three cutaneous stages characterized by marked changes in the skin color, does not involve osseous tissue or viscera, and causes no disability other than that associated with cosmetic disfigurement.

The initial lesion is a small papule which appears 7 to 30 days after exposure and is located most often on the extremities, face, neck, or buttocks. It increases in size slowly by peripheral extension and by coalescing with smaller satellite papules. Regional lymphadenopathy occurs. A secondary eruption not associated with generalized lymphadenopathy appears 1 month to 1 year after the appearance of the initial lesion. The secondary lesions are termed *pintides*, may be numerous, and evolve into a psoriatic or circinate configuration. Pintides are initially red but become deeply pigmented, reaching a slate-blue color after a period of time which is related to exposure to sun. Pigmentation occurs most rapidly on the exposed parts of the body. These pigmented lesions are known as dyschromic macules and contain treponemes which are located principally in the epidermis in older lesions. Histologically there is deposition of pigment in the dermis with decreased melanin pigment in the basal cell layer. Within 3 months to a year, most of the pintides show varying degrees of depigmentation, becoming brown and finally white and giving the skin a mottled appearance. The porcelain-white achromic lesions represent the "late" stage of the disease in which the epidermis is atrophic, and melanocytes and melanin are absent. *T. carateum* can be demonstrated in transudates from initial, early secondary, or dyschromic lesions. Reaginic and antitreponemal antibody tests are positive, but may take four times longer to become positive in pinta than in venereal syphilis.

TREATMENT Treatment is similar for all the endemic treponematoses. Intramuscular injection of 2.4 million units of benzathine penicillin G in adults and half this dose in children results in rapid resolution of lesions and prevents recurrence. Procaine penicillin G in oil and 2% aluminum monostearate (PAM) has been used extensively. In persons who are allergic to penicillin, tetracycline hydrochloride in a dose similar to that used for infectious syphilis (see Chap. 128) is effective. In areas where less than 5 percent of the population has active disease, cases are managed on an individual basis, and all contacts of infected persons are treated with antibiotics.

PREVENTION Although the nonvenereal treponematoses are less amenable to eradication than smallpox, the resurgence of yaws has led some authorities to suggest that the application of *selective epidemiologic control* as used in smallpox eradication be applied to yaws control. This strategy would emphasize ongoing active surveillance, investigation of outbreaks, and treatment of active cases and their contacts rather than mass treatment.

REFERENCES

BURKE JP et al (eds): International symposium on yaws and other endemic treponematoses. Rev Infect Dis 7:S217, 1985

FOHN MJ et al: Specificity of antibodies from patients with pinta for antigens of *T. pallidum* ssp. *pallidum*. J Infect Dis 157:32, 1988.

GUTHE T: Clinical, serological and epidemiological features of framboesia tropica (yaws) and its control in rural communities. Acta Derm Venereol 49:343, 1969

HOPKINS DR: Yaws in the Americas, 1950–1975. J Infect Dis 136:548, 1977

PERINE PL et al: *Handbook of Endemic Treponematoses*. WHO, Geneva, 1984

Treponematoses Research: Report of a WHO Scientific Group, WHO Technical Report Series 674, 1982

WORLD HEALTH ORGANIZATION: Endemic treponematoses. Week Epidem Rec 61:198, 1986

130 LEPTOSPIROSIS

JAY P. SANFORD

DEFINITION *Leptospirosis* is a term applied to disease caused by all leptospiras regardless of specific serotype. Correlation of clinical syndromes with infection by differing serotypes leads to the conclusion that a single serotype of *Leptospira* may be responsible for a variety of clinical features; conversely, a single syndrome, e.g., aseptic meningitis, may be caused by multiple serotypes. Hence there is a preference for the general term leptospirosis rather than the synonyms such as Weil's disease and canicola fever.

ETIOLOGY The genus *Leptospira* contains only one species, *L. interrogans*, which may be subdivided into two complexes, interrogans and biflexa. The interrogans complex includes the pathogenic strains, while the biflexa complex includes saprophytic strains. Within each complex the organisms show antigenic variations that are stable and allow them to be classed as serotypes (serovars). Serotypes with common antigens are arranged in serogroups (varieties). Despite contrary common usage, an example of the correct designation of *Leptospira* is as follows: Pomona serogroup of *L. interrogans* or *L. interrogans* var. pomona, not *L. pomona*. The interrogans complex now contains about 170 serotypes arranged in 18 serogroups (the number in parentheses refers to number of serotypes within the serogroup): Icterohemorrhagiae (18), Hebdomadis (30), Autumnalis (17), Canicola (12), Australis (12), Tarassovi (17), Pyrogenes (12), Bataviae (10), Javanica (8), Pomona (8), Ballum (3), Cynopteri (3), Celledoni (3), Grippotyphosa (5), Panama (2), Shermani (1), Ranarum (2), and Bufonis (1). At least 27 serotypes of *Leptospira* occur naturally in the United States.

EPIDEMIOLOGY Leptospirosis is thought to be the most widespread zoonosis in the world. Cases are regularly reported from all continents except Antarctica and are especially prevalent in the tropics. Although leptospirosis is not a common disease, it has been reported from all regions of the United States including arid areas such as Arizona. Between 1985 and 1988, 41 to 57 cases were reported annually. Infection in humans is an incidental occurrence and is not essential to the maintenance of leptospirosis. The disease occurs in a wide range of domestic and wild animal hosts, including poikilothermic vertebrates. In many species, such as opossums, skunks, raccoons, and foxes, infectivity ratios in the range of 10 to 50 percent are not unusual. Interspecies spread of specific serotypes of leptospiras between animal hosts is frequent, e.g., Pomona, a serotype principally associated with livestock, has been demonstrated in dogs. Infection in animals may vary from inapparent illness to severe fatal disease. Even asymptomatic animals may carry high numbers ($>10^{10}$ organisms per gram) in their kidneys. The carrier state, in which the host may shed leptospiras in its urine for months to years, may develop in many animals. Immunization of dogs may not prevent the carrier, or shedder, state.

Survival of pathogenic leptospiras in nature is governed by factors including pH of the urine of the host, pH of soil or water into which they are shed, and ambient temperature. Leptospiras in most "urine spots" in soil retain infectivity for 6 to 48 h. Acid urine permits only limited survival; however, if the urine is neutral or alkaline and is shed into a similar moist environment which has low salinity, is not badly polluted with microorganisms or detergents, and has a temperature above 22°C, leptospiras may survive for several weeks. Human infections can occur either by direct contact with urine or tissue of an infected animal or indirectly through contaminated water, soil, or vegetation. The usual portals of entry in humans are abraded skin, particularly about the feet, and exposed conjunctival, nasal, and oral mucous membranes. The previously held concept that organisms could penetrate intact skin has been questioned. While leptospiras have been isolated from ticks, these arthropods appear to be unimportant in transmission.

With the ubiquitous infection of animals, leptospirosis in human beings can occur in all age groups, at all seasons, and in both sexes. However, it is primarily a disease of teenage children and young adults (about one-half of patients are between the ages of 10 and 39), occurs predominantly in males (80 percent), and develops most frequently in hot weather (in the United States one-half of infections occur from July to October). The wide spectrum of animal hosts results in both urban and rural human disease. Leptospirosis has been considered an occupational disease; however, improved methods of rat control and better standards of hygiene have reduced the incidence among occupational groups such as coal miners and people who work in sewers. The epidemiologic pattern has changed; in the United States and the United Kingdom, water-associated and cattle-associated leptospirosis is most common. Less than 20 percent of patients have had direct contact with animals; they are mostly farmers, trappers, or abattoir workers. In the majority of patients exposure is incidental; two-thirds of cases occur in children, students, or housewives. Swimming or partial immersion in contaminated water, e.g., riding motorcycles through contaminated pools of water, has been implicated in one-fifth of patients and has accounted for most of the recognized common-source outbreaks. In Hawaii, one-fourth of cases have been associated with aquaculture industries, while in Italy leptospirosis remains common in the rice-growing areas of the Po River Valley.

PATHOLOGY   In patients who have died with hepatorenal involvement (Weil's syndrome), the significant gross changes include hemorrhages and bile staining of tissues. The hemorrhages, which vary from petechial to ecchymotic, are widespread and are most prominent in skeletal muscle, kidneys, adrenals, liver, stomach, spleen, and lungs.

In skeletal muscle, focal, necrotic, and necrobiotic changes typical of leptospirosis occur. Biopsies early in the illness demonstrate swelling and vacuolation. Leptospiral antigen has been demonstrated in these lesions by the fluorescent antibody technique. Healing ensues by the formation of new myofibrils with minimal fibrosis. The renal lesions in the acute phase involve predominantly the tubules and vary from simple dilatation of distal convoluted tubules to degeneration, necrosis, and basement membrane rupture. Interstitial edema and cellular infiltrates consisting of lymphocytes, neutrophilic leukocytes, histiocytes, and plasma cells are uniformly present. Glomerular lesions either are absent or consist of mesangial hyperplasia and focal foot process fusion which are interpreted as representing nonspecific changes associated with acute inflammation and protein filtration. Microscopic alterations in the liver are not diagnostic and correlate poorly with the degree of functional impairment. The changes include cloudy swelling of parenchymal cells, disruption of liver cords, enlargement of Kupffer cells, and bile stasis in biliary canaliculi. The changes in the brain and meninges are also minimal and are not diagnostic. Microscopic evidence of myocarditis has been recorded. Pulmonary findings consist of a patchy, localized hemorrhagic pneumonitis. Special staining techniques utilizing silver impregnation methods have demonstrated organisms in the lumina of renal tubules but rarely in other organs.

CLINICAL MANIFESTATIONS   General features   The incubation period following immersion or accidental laboratory exposure has shown extremes of 2 to 26 days, the usual range being 7 to 13 days and the average 10 days.

Leptospirosis is a typically biphasic illness. *During the leptospiremic* or *first phase,* leptospiras are present in the blood and cerebrospinal fluid. The onset is typically abrupt, and initial symptoms include headache, which is usually frontal, less often retroorbital, but occasionally may be bitemporal or occipital. Severe muscle aching occurs in most patients, the muscles of the thighs and lumbar areas being most prominently involved, and often is accompanied by severe pain on palpation. The myalgia may be accompanied by extreme cutaneous hyperesthesia (causalgia). Chills followed by a rapidly rising temperature are prominent. Following the abrupt onset, the leptospiremic phase typically lasts 4 to 9 days. Features during this interval include recurrent chills, high spiking temperatures [usually

38.9°C (102°F) or greater], headache, and continued severe myalgia. Involvement of one organ system may predominate, often leading to initial misdiagnosis. Such symptom complexes most commonly include hepatitis, nephritis, atypical pneumonia, influenza, or "viral" gastroenteritis. Anorexia, nausea, and vomiting are encountered in one-half or more of the patients. Occasional patients have diarrhea. Pulmonary manifestations, usually either cough or chest pain, have varied in frequency of occurrence from less than 25 percent to 86 percent. Hemoptysis occurs but is rare. Examination during this phase reveals an acutely ill, febrile patient, with a relative bradycardia and normal blood pressure. Disturbances in sensorium may be encountered in up to 25 percent of patients. Transient cerebral ischemic attacks in children associated with leptospiral arteritis have been reported from China.

The most characteristic physical sign is conjunctival suffusion, which usually first appears on the third or fourth day. It may be lacking in some patients but more often is overlooked. It may be associated with photophobia, but serous or purulent secretion is unusual. Less common findings may include pharyngeal injection, cutaneous hemorrhages, and skin rashes that are usually macular, maculopapular, or urticarial and usually occur on the trunk. Uncommon findings are splenomegaly, hepatomegaly, lymphadenopathy, or jaundice. The first phase terminates after 4 to 9 days, usually with defervescence and improvement in symptoms. This coincides with the disappearance of leptospiras from the blood and cerebrospinal fluid.

The second phase has been characterized as the "immune" phase and correlates with the appearance of circulating IgM antibodies; the concentration of C3 in serum remains normal. The clinical manifestations of this phase show greater variability than those during the first phase. After a relatively asymptomatic period of 1 to 3 days, the fever and earlier symptoms recur and meningismus may develop. The fever rarely exceeds 38.9°C (102°F) and is usually of 1 to 3 days' duration. It is not uncommon for fever to be absent or quite transient. Even when symptoms or signs of meningeal irritation are absent, routine examination of cerebrospinal fluid after the seventh day has revealed pleocytosis in 50 to 90 percent of patients. Less common features include iridocyclitis, optic neuritis, and other nervous system manifestations, including encephalitis, myelitis, and peripheral neuropathy. Leptospirosis during pregnancy may be associated with an increased risk of fetal loss.

Specific features   WEIL'S SYNDROME   Weil's syndrome, which may be due to serotypes other than Icterohemorrhagiae, is defined as severe leptospirosis with jaundice, usually accompanied by azotemia, hemorrhages, anemia, disturbances in consciousness, and continued fever. There is uncertainty as to the pathogenesis of the syndrome, i.e., whether it represents direct toxic damage due to leptospiras or whether it is the consequence of immune response to leptospiral antigens. The consensus favors toxic damage.

The onset and first stage are identical with the less severe forms of leptospirosis. The distinctive features of Weil's syndrome appear from the third to the sixth days but do not reach their peak until well into the second stage. As in milder forms of leptospirosis, there is a tendency for defervescence about the seventh day; however, with recurrence, fever is marked and may persist for several weeks. Either renal or hepatic manifestations may predominate. Hepatic disturbances include tenderness in the right upper quadrant and hepatic enlargement, both of which are common when jaundice is present. Serum glutamic oxaloacetic transaminase (SGOT) values are rarely increased more than fivefold regardless of the degree of hyperbilirubinemia, which is predominantly conjugated. The predominant mechanism appears to be an intracellular block to bilirubin excretion.

HEMORRHAGIC FEVER WITH RENAL SYNDROME   Studies on the epidemiology of Hantavirus (Chap. 148) have shown that for the initial 24 to 72 h there is significant overlap in the clinical features of leptospirosis, hemorrhagic fever with renal syndrome (HFRS), and scrub typhus (H.W. Lee, personal communication). In Korea, where all three diseases are prevalent, of the blood samples submitted for

Hantavirus serology 21 percent had antibody to *Leptospira* antigens and 6 percent to *Rickettsia tsutsugamushi*. Conversely, among 261 patients in Singapore clinically suspected of having leptospirosis, 3 percent had serologic evidence of Hantavirus infection. Hantavirus disease, which varies from mild (nephropathica epidemica) to severe (Balkan nephropathy), is common in Europe and Scandinavia. Because of the similarity in epidemiology and clinical presentation and the potential for dual infections, it has been recommended that blood be submitted for Hantavirus serology in all cases of suspected leptospirosis. Clinically the term *lepthangamushi syndrome* has been used to describe this overlap syndrome.

Renal manifestations of Weil's syndrome consist primarily of proteinuria, pyuria, hematuria, and azotemia. Dysuria is rare. Serious renal damage usually occurs in the form of acute tubular necrosis associated with oliguria. The peak elevation of blood urea nitrogen usually is seen on the fifth to seventh day. Hemorrhagic manifestations are most prevalent in this group of patients and include epistaxis, hemoptysis, gastrointestinal bleeding, hemorrhage into the adrenal glands, hemorrhagic pneumonitis, and subarachnoid hemorrhage. These have been explained on the basis of diffuse vasculitis with capillary injury. In addition, in some patients hypoprothrombinemia and thrombocytopenia have been observed.

ATYPICAL PNEUMONIA SYNDROME Pulmonary symptoms and signs are common in patients with leptospirosis; even the adult respiratory distress syndrome (ARDS) has been reported. While not fully appreciated in the United States, in other parts of the world leptospirosis is recognized as an important differential diagnostic consideration in the patient with fever, chills, headache, severe myalgia, and bilateral bronchopneumonia, with or without an associated "active" urine sediment. In Italy, respiratory or influenza-like symptoms were the only clinical signs of illness in 21 percent of over 300 patients with confirmed leptospirosis. Of 15 patients with leptospirosis reported from the Republic of Korea, 5 presented with bilateral pulmonary infiltrates. Given appropriate epidemiologic circumstances, leptospirosis should be added to the differential diagnosis of "atypical" pneumonia.

ASEPTIC MENINGITIS A leptospiral etiology has been incriminated in 5 to 13 percent of sporadic cases of aseptic meningitis. Pleocytosis is not present before the immune phase, but then develops rapidly. There are usually tens to hundreds of leukocytes, occasionally 1000, per microliter, among which neutrophils or mononuclear cells may predominate. CSF glucose concentration is almost always normal, but occasional instances of lowered glucose levels have been recorded. CSF protein may exceed 1 g/L (100 mg/dL) early in the course. Xanthochromic cerebrospinal fluid has been observed in the presence of jaundice. Each of the serotypes of leptospiras that are pathogenic for humans is probably capable of causing aseptic meningitis. The most prevalent serotypes have been Canicola, Icterohemorrhagiae, and Pomona.

MYOCARDITIS Cardiac arrhythmias including paroxysmal atrial fibrillation, atrial flutter, ventricular tachycardia, and premature ventricular contractions have been described but are usually of little clinical significance. However, on rare occasions definite cardiac dilatation with acute left ventricular failure has been observed. Associated manifestations have included jaundice, pulmonary infiltrates, arthritis, and skin rashes. The serotypes thus far incriminated have included Icterohemorrhagiae, Pomona, and Grippotyphosa.

CHILDREN Several clinical features which are not seen or are very rare in adults occur in children: hypertension, acalculous cholecystitis (five of nine children in one series), pancreatitis, abdominal causalgia, and peripheral desquamation of a rash that may be associated with gangrene and cardiopulmonary arrest. The features of desquamation, myocardial involvement, and hydrops of the gallbladder suggest Kawasaki syndrome [mucocutaneous lymph node syndrome (see Chap. 63)].

LABORATORY FEATURES Leukocyte counts vary from leukopenic levels to mild elevations in the anicteric patients. In patients with jaundice, leukocytosis as high as 70,000 cells per microliter

may be present. However, regardless of the total leukocyte count, neutrophilia of greater than 70 percent is very frequently encountered during the first stage.

Hemolytic substances have been demonstrated in cultures of pathogenic leptospiras. In contrast to many hemolysins of bacterial origin which are not hemolytic in vivo, the leptospiral hemolysins appear to be active in vivo. In patients with jaundice, anemia may be severe and is most characteristically due to intravascular hemolysis. Other mechanisms of anemia include azotemia and blood loss secondary to hemorrhage. Anemia due to leptospirosis is unusual in anicteric patients.

Thrombocytopenia sufficient to be associated with bleeding (less than 30,000 platelets per microliter) may be encountered. Additional hematologic abnormalities include elevation of the erythrocyte sedimentation rate in over one-half of patients (usually less than 50 mm/h).

Urinalysis during the leptospiremic phase reveals mild proteinuria, casts, and an increase in cellular elements. In anicteric infections, these abnormalities rapidly disappear after the first week. Proteinuria and abnormalities in the urine sediment usually are not associated with elevations in blood urea nitrogen. Since the anicteric form of the disease often has gone undiagnosed, estimates of the frequency of azotemia and jaundice are probably high. Azotemia has been reported in approximately one-fourth of patients. In three-fourths of these patients, the blood urea nitrogen is less than 36 mmol/L (100 mg/dL). Azotemia is usually associated with jaundice. The serum bilirubin levels may reach 1110 μmol/L (65 mg/dL); however, in two-thirds of patients the levels are less than 340 μmol/L (20 mg/dL). During the first phase, one-half of the patients have increased serum creatine phosphokinase (CK) levels, with mean values of five times normal. Such increases are not seen in viral hepatitis, and a slight increase in transaminase with a definite increase in CK suggests leptospirosis rather than viral hepatitis.

DIAGNOSIS Diagnosis is based upon culture of the organism or serologic proof of its existence. The most common initial diagnostic impressions in patients with leptospirosis are meningitis, hepatitis, nephritis, fever of undetermined origin (FUO), influenza, Kawasaki syndrome, toxic shock syndrome, and Legionnaires' disease. Leptospiras may be isolated quite readily during the first phase from blood and cerebrospinal fluid or during the second phase from the urine. Leptospiras may be excreted in the urine for up to 11 months after the onset of illness and may persist despite antimicrobial therapy. Whole blood should be inoculated immediately into tubes containing semisolid medium, such as Fletcher's or EMJH medium. If culture medium is not available, leptospiras reportedly will remain viable up to 11 days in blood to which anticoagulants, preferably sodium oxalate, have been added. Animal inoculation (preferably either suckling hamsters or guinea pigs) may be used and is of particular value if specimens are contaminated. Direct examination of blood or urine by dark-field methods has been employed; *however, this method so frequently results in failure or misdiagnosis that it should not be employed.* Serologic methods are applicable during the second phase; antibodies appear from the sixth to the twelfth days of illness. Two serologic methods are commonly used: a macroscopic or slide agglutination test which is easy to perform but lacks specificity and sensitivity, and hence is suitable for screening only, and the microscopic agglutination test, which is more complicated but also more specific. An IgM-specific dot-ELISA (enzyme-linked immunosorbent assay) has been effective in diagnosing leptospirosis in an endemic area. Serologic criteria for diagnosis include a fourfold or greater rise in titer during the course of illness. Cross-agglutination reactions between various serotypes commonly occur so that the infection serotype often cannot be determined with certainty without isolation of leptospiras.

PROGNOSIS The prognosis is dependent upon both the virulence of the organism and the general condition of the patient. The mortality rate in reported cases in the United States has varied annually between 2.5 and 16.4 percent, averaging 7.1 percent. Age is the most significant host factor related to increased mortality. In a representative series, the mortality rate rose from 10 percent in men less than 50 years of age to 56 percent in those over 51 years of age. The virulence of the infecting leptospiras correlates best with the development of jaundice. In anicteric patients, mortality is extremely rare, but with the development of jaundice, the mortality rate in various series has ranged from 15 to 48 percent. The long-term prognosis following the acute renal lesion of leptospirosis is good. Glomerular filtration rates have returned to normal, usually within 2 months; however, a few patients show residual tubular dysfunction such as a defect in concentrating capacity.

TREATMENT A variety of antimicrobial drugs, including penicillin, streptomycin, the tetracycline congeners, chloramphenicol, and erythromycin, have been effective in vitro and in experimental leptospiral infections. Data concerning the efficacy of antibiotics in human beings have been conflicting. Within 4 to 6 h after initiation of penicillin G therapy, a Jarisch-Herxheimer type of reaction, which suggests antileptospiral activity, may occur. A controlled trial of intravenous penicillin (1.5 million units every 6 h for 7 days) clearly demonstrated shortening of duration of fever and creatinine elevation, shortening of hospitalization, and prevention of leptospiruria, even when treatment was started after the fifth day of illness. Doxycycline (100 mg orally taken twice daily for 7 days), when started within 4 days of onset of symptoms, significantly shortened the duration of fever and most other symptoms and decreased the frequency of leptospiruria in patients with mild illness. Doxycycline (200 mg orally taken once per week) is also highly effective in preventing disease in an area of high prevalence. Azotemia and jaundice require meticulous attention to fluid and electrolyte therapy. Since the renal damage is reversible, patients with azotemia should be considered for peritoneal hemodialysis. Exchange transfusion may be beneficial in the management of patients with extreme hyperbilirubinemia.

REFERENCES

CHUN SH et al: 15 cases of leptospirosis in the northern part of Kyoung Ki Do. Korean J Intern Med 32:76, 1987

CICERONI L et al: Recent trends in human leptospirosis in Italy. Eur J Epidemiol 4:49, 1988

FEIGIN RD, ANDERSON DC: Human leptospirosis. CRC Crit Rev Clin Lab Sci 5:413, 1975

GILKS CF et al: Failure of penicillin prophylaxis in laboratory acquired leptospirosis. Postgrad Med J 64:236, 1988

JOHNSON RC: The Biology of Parasitic Spirochetes. New York, Academic, 1976

JOHNSON WD JR et al: Serum creatine phosphokinase in leptospirosis. JAMA 233:981, 1975

KUDESIA G et al: Dual infection with Leptospira and Hantavirus. Lancet 1:1397, 1988

McCLAIN JB et al: Doxycycline therapy for leptospirosis. Ann Intern Med 100:696, 1984

TAKAFUJI ET et al: An efficacy trial of doxycycline chemoprophylaxis against leptospirosis. N Engl J Med 310:497, 1984

WATT G et al: Placebo-controlled trial of intravenous penicillin for severe and late leptospirosis. Lancet 1:433, 1988

——— et al: Rapid diagnosis of leptospirosis: Prospective comparison of dot-ELISA and genus specific microscopic agglutination test at different stages of illness. J Infect Dis 157:840, 1988

WINEARLS CG et al: Acute renal failure due to leptospirosis: Clinical features and outcome in six cases. Q J Med 53:487, 1984

WONG ML et al: Leptospirosis: A childhood disease. J Pediatr 90:532, 1977

WORLD HEALTH ORGANIZATION: Tick-borne encephalitis and hemorrhagic fever with renal syndrome in Europe. EURO Reports and Studies No 104, Copenhagen 1986

131 RELAPSING FEVER

PETER L. PERINE

DEFINITION Relapsing fevers are a group of acute infections characterized by recurrent cycles of pyrexia which are separated by asymptomatic intervals of apparent recovery. They are caused by spirochetes of the genus Borrelia and occur in two epidemiologic varieties—louse-borne and tick-borne.

ETIOLOGY Borreliae are slender, helical-shaped, motile organisms measuring 7 to 20 μm long and 0.7 μm in diameter. Unlike other spirochetes, they are readily stained by aniline dyes. They are microaerophilic, and tick-borne strains grow well in Kelly's medium. Tick-borne Borrelia strains are named after their tick vectors, which in the United States include B. hermsi, B. parkeri, and B. turicate.

EPIDEMIOLOGY Louse-borne relapsing fever is transmitted from person to person solely by human body lice, which ingest blood infected with B. recurrentis. The spirochetes penetrate the wall of the intestine of the louse and multiply in its body cavity. Infection occurs when the louse is crushed against the bite site or an abrasion is caused by scratching. There is no known animal reservoir. The disease is endemic in remote areas of central and east Africa, the Peruvian Andes, and China, where poverty and crowding promote louse infestation. Like typhus, it is now present among the famine refugees in Ethiopia and Sudan. An occasional case of louse-borne relapsing fever has been imported into Europe and North America.

The tick vectors of relapsing fever belong to several species of the genus Ornithodorus. These long-lived, soft-shelled (argasid) ticks are reclusive, nocturnal biters which usually feed on ground squirrels and other small rodents. Their bite is painless and lasts for less than an hour. A small pruritic eschar may appear for a few days at the bite site. Ticks of both sexes are potentially infectious, and the spirochetes are transmitted by the female to her progeny. A rodent-tick reservoir of relapsing fever can persist near human dwellings or habitats for decades. Transmission to human beings occurs if the infected tick's saliva or coxial fluid contaminates its feeding site. Most cases in the United States occur during the spring and summer when ticks and rodents are active, particularly in western mountain states, from Texas to Colorado, Washington, Montana, and Idaho. Clusters of cases have often been linked to a tick-infested dwelling visited by travelers from different parts of the country.

PATHOGENESIS AND PATHOLOGY Once inoculated into a human, the borreliae reach the bloodstream, producing spirochetemia. Although most organs and tissues are invaded, the organisms remain and multiply primarily in the vascular system. Fever, the first manifestation of the disease, appears 3 to 12 days after infection. The severity of the fever and tissue injury is roughly correlated with the number of circulating spirochetes. Endothelial injury by borreliae is widespread, and subacute disseminated intravascular coagulation with thrombocytopenia and extravasation of blood into serosal membranes and skin is common. Immobilizing (opsonizing) antibodies appear after 3 to 5 days, and the organisms are rapidly cleared from the bloodstream by leukocyte phagocytosis, inducing a febrile crisis of short duration. Fever resolves, but a small number of a new antigenic variant of the spirochete survive in the blood or are sequestered in tissues. A new variant occurs spontaneously by genetic mutation with a frequency of once every 10^3 to 10^4 spirochetes and possesses surface proteins that are different from the infecting or preceding serotypes. They multiply and are detectable in the peripheral blood after a latent period of approximately 1 week, causing a second paroxysm of fever. The number of relapses is fewer in louse-borne than in tick-borne infections and is probably limited by the production of host antibodies directed against common, integral proteins possessed by each new variant.

MANIFESTATIONS Symptoms and signs are usually of greater severity in louse-borne relapsing fever and may vary in tick-borne infections depending on the particular species. After an incubation period of 3 to 18 days, the disease begins abruptly with the onset of high fever (39 to 40°C) which remains until the time of crisis. Patients appear acutely distressed, with some alteration in mental status. They complain of headache, muscle and joint pains, weakness, and anorexia. Nausea, vomiting, upper abdominal pain, and nonproductive cough are common. The pulse is increased in proportion to fever. Meningismus occurs in about 40 percent of patients. The liver and spleen are tender and enlarged in the majority of patients, especially in those with louse-borne disease. Jaundice, secondary to hepatocellular injury, occurs in between 10 and 80 percent of cases, appears late in the course of infection, and is more common in louse-borne disease.

Bleeding is common in both types of relapsing fever. In 10 to 60 percent of cases, a petechial or ecchymotic rash is present. Later, with the development of hepatitis, severe and prolonged epistaxis occurs in 25 percent of patients with louse-borne disease. Less common are hemoptysis, hematuria, and subconjunctival and retinal hemorrhages. Cerebral and gastrointestinal hemorrhage may occur as terminal events in fatal cases. Transient focal neurologic signs may be present without intracranial bleeding. Photophobia is common, and iritis or iridocyclitis leading to permanent visual impairment may develop in patients with tick-borne disease after several relapses.

Three to six days after the onset of symptoms, the attack resolves by crisis. It begins with a brief period of shaking chills which is followed by a transient but pronounced rise in temperature, heart rate, respiratory rate, and systolic blood pressure. This, in turn, is followed by reductions in temperature and peripheral vascular resistance, producing a hypotensive episode of several hours' duration. Most patients recover with return of vital signs to normal within 24 h, leaving the patient weak but comfortable. An identical crisis—the Jarisch-Herxheimer-like reaction—is precipitated by antibiotic therapy. The mediators of the crisis have not been identified, but phagocytosis of opsonized or antibiotically damaged spirochetes is the initiating event. An afebrile period of apparent recovery lasting 5 to 7 days ensues before the patient relapses with fever. In relapse, the symptoms are milder, shorter, and the crisis less severe than in the first attack. While only one or two relapses occur in louse-borne disease, multiple relapses over a period of several weeks are characteristic of tick-borne disease.

LABORATORY FINDINGS A moderate anemia is common. The leukocyte count is usually normal except for leukopenia at the peak of the crisis. The erythrocyte sedimentation rate is elevated. Thrombocytopenia with platelet counts below 150,000 per microliter and a prolonged bleeding time are seen regularly. Elevated serum aminotransferases, bilirubin, and prolonged prothrombin and partial thromboplastin times are common. Azotemia unrelated to extracellular fluid volume occurs in most patients with louse-borne disease. Electrocardiogram abnormalities include a prolonged QTc interval. The majority of patients with louse-borne and about 30 percent of those with tick-borne relapsing fever develop agglutinins to *Proteus* OXK antigens.

The definitive diagnosis is made by demonstrating borreliae in peripheral blood during a febrile episode by examining blood films stained with Giemsa's or Wright's stains. Repeated examinations may be required. Motile spirochetes can be visualized in wet mounts of freshly drawn blood by dark-field or phase-contrast microscopy. If direct methods are negative and tick-borne disease is suspected, blood may be injected into mice or rats and their blood examined frequently for the presence of spirochetes.

DIFFERENTIAL DIAGNOSIS Many acute febrile illnesses, including Lyme disease, rat-bite fever, salmonellosis, typhus, and Weil's disease, must be considered. Practically, there is seldom confusion if the travel history of the patient is considered and if blood films are examined carefully.

TREATMENT The peripheral blood is quickly cleared of spirochetes by treatment with penicillin, tetracyclines, erythromycin, or chloramphenicol. The first dose of any of these antimicrobial drugs usually provokes a Jarisch-Herxheimer-like reaction beginning 1 to 2 h after treatment is initiated. The severity of the reaction is greater and more predictable in louse-borne than in tick-borne relapsing fever, where it is potentially fatal. Treatment should be given in a hospital where supportive care can be given and vital signs can be monitored carefully. The hyperpyrexia can be treated with acetaminophen and tepid sponging. Most patients are hypovolemic and require 4 or more liters of isotonic saline during the first 24 h. Those with bleeding and jaundice should be given vitamin K; heparin is not effective in controlling the coagulopathy and should not be given.

The treatment of choice in louse-borne relapsing fever is tetracycline, chloramphenicol, or erythromycin stearate, 500 mg in a single oral or intravenous dose.

Tetracycline hydrochloride, 500 mg orally every 6 h for 10 days, is the recommended treatment for tick-borne relapsing fever. Doxycycline, 100 mg twice daily, is also effective. The dosage is halved for children under 12 years of age. Erythromycin stearate or chloramphenicol, 500 mg orally every 6 h for 10 days, can be given to patients who are allergic to tetracycline.

PROGNOSIS The untreated mortality rate in epidemics of louse-borne disease is between 30 to 70 percent. Appropriate treatment lowers mortality to less than 1 percent. Adverse signs are deep jaundice, delirium or coma, uncontrolled bleeding, and a marked prolongation of the QTc interval. Typhus, malaria, and enteric fever may occur simultaneously with louse-borne relapsing fever, and they probably contribute to the mortality rate, particularly during epidemics.

REFERENCES

BURGDORFER W: The enlarging spectrum of tick-borne spirotrichosis, RR Parker Memorial Address. Rev Infect Dis 8:932, 1986

HORTON JM, BLASER MJ: The spectrum of relapsing fever in the Rocky Mountains. Arch Intern Med 145:871, 1985

JUDGE DM et al: Louse-borne relapsing fever in man. Arch Pathol 97:136, 1974

PERINE PL, TEKLU B: Antibiotic treatment of relapsing fever in Ethiopia: A report of 377 cases. Am J Trop Med Hyg 32:1096, 1983

TEKLU B et al: Meptazinol diminishes the Jarisch-Herxheimer reaction of relapsing fever. Lancet 1:835, 1983

WARRELL DM et al: Pathophysiology and immunology of the Jarisch-Herxheimer-like reaction in louse-borne relapsing fever: Comparison of tetracycline and slow release penicillin. J Infect Dis 147:898, 1983

132 LYME BORRELIOSIS

ALLEN C. STEERE

DEFINITION Lyme borreliosis, a tick-transmitted spirochetal illness, usually begins with a characteristic expanding skin lesion, erythema migrans (EM), accompanied by "flulike" or "meningitis-like" symptoms (stage 1). This phase of the disorder may be followed by frank meningitis, cranial or peripheral neuritis, carditis, or migratory musculoskeletal pain (stage 2), or by intermittent or chronic arthritis or chronic neurologic or skin abnormalities (stage 3).

ETIOLOGY *Borrelia burgdorferi*, the causative agent of the disease, is 11 to 39 μm long. Organisms have 7 to 11 flagella, and their cytosine/guanine ratio is 27.3 to 30.5 percent. Like other *Borrelia*, they grow in Barbour, Stoenner, Kelly (BSK) medium. Isolates of *B. burgdorferi* have four to seven plasmids, one of which encodes for the organism's two major outer membrane proteins, the 31-kDa OspA protein and the 34-kDa OspB protein. These proteins appear to undergo antigenic variation during the course of the disease.

EPIDEMIOLOGY Lyme disease has worldwide distribution that correlates primarily with the geographic ranges of certain ixodid ticks—*Ixodes dammini*, *I. pacificus*, *I. ricinus*, and *I. persulcatus*. *I. dammini* is the principal vector in the northeastern United States from Massachusetts to Maryland and in the midwest in Wisconsin and Minnesota. In surveys of *I. dammini* in these states, 20 percent or more of the ticks have been infected with *B. burgdorferi*, and most of the cases of Lyme disease in the United States have occurred in these areas. *I. pacificus* is the vector in the western United States. The disease may be acquired throughout Europe—from Great Britain to Scandinavia to Russia—where *I. ricinus* is the vector; in Asia, where *I. persulcatus* is the vector; and in Australia. The ticks have different reservoirs; for *I. dammini*, the white-footed mouse is the preferred reservoir of the immature tick and the white-tailed deer of the mature tick.

Most new cases have onsets during the summer months. Cases have occurred in association with hiking, camping, or hunting trips or among people living in wooded or rural areas. Patients of any age and both sexes are affected. Cases have been reported in 33 states, and more than 1000 people now acquire the infection in the United States each summer.

PATHOGENESIS After injection into the skin, *B. burgdorferi* may migrate outward in the skin, producing EM, and may spread hematogenously to other organs. The spirochete has been cultured from blood, skin (EM), cerebrospinal fluid, and joint fluid and has been seen in most affected tissues. These findings and the response of all stages of the disease to antibiotic therapy suggest that the organism invades and persists in affected tissues throughout the illness.

Initially, the immune response seems to be suppressed. The mononuclear cells of patients respond minimally to *B. burgdorferi* antigens and less than normally to mitogens. Suppressor cell activity is greater than normal. After the first several weeks of infection, mononuclear cells generally have heightened responsiveness to *B. burgdorferi* antigens and to mitogens, less suppressor cell activity than normal, and evidence of B-cell hyperactivity—elevated total serum IgM levels, cryoprecipitates, and circulating immune complexes. The specific antibody response to the spirochete develops gradually over months to years and to an increasing array of spirochetal polypeptides. Specific IgM antibody titers to *B. burgdorferi* peak between the third and sixth week after disease onset; specific IgG antibody titers rise slowly and are generally highest months or years after when arthritis is present. By that time, antigen-reactive mononuclear cells and immune complexes are found in the fluid. Patients with chronic arthritis have an increased frequency of the B-cell alloantigens DR3 and DR4.

CLINICAL MANIFESTATIONS As with other spirochetal illnesses, Lyme disease occurs in stages, with remissions and exacerbations and different clinical manifestations at each stage. Stage 1 generally lasts for several weeks, stage 2 occurs during the following several months, and stage 3 occurs months to years after the onset of infection. Marked variation is possible in the clinical expression of the disease. Some patients without EM have the nonspecific symptoms associated with stage 1. In other patients, neurologic, cardiac, or joint involvement is the presenting sign of the illness. Antibiotic treatment at any point may modify or completely suppress the development and evolution of the characteristic stages.

Stage 1 After an incubation period of 3 to 32 days, EM, which occurs at the site of the tick bite, usually begins as a red macule or papule that expands to form a large annular lesion, usually with a bright red outer border and partial central clearing. Because of the small size of ixodid ticks, most patients do not remember the preceding tick bite. The center of the lesion sometimes becomes intensely erythematous and indurated, vesicular, or necrotic. In other instances, the expanding lesion remains an even, intense red; several red rings are found within the outside one; or the central area turns blue before it clears. Although the lesion can be located anywhere, the thigh, groin, and axilla are particularly common sites. The lesion is warm, but not often painful. Skin biopsies show perivascular infiltrates or lymphocytes and histiocytes. In some patients, the Lyme spirochete remains localized to this skin lesion and to regional lymph nodes and is sometimes accompanied by minor constitutional symptoms. In others, the organism spreads hematogenously to many different sites. Within days after the onset of EM, such patients often develop secondary annular skin lesions, which are similar in appearance to the initial lesion. Additional dermatologic manifestations include malar rash, diffuse erythema, urticaria, or evanescent lesions. Skin involvement is frequently accompanied by severe headache, mild neck stiffness, fever, chills, migratory musculoskeletal pain, arthralgias, and profound malaise and fatigue. Less common manifestations include generalized lymphadenopathy or splenomegaly, hepatitis,

sore throat, nonproductive cough, conjunctivitis, iritis, or testicular swelling.

Except for fatigue and lethargy, which are often constant, the early signs and symptoms of Lyme disease are typically intermittent and changing. Even in untreated patients, the early symptoms usually improve or disappear within several weeks. However, fatigue and lethargy and sometimes vague musculoskeletal pain may last for months after the skin lesions have disappeared.

Stage 2 Symptoms suggestive of meningeal irritation may occur early in Lyme disease when EM is present but are usually not associated with a spinal fluid pleocytosis or objective neurologic deficit. After several weeks to months, about 15 percent of patients develop frank neurologic abnormalities, including meningitis, subtle encephalitic signs, cranial neuritis (including bilateral facial palsy), motor or sensory radiculoneuropathy, mononeuritis multiplex, chorea, or myelitis, alone or in various combinations. The usual pattern consists of fluctuating symptoms of meningitis accompanied by facial palsy and peripheral radiculoneuropathy. Cerebrospinal fluid shows a lymphocytic pleocytosis (about 100 cells per microliter), often with elevated protein, and normal or slightly low glucose. Neurologic abnormalities usually resolve completely within months, but chronic neurologic disease may occur later.

Within several weeks after the onset of illness, about 8 percent of patients develop cardiac involvement. The most common abnormality is fluctuating degrees of atrioventricular block (first-degree, Wenckebach, or complete heart block). Some patients have more diffuse cardiac involvement, including electrocardiographic changes of acute myopericarditis, left ventricular dysfunction on radionuclide scans, or, rarely, cardiomegaly or pancarditis. Cardiac involvement usually lasts only a few weeks but may recur.

During this stage, musculoskeletal pain is common. The typical pattern is migratory pain in joints, tendons, bursae, muscle, or bone, usually without joint swelling.

Stage 3 Within weeks to 2 years after the onset of infection, about 80 percent of patients in the United States who have received no antibiotic treatment develop joint symptoms ranging from subjective joint pain, to intermittent attacks of arthritis, to chronic erosive synovitis. Marked joint swelling does not usually begin until months after the onset of the illness. The typical pattern is intermittent attacks of oligoarticular arthritis in large joints, especially knees, lasting weeks to months in a given joint. Small joints and periarticular sites may also be affected. The total number of patients who continue to have recurrent attacks decreases by about 10 to 20 percent each year, but patients have been known to have recurrence for as long as 8 years. In a small percentage of patients, involvement in large joints becomes chronic, with erosion of cartilage and bone.

Joint fluid white cell counts range from 500 to 110,000 cells per microliter (average, 25,000 cells per microliter), mostly polymorphonuclear leukocytes. Tests for rheumatoid factor or antinuclear antibodies are usually negative. Synovial biopsies show fibrin deposits, villous hypertrophy, vascular proliferation, microangiopathic lesions, and a heavy infiltration of lymphocytes and plasma cells.

Although less common, chronic neurologic or skin involvement (acrodermatitis chronica atrophicans) may also occur months to years after the onset of infection. Some patients may have intermittent tingling paresthesias of their extremities for years. In severe cases, *B. burgdorferi* may cause slowly progressive encephalomyelitis, organic brain syndromes, spastic parapareses, transverse myelitis, or dementia. Acrodermatitis begins with red-violaceous lesions that become sclerotic or atrophic over a period of years.

TREATMENT For early Lyme disease, tetracycline, 250 mg four times a day, is effective therapy in adults. In vitro, *B. burgdorferi* is as sensitive to doxycycline and amoxicillin as to tetracycline. Phenoxymethylpenicillin, 500 mg four times a day, or erythromycin, 250 mg four times a day, are second- and third-choice alternatives. Therapy should be given for at least 10 days, and for up to 30 days, if symptoms persist or recur. In children, amoxicillin or phenoxymethylpenicillin are effective (50 mg/kg per day, but not more than

2g/d) in divided doses for the same duration, or, in cases of penicillin allergy, erythromycin, 30 mg/kg per day, in divided doses for 15 to 20 days, should be used. Approximately 15 percent of patients experience a Jarisch-Herxheimer-like reaction during the first 24 h of therapy.

Later in the illness, parenteral antibiotic therapy may be necessary. In patients with frank meningitis and cranial or peripheral neuropathies, intravenous penicillin G, 20 million units per day in divided doses for 14 days or intravenous ceftriaxone, 2 g/d, are usually effective. In patients with high-degree atrioventricular block or a PR interval of greater than 0.3 s, intravenous penicillin, 10 to 20 million units per day, or intravenous ceftriaxone, 2 g/d, for at least 10 days, and cardiac monitoring are recommended. In patients with complete heart block or congestive heart failure, glucocorticoids may be of benefit if the patient does not improve on antimicrobial therapy alone within 24 h. For established arthritis, doxycycline, 100 mg twice a day, or amoxicillin and probenecid, each 500 mg four times a day, given for 30 days, are effective in about 70 percent of patients. However, the response to therapy is frequently slow, and a repeat course of oral therapy or of intravenous penicillin or ceftriaxone may need to be given. A small percentage of patients with arthritis, particularly those with DR3 and DR4 HLA antigen, do not respond to antimicrobial therapy. Synovectomy may be successful in such patients.

PROGNOSIS The response to treatment is best early in the illness. When treated later, convalescence often requires months. Nearly half the patients with Lyme disease irrespective of the antibiotic given have minor recurrences of headaches, musculoskeletal pain, or lethargy. The recrudescences correlate significantly with the severity of the initial illness. Eventually, complete recovery ensues in the majority of patients.

REFERENCES

BARBOUR AG, HAYES SF: Biology of *Borrelia* species. Microbiol Rev 50:381, 1986
HALPERIN JJ et al: Lyme disease. Cause of treatable peripheral neuropathy. Neurology 37:1700, 1987
PACHNER AR, STEERE AC: The triad of neurologic manifestations of Lyme disease: Meningitis, cranial neuritis, and radiculoneuritis. Neurology 35:47, 1985
STEERE AC: Lyme borreliosis, in *Principles and Practice of Infectious Diseases*, 3d ed, GL Mandell et al (eds). New York, Churchill-Livingstone, 1990
——: Lyme disease. N Engl J Med 321:586, 1989
—— et al: Lyme carditis: Cardiac abnormalities of Lyme disease. Ann Intern Med 93:8, 1980
—— et al: The spirochetal etiology of Lyme disease. N Engl J Med 308:733, 1983
—— et al: The early clinical manifestations of Lyme disease. Ann Intern Med 99:76, 1983
—— et al: Treatment of the early manifestations of Lyme disease. Ann Intern Med 99:22, 1983
—— et al: The clinical evolution of Lyme arthritis. Ann Intern Med 107:725, 1987

section 8   Viral diseases

---

133   THE BIOLOGY OF VIRUSES

BERNARD N. FIELDS

STRUCTURE AND CLASSIFICATION OF VIRUSES A typical virus particle (*virion*) contains a core of nucleic acid of either DNA or RNA. There is considerable variability in the structure and size of viral nucleic acids (Table 133-1). The smallest molecular weight genomes, such as those of the parvoviridae, encode three or four proteins, whereas the larger genomes, such as those of the poxviridae, encode more than 50 structural proteins and enzymes. The number of proteins encoded by a viral genome may be greater than predicted from the genome's molecular weight because of the presence of multiple open reading frames and/or the presence of overlapping regions of nucleic acid that can be transcribed into several distinct mRNAs. Extensive nucleotide sequence data are available for part or all of the genomes of many viruses.

The viral nucleic acid is surrounded by either a single or double protein shell (*capsid*). The viral nucleic acid plus the capsid are referred to as the *nucleocapsid*. The viral capsids are composed of smaller repetitive subunits (*capsomers*) arranged in symmetric constructions. The repeating subunits facilitate assembly of viral proteins into mature virions and reduce the amount of genomic information required to encode structural proteins. Capsids are formed by self-assembly of their structural subunits.

The two fundamental patterns of capsid structural symmetry are icosahedral and helical. Some of the largest viruses, such as the poxviruses, have more complex structural patterns. The retroviruses appear to have icosahedral capsid symmetry and helical core symmetry. Viruses with icosahedral capsid symmetry generally follow principles of physical organization that specify the total allowable number of structural subunits. The nucleic acid in icosahedral viruses is usually in a condensed form and is geometrically independent of the surrounding capsid structure.

Animal viruses with helical symmetry have RNA genomes. A general feature of animal viruses is the binding of protein subunits of the capsid in a regular, periodic fashion along the viral RNA. This close interaction between the capsid proteins and nucleic acid is in sharp contrast to the loose interactions in viruses with icosahedral symmetry and imposes different constraints for viral assembly.

Many viruses have an envelope surrounding the nucleocapsid. The viral envelope is composed of viral-specific proteins and of lipids and carbohydrates derived from host cell membranes. The host cell components are added as the virus buds through the host cell nuclear membrane, endoplasmic reticulum, Golgi apparatus, or cytoplasmic membrane. Different viruses utilize distinctive types of host cell membranes for budding. The factors that determine this specificity are incompletely understood. In some cases viral-specific envelope proteins may include a matrix protein (*M protein*) which lines the inner side of the envelope and is in contact with the nucleocapsid. Viral-specific glycoproteins protrude from the outer surface of the envelope (e.g., as "spikes") and may in some cases contain hydrophobic domains, which span the lipid bilayer of the envelope, as well as internal domains which may contact the M proteins.

Viral proteins, referred to as *structural* or *virion proteins*, can form the viral capsid, can be a major component of viral envelopes, or can be associated with the viral nucleic acid (*core proteins*). A number of viruses contain surface glycoproteins that agglutinate red blood cells (*hemagglutinins*) by binding to receptors on the red cell surface. Many viruses contain proteins with enzymatic activity. In many cases these enzymes are required for the synthesis of messenger

TABLE 133-1   Structure of viral nucleic acid

Family	Example	Type of nucleic acid	Genome size, kilobases or kilobase pairs	Envelope	Capsid symmetry
Picornaviridae	Poliovirus	ss(+)RNA	7.2–8.4	No	I
Caliciviridae	Norwalk virus	ss(+)RNA	8	No	I
Togaviridae	Rubella virus	ss(+)RNA	12	Yes	I
Flaviviridae	Yellow fever virus	ss(.+)RNA	10	Yes	UNK
Coronaviridae	Coronaviruses	ss(+)RNA	16–21	Yes	H
Rhabdoviridae	Rabies virus	ss(−)RNA	13–16	Yes	H
Filoviridae	Marburg virus	ss(−)RNA	13	Yes	H
Paramyxoviridae	Measles virus	ss(−)RNA	16–20	Yes	H
Orthomyxoviridae	Influenza viruses	8 ss(−)RNA segments*	14	Yes	H
Bunyaviridae	California encephalitis virus	3 circular ss(−)RNA segments	13–21	Yes	H
Arenaviridae	Lymphocytic choriomeningitis virus	2 circular ss(−)RNA segments	10–14	Yes	H
Reoviridae	Rotaviruses	10–12 dsRNA† segments	16–27	No	I
Retroviridae	HIV-1	2 identical ss(+)RNA segments	3–9	Yes	I-capsid H-nucleocapsid (probable)
Hepadnaviridae	Hepatitis B	dsDNA with ss portions	3	Yes	UNK
Parvoviridae	Human parvovirus B-19	ss(+) or (−) DNA	5	No	I
Papovaviridae	JC virus	Circular dsDNA	8	No	I
Adenoviridae	Human adenoviruses	dsDNA	36–38	No	I
Herpesviridae	Herpes simplex virus	dsDNA	120–220	Yes	I
Poxviridae	Vaccinia	dsDNA with covalently closed ends	130–280	Yes	Complex

* Influenza C = 7 segments.
† Reovirus, orbivirus = 10 segments; rotavirus = 11 segments; Colorado tick fever = 12 segments.
NOTE: ds = double-stranded; ss = single-stranded; (+) message sense; (−) anti-message sense; I = icosahedral; H = helical; UNK = unknown.
SOURCES: FA Murphy, in *Fundamental Virology*, BN Fields, DM Knipe (eds), New York, Raven, 1986, and KL Tyler, BN Fields, in *Laboratory Diagnosis of Infectious Diseases*, vol 2, EH Lennette et al (eds), New York, Springer-Verlag, 1988.

RNA (mRNA) of the appropriate (+) polarity for translation into protein or for replication of the viral genome. An RNA-dependent RNA polymerase activity is found in all (−) polarity RNA viruses. Poxviruses contain a DNA-dependent RNA polymerase. Retroviruses contain an RNA-dependent DNA polymerase commonly referred to as *reverse transcriptase*. Some viruses, including the poxviruses, reoviruses, paramyxoviruses, and rhabdoviruses, have RNA "capping enzymes" which modify viral mRNAs at their 5' end by adding a 7-methylguanosine cap in 5'-5'-triphosphate linkage. Enzymes which polyadenylate the 3' end of viral mRNAs may also be virally encoded. Additional virally encoded enzymes include protein kinases, nucleoside triphosphate phosphohydrolases, endonucleases, and RNAses.

The earliest classifications of viruses were based solely on their ability to pass through filters with small pore sizes. Subsequent classifications stressed pathogenic properties, specific organ tropisms (e.g., enteroviruses), or epidemiologic characteristics (e.g., arboviruses). Current classifications of viruses are based on a combination of genetic, physicochemical, and biologic factors. These include the type and structure of the viral nucleic acid, the nature of virion ultrastructure including size, type of capsid symmetry, capsid composition, and the presence or absence of an envelope, as well as the strategy used by the virus for genome replication. The reliance on morphologic criteria often means that electron-micrographic studies provide sufficient information to identify both the family and the genus to which a virus belongs. Subdivisions within major viral taxonomic groups may be based on immunologic, cytopathologic, pathogenetic, or epidemiologic features. The application of recombinant DNA techniques will require revision of these classifications based on degrees of genetic relatedness.

REPLICATION   Replication refers to the process by which viruses infect susceptible cells, reproduce their genomic material and proteins, and assemble and release infectious progeny. The diversity among viruses in terms of structure and type of genomic material is reflected by the large number of replicative strategies.

The first stage of viral infection of target cells begins with adsorption of the virus particles and ends with the onset of formation of infectious progeny virus. This stage is often referred to as the *eclipse period* and varies from 1 to 5 h (e.g., picornaviruses, togaviruses, rhabdoviruses, orthomyxoviruses, herpesviruses) to 8 to 14 h (adenoviruses, papovaviruses). During this period there is a dramatic drop in the amount of infectious virus that can be recovered from disrupted cells.

Adsorption appears to be a process that is initially reversible, resulting from random collisions between viruses and target cells. It has been estimated that only one in 10^3 to 10^4 such collisions leads to tighter binding (*attachment*). Attachment is facilitated by the appropriate ionic and pH conditions but is largely temperature-independent and does not require energy. Adsorption of virus to a target cell may involve specific binding of viral proteins to receptors on the cell surface (also called attachment). The virion structure mediating cell attachment has been identified for a number of viruses. For enveloped viruses the viral attachment protein is typically one of the "spikes" inserted on the outer surface of the viral envelope such as the hemagglutinin (HA) of influenza viruses. Some enveloped viruses, such as the herpesviruses and vaccinia, may have more than one type of cell attachment protein. In nonenveloped viruses, surface polypeptides, such as the fiber protein of adenovirus and the hemagglutinin (σ1) protein of reovirus, often function as the viral attachment proteins.

The exact nature of the cellular receptors for animal viruses is known in only a few specific cases. Even when the specific receptor is still unknown, it has been possible to identify "families" or classes of viral receptors using competition binding studies. Viruses of the same species, but different serotypes, may compete for the same receptor class (e.g., poliovirus serotypes 1, 2, 3) or for different receptor classes (e.g., human rhinovirus 2 and 14). Viruses from different families (e.g., coxsackievirus B3 and adenovirus 2) may also compete for the same class of receptor. These types of binding studies suggest that there are generally 10^4 to 10^6 viral binding sites (receptors) per cell.

Once attachment has occurred, the entire virion or a substructure containing the viral genome and any virion polymerases required for its initial transcription must be translocated across the plasma membrane of the cell. The rate of penetration varies depending on the nature of the virus, the type of cells being infected, and environmental factors such as temperature. Some nonenveloped viruses such as poliovirus and reovirus undergo a process of receptor-mediated endocytosis (*viropexis*) and appear in the cytoplasm inside endocytic vesicles. Other nonenveloped viruses may be able to cross the plasma membrane directly and appear free in the cytoplasm without entering endocytic vesicles.

Enveloped viruses also utilize at least two strategies for penetration. The first is exemplified by Semliki Forest virus (SFV). SFV, a togavirus, binds to specific cell surface receptors, which then aggregate at distinct sites on the plasma membrane (*coated pits*) and are internalized by receptor-mediated endocytosis. They subsequently appear inside clathrin-coated vesicles within the cell cytoplasm. Fusion between the viral envelope and the endosomal membrane causes release of the viral nucleocapsid into the cytoplasm. A second mechanism for penetration of enveloped viruses occurs with paramyxoviruses (e.g., Sendai). The viral envelope fuses directly with the cell plasma membrane, and the viral nucleocapsid is discharged free into the cytoplasm.

Uncoating is the process of removing or disaggregating part or all of the viral protein capsid in preparation for transcription and translation of the viral genome. In many cases penetration and uncoating are part of a single process. Some picornaviruses, for example, seem to undergo an alteration in capsid structure and integrity and loss of an internal protein as they are translocated across the plasma membrane. The structural alterations associated with loss of the protein may facilitate entry of the viral RNA into the cytoplasm.

Nonenveloped viruses which enter endosomes, such as adenovirus, may induce fusion of lysosomes with the endosome and have their capsid removed by lysosomal enzymes. In the case of reoviruses, intraendosomal proteases sequentially remove the three outer capsid proteins to produce a "subviral particle," a process which leads to activation of the viral transcriptase. Uncoating of poxviruses, such as vaccinia, first involves degradation of the outer protein coat by intraendosomal enzymes and then of the remaining "core," liberating the viral DNA. This step appears to require the synthesis of a virus-specified "uncoating protein."

A number of strategies have evolved for *transcription* of viral genomes into mRNA and *translation* of mRNA into protein. One approach is for viruses to contain mRNA that is translated into a large precursor polyprotein, which is then cleaved to produce the various virion proteins. This approach is exemplified by viruses such as the picornaviruses and togaviruses in which the nucleic acid is in the form of (+) polarity, single-stranded RNA (ssRNA) and serves as mRNA. It binds to large polyribosomes and is fully translated (5′ → 3′) to produce a single large polyprotein, which is then cleaved in a series of steps to produce the nonstructural, core, and capsid proteins. In the case of both the picornaviruses and the togaviruses a virally encoded RNA polymerase synthesizes a complementary RNA using the genomic RNA as template. In turn, the newly synthesized RNA serves as template for the synthesis of more genomic RNA. The new genomic RNAs may serve as mRNAs or as precursor RNA for progeny virions.

Viruses which contain linear or segmented RNA produce unique mRNAs for each viral protein rather than a single large mRNA molecule. A transcriptase enzyme contained in the virion (the virion

polymerase) is required to produce mRNAs from the genomic RNA. The presence of multiple mRNAs allows regulation of the amount of each protein synthesized. A single region of genomic RNA may have multiple reading frames, each of which is transcribed into unique mRNAs, which are in turn translated into distinct proteins. Genomic (−)ssRNA is replicated via a (+)ssRNA intermediate, which then serves as a template to synthesize more (−)ss genomic RNA.

Reoviruses contain a RNA-dependent RNA polymerase that transcribes (+)ssRNAs from the (−) strand of each double-stranded (ds) RNA segment. These (+)ssRNAs are extruded from the viral core through channels in the core spike, and serve as mRNAs for translation into viral proteins. The viral RNA polymerase also synthesizes (+)ssRNAs, which in turn serve as templates for the complementary (−) strand during replication of the viral genome.

The retroviruses utilize a unique replicative strategy. Viral (+)ssRNA serves as a template for the virion RNA-dependent DNA polymerase (reverse transcriptase) and primer transfer RNAs (tRNAs). A ssDNA copy is produced which is initially hydrogen bonded to its complementary (+)ssRNA. A virally encoded ribonuclease digests the ssRNA, and a complementary DNA strand is synthesized. Then dsDNA is integrated into chromosomal DNA in the host cell nucleus. Transcription of this integrated viral DNA is under the control of the host cell transcriptases.

DNA-containing viruses are capable of using strategies similar to those in eukaryotic cells for replication during lytic infection. Papovaviruses, adenoviruses, and herpesviruses use replicative strategies in which transcription of viral DNA into mRNA occurs in the nucleus of the host cell and depends on host cell enzymes. In the case of papovaviruses (e.g., SV40), the initial proteins produced after infection are the *T antigens* (tumor antigens or *early proteins*). Some of the T-antigen proteins appear to interact with the viral genomic dsDNA by binding near the site of initiation of DNA replication. This binding facilitates DNA replication. Subsequently, mRNAs encoding the capsid polypeptides are transcribed (*late proteins*). The early mRNAs are all derived from only one of the two viral DNA strands (referred to as the E or *E*arly strand), and the late mRNAs from the other (the L or *L*ate strand). Adenoviruses also have early and late genes, but they are intermixed along both strands of the viral DNA rather than on separate strands.

In the replication of both papovaviruses and adenoviruses, early proteins appear to be primarily regulatory in nature and often pleiotropic in function. Late proteins include structural proteins. The individual mRNAs for both early and late proteins are often complementary to dispersed segments of the viral DNA, indicating that extensive splicing, with removal of intervening regions, has occurred. In many cases mRNAs are synthesized from overlapping regions of the viral DNA. This type of redundancy reduces the amount of viral DNA needed to encode viral proteins.

Poxviruses are the most complicated of the known animal viruses, and their replicative cycle is correspondingly complex. All the initial steps of transcription and translation appear to occur in the host cell cytoplasm, which requires that the virus contain its own DNA-dependent RNA polymerase to initiate transcription. One of the virus-encoded early proteins is responsible for the second stage of uncoating which makes the viral DNA fully accessible for transcription and replication. Replication, transcription, and later viral assembly all occur in virus-initiated "factories" within the host cell cytoplasm. Sequential groups of virus-specified proteins can be detected in infected cells. Early proteins include a number of enzymes (e.g., a DNA polymerase and a thymidine kinase), as well as some structural proteins. As infection proceeds, DNA replication begins, the synthesis of the early nonstructural proteins ceases, and the synthesis of late proteins begins. Many of the late proteins are structural proteins; other late proteins include enzymes and proteins that may play a role in viral assembly.

Once replication of the viral genome and synthesis of the viral proteins have been completed, intact virions must then be assembled and released from the host cells. Assembly of the nonenveloped viruses and the nucleocapsid of enveloped viruses often appears to proceed in a crystallization-like fashion which depends on the self-assembly of viral capsomers.

In most cases nonenveloped virions accumulate within the infected cell and are released together when the cell lyses. The events leading to cell disruption include inhibition of the synthesis of host cell protein, lipid, and nucleic acids, disorganization of the host cell cytoskeleton, and alteration of host cell membrane structure. Membrane disruption may result in increased cell permeability and in the release of proteolytic enzymes from lysosomes. The failure to replenish energy-rich substrate molecules inhibits the function of ion transport pumps and disturbs transport of essential nutrients and cellular waste products.

Enveloped viruses are typically released from infected cells by budding. This process may be lethal to the cell. In all cases virus-specified proteins are inserted into host cell membranes in a fashion that restructures the membrane by displacing some of its normal protein components. Viral capsids may then bind to virus-specified matrix proteins which line the cytoplasmic side of these altered patches of membrane. In the case of the smallest enveloped viruses, the togaviruses, the capsids bind to the intracytoplasmic domains of viral proteins inserted in the host cell membrane rather than to matrix proteins.

PATHOGENESIS The signs and symptoms of disease are the result of the culmination of a series of interactions between the virus and the host. A virus must first be able to enter the host, then undergo a period of primary replication, followed by spread to its final target tissue. Once a virus reaches its target organs, it must then infect and successfully replicate in a susceptible population of host cells. The outcome of this last step may be a productive infection with or without cell injury, latent infection, or persistent infection. To transmit infectious virus to the next host the virus must successfully avoid or overcome the host immune response and a wide variety of other host defense mechanisms. A great deal of viral replication can occur before any signs or symptoms of clinical illness are detectable. This "incubation period" can vary from a few days (e.g., influenza), to weeks (e.g., measles, varicella), to months (rabies, hepatitis), to years (slow viruses).

Most viral diseases result from exposure to exogenous virus. However, in some cases disease results from the reactivation of endogenous virus, which has been latent within specific host cells. Examples of infections caused by reactivated endogenous viruses include shingles (herpes zoster), progressive multifocal leukoencephalopathy (JC or BK papovaviruses), recurrent labial and genital herpes (herpes simplex), and some types of cytomegalovirus (CMV) infections.

In the majority of cases, transmission of viral illnesses occurs between members of a susceptible host population (*horizontal spread*). *Vertical spread* of infection occurs when the fetus becomes infected in utero through virus carried in the germ cell line, virus infecting the placenta, or virus in the maternal birth canal. Rubella virus, CMV, herpes simplex virus, varicella-zoster virus, and hepatitis B virus can all produce vertically transmitted congenital infections.

The age and genetic background of the host can have important implications for the outcome of viral infections. Newborns, for example, are particularly susceptible to severe, disseminated herpes simplex virus infections. In contrast, many of the exanthematous illnesses, poliovirus infection, and Epstein-Barr virus (EBV) infection are typically more severe in older individuals than in children. In mice, specific genes help determine susceptibility to certain viral infections. These genes may act through effects on the immune system, interferon production, or viral receptors. Inadequate host nutritional status may increase susceptibility to infections such as measles, perhaps by depressing cell-mediated immunity. The host can also influence viral infections in ways that are still poorly understood. Stress may trigger recurrent herpes labialis. Strenuous exercise may have an adverse effect on the course of polio.

Viral infection begins with *entry* into the host, which may occur via a number of routes. The stratum corneum of the skin provides both a physical barrier and a biologic barrier against the entry of viruses. Some viruses overcome the skin barrier by being directly inoculated via insect or animal bites or mechanical devices such as needles. The arthropod-borne viruses are directly inoculated into the bloodstream when an infected tick or mosquito takes a blood meal. Rabies virus and herpesvirus simiae (monkey B virus) enter tissues after an animal bite. Iatrogenic inoculation allows entry of a large number of viruses. Hepatitis B virus, CMV, and human immunodeficiency virus (HIV-1) may all be present in contaminated blood products used for transfusion. Infected corneal transplants, infected instruments used in neurosurgical procedures, and infected pituitary tissues used to prepare growth hormone have been implicated as causes of Creutzfeldt-Jakob disease. Parenteral vaccination using live attenuated virus represents another category of iatrogenic inoculation.

A large number of viruses enter the host by crossing mucosal barriers in the respiratory and gastrointestinal tracts. Respiratory infection can be either by means of aerosol droplets, nasal secretions, or saliva. Entry via either the respiratory or enteric routes requires that the virus overcome a formidable series of host defenses. In the lung, immunologic defenses include secretory IgA, natural killer (NK) cells, and macrophages. Nonspecific glycoprotein viral inhibitors are present in tracheobronchial mucus. Ciliated respiratory epithelial cells continually move mucus away from the lower respiratory tract. The harsh acidic environment of the stomach inactivates acid-labile viruses such as rhinoviruses. Bile salts, present in the lumen of the small intestine, can destroy the lipid envelope of many viruses and may account for the fact that entry via the gastrointestinal route is limited largely to nonenveloped viruses. Proteolytic enzymes and secretory IgA contribute to host antiviral defenses in the gastrointestinal tract. Specific viral capsid proteins may allow some viruses to withstand proteolytic digestion in the gut.

For some enteric viruses, passage across the mucosal barrier of the gut is mediated by a specific population of cells overlying Peyer's patches known as microfold (M) cells. These cells, and perhaps their analogues in bronchial lymphoid tissue, seem to facilitate transport of some viruses, including reoviruses and possibly enteroviruses, to the abluminal surface of the small intestine.

Venereal transmission with entry across the genitourinary or rectal mucosa appears to be important for herpes simplex virus type 2, CMV, hepatitis B virus, and HIV-1.

For some viruses, the processes of entry, primary replication, and tissue tropism all occur at the same anatomic site. Examples of this type of viral illness include the upper and lower respiratory infections caused by the rhinoviruses, ortho- and paramyxoviruses; the enteritis caused by rotaviruses; and the dermatologic lesions induced by human papillomavirus (warts) and paravaccinia virus (milker's nodules). In other cases a virus enters at one site and must subsequently spread to a distant area, such as the central nervous system, to produce disease. Enteroviruses enter via the gastrointestinal tract but must spread to the CNS to produce meningitis, encephalitis, and poliomyelitis. Measles virus and varicella virus enter the body through the respiratory tract but then spread to produce skin disease (exanthem) and often generalized organ involvement.

Neural, hematogenous, and lymphatic pathways are all utilized by viruses to spread to target tissues. Rabies virus, herpes simplex virus, herpesvirus simiae (monkey B), varicella-zoster virus, and the scrapie agent spread via nerves. Herpes simplex virus appears to enter nerves via receptors located primarily near synaptic endings rather than on the nerve cell body. Rabies virus accumulates at the motor end plate of the neuromuscular junction (NMJ) and may utilize the acetylcholine receptor (AChR) or a closely related structure to enter the distal axons of motor neurons. Other viruses including La Crosse bunyavirus and the togavirus Sindbis also accumulate at the NMJ, although their receptor molecules have not been identified. Rabies virus also infects muscle and spreads via motor and sensory nerves to the spinal cord. The kinetics of neural spread for rabies, herpes simplex, and polio strongly suggest that these agents utilize intraneuronal mechanisms involved with fast axonal transport. The scrapie agent, which appears to spread slowly along neural pathways, may be an example of movement via slow axonal transport. Infection of Schwann cells may provide another "neural" pathway to the CNS. Neural spread may be important not only as a pathway to the CNS but also for spread within the CNS and from the CNS to the periphery.

The olfactory pathway represents a special category of neural spread. The rod processes of olfactory receptor cells lie exposed in the olfactory mucosa. These cells synapse directly with the mitral cells in the olfactory bulb within the CNS. Under experimental conditions, intranasal or aerosol inoculations of rabies virus, herpes simplex virus, poliovirus, and some togaviruses can lead to CNS infection via the olfactory route. This route may provide a pathway to the CNS in humans for rabies, and possibly other viruses, in circumstances, such as in caves occupied by large numbers of rabid bats or in accidental laboratory-acquired infections, where high-titer aerosols are present. An olfactory route of spread might be one explanation for the localization of herpes simplex virus to the orbitofrontal and medial temporal cortex in cases of herpes simplex encephalitis.

Hematogenous spread is important for many viruses. A period of primary replication usually precedes the initial viremia and can be asymptomatic or result in prodromal symptoms. For enteric viruses, primary replication occurs in Peyer's patches and peritonsillar lymphatic tissue. Primary replication of respiratory viruses occurs in epithelial or alveolar cells and for many enteroviruses and togaviruses in skeletal muscle. In some cases virus travels from the site of initial multiplication via lymphatics to regional lymph nodes before entering the bloodstream. The initial (*primary*) viremia often disseminates virus to tissues such as the spleen and liver where continued multiplication in parenchymal cells leads to an amplified secondary viremia. Growth in endothelial cells may help sustain the viremic phase in some togavirus infections. Sustained secondary amplification of the viremia is required if a virus is to overcome clearance by reticuloendothelial cells.

Blood-borne virus can travel free or in association with cellular elements. Hepatitis B virus, picornaviruses, and togaviruses all travel free within plasma; Colorado tick fever virus and Rift valley fever virus are associated with red blood cells; EBV, CMV, rubella, and HIV are lymphocyte- or monocyte-associated.

In some cases viruses use different pathways of spread at different stages in the infectious cycle. Varicella-zoster virus disseminates to the skin by the hematogenous route to produce "chickenpox." The virus then spreads centripetally along nerves from the skin to neurons in the dorsal root ganglion where it remains latent. Reactivation results in centrifugal spread of virus down sensory nerves to their skin dermatome and the production of "shingles" (zoster). Neural spread of virus presumably accounts for recurrent episodes of oral and genital infection caused by herpes simplex virus. Poliovirus represents an example of a virus capable of spreading by both hematogenous and neural routes. The hematogenous route is generally accepted as the primary pathway to the CNS, although the virus may spread to the CNS via autonomic nerves in the gut. Axonal transport may play a role in the spread of poliovirus within the CNS.

Once a virus has spread from its site of primary replication to a target organ, it must infect a population of susceptible cells. This requires the interaction between specific viral structures (*viral attachment proteins*) and viral receptors on cells. Virus-encoded tissue-specific enhancers may in part mediate viral injury to specific cell populations. Lytic infection also requires that all of the subsequent steps in the viral replicative cycle be successfully completed.

HOST FACTORS **The antibody response** Most viruses make good antigens for stimulating the immune response because they contain a large number of foreign proteins, each of which may contain multiple antigenic sites. In addition, although the amount of viral antigenic material may initially be quite small, there is amplification in its quantity due to viral replication. Few of the antibodies play a significant role in protecting the host against

infection, and in some cases they may themselves be implicated in disease pathogenesis.

The immunogenicity of viruses depends on the nature of the virus itself and on a variety of host factors. The slow virus agents responsible for kuru and Creutzfeldt-Jakob disease do not appear to provoke any detectable immune response in the host. The route of viral infection may also play a role in immunity. In experimental influenza infections, intravenous inoculation is more immunogenic than intraperitoneal inoculation, which in turn exceeds the subcutaneous route.

Antibodies which protect the host by destroying the infectivity of virus are referred to as neutralizing antibodies (Nab). Nabs usually are directed against epitopes present on viral proteins located on the surface of the virus particle. The binding of Nab to virus is generally a reversible reaction. Viral infectivity may be reduced because Nab inhibits attachment, penetration, or uncoating of virus; produces aggregation of virions; accelerates viral degradation in vesicles, or enhances viral opsonization and subsequent phagocytosis. In the case of poliovirus, Nab binding appears to induce a conformational rearrangement of the viral outer capsid which blocks viral uncoating but not attachment.

Complement Viruses can trigger activation of both the alternate and classic pathways of complement activation in the absence of an antibody response. Activated complement components (e.g., C3b) may act as opsonins that enhance phagocytosis of viruses. Activation of the alternate complement pathway, in combination with antibody, may produce lysis of enveloped viruses or virus-infected cells. Although the complement system plays a role in the protection against viral infection in animals, human complement deficiency states are not typically associated with an increase in the frequency or severity of viral illnesses.

Cell-mediated immunity Virus-infected cells can be lysed by lymphocytes and other cells through both antibody-dependent and antibody-independent pathways. NK cells are large granular lymphocytes that bind to infected target cells and then secrete cytotoxic molecules contained in azurophilic granular vesicles. NK activity is increased by interferons and possibly by some viral glycoproteins, and does not require antibody. NK cytotoxicity provides one of the earliest host defenses against viral infection (peak activity at 2 to 3 days) and precedes the appearance of antibody (7 days), cytotoxic T lymphocytes (CTL), and delayed type hypersensitivity (DTH). Activated NK cells have been identified in human viral infections caused by CMV, EBV, measles, and mumps virus.

Antibody-dependent lysis of infected cells can occur via antibody-dependent cell-mediated cytotoxicity (ADCC) or via antibody-independent CTLs. In ADCC reactions, virus-specific antibody bound to antigens on an infected cell interacts with Fc receptors for IgG on the surface of specialized lymphocytoid cells ["killer" (K) cells]. The binding of IgG to the Fc receptor activates the K cell and results in target cell killing. Macrophages, lymphocytes, and PMNs also have Fc receptors and may also participate in ADCC.

Lysis of infected cells mediated by CTLs is typically class I histocompatibility antigen restricted, although examples of class II restricted CTLs have been described. CTLs must be activated by antigen presented by macrophages or other antigen-presenting cells (APCs). The nature of the specific epitopes expressed on the surface of infected cells that CTLs recognize has been defined for some viruses, such as influenza. In contrast to the specificity of neutralizing antibodies, which typically recognize epitopes on intact viral surface proteins, CTLs recognize protein fragments derived from both viral surface and internal proteins. The pathways by which these peptides are processed, appear on the surface of infected cells, and interact with MHC antigens are subjects of active investigation.

Interferons Leukocytes produce more than a dozen alpha ("leukocyte") interferons that share about 70 percent amino acid sequence homology. Beta ("fibroblast") interferon is produced by fibroblasts and epithelial cells and has 30 percent homology to α-interferons. Both α- and β-interferons are acid-stable (pH = 2) and relatively heat resistant. "Immune" (γ-) interferon is produced by both sensitized and unsensitized T lymphocytes, has different physico-chemical properties and different inducers, and uses a different cellular receptor from α- and β-interferons. Genes encoding interferons are located on human chromosomes 9(α and β), 2(β), 5(β), and 12(γ).

Interferons can be induced by both active and inactivated viruses, by double-stranded RNA, and by a number of other compounds. The amount of interferon produced may vary with different viruses. All the interferons have extremely high specific activity and are generally most active in cells of the species in which they are induced ("species-specific"), presumably because of variation in the nature of the interferon receptor. Interferon production appears to involve a de-repression of cellular genes induced by the presence of viral nucleic acid in the host cell cytoplasm. This results in the rapid production of mRNAs for interferon and subsequent interferon synthesis.

Newly produced interferon is released into extracellular fluid and then binds to a specific receptor on adjacent cells. The gene encoding the glycoprotein receptor for α- and β-interferon appears to be on human chromosome 21. Binding of interferon to this receptor results in a complex variety of subsequent events. A protein kinase is synthesized which phosphorylates a protein synthesis initiation factor, resulting in inhibition of initiation complex formation and hence of viral protein synthesis. An induced 2,5-oligoisoadenylate synthetase produces 2,5-oligoadenylates, which in turn activate a cellular endonuclease (RNase L) which degrades viral mRNA. Methyltransferase reactions are inhibited, which decreases methylation of mRNAs and thereby interferes with viral protein synthesis. In addition to these actions there are changes in target cell surface antigens, resulting in enhanced expression of both class I and class II histocompatability antigens. Interferons also increase the activity of NK cells, CTLs, and cells involved in ADCC reactions. The relative importance of each of these activities in creating the interferon-induced antiviral state is not established.

Virus-induced immunopathology Viruses can combine with virus-specific antibodies to produce circulating immune complexes which may be involved in immunopathogenesis. Virus stimulation of B lymphocytes may result in the production of polyclonal antibodies to antigens unrelated to the inciting virus. Viruses can also induce cross-reacting antibodies to normal host structures which contain antigenic regions similar to those of the virus (*molecular mimicry*). These types of autoantibodies may also lead to immune-complex formation. Immune complexes can become trapped in basement membranes at a variety of sites including the skin, the kidney, the choroid plexus, and the walls of blood vessels. These immune complexes result in tissue injury by attracting and activating a variety of inflammatory mediators.

Autoantibodies produced by virus infection may also result in direct tissue injury. Autoantibodies to lymphocytes, platelets, smooth muscle, intermediate filaments, immunoglobulins and myelin basic protein are usually transient and of low titer. These autoantibodies could result from a variety of mechanisms including (1) incorporation of host antigens into viral structures or virus-induced alteration of host antigens, (2) virus-induced alterations in immunoregulatory systems, (3) cross-reactivity between virus antigens and normal host cell structures (molecular mimicry), and (4) eliciting anti-idiotypic antibodies which stimulate host cell receptors.

EPIDEMIOLOGY Viral epidemiology includes the study of the causes, distribution, frequency, modes of transmission, and spread of viral diseases. Accurate enumeration of the incidence and prevalence of viral diseases is an important aspect of epidemiology. Incidence can be defined as the number of *new* cases of a particular disease that appear during a defined period of time, and prevalence as the *total* number of cases. It is often useful to refer to incidence and prevalence *rates*, which are obtained by dividing incidence or prevalence numbers by the size of the total population at risk. Terms such as "epidemic" and "outbreak" are arbitrary and simply indicate that a greater than expected number of cases of a particular disease

has occurred in a specific population, geographic location, or time period.

The appearance of an acute viral disease indicates that an infected host has come into contact with a susceptible individual under conditions that permit the transmission of a particular viral agent. The time interval between exposure to a virus and the development of signs and symptoms of disease is referred to as the "incubation period" and can vary from a few days (e.g., influenza) to years (slow virus diseases). Viral infection does not always lead to overt clinical disease. The percentage of those infected who develop overt disease ranges from 100 percent (e.g., rabies, measles) to 0 percent (BK, JC papovaviruses). In most cases symptomatic disease is less common in children than in adults (e.g., EBV mononucleosis, paralytic poliomyelitis, hepatitis A virus).

Transmission of a virus from an infected host to a susceptible individual can take a variety of forms. Human-to-human transmission can occur from an acutely ill individual, from a chronic carrier, or from mother to fetus. The method of spread can involve respiratory aerosols, fecal-oral contamination, sexual contact, or direct inoculation via infected needles or blood products.

Respiratory aerosolization usually occurs via coughing or sneezing. A sneeze may generate up to 2 million aerosol particles and a cough up to 90,000. The fate of these particles depends both on ambient environmental conditions (e.g., humidity, wind currents) and particle size. Small particles remain airborne longer and can escape the filtering action of the nose, which traps particles larger than 6 μm in diameter. The number of viral particles aerosolized may vary for different strains of the same virus.

For most viruses it is unclear how many viral particles are required to initiate a respiratory infection. For influenza A, adenovirus, or coxsackie A21, as few as 10 particles may be sufficient. Aerosolization is not the only possible route of respiratory transmission. EBV is typically spread by saliva during kissing. A critical pathway of spread for rhinoviruses, which cause the common cold, is from hands to eyes, nose, or mouth—a cycle which can be interrupted by hand washing.

Gastrointestinal transmission occurs when virus shed in feces contaminates food or water and is then ingested by a susceptible individual ("fecal-oral spread"). Stool-tainted hands, resulting from poor personal hygiene, provide another vehicle of spread for enteric viruses. The high incidence of enteric virus infections in infant day-care centers and institutions for the mentally retarded reflect the difficulty of maintaining hygiene in these settings.

In many types of viral disease the vector is an insect or infected animal. In dengue fever there is a continuing cycle between humans and infected mosquitoes. Dengue virus multiplies in the gut of the *Aedes aegypti* mosquito, spreads to its salivary glands, and is injected into a human during the mosquito's blood meal. The infected person develops a high-titer viremia which is sufficient to transmit virus to an uninfected mosquito during biting. In other arbovirus infections the human being is a "dead-end host" because the degree of viremia in infected individuals is insufficient to transmit infection to a new group of insect vectors. Examples of this type of cycle are provided by togaviruses, such as eastern, western, and St. Louis encephalitis viruses. The normal animal reservoirs for arboviruses include small birds and mammals. The horse, like humans, is usually a dead-end host, although in Venezuelan equine encephalitis, horses may be a reservoir of virus.

Some arthropod-borne infections do not require a viremic vertebrate intermediate host. Virus can be passed in transovarian fashion to the progeny of an infected tick or mosquito or by venereal transmission between male and female mosquitoes. Transovarian transmission may allow survival of arthropod viruses through the winter months.

Zoonotic infections illustrate another mechanism of disease transmission. In the case of rabies, transmission results from the bite of an infected animal. Many human infections occur when humans are exposed to the excreta (feces, urine, saliva) of infected rodents.

Examples include arenavirus infections and the hemorrhagic fevers with renal disease caused by the bunyaviruses.

Defective agents, such as the adeno-associated human parvoviruses (AAHP) and the delta hepatitis virus (hepatitis D), require coinfection with a "helper" virus. Infection with the delta virus is dependent on coincident infection with hepatitis B virus (HBV) and does not occur in its absence. Many details of the epidemiology of these viruses remain to be established. The defective adeno-associated human parvoviruses do not appear to alter significantly the disease produced by the helper adenovirus alone. Conversely, coinfection with HBV and the delta antigen frequently results in fulminant hepatitis.

DIAGNOSIS OF VIRAL DISEASES A reasonably accurate diagnosis of some viral illnesses, such as measles, can be made on clinical grounds alone. In other cases the best that can be done clinically is to identify a group of viruses that are likely pathogens for specific categories of illness. More definitive diagnosis is often necessary because of availability of antiviral agents with activity limited only to certain types of viruses. Definitive diagnosis requires isolation of the virus in animals or in tissue culture, identification of the virus or detection of virus-specified antigens or viral nucleic acids in tissues or body fluids, or documentation of specific serologic responses. The physician must ensure that the appropriate specimens are obtained for diagnostic studies during a suitable phase of the illness, that they are rapidly transported, and that adequate clinical information is provided to the diagnostic laboratories.

In the case of diarrheal or gastrointestinal illness where a viral etiology is suspected, a fresh stool sample is the specimen of choice for virus isolation. In diseases of the respiratory system, including pharyngitis, croup, bronchiolitis, and pneumonia, nasopharyngeal or tracheal *aspirates* provide the best specimens. Nasopharyngeal and throat *swabs* are less satisfactory. When a vesicular rash is present, a needle aspirate of vesicular fluid provides the optimum specimen. When the rash is petechial or maculopapular, both nasopharyngeal aspirates and a stool sample should be obtained. In patients with CNS diseases of suspected viral etiology, including meningitis, encephalitis, myelitis, and Guillain-Barré syndrome, a nasopharyngeal aspirate and stool and cerebrospinal fluid specimens should be obtained. A urine sample may be helpful when infection due to CMV, measles, mumps, or papovaviruses is suspected. Blood specimens may be useful for the detection of some arboviruses, herpesviruses, and LCM. Saliva has been used for the detection of rabies and mumps viruses. A brain biopsy specimen is often required for the definitive diagnosis of herpes simplex encephalitis, progressive multifocal leukoencephalopathy, subacute sclerosing panencephalitis (SSPE), progressive rubella panencephalitis, and slow virus diseases such as Creutzfeldt-Jakob disease.

Nasopharyngeal or rectal swab specimens should be placed in an appropriate transport medium. In general this consists of a few milliliters of a neutral isotonic salt solution to which a small amount of protein or animal serum has been added. Antibiotics should be added to inhibit bacterial contaminants. Specimens can be placed in a thermos flask filled with crushed ice if any delay in transport is anticipated. Ideally, specimens should be inoculated into the appropriate culture systems on arrival in the virology laboratory. Storage up to 48 h can often be safely done at refrigerator temperature (4°C), and longer storage should be at −70°C. Many viruses quickly lose infectivity if repeatedly frozen and thawed.

Isolation of virus from clinical specimens is done in cell cultures, embryonated eggs, and animals such as suckling mice. Cell culture techniques involve the use of primary cultures of cells prepared from organs of freshly killed animals (e.g., monkey kidney cells); human diploid cell lines such as WI-38 embryo fibroblasts; and continuous (heterodiploid) cell lines such as HeLa, HEp-2, BHK-21, and vero. Some viruses grow better on certain cell lines than others. Inoculation into the amniotic cavity or the allantoic cavity of embryonated chicken eggs is useful in the isolation of influenza virus. Intraperitoneal and intracerebral inoculation into neonatal mice may be necessary for

isolation of coxsackie A viruses and may help in the isolation of many arboviruses, rabies virus, arenaviruses, and orbiviruses. Adult mice or guinea pigs can be used to isolate LCM virus. Identification of the agent responsible for slow virus diseases such as kuru and Creutzfeldt-Jakob disease may require intracerebral inoculation of higher primates such as chimpanzees. Special isolation techniques using brain tissue explants are required to identify measles virus in cases of SSPE, or rubella virus in patients with progressive rubella panencephalitis.

Once cell culture inoculation has been performed, the specimens are examined for distinctive patterns of cytopathic effect (CPE). Viruses such as HSV and many enteroviruses produce early CPE, whereas cultures may need to be followed for weeks and even subcultured to detect CPE due to CMV, rubella, and some adenoviruses. Cultured cells are examined for cell lysis and vacuolization. The presence of syncytia suggests HSV, RSV, measles, or mumps virus. Cytomegaly is seen with HSV, varicella-zoster virus (VZV), and CMV. Detection of inclusion bodies is aided by the use of Giemsa or other stains. Immunocytochemical staining of cell cultures to detect viral antigens using fluorescein or enzyme-conjugated specific antiviral antibodies can aid in the detection and identification of many viruses. Some viruses produce minimal or no detectable CPE. Ortho- and paramyxoviruses (influenza, parainfluenza, measles, mumps) can be detected by the ability of infected cultures to adsorb certain red blood cells (*hemadsorption*). Infection with rubella can be detected by the ability of infected cultures to block the CPE produced by infection with a second challenge virus (*interference*).

Identification of virus particles or antigens in tissue specimens provides another important method of viral diagnosis. Skin scrapings from the base of vesicles can be stained with Wright or Giemsa stain according to the Tzanck method to help identify HSV or VZV. Similar techniques may help identify CMV-infected cells in urine sediment or measles-infected cells in scrapings from Koplik spots. In some cases, examination of appropriately prepared specimens by electron microscopy (EM) is of diagnostic value; high concentrations of virus must be present. A special technique which concentrates virus in specimens by adsorbing excess fluid and salts on an agarose surface may enable detection of as few as 10^4 particles per milliliter (pseudoreplica technique). EM easily distinguishes between vaccinia and varicella-zoster viruses in vesicular fluid negatively stained with phosphotungstic acid, and may be extremely useful in identifying skin viruses such as human papilloma virus, orf virus, and molluscum contagiosum. The use of specific antisera to aggregate virus in prepared stool specimens facilitates EM detection of rotaviruses, hepatitis A virus, and the Norwalk agent. EM examination of brain biopsy specimens may allow identification of herpes simplex encephalitis, PML, and SSPE.

Detection of virus-specific antigens is facilitated by immunofluorescence and immunocytochemical techniques. These procedures are particularly valuable in diagnosing rabies, herpes infection, PML, and SSPE in brain biopsy specimens; herpes keratitis from corneal scrapings; HSV, VZV, and vaccinia infections from vesicle scrapings; parainfluenza, influenza, and RSV infections from nasopharyngeal aspirates; hepatitis B infections in liver biopsy specimens; and Colorado tick fever virus infection from blood clots. Viral antigens can be detected in these tissue specimens using virus-specific antibodies directly or indirectly coupled with fluorescein isothiocyanate (FITC), or enzymes including horseradish peroxidase (HRP), alkaline phosphatase (AP), and glucose oxidase (GO). Enzyme-linked antibody techniques offer the advantage of increased sensitivity, preservability of stained specimens, and detectability with conventional light microscopy. Coupling a biotin-linked antibody with avidin-linked FITC or enzymes promises to improve immunocytochemical techniques. Radioimmunoassays and immunoassays, in which viral antibody coupled to a solid support (ELISA) is used to detect viral antigens, have proved useful in the diagnosis of hepatitis A and B virus, rotavirus, and adenovirus infections.

The detection of a fourfold or greater increase in antibody titer to a specific viral agent in a patient's acute and convalescent (3 to 4 weeks later) sera can usually be considered diagnostic of acute infection. A single serum specimen is only occasionally useful in viral diagnosis. A high antibody titer against a rare agent in a typical clinical setting or a distinct pattern of antibody titers to viral antigens of specific types may provide presumptive evidence of acute infection. Blood for serology should be collected in anticoagulant- and preservative-free glass tubes, and allowed to clot. Serum should be separated out and stored frozen. A number of different types of antibodies including neutralizing (N), complement-fixing (CF), and hemagglutination-inhibiting (HI) antibodies are routinely assayed. The time course of these antibody responses and their sensitivity and specificity differ greatly.

Restriction enzyme analysis of the genomes of DNA viruses (e.g., HSV, VZV, CMV) and oligonucleotide fingerprinting of ribonuclease T_1 cleaved genomes of RNA viruses (e.g., influenza, dengue enteroviruses) are valuable in epidemiologic studies and in establishing the origin of certain types of viral isolates. In situ hybridization and the polymerase chain reaction technique may enable the detection of even single copies of virus genomes in tissue samples or cells from body fluids.

PREVENTION OF VIRAL ILLNESS   Vaccines   Currently available vaccines utilize inactivated virus, attenuated virus, or virus subunits to induce active immunization. Formalin- or β-propiolactone–inactivated vaccines are available for rabies, influenza, and polio. Strains used in the inactivated influenza whole-virus vaccine are specified yearly by the FDA. The vaccine is composed of formalin-inactivated natural isolates of influenza virus and laboratory-designed reassortant strains containing the hemagglutinin and neuraminidase genes of the influenza viruses that are currently circulating. As many as 60 to 80 percent of those immunized show a reduction in the frequency or severity of influenzal illness. Guillain-Barré syndrome occurred in 1 in 100,000 individuals vaccinated with the swine influenza vaccine in 1976 to 1977 but has not been associated with subsequent influenza vaccine preparations. Killed polio vaccine is used in Sweden, Finland, and the Netherlands, and in combination with live vaccine in Denmark, but has been supplanted by the Sabin live oral vaccine in the United States, except for use in immunodeficient individuals.

Inactivated virus vaccines have advantages and disadvantages compared to live vaccines. The absence of live virus results in immunization without active infection. Since there is no live virus present, reversion to virulence does not occur, although improperly prepared vaccines can contain virulent virus or adventitious viral contaminants (e.g., SV40, avian leukosis virus). Effective local immunity does not develop, so vaccinated individuals may still transmit virus to the community. In rare cases (measles, RSV), inactivated vaccines have resulted in atypical immunologic responses which potentiated rather than prevented subsequent natural infections.

The attenuated virus vaccines in current use have been developed from either naturally occurring attenuated viruses (e.g., poliovirus type 2 strain 712) or from viruses after serial passage in tissue culture cells or embryonated eggs. These passage-selected viruses have mutations when compared to their wild type parents. For example, the vaccine strain of poliovirus type 1 differs in 21 amino acids from the original parent virus. On some vaccine viruses, the largest number of mutations are located in genes coding for viral surface proteins such as VP1 (polio) or V3 (yellow fever). However, in the case of the type 1 polio vaccine strain, mutations responsible for attenuation appear to be distributed throughout the viral genome. In other cases (e.g., mumps) a clear marker for the vaccine virus strain has not been identified.

Following immunization with the oral Sabin polio vaccine, the vaccinated person excretes virus which can infect other individuals in the community. In rare cases, the excreted virus appears to be more virulent than the vaccine strain, and may account for some of the rare cases of paralytic polio in close contacts of vaccinees. Reversion to virulence by the vaccine strain of virus may also cause paralytic polio in vaccinees. Approximately 1 in 10 million vaccinated individuals develops paralytic polio, and there are 3 cases of paralytic polio per 10 million household and community contacts of recent vaccinees. These risks are small and are probably overestimates which include coincidental as well as causal associations. In rare settings, where exposure to polio occurs at a very young age, a combined program using both inactivated (killed) and attenuated vaccines may be of benefit (see also Chap. 144).

Live attenuated measles, mumps, and rubella vaccines can be administered together (MMR) without any loss in immunizing capacity (>90 percent). Of individuals who receive the measles vaccine alone (Schwarz strain), 10 to 30 percent have mild clinical reactions, and there are rare cases of encephalitis. It is not clear that the very rare cases of encephalitis in recipients of measles vaccine are related to the vaccine virus. On the contrary, by preventing natural measles, measles vaccine has been associated with a dramatic reduction in the incidence of SSPE. The attenuated Jeryl Lynn B strain is used in the live mumps virus vaccine. Adverse effects are rare and include allergic reactions as well as CNS complications. The most commonly used rubella vaccine strain (RA 27/3) was attenuated by multiple passages through the WI-38 line of cultured human diploid fibroblasts. The most notable complications are transient arthralgia and rare cases of arthritis.

A live attenuated vaccine for yellow fever has been prepared using virus derived from passage through chicken embryos. Of those vaccinated intradermally, 95 percent develop an immune response. Serious adverse reactions occur in fewer than 1 in 1 million cases.

A novel approach to vaccination is illustrated by the adenovirus vaccine. In this case the live vaccine virus strains (4, 7) are not attenuated, but the route of administration (via oral ingestion of an enteric coated tablet) results in an asymptomatic infection with subsequent immunity. Ingested virus does not reach the respiratory tract, but produces an intestinal infection that stimulates an immune response against subsequent adenovirus-induced respiratory infections.

Two vaccines utilize virus subunits rather than whole virus to induce immunity. The influenza subunit vaccine is composed of purified envelope glycoproteins. It appears to be less toxic than live whole virus vaccine but also less antigenic. The hepatitis B vaccine uses a formalin-treated antigen as an immunogen. Purified proteins from cloned viral DNA are used in hepatitis B vaccine that may be useful in a herpes vaccine. Synthetic polypeptides analogous to major antigenic sites on viral structural proteins may be of value either as vaccines or as primers that induce a primary immune response that requires a subsequent boost.

ANTIVIRAL THERAPY   Immune globulins   The role in antiviral therapy of immunoglobulins extracted from pooled lots of adult plasma is limited. Antibody titers to specific viruses in different pooled lots of gamma globulin vary over a tenfold range. Intramuscular administration of immune globulin at the time of exposure to hepatitis A virus can prevent infection or decrease the severity of subsequent illness. A similar beneficial effect has been reported for measles infection and possibly for hepatitis B infection.

Specific immune globulins are made from plasma with high antibody titer against specific viruses. When given within 72 h of exposure to varicella-zoster virus, varicella-zoster immune globulin can prevent or modify subsequent infection. Such therapy is of value in exposed immunocompromised individuals, pregnant women, infants of mothers who develop chickenpox, and newborns of nonimmune mothers exposed to chickenpox. Hepatitis B immune globulin is useful in preventing infection of individuals exposed to HBsAg-positive material (e.g., a needle stick) or of infants exposed to hepatitis B–infected mothers. Rabies immune globulin is an integral part of postexposure prophylaxis of rabies. Other immune globulins are available but are not widely used.

Antiviral chemotherapy   See Chap. 86.

REFERENCES

Evans AS (ed): *Viral Infections of Humans: Epidemiology and Control*, 2d ed. New York, Plenum, 1984

Fields BN et al (eds): *Virology.* New York, Raven, 1985

Galasso GJ et al (eds): *Antiviral Agents and Chemotherapy*, 2d ed. New York, Raven, 1984

Johnson RT: *Viral Infections of the Nervous System.* New York, Raven, 1982

Lennette EH, Halonen P, Murphy FA (eds): *Laboratory Diagnosis of Infectious Diseases, Principles and Practice*, vol 2, *Viral, Rickettsial, and Chlamydial Diseases.* New York, Springer-Verlag, 1988

Mims CA, White DO: *Viral Pathogenesis and Immunology.* Oxford, Blackwell, 1984

Notkins AL, Oldstone MBA (eds): *Concepts in Viral Pathogenesis.* New York, Springer-Verlag, 1984

————: *Concepts in Viral Pathogenesis II.* New York, Springer-Verlag, 1986

134 THE HUMAN RETROVIRUSES

ROBERT C. GALLO / ANTHONY S. FAUCI

Retroviruses were first described at the beginning of the century as filterable agents that caused transmissible tumors in chickens; the first recognized mammalian retroviruses were isolated from mice with leukemia in the 1950s. However despite extensive investigation the first human retrovirus, HTLV-I, was not isolated until 1978. This became possible only after the discovery of RNA-to-DNA transcription by viruses and through the use of reverse transcriptase (RT) as a sensitive "footprint" for these viruses. In addition the obligate requirement of a T-cell growth factor, interleukin 2 (IL-2) (see Chap. 13), for growth of T cells in culture helped make isolation possible. There are now four human retroviruses belonging to two distinct groups: the human T-cell leukemia retroviruses, HTLV-I and HTLV-II, and the human immunodeficiency viruses, HIV-1 and HIV-2.

Although retroviruses are sometimes categorized as oncogenic viruses, lentiviruses, and spumaviruses, they may also be grouped by the disease they cause, their electron-microscopic appearance, and their biologic effects. In contrast to the infectious retroviruses some, called endogenous retroviruses, are transmitted in the germ line. Although there is limited homology of the genomes of animal retroviruses to some sequences in the human genome, there are no known human endogenous viruses. The spumaviruses are known for their ability to produce a characteristic foamy cytopathic effect in tissue culture, but their existence and biologic role in human beings is uncertain. The lentiviruses, first recognized in ungulates, are so far associated only with nonmalignant disease, particularly neurologic disorders (visna), immune-complex disease (equine infectious anemia virus), and encephalitis and arthritis (caprine arthritis encephalitis virus). These viruses are "slow-acting" only by comparison with viruses that cause acute infections such as influenza virus but not by comparison with other retroviruses. Retroviruses associated with malignant disease include HTLV-I and HTLV-II, some of the closely related simian viruses (STLV-I), feline leukemia virus (FeLV), bovine leukemia virus (BLV), gibbon ape leukemia virus (GaLV), and many avian and murine viruses. These viruses may also induce nonmalignant disease. For example, FeLV, which can cause T-cell leukemia, more frequently causes immunodeficiency in cats, mimicking the acquired immune deficiency syndrome (AIDS) of human beings. It appears that a change in the envelope of the virus is correlated with a change in the kind of disease induced by the virus.

GENERAL BIOLOGY OF RETROVIRUSES Retroviruses are enveloped viruses, usually about 100 nm in diameter, that form by budding from cell membranes (Fig. 134-1). An electron-dense central core surrounds two identical copies of the single-stranded viral RNA genome, making retroviruses diploid, which is unusual among viruses (see Chap. 133). However, it is the DNA polymerase, known as reverse transcriptase, that is the distinguishing feature of a retrovirus.

Complexed to an RNA in the viral core, this enzyme catalyzes the transcription of the RNA genome into a double-stranded DNA form that migrates from the cytoplasm to the nucleus and integrates into the host cell DNA. In this form, known as the provirus, the viral genes remain integrated for the lifetime of the cell. They are duplicated with the cell DNA during the S phase of the cell cycle. Therefore, once established, infection of an organism is generally lifelong. When the provirus is expressed, viral RNA and proteins are found in the cell cytoplasm and assembled at the cell membrane, where budding and release of infectious virions completes the replication cycle (Fig. 134-2).

The molecular mechanisms by which retroviruses alter the life cycle of infected cells are strikingly diverse and often depend on the organization of the viral genome. All retroviruses contain three essential genes for virus replication: *gag*, *pol*, and *env* (Fig. 134-3). *Gag* codes for a polyprotein precursor that is cleaved by a viral protease into three or four structural proteins; *pol* codes for RT and the viral protease and integrase; *env* codes for the transmembrane and outer glycoprotein of the virus. The properties of the envelope have a major influence on the kind of cell the virus can infect, and production of antibodies against the envelope is one of the essential features sought in a vaccine. At either end of the provirus the long terminal repeats (LTR) are covalently joined to the cellular DNA;

FIGURE 134-1 Electron micrographs of the characterized human retrovirus. The viruses are shown as they replicate by budding from a cell membrane (*upper panels*) and as the mature infectious extracellular virion (*lower panels*).

HTLV-I

HTLV-II

HIV-1

HIV-2

FIGURE 134-2   Life cycle of a retrovirus (as represented by HIV-1). Intact virions are endocytosed via a specific cellular receptor. The uncoated viral single-stranded RNA is then transcribed into double-stranded DNA, enters the cell nucleus, and integrates into the host genome. The DNA provirus in some conditions is unexpressed. In other cases it is transcribed, giving rise to viral RNA encoding viral proteins and genome-length viral RNA molecules which then reassemble with viral proteins to make complete virions. These progeny are released by budding from the cell membrane. All known infectious retroviruses follow these steps. The specific molecules described pertain only to HIV-1 (the CD4 receptor with *vif*, *tat*, and *rev* viral proteins).

they contain regulatory elements that influence the expression of the viral genes and sometimes nearby cellular genes. The LTR shares features in common with movable genetic elements such as retrotransposons.

Examples of chronic leukemia viruses, which contain only these three genes, are FeLV, murine leukemia virus (MuLV), GaLV, and avian leukosis virus (ALV). These viruses are replication competent, take a long time to cause disease, and are relatively common in nature. There is some evidence that they cause leukemia by integration into a specific region of a chromosome so that the associated LTRs act to promote continual expression of a nearby cellular gene involved

in growth (a proto-oncogene) (see Chaps. 9 and 10). The best studied example of this *cis* mechanism is in chickens, where the LTR of avian leukosis virus promotes expression of the cellular proto-oncogene *myc*, believed to be the first step in the induction of B-cell leukemia by this virus. Since integration by retroviruses is random, a high rate of replication favors the chance of integration into regions sufficiently near the cellular oncogene as to effect its expression. There are no known human viruses of this type.

When a retrovirus acquires a host cell gene that rapidly transforms cells and induces acute malignancies, the virus is often called an *acute leukemia* or *sarcoma virus*, and the acquired gene (i.e., host

FIGURE 134-3   Genomic structure of human retroviruses. Viral proteins may be translated in each of three reading frames. RNA is transcribed from viral DNA and processed by viral and cellular enzymes giving rise to both genomic viral RNA and mRNA. Arrows indicate double spliced mRNA. LTR, long terminal repeat; *gag*, core proteins; *pol*, polymerase (RT); *env*, envelope. Viral genes shown in color code for regulatory proteins.

proto-oncogene) is called a *viral onc gene*. This type of change almost always leads to an incomplete viral genome which forms defective viral particles. The virus then needs the addition of a helper virus and in vitro manipulation for its propagation. Viruses with *onc* genes are thought to be rare in nature and are of interest in animals chiefly for investigating mechanisms of neoplastic transformation rather than as causes of naturally occurring cancer. An example of this appears with FeLV. In addition to the mechanism of specific integration near a proto-oncogene and subsequent activation of this gene, FeLV may cause malignancies by the relatively frequent acquisition of cell-derived oncogenes. Every cell infected by these viruses can be transformed (giving rise to polyclonal tumors) because the product of the viral *onc* gene directly transforms the cells. Therefore, a common site of integration or a second genetic event to trigger transformation is not needed. The development of the malignancy is usually rapid and sometimes occurs within months of infection. Human viruses of this type have never been found.

FEATURES OF HUMAN RETROVIRUSES The known human and some related animal retroviruses can be regarded as unique categories of retroviruses. Human T-lymphotropic (or leukemia) viruses (HTLV-I and HTLV-II) transform cells in culture, while human immunodeficiency viruses (HIV-1 and -2) are cytopathic in culture. While the two groups have little sequence homology, they have some striking similarities and differences.

In addition to the usual viral structural genes, all of the human retroviruses contain extra genes that provide regulatory signals essential to virus replication and to the biologic activities of the virus. Such genes were first found in HTLV-I and HTLV-II and more recently in HIV-2 and HIV-1, the well-known cause of AIDS.

One of these, called *tax-1* in HTLV-I and *tat-1* in HIV-1, codes for proteins that activate the expression of viral and some cellular genes. Another gene, *rex* in HTLV-I and *rev* in HIV-1, codes for proteins that favor the formation of unspliced or single-spliced viral mRNA; in their absence only small doubly spliced mRNAs are made. The *rev* protein is localized in the nucleus and appears to increase transport of the larger mRNA, which encodes for structural proteins, to the cytoplasm. Conversely, it diminishes the availability of the mRNA for *rev* itself and for the other regulatory proteins. For each virus these proteins are structurally distinct but have similar functions.

HIV-1 follows many of the same regulatory strategies as HTLV-1, but its genome is even more complex. By deletion analysis the function of several other genes has been evaluated. The *nef* gene product appears to be a negative regulator of viral production, while the *vif* gene affects the ability of virus particle(s) to infect target cells but does not affect viral replication. The *vpu* gene has been reported to enhance modestly the maturation and exit of virus from the cell in vitro, and the *vpr* gene has been reported to stimulate the promoter region of the virus. In reality, the functions of these genes are poorly understood and their in vivo relevance is unclear.

All of the four known human retroviruses preferentially infect the T4 lymphocyte, and the diseases they cause involve this cell, often resulting in profound biologic consequences. Ironically, the cellular receptor for HIV is the CD4 molecule itself (Fig. 134-2) (see Chap. 13 for discussion of the function of CD4.) The remarkably high affinity of gp120 envelope protein for this molecule probably determines the host range of the virus, the nature of cell target populations, the mode and ability of the virus to be efficiently transmitted, and contributes to the cytopathic effect both through the formation of syncytia and through effects upon virus production. A region of the transmembrane protein gp41 facilitates entry of the virus into the cell by helping to fuse the virus coat with the target cell membrane. The cellular receptor(s) for the HTLVs is not known, but its gene is on chromosome 17. HTLV-I can usually be transmitted only by cell-to-cell contact while the HIVs can be transmitted in this manner and as extracellular virus.

The monocyte-macrophage is also a major target for HIV-1. As for lymphocytes, entry requires attachment to CD4 molecules expressed on the cell surface and may be enhanced by Fc-receptor-mediated endocytosis. Infected monocytes are believed to play a major role in the disease by acting as reservoirs for the virus and as vehicles for its spread. Related cells are infected in the brain, lymph node, skin, lung, and gastrointestinal tract. Cytokine production by infected monocytes and T cells may play a direct role in the induction of malignancy, neurologic disease, and perhaps other clinical manifestations such as enteritis and lymphoid interstitial pneumonitis.

DISEASES ASSOCIATED WITH HTLV-I INFECTION HTLV-I rapidly induces transformation of human T cells in vitro; it has neither an *onc* gene nor a single integration site, yet results in monoclonal malignancies. The majority of HTLV-I–induced leukemias or lymphomas involve the T4+ cell. Infection of T4+ cells by HTLV-I or HTLV-II leads to the transformation of some of the infected cells, and the properties of such transformed cells are similar. The infected cells often exhibit extensive "cerebriform" lobulation of the nuclei and form giant multinucleated cells in culture. They constitutively express increased numbers of receptors for IL-2 (IL-2R) which can be found on circulating T4+ cells. This may be due to the *tax* gene product, which can up-regulate the receptor, transform T cells when transfected, and induce tumors in transgenic animals. The maintenance of malignancy is not believed to require additional viral gene products since the HTLV-I genes are usually not expressed in the leukemic cells in vivo by the time the leukemia is clinically evident. The reason that only some individuals develop malignancy is not known. Since cells other than T4 lymphocytes can be infected, the reason for the frequency of transformation of the T4+ cell is unclear. The relatively high incidence of adult T-cell leukemia/lymphoma (ATLL) (lifetime risk of 1 to 3 percent) independent of geographic location suggests that a specific environmental cofactor is not necessary to produce disease. In contrast, the development of lymphoma associated with EBV occurs at a much lower rate and only in certain areas such as the "Burkitt lymphoma belt" in Africa where specific environmental cofactors are present.

Leukemias/lymphomas caused by HTLV-I are characterized by an aggressive course, frequent hypercalcemia (associated with tumor necrosis factor β secretion), opportunistic infection and, in over one-half of the cases, leukemic skin infiltrates. HTLV-I may also be involved in T4 cell leukemias/lymphomas that exhibit a more chronic course (15 to 20 percent of cases) involving progression from polyclonal T-cell proliferation to an expansion of a particular clone to frank clinical malignancy. These malignancies may be indistinguishable pathologically or clinically from chronic T-cell lymphocytic leukemia (CLL), diffuse histiocytic lymphoma, large and mixed cell lymphomas, and mycosis fungoides or Sézary leukemias (see Chaps. 296 and 302). Typical ATL cases recognized worldwide are almost always HTLV-I-positive. In the United States only a small percentage of T-cell malignancies are HTLV-I-positive. In contrast, in endemic areas almost all T4 cell malignancies are virus-positive.

In areas of the world where HTLV-I is endemic, some B-cell lymphoid malignancies and certain other cancers are associated with HTLV-I infection more frequently than expected from the prevalence of the virus in the general population. In contrast to virus-positive T-cell leukemias, where the viral genes are integrated into the DNA of the leukemic cell, HTLV-I is not found in the DNA of these B-cell tumors. Instead, the virus is present in the normal T cells of these patients, and the role of the virus must be indirect. Several of these B-cell neoplasms have been shown to make specific antibody against HTLV-I, suggesting that years of stimulation of some B-cell populations by HTLV-I proteins may be involved in their malignant transformation.

The etiologic association of HTLV-I with ATL was firmly established by the epidemiology and serology in endemic areas and by the presence of proviral DNA integrated in a monoclonal manner in the tumor. This indicated that the first transformed cell contained the provirus rather than being infected later as an opportunistic infection. The ability of HTLV-I to immortalize target T cells in vitro is also consistent with its role in vivo as a transforming virus. Considerable data in animals show that exogenous type C retroviruses are usually leukemogenic. This finding predicted that HTLVs would also be leukemogenic in human beings.

A new aspect of HTLV-I has been revealed by the discovery of the association of this virus with a demyelinating disorder, tropical spastic paraparesis (TSP) (see Chap. 355). This syndrome has also been referred to as HTLV-I–associated myelopathy (HAM). It is a chronic progressive encephalomyelopathy with symmetric upper motor neuron disease, prominent lower extremity weakness, and hyperreflexia, with sphincter and sensory abnormalities that may resemble a spinal cord variant of multiple sclerosis. Central nervous system lesions are seen on MRI scans. The pathogenesis is not known, but high antibody responses to HTLV-I and improvement with glucocorticoids suggest an autoimmune disease mechanism. A few individuals have both ATL and neurologic disease. While the lifetime risk of developing ATL appears to be between 1 and 3 percent in HTLV-I–infected individuals, the attack rate of TSP in some areas such as Colombia may be higher. Several other neurologic diseases may be associated with HTLV-I infection in endemic areas including polymyositis, Bell's palsy, and Guillain-Barré syndrome.

Treatment   There are two major considerations in the treatment of HTLV-I infection. First, the time from infection to disease may be 20 years or more. Second, when ATL develops, the virus is transcriptionally silent in the peripheral blood leukemic cells. Treatment for asymptomatic seropositive individuals at present is limited to periodic evaluation for neurologic and hematologic disease, screening family members at risk, and avoiding infection by breast feeding, sexual transmission, and transfusion donation. Thus far, no regimen of chemotherapy has been demonstrated to increase survival in ATL. Clinical trials with several experimental approaches are currently being evaluated including targeting of the IL-2 receptor on leukemic cells with toxin-coupled antibody. Since virus is not replicating, antiviral chemotherapy seems unlikely to be effective. Several reports have indicated that high-dose glucocorticoids benefit TSP patients, but well-controlled trials have not been done.

ORIGIN AND EPIDEMIOLOGY OF HTLV-I AND HTLV-II   HTLV-I was originally discovered in two black patients with T-cell malignancies in the United States, and within 1 year it was associated with clusters of a newly described T-cell malignancy (ATL) in some southwestern islands of Japan and in Caribbean-born blacks. It may have been brought to both areas from Africa centuries ago by merchants and slave traders. HTLV-I occurs worldwide but tends to be highly geographically restricted or clustered. In endemic areas the fraction of infected individuals ranges from 5 to 25 percent. Transmission is by intimate contact, by blood or blood products, and by nursing mothers (and perhaps by infection of the developing fetus in utero). Because of increased travel, changes in sexual habits, intravenous drug abuse (blood-contaminated needles), and wide use of blood and blood products, the prevalence of HTLV in nonendemic areas may be increasing.

HTLV-II was originally isolated from a cell line derived from a patient with a T-cell variant of hairy cell leukemia and can be distinguished from HTLV-I by competition radioimmunoassay. The virus has subsequently been isolated from several patients with more chronic forms of T-cell malignancies. Overall it is about 55 percent identical at the nucleotide level to HTLV-I, and only a few biologic differences have been found between the two viruses.

Current routine serologic tests do not distinguish between antibodies to HTLV-I and HTLV-II. Seropositivity to HTLV-I has been found in surprisingly high frequency in drug addict populations also at risk for HIV infection. The risk of being HTLV-I–positive correlates with geographic location. In many areas of the country the dominant HTLV virus in the drug addict population is HTLV-II. At the present time, the role of HTLV-II in disease is unclear; there are suggestions that dual infection with HIV and one of the HTLVs may lead to accelerated emergence of AIDS.

DISEASES ASSOCIATED WITH HIV INFECTION (See also Chap. 264)   The etiologic agent of AIDS is a retrovirus called HIV-1 (formerly HTLV-III/LAV). As the discovery of the tuberculosis

bacillus or the spirochete of syphilis unified diverse disease manifestations, the spectrum of disease associated with AIDS has been interpreted in the context of the biology and epidemiology of HIV-1 infection. HIV-2, the most recently described human retrovirus, has about 40 percent genetic identity with HIV-1. It is even more closely related to some members of a group of viruses causing immune deficiency in simians [simian immune deficiency virus (SIV)]. It has been isolated from patients with immunodeficiency and has been detected serologically in western Africa in populations different from those with HIV-1 infection in whom AIDS is not endemic. It appears to be a relatively uncommon and inefficient cause of AIDS and is not spreading with the rapidity of HIV. Cofactors that increase virus replication or enhance T-cell killing are being investigated for their role in the progression of disease. Particular factors include viruses such as HTLV-I, human herpes virus (HHV-6), and cytomegalovirus (CMV) which can promote HIV expression and also directly infect T cells. HHV-6, a new herpes virus, can also kill T4 lymphocytes. However, only in the case of HTLV-I is more rapid progression to AIDS supported by epidemiologic data.

HIV-1–associated Kaposi's sarcoma (KS)   HIV-1–infected patients have an increased incidence of certain B-cell lymphomas, Hodgkin's disease, certain carcinomas, and KS. The reason for the increase in these malignancies is not understood, but it is not necessarily associated with the degree of immune impairment. HIV-1 is not the direct cause of any of these tumors because viral sequences are not found in the DNA from the majority of tumor cells. For the B-cell lymphomas, the mechanism may be similar to the indirect role described above for HTLV-I. Direct culture of tissue from KS lesions suggests that the role of HIV in KS may be the induction of a growth factor produced by infected CD4+ cells. This factor activates vascular cells which release several cytokines; the continuous release of these cytokines may result in the mixed cell population of KS. Additional support for this model is the appearance of KS-like lesions in transgenic male mice expressing the *tat* protein.

MOLECULAR HETEROGENEITY OF HIV   Analysis at the molecular level of various HIV isolates reveals variation of nucleotide sequences of certain parts of the genome, especially in the envelope gene. In different isolates the amino acid sequence of the envelope proteins ranges from very closely related (1 to 2 percent variation) to those that vary 25 to 30 percent. A single individual (and perhaps intimate contacts) is usually infected with a "swarm" of closely related viruses that may constitute a single "strain." Even a very small difference, called "microheterogeneity," may exert a profound influence on the biology of the virus. Variation probably develops with successive infections and does not occur during prolonged tissue culture of a single molecularly cloned virus, suggesting that these changes occur during transcription of the viral RNA genome to the DNA form and/or during the recombinational process when the DNA provirus integrates into the host cell DNA. RT tends to be error prone because, unlike cellular DNA polymerases, RT lacks a proofreading mechanism. The RT of HIV may be particularly error prone. Variation of other genes is generally far less than that of the envelope. It is possible that strain variation may account for a difference in the clinical course of an HIV infected person; experimental studies have revealed significant biologic variations among strains, including target cell tropism and response to neutralizing antibody. A variant that can avoid elimination by antibodies or cytotoxic T8+ cells could lead more easily to progressive disease. For example, selection pressure on cultured virus in the presence of human neutralizing antisera has resulted in a virus with one amino acid change that is no longer neutralized by the selecting sera.

PREVENTION AND TREATMENT OF RETROVIRUS INFECTION   There are three major approaches to the control of human retroviral disease: vaccination; antiviral therapy; and education and public health measures (see Chap. 264). Vaccines have proved to be the least costly and most effective way of preventing infectious disease, especially those caused by viruses, but there are special problems with HIV: (1) Because of the integration of viral genes, a limited number of viral particles may be sufficient to establish infection, and therefore the demands on a vaccine may be very stringent. (2) T cells are the principal cells involved in protection against a virus, and these are the cells destroyed by the virus. (3) Envelope heterogeneity allows the escape from neutralizing antibodies; there are several conserved areas of the envelope gene which are being actively studied as subunit vaccines. (4) The nature of the protective immune response is not yet clear. Most infected individuals develop progressive disease despite the presence of neutralizing antibodies and cytotoxic T cells. The expectation is that immunization prior to infection may prevent disease. Some encouragement comes from the finding that for most infections of a single individual only one strain of the virus has been found. This suggests that an individual is infected only once despite repeated exposure. And (5) animal models for vaccine development against HIV are limited, but the development of animal systems with SIV, the related African green monkey virus that can produce AIDS in macaques, is likely to be very helpful.

Antiviral therapy is based on a detailed understanding of the viral replication cycle, and almost every definable step offers the possibility of interfering with replication of virus (see Chap. 264). Approaches are available beginning with HIV binding to the cell. Recombinant CD4 is being tested that acts as a ''molecular decoy'' for the virus by competing with cellular receptors for binding viral gp120 envelope proteins. Early studies in animals and humans have been encouraging with regard to toxicity, but no beneficial effects have as yet emerged. The most successful agents to date affect the next stage, formation of the DNA provirus, by inhibiting RT. These agents include AZT and other nucleoside analogues such as dideoxycytodine (ddC) and dideoxyinosine (ddI). The next targets are the synthesis, maturation, and transport from nucleus to cytoplasm of viral RNA from proviral DNA, for which inhibitors of *tat* and *rev* function are being studied. Viral mRNA must be translated, and on an experimental basis this step can be specifically inhibited with antisense DNA. Lastly, viral proteins must assemble to form new virus, and this depends on a specific viral protease. This protein has been crystallized, and inhibitors are under study.

Because infection with HIV probably always means integration of the viral genes into the DNA of the infected cells, it is likely that lifelong treatment will be required. To minimize toxicity and reduce the chance for viral resistance, it may be necessary to use a combination of compounds with different mechanisms of action. Another approach would be to kill infected cells; success would depend upon elimination of all infected cells. However, this may not be possible with human retroviruses because most infected cells do not express viral proteins and are therefore not distinguishable from uninfected cells. Moreover, infected macrophages appear to act as reservoirs for the virus and may release additional virions from intracellular vacuolar membranes when killed.

OTHER DISEASES ASSOCIATED WITH HUMAN RETROVIRAL INFECTION

The possibility that several well-described human diseases are associated with retroviral infection should be carefully considered. While the promise of many candidate viruses has not been fulfilled, the number of retroviruses with diverse mechanisms of disease found in other species suggests a wide range of possibilities. A report of RT activity in non-A, non-B hepatitis has not been substantiated since a new flavivirus has been discovered as the probable cause. RT activity has been detected in patients with Kawasaki disease, but neither a virus nor viral sequences have been found and there has been no confirmation of the original reports. Mammary tumors in mice have been transmitted via breast milk infected with mammary tumor virus. Despite sporadic reports of electron-micrographic evidence of virus in human tumors, no human equivalent has been isolated and characterized. The presence of a retrovirus in some patients with mycosis fungoides that differs from HTLV-I–associated tumors has been reported as HTLV-V. Verification awaits further characterization of the candidate virus. Retroviruses are known to produce neurologic disease in some species (e.g., visna in sheep and MuLV in some mice); HIV-1 infects the central nervous system; and

HTLV-I is associated with a demyelinating disease. A possible retroviral etiology of multiple sclerosis has been considered. Sequences related to HTLV-I have been reported in the peripheral blood of patients with multiple sclerosis by in situ hybridization or polymerase chain reaction. Differentiation of these sequences from those endogenous to cells and recovery of intact virus are needed to confirm the significance of these associations.

The discovery of the HTLV-I occurred at a time when many thought that there would be no human retroviruses. In the ensuing decade, four human retroviruses have been discovered and associated with several human diseases. These viruses have provided major insights into the pathogenesis of neoplastic, immunosuppressive, and neurologic disorders as well as some of the most difficult medical, social, and scientific challenges of the late twentieth century.

REFERENCES

BARRE-SINOUSSI F et al: Isolation of a T lymphotropic retrovirus from a patient at risk for acquired immune deficiency syndrome (AIDS). Science 220:868, 1983

BLATTNER W: Retroviruses, in *Viral Infections of Humans,* AS Evans (ed). New York, Plenum, 1989, pp 545–592

BRODER S, GALLO R: A pathogenic retrovirus (HTLV-III) linked to AIDS. N Engl J Med 311:1292, 1984

FAUCI AS: The human immunodeficiency virus: Infectivity and mechanisms of pathogenesis. Science 239:617, 1988

GALLO RC: The first human retrovirus. Sci Am 255:88, 1986

———, MONTAGNIER L: AIDS in 1988. Sci Am 259:41, 1988

——— et al: Frequent detection and isolation of cytopathic retroviruses (HTLV-III) from patients with AIDS and at risk for AIDS. Science 224:500, 1984

SALAHUDDIN SZ et al: Angiogenic properties of Kaposi's sarcoma-derived cells after long-term culture *in vitro.* Science 242:430, 1988

VARMUS H: Retroviruses. Science 240:1427, 1988

135 HERPES SIMPLEX VIRUSES

LAWRENCE COREY

DEFINITION Herpes simplex viruses (HSV-1, HSV-2) (*Herpesvirus hominis*) produce a variety of infections involving mucocutaneous surfaces, the central nervous system, and occasionally visceral organs. The advent of effective antiviral chemotherapy for HSV infections has made prompt recognition of these syndromes of clinical importance.

ETIOLOGY The genome of herpes simplex virus is a linear, double-stranded DNA molecule (about 100×10^6 in molecular weight) large enough to encode in excess of 60 gene products. The structure of the genome is unusual among DNA viruses because two unique nucleotide sequences are flanked by inverted repeated sequences. The two components can invert relative to each other, so that DNA isolated from the virus consists of four isomers differing in their orientation of the two components. The genomes of the HSV-1 and HSV-2 viruses are about 50 percent homologous. The homologous sequences are distributed over the entire genome map, and most (if not all) of the polypeptides specified by one viral type are antigenically related to polypeptides of the other viral type. Restriction endonuclease analysis of viral DNA can be utilized to distinguish between the two subtypes and among strains of the two subtypes. The variability of nucleotide sequences from clinical strains of HSV-1 and HSV-2 are such that HSV isolates obtained from two individuals can be differentiated by restriction enzyme patterns unless the isolates are from epidemiologically related sources such as sexual partners, mother-infant pairs, or common source outbreaks.

The viral genome is packaged within a regular icosahedral protein shell (capsid) composed of 162 capsomers. The outer covering of the virus is a lipid-containing membrane (envelope) derived from modified cell membrane, acquired as the DNA-containing capsid buds through the inner nuclear membrane of the host cell. Between the capsid and lipid bilayer of the envelope is the tegument, composed of a number of viral proteins whose properties and functions are largely unknown. Viral replication has both nuclear and cytoplasmic phases. The initial steps of replication include attachment, fusion between the viral envelope and a cell membrane to liberate the nucleocapsid into the cytoplasm of the cell, and disassembly of the nucleocapsid to release the viral DNA. Three classes of HSV genes have been defined. The genes designated α are expressed earliest in infection without any requirement for prior viral protein synthesis. Some of the α genes transcribe in latently infected cells. The HSV genes designated β require prior synthesis of an α protein but not viral DNA replication. The β proteins include regulatory proteins and enzymes required for DNA replication. Most current antiviral drugs interrupt β proteins such as the viral DNA polymerase enzyme. The third (γ) class of HSV genes require viral DNA replication for expression, and most of the structural proteins specified by the virus are γ proteins.

Following replication of the viral genome and synthesis of structural proteins, nucleocapsids are assembled in the nucleus of the cell. Envelopment occurs as the nucleocapsids bud through the inner nuclear membrane into the perinuclear space. In some cells, viral replication within the nucleus forms two types of inclusion bodies, type A basophilic Feulgen-positive bodies that contain viral DNA, and an eosinophilic inclusion body which is devoid of viral nucleic acid or protein, representing a "scar" of viral infection. Virions are then transported via the endoplasmic reticulum and the Golgi apparatus to the cell surface.

HSV infection of some neuronal cells does not result in cell death. Instead, viral genomes are maintained by the cell in a repressed state compatible with survival and normal activities of the cell, a process called *latency*. Subsequently, activation of the viral genome may occur resulting in viral replication and, in some cases, the redevelopment of herpetic lesions, a process termed *reactivation*. Whereas infectious virus rarely can be recovered from sensory or autonomic nervous system ganglia dissected from cadavers, maintenance and growth of the neural cells in tissue culture result in production of infectious virions, a process called *explantation,* and subsequent permissive infection of susceptible cells, a process called *cocultivation*. Virus replication was first detected in neurons during reactivation in vitro, suggesting that the neuron harbors the latent virus in vivo. Subsequently, viral DNA has been found in neural tissue at times when infectious virus cannot be isolated. HSV DNA extracted from latently infected neural tissue differs from HSV DNA in cells actively replicating virus. In latently infected cells only partial transcription of viral proteins occurs. Two RNA transcripts which overlap the immediate early (α) gene product, called ICP-o, are found in abundance in the nuclei of latently infected neurons. These RNA transcripts code in an "antisense" direction, suggesting that they may be a factor in inhibiting the subsequent transcription of β and γ proteins. Deletion mutants of this region have been made. While these viruses can become latent, the efficiency of their subsequent reactivation is reduced, suggesting that the "antisense" transcripts may play a role in maintaining rather than in establishing latency. Understanding molecular mechanisms of latency may lead to new therapies to prevent reactivation of HSV.

PATHOGENESIS Exposure to virus at mucosal surfaces or abraded skin permits entry of virus and initiation of replication in cells of the epidermis and dermis. Whether or not clinically apparent lesions develop, sufficient viral replication to permit infection of either sensory or autonomic nerve endings may occur. Whether latency always results from peripheral mucosal infection is unclear. Virus, or more likely, nucleocapsid, is then thought to be transported intraaxonally to the nerve cell bodies in ganglia. In humans, the time from inoculation of virus in peripheral tissue to spread to the ganglia is unknown. During the initial phase of infection, viral replication occurs in ganglia and contiguous neural tissue. Virus then spreads to other mucosal skin surfaces through centrifugal migration of infectious virions via peripheral sensory nerves. This spread of virus to the skin

from peripheral sensory nerves helps explain the large surface area, the high frequency of new lesions distant from the initial crop of vesicles which are characteristic in patients with primary genital or oral-labial HSV, and the recovery of virus from neural tissue distant from neurons innervating the inoculation site. Contiguous spread of locally inoculated virus may also occur and allow further mucosal extension of disease.

Following resolution of primary disease, infectious virus can no longer be recovered in the ganglia, and the surface viral proteins are not expressed in detectable amounts. The mechanisms by which various stimuli cause reactivation of HSV infection are unknown. Ultraviolet light, immunosuppression, and trauma to the skin or ganglia are associated with reactivation.

Analysis of the HSV DNA from sequentially isolated strains of HSV or from multiple infected ganglia in any one individual has revealed identical restriction endonuclease patterns in most persons. Occasionally, and more frequently in immunocompromised persons, multiple strains of the same viral subtype can be detected in the same person, suggesting that exogenous infection with different strains of the same subtype is possible.

IMMUNITY Host responses to infection influence the acquisition of disease, severity of infection, resistance to development of latency, maintenance of latency, and frequency of HSV recurrences. Both antibody-mediated and cell-mediated reactions are clinically important. Immunocompromised patients with defects in cell-mediated immunity experience more severe and extensive HSV infections than those with deficits in humoral immunity such as agammaglobulinemia. Experimental ablation of lymphocytes indicates that T cells play a major role in preventing lethal disseminated disease, although antibodies help reduce virus titers in neural tissue. Some aspects of the pathogenesis of disease may also be related to the host immune response, e.g., stromal opacities associated with recurrent herpetic keratitis. The surface viral glycoproteins have been shown to be antigens recognized by antibodies mediating neutralization and immune-mediated cytolysis (antibody-dependent cell-mediated cytotoxicity, ADCC). Monoclonal antibodies specific for each of the known viral glycoproteins have, in experimental infections, conferred protection against subsequent neurologic disease or ganglionic latency. Multiple cell populations including natural killer (NK) cells, macrophages, a variety of T-lymphocyte populations, and lymphokines generated by these cells play a role in host defenses to HSV infections. In animals passive transfer of primed lymphocytes confers protection from subsequent challenge. Maximum protection usually requires the activation of multiple T-cell subpopulations including cytotoxic T cells and T cells responsible for delayed hypersensitivity. The latter cells may confer protection by the antigen-stimulated release of lymphokines (e.g., interferons) which may have a direct antiviral effect or activate other nonspecific effector cells. In humans the viral proteins to which the responses of cytotoxic T cells are directed are unknown.

EPIDEMIOLOGY Seroepidemiologic studies have shown that HSV infections are found worldwide. Much of the humoral immune response to HSV is to type-common antigenic determinants, making it difficult to detect HSV-2 antibodies in persons with prior HSV-1 infection and HSV-1 antibodies in those with prior HSV-2 infections. Serologic assays which utilize whole-virus antigen preparations such as complement fixation, neutralization, indirect immunofluorescent (IFA), passive hemagglutination (PHA), radioimmunoassay (RIA), and enzyme-linked immunosorbent assay (ELISA) do not reliably identify persons who are infected with both viral subtypes. Recently, serologic assays which identify antibodies to type-specific surface proteins of the two viruses have been developed. These assays can reliably distinguish the human antibody response between HSV-1 and HSV-2. These assays are based upon demonstrating antibodies to type-specific epitopes of the glycoprotein G of HSV-1 (gGl) and HSV-2 (gG2).

Infection with HSV-1 is acquired more frequently and earlier than infection with HSV-2. Over 90 percent of adults have antibodies to

HSV-1 by the fourth decade. In lower socioeconomic populations most persons will acquire HSV-1 infection before the third decade.

Antibodies to HSV-2 are not routinely detected until puberty, and antibody prevalence rates correlate with past sexual activity. Antibodies to HSV-2 are detected in 10 to 40 percent of the general U.S. population. In most routine obstetrical clinics 20 to 30 percent of pregnant women possess HSV-2 antibodies, although only 10 percent report a history of genital lesions. As many as 50 percent of heterosexual adults attending STD clinics possess HSV-2 antibodies. Antibody prevalence rates average about 5 percent higher in women than men.

HSV infections occur throughout the year. The incubation period ranges from 1 to 26 days (median 6 to 8 days). Contact with active ulcerative lesions or asymptomatically excreting patients can result in transmission. Asymptomatic salivary excretion of HSV-1 has been reported in 2 to 9 percent of adults and 5 to 8 percent of children. HSV-2 has been isolated from the genital tract of from 0.3 to 6 percent of males and 1.5 to 13 percent of females attending sexually transmitted disease clinics. The titer of HSV in cultures from lesions is 100 to 1000 times higher than from salivary or genital tract secretions in asymptomatically excreting persons. The efficiency of transmission is greater during symptomatic versus asymptomatic periods of viral excretion.

CLINICAL SPECTRUM HSV has been isolated from nearly all visceral or mucocutaneous sites. The clinical manifestations and course of HSV depend on the anatomic site of the infection, the age and immune status of the host, and the antigenic type of the virus. First episodes of HSV disease, especially primary infection (that is, first infections with either HSV-1 or HSV-2 in which the host lacks HSV antibodies in acute phase sera), are frequently accompanied by systemic signs and symptoms, involve both mucosal and extramucosal sites, have a longer duration of symptoms, a longer time from which virus is isolated from lesions, and a higher rate of complications than recurrent episodes of disease. Both viral subtypes can cause genital and oral-facial infections, and these infections are clinically indistinguishable. However, the frequency of future reactivations of infection is influenced by the anatomic site and virus type. Genital HSV-2 infection is twice as likely to reactivate and will recur 8 to 10 times more frequently than genital HSV-1 infection. Conversely, oral-labial HSV-1 infections will recur more frequently than oral-labial HSV-2 infections.

Oral-facial HSV infections Gingivostomatitis and pharyngitis are the most frequent clinical manifestations of first-episode HSV-1 infection, while recurrent herpes labialis is the most frequent clinical manifestation of reactivation HSV infection. HSV pharyngitis and gingivostomatitis usually result from primary infection and are most commonly seen in children and young adults. Clinical symptoms and signs include fever, malaise, myalgias, inability to eat, irritability, and cervical adenopathy, which may last from 3 to 14 days. Lesions may involve the hard and soft palate, gingiva, tongue, lip, and facial area. HSV-1 or HSV-2 infection of the pharynx usually results in exudative or ulcerative lesions of the posterior pharynx and/or tonsillar pillars. Concomitant lesions of the tongue, buccal mucosa, or gingiva may occur later in the course in one-third of cases. Fever lasting from 2 to 7 days and cervical adenopathy are common. The clinical differentiation of HSV pharyngitis from bacterial pharyngitis, *Mycoplasma pneumoniae* infections, and noninfectious causes of pharyngeal ulcerations such as Stevens-Johnson syndrome may be difficult. No substantial evidence suggests that reactivation oral-labial HSV infection is associated with symptomatic recurrent pharyngitis.

Reactivation of HSV from the trigeminal ganglia may be associated with asymptomatic excretion in the saliva, development of intraoral mucosal ulcerations, or herpetic ulcerations on the vermilion border of the lip or external facial skin. About 50 to 70 percent of seropositive patients undergoing trigeminal nerve root decompression and 10 to 15 percent of those undergoing dental extraction will develop oral-labial HSV infection a median of 3 days after these procedures.

In immunosuppressed patients infection may extend into mucosal and deep cutaneous layers. Friability, necrosis, bleeding, severe pain, and inability to eat or drink may result. HSV mucositis is clinically similar to mucosal lesions due to cytotoxic drug therapy, trauma, or fungal or bacterial infections. Persistent ulcerative HSV infections are one of the most common in patients with AIDS. Concomitant HSV and *Candida* infection also occur commonly. Systemic acyclovir therapy speeds the rate of healing and relieves the pain of mucosal HSV infections in immunosuppressed patients. Patients with atopic eczema may also develop severe oral-facial HSV infections (eczema herpeticum) which may rapidly involve extensive areas of skin and occasionally disseminate to visceral organs. Prompt resolution of extensive eczema herpeticum has been achieved with the administration of intravenous acyclovir. Erythema multiforme (EM) may also be associated with HSV infections, and some evidence suggests that it is the precipitating event in about 75 percent of cases of cutaneous EM. HSV antigen has been demonstrated in both circulatory immune complexes and in skin lesion biopsy of these patients. Patients with severe HSV-associated erythema multiforme may be candidates for chronic suppressive oral acyclovir therapy.

Genital HSV infections First-episode primary genital herpes is characterized by fever, headache, malaise, and myalgias. Pain, itching, dysuria, vaginal and urethral discharge, and tender inguinal lymph adenopathy are the predominant local symptoms. Characteristically widely spaced bilateral lesions of the external genitalia are seen. Lesions may be present in varying stages including vesicles, pustules, or painful erythematous ulcers. Involvement of the cervix and urethra are seen in over 80 percent of women with first-episode infections. First episodes of genital herpes in patients who have had prior HSV-1 infection are associated with less frequent systemic symptoms and faster healing than primary genital herpes. The clinical courses of acute first-episode genital herpes among patients with HSV-1 and HSV-2 infections are similar. However, the recurrence rates of genital disease differ. About 90 percent of patients with first-episode HSV-2 infection will have a recurrence within 12 months (median number of recurrences, four) compared to 55 percent of those with primary HSV-1 infections (median number of recurrences, less than one). Recurrence rates of genital HSV-2 infections vary greatly between individuals and over time within the same individual. HSV has been isolated from the urethra and urine of men and women without concomitant external genital lesions. A clear mucoid discharge and dysuria are characteristics of symptomatic HSV urethritis. HSV has been isolated from the urethra of 5 percent of women with the dysuria-frequency syndrome. Occasionally, genital tract disease manifested by HSV endometritis and salpingitis in women and HSV prostatitis in men may occur.

Rectal and perianal HSV infections due to HSV-1 and HSV-2 may be seen, especially among homosexual men and/or heterosexual women who engage in anorectal intercourse. Symptoms of HSV proctitis include anorectal pain, anorectal discharge, tenesmus, and constipation. Sigmoidoscopy reveals ulcerative lesions of the distal 10 cm of the rectal mucosa. Rectal biopsies show mucosal ulceration, necrosis, polymorphonuclear and lymphocytic infiltration of the lamina propria, and occasionally multinucleated intranuclear inclusion–bearing cells. Perianal herpetic lesions are also seen in immunosuppressed patients receiving cytotoxic therapy. HSV-1 strains, usually identical to those found in the oropharynx, are obtained from these lesions, suggesting the mode of spread is autoinoculation of the perianal area from HSV-infected saliva and/or finger lesions. Extensive perianal herpetic lesions and/or HSV proctitis may occur in patients with AIDS.

Herpetic whitlow Herpetic whitlow, HSV infection of the finger, may occur as a complication of primary oral or genital herpes by inoculation of virus via a break in the epidermal surface or by direct introduction of virus into the hand through occupational or other exposure. Clinical signs and symptoms include the abrupt onset of edema, erythema, and localized tenderness of the infected finger. Vesicular or pustular lesions of the fingertip indistinguishable from pyogenic bacterial infection are seen. Fever, lymphadenitis, and epitrochlear and axillary lymphadenopathy are common. Recurrences may occur. Prompt diagnosis to avoid unnecessary and potentially exacerbating surgical therapy and/or transmission is essential.

Herpetic eye infections HSV infection of the eye is the most frequent cause of corneal blindness in the United States. HSV keratitis presents with acute onset of pain, blurring of vision, chemosis, conjunctivitis, and characteristic dendritic lesions of the cornea. Use of topical corticosteroids may exacerbate symptoms and lead to involvement of deep structures of the eye. Debridement, topical antiviral, and/or interferon therapy hasten healing. However, recurrences are common and immunopathologic injury of the deeper structures of the eye may occur. Chorioretinitis, usually as a manifestation of disseminated HSV infection, may occur in neonates or those with AIDS. Acute necrotizing retinitis due to HSV is an uncommon but severe manifestation of HSV infection.

Central and peripheral nervous system infections with HSV-1 and HSV-2 HSV encephalitis is the most common identified cause of acute, sporadic viral encephalitis in the United States, comprising 10 to 20 percent of all cases. The estimated incidence is about 2.3 cases per million persons per year. Cases are distributed throughout the year, and the age distribution appears biphasic with peaks at between 5 and 30 and greater-than-50 years of age. HSV-1 accounts for more than 95 percent of cases. The pathogenesis of HSV encephalitis varies. In children and young adults primary HSV infection may result in encephalitis; presumably exogenously acquired virus enters the CNS by neurotropic spread from the periphery via the olfactory bulb. However, most adults with HSV encephalitis have clinical or serologic evidence of mucocutaneous HSV-1 infection prior to the onset of the CNS symptoms. In about 25 percent of the cases examined, the HSV-1 strains from the oropharynx and brain tissue of the same patient differ, suggesting that some cases may result from reinfection with another strain of HSV-1 that reached the CNS. Two theories have been proposed to explain the development of actively replicating HSV in localized areas of the CNS in persons from whom the ganglionic and CNS isolates are similar. Reactivation of latent trigeminal or autonomic nerve root HSV-1 infection may be associated with extension of virus into the CNS via nerves innervating the middle cranial fossa. HSV DNA has been demonstrated by DNA hybridization in human autopsy brain tissue. Reactivation of long-standing latent CNS infection may be another potential mechanism for the development of HSV encephalitis.

The clinical hallmark of HSV encephalitis has been the acute onset of fever and focal neurologic, especially temporal lobe, symptoms. To date no reliable noninvasive radiologic or virologic technique has been developed to diagnose HSV encephalitis during its early clinical stages, and differentiation of HSV encephalitis from other viral encephalitides and other focal infections and noninfectious processes is difficult. An increase in CSF and serum antibodies to HSV does occur with most cases of HSV encephalitis. However, these antibody rises rarely are present prior to 10 days into the illness and, while useful retrospectively, are not helpful in establishing the clinical diagnosis early in the course of disease. Brain biopsy because of its high sensitivity, low complication rate, and ability to establish alternative potentially treatable diagnoses has been felt to be the most expeditious method to diagnose HSV encephalitis, but newly developed assays for HSV antigens or DNA in CSF may supplant it. Antiviral chemotherapy reduces the mortality of HSV encephalitis, and intravenous acyclovir is more effective than vidarabine. Even with therapy, however, neurologic sequelae are frequent.

HSV has been isolated from the cerebrospinal fluid of 0.5 to 3 percent of patients presenting to the hospital with aseptic meningitis. HSV meningitis is usually seen in association with primary genital HSV infection. HSV meningitis is an acute self-limited disease manifested by headache, fever, and mild photophobia, which lasts from 2 to 7 days. A lymphocytic pleocytosis in the CSF is characteristic. Neurologic sequelae are rare. Recurrent bouts of aseptic meningitis related to reactivation of HSV have been reported.

Autonomic nervous system dysfunction, especially of the sacral region, has been reported in association with both HSV and varicella-zoster infections. Numbness, tingling of the buttock or perineal areas, urinary retention, constipation, cerebrospinal fluid pleocytosis, and impotence in males may occur. Symptoms appear to resolve slowly over a period of days to weeks. Occasionally hypesthesia and/or weakness of the lower extremities may persist for many months. Rarely transverse myelitis manifested by a rapidly progressive symmetric paralysis of the lower extremities or a Guillain-Barré syndrome may occur after HSV infection. Similarly, peripheral nervous system involvement [idiopathic facial paralysis (Bell's palsy)] or cranial polyneuritis may also be related to reactivation of HSV-1 infection. Transitory hypesthesia of the area of skin innervated by the trigeminal nerve and vestibular system dysfunction as measured by electronystagmography are the predominant signs of disease. Studies to determine if antiviral chemotherapy may abort or alleviate the frequency and severity of these signs are unavailable.

Visceral infections HSV infection of visceral organs usually results from viremia, and multiple organ involvement is common. Occasionally, however, the clinical manifestations of HSV infections may involve only the esophagus, lung, or liver. HSV esophagitis may result from direct extension of oral-pharyngeal HSV infection into the esophagus or may occur de novo by reactivation of HSV and spread of virus to the esophageal mucosa via the vagus nerve. The predominant symptoms of HSV esophagitis are odynophagia, dysphagia, substernal pain, and weight loss. There are multiple oval ulcerations on an erythematous base with or without a patchy white pseudomembrane. The distal esophagus is most commonly involved. With extensive disease diffuse friability may spread to the entire esophagus. Neither endoscopic nor barium examination can differentiate HSV from Candida esophagitis, or from esophageal ulcerations due to thermal injury, radiation, and corrosives. Endoscopically obtained secretions for cytologic examination and culture provide the most accurate material for diagnosis. Anecdotal observations suggest resolution of the symptoms of HSV esophagitis with systemic antiviral chemotherapy.

HSV pneumonitis is uncommon except in severely immunosuppressed patients and may result from extension of herpetic tracheobronchitis into lung parenchyma. Focal necrotizing pneumonitis usually results. Hematogenous dissemination of virus from oral or genital mucocutaneous disease may also occur and produce a bilateral interstitial pneumonitis. Concomitant bacterial, fungal, and parasitic pathogens are common in HSV pneumonitis. As the mortality of HSV pneumonia in immunosuppressed patients is high (>80 percent), these patients should be candidates for antiviral chemotherapy. HSV has also been isolated from the lower respiratory tract of persons with acute respiratory distress syndrome (ARDS). However, the relationship between isolation of HSV and the pathogenesis of the respiratory distress syndrome is unclear.

HSV is an uncommon cause of hepatitis in immunocompetent patients. HSV infection of the liver is associated with fever, abrupt elevations of the bilirubin and serum transaminases, and leukopenia (white blood cells <4000 per microliter). Disseminated intravascular coagulation may also be present.

Other isolated but reported complications of HSV include monarticular arthritis, adrenal necrosis, idiopathic thrombocytopenia, and glomerulonephritis. Disseminated HSV infection in the immunocompetent patient is rare. In immunocompromised, burn, or malnourished patients, dissemination of HSV to other visceral organs such as adrenal glands, pancreas, small and large intestine, and bone marrow may occur occasionally. Rarely, primary HSV infection in pregnancy may disseminate and may be associated with mortality in both mother and fetus. This uncommon event is usually associated with acquisition of primary infection in the third trimester.

NEONATAL HSV INFECTION Neonates (<6 weeks of age) have the highest frequency of visceral and/or CNS infection of any HSV-infected patient population. Untreated, over 70 percent of neonatal herpes cases will disseminate or develop CNS infection. Without therapy, the overall mortality of neonatal herpes is 65 percent, and less than 10 percent of neonates with CNS infection experience normal development. While skin lesions are the most commonly recognized features of disease, many infants do not develop lesions until well into the course of disease. Seventy percent of neonatal HSV cases are caused by HSV-2 infection, almost all of which result from contact via infected genital secretions at the time of delivery. However, congenitally infected infants have been reported, usually from mothers who acquired primary HSV infection during pregnancy. Neonatal HSV-1 infections are usually acquired postnatally through contact with immediate family members with symptomatic or asymptomatic oral-labial HSV-1 infection or from nosocomial transmission within the hospital. Antiviral chemotherapy has reduced the mortality of neonatal herpes to 25 percent. However, the morbidity, especially in infants with HSV-2 CNS involvement, is still very high.

DIAGNOSIS Both clinical and laboratory criteria are useful for establishing the diagnosis of HSV infections. Clinical diagnosis can be made accurately where characteristic multiple vesicular lesions on an erythematous base are present. Scrapings of the base of the lesions and subsequent staining with Wright, Giemsa (Tzanck preparation), or Papanicolaou's stain will demonstrate characteristic giant cells or intranuclear inclusions of a herpesvirus infection. These cytologic techniques are often useful as a quick office procedure to confirm the diagnosis. Limitations of this method are that it does not differentiate between HSV and varicella-zoster infections and is only about 60 percent as sensitive as viral isolation. The laboratory confirmation of HSV infection is best performed by isolation of virus in tissue culture. HSV causes a discernible cytopathic effect in a variety of cell culture systems, and most specimens can be identified within 48 to 96 h after inoculation. Spin-amplified culture with subsequent staining for HSV antigen has shortened the time needed to identify HSV to less than 24 h. The sensitivity of viral isolation varies with the stage of lesions (higher in vesicular than in ulcerative lesions), whether the patient has a first or recurrent episode of the disease (higher in first episodes), and whether the sample is from an immunosuppressed or immunocompetent patient (more antigen in immunosuppressed). Immunofluorescent assays using monoclonal antibodies and some DNA hybridization procedures have approached the sensitivity of viral isolation for detecting HSV from genital or oral-labial lesions, but appear only about 50 percent as sensitive as viral isolation for the detection of asymptomatic HSV in cervical or salivary secretions. Laboratory confirmation allows for subtyping the virus, which may be useful epidemiologically as well as in helping to predict the frequency of reactivation after first-episode oral-labial or genital HSV infection. Restriction endonuclease analysis of viral DNA can also be used to differentiate between HSV-1 and HSV-2 as well as to differentiate between strains within the same subtypes, information which may be very useful in identifying common source outbreaks of HSV.

Acute and convalescent serum can be useful in documenting seroconversion during primary HSV-1 or HSV-2 infection. However, only 5 percent of patients with recurrent mucocutaneous HSV infections show a fourfold or greater rise in anti-HSV antibodies between acute and convalescent sera. Serologic assays have little utility in diagnosing acute mucocutaneous HSV infection and are best used to identify persons with past infection. Newly developed type-specific serologic assays can be utilized to identify asymptomatic carriers of HSV-1 or HSV-2 infection.

THERAPY Many aspects of mucocutaneous and visceral HSV infections are amenable to treatment with antiviral chemotherapy. For mucocutaneous infections acyclovir has been the mainstay of therapy. Several antivirals are available for topical use in HSV eye infections: idoxuridine, trifluorothymidine, and topical vidarabine. For HSV encephalitis, intravenous acyclovir is the treatment of choice. For neonatal HSV infections high-dose intravenous vidarabine and acyclovir are effective.

Acyclovir has been shown to be effective in shortening symptoms and the duration of lesions of mucocutaneous HSV infections in immunocompromised patients and first-episode genital herpes in immunocompetent patients (Table 135-1). Intravenous and oral acyclovir will also prevent reactivation of HSV in seropositive immunocompromised patients who are undergoing induction chemotherapy for acute leukemia or in the immediate posttransplant period.

Oral acyclovir has also been shown to speed the healing and resolution of symptoms in first and recurrent episodes of genital HSV-1 and HSV-2 infections. The benefit of treating acute episodes of recurrent genital disease with oral acyclovir is modest, and as such, routine use for recurrent episodes of disease, especially for mild episodes, is not recommended. Chronic daily suppressive therapy may be useful in reducing the frequency of reactivation disease among patients with very frequent genital herpes. Chronic suppressive oral acyclovir does not eliminate sacral ganglionic latency, and reactivation of genital herpes occurs after discontinuing therapy. Oral acyclovir is of benefit in primary gingivostomatitis but has limited benefit in the treatment of recurrent oral-labial lesions; lesions are not aborted and total healing time is not reduced. If started early, the duration of the ulcerative stage of the lip lesion may be reduced.

TABLE 135-1 Current antiviral chemotherapy of HSV infection

I Mucocutaneous HSV infections
  A Immunosuppressed patients
    1 Acute symptomatic first or recurrent episodes: IV acyclovir (5 mg/kg every 8 h) or oral acyclovir (400 mg PO 4 times per day for 7 to 10 days) relieves pain and speeds healing. With localized external lesions 5% topical acyclovir ointment applied 4 to 6 times daily may be beneficial.
    2 Suppression of reactivation disease: IV (5 mg/kg every 8 h) or oral acyclovir (400 mg PO 3 to 5 times per day) will when taken daily prevent recurrences during high-risk period, e.g., immediate posttransplantation period.
  B Immunocompetent patients
    1 Genital herpes
      a First episodes: Oral acyclovir (200 mg PO 5 times per day for 10 to 14 days) is the treatment of choice. IV acyclovir (5 mg/kg every 8 h for 5 days) is given for severe disease or neurologic complications such as aseptic meningitis. Topical 5% ointment or cream applied 4 to 6 times daily for 7 to 10 days may be beneficial in patients without cervical, urethral, or pharyngeal involvement.
      b Symptomatic recurrent genital herpes: Oral acyclovir (200 mg PO 5 times per day for 5 days) has modest benefit in shortening lesions and viral excretion time. Routine use for all episodes not recommended.
      c Suppression of recurrent genital herpes: Daily oral acyclovir 200-mg capsules, 2 to 3 times daily or 400 mg PO 2 times per day will prevent reactivation of symptomatic recurrences; use at present limited to 6-month course in frequent recurrers.
    2 Oral-labial HSV
      a First episode: Oral acyclovir 200 mg 4–5 times per day.
      b Recurrent episodes: Topical acyclovir ointment is of no clinical benefit. Oral acyclovir has minimal benefit.
    3 Herpetic whitlow: Oral acyclovir 200 mg 5 times daily for 7–10 days.
    4 HSV proctitis: Oral acyclovir (400 mg PO 5 times per day) is useful in shortening course of infection. In immunosuppressed patients or in severe infection, IV acyclovir 5 mg/kg every 8 h may be useful.
  C Herpetic eye infections
    1 Acute keratitis: Topical trifluorothymidine, vidarabine, idoxuridine, acyclovir, and interferon are all beneficial. Debridement may be required; topical steroids may worsen disease.
II CNS HSV infection
  A HSV encephalitis: Intravenous acyclovir 10 mg/kg every 8 h (30 mg/kg per day) for 10 days or vidarabine (15 mg/kg per day) decrease mortality; acyclovir is the preferred agent.
  B HSV aseptic meningitis: No studies of systemic antiviral chemotherapy. If therapy is to be given IV, acyclovir at 15 to 30 mg/kg per day should be utilized.
  C Autonomic radiculopathy: No studies are available.
III Neonatal HSV infection: Intravenous vidarabine (30 mg/kg per day) or acyclovir (30 mg/kg per day). Neonates appear to tolerate this high dose of vidarabine.
IV Visceral HSV infections
  A HSV esophagitis: Systemic acyclovir (15 mg/kg per day) or vidarabine (15 mg/kg per day) should be considered.
  B HSV pneumonitis: No controlled studies. Systemic acyclovir (15 mg/kg per day) or vidarabine (15 mg/kg per day) should be considered.
V Disseminated HSV: No controlled studies, intravenous acyclovir or vidarabine should be attempted. No definite evidence that therapy will decrease mortality.
VI Erythema multiforme associated with HSV: Anecdotal observations suggest oral acyclovir capsules 2 to 3 times daily will suppress EM.

Both intravenous vidarabine 15 mg/kg per day over 12 h daily and intravenous acyclovir 30 mg/kg per day given as 10 mg/kg infusion over 1 h at 8-hourly intervals have been shown to be effective in reducing the mortality of HSV encephalitis. Primary determinants of outcome include young age and early therapy. Comparative trials of the two drugs for the treatment of HSV encephalitis have indicated a lower mortality rate and fewer neurologic sequelae with intravenous acyclovir. The major side effect associated with intravenous acyclovir is transient renal insufficiency usually due to crystallization of the compound in the renal parenchyma. This can be avoided if the medication is given slowly over 1 h and the patient is well-hydrated. Because CSF levels of acyclovir average only 30 to 50 percent of plasma levels, the dosage of acyclovir used for treatment of CNS infection (30 mg/kg per day) is double that used for treatment of mucocutaneous or visceral disease (15 mg/kg per day). Vidarabine at doses of 15 mg/kg per day tends to produce more hematopoietic and hepatic toxicity than acyclovir, but this is usually not a limiting problem in treating severe neonatal or CNS infections.

Acyclovir-resistant strains are being identified with increasing frequency. Almost all clinically significant acyclovir resistance has been seen in immunocompromised patients who have received multiple intermittent courses of therapy. Increasingly, patients with human immunodeficiency virus infection are noted to have persistent mucocutaneous HSV infection which is unresponsive to even very high dose acyclovir therapy. Most acyclovir-resistant strains of HSV have an altered substrate specificity for phosphorylating acyclovir. The frequent reactivation of virus and high virus titers in the lesions of immunocompromised patients in combination with the use of the medication selects out these resistant variants. In some patients, higher doses of acyclovir will be associated with clearing of lesions. In others, clinical disease will progress despite high-dose therapy. Therapy with an antiviral with another mechanism of action such as foscarnate or vidarabine may be useful (see Chap. 86).

PREVENTION   The large reservoir of persons with asymptomatic HSV-1 and HSV-2 infections indicates that control of HSV disease through suppressive antiviral chemotherapy and/or educational programs will be limited. Control of HSV infection will require prevention of infection, a goal most likely achievable by vaccination. Effective HSV vaccines are not currently available. Heterologous vaccines such as smallpox, bacillus Calmette-Guérin, and influenza, which have been used as therapies for genital HSV infection, have been ineffective.

Barrier forms of contraception, especially condoms, may decrease transmission of disease especially during periods of asymptomatic viral excretion. Transmission of disease when lesions were present despite the use of a condom may still occur, and patients should be instructed to avoid sexual activity when genital lesions are present.

REFERENCES

COREY L: Genital herpes simplex virus infections: Clinical manifestations, course, and complications. Ann Intern Med 98:958, 1983

————, SPEAR P: Infections with herpes simplex viruses. N Engl J Med 314:686, 749, 1986

———— et al: Differences between herpes simplex virus type 1 and type 2 neonatal encephalitis in neurological outcome. Lancet 2:1, 1988

DORSKY DI, CRUMPACKER CS: Drugs five years later: Acyclovir. Ann Intern Med 107:859, 1987

DOUGLAS JM et al: A double-blind study of oral acyclovir for suppression of recurrences of genital herpes simplex virus infection. N Engl J Med 310:1551, 1984

ERLICH KS et al: Acyclovir-resistant herpes simplex virus infections in patients with the acquired immunodeficiency syndrome. N Engl J Med 320:293, 1989

SHEPP DH et al: Oral acyclovir therapy for mucocutaneous herpes simplex infections in immunocompromised marrow transplant recipients. Ann Intern Med 102:783, 1985

SPRUANCE SL et al: Early application of topical 15% idoxuridine in dimethyl sulfoxide shortens the course of herpes simplex labialis: A multicenter placebo-controlled trial. J Infect Dis 161:191, 1990

STRAUSS SE et al: Herpes simplex virus infection: Biology, treatment, and prevention. Ann Intern Med 103:404, 1985

136   VARICELLA-ZOSTER VIRUS INFECTIONS

RICHARD J. WHITLEY

DEFINITION   Varicella-zoster virus (VZV) causes two distinct clinical entities: varicella, or chickenpox, and herpes zoster, or shingles. Chickenpox, a ubiquitous and extremely contagious infection, is usually a benign illness of childhood characterized by an exanthematous, vesicular rash. With reactivation of latent VZV, more common after the sixth decade of life, the disease presents as a dermatomal, vesicular rash which is usually associated with severe pain.

ETIOLOGY   A clinical association between varicella and herpes zoster has been recognized for nearly 100 years. Early in the twentieth century, similarities in the histopathologic findings of skin lesions resulting from varicella and herpes zoster were demonstrated. Viral isolates from patients with chickenpox and herpes zoster demonstrated similar alterations in tissue culture, specifically the appearance of eosinophilic intranuclear inclusions and multinucleated giant cells, suggesting that the viruses were biologically similar. Restriction endonuclease analysis of viral DNA from a patient with chickenpox who subsequently developed herpes zoster verified the molecular identity of the two viruses responsible for these differing clinical presentations. Varicella-zoster virus is a member of the herpesvirus family, sharing such similar structural characteristics as a lipid envelope, surrounding a nucleocapsid with icosahedral symmetry, a total size of approximately 150 to 200 nm, and centrally located double-stranded DNA with a molecular weight of approximately 80 million. Only enveloped virions are infectious.

PATHOGENESIS AND PATHOLOGY   Primary infection   Transmission is likely by the respiratory route, followed by localized replication at an undefined site, and leading to seeding of the reticuloendothelial system with, ultimately, viremia. The occurrence of viremia in patients with chickenpox is supported by the diffuse and scattered nature of the skin lesions and can be verified in selected cases by the recovery of virus from the blood. Vesicles involve the corium and dermis with degenerative changes characterized by ballooning, multinucleated giant cells, and eosinophilic intranuclear inclusions. Infection may involve localized blood vessels of the skin, resulting in necrosis and epidermal hemorrhage. With disease evolution, vesicular fluid becomes cloudy with the recruitment of polymorphonuclear leukocytes, degenerated cells, and fibrin. Ultimately, the vesicles rupture and release their fluid contents, which include infectious virus, or are gradually reabsorbed.

Recurrent infection   The mechanism of reactivation of VZV that results in herpes zoster is unknown. It is presumed that virus infects the dorsal root ganglia during chickenpox where it remains latent until reactivated. Histopathologic examination of the representative dorsal root ganglia during active herpes zoster demonstrates hemorrhage, edema, and lymphocytic infiltration.

Involvement with active VZV replication in other organs, such as the lung or brain, can occur during either chickenpox or herpes zoster but is uncommon in the immune-competent host. Lung involvement is characterized by interstitial pneumonitis, multinucleated giant cell formation, intranuclear inclusions, and pulmonary hemorrhage. Central nervous system (CNS) infection leads to histopathologic evidence of perivascular cuffing similar to that encountered with measles and other viral encephalitides. Focal hemorrhagic necrosis of the brain, characteristic of herpes simplex virus encephalitis, is uncommon with VZV infection.

EPIDEMIOLOGY AND CLINICAL PRESENTATION   Chickenpox   Humans are the only known reservoir for VZV. Chickenpox is highly contagious with an attack rate of at least 90 percent among susceptible or seronegative individuals. Both sexes and individuals of all races are infected equally. The virus is endemic in the population at large;

however, it becomes epidemic among susceptible individuals during seasonal periods, namely, late winter and early spring in the temperate zone. Children between the ages of 5 and 9 are most commonly affected and account for 50 percent of all cases. Most other cases occur between the ages of 1 to 4 and 10 to 14. Over the age of 15, approximately 10 percent of the population of the United States is susceptible to infection.

The incubation period of chickenpox ranges between 10 and 21 days but is usually between 14 and 17 days. Secondary attack rates in susceptible siblings within a household are between 70 and 90 percent. Patients are infectious approximately 48 h prior to the onset of the vesicular rash, during the period of vesicle formation, generally 4 to 5 days, and until all vesicles are crusted.

Clinically, chickenpox presents with a rash, low-grade fever, and malaise, although a few patients will develop a prodrome 1 to 2 days prior to the onset of the exanthem. In the immune-competent, this is usually a benign illness that is associated with lassitude and fever from 37.8 to 39.4°C (100 to 103°F) of 3 to 5 days' duration. The skin lesions, the hallmark of the infection, consist of maculopapules, vesicles, and scabs in varying stages of evolution. The evolution of lesions from maculopapules to vesicles occurs over a matter of hours to days. The lesions appear on the trunk and face and rapidly involve other areas of the body. Most are small and have an erythematous base with a diameter of 5 to 10 mm. Successive crops appear over a 2- to 4-day period. Lesions can also be found on the mucosa of the pharynx or the vagina. Their severity varies from individual to individual. Some individuals have very few lesions, while others can have as many as 2000. Younger children tend to have fewer vesicles compared to older individuals. Immunocompromised individuals, both children and adults, particularly those with leukemia, have more numerous lesions, often with a hemorrhagic base, and the lesions take longer to heal. These individuals also are at greater risk for visceral complications, which occur in 30 to 50 percent of cases and which are fatal in 15 percent.

The most common infectious complication of varicella is secondary bacterial superinfection of the skin, which is usually caused by *Streptococcus pyogenes* or *Staphylococcus aureus*. This may result from excoriation of skin lesions following scratching. Gram's stain of skin lesions should help clarify the etiology of unusually erythematous and pustulated lesions.

The most common extracutaneous site of involvement in children is the central nervous system and consists of acute cerebellar ataxia which generally appears approximately 21 days after the onset of the rash and rarely occurs in the preeruptive phase. The most prominent clinical finding is ataxia and meningeal irritation. The cerebrospinal fluid contains lymphocytes and elevated levels of protein. This is a benign complication of VZV infection in children and does not generally require hospitalization. Aseptic meningitis, encephalitis, transverse myelitis, and Reye's syndrome can also occur. Encephalitis is reported in 0.1 to 0.2 percent of children with chickenpox. No specific therapy is available for patients with central nervous system involvement caused by VZV.

Varicella pneumonia is the most serious complication following chickenpox, occurring more commonly in adults (up to 20 percent) than in children. It usually appears 3 to 5 days into the course of illness and is associated with tachypnea, cough, dyspnea, and fever. Cyanosis, pleuritic chest pain, and hemoptysis are frequent. Roentgenographic evidence of disease consists of nodular infiltrates and an interstitial pneumonitis. Resolution of pneumonitis parallels improvement of skin rash; however, patients may have persistent fever and compromised pulmonary function for weeks.

Other complications of chickenpox include myocarditis, corneal lesions, nephritis, arthritis, bleeding diatheses, acute glomerulonephritis, and hepatitis. Hepatic involvement, distinct from Reye's syndrome, is common in chickenpox and is usually characterized by an elevation of liver enzymes, particularly serum glutamic oxaloacetic transaminase (SGOT) and serum glutamic pyruvic transaminase (SGPT). Hepatic involvement is usually asymptomatic.

Perinatal varicella is associated with a high mortality rate when maternal disease develops within 5 days before delivery and 48 h post partum. Because the newborn does not receive protective transplacental antibodies and has an immature immune system, illness may be exaggerated. The mortality rate has been reported as high as 30 percent in this group. Congenital varicella with clinical manifestations at birth is extremely uncommon.

Herpes zoster Herpes zoster, a sporadic disease, is the consequence of reactivation of latent virus from the dorsal root ganglia. It occurs at all ages but mainly among the elderly. Most patients have no history of exposure to other individuals with VZV infection. The highest incidence is between 5 and 10 cases per 1000 persons for individuals in the sixth through the eighth decades of life. Approximately 2 percent of herpes zoster patients who do not receive immunosuppressive therapy will develop a second episode of infection. This figure is at least fivefold higher in immunocompromised individuals.

Herpes zoster, or "shingles," is characterized by a unilateral vesicular eruption within a dermatome, often associated with severe pain. The dermatomes from T3 to L3 are most frequently involved. If the ophthalmic branch of the trigeminal nerve is involved, zoster ophthalmicus results. The factors responsible for reactivation of virus are not known. In children, reactivation is usually benign, whereas in adults, acute neuritis and postherpetic neuralgia can be particularly debilitating. The onset of disease is heralded by pain within the dermatome that may precede lesions by 48 to 72 h, followed by an erythematous maculopapular rash which evolves rapidly to vesiculate. In the normal host, these lesions may remain few in number and continue to form only for a period of 3 to 5 days. The total duration of disease is generally between 7 and 10 days; however, it may take as long as 2 to 4 weeks before the skin returns to normal. In a few patients, characteristic localization of pain to a dermatome with serologic evidence of herpes zoster has been reported in the absence of skin lesions. When branches of the trigeminal nerve are involved, lesions may appear on the face, in the mouth, in the eye, or on the tongue. Lesions appear on the ear canal and tongue when the sensory branch of the facial nerve is involved (Ramsay Hunt syndrome).

The most debilitating complication of herpes zoster, both in the normal and in the immunocompromised host, is pain associated with acute neuritis and postherpetic neuralgia. Postherpetic neuralgia is uncommon in young individuals; however, at least 50 percent of patients over age 50 with zoster will report pain in the involved dermatome months after resolution of cutaneous disease. Changes in sensation within the dermatome, resulting in either hypo- or hyperesthesia, are common.

Central nervous system involvement following localized herpes zoster may occur. Many patients without signs of meningeal irritation will have cerebrospinal fluid pleocytosis and moderately elevated levels of CSF protein. Symptomatic meningoencephalitis is characterized by headache, fever, photophobia, meningitis, and vomiting. A rare manifestation of CNS involvement is granulomatous angiitis with contralateral hemiplegia, which can be diagnosed by cerebral arteriography. Other neurologic manifestations include transverse myelitis with or without motor paralysis.

As with chickenpox, herpes zoster in the immunocompromised host is more severe than in the normal individual. Lesion formation continues for over a week, and total scabbing does not develop in the majority of patients until 3 weeks into the course. Patients with Hodgkin's disease and non-Hodgkin's lymphoma are at greatest risk for progressive herpes zoster because cutaneous dissemination develops in about 40 percent of these patients. Among patients with cutaneous dissemination, there is a 5 to 10 percent increased risk of pneumonitis, meningoencephalitis, hepatitis, and other serious complications. However, even in immunocompromised patients disseminated zoster is rarely fatal.

Patients who have had a bone marrow transplant are at a particular risk of VZV infection. Thirty percent of cases of posttransplant VZV infection occur within 1 year (50 percent of these within 9 months), and 45 percent of such patients have cutaneous or visceral dissemination. The mortality rate is 10 percent, and postherpetic neuralgia, scarring, and bacterial superinfection are more frequent in VZV infections occurring within 9 months of a transplant. Among infected patients, concomitant graft-versus-host disease increases the chance for dissemination and/or a fatal outcome.

DIFFERENTIAL DIAGNOSIS   The diagnosis of chickenpox is not difficult. The characteristic rash of chickenpox and the epidemiologic history of recent exposure should lead to prompt diagnosis. Other viral infections which can mimic chickenpox include disseminated herpes simplex virus infection in patients with atopic dermatitis, and the disseminated vesiculopapular lesions sometimes associated with coxsackievirus, echovirus, or atypical measles infections. These rashes are more commonly morbilliform with a hemorrhagic component rather than vesicular or vesiculopustular. Rickettsialpox can be confused with chickenpox; however, it can be easily distinguished by finding the ''herald spot'' at the site of the mite bite and a more pronounced headache. The serologic test is also useful in differentiating rickettsialpox from varicella.

Unilateral vesicular lesions in a dermatomal pattern should lead rapidly to the diagnosis of herpes zoster. Both herpes simplex virus infections and coxsackievirus infections can be a cause of dermatomal vesicular lesions. In such situations, a Tzanck smear with supportive diagnostic virology will be helpful in ensuring the proper diagnosis. In the prodromal stage of herpes zoster, the diagnosis can be exceedingly difficult and may only be achieved once lesions have appeared, or by retrospective serologic assessment.

LABORATORY FINDINGS   Unequivocal confirmation of the diagnosis is possible only through the isolation of virus in susceptible tissue culture cell lines or by the demonstration of seroconversion or a fourfold or greater antibody rise when comparing acute and convalescent specimens. A rapid impression can be obtained by a Tzanck smear, performed by scraping the base of the lesions in an attempt to demonstrate multinucleated giant cells. Direct immunofluorescent staining of cells from the skin base or detection of viral antigens by other assays (immunoperoxidase) can also be utilized, although such tests are not commercially available. The most frequently employed serologic tools for assessing host response are immunofluorescent detection of antibodies to VZV membrane antigens, fluorescent antibody to membrane antigen (FAMA) test, immune adherence hemagglutination, or enzyme-linked immunosorbent assay (ELISA). The FAMA and ELISA tests appear to be the most sensitive.

PROPHYLAXIS   In the normal host, prophylaxis and treatment of chickenpox are of little relevance since the disease is usually benign. However, because the immunocompromised individual is at significant risk for developing progressive varicella, modalities of prevention include passive immunization or experimental administration of a live attenuated vaccine. Immune prophylaxis can be accomplished by the administration of specific zoster immune globulin (ZIG), derived from patients with herpes zoster, varicella-zoster immune globulin (VZIG), or the intravenous formulation of zoster immune plasma (ZIP). Both ZIG and VZIG should be given within 96 h, but preferably within 72 h, of exposure in order to be effective. It is likely that ZIP can be given somewhat later. Indications for the administration of ZIG or VZIG are summarized in Table 136-1. VZIG should be administered to immunodeficient patients under 15 who have a negative or unknown history of chickenpox, who have not been vaccinated against VZV, and who have had a contact in a household, with a playmate for more than 1 h indoors, or in a shared hospital room. It should also be administered to the newborn whose mother had an onset of chickenpox within less than 5 days before delivery and 48 h post partum. The use of VZIG for susceptible individuals over 15 must be evaluated on an individual basis. There is no evidence that VZIG is useful for adults with chickenpox, including pregnant women.

Clinical trials in Japan and the United States have demonstrated the efficacy of live attenuated vaccine both in normal individuals and

---

TABLE 136-1   Recommendations for VZIG utilization

I Exposure:
  A Both exposure to person with chickenpox or zoster as:
    1 Continuous household contact
    2 Playmate of >1-h duration indoors
    3 Hospital contact (same room or prolonged face-to-face)
    4 Newborn exposure whereby mother had onset of chickenpox <5 days before delivery to 48 h post partum
  B And time elapsed ≤96 h (preferably sooner)
II Candidates should:
  A Have significant exposure (see *I* above)
  B Be susceptible to VZV infection
  C Be <15 years of age (older immunocompromised patients require individual decision)
  D Have one of the following conditions:
    1 Leukemia or lymphoma
    2 Congenital or acquired immune deficiency
    3 Immunosuppressive treatment
    4 Newborn defined above (see *IA4*)

---

in immunocompromised hosts. A live attenuated VZV vaccine may be licensed in the United States in the future.

TREATMENT   Medical management of chickenpox in the normal host is directed toward preventing avoidable complications. Obviously, good hygiene should include daily bathing and soaks. Secondary bacterial infection of the skin can be avoided by meticulous skin care, particularly with close cropping of fingernails. Pruritus can be decreased with topical dressings or the administration of antipruritic drugs. Tepid water baths and wet compresses are better than drying lotions for the relief of itching. Domeboro soaks for the management of herpes zoster can be both soothing and cleansing. Administration of aspirin should be avoided in children with chickenpox because of the recent association between aspirin derivatives and the development of Reye's syndrome.

Patients with varicella pneumonia may require removal of bronchial secretions and ventilatory support. Zoster ophthalmicus should be referred promptly and immediately to an ophthalmologist. Therapy consists of administration of analgesics for severe pain and the use of atropine. The role of parenteral administration of antivirals for the management of zoster ophthalmicus remains unclear, although both acyclovir and vidarabine have been utilized (see Chap. 86).

Both chickenpox and herpes zoster in the immunocompromised host can be treated successfully with intravenous vidarabine or acyclovir. When the former drug is administered to patients with either disease, healing of skin lesions is accelerated and visceral complications are likely to be decreased. For patients with herpes zoster, intravenous vidarabine therapy will also accelerate resolution of acute neuritis and decrease both the duration of postherpetic neuralgia and the frequency of cutaneous dissemination. The dose is 15 mg/kg per day once daily intravenously over 12 h at a concentration of 0.5 mg of standard intravenous fluids. While acyclovir is not yet approved for this indication by the Food and Drug Administration, it is used preferentially over vidarabine because of decreased toxicity, especially in immunocompromised patients. Intravenous acyclovir leads to the decreased occurrence of visceral complications but has no effect on healing of skin lesions or pain. The treatment of herpes zoster with oral acyclovir is experimental. Concomitant with the administration of intravenous acyclovir to the immunosuppressed host, it is desirable to attempt to wean patients from immunosuppressive treatment.

Management of acute neuritis and/or postherpetic neuralgia can be particularly difficult. In addition to the judicious use of analgesics, ranging from nonnarcotic to narcotic derivatives, drugs such as amitriptyline hydrochloride and fluphenazine hydrochloride have been reported to be beneficial for pain relief. Glucocorticoids have been reported in some studies to be useful when administered early in the course for prevention of postherpetic neuralgia. This approach remains controversial.

REFERENCES

BRUNELL PA et al: Prevention of varicella by zoster immune globulin. N Engl J Med 280:1191, 1969

ESSMAN V et al: Prednisone does not prevent postherpetic neuralgia. Lancet 2:126, 1987

GERSHON AA et al: Live attenuated varicella vaccine. JAMA 252:355, 1984

HOPE-SIMPSON RE: The nature of herpes zoster: A long-term study and a new hypothesis. Proc R Soc Med 58:9, 1965

LOCKSLEY RM et al: Infection with varicella zoster virus after marrow transplantation. J Infect Dis 152:1172, 1985

PROBER CG et al: Acyclovir therapy of chickenpox in immunosuppressed children—a collaborative study. J Pediatr 101:622, 1982

SHEPP D et al: Treatment of varicella-zoster virus in severely immunocompromised patients: A randomized comparison of acyclovir and vidarabine. N Engl J Med 314:208, 1987

WEIBEL RE et al: Live attenuated varicella versus vaccine: Efficacy trial in healthy children. N Engl J Med 310:1409, 1984

WELLER TH: Varicella and herpes zoster: Changing concepts of the natural history, control, and importance of a not-so-benign virus. N Engl J Med 309:1362, 1434, 1983

WHITLEY RJ et al: Early vidarabine therapy to control the complications of herpes zoster in immunosuppressed patients. N Engl J Med 307:971, 1982

———: Vidarabine therapy of varicella in immunosuppressed patients. J Pediatr 1:125, 1982

———: Varicella-zoster virus infections, in *Antiviral Agents and Viral Diseases of Man 2*, GJ Galasso et al (eds). New York, Raven, 1984, pp 517–542

ZAIA JA et al: Evaluation of varicella-zoster immune globulin: Protection of immunosuppressed children after household exposure to varicella. J Infect Dis 147:737, 1983

137 EPSTEIN-BARR VIRUS INFECTIONS, INCLUDING INFECTIOUS MONONUCLEOSIS

ROBERT T. SCHOOLEY

DEFINITION Epstein-Barr virus (EBV) is a B lymphotropic human herpesvirus which is worldwide in distribution. Primary infection with EBV during childhood is usually subclinical. Between 25 and 70 percent of adolescents and adults who undergo a primary EBV infection develop the clinical syndrome of infectious mononucleosis. Infectious mononucleosis is defined by the clinical triad of fever, lymphadenopathy, and pharyngitis combined with the transient appearance of heterophil antibodies and an atypical lymphocytosis. EBV is also associated with nasopharyngeal carcinoma and certain B-cell lymphomas.

EPIDEMIOLOGY OF EBV INFECTIONS EBV is a ubiquitous agent that has been found in all population groups surveyed to date. The virus was initially described by Epstein, Achong, and Barr who noted, by electron microscopy, the presence of particles similar in morphology to herpes simplex virus in continuous cell lines which had arisen from tumor tissue obtained from patients with Burkitt's lymphoma. Following an observation by the Henles of antibodies to EBV in a patient with infectious mononucleosis, large-scale serologic surveys confirmed EBV as the etiologic agent for infectious mononucleosis.

EBV is transmitted primarily in saliva, or, less commonly, by blood transfusion. Primary infection tends to occur at an earlier age among lower socioeconomic groups and in developing countries. In industrialized countries approximately 50 percent of individuals have experienced a primary EBV infection by adolescence. These early infections are usually mild and nonspecific or clinically inapparent. A second wave of seroconversions to EBV occurs with the onset of the social activity associated with adolescence and young adulthood. Primary EBV infection among this age group accounts for most cases of infectious mononucleosis. The peak incidence of infectious mononucleosis occurs between 14 and 16 years of age for girls, and between 16 and 18 years of age for boys. By adulthood most individuals are EBV-seropositive.

EBV is shed from the oropharynx for up to 18 months following primary infection; thereafter it is shed intermittently by all EBV-seropositive individuals in the absence of a clinical illness. EBV can be isolated from the oropharyngeal washings of 15 to 25 percent of healthy EBV-seropositive individuals. Immunosuppressed individuals shed the virus more frequently. EBV can be isolated from 25 to 50 percent of the oropharyngeal washings obtained from renal allograft recipients and from virtually all patients with the acquired immunodeficiency syndrome (AIDS). Asymptomatic shedding of EBV by healthy individuals accounts for most of the spread to uninfected members of the population despite the fact that it is not highly contagious. Transmission is largely dependent on salivary contact (e.g., kissing). It is not likely to be transmitted by aerosol or fomites. Thus, isolation restrictions on patients with mononucleosis or individuals likely to be shedding EBV are not appropriate.

ETIOLOGY AND PATHOGENESIS OF INFECTIOUS MONONUCLEOSIS By electron microscopy the EB virus appears as an icosahedral nucleocapsid surrounded by a complex envelope and is indistinguishable from other members of the human herpesvirus group. The double-stranded EBV DNA has a molecular weight of approximately 101×10^6 and encodes for at least 30 polypeptides. There is no convincing evidence that there are strain differences among EBV isolates which account for the wide range of clinical conditions associated with EBV infection.

When EBV is transmitted by saliva, the initial site of replication is the oropharynx. EBV grows productively in B lymphocytes and oropharyngeal epithelial cells of patients with infectious mononucleosis; both cell types have specific surface receptors for EBV. During the acute phase of the illness, EBV antigens can be demonstrated within the nuclei of up to 20 percent of circulating B lymphocytes. After the infection subsides, the virus can be isolated from a small number of B lymphocytes of EBV-seropositive individuals and also resides within nasopharyngeal epithelial cells.

Virus-host interactions EBV infection has both direct and indirect effects on the cellular and humoral immune responses. Within 18 to 24 h after entry of EBV into B lymphocytes by means of the C3d receptor (also known as CD21), Epstein-Barr nuclear antigens (EBNA) are detectable within the nucleus of the infected cell. Expression of EBNA corresponds to the acquisition of the transformed or immortalized phenotype. EBV-infected B lymphocytes also express lymphocyte-determined membrane antigens (LYDMA) which serve as the putative target for the cellular immune response to virus-infected B lymphocytes. Immortalized B lymphocytes can be propagated continuously in vitro and are polyclonally stimulated by EBV to produce immunoglobulin. Antibodies reactive with sheep red blood cells (heterophil) and antibodies with several other specificities are manifestations of polyclonal immunoglobulin production and may mediate several of the complications of infectious mononucleosis. A minority of EBV-infected B lymphocytes enter the lytic cycle (production of mature progeny virus and death of the host cell) and produce EBV antigens that are detected during virus replication. These are divided into the early antigen complex (EA) and viral capsid antigens (VCA). The early antigen complex consists of two groups of antigens; (1) diffuse (EA-D), which are detectable in both the cytoplasm and the nucleus of cells in the lytic cycle, and (2) restricted (EA-R), which are demonstrable only in the cytoplasm. These antigens serve as markers of infection at the cellular level; the pattern of the antibody response to these antigens is useful diagnostically in the identification of EBV-associated disease states (Table 137-1). After the appearance of VCA the host cell dies and virions are released, which can infect and transform additional B lymphocytes.

An effective immune response to EBV involves humoral and cellular components. Neutralizing antibodies which inactivate cell-free virus and antibodies to VCA and EBNA appear during primary infection in all patients; antibodies to EA-D appear in most patients. The cellular immune response is largely responsible for controlling B-cell proliferation and polyclonal immunoglobulin production trig-

TABLE 137-1 EBV-specific antibodies

Antibody specificity	Time of appearance in IM	Persistence	Percent of IM patients with antibody	Comments
VCA:				
IgM	At clinical presentation	1–2 months	100	Best indicator of primary infection; not present with reactivation
IgG	At clinical presentation	Lifelong	100	Standard "EBV titer" reported by most commercial and state labs; major utility is as a marker for prior or current infection in epidemiologic studies
EA:				
EA-D	Peaks 3–4 weeks after onset	3–6 months	70	Presence correlates with more severe disease in patients with IM; present in nasopharyngeal carcinoma; IgA anti-EA-D antibodies useful for prediction of NPC in high-risk populations
EA-R	Several weeks after onset	Months to years		Present in high titer in African Burkitt's lymphoma; may be useful as an indicator of reactivation of EBV in immunosuppressed patients
EBNA	3–6 weeks after onset	Lifelong	100	Late appearance of anti-EBNA antibodies in IM makes seroconversion a useful marker for primary infection if IgM anti-VCA antibody studies are not available

NOTE: IM = infectious mononucleosis; VCA = viral capsid antigen; EA = early antigens; EA-D = diffuse early antigens; EA-R = restricted early antigens; EBNA = Epstein-Barr nuclear antigens; NPC = nasopharyngeal carcinoma.

gered by EBV and is composed primarily of T lymphocytes having functional and surface phenotypic characteristics of activated, suppressor-cytotoxic T lymphocytes (CD8+, Ia+). As the illness progresses, memory T lymphocytes capable of limiting proliferation of autologous EBV-infected B lymphocytes are demonstrable. These memory T lymphocytes persist for life. However, latent EBV remains in a small proportion of B lymphocytes and also in epithelial cells in the oropharynx.

During the primary immune response to EBV, global cellular immune hyporesponsiveness is readily demonstrable. This resolves after resolution of the illness, but reactivation of EBV is facilitated by conditions which interfere with the cellular immune response (immunosuppressive drugs, especially cyclosporin A, and disorders associated with cellular immunodeficiency, e.g., AIDS). EBV and cytomegalovirus (CMV) reactivation in immunosuppressed patients are frequently associated with a return of the immunoregulatory abnormalities characteristic of the primary immune response to these viruses. In the case of CMV, particularly, this hyporesponsiveness may contribute to many of the superinfections which frequently accompany CMV infections in immunocompromised hosts. The cellular hyporesponsiveness associated with EBV reactivation is generally less intense and less prolonged than that associated with CMV but may also contribute to morbidity in immunocompromised individuals.

CLINICAL MANIFESTATIONS Symptoms and signs After an incubation period of 4 to 8 weeks, prodromal symptoms of malaise, anorexia, and chills frequently precede the onset of pharyngitis, fever, and lymphadenopathy by several days. Severe pharyngitis is the symptom which most frequently prompts patients to seek medical attention. Occasionally patients will note only fever or lymphadenopathy or will present with one of the complications of infectious mononucleosis. Most patients also complain of headache and malaise. Abdominal pain is infrequent in the absence of splenic rupture.

Physical examination Fever is present in 90 percent of patients and may reach 39 to 40°C. Periorbital edema may be seen. The pharyngitis is usually diffuse; an exudate is observed in one-third of the cases. Palatal petechiae may also be observed. Posterior and/or anterior cervical adenopathy is noted in 90 percent of patients with infectious mononucleosis. Individual nodes are rarely painful but may be moderately tender to palpation. Hepatomegaly is infrequent, although mild hepatic tenderness is present in up to half the patients. Approximately half of all patients have splenomegaly, which is usually maximal in the second or third week of illness. In 5 percent of patients a macular, petechial, scarlatiniform, urticarial, or erythema multiforme-like rash may appear. Administration of ampicillin results in a pruritic, maculopapular eruption in 90 to 100 percent of patients.

Clinical course Infectious mononucleosis is a self-limited illness in the vast majority of cases. The pharyngitis is maximal for 5 to 7 days and then resolves over the subsequent 7 to 10 days. Fever usually persists for 7 to 14 days, but occasionally may continue somewhat longer. The course of the lymphadenopathy is variable, but rarely exceeds 3 weeks. The most persistent symptom is malaise. Most patients are well enough to return to work or school within 3 to 4 weeks, but occasional patients remain exhausted, have difficulty concentrating, and are unable to return to full activities for months. This subgroup is often found among those who present with a less acute onset without severe pharyngitis and high fever.

Occasional patients have been reported in which recurrent pharyngitis and fever is accompanied by persistent or resurgent heterophil antibodies. A group of patients has been described with nonspecific symptoms which may include malaise, fatigue, pharyngitis, fever, lymphadenopathy, and difficulty with higher cognitive function. These patients are usually heterophil-negative. The demonstration that some of these patients have anti-VCA and EA-R titers which are higher, and anti-EBNA titers which are lower, than median titers for the general population has led to the speculation that this symptom complex may be a manifestation of ongoing replication of EBV. However, healthy members of the general population not infrequently have antibodies to EA-R antigens, and one should be cautious about applying the diagnosis of chronic active EBV infection to patients with these nonspecific symptoms simply on the basis of the presence of anti-EA-R antibodies. Several studies have demonstrated the lack of utility of EBV-specific antibodies in the evaluation of most patients with chronic fatigue and malaise. A blinded placebo-controlled crossover study demonstrated no benefit from acyclovir therapy in this patient population. Occasional patients have been reported in whom mortality or severe morbidity (pneumonitis, fever, pancytopenia) is associated with evidence of ongoing EBV replication. Such patients are extremely rare, and specific antiviral therapy may be useful in their management.

Complications Complications of infectious mononucleosis occur infrequently but may be so dramatic as to be the predominant manifestation of the illness (Table 137-2). Hematologic complications include autoimmune hemolytic anemia, which may be mediated by

TABLE 137-2   Complications of infectious mononucleosis

Hematologic complications:
   Autoimmune hemolytic anemia
   Thrombocytopenia
   Granulocytopenia
Splenic rupture
Neurologic complications:
   Encephalitis
   Cranial nerve palsies, especially Bell's palsy
   Meningoencephalitis
   Guillain-Barré syndrome
   Seizures
   Mononeuritis multiplex
   Transverse myelitis
   Psychosis
Hepatic complications:
   Hepatitis
Cardiac complications:
   Pericarditis
   Myocarditis
Pulmonary complications:
   Airway obstruction
   Interstitial pneumonitis

IgM antibodies with anti-i specificity. Hemolytic anemia usually subsides over a 1- to 2-month period. Mild thrombocytopenia occurs in up to 50 percent of cases; profound thrombocytopenia is a rare, but well-recognized, complication and is frequently antibody-mediated. Mild granulocytopenia is frequently observed in uncomplicated infectious mononucleosis, and severe granulocytopenia associated with infection or death has been reported. Antibodies which react with granulocytes have been detected in up to 80 percent of patients and may contribute to the profound granulocytopenia which is occasionally observed. Both the thrombocytopenia and the granulocytopenia are usually self-limited and resolve over 3 to 6 weeks. Glucocorticoids have been advocated for treatment of both hemolytic anemia and thrombocytopenia associated with infectious mononucleosis, but efficacy has not been proved in controlled studies. Splenic rupture is an infrequent complication of infectious mononucleosis, often accompanied by the insidious or abrupt onset of abdominal pain, and is usually observed during the second or third week of illness. Surgery, usually splenectomy or splenorrhaphy, is the only effective management.

Neurologic complications of infectious mononucleosis may be the presenting or sole manifestation of the illness. Heterophil antibodies may be absent, and atypical lymphocytes may not be present at the onset of the neurologic event. The most frequent neurologic complications are cranial nerve palsies and encephalitis which may present initially with cerebellar findings. The onset of the encephalitis is usually abrupt. Cerebrospinal fluid findings are not diagnostic, and localization by noninvasive neurodiagnostic studies may suggest herpes simplex encephalitis. Eighty-five percent of patients with EBV-associated neurologic findings recover spontaneously.

Hepatitis is a common component of infectious mononucleosis. Almost 90 percent of patients have mild elevation of hepatic transaminases. Although more serious hepatic sequelae have been reported, severe or permanent hepatic dysfunction is exceedingly rare.

Cardiac abnormalities are uncommon but may include pericarditis, myocarditis, coronary artery spasm, or electrocardiographic abnormalities.

Airway obstruction from pharyngeal or paratracheal adenopathy can occur. This may require surgical intervention but is usually quite sensitive to glucocorticoid therapy. Pulmonary parenchymal abnormalities such as interstitial infiltrates are noted infrequently in adults but appear to be more common among children.

Infectious mononucleosis is rarely fatal. Neurologic complications, airway obstruction, and splenic rupture are the most frequent causes of death in previously healthy individuals with primary EBV infection. Sporadic or X-linked cases of overwhelming EBV infection accompanied by lymphoproliferation and hepatic dysfunction have been reported.

The X-linked condition, known as *X-linked lymphoproliferative (XLP) or Duncan's syndrome* (see Chap. 263), results in the death of 40 percent of affected males during primary EBV infection. In addition to overwhelming lymphoproliferation, XLP patients may manifest severe immunologic or hematologic sequelae such as agammaglobulinemia, aplastic anemia, or lymphocytic lymphoma. The pathophysiology of the XLP syndrome has not yet been completely elucidated, but an X-linked defect in the immune response to EBV may result in failure to control EBV replication or in disordered immunoregulation which leads to the other immunologic sequelae observed in this syndrome.

LABORATORY MANIFESTATIONS Heterophil antibodies Antibodies to sheep erythrocytes which can be removed by prior absorption with beef red blood cells, but not with guinea pig kidney, are termed heterophil antibodies. Heterophil antibodies are demonstrated in 50 percent of children and 90 to 95 percent of adolescents and adults with mononucleosis. Although the classic tube heterophil titer is still performed in many laboratories, the "monospot" test using a commerical kit is sensitive, specific, easily performed, and more routinely employed. The frequency of heterophil positivity associated with infectious mononucleosis depends upon the test used, the age of the patient population, and the time during the illness at which the test is performed. Monospot tests may be slightly more sensitive than heterophil titers. Ten to fifteen percent of patients with mononucleosis may be heterophil-negative if tested only during the first week of the illness. If the clinical suspicion of mononucleosis is high enough, retesting for heterophil antibodies during the second or third week of illness is warranted. Heterophil antibodies decline in titer after the acute illness has resolved but may be detectable for up to 9 months after the onset of the illness.

Atypical lymphocytosis A relative and absolute lymphocytosis is present in about 75 percent of cases of infectious mononucleosis. The lymphocytosis usually peaks in the second or third week of illness and is characterized by cells with atypical morphology. These atypical lymphocytes, which are primarily activated T lymphocytes, are larger than mature lymphocytes and often contain eccentrically placed lobulated nuclei with nucleoli, and vacuolated cytoplasm with rolled up edges. Mild neutropenia and thrombocytopenia are frequent. Other laboratory abnormalities include a mild polyclonal increase in immunoglobulins of the IgM, IgG, and IgA classes, and mild elevations of hepatocellular enzymes.

EBV-specific antibody response Antibodies to several EBV-specific antigens arise during primary EBV infection (Table 137-1). Proper utilization of EBV-specific antibody studies may facilitate the diagnosis of primary EBV infection in clinically atypical or heterophil-negative cases. IgM antibodies to the VCA are diagnostic of a primary EBV infection. IgG anti-VCA antibodies are present at clinical presentation in almost all patients and remain detectable for life. IgG anti-VCA antibodies are useful mainly as a test for susceptibility to EBV and are not useful for the diagnosis of primary infection. Approximately 70 percent of patients with infectious mononucleosis make antibodies to EA-D. Anti-EA-D antibodies usually peak 3 to 4 weeks after the onset of illness and usually disappear after recovery. Antibodies to EBNA appear 6 to 8 weeks into the illness and persist for life. The presence of IgM anti-VCA antibodies, and seroconversion to EBNA is diagnostic of a primary EBV infection. Patients with defects in cellular immunity may fail to make antibodies to EBNA.

DIAGNOSIS The diagnosis of infectious mononucleosis is not difficult in the vast majority of cases. The constellation of fever, pharyngitis, and lymphadenopathy coupled with an atypical lymphocytosis and heterophil antibodies is virtually always due to primary EBV infection and requires no further laboratory studies. Certain patients with EBV-induced mononucleosis, particularly preadolescents, or those with neurologic complications may be heterophil-negative or may lack an atypical lymphocytosis. Primary EBV infection can be diagnosed with certainty in these patients with the proper use of EBV-specific serologic studies (see above). Culturing EBV from oropharyngeal washings or peripheral blood mononuclear cells is laborious, and because of the ubiquity of the virus among EBV-seropositive individuals, it is not diagnostic of primary EBV infection.

Primary CMV infection is the illness most frequently confused with EBV-induced infectious mononucleosis. About two-thirds of adults with heterophil-negative mononucleosis have CMV-induced mononucleosis. Patients with CMV mononucleosis are, on the average, slightly older than those with EBV-induced infectious mononucleosis and usually have an illness characterized predominantly by fever and malaise. Pharyngitis and lymphadenopathy are less common than with infectious mononucleosis. CMV-induced mononucleosis is usually more insidious in onset and slower to resolve than EBV-induced mononucleosis. The diagnosis can be made by the isolation of CMV from the peripheral blood, and the demonstration of seroconversion or a fourfold or greater rise in antibody titer to CMV. Although CMV is also shed in saliva and urine by patients with CMV mononucleosis, demonstration of the agent in the blood is a more specific, but less sensitive, indicator of CMV-induced morbidity.

Severe pharyngitis may also be caused by another virus (e.g., herpes simplex) or by group A beta-hemolytic streptococci. Since group A beta-hemolytic streptococci can be isolated from the throat of up to 30 percent of patients with infectious mononucleosis, isolation of this organism does not rule out the diagnosis of infectious mononucleosis. Atypical lymphocytes may also be observed in a number of other conditions including rubella, hepatitis, toxoplasmosis, mumps, and drug reactions. These conditions rarely pose major differential diagnostic problems when careful attention is paid to the other clinical and laboratory features of these illnesses.

TREATMENT   Infectious mononucleosis usually requires only supportive management. Patients should be advised to obtain adequate rest; there is no evidence that forced bed rest hastens recovery. Fever and pharyngitis are usually ameliorated by acetaminophen. Because of the infrequent complication of splenic rupture, patients should be advised to avoid contact sports for 6 to 8 weeks after the onset of illness. The timing of return to school or work is determined solely by symptoms. Patients with mild illness may not require any major changes in routine. Occasional patients with protracted illness may not return to a full school or work schedule for several months. Recovery from mononucleosis is often gradual and the malaise may wax and wane for some time.

Although glucocorticoids may hasten defervescence and the resolution of pharyngitis, they are indicated only for certain specific complications of mononucleosis; airway obstruction usually responds dramatically to parenteral glucocorticoids. Glucocorticoids may also hasten the recovery of patients with severe hemolytic anemia or thrombocytopenia. There is no evidence that glucocorticoids are beneficial for the neurologic complications of the illness. Occasional selected patients with protracted illness may benefit from a short course of prednisone, but glucocorticoids should be avoided in the majority of patients with infectious mononucleosis.

Acyclovir, interferon alpha, and 9-[2-hydroxy-1-(hydroxymethyl)ethoxy]methyl guanine (ganciclovir) are active inhibitors of EBV replication in vitro. Interferon alpha has antiviral activity and can decrease shedding of EBV by renal allograft recipients treated with antithymocyte globulin. Administration of intravenous or high-dose oral acyclovir halts oropharyngeal shedding of EBV in patients with acute infectious mononucleosis; however, clinical benefits are minimal or inapparent.

EBV-ASSOCIATED MALIGNANCY   Since the initial description of EBV in patients with African Burkitt's lymphoma, the virus has been detected in association with several other malignancies. EBV DNA sequences have been detected in tumor tissue from more than 90 percent of patients with African Burkitt's lymphomas. American Burkitt's lymphoma, which often affects older children, and more often presents as an intraabdominal tumor, is EBV-associated in only 15 percent of cases. Anaplastic nasopharyngeal carcinoma, a common neoplasm in southeast China, is highly associated with EBV; virtually all adequately studied patients with this malignancy have evidence of EBV in tumor tissue.

There is increasing evidence that implicates EBV in the pathogenesis of certain cases of lymphocytic lymphoma in the immunoincompetent host (see Chap. 302). B-cell lymphoma is greatly overrepresented among malignancies developing in immunosuppressed individuals such as organ allograft recipients, patients with ataxia telangiectasia, and patients with AIDS. Immunologically privileged areas such as the central nervous system also appear to be particularly susceptible to B-cell lymphomas. Cardiac allograft recipients treated with cyclosporin A appear to be particularly susceptible to B-cell lymphoma. EBV sequences are detectable in up to half of the B-cell malignancies encountered in immunosuppressed individuals. Controversy exists as to whether the B-cell lymphoproliferation, which is initially polyclonal and may be driven by EBV reactivated in the setting of cellular immunodeficiency, is the first step in the development of these malignancies. The process, which is thought to be polyclonal initially, becomes oligoclonal or monoclonal with a second-step chromosomal translocation made more likely by the increased number of proliferating B lymphocytes. The biologic behavior of these tumors does not always correlate with clonality as defined by conventional techniques. Patients have been described who have succumbed to lymphoproliferative processes which appear to be polyclonal by surface immunoglobulin studies. More sensitive techniques of defining clonality, such as that utilizing immunoglobulin gene rearrangement, may reveal that a larger proportion of the polyclonal lymphomas are in fact oligo- or monoclonal. The response of these B-cell lymphomas to conventional chemotherapy is often disappointing. Some have advocated acyclovir therapy; others feel many of these lymphoproliferative syndromes are reversible if the immunosuppression is decreased. Studies of larger numbers of these patients for the presence of EBV sequences and for the progression from a polyclonal to an oligoclonal or monoclonal disorder will shed more light on the role of EBV in oncogenesis in both immunoincompetent and immunologically normal hosts.

REFERENCES

ANDIMAN W et al: Use of cloned probes to detect Epstein-Barr viral DNA in tissues of patients with neoplastic and lymphoproliferative diseases. J Infect Dis 148:967, 1983

GROSE C et al: Primary Epstein-Barr virus infections in acute neurologic diseases. N Engl J Med 292:392, 1975

HANTO DW et al: Epstein-Barr virus induced B-cell lymphoma after renal transplantation. Acyclovir therapy and transition from polyclonal to monoclonal B-cell proliferation. N Engl J Med 306:913, 1982

HENLE W et al: Epstein-Barr virus specific diagnostic tests in infectious mononucleosis. Hum Pathol 5:551, 1974

HOLMES GP et al: Chronic fatigue syndrome: A working case definition. Ann Intern Med 108:387, 1989

MILLER G et al: Selective lack of antibody to a component of EB nuclear antigen in patients with chronic active Epstein-Barr virus infection. J Infect Dis 156:26, 1987

SCHOOLEY RT et al: Chronic Epstein-Barr virus infection associated with fever and interstitial pneumonitis. Ann Intern Med 104:636, 1986

SIXBY JW et al: Epstein-Barr virus replication in oropharyngeal epithelial cells. N Engl J Med 310:1225, 1984

STRAUS SE et al: Treatment of the chronic fatigue syndrome with acyclovir: Lack of efficacy in a placebo-controlled trial. N Engl J Med 319:1692–1698, 1988

THORLEY-LAWSON, DA: Immunological responses to Epstein-Barr virus infection and the pathogenesis of EBV-induced diseases. Biochem Biophys Acta 948:263, 1988

138   CYTOMEGALOVIRUS INFECTION

MARTIN S. HIRSCH

DEFINITION   Cytomegalovirus (CMV), which was initially isolated from patients with congenital cytomegalic inclusion disease, is now recognized as an important pathogen in all age groups. In addition to inducing severe birth defects, CMV causes a wide spectrum of disorders in older children and adults, ranging from an asymptomatic, subclinical infection to a mononucleosis syndrome in healthy individuals to disseminated disease in the immunocompromised. Human CMV is one of several related species-specific viruses that cause similar diseases in various animals. All are associated with the production of characteristic enlarged cells; hence the name cytomegalovirus.

ETIOLOGY CMV is a member of the herpesvirus group and contains double-stranded DNA, a protein capsid, and a lipoprotein envelope. Like other members of the herpesvirus group, CMV demonstrates icosahedral symmetry, replicates in the cell nucleus, and can cause either a lytic and productive or a latent infection. CMV can be distinguished from other herpesviruses by certain biologic properties such as host range and the type of cytopathology induced. Virus replication is associated with the production of large intranuclear inclusions and smaller cytoplasmic inclusions. The virus appears to replicate in a variety of cell types in vivo; in tissue culture it grows preferentially in fibroblasts. It is unclear whether CMV is oncogenic in vivo. However, the virus can rarely transform fibroblasts and genomic transforming fragments have been identified.

EPIDEMIOLOGY CMV has a worldwide distribution. Approximately 1 percent of newborns in the United States are infected with CMV, and the percentage is higher in many less-developed countries. Communal living and poor personal hygiene facilitate early spread. Perinatal and early childhood infections are common. Virus may be present in milk, saliva, feces, and urine. Transmission of CMV has been identified among young children in day-care centers and has been traced by restriction endonuclease techniques from infected toddler to pregnant mother to developing fetus.

The virus is not readily spread by casual contact but requires repeated or prolonged intimate exposure for transmission. In late adolescence and young adulthood, CMV is often transmitted sexually, and asymptomatic viral carriage in semen or cervical secretions is common. CMV antibody titers approach 100 percent in female prostitutes and in sexually active homosexual men. Sexually active adults may harbor several strains of CMV simultaneously. Transfusion of whole blood or certain blood products containing viable leukocytes may also transmit CMV with a frequency of 0.14 to 10 percent per unit transfused.

Once infected, an individual probably carries the virus for life. Most commonly these infections remain latent. However, with compromise of T-lymphocyte-mediated immunity, as occurs following organ transplantation or in association with lymphoid neoplasms and certain acquired immunodeficiencies in particular that caused by infection with the human immunodeficiency virus (HIV) (see Chap. 264), CMV reactivation syndromes develop frequently.

PATHOGENESIS Congenital CMV infection can follow either primary or reactivation infection of the mother. However, clinical disease in the fetus or newborn is almost exclusively limited to primary maternal infections. Factors determining the severity of congenital infection are unknown; a deficient capacity to produce precipitating antibodies and to mount T-cell responses to CMV are associated with more severe disease.

Primary infection in late childhood or adulthood is often associated with a vigorous T-lymphocyte response that may contribute to the development of a mononucleosis syndrome similar to that observed following Epstein-Barr virus infection (see Chap. 137). The hallmarks of such infections are the appearance of atypical lymphocytes in the peripheral blood; these cells are predominantly activated T lymphocytes of cytotoxic-suppressor phenotype. Polyclonal activation of B cells by the virus contributes to the development of rheumatoid factors and other autoantibodies during CMV mononucleosis.

Once acquired during symptomatic or asymptomatic primary infection, CMV persists indefinitely in tissues of the host. The sites of persistent or latent infection are unclear, but probably involve multiple cell types and various organs. Transmission following blood transfusion or organ transplantation is due to silent infections in these tissues. Autopsy studies suggest that lungs, salivary glands, and bowel may also be areas of latent infection.

If T-cell responses of the host become compromised by disease or by iatrogenic immunosuppression, latent virus can be reactivated to cause a variety of syndromes. Chronic antigenic stimulation, as occurs following tissue transplantation, in the presence of immunosuppression, appears to be an ideal setting for CMV activation and CMV-induced disease. Certain particularly potent suppressants of T-cell immunity, such as antithymocyte globulin, are associated with a high rate of clinical CMV syndromes, which may follow either primary or reactivation infection. CMV may itself contribute to further T-lymphocyte hyporesponsiveness, which often precedes superinfection with other opportunistic pathogens, such as *Pneumocystis carinii*. CMV and pneumocystis are frequently found together in immunosuppressed patients with severe interstitial pneumonia. CMV may function as a cofactor to activate latent HIV infection.

PATHOLOGY Cytomegalic cells in vivo are presumed to be infected epithelial cells. They are two to four times larger than surrounding cells and often contain an 8- to 10-μm intranuclear inclusion that is eccentrically placed and surrounded by a clear halo, resulting in an "owl's eye" appearance. Smaller granular cytoplasmic inclusions may also be demonstrated occasionally. Cytomegalic cells are found in a wide variety of organs including salivary glands, lung, liver, kidney, intestines, pancreas, adrenal glands, and the central nervous system.

The cellular inflammatory response to infection consists of plasma cells, lymphocytes, and monocyte-macrophages. Granulomatous reactions are occasionally observed, particularly in the liver. Immunopathologic reactions may contribute to CMV disease. Immune complexes have been described in infected infants, sometimes associated with CMV-related glomerulopathies. Immune-complex glomerulopathy has been observed in some CMV-infected patients following renal transplantation.

CLINICAL MANIFESTATIONS **Congenital CMV infection** Fetal infections range from inapparent to severe and disseminated. Cytomegalic inclusion disease develops in approximately 5 percent of infected fetuses and is seen almost exclusively in infants born to mothers who develop primary infections during pregnancy. Petechiae, hepatosplenomegaly, and jaundice are the most common presenting features (60 to 80 percent). Microcephaly with or without cerebral calcifications, intrauterine growth retardation, and prematurity are noted in 30 to 50 percent of patients. Inguinal hernias and chorioretinitis are observed less commonly. Laboratory abnormalities in decreasing order of frequency include increased serum IgM above 0.20 g/L (20 mg/dL), atypical lymphocytosis, elevated liver transaminases, thrombocytopenia, hyperbilirubinemia, and increased cerebrospinal fluid protein above 0.20 g/L (20 mg/dL). Prognosis among severely infected infants is poor, with mortality rates of 20 to 30 percent; few patients escape intellectual or hearing difficulties in later years. Differential diagnoses of cytomegalic inclusion disease in infants include syphilis, rubella, toxoplasmosis, herpes simplex or enterovirus infection, and bacterial sepsis. *TORCHES*

Most congenital CMV infections are clinically inapparent at birth. Between 5 to 25 percent of asymptomatically infected infants develop significant psychomotor, hearing, ocular, or dental abnormalities over the next several years.

Perinatal CMV infection The newborn may acquire CMV at the time of delivery by passage through an infected birth canal or by postnatal contact with maternal milk or other secretions. Approximately 40 to 60 percent of infants who are breast-fed for over 1 month by seropositive mothers will become infected. Iatrogenic transmission can also result from neonatal blood transfusion. Screening of blood products prior to transfusion into low-birth-weight seronegative infants or seronegative pregnant women will decrease the risk of infection. The great majority of infants infected at or after delivery will remain asymptomatic. However, protracted interstitial pneumonitis has been associated with perinatally acquired CMV infection, particularly in premature infants, occasionally associated with *Chlamydia trachomatis*, *P. carinii*, or *Ureaplasma urealyticum* infections. Poor weight gain, adenopathy, rash, hepatitis, anemia, and atypical lymphocytosis may also be present, and CMV excretion often persists for months to years.

CMV mononucleosis The most common clinical manifestation of CMV infection in normal hosts beyond the neonatal period is a heterophil-antibody negative mononucleosis syndrome. This may occur spontaneously or following the transfusion of leukocyte-containing blood products. Although the syndrome occurs at all ages, sexually active young adults are most often involved. Incubation periods range from 20 to 60 days, and the illness generally lasts 2 to 6 weeks. Prolonged high fevers, sometimes accompanied by chills, profound fatigue, and malaise characterize this disorder. Myalgias, headache, and splenomegaly are frequent, but exudative pharyngitis and cervical lymphadenopathy are rare, in contrast to infectious mononucleosis caused by Epstein-Barr virus. Occasional patients will develop rubelliform rashes, often after exposure to ampicillin. Less commonly observed are interstitial or segmental pneumonia, myocarditis, pleuritis, arthritis, or encephalitis. Rarely, Guillain-Barré syndrome may complicate CMV mononucleosis. The characteristic laboratory abnormality is a peripheral blood relative lymphocytosis with greater than 10 percent atypical lymphocytes. Total leukocyte counts may be low, normal, or markedly elevated. Although significant jaundice is uncommon, moderately elevated serum transaminase and alkaline phosphatase levels are often present. Heterophil antibodies are absent; however, transient immunologic abnormalities are common. These may include the presence of cryoglobulins, rheumatoid factors, cold agglutinins, and antinuclear antibodies. Rarely, hemolytic anemia, thrombocytopenia, and granulocytopenia complicate recovery.

Most patients recover without sequelae, although postviral asthenia may persist for months. CMV excretion in urine, genital secretions, or saliva often continues for months to years. Rare patients have recurrent episodes of fever and malaise, sometimes associated with autonomic nervous system dysfunction, e.g., attacks of sweating or flushing.

CMV infection in the immunocompromised host CMV appears to be the most frequent and important viral pathogen complicating organ transplantation. In renal, cardiac, and liver transplant recipients, CMV induces a variety of syndromes including fever and leukopenia, hepatitis, pneumonitis, colitis, and retinitis. The maximal period of risk appears between 1 to 4 months after transplantation, although retinitis is often a later complication. The risk of disease appears greater following primary infection. In addition, restriction endonuclease studies indicate that seropositive transplant recipients are susceptible to reinfection with donor-derived CMV, often resulting in disease. Reactivation infection, although frequent, is less likely to be important clinically. Clinical disease is related to the degree of immunosuppression; patients receiving certain immunosuppressive agents, such as antithymocyte globulin, appear more likely to have severe infections than those receiving other agents, such as cyclosporine A.

CMV pneumonia occurs in nearly 15 to 20 percent of bone marrow transplant recipients, with a case fatality rate of 84 to 88 percent. The risk is greatest between 5 to 13 weeks after transplant, and several risk factors have been identified. These include type of immunosuppression, acute graft-versus-host disease, older age, viremia, seropositivity before transplantation, and granulocyte transfusions.

CMV has become recognized as an important pathogen in patients with the acquired immunodeficiency syndrome (AIDS) (see Chap. 264). CMV infection is nearly ubiquitous in this disorder and often causes retinitis or disseminated disease, contributing to death. CMV-induced immunosuppression probably also contributes to the T-lymphocyte deficiency initiated by the etiologic retrovirus.

CMV syndromes in the immunocompromised host often begin with prolonged fever, malaise, anorexia, fatigue, night sweats, and arthralgias or myalgias. Liver function abnormalities, leukopenia, thrombocytopenia, and atypical lymphocytosis may be observed during these episodes. The development of tachypnea, hypoxia, and unproductive cough signals respiratory involvement. Radiologic examination of the lung often demonstrates bilateral interstitial or reticulonodular infiltrates, beginning in the periphery of the lower lobes and spreading centrally and superiorly; localized segmental, nodular, or alveolar patterns are less commonly observed. Diagnosis requires lung biopsy, since neither peripheral virus excretion nor high antibody titers provides sufficient information to prove etiology. The differential diagnoses include *P. carinii*, other viral, bacterial, or fungal pathogens, pulmonary hemorrhage, and injury secondary to radiation or cytotoxic drugs.

Gastrointestinal CMV involvement may be localized or extensive and occurs almost exclusively in compromised hosts. Ulcers of the esophagus, stomach, small intestine, or colon may result in bleeding or perforation. CMV infection may lead to exacerbations of underlying ulcerative colitis. Hepatitis occurs frequently, and CMV-associated acalculous cholecystitis has been described.

CMV rarely causes meningoencephalitis in otherwise healthy individuals. Although CMV antigens and inclusions are observed occasionally in brains of patients dying from AIDS encephalopathy, the relative roles and interactions of CMV and HIV in this disorder are unclear.

CMV retinitis is an important cause of blindness in immunocompromised patients, including patients with AIDS and organ transplant recipients. Early lesions consist of small, opaque, white areas of granular retinal necrosis that spread in a centrifugal manner and are later accompanied by hemorrhages, vessel sheathing, and retinal edema (see Fig. A4-14). CMV must be distinguished from other causes of retinopathy including toxoplasmosis, candidiasis, and herpes simplex virus.

Fatal infections are often associated with persistent viremia and multiple organ system involvement. Progressive pulmonary infiltrates, pancytopenia, hyperamylasemia, and hypotension are characteristic, often with a terminal bacterial, fungal, or protozoan superinfection. Extensive adrenal necrosis with CMV inclusions is present at autopsy, as well as CMV involvement of many other organs.

In the renal transplant recipient, CMV also contributes to graft dysfunction by mechanisms other than direct viral cytopathic effects. An immune-complex glomerulopathy may accompany CMV infection and should be differentiated from true graft rejection, since the former does not respond well to increased immunosuppression. In addition, a protein encoded by the CMV genome contains sequence homology and immunologic cross-reactivity with a conserved domain of the HLA-DR antigen, suggesting an alternative mechanism for increased graft dysfunction associated with infection.

DIAGNOSIS The diagnosis of CMV infection cannot be made reliably on clinical grounds alone. Virus isolation from appropriate clinical specimens, together with demonstration of a fourfold or greater antibody rise or persistently elevated antibody titers, is the preferred diagnostic approach. Virus excretion or viremia is readily detected by culture of appropriate specimens on human fibroblast monolayers. If virus titers are high, as is frequently the case in congenital disseminated infection or in patients with AIDS, characteristic cytopathic effects may be detected within a few days. However, in some situations, e.g., CMV mononucleosis, virus titers are low and cytopathic effects may take several weeks to appear. Many laboratories expedite diagnosis by using an overnight tissue culture method (shell vial assay) with an immunofluorescence detection technique employing monoclonal antibodies to an immediate early CMV antigen. Virus isolation from urine or saliva by itself does not necessarily imply acute infection since excretion from these sites may continue for months to years following illness. Detection of CMV viremia is a better predictor of acute infection. Direct detection of CMV DNA or antigens in tissues or secretions does not yet appear of sufficient sensitivity or specificity to replace virus culture.

A variety of serologic assays (complement fixation, immunofluorescence, indirect hemagglutination, enzyme-linked immunosorbent assay) are available to detect antibody rises to CMV antigens. Antibody rises may not be detectable for up to 4 weeks after primary infection, and titers often remain high for years after infection. For this reason, single-sample antibody determinations are of no value in assessing the acuteness of infection. Detection of CMV-specific IgM is sometimes useful in the diagnosis of recent or active infection; circulating rheumatoid factors may result in occasional false-positive IgM tests.

PREVENTION AND TREATMENT Several prophylactic measures are useful to prevent CMV infection in patients at high risk. The use of blood from seronegative donors or blood that was frozen, thawed, and deglycerolized greatly decreases transfusion-associated transmission of CMV. Similarly, matching of kidney or bone marrow transplants by CMV serology, using only organs from seronegative donors for seronegative recipients, reduces primary infections following transplantation.

CMV immune globulin has been reported to reduce CMV-associated syndromes and fungal or parasitic superinfections in seronegative renal transplant recipients. Similar studies in bone marrow transplant recipients have been conducted; most, but not all, studies have shown benefit from prophylactic CMV immune globulin. Prophylactic acyclovir has been demonstrated to reduce CMV infection and disease in seronegative renal transplant recipients; acyclovir is not effective in treatment of active CMV disease, however.

Ganciclovir or DHPG (dihydroxypropoxymethylguanine) is a guanosine derivative with considerably more activity against CMV than its congener, acyclovir. Several trials in immunocompromised patients with life- or sight-threatening CMV infections suggested beneficial effects of intravenous ganciclovir, and it is now approved by the Federal Drug Administration in the United States for patients with CMV retinitis. Response rates of CMV retinitis or colitis range from 70 to 90 percent. CMV pneumonitis, particularly in bone marrow transplant recipients, responds less well, with improvement noted in ≤30 percent when ganciclovir is used alone; when ganciclovir is used in combination with CMV immune globulin, response rates of 50 to 70 percent have been noted. Peripheral blood neutropenia is the major toxic effect of ganciclovir and is sometimes dose-limiting. In many patients, particularly those with AIDS, clinical and virologic relapses of CMV infection occur once ganciclovir is discontinued. Therefore, prolonged maintenance regimens are recommended. Usual induction courses are 5 mg/kg twice daily for 14 days with maintenance regimens of 5 mg/kg for 5 to 7 days per week.

Phosphonoformate (foscarnet) also shows promise against CMV retinitis in patients with AIDS. Both foscarnet and ganciclovir are undergoing further evaluation in severe CMV infections.

REFERENCES

Balfour HH et al: A randomized, placebo-controlled trial of oral acyclovir for the prevention of cytomegalovirus disease in recipients of renal allografts. N Engl J Med 320:1381, 1989

Bowden RA et al: Cytomegalovirus immune globulin and seronegative blood products to prevent primary cytomegalovirus infection after marrow transplantation. N Engl J Med 314:1006, 1986

Buhles WC et al: Ganciclovir treatment of life- or sight-threatening cytomegalovirus infection: Experience in 314 immunocompromised patients. Rev Infect Dis 10:S495, 1988

Chandler SH et al: Isolation of multiple strains of cytomegalovirus from women attending a clinic for sexually transmitted diseases. J Infect Dis 155:655, 1987

Drew WL: Diagnosis of cytomegalovirus infection. Rev Infect Dis 10:S468, 1988

Dummer JS et al: Morbidity of cytomegalovirus infection in recipients of heart or heart-lung transplants who received cyclosporine. J Infect Dis 152:1182, 1985

Emmanuel D et al: Cytomegalovirus pneumonia after bone marrow transplantation successfully treated with the combination of ganciclovir and high-dose intravenous immunoglobulin. Ann Intern Med 109:777, 1988

Felsenstein D et al: Treatment of cytomegalovirus retinitis with 9-[2-hydroxy-1-(hydroxymethyl)ethoxymethyl] guanine (BWB759U). Ann Intern Med 103:377, 1985

Grundy JE et al: Symptomatic cytomegalovirus infection in seropositive kidney recipients: Reinfection with donor virus rather than reactivation of recipient virus. Lancet 2:132, 1988

Ho M: *Cytomegalovirus: Biology and Infection.* New York, Plenum, 1982

Horwitz CA et al: Clinical and laboratory evaluation of cytomegalovirus-induced mononucleosis in previously healthy patients. Medicine 65:124, 1986

Jacobson MA, Mills J: Serious cytomegalovirus disease in the acquired immunodeficiency syndrome (AIDS). Ann Intern Med 108:585, 1988

Meyers JD et al: Risk factors for cytomegalovirus infection after human marrow transplantation. J Infect Dis 153:478, 1986

Onorato IM et al: Epidemiology of cytomegaloviral infections: Recommendations for prevention and control. Rev Infect Dis 7:479, 1985

Pass RF et al: Young children as a probable source of maternal and congenital cytomegalovirus infection. N Engl J Med 316:1366, 1987

Preiksaitis JK et al: The risk of cytomegalovirus infection in seronegative transfusion recipients not receiving exogenous immunosuppression. J Infect Dis 157:523, 1988

Reed EC et al: Treatment of cytomegalovirus pneumonia with ganciclovir and intravenous cytomegalovirus immunoglobulin in patients with bone marrow transplants. Ann Intern Med 109:783, 1988

Schooley RE et al: Association of herpesvirus infections with T-lymphocyte subset alterations, glomerulopathy, and opportunistic infections after renal transplantation. N Engl J Med 308:307, 1983

Skolnik PR, Hirsch MS: Therapy and prevention of cytomegalovirus infections. In DeClerq E (ed): *Clinical Use of Antiviral Drugs.* Boston, Martinus Nijhoff 1988

Snyderman DR et al: Use of cytomegalovirus immune globulin to prevent cytomegalovirus disease in renal transplant recipients. N Engl J Med 317:1049, 1987

139 INFLUENZA

RAPHAEL DOLIN

DEFINITION Influenza is an acute respiratory illness caused by infection with influenza viruses. The illness affects the upper and/or lower respiratory tracts, and is often accompanied by systemic signs and symptoms such as fever, headache, myalgia, and weakness. Outbreaks of illness of variable extent and severity occur nearly every winter. Such outbreaks result in significant morbidity in the general population and in increased mortality rates in certain "high-risk" patients, predominantly as a result of pulmonary complications.

ETIOLOGY Influenza viruses are members of the Orthomyxoviridae family. Influenza A and B viruses constitute one genus, and influenza C is the other genus. The designation of influenza viruses as types A, B, or C is based on antigenic characteristics of the nucleoprotein (NP) and matrix (M) protein antigens. Influenza A viruses are further subdivided (subtyped) on the basis of the surface hemagglutinin (H) and neuraminidase (N) antigens (see below). Individual strains are also designated according to the site of origin, isolate number, year of isolation, and subtype (e.g., influenza A/Victoria/3/79 H3N2). Influenza B and C viruses are similarly designated, but H and N antigens from these viruses do not receive subtype designations, since intratypic variations in H and N antigens of influenza B and C viruses are less extensive.

Most of the information regarding the molecular biology of influenza viruses has been generated from studies of influenza A viruses, and less is known about the replicative cycle of influenza B and C viruses. Morphologically, influenza viruses A, B, and C are similar. The virions are irregularly shaped spherical particles, 80 to 120 nm in diameter, and contain a lipid envelope from whose surface the hemagglutinin and neuraminidase glycoproteins project. The hemagglutinin serves as the site by which virus binds to cell receptors, while the neuraminidase degrades the receptor and probably plays a role in release of virus from infected cells after replication has taken place. Antibodies directed against the H antigen are the major determinants of immunity against influenza virus, while antineuraminidase antibodies limit viral spread and contribute to reduction of the infection. The inner surface of the lipid envelope contains the matrix proteins (M1 and M2), whose functions are incompletely understood but which may be involved in virus assembly and stabilization of the lipid envelope. The virion also contains the nucleoprotein (NP) with which the genome of the virus is associated, as well as three polymerase (P) proteins which are essential for transcription and synthesis of viral RNA. Three nonstructural (NS) proteins of unknown function are also present in infected cells.

The genome of influenza A virus consists of eight single-stranded segments of viral RNA, which code for the structural and nonstructural proteins. Because the genome is segmented, the opportunity for reassortment of genes during infection is high, and reassortment has been noted to occur frequently during infection of cells with more than one influenza A virus.

TABLE 139-1 Emergence of antigenic subtypes of influenza A associated with pandemic or epidemic disease

1889–90	H2N8*	Severe pandemic
1900–03	H3N8*	?Moderate epidemic
1918–19	H1N1† (formerly HswN1)	Severe pandemic
1933–35	H1N1† (formerly H0N1)	Mild epidemic
1946–47	H1N1	Mild epidemic
1957–58	H2N2	Severe pandemic
1968–69	H3N2	Moderate pandemic
1977–78‡	H1N1	Mild pandemic

* As determined by retrospective serologic survey of individuals alive during those years ("seroarcheology").

† Hemagglutinins formerly designated as Hsw and H0 are now classified as variants of H1.

‡ From this time until the present (1988–89), new antigenic subtypes of influenza A have not emerged. Rather, viruses of H1N1 or H3N2 subtypes have circulated either in alternating years or concurrently.

EPIDEMIOLOGY Influenza outbreaks occur virtually every year, although the extent and severity of such outbreaks vary widely. Localized outbreaks occur at variable intervals, usually every 1 to 3 years. Global epidemics or pandemics have occurred approximately every 10 to 15 years since the 1918–1919 pandemic (Table 139-1).

The most extensive and severe outbreaks are caused by influenza A viruses. In part, this is a result of the remarkable propensity of the hemagglutinin and neuraminidase antigens of influenza A virus to undergo periodic antigenic variation. Major antigenic variations are referred to as "antigenic shifts," which most likely occur from reassortment of genome segments between viral strains. Antigenic shifts may be associated with pandemics and are restricted to influenza A viruses. Minor variations are called "antigenic drifts" and likely arise from point mutations. These antigenic changes may involve the hemagglutinin alone, or both the hemagglutinin and the neuraminidase. In human infections, three major antigenic subtypes of hemagglutinins (H1, H2, and H3) and two neuraminidases (N1, N2) have been recognized. The hemagglutinins formerly designated as H0 and Hsw1 are now classified as variants of H1. An example of an antigenic shift which involved both the hemagglutinin and neuraminidase occurred in 1957, when the predominant influenza A virus subtype shifted from H1N1 to H2N2, and resulted in a severe pandemic, with an estimated 70,000 excess deaths in the United States alone. In 1968, an antigenic shift occurred which involved only the hemagglutinin (H2N2 to H3N2), and the subsequent pandemic was less severe than that seen in 1957. In 1977, an A/H1N1 virus emerged which caused a pandemic that primarily affected younger individuals, i.e., those born after 1957. As can be seen in Table 139-1, H1N1 viruses circulated from 1918 to 1956, so that individuals born prior to 1957 would be expected to possess some degree of immunity to H1N1 viruses. During most outbreaks of influenza A, a single subtype has circulated at a time. However, since 1977 both A/H1N1 and A/H3N2 viruses have circulated simultaneously resulting in outbreaks of varying severity. In some outbreaks influenza B viruses also circulated simultaneously with influenza A viruses.

The origin of pandemic strains is unknown. Because of the marked differences between the primary structures of the hemagglutinins of different subtypes of influenza A viruses (H1, H2, or H3), it is believed unlikely that antigenic shifts result from spontaneous mutations in the hemagglutinin gene. Because the segmented genome of influenza viruses may result in high rates of reassortment, it has been suggested that pandemic strains may emerge by reassortment of genes between human and animal influenza viruses. Influenza B viruses do not have an animal reservoir and do not undergo antigenic shifts, although antigenic drifting occurs.

Although pandemics provide the most dramatic evidence of the impact of influenza, illnesses that occur in between pandemics account for an even greater total in mortality and morbidity, albeit over a longer period of time. Since 1957, interpandemic illness has been associated with 10,000 or more "excess deaths" on 19 occasions in the United States, resulting in an accumulated mortality of more than 500,000 over that period of time. Influenza A viruses that circulate in between pandemics demonstrate antigenic drifts in the hemagglutinin antigen. These antigenic drifts apparently result from point mutations which involve the RNA segment which codes for the hemagglutinin. Amino acid analysis of "drifted" hemagglutinins indicates that changes in a single amino acid have little effect on the antigenic properties of the hemagglutinin. Epidemiologically significant strains, i.e., those which have potential for causing widespread outbreaks, have changes in amino acids in at least two of the four major antigenic sites in the HA molecule. Since two-point mutations are unlikely to occur simultaneously, it is believed that antigenic drifts result from point mutations which occur sequentially during the spread of virus from person to person. Antigenic drifts have occurred nearly annually since 1977 for A/H1N1 viruses, and since 1968 for A/H3N2 viruses.

Influenza A epidemics begin abruptly, reach a peak over a 2- to 3-week period, generally last for 2 to 3 months, and often subside almost as rapidly as they began. The first indication of influenza activity in a community is an increase in the number of children with febrile respiratory illnesses who present for medical attention. This is followed by increases in influenza-like illnesses among adults, and eventually by an increase in hospital admissions for patients with pneumonia, worsening of congestive heart failure, and exacerbations of chronic pulmonary disease. Rises in industrial and school absenteeism also occur at this time. An increase in the number of deaths caused by pneumonia and influenza ("excess mortality") is generally a late observation in an outbreak. Attack rates have been highly variable from outbreak to outbreak but most commonly are in the range of 10 to 20 percent of the general population. During the pandemic of 1957, it was estimated that the attack rate of clinical influenza exceeded 50 percent in urban populations, and that an additional 25 percent or more may have been subclinically infected with influenza A virus. Among institutionalized populations and in semiclosed settings where a large number of susceptible individuals are present, even higher attack rates have been reported.

Epidemics of influenza occur almost exclusively during the winter months in the northern and southern hemispheres. It is highly unusual to detect influenza A virus at times other than those in which an outbreak occurs, although rarely serologic rises have been noted at other times of the year. Where or how influenza A virus persists in between outbreaks is unknown. A possible explanation is that influenza A viruses are maintained in the human population on a worldwide basis by person-to-person transmission, and that large population clusters might be able to support a low level of interepidemic transmission. Alternatively, human strains may persist in animal reservoirs, but convincing evidence to support either explanation is not available. In the modern era, rapid modes of transportation may contribute to the transmission of viruses from widespread geographic locales.

The factors which result in the inception and termination of outbreaks of influenza are also incompletely understood. A major determinant of the extent and severity of an outbreak is the level of immunity present in the population at risk. When an antigenically novel influenza virus emerges to which little or no antibody is present in a community, extensive outbreaks may occur. When the absence of antibody is worldwide, epidemic disease may spread around the globe, resulting in a pandemic. Such pandemic waves can occur for several years, until immunity in the population reaches a high level. In the years following pandemic influenza, antigenic drifts among influenza viruses result in outbreaks of variable severity in populations that have high levels of immunity to the pandemic strain which circulated earlier. This situation persists until another antigenically novel pandemic strain emerges. On the other hand, outbreaks may also terminate despite the persistence of a large pool of susceptible individuals in the population. Occasionally, the emergence of a significantly different antigenic variant will result only in a localized outbreak. The "swine influenza outbreak" of 1976 in the United

States may be considered to be an example of this, although this outbreak may simply represent the introduction of a swine influenza virus into a crowded human population without spread beyond that setting. It has also been suggested that certain viruses, such as recently circulating A/H1N1 strains, may be intrinsically less virulent and cause less severe disease, even in immunologically virgin subjects, suggesting that other undefined factors besides the level of preexisting immunity play a role in the epidemiology of influenza.

Influenza B causes outbreaks which are generally less extensive and are associated with less severe disease than those caused by influenza A virus. The hemagglutinin and neuraminidase of influenza B virus undergo less frequent and less extensive variation than is seen in influenza A viruses, which may account, in part, for the observation of less extensive disease. Influenza B outbreaks are seen most frequently in schools and military camps, although occasional outbreaks in institutions in which elderly individuals reside have also been noted. The most serious complication of influenza B virus infection is Reye's syndrome (see below). Influenza C has been infrequently associated with human disease, although infection with influenza C virus is widespread.

The morbidity and mortality of influenza outbreaks continue to be substantial. Mortality occurs primarily in individuals with underlying diseases who have been characterized as being at "high risk" for complications of influenza. Excess hospitalizations for adults with "high risk" medical conditions have reached rates of 800 per 100,000 during recent outbreaks of influenza. These high-risk conditions are primarily chronic cardiac and pulmonary diseases, as well as increased age. Increased mortality rates have also been observed among individuals with chronic metabolic, renal, and certain immunosuppressive diseases, although to a lesser extent than among those with chronic cardiopulmonary diseases. In addition to the excess mortality, the morbidity of influenza in the general population is also extensive. For each of three outbreaks in the United States that were studied during the 1960s, it has been estimated that direct and indirect economic costs ranged from 1.5 to 3.5 billion dollars, and that today, such costs would be much greater.

PATHOGENESIS The initial event in influenza is infection of the respiratory epithelium with influenza virus, which is acquired from respiratory secretions of acutely infected individuals. In all likelihood, this occurs via aerosols generated by coughs and sneezes, although hand to hand, other personal contact, and even fomite transmission may occur. Experimental evidence suggests that infection by small-particle aerosol (less than 10 μm in diameter) is more efficient than that produced by larger droplets. Initially, viral infection involves the ciliated columnar epithelial cells, but it may also involve other respiratory tract cells, including alveolar cells, mucous gland cells, and macrophages. In infected cells, virus replication takes place within 4 to 6 h, after which infectious virus is released to infect adjacent or nearby cells. This results in spread of infection from a few foci to a large number of respiratory cells over several hours. In experimentally induced infection, the incubation period of illness has ranged from 18 to 72 h, depending on the size of the virus inoculum. Histopathologically, degenerative changes can be seen in infected ciliated cells, including granulation, vacuolization, swelling, and pyknotic nuclei. The cells eventually become necrotic and desquamate, and in some areas, previously columnar epithelium is replaced by flattened and metaplastic epithelial cells. The severity of illness is correlated with the quantity of virus shed in secretions, suggesting that the degree of viral replication itself may be an important mechanism in the pathogenesis of illness. Despite the frequent presence of systemic signs and symptoms such as fever, headache, and myalgias, influenza virus has only rarely been detected in extrapulmonary sites, including the bloodstream, and the pathogenesis of systemic symptoms in influenza remains unknown.

The host response to influenza infections involves a complex interplay of humoral antibody, local antibody, cell-mediated immune responses, interferon, and other host defenses. Serum antibody responses may be measured by a variety of techniques and can be detected by the second week after primary infection with influenza virus. Such antibodies may be measured by hemagglutination inhibition (HAI), complement fixation (CF), neutralization, enzyme-linked immunosorbent assays (ELISA), and antineuraminidase antibody assays. Antibodies directed against the hemagglutinin appear to be the most important mediators of immunity, and in several studies, HAI titers of 40 or greater have been associated with protection from infection. Secretory antibodies produced in the respiratory tract are predominantly of the IgA class, and also play a major role in protection against infection. Secretory antibody neutralization titers of 4 or higher have also been associated with protection. A variety of cell-mediated immune responses, both antigen-specific and nonantigen-specific, can be detected early after infection, depending upon prior immunity of the host. These responses include T-cell proliferative, T-cell cytotoxic, and natural killer cell activity. Interferons have been detected in respiratory secretions shortly after shedding of virus has begun, and rises in interferon titers coincide with decreases in virus shedding.

The host defense factors responsible for cessation of virus shedding and resolution of illness have not been defined specifically. Virus shedding generally stops within 2 to 5 days after symptoms first appear, at a time when serum and local antibody responses are often not detectable by conventional techniques, although antibody rises may be detected earlier by use of highly sensitive techniques, particularly in individuals with previous immunity to the virus. It has been suggested that interferon, cell-mediated immune responses, or nonspecific inflammatory responses may be important in the resolution of illness.

MANIFESTATIONS Influenza has been most frequently described as an illness characterized by the abrupt onset of systemic symptoms such as headache, feverishness, chilliness, myalgia, or malaise, accompanied by respiratory tract signs, particularly cough and sore throat. In many cases, the onset is so abrupt that patients can recall the precise time of the onset of illness. A typical case of naturally occurring influenza is depicted in Fig. 139-1. However, a wide spectrum of clinical presentations may occur. These can range from mild, afebrile respiratory illnesses similar to the common cold, with

FIGURE 139-1 Clinical characteristics of a naturally occurring case of influenza A in an otherwise healthy 28-year-old male. (*From R Dolin, Am Fam Phys 14:74, 1976.*)

either gradual or abrupt onset, to illnesses in which severe prostration with relatively few respiratory signs and symptoms may be present. In the majority of cases which come to a physician's attention, fever is present and can range from 38°C to as high as 41°C. The temperature rises rapidly within the first 24 h of illness, and is generally followed by a gradual defervescence over a 2- to 3-day period, although, on occasion, fever may last for as long as a week. Patients complain of a feverish feeling and chilliness, but true rigors are rare. Headache, either generalized or frontal, is often a particularly troublesome complaint. Myalgias may involve any part of the body, but are most common in the legs and lumbosacral area. Arthralgias may also be present.

Respiratory complaints often become more prominent as systemic symptoms subside. Many patients complain of a sore throat or persistent cough which may last for a week or more, and which is often accompanied by substernal discomfort. Ocular signs and symptoms include pain on motion of the eyes, photophobia, and burning of the eyes.

Physical findings are usually minimal in cases of uncomplicated influenza. Early in the illness, the patient appears flushed and the skin is hot and dry, although diaphoresis and mottled extremities, particularly in older patients, may occur. Examination of the pharynx may be surprisingly unremarkable despite a severe sore throat, but injection of the mucous membranes and postnasal discharge can be present. Mild cervical lymphadenopathy may be noted, particularly in younger individuals. Chest examination is largely negative in uncomplicated influenza, although rhonchi, wheezes, and scattered rales have been reported with variable frequency in different outbreaks. Frank dyspnea, hyperpnea, cyanosis, diffuse rales, or signs of consolidation are evidence of pulmonary complications. Patients with apparently uncomplicated influenza have been reported to have a variety of mild ventilatory defects and increased alveolar-capillary diffusion gradients, indicating that subclinical pulmonary involvement may be more frequent than is appreciated.

In uncomplicated influenza, the acute illness generally resolves over a 2- to 5-day period, and most patients have largely recovered in 1 week. In a significant minority, however, symptoms of weakness or lassitude ("postinfluenzal asthenia") may persist for several weeks, particularly in the elderly, and may prove troublesome for those who wish to return to full activity promptly. The pathogenetic basis for this "asthenia" is unknown, although pulmonary function abnormalities may persist for several weeks after uncomplicated influenza.

COMPLICATIONS OF INFLUENZA
The most common complication of influenza is pneumonia, which may occur either as "primary" influenza viral pneumonia, secondary bacterial pneumonia, or mixed viral and bacterial pneumonia. Primary influenza viral pneumonia is the least common but most severe of the pneumonic complications. It presents as acute influenza which does not resolve, but instead relentlessly progresses with persistent fever, dyspnea, and eventual cyanosis. Sputum production is generally scanty but can contain blood, and few physical signs may be present early in the illness. In more advanced cases, diffuse rales may be noted, and chest x-ray findings consistent with diffuse interstitial infiltrates and/or acute respiratory distress syndrome may be present. In such cases arterial blood gases show marked hypoxia. Viral cultures, particularly if taken early in illness, show high titers of virus in respiratory secretions and in the lung parenchyma. Histopathology of fatal cases of primary viral pneumonia shows a marked inflammatory reaction in the alveolar septa, with edema and infiltration with lymphocytes, macrophages, occasional plasma cells, and variable numbers of neutrophils. Fibrin thrombi in alveolar capillaries, along with necrosis and hemorrhage, have also been noted. Eosinophilic hyaline membranes can also be found lining alveoli and alveolar ducts.

Primary influenza viral pneumonia has a predilection for individuals with cardiac disease, particularly those with mitral stenosis, but has also been reported in otherwise healthy young adults, as well as in older individuals with chronic pulmonary disorders. In some epidemics of influenza (notably 1918 and 1957), pregnancy increased the risk of the development of primary influenza pneumonia.

Secondary bacterial pneumonia is a complication in which bacterial infection develops following a case of acute influenza. With this illness, patients experience a period of improvement for 2 to 3 days after acute influenza, followed by a reappearance of fever, along with clinical signs and symptoms of bacterial pneumonia. These include cough, production of purulent sputum, and physical and x-ray signs of consolidation. The most common bacterial pathogens in this setting are *Streptococcus pneumoniae*, *Staphylococcus aureus*, or *Haemophilus influenzae*, organisms that can colonize the nasopharynx and that cause infection in the wake of changes in bronchopulmonary defenses. The etiology can often be determined by Gram stain and culture of an appropriately obtained sputum specimen. Secondary bacterial pneumonia occurs most frequently in high-risk individuals with chronic pulmonary and cardiac disease and in elderly individuals. Patients with secondary bacterial pneumonias will often respond to antibiotic therapy when it is instituted promptly.

Perhaps the most common of the pneumonic complications that occur during outbreaks of influenza are mixed viral and bacterial pneumonias. The clinical course of this complication contains features of both primary and secondary pneumonias. Patients may have a gradual progression of their acute illness, or may show a transient improvement followed by a clinical worsening, with eventual manifestion of the clinical features of a bacterial pneumonia. Sputum cultures may contain both influenza A virus and one of the bacterial pathogens described above. Patchy infiltrates or areas of consolidation may be noted by physical examination and chest x-ray. Patients with mixed viral and bacterial pneumonias generally have less widespread involvement of the lung than those with primary viral pneumonia, and their bacterial infections may respond to appropriate antibiotics. Mixed viral and bacterial pneumonias occur primarily in patients with chronic cardiovascular and pulmonary diseases.

In addition to the pulmonary complications of influenza, a number of extrapulmonary complications may occur. Reye's syndrome is a serious complication of influenza B, and to a lesser extent of influenza A virus infection, as well as of varicella-zoster virus infection. It occurs in children most commonly between the ages of 2 and 16, and follows several days after a generally unremarkable viral illness. Reye's syndrome is marked by the onset of nausea and vomiting for 1 to 2 days, after which central nervous system symptoms appear. These are most frequently changes in mental status, ranging from lethargy to coma, and can include delirium and seizures. Hepatomegaly is noted, along with a marked elevation of SGOT, SGPT, and LDH levels. Bilirubin values are only moderately elevated, so that the children are not jaundiced, but blood ammonia levels are elevated in virtually all patients. Hypoglycemia can occur, especially after varicella-zoster virus infection or after viral gastrointestinal illnesses. Children are usually afebrile, and while lumbar puncture generally shows an elevated pressure, the cerebrospinal fluid is quite unremarkable, indicating that an encephalopathy rather than a meningoencephalitis is present. The mortality of the syndrome is related to the state of consciousness on admission and has decreased from more than 40 percent, when the syndrome was originally described, to approximately 10 percent, reflecting earlier recognition and improved management of cerebral edema and hypoglycemia. Histopathology demonstrates little in the way of inflammatory changes in either the liver or the central nervous system. Liver biopsy shows diffuse fatty infiltration of hepatocytes, and swelling and pleomorphism in mitochondria. Cerebral edema and anoxic changes in neurons are the only pathologic changes detected in the central nervous system. The pathogenesis of Reye's syndrome is unknown, but the virus is almost never found in the affected liver and brain. An epidemiologic association with aspirin therapy for the antecedent viral infection has been noted, and the incidence of Reye's syndrome has decreased markedly with widespread warnings regarding the use of aspirin in children with acute viral respiratory infections.

Myositis, rhabdomyolysis, and myoglobinuria have also been reported as occasional complications of influenza infection. Although myalgias are exceedingly common in influenza, true myositis is rare. Patients with acute myositis have exquisite tenderness of the affected muscles, most commonly in the legs, and may not be able to tolerate even the slightest pressure, such as the touch of bed sheets. In the most severe cases, there is frank swelling and bogginess of muscles. Markedly elevated serum creatine phosphokinase and aldolase levels are present, and an occasional patient has developed renal failure from myoglobinuria. The pathogenesis of influenza-associated myositis is also unclear, although the presence of influenza virus in affected muscles has been reported.

Myocarditis and pericarditis in association with influenza virus infection was reported during the 1918–1919 pandemic, based largely on histopathologic findings, and has been infrequently documented since that time. ECG changes during acute influenza are commonly noted in patients who have cardiac disease but these have been most often ascribed to exacerbations of the underlying cardiac disease rather than to direct involvement of the myocardium with influenza virus.

Central nervous system disease has also been reported during influenza, including encephalitis, transverse myelitis, and Guillain-Barré syndrome. The etiologic relationship of influenza virus to such CNS illnesses remains unestablished.

In addition to complications involving the specific organ systems described above, every influenza outbreak includes a number of elderly and other high-risk individuals who develop influenza, and who subsequently experience a gradual deterioration of underlying cardiovascular, pulmonary, or renal function, occasionally leading to irreversible changes and death. These fatalities contribute to the overall toll of excess mortality associated with influenza A outbreaks.

LABORATORY FINDINGS   Laboratory diagnosis is accomplished during the acute illness by isolation of virus from throat swabs, nasopharyngeal washes, or sputum. Virus is usually detected in tissue culture or less commonly in the amniotic cavity of chick embryos within 48 to 72 h after inoculation. Viral antigens may be detected somewhat earlier by use of immunodiagnostic techniques in tissue culture, or directly in exfoliated nasopharyngeal cells obtained by washings, although this technique is less sensitive than isolation of virus in tissue culture. The type of influenza virus (A or B) may be identified by either immunofluorescence or hemagglutination inhibition techniques, and the hemagglutinin subtype of influenza A virus (H1, H2, or H3) may be identified by hemagglutination inhibition using subtype-specific antisera. Serologic methods for diagnosis require comparison of antibody titers in sera obtained during the acute illness with those obtained 10 to 14 days after the onset of illness and are useful primarily in retrospect. Fourfold or greater rises as detected by hemagglutination inhibition, complement fixation, or significant rises by ELISA techniques are diagnostic of acute infection. Complement fixation tests are generally less sensitive than other serologic techniques, but since they detect type-specific antigens, they may be particularly useful when subtype-specific reagents are not available.

The remainder of other laboratory tests are generally not helpful in making a specific diagnosis of influenza virus infection. Leukocyte counts are variable, being frequently low early in illness, and normal or slightly elevated later. Severe leukopenia has been described in overwhelming viral or bacterial infection, while leukocytosis with counts of greater than 15,000 cells per microliter should raise the suspicion that secondary bacterial infection is present.

DIFFERENTIAL DIAGNOSIS   On clinical grounds alone, an individual case of influenza may be difficult to differentiate from an acute respiratory illness caused by a variety of respiratory viruses or by *Mycoplasma pneumoniae*. Severe streptococcal pharyngitis or early bacterial pneumonia may mimic acute influenza, although bacterial pneumonias generally do not run a self-limited course. The presence of purulent sputum in which a bacterial pathogen can be detected by Gram stain is an important diagnostic feature in bacterial pneumonia. The fact that influenza occurs in characteristic outbreaks during the winter months may be helpful in making a clinical diagnosis. When local health authorities indicate that influenza activity is present in the community, the etiology of an acute febrile respiratory illness can be attributed to influenza with a high degree of certainty, particularly if the typical features of abrupt onset and systemic symptoms are present.

TREATMENT   In uncomplicated cases of influenza, symptomatic therapy for headache, myalgia, and fever may be considered, employing either acetaminophen or salicylates, but salicylates should be avoided in children below 18 years of age because of the possible association of salicylates with Reye's syndrome. Since cough is ordinarily self-limited, treatment with cough suppressants generally is not indicated, although codeine-containing compounds may be employed if the cough is particularly troublesome. Patients should be advised to rest and maintain hydration during acute illness, and should return to full activity only gradually after the illness has resolved, particularly if illness has been severe.

The only specific antiviral therapy available for influenza is amantadine. Amantadine is active only against influenza A viruses and has been licensed for the prophylaxis and therapy of influenza A virus infections in the United States. If begun within 48 h of the onset of illness, amantadine reduces the duration of systemic and respiratory symptoms of influenza by approximately 50 percent, and in one study, was superior to aspirin. From 5 to 10 percent of individuals who receive amantadine will experience mild CNS side effects, primarily jitteriness, anxiety, insomnia, or difficulty in concentrating. These side effects disappear promptly upon cessation of the drug. The dose of amantadine for adults is 200 mg per day for 3 to 5 days or up to 48 h after illness has resolved. Because amantadine is excreted almost entirely by the kidneys, the dose should be reduced in individuals with renal insufficiency. Rimantadine, an experimental drug which is a closely related analogue of amantadine, appears to be equally efficacious and is associated with less frequent CNS side effects than is amantadine. Ribavirin, a nucleoside analogue with activity against a variety of viral agents, has been reported to be effective against both influenza A and B virus infections when administered as an aerosol, although it is relatively ineffective when administered orally.

Studies demonstrating the therapeutic efficacy of antiviral compounds in influenza have been carried out almost exclusively in uncomplicated disease in young adults, and it is not known whether such compounds are effective in the treatment of complications such as influenza pneumonia. Therapy for primary influenza pneumonia is directed at maintaining oxygenation and is most appropriately managed in an intensive care unit, with aggressive respiratory and hemodynamic support as needed. Bypass membrane oxygenators have been employed in this setting with variable results. When an acute respiratory distress syndrome develops, fluids must be administered cautiously, with close monitoring of blood gases and hemodynamic function.

Antibacterial drugs should be reserved for the therapy of bacterial complications of acute influenza such as secondary bacterial pneumonia. The choice of antibiotics should be guided by Gram stain and culture of appropriate specimens of respiratory secretions, such as sputum or transtracheal aspirates. If the etiology of a bacterial pneumonia is unclear from examination of respiratory secretions, empiric antibiotics should be selected which are effective against the most common bacterial pathogens in this setting, namely, *S. pneumoniae*, *S. aureus*, and *H. influenzae* (see Chaps. 99, 100, 115).

PROPHYLAXIS   The major public health measure for prevention of influenza has been the use of inactivated influenza vaccines. These vaccines are derived from influenza A and B viruses which circulated during the previous influenza season. If the vaccine and currently circulating viruses are closely related, such vaccines would be expected to provide 50 to 80 percent protection against influenza. Currently available vaccines have been highly purified and are associated with few reactions. Up to 5 percent of individuals will experience low-grade fever and mild systemic symptoms 8 to 24 h after vaccination, and up to one-third may have mild redness or tenderness at the vaccination site. Since the vaccine is produced in eggs, individuals with true hypersensitivity to egg products should either be desensitized or should not receive vaccine. Although the 1976 swine influenza vaccine appears to have been associated with an increased frequency of Guillain-Barré syndrome, influenza vaccines administered since 1976 have not been associated with Guillain-Barré syndrome. Live attenuated ("cold-adapted") influenza A vaccines have also been developed and appear to be promising in ongoing studies in adults and children. Such vaccines are administered intranasally and stimulate local antibody production more efficiently than conventional inactivated vaccines.

The U.S. Public Health Service recommends influenza vaccination for any individual older than 6 months who is at an increased risk for complications of influenza. These include individuals with chronic cardiovascular or pulmonary disorders (including asthma) and residents of nursing homes and other chronic care facilities. Other populations for whom the vaccine is recommended include otherwise healthy individuals over 65 years of age and individuals who have required regular medical attention for diabetes mellitus, renal disease, hemoglobinopathies, or immunosuppression. Individuals who provide care for high-risk patients or who come into frequent contact with such patients should also receive vaccine to reduce the likelihood of transmission of infection. Since commercially available vaccines are inactivated ("killed"), they may be administered safely to immunocompromised patients. Influenza vaccination is not associated with exacerbations of chronic nervous system diseases such as multiple sclerosis. Vaccination should be administered early in the autumn before influenza outbreaks occur, and should be administered on an annual basis to maintain immunity against the most current influenza virus strains.

Amantadine and rimantadine have also been demonstrated to be effective in the prophylaxis of influenza A. Studies have demonstrated 70 to 100 percent effectiveness of these drugs in preventing illness associated with influenza A virus infection. The major use for prophylaxis with amantadine or rimantadine is likely to be for high-risk individuals who have not received influenza vaccine, or when the vaccines previously administered are relatively ineffective because of antigenic changes in the circulating virus. If vaccination is performed during an outbreak, amantadine can be administered simultaneously with inactivated vaccine, since it will not interfere with an immune response to the vaccine. There is also evidence that the protective effects of amantadine and vaccine may be additive. Amantadine has also been employed to control nosocomial outbreaks of influenza A. For prophylaxis, amantadine, or rimantadine should be instituted promptly when influenza A activity is detected and must be administered daily for the duration of the outbreak. The dosage most frequently employed has been 200 mg per day for adults, but the dose of amantadine should be reduced in patients with renal insufficiency and in the elderly.

REFERENCES

CENTERS FOR DISEASE CONTROL: Prevention and control of influenza. Morb Mort Week Rep 38:297, 1989

DOLIN R et al: A controlled trial of amantadine and rimantadine in the prophylaxis of influenza A infection. N Engl J Med 307:580, 1982

DOUGLAS RG JR (ed): Prevention, management, and control of influenza: A mandate for the 1980s. Am J Med 82 (suppl 6A), 1987

GLEZEN, WP: Serious morbidity and mortality associated with influenza epidemics. Epidemiol Rev 4:25, 1982

LAMONTAGNE JR et al: Summary of clinical trials of inactivated influenza vaccines, 1978. Rev Infect Dis 5:723, 1983

MURPHY BR, WEBSTER RG: Orthomyxoviruses, in Virology, 2d ed, BN Fields (ed). New York, Raven, 1989, pp 1091-1152

140 COMMON VIRAL RESPIRATORY INFECTIONS

RAPHAEL DOLIN

GENERAL CONSIDERATIONS Acute viral respiratory illnesses are among the most common of human diseases, accounting for one-half or more of all acute illnesses. The incidence of acute respiratory disease in the United States is from 3 to 5.6 cases per person per year. The highest rates occur in children under 1 (6.1 to 8.3 cases per year) and the rates remain high until age 6, when a progressive decrease is noted. Adults have three to four illnesses per person per year. Morbidity from acute respiratory illnesses accounts for 30 to 50 percent of time lost from work by adults and from 60 to 80 percent of time lost from school by children.

It has been estimated that two-thirds to three-fourths of cases of acute respiratory illnesses are caused by viruses. More than 200 antigenically distinct viruses from 8 different genera have been reported to cause acute respiratory illness, and it is likely that additional agents will be described in the future. The vast majority of these viral infections involve the upper respiratory tract, but lower respiratory tract disease can also occur, particularly in younger age groups and in certain epidemiologic settings.

The illnesses caused by respiratory viruses traditionally have been divided into multiple distinct syndromes, such as the "common cold," pharyngitis, croup (laryngotracheobronchitis), tracheitis, bronchiolitis, bronchitis, and pneumonia. These general categories of illnesses have a certain epidemiologic and clinical utility, e.g., croup occurs exclusively in very young children and has a characteristic clinical course. Some types of respiratory illnesses are more likely to be associated with certain viruses, e.g., the "common cold" with rhinoviruses, while others occupy characteristic epidemiologic niches, such as adenoviruses in military recruits. The syndromes most commonly associated with infection with the major respiratory virus groups are summarized in Table 140-1. Despite these associations, it is clear that most respiratory viruses have the potential to cause more than one type of respiratory illness, and frequently features of several types of illness may be present in the same patient. Moreover, the clinical illnesses induced by these viruses are rarely sufficiently distinctive to enable an etiologic diagnosis to be made on clinical grounds alone, although the epidemiologic setting increases the likelihood that one group of viruses rather than another may be involved. In general, laboratory methods must be relied upon to establish a specific viral diagnosis.

This chapter will review viral infections caused by five of the major groups of respiratory viruses: rhinoviruses, coronaviruses, respiratory syncytial viruses, parainfluenza viruses, and adenoviruses. Influenza viruses, which are a major cause of mortality as well as morbidity, are reviewed in Chap. 139. Herpesviruses, which occasionally cause pharyngitis and which also cause lower respiratory tract disease in immunosuppressed patients, are reviewed in Chap. 135. Enteroviruses, which account for occasional respiratory illnesses during the summer months, are reviewed in Chap. 144.

RHINOVIRUS INFECTIONS

ETIOLOGY Rhinoviruses are members of the Picornaviridae family, which are small (15 to 30 nm), nonenveloped viruses which contain a single-stranded RNA genome. In contrast to other members of the picornavirus family, such as enteroviruses, rhinoviruses are acid-labile and are almost completely inactivated at pH 3 or lower. Rhinoviruses grow preferentially at 33 to 34°C, which is the temperature of nasal passages in humans, rather than the higher temperature (37°C) of the lower respiratory tract. One hundred distinct serotypes of rhinoviruses are recognized.

TABLE 140-1 Illnesses associated with respiratory viruses

Frequency of respiratory syndromes associated with virus groups

Virus	Most frequent	Occasional	Infrequent
Rhinoviruses	Common cold	Exacerbation of chronic bronchitis and asthma	Pneumonia (children)
Coronaviruses	Common cold	Exacerbation of chronic bronchitis and asthma	Pneumonia and bronchiolitis
Respiratory syncytial virus	Pneumonia and bronchiolitis in young children	Common cold in adults	Pneumonia in elderly
Parainfluenza viruses	Croup and lower respiratory tract disease in young children	Pharyngitis and common cold	Tracheobronchitis in adults
Adenoviruses	Common cold and pharyngitis in children	Outbreaks of ARD in military recruits	Pneumonia in children and immunosuppressed patients
Influenza A viruses	"Influenza-like illness"†	Pneumonia and excess mortality in "high-risk" patients	Pneumonia in healthy individuals
Influenza B viruses	"Influenza-like illness"†	Rhinitis and pharyngitis alone	Pneumonia
Enteroviruses	Acute undifferentiated febrile illnesses‡	Rhinitis and pharyngitis	Pneumonia
Herpes simplex viruses	Gingivostomatitis‡ (children) Pharyngotonsillitis (adults)	Tracheitis and pneumonia in immunocompromised patients	Disseminated infection in immunocompromised patients

* Serotypes 4 and 7.
† Fever, cough, myalgia, malaise.
‡ May or may not have a respiratory component.

EPIDEMIOLOGY Rhinoviruses are a major cause of the common cold and have been isolated from 15 to 40 percent of adults with common cold–like illnesses. Infection rates are higher among infants and young children and decrease with increasing age. Rhinovirus infections occur throughout the year, but seasonal peaks occur in early fall and spring in temperate climates. Rhinovirus infections are most often introduced into families by preschool or grade school children below 6 years of age. Between 25 and 50 percent of initial illnesses in family settings are followed by secondary cases, with the highest attack rates occurring in the youngest siblings at home. Attack rates also increase with increasing size of families.

The spread of rhinoviruses appears to be by direct contact with infected secretions, usually respiratory droplets. In volunteer studies, transmission was most efficient by hand-to-hand contact, with subsequent self-inoculation of the conjunctival or nasal mucosa. Transmission appears to be much less efficient following exposure to large or small aerosolized particles. Virus can also be recovered from plastic surfaces inoculated 1 to 3 h previously, suggesting that environmental surfaces may also contribute to transmission. In studies conducted in married couples in which serum antibody was not present in either partner, transmission was associated with prolonged contact (122 h or more) during a 7-day period. Transmission was infrequent unless virus was recoverable from the donor's hands and nasal mucosa, at least 1000 TCID$_{50}$ of virus was present in nasal washes of the donor, and the donor was at least moderately symptomatic with the "cold." Despite anecdotal observations, exposure to cold temperatures, fatigue, or sleep deprivation has not been associated with increased rates of rhinovirus-induced illness in human volunteers.

Infection with rhinoviruses is worldwide in distribution, and by the time they reach adulthood, nearly all individuals have neutralizing antibodies to multiple serotypes, although the prevalence of antibody to any one serotype varies widely. Multiple serotypes circulate simultaneously, and generally no single serotype or group of serotypes has emerged as being more prevalent than others.

PATHOGENESIS Rhinoviruses infect cells via attachment to specific cellular receptors. Relatively limited information is available on the histopathology and pathogenesis of acute rhinovirus infections in humans. Biopsies performed in experimentally induced and in naturally occurring illness indicate that the nasal mucosa is edematous, often hyperemic, and during acute illness, is covered by a mucoid discharge. There is a mild infiltrate with inflammatory cells, including neutrophils, lymphocytes, plasma cells, and eosinophils. Mucus-secreting glands in the submucosa appear hyperactive; the nasal turbinates are engorged, which may lead to obstruction of nearby openings of sinus cavities.

The incubation period for rhinovirus illness is short, and generally ranges from 1 to 2 days. Virus shedding coincides with the onset of illness or may begin shortly before symptoms develop. The mechanisms of immunity to rhinovirus are not well worked out. In some studies, the presence of homotypic antibody significantly reduced the rates of subsequent infection and illness, but conflicting data exist as to the relative importance of serum and local antibody in protection from rhinovirus infection.

CLINICAL MANIFESTATIONS The most common clinical manifestations of rhinovirus infections are those of the common cold. Initially, illness begins with rhinorrhea and sneezing, accompanied by nasal congestion. Sore throat is frequently present and in some cases may be the initial complaint. Systemic signs and symptoms, such as malaise and headache, are mild or absent and fever is unusual. Illness generally lasts for 4 to 9 days, and resolves spontaneously without sequelae. In children, lower respiratory tract involvement may be seen, including bronchitis, bronchiolitis, and, on occasion, bronchopneumonia. Rhinoviruses may also cause exacerbations of asthma and chronic pulmonary disease in adults. The vast majority of rhinovirus infections resolve without sequelae, but complications related to obstruction of the eustachian tubes or sinus ostia, including otitis media or acute sinusitis, can occur.

DIAGNOSIS Although rhinoviruses are the most frequently recognized cause of the common cold, similar illnesses may be caused by a variety of other viruses, and the etiologic diagnosis cannot be made on clinical grounds alone. The diagnosis of rhinovirus infection is made by isolation of virus from nasal washes or nasal secretions in tissue culture. In practice, this procedure is rarely carried out because of the benign, self-limited nature of the illness. Because of the large number of serotypes of rhinovirus, diagnosis of rhinovirus infections by serum antibody tests is currently not practical. Common laboratory tests such as white cell count and sedimentation rate are not helpful in the diagnosis of rhinovirus infection.

TREATMENT AND PREVENTION Rhinovirus infections are generally mild and self-limited so that treatment is not necessary. Some patients may benefit from the use of analgesics and nasal decongestants, and reduction of activity is prudent if significant discomfort or fatigability is present. Specific antiviral therapy is not available. Application of interferon sprays intranasally has been effective in the prophylaxis of rhinovirus infections, but is also associated with local irritation of nasal mucosa. Prevention of rhinovirus infection by antibodies directed against rhinovirus receptors or by the use of the purified receptors themselves is under study. Experimental vaccines to certain rhinovirus serotypes have been prepared, but their utility is questionable because of the existence of the large number of serotypes and the uncertainty regarding the mechanisms of immunity. Thorough hand washing or barrier protection against autoinoculation may help to reduce transmission of infection.

CORONAVIRUS INFECTIONS

ETIOLOGY   Coronaviruses are pleomorphic, single-stranded RNA viruses, 80 to 160 nm in diameter, with clublike projections emanating from the virus envelope, resulting in an appearance which resembles that of the solar "corona" from which their name is derived. Three distinct coronavirus serotypes, designated B814, 229E, and OC43, have been isolated from humans. Coronaviruses are fastidious and are difficult to culture in vitro. Some strains will grow only in human tracheal organ cultures rather than in tissue culture.

EPIDEMIOLOGY   Only limited seroepidemiologic studies have been carried out in coronavirus infections. Seroprevalence studies of two of the serotypes, 229E and OC43, have yielded variable rates of serum antibodies, ranging from 12 to 80 percent in various populations. Overall, coronaviruses account for 10 to 20 percent of common colds. Coronavirus infections appear to be particularly prevalent in late fall, winter, and early spring, at a time when rhinovirus infections are less common. Depending on the serotype, a cyclical pattern for outbreaks of coronavirus infection has been suggested, which ranges from every 2 years for OC43, to every 2 to 4 years with 229E.

CLINICAL FEATURES   The clinical features of illness caused by coronaviruses are similar to those caused by rhinoviruses. In volunteer studies, the mean incubation period of illness induced by coronaviruses (3 days) is somewhat longer than that caused by rhinoviruses, and the duration of illness is somewhat shorter, with a mean of 6 to 7 days. In some studies, the amount of nasal discharge was somewhat greater in colds induced by coronaviruses compared to those induced by rhinoviruses. Coronaviruses have also been recovered from infants with pneumonia and from military recruits with lower respiratory tract disease and have also been associated with worsening of chronic bronchitis. However, the overall significance of coronaviruses in lower respiratory tract disease in humans is unclear.

TREATMENT AND PREVENTION   The approach to the treatment of common colds caused by coronaviruses is similar to that discussed above for rhinovirus-induced illnesses. Because of the uncertainty regarding the number and relative importance of coronavirus serotypes and the mechanisms of immunity, vaccines against coronaviruses have not been developed.

RESPIRATORY SYNCYTIAL VIRUS INFECTIONS

ETIOLOGY   Respiratory syncytial virus (RSV) is a member of the Paramyxoviridae family and comprises the genus *Pneumovirus*. RSV is an enveloped virus approximately 150 to 300 nm in size, so named because virus replication leads to fusion of neighboring cells into large multinucleated syncytia. The single-stranded RNA genome codes for 10 virus-specific proteins. Viral RNA is contained in a helical nucleocapsid surrounded by a lipid envelope bearing two glycoproteins, one of which is the G protein by which the virus attaches to cells, and the other is the fusion protein which facilitates entry of virus into the cell by fusing host and viral membranes. Respiratory syncytial viruses have been considered to be of a single antigenic type, but it has been found that two distinct subtypes (A and B) exist. The epidemiologic and clinical significance of subtype differences are being investigated.

EPIDEMIOLOGY   RSV is the major respiratory pathogen of young children and is the major cause of lower respiratory disease in infants. Infection with RSV is seen throughout the world, in annual epidemics which occur in either late fall, winter, or spring, and can last up to 5 months. The virus is rarely encountered during the summer. The highest rates of illness occur in infants between 1 and 6 months of age, with peak rates occurring between 2 and 3 months of age. The attack rates among susceptibles are extraordinarily high, approaching 100 percent in settings such as day-care centers where large numbers of susceptible infants are present. RSV accounts for 20 to 25 percent of hospital admissions for pneumonia of young infants and children, and up to 75 percent of cases of bronchiolitis in this age group. It

has been estimated that more than half of infants who are at risk will become infected during an RSV epidemic.

In older children and adults, reinfection with RSV is frequent, but disease is milder than in infancy. A "common cold–like syndrome" is the illness most commonly associated with RSV infection in adults. Severe lower respiratory tract disease with pneumonitis can occur in elderly, often institutionalized, adults or those with immunocompromising disorders or treatment. RSV infection is more severe and prolonged in immunocompromised children. RSV is also an important nosocomial pathogen and can infect pediatric patients and up to 25 to 50 percent of the staff on pediatric wards during an RSV outbreak. The spread of virus among families is also efficient, and up to 40 percent of siblings may become infected when RSV is introduced into the family setting.

RSV is transmitted primarily by close contact with contaminated fingers or fomites, and by self-inoculation of the conjunctiva or anterior nares. Virus may also be spread by coarse aerosols produced by coughing or sneezing but is inefficiently spread by fine-particle aerosols. The incubation period of illness is approximately 4 to 6 days, and virus shedding may last for 2 weeks or longer in children and for shorter periods of time in adults.

PATHOGENESIS   The characteristics of the immune response to RSV are not well elucidated. Because reinfection occurs frequently and is often associated with illness, the immunity that develops after single episodes of infection is not complete or long-lasting. However, the cumulative effect of multiple reinfections ameliorates subsequent disease and provides some temporary measure of protection against infection. Studies of experimentally induced disease in normal volunteers indicate that the presence of nasal IgA neutralizing antibody correlates more closely with protection than does the presence of serum antibody. Studies in infants, however, suggest that maternally acquired antibody provides some protection from lower respiratory tract disease, although severe illness may also occur in infants who have moderate levels of maternally derived serum antibody.

CLINICAL MANIFESTATIONS   RSV infection leads to a wide spectrum of respiratory illnesses. In infants, 25 to 40 percent of infections result in lower respiratory tract involvement, including pneumonia, bronchiolitis, and tracheobronchitis. In infants, illness begins most frequently with rhinorrhea, low-grade fever, and mild systemic symptoms, often accompanied by cough and wheezing. Most patients gradually recover in 1 to 2 weeks. In more severe illness, tachypnea and dyspnea develop, and eventually frank hypoxia, cyanosis, and apnea can ensue. Physical examination may reveal diffuse wheezing, rhonchi, and rales. Chest x-ray shows hyperexpansion, peribronchial thickening, and variable infiltrates ranging from diffuse interstitial infiltrates to segmental or lobar consolidation. Illness may be particularly severe in children with congenital cardiac disease, bronchopulmonary dysplasia, or immunosuppression. One study documented a 37-percent mortality rate for infants with RSV pneumonia and congenital cardiac disease.

In adults, the most common symptoms of RSV infection are those of the common cold, with rhinorrhea, sore throat, and cough. Illness may occasionally be associated with moderate systemic symptoms such as malaise, headache, and fever. RSV has also been reported to cause febrile lower respiratory tract disease in adults, including severe pneumonia in the elderly.

LABORATORY FINDINGS AND DIAGNOSIS   The diagnosis of RSV infection can be suspected on the basis of the epidemiologic setting, i.e., severe illness in infants during an outbreak of RSV in the community. Infections in older children and adults cannot be differentiated with certainty from those caused by other respiratory viruses. The specific diagnosis is established by isolation of RSV from respiratory secretions, including sputum, throat swabs, or nasopharyngeal washes. Virus is detected in tissue culture and identified specifically by immunologic reactions, employing immunofluorescence, enzyme-linked immunosorbent assay (ELISA), or other techniques. Immunofluorescence microscopy of nasal scrapings or washings provides a rapid diagnostic method that is in use in many diagnostic virology laboratories. Serologic tests which depend on fourfold or greater rises in complement fixing or neutralizing antibody titers are useful for diagnosis in older children and adults but are less sensitive in children under 4 months of age. Compared to complement fixation or neutralization tests, ELISA detects serum antibody with more sensitivity. As with other serologic tests, diagnosis requires comparison of acute and convalescent serum specimens and is therefore not useful during the acute illness.

TREATMENT AND PREVENTION Treatment of upper respiratory tract RSV infection consists primarily of symptomatic therapy similar to that for other upper respiratory tract viral infections. For lower respiratory tract infections, treatment consists of respiratory therapy, including hydration, suctioning of secretions, administration of humidified oxygen, and antibronchospastic agents as needed. If severe hypoxia is present, intubation and ventilatory assistance may be required. Studies of infants with RSV infection who were given aerosolized ribavirin, a nucleoside analogue which is active in vitro against RSV, have demonstrated a beneficial effect on the resolution of lower respiratory tract illness, including improvement of blood gases. Similar studies have not been performed in adults with RSV pneumonitis and its benefit in these patients is questionable.

Considerable interest exists in the development of an effective vaccine against RSV. Inactivated whole virus vaccines have been either ineffective or, in one study, potentiated the disease in infants. Other approaches to vaccine development include immunization with purified F and G surface glycoproteins of RSV, or generation of stable, live attenuated virus vaccines. In the settings where high rates of transmission occur, such as pediatric wards, barrier methods of protection of hands and conjunctiva may be useful in reducing the spread of virus.

PARAINFLUENZA VIRUS INFECTIONS

ETIOLOGY Parainfluenza viruses are members of the Paramyxoviridae family and comprise the genus *Paramyxovirus*. Parainfluenza viruses are 150 to 250 nm in diameter, enveloped, and contain a single-stranded RNA genome. The envelope is studded with two glycoproteins, one of which possesses both hemagglutinin and neuraminidase activity, while the other glycoprotein contains the fusion activity. The viral RNA genome is enclosed in a helical nucleocapsid and codes for seven virus-specific proteins. There are four distinct serotypes of parainfluenza viruses, all of which share certain common antigens with other members of the Paramyxoviridae family, including mumps and Newcastle disease virus.

EPIDEMIOLOGY Parainfluenza viruses are distributed throughout the world, although type 4 has been reported less widely, probably because it is more difficult to grow in tissue culture. Infection occurs in early childhood so that by 8 years of age, most children show antibodies to serotypes 1, 2, and 3. Parainfluenza types 1 and 2 cause epidemics during the fall, primarily in odd-numbered years. Type 3 infection has been detected during all seasons of the year, but epidemics of type 3 virus have occurred annually in the spring.

The contribution of parainfluenza infections to respiratory disease are variable according to both the location and year. In studies carried out in the United States, parainfluenza virus infections accounted for 4.3 to 22 percent of respiratory illnesses in children. In adults, parainfluenza infections are generally mild and account for less than 5 percent of respiratory illnesses. The major importance of parainfluenza viruses is as a cause of respiratory illness in young children, where they are second only to RSV as causes of lower respiratory tract illness. Like RSV, but unlike parainfluenza types 1 and 2, parainfluenza type 3 frequently causes illness during the first month of life, while passively acquired maternal antibody is still present. In contrast, parainfluenza type 1 is the most frequent cause of croup (laryngotracheobronchitis) in children, while serotype 2 causes sim-

ilar, although generally less severe, disease. Parainfluenza type 3 is an important cause of bronchiolitis and pneumonia in infants, while illnesses associated with parainfluenza type 4 have been generally mild. Parainfluenza viruses are spread through infected respiratory secretions, primarily by person-to-person contact and/or by large droplets. In experimental studies, the incubation period has varied from 3 to 6 days but may be somewhat shorter in naturally occurring disease in children.

PATHOGENESIS Immunity to parainfluenza viruses is incompletely understood, but there is suggestive evidence that immunity to types 1 and 2 infections is mediated by local IgA antibodies in the respiratory tract. Passively acquired serum-neutralizing antibodies also confer some protection against infection with parainfluenza viruses types 1, 2, and, to a lesser degree, type 3.

CLINICAL MANIFESTATIONS Parainfluenza virus infections occur most frequently in children, in whom initial infection with serotypes 1, 2, and 3 is associated with an acute febrile illness in 50 to 80 percent of cases. Children may present with coryza, sore throat, hoarseness, and cough, which may or may not be croupy. In severe croup, fever persists, with worsening coryza and sore throat. A brassy or barking cough may be noted and may progress to frank stridor. In most children, recovery will occur over the next 1 to 2 days, although progressive airway obstruction and hypoxia may ensue occasionally. If bronchiolitis or pneumonia develops, progressive cough accompanied by wheezing, tachypnea, and intercostal retractions may be present. In this setting, a moderate increase in sputum production can be seen. Physical examination shows nasopharyngeal discharge and oropharyngeal injection, along with rhonchi, wheezes, or coarse breath sounds. Chest x-rays can show air trapping and, occasionally, interstitial infiltrates.

In older children and adults, parainfluenza infections tend to be milder, presenting most frequently as the common cold or hoarseness, with or without cough. Lower respiratory tract involvement in older children and adults is uncommon, but tracheobronchitis in adults has been reported. More severe and prolonged parainfluenza infection has been reported in children with severe immunosuppression.

LABORATORY FINDINGS AND DIAGNOSIS As with other respiratory viral diseases, the clinical syndromes caused by parainfluenza viruses are not sufficiently distinctive to permit a diagnosis to be made on clinical grounds alone, with the possible exception of croup in young children. A specific diagnosis is established by detection of virus in respiratory tract secretions, throat swabs, or nasopharyngeal washings. Virus is detected by growth in tissue culture, either by hemagglutination or by cytopathic effect, or by immunofluorescence of viral antigens in exfoliated cells from the respiratory tract. Serologic diagnosis can be made by fourfold or greater rises in acute and convalescent serum specimens as detected by hemagglutination inhibition, complement fixation, or neutralization tests. However, frequent heterotypic responses occur among the parainfluenza serotypes, so that identification of the serotype which causes the illness often cannot be made by serologic techniques alone.

Acute epiglottitis caused by *Haemophilus influenza*, type B (bacterial croup), must be differentiated from viral croup. Influenza A virus also is a common cause of croup during epidemic periods.

TREATMENT AND PREVENTION For upper respiratory tract illness, symptomatic therapy can be employed as discussed for other viral respiratory tract illnesses. If complications such as sinusitis, otitis, or superimposed bacterial bronchitis develop, appropriate antibiotics should be administered. Mild cases of croup should be treated with bed rest and moist air as generated by vaporizers. More severe cases require hospitalization and close observation for the development of respiratory distress. If acute respiratory distress develops, humidified oxygen and bronchodilators should be employed. There is no specific antiviral therapy available, although ribavirin has activity against parainfluenza viruses in vitro and is being evaluated clinically. Effective vaccines against parainfluenza viruses have not been developed.

ADENOVIRUS INFECTIONS

ETIOLOGY Adenoviruses are complex DNA viruses which are 70 to 80 nm in diameter. Human adenoviruses belong to the genus *Mastadenovirus*, of which 41 serotypes are recognized. Adenoviruses have a characteristic morphology consisting of an icosahedral shell composed of 20 equilateral triangular faces and 12 vertices. The protein coat (''capsid'') consists of hexon subunits with group-specific and type-specific antigenic determinants, and penton subunits at each vertex primarily containing group-specific antigens. From each penton, a fiber with a knob at the end projects, which contains type-specific and some group-specific antigens. Adenoviruses have been divided into six or seven subgroups based on the homology of DNA genomes. The adenovirus genome is a linear double-stranded DNA which codes for structural and nonstructural polypeptides. The replicative cycle of adenovirus may result in either lytic infection of cells, or in the establishment of a latent infection (primarily involving lymphoid cells). Some adenovirus types can induce oncogenic transformation, and tumor formation has been observed in rodents, but despite intensive investigation, adenoviruses have not been associated with tumors in humans.

EPIDEMIOLOGY Adenovirus infections occur most frequently in infants and children. Infections occur throughout the year but are most commonly noted from fall to spring. Large-scale surveys have shown that adenoviruses account for 3 to 5 percent of acute respiratory infections in children. Infections are less frequent in adults and account for less than 2 percent of respiratory illness in civilians. Nearly 100 percent of adults have serum antibody against multiple serotypes, indicating that infection is common in childhood. Types 1, 2, 3, and 5 are the most frequent isolates obtained from children. Certain adenovirus serotypes, particularly 4 and 7, but also 3, 14, and 21, are associated with outbreaks of acute respiratory disease (ARD) in military recruits which occur in winter and spring. Transmission of adenovirus infection can occur by inhalation of aerosolized virus, by inoculation of virus in conjunctival sacs, and probably occurs by the fecal-oral route as well. Type-specific antibody generally develops after infection and is associated with protection against infection with the same serotype.

CLINICAL MANIFESTATIONS In children, adenoviruses cause a variety of clinical syndromes. The most common is an acute upper respiratory tract infection, with prominent rhinitis. On occasion, lower respiratory tract disease, including bronchiolitis and pneumonia, can also be seen. Adenoviruses, particularly types 3 and 7, cause pharyngoconjunctival fever, a characteristic acute febrile illness of children which occurs in outbreaks, most often in summer camps. The syndrome is marked by bilateral conjunctivitis in which the bulbar and palpebral conjunctiva have a granular appearance. Low-grade fever is frequently present, along with rhinitis, sore throat, and cervical adenopathy. The illness generally lasts for 1 to 2 weeks and resolves spontaneously. Febrile pharyngitis without conjunctivitis has also been associated with adenovirus infection. Adenoviruses have also been isolated from cases of whooping cough with or without *Bordetella pertussis;* the significance of adenovirus in that disease is unknown.

In adults, the most frequently reported illness has been ARD in military recruits caused by adenovirus types 4 and 7. This illness is marked by a prominent sore throat and the gradual onset of fever, often reaching 39°C on the second or third day of illness. Cough is almost always present, and coryza and regional lymphadenopathy are also frequently seen. Physical examination may show pharyngeal edema, injection, and tonsillar enlargement with little or no exudate. If pneumonia is present, auscultation of the chest and x-ray may indicate areas of patchy infiltration.

Adenoviruses have also been associated with a number of non-respiratory tract diseases, including acute diarrheal illness in young children caused by adenovirus types 40 and 41, and hemorrhagic cystitis caused by adenoviruses 11 and 21. Epidemic keratoconjunctivitis, caused most frequently by adenovirus types 8, 19, and 37,

has been associated with contaminated common sources such as ophthalmic solutions and roller towels. Adenoviruses have also been associated with disseminated disease and pneumonia in immunosuppressed patients, including patients with acquired immunodeficiency syndrome (AIDS).

LABORATORY FINDINGS AND DIAGNOSIS Adenovirus infection should be suspected in the epidemiologic setting of ARD and in certain of the clinical syndromes such as pharyngoconjunctival fever or epidemic keratoconjunctivitis in which outbreaks of characteristic illnesses occur. In the majority of cases, however, illnesses caused by adenovirus infection cannot be differentiated from those caused by a number of other viral respiratory agents and *Mycoplasma pneumoniae*. A definitive diagnosis of adenovirus infection is established by culture or detection of virus from sites such as the conjunctiva and oropharynx or from sputum, urine, or stool. Virus may be detected in tissue culture by cytopathic changes, and specifically identified by immunofluorescence or other immunologic techniques. Adenovirus types 40 and 41, which have been associated with diarrheal disease in children, require special tissue culture cells for isolation, and these serotypes are most commonly detected by direct ELISA of stool. Serum antibody rises can be demonstrated by complement fixation, neutralization, ELISA, or radioimmunoassays. Hemagglutination inhibition tests may also be done for those adenoviruses which hemagglutinate red cells.

TREATMENT AND PREVENTION Only symptomatic and supportive therapy is available for adenovirus infections, and no clinically useful antiviral compounds have emerged. Live vaccines have been developed against adenovirus types 4 and 7 and are widely utilized to control this illness in military recruits. These vaccines consist of live, unattenuated virus which is administered in enteric coated capsules. Infection of the gastrointestinal tract with types 4 and 7 does not cause disease but stimulates local and systemic antibodies which protect against subsequent ARD with those serotypes. Vaccines prepared from purified subunits of adenovirus are currently under investigation.

REFERENCES

Rhinoviruses

D'ALESSIO DJ et al: Short-duration exposure and the transmission of rhinoviral colds. J Infect Dis 150:189, 1984
GWALTNEY JM: Rhinoviruses, in *Viral Infections of Humans*, AS Evans (ed). New York, Plenum, 1982, pp 491–517
ROSSMAN MG et al: Structure of a human common cold virus and functional relationships to other picornaviruses. Nature 317:145, 1985
TYRRELL DAJ: Common colds. Intervirology 25:177, 1986

Coronaviruses

LARSON HE et al: Isolation of rhinoviruses and coronaviruses from 38 colds in adults. J Med Virol 5:221, 1980
MCINTOSH K: Coronaviruses, in *Virology*, 2d ed, BN Fields (ed). New York, Raven, 1989

Respiratory syncytial virus

ENGLUND JA et al: Respiratory syncytial virus infection in immunocompromised adults. Ann Intern Med 109:203, 1988
GLEZEN WP et al: Risk of primary infection and reinfection with respiratory syncytial virus. Am J Dis Child 140:543, 1986
HALL CB et al: Aerosolized ribavirin treatment of infants with respiratory syncytial viral infection. A randomized double blind study. N Engl J Med 308:1443, 1983
HENDERSON FW et al: Respiratory syncytial virus infections, reinfections and immunity. N Engl J Med 300:530, 1979
MUFSON MA et al: Respiratory syncytial virus epidemics: Variable dominance of subgroups A and B strains among children, 1981–1986. J Infect Dis 1:143, 1988

Parainfluenza viruses

DENNY FW et al: Croup: An 11 year study in a pediatric practice. Pediatrics 71:871, 1983
TYERYAR FJ: Report of a workshop on respiratory syncytial virus and parainfluenza viruses. J Infect Dis 148:528, 1983
WRIGHT PF: Parainfluenzaviruses, in *Textbook of Human Virology*, RB Belshe (ed). Littleton, MA, PSG Publishing, 1985, pp 1241–1255

Adenoviruses

BAUM SG: Adenoviruses, in *Principles and Practice of Infectious Diseases*, 3d ed, G Mandell et al (eds). New York, Wiley, 1990

Fox JP et al: The Seattle virus watch. VII. Observations of adenovirus infections. Am J Epidemiol 105:362, 1977

WIGAND R et al: Adenoviridiae: Second report. Intervirology 18:169, 1982

ZAHRADNIK JM et al: Adenovirus infection in the immunosuppressed patient. Am J Med 68:725, 1980

141   MEASLES (RUBEOLA)

C. GEORGE RAY

DEFINITION   Measles, or rubeola, is an acute febrile eruption which has been one of the most common diseases of civilization. Despite the development of an effective vaccine it remains a worldwide health problem.

ETIOLOGY   The measles virion is composed of a central core of ribonucleic acid with a helically arranged protein coat surrounded by a lipoprotein envelope with small, spikelike structures. The virion is 120 to 200 nm in diameter and is classified as a morbillivirus in the paramyxovirus family.

EPIDEMIOLOGY   Measles occurs naturally only in human beings, although infection with the virus can be demonstrated in laboratory colonies of monkeys exposed to infected individuals. Before active immunization was available, epidemics of measles occurred in 2- to 3-year cycles, usually during the spring months, and about 95 percent of urban dwellers developed the disease before the age of 15. The virus is transmitted by transfer of nasopharyngeal secretions, either directly or in airborne droplets, to the respiratory mucous membranes or conjunctivae of susceptible individuals. Persons infected with the virus may transmit the disease during a period which extends from 5 days after exposure until 5 days after skin lesions have appeared. The virus is highly contagious, with secondary attack rates among susceptible household contacts usually exceeding 90 percent; asymptomatic primary infections are rare. Measles is typically a disease of childhood in populous areas, but may occur at any age in remote isolated communities if the disease is introduced. In the United States, there has been a distinct shift in age-specific attack rates, with outbreaks most usually occurring among teenagers and young adults. Infants are uncommonly affected under the age of 6 to 8 months, presumably because of the persistence of maternal antibody acquired by transplacental transmission. With increasingly effective attempts at control, the incidence of measles in the United States fell to the lowest level ever recorded in 1983. However, this trend was sharply reversed from 1984 to 1987, with increasing reports of outbreaks primarily among the 5- to 19-year age group. Transmission has occurred even though vaccination levels have exceeded 98 percent.

PATHOGENESIS AND PATHOLOGY   It is probable that, after infection, measles virus multiplies in the epithelium of the respiratory tract and is disseminated by way of the blood to distant sites. For a few days before the rash appears, and for 1 or 2 days after, the virus can be isolated from blood or washed white blood cells, conjunctivae, lymphoid tissue, and respiratory mucous membranes and secretions. The virus can be obtained from urine for as long as 4 days after the onset of the eruptions. Virus replication in thymic Hassall's corpuscles, capillary endothelium, and hepatic duct epithelium also occurs.

The mucous membrane lesions (Koplik's spots) consist of vesicle formation and epithelial necrosis. Histology of the Koplik's spots reveals cytoplasmic and intranuclear inclusions, giant cells, and intercellular edema. Virion components can be detected in biopsy specimens of Koplik's spots and vascular endothelial cells in the areas of skin rash, suggesting that both the exanthem and enanthem are associated with local viral replication. Large multinucleated epithelial giant cells that show inclusion bodies within the nucleus and cytoplasm can be found during the prodrome and acute stages of illness in the buccal mucosa, pharynx, tracheobronchial mucosa, and occasionally in the urine. In addition, reticuloendothelial giant cells (Warthin-Finkeldey cells) are found in hyperplastic lymphoid tissues, including lymph nodes, tonsils, spleen, and thymus. During the viremic phase measles infects T and B lymphocytes, circulating monocytes, and polymorphonuclear leukocytes without producing lytic changes. There are transient suppression of immunoglobulin synthesis, impaired natural killer cell activity, and diminished capability of polymorphonuclear leukocytes to generate oxygen radicals. The epithelium of the respiratory passages may become necrotic and slough off, leading to secondary bacterial infection; interstitial pneumonia with giant cell infiltration may be observed. Changes in the brain of patients with encephalitis resemble those seen in other postviral encephalitides and consist of focal hemorrhage, congestion, and perivenous demyelination. The pathogenesis is probably similar to experimental allergic encephalomyelitis.

MANIFESTATIONS   The time from exposure to the development of the first symptoms of measles infection is usually 9 to 11 days, and from exposure to the appearance of rash about 2 weeks. The initial manifestations of the disease are malaise, irritability, fever as high as 40.6°C (105°F), conjunctivitis with excessive lacrimation, edema of the eyelids and photophobia, moderately severe hacking cough, and nasal discharge. The prodromal period usually lasts 3 to 4 days, with a range of 1 to 8 days before the onset of a rash. Koplik's spots—small, red, irregular lesions with blue-white centers—appear 1 or 2 days before the onset of the rash on the mucous membranes of the mouth and occasionally on the conjunctiva or intestinal mucosa. The findings of the prodromal illness subside or disappear within 1 or 2 days after the appearance of skin lesions, although the cough may persist throughout the course of the disease.

The red maculopapular rash of measles breaks out first on the forehead, spreads downward over the face, neck, and trunk, and appears on the feet on the third day. The density of lesions is greatest on the forehead, face, and shoulders, where coalescence of individual spots usually occurs. The lesions in each area persist for about 3 days and disappear in the same order in which they appeared, resulting in total duration of rash of about 6 days. As the maculopapules fade, a brown discoloration of the skin may be noticed, and finely granular desquamation may occur. In adults the duration of fever may be longer, the rash more prominent, and the incidence of complications higher.

The course of measles can be altered by the administration of gamma globulin soon after exposure. The incubation period may be prolonged for as long as 20 days. The prodromal period of the modified disease may be shorter; the fever, respiratory symptoms, and conjunctivitis milder; and the rash less marked; Koplik's spots may not be present. Rarely, an atypical, severe form of measles is seen in some persons who received inactivated measles vaccine several years before exposure. The prodromal period with prominent fever, headache, myalgias, and abdominal pain lasts for 1 or 2 days and is followed by an eruption which may be urticarial, maculopapular, hemorrhagic, and/or vesicular. In contrast to natural measles, the rash begins on the hands and feet and progresses toward the head. The rash is especially prominent on the legs and in the body creases. Peripheral edema and pneumonia have been prevalent in this form of atypical measles. The pneumonia is lobar or segmental; hilar lymphadenopathy and pleural effusion are frequent. Ill-defined nodular shadows may persist at the periphery of the lung for as long as 1 to 2 years.

COMPLICATIONS   Measles, usually a benign self-limited disease, may be complicated by a number of illnesses. Viral involvement of the respiratory tract may lead to croup, bronchitis, bronchiolitis, or rarely to *interstitial giant cell pneumonia,* which is seen most often in children suffering from severe systemic disease such as leukemia, congenital or acquired immunodeficiency, or severe malnutrition, and which is characterized by severe respiratory symptoms, pulmonary infiltrations, and multinucleated giant cells in the pulmonary parenchyma. Pneumonitis may occur in the absence of the typical measles exanthem. _Conjunctivitis_, which is seen regularly in the course of uncomplicated measles, may occasionally progress to corneal ulceration, keratitis, and blindness. _Myocarditis_, characterized by transient changes in the electrocardiogram, occurs in about 20 percent of patients with measles, but clinical evidence of cardiac dysfunction is rare. Viral involvement of the mesenteric lymph nodes and appendix may result in abdominal pain and signs of peritoneal inflammation so severe that surgical exploration is considered. The situation is especially confusing if the evidence of appendiceal involvement becomes manifest during the preeruptive phase of the disease. _Hepatitis_, usually without clinical signs, also frequently occurs. It is usually detected by the presence of a transient elevation of SGOT or SGPT values during the acute phase of illness. _Acute glomerulonephritis_ has also been transiently observed during the acute phase of illness. In adults, mild to moderate hypocalcemia and musculoskeletal symptoms with elevated CPK levels have each been reported to occur in one-third or more of cases. Measles infection of pregnant women results in death of the fetus in about 20 percent of the cases; however, a teratogenic effect such as that observed in rubella has not been demonstrated.

Superimposed bacterial pneumonia caused by streptococci, pneumococci, staphylococci, or _Haemophilus influenzae_ is considerably more common than giant cell pneumonia and occasionally may progress to empyema or lung abscess. Bacterial otitis media is a frequent sequel of measles infection in children. In tropical areas, stomatitis, probably of bacterial origin, progressing to cancrum oris may be encountered during the course of the disease.

Clinically apparent _encephalomyelitis_ occurs in 1 of 1000 patients with measles. It usually begins 4 to 7 days after the appearance of the eruption, but may precede the rash by 10 days or follow it by 24 days. It is characterized by high fever, headache, drowsiness, and coma, and in some patients by focal brain or spinal cord involvement. Death occurs in about 10 percent of affected individuals, and persistent signs of central nervous system damage, including mental changes, epilepsy, and paralysis, are encountered. Electroencephalographic abnormalities without other signs of central nervous system dysfunction may be demonstrated in 50 percent of patients with otherwise uncomplicated measles. A progressive, fatal encephalitis has been described in children with lymphatic malignancies treated with immunosuppressive drugs, with onset 1 to 6 months after an episode of measles. Other, more unusual neurologic complications include transverse myelitis and ascending myelitis. An extremely rare condition, _subacute sclerosing panencephalitis_ (see Chap. 355), is probably a late complication of measles. _Thrombocytopenia_ may occur 3 to 15 days after the onset of symptoms and results in purpura as well as bleeding from mouth, intestine, and genitourinary tract. Measles is also associated with transient suppression of delayed hypersensitivity to tuberculin, exacerbation of existing tuberculosis, and an increased incidence of new tuberculous infections.

LABORATORY FINDINGS Leukopenia is frequent in the prodromal phase of measles, and the appearance of leukocytosis suggests bacterial superinfection or another complication. Extreme lymphopenia (less than 2000 lymphocytes per microliter) is considered to be a poor prognostic sign. During the prodrome and in the early eruptive phase, multinucleated giant cells can be identified in stained preparations of sputum, nasal secretions, or urine, and the measles virus can be isolated by inoculation of the same materials onto appropriate cell cultures. Measles antigen can often be detected quickly by fluorescent antibody staining of infected respiratory or urinary epithelial cells. Complement fixation, enzyme immunoassay, immunofluorescent, and hemagglutination inhibition tests are available for serologic confirmation of measles. Spinal fluid protein of patients with encephalomyelitis ranges from 48 to 240 mg/dL, and lymphocyte counts are usually in a range of 5 to 99 per microliter, although counts as high as 1000 per microliter have been reported. Bacterial infection can be identified by appropriate cultures.

DIFFERENTIAL DIAGNOSIS With its prodrome, Koplik's spots, and characteristic rash, measles is infrequently confused with other diseases. Rubella is a milder disease of shorter duration with mild or no respiratory complaints. Infectious mononucleosis and toxoplasmosis can be identified by the presence of atypical lymphocytes and by serologic tests. Secondary syphilis may show skin lesions similar to the measles rash. Other infections which can sometimes mimic measles include those caused by adenoviruses, enteroviruses, _Mycoplasma pneumoniae_, _Staphylococcus aureus_ (toxic shock syndrome), and _Streptococcus pyogenes_ (scarlet fever). Drug reactions, particularly those associated with ampicillin and phenytoin, and Kawasaki syndrome can also produce a morbilliform rash. The atypical form of measles in patients previously immunized with inactivated vaccine may suggest Rocky Mountain spotted fever, varicella, scarlet fever, or meningococcemia.

PROPHYLAXIS Measles can be prevented by the administration of 0.25 mL/kg gamma globulin within 6 days of exposure. Passive immunization should be considered for any susceptible person exposed to the disease, but is especially important for children under 3 years of age, for pregnant women, for patients with tuberculosis, and for those patients in whom immune mechanisms are impaired. In this instance, a dose of 0.5 mL/kg gamma globulin (maximum of 15 mL) may be necessary. Prophylactic administration of antibiotics does not decrease the frequency or severity of bacterial superinfections.

Active immunity can be induced by the use of live, attenuated measles virus without spread to contacts of vaccinated individuals. Attenuated vaccine (Schwarz, Attenuvax) is associated with few local or systemic reactions. Vaccination induces antibody formation in more than 95 percent of susceptible individuals inoculated at age 15 months or older. The vaccine can induce protection if given before, or within 3 days after, exposure. Vaccination results in protection for at least 23 years, but the total duration of immunity is not known. Live measles vaccine should not be given to pregnant women, to patients with untreated tuberculosis, to patients with leukemia or lymphoma, or to those whose immune responsiveness is depressed. All children infected with human immunodeficiency virus should be immunized on schedule; the degree of protection is uncertain. Hypersensitivity reactions to the vaccine even among egg-sensitive individuals have been rare; however, the vaccine should not be given to persons known to be hypersensitive to vaccine components, such as trace amounts of antibiotics, and extreme caution should be observed in persons with a history of anaphylactic reactions following egg ingestion. Except in unusual circumstances, vaccination should not be given in the first 13 months of life. However, if epidemiologic circumstances suggest a risk to infants less than 15 months of age (where risk is defined as a county reporting more than 5 cases of measles among preschool-aged children each of the previous 5 years), the following is recommended: monovalent vaccine at 9 months of age or the first visit thereafter, followed by a dose of mumps-measles-rubella vaccine at 15 months of age. Measles vaccination has been very effective in decreasing the incidence of infection in the United States without producing serious side effects; however, there have been vaccine failures. These failures are related, in part, to early vaccination of infants who still have maternal neutralizing antibody, and perhaps to less-than-optimal vaccine storage and handling. There is evidence that vaccine manufactured before a new stabilizer was used in 1979 may have greater lability. It is therefore recommended that school-outbreak control measures include revaccination of all persons who received their most recent vaccination before 1980. If this is not practical, children vaccinated before 15 months of age should be revaccinated.

There is no indication for the use of _inactivated_ vaccine because of severe atypical measles, which has been observed in persons immunized with it (see "Manifestations" above).

TREATMENT No therapy is indicated for uncomplicated measles. Gamma globulin, although effective in prophylaxis, is of no value once symptoms are evident. In countries where nutritional deficiencies are common, vitamin A supplementation on two successive days as soon as measles is diagnosed may reduce delayed mortality and blindness. Patients should be monitored for the development of bacterial superinfections, which require appropriate antibiotics on the basis of clinical and bacteriologic findings.

REFERENCES

Bloch AB et al: Measles outbreak in a pediatric practice: Airborne transmission in an office setting. Pediatrics 75:676, 1985

Centers for Disease Control: Measles prevention. Recommendation of the Immunization Practices Advisory Committee. Morb Mort Week Rep 36:409, 1987
   · Measles prevention: Supplementary statement. Morb Mort Week Rep 38:11, 1989

Fulginiti VA, Helfer RE: Atypical measles in adolescent siblings 16 years after killed measles virus vaccine. JAMA 244:804, 1980

Gavish D et al: Hepatitis and jaundice associated with measles in young adults. Arch Intern Med 143:674, 1983

Giladi M et al: Measles in adults: A prospective study of 291 consecutive cases. Brit Med J 295:1314, 1987

Gustafson TL et al: Measles outbreak in a fully immunized secondary-school population. N Engl J Med 317:771, 1987

Johnson RT et al: Measles encephalomyelitis—clinical and immunologic studies. N Engl J Med 310:137, 1984

Krause PH et al: Epidemic measles in young adults. Ann Intern Med 90:873, 1979

Lampe RM et al: Measles reimmunization in children immunized before 1 year of age. Am J Dis Child 139:33, 1985

Markowitz LE et al: Patterns of transmission in measles outbreaks in the United States, 1985–1986. N Engl J Med 320:75, 1989

Moench TR et al: Acute measles in patients with and without neurological involvement: Distribution of measles virus antigen and RNA. J Infect Dis 158:433, 1988

Mouallem M et al: Measles epidemic in young adults. Arch Intern Med 147:1111, 1987

Vitamin A for measles, editorial. Lancet 1:1067, 1987

142 RUBELLA ("GERMAN MEASLES") AND OTHER VIRAL EXANTHEMS

C. GEORGE RAY

RUBELLA

DEFINITION Rubella ("German measles," "3-day measles") is usually a benign febrile exanthem, but when it occurs in pregnant women it may lead to serious chronic fetal infection and malformations.

ETIOLOGY In the late 1930s and 1940s rubella was transmitted to humans and monkeys, and in 1962 a viral agent was recovered in cell cultures inoculated with nasopharyngeal secretions of infected persons. The rubella virion, 60 to 70 nm in diameter, is a somewhat spheroidal RNA virus which has been classified in the togavirus family.

PATHOGENESIS AND PATHOLOGY Rubella can be induced in susceptible persons by the instillation of virus into the nasopharynx, and natural infection is probably induced in the same way. Virus is present in blood, throat washings, and occasionally feces for several days before the exanthem becomes apparent. It can be detected in blood for 1 to 2 days, and in throat washings for as long as 7 days before appearance of rash, to 2 weeks after onset. Lymph nodes show edema and hyperplasia.

Congenital rubella results from transplacental transmission of virus to the fetus from an infected mother, and may be associated with growth retardation, infiltration of liver and spleen by hematopoietic tissue, interstitial pneumonia, a decreased number of megakaryocytes in the bone marrow, and various structural malformations of the cardiovascular and central nervous systems. The virus can persist in the fetus during intrauterine life and may be excreted for 6 to 31 months after birth.

EPIDEMIOLOGY Rubella is not as contagious as measles, and immunity to the disease is not so widespread. Estimates of susceptibility to rubella among unimmunized women of childbearing age range from 10 to 25 percent. Before the routine introduction of vaccine in 1969, epidemics occurred at 6- to 9-year intervals; however, this cyclical pattern is no longer seen. In 1964 more than 1.8 million cases of rubella were reported in the United States; in 1986, only 551 cases, an all-time low, were reported. Rubella was once most frequent among children 5 to 9 years of age, but with the advent of immunization programs often directed primarily at this age group as well as at preschoolers, a greater proportion of cases is now being reported among older schoolchildren (15 to 19 years) and young adults (20 to 24 years).

MANIFESTATIONS The time from exposure to the appearance of the rash of rubella is 14 to 21 days, usually about 18 days. In adults there may be a prodromal illness preceding the exanthem by 1 to 7 days. The prodrome consists of malaise, headache, fever, mild conjunctivitis, and lymphadenopathy. In children the rash may be the first manifestation of disease. It is apparent from serologic studies that 25 to 50 percent of infections are subclinical, or may result in only lymph node enlargement without skin lesions; however, rash without lymphadenopathy is uncommon. Respiratory symptoms are mild or absent. Small, red lesions (Forchheimer's spots) occasionally may be seen on the soft palate but are not pathognomonic of the disease.

The rash begins on the forehead and face and spreads downward to the trunk and extremities. The small maculopapular lesions, of lighter hue than those of measles, are usually discrete but may coalesce to form a diffuse erythema suggestive of scarlet fever. The rash may last from 1 to 5 days, but is most commonly present for 3 days. Enlarged, tender lymph nodes appear before the rash, are most impressive during the early eruptive phase, and may persist several days after the rash has disappeared. Splenomegaly or generalized lymphadenopathy may occur, but the postauricular and suboccipital nodes are most strikingly involved. Arthralgias and slight joint swellings may be a complication of rubella, especially in young women. The pain and swelling, involving wrists, fingers, and knees, are most marked during the period of rash and may persist for 1 to 14 days after other manifestations of rubella have disappeared. Recurring joint symptoms for a year or more have also been reported. Purpura with or without thrombocytopenia may occur and may be associated with hemorrhage. Encephalomyelitis following rubella resembles other postinfectious encephalitides and is much less common than encephalitis following measles. Testicular pain is also occasionally reported in young adults.

Congenital rubella The syndrome of congenital rubella has conventionally been thought to consist of heart malformations—patent ductus arteriosus, interventricular septal defect, or pulmonic stenosis; eye lesions—corneal clouding, cataracts, chorioretinitis, and microphthalmia; microcephaly; mental retardation; and deafness. In the American epidemic of 1964, thrombocytopenic purpura, hepatosplenomegaly, intrauterine growth retardation, interstitial pneumonia, myocarditis or myocardial necrosis, and metaphyseal bone lesions were encountered frequently in association with the previously recognized manifestations, leading to the term *expanded rubella syndrome*. Some infants have also been found to have significant humoral and/or cellular immunodeficiency, which generally resolves as chronic viral excretion diminishes and eventually ceases. Any combination of lesions may be seen in an individual infant, and the severity is highly variable.

Later complications include an apparent higher risk of subsequent development of diabetes mellitus. There are reports of patients with congenital rubella who develop a progressive, subacute panencephalitis, with onset in the second decade of life. It is characterized by intellectual deterioration, ataxia, seizures, and spasticity. T-cell abnormalities occur persisting into adulthood and are characterized by slightly decreased T4/T8 ratios and other minor subset defects.

Congenital rubella is usually the result of maternal infection during the first trimester of pregnancy, although well-documented cases have resulted from infection several days before conception; deafness may occur as a result of infection in the fourth month. The greatest risk to the fetus is when maternal infection develops 3 to 6 weeks after conception. Serologically identified, asymptomatic maternal rubella can also result in severe fetal disease. It is therefore desirable to ascertain the immune status of every woman, either before conception or as early in the pregnancy as possible, by history of previous immunization or by serologic testing. If rubella antibodies are present before or within 10 days after exposure, the patient is considered immune, and the risk of fetal damage is virtually nil. If antibodies are not detectable and exposure has occurred, acute and convalescent antibody titers should be determined simultaneously on serums obtained 2 to 4 weeks apart, depending upon the time after exposure when the acute sample was drawn.

DIAGNOSIS Rubella is frequently confused with other diseases associated with maculopapular exanthems, with infectious mononucleosis (see Chap. 137), as well as with drug eruptions and scarlet fever. *A certain diagnosis of rubella can be made only by virus isolation and identification, or by changes in antibody titers.* Rubella hemagglutination-inhibiting antibodies may be present by the second day of rash and increase in quantity over the next 10 to 21 days. Other serologic tests which are used for diagnosis or determination of immunity include complement fixation (CF), enzyme-linked immunosorbentassay (ELISA), fluorescence immunoassay (FIA), radioimmunoassay (RIA), and a variety of IgM-specific antibody tests. In addition, there are several inexpensive and rapid semiquantitative screening tests to determine immunity: latex agglutination, passive hemagglutination (PHA), and single radial hemolysis. Antibodies detected by ELISA, FIA, and RIA tend to parallel the hemagglutination-inhibiting antibodies, while the appearance of CF antibody lags behind the others by a period of 3 to 7 days and often does not disappear until 1 or 2 years after infection. The PHA antibody first appears even later (14 to 21 days after rash onset), but persists thereafter. The presence of IgM-specific antibodies suggests recent rubella infection (within 2 months); however, they have been known to persist as long as 1 year in some cases. There are no other laboratory findings helpful in the diagnosis of rubella, although lymphocytosis with atypical lymphocytes may occur.

Patients with the congenital rubella syndrome may lose antibodies at age 3 or 4 years. Therefore a negative serologic test in a child over 3 years does not exclude the possibility of congenital rubella. Congenital rubella should be differentiated by appropriate serologic tests from congenital syphilis (see Chap. 128), toxoplasmosis (see Chap. 162), and cytomegalic inclusion virus disease (see Chap. 138). IgM-specific antibodies are often found early in the first year of life in infants with congenital rubella, but virus isolation is the most reliable way to confirm the diagnosis.

PREVENTION In adults and children rubella is usually a mild disease with infrequent complications. However, the severity of congenital infection has prompted efforts to prevent the disease. Administration of gamma globulin to exposed persons can abort the clinical disease, but seroconversion and transmission of the disease from mother to fetus may occur despite the administration of large amounts of gamma globulin soon after exposure.

Active immunization with live attenuated rubella vaccines has been practiced in this country since 1969, especially among young children. The aim has been to decrease the frequency of the infection in the population and to decrease the chance that susceptible pregnant women will be exposed. Because of concern for a possibly enlarging pool of susceptible adolescents and adults, there has been increasing enthusiasm for serologic screening of pubertal females with no history of immunization, followed by selective immunization of those who are seronegative, with appropriate precautions, as noted below. Persons working in hospitals or clinics who might contract rubella from infected patients or who, if infected, might transmit the infection to pregnant patients should be required to have proof of immunity (either documented immunization or presence of serum antibody).

The attenuated virus can be detected in the respiratory secretions of vaccinees for as long as 4 weeks after immunization, but transmission to other susceptible individuals rarely, if ever, occurs, even in households where susceptible pregnant women are in contact with children who are being vaccinated. The vaccine induces detectable antibodies that persist for at least 16 years and probably longer, in about 95 percent of recipients. After heavy exposure in closed populations, vaccinated individuals sometimes develop subclinical infections (diagnosed by antibody rises and virus isolation). However, viremia has not been demonstrated in immunized persons, which suggests that previously vaccinated pregnant women will not infect their fetuses even if they acquire subclinical rubella.

Side effects of fever, rash, lymphadenopathy, polyneuropathy, or arthralgias occur very seldom in vaccinated children; joint pain and swelling or paresthesias are seen in less than 2 percent of women with vaccines prepared in human embryonic fibroblast cell cultures (RA 27/3 vaccine). The joint symptoms usually begin 1 to 3 weeks after vaccination, and may be confused with other forms of arthritis. *Rubella vaccine must never be given to pregnant women or to those who may become pregnant within 3 months of immunization.* Although no infant with the congenital rubella syndrome has been reported to have been born to a woman inadvertently vaccinated during pregnancy, the theoretical risk of vaccine virus–induced fetal damage remains. Vaccine is contraindicated in patients with immune-deficiency diseases other than children with HIV infection or who are taking immunosuppressive drugs.

OTHER VIRAL EXANTHEMS

In addition to the diseases such as measles, rubella, and chickenpox which historically have been associated with prominent skin lesions there are other virus infections in which skin manifestations may occur. Table 142-1 lists the most commonly recognized causes of maculopapular eruptions. Some of them, particularly the enteroviruses, can also occasionally cause papulovesicular or petechial rashes; others are capable of provoking erythema multiforme–like eruptions. One helpful aspect of the physical examination is the observation that viral-caused maculopapular (not vesicular) exanthems usually *relatively* spare the palms and soles. This is in contrast to eruptions associated with drug reactions, bacteria, *Mycoplasma,* and *Rickettsia,* in which a prominent palmar or plantar eruption is often noted.

EXANTHEM SUBITUM (ROSEOLA INFANTUM) Exanthem subitum is a benign disease of infants 6 months to 4 years of age that is characterized by a high fever and rash. The disease can be transmitted to humans and monkeys by the transfer of blood obtained from a patient during the first few days of illness. Several different agents, such as enteroviruses and adenoviruses, may produce a similar illness; however, human herpesvirus type 6 (HHV-6) has also been implicated as a major cause. The first manifestations of disease, after an estimated incubation period of 5 to 15 days, are the abrupt onset of irritability and fever, which last for 3 to 5 days; the temperature may be as high

TABLE 142-1 Causes of maculopapular eruptions

Viral	Other
Measles	*Mycoplasma pneumoniae*
Rubella	Syphilis
Exanthem subitum	Typhoid fever
Erythema infectiosum: human parvovirus B19	Bacterial toxins: streptococci and staphylococci
Enteroviruses: coxsackievirus, echovirus	Rat-bite fever
Infectious mononucleosis	*Rickettsia*
Adenoviruses	Live-virus vaccines
Reoviruses	Drug eruptions
Arboviruses	Mucocutaneous lymph node syndrome

as 40.6°C (105°F). There may be mild pharyngitis and slight lymph node enlargement; convulsions may occur during the height of the fever. On the fourth to fifth day of illness, there is a sudden drop in temperature to normal or below normal; several hours before or after defervescence the rash suddenly and surprisingly appears. It is characterized by faint 2- to 3-mm macules or maculopapules over the neck and trunk and may extend to the thighs and buttocks; it may last for only a few hours or may be present for a day or two. Leukopenia is frequently noted later in the febrile period. The disease is benign and not associated with complications, although rarely an infant may show sequelae as a result of febrile convulsions. In the early, preeruptive phase, the disease may be difficult to differentiate from an acute bacteremia, particularly from one associated with *Streptococcus pneumoniae.* Though a leukocytosis with an increase in band forms is often seen in bacteremias presenting in this fashion, blood cultures are necessary to make the diagnosis.

ERYTHEMA INFECTIOSUM (FIFTH DISEASE) Erythema infectiosum is a mild febrile exanthematous disease with little or no prodrome. The mean incubation period is estimated as approximately 4 to 12 days (median 7 days). The first manifestations are low-grade fever with varying degrees of conjunctivitis, upper respiratory complaints, cough, myalgia, itching, nausea, and diarrhea, followed in many cases by the appearance of indurated, confluent erythema over the cheeks, giving a "slapped face" appearance. A day or so later, a bilaterally symmetric eruption is seen on the arms, legs, and trunk, but rarely on the palms or soles. The lesions are maculopapular and tend to be confluent, forming slightly raised blotchy areas and reticular or lacy patterns. When it occurs, the rash usually lasts about a week, and during this time it may disappear, only to reappear in the same areas a few hours later. The waxing and waning eruption may occasionally persist for several weeks, and can be brought on by fever, heat, exercise, sunlight exposure, or emotional stress. Occasionally a hemorrhagic exanthem and enanthem with pustules and pseudopustules occur. Mild joint pain and swelling have been observed in a large proportion of adults with the disease, and some have had symptoms lasting from a few months to over 4 years. Some adults have had transient elevations in rheumatoid factor or ANA antibody tests. Erythema infectiosum affects all ages but is most common in children of school age and may occur in epidemic form. The etiologic agent has now been identified as a human parvovirus (B19) which also is considered to be the primary cause of aplastic crises in patients with chronic hemolytic anemias such as sickle cell disease and hereditary spherocytosis. This may be a result of the fact that the site of replication is the nucleus of an immature cell in the erythrocyte lineage, resulting in an impairment of normal erythrocyte development. Like rubella, active transplacental transmission of B19 virus can occur during primary infections, sometimes resulting in severe fetal anemia with hydrops fetalis. The frequency of this occurrence is as yet undetermined. The route of transmission of the natural disease is probably respiratory. Subclinical infection is common. Antibody to the virus has been demonstrated in 30 to 50 percent of healthy adults. Specific diagnosis is accomplished by detection of the virus particles in early acute-phase serum by electron microscopy, by demonstration of specific viral DNA in serum or pharyngeal secretions, or, more commonly, by detection of IgM-specific antibodies in sera collected in the acute or early convalescent phase of illness. A clinical diagnosis of this disease should be made with caution, since rubella and some enteroviruses have also been shown at times to cause a nearly identical syndrome.

ENTEROVIRAL EXANTHEMS Many individual enteroviruses have been associated with rash. Of these, polioviruses are rarely implicated. More commonly, echovirus serotypes 1 through 7, 9, 11, 12, 14, 16, 18, 19, 20, 25, and 30, coxsackievirus serotypes A4, A5, A6, A9, A10, A16, and B2, B3, and B5 have all been implicated. With the exception of hand-foot-and-mouth disease, usually associated with coxsackievirus A16 or enterovirus 71 infection (see Chap. 144), there is no set of clinical or epidemiologic features that aids in differentiating the specific enteroviral agent involved in a specific

case. All are capable of producing maculopapular rashes which vary in intensity and duration, and can also occasionally produce petechial or papulovesicular exanthems and enanthems. In community and household outbreaks, younger children and infants are usually more likely to have exanthems, while other features of enteroviral infection, such as fever, myalgia, and aseptic meningitis, are more prominent among older children and young adults. Two enterovirus serotypes that have been particularly associated with outbreaks of febrile exanthems are echoviruses 9 and 16.

REFERENCES

ANDERSON MJ et al: Experimental parvoviral infection in humans. J Infect Dis 152:257, 1985

ASANO Y et al: Viremia and neutralizing antibody response in infants with exanthem subitum. J Pediatr 114:535, 1989

CENTERS FOR DISEASE CONTROL: Risks associated with human parvovirus B19 infection. Morb Mort Week Rep 38:81, 1989

CHU SY et al: Rubella antibody persistence after immunization. JAMA 259:3133, 1988

CLARKE WL et al: Autoimmunity in congenital rubella syndrome. J Pediatr 104:370, 1984

ENDERS G et al: Outcome of confirmed periconceptional rubella. Lancet 1:1445, 1988

HERRMANN KL: Available rubella serologic tests. Rev Infect Dis 7:S108, 1985

HILL HR, RAY CG: The differential diagnosis of viral exanthems and enanthems, in *Infections in Children,* RJ Wedgwood et al (eds). Philadelphia, Harper & Row, 1982, p 235

KONNEY JS et al: Risk of adverse outcomes of pregnancy after human parvovirus B19 infection. J Infect Dis 157:663, 1988

KURTZMAN GJ et al: Chronic bone marrow failure due to persistent B19 parvovirus infection. N Engl J Med 317:287, 1987

NAIDES SJ et al: Human parvovirus B19–induced vesiculopustular skin eruption. Am J Med 84:968, 1988

PLUMMER FA et al: An erythema infectiosum-like illness caused by human parvovirus infection. N Engl J Med 313:74, 1985

RABINOWE SL et al: Congenital rubella. Monoclonal antibody–defined T cell abnormalities in young adults. Am J Med 81:779, 1986

REID DM et al: Human parvovirus-associated arthritis: A clinical and laboratory description. Lancet 1:422, 1985

SEMBLE EL et al: Human parvovirus arthropathy in two adults after contact with childhood erythema infectiosum. Am J Med 83:560, 1987

THURN J: Human parvovirus B19: Historical and clinical review. Rev Infect Dis 10:1005, 1988

TINGLE AJ et al: Failed rubella immunization in adults: Association with immunologic and virological abnormalities. J Infect Dis 151:330, 1985

TOWNSEND JJ et al: Progressive rubella panencephalitis: Late onset after congenital rubella. N Engl J Med 292:990, 1975

143 SMALLPOX, VACCINIA, AND OTHER POXVIRUSES

HARVEY M. FRIEDMAN

INTRODUCTION Poxviruses that infect humans share the common feature of producing cutaneous vesicular eruptions. They are brick-shaped, double-stranded DNA viruses and are the largest of the animal viruses. Human pathogens include variola, vaccinia, monkeypox, cowpox, milker's node virus, and molluscum contagiosum. These viruses can be distinguished from one another by antigenic differences, clinical manifestations of infection, and pox morphology when inoculated onto chick embryo chorioallantoic membranes. Global eradication of smallpox and the concomitant reduction in smallpox vaccination programs have changed the epidemiology of variola and vaccinia and modified their importance in modern medicine.

SMALLPOX

DEFINITION Smallpox (variola major) is a highly contagious disease characterized by fever, a vesicular and pustular eruption, and a high mortality rate. A milder form (variola minor) may be caused by the same virus.

The global eradication of smallpox was officially announced in 1979, marking one of the greatest achievements of modern medicine. Over the past decade, smallpox has not reappeared. If this pattern persists, a disease that once accounted for 10 percent of all deaths will become an illness mainly of historical interest. Although smallpox may eventually disappear as a topic in future editions of textbooks of medicine, it seems prudent to continue to be prepared to recognize the disease and prevent its spread.

ETIOLOGY Variola virus, the causative agent of smallpox, is an orthopoxvirus within the Poxviridae family. Variola is a large (200 to 400 nm) DNA virus differing from other DNA viruses in that it lacks icosahedral symmetry. When viewed by electron microscopy it has a complex structure and appears brick-shaped. It has an outer membrane, two lateral bodies, and a dumbbell-shaped core that contains a single molecule of double-stranded DNA.

PATHOGENESIS AND PATHOLOGY The oropharynx of infected patients serves as the main source for virus spread. Contacts become infected by inhaling virus which enters the respiratory tract and multiplies locally, probably within macrophages. Virus is carried within macrophages into the circulation and to regional lymph nodes. Multiplication occurs within lymphoid organs and a secondary viremia develops. Virus localizes within small dermal blood vessels, leading to dilatation of capillaries, endothelial swelling, and mononuclear cell infiltration. Epidermal cells enlarge, and intraepidermal vesicles form in skin and mucous membranes. The vesicles rupture to form shallow ulcers, while the epidermal cells enlarge and extend into the corium. When stained with hematoxylin and eosin, the cytoplasm of infected cells contains faintly basophilic or acidophilic inclusions (Guarnieri bodies). Infiltration by granulocytes changes the vesicle into a pustule, which heals either by rupture or resorption. Extension of infection into the corium and sebaceous glands produces pockmarks, or scars, which, upon healing, are characteristic of smallpox infection. Focal infiltration of the liver, spleen, and lymph nodes with macrophages may occur.

Virus infection stimulates cytotoxic T-cell responses, neutralizing antibodies, and the production of interferons. These responses restrict viral replication and induce prolonged immunity if the patient recovers. The infection is likely to be most severe in impaired hosts, particularly those with T-cell deficits. Milder forms of the infection have been observed in immunized patients, although it remains unclear why variola minor may be produced by the same virus in the unimmunized.

EPIDEMIOLOGY Smallpox was described in Asia during the first century A.D. and in Europe and Africa around 700 A.D. Infection was carried to Central, South, and North America during the sixteenth and seventeenth centuries. Endemic variola major was eradicated from the United States in 1926, and variola minor during the 1940s. Eradication was slower in Asia, Africa, and parts of the Americas. The last naturally occurring smallpox infection occurred in Somalia, Africa, in October 1977. The last known case developed 1 year later in Birmingham, England, in September 1978 and was the result of a laboratory accident. Over the past decade smallpox has not reappeared. The ability to eradicate this disease by an effective worldwide vaccination program appears to be centrally related to the facts that man was the only known reservoir for the variola virus; that no asymptomatic carrier state existed, facilitating surveillance; and that early diagnosis and prevention of disease or modification of the course by rapid vaccination of contacts were possible.

In temperate climates, endemic smallpox occurred in winter and spring. It was mainly a disease of children and young adults. Spread in unvaccinated family contacts was approximately 58 percent compared with 4 percent in vaccinees. Patients were usually severely ill and confined to bed, which restricted transmission to immediate family contacts. Index cases rarely infected more than five patients, most commonly those sharing living quarters. Transmission intervals were 2 to 3 weeks apart, and new cases would appear in a community or region over many months.

CLINICAL FEATURES Smallpox was endemic in every country of the world and existed as two forms, variola major, which was a serious illness with a mortality rate of >20 percent in the unvaccinated, and variola minor, which was a milder infection with a mortality of <1 percent. Both were caused by the same virus. On an individual case basis, it may be difficult to distinguish variola minor from a mild case of variola major. The severity of an entire outbreak is generally required to differentiate the two. The evolution of rash in variola minor is more rapid, similar to accelerated smallpox.

Variola major has been classified into five clinical categories:

1 *Ordinary type:* This comprised >70 percent of cases. It is characterized by raised pustular skin lesions which can be divided into three categories: (a) *Confluent* rash present on face and forearms; (b) *semiconfluent* rash present on face with discrete rash elsewhere; (c) *discrete* rash on all involved areas with normal skin between pustules. In unvaccinated patients, mortality was 62 percent for confluent infection, 37 percent for semiconfluent, and 9 percent for discrete infection.

2 *Modified type:* This form of smallpox is similar to ordinary disease, except that the course is accelerated, and pustular lesions are smaller. Modified smallpox was common in vaccinated patients who developed lesions, in health care workers exposed by accidental inoculation, and in those intentionally infected by variolation, a procedure once widely used as a method of vaccination.

3 *Variola sine eruptione:* Patients have fever but no rash. This was seen in vaccinated patients or those previously infected. Laboratory testing is required for confirmation of the diagnosis.

4 *Flat type:* Pustules remain flat and are usually confluent or semiconfluent in distribution. This form of infection occurred mainly in children and was often fatal.

5 *Hemorrhagic type:* Skin lesions and mucous membranes become hemorrhagic. Pregnant women were predisposed to this form of smallpox, which was rare but severe. Profound prostration, heart failure, diffuse bleeding, and bone marrow suppression resulted, and most infections were fatal within 3 to 4 days, earning the name "sledgehammer smallpox."

In a typical case of ordinary type smallpox, the incubation period is 7 to 19 days, with a mean of 12. A preeruptive phase lasting 2 to 4 days is characterized by sudden onset of fever, severe headache, backache, and malaise. Vomiting occurs in 50 percent, and diarrhea in 10 percent of patients. The rash first appears as minute red spots on the tongue and palate and as small macules (herald spots) on the face. Spread is centrifugal, involving the face, proximal extremities, trunk, and then distal extremities. Intraoral rash evolves from papules to vesicles, which break down and release large amounts of virus. The enanthem is an important source of virus spread. On the skin, macules evolve to papules by day 2, vesicles by days 4 to 5, and pustules by day 7 of rash. Fever may recur during the pustular phase. Lesions, which range from few to thousands, have a shotty, hard feel to them. Crusts develop by day 14 and heal leaving depigmented areas.

LABORATORY FINDINGS **Virus isolation** Virus can be isolated from skin lesions (until scabs form), oropharynx, conjunctiva, and urine. Viremia precedes the rash and clears in most patients when the rash appears. Virus particles can be seen by negative-staining electron microscopy performed on fluid obtained from skin lesions. This form of diagnosis was used to identify cases during the intensified eradication programs carried out in the 1960s and 1970s.

Serology Antibodies appear by days 6 to 8 of infection. Antibody titer rises can be detected by testing paired serum samples drawn 2 to 3 weeks apart. Various methods have been used to measure antibodies, including hemagglutination inhibition, complement fixation, neutralization, and gel precipitation.

Hematology Granulocytopenia, thrombocytopenia, and lymphocytosis are common during the prodromal and early rash phase. Leukocytosis occurs with pustulation of the vesicles. A profile consistent with disseminated intravascular coagulation is seen in patients with hemorrhagic smallpox.

DIFFERENTIAL DIAGNOSIS Distinguishing varicella from smallpox was particularly difficult during epidemics of variola minor or when mild smallpox infection developed in vaccinated patients. Dense rash on the trunk and appearance of lesions in crops are features of varicella not seen in smallpox. Human monkeypox, seen in western and central Africa, is difficult to distinguish from smallpox. Monkeypox is associated with more lymphadenopathy than smallpox. In the past, virus isolation was required to differentiate the two. On occasion, virus isolation was also required to distinguish disseminated vaccinia infection from smallpox.

COMPLICATIONS AND SEQUELAE Complications include secondary bacterial infections of the skin, keratitis and corneal ulcerations, viral arthritis and osteomyelitis, bacterial pneumonia, orchitis, and encephalitis. Sequelae include blindness from corneal scarring, limb deformities, and pockmarks, which appear hypopigmented in dark-skinned individuals and hyperpigmented in light-skinned patients.

TREATMENT AND OUTCOME In the past, mortality was highest in infants and the elderly. Infection in pregnant women led to abortion rates of >60 percent. Vaccination during the first week of incubation modified the course of disease by protecting many and reducing the severity of infection in others. This constituted an important method for control of smallpox. Immunotherapy with vaccinia immune globulin given during the incubation period of infection modified disease; however, supplies were too limited for this form of therapy to be widely applicable. Several different thiosemicarbazones, a class of antiviral compounds, were tried for treatment, but no benefit was detected in controlled human trials. One thiosemicarbazone, metisazone, was found to be useful as preventive therapy following exposure. Vaccinia immune globulin was also effective in postexposure prophylaxis without the side effects of metisazone. The mainstay of treatment was good nursing care, which was often provided by family members at home or in hospitals.

CONTROL Attempts at control of smallpox began once it was noted that accidental exposure to smallpox by scratch on the skin resulted in less severe infection. This led to the practice of variolation, which began in China and India in the tenth century. Variolation involved intentional administration of pustular fluids or scabs to uninfected persons. In 1796, Edward Jenner showed that inoculation with cowpox virus protected against smallpox and carried less risk of illness than variolation. Subsequently, vaccination was modified to use of vaccinia virus for smallpox control. The origins of vaccinia virus are uncertain, but many strains existed which were apparently derived from either variola or cowpox virus. Successful vaccination provided high levels of protection for 5 years and some protection for 20 years. Periodic revaccination was necessary for optimal protection. Postexposure vaccination lowered the incidence and reduced the severity of infection when administered within 1 week after exposure.

In 1959, the World Health Assembly adopted a program aimed at global eradication of smallpox. The development of stable freeze-dried vaccine meant that vaccination programs could reach less developed tropical countries. Efforts were intensified by 1967 and were built on the principles of surveillance and containment involving case detection, quarantine of infected patients, and vaccination of contacts and others living in the immediate area. Surveillance and contact vaccination were extremely important for the eventual success of the program. This approach was successful because smallpox has a long incubation period that allows vaccination to modify the course of the illness. The lack of a reservoir for variola, other than humans, the ease of clinical diagnosis, and the fact that variola does not establish latent or persistent infection were important contributors to the success of the eradication program.

VACCINIA

DEFINITION AND ETIOLOGY Vaccinia is a localized skin infection caused by inoculation of vaccinia virus. In immunosuppressed patients it may occasionally disseminate and produce severe disease. Vaccinia virus is thought to be derived from either variola, cowpox, or perhaps a hybrid of the two. "Vaccination" with vaccinia induces immunity to variola and was the method used to control or prevent smallpox. Endemic smallpox was eradicated from the United States in 1949, which led to the eventual discontinuation of routine childhood immunization by 1972. Evidence of immunization against smallpox is no longer required for international travel. As a result, physicians today have little experience with vaccinia immunization or its complications.

COMPLICATIONS OF VACCINATION Vaccine is applied to the skin, which is punctured several times by a sterile needle to penetrate the epidermis. Primary vaccination results in formation of a papule in 4 to 5 days that becomes a vesicle 2 to 3 days later. Mild fever and localized lymphadenopathy are often present at this stage. Within 2 weeks a scab forms that leaves a scar when healing is complete. The response during revaccination is accelerated and generally is not associated with fever or lymphadenopathy.

Vaccinia virus never underwent controlled trials to establish safety and efficacy before licensing. Nevertheless, the vaccine was highly effective, despite considerable adverse effects. *Complications* included: (1) *Progressive vaccinia* (vaccinia gangrenosum) developed in patients who were agammaglobulinemic, T-cell deficient, or receiving immunosuppressive therapy. Destruction of local areas of skin, subcutaneous tissue, and other underlying structures occurred, with metastatic lesions appearing at other cutaneous sites and in viscera and bone. This complication developed in approximately 1 patient per million during primary or revaccination and was usually fatal over a period of several months. (2) *Eczema vaccinatum* involved wide cutaneous spread of vaccinia virus in vaccinees and their contacts who had eczema or other chronic skin diseases. It developed in 1 per 100,000 primary vaccinations or 1 per million revaccinations and was sometimes fatal; bacterial superinfection often complicated eczema vaccinatum. (3) *Generalized vaccinia,* characterized by satellite lesions around the inoculation site or more widely disseminated pox, occasionally occurred in immunocompetent individuals and developed in 3 per 100,000 primary vaccinations or 1 per million revaccinations. This complication had a good prognosis. (4) *Accidental inoculation,* especially of eyelids, perineum, and vulva, occurred in 3 per 100,000 to 1 million vaccinees. The consequences were generally not serious. (5) *Postvaccinial encephalitis* was a serious complication which occurred in 3 per 1 million patients after primary vaccination. It usually developed 6 to 15 days after vaccination and had a violent onset. Features included convulsions, hemiplegia, and aphasia. Spinal fluid analysis was normal except for increased pressure. Recovery was often incomplete, and neurologic sequelae ensued.

Contraindications to vaccination include B- or T-cell immune disorders, neoplasms of the reticuloendothelial system, concomitant use of immunosuppressive drugs, eczema, pregnancy, and disorders of the central nervous system. When complications developed due to uncontrolled or progressive vaccinia infection, some were treated effectively with vaccinia immune globulin. This treatment is not effective for postvaccinial encephalitis. A role for antivirals, such as thiosemicarbazones, has not been definitely established.

Interest has reemerged in vaccinia as a vehicle for vaccination. Genes from herpes simplex virus, hepatitis B virus, human immunodeficiency virus, and malaria have been introduced into the vaccinia genome. Proteins encoded by these genes are expressed in vitro during vaccinia infection, which indicates that this virus potentially could serve as a vector for multiple vaccines. Should this approach prove successful, then the same precautions should be followed as in vaccination to prevent smallpox.

OTHER POXVIRUSES

HUMAN MONKEYPOX The monkeypox virus is a member of the orthopox genus. Human monkeypox is a rare zoonosis that occurs in tropical rain forests of west and central Africa. This disease was first recognized in the 1960s during smallpox eradication efforts. Identification resulted from attempts to confirm suspected cases of smallpox by laboratory methods. Infection does not spread from person to person, which accounts for the low number of cases, less than 100, identified so far. The clinical features of infection are similar to smallpox, except that cervical and inguinal lymphadenopathy are more prominent in human monkeypox. The diagnosis can be established by the characteristic pox morphology when virus is inoculated onto chorioallantoic membrane cultures.

COWPOX Cowpox virus is another member of the genus *Orthopoxvirus*. Infection develops by hand contact with infected ulcers on the teats of cows. The virus is also found in wild rodents, which may serve as a reservoir for some human infections. After exposure, one or more skin lesions develop, most often on the hands. The evolution of a lesion is similar to that seen during primary smallpox vaccination: a vesicle progresses to a pustule that later scabs. The rash does not become generalized. It is often associated with lymphangitis and localized lymphadenopathy. The disease may be confused with milker's nodule (see below). Laboratory confirmation can be established by the characteristic pox that develop when virus is isolated on chorioallantoic membranes.

MILKER'S NODE VIRUS This infection is caused by a parapoxvirus and is sometimes referred to as pseudocowpox or paravaccinia. It is acquired by contact with infected cows. Lesions appear as red nodules that progress to firm purple papules. The lack of vesicles or pustules distinguish it from cowpox. Lesions are relatively painless and generally resolve in 4 to 6 weeks.

ORF This is a disease of sheep that is sometimes referred to as contagious pustular dermatitis. It is caused by a parapoxvirus. Human infection is acquired by contact with sheep infected around the mouth, nose, or eyes. Human infection usually occurs at abrasion sites on the hands. Single or multiple painful large vesicles develop and are often associated with lymphadenopathy. Resolution occurs within several weeks.

MOLLUSCUM CONTAGIOSUM This infection occurs only in humans and is caused by an unclassified poxvirus that cannot be cultured in vitro. Lesions occur anywhere on the body, except on the palms and soles, and appear as pearly, flesh-colored, raised, umbilicated nodules 2 to 5 mm in diameter. Lesions develop in crops, are painless, and resolve over a period of weeks to several years. Spread is probably by direct contact, which accounts for the commonly observed genital distribution of lesions in sexually active adults. An increased incidence of molluscum contagiosum is seen in patients infected with the human immunodeficiency virus. No specific therapy is available, although lesions can be removed by curettage.

REFERENCES

Baxby D: The origins of vaccinia virus. J Infect Dis 136:453, 1977

Breman JG, Arita I: The confirmation and maintenance of smallpox eradication. N Engl J Med 303:1263, 1980

Fenner F: Poxviruses, in *Virology*, 2d ed, BN Fields et al (eds). New York, Raven, 1990, pp 2113–2133

Fenner F et al: *Smallpox and Its Eradication*. World Health Organization, Geneva, 1988

Moss B: Poxviridae and their replication, in *Virology*, 2d ed, BN Fields et al (eds). New York, Raven, 1990, pp 2079–2111

144 ENTEROVIRUSES AND REOVIRUSES

C. GEORGE RAY

GENERAL CONSIDERATIONS

Enteroviruses consist of a major subgroup of picornaviruses that include the polioviruses, coxsackieviruses, echoviruses, and more recently discovered agents that are simply designated enteroviruses. The number of serotypes that infect humans is nearly 70, and more are likely to be found in the future. Their name is derived from their ability to infect intestinal tract epithelial and lymphoid tissues and to be shed into the feces.

Enteroviruses can cause paralytic disease, encephalitis and acute aseptic meningitis syndromes, pleurodynia, exanthems, pericarditis, myocarditis, nonspecific febrile illness, and occasional fulminant disease in the newborn. The spectrum of disease may be even broader. Some infections can lead to permanent damage, and others may trigger chronic, active disease processes.

Since these viruses have many features in common, they will first be considered as a group. Some of the special features of important serotypes will be discussed in detail later in this chapter.

CHARACTERISTICS OF ENTEROVIRUSES As a group, the picornaviruses are extremely small (22 to 30 nm in diameter), single-stranded RNA viruses with icosahedral symmetry. In contrast to the rhinoviruses, the enterovirus subgroup is resistant to ether, acid pH (3.0), and bile. Another feature is cationic stability; in the presence of magnesium chloride, the viruses become more resistant to thermal inactivation. They can survive for prolonged periods in sewage and even in chlorinated water if sufficient organic debris is present. Although some of the enterovirus serotypes share antigens, there are no significant serologic relationships between the major classes listed in Table 144-1; however, a single, highly conserved epitope may be shared by virtually all serotypes except enterovirus 72. Genetic variation within specific strains occurs, and mutants which exhibit antigenic drift and altered tropism for specific cell types have been recognized. Definitive identification of isolates usually requires neutralization tests.

Most of these agents can be isolated in primate (human or simian) cell cultures; however, some strains, such as several coxsackievirus group A serotypes, are grown with difficulty in cell cultures, and inoculation of newborn mice may be necessary for detection. Inoculation of newborn mice was one basis for the original classification of group A and B coxsackieviruses. After the mice have been inoculated, at 24 h of age or less, and observed for 2 to 12 days, group A viruses primarily have a widespread, inflammatory, necrotic effect on skeletal muscle, leading to flaccid paralysis and usually death; similar inoculation of group B viruses causes encephalitis, resulting in spasticity and occasionally convulsions. Other organs are variably affected, and histopathologic examination is sometimes helpful in distinguishing the two. Echoviruses and polioviruses rarely have an adverse effect on mice, unless special adaptation procedures are employed. The higher-numbered enteroviruses (types 68 to 72),

TABLE 144-1 Enteroviruses that infect humans

Class	Number of serotypes
Poliovirus	3
Coxsackievirus	
Group A	23*
Group B	6
Echovirus	31
Enterovirus	Types 68–72†

* Includes several subtypes; coxsackievirus A23 is the same as echovirus 9.

† The classification of the more recently described enteroviruses is based on overlapping biologic characteristics. These are identified numerically. Enterovirus 72 is hepatitis A virus.

which have overlapping growth and host characteristics, have been classified separately. Hepatitis A virus has been classified as enterovirus 72 and is discussed in Chap. 252.

Humans are the major natural host for the polioviruses, coxsackieviruses, and echoviruses. There are enteroviruses of other animals with a limited host range that does not appear to extend to humans. Conversely, viruses thought to be identical or related to human enteroviruses have been isolated from dogs and cats. Whether these agents cause disease in these animals is debatable, and there is no evidence of spread from animals to humans.

EPIDEMIOLOGY The enteroviruses have a worldwide distribution, and asymptomatic infection is common. The proportion of infected individuals who will develop illness varies from 2 to 100 percent, depending upon the serotype or strain involved, prior immune status, and the age of the patient. Secondary infections in households are common and range as high as 40 to 70 percent, depending upon factors such as family size, crowding, and sanitary conditions.

There is a seasonal predilection; epidemics are usually observed during the summer and fall. In subtropical and tropical climates, the duration of greatest transmission sometimes extends into the winter. In some years, certain serotypes emerge as dominant strains; they then may wane, only to reappear in epidemics years later. The emergence of dominant serotypes is unpredictable from year to year.

Direct or indirect fecal-oral transmission is considered the most common mode of spread. After infection, the virus persists in the oropharynx for 1 to 4 weeks, and it can be shed in the feces for 1 to 18 weeks. Sewage-contaminated water, contaminated foods, or insect vectors (flies, cockroaches) may occasionally be the source of infection. More commonly, however, spread is directly from person to person. Approximately two-thirds of all isolates are from children 9 years of age or younger.

Incubation periods vary, but relatively short intervals (2 to 10 days) are the rule. Illness is often seen concurrently in more than one family member, and the clinical features may vary within the household.

PATHOGENESIS AND PATHOLOGY After primary replication in the epithelial cells and lymphoid tissues in the upper respiratory and gastrointestinal tracts, viremic spread to other sites can occur. Potential target organs vary according to the virus strain and its tropism, but may include the central nervous system, heart, vascular endothelium, liver, pancreas, gonads, lungs, skeletal muscles, synovial tissues, skin, and mucous membranes. Histopathologic findings include cell necrosis and mononuclear cell inflammatory infiltrates; in the central nervous system, the inflammatory cells are localized most prominently in perivascular sites. The initial tissue damage is thought to result from the lytic cycle of virus replication. Viremia is usually undetectable by the time symptoms appear, and termination of virus replication commences with the appearance of circulating interferon, neutralizing antibody, and mononuclear cell infiltrations of infected tissue. The early antibody response is mainly immunoglobulin M–specific, and usually wanes 6 to 12 weeks after onset to be replaced by IgG-specific antibodies. The important role of antibodies in the termination of infection is supported by persistent enterovirus replication in patients with antibody-deficiency diseases.

Although initial acute tissue damage may be caused by the lytic effects of the virus on the cell, many of the secondary sequelae appear to be immunologically mediated. Enterovirus-caused poliomyelitis, disseminated disease of the newborn, aseptic meningitis, encephalitis, exanthems, and acute respiratory illnesses, thought to represent primary lytic infections, can usually be identified through routine methods of virus isolation and determination of specific antibody titer changes. On the other hand, syndromes such as myopericarditis, nephritis, and myositis have been associated with enteroviruses primarily by serologic evidence, and the use of cDNA probes to detect viral RNA in tissues. Viral isolation is the exception. The pathogenesis of these illnesses may be a cell-mediated immunologic response to tissue injury by the virus or to viral or virus-induced antigens that persist in the affected tissues.

Infection by a specific serotype in an immunologically normal host is followed by a humoral antibody response, which can often be detected by neutralization methods for many years thereafter. There is relative immunity to reinfection by the same serotype; however, reinfection has been reported, usually resulting in subclinical infection or mild illness. Although there is some antigenic sharing between serotypes in some of the enterovirus classes (for example, group B coxsackieviruses), there is no evidence of significant heterotypic immunity to infection by different serotypes.

LABORATORY DIAGNOSIS In acute enteroviral infections, the diagnosis is most readily established by virus isolation from throat swabs, stool or rectal swabs, body fluids, and occasionally tissues. Except in young infants, viremia is usually undetectable by the time symptoms appear. When there is central nervous system involvement, cerebrospinal fluid cultures taken during the acute phase of the disease may be positive in 10 to 85 percent of cases (except in poliovirus infections, in which virus recovery from this site is rare), depending upon the stage of illness and the serotype involved. Direct isolation of virus from affected tissues or body fluids in enclosed spaces (for example, pleural, pericardial, or cerebrospinal fluid) usually confirms the diagnosis. Isolation of an enterovirus from the throat is suggestive of an etiologic association because the virus is usually detectable at this site for only 2 days to 2 weeks after infection; isolation of virus from fecal specimens only must be interpreted more cautiously because asymptomatic shedding from the bowel may persist for as long as 4 months.

The diagnosis may be further supported by a fourfold or greater increase in neutralizing antibody titer in paired acute and convalescent serum samples. This method is expensive and cumbersome, requiring careful selection of serotypes for use as antigens. Serodiagnosis is generally reserved for critical situations in which the etiology is questionable, such as isolation of a virus only from a peripheral source such as the feces, or in illnesses such as myopericarditis, in which the yield on routine culture is low and the number of serotypes that might be expected to be involved is limited. Quantitative interpretations of antibody titers on single serum samples are rarely helpful because of the high prevalence and wide range of titers to different serotypes that can be found in healthy individuals. In acute poliovirus infections, complement-fixing antibody titer determinations on acute and convalescent sera can aid in diagnosis.

White blood cell counts and the erythrocyte sedimentation rates are usually only mildly elevated. If there is necrosis (e.g., liver, lung), a neutrophilic reaction may be noted. Hyperbilirubinemia and elevated transaminase and alkaline phosphatase levels may be seen in patients with hepatitis. Albuminuria often occurs transiently, but hematuria is rare.

PROPHYLAXIS AND TREATMENT Vaccines, which are available only for the prevention of poliovirus infections, will be discussed in detail below. Although proper disposal of feces and careful personal hygiene are recommended, the usual quarantine or isolation measures are relatively ineffective in controlling the spread of enteroviruses in the family or community.

None of the currently available antiviral agents or immune serum globulins has been effective in treatment or prophylaxis of enterovirus infections. The only exception may be the intravenous or intraventricular use of high-titered immunoglobulin in the treatment of chronic enteroviral encephalitis in antibody-deficient patients. Otherwise, treatment is entirely symptomatic and supportive. Glucocorticoids are contraindicated.

POLIOVIRUS INFECTIONS

The most important enteroviruses are the three poliovirus serotypes (types 1, 2, and 3). They first emerged as important causes of disease in developed temperate-zone countries during the latter part of the nineteenth century, and they continue to be a serious public health problem in developing countries.

The particular tropism of polioviruses for the central nervous system, which they usually reach by passage across the blood-CNS barrier, is perhaps favored by reflex dilatation of capillaries supplying the affected motor centers of the anterior horn of the brainstem or spinal cord. An alternate pathway may be via entry into motor neurons at peripheral neuromuscular junctions. Motor neurons are particularly vulnerable to infection and variable degrees of destruction. The histopathologic findings in the brainstem and spinal cord include necrosis of neuronal cells and perivascular "cuffing" by infiltration with mononuclear cells, primarily lymphocytes.

CLINICAL MANIFESTATIONS Most infections (perhaps 90 percent) are either subclinical or extremely mild. When disease does result, the incubation period can be from 4 to 35 days, but is usually between 7 and 14 days. The disease falls into three classes: The first, abortive poliomyelitis, is a nonspecific febrile illness of 2- to 3-day duration with no signs of CNS localization. A second group of patients will additionally develop aseptic meningitis. Recovery is rapid and complete, usually within a few days. The third class, paralytic poliomyelitis, is the major possible outcome of infection and is often preceded by a period of fever and "minor illness." Classically, after several days, symptoms disappear. In 5 to 10 days fever recurs, and signs of meningeal irritation and asymmetric flaccid paralysis ensue. Cramping muscle pain and spasm as well as coarse twitching in affected parts follows. The maximum extent of involvement is apparent within a few days after first paralysis. In children under 5 years, paralysis of one leg is most common. In patients 5 to 15 years of age, weakness of one arm or paraplegia is frequent, while in adults quadriplegia is more likely to occur. Urinary bladder and respiratory muscle dysfunction are also frequent in adults. Encephalitis is rare.

Tendon reflexes are diminished or absent. Sensation is intact, in contrast to the usually symmetric paralysis and mild sensory disturbance of the Guillain-Barré syndrome. Paralysis due to heavy metal poisoning may also be difficult to distinguish clinically from poliomyelitis.

Among paralytic cases, 6 to 25 percent may be bulbar. Myocarditis, hypertension, pulmonary edema, shock, nosocomial gram-negative or staphylococcal pneumonias, urinary tract infections, and emotional problems are among the complications of severe paralytic disease. Treatment is supportive. About 2 to 5 percent of children and 15 to 30 percent of adults with paralyzing infection die. As temporarily damaged neurons regain their function, recovery begins and may continue for as long as 6 months. Paralysis persisting beyond that time is permanent, and may be associated with complaints of severe pain in the affected areas which sometimes recur years after the illness.

Some patients develop progressive muscle weakness, usually beginning 20 to 30 years later. This is called post-poliomyelitis neuromuscular atrophy, or the "post-polio syndrome." Symptoms vary from mild to moderate deterioration of function, with fatigue, joint pain, and weakness that may stabilize or progress to muscle atrophy. It is not considered to be life-threatening. The pathogenesis appears to involve a dysfunction of surviving motor neurons with slow disintegration of axon terminals, leading to late denervation of muscle.

PREVENTION Two types of poliovirus vaccines are currently licensed in the United States: inactivated polio vaccine and live, oral, attenuated virus vaccine. Each contains the three serotypes of poliomyelitis virus.

Inactivated polio vaccine (IPV) remains the only vaccine used in some countries, notably Sweden, Finland, and the Netherlands, and its efficacy has been excellent. The current product is considered safe, with no significant deleterious side effects. In 1987, a more potent IPV, which is produced in human diploid cells, was licensed. This enhanced-potency IPV has been shown to produce 99 to 100 percent seropositivity for all three poliovirus types after two doses in infants. Primary vaccination with three subcutaneous doses (two doses 4 to 8 weeks apart, and the third 6 to 12 months later) is recommended for unimmunized children and adults. A booster dose at the time of school entry is recommended for children. The duration of protection is at least 5 years, and may be considerably longer.

Oral polio vaccine (OPV) is composed of live, attenuated viruses. The vaccine is given as a primary series of three doses (the first two doses usually 6 to 8 weeks apart, and the third 8 to 12 months later) and produces antibodies to all three serotypes in more than 95 percent of recipients. As with IPV, recall boosters are recommended to maintain adequate antibody levels. Like wild poliovirus, OPV viruses infect and replicate in the oropharynx and intestinal tract, and may be shed into the feces for 6 weeks or longer.

One disadvantage of OPV is the remote risk of vaccine-associated paralytic disease in some recipients, such as immunocompromised persons; susceptible adults are at a slightly higher risk than children. The incidence of vaccine-associated paralytic poliomyelitis is estimated at approximately 1 per 2.6 million doses distributed, and one per 520,000 after the first dose. Of the 138 cases of paralytic poliomyelitis reported in the United States from 1973 through 1984, 105 were vaccine-associated (35 in healthy recipients, 50 in close contacts, 14 with immune-deficiency conditions, and 6 with no history of vaccination or contact).

The major advantages of OPV include ease of administration and secondary immunization of nonimmune contacts through shedding of vaccine virus into the intestinal tract, resulting in more widespread immunity in the population. It is also theorized that during outbreaks, transient vaccine virus colonization results in the induction of mucosal immunity (primarily through secretory IgA), which may interfere with subsequent acquisition and spread of wild poliovirus.

The choice between IPV and OPV for routine primary immunization is widely debated; however, it is clear that both are highly effective vaccines, and that routine immunization with one or the other is important in the prevention of disease. Ideally, immunization should commence in infancy. A susceptible adult at risk of exposure to infection because of travel to an endemic area should receive complete immunization. Persons with immunodeficiency or altered immune status should not be exposed to OPV, either directly or by household contact, because of the increased risk of vaccine-associated paralysis.

Although there are no currently recognized areas of wild poliovirus prevalence in the United States, importation of these strains can readily occur from endemic areas in contiguous countries as well as from developing nations abroad. Once introduced into a community, the virus can spread rapidly among susceptible individuals. For this reason, continuing immunization programs are of utmost importance in preventing spread of this disease.

COXSACKIEVIRUSES AND ECHOVIRUSES

The coxsackieviruses and echoviruses are widespread throughout the world. The basic features of their epidemiology and pathogenesis appear to be the same as those of the polioviruses. Unlike polioviruses, they have a greater tendency to affect the meninges and occasionally the cerebrum, and only rarely do they affect anterior horn cells.

The consequences of infection with these agents are highly variable and related only in part to virus subgroup and serotype. Up to 60 percent of infections are subclinical. The main interest in these agents stems from their ability to cause more serious illness, which becomes most evident during epidemics.

Inapparent infection is common, but varies with the infecting strain and the host involved. The manifestations of illness range from mild to lethal and from acute to chronic. Table 144-2 lists the major syndromes and serotypes commonly associated with each. Considerable overlap occurs, however, and it is not surprising to find an enteroviral serotype associated with a specific syndrome which differs from that most often encountered. The group B coxsackieviruses generally have the greatest latitude with regard to tissue tropism.

ASEPTIC MENINGITIS (See Chap. 355) In terms of relative frequency, aseptic meningitis is the most important illness associated

TABLE 144-2 Clinical syndromes reported to be commonly associated with enterovirus serotypes

Syndrome	Coxsackievirus Group A	Group B	Echovirus and enterovirus (E)
Aseptic meningitis, encephalitis	2,4,7,9,10	1,2,3,4,5	4,6,9,11,16,30;E70,E71
Muscle weakness and paralysis (poliomyelitis-like disease)	7,9	2,3,4,5	2,4,6,9,11,30;E71
Cerebellar ataxia	2,4,9	3,4	4,6,9
Generalized disease (infants)	———	1,2,3,4,5	3,6,9,11,14,17,19
Exanthems and enanthems	4,5,6,9,10,16	2,3,4,5	2,4,5,6,9,11,16,18,25;E71
Pericarditis, myocarditis	4,16	2,3,4,5	1,6,8,9,19
Epidemic myalgia (pleurodynia), orchitis	9	1,2,3,4,5	1,6,9
Respiratory symptoms	9,16,21,24	1,3,4,5	4,9,11,20,25
Conjunctivitis	24	1,5	7;E70

with enterovirus infections. This syndrome can be mild and self-limiting; however, it is occasionally accompanied by encephalitis, which can lead to permanent sequelae, particularly in infants. Overall, enteroviruses cause the majority of all nonbacterial CNS infections now observed in the United States.

There may be a mild prodromal malaise, but major illness usually begins with fever, headache, and stiff neck. Kernig's and Brudzinski's signs may be present. Localizing sensory or motor deficits are unusual. Confusion and delirium are common. These acute findings may persist for 4 to 7 days. Cerebrospinal pleocytosis is usually less than 500 cells per microliter. Early, there may be as many as 90 percent polymorphonuclear leukocytes, but within 48 h the cellular response becomes completely mononuclear. Persistence of polymorphonuclear leukocytes in the cerebrospinal fluid suggests pyogenic meningitis or intracerebral, subdural, or epidural abscess. Gram's stain and appropriate spinal fluid cultures must be done to exclude bacterial meningitis, tuberculosis, or mycotic meningitis. Protein concentration in the cerebrospinal fluid is moderately elevated, but glucose is usually normal. Early in the illness enteroviruses may be isolated from spinal fluid, even in the absence of significant pleocytosis. It usually takes several weeks before the cerebrospinal fluid reverts to normal. An occasional patient may develop a transient syndrome of inappropriate secretion of antidiuretic hormone. In hypo- or agammaglobulinemic syndromes echoviruses have persisted in CSF for months to years, producing a progressive encephalitis or polymyositis.

For attempts at virus isolation, throat, stool, and cerebrospinal fluid specimens should be collected as early in the course as possible. Acute and convalescent sera can also be studied for rises in type-specific neutralizing antibodies in patients in whom viral isolation results are negative or equivocal.

It is not possible to distinguish clinically between aseptic meningitis due to various enteroviruses, arboviruses, Epstein-Barr virus, and mumps. Localizing findings, hemiplegia, oculogyric crises, coma, and bloody spinal fluid favor the diagnosis of type 1 herpes simplex virus encephalitis (see Chap. 135). Although enterovirus aseptic meningitis most often is self-limited and recovery in persons afflicted after the first year of life is usually complete, about 10 percent of patients have more serious involvement of the central nervous system. Minor muscle weakness with reflex changes may persist for weeks to months, but over 90 percent of patients recover completely within a year. Occasionally, choreiform movements, ataxia, nystagmus, transverse myelitis, Guillain-Barré syndrome, poliomyelitis-like symptoms, coma, bulbar involvement, and death occur.

OTHER ENTEROVIRAL ILLNESSES *Generalized disease of the newborn* is a highly lethal expression of enteroviral infection, in which the infant may be overwhelmed by simultaneous virus infection of the heart, liver, adrenals, brain, and other organs.

Acute myocarditis and/or pericarditis can be caused by a variety of viral agents; however, it is estimated that as many as 50 percent of cases are associated with infection by coxsackie B viruses. Such

infections are usually self-limited, but can lead to a fatal outcome (arrhythmia or heart failure) or cause chronic heart disease (see Chaps. 192 and 193).

The exanthems may or may not be associated with CNS inflammation. The rashes usually resemble rubella, roseola infantum, or adenovirus macular or maculopapular exanthems, but may also appear as vesicular or hemangioma-like lesions. Hand-foot-and-mouth disease usually affects children and is characterized by a vesicular eruption over the extremities and the anterior oral cavity. Coxsackievirus A16 is the specific agent most frequently implicated, but others, such as enterovirus 71, can cause a similar illness.

Herpangina is an enanthematous (mucous membrane) disease characterized by the acute onset of fever and sore throat. Characteristic small vesicles or white papules (lymphonodules) surrounded by a red halo are seen over the posterior half of the palate, pharynx, and tonsillar areas. This mild, self-limiting (1 to 2 weeks) illness has usually been associated with infection by several different group A coxsackievirus serotypes.

Epidemic myalgia (pleurodynia, or Bornholm disease) is characterized by fever and sudden onset of intense upper abdominal or lower thoracic pain, often accompanied by a frontal headache. The pain may be aggravated by movement, such as breathing or coughing, and usually persists for 3 to 14 days. Coxsackie B viruses are most frequently implicated.

A variety of other illnesses may also result from infections by this subgroup. Epidemic acute hemorrhagic keratoconjunctivitis associated with enterovirus 70 has been reported in Asia and the United States, and disease resembling paralytic poliomyelitis caused by enterovirus 71 infection has occurred in Bulgaria, Australia, and the United States. There is some evidence that certain enteroviruses may participate in the pathogenesis of at least some cases of insulin-dependent diabetes mellitus, acute arthritis, polymyositis, hemolytic-uremic syndrome, and idiopathic acute nephritis.

REOVIRUS INFECTIONS

The reoviruses (respiratory enteric orphans) are naked virions that contain double-stranded RNA. They are extremely ubiquitous and have been found in humans, simians, cattle, rodents, and a variety of other hosts. Three serotypes are known to infect humans; however, their role and relative importance in causing disease remains uncertain. Sporadic cases of febrile upper respiratory infections, exanthems, pneumonia, hepatitis, encephalitis, and gastroenteritis have all been reported to be associated with these viruses. Reovirus type 3 has also been implicated as a possible cause of biliary atresia and neonatal hepatitis, but this relationship remains uncertain. Asymptomatic shedding of reoviruses also occurs, which makes it difficult to prove association with disease. Reoviruses can be isolated in cell cultures, particularly primary monkey kidney or human kidney monolayers.

REFERENCES

BOWLES NE et al: Detection of coxsackie-B-virus-specific RNA sequences in myocardial biopsy samples from patients with myocarditis and dilated cardiomyopathy. Lancet 1:1120, 1986

——— et al: Dermatomyositis, polymyositis, and coxsackie-B-virus infection. Lancet 1:1004, 1987

BROWN WR et al: Lack of correlation between infection with reovirus 3 and extrahepatic biliary atresia or neonatal hepatitis. J Pediatr 113:670, 1988

CASHMAN NR et al: Late denervation in patients with antecedent paralytic poliomyelitis. N Engl J Med 317:7, 1987

CHEMTOB S et al: Syndrome of inappropriate secretion of antidiuretic hormone in enteroviral meningitis. Am J Dis Child 139:292, 1985

CRENNAN JM et al: Echovirus polymyositis in patients with hypogammaglobulinemia. Failure of high-dose intravenous gamma-globulin therapy and review of the literature. Am J Med 81:35, 1986

DALAKIS MC et al: A long-term follow-up study of patients with post-poliomyelitis neuromuscular symptoms. N Engl J Med 314:959, 1986

JOSSELSON J et al: Acute rhabdomyolysis associated with an echovirus infection. Arch Intern Med 140:1671, 1980

KAPLAN MH et al: Group B coxsackievirus infections in infants younger than three months of age: A serious childhood illness. Rev Infect Dis 5:1019, 1983

MCBEAN AM et al: Serological response to oral polio vaccine and enhanced-potency inactivated polio vaccine. Am J Epidemiol 128:615, 1988

MCKINNEY RE JR et al: Chronic enteroviral meningoencephalitis in agammaglobulinemia patients. Rev Infect Dis 9:334, 1987

NKOWANE BM et al: Vaccine-associated paralytic poliomyelitis. JAMA 257:1335, 1987

SHARPE AH, FIELDS BN: Pathogenesis of viral infections: Basic concepts derived from the reovirus model. N Engl J Med 312:486, 1985

145 VIRAL GASTROENTERITIS

HARRY B. GREENBERG

INTRODUCTION In less developed countries, acute infectious diarrheal disease is a leading cause of morbidity in all age groups, and of mortality in infants and young children. In developed countries, acute diarrheal illness remains an important cause of morbidity among both children and adults. Two distinct groups of viruses—the rotaviruses and the Norwalk viruses—as well as a variety of bacterial pathogens (see Chap. 92) have emerged as important etiologic agents of gastroenteritis. The rotaviruses are primarily pathogens of young children. The Norwalk and related small round viruses affect predominantly older children and adults.

ROTAVIRUS Classification and characterization Rotaviruses are members of the Reoviridae family. The rotavirus virion consists of a 70-nm double-shelled icosahedral capsid which surrounds a genome composed of 11 segments of double-stranded RNA. The virus has two surface proteins which are both involved with viral neutralization. Because rotaviruses have a segmented genome, they are capable of undergoing gene reassortment at very high frequency. The role of gene reassortment in generating rotavirus antigenic diversity is not known. In humans, rotavirus infection is characterized by replication that is localized exclusively in the small intestinal epithelial cells.

Epidemiology Rotavirus infection occurs worldwide. By the age of 3, virtually every individual has been infected by rotaviruses at least once. In areas with a temperate climate, rotavirus infection is seasonal, occurring in the cooler winter months. In tropical areas rotavirus infection tends to occur throughout the year, with some increase in incidence during the cooler rainy season. Rotaviruses are the single most important cause of severe dehydrating diarrhea in infants and young children under 3 in both developed and less developed countries, and account for between 30 and 50 percent of all cases of diarrhea requiring hospitalization or intensive rehydration therapy. Although rotavirus infections are primarily confined to infants and small children, they are frequently associated with diarrhea in adults, particularly family members of affected infants, geriatric patients, and immunocompromised hosts. They account for up to 25 percent of traveler's diarrhea (see Chap. 92). Rotaviruses may also be responsible for some cases of acute and chronic diarrhea in patients with AIDS. Subclinical infections or mild gastrointestinal illnesses which do not require hospitalization account for the majority of rotavirus infections. Subclinical infections have also been documented in neonates; these infections were shown to protect against severe rotavirus gastroenteritis for up to 3 years. At least five distinct serotypes of human rotavirus have been described. The relationship of the frequency of infection with these serotypes to host immune status is unclear. A large variety of other mammals and avian species can be infected by rotavirus, but it does not appear that these animal rotavirus strains cause disease in humans under natural conditions. Rotaviruses are shed in very large numbers (up to 10^{10} particles per gram of feces) in the stool; it is presumed that transmission occurs via fecal-oral spread.

Pathophysiology Rotavirus infects and kills the mature villus tip cells of the small intestine. The mature epithelial cells are replaced by immature absorptive cells that cannot absorb carbohydrates or other nutrients efficiently. Rotavirus infection leads to an osmotic diarrhea due to nutrient malabsorption. Changes in intracellular cyclic adenosine monophosphate or guanosine monophosphate are not involved in the etiology of rotavirus diarrhea.

Manifestations These range from subclinical infections to mild diarrhea to severe, occasionally fatal, illness. Most information concerning the signs and symptoms of rotavirus infection has been derived from studies of hospitalized young children. The onset of illness is usually abrupt. Vomiting, followed by diarrhea, occurs in over 80 percent of affected children. About one-third of hospitalized children will have a temperature greater than 39°C (102.2°F). Gastrointestinal symptoms usually last between 2 and 6 days. Mucus is commonly found in the stool but white and red blood cells are present in less than 15 percent of cases. Rotavirus infection frequently occurs in conjunction with respiratory tract symptoms, but there is little evidence to indicate that rotavirus replicates in the respiratory tract. Rotavirus infection has been observed in association with a wide variety of other clinical syndromes, including sudden infant death syndrome, Reye's syndrome, encephalitis, aseptic meningitis, pneumonia, exanthem subitum, Kawasaki's syndrome, necrotizing enterocolitis, gastroenteritis (which may be accompanied by hemorrhage), intussusception, Henoch-Schönlein purpura, hemolytic uremic syndrome, disseminated intravascular coagulation, and Crohn's disease. The etiologic relationship between these clinical syndromes and rotavirus infection is probably coincidental rather than causal. Rotavirus infection may be especially severe, and even fatal, in immunocompromised children.

Clinical immunity Relative immunity to rotavirus illness is acquired following infection early in childhood. Immunity is not complete, and adults with low levels of antibody can be symptomatically infected. Local immunity appears to be the critical determinant in protection.

Diagnosis Because rotavirus is shed in large amounts in the stool, detection is relatively easy. A variety of specific commercial immunoassays are available to detect rotavirus antigen in fecal specimens. DNA probe diagnosis also appears to be sensitive and specific. There are no pathognomonic signs or symptoms of rotavirus infection, but rotavirus infection is more frequently associated with severe dehydration than other enteric bacterial or viral pathogens.

Treatment and prevention Despite the fact that rotavirus diarrhea is caused by intestinal epithelial cell lysis and death, it can be adequately treated by standard oral rehydration therapy. Only rarely is intravenous rehydration required. Since rotavirus infections have persisted in developed countries with advanced sanitation facilities and widely available clean water, it is unlikely that the viral infection will be preventable by hygienic measures alone. Progress with a number of candidate live attenuated vaccines suggests that prevention through vaccination may be feasible in the future.

NORWALK AND RELATED SMALL ROUND VIRUSES Classification and characterization A variety of round 27- to 32-nm particles, some with clearly defined ultrastructure, have been identified in the stools of individuals with acute nonbacterial gastroenteritis. These agents have not been definitely classified because they are shed in the stool in small amounts for only a few days, and they have not been adapted to cell culture or to animal models. The Norwalk virus represents the most extensively studied and best characterized member of this group of agents, which also includes such serologically distinct viruses as the Hawaii agent, the Snow Mountain agent, the W-Ditchling agent, and a number of agents described as either astrovirus-like or calicivirus-like. The Norwalk virus and the Snow Mountain virus appear to have a protein structure similar to typical caliciviruses, and it is likely that most of these 27-nm gastroenteritis agents will prove to be plus-stranded RNA viruses.

Epidemiology Norwalk infection occurs year-round and is common. From 58 to 70 percent of adults in both developed and less developed countries have antibodies to this virus. Antibody acquisition occurs at a considerably younger age in children in less developed countries than in those in developed areas, consistent with the presumption that Norwalk virus is spread by the fecal-oral route. In developed countries, the virus is responsible for approximately one-third of all epidemics of nonbacterial gastroenteritis. Norwalk virus has been incriminated in a variety of food-borne epidemics, and transmission vehicles have included oysters, green salad, and chocolate icing. The virus is a common cause of waterborne epidemics of gastroenteritis and has been shown to be the etiologic agent in nursing home, cruise ship, and institutional (summer camps and schools) outbreaks.

In less developed countries, the role of Norwalk virus infection in the etiology of diarrhea has not been thoroughly investigated. Preliminary studies indicate that Norwalk virus can cause mild diarrhea in young children, but it does not appear to cause severe illness in infants in either developed or less developed countries. The other serologically distinct small round gastroenteritis viruses must be studied in more detail before their epidemiology can be distinguished from Norwalk infection. It appears, however, that astroviruses and typical human caliciviruses are primarily pathogens of young children rather than adults.

Pathophysiology Following infection with Norwalk or Hawaii viruses, the proximal small intestinal architecture is altered with villus shortening, crypt hyperplasia, and lamina propria infiltration by polymorphonuclear and mononuclear cells. Changes are not observed in the stomach or colon. The cells in which viral replication occurs have not been identified. The histologic alterations are accompanied by mild steatorrhea, carbohydrate malabsorption, and decreased levels of some brush border enzymes. Changes in adenylate cyclase activity have not been observed.

Manifestations Norwalk illness has an incubation period of between 18 and 72 h. Disease is characterized by the abrupt onset of nausea and abdominal cramps followed by vomiting and/or diarrhea. Vomiting occurs more frequently in children than adults. Low-grade fever [above 37.5°C (99.5°F)] is seen in about half of affected individuals. Headache, myalgias, and abdominal pain are common. The white blood cell count is normal; rarely there is leukocytosis with a relative lymphopenia. Red and white cells are not found in the stool. The illness is usually mild and self limited, lasting 24 to 48 h.

Clinical immunity For most people long-term (2 years or greater) resistance to Norwalk reinfection does not occur. In volunteers, there is a paradoxical relationship between the level of antibody to Norwalk virus and susceptibility to illness. Low levels of Norwalk antibody in the serum and intestine are associated with clinical resistance to illness. It appears, therefore, that immune mechanisms are not the primary determinants of protection from Norwalk virus.

Diagnosis, treatment, and prevention Radioimmunoassays and an enzyme-linked immunosorbentassay (ELISA) have been developed for Norwalk virus and several other 27- to 30-nm gastroenteritis agents. These tests are not yet available commercially. Norwalk illness is acute and self-limited; treatment is not usually required. In the rare case of severe vomiting or diarrhea, oral or intravenous rehydration is indicated. Because long-term immunity to Norwalk illness does not usually follow natural infection, it seems unlikely that a vaccine will be developed.

MISCELLANEOUS ENTERIC VIRAL PATHOGENS Enteric adenoviruses are a minor (~10 percent) cause of diarrheal illness in infants and children. These viruses differ from other adenovirus strains in a variety of ways including neutralization serotype, restriction endonuclease digestion pattern, and their ability to grow in tissue culture. The role of enteric adenovirus illness in adults or in less developed countries is not known.

Several strains of antigenically distinct rotaviruses, presently called "atypical rotaviruses" or group B and C rotaviruses, have been identified as the cause of occasional episodes of diarrhea in humans and animals.

Corona viruses are frequent causes of diarrheal disease in a variety of animals. Several investigators, using electron microscopy, have identified putative corona virus–like particles in the stools of patients with diarrhea. In most cases, however, these particles do not have the typical morphologic features of corona viruses and may represent bacterial breakdown products or cellular fragments.

REFERENCES

BLACK RE et al: A two-year study of bacterial, viral and parasitic agents associated with diarrhea in rural Bangladesh. J Infect Dis 142:660, 1980

BRANDT CD et al: Pediatric viral gastroenteritis during eight years of study. J Clin Microbiol 18:71, 1983

KAPIKIAN AZ et al: Rotaviruses, in *Virology*, B Fields (ed). New York, Raven Press, 1985, pp 863–906

——— et al: Norwalk group of viruses, in *Virology*, B Fields (ed). New York, Raven Press, 1985, pp 1495–1518

KAPLAN JE et al: Epidemiology of Norwalk gastroenteritis and the role of Norwalk virus in outbreaks of acute non-bacterial gastroenteritis. Ann Intern Med 96:756, 1982

MORSE DL et al: Widespread outbreaks of clam- and oyster-associated gastroenteritis. Role of Norwalk virus. N Engl J Med 314:678, 1986

VESIKARI T et al: Protection of infants against rotavirus diarrhea by RIT 4237 attenuated bovine rotavirus strain vaccine. Lancet 1:977, 1984

146 MUMPS

C. GEORGE RAY

DEFINITION Mumps is an acute communicable disease of viral origin characterized by painful enlargement of the salivary glands and sometimes by involvement of the gonads, meninges, pancreas, and other organs.

ETIOLOGY The causative agent of mumps is a paramyxovirus of intermediate size (120 to 200 nm in diameter). It has a tight helical inner core (RNA) enclosed in an outer envelope of lipid and protein. The virus of mumps has two components capable of fixing complement. These are the soluble, or S, antigens derived from the nucleocapsid, and the V antigen derived from the surface hemagglutinin. The virus can be cultivated in chick embryos and in a variety of mammalian cell cultures.

EPIDEMIOLOGY Human beings are the only natural host for mumps. The disease is worldwide and is endemic in urban communities. Epidemics are relatively infrequent and are usually confined to closely associated groups who live in orphanages, army camps, or schools. The disease is most frequent in the spring, particularly during April and May. Although mumps is generally considered less "contagious" than measles and chickenpox, this difference may be more apparent than real because many mumps infections (at least 25 percent) tend to be inapparent clinically. In some surveys, 80 to 90 percent of an adult population had serologic evidence of previous infection with mumps. By 1985, the incidence of mumps in the United States had reached its lowest point since reporting began

(2982 cases). However, an alarming resurgence took place in the ensuing 2 years and almost 12,900 cases were reported in 1987.

Infections are rare before the age of 2 years and then increase in frequency, peaking at ages 10 to 19. Clinical mumps may be more common in males than in females. The virus is transmitted in infected salivary secretions, although its isolation from urine suggests that it may also spread via this route. Mumps virus is rarely isolated from stool. The saliva is infectious for approximately 6 days prior to the onset of parotitis, and virus has been recovered from this site for as long as 2 weeks after onset of parotid swelling. Viruria also persists for 2 to 3 weeks in some patients. Despite this prolonged secretion of virus, the peak of infectivity occurs a day or two before onset of parotitis and subsides rapidly after the appearance of glandular enlargement.

One attack of clinical or subclinical mumps confers lasting immunity, and second attacks are most unusual. Unilateral parotitis affords protection just as effectively as does bilateral disease.

PATHOGENESIS The virus enters via the respiratory route; during the incubation period of 12 to 25 days it presumably replicates in the upper respiratory tract and cervical lymph nodes, from which it is disseminated via the bloodstream to other organs, including the meninges, gonads, pancreas, breasts, thyroid, heart, liver, kidneys, and cranial nerves. The salivary adenitis is thought by many to be secondary to viremia, but primary spread from the respiratory tract has not been ruled out as an alternative mechanism.

MANIFESTATIONS Salivary adenitis The onset of parotitis is usually sudden, although it may be preceded by a prodromal period of malaise, anorexia, chilly sensations, feverishness, sore throat, and tenderness at the angle of the jaw. In many cases, however, parotid swelling is the first indication of illness. The glands enlarge progressively over a period of 1 to 3 days, and the swelling resolves within a week after maximal enlargement. The swollen gland extends from the ear to the lower portion of the mandibular ramus and to the inferior portion of the zygomatic arch, often displacing the ear upward and outward. The skin over the gland is usually not warm or erythematous, in contrast to bacterial parotitis. There may be reddening and pouting of the orifice of Stensen's duct. Usually, pain and tenderness are marked, although at times they are absent. The edema of mumps has been described as ''gelatinous,'' and when the involved gland is tweaked, it rolls like jelly. Swelling may involve only the submaxillary and sublingual glands and may extend over the anterior part of the chest, producing *presternal edema.* Involvement of submaxillary glands alone can cause difficulty in distinguishing mumps from acute cervical adenitis. Swelling of the glottis occurs rarely but may require tracheostomy. Parotitis is bilateral in two-thirds of cases and remains confined to one side in the remainder. The second gland tends to swell as the first is subsiding, usually 4 to 5 days after onset. In general, parotitis is accompanied by a temperature of 37.8 to 39.4°C (100 to 103°F), malaise, headache, and anorexia, but systemic symptoms may be virtually absent, particularly in children. In most patients, the chief complaints refer to difficulty in eating, swallowing, and talking.

Epididymoorchitis Mumps is complicated by orchitis in 20 to 35 percent of postpubertal males. Testicular involvement usually appears 7 to 10 days after onset of parotitis, although it may precede it or appear simultaneously. Occasionally, orchitis occurs in the absence of parotitis. Gonadal involvement is bilateral in 3 to 17 percent of patients. Orchitis is heralded by recrudescence of malaise and appearance of chilly sensations, headache, nausea, and vomiting. Shaking chills and high fevers, with temperatures between 39.4 to 41.1°C (103 and 106°F), are frequent. The testicle becomes greatly swollen and acutely painful. The epididymis is often palpable as a swollen tender cord. Occasionally there may be epididymitis without orchitis. Swelling, pain, and tenderness persist for 3 to 7 days and gradually subside; lysis of fever usually parallels abatement of swelling. Occasionally, the temperature falls by crisis. Mumps orchitis is followed by progressive atrophy of the testicle in one-half the cases. Even after bilateral orchitis, sterility is unusual, provided no

significant atrophy has taken place. However, if bilateral testicular atrophy occurs after mumps, sterility or subnormal sperm counts are quite common. Plasma testosterone levels are depressed during acute orchitis but return to normal with recovery. *Pulmonary infarction* has been noted to follow mumps orchitis. This may be the result of thrombosis of the veins in the prostatic and pelvic plexuses in association with the testicular inflammation. Priapism is a rare but painful complication of mumps orchitis.

Pancreatitis Pancreatic involvement is a potentially serious manifestation of mumps, which may rarely be complicated by shock or pseudocyst formation. It should be suspected in patients with abdominal pain and tenderness together with clinical or epidemiologic evidence of mumps. It is difficult to document, since hyperamylasemia, the hallmark of pancreatitis, is also often present in parotitis. Many times the symptoms resemble those of gastroenteritis. Although diabetes or pancreatic insufficiency rarely follows mumps pancreatitis, several children have developed ''brittle'' diabetes a few weeks after mumps.

Central nervous system involvement Approximately 60 percent of patients with clinical mumps have an increased number of cells, usually lymphocytes, in the cerebrospinal fluid (CSF), while 10 percent will have symptoms of meningitis: stiff neck, headache, and drowsiness. In typical cases, the onset of overt central nervous system signs and symptoms occurs 3 to 10 days after the onset of parotitis; however, CNS mumps may develop prior to the parotitis or 2 to 3 weeks later. In approximately 30 to 40 percent of laboratory-proven cases, there is *no* associated salivary gland involvement at any time in the course of illness. The CSF protein is moderately elevated, and CSF glucose tends to be normal, although in as many as 10 percent of patients low CSF glucose concentrations, in the range of 1.1 to 2.8 mmol/L (20 to 50 mg/dL), may be seen. True encephalitis is unusual, although it is responsible for most of the central nervous system sequelae, including behavioral disturbances, headaches, seizures, deafness (usually unilateral), and visual disturbances. Rarely, aqueductal stenosis and hydrocephalus have been reported as possible late sequelae to mumps encephalitis, but the association remains unproven. Mumps should also be recognized as capable of presenting a picture of mild paralytic poliomyelitis; definition of the cause depends on isolation of virus or serologic confirmation of mumps in the absence of changing antibody titers to poliomyelitis viruses. Rarely, mumps may produce a transverse myelitis, cerebellar ataxia, or the Guillain-Barré syndrome. Mumps meningitis, without clinical encephalitis, is generally thought to be benign.

Other manifestations Mumps virus tends to involve glandular tissues; inflammation of the lacrimal glands, thymus, thyroid, breasts, and ovaries occurs occasionally. *Oophoritis* may be recognized by persistence of pain in the lower part of the abdomen and fever. It does not result in sterility. Mumps virus has been implicated in the causation of subacute thyroiditis; the diagnosis can be made serologically, and occasionally the virus can be isolated from the thyroid gland. Myxedema following mumps thyroiditis has been reported. Ocular manifestations of mumps include dacryoadenitis, optic neuritis, keratitis, iritis, conjunctivitis, and episcleritis. Although these conditions may transiently interfere with vision, complete resolution is the rule. Mumps *myocarditis,* evidenced primarily by transient abnormalities in the electrocardiogram, is relatively common. On rare occasions it can be fatal but it does not usually produce symptomatic disease or impair cardiac function. Similarly, *hepatic* involvement may be manifested by mild abnormalities in liver function, but icterus and other clinical signs of hepatic damage are extremely rare. *Thrombocytopenic purpura* as a complication of mumps has been described, and an occasional patient has a leukemoid reaction involving predominantly lymphocytes. Tracheobronchitis and interstitial pneumonia have also been associated with mumps infection, particularly among young children.

A rare but interesting manifestation of mumps is *polyarthritis which is often migratory.* It is most common in males between the ages of 20 and 30. Joint symptoms begin 1 to 2 weeks after subsidence of parotitis; usually the large joints are involved. The illness lasts 1 to 6 weeks, and complete recovery is the rule. It is not clear whether arthritis is due to viremia or whether it is a "hypersensitivity reaction."

Acute hemorrhagic glomerulonephritis in the absence of streptococcosis has been reported after mumps. The relationship of these two diseases is not clear.

Late complications With the exception of the rare central nervous system complications and occasional patients who become sterile following bilateral testicular involvement, mumps leaves no sequelae. However, persistent mumps infection may be a cause of inclusion body myositis, a chronic inflammatory myopathy that occurs primarily in the sixth decade. There is no firm evidence that offspring with congenital defects are more common among mothers who have mumps during pregnancy. Likewise, the causal relationship between intrauterine mumps infection and endocardial fibroelastosis has not been clearly established. Mumps illness during the first trimester of pregnancy has been associated with an increased risk of spontaneous abortion.

LABORATORY FINDINGS In uncomplicated parotitis, the blood leukocyte count is normal, although there may be mild leukopenia with relative lymphocytosis. Patients with mumps orchitis, however, may have a marked leukocytosis with a shift to the left. In meningoencephalitis, the white blood cell count is usually within normal limits. The erythrocyte sedimentation rate is usually normal but may rise with testicular or pancreatic involvement. The serum amylase level is elevated both in pancreatitis and in salivary adenitis. It may also be elevated in some patients in whom the sole evidence of mumps is meningoencephalitis, and probably reflects subclinical involvement of the salivary glands. In contrast to the amylase, the serum lipase level is elevated only in pancreatitis, in which hyperglycemia and glucosuria also may occur. The cerebrospinal fluid contains 0 to 2000 cells per microliter, almost all mononuclear, although occasionally polymorphonuclear cells will predominate in the early stages. The pleocytosis in mumps meningitis tends to be greater than in aseptic meningitides caused by the polio-, coxsackie-, and echoviruses. There is no relationship between the cell count and the severity of central nervous system involvement. Transient hematuria and mild reversible abnormalities in renal function, including inability to concentrate the urine maximally and to clear creatinine, occur in association with the viruria of mumps.

DIAGNOSIS The definitive diagnosis of mumps depends on isolation of the virus from blood, throat swabs, secretions from Stensen's duct, cerebrospinal fluid, or urine. Immunofluorescence methods can detect positive cell cultures in 2 to 3 days rather than the 6 days required with standard methods. In addition, immunofluorescence can be utilized for rapid detection of the viral antigen directly in oropharyngeal cells. Serologic determination of acute infection or susceptibility can be done by a variety of methods. The best test is the enzyme-linked immunosorbent assay (ELISA). Immunofluorescent assays are also commonly available, and can be used for identification of IgM- and IgG-specific antibody responses. The complement fixation test can be employed to quantitate antibody responses to the S and V antigenic components for the diagnosis of acute or recent mumps infection. Antibodies to the S antigen develop rather rapidly, often reaching a peak within 1 week after the onset of symptoms, and usually disappear in 6 to 12 months. Complement-fixing antibodies to the V antigen reach a peak titer within 2 to 3 weeks after onset, remain elevated for at least 6 weeks, and then persist at lower levels for years afterward. Paired serums obtained 2 to 3 weeks apart are recommended. A fourfold increase in titer by any standard assay confirms recent infection. When an acute serum is not obtained until later in the course of illness, an elevation of antibodies to the S antigen which exceeds the V antibody titer or the presence of IgM-specific antibody suggests recent infection. The *skin test* consists of intradermal injection of killed mumps virus; previous exposure will result in a delayed reaction of the tuberculin type and an anamnestic antibody titer rise to mumps. The skin test is unreliable when used alone in determining the immune status of an individual,

is useless in the diagnosis of acute mumps, and is no longer commercially available in the United States.

The diagnosis of mumps during an epidemic is usually obvious. Sporadic cases, however, must be distinguished from other causes of parotid enlargement. Parotitis may be caused by other viruses, notably parainfluenza, influenza, and coxsackieviruses. *Bacterial parotitis* usually occurs in debilitated patients with severe underlying diseases, such as uncontrolled diabetes mellitus, cerebrovascular accidents, or uremia. It may also follow surgical operations. The parotid glands are swollen, warm, and tender, and pus can be expressed from the orifices of Stensen's ducts. Marked polymorphonuclear leukocytosis is present. The disease is usually acquired in the hospital, and *Staphylococcus aureus* is the usual causative organism. Dehydration followed by inspissation of secretions in the salivary ducts is an important predisposing factor. *Calculus* in a salivary duct is usually detectable by palpation or by injection of radiopaque media into Stensen's duct. *Drug reactions* may produce tender swelling of the parotid and other salivary glands. "Iodine mumps" is the most common type; it may follow such procedures as intravenous urography. The antihypertensive agent guanethidine may also cause parotid enlargement and tenderness. A careful history usually serves to clarify the cause of these reactions. *Cervical adenitis* caused by streptococci, "bullneck" diphtheria, infectious mononucleosis, cat-scratch disease, sublingual cellulitis (Ludwig's angina), and cellulitis of the external auditory canal are usually easy to distinguish from mumps by careful examination. Parotid tumors and chronic infections such as actinomycosis tend to follow a more indolent course, with slowly progressive swelling. The common "mixed tumor" of the parotid is well-circumscribed, nontender, and very firm, almost cartilaginous on palpation. Parotid swelling and fever, often accompanied by lacrimal adenitis and uveitis (Mikulicz's syndrome), may occur in tuberculosis, leukemia, Hodgkin's disease, and lupus erythematosus. The onset may be sudden, but the process is usually painless and of long duration. "Uveoparotid fever" of similar type may be the first manifestation of sarcoidosis; in this disease parotid swelling is frequently accompanied by single or multiple palsies of cranial nerves, particularly the facial nerve, and is referred to as Heerfordt's syndrome. Presternal edema may also be a manifestation of malignant lymphoma involving retrosternal lymph nodes. Bilateral painless parotid swelling unassociated with fever is found in patients with Laennec's cirrhosis, chronic alcoholism, malnutrition, diabetes mellitus, pregnancy and lactation, and hypertriglyceridemia.

Sjögren's syndrome (see Chap. 273) is a chronic inflammation of the parotid and other salivary glands which is often associated with atrophy of the lacrimal glands and occurs most commonly in women past the menopause. With cessation of lacrimal and salivary function, there may be striking dryness of the conjunctiva and the cornea (keratoconjunctivitis sicca) and of the mouth (xerostomia). These patients may also have a variety of systemic manifestations, including rheumatoid arthritis, splenomegaly, leukopenia, and hemolytic anemia. The chronicity of the process and its occurrence in elderly women make confusion with mumps unlikely. Finally, benign hypertrophy of both masseter muscles, presumably due to habitual clenching and grinding of teeth, may be confused with painless parotid swelling.

The causes of aseptic meningitis are discussed in Chap. 355.

Orchitis occurring in the absence of parotitis is likely to remain undiagnosed. Serologic testing may later confirm the diagnosis of mumps. Orchitis may occur in association with acute bacterial prostatitis and seminal vesiculitis. It is a rare complication of gonorrhea. Occasionally testicular inflammation accompanies pleurodynia, leptospirosis, melioidosis, tuberculosis, relapsing fever, chickenpox, brucellosis, and lymphocytic choriomeningitis. *Chlamydia trachomatis* should also be considered in the differential diagnosis of epididymitis.

TREATMENT There is no specific treatment for infections with the mumps virus. Patients with parotitis should receive mouth care, analgesics, and a bland diet. Bed rest is advisable only as long as the patient is febrile; contrary to popular belief, physical activity has no influence on the development of orchitis or other complications. Patients with epididymoorchitis may be acutely ill and in great pain. Many forms of treatment, including surgical decompression of the testicle, infiltration of the spermatic cord with local anesthetics, estrogens, convalescent serum, and broad-spectrum antibiotics, have not been regularly effective. Despite failure to document their effectiveness in controlled studies, glucocorticoids have been of considerable benefit in diminishing fever and testicular pain and swelling, and in restoring the sense of well-being in a number of patients. It is important to give a large initial daily dose corresponding to 60 mg prednisone. Subsequently, administration of the hormone can be tapered over 7 to 10 days. Glucocorticoids have not exerted an adverse effect on concomitant pancreatitis or meningitis, although they have not benefited patients with meningeal involvement, and their withdrawal has usually been accompanied by a recrudescence of symptoms. They have not prevented the appearance of parotid involvement on the contralateral side. Mumps arthritis is usually mild and requires no treatment. Mumps thyroiditis may subside spontaneously, but excellent relief has been obtained with glucocorticoids.

PREVENTION   A live attenuated mumps virus vaccine (Jeryl Lynn strain) has been highly effective in producing significant rises in mumps antibody in individuals who are seronegative prior to vaccination, and has afforded 75 to 95 percent protection to individuals subsequently exposed to mumps. The vaccine also has boosted antibody levels in vaccinated individuals who are seropositive. The vaccine produces an inapparent, noncommunicable infection. Parotitis after vaccination has been reported only rarely, and central nervous system dysfunction has not been proved to be a complication. It has conferred excellent protection for at least 17 years and has not interfered with vaccines against measles, rubella, and poliomyelitis or with smallpox vaccination given simultaneously. Protection has been demonstrated in both children and adults.

Live mumps vaccine can be administered at any time after 1 year of age, and should be considered particularly for children approaching puberty, adolescents, and adults born after 1956 who have not had clinical mumps or live mumps vaccine in the past. Individuals living in groups or in institutions should be vaccinated, particularly because it has been shown that physical isolation of mumps patients does not effectively prevent transmission of the infection.

Vaccination is contraindicated in babies under the age of 1 year because of the interfering effect of maternal antibody; in individuals with a history of hypersensitivity to vaccine components; in patients with febrile illnesses, leukemia, lymphoma, or generalized malignancies; in those receiving glucocorticoids, alkylating drugs, antimetabolites, or irradiation; and during pregnancy.

It is not known whether the vaccine will prevent infection when administered after exposure, but no contraindication to its use in this situation exists. Neither mumps immune globulin nor ordinary gamma globulin has been shown to be effective in postexposure prophylaxis, and neither is recommended.

REFERENCES

BEARD CM et al: The incidence and outcome of mumps orchitis in Rochester Minnesota 1935 to 1974. Mayo Clin Proc 52:3, 1977

CHOU SM: Inclusion body myositis: A chronic persistent mumps myositis? Hum Pathol 17:765, 1986

COCHI SL et al: Perspective on the relative resurgence of mumps in the United States. Am J Dis Child 142:499, 1988

GORDON SC, LAUTER CB: Mumps arthritis: Unusual presentation as adult Still's disease. Ann Intern Med 97:45, 1982

KAPLAN KM et al: Mumps in the workplace. JAMA 260:1434, 1988

LEVITT LP et al: Central nervous system mumps: A review of 64 cases. Neurology 20:829, 1970

SHEHAB ZM et al: Epidemiological standardization of a test for susceptibility to mumps. J Infect Dis 149:810, 1984

147   RABIES, RHABDOVIRUSES, AND MARBURG-LIKE AGENTS

LAWRENCE COREY

RABIES

DEFINITION   Rabies is an acute viral disease of the central nervous system that affects all mammals and that is transmitted by infected secretions, usually saliva. Most exposures to rabies are through the bite of an infected animal, but on occasion a virus aerosol or the ingestion or transplantation of infected tissues may initiate the disease process.

ETIOLOGY   The rabies virus is a bullet-shaped, enveloped, single-stranded ribonucleic acid virus of 75- to 80-nm diameter belonging to the rhabdovirus group. The envelope glycoproteins are arranged in knoblike structures, which cover the surface of the virion. The viral glycoproteins bind to acetylcholine receptors, contribute to the neurovirulence of rabies virus, elicit neutralizing and hemagglutination-inhibiting antibodies, and stimulate T-cell immunity. The nucleocapsid antigen induces a complement-fixing antibody. Neutralizing antibodies to the surface glycoproteins appear to be protective. Antirabies antibodies used in diagnostic immunofluorescent assays are generally directed against the nucleocapsid antigens. Isolates of rabies virus from different animal species and locales differ in their antigenic and biologic properties. These variations may account for differences in virulence between isolates. Interferon is induced by rabies virus, particularly in those tissues with high virus concentrations, and may play some role in retarding progressive infection.

EPIDEMIOLOGY   Rabies exists in two epidemiologic forms: urban, propagated chiefly by unimmunized domestic dogs and/or cats, and sylvatic, propagated by skunks, foxes, raccoons, mongooses, wolves, and bats. Infection in domestic animals usually represents a "spillover" from sylvatic reservoirs of infection, and human beings can be infected by either. Hence, human infection tends to occur in locales where rabies is enzootic or epizootic, where there is a large population of unimmunized domestic animals, and where human contact with the outdoors is common. While only about 1000 rabies deaths are reported to the World Health Organization (WHO) each year, the worldwide incidence of rabies is approximated at over 30,000 cases per year. Southeast Asia, the Philippines, Africa, the Indian subcontinent, and tropical South America are areas where the disease is especially common. In some endemic areas 1 to 2 percent of autopsied patients show evidence of rabies. Increased spread of terrestrial rabies and increased travel to countries where urban rabies is present has made recognition of clinical rabies and its prevention of increasing importance. In the United States human rabies is exceedingly rare, and only 9 cases have been reported since 1980, 5 of which originated from exposures in countries where canine rabies was endemic.

In most areas of the world, the dog is the important vector of rabies virus for humans. However, the wolf (eastern Europe, arctic regions), the mongoose (South Africa, the Caribbean), the fox (western Europe), and the vampire bat (Latin America) may also be prominent vectors of the disease. Rodents and lagomorphs are rarely infected with rabies. In the United States, rabies in wildlife accounts for about 85 percent of the reported animal rabies, with dogs and cats comprising only about 2 and 3 percent, respectively. However, most cases of postexposure prophylaxis are associated with dog bites. Many human cases of rabies in U.S. citizens have resulted from domestic animal bites that occurred outside the country.

Several cases of human-to-human transmission of rabies through corneal transplantation have been documented.

PATHOGENESIS   The first event is the introduction of live virus through the epidermis or onto a mucous membrane. Initial viral replication appears to occur within striated muscle cells at the site of inoculation. The peripheral nervous system is exposed at the neuromuscular and/or neurotendinal spindles. The virus then spreads centripetally up the nerve to the central nervous system, probably via peripheral nerve axoplasm. Experimentally, viremia has been shown to occur, but is not thought to play a role in naturally acquired disease. Once the virus reaches the central nervous system, it replicates almost exclusively within the gray matter and then passes centrifugally along autonomic nerves to reach other tissue—the salivary glands, adrenal medulla, kidney, lung, liver, skeletal muscle, skin, and heart. Passage into the salivary glands facilitates further transmission of the disease via infected saliva. The incubation period of rabies is exceedingly variable, ranging from 10 days to over 1 year (mean 1 to 2 months). The time period appears to depend upon the amount of virus introduced, the amount of tissue involved, host defense mechanisms, and the actual distance that the virus has to travel from the site of inoculation to the central nervous system. Host immune responses and viral strains may also influence disease expression. Cell-mediated immune responses were noted in patients with rabies encephalitis but were absent in patients with paralytic rabies.

The neuropathology of rabies resembles other viral diseases of the central nervous system: hyperemia, varying degrees of chromatolysis, nuclear pyknosis, and neuronophagia of the nerve cells; infiltration by lymphocytes and plasma cells of the Virchow-Robin space; microglial infiltration, and parenchymal areas of nerve cell destruction. The pathognomonic lesion of rabies is the Negri body. This eosinophilic mass, approximately 10 nm in size, is made up of a finely fibrillar matrix and rabies virus particles. Negri bodies are distributed throughout the brain, particularly in Ammon's horn, the cerebral cortex, the brainstem, the Purkinje cells of the cerebellum, and the dorsal spinal ganglia. Negri bodies are not demonstrated in at least 20 percent of rabies, and their absence in brain material does not rule out the diagnosis.

MANIFESTATIONS The clinical manifestations of rabies can be divided into four stages: (1) a nonspecific prodrome, (2) an acute encephalitis similar to other viral encephalitides, (3) a profound dysfunction of brainstem centers which produces the classic features of rabies encephalitis, and (4) rarely, recovery.

The prodromal period usually persists for 1 to 4 days and is marked by fever, headache, malaise, myalgias, increased fatigability, anorexia, nausea and vomiting, sore throat, and a nonproductive cough. The prodromal symptom suggestive of rabies is the complaint of paresthesias and/or fasciculations at or about the site of inoculation of virus and may be related to the multiplication of virus in the dorsal root ganglion of the sensory nerve supplying the area of the bite. This symptom is present in 50 to 80 percent of patients.

The encephalitic phase is usually ushered in by periods of excessive motor activity, excitation, and agitation. Quickly, confusion, hallucinations, combativeness, bizarre aberrations of thought, muscle spasms, meningismus, opisthotonic posturing, seizures, and focal paralysis appear. Characteristically, the periods of mental aberration are interspersed with completely lucid periods, but as the disease progresses, the lucid periods get shorter until the patient lapses into coma. Hyperesthesia, with excessive sensitivity to bright light, loud noise, touch, and even gentle breezes, is very common. On physical examination the temperature may be found to be as high as 40.6°C (105°F). Abnormalities of the autonomic nervous system include dilated, irregular pupils, increased lacrimation, salivation, perspiration, and postural hypotension. Evidence of upper motor neuron paralysis with weakness, increased deep tendon reflexes, and extensor plantar responses is the rule. Paralysis of the vocal cords is common.

The manifestations of brainstem dysfunction begin shortly after the onset of the encephalitic phase. Cranial nerve involvement causes diplopia, facial palsies, optic neuritis, and the characteristic difficulty with deglutition. The combination of excessive salivation and difficulty in swallowing produces the traditional picture of "foaming at the mouth." Hydrophobia, the painful, violent involuntary contraction of the diaphragm, accessory respiratory, pharyngeal, and laryngeal muscles initiated by swallowing liquids, is seen in about 50 percent

of cases. Involvement of the amygdaloid nucleus may result in priapism and spontaneous ejaculation. The patient lapses into coma, and involvement of the respiratory center produces an apneic death. The prominence of early brainstem dysfunction distinguishes rabies from other viral encephalitides and accounts for the rapid downhill course. The median survival after the onset of symptoms is 4 days, with a maximum of 20, unless artificial supporting measures are instituted.

If intensive respiratory support is used, a number of late complications may appear and include inappropriate secretion of antidiuretic hormone, diabetes insipidus, cardiac arrythmias, vascular instability, adult respiratory distress syndrome, gastrointestinal bleeding, thrombocytopenia, and paralytic ileus. Recovery is very rare, and when it occurs, has been gradual.

Occasionally, rabies may present as an ascending paralysis resembling the Landry-Guillain-Barré syndrome (dumb rabies, *rage tranquille*). This clinical pattern occurs most frequently in those bitten by vampire bats or who have received postexposure rabies prophylaxis.

The difficulty of suspecting rabies when it is associated with ascending paralysis is illustrated by the documentation of person-to-person transmission of the virus by tissue transplantation. Corneal transplants from donors who died of presumed Landry-Guillain-Barré syndrome have produced clinical rabies and death in the recipient. Retrospective pathologic examinations of the brains of both patients demonstrated Negri bodies, and rabies virus was subsequently isolated from each donor's frozen eye.

LABORATORY FINDINGS Early in the disease the hemoglobin and routine blood chemistries are normal, but abnormalities occur as hypothalamic dysfunction, gastrointestinal bleeding, and other complications ensue. The peripheral white blood cell count is usually slightly elevated (12,000 to 17,000 per microliter) but may be normal or as high as 30,000 per microliter.

As in any viral infection, the specific diagnosis of rabies depends upon (1) the isolation of virus from infected secretions [saliva, rarely cerebrospinal fluid (CSF), or tissue (brain)], (2) the serologic demonstration of acute infection, or (3) the demonstration of viral antigen in infected tissue, e.g., corneal impression smears, skin biopsies, or brain. Samples of brain obtained either on postmortem examination or from brain biopsy should be subjected to (1) mouse inoculation studies for virus isolation, (2) fluorescent-antibody (FA) staining for viral antigen, and (3) histologic and/or electron-microscopic examination for Negri bodies. While the mouse inoculation studies for virus isolation and direct FA staining for viral antigen are quite reliable and sensitive, if the patient's life has been prolonged and high levels of neutralizing antibody are present in serum and CSF, "autosterilization" may occur, and these tests may be negative. The use of FA staining of skin biopsies, corneal impression smears, and saliva for evidence of rabies antigen has been helpful in diagnosing rabies during life. Confirmation of these findings either serologically or by demonstration of virus in brain should be sought.

If the patient has not received antirabies immunization, a fourfold rise in neutralizing antibody to rabies virus in serial serum samples is diagnostic. If the patient has received rabies vaccination, a clue to the diagnosis may be obtained from the absolute titers of serum-neutralizing antibody and the presence of neutralizing antibody to rabies in CSF. Postexposure rabies prophylaxis rarely produces CSF-neutralizing antibody to rabies. If present, it is usually in low titer, e.g., less than 1:64, whereas CSF titers in human rabies may vary from 1:200 to 1:160,000.

DIFFERENTIAL DIAGNOSIS There is little to distinguish rabies from other viral encephalitides, and the most helpful point in diagnosis is the history of exposure. Other problems to be considered include hysterical reactions to animal bites (pseudohydrophobia), Landry-Guillain-Barré syndrome, poliomyelitis, and allergic encephalomyelitis to rabies vaccine. The latter occurs most commonly after use of nerve tissue–derived vaccine and usually begins 1 to 4 weeks after vaccination.

PREVENTION AND TREATMENT Each year more than 1 million Americans are bitten by animals. In each instance, a decision must be made whether to initiate postexposure rabies prophylaxis. When deciding whether to institute rabies prophylaxis, the following considerations apply: (1) whether the individual came into physical contact with saliva or another substance likely to contain rabies virus; (2) whether rabies is known or suspected in the species and area associated with the exposure (e.g., all persons within the continental United States bitten by a bat that then escapes should receive postexposure prophylaxis); (3) the circumstances surrounding the exposure; and (4) the treatment alternative and complications. A guide for postexposure rabies prophylaxis is illustrated in Fig. 147-1.

If rabies is known to be present or suspected to be present in the animal species involved in a human exposure, the animal should be captured, if possible. Wild animals or any ill, unvaccinated, or stray domestic animal involved in a rabies exposure, particularly any animal involved in an unprovoked bite, exhibiting abnormal behavior, or suspected of being rabid, should be killed, and the head should be sent immediately to an appropriate laboratory for rabies FA examination. If examination of the brain by the FA technique is negative for rabies, it can be assumed that the saliva contains no virus, and the exposed person need not be treated. Persons exposed to escaped wild animals capable of carrying rabies (bats, skunks, coyotes, foxes, raccoons, etc.) in an area where rabies is known or suspected to be present should receive both passive and active immunization against rabies.

If a healthy dog or cat bites a person, the animal should be captured, confined, and observed for 10 days. If any illness or abnormal behavior develops in the animal during the observation period, it should be killed for FA examination.

Postexposure prophylaxis Once a decision regarding the necessity to initiate postexposure rabies prophylaxis has been made, the general principle of postexposure therapy is to minimize the amount of virus at the site of inoculation with local treatment of the wound and to establish an early and long-lasting neutralizing antibody titer to rabies virus. In most instances, this includes administration of globulin and vaccines. The following is a therapeutic regimen:

1 *Local wound therapy.* This is an important part of rabies prevention. The wound should be scrubbed with soap and then flushed with water. Both mechanical and chemical cleansing are important. Quaternary ammonium compounds such as 1 to 4% benzalkonium chloride or 1% cetrimonium bromide are useful because they inactivate the rabies virus. However, 0.1% benzalkonium solutions are less effective than 20% soap solutions. Usually tetanus toxoid and antibiotics should be administered.

2 *Passive immunization with antirabies antiserum* of either equine or human origin. Human rabies immune globulin (RIG) is preferred because equine antiserum may cause serum sickness. Fifty percent of the total dose of 20 units per kilogram for RIG and 40 units per kilogram for the equine antiserum is given by local infiltration of the wound, and the rest is administered intramuscularly into the gluteal region.

3 *Active immunization with antirabies vaccine.* Human diploid cell vaccine (HDCV) is the recommended rabies vaccine. HDCV is an inactivated whole-virus vaccine prepared from a laboratory strain of rabies virus grown in human diploid cell cultures. Severe reactions to HDCV are uncommon. Immediate hypersensitivity responses such as urticaria have been reported in approximately 1 in 650 recipients. Systemic reactions such as fever, headache, and nausea are generally mild and are reported in 1 to 4 percent of recipients. Local reactions such as swelling, erythema, and induration at the injection site occur in 15 to 20 percent of vaccinees.

Five 1-mL doses of HDCV are given intramuscularly as soon as possible after exposure. The first dose (day 0) should also be accompanied by antirabies serum (RIG) in the gluteal area. HDCV

FIGURE 147-1 Postexposure rabies prophylaxis algorithm.

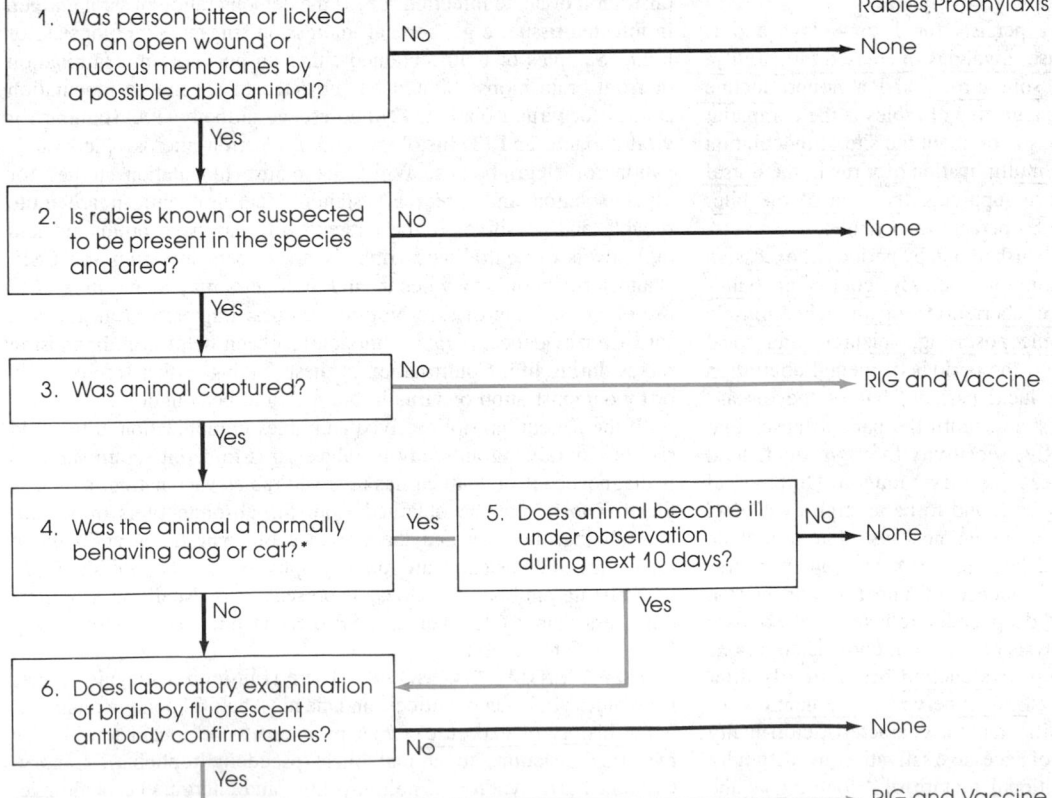

*Livestock exposure and normally behaving unvaccinated dogs or cats should be considered individually and local and state public health officials should be consulted.

should be given intramuscularly in the deltoid area; five doses should be administered within 28 days on the following schedule: days 0, 3, 7, 14, and 28. The WHO also recommends a 21- and 90-day course.

The combination of RIG and HDCV produces high titers of neutralizing antibodies in almost all recipients. Only rarely has this regimen proved unsuccessful in preventing the subsequent development of rabies. The administration of vaccine alone appears to be associated with a higher failure rate than RIG and HDCV, especially in severe bite exposures. The combination of RIG plus 0.1-mL intradermal doses at eight sites on day 0, four sites on day 7, and one site on days 28 and 91 produces good antibody responses, although the clinical experience with this regimen is less than with intramuscular administration.

Preexposure prophylaxis Individuals with a high risk of contact with rabies virus—veterinarians, cave explorers, laboratory workers, and animal handlers—should have preexposure prophylaxis with rabies vaccine. HDCV is the preferred vaccine for preexposure prophylaxis; three IM or three 0.1-mL intradermal injections on days 0, 7, and 28 should be administered. A neutralizing antibody titer should be checked after vaccination. Concomitant chloroquine administration interferes with the antibody response to vaccine. Booster doses may be administered either as a single 1-mL intramuscular or 0.1-mL intradermal injection. Postexposure prophylaxis in individuals previously given preexposure therapy consists of HDCV vaccine alone (two IM doses of HDCV on days 0 and 3 are usually adequate).

Booster doses of HDCV are associated with fever, headache, muscle aches, and joint pains in about 20 percent of recipients. Up to 6 percent of persons receiving IM booster doses of HDCV have developed an immune-complex-like reaction characterized by urticaria, arthritis, nausea, vomiting, and, occasionally, angioedema. These reactions have been self-limited and appear to be less with infrequent administration of booster doses. Persons who work in high-risk areas should undergo periodic measurement of antibodies, and booster doses are recommended for those with low antibody titers. Those at very low risk may elect not to receive routine booster doses but only to receive active immunization with any substantive exposure.

MOKOLA VIRUS

Mokola virus was first isolated from wild shrews captured in Nigeria and subsequently was shown to be related morphologically and serologically to rabies. However, neither of the two reported cases of human disease (both children) demonstrated classic clinical features of rabies. One patient had a nonfatal illness characterized by fever, pharyngitis, and convulsions. Mokola virus was recovered from her cerebrospinal fluid. The second patient initially had fever, cough, and vomiting, followed in several days by drowsiness, confusion, and generalized flaccid weakness. Her cerebrospinal fluid was normal. She progressed to deep coma and died within 10 days of onset. Mokola virus was isolated from her brain, and histopathologic sections revealed finely granular cytoplasmic inclusions that were distinguishable from Negri bodies in many neurons.

VESICULAR STOMATITIS VIRUS

Vesicular stomatitis is a viral illness of animals which can occasionally infect humans. It presents as an acute self-limited influenza-like disease. The disease in animals is found in the United States and South America and affects chiefly domestic cattle, horses, swine, wild deer, raccoons, skunks, and bobcats.

In animals, vesicular stomatitis is characterized by the development of vesicles on the oral mucosa, particularly the tongue, udders, and heels. The mode of spread is probably by direct contact; however, epidemics tend to occur in warm weather, and the virus has been isolated from *Phlebotomus* sandflies in Panama and *Äedes* species in New Mexico, suggesting these as possible vectors. Two distinct serotypes, New Jersey and Indiana, have been recognized, and most of the outbreaks in North America have been attributed to the New Jersey strain. The disease is most common in laboratory workers, and in one report three-fourths of laboratory personnel handling experimentally infected animals or manipulating the virus developed neutralizing antibodies. The disease is transmissible, however, under natural conditions among workers having direct contact with infected animals, especially cattle. The incubation period ranges from 1 to 6 days. This is followed by the sudden onset of fever up to 40°C (104°F), chills, profuse sweating, myalgias, malaise, headache, and pain on ocular movement. One-third to one-half of patients have sore throat and cervical and/or submandibular adenopathy. Small raised vesicular lesions may appear on the buccal mucosa. Conjunctivitis and coryza are present in about 20 percent of cases. Occasionally, small subcorneal, intraepithelial vesicles may appear on the fingers, usually associated with direct inoculation of the virus. Symptoms generally last 3 to 4 days, but occasionally a diphasic course may occur. Inapparent infection is common, and among laboratory workers with serologic evidence of infection, only about one-half reported clinical symptoms. In some areas of Panama, 17 to 35 percent of the population have neutralizing antibodies against vesicular stomatitis virus.

The differential diagnosis includes hand-foot-and-mouth disease, herpangina, primary herpetic pharyngitis and other mucocutaneous syndromes, and influenza. Viral isolation from patients is not common; however, a rise in complement fixation and/or neutralizing antibodies to vesicular stomatitis virus between acute and convalescent serums will help to confirm the diagnosis. Treatment is nonspecific.

MARBURG VIRUS DISEASE

DEFINITION Marburg virus causes an acute systemic febrile illness characterized by the abrupt onset of headache, myalgias, pharyngitis, rash, and hemorrhagic manifestations. It was recognized first in 1967 when it caused simultaneous outbreaks in the Federal Republic of Germany and Yugoslavia among laboratory workers exposed to imported African green monkeys (*Cercopithecus aethiops*). Outbreaks have been reported from Kenya. The clinical manifestations are similar to other hemorrhagic fevers of the arenavirus class or flavivirus group (Argentina and Bolivian hemorrhagic fever, Chap. 149). The high case fatality rate and demonstrated ability for nosocomial spread has made recognition of this rare agent an important worldwide public health concern.

ETIOLOGY The Marburg virus has been isolated in guinea pig and various cell culture systems such as vervet monkey kidney. The virus particle contains lipid and RNA, and under the electron microscope the virus appears as an 80- to 100-nm elongated filamentous particle with occasional "blister-like excrescences." Marburg and Ebola viruses have been included in a new family of viruses called Filoviridae. These viruses are biosafety level 4 pathogens, and maximum biologic containment facilities are recommended.

EPIDEMIOLOGY The initial outbreak affected 31 patients in Marburg and Frankfurt, Germany, and Belgrade, Yugoslavia, and was epidemiologically linked to monkeys imported from the same source in Uganda. Virus was isolated from the blood and tissue of these monkeys. Of the 25 primary infections, there were seven deaths. Six secondary cases, involving two physicians, one nurse, a postmortem attendant, and the wife of a veterinarian, occurred. Person-to-person transmission was felt to take place via accidental needle sticks or abrasions, although respiratory and conjunctival infection could not be ruled out. The wife of one patient developed Marburg virus disease. Marburg virus was demonstrated in semen of the original patient, despite the presence of circulating antibody, and this secondary case is believed to have been acquired through sexual intercourse. The natural reservoir of Marburg virus is unknown.

Serologic survey for virus showed primates and guinea pigs to be susceptible to infection.

PATHOLOGY Marburg virus appears "pantropic" and produces lesions in almost all organs including lymphoid tissue, liver, spleen, pancreas, adrenals, thyroid, kidney, testes, skin, and brain. In lymphoid tissue focal necrosis with degeneration of lymphoid tissue is apparent. In the liver, eosinophilic cytoplasmic bodies resembling the Councilman bodies of yellow fever have been noted. The lungs may show interstitial pneumonitis, as well as vascular lesions in small arterioles indicative of endarteritis. Neuropathologic changes consist of multiple small hemorrhagic infarcts with glial proliferation.

CLINICAL MANIFESTATIONS After an incubation period of 3 to 9 days, patients develop the abrupt onset of frontal and temporal headache, malaise, myalgias, especially in the lumbar area, nausea, and vomiting. Fever of 39.4 to 40°C (103 to 104°F) is characteristic, and about half the patients have conjunctivitis. Between 1 and 3 days after onset, watery diarrhea, which is often severe, lethargy, and a change in mentation are noted. An enanthem of the palate and tonsils and cervical lymphadenopathy may also be noted during the first week of illness. The most reliable clinical feature is the appearance of nonpruritic maculopapular rash which begins on the fifth to seventh day on the face and neck and spreads centrifugally to involve the extremities. A fine desquamation of the affected skin, especially the palms and soles, appears 4 to 5 days later. Hemorrhagic manifestations, including gastrointestinal, renal, vaginal, and/or conjunctival hemorrhages, generally develop between days 5 and 7 of disease.

During the first week, the temperature continues in the vicinity of 40°C (104°F), falling by lysis during the second week, to increase again between the twelfth and fourteenth days. Other clinical signs apparent in the second week of disease include splenomegaly, hepatomegaly, facial edema, and scrotal or labial reddening. Complications include orchitis, which may lead to testicular atrophy, myocarditis with irregular pulse and electrocardiographic abnormalities, and pancreatitis. The overall case fatality rate has been about 25 percent, with death usually occurring during the eighth to sixteenth days of illness. Recovery is often protracted over a 3- to 4-week period, and during this period loss of hair, intermittent abdominal pain, poor appetite, and prolonged psychotic disturbances have been noted. Late sequelae including transverse myelitis and uveitis have been reported. Marburg virus has been isolated from the anterior eye chamber and semen nearly 3 months after onset of disease.

LABORATORY FINDINGS Abnormalities in granulocyte function are found, and leukopenia is detected as early as the first day, with leukocyte counts as low as 1000 per microliter and a neutrophilia by the fourth day. Subsequently, atypical lymphocytes, as well as neutrophils exhibiting the characteristic of the Pelger-Huet anomaly, may appear. Thrombocytopenia appears early and is most marked, often less than 10,000 cells per microliter, between the sixth and twelfth days. In fatal cases, evidence of disseminated intravascular coagulation can be demonstrated. Hypoproteinemia, proteinuria, and azotemia may occur. Elevations in serum glutamic oxaloacetic transaminase (SGOT) and alanine aminotransferase (SGPT) are usual. Lumbar puncture may be normal or reveal a minimal pleocytosis. The erythrocyte sedimentation rate is usually low.

DIAGNOSIS The characteristic clinical course and epidemiologic features are the basis of the diagnosis. Specific diagnosis requires isolation of the virus or serologic evidence of infection in paired serum samples. Viremia coincides with the febrile state of disease, and virus has been isolated from tissue as well as urine, semen, throat, and rectal swabs. Attempts to isolate virus must be carried out only in *specialized high-security laboratories*. All patients should be kept in strict isolation, and all specimens should be handled and shipped according to World Health Organization guidelines.

TREATMENT Patients have received a multiplicity of drugs without apparent influence on the course of the illness. Convalescent serum was administered to four patients, whose subsequent disease followed a mild course. However, similarly benign outcomes were observed in patients who did not receive serum.

EBOLA VIRUS

Between July and November 1976 simultaneous outbreaks of an acute febrile hemorrhagic disease occurred in southern Sudan and northern Zaire. "Secondary and tertiary" spread of infection, particularly among hospital staff, was noted. In the Sudan over 300 cases with 151 deaths and in Zaire 237 cases with 211 fatalities were reported. The virus isolated from these patients was morphologically similar to but antigenically distinct from the Marburg agent. The name Ebola virus, after the river in Zaire located near the epidemic, has been proposed. Biologic and antigenic differences between strains of Ebola viruses isolated in Zaire and Sudan may account for the differences in mortality between the two outbreaks. Sporadic cases of disease also appear to occur, and a serosurvey revealed a prevalence rate of 7 percent for antibodies to Ebola virus in endemic areas. As with other hemorrhagic fevers, neutrophil leukocytosis, hypofibrinogenemia, thrombocytopenia, and microangiopathic hemolytic anemia are features of the illness.

Ebola virus has been propagated in tissue culture (vero cells) and in suckling mice and guinea pigs. The source of the outbreak in both the Sudan and Zaire is unknown; however, as with other viral hemorrhagic fevers, peridomestic rodents are suspected as being a reservoir of the infection, and serologic evidence of Ebola virus infection was detected in a domestic guinea pig trapped in Zaire. Once established, nosocomial as well as community-acquired cases occur, especially among those with close and prolonged contact. Parenteral exposure to the virus through disinfected rather than sterilized needles may have played a role in transmission. Barrier nursing and strict isolation precautions using protective clothing appeared to decrease the number of nosocomial cases.

CLINICAL MANIFESTATIONS Clinically, the disease is similar to Marburg virus disease. The incubation period ranges from 4 to 6 days (mean is 7 days). Patients usually present on the fifth day of illness with a history of abrupt onset of headache, malaise, myalgias, high fever, diarrhea, abdominal pain, dehydration, and lethargy. Pleuritic chest pain, a dry hacking cough, and a pronounced pharyngitis were also noted. A maculopapular eruption develops between days 5 to 7 of illness. On black skins the rash is often faint and not recognized until desquamation occurs. Hematemesis, melena, and bleeding from the nose, gums, and vagina are common. Abortion and massive metrorrhagia was a frequent complication among pregnant women. Death usually occurs in the second week of illness and is preceded by severe blood loss and shock.

TREATMENT Patients should be isolated until virologic studies indicate they are free of virus, usually 21 days from onset of illness. Malaria parasites were frequently found in blood films of patients with Ebola virus infection in the Sudan indicating that the presence of parasitemia does not rule out concomitant viral illness. Treatment with plasma containing Ebola virus–specific antibodies has resulted in diminished levels of viremia; however, further tests are required to establish the effectiveness of this form of therapy. Requests for viral isolation as well as convalescent plasma should be addressed to WHO Regional Centers in Atlanta or Geneva.

REFERENCES

Rabies

BAER GM: Research towards rabies prevention: Overview. Rev Infect Dis 10 (Suppl 4):S576, 1988

———, Fishbein DB: Rabies post exposure prophylaxis. N Engl J Med 316:1270, 1987

BERNARD KW et al: Preexposure immunization with intradermal human diploid cell rabies vaccine. JAMA 257:1059, 1987

HOUFF SA et al: Human-to-human transmission of rabies virus by a corneal transplant. N Engl J Med 300:603, 1979

PAPPAIVANOU M et al: Antibody response to preexposure diploid-cell rabies vaccine given concurrently with chloroquine. N Engl J Med 314:280, 1986

Recommendations of the Public Health Service, Immunization Practices Advisory Committee (ACIP): Rabies prevention. United States. MMWR 38(13):205, 1989

SHILL M et al: Fatal rabies encephalitis despite appropriate post exposure prophylaxis. N Engl J Med 316:1257, 1987

WARRELL DA, WARRELL MJ: Human rabies and its prevention: An overview. Rev Infect Dis 10 (Suppl 4):S726, 1988

Mokola virus

FAMILUSI JB: Fatal human infection with Mokola virus. Am J Trop Med Hyg 21:959, 1972

Marburg virus

SIMPSON DH: Marburg and ebola virus infections: A guide for their diagnosis, management and control. Geneva, WHO Offset Publication 36, 1977

SMITH DH et al: Marburg-virus disease in Kenya. Lancet 1:816, 1982

Ebola virus

MCCORMICK JB et al: Biologic differences between strains of Ebola virus from Zaire and Sudan. J Infect Dis 147:264, 1983

STANSFIELD SK: Antibody to Ebola virus in guinea pigs: Tandala, Zaire. J Infect Dis 146:483, 1982

148 ARBOVIRUS INFECTIONS

JAY P. SANFORD

Most viral infections in humans are either asymptomatic or present as undifferentiated illnesses characterized by fever, malaise, headache, and generalized myalgia. The similarities in clinical features between infections caused by viruses as dissimilar as the myxoviruses (e.g., influenza), the enteroviruses (e.g., poliovirus, coxsackievirus, echovirus), some of the herpesviruses (e.g., cytomegalovirus), and the arboviruses usually preclude an etiologic diagnosis based entirely on clinical manifestations without ancillary information regarding epidemiologic features and serologic findings. The purpose of this chapter is to define viral illness transmitted to humans by biting insects. Because the number of agents is large, mention will be made of those which have been best documented, have demonstrated unusual features, or seem to be of greatest potential public health importance.

DEFINITION AND CLASSIFICATION The definition of an arthropod-borne virus (arbovirus) was published in 1967 by the World Health Organization:

Arboviruses are viruses which are maintained in nature principally, or to an important extent, through biological transmission between susceptible vertebrate hosts by hematophagous arthropods; they multiply and produce viremia in the vertebrates, multiply in the tissues of arthropods, and are passed on to new vertebrates by the bites of arthropods after a period of extrinsic incubation.

From this definition it can be appreciated that the term *arbovirus* is used in the ecologic sense. Transmission by vectors is not correlated with virus architecture. Current approaches to taxonomy are based upon viral morphology, structure, and function. As a result, for taxonomic purposes, the term *arbovirus* has been eliminated.

The more than 250 antigenically distinct "arboviruses" are now grouped into six families (Table 148-1). The majority of agents contain single-stranded RNA, although some, such as the Reoviridae, contain double-stranded RNA.

"Arboviruses" are of importance in both temperate and tropical zones. Representative viruses have been isolated in almost every geographic area outside the polar regions.

"Arbovirus" infection of vertebrates is usually asymptomatic. The viremia stimulates an immune response which sharply limits the duration of the viremia. In "arbovirus" infections other than urban yellow fever, phlebotomus fever, chikungunya, o'nyong-nyong, mayaro, oropouche, dengue, and possibly Ross River virus, infection of humans represents an incidental occurrence which is tangential to the basic maintenance cycle of the virus. Hence, the isolation of

TABLE 148-1 Virus taxonomy and arboviruses-arenaviruses*

Family	Genus	Virus "English vernacular name"†
Reoviridae	Orbivirus	Colorado tick fever‡ Orongo Kemerovo

Togaviridae	Alphavirus (group A)	Eastern equine encephalitis‡
		Venezuelan encephalitis‡
		Western equine encephalitis‡
		Sindbis
		Semliki Forest complex
		  Chikungunya‡
		  O'nyong-nyong
		  Ross River†
		  Mayaro

	Flavivirus (group B)	*Associated with encephalitis*
		St. Louis encephalitis‡
		Japanese encephalitis‡
		Murray Valley encephalitis‡
		Tick-borne encephalitis complex‡
		  Russian spring-summer encephalitis
		  Central European encephalitis
		  Negishi
		  Powassan‡
		  Louping-ill
		Rocio
		
		Associated with fever-arthralgia-rash
		Dengue fever‡
		West Nile fever‡
		Nine other agents–not of major public health importance
		
		Associated with hemorrhagic fever
		Yellow fever‡
		Dengue fever‡
		Omsk hemorrhagic fever
		Kyasanur Forest disease

Rhabdoviridae	Vesiculovirus	Vesicular stomatitis Indiana‡ Vesicular stomatitis New Jersey‡ Cocal Chandipura Piry Isfahan
	Lyssavirus	Rabies‡ Mokola Duvenhage
Filoviridae		Marburg‡ Ebola‡

Bunyaviridae	Bunyavirus (16 serogroups)	Twenty-four agents may cause fever, fever-rash. None cause death. None in United States.
		California serogroup
		  LaCrosse‡
		  Snowshoe hare
		  Jamestown Canyon
		  California encephalitis
		  Tahyna
		  Inkoo

	Phlebovirus	Thirty-seven phleboviruses isolated from human beings; none cause death except Rift Valley fever virus. Sandfly fever–Naples‡ Sandfly fever–Sicilian‡ Rift Valley fever‡
	Nairovirus	Crimean-Congo hemorrhagic fever‡
	Not yet established	Hantaan‡ Puumala‡ Prospect Hill‡ Tchoupitoulas‡
Arenaviridae	Arenavirus	Lymphocytic choriomeningitis‡ Lassa‡ Machupo‡ Junin‡

* Only agents which have been shown to naturally infect humans are tabulated.
† Virus species have not yet been designated formally. The International Committee on Taxonomy of Viruses lists species under the term "English vernacular name."
‡ Viruses found in the United States and/or of major public health importance.

TABLE 148-2 Major clinical syndromes,* associated arboviruses-arenaviruses, and major geographic distribution

Virus	Geographic distribution
FEVER, ARTHRALGIA, RASH	
Chikungunya	Africa, southeast Asia
O'nyong-nyong	East Africa
Ross River	Australia, Fiji, Samoa, Cook Islands, New Guinea
Sindbis	Africa, U.S.S.R., Finland, Sweden
Mayaro	South and Central America
Dengue fever	Tropical Asia, Oceania, Africa, Australia, Americas
West Nile fever	Africa, Middle East, U.S.S.R., France, India, Indonesia
Lymphocytic choriomeningitis	United States, Germany, Hungary, Argentina
ENCEPHALITIS/ASEPTIC MENINGITIS	
Kemerovo	Central Europe
Eastern equine encephalitis	Atlantic, Gulf coasts, United States, upper New York, Caribbean, western Michigan
Venezuelan equine encephalitis	Northern South America, Central America, Mexico, Florida
Western equine encephalitis	United States, Canada, Central and South America
Semliki Forest	Africa
St. Louis encephalitis	United States, Caribbean
Japanese encephalitis	Japan, Korea, China, India, Philippines, southeast Asia, eastern U.S.S.R.
Murray Valley encephalitis	Australia
Rocio	Brazil
Omsk hemorrhagic fever	U.S.S.R.
Kyasanur Forest disease complex	India
Negishi	Japan
Powassan	New York, eastern Canada
Louping ill	United Kingdom, Ireland
Russian spring-summer encephalitis	U.S.S.R.
Central European encephalitis	Eastern Europe, Scandinavia, France, Switzerland
California group	North America
Tahyna	Europe
Inkoo	Europe
Phlebotomus fever	Mediterranean basin, Balkans, Near and Middle East, east Africa, central Asia, Pakistan, parts of India, southern China, Panama, Brazil
Rift Valley fever	South and east Africa
Lymphocytic choriomeningitis	United States, Germany, Hungary, Argentina
HEMORRHAGIC FEVER	
Yellow fever	South America, Africa
Dengue	Caribbean, southeast Asia
Chikungunya	Southeast Asia
Kyasanur Forest disease	India
Omsk hemorrhagic fever	U.S.S.R.
Crimean-Congo hemorrhagic fever	Africa, eastern Europe, Middle East, Asia
Hantaan	Korea, Japan, Scandinavia, U.S.S.R., central Europe
Marburg	Uganda, Kenya, Zimbabwe
Ebola	Zaire, Sudan
Lassa fever	West Africa
Machupo	Bolivia
Junin	Argentina

* Most agents are more often associated with undifferentiated febrile illness than with the specific syndromes. See text for exceptions.

virus from arthropod vectors or the detection of infection in the natural vertebrate host may provide a means for early detection and enable control of epizootic infection before significant spread to humans occurs.

Most human "arbovirus" infections are asymptomatic. When disease is produced, the spectrum of clinical illness is varied both in predominant features and in severity. Most commonly, disease is self-limited with symptoms of fever, headache, malaise, and myalgia.

Associated lymphadenopathy may be a feature. "Arboviruses" which may cause three major clinical syndromes—arthralgia-arthritis, encephalitis–aseptic meningitis, or hemorrhagic disease—are tabulated in Table 148-2.

"ARBOVIRUS" INFECTIONS PRESENTING CHIEFLY WITH FEVER, MALAISE, HEADACHE, AND MYALGIA

PHLEBOTOMUS FEVER Phlebotomus (sandfly, pappataci, or 3-day) fever is an acute, relatively mild, self-limited infection caused by at least five immunologically distinct phleboviruses (Naples, Sicilian, Punta Toro, Chagres, and Candiru). Serologic evidence of human infection has been demonstrated for four additional agents (Bujaru, Cacao, Karimabad, and Salehabad). Humans, the only known host, probably serve as a dead-end host. Voles are suspected of being an endemic host in the Middle East.

Prevalence The disease occurs throughout the Mediterranean basin, the Balkans, the Near and Middle East, the eastern part of Africa, the Soviet republics of central Asia, Pakistan, parts of India, Panama, Brazil, and possibly certain parts of southern China. In the Middle East and central Asia native populations acquire the disease at an early age and develop and maintain high levels of immunity. Cases in Panama and Brazil are sporadic, occurring mainly in persons entering the forest. The apparent absence of phlebotomus fever in indigenous adult populations residing in areas where sandflies are abundant may present a deceptive picture of the actual risk to susceptible persons.

Epidemiology In the Middle East and central Asia, the disease occurs during the hot, dry season (summer or autumn months) and is transmitted to human beings by the bite of infected sandflies (*Phlebotomus papatasii*), which are small (2- to 3-mm) urban flies that can penetrate ordinary house screens. Only the female bites and usually does so during the night. In persons who are not sensitive, there is neither pain nor local irritation after the bite; hence only about 1 percent of patients will remember having been bitten. In contrast, most of the human-biting sandflies (*Lutzomyia* sp.) of tropical America are sylvan in their habits. Transovarial and transstadial transmission of the virus has been demonstrated and in view of the low-titered and transient viremia in humans suggests the phlebotomine fly is both vector and reservoir. In humans, the incubation period averages 3 to 5 days. Viremia is present for at least 24 h before the onset of fever, but is not detectable for more than 2 days after the onset of illness.

Clinical manifestations The onset of symptoms is abrupt in over 90 percent of patients, with the temperature rapidly rising to its highest point, which may vary from 37.8 to 40.1°C (100 to 105°F). Headache is nearly always present and often is accompanied by pain on moving the eyes and by retroorbital pain. Myalgia is common and may be localized to the chest, resembling pleurodynia, or to the abdomen. Other symptoms may include vomiting, photophobia, giddiness, neck stiffness, alteration or loss of taste, and arthralgia. Conjunctival injection is present in approximately one-third of patients. Small vesicles may be seen on the palate, and macular or urticarial rashes occur. The spleen is rarely palpable, and lymphadenopathy is absent. The pulse rate may be elevated in proportion to the temperature on the first day; thereafter bradycardia is often present. The fever persists 3 days in most patients, with gradual defervescence. Giddiness, weakness, and feelings of depression are frequently encountered during convalescence. Second attacks 2 to 12 weeks after the first occur in 15 percent of cases.

In common with other "arbovirus" infections, phlebotomus fever may be associated with *aseptic meningitis*. In one series, 12 percent of patients had symptoms and signs sufficient to warrant a lumbar puncture. Findings in these patients included pleocytosis, with an average cell count of 90 per microliter and a predominance of either polymorphonuclear or mononuclear leukocytes. Spinal fluid protein concentration ranged from 0.2 to 1.3 g/L (20 to 130 mg/dL). In another series mild papilledema was observed in a few patients with severe illness.

Laboratory findings The changes in leukocyte count constitute the only positive laboratory findings. Total leukocyte counts of less than 5000 per microliter are observed in 90 percent of patients if daily counts are done during the febrile period and convalescence. The leukopenia may not appear until the last day of fever or even after defervescence. The differential leukocyte count will reveal an absolute decrease in lymphocytes on the first day, accompanied by an increase in nonsegmented neutrophils. During the second or third day, the number of lymphocytes begins to return to normal and may constitute 40 to 65 percent of the total count. Concurrently, there is a reversal in proportion of segmented and band neutrophils. The differential count usually returns to normal within 5 to 8 days after defervescence. Erythrocyte values and urinalyses are usually normal.

Diagnosis In the absence of a specific serologic test, the diagnosis must be made on clinical and epidemiologic grounds.

Treatment The disease is self-limited, and no specific therapy is available. Symptomatic care, including bed rest, adequate fluid intake, and analgesia with aspirin, is recommended. Convalescence may require a week or longer.

Prognosis No fatalities have been recorded among tens of thousands of cases.

COLORADO TICK FEVER Colorado tick fever is one of the two tick-transmitted virus diseases of humans recognized in the United States and Canada, Powassan virus being the other. Though "mountain fever" had been described ever since the advent of immigrants to the Rocky Mountain region, it must be differentiated from mild Rocky Mountain spotted fever. Once the clinical picture of disease had been established, it was renamed Colorado tick fever. A second serotype of the Colorado tick fever serogroup (Eyach virus) was isolated from *Ixodes ricinus* ticks near the village of Eyach in West Germany.

Etiology Colorado tick fever virus is grouped as an "arbovirus" because it replicates in ticks. It is a double-stranded RNA virus belonging to the orbivirus genus of the Reoviridae family (see Table 148-1).

Prevalence The disease has been contracted in Colorado, Idaho, Nevada, Wyoming, Montana, Utah, eastern Oregon, Washington, California, northern Arizona and New Mexico, and Alberta and British Columbia. The possibility exists that Colorado tick fever may occur over a wider geographic area. Mild and clinically inapparent forms of the disease occur. Up to 15 percent of perennial campers have neutralizing antibodies. The number of cases of Colorado tick fever reported in Colorado is 20 times greater than that of Rocky Mountain spotted fever. In fact, almost one-half of the patients diagnosed as having Rocky Mountain spotted fever in Utah were subsequently shown to have Colorado tick fever.

Epidemiology Colorado tick fever is transmitted to humans by the adult hard-shelled wood tick, *Dermacentor andersoni*. The virus has been found in as many as 14 percent of this species of ticks collected in endemic areas. Transovarial transmission of the virus in the tick has been established. Illness occurs from late March through September, mostly in May and June. Virus can be recovered from blood for 2 weeks in most patients, for at least 1 month in nearly one-half, and from spinal fluid during the acute illness. The virus persists within erythrocytes of convalescent patients for as long as 120 days and can be readily isolated from washed erythrocytes 100 days following infection. Transfusion-associated Colorado tick fever has been reported.

Clinical manifestations The incubation period is usually 3 to 6 days, and in 90 percent a history of tick contact within 10 days of onset of illness can be obtained. Failure to obtain such a history militates against the diagnosis. Persons affected usually are those whose occupational or recreational activities bring them in contact with ticks. The disease may occur at any age, although 40 percent

in one series were 20 to 29 years of age. The clinical picture is characterized by the sudden onset of severe aching of the muscles of the back and legs, chilliness without true rigors, a rapid increase in temperature, which usually reaches 38.9 to 40°C (102 to 104°F), headache with pain on ocular movement, retroorbital pain, and photophobia. Abdominal pain and vomiting occur in one-fourth of patients; diarrhea is rare. The physical findings are not specific. Tachycardia in proportion to the temperature, flushed facies, and variable conjunctival injection may be present. Occasionally the spleen is palpable. Rash occurs in only 5 percent of patients, but on occasion a petechial rash involving primarily the arms and legs or a maculopapular rash over the entire body may occur. Rarely, punched-out ulcers may form at the site of tick bite. The fever with the associated symptoms lasts about 2 days, then abruptly lyses to normal or subnormal, leaving the patient very weak. After an afebrile period of about 2 days, the fever recurs, may be higher than in the first phase, and may last as long as 3 days. One-half of patients show this saddleback pattern of temperature. Rarely there may be three febrile phases. Convalescence of more than 3 weeks is reported in 70 percent of patients over age 30, while symptoms last less than 1 week in 60 percent of patients under 20. Prolonged convalescence has no relationship to persistent viremia.

Evidence of central nervous system involvement has been recorded in a few patients. The findings are those of either an aseptic meningitis with stiffness of the neck or encephalitis with clouding of the sensorium, delirium, and coma. Rarer complications include epididymoorchitis and patchy pneumonitis.

Laboratory findings The most important laboratory feature is moderate to marked leukopenia, although in one-third of confirmed cases leukocyte counts remain about 4500 per microliter. On the first day of illness, the total leukocyte count may be at normal levels, but usually by the fifth or sixth day there has been a decrease to 2000 to 3000 per microliter. Characteristically there is a proportionate decrease in lymphocytes and granulocytes. Toxic changes in neutrophils are often conspicuous, and "virocyte" types of lymphocytes are frequently observed. Bone marrow examination reveals "maturation arrest" in the granulocytic series. Erythrocyte values remain normal. The blood picture returns to normal within a week after the fever subsides.

Diagnosis The diagnosis of Colorado tick fever is suspected on the basis of the epidemiologic history and clinical findings. Because of the infrequency of rash, patients who develop fever and rash after tick bites should be suspected of having Rocky Mountain spotted fever. The usual methods for confirming Colorado tick fever are mouse inoculation and fluorescent antibody (FA) staining of patients' erythrocytes; a combination of the two is best. Special handling of blood is not necessary for the FA test which remains positive for several weeks after clinical illness.

Treatment Treatment is entirely symptomatic.

Prognosis The prognosis is excellent.

Prevention Active immunity with an attenuated virus has been produced, but the immunization itself frequently produced mild disease. Colorado tick fever is best prevented by avoiding contact with the wood tick. Convalescent individuals should be excluded as blood donors for at least 6 months.

VENEZUELAN EQUINE ENCEPHALITIS Venezuelan equine encephalitis (VEE) was first noted in equines in Colombia in 1935.

Etiology Like other alphaviruses, the causative agent of VEE is a 40- to 45-nm, single-stranded RNA virus. Based on serologic tests and oligonucleotide fingerprints a complex of Venezuelan encephalitis viruses has been established: VE subtypes IA to IE, II (Everglades), III (Mucambo), and IV (Pixuna). IA was the original epidemic strain which occurred in Venezuela, and IB, which was recognized in Ecuador in 1963, spread through Central America into Mexico and was responsible for the epidemic in Mexico in 1971 which spread into southern Texas, with the occurrence of at least 76 laboratory-confirmed human cases. In early 1973, almost 4000 cases occurred in Peru.

Epidemiology VEE has been primarily a disease of equines and other mammals, although occasionally the agent has infected humans. Evidence of human infection (virus isolation or specific neutralizing antibodies) has been found in Colombia, Ecuador, Panama, Surinam, Guyana, French Guiana, Mexico, Brazil, Curaçao, Trinidad, Argentina, Peru, Florida, and Texas. Each subtype of VE virus is unique to its enzootic vector and does not replicate well in other vectors. Most common is an enzootic cycle between *Culex* mosquitoes and forest rodents. Enzootic VEE infects people who enter the rain forest or swamps, rubber tappers, forestry workers, and military personnel on jungle maneuvers. During an epizootic, many species of mosquitoes can transmit virus, especially *Aëdes, Mansonia,* and *Psorophora.* The virus has a wide host range in wild mammals, with at least 20 genera, including capuchin monkeys, rats, mice, opossum, jackrabbit, fox, and bats, being naturally infected. Domestic animals other than equines which have been shown to be infected include cattle and pigs in Mexico and goats and sheep in Venezuela. VEE appears to multiply well in mammals with high titers of virus in the blood; e.g., infected horses may have titers of up to $10^{7.5}$ mouse intraperitoneal lethal doses per milliliter of blood. Though 29 species of wild birds have been shown to be naturally infected with VEE (20 percent of which are colonial nestling herons and related species), whether the VEE-viremia levels in birds are high enough to infect vector mosquitoes is not known. During the initial 3 days of illness, viremia has been detected in approximately two-thirds of patients. The levels of viremia are sufficiently high that humans could serve as a reservoir. VEE virus also has been isolated by pharyngeal swab in a few patients, suggesting the potential for person-to-person transmission. The available observations make it reasonable to consider that the natural vector is a mosquito, with the primary reservoir being either wild or domestic terrestrial mammals. However, natural infection can probably take place without an arthropod vector. Laboratory infections have occurred and are probably due to inhalation of aerosols.

Clinical manifestations In humans, infection with VEE virus usually results in a mild acute febrile illness without neurologic complications. No age is spared, and there is no sex preponderance. The incubation period is 2 to 5 days, followed by the abrupt onset of headache, fever often associated with rigors, malaise, and myalgia. Other common symptoms may include nausea, vomiting, diarrhea, and sore throat. Uncommon features include photophobia, seizures, mental confusion, coma, tremors, and diplopia. Lymphadenopathy occurs in one-third of patients. On laboratory examination initial leukocyte counts are normal with 80 percent neutrophils. By the third day leukopenia occurs in two-thirds of patients. The cerebrospinal fluid may reveal pleocytosis with modest increases in protein and normal glucose concentration. Virus may be isolated both from blood and from cerebrospinal fluid. The symptoms usually last 3 to 5 days in mild cases and up to 8 days in more severe cases. A biphasic course of illness may be encountered, with recrudescence of symptoms on the sixth to the ninth day. In an epidemic in Venezuela in 1962, almost 16,000 cases of acute disease were evaluated; 38 percent were classified as encephalitis, but only 3 to 4 percent had severe neurologic abnormalities: convulsions, nystagmus, drowsiness, delirium, or meningitis. The mortality rate was estimated to be less than 0.5 percent, and nearly all deaths occurred in young children.

RIFT VALLEY FEVER Rift Valley fever is an acute disease principally of livestock, sheep, goats, cattle, and camels which is widespread throughout east and South Africa. It was first described in humans during an extensive epizootic of hepatitis in sheep in the Rift Valley in Kenya. During an epizootic in South Africa in 1950–1951, an estimated 20,000 humans became infected. Fatal human disease, four cases of hemorrhagic illness and hepatitis, was first reported during an epizootic in South Africa in 1975. In 1977 Rift Valley fever jumped the Sahara to Egypt with a major outbreak. Cases occurred in subsequent years until 1980; an estimated 200,000 cases with 598 reported deaths occurred in 1977.

Virus has been found in several species of mosquitoes: *Culex pipiens, Eretmapodites chrysogaster, Aëdes caballus, Aëdes circumluteolus,* and *Culex theileri. Culex pipiens* has been suggested as the vector in Egypt. While antibodies to Rift Valley fever have been found in wild field rats in Uganda, the reservoir is unknown. It has been suggested that the virus may be maintained by transovarial transmission in floodwater *Aëdes.* Although humans presumably can be infected by arthropods, many infections occur as a result of handling infected animal tissues. In addition, laboratory-acquired infections have been common, suggesting a respiratory route of transmission.

The incubation period is usually 3 to 6 days. The onset is abrupt, with malaise, chilly sensation or rigors, headache, retroorbital pain, and generalized aching and backache. The temperature rises rapidly to 38.3 to 40°C (101 to 104°F). Later complaints include anorexia, loss of taste, epigastric pain, and photophobia. Findings on examination are usually unremarkable except for flushing of the face and conjunctival injection. The temperature curve is often saddleback in type, with an initial elevation lasting 2 to 3 days, followed by a remission and second febrile period. Convalescence is typically rapid. Prior to the outbreak in Egypt, Rift Valley fever was a benign illness with almost no fatalities. In Egypt, approximately 1 percent of patients developed severe complications, such as encephalitis, retinopathy, or hemorrhagic manifestations. Encephalitis appeared as the acute infection waned and was severe with serious residua in some survivors. Generalized hemorrhages and icterus appeared as the disease evolved. Deaths from massive hepatic necrosis occurred 7 to 10 days after onset of illness. The fatality rate in severely ill patients may exceed 50 percent. Visual loss, including light perception, occurred 2 to 7 days after the onset of fever. Macular edema, hemorrhage, vasculitis, retinitis, and vascular occlusion were noted. One-half of patients had some permanent loss of visual acuity. A characteristic finding is an initial normal total leukocyte count followed by leukopenia with a decrease in neutrophils associated with an increase in band forms. The diagnosis is made by isolating the virus from the blood by inoculation of mice. Three-fourths of patients are viremic (up to 10^8 mouse intraperitoneal lethal doses per milliliter blood) when first seen. Neutralizing antibodies have been demonstrated as early as 4 days after onset. There is no specific treatment. A killed vaccine which had been stockpiled in the United States is being utilized.

ZIKA VIRUS Zika virus was first isolated from a captive rhesus monkey in Uganda and subsequently from wild mosquitoes. Serologic surveys reveal a prevalence of human infection up to 50 percent in central Africa and parts of Asia (Indonesia), but human disease is rarely reported. During investigation in eastern Nigeria of an outbreak of jaundice that was suspected of being yellow fever, Zika virus was isolated from one patient and two others had a rise in neutralizing antibodies. The symptoms in these patients included fever, arthralgia, and headache with retroorbital pain. Other findings were jaundice and albuminuria. The clinical syndrome appears to simulate mild yellow fever.

BUNYAVIRUSES The family Bunyaviridae consists almost entirely of viruses transmitted to vertebrate animals by arthropods. There are more than 200 viruses in the family, classified into five genera: Bunyavirus (formerly the Bunyamwera supergroup), Uukuvirus, Nairovirus, Phlebovirus, Hantavirus (Table 148-1). Most Bunyaviruses have not been associated with human infection or disease but 24 Bunyaviruses have been associated with febrile human disease which may or may not be associated with rashes. This includes the C group, Bunyamwera and Oropouche. The geographic distribution of C-group viruses includes Brazil, Trinidad, and Panama. Isolates have been obtained mostly from forest workers and laboratory technicians. Epidemics have not been recognized. The disease begins with headache, fever [with temperature up to 40.6°C (105°F)], and myalgia. Additional symptoms include malaise, photophobia, vertigo, and nausea. Illness is generally mild, lasting 2 to 4 days, and is occasionally followed by a relapse. No fatalities have been reported. Occasionally a prolonged period of convalescence ensues. Leukopenia, with total leukocyte counts as low as 2600 per microliter, is a common finding. Diagnosis has been established mainly by virus isolation.

Representative viruses of the Bunyamwera group are found in all inhabited continents except Australia. Only five viruses of the group—Bunyamwera itself, Germiston, Ilesha, Guaroa, and Wycomyia—have been associated with clinical disease. Serologic surveys give evidence of a high prevalence of inapparent infection in some areas. Clinical illness is characterized by low-grade fever, headache, and myalgia which last several days, and may be followed by weakness during convalescence. Infection due to Bunyamwera virus is associated often with arthralgia and sometimes with a rash. Since 1962 seven epidemics of Oropouche disease involving thousands of persons in Brazil, in the populated regions south of the Amazon River, have occurred during the rainy season. The epidemic vector is the midge of *Culicoides paraensis*. The incubation period is 4 to 8 days. Clinical features include abrupt onset of fever, usually to 39 to 40°C (102 to 104°F), with rigors. Symptoms, which include headache, photophobia, dizziness, myalgia, anorexia, nausea, and vomiting, last 2 to 5 days. Lymphadenopathy, splenomegaly, or rash have not been features. Laboratory findings include leukopenia with relative lymphocytosis. Urinalyses are normal. Mild elevations of transaminase may occur. Fatalities have not been reported.

"ARBOVIRUS" INFECTIONS PRESENTING CHIEFLY WITH FEVER, MALAISE, ARTHRALGIA, AND RASH

CHIKUNGUNYA In 1952 an epidemic of a disease occurred in Tanzania, which was given the name *chikungunya* ("that which bends up") because of the sudden onset of joint pains. An alphavirus of the Semliki Forest complex was isolated in 1956 both from serum of patients ill with the disease and from a pool of *A. aegypti* mosquitoes.

Chikungunya virus is responsible for a dengue-like illness in Africa, India, southeast Asia, New Guinea, and Guam, as well as for a rather mild form of hemorrhagic fever in Asian children. Outbreaks have been associated with high attack rates, with as many as 80 percent of inhabitants in some settlements becoming ill. In large epidemics, *Aëdes aegypti* is the vector. In Africa, virus is transmitted among monkeys and baboons by forest *Aëdes* mosquitoes, *A. africanus*. The cycle in southeast Asia has not been clearly defined, but humans may be the host.

After an incubation period of 3 to 12 days, the onset is typically abrupt, with a rapid rise in temperature to 38.9 to 40.6°C (102 to 105°F), often associated with a rigor and headache. Pain in large joints occurs early, incapacitating some individuals within a few minutes of onset. The arthralgia is often associated with objective arthritis. Sites of involvement include knees, ankles, shoulders, wrists, or proximal interphalangeal joints. Myalgia, especially backache, and malaise occur frequently. In 60 to 80 percent of patients a maculopapular eruption, which may appear at any time during the febrile course, is noted on the trunk or on the extensor surfaces of the extremities. Mild lymphadenopathy, predominantly in the axillary or inguinal areas, may be evident. Pharyngitis and conjunctival suffusion may be observed in a few patients. Fever continues for 1 to 10 days, and in some patients an afebrile interval of 1 to 3 days is followed by a second rise in temperature. The joint pains may continue after the temperature has returned to normal. In a few individuals joint pains have persisted for up to 4 months. Hematocrit values remain normal. Total leukocyte counts may be less than 5000 per microliter in some patients, while in others they remain normal. Urinalyses are normal. There is no specific antiviral treatment. Antiinflammatory agents such as aspirin or indomethacin have been utilized. No second attacks have been recognized, and in the absence of the hemorrhagic fever syndrome, no deaths have been described.

MAYARO VIRUS DISEASE Outbreaks involving a number of persons have occurred in Brazil and Bolivia. Survey for antibodies in serums obtained from residents in Rio de Janeiro showed that almost one-third were positive. Mayaro virus has been isolated from a wild mosquito, *Mansonia venezuelansis*, and can be maintained serially in *A. aegypti* and *Anopheles quadrimaculatus*.

The incubation period has not been clearly defined but is about 1 week. Ages of patients have ranged from 2 to 62 years, with both sexes involved. Illness begins abruptly with fever, chills, severe frontal headache, myalgia, and dizziness. Temperatures usually exceed 40°C (104°F). Arthralgia occurs uniformly and is very prominent, occasionally incapacitating, and in some patients precedes the fever by a few hours. Involvement of the wrists, fingers, ankles, and toes predominates. Other initial symptoms (in less than one-third of patients) include nausea, vomiting, and diarrhea. Initial examination reveals inguinal lymphadenopathy (one-half of cases), swelling of affected joints (one-quarter of cases), and occasional conjunctival congestion. The initial clinical features last 3 to 5 days except the arthralgia, which may persist for 2 months. On about the fifth day a maculopapular rash develops over the chest, back, arms, and legs. Rash appeared in 90 percent of children and in one-half of adults and lasted about 3 days.

Laboratory findings include leukopenia with leukocyte counts as low as 2500 per microliter during the first week. Urinalysis revealed albuminuria (2+) in one-fourth of patients. Some patients showed slight elevations in serum glutamic oxaloacetic transaminase levels.

In Brazil, no relapses were observed and no deaths have been recognized. In Bolivia, more severe illness and several fatalities have been reported.

O'NYONG-NYONG FEVER O'nyong-nyong fever was first noted as an epidemic illness characterized by joint pains, rash, and lymphadenopathy in the northern province of Uganda in 1959. The agent is an alphavirus which shows close antigenic relationships with chikungunya viruses. The original outbreak was associated with an explosive epidemic which spread to Tanzania and other areas in east Africa. By 1961, 2 million cases were recorded. In some areas, 90 percent of the population had either clinical disease or inapparent infection. Local outbreaks extended over the entire year. All age groups were affected. The most likely vector is *Anopheles funestus*. The clinical features are similar to those of chikungunya virus infection. The disease disappeared in 1962. While the virus was isolated from *A. funestus* in Kenya in 1978, no further outbreaks have been recognized.

SINDBIS VIRUS Sindbis virus, once thought rarely to present as clinical disease, has been recognized in Africa (Uganda, Republic of South Africa), Australia, and Europe (U.S.S.R., Finland, and Sweden). In the U.S.S.R. it is known as Karelian fever, in Sweden as Okelbo disease, and in Finland as Pogosta disease. Clinically, fever is low-grade and accompanied by malaise, myalgia, and arthralgia involving joints and tendons. The most striking feature is a maculopapular rash appearing on the trunk and extremities but usually sparing the face. Unlike the rash of chikungunya or o'nyong-nyong, the rash often becomes vesicular, especially on the feet and hands.

ROSS RIVER VIRUS Epidemics of polyarthritis associated with rashes have been observed in Australia since 1928. Outbreaks occur almost entirely in the period December to June. Ross River virus infection was limited to Australia, New Guinea, and the Solomon Islands until 1979 when a major outbreak occurred in Fiji which spread to the Samoan, Cook, and some Melanesian Islands. In the Fiji outbreak in 1979, infection rates were equal at all ages and in both sexes, but clinical attack rates were 4 percent in patients under 20 years and 42 percent in adults, and the clinical attack rate of males to females was 1:1.7. The onset is characterized by headache, mild catarrh, and occasionally tenderness of the palms and soles. Initially fever may be absent or minimal [highest 38°C (100.4°F)]. In about one-half of patients, arthritis, involving mainly the small joints, wrists, and ankles and sometimes associated with swelling, and paresthesias precede a rash by 1 to 15 days. In the other half, the rash precedes the arthralgia. The rash, which lasts 2 to 10 days, is usually maculopapular, appears on the cheeks and forehead, occasionally spreads to the trunk, or may be restricted to the limbs.

The rash may be pruritic. Vesicles occur rarely. Tender lymphadenopathy occurs in one-fifth of the patients. Joint symptoms persist for 3 weeks to 3 months. The virus has been isolated from *Culex annulirostris* and *Aëdes vigilax*. Animals may serve as reservoir hosts in Australia. In the Pacific, person-mosquito-person transmission seems likely.

"ARBOVIRUS" INFECTIONS PRESENTING CHIEFLY WITH FEVER, MALAISE, LYMPHADENOPATHY, AND RASH

DENGUE FEVER Dengue is endemic over large areas of the tropics and subtropics, southeast Asia, the South Pacific, and Africa. Outbreaks of dengue have occurred in the Caribbean including Puerto Rico and the U.S. Virgin Islands since 1969. Approximately 3000 cases were reported in Mexico in 1979. Indigenous infection occurred in the United States for the first time in 35 years in 1980. Eleven cases have been recognized in residents of the Rio Grande valley of Texas. In the summer of 1981, 79,000 cases of dengue-like illness with 31 deaths were reported from Cuba. *Aëdes aegypti,* the vector, has reappeared along the U.S. Gulf Coast; hence, the threat of dengue along the Gulf Coast is real.

Etiology There are four distinct serogroups of dengue viruses, all of which are flaviviruses. In the Caribbean, type 1 was associated with the 1977–1978 outbreak, type 2 in 1968–1969, type 3 in 1963–1964, and type 4 was documented in the western hemisphere for the first time in 1981.

Epidemiology Dengue infections in nature involve primarily humans and *Aëdes* mosquitoes. Dengue transmission involving monkeys and forest *Aëdes* spp. has been documented in Malaysia and West Africa. *Aëdes aegypti* is the most important worldwide vector species. This species, as well as the less common vector species, is peridomestic, biting humans readily or even preferentially and breeding in small collections of water such as cisterns and backyard litter. Surveys in Texas have revealed containers with water in which *A. aegypti* were breeding in up to 25 percent of premises. They fly during the day. Humans appear to be uniformly susceptible, and susceptibility is not influenced by age, sex, or race. During outbreaks, attack rates may be very high; in Puerto Rico and the U.S. Virgin Islands, the overall rate of clinical illness was 20 percent, with infection rates as determined by serologic survey as high as 79 per 100.

Clinical manifestations Dengue viruses frequently produce inapparent infections in humans. When symptoms develop, three broad clinical patterns may be encountered: classic dengue, hemorrhagic fever (see below), and a mild atypical form. Classic dengue (breakbone fever) occurs primarily in nonimmune individuals, specifically nonindigenous adults and children. The usual incubation period is 5 to 8 days. Prodromal symptoms such as mild conjunctivitis or coryza may occur, followed in hours by the abrupt onset of a severe splitting headache, retroorbital pain, backache, especially in the lumbar area, and leg and joint pains. The headache is aggravated by movement. At least three-fourths of patients have ocular soreness, with pain on moving the eyes. A few have mild photophobia. Though true rigors are common during the course, they are usually not present at the onset. Additional symptoms include insomnia, anorexia with loss of taste or bitter taste, and weakness. Mild transient rhinopharyngitis occurs in as many as one-quarter of the individuals. Cough is almost never seen. Epistaxis has been observed. Examination reveals scleral injection (90 percent), tenderness upon pressure on the ocular globe, and nontender posterior cervical, epitrochlear, and inguinal lymphadenopathy. Over one-half of patients have an enanthem characterized initially by pinpoint-sized vesicles over the posterior half of the soft palate. The tongue is often coated. Skin rashes, varying from diffuse flushing to scarlatiniform and morbilliform, are frequently present over the thorax and inner aspects of the arms. These are transient and fade, only to be followed by a more definite maculopapular rash which appears on the trunk on the third to the fifth day and spreads peripherally. The rash may be pruritic and generally terminates with desquamation. Extreme bradycardia is not observed. Within 2 to 3 days after the onset, the temperature may decrease to nearly normal and other symptoms disappear. The remission typically lasts 2 days and is followed by return of fever and the other symptoms, although they are generally less severe than during the initial phase. This saddleback diphasic febrile course is considered characteristic, but often is not encountered. The febrile illness usually lasts 5 to 6 days and terminates abruptly. Complaints of fatigue for several weeks after infection are common.

In addition to this "classic" syndrome, an atypically mild illness may occur. Symptoms include fever, anorexia, headache, and myalgia. On examination, evanescent rashes may be seen, but lymphadenopathy is usually absent. The course is usually less than 72 h in duration.

At the onset both in classic and in mild dengue, the leukocyte counts may be low or normal; however, by the third to the fifth day, leukopenia, usually with counts of less than 5000 leukocytes per microliter, and neutropenia are the rule. Occasionally albuminuria of moderate degree occurs.

Diagnosis Inoculation of blood obtained within the first 3 to 5 days onto mosquito tissue cell cultures or inoculation into mosquitoes is used for primary viral isolation. Diagnosis can be made by serologic tests employing paired serums for hemagglutination inhibition tests and complement fixation tests. IgM antibodies are produced in primary dengue infections. Specific serologic diagnosis is complicated by cross-reactions with other flavivirus antibodies such as those following immunization with yellow fever vaccine.

Treatment Treatment is entirely symptomatic.

Prognosis In the absence of the dengue hemorrhagic fever or dengue shock syndrome, mortality is nil.

Prevention An attenuated vaccine for dengue type 2 is undergoing experimental evaluation. Control depends upon mosquito abatement.

WEST NILE FEVER West Nile virus is distributed throughout Africa, the Middle East, parts of Europe (Camargue, France), U.S.S.R., India, and Indonesia. It produces a clinical picture closely resembling dengue. Outbreaks of disease involving several hundred patients occurred in Israel in 1950 to 1952. In one outbreak, over 60 percent of the population developed overt disease.

Epidemiology The disease is highly endemic in Egypt but goes largely unrecognized. Presumably most of the adult population is immune, and the infection in childhood is an undifferentiated mild febrile illness, whereas in Israel it mainly affects adults. The infection occurs in the summer both in Israel and in Egypt. The transmission cycle in the Middle East is bird-mosquito-bird, with *Culex univittatus* and *Culex pipiens molestus* being the principal vectors. *Culex tritaeniorhynchus* is an important vector in Asia. Although humans and a variety of other vertebrates are infected by the virus, their involvement is tangential.

Clinical manifestations The incubation period is 1 to 6 days. Most of the patients in Israel have been young adults, with neither sex predominating. The onset is usually abrupt and without prodromal symptoms. The temperature quickly rises to 38.3 to 40°C (101 to 104°F), with chills occurring in one-third of patients. Symptoms include drowsiness, severe frontal headache, ocular pain, and pain in the abdomen and back. A small number of patients have anorexia, nausea, and dryness of the throat. Cough is uncommon. There are flushing of the face, conjunctival injection, and coating of the tongue. The prominent finding is general enlargement of lymph nodes, which are of moderate size but are not hard and are only slightly tender. Occipital, axillary, and inguinal nodes are usually involved. The spleen and liver are slightly enlarged in a small proportion of patients. In one-half of patients a rash may appear from the second to the fifth day of illness and may persist for several hours or until defervescence. The rash occurs predominantly over the trunk and consists of pale roseolar maculopapular lesions. The illness is self-limited and lasts 3 to 5 days in 80 percent of patients.

In a few patients, transitory meningeal involvement may be encountered. Spinal fluid examinations may reveal a pleocytosis and some increase in protein concentration.

Leukopenia occurs in the majority of patients, and total leukocyte counts are lower than 4000 per microliter in one-third. Differential counts vary from a moderate shift to the left to a slight lymphocytosis.

Convalescence is often prolonged, lasting 1 to 2 weeks, with prominent symptoms of fatigue. Enlargement of lymph nodes subsides over several months. Only rarely have complications, sequelae, or fatalities been seen in natural infections, although in one outbreak in a group of elderly patients a high proportion of patients developed meningoencephalitis, and four fatalities ensued.

Accurate diagnosis rests on virus isolation, which can be accomplished because viremia persists for as long as 6 days, or the demonstration of a rising specific antibody titer.

The treatment is symptomatic.

"ARBOVIRUS" INFECTIONS PRESENTING CHIEFLY WITH CENTRAL NERVOUS SYSTEM INVOLVEMENT

Four "arboviruses" are presently recognized as numerically important causes of central nervous system disease in the United States: St. Louis encephalitis virus (SLE), eastern equine encephalitis virus (EEE), western equine encephalitis virus (WEE), and the California serogroup (CE) viruses. The spectrum of infection caused by these agents includes inapparent infection, fever with headache, aseptic meningitis, and encephalitis. Some 1500 to 2000 cases of encephalitis are reported in the United States each year. In the absence of epidemics, 5 to 10 percent of these (75 to 200 cases) are confirmed as "arboviral" in etiology. In nonepidemic years, California serogroup viruses (predominantly LaCrosse virus) represent two-thirds to three-fourths of the cases. Because of epidemics of St. Louis and western equine encephalitis, which contribute a larger number of cases, the overall distribution in the 30 years between 1955 and 1984 has been: SLE 65 percent, CE 20 percent, WEE 13 percent, and EEE 2 percent.

Etiology Despite the diversity of specific viral etiologies (see Table 148-2), in individual patients the clinical manifestations of aseptic meningitis and encephalitis are very similar, and preclude an etiologic diagnosis without ancillary information regarding epidemiologic and serologic features (see Table 148-3). The clinical features of aseptic meningitis due to "arboviruses" are indistinguishable from those due to the more prevalent enteroviruses. Since transmission to humans in the United States and Canada involves arthropods, specifically mosquitoes, except for Powassan and Colorado tick fever, indigenously acquired disease occurs at times when mosquitoes are prevalent, such as late spring through early fall.

Clinical manifestations The clinical features of "arbovirus" encephalitis differ among age groups. In infants under 1 year of age, the only consistently noted symptoms are sudden onset of fever, which is often accompanied by convulsions. Convulsions may be either generalized or focal. Typically the fever ranges between 38.9 and 40°C (102 and 104°F). Other physical findings may include bulging of the fontanelle, rigidity of the extremities, and abnormalities in reflexes.

In children between 5 and 14 years of age, subjective symptoms are more easily elicited. Headache, fever, and drowsiness of 2 to 3 days' duration before medical attention is sought are common. The symptoms may then subside or become more intense and may be associated with nausea, vomiting, muscular pain, photophobia, and, less frequently, convulsions (less than 10 percent except in California encephalitis). The child is found to be acutely ill, febrile, and lethargic. Nuchal rigidity and intention tremors are often present, and on occasion muscular weakness can be demonstrated.

In adults, the initial symptoms commonly include the fairly abrupt onset of fever, nausea with vomiting, and severe headache. The headache is most often frontal but may be occipital or diffuse. Mental aberrations, represented by confusion and disorientation, usually appear within the subsequent 24 h. Other symptoms may include diffuse myalgia and photophobia. The abnormalities found on physical examination predominantly relate to the neurologic examination, although conjunctival suffusion is frequently seen and skin rashes may occur. Disturbances in mentation are among the most outstanding clinical features. These range from coma through severe disorientation to subtle abnormalities detected only by cerebral function tests such as the subtraction of serial 7s. A small proportion of patients show only lethargy, lying quietly, apparently asleep unless stimulated. Tremor is common and is observed more frequently in individuals over 40 years of age. The tremors vary in location and may be continuous or intention in type. Cranial nerve abnormalities resulting in oculomotor muscle paresis and nystagmus, facial weakness, and difficulty in deglutition may occur and are usually present within the initial several days. Objective sensory changes are unusual. Hemiparesis or monoparesis may occur. Reflex abnormalities are also common; these include exaggerated palmomental reflexes, and suck and snout reflexes. Superficial abdominal and cremasteric reflexes are usually absent. Changes in the tendon reflexes are variable and inconstant. The plantar response may be extensor and fluctuates almost hourly. Dysdiadochokinesia often exists.

The duration of the fever and neurologic symptoms and signs varies from several days to a month but usually ranges from 4 to 14 days. Clinical improvement generally follows the subsidence of the fever within several days unless irreversible anatomic changes have occurred.

Laboratory findings Erythrocytes are usually normal. Total leukocyte counts often reveal both a slight to moderate leukocytosis (occasionally greater than 20,000 leukocytes per microliter) and neutrophilia. Examination of the cerebrospinal fluid usually reveals several hundred cells per microliter, but on occasion cloudy cerebrospinal fluid with cells in excess of 1000 per microliter may be seen. Within the first several days of illness, polymorphonuclear neutrophils may predominate. The initial cerebrospinal fluid protein is usually

TABLE 148-3 Features of arboviral encephalitides common in the United States

Etiology	Geographic predominance in the United States	Urban/rural	Age, years	Sex	Unique clinical features	Mortality, %	Residua
California encephalitis	Midwest	Rural	5–10	M	Seizures	2	Seizures (one-fourth who had them in acute phase), behavioral problems (15%)
Eastern equine encephalitis	Eastern seaboard	Both	<5 >55	=	CSF may have >1000 WBC/μL	50	Children <10 years have emotional lability, retardation, convulsions
St. Louis encephalitis	Eastern and midwest	Both	>35	=	Dysuria	2–12	Ataxia, speech difficulties (5%)
Western equine encephalitis	Entire	Both	<1 >55	=	None	3	Children <3 months have behavioral problems, convulsions

only slightly elevated but on occasion may exceed 1.0 g/L (100 mg/dL). The level of spinal fluid sugar is normal; a significant decrease should raise serious consideration of an alternative diagnosis. As the illness progresses, mononuclear cells in the cerebrospinal fluid tend to increase so that they predominate and the protein concentration may increase. Other laboratory studies have been reported only sporadically, but abnormalities may include hyponatremia, often due to the inappropriate secretion of antidiuretic hormone, and elevations in serum creatine phosphokinase.

Diagnosis   Specific diagnosis requires the isolation of the virus or detection of antibodies with a rising titer between the acute phase of disease and convalescence. Antibodies can be detected by hemagglutination inhibition, complement fixation, or virus neutralization techniques.

Treatment   Treatment is entirely supportive and requires meticulous attention in the comatose patient.

LACROSSE ENCEPHALITIS   A previously undescribed virus was isolated in 1943 from mosquitoes in Kern County, California. Since 1963, a large number of agents now designated as the California group of viruses have been isolated (Table 148-1). LaCrosse, snowshoe hare, Jamestown Canyon, and California encephalitis viruses cause human encephalitis in North America. Tahyna and Inkoo viruses are associated with febrile and, rarely, encephalitic disease in Europe. Since 1966 in the midwest United States, LaCrosse virus (California) encephalitis has been incriminated in 5 to 6 percent of cases of acute central nervous system disease, ranking above all agents except the enteroviruses.

Epidemiology   LaCrosse virus infection occurs in the north central states, New York, in wooded areas of eastern Texas and Louisiana, and along the eastern seaboard. The virus is maintained by transovarial transmission in woodland mosquitoes, *Aëdes triseratus*, which breed in tree holes in hardwood forests and have adapted to discarded tires. The virus is present in seminal fluid of male mosquitoes and transmitted to the female. The virus overwinters in eggs of *A. triseratus*. Chipmunks and gray squirrels serve as amplifier hosts. LaCrosse virus (California) encephalitis occurs during the summer months (June to October), most often involving boys (60 percent) 5 to 10 years of age (60 percent) who live in rural areas.

Clinical manifestations   Two clinical patterns of LaCrosse virus disease have been defined. One is a mild form with a 2- to 3-day prodrome of fever, headache, malaise, and gastrointestinal symptoms. About the third day the temperature increases to 40°C (104°F), and the patient becomes lethargic and develops meningeal signs. These findings abate gradually over a 7- to 8-day period without overt sequelae. The second pattern, a severe form which occurs in at least one-half of the patients, begins abruptly with fever, headache, and vomiting, followed shortly by lethargy and disorientation. During the first 2 to 4 days the course is rapidly progressive with the occurrence of seizures (50 to 60 percent), focal neurologic signs (20 percent), pathologic reflexes (10 percent), and coma (10 percent). Focal neurologic signs may include asymmetric flaccid paralysis. Uncommon findings have included arthralgia and rash. Clinical laboratory features include peripheral leukocyte counts ranging from 7000 to 30,000 per microliter (median 16,000 per microliter) with neutrophilia. Cerebrospinal fluid examination reveals 10 to 500 cells per microliter, usually with a predominance of mononuclear cells, protein concentrations of less than 1.0 g/L (100 mg/dL), and normal sugar concentrations. Electroencephalograms (EEGs) are abnormal in at least 80 percent of patients, revealing slow delta-wave activity. In one-half of the patients the abnormality is asymmetric, suggesting focal destructive lesions. Brain scans using [^{99}Tc]pertechnetate and computed tomography (CT) also may be abnormal, and temporal lobe localization has been observed. Beginning about the fourth day and proceeding over the next 3 to 7 days, there is progressive improvement, with almost all patients becoming afebrile, seizure-free, and ready for discharge from the hospital within 2 weeks after onset.

Diagnosis   Serum and CSF should be tested for LaCrosse virus IgM antibodies. Serum capture IgM enzyme-linked immunosorbent assay (ELISA) tests detected 83 percent of cases on admission in LaCrosse encephalitis. Early specific diagnosis eliminates the need for brain biopsy to exclude herpes encephalitis which is suggested by the temporal lobe localization.

Treatment   Initial seizure activity is frequently prolonged and difficult to control. The most effective anticonvulsant medication has been parenteral diazepam. Patients with the severe form of disease should be discharged on anticonvulsants such as phenobarbital for 6 to 12 months.

Prognosis   The case fatality ratio is low (2 percent or less); however, one-third of patients may have abnormal neurologic findings at the time of discharge. During the early convalescent period, emotional lability and irritability are common. In one series, recurrent seizures occurred in one-quarter of the patients who had seizures during the acute phase. In this same series EEGs were abnormal in one-third of patients evaluated 1 to 8 years after their acute illness. In another series, 15 percent had sequelae, predominantly personality or behavioral problems.

OTHER CALIFORNIA GROUP ENCEPHALITIDES   Jamestown Canyon encephalitis is uncommon, but in contrast to LaCrosse encephalitis usually occurs in adults. Snowshoe hare virus has been isolated from mosquitoes throughout Canada and from Alaska. Encephalitis has been reported from the eastern provinces. Clinical features of Tahyna virus disease, which has been seen in children in Europe, include fever, pharyngitis, pneumonitis, gastrointestinal symptoms, and aseptic meningitis. Neither mortality nor sequelae are reported.

EASTERN EQUINE ENCEPHALITIS   Eastern equine encephalitis (EEE), an alphavirus, was first isolated in 1933 from the brain tissue of horses during an outbreak of equine illness in New Jersey. The first recognized human outbreak occurred in Massachusetts in 1938.

Epidemiology   The virus is distributed along the eastern coast of the Americas from northeastern United States to Argentina. Foci have been found in the Syracuse region of New York, Ontario, Canada, western Michigan, and South Dakota. Viral isolations also have been reported in the Philippines, Thailand, Czechoslovakia, Poland, and the U.S.S.R., but the question of type specificity has not been resolved. In the northeastern United States, epidemics occur in the late summer and early fall. Epizootics in horses precede the occurrence of human cases by 1 to 2 weeks. The disease affects mainly infants, children, and adults over 55 years of age. There is no sex preponderance. Inapparent infection occurs in all age groups, suggesting that the decreased likelihood of developing overt infection in the 15- to 54-year age group is not the result of decreased exposure. The ratio of inapparent infection to overt encephalitis approximates 25:1.

The transmission of EEE involves *Culiseta melanura* mosquitoes and swamp-dwelling birds, e.g., red-winged blackbirds, sparrows, pheasants. Transmission by pecking has been shown in domestic pheasant flocks. *C. melanura* rarely feed on horses or humans, and other mosquitoes, especially *Aëdes sollicitans*, a salt-marsh mosquito which is an avid human feeder, have been postulated as the epidemic vector. The epidemiology of overwintering and maintenance between outbreaks remains unknown. Equine animals and human beings are "dead ends" in the transmission cycle, and infection in them is accidental.

Clinical manifestations   Though human infections have been thought usually to result in serious, if not fatal, central nervous system involvement, the detection of inapparent infection as well as relatively mild disease establishes the occurrence of milder forms. In many patients, the cerebrospinal fluid is cloudy and contains in excess of 1000 cells per microliter.

Diagnosis   ELISA tests for the detection of specific IgM antibodies in CSF or serum permit early diagnosis, although absence of IgM does not exclude infection. Confirmation can be obtained by a fourfold or more rise or fall in complement fixation (CF), hemagglutination inhibition, or virus neutralization tests.

Prognosis The mortality rate in clinical infection exceeds 50 percent. In the most severe cases, death occurs between the third and fifth days. Children under 10 years of age have a greater likelihood of surviving the acute illness, but they also have a greater likelihood of developing severe disabling residuals: mental retardation, convulsions, emotional lability, blindness, deafness, speech disorders, and hemiplegia.

ST. LOUIS ENCEPHALITIS St. Louis encephalitis (SLE) was first recognized as an entity during a major outbreak in St. Louis, Missouri, and the surrounding area in 1933. Subsequently, sporadic, unpredictable outbreaks have occurred in Houston (1964), Dallas (1966), Memphis (1974), northern Mississippi and Illinois (1975). The attack rate in Greenville, Mississippi, in 1975 was the highest which has been encountered, 10 per 10,000 population.

Epidemiology In the United States, epidemics of SLE fall into two epidemiologic patterns. One pattern is found in the west, where mixed outbreaks of western equine encephalitis and SLE have occurred primarily in isolated rural areas. The vector has been *Culex tarsalis*. The second pattern occurred in the original St. Louis outbreak and the numerous subsequent epidemics in the midwest, Texas, New Jersey, and Florida. These outbreaks have been more urban in location and are characterized by occurrence of encephalitis in older persons. In such urban-suburban epidemics, the epidemic vectors have been mosquitoes of the *Culex pipiens-quinquefasciatus* complex with the exception of the Florida epidemic, in which *Culex nigripalpus* was incriminated. The presence of SLE virus outside the United States has been proved by isolations in Trinidad, Panama, Jamaica, Brazil, and Argentina. However, except for Jamaica, SLE has not been reported outside the United States. The basic transmission cycle is that of wild bird–mosquito–wild bird. The virus survives the winter in female mosquitoes which ingest a blood meal from a viremic bird before overwintering. The disease in humans usually appears in midsummer to early fall. In urban epidemics, there is no sex predominance while among sporadic cases in the west, men predominate 2:1 due to greater occupational exposure. The human represents an accidental host and plays no role in the basic transmission cycle. Serologic studies following most urban epidemics indicate that infection rates are similar in all age groups, and that the increasing age-specific attack rate for clinical encephalitis which is typical of urban St. Louis encephalitis is probably due to age differences in host susceptibility to overt disease rather than to a higher rate of infection.

Clinical manifestations Infection with SLE virus most commonly results in an inapparent infection. Of the patients with confirmed disease, approximately three-fourths have clinical encephalitis; the remainder present with aseptic meningitis, febrile headaches, or nonspecific illness. Virtually all patients over 40 years have encephalitic manifestations. Urinary frequency and dysuria have been symptoms in approximately 20 percent of patients despite sterile routine aerobic urine cultures. SLE virus antigen has been demonstrated in urine; this may account for the occurrence of urinary tract symptoms.

Diagnosis The occurrence of either encephalitis or aseptic meningitis as manifested by febrile illness with cerebrospinal fluid pleocytosis in the months of June through September in an adult, especially over 35 years of age, should raise the suspicion of St. Louis encephalitis. Because approximately 40 percent of patients with SLE have antibodies detectable by hemagglutination inhibition at the onset of illness, acute serum for serologic studies should be submitted promptly to a competent laboratory. ELISA tests for the detection of specific IgM antibodies in CSF or serum provide a means of early specific diagnosis.

Prognosis The case fatality ratio in the original St. Louis epidemic was 20 percent. In most subsequent outbreaks the mortality rate has varied from 2 to 12 percent. Subjective complaints, including

nervousness, headaches, and easy fatigability and excitability, appear to be the most common residuals. Late organic defects such as speech defects, difficulty in walking, and disturbances in vision were demonstrated in approximately 5 percent of patients 3 years following infection.

WESTERN EQUINE ENCEPHALITIS Western equine encephalitis (WEE) virus is an alphavirus that was isolated in 1930 in California from horses with encephalitis. In 1938 it was recovered from a fatal human infection.

Epidemiology WEE virus has been isolated in the United States, Canada, Brazil, Guyana, and Argentina. Human disease has been diagnosed in the United States, Canada, and Brazil. In the United States, the virus is found in virtually all geographic areas. The central valley of California represents an important endemic area. The disease occurs mainly in early summer and midsummer. Wild birds, which develop viremia of sufficiently high titer to be able to infect mosquitoes that feed on them, are the basic reservoir. *Culex tarsalis* is the principal vector in the western United States. In areas east of the Appalachian Mountains, another vector may be operative. The virus has been repeatedly isolated from *Culiseta melanura;* however, the importance of this species has been questioned, since it is not primarily a human-biting mosquito. The overwintering mechanism is not known. The ratio of inapparent infection to disease, as evidenced by serologic survey studies, varies from 58:1 in children to 1150:1 in adults. Approximately one-fourth of patients are less than 1 year of age. The highest attack rates occur in persons 55 years or older.

Prognosis The fatality rate approximates 3 percent in laboratory-confirmed cases. The incidence and severity of sequelae are related to age. Sequelae among very young infants are frequent (appearing in 61 percent of a group of patients less than 3 months old) and severe; they consist of upper motor neuron impairment, involving the pyramidal tracts, extrapyramidal structures, and cerebellum, and result in behavioral problems and convulsions. Both the incidence and severity of sequelae diminish rapidly after 1 year of age. Adults may complain of nervousness, irritability, easy fatigability, and tremulousness for 6 months or longer after the acute illness. Probably not more than 5 percent of adults have sequelae which are sufficiently severe to be of practical significance. Postencephalitic seizures are rare.

JAPANESE ENCEPHALITIS The name Japanese B encephalitis was employed during an epidemic which occurred in 1924 to distinguish it from von Economo's disease, which was designated as type A encephalitis. The designation as Japanese B no longer seems useful, and the term Japanese encephalitis (JE) will be employed.

Epidemiology Japanese encephalitis virus infection is known to occur in eastern Siberia, China, Korea, Taiwan, Japan, Malaya, Vietnam, Thailand, Singapore, Guam, and India. Since the late 1960s JE has declined in Japan and China. JE remains a major problem in northern Thailand. In temperate climates, the disease shows a late-summer–early-fall seasonal incidence. In tropical climates there is no seasonal variation. The mosquito *Culex tritaeniorhynchus* is the major vector species. It is a rural mosquito which breeds in rice fields and preferentially bites large domestic animals, such as pigs, but also feeds on birds and humans. The human is an accidental host in the transmission cycle. In endemic areas, children ages 3 to 15 are primarily affected. Epidemics in nonendemic areas have affected all age groups, but young children and older adults predominate. The ratio of inapparent infection, as evidenced by a serologic survey study of Australian troops in Vietnam, was 210:1.

Clinical manifestations The incubation period is 5 to 15 days. As with SLE, illness may present as encephalitis, aseptic meningitis, or febrile headache. The occurrence of severe rigors at the onset has been noted in almost 90 percent of patients. On admission, most patients are alert, but deterioration of mental status occurs in about three-fourths of patients within 3 to 4 days. Localized paresis is found more often than with other "arboviral" encephalitides, e.g., in 31 percent of cases, with predominantly upper extremity involvement; however, it resolves rapidly with defervescence. Convulsions are frequent in children, but occur in less than 10 percent of adults. Severe hyperthermia may occur and require treatment. A peripheral leukocytosis with 50 to 90 percent neutrophils is common. Weight loss has been very striking. The failure of the temperature to lyse, appearance of diaphoresis, tachypnea, and the accumulation of bronchial secretions are grave prognostic signs.

Prognosis The immediate mortality rate has varied from 7 to 33 percent or higher. The occurrence of sequelae varies inversely with the fatality rate; in those series with high fatality rates (33 percent), sequelae occurred in 3 to 14 percent. In another series with a fatality rate of 7.4 percent, the rate of adverse sequelae was 32 percent. Individuals who had neurologic abnormalities during the acute phase but survived have no more than an 80 percent chance for complete recovery. Sequelae consist of seizures, persistent paralysis, ataxia, mental retardation, and behavioral disorders.

OTHER "ARBOVIRUSES" WITH CENTRAL NERVOUS SYSTEM INVOLVEMENT A large group of additional "arboviruses" have been associated with encephalitis or aseptic meningitis. Some of these agents are listed in Table 148-2. Though the epidemiologic picture of each of these agents is unique, the general features are sufficiently similar to require laboratory support for their differentiation.

"ARBOVIRUS" DISEASES PRESENTING CHIEFLY WITH HEMORRHAGIC MANIFESTATIONS

For 300 years, yellow fever was the only epidemic viral disease known to be accompanied by grave hemorrhagic manifestations. Since the 1930s diverse viral etiologies of the hemorrhagic fever syndrome have been recognized (Table 148-2). Additional agents include members of several families and genera: flavivirus, Filoviridae, phlebovirus, Nairovirus, Hantavirus, and arenavirus (see Chap. 149). Despite diverse etiologies, there are many similar clinical manifestations. The onset is usually sudden, with headache, backache, generalized myalgia, conjunctivitis, and prostration. From approximately the third day, the initial stage is followed by hypotension, and hemorrhagic manifestations may occur; these are characterized by bleeding gums, epistaxis, hemoptysis, hematemesis, melena, petechiae, ecchymoses, and hemorrhages into most visceral organs. Mild leukopenia develops early, but with the appearance of hemorrhagic manifestations, leukocytosis may occur. The pathophysiology of the cardinal signs is attributable to hematopoietic and capillary damage, with variable localization of lesions. On the basis of limited confirmatory observations, variable degrees of disseminated intravascular coagulation may be in part responsible for the pathophysiology of the hemorrhagic fever syndromes. Death usually occurs in the second week of disease, at which time a high titer of antibody has developed and the patient may have become afebrile. Death is usually associated with coma, which is due not to encephalitis but to an encephalopathy. The pathologic changes may be similar despite diverse viral etiologies, with midzonal hepatic necrosis and acidophilic cytoplasmic inclusions similar to the Councilman bodies of yellow fever.

YELLOW FEVER Yellow fever is an acute infectious disease of short duration and extremely variable severity; it is caused by a flavivirus and is followed by lifelong immunity. The classic triad of symptoms—jaundice, hemorrhages, and intense albuminuria—is present only in severe infections, which make up only a small proportion of the total.

Prevalence For more than 200 years, after the first identifiable outbreak occurred in Yucatan in 1648, yellow fever was one of the great plagues of the world. As late as 1905, New Orleans and other southern United States ports experienced at least 5000 cases and 1000 deaths. Because of the existence of the sylvatic form of the disease, protective measures must be maintained against human disease, as demonstrated by outbreaks in Central America from 1948 to 1957.

In southern Ethiopia from 1962 to 1964 there were over 100,000 cases with some 30,000 deaths. From 1978 to 1980 there were outbreaks in Bolivia, Brazil, Colombia, Ecuador, Peru, and Venezuela. In 1979, yellow fever reappeared in Trinidad. During the same time period extensive epidemics were seen in Nigeria, Ghana, Senegal, and Gambia. In Gambia the attack rate was 2.6 to 4.4 percent with a case fatality rate of 19 percent. In 1983, epidemics occurred in Burkino Faso (formerly Upper Volta) and Ghana.

Epidemiology Human infection results from two basically different cycles of virus transmission, urban and sylvatic. The urban cycle is human-mosquito-human, i.e., *Aëdes aegypti*–transmitted yellow fever. After a 2-week extrinsic incubation period, mosquitoes can transmit infection. Sylvan yellow fever differs under various ecologic circumstances. In the rain forests of South and Central America, species of treetop *Haemagogus* or *Sabethes* mosquitoes maintain transmission in wild primates. Once infected, the mosquito vector remains infectious for life; hence it may serve as a reservoir as well as a vector. When humans come into proximity with the forest-canopy mosquitoes, sporadic cases or focal outbreaks may occur. With sylvan yellow fever, males predominate. Focal outbreaks may be quite extensive; in Brazil in 1973 at least 21,000 persons out of 1.5 million (1.4 percent) were infected. In east Africa, the mosquito-primate cycle is maintained by the forest-canopy mosquito, *A. africanus,* which seldom feeds on humans. The peridomestic mosquito *A. simpsoni* feeds upon primates entering the village gardens and can then in turn transmit the virus to humans. Once yellow fever is reintroduced into urban areas, the urban cycle can be reinitiated, with the potential for epidemic disease.

Clinical manifestations The incubation period is usually 3 to 6 days. In accidental laboratory- or hospital-acquired infections longer incubation periods (10 to 13 days) have been reported. In mild yellow fever the only symptoms may be the abrupt onset of fever and headache. Additional symptoms may include nausea, epistaxis, relative bradycardia known as Faget's sign [e.g., with a temperature of 38.9°C (102°F) the pulse may be only 48 to 52 beats per minute], and slight albuminuria. The mild illness lasts only 1 to 3 days and resembles influenza except that coryzal symptoms are lacking.

Moderately severe and malignant attacks of yellow fever are characterized by three distinct clinical periods: the period of infection, the period of remission, and the period of intoxication. Prodromal symptoms are usually absent. The onset is characteristically sudden, with headache, dizziness, and temperature elevations to 40°C (104°F) without a relative bradycardia. Young children may have febrile convulsions. The headache is followed quickly by pains in the neck, back, and legs. Often there is nausea with vomiting and retching. Examination reveals a flushed face and injection of the conjunctivae. The congestion of the eyes persists until the third day. The tongue characteristically shows bright-red margins and tip and a white furred center. Faget's sign appears by the second day. Epistaxis and gingival bleeding are common. On the third day of illness, the fever may fall by crisis and the patient enters remission, or, in the malignant form, copious hemorrhages, anuria, or delirium may occur. The stage of remission lasts from several hours to several days. In the third stage, the "classic" symptoms develop; the fever returns but the pulse remains slow. Jaundice becomes detectable about the third day; however, jaundice often is not prominent even in fatal illnesses. Increased epistaxis, melena, and uterine hemorrhages are common, but gross hematuria is rare. Of the classic signs, "black vomit" is more characteristic than is jaundice. Hematemesis usually does not occur before the fourth day and is often associated with a fatal outcome. Albuminuria, which rarely develops before the third day, occurs in 90 percent of patients and may be quite marked (3 to 20 g albumin per liter). In spite of this massive albuminuria, edema or ascites has not been reported. In malignant infections, coma frequently occurs 2 to 3 days before death. Shortly before death, which usually occurs between the fourth and the sixth days, the patient becomes delirious and wildly agitated. Though the duration of fever in the third stage is usually 5 to 7 days, the period of intoxication is the most variable of the stages and may last up to 2 weeks. Yellow fever is relatively free from complications, suppurative parotitis being the most striking of those which do occur. Clinical relapses are not characteristic of yellow fever.

Laboratory findings Early in the disease, progressive leukopenia may occur. By the fifth day, total leukocyte counts of 1500 to 2500 per microliter often are found, the decrease being due mostly to a decrease in neutrophils. Total leukocyte counts return to normal by the tenth day, and in fatal cases there may be a marked terminal leukocytosis. Hemoglobin values remain normal except terminally, when hemoconcentration or bleeding may occur. Platelet counts are normal or decreased. Prolongation of clotting, prothrombin, and partial thromboplastin times is marked in patients with jaundice. Increases in total and conjugated bilirubin occur. In icteric patients, marked elevations of serum glutamic oxaloacetic transaminase occur. Hypoglycemia has been seen in patients with severe hepatic damage. Electrocardiograms may show T-wave changes. The cerebrospinal fluid is normal.

Diagnosis Inoculation onto mosquito cell cultures or intrathoracically into mosquitoes are methods of choice for virus isolation from blood. Isolation is most likely from specimens obtained during the first 3 days of illness. Serologic methods include plaque reduction neutralization tests on paired sera and detection of yellow fever IgM antibodies and antigen usually by ELISA methods. The ELISA method enables confirmation in the field within 3 h.

Treatment The management has been symptomatic and supportive and should be based upon assessment and correction of the circulatory abnormalities. If evidence of disseminated intravascular coagulation is present, the administration of heparin should be considered. Close attention to fluids and electrolytes is essential. As with all of the hemorrhagic fevers, aspirin is contraindicated.

Prognosis The overall fatality rate in yellow fever is between 5 and 10 percent of clinical cases; it may be even less since many infections are mild or inapparent.

Prevention Effective control measures are available. Immunization has been effective in the prevention of outbreaks. With the occurrence of sylvatic outbreaks, work in the area of epizootic activity should be discontinued and intensive mosquito abatement measures should be instituted. These measures may provide the time necessary for a mass immunization program.

DENGUE HEMORRHAGIC FEVER All four dengue virus serotypes can cause dengue hemorrhagic fever (DHF) and dengue shock syndrome (DSS). Infection with dengue 1, 3, or 4 followed within a few years by dengue 2 may be especially important in the pathogenesis. There is consensus that DHF is an immunologically mediated disease. Enhanced growth of dengue 2 virus occurs in peripheral blood mononuclear phagocytes obtained from dengue immune donors or in cells from normal donors in the presence of subneutralizing concentrations of dengue or cross-reacting heterotypic flavivirus antibodies. Infectious virus-antibody complexes attach and enter mononuclear phagocytes by way of Fc receptors. Increased replication of virus in these cells may be followed by a secondary set of reactions: complement activation, mast cell degranulation, and activation of the kinin system.

Prevalence The reasons for the apparent sudden "appearance" of the syndrome in the past 30 years are completely obscure. However, during the 1922 epidemic of dengue fever in Louisiana, hemorrhagic manifestations, including epistaxis, bleeding gums, melena, menorrhagia, and even "black vomit," were observed. DHF is now a leading cause of morbidity and mortality in tropical Asia. Over 500,000 cases of DHF have been officially reported with major epidemics in the People's Republic of China, Vietnam, Indonesia, Thailand, and Cuba. In the Cuban outbreak in 1981, almost 350,000 persons developed dengue, approximately 10,000 had hemorrhagic manifestations, and 158 died (1.6 percent mortality). DHF in Asia is a disease of childhood with one peak observed in children under 1 year, and a second in children ages 3 to 5. The disease in infants is associated with primary infection in the presence of maternal

antibody. Studies in Thailand have estimated the frequency of DSS as 11 cases per 1000 secondary dengue infections. DSS occurs more frequently in girls than boys. Dengue hemorrhagic fever occurs almost exclusively in indigenous populations; it has been observed only rarely in whites of European descent despite the frequent occurrence of classic dengue in this group.

Clinical manifestations Illness begins abruptly with a minor stage characterized by fever, cough, pharyngitis, headache, anorexia, nausea, vomiting, and abdominal pain which is often severe. This continues for 2 to 4 days. In contrast to classic dengue, myalgia, arthralgia, and bone pain are unusual. Physical signs include fever varying from 38.3 to 40.6°C (101 to 105°F), injection of the tonsils and pharynx, and palpable lymph nodes and liver. The initial state is followed by abrupt deterioration, with the rapid onset of lassitude and weakness (Table 148-4). On examination the child is found to be restless and to have cold clammy extremities with a warm trunk and a pallid face with circumoral cyanosis. Petechiae, most frequently located on the forehead and distal extremities, are seen in half the cases. Occasionally there may be a macular or maculopapular rash. The extremities are frequently cyanotic. Hypotension, with narrowing of the pulse pressure, and tachycardia occur. Pathologic reflexes may be present. Most fatalities occur in the fourth or fifth day of illness; melena, hematemesis, coma, or unresponsive shock are poor prognostic signs. Cyanosis, dyspnea, and convulsions are terminal manifestations. Following this critical period, survivors show steady and rapid improvement.

Laboratory findings In one study, hemoconcentration was found in one-fifth of the children. The majority had leukocyte counts between 5000 and 10,000 per microliter, with one-third showing a leukocytosis. Only 10 percent of children had a true leukopenia. The most characteristic findings were thrombocytopenia, rarely with blood platelets under 75,000 per microliter, positive tourniquet test, and prolonged bleeding time. Prothrombin time and partial thromboplastin times were usually near normal values. Depression of clotting factors V, VII, IX, and X may be present. Bone marrow examination may reveal maturation arrest of megakaryocytes. In Manila or Bangkok, hematuria has been infrequent even with other serious bleeding manifestations; however, in Tahiti, gross hematuria was common. Cerebrospinal fluid examinations are usually normal. Other abnormal laboratory findings may include hyponatremia, acidosis, elevated blood urea nitrogen levels, elevation in serum glutamic oxalacetic transaminase levels, mild hyperbilirubinemia, and hypoproteinemia. Electrocardiograms may reveal diffuse myocardial abnormalities. Two-thirds of patients have radiologic evidence of bronchopneumonia, with many showing pleural effusions.

Diagnosis The World Health Organization (WHO) has established criteria for the diagnosis of DHF: fever—acute onset, high, continuous, and lasting for 2 to 7 days; hemorrhagic manifestations including at least a positive tourniquet test and any of the following: petechiae, purpura, ecchymoses, epistaxis, bleeding gums, hematemesis, or melena; enlargement of the liver; thrombocytopenia, ≤100,000 per microliter; hemoconcentration, hematocrit increased by ≥20 percent. Criteria for DSS are a rapid, weak pulse with

TABLE 148-4 World Health Organization's clinical classification of dengue hemorrhagic fever

	Grade	Clinical features	Laboratory findings
DHF*	I	Fever, constitutional symptoms, positive tourniquet test	Hemoconcentration Thrombocytopenia
	II	Grade I plus spontaneous bleeding (e.g., skin, gums, gastrointestinal tract)	Hemoconcentration Thrombocytopenia
DSS*	III	Grade II plus circulatory failure, agitation	Hemoconcentration Thrombocytopenia
	IV	Grade II plus profound shock (blood pressure = 0)	Hemoconcentration Thrombocytopenia

* DHF, dengue hemorrhagic fever; DSS, dengue shock syndrome.

narrowing of the pulse pressure (≤20 mmHg) or hypotension with cold, clammy skin and restlessness. The WHO classification includes a grading of severity (Table 148-4). Minor hemorrhagic manifestations may be seen during the course of classic dengue fever without meeting WHO criteria for DHF. These cases should be termed dengue fever with hemorrhage, not DHF.

Treatment   The mainstay is correction of circulatory collapse while avoiding fluid overload. Administration of 5% glucose in 0.5 N saline at a rate of 40 mL/kg restored blood pressure within 1 to 2 h in one-half of patients. When stable, the rate of administration of intravenous fluids was slowed to 10 (mL/kg)/h. If improvement did not occur, plasma or a plasma expander (20 mL/kg) was administered. Transfusion of whole blood is not recommended. Oxygen should be administered. Glucocorticoids have been used, but doses of 25 mg/kg have not resulted in significant improvement. Since the evidence for severe disseminated intravascular coagulation is questionable, use of heparin is not clear-cut, although in a group of Filipino children with type 3 dengue virus, administration of heparin (1 mg sodium heparin per kilogram) was associated with a dramatic rise in number of platelets and level of plasma fibrinogen. Antibiotics are not indicated; sympathomimetic amines and salicylates are contraindicated. Recovery from vascular collapse usually occurs within 24 to 48 h, at which time diuretics and digitalis may be necessary. An uncontrolled trial of interferon was conducted during the 1981 epidemic in Cuba with some indication of efficacy.

Prognosis   Mortality has varied from 1 to 23 percent. Deaths have been most common in infants under 1 year of age.

Prevention   At present, vector control is the only method available to prevent hemorrhagic fever.

TICK-BORNE HEMORRHAGIC FEVERS   Crimean-Congo hemorrhagic fever   At the close of World War II, a new disease entity was recognized in the Crimea region of the U.S.S.R. Retrospective studies demonstrated that an almost identical syndrome had been recognized in the south central Asian republics of the U.S.S.R. for many years. Soviet workers repeatedly isolated virus strains during 1967 to 1969.

The virus of Crimean hemorrhagic fever (CHF) is antigenically identical with Congo virus, which was isolated from patients, cattle, and ticks in Kenya, Uganda, Zaire, and Nigeria. Crimean-Congo hemorrhagic fever (CCHF) virus is now known in South Africa, throughout most of subsaharan Africa, eastern Europe, the Middle East, and Asia as far as the Xinjiang province of China. CCHF occurs where *Hyalomma* ticks are found.

Approximately 30 cases of CCHF have been recorded annually in each of the known areas of occurrence in the U.S.S.R. The cases occur between April and September. The sex distribution of CCHF is equal, and 80 percent of the cases occur in the 20- to 60-year age group, with the majority occurring in dairy and agricultural workers. The major arthropod vectors for transmission to humans are ticks which belong to the genus *Hyalomma*. Cattle and wild hares appear to be important reservoirs, and rooks and other birds have been implicated. Once a case of human CCHF occurs, person-to-person transmission is possible. Nosocomial outbreaks have occurred in the U.S.S.R., Pakistan, India, and Iraq. Transmission is presumed to occur through direct contact with infected blood. There are no data to suggest airborne transmission.

After an incubation period of 3 to 6 days, the onset is abrupt, with temperatures to 40°C (104°F), dizziness, headache, and diffuse myalgia. The course of fever is occasionally biphasic, with an average duration of 8 days. Findings include flushing of the face, conjunctival injection, vomiting, and, on occasion, epigastric pain. Hepatomegaly occurs in half the patients. Splenomegaly has been reported in 2 to 25 percent of patients. Respiratory symptoms or signs are unusual. Hemorrhagic manifestations generally begin on the fourth day with petechiae on the oral mucosa and skin, epistaxis, gingival bleeding, hematemesis, and melena. Neurologic abnormalities, seen in 10 to 25 percent of patients, include nuchal rigidity, excitation, and coma. Laboratory findings show leukopenia, with the number of white blood

cells falling as low as 1000 per microliter, and thrombocytopenia, which is often severe. Proteinuria and microscopic hematuria are common, but azotemia and oliguria are not. Convalescence may be prolonged. Death is usually attributed to shock or intercurrent infection. Sequelae include transient alopecia and mono- or polyneuritis.

The major approach to therapy has been supportive. Convalescent immune serum has shown promise if administered during the first 3 days of illness. Patients should be isolated with contact restricted to hospital staff and immediate family. Masks and gowns should be worn, and blood and body fluids handled as infectious. The reported mortality rate has varied between 9 and 50 percent.

Omsk hemorrhagic fever   Omsk hemorrhagic fever (OHF) is an acute febrile disease which occurs in the Omsk and Novosibirsk oblasts in the U.S.S.R. and is caused by a flavivirus. The seasonal occurrence of OHF shows a biphasic pattern with peaks in May and August. The transmission cycle is uncertain. OHF is transmitted to humans either by the bite of infected ticks, *Ixodes apronophorus*, or by the handling of infected muskrats. The natural reservoir includes muskrats, other rodents, especially water voles, and ticks. Epidemics occurred from 1945 to 1948, but recently the disease has been less prevalent.

Following an incubation interval of 3 to 8 days, illness begins abruptly with fever, headache, and hemorrhagic manifestations, which include epistaxis and gastrointestinal and uterine bleeding. Rarely, neurologic abnormalities may occur. Laboratory features include leukopenia. In contrast to many of the other hemorrhagic fevers, OHF has a low case fatality rate (0.5 to 3.0 percent).

Kyasanur Forest disease   Kyasanur Forest disease was first recognized in south India in 1957 as a discrete clinical entity shown to be due to a flavivirus. Kyasanur Forest disease occurs following occupational exposure to *Haemaphysalis spinigera* ticks in the tropical forests of western Mysore in southern India. The silent reservoir cycle which infects the primate- and bird-feeding *Haemaphysalis* ticks is now believed to be *Ixodes* ticks transmitted among small forest mammals, especially the shrew. Laboratory-associated infections have been common.

The major symptoms include abrupt onset of fever, headache, fatigue, myalgia (especially of the lumbar area and calf muscles), and retroorbital pain. Cough and abdominal pain occur in half the patients. Additional symptoms may include photophobia and polyarthralgia. Epistaxis and hematemesis are observed in some patients. On examination, findings include relative bradycardia, conjunctival injection, and generalized lymphadenopathy. Fine and coarse rales are frequently heard. Hepatosplenomegaly has been encountered occasionally. During the initial phase, generalized hyperesthesia of the skin occurs occasionally. The fever usually lasts from 6 to 11 days. After an afebrile period of 9 to 21 days, approximately half the patients may develop a second phase, which lasts from 2 to 12 days. This is manifested by recurrence of fever, severe headache, neck stiffness, mental disturbance, coarse tremors, giddiness, and abnormalities in reflexes, as well as by recurrence of many of the initial symptoms. No sequelae have been observed, but convalescence is often prolonged.

Only limited laboratory studies have been reported. During the initial phase, leukopenia is a constant feature, with a total leukocyte count of fewer than 3000 per microliter by the fourth to sixth day. The leukopenia is associated with neutropenia. During the second phase there is a mild leukocytosis. Lumbar puncture during the second phase has shown a pattern of aseptic meningitis. Diagnosis is based upon virus isolation from blood; this is readily accomplished, since viremia is prolonged. Serologic tests of paired serums also can be performed. The management is supportive. The mortality rate is approximately 5 percent.

HEMORRHAGIC FEVER WITH RENAL SYNDROME

Synonyms for this disease (HFRS) include Korean hemorrhagic fever, Far Eastern hemorrhagic fever, endemic or epidemic nephrosonephritis, Manchurian epidemic hemorrhagic fever, Songo fever, and Churilov's disease. A similar but milder disease in Scandinavia has been called nephropathia epidemica or epidemic nephritis (EN).

ETIOLOGY In 1976, the antigen of HFRS was reported in the lungs of the rodent *Apodemus agrarius coreae*. Diagnostic increases in immunofluorescent antibodies were demonstrated in 113 of 116 cases of severe HFRS. The agent designated Hantaan virus is a single-stranded RNA virus belonging to the family Bunyaviridae, genus Hantavirus (Table 148-1). The genus consists of at least four species: Hantaan virus (Korean hemorrhagic fever), Seoul virus, Puumala virus (nephropathia epidemica), and Prospect Hill virus (isolated from meadow voles in Maryland and associated with human diseases).

PREVALENCE In Korea between April 1951 and January 1953, 2070 cases of epidemic hemorrhagic fever were reported among United Nations personnel. The disease usually occurs as an isolated event; hence, overall attack rates have relatively less meaning. With this reservation, attack rates in two United States Army divisions stationed in Korea varied between 1.9 and 2.9 cases per 1000 persons per epidemic season. Approximately 800 cases per year have continued to occur; however, most cases are now seen in Korean civilians and military with less than 10 cases per year in U.S. military personnel. During the past 15 years, the disease has increased in prevalence in Korea, urban Japan, and in China. In the People's Republic of China over 100,000 cases of HFRS are reported annually; the incidence is increasing. Hundreds of cases of EN have occurred annually in Finland and other Scandinavian countries since the 1930s. In 1953 a severe form of HFRS was recognized in the Balkan countries, and in 1982 in Greece and France. Antibody studies indicate worldwide distribution. Antibodies in human sera have been found in Argentina, Brazil, Colombia, Europe, Canada, the United States, including Hawaii and Alaska, southeast Asia, Egypt, and central Africa.

EPIDEMIOLOGY The majority of cases occur in May to June and in October to November. These peaks coincide with rodent density population. Hantaan virus is present in rodent urine, feces, and saliva in high titer. Transmission from rodent to rodent is primarily respiratory, with transmission to people through inhalation of virus-containing dried excreta. There is no evidence for person-to-person transmission. The urban reservoir appears to be the house rat. Laboratory-acquired cases have occurred in the U.S.S.R., Korea, Japan, and Europe with rats implicated in Korea, Japan, and the U.K.

CLINICAL MANIFESTATIONS There are two forms of disease, a mild illness characteristically diagnosed in Scandinavia as epidemic nephritis (EN) and the more severe Far Eastern form, epidemic hemorrhagic fever.

EN is characterized by sudden onset of high fever, backache, headache, and abdominal pain. On the third or fourth day, hemorrhagic manifestations may occur and conjunctival hemorrhages, palatine petechiae, and a petechial rash appear on the trunk. About one patient in five is "toxic" and mentally obtunded. Oliguria and azotemia develop. Urinalysis reveals proteinuria, hematuria, and leukocyturia. After about 3 days the rash subsides, the patient develops polyuria, and recovers in several weeks.

Epidemic hemorrhagic fever The incubation period in epidemic hemorrhagic fever (EHF) is usually 10 to 25 days, with possible extremes of 7 and 36 days. Visitors who contract the disease in an endemic area may not develop illness until after their return home.

The clinical course of EHF may be divided into phases on the basis of the underlying physiologic aberrations: febrile, hypotensive, oliguric, diuretic, and convalescent. There is considerable variation among patients in the severity of the illness. In one study two-thirds of the 264 cases studied were classified as mild, while 14 percent were termed severe.

FEBRILE (INVASIVE) PHASE From 10 to 20 percent of patients describe vague prodromal symptoms resembling mild upper respiratory infections. The onset is then usually abrupt, often initiated by a chill and accompanied by fever, headache, backache, abdominal pain, and generalized myalgia. Anorexia and thirst are almost universal, while nausea and vomiting are common although not constant symptoms. The headache is most commonly frontal or retroorbital. Eye symptoms, especially mild photophobia and pain on movement of the eyes, are characteristic. Diarrhea is not a feature. Fever is present in almost all patients; the temperature ranges from 37.8 to 41.1°C (100 to 106°F), reaches a peak on the third or fourth day after onset, and falls by lysis on the fourth to seventh day. There is a relative bradycardia. Initially the blood pressure is normal. One of the most typical early findings is a diffuse reddening of the skin, most marked over the face and V area of the neck that may resemble a severe sunburn. The erythema blanches on pressure. Dermographism can be demonstrated in over 90 percent of patients at the same time as the flush. Slight edema of the upper eyelids causes a bleary-eyed appearance. Bulbar and palpebral conjunctivas show injection. Conjunctival petechiae may develop by the third or fifth day of illness. Subconjunctival hemorrhages may be striking. Intense pharyngeal reddening without significant sore throat is typical. The first location for petechiae is usually the palate, where they occur in half the patients. Within 12 to 24 h, petechiae appear at pressure areas such as the axillary folds, lateral chest wall, belt line, hips, and thighs. Retinal hemorrhages occur rarely. Cervical, axillary, and inguinal nodes are moderately enlarged but nontender. Abdominal and costovertebral tenderness is almost a constant finding. Splenomegaly is unusual and in Korea was generally attributable to malaria with which EHF coexisted in about 1 percent of patients. The degree of flush, fever, and conjunctival injection and the number of petechiae correlate quite well with the overall severity of illness.

Laboratory studies during this phase are often not striking. Initial hemoglobin and hematocrit values are usually normal. Prior to the fourth day, leukocyte counts range from 3600 to 6000 per microliter but are associated with neutrophilia. Early in the course urine specific gravity may be high. Albuminuria, which is an almost universal finding, appears, often abruptly, between the second and fifth days of illness. The urinary sediment reveals microscopic hematuria and hyaline, granular, red blood cell casts, and/or white blood cell casts. Erythrocyte sedimentation rates are normal during the first week. Capillary fragility tests are usually positive at the time of admission and become most abnormal by the ninth day. Electrocardiographic abnormalities may be seen in 15 to 30 percent of patients; these include sinus bradycardia and low or inverted T waves. Lumbar punctures may reveal gross blood in the spinal fluid.

HYPOTENSIVE PHASE On about the fifth day of illness, during the last 24 to 48 h of the febrile phase, hypotension or shock may occur. In mild cases, only a transient fall in blood pressure occurs; among moderately and severely ill patients shock may persist for 1 to 3 days. In 828 patients, 16.5 percent had clinical shock, and another 14 percent had hypotension without shock. Headache often diminishes, but thirst persists. In the beginning of the hypotensive phase, most patients have warm, dry skin and extremities. As the systolic blood pressure decreases and pulse pressure narrows, the skin becomes cool and moist. Tachycardia replaces the relative bradycardia.

At this stage, an increase in hematocrit with no change in total serum protein level is found. This is thought to reflect a loss of plasma through damaged capillaries. On about the fifth day, all patients develop marked proteinuria. The previously normal urine specific gravity begins to fall and in 2 to 3 days is usually around 1.010. Blood urea nitrogen concentrations begin to increase. Other laboratory findings include leukocytosis with white blood cell counts of 10,000 to 56,000 per microliter with neutrophilia and toxic granulation. The number of platelets often decreases to less than 70,000 per microliter.

OLIGURIC PHASE (HEMORRHAGIC OR TOXIC PHASE) About the eighth day of illness, blood pressure returns to the normal range and in some instances increases to hypertensive levels. While oliguria may have appeared during the shock phase, it now becomes a prominent feature. Oliguria develops even though hypotension was not recognized. Symptomatically patients continue to feel weak and thirsty and have more severe backache. Protracted vomiting and hiccups may ensue.

Blood urea nitrogen levels increase rapidly and are associated with hyperkalemia, hyperphosphatemia, and hypocalcemia. Metabolic acidosis is rarely severe. Although platelets begin to return to normal, hemorrhagic manifestations become more prominent and include petechiae, hematemesis (analogous to "black vomit" in yellow fever), melena, hemoptysis, gross hematuria, and hemorrhages into the central nervous system. The enlarged lymph nodes may now become tender.

With the onset of diuresis on about the seventh day in moderately ill patients and the ninth to eleventh day in severely ill patients, symptoms of fluid and electrolyte abnormalities and central nervous system or pulmonary complications may appear. Central nervous system symptoms include disorientation, extreme restlessness, lethargy, paranoid delusions, and hallucinations. Grand mal seizures, pulmonary edema, and pulmonary infection occur in some patients.

DIURETIC PHASE   With the onset of diuresis, progressive improvement is the rule. Most patients begin to eat and regain their strength. In fatal cases the diuretic phase is associated with a daily urine output of less than 4 liters and often less than 2 liters, in contrast to larger volumes in surviving patients.

CONVALESCENT PHASE   The convalescent phase lasts 3 to 6 weeks. Weight is regained slowly. Complaints include muscular weakness, intention tremor, and lack of stamina. Hyposthenuria and polyuria are present; however, within 2 months most patients are able to concentrate their urine to a specific gravity of 1.023 or greater after a 12-h period of water deprivation.

DIAGNOSIS   Diagnosis is based on demonstration of specific IgM antibodies by ELISA or a fourfold change in immune adherence hemagglutination titers in paired sera. Studies on the epidemiology of Hantavirus have shown that during the initial 24 to 72 h (febrile phase) there is significant overlap in the clinical features of leptospirosis, HFRS, and scrub typhus. In Korea where all three diseases are prevalent, of blood samples submitted for Hantavirus serology, 21 percent had antibody to leptospira antigens and 6 percent to *Rickettsia tsutsugamushi*. Because of the similarity in epidemiology and clinical presentation and the potential for dual infections, it has been recommended that blood be submitted for Hantavirus serology in all cases of suspected leptospirosis (see Chap. 130).

TREATMENT   Clinical management primarily revolves around meticulous supportive care. Trials with a variety of agents including antibiotics, glucocorticoids, antihistamines, convalescent serum, and alpha interferon were without significant beneficial effect during the Korean epidemics. In a controlled U.S./Chinese clinical trial in the People's Republic of China, ribavirin was shown to have efficacy.

PROGNOSIS   The Soviet experience indicates a mortality rate of 3 to 32 percent; in China, the case fatality ratio was 7 to 15 percent. Between April 1951 and December 1976 the overall case fatality ratio in Korea was 6.6 percent.

Residua are uncommon. Of 783 surviving patients cared for at the Hemorrhagic Fever Center in Korea between April and December 1952, only 16 were unable to return to duty within a period of 4 months. Fifteen of these individuals still had hyposthenuria. Follow-up studies on former EHF patients 3 to 5 years later showed that they had many more subsequent hospital admissions for urologic problems than did a control group and that the relative frequency correlated with the severity of the acute episode of EHF.

REFERENCES

"Arboviruses": Definition and classification

FIELDS BN et al (eds): *Virology*. New York, Raven, 1985

"Arbovirus" infections characterized by fever, malaise, headaches, and myalgia

BOWEN GS et al: Clinical aspects of human Venezuelan equine encephalitis in Texas, 1971. Bull Pan Am Health Org 10:46, 1976

BRICENO ROSSIE AL: Rural epidemic encephalitis in Venezuela caused by a group A arbovirus (VEE). Prog Med Virol 9:176, 1967

CALISHER CH et al: Rio Grande—a new phlebotomus fever group virus from south Texas. Am J Trop Med Hyg 26:997, 1977

DIETZ WH JR et al: Ten clinical cases of human infection with Venezuelan equine encephalomyelitis virus, subtype I-D. Am J Trop Med Hyg 28:329, 1979

FLEMING J et al: Sandfly fever. Review of 664 cases. Lancet 1:443, 1947

GOODPASTURE HC et al: Colorado tick fever: Clinical, epidemiologic and laboratory aspects of 228 cases in Colorado in 1973–1974. Ann Intern Med 88:303, 1978

HUGHES LE et al: Persistence of Colorado tick fever virus in red blood cells. Am J Trop Med Hyg 23:530, 1974

LAUGHLIN LW et al: Epidemic Rift Valley fever in Egypt: Observations of the spectrum of human illness. Trans R Soc Trop Med Hyg 73:630, 1979

LENNETTE EH, KOPROWSKI H: Human infection with Venezuelan equine encephalomyelitis virus. JAMA 123:1088, 1943

SCHERER WF et al: Ecologic studies of Venezuelan encephalitis virus in Southeastern Mexico: VII. Infection of man. Am J Trop Med 21:79, 1972

SIAM AL et al: Rift Valley fever ocular manifestations: Observations during 1977 epidemic in Egypt. Br J Ophthalmol 64:366, 1980

VAN VELDEN et al: Rift Valley fever affecting humans in South Africa: A clinicopathologic study. S Afr Med J 29:867, 1977

"Arbovirus" infections presenting chiefly with fever, malaise, arthralgia, and rash

AASKOV JG et al: An epidemic of Ross River virus infection in Fiji, 1979. Am J Trop Med Hyg 30:1053, 1981

CLARK JA et al: Annually recurrent epidemic polyarthritis and Ross River virus activity in a coastal area of New South Wales. I. Occurrence of the disease. Am J Trop Med Hyg 22:543, 1973

DELLER JJ JR, RUSSELL PK: Chikungunya disease. Am J Trop Med 17:107, 1968

PINHEIRO FP et al: An outbreak of Mayaro virus disease in Belterra, Brazil: I. Clinical and virological findings. Am J Trop Med Hyg 30:674, 1981

ROBINSON MC: An epidemic of virus disease in Southern Province, Tanganyika territory in 1952–53: I. Clinical features. Trans R Soc Trop Med Hyg 49:28, 1955

SHORE H: O'nyong-nyong fever: An epidemic virus disease in East Africa: III. Some clinical and epidemiological observations in the Northern Province of Uganda. Trans R Soc Trop Med Hyg 55:361, 1961

"Arbovirus" infections presenting chiefly with fever, malaise, lymphadenopathy, and rash

ALVAREZ MD, RAMÍREZ-RONDA CH: Dengue and hepatic failure. Am J Med 79:670, 1985

CENTERS FOR DISEASE CONTROL: Dengue in the United States, 1983–1984. CDC Surveillance Summaries 34(255):555, 1985

MICKS DW, MOON WB: *Aëdes aegypti* in a Texas coastal county as an index of dengue fever receptivity and control. Am J Trop Med Hyg 29:1382, 1980

"Arbovirus" infections presenting chiefly with central nervous system involvement

BALFOUR HH JR et al: California arbovirus (LaCrosse) infections. Pediatrics 52:680, 1973

CENTERS FOR DISEASE CONTROL: Arboviral infections of the central nervous system—United States, 1987. Morb Mort Week Rep 37:506, 1988

DICKERSON RB et al: Diagnosis and immediate prognosis of Japanese B encephalitis. Observations based on more than 200 patients with detailed analysis of 65 serologically confirmed cases. Am J Med 12:277, 1952

EDELMAN R, PARYANONDA A: Human immunoglobulin M antibody in the serodiagnosis of Japanese encephalitis virus infections. Am J Epidemiol 98:29, 1973

FINLEY KH et al: Western equine and St. Louis encephalitis. Preliminary report of a clinical follow-up study in California. Neurology 5:223, 1955

GRABOW JD et al: The electroencephalogram and clinical sequelae of California arbovirus encephalitis. Neurology 19:394, 1969

HILTY MD et al: California encephalitis in children. Am J Dis Child 124:530, 1972

HOKE CH et al: Protection against Japanese encephalitis by inactivated vaccines. N Engl J Med 319:608, 1988

KETEL WB, OGNIBENE AJ: Japanese B encephalitis in Vietnam. Am J Med Sci 261:271, 1971

LUBY JP et al: The epidemiology of St. Louis encephalitis (SLE): A review. Ann Rev Med 20:329, 1969

——: Antigenemia in St. Louis encephalitis. Am J Trop Med Hyg 29:265, 1980

SCHNEIDER RJ et al: Clinical sequelae after Japanese encephalitis: One year follow-up study in Thailand. Southeast Asian J Trop Med Public Health 5:560, 1974

"Arbovirus" diseases presenting primarily with hemorrhagic manifestations

BURNEY MI et al: Nosocomial outbreak of viral hemorrhagic fever caused by Crimean hemorrhagic fever—Congo virus in Pakistan, January 1976. Am J Trop Med Hyg 29:941, 1980

CENTERS FOR DISEASE CONTROL: Viral hemorrhagic fever. Initial management of suspected and confirmed cases. Ann Intern Med 101:73, 1984

——: Korean hemorrhagic fever. JAMA 259:1622, 1988

DENNIS LH et al: The original hemorrhagic fever: Yellow fever. Blood 30:858, 1967

GARTNER L: Hantaan virus infection (Korean hemorrhagic fever) as a cause of acute renal failure. Dtsch Med Wochenschr 113:937, 1988

GUI XE et al: Hemorrhagic fever with renal syndrome: Treatment with recombinant alpha interferon. J Infect Dis 155:1047, 1987

HALSTEAD SB, O'ROURKE EF: Dengue viruses and mononuclear phagocytes: I. Infection enhancement by non-neutralizing antibody. J Exp Med 146:201, 1977

——: The pathogenesis of dengue: Molecular epidemiology in infectious disease. Am J Epidemiol 114:632, 1981

KLIKS SC et al: Antibody-dependant enhancement of dengue virus growth in human monocytes as a risk factor for dengue hemorrhagic fever. Am J Trop Med Hyg 40:444, 1989

KUDESIA G et al: Dual infection with leptospira and Hantavirus. Lancet 1:1397, 1988

LEE HW et al: Isolation of the etiologic agent of Korean hemorrhagic fever. J Infect Dis 137:298, 1978

MONATH TP et al: Yellow fever in the Gambia, 1978–1979: Epidemiologic aspects with observations on the occurrence of Orongo virus infections. Am J Trop Med Hyg 29:912, 1980

NELSON ER: Hemorrhagic fever in children in Thailand: Report of 69 cases. J Pediatr 56:101, 1960

PINHEIRO FP et al: An epidemic of yellow fever in Central Brazil 1972–1973: I. Epidemiological studies. Am J Trop Med Hyg 27:125, 1978

WORLD HEALTH ORGANIZATION: Dengue hemorrhagic fever: Diagnosis, treatment and control. Geneva, 1986

——: Hemorrhagic fever with renal syndrome: Memorandum from a WHO meeting. Bull WHO 61:269, 1983

149 ARENAVIRUS INFECTIONS

JAY P. SANFORD

DEFINITION AND CLASSIFICATION The term *arenavirus* is the proposed designation for a group of RNA viruses which have unique morphology. The virions are round, oval, or pleomorphic, with diameters between 60 and 350 nm, and contain an electron-dense membrane with projections and 2 to 10 inclusion-like dense particles (resembling ribosomes) that give the virion an appearance of having been sprinkled with sand (Latin *arenaceus*, "sandy"). Eleven distinct arenaviruses have been described (Table 149-1). All except Tacaribe are parasites of rodents, and most are unique to tropical America. A special property of arenaviruses that cause disease in humans, especially Machupo and lymphocytic choriomeningitis, is their capacity to induce persistent infection in their reservoir hosts with no ill effects and in the absence of an immune response.

LYMPHOCYTIC CHORIOMENINGITIS The first-recognized arenavirus was lymphocytic choriomeningitis (LCM) virus. It was recognized early that LCM was carried by apparently healthy laboratory mice. Clinically LCM has been considered primarily in the context of aseptic meningitis; however, it is associated with at least two clinical syndromes in humans: central nervous system and influenza-like illness which may be associated with rash, arthritis, or orchitis. LCM virus has provided a valuable model for the study of chronic, persistent, and generally symptomless viral infections in laboratory animals.

Prevalence In the United States human infection with LCM virus is rare; however, seroepidemiologic studies on specimens obtained in 1935 to 1940 from persons with no history of central nervous system disease from all parts of the United States revealed neutralizing antibodies in 10 to 28 percent. In recent years, the prevalence of infection seems to have decreased markedly.

Epidemiology The virus of LCM is worldwide in distribution. Foci of LCM virus have been defined in Germany, Hungary, and elsewhere in Europe. Scandinavia appears to be LCM virus–free as are most of the Americas except Argentina. Although infection can be induced in a variety of animals, mice are the major natural reservoir as well as the primary host in which latent, asymptomatic infection occurs. The latency of infection in the mouse depends upon immunologic tolerance. Animals infected in utero or shortly after birth excrete LCM virus for life without overt disease. Human infections are secondary to contact with an infected rodent. The mode of transmission is thought to be via airborne spread or contact with excrement from infected animals. In the past, most cases have arisen in persons living in rodent-infested houses, but lately outbreaks of LCM virus disease in humans have been reported from Germany and from the United States in which the source of infection was traced to laboratory animals and household pets, specifically hamsters which, like mice, can shed LCM virus in urine and stool. LCM occurs throughout the year but has been more frequent in the colder months. Person-to-person transmission has not been demonstrated.

Pathogenesis In natural infection, the portal of entry of the LCM virus is probably through the respiratory tract. Virus multiplication occurs initially in the respiratory epithelium, and an influenza-like illness develops. Dissemination of virus to extrapulmonary sites, presumably to reticuloendothelial cells with multiplication, and viremia occur. LCM virus crosses the blood-brain barrier. In mice, the resulting meningitis is attributed to a cell-mediated immune reaction. Support for this hypothesis derives from observations that disease but not infection can be prevented in experimental animals by neonatal thymectomy, irradiation, or immunodepressant drugs such as cyclophosphamide. Similar pathogenetic mechanisms may operate in humans, although isolation of LCM virus from the CSF of patients with aseptic meningitis is quite common.

Clinical manifestations The exact incubation period is not known. Following experimental inoculation of LCM virus into volunteers, fever occurred in $1\frac{1}{2}$ to 3 days, while an influenza-like constellation of symptoms developed 5 to 10 days after exposure. An influenza-like illness is the commonest clinical pattern. In some patients the illness may be biphasic with subsequent aseptic meningitis or encephalomyelitis. Fever, usually from 38.3 to 40°C (101 to 104°F), associated with rigors, is uniformly noted. Other symptoms which are encountered in over one-half of patients include malaise, weakness, myalgia (especially lumbar aching), retroorbital headache, photophobia, anorexia, nausea, and light-headedness. Symptoms which occur in one-fourth to one-half of patients include sore throat, vomiting, and dysesthesias. Later, arthralgias, especially in the hands, occur. Less common complaints (up to one-quarter of patients) include aching pain in the chest, associated with pneumonitis; increased hair loss progressing to generalized alopecia, 2 or 3 weeks after the onset of illness; testicular pain or frank orchitis, usually unilateral, 1 to 3 weeks after onset; and parotid pain, which may lead to a misdiagnosis of mumps. Physical findings in the first week of illness are few. Patients often have a relative bradycardia. Pharyngeal injection without exudate is common (60 percent). Mild

TABLE 149-1 Classification of arenaviruses

Virus	Clinical disease	Reservoir	Known geographic range
Lymphocytic choriomeningitis	Aseptic meningitis, meningoencephalitis, influenzal syndrome, orchitis, arthritis	Mice, hamsters	Worldwide except Australia
Tacaribe		Bats	Trinidad
Junin	Argentinian hemorrhagic fever	*Calomys musculinus*	Argentina
Machupo	Bolivian hemorrhagic fever	*Calomys callosus*	Northeast Bolivia
Amapari			Brazil
Latino			Bolivia
Parana			Paraguay
Pichinde			Colombia
Tamiami			Florida
Lassa	Lassa fever	*Mastomys natalensis*	Nigeria, Liberia, Sierra Leone, Republic of Guinea, Central African Republic
Flexal		*Orzomys* sp.	Brazil

nontender cervical or axillary lymphadenopathy may occur. The initial phase lasts from 5 days to 3 weeks followed by improvement. After a remission of 1 to 2 days many patients relapse with recurrent fever and more prominent headache. Physical signs may include skin rashes, swelling of metacarpophalangeal and proximal interphalangeal joints, meningeal signs, orchitis, parotitis, and alopecia. Convalescence generally is of 1 to 4 weeks' duration, characterized by easy fatigability, an excessive need for sleep, dysesthesias, and occasional dizziness. Patients with aseptic meningitis almost always recover without sequelae. With encephalitis, 25 to 30 percent of patients have neurologic residua.

Laboratory findings   Leukopenia and thrombocytopenia are almost uniform during the first week of illness. Although leukocyte counts usually vary between 2000 and 3000 per microliter, counts as low as 600 per microliter have been recorded. Differential counts generally show slight relative lymphocytosis. Platelet counts are usually between 50,000 and 100,000 per microliter. Anemia is not encountered. The erythrocyte sedimentation rate often is normal. Mild elevations of serum glutamic oxaloacetic transaminase (SGOT) and lactic dehydrogenase (LDH) may occur. Chest radiographs may suggest basilar pneumonias. In patients with meningeal signs, examination of the cerebrospinal fluid usually reveals several hundred cells per microliter, although cell counts in excess of 1000 per microliter are reported in half the patients in some series. Lymphocytes predominate (greater than 80 percent) even early. The initial cerebrospinal fluid protein is usually slightly elevated, but on occasion levels may exceed 1.5 g/L (150 mg/dL). Although a normal cerebrospinal fluid glucose level is considered the hallmark of viral meningitides, low CSF glucose has been observed in up to 27 percent of patients with LCM.

Diagnosis   The diagnosis of LCM can be established with certainty by recovery of the virus from blood or spinal fluid. Complement-fixing antibodies are usually detectable 1 to 2 weeks after the onset of infection, peak at 5 to 8 weeks, and are gone by 6 months. Neutralizing antibodies appear after 6 to 8 weeks, increase in titer slowly, and remain high for years. Immunofluorescent studies have detected antibody to LCM virus earlier in the course of illness, and its appearance seems to parallel the development of the neurologic phase. The clinical manifestations of LCM cannot be differentiated from those produced by numerous other viruses.

Treatment   There is no specific treatment.

ARGENTINIAN AND BOLIVIAN HEMORRHAGIC FEVERS   The first cases of a new American hemorrhagic disease were seen near the Argentinian town of Junin near Buenos Aires in 1953. A virus was isolated from patients' blood and from local rodents and their mites. In 1959, cases of a disease thought to resemble severe epidemic typhus were noted among rural workers in northeastern Bolivia. The similarity between these syndromes was recognized. In 1963, the causal virus was isolated from patients and rodents and named the Machupo virus. Machupo virus is serologically related to but distinct from Junin virus.

Prevalence   Junin virus infections have occurred in epidemic form since 1958 with between 100 and 3500 cases reported annually. The hemorrhagic disease in Bolivia has been particularly severe.

Epidemiology   Argentinian hemorrhagic fever (AHF) occurs in sharply endemic seasonal form (February to August), mostly among male rural workers, especially those exposed to fields at the time of the maize harvest. Virus is transmitted in the urine of rodents with chronic infection and viruria. Humans acquire the virus through contact with items or foodstuffs which have been contaminated with infected rodent urine. The main reservoir is two species of cricetidae, *Calomys laucha* and *C. musculinus*.

Bolivian hemorrhagic fever (BHF) is similarly transmitted by the urine of *C. callosus* (a mouselike rodent) chronically infected with Machupo virus. Direct person-to-person transmission is possible and may have occurred in the outbreak in Cochabamba. Disease has not occurred in medical personnel attending infected patients.

Clinical features   Argentinian hemorrhagic fever presents manifestations of renal, cardiovascular, and hematologic involvement. Inapparent infections are rare. The incubation period is estimated to be 7 to 16 days, followed by a gradual onset of chills, fever, headache, malaise, myalgia, anorexia, nausea, and vomiting. The temperature reaches 38.9 to 40°C (102 to 104°F), facial flushing may be prominent, and there is a painless enanthem of the pharynx. Lymphadenopathy and splenomegaly are not present. From 3 to 5 days after the onset, the signs and symptoms worsen, with the appearance of dehydration, hypotension to 50 to 100 mmHg, oliguria, and relative bradycardia. In the more severe cases, hemorrhagic manifestations, including bleeding from the gums, hematemesis, hematuria, and melena, occur. Progressive oliguria and tremor of the tongue and extremities may develop. Some patients develop psychic manifestations, with agitation, delirium, or stupor. Progressive shock, hypothermia, gallop rhythm, or gastrointestinal bleeding may occur from the seventh to tenth days. In fatal cases, pulmonary edema usually is the cause of death. During convalescence temporary alopecia has been noted. Erythrocyte counts are normal or elevated. The total leukocyte count drops to 1200 to 3400 blood cells per microliter. Thrombocytopenia may occur. Disseminated intravascular coagulation does not seem to be the mechanism responsible for the hemorrhagic manifestations. Complement components C2, C3, and C5 are decreased. The urine is dark with intense proteinuria. Blood urea nitrogen levels rise rapidly.

The clinical picture of Bolivian hemorrhagic fever is similar to Argentinian, although epistaxis and hematemesis at the onset is more common.

Diagnosis   Antibody responses, including IgM antibodies, do not occur before 10 to 20 days.

Treatment   Treatment consists of supportive measures, including peritoneal dialysis or hemodialysis-filtration to correct both the azotemia and the pulmonary edema. In AHF, a double-blind trial with immune plasma reduced mortality from 16 to 1 percent. However, fever and cerebellar signs occurred in patients treated with immune plasma. Preliminary studies suggest that ribavirin may be effective in experimental BHF in rhesus monkeys.

Prognosis   The mortality rate among patients with Argentinian hemorrhagic fever is usually 3 to 15 percent, while that in Bolivian hemorrhagic fever is 5 to 30 percent.

Prevention   In Bolivia, rodent control measures directed primarily against *C. callosus* populations in the houses has resulted in a prompt and dramatic cessation of human cases. In Argentina, the wide dispersal of infected hosts renders rodent control measures futile.

LASSA FEVER   A virus disease which is both highly contagious and virulent occurred in a missionary nurse in Lassa, a town in northeast Nigeria, in 1969.

Epidemiology   Since the initial outbreak at Lassa in 1969, during which one of the patients was transferred to New York City, there have been other outbreaks near Jos in northern Nigeria in 1970 (32 suspected cases with 10 deaths), in Zorzor, Liberia, in 1972 (11 cases with 4 deaths), and in the eastern province of Sierra Leone with 63 suspected cases admitted to two hospitals between 1970 and 1972. Lassa fever occurs as an endemic disease in eastern Sierra Leone. Population surveys showed more than one-half of older adults had antibodies. Other countries in west Africa having clinical or serologic evidence of Lassa fever include Senegal, Gambia, Guinea, Ghana, Burkina Faso (formerly Upper Volta), Mali, and Ivory Coast. Lassa-related viruses (Mopeia, Mobala) have been isolated from rodents in Mozambique, Zimbabwe, and the Central African Republic; however, they have not been associated with human illness. In Jos and Zorzor, outbreaks apparently resulted from person-to-person nosocomial spread from the index case to hospital workers or other patients. In Sierra Leone, the great majority of cases were acquired outside the hospital, although hospital workers were at risk. *Mastomys natalensis,* a multimammate rat widespread in Africa, is the animal reservoir, and primary human cases result from contamination of foodstuffs with rodent urine. Human-to-human transmission may occur through contact with urine, feces, vomitus, or saliva through droplets, and particularly through wounds contaminated with blood. Intrafamilial outbreaks have occurred around several cases. There are a number of cases which have been acquired through accidental autoinoculation with needles while starting intravenous fluids. At least one laboratory-acquired infection has occurred. In Sierra Leone 6 percent of the population surveyed had complement-fixing antibody against Lassa virus, while only 0.2 percent had recognized disease, suggesting mild disease or inapparent infection. In Liberia 10 percent of hospital personnel had antibodies.

Clinical features   The incubation period is 1 to 24 days, and was 10 days following accidental inoculation. Patients have ranged from 5 months to 46 years of age; approximately two-thirds are women. Three of eight women in one series were 22 to 28 weeks pregnant during their illness. The apparent predilection for women may relate to exposure to contaminated food or work in hospitals rather than to differences in susceptibility. The onset of illness was described by most patients as insidious. The most frequent initial symptoms were fever (100 percent), chilliness and true rigors, headache (50 percent), malaise (100 percent), and myalgia (50 percent). Most patients did not seek medical attention for 4 to 9 days after onset. Symptoms of a systemic viral illness then developed with anorexia, nausea, vomiting, myalgia, and pain in the chest, epigastrium, and lumbar area. Headache was usually present. Early examination revealed fever and flushing of the face and V area of the neck. Pharyngitis developed early and became progressively more severe during the first week; examination in some cases revealed raised patches of whitish exudate occurring on the palatine arches, which occasionally coalesced into a pseudomembrane. Oral ulcerations have been noted in up to one-half of cases. Generalized nontender lymphadenopathy occurred in one-half of patients. During the second week severe lower abdominal pain and intractable vomiting were common, and facial and neck swelling with conjunctival edema and infection frequently developed. Occasionally patients had tinnitus, epistaxis, bleeding from the gums and venipuncture sites, maculopapular rashes, cough, and dizziness. During the acute stage, systolic blood pressures of less than 90 mmHg, with pulse pressures less than 20 mmHg, occurred in 60 to 80 percent of patients. Initially, relative bradycardia was common. During the second week, the patients who recovered defervesced while the patients who died often developed signs of shock, clouding of the sensorium, rales, signs of pleural effusion, agitation and, on occasion, grand mal seizures. The duration of illness in surviving patients ranged from 7 to 31 days (average 15 days), while that in fatal cases was 7 to 26 days (average 12 days). The mortality rates in Jos and Zorzor were 52 percent and 36 percent, respectively, while in Sierra Leone the rate was 8 percent. During convalescence occasional flurries of rapid involuntary eye movements (oculogyric crises) occurred. Late sequelae include deafness and alopecia.

Laboratory features   The hematologic findings include relatively normal hematocrit values and early leukopenia (less than 4000 cells per microliter in 36 percent) with a relative neutrophilia and immature forms of leukocytes. In two cases in which it was recorded, the erythrocyte sedimentation rate was normal. Urinalyses revealed proteinuria, which was often massive. Chest radiographs may suggest basilar pneumonitis and pleural effusions. Electrocardiographic abnormalities compatible with diffuse myocardial disease have been encountered. Levels of serum enzymes, SGOT, creatinine phosphokinase (CPK), and LDH have been elevated. Lassa virus may be recovered from cerebrospinal fluid.

Diagnosis   Diagnosis can be made by demonstrating a fourfold rise in antibody titer to Lassa virus between acute phase and convalescent phase serum specimens with the indirect fluorescent antibody technique or with Lassa IgM antibodies. The diagnosis is unlikely if IgM antibodies are absent by the fourteenth day of illness.

Treatment   The management has been supportive. Infusion of immune plasma from convalescent patients resulted in a dramatic effect in three of four patients. Because of the self-limited nature of the disease, these results cannot be assessed easily. In a study of the antiviral agent ribavirin, 19 of 20 patients treated intravenously within 6 days of onset with a 2.0-g loading dose, followed by 1.0 g every 6 h for 4 days, then 0.5 g every 8 h for another 6 days, survived, whereas 11 of 18 who received no therapy, and 10 of 16 who received convalescent plasma died. In view of the hospital association and the presence of virus in pharyngeal secretions and urine, respiratory and enteric isolation and blood precautions are required. With reasonable isolation practices, nosocomial spread need not be as feared as previously.

OTHER HEMORRHAGIC FEVERS   Ebola hemorrhagic fever and Marburg virus disease are caused by members of the family Filoviridae and are discussed in Chap. 147 and summarized in Table 148-1.

REFERENCES

BAUM SG et al: Epidemic non-meningitic lymphocytic-choriomeningitis virus infection. N Engl J Med 274:934, 1966

CASALS J: Arenaviruses. Yale J Biol Med 48:115, 1975

CENTERS FOR DISEASE CONTROL: Viral hemorrhagic fever. Initial management of suspected and confirmed cases. Ann Intern Med 101.73, 1984

FIELDS BN et al (eds): Virology. New York, Raven, 1985

FRAME JD et al: Lassa fever, a new virus disease of man from West Africa: I. Clinical description and pathological findings. Am J Trop Med Hyg 19:670, 1970

JOHNSON KM et al: Hemorrhagic fever of Southeast Asia and South America. A comparative approach. Prog Med Virol 9:105, 1967

McCORMICK JB et al: Lassa fever: Effective therapy with ribavirin. N Engl J Med 314:20, 1986

McKEE KT JR et al: Ribavirin prophylaxis and therapy for experimental Argentine hemorrhagic fever. Antimicrob Agents Chemother 32:1304, 1988

MACKENZIE RB et al: Epidemic hemorrhagic fever in Bolivia: 1. A preliminary report of the epidemiologic and clinical findings in a new epidemic area in South America. Am J Trop Med Hyg 13:620, 1964

MERTENS PE et al: Clinical presentation of Lassa fever cases during the hospital epidemic at Zorzor, Liberia, March–April 1972. Am J Trop Med Hyg 22:780, 1973

MONATH TP et al: Lassa fever in the Eastern Province of Sierra Leone, 1970–1972: II. Clinical observations and virological studies on selected hospital cases. Am J Trop Med Hyg 23.1140, 1974

VANZEE BE et al: Lymphocytic choriomeningitis in University hospital personnel. Clinical features. Am J Med 58:803, 1975

150   HUMAN PAPILLOMAVIRUS INFECTIONS

RICHARD C. REICHMAN

DEFINITION   Human papillomaviruses (HPV) selectively infect the epithelium of skin or mucous membranes. These infections may be asymptomatic, produce warts, or be associated with a variety of both benign and malignant neoplasias.

ETIOLOGY   HPV, members of the A genus of the family Papovaviridae, are nonenveloped viruses, 50 to 55 nm in diameter, with icosahedral capsids composed of 72 capsomeres. They contain a double-stranded, circular DNA genome of about 7900 base pairs. Papillomaviruses (PV) appear to be species specific, and HPV have not been propagated in tissue culture or in standard experimental animals. Significant quantities of virus are difficult to obtain, and HPV are incompletely characterized. Suitable HPV antigens have not been available, and work on the epidemiology, pathogenesis, immunology, and treatment of HPV-induced disease has been difficult to carry out. Structural viral proteins make up 88 percent of the mass of PV virions. A major capsid protein with a molecular weight of 56,000 and a minor capsid protein which migrates at 76,000 have been identified by sodium dodecyl sulfate polyacrylamide gel elec-

TABLE 150-1   Correlation of human papillomavirus (HPV) type with disease

Disease	Associated HPV types*
Deep plantar warts	1, 4
Common warts	1, 2, 4, 41
Common warts of meat handlers	7
Flat warts	3, 10, 27, 41
Intermediate warts	10, 26, 28
Epidermodysplasia verruciformis	5, 8, 9, 12, 14, 15, 17, 19–25, 36, 46, 47
Condylomata acuminata	6, 11, 40–45, 51
Intraepithelial neoplasias, unspecified	33, 35, 42–45, 51
Bowen's disease	16, 31
Bowenoid papulosis	16, 34, 39, 42
High-grade dysplasias	16, 18
Low-grade dysplasias	6, 11, 31, 45
Laryngeal papillomas	6, 11, 30
Focal epithelial hyperplasia of Heck	13, 32
Conjunctival papillomas	6, 11
Others	37, 38

*Types 29, 48–50, 52–60 have been identified but not published (data kindly supplied by Ethel-Michele de Villiers; HPV Reference Center, Heidelberg, FRG).

trophoresis. Four cellular histones are associated with the viral DNA. Type-specific antigenic determinants appear to be located on the virion surface and genus-specific determinants internally. Antisera produced by immunization of experimental animals with disrupted PV virions are broadly cross-reactive.

The genomic organization of all PV is similar. Types and subtypes are defined by degree of DNA hybridization under stringent conditions. DNA of a distinct PV type cross-hybridizes less than 50 percent with DNAs of other classified viruses. At least 60 types of HPV are recognized. Individual types are associated with specific kinds of warts (Table 150-1).

EPIDEMIOLOGY   Seroepidemiologic studies of HPV infections have been hampered severely by lack of appropriate antigens, and there are few good studies of the incidence or prevalence of human warts in well-defined populations. Common warts are found in as many as 25 percent of some groups, and are most prevalent among young children. Plantar warts are also widely prevalent and occur most commonly among adolescents and young adults. The incidence of venereal warts (condylomata acuminata) has risen dramatically in the last 15 to 20 years, and condyloma acuminatum is one of the most common sexually transmitted diseases in the United States. HPV infection of the uterine cervix produces the most commonly detected squamous cell abnormalities on Papanicolaou smears.

CLINICAL MANIFESTATIONS   Until the mid-1970s, it was generally believed that there was only one HPV and that clinical and pathologic differences among warts were a function of the nature of the squamous epithelium at the site of infection. With the discovery of multiple HPVs, it has become clear that the specific HPV is an important determinant of the nature of the lesion. Thus, clinical manifestations of HPV infection depend upon location of lesions and virus type. Common warts (verrucae vulgaris) usually occur on the hands, and are flesh-colored to brown, exophytic, hyperkeratotic papules. Plantar warts (verrucae plantaris) differ from most other warts by growing inward. They may be quite painful, and can be differentiated from callus by paring the surface to reveal thrombosed capillaries that bleed easily. Flat warts (verrucae plana) are most common among children and occur on the face, neck, chest, and flexor surfaces of forearms and legs.

Anogenital warts (condylomata acuminata, or venereal warts) occur on skin and mucosal surfaces of external genitalia and perianal areas. The differential diagnosis of anogenital warts includes condylomata lata of secondary syphilis, molluscum contagiosum, pearly penile papules, fibroepitheliomas, and a variety of benign and malignant mucocutaneous neoplasms. Anogenital warts are sexually transmitted, and have an incubation period of 1 to 6 months. In men, condylomata are found most frequently at the frenum or coronal

sulcus, but they may affect any part of the penis. They occur commonly at the urethral meatus, and may extend proximally. Perianal warts are common among homosexual men, but appear in heterosexual men as well. In women, warts appear first at the posterior introitus and adjacent labia. They then spread to other parts of the vulva and commonly involve the perineum and anus. Condylomata frequently involve the vagina and cervix. These lesions may be present in the absence of external warts. Respiratory papillomatosis is uncommon, occurs predominantly in preschool children, and may result from acquisition of virus at the time of delivery through an infected birth canal. These lesions are typically multiple and may produce life-threatening airway obstruction. Disease in adults may be acquired by orogenital sexual contact.

Immunosuppressed patients, particularly those undergoing organ transplantation, often develop pityriasis versicolor–like lesions from which DNA of several HPV types has been extracted. Occasionally, such lesions appear to undergo malignant transformation.

Epidermodysplasia verruciformis is a rare, autosomal recessive disease characterized by the inability to terminate HPV infection and later development of cutaneous squamous cell malignancies. Lesions resemble flat warts or macules similar to those of pityriasis versicolor.

Complications of warts include itching and occasionally bleeding. Rarely, they may become secondarily infected with bacteria or fungi. Large masses of warts may produce mechanical problems such as obstruction of the birth canal. Epidemiologic, cytopathologic, virologic, and histologic data suggest an association of HPV infection with dysplasia and carcinoma of the uterine cervix. HPV nucleic acid sequences have been detected in cervical scrapings and biopsy specimens from most patients with these pathologic findings. Sequences homologous to certain HPV types have been found in 70 to 90 percent of specimens of cervical cancer tissue from patients in several geographic areas. Other genital tract malignancies have also been associated with these viruses.

PATHOGENESIS   HPV infection is transmitted by close personal contact and is facilitated by minor trauma at the site of inoculation. It may result from direct contact with another individual, or, less commonly, by autoinoculation or via fomites. All types of squamous epithelium may be infected by HPV, and gross and histologic appearances of individual lesions vary with site of infection and virus type. Exophytic warts are characterized by papillomatosis, hyperkeratosis, and parakeratosis. Acanthosis, an increase in cellularity, occurs in the prickle cell layer in association with viral DNA synthesis. Late gene expression, manifested by appearance of structural proteins and assembled virions, is evident within nuclei of cells in the granular layer, where koilocytosis develops. Koilocytes are large round cells with pyknotic nuclei and large areas of perinuclear vacuolization surrounded by a ring of dense amphophilic cytoplasm. Histologically normal epithelium may contain HPV DNA. The presence of residual DNA after treatment often leads to recurrent disease.

Host defense responses to HPV infection are poorly understood. Most immunologic studies are difficult to interpret because crude and poorly characterized preparations have been employed as antigens. The potential importance of type-specific responses has not been adequately evaluated because appropriate antigenic materials are not widely available. Virus-specific IgM and IgG antibodies have been demonstrated in patients with and without clinical evidence of active infection. Cell-mediated immune responses to HPV antigens have also been measured, and patients with defects in cell-mediated immunity appear to be more susceptible than normals to HPV infections. Such patients occasionally develop extensive HPV disease.

DIAGNOSIS   Most warts that are visible to the naked eye can be diagnosed correctly by history and physical examination alone. Colposcopy is invaluable in assessing vaginal and cervical lesions and is helpful in the diagnosis of oral and cutaneous HPV disease as well. Papanicolaou smears prepared from cervical scrapings often show cytologic evidence of HPV infection. Persistent or atypical lesions should be biopsied and examined by routine histologic methods. In addition, the genus-specific capsid antigen can be identified in tissue sections using immunologic techniques, and virus type can be determined by nucleic acid hybridization.

TREATMENT Therapy should be initiated with the knowledge that no treatment of proven safety and efficacy is currently available, and that many HPV lesions resolve spontaneously. Frequently used therapies include cryosurgery, application of caustic agents, electrodesiccation, surgical excision, and ablation with laser. Topical antimetabolites such as 5-fluorouracil have been used also. Failure as well as recurrence have been well-documented following all these methods of treatment. The high frequency of recurrence may be explained by the presence of HPV DNA in normal-appearing tissue adjacent to lesions, and in previously involved areas during periods of remission. For many years, topically applied podophyllum preparations have been used in treatment of condyloma acuminatum. However, use of these compounds is associated with resolution rates of less than 50 percent, and initial treatment of venereal warts with cryosurgery is preferable. Promising results have been observed in the treatment of respiratory papillomatosis and condyloma acuminatum with different interferon preparations.

At the present time, no effective methods of prevention are available for HPV infections other than avoiding contact with infectious lesions. Barrier methods of contraception may be helpful in preventing transmission of condyloma acuminatum and other HPV-associated diseases of the genital tract.

REFERENCES

HEALY G et al: Treatment of recurrent respiratory papillomatosis with human leukocyte interferon. N Engl J Med 319:401, 1988

HOWLEY PM: The role of papillomaviruses in human cancer, in *Important Advances in Oncology*, V de Vita, S Hellman, SA Rosenberg (eds). Philadelphia, Lippincott, 1987, pp 55–73

KOUTSY LA et al: Epidemiology of genital human papillomavirus infection. Epidemiologic Rev 10:122, 1988

McCANCE DJ et al: Human papillomavirus type 16 alters human epithelial cell differentiation in vitro. Proc Natl Acad Sci USA 85.7169, 1988

REEVES WC et al: Human papillomavirus infection and cervical cancer in Latin America. N Engl J Med 320:1437, 1989

REICHMAN RC, BONNEZ W: Papillomaviruses, in *Principles and Practice of Infectious Diseases*, GL Mandell et al (eds) New York, Wiley 1990

——— et al: Treatment of condyloma acuminatum with three different interferons administered intralesionally. A double-blind, placebo-controlled trial. Ann Intern Med 108:675, 1988

SCHREIER AA et al: Prospects for human papillomavirus vaccines and immunotherapies. J Natl Cancer Inst 80:896, 1988

STEINBERG BM et al: Persistence and expression of human papillomavirus during interferon therapy. Arch Otolaryngol Head Neck Surg 114:27, 1988

STRIKE DG et al: Expression in *Escherichia coli* of seven DNA segments comprising the complete L1 and L2 open reading frames of human papillomavirus type 6b and localization of the "common antigen" region. J Gen Virol 70:543, 1989

ZUR HAUSEN H: Genital papillomavirus infections. Prog Med Virol 32:15, 1985

section 9 Infection caused by fungi and higher bacteria

151 FUNGAL INFECTIONS

JOHN E. BENNETT

INTRODUCTION Actinomycetes and fungi are considered together in this section, but this should not obscure profound differences between these two groups of organisms. The agents of actinomycosis, nocardiosis, and actinomycetoma are actinomycetes. These organisms are gram-positive higher bacteria that branch but have the diameter, antibiotic susceptibility, and ability to induce the neutrophilic inflammatory response of other bacteria. Actinomycetes resemble fungi in causing infections that may be extremely chronic and that are poorly transmissible from person to person. Few other similarities exist between fungi and actinomycetes. This introductory section will concern mycoses.

The diagnosis of a mycosis requires demonstration of the pathogenic fungus in appropriate patient specimens. Visualization of the fungus by smear or histology is a less precise and less sensitive diagnostic method than culture but is more rapid. Culture allows definitive identification of the pathogen and can detect a small number of organisms. False-positives occur with both methods. Artifacts may be mistaken for fungi in smears or histologic sections. *Candida albicans* can be isolated from the mouth, vagina, sputum, urine, or stool in the absence of candidiasis. *Aspergillus* and, occasionally, *Cryptococcus neoformans* appear in sputum of patients without a mycosis. Histology has the uniquely valuable potential of demonstrating the fungus within the area of inflammation. Only this method can show whether *Aspergillus* in the lung or paranasal sinus tissue exists as a pathogen or merely as a saprophyte growing in pooled secretions. Demonstration of fungi in tissue section usually requires special stains, such as methenamine silver.

Skin testing with fungal antigens has little diagnostic value in active infection. Serologic testing is very helpful in diagnosing coccidioidomycosis and cryptococcosis, as well as in following response to therapy of these mycoses. In histoplasmosis and paracoccidioidomycosis, serologic tests are useful in adding some support to the clinical diagnosis.

THE DEEP MYCOSES

CRYPTOCOCCOSIS Etiology Cryptococcosis is an infection caused by the yeastlike fungus *Cryptococcus neoformans*. *C. neoformans* reproduces by budding and forms round, yeastlike cells 4 to 6 μm in diameter. Within the host and on certain culture media, a large polysaccharide capsule surrounds each yeast cell. The fungus grows well as smooth, creamy white colonies on Sabouraud's or other simple media at 20 to 37°C. Certain culture media for ringworm contain cycloheximide, which inhibits *C. neoformans*. Identification is based on gross and microscopic appearance, biochemical tests, and growth at 37°C. The fungus has four capsular serotypes, designated A, B, C, and D.

Pathogenesis and pathology Infection is thought to be acquired by inhalation of fungus into the lungs. Pulmonary infection has a tendency toward spontaneous resolution and is frequently asymptomatic. Silent hematogenous spread to the brain leads to clusters of cryptococci in the perivascular areas of cortical gray matter, basal ganglia, and, to a lesser extent, other areas of the central nervous system. Inflammatory response around these foci is usually scant. In the more chronic cases, a dense basilar arachnoiditis occurs. Lung lesions show an intense granulomatous inflammation. Cryptococci are best seen in tissue by staining with methenamine silver or periodic acid Schiff. A strongly positive mucicarmine stain of the organism in tissue is diagnostic, but staining varies from intense to absent.

Cryptococcus neoformans has been isolated from several sites in nature, particularly weathered pigeon droppings. Patients are usually unaware of any unusual exposure to pigeon droppings. No significant case clustering, highly endemic areas, or racial or occupational predisposition is known. Infection before puberty is uncommon. The male/female ratio is about 2:1. Approximately three-fourths of the patients have a predisposing condition, such as lymphoma or sarcoidosis, or are receiving supraphysiologic doses of glucocorticoids. Approximately 7 percent of patients with the acquired immunodeficiency syndrome (AIDS) develop cryptococcosis. In these patients the mycosis disseminates and is difficult to cure. Neither neutropenia nor hypogammaglobulinemia seems to increase susceptibility to cryptococcosis. Transmission from animals to humans or from person to person has not been documented.

Clinical manifestations The majority of patients have meningoencephalitis at the time of diagnosis. This form of the infection is invariably fatal without appropriate therapy, and death occurs anywhere from 2 weeks to several years from onset of symptoms. Early manifestations include headache, nausea, staggering gait, dementia, irritability, confusion, and blurred vision. Both fever and nuchal rigidity are often mild or absent. Papilledema is present in one-third of the patients at the time of diagnosis. Cranial nerve palsies, typically asymmetric, occur in about one-fourth of the patients. Other lateralizing signs are rare. With progression of the infection, deepening coma and signs of brainstem compression appear. Autopsy often reveals cerebral edema in the more acute cases or hydrocephalus in more chronic cases.

Pulmonary cryptococcosis causes chest pain in about 40 percent of patients and cough in 20 percent. Chest x-ray shows one or more dense infiltrates, which are often well circumscribed. Cavitation, pleural effusions, or hilar adenopathy are infrequent. Calcification is not present, and fibrotic stranding is rarely noticeable.

Skin lesions are present in 10 percent of patients with cryptococcosis and the vast majority of patients with skin lesions have disseminated infection. One or a few asymptomatic tiny papular lesions appear, slowly enlarge, and tend to show central softening leading to ulceration. Osteolytic bone lesions occur in 4 percent of patients and usually present as a cold abscess. Rare manifestations of cryptococcosis include prostatitis, endophthalmitis, hepatitis, pericarditis, endocarditis, and renal abscess.

Diagnosis Cryptococcal meningoencephalitis must be distinguished from tuberculosis, neoplasm, coccidioidomycosis, histoplasmosis, candidiasis, viral meningitis, and sarcoidosis. Computed tomography (CT) scan or magnetic resonance imaging will occasionally show one or two focal areas of decreased density with contrast-enhancing margins. Lumbar puncture is the single most useful test. An india ink smear of centrifuged spinal fluid sediment reveals encapsulated yeast in one-half the cases, but artifacts resembling cryptococci may cause confusion. Cerebrospinal fluid glucose is reduced in half the cases, protein concentration is usually increased, and 20 to 600 leukocytes per microliter are typically present and consist predominantly of lymphocytes. Approximately 90 percent of patients with cryptococcal meningoencephalitis, including all those with a positive cerebrospinal fluid smear, will have capsular antigen detectable in cerebrospinal fluid or serum by latex agglutination. False-positive tests occur occasionally, making culture the definitive diagnostic test. *C. neoformans* is often present in urine from patients with meningoencephalitis. Fungemia occurs in 10 to 30 percent of patients, and is particularly common in AIDS patients.

Pulmonary cryptococcosis mimics malignancy by x-ray and symptoms. Sputum culture is positive in only 10 percent, and serum antigen tests are positive in only a third. Occasionally, *C. neoformans* appears in one or multiple sputum specimens as an endobronchial saprophyte. Biopsy is usually required for diagnosis of pulmonary cryptococcosis. Cutaneous cryptococcosis may be mistaken for a comedo, basal-cell carcinoma, or sarcoidosis. In AIDS patients, skin lesions may be numerous and mistaken for molluscum contagiosum.

Biopsy reveals a myriad of cryptococci. Osseous cryptococcosis resembles tuberculosis.

Treatment Cryptococcal meningoencephalitis may be treated either with amphotericin B alone or in combination with flucytosine. Amphotericin B is given as 0.5 to 0.6 mg/kg per day when used alone or as 0.3 mg/kg per day in combination therapy. With either regimen, double-dose therapy on alternate days may be employed. Flucytosine is given initially as 37.5 mg/kg every 6 h to patients with normal renal function. Although nomograms are available for adjusting flucytosine dosage in the presence of reduced renal function, frequent measurement of serum levels and maintenance between 50 and 100 μg/mL offer the best chance of preventing toxicity. Even with this precaution, the problems of leukopenia, thrombocytopenia, diarrhea, and rash have been so common in AIDS patients that amphotericin B is usually given alone.

Duration of therapy is based upon the results of lumbar punctures. These are best done weekly until culture conversion is clearly documented. Six weeks of therapy may be adequate for patients with at least four weekly cultures of 2 to 4 mL CSF, whose india ink smear has become negative, and whose CSF glucose is normal. Approximately 50 to 70 percent of patients are cured. AIDS patients have proven so difficult to cure that most receive an intensive course of amphotericin B until CSF cultures are negative, and then require weekly intravenous injections of 1 mg/kg amphotericin B for the remainder of their lives. Average survival of AIDS patients after diagnosis of cryptococcosis has been about 8 months.

Hydrocephalus may be an early or late complication of cryptococcosis. Blindness, dementia, and personality change are other sequelae.

Patients with extraneural cryptococcosis most often require intravenous amphotericin B, with or without flucytosine. Observation or excision of lesions may suffice for some patients who are previously normal, who have a single focus in lung, skin, or bone, and who have no cryptococci in the cerebrospinal fluid, urine, or blood.

BLASTOMYCOSIS **Etiology** *Blastomyces dermatitidis* is a dimorphic fungus, growing at room temperature as a white or tan mold but growing within the host or at 37°C as budding, round yeastlike cells. The fungus is identified by its appearance, its dimorphism, and the appearance of small spores borne on hyphae of the mold form. When isolates of the two opposite mating types are grown closely together on specialized culture media, sporulating structures appear which characterize the perfect form, *Ajellomyces dermatitidis*.

Pathogenesis and pathology The infection is restricted by geography and age. Blastomycosis is uncommon in any locality, but the majority of cases occur in the southeast, central, and midatlantic areas of the United States, with occasional cases in other localities in the United States and Canada. Cases have also been encountered in Africa, Mexico, Central America, and, rarely, South America. Most patients are between 20 and 69 years old. The male/female ratio is about 10:1. There is no occupational predisposition.

Infection appears to be acquired by inhalation of the fungus from soil, decomposed vegetation, or rotting wood. Several case clusters have occurred during recreational activities in wooded areas along waterways. Infection is not transmissible from person to person. The initial pulmonary infection may heal spontaneously or become chronic. Spread to other portions of the lung, cavitation, or endobronchial lesions may appear in chronic cases. Whether or not the lung lesion resolves spontaneously, infection commonly spreads hematogenously to skin, subcutaneous tissue, bone, prostate, epididymis, or mucosa of the nose, mouth, or larynx. Less commonly, infection spreads to the brain, meninges, liver, lymph nodes, or spleen. Dissemination may not be evident for weeks or years after the appearance of the lung lesion. Progressive infection is only rarely attributable to an underlying disease or immunosuppressive treatment. The inflammatory response includes lymphocytes, giant cells, and neutrophils. Pseudoepitheliomatous hyperplasia may be striking and lead to a mistaken diagnosis of squamous cell carcinoma.

Clinical manifestations A small number of patients have an acute, self-limited pneumonia. Fever, productive cough, myalgia, and malaise usually have resolved within a month. Pulmonary infiltrates have cleared slowly as *B. dermatitidis* disappeared from the sputum.

The vast majority of patients with blastomycosis have an indolent onset and a chronically progressive course. Fever, cough, weight loss, lassitude, skin lesions, and chest ache are common symptoms. Skin lesions favor exposed areas and enlarge over many weeks from a pimple to a well-circumscribed, verrucous, crusted, or ulcerated lesion. Pain and regional lymphadenopathy are minimal. Large chronic lesions may show central healing with scarring and contracture. Mucous membrane lesions resemble squamous cell carcinoma. Chest x-ray is abnormal in two-thirds of cases, with one or more pneumonic or nodular infiltrates. Calcification, hilar adenopathy, and large pleural effusions are rare. Osteolytic lesions may occur in nearly any bone and present as cold abscess or a draining sinus. Extension to a contiguous joint may cause indolent swelling, pain, and restricted motion. Prostatic and epididymal lesions resemble tuberculosis clinically.

Diagnosis The diagnosis is made by demonstrating the fungus in culture of sputum, pus, or urine. In experienced hands, diagnosis by appearance of the organism in wet smear or histopathologic section is adequate. The fungus may be visible in a sputum cytology smear but is easily overlooked.

Treatment A few patients have been observed with transitory lung lesions, but no guidelines are known to distinguish these patients from those whose disease will progress locally or disseminate. Therefore, every patient should receive treatment. Intravenous amphotericin B is the drug of choice for patients with rapidly progressive infections, severe illness, or meningitis. Skin and noncavitary lung lesions should be treated for about 8 to 10 weeks. The recommended total dose for an adult is about 2.0 g. Cavitary lung disease or infection beyond the lung and skin should be treated for about 10 to 12 weeks with 2.5 g or more. Ketoconazole is an effective drug in patients with indolent nonmeningeal blastomycosis of mild to moderate severity and who take the drug reliably. The initial adult dose is 400 mg once daily, raised after a month to 600 or 800 mg daily if improvement is suboptimal. Therapy is continued for 6 to 12 months. The mortality rate in appropriately treated cases is 15 percent or less.

HISTOPLASMOSIS Etiology *Histoplasma capsulatum* is a dimorphic fungus that grows as a mold in nature or on Sabouraud's agar at room temperature. Hyphae bear both large and small spores, which are used for identification. *H. capsulatum* grows as a small budding yeast in host tissue and on enriched agar, such as blood cysteine glucose, at 37°C. Despite the name, the fungus is unencapsulated.

Pathogenesis and pathology Infection with *H. capsulatum* has been encountered in many areas of the world but is much more frequent in certain areas. Within the United States infection is most common in the southeastern, midatlantic, and central states. Endemic areas are probably determined by the availability of proper conditions in nature for growth of the fungus. *H. capsulatum* prefers moist surface soil, particularly when it is enriched by droppings of certain birds and bats. The fungus has not only been isolated repeatedly from such sites but many case clusters have occurred 5 to 18 days after groups were exposed to such dust, for example, by raking, cleaning dirt-floored chicken coops, bulldozing, or cave exploring. Judging by skin test reactivity in many endemic areas, 80 percent or more of residents over age 16 have been exposed.

Microconidia, or small spores, of *H. capsulatum* are small enough to reach the alveoli on inhalation and are transformed to budding forms. With time, an intense granulomatous reaction occurs. Caseation necrosis or calcification may mimic tuberculosis. The primary infection in children usually heals completely but may leave spotty calcification in the hilar nodes or lung. Transient dissemination may leave calcified granulomas in the spleen. In adults, a rounded mass of scar tissue, with or without central calcification, may remain in the lung. This has been called a *histoplasmoma*. Previous exposure is thought to confer some protection against reinfection, but infection in persons with prior positive skin tests clearly has occurred.

In a small proportion of patients, histoplasmosis becomes a progressive, potentially fatal infection. The disease occurs either as chronic fibrocavitary pneumonia or, less commonly, as disseminated infection. Patients with either form lack a history of acute primary pulmonary histoplasmosis. Chronic pulmonary infection favors otherwise healthy males over the age of 40. A history of cigarette use can be elicited from nearly all patients with chronic progressive pulmonary histoplasmosis. An acute, rapidly fatal course is most likely to be encountered in young children and immunosuppressed patients, including those with AIDS. A more chronic but equally lethal disseminated infection is more common in previously healthy adults.

Clinical manifestations The vast majority of infections are either asymptomatic or mild, and the diagnosis is elusive. Cough, fever, malaise, and chest x-ray findings of hilar adenopathy with or without one or more areas of pneumonitis occur. Erythema nodosum and erythema multiforme have been reported in a few outbreaks. Hilar adenopathy may cause temporary compression of the right middle lobe bronchus in children and young adults. Subacute pericarditis may occur, probably by extension from contiguous lymph nodes. Rarely, hilar nodes undergo a caseous, granulomatous reaction with perinodal fibrosis. Mediastinal structures become encased by progressive fibrosis, and, over many years, compression of the pulmonary veins, superior vena cava, pulmonary arteries, and esophagus may occur. Late in mediastinal disease only rare nonviable histoplasma can be found in caseous residua of lymph nodes.

Patients with *chronic pulmonary histoplasmosis* have a gradual onset over weeks or months of increasing productive cough, weight loss, and sometimes night sweats. Chest x-ray reveals uni- or bilateral fibronodular apical infiltrates. Approximately one-third of cases will stabilize or improve spontaneously early in the course. The remainder show insidious progression. Retraction and cavitation of the upper lobes occur with spread to the apex of the lower lobes and other areas of the lung. Emphysema and bullae formation further compromise pulmonary function. Death from cor pulmonale, bacterial pneumonia, or histoplasmosis occurs after months or years.

Acute disseminated histoplasmosis may be mistaken for miliary tuberculosis (see Chap. 125). Common findings include fever, emaciation, hepatosplenomegaly, lymphadenopathy, jaundice, anemia, leukopenia, and thrombocytopenia. All these features may occur in chronic dissemination as well, but the disease tends to be more localized. Indurated ulcers of the mouth, tongue, nose, or larynx occur in about a fourth of patients. Other focal findings include granulomatous hepatitis, Addison's disease, gastrointestinal ulceration, endocarditis, and chronic meningitis. Chest x-ray abnormalities occur in half the cases and show discrete nodules or a miliary pattern.

The presumed *ocular histoplasmosis* syndrome is a distinct clinical form of uveitis. Although a positive histoplasmin skin test is a requisite for diagnosis, none of these patients has had active histoplasmosis.

Diagnosis Histoplasmosis may be suspected by serologic tests and clinical manifestations, but definitive diagnosis requires demonstration of the organism by culture or histology. Serologic tests are performed on serum or CSF using either a culture filtrate called histoplasmin or whole yeast form cells. The results are interchangeable. Complement fixation is quantifiable and is the best test. An agar gel diffusion test with histoplasmin is useful but not quantifiable. An H band on agar gel testing is more diagnostic of active histoplasmosis than an M band. Frequent false-negatives and false-positives limit all current serologic tests. Serologic conversion is helpful but occurs rarely except in acute pulmonary histoplasmosis. High complement fixation titers, such as 1:32 or greater, are suggestive of the diagnosis, but no titer is diagnostic. Cross reactions with serologic tests for blastomycosis are common. A 5-mm or more diameter area of induration 24 to 48 h after skin testing with histoplasmin has been very helpful in identifying prior exposure to *Histoplasma*, but false-negatives and false-positives are so frequent that skin testing has little value in the study of ill patients. Further, a positive skin test can cause seroconversion.

Culture of *H. capsulatum* from sputum is difficult but is the procedure of choice in chronic pulmonary histoplasmosis. Digestion by proteolytic enzymes and centrifugation of sputum are helpful. In disseminated histoplasmosis, cultures of bone marrow, blood, centrifuged urine sediment, and biopsy specimens are most often positive. Lysis centrifugation is the best method for blood culture. Histologic sections of bone marrow, liver, lymph node, lung, and mucosal lesions may yield the diagnosis.

Treatment Acute pulmonary histoplasmosis requires no therapy. Mediastinal fibrosis may benefit by surgery, but the ultimate prognosis is poor. All patients with disseminated or chronic fibronodular pulmonary histoplasmosis should receive chemotherapy. The indications for using ketoconazole, as well as the treatment regimen, are the same as those given in the section on "Blastomycosis." Amphotericin B is given as 0.4 to 0.5 mg/kg per day or double that on alternate days, and is continued for at least 10 weeks. AIDS patients with disseminated histoplasmosis respond poorly to ketoconazole and should be treated with amphotericin B. After an initial intensive course, these patients are often given weekly therapy with amphotericin B to prevent relapse. In chronic pulmonary histoplasmosis, chest x-ray abnormalities improve somewhat, but pulmonary function improves very little. Successful therapy prevents progression. Addisonian crisis is a preventable cause of death in disseminated histoplasmosis.

African histoplasmosis Patients have been encountered in Africa who seem to be infected with *H. capsulatum* except that the yeast form is larger. Clinical manifestations resemble blastomycosis more than histoplasmosis because skin and bone lesions are very common.

COCCIDIOIDOMYCOSIS **Etiology** *Coccidioides immitis* has two forms, growing as a white fluffy mold on most culture media but as a nonbudding spherical form, a spherule, in host tissue or under specialized conditions. Reproduction in the host tissue is by formation of small endospores within mature spherules. After rupture of the spherule, the released endospores enlarge, become spherules, and repeat the cycle. The fungus is identified by its appearance and by formation of thick-walled, barrel-shaped spores, called *arthrospores*, in the hyphae of the mold form.

Pathogenesis and pathology *C. immitis* is a soil saprophyte in certain arid regions of the United States, Mexico, Central America, and South America. Within the United States, most cases are acquired in California, Arizona, west Texas, and New Mexico. A few cases are acquired in bordering areas and by exposure to fomites from endemic areas, such as in cotton bales.

Infection in humans and animals results from inhalation of windborne arthrospores arising from soil sites. This primary pulmonary infection is symptomatic in only 40 percent of individuals, with symptoms ranging from a mild, influenza-like illness to severe pneumonia. Mild, self-limited infections may come to medical attention because of case clusters or hypersensitivity reactions: erythema nodosum, erythema multiforme, toxic erythema, arthralgia, arthritis, conjunctivitis, or episcleritis. Case clusters occur 10 to 14 days after a group of susceptible individuals is exposed to dust in an endemic area through such activities as unearthing Indian relics, rock hunting, military maneuvers, or construction. Wind storms can carry spores to adjacent nonendemic areas and cause case clusters. The usual course of primary pulmonary infection is complete healing, though an area of pneumonitis on x-ray may heal by forming a coinlike lesion, or coccidioidoma. Less commonly, a single thin-walled cavity remains as a chronic sequela in the area of consolidation. The consolidation may persist as a chronic pneumonia or progress to fibronodular, cavitary disease.

Pleural effusion may be the only manifestation of primary infection. Self-healing of this form is common.

An uncommon but dreaded complication of coccidioidomycosis is dissemination beyond the lung and hilar lymph nodes. Dissemination is more frequent in blacks, Filipinos, Native Americans, Mexican-Americans, and pregnant or immunosuppressed patients, including those with AIDS.

C. immitis incites a chronic granulomatous reaction in host tissue, often with caseation necrosis. Lung and hilar node lesions may show calcification. Both IgM and IgG antibodies against *C. immitis* are induced by infection but neither appears protective. The amount of specific IgG antibody is a rough measure of the antigenic mass, i.e., of the amount of infection, and a high titer is a poor prognostic sign. Appearance of delayed hypersensitivity to antigens of *C. immitis* is most common in those clinical forms of disease with a good prognosis, such as self-limited primary pulmonary disease. Negative skin tests to *Coccidioides* antigens occur in roughly half the patients with disseminated disease and portend a poor prognosis.

Clinical manifestations Symptomatic primary pulmonary infection is manifested by fever, cough, chest pain, malaise, and sometimes hypersensitivity reactions. Chest x-ray may show an infiltrate, hilar adenopathy, or pleural effusion. Peripheral blood may show a mild eosinophilia. Spontaneous improvement begins after several days to 2 weeks of illness and usually culminates in complete recovery.

The symptoms of a chronic thin-walled cavity include cough or hemoptysis in half the cases; the other patients are asymptomatic. Chronic progressive pulmonary coccidioidomycosis produces cough, sputum, variable degrees of fever, and weight loss. The first indications of dissemination usually appear during the primary infection. Reactivation with dissemination in later years occurs occasionally, especially if Hodgkin's disease, non-Hodgkin's lymphoma, renal transplantation, AIDS, or other immunosuppression has supervened. Dissemination should be suspected when fever, malaise, hilar or paratracheal lymphadenopathy, elevated sedimentation rate, and high complement fixation titers show abnormal persistence in patients with primary pulmonary coccidioidomycosis. With time, lesions appear in the bone, skin, subcutaneous tissue, meninges, joints, and other sites. Without therapy, dissemination may progress rapidly to death or wax and wane for years.

Diagnosis When coccidioidomycosis is suspected, sputum, urine, and pus should be examined for *C. immitis* by wet smear and culture. *The laboratory request should indicate clearly that coccidioidomycosis is suspected because the mold form must be handled with extreme care to prevent infection of laboratory personnel.* On biopsy, smaller spherules must be distinguished from nonbudding forms of *Blastomyces* and *Cryptococcus*, but appearance of the mature spherule is diagnostic.

Serologic tests are very helpful in coccidioidomycosis. Latex agglutination and agar gel diffusion tests are useful in screening sera for antibody to *Coccidioides*. The complement fixation test is used on cerebrospinal fluid and to confirm and quantitate serum antibody detected by screening tests. The number of cases with a positive complement fixation test will depend upon the severity of disease and upon the laboratory performing the test. Positive tests are least common in patients with solitary pulmonary cavities or primary pulmonary infection, while sera from patients with multiorgan disseminated disease are nearly all positive. Seroconversion is helpful in primary pulmonary coccidioidomycosis but may not occur for up to 8 weeks after onset. A positive complement fixation test in unconcentrated cerebrospinal fluid is diagnostic of meningitis. Rarely, a parameningeal focus will cause a positive CSF serology.

Conversion of the skin test from negative to positive (≥ 5 mm induration at 24 or 48 h) with either coccidioidin or spherulin, the two commercially available antigens, may occur between the third and twenty-first days of symptoms in primary pulmonary coccidioidomycosis. Skin testing can also be helpful in epidemiologic studies, such as investigation of case clusters or definition of endemic areas.

The utility of skin testing as a diagnostic tool is limited by the presence of persistent positive tests resulting from remote exposures to *Coccidioides* and by the frequency of negative skin tests in many patients with either thin-walled cavities or disseminated coccidioidomycosis.

Treatment Primary pulmonary coccidioidomycosis usually resolves spontaneously. Some physicians give a few weeks of intravenous amphotericin B when patients show an unusually severe or protracted primary infection, hoping to abort disseminated or chronic pulmonary disease. There is no solid evidence to support this practice, but the stronger the suspicion of dissemination becomes in any given patient, the more logical this approach appears. Once evidence for dissemination becomes incontrovertible, amphotericin B may be palliative rather than curative. Incomplete recovery and relapse after apparent cure with amphotericin B have been distressingly common in both disseminated and chronic progressive pulmonary infection. The low toxicity and possibility of long-term oral therapy with ketoconazole have encouraged study of this drug in nonmeningeal coccidioidomycosis. Doses of 200 to 400 mg/d have resulted in improvement of some patients with skin, bone, and lung lesions. Patients failing to respond to this dose should have the dose escalated gradually in the 10 to 20 mg/kg per day range to assess clinical response and toxicity. Treatment is continued 12 months or more. A seriously ill or rapidly deteriorating patient should not be treated with ketoconazole. Such patients are given intravenous amphotericin B 0.5 to 0.7 mg/kg daily or 1.0 mg/kg on alternate days until infection appears relatively quiescent, often 10 or 12 weeks later. More prolonged courses may be changed to 1.0 mg/kg three times a week. Surgical debridement of bone lesions and drainage of abscesses contribute to cure. Resection of chronic progressive pulmonary lesions is a helpful adjunct to chemotherapy when infection is confined to the lung and to one lobe. A single thin-walled cavity tends to close spontaneously and ordinarily is not resected. Such a cavity responds poorly to chemotherapy. Coccidioidal meningitis is treated with long-term intrathecal amphotericin B. Hydrocephalus, a frequent complication, renders this therapy less effective. Fluconazole, an investigational agent, may be useful in such patients. The prognosis in all forms of chronic progressive coccidioidomycosis must be guarded.

THE OPPORTUNISTIC DEEP MYCOSES

CANDIDIASIS Etiology *Candida albicans* is the most common cause of candidiasis, but *C. tropicalis, C. parapsilosis, C. guilliermondii, C. krusei,* and a few other species can cause candidiasis and may even be fatal. *C. parapsilosis* is particularly notable for its ability to cause endocarditis. All *Candida* species pathogenic for humans are also encountered as commensals of humans, particularly in the mouth, stool, and vagina. These species grow rapidly at 25 to 37°C on simple media as oval budding cells. In specialized culture media, hyphae or elongated branching structures called *pseudohyphae* are formed. *C. albicans* can be identified presumptively by its ability to form germ tubes in serum or by the formation of thick-walled large spores, called *chlamydospores*. Final identification of all species requires biochemical tests.

Pathogenesis and pathology Either local or systemic factors may lead to tissue invasion by *Candida*. Chronic maceration predisposes to cutaneous candidiasis, as in diaper rash, intertrigo in obese patients, or paronychia in bartenders or cannery workers. Age is important because neonatal colonization often leads to oral candidiasis (thrush). Women in the third trimester of pregnancy are prone to vulvovaginal thrush. Patients with diabetes mellitus, AIDS, or hematologic malignancy, or who are receiving broad-spectrum antibiotics or high doses of adrenal corticosteroids, are especially susceptible to candidiasis. Breaks in the integrity of the skin or mucous membranes may provide access to deeper tissues. Examples include perforation of the gastrointestinal tract by trauma, surgery,

and peptic ulceration; indwelling catheters for intravenous alimentation, peritoneal dialysis, and urinary tract drainage; severe burns; and intravenous drug abuse.

Candida grows within tissues in both yeast and pseudohyphal forms. Rarely, only one form is present. Visceral lesions are characterized by necrosis and a neutrophilic inflammatory response. Neutrophils kill *Candida* yeast cells and damage segments of pseudohyphae in vitro, and visceral candidiasis complicates neutropenia, chronic granulomatous disease, and myeloperoxidase deficiency, suggesting a major role for the neutrophil in host defense against this fungus. Visceral lesions show a preference for kidney, brain, spleen, heart, and liver.

Clinical manifestations Oral thrush presents as discrete and confluent adherent white plaques on the oral and pharyngeal mucosa, particularly in the mouth and tongue. These lesions are usually painless, but fissuring at the corners of the mouth can be painful. *Cutaneous candidiasis* presents as red, macerated intertriginous areas, paronychia, balanitis, or pruritus ani. Candidiasis of the perineal and scrotal skin may be accompanied by discrete pustular lesions on the inner aspects of the thighs. *Chronic mucocutaneous candidiasis* or *Candida granuloma* typically presents as circumscribed hyperkeratotic skin lesions, crumbling dystrophic nails, partial alopecia in areas of scalp lesions, and both oral and vaginal thrush. Systemic infection is very rare, but disfigurement of the face and hands can be severe. Other findings may include chronic epidermophytosis, dental dysplasia, and hypofunction of the parathyroid, adrenal, or thyroid glands. A variety of defects in T-cell function have been described in these patients. Vulvovaginal thrush causes pruritus, discharge, and sometimes pain on intercourse or urination. Speculum examination reveals an inflamed mucosa and a thin exudate, often with white curds.

From one to multiple small shallow ulcerations due to *Candida* may appear in the esophagus or gastrointestinal tract. Esophageal lesions favor the distal third and may cause dysphagia or substernal pain. Other such lesions tend to be asymptomatic but assume importance in the leukemic patient as a portal for disseminated candidiasis. Within the urinary tract, the most common lesions are either hematogenous renal abscesses, which can cause azotemia, or bladder thrush. Bladder invasion usually follows catheterization or instrumentation of a patient with diabetes mellitus or who is receiving broad-spectrum antibiotics. This lesion generally is asymptomatic and benign. Rarely, retrograde invasion of the renal pelvis leads to renal papillary necrosis.

Hematogenous dissemination of Candida presents with fever and toxicity but with few localizing findings. One or more retinal abscesses may appear and extend slowly into the vitreous humor. The patient may note orbital pain, blurred vision, scotoma, or opacities floating across the visual field. Pulmonary candidiasis is almost always hematogenous and is visible on chest x-ray only when the abscesses are numerous enough to cause a diffuse, vaguely nodular infiltrate. Candidiasis of the endocardium or around intracardiac prostheses resembles bacterial infection of these sites. Chronic *Candida* meningitis or arthritis may occur, from either disseminated disease or insertion of a prosthesis in the case of arthritis. Rare focal manifestations of disseminated disease include osteomyelitis, pustular skin lesions, myositis, and brain abscess.

Diagnosis Demonstration of pseudohyphae on wet smear with confirmation by culture is the procedure of choice for diagnosing superficial candidiasis. Scrapings for the smear may be obtained from skin, nails, and oral and vaginal mucosa. Culture alone is not diagnostic; however, recovery of *Candida* species from multiple superficial sites in immunosuppressed patients may portend visceral invasion.

Deeper lesions of *Candida* may be diagnosed by histologic section of biopsy specimens or by culture of cerebrospinal fluid, blood, joint fluid, or surgical specimens. Blood cultures in vented bottles or concentrated by lysis-centrifugation are very useful in *Candida* endocarditis and intravenous catheter-induced sepsis but are positive less often in other forms of disseminated disease. Serologic tests for antibody or antigen are not useful.

Treatment   Cutaneous candidiasis of macerated areas responds to measures which reduce moisture and chafing plus a topically applied antifungal agent in a nonocclusive base. Nystatin, ciclopirox, and the imidazole creams such as clotrimazole and miconazole appear roughly equivalent. Nystatin and some imidazoles are available also for vaginal application. Oral candidiasis should be treated with clotrimazole troches or a nystatin suspension. Swallowing nystatin suspension, sucking on clotrimazole troches, or taking ketoconazole, 200 to 400 mg/d, may improve symptoms of esophageal candidiasis. When esophageal symptoms are pronounced, a 5- to 10-day course of intravenous amphotericin B, 0.3 mg/kg per day, may be beneficial. Bladder thrush responds to bladder irrigations with amphotericin B, 50 μg/mL for 5 days. In all forms of skin and mucosal candidiasis, relapse after successful treatment is common.

Intravenous amphotericin B is the drug of choice in disseminated candidiasis. The drug is usually given as 0.4 to 0.5 mg/kg every day or as a double dose on alternate days for several weeks. In patients with no contraindication to the use of flucytosine, administration of that drug in dosage of 100 to 150 mg/kg per day plus amphotericin B, 0.3 mg/kg per day, is an effective alternative. Ketoconazole in an adult dose of 200 mg daily is probably the drug of choice for chronic mucocutaneous candidiasis.

Candida isolated from a properly obtained blood culture should be considered significant; true false-positives are rare. Whether a patient with candidiasis should receive antifungal therapy will depend on the degree of illness and the likelihood of spontaneous recovery. For example, a febrile, severely immunosuppressed patient with one positive blood culture should receive prompt therapy because a rapidly fatal course is common. A nonimmunosuppressed patient acquiring candidiasis from an indwelling intravenous plastic catheter may recover spontaneously if the catheter is removed promptly. The species of *Candida* is irrelevant to this decision. Patients with candidiasis in whom antifungal therapy is withheld should be observed carefully for the development of endophthalmitis, endocarditis, arthritis, osteomyelitis, or other visceral lesions that require therapy.

ASPERGILLOSIS   Etiology   *Aspergillus fumigatus* is the most common pathogen, but *A. flavus, A. niger,* and several other species can cause disease. *Aspergillus* is a mold with septate hyphae about 2 to 4 μm in diameter. The fungus is identified by its gross and microscopic appearance in culture.

Pathogenesis and pathology   All the common species of *Aspergillus* which cause disease in humans are ubiquitous in the environment, growing on dead leaves, stored grain, compost piles, hay, and other decaying vegetation. Inhalation of *Aspergillus* spores must be extremely common, but disease is rare. Invasion of lung tissue is almost entirely confined to immunosuppressed patients. Roughly 90 percent will have two of these three conditions: less than 500 granulocytes per microliter of peripheral blood, supraphysiologic doses of adrenal corticosteroids, and a history of cytotoxic drugs such as azathioprine. Infection in such patients is characterized by hyphal invasion of blood vessels, thrombosis, necrosis, and hemorrhagic infarction. Chronic granulomatous disease of childhood also predisposes to invasive pulmonary aspergillosis, but here the inflammatory response is granulomatous and blood vessel invasion is rare.

Massive inhalation of *Aspergillus* spores by normal persons can lead to an acute, diffuse, self-limited pneumonitis. Epithelioid granulomas with giant cells and central pyogenic areas containing hyphae are seen. Spontaneous recovery taking several weeks is the usual course.

Aspergillus can colonize the damaged bronchial tree, pulmonary cysts, or cavities of patients with underlying lung disease. Balls of hyphae within cysts or cavities may reach several centimeters in diameter and be visible on chest x-ray. Tissue invasion does not occur. The term *allergic bronchial aspergillosis* denotes the condition of patients with preexisting asthma who have eosinophilia, IgE

antibody to *Aspergillus,* and fleeting pulmonary infiltrates from bronchial plugging (see Chap. 205).

Clinical manifestations   *Endobronchial pulmonary aspergillosis* presents as chronic productive cough and often hemoptysis in a patient with prior chronic lung disease, such as tuberculosis, sarcoidosis, bronchiectasis, or histoplasmosis. *Aspergilloma* refers to a ball of hyphae within a lung cyst or cavity, usually in the upper lobe. *Aspergillus* may be spread from its endocavitary or endobronchial site to the pleura during the course of bacterial lung abscess or surgery.

Invasive aspergillosis in the immunosuppressed host presents as an acute pneumonia and has a tendency to cavitation. Infection progresses by hematogenous spread as well as extension to surrounding lung and other contiguous structures. Occasionally the portal of infection in the immunosuppressed host is the paranasal sinus, gastrointestinal tract, skin, or palate.

Aspergillus sinusitis in nonimmunosuppressed patients may take two forms. A ball of hyphae may form in a chronically obstructed paranasal sinus, without tissue invasion. Much less commonly, a chronic, fibrosing granulomatous inflammation with *Aspergillus* hyphae within tissue may begin in the sinus and spread slowly to the orbit and brain.

Growth of *Aspergillus* on cerumen and detritus within the external auditory canal is termed *otomycosis.* Trauma to the cornea may cause chronic *Aspergillus* keratitis. Endophthalmitis follows introduction of *Aspergillus* into the globe by trauma or surgery. *Aspergillus* may infect intracardiac or intravascular prostheses.

Diagnosis   Repeated isolation of *Aspergillus* from sputum or demonstration of hyphae in sputum or bronchial brushing specimens suggests endobronchial colonization or infection. Even a single isolation of *Aspergillus* from the sputum of a neutropenic patient with pneumonia, particularly a child or nonsmoker, suggests the diagnosis of invasive aspergillosis. Fungus ball of the lung is usually detectable by chest x-ray. Antibody of the IgG class to *Aspergillus* antigens is demonstrable in the serum of many colonized patients and of virtually all patients with fungus ball.

Biopsy is usually required to diagnose invasive aspergillosis of the lung, paranasal sinus, or sites of dissemination. Blood cultures are rarely positive, even in patients with infected cardiac prosthetic valves. *Aspergillus* hyphae can be identified presumptively by histology, but culture is required for confirmation and determination of species.

Treatment   Patients with severe hemoptysis due to fungus ball of the lung may benefit by lobectomy. Poor pulmonary function in residual lung and dense pleural adhesions around the lesion can complicate the resection. Systemic chemotherapy is of no value in endobronchial or endocavitary aspergillosis.

Intravenous amphotericin B has resulted in arrest or cure of invasive aspergillosis when immunosuppression is not severe. Combined flucytosine–amphotericin B may be useful in nonneutropenic patients with invasive aspergillosis.

MUCORMYCOSIS (ZYGOMYCOSIS, PHYCOMYCOSIS)   Etiology   Species of *Rhizopus, Rhizomucor,* and *Cunninghamella* are most common, but species of *Apophysomyces, Saksenaea, Mucor,* and *Absidia* occasionally cause mucormycosis. These molds have broad, rarely septate hyphae of uneven diameter, ranging from 6 to 50 μm. The fungus is inexplicably difficult to grow from infected tissue. When it occurs, growth is rapid and profuse on most media at room temperature. Identification is based upon gross and microscopic appearance of the mold.

Pathogenesis and pathology   *Rhizopus* and *Rhizomucor* species are ubiquitous, appearing on decaying vegetation, dung, and foods of high sugar content. Infection is uncommon and is largely confined to patients with serious preexisting diseases. Mucormycosis originating in the paranasal sinuses and nose occurs predominantly in patients with poorly controlled diabetes mellitus. Patients with organ transplantation, hematologic malignancy, or who are receiving long-term deferoxamine therapy are predisposed to mucormycosis of either sinus or lung. Gastrointestinal mucormycosis occurs in a variety of conditions, including uremia, severe malnutrition, and diarrheal diseases. Infection is acquired from nature, with no person-to-person spread. In all forms of mucormycosis, vascular invasion by hyphae is prominent. Ischemic or hemorrhagic necrosis is the predominant histologic finding.

Clinical manifestations Mucormycosis originating in the nose and paranasal sinuses produces a characteristic clinical picture. Low-grade fever, dull sinus pain, and sometimes nasal congestion or a thin, bloody nasal discharge are followed in a few days by double vision, increasing fever, and obtundation. Examination reveals a unilateral generalized reduction of ocular motion, chemosis, and proptosis. The nasal turbinates on the involved side may be dusky red or necrotic. A sharply delineated area of necrosis, strictly respecting the midline, may appear in the hard palate. The skin of the cheek may become inflamed. Fungal invasion of the globe or ophthalmic artery leads to blindness. Opacification of one or more sinuses is found on CT scan or by NMR imaging. Carotid arteriogram may show invasion or obstruction of the carotid siphon. Coma is due to direct invasion of the frontal lobe. Early symptoms mimic bacterial sinusitis. Clouding of the sensorium may be attributed to diabetic acidosis. Cavernous sinus thrombosis may be considered when orbital invasion occurs. Without treatment, death may occur in a few days to a few weeks.

Pulmonary mucormycosis is a progressive severe pneumonia, accompanied by high fever and toxicity. The necrotic center of large infiltrates may cavitate. Hematogenous spread to other areas of the lung, as well as to brain and other organs, is common. Survival beyond 2 weeks is unusual. Gastrointestinal invasion presents as one or more ulcers which tend to perforate. Hematogenous dissemination can originate from the gastrointestinal tract, lung, or paranasal sinuses. Sometimes no portal of entry can be found.

Diagnosis Lesions of the lung and craniofacial structures are best diagnosed by biopsy and histologic section. Cultural confirmation should be attempted. Wet smear of crushed tissue can provide rapid diagnosis. Cultures of blood and cerebrospinal fluid are negative. Smear and culture of sputum may be positive during cavitation of a lung lesion.

Treatment Regulation of diabetes mellitus and decreasing the dose of immunosuppressive drugs aid in the treatment. Extensive debridement of craniofacial lesions appears to be very important. Orbital exenteration may be required. Intravenous amphotericin B is clearly of value in craniofacial mucormycosis and should be employed in the other forms of mucormycosis as well. Maximum tolerated doses are given until progression is halted. The drug is continued for a total of 10 to 12 weeks. Appropriate management results in cure of about half of the craniofacial infections. Survival of patients with pulmonary, gastrointestinal, or disseminated mucormycosis is rare.

SPOROTRICHOSIS Etiology *Sporothrix schenckii* lives as a saprophyte on plants in many areas of the world. In nature and on culture at room temperature the fungus grows as a mold, but within host tissue or at 37°C on enriched media it grows as a budding yeast. Identification is by appearance of the fungus in mold and yeast forms.

Pathogenesis and pathology Infection results when minor trauma inoculates the fungus into subcutaneous tissue. Nursery workers, florists, and gardeners acquire the illness from roses, sphagnum moss, and other plants. Infection may be limited to the site of inoculation (plaque sporotrichosis) or extend along proximal lymphatic channels (lymphangitic sporotrichosis). Spread beyond an extremity, the usual site of infection, is rare, and hematogenous dissemination from the skin remains unproven. The portal for osteoarticular, pulmonary, and other extracutaneous forms of sporotrichosis is unknown but is likely the lung.

Untreated sporotrichosis shows little evidence of self-healing and is capable of extreme chronicity. The inflammatory response contains both clusters of neutrophils and a marked granulomatous response with epithelioid cells and giant cells.

Clinical manifestations Lymphangitic sporotrichosis, by far the most common manifestation, forms a nearly painless red papule at the site of inoculation. Over the next several weeks, similar nodules form along proximal lymphatic channels. Nodules intermittently discharge small amounts of pus. Ulceration may occur. The proximal extension of these lesions, often with skip areas, is quite distinctive but may be mimicked by lesions of *Nocardia brasiliensis*, *Mycobacterium marinum*, or, on rare occasions, by *Leishmania brasiliensis* or *M. kansasii*.

Plaque sporotrichosis is a nontender red maculopapular granuloma confined to the site of inoculation. Osteoarticular sporotrichosis presents as mono- or polyarticular arthritis of indolent onset and progression over months or years, involving the elbows, knees, wrists, ankles, and, rarely, smaller joints of the extremities. Periarticular bone develops areas of demineralization on x-ray, and draining sinuses may appear over joints and bursae. Hematogenous spread to the skin may be observed during polyarticular disease, but none of the skin lesions shows lymphangitic spread. Immunosuppression predisposes to hematogenous spread. Pulmonary sporotrichosis usually presents as a single chronic cavitary upper-lobe lung lesion.

Diagnosis Culture of pus, joint fluid, sputum, or skin biopsy specimen is the preferred method of diagnosis. Appearance of *S. schenckii* in tissue is quite variable. In skin lesions, the organisms are hard to find.

Treatment Cutaneous sporotrichosis can be cured with oral administration of a saturated solution of potassium iodide, given in increasing divided daily doses up to 4.5 to 9 mL/d for adults, as tolerated. Gastrointestinal disturbance or acneiform rash over the cape area and face are common, but therapy should be continued for 1 month after resolution of all lesions. Patients with serious allergic reactions to iodides may respond to local heat, particularly when plaque sporotrichosis is the only form of disease. Itraconazole, an experimental drug, may be of value. Extracutaneous sporotrichosis rarely responds to iodides, but cures have been obtained in over half such patients with prolonged courses of intravenous amphotericin B.

RARER DEEP MYCOSES

PARACOCCIDIOIDOMYCOSIS Etiology Formerly called *South American blastomycosis*, this is the mycosis caused by *Paracoccidioides brasiliensis*. A dimorphic fungus, *P. brasiliensis* grows as a budding yeast but may be grown as either yeast or mold on a culture medium. Identification is by gross and microscopic appearance. A superficial resemblance to *Blastomyces dermatitidis* may cause misdiagnosis.

Pathogenesis and pathology Infection is thought to be acquired by inhalation of spores from environmental sources, but the reservoir in nature remains obscure. Pulmonary infection produces few symptoms initially. Hematogenous spread to the mucous membranes of the mouth and nose, the lymph nodes, and other sites brings the patient to medical attention. Fatal cases show spread to the adrenal, the gastrointestinal tract, and many other viscera.

Clinical manifestations Common symptoms include indurated ulcers of the mouth, oropharynx, larynx, and nose, enlarged and draining lymph nodes, lesions of the skin and genitalia, productive cough, weight loss, dyspnea, and sometimes fever. Acquisition of infection is restricted to South America, Central America, and Mexico, but the extreme indolence of this infection may lead to recognition many years after the patient has left the endemic area. Chest x-ray most often shows a bilateral patchy pneumonia.

Diagnosis Cultures of sputum, pus, and mucosal lesions are often diagnostic. The diagnosis can be made by smear or histologic section, though confirmation by culture is preferable. Serologic tests are useful in suggesting the diagnosis and monitoring therapy.

Treatment   Milder cases may be cured by one year's treatment with oral ketoconazole, 200 to 400 mg daily. Itraconazole appears to give comparable results. More advanced cases are given intravenous amphotericin B, followed by ketoconazole.

PSEUDALLESCHERIASIS   Etiology   Also called *Petriellidium boydii, Pseudallescheria boydii* is a mold frequently found in soil. When the fungus is isolated in the imperfect state, it is called *Scedosporium apiospermum.*

Pathogenesis and pathology   Wind-borne spores of *P. boydii*, arising in soil, are the presumed source of infection. The fungus grows as a mold within tissue, causing necrosis and abscess formation.

Clinical manifestations   *P. boydii* resembles *Aspergillus* in its ability to colonize the endobronchial tree, to form fungus balls in the lung or paranasal sinuses, and to invade the cornea or globe following trauma or surgery and by its propensity to invade the immunosuppressed host. Hyphae of *P. boydii* in tissue may be difficult to distinguish from *Aspergillus*. Infection with *P. boydii* is much less common than with *Aspergillus*. *P. boydii* is the single most common cause in the United States of mycetoma. Intravascular hyphae, a hallmark of invasive aspergillosis, also can be found in pseudallescheriasis. Occasional normal patients have developed necrotizing pneumonia or abscesses in brain or other organs due to *P. boydii*.

Diagnosis   Demonstration of hyphae in tissue and culture confirmation are required for diagnosis.

Treatment   Intravenous miconazole or ketoconazole is recommended, but therapeutic response to all drugs has been poor.

TORULOPSOSIS   Etiology   *Torulopsis glabrata (Candida glabrata)* is a small yeast-like fungus, the same size as the yeast form of *Histoplasma capsulatum*. *T. glabrata* does not form hyphae or pseudohyphae. Identification is by biochemical tests.

Pathogenesis and pathology   *T. glabrata* is a normal inhabitant of the human gastrointestinal tract and vagina. Within tissue, *T. glabrata* causes abscess formation with a neutrophilic inflammatory response. In immunosuppressed patients, a scanty or mononuclear inflammatory response may be seen.

Clinical manifestations   Torulopsosis mimics many of the manifestations of candidiasis, but infection is less common and often less severe. Clinical entities include intravenous catheter–induced sepsis or endocarditis, gastrointestinal and disseminated infection in immunosuppressed patients, and retrograde infection of the urinary tract.

Diagnosis   *Torulopsis* may be difficult to distinguish from yeast cells of *Candida* in histologic section. Culture is the most reliable diagnostic tool.

Treatment   Therapeutic measures used in candidiasis appear appropriate for torulopsosis.

MYCETOMA   Etiology   *Actinomycetoma* refers to infection by actinomycetes of the genera *Nocardia, Streptomyces*, and *Actinomadura*. *Eumycetoma* is caused by true fungi of many different genera. The most common agent varies with the locality.

Pathogenesis and pathology   The pathogens live in the soil and enter the skin through minor trauma. The most common site of infection is the foot. Infection runs a relentless course over many years, with destruction of contiguous bone and fascia. Grains are found in purulent foci, surrounded by fibrosis and a mononuclear cell inflammatory response.

Clinical manifestations   *Mycetoma* is a chronic suppurative infection originating in subcutaneous tissue and characterized by the presence of grains, which are tightly clumped colonies of the causative agent. The infected site shows painless swelling, woody induration, and sinus tracts which discharge pus intermittently. Systemic symptoms and spread to distant sites in the body are not seen.

Diagnosis   The clinical picture is characteristic, but confusion with chronic osteomyelitis or botryomycosis may occur. The diagnosis requires demonstration of grains in pus from the draining sinus or in biopsy sections. Many histologic sections may need to be examined to locate a grain.

Treatment   Actinomycetoma may respond to prolonged combination chemotherapy, such as streptomycin and either dapsone or trimethoprim-sulfamethoxazole. Eumycetoma rarely has responded to chemotherapy. As a possible exception, some cases infected with *Madurella mycetomatis* have appeared to respond to ketoconazole.

CHROMOMYCOSIS   This chronic subcutaneous mycosis is rarely seen in the United States but presents as a verrucoid, ulcerated, or crusted skin lesion. Disease originates when thorns or bits of vegetation introduce the fungus into the subcutaneous tissue. Infection spreads over ensuing months and years to contiguous tissue, causing very few symptoms. Appearance of the thick-walled dark-colored rounded forms ("copper pennies") in tissue is diagnostic. No satisfactory treatment is available.

DERMATOPHYTOSIS

Definition   Dermatophytosis, also known as ringworm or tinea, is a chronic fungal infection of the skin, hair, or nails.

Etiology   Species of *Trichophyton, Microsporum*, and *Epidermophyton* are called *dermatophytes*. They grow in and remain confined to the keratinous structures of the body. Other mycoses can show fungal invasion of keratinous structures, such as candidiasis, pityriasis versicolor, and tinea nigra, but are traditionally not termed *dermatophytoses*.

Pathology and pathogenesis   Dermatophyte species are called anthropophilic, zoophilic, or geophilic, depending on whether their usual reservoir within nature appears to be humans, animals, or soil. Infectivity of all those sources is low, and group outbreaks are largely confined to an occasional case clustering of scalp infections in children. Acquisition of a dermatophytosis appears to be favored by minor trauma, maceration, and poor hygiene of the skin. Infection does not seem to confer solid immunity. Repeated infection with the same species is commonplace, particularly with anthropophilic species. Infrequency of scalp infection in adults has been attributed to local factors rather than immunity.

Invasion of the stratum corneum by dermatophytes may cause little inflammation, or, particularly with zoophilic fungi, inflammation can be intense. Shedding of the stratum corneum is increased by inflammation. To the extent that fungal growth cannot keep up with shedding, inflammation may help terminate infection. Conversely, infection is probably favored when shedding is reduced by glucocorticoids and cytotoxic drugs. Antifungal drugs interfere with the ability of fungal growth to keep up with shedding.

Clinical manifestations   The disease varies with the site of infection and fungal species. Foot infection (athlete's foot, tinea pedis) may present as fissuring of the toe webs, scaling of the plantar surfaces, or vesicles around the toe webs and soles. Interdigital lesions may be pruritic or, when bacterial superinfection occurs, may be painful. Hand infection is less common but resembles foot infection. Scalp dermatophytosis (tinea capitis) is characterized by areas of alopecia and scaling. In so-called endothrix infection, the hair shaft breaks off at the skin surface, leaving the hairs visible as black dots in the scalp. With some forms of scalp infection an intense boggy suppuration occurs, called a *kerion*. Dermatophytosis of the glabrous skin (tinea corporis) presents as circumscribed lesions with a wide variety of appearances. Scales, vesicles, or pustules may appear. Inflammation may be minimal or intense. Central healing of less inflamed lesions may be seen. The serpiginous border of inflammation is the source of the name *ringworm*. Dermatophytosis of the bearded area (tinea barbae) appears as a pustular folliculitis. Onychomycosis (tinea unguium) presents as white discolored nails or thickened, chalky crumbling nails. Peeling and fissuring of the paronychia or keratotic debris under the nail edge may also be seen.

Diagnosis   Discolored hairs, scales, and keratotic debris under infected nails should be collected for KOH smear and culture. In the scraping of skin lesions, a drop of water on the skin site may keep the removed scales from flying off and aid in their collection. Culture is important in distinguishing dermatophytes from *Candida* and fungal saprophytes growing in keratinaceous debris.

Treatment Mild or moderately severe lesions of the trunk, groin, and feet often respond to topical therapy with an imidazole or one of the other agents mentioned earlier in this chapter. Hyperkeratotic lesions of the palms and soles respond less well. Ringworm that is moderately severe or severe, that is unresponsive to topical therapy, or that involves the scalp, nails, or bearded area should be treated systemically. The drug of choice is griseofulvin. Either 500 mg of the microcrystalline form or 375 mg of the ultramicrocrystalline form is given once daily or divided into two doses, given with meals. Double this amount has been recommended for refractory infections. Treatment must be continued until all infected keratin is gone. Cutting of infected hair, epilating nails, and cleansing interdigital webs can expedite cure. Secondary bacterial infection of the foot may require soaks or antibacterial agents. Relapse of dermatophyte foot infections may be decreased by measures to keep the feet clean and dry. Griseofulvin-resistant cases may respond to oral ketoconazole, 200 to 400 mg daily.

REFERENCES

Therapy

DAMESHMEND TK, WARNOCK DW: Clinical pharmacokinetics of ketoconazole. Clin Pharmacokinetics 14:13, 1988

HEIDEMANN HT et al: Amphotericin B nephrotoxicity in humans decreased by salt repletion. Am J Med 75:476, 1983

KERRIDGE D: Present status of antimycotics. Microbiol Sci 2:83, 1985

NIAID MYCOSES STUDY GROUP: Treatment of blastomycosis and histoplasmosis with ketoconazole. Ann Intern Med 103:861, 1986

SAAG MS, DISMUKES WE: Azole antifungal agents: Emphasis on new triazoles. Antimicrob Agents Chemother 32:1, 1988

Cryptococcosis

DISMUKES WE: Cryptococcal meningitis in patients with AIDS. J Infect Dis 157:624, 1988

——— et al: Treatment of cryptococcal meningitis with combination amphotericin B and flucytosine for four as compared with six weeks. N Engl J Med 317:334, 1987

GAL AA et al: The pathology of pulmonary cryptococcal infections in the acquired immunodeficiency syndrome. Arch Pathol Lab Med 110:502, 1986

KOVACS JA et al: Cryptococcosis in the acquired immunodeficiency syndrome. Ann Intern Med 103:533, 1985

Blastomycosis

CAMPBELL GD, CHAPMAN SW: Blastomycosis. Semin Respir Med 9:164, 1987

KLEIN BS et al: Two outbreaks of blastomycosis along rivers in Wisconsin: Isolation of *Blastomyces dermatitidis* from riverbank soil and evidence of its transmission along waterways. Am Rev Respir Dis 136:1333, 1987

Histoplasmosis

GOODWIN RA et al: Histoplasmosis in normal hosts. Medicine 60:231, 1981

JOHNSON PC et al: Progressive disseminated histoplasmosis in patients with acquired immunodeficiency syndrome. Am J Med 85:152, 1988

WHEAT LJ et al: Cavitary histoplasmosis occurring during two large urban outbreaks. Analysis of clinical, epidemiologic, roentgenographic, and laboratory features. Medicine 63:201, 1984

Coccidioidomycosis

BOUZA E et al: Coccidioidal meningitis. An analysis of thirty-one cases and review of the literature. Medicine 60:139, 1980

BRENNIMAN DA et al: Coccidioidomycosis in the acquired immunodeficiency syndrome. Ann Intern Med 106:372, 1987

DRUTZ DJ: Amphotericin B in the treatment of coccidioidomycosis. Drugs 26:337, 1983

GALGIANI JN et al: Ketoconazole therapy of progressive coccidioidomycosis. Comparison of 400 and 800 mg doses and observations at higher doses. Am J Med 84:603, 1988

Candidiasis

DUPONT B, ROUHET E: Cutaneous, ocular, and osteoarticular candidiasis in heroin addicts: New clinical and therapeutic aspects in 38 patients. J Infect Dis 152:577, 1985

HARON E et al: Hepatic candidiasis: An increasing problem in immunocompromised patients. Am J Med 83:17, 1987

KLEIN RS et al: Oral candidiasis in high-risk patients as the initial manifestation of the acquired immunodeficiency syndrome. N Engl J Med 311:354, 1984

LEVINE MS et al: *Candida* esophagitis: accuracy of radiographic diagnosis. Radiology 154:581, 1985

ODD FC: *Candida and Candidosis*. Baltimore, Saunders, 1988

THALER M et al: Hepatic candidiasis in cancer patients: The evolving picture of the syndrome. Ann Intern Med 198:88, 1988

Aspergillosis

GERSON SL et al: Prolonged granulocytopenia: The major risk factor for invasive pulmonary aspergillosis in patients with acute leukemia. Ann Intern Med 100:345, 1984

KUHLMAN JE et al: Invasive pulmonary aspergillosis in acute leukemia: Characteristic findings on CT, the CT halo sign, and the role of CT in early diagnosis. Radiology 157:611, 1985

WALSH TJ et al: *Candida* suppurative peripheral thrombophlebitis: Recognition, prevention, and management. Infect Control 7:16, 1986

YU VL et al: Significance of isolation of *Aspergillus* from the respiratory tract in diagnosis of invasive pulmonary aspergillosis. Am J Med 81:249, 1986

Mucormycosis

BRENNAN RO et al: Cunninghamella: A newly recognized cause of rhinocerebral mucormycosis. Am J Clin Pathol 80:98, 1983

LEHRER RI et al: Mucormycosis. Ann Intern Med 93:93, 1980

MANIGLIA AL et al: Cephalic phycomycosis: A report of eight cases. Laryngoscope 92:755, 1982

WINDUS DW et al: Fetal *Rhizopus* infections in hemodialysis patients receiving deferoxamine. Ann Intern Med 107:678, 1987

Sporotrichosis

BULLPITT P, WEEDON D: Sporotrichosis: A review of 39 cases. Pathology 10:249, 1978

ENGLAND DM, HOCHHOLZER L: Primary pulmonary sporotrichosis. Am J Surg Pathol 9:193, 1985

FRIEDMAN SJ, DOYLE JA: Extracutaneous sporotrichosis. Int J Dermatol 22:171, 1983

PLUSS JL, OPAL SM: Pulmonary sporotrichosis: Review of treatment and outcome. Medicine 65:143, 1986

URABE H, HONBO B: Sporotrichosis. Int J Dermatol 25:255, 1986

Paracoccidioidomycosis

LONDERO AT, SEVERO LC: The gamut of progressive pulmonary paracoccidioidomycosis. Mycopathologia 75:65, 1981

RESTREPO A et al: Itraconazole in the treatment of parracoccidioidomycosis. A preliminary report. Rev Infect Dis 9(Suppl 1):51, 1987

SUGAR AM et al: Paracoccidioidomycosis in the immunosuppressed host: Report of a case and review of the literature. Am Rev Respir Dis 129:340, 1984

Pseudallescheriasis

ALSIP SG, COBBA CG: *Pseudallescheria boydii* infection of the central nervous system in a cardiac transplant recipient. South Med J 79:383, 1986

GALGIANI JN et al: *Pseudallescheria boydii* infections treated with ketoconazole. Chest 86:219, 1984

TRAVIS LB et al: Clinical significance of *Pseudallescheria boydii*: A review of 10 years' experience. Mayo Clin Proc 60:531, 1985

YOO D et al: Brain abscesses due to *Pseudallescheria boydii* associated with primary nonHodgkin's lymphoma of the central nervous system: A case report and literature review. Rev Infect Dis 7:272, 1985

Torulopsosis

KAUFFMAN CA, TAN JS: *Torulopsis glabrata* renal infection. Am J Med 57:217, 1974

VALDIVIESO M et al: Fungemia due to *Torulopsis glabrata* in the compromised host. Cancer 38:1750, 1976

Mycetoma

GUMAA SA et al: Mycetoma of the head and neck. Am J Trop Med Hyg 35:594, 1986

TIGHT RR, BARTLETT MS: Actinomycetoma in the United States. Rev Infect Dis 3:1139, 1981

Chromomycosis

LONDERO AT, RAMOS DC: Chromomycosis: A clinical and mycologic study of thirty-five cases observed in the hinterland of Rio Grande Do Sul, Brazil. Am J Trop Med Hyg 25:132, 1976

Dermatophytosis

ROBERTSON MH et al: Ketoconazole in griseofulvin-resistant dermatophytosis. J Am Acad Dermatol 6:224, 1982

——— et al: Ketoconazole in griseofulvin-resistant dermatophytosis. J Am Acad Dermatol 6:224, 1982

WEISMANN K et al: White nails in AIDS/ARC due to *Trichophyton rubrum* infection. Clin Exp Dermatol 13:24, 1988

152   ACTINOMYCOSIS AND NOCARDIOSIS

JOHN E. BENNETT

ACTINOMYCOSIS

DEFINITION   Actinomycosis is an indolent suppurative infection caused by certain anaerobic actinomycetes. The microorganisms grow within the tissue as grossly visible, tightly knit clusters, called *grains*.

ETIOLOGY   *Actinomyces israelii* is the usual pathogen, with occasional cases due to other species of *Actinomyces* (*A. naeslundii, A. viscosus, A. odontolyticus, A. meyeri*) or *Arachnia propionica*. All can form branching gram-positive hyphae and are the same width as bacteria. Most species grow best in an atmosphere that is either anaerobic or contains 6 to 10% CO_2. Isolation of the causative agent is made difficult by the mixed flora usually present in actinomycotic abscesses.

PATHOLOGY AND PATHOGENESIS   All agents of actinomycosis are commensals in the mouth and gastrointestinal tract of humans. The portal of entry appears to be either a break in the integrity of the mucosa or aspiration into the lung. Poor dental hygiene and dental abscess predispose to cervicofacial lesions. Within the gastrointestinal tract, the appendiceal area is the most common site. Infection presents as a chronic suppurative inflammation, usually in the cervicofacial, thoracic, or abdominal area. In histopathologic section, each grain is typically surrounded by polymorphonuclear neutrophils. The adjacent tissue shows subacute or chronic inflammation with extensive fibrosis and formation of sinus tracts. Giant cells are infrequent. Grains are a few millimeters in diameter. Several sections may have to be searched to find a grain. Grains may be observed grossly in pus or on bandages covering draining sinuses. These pale yellow, cheeselike particles can be crushed on a microscope slide and Gram-stained. Demonstration of gram-positive filaments in a smear of crushed grains or in histologic section helps distinguish actinomycosis from botryomycosis or eumycetoma.

Infection spreads by direct extension and hematogenously. Direct extension through the skin causes one or more chronic draining sinuses to appear in the abdomen, chest, or cervicofacial area. Hematogenous foci may appear in bone, brain, liver, or other organs.

CLINICAL MANIFESTATIONS   *Cervicofacial actinomycosis* presents as a red or purplish, firmly indurated subcutaneous mass, typically in the submandibular area or in the anterior cervical triangle near the angle of the mandible. One or more draining sinuses may be present. Tenderness is slight or absent. Lethargy, weight loss, variable low-grade fever, anemia, and leukocytosis are infrequent in cervicofacial actinomycosis but common in *thoracic* and *abdominal actinomycosis*. Localizing findings in the latter forms include draining sinuses and, in thoracic actinomycosis, cough and purulent sputum. Pulmonic lesions may extend through the chest wall and present as an indolent subcutaneous abscess. Pain or a palpable mass may appear in abdominal actinomycosis. *Pelvic actinomycosis* may originate from either the female reproductive tract or the intestine, particularly the appendix. Women with an intrauterine device in place for more than 2 years appear to be at a slightly increased risk of pelvic actinomycosis. Tuboovarian abscess, ureteral obstruction, or, rarely, hepatic abscess have been reported. The indolent onset, variable low-grade fever, abdominal pain, and adnexal mass may lead to an erroneous diagnosis of pelvic inflammatory disease or tumor. In all forms of actinomycosis, disease typically has been present for weeks or months at time of diagnosis.

Chest x-ray may reveal an area of dense pneumonitis. Fibrosis, empyema, or cavitation may be seen. Periappendiceal abscess may appear as an extrinsic mass on barium enema or may be detected by ultrasonography or CT scan.

DIAGNOSIS   Laboratory tests other than culture or histologic section are not helpful. Blood cultures are rarely positive. Isolation of *Actinomyces* or *Arachnia* species from the mouth, sputum, stool, or feculent draining sinuses is not diagnostic. Demonstration of a grain in pus or deep tissue is diagnostic if botryomycosis and mycetoma can be excluded. Nocardiosis can be distinguished by the absence of grains, identification of the organism in culture, and, usually, by the weak acid-fast staining of *Nocardia*.

TREATMENT   Milder cases of actinomycosis, including most cervicofacial infections, respond well to penicillin V (2 to 4 g/d for adults) or one of the tetracyclines. Sulfonamides, metronidazole, oral cephalosporins, and oral antistaphylococcal penicillins are not recommended. More severe cases, including most thoracic and abdominal infections, should receive parenteral penicillin G for roughly 6 weeks (in adults 2 to 6 million units per day) followed by prolonged therapy with oral penicillin V or one of the tetracyclines. The likelihood of relapse is reduced if the total duration of therapy is 2 to 4 months in mild cases and up to 6 to 12 months in severe ones. Drug resistance has not been encountered in relapses. Curettage of bone lesions, surgical resection of necrotic tissue, and drainage of empyema, brain abscess, or other large collections of pus facilitate recovery but are usually not curative by themselves.

It is common in actinomycosis to isolate microbes other than actinomycetes from pus. In general, the antibiotic susceptibility of these secondary organisms does not have to be considered in the selection of therapeutic agents.

NOCARDIOSIS

DEFINITION   Nocardiosis is an acute, subacute, or chronic infection, most often beginning in the lung.

ETIOLOGY   *Nocardia asteroides, N. brasiliensis,* and *N. caviae* are the etiologic agents of two different diseases, nocardiosis and mycetoma. In the latter infection, the organism enters the skin by trauma, forms grains within tissue, and spreads slowly to contiguous tissue (see Chap. 151). While nocardiosis can result from local trauma, the organism usually enters via the lung, does not form grains, and is prone to hematogenous spread. Even though the etiologic agents of these diseases do overlap, *N. asteroides* causes most cases of nocardiosis and *N. brasiliensis* is the species usually isolated from mycetoma. *Nocardia otitidiscaviarum* is a rare cause of either disease. *Nocardia brasiliensis* and perhaps *N. asteroides* can also cause a lymphocutaneous disease closely resembling sporotrichosis; this infection differs from mycetoma by its lymphangitic spread and by the absence of grains.

Nocardia species are aerobic actinomycetes with branching hyphae the same width as bacteria. Hyphae are weakly gram-positive and weakly acid-fast. Growth appears in 2 to 5 days on blood agar, Sabouraud's agar, or other simple media. Incorporation of antibiotics into media to inhibit bacterial growth usually inhibits *Nocardia* as well. Colonies become rough and chalky with an orange or yellow hue. Identification of *Nocardia* species, including distinction between *Streptomyces, Actinomadura,* and *Nocardia,* is difficult and best assigned to a reference laboratory.

PATHOGENESIS AND PATHOLOGY   *Nocardia* is a soil saprophyte widely distributed throughout the world. Infection is acquired from sites in nature, never from infected persons or animals. Males are infected two to three times more commonly than females. No age or exposure is known to predispose to nocardiosis. Many patients have serious preexisting conditions, such as adrenal corticosteroid therapy, cancer, pulmonary alveolar proteinosis, AIDS, or chronic granulomatous disease of childhood.

Lesions of nocardiosis show suppuration, necrosis, and abscess formation. Neutrophils are the predominant inflammatory cell. Branching hyphae are scattered throughout the lesion without formation of grains. Tissue Gram stain or overstained methenamine silver demonstrates the hyphae best. A modified Fite-Faraco stain of histologic sections can be used to demonstrate acid-fastness.

CLINICAL MANIFESTATIONS *Nocardia* pneumonia presents with fever and productive cough of several days' or up to several months' duration. The initial illness may resemble a bacterial pneumonia, but slow radiologic progression continues despite antibiotic therapy, often with cavitation of radiodense central areas. Hematogenous dissemination to brain and subcutaneous tissue is frequent. A pulmonary portal is usually but not always detectable clinically. Brain lesions are typically multiple abscesses. Purulent meningitis may result from rupture of an abscess into the ventricle. The subcutaneous lesion typically consists of one or a few indolent abscesses. Hematogenous dissemination to other organs occurs but is rarely detectable clinically.

DIAGNOSIS A progressive pneumonia with purulent sputum should suggest the diagnosis of nocardiosis, particularly if cavitation or spread to brain or subcutaneous tissue occurs. Sputum, pus, or bronchial lavage specimens should be examined by Gram stain and modified acid-fast stain. On Gram stain the hyphae are usually branching, beaded, and refractile. They are not strongly gram-positive but take the red counterstain even less well. Conventional acid-fast staining procedures such as Ziehl-Neelsen or a fluorochrome often do not stain *Nocardia*. Identification of branching, weakly acid-fast organisms in histologic section or smear of pus or sputum is sufficient to establish the diagnosis of nocardiosis. Cultural confirmation is highly desirable, but isolation of *Nocardia* from heavily contaminated specimens is difficult. Isolation of *Nocardia* from otherwise sterile pus is readily accomplished. *Nocardia* is rarely isolated from blood, but diphasic culture media or lysis centrifugation techniques facilitate isolation. When *Nocardia* is isolated from sputum, the diagnosis of nocardiosis should be suspected, but occasionally no disease can be detected.

TREATMENT Surgical drainage of empyema and abscesses in brain or subcutaneous tissue is helpful but not sufficient to achieve cure. Virtually all patients should receive prolonged chemotherapy. The treatment of choice is sulfisoxazole or trimethoprim-sulfamethoxazole. Sulfisoxazole therapy is begun orally or intravenously at 100 mg/kg per day in four divided doses. The dose is then adjusted downward to achieve a peak blood concentration of 10 to 15 mg/dL (100 to 150 μg/mL). Alternatively, trimethoprim-sulfa-

methoxazole can be given orally or intravenously as 50 mg/kg per day of the sulfamethoxazole component, divided into two doses per day. With either regimen, therapy is continued for 6 to 12 months, depending on the severity of the infection and the presence of immunosuppression. Addition of other antibiotics to sulfa drugs may be indicated in patients who show continued deterioration. Ampicillin 150 mg/kg per day, amikacin, imipenem, and minocycline have been used. In sulfa-allergic patients, minocycline has sometimes been successful in the absence of central nervous system involvement.

Survival has been reported in 92 percent of cases with isolated pulmonary nocardiosis compared to 52 percent in cases with brain abscess. Concomitant use of immunosuppressive therapy seems to impair the therapeutic response in nocardiosis.

REFERENCES

Actinomycosis

BARTELS LJ, VRABEC DP: Cervicofacial actinomycosis—A variable disorder. Arch Otolaryngol 104:705, 1978

BENHOF DF: Actinomycosis: Diagnostic and therapeutic considerations and a review of 32 cases. Laryngoscope 94:1198, 1984

JACKSON AE et al: Ureteric obstruction secondary to pelvic actinomycosis. Br J Urol 62:85, 1988

PERSSON E: Genital actinomycosis and *Actinomyces israelii* in the female genital tract. Adv Contracept 3:115, 1987

SMEGO RA JR: Actinomycosis of the central nervous system. Rev Infect Dis 9:855, 1987

WEESE WC, SMITH IM: A study of 57 cases of actinomycosis over a 36-year period. Arch Intern Med 135:1562, 1975

Nocardiosis

ADAIR JC et al: Nocardial cerebral abscess in the acquired immunodeficiency syndrome. Arch Neurol 44:548, 1987

DEWSNUP DH, WRIGHT CN: In vitro susceptibility of *Nocardia asteroides* to 25 antimicrobial agents. Antimicrob Agents Chemother 25:165, 1984

GALLIS HA: The clinical spectrum of *Nocardia brasiliensis* infection in the United States. Rev Infect Dis 6:164, 1984

GOMBERT ME et al: Therapy of experimental cerebral nocardiosis with imipenem, amikacin, trimethoprim-sulfamethoxazole and minocycline. Antimicrob Agents Chemother 30:270, 1986

PETERSEN EA et al: Minocycline treatment of pulmonary nocardiosis. JAMA 250:930, 1983

SMEGO RA et al: Trimethoprim-sulfamethoxazole therapy for *Nocardia* infections. Arch Intern Med 143:711, 1983

section 10 Rickettsia, *Mycoplasma*, and *Chlamydia*

153 RICKETTSIAL DISEASES

THEODORE E. WOODWARD

INTRODUCTION The rickettsial diseases of humans consist of a variety of clinical entities caused by microorganisms of the family Rickettsiaceae. The rickettsias are obligate intracellular parasites about the size of bacteria and are usually seen microscopically as pleomorphic coccobacilli. Each of the rickettsias pathogenic for humans is capable of multiplying in one or more species of arthropod as well as in animals and humans. Indeed, the majority of the rickettsias are maintained in nature by a cycle which involves an insect vector and an animal reservoir, and infection of humans is unimportant in the cycle. Epidemic typhus presents a number of points of dissimilarity to most of the other rickettsioses. Until recently,

the natural cycle of infection was thought to involve only humans and lice. The finding of a sylvatic reservoir in flying squirrels associated with a human illness which resembles classic typhus emphasizes that there are other mechanisms.

A compendium of information of the rickettsial diseases is given in Table 153-1.

Of all the afflictions of the human race the rickettsial diseases, particularly epidemic typhus, rank among the foremost as a cause of suffering and death. The record of deaths from epidemic typhus in this century in the Balkan countries and in Poland and Russia reached astounding figures. Typhus ravaged Russia and eastern Poland from 1915 to 1922, infecting 30 million inhabitants and causing an estimated 3 million deaths.

The past two decades have seen the development of excellent methods for the prevention and treatment of rickettsioses. In fact, these measures have been so successful that the rickettsioses have become of minor importance in the United States and in many other

TABLE 153-1   Rickettsial diseases

Disease Type	Agent	Geographic distribution	Natural cycle Arthropod	Mammal	Principal means of transmission to humans	Serologic diagnosis Weil-Felix reaction	CF, MA, and IFA reactions*
SPOTTED FEVER GROUP							
Rocky Mountain spotted fever	R. rickettsii	Western hemisphere	Ticks	Wild rodents, dogs	Tick bite	Positive OX-19 OX-2	Positive group- and type-specific
Boutonneuse fever	R. conorii	Africa, Europe, Middle East, India					
Queensland tick typhus	R. australis	Australia		Marsupials, wild rodents			
North Asian tick-borne rickettsiosis	R. sibirica	Siberia, Mongolia		Wild rodents			
Rickettsial-pox	R. akari	United States, Russia, Africa(?)	Blood-sucking mite	House mouse, other rodents	Mite bite	Negative	
TYPHUS GROUP							
Endemic (murine)	R. typhi	Worldwide	Flea	Small rodents	Infected flea feces into broken skin	Positive OX-19	Positive group- and type-specific
Epidemic	R. prowazekii	Worldwide	Body louse	Humans Flying squirrels	Infected louse feces into broken skin	Positive OX-19	
	R. Canada	North America	Ticks			Positive OX-19	
Brill-Zinsser disease	R. prowazekii	Worldwide	Recurrence years after original attack of epidemic typhus			Usually negative	
Scrub	R. tsutsuga-mushi	Asia, Australia, Pacific islands	Trombiculid mites	Wild rodents	Mite bite	Positive OX-K	Positive in about 50% of patients
OTHER RICKETTSIAL DISEASES							
Q fever	R. burnetii	Worldwide	Ticks	Small mammals, cattle, sheep, goats	Inhalation of dried infected material	Negative	Positive
Trench fever	R. quintana†	Europe, Africa, North America	Body louse	Humans	Infected louse feces into broken skin	Negative	None available

* CF = complement fixation; MA = microscopic agglutination; IFA = immunofluorescent antibody.
† Some authorities no longer place the agent in the genus *Rickettsia* because it can be cultured on artificial media.

countries. Although conquered, these infections have not been eliminated, and they could again become rampant if the will to control them, the present high standards of sanitation, and the necessary industrial capacities for production of effective insecticides and therapeutic agents should be compromised.

PATHOGENESIS Rickettsial diseases develop after infection through the skin or the respiratory tract. Agents of the typhus and spotted fever group are introduced through the bite of the infected arthropod vector. Ticks and mites, which transmit the agents of spotted fever and scrub typhus, inoculate the rickettsias directly into the dermis during feeding. The louse and flea, which transmit epidemic and murine typhus, respectively, deposit infected feces on the skin; infection occurs when organisms are rubbed into the puncture wound made by the arthropod. The rickettsias of Q fever gain entry through the respiratory tract when infected dust is inhaled; the respiratory route is also occasionally implicated in epidemic typhus when infection results from inhalation of dried infected louse feces.

Although organisms probably multiply at the original site of entry in all instances, local lesions appear with regularity only in certain diseases, namely, the initial cutaneous lesions of scrub typhus, rickettsialpox, and boutonneuse fever, and the pneumonitis which develops in about half the persons with Q fever.

Volunteers infected with either scrub typhus or Q fever develop rickettsemia late in the incubation period, often some hours before

the onset of fever. Similar events probably occur in all the rickettsial diseases; circulating rickettsias can be detected during the early febrile period in practically all patients. Little is known about the pathogenesis of infection during the midportion of the incubation period. However, it is reasonable to assume that during this time, in patients with typhus or spotted fever, a transient low-grade rickettsemia results from release of organisms multiplying at the initial site of infection and that this seeds infection in the endothelial cells of the vascular tree. Vascular lesions developing at such sites account for the pathologic changes, including the rash.

Rickettsias apparently invade and proliferate in the endothelial cells of small blood vessels. Endothelial cell destruction occurs from the proliferation of organisms and eventual disruption. Rickettsias may exert a cytotoxic effect on endothelial cells; in mice the rickettsial toxin causes remarkable increase in capillary permeability, independent of proliferation. The anatomic localization of multiple microscopic-sized lesions and the numerous foci of rickettsial vascular changes with rickettsias present coincide well with the organs examined microscopically such as the kidney, lung, heart, and liver. These findings confirm Wolbach's original conclusion that "the lesions of the blood vessel are due to the presence of the parasite." Absence of inflammatory cell reactions in fulminant Rocky Mountain spotted fever tends to exclude several host-mediated immunopathogenic mechanisms. The underlying cause of the toxic-febrile state which characterizes the rickettsial diseases remains unknown. Several rickettsial species contain type-specific toxins which are lethal for mice, and these may play a role in humans.

PATHOLOGIC PHYSIOLOGY Peripheral vascular collapse results in death in fulminating cases during the first week, with capillary dilatation and pooling of blood without increased capillary permeability or loss of fluid into extravascular spaces. Proliferative and thrombotic lesions develop in small vessels, resulting in necrosis and increased capillary permeability, with loss of water, electrolytes, proteins, and erythrocytes. This in turn results in a decrease in blood volume, together with an increase in the extravascular space and clinical edema. Edema, anoxia of the myocardium, and histologic evidence of myocarditis are disclosed by electrocardiographic abnormalities, including serious arrhythmias. Liver function is impaired. The azotemia which develops in seriously ill patients appears to be prerenal. Clinical manifestations resulting from the peripheral vascular collapse are oliguria and anuria, azotemia, anemia, hypoproteinemia, hyponatremia, edema, and coma. In spotted fever and typhus patients with hemorrhagic skin lesions, consumptive coagulopathy is present. All these alterations are absent or minimal in mild cases or in those who are given specific treatment early.

PATHOLOGY The basic changes in the spotted and typhus fever groups are vascular, with resultant widespread lesions in adjacent parenchymatous organs. They are most common in the skin, muscles, heart, lung, and brain. The most conspicuous and diverse are found in Rocky Mountain spotted fever, where swelling, proliferation, and degeneration of the endothelial cells occur, frequently with thrombus formation which partially or completely occludes the lumen. The muscle cells of the arterioles undergo swelling and fibrinoid changes. The adventitial tissues are infiltrated with mononuclear leukocytes, lymphocytes, and plasma cells. The vascular damage is scattered along arteries, veins, and capillaries, with normal architecture prevailing throughout most of the vascular bed. The changes in murine, epidemic, and scrub typhus fevers resemble those in Rocky Mountain spotted fever, but thrombosis is uncommon and involvement of the musculature is rare.

Interstitial myocarditis occurs in each of these diseases but is usually most extensive in Rocky Mountain spotted fever and in scrub typhus. In the brain glial nodules are found in all members of the group, but microinfarcts in the brain tissue or in the myocardium are most often observed in spotted fever.

Rickettsial pneumonitis occurs, at least to some extent, in many patients with spotted or typhus fever and is characteristic in patients with Q fever. The process is patchy and consists microscopically of areas of congestion and edema. Within the consolidated areas the alveoli are filled with compact fibrinocellular exudate containing lymphocytes, plasma cells, large mononuclear cells, and erythrocytes, but few, if any, polymorphonuclear leukocytes.

Rickettsias can occasionally be observed microscopically in sections of tissue. Failure to demonstrate them is of no diagnostic significance. They are readily identifiable by the immunofluorescent technique.

LABORATORY DIAGNOSIS Diagnostic procedures which depend on isolation of the etiologic agent from blood or other clinical material are expensive, time-consuming, and hazardous to laboratory personnel. Primary isolation of rickettsias by chick embryo inoculation or tissue culture usually fails because of the small number of organisms in the patient's blood. Rickettsias have been identified in stained cultured monocytes of infected monkeys and by direct or indirect immunofluorescence of infected animal tissues. Except in unusual circumstances, however, currently available serologic tests are adequate for laboratory confirmation of the clinical diagnosis in each of the rickettsial diseases. The demonstration of a rise in titer of specific antibody during convalescence is of prime importance in establishing laboratory confirmation. Table 153-2 summarizes the serologic results usually encountered in persons who have rickettsial diseases in the United States. The Weil-Felix test employing *Proteus* strains OX-19 and OX-2 gives positive results in patients with spotted fever and murine typhus and negative results in those with rickettsialpox and Q fever. It is useful as a screening procedure but cannot be relied upon to differentiate spotted fever from murine typhus. In patients with Brill-Zinsser disease the *Proteus* OX-19 reaction is usually negative or low in titer.

Serologic tests employing group-specific rickettsial antigens provide data which clearly differentiate the most common infections, i.e., epidemic typhus, murine typhus, Rocky Mountain spotted fever, and Q fever. Type-specific rickettsial antigens generally make it possible to distinguish rickettsialpox from spotted fever and Brill-Zinsser disease from murine typhus.

The type of immunoglobulin in acute (IgM) and late or recurrent (IgG) illness is helpful in identifying recrudescent typhus (Brill-Zinsser disease). In general, the Weil-Felix and complement fixation tests are useful for routine diagnosis; microscopic agglutination, immunofluorescent antibody, and hemagglutination reactions are valuable for specific identification.

Specific antibiotic therapy has little effect on the time of appearance of antibodies or on their ultimate titer, provided treatment is instituted some days after onset of the illness. However, if the illness is cut short by early and vigorous treatment, antibody production may be delayed for a week or so, and the maximum titers attained may be below those illustrated in Table 153-2. Under these circumstances a sample of blood taken 4 to 6 weeks after onset of illness should also be tested.

TABLE 153-2 Serologic diagnosis of rickettsial diseases in the United States

Group	Disease	Proteus	Weil-Felix reaction Illustrative titer 10th day	20th day	Cases with diagnostic titer	Rickettsial antigen	Complement fixation tests with type-specific antigen Illustrative titer 10th day	20th day	30th day	Cases with diagnostic titer
Spotted fever	Rocky Mountain spotted fever	OX-19 OX-2	40 20	320 160	Most	*R. rickettsii*	20	160	80	Most
	Rickettsialpox	OX-19 OX-2	0 0	0 0	None	*R. akari*	0	64	128	Most
Typhus	Murine typhus	OX-19 OX-2	160 10	640 40	Most	*R. typhi*	0	160	160	Most
	Epidemic typhus, squirrel related	OX-19 OX-2	160 10	640 40	Most	*R. prowazekii*	0	160	160	Most
	Brill-Zinsser disease	OX-19 OX-2	160 0	20 0	Infrequent	*R. prowazekii*	1280	640	320	Most
	Q fever	OX-19 OX-2	0 0	0 0	None	*R. burnetii*	10	80	160	Most

The immunofluorescent antibody test is very useful for detecting rickettsia in the tissues of patients with the typhus group of rickettsioses, the spotted fevers, and Q fever. Identifiable rickettsias have been visualized in skin lesions of patients with Rocky Mountain spotted fever as early as the fourth day of illness and as late as the tenth day. Rickettsias may be visualized in human tissues several days after administration of chloramphenicol or tetracycline. The technique also visualizes rickettsias in ticks and in animal tissues, including those fixed with paraffin.

Normochromic anemia occurs in patients severely ill with rickettsial diseases. The white blood cell count in Rocky Mountain spotted fever, rickettsialpox, murine and epidemic typhus, Brill-Zinsser disease, Q fever, and other rickettsial diseases is usually within the normal range; 6000 to 10,000 cells per microliter. Leukopenia is occasionally observed, and in the presence of complications, such as superimposed infections and extensive vascular lesions, moderate leukocytosis occurs. The differential blood cell count is usually normal. Thrombocytopenia occurs in severely ill spotted and scrub typhus fever patients with extensive vascular lesions; hypofibrinogenemia, prolonged prothrombin and partial thromboplastin times, and other clotting abnormalities occur.

TREATMENT Patients seriously ill with one of the diseases of the typhus–spotted fever group may show circulatory collapse, coma, oliguria and anuria, azotemia, anemia, hypoproteinemia, hypochloremia and hyponatremia, and edema. These alterations are often absent in the mildly ill, and in them management is much less complicated. The therapeutic principles necessary for treatment of all rickettsioses are (1) specific chemotherapy and (2) supportive care. Attention to both is mandatory for the seriously ill patient first recognized late in the disease. During the first week in the moderately ill patient, supportive therapy may need to be less energetic, because specific chemotherapy usually suffices. The early mild case may be successfully treated at home; more severely ill patients should receive hospital care.

Specific therapy Specific therapy is most effective when initiated during the early stages of disease coincident with the appearance of the rash. When therapy is delayed until the rash has become hemorrhagic and widespread, the response is less dramatic. The antibiotics of choice are chloramphenicol and the tetracyclines, which are effective because of their rickettsiostatic properties. They are not rickettsiocidal.

The following antibiotic regimen is considered optimal: for chloramphenicol, an initial dose of 50 mg per kilogram of body weight, and for tetracycline, 25 mg/kg. Subsequent daily doses are the same as the initial loading dose, with the requirement divided equally and given at 6- to 8-h intervals. Antibiotic treatment is continued until the patient has improved and has been afebrile approximately 24 h. In patients too ill to take oral medication, an intravenous preparation of one of the antimicrobials should be employed.

Adrenal cortical hormones may be needed for their antitoxemic effects in patients first observed late in the course of severe illness. Large doses for brief periods of about 3 days, in combination with specific antibiotics, are recommended in critically ill patients.

In uncomplicated cases of spotted fever, there is symptomatic improvement within 24 h and the temperature becomes normal in 60 to 72 h.

Supportive care Frequent turning of the patient relieves pressure from prominent bony parts and also militates against the development of aspiration pneumonia. Proper mouth care, with frequent swabbing of the oral cavity, may avert the development of parotitis and gingivitis. Sucking of the juice of a lemon or the oral use of glycerin or mineral oil is helpful. Usually food is well tolerated by patients with rickettsial disease, and the daily diet should provide 1 to 2 g protein per kilogram of normal body weight; the diet may need to be supplemented with oral or parenteral hyperalimentation (see Chap. 75).

When indicated, red cell transfusions given slowly are helpful.

The support of the hypotensive patient with rickettsial disease is similar to other patients with shock (see Chap. 89). Dialysis is indicated when there is clear-cut evidence of acute renal failure.

ROCKY MOUNTAIN SPOTTED FEVER Definition Rocky Mountain spotted fever is an acute febrile illness caused by *Rickettsia rickettsii*. It is transmitted to humans by ticks. The disease is characterized by sudden onset with headache and chills and by fever which persists for 2 to 3 weeks. A characteristic exanthem appears on the extremities and trunk about the fourth day of illness. Delirium, shock, and renal failure occur in severely ill patients.

Etiology and epidemiology The causative microbe, *R. rickettsii*, is the prototype for the rickettsial group of agents. The minute organisms are purple when stained by Giemsa's method or red by Macchiavello's technique; most of them are gram-negative. These organisms often occur in pairs and possess a cell wall similar in structure and chemical composition to that of gram-negative bacteria; there are a cell membrane, cytoplasmic granules corresponding to ribosomes, and prokaryotic organization of nuclear material. The cell membrane is selectively permeable; the cell wall is the focus of important antigens and an endotoxin-like substance.

The rickettsias grow in the nucleus and the cytoplasm of infected cells of ticks, mammals, and embryonated eggs; the intranuclear situation of the organisms is shared by the other members of the spotted fever group, but not by rickettsias of the typhus group. *Rickettsia rickettsii* is readily distinguishable from the agents of the typhus fevers by cross-immunity tests in guinea pigs and by complement fixation tests employing antigens prepared from infected yolk sac tissues. The differentiation of *R. rickettsii* from closely related members of the spotted fever group frequently requires elaborate procedures. Strains of the agent of Rocky Mountain spotted fever vary considerably in their virulence for humans and animals.

The first reports of spotted fever in Idaho and Montana during the final decade of the last century led to the name Rocky Mountain spotted fever. However, the disease has been reported from all states (except Maine, Alaska, and Hawaii), as well as from Canada, Mexico, Colombia, and Brazil. Although related diseases are found on other continents, this particular infection is limited to the western hemisphere. In the years 1981, 1982, 1983, 1984, 1985, 1986, and 1987 there were 1176, 976, 1126, 848, 714, 760, and 604 cases reported. Why this decrease has occurred is not known. The mortality rate was about 20 percent in the days before specific therapy but has decreased to about 7 percent. More than half the cases occur in the south Atlantic and south central states, with the greatest number in North Carolina, Virginia, Georgia, Maryland, Tennessee, and Oklahoma.

An unusual outbreak of "urban" spotted fever occurred in New York City's Bronx borough during the summer of 1987. Eight percent of dog ticks were positive for *R. rickettsii*.

A number of species of ticks are found infected with *R. rickettsii* in nature, but only two are important in transmitting spotted fever to humans. These are *Dermacentor andersoni*, the wood tick, which is the principal vector in the west, and *D. variabilis*, the dog tick, which assumes this role in the east. *Amblyomma americanum*, the lone star tick, and *D. variabilis* are the common vectors in the west south central states. Infected female ticks transmit the agent transovarially to at least some of their offspring. Ticks which become infected, either through the egg or at one of the stages during their development cycle by feeding on an infected mammal, harbor the rickettsias throughout their lifetime, which may be several years, making the tick a reservoir as well as a vector. Small wild mammals are suspected of playing an important role in spreading the rickettsias in nature by infecting ticks which feed on them during rickettsemia.

Disease in humans is generally acquired from the bite of an infected tick. Transmission is unlikely unless the tick remains attached for a number of hours. Infection may also be acquired through abrasions in the skin which become contaminated with infected tick feces or tissue juices; hence, the hazard associated with crushing ticks between the fingers when removing them from persons or animals. The agent of Rocky Mountain spotted fever has been transmitted accidentally to humans by transfusion of blood taken from a donor just before onset of illness.

There are seasonal variations in the incidence of cases of spotted fever, as well as differences in age and sex distribution of cases. In each instance these differences are related to exposure to ticks. Most cases are seen during the period of maximal tick activity, i.e., April to September, and 60 percent of cases occur in individuals under 20 years of age. This age distribution is undoubtedly influenced by propinquity to the wood and dog ticks. The mortality rate increases with the age of the patient.

Rocky Mountain spotted fever has been acquired by laboratory workers via aerosol transmission, and special precautions are necessary when the agent is handled in the laboratory.

Clinical manifestations INCUBATION PERIOD AND PRODROMATA A history of tick bite is elicited in approximately 80 percent of patients. The incubation period varies between 3 and 12 days with a mean of 7 days. A short incubation period usually indicates a more serious infection.

ONSET In nonvaccinated persons, the onset is usually abrupt, with severe headache, a sudden shaking rigor, prostration, generalized myalgia, especially in the back and leg muscles, nausea with occasional vomiting, and fever which reaches 39.4 to 40°C (103 to 104°F) within the first 2 days. Pain in the abdominal muscles may be severe, and arthralgia is not uncommon. Deep muscle palpation often elicits tenderness. Occasionally the debut of illness in children and adults is mild, accompanied by lethargy, anorexia, headache, and low-grade fever. These symptoms are similar to those of many acute infectious diseases, making specific diagnosis difficult during the first few days.

PYREXIA Fever continues for approximately 15 to 20 days in untreated cases. The febrile course in children may be shorter. Hyperthermia of 40.5°C (105°F) or greater is of unfavorable prognostic significance, although fatalities may occur when the patient is hypothermic, with concurrent vasomotor collapse. Fever generally terminates by lysis over a period of several days, but rarely does so by crisis. Recurrent fever is uncommon except in the presence of secondary pyogenic complications.

The *headache* is generalized and excruciating, and frequently most intense over the frontal area. It persists throughout the first and second weeks of illness in untreated cases. Occasionally headache is mild. Malaise continues for the first week; irritability is notable, and the patient shuns distractions such as questioning and examination.

CUTANEOUS MANIFESTATIONS The rash which is present in practically all cases is the most characteristic and helpful diagnostic sign. It usually appears on the fourth febrile day; the range is 2 to 6 days. Faint-pink macules which fade on pressure have been noted on the first febrile day. The initial lesions are on the wrists, ankles, palms, soles, and forearms. The first lesions are macular, nonfixed, pink, irregularly defined, and measure 2 to 6 mm. A warm compress applied to the extremity accentuates the rash in the early stages. The exanthem is most prominent when the temperature is elevated. After 6 to 12 h, the rash extends centripetally to the axilla, buttocks, trunk, neck, and face. (This is in contrast to the eruption of typhus fever, which begins on the trunk and spreads centrifugally, rarely involving the face, palms, or soles.) The rash becomes maculopapular after 2 to 3 days (it may be felt by light palpation) and assumes a deeper red hue. By about the fourth day it is petechial and fails to fade on pressure. Not uncommonly, the hemorrhagic lesions coalesce to form large ecchymotic blemishes; these lesions tend to form over bony prominences and may ultimately slough to form indolent, slow-healing ulcers. Patients who have had the typical rash show brownish discolorations at the site for several weeks during convalescence. In milder cases, the rash does not become purpuric and may disappear within a few days. Antibiotic therapy may abort the early exanthem; the later fixed lesion fades less rapidly with specific therapy. Occasionally, a rash does not occur or is unnoticed, particularly in dark-skinned patients.

The application of tourniquets for several minutes, or the occasional taking of the blood pressure may provoke additional petechiae (Rumpel-Leede phenomenon), further evidence of capillary abnormalities.

CARDIOVASCULAR AND RESPIRATORY FEATURES During the early stages, the pulse is full and regular and is accelerated in proportion to the height of the temperature, and the blood pressure is well sustained. During the peak of illness in seriously ill patients, the pulse is rapid and feeble, and hypotension of 90 mmHg or less is common. If circulatory failure is sustained, the resultant hypoxia and shock lead to agitation and delirium and contribute to the formation of ecchymoses and gangrene of fingers, toes, genitalia, buttocks, earlobes, and nose. Cyanosis of the peripheral parts of the body is common. A reduction of the total blood volume is found occasionally. The ECG shows low voltage, minor ST-segment deflections, and, occasionally, delay in atrioventricular conduction. These changes are transient and nonspecific. Severely ill patients have a puffy appearance of the face, hands, ankles, feet, and lower parts of the sacrum. Occasionally a severe arrhythmia associated with myocarditis results in sudden death.

Respirations are either normal or slightly accelerated. Cough may be harassing and nonproductive, and localized pneumonitis may occur, but pulmonary consolidation is extremely rare. Pulmonary edema may develop after injudicious use of intravenous fluids.

HEPATIC AND RENAL MANIFESTATIONS In the majority of patients, there is little alteration in renal or hepatic function. The liver may be enlarged, but jaundice is unusual. Oliguria and anuria commonly occur in seriously ill patients. Azotemia is common; when marked, it is a very unfavorable sign. Abnormalities in liver function include hypoproteinemia, with reduction in the albumin fraction.

NEUROLOGIC MANIFESTATIONS The principal neurologic manifestations are headache, restlessness, and varying degrees of insomnia. Stiffness of the back is common. The cerebrospinal fluid is clear, with normal dynamics and normal chemical constituents. Occasionally, the CSF pressure is elevated; there may be a slight increase in mononuclear cells. Coma and muscular rigidity may occur. Athetoid movements, convulsive seizures, and hemiplegia are grave manifestations. Deafness during the active stages of the disease is not uncommon. As a rule, all neurologic signs abate without residua. Findings based upon follow-up examinations and electroencephalograms may be interpreted as indicative of minor residual brain damage for a year or more following recovery of some patients from Rocky Mountain spotted fever.

OTHER PHYSICAL MANIFESTATIONS Patients become dehydrated, with extreme dryness of lips, gums, tongue, and pharynx. The skin is hot and dry, the conjunctivas are frequently injected, and the eyes suffused. Photophobia is common in the early stages of illness. Petechial hemorrhages may be noted in the conjunctivas or in the retina. The spleen is enlarged in approximately one-half the cases and is firm and nontender. Usually there is abdominal distention and some degree of intestinal ileus. Occasionally the severity of abdominal discomfort may suggest the diagnosis of appendicitis or cholecystitis.

Course In patients with mild and moderately severe cases who are given no specific antibiotic therapy, the disease abates within 2 weeks, and convalescence is rapid. In fatal cases death usually occurs during the latter part of the second week as a result of toxemia, vasomotor collapse and shock, or renal failure. In a few patients, the course is fulminant with death occurring as early as the sixth day of illness.

In vaccinated individuals who contract the disease, the illness is mild, with a short febrile course and an atypical rash.

Prognosis If the serious manifestations of spotted fever are regarded as intrinsic parts of the disease, then complications are uncommon and consist mainly of secondary bacterial infections such as bronchopneumonia, otitis media, and parotitis. Thrombosis of major blood vessels may result in gangrene of a portion of an extremity. Hemiplegia and peripheral neuritis are rare sequelae.

The overall mortality rate for spotted fever was formerly about 20 percent. Death occurred in more than half of persons over 40 years of age, but the mortality rate was much lower in children and young adults. Since the introduction of the broad-spectrum antibiotics and the development of more precise knowledge regarding correction of the physiologic abnormalities which develop during the disease, fewer deaths occur. Some of the fatalities can be attributed to failure to consider spotted fever in the differential diagnosis and resultant delay in instituting appropriate treatment.

Differential diagnosis During the early stages of infection before the rash has appeared, differentiation from other acute infections is difficult. A history of tick bite while living or traveling in wooded or bushy sites known to be in a highly endemic area is helpful. The rash of meningococcemia (see Chap. 109) resembles Rocky Mountain spotted fever in certain aspects, because it is macular, maculopapular, or petechial in the chronic form, and petechial, confluent, or ecchymotic in the fulminant type. The meningococcal skin lesion is tender and develops with extreme rapidity in the fulminant form, whereas the rickettsial rash occurs on about the fourth day of disease and gradually becomes petechial. *Spotted fever is often confused with measles.* The exanthem of rubeola rapidly becomes confluent, while that of rubella *usually remains discrete.*

Murine typhus is a milder disease than Rocky Mountain spotted fever; the rash is less extensive, nonpurpuric, and nonconfluent, and renal and vascular complications are uncommon. Not infrequently differentiation of these two rickettsial infections must await the results of specific serologic tests. Epidemic typhus fever is capable of causing all the pronounced clinical, physiologic, and anatomic alterations seen in patients with Rocky Mountain spotted fever, i.e., hypotension, peripheral vascular collapse, cyanosis, skin necrosis and gangrene of digits, renal failure and azotemia, and neurologic manifestations. However, the rash of classic typhus is noted initially in the axillary folds of the trunk and later extends peripherally, rarely involving the palms, soles, or face. The serologic patterns in these two diseases are distinctive when specific rickettsial antigens are employed. Moreover, louse-borne typhus is now recognized in the United States as a flying squirrel–related illness which occurs sporadically and as Brill-Zinsser disease (recrudescent typhus fever). Rickettsialpox, although caused by a member of the spotted fever group, is usually readily differentiated from Rocky Mountain spotted fever by the initial lesion, the relative mildness of the illness, and the early vesiculation of the maculopapular rash. The Weil-Felix reaction is positive in Rocky Mountain spotted fever and in murine and epidemic typhus, but is negative in rickettsialpox. Agglutinins against *Proteus* OX-19 and OX-2 appear in the serum of patients with spotted fever, but only those against OX-19 are generally found in murine and epidemic typhus.

Complications *Pyogenic complications,* including otitis media and parotitis, are encountered in patients severely ill with Rocky Mountain spotted fever and other rickettsioses. These localized infections respond to therapy with appropriate antibiotics combined with surgical measures.

Pneumonitis may develop as a result of specific rickettsial action or as a bacterial superinfection. The sputum is scanty and should be examined to determine whether superimposed bacterial infection is present. Specific therapy is guided by the results of these laboratory studies. The pneumonitis generally responds to the antibiotic therapy the patient is receiving, but if staphylococcal pneumonia is suspected, a penicillinase-resistant penicillin or a cephalosporin should be added to the tetracycline or chloramphenicol.

Circulatory failure of peripheral or central origin is treated with careful administration of plasma expanders and fluids (see Chaps. 39 and 89). When the clinical signs reveal unmistakable evidence of cardiac failure, digitalis, diuretics, and other cardiac drugs should be employed as indicated (see Chap. 182).

Prevention Prevention is attained primarily by avoidance of tick-infested areas. When this is impractical, prophylactic measures include (1) spraying the ground with dieldrin or chlordane for area control of ticks (though there are environmental objections to the use of residual insecticides in area control of ticks, under special conditions

such procedures may be warranted); (2) application of repellents such as diethyltoluamide or dimethylphthalate to clothing and exposed parts of the body, or in very heavily infested areas the wearing of clothing which interferes with the attachment of ticks, i.e., boots and a one-piece outer garment, preferably impregnated with repellent; and (3) daily inspection of the entire body, including the hairy parts, to detect and remove attached ticks. In removing attached ticks great care should be taken to avoid crushing the arthropod with resultant contamination of the bite wound. Gentle traction with tweezers applied close to the mouth parts may be necessary; the skin area should be disinfected with soap and water or other antiseptics. Similarly, precautions should be employed in removing engorged ticks from dogs and other animals, because infection through minor abrasions on the hands is possible. Improved vaccines containing inactivated *R. rickettsii* are under development and when available commercially should be used for those at great risk, namely, persons frequenting highly endemic areas and laboratory workers exposed to the agent. Because the broad-spectrum antibiotics are such excellent therapeutic agents in spotted fever, there has been less impetus for vaccination of persons who run only a minor risk of infection.

After a tick bite in a known endemic area, an exposed person should be observed for signs of fever, headache, prostration, and rash; therapy is very effective early in the infection.

MURINE (ENDEMIC) TYPHUS FEVER Definition Murine typhus fever is an acute febrile disease caused by *Rickettsia typhi (mooseri)* and transmitted to humans by fleas. The clinical illness is characterized by fever of 9 to 14 days, headache, a maculopapular rash appearing on the third to fifth day, and myalgia.

Etiology and epidemiology *R. typhi* resembles other rickettsias in morphologic properties, staining characteristics, and intracellular parasitism. Under the electron microscope *R. typhi* is seen to contain dense masses of nuclear material in a less dense homogeneous protoplasmic substance, the whole of which is surrounded by a limiting membrane. It differs from *R. rickettsii* in that it always multiplies within the cytoplasm of cells, in contrast to the intranuclear and cytoplasmic positions of spotted fever rickettsias.

Invasion of the body by *R. typhi* provokes specific and nonspecific immunologic responses. Utilizing highly purified antigens, specific antibodies may be demonstrated readily by complement fixation, microscopic agglutination, and immunofluorescent antibody reactions. The positive Weil-Felix reaction that occurs in this disease is nonspecific, because it is attributable to the presence of common carbohydrate antigens.

The common vector of *R. typhi* for rats and humans is the rat flea (*Xenopsylla cheopis*). In nature, the rat louse (*Polyplax spinulosis*) may transmit the agent among rodents. Customarily, rat fleas become infected on ingestion of blood from diseased rats; the rickettsias multiply within the intestinal cells of the arthropod and are excreted in the feces. Infection in humans occurs after the flea bite and contamination of the broken skin by rickettsia-laden feces. Dried flea feces may also infect via the conjunctivas or the upper part of the respiratory tract.

Rats and mice are naturally infected with murine typhus, and although the rodent disease is nonfatal, viable rickettsias persist in the brain for variable periods.

Murine typhus is one of the most benign and widespread of the rickettsioses in the United States. Prevalent in the southeastern and Gulf Coast states, it has been identified in most of the other states and in harbor centers throughout the world wherever rats and fleas abound. In the early 1940s, 2000 to 5000 cases of murine typhus were reported annually. This contrasts to 67 and 69 cases reported in the United States in 1986 and 1987, respectively. This sharp reduction was achieved by control of rats and their fleas in known areas of high prevalence. In urban areas the disease is more prevalent during the summer and fall and occurs predominantly among persons working in proximity to granaries or food depots. There has been an extension to certain rural areas when changing agricultural practices have provided rats with ready access to adequate food supplies. Endemic typhus has been reported in laboratory workers. This emphasizes the importance of taking special precautions when working with rickettsial organisms in the laboratory.

Clinical manifestations INCUBATION PERIOD AND PRODROMATA The incubation period ranges from 8 to 16 days, with a mean of 10 days. Common prodromata are headache, backache, arthralgia, and chilly sensations. Nausea, malaise, and transient temperature rises may precede the true onset of disease.

ONSET AND GENERAL SYMPTOMS A frank shaking chill and repeated rigors are present at the onset, associated with a severe frontal headache and fever. This triad of headache, chill, and pyrexia is usually followed within a few hours by nausea and vomiting. Prostration, malaise, and weakness are sufficient to enforce cessation of activity in adults, in contrast to children, whose illness is less severe. Occasionally, mild symptoms make it difficult to define the actual onset.

PYREXIA The usual febrile course in murine typhus lasts for about 12 days in adults; the temperature ranges from 38.8 to 40°C (102 to 104°F) but may reach 40.5 to 41.1°C (105 to 106°F) in children. The temperature may reach high levels abruptly after onset or ascend in a stepwise manner during the first few days. With the appearance of the rash, fever is usually sustained, with partial daily remissions which occasionally reach normal levels in the morning. Defervescence is generally by lysis over several days but sometimes occurs by crisis. Transient mild fever of 37.7°C (100°F) is not uncommon during early convalescence. A few patients experience only low-grade fever throughout, but this does not necessarily connote a mild illness.

CUTANEOUS MANIFESTATIONS The early lesions, which are sparse and discrete, are hidden in the axillae and inner surface of the arm. Most patients then develop with surprising suddenness a generalized, dull-red macular rash of the upper part of the abdomen, shoulders, chest, arms, and thighs. The individual lesions are discrete and pea-sized, with an ill-defined border, and fade on pressure during the first 24 h. They later become maculopapular, in contrast to the exanthem of epidemic typhus, which is persistently macular. The distribution over the trunk with sparse involvement of the extremities, palms, soles, and face differs from the peripheral distribution and facial involvement of Rocky Mountain spotted fever. The murine rash generally appears initially on the fifth febrile day, but rarely it is seen concurrently with the onset of fever or develops as late as the seventh day.

Eighty percent of patients develop a rash which persists for 4 to 8 days and fades before defervescence. The cutaneous manifestations vary greatly in intensity and duration and may be fleeting. They are readily overlooked in dark-skinned patients, in whom they should be sought by light palpation and indirect lighting.

CARDIOVASCULAR AND RESPIRATORY FEATURES An irritating, nonproductive cough is frequent and is occasionally associated with moderate hemoptysis. Early in the second week, rales may be detected in the basilar lung areas. These changes are generally rickettsial rather than bacterial in origin and respond to the broad-spectrum antibiotics. Pulmonary congestion occurs in extremely ill and elderly patients.

Accelerated pulse and hypotension occur, although less frequently than in patients with epidemic typhus or Rocky Mountain spotted fever.

NEUROLOGIC MANIFESTATIONS Headache is the most common neurologic manifestation of murine typhus and may dominate the clinical picture. It is frontal and continues into the second week of illness. Stupor and prostration may occur in the second week, and in severe cases there may be delirium, extreme agitation, or coma. Coma in elderly patients after 2 weeks of illness presages death. Nuchal rigidity and general spasticity often suggest meningitis, although the spinal fluid is normal except for slight increases in pressure and the presence of lymphocytes (5 to 30 per microliter). Transient partial deafness occurs occasionally, but rarely is there

localized neuritis or hemiplegia. Neurologic sequelae are unusual. Children experience minimal neurologic changes.

OTHER PHYSICAL MANIFESTATIONS During the first 2 days of illness the patient may be nauseated and vomit, but vomiting later in the illness should arouse suspicion of a complication. Abdominal pain is bothersome; when associated with diarrhea or ileus, it responds to intravenous alimentation. Hepatomegaly and jaundice are unusual. There is splenomegaly in approximately 25 percent of patients.

Photophobia, retroocular pain, and suffusion of the conjunctivas are common but are less severe than in the other typhus and spotted fevers.

Renal function is usually unaltered except in elderly patients with prolonged hypotension. Under these circumstances, azotemia may develop to the degree observed in epidemic typhus. In severe murine typhus, as in the epidemic typhus, hyponatremia and hypoalbuminemia are encountered.

Course After defervescence, murine typhus patients recover rapidly. Fatalities occur between the ninth and twelfth days in elderly or debilitated patients, usually as a result of circulatory and renal failure or intercurrent bacterial infection.

Prognosis The mortality rate in murine typhus was low even before the introduction of specific therapy (<1 percent).

Differential diagnosis Because murine typhus and Rocky Mountain spotted fever occur in many of the same states, the problem of differential diagnosis often arises. Flea-borne murine typhus, which is predominantly an urban disease, is more likely to occur in late summer and autumn. In contrast, spotted fever is a rural and suburban disease in which exposure to ticks is important. Most cases occur in the spring and summer.

Treatment and prevention Both chloramphenicol and the tetracycline antibiotics have controlled the disease (see above). Prevention of murine typhus in humans is attained by reducing the natural reservoir and vector by applying measures for eliminating rodents and employing appropriate insecticides in rat-infested areas to control fleas. Spraying of rat burrows with DDT effectively reduces the population of the vector.

EPIDEMIC (LOUSE-BORNE) TYPHUS FEVER **Definition** Classic epidemic typhus is a severe, febrile disease caused by R. prowazekii and transmitted to humans by the body louse. Intense headache, continuous pyrexia of about 2 weeks, a macular skin eruption appearing on about the fifth febrile day, malaise, and vascular and neurologic disturbances represent the principal clinical features. Confirmation of the diagnosis is made by demonstration of Proteus OX-19 agglutinins and of specific complement-fixing antibodies in convalescence. The broad-spectrum antibiotics are specific therapeutic agents.

Etiology and epidemiology The causative microbe, R. prowazekii, is closely related to R. typhi, which causes murine typhus; indeed, the two have a number of common antigens.

Human beings generally are infected when rickettsia-laden louse feces are rubbed into the broken skin; scratching the louse bite facilitates this process. Pediculus humanus corporis, which is peculiarly adapted to humans, is the only important vector of epidemic typhus. It dies of its infection and fails to transmit rickettsias to its offspring. R. prowazekii has been isolated from flying squirrels, and the organism probably infests their ectoparasites. Generally, however, the organism is maintained by a cycle involving human-louse-human. New epidemics apparently originate from patients with Brill-Zinsser disease (recurrent epidemic typhus). Flying squirrels can serve as a potential host to initiate an outbreak of epidemic typhus provided an avid human vector, such as the body louse, is prevalent. Pathogenic rickettsias reside for long periods in patients with epidemic typhus as well as Rocky Mountain spotted fever and scrub typhus. Lice readily become infected when fed on patients with recurrent typhus. Inhalation of dust containing dried louse feces may cause infection. An established nonhuman reservoir such as flying squirrels poses a serious threat.

If uncontrolled, epidemic typhus behaves as a cyclic disease in a susceptible population, extending over a 3-year period. During the first year there is a gradual seeding of cases throughout the group; during the second there is epidemic spread; and during the third the epidemic tapers off, because the majority of persons have become immune. Outbreaks of epidemic typhus last occurred in the United States in the nineteenth century, and its presence is now recognized in the form of Brill-Zinsser disease and flying squirrel–related typhus.

Clinical manifestations Epidemic typhus resembles murine typhus but is more severe. After an incubation period of about 7 days an abrupt onset of headache, chill, and rapidly mounting fever ushers in the illness. Headache, malaise, and prostration continue unabated until the rash appears on the fifth febrile day. It is initially macular in the axillary folds but ultimately invades the trunk and extremities as a pink, irregular macular lesion, which becomes fixed, petechial, and confluent in the later stages.

Neurologic features range from headache and general spasticity to extreme agitation, stupor, and coma. Circulatory disturbances consisting of tachycardia, hypotension, and cyanosis are more profound than those observed in murine typhus and are almost as severe as in Rocky Mountain spotted fever. Ultimately, in untreated cases, azotemia often reaches high levels as a result of vascular and renal failure, and death occurs late in the second week of illness. Thrombosis of major blood vessels and cutaneous gangrene develop in a manner similar to that seen in the virulent form of Rocky Mountain spotted fever.

The complications and sequelae of epidemic typhus are more severe than those in murine typhus, but not as severe as those in Rocky Mountain spotted fever. However, during certain outbreaks, epidemic typhus was fatal in 60 percent of those infected, and convalescence in survivors was prolonged. The use of chloramphenicol or tetracycline has almost eradicated mortality in this dread disease, provided therapy is instituted before irreversible organ system changes occur.

Differential diagnosis Differentiation of epidemic typhus from the various rickettsioses and other diseases with which it may be confused was described above. The disease is not known to occur in epidemic form in the absence of louse infestation in the general population. Under the conditions in which typhus epidemics are likely to occur, other diseases which may cause confusion include malaria, relapsing fever, pneumonia, and tuberculosis. Classic typhus contracted by a previously vaccinated person is usually mild and may be clinically indistinguishable from murine typhus except by serologic methods.

Treatment and prevention Both chloramphenicol and the tetracycline antibiotics have been found to be highly efficient therapeutic agents in epidemic typhus. Usually the patient becomes afebrile after 2 days of treatment. Under field conditions, 100 mg doxycycline in a single oral dose resulted in abatement of clinical manifestations and defervescence in epidemic typhus.

The most effective measures for controlling epidemic typhus are those which eliminate lice. DDT or lindane powder when dusted into clothing is suitable for this purpose. If resistant lice are found, malathion or carbaryl may prove effective.

A commercially available vaccine prepared from formalin-treated suspensions of infected yolk sac tissue is an effective immunizing agent.

BRILL-ZINSSER DISEASE (RECRUDESCENT TYPHUS) Brill-Zinsser disease is a recrudescent episode of epidemic typhus fever that occurs years after the initial attack. *R. prowazekii* have been isolated from lice fed on patients during the active stages of illness.

The clinical entity, not always mild, resembles epidemic typhus in the character of the rash, circulatory disturbances, and hepatic, renal, and nervous system changes. Recovery is the rule. The Weil-Felix reaction with the various *Proteus* antigens is usually negative, or positive in very low titer. The specific complement fixation, microscopic agglutination, and immunofluorescent antibody reactions are valuable in establishing the diagnosis. In Brill-Zinsser disease the specific complement-fixing antibodies appear as early as the fourth

day after the onset of illness; antibodies are IgG, and the peak response is attained by the eighth to tenth days. Specific antibody titers in the primary attack of epidemic typhus begin later, about the eighth to twelfth day, with maximum titers on about the sixteenth day after onset. Treatment is the same as for other rickettsial infections.

SCRUB TYPHUS Definition Scrub typhus is limited to eastern and southeastern Asia, India, northern Australia, and the adjacent islands. It is caused by *R. tsutsugamushi* and is characterized by a primary lesion at the site of the bite of an infected mite, a fever of about 2 weeks' duration, a cutaneous rash which develops about the fifth day, and the appearance late in the second week of agglutinins against the OX-K strain of *Proteus* bacillus. The broad-spectrum antibiotics are specific therapeutic agents.

Etiology The agent of scrub typhus resembles other rickettsias in its physical properties but differs from them in antigenic structure, vector, and reservoir. The disease is transmitted by larvae of several species of mites, especially *Leptotrombidium (Trombicula) akamushi* and *L. deliense*. These tiny chiggers attach themselves to the skin and during the process of obtaining a meal of tissue juice may acquire infection from the host or transmit rickettsias to the vertebrate. The infection is maintained in nature by a cycle involving mites and small rodents and by transovarial transmission in mites; human infection represents an accident attributable to propinquity.

Clinical manifestations About 10 to 12 days after infection, illness begins abruptly with chilliness, severe headache, fever, conjunctival injection, and moderate generalized lymphadenopathy, which is most prominent in the nodes draining the area of the primary lesion. The initial lesion at the beginning of fever is evidenced by an erythematous indurated area 1 cm in diameter, surmounted by a multiloculated vesicle; within a few days the vesicle ulcerates and becomes covered with a black crust.

Fever increases progressively during the first week, generally reaching 40 to 40.5°C (104 to 105°F), but the pulse remains relatively slow, 70 to 100 beats per minute. The red macular rash, which begins on the trunk about the fifth day and spreads to the extremities, sometimes becomes maculopapular but usually fades in a few days. The course of the disease and the complications resemble those of endemic and epidemic typhus; however, interstitial myocarditis is more prominent than in the other typhus fevers.

Prognosis Before the introduction of chloramphenicol and tetracycline the mortality rate varied from 1 to 60 percent, depending on the geographic area and the virulence of the local strains of *R. tsutsugamushi*, and convalescence was prolonged. With modern therapeutic methods, deaths are rare and convalescence is short.

Differential diagnosis Scrub typhus must be differentiated from the other members of the typhus and the spotted fever group of diseases as well as from measles, typhoid fever, and the meningococcal infections. The geographic localization of scrub typhus, the primary lesion, and the occurrence of OX-K agglutinins are especially useful in establishing the diagnosis.

Treatment and prevention Chloramphenicol and the tetracycline antibiotics are extremely effective in scrub typhus. Scrub typhus is more amenable to drugs than are the other rickettsial infections, and patients with this disease regularly become afebrile and are decidedly improved within 24 to 36 h after beginning treatment, irrespective of the stage of disease. Antibiotic treatment may be discontinued after several afebrile days.

Relapse of clinical illness is unusual unless specific treatment is initiated early, such as before the fifth febrile day. Under these circumstances, recrudescence is obviated by giving the antibiotic for several days and resuming treatment about 5 days after cessation of the initial course of therapy.

Prevention of disease in the individual is accomplished by the application of miticidal chemicals (dibutyl phthalate, benzyl benzoate, diethyltoluamide, and others) to clothing and the skin. There is no satisfactory vaccine. Chemoprophylactic studies conducted in highly endemic infested areas of scrub typhus showed that single oral doses of chloramphenicol or tetracycline given every 5 days for a total of

35 days (seven doses with 5-day nontreatment intervals) prevent scrub typhus and result in active immunity. This procedure is recommended under special circumstances. A long-acting tetracycline (doxycycline) serves the same purpose.

TRENCH FEVER Trench fever is a rare febrile disease transmitted between humans by the body louse, *Pediculus humanus corporis*. It is characterized by a sudden onset with headache and severe pain in the muscles, bones, and joints. In most cases, the fever and other symptoms assume a relapsing character. Fatalities are rare. The disease is also known as shin bone fever, Volhynia fever, His-Werner disease, and quintan fever. Because of its rarity in the United States, textbooks of rickettsiology should be consulted for a detailed description.

RICKETTSIALPOX Definition Rickettsialpox is a mild, nonfatal, self-limited, febrile illness caused by *R. akari*, which is transmitted from mice to humans by mites. It is characterized by an initial skin lesion at the mite bite, a week's febrile course, and a papulovesicular rash.

Etiology and epidemiology Rickettsialpox was first recognized in New York City in 1946, and about 180 cases were reported annually for several years thereafter. It has been diagnosed in several other areas of the United States, and outbreaks have been reported in European Russia. The vector is a small, colorless mite, *Allodermanyssus sanguineus* (Hirst), which infests small mice and rodents. House mice serve as the reservoir of infection.

R. akari is morphologically and biologically similar to other rickettsias and is antigenically related to, but distinct from, *R. rickettsii*, the cause of Rocky Mountain spotted fever.

Clinical manifestations The initial skin lesion appears about 7 to 10 days after the mite bite as a firm red papule 1 to 1.5 cm in diameter. In a few days, the center vesiculates, and the papule is surrounded by an area of erythema. The regional lymph glands are moderately enlarged. The primary lesion, which is not painful, becomes covered with a black scab; it heals slowly, and a small scar is visible on separation of the crust.

The febrile phase begins 3 to 7 days after the initial lesion, and an exanthem may accompany the fever or begin several days later. The onset of fever is sudden, with chilly sensations or frank chills, headache, sweats, myalgia, anorexia, and photophobia. The pyrexia ranges from 39.4 to 40°C (103 to 104°F) and continues for about a week, occasionally with morning remissions.

The exanthem is maculopapular-vesicular, generalized in distribution, and may be abundant or scant. The lesions may involve the oral cavity but not the palms or soles. In a week, the vesicles dry and form scabs which eventually scale but leave no scar.

The constitutional symptoms are generally mild, and the course of illness is uncomplicated. No fatal cases have been reported.

The disease may be confused with chickenpox, which is different because it occurs usually in childhood and has no initial lesion and the papular cutaneous lesion is entirely transformed into a vesicle. Variola (smallpox) is accompanied by a more severe constitutional reaction, and the vesicles become pustules. The skin lesions of the other rickettsioses differ in their lack of vesiculation. The Weil-Felix reaction is usually negative in this rickettsial disease, but specific complement fixation, microscopic agglutination, and immunofluorescent antibody reactions are useful diagnostic aids even though there is considerable antigenic crossing with Rocky Mountain spotted fever.

Treatment and prevention Chloramphenicol and the tetracycline antibiotics are all effective for treating patients with rickettsialpox. The temperature reaches normal levels in about 2 days, and recovery is rapid.

Control measures should be directed toward elimination of house mice and the vector mites responsible for transmitting the disease.

OTHER TICK-BORNE RICKETTSIAL DISEASES Definition Boutonneuse fever, North Asian tick-borne rickettsiosis, and Queensland tick typhus, three diseases occurring in the eastern hemisphere, are caused by rickettsias closely related to one another and to the agent of Rocky Mountain spotted fever. Each is transmitted by the bite of

an ixodid tick. These mild to moderately severe illnesses are characterized by an initial lesion (called *tache noire* in boutonneuse fever), a fever of several days to 2 weeks, and a generalized maculopapular erythematous rash which appears on about the fifth day and usually involves the palms and soles. Specific complement-fixing antibodies appear in the patients' sera during convalescence, but agglutinins to *Proteus* OX-19 (Weil-Felix reaction) are frequently found only in low titer.

Etiology and epidemiology The etiologic agents of these three diseases are all members of the spotted fever group of rickettsias. Together with *R. rickettsii* and *R. akari* they possess common group antigens which are readily demonstrated by agglutination, complement fixation, microscopic agglutination, and immunofluorescent antibody reactions.

Boutonneuse fever, which may be regarded as the prototype of the three, is caused by *R. conorii*. Modern serologic methods employing specific rickettsial antigens have shown this rickettsia to be the causative agent for a single widely disseminated disease known by various local names. Information on the distribution and etiology of the various tick-borne rickettsial diseases is contained in Table 153-1.

In general, the epidemiology of these tick-borne rickettsioses resembles that of spotted fever in the western hemisphere. Ixodid ticks and small wild animals maintain the rickettsias in nature; if humans intrude accidentally into the cycle, they become a dead end in the transmission chain. In certain areas, the cycle of boutonneuse fever involves domiciliary environments, with the brown dog tick, *Rhipicephalus sanguineus*, as the dominant vector.

Clinical manifestations These three tick-borne rickettsioses resemble one another closely. The clinical course is usually milder than that of spotted fever, with a shorter febrile period and fewer severe complications; fatalities are rare and generally limited to the aged and debilitated. The initial lesion, which is present in most cases at the onset of fever, heals slowly; the regional lymph nodes are enlarged. The rash usually remains papular and only in severe cases becomes hemorrhagic.

The clinical picture (including the primary lesion), the geographic location, and epidemiologic considerations are helpful in establishing the diagnosis. The typhus fevers, meningococcal infections, leptospirosis, and measles must be considered in the differential diagnosis; the Weil-Felix and complement fixation tests are of value here.

Treatment and prevention Chloramphenicol and the tetracyclines are effective therapeutic agents; patients generally become afebrile after 2 to 3 days of treatment, and recovery is rapid.

The major effective methods of control are concerned with avoidance of tick bites; these include application of repellents and prompt removal of attached ticks. Effective vaccines are not available commercially.

Q FEVER Definition Q fever is an acute infectious disease caused by *Coxiella burnetii* and characterized by a sudden onset of fever, malaise, headache, weakness, anorexia, and interstitial pneumonitis. Rickettsemia occurs during the febrile period, and specific complement-fixing antibodies are present during convalescence. In contrast to the other rickettsioses, the disease is not associated with a cutaneous exanthem or agglutinins for the *Proteus* bacteria (Weil-Felix reaction).

Etiology and epidemiology *C. burnetii* possesses the general properties of other rickettsias but is somewhat more resistant to inactivation in unfavorable environments and more pleomorphic than the others. Its infectivity after drying under natural conditions is of importance in the spread of infection to humans. *C. burnetii* has a wide host range in nature, but guinea pigs and embryonated eggs are the common laboratory hosts employed for its propagation.

C. burnetii undergoes antigenic phase variation similar to the rough-smooth dissociation of bacteria. Phase I organisms are found in nature; they possess a cell-wall-associated surface antigen that is probably related to virulence and is antiphagocytic. The phase II variant is a laboratory artifact that follows adaptation of phase I in chick embryos. Complement-fixing antibodies to phase I antigen reflect a recent acute infection; they appear in 7 to 10 days, peak at about 20 days, and slowly decline.

Human Q fever is contracted by inhalation of infected dusts, by handling infected materials, possibly by drinking milk contaminated with *C. burnetii*, and, in one instance, by blood transfusion. The disease in Australia is enzootic in animals, especially bandicoots, and is transmitted in nature by ticks. Rickettsia-laden tick feces may contaminate cattle hides, and inhalation of this material has caused infection in humans. In the United States, a number of species of ticks are naturally infected, among them *Dermacentor andersoni* and *Amblyomma americanum*, and in North Africa transovarial transmission of the agent in indigenous ticks has been demonstrated. Sheep, goats, and cows have been found to be naturally infected in North America and in Europe, and *C. burnetii* has been recovered from the milk of such animals. Milk, as well as infected excretions from livestock, probably accounts for certain outbreaks of human disease following inhalation by cows of infected dust from barns and pens. The airborne route of dried contaminated material is the most likely method of spread. A number of epidemics have occurred among laboratory workers engaged in studies on *C. burnetii*. The disease is not transmitted between humans.

Slaughterhouse workers are often exposed to infected aerosols; in 1985, five cases of hepatitis occurred at a meat packing plant that processed sheep in California. A serologic survey of approximately 100 employees, conducted to identify the extent of the outbreak, revealed a total of 31 persons with evidence of infection. The primary reservoirs of *C. burnetti* are cattle, sheep, goats, and ticks. Many wild and domestic animals are susceptible to infection. In Uruguay, there were 14 outbreaks of Q fever between 1975 and 1985, comprising 1358 clinically suspected cases, all of which occurred in workers at meat processing plants; 814 were serologically confirmed.

An "urban" outbreak of Q fever occurred in 12 poker players in Halifax, Nova Scotia. Presumably the disease was transmitted by a parturient cat.

Clinical manifestations   After incubation of approximately 19 days (range 14 to 26 days), the disease begins with headache, chilly sensations, fever, malaise, myalgia, and anorexia. For several days, the temperature ranges from 38.3 to 40°C (101 to 104°F); the entire course rarely exceeds 2 weeks and usually ranges from 3 to 6 days. There may be wide fluctuations in the fever. Respiratory and gastrointestinal symptoms are not conspicuous in the early stages. Headache and fever predominate. A dry cough and chest pain occur after about 5 days, when rales are usually audible. Roentgenographic findings indistinguishable from those of primary atypical pneumonia are present usually by the third to fourth day of disease, first as patchy areas of consolidation involving a portion of one lobe, giving a homogeneous ground-glass appearance. Occasionally, a homogeneous localized infiltration may resemble a tumor mass. These manifestations persist beyond the febrile period and may appear in patients who are unaware of pulmonary involvement. Complications are rare, and coincident with defervescence the appetite begins to return. Convalescence progresses slowly for several weeks, during which time the principal disability is weakness. It is not uncommon for patients to lose 7 to 9 kg during the active stages of disease. The disease may be protracted in approximately 20 percent of cases, with fever persisting for longer than 4 weeks, particularly in elderly patients. Occasionally relapse occurs, especially in patients treated with antibiotics during the first several days of disease.

Hepatitis, with the development of clinically detectable icterus, occurs in approximately one-third of patients with the protracted form. This form of Q fever is characterized by fever, malaise, absence of headache or respiratory signs, and hepatomegaly with right upper quadrant pain. Liver biopsy specimens show diffuse granulomatous changes with multinucleated giant cells and scattered infiltrations of polymorphonuclear leukocytes, lymphocytes, and macrophages. *C. burnetii* may be demonstrated in such specimens with the fluorescent antibody technique. Q fever must be included in the differential diagnosis of patients with hepatitis and those with hepatic granulomas such as tuberculosis, sarcoidosis, histoplasmosis, brucellosis, tularemia, syphilis, and others.

Endocarditis with *C. burnetii* has been identified by smear and isolation of the rickettsia in vegetations on the heart valves obtained at operation or autopsy. The aortic valve is most commonly involved, often with large vegetations. It is important to suspect the possibility of Q fever in cases of apparent subacute bacterial endocarditis with persistently negative blood cultures. Operative intervention with replacement of damaged valves is usually necessary for recovery because the available antibiotics are not rickettsicidal. In some instances long-term antibiotic therapy has been successful.

A high complement-fixing antibody titer to phase I antigen is present in patients with endocarditis and granulomatous hepatitis.

Prognosis   Few fatalities have been recorded and, except for the patient with protracted illness and hepatic involvement or endocarditis, the course of disease is generally uncomplicated and benign.

Treatment and control   The tetracycline antibiotics and chloramphenicol are effective in the treatment of patients with Q fever. Most patients, when treated early in the course of disease, respond promptly and recover without relapses. The therapeutic procedures are comparable to those used in spotted fever.

Control of Q fever depends primarily on immunization of susceptible persons with specific vaccines. Vaccines made from phase I rickettsias are potent and afford considerable protection to slaughterhouse and dairy workers, herders, rendering-plant workers, woolsorters, tanners, laboratory workers, and others at risk. To avoid side reactions it is important that the vaccine be given only to persons who are skin test negative. Measures should be taken to avoid exposure to infected aerosols; milk from infected domestic livestock must be pasteurized or boiled.

REFERENCES

ANDREW R et al: Tick typhus in North Queensland. Med J Aust 2:253, 1946

BOZEMAN FM et al: Serologic evidence of *Rickettsia canada* infection in man. J Infect Dis 121:367, 1970

——— et al: Epidemic typhus rickettsiae isolated from flying squirrels. Nature 255:545, 1975

CENTERS FOR DISEASE CONTROL: Summary of notifiable diseases, United States, 1987. Morb Mort Week Rep 36:54, 1987

DERRICK EH: The epidemiology of Q fever: A review. Med J Aust 1:245, 1953

DESHAZO RD et al: Early diagnosis of Rocky Mountain spotted fever. Use of primary monocyte culture technique. JAMA 235:1353, 1976

FERGUSON IC et al: Clinical, virological and pathological findings in a fatal case of Q fever endocarditis. Br J Clin Pathol 15:235, 1962

GAMBRILL MR, WISSEMAN CL JR: Mechanisms of immunity in typhus infections. Infect Immun 8:519, 1973

HARRELL GT: Rickettsial involvement of the nervous system. Med Clin North Am 37:395, 1953

HATTWICK MAW et al: Rocky Mountain spotted fever: Epidemiology of an increasing problem. Ann Intern Med 84:732, 1976

KOSTER FT et al: Cellular immunity in Q fever: Specific lymphocyte unresponsiveness in Q fever endocarditis. J Infect Dis 152:1283, 1985

LANGLEY J et al: Poker player's pneumonia: An urban outbreak of Q fever following exposure to a parturient cat. N Engl J Med 319:354, 1988

MOULTON FR (ed): *The Rickettsial Diseases of Man.* Washington, DC, American Association for the Advancement of Science, 1948

MURRAY ES et al: Brill's disease: I. Clinical and laboratory diagnosis. JAMA 142:1059, 1950

———, SNYDER JC: Brill's disease: II. Etiology. Am J Hyg 53:22, 1951

ORMSBEE RA et al: The influence of phase on the protective potency of Q fever vaccine. J Immunol 92:404, 1964

——— et al: Serologic diagnosis of epidemic typhus fever. Am J Epidemiol 105:261, 1977

OSTER CN et al: Laboratory acquired Rocky Mountain spotted fever: The hazard of aerosol transmission. N Engl J Med 297:859, 1977

PEDERSEN CE et al: Demonstration of *Rickettsia rickettsii* in Rhesus monkeys by immune fluorescence microscopy. J Clin Microbiol 2:121, 1975

PHILIP RN et al: A comparison of serologic methods for diagnosis of Rocky Mountain spotted fever. Am J Epidemiol 105:56, 1977

ROSE HM: The clinical manifestations and laboratory diagnosis of rickettsialpox. Ann Intern Med 31:871, 1949

SALGO MP et al: A focus of Rocky Mountain Spotted Fever within New York City. N Engl J Med 318:345, 1988

SMADEL JE: Influence of antibiotics on immunologic responses in scrub typhus. Am J Med 17:246, 1954

——— (ed): *Symposium on Q Fever*, Medical Science Publication 6. Washington, DC, Walter Reed Army Institute of Research, 1959

SOMENSHINE DE et al: Epizootiology of epidemic typhus (*Rickettsia prowazekii*) in flying squirrels. Am J Trop Med Hyg 27:339, 1978

SOMMA-MOREIRA RE et al: Analysis of Q fever in Uruguay. Rev Infect Dis 9:386, 1987

VINSON JW: Etiology of trench fever in Mexico, in *Industry and Tropical Health*, vol V. Boston, Harvard School of Public Health, 1964, p 109

WALKER DH, CAIN BG: A method for specific diagnosis of Rocky Mountain spotted fever on fixed, paraffin-embedded tissue by immunofluorescence. J Infect Dis 137:206, 1978

———, BRADFORD WD: Rocky Mountain spotted fever in childhood, in *Perspectives in Pediatric Pathology*, vol 6, HS Rosenberg, J Bernstein (eds). New York, Masson Publishing, 1981, pp 35–61

WOODWARD TE: A historical account of the rickettsial diseases with a discussion of unsolved problems. J Infect Dis 127:583, 1973

———: Identification of *Rickettsia* in skin tissues. J Infect Dis 134:297, 1976

154 MYCOPLASMA INFECTIONS

WALLACE A. CLYDE, JR.

INTRODUCTION The mycoplasmas are a heterogeneous group of unusual bacteria belonging to microbial class Mollicutes ("soft skin"). They differ from classical bacteria by lacking rigid cell wall structures, being contained instead by trilaminar unit membranes. This property confers on mycoplasmas an inability to react with organic dyes, such as those in the Gram stain, and an absolute insensitivity to the penicillins, since there are no cell wall receptor sites for these antibiotics. The mycoplasma genome is roughly one-sixth the size of that in *Escherichia coli*, making them fastidious species requiring many precursor substances for growth in artificial media. With maximum dimensions of 0.15 to 0.5 μm, less than some of the larger viruses, mycoplasmas are the smallest organisms known that are capable of extracellular existence.

Mycoplasmas are ubiquitous in nature and cause a wide variety of diseases among animals, birds, plants, and insects. In humans the most important pathogen is *Mycoplasma pneumoniae*, a common cause of respiratory tract infections. *M. hominis* and *Ureaplasma urealyticum* also are implicated in disease involving mainly the genitourinary system. A newly described species having many pathogenic properties, *M. genitalium*, is of uncertain significance. In addition to these organisms there are eight other distinct species that are components of the normal microflora on the oropharyngeal and genital mucosal surfaces.

MYCOPLASMA PNEUMONIAE

DEFINITION *M. pneumoniae* produces an influenza-like respiratory illness of gradual onset with headache, malaise, fever, and cough. When pneumonia is present, physical findings may be minimal despite extensive changes seen in chest x-rays. Synonyms include Eaton agent pneumonia, cold hemagglutinin–positive pneumonia, atypical or primary atypical pneumonia, and "walking" pneumonia. Asymptomatic infections also occur, especially in young children and partially immune adults.

ETIOLOGY *M. pneumoniae* was discovered by Eaton in 1941 and related to the syndrome of atypical pneumonia. It is a minute, motile filament, measuring approximately 0.1 by 2 μm, that has one differentiated pole where a specialized adhesin (P1) mediates attachment to respiratory epithelial cells. Production of peroxide and an inhibitor of host cell catalase are thought to be major mediators of parasitized cell injury. The organism may be isolated from respiratory secretions using complex artificial media, requiring usually 1 to 3 weeks or more for growth and identification procedures. New rapid diagnostic techniques, based on antigen detection or nucleic acid probes used directly on specimens, appear promising.

EPIDEMIOLOGY Communicability of *M. pneumoniae* infections is thought to be via large droplets of respiratory secretions; close indoor contact such as in household, institutional, or dormitory settings facilitates spread. The incubation period has been estimated at 2 to 3 weeks. Disease occurs most commonly in elementary school children, adolescents, and young adults. Infections can be found during any season of the year, although epidemic disease tends to occur during the fall and early winter months in temperate countries. Many studies have shown a periodicity of 3 to 5 years in the occurrence of major outbreaks. In Seattle, Washington, it was found that the average incidence of disease across all years and age groups was 2/1000 population per year. This occurrence doubled during epidemic years and was higher in the age groups between 5 and 40 years. In adolescent patients, 15 to 20 percent of all pneumonias could be attributed to *M. pneumoniae*. The organism has been implicated in up to 50 percent of pneumonia episodes in college students and in 20 to 30 percent of cases occurring in military recruits.

CLINICAL MANIFESTATIONS The most common clinical syndrome associated with *M. pneumoniae* infections is that of an acute or subacute tracheobronchitis. Symptoms appearing over several days' time include headache, malaise, feverishness, scratchy sore throat, and dry cough. The cough may be paroxysmal, often disturbing sleep, and gradually becomes productive of mucoid or mucopurulent sputum. Physical findings may be minimal, other than temperature elevation rarely exceeding 38.9°C (102°F). If pneumonia is present, isolated crackles or areas of wheezing may be heard usually over one of the lower lobes. Areas of subsegmental atelectasis and small pleural effusions that rarely may be seen on chest x-rays are detectable by physical examination.

Most *M. pneumoniae* disease is mild and self-limited, running its course in 2 to 4 weeks without treatment. Appropriate antibiotics in controlled clinical trials have been shown to shorten significantly the duration of fever, days of hospitalization required, and x-ray manifestations. Rarely, severe, life-threatening, or fatal episodes can occur.

A wide variety of respiratory and nonrespiratory tract complications may be encountered. Otitis media may be seen in children, while sinusitis is commonly present in adults. Occasional patients develop the syndrome of bullous myringitis. Nondescript maculopapular skin rashes are frequent in children, and *M. pneumoniae* infections have been associated with erythema multiforme and the Stevens-Johnson syndrome. Central nervous system complications of meningoencephalitis, cerebellar ataxia, and various radiculopathies have been described. Other rare complications include monarticular arthritis, myocarditis, pericarditis, coagulopathies, hemolytic anemia, and noncardiogenic pulmonary edema.

ROENTGENOGRAPHIC FINDINGS X-ray manifestations of *M. pneumoniae* pneumonia are protean and nonspecific. The most frequent pattern is one of bronchial thickening with areas of interstitial infiltration and subsegmental atelectasis involving one of the lower lobes. Another common finding is the occurrence of "platelike" atelectasis, often seen to best advantage on lateral views. Other changes include areas of small nodular densities, which can be confused with tuberculosis, and hilar adenopathy suggesting a variety of other entities. Lobular or lobar consolidation and massive pleural effusions are uncommon.

LABORATORY FINDINGS Total blood leukocyte and differential cell counts are usually normal, but the erythrocyte sedimentation rate is often elevated and C-reactive proteins may be demonstrated. There are no characteristic findings in urinalysis, liver or renal function tests, serum electrolytes, or electrocardiograms, although abnormalities may be seen with some of the disease complications. Specific diagnostic tests include recovery of *M. pneumoniae* from respiratory secretions, or demonstration of fourfold titer changes between paired sera using a variety of methods of which the complement fixation technique is the most widely available. However, these test results are not available promptly enough to assist therapeutic decision making. New rapid diagnostic tests of two types have been marketed:

one depends upon detection of *M. pneumoniae* rRNA by a nucleic acid hybridization technique; a second detects a major protein present in the organisms. The usefulness of these rapid tests will be determined as greater clinical experience with them accrues. Another helpful test is cold hemagglutination serology, because of its rapidity and simplicity. These IgM class antibodies directed toward the I antigen of erythrocyte membranes develop during the first or second week of illness in up to 70 percent of patients with pneumonia, and may be present in high or rising titers when patients first present. Single titers of or above 64, or fourfold or greater titer changes in sera collected 5 or more days apart, are considered significant. "False"-positive cold hemagglutinin reactions may be seen in rubeola, infectious mononucleosis, adenovirus pneumonias, several tropical diseases, and, more rarely, in collagen vascular disease. As in some of these entities, polyclonal B-lymphocyte activation and T-cell suppression occurs during *M. pneumoniae* infections, which may explain the appearance of various host tissue autoantibodies and of transient anergy in some patients.

DIFFERENTIAL DIAGNOSIS   Because of its common occurrence, *M. pneumoniae* should be considered in all cases of pneumonia. Generally patients with mycoplasma pneumonia have milder illnesses than those caused by classical bacteria, less dense pulmonary infiltrations on x-rays, and normal blood leukocyte values. Epidemiologic data are especially useful: age (5 to 40 years); season (fall months predominantly); year (3- to 5-year epidemic cycles); and contact history with other cases. Other infections requiring special consideration are influenza virus pneumonia or its secondary bacterial complications (during epidemic periods) (see Chap. 139), adenovirus pneumonias (see Chap. 140) (particularly in military recruits), and mild forms of community-acquired *Legionella pneumophilia* (see Chap. 124) pneumonia. A newly recognized agent, tentatively named *Chlamydia pneumoniae* (TWAR), may produce disease clinically indistinguishable from that due to *M. pneumoniae*.

TREATMENT   Erythromycin and tetracycline derivatives are effective in reducing the morbidity of *M. pneumoniae* disease. For adults, erythromycin (0.5 g every 6 h orally), tetracycline (250 mg every 6 h orally), or doxycycline (100 mg once daily orally), in 10- to 14-day courses are usually prescribed. In severely ill patients intravenous erythromycin may be selected, but tetracycline is not recommended by this route. For children less than 8 to 10 years old erythromycin (30 to 50 mg/kg per day orally for 14 days) is the primary choice; tetracycline or doxycycline are alternatives for older patients. Relapses occasionally occur upon cessation of therapy but respond to retreatment. In cases where *Legionella* infection cannot be excluded, erythromycin should be chosen for therapy. If *Chlamydia pneumoniae* pneumonia is a consideration, the use of tetracycline or doxycycline is recommended.

OTHER MYCOPLASMAL INFECTIONS

A growing body of literature documents evidence of other human mycoplasma infections, including a variety of genitourinary syndromes in both sexes and in perinatal diseases. Mycoplasma infection should be considered in suppurative processes where classical bacterial cultures are negative; examples include urethritis, salpingitis, amnionitis, pyelonephritis, postpartum sepsis, and neonatal pneumonia or meningitis. Mycoplasmal abcesses or arthritis may occur in immunocompromised patients. Sexually transmitted diseases associated with mycoplasmas are considered in Chaps. 93 and 94.

In these infections the species most commonly encountered are *M. hominis* and *U. urealyticum*. Standard bacteriologic media may support growth of *M. hominis* as minute colonies, especially media for anaerobic bacteria that are incubated for several days. Selective media for *Ureaplasma* species are available that may permit their identification in 24 to 48 h. Cultural facilities for *Mycoplasma* species are available in some diagnostic microbiology laboratories, whereas serodiagnosis of infections other than those due to *M. pneumoniae*

are not routine. Specimens may be transported on wet ice (within 24 h) or dry ice (greater than 24 h) to reference laboratories for assistance. For *M. hominis* infections, tetracycline or clindamycin are effective antibiotics; this species is insensitive to erythromycin. Erythromycin or tetracycline may be used for *Ureaplasma* infections. Resistance of both species to the recommended antibiotics occurs and is a problem requiring special laboratory guidance.

REFERENCES

BROUGHTON RA: Infections due to *Mycoplasma pneumoniae* in childhood. Ped Infect Dis J 5:71, 1986
CASSELL GH (ed): Ureaplasmas of humans: With emphasis upon maternal and neonatal infections. Ped Infect Dis J 5:S221, 1986
CLYDE WA JR: Mycoplasmal infections, in *Diagnostic Procedures for Bacterial Infections*, 7th ed, BB Wentworth (ed). Washington, DC, American Public Health Association, 1987, pp 391–405
GRAYSTON JT et al: A new *Chlamydia psittaci* strain, TWAR, isolated in acute respiratory tract infections. N Engl J Med 315:161, 1986
MÅARDH P-A et al (eds): International symposium on *Mycoplasma hominis*—a human pathogen. Sex Trans Dis 10(Suppl):225, 1983
MCCRACKEN GH JR: Current status of antibiotic treatment for *Mycoplasma pneumoniae* disease. Ped Infect Dis J 5:167, 1986
NAGAYAMA Y et al: Isolation of *Mycoplasma pneumoniae* from children with lower-respiratory-tract infections. J Infect Dis 157:911, 1988

155   CHLAMYDIAL INFECTIONS

WALTER E. STAMM / KING K. HOLMES

The genus *Chlamydia* contains three species, *C. psittaci*, *C. trachomatis*, and *C. pneumoniae* (formerly the TWAR agent). *C. psittaci* is widely distributed in nature, producing genital, conjunctival, intestinal, or respiratory infections in many mammalian and avian species. Genital infections with *C. psittaci* have been well characterized in several species and cause complications such as abortion and infertility. Although mammalian strains of *C. psittaci* are not known to infect humans, avian strains occasionally infect humans, causing pneumonia. *C. pneumoniae* is a fastidious chlamydial species that appears to be a frequent cause of upper respiratory tract infection and pneumonia, primarily in children and young adults. No animal reservoir has been identified for *C. pneumoniae*, and it appears to be a human pathogen spread by close personal contact.

C. trachomatis is exclusively a human pathogen and was recognized as the cause of trachoma in the 1940s. Since then, *C. trachomatis* has been recognized as a major sexually transmitted and perinatal infection.

Chlamydiae are obligate, intracellular parasites. They possess both DNA and RNA, have a cell wall and ribosomes similar to those of gram-negative bacteria, and are inhibited by antibiotics such as tetracycline. Chlamydiae are classified as bacteria belonging to their own order (Chlamydiales) and genus (*Chlamydia*).

A unique feature of all chlamydia is their complex reproductive cycle. Two forms of the microorganism—the extracellular elementary body and the intracellular reticulate body—participate in this cycle. The elementary body is adapted for extracellular survival and is the infective form transmitted from one person to another. Elementary bodies attach to susceptible target cells (usually columnar or transitional epithelial cells) via specific receptors and enter the cell within a phagosome. Within 8 h, the elementary bodies reorganize into reticulate bodies. These forms are adapted to intracellular survival and multiplication. They undergo binary fission, eventually producing numerous replicates contained within the membrane-bound "inclusion body" which occupies much of the infected host cell. Chlamydial inclusions resist lysosomal fusion until late in the developmental cycle. After 24 h, the reticulate bodies condense and form elementary bodies still contained within the inclusion. The inclusion then ruptures, releasing elementary bodies from the cell to initiate infection of adjacent cells.

C. psittaci, C. pneumoniae, and *C. trachomatis* share a genus-specific or group antigen. Antibody against this antigen is measured in the complement-fixation serologic test available in most state health departments. With a microimmunofluorescence test, *C. trachomatis* strains can be further characterized serologically on the basis of antibody produced against their major outer membrane protein. Using the serovar classification of Wang and Grayston, strains associated with trachoma have generally been those of the A, B, Ba, and C serovars, while serovars D through K have been largely associated with sexually transmitted and perinatally acquired infections. Serovars L₁, L₂, and L₃ produce lymphogranuloma venereum (LGV) and hemorrhagic proctocolitis. These LGV strains demonstrate unique biologic behavior in that they are more invasive than the other serovars, produce disease in lymphatic tissue, grow readily in cell culture systems and macrophages, and are fatal when inoculated intracerebrally in mice and monkeys. Non-LGV strains of *C. trachomatis* characteristically produce superficial infections involving the columnar epithelium of the eye, genitalia, and respiratory tract.

SEXUALLY TRANSMITTED AND PERINATAL *C. TRACHOMATIS* INFECTIONS

SPECTRUM OF *C. TRACHOMATIS* GENITAL INFECTIONS Genital infections caused by *C. trachomatis* are the most common sexually transmitted disease (STD) in the United States. An estimated 3 to 4 million cases occur each year. In adults the clinical spectrum of sexually transmitted *C. trachomatis* infections parallels the spectrum of gonococcal infections (Table 155-1). Chlamydial and gonococcal infections have been associated with urethritis in both sexes, with epididymitis, mucopurulent cervicitis, acute salpingitis, bartholinitis, proctitis, and the Fitz-Hugh–Curtis syndrome (perihepatitis), and both can be associated with systemic complications, particularly with arthritis. Simultaneous infection with *C. trachomatis* occurs in 30 to 50 percent of women with cervical gonococcal infection and in about 25 percent of heterosexual men with gonococcal urethritis.

EPIDEMIOLOGY Genital infections other than LGV are caused by *C. trachomatis* serovars D through K. The incidence of nongonococcal urethritis (NGU) increased dramatically during the 1960s and 1970s. During the 1980s, the incidence of NGU stabilized in the United States, even as the incidence of gonococcal urethritis fell, probably reflecting the relative lack of implementation of programs to control chlamydial infections.

C. trachomatis has consistently been isolated from 30 to 50 percent of men with NGU. The peak age incidence of genital *C. trachomatis* infections is in the late teens and early twenties, resembling other sexually transmitted infections. The prevalence of chlamydial urethral infection in young men ranges from 3 to 5 percent of men seen in general medical settings, to over 10 percent of asymptomatic soldiers undergoing routine physical examination, to 15 to 20 percent of heterosexual men seen in STD clinics. Among homosexual men, urethral infection is less common than in heterosexual men, but rectal infections occur in homosexual men who practice receptive anorectal intercourse without condoms. The ratio of chlamydial to gonococcal urethritis is highest for heterosexual men and those with high socioeconomic status and lowest for homosexual men and indigent populations.

Cervical infection in women has ranged from approximately 5 percent of asymptomatic college students or prenatal patients in the United States, to over 10 percent of women seen in family planning clinics, to over 20 percent of women seen in STD clinics. In the United States, the prevalence of *C. trachomatis* in the cervix of pregnant women is 5 to 10 times higher than that of *Neisseria gonorrhoeae*. The prevalence of genital infection with either agent is highest in individuals who are single, nonwhite or Asian, and between ages 18 and 24. The proportion of infections that are asymptomatic appears to be higher for *C. trachomatis* than for *N. gonorrhoeae*, and symptomatic *C. trachomatis* infections are clinically less severe. It is suspected that mild or asymptomatic chlamydial infections of the fallopian tubes may nonetheless cause ongoing tubal damage and infertility. Furthermore, because the total number of *C. trachomatis* infections exceeds that of *N. gonorrhoeae* infections in industrialized countries, the total morbidity caused by *C. trachomatis* genital infections equals or exceeds that caused by *N. gonorrhoeae*. The prevalence of *C. trachomatis* is higher than that of *N. gonorrhoeae* in industrialized countries, in part because measures such as treatment of sex partners and routine cultures for case detection in asymptomatic individuals have been applied much more effectively for gonorrhea than for control of *C. trachomatis* infection.

CLINICAL MANIFESTATIONS **Nongonococcal and postgonococcal urethritis** Nongonococcal urethritis is a diagnosis of exclusion that is applied to men with symptoms and/or signs of urethritis who do not have gonorrhea. Postgonococcal urethritis (PGU) refers to nongonococcal urethritis which develops 2 to 3 weeks after treatment of gonococcal urethritis in men. *C. trachomatis* causes 30 to 50 percent of the cases of NGU and PGU in heterosexual men but is less commonly isolated from homosexual men with these syndromes. The cause of the remaining cases is uncertain, although considerable evidence suggests that *Ureaplasma urealyticum* causes some of these infections.

Nongonococcal urethritis is diagnosed by documentation of a leukocytic urethral exudate and by exclusion of gonorrhea by Gram's stain or culture. *C. trachomatis* urethritis is generally less severe than gonococcal urethritis, although in an individual patient these two forms of urethritis cannot be differentiated solely on clinical grounds. Symptoms include urethral discharge, dysuria (often whitish and mucoid rather than frankly purulent), and urethral itching. The examination may show meatal erythema and tenderness and a urethral exudate which is often demonstrable only by stripping the urethra. About one-third of male STD patients who have *C. trachomatis* urethral infection have no demonstrable signs or symptoms of urethritis. Asymptomatic chlamydial urethritis has been demonstrated in 5 to 10 percent of sexually active adolescent males screened in teen clinics. Such patients frequently have first-glass pyuria (15 leukocytes per 400× microscopic field in the sediment of first-voided urine), a positive leukocyte esterase test, or an increased number of leukocytes on gram-stained smear prepared from a urogenital swab inserted 1 to 2 cm into the anterior urethra. The smear is first scanned

TABLE 155-1 Clinical parallels between sexually transmitted infections due to *Neisseria gonorrhoeae* and *Chlamydia trachomatis*

	Resulting clinical syndrome	
Site of infection	*N. gonorrhoeae*	*C. trachomatis*
MEN		
Urethra	Urethritis	NGU, PGU
Epididymis	Epididymitis	Epididymitis
Rectum	Proctitis	Proctitis
Conjunctiva	Conjunctivitis	Conjunctivitis
Systemic	Disseminated gonococcal infection (DGI)	Reiter's syndrome
WOMEN		
Urethra	Acute urethral syndrome	Acute urethral syndrome
Bartholin's gland	Bartholinitis	Bartholinitis
Cervix	Cervicitis	Cervicitis
Endometrium	Endometritis	Endometritis
Fallopian tube	Salpingitis	Salpingitis
Conjunctiva	Conjunctivitis	Conjunctivitis
Liver capsule	Perihepatitis	Perihepatitis
Systemic	DGI	Reiter's syndrome

at low power to identify areas of the slide containing the highest concentration of leukocytes. These areas are then examined under oil immersion (1000×). An average of four or more leukocytes in at least three of five 1000× (oil immersion) fields is indicative of urethritis and correlates with recovery of *C. trachomatis*. To differentiate between true urethritis and functional symptoms among symptomatic patients, or to make a presumptive diagnosis of *C. trachomatis* infection in asymptomatic men (e.g., male patients in STD clinics, sex partners of women with nongonococcal salpingitis or mucopurulent cervicitis, fathers of children with inclusion conjunctivitis), the examination of an endourethral specimen for increased leukocytes is useful if specific diagnostic tests for chlamydia are not available. Alternatively, noninvasive screening for urethritis can be accomplished by testing a first-void urine for pyuria either by microscopy or by the leukocyte esterase test.

Epididymitis *C. trachomatis* is the major cause of epididymitis in sexually active heterosexual men under 35 years of age who present with epididymitis. Coliform bacteria and *Pseudomonas aeruginosa* are the most common causes of epididymitis in men over 35. In homosexual men, sexually transmitted coliform infection acquired via rectal intercourse may cause epididymitis. Testicular torsion should be promptly excluded by radionuclide scan, Doppler flow study, or surgical exploration in a teenager or young adult who presents with acute unilateral testicular pain without urethritis. Testicular tumor or chronic infection (e.g., tuberculosis) should be excluded in the patient with unilateral intrascrotal pain and swelling who does not respond to appropriate antimicrobial therapy.

Reiter's syndrome *C. trachomatis* has been recovered from the urethra of up to 70 percent of men with untreated nondiarrheal Reiter's syndrome and associated urethritis. The syndrome consists of conjunctivitis, urethritis (or cervicitis in females), arthritis, and characteristic mucocutaneous lesions (see Chap. 274). In the absence of overt urethritis, it is important to exclude subclinical urethritis.

Proctitis *C. trachomatis* of either the genital immunotypes D through K or the LGV immunotype L₂ causes proctitis in homosexual men and heterosexual women who practice receptive anorectal intercourse. Either asymptomatic infection or mild proctitis not unlike gonococcal proctitis results from infection with immunotypes D through K. Clinically, these patients present with mild rectal pain, mucus discharge, tenesmus, and, occasionally, bleeding. Nearly all have neutrophils in their rectal Gram stain. Sigmoidoscopy in these non-LGV cases of chlamydial proctitis reveals mild, patchy mucosal friability and mucopurulent discharge, and the disease process is limited to the distal rectum. LGV strains produce a more severe ulcerative proctitis or proctocolitis which can be confused clinically with herpes simplex virus proctitis and which histologically resembles Crohn's disease in that giant-cell formation and granulomas can be seen (see Chap. 241).

Mucopurulent cervicitis *C. trachomatis* has been isolated from the cervix of 30 to 60 percent of women with gonorrhea or a history of contact with gonorrhea, from 30 to 70 percent of women whose male partners have nongonococcal urethritis, and from 10 to 20 percent of women attending STD clinics who do not have a history of contact with a partner with urethritis. Women who have cervical ectopy or who use oral contraceptives appear to have an increased prevalence of cervical infection with *C. trachomatis*.

Although some women with *C. trachomatis* infection of the cervix have no symptoms or signs, careful speculum examination shows that many have mucopurulent cervicitis. As discussed more fully in Chap. 94, mucopurulent cervicitis is associated with yellow mucopurulent discharge from the endocervical columnar epithelium, and with ≥30 neutrophils per 1000× microscopic field within strands of cervical mucus on a thinly smeared, Gram-stained preparation of endocervical exudate. Other characteristic findings include edema of the zone of cervical ectopy and a propensity of the mucosa to bleed on minor trauma as happens when specimens are collected with a swab. Pap smear shows increased neutrophils, as well as a characteristic pattern of mononuclear inflammatory cells, including plasma cells, transformed lymphocytes, and histiocytes. Cervical biopsy shows predominantly a mononuclear infiltrate of the subepithelial stroma, often with a follicular cervicitis.

Pelvic inflammatory disease (PID) *C. trachomatis* plays an important causative role in salpingitis. *C. trachomatis* infection has been demonstrated in laparoscopically verified salpingitis, recovered from the fallopian tubes in the absence of other pathogens, and serologic evidence of recent *C. trachomatis* infection has been found in women with PID. In the United States *C. trachomatis* has been identified in the fallopian tubes or endometrium in up to 50 percent of women with PID, and its role as an important etiologic agent in this syndrome is well accepted.

Pelvic inflammatory disease occurs via ascending intraluminal spread of *C. trachomatis* from the lower genital tract. Mucopurulent cervicitis is followed by endometritis, endosalpingitis, and finally pelvic peritonitis. Evidence of mucopurulent cervicitis is usually present in women with laparoscopically verified salpingitis. Similarly, endometritis, demonstrated by endometrial biopsy showing plasma cell infiltration of the endometrial epithelium, is present in most women with laparoscopically verified chlamydial (or gonococcal) salpingitis. Chlamydial endometritis also occurs in the absence of clinical evidence of salpingitis: approximately 40 to 50 percent of women with mucopurulent cervicitis have plasma cell endometritis. Histologic evidence of endometritis has been correlated with an "endometritis syndrome," consisting of vaginal bleeding, lower abdominal pain, and uterine tenderness in the absence of adnexal tenderness, and with peripheral blood leukocytosis. Since laparoscopy was not performed in these patients, it is not known what proportion of those with chlamydial endometritis without adnexal tenderness had salpingitis. However, chlamydial salpingitis apparently produces milder symptoms then does gonococcal salpingitis and is associated with less marked adnexal tenderness. The presence of mild adnexal or uterine tenderness in sexually active women with cervicitis should suggest PID.

Infertility associated with fallopian tube scarring has been strongly linked to antecedent *C. trachomatis* infection in serologic studies. Since many infertile women with tubal scarring and antichlamydial antibody in these studies had no history of prior PID, subclinical tubal infection may produce scarring. Ectopic pregnancy, which occurs in over 70,000 women in the United States annually, is also thought to be related to chlamydia-induced tubal scarring in many cases.

Perihepatitis, or the Fitz-Hugh–Curtis syndrome, was originally described as a complication of gonococcal PID. However, cultural and/or serologic evidence of *C. trachomatis* infection is found in three-quarters of women with this syndrome. *C. trachomatis* has also been cultured from exudate on the hepatic capsule in laparoscopically verified cases. This syndrome should be suspected whenever a young, sexually active woman presents with an illness resembling cholecystitis (fever and right upper quadrant pain of subacute or acute onset). Symptoms and signs of salpingitis may be minimal.

Urethral syndrome in women *C. trachomatis* has been found to be the most common pathogen isolated from college women with dysuria, frequency, and pyuria in the absence of uropathogens such as coliforms or *Staphylococcus saprophyticus* in *any* concentration in a clean-catch midstream urine specimen (see Chap. 95). *Chlamydia* can also be isolated from the urethra of women without symptoms of urethritis, and up to 25 percent of female STD clinic patients have had positive *C. trachomatis* cultures from the urethra only.

C. trachomatis infection in pregnancy *C. trachomatis* in pregnancy has been associated in some studies (but not in others) with premature delivery and with postpartum endometritis. Whether these complications are in part attributable to *C. trachomatis* is not clear.

PERINATAL INFECTIONS: INCLUSION CONJUNCTIVITIS AND PNEUMONIA

EPIDEMIOLOGY Studies in the United States have demonstrated that 5 to 25 percent of pregnant women have *C. trachomatis* infections of the cervix. In these studies, approximately one-half to two-thirds of the children who were exposed during birth eventually showed laboratory evidence of *C. trachomatis* infection. Roughly half of the infants who developed laboratory evidence of infection (or 25 percent of the group exposed) developed clinical inclusion conjunctivitis. In addition to eye infection, *C. trachomatis* has been isolated frequently and persistently from the nasopharynx, the rectum, and the vagina, occasionally for periods exceeding 1 year in the absence of treatment. Pneumonia occurs in about 10 percent of children infected perinatally, and otitis media may in some cases result from perinatally acquired chlamydial infection.

INCLUSION CONJUNCTIVITIS OF THE NEWBORN (NEONATAL CHLAMYDIAL CONJUNCTIVITIS)   In the newborn, chlamydial conjunctivitis generally has a longer incubation period than gonococcal conjunctivitis (usually 5 to 14 days vs. 1 to 3 days), but this is not reliable in the individual patient. The other common causes of conjunctivitis in newborns include *Staphylococcus aureus, Haemophilus influenzae, Streptococcus pneumoniae,* and herpes simplex virus. Neonatal chlamydial conjunctivitis has an acute onset and often produces a profuse mucopurulent discharge. However, it is impossible to differentiate chlamydial conjunctivitis from other forms of neonatal bacterial conjunctivitis clinically, and laboratory diagnosis is required. Inclusions within epithelial cells often can be demonstrated in Giemsa-stained conjunctival smears, but these smears are less sensitive than cultures or antigen detection tests. Similarly, Gram-stained smears may show gonococci, or occasional small gram-negative coccobacilli in *Haemophilus* conjunctivitis, but smears should be accompanied by cultures for these agents. Very rarely a trachoma-like eye disease occurs in children with chlamydial infection living in areas that do not have endemic trachoma. If neonatal chlamydial conjunctivitis is not treated appropriately with oral antimicrobials, it may be followed by chlamydial pneumonia.

INFANT PNEUMONIA   *C. trachomatis* causes a distinctive pneumonia syndrome in infants. For details, standard textbooks of pediatrics should be consulted.

LYMPHOGRANULOMA VENEREUM

DEFINITION   Lymphogranuloma venereum (LGV) is a sexually transmitted infection caused by *C. trachomatis* strains of the L_1, L_2, or L_3 serovars. Most cases are caused by L_2 infections. The acute disease in heterosexual men is characterized by a transient primary genital lesion followed by multilocular suppurative regional lymphadenopathy. Women, homosexual men, and, occasionally, heterosexual men may develop hemorrhagic proctitis with regional lymphadenitis. Acute LGV is almost always associated with systemic symptoms such as fever and leukocytosis and rarely with systemic complications such as meningoencephalitis. After a latent period of years, late complications include genital elephantiasis due to lymphatic involvement, strictures, and fistulas of the penis, urethra, and rectum.

EPIDEMIOLOGY   LGV is usually sexually transmitted, but occasional transmission by nonsexual personal contact, fomites, or laboratory accidents has been documented. Laboratory work involving creation of aerosols of this organism (e.g., sonication, homogenization) must be conducted with appropriate biologic containment.

The peak incidence of LGV corresponds to the age of greatest sexual activity, the second and third decades of life. The worldwide incidence of LGV is falling, but the disease is still endemic and a major cause of morbidity in Asia, Africa, and South America. Only 303 cases were reported in the United States in 1987.

The frequency of infection following exposure is believed to be much less than that associated with gonorrhea and syphilis. Early manifestations are recognized far more often in men than in women, who usually present with late complications. In the United States, where the reported sex ratio is 3.4 males to 1 female, most cases have involved homosexually active men; travelers, seamen, and military personnel returning from abroad; and individuals of low

socioeconomic status living in areas of low but continuing endemicity in the southeast. The main reservoir of infection is presumed to be asymptomatically infected individuals, although this has not been directly demonstrated.

CLINICAL MANIFESTATIONS   In heterosexuals, a *primary genital lesion* occurs from 3 days to 3 weeks after exposure. It is a small, painless vesicle or nonindurated ulcer or papule located on the penis in men or on the labia, posterior vagina, or fourchette in women. The primary lesion is noticed by less than one-third of men with LGV and only rarely by women. It heals in a few days without scarring and even when noticed is usually not recognized as LGV except in retrospect. LGV strains of *C. trachomatis* have occasionally been recovered from genital ulcers, and also from the urethra of men and the endocervix of women who present with inguinal adenopathy, suggesting that these areas may be the primary site of infection in some cases.

In women and homosexual men, *primary anal or rectal infection* occurs following receptive anorectal intercourse. In women, rectal infection with LGV (or non-LGV) strains of *C. trachomatis* presumably can also arise either via contiguous spread of infected secretions along the perineum (as with rectal gonococcal infection in women) or perhaps by spread to the rectum via the pelvic lymphatics. From the site of the primary urethral, genital, anal, or rectal infection, the organism spreads via the regional lymphatics. Penile, vulvar, and anal infection can lead to inguinal and femoral lymphadenitis. Rectal infection produces hypogastric and deep iliac lymphadenitis. Upper vaginal or cervical infection results in enlargement of the obturator and iliac nodes. The most common presenting picture in heterosexual men is the *inguinal syndrome,* which is characterized by painful inguinal lymphadenopathy beginning 2 to 6 weeks after presumed exposure; rarely the onset occurs after a few months. The inguinal adenopathy is unilateral in two-thirds of cases, and palpable enlargement of the iliac and femoral nodes is often present on the same side as the enlarged inguinal nodes. The nodes are initially discrete, but progressive periadenitis results in a matted mass of nodes which become fluctuant and suppurative. The overlying skin becomes fixed, inflamed, and thinned and finally develops multiple draining fistulas. Extensive enlargement of chains of inguinal nodes above and below the inguinal ligament ("the sign of the groove") is common but is not specific, and is present in only a minority of cases. Histologically, infected nodes initially show characteristic small stellate abscesses surrounded by histiocytes. These abscesses coalesce to cause large, necrotic, suppurative foci. Spontaneous healing usually occurs after several months, leaving inguinal scars or granulomatous masses of varying size which persist for life. Massive pelvic lymphadenopathy in women or homosexual men may lead to exploratory laparotomy.

As cultures and serology for *C. trachomatis* are being used more often, increasing numbers of cases of LGV proctitis are being recognized in homosexual men. Such patients present with anorectal pain and mucopurulent, bloody rectal discharge. Although patients may complain of diarrhea, this usually represents frequent, painful, unsuccessful attempts at defecation (tenesmus). Sigmoidoscopy reveals ulcerative proctitis or proctocolitis, with purulent exudate and mucosal bleeding. Since the LGV agent is an obligate intracellular pathogen, the histopathologic findings in the rectal mucosa include granulomas with giant cells, along with crypt abscesses and extensive inflammation. These clinical, sigmoidoscopic, and histopathologic findings may closely resemble Crohn's disease of the rectum.

Constitutional symptoms are common during the stage of regional lymphadenopathy and, in the presence of proctitis, may include fever, chills, headache, meningismus, anorexia, myalgias, and arthralgias. These findings in the presence of lymphadenopathy are sometimes mistaken for malignant lymphoma. Other systemic complications are infrequent but include arthritis with sterile effusion, aseptic meningitis, meningoencephalitis, conjunctivitis, hepatitis, and erythema nodosum. Chlamydiae have been recovered from the cerebrospinal fluid, and in one case from the blood in a patient with severe constitutional symptoms, indicating the occurrence of disseminated infection. Laboratory infections due to suspected inhalation of aerosols have been associated with mediastinal lymphadenitis, pneumonitis, and pleural effusion.

Complications of untreated anorectal infection include perirectal abscess, fistula in ano, and rectovaginal, rectovesical, and ischiorectal fistulas. Secondary bacterial infection probably contributes to these complications. Rectal stricture is a late complication of anorectal infection and usually occurs 2 to 6 cm from the anal orifice, within reach on digital rectal examination. The stricture may extend proximally for several centimeters, leading to a mistaken clinical and radiographic diagnosis of carcinoma.

A small percentage of cases of LGV in men presents with chronic progressive infiltrative, ulcerative, or fistular lesions of the penis, urethra, or scrotum. Associated lymphatic obstruction may produce elephantiasis. Urethral stricture may occur and usually involves the posterior urethra, causing incontinence or difficulty with micturition.

APPROACH TO THE DIAGNOSIS AND TREATMENT OF C. TRACHOMATIS OCULOGENITAL INFECTIONS

Four types of laboratory procedures are available to confirm *C. trachomatis* infection. These are direct microscopic examination of tissue scrapings for typical intracytoplasmic inclusions, isolation of the organism, detection of chlamydial antigens by immunologic methods, and detection of antibody in the serum or in local secretions.

Except in conjunctivitis, direct microscopic examination of Giemsa-stained cell scrapings for typical inclusion has an unacceptably low sensitivity and false-positive interpretations by inexperienced observers are common.

Cell culture techniques have replaced the yolk sac of embryonated eggs for isolation of *C. trachomatis.* While LGV strains grow well in many cell lines, the other *C. trachomatis* strains are much more difficult to culture. Although culture remains the "gold standard" for diagnosis of chlamydial infection, it is expensive, technically demanding, and not widely available. Therefore, antigen detection methods have been developed that can be used instead of cultures. In the immunofluorescent slide test, potentially infected genital or ocular secretions are smeared on a slide, fixed, and stained with fluorescein-conjugated monoclonal antibody. When viewing the slide using a fluorescence microscope, the presence of fluorescing elementary bodies confirms the diagnosis. Compared with culture, this test is 85 to 90 percent sensitive and quite specific when used for confirmation of urethral, cervical, or ocular infection in high-risk patients with suspected *C. trachomatis* infection. The sensitivity of the test appears lower in low-risk populations. This plus the relatively labor-intensive nature of the test limit its value as a screening test. An enzyme-linked immunosorbent assay (ELISA) technique for chlamydial antigen detection has also been developed and provides another alternative to culture. Reported sensitivity and specificity of this test for genital infections has been 70 to 95 percent and 92 to 97 percent in high-risk populations. This test is well-suited to screening because large numbers of specimens can be easily processed.

Serologic tests have limited usefulness in the diagnosis of chlamydial oculogenital infections. The complement fixation (CF) test with the heat-stable genus-specific antigen has been used to diagnose LGV with some success, but it is insensitive in non-LGV *C. trachomatis* infections. The microimmunofluorescence (micro-IF) test with *C. trachomatis* antigens is more sensitive but is generally available only in research laboratories. The test measures antibodies by serovar specificity and by immunoglobulin class (IgM, IgG, IgA, secretory IgA) in both serum and local secretions. Serologic diagnosis using the micro-IF test may be useful in infant pneumonia (high-titer IgM antibody and/or fourfold titer rises can often be demonstrated), in women with chlamydial salpingitis (especially with Fitz-Hugh–Curtis syndrome), and in LGV.

Table 155-2 summarizes the diagnostic tests of choice for patients with suspected chlamydial infection. With few exceptions, the most suitable method for diagnosis is demonstration of the agent in tissue-cell culture or by antigen detection methods. Selection of the most appropriate of these tests depends upon local availability and expertise. Since *C. trachomatis* is an intracellular pathogen, adequate specimens for chlamydial culture must include epithelial cells. Cultures of pus result in fewer isolations of the organism. In urethritis, a thin-shafted urogenital swab should be inserted at least 2 cm into the urethra to obtain an appropriate specimen. When a cervical culture is taken, the external os should first be cleaned of debris and purulent material, and a plastic-shafted swab then inserted into the cervix, rotated slowly several times, and withdrawn. When conjunctival specimens are sought, the epithelium should be swabbed to remove cells, rather than simply purulent material. All specimens for chlamydial culture should be placed immediately into a transport medium and then either refrigerated if they will reach the laboratory within 12 to 18 h or frozen at −70°C if longer storage is anticipated. A major advantage of antigen detection techniques is their less rigid transport requirements.

From a public health viewpoint, the most effective use of chlamydia diagnostic testing has not been established and will vary depending upon clinical population, local resources, and laboratory expertise. The Centers for Disease Control have recommended empiric treatment (without diagnostic testing if resources are not available for testing) of selected high-risk groups. These include men with NGU or sexually transmitted epididymitis; women with mucopurulent cervicitis (MPC) or PID; asymptomatic sex partners of patients with these syndromes; women and heterosexual men with gonorrhea (because of the high proportion of these patients who will also have *C. trachomatis* infection); and contacts of men or women with gonorrhea. Where funds for diagnostic testing are limited (e.g., in public clinics serving indigent patients), it has been rationalized that these groups will receive empiric therapy in any event, and hence diagnostic testing is not absolutely essential. However, it has several potential benefits in these patients, including confirmation of infection and support of the clinical diagnosis (especially in women with MPC and PID), enhancement of sex partner referral and compliance with drug therapy, determination of prognosis, and education of physicians (ability to correlate signs and symptoms with culture results). Where diagnostic testing must be rationed because of limited resources, highest priority should be given to screening asymptomatic high-risk women, especially those seen in high-risk settings (i.e., STD clinics, abortion clinics, family planning clinics), or individuals with a high-risk profile (young, multiple sex partners, lower socioeconomic status).

ANTIMICROBIAL SUSCEPTIBILITY In laboratory tests, death of inoculated mice and chick embryos, as well as growth in cell cultures, is prevented or inhibited by tetracyclines, erythromycin, rifampin (rifampicin), and certain of the fluoroquinolones; sulfonamides, clindamycin, and cycloserine are also active against *C. trachomatis*, but bacitracin and polymyxin B are less effective; penicillin and ampicillin suppress *Chlamydia* multiplication but do not eradicate the organism in vitro. The cephalosporins also appear relatively ineffective against *C. trachomatis*. Streptomycin, gentamicin, neomycin, kanamycin, vancomycin, ristocetin, spectinomycin, and nystatin are not effective at concentrations inhibitory for most bacteria and fungi. For treatment of human *C. trachomatis* infection, the tetracyclines, erythromycin, and sulfonamides are most useful.

TREATMENT In general, chlamydial infections cannot be eradicated by single-dose or short-term antimicrobial regimens. In most situations, at least 7 days and sometimes 2 to 3 weeks of antibiotic should be given. Failure after treatment of genital infections with a tetracycline usually indicates inadequate therapy, poor compliance, or reinfection. Tetracycline-resistant strains of *C. trachomatis* have not been described.

Therapy of *C. trachomatis* urethritis is more effective than therapy of other forms of NGU. *C. trachomatis* is eradicated from the urethra by treatment with tetracycline hydrochloride, 500 mg qid for 7 days, or doxycycline, 100 mg by mouth bid for 7 days. An effective alternative regimen is erythromycin, 500 mg qid for 7 days.

TABLE 155-2 Diagnostic tests in *C. trachomatis* infection

Infection	Suggestive signs/symptoms	Presumptive diagnosis*	Confirmatory test of choice
ADULT MALES			
Nongonococcal urethritis, postgonococcal urethritis	Discharge, dysuria	Gram stain with more than four neutrophils per oil immersion field, no gonococci	Urethral culture or antigen detection test for *C. trachomatis*
Epididymitis	Unilateral intrascrotal swelling, pain, tenderness; fever; nongonococcal urethritis	Gram stain with more than four neutrophils per oil immersion field, no gonococci	Urethral culture or antigen detection test for *C. trachomatis*
ADULT FEMALES			
Cervicitis	Mucopurulent cervical discharge, cervical edema, ectopy, bleeding	Cervical Gram stain with ≥30 neutrophils per oil immersion field in cervical mucus	Cervical culture or antigen detection test for *C. trachomatis*
Salpingitis	Evidence of pelvic inflammatory disease on examination	*C. trachomatis* should always be suspected in salpingitis	Cervical culture or antigen detection test for *C. trachomatis*
Urethritis	Dysuria and frequency without urgency or hematuria	Mucopurulent cervicitis, sterile pyuria, negative routine urine culture	Urethral and cervical cultures or antigen detection test for *C. trachomatis*
ADULTS OF EITHER SEX			
Proctitis	Rectal pain, discharge, tenesmus, blood; receptive anorectal intercourse	Negative gonococcal culture and Gram stain; ≥1 neutrophils in rectal Gram stain	Rectal culture or direct immunofluorescence test for *C. trachomatis*
Reiter's syndrome	Nongonococcal urethritis, arthritis, conjunctivitis, typical skin lesions	Gram stain with more than four neutrophils per oil immersion field, no gonococci	Urethral culture or antigen detection test for *C. trachomatis*
LGV	Regional adenopathy, primary lesion, proctitis, systemic symptoms	None	Isolation of LGV strain from node, rectum, occasionally from urethra or cervix; LGV CF-titer ≥1:64; micro-IF titer ≥1:512
NEONATES			
Conjunctivitis	Purulent conjunctival discharge 6 to 18 days postdelivery	Negative cultures and gram stains for gonococci, *Haemophilus* sp., pneumococci, staphylococci	Conjunctival culture or antigen detection test for *C. trachomatis;* Giemsa-stained scraping of conjunctival material can provide more rapid diagnosis but is less sensitive
Infant pneumonia	Afebrile, staccato cough, diffuse rales, bilateral hyperinflation, interstitial infiltrates	None	Chlamydial culture of sputum, pharynx, eye, rectum; micro-IF antibody to *C. trachomatis*—fourfold change in IgG or IgM antibody

* Although a presumptive diagnosis of chlamydial infection is often made in the syndromes listed when gonococci are not found, a positive test for *Neisseria gonorrhoeae* does not exclude *C. trachomatis*, which is very often also present in patients with gonorrhea.

Eradication of *C. trachomatis* from the cervix has been demonstrated with similar doses and durations of tetracycline, doxycycline, and erythromycin. Erythromycin base, 500 mg qid for 10 to 14 days, is the regimen of choice for pregnant women with *C. trachomatis* infection. Amoxicillin, 500 mg tid for 10 days, has also been used successfully in one study of pregnant women. Tetracycline hydrochloride, 500 mg qid for 14 days, produces clinical and microbiologic cure of epididymitis associated with *C. trachomatis* infection.

Treatment of sex partners Genital *C. trachomatis* infections have continued to increase in incidence, whereas gonococcal infections have steadily fallen in incidence over the same period. The increase in chlamydial infection probably is due to the inability to diagnose asymptomatic infection and also failure to diagnose and treat *C. trachomatis* infections in symptomatic patients or their sex partners. Cases of NGU, epididymitis, Reiter's syndrome, and mucopurulent endocervicitis are sometimes not treated with antimicrobials, and sex partners are treated even less often. *C. trachomatis* urethral or cervical infection has been well-documented in a high proportion of the sex partners of patients with NGU, epididymitis, Reiter's syndrome, salpingitis, or endocervicitis. This is analogous to the problem of asymptomatic gonococcal infection in sex partners of patients with gonorrhea. Confirmatory laboratory tests for *Chlamydia* should be obtained if possible, but antigen detection tests may be less sensitive in asymptomatic carriers. Even those without evidence of clinical disease who have been recently exposed to proven or possible chlamydial infection (for example, NGU) should be offered therapy.

In neonates with conjunctivitis or infants with pneumonia, erythromycin ethylsuccinate or estolate can be given orally in a dose of 50 mg/kg per day, preferably as 12.5 mg/kg qid, for 2 weeks. Careful attention must be given to compliance with therapy—a frequent problem. Relapses of eye infection are common following treatment with topical erythromycin or tetracycline ophthalmic ointment and may occur after oral erythromycin therapy also, so that follow-up cultures should be obtained after treatment. Both parents should be examined for *C. trachomatis* infection and, if diagnostic tests are not readily available, should be treated with a tetracycline.

TRACHOMA AND ADULT INCLUSION CONJUNCTIVITIS

DEFINITION Trachoma is a chronic conjunctivitis associated with infection by *C. trachomatis* serovars A, B, and C. It has produced an estimated 20 million cases of blindness throughout the world and remains an important preventable cause of blindness. Inclusion conjunctivitis is an acute ocular infection caused by sexually transmitted *C. trachomatis* strains (usually serovars D through K) in adults exposed to infected genital secretions and in their newborn offspring.

EPIDEMIOLOGY Epidemiologically, two types of eye disease are caused by *C. trachomatis*. In trachoma-endemic areas where the classic eye disease is seen, transmission is from eye to eye, via hands, towels, flies, and other fomites, and usually involves serovars A, B, or C. In nonendemic areas, organisms of serovars D through K can be transmitted from the genital tract to the eye, usually causing only the inclusion conjunctivitis syndrome with or without keratitis. Rarely the eye disease acquired in this way progresses with the development of pannus and scars similar to endemic trachoma. These cases may be referred to as paratrachoma to differentiate them epidemiologically from eye-to-eye transmitted endemic trachoma.

The worldwide incidence and severity of trachoma have decreased dramatically during the past 30 years in areas with improving hygienic and economic conditions. Endemic trachoma is still the major cause of preventable blindness in north Africa, sub-Saharan Africa, the Middle East, and parts of Asia. Transmission of the endemic disease occurs primarily through close personal contact, particularly among young children in rural communities. In endemic areas, trachoma is associated with repeated exposure and reinfection, but the infection can also be latent. In the United States a mild form of endemic trachoma still occurs in Mexican Americans as well as in immigrants from areas where trachoma is endemic. Acute relapse of old trachoma has been seen occasionally following treatment with cortisone eye ointment or in very old persons exposed in their youth.

CLINICAL MANIFESTATIONS Both endemic trachoma and adult inclusion conjunctivitis present initially as a conjunctivitis characterized by small lymphoid follicles in the conjunctiva. In regions with hyperendemic classic blinding trachoma, the disease usually starts insidiously before the age of 2 years. Reinfection is common and probably contributes to the pathogenesis of trachoma.

The cornea becomes involved with inflammatory leukocytic infiltration and superficial vascularization (pannus formation). As the inflammation continues, there is conjunctival scarring that eventually distorts the eyelids, causing them to turn inward so that the inturned lashes constantly abrade the eyeball (trichiasis and entropion); eventually the corneal epithelium is abraded and may then ulcerate with subsequent corneal scarring and blindness. Destruction of the conjunctival goblet cells, lacrimal ducts, and lacrimal gland may produce a "dry-eye" syndrome with resultant corneal opacity due to drying (xerosis) or secondary bacterial corneal ulcers.

Communities with blinding trachoma often experience seasonal epidemics of bacterial conjunctivitis with *Haemophilus influenzae* which contribute to the intensity of the inflammatory process. In such areas the active infectious process usually resolves spontaneously in affected persons between 10 and 15 years of age, but the conjunctival scars continue to shrink, producing trichiasis and entropion and subsequent corneal scarring in adults. In areas with milder and less prevalent disease the process may be much slower, with active disease continuing into adulthood; blindness is rare in these cases.

Eye infection with genital *C. trachomatis* strains, usually in sexually active young adults, presents with acute onset of unilateral follicular conjunctivitis and preauricular lymphadenopathy similar to acute adenovirus or herpesvirus conjunctivitis. If untreated, the disease may persist for 6 weeks to 2 years. It is frequently associated with corneal inflammation in the form of discrete opacities ("infiltrates"), punctate epithelial erosions, and minor degrees of superficial corneal vascularization. Very rarely conjunctival scarring and eyelid distortion occur, particularly in patients treated for many months with topical corticosteroids. Recurrent eye infections occur most often in patients whose sexual consorts are not treated with antimicrobials.

DIAGNOSIS The clinical diagnosis of classic trachoma can be made if two of the following signs are present:

1 Lymphoid follicles on the upper tarsal conjunctiva
2 Typical conjunctival scarring
3 Vascular pannus
4 Limbal follicles or their sequelae, Herbert's pits

The clinical diagnosis of endemic trachoma should be confirmed by laboratory tests in children with more marked degrees of inflammation. Intracytoplasmic chlamydial inclusions occur in 10 to 60 percent of Giemsa-stained conjunctival smears in such populations, but isolation in cell cultures is more sensitive. Follicular conjunctivitis in adult Europeans or Americans living in trachomatous regions is rarely trachoma.

Sporadic cases of adult inclusion conjunctivitis must be differentiated from adenovirus and herpes simplex virus keratoconjunctivitis during the first 15 days after onset, and later from other forms of chronic follicular conjunctivitis. Demonstration of chlamydial infection by Giemsa- or immunofluorescent-stained smears or by isolation in cell cultures constitutes definitive evidence of infection. Genital examination and tests for genital chlamydial infection are indicated. Serum antibody does not constitute evidence of chlamydial eye infection since many sexually active adults have serum antibody. A practical diagnostic procedure in cases with chronic follicular conjunctivitis is treatment for 6 days with an oral tetracycline or erythromycin; a marked symptomatic response within 3 to 4 days is highly suggestive of inclusion conjunctivitis, and treatment should be continued for at least 3 weeks.

DIFFERENTIAL DIAGNOSIS OF CONJUNCTIVITIS AND KERATOCONJUNCTIVITIS The eye and its adnexa may be infected during the course of many cutaneous and systemic viral diseases. Sometimes these ocular infections produce minor manifestations, such as the transient loss of accommodation in dengue and the milder forms of conjunctivitis in systemic adenovirus infections. Other virus infections, however, such as herpes simplex (see Chap. 135), herpes zoster (see Chap. 136), measles (see Chap. 141), and vaccinia (see Chap. 143), occasionally produce serious and permanent visual loss. In addition, congenital infections are an important cause of blindness, particularly rubella, which leads to cataracts and microphthalmus, cytomegalic inclusion disease with retinal involvement, and syphilis with interstitial keratitis. Among the viral infections limited to the outer eye and manifested as a follicular conjunctivitis are epidemic keratoconjunctivitis (EKC), herpes simplex keratoconjunctivitis, Newcastle disease virus (NDV) conjunctivitis, and acute hemorrhagic conjunctivitis.

TREATMENT Public health control programs for endemic trachoma have consisted of the mass application of tetracycline or erythromycin ointment to the eyes of all children in affected communities for 21 to 60 days or on an intermittent schedule. These programs also include surgical correction of inturned eyelids by a mobile surgical team that visits each locality. Oral erythromycin, but not oral tetracyclines, offers an alternative method of mass antibiotic treatment for trachoma of young children and pregnant women.

Adult inclusion conjunctivitis responds well to treatment with full doses of systemic tetracycline or erythromycin for 3 weeks. Treating all sexual consorts of the patient simultaneously is also necessary to prevent ocular reinfection and to avoid the genital diseases due to chlamydial infection. Topical antibiotic treatment is not required in patients treated with systemic antibiotics.

PREVENTION Efforts to develop a trachoma vaccine have not yet been successful. General hygienic measures associated with improved living standards are effective in the elimination of endemic trachoma. Adequate water supply for personal cleanliness may be a key factor. In some areas the reduction of flies in the household is important.

OTHER INFECTIONS CAUSED BY *C. TRACHOMATIS* IN ADULTS

C. trachomatis has been reported as an infrequent cause of subacute endocarditis, peritonitis, pleuritis, and possibly appendicitis, and may cause respiratory infections in older children and adults. Immunosuppressed patients with pneumonia have had, in some cases, either serologic or cultural evidence of *C. trachomatis* infection, but more data are necessary to define the role of *Chlamydia* in these patients.

PSITTACOSIS

DEFINITION Psittacosis is primarily an infectious disease of birds caused by *Chlamydia psittaci*. Transmission of infection from birds to humans results in a febrile illness characterized by pneumonitis and systemic manifestations. Inapparent infections or mild influenza-like illnesses may also occur. The term *ornithosis* is sometimes applied to infections contracted from birds other than parrots or parakeets, but *psittacosis* is the preferred generic term for all forms of the disease.

EPIDEMIOLOGY Almost any avian species can harbor *C. psittaci*. Psittacine birds (parrots, parakeets, budgerigars) are most commonly infected, but human cases have been traced to contact with pigeons, ducks, turkeys, chickens, and many other birds. Psittacosis may be considered an occupational disease of pet-shop owners, poultry workers, pigeon fanciers, taxidermists, veterinarians, and zoo attendants. Since 1973, there has been a steady increase in incidence, with cases occurring primarily among employees of poultry processing plants. It is suspected that many cases are undiagnosed and not reported. The disease appears to be more common in England, where budgerigars are popular household pets and where restrictions on the importation of these birds have been eased.

The agent is present in nasal secretions, excreta, tissues, and feathers of infected birds. Although the disease can be fatal, infected birds frequently show only minor evidence of illness, such as ruffled feathers, lethargy, and anorexia. Asymptomatic avian carriers are common, and complete recovery may be followed by continued shedding of the organism for many months.

Psittacosis is almost always transmitted to humans by the respiratory route. On rare occasions the disease may be acquired from the bite of a pet bird. Prolonged contact is not essential for transmission of the disease; a few minutes spent in an environment previously occupied by an infected bird has resulted in human infection. The severity of the disease in humans bears no apparent relationship to closeness or duration of contact, although sick birds are more likely to transmit infection than healthy ones. Transmission of a psittacosis-like agent between humans has occurred among hospital personnel, with severe and sometimes fatal infections. There is evidence that these "human" strains are more virulent than native avian organisms. There is no record of infection acquired by eating poultry products.

PATHOGENESIS The psittacosis agent gains entrance to the body through the upper part of the respiratory tract, spreads via the bloodstream, and eventually localizes in the pulmonary alveoli and in the reticuloendothelial cells of the spleen and liver. Invasion of the lung probably takes place by way of the bloodstream rather than by direct extension from the upper air passages. A lymphocytic inflammatory response occurs on both the interstitial and respiratory surfaces of the alveoli as well as in the perivascular spaces. The alveolar walls and interstitial tissues of the lung are thickened, edematous, necrotic, and occasionally hemorrhagic. Histologically, the affected areas show alveolar spaces filled with fluid, erythrocytes, and lymphocytes. The picture is not pathognomonic of psittacosis unless macrophages containing characteristic cytoplasmic inclusion bodies (LCL bodies) can be identified. The respiratory epithelium of the bronchi and bronchioles usually remains intact.

CLINICAL MANIFESTATIONS The clinical manifestations and course of psittacosis are extremely variable. After an incubation period of 7 to 14 days or longer, the disease may start abruptly with shaking chills and fever ranging as high as 40.5°C (105°F), but the onset is often gradual with increasing fever over a 3- to 4-day period. Headache is almost always a prominent symptom; it is usually diffuse and excruciating and often the patient's chief complaint.

Many patients present with a dry hacking cough which is usually nonproductive, but small amounts of mucoid or bloody sputum may be raised as the disease progresses. Cough may appear early in the course of the disease or as late as 5 days after the onset of fever. Chest pain, pleurisy with effusion, or a friction rub may all occur but are rare. Pericarditis and myocarditis have been reported. Most patients have a normal or slightly increased respiratory rate; marked dyspnea with cyanosis occurs only in severe psittacosis with extensive pulmonary involvement. In psittacosis, as in most nonbacterial pneumonias, the physical signs of pneumonitis tend to be less prominent than symptoms and x-ray findings would suggest. The initial examination may reveal fine, sibilant rales, or clinical evidence of pneumonia may be completely lacking. Rales usually become audible and more numerous as the illness progresses. Signs of frank pulmonary consolidation are usually absent. Symptoms of upper respiratory tract infection are not prominent, although mild sore throat, pharyngitis, and cervical adenopathy are often present; on occasion they may be the only manifestations of illness. Epistaxis is encountered early in the course of nearly one-fourth of the cases. Photophobia is also a common complaint.

There is commonly a complaint of generalized myalgia, and spasm and stiffness of the muscles of the back and neck may lead to an erroneous diagnosis of meningitis. Lethargy, mental depression, agitation, insomnia, and disorientation have been prominent features of the illness in some epidemics, but not in others; delirium and stupor occur near the end of the first week in severe cases. Occasional patients are comatose when first seen, and the diagnosis of psittacosis may be missed. Gastrointestinal complaints such as abdominal pain, nausea, vomiting, or diarrhea are present in some cases; constipation and abdominal distention sometimes occur as late complications. Icterus, the result of severe hepatic involvement, is a rare and ominous finding. A faint, macular rash (Horder's spots) simulating the rose spots of typhoid fever has been described.

Patients without cough or other clinical evidence of respiratory involvement present as fever of unknown origin (see Chap. 20). The pulse rate is slow in relation to the fever. When splenomegaly is present in a patient with acute pneumonitis, psittacosis should be considered; the reported incidence of splenomegaly ranges from 10 to 70 percent. Nontender hepatic enlargement also occurs, but jaundice is rare. Thrombophlebitis is not unusual during convalescence; indeed, pulmonary infarction is sometimes a late complication and may be fatal.

In untreated cases of psittacosis, sustained or mildly remittent fever persists for 10 days to 3 weeks, or occasionally as long as 3 months. Over this period, the respiratory manifestations gradually abate. Psittacosis contracted from parrots or parakeets is more likely to be a severe, prolonged illness than infections acquired from pigeons or barnyard fowl. Relapses occur but are rare. Occasional patients develop endocarditis, and *C. psittaci* infection should be considered in cases of culture-negative endocarditis. Secondary bacterial infections are uncommon. Immunity to reinfection is probably permanent.

LABORATORY FINDINGS The chest x-ray in psittacosis mimics that in a great variety of pulmonary diseases. The pneumonic lesions are usually patchy in appearance but can be hazy, diffuse, homogeneous, lobar, atelectatic, wedge-shaped, nodular, or miliary. The white blood cell count is normal or moderately decreased in the acute phase of the disease but may rise in convalescence. The erythrocyte sedimentation rate is frequently not elevated. Transient proteinuria is common. The cerebrospinal fluid sometimes contains a few mononuclear cells but is otherwise normal. Despite hepatomegaly, liver function tests are generally normal.

The diagnosis can be confirmed only by isolation of the causative microorganism or by serologic studies. The agent is present in the blood during the acute phase of the disease and in the bronchial secretions for weeks or sometimes years after infection, but it is difficult to isolate. Psittacosis is most readily diagnosed by the demonstration of a rising titer of complement-fixing antibody in serum. An acute and convalescent specimen should always be tested. *C. trachomatis*, *C. psittaci*, and *C. pneumoniae* share a common genus-specific "group" antigen, which is the basis of the complement fixation test and can lead to cross reactions in the micro-IF test as well. These three species have different protein antigens that are principal antigens in the micro-IF test. The prompt initiation of treatment with tetracycline has been shown to delay antibody rise in convalescence for several weeks or months. Interpretation of a single complement fixation test may be difficult because of the antigenic cross reaction between *C. psittaci, C. pneumoniae,* and *C. trachomatis.*

DIFFERENTIAL DIAGNOSIS   A history of exposure to birds may be the only clinical basis for differentiating psittacosis from a great variety of infectious and noninfectious febrile disorders. A partial list of pulmonary diseases that may be confused with psittacosis includes *Mycoplasma* pneumonia, *C. pneumoniae* pneumonia, legionellosis (see Chap. 124), viral pneumonia, Q fever, coccidioidomycosis, tuberculosis, enteroviral infection, carcinoma of the lung with bronchial obstruction, and common bacterial pneumonias. In the early stages, before pneumonitis appears, psittacosis may be mistaken for influenza, typhoid fever, miliary tuberculosis, and infectious mononucleosis.

TREATMENT   The tetracyclines are consistently effective in the treatment of psittacosis. Defervescence and alleviation of symptoms usually occur in 24 to 48 h after instituting therapy with 2 g daily in four divided doses. To avoid relapse, treatment should probably be continued for at least 7 days after defervescence. In severe cases, hospitalization and pulmonary intensive care may be indicated. Sulfonamides are not active against *C. psittaci.*

C. PNEUMONIAE INFECTIONS

A third and previously unrecognized chlamydial species, *C. pneumoniae,* has been described by Grayston and coworkers. *C. pneumoniae* shares genus-specific antigens with *C. trachomatis* and *C. psittaci* but is otherwise serologically distinct. *C. pneumoniae* can also be distinguished from the other two species on the basis of DNA hybridization and restriction endonuclease analyses. Although *C. pneumoniae* can be grown in a variety of cell cultures, it is considerably more difficult to culture than other chlamydiae, especially from clinical specimens. Fewer than 50 isolates have been obtained from patients worldwide.

Knowledge of the epidemiology of *C. pneumoniae* infections has been derived primarily from serologic studies. Infections begin to occur in late childhood and adolescence and continue to develop throughout adult life. Seroprevalence in many adult populations that have been tested throughout the world exceeds 40 percent and suggests that *C. pneumoniae* infections are ubiquitous. Secondary infections appear to occur in older adults. In Scandinavia, *C. pneumoniae* produces epidemics of pneumonia and respiratory illness followed by periods of infrequent infection. The incidence of infections that occur outside of epidemics remains poorly defined. Transmission is presumed to be from person to person.

The clinical spectrum of *C. pneumoniae* infection includes acute pharyngitis, sinusitis, bronchitis, and pneumonitis, primarily in young adults. The pneumonitis resembles *Mycoplasma pneumoniae* pneumonia because patients often have prominent antecedent upper respiratory tract symptoms, fever, nonproductive cough, mild to moderate degree of illness, absence of leukocytosis, minimal findings on chest auscultation, and small segmental infiltrates on chest x-ray. In elderly patients, pneumonia due to *C. pneumoniae* can be more severe and may necessitate hospitalization and respiratory support.

Diagnosis of *C. pneumoniae* is uncertain because cell culture techniques are probably too insensitive for routine clinical use and noncultural tests using antigen detection methods or DNA probes have not been developed. Acute and convalescent sera can be tested for chlamydial CF antibody to make a retrospective diagnosis. However, this test does not distinguish *C. pneumoniae* infection from infection due to *C. trachomatis* or *C. psittaci.* Although controlled treatment trials have not been conducted, *C. pneumoniae* is inhibited in vitro by erythromycin and tetracycline. Recommended therapy is 2 g/d of either agent for 10 to 14 days.

REFERENCES

ADGER H et al: Screening for *Chlamydia trachomatis* and *Neisseria gonorrhoeae* in adolescent males: Values of first catch urine examination. Lancet 2:944, 1984
ALEXANDER ER, HARRISON HR: Role of *Chlamydia trachomatis* in perinatal infection. Rev Infect Dis 5:713, 1983
BRUNHAM RC et al: Mucopurulent cervicitis—the ignored counterpart in women of urethritis in men. N Engl J Med 311:1, 1984
CENTERS FOR DISEASE CONTROL: *Chlamydia trachomatis* infections: Policy guidelines for prevention and control. Morb Mort Week Rep 34:535, 1985
COULTS II et al: Clinical and radiographic features of psittacosis infection. Thorax 40:530, 1985
GRAYSTON JT: *Chlamydia pneumoniae,* strain TWAR. Chest 95:664, 1989
——— et al: A new *Chlamydia psittaci* strain, TWAR, isolated in acute respiratory tract infections. N Engl J Med 315:161, 1986
HANDSFIELD HH et al: Criteria for selective screening for *Chlamydia trachomatis* infection in women attending family planning clinics. JAMA 255:1730, 1986
MÄRDH PA: Ascending chlamydial infection in the female tract, in *Chlamydial Infections,* D Oriel et al (eds). London, Cambridge University Press, 1986
McCORMACK WM: Chlamydial infections in men, in *Chlamydial Infections,* D Oriel et al (eds). London, Cambridge University Press, 1986
SCHACHTER J et al: Experience with the routine use of erythromycin for chlamydial infections in pregnancy. N Engl J Med 314:276, 1986
STAMM WE: Diagnosis of *Chlamydia trachomatis* genitourinary infections. Ann Intern Med 108:710, 1988
——— et al: *Chlamydia trachomatis* urethral infections in men. Prevalence, risk factors, and clinical manifestations. Ann Intern Med 100:47, 1984

section 11 Protozoal and helminthic infections

156 THE IMMUNOLOGY OF PARASITES

JOHN R. DAVID

During the past decade interest in parasitic diseases of humans and in new approaches to their control has increased steadily. One reason for this is the enormous scope of the problem. Over a billion people in the world are affected by parasitic diseases. Although accurate statistics are difficult to obtain, it is estimated that over 200 million people have malaria, the most serious protozoan disease of humans, and that more than a million children die of malaria each year in Africa alone. Schistosomiasis, a disease caused by helminths that are transmitted by snails, affects 200 to 300 million persons. Filarial parasites affect an equal number of people, and one of these, *Onchocerca volvulus,* is the second major cause of blindness in the world. *Trypanosoma cruzi,* another protozoan, is the major cause of heart disease in South America, and hookworm infects over 800 million persons.

With the modernization of developing countries, many of these diseases are becoming more prevalent. For example, the pressure to provide energy for industrialization leads to building dams which have brought about profound changes in the local environment; the lake behind the Volta Dam has increased the coastline by 4000 miles, and the snails on its banks infected with schistosomes have increased the prevalence of schistosomiasis in people living on the lake's borders from a few percent to almost 100 percent. Improvement schemes for agriculture often involve extension of irrigation for the cultivation of rice. Some of these projects have been associated with increases in transmission of malaria by mosquitoes, which breed in the irrigation ditches. Another example of the unanticipated effects of progress can be seen in the Amazon basin, where the clearing of the forests in order to reclaim the land for industry and agriculture has greatly increased human contact with sandflies which live in these areas and transmit leishmaniasis.

Another reason for the increasing focus on these diseases by scientists and physicians is that the classic control measures are less than adequate. The most telling example of this is malaria. After World War II, there was great optimism that this disease could be eradicated by spraying homes with DDT and by treating the disease in humans with chloroquine. After an extensive eradication program was instituted in the early 1960s in Sri Lanka, only 18 cases of malaria were reported in that country. However, 5 years later there were over a half million cases. The failure of malaria eradication was due to at least three factors: (1) the surveillance stage of the eradication effort was not maintained; (2) mosquitoes became resistant to DDT; and (3) the parasite became resistant to chloroquine. Moreover, the cost of these control measures proved to be enormous.

The large number of people affected by parasitic diseases, the increasing environmental changes in the developing world, and the failure of classic control programs have stimulated the search for new approaches for the control of these disorders. One of these approaches is immunologic. Currently, immunologists are studying several aspects of parasites' interaction with the host. They are trying to delineate the mechanisms that parasites have evolved to evade the immune response of the host, to define which immune mechanisms they do not escape, and to learn which immune responses are the basis for the pathologic lesions. Immunology is also providing diagnostic tests and ultimately, it is hoped, will provide effective vaccines for some of these diseases. At present, there is not a single vaccine available to protect humans against parasites, despite the availability of several effective vaccines against animal parasitic diseases. For the purposes of this discussion, the most useful way to present the problems of vaccine development in these complex diseases is to give a relatively detailed description of what is being done in one disease, malaria, rather than a cursory summary of many.

MALARIA VACCINE Although investigators are trying to produce vaccines to many parasites, especially intensive work is under way on vaccines for *Plasmodium falciparum*, the most malignant malaria parasite. In order to understand the various approaches that are being pursued, it is necessary to review briefly the life cycle of the malaria parasite (see Chap. 159). When an infected mosquito bites a human, it injects the motile sporozoite, which is in its salivary gland. In less than half an hour, the sporozoite leaves the blood and invades the liver. It then goes through the exoerythrocytic cycle, undergoing asexual division by schizogony and producing many merozoites. These burst out of the liver cells into the blood and invade erythrocytes. Here, they differentiate into trophozoites, undergo division by schizogony, and burst, liberating more merozoites, which reinvade erythrocytes and continue the cycle. Some of the merozoites develop into the sexual stages, the gametocytes. When a mosquito bites an infected person, the gametocytes are taken up in the blood meal and rapidly come out of the erythrocytes. The male microgametes then fertilize the female macrogametes, forming the ookinete and then the oocyst. Further division within the oocyst leads to the infective stage, the sporozoite. Several of these stages can be targeted for immunologic attack by a vaccine.

Sporozoite vaccine Persons can become immune to *P. falciparum* via the sporozoite stage. This has been shown by allowing irradiated infected mosquitoes (containing irradiated sporozoites which cannot divide) to bite humans. Investigations have resulted in the characterization of a single sporozoite antigen. Monoclonal antibodies to this antigen can passively transfer resistance to malaria in rodents and monkeys. Using recombinant DNA technology, the gene coding for the protective sporozoite antigen of *P. falciparum* has been cloned. The protective epitope is made up of four amino acids repeated 23 times. Two trials of recombinant or synthetic sporozoite vaccines in humans had disappointing results; in general, the vaccines elicited poor antibody responses, and parasitemia was prevented in only a few individuals who had high titers of antibody. Studies suggest that the repeat portion of the circumsporozoite antigen may have limited immunogenicity; efforts are being made to improve immunogenicity by combining the repeat sequence with potent T-cell epitopes found elsewhere in the molecule. T-cell epitopes need to be used not only to enhance the antibody response but also because both γ-interferon, a T-cell lymphokine, and CD8 cytotoxic T cells play a protective role in the early stages of malaria in mice. Such epitopes should be on the natural molecule and not on an artificial carrier if the immunity from the vaccine is to be boosted in nature. The possibility of genetic restriction to these T-cell epitopes may complicate the development of an effective vaccine. Immunomodulators incorporated into the vaccine may be helpful in enhancing the immune response. The advantages of the sporozoite vaccine are that it may protect against different strains of *P. falciparum* and that it inhibits the early liver stages of the parasite. The disadvantage is that it may be an all-or-none phenomenon; if a few sporozoites evaded the immune response, the person might get malaria.

Blood-stage vaccine The host encounters merozoites for short periods as they leave one erythrocyte and invade another. Erythrocytes infected by parasites develop new antigens of parasite origin on their surfaces. Both merozoites and infected erythrocytes can be targets for a vaccine. Monoclonal antibodies to this stage in rodent malaria confer partial protection when transferred passively, and antigens isolated by means of these antibodies can induce protective immunity. There has been some success in protecting primates with blood-stage vaccines using recombinant or synthesized antigens combined with complete Freund's adjuvant. One study reported partial protection of humans using a combination of several synthetic peptides polymerized together. T cells have also been shown to play a role in immunity in mice during the blood stage.

Blood-stage vaccines have the advantage that they act against the parasite at the merozoite stage, which involves a longer interaction with the host than the sporozoite stage and also causes the symptoms and the pathology. Their disadvantages are that adjuvants are necessary in most cases, the vaccines may be strain-specific, and some of these antigens may exhibit variation.

Gamete vaccine If antibodies are raised against gametes in an animal, they will be taken up with the gametes when the mosquito bites and will then neutralize the gametes escaping from the erythrocytes in the mosquito. Several gamete antigens have been isolated, and some have been cloned. Monoclonal antibodies to these will prevent the fertilization of the gametes in the mosquito, thus blocking transmission. Studies suggest that natural antigamete antibodies to *P. vivax* may play a part in limiting the transmission of malaria. Because the antigamete vaccine would not protect the individual but might reduce transmission, it could be incorporated into a multivalent vaccine.

IMMUNE EVASION BY PARASITES Parasites have developed a variety of ingenious ways of evading the immune response of the host. Some of these are listed in Table 156-1. The most fascinating mechanism is that of antigenic variation by African trypanosomes, the flagellated protozoa transmitted by the tsetse fly that is the cause of sleeping sickness (see Chap. 161). The trypanosome has a thick surface coat, which is made up of many molecules of a single antigenic glycoprotein. When cloned organisms, all having the same surface antigen, are injected into certain animals, successive waves of parasitemia ensue similar to those seen when a human is bitten by an infected tsetse fly. The peak of each wave consists of organisms expressing a single variant surface glycoprotein antigen (VSG), and this VSG is different from VSGs expressed by organisms in previous peaks in the same animal. A cloned organism can produce over 100

TABLE 156-1   Some mechanisms of immune evasion

Parasite	Mechanism
Trypanosoma brucei	Antigenic variation
Toxoplasma	Lysosome-phagosome fusion prevented
Malaria, Babesia	Escape into host cells
Schistosomes	Host molecule acquisition
	Loss of surface antigens
	Intrinsic membrane changes
	Immune-complex blockade
Filaria, Leishmania	Specific T-cell suppression
Taenia, amebae	Inactivation of mediators of inflammation

different VSGs! Each peak of parasitemia induces soluble antibody directed at the major VSG. Presumably the antibody eliminates the organism with that specific VSG, but trypanosomes that can switch to another VSG escape. Analysis of the amino acid sequence of a number of VSGs indicates that they do not differ by only a few substitutions, which could be explained by point mutations; on the contrary, the amino acid sequence of each VSG is quite different.

Studies of the genes encoding the VSGs have shown that each VSG is encoded by a distinct gene. Every trypanosome, regardless of the VSG it is expressing, contains a copy of each VSG gene. Trypanosomes have several mechanisms for expressing a VSG. For example, the organism expressing a particular VSG gene may have an additional, duplicate copy of that gene; this is referred to as the *expression-linked copy*. Studies using restriction enzymes indicate that the expression-linked copy is moved to a new site in the trypanosome near the telomere that is gene-specific for expression. If each gene is visualized as a tape cassette in a library, to express the VSG the cassette is duplicated, the duplicate is removed from the library, inserted into a genetic tape deck, and expressed. Although recent studies have revealed alternatives to the formation of an expression-linked copy for VSG gene activation, the molecular mechanism of gene expression is still unclear.

It was thought initially that the driving force for antigenic variation was antibody to that antigen; however, it has been shown that antigenic variation can be triggered in the absence of antibody both in vitro and in vivo.

Some organisms have developed multiple ways of evading the immune response. Schistosomes, for instance, can lose surface antigens after they enter the host, can take up host antigens and masquerade as host tissue, can develop certain intrinsic membrane changes making them resistant to attack even when surface antigens are present, and can shed antigens which may block effector cells and antibodies. A number of parasites, *Toxoplasma* being one example, when engulfed by a macrophage, prevent the fusion of the phagosome with the lysosomes. Others, such as *Leishmania*, do not prevent fusion when engulfed but are resistant to toxic substances in the lysosomes of the macrophage. A lipophosphoglycan (LPG) molecule on the surface of *Leishmania* is thought to play a role in this immune evasion. Indeed, the length of the carbohydrate chains on the LPG molecule may determine whether the organism can resist lysis by the alternate complement pathway. Still other parasites, such as *Trypanosoma cruzi*, escape from the lysosomes into the cytoplasm.

A number of parasites such as filaria, *Leishmania*, and *Plasmodium* induce strong suppressor mechanisms, including T suppressor cells, which dampen or eliminate the host's effective immune response. Organisms evade lysis by the alternative complement pathway by a number of means, including the presentation of surface glycoproteins that bind the inactive fragment, iC3b, rather than the hemolytically active C3b. Some parasites can destroy mediators of inflammation involved in an effective immune response. For example, *Taenia* destroys complement components, and amebae produce factors that neutralize chemotaxins for macrophages. Other parasites such as *Ascaris* appear to have a surface coat that is antigenic and can induce an immune response but is, nevertheless, resistant to immune system attack.

Although some parasites can evade the immune response, they can induce an effective protective immune response to a subsequent infection by the same species. This is called *concomitant immunity* or *premunition*.

EFFECTOR MECHANISMS AGAINST PARASITES   Mechanisms that may be effective against parasites include the following: antibodies, cells including cytotoxic T cells, T-cell–induced activated macrophages, natural killer cells, and a variety of cells that mediate antibody-dependent cell-mediated cytotoxicity. Amplifiers of the immune system such as lymphokines and complement are also involved.

Immunity against several parasites such as malaria, schistosomes, and *Trypanosoma cruzi* can be transferred by antibodies. Nevertheless, evidence obtained in a number of animal models suggests that cell-mediated immunity is also involved against these and other parasites, including the organisms causing malaria, leishmaniasis, toxoplasmosis, schistosomiasis, filariasis, and trichinosis. Studies in mice have shown that protective immunity to *Leishmania* is generally associated with the T-cell subset T_{H1}, which produces interleukin 2 (IL-2) and γ-interferon, whereas the T_{H2} subset, which produces IL-4 and IL-5, usually exacerbates the disease. It is less clear whether protective immunity develops against amebae, African trypanosomes, or hookworm. There appears to be no naturally acquired immunity to *Ascaris*, guinea worm, or pinworm.

Two immune mechanisms have been described which appear to be unique for helminths. These involve eosinophils in one case and IgE in the other.

EOSINOPHILS AND ANTIBODY-DEPENDENT CELL-MEDIATED CYTOTOXICITY (ADCC)   It has been known for over 100 years that eosinophils are associated with helminth infections, but only in the past few years has it become known that these cells can function as killer cells. Specifically, highly purified preparations of eosinophils, when mixed with antibody-coated schistosomula of *Schistosoma mansoni* in vitro, killed the larvae. The antibody formed is of the IgG class, and the eosinophils attach to the Fc portion of the IgG by the cells' Fc receptor. Immune complexes or staphylococcal protein A, which can interfere with the binding of eosinophils to the Fc portion of the antibody, inhibit the reaction. Incubation at 37°C makes the interaction between eosinophils and antibody-coated schistosomula become irreversible. This is associated with degranulation and the release of major basic protein (MBP), the most abundant protein in the eosinophil granule, and eosinophil cationic protein (ECP) over the surface of the schistosomula. MBP and ECP, in turn, are toxic to the larvae. Eosinophils can also kill other helminths such as *Trichinella spiralis*, presumably by a similar mechanism.

Eosinophils from patients with eosinophilia exhibit an enhanced ability to kill antibody-coated schistosomula in vitro; they act as if they were activated. Moreover, a number of soluble substances such as granulocyte-monocyte colony stimulating factor (GM-CSF), tumor necrosis factor (TNF), and a monocyte-derived eosinophil cytotoxic enhancing factor (ECEF) can increase the eosinophil's capacity to kill in vitro. Eosinophils are activated in cancer patients treated with IL-2 and lymphokine-activated killer cells generated by IL-2. IL-5 stimulates eosinophilia. In mice, this lymphokine is produced by the T_{H2} subset of T cells. Mice given anti-IL-5 antibodies have very few eosinophils, providing a good model for studying the role of eosinophils in immunity.

ROLE FOR IgE   The observation that IgE levels are elevated in some persons in the tropics, notably those infected with helminths, suggests that IgE may act to protect the host against parasites. The mediators released by triggered mast cells could affect the parasites directly, or, by increasing vascular permeability and releasing eosinophil chemotactic factors, they could lead to the accumulation of necessary antibodies (IgG) and cells to attack the parasite. IgE immune complexes can induce macrophage-mediated cytotoxicity to schistosomula. Rats made specifically IgE-deficient by the repeated injection of antiepsilon chain antibodies show markedly impaired resistance to *Trichinella* infection. IgE also plays an important role in pathology associated with parasites, such as in the tropical eosinophilia syndrome associated with filariasis; it mediates immediate hypersensitivity reactions triggered by parasites.

IMMUNOPATHOLOGY Immune mechanisms play a major role in the pathology induced by many parasites. Such mechanisms are the cause of the granulomatous reaction to eggs of *S. mansoni* which is the basis of the immunopathology of this disease; immune-complex renal disease in malaria and visceral leishmaniasis; heart disease due to *T. cruzi;* the obstructive and ocular disease in filariasis and onchocerciasis; the muscle pathology in trichinosis; the allergic reactions to ruptured hydatid cyst fluid; and the pulmonary complications to migrating nematode larvae. Just as suppressor mechanisms are involved in damping protective immunity, they are also involved in modulating the immunopathology. An example of this is the modulation of *S. mansoni* granulomas by T suppressor cells. Anti-idiotypic antibodies (see next section) can modify the host's response to the parasite. Some patients, including infants born to mothers with schistosomiasis, have anti-idiotypic T cells which react to antiegg antibodies. The precise role played by anti-idiotypic T cells and/or antigen transferred from mother to infant in the modulation of the child's immune response to the parasites needs further clarification.

MONOCLONAL AND ANTI-IDIOTYPIC ANTIBODIES Monoclonal antibodies to various stages of malaria parasites have been used to detect antigens that can induce protective immunity. In addition, passive protection has been demonstrated with monoclonal antibodies to the promastigote stage of *Leishmania mexicana* and to schistosomula of *S. mansoni.* Because of their specificity, monoclonal antibodies can also be used for diagnosis because they can be selected not to show the multiple cross-reactions with other parasites that are frequently found with sera from infected animals. For example, species-specific monoclonal antibodies have been developed which can distinguish between five different species of South American *Leishmania* without cross-reacting with *T. cruzi.* Antibodies in the serum of an infected patient will usually cross-react with all these parasites. Diagnostic tests using these antibodies have been developed.

An antibody to an antigen has a specific antigen unique to itself on the immunoglobulin. This antigen is called the *idiotype,* which is the unique amino acid sequence and configuration of the antigen-binding site of that antibody. For instance, it is possible to make an antibody to a particular monoclonal antibody; that antibody will then recognize the idiotype and is called an *anti-idiotypic antibody.* The monoclonal antibody will bind to the anti-idiotype or to the original antigen. If a monoclonal antibody to a parasite were used to induce an anti-idiotypic antibody, it should be possible to induce protective immunity with this anti-idiotype instead of using the antigen. This would have the advantage of bypassing the need to purify antigens and then to produce them in large quantities. This novel strategy for the production of a vaccine is under study. It has proved successful in producing immunity to schistosomiasis in rats.

The rapidly accelerating pace of discovery and definition of the regulatory systems of the immune response, together with the revolution in technology, may soon make it possible to induce stronger protective immunity artificially than that which is acquired naturally, and the prediction that vaccines can be produced against the diseases caused by a number of parasites is based on this assumption.

REFERENCES

DAVID JR: Host-parasite interface: Immune evasion, in *Tropical and Geographical Medicine,* 2d ed, KS Warren, AF Mahmoud (eds). New York, McGraw-Hill, 1990, p 117

DONELSON JE, TURNER MJ: How the trypanosome changes its coat. Sci Am 252(2):44, 1985

ENGLUND PT, SHER A (eds): *The Biology of Animal Parasitism.* New York, Plenum, 1986

HOMMELL M: Antigenic variation in malaria parasites. Immunol Today 6:28, 1985

MILLER LH et al: Research toward malaria vaccines. Science 234:1349, 1986

SILBERSTEIN DS, DAVID JR: The regulation of human eosinophil function by cytokines. Immunol Today 8:380, 1987

TRAGER W: *Living Together. The Biology of Animal Parasitism.* New York, Plenum, 1986

157 DIAGNOSIS OF PARASITIC INFECTIONS

JAMES J. PLORDE

SIGNIFICANCE OF PARASITIC INFECTIONS Parasitic diseases such as malaria, trypanosomiasis, leishmaniasis, schistosomiasis, and filariasis remain among the major causes of human sickness and death in the world. A number of technical, social, economic, and political phenomena have combined to produce a dramatic increase in the prevalence of some of these illnesses. This has been most devastating in the case of malaria. Growing resistance of the mosquito vector to insecticides, development of drug-resistant strains of *Plasmodium falciparum,* and cutbacks in many malaria control programs have led to a worldwide resurgence of this disease. At present, over 1 billion people reside in endemic areas; between 125 and 200 million of these are infected at any given time. In Africa, where the intensity of parasite transmission defies current control measures, malaria kills over 1 million children annually. The resurgence of malaria together with an increase in international travel has resulted in an upsurge in the number of infected patients who enter the United States. From 1969 to 1980 civilian malaria cases reported annually to the Centers for Disease Control have increased from 151 to 1864; in the seven subsequent years, the number has averaged 1000 cases annually. Over the same 18-year period, the number of infections involving U.S. citizens has climbed steadily from 90 to 421.

In Africa, from the Sahara in the north to the Kalahari Desert in the south, human strains of *Trypanosoma brucei* cause one of the most lethal of all human diseases, sleeping sickness. Animal strains of this species limit food supply in the same area through their impact on animal husbandry. In South America, a related organism, *T. cruzi,* infects several million people, leaving many with severe heart and gastrointestinal lesions (Chagas' disease).

Leishmaniasis is found in parts of Europe, Asia, Africa, and South and Central America where it may present as a chronic, highly lethal infection of the reticuloendothelial system (kala azar), a mutilating mucocutaneous infection (espundia), or a self-limiting skin ulcer (oriental sore).

Schistosomiasis is the most serious of the helminthic infections, affecting an estimated 200 million individuals living between the tropics of Cancer and Capricorn. In many it produces bladder, intestinal, and/or liver disease which can eventually result in death. In many countries irrigation schemes have resulted in the dissemination of the disease to previously uninvolved areas, mitigating the economic gains of these projects. Although not transmitted in the continental United States, exogenously acquired schistosomiasis involves nearly a half million people now residing in this country.

Wuchereria bancrofti and *Brugia malayi,* two closely related filarial worms, obstruct lymphatic circulation and produce grotesque swellings of the legs, arms, and genitals in tropical populations. Onchocerciasis, another filarial infection, affects millions of people in Africa, leaving thousands blind.

Toxoplasmosis, pneumocystosis, giardiasis, cryptosporidiosis, and trichomoniasis are five cosmopolitan protozoan infections well known in the United States. The first infects perhaps one-third of the world's population. Although it is usually asymptomatic, congenital toxoplasmosis may result in abortion, stillbirth, prematurity, or severe neurologic defects. Even when there are no obvious signs at birth, chorioretinitis with visual impairment may occur years later. Mild or asymptomatic toxoplasma, pneumocystis, and cryptosporidia infections can result in fatal illness later in life during periods of immunosuppression.

In contrast, giardiasis and trichomoniasis seldom result in severe disability; nevertheless they cause morbidity in millions of otherwise healthy individuals. Both appear to be increasing in incidence, apparently the result of changing American lifestyles. Giardiasis is particularly frequent among day-care center attendees, hikers and campers in western states, and male homosexuals who practice anilingus, while the incidence of trichomoniasis is closely tied to the level of promiscuous heterosexual activity.

DIAGNOSIS Although some of the diseases mentioned above are uncommon in the United States, the continuous arrival of travelers and immigrants from endemic areas of the world makes it necessary to consider them in the differential diagnosis of many illnesses. Typically, neither the clinical manifestations nor the general laboratory findings observed in patients suffering from parasitic infections are sufficiently unique to raise this possibility in the mind of the clinician. Although eosinophilia has long been recognized as a clue to the presence of a hidden parasite, this phenomenon is characteristic only of helminthic infections. Even here its absence does not preclude this diagnosis. The eosinophilia reflects the terminal step in the host's immunologic response to worm antigens mounted during the stage of tissue migration and invasion. Once migration ceases and the worm matures to adulthood, eosinophilia may diminish or disappear.

PARASITE RECOVERY AND IDENTIFICATION Unless a careful travel, transfusion, and socioeconomic history is taken, the correct diagnosis may never be entertained. Once considered, however, the presence of a parasitic disease is easily confirmed. Most commonly, this is accomplished by the recovery and morphologic identification of the parasite in the stool, urine, sputum, blood, or tissues of the patient.

In intestinal infections, examination of a wet-mount and/or stained smear of the stool is usually adequate. Because many parasites are passed intermittently or in fluctuating numbers, the examination of a single stool specimen may detect only one-third to one-half of involved patients. The testing of three such specimens collected at intervals of 2 or 3 days will improve this yield substantially. Alternatively, a saline cathartic may be administered to evacuate the cecal area, where many protozoa are concentrated, and the entire purge examined. The stool must be free of interfering substances such as antidiarrheal or contrast agents, antacids, and antibiotics. If the appropriate specimens cannot be obtained prior to administration of such substances, testing should be performed 1 week or, in the case of antimicrobial agents, 3 weeks after their discontinuation. Occasionally, specimens other than stool must be examined. In small-bowel infections such as giardiasis and strongyloidiasis, the diagnosis, at times, can be established only by sampling the duodenal contents or by performing a jejunal biopsy. Similarly, eggs of *Enterobius* (pinworm) and *Taenia* (tapeworm) are frequently found on the perianal skin when absent from the feces. Recovery of large-bowel parasites such as *Entamoeba histolytica* and *Schistosoma mansoni* may require colonic intubation with aspiration or biopsy of suspect lesions. Whenever intestinal aspirates or soft to watery fecal specimens are collected, they should be immediately placed in a preservative such as polyvinyl alcohol (PVA) to prevent rapid disintegration of fragile protozoan trophozoites and allow the preparation of permanently stained smears. Protozoan cysts and helminthic ova found in formed stool will survive for 1 to 2 days at room temperature and indefinitely if placed in 5% formaldehyde.

Direct examination of the blood is useful for the detection of malaria parasites, leishmania, trypanosomes, and microfilaria. Preferably, fresh capillary blood should be used to prepare thin and thick blood smears and, when appropriate, wet mounts. Only specially prepared glass slides should be used, as traces of soda lime or potash on uncleaned slides may alter the pH of the stain, making recognition of parasites difficult. If an experienced technologist is not available to assist in the bedside preparation of smears, it is preferable to collect venous blood in an EDTA Vacutainer and send it to the laboratory. As in the case of intestinal parasites, organisms in the peripheral blood may fluctuate, requiring the collection of multiple specimens over a period of several days. Parasites dwelling within the tissues of the host are more difficult to identify. Some discharge their offspring into the sputum (lung flukes) where they can be found with appropriate concentration procedures. In others, larvae can be recovered with skin (*Onchocerca volvulus*) or muscle (*Trichinella spiralis*) biopsies.

Diagnostic procedures based on the recovery and morphologic identification of the parasite suffer from a number of limitations. The relative insensitivity of the techniques involved, the absence of diagnostic forms in excreta, blood, or tissue during the early stages of infection, and their irregular shedding thereafter often dictate the need for repetitive testing. In strongyloidiasis, for example, a dozen or more stool examinations may be required before rhabditiform larvae are eventually detected microscopically. Recovery of pathogens such as *Toxoplasma gondii* or *Taenia solium* from the central nervous system or other deep tissues may be difficult or even dangerous. The procedures themselves are labor intensive and require a level of technical expertise frequently unavailable to small clinical laboratories. Immunodiagnostic and nucleic acid hybridization techniques have begun to provide alternatives to these traditional methods.

Detection of circulating antibodies Although immunodiagnostic tests have long been available for a number of parasitic diseases, they have lacked the sensitivity and specificity of those developed for viral and bacterial agents. This has been particularly true for infections caused by helminths which are broadly cross-reactive with one another. Replacement of antigenically complex worm extracts and cryosections with highly purified stage- or fraction-specific antigens has improved the specificity of many of the tests for circulating antibodies. In malaria, as well as a few other diseases, synthesized, immunologically reactive peptides have been employed as test antigens. The use of such antigens in highly reactive test systems including enzyme-linked immunosorbent assays (ELISA), kinetic enzyme immunoassays (k-ELISA, FAST-ELISA), antibody capture ELISA, and immunoblot assays has provided a new generation of serologic tests with exquisite sensitivity and specificity. Currently, they are available through a limited number of reference laboratories. Table 157-1 lists the tests offered by the Centers for Disease Control (CDC). In Table 157-2, the diagnostic endpoint, sensitivity, and specificity of the most frequently requested CDC procedures are given.

Antigen detection Soluble antigens have been detected in the blood, body fluids, tissues, and excreta of a number of protozoan and helminthic diseases (Table 157-3). Early attempts at developing diagnostically useful antigen detection procedures focused on enteric protozoan infections, as microscopic examination of the stool for the causative agents is always tedious and frequently unsuccessful. Commercial immunofluorescent kits have been marketed for the detection of *Giardia* and *Cryptosporidium* in the stool and *Trichomonas vaginalis* in genitourinary secretions. Visually read enzyme immunoassays may soon be available for these and other enteric pathogens such as *Entamoeba histolytica*, circumventing the need for the highly trained technologists and expensive laboratory equipment that are required for immunofluorescent procedures. Although early studies indicate that the sensitivity and specificity of such tests is high, a number of technical problems remain to be addressed

TABLE 157-1 Parasitic diseases for which serology is available

Taxonomic group	Diagnostic usefulness	
	High	Marginal
Protozoan	Amebiasis*	Malaria*
	Babesiosis*	Giardiasis
	Chagas' disease*	Pneumocystosis
	Leishmaniasis*	
	Toxoplasmosis*	
Helminthic	Cysticercosis*	Ascariasis
	Echinococcosis*	Clonorchiasis
	Paragonimiasis*	Dracunculiasis
	Toxocariasis*	Filariasis
	Trichinosis*	Schistosomiasis*
		Strongyloidiasis*

* Available at the Centers for Disease Control, Atlanta, Ga.

TABLE 157-2 Interpretation of tests frequently performed at the Centers for Disease Control

Disease	Test*	Diagnostic endpoint	Sensitivity†	Specificity†	Comments
Invasive amebiasis	IHA	≥1:256	70,[1] 95[2]	90[3]	1 Intestinal infection 2 Extraintestinal infection. 3 Titers may persist for years.
Cysticercosis	WBA[1]	+ or −	98[2]	100[2]	1 7 major bands. 2 Serum and CSF results identical.
Echinococcosis	IHA	≥1:256	60,[1] 88[2]	90–95[3,4]	1 Lung or calcified cyst. 2 Liver or peritoneal. 3 Cross-reacts with cysticercosis. 4 Titer may persist for years. 5 8-kDa antigen. 6 Cross-reacts with *E. multilocularis*.
	WBA[5]	+ or −	91[5]	100[6]	
Paragonimiasis	WBA[1]	+ or −	96	99	1 8-kDa protein, Chaffee antigen.
Schistosomiasis	FAST-ELISA[1]	≥10 U/μl	99,[2] 50[3]	99	1 *S. mansoni* adult microsomal antigen. 2 *S. mansoni* infections. 3 *S. japonicum* infections.
	WBA[1]	+ or −	High	High	1 Separate antigens for Sm, Sh, Sj.
Strongyloidiasis	ELISA	≥1:8	71[1]	80[2,3]	1 *S. stercoralis* larval antigen. 2 No absolute reference standard 3 Cross-reacts with filariasis, ascariasis.
Toxocariasis					
Visceral	ELISA	≥1:32	78	92[1,2]	1 Cross-reaction with ascariasis eliminated by preabsorption. 2 In children. 3 Patients with ocular disease.
Ocular	ELISA	≥1:8	90	91[3]	
Toxoplasmosis	IFA-IgG	≥1:16	High[1,2]	High[1,2]	1 No absolute reference standard. 2 Antibodies may persist for years. 3 Antibodies may persist for months. 4 May be negative in immunocompromised patients.
	Capture ELISA-IgM	≥1:4	High[1,3,4]	High[1,3]	
Trichinosis	BFT	≥1:5	97[1]	90[2]	1 Detected after third week of illness. 2 Titers may persist for years.

* IHA = Indirect hemagglutination; WBA = Western blot assay; ELISA = enzyme-linked immunosorbent assay; IFA = indirect fluorescent assay; BFT = bentonite flocculation.
† Superscript numbers refer to comments at right.
SOURCE: Division of Parasitic Diseases, CDC, 1989.

Rheumatoid factor and other copro-antibodies may produce false-positive results in some specimens. Antigens are rapidly destroyed by a variety of stool enzymes, restricting the use of these methods to fresh stool. Immunologic reagents may cross-react with one or more of the diverse complex of stool components. In solid-phase test systems, antibodies may desorb from plastic surfaces, affecting test sensitivity. There are a number of potential solutions to each of these problems, and it is expected that highly sensitive, specific, visually read immunoassays will be commercially available in the near future. A number of systems have been developed for the detection of malaria antigens in blood and *Toxoplasma gondii* antigens in tissue. Most of the malaria systems are less sensitive than the examination of a thick smear by a skilled technologist.

DNA probes Parasites, like other microorganisms, may be detected and identified in a clinical specimen by documenting the presence of genetic sequences unique to the parasite in question. The detection device is a DNA probe, a labeled nucleotide sequence complementary to a segment of parasitic genome unique to a particular strain, species, or genus. Addition of the probe to a positive specimen results in hybridization of the probe and parasite DNA with accompanying specimen labeling. The technology is highly specific, repro-ducible, inexpensive, and technically simple. Unlike immunodiagnostic tests, the effectiveness of DNA probes is not influenced by environmental or life-stage-dependent variations in antigenic expression. As the genome generally remains stable throughout the parasitic cycle, a single probe can often be used to identify any life stage of the pathogen.

The effectiveness of DNA probes has been facilitated by the large number of short nucleotide sequences that are randomly repeated, often millions of times, throughout the parasitic genome. Those specific to the parasite sought can be cloned or synthesized. As probe sensitivity depends upon the copy number of the target sequences, highly repeated sequences are more likely to be detected in specimens containing small amounts of parasitic DNA. Methods of in vitro amplification of DNA sequences, as well as improvements in labeling techniques, will soon allow further increases in the sensitivity of individual probes.

DNA probes are available for the detection of *P. falciparum*, *Trypanosoma cruzi*, *T. brucei*, *Onchocerca* spp., and etiologic agents of lymphatic filariasis. Although used primarily by field epidemiologists for the detection of infected insect vectors, they are being increasingly applied to the detection of the parasites in vertebrate hosts. A diagnostic probe for *P. falciparum* has demonstrated a sensitivity that approaches that achieved by the traditional thick smear technique; filarial probes have been developed that can detect a single parasite in a DNA blot. The major limitations of DNA probes as diagnostic tools relate to technical aspects of the hybridization procedure itself, but these should be overcome in the near future.

TABLE 157-3 Diseases for which antigen detection procedures have been described

Protozoan diseases	Helminthic diseases
Amebiasis	Cysticercosis
Amebic meningoencephalitis	Echinococcosis
Chagas' disease	Lymphatic filariasis
Giardiasis	Onchocerciasis
Malaria	Schistosomiasis
Pneumocystosis	
Toxoplasmosis	
Trichomoniasis	

SOURCE: After Smith and Walls.

REFERENCES

GAM AA et al: Comparative sensitivity and specificity of ELISA and IHA for serodiagnosis of strongyloidiasis with larval antigens. Am J Trop Med Hyg 37:157, 1987

HANCOCK K, TSANG VCW: Development and optimization of the FAST-ELISA for detecting antibodies to *Schistosoma mansoni*. J Immunol Methods 92:167, 1986

HERBRINK P et al: Interlaboratory evaluation of indirect enzyme-linked immunosorbent assay, antibody capture enzyme-linked immunosorbent assay, and immunoblotting for detection of immunoglobulin M antibodies to *Toxoplasma gondii*. J Clin Microbiol 25:100, 1987

MADDISON SE: Parasitic infections, in *Microbial Antigenodiagnosis*, Boca Raton, CRC Press, 2:110, 1987, vol 2

———— et al: A specific diagnostic antigen of *Echinococcus granulosus* with an apparent molecular weight of 8 kDa. Am J Trop Med Hyg 40:377, 1989

POST RJ, CRAMPTON JM: Probing the unknown. Parasitology Today 3:380, 1987

SLEMENDA SM et al: Diagnosis of paragonimiasis by immunoblot. Am J Trop Med Hyg 39:469, 1988

SMITH JW, WALLS KW: Rapid immunologic diagnosis of parasitic infections. Clin Microbiol Newsletter 10:89, 1988

TSANG VCW et al: An enzyme-linked immunoelectrotransfer blot assay and glycoprotein antigens for diagnosing human cysticercosis (*Taenia solium*). J Infect Dis 159:50, 1989

158   AMEBIASIS

JAMES J. PLORDE

DEFINITION Amebiasis is an infection of the large intestine produced by *Entamoeba histolytica*. It is an asymptomatic carrier state in most individuals, but diseases ranging from chronic, mild diarrhea to fulminant dysentery may occur. Among extraintestinal complications, the most common is hepatic abscess, which may rupture into peritoneum, pleura, lung, or pericardium.

ETIOLOGY There are seven species of ameba that naturally parasitize the human mouth and intestine, but of these only *E. histolytica* causes disease. *Entamoeba coli* and *E. hartmanni* are the two species with which it is most likely to be confused in examination of stools.

E. histolytica exists in two forms: the motile trophozoite and the cyst. The trophozoite is the parasitic form and dwells in the lumen and/or wall of the colon, divides by binary fission, grows best under anaerobic conditions, and requires the presence of either bacteria or tissue substrates to satisfy its nutritional requirements. When diarrhea occurs, the trophozoites are passed unchanged in the liquid stool, where they can be distinguished by their size (10 to 20 μm in diameter), directional motility, sharply demarcated clear ectoplasm with slender finger-like pseudopodia, and finely granular endoplasm. In dysentery, the trophozoites are larger (up to 50 μm in diameter), and often contain ingested erythrocytes. In the absence of diarrhea, the trophozoites usually encyst before leaving the gut. The cysts have a chitinous wall which renders them highly resistant to environmental changes, chlorine concentrations found in water purification systems, and gastric acid. With rare exception they are responsible for transmission of disease. Young cysts have a single nucleus, a glycogen vacuole, and sausage-shaped collections of ribosomes known as chromatoid bodies. As the cyst matures, it absorbs its cytoplasmic inclusions and becomes quadrinucleate. The cysts of *E. histolytica* can be distinguished from those of *E. hartmanni* by their larger diameter (10 μm) and from those of *Entamoeba coli* by the presence of one to four nuclei with small centric karyosomes and fine peripheral chromatin and by their thick chromatoid bodies with round ends.

The electrophoretic mobility patterns of four enzymes found in trophozoites have been used to define 22 *E. histolytica* zymodemes. Amebas recovered from patients with invasive disease belong to just 9; all are characterized by the presence of advanced, paired hexokinase bands and/or a beta phosphoglucomutase without an accompanying alpha-phosphoglucomutase band. Although conversion between pathogenic and nonpathogenic zymodemes has been reported in cloned cultures, the zymodemes appear to be clinically stable markers of virulence.

Entamoeba histolytica can be cultivated in artificial media, a procedure that is essential for the determination of isoenzyme patterns

and preparation of the purified antigens used in serologic testing. Its diagnostic value remains uncertain.

EPIDEMIOLOGY Although *E. histolytica* can sometimes infect animals, humans are the principal hosts and reservoir. Because trophozoites die rapidly after leaving the intestine, the asymptomatic cyst passer is the source of new infections; a chronic carrier may excrete several million organisms daily. The infective dose usually exceeds 10^3, but infection has followed the ingestion of a single cyst. These structures are transmitted by the fecal-oral route, usually through direct person-to-person contact. Poverty, ignorance, mental retardation, and other factors which impair personal hygiene facilitate the spread of the parasite. Oral-anal sexual contact produces high infection rates in male homosexuals. Food- and waterborne transmission occur in areas of the world with poor sanitation, including certain southern rural communities, Indian reservations, and migrant farm camps in the United States. Occasionally this results in common source outbreaks; these epidemics, however, are never as explosive as those produced by pathogenic intestinal bacteria. Symptomatic amebiasis is unusual below the age of 10 years in temperate climates, and both intestinal and hepatic lesions predominate in adult males to an extent that is not readily explainable on the basis of different rates of exposure to infection.

It has been estimated that 50 percent of inhabitants of some less well-developed nations, 10 percent of the world's population as a whole, and 1 percent of Americans are infected with *E. histolytica*. Invasive amebiasis, which produces an estimated 40 million disabling infections and 40,000 deaths annually, is concentrated in comparatively few parts of the world, most notably Mexico, western South America, south Asia, and west and southeastern Africa. This is presumably related to the concurrent presence in these geographic areas of virulent strains of *E. histolytica*, the hygienic and sanitary conditions necessary for their transmission, and, perhaps, malnutrition and immunodeficiency. Even in areas endemic for invasive disease, however, only 10 percent of infected patients harbor virulent zymodemes of *E. histolytica*. A minority of these experience clinical disease. In the United States the incidence of invasive amebiasis dropped sharply in the four decades preceding the 1970s. Between 1971 and 1974, an average of 3500 cases were reported annually to the Centers for Disease Control; since then the numbers have steadily increased. Isoenzyme studies of *E. histolytica* strains isolated from male homosexuals and inmates of mental hospitals in Great Britain indicate the overwhelming majority belong to nonpathogenic zymodemes, suggesting that virulent strains are now uncommon in developed countries. Although patients with dysentery and liver abscess can still be found in the impoverished segments of the American population, the bulk of the invasive disease diagnosed in the United States is now acquired outside the United States.

IMMUNITY Repeated intestinal infections are common. However, there are data suggesting the presence of protective immunity, particularly following invasive liver disease. There is no correlation between the presence of circulating antibodies and resistance to reinfection. It is likely that immunity is incomplete, develops only after recovery from invasive disease, and is cell-mediated.

PATHOGENESIS AND PATHOLOGY After ingestion, cysts undergo further nuclear division. In the small intestine, the cyst wall disintegrates, and trophozoites are released. The immature amebas are carried to the large intestine, where they live in the lumen of the gut feeding on bacteria and debris. Organisms belonging to nonpathogenic zymodemes are seldom responsible for sustained tissue invasion and destruction. In contrast, the almost universal presence of specific humoral antibodies in carriers of pathogenic zymodemes suggests that tissue invasion by these strains is the rule. Only in the minority, however, is this sufficiently extensive to produce symptoms. The factors modulating invasion are not completely understood, but the state of the host and the virulence of the infecting organism both play roles. High carbohydrate intake, corticosteroids, protein malnutrition, pregnancy, HIV infection, and other immunosuppressed states render the host more susceptible. High-molecular-weight glycoproteins present in colonic mucus bind avidly to an adhesion molecule on the surface of *E. histolytica* trophozoites, blocking their attachment to host cells. Changes in the composition or production of mucus may, therefore, alter the host's susceptibility to amebic invasion. Trophozoite virulence is enhanced by rapid animal passage; presumably, a similar phenomenon occurs in epidemiologic settings conducive to rapid spread of the protozoan from human to human. Direct association with certain strains of bacteria may also enhance the virulence of pathogenic strains, possibly by protecting the ameba from oxidant stress or through the exchange of genetic material.

The precise pathogenic mechanisms responsible for tissue invasion are not fully understood. The invasiveness of a strain correlates well with its phagocytic prowess, production of collagenase and an immunogenic cytotoxic protein, resistance to the host's inflammatory response, and, perhaps most importantly, its capacity to induce histolysis following direct cell-to-cell contact with host tissue. The latter phenomenon is initiated by a lectin-mediated adherence of the trophozoite to a target cell. Amebapore, a pore-forming protein, is released and polymerizes in the target cell membrane, forming large membrane holes. Cytolysis, which appears to require both intact microfilament function and amebic phospholipase A enzymes, rapidly follows. The lysis of neutrophils, which are attracted to, and killed by, *E. histolytica* trophozoites, may amplify tissue damage.

Amebic ulceration of the intestinal wall is characteristic. A small mucosal defect overlies a larger, burrowing area of necrosis in the submucosa and muscularis, producing a bottle-shaped lesion. There is little acute inflammatory response, and in contrast to the picture in bacillary dysentery, the mucosa between ulcers is normal. The sites of involvement in order of frequency are cecum and ascending colon, rectum, sigmoid, appendix, and terminal ileum. Involvement of the colonic musculature may lead to the formation of large masses of granulation tissue or *amebomas*. Amebas can enter the portal circulation and lodge in venules; liquefaction necrosis of liver tissue leads to the formation of an abscess cavity. Rarely, embolization results in lung, brain, or splenic abscess.

A soluble protein product of invasive strains of *E. histolytica* has been shown to induce HIV replication in infected lymphocytes. Conceivably, individuals infected with both pathogens might experience the accelerated development of AIDS (see Chap. 264).

CLINICAL MANIFESTATIONS **Asymptomatic cyst passer** In the majority of patients with this common form of amebiasis, *E. histolytica* probably lives as a commensal in the bowel lumen. Individuals infected in temperate climates are unlikely to harbor virulent strains. However, as invasion can occasionally occur, treatment of all cyst passers is warranted.

Symptomatic intestinal amebiasis In some patients there is intermittent diarrhea consisting of one to four foul-smelling loose or watery stools daily. The stools sometimes contain mucus and blood. Loose stools alternate with periods of relative normality and may persist for months or years. Flatulence and abnormal cramping are frequent. The only physical findings are occasional tender hepatomegaly and slight pain when the cecum and ascending colon are palpated. Sigmoidoscopy sometimes reveals typical ulcerations with areas of normal mucosa interspersed. The diagnosis depends upon finding the organism in the feces or in ulcers.

Fulminating attacks of amebic dysentery are less common. Waterborne outbreaks may occur, but fulminating dysentery is more likely to occur spontaneously in debilitated or immunocompromised individuals. Attacks may be precipitated by pregnancy or corticosteroids. The onset in half the cases is abrupt with high fever, between 40 and 40.6°C (104 and 105°F), severe abdominal cramps, and profuse, bloody diarrhea with tenesmus. There is diffuse abdominal tenderness, often so severe that peritonitis is suspected. Hepatomegaly is very frequent, and sigmoidoscopy almost always demonstrates extensive rectosigmoid ulceration. Trophozoites are numerous in stools and in material obtained directly from the ulcers.

In some cases there may be extensive destruction of the colonic mucosa and submucosa, massive hemorrhage or perforation of the bowel wall, with resultant peritonitis. Repeated severe attacks of intestinal amebiasis can lead to an ulcerative postdysenteric colitis. Penetration of trophozoites through the muscle wall of the bowel may result in the development of large masses of granulation tissue. When the entire circumference of the intestine is involved, there may then be partial obstruction, and a movable, tender, sausage shaped mass is often palpable. This lesion, or ameboma, is most frequently seen in the cecum, where a palpable mass and radiologic demonstration of a ragged encroachment of the lumen may lead to a mistaken diagnosis of adenocarcinoma.

Hepatic amebiasis The term *amebic hepatitis* is used for a syndrome of tender hepatomegaly, right upper quadrant pain, fever, and leukocytosis in patients with amebic colitis. Hepatic biopsy reveals nonspecific periportal inflammation. The absence of ameba within the areas of inflammation, the rarity with which the syndrome is followed by an amebic liver abscess, and the resolution of the liver signs following treatment of the intestinal disease with luminal amebicides indicate that these manifestations are not secondary to spread of trophozoites from the intestine, but are rather a nonspecific accompaniment of amebic colitis.

Hepatic abscess may develop insidiously, with fever, sweats, weight loss, and no local signs other than painless or slightly tender hepatomegaly. In immunologically naive patients, there is more often an abrupt onset, with chills, fever to 40.6°C (105°F), nausea, vomiting, severe upper abdominal pain, and polymorphonuclear leukocytosis. Initially, cholecystitis, perforated ulcer, or acute pancreatitis may be suspected. Over 80 percent of patients with an insidious onset and half of those presenting with acute manifestations have a single abscess. Most commonly, this is localized in the posterior portion of the right lobe of the liver, because this lobe receives most of the blood draining the right colon through the "streaming" effect in portal vein flow. This location is responsible for several features that aid in diagnosis. *Point tenderness* in the posterolateral portion of a lower right intercostal space is frequent even in the absence of diffuse liver pain. Most abscesses enlarge upward, producing a bulge in the diaphragmatic dome, obliteration of the costophrenic gutter, small hydrothorax, basilar atelectasis, and pain referred to the right shoulder.

Liver function tests may be mildly to moderately disturbed and provide little diagnostic aid; the level of the serum glutamic oxaloacetic transaminase (SGOT), however, is of clinical value as it directly reflects the severity of disease. Jaundice is uncommon, and when present implies a grave prognosis. Radiologically, unruptured abscesses do not show a fluid level, and calcification of the liver parenchyma is very rare. Isotope liver scan utilizing two, or preferably three, projections is invaluable in confirming the presence and location of a liver abscess. It becomes positive within the first days of illness, often prior to other imaging techniques. Presumably these early changes reflect either a focal decrease in blood supply or injury to the Kupffer cells rather than liquefaction necrosis. Ultrasonic scanning and computed tomography, although becoming positive slightly later in the course of the disease, are ultimately as sensitive as isotopic scanning and provide confirmation of the cystic nature of the lesion. The defect seen on imaging commonly persists for several months after the complete recovery of the patient. Serologic tests are positive in over 90 percent of cases.

Needle puncture results in the withdrawal of "pus" which consists of liquefied, necrotic liver. Typically, it is thick and odorless, resembling "chocolate syrup" or "anchovy paste." It may, however, be thin in consistency and yellow or green in color. The pus contains no polymorphonuclear leukocytes (barring secondary bacterial infection) and, usually, no amebas. The parasites are localized in the cyst wall and may be demonstrated in the terminal portion of the aspirate or, at times, by a Vim-Silverman needle biopsy of the cyst wall following aspiration of the abscess.

Hepatic abscess complicates asymptomatic infection of the colon more often than symptomatic intestinal disease, another factor making recognition difficult. Trophozoites or cysts are demonstrable in the feces of only about one-third of patients with abscess, and fewer than one-half can recall significant diarrheal illness.

Pleuropulmonary amebiasis   The right pleural cavity and lung are involved by direct extension from the liver in 10 to 20 percent of patients with liver abscess. Rarely, amebic lung abscess has resulted from embolization rather than direct extension. Manifestations are those of a consolidating pneumonia or lung abscess. If perforation into a bronchus occurs, patients expectorate large amounts of the typical exudate, some patients even commenting that the sputum "tastes like liver." Cough, pleural pain, fever, and leukocytosis are the rule, and secondary bacterial infection is frequent. Rupture into the free pleural space results in a massive pleural effusion; aspiration of "chocolate" fluid is diagnostic.

Other extraintestinal lesions   Extension of an abscess from the left lobe of the liver to the pericardium is the most dangerous complication of hepatic abscess. It may be mistaken for tuberculous pericarditis or congestive cardiomyopathy. Less frequently, rapid cardiac tamponade occurs with ensuing dyspnea, shock, and death. Peritonitis is a result of perforation of colonic ulcer or rupture of liver abscess. Painful ulcers or condylomata of the genitalia, perianal skin, or abdominal wall (draining sinuses) are unusual complications which may be mistaken for syphilitic, tuberculous, or neoplastic lesions. They usually result from direct extension of intestinal disease; some are thought to result from sexual transmission. Metastatic brain abscess is rare, and an etiologic diagnosis is seldom made clinically. Splenic abscess has been reported but is very unusual.

DIFFERENTIAL DIAGNOSIS   **Intestinal amebiasis**   Patients with nondysenteric amebiasis are often misdiagnosed as having irritable bowel syndrome, diverticulitis, or regional enteritis. Ameboma may mimic colonic carcinoma or granulomatous disease, while the clinical spectrum of amebic dysentery overlaps those of shigellosis, salmonellosis, ulcerative colitis, and, in endemic areas, schistosomiasis. The invasive bacterial infections are usually more acute, severe, and self-limited than amebiasis. Stools from patients with shigellosis, salmonellosis, and ulcerative colitis contain large numbers of polymorphonuclear leukocytes, while those in amebic infection do not. Nevertheless, amebiasis may closely resemble any of the above diseases both clinically and radiologically and must be considered in the differential diagnosis of any chronic diarrhea or dysentery.

The identification of E. histolytica in the stool, however, does not eliminate other diagnostic possibilities. Amebic infection is often superimposed on or exacerbated by other colonic disease including schistosomiasis and cecal carcinoma. For this reason, patients with intestinal amebiasis and abdominal complaints still require stool culture, sigmoidoscopy, and a barium enema.

Hepatic abscess   Once a filling defect has been demonstrated by isotope liver scanning, the differential diagnosis includes hepatic neoplasm, hydatid cyst, and pyogenic abscess. Neoplasms can usually be differentiated on the basis of their ultrasonic scanning characteristics, while the lack of constitutional manifestations and presence of an appropriate epidemiologic history is helpful in recognizing echinococcosis. The most difficult problem lies in the exclusion of a pyogenic abscess. An insidious onset in an adult male, a history of chronic diarrhea, significant pleuritic chest pain, and a single right lobe lesion favors the diagnosis of amebiasis. High fever, hyperbilirubinemia, multiple hepatic filling defects, and foul-smelling hepatic aspirate are more suggestive of pyogenic disease. Ultimately, the separation of the two diseases rests upon laboratory procedures.

LABORATORY DIAGNOSIS   The diagnosis of intestinal amebiasis depends upon identification of the organism in the stool or tissues. Formed stools are microscopically examined initially in saline and iodine mounts for amebic cysts; concentration methods such as the formalin-ether technique increase the yield two- to threefold. Liquid or semiformed stools should be examined immediately in saline solution for the presence of motile hematophagous trophozoites. The addition of a supravital stain such as buffered methylene blue to the saline enhances nuclear detail and minimizes the possibility of confusing fecal leukocytes with amebic trophozoites. If there is any

delay in examination of the stool, a portion of the specimen may be refrigerated for a few hours at 4°C, or placed in polyvinyl alcohol and 10% formalin. Definitive identification of E. histolytica requires the examination of permanently stained slides prepared from the material preserved with polyvinyl alcohol. An ocular micrometer is necessary to separate E. hartmanni from its larger relative. Four to six stool specimens may be required for diagnosis. If possible, the stool should be examined before the administration of antimicrobial, antidiarrheal, or antacid preparations because all these agents may interfere with the recovery of amebas. Likewise, enemas and radiographic procedures utilizing barium sulfate are best postponed until after a thorough search for E. histolytica has been made. A number of nonmicroscopic techniques have been developed for the rapid detection of E. histolytica in the stool. They include enzyme-linked immunosorbent and immunofluorescent assays for trophozoite and/or cyst antigens and DNA hybridization probes to tandemly repeated parasite nucleotide sequences. If commercially developed, they could provide a useful alternative to microscopic examination.

Sigmoidoscopy is of value in symptomatic cases. The mucosal lesions should be aspirated and the material examined for trophozoites as described above. Biopsy material obtained from such lesions and stained with periodic acid Schiff solution also will frequently reveal trophozoites.

The diagnosis of extraintestinal amebiasis is difficult. The parasite usually cannot be recovered from stool or tissue. Cultivation of amebas from feces or pus is possible but is not practical in most laboratories. Serologic tests employing purified antigens are positive in nearly all patients with proven amebic liver abscess and in a great majority of those with acute amebic dysentery. The persistence of significant antibody titers for months to years after complete cure makes serology, particularly in endemic areas, of more value in excluding the diagnosis than in confirming it. Of the available tests, the indirect hemagglutination and enzyme-linked immunosorbent assays appear to be the most sensitive; average time to positivity is 3 and 2 weeks, respectively. Indirect immunofluorescence, countercurrent electrophoresis, and agar gel diffusion are also highly reliable. A number of these testing procedures are now available as commercial kits, making serologic testing feasible for most laboratories.

TREATMENT   Treatment should be aimed at relief of symptoms, replacement of fluid, electrolyte, and blood losses, and eradication of the organism. Amebas may be found in the lumen of the bowel, in the intestinal wall, or extraintestinally. Most amebicides are not effective at all sites or when used alone, and a combination of drugs is often necessary to achieve cure. The available drugs based on their site of action fall into two categories.

Luminal amebicides   These oral agents act by direct contact with trophozoites dwelling in the bowel lumen but are ineffective against amebas in tissue. Of the large number of available drugs, diloxanide furoate is one of the most effective and well tolerated but is presently available in the United States only through the Centers for Disease Control. A response rate of 80 to 85 percent has been noted; flatulence appears to be the only major side effect.

Iodoquinol has been effective in 60 to 70 percent of cases. As with its analogue iodochlorhydroxyquin, myelooptic neuropathy has been reported after long-term use. However, no such case has been noted when the dosage was limited to that given in Table 158-1. The drug should not be used in patients with thyroid disease or preexisting optic neuropathy.

Tissue amebicides   Chloroquine phosphate is a systemic amebicide which is useful in hepatic disease because of its high concentration in the liver. It has little activity elsewhere.

Emetine is an alkaloid derivative of ipecac. When given intramuscularly, it is highly effective in destroying trophozoites in tissue including those in the wall of the intestine. It is ineffective against luminal amebas. Emetine is relatively toxic and may produce vomiting, diarrhea, abdominal cramping, weakness, muscle pain, tachycardia, hypotension, precordial pain, and electrocardiographic abnormalities. The common ECG changes include T-wave inversion and prolongation

TABLE 158-1 Drug therapy of amebiasis

	Dosage
ASYMPTOMATIC INTESTINAL CARRIER	
Iodoquinol*	650 mg tid for 20 days
or diloxanide furoate†	500 mg tid for 10 days
MILD TO MODERATE INTESTINAL DISEASE	
Metronidazole	750 mg tid for 5–10 days
plus iodoquinol	As above
or diloxanide furoate	As above
or tetracycline	500 mg qid for 5 days
SEVERE INTESTINAL DISEASE	
Above regimen	
plus dehydroemetine†	1.0–1.5 mg/kg IM per day (maximum 90 mg/d) up to 5 d
or emetine	1 mg/kg IM per day (maximum 60 mg/d) for up to 5 days
EXTRAINTESTINAL DISEASE	
Metronidazole	As above
plus iodoquinol	
or chloroquine phosphate	1 g/d for 2 days, then 500 mg/d for 4 weeks
plus dehydroemetine†	As above for 10 days
or emetine	As above for 10 days

* Glenwood Laboratories, Inc, 83 North Summit St, Tenafly, NJ 07670.
† Investigational drug available through the Parasitic Drug Service, Centers for Disease Control, Atlanta, Ga, (404) 639-3670, nights and weekends 639 2888.

of the QTc interval. Rarely arrhythmias and prolongation of the QRS complex are seen. A synthetic derivative, dehydroemetine, is thought to be less toxic by virtue of its more rapid excretion and lower concentration in myocardial tissue. It is not free of toxicity, however, and patients treated with either drug should be at bed rest with ECG monitoring. Neither drug should be used in patients with renal, cardiac, or muscle disease, during pregnancy, or in children, unless other drugs fail.

Metronidazole is unique because it is effective against trophozoites at all sites, intestinally and extraintestinally. For intestinal amebiasis it is given in dosage of 750 mg three times daily for 5 to 10 days. Smaller doses are effective in hepatic amebiasis. Metronidazole has an Antabuse-like action, and alcohol should be avoided during its administration. The evidence that this drug is carcinogenic and possibly teratogenic in animals when given in large doses is disturbing but lacks confirmation in humans. Metronidazole should not be given in the first trimester of pregnancy.

Specific antiprotozoal therapy is outlined in Table 158-1.

In extraintestinal amebiasis including hepatic abscess, metronidazole is the drug of choice. In cases of relapse, impending rupture of an abscess, or in situations where the patient is unable to take oral medication, therapy with dehydroemetine or emetine should be instituted, and oral chloroquine added as soon as possible. Most authors prefer to add luminal amebicides to both the metronidazole and chloroquine-emetine programs. Treatment failures have been reported for both emetine-chloroquine and metronidazole. They appear to be unrelated to the organism's resistance.

There is debate over the value of routine aspiration of amebic liver abscesses. Certainly, if there is localized swelling over the liver, marked elevation of the diaphragm, severe localized liver tenderness, and failure to respond to systemic amebicides within 72 h, it should be done. Adequate drainage can usually be accomplished by needle alone, and surgical drainage is rarely necessary. The greatest hazard in needling an abscess is secondary bacterial infection.

PROGNOSIS Intestinal amebiasis usually responds readily and completely to appropriate drugs. Parasitologic relapses sometimes occur, and posttreatment stools should be checked monthly for 6 months. Repeated relapses, however, are usually a manifestation of reinfection, complicating illness, inadequate therapy, or incorrect diagnosis. The fatality rate is less than 5 percent.

Hepatic and pulmonary amebiasis are still accompanied by an appreciable mortality, but no reliable figures are available.

PREVENTION For the individual, avoidance of contaminated food and water, scalding of vegetables, and the use of iodine-releasing tablets in drinking water (chlorine, in the form of halazone, is ineffective) are important measures. Globaline tablets, containing tetraglycine hydroperiodide, are convenient and effective.

Improvements in general sanitation and the detection of cyst passers and their removal from food-handling duties are general measures in prophylaxis, but such segregation of carriers is rarely practiced. Community control of amebic disease by periodic mass treatment with metronidazole and diloxanide furoate has been successful in some areas. Personal chemoprophylaxis for travelers is not recommended.

PRIMARY AMEBIC MENINGOENCEPHALITIS AND KERATITIS

Primary amebic meningoencephalitis is caused by free-living amebas of the genus Naegleria or Acanthamoeba. The former most often affects children and young adults, appears to be acquired by swimming in fresh, warm water, and is almost invariably fatal. Acanthamoeba infections involve older immunocompromised individuals, and spontaneous recovery is sometimes seen.

Free-living amebas are ubiquitous in nature where they are commonly found in soil and water. Although generally considered harmless, some varieties are clearly pathogenic for the central nervous system of mammals. In those instances of human meningoencephalitis where the responsible organism has been isolated and cultured, it is usually an amoeboflagellate, Naegleria fowleri.

Over 140 Naegleria cases have been reported from different parts of the world. Serologic studies suggest that inapparent infections are much more common. Most of the 50 cases recognized in the United States have occurred in the southeastern states, particularly Florida, Georgia, and Virginia. Characteristically the patients have fallen ill during the summer months approximately 1 week after swimming in fresh or brackish water. The 16 Czechoslovakian cases followed swimming in an indoor pool with chlorinated water maintained at 24°C, and 6 cases have been acquired apparently after bathing in hot mineral water. In sub-Saharan Africa, cases appear to follow inhalation of airborne cysts during the dry, windy harmattan season. Histologic evidence suggests that the amebas reach the central nervous system directly via the nasal mucosa at the level of the cribriform plate. Clinically, the illness is rapid in onset, brief in duration, and inexorable in course. The initial symptom is a severe, persistent, frontal headache followed by nausea, vomiting, fever, and nuchal rigidity. Unusual tastes or smells may be noted. Later, drowsiness, confusion, convulsions, and coma appear. Focal neurologic findings may occur late in the course of the illness.

A more benign, chronic form of meningoencephalitis is produced by organisms of the genus Acanthamoeba. They appear to be disseminated to the brain and skin from the nasal sinuses or lungs. Clinical manifestations include cognitive abnormalities, focal neurologic findings, and coma. Patients with this clinical syndrome are frequently older, are immunocompromised, lack a history of freshwater swimming, and may recover spontaneously. Pathologically, the disease can be distinguished from Naegleria infections by the granulomatous nature of the inflammatory reaction and the presence of both trophozoites and cysts in the tissues. Unfortunately, the responsible organisms have seldom been recovered by culture and identified. It is possible that the free-living amebas of several species are involved. An increasing number of patients with Acanthamoeba keratitis have been reported. Infection usually follows eye trauma or prolonged use of soft contact lenses. The chronic progressive ulcerative disease can be distinguished from herpes simplex keratitis by a paracentral ring infiltrate, recurrent epithelial breakdown, severe pain, Progressive corneal damage usually results in blindness and/or corneal prolapse.

A careful examination of the cerebrospinal fluid is the single most helpful diagnostic procedure in patients with clinical evidence of meningitis. In *Naegleria* infections the fluid is usually bloody or sanguinopurulent and demonstrates an intense neutrophilic response. The protein is elevated and the glucose diminished. No organisms are demonstrated on Gram's stain or routine culture. Early examination of a wet preparation of unspun spinal fluid will usually reveal viable trophozoites. They are 10 to 20 μm in diameter, possess a granular cytoplasm, a distinct ectoplasm, and bulbous pseudopodia. If the specimen is allowed to cool, the trophozoites may become immobile and more difficult to recognize. The diagnosis is confirmed with direct fluorescent antibody (DFA) stains. Although the amebas may be easily grown on ordinary culture media which have been seeded with coliform bacteria, this is not helpful in clinical management, so rapidly progressive is the disease. In contrast, the spinal fluid in *Acanthamoeba* infections usually demonstrates a mononuclear response. Trophozoites have seldom been cultured or seen on wet mounts. A positive DFA stain has been seen in a few cases. Brain biopsy is diagnostic in approximately 75 percent of cases. *Acanthamoeba* keratitis is confirmed by demonstrating the typical double wrinkled wall cyst in corneal scrapings or biopsies. Culture, when available, is usually successful. Treatment with standard antiprotozoal agents seems completely ineffective. *Naegleria*, however, is highly sensitive to amphotericin B, miconazole, tetracycline, and rifampin. To date only four patients have survived a *Naegleria* infection. All were diagnosed early and treated, three with amphotericin B and the other with amphotericin B, miconazole, and rifampin. Intracisternal, as well as intravenous, administration of amphotericin is probably essential to rapidly obtain effective levels in the cerebrospinal fluid. The intraventricular dose is 0.5 to 1 mg for the first few days. The intravenous dose is similar to that for cryptococcal meningitis (see Chap. 87). *Acanthamoeba* are sensitive to sulfonamides, clotrimazole, 5-FC, and polymyxin B, in vitro but not clinically. Keratitis has responded to topical miconazole, propamidine isethionate (Brolene), and antibiotics followed by keratoplasty.

If the source of the infection can be determined, further *Naegleria* cases might be prevented by closing the area to bathing.

REFERENCES

Amebiasis

ADAMS EB, MACLEOD IN: Invasive amebiasis. Medicine 56:315, 1977

DENIS M, CHADEE K: Immunopathology of *Entamoeba histolytica* infections. Parasitology Today 4:247, 1988

KATZENSTEIN D et al: New concepts of amebic liver abscess derived from hepatic imaging, serodiagnosis, and hepatic enzymes in 67 consecutive cases in San Diego. Medicine 61:237, 1982

KNOBLOCH J, MANNWEILER E: Development and persistence of antibodies to *Entamoeba histolytica* in patients with amebic liver abscess: Analysis of 216 cases. Am J Trop Med Hyg 32:727, 1983

MARTINEZ-PALOMO A: The pathogenesis of amoebiasis. Parasitology Today 3:111, 1987

PROCTOR EM et al: The electrophoretic isoenzyme patterns of strains of *Entamoeba histolytica* isolated in two major cities in Canada. Am J Trop Med Hyg 37:296, 1987

RAVDIN JI: Pathogenesis of disease caused by *Entamoeba histolytica*: Studies of adherence, secreted toxins, and contact-dependent cytolysis. Rev Infect Dis 8:247, 1986

SALATA RA, RAVDIN JI: Review of the human immune mechanisms directed against *Entamoeba histolytica*. Rev Infect Dis 8:261, 1986

THOMPSON JE et al: Amebic liver abscess: A therapeutic approach. Rev Infect Dis 7:171, 1985

WALSH J: Problems in recognition and diagnosis of amebiasis: Estimation of the global magnitude of morbidity and mortality. Rev Infect Dis 8:228, 1986

Primary amebic meningoencephalitis

AURAN JD et al: *Acanthamoeba* keratitis. A review of the literature. Cornea 6:2, 1987

SEIDEL JS et al: Successful treatment of primary amebic meningoencephalitis. N Engl J Med 306:346, 1982

STEHR-GREEN JK et al: *Acanthamoeba* keratitis in soft contact lens wearers. JAMA 258:57, 1987

WILEY CA et al: *Acanthamoeba* meningoencephalitis in a patient with AIDS. J Infect Dis 155:130, 1987

159 MALARIA

NICHOLAS J. WHITE / JAMES J. PLORDE

INTRODUCTION Malaria is a protozoan disease transmitted by the bite of *Anopheles* mosquitoes. It is the most important of the parasitic diseases of human beings, affecting approximately 200 million people and causing over 1 million deaths each year. Malaria has now been eradicated from North America, Europe, and Russia, but despite enormous control efforts, there has been a resurgence of the disease in many parts of the tropics. Added to this are the increasing problems of drug resistance. Malaria remains today, as it has for centuries, a major burden on tropical communities and a danger to travelers.

ETIOLOGY Four species of the genus *Plasmodium* infect humans (although occasional infections with primate malarias may occur). These are *P. vivax*, *P. ovale*, *P. malariae*, and *P. falciparum* (Table 159-1). Almost all deaths are caused by falciparum malaria. Human infection begins when a female anopheline mosquito inoculates plasmodial sporozoites from its salivary gland during a blood meal. These small motile forms are carried rapidly via the bloodstream to the liver where they target hepatic parenchymal cells, invade, and begin a period of asexual reproduction. By this process (known as intrahepatic or preerythrocytic schizogony), a single sporozoite eventually produces several thousand daughter merozoites. The swollen liver cell eventually bursts, discharging merozoites into the bloodstream, beginning the symptomatic blood stage of the infection. In *P. vivax* and *P. ovale* infections a proportion of the intrahepatic forms do not divide immediately, but remain dormant for months before reproduction begins. These sleeping forms, or hypnozoites, are the cause of the relapses that characterize infection with these two species.

After entry into the bloodstream merozoites rapidly invade erythrocytes. Attachment is mediated via a specific erythrocyte surface receptor. In *P. vivax* this is related to the Duffy blood group antigen Fy^a or Fy^b. Most west Africans, or people with origins in that region, carry the Duffy-negative FyFy phenotype and are therefore resistant to *P. vivax* malaria. The glycophorins, a family of membrane sialoglycoproteins, have been implicated as the red cell attachment sites for the merozoites of *P. falciparum*. During invasion the merozoite first orientates so that its apical end is apposed to the erythrocyte surface and then interiorizes itself so as to lie within an intraerythrocytic parasitophorous vacuole. During the early stage of development the small "ring forms" of the four parasite species appear similar under light microscopy. As the trophozoites enlarge, species-specific characteristics become evident, pigment becomes visible, and the parasite assumes an irregular or ameboid shape. By the end of the 48-h cycle (72 h for *P. malariae*) the parasite has grown to occupy most of the red cell. Multiple nuclear fission then takes place (schizogony), and the red cell ruptures to release from 6 to 24 daughter merozoites. Each of these is capable of invading a new red cell and repeating the cycle. After a series of such asexual cycles some of the parasites develop into morphologically distinct sexual forms (gametocytes) which are long-lived and relatively inert.

Following ingestion in the blood meal of a biting female anopheline mosquito, the male and female gametocytes fuse in the insect's midgut to form a zygote. This matures to form an ookinete, which penetrates and encysts in the mosquito gut wall. The resulting oocyst expands by asexual division until it bursts to liberate myriads of motile sporozoites, which then migrate to the salivary gland to await inoculation into another human at the next feeding.

The disease in human beings is caused by the direct effects of red cell invasion and destruction and the host reaction to this process.

EPIDEMIOLOGY Malaria occurs throughout most of the tropical regions of the world. *P. falciparum* predominates in Africa, New Guinea, and Haiti; *P. vivax* is more common in Central America and

TABLE 159-1   Human malaria parasites

	P. falciparum	*P. vivax*	*P. ovale*	*P. malariae*
Duration of intrahepatic phase (days)	5½	8	9	15
Number of merozoites released per infected hepatocyte	30,000	10,000	15,000	15,000
Duration of erythrocytic cycle (hours)	48	48	50	72
Red cell preference	Younger cells but can invade cells of all ages.	Reticulocytes	Reticulocytes	Older cells
Morphologic characteristics	Usually only ring forms. Parasitemia may exceed 2 percent with multiple infections of a single erythrocyte. Banana-shaped gametocytes.	Irregular-shaped large rings and trophozoites. Enlarged erythrocytes. Schüffner's dots.	Infected erythrocytes enlarged and oval. Schüffner's dots.	Band or rectangular forms of trophozoites common.
Pigment color	Black	Yellow-brown	Dark brown	Brown/black
Relapses	No	Yes	Yes	No

the Indian subcontinent. The prevalence of both species is approximately equal in South America, east Asia, and Oceania. *P. malariae* is found in most areas, but is much less common. *P. ovale* is relatively unusual outside Africa.

The epidemiology of malaria is complex and may vary considerably even within relatively small geographic areas. Endemicity is traditionally defined in terms of spleen rates in children (i.e., percentage of children with a palpable spleen) as hypoendemic < 10 percent, mesoendemic 11 to 50 percent, hyperendemic 51 to 75 percent, and holoendemic > 75 percent. In holo- and hyperendemic areas (Fig. 159-1) such as much of tropical Africa or coastal New Guinea, where there is intense *P. falciparum* transmission, people are infected repeatedly throughout their lives. There is considerable morbidity and mortality during childhood. Immunity is hard won, but by the time of adulthood malaria infections are largely asymptomatic. In areas where transmission is low, erratic, or focal, the chance of one

infected person transmitting malaria to another is relatively small, full immunity is not acquired, and symptomatic disease may occur at all ages. This is termed "unstable malaria" in contrast to the "stable" malaria in holo- and hyperendemic areas. Even in areas with stable malaria, there is often seasonal variation coinciding with increased mosquito breeding during the rainy season. Malaria can behave like an epidemic disease in some areas, such as in north India and southeast Asia. This occurs when there are migrations (usually of refugees or workers) from a nonmalarious region to areas of high transmission. This usually produces considerable mortality at all ages.

The principal determinants of malaria epidemiology are the biting habits, longevity, and number (density) of the anopheline mosquito vectors. As a general approximation, malaria transmission is directly proportional to the density of the vector, the square of the number of human bites per day per mosquito, and the tenth power of the probability of the mosquito surviving for 1 day. Mosquito longevity

FIGURE 159-1   Distribution of chloroquine-resistant *Plasmodium falciparum*, 1988. Shaded area denotes regions where malaria occurs or might occur. *(Courtesy of Malaria Section, Centers for Disease Control.)*

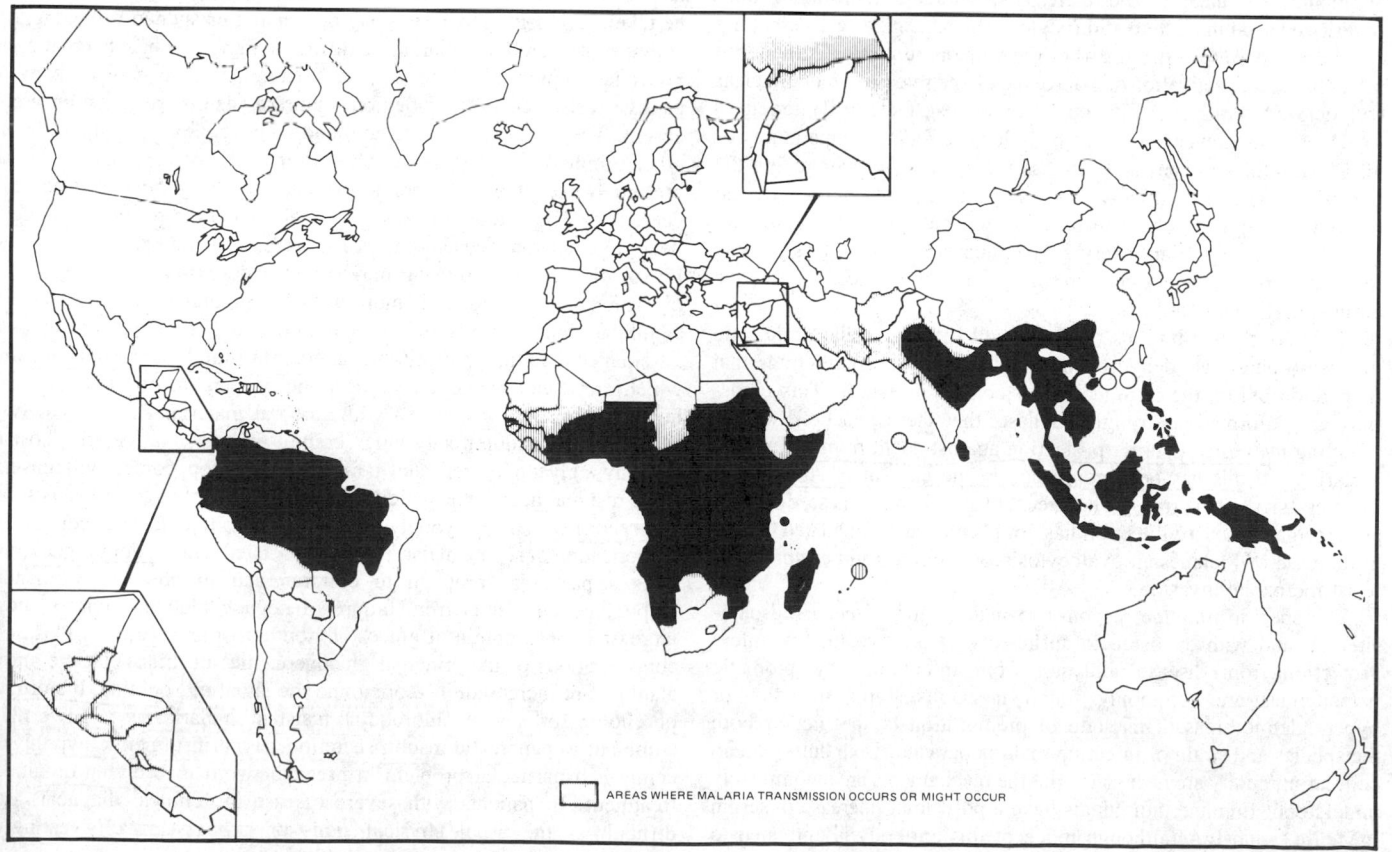

AREAS WHERE MALARIA TRANSMISSION OCCURS OR MIGHT OCCUR

is particularly important, because the extrinsic cycle from sporozoite ingestion to subsequent inoculation takes a minimum of 7 days (depending on ambient temperature) and in order to transmit malaria the mosquito must survive for longer than this. Therefore the most effective mosquito vectors are those (such as *A. gambiae* in west Africa) which are long-lived, occur in high densities, and bite humans frequently.

ERYTHROCYTE CHANGES   After invasion, the growing parasite progressively consumes and degrades intracellular proteins, principally hemoglobin, and also alters the red-cell membrane by changing its transport properties, exposing cryptic surface antigens, and inserting new parasite-derived proteins. The red cell becomes more spherical and less deformable. In *P. falciparum* infections membrane protuberances appear on the erythrocyte surface in the second 24 h of the asexual cycle. These "knobs" overlie accretions of electron-dense, histidine-rich parasite proteins and extrude a high-molecular-weight, strain-specific, adhesive protein which mediates attachment to receptors on venular and capillary endothelium. These receptors are related to thrombospondin, its natural receptor, platelet glycoprotein 4, and other unidentified proteins. This process of "cytoadherence" is central to the pathogenesis of falciparum malaria. It results in sequestration of mature forms of the parasite in vital organs (particularly the brain and heart) where they interfere with microcirculatory flow and metabolism and continue development away from the principal host defense, i.e., by splenic processing and filtration. As a consequence, only the younger ring forms of the asexual parasites are seen in the peripheral blood in falciparum malaria, and the peripheral parasitemia is an underestimate of the true number of parasites within the body. In the other three "benign" malarias sequestration does not occur, and all stages of parasite development may be seen on peripheral blood smears. Whereas these species show a marked predilection for either old red cells or reticulocytes and parasitemias seldom exceed 2 percent, *P. falciparum* can invade erythrocytes of all ages, and very high parasitemias may occur.

HOST RESPONSE   The initial response to infection in the nonimmune subject is the activation of nonspecific host defense mechanisms. Splenic immunologic and filtrative clearance functions are augmented in malaria, and there is accelerated removal of both parasitized and uninfected erythrocytes. The parasitized cells escaping splenic removal are destroyed when the schizont ruptures. The material released induces activation of macrophages and release of mononuclear cell–derived cytokines (including tumor necrosis factor and interleukin 1) which cause fever and other pathologic effects. Temperatures of 40°C are schizonticidal, and this has the effect of synchronizing the parasite cycle and eventually producing the regular fever spikes and rigors that originally characterized the different malarias (quotidian, daily fever spike; tertian, every 2 days; quartan, every 3 days). These fever patterns are seldom seen in patients who receive effective antimalarial treatment.

The global distributions of sickle cell disease, thalassemia, and glucose-6-phosphate dehydrogenase deficiency closely resemble that of malaria before the introduction of control measures. This epidemiologic information strongly suggests that these genetic disorders affecting the red cell confer protection against death from falciparum malaria, and this has been confirmed in the case of HbA/S heterozygotes (sickle cell trait). The mechanism whereby these disorders protect against severe infection has not been clearly elucidated except in the case of Melanesian ovalocytosis, where the rigid erythrocytes resist merozoite invasion.

The specific immune response to malaria limits the rising parasitemia, and with exposure to sufficient strains, eventually confers protection from disease, but not from infection. Asymptomatic parasitemias are commonly found in adults living in holo- or hyperendemic areas. This state of premunition is specific for both the species and strain of infecting malaria parasite. Both humoral and cellular immunity are necessary, but the mechanisms are incompletely understood. Immune individuals have a polyclonal increase in serum IgM, IgG, and IgA (although much of this antibody is unrelated to

protection). Antibodies against a variety of parasite stage–specific antigens (particularly those related to the red cell surface cytoadherence protein) presumably act in concert to limit in vivo parasite replication. Passively transferred IgG from immune adults has been shown to reduce parasitemia in children, and passive transfer of maternal antibody also presumably contributes to the relative protection from severe malaria in the first months of life. Several factors retard the development of cellular immunity. These include the absence of major histocompatibility antigens on the surface of infected red cells, which precludes direct T-cell recognition; malaria antigen–specific immune unresponsiveness; and the enormous strain diversity of malaria parasites and their ability to express variant antigens on the erythrocyte surface which change during the period of infection. Immunity against all strains is never achieved. Parasites may persist in the blood for months and, in the case of *P. malariae*, for many years if treatment is not given. The complexity of the immune response in malaria, the sophistication of the parasites' evasive mechanisms, and the lack of a good in vitro correlate with clinical immunity have all contributed to the slow progress toward an effective vaccine.

CLINICAL FEATURES   The first symptoms of malaria are nonspecific; lack of well-being, headache, fatigue, and muscle aching followed by fever are all similar to those of a minor viral illness. In some patients headache, chest pain, abdominal pain, arthralgia, myalgia, or diarrhea may be prominent and suggest an alternative diagnosis. The classic malarial paroxysms in which fever spikes, chills, and rigors occur at regular intervals are rare. The fever is irregular at first and in nonimmune individuals or children often rises over 40°C accompanied by an appropriate tachycardia and, in some cases, delirium. Nausea, vomiting, and orthostatic hypotension are common. Although many clinical abnormalities have been described in acute malaria, most patients with uncomplicated infections have few abnormal findings other than mild anemia and, in some cases, a palpable spleen.

Severe falciparum malaria   CEREBRAL MALARIA   Coma is a characteristic and ominous feature of falciparum malaria and is associated with a mortality of 20 percent despite treatment. Lesser degrees of obtundation, delirium, or abnormal behavior should also be taken seriously. The onset may be gradual or sudden following a convulsion. Cerebral malaria is a diffuse symmetric encephalopathy. Focal neurologic signs are unusual. Although there may be some passive resistance to head flexion, signs of meningeal irritation are absent. The eyes may be divergent and a pout reflex is common, but other primitive reflexes are usually absent. The corneal reflexes are preserved except in deep coma. Muscle tone may be increased or decreased. The tendon reflexes are variable, and the plantars may be flexor or extensor. The abdominal and cremasteric reflexes are absent. Flexor or extensor posturing may occur. Approximately 15 percent of patients have retinal hemorrhages. Less than 5 percent have significant bleeding or other clinical evidence of disseminated intravascular coagulation. Anemia and jaundice are common. Convulsions, which are usually generalized, occur in 50 percent of adults and a higher proportion of children with cerebral malaria. Approximately 10 percent of children surviving cerebral malaria, particularly those with hypoglycemia, repeated seizures, and deep coma, will have some residual neurologic deficit following recovery of consciousness.

HYPOGLYCEMIA   Hypoglycemia is an important and common complication of severe malaria and is associated with a poor prognosis. It is a particular problem in children and in pregnant women. Hypoglycemia results from failure of hepatic gluconeogenesis and increased consumption of glucose by both host and parasite. Plasma concentrations of the principal gluconeogenic substrates, lactate and alanine, are increased. To compound the situation, quinine, the drug of choice for severe chloroquine-resistant malaria, is a powerful stimulant to pancreatic insulin secretion. Hyperinsulinemic hypoglycemia is a particular problem in pregnant women receiving quinine treatment. In patients with severe disease the clinical diagnosis is difficult as the usual physical signs of hypoglycemia (sweating, gooseflesh, tachycardia) are absent and neurologic impairment cannot be distinguished from that caused by malaria.

LACTIC ACIDOSIS Lactic acidosis commonly coexists with hypoglycemia. Anaerobic glycolysis in tissues where sequestered parasitized erythrocytes interfere with microcirculatory flow, parasite lactate production, and a failure of hepatic lactate clearance combine to raise plasma lactate concentrations. The prognosis is poor. Hyperventilation is usually followed by circulatory failure refractory to volume expansion or inotropic drugs.

NONCARDIOGENIC PULMONARY EDEMA This may develop in adults with severe falciparum malaria even after several days' antimalarial therapy. The pathogenesis of this variant of the adult respiratory distress syndrome is unclear. The mortality is over 80 percent.

RENAL IMPAIRMENT This is common in adults with severe falciparum malaria but rare in children. It is a marker of severe disease and carries a high mortality. The pathogenesis of renal failure is unclear, but may be related to parasitized erythrocyte sequestration which interferes with renal microcirculatory flow and regional metabolism. Clinically and pathologically this syndrome behaves like acute tubular necrosis, and provided the acute phase of the disease can be overcome, renal function returns over a period of days or weeks (see Chap. 223).

HEMATOLOGIC ABNORMALITIES The pathophysiology of anemia in malaria is multifactorial. There are accelerated red cell destruction and removal by the spleen and bone marrow suppression with ineffective erythropoiesis. In severe malaria anemia develops rapidly, and transfusion is often required. Slight coagulation abnormalities are common in falciparum malaria, and mild thrombocytopenia is usual. In a small number of cases (less than 5 percent of patients with cerebral malaria) significant bleeding occurs with evidence of disseminated intravascular coagulation. Hematemesis, presumably from stress ulceration or acute gastric erosions, may also occur.

OTHER COMPLICATIONS Aspiration pneumonia following convulsions is an important cause of death in cerebral malaria. Malaria predisposes to bacterial superinfection. Catheter-induced urinary infections are common. Spontaneous gram-negative septicemia may occur in severe malaria, and Salmonella septicemias have been associated with P. falciparum infections in endemic areas.

Malaria in pregnancy Falciparum malaria is an important cause of fetal death. In hyper- and holoendemic areas malaria is associated with low birth weight, but in general the mothers remain asymptomatic despite intense parasitization of the placenta (due to sequestration of parasitized erythrocytes in the placental microcirculation).

In areas with unstable transmission, pregnant women are prone to severe infections, and are particularly vulnerable to develop high parasitemias with anemia, hypoglycemia, and acute pulmonary edema. Fetal distress, premature labor, and stillbirth commonly ensue, and congenital malaria can develop in the newborn.

Malaria in children Most of the estimated 1 million deaths from falciparum malaria each year occur in children. Convulsions, coma, hypoglycemia, metabolic acidosis, and severe anemia are relatively common in children with severe malaria, whereas acute renal failure and acute pulmonary edema are unusual. In general, children tolerate the antimalarial drugs well and respond rapidly to treatment.

Transfusion malaria Malaria can be transmitted by blood transfusion or needle sharing with infected intravenous drug addicts. P. malariae and P. falciparum have been the most common causes. The incubation period is often short because there is no preerythrocytic development. Clinical features and management are as in naturally acquired infections. Radical chemotherapy with primaquine in P. vivax and P. ovale infections is unnecessary.

CHRONIC COMPLICATIONS OF MALARIA Tropical splenomegaly (hyperreactive malarial splenomegaly) Chronic or repeated malaria infections produce hypergammaglobulinemia, a normochromic normocytic anemia, and, in certain situations, splenomegaly. Some residents of malaria-endemic areas exhibit an abnormal im-

munologic response to repeated infections which results in massive splenomegaly, hepatomegaly, marked elevations in serum IgM and malaria antibody, hepatic sinusoidal lymphocytosis, and, in Africa, peripheral (B-cell) lymphocytosis. On Flores Island, Indonesia, the condition is associated with the production of cytotoxic IgM antisuppressor lymphocyte (CD8+) antibodies. This leads to uninhibited B-cell production of IgM and the formation of cryoglobulins (IgM aggregates and immune complexes), which stimulates reticuloendothelial hyperplasia and clearance activity and eventually produces splenomegaly. Patients with hyperreactive malarial splenomegaly (HMS) present with an abdominal mass or complaints of a dragging sensation in the abdomen and occasional sharp abdominal pains suggesting perisplenitis. There is usually anemia and some degree of pancytopenia, but in most cases malaria parasites cannot be found in peripheral blood smears. There is increased vulnerability to respiratory and skin infections, and many patients die of overwhelming sepsis. HMS usually responds to effective antimalarial prophylaxis.

Quartan malaria nephropathy Chronic or repeated infections with P. malariae may cause soluble immune-complex injury to the renal glomeruli resulting in nephrotic syndrome. Other unidentified factors must be contributory, because only a very small proportion of infected patients develop renal disease. The histologic appearance is of a focal or segmental glomerulonephritis with splitting of the capillary basement membrane. Subendothelial dense deposits are seen on electron microscopy, and immunofluorescence reveals deposits of complement and immunoglobulins; in children P. malariae antigens can often be seen. Patients with a coarse granular pattern of basement membrane immunofluorescent deposits (predominantly IgG3) and selective proteinuria have a better prognosis than those with a fine granular, predominantly IgG2 pattern and nonselective proteinuria. Quartan nephropathy usually responds poorly to treatment with either antimalarials or glucocorticoids and cytotoxic drugs.

DIAGNOSIS The diagnosis of malaria rests on the demonstration of asexual forms of the parasite in peripheral blood smears stained with one of the Romanowsky stains (Wright's, Field's, Leishman's, or Giemsa at pH 7.2). Both thin and thick blood smears should be examined. The thin smear should be air-dried rapidly, fixed in anhydrous methanol, and stained, and the red cells in the tail of the film examined under oil immersion. The parasitemia is expressed as the number of parasitized erythrocytes in 1000 cells and then converted to the number per microliter. The relationship between parasitemia and prognosis is complex; in general, patients with parasitemias in excess of 10^5 per microliter are at an increased risk of a fatal outcome, but nonimmunes may die with much lower counts, and semi-immunes may tolerate parasitemias of three times this value with only minor symptoms.

The thick film should be of uneven thickness. The smear should be dried thoroughly and stained *without* fixing. As many layers of erythrocytes overlie each other and are then lysed during the staining procedure, the thick film has the advantage of concentrating the parasites, and therefore increasing the sensitivity of diagnosis. Both parasites and white cells are counted and the number of parasites per unit volume calculated from the total leukocyte count. A minimum of 200 white cells should be counted. Interpretation of thick films requires some experience because artifacts are common. Phagocytosed malaria pigment may be seen inside peripheral blood monocytes or polymorphonuclear leukocytes and may provide a clue to recent infection if malaria parasites are not seen. Occasionally parasites and pigment are evident in bone marrow aspirates or smears obtained from fluid expressed after intradermal puncture, but not on peripheral blood smears. Considerable advances have been made with DNA probes and flow cytometry in the diagnosis of malaria, and their sensitivity is approaching that of a trained microscopist.

Laboratory findings A normochromic normocytic anemia is usual. The leukocyte count is low to normal, although it may be raised in very severe infections. The erythrocyte sedimentation rate, plasma viscosity, and C-reactive protein levels are high. The platelet count is usually moderately reduced. In severe infections there may be prolongation of the prothrombin and partial thromboplastin times. Antithrombin III levels are reduced even in mild infection. In uncomplicated malaria, plasma concentration of electrolytes, blood urea nitrogen, and creatinine are usually normal. In severe malaria there may be a metabolic acidosis with low plasma concentrations of glucose, sodium, bicarbonate, calcium, magnesium, and albumin together with elevations in lactate, BUN, creatinine, muscle and liver enzymes, and conjugated and unconjugated bilirubin. Hypergammaglobulinemia is usual in immune and semi-immune subjects. Urinalysis is usually normal.

PREVENTION In most of the rural tropics, eradication of malaria is not feasible. Where possible, the disease is contained by judicious use of insecticides to kill the mosquito vector, and chemoprophylaxis in high-risk groups. All pregnant women at risk should receive prophylaxis, and prophylactic antimalarials should be given to children between the ages of 1 and 4 in areas where malaria causes high childhood mortality. Widespread use of bed nets, particularly if treated with permethrin (a residual pyrethroid), will considerably reduce the incidence of malaria. Despite massive investment toward development of a malaria vaccine, a safe, effective, and long-lasting vaccine is unlikely soon (see Chap. 156).

PERSONAL PROTECTION AGAINST MALARIA Simple measures to reduce the frequency of mosquito bites in malarious areas are very important. These include avoiding exposure at peak feeding times (usually dusk and dawn), and use of insect repellants, suitable clothing, and impregnated bed nets.

Chemoprophylaxis (Table 159-2) Few areas of therapeutics are as controversial as antimalarial drug prophylaxis. Recommendations for prophylaxis depend on a knowledge of local parasite drug sensitivity and the likelihood of acquiring malaria infection. Chemoprophylaxis is never entirely reliable, and malaria should always be considered in the differential diagnosis of fever in patients who have taken prophylactic antimalarial drugs. Chloroquine [5 mg base per kilogram per week (300 mg maximum) weekly] remains the drug of choice for the prevention of drug-sensitive *P. falciparum* and the other human malarias. It is generally well tolerated, although some patients are unable to take the drug because of dysphoria, headache, or, in dark-skinned patients, pruritus. It is considered relatively safe in pregnancy. With chronic administration a characteristic dose-related retinopathy develops; in adults cumulative doses over 100 g are associated with significant risk. Individuals receiving long-term chloroquine prophylaxis should therefore have regular ophthalmologic examinations. Idiosyncratic or allergic reactions are rare. Skeletal and cardiac myopathy may also occur but are more likely with the high doses used in the treatment of rheumatoid arthritis. Neuropsychiatric reactions and skin rashes are unusual. The related aminoquinoline amodiaquine has also been used, but is associated with a high risk of agranulocytosis and is not recommended. In the past the dihydrofolate reductase inhibitors pyrimethamine and proguanil (chloroguanide) have been used widely, but resistant strains of both *P. falciparum* and *P. vivax* have limited their use. Whereas the quinoline antimalarials such as chloroquine act on the erythrocyte stage of parasite development, the dihydrofolate reductase inhibitors also inhibit preerythrocytic growth (causal prophylactics) and development in the mosquito (sporontocidal activity). There has been a resurgence of interest in proguanil [1.5 to 3 mg/kg (200 mg maximum) daily] because it may retain efficacy against pyrimethamine-resistant strains of *P. falciparum,* and apart from rare cases of mouth ulceration, it is safe and well tolerated. Proguanil is considered the safest antimalarial prophylactic in pregnancy. The prophylactic use of the combination of pyrimethamine and sulfadoxine is not recommended because of an unacceptable incidence of severe toxicity, principally exfoliative dermatitis and other skin rashes, agranulocytosis, hepatitis, and pulmonary eosinophilia.

The combination of pyrimethamine with dapsone [0.2/1.5 mg/kg (25/200 mg maximum) weekly] is widely used in areas with chloroquine-resistant *P. falciparum* and is generally well tolerated, although there is increasing resistance and dapsone may cause methemoglobinemia, allergic reactions, and, with higher doses, a significant risk of agranulocytosis. In areas with multi-drug-resistant falciparum malaria there is no satisfactory, generally available prophylactic. Daily doxycycline (100 mg maximum) is effective and also has causal prophylactic activity. It is generally well tolerated but may cause *Monilia* infections, diarrhea, and photosensitivity and cannot be used in children or in pregnancy. Faced with the problems of variable drug resistance and the lack of safe and effective prophylactic antimalarials, the Centers for Disease Control have opted for pragmatism adopting a strategy of presumptive treatment for those at risk

TABLE 159-2 Prophylaxis and treatment of malaria

	Chloroquine-sensitive *P. falciparum, P. vivax, P. malariae,* and *P. ovale*	Chloroquine-resistant *P. falciparum*
Prophylaxis	Chloroquine 5 mg base/kg/wk (300 mg maximum) or proguanil 3 mg/kg/d (200 mg maximum). Mefloquine: See discussion on p. 788.	No safe and reliable drug for all geographic areas. Strategies include combined chloroquine & proguanil or: 1. Chloroquine 10 mg base/kg/wk (600 mg maximum). 2. Doxycycline 1.5 mg/kg/d (100 mg maximum). 3. Presumptive treatment with either sulfadoxine-pyrimethamine or quinine.
Treatment of uncomplicated infections	Chloroquine 10 mg base/kg (600 mg maximum) stat followed by 5 mg/kg at 6 (600 mg maximum), 24, and 48 h (or 10 mg/kg daily for 3 days).	Quinine 10 mg salt/kg (650 mg maximum) q8h PO (5–7 days) together with tetracycline* 4 mg/kg (250 mg maximum) q6h (7 days), or in some areas pyrimethamine 1 mg/kg + sulfadoxine 20 mg/kg stat (75/1500 mg maximum).
Treatment of severe malaria†	Chloroquine 10 mg base/kg (600 mg maximum) infused IV at a constant rate over 8 h followed by 15 mg base/kg (900 mg maximum) infused over 24 h.	Quinine‡,§ 7 mg salt/kg (400 mg maximum) infused IV at a constant rate over 30 min, followed immediately by 10 mg salt/kg (600 mg maximum) over 4 h, and then, after an interval of 4 h, by infusions of 10 mg salt/kg (600 mg maximum) q8h for 7 days. (Infusion times 2–8 h.)
Hospital and nursing facilities Rural clinic without nursing facilities	Chloroquine 3.5 mg/kg base (200 mg maximum) q6h or 2.5 mg base q4h (150 mg maximum) by either SC or IM injection. Total dose 25 mg/kg (1500 mg maximum).	Quinine 20 mg salt/kg (1200 mg maximum) stat followed by 10 mg salt/kg q8h given by deep IM injection. The quinine concentration should be 60 mg salt/mL, and the first dose should be split into two, e.g., half the dose into each thigh.

* Tetracycline should not be given in pregnancy or to children under 8 years.
† Oral treatment should be substituted as soon as the patient recovers sufficiently to take fluids by mouth. Nasogastric administration of oral antimalarials should be attempted if patients are first seen in a situation where parenteral treatment is not possible pending transfer to hospital.
‡ Quinidine gluconate may be substituted if quinine is not available but electrocardiographic monitoring is advisable, and quinine should be substituted when possible. Loading dose 10 mg salt/kg infused over 1 h followed by continuous infusion given at rate of 0.02 mg/kg/min for 3 days.
§ A loading dose should not be given if quinine or quinidine has been given in the previous 24 h.

from multi-drug-resistant malaria. Adult travelers are advised to take three 25/500 mg tablets of sulfadoxine-pyrimethamine if they develop fever and have no recourse to medical facilities. Alternatives are weekly chloroquine and daily proguanil (Table 159-2), or weekly chloroquine and pyrimethamine-dapsone, with appropriate medical advice in case of fever.

Travelers should start taking antimalarial drugs at least 1 week before departure in order to detect untoward reactions and to provide therapeutic antimalarial blood concentrations when needed in the endemic area. Those persons starting chloroquine immediately before departure should take a loading dose [10 mg base per kilogram (600 mg maximum)]. Antimalarial prophylaxis should continue for 6 weeks after leaving an endemic area.

TREATMENT Patients in or from malarious areas who present with fever should have a blood smear to confirm the diagnosis and identify the species of infecting parasite. In endemic areas uncomplicated infections may be treated on an outpatient basis. Regimens for FDA-approved drugs are detailed in Table 159-2, and characteristics of various agents in Table 159-3. Three additional drugs yet to be approved for antimalarial use in the United States deserve mention; two are quinine analogues that can be substituted for that agent in some circumstances. The antiarrhythmic quinidine gluconate appears to be as rapidly schizonticidal as quinine and is more readily available. However, because it appears to be more cardiotoxic than quinine, its administration must be closely monitored if inadvertent arrhythmia and/or hypotension are to be avoided. Blood levels in excess of 6 μg/mL, QT interval greater than 0.6 s, or QRS widening beyond 25 percent of baseline are indications for slowing infusion rates. If arrhythmia or saline-unresponsive hypotension develop, the drug should be discontinued. Dosage is provided in Table 159-2. As the agent has not been approved for malaria, informed consent should be obtained prior to administration. Mefloquine, a newly developed oral 4-quinolinemethanol, also displays rapid schizonticidal activity against chloroquine-resistant strains of *P. falciparum*. Although effective as a prophylactic agent, there is concern that widespread use will accelerate the development of resistant strains and shorten its period of usefulness as a therapeutic agent in chloroquine-resistant falciparum infections. Its ease of administration and relative lack of toxicity has led to its replacement of quinine in some endemic areas. The third agent, halofantrine, is a well-tolerated, oral phenanthrenemethanol that is used in some parts of Africa. It is effective against both chloroquine-sensitive and chloroquine-resistant strains of falciparum malaria. Acetaminophen lowers fever and provides symptomatic relief and thereby reduces the propensity to vomit the oral antimalarial drugs. Pregnant women, young children, patients unable to tolerate oral therapy, and nonimmune subjects (e.g., travelers) with suspected malaria should be hospitalized.

If there is any doubt as to the identification of the malaria species, treatment for falciparum malaria should be given. If the smear is negative, this does not rule out malaria, and thick blood films should be checked 1 and 2 days later to exclude the diagnosis. Nonimmune subjects with malaria should have daily parasite counts performed until thick films are negative (parasite clearance). If the parasitemia does not fall below 25 percent of the admission value in 48 h, or has not cleared by 7 days, drug resistance should be suspected and treatment should be changed. If falciparum malaria has been contracted in an area of known drug sensitivity, chloroquine or sulfadoxine-pyrimethamine are preferable because they are better tolerated and simpler than quinine and tetracycline. If there is doubt about drug sensitivity, the latter combination should be prescribed.

Primaquine [0.2 mg base per kilogram (15 mg maximum)] should be given daily for 14 days in patients with *P. vivax* or *P. ovale*

TABLE 159-3 Antimalarial drugs

Drug	Pharmacokinetic properties	Antimalarial activity	Minor toxicity	Major toxicity
Quinine	Absorption: Oral: good Intramuscular: good Cl* ↓ and Vd† ↓ but plasma protein binding ↑ (90%) in malaria t½: 16 h in malaria, 11 h in health	Rapid "schizonticide" Gametocytocidal against *P. vivax*, *P. ovale*, and *P. malariae*; no action on liver stages	Bitter-tasting Common: "cinchonism," tinnitus, high-tone hearing loss, nausea, vomiting, dysphoria, postural hypotension; prolongation of ECG QTc interval Rare: diarrhea, visual disturbance, rashes	Common: hypoglycemia Rare: hypotension, blindness, deafness, cardiac arrhythmias, thrombocytopenia, hemolysis, cholestatic hepatitis, neuromuscular paralysis
Chloroquine	Absorption: Oral: good Intramuscular: very rapid Subcutaneous: very rapid Complex pharmacokinetics Enormous Cl* and Vd† (unaffected by malaria) Distribution processes determine blood concentration profile in malaria t½: 1–2 months	Rapid "schizonticide" Gametocytocidal against *P. vivax*, *P. ovale*, and *P. malariae*; no action on liver stages	Bitter-tasting Well-tolerated Common: nausea, dysphoria, pruritus in dark-skinned patients; postural hypotension Rare: accommodation difficulties, rash	Acute: hypotension shock (parenteral); cardiac arrhythmias; neuropsychiatric reactions Chronic: retinopathy (cumulative dose >100 g); skeletal and cardiac myopathy
Mefloquine:	See discussion on p. 788.			
Pyrimethamine	Absorption: Oral: good Intramuscular: insufficient data t½: 4 days	Speed of action depends on stage of parasite development	Well-tolerated	Megaloblastic anemia Pancytopenia Pulmonary infiltration
Proguanil (chloroguanide)	Absorption: Oral: good Biotransformed to active metabolite cycloguanil t½: 16 h	Causal prophylactic; not used for treatment	Well-tolerated Rare: mouth ulcers	Megaloblastic anemia in renal failure
Primaquine	Absorption: Oral: complete Active compound not known t½: 7 h	Radical cure Eradicates exoerythrocytic forms of *P. vivax* and *P. ovale* Gametocytocidal against *P. falciparum*	Nausea, vomiting diarrhea, abdominal pain; hemolysis; methemoglobinemia	Massive hemolysis in subjects with severe G6PD deficiency

*Cl = systemic clearance.
†Vd = total apparent volume of distribution.

infections after laboratory tests for G6PD deficiency have proved negative. If the patient has one of the mild variants of G6PD deficiency, the primaquine can be given in a dose of 0.6 mg base per kilogram (45 mg maximum) once weekly for 6 weeks.

Severe falciparum malaria is a medical emergency requiring intensive nursing care and careful management. Patients should be weighed and, if comatose, nursed on their side and given a single parenteral dose of phenobarbital (3.5 to 5 mg/kg) to prevent convulsions. The immediate management is outlined in Table 159-4. Frequent evaluation is essential. Ancillary drugs such as high-dose glucocorticoids, mannitol, urea, heparin, and dextran are of no value. The choice of antimalarial drug depends on knowledge of the prevailing sensitivity of *P. falciparum* to antimalarials. If there is any doubt, quinine (or if not available, quinidine) should be given. Systemic clearance and apparent volume of distribution of these drugs are markedly reduced in severe malaria, and blood concentrations for a given dose are consequently higher. The optimum therapeutic range of quinine in severe malaria is not known with certainty, but plasma concentrations between 0.8 and 1.5 mg/dL are effective and do not cause serious toxicity. An initial loading dose is given to provide therapeutic concentrations as soon as possible but is not necessary if the patient has already started quinine treatment before admission to the hospital. If the patient remains seriously ill or in acute renal failure for 3 days, the maintenance doses should be reduced by one-third to one-half to prevent accumulation of quinine to toxic concentrations. The initial doses should never be reduced. If chloroquine is given, dose reduction is unnecessary even in the face of renal failure.

In unconscious patients the blood glucose should be measured every 6 h and blood glucose values below 2.2 mmol/L (40 mg/dL) treated with intravenous dextrose. Patients treated with intravenous quinine should receive a continuous infusion of dextrose. The parasite count and hematocrit should be measured every 12 h. Anemia develops rapidly; if the hematocrit falls below 20 percent, then whole blood (preferably fresh) or packed cells should be transfused slowly with careful attention to circulatory status and judicious use of small doses of a diuretic to prevent fluid overload. Renal function should be checked daily. Management of fluid balance is difficult in severe malaria because there is a thin dividing line between overhydration, leading to pulmonary edema, and underhydration, contributing to renal impairment. If necessary, pulmonary artery wedge pressure should be measured and maintained in the low-normal range. As soon as the patient can take fluids, oral antimalarials are substituted.

MEFLOQUINE   Approved by the FDA in 1989 for prevention and treatment of *P. falciparum* and *P. vivax* malaria, the drug is active against all species including strains resistant to chloroquine and fansidar (some *P. falciparum* strains are resistant). Mefloquine

Lariam (Roche)

HCl is well absorbed from the GI tract, metabolized in the liver, and excreted in the bile and feces. Doses of 500 to 1000 mg are effective, even against strains resistant to multiple drugs. Adverse effects are dose related and include vertigo, nausea, and lightheadedness. Confusion, convulsions, and psychosis have been reported. The drug may prolong cardiac conduction and is contraindicated in patients taking beta blockers and calcium channel blockers. It should not be used with quinine or quinidine nor by children or pregnant women. The dose for prophylaxis is one 250-mg tablet weekly for 4 weeks (beginning 1 week before travel), then one tablet every other week during a stay in a malarious area and for two doses afterward. For acute uncomplicated *P. falciparum* malaria treatment is a single oral dose of 1250 mg with 8 oz. of water.

COMPLICATIONS   Acute renal failure   If there is a rising blood urea nitrogen or creatinine level despite adequate rehydration, fluid administration should be restricted to keep pulmonary arterial wedge pressures from rising. The indications for dialysis are the same as those in other forms of hypercatabolic acute renal failure (see Chap. 223). Although peritoneal dialysis is adequate, secondary bacterial infections are common in the tropics, and hemodialysis is preferable. Some patients will pass small volumes of urine sufficient to allow control of fluid balance and may be managed conservatively if other indications for dialysis do not arise. Renal function usually improves in days, but may take weeks to recover fully.

Acute pulmonary edema   Patients should be nursed at 45° and given oxygen and intravenous diuretics. Pulmonary artery wedge pressures may be normal, indicating increased pulmonary capillary permeability. Positive pressure ventilation should be instituted if these immediate measures fail (see Chap. 219).

Hypoglycemia   An initial slow infusion of 50% dextrose (0.5 g dextrose per kilogram per hour) should be followed by an infusion of 10% dextrose (0.10 g dextrose per kilogram per hour). The blood glucose should be checked regularly thereafter, as recurrent hypoglycemia is common, particularly in patients receiving quinine or quinidine. In severely ill patients hypoglycemia commonly occurs together with a metabolic (lactic) acidosis, and may prove fatal.

Other complications   Patients who develop spontaneous bleeding should be given fresh blood and intravenous vitamin K. Convulsions should be treated with intravenous (or rectal) diazepam. Aspiration pneumonia should be suspected in any unconscious patient with convulsions, particularly if there is persistent hyperventilation. Intravenous antimicrobials, pulmonary toilet, and oxygen should be administered. Hypoglycemia or gram-negative septicemia should be suspected in any patient who suddenly deteriorates for no immediately obvious reason while receiving antimalarial treatment.

TABLE 159-4   Immediate management of severe malaria

1. Weigh.
2. Check airway, nurse patient on side.
3. Make rapid clinical assessment.
4. Take venous blood for quantitative parasite count, hematocrit, blood glucose, blood urea nitrogen (or creatinine), blood culture, and blood group.
5. Take arterial blood for pH and gases if clinically indicated.
6. Start controlled-rate infusion of antimalarial.
7. Make brief clinical examination; assess state of hydration.
8. Check urine output and consider need for hemodynamic monitoring.
9. If core temperature exceeds 38.5°C, give rectal acetaminophen suppository and start tepid sponging and fanning.
10. If patient is comatose, perform diagnostic lumbar puncture and give single intravenous or intramuscular dose of phenobarbital (3.5 to 5 mg/kg).
11. Consider need for blood transfusion and treatment of complications such as hypoglycemia, bacterial superinfections, bleeding, etc.

REFERENCES

Bray RS, Garnham PCC: Life cycle of primate malaria parasites. Br Med Bull 38:117, 1982

David PH et al: Parasite sequestration in *Plasmodium falciparum* malaria: Spleen and antibody modulation of cytoadherence of infected erythrocytes. Proc Nat Acad Sci USA 80:5075, 1983

Galbraith RM et al: The human materno-fetal relationship in malaria. Trans R Soc Trop Med Hyg 74:52, 61, 1980

Hoffman SL et al: Reduction of suppressor T lymphocytes in the tropical splenomegaly syndrome. N Engl J Med 310:337, 1984

Molineau XL, Gramiccia G: *The Garki Project. Research on the Epidemiology and Control of Malaria in the Sudan Savannah of West Africa*. Geneva, WHO, 1980

Pasvol G: Receptors on red cells for *Plasmodium falciparum* and their interaction with the merozoite. Philos Trans R Soc 307:189, 1984

Phillips RE et al: Intravenous quinidine for the treatment of severe falciparum malaria. Clinical and pharmacokinetic studies. N Engl J Med 312:1273, 1985

Spitz S: Pathology of acute falciparum malaria. Military Med 99:555, 1946

Warrell DA et al: Dexamethasone proves deleterious in cerebral malaria. A double blind trial in 100 comatose patients. N Engl J Med 306:313, 1982

White NJ: Drug treatment and prevention of malaria. Eur J Clin Pharmacol 34:1, 1988
——— et al: Severe hypoglycemia and hyperinsulinaemia in falciparum malaria. N Engl J Med 309:61, 1983

World Health Organization, Malaria Action Programme: Severe and complicated malaria. Trans R Soc Trop Med Hyg 80(Suppl):1,1986

160 LEISHMANIASIS

RICHARD M. LOCKSLEY

DEFINITION Leishmaniasis denotes disease caused by any of the number of species of protozoa in the genus *Leishmania*. There are four major clinical syndromes—visceral leishmaniasis (kala azar), cutaneous leishmaniasis of the old and new worlds, mucocutaneous leishmaniasis (espundia), and diffuse cutaneous leishmaniasis. Most commonly, these parasites are transmitted from animal reservoirs to human hosts by the bite of phlebotomine sandflies.

ETIOLOGY Different *Leishmania* species appear identical and are generally distinguished by clinical and geographic characteristics. Traditionally, speciation required determination of isoenzyme patterns, kinetoplast DNA buoyant densities, or specific phlebotomine vectors. Monoclonal antibodies, DNA hybridization, DNA restriction endonuclease fragment analysis, and chromosomal karyotyping using pulse-field electrophoresis are powerful new methods for distinguishing these parasites.

In the sandfly and in culture media, *Leishmania* exist as motile, spindle-shaped promastigotes (1.5 to 4 μm by 14 to 20 μm) with a single anterior flagellum. On inoculation into a mammalian host, the organisms enter mononuclear phagocytes, lose their flagella, and multiply as small (2 by 5 μm), oval, intracellular amastigotes (Leishman-Donovan bodies). In stained preparations a dark, slightly flattened nucleus and rod-shaped kinetoplast may be discerned.

EPIDEMIOLOGY Leishmaniasis is a zoonotic infection which involves the rodents, canines, and various forest mammals of every inhabited continent except Australia. The disease is spread when female sandflies of the genus *Phlebotomus* (old world) or *Lutzomyia* (new world) ingest amastigotes while taking a blood meal from an infected mammal. These transform into promastigotes within the insect's gut, migrate to the proboscis, and are deposited on the skin of the new host when the insect next engorges. Phlebotomines breed in warm, humid microclimates and are typically found in rodent burrows, termite hills, and rotting vegetation. Humans may acquire the disease when they encroach upon this sylvatic cycle. Establishment of infection in the domestic dog provides an important urban reservoir of leishmaniasis. Person-to-person transmission is infrequent except in the Indian form of kala azar. Rarely, transmission can occur by blood transfusion, contact inoculation, and coitus. It is estimated that worldwide over 12 million people are infected.

PATHOGENESIS Promastigotes are deposited on the skin into a small pool of blood drawn by the probing sandfly. Products from the fly salivary gland promote infectivity, in part via peptides that deactivate host macrophages. Complement is activated by the classical and/or alternative pathways, depending upon the species, and is deposited onto the major outer membrane molecules of the promastigote—a 63-kDa molecular weight glycoprotein (gp63) or lipophosphoglycan (LPG). LPG and gp63 either directly or through bound C3b or C3bi target the organisms to macrophages via the complement receptors CR3 and CR1. The promastigotes transform into amastigotes within phagolysosomes and replicate by binary fission. They eventually rupture the cell and invade adjacent macrophages.

The course of the subsequent disease is determined by the host's cellular immunity as well as the species of the parasite. In cutaneous leishmaniasis, there is a marked lymphocytic infiltration associated with a reduction in the number of parasites, the development of a delayed skin (leishmanin) reaction, and, frequently, spontaneous cure. In mucocutaneous disease, the complete or partial resolution of the primary lesion may be followed by metastatic mucocutaneous lesions at a later date. The destructiveness of the metastatic lesions is attributed to the development of hypersensitivity to parasite antigens. In diffuse cutaneous leishmaniasis there is no infiltration by lymphocytes or reduction in the number of parasites, the leishmanin reaction remains negative, and the skin lesions become chronic, progressive,

and disseminated. The patients have a selective anergy to *Leishmania* antigens that is mediated at least in part by adherent suppressor cells. In visceral leishmaniasis the parasites spread to macrophages throughout the body, perhaps due to the greater resistance of *L. donovani* to the spontaneous cidal activity present in normal serum. Although antibodies are present, they are nonprotective. The ability of the organism to cause progressive disease may be related to the development in the host of suppressor T lymphocytes. Cure of leishmaniasis requires activation of infected macrophages by lymphokines released from sensitized T cells and confers immunity to the infecting strain.

DIAGNOSIS Diagnosis of leishmaniasis requires demonstrating the organism by smear or culture of aspirates or tissue. Although Novy-MacNeal-Nicolle (NNN) medium traditionally has been used to culture *Leishmania*, several commercially available liquid media offer improved storage capability and enhanced recovery of organisms. Cultures are maintained at 22 to 28°C for 21 days and examined microscopically for the presence of the motile promastigotes. Inoculation of hamsters with infected clinical material results in infections after a period of weeks.

Species-specific diagnosis of human cutaneous new world isolates has been achieved by hybridization of tissue touch blots with radiolabeled kinetoplast DNA probes, but the method is not readily available.

Antibodies are detectable in all forms of leishmaniasis. The direct agglutination test detects IgM antibody and is a sensitive indicator of acute disease. The test is group-specific, but the titer is generally greatest to the homologous strain. A positive test (> 1:32) varies from 97 percent in visceral leishmaniasis to 81 percent in new world cutaneous leishmaniasis. Direct agglutination antibodies decline and may disappear with cure. Complement fixation (positive > 1:8) and indirect immunofluorescence (positive > 1:16) titers[1] may persist for years after resolution of disease. Other serologic tests are less available.

VISCERAL LEISHMANIASIS (KALA AZAR) *Leishmania donovani* causes kala azar, a disease that may be endemic, epidemic, or sporadic. Although the characteristics of the disease are similar throughout the world, certain local peculiarities in its behavior justify the classification of visceral leishmaniasis into three main types. These differences are attributed principally to the length of time that the disease has been endemic in a population.

African kala azar is found in the eastern half of Africa from the Sahara in the north to the equator in the south. Sporadic cases have been reported from west Africa. It is a disease of older children and young adults (10 to 25 years); males are involved more commonly than females. It is endemic in dogs and several wild carnivores in many areas and is more resistant to therapy with antimony compounds than the forms of kala azar found in the rest of the world.

Mediterranean, or infantile, kala azar is seen primarily in the Mediterranean area, China, U.S.S.R., and Latin America. It is a disease of children under the age of 4, but adults, particularly travelers to endemic areas, are not spared. Dogs, jackals, and foxes serve as reservoirs. Rats have been identified as a potential reservoir in Italy. The strains responsible for the Eurasian and American disease are sometimes referred to as *L. infantum* and *L. chagasi*, respectively.

Indian kala azar has an age and sex distribution similar to African kala azar. Humans are the only known reservoir, and transmission is carried out by anthropophilic sandflies.

Manifestations The incubation period is generally about 3 months (3 weeks to 18 months). A primary cutaneous lesion (leishmanioma) is not uncommon in Africa. The onset of disease may be insidious or abrupt; the latter occurs more frequently in individuals from nonendemic areas. Failure to thrive is common among infected infants and children. Fever, typically nocturnal and occasionally double-quotidian, is almost universal and is accompanied by tachycardia without signs of toxemia. Diarrhea and cough are frequent. Nontender splenomegaly becomes dramatic by the third month. The liver enlarges

---

[1]Available from the Centers for Disease Control, Atlanta, Georgia.

less conspicuously. Cirrhosis and portal hypertension occur in about 10 percent of patients. Lymphadenopathy accompanies some cases of African kala azar. Asymptomatic and prolonged, subclinical forms of infection are common in endemic areas; malnutrition is a risk factor for the progression to full-blown disease. Fulminant kala azar has been described in patients with AIDS.

Pancytopenia is characteristic. Anemia is multifactorial: autoimmune hemolysis, splenomegaly, and gastrointestinal blood loss all contribute. The latter is exacerbated by thrombocytopenia. Agranulocytosis, cancrum oris, and superinfections complicate untreated cases. Extensive leishmanial infiltration of the gastrointestinal tract may lead to malabsorption. Hypoalbuminemia and polyclonal hypergammaglobulinemia (IgG and IgM) are constant features. Circulating immune complexes are frequently present. Immune-complex glomerulonephritis and interstitial nephritis have been described. Amyloidosis may occur in patients with chronic infections. Edema, cachexia, and hyperpigmentation (kala azar means "black fever") are late manifestations. Without treatment death occurs within 3 to 20 months in 90 to 95 percent of adults and 75 to 85 percent of children, usually from superinfections or gastrointestinal hemorrhage.

After successful treatment, 3 percent of African cases and up to 10 percent of Indian cases develop post–kala azar dermal leishmaniasis (PKDL), characterized by a spectrum of lesions ranging from depigmented macules to wartlike nodules over the face and extensor surfaces of the limbs. PKDL appears shortly after symptoms subside in African cases and typically disappears after several weeks. In the Indian disease, PKDL appears after a latent period of 1 to 2 years and may last for years, creating a persistent human reservoir.

Diagnosis   Buffy coat preparations may demonstrate the parasite, particularly in Indian kala azar (90 percent). Bone marrow aspirate and biopsy are positive in over 85 percent of cases. In Kenya, splenic aspiration (95 percent) has proved quite safe and has been used serially to assess the response to therapy. In general, however, aspiration of the spleen or liver (75 percent) is not recommended because of the risk of hemorrhage. Aspirates or biopsy of enlarged lymph nodes will show parasites in 60 percent of cases. Suspicious skin lesions should be biopsied as well. The direct agglutination test is positive early in the disease. The leishmanin skin test becomes positive 6 to 8 weeks after recovery.[2] Other causes of fever in the tropics, including malaria, brucellosis, tuberculosis, typhoid, and hepatic abscess, can be distinguished by appropriate testing. PKDL must be differentiated from leprosy, syphilis, and yaws.

Treatment   Transfusions and treatment of complicating superinfections must supplement specific therapy. Pentavalent antimonials are highly effective against *Leishmania* and are relatively nontoxic. Sodium antimony gluconate (Pentostam[1]; 100 mg Sb^{5+} per milliliter) is given intravenously or intramuscularly in a single daily dose of 10 mg/kg for adults and 20 mg/kg for patients under 18 years of age. Treatment should be given for at least 20 days in Indian kala azar and 30 days in other forms. Meglumine antimoniate (Glucantime; 85 mg Sb^{5+} per milliliter) can also be used. Therapy should be repeated using 20 mg/kg for 40 to 60 days in patients with relapses or incomplete responses. Periodic electrocardiographic monitoring is recommended during prolonged therapy. The addition of oral allopurinol (20 to 30 mg/kg per day in three divided doses) has been effective. Resistant cases must be treated with intravenous amphotericin B (0.5 to 1 mg/kg on alternate days) or pentamidine (3 to 4 mg/kg three times per week for 5 to 25 weeks, depending on the response). Adjunctive splenectomy has been successful in some cases of drug-resistant kala azar. Mortality remains 15 to 25 percent in advanced cases, although the cure rate is over 90 percent when therapy is given early. Follow-up at 3 and 12 months is recommended to detect relapses. PKDL should be treated in the same fashion as the initial illness. Recombinant human interferon-γ has shown promise as adjunctive therapy with pentavalent antimony in previous treatment failures or in seriously ill patients with kala azar.

[2]The leishmanin skin test (Montenegro test), performed by the intradermal injection of promastigote antigens, is nonstandardized and generally unavailable.

Prevention   Preventive measures include early treatment of human cases, elimination of diseased dogs, and the use of DDT against sandflies. Application of insect repellents and the use of fine netting are important for travelers. There are no useful prophylactic agents.

CUTANEOUS AND MUCOCUTANEOUS LEISHMANIASIS   This form of leishmaniasis is caused by a number of species in both the old world and the new world. Disease is characterized by the development of single or multiple localized lesions on exposed areas of skin that typically ulcerate. Although spontaneous healing is the rule for old world cutaneous leishmaniasis, this is less common in new world disease.

Old world cutaneous leishmaniasis   *L. tropica* causes anthroponotic (urban, chronic, dry) cutaneous leishmaniasis, an endemic disease of children and young adults in areas bordering the Mediterranean, the Middle East, the southern U.S.S.R., and India. The principal reservoirs are humans, although domestic dogs are synanthropic hosts. The incubation period ranges from 2 to 24 months. Usually the lesion begins as a single, red pruritic papule on the face (oriental sore). The central area ulcerates and slowly enlarges centrifugally, reaching a size of approximately 2 cm. Lymphadenopathy is unusual. Healing occurs over 1 to 2 years and leaves a small depigmented scar. The disease can be complicated by the development of leishmaniasis recidiva, a condition marked by persistent facial lesions containing a scant number of parasites and by an exaggerated delayed hypersensitivity response to parasite antigens. Rarely, the organism may spread to the viscera.

L. major causes zoonotic (rural, acute, moist) cutaneous leishmaniasis, which is endemic to the desert areas of the Middle East, the southern U.S.S.R., and Africa. The reservoir is maintained in burrowing rodents. The incubation period ranges from 2 to 6 weeks. The initial lesions are often multiple and located on the lower extremities. Regional lymphadenopathy and satellite lesions are common. Healing with scarring occurs within 3 to 6 months. *L. major* has been implicated in cases of mucocutaneous leishmaniasis in Saudi Arabia. Although *L. major* confers immunity to *L. tropica*, the converse is not true.

L. aethiopica, maintained in rock hyraxes of the Ethiopian and Kenyan highlands, causes cutaneous leishmaniasis which may pursue a relatively prolonged course and can be complicated by the development of diffuse cutaneous leishmaniasis (see below).

DIAGNOSIS   Lesions should first be cleansed with alcohol to reduce bacterial contamination, which hinders recovery of the organisms. Aspirates should be obtained from the outer edge of the ulcer. If the aspirated smears are negative, full-thickness skin biopsies from the ulcer margin should be taken for touch smears, histology, and culture. The direct agglutination test and the leishmanin skin test become positive within 4 to 6 weeks.

TREATMENT   Specific therapy should be withheld in endemic areas until ulceration takes place, thereby conferring immunity. Exceptions include disfiguring or disabling lesions and lesions persisting for longer than 6 months. Treatment is with antimonials as described for kala azar, although shorter courses (10 days) are effective. Higher doses of antimony may be required for *L. aethiopica* infections (20 mg/kg twice a day for 30 days). Ulcers should be covered to prevent infection of vectors and other canine and human hosts.

New world cutaneous and mucocutaneous leishmaniasis   Leishmania causing new world cutaneous disease is divided into subspecies within the *L. mexicana* and *L. braziliensis* groups. The natural reservoirs for these organisms include a wide variety of mammals inhabiting the forests of South and Central America. Organisms are transmitted to humans entering the jungle to gather chicle or to clear land. Disease is most prevalent in the Amazon basin but occurs in most countries of the area. *L. mexicana* species are endemic in south-central Texas.

L.m. mexicana causes chiclero's ulcer, or bay sore. Chicle gatherers who work in forests during the rainy season when sandflies are abundant develop isolated cutaneous lesions on the hand or head.

These show little tendency to ulcerate and generally heal spontaneously within 6 months. Ear lesions, however, persist for years and may cause extensive destruction of the pinna.

L.m. venezuelensis causes indolent nodular lesions, *L.m. garnhami* causes ulcerating lesions that usually heal spontaneously, and *L.m. amazonensis* causes persistent lesions that may be multiple and seldom heal spontaneously. *L.m. amazonensis* less frequently causes diffuse cutaneous leishmaniasis (see below) and, rarely, visceral leishmaniasis.

L.b. peruviana causes uta, a disease consisting of single or multiple ulcers typically on the face. Spontaneous healing within 3 months to a year is the rule. The reservoir is the domestic dog. The disease occurs on the western slopes of the Peruvian Andes at altitudes above 600 m (2000 ft). With widespread use of insecticides, the disease has become uncommon.

Mucocutaneous leishmaniasis, or espundia, is caused primarily by *L.b. braziliensis,* which typically produces one or several lesions on the lower extremities that undergo extensive ulceration; complete healing seldom occurs spontaneously. After months to years, metastatic lesions may appear in the nasopharynx in 2 to 5 percent of patients. Less frequently, lesions occur in the perineum. Multiple, large antecedent skin lesions and insufficient antimony therapy for the primary infection are risk factors. Nasal obstruction and epistaxis are frequent presenting symptoms. Extensive destruction of soft tissue structures ensues, with painful mutilating erosions (espundia). Fever, anemia, and weight loss are common. Death is caused by bacterial infection, inanition, aspiration, and respiratory obstruction.

L.b. panamensis causes nonhealing ulcerative lesions and *L.b. guyanensis* causes nodular lesions that persist and metastasize along lymphatics (pian bois). These strains may cause mucocutaneous leishmaniasis in Colombia.

DIAGNOSIS Speciation of the infecting organism should be attempted because of the marked differences in outcome. Skin biopsies are the preferred means of obtaining tissue for stains and culture. Parasites may be scant, particularly in mucocutaneous lesions. The direct agglutination test and the leishmanin skin test become positive within 4 to 6 weeks. Syphilis, yaws, blastomycosis, paracoccidiodomycosis, sporotrichosis, leprosy, and carcinoma must be considered in the differential diagnosis.

TREATMENT Inconspicuous lesions due to *L.b. peruviana* or *L. mexicana* subspecies other than *L.m. amazonensis* may heal spontaneously or be treated with intralesional injections of antimonials. Local heat (40 to 41°C) may accelerate healing. Disfiguring or disabling lesions, cartilaginous involvement or lymphatic spread, and lesions due to *L.m. amazonensis* or other *L. braziliensis* subspecies should be treated with systemic antimonials as described for kala azar.

Espundia should be treated with antimonials (20 mg/kg per day) for at least 30 days. Cases that fail to respond should be treated with amphotericin. Reconstructive facial prostheses should not be used until the disease has been in remission for at least 1 year without therapy. A rising antibody titer may predict relapse and indicate that further therapy is required.

Diffuse cutaneous leishmaniasis Diffuse cutaneous leishmaniasis is found in Venezuela, Brazil, and the Dominican Republic in the new world and in Ethiopia in the old world. Patients display a specific deficiency of cell-mediated immunity to leishmanial antigens. *L.m. pifanoi* (Venezuela), *L.m. amazonensis* (Brazil), members of the *L. mexicana* complex (Dominican Republic), and *L. aethiopica* (Africa) are responsible. Disease is characterized by massive dissemination of skin lesions without visceral involvement. The clinical picture often bears a striking resemblance to lepromatous leprosy. The diagnosis is not difficult, because the lesions contain large numbers of organisms. In contrast to all other types of cutaneous leishmaniasis, the leishmanin skin test remains negative. The disease is progressive and very refractory to treatment. High doses of antimony (20 mg/kg twice a day for 30 days) and multiple courses of amphotericin or pentamidine are often required to produce remission, but cures are rare.

REFERENCES

BADARO R et al: New perspectives on a subclinical form of visceral leishmaniasis. J Infect Dis 154:1003, 1986

——— et al: Treatment of visceral leishmaniasis with pentavalent antimony and interferon gamma. N Engl J Med 322:16, 1990

BALLOU WR et al: Safety and efficacy of high-dose sodium stibogluconate therapy of American cutaneous leishmaniasis. Lancet 2.13, 1987

BERENGUER J et al: Visceral leishmaniasis in patients infected with human immunodeficiency virus (HIV). Ann Intern Med 111:129, 1989

BERMAN JD: Chemotherapy for leishmaniasis: Biochemical mechanisms, clinical efficacy and future strategies. Rev Infect Dis 10:560, 1988

MARSDEN PD: Mucosal leishmaniasis ("espundia" Escomel, 1911). Trans R Soc Trop Med Hyg 80:859, 1986

PETERS W, KILLICK-KENDRICK R (eds): *The Leismaniases in Biology and Medicine.* London, Academic, 1987, vols I and II

WIRTH DF et al: Leishmaniasis and malaria: New tools for epidemiologic analysis. Science 234:975, 1986

161 TRYPANOSOMIASIS

LOUIS V. KIRCHHOFF

CHAGAS' DISEASE

DEFINITION Chagas' disease, or American trypanosomiasis, is a zoonosis caused by the protozoan parasite *Trypanosoma cruzi*. Acute Chagas' disease is generally a mild, febrile illness that results from initial infection with the organism. Following spontaneous resolution of the acute illness, most infected individuals remain for life in the indeterminate phase of chronic Chagas' disease, which is characterized by subpatent parasitemia, high levels of anti-*T. cruzi* antibodies, and an absence of symptoms. In a minority of chronically infected individuals, cardiac and gastrointestinal lesions result in serious morbidity and death.

LIFE CYCLE AND TRANSMISSION *Trypanosoma cruzi* is transmitted among its mammalian hosts by hematophagous triatomine insects, or reduviid bugs. The insects become infected by sucking blood from animals or humans who have circulating parasites. The ingested organisms multiply in the gut of the reduviids, and infective forms are discharged with the feces at the time of subsequent blood meals. Transmission to a second vertebrate host occurs when breaks in the skin, mucous membranes, or conjunctivae are contaminated with bug feces that contain infective parasites. *Trypanosoma cruzi* can also be transmitted by transfusion of blood donated by infected individuals, and congenital infection occurs as well.

PATHOLOGY An indurated inflammatory lesion, called a chagoma, often appears at the site of the parasite's entry. Local histologic changes include intracellular parasites in leukocytes and cells of subcutaneous tissues, interstitial edema, lymphocytic infiltration, and reactive hyperplasia of adjacent lymph nodes. After dissemination, muscles, including the myocardium, may be heavily parasitized. The characteristic pseudocysts seen in sections of infected tissues are intracellular aggregates of multiplying parasites.

The pathogenesis of chronic Chagas' disease is poorly understood. The heart is the organ most commonly affected, and changes include biventricular enlargement, thinning of the ventricular walls, apical aneurysms, and mural thrombi. Widespread lymphocytic infiltration, diffuse interstitial fibrosis, and atrophy of myocardial cells are often present, but parasites are rarely demonstrated in myocardial tissue. Conduction system involvement most frequently affects the right branch and the left anterior branch of the bundle of His. In chronic Chagas' disease of the gastrointestinal tract (megadisease), the esophagus and colon may be enormously dilated and hypertrophied. On microscopic examination focal inflammatory lesions with lymphocytic infiltration are seen, and the number of neurons in the myenteric plexus is reduced.

EPIDEMIOLOGY *Trypanosoma cruzi* is found only in the Americas. Wild and domestic mammals harboring *T. cruzi* and infected reduviids are found in spotty distributions from the southern United States to southern Argentina. Humans become involved in the cycle of transmission when infected vectors take up residence in the thatched roofs and walls of primitive wood and adobe houses common in much of Latin America. Thus, human. *T. cruzi* infection is primarily a health problem among the poor in rural areas of Central and South America. Most new *T. cruzi* infections in rural settings occur in children, but the incidence is unknown because most go undiagnosed. Thousands of individuals also become infected every year through blood transfusions in urban areas. It is estimated that 10 to 12 million people are chronically infected with *T. cruzi*, more than half of whom live in Brazil. Chronic Chagas' disease is a major cause of morbidity and mortality in many areas of Latin America, including Mexico, since many chronically infected individuals eventually develop symptomatic cardiac lesions or gastrointestinal disease.

Acute Chagas' disease is rare in the United States. Three cases of autochthonous transmission have been described, and two instances of transmission by blood transfusion have occurred. In addition, between 1971 and 1989, six laboratory-acquired infections and nine imported cases of acute Chagas' disease were reported to the Centers for Disease Control (CDC). In contrast, the prevalence of chronic *T. cruzi* infections in the United States has increased. Since the mid-1970s an enormous number of Central Americans have emigrated to the United States, and in one study in Washington, D.C., 5 percent of Salvadoran and Nicaraguan immigrants were found to have chronic *T. cruzi* infections. Conservative estimates place the total number of infected immigrants at more that 50,000. The presence of these carriers of *T. cruzi* poses a significant risk of transmission by blood transfusion, as evidenced by the occurrence of the two transfusion-associated cases.

CLINICAL COURSE The first signs of acute Chagas' disease occur at least 1 week after invasion by the parasites. When the organisms have entered through a break in the skin, an indurated area of erythema and swelling, a chagoma, accompanied by local lymphadenopathy may appear. Romaña's sign, the classic finding in acute Chagas' disease, consists of unilateral painless edema of the palpebrae and periocular tissues that can result when the conjunctiva is the portal of entry. These initial local signs are followed by malaise, fever, anorexia, and edema of the face and lower extremities. Generalized lymphadenopathy and mild hepatosplenomegaly may appear. Severe myocarditis develops rarely, and most deaths in acute Chagas' disease are due to heart failure. Neurologic signs are uncommon, but meningoencephalitis has been reported. The acute symptoms resolve spontaneously in virtually all patients, who then enter the asymptomatic or indeterminate phase of chronic *T. cruzi* infection.

Symptomatic chronic Chagas' disease becomes apparent years or decades after the initial infection. The heart is commonly involved, and symptoms are due to rhythm disturbances, cardiomyopathy, and thromboembolism. Right bundle branch block is the most common ECG abnormality, but other types of AV block, premature ventricular contractions, and tachy- and bradyarrhythmias are seen frequently. Cardiomyopathy often results in right-sided or biventricular heart failure, and embolization of mural thrombi to the brain or other areas may occur. Patients with megaesophagus suffer from dysphagia, odynophagia, chest pain, and regurgitation. Aspiration can occur, especially during sleep, and repeated episodes of aspiration pneumonitis are common. Weight loss, cachexia, and pulmonary infection can result in death. Patients with megacolon are plagued by abdominal pain and chronic constipation, and advanced megacolon can cause obstruction, perforation, septicemia, and death.

DIAGNOSIS The diagnosis of acute Chagas' disease is made by detecting parasites. Microscopic examination of fresh anticoagulated blood or of the buffy coat is the simplest way to see the motile organisms. Parasites can also be seen in Giemsa-stained thin and thick blood smears. When repeated attempts to visualize the organisms are unsuccessful, mouse inoculation and culture of blood on specialized media should be performed. As a last resort, xenodiagnosis

should be attempted. In this technique, uninfected reduviid bugs are allowed to feed on the patient's blood. Approximately 30 days after the blood meal, the intestinal contents of the bugs are examined for parasites. When done properly, this method is positive in virtually all patients with acute Chagas' disease and in approximately half of those with chronic infections. Since early treatment of acute Chagas' disease is extremely important, however, the decision to initiate anti-*T. cruzi* therapy in a patient with negative wet preparations and smears must be made on clinical and epidemiologic grounds before the results of these indirect methods become available. Serologic testing is of limited usefulness in diagnosing acute Chagas' disease.

The diagnosis of chronic Chagas' disease is made by detecting serum antibodies that bind to *T. cruzi* antigens. Demonstration of the parasite is not of primary importance. A number of highly sensitive serologic tests for the detection of anti-*T. cruzi* antibodies are available, including complement fixation and immunofluorescence assays, and enzyme-linked immunosorbent assay (ELISA). However, a persistent problem with these conventional assays is the occurrence of false-positive reactions, typically with sera from patients with diseases such as leishmaniasis. For this reason, it is generally recommended that positivity in one assay be confirmed in two other tests, and that well-characterized positive and negative comparison sera be included in each run. A highly sensitive and specific method for detecting anti-*T. cruzi* antibodies that employs immunoprecipitation of radiolabeled *T. cruzi* antigens has been described. This assay effectively deals with the problem of false-positive reactions and is available as a confirmatory test in the author's laboratory, but it has not been adapted for mass screening.

TREATMENT Therapy for Chagas' disease is unsatisfactory. Nifurtimox is the only drug active against *T. cruzi* that is available in the United States. In acute Chagas' disease, nifurtimox markedly reduces the duration of symptoms and parasitemia and decreases mortality. Nevertheless, its ability to eradicate parasites is limited, since patients treated with nifurtimox during the acute phase may have positive xenodiagnoses after full courses of the drug. Nifurtimox treatment should be initiated as early as possible in the acute disease. Moreover, when laboratory accidents occur in which it appears likely that *T. cruzi* infection could become established, nifurtimox therapy should be initiated without waiting for clinical or parasitologic indications of infection.

The usefulness of nifurtimox in individuals with indeterminate phase or symptomatic chronic Chagas' disease has not been established. There is no evidence that patients in the indeterminate phase are less likely to develop symptomatic disease after treatment with nifurtimox, and likewise it has not been shown that it has any effect on symptomatic chronic disease. Moreover, posttreatment xenodiagnoses are also positive in many chronically infected patients given this drug. Hence, there is no indication for treating individuals with chronic *T. cruzi* infections with nifurtimox.

Common side effects of nifurtimox include abdominal pain, anorexia, nausea, vomiting, and weight loss. Neurologic symptoms may include restlessness, disorientation, insomnia, twitching, paresthesias, polyneuritis, and seizures. These symptoms usually disappear when the dosage is reduced or treatment is discontinued. The recommended dosage for adults is 8 to 10 mg/kg body weight per day. The dose for adolescents is 12.5 to 15 mg/kg body weight per day and for children 1 to 10 years of age is 15 to 20 mg/kg body weight per day. The drug should be given by mouth in four divided doses each day, and therapy should be continued for 90 to 120 days. In the United States, nifurtimox is available from the Drug Service of the CDC, Atlanta, Georgia [telephone no. 404-639-3670 (days), 404-639-2888 (nights)].

Benznidazole is a second agent used to treat Chagas' disease. Its efficacy is similar to that of nifurtimox, and side effects include peripheral neuropathy, rash, and granulocytopenia. The recommended oral dosage is 5 mg/kg body weight per day for 60 days. Benznidazole is used widely in Latin America, but it is not available in the United States.

PREVENTION Since drug therapy is unsatisfactory and vaccines are not available, the control of *T. cruzi* transmission in endemic countries must depend on reduction of domiciliary vector populations by spraying of insecticides and improvement in rural housing. Also, in endemic areas, expansion and improvement of programs for screening donated blood for the presence of *T. cruzi* are necessary to reduce transmission by transfusion. Tourists traveling in endemic areas should avoid sleeping in dilapidated houses or in dwellings with thatched roofs. Mosquito nets and insect repellent provide additional protection.

In the United States, blood donations should not be accepted from immigrants from regions in which Chagas' disease is endemic, unless serologic assays indicate that the donor is not infected with *T. cruzi*. Moreover, immigrants from endemic regions should be screened for serologic evidence of infection with the parasite. Identification of infected individuals in this group is important, not only to prevent transmission by blood transfusion, but also to enable physicians who care for these patients to undertake appropriate diagnostic monitoring and supportive therapy. Laboratory personnel should wear gloves and eye protection when working with *T. cruzi* and with infected vectors.

SLEEPING SICKNESS

DEFINITION Sleeping sickness, or African trypanosomiasis, is caused by flagellated protozoan parasites belonging to the *Trypanosoma brucei* complex and are transmitted to humans by tsetse flies. In untreated patients the trypanosomes first cause a febrile illness that is followed months or years later by progressive neurologic impairment and death.

THE PARASITES AND THEIR TRANSMISSION The east African (*rhodesiense*) and the west African (*gambiense*) forms of sleeping sickness are caused by two trypanosome subspecies, *T. brucei rhodesiense* and *T. brucei gambiense*. These subspecies are indistinguishable morphologically but cause illnesses that are epidemiologically and clinically distinct. The parasites are transmitted by blood-sucking tsetse flies of the genus *Glossina*. The insects acquire the infection when they ingest blood from infected mammalian hosts. After many cycles of multiplication in the midgut of the vector, the parasites migrate to the salivary glands, and transmission takes place when they are inoculated during a subsequent blood meal. The injected trypanosomes multiply in the blood and other extracellular spaces and evade immune destruction in mammalian hosts for long periods because they undergo antigenic variation, a process by which the antigenic structure of the surface coat of glycoproteins changes periodically.

PATHOGENESIS AND PATHOLOGY A self-limited inflammatory lesion (trypanosomal chancre) may appear a week or so after the bite of an infected tsetse fly. A systemic febrile illness then evolves as the parasites are disseminated through the lymphatics and bloodstream. Systemic African trypanosomiasis without central nervous system (CNS) involvement is generally referred to as stage I disease. In this stage, there is widespread lymphadenopathy and splenomegaly, reflecting marked lymphocytic and histiocytic proliferation and invasion of morular cells, which are plasmacytes that may be involved in the production of IgM. An endarteritis with perivascular infiltration of both parasites and lymphocytes may develop in lymph nodes and spleen. Myocarditis is common in stage I disease, especially with *T. b. rhodesiense* infection.

Hematologic manifestations in stage I trypanosomiasis include moderate leukocytosis, thrombocytopenia, and anemia. High levels of immunoglobulins, primarily polyclonal IgM, are a constant feature, and heterophile antibodies, anti-DNA antibodies, and rheumatoid factor are often detected. High levels of antigen-antibody complexes may play a role in the tissue damage and increased vascular permeability that facilitate dissemination of the parasites.

Stage II trypanosomiasis involves invasion of the CNS. The presence of trypanosomes in perivascular areas is accompanied by intense infiltration of mononuclear cells. Cerebrospinal fluid (CSF) abnormalities include increased pressure, elevated total protein concentration, and pleocytosis. Trypanosomes also are frequently present in the CSF.

EPIDEMIOLOGY The trypanosomes that cause sleeping sickness are found only in Africa. Approximately 50 million people are at risk for acquiring African trypanosomiasis, and about 20,000 new cases are reported each year. Humans are the major reservoir of *T. b. gambiense*, and infections occur in tropical rain forests of central and West africa. Gambiense trypanosomiasis is primarily a problem in rural populations, and tourists rarely become infected. Antelope species in savanna and woodland areas of central and east Africa are the principal reservoir of *T. b. rhodesiense*. Cattle also can become infected but generally succumb to the parasite. Humans acquire *T. b. rhodesiense* infection only incidentally, for the most part from contact with the tsetse flies that feed on wild animals. Thus, the disease is an occupational hazard for individuals who work in areas where infected game and vectors are present. In addition, occasional cases of *T. b. rhodesiense* infection occur among visitors to game parks in east Africa. During the past two decades 15 cases of imported African trypanosomiasis have been reported in the United States, most of which were caused by *T. b. rhodesiense*.

CLINICAL COURSE A painful trypanosomal chancre appears in some patients at the site where parasites were inoculated. Hematogenous and lymphatic dissemination (stage I disease) is marked by the onset of fever, and, typically, bouts of high temperatures lasting several days are separated by afebrile periods. Lymphadenopathy is prominent in gambiense trypanosomiasis. The nodes are discrete, movable, rubbery, and nontender. Cervical nodes are often visible, and enlargement of the nodes of the posterior cervical triangle, or Winterbottom's sign, is a classic finding in individuals infected with *T. b. gambiense*. Pruritus is frequent, and a circinate rash is often present. Inconstant findings include malaise, headache, arthralgias, weight loss, edema, hepatosplenomegaly, and tachycardia.

Central nervous system invasion (stage II disease) is characterized by the insidious development of protean neurologic manifestations, accompanied by progressive abnormalities in the CSF. A picture of progressive indifference and daytime somnolence (sleeping sickness) sometimes alternates with restlessness and insomnia at night. A listless gaze accompanies a loss of spontaneity, and speech may become halting and indistinct. Extrapyramidal signs may include choreiform movements, tremors, and fasciculations. Ataxia is frequent, and the patient may appear to have Parkinson's disease with a shuffling gait, hypertonia, and tremors. In the final phase, progressive neurologic impairment ends in coma and death.

The most striking difference between the west African and east African trypanosomiasis is that the latter illness tends to follow a more acute course. Typically in tourists, systemic signs of infection such as fever, malaise, and headache may appear before the end of the trip or shortly after return home. Persistent tachycardia unrelated to fever is common early in the course of rhodesiense trypanosomiasis, and death may result from arrhythmias and congestive heart failure before CNS disease develops. In general, untreated east African trypanosomiasis leads to death in a matter of weeks to months, often without a clear distinction between the lymphatic and CNS stages.

DIAGNOSIS A definitive diagnosis requires detection of the parasite. If a chancre is present, fluid should be expressed and examined directly under light microscopy for the highly motile trypanosomes. The fluid should also be fixed and stained with Giemsa. Material obtained by needle aspiration of lymph nodes early in the course of the illness should be examined similarly. Examination of wet preparations and of Giemsa-stained thin and thick films of serial samples of peripheral blood is also useful. If parasites are not found by these methods, the buffy coat from 10 to 15 mL of anticoagulated blood or the pellet obtained by centrifugation of the eluate from 25 to 50 mL of blood passed through a DEAE-cellulose column should be examined. Trypanosomes may also been seen in material aspirated from the bone marrow, and the aspirate can be inoculated into liquid culture medium, as can blood, lymph node aspirates, and CSF. Finally, *T. b. rhodesiense* infection can be detected by inoculation of these specimens into mice or rats, resulting in patent parasitemias in 1 to 2 weeks. This is a highly sensitive method for the detection of *T. b. rhodesiense*, but due to host specificity, *T. b. gambiense* cannot be detected by this technique.

Examination of the CSF is mandatory in all patients suspected of having African trypanosmiasis. An increase in the CSF cell count is the first abnormality to be detected, and increased opening pressure, total protein, and IgM levels develop later. Trypanosomes may be seen in the sediment of centrifuged CSF. Any CSF abnormality in an individual in whom trypanosomes have been found in specimens from other sites must be viewed as pathognomonic for CNS involvement, and specific treatment for CNS disease must be given.

A number of serologic assays are available to aid in the diagnosis of African trypanosomiasis, but their variable sensitivity and specificity mandates that treatment decisions be based on demonstration of the parasite. Such tests are of value for epidemiologic surveys.

TREATMENT The drugs traditionally used for treatment of African trypanosomiasis are suramin, pentamidine, and organic arsenicals. In addition, eflornithine has shown promise in the therapy of west African trypanosomiasis. Gambiense and rhodesiense trypanosomiases are treated similarly, and the type of therapy is determined by the presence or absence of CNS disease, side effects, and occasionally drug resistance. Suramin and pentamidine do not penetrate the CNS well, and the more toxic arsenicals must be used in patients with CNS involvement. Eflornithine penetrates the CNS well. In the United States, these drugs can be obtained from the CDC.

The drug of choice for treatment of patients with stage I African trypanosomiasis and normal CSF is suramin. A 100- to 200-mg test dose should be administered to detect hypersensitivity. The dosage for adults is 1 g intravenously on days 1, 3, 7, 14, and 21. The regimen for children is 20 mg/kg body weight intravenously on days 1, 3, 7, 14, and 21. The drug is given by slow intravenous infusion of a freshly prepared 10% aqueous solution. Suramin can cause serious side effects and must be administered under the close supervision of a physician. Approximately 1 patient in 20,000 has an immediate, severe, and potentially fatal reaction to the drug consisting of nausea, vomiting, shock, and seizures. Less severe reactions include fever, photophobia, pruritus, arthralgias, and skin eruptions. Renal damage is the most common, important side effect of suramin. Transient proteinuria often appears during treatment. Urinalysis should be done before each dose, and the drug should be discontinued if proteinuria increases or casts and red cells appear in the sediment. Suramin should not be used in patients with renal insufficiency.

Pentamidine isethionate is the alternative drug for patients with stage I trypanosomiasis. It is effective in the early stages of gambiense trypanosomiasis, but it has a lower cure rate than suramin. In addition, some *T. b. rhodesiense* infections are unresponsive to pentamidine. The dose for both adults and children is 4 mg/kg body weight per day intramuscularly or intravenously for 10 days. Frequent, immediate side effects include nausea, vomiting, tachycardia, and hypotension. These reactions are usually transient and do not warrant cessation of therapy. Other adverse reactions include nephrotoxicity, abnormal liver function tests, neutropenia, rashes, hypoglycemia, and sterile abscesses.

An arsenical, melarsoprol, is the drug of choice for African trypanosomiasis with CNS involvement. Melarsoprol will cure both stages of the disease, and thus it is also indicated for treatment of stage I patients in whom suramin and/or pentamidine have failed or are not tolerated. However, melarsoprol should never be the first choice for therapy of stage I disease, because of its relatively high toxicity. In adults the drug should be given in 3 courses of 3 days each. The dosage is 2 to 3.6 mg/kg body weight per day intravenously in 3 divided doses for 3 days, followed 1 week later by 3.6 mg/kg body weight per day, also in 3 divided doses for 3 days. The latter course is then repeated 10 to 21 days later. In debilitated patients, 2

to 4 days of suramin treatment is administered before starting melarsoprol, and an 18-mg initial dose of the latter drug, followed by progressive increases to the standard dose, has been recommended. For children, 18 to 25 mg/kg body weight total should be given over 1 month. A starting dose of 0.36 mg/kg body weight intravenously should be increased gradually to a maximum of 3.6 mg/kg at 1 to 5 day intervals for a total of 9 to 10 doses.

Melarsoprol is highly toxic and should be administered with great care. The incidence of reactive encephalopathy has been reported to be as high as 18 percent in some series. Clinical manifestations of reactive encephalopathy include high fever, headache, tremor, impaired speech, seizures, and even coma and death. Melarsoprol should be discontinued at the first sign of encephalopathy, but may be restarted cautiously with small doses a few days after the signs have resolved. Extravasation of the drug results in intense local reactions, and vomiting, abdominal pain, nephrotoxicity, and myocardial damage can occur.

The combination of the arsenical, tryparsamide, and suramin is the alternative treatment for patients with stage II disease who cannot tolerate melarsoprol. Tryparsamide is effective against *T. b. gambiense* but not *T. b. rhodesiense*. The dose of tryparsamide is one injection of 30 mg/kg body weight every 5 days for a total of 12 injections, and that for suramin is 10 mg/kg body weight intravenously every 5 days, also for a total of 12 injections. Tryparsamide can cause encephalopathy, fever, vomiting, abdominal pain, rash, tinnitus, and a variety of ocular symptoms.

Eflornithine is an experimental drug being used to treat gambiense trypanosomiasis. When given intravenously, it appears to be effective in both stages of the disease. The dosage is 20 to 30 g/d intravenously in 4 doses for 6 to 8 weeks. Eflornithine is also available as an oral preparation, but optimal dosage and duration of therapy have not been established. Side effects include diarrhea, anemia, thrombocytopenia, and seizures and hearing loss. The efficacy of eflornithine in *T. b. rhodesiense* has not been determined. The high dosage and long duration of therapy required are disadvantages that may make widespread use difficult.

PREVENTION The trypanosomiases constitute complex public health and epizootic problems in Africa. Considerable progress has been made in some areas through control programs that focus on eradication of vectors and drug treatment of infected humans, but there is no consensus on the best approach to solving the overall problem. Individuals can reduce the risk of acquiring trypanosomiasis by avoiding areas known to harbor infected insects, by wearing protective clothing, and by using insect repellent. Chemoprophylaxis is not recommended, and no vaccine is available to prevent transmission of the parasites.

REFERENCES

Chagas' disease

BRENER Z: Biology of *Trypanosoma cruzi*. Ann Rev Microbiol 27:347, 1973

GOLDSMITH RS et al: Clinical and epidemiologic studies of Chagas' disease in rural communities in Oaxaca state, Mexico, and a seven-year follow up: I. Cerro de Air. Bull Pan Am Health Organ 19:120, 1985

KIRCHHOFF LV: Is *Trypanasoma cruzi* a new threat to our blood supply? Ann Intern Med 111:773, 1989

——— et al: American trypanosomiasis (Chagas' disease) in Central American immigrants. Am J Med 82:915, 1987

——— et al: Increased specificity of serodiagnosis of Chagas's disease by detection of antibody to the 72 and 90 kDa glycoproteins of *Trypanosoma cruzi*. J Infect Dis 155:561, 1987

MARR JJ, DOCAMPO R: Chemotherapy for Chagas' disease: A perspective of current therapy and considerations for future research. Rev Infect Dis 8:884, 1986

SCHIFFLER RJ et al: Indigenous Chagas' disease (American trypanosomiasis) in California. JAMA 251:2983, 1984

SCHMUNIS GA: Chagas' disease and blood transfusion, in *Infection, Immunity and Blood Transfusion*, RY Dodd, LF Barker (eds). New York, Alan R. Liss, 1984, pp 127–145

Sleeping sickness

DONELSON JE: Antigenic variation in African trypanosomes. Contrib Microbiol Immunol 8:138, 1987

JORDAN AM: *Trypanosomiasis Control and African Rural Development*. London, Longmans, 1986

POLTERA AA: Pathology of human African trypanosomiasis with reference to experimental African trypanosomiasis and infections of the central nervous system. Br Med Bull 41:169, 1985

SCHECHTER PJ et al: Therapeutic utility of selected enzyme-activated irreversible inhibitors, in *Enzymes as Targets for Drug Design*, MG Palfreyman et al (eds). San Diego, Academic Press, 1989, pp 201–210

VICKERMAN K: Development cycles and biology of pathogenic trypanosomes. Br Med Bull 41:105, 1985

162 TOXOPLASMOSIS

HENRY W. MURRAY

DEFINITION Toxoplasmosis is defined by the presence of clinical and/or pathologic evidence of *active* infection caused by the obligate intracellular protozoan *Toxoplasma gondii*. Using this definition, toxoplasmosis can and should be differentiated from the much more common asymptomatic infection typically associated with exposure to this pathogen.

THE ORGANISM AND ITS LIFE CYCLE *T. gondii* exists in three forms: trophozoite (tachyzoite), tissue cyst, and oocyst. The ingested cyst and oocyst contain thousands of trophozoites which are released in the gastrointestinal tract, initiate tissue infection, and are responsible for acute toxoplasmosis. Years later, trophozoites may be liberated in the tissues by cyst rupture leading to reactivated infection.

Trophozoites are oval or crescent-shaped and measure 3 by 7 µm. The trophozoite is an obligate intracellular form which requires a host cell for growth and, therefore, cannot survive or multiply extracellularly nor be maintained in culture medium alone. Trophozoites can invade and rapidly replicate within cytoplasmic vacuoles of any nucleated cell. After several rounds of intravacuolar division by endodyogeny, trophozoites rupture free from the host cell and proceed to infect adjacent cells. The proliferating trophozoites are responsible for and define acute infection. Intracellular replication and the parasitization of new cells do not slow until an effective immune response develops.

Cysts arise within host cells, range from 10 to 200 µm in diameter, and are filled with viable trophozoites. Cysts may form within as short a time as 1 week after infection; therefore, their initial development is probably not dependent on either the host's humoral or cellular immune response. In contrast, antigen-sensitized T cells appear critical for maintenance of the organism in the cyst form and for effective control over trophozoites potentially liberated in the tissues from periodic cyst breakdown. Cysts persist for life in the mammalian host and can be found in virtually any tissue, most commonly skeletal muscle, myocardium, and brain. Cysts are the pathologic hallmark of chronic (latent) infection and remain clinically silent in immunologically normal hosts. In contrast, cysts provide a ready endogenous source of trophozoites in patients who become immunosuppressed or T cell–deficient (AIDS), putting them at particular risk for developing reactivated infection (see Chap. 264). Trophozoites released from tissue cysts in immunologically intact individuals can create retinochoroiditis and rare cases of recurrent or persistent parasitemia.

Oocysts, 10 to 12 µm in diameter, are formed exclusively by a sexual cycle in the intestinal mucosal cells of cats which have ingested either cysts in poorly cooked meat or animal tissue or oocysts shed by other cats. Three to five days after such exposure, cats develop systemic infection and also begin to excrete up to millions of oocysts per day for as long as 3 weeks. After a cat has stopped shedding oocysts in its feces, the process seldom resumes. For oocysts to become infectious after excretion, they must first sporulate, a temperature-dependent process which requires several days at room temperature and fails to occur in the cold (4°C) or heat (37°C).

Oocysts may persist in the environment in an infectious state for a year or more, however, if the conditions are favorable (e.g., in moist, warm soil).

EPIDEMIOLOGY Cats, small mammals, and birds serve as the likely natural reservoirs of *T. gondii*, but virtually any animal that has access to and ingests material contaminated by oocysts or cyst-containing tissue can become infected. Cysts can be found, for example, in 10 to 25 percent of lamb and 25 percent of pork prepared for human consumption and less often in beef. If meat is not properly heated during cooking to 60°C or frozen to below −20°C, cysts remain fully viable. The prevalence or frequency of *T. gondii* infection in humans varies considerably depending upon age and other factors including dietary habits, climate, and proximity to cats. In this country, positive serologic results increase with age at the rate of about 1 percent per year making 20 to 50 percent of adults seropositive depending upon the locale. In contrast, >90 percent of adults 30 to 40 years old may be seropositive to *T. gondii* in Central America, certain islands in the South Pacific, and France, where cats are plentiful or eating rare meat is customary. Outbreaks among families or closed groups may develop after a common source exposure, but human-to-human transmission does not occur.

TRANSMISSION There are three principal modes of transmission of *T. gondii*: ingestion of oocysts or cyst-containing material, transplacental spread, and inadvertent direct administration.

Ingestion of poorly cooked lamb, pork, or beef is the most likely mechanism of transmission in developed countries where cats are confined indoors and fed processed foods and where efforts are made to cover and refrigerate food. However, outdoor cats can ingest oocysts excreted by other cats or kill and eat infected small animals, acquire infection, and then shed oocysts in areas inside and outside the home that are accessible to both children and adults. Uncovered food may also become contaminated with oocysts transferred by insects such as flies or cockroaches.

Congenital toxoplasmosis in the fetus occurs if the mother acquires the infection during pregnancy. Maternal infection acquired during the 6 months prior to conception poses a possible but very low risk to the fetus; infection acquired more than 6 months before conception presents no risk. The likelihood that acute infection in a pregnant woman will be transmitted to the fetus increases with each trimester: 15 percent in the first, 30 percent in the second, and 60 percent in the third trimester. Congenital toxoplasmosis is most severe if acquired early on in the first trimester; most infants infected in the third trimester are asymptomatic at birth. Only 20 percent of pregnant women acutely infected with *T. gondii* show clinical signs of infection; most often the diagnosis is first suggested by the results of routine post-conception serologic testing which show high titers of specific antibody.

On rare occasions, *T. gondii* has also been transmitted by needle stick injury, laboratory or autopsy room accident, transplantation of infected organs (heart or kidney) into seronegative recipients, or by transfusion of whole blood, leukocytes, or platelets. Certain immunocompromised patients, such as those with chronic myelogenous leukemia, and, rarely, normal individuals may have recurrent asymptomatic parasitemia and transmit infection by donation of their blood products. In these patients, parasitemia may develop despite the presence of high titers of circulating specific antibody. *T. gondii* can survive for up to 50 days in refrigerated anticoagulated blood.

PATHOGENESIS AND PATHOLOGY Following ingestion of cysts or oocysts, trophozoites are released in the gastrointestinal tract and invade and multiply within mucosal cells. These cells are eventually disrupted by replicating organisms, the mucosal barrier is breached, and trophozoites disseminate lymphohematogenously to infect virtually any tissue or organ. Lymph nodes, skeletal muscle, myocardium, brain, the retina, and the placenta are particularly frequent and/or clinically important target organs. In infected tissues, trophozoites enter a variety of host cells (parenchymal, endothelial, epithelial, and macrophages), replicate in the cytoplasm, rupture the cell, and proceed to infect adjacent cells. In the immunologically intact individual, acute infection in all tissues is quite rapidly brought under control with the emergence of both humoral and cellular immune responses, trophozoites disappear, and the organisms encyst. However, in immunosuppressed or T cell–deficient patients (and, rarely, in otherwise healthy individuals), acute infection is not well controlled, and retinochoroiditis and potentially fatal encephalitis, pneumonitis, or myocarditis may develop.

Focal necrosis surrounded by an intense and largely mononuclear cell inflammatory response is seen in any tissue where constantly proliferating trophozoites have caused cell destruction. Larger and more destructive lesions are typically present in congenital infection, acute infection in immunodeficient patients, and in the unusual immunologically intact individual who develops progressive disseminated disease. In contrast to the histopathologic effects provoked by replicating trophozoites, the cyst form of *T. gondii* elicits no tissue inflammatory response.

In the immunocompetent individual, pathologic data concerning acute infection have been derived principally from lymph node examination since there is seldom an indication for biopsy or removal of other involved organs. Lymphadenitis resulting from *T. gondii* produces a characteristic and near-diagnostic histologic reaction consisting of exuberant follicular hyperplasia and irregular clusters of epithelioid histiocytes (macrophages) with eosinophilic cytoplasm which encroach upon the margins of germinal centers. Granulomas are typically not present. Trophozoites or cysts are seldom demonstrated in involved lymph nodes; however, mice inoculated with infected lymph node may subsequently yield the organism. Involvement of the eye produces single or multiple necrotic lesions in which both cysts and trophozoites are present along with inflammatory infiltrates made up of monocytes, lymphocytes, and plasma cells. Complications of the necrotizing retinitis occur largely in the posterior chamber, and include granulomatous choroiditis, iridocyclitis, cataracts, and glaucoma. Retinochoroiditis is probably initiated by trophozoites released from ruptured retinal cysts; a hypersensitivity reaction directed at retinal tissue has also been proposed.

Infection in immunocompromised patients, fetuses, and in infants with severe congenital disease has provided additional histopathologic data. Findings vary greatly from scattered cysts in virtually any organ to widespread areas of inflammation and necrosis with cysts and intra- and extracellular trophozoites often found at the periphery of destructive lesions. In disseminated disease associated with either primary or reactivated infection, the brain, heart, lungs, kidneys (glomerulonephritis), pancreas, spleen, and muscle may all be involved with single or multiple necrotic lesions approaching several centimeters in diameter. Central nervous system infection is accompanied by a mononuclear cell infiltrate and microglial nodule formation and can be associated with focal or diffuse necrotizing encephalitis, meningitis, or necrotic mass lesions (abscesses) with edema. Vasculitis and necrosis in periaqueductal and periventricular areas which may calcify are typical in congenital toxoplasmosis and may result in hydrocephalus.

HOST DEFENSE IMMUNOLOGIC RESPONSE In the healthy individual, *T. gondii* infection rapidly provokes both humoral and cellular immune responses which can be detected in the serum (specific IgM and IgG antibody) and in vitro by assays which measure T-cell responsiveness to *T. gondii* antigen. Both types of immune responses appear critical for the induction of initial control over the proliferating organism, and virtually all symptomatic patients with acute infection are seropositive when first seen. Activation of T cells also probably occurs soon after acute infection, but laboratory detection of specific reactivity to *T. gondii* antigen may require 6 to 8 weeks or longer. Specific IgG antibody lyses extracellular trophozoites in the presence of the alternative complement pathway, and opsonized organisms are susceptible to killing upon ingestion by mononuclear phagocytes. Experimental evidence also suggests that soluble products (lymphokines) secreted by antigen-sensitized CD4-positive helper T cells including interleukin 2 (IL-2) and interferon-gamma (IFN-γ) are crucial components of the successful response to

T. gondii infection (see Chap. 13). IL-2 expands T-cell populations, activates T cells and natural killer cells, and stimulates the generation of IFN-γ. IFN-γ has pleiotropic and amplifying effects including the capacity to induce otherwise susceptible cells (e.g., the tissue macrophage and probably most parenchymal cells) to kill or inhibit the intracellular replication of *T. gondii* trophozoites. In vitro, peripheral blood T cells from healthy seropositive immune individuals readily proliferate and produce IL-2 and IFN-γ after stimulation with *T. gondii* antigen; cells from T cell–deficient seropositive AIDS patients with reactivated toxoplasmosis secrete neither lymphokine. In an animal model, treatment with either IL-2 or IFN-γ protects against acute toxoplasmosis, and conversely, administration of a neutralizing anti-IFN-γ monoclonal antibody converts an avirulent to a virulent infection. The critical role of such T-cell–dependent mechanisms has been clearly reemphasized by the reactivation of latent infection in iatrogenically immunosuppressed patients and in patients with AIDS despite the presence of circulating specific antibody. In otherwise healthy individuals, acute *T. gondii* infection may also induce substantial quantitative alterations in peripheral blood T-cell subsets, including depression of CD4-positive helper cells, increases in CD8-positive suppressor cells, and reduction in the CD4/CD8 cell ratio. Although such changes may be more pronounced in symptomatic patients and persist for 6 months or longer, their clinical significance is unclear since almost all healthy patients rapidly and spontaneously recover with no sequelae.

CLINICAL MANIFESTATIONS Data from serologic surveys indicate that acute, acquired toxoplasmosis probably goes unrecognized in 80 to 90 percent of healthy adults and children, and therefore is largely a self-limited, symptom-free infection. In immunologically intact individuals, the subsequent lifelong latent infection is of no consequence unless retinal cysts break down (retinochoroiditis) or protective T cell–dependent mechanisms become impaired permitting tissue infection to reactivate in any cyst-containing organ. Although fewer than 20 percent of pregnant women with acute toxoplasmosis are symptomatic or develop lymphadenopathy, transmission via placental infection to the fetus occurs relatively frequently (depending upon the trimester) and may produce congenital toxoplasmosis. The manifestations of the congenital disease are diverse and range from simply being seropositive at birth (but at risk for late neurologic sequelae or subsequent episodes of retinochoroiditis) to overt multiorgan dysfunction and congenital malformations, to prematurity and intrauterine death. The diagnosis and management of acute toxoplasmosis during pregnancy and the treatment of both symptomatic and asymptomatic congenital toxoplasmosis require special expertise.

Acute infection in the immunocompetent adult From 7 to 21 days after exposure, up to 20 percent of patients develop lymphadenopathy which may be asymptomatic or accompanied by a brief, systemic flulike illness. Cervical lymphadenopathy is the most common manifestation of *T. gondii* infection. Enlargement may involve one or several nodes, which are usually nontender. Anterior and posterior cervical and postauricular lymphadenopathy is most frequent, but any single node or node group may be enlarged including those in mediastinum and retroperitoneum. Generalized lymphadenopathy and splenomegaly occur in less than 30 percent of symptomatic patients. Although the majority of individuals with lymphadenopathy have no symptoms or other signs, between 20 and 40 percent have low-grade fever, headache, malaise, and fatigue. Fewer than 20 percent have arthralgias, myalgias, sore throat, abdominal pain, rash, or hepatomegaly. Unusual manifestations or complications in the normal host include high or prolonged fever and unilateral retinochoroiditis; transient pneumonitis and pleural effusion, hepatitis, pericarditis, myocarditis, Guillain-Barré syndrome, intracerebral mass lesions, and meningoencephalitis are all rare. Other than fatigue and minimal to moderate lymphadenopathy, both of which can persist or recur for months, the signs and symptoms of acute toxoplasmosis typically resolve within 1 to 3 weeks. A chronic syndrome of symptomatic lymphadenopathy occurs very infrequently.

Routine laboratory studies typically indicate a normal hemoglobin and white blood cell count, a modest lymphocytosis, <6 percent atypical lymphocytes, and either normal or only modest elevations in the sedimentation rate and hepatic transaminases. A Coombs-negative hemolytic anemia, striking atypical lymphocytosis (up to 40 to 50 percent), and electrocardiographic changes are seen only occasionally. The clinical manifestations of acute toxoplasmosis are not distinctive, and may be mimicked by a variety of disorders including lymphoma, mononucleosis due to Epstein-Barr virus or cytomegalovirus, tuberculosis, sarcoidosis, cat-scratch disease, AIDS, metastatic cancer, and virtually any disease associated with lymphadenopathy. Not infrequently, the diagnosis of toxoplasmosis is first made by lymph node biopsy in patients believed to have Hodgkin's disease.

Ocular infection Up to 35 percent of cases of chorioretinitis in all age groups is thought to be caused by *T. gondii* infection, and almost always but not exclusively reflects a late sequel of congenital infection. Ocular disease is characteristically associated with bilateral retinal lesions and usually occurs in individuals 10 to 30 years old; retinochoroiditis is unusual after the age of 40. The location and extent of retinal involvement determine both the degree of visual impairment (macular lesions) and symptoms which may include blurred vision, ocular pain, photophobia, scotoma, and epiphora. Funduscopic lesions are usually multiple, ill-defined yellow-white patches centrally located at the posterior pole. Separate lesions in clusters may be in various stages of development and simultaneously show yellow-white patches, pale atrophic gray plaques, or black pigmented scars. Panuveitis, papillitis, and optic atrophy may also be present. With treatment, inflammation subsides, but recovery of visual acuity may be incomplete, relapses are common up until the age of 40 years, and with relapses visual loss may be progressive. Other infections or inflammatory disorders which may cause somewhat similar types of ocular disease include cytomegalovirus, tuberculosis, syphilis, histoplasmosis, *Herpes simplex,* leprosy, and sarcoidosis.

Toxoplasmosis in the immunosuppressed and T cell–deficient patient Although acute *T. gondii* infection can occur in any immunocompromised patient who inadvertently ingests cysts or oocysts, reactivation of previously acquired (latent) infection is the pathogenetic mechanism usually encountered. Patients with Hodgkin's disease, any individual receiving corticosteroid or immunosuppressive agents (e.g., organ transplant recipients, those with hematologic malignancies), and patients with AIDS are at particular risk (see Chap. 264). In such settings, *acute* toxoplasmosis may be associated with a widely disseminated and rapidly fatal infection characterized by high fever, pneumonia, rash, hepatosplenomegaly, myocarditis, myositis, orchitis, and especially central nervous system involvement with intracerebral mass lesions or meningoencephalitis. Lymphadenopathy may not be present.

The signs and symptoms of *reactivated* toxoplasmosis in the immunodeficient patient depend upon the location(s) of cyst breakdown and the intensity of the resultant inflammatory response. Although liberated trophozoites may be found simultaneously in a variety of areas (e.g., lung, myocardium, muscle, testes, skin, ascitic fluid) and produce signs of organ dysfunction (pneumonitis, retinitis, orchitis), clinically apparent reactivated disease is largely limited to the central nervous system. This observation has been shown repeatedly by AIDS patients seropositive for *T. gondii* in whom intracerebral toxoplasmosis appears almost entirely due to reactivated infection and not infrequently is the first manifestation of AIDS. Up to 30 percent of patients infected with human immunodeficiency virus who have antibody to *T. gondii* have developed reactivated toxoplasmosis; conversely, between 25 and 80 percent of cases of encephalitis or brain abscess in AIDS patients are caused by *T. gondii*. Immunosuppressed non-AIDS patients may be more prone to develop reactivated infection outside the brain.

Intracerebral toxoplasmosis typically presents in a subacute fashion with headache, focal neurologic signs, seizures, or altered mental status which can progress to coma. Fever is not always present. In intracerebral toxoplasmosis associated with either acute or reactivated

FIGURE 162-1 *Left:* Brain CT scan showing contrast-enhancing right cerebral lesion in a 35-year-old homosexual man. Biopsy demonstrated *T. gondii* cysts and free trophozoites on histologic examination. *Right:* Histologic appearance of replicating intracellular *T. gondii* trophozoites (*arrows*) in the brain biopsy of mass lesion in a patient with AIDS and neurologic signs (H & E, 600x).

infection, computed tomography (CT) of the brain may suggest encephalitis but more often shows single (Fig. 162-1) or numerous contrast-enhancing mass lesions of <2 cm in diameter with a predilection for the basal ganglia. Lesions can occur at any site in the brain, however, and may not show enhancement with contrast injection. Occasionally, the standard CT scan is normal early, in which case a follow-up scan, a double-dose-delay CT study, or magnetic resonance imaging (MRI) usually demonstrates the lesions. Cerebrospinal fluid changes include a modest mononuclear pleocytosis, moderately elevated protein, and only rarely a reduced glucose level. The diagnostic possibilities other than toxoplasmosis in an immunocompromised patient with intracerebral lesions are diverse: lymphoma, progressive multifocal leukoencephalopathy, histoplasmosis, mycobacterial infection, cryptococcosis, and encephalitis caused by cytomegalovirus and HIV. Therefore, brain biopsy (Fig. 162-1) should always be undertaken if clinically feasible. Stereotactic CT-guided needle biopsies provide a relatively safe approach with a high diagnostic yield, although excisional biopsies are usually more definitive. In AIDS patients a trial of anti-*Toxoplasma* treatment to assess response is appropriate before proceeding to brain biopsy.

DIAGNOSIS Infection with *T. gondii* is most frequently established by serologic testing for specific antibody; other methods include isolating the protozoan from clinical materials inoculated into tissue culture or mice, finding characteristic histopathologic changes (lymph node), and directly demonstrating trophozoites in either body fluids or cysts or in tissue sections. The presence of IgG antibody in the serum or cysts in the tissues may simply indicate prior infection and therefore does not imply any causal relationship to current signs or symptoms.

Serology Specific anti-*Toxoplasma* IgG antibody can be detected in the serum using the time-honored Sabin-Feldman dye test (SFDT), an indirect fluorescent antibody (IFA) test, or a complement fixation (CF) assay. Other techniques to measure IgG antibody are either not in general use or have not proved to be of particular value. In both the SFDT and IFA, positive titers ($\geq$1:4) may be detected as early as 1 to 2 weeks after infection, are at or near their peak ($\geq$1:1024, up to 1:64000 or greater) within 4 to 8 weeks, and begin to slowly decline after 6 to 12 months. IgG titers persist at low levels (1:16 to 1:256) for life. The rapid rise and peaking of SFDT and IFA titers accounts for the observation that 90 to 95 percent of symptomatic patients or those with lymphadenopathy have high titers ($\geq$1:1024) when they first seek attention and also explains why diagnostic fourfold increases in SFDT or IFA titer can only be demonstrated in 20 percent of cases. Antibody detected by the CF test is generated less rapidly, appears in the serum 3 to 8 weeks after infection, rises over the next 2 to 8 months, and then declines to low or undetectable levels within a year. Therefore, although seroconversion or a fourfold increase in titer may be more readily detected using the CF test, titers may be absent both early in acute infection and in chronic (latent) infection. Up to 60 percent of AIDS patients with intracerebral toxoplasmosis have detectable IgG antibody to *T. gondii* in the cerebrospinal fluid, and in the majority of these patients, intrathecal antibody production can be demonstrated. This finding may support but does not prove that active toxoplasmosis is present.

Specific anti-*Toxoplasma* IgM antibody can be detected in the serum using an IgM fluorescent antibody (IgM-IFA) assay or a more sensitive and specific double-sandwich enzyme-linked immunosorbent technique (DS-IgM-ELISA). Testing for IgM antibody has not been well-standardized in many commercial laboratories. Since IgM titers appear earlier (within the first week after infection) and disappear more rapidly than IgG antibodies, testing for IgM is often useful in patients suspected of having acute infection. Within the first 6 months after the appearance of lymphadenopathy, sera from up to 80 percent of immunocompetent individuals show antibody in the IgM-IFA assay, and 90 percent are positive in the DS-IgM-ELISA. The absence of IgM antibody, however, does not exclude acute infection because 10 to 20 percent of patients with biopsy-proven acute-*Toxoplasma* lymphadenitis are seronegative for IgM. Between 4 and 6 months after infection, IgM-IFA titers decline to low or negative levels in 80 percent of cases. However, 50 percent of sera from acutely infected patients are still IgM antibody–positive 7 to 12 months later using the DS-IgM-ELISA, limiting the usefulness of an isolated positive titer in this test. Irrespective of the IgM or IgG test selected, acute and convalescent (4 weeks later) sera should always be obtained, frozen, and simultaneously assayed together for both IgM and IgG in the same laboratory. The presence of rheumatoid factor or antinuclear antibodies may cause false-positive reactions in both the IFA and the IgM-IFA tests.

In the immunologically intact individual, a serologic diagnosis of acute (recent) toxoplasmosis is suggested by a SFDT or IFA titer of ≥1:1024 and preferably confirmed by a fourfold rise in SFDT, IFA, or CF titer and a positive test for IgM antibody. In reactivated infection (retinochoroiditis in the normal host, intracerebral or disseminated disease in the immunosuppressed or HIV-infected patient), *low* serum titers (<1:1024) in the SFDT and IFA tests and absent CF and IgM titers are common. In these clinical settings, the role of serologic testing is primarily to document prior exposure to *T. gondii* by the presence of IgG antibodies. In a French study, however, sera from 20 percent of AIDS patients with *Toxoplasma* encephalitis contained IgM antibody, suggesting recent infection. These data directly contrast with the United States experience with AIDS patients (IgM antibody almost always absent) and presumably reflect the high prevalence of *T. gondii* infection (80 to 90 percent) in France. A negative (<1:4) SFDT or IFA test excludes *T. gondii* as the cause of ocular or intracerebral disease or other organ dysfunction. In congenital toxoplasmosis, maternal IgG antibody is readily passed to the fetus. However, stable or rising SFDT or IFA titers or a positive IgM test in an infant at risk or with consistent signs or symptoms strongly suggest congenital infection.

Isolation   The isolation of *T. gondii* can be accomplished by injecting mice intraperitoneally with human material suspected of being infected—body fluids, buffy coat leukocytes, fetal blood clot, bone marrow, and homogenates of tissue including brain and placenta. The peritoneal fluid of inoculated mice is examined microscopically 1 to 2 weeks later for the presence of trophozoites; if none are found, mice are examined after 4 to 6 weeks for serum IgG antibody to *T. gondii* and brain cysts. In some laboratories, tissue cell cultures are also inoculated with clinical samples and examined for replicating trophozoites. Although asymptomatic parasitemia persisting for up to a year has been rarely reported, the isolation of *T. gondii* from blood or body fluids (cerebrospinal, amniotic, ascites) is considered diagnostic of acute toxoplasmosis. In contrast, the isolation of *T. gondii* from tissue homogenates does not necessarily confirm acute

infection because such a result may simply reflect the presence of tissue cysts and latent infection.

Histologic diagnosis   The finding of free or intracellular trophozoites (but not cysts) in tissue sections (Fig. 162-1), impression smears of tissue biopsies, or cytocentrifuge specimens of any fluid confirms the presence of acute infection. Cysts are also typically found in tissue sections, and if numerous, suggest but do not prove recent infection. Since trophozoites may be difficult to locate microscopically in conventionally stained sections, tissue likely to be infected should also be analyzed histocytochemically (immunoperoxidase assay) for the detection of trophozoites or cells bearing *T. gondii* antigen. In patients with lymphadenitis, the organism is seldom visualized; however, the histologic appearance of the lymph node tissue alone is sufficiently characteristic to permit an experienced pathologist to make the diagnosis. By itself, the inflammatory reaction in other tissues is not specific for *T. gondii* infection.

TREATMENT   Pyrimethamine plus sulfadiazine   The synergistic combination of pyrimethamine plus sulfadiazine, both of which inhibit folate synthesis, is active against trophozoites and is effective in treating patients with acute, reactivated, or congenital toxoplasmosis. The tissue cyst, however, is resistant to all currently available agents, and persists despite clinical responses to therapy. Once treatment is discontinued in the immunodeficient patient, relapse is common presumably because of continued breakdown of tissue cysts. In adults, oral pyrimethamine is initially administered as a 100 mg/d loading dose for 2 days and then continued at 25 mg/d given once daily thereafter. Because of its long half-life (4 to 5 days), pyrimethamine can be given every other day; however, in most immunodeficient patients, it is used daily and often increased to 50 to 75 mg/d for severe infections. Sulfadiazine is adminstered with an oral loading dose of 75 mg/kg (up to 4 g) given once followed by a total daily dose of 100 mg/kg (up to 8 g/d) administered orally in two or four divided doses. Trisulfapyrimidines in the same dosages can be substituted for sulfadiazine; other sulfonamides including sulfamethoxazole are less active. The most common adverse reaction to pyrimethamine is dose-related bone marrow suppression which may be exacerbated by sulfonamides but can be ameliorated by oral folinic acid (calcium leucovorin, 5 to 20 mg/d). Complete blood counts and platelet counts should be performed at least once or twice each week in all treated patients. Complications of sulfonamide therapy include hypersensitivity reactions (fever, rash, hepatitis) which are distressingly frequent in patients with AIDS, leukopenia, and crystalluria with potential urinary stone formation. An increased intake of fluids and high urine flow is important in sulfonamide-treated patients.

Other agents   There are no uniformly accepted or clearly effective therapeutic alternatives to pyrimethamine plus sulfadiazine for the treatment of toxoplasmosis. Clindamycin, spiramycin, and trimethoprim-sulfamethoxazole each show either in vitro or in vivo anti-*Toxoplasma* effects, but are all less active and have not been systematically evaluated. However, accumulating clinical evidence suggests that clindamycin and spiramycin probably exert beneficial effects in reactivated and congenital toxoplasmosis, respectively (see below).

Indications for treatment   Immunologically intact children or adults including those with lymphadenitis seldom require specific treatment for acute, acquired *T. gondii* infection. In the unusual, otherwise healthy individual with prolonged symptoms or signs suggesting vital organ involvement, 4 to 6 weeks of therapy is reasonable. Infections acquired by inadvertent direct inoculation (transfusion, laboratory accident) should also probably be similarly treated.

Retinochoroiditis   Although ocular disease may remit spontaneously without specific therapy, 4 weeks of treatment with pyrimethamine and sulfadiazine results in demonstrable improvement in 70 percent of patients. Repeated courses of therapy may be required. Clindamycin, often recommended by ophthalmologists, is concentrated in the choroid and may also be effective. Control over retinal inflammation is critical in the presence of macular lesions, and systemic glucocorticoids are frequently used.

Acquired infection in pregnant women The incidence but not necessarily the severity of fetal infection can be reduced up to two- to threefold by treating pregnant women with acute toxoplasmosis. Although no one regimen has been proven to be superior, oral spiramycin (2 to 4 g/d), sulfadiazine alone, or alternating 3-week cycles of spiramycin and then sulfadiazine plus pyrimethamine (pyrimethamine is teratogenic and should only be used after the first trimester of pregnancy) all are probably effective in reducing transmission to and infection of the fetus. Some women opt for a therapeutic abortion. Irrespective of the presence of signs or symptoms of congenital toxoplasmosis, all infected infants should probably be treated to control active or subclinical infection and reduce the high likelihood of subsequent manifestations of symptomatic toxoplasmosis.

The immunodeficient patient Newly acquired or more likely reactivated toxoplasmosis always requires specific therapy in the immunosuppressed or T cell–deficient patient. For AIDS patients treated with pyrimethamine and sulfadiazine, between 60 and 80 percent show clear and rapid improvement and more than one-half of responding patients show complete resolution of clinical manifestations and brain CT scan abnormalities. In patients in whom immunosuppression can be relieved (e.g., discontinuing corticosteroid therapy), treatment is usually given for at least 4 weeks after all manifestations have resolved, which may take several months. Since the T cell–deficient state cannot be reversed in patients with AIDS, and at least 50 percent of these patients relapse once treatment is discontinued, anti-*Toxoplasma* therapy should be continued probably at full doses for life. The extraordinarily frequent drug toxicity observed in AIDS patients treated with pyrimethamine and sulfonamides often necessitates discontinuing the sulfonamide. In such cases, anecdotal information suggests that clindamycin (2.7 g/d intravenously, 1.2 to 1.8 g/d orally) can be given along with an increased dose of pyrimethamine (50 to 75 mg/d) to induce or maintain a clinical response. Relapses have occurred in patients treated with pyrimethamine or spiramycin alone, and there is insufficient experience to recommend clindamycin or trimethoprim-sulfamethoxazole alone. Addition of glucocorticoids is indicated only to reduce cerebral edema in patients with mass lesions; overall, their use has been neither beneficial nor apparently harmful. However, in patients with intracerebral disease thought but not proven to be caused by *T. gondii* (e.g., an AIDS patient seropositive to *T. gondii*, no brain biopsy), the clinical improvement induced by the use of glucocorticoids may obscure what is presumed to be a "diagnostic" response to anti-*Toxoplasma* therapy. Anti-seizure medications (e.g., phenytoin) are commonly added to treatment. Given the frequency with which toxoplasmosis develops in HIV-infected patients who have previously acquired (latent) *T. gondii* infection, it is essential to determine the efficacy of prophylactic agents (e.g., pyrimethamine-sulfadoxine) in preventing disease reactivation.

PREVENTION For seronegative pregnant women and immunodeficient patients, prevention of toxoplasmosis is important, and warnings to avoid eating undercooked meat and exposure to oocyst-containing materials are important. For seronegative immunodeficient patients as well as seronegative transplant recipients, it also seems reasonable to attempt to avoid direct inoculation by screening blood and organ donors for antibody to *T. gondii*. Although not universally accepted, recommendations for screening women two to three times during pregnancy if they are initially seronegative are also reasonable given the availability of therapy and consequences of untreated congenital infection.

REFERENCES

Brooks RG et al: Role of serology in the diagnosis of toxoplasmic lymphadenopathy. Rev Infect Dis 9:1055, 1987

Daffos F et al: Prenatal management of 746 pregnancies at risk for congenital toxoplasmosis. N Engl J Med 318:271, 1988

Dorfman RF, Remington JS: Value of lymph node biopsy in the diagnosis of acute acquired toxoplasmosis. N Engl J Med 289:878, 1973

Israelski DM, Remington JS: Toxoplasmic encephalitis in patients with AIDS. Infect Dis Clin North Am 2:429, 1988

Leport C et al: Treatment of central nervous system toxoplasmosis with pyrimethamine/sulfadiazine combination in 35 patients with the acquired immunodeficiency syndrome. Efficacy of long-term continuous therapy. Am J Med 84:94, 1988

Luft BJ, Remington JS: Toxoplasmic encephalitis. J Infect Dis 157:1, 1988

Masur H et al: Outbreak of toxoplasmosis in a family and documentation of acquired retinochoroiditis. Am J Med 66:396, 1978

McCabe RE et al: Clinical spectrum in 107 cases of toxoplasmic lymphadenopathy. Rev Infect Dis 9:754, 1987

————, Remington JS: Toxoplasmosis: The time has come. N Engl J Med 318:313, 1988

Murray HW: Gamma interferon, the activated macrophage, and host defense against microbial challenge. Ann Intern Med 108:595, 1988

O'Connor GR: Manifestations and management of ocular toxoplasmosis. Bull NY Acad Med 50:192, 1974

Ruskin J, Remington JS: Toxoplasmosis in the compromised host. Ann Intern Med 84:193, 1976

163 PNEUMOCYSTIS CARINII PNEUMONIA

PETER D. WALZER

DEFINITION *Pneumocystis carinii* is an opportunistic pathogen whose natural habitat is the lung. The organism is an important cause of pneumonia in the compromised host.

ETIOLOGY The taxonomy of *P. carinii* is unsettled, but analysis of the organism's ribosomal RNA suggests that *P. carinii* is more closely related to fungi than to protozoa. Major developmental stages of the organism include the small (1- to 4-μm), pleomorphic trophozoite or trophic form; the 5- to 8-μm cyst, which has a thick cell wall and contains up to eight intracystic bodies; and the precyst, an intermediate stage. The life cycle of *P. carinii* probably involves asexual replication by the trophic form and sexual reproduction by the cyst which ends in release of the intracystic bodies; an intracellular stage has not been identified. Modest propagation of *P. carinii* of animal origin has been achieved in tissue culture. Ultrastructurally, *P. carinii* has a primitive organelle system, but little is known about its metabolism.

EPIDEMIOLOGY *P. carinii* has a worldwide distribution among humans and has been found in a variety of animals. Organisms for these hosts are morphologically identical, but species or strain differences exist. Data about environmental sources of *P. carinii* are lacking. Serologic surveys indicate that most normal children have been exposed to the organism by 3 to 4 years of age. Animal model experiments have demonstrated that *P. carinii* is transmitted by the airborne route. Human-to-human transmission has been suggested by the occurrence of outbreaks of pneumocystosis among institutionalized debilitated infants and in hospitals caring for immunosuppressed patients. Based on animal studies, the incubation period is thought to be 4 to 8 weeks.

PATHOGENESIS *P. carinii* pneumonia occurs in the following hosts: premature, malnourished infants; children with primary immunodeficiency diseases; patients receiving immunosuppressive therapy (particularly corticosteroids) for cancer, organ transplantation, and other disorders; and patients with the acquired immunodeficiency syndrome. AIDS is by far the most common underlying disease for *P. carinii*; conversely, *P. carinii* is the most common opportunistic infection in AIDS, occurring in at least 60 percent and perhaps up to 80 to 90 percent of patients during their lifetime (see Chap. 264).

Available data suggest that impaired cellular immunity is the major host predisposing factor in the development of pneumocystosis.

Antibodies are produced locally and systemically in response to exposure to *P. carinii*, but do not appear to have a protective role. *P. carinii* pneumonia which develops with the use of immunosuppressive drugs probably represents reactivation of latent infection. In some reports the incidence of the disease has been related to the intensity of the immunosuppression. *P. carinii* pneumonia which develops in patients with primary immunodeficiency diseases and AIDS either could arise from latent infection with the progressive breakdown of host defenses or could be acquired by contagion.

PATHOLOGY The histopathologic features of *P. carinii* pneumonia in humans and experimental animals are identical. Early in the infection the organisms line up along walls of alveoli in close apposition to the type I pneumocyte. The interaction of *P. carinii* with this alveolar cell plays a major role in the host-parasite relationship in the infection. The organisms propagate slowly and, as seen on methenamine silver–stained lung sections, gradually fill the alveolar spaces. With hematoxylin and eosin staining there is the typical foamy, vacuolated alveolar exudate which consists of organisms, host serum proteins, debris, and surfactant. On electron microscopy in the animal model there is a series of changes in alveolar microenvironment which culminate in damage to the type I cell.

The host inflammatory changes are mild and nonspecific, even with extensive infection. Hypertrophy of alveolar type II cells can frequently be found and has been interpreted as a reparative response. Alveolar macrophages are present but usually not prominent in phagocytosis of the organism. In most compromised hosts there is a mild mononuclear cell interstitial cell infiltrate; however, malnourished infants display an intense interstitial plasma cell infiltrate which was responsible for the disease's early name of "interstitial plasma cell pneumonia." Very rarely *P. carinii* can be found in tissue other than the lungs.

CLINICAL FEATURES Patients with *P. carinii* pneumonia complain of dyspnea, fever, and nonproductive cough. When corticosteroids have been administered, symptoms frequently begin after the dose has been tapered. The duration of illness until diagnosis is typically 1 to 2 weeks in non-AIDS patients, although considerable variation exists. Pneumocystosis in AIDS usually follows a more chronic and indolent course. Patients typically are ill for several weeks but sometimes may experience subtle respiratory symptoms for several months. As a consequence, *P. carinii* can be easily overlooked unless a careful history is taken. Physical findings include tachypnea, tachycardia, and cyanosis, but lung auscultation reveals few abnormalities. The white blood count is variable and usually governed by the patient's underlying disease. Arterial blood gases demonstrate hypoxemia, increased alveolar-arterial oxygen gradient ($PA_{O_2} - Pa_{O_2}$), and respiratory alkalosis; changes in pulmonary function tests (e.g., vital capacity, diffusing capacity) are also present. These laboratory abnormalities are usually less severe in AIDS patients. The classic findings on chest radiograph consist of bilateral diffuse infiltrates beginning in the perihilar regions; with time, air bronchograms develop. Variants (e.g., nodular densities, unilateral infiltrates) to this picture have also been reported. Some patients may have a normal chest radiograph early in the course of the disease but demonstrate increased uptake on gallium scan.

DIAGNOSIS Since the clinical picture of *P. carinii* can be produced by many different infectious and noninfectious agents, diagnosis must be made by specific identification of the organism. Culture of human *P. carinii* is not yet feasible, and serology, whether based on antibody or antigen detection, is not reliable. Definitive diagnosis is made by histopathologic staining. Stains which selectively stain the cell wall of *P. carinii* cysts are the most popular. Methenamine silver is the prototype; but toluidine blue and cresyl echt violet are simpler, more rapid alternatives. Stains such as Giemsa's or Diff Quik stain both the trophozoite and cyst forms of *P. carinii;* these reagents also stain host tissues, and hence require a greater degree of experience for proper interpretation. *P. carinii* can also be stained by immunofluorescence and immunoperoxidase techniques.

Previously, *P. carinii* has been found infrequently in sputum;

however, it has been shown that pneumocystosis can be diagnosed frequently in AIDS patients by examination of sputum induced by inhalation of a saline mist. This probably reflects the higher organism burden in AIDS patients as well as the improved proficiency of clinical laboratories. Fiberoptic bronchoscopy with bronchoalveolar lavage and/or transbronchial biopsy is the most commonly used procedure and has a high diagnostic yield in AIDS and non-AIDS patients. Open-lung biopsy, the most invasive technique, is usually performed when bronchoscopy is nondiagnostic or when infection with an additional organism is suspected.

COURSE AND PROGNOSIS Pneumocystosis is usually confined to the lungs, although cases of disseminated infection are receiving increasing attention. In the typical case of untreated *P. carinii* pneumonia, there is progressive respiratory embarrassment leading ultimately to death. Therapy is most effective when it is instituted early in the course of the disease before there is extensive alveolar damage. Prognosis is influenced by such factors as the patient's underlying disease and immune function, nutritional status, $PA_{O_2} - Pa_{O_2}$, and concomitant infection with other opportunistic pathogens.

TREATMENT The two major drugs used in the treatment of *P. carinii* pneumonia have been trimethoprim-sulfamethoxazole (TMP-SMX) and pentamidine isethionate. These agents are equally effective, with an overall success rate of 70 to 80 percent. TMP-SMX acts by inhibiting folic acid synthesis, but the mode of action of pentamidine against *P. carinii* is unclear. TMP-SMX is administered orally or intravenously in a dose of 20 mg/kg per day TMP and 100 mg/kg per day SMX in four divided doses; this regimen should be modified to achieve optimum serum levels of 5 to 8 µg/mL TMP and 100 to 150 µg/mL SMX in adults. Pentamidine is given intramuscularly or by slow intravenous infusion in a dose of 4 mg/kg per day. Both drugs are administered for 14 days in non-AIDS patients and for 21 days in persons with AIDS.

TMP-SMX is well tolerated by non-AIDS patients, but over half of the AIDS patients experience serious adverse reactions including fever, rash, neutropenia, thrombocytopenia, and hepatitis. Pentamidine is a toxic drug for all recipients; major side effects include cardiovascular abnormalities, dysglycemias, azotemia, neutropenia, and sterile abscesses with intramuscular injection.

Clinical improvement usually begins after several days of therapy and is characterized by changes in fever, respiratory symptoms, and blood gases. Since persons with AIDS may respond even more slowly, it is prudent to wait at least 7 days in these patients before switching to another drug. The combination of TMP-SMX and pentamidine does not improve efficacy and may increase the risk of toxicity. Important general supportive measures include maintaining adequate oxygenation, nutrition, fluid and electrolyte balance, and tapering immunosuppressive drugs in non-AIDS patients to as low a dose as possible to control the underlying disease. The use of mechanical ventilation and other life support systems in persons with AIDS has provoked considerable debate and is best handled on an individualized basis. In cases of severe *P. carinii* pneumonia not responding to conventional therapy, glucocorticoids (e.g., methyl prednisolone) can be added with caution.

Alternative forms of therapy of pneumocystosis appear promising, but at the present time must be considered investigational. These include administration of pentamidine via aerosol, which results in high concentrations of the drug in the lungs with minimal systemic absorption; the use of trimetrexate, which is more active than TMP against *P. carinii* dihydrofolate reductase; dapsone, a sulfone which may be less toxic than SMX; α-difluoromethylornithine, which inhibits polyamine synthesis; and the combination of clindamycin and primaquine.

PREVENTION All patients who recover from pneumocystosis are at risk for recurrent episodes of the disease as long as the underlying immunosuppressive conditions persist. Persons with AIDS have the highest recurrence rate (about 50 percent at 1 year) despite the introduction of azidothymidine therapy; the mechanisms of these recurrences (i.e., relapse or reinfection) and their relationship to persisting organisms which are frequently present in follow-up bronchoscopy are unclear. TMP-SMX in the dose of 5 mg/kg per day TMP and 25 mg/kg per day SMX administered daily or three times a week has been highly effective in preventing *P. carinii* in non-AIDS patients; however, its use in AIDS patients has been limited by the high frequency of side effects. Aerosolized pentamidine is recommended as (secondary) prophylaxis for patients with previous bouts of *P. carinii* pneumonia as well as for patients with no history of pneumonia but with CD4+ T cells <200 per microliter. Other regimens including dapsone and pyramethamine-sulfadoxine are undergoing clinical evaluation and appear promising. Since none of these agents are lethal for *P. carinii*, they are only effective in chemoprophylaxis as long as they are being given. Specific environmental measures have not yet been developed, but it is prudent to separate patients with *P. carinii* infection from direct contact with other susceptible hosts.

REFERENCES

BRENNER M et al: Prognostic factors and life expectancy of patients with acquired immunodeficiency syndrome and *Pneumocystis carinii* pneumonia. Am Rev Respir Dis 136:1199, 1987

CARTER TR et al: *Pneumocystis carinii* infection of the small intestine in a patient with the acquired immunodeficiency syndrome. Am J Clin Pathol 89:679, 1988

CUSHION MT et al: Analysis of the developmental stages of *Pneumocystis carinii* in vitro. Lab Invest 58:324, 1988

EDMAN JC et al: Ribosomal RNA sequence shows *Pneumocystis carinii* to be a member of the fungi. Nature 334:519, 1988

FISCHL MA et al: Safety and efficacy of sulfamethoxazole and trimethoprim chemoprophylaxis for *Pneumocystis carinii* pneumonia in AIDS. JAMA 259:1185, 1988

HAGLER DN et al: Blastogenic responses to *Pneumocystis carinii* among patients with human immunodeficiency virus (HIV) infection. Clin Exp Immunol 74:7, 1988

KOVACS JA, MASUR H: *Pneumocystis carinii* pneumonia: Therapy and prophylaxis. J Infect Dis 158:254, 1988

MONTGOMERY AB et al: Aerosolized pentamidine as sole therapy for *Pneumocystis carinii* pneumonia in patients with acquired immunodeficiency syndrome. Lancet 2:480, 1987

MURRAY JF et al: Pulmonary complications of the acquired immunodeficiency syndrome: An update. Am Rev Respir Dis 135:504, 1987

SANKARY RM et al: Alveolar-capillary block in patients with AIDS and *Pneumocystis carinii* pneumonia. Am Rev Respir Dis 137:443, 1988

SATTLER FR et al: Trimethoprim-sulfamethoxazole compared with pentamidine for treatment of *Pneumocystis carinii* pneumonia in the acquired immunodeficiency syndrome. Ann Intern Med 109:280, 1988

STRINGER SL et al: *Pneumocystis carinii*: Sequence from ribosomal RNA implies a close relationship with fungi. Exp Parasitol 68:450, 1989

WALZER PD et al: *Pneumocystis carinii*, in *Parasitic Infections in the Compromised Host*, PD Walzer, RM Genta (eds). New York, Dekker, 1989, pp 83–178

164 BABESIOSIS

JAMES J. PLORDE

DEFINITION AND HISTORY Known since biblical times, this cosmopolitan infection of domestic and wild animals is caused by protozoa of the genus *Babesia*. These organisms are transmitted by ticks, multiply in red blood cells, and produce an acute febrile hemolytic anemia, the most prominent manifestation of which is hemoglobinuria.

EPIDEMIOLOGY AND CLINICAL MANIFESTATIONS The first human infection was described in Yugoslavia by Skrabalo in 1957. This and six other European cases were particularly severe with high fever, hemoglobinuria, jaundice, and renal failure. Both in their clinical presentation and in the presence of small intraerythrocytic parasites they closely resembled falciparum malaria with which they were originally confused. All seven occurred in splenectomized patients, and five ended fatally. The causative agents were bovine parasites (*B. bovis*, *B. divergens*). Some 120 cases have now been documented in the United States. Two California cases resembled the European infections and were thought to be caused by equine babesia. With the exception of single cases in Georgia and Wisconsin, all others have been acquired during the summer months on Cape Cod and the offshore islands lying between New York and Massachusetts, including Long Island, Fire Island, Shelter Island, Nantucket, and Martha's Vineyard. All of the New England and the single Wisconsin infection were caused by a rodent parasite, *B. microti*, and approximately 80 percent occurred in patients with intact spleens. The patients experienced an illness of several weeks characterized by the insidious onset of fever, chills, sweating, myalgia, and mild to moderate hemolytic anemia presumably caused by direct, parasite-induced damage to the erythrocytic membrane. The physical examination was usually negative except for occasional splenomegaly. In general, clinical manifestations have been more severe in asplenic subjects. Most patients were over 50 years of age, and all but two recovered. The carrier state persisted for weeks to months in some patients and in four resulted in subsequent transfusion-induced infections. Three of the four recipients were asplenic; the fourth was an elderly individual who represents the only fatality in the series. Serologic studies suggest that most patients infected with *B. microti* are asymptomatic; seroconversion rates of nearly 6 percent and point prevalence rates of 2 to 4.4 percent have been noted in endemic areas. All age groups seem equally susceptible. Like their symptomatic counterparts, patients with subclinical infections may remain parasitemic for several months.

B. microti has been found in field moles and deer mice in New York State, Wisconsin, Utah, and California. On the offshore islands of New England, however, the principal reservoir is the white-footed mouse. The northern deer tick, *Ixodes dammini*, which also serves as the vector in Lyme disease, is responsible for the transmission of *B. microti*. This hard-bodied tick takes a blood meal during each of its three developmental stages: larva, nymph, and adult. Rodents are the principal hosts of the first two stages while deer host the adult ticks. Only the nymphs, which feed from May through September, are capable of transmitting *B. microti* to humans. Since the engorged nymph measures 2 mm in diameter, infested patients may be oblivious to its presence. Transovarial transmission does not occur.

DIAGNOSIS The diagnosis depends on the demonstration of the intraerythrocytic parasite in Giemsa-stained peripheral blood smears. Like malaria parasites, these organisms measure 2 to 3 μm in diameter and demonstrate red-staining nuclear material with blue cytoplasm. In contrast to malaria parasites, however, neither gametocytes nor pigment are seen. As the parasites multiply by a nonsynchronous budding process, the organism displays marked pleomorphism; a single red cell may contain multiple parasites in different developmental stages. Unique basket shapes, tetrads, and trophozoites with multiple chromatin dots are helpful distinguishing features. In heavy infections, organisms can be seen outside red blood cells. Serologic diagnosis can be made with the indirect fluorescent antibody test or enzyme-linked immunosorbent assay. Because the disease is insidious in onset, most infected patients have titers ≥1024 at the time they present for medical care. There is no correlation between disease severity and the titer level; cross reactions with other *Babesia* species and malaria may be seen, but titers with homologous antigens are generally higher. Over 50 percent of patients with babesiosis have IgG- and IgM-specific antibodies to *Borrelia burgdorferi*, suggesting that simultaneous infections with these two organisms are more common than the limited number reported to date. Active infections have been demonstrated in smear-negative, serology-positive infections by inducing infection in experimental animals.

TREATMENT Mild disease should be managed symptomatically with antipyretics. If significant hemolysis ensues, transfusion may be warranted. In more severe infections specific therapy should be attempted. Although chloroquine provides symptomatic improvement, it appears to have little activity against this parasite. Oral quinine (650 mg tid for 7 days) plus clindamycin (600 mg tid for 7 days) has been successful in several patients. Antitrypanosomal agents also appear effective, and, in life-threatening infections, pentamidine should be considered. This agent appears to be effective in controlling the clinical manifestations of babesiosis and decreasing parasitemia; it may not eradicate the organism. Exchange transfusions are helpful in fulminant infections.

PREVENTION   The prevention of *B. microti* infections in humans is difficult. Individuals summering on the offshore islands of New England should consider the use of insect repellents containing diethyltoluamide and examine themselves daily for the presence of the 2- to 3-mm nymphs. A pilot tick control program has been initiated on one of the islands. Asplenic patients should be advised to avoid endemic areas. To avoid transfusion-transmitted babesiosis, blood donors should be screened serologically for evidence of *B. microti* infection.

REFERENCES

BENECH JL et al: Serologic evidence for simultaneous transmission of Lyme disease and babesiosis. J Infect Dis 152:473, 1985

CHISHOLM ES et al: Indirect immunofluorescence test for human *Babesia microti* infection: Antigenic specificity. Am J Trop Med Hyg 35:921, 1986

JACOBY GA et al: Treatment of transfusion-transmitted babesiosis by exchange transfusion. N Engl J Med 303:1098, 1980

MARCUS LC et al: Fatal pancarditis in a patient with coexistent Lyme disease and babesiosis. Ann Intern Med 103:374, 1985

ROSNER F et al: Babesiosis in splenectomized adults: Review of 22 reported cases. Am J Med 76:696, 1984

RUEBUSH TK II et al: Development and persistence of antibody in persons with *Babesia microti*. Am J Trop Med Hyg 30:291, 1981

STEKETEE RW et al: Babesiosis in Wisconsin: A new focus of disease transmission. JAMA 253:2675, 1985

SUN T et al: Morphologic and clinical observations in human infection with *Babesia microti*. J Infect Dis 148:239, 1983

WITTER M et al: Successful chemotherapy of transfusion babesiosis. Ann Intern Med 96:601, 1982

165   GIARDIASIS

JAMES J. PLORDE

ETIOLOGY AND EPIDEMIOLOGY   *Giardia lamblia* is a pear-shaped multiflagellar protozoan that parasitizes the human duodenum and the jejunum of humans and other animals, where it multiplies by longitudinal fission. Under a microscope, its pyriform shape, two nuclei, and central parabasal body give the organism the appearance of a face with two large eyes. It may actively browse the unstirred mucous layer at the bases of the microvilli or attach to the intestinal mucosa by means of a large ventral sucking disk. Unattached trophozoites may be carried in the fecal stream to the large bowel. If their passage through the gut is hurried, they will exit unchanged in the liquid stool and perish rapidly. With normal colonic transit times, however, the organisms retract their flagella, envelop themselves in a protective membrane, and undergo nuclear division. The resulting quadrinucleate cysts are infectious and may be transmitted to new hosts by a number of fecal-oral routes. Cysts deposited in cold water can survive for more than 2 months and have been shown to be resistant to chlorine concentrations (0.4 mg/L) routinely used in community purification systems. The ingestion of water contaminated with as few as 10 cysts is sufficient to establish human infection. Not surprisingly, waterborne outbreaks in humans have been documented repeatedly during the past two decades. In fact, *G. lamblia* is now the single most frequently defined cause of waterborne outbreaks of diarrhea in the United States. They have involved campers who have drunk from remote surface waters, skiers who have used well water, and ordinary citizens served by municipal systems with no or inadequate filtration equipment. Contamination of the water supply with raw sewage has been found in several outbreaks. In others, *G. lamblia*–infected beavers were located within the watershed, suggesting that these mammals may serve as alternate reservoirs. There have been two reports of *Giardia* transmission

among swimming pool attendees. Waterborne cysts are also thought to be responsible for the high incidence of giardiasis in travelers returning from third-world countries. Food may also serve as a transmission vehicle in these areas as well.

Direct person-to-person spread occurs with some frequency. This is most dramatically evident among male homosexuals practicing anilingus, children attending day care centers, and the secondary cases seen in families of infected children. It may also explain apparent transmission from dogs to their masters.

Giardiasis is a cosmopolitan infection that is particularly common in areas with poor sanitation and among populations unable to maintain adequate levels of hygiene. The prevalence of giardiasis often exceeds 20 percent in developing countries. In the United States prevalence rates of 1 to 6 percent have been reported. Young children are three times more likely to be involved than adults, and among the institutionalized retarded, rates exceeding 50 percent have been reported. Giardiasis is also frequent in individuals with immunoglobulin deficiencies. It has been suggested that the parasite is able to persist in such patients because of a relative deficiency of secretory IgA. Similarly, the immune deficiencies accompanying protein-calorie malnutrition are thought to enhance the susceptibility of involved individuals to parasitization with *G. lamblia*.

Among adults, parasitism is common in parents of infected children, travelers to endemic areas, and campers who ingest untreated water, but the precise prevalence in these populations is unknown. Achlorhydric individuals may be more susceptible to infection. Several studies have emphasized the association between male homosexuality and intestinal parasitosis; infection rates for *G. lamblia* and/or *Entamoeba histolytica* have ranged from 11 to 40 percent.

PATHOLOGY AND PATHOGENESIS   Clinical manifestations appear to be caused by an impairment of the absorptive capacity of the gut, particularly for fat and carbohydrates. The mechanism responsible for these changes is unknown. Mechanical blockage of the intestinal mucosa by large numbers of trophozoites, competition for essential nutrients, altered jejunal mobility with or without overgrowth of enteric bacteria or yeasts, pancreatic or biliary dysfunction, and organism-induced deconjugation of bile salts have been implicated. None, however, correlates well with disease severity, and eradication of associated microorganisms does not uniformly result in clinical improvement. Disaccharidase deficiency with lactose intolerance, altered levels of peptide hydrolyase and enteropeptidase, and decreased vitamin B_{12} absorption indicate that *G. lamblia* produces direct or indirect damage to the microvillar structure of the small bowel. Mechanical irritation of the fuzzy coat by the trophozoite's sucking disk might induce an accelerated turnover of the mucosal epithelium, resulting in functional immaturity of the transport systems. Excretion of a soluble toxin that interacts with the epithelial cell has been hypothesized, but never documented. Mucosal invasion may provoke a T cell–mediated insult to the jejunal mucosa. In experimentally infected nude mice immunologic reconstitution with lymphoid cells from previously infected animals results in marked mucosal changes including cellular infiltration and a decreased villus/crypt ratio. Similar pathologic findings have been reported in humans with giardial malabsorption. Both the structural changes and the malabsorption are reversible with specific therapy.

Although reinfection is common, the frequent occurrence of giardiasis in patients with immunologic defects, and the rarity with which it is seen in older adults, suggest that protective immunity, albeit incomplete, does develop with time. The diversity of surface antigens, secretory products, and DNA banding patterns in *Giardia* isolates could influence the effectiveness of the host immune response in preventing reinfection.

CLINICAL MANIFESTATIONS   In endemic situations, over two-thirds of infected patients may be asymptomatic. This ratio is usually reversed in point-source outbreaks. From 1 to 3 weeks after exposure, the patient notes the explosive onset of watery diarrhea. The stool is foul smelling, greasy in appearance, and floats. There is neither blood nor mucus. Epigastric abdominal cramping is present. The formation of large quantities of intestinal gas produces distention, sulfuric eructation, and flatulence. Anorexia, nausea, vomiting, and low-grade fever may be present. Typically, acute symptoms continue for at least 5 to 7 days. In an occasional patient, they may persist for months, leading to significant malabsorption and weight loss. More commonly, the illness resolves spontaneously in 1 to 4 weeks or lapses into a chronic phase characterized by intermittent bouts of flatulence, epigastric pain, and the passage of mushy stools. It is not unusual for patients to present in this fashion without having experienced the more acute manifestations described above. Chronic giardiasis is associated with reduced growth in preschool children. Eventually, both parasites and symptoms disappear. Lactose intolerance, however, may persist, producing a clinical picture easily confused with the parasitologic disease and may result in unnecessary therapy.

DIAGNOSIS   The diagnosis is made by identifying the cyst in formed feces or the trophozoite in diarrheal stools, duodenal secretions, or jejunal biopsies. In the majority of acute cases, the parasite can be demonstrated easily in a series of stool specimens collected and examined in the manner described for amebiasis (see Chap. 158). In acute illness, the onset of clinical manifestations may antedate the excretion of organisms by 5 to 7 days while in chronic infections the discharge of parasites is often scanty or intermittent, making laboratory confirmation more difficult. Many of these patients, however, can be diagnosed by examining specimens collected at weekly intervals for a period of 4 to 5 weeks. Alternatively, the duodenal contents can be sampled with a nylon string (Entrotest) or gastric tube and cultured by direct wet-mount preparation. Occasionally, jejunal biopsy is required to establish the diagnosis in patients with typical clinical manifestations. Immunodiagnostic methods for the rapid detection of *Giardia* antigen in feces appear both highly sensitive and specific, but are not commercially available. Enzyme-linked immunosorbent and indirect fluorescent serologic tests using axenically cultured *G. lamblia* have been developed. Their diagnostic usefulness remains to be established.

TREATMENT   Treatment is usually carried out with quinacrine hydrochloride or metronidazole. Tinidazole, a more effective agent, is presently not available in the United States. Quinacrine, 0.1 g given three times daily for 5 days, eliminates the organisms in 70 to 95 percent of cases. Although the drug is usually well tolerated, it may produce gastrointestinal disturbances, exacerbate psoriasis, and, rarely, produce toxic psychosis. Metronidazole appears to be better tolerated and equally effective. A single oral dose of 2.0 g given on 3 consecutive days, 750 mg tid for 5 days, and 250 mg tid for 5 days give cure rates of 95, 95, and 70 percent, respectively. However, this drug is not currently licensed for giardiasis, and there is concern over its mutagenicity. Household contacts and sexual partners of infected patients should be examined; individuals harboring the parasite should be treated even if asymptomatic to prevent the spread to others. Pregnant women, however, should receive therapy only if severely symptomatic and never in the first trimester. Because parasitologic and clinical relapse can occur up to 7 weeks after the completion of therapy, long-term follow-up is essential.

PREVENTION   Chemoprophylactic drugs are not effective in preventing the acquisition of giardiasis. Individuals visiting endemic areas should avoid the ingestion of potentially contaminated food and water. The latter may be made potable by boiling or by treating with a suitable halogen disinfectant. Most of the commercially available tablets appear effective when appropriate concentrations and contact times are utilized; they are temperature-dependent, and their dose should be increased when dealing with cold water. Custodial institutions for children should screen new admissions for the presence of *G. lamblia* and treat those found to be positive. Handwashing by children and staff must be emphasized. Community water purification systems should provide for adequate filtration as well as disinfection. Breast feeding appears to protect infants from giardiasis; this may be related to the known presence of antigiardial substances, including specific IgA antibodies, in breast milk.

REFERENCES

BLACK RE et al: Giardiasis in day-care centers—Evidence of person to person transmission. Pediatrics 60:486, 1977

DYKES AC et al: Municipal waterborne giardiasis: An epidemiologic investigation. Ann Intern Med 93:165, 1980

GUPTA MC, URRUTIA JJ: Effect of periodic antiascaris and antigiardia treatment on nutritional status of preschool children. Am J Clin Nutr 36:79, 1982

JARROLL EL JR et al: *Giardia* cyst destruction: Effectiveness of six small-quantity water disinfection methods. Am J Trop Med Hyg 29:8, 1980

NASH TE et al: Experimental human infections with *Giardia lamblia*. J Infect Dis 156:974, 1987

PETERSEN LR et al: A food-borne outbreak of *Giardia lamblia*. J Infect Dis 157:846, 1988

PICKERING LK, ENGELKIRK PG: *Giardia lamblia*. Ped Clin North Am 35:565, 1988

STEVENS DP: Giardiasis: Host-pathogen biology. Rev Infect Dis 4:851, 1982

———. Selective primary health care. Strategies for control of disease in the developing world. XIX. Giardiasis. Rev Infect Dis 7:530, 1985

166   CRYPTOSPORIDIOSIS

JAMES J. PLORDE

DEFINITION   Cryptosporidiosis is a diarrheal disease of vertebrates produced by protozoa of the genus *Cryptosporidium*. These parasites inhabit the microvillous border of the intestinal epithelium, where they produce clinical illness ranging from an acute, self-limited, watery diarrhea in normal individuals to chronic, severe, life-threatening gastroenteritis in the immunocompromised. Unknown as human pathogens prior to 1976, cryptosporidia now rank with *Salmonella*, *Shigella*, *Campylobacter*, enterotoxigenic *Escherichia coli*, rotavirus, and *Giardia lamblia* as major enteric pathogens of humans.

ETIOLOGY   Regardless of animal host, most strains of this tiny parasite appear morphologically similar. Those capable of infecting humans and most domestic mammals have oocysts which measure 5 μm in diameter and are known as *C. parvum*. Cryptosporidia exhibit alternating cycles of sexual and asexual reproduction and are thereby classified as sporozoan protozoa. As is true for *Toxoplasma*, *Isospora*, and other members of the sporozoan subgroup known as Coccidia, both cycles are completed within the gastrointestinal tract of a single host. The infective forms or oocysts are shed into the intestinal lumen of the parasitized animal. These hardy structures are resistant to most disinfectants, chlorine concentrates generally present in municipal water supplies, and temperatures between −20°C and 60°C. In cool moist environments they may survive for months. Unlike those of *Toxoplasma* and *Isospora*, cryptosporidia oocysts are fully mature and immediately infective upon passage in the feces. Following ingestion by another animal, *sporozoites* are released from the oocyst, attach themselves to the epithelial surface, and begin a series of developmental changes. Although excluded from the cytoplasm of the epithelial cell, *trophozoites* and all subsequent developmental stages are surrounded by a double membrane of host origin and are, by definition, intracellular parasites. The trophozoites divide asexually by a process of multiple fission (*schizogony*) to form *meronts* containing eight daughter cells known as type I *merozoites*. Upon release from the meront, each merozoite attaches itself to another epithelial cell, where it repeats the schizogony cycle, producing another generation of type I merozoites. Eventually, meronts containing only four daughter cells are seen. Incapable of continued asexual reproduction, these type II merozoites are transformed into male (*microgamete*) and female (*macrogamete*) sexual forms. Following fertilization, the resulting *zygote* develops into an oocyst. The majority possess a thick, double-layered protective cell wall which ensures their intact passage in the feces and survival in the external environment. Approximately 20 percent of the oocysts, however, fail to develop such a wall. Their thin single cell membrane ruptures, releasing infective sporozoites directly into the intestinal lumen and initiating a new "autoinfective" cycle within the original host. In the normal host, the presence of innate or acquired immunity dampens both the cyclic production of type I merozoites and the formation of thin-walled oocysts, halting further parasite multiplication and terminating the acute infection. In the immunocompromised both presumably continue, explaining why such individuals develop severe, persistent infections in the absence of repeated reinfections.

EPIDEMIOLOGY Cryptosporidiosis appears to involve most vertebrate groups; the available prevalence studies demonstrate that although rare in adult animals, infection rates can be high in immature pets and farm stock. Experimental transmission of human *Cryptosporidium* strains to rodents, kittens, and puppies, and an outbreak of infection in human handlers of infected calves clearly suggest that domestic animals constitute an important reservoir of disease for humans. Disease outbreaks in day-care centers, hospitals, and urban family groups, however, indicate that most human infections result from person-to-person transmission rather than zoonotic spread. As in animals, human disease is more common in the young. In western countries, 0.6 to 4.3 percent of small children presenting to medical centers with gastroenteritis have been shown to harbor cryptosporidia oocysts; in third world countries the rates have varied from 3 to 30 percent. Up to 63 percent of children attending day-care centers during outbreaks of diarrhea have had oocysts detected in their stool. Infection rates in adults suffering from gastroenteritis are approximately one-third those reported for children and have been highest in family members of infected children, medical personnel caring for patients with cryptosporidiosis, AIDS patients, and travelers to foreign countries. Asymptomatic carriage is uncommon in the United States and Europe. However, in less well developed nations, oocysts have been found in up to 10 percent of diarrhea-free children, suggesting that early, repeated exposure may produce clinical immunity with persistent oocyst excretion. Other enteric pathogens, particularly *Giardia lamblia*, are recovered from a significant minority of infected patients. Since oocysts are found almost exclusively in stool, the principal transmission route is undoubtedly fecal-oral. In day-care centers and among male homosexual groups the spread is probably direct. The recovery of oocysts from both surface and drinking water and the documentation of at least two waterborne outbreaks makes it likely that indirect transmission via water, and possibly food and fomites, is not uncommon. The increase in infection rates seen during the summer months is compatible with this hypothesis. On rare occasions oocysts have been recovered from the pharynx or found in expectorated sputum, raising the possibility that cryptosporidiosis may be acquired through contact with the respiratory secretions of infected patients.

PATHOGENESIS AND PATHOLOGY Although the jejunum is most heavily involved, cryptosporidia have been found in the pharynx, bronchi, esophagus, stomach, duodenum, gallbladder, ileum, appendix, colon, and rectum of immunocompromised subjects. They appear as small, basophilic, spherical structures arranged in rows or clusters along the brush border of the epithelial cells. They color readily with Giemsa and hematoxylin-eosin, but not with acid-fast stains; they may be mistaken for epithelial blebs. Electron microscopy reveals the entire gamut of developmental forms including trophozoites, meronts, merozoites, and macrogametes. All are covered by a double membrane derived from the reflection, fusion, and attenuation of the microvilli over the parasite. By light microscopy, bowel changes appear minimal, consisting of mild-to-moderate villous atrophy, crypt enlargement, and a mononuclear infiltrate of the lamina propria.

The pathophysiology of the diarrhea that accompanies cryptosporidiosis is unknown, but malabsorption of fat and carbohydrate has been reported, particularly in AIDS patients, suggesting damage to the brush border. The profuse, watery diarrhea characteristic of the clinical disease raises the possibility of an enterotoxin, but none has been identified. The deep, intracellular location of some parasites may facilitate antigen processing with resultant immune-mediated damage. The vital role played by the host's immune status in the pathogenesis of the disease is further indicated by the enhanced susceptibility of the young to infection, the frequency with which clinical infection occurs during measles, and the prolonged, severe clinical disease seen in inmmunocompromised patients. Animal studies suggest that resistance to reinfection is mediated by T lymphocytes while the severity and duration of the primary infection are influenced by both cellular and humoral mechanisms.

CLINICAL MANIFESTATIONS Immunocompetent hosts Following an incubation period of 4 to 14 days, the patient notes the onset of an explosive, profuse, watery diarrhea accompanied by abdominal cramping. Typically, these manifestations persist for 5 to 11 days before rapidly abating; rarely, purging may continue for up to 4 weeks. When this happens, mild malabsorption with weight loss may be seen. Its shorter duration, more prominent abdominal pain and relative lack of flatulence help to distinguish cryptosporidiosis from the clinically similar *Giardia lamblia* infection. A small percentage of patients describe nausea, anorexia, low-grade fever, or vomiting. Routine laboratory work is unremarkable. Radiographic and endoscopic examinations of the gut either are normal or demonstrate mild, nonspecific abnormalities. Recovery is complete, and neither relapse nor reinfection has been reported.

Immunocompromised hosts Cryptosporidiosis has been described in patients with a broad range of immunodeficiencies. In third world countries, marasmus and other forms of childhood malnutrition have been most common. In the United States, AIDS, congenital hypogammaglobulinemia, measles, cancer chemotherapy, and immunosuppressive management of organ transplantation patients have been the abnormalities noted most frequently. In patients with these conditions, cryptosporidiosis is usually indolent in onset and prolonged in duration. The abdominal cramping and systemic manifestations are similar to those seen in normal hosts. The diarrhea, however, is characteristically more severe; fluid losses of up to 17 liters a day have been described. Unless the patient's immunologic defect is reversed, the disease usually continues in a persistent or remittent fashion for the duration of life. In two-thirds of patients, the diarrhea has lasted for more than 4 months; in a few it has persisted unabated for a number of years. Weight loss is often prominent. Patients occasionally experience cough and organisms have been identified on the bronchial epithelium of a few patients with progressive pneumonia. The prognosis depends upon the nature of the underlying immunologic abnormality; the 6-month survival rate in patients with AIDS is 50 percent. Although other intercurrent infections are usually the direct cause of death, malnutrition and complications of parenteral nutrition are often thought to play a contributory role.

DIAGNOSIS The diagnosis of cryptosporidiosis must be pursued in any immunocompromised patient who develops diarrhea. Before 1978, the diagnosis required small-bowel biopsy. The development of effective concentration and staining techniques, as well as the growing laboratory experience with this parasite, have made the recovery and identification of cryptosporidia oocysts from the stool the procedure of choice. Oocyst excretion is most intense during the first 4 or 5 days of illness, tapers during the second week, and generally stops within 1 or 2 weeks of the cessation of diarrhea; oocysts are rarely recovered from solid stool. Specimens should be examined immediately after passage or preserved in 2.5% potassium dichromate or 10% buffered formalin. Fresh and dichromate-preserved specimens are infectious and must be handled with care. The specimen may contain small amounts of mucus, but fecal erythrocytes or white cells are uncommon. Initially, an iodine wet mount can be made from the unconcentrated specimen and examined microscopically; the spherical 5-μm oocysts are differentiated from yeasts, which they resemble in size and morphology, by their failure to take up the iodine. As cryptosporidia oocysts are one of the few acid-fast particles found in feces, a presumptive identification can be made with any one of the many acid-fast staining procedures developed for mycobacteria. If the direct examinations are negative, the stool should be concentrated using either Sheather's sugar flotation or Ritchie's formalin-diethylacetate sedimentation procedure. The two are equally sensitive; use of both will improve yield in specimens with few oocysts. Supernatant from the former is examined by light or phase microscopy for the typical pink-tinged, refractile oocysts. Sediment from the formalin-diethylacetate procedure is acid-fast–stained before examination. Definitive identification of oocysts visualized by the methods described above can be afforded with commercially available, indirect immunofluorescent procedures utilizing crytosporidium-specific antibodies.

Highly sensitive and specific indirect immunofluorescent and enzyme-linked immunosorbent (ELISA) assays have been developed. IgG seroconversion occurs within 60 days of acute infection in both immunocompetent patients and those with AIDS; antibodies persist for at least 1 year. IgM antibodies rise and fall more quickly, but do not uniformly develop in patients with AIDS. Seroprevalence studies in developing nations have demonstrated that two-thirds of the population have detectable levels of specific IgG, indicating past infection. Positivity rates rose with advancing age, reaching a plateau in late childhood. The usefulness of such tests for the diagnosis of acute infection remains undetermined.

TREATMENT AND PREVENTION In the immunocompetent patient, the disease is self-limited, and attempts at specific antiparasitic therapy are not warranted. Oral, and occasionally parenteral, rehydration may be required in small children. In the immunocompromised host, the severity and chronicity of the diarrhea warrants therapeutic intervention. The only uniformly successful approach has been the reversal of underlying immunologic abnormalities. Withdrawal of cancer chemotherapy agents, discontinuation of immunosuppressive drugs, and successful bone marrow transplantation have all resulted in cure. Specific anticryptosporidial therapy has been attempted with a large number of drugs; most have been ineffective. Some patients have experienced an amelioration or complete resolution of symptoms following treatment with spiramycin, alpha-difluoromethylornithine (DFMO), oral bovine transfer factor, or trimetrexate, a folate antagonist; however, clinical failures have been common, and parasitologic cures have been reported in few. In patients who responded clinically but continued to excrete oocysts, relapses have followed discontinuation of the therapeutic agent. Because spontaneous remissions can occur, the value of these drugs in the treatment of cryptosporidiosis remains uncertain.

The stools of patients with cryptosporidiosis are infectious. Stool precautions should be instituted at the time the diagnosis is first suspected; for the immunosuppressed patient this should be whenever diarrhea, regardless of presumed etiology, is first noted. This is particularly important in cancer chemotherapy and transplantation units, where spread of the disease, directly or indirectly, from a symptomatic patient to other immunosuppressed patients can have life-threatening consequences.

REFERENCES

CURRENT WL: The biology of *cryptosporidium*. ASM News 54:605, 1988

D'ANTONIO RG et al: A waterborne outbreak of cryptosporidiosis in normal hosts. Ann Intern Med 103:886, 1985

HAYES EB et al: Large community outbreak of cryptosporidiosis due to contamination of a filtered public water supply. N Engl J Med 320:1372, 1989

JANOFF EN, RELLER LB: *Cryptosporidium* species, a protein parasite. J Clin Microbiol 25:967, 1987

KOCH KL et al: Cryptosporidiosis in hospital personnel. Evidence for person-to-person transmission. Ann Intern Med 102:593, 1985

ROBERTS WG et al: Prevalence of cryptosporidiosis in patients undergoing endoscopy: Evidence for an asymptomatic carrier state. Am J Med 87:537, 1989

SOAVE R: Cryptosporidiosis and isosporiasis in patients with AIDS. Infect Dis Clin North Am 2:485, 1988

TZIPORI S: Cryptosporidiosis in perspective. Adv Parasitol 27:63, 1988

UNGER BLP et al: Seroepidemiology of *cryptosporidium* infection in two Latin American populations. J Infect Dis 157:551, 1988

167 TRICHOMONIASIS AND OTHER PROTOZOAN INFECTIONS

JAMES J. PLORDE

TRICHOMONIASIS

Trichomoniasis is a venereal infection caused by the protozoan *Trichomonas vaginalis*. Of the many members of the genus *Trichomonas*, three are parasites of human beings: *T. hominis* in the intestine, *T. tenax* in the oral cavity, and *T. vaginalis*, the only established pathogen, in the vagina, urethra, and prostate. All three exist only in the trophozoite stage and resemble one another morphologically. *Trichomonas vaginalis* is the largest, however, and confusion in diagnosis is rare because of the anatomic specificity of their habits. Strains varying in size, growth rates, virulence, and antigenic characteristics have been described.

Trichomonas vaginalis is transmitted by sexual intercourse. Although the organism is viable for up to 24 h in urine, semen, and water and may survive on moist washcloths for a few hours, transmission by fomites is probably uncommon. Approximately 5 percent of children born to infected mothers acquire the infection. The parasite is cosmopolitan in its distribution. It is estimated that 3 million women in the United States and 180 million worldwide are infected annually; 30 to 70 percent of their male sexual partners are parasitized, at least transiently. Prevalence correlates directly with the number of sexual contacts. The incidence in adult virgins is zero; rates as high as 70 percent have been seen in prostitutes, individuals with other venereal disease, and sexual partners of infected patients. Women with trichomoniasis are, on the average, a decade older than those with gonorrhea. Although the peak incidence is between 16 and 35 years, there is a relatively high prevalence among the 30- to 40- and 40- to 50-year-old age groups.

In the female, trichomoniasis usually presents as a persistent vaginitis. It is estimated that half of women with *Trichomonas* are asymptomatic when first diagnosed. A third, however, go on to develop clinical manifestations within 6 months. In approximately two-thirds a discharge is present and is frequently accompanied by vulvar itching (50 percent), dyspareunia (50 percent), odor (10 percent), and dysuria. This acute stage may persist for a week or months, often fluctuating in intensity; it may worsen following menstruation. Eventually the discharge and other symptoms subside and may actually disappear completely, even though the patient still harbors trichomonads. Examination shows inflammation ranging from mild hyperemia of the vaginal vault and endocervix to extensive erosion, petechial hemorrhages, and perianal intertrigo. The finding of a granular, friable, reddened endocervix (strawberry cervix) is a highly characteristic, although uncommon, finding. A discharge, typically thin, gray to yellow, and frothy in nature, is found pooled in the posterior vaginal fornix.

The prostate and urethra are the usual sites of infection in the male. Most commonly the infection is completely asymptomatic, but may present as persistent or recurring nonspecific urethritis. Approximately 5 to 15 percent of all episodes of nongonococcal urethritis in males is caused by *T. vaginalis*. The prevalence is higher among those failing tetracycline therapy. Acute purulent urethritis occurs rarely.

The diagnosis is made by examining vaginal, prostatic, or urethral secretions for the presence of *Trichomonas*. The organism may also be found in the sedimented urine. A wet mount reveals squamous epithelial cells, polymorphonuclear nucleocytes, and *T. vaginalis* with its characteristic twitching motility; although highly specific when positive, it is often negative in asymptomatic women and in patients who have douched in the previous 24 h. Stained smears provide little additional help. Culture is more sensitive but is not generally available. Sensitive and specific latex agglutination, immunofluorescent, and enzyme immunoassays for *T. vaginalis* antigen that may prove useful in routine diagnostic laboratories have been developed.

Trichomonas is sometimes responsible for confusing changes in the cytologic pattern of exfoliated vaginal cells. Moreover, ordinary Papanicolaou preparations are not well suited to the diagnosis, and when trichomoniasis is suspected, fresh material should be looked at immediately.

Oral metronidazole (Flagyl), given either in dosage of 250 mg three times daily for 7 days or in a single 2-g dose, is an extremely effective therapeutic agent. Concurrent treatment of sexual partners is very important, particularly when single-dose therapy is given, if recurrent infection is to be avoided. A small number of *T. vaginalis* strains with high levels of resistance to metronidazole have been isolated from patients failing multiple courses of therapy.

The evidence that metronidazole is carcinogenic in rodents and mutagenic in bacteria mandates that the drug should not be used in the first trimester of pregnancy until further information on its teratogenicity is available. Because of the agent's antabuse-like action, alcohol consumption is contraindicated during therapy and for 24 h following its completion. Topical therapy with clotrimazole, an imidazole antifungal agent, can be employed in situations where systemic metronidazole therapy is contraindicated. The drug is applied intravaginally, in a dose of 100 mg daily for 6 days.

ISOSPORIASIS

This is an infrequently recognized disease characterized by fever, diarrhea, abdominal pain, and weight loss which results from ingestion of the oocysts of coccidia belonging to the genus *Isospora*. These sporozoan protozoa are widespread in the animal kingdom. *Isospora belli* and *Sacrocystis* (formerly *Isospora*) *hominis* have been shown to infect humans. Parasitization is much more common in children and is worldwide in distribution, particularly in tropical areas. In this country, a disproportionately large percentage of reported cases have occurred in patients with acquired immunodeficiency syndrome (AIDS).

Like the related plasmodia, there is both an asexual and sexual stage of multiplication in *I. belli* infections. However, both occur within a single host. Following the ingestion of an oocyst, *sporozoites* are released which invade the epithelial cells of the intestine to become trophozoites. These multiply asexually producing a large number of *merozoites*, which in turn invade other epithelial cells to continue the cycle. In some cells sexual gametocytes are produced. With the fertilization of the female gametocyte, an oocyst is formed which is then passed in the stool. Transmission is by the fecal-oral route. Volunteers develop symptoms about 1 week after the ingestion of viable oocysts. The illness usually has an acute onset with fever, headache, abdominal cramps, and diarrhea. Stools are often fatty and weight loss is common. Isosporiasis may be associated with a malabsorption syndrome and abnormalities of the mucosa in the small bowel. Symptoms, which presumably continue as long as the asexual cycle of multiplication continues, usually subside spontaneously within a few weeks. In the immunocompromised host, however, they are often severe, and may persist for months or even years, eventually resulting in death. Dissemination to the mesenteric and tracheobronchial lymph nodes with associated granulomatous inflammation has been reported in a patient with AIDS and cytomegalovirus enteritis.

A peripheral eosinophilia occurs in approximately half of the infected patients. The diagnosis can be made by examination of stool for oocysts. These are often scanty, and concentration techniques such as zinc sulfate flotation or the formol-ether method must usually be employed. Incubation of the stool for 2 days at room temperature improves the recovery rate. Duodenal aspiration and jejunal biopsy are less cumbersome and more reliable. The oocysts stain well with the acid-fast techniques described for the closely related *Cryptospo-*

ridium species (see Chap. 166). *Isospora belli* infections have been successfully treated with combinations of pyrimethamine-sulfonamide and trimethoprim-sulfamethoxazole. The dose for the latter combination is 160/800 mg four times daily for 10 days, then three times daily for 3 weeks. In patients with AIDS or sulfonamide allergy, pyrimethamine alone, in the dose of 75 mg/d, can be used. Relapses in AIDS patients can be prevented by the daily administration of 25 mg.

Sarcocystis hominis oocysts are believed to be infectious only for pigs and cattle in which it produces tissue sarcocysts. Humans become infected by eating undercooked pork or beef containing the cysts. These liberate trophozoites which invade intestinal epithelial cells to undergo gametogony with the formation of new oocysts. The disease in humans is usually asymptomatic, but mild self-limited gastrointestinal manifestations have been described. Therapy is not required. The disease can be prevented by freezing raw beef and pork at −20°C (−4°F) for 24 h or cooking to an internal temperature of 65°C (150°F).

BALANTIDIASIS

Balantidium coli, the largest protozoan of human beings, inhabits the large intestine. In addition to producing an asymptomatic carrier state, it elicits disease ranging from mild recurrent diarrhea to fulminant ulceration with perforation and death. In many respects the disease is similar to amebiasis in its range of manifestations, exclusive of spread to the liver.

The illness has been reproduced by feeding the organism to volunteers. The diagnosis is made by finding the trophozoite or cyst in the stool, but repeated examinations may be required because shedding of *Balantidium* is intermittent. The disease is more likely to occur in tropical areas, particularly in Iran, New Guinea, and several Pacific islands. At least 60 cases have been reported in the United States. Swine and rats are frequent carriers of *B. coli* and may play an important role in the spread of the disease to humans. Outbreaks have been noted in mental institutions where coprophagy implicated direct person-to-person transmission.

The tetracyclines in ordinary doses are highly effective in treatment, as is iodoquinol (diiodohydroxyquinoline, INN) given in the dosage of 650 mg three times daily for 20 days. Metronidazole in the dosage used for amebiasis has also been effective (see Chap. 158).

DIENTAMEBIASIS

Dientamebiasis is an intestinal infection produced by a flagellated ameba, *Dientamoeba fragilis*. The genus and species names derive, respectively, from the binucleate nature of the trophozoite and the fragmented appearance of its nuclear chromatin. Like the related *Trichomonas* genus, the protozoan lacks a cyst stage. By virtue of its location in the large bowel, it has been thought to be spread from person to person by the fecal-oral route. However, the prevalence of the organism does not parallel that of other intestinal protozoa, its incidence in homosexual men does not correlate with the frequency of oral-anal sex, and the trophozoite is rapidly destroyed in both water and gastric juice. A mechanism of transmission compatible with these facts was suggested when *D. fragilis*–like structures were noted inside the eggs of pinworms. Several studies have demonstrated that coinfection with these two intestinal parasites is 9 to 20 times higher than that expected by random occurrence, reinforcing the possibility that the helminth eggs may serve as a vector for the protozoan trophozoite. *Dientamoeba fragilis* is a cosmopolitan parasite. Studies in this country report prevalence rates ranging from 1.4 to 18.6 percent. Rates are highest among children between 0 and 10 years of age, institutionalized individuals, communal groups, and missionaries serving in tropical areas. While *D. fragilis* was thought to be a harmless commensal of the colonic mucosal crypts, and probably is not capable of tissue invasion, it may act as a chronic irritant producing excess mucous secretion and hypermotility. Pathologic studies of surgically removed appendices shown to harbor *D. fragilis* demonstrated fibrosis that encroached upon the mucosal lymphoid tissue. Patients free of intestinal pathogens other than *D. fragilis* have reported a variety of clinical manifestations including diarrhea (58 percent) with blood or mucus (11 percent), abdominal pain (54 percent), and anal pruritus (11 percent).

The diagnosis is established by the identification of the parasite in stool. As the number of organisms varies greatly from day to day, at least three stool samples should be collected over a period of 3 to 6 days. Because the trophozoites are rapidly destroyed in the external environment, the stool should be examined immediately or preserved in polyvinyl alcohol. The use of permanent stains increases both the yield and identification accuracy of the examination. Tetracycline, iodoquinol, or metronidazole in the doses recommended for *Entamoeba histolytica* infections (see Chap. 158) have all been used. There are little data available on their relative efficacy.

BLASTOCYSTIS HOMINIS INFECTION

Previously considered a commensal yeast, it now appears that *Blastocystis hominis* is a protozoan that, at least on occasion, may act as an agent of human disease. Evidence of its protozoan nature includes the lack of a cell wall, the capacity for pseudopod formation and particulate matter ingestion, multiplication by binary fission or sporulation, and possession of a well-demarcated smooth and rough endoplasmic reticulum, membrane-bound central body, and protozoan-like mitochondria and Golgi apparatus. Physiologically the organism is a strict anaerobe that requires the presence of bacteria for growth; it grows best at a neutral pH and a temperature of 37°C (98.6°F). The organism is resistant to high concentrations of amphotericin B.

Surveys have generally found small numbers of this organism in 10 to 20 percent of human stools submitted for parasitologic studies; higher positivity rates and organism numbers have been reported in stools of AIDS patients and patients with other immunosuppressive diseases. Evidence of pathogenicity rests on the experimental induction of diarrhea in guinea pigs, its assocation with diarrhea in nonhuman primates, and a small number of reports describing human diarrheal disease, one fatal, for which no other cause could be established. Several studies attempting to evaluate the pathogenicity and clinical relevance of *B. hominis* have reported conflicting data on the rate of symptomatic enteritis in stool-positive patients, the frequency with which alternative explanations for diarrhea were available, the response of infected patients to therapy, and the correlation between resolution of symptoms and the disappearance of *B. hominis* from the stool. In the one study utilizing age- and sex-matched controls, the carriage of *B. hominis* was strongly associated with recent travel and the consumption of untreated water. Over 90 percent of patients without other enteric pathogens or apparent disease had gastrointestinal manifestations. Patients with high concentrations of *B. hominis* were significantly more likely to present with acute manifestations. Patients demonstrating a decrease in number, or a complete loss, of the parasite improved or became totally asymptomatic significantly more frequently than patients without a change in their parasite load. However, patients improved both parasitologically and clinically without therapy.

Routine stool examinations utilizing concentration and permanent staining procedures are adequate for the identification of *B. hominis*. Some authorities recommend treating symptomatic patients shown to have more than five organisms per oil immersion field if other causes of disease cannot be identified. Metronidazole and iodoquinol, used in the doses described for *E. histolytica* (see Chap. 158), appear to be suitable agents.

REFERENCES

Balantidiasis

GRAINGER CR: Endemic balantidiasis in the Seychelles. J R Soc Health 106:13, 1986
KNIGHT R: Giardiasis, isosporiasis and balantidiasis. Clin Gastroenterol 7:31, 1978
SCHMUTZHARD E, RAINER J: Acute balantidial dysentery associated with cholera: A case report. East Afr Med J 64:790, 1987

Blastocystis hominis infection

GARCIA LS et al: Clinical relevance of *Blastocystis hominis*. Lancet 1:1233, 1984
KAIN KC et al: Epidemiology and clinical features associated with *Blastocystis hominis* infection. Diagn Microbiol Infect Dis 8:235, 1987
MARKELL EK, UDKOW MP: *Blastocystis hominis:* Pathogen or fellow traveler. Am J Trop Med Hyg 35:1023, 1986
MILLER RA, MINSHEW BH: *Blastocystis hominis:* An organism in search of a disease. Rev Infect Dis 10:930, 1988

Dientamebiasis

SHEIN R, GELB A: Colitis due to *Dientamoeba fragilis*. Am J Gastroenterol 78:634, 1983
SPENCER MJ et al: *Dientamoeba fragilis*. Gastrointestinal protozoan infection in adults. Am J Gastroenterol 77:565, 1982
TURNER JA: Giardiasis and infections with *Dientamoeba fragilis*. Pediatr Clin North Am 32:865, 1985

Isosporiasis

COOK GC: Small-intestinal coccidiosis: An emergent clinical problem. J Infect Dis 16:213, 1988
DEHOVITZ JA et al: Clinical manifestations and therapy of *Isospora belli* infection in patients with the acquired immunodeficiency syndrome. N Engl J Med 315:87, 1986
RESTREPO C et al: Disseminated extraintestinal isosporiasis in a patient with acquired immune deficiency syndrome. Am J Pathol 87:536, 1987
WEISS LM et al: *Isospora belli* infection: Treatment with pyrimethamine. Ann Intern Med 109:474, 1988

Trichomoniasis

KRIEGER JN et al: Geographic variation among isolates of *Trichomonas vaginalis:* Demonstration of antigenic heterogeneity by using monoclonal antibodies and the indirect immunofluorescence technique. J Infect Dis 152:979, 1985
REIN MF, MÜLLER M: *Trichomonas vaginalis*, in *Sexually Transmitted Diseases*, 2d ed, KK Holmes et al (eds). New York, McGraw-Hill, 1990, pp 481–492
SEARS SD, O'HARE J: In vitro susceptibility of *Trichomonas vaginalis* to 50 antimicrobial agents. Antimicrob Agents Chemother 32:144, 1988
WLNER-HANSSEN P et al: Clinical manifestations of vaginal trichomoniasis. JAMA 261:571, 1989

168 TRICHINOSIS

JAMES J. PLORDE

DEFINITION Trichinosis is an intestinal and tissue infection of humans and other mammals caused by the nematode *Trichinella spiralis*. The disease is characterized by diarrhea during the development of the adults in the intestine and by myositis, fever, prostration, periorbital edema, eosinophilic leukocytosis, and, occasionally, evidence of myocarditis, pneumonitis, or encephalitis during the stage of larval migration in tissue.

ETIOLOGY Trichinosis in humans is contracted by ingestion of meat containing the encysted larvae of *T. spiralis*. The meat has almost always been domestic pork, but for the past several years about one-third of cases reported in this country have been attributed to feral meat, usually wild boar, bear, or walrus. This has been particularly frequent in the northern and western states. There are no intermediate hosts, and both the adult and larval stages develop in the same animal. Infection has been produced or observed in the bear, wild boar, wolf, coyote, fox, muskrat, horse, cow, dog, cat, rabbit, guinea pig, mouse, and marine mammals, in addition to the rat and the pig. Humans are particularly susceptible. Among pigs, infection is contracted following the feeding of uncooked scraps, less often by eating infected rats or the flesh of dead pigs. The incidence of infection in pigs has been reduced by laws requiring that garbage be cooked thoroughly before being fed. Rats also feed on uncooked pork scraps and, in addition, maintain a high incidence of infection by their cannibalism.

Soon after ingestion, the larvae are liberated from their cysts by gastric digestion and migrate into the intestinal mucosa, where maturation occurs. Following copulation the male dies, and within a week, the viviparous female is discharging larvae (100 by 6 μm), which enter the mucosal vascular channels and are distributed throughout the body. Larviposition continues for about 4 to 6 weeks, each female producing approximately 1500 offspring. The larvae enter skeletal muscle, coil, grow, and begin encysting within 3 weeks; calcification of cysts begins in 6 to 18 months. The life span of the encysted organism has been estimated at 5 to 10 years. The muscles of the diaphragm, tongue, and eye, and the deltoid, pectoral, gastrocnemius, and intercostal muscles are most often affected. Larvae carried to sites other than skeletal muscles do not encyst but disintegrate, often stimulating a granulomatous inflammatory reaction. The life cycle can be carried further only if a new host ingests the encysted larvae.

The description of a fatal case of trichinosis in an immunosuppressed patient emphasizes the importance of the immune response in limiting the intensity of infection. Apparently, it does so by acting directly on circulating larvae, inhibiting the reproduction of the female worms, and accelerating the expulsion of the adult parasites from the intestine. Eosinophils as well as B- and T-cell lymphocytes are involved in the response. The T cells appear to have a "helper" function in promoting the production of IgG and IgM antibodies which, in collaboration with eosinophils, induce fracture of the larval cuticle and disintegration of its internal structures. Once safely encysted in striated muscle, the larvae appear resistant to immunologic attack.

EPIDEMIOLOGY Trichinosis is particularly common in Europe and North America, but with the exception of Australia, India, and New Zealand, it is found worldwide. In the United States its prevalence as measured by finding cysts in human diaphragms at autopsy declined from 16.1 to 4.2 percent between 1930 and 1970. In the 1970 survey it was 1.8 percent in people under 45. The prevalence appears highest in the New England and mid-Atlantic states, Hawaii, and Alaska. It is estimated that 1.5 million Americans carry live trichinae in their musculature and that several thousand acquire new infections annually. The overwhelming majority of these infections are asymptomatic, and many of those that become clinically manifest are never correctly diagnosed. In 1986 only 51 cases were officially reported in the United States; over the last decade the case fatality rate has been 0.6 per 1000. Although pork products are not currently inspected for trichinosis, ready-to-eat products inspected by the U.S. Department of Agriculture are processed in a manner designed to destroy trichina larvae. Large outbreaks are usually caused by consumption of ready-to-eat pork sausage prepared in small commercial facilities or at home. The incidence appears highest among Americans of Italian, German, Polish, or Portuguese descent, presumably because of their inclination to make and eat pork sausage over the holiday season. Outbreaks have been reported among southeast Asian refugees living in the United States following the ingestion of undercooked pork obtained from private farms. Notable epidemics have also followed the ingestion of trichinae-infected wild pig in Hawaii and California and walrus in Alaska, the Canadian Arctic, and Greenland. Each year, a few cases are acquired from ground beef, attesting to the frequency with which this meat is adulterated with pork. Horsemeat has been implicated in several large outbreaks in France and Italy.

PATHOLOGY The adult female induces hyperemia, edema, and an eosinophilic inflammatory response in the submucosa of the small bowel. The most striking lesions are in the skeletal muscles, where there is a severe myositis with basophilic granular degeneration of the invaded muscle fiber. Adjacent fibers exhibit hyaline or hydropic degeneration, and the focus becomes infiltrated with neutrophilic and eosinophilic leukocytes, some lymphocytes, and mononuclear mac-

rophages. Hyperemia, edema, and hemorrhages are constant features. Larvae do not encyst in cardiac muscle, but an intense myocarditis with eosinophilic infiltrates and focal necrosis has been observed in fatal cases. In cases of central nervous system involvement, there may be granulomatous nodules and vasculitis involving small arterioles and capillaries of the brain meninges, and eye. Although larvae may be present, encystment is unusual.

CLINICAL MANIFESTATIONS The severity of the clinical manifestations relates to the host's immune status, prior infection, and to the number of larvae disseminated to the tissues. Patients with severe disease usually harbor 50 to 100 larvae per gram of muscle, while those with 10 or less are often asymptomatic. The first symptoms usually appear within 1 to 2 days after ingestion of the uncooked or undercooked meat containing encysted larvae. At that time diarrhea, abdominal pain, nausea, and sometimes prostration and fever develop. Although generally brief, the intestinal phase appears to be common, severe, and prolonged in infections produced by arctic strains of trichina (T. spiralis var. nativa). The next stage, that of muscular invasion, is attenuated in T. s. nativa infections. Typically the muscular stage begins about the end of the first week and may last as long as 6 weeks. During this period, patients have fever, periorbital edema, conjunctivitis, muscle pain and tenderness, and often severe weakness. There may be a maculopapular rash which lasts for several days and subungual, subconjunctival, and retinal hemorrhages. More serious manifestations accompany lung, heart, or central nervous system invasion. Lung involvement is manifested by hemoptysis and consolidation on chest x-rays. Central nervous system involvement may be evident as polyneuritis, poliomyelitis, myasthenia, meningitis, encephalitis, focal or diffuse pareses, delirium, psychosis, and coma. Despite the severity of central nervous system involvement in some patients, the cerebrospinal fluid remains normal.

Myocarditis is characterized by persistent tachycardia or development of congestive heart failure. There are marked electrocardiographic alterations, including ST-T wave changes and conduction abnormalities in 20 percent of patients. High levels of circulating eosinophils may produce damage to the ventricular endothelium with superimposed thrombosis. A causal relationship between trichinosis and polyarteritis nodosa has been reported, presumably related to the presence of circulating immune complexes.

LABORATORY FINDINGS The most constant finding, and one of significance early in the course of the disease, is the eosinophilic leukocytosis (over 500 eosinophilic leukocytes per microliter) which generally appears before the end of the second week. In cases of moderate severity, the proportion of eosinophilic leukocytes peaks between 15 and 90 percent in the third or fourth week of illness. In severe cases, particularly terminally, the eosinophilic leukocytosis may disappear entirely. In severe trichinosis there may be marked hypoalbuminemia, probably because of protein leakage from damaged capillaries. During the fourth, fifth, and sixth weeks of the disease, concomitant with a rise in antibody, diffuse hypergammaglobulinemia occurs. Elevated levels of circulating IgE have been reported. There may be moderate rises in serum glutamic oxaloacetic transaminase, lactic dehydrogenase, aldolase, and creatine phosphokinase; electromyography may show evidence of altered motor function. Typically the sedimentation rate is slow.

The skin test to larval antigen becomes positive early in the third week of infection and may remain so for up to 20 years. The usual positive response is a wheal of 5 mm or more appearing within 30 min. The commercially available skin test preparations are not reliable and should not be used.

There are a variety of serologic tests for trichinosis, including the countercurrent electrophoresis test, the complement fixation test, the indirect hemagglutination test, the indirect fluorescent antibody test, and the bentonite flocculation test, which is probably the most widely used. A commercially available latex agglutination test is as sensitive but is less specific. These serologic tests all become positive during the third week of the disease and may remain positive for a few years. The highly sensitive enzyme-linked immunosorbent test is increasingly being used to detect specific antibody in the first week of infection. Since each may occasionally be falsely negative, two or more tests should be used; false negative results may be more common in *T. s. nativa* infections. The serologic tests are most valuable if they are negative initially and then turn positive or if there is a change in titer.

Muscle biopsy when carried out during the third week of infection remains the most useful test for demonstration of larvae or cysts. The deltoid or gastrocnemius muscles are the most useful sites for biopsy. A 1-g portion of the excised muscle should be compressed between glass slides and examined under a low-power microscope for the presence of larvae. Calcified cysts or larvae represent an old infection. The remainder of the biopsy should be submitted for routine processing because myositis is a significant finding even in the absence of larvae or cysts.

DIFFERENTIAL DIAGNOSIS Trichinosis must be differentiated from diseases that are characterized by eosinophilia (such as Hodgkin's disease, eosinophilic leukemia, and periarteritis nodosa) and from entities that are characterized by myopathy, such as dermatomyositis. When the central nervous system is involved, the diagnosis may be very difficult.

TREATMENT Thiabendazole (tiabendazole), in dosage of 25 mg/kg bid for 5 to 7 days (maximum 3 g/d), has resulted in apparent improvement in a number of patients, with relief of muscle pain and tenderness and with lysis of fever. The results have not been uniform and the drug may not be larvicidal. Moreover, the use of this drug in trichinosis has been associated with nausea, vomiting, abdominal discomfort, dermatitis, and drug fever. Mebendazole, given in the dosage of 400 mg tid for 2 weeks, appears to kill both adult worms and their larval offspring. Its side effects are minimal, but this drug should not be used in children or pregnant women.

Patients with "allergic" manifestations of trichinosis, including angioedema and urticaria as well as myocardial or central nervous system involvement, should be treated with prednisone in dosage of 20 to 60 mg per day. Response to steroids usually has been prompt, particularly in central nervous system trichinosis. Because steroids appear to prolong larval production, they should be given in conjunction with anthelmintics. Other measures should be directed at relief of pain and maintenance of adequate caloric and fluid intake.

PROGNOSIS The prognosis in trichinosis has improved markedly, and even when the central nervous system is involved, the mortality rate has fallen to under 10 percent. The overall mortality rate is now less than 1 percent.

PREVENTION The responsibility for control rests with the consumer. Adequate cooking of pork involves heating all portions of the meat to 77°C (170°F). Internal heating in microwave ovens is often uneven, allowing survival of larvae in apparently well-cooked meat. Meat demonstrating visibly pink juice has not been cooked adequately. Freezing procedures to kill porcine larvae require a temperature of −15°C for 20 days or −32°C for 24 h. Larvae isolated from arctic animals are more resistant to freezing. Proper smoking and pickling will also destroy the larvae. Important in control is the cooking of garbage fed to hogs. The enzyme-linked immunosorbent procedure described above is sufficiently sensitive, specific, and simple to be used for the routine inspection of pigs brought to slaughter. However, such screening tests have not been made mandatory.

REFERENCES

BAILY TM, SCHANTZ PM: Trichinosis surveillance, United States, 1986. MMWR CDC Surveill Summ 37:1, 1988

CAMPBELL WC (ed): *Trichinella and Trichinosis*. New York, Plenum, 1983

FOURESTIE V et al: Randomized trial of albendazole versus tiabendazole plus flubendazole during an outbreak of human trichinellosis. Parasitol Res 75:36, 1988

FRAYHA RA: Trichinosis-related polyarteritis nodosa. Am J Med 71:307, 1981

KAZURA JW, AIKAWA M: Host defense mechanisms against *Trichinella spiralis* infection in the mouse: Eosinophil mediated destruction of newborn larvae *in vitro*. J Immunol 124:355, 1980

KOLATA G: Testing for trichinosis: A new serological test should make it quick and easy to detect trichinosis in meat—a feat of no small economic importance. Science 227:621, 1985

MACLEAN JD et al: Trichinosis in the Canadian Arctic. Report of five outbreaks and a new clinical syndrome. J Infect Dis 160:513, 1989

METZLER MH et al: Second-degree atrioventricular block in acute trichinosis. Am J Dis Child 124:598, 1972

STEHR-GREEN JK, SHANTZ PM: Trichinosis in Southeast Asian refugees in the United States. Am J Pub Health 76:1238, 1986

---

169 FILARIASIS

BRUCE M. GREENE

Human filarial parasites infect an estimated 200 million persons and cause a range of disease manifestations that are relatively characteristic for individual parasite species. These include lymphadenitis, lymphangitis, elephantiasis, and other obstructive manifestations in the case of lymphatic filariasis, and blindness and dermatitis in the case of onchocerciasis. *Loa loa* causes transient subcutaneous swelling.

Although not associated with a high mortality rate, chronic filarial infection causes enormous suffering in a widely distributed population, and the socioeconomic impact due to long-term debility is extraordinarily great.

Adult filarial worms are threadlike, live in the subcutaneous tissues and lymphatics (or the peritoneum), and reproduce sexually to produce microfilariae, the first larval stage. Microfilariae are ingested by hematophagous arthropods, in which they develop into infective, or third-stage, larvae. Infective larvae molt in the vertebrate host and mature into male or female adult worms.

LYMPHATIC FILARIASIS

The three filarial parasites of humans that are associated with lymphatic filariasis are *Wuchereria bancrofti*, *Brugia malayi*, and *Brugia timori*, the latter being far less important than the other two. The threadlike adult parasites reside in the afferent lymphatic channels or lymph nodes, where they reproduce sexually to yield vast numbers of microfilariae, some of which circulate in the bloodstream. The adult females of *W. bancrofti* and *B. malayi* are approximately 4 to 10 cm in length. Bancrofti females are larger than the males; they measure about 4 and 1.5 cm, respectively. The adult parasites are quite thin, the females being approximately 250 to 150 μm in width. Adult parasites of *Brugia timori* are considerably smaller. Microfilariae are approximately 200 to 300 μm in length, and in all three species are sheathed. Infection is transmitted from person to person by mosquitoes, which ingest microfilariae while taking a blood meal. Microfilariae work their way through the wall of the proventriculus and midgut and penetrate into the thoracic muscles. They undergo two molts and over a period of approximately 2 weeks develop into infective larvae which then migrate to the tip of the labella, through which they escape at the time the blood meal is being taken. The infective larvae migrate into the tissues, and subsequently to the peripheral lymphatics, where they reside and develop into adult worms. Within the lymphatics, the male and female filariae mate, and microfilariae are discharged into the blood after 6 to 12 months. The adult parasites can live for decades in the human host.

EPIDEMIOLOGY *Wuchereria bancrofti* is the most widely distributed filarial parasite of humans, with distribution through equatorial Africa, the Indian subcontinent, southeast Asia, the western Pacific, the eastern Mediterranean region, and parts of South and Central America, as well as the Caribbean. The total number of persons infected with *W. bancrofti* is estimated to be 80 million. *B. malayi* has a much more restricted distribution, primarily involving southeast Asia and the western Pacific, with an additional focus in the southwestern coastal region of India. The total number of persons infected with the latter has been estimated at 9 million. *W. bancrofti* shows a markedly exaggerated concentration of microfilariae in the blood late at night (nocturnal periodicity) and is transmitted by *Culex* and, in urban areas, by *Anopheles* and *Aëdes* mosquitoes. There is also a subperiodic form (with less exaggerated fluctuations in microfilarial blood density) that occurs mainly in the eastern Pacific. *B. malayi* also demonstrates nocturnal periodicity and is transmitted primarily by *Anopheles* and *Mansonia* mosquitoes. A less common subperiodic form associated with an animal reservoir is transmitted by *Mansonia* and *Coquillettidia*. *B. timori* is nocturnally periodic and transmitted by *Anopheles* in Indonesia. Animal reservoirs are not thought to play a major role in epidemiology of lymphatic filariasis, although in Indonesia and Malaysia nonhuman primates may constitute an important reservoir of zoonotic filariasis that does play a part in human disease.

PATHOLOGY The principal pathologic changes in lymphatic filariasis result from chronic inflammatory damage to the lymphatics. Adult worms live in the afferent lymphatics or sinuses of the lymph nodes, and over a period of time, the lymphatics become thickened and tortuous and the lymph valves become damaged and incompetent. Histologically, there is infiltration with plasma cells, eosinophils, and macrophages in and around the affected vessels. There is endothelial and connective tissue proliferation, and eventually total lymphatic obstruction may occur. The overlying skin shows lymphedema, and chronic stasis changes with hard or brawny edema. Death of adult worms may hasten lymphatic obstruction.

PATHOGENESIS The presence of filarial parasites in the lymphatics elicits an inflammatory response. It is believed that most of the pathologic consequences of lymphatic filariasis relate to the immune response directed against the parasite, and the host immune response appears to be the major determinant of disease. In the lymphatics many highly immunogenic adult worm and microfilarial antigens are liberated; they are believed to cause the granulomatous and proliferative process that precedes obstruction. Whether microfilarial, adult worm, or infective larval antigens are of most importance in eliciting lymphatic inflammation is unknown. Superimposed bacterial infection may accelerate lymphatic blockage.

CLINICAL MANIFESTATIONS The major clinical presentation of lymphatic filariasis includes filarial fevers and lymphatic obstruction. In addition, asymptomatic individuals may be found to be microfilaremic. Tropical pulmonary eosinophilia is an uncommon presentation of infection by these parasites.

Filarial fevers are usually low-grade, but occasionally are severe and accompanied by chills. Other symptoms may include general malaise, headache, and vague pain. If the lymphangitis is superficial, pain along the lymphatics may be the predominant symptom. These episodes may occur several times a year, lasting up to a week at a time. Lymphadenitis often accompanies lymphangitis. On examination, the lymphatics are tender, thickened, firm, and red; the overlying skin is tender.

There are major differences in the clinical presentations most commonly seen in *W. bancrofti* versus *Brugia* infection. In bancroftian filariasis, the acute episodes most commonly affect the male genitalia leading to funiculitis, epididymitis, or orchitis. In contrast, lymphadenitis and lymphangitis of the extremities are more common in brugian than in bancroftian filariasis. This difference relates to the predilection that brugian filariasis has for involving the superficial inguinal nodes, typically one at a time, often with some concurrent lymphedema of the extremity. Occasional involvement of the upper extremities and, much less commonly, the breast and other areas is seen with both forms of lymphatic filariasis.

Chronic lymphatic obstruction leads to brawny edema, with thickening and hyperkeratosis of the skin. The skin becomes friable, easily abraded, and is subject to superinfection with bacteria and skin-dwelling fungi. Elephantiasis of the lower extremities in bancroftian filariasis typically involves the entire leg, while in brugian filariasis, the leg above the knee typically has a normal

contour. Marked elephantiasis of the scrotum is a characteristic finding in bancroftian filariasis but tends not to occur in brugian filariasis.

Following the onset of patency, a number of individuals demonstrate asymptomatic microfilaremia. Such an individual may remain asymptomatic and spontaneously clear infection, or may develop the acute phase with recurrent lymphangitis and lymphadenitis described above.

Another category of illness associated with lymphatic filariasis is tropical eosinophilia, which is manifested primarily by respiratory symptoms including asthma, low-grade fever, and cough. This syndrome is found primarily in infected individuals from the Indian subcontinent. Marked eosinophilia, very high levels of serum IgE, and infiltrates on chest x-ray are characteristic. These individuals appear to be manifesting an abnormal immune response against the parasite, with trapping and destruction of microfilariae in the pulmonary capillaries. Pulmonary function testing demonstrates restrictive and sometimes obstructive defects.

DIAGNOSIS The diagnosis of lymphatic filariasis is made by finding microfilariae in the blood or, in the case of obstructive disease, by the clinical presentation. Usually microfilariae are not found in the latter setting. Other suggestive laboratory data include eosinophilia, particularly in association with acute symptoms and elevated titers of antifilarial antibodies. In addition to blood, microfilariae can occasionally be found in hydrocele fluid or urine. Chyluria is suggestive of bancroftian filariasis. The most efficient method for concentrating microfilariae in tissue fluids is by filtration through a 3- to 5-μm filter, through which blood cells pass freely but microfilariae are retained. Adult worms in the lymphatics are rarely found, except at autopsy.

In tropical eosinophilia, microfilariae are usually not found despite the presence of symptoms. High-titer antifilarial antibodies and the other clinical features mentioned above are usually present, and there is usually a response to diethylcarbamazine therapy (see below).

TREATMENT The treatment of choice for lymphatic filariasis is diethylcarbamazine citrate (DEC), 5 mg/kg daily in divided doses for 3 weeks. This treatment rapidly eliminates microfilariae from the blood and is partially effective against adult worms. However, side effects are quite common and may be severe. Systemic symptoms include malaise, myalgias, fever, chills, headache, dizziness, and arthralgias. Nausea and vomiting may occur. These side effects appear to be related to massive killing of microfilariae and are most prominent within the first 2 days following treatment. With heavy infection, a test dose of 25 to 50 mg DEC should be given. Because of the frequent adverse effects associated with DEC, other drugs are being actively investigated. Ivermectin, the drug of choice for onchocerciasis, also appears promising in treating lymphatic filariasis.

A course of treatment with DEC will eliminate microfilariae from the bloodstream, usually for several months. However, a single course of DEC usually does not eradicate adult worms, which may require long-term or repeated treatment. This may be indicated particularly in individuals who have left an endemic area and will not be subjected to continued reexposure.

Treatment of chronic lymphatic obstruction is difficult, but considerable improvement can be obtained in many individuals. Chronic therapy with 3 to 5 mg/kg per day of DEC is indicated to avoid further infection and to attempt to eradicate existing adult worms. In addition, surgical bypass shunts may be used to decompress the obstructed limb. Repeated bacterial infections should be avoided by meticulous skin care, and early treatment is essential. Surgical management of hydrocele frequently achieves marked success. The psychological trauma to the individual is frequently the overriding concern and should be dealt with positively.

Acutely inflamed lymph nodes may occasionally suppurate, but usually the ulceration heals spontaneously over approximately a week's time.

PREVENTION Avoidance of mosquito bites is usually not possible for residents of endemic areas, but visitors should make use of repellents and mosquito nets. Chronic administration of diethylcarb-amazine has been effective in preventing disease.

ONCHOCERCIASIS

Onchocerciasis (river blindness) is caused by the filarial nematode *Onchocerca volvulus*. An estimated 20 million persons, located largely in equatorial Africa and Latin America, are infected by *O. volvulus*. Onchocerciasis is one of the four leading causes of blindness worldwide; in addition, it causes great suffering and disfiguration from dermatitis.

ETIOLOGY AND EPIDEMIOLOGY Infection in humans begins with inoculation of infective larvae into the skin by the bite of the female blackfly (*Simulium* species). Infective larvae develop into adult worms over a period estimated to be several months; the adult worms then coil up into roughly spherical bundles, typically containing two to three females and one to two males. After a prepatent period of from 7 to 34 months following introduction of infective larvae, the gravid female releases microfilariae, which then migrate out of the nodule and throughout the tissues of the host, concentrating in the dermis. Transmission of infection to other individuals is initiated by the bite of a female fly, which, along with a blood meal, ingests microfilariae from the host skin, some of which develop into infective larvae over a period of 6 to 8 days. Infective larvae are about 600 μm in length. Adult *O. volvulus* females are about 40 to 60 cm in length, and adult males 3 to 6 cm. *O. volvulus* microfilariae are unsheathed and measure 210 to 320 μm in length.

Simulium damnosum and its subspecies represent the predominant vector in most of the endemic areas of Africa and in south Arabia. In Central America, *S. ochraceum* is the principal vector.

Simuliids (blackflies) oviposit into free-flowing rivers and streams, particularly in rapids. The gravid female deposits eggs on sticks, rocks, and trailing vegetation or other superficial debris. Eggs hatch into larvae in 2 days; these migrate downstream and develop into pupae in 8 to 10 days. Pupae remain fixed to some stucture in the stream of water, and the adult fly emerges from the pupal shell in 2 days. Adult females are hematophagous, requiring a blood meal for initiation of a gonotrophic cycle. Female blackflies generally restrict their flight to within a few kilometers of larval and pupal habitats (commonly termed breeding sites) and bite most intensely in the immediate vicinity. However, blackflies can be carried long distances, perhaps hundreds of kilometers, in association with monsoon winds. There are an estimated 20 million persons worldwide infected with *O. volvulus*, the vast majority in equatorial Africa in a belt that extends for more than 6000 km from the far western Atlantic coast to the Red Sea. In Guatemala and Mexico there are about 70,000 infected persons, located at altitudes of 500 to 1500 m on the Pacific slope of the Sierra Madre; in Venezuela there are about 20,000 infected persons. Smaller foci have been found in Colombia, Brazil, Ecuador, Yemen, and Saudi Arabia. The occurrence of onchocerciasis is determined by the relation of the population to *Simulium* breeding sites. The level of endemicity depends upon distance from larval and pupal habitats, the hyperendemic zones lying within a few kilometers.

PATHOGENESIS The pathogenesis of the manifestations in onchocerciasis is largely unknown. The only exception is punctate keratitis, which on biopsy has been shown to represent an inflammatory focus surrounding dead or dying microfilariae. However, these lesions are transitory and resolve completely, and any direct relation of microfilariae to other tissue lesions remains speculative. Nevertheless, because of their vast number and wide distribution throughout the body, as well as the clinical correlation between microfilaria counts and complications, microfilariae are thought to cause, directly or indirectly, most of the disease manifestations. It is believed that the host immune response, including a contribution of immediate hyper-sensitivity (e.g., eosinophil degranulation), immune-complex deposition, products of activated lymphoid cells, and perhaps autoanti-bodies and cytotoxic T cells, is largely responsible for the disease.

CLINICAL MANIFESTATIONS The major disease manifestations are dermatitis, onchocercomata, lymphadenitis, and visual impairment or blindness. The frequency of these features varies according to duration and intensity of exposure and geographical location.

Skin The most frequent manifestation of onchocercal dermatitis is pruritus. The pruritus can be unrelenting and incapacitating, even though microfilariae in the skin may be sparse. In addition, transitory localized areas of edema and erythema may occur in any part of the body. Over a period of years, most persons with significant infections will develop premature and exaggerated wrinkling of the skin, which has been associated with accelerated loss of elastic fibers. Atrophy of the epidermis with loss of elastic fibers can lead to loose, redundant skin. Hypo- or hyperpigmentation may also occur.

A localized eczematoid dermatitis with hyperkeratosis, scaling, and pigmentary changes occurs with variable severity. Such lesions are commonly seen in the lower extremities but in some cases are quite extensive. They can become superinfected, particularly with repeated trauma or excoriation.

Onchocercomata These subcutaneous nodules, which may be visible or palpable, contain the adult worms. In Africa, they are found particularly over the coccyx and sacrum, the trochanter of the femur, and the lateral and anterior iliac crests. Other common locations include various bony prominences. In American onchocerciasis, nodules tend to be distributed preferentially about the head, neck, and shoulders. Nodules vary in size from barely palpable, measuring a few millimeters, to several centimeters in diameter. They are firm, nontender, and have variable mobility.

Lymph nodes In Africans, mild to moderate lymphadenopathy is frequent, particularly in the inguinal and femoral areas. Enlarged inguinal or femoral nodes and surrounding fluid may become dependent ("hanging groin") and may predispose to inguinal and femoral hernias.

Ocular tissues Visual impairment is the major complication of onchocerciasis and is usually seen only in persons with moderate or heavy levels of infection. Lesions occur in all parts of the eye. Conjunctivitis with photophobia is a common early finding, particularly in young persons. In the cornea, punctate keratitis occurs as an acute inflammatory infiltrate surrounding dying microfilariae, manifest as "snowflake" opacities. These lesions occur most frequently in younger age groups and resolve without apparent sequelae. Sclerosing keratitis occurs in approximately 5 percent of persons infected with savannah strains and 1 percent of those with the forest strain. Sclerosing keratitis is the leading cause of onchocercal blindness in the savannah areas of Africa. Sclerosing keratitis begins at the limbus and progresses inward, leading to irreversible visual impairment. Anterior uveitis and iridocyclitis occur in roughly 5 percent of all infected persons in Africa. In Central American onchocerciasis complications of anterior uveal tract involvement (e.g., pupillary deformity) are particularly prominent relative to other causes of visual impairment. Secondary glaucoma may occur. Characteristic chorio-retinal lesions occur with atrophy of the retinal pigment epithelium and of the choriocapillaris and hyperpigmentation of the pigment epithelial layer. Chorioretinal lesions are more frequently a cause of blindness in the forest areas of Africa than is sclerosing keratitis. Constriction of the visual fields and frank optic atrophy may occur as part of the disease. Primary changes in the optic disk related to *O. volvulus* infection occur in about 2 percent of infected persons in Africa.

Systemic manifestations Some heavily infected individuals show wasting and generalized weakness, with loss of adipose tissue and muscle mass. In adults who become blind, there is a three- to fourfold increased mortality rate.

DIAGNOSIS Diagnosis of onchocerciasis is usually based on demonstration of microfilariae. A sclerocorneal punch is used to obtain an essentially blood-free skin biopsy which extends just below the epidermis to the tips of the dermal papillae. The biopsy tissue is weighed and incubated in tissue-culture medium or in saline in a flat-bottomed microtiter plate or on a glass slide. Emergent microfilariae are counted after 2 to 4 h or an overnight incubation. The skin-snip examination can provide both a definitive diagnosis and some quantification of the intensity of infection. One hundred or more microfilariae per milligram of skin indicates heavy infection and implies a significant risk of serious complications. Histopathologic examination of an excised nodule can yield the diagnosis, and a small percentage of individuals with negative skin biopsies will have palpable nodules which can be excised. Several serodiagnostic tests for onchocerciasis have been described, but their potential utility is unclear.

TREATMENT AND PREVENTION The major goals of therapy of infected individuals are to prevent irreversible ocular and skin lesions and to alleviate distressing symptoms, particularly pruritus.

Ivermectin, a semisynthetic macrocyclic lactone, has been extensively tested in human onchocerciasis over the past few years and is now considered the drug of choice. The advantages of this drug over DEC are: (1) it can be given in a single dose orally; (2) it causes little or no systemic and ocular reaction; and (3) it appears to suppress microfilariae in the skin and eye longer than does DEC, and therefore, can be given on a yearly basis.

Ivermectin (available from the Centers for Disease Control) is given orally on an empty stomach at least 2 h before the next meal in a single dose of 150 µg/kg. Following treatment, most persons have little or no reaction. Approximately 1 to 10 percent of persons will develop cutaneous edema and pruritus, with or without a maculopapular rash characteristic of the so-called Mazzotti reaction. Symptomatic hypotension develops in about one person in 10,000, and rarely may require intravenous fluids and additional supportive measures. Significant ocular reactions are rare.

Contraindications to ivermectin treatment include pregnancy; breast feeding within the first 3 months following delivery, central nervous system disorders including, in particular, meningitis or other illnesses that may increase penetration of ivermectin into the central nervous system; allergy to the drug; and age less than 5 years.

Diethylcarbamazine citrate (DEC) treatment results in rapid and massive killing of a majority of microfilariae over a period of a few days. In association with this microfilaricidal action, most individuals experience a number of adverse effects and, in some cases, serious complications. The early side effects (Mazzotti reaction) include pruritus, painful swelling of lymph nodes (particularly femoral, inguinal, and axillary nodes), fever, headache, rash, nausea and vomiting, and occasionally vertigo, arthralgias, and myalgias. Cardiovascular collapse has also been described. Frequent early ocular effects include conjunctivitis, punctate keratitis, limbitis, and anterior uveitis.

Because of the severity of the DEC reaction it is best to begin therapy with a test dose, e.g., 25 to 50 mg on the first day. If the test dose is tolerated, DEC is then continued for 2 weeks at 3 to 4 mg/kg per day in two daily doses. Moderate doses of corticosteroids, when started 24 to 48 h before therapy, significantly blunt the reaction. Because of the side effects and complications associated with DEC, it should be given only if ivermectin is contraindicated or unavailable and there is a clear need for treatment.

Suramin is a proven and potent macrofilaricidal agent, but it has major toxicity and must be given intravenously in repeated doses. Therefore, its use is restricted to the rare individual with moderate to heavy levels of infection who is leaving the endemic area and who cannot take repeated doses of ivermectin or DEC.

The potential of vector control as a means of containment of onchocerciasis is dependent on a number of local factors. These include the size, number, and accessibility of larval and pupal habitats; the proximity of other foci of onchocerciasis which may serve as a source of reinvading flies; the topography and vegetation; rainfall patterns; and the dynamics of transmission. Although vector control may be quite beneficial over a period of time in areas of high endemicity with breeding sites which are vulnerable to attack, a large proportion of endemic areas are not suited to this means of control based on current technology. It is possible to minimize *Simulium*

bites by avoiding fly-infested areas in the morning and evening and by wearing protective garments. However, it is unlikely that such measures will achieve significant success for the indigenous populations in the near future.

There is no drug that has been shown to prevent infection with *O. volvulus*.

LOAISIS

Loa loa adult worms live in the subcutaneous tissues and evoke a characteristic edematous reaction. The adult females are approximately 4 to 7 cm in length and the males 3 cm. Microfilariae (sheathed) appear in the blood in maximal concentrations around midday. The infection is transmitted by biting *Chrysops* species. The disease is endemic across central Africa and is particularly prevalent in coastal west Africa around Nigeria and Cameroon.

The major disease manifestation in transient subcutaneous swelling (Calabar swelling), which characteristically affects the distal extremities or the soft tissues surrounding the eyes. This phenomenon is associated with migration of adult worms through the tissues. The swelling can be painful, but typically resolves in 1 to 2 days. A spectacular occurrence is the migration of an adult worm across the scleral or conjunctival tissues. In nonresidents of endemic areas, fever, urticaria, and marked eosinophilia occur, while residents tend to have less exaggerated reactions.

Treatment is surgical removal of migrating adult worms if accessible, or high doses of diethylcarbamazine citrate (400 to 600 mg/d for 3 weeks). Repeat dosing with diethylcarbamazine may be necessary. Because of occasional severe reactions to diethylcarbamazine, a test dose (e.g., 25 mg) is suggested. Once-weekly diethylcarbamazine (300 mg) has been demonstrated to prevent infection.

MANSONELLA INFECTIONS

MANSONELLA PERSTANS This parasite is widely distributed in tropical Africa and coastal South America, and is transmitted by *Culicoides* mosquitoes. The adult worms live in serosal cavities, primarily the peritoneal or, less commonly, the pleural cavity, and measure 4 to 8 cm in length. Microfilariae are unsheathed, with a predilection for nocturnal appearance in the blood (i.e., they are subperiodic). The infection may be associated with eosinophilia, but is not believed to cause definite symptomatology in many infected humans. However, particularly in visitors to endemic areas who become infected, edema, inflammation in serosal cavities, and fever may occur. Treatment with high-dose diethylcarbamazine as recommended for loaiasis may lead to cure. Mebendazole (100 mg bid for 30 days) has also been reported to be effective.

MANSONELLA STREPTOCERCA This filarial infection occurs in west Africa. The microfilariae may be found in the skin or blood and are 200 µm in length and unsheathed. The adult worms live in the dermis and measure approximately 3 cm. This infection may cause hypopigmented macules which resemble those of leprosy but are not anesthetic. Furthermore, pruritus due to *M. streptocerca* may suggest onchocerciasis, and the smaller microfilariae of *M. streptocerca* must be distinguished from *O. volvulus* on skin snips (see above). Treatment with diethylcarbamazine citrate (6 mg/kg for 10 days) is usually effective against microfilariae and adult worms.

MANSONELLA OZZARDI This parasite occurs in South and Central America and the Caribbean. Adult worms appear to live in the peritoneal cavity. Microfilariae are unsheathed and nonperiodic. There are few symptoms, although the occurrence of upper extremity and shoulder arthralgias has been reported in association with this infection. No drug has been proven effective.

DIROFILARIA IMMITIS Humans become infected with *D. immitis* (dog heartworm) as accidental hosts; the dog is the natural reservoir. Mosquitoes infected with *D. immitis* larvae are quite common in many urban areas throughout the United States, although the highest-intensity transmission occurs in the southeastern United States. This parasite is also found in Africa, Asia (including Japan), Australia, the Pacific Islands, and primarily southern Europe. The adult worms do not develop fully in humans, and circulating microfilariae are extremely rare. In humans, the infection may lead to cough, fever, and chest pain, signaling pulmonary infarction. A frequent radiographic finding is a solitary nodule resembling a neoplasm on chest x-ray. The diagnosis is usually made histopathologically after thoracotomy, when degenerating nematodes are found. No further treatment is necessary.

REFERENCES

ANDERSON J et al: Studies on onchocerciasis in the United Cameroon Republic: II. Comparison of onchocerciasis in rain-forest and sudan-savanna. Trans R Soc Trop Med Hyg 68:209, 1974

BAIRD JK et al: Adult *Mansonella perstans* in the abdominal cavity in nine Africans. Am J Trop Med Hyg 37:578, 1987

Ciba Foundation Symposium No. 127: *Filariasis*. Singapore, Wiley, 1987

CLARKE VDV et al: Filariasis: *Dipetalonema perstans* infections in Rhodesia. Cen African J Med 17:1, 1971

GREENE BM et al: Comparison of ivermectin and diethylcarbamizine in the treatment of onchocerciasis. N Engl J Med 313:133, 1985

KOCHAR AS et al: Human pulmonary dirofilariasis. Report of three cases and brief review of the literature. Am J Clin Pathol 84:19, 1985

MARINKELLE CH, GERMAN E et al: Mansonelliasis in the Comisaria del Vaupes of Columbia. Trop Geogr Med 22:101, 1970

MEYERS WM et al: Human streptocerciasis. Am J Trop Med Hyg 21:528, 1972

NUTMAN TB et al: Diethylcarbamazine prophylaxis for human loaisis. Results of a double-blind study. N Engl J Med 319:752, 1988

WHITE AT et al: Controlled trial and dose-finding study of ivermectin for treatment of onchocerciasis. J Infect Dis 156:463, 1987

WHO Expert Committee on Onchocerciasis: *Third Report*, Technical Report Series 752. Geneva, World Health Organization, 1987

YOGESHWAR D, NEAFIE RC et al: Human pulmonary dirofilariasis. A case report and review of the literature. Am Rev Respir Dis 112:437, 1975

170 SCHISTOSOMIASIS

THEODORE E. NASH

Three major schistosome species, *Schistosoma mansoni, Schistosoma haematobium,* and *Schistosoma japonicum,* and a number of less prevalent species of the genus *Schistosoma* infect humans. Both *S. mansoni* and *S. japonicum* adults reside in the venules of the intestine, and the major disease manifestations of these parasites are hepatic. *S. mansoni* is found in parts of South America (Brazil, Venezuela, and Surinam), some Caribbean islands, Africa, and the Middle East while infections with *S. japonicum* occur in the Far East, mostly in China and the Philippines. *S. haematobium* adults are found mostly in the venules of the urinary tract and cause lesions primarily of the ureters and bladder. Infections with this species occur in Africa and the Middle East. Of lesser importance are *S. mekongi,* a newly recognized parasite related to *S. japonicum* which is found along the Mekong River in Indochina, and *S. intercalatum,* found in certain areas of central West Africa. Worldwide, as many as 200 million persons may be infected, and infection of entire communities is common. However, most infected persons experience few, if any, signs and symptoms, and only a small minority develop significant disease.

LIFE CYCLE   The schistosome species infecting humans all share the same basic life cycle but are unique in ways which account for some of the different clinical and pathologic findings. Important differences include the length of time before egg laying begins (prepatent period), location of the adult worms, number of eggs produced by each pair of worms, response by the host to the ova, and eventual fate of retained eggs. The morphology of the parasites and the types of intermediate host snail are also distinct. Humans become infected after contact with water containing the infective stage of the parasite, called a cercaria, which is a microscopic form of the schistosome possessing a forked tail used for swimming and a head which is the anlage of the worm. Cercariae penetrate the unbroken skin, with the help of secreted enzymes, and in the skin transform into schistosomules or developing schistosomes. After 2 to 3 days the schistosomules migrate to the lungs and then to the portal vein, probably by an intravascular route. In the portal vein the maturing male and female schistosomes pair and migrate to the venules of the mesentery, bladder, or ureters, depending on the species of schistosome, and begin to deposit eggs. The time spent in migration and maturation differs. *S. mansoni* and *S. japonicum* begin depositing eggs around 4 to 5 weeks after infection, while egg deposition begins after 2 to 3 months for *S. haematobium.* Adult worms are about 1 to 2 cm in length and migrate in the blood vessels without eliciting a local inflammatory reaction. Adult worms do not multiply in humans, and immunosuppressive therapy does not result in increased numbers of worms. Once released, eggs are either retained in the tissues at the site of deposition or swept back, mostly to the liver, by way of the venous portal system in the case of the intestinal schistosomes. Eggs are deposited mainly in the bladder and ureters by *S. haematobium.* A portion of the mature schistosome ova are extruded into the lumen of the intestines, bladder, or ureters and after contact with water, hatch, releasing a miracidium. This free-swimming ciliated stage seeks out the proper intermediate snail vector and burrows into the soft tissues of the snail. After 1 to 2 months, depending on the species, the miracidium develops into a primary and then secondary sporocyst which, after further development, begins releasing cercariae into the surrounding water. Thousands of cercariae can be released daily from each infected snail. Therefore one miracidium produces many cercariae, and this amplifies the number of infective parasites and the risk of infection. Cercariae are most infectious immediately after shedding and are not viable 48 h after release so storing water for 48 h before contact prevents exposure and infection. Unlike most other trematodes the sexes are separate in schistosomes, but this is only evident in the adult stage. Ova are laid only when males and females infect the same individual.

PATHOPHYSIOLOGY   A number of factors govern the disease manifestations. These include the duration and intensity of infection, location of egg deposition, host genetics, concurrent infections, and other still undefined factors.

In individuals from endemic areas initial infection goes unnoticed. There are a number of possible reasons for this, including age of initial exposure, manner of exposure, and transfer of antigens, antibodies, and anti-idiotypes from the mother. In visitors to endemic areas initial infection with schistosomes commonly results in an acute febrile illness (Katayama fever or acute schistosomiasis) which is most likely a manifestation of the immune response to the developing schistosomes and eggs. There is a vigorous hypersensitivity response which becomes modulated. These individuals have elevated levels of eosinophils and immune complexes and react markedly to schistosome antigens as measured by lymphocyte blastogenesis. Despite ongoing infection, symptoms subside, as do blastogenic responses to schistosome antigens but not to unrelated antigens such as purified protein derivative of tuberculin (PPD). The exudative acute granulomatous response to schistosome eggs is also modulated.

A major factor in determining the development of disease in humans is the worm burden of the host, which determines the number of eggs produced. The inflammatory and fibrotic response to these eggs is responsible for most of the morbidity and mortality associated with schistosomiasis. Factors which limit parasite survival will limit the development of disease. In human schistosome infections it has not been clearly established that protective immunity develops, but immunity exists in experimental animals. In the first few days after infection the schistosomule is relatively susceptible to immune attack. A number of systems employing antibody and/or eosinophils, neutrophils, macrophages, and complement have been used to kill schistosomules in vitro. However, as the schistosomules mature, they become refractory to these immune responses. In addition, schistosomes coat their tegument with host proteins and evade recognition by the host. A number of antibodies which block effective killing may also result in enhanced parasite survival. Schistosomule and adult antigens have been defined with the hope of developing vaccines; the administration of murine monoclonal antibodies to some of these antigens has reduced worm burdens in challenge infections by about 50 percent, and immunization with one antigen has produced similar levels of protection. Successful vaccination with anti-idiotypes has also been reported.

All schistosome eggs elicit a granulomatous response which is best understood in *S. mansoni* infections. The host becomes sensitized to the egg proteins by a T-cell-mediated mechanism which induces a larger granuloma. However, with continued infection the granuloma decreases in size due to the recruitment of suppressor T cells, while antibody has no effect on granuloma size. The regulation of granulomas due to *S. japonicum* eggs differs from that of granulomas from *S. mansoni* eggs. Immune modulation is mediated by serum factors, including anti-idiotype networks, at least in the chronic stage of infection. Both eggs and granulomas release factors which induce fibroblast proliferation in vitro. The early cellular response induced by granulomas is followed by fibrosis in vivo; however, liver fibrosis in humans probably involves more than simple fusion of fibrotic granulomas. After years of continued infection, some heavily infected individuals develop end-stage fibrotic lesions, mainly portal fibrosis (Symmers' fibrosis), sometimes resulting in esophageal varices and splenomegaly in *S. mansoni*, *S. japonicum*, and *S. mekongi* infections, and fibrosis of the ureters and bladder in *S. haematobium* infections. After the development of portal fibrosis, eggs are shunted to the lungs via portal-systemic collateral veins resulting in cor pulmonale in about 15 percent of patients with Symmers' fibrosis. Immune complexes shunted to the systemic circulation cause glomerulonephritis.

Host genetic factors have been found to influence the development of Symmers' fibrosis although there is no general agreement as to which are important. Schistosomes even of the same species are also genetically diverse, as shown by endonuclease restriction analysis, but the effect of this on disease in humans is unknown.

CLINICAL SYNDROMES (See Table 170-1) **Acute schistosomiasis** Acute schistosomiasis, or Katayama fever, occurs following initial exposure and infection with *S. mansoni* and *S. japonicum*. It rarely follows infection with *S. haematobium*. Acute schistosomiasis is seldom recognized in endemic populations and therefore is noted primarily in visitors to endemic areas. Immediately following exposure, patients frequently complain of intense transient itching. From 2 to 6 weeks or longer after exposure the patient may complain of a variety of symptoms including fever, chills, headache, hives or angioedema, weakness, weight loss, nonproductive cough, abdominal pain, and diarrhea. Sometimes symptoms abate but return with increased intensity about the time egg laying commences. These symptoms gradually diminish but may last as long as 2 to 3 months. Other newly infected individuals may be asymptomatic or have only minimal symptoms. In these individuals the diagnosis is established only after further evaluation prompted by suggestive laboratory test results or exposure history. More severe symptoms occur with heavier infections, but light infections may cause severe illness. Central nervous system lesions may occur during acute schistosome infection. The diagnosis of acute schistosomiasis is suggested by the clinical findings and the presence of eosinophilia, which is sometimes greater than 50 percent. Leukocytosis, increased immune complexes, and elevated IgM, IgG, and IgE immunoglobulins are found commonly. Although immune complexes have been suggested to play a role in the pathophysiology of acute schistosomiasis, glomerulonephritis and vasculitis are not present. The specific diagnosis can be established, even before the shedding of ova, by the detection of antibodies to adult schistosome gut antigens, or after egg excretion (5 to 6 weeks following exposure), by appropriate serologic testing and the finding

TABLE 170-1 Clinical manifestations of schistosomiasis from various *Schistosoma* species*

Manifestation	*S. mansoni*	*S. japonicum*	*S. haematobium*
Acute toxemic schistosomiasis	+	+	+
Chronic asymptomatic schistosomiasis	+	+	+
Hepatosplenic schistosomiasis	+	+	0
Cor pulmonale	+	+	±
Glomerulonephritis (clinically significant)	+	+	0†
Colonic polyposis	+	+	±
Ectopic lesions			
Brain	±	+	±
Spinal cord	+	±	+
Skin	+	+	+
Chronic cystitis and ureteritis	0	0	+
Mass lesions, bladder and ureters	0	0	+
Bladder cancer	0	0	+
Association with salmonella	+	+	+
Prolonged fever	+	+	+
Urinary carrier stage	?	?	+
Swimmer's itch‡	+	+	+

* + = recognized complications of infections by this species; ± = findings much less prominent in individuals infected by this species; 0 = complications not present in infections by this species.
† Except with associated salmonella infections.
‡ Usually from schistosomes that do not infect humans.

of eggs in the stool or rectal biopsy. Clinically, acute schistosomiasis is frequently misdiagnosed as typhoid fever but can be confused with any prolonged febrile illness. Although these patients seem to tolerate chemotherapy well, whether therapy shortens the course of disease or decreases symptoms is unclear. Glucocorticoids may be useful, but this has not been demonstrated in controlled studies.

Liver fibrosis The most important complication of intestinal schistosome infection is the development of periportal or Symmers' fibrosis and portal hypertension (hepatosplenic schistosomiasis). This pathognomonic finding occurs in *S. mansoni*, *S. japonicum*,·and *S. mekongi* infections but has been best studied in *S. mansoni* infections, where it normally develops after 10 to 15 years of prolonged exposure and infection. The liver may be enlarged but in many cases is small, firm, and nodular, and the left lobe is characteristically prominent. Macroscopically, finger-sized bands of fibrosis ("pipe-stem" fibrosis) encompass the large portal tracts. The portal venous tracts are replaced with fibrous tissue sometimes leading to presinusoidal blockage, portal hypertension, splenomegaly, and esophageal and gastric varices. The intrahepatic pressure is normal. Hepatic function is generally well preserved, and patients commonly present with hematemesis and/or signs and symptoms of splenomegaly. Ascites, hepatic coma, edema, spider angiomas, gynecomastia, and other signs of liver failure occur less frequently than in alcoholic and postnecrotic cirrhosis. Despite repeated episodes of hematemesis, patients may do reasonably well.

In the past, the diagnosis of periportal fibrosis required a wedge biopsy of the liver; needle biopsy specimens are frequently inadequate. Ultrasonograms of the liver show characteristic findings. The fibrotic bands appear as dense echogenic areas surrounding the portal vein and its tributaries. Studies comparing wedge biopsies of the liver to ultrasonographic examination showed that the latter technique had a specificity and sensitivity of 100 percent. Ultrasonography should replace invasive biopsies as the method of choice to diagnose hepatic schistosomiasis.

Ultrasonographic evaluation of *S. mansoni*–infected populations in the Sudan revealed a much higher prevalence of periportal fibrosis than could be determined by physical examination. As many as half of the group studied lacked palpable splenomegaly, and a majority did not give a history of hematemesis.

Patients with periportal fibrosis may not have schistosome eggs in the feces because of previous treatment and/or attrition of adult worms without subsequent reinfection. Since schistosome infections are practically universal in many populations, the mere presence of schistosome eggs in the feces does not establish the diagnosis of schistosomal periportal fibrosis; other liver diseases may be present. It is not clear whether there is any benefit from shunting procedures or splenectomy although these procedures are used commonly. The mortality of patients with portal fibrosis has not been well studied, but in one group was 8.2 percent after 3.6 years.

Glomerulonephritis and pulmonary hypertension These two complications occur almost exclusively in patients with periportal fibrosis and portal hypertension. Pulmonary hypertension appears to be due to obliteration of pulmonary arterioles by granulomatous inflammation induced by shunted and embolized schistosome eggs. This is most frequently recognized with *S. mansoni* and *S. japonicum* infections but also occurs with *S. haematobium*. The association of glomerulonephritis and schistosomiasis has been noted in humans and in experimentally infected animals. This complication is manifested clinically as proteinuria and/or renal failure. Schistosome-specific antibodies and antigens have been detected in the glomeruli of infected patients.

Other complications Focal dense deposits of eggs of *S. mansoni* in the large intestine (and less commonly of *S. haematobium* and probably of *S. japonicum*) incite an exudative granulomatous response resulting in the formation of inflammatory polyps. Histologically, these consist of masses of eggs, inflammatory cells, and fibrosis. The major clinical presentation is bloody diarrhea, sometimes associated with protein-losing enteropathy and anemia. This type of involvement of the bowel is recognized primarily in Egypt and the Sudan. Gastrointestinal symptoms are not increased in most chronically infected patients compared to control populations, although blood in the stool is found more frequently in some studies. Granulomatous masses involving the bowel wall may mimic carcinoma of the bowel. Central nervous system (CNS) involvement with *S. mansoni* and *S. haematobium* has a predilection for the spinal cord, while the brain is involved more commonly in *S. japonicum* infections.

Patients infected with the three major species of schistosomes and subsequently infected with salmonella may develop a prolonged intermittent febrile illness. In *S. haematobium* infections prolonged excretion of salmonella in the urine is common. Many times treatment of the salmonella infection alone is not effective, and specific antischistosomal chemotherapy is also required. Salmonella may be protected from host immune responses by residing in schistosome gut or by adhering to the surface of the schistosome.

SCHISTOSOMA MANSONI Epidemiology and manifestations *S. mansoni* is found in South America and certain islands of the Caribbean, Africa, and the Middle East. The prepatent period is about 4 to 5 weeks. The intermediate hosts are various species in the genus *Biomphalaria*.

Although infection is frequent and sometimes universal in endemic areas, the development of disease is relatively uncommon and depends on a number of factors which include the duration and intensity of infection. In endemic populations chronic infections are usual, many times lasting decades, and disease manifestations develop in a predictable manner. For the most part, the initial infection of persons living in endemic areas goes unnoticed. In endemic populations, throughout the first decade of life the intensity of infection as measured by the number of eggs excreted in the feces increases, and prevalence rates often approach 100 percent in highly endemic communities. Few if any symptoms are attributable to schistosomiasis during this time. The liver, particularly the left lobe, gradually enlarges and becomes firm. Between 10 and 15 years of age, some heavily infected persons develop splenomegaly which partly reflects the presence of portal fibrosis and portal hypertension. About the same time, the number of eggs in the feces decreases, and there is

evidence to suggest that immune factors as well as decreased water contact are responsible for this. During the next three decades, persons with portal fibrosis and hypertension may experience repeated bouts of hematemesis secondary to esophageal varices or symptoms secondary to a massively enlarged spleen. Not infrequently, because of prior chemotherapy, decreased exposure, or increased host immunity, patients with end-stage portal fibrosis no longer excrete eggs. Adult schistosomes can survive 20 years or more in the human host but usually live 5 to 8 years. The prognosis and the potential for reversing complications of infection after appropriate chemotherapy depend on the stage of disease. Some regression of periportal fibrosis occurs after chemotherapy as judged by ultrasound examination, but in most individuals with periportal fibrosis and clinical manifestations, regression does not occur. Glomerulonephritis and cor pulmonale secondary to schistosomiasis occur exclusively in patients with portal fibrosis. Central nervous system involvement can occur at any stage of the infection and is not related to the intensity of infection.

Diagnosis The diagnosis of *S. mansoni* is established by identification of ova in the feces or tissues. The ova are 114 to 175 μm in length and 45 to 68 μm in width and have a prominent lateral spine. In light infections with less than 50 eggs per gram of feces, ova may not be detected in the stool without the use of techniques which sample large quantities of stool. Even in light infections, ova can usually be detected in rectal biopsies and are best identified by squashing a small amount of tissue between two glass slides and searching for ova microscopically.

Many serologic tests have been employed in the diagnosis of schistosomiasis. These tests are not standardized and differ in sensitivity and specificity. Most current tests have greater than 90 percent sensitivity, and a positive serology is indicative of a present or past infection. An immunofluorescent antibody test employing sections of adult schistosomes to determine the presence of antibodies to schistosome gut antigens has been extremely useful in identifying recently infected persons or those with acute schistosomiasis.

Treatment In the past, chemotherapy was offered only to more heavily infected individuals who were more likely to develop disease. Although the risks of continued infection have not been clearly defined, with the availability of easily administered and safe drugs, most infected persons are likely to benefit from treatment. Patients with active infections have live eggs, which can be identified microscopically by experienced parasitologists or by the presence of flame cells, or by their ability to hatch after contact with water. Although a number of drugs are available for the treatment of schistosomiasis mansoni, praziquantel and oxamniquine are the drugs of choice (Table 170-2). Both drugs are equally safe and effective in schistosomiasis mansoni found in the Caribbean and South America. Because some strains of *S. mansoni* in Africa are relatively resistant to oxamniquine, praziquantel is the better drug. Both drugs can be used in patients with portal fibrosis. The side effects of praziquantel and oxamniquine are frequent but transient and mild. For praziquantel they include abdominal pain, lethargy, diarrhea, and fever and for oxamniquine, dizziness, tiredness, nausea and vomiting, neuropsychiatric manifestations, and rarely convulsions.

SCHISTOSOMA JAPONICUM Epidemiology and clinical manifestations *Schistosoma japonicum* is found in southeast Asia and is an important health concern in areas of China and the Philippines. The intermediate hosts are amphibious snails of the genus *Oncomelania*. Besides humans, numerous mammals such as cattle and water buffalo are naturally infected and serve as reservoirs of infection. The prepatent period is about 4 weeks.

The course of infection and clinical manifestations of *S. japonicum* are similar to those of *S. mansoni*, but the epidemiology and disease manifestations are less well studied. Experimental infections are more virulent, probably because each worm pair produces 10 times as many eggs as *S. mansoni*. The granulomas contain clusters of eggs and are larger and frequently show central necrosis. As in *S. mansoni* infections, periportal fibrosis is the major clinical manifestation. The other clinical syndromes described in *S. mansoni* also occur as

TABLE 170-2   Treatment of schistosomiasis

Species	Drug	Total dose* (mg per kilogram body weight)	Regimen
S. haematobium	Praziquantel	40	Single dose or two 20 mg/kg doses
	Metrifonate†	22.5–30	Single dose of 7.5 to 10 mg/kg body weight given every other week × 3
S. mansoni			
Americas and Caribbean	Oxamniquine	15	Single oral dose with food
	Praziquantel	40	Single or two 20 mg/kg doses 4 h apart with food
Africa and Middle East	Oxamniquine	60	15 mg/kg body weight twice a day for 2 days with food
	Praziquantel	40	Single dose or two 20 mg/kg doses 4 h apart with food
S. japonicum or S. mekongi	Praziquantel	60	20 mg/kg body weight every 4 h with food

* All recommended drugs are given orally.
† Available from the Parasitic Diseases Division, Centers for Infectious Diseases, Centers for Disease Control, Atlanta, GA 30333.

complications of this infection. However, there are some notable differences in disease manifestations, particularly CNS involvement. In acute schistosomiasis associated with *S. japonicum* infections, about 2 to 3 percent of patients experience CNS symptoms and signs that mimic acute encephalitis or a focal neurologic process. Computed tomography shows multiple enhancing lesions. In chronic infections, patients may present with focal lesions of the brain which mimic brain tumors. These lesions contain masses of eggs and granulomas. Uncontrolled studies suggest that treatment with antischistosomal drugs and glucocorticoids is effective.

Diagnosis The principles of diagnosis are similar to those of *S. mansoni* and require the demonstration of the typical ova in the tissues or feces of infected individuals. The eggs are oval in shape, 70 to 100 μm by 50 to 65 μm, and have a vestigial spine. Old, calcified, dead eggs are commonly retained in the tissues for long periods of time and do not indicate active infection.

Treatment Most infected persons should be treated. The only safe and effective therapy for *S. japonicum* infections is praziquantel (Table 170-2).

SCHISTOSOMA MEKONGI *Schistosoma mekongi* occurs in the Mekong River in Indochina (Laos, Cambodia, and Thailand). The intermediate host is an aquatic snail, *T. aperta*. The eggs are similar to *S. japonicum*'s but are slightly smaller and round, about 56 μm by 64 μm. Dogs and human beings are frequently naturally infected. The prepatent period is about 5 weeks. The disease manifestations appear to be similar to those of *S. japonicum* but are not fully documented. Praziquantel is effective therapy for this infection (Table 170-2).

SCHISTOSOMA HAEMATOBIUM Epidemiology and clinical manifestations *S. haematobium* infections occur in extensive areas of Africa and in the Middle East. The intermediate hosts are of the genus *Bulinus*. The prepatent period is 2 to 3 months. Natural infection is primarily limited to human beings.

As in *S. mansoni* infections, the prevalence and intensity of infection in endemic areas increases until 10 to 15 years of age. Thereafter, the intensity decreases markedly while the prevalence rate falls moderately. The signs and symptoms due to *S. haematobium*, owing to its predilection for the veins of the urinary tract, result from involvement of the ureters and bladder. In contrast to the asymptomatic period following initial infection with the intestinal schistosomes, dysuria and hematuria are frequently noted 2 to 3 months after infection. These findings may continue throughout the course of active infection. Initially, the eggs evoke an intense inflammatory and granulomatous response which may cause anatomic and/or functional obstruction, hydroureter and hydronephrosis, and masses in the bladder or ureters. Cystoscopic examination may reveal friable masses extending into the bladder, ulceration, petechiae, and granulomas. These early lesions are reversible after antischistosomal chemotherapy. Eggs shed into the urine are usually easily demonstrable. As the infection progresses, the inflammatory component lessens, possibly due to a modulating effect of the host's immune response, and fibrosis increases, most likely due to the accumulation of many old and some new lesions. Later most lesions consist of masses of dead and calcified eggs in fibrous tissue. When the concentration of calcified eggs in the tissues is large enough, radiographic opacification of the affected areas of the urinary tract becomes evident. Fibrotic lesions which cause hydroureter and hydronephrosis are not reversible by antischistosomal chemotherapy. Renal failure occurs in a surprisingly small proportion of infected individuals.

Portal fibrosis and clinically significant glomerulonephritis are not complications of this infection, but passage of eggs into the lungs may result in pulmonary hypertension. Prolonged excretion of salmonella in the urine and intermittent bacteremias are well documented. Urinary tract infections with other bacteria do not appear to be increased in frequency unless there is instrumentation of the urinary tract; however, they may be difficult to eradicate once established. Central nervous system infection most commonly involves the spinal cord, as in *S. mansoni* infections. Although eggs of *S. haematobium* are frequently detected in the feces in low numbers and are often found in rectal biopsies, intestinal polyposis is uncommon. In certain geographic areas squamous cell cancer of the bladder is felt to be associated with *S. haematobium* infection and is a significant cause of morbidity and mortality.

Diagnosis The diagnosis of *S. haematobium* is established by demonstrating the characteristic eggs in the tissues or urine. These are 112 to 170 μm by 40 to 70 μm, have a prominent terminal spine, and are easily seen in the urine. An increased number of eggs is excreted around midday, and microscopic examination of a centrifuged urine specimen collected at this time usually reveals ova. In light infections, examination of increased quantities of urine is sometimes required. Gross or microscopic hematuria is common in endemic populations, and its presence should always suggest the diagnosis in exposed individuals. Antibodies to *S. haematobium* can be detected using *S. mansoni* antigen preparations.

Treatment Infected persons should be treated. Dead and calcified eggs are common in tissue, are often seen in urine specimens, and should be differentiated from viable eggs. Although a number of drugs have been used to treat *S. haematobium*, praziquantel is the treatment of choice (Table 170-2). Metrifonate, a safe, orally administered agent, is also effective. Its major advantage is low cost, and the major disadvantage is that in order to cure infection it needs to be given in three doses 2 weeks apart.

SCHISTOSOMA INTERCALATUM *Schistosoma intercalatum* infection is limited to areas of West Africa. Eggs, 140 to 240 μm by 50 to 85 μm, are found in the stool and have a terminal spine. Few symptoms are attributable to this infection, and no cases of portal fibrosis have been reported. Praziquantel is effective treatment (Table 170-2).

SCHISTOSOME DERMATITIS (SWIMMER'S ITCH) When cercariae penetrate the skin, they may provoke a reaction known as schistosome dermatitis. Symptoms occur most commonly after penetration of nonhuman schistosomes of birds and mammals. In previously unexposed persons, the initial invasion causes transient itching and uncommonly urticaria followed by the development of macules within 24 h and papules after 24 h. Following repeated exposures, the signs and symptoms increase dramatically and occur earlier. Large pruritic, erythematous papules and, uncommonly, vesicles develop within 24 h. The lesions are most intense 2 to 3 days following exposure and subside after a few days. These lesions represent a delayed hypersensitivity reaction to the invading schistosome. Nonhuman schistosomes do not fully develop in humans, and the signs and symptoms are limited to the skin. A similar dermatitis also occurs after infection with human schistosomes.

Schistosome dermatitis occurs after exposure to fresh water in many areas of the world but is particularly common in the north central and western United States. A dermatitis following seawater exposure (clam digger's itch) has also been described.

Treatment is symptomatic. Since cercariae need some time to invade the skin (15 min or less), rapid removal of cercariae-containing droplets after water contact will decrease exposure. Limiting the numbers of the intermediate host snail in frequented areas can effectively control exposure.

CONTROL OF SCHISTOSOMIASIS Theoretically, schistosome infections can be controlled by a variety of methods, but their application has generally been only partially successful. Simple and effective health education measures such as the elimination of indiscriminate urination and defecation are difficult to implement in endemic areas. Elimination of the intermediate molluscan host can be accomplished with the use of molluscicides or by destroying the habitat of the snail. Both methods require dedication of resources and personnel often not readily available. Mass chemotherapy of populations has been tried, and repeated treatments will be needed depending on the degree of reinfection. Some advocate the treatment of those likely to develop serious disease (e.g., those heavily infected). The methods employed will depend on the nature of the endemic area and the resources available.

REFERENCES

CHEEVER AW, ANDRADE ZA: Pathological lesions associated with *Schistosoma mansoni* infection in man. Trans R Soc Trop Med Hyg 61:626, 1968

DAVIS A, WEGNER DHG: Multicenter trials of praziquantel in human schistosomiasis: Design and techniques. Bull WHO 57:767, 1979

FORSYTH DM: A longitudinal study of endemic urinary schistosomiasis in a small East African community. Bull WHO 40:771, 1969

HIAT RA et al: Factors in the pathogenesis of acute schistosomiasis mansoni. J Infect Dis 139:659, 1979

HOMEIDA M et al: Morbidity associated with *Schistosoma mansoni* infection as determined by ultrasound: A study in Gezira, Sudan. Am J Trop Med Hyg 39:196, 1988

————: Diagnosis of pathologically confirmed Symmers' periportal fibrosis by ultrasonography: A prospective blinded study. Am J Trop Med Hyg 39:86, 1988

JORDAN P, WEBBE G (eds): *Schistosomiasis, Epidemiology, Treatment and Control.* London, Heinemann Medical, 1982

LEHMAN JS et al: Urinary schistosomiasis in Egypt: Clinical, radiological, bacteriological, and parasitological correlations. Trans R Soc Trop Med Hyg 67:384, 1973

McCUTCHAN TF et al: Differentiation of schistosome by species, strain, and sex by using cloned DNA markers. Proc Natl Acad Sci USA 81:889, 1984

NASH TE et al: Schistosome infections in humans: Perspective and recent findings. Ann Intern Med 97:740, 1982

———— et al: Treatment of *Schistosoma mekongi* with praziquantel: A double-blinded study. Am J Trop Med Hyg 3:977, 1982

ROLLINSON O, SIMPSON AJG (eds): *The Biology of Schistosomes. From Genes to Latrines.* New York, Academic, 1987

NEMATODES, CESTODES, AND HERMAPHRODITIC TREMATODES

JAMES J. PLORDE / PAUL G. RAMSEY

INTESTINAL NEMATODE INFECTIONS

ENTEROBIASIS Definition Enterobiasis (pinworm, seatworm, or threadworm infection, oxyuriasis) is an intestinal infection of humans caused by *Enterobius vermicularis* and characterized by perianal pruritus. It has been estimated that the worm infects 200 million people, 30 to 40 million of them in the United States and Canada.

Etiology The female averages 10 mm in length, the male 3 mm. They live with their heads attached to the mucosa of the cecum, appendix, and adjacent parts of the bowel. On average, an infected individual harbors 50 worms, but in areas of intense transmission thousands may be present. The gravid female migrates through the anal canal at night, deposits her 10,000 eggs on the perianal skin, and dies. In female patients the worm may enter the vagina and occasionally gain access to the peritoneal cavity through the fallopian tubes. Each egg contains an embryo which, within a few hours, develops into an infective larva. After the egg has been ingested, the larva is released in the small intestine and migrates down the bowel lumen to the cecum. In less than 1 month from the time of ingestion, newly developed gravid females are again discharging eggs. They are planoconvex and measure approximately 20 by 50 μm. The shell is clear and doubly contoured.

Epidemiology Humans are usually infected by the direct transfer of eggs from the anus to the mouth by way of contaminated fingers. Retroinfection, which is seen primarily in adults, may occasionally take place when eggs hatch in the perianal area and the larvae migrate back into the bowel to mature. The eggs, which are relatively resistant to desiccation, also contaminate nightclothes and bed linen, where they remain viable and infective for 2 to 3 weeks. Airborne transmission is possible, and spread within family and children's groups occurs readily. Prevalence rates in North America have been estimated at 30 percent, but may be higher in institutionalized individuals. The disease may be sexually transmitted among homosexuals. Enterobiasis is found in all climates.

Clinical manifestations Many infections are asymptomatic. The most common complaint is pruritus ani, which is most troublesome at night, being related to the migration of the gravid female worms. Irritability, insomnia, enuresis, and other minor complaints are probably secondary to the pruritus. Scratching may lead to perianal eczema or pyogenic infection. Vaginal discharge has been reported, and rarely a chronic granulomatous salpingitis or endometritis results from the presence of ectopic adults. An association between enterobiasis and cystitis in young females has been reported. This may result from the transport of enteric bacteria into the bladder by the migrating worm. Other rare ectopic locations include the lung, liver, and peritoneum. The worms can penetrate the bowel wall only if its continuity has been compromised by some other disease.

Laboratory findings Examination for ova of material obtained from the perianal skin by means of a cellophane tape swab is the preferable method for the detection of enterobiasis. The tape is folded sticky-side out over the end of a tongue blade, pressed firmly against the perianal area, and then spread on a glass slide and examined under the lower power of a microscope. The swab should be taken at home by the patient on three to five consecutive mornings prior to bathing and brought to the laboratory for examination. The diagnosis is sometimes made by finding adult worms in the perianal area or in the feces following a laxative or an enema. There is a strong association between infection with *Dientamoeba fragilis* and pinworm; discovery of this parasite in the stool should stimulate a search for pinworm.

Treatment All infected individuals in a family or communal group should be treated simultaneously. The frequently recommended sanitary measures aside from daily bathing and hand washing before meals and after stools are of dubious benefit. It is relatively easy to eradicate the worms, but reinfection is frequent. Retreatment does not appear necessary unless symptoms recur.

Two highly satisfactory drugs are available. Pyrantel pamoate given in a single oral dose of 11 mg/kg (maximum 1.0 g) is probably the drug of choice. Alternatively, a single 100-mg oral dose of mebendazole can be used. This drug is not recommended for infants or pregnant women. Pyrvinium pamoate is equally effective but less convenient. It is given orally as a single dose of 5 mg/kg in tablet or liquid form. This compound turns the stool red and may stain bedclothes or undergarments. In heavily contaminated environments, treatment with the above drugs may be repeated after an interval of 2 weeks to eliminate any new infections.

Prevention Methods of preventing autoinfection and dissemination within a group involving children are extremely difficult to enforce. Personal environmental hygiene should be stressed, and anthelmintic and symptomatic treatment of pruritus ani should be instituted. To control infection within a group, simultaneous treatment of all cases is mandatory.

TRICHURIASIS Definition Trichuriasis (whipworm infection, trichocephaliasis) is an intestinal infection of humans caused by *Trichuris trichiura* and is characterized by invasion of the colonic mucosa by the adult trichuris. Five to eight hundred million persons are thought to be infected with this parasite including 2.4 million in the United States. It may be the most commonly encountered helminthic infection in Americans returning from subtropical and tropical areas, where prevalence rates up to 80 percent have been reported.

Etiology The adult whipworms are found in the large intestine with their anterior ends deeply embedded in the mucosa. They are 30 to 50 mm in length and possess a threadlike anterior two-thirds with a stouter posterior third, giving them a whiplike structure. The female produces about 5000 eggs each day. They are characteristically football-shaped (20 to 50 μm), brown, thick-walled, with translucent knoblike ends. The eggs, like those of *Ascaris*, must incubate at least 3 weeks in soil before they become infective. After ingestion, the eggs hatch in the small intestine and the larvae become embedded in the intestinal villi. After several days they migrate to the large intestine where they mature in about 3 months. The adult worms may live for 4 to 8 years.

Epidemiology Whipworm is a cosmopolitan parasite but is most commonly found in the tropics, where the level of sanitation is low and environmental conditions necessary for the incubation of the eggs are optimal. In the United States, it is found throughout the rural areas of the southeast. Its distribution is similar to that of *Ascaris* and hookworm, but the eggs are less resistant to sunlight and drying than those of *Ascaris*. Because of their general lack of sanitary habits, children and the mentally retarded have the highest incidence of infection.

Pathogenesis and clinical manifestations Petechiae (subepithelial hemorrhages and superficial mucosal infiltration of eosinophilic lymphocytes) and plasma cells are seen at worm attachment sites in the gut. It has been estimated that infected patients lose 0.005 mL blood per worm per day. Symptomatic infection generally requires the presence of large numbers of adult whipworms and may be correlated in part with the degree of mucosal involvement. Typically, worm burdens sufficient to produce clinical disease are limited to 10 to 15 percent of infected individuals, primarily children 2 to 10 years of age. Burdens of 200 trichuris can produce growth retardation and three to four unformed stools daily, occasionally with mucus and blood. Infections with more than 800 worms often result in anemia, finger clubbing, abdominal pain, and dysentery. In heavier infections, the distribution of worms throughout the colon and rectum may result in rectal prolapse while straining at stool. Some investigators also feel that *Trichuris* infections predispose to amebic dysentery and bacterial gastroenteritis.

Laboratory findings In symptomatic infection, large numbers of eggs are present in the feces, and there may be eosinophilic leukocytosis and anemia. In light infections, concentration techniques may be necessary to recover the eggs. Quantitation of egg output is helpful since only counts above 3000 eggs per gram of feces are likely to be associated with symptoms. Stools should be cultured for bacterial pathogens and examined for the presence of *Entamoeba histolytica*.

Treatment Mebendazole in the oral dose of 100 mg twice daily for 3 days is the drug of choice. Its cure rate is 60 to 70 percent, and it achieves a 90 percent reduction in egg burden. The dose may have to be repeated in patients with heavy infections. It is not recommended for children under the age of 2 or pregnant women.

Prognosis Whipworm infection, unless characterized by severe diarrhea, blood loss, and systemic reaction, usually responds well to treatment. Posttreatment growth rates of children with heavy worm burden accelerate dramatically, even in the absence of nutritional supplements.

Prevention Measures recommended for ascariasis apply also to trichuriasis.

ASCARIASIS Definition Ascariasis is an infection of humans caused by *Ascaris lumbricoides* and characterized by an early pulmonary phase related to larval migration and a later, prolonged intestinal phase. It is estimated that 25 percent of the world's population, including 4 million Americans, are infected with this nematode.

Etiology The adult ascarids are large (15 to 40 cm in length), cylindric worms with blunt ends; they maintain themselves in the lumen of the jejunum by virtue of their muscular activity. Despite a life span of only 6 to 18 months, the female releases millions of eggs, both fertile and infertile, into the fecal stream; the daily output is estimated to be 200,000 per worm. Fertilized eggs are elliptic (30 to 40 μm by 50 to 60 μm) with an irregular, dense outer shell and a regular, translucent inner shell. They require a period of soil incubation before they become infective. Under optimum conditions of warmth and moisture this occurs in 2 to 3 weeks. The eggs may then remain viable for up to 6 years in temperate climates and may survive freezing. When an infective egg is ingested, the larva is liberated in the small intestine. It migrates through the wall and is carried by the bloodstream or lymphatics to the lung. After about 10 days in the pulmonary capillaries and alveoli, the larvae pass in turn up the bronchioles, bronchi, trachea, and epiglottis, are swallowed, and return to the jejunum. There they develop into mature adult worms within 2 to 3 months of ingestion. *Ascaris suum*, a roundworm of pigs, may occasionally complete a similar life cycle in humans.

Epidemiology Infection follows the ingestion of the embryonated eggs contained in contaminated food, or, more commonly, the introduction of the eggs into the mouth by the hands after contact with contaminated soil. Geophagia may produce massive infections. In endemic areas, the infection is maintained primarily by small children who defecate indiscriminately in the area of the home. In dry, windy climates, eggs may become airborne, get into the mouth, and be swallowed. Since the eggs are relatively resistant to desiccation and wide variations in temperature, the disease occurs worldwide. In the developing areas of the world where the lack of sanitary facilities exposes populations to the greatest risk, the prevalence of infection may be as high as 80 to 90 percent. Children are almost universally infected in these areas, with peak infection rates achieved by age 5. In temperate areas, the infection occurs in family clusters.

Pathogenesis and clinical manifestations Because of the extensive migration of which both the larvae and adults are capable, the manifestations may be diverse. Bronchopneumonia characterized by fever, cough, dyspnea, wheeze, eosinophilic leukocytosis, and migratory pulmonary infiltrates may occur during the passage of the larvae through the lung. This is most commonly seen in communities where *Ascaris* transmission is seasonal. The severity of symptoms is apparently related to both intensity of infection and the degree of sensitization resulting from previous exposures. Significant arterial oxygen desaturation and, rarely, death may occur. Adult worms may produce no symptoms if the infection is light and may be detected accidentally when the adult worm is vomited or passed in the stool. Heavier infections may cause abdominal pain and malabsorption of fat, protein, carbohydrate, and vitamins. In marginally nourished children this may produce growth retardation. Occasionally a bolus of worms may result in volvulus, intussusception, or intestinal obstruction in the ileocecal area. Children are most likely to have these complications because of their anatomically smaller intestine and larger worm loads. Up to 2000 worms have been found in children, although the usual load is less than 20. In the United States, where worm loads are usually modest, the incidence of obstruction is 2 per 1000 infected children per year. It often follows a febrile illness, spicy meal, anesthesia, or drug therapy which stimulates the worms to increase motility. Rarely, an adult worm will migrate into the appendix, bile ducts, or pancreatic ducts, causing obstruction and inflammation of these organs. Biliary tract obstruction may be associated with bacterial cholangitis and liver abscess. Worms may also penetrate the intestinal wall, particularly at a site of surgical anastomosis, and patients should be dewormed prior to elective surgery. Migration of the worms into the oral pharynx and mouth may lead to acute respiratory distress.

Laboratory findings The diagnosis is usually made by finding the ova in the feces. The fertilized eggs are usually numerous, characteristic, and not easily confused with those of other helminths. The occasional unisexual infection may pose diagnostic problems. The male produces no eggs, and the unfertilized ova produced by a single female may be atypical and difficult to recognize. Occasionally the worms may be seen after a barium meal, either as negative images or after ingesting barium themselves. In biliary ascariasis an intravenous cholangiogram will often demonstrate dilatation of the common duct and/or the negative image of the parasite. Ascaris pneumonia may be diagnosed by finding larvae and eosinophils in the sputum or gastric aspirate. Eggs will usually not be found until after the larvae have matured in the intestine. Eosinophilic leukocytosis is usually noted during larval migration, but diminishes and often disappears during the chronic intestinal phase of infection.

Treatment Only symptomatic treatment can be used during the period of pulmonary involvement by the migrating larvae. For removal of the adult worms from the intestines, either pyrantel pamoate or mebendazole should be used. Pyrantel is given as a single oral dose of 11 mg/kg (maximum 1.0 g). Mebendazole is given as described for trichuriasis and is the preferred agent if both *Ascaris* and *Trichuris* are present. An older agent, piperazine citrate, is highly effective, less expensive, but slightly more toxic than the above two agents. It is given in a single dose (75 mg/kg, maximum 3.5 g) after breakfast on two successive days. The drug must be administered with caution to patients with renal insufficiency and epilepsy, because impaired elimination may produce neurotoxic signs. In intestinal obstruction, nasogastric suction should be initiated. After vomiting is controlled, piperazine should be given through the nasogastric tube every 12 to 24 h in dosage of 65 mg/kg (maximum 1.0 g) for six doses. Usually surgery is not required.

Prognosis The prognosis in intestinal infection is generally good. When acute or chronic obstruction of ducts or hollow viscera has occurred, the immediate prognosis is determined by the promptness of diagnosis and treatment. The case fatality rate of intestinal obstruction in the United States is 3 percent. However, world-wide an estimated 20,000 people die of ascariasis annually.

Prevention Ascariasis is primarily a household infection of rural areas. All infections should be treated, personal hygiene stressed, and adequate toilet facilities provided. Mass therapy administered at 6-month intervals may be effective in controlling ascariasis in small communities.

TOXOCARIASIS (VISCERAL LARVA MIGRANS) Definition

This is a human infection with the dog ascarid, *Toxocara canis*. *Bayliascaris procyonis*, an ascarid of raccoons, occasionally produces particularly severe human infection. These animal parasites are usually unable to complete their life cycle in humans, but may disseminate widely in the body, producing a variety of clinical manifestations, collectively referred to as *visceral larva migrans*.

Etiology and epidemiology The large adult toxocaral worms live in the intestine of dogs. Their eggs must be passed in the stool and incubate in soil for 2 to 3 weeks before they become infective. When ingested by a mammal, larvae are liberated in the intestine, penetrate the wall, and are carried in the blood to the liver, where most remain, and to the lung. If the host is a young puppy, the larvae burst into the alveoli and complete their life cycle in a manner analogous to *A. lumbricoides* in humans. In humans and fully grown dogs, *Toxocara* larvae, which are approximately one-half the size of those of *A. lumbricoides,* pass through the pulmonary capillaries to reach the systemic circulation. Larvae leave the circulatory system when their gradually increasing size approaches the diameter of the vessel through which they are traveling. They migrate extensively in the surrounding tissue; some may become dormant for years, only to resume migration at a later time. *Toxocara* infections of dogs are common and widespread. Transplacental and transmammary migration of larvae account for infection rates of 80 percent or more in young puppies; they can shed a large number of ova within 4 weeks of birth. Viable ova were found in 25 percent of soil samples taken from public parks in the United States and Great Britain. Although most of the 2000 documented human infections have occurred in the United States and Europe, cases have been reported from 48 countries around the world. Children from the age of 2 to 5 years, because of their sanitary habits, predilection to geophagia, and intimate association with domestic pets, are most frequently involved. The seroprevalence of childhood *Toxocara* infection in the United States varies from 3 to 25 percent; the rates are highest in the south and northeast.

Pathogenesis and clinical manifestations The larvae migrate freely in tissues, causing hemorrhage, necrosis, eosinophilic inflammatory reaction, and eventually granuloma formation. The most frequently involved organs are the liver, lungs, brain, eye, heart, and skeletal muscles. Symptoms and signs are related to the number and location of the granulomas as well as sensitization to the parasite antigen. Commonly, only asymptomatic eosinophilia marks the presence of infection. Symptomatic patients most frequently present with fever and tender hepatomegaly. Splenomegaly, skin rash, and recurrent pneumonitis with wheezing respirations may occur in more severe infections. Respiratory failure with death has been reported. Most fatalities, however, result from involvement of the myocardium or central nervous system; the latter may result in convulsions, behavior disorders, or focal neurological defects. There is often a history of dirt eating and contact with puppies. Leukocytosis with eosinophilia to high levels (over 60 percent) and hypergammaglobulinemia with raised levels of IgG, IgM, and IgE are common. These manifestations may persist for months or years. At surgery or autopsy the liver may be studded with small granulomas. An exudative or granulomatous endophthalmitis, which may be mistaken for retinoblastoma, is observed in older children and adults. Typically, this is unilateral and occurs in the absence of other clinical manifestations of visceral larva migrans. Decreased visual acuity, strabismus, or eye pain brings the patient to medical attention.

Diagnosis The diagnosis can usually be made on the basis of clinical findings. Infections with *A. lumbricoides*, hookworm, and *Strongyloides stercoralis*, as well as other nonhuman nematodes, may also on occasion present as visceral larva migrans, making the etiologic diagnosis difficult. Eosinophilic leukemia, trichinosis, trematode infections, and periarteritis nodosa must be ruled out. The adaptation of larval antigens to the enzyme-linked immunosorbent assay (ELISA) has provided a serologic test of diagnostic value. In one study, the sensitivity and specificity were 78 and 92 percent, respectively. A definitive diagnosis depends on the identification of the larvae in sputum or tissue granuloma. Biopsy of the liver with serial sections of the specimen may reveal eosinophilic granulomas or a *Toxocara* larva.

Treatment No uniformly effective therapy is available. Diethylcarbamazine as used in Bancroftian filariasis (see Chap. 169) is probably the drug of choice. Thiabendazole (tiabendazole) in dosage of 25 to 50 mg/kg for 7 to 10 days may be helpful. Glucocorticoids may be beneficial when respiratory difficulty is pronounced. Ocular larvae close to the macula may be destroyed with laser photocoagulation. Control measures are directed toward preventing ingestion of eggs. Removal and repeated worming of infected dogs must be considered. Animals less than 6 months of age should be wormed monthly; older ones every 2 or 3 months. Keeping raccoons as pets should be discouraged.

ANISAKIASIS Ascarids belonging to the family Anisakidae infect seals, dolphins, porpoises, whales, and other large sea mammals. Their larval stages are found in the flesh of squid and several marine fish including mackerel, herring, and salmon. The ascarids of the *Pseudoterranova* genus, however, are more commonly seen in bottom fish such as cod, halibut, and "Pacific red snapper." Humans are infected by eating raw, pickled, or slightly salted fish delicacies such as "green herring," sushi, sashimi, sunomono, ceviche, and gravlax, which contain the third-stage larvae. *Pseudoterranova* infections are usually confined to the stomach; they may be asymptomatic and noted only when the worm is coughed or vomited up. More characteristically, the larvae burrow into the mucosa of the stomach. Here they produce eosinophilic granulomatous tumors with edema, thickening, and induration which may be mistaken for gastric carcinoma or regional enteritis. The pathologic changes are thought to be the result of a hypersensitivity reaction. The patient develops recurrent waves of severe epigastric pain, nausea, and vomiting within a few hours of ingesting infected fish. Some patients note urticaria and tingling in the throat. Gastroscopically, 2- to 4-cm larvae can be seen penetrating the mucosa and can sometimes be removed. *Anisakis* larvae most frequently involve the intestine. Patients develop sudden abdominal pain 1 to 5 days after fish ingestion. The clinical picture may be severe enough to simulate an acute surgical abdomen. More commonly, colicky pain, diffuse abdominal tenderness, fever, and leukocytosis are seen. Occasionally, larvae may penetrate the intestinal wall to involve other abdominal organs. Perforations of the bowel with peritonitis have also been described. Peripheral eosinophilia is not always present, and a definitive diagnosis can be made only by the identification of larvae in tissue. Serologic tests are neither highly reliable nor generally available. The disease usually subsides spontaneously with conservative therapy. Occasionally, a chronic illness develops which requires surgical resection of the lesion.

Over 1000 cases have been recognized in the Netherlands and Japan; approximately 30 have been reported from North America, primarily following the ingestion of salmon or red snapper. The disease can be prevented by storing marine fish at −20°C for a single day or by cooking it at normal cooking temperatures.

HOOKWORM DISEASE Definition Hookworm disease is a symptomatic infection caused by *Necator americanus, Ancylostoma duodenale*, or, less commonly, *A. ceylanicum*. Asymptomatic infection may be termed simply *hookworm infection*, and the individual with such infection is called a *carrier*.

Etiology *Ancylostoma duodenale*, also known as the "old world" hookworm, possesses four prominent hooklike teeth in its adult stage. The adults are about 1 cm long and inhabit the upper part of the human small intestine, where they attach to the mucosa by means of their mouth parts and suck blood. Each adult extracts approximately 0.20 mL blood daily. The adults migrate within the small intestine, and each site of attachment persists temporarily as a bleeding point. Following fertilization, the female liberates approximately 20,000 eggs per day. They measure about 40 by 60 μm and are usually in the two- to four-cell stage when discharged in the feces.

Necator americanus, the "new world" hookworm, has a buccal capsule containing dorsal and ventral plates rather than teeth. It is slightly smaller, deposits fewer eggs, and causes much less blood loss than *A. duodenale*. *Ancylostoma ceylanicum*, a hookworm of cats found in the Far East, may occasionally reach maturity in humans.

The life cycles of the hookworms are similar. Under appropriate conditions, the eggs hatch in 24 to 48 h, releasing free-living or rhabditiform larvae. Within a few days, these develop into infective or filariform larvae which may remain viable in the soil for several weeks. These, in turn, penetrate the skin to enter vessels which carry them to the lungs. The larvae leave the alveolar capillaries, enter the alveoli, ascend the respiratory tree, enter the pharynx, and are swallowed. They reach the intestine about 1 week after penetration of the skin and mature within 5 weeks. Larval development of *Ancylostoma* may be arrested or retarded in the human host. This may result in a prolonged latent period between the onset of infection and the appearance of gravid females in the intestine. Adults have been known to survive in the human intestine for as long as 14 years, but *A. duodenale* seldom persists beyond 6 to 8 years, and most *N. americanus* infections are eliminated within 2 to 4 years.

Epidemiology It has been estimated that hookworms infect 900 million people and cause the loss of 9 million liters of blood daily throughout the world from 45°N to 30°S latitude. *Necator americanus* is found predominantly in the tropical areas of Africa, Asia, and the Americas, while *A. duodenale* occurs in the Mediterranean Basin, the Middle East, northern India, China, and Japan. In many areas both species are found. In general, *Ancylostoma* presents a greater public health hazard than *N. americanus*, the species which is most prevalent in the southern United States, because it is more persistent in the environment, more harmful to the host, and less amenable to treatment. Conditions conducive to the development of the hookworm egg into infective filariform larvae are a mean temperature between 23 and 33°C, abundant rainfall, shade, and well-drained sandy soil. Hookworm infection occurs where there is opportunity for direct contact of the skin with soil contaminated by promiscuous defecation. *A. duodenale* disease may also be acquired by oral ingestion of infective larvae. Transmammary and transplacental transmission may also occur with this species; presumably this results from the activation of larvae whose development within the tissues of the host has been arrested or retarded. Because of greater exposure, males show a higher incidence of infection than females. Infections are particularly common in closed, heavily populated communities such as coffee or tea plantations.

Repeated infections of hookworm in dogs result in immunity and elimination of the parasite. It seems probable that a similar phenomenon occurs in human infections. When the possibility of reinfection is eliminated, the majority of worms is eliminated spontaneously within 1 or 2 years.

Pathogenesis and clinical manifestations During the invasion of the exposed skin by the larvae, there may be an erythematous maculopapular skin rash and edema with severe pruritus. These manifestations, which may persist for several days, are more marked in *N. americanus* infection. The lesions are most common about the feet, particularly between the toes, and have been termed "ground itch."

During migration through the lungs, cough, pneumonia, and, in severe infections, fever may occur. Usually, however, pulmonary involvement does not give rise to clinical symptoms.

Various gastrointestinal symptoms, ranging from vague epigastric distress and pica to typical ulcer pain, have been reported in association with hookworm infection. Roentgenographic studies may reveal nonspecific changes such as excessive peristalsis and "puddling," particularly in the proximal jejunum. However, gross and microscopic examination of the bowel itself reveals conspicuously little damage.

The major clinical manifestations of hookworm disease clearly are those of iron-deficiency anemia and hypoalbuminemia consequent to chronic intestinal blood loss. Whether anemia develops and how severe it becomes depends on the balance between iron lost in the gut and iron absorbed from the diet. The severity of the disease and the prognosis depend on the age of the patient, the magnitude of the worm burden, and the duration of the disease. Young children often have extreme anemia, with cardiac insufficiency and anasarca. These conditions may precipitate kwashiorkor. Those who survive to puberty show retarded physical, mental, and sexual development. Milder degrees of the disease, as seen in older children and adults, are characterized by lassitude, dyspnea, palpitation, tachycardia, constipation, and pallor of the skin and mucous membranes.

Asymptomatic infections outnumber symptomatic infections, considering all age groups, 20 to 40 times in endemic areas. The worm burden is small in asymptomatic infections, and the carrier state may be indicative of some degree of acquired host resistance.

Laboratory findings In symptomatic infection, hookworm eggs are usually numerous enough to be detected by microscopic examination of a direct or concentrated fecal smear. A quantitative egg count, using the cellophane thick smear (Kato) technique, allows an estimation of the intensity of infection. If a stool specimen is allowed to stand for several hours before examination, the eggs may hatch, releasing larvae which are easily confused with those of *Strongyloides*. The species of hookworm may be determined by the identification of the adult worm passed in the stool following treatment or by culturing the feces and identifying the third-stage larvae. This is seldom important in clinical practice. Abdominal and pulmonary symptoms appear before the eggs are discharged, although a presumptive diagnosis may be made on the basis of the clinical history and the eosinophilic leukocytosis.

Generally, the leukocyte count is normal. However, in some early cases, leukocytosis may be marked, with an eosinophilia as high as 70 or 80 percent. The anemia is characteristically hypochromic and microcytic.

Treatment In areas where reinfection is likely, administration of anthelmintics to patients with light infections (less than 2000 eggs per milliliter of feces) is probably not beneficial. A number of satisfactory anthelmintic agents are available, but two, pyrantel pamoate (see "Ascariasis" above) and mebendazole (see "Trichuriasis" above) are currently favored. Treatment can be repeated in a week if complete cure is desired and has not been accomplished. This is seldom necessary in endemic areas, where the aim of therapy is reduction of the worm load to an asymptomatic level.

The anemia requires iron replacement. When anemia is severe and there is malnutrition with anasarca, blood transfusions and a high-protein diet should be given before drug treatment is begun. Blood should be given in an amount sufficient to raise the hemoglobin level to 100 g/L (10 g/dL). In advanced cases it may be necessary to delay drug treatment for 2 to 3 weeks.

Prognosis The immediate prognosis is good. When opportunity for reinfection persists and nutrition cannot be maintained, a state of chronic debility develops. Maturation of children is impaired, and intercurrent disease is a serious problem in adults.

Prevention Many of the measures required are obvious but difficult to apply on a large scale. Even if facilities for proper disposal of feces are provided, it is no simple matter to sustain their use. Soil pollution must be eliminated. Avoidance of direct skin contact with the soil (by wearing shoes) is often not practical in endemic areas. Periodic mass treatment of the population has been used in some hookworm control programs. Dietary iron supplementation can prevent the development of anemia.

CUTANEOUS LARVA MIGRANS (CREEPING ERUPTION)

Definition Creeping eruption is an infection of human skin caused by the larvae of the dog and cat hookworm, *A. brasiliense*. The other dog hookworms, *A. caninum* and *Uncinaria stenocephala,* as well as the human parasites, *Strongyloides stercoralis* and *Necator americanus,* may also produce the disease. The larvae of *Gnathostoma spinigerum,* a nematode found in the Orient, and *Gasterophilus,* the horse botfly, may produce a similar cutaneous infection.

Etiology *Ancylostoma brasiliense* reaches adulthood regularly only in the dog and cat. The larvae emerging from eggs discharged in the feces develop to the filariform stage and then are capable of penetrating the skin. In humans, the larvae usually remain in the epidermis and migrate, producing an irregular erythematous tunnel visible on the skin surface.

Epidemiology and distribution Transmission to humans requires environmental temperature and humidity appropriate for development of the egg to the infective filariform larva stage. Beaches and other moist, sandy areas are hazardous, because animals choose such areas for defecation, and the *A. brasiliense* eggs develop well in such soil. In the United States infection is found in the southern Atlantic and Gulf states.

Pathogenesis and clinical manifestations The site of penetration of the skin by the larvae becomes apparent in a few hours. The migration of the larvae in the skin is accompanied by severe itching. Scratching may lead to bacterial infection. In the course of 1 week, the initial red papule develops into an irregular, erythematous, linear lesion which may attain a length of 15 to 20 cm. The larvae may persist for weeks to months without treatment.

Loeffler's syndrome has been observed in 26 of 52 cases of creeping eruption. Transient, migratory pulmonary infiltrations associated with an increased number of eosinophils in the blood and sputum were interpreted as an allergic reaction to the helminthic infection but may have reflected pulmonary migration of the larvae.

Laboratory findings Eosinophils occur in the lesion, but eosinophilic leukocytosis is slight, except when Loeffler's syndrome appears. The percentage of eosinophils in the blood may then rise to 50 percent and in the sputum to 90 percent. Only rarely are larvae found on skin biopsy.

Treatment Thiabendazole is the drug of choice; it should be given orally in the dosage suggested for strongyloidiasis (see below). It may be repeated if necessary. Alternatively, it may be applied topically as a 10% aqueous suspension. Topical administration avoids systemic toxicity. Superficial bacterial infections are improved by the application of wet dressings and elevation of the extremity. For intense itching, oral antihistaminics may be helpful.

Prognosis Untreated infections last several months. Treatment, which is usually sought because of severe pruritus, is usually successful.

Prevention Dogs and cats should be prevented from contaminating recreation areas and children's sandboxes.

TRICHOSTRONGYLIASIS Trichostrongyliasis is an intestinal infection of herbivorous animals, and incidentally humans, throughout the world. The disease is most common in Asia, the Middle East, and South America. In view of the high frequency of animal infections in the United States, the low incidence of human infections here is difficult to understand. The ova resemble those of the hookworm but are larger, have more pointed ends, and, when observed in a fresh fecal specimen, show a more advanced stage of segmentation (16- to 32-cell stage). Infection is acquired by ingestion of green leafy plants contaminated with third-stage larvae. On reaching the small intestine, they attach themselves to the mucosa and develop into adult worms within 4 weeks. The adult at that time sucks blood and maintains residence in the intestine for long periods. Most infections are asymptomatic, but massive infections may result in epigastric distress and anemia. The parasite owes its importance primarily to the resemblance of its ova to those of the hookworms. Moreover, because the trichostrongylidae do not respond to some of the anthelmintics effective in hookworm infection, it may be assumed incorrectly that refractory hookworm infection is present. The diagnosis depends on the finding of the ova in the feces. Since they are few, they are usually found only when a concentration method is used. In symptomatic infections, there may be leukocytosis with marked eosinophilia (80 percent). Thiabendazole 25 mg/kg twice daily for 2 or 3 days, or pyrantel pamoate as used in hookworm infections, is effective in symptomatic infections. Both are considered investigational drugs for this condition by the U.S. Food and Drug Administration.

STRONGYLOIDIASIS **Definition** Strongyloidiasis is an intestinal infection of humans caused by *Strongyloides stercoralis* or, on occasion, the primate species, *S. fuelleborni*. Extraintestinal involvement may occur in severe cases.

Etiology The tiny (2 mm in length) adult female resides and lays her eggs in the mucosa of the upper part of the jejunum. In heavy infections, the biliary and pancreatic ducts, the entire small bowel, and the colon may be parasitized. The eggs quickly hatch, releasing rhabditiform larvae which enter the lumen of the bowel and are passed in the feces. On reaching the soil, the larvae develop into the infective filariform stage. There, as in the case of the filariform larvae of hookworm, they penetrate the skin and small blood vessels of humans. They are then carried to the lungs where they leave the alveolar capillaries, ascend the respiratory tree, enter the pharynx, and are swallowed. On reaching the small intestine, they mature and burrow into the jejunal mucosa. Parasitic males have not been observed and it is likely that females reproduce parthenogenetically. Oviposition (up to 40 eggs per day) begins 17 to 28 days after the initial infection. In addition to the *direct* host-soil-host cycle, *Strongyloides* has two alternative cycles. In the first, or *indirect*, cycle, the rhabditiform larvae, after passing from the host, develop into free-living male and female adults which reside and reproduce in the soil, thus creating a reservoir of infection independent of the human host. Under certain environmental conditions, the free-living larvae are capable of transforming back into filariform larvae which initiate a new cycle in humans. In the second, or *autoinfection,* cycle, the rhabditiform larvae develop into filariform larvae before they are passed in the stool. They may then invade the intestinal mucosa or perianal skin of the same host without first going through a soil phase. This may explain the long persistence (20 to 30 years) of strongyloidiasis in patients who have left endemic areas and may also account for the extremely heavy worm loads in some individuals. Autoinfection appears to occur frequently in patients with achlorhydria, delayed intestinal transit time, and blind loops or diverticula. Contamination of the perianal area, clothing, or bedding with feces permits development of filariform larvae outside of the body and invasion of the perianal skin of the host or transmission to others by direct physical contact. The transformation of the filariform larvae outside the body is probably responsible for the frequency with which strongyloidiasis is seen in crowded, unsanitary institutions for the mentally retarded.

Epidemiology The usual mode of infection is the penetration of the skin by larvae. Some infections may result from ingestion of contaminated food and drink, and some are transmitted by contact. Transmission between sexual partners, however, appears to be uncommon. Transmammary passage in humans has been demonstrated for *S. fuelleborni*. The majority of the 80 million infected individuals reside in the tropics, where the warmth, moisture, and lack of sanitation favor its spread. Sporadic cases appear among Puerto Ricans and throughout the rural south of the continental United States. Homosexual men may be at increased risk. Chronic strongyloidiasis has been reported in Vietnam veterans.

Pathogenesis and clinical manifestations The initial cutaneous penetration of the filariform larvae usually produces no symptoms. However, *larva currens,* transitory skin eruptions characterized by blotchy erythema, serpiginous lesions, and urticaria, may be seen during episodes of autoinfection. These may recur at irregular intervals and are particularly common following recovery from an acute febrile illness. In these situations the lesions are generally found over the lower back and buttocks. Cough, dyspnea, gross hemoptysis, and bronchospasm may accompany migration through the lungs. Chest x-rays may show pulmonary infiltration at this time. The intestinal infestation is usually asymptomatic or productive only of vague abdominal complaints. In heavier infections, epigastric pain and tenderness, nausea, flatulence, vomiting, and diarrhea alternating with constipation may be observed. Peptic ulcer may be simulated, but food often aggravates the pain. The mucosal inflammation may be severe enough to produce subacute obstruction, segmental ileus,

and impaired absorption. Chronic, relapsing intestinal and pulmonary manifestations have been noted in a few patients. A severe form of ulcerative colitis, accompanied by intestinal perforation and peritonitis, has also been encountered. In debilitated, immunodepressed, steroid-treated, alcoholic, and hemodialyzed patients, massive autoinfection with widespread dissemination of larvae to the extraintestinal organs including the central nervous system may occur. This hyperinfection is usually abrupt in onset with fever and severe abdominal pain; it is often associated with shock, pulmonary manifestations, severe enterocolitis, persistent gram-negative bacteremia, and occasionally gram-negative meningitis. Unrecognized, it usually leads to death. Disseminated strongyloidiasis should be considered in any compromised host with unexplained gram-negative bacteremia, abdominal complaints, and pulmonary infiltrates with or without eosinophilia.

Laboratory findings The definitive diagnosis can be made by identification of the larvae in the stool. Fresh fecal specimens should be examined to avoid confusion with hookworm infection; generally, fresh specimens contain *larvae* in strongyloidiasis infections, while in hookworm infection they contain *eggs*. Since the number of larvae in the stool is small and varies from day to day, several samples should be checked, using concentration and culture techniques. Microscopic examination of the duodenal aspirates and jejunal biopsies may also establish the diagnosis. Alternatively, a weighted string can be passed into the duodenum, allowed to remain for a short time, and then withdrawn. The bile-stained section of the string is stripped of fluid which is then examined for the presence of larvae. If pulmonary involvement is present, the sputum should be examined for larvae. An ELISA utilizing *S. stercoralis* larval antigens was shown to be positive in approximately 80 to 90 percent of patients and may have some diagnostic utility.

Eosinophilic leukocytosis is common, except in very severe cases. When eosinophilia occurs in association with peptic ulcer symptoms, strongyloidiasis should be suspected.

Treatment All infected patients should be treated to prevent the occurrence of severe invasive disease. The drug of choice is thiabendazole, which should be given orally in dosage of 25 mg/kg twice a day for 2 or 3 days. In disseminated strongyloidiasis, treatment should be continued for 7 days or more. Lightheadedness, nausea, and vomiting are common accompaniments of therapy with this agent. Delayed aminophylline excretion may result in toxicity. Hypersensitivity reactions may occur but usually respond to treatment with antihistamines. The stools should be rechecked at intervals of 3 months because the parasite is not easily eradicated and retreatment may be necessary.

Prognosis In the usual case, the prognosis is good. Since the occurrence of hyperinfection is unpredictable, every effort should be made to eradicate the infection in each case. In severe cases with hyperinfection, the prognosis is poor.

Prevention In general, the measures are those for the control of hookworm infection. In addition, it is well to remember that infection may be contracted by ingestion of contaminated food (especially uncooked vegetables) or of contaminated drinking water and by contact. Patients who have a history of residence in an endemic area or eosinophilia should be carefully checked for the presence of the parasite prior to the initiation of steroid or immunosuppressive therapy. Because the larvae may not appear in the stool for several weeks after the initiation of such therapy, repeated examinations of stool and upper intestinal aspirates are indicated. Since sputum, vomitus, stool, and body fluids of patients with disseminated disease may contain infective filariform larvae, gloves and gowns should be worn by hospital personnel caring for such patients.

INTESTINAL CAPILLARIASIS **Definition** Intestinal capillariasis is an infection of humans caused by the roundworm *Capillaria philippinensis* that is characterized by intractable diarrhea with a high mortality rate.

Etiology Adult *C. philippinensis* are small, measuring 2 to 4 mm in length. The peanut-shaped eggs have flattened bipolar plugs and an average size of 42 by 20 μm. The adults inhabit the mucosa of the small intestine, especially the jejunum. Adults, larval forms, and eggs are found in the stool.

Epidemiology The infection has been found almost exclusively in persons residing along the north and west coastal areas of Luzon, Philippines. Several cases from Thailand have also been reported. Since 1966 the disease has occurred in epidemic form, and more than 2000 cases and 100 deaths have been reported.

The mode of transmission and life cycle of the parasite are incompletely understood. The adult worm is thought to parasitize the gut of birds. Eggs passed in their excrement presumably embryonate in fresh water before being ingested by an intermediate fish or crustacean host. When humans ingest an infected intermediate host in the raw state, the first-stage larvae are released and develop to adulthood within their intestinal lumina. These rapidly produce new larvae which mature to a second generation of adults. Most of the females from this generation are oviparous, the resulting eggs passing in the stool. Some, however, remain larviparous, leading to another generation of intestinal adults.

Pathogenesis and manifestations Adult worms in large numbers invade the small-intestinal mucosa and cause a severe protein-losing enteropathy and malabsorption. Hypokalemia, hypocalcemia, and hypoproteinemia are the rule. Autopsy studies have failed to show extraintestinal spread of the parasite. Initial symptoms of intestinal "gurgling" (borborygmi) and recurrent vague abdominal pain are followed, usually within 2 to 3 weeks, by a voluminous watery diarrhea. Other findings, consistent with the basic pathophysiologic process, are anorexia, vomiting, weight loss, muscle wasting and weakness, hyporeflexia, and edema. Abdominal tenderness and distention may occur. The period between onset of symptoms and death is usually 2 to 3 months. Subclinical infection has not been noted.

Diagnosis The diagnosis is made by finding ova in the stool. The ova of *C. philippinensis* must be differentiated from those of *T. trichiura*, which are similar. Care must be taken that capillaria are not overlooked in patients with *Trichuris* infections because in the endemic area most patients with capillariasis have coexistent *Trichuris* infection.

Treatment Administration of mebendazole combined with fluid and electrolyte replacement leads to dramatic improvement; 400 mg per day in divided dosage should be given for 20 days to prevent relapse. Alternatively, thiabendazole, 25 mg/kg per day for 30 days, can be given.

TISSUE NEMATODE INFECTIONS

ANGIOSTRONGYLIASIS CANTONENSIS Definition *Angiostrongylus cantonensis,* the rat lungworm, is the etiologic agent of the common form of *eosinophilic meningitis* found in southeast Asia and the tropical areas of the Pacific.

Etiology The delicate filariform adults (20 mm in length) reside and lay their eggs in the pulmonary arterioles of rats and certain other rodents. After hatching, the larvae break into the alveoli, migrate up the respiratory tract, are swallowed, and pass in the feces. They develop into infective third-stage larvae within snails and slugs, their natural intermediate host. Viable third-stage organisms may also be found in land planarians, crabs, and freshwater prawns, which acquire the larvae by feeding on the tissues of infected mollusks. Humans, like rodents, become parasitized when they ingest raw intermediate or carrier hosts containing the infective stage. In rodents the larvae migrate to the brain where they grow into young adults. After a period of further maturation, the worms travel to the lungs and begin to deposit eggs. The nematode does not complete its life cycle in humans and dies after reaching the central nervous system.

Epidemiology The majority of human infections with *A. cantonensis* have been found in Thailand, Vietnam, Cambodia, Indonesia, the Philippines, Taiwan, Hawaii, and several smaller Pacific islands

from Okinawa in the north to Tahiti in the south. Cases have been described in Puerto Rico, Cuba, Egypt, and the Ivory Coast.

Pathology and pathogenesis The nematode can produce extensive tissue damage by moving through the brain when alive and provokes a marked inflammatory reaction when dead. The pathologic lesions are characterized by (1) marked lymphocyte and eosinophilic infiltration of the meninges, (2) hemorrhagic worm tracts through the brainstem and spinal cord, (3) granuloma formation around dead parasites and necrotic debris which sheathes the worm, and (4) engorgement of almost all blood vessels, particularly the veins. Necrosis of vessel walls, aneurysmal dilatation of arteries, and perivascular hemorrhages have been noted. Living worms have been removed from the eyes of patients without central nervous system involvement.

Clinical manifestations The eosinophilic meningitis usually presents as severe headache of acute or insidious onset. Fever is usually mild or absent, and only 15 percent of patients show signs of meningeal irritation. Patients frequently complain of visual impairment and, in a majority of these, visual defects or blurring of the optic disk can be demonstrated. Paresthesias and exquisite pains of the trunk and lower extremities are a common complaint, and paralysis of the sixth and seventh nerves is seen in 3 to 7 percent of cases. Paralysis of the limbs, convulsions, and loss of consciousness are rare. Although some patients have experienced significant neurologic residua, the disease usually ends in complete spontaneous recovery. Death is rare. The cerebrospinal fluid contains several hundred cells per cubic millimeter and many eosinophils, and the protein is elevated. There may or may not be an eosinophilia in the peripheral blood.

Diagnosis The diagnosis is entertained on the basis of the clinical manifestations in an endemic area. Small areas of attenuation with surrounding hypodense collars may be seen on computed tomography (CT) scan of the brain. Rarely, the adult worm is found in the cerebrospinal fluid. Angiostrongyliasis must be differentiated from other ectopic worm infections of the central nervous system including strongyloidiasis, filariasis, paragonimiasis, hydatid disease, schistosomiasis japonicum, trichinosis, cysticercosis, toxocariasis, and gnathostomiasis. A case of visceral larva migrans with eosinophilic meningitis has been described, in which the raccoon ascarid, *Baylisascaris procyonis,* was implicated. The diagnosis can be confirmed with an ELISA for circulating antibodies.

Treatment and prevention Mebendazole, in the dose of 100 mg, is often administered twice daily for 5 days, but is of uncertain efficacy. Anthelmintic therapy has been thought by some authors to be dangerous since the simultaneous death of many worms might produce a severe inflammatory reaction. Steroids may be beneficial in severe cases. Prevention depends upon avoidance or proper cooking of such foods as snails, prawns, and crabs. Raw vegetables should be carefully inspected for the presence of planarians and mollusks before they are eaten. Freezing of crustaceans and mollusks at −15°C for 12 h will destroy infective larvae of *A. cantonensis*.

ANGIOSTRONGYLIASIS COSTARICENSIS *Angiostrongylus costaricensis* is a nematode that dwells in the mesenteric arteries of Central and South American rats. Larvae pass in the stool and develop in slugs, the intermediate hosts. Rats, and incidentally humans, are infected when they ingest slugs or vegetables contaminated with third-stage larvae deposited in the mucous trail of these mollusks. The larvae mature in the lymphatics and move to the mesenteric radicals of the cecum. Here they may cause arterial thrombosis, ischemic necrosis, ulceration, and eosinophilic granuloma formation. Infected patients present with fever, eosinophilic leukocytosis, abdominal pain, and a right lower quadrant mass. Occasionally, perforation of the bowel and generalized peritonitis occur. The fever may persist for up to 2 months. Children are more frequently involved than adults. Neither larvae nor eggs are seen in the stool of the human host. The diagnosis is usually established at the time of surgery. The value of specific anthelmintic therapy has not been established.

GNATHOSTOMIASIS Definition Gnathostomiasis is a tissue infection of humans caused by *Gnathostoma spinigerum*. Clinically it is manifest as cutaneous or visceral larva migrans, ocular infection, or a lethal eosinophilic meningitis.

Etiology and epidemiology The parasite, which is found throughout the Far East, lives encysted in the gastric mucosa of dogs, cats, and wild felines. The ova are passed to the external environment via the feces, hatch in water, and are ingested by *Cyclops,* the first intermediate hosts. These in turn are eaten by freshwater fish, frogs, snakes, and eels in whose flesh the infective third-stage larvae develop. Ducks and chickens fed on these second intermediate hosts may also come to harbor infective larvae. Human infections, which are most commonly seen in Thailand and Japan, occur when humans ingest infected uncooked fish (somfak, sashimi), duck, or chicken.

Pathogenesis and manifestations The parasite cannot complete its cycle in humans, and the immature worms migrate through the abdominal and thoracic organs producing localized areas of inflammation and hemorrhage. Clinically, this is manifest as fever, eosinophilic leukocytosis, urticaria, and pain. Typically, the systemic manifestations subside within a month as the worms make their way to the subcutaneous tissues. Here, their continued migration results in the production of transient serpiginous pruritic swellings, subcutaneous tunnels, and abscesses. If the worm invades the epidermis, the resulting lesions closely resemble those of cutanea larva migrans. Not uncommonly, the eye may be involved with orbital cellulitis, iritis, or uveitis. Migration into the central nervous system results in a lethal eosinophilic meningitis (see ''Angiostrongyliasis Cantonensis'' above). This presents as a radiculomyeloencephalitis with limb pain and paresis. The cerebrospinal fluid eosinophilic leukocytosis is present but less marked than in *Angiostrongylus* infections. The fluid is often xanthochromic. Death may occur from cerebral hemorrhage or destruction of vital centers.

Diagnosis and treatment Painless, recurrent migratory subcutaneous swellings and eosinophilic leukocytosis occurring in an endemic area make the diagnosis likely. It must be differentiated from cutanea larva migrans, however, and from angiostrongyliasis cantonensis when the central nervous system is involved. Areas of CNS hemorrhage appear as hyperdense areas on brain CT. Definitive diagnosis depends upon the removal and identification of the worm. The ELISA appears to be a useful diagnostic adjunct. Other than excision, there is no specific therapy of documented efficacy. However, mebendazole, 200 mg every 3 h for 6 days, is frequently administered with glucocorticoids in CNS disease. The disease can be prevented by the adequate cooking of fish, chicken, and duck in endemic areas.

DRACUNCULIASIS Definition Dracunculiasis is an infection of human connective and subcutaneous tissues by the guinea worm, *Dracunculus medinensis.*

Etiology and epidemiology Dracunculiasis affects about 10 million people in Africa, the Middle East, and the Indian subcontinent. Humans acquire the parasite when they ingest raw drinking water containing infected copepods (*Cyclops* spp.) which serve as the intermediate host. Shallow ponds, cisterns, and wells are the usual habitat of these crustaceans. In the stomach the copepod is digested and the larvae are released. The larva penetrates the intestinal wall and matures in the connective tissue of the retroperitoneal space. The adult male is small, seldom seen, and presumably dies after mating. In contrast, the female *Dracunculus* is one of the largest nematodes known—1 to 2 mm in diameter and 300 to 800 mm in length. The female reaches gravidity in approximately one year and then migrates to the subcutaneous tissue of the lower extremities. When the anterior end of the worm approaches the skin, a blister forms. This breaks down in a few days, forming a superficial ulcer. When the protruding portion of the worm comes in contact with water, the uterus prolapses through the body and discharges large numbers of motile rhabditiform larvae. Following ingestion by one of several species of *Cyclops,* the larvae undergo further development, becoming infective in 10 to 12 days. Mammals other than humans may be infected, but their importance as a disease reservoir is uncertain.

Pathogenesis and manifestations The infection is asymptomatic until the gravid female appears in the subcutaneous tissues, where it may, on occasion, be palpable. A few days before the formation of the blister, the patient frequently has fever, generalized urticaria, periorbital edema, and wheezing. Blister formation is accompanied by intense local pain and pruritus; like the systemic manifestations, this is thought to represent an allergic reaction to prematurely liberated larvae. The local lesion is usually found over the feet and ankles, making walking difficult, but may occur on the trunk or the upper extremities. Multiple infections are common. With the rupture of the blister and the release of embryos, the systemic manifestations abate, and the worm is slowly extruded over a period of 4 to 5 weeks. Secondary infection and cellulitis are common, particularly if the worm is ruptured during the process of extraction. In Nigeria, guinea worm ulcers are a common portal of entry for the spores of *Clostridium tetani.* The female worm often fails to reach the surface and discharge her larvae. In most of these cases, it dies without producing symptoms. The calcified appearance on roentgenograms is characteristic. Occasionally the worm may invade the deep tissues, causing serious symptoms, and sterile abscesses may follow the release of embryos. Invasion of joint spaces by the adult worm or larvae results in arthritis.

Diagnosis The clinical picture is characteristic. Placing a small amount of water on the worm results in discharge of larvae, which can then be examined microscopically.

Treatment and prevention If the outline of the worm can be clearly seen or palpated, it may sometimes be completely removed with a single incision. The gradual extraction of the worm can be accomplished by winding a few centimeters onto a stick each day. Thiabendazole in dosage of 25 mg/kg twice daily for 3 days or metronidazole 250 mg three times a day for 10 days is effective in the relief of symptoms, but there is serious question whether either agent hastens worm extrusion or death. Dracunculiasis can be prevented by the chemical treatment of drinking water or the provision of piped water.

CESTODE INFECTIONS

The tapeworms, or cestodes, are ribbon-shaped segmented hermaphroditic worms which inhabit the intestinal tract of many vertebrates. Unlike other helminths, they lack a digestive tract but absorb food through their entire surface. Tapeworms have a primitive nervous system, a muscular system, and excretory canals. Attachment to the host's intestinal mucosa is accomplished by sucking cups or grooves located on the head, or *scolex.* In some species, attachment is aided by hooklets located on the scolex. Behind the globular scolex lies a short, narrow neck from which segments or *proglottides* develop to form the chainlike *strobila* of the worm. The proglottides progressively mature as they are displaced further from the neck by new segments. As each section becomes gravid, eggs are released either through a uterine pore, by splitting open, or by disintegrating. Because the eggs of many tapeworms appear identical, species identification depends on the morphologic characteristics of the scolex or gravid proglottides.

Except for *Hymenolepis nana* the human tapeworms require one or more intermediate hosts for larval development. After ingestion by a susceptible intermediate host, eggs develop into larvae or *oncospheres* which are capable of penetrating the intestinal mucosa, migrating in tissues, and developing into encysted forms. A cyst with a single scolex is called a *cysticercus* or *cysticercoid* in the case of *H. nana.* A *coenurus* is a cyst which contains several scolices, and a *hydatid* is a structure with daughter cysts each containing several scolices. Ingestion of tissues containing cysts with viable scolices by a definitive host allows development of the larval stage into an adult tapeworm. Cestodes in the *Diphyllobothrium* genus have a more complex life cycle involving two intermediate hosts (see below).

Human tapeworm infections may be divided into two major clinical groups. In the first, humans act as the definitive host and harbor the adult tapeworm in their intestines. The important species in this group are *Taenia saginata*, *Diphyllobothrium* species, *Hymenolepis* species, and *Dipylidium caninum*. In the second group, humans are intermediate hosts and harbor the larval forms in their tissues. This is exemplified by echinococcosis, sparganosis, and coenurosis. *Taenia solium* is unique because humans may act as both the definitive and intermediate hosts.

TAENIASIS SAGINATA Epidemiology Intestinal infection in humans with *Taenia saginata* occurs in all countries where raw or undercooked beef is eaten. It is particularly prevalent in Ethiopia, Kenya, Yugoslavia, the Middle East, Mexico and parts of South America, and the U.S.S.R. Indigenously acquired infection is uncommon in the United States except in areas where cattle and humans are concentrated such as around feedlots in the southwest.

Etiology and pathogenesis Humans are the only definitive host for the adult stage of *T. saginata*, which inhabits the upper jejunum for as long as 25 years. The cestode is 3 to 10 m long and has a small, unarmed scolex with four prominent suckers and 1000 to 2000 proglottides. The gravid segments are longer than they are wide (5 by 20 mm) and have 15 to 30 lateral uterine branches (*T. solium* has 8 to 12). The eggs, which are indistinguishable from *T. solium* eggs, measure 30 by 40 μm, have a thick brown radially striated shell, and contain a fully developed embryo with three pairs of hooklets. After the egg-containing proglottides are deposited on soil or vegetation, they are ingested by cattle or other herbivores. The embryo is released in the intestine, invades the intestinal wall, and is carried by vascular channels to striated muscle in the hind limbs, diaphragm, and tongue, where it is transformed over a period of 3 to 4 months into an ovoid bladder worm, or cysticercus. This form, which may be viable for 1 to 3 years, measures about 5 by 10 mm and consists of one scolex suspended in a fluid-filled sac. After ingestion of the cyst in raw or undercooked beef by humans, an adult worm develops in the intestine in about 2 months.

Clinical manifestations Most patients have minimal or no symptoms. Mild epigastric discomfort, nausea, flatulence, or hunger sensations may occur. Weight loss, diarrhea, irritability, and an increase in appetite are more unusual. Movements of the worm are sometimes apparent, and occasionally proglottides may crawl through the anus, appearing in the bed linen or underclothing of the distraught host. Rarely, segments become impacted in the appendix or cystic or pancreatic duct, producing obstruction and inflammation of these organs.

Diagnosis After the adult tapeworm has been established for 2 to 3 months, several proglottides are shed daily in the stool. Eggs also may be found in the stool or on the perianal area if a proglottid ruptures during defecation. If proglottides or eggs are not found in the stool, the perianal region should be examined using a cellophane tape swab as for pinworm infection. Since egg morphology is not diagnostic, however, examination of mature proglottides or the scolex is still necessary to identify the tapeworm species correctly. Reliable serologic tests are not available.

Treatment Niclosamide (Yomesan) is a highly effective taenicide which kills the scolex and immature segments of the worm on contact. Four 0.5-g tablets are thoroughly chewed at one time and swallowed with a small amount of water. No preparation or purge is necessary, and few side effects have been reported. As the worm is digested before it is passed in the stool, no attempt should be made to recover the scolex. Stool should be examined at 3 and 6 months for test of cure. Alternatively, a single dose of praziquantel (10 mg/kg) is effective, but this agent has not been approved for treating taeniasis in the United States.

Prevention Thorough cooking of beef is the major means of preventing taeniasis saginata. Temperatures as low as 56°C for as little as 5 min will destroy cysticerci. Refrigeration and salting for prolonged periods or freezing at −10°C for 9 days also destroys the cysticercus. General preventive measures include adequate meat inspection and proper disposal of human feces.

TAENIASIS SOLIUM AND CYSTICERCOSIS *Taenia solium*, the pork tapeworm, inhabits the intestinal lumen of humans, its only definitive host. The hog is the usual intermediate host, although humans, dogs, cats, and sheep may harbor the larval form. When human tissue is invaded by the larval form, the condition is referred to as *cysticercosis*.

Epidemiology Taeniasis solium is worldwide but is most common in Mexico, Africa, southeast Asia, eastern Europe, and South America. *T. solium* has been found in swine in Colorado and New Mexico, and autochthonously acquired human disease has been recognized in the United States. Cysticercosis is more frequent in industrialized nations due to migration of infected persons from endemic areas.

Etiology and pathogenesis The adult worm is about 3 m in length, resides in the upper jejunum, and may live for decades. The globular scolex contains a rostellum with two rows of hooklets. There are usually fewer than 1000 proglottides. The gravid proglottid is about 6 by 12 mm and contains a uterus with 8 to 12 lateral branchings. The eggs are infective for both human and hog. Infection usually occurs by the fecal-oral route, but humans may be autoinfected when gravid segments are returned to the stomach by reverse peristalsis. In the intermediate host, the embryo is released from the egg, penetrates the intestinal wall, and is carried by vascular channels to all parts of the body. Localization with development over 60 to 90 days to the encysted larval stage ("bladder worm") occurs primarily in striated muscle of the tongue, neck, and trunk. *Cysticerci cellulosae* are ovoid, gray-white opalescent structures about 1 cm in diameter, and *cysticerci racemosus* are irregular-shaped structures about 3 to 6 cm in diameter. Cysticerci can survive for 5 years. Humans become infected with the adult stage following ingestion of undercooked pork containing cysticerci.

Clinical manifestations Clinical manifestations of adult worm infestation resemble those with *T. saginata*. When humans serve as the intermediate host (cysticercosis), the clinical picture is entirely different. Cysticerci develop in the subcutaneous tissues, in muscles, in viscera, and, most importantly, in the eye and brain. Only a moderate tissue reaction occurs while the scolex is viable, but the dead larvae invoke a marked tissue response with muscular pains, weakness, fever, and eosinophilia. More inflammatory response is seen with racemose-type cysticerci than with cellulose-type. Symptoms in neurocysticercosis may be due to an acute encephalitic stage or due to brain cysts that are usually located in the cerebrum, ventricles, or subarachnoid space. The cerebral cysts are often less than 2 cm in diameter but may rarely be as large as 6 cm with the racemose type. Cerebral calcifications are seen in patients with dead parasites. Patients may have symptoms and signs of meningoencephalitis, including an eosinophilic cerebrospinal fluid pleocytosis, with the acute encephalitic stage or if cysticerci are widely distributed. Epilepsy, brain tumors, and other types of neurologic or psychiatric disorders may also be simulated. Clinical findings may change during the course of infection due to changes in the inflammatory response.

Diagnosis Infection with the adult worm can be detected by finding eggs in perianal scrapings or in the feces. To differentiate *T. solium* from *T. saginata*, proglottides or the scolex must be examined. Cysticercosis should be suspected in an individual who has lived in a hyperendemic area and who develops neurologic findings. Subcutaneous cysts may be found in approximately 50 percent of patients, and roentgenograms of soft tissue may show typical calcifications later in the course of cysticercosis. Contrast-enhanced CT scans and magnetic resonance imaging (MRI) are valuable for identifying brain lesions, which may appear as solid nodules or cystic or calcified lesions. In patients with the acute encephalitic stage, only hydrocephalus may be seen. Cerebrospinal fluid is often abnormal but not diagnostic. ELISA of serum and cerebrospinal fluid provides a sensitive serologic test for diagnosis of cysticercosis, but cross-reactive antibodies occur in some patients with other infections. Brain, subcutaneous nodule, or skin biopsy specimens permit a specific diagnosis.

Treatment   The stage and location of the parasite determine the prognosis and treatment. For removal of the adult worm in the human intestine, niclosamide or praziquantel may be given as for *Taeniasis saginata*. However, because these drugs cause maceration of the proglottides with release of ova, cysticercosis could theoretically occur. To prevent this, some authorities recommend that a saline purge be administered 1 h after the medication.

Praziquantel has been used to treat neurocysticercosis associated with hydrocephalus with promising results, although the drug is not approved for this use in the United States. A dose of 50 mg of praziquantel per kilogram given daily in three divided doses for 15 days has been recommended. Treatment of neurocysticercosis with praziquantel may be associated with an exacerbation of symptoms in 90 percent of patients. Glucocorticoids have been used to ameliorate the exacerbations which presumably occur secondary to an inflammatory response to dying cysticerci. Other drugs including albendazole, flubendazole, and metrifonate may also be effective for neurocysticercosis. The optimal dose and duration of these agents, the long-term side effects, and the need for concomitant glucocorticoid treatment have not been studied adequately. There are two groups of patients with cysticercosis for whom praziquantel should not be considered. Treatment of ocular cysticercosis should be surgical. Patients with a seizure disorder, only calcifications on CT scan, and normal cerebrospinal fluid examination should be treated only with anticonvulsant medication.

HYMENOLEPIASIS NANA   Epidemiology   *Hymenolepis nana* (dwarf tapeworm) infection has been reported in temperate and tropical regions around the globe. It is the most common autochthonously acquired tapeworm in the United States, most of the infections occurring in the southern states. The infection is spread by the direct fecal-oral route and is particularly common in children and institutional populations.

Etiology and pathogenesis   The life cycle is unique because both the larval and adult phases occur in the same host. The adult worm is small, about 2 cm, and lives for only a few weeks in the proximal ileum. Its proglottides are very small and are rarely seen in the stool. The gravid segments break apart in the fecal stream releasing spherical eggs. These measure 30 to 44 μm in diameter and have a double membrane enclosing the embryo which has six hooklets. The inner vitelline membrane has four to eight slender filaments arising from each pole. The eggs are immediately infective, and when ingested by a new host, the freed oncospheres penetrate the intestinal villi, becoming cysticercoids. Larvae migrate back into the intestinal lumen, attach to the mucosa, and mature into adult worms. The eggs may also hatch before passing in the stool, causing internal autoinfection with gradually increasing numbers of worms in the host.

Clinical manifestations   Dwarf tapeworm infection may be asymptomatic even with many adult worms in the intestine. When infection is massive, abdominal cramps and diarrhea occur. Rarely, dizziness or seizures have been seen in children and have been attributed to a neurotoxic product of the worms.

Treatment   Niclosamide, 2 g per day, must be given for 5 to 7 consecutive days. The dosage for children must be adjusted for body weight. The longer treatment course is necessary because niclosamide is not effective against the cysticercoid stage, and the encysted larvae continue to release organisms for 4 days. A repeat treatment course may be required in 2 weeks for patients with heavy infections. A single dose of praziquantel (25 mg/kg) may be more effective, but has not been licensed in the United States for this purpose.

Prevention   With a single host involved and the eggs being immediately infective, eradication of the disease presents problems similar to those encountered with enterobiasis. Personal hygiene is imperative. In an institution, epidemics can be avoided by proper screening programs.

HYMENOLEPIASIS DIMINUTA   *Hymenolepis diminuta* is a cestode of rats and mice that occasionally infects small children. Larval development occurs in a wide variety of insects including fleas and mealworms. Humans become infected with the adult worm when they ingest uncooked cereal foods contaminated by these insects. Infection is usually asymptomatic, and the diagnosis is made only when characteristic eggs are found in the stool. The eggs resemble those of *H. nana* but are longer and lack polar filaments. Niclosamide, as prescribed for *H. nana*, results in approximately a 90 percent cure rate.

DIPYLIDIASIS CANINUM   *Dipylidium caninum* is the common tapeworm of cats and dogs. The orange-brown proglottid, which resembles a pumpkin seed, is often passed intact in the stool or migrates through the anal canal. This may cause animals harboring the parasite to drag their buttocks across the floor. The characteristic egg packets are then expelled by the proglottides and ingested by fleas to develop into infective larval forms. The definitive host becomes infected by swallowing involved fleas. Human infections occur primarily in small children who ingest fleas while playing with their pets. The diagnosis is made by recovering the characteristic proglottid or egg packet. Treatment is the same as for *T. saginata* described above. Periodic deworming of pets provides the best prevention.

DIPHYLLOBOTHRIASIS   Epidemiology   *Diphyllobothrium latum* and *Diphyllobothrium* species are common in the Baltic and Scandinavian countries, Japan, U.S.S.R., Switzerland, Italy, Chile, and central Africa. The infection occurs in the north central United States, Florida, and along the Pacific coast. Its prevalence is enhanced by the disposal of raw sewage into freshwater lakes. Anadromous Alaskan salmon have been implicated in an outbreak along the west coast. The popularity of raw fish dishes such as Japanese sushi and sashimi may lead to increased prevalence of the disease in the United States.

Etiology and pathogenesis   The adult worm lies attached to the mucosa of the ileum and occasionally the jejunum by a pair of sucking grooves located on the scolex. It can live 20 years and achieve a length of more than 10 m. The 3000 to 4000 proglottides are wider than they are long. Unlike *Taenia*, the gravid segments are retained by the worm, and each day a million operculated ova are passed directly in the stool. On reaching water, the egg hatches, releasing a free-swimming embryo. This is eaten by small freshwater crustaceans belonging to the species *Cyclops* or *Diaptomus*, in which it develops into a *procercoid*. When the infected crustacean is swallowed by a fish, the larva migrates into the flesh and grows into a *plerocercoid*, or *sparganum*, larva. Humans acquire disease by ingesting raw infected fish. In 3 to 5 weeks the tapeworm matures in the intestine into an adult capable of discharging eggs. Several *Diphyllobothrium* species can infect humans, and *D. latum* cannot be distinguished from other species by its eggs or proglottides. Species determination requires examination of the scolex.

Clinical manifestations   Most infections are asymptomatic or produce slight, transient abdominal discomfort. Rarely, there may be severe cramping abdominal pain, diarrhea or constipation, vomiting, weakness, and loss of weight. Intestinal obstruction has been reported in multiple infections. In 0.1 to 2 percent of infected patients, an anemia develops, and about 40 percent of fish tapeworm carriers will have low serum vitamin B_{12} levels. The anemia appears to result from the ability of the tapeworm to compete successfully with its host for vitamin B_{12} and resembles pernicious anemia including central nervous system involvement. A worm located high in the jejunum may take up 80 to 100 percent of labeled vitamin B_{12} ingested by a patient with anemia. These patients tend to be elderly, have diminished production of intrinsic factor, and have worms located in the proximal small bowel. Folate absorption may also be decreased and contribute to the anemia. Lysolecithin, a product of the tapeworm, may contribute to the severity of the disease. Neurologic manifestations are more common than in pernicious anemia and may occur in the absence of hematologic findings. Typically, they include paresthesias, impaired vibration sense, numbness, weakness, and, less commonly, central scotomas secondary to optic atrophy. These findings are reversible with proper treatment.

Diagnosis The characteristic eggs are present in the stool in large numbers, making the diagnosis easy. They measure 55 to 76 by 41 to 56 μm and possess a single shell with an operculum at one end and a knob on the other. Mild eosinophilia may be present.

Treatment Niclosamide or praziquantel as prescribed for taeniasis saginata will cure most infections. In the presence of macrocytic anemia, parenteral vitamin B_{12} should be given.

Prevention Fish tapeworm infection can be prevented by cooking to a temperature of at least 56°C for 5 min. Freezing at −10°C for 72 h or placing the fish in a brine solution with appropriate salt concentration and exposure time can also prevent disease. Commercially prepared lox is usually brined appropriately before smoking.

SPARGANOSIS The *sparganum,* or plerocercoid larva, of *Diphyllobothrium*-related tapeworms belonging to the genus *Spirometra* will develop in humans following ingestion (usually in drinking water) of a *Cyclops* bearing the procercoid larva. Sparganosis also follows ingestion of infected fish, snakes, or frogs or application of infected flesh as a poultice. The frog tissues contain the sparganum, which is capable of invading human tissues. The dog and cat are definitive hosts for *Spirometra*. The infection often presents as a painful subcutaneous swelling. Periorbital tissues may be involved with marked palpebral edema and destruction of the globe. A marked eosinophilia is usually present. The location of the larvae determines the prognosis of the infection in humans. Surgery and injection of ethyl alcohol with epinephrine-free procaine to kill worms is the preferred method of treatment.

COENUROSIS This is a rare infection of humans by the larval stage, or coenurus, of the dog tapeworm *Taenia multiceps*. As in cysticercosis, the subcutaneous tissue, eye, and central nervous system may be involved. In tropical areas the brain has often been invaded, and the cases have been fatal. The clinical presentation is that of a slowly growing space-occupying lesion. Diagnosis and treatment both rely on surgical excision of the lesion. Treatment with drugs including mebendazole has not been effective.

ECHINOCOCCIASIS Echinococciasis is a tissue infection of humans caused by the larval stage of *Echinococcus granulosus* or *E. multilocularis*. These species of echinococcus are distinct morphologically and biologically. In humans, *E. granulosus* produces cystic lesions primarily involving the liver and lungs, whereas *E. multilocularis* causes multilocular (alveolar) lesions that are locally invasive. A "sylvatic" form of *E. granulosus* differs in clinical findings from a "pastoral" form.

Epidemiology Canines are the definitive hosts for *E. granulosus*. Sheep, cattle, and, in the Middle East, camels are the common intermediates for the pastoral form. This form of the disease has its highest incidence in countries where sheep and cattle raising is carried out with the help of dogs, particularly in the Middle East, Australia, New Zealand, east and south Africa, South America, and central Europe. Approximately 200 cases per year of echinococciasis are diagnosed in the United States, but most are imported. Autochthonously acquired cases have been reported from a few well-defined populations, including Basque sheep farmers in California, southwestern Indians, and sheep raisers in Utah.

The sylvatic focus of *E. granulosus* exists primarily in Alaska and western Canada, where wolves act as the definitive host and caribou and moose as the intermediate. A second sylvatic cycle involving deer and coyotes has been reported from California. A domestic cycle can be established when humans kill the herbivores and feed their viscera to dogs.

In *E. multilocularis* infections, rodents such as deer mice are the natural intermediate hosts, while wolves, foxes, coyotes, and domestic dogs and cats may serve as definitive hosts. An urban cycle involving the cat and common house mouse has been described. Human

infection in the United States is most common in Alaska but has also been described in Minnesota. Large series of patients with *E. multilocularis* have been reported from Siberia and Switzerland.

Etiology The adult *E. granulosus* is a small (5 mm) worm which resides in the jejunum of canines for 5 to 20 months. In addition to the scolex and neck, it has three proglottides, one immature, one mature, and one gravid. The gravid segment splits, either before or after passage in the stool, to release eggs which appear identical with those of *T. saginata*. When ingested by an appropriate intermediate host, the embryos escape from the eggs, penetrate the intestinal mucosa, and enter the portal circulation. Most are filtered out by the liver or lung, but some escape into the general circulation to involve brain, kidney, bones, and other tissues. The larvae that are not phagocytosed and destroyed develop into hydatid cysts which are unilocular and consist of an external laminated cuticula and an inner germinal layer. The laminated membrane in the sylvatic form may be semitranslucent in appearance and more fragile than in the pastoral type. Fluid fills and distends the cyst. Brood capsules and second- or third-generation daughter cysts develop from the germinal layer. "Hydatid sand" found in the cyst consists of scolices liberated from ruptured brood capsules. The cysts grow slowly over a period of years. In the pastoral type cysts often reach a diameter of over 10 cm, while cysts in the sylvatic form are usually only 3 to 5 cm. When the hydatid cyst is ingested by a canine, the cycle is complete.

The life cycle of *E. multilocularis* is similar except that small rodents serve as the natural intermediate host. However, the cyst is quite different. Humans do not provide optimal conditions for development of *E. multilocularis*, and the larval form remains in the proliferative phase. The hydatid cyst is always multilocular or alveolar in type. Its vesicles progressively invade the host tissue, usually the liver, by extension of processes from the germinal layer. In general, the growth pattern is like a neoplasm, and the lesions may metastasize when growth extends into blood vessels.

Clinical manifestations Echinococciasis is usually acquired in childhood, but a latent period of 5 to 20 years occurs before diagnosis. In one patient the latent period of a hepatic cyst was 75 years. Enlarging cysts usually produce tissue damage by mechanical means. The resulting symptoms depend upon the site, type, and rate of growth of the cystic lesions.

Patients with the sylvatic form of *E. granulosus* are usually asymptomatic at the time of diagnosis. Approximately 60 percent of the cysts are found in the lung and 40 percent in the liver. The cysts are diagnosed as an incidental finding on routine x-ray. Rarely, a patient may present with hemoptysis or a palpable mass in the liver. Morbidity and mortality are almost never seen.

With the pastoral type the ratio of pulmonary to liver cysts is reversed, and the hydatids may reach enormous size. In as many as 20 percent of patients, the pulmonary hydatid may rupture producing cough, chest pain, or hemoptysis. Hepatic lesions often present as abdominal pain or a palpable mass. Rupture through the diaphragm or into the peritoneal cavity can occur. Intrabiliary extrusion of calcified hepatic cysts has been reported in 5 to 15 percent of affected patients and mimics recurrent cholecystitis. Obstruction of the bile duct may result in jaundice. Rupture of a hydatid into the bile duct, peritoneal cavity, lung, pleura, or bronchus may produce fever, pruritus, urticarial rash, or an anaphylactoid reaction which may be fatal. Release of the numerous scolices leads to disseminated infection. Most patients initially have one or more hydatids in a single site, but in about 10 percent other tissues are involved. In bone, the cysts are semisolid, invade the medullary cavity, and slowly erode bone, producing pathologic fractures. Central nervous system involvement may produce epilepsy or blindness. Cardiac cysts can lead to conduction defects, pericarditis, and ventricular rupture. Hydatid antigen has been shown by fluorescent antibody in the glomerulus and has been related to membranous glomerulonephritis. Many other sites can be involved including spleen, ovary, prostate, and thyroid.

The alveolar cyst of *E. multilocularis* usually presents as a slowly growing hepatic tumor, with a minority of patients having metastatic disease to lung, brain, or other tissues. The natural course is one of malignant growth with massive destruction of the liver and extension into vital structures. If untreated, the disease is often fatal, but there is considerable individual variation in the course of the disease.

Diagnosis If a hydatid cyst ruptures or leaks fluid, an anaphylactoid reaction associated with eosinophilia and increased IgE levels may suggest the diagnosis. However, the clinical picture is usually not characteristic, and eosinophilia is seen in fewer than 25 percent of cases. Echinococciasis is most commonly discovered by routine x-ray. Pulmonary lesions usually are round, somewhat irregular masses of uniform density. They do not calcify. In contrast, hepatic cysts of *E. granulosus* show a smooth rim of calcification in about 50 percent of cases. Diffuse radiolucencies (2 to 4 mm) outlined by calcific densities may be seen in the liver with *E. multilocularis*. CT and ultrasound can be useful in demonstrating more details of the hydatid. In some cases of *E. granulosus*, simple, fluid-filled cysts indistinguishable from benign hepatic cysts are seen. In others, the findings of daughter cysts and hydatid sand strongly suggest echinococciasis. Thin eggshell calcification may indicate active disease. With alveolar hydatids, CT reveals indistinct solid masses, often with central necrosis, and plaque-like calcification. Angiography may be necessary prior to surgical therapy.

Specific diagnosis is best accomplished by histologic examination. In general, however, diagnostic aspiration should not be attempted because of potential anaphylactoid reactions to leakage of cyst fluid. Occasionally scolices may be found in sputum, stool, or urine and are shown by trichrome, Ziehl-Neelsen, and other stains. Serologic tests including indirect hemagglutination and latex agglutination are useful if positive, but many cyst carriers will not develop an immune response. Indirect hemagglutination should be positive in 90 percent of patients with hepatic cysts but in only 50 to 60 percent of those with pulmonary hydatids. ELISA provides the most sensitive and specific serologic diagnosis of hydatid disease. Following surgical removal of cysts, serologic tests may be helpful in screening for residual or recurrent disease.

Treatment Surgical treatment remains the standard therapy. Patients with small calcified hepatic cysts and pulmonary hydatids of the sylvatic type need to be operated on only if the cysts are symptomatic or enlarge dramatically over time. All others should have their cysts excised if possible, or sterilized and drained. With a large cyst, the contents should be sterilized with hypertonic saline before an attempt is made to open it. The entire endocyst should then be removed if possible, and all biliary or bronchial fistulas carefully closed. The residual space must be obliterated to prevent postoperative infection or prolonged drainage. Aspergillomas have been seen in residual cavities of pulmonary cysts.

Medical therapy with "high-dose" mebendazole (40 to 50 mg/kg per day in three divided doses) may be considered in patients with other medical problems that preclude surgery or in patients with extensive disease that makes surgical cure impossible. In selected patients, it may also be considered in conjunction with definitive surgery to reduce the risk of metastatic spread of viable organisms. In animal models, mebendazole is larvacidal for *E. granulosus* but not for *E. multilocularis*. In human trials, all forms of echinococciasis appear to respond to the agent, although the experience with *E. multilocularis* is limited. Significant side effects including neutropenia have been reported. The agent should be used only with the patient's informed consent. The absorption is erratic and drug levels should be followed. The drug is contraindicated in pregnancy. Other benzimidazoles such as flubendazole and albendazole also appear to be effective for echinococciasis.

Prevention The incidence of echinococciasis can be reduced by appropriate control measures as demonstrated in Iceland. Contact with infected dogs must be avoided, infected carcasses and offal should be burned or buried, and infected dogs should be treated with niclosamide or arecoline.

HERMAPHRODITIC TREMATODE INFECTIONS

The trematodes of humans are long-lived parasites that produce progressive damage to the tissues of their hosts. With the exception of schistosomes, they are similar in morphology and life cycle. The adult flukes are flat, leaflike hermaphrodites that vary in length from a few millimeters to several centimeters. Their digestive tract, unlike that of the nematodes, ends blindly. As their name indicates, they have two "holes" in the form of oral and ventral suckers which are used as organs of attachment and locomotion. The operculated eggs, which are passed in the feces or sputum, hatch in the water to produce a ciliated, free-swimming *miracidium*. The miracidium reaches and penetrates the tissue of an intermediate snail host to undergo a period of development, eventuating in the release of swarms of free-living *cercariae* from the snail. These thousands of tail-bearing larvae must, in turn, reach a second intermediate host, usually an aquatic animal or vegetation, where they encyst forming *metacercariae*. The definitive host is infected when he or she ingests the parasitized second intermediate host. The distribution of flukes is usually limited by the location of their molluscan intermediate host. With the exception of *Opisthorchis* and *Fasciola*, most hermaphroditic flukes are found only in tropical or subtropical areas.

PARAGONIMIASIS Definition Paragonimiasis (endemic hemoptysis) is a chronic infection of the lung caused by trematodes of the genus *Paragonimus*. Clinically, the disease is characterized by cough and hemoptysis. Ectopic worms may cause a variety of other manifestations.

Etiology and epidemiology Although *P. westermani*, which is widely distributed in the Far East, is the most common cause of human paragonimiasis, over 30 species, including *P. skrjabini*, *P. heterotremus* (China), *P. africanus* (central and west Africa), *P. mexicanus*, *P. ecuadoriensis*, and *P. caliensis* (Central and South America), may cause the disease. The short, plump adults (7 to 12 mm in length, 4 to 6 mm in width) have a life span of 4 to 5 years which they typically spend encysted, in pairs, within the lung parenchyma of the host. Their golden-brown operculated eggs (50 by 90 μm) reach the bronchioles from where they are coughed up and excreted in the sputum or swallowed and passed in the feces. They must embryonate several weeks in fresh water before hatching to release the miracidia.

The infection is acquired by ingestion of cysts in the second intermediate host, a freshwater shrimp, crab, or crayfish. The metacercariae excyst in the duodenum, burrow through the intestinal wall into the peritoneal cavity, and then usually migrate through the diaphragm and into the lung. The worms also may be found in the intestinal wall, liver, pancreas, kidney, epididymis, mesentery, skeletal muscle, subcutaneous tissues, and central nervous system, particularly the brain. The dog, cat, pig, rat, and wild carnivores are definitive hosts for the parasite in addition to humans. In some of these, very young adults can be found in their striated muscles. Human infection has been reported following the ingestion of this undercooked flesh.

It is estimated that there are over 3 million human infections, the vast majority in Asia, particularly China, Korea, Japan, Taiwan, the Philippines, and Southeast Asia. Approximately 1 percent of Indochinese immigrants to the United States harbor the trematode. Infections have also been reported from the Indian subcontinent, West Africa, Latin America, and the Pacific, including Samoa and the Solomon Islands. The incidence of paragonimiasis is often affected by food shortages or local customs. The metacercariae survive in vinegar, and lightly pickled or inadequately cooked food usually serves as the source of infection in the Far East. Children may acquire the disease in endemic areas while handling or eating raw crabs during play.

Pathogenesis and clinical manifestations During the migration of larvae, patients may experience fever, urticaria, abdominal pain, or diarrhea. An eosinophilic granuloma forms about the adult worm, eventually leading to the formation of a fibrous cyst. The pulmonary lesions which measure up to 1 cm in diameter frequently communicate with a bronchiole, resulting in secondary bacterial infection. Small, fibrous nodules representing reaction around deposited eggs also occur. Clinically the picture is one of chronic bronchitis and bronchiectasis with production of brownish sputum, hemoptysis, weight loss, nightsweats, low-grade fever, and occasionally finger clubbing. A poorly resolving pulmonary infiltrate, lung abscess, or pleural effusion may be present in heavy infections. Effusions are often large, may occur in the absence of parenchymal disease, and are typically exudative with eosinophils and cholesterol crystals. The roentgenographic findings vary with the stage of infection. Initially diffuse or segmental infiltrates, with or without pleural effusions, may be seen in lower or midlung fields. These are then gradually replaced by round 2- to 4-cm nodules which not infrequently cavitate. Eventually, cystic rings, fibrosis, and calcification occur, presenting a picture closely resembling tuberculosis, a disease which often coexists with paragonimiasis.

An abdominal mass, pain, and dysentery characterize intestinal or peritoneal infections. Ectopic worms in the liver or spleen may produce clinical manifestations of abscess formation. Involvement of the central nervous system usually presents acutely as a meningoencephalitis. Chronically, paralysis and epilepsy occur, usually the result of temporal or occipital lobe involvement. Homonymous hemianopsia, optic atrophy, and papilledema are common. The cerebrospinal fluid usually shows an eosinophilic leukocytosis and elevated protein. Cerebral calcifications are seen on x-ray in 50 percent of cases. *Paragonimus skrjabini* and, perhaps, *P. ecuadoriensis* infections are characterized by migratory subcutaneous nodules that contain adult flukes and that frequently ulcerate.

Laboratory findings   Eosinophilia is a constant finding. CT scans of the head, chest, and abdomen provide the best demonstration of parasite cavities. Definitive diagnosis depends upon finding the characteristic operculated ova in the sputum, stool, pleural fluid, or tissue. Eggs may be rare or totally absent from the sputum during the first 3 months of infection but are eventually found in 75 to 85 percent of infected patients. Their presence correlates well with the roentgenographic appearance of cavities. Even later, however, repeated examinations using concentration techniques may be required for their recovery. Ziehl-Neelsen staining, often carried out for suspected tuberculosis, usually will not demonstrate the eggs. In fact, the sputum concentration techniques for tuberculosis may destroy the eggs that are present. Since many patients have concomitant tuberculosis, the diagnosis may be overlooked. Stool examination is frequently helpful in children. A number of serologic tests, including complement fixation, counterimmunoelectrophoresis, ELISA, and latex agglutination tests, are available; the results correlate well with active infection. They are particularly useful in extrapulmonary infections. The skin test does not distinguish present and past infections and is used primarily for epidemiologic purposes.

Treatment and prevention   Praziquantel is the drug of choice. A total of 75 mg/kg is given in three divided doses for 1 or 2 days. Alternatively, bithionol may be administered. From 30 to 40 mg/kg in divided doses should be given every other day for a total of 10 to 15 treatment days. The symptoms disappear rapidly, and most infiltrates resolve within 3 months. Side effects are minor and consist of nausea, vomiting, and urticaria. Concomitant bacterial infection must be treated. Prevention of superinfection by the same parasite is important, because the disease is self-limiting.

The most practical control measure is the adequate cooking of all shellfish before they are eaten. Cooks should refrain from tasting shellfish during preparation and should wash their hands thoroughly thereafter.

CLONORCHIASIS   Definition   Clonorchiasis is an infection of the biliary passages caused by *Clonorchis sinensis,* the most important liver fluke of humans. Although the infection is usually asymptomatic, heavy worm loads may produce manifestations of biliary obstruction.

Etiology and epidemiology   *Clonorchis sinensis* is a small fluke (5 by 15 mm) that lives as long as 50 years in the biliary tree of its host. Here the flukes feed on mucosal secretions and pass operculated eggs into the feces. On reaching fresh water, the eggs are ingested by the intermediate snail host. After multiplication and development within the snail, the cercariae are released and penetrate freshwater fish. Infections result from ingestion of the raw, dried, salted, or pickled flesh of freshwater fish containing encysted metacercariae. The larva is released in the duodenum. It enters the common bile duct and migrates to the second-order bile ducts, where it develops into the adult form in about 1 month. In addition to humans, dogs, cats, pigs, and rats serve as disease reservoirs. The main endemic areas are Korea, Japan, Taiwan, Hong Kong, southern China, and Vietnam where, in previous years, clonorchiasis was perpetuated by the practice of fertilizing fish ponds with manure and human feces. Improvements in the disposal of human feces have dramatically decreased transmission in most areas, but the infection rate has remained high due to the prolonged life span of the adult worm. Twenty-five percent of the population of Hong Kong and a small proportion of Chinese and southeast Asian immigrants to this country have been shown to be infected. The disease may also be acquired in the United States by the ingestion of infected, dried, frozen, or pickled fish imported from the Far East. Clinically apparent cases are restricted to the adult population in whom the accumulated worm load eventually produces pathologic effects.

Pathogenesis and clinical manifestations   Light infections are usually asymptomatic, but worm loads of 500 to 1000 flukes often result in clinical manifestations. During the migration of the larvae, the patient may have fever, chills, tender hepatomegaly, mild jaundice, and eosinophilia. The mature worm causes proliferation of the biliary epithelium, increased mucin production, adenoma formation, chronic pericholangitis, and periductal fibrosis. Hepatic parenchymal damage and portal hypertension are not seen in uncomplicated infections. Recurrent attacks of suppurative cholangitis with or without intrahepatic choledocholithiasis may follow biliary obstruction with dead flukes. Hypoglycemic coma is a rare presenting manifestation. The occurrence of biliary stones in clonorchiasis is associated with an increased incidence of chronic *Salmonella typhi* carriage. Cholangiocarcinoma may occur in patients with severe, long-standing infections. The adult worms may infest the pancreatic ducts, where they can cause squamous metaplasia, periductal fibrosis, and acute pancreatitis.

Laboratory diagnosis   Clinical and epidemiologic findings often suggest the diagnosis. There may be elevation of the alkaline phosphatase, transaminase, and bilirubin levels during the acute phase of the disease, resulting in confusion with acute viral hepatitis. Eosinophilia is variable. Occasionally, a plain film of the abdomen will demonstrate intrahepatic calcification. Liver scan is usually negative in asymptomatic infections but may show multiple areas of diminished uptake in acute symptomatic disease. Percutaneous transhepatic cholangiography, sonography, and CT scans in these patients often reveal dilatation of the peripheral intrahepatic bile ducts and, on occasion, cholangiocarcinoma. The adult worms appear as round filling defects several millimeters in diameter. Definitive diagnosis depends on the demonstration of the eggs in the feces or the duodenal contents. They measure 29 by 16 μm, possess a conspicuous opercular rim as well as a posterior knob, and can be distinguished from the eggs of *Metagonimus, Heterophyes,* and *Opisthorchis* only with difficulty. An antigen extracted from adult worms can be used in a complement fixation or enzyme-linked immunosorbent test for the detection of the host's antibody response, but its diagnostic usefulness is questionable.

Treatment and prevention   Praziquantel is an effective chemotherapeutic agent for clonorchiasis. It is administered in a dosage of 25 mg/kg tid for a single day. Acute cholangitis can usually be managed medically with antimicrobial agents. If obstruction persists, surgery with physical removal of worms and/or stones may be required. Thorough cooking of freshwater fish will prevent infection.

OPISTHORCHIASIS Opisthorchiasis is caused by *Opisthorchis felineus* or *O. viverrini* and is characterized by hepatic lesions produced by adult worms in the larger bile ducts. The life cycle resembles that of *C. sinensis*. The geographic distribution differs in that *O. felineus* is endemic in eastern and central Europe and in Siberia and occurs in some parts of Asia, while *O. viverrini* is found in Thailand and Laos. Cats and wild carnivores act as the principal reservoir hosts, and the infection is found most commonly along rivers and lakes which harbor an abundant fish life. Up to 90 percent of inhabitants of some villages in northeastern Thailand are purported to carry the parasite. The clinical picture is similar to that seen in clonorchiasis except that gallstones are rare. Cholangiocarcinoma occurs in approximately 50 percent of infected patients who come to autopsy. The diagnosis usually is based on the finding of the eggs in the feces or duodenal contents. Treatment as recommended for clonorchiasis may be used. Infection can be prevented by eating only well-cooked fish.

FASCIOLIASIS Fascioliasis is caused by *Fasciola hepatica*, which, like *Clonorchis*, inhabits the bile ducts of the definitive host. When fully matured, the adult measures about 3 by 1 cm and discharges large operculate eggs 140 by 70 μm which must embryonate in fresh water before hatching.

Fascioliasis produces so-called liver rot in sheep, the principal definitive host. The disease is most common in sheep- and cattle-raising countries but has been reported from many parts of the world. In North America it occurs in the southern and western United States, Central America, and in the Caribbean Islands, including Puerto Rico.

Infection is contracted by ingestion of the encysted forms of the fluke attached to edible aquatic plants such as watercress. The larvae excyst in the duodenum, migrate through the intestinal wall, pass into the peritoneal cavity, penetrate the liver capsule, and finally reach the bile ducts, where they mature. Occasionally larvae may migrate to and mature in ectopic locations including the pancreas, subcutaneous tissue, chest cavity, or brain.

Early clinical manifestations are related to the migration of the larval form to and within the liver. Epigastric pain, fever, diarrhea, jaundice, urticaria, pruritus, arthralgia, and eosinophilia may be observed during this stage. Fibrosis of the liver similar to that found in clonorchiasis appears only after prolonged residence of many adult worms in the bile ducts. Obstruction of the bile duct occurs frequently and may be the presenting manifestation of disease.

The diagnosis usually is based on the finding of the eggs in the feces or in the duodenal contents. It is difficult to distinguish the eggs from those of *Fasciolopsis buski*. Complement fixation, hemagglutination, and precipitin tests have been reported to be helpful. A skin test is also available.

Bithionol, as administered for paragonimiasis, appears to be superior to praziquantel for treatment.

To prevent infection, aquatic plants such as watercress should not be eaten, vegetables grown in fields irrigated with polluted water should be boiled, and safe drinking water should be provided.

FASCIOLOPSIASIS Fasciolopsiasis is caused by the large intestinal fluke *F. buski*, which inhabits the upper part of the intestine of its definitive host. The principal definitive host is the pig. China, Thailand, India, and other areas in the Far East are the major endemic loci. Infection of humans occurs following ingestion, or peeling with the teeth, of water chestnuts, water lotus, and other edible aquatic plants. The large adults attach themselves to the intestinal mucosa, and these sites may later ulcerate. The infection is usually asymptomatic. In heavy infections, diarrhea, abdominal pain, gastrointestinal hemorrhage, and intestinal obstruction may appear early. Later, asthenia with ascites and anasarca occurs. Diagnosis is based upon the history and the finding of eggs in the feces. The eggs resemble those of *Fasciola hepatica*. The prognosis in untreated heavy infections, especially in children, is poor. Praziquantel as given for clonorchiasis is the treatment of choice.

HETEROPHYIASIS AND METAGONIMIASIS *Heterophyes heterophyes* and *Metagonimus yakagawa* are small intestinal flukes of humans and other fish-eating mammals. They are found in the Far East and, in the case of *Heterophyes*, in the Philippines, India, Egypt, and Tunisia. Both are acquired by ingesting the raw or undercooked flesh of metacercarial-infected freshwater fish. The 2- to 3-mm adults attach themselves to the mucosa of the small intestine. If present in sufficient numbers, they may cause abdominal pain and/or diarrhea. Rarely the eggs have been found in sites such as the brain, spinal cord, or heart where they produce granulomatous lesions. Most commonly, they are passed in the stool where they very closely resemble those of *Clonorchis*. Both species can be treated with praziquantel as described for clonorchiasis. As the life span of these trematodes is limited to a year or less, treatment is not indicated unless the patient is symptomatic.

REFERENCES

Intestinal nematodes

Anisakiasis

KLIKS MM: Anisakiasis in the western United States: Four new case reports from California. Am J Trop Med Hyg 32:526, 1983
OSHIMA T: Anisakiasis—is the sushi bar guilty? Parasitology Today 3:44, 1987

Ascariasis

ARFAA F: Selective primary health care: Strategies for control of disease in the developing world. XII. Ascariasis and trichuriasis. Rev Infect Dis 6:364, 1984
PAWLOWSKI Z: Ascariasis: Host-parasite biology. Rev Infect Dis 4:806, 1982

Capillariasis

BASACA-SEVILLA V, CROSS JH: Attempts to modify treatment of intestinal capillariasis. Southeastern Asian J Trop Med Public Health 16:546, 1985

Enterobiasis

VERMUND SH, MACLEOD S: Is pinworm vanishing? Laboratory surveillance in a New York City medical center from 1971–1986. Am J Dis Child 142:566, 1988
WAGNER ED, EBY WC: Pinworm prevalence in California elementary school children, and diagnostic methods. Am J Trop Med Hyg 32:998, 1983

Hookworm

GILLIS HM: Selective primary health care: Strategies for control of disease in the developing world. XVII. Hookworm infection and anemia. Rev Infect Dis 7:111, 1985
LITTLE MD et al: *Ancylostoma* larva in a muscle fiber of man follow cutaneous larva migrans. Am J Trop Med Hyg 32:1285, 1983

Strongyloidiasis

IRGA-SIEGMAN Y et al: Syndrome of hyperinfection with *Strongyloides stercoralis*. Rev Infect Dis 3:397, 1981
NEVA FA et al: Biology and immunology of human strongyloidiasis. J Infect Dis 153:397, 1986
PELLETIER LL JR: Chronic strongyloidiasis in World War II Far East ex-prisoners of war. Am J Trop Med Hyg 33:55, 1984

Toxocariasis

GLICKMAN LT, SCHANTZ PM: Epidemiology and pathogenesis of zoonotic toxocariasis. Epidemiol Rev 3:230, 1981
TAYLOR MRH et al: The expanded spectrum of toxocaral disease. Lancet 1:692, 1988
WORLEY G et al: *Toxocara canis* infection: Clinical and epidemiological association with seropositivity in kindergarten children. J Infect Dis 149:591, 1984

Trichuriasis

COOPER ES, BUNDY DAP: *Trichuris* is not trivial. Parasitology today 4:301, 1988
FISHMAN JA, PERRONE TL: Colonic obstruction and perforation due to *Trichuris trichuria*. Am J Med 77:154, 1984

Miscellaneous tissue nematodes

Angiostrongyliasis

ANDERSON E et al: First report of *Angiostrongylus cantonensis* in Puerto Rico. Am J Trop Med Hyg 35:319, 1986
BIA F, BARRY M: Parasitic infections of the central nervous system. Neurologic Clinics 4:171, 1986
LORIA-CORTES R, LOBO-SANAHUJA JF: Clinical abdominal angiostrongylosis. A study of 116 children with intestinal eosinophilic granuloma caused by *Angiostrongylus costaricensis*. Am J Trop Med Hyg 29:538, 1980

WITTNER M et al: Eustrongylidiasis—a parasitic infection acquired by eating sushi. N Engl J Med 320:1124, 1989

Dracunculiasis

HOPKINS DR: Dracunculiasis eradication: A mid-decade status report. Am J Trop Med Hyg 37:115, 1987

Cestodes

Coenurosis

BENGER A et al: A human coenurus infection in Canada. Am J Trop Med Hyg 30:638, 1981

Cysticercosis

EARNEST MT et al: Neurocysticercosis in the United States: 35 cases and a review. Rev Infect Dis 9:961, 1987
NASCIMENTO E et al: Immunodiagnosis of human cysticercosis (*Taenia solium*) with antigens purified by monoclonal antibodies. J Clin Microbiol 25:1181, 1987
RAMOS DM et al: Diagnosis of neurocysticercosis by magnetic resonance imaging. Pediatr Infect Dis 5:470, 1986
RANGEL R et al: Cysticercotic encephalitis: A severe form in young females. Am J Trop Med Hyg 36:387, 1987

Echinococciasis

HIRA PR et al: Diagnosis of cystic hydatid disease: Role of aspiration cytology. Lancet 2:655, 1988
LANGER JL et al: Diagnosis and management of hydatid disease of the liver. A 15 year North American experience. Ann Surg 199:412, 1984
LANIER AP et al: Comparison of serologic tests for the diagnosis and follow-up of alveolar hydatid disease. Am J Trop Med Hyg 37:609, 1987
SCHANTZ PM: Effective medical treatment for hydatid disease? JAMA 253:2095, 1985
WILSON JF, RAUSCH RL: Alveolar hydatid disease. A review of clinical features of 33 indigenous cases of *E. multilocularis* infection in Alaskan Eskimos. Am J Trop Med Hyg 29:1340, 1980

Hermaphroditic trematodes

Clonorchiasis and Opisthorchiasis

FLAVELL DJ: Liver-fluke infection as an aetiologic factor in bile-duct carcinoma of man. Trans R Soc Trop Med Hyg 75:814, 1981
KOOMPIROCHANA C et al: Opisthorchiasis: A clinicopathologic study of 154 autopsy cases. Southeastern Asian J Trop Med 9:60, 1978
RIM H-J: The current pathobiology and chemotherapy of clonorchiasis. Korean J Parasitol 24 (suppl: Monograph Series 3):1, 1986
YANGCO BG et al: Clinical study evaluating efficacy of praziquantel in clonorchiasis. Antimicrob Agents Chemother 31:135, 1987

Fascioliasis and Fasciolopsiasis

FARID Z et al: Unsuccessful use of praziquantel to treat acute fascioliasis in children. J Infect Dis 154:920, 1986
JONES EA et al: Massive infection with *Fasciola hepatica* in man. Am J Med 63:842, 1977
PLANT AG et al: A clinical study of *Fasciolopsis buski* in Thailand. Trans R Soc Trop Med Hyg 63:470, 1969

Paragonimiasis

JOHNSON RJ et al: Paragonimiasis: Diagnosis and the use of praziquantel in treatment. Rev Infect Dis 7:200, 1985
YOKOGAWA M: *Paragonimus* and paragonimiasis, in *Advances in Parasitology*, B Dawes (ed). London, Academic, 1969, vol 7, p 375

172 SCABIES, CHIGGERS, AND OTHER ECTOPARASITES

JAMES J. PLORDE

SCABIES Scabies is a cosmopolitan skin infection commonly referred to as the "seven-year itch." It is caused by a burrowing mite, *Sarcoptes scabiei* var. *hominis,* and is transmitted from person to person by close bodily contact, particularly among family members and bed partners. The survival of mites for 2 or 3 days in bedding, clothing, and house dust makes it possible that fomite-spread disease occurs, at least occasionally. Although the disease is more common in the poor and unclean, sporadic cases involve individuals of all socioeconomic groups. Children under 15 years of age have the highest prevalence of scabies and are usually the first members of families to contract the disease. Those who spend nights with friends or exchange clothing with others are at increased risk. Institutional outbreaks in hospitals, nursing homes, mental institutions, and aboard naval vessels have been reported. There has been a worldwide resurgence of this infection over the past 20 years, and in the United States it currently involves 2 to 4 percent of patients seen by dermatologists.

The turtle-shaped female measures 0.4 mm in length and possesses four pairs of legs. With the help of the two anterior pairs and her mouth, she burrows into the superficial layer of the epidermis. Here she deposits two or three enormous eggs daily until she dies 30 to 60 days later. The newly hatched larvae mature to adulthood on the skin surface within 2 weeks to continue the cycle of infection. Although an involved person may harbor thousands or occasionally millions of adult mites, the average number of adult females per infection is 11.

Two-thirds of the burrows are found in the upper extremities, particularly on the interdigital spaces of the hands and the flexor surface of the wrists. In heavy infections, other sites are typically involved. These include the dorsal surfaces of the elbows, anterior axillary folds, female breasts, periumbilical area, penis, scrotum, and buttocks. In bedridden patients, lesions are often concentrated over pressure points. The face, head, palms, and soles are seldom involved in adults; in infants, any area of the skin can be involved. Characteristically, a burrow appears as a short dark wavy line which may end in a small vesicle, the site of the adult female.

Sensitization (type IV) to the mites and their products begins approximately 1 month after infection and results in a papular or eczematous reaction at the sites of involvement. Itching is often severe and tends to be more marked at night or after a hot bath. Scratching frequently leads to secondary infection with pustulation and lichenification. Acute glomerulonephritis has followed infection with nephritogenic strains of streptococci. Occasionally, reddish pruritic nodules are seen in the groin and axillary regions. Infected individuals with good personal hygiene usually have few lesions, and burrows may be difficult to identify. In mentally retarded, debilitated, or immunosuppressed patients, a particularly virulent infection known as *crusted (Norwegian) scabies* is sometimes seen. Millions of mites may be present, producing a highly infectious exfoliative dermatitis; crusted, psoriasiform plaques are common. Itching is often mild or absent. Scabies usually terminates spontaneously in a few months, but chronic cases occur.

The diagnosis should be considered in any patient presenting with a pruritic eruption, particularly if it involves several members of a living group. The occurrence of symmetric lesions at the sites of predilection should initiate a search for the characteristic burrows. These should be vigorously scraped with a sterile needle or scalpel blade, and the scrapings transferred to a drop of 10% potassium hydroxide on a glass slide. A coverslip is placed over the top, and the preparation examined for adults, larvae, and eggs. The diagnosis can also be made on histologic sections prepared from a punch biopsy. Considering the mode of disease transmission, adults shown to have scabies should also be checked for venereal disease.

All sexual contacts and household members should be treated simultaneously with the patient to prevent the occurrence of "ping-pong infections." The therapeutic agents are applied topically, covering the skin thinly but completely from the neck down. Although the patient is rendered noninfectious within 24 h, up to 2 months may be required for the clinical manifestations of the disease to disappear completely. Needless retreatment during this period can lead to contact dermatitis. Bed linen and clothes used by the patient the day prior to therapy should be washed in hot water.

A number of effective agents are available for use. Lindane

(gamma benzene hexachloride) is left on for 8 to 12 h and then thoroughly washed off. Care must be taken to keep it away from eyes and mucous membranes. It should not be used in infants or pregnant adults. Crotamiton (Eurax) is massaged into the skin, and a second dose applied 24 h later. Benzyl benzoate (25%) is administered in a similar fashion. Antihistamines or salicylates are helpful in counteracting pruritus. Topical steroids may potentiate the infection and should not be used. Antibiotics are required occasionally when there is a significant bacterial superinfection.

CHIGGER AND OTHER MITES   The term *chigger* is used to refer to larvae of harvest mites belonging to the family Trombiculidae. The cosmopolitan adults feed on vegetable matter and deposit their eggs upon the ground. The tiny (0.4 mm) emergent larvae crawl along the ground and upward onto vegetation. Here, they await the passage of a vertebrate host, upon which they must feed before again dropping to the ground and molting. In humans, the chigger usually attaches about the ankles, but some advance along the skin until they are stopped by tight-fitting clothing. It then pierces the skin, releases a digestant to liquefy tissue cells, and feeds for 3 or 4 days. Within a few hours, the chigger's secretions have produced an intensely pruritic papule 0.5 to 2 cm in diameter. This usually vesiculates, resulting in a chickenpox-like lesion. Occasionally, subcutaneous bleeding results in a surrounding area of ecchymosis. The lesion and itching may persist for several weeks. In the United States, most clinical cases are seen during the summer months; in warm climates, the seasonal pattern is missing.

Grain mites as well as those of cats, dogs, fowl, and rodents may also feed on humans. Because these species are very small and the resulting skin lesions variable, diagnosis depends on the history of contact with the mite source. Treatment is directed at the relief of itching and the prevention of secondary infections. Insect repellents are highly effective prophylactic agents. Fumigation of mite sources may prevent recurrences.

FLEAS   Fleas are small wingless laterally compressed ectoparasites of humans and other warm-blooded animals. They tend to be found on the hairy portions of the host where they feed and deposit their eggs. The active larvae, which hatch in 3 days, can be found on the host, in its nest, or in dust. They eventually pupate and may remain dormant for weeks or months before completing their development to adults. Medically, fleas serve as both vectors and agents of disease. Rodent fleas of the genus *Xenopsylla* are the most important. They are responsible for the transmission of both plague (*Yersinia pestis*) and murine typhus (*Rickettsia mooseri*) from animal reservoirs to humans. Humans may also acquire the rat tapeworm *Hymenolepis diminuta* by swallowing fleas containing the cysticeroid. The dog tapeworm *Dipylidium caninum* may be transmitted in a similar fashion. The bites of these and other species of fleas belonging to the family Pulicidae can induce an irritating dermatitis. In addition, the tungidae (*Tunga penetrans*) may burrow into the subcutaneous tissues, producing a painful and debilitating disease.

Flea dermatitis   The fleas of humans (*Pulex irritans*), cats and dogs (*Cetenocephalides*), and rodents (*Xenopsylla*) may all induce dermatitis. In many individuals, the bites seem completely innocuous, but in sensitive persons, the saliva induces an erythematous raised pruritic papule. Repeated scratching may result in secondary infection with pustulation or ulceration. The intense pruritus, the ability of the flea to escape capture by virtue of its prodigious jumping ability, and the difficulty involved in crushing their hard chitinous bodies has led to many a frustrating nocturnal safari dedicated to the destruction of this unwanted bed partner. Control is effected by the use of frequent vacuuming to remove eggs, larvae, pupae, and adults from the environment. Insecticide sprays and dusting powders are also of help, but fleas have developed resistance to many of these. Dogs and cats should be washed, flea collars applied, and kennels dusted or sprayed with DDT or malathion. If rat runs can be located, they should also be dusted.

Tunga penetrans, sometimes referred to as a *jigger* or *chigoe flea*, is a burrowing flea found in the tropical areas of the Caribbean, South America, and Africa. These small (1 mm) free-living insects reside in sandy soil. The fertilized female burrows into the skin of the first warm-blooded animal encountered. In humans, they usually embed on the sole of the foot or under a toenail with only their anal pore exposed to the outside. Multiple infections are common. As the female becomes engorged with blood and eggs, a painful and pruritic pea-sized swelling is produced. Eventually, the overlying skin ulcerates, the flea dies, and the eggs are extruded. Secondary bacterial infections including tetanus and gas gangrene occur commonly. Autoamputation of the toes has been reported from Africa. The intact flea can usually be extracted by gently enlarging the entrance hole with a sterile needle and then applying pressure from the side. Alternatively, the lesion can be soaked in Lysol, the flea penetrated with a needle, and the lesion resoaked to kill the eggs and sterilize the wound. Antibiotics may be required to treat secondary bacterial infections.

PEDICULOSIS   Lice are obligate human ectoparasites that complete their entire 30- to 40-day life cycle on the body of the host. *Pediculus humanus* var. *capitis* infests the head, *P. humanus* var. *corporis* the body and clothing, and *Phthirius pubis* (crab lice) the genital and occasionally other hairy areas of the body. All three are flattened dorsoventrally and measure 2 to 3 mm in length. The crab louse is broader and flatter than *Pediculus* and possesses powerful claws on its second and third legs, with which it clings to the pubic hair. The females lay five or six eggs daily, which they firmly attach to the hairs or, in the case of the body louse, the clothing of the host. These clearly visible tiny white nits hatch in 8 to 10 days. The resulting nymph matures to adulthood in an additional 2 weeks. Both the larvae and adults take two blood meals daily, leaving behind a small purpuric puncture site. With repeated exposure, the host develops an inflammatory hypersensitivity reaction manifested as a small red papule at each new feeding site. Pruritus results in scratching, a weeping dermatitis, and secondary infection. Chronic infections of the scalp may result in a fetid mass of matted hair and exudate. On the body and genital areas, the lesions may become lichenified and pigmented—so-called vagabond disease. Heavy infections with *P. pubis* may involve the eyebrows and eyelids leading to blepharitis.

Lice can be transferred from person to person by direct contact or via discarded clothing in which the body louse can survive for up to a week. Migration is stimulated by fever, making *P. humanus* var. *corporis* an efficient vector of relapsing fever (*Borrelia recurrentis*), typhus (*R. prowazekii*), and trench fever (*R. quintana*). *Phthirius pubis* is not known to be a vector of human disease.

Pediculosis corporis is typically seen in the poor and transient who are unable to maintain even minimal levels of personal hygiene. In contrast, head and pubic lice are found on patients of all socioeconomic classes and are currently enjoying a resurgence in the United States. *P. capitis* most frequently infests white schoolchildren; blacks are seldom involved. Pubic lice are more common among the sexually active; their presence should stimulate a search for venereal disease.

The diagnosis is suggested by the typical dermatitis and confirmed by finding the adults or nits on the hair or clothing of the patient. Treatment may be carried out with 1% pyrethrin (Nix—approved for head lice only), with piperonyl butoxide (RID), or lindane (1% gamma benzene hexachloride, Kwell). The latter agent may be absorbed through the skin, resulting in CNS toxicity if applied inappropriately. It should not be used in infants and pregnant women. In head infections, the hair should first be shampooed with ordinary soap. RID or Nix are then rubbed in for at least 10 min (Kwell shampoo, 4 min), the hair is rinsed, dried, and combed with a fine-tooth comb to remove the nits. If RID or Kwell have been used, the process should be repeated in 7 days. Combs and brushes should be heated in water to 65°C for 5 min or soaked in 2% Lysol. The clothing and bedding of the patient with body lice are heat-sterilized. The patient's body should be lathered for 10 min with RID or 4 min with Kwell and then rinsed thoroughly. The therapy may be repeated in 7 days. In crab louse infestations, RID or Kwell cream or lotion should be used on the involved areas and left for 24 h. In hirsute individuals, the treatment can be repeated in 1 week. If the eyelashes are involved, 0.25% physostigmine ophthalmic ointment is applied twice daily for 10 days. Lice and nits are carefully removed with a cotton-tipped applicator. Narrow-angle glaucoma should be ruled out before the physostigmine is used.

MYIASIS Infections with maggots or fly larvae are seen worldwide in a variety of animals. Human involvement occurs most frequently where people live in close contact with domestic animals. Many different species of flies are involved. In some, an animal host is required for larval development; in these, the larvae are capable of invading normal tissue or enter the body through the nose, mouth, or ears. Others are opportunists, depositing their eggs or larvae in the open wounds of debilitated patients. The clinical manifestations vary with the species of fly and site of involvement. Four of the more common clinical syndromes are described below.

Localized cutaneous myiasis In tropical America the lesions are produced by *Dermatobia hominis,* the human botfly. This remarkable forest-dwelling Diptera captures a mosquito or other blood-feeding insect on which to deposit its packet of eggs. When this unwilling vector then lands on a warm-blooded animal to feed, the eggs hatch and penetrate the feeding site. Within the skin of the host, the larva develops for 2 or 3 months. Finally, it emerges, drops to the ground, and pupates. The lesions are most frequently seen on unprotected areas of the body including the hands, feet, head, and neck. During the first week of infection, the pruritic lesion closely resembles a mosquito bite. As the larva grows and begins to move, it produces severe pain and itching. Tissue destruction and inflammation results in the development of a furuncle-like lesion. Generally, a central opening is present through which the posterior end of the larva protrudes. A dark serosanguinous discharge containing the feces of the insect may be noted.

In Africa, a similar lesion is produced by *Cordylobia anthropophaga* (tumbu fly). These flies deposit their eggs on sandy soil or laundry laid out to dry. The larvae hatch and invade the unbroken skin of humans or wild rodents, where they mature in 8 or 9 days. In either case, the larvae can be surgically extracted without difficulty. In tumbu fly infections, letting the larvae mature and drop off spontaneously may be appropriate. This process can occasionally be hastened by applying mineral oil to the central opening. This results in the suffocation of the larva and stimulates its early exodus.

Cutanea larva migrans This is usually caused by the large (1 to 2 cm) horse botflies belonging to the genus *Gasterophilus.* When the larvae hatch on the skin, they penetrate to the lower epidermis. Because they do not mature in humans, they may migrate in the skin for several months. Clinically, the infection presents as a pruritic serpiginous band of erythema closely resembling cutanea larva migrans produced by *Ancylostoma braziliense.* The diagnosis can be made by placing a small drop of mineral oil on the skin just in advance of the worm tract. This allows visualization of black backward-directed spines on its body segments. The parasite can be easily removed with a sharp needle. Occasionally, the larvae may penetrate the eye. A similar clinical picture is sometimes produced by the larvae of *Hypoderma* spp. (cattle botfly). These, however, often penetrate deeply into the subcutaneous tissue and produce more pain and less pruritus than *Gasterophilus* larvae.

Deep-tissue myiasis Screwflies of several genera can deposit large batches of eggs on unbroken skin or in wounds, ears, or the nose. After hatching, the larvae burrow into the tissues and develop for 2 or 3 weeks. The mature 1- to 2-cm larvae then drop to the ground and pupate. At times, they penetrate deep tissues, including the eye, nasal sinuses, and cranium, where they produce destructive foul-smelling lesions. Bacterial superinfection is common. In India and Africa, the flies are usually of genus *Chrysomyia.* In the western hemisphere, *Callitroga* spp. are involved. The occurrence of human cases in the United States often accompanies epizootics of screwworm activity. Flesh flies of the family Sarcophagidae have also been implicated in deep-tissue myiasis both in the United States and

elsewhere. In all the above infections, the lesions should be surgically incised and debrided, the larvae removed, and secondary infections treated.

Intestinal myiasis When humans ingest food contaminated with the eggs or larvae of several genera of flies, some survive passage through the stomach and later mature in the intestine before they are extruded in the stool. In the United States, *Tubifera tenax* is the most frequently implicated species. Invasion of the intestinal mucosa may occur with *Sarcophaga* infections.

PENTASTOMIASIS Pentastomes, invertebrate endoparasites of reptiles, birds, and mammals, share a number of morphologic similarities with both the worms and arthropods. Although previously classified with each, they are now thought to constitute a phylum distinct from both, the Pentastomida. Adult worms resemble nematodes with an elongated, nonsegmented body varying in length from a few millimeters to several centimeters; separate sexes whose reproductive organs occupy the bulk of the body cavity; a straight, tubelike gut; and a chitinous cuticle. Their name ("five-mouthed") resulted from the early misidentification of the four hooklets surrounding the mouth projection as additional mouths.

Adult worms are found in the respiratory tract of carnivores where they attach by their hooklets and feed on the host's epithelial cells, blood, and tissue fluid. Eggs released by the female are passed to the external environment in nasal discharge, saliva, or feces. Once ingested by herbivores, the eggs hatch in the gut of these intermediate hosts, releasing mitelike first-stage larvae; these penetrate the gut wall and encyst in a variety of tissues. After a series of molts, the third-stage larvae exit from the tissue cysts and return to the peritoneal cavity. When the definite host feeds on the tissues of the intermediate host, ingested third-stage larvae migrate to the respiratory tract where they mature to adulthood.

Most human infections are caused by one of two species, *Armillfer armillatus* and *Linguatula serrata.* The African python is the definite host of the first. Humans come in contact with the eggs while handling pythons or by ingesting contaminated drink or food. The larvae do not develop into adult worms in the human intermediate host and most infections remain asymptomatic. Occasionally, the enlargement of larval cysts, during the molting stage, produces mechanical pressure on vital organs, resulting in obstruction of bile ducts, gut, or bronchi. Migrating third-stage larvae may penetrate organs, inducing pneumonitis, pericarditis, meningitis, peritonitis, and prostatitis. The diagnosis is generally made at autopsy when the cysts are discovered in the liver, peritoneum, mesentery, or lung hilum. Dead, calcified larvae produce distinctive, 1-cm radiopaque lesions, shaped like cashew nuts, which may be apparent in abdominal or chest radiographs. Although serologic tests have been developed, their usefulness is uncertain. Treatment is indicated only when mechanical pressure on vital organs requires surgical removal of the larval cysts.

Human infection with *L. serrata* is found primarily in the Middle East, but isolated cases have been reported from Africa, Europe, and the Americas. The parasite is acquired when third-stage larvae are ingested in raw liver or lymph nodes of sheep or goats, generally at times of religious feasts. The larvae migrate to the nasopharynx where they produce pain and itching of the throat and ears, nasal discharge, lacrimation, hoarseness, dyspnea, dysphagia, cough, hemoptysis, and vomiting—a syndrome known as *halzoun* in the Middle East and *marrara* in the Sudan. Manifestations begin within minutes to hours of ingesting the infested tissues and usually persist for 7 to 10 days. Occasionally, respiratory obstruction requiring tracheostomy develops. Eustachian tube abscess, facial paralysis, and invasion of the ocular globe have also been reported. Rarely, the larvae mature to adulthood, producing nasal pressure, sneezing, and recurrent epistaxis. The diagnosis is established by demonstrating the 0.5- to 1.0-cm third-stage larvae in nasal discharge, sputum, or vomitus or, rarely, by the recovery of the adult worm following a violent attack of sneezing. Treatment is directed to the protection of the airway and antibiotic therapy of secondary bacterial infections.

A third species, *Reighardia sternae,* is thought to produce a cutanea larva migrans–like syndrome in Southeast Asians who ingest live lizards.

REFERENCES

CARSON DS et al: Pyrethrins combined with piperonyl butoxide (RID) vs 1% permethrin (NIX) in the treatment of head lice. Am J Dis Child 42:768, 1988

DRABICK JJ: Pentastomiasis. Rev Infect Dis 9:1087, 1987

HARWOOD RB, JAMES MT: Mylasis, in Entomology in Human and Animal Health. New York, Macmillan, 1979

KRINSKI WL: Dermatoses associated with the bites of mites and ticks (Arthropodia: Acari). Int J Dermatol 22:75, 1983

MAUNDER JW: Insecticides in pediculosis capitis. Arch Dis Child 64:69, 1989

REEVES JRT: Head lice and scabies in children. Pediatr Infect Dis J 6:598, 1987

SHELLEY WB et al: Staphylococcus aureus colonization of burrows in erythrodermic Norwegian scabies. A case study of iatrogenic contagion. J Am Acad Dermatol 19:673, 1988

VAN NESTE DJ: Human scabies in perspective. Int J Dermatol 27:10, 1988

PART SIX

Disorders of the heart

173 CELLULAR AND MOLECULAR BIOLOGY OF CARDIOVASCULAR DISEASE

EUGENE BRAUNWALD

Because the principal function of the heart is to serve as a pump, clinical cardiology, since the era of William Harvey, has been deeply rooted in physiology and hemodynamics. The development of electrocardiography at the beginning of this century and the recognition of clinical disturbances of cardiac rhythm led to increasing interest in electrophysiology. Since both the mechanical and the electrical properties of the heart can be altered profoundly by drugs, pharmacology has also provided strong scientific underpinnings to clinical cardiology.

A fuller understanding of cardiac function and dysfunction will ulimately require studies at the cellular, molecular, and genetic levels. However, such investigations have been retarded by the absence of any cell line of adult, fully differentiated myocytes that can be readily grown in vitro, manipulated, and studied. Perhaps for this reason, cellular biology and molecular genetics have been slower to impact on cardiovascular disease than on some other branches of medicine, such as hematology, oncology, endocrinology, and infectious diseases. However, application of these techniques to cardiovascular science has now gained momentum, and these efforts are beginning to influence the care of patients with cardiovascular disease. Several examples of this influence are considered in this chapter and include advances in understanding myocardial cells, specifically the process of myocardial hypertrophy, the constituents of the bloodstream, such as apoproteins, and noncardiac cells, including vascular smooth-muscle cells, endothelial cells, and platelets. Discussed elsewhere (Chap. 289) are advances in thrombolytic therapy which have also resulted from studies at the cellular and molecular levels. The prominence of noncardiac cells in this discussion reflects the fact that the most prevalent forms of cardiovascular disease, hypertensive and ischemic heart disease, are diseases of the blood vessels, the myocardium itself being secondarily affected, as an "innocent bystander."

HYPERTROPHY

MYOCARDIAL HYPERTROPHY One of the most remarkable and important capacities of the heart is to adapt both acutely and chronically to changes in hemodynamic load. *Acute* adaptations are mediated by the two mechanisms discussed in Chap. 181: (1) an alteration in the number of cross-bridges that cycle between the actin and myosin myofilaments, depending on the length of the myocardial sarcomeres (this adaptation expresses, at the molecular level, Starling's law of the heart) and (2) changes in contractility mediated by the adrenergic neurotransmitter norepinephrine via beta-adrenergic receptors. The degree of activation of these receptors ultimately regulates the concentration of calcium ions around the contractile proteins and, thereby, myocardial contractility. In contrast, with *chronic* hemodynamic overload, as in hypertension, valvular heart disease, and many forms of congenital heart disease, *myocardial hypertrophy* is the major adaptive response. As the ventricle hypertrophies, new sarcomeres are added to each myocyte, protein synthesis is augmented, and sometimes protein degradation declines. The fraction of total cardiac protein composed of myofibrillar proteins increases in hypertrophy and subsequently declines as heart failure supervenes.

The mechanism responsible for the development of myocardial hypertrophy is the subject of intense investigation. The imposition of a pressure load on the ventricle is accompanied by an increase in the expression of messenger RNA (mRNA) that codes for various contractile proteins, and these increased levels of mRNA are responsible for the increase in myocardial protein synthesis. Proteins often occur in families of closely related isoforms, the expression of which is regulated in a tissue-specific and developmentally specific manner. In experimental animals the hypertrophic response involves the reappearance in the adult heart of contractile protein isoforms characteristic of the fetus such as the V_3 form of beta-myosin heavy chain ("slow myosin"), which has a low ATPase activity and promotes a slower, more sustained contraction requiring less energy than the V_1 form ("fast myosin"). The fetal isoforms of alpha-actin and tropomyosin and the mRNA of atrial natriuretic peptide (ANP, see later) are also reexpressed when left ventricular hypertrophy is induced. This reexpression of fetal protein genes appears to represent a general adaptive response.

In contrast to the cardiac hypertrophy resulting from hemodynamic overload, the hypertrophy of hyperthyroidism is *not* accompanied by the induction of fetal forms of contractile protein genes or of the ANP gene. Thyroid hormone acts directly via nuclear receptors to regulate myosin heavy chain gene expression at the transcriptional level, causing an accumulation of alpha-myosin heavy chain mRNA, and inhibits the expression of beta-myosin heavy chain mRNA, thereby increasing the level of myosin isoenzyme V_1 and bringing about a more rapid contraction. Hypothyroid hearts have higher levels of beta-myosin heavy chain mRNA and the V_3 myosin isoform, and lower levels of the mRNA encoding Ca^{2+} ATPase of sarcoplasmic reticulum.

Some of the changes in gene expression in ventricular hypertrophy involve proto-oncogenes, which are normal cellular homologues of transforming genes carried by oncogenic retroviruses (Chap. 10), and a gene that encodes one of the heat shock proteins (which appears to play a protective role during stress). Three major classes of proto-oncogenes are induced by pressure overload and are responsible for the acceleration of protein synthesis and of fetal isoforms: (1) one class encodes peptide growth factors, e.g., the c-*sis* proto-oncogene that encodes the beta chain of platelet-derived growth factor (PDGF, see later); (2) proto-oncogenes such as c-*myc* and c-*fos*, which code for nuclear proteins that regulate transcription of a variety of genes which influence the cell cycle; and (3) proto-oncogenes such as c-*ras*, which code for cytoplasmic proteins that bind to guanine nucleotides and regulate other intracellular signaling systems. The reinduction of genes normally expressed in fetal life, such as the fetal isoforms of myosin and ANP (in the ventricle), is a later event.

Stimuli that increase intracellular cyclic AMP and intracellular Ca^{2+} or alpha-adrenergic agonists that enhance the turnover of inositol phospholipids regulate the expression of the c-*fos* gene. The protein expressed by this gene may play a role in modulation of the response to neurotransmitters and drugs that affect the function of the heart acutely in the development of cardiac hypertrophy. Norepinephrine augments c-*myc* and c-*fos* mRNA expression, and stimulation of primary cultured neonatal cardiac myocytes by alpha$_1$-adrenergic agents causes their hypertrophy and induces the fetal isoforms of actin and myosin synthesis, possibly by increasing the expression of the c-*myc* and c-*fos* proto-oncogenes. This action of the alpha-adrenergic receptor on c-*myc* and c-*fos* may occur through an increase of phosphoinositide turnover and the activation of protein kinase C.

In addition to the growth of myocytes, the interstitium also participates in pressure overload hypertrophy, which is associated with hyperplasia of fibroblasts and the deposition of excess and altered types of extracellular collagen. The relief of hemodynamic overload, either surgical or pharmacologic, usually results in partial regression of myocyte hypertrophy, but not necessarily in regression of interstitial proliferation. Exactly how mechanical load is converted into growth, a process that might be termed *mechanogrowth coupling,* is poorly understood. When myocytes are stretched in vitro an increase in mRNA and protein synthesis takes place. Thus, myocytes appear to be able to *sense* external load and to undergo hypertrophy, perhaps triggered by the activation of *stretch-activated* channels through which an influx of cations occurs.

There are many potential applications to cardiology of the growing understanding of the mechanisms involved in myocyte hypertrophy. For example, the c-*myc* proto-oncogene is expressed in the heart of the Syrian hamster with hereditary idiopathic cardiomyopathy. Since this animal model resembles the human disorder, it will be of great interest to determine if the same might be true in the latter. Investigation of this phenomenon might also reveal the mechanism by which compensatory hypertrophy may lead to myocardial failure and could suggest measures to prevent this complication. Ultimately, this knowledge could also lead to the development of a method for stimulating myocardial hypertrophy or even myocyte hyperplasia after cell death has occurred consequent to myocardial infarction, viral myocarditis, and other conditions causing myocyte necrosis.

Efforts are also under way to identify genes causing hereditary forms of cardiomyopathy or cardiac hypertrophy using the technique of genetic linkage (or cosegregation) analysis (see Chap. 6). This technique allows identification of the genetic region responsible for a disease. It is used to map the loci of genes that are tightly linked to a specific phenotype by making use of restriction fragment length polymorphisms (RFLPs), which are due to DNA sequence differences between individuals. Such an approach has been used to localize the gene responsible for Duchenne's muscular dystrophy (Chap. 365) and for cystic fibrosis (Chap. 209), and the genes for these conditions, which often affect the heart directly or indirectly, have been cloned. A high-molecular-weight protein (dystrophin) is absent from the transverse tubules of skeletal muscle of patients with Duchenne's muscular dystrophy. Presumably its absence in the myocardium is responsible for the cardiomyopathy that frequently occurs in this condition. Similarly, a gene responsible for familial hypertrophic cardiomyopathy (Chap. 192) has been mapped to chromosome 14 using genetic linkage analyses. This should allow early (including prenatal) diagnosis.

VASCULAR WALL   The renin-angiotensin system in the vascular wall may be involved in the development of hypertrophy of vascular smooth muscle. Angiotensinogen mRNA in blood vessel walls may be elevated in chronic hypertension. The addition of angiotensin II to cultures of vascular smooth-muscle cells causes the rapid activation of the c-*fos* proto-oncogene, which may mediate angiotensin II–induced hypertrophy in smooth-muscle cells in vivo. Indeed, angiotensin II induces hypertrophy of arterial smooth-muscle cells in vitro, in association with rapid induction in c-*fos*, c-*myc*, and c-*jun* mRNA levels followed by marked increases in the expression of the α chain of PDGF. This hypertrophy of vascular smooth muscle can be blocked by angiotensin-converting enzyme inhibitors. The gene for the PDGF receptor has been cloned; the PDGF receptor mediates the mitogenic effects of this substance on vascular smooth-muscle (and other) cells. The PDGF receptor has a structure similar to a family of growth factor receptors that have tyrosine kinase activity. The PDGF receptor interacts with the c-*ras* proto-oncogene product and activates phospholipase C.

Many growth factors in the cardiovascular system, such as angiotensin II, vasopressin, PDGF, and epidermal growth factor, are also vasoconstrictors. These considerations may be of significance in selecting or designing antihypertensive drugs. Indeed, angiotensin-converting enzyme inhibitors are more potent in causing regression of left ventricular hypertrophy than are direct-acting vasodilators such as hydralazine.

SPECIALIZED SARCOLEMMAL PROTEINS

ADRENERGIC AND MUSCARINIC RECEPTORS AND G PROTEINS (Fig. 173-1)   Plasma membrane receptors mediate the interaction between ligands, including drugs, neurotransmitters, and cells, and basically constitute key transmembrane signalling systems (see Chaps. 11 and 68). There are important functional and topographic analogies and amino acid sequence homologues between the beta-adrenergic receptor, the muscarinic cholinergic receptor, and rhodopsin, the light receptor in the rods of the retina. These receptors are all glycoproteins with seven membrane-spanning domains (Fig. 173-2). A reduction in the density of beta$_1$-adrenergic receptors ("down-regulation") occurs in chronic heart failure (Chap. 181) consequent to the heart's chronic exposure to the adrenergic agonist norepinephrine. Agonist-occupied receptors are preferentially phosphorylated, which leads to their dissociation from the sarcolemma and internalization in the myocyte.

After an agonist binds to a beta-adrenergic receptor, the receptor associates tightly with the G (guanine nucleotide regulatory) protein (Fig. 173-1), which in turn activates effectors such as adenylate cyclase or calcium channels (see also Chap. 68). Structure-function analyses of the beta-adrenergic receptor have defined the regions of the receptor involved in (1) binding ligands (drugs and neurotransmitters); (2) coupling to G proteins; and (3) desensitization. The ligand binding portion of the molecule lies in the transmembrane domains, and the third intracellular loop of the protein appears to be critical to the attachment of the receptor to the G protein. Beta-adrenergic and alpha$_1$-adrenergic receptors are coupled to different classes of G proteins. These proteins couple alpha$_1$ receptors to the activation of phospholipase C, which in turn breaks down a cell membrane phospholipid (PIP$_2$) into inositol trisphosphate (IP$_3$) and diacylglycerol; IP$_3$ liberates calcium from intracellular sites (see Chap. 11). G proteins may either augment or reduce the formation of the second messenger cyclic AMP. A stimulatory G protein (G$_s$) couples the beta-adrenergic receptor to adenylate cyclase, while an inhibitory G protein (G$_i$) causes inhibition of this enzyme (and therefore the formation of cyclic AMP) when muscarinic and adenosine receptors are stimulated. There is evidence that alterations in G proteins (reduced levels of G$_s$ and increased levels of G$_i$) may play a role in the pathogenesis of heart failure; the mechanism responsible for these alterations remains to be elucidated.

Five muscarinic receptor cDNAs (complementary DNAs) have

FIGURE 173-1 Ion transport through the sarcolemma of a myocyte. The Na$^+$ channel of the heart muscle cell opens briefly at the start of an action potential, permitting an influx of Na$^+$. The Na$^+$ channel can be blocked by tetrodotoxin (TTX) or by type I antiarrhythmic agents (see Chap. 185). Depolarization of the sarcolemma leads to Ca^{2+} influx through the Ca^{2+} channel, which is sensitive to the change in potential. The Ca^{2+} channel can be blocked by the calcium entry blockers. D, diltiazem; V, verapamil; DHP, dihydropyridines. Repolarization of the membrane results principally from the opening of K$^+$ channels and the efflux of K$^+$. Ca^{2+} is removed from the cell by the Na$^+$/Ca^{2+} exchanger and by a Ca^{2+}-ATPase (an energy-requiring process). The Na$^+$ pump (Na$^+$,K$^+$-ATPase) removes Na$^+$ which has flowed into the cell and returns K$^+$ to the cell by an energy-requiring process; it may be blocked by digitalis (DIG).

Two types of receptors modulate ionic pathways. Beta-adrenergic receptors (which are one kind of type 2 receptor) stimulate the production of the second messenger cyclic AMP which by causing phosphorylation (P) allows the Ca^{2+} channel to open. Muscarinic cholinergic receptors (one kind of type 1 receptor) inhibit cyclic AMP production and also activate phospholipase C, the enzyme producing the second messenger inositol trisphosphate (IP$_3$), which in smooth-muscle cells mobilizes intracellular calcium.

DIG, digitalis glycoside (Na$^+$,K$^+$-ATPase inhibitor); R$_1$ and R$_2$, binding proteins for the respective receptor types; AC, adenylate cyclase; Ni (AC-inhibiting) and Ns (AC-stimulating) nucleotide binding G proteins (G$_i$ and G$_s$, respectively); PhC, phospholipase C; PIP$_2$, phosphotidylinositol diphosphate, a membrane phospholipid; P, phosphate. (*Reproduced with permission from U Ruegg, Sandorama, 2:5, 1987.*)

been cloned. These fall into two groups: the M$_1$ subtype predominates in the vasculature and neurons and the M$_2$ subtype, linked to adenylate cyclase, predominates in the heart.

The gene for the human beta$_2$-adrenergic receptor has been cloned; it is unusual in that it lacks introns within the coding region and in

FIGURE 173-2 Structure of the human beta$_2$-adrenergic receptor as it may be organized within the membrane. Open circles represent amino acids that are identical to those of hamster beta$_2$-adrenergic receptor. (*Reproduced with permission from Dohlman et al, Biochemistry 26:2664, 1987.*)

this respect it resembles the proto-oncogene c-*mas*, which also encodes the angiotensin II receptor. The large family of receptors that are coupled to G proteins probably arose from a common ancestral gene.

An understanding of the molecular structure of cardiac receptors and of the genes which encode them is likely to lead to more rational design of drugs that can modify cardiac function by acting on these receptors.

CALCIUM CHANNELS Calcium ions play a unique role in a variety of cellular functions, in particular, contraction of cardiac and vascular smooth muscle (Chap. 181). Calcium enters cardiac cells through voltage-sensitive calcium channels (Fig. 173-1) that are controlled by transmembrane electrical potentials and open during depolarization of the sarcolemma. The catalytic subunit of cyclic AMP–dependent protein kinase enhances the opening of calcium channels, thereby increasing influx of calcium into myocytes and enhancing the force of cardiac contraction. This explains, in part, the positive inotropic actions of the beta-adrenergic agonists and of the phosphodiesterase inhibitors, both of which enhance activity of cyclic AMP.

The (L-type) cardiac calcium channels appear to be large aqueous pores through which the calcium ions move, probably in single file. Their primary structure has been elucidated by cDNA cloning. These channels are quite selective for calcium ions under physiologic conditions and are composed of several subunits, the largest of which has a molecular weight of 243,000 Da and binds calcium channel antagonists. Prolongation of the action potential occurs often in hypertrophied myocytes and may be responsible for arrhythmias in patients with heart failure. This prolongation may be due to delays in the inactivation of the L type calcium channels. Three physically associated, but distinct sites in the channels bind the three classes of calcium antagonists—nifedipine, verapamil, and diltiazem (Chap. 190). The cDNAs (DNAs complementary to their mRNA) encoding the calcium channels have been cloned, and their predicted sequences have been determined. This information should make possible the design of drugs to influence the function of these channels with greater specificity, thereby increasing the ability to control function of the myocardium and of vascular smooth muscle.

SARCOLEMMAL ATPase   One of the most important membrane proteins is the Na$^+$,K$^+$-ATPase (Fig. 173-1) which plays a critical role in establishing sodium and potassium gradients across cell membranes. This enzyme catalyzes the reaction that extrudes sodium and transports potassium into the cell against concentration gradients. This process requires the hydrolysis of ATP and is critical to the function of cardiac (and other excitable) tissue by controlling membrane potentials. Phosphorylation and ATP binding sites are on the cytoplasmic component of the enzyme, and the cardiac glycoside binding site is located on the extracellular component. Knowledge of the primary structure of the enzyme may allow the design of inhibitors perhaps more potent and/or more selective than the cardiac glycosides.

ATRIAL NATRIURETIC PEPTIDE

In 1979 de Bold and his collaborators reported that extracts from atrial myocytes had potent vasodilatory and natriuretic properties. Subsequently it was shown that the active factor is a 28-amino-acid polypeptide named atrial natriuretic peptide (ANP). ANP is released from granules in atrial myocytes during atrial stretch and binds to receptors on the surfaces of cells in the kidney (renal vessels, glomeruli, and medulla), vascular bed, and adrenal gland. In the central nervous system, ANP acts in areas known to be involved in the control of vascular resistance and in the regulation of salt and water balance.

The interaction of ANP with its receptors activates plasma membrane–associated (particulate) guanylate cyclase leading to the accumulation of cyclic GMP, which in turn activates cyclic GMP–dependent protein kinases and thereby instigates the phosphorylation of a number of intracellular proteins. In vascular smooth muscle cyclic GMP causes relaxation by phosphorylating myosin light chains, while in renal tubular epithelial cells it inhibits the activity of sodium channels. In smooth-muscle cells, by stimulating cyclic GMP–dependent protein kinase, ANP enhances the activity of a Ca^{2+}-ATPase, thereby increasing the removal of ionic calcium and promoting vascular relaxation. ANP also inhibits basal and hormone-stimulated adenylate cyclase activity in vascular smooth-muscle and renal glomerular cells.

ANP reduces cardiac output, in part by inhibiting sympathetic stimulation of the heart and in part by reducing cardiac preload. The latter results from a reduction of intravascular volume consequent to a redistribution of fluid from the vascular to the interstitial compartments, perhaps as a result of increased capillary permeability. ANP induces natriuresis and diuresis by increasing glomerular filtration rate, inhibiting Na$^+$ reabsorption in the proximal tubule and the collecting duct, and reducing aldosterone secretion; the latter results from suppression of renin secretion and from inhibition of the biosynthesis and secretion of aldosterone by the glomerulosa cells of the adrenal cortex.

Collectively, these actions serve to reduce arterial and venous pressures and blood volume. As a consequence, ANP appears to play a role as a counterregulatory hormone in many disorders characterized by volume expansion, including congestive heart failure, acute and chronic renal failure, and nephrotic syndrome, hypertension, and hepatic disease.

The biosynthetic mechanisms for ANP have been defined (Fig. 173-3). The precursor of ANP in human atrial tissue is *preproANP*, a 151-amino-acid polypeptide encoded by a gene on the short arm of chromosome 1.

Factors that stimulate ANP secretion enhance the transcription of preproANP mRNA. Cleavage of the signal peptide from preproANP results in proANP, a 126-amino-acid peptide, which is the storage form of ANP and is converted to the active hormone at the time of its secretion from the atrial myocyte; the 28-amino-acid biologically active peptide is cleaved from the C-terminus of the storage form. ANP is synthesized in adult atrium, in normal fetal ventricle, and in adult ventricle which has been stimulated by glucocorticoids or stressed by left ventricular hypertrophy. As already described at the beginning of the chapter, such diseased ventricles have increased expression of ANP mRNA.

Additional stimuli affect the production and secretion of ANP. Glucocorticoids play a significant role in stimulating the secretion of

FIGURE 173-3   Schematic representation of the ANP gene, messenger RNA (mRNA), and precursor (pro-ANP). Arabic numerals indicate the positions of coding sequences to the respective amino acids in pro-ANP. The gene contains three coding regions or exons (I, II, III) and two intervening sequences (introns), as well as a typical iniation site (T) and poly-A tail (A). A putative glucocorticoid recognition site (GR) exists in the second intron. The mRNA contains untranslated regions (ut) at the 5′ and 3′ ends and also codes for a signal peptide (hatched region) which is typical for secreted proteins and is presumably cleaved cotranslationally. ANP (shaded region) is derived from the C-terminus (COOH) of pro-ANP, following hydrolytic cleavage between residue 98 and 99 in the heart but possibly at other points in extracardiac tissues. (*Reproduced with permission from SA Atlas, Recent Prog Horm Res 42:207–249, 1986.*)

ANP. There appears to be a glucocorticoid regulatory element near the ANP gene, and glucocorticoids increase its rate of transcription. Endothelin (see later), a potent vasoconstrictor released by endothelial cells, also increases the release of ANP from atrial myocytes; this may serve as a counterregulatory influence to the vasoconstrictor.

The elucidation of the structure of the ANP gene and the understanding of the mechanism by which ANP is synthesized, processed, and released represents a major advance in understanding the control of the circulation and regulation of blood volume. Analogues of ANP or substances that influence its synthesis and release or mimic its actions are being developed and should be useful in the treatment of a broad array of pathophysiologic states.

APOPROTEINS AND ATHEROGENESIS

Abnormalities in the number or function of the low-density lipoprotein (LDL) receptors are responsible for some forms of atherosclerosis (Chaps. 195 and 326). Abnormalities of the *apoproteins,* many of which are genetic, may play more frequent roles in atherogenesis. At least 10 apoproteins are embedded in the surface of the spherical lipoprotein particles that carry the lipids in the bloodstream and are encoded by genes localized to chromosomes 1, 2, 6, 11, and 19 (the LDL receptor gene is also on chromosome 19). Amino acid sequences suggest that several of these apoproteins are derived from a common ancestral gene. The major functions of apoproteins are to serve as (1) ligands that interact with cellular receptors for the lipoprotein particles, (2) cofactors of enzymes involved in lipid metabolism, and (3) structural components of the lipoproteins.

High-density lipoproteins (HDL) take up excess cholesterol from cells, and the concentration of circulating HDL is related inversely to the risk of the development of ischemic heart disease (Chaps. 195 and 326). Apoproteins AI, CIII, and AIV are three HDL apoproteins encoded by genes clustered on chromosome 11. Several disorders are associated with mutations of these apoproteins, leading to a defect in the synthesis or function of HDL and the development of premature atherosclerosis. For example, apo AI serves as a cofactor for the enzyme lecithin cholesterol acyl transferase (LCAT) which catalyzes the reaction that converts cholesterol taken up by the HDL particle into the form in which it is transported, i.e., cholesteryl ester. Some variants of apo AI are defective for this cofactor activity, thereby preventing the normal function of HDL and causing premature atherosclerosis.

Apo E is one of the principal constituents of very low density lipoproteins (VLDL) and of chylomicron remnants, the latter particles having great atherogenic activity. Three alleles of the apo E gene have been described. Subjects who are homozygous for the *e2* allele, which encodes apo E2, have decreased clearance of VLDL and chylomicron remnants from the circulation, presumably because apo E2 fails to bind normally to lipoprotein receptors. As a consequence, the *e2* allele plays a permissive role in the development of type III hyperlipoproteinemia, a condition associated with the development of xanthomas and premature atherosclerosis (Chap. 195). Patients who are homozygous for the *e4* allele, encoding for apo E4, have a reduced catabolism of LDL and premature atherosclerosis.

Elevation of the plasma concentration of Lp(a) (referred to as "lipoprotein little a") is another important risk factor for the development of premature atherosclerosis. Its protein components consist of apo B100 linked to apo(a). Six inherited apo(a) isoproteins and a series of alleles at a single gene locus control the apo(a) phenotypes and appear to determine the Lp(a) concentration. An interesting clue to the mechanism by which Lp(a) accelerates atherosclerosis has recently emerged. Through cDNA cloning and the deduced protein structure, it has been shown that apo(a) is a deformed relative of plasminogen, the precursor of the proteolytic enzyme plasmin, which dissolves fibrin clots (Chap. 288). Apo(a) contains 37 copies of kringle 4 (a portion of the plasminogen molecule in the shape of the Danish pastry known as *kringle*) followed by kringle 5

and the protease domain. This strong resemblance between a lipoprotein and plasminogen may provide a link between lipids, the clotting system, and atherogenesis. Microthrombi containing fibrin on the vessel wall become incorporated into atherosclerotic plaques. Kringle 4 of plasminogen normally binds to fibrin during fibrinolysis. Apo(a), with many copies of this kringle, could also bind to fibrin in microthrombi in the vessel wall. Following endothelial damage, Lp(a) may insinuate itself into the arterial wall, inhibiting the cleavage of fibrin in microthrombi by competing with plasminogen for access to fibrin.

Discussed above are three examples of how the genes encoding apolipoproteins can play a critical role in determining the risk for the development of atherosclerosis. It may prove to be cost-effective to attempt to identify genetic defects of apoproteins (as well as of the LDL receptor) in childhood and to use a preventive approach *selectively* on subjects identified by such genetic analyses, as opposed to the broad *shotgun* preventive approach that is currently in vogue and that is directed nonselectively at the entire population.

PLATELETS

Platelets (see Chap. 287) are intimately involved in three critical aspects of coronary artery disease: (1) they participate in the progression of the underlying atherogenic process; (2) they form the nidus of the coronary thrombus responsible for acute myocardial infarction; and (3) they may release vasoactive substances that can cause coronary vasoconstriction. Activated platelets secrete alpha granules that contain platelet factor 4, a procoagulant that neutralizes the action of heparin and several growth factors, including alpha and beta fibroblast growth factors and PDGF (see Chap. 9). The latter, a 30,000-Da protein, is also generated by macrophages and endothelial cells. PDGF acts on at least two specific membrane receptors which have been cloned. It is a powerful vasoconstrictor and a potent growth factor that stimulates DNA synthesis and proliferation of arterial smooth-muscle cells, an important step in atherogenesis.

PDGF may also be involved in malignant transformation. Its amino acid sequence is almost identical to that of a segment of transforming factor of the simian sarcoma virus (SSV), an acute transforming virus that induces the cells it invades to produce viral proteins, one of which, the v-*sis* gene product, causes monkey cells to undergo malignant transformation (Chap. 9).

Other substances released from aggregating platelets possess potent vasoactive properties; serotonin and thromboxane A_2 cause vasoconstriction, while ATP and ADP cause relaxation (through release of endothelium-derived relaxing factor, see below). The net effect of these influences depends on the presence of intact endothelium. In the normal endothelium the vasodilator influences dominate, while in the dysfunctional endothelium, as discussed below, the vasoconstrictor influences prevail.

ENDOTHELIUM

For many years the endothelium, the monolayer of cells in direct contact with blood, was considered to be a relatively inert, smooth boundary between the blood and the vascular wall (Fig. 173-4). In fact, endothelial cells are quite active metabolically and normally produce a number of substances that affect the vascular lumen as well as platelets.

The first and best known of the endothelial vasodilators is prostacyclin (PGI_2) (see Chap. 69), which also inhibits the adhesion and aggregation of platelets. The action of PGI_2 involves the activation of adenylate cyclase and formation of cyclic AMP. When stimulated by a large number of substances, including ATP and ADP, acetylcholine, thrombin, neurotransmitters, and serotonin, the normal endothelium also releases a labile, highly diffusible vasodilator, termed endothelium-derived relaxing factor (EDRF), which appears

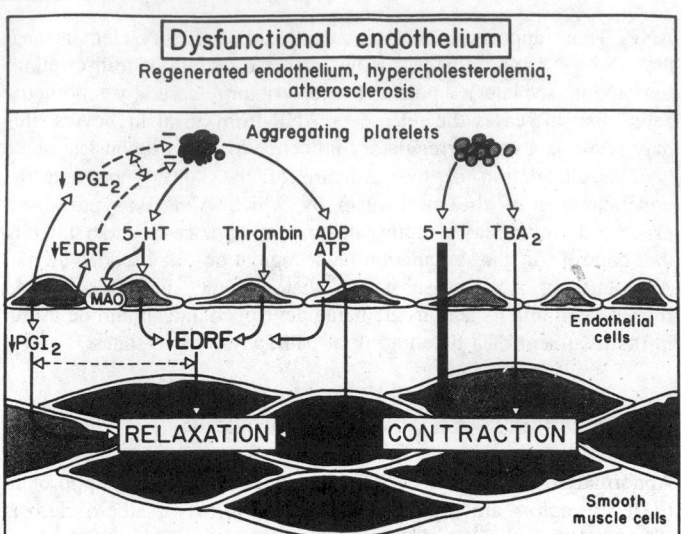

FIGURE 173-4 Current concepts of endothelium-derived factors and their modulation of vascular smooth-muscle contraction: Endothelium-derived relaxing factor (EDRF), a potent vasodilator of the underlying smooth muscle, increases cyclic GMP (cGMP) levels through activation of soluble guanylate cyclase. Prostacyclin (PGI₂) is another vasodilator released from the endothelium but whose effects depend on elevation of cyclic AMP (cAMP) through activation of adenylate cyclase. EDRF and PGI₂ may act synergistically in relaxing vascular smooth muscle and inhibiting platelet aggregation. The endothelial cells also secrete a hyperpolarizing factor (EDHF), the exact nature of which is unknown and which also has a vasodilator action. There are at least two endothelium-derived contracting factors; one is indomethacin-insensitive (EDCF₁) and may be endothelin, while the other is indomethacin-sensitive (EDCF₂) and may be superoxide anion. ACh, acetylcholine; 5-HT, 5-hydroxytryptamine (serotonin); ADP, adenosine diphosphate; AA, arachidonic acid; +, synergism or facilitation; −, inhibition; ?, exact nature unknown; M, muscarinic receptor; S, serotonergic receptor; P, purinergic receptor; T, thrombin receptor; V, vasopressinergic receptor. (*Reproduced with permission from P Vanhoutte and Shimokawa, Circulation 80:1, 1989.*)

FIGURE 173-5 Responses of dysfunctional endothelium. The endothelium is dysfunctional when it is in a regenerated state, in the presence of hypercholesterolemia, hypertension, or atherosclerosis, releasing less endothelium-derived relaxing factor (EDRF), whereas the ability of the smooth muscle to contract is unaltered. As a result, in endothelial dysfunction smooth-muscle contraction predominates. In atherosclerosis, the production of both EDRF and prostacyclin (PGI₂) are reduced, and their synergistic actions against aggregating platelets may not occur, enhancing platelet aggregation. This may lead to thrombus formation, enhanced vascular contraction, and atherogenesis. 5-HT, 5-hydroxytryptamine (serotonin); ADP, adenosine diphosphate; ATP, adenosine triphosphate; TBA2, thromboxane A₂; MAO, monomine oxidase; ms, inhibition; +, synergism. (*Reproduced with permission from Vanhoutte and Shimokawa, Circulation 80:1, 1989.*)

to be nitric oxide (NO). Normal endothelium also releases EDRF when stimulated by the shear stress of flowing blood, thereby controlling the lumen of arteries and arterioles in relation to the blood flow through the vessel. EDRF stimulates soluble guanylate cyclase, which catalyzes the formation of cyclic GMP, which in turn relaxes vascular smooth muscle. EDRF also inhibits adhesion and aggregation of platelets, an action apparently also mediated by cyclic GMP. EDRF and prostacyclin interact synergistically to dilate blood vessels and inhibit platelet aggregation.

When the endothelium is destroyed or damaged (Fig. 173-5), as in atherosclerotic plaques, EDRF production may be impaired, thereby permitting coronary vasoconstriction in the vicinity of such plaques. Moreover, subtle damage to the endothelium, as in hypertension, some forms of hyperlipidemia, reperfusion after ischemia, and in regenerating endothelium after mechanical trauma, leads to defective release of EDRF. On the other hand, the eicosapentanoic acid in fish oils stimulates the production of EDRF, perhaps explaining the putative antiatherogenic properties of these substances.

Endothelium also synthesizes thrombomodulin, a glycoprotein with a molecular weight of 105,000 whose gene has been isolated. Thrombomodulin serves as an endothelial receptor for thrombin. When thrombin is bound to thrombomodulin, which is located on the luminal side of the vascular endothelium, it loses its procoagulant activity (conversion of fibrinogen to fibrin, stimulation of platelets), the rate at which it is inactivated by antithrombin III is accelerated, and its activation of protein C, an anticoagulant, is enhanced.

Endothelium also releases at least two vasoconstrictors, one a product of cyclooxygenase activity that appears to be responsible for hypoxia-induced vascular contraction. The other is a 21-amino-acid peptide called *endothelin*, an extremely potent vasoconstrictor. The

expression of the gene for endothelin appears to be inhibited by the shear stress of flowing blood, a mechanism that appears to act in concert with the release of EDRF by the same stimulus to enhance vessel diameter as flow increases. In hypertension, EDRF release is impaired, whereas the release of endothelial-derived contracting factor(s) may be augmented, presumably aggravating this condition. Like PDGF, endothelin is both a vasoconstrictor and a smooth-muscle mitogen.

In early atherosclerosis, dysfunction of a G protein in endothelial cells may play a role in the failure of EDRF release. Endothelial injury or dysfunction also enhances platelet deposition on the arterial wall. If unopposed by EDRF and prostacyclin, serotonin and thromboxane A₂ released from the deposited platelets cause arterial constriction and spasm in the coronary arterial system. The adhesion and aggregation of platelets consequent to the defective production of EDRF enhances further the atherosclerotic process.

ANGIOGENESIS

Endothelial cells also secrete a group of growth factors that are mitogenic for endothelium and can induce formation of new blood vessels (angiogenesis). Angiogenic stimuli cause the elongation and proliferation of endothelial cells and the generation of new vessels. A group of angiogenic mitogens, which are heparin-binding peptides related to endothelial cell growth factors, have been identified. The amino acid sequences of several of these growth factors have been deduced by cloning and analysis of their genes.

Angiogenesis is of considerable pathogenetic significance. Folkman has postulated that the growth of tumors depends on an adequate blood supply, which in turn is dependent on the growth of new vessels into the tumors; the latter is stimulated by angiogenesis factors(s) secreted by the tumor. Inhibition of angiogenesis can cause tumor regression in animal models. Abnormal angiogenesis may be involved in diverse disease states, including diabetic retinopathy, neovascular glaucoma, rheumatoid arthritis, and psoriasis.

The development of new vessels in the heart, i.e., of the coronary collateral circulation, is of critical importance in protecting the myocardium from the consequences of coronary obstruction. The extent of the collateral circulation varies enormously among patients with similar degrees of coronary arterial narrowing, and this difference may be related in part to differences in the production of angiogenic factors. It has been speculated that the introduction of purified angiogenic factors directly into ischemic myocardium might enhance the development of collaterals, accelerate the healing of the necrotic tissue, and prevent infarct expansion and cardiac dilatation. Angiogenesis may also be deleterious. Coronary atheroma are highly vascularized by a fragile capillary network, and rupture of these newly formed capillaries when they are exposed to high intravascular pressures may lead to hemorrhage into atherosclerotic plaques and coronary occlusion.

CONCLUSIONS

The applications of cellular and molecular biology to studies of the myocardium, vascular wall, platelets, and lipoproteins have already increased greatly our understanding of the fundamental abnormalities in cardiovascular disease. In the future these approaches are likely to improve the diagnosis of patients with genetic disorders causing cardiac disease, help to identify individuals at risk of developing these disorders, thereby leading to the institution of preventive measures, and provide new agents for the treatment and prevention of cardiovascular diseases.

REFERENCES

BRAUNWALD E: On future directions for cardiology: The Paul Dudley White lecture. Circulation 77:1:13, 1988

BRENNER BM et al: The diverse biological actions of atrial natriuretic peptide. Physiol Rev (in press)

CATTERALL WA: Structure and function of voltage-sensitive ion channels. Science 242:50, 1988

CHIEN KR, KNOWLTON KU: Cardiovascular molecular biology. Circulation 80:2:219, 1989

FOLKMAN J, WEISZ PD: Control of angiogenesis, in Biocatalysis and Biometrics, JD Burrington, DS Clark (eds). Washington, DC, American Chemical Society, ACS Symposium Series 392, 1989, pp 19–32

FURCHGOTT RF, VANHOUTTE PM: Endothelium-derived relaxing and contracting factors. FASEB J 3:2007, 1989

HATHAWAY DR, MARCH KL: Molecular biology: New avenues for the diagnosis and treatment of cardiovascular disease. J Am Coll Cardiol 13:265, 1989

JARCHO JA et al: Mapping a gene for familial hypertrophic cardiomyopathy to chromosome 14ql. N Engl J Med 321:1372, 1989

KATZ AM: Molecular biology in cardiology, a paradigmatic shift. J Mol Cell Biol 20:355, 1988 (editorial)

VANHOUTTE PM, SHIMOKAWA H: Endothelium-derived relaxing factor and coronary vasospasm. Circulation 80:1, 1989

VENTER JC, TRIGGLE D (eds): Structure and Physiology of the Slow Inward Calcium Channel. New York, Alan R. Liss, 1987

174 APPROACH TO THE PATIENT WITH HEART DISEASE

EUGENE BRAUNWALD

The symptoms caused by heart disease result most commonly from myocardial ischemia, from disturbance of the contraction or relaxation of the myocardium, or from an abnormal cardiac rhythm or rate. Ischemia is manifest most frequently as chest discomfort, while reduction of the pumping ability of the heart commonly leads to

weakness and fatigability or, when severe, produces cyanosis, hypotension, syncope, and elevated intravascular pressure behind a failing ventricle; the latter results in abnormal fluid accumulation, which in turn leads to dyspnea, orthopnea, and edema. Cardiac arrhythmias often develop suddenly, and the resulting signs and symptoms—palpitation, dyspnea, angina, hypotension, and syncope—generally occur abruptly and may disappear as rapidly as they develop.

A cardinal principle useful in the evaluation of the patient with suspected heart disease is that myocardial or coronary function which may be adequate at rest may be inadequate during exertion. Thus, a history of chest discomfort and/or dyspnea which appears only during activity is characteristic of heart disease, while the opposite pattern, i.e., the appearance of these symptoms at rest and their remission during exertion, is rarely observed in patients with organic heart disease.

Patients with cardiocirculatory disease may also be asymptomatic, both at rest and during exertion, but may present an abnormal physical finding, such as a heart murmur, elevated systemic arterial pressure, or an abnormality of the electrocardiogram or of the cardiac silhouette on the chest roentgenogram. Increasingly, patients are discovered to have asymptomatic ischemia on an exercise stress test or an ambulatory electrocardiogram.

Diseases of the heart and circulation are so common and the laity is so well acquainted with the major symptoms resulting from these disorders that patients, and occasionally physicians, erroneously attribute many noncardiac complaints to organic cardiovascular disease. Furthermore, the combination of the widespread fear of heart disease in the western world with the deep-seated emotional connotations concerning this organ's function results in the frequent development in persons with normal cardiovascular systems of symptoms which mimic those of organic disease. Sometimes it is difficult to interpret correctly the symptoms of patients with recognized organic cardiovascular disturbances. Such patients, in addition to having symptoms resulting from their disease, may also develop functional complaints referable to the cardiovascular system. The unraveling of symptoms and signs due to organic heart disease from those which are not directly related is an important and challenging task in these patients.

It must be recognized that dyspnea, one of the cardinal manifestations of diminished cardiac reserve, is not limited to disease of the heart, but is also characteristic of conditions as diverse as pulmonary disease, marked obesity, and anxiety (Chap. 36). Similarly, chest discomfort (Chap. 16) may result from a variety of causes other than myocardial ischemia. Whether heart disease is responsible for these symptoms can frequently be determined by carrying out a detailed clinical examination. Noninvasive testing using electrocardiography at rest and during exercise (Chap. 176), roentgenography, and echocardiography (Chap. 177) usually provide important additional information to permit the correct interpretation of symptoms; more specialized invasive examinations (catheterization and angiography) are occasionally necessary.

DIAGNOSIS In every branch of medicine the establishment of the prognosis and the development of a rational plan of management are based on a correct diagnostic appraisal. In patients with disorders of the cardiocirculatory system, particular care must be taken to establish not only a correct but also a *complete* diagnosis. As outlined by the New York Heart Association, the elements of a complete cardiac diagnosis include consideration of

1 *The underlying etiology.* Is the disease congenital, rheumatic, hypertensive, or ischemic in origin?
2 *The anatomic abnormalities.* Which chambers are enlarged? Which valves are affected? Is there pericardial involvement? Has there been a myocardial infarction?
3 *The physiologic disturbances.* Is an arrhythmia present? Is there evidence of congestive heart failure or of myocardial ischemia?
4 *The extent of functional disability.* How strenuous is the physical

activity required to elicit symptoms? The latter should be evaluated in the light of the intensity of therapy.

Two simple examples may serve to illustrate the importance of establishing a complete diagnosis: (1) The identification of myocardial ischemia as the cause of exertional chest discomfort is of great clinical importance. However, this diagnosis is insufficient to develop either a strategy of specific treatment or prognosis until the underlying disease process, e.g., coronary atherosclerosis or aortic stenosis, which is responsible for the myocardial ischemia, is identified and a judgment made as to whether severe anemia, thyrotoxicosis, or supraventricular tachycardia plays a contributory role. (2) Determining that heart disease is congenital provides an important starting point, but the decision about whether surgical treatment is advisable depends upon the specific anatomic defect present and often upon the nature of the physiologic disturbance and the functional impairment as well.

The establishment of a correct and complete cardiac diagnosis often requires the use of six different methods of examination: (1) history, (2) physical examination (Chap. 175), (3) electrocardiogram (Chap. 176), (4) chest roentgenogram (Chap. 177), (5) noninvasive graphic examinations (echocardiogram, radionuclide scanning techniques, and other newer "noninvasive" imaging techniques, Chaps. 177 and 178), and occasionally (6) specialized "invasive" examinations, such as cardiac catheterization, angiocardiography, and coronary arteriography (Chap. 179). In order to be most effective, the results obtained from each of these six modalities should be analyzed independently of one another as well as with the information derived from the other methods clearly in mind. Only in this way can one avoid overlooking a subtle, though extremely significant, finding. For example, an electrocardiogram should be obtained in every patient suspected of having heart disease. It may provide the critical clue in establishing the correct diagnosis, e.g., the finding of a moderate atrioventricular conduction disturbance in a patient with unexplained syncope, even when all other methods of examination reveal no abnormal findings. On the other hand, when combined intelligently with the results of other methods of examination, the electrocardiogram may provide essential confirmatory data. Thus, the knowledge that a patient has an apical diastolic rumbling murmur may direct particular attention to the P waves, and the recognition of left atrial enlargement electrocardiographically supports the suggestion that the murmur is caused by mitral stenosis. Under these circumstances the additional finding on the electrocardiogram of right ventricular hypertrophy suggests that pulmonary hypertension is present and that the mitral stenosis is severe.

Although the electrocardiogram is an invaluable aspect of every cardiovascular examination, with the exception of the identification of arrhythmias it rarely permits establishment of a specific diagnosis. In the absence of other abnormal findings, electrocardiographic changes must not be overinterpreted. The range of normal electrocardiographic findings is wide, and the tracing can be affected significantly by many noncardiac factors, such as age, body habitus, and serum electrolyte concentrations.

In obtaining the history of the patient with known or suspected cardiovascular disease, particular attention should be directed to the family history. Familial clustering is common in many forms of heart disease. Genetic transmission may occur, as in hypertrophic cardiomyopathy (Chap. 192) or Marfan's syndrome (Chap. 333). In patients with essential hypertension or coronary atherosclerosis the genetic component may be less obvious but is also of considerable importance. Familial clustering of cardiovascular diseases may occur not only on a genetic basis but may also be related to familial dietary or behavior patterns, such as excessive injection of salt or calories, or cigarette smoking.

When an attempt is made to ascertain the severity of functional impairment in a patient with heart disease, it is essential to determine the precise extent of activity and the rate at which it is performed before symptoms develop. Thus, breathlessness which occurs after running up two long flights of stairs denotes far less functional impairment than similar symptoms occurring after taking a few steps on the level. Also, the degree of customary physical activity at work and during recreation should be considered. The development of two-flight dyspnea in a marathon runner may be far more significant than the development of one-flight dyspnea in a previously sedentary person. Similarly, the history must include a detailed consideration of the patient's therapeutic regimen. For example, the persistence or development of edema, breathlessness, and other manifestations of heart failure in a patient whose diet is rigidly restricted in sodium content and who is receiving optimum doses of diuretics must be interpreted quite differently from the finding of edema in the absence of these measures. In an effort to ascertain the rate of progression of symptoms, and thereby of the severity of the underlying illness, it may be useful to ascertain what, if any, specific tasks the patient could carry out 1 year earlier which he or she cannot carry out now.

PITFALLS IN CARDIOVASCULAR MEDICINE Increasing subspecialization in internal medicine and the perfection of advanced diagnostic techniques in cardiology may sometimes be accompanied by several undesirable consequences, which can be summarized as follows:

1 Failure by the *noncardiologist* to recognize cardiac manifestations of systemic illnesses. The latter include but are not limited to (a) the Down syndrome (associated with endocardial cushion defect); (b) gonadal dysgenesis, i.e., Turner's syndrome (associated with a variety of congenital cardiovascular defects, particularly coarctation of the aorta); (c) bony abnormalities of the upper extremities (associated with atrial septal defect), the Holt-Oram syndrome; (d) muscular dystrophies (associated with cardiomyopathy); (e) hemochromatosis and glycogen storage disease (associated with myocardial infiltration); (f) congenital deafness (associated with prolonged QT interval and serious cardiac arrhythmias); (g) Raynaud's disease (associated with primary pulmonary hypertension and coronary vasospasm); (h) connective tissue disorders, i.e., Marfan's syndrome, Ehlers-Danlos syndrome, Hurler's syndrome, and related disorders of mucopolysaccharide metabolism (aortic dilatation, prolapsed mitral valve, a variety of arterial abnormalities); (i) chronic hemolytic anemia (cardiac dilatation); (j) Refsum's disease (myocardial failure and conduction defects); (k) acromegaly (accelerated coronary atherosclerosis, conduction defects, cardiomyopathy); (l) hyperthyroidism (heart failure, atrial fibrillation); (m) hypothyroidism (pericardial effusion, coronary artery disease); (n) rheumatoid arthritis (pericarditis, aortic valve disease); (o) Whipple's disease (pericarditis and endocarditis); (p) scleroderma (cor pulmonale, myocardial fibrosis, pericarditis); (q) systemic lupus erythematosus (valvulitis, myocarditis, pericarditis); (r) polymyositis (pericarditis, myocarditis); (s) sarcoidosis (arrhythmias, cardiomyopathy); (t) Fabry's disease (myocardial ischemia, heart failure); and (u) exfoliative dermatitis (high-output heart failure). In patients in whom these and other systemic disorders in which cardiovascular involvement may occur, a detailed cardiovascular examination should be carried out.

2 Failure by the cardiac specialist to recognize an underlying systemic illness, such as those listed above, among patients with a cardiac disorder. Patients known or suspected of having heart disease require a detailed general assessment and a search for the frequent noncardiac manifestations of systemic disorders with cardiovascular manifestations. Indeed, the cardiovascular abnormality may provide the clue critical to the recognition of these systemic disorders. Closely related is the failure to appreciate the profound effects of stress, such as that resulting from an intercurrent infection, from pregnancy, or from emotional disturbances, on cardiovascular performance and symptoms.

3 Overreliance on and overutilization of laboratory tests, particularly specialized invasive techniques for the examination of the cardiovascular system. Catheterization of the right and left sides of the heart, selective angiography, and coronary arteriography (Chap. 179) provide precise diagnostic information under many circum-

stances. For example, they aid in establishing a specific anatomic diagnosis and in determining the physiologic consequences of the abnormalities in patients with congenital heart disease and in patients with chest pain of uncertain etiology in whom coronary artery disease is suspected, and in determining the functional significance of valvular abnormalities in patients with rheumatic heart disease being considered for surgical treatment. Although a great deal of attention has been lavished on the newer specialized laboratory examinations, it should be recognized that they serve to *supplement,* not *supplant,* a careful examination carried out by clinical and noninvasive examination. There is an unfortunate tendency to carry out procedures such as coronary arteriography in patients with chest pain suspected of having coronary artery disease instead of taking a detailed and thoughtful history; although it may be established whether the coronary arteries are obstructed, the results often do not provide a definite answer to the question of whether a patient's complaint of chest pain is clearly attributable to coronary arteriosclerosis. Coronary arteriography is often carried out unnecessarily in patients with mild symptoms and signs of myocardial ischemia during exertion with normal left ventricular function who are not likely to be candidates for coronary bypass surgery. Similarly, catheterization of the left side of the heart is all too frequently employed to determine whether operative treatment of valvular disease is indicated, even before the patient has had a trial of medical therapy. Despite their enormous value, it must not be overlooked that these specialized examinations entail some small risk to the patient, involve discomfort and substantial cost, and place a strain on existing medical facilities. Therefore, *they should be carried out not as part of a "fishing expedition" or as evidence to the patient and the family that "everything is being done," but only if, after detailed clinical examination and assessment by noninvasive tests, the results of the invasive examination can be expected to modify or aid in the patient's management.*

TREATMENT   After a complete diagnosis has been established, a number of therapeutic options are usually available. Several examples may be used to demonstrate some of the principles of modern cardiovascular therapeutics:

1 In the absence of evidence for the existence of heart disease a clear, definitive statement to that effect should be made and the patient should *not* be asked to return at intervals for repeated examinations. If there is no evidence for disease, such attention may lead to the patient developing an inappropriate and abnormal fixation on the heart.

2 If there is no evidence of cardiovascular disease but the patient has one or more risk factors for the development of ischemic heart disease (Chap. 195), a plan for their reduction should be developed and the patient should be retested at intervals to assess that he or she is complying and that these risk factors are in fact being reduced.

3 Asymptomatic or mildly symptomatic patients with established organic heart disease, e.g., valvular heart disease, should be evaluated periodically, e.g., every 6 to 12 months, by clinical and noninvasive examinations (Chap. 177). Early warning signs of deterioration of ventricular function can be detected in this manner and in appropriate patients may signify the need for cardiac catheterization and surgical treatment before the development of disabling symptoms, irreversible myocardial damage, and an excessive risk of surgical treatment (Chap. 188).

4 It is critical for the physician to establish clear criteria for deciding on the form of treatment (medical, angioplasty, or surgical revascularization) in patients with ischemic heart disease (Chap. 190). Surgical treatment represents a major therapeutic advance in the treatment of this most common form of heart disease, but operation has probably been employed too widely in the United States; the mere presence of angina pectoris and/or the demonstration of coronary arterial narrowing at angiography should not reflexly

evoke a decision to treat the patient surgically. Instead, this form of treatment should be limited to those patients with ischemic heart disease in whom it has been demonstrated that surgical treatment is superior to medical treatment.

REFERENCES

BRAUNWALD E (ed): *Heart Disease,* 3d ed. Philadelphia, Saunders, 1988

FOWLER NO: *Cardiac Diagnosis and Treatment,* 3d ed. Hagerstown, Harper & Row, 1980

HORWITZ LD, GROVES BM (eds): *Signs and Symptoms in Cardiology.* Philadelphia, Lippincott, 1985

HURST JW et al (ed): *The Heart,* 7th ed. New York, McGraw-Hill, 1990

KANNEL WB: Contribution of the Framingham Study to preventive cardiology. *J Am Coll Cardiol* 15;1:206, 1990

NEW YORK HEART ASSOCIATION, INC, CRITERIA COMMITTEE: *Nomenclature and Criteria for Diagnosis of Diseases of the Heart and Great Vessels,* 8th ed. Boston, Little, Brown, 1981

PERLOFF JK (ed): *Physical Examination of the Heart and Circulation,* 2d ed. Philadelphia, Saunders, 1990

175 PHYSICAL EXAMINATION OF THE CARDIOVASCULAR SYSTEM

ROBERT A. O'ROURKE / EUGENE BRAUNWALD

An attentive physical examination remains a cost-effective method for assessing the status of the cardiovascular system and often provides important information relative to the appropriate selection of additional tests. The general physical appearance should first be assessed. The patient may appear tired because of a chronic low cardiac output; the respiratory rate may be rapid, indicating pulmonary venous congestion. Central cyanosis, often associated with clubbing of the fingers and toes, indicates right-to-left cardiac or extracardiac shunting or inadequate oxygenation of blood by the lungs. Cyanosis in the distal extremities, cool skin, and increased sweating result from vasoconstriction in patients with severe heart failure (Chap. 37). Noncardiovascular details can be equally important. For example, the diagnosis of infective endocarditis is highly likely in patients with petechiae, Osler's nodes, and Janeway lesions (Chap. 90).

The blood pressure should be taken in both arms and with the patient supine and upright; the heart rate should be timed for 1 min. Orthostatic hypotension and tachycardia may indicate a reduced blood volume, while resting tachycardia may be a clue to the presence of severe heart failure.

Careful examination of the optic fundi is essential (Chap. 196), and the retinal vessels may show evidence of systemic hypertension, arteriosclerosis, or embolism. The latter may result from atherosclerosis in larger arteries (e.g., carotid) or may represent a complication of valvular heart disease (e.g., endocarditis).

Palpation of the peripheral arterial pulses in the upper and lower extremities is necessary to define the adequacy of systemic blood flow and to detect the presence of occlusive arterial lesions. It is also important to examine both legs for evidence of edema, varicose veins, or thrombophlebitis (Chap. 198). The cardiovascular examination includes careful evaluation of both the carotid arterial and the jugular venous pulses, as well as deliberate precordial palpation and attentive cardiac auscultation. An understanding of the events of the cardiac cycle is vital to performing an accurate cardiovascular examination.

ARTERIAL PRESSURE PULSE   The normal central aortic pulse wave is characterized by a fairly rapid rise to a somewhat rounded peak (Fig. 175-1). The anacrotic shoulder, present on the ascending limb, occurs at the time of peak rate of aortic flow just before maximum pressure is reached. The less steep descending limb is interrupted by a sharp downward deflection, synchronous with aortic valve closure, called the *incisura.* As the pulse wave is transmitted peripherally, the initial upstroke becomes steeper, the anacrotic

FIGURE 175-1 *A.* Schematic representation of electrocardiogram, aortic pressure pulse (AOP), phonocardiogram recorded at the apex, and apexcardiogram (ACG). On the phonocardiogram, S_1, S_2, S_3, and S_4 represent the first through fourth heart sounds; OS represents the opening snap of the mitral valve, which occurs coincident with the O point of the apexcardiogram. S_3 occurs coincident with the termination of the rapid-filling wave (RFW) of the ACG, while S_4 occurs coincident with the a wave of the ACG. *B.* Simultaneous recording of electrocardiogram, indirect carotid pulse (CP), phonocardiogram along the left sternal border (LSB), and indirect jugular venous pulse (JVP). ES, ejection sound; SC, systolic click.

shoulder becomes less apparent, and the incisura is replaced by the smoother dicrotic notch. Accordingly, palpation of a peripheral arterial pulse (e.g., radial) frequently gives less information than examination of a more central pulse (e.g., carotid) regarding alterations in left ventricular ejection or aortic valve function. However, certain findings such as the hyperkinetic pulse of aortic regurgitation or pulsus alternans are more readily evident in peripheral than in central arteries (Fig. 175-2). The carotid pulse usually is best examined with the sternocleidomastoid muscle relaxed and with the head rotated slightly toward the examiner. In examining the brachial arterial pulse, the examiner can support the subject's relaxed elbow with his or her right arm while compressing the brachial pulse with the thumb. The usual technique for palpating the pulse is to compress the artery with the thumb or forefinger until the maximum pulse is sensed. The examiner should apply varying degrees of pressure while concentrating on the separate phases of the pulse wave. This method, known as *trisection*, is useful for assessing the sharpness of the upstroke, systolic peak, and diastolic slope of the arterial pulse. In most normal persons a dicrotic wave is not palpable.

A small weak pulse, *pulsus parvus*, is frequently present in conditions with a diminished left ventricular stroke volume, a narrow pulse pressure, and increased peripheral vascular resistance (Fig. 175-2). A *hypokinetic* pulse may be due to hypovolemia, to left ventricular failure secondary to myocardial disease or myocardial

FIGURE 175-2 Schematic representation of arterial pulse waveforms that occur with alterations in cardiac hemodynamics which may result from normal physiologic responses or may be due to cardiac disease. S, systole; D, diastole. (*Modified from RA O'Rourke, in JW Hurst et al, eds. The Heart, 7th ed, New York, McGraw-Hill, 1990, with permission.*)

A. Hypokinetic Pulse   B. Parvus et Tardus Pulse   C. Hyperkinetic Pulse

D. Bisferiens Pulse   E. Dicrotic Pulse + Alternans

infarction, to restrictive pericardial disease, or to mitral valve stenosis. In aortic valve stenosis the delayed systolic peak, *pulsus tardus*, is the result of mechanical obstruction to left ventricular ejection and is often accompanied by the transmission of a coarse systolic thrill. In contrast, a large bounding or *hyperkinetic* pulse is usually associated with an increased left ventricular stroke volume, a wide pulse pressure, and a decrease in peripheral vascular resistance. This occurs characteristically in patients with abnormally elevated stroke volumes as in complete heart block, hyperkinetic circulation due to anxiety, anemia, exercise, or fever, or in patients with an abnormally rapid runoff of blood from the arterial system (patent ductus arteriosus, peripheral arteriovenous fistula). Patients with mitral regurgitation or a ventricular septal defect may also have a bounding pulse, since vigorous left ventricular ejection produces a rapid upstroke in the arterial pulse even though the duration of systole and the forward stroke volume may be diminished. In aortic regurgitation the rapidly rising, bounding arterial pulse results from increased left ventricular stroke volume and the associated increased rate of ventricular ejection.

The *bisferiens pulse*, which consists of two systolic peaks, is characteristic of aortic regurgitation (with or without accompanying stenosis) and of hypertrophic cardiomyopathy (Chap. 192). In the latter the pulse wave upstroke rises rapidly and forcefully, producing the first systolic peak ("percussion wave"). A brief decline in pressure follows because of the sudden decrease in the rate of left ventricular ejection during midsystole, when severe obstruction often develops. This pressure trough is followed by a smaller and more slowly rising positive pulse wave ("tidal wave") produced by continued ventricular ejection and by reflected waves from the periphery. The *dicrotic pulse* has two palpable waves, one in systole and one in diastole. It occurs most frequently in patients with a very low stroke volume, particularly in those with dilated (congestive) cardiomyopathy.

Pulsus alternans refers to a pattern in which there is regular alteration of the pressure pulse amplitude, despite a regular rhythm (Fig. 175-2). It is due to alternating left ventricular contractile force, usually denotes severe left ventricular decompensation, and commonly occurs in patients who also have a loud third heart sound. Pulsus alternans may also occur during or following paroxysmal tachycardia or for several beats following a premature beat in patients without heart disease. In *pulsus bigeminus* there is also regular alteration of pressure pulse amplitude, but it is caused by a premature ventricular contraction that follows each regular beat. *Pulsus paradoxus* is an accentuation of the decrease in systolic arterial pressure accompanying the reduced amplitude of the arterial pulse which normally occurs during inspiration. In patients with pericardial tamponade (Chap. 193), airway obstruction, or superior vena cava obstruction, the decrease in systolic arterial pressure frequently exceeds the normal of 10 mmHg (1.33 kPa) and the peripheral pulse may disappear completely during inspiration.

Simultaneous palpation of the radial and femoral arterial pulses, which normally are virtually coincident, is important to rule out aortic coarctation, in which the latter is weaker and delayed (Chap. 186).

JUGULAR VENOUS PULSE (JVP)   The two main objectives of the bedside examination of the neck veins are inspection of their waveform and estimation of the central venous pressure (CVP). In most patients, the right internal jugular vein is superior for both purposes, but occasionally examination of the other jugular vein or the venous pulsations in the supraclavicular fossae may yield more information. Usually, the maximum pulsation of the internal jugular vein is observed when the trunk is inclined by less than 30°. In patients with elevated venous pressure it may be necessary to elevate the trunk further, sometimes to as much as 90°. When the neck muscles are relaxed, shining a beam of light tangentially across the skin overlying the vein exposes the pulsations of the internal jugular vein. Simultaneous palpation of the left carotid artery aids the examiner in deciding which pulsations are venous and in relating the venous pulsations to their timing in the cardiac cycle.

The normal JVP reflects phasic pressure changes in the right

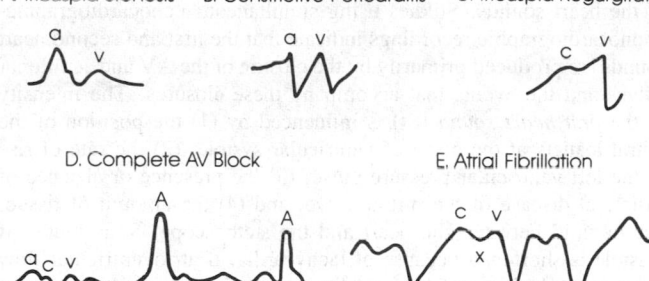

A. Tricuspid Stenosis   B. Constrictive Pericarditis   C. Tricuspid Regurgitation

D. Complete AV Block   E. Atrial Fibrillation

FIGURE 175-3 Abnormal jugular venous pulse waveforms commonly present in patients with cardiac disease and/or arrhythmias. See text. (*Modified from RA O'Rourke, in JW Hurst et al, eds. The Heart, 7th ed, New York, McGraw-Hill, 1990, with permission.*)

atrium and consists of two or sometimes three positive waves and two negative troughs (Fig. 175-1). The positive presystolic *a* wave is produced by venous distention due to right atrial contraction and is the dominant wave in the JVP, particularly during inspiration. Large *a* waves indicate that the right atrium is contracting against an increased resistance (Fig. 175-3), such as occurs with obstruction at the tricuspid valve (tricuspid stenosis) or more commonly with increased resistance to right ventricular filling (pulmonary hypertension or pulmonic stenosis). Large *a* waves also occur during arrhythmias whenever the right atrium contracts while the tricuspid valve is closed by right ventricular systole. Such "cannon" *a* waves may occur regularly (as during junctional rhythm) or irregularly (as in atrioventricular dissociation with ventricular tachycardia or complete heart block). The *a* wave is absent in patients with atrial fibrillation, and there is an increased temporal delay between the *a* wave and the carotid arterial pulse in patients with first-degree atrioventricular block.

The *c* wave, often but not invariably observed in the JVP, is a positive wave produced by the bulging of the tricuspid valve into the right atrium during right ventricular isovolumetric systole and by the impact of the carotid artery adjacent to the jugular vein. The *x* descent is due to a combination of atrial relaxation and the downward displacement of the tricuspid valve during ventricular systole. In patients with constrictive pericarditis (Fig. 175-3), there is often increased prominence of the *x* descent wave during systole, but this wave is reduced with right ventricular dilatation and often is reversed in tricuspid regurgitation. The positive, late systolic *v* wave results from the increasing volume of blood in the venae cavae and right atrium during ventricular systole when the tricuspid valve is closed. With mild tricuspid regurgitation the *v* wave becomes more prominent, and when tricuspid regurgitation becomes severe, the prominent *v* wave and the obliteration of the *x* descent result in a single large positive systolic wave ("ventricularization"). After the peak of the *v* wave is reached, the right atrial pressure diminishes because of the decreased bulging of the tricuspid valve into the right atrium as right ventricular pressure declines and the tricuspid valve opens (Fig. 175-3).

Following the summit of the *v* wave there is a negative descending limb, referred to as the *y* descent or "diastolic collapse," which is produced mainly by the tricuspid valve opening and the rapid inflow of blood into the right ventricle. A rapid, deep *y* descent in early diastole occurs with severe tricuspid regurgitation. A venous pulse characterized by a sharp *y* descent, a deep *y* trough, and a rapid ascent to the baseline is seen in patients with constrictive pericarditis or with severe failure of the right side of the heart and a high venous pressure. A slow *y* descent in the JVP suggests an obstruction to right ventricular filling, as occurs with tricuspid stenosis or right atrial myxoma.

For accurate estimation of the CVP, the right internal jugular vein is best utilized, with the sternal angle as the reference point, since in the average patient the center of the right atrium lies approximately 5 cm below the sternal angle, regardless of body position. The patient is examined at the optimum degree of trunk elevation for visualization of venous pulsations. The vertical distance between the top of the oscillating venous column and the level of the sternal angle is determined and generally found to be less than 3 cm (3 cm + 5 cm = 8 cm blood). The most common cause of an elevated venous pressure is an elevated right ventricular diastolic pressure. In patients suspected of having right ventricular failure who have a normal CVP at rest, the abdominojugular reflux test may be helpful. The palm of the hand is placed over the abdomen and firm pressure is applied for 10 s or more. Normally, the jugular venous pressure is not significantly altered, but with impaired function of the right side of the heart the upper level of venous pulsation usually increases. A positive abdominojugular test is best defined as an increase in JVP during 10 s of firm midabdominal compression followed by an abrupt drop in pressure of 4 cm blood upon release of the compression. The most common cause of a positive test is right heart failure secondary to elevated left heart filling pressures. Also, abdominal compression may elicit the typical JVP of tricuspid regurgitation when the resting pulse wave is normal. Kussmaul's sign, an increase rather than the normal decrease in the CVP during inspiration, is most commonly caused by severe right-sided heart failure; it is a frequent finding in patients with constrictive pericarditis or right ventricular infarction.

PRECORDIAL PALPATION The location, amplitude, duration, and direction of the cardiac impulse can usually be best appreciated by using the fingertips. The normal left ventricular apex impulse is located at or medial to the left midclavicular line in the fourth or fifth intercostal space and is a tapping, early systolic outward thrust localized to a point not more than 3 cm in diameter. It is due primarily to recoil of the heart as blood is ejected and should be evaluated with the patient supine and in the left lateral decubitus position. Left ventricular hypertrophy results in an exaggerated amplitude, duration, and often size of the normal left ventricular thrust. The impulse may be displaced laterally and downward into the sixth or seventh interspace, particularly in patients with a left ventricular volume load such as occurs in aortic regurgitation and in those with a dilated cardiomyopathy.

Additional abnormal features of the left ventricular apex include marked presystolic distention of the left ventricle, often accompanying a fourth heart sound in patients with an excessive left ventricular pressure load or myocardial ischemia/infarction, and a prominent early diastolic rapid-filling wave, often accompanying a third heart sound in patients with left ventricular failure or mitral valve regurgitation (Fig. 175-1). A double systolic impulse is frequently palpable in patients with hypertrophic cardiomyopathy.

Right ventricular hypertrophy results in a sustained systolic lift at the lower left parasternal area which starts in early systole and is synchronous with the left ventricular apical impulse. In patients with chronic obstructive pulmonary disease a right ventricular impulse may often be detected by sliding the fingers up under the rib cage just beneath the sternum. The enlarged right ventricle strikes the ends of the fingertips as an inferiorly directed movement.

Abnormal precordial pulsations occur during systole in patients with left ventricular dyssynergy due to ischemic heart disease or to diffuse myocardial disease from some other cause. These pulsations often occur in patients with a recent transmural myocardial infarction and may be present in some patients only during episodes of anginal pain. They are most commonly felt in the left midprecordium one or two interspaces above and/or 1 to 2 cm medial to the left ventricular apex. When a systolic bulge occurs in the region of the apex, it is difficult to distinguish it from the impulse of left ventricular hypertrophy.

A left parasternal lift is present frequently in patients with severe mitral regurgitation. This pulsation occurs distinctly later than the left ventricular apical impulse, is synchronous with the *v* wave in left atrial pressure curve, and is due to anterior displacement of the right ventricle by an enlarged, expanding left atrium. A similar impulse occurs to the right of the sternum in some patients with severe tricuspid regurgitation and a giant right atrium. Pulsation of the right sternoclavicular joint may indicate a right-sided aortic arch or aneurysmal dilatation of the ascending aorta. Pulmonary artery pulsation is often visible and palpable in the second left intercostal space and may be normal in children or thin young adults. However, this pulsation usually denotes pulmonary hypertension, increased pulmonary blood flow, or poststenotic pulmonary artery dilatation.

Thrills are palpable, low-frequency vibrations associated with heart murmurs. The diastolic rumble of mitral stenosis and the systolic murmur of mitral regurgitation may be palpated at the cardiac apex. When the palm of the hand is placed over the precordium, the thrill of aortic stenosis crosses the palm of the hand toward the right side of the neck, while the thrill of pulmonic stenosis radiates more often to the left side of the neck. The thrill due to a ventricular septal defect is usually located in the third and fourth intercostal spaces near the left sternal border.

Percussion should be performed in each patient to identify normal or abnormal position of the heart, stomach, and liver. However, in patients with a normal cardiac situs, percussion adds little to careful inspection and palpation in the recognition of cardiac enlargement.

CARDIAC AUSCULTATION

To obtain maximal information from cardiac auscultation, the observer should keep in mind several principles: (1) It should be carried out in a quiet room to avoid the distractions caused by the noises of normal activity. (2) In order to hear a faint heart sound or murmur, attention must be focused on that phase of the cardiac cycle during which the auscultatory event may be expected to occur. (3) The accurate timing of a heart sound or murmur necessarily involves determining its relation to other observable events in the cardiac cycle—the carotid arterial pulse, the JVP, or the apical impulse. (4) To define the significance of a cardiac sound or murmur, it is often necessary to observe alterations in its timing or intensity during various physiologic and/or pharmacologic interventions (Table 175-1).

HEART SOUNDS The major components of heart sounds are vibrations associated with the abrupt acceleration or deceleration of blood within the cardiovascular system, but there is continuing controversy regarding the relative significance of the vibrations of

valves, muscles, vessels, and supporting structures in the production of the heart sounds. Studies using simultaneous echocardiographic-phonocardiographic recordings indicate that the first and second heart sounds are produced primarily by the closure of the AV and semilunar valves and the events that accompany these closures. The intensity of the *first heart sound* (S_1) is influenced by (1) the position of the mitral leaflets at the onset of ventricular systole, (2) the rate of rise of the left ventricular pressure pulse, (3) the presence or absence of structural disease of the mitral valve, and (4) the amount of tissue, air, or fluid between the heart and the stethoscope. S_1 is louder if diastole is shortened because of tachycardia, if atrioventricular flow is increased because of high cardiac output or prolonged because of mitral stenosis, or if atrial contraction precedes ventricular contractions by a short PR interval. The loud S_1 in mitral stenosis usually signifies that the valve is pliable and that it remains open at the onset of isovolumetric contraction because of the elevated left atrial pressure. A reduction in the intensity of S_1 may be due to poor conduction of sound through the chest wall, a slow rise of the left ventricular pressure pulse, a long PR interval, or imperfect closure due to reduced valve substance, as in mitral regurgitation. S_1 is also soft when the anterior mitral leaflet is immobile because of rigidity and calcification even in the presence of predominant mitral stenosis.

Splitting of the two high-pitched components of S_1 by 10 to 30 ms is a normal phenomenon (Fig. 175-1). The first component of S_1 normally is attributed to mitral valve closure and the second to tricuspid valve closure. A widened split of S_1 is most often due to complete right bundle branch block and the resulting delay in onset of the right ventricular pressure pulse. Reversed splitting of the S_1 with the mitral component following the tricuspid component has occasionally been noted in complete left bundle branch block and frequently is present in patients with severe mitral stenosis or a left atrial myxoma.

Splitting of S_2 into audibly distinct aortic (A_2) and pulmonic (P_2) components occurs normally during inspiration when augmented inflow into the right ventricle increases its stroke volume and ejection period and delays closure of the pulmonic valve. P_2 is coincident with the incisura of the pulmonary artery pressure curve, which is separated from the right ventricular pressure tracing by an interval termed the "hangout time." The absolute value of this interval reflects the resistance to pulmonary blood flow and the impedance characteristics of the pulmonary vascular bed. This interval is prolonged, and physiologic splitting of S_2 is accentuated in conditions associated with right ventricular volume overload and a distensible

TABLE 175-1 Effects of physiologic and pharmacologic interventions on the intensity of heart murmurs and sounds*

Intervention	Changes in heart murmurs and sounds
Respiration	Systolic murmurs due to TR or pulmonic blood flow through a normal or stenotic valve and diastolic murmurs of TS or PR generally increase with inspiration as do right-sided S_3 and S_4. Left-sided murmurs and sounds usually are louder during expiration.
Valsalva maneuver	Most murmurs decrease in length and intensity. Two exceptions are the systolic murmur of HCM, which usually becomes much louder, and that of MVP, which becomes longer and often louder. Following release of the Valsalva, right-sided murmurs tend to return to control intensity earlier than left-sided murmurs.
Post VPB or AF	Murmurs originating at normal or stenotic semilunar valves increase in the cardiac cycle following a VPB or in the cycle after a long cycle length in AF. By contrast, systolic murmurs due to AV valve regurgitation do not change, diminish (papillary muscle dysfunction), or become shorter (MVP).
Positional changes	With *standing* most murmurs diminish, two exceptions being the murmur of HCM, which becomes louder, and that of MVP, which lengthens and often is intensified. With *squatting* most murmurs become louder but those of HCM and MVP usually soften and may disappear.
Exercise	Murmurs due to blood flow across normal or obstructed valves (e.g., PS, MS) become louder with both isotonic and submaximal isometric (handgrip) exercise. Murmurs of MR, VSD, and AR also increase with handgrip exercise. However, the murmur of HCM often decreases with near maximum handgrip exercise. Left-sided S_4 and S_3 are often accentuated by exercise, particularly when due to ischemic heart disease.
Pharmacologic interventions	During the initial relative hypotension following amyl nitrite inhalation, murmurs of MR, VSD, and AR decrease while murmurs of aortic stenosis or sclerosis increase. During the later tachycardia phase, murmurs of MS and right-sided lesions also increase. The response in MVP often is biphasic (softer then louder than control). The arterial constrictor phenylephrine tends to produce the opposite effects.
Transient arterial occlusion	Transient external compression of both arms by bilateral cuff inflation to 20 mmHg > peak systolic pressure augments the murmurs of MR, VSD, and AR but not murmurs due to other causes.

* TR, tricuspid regurgitation; TS, tricuspid stenosis; PR, pulmonic regurgitation; HCM, hypertrophic cardiomyopathy; MVP, mitral valve prolapse; PS, pulmonic stenosis; MS, mitral stenosis; MR, mitral regurgitation; VSD, ventricular septal defect; AR, aortic regurgitation; VPB, ventricular premature beat; and AF, atrial fibrillation.

pulmonary vascular bed. However, in patients with an increase in pulmonary vascular resistance, the hangout time is markedly reduced and narrow splitting of S_2 is present. Splitting that persists with expiration, heard best at the pulmonic area or left sternal border, is usually abnormal when the patient is in the upright position. Such splitting may be due to delayed activation of the right ventricle (right bundle branch block), to prolongation of right ventricular contraction with an increased right ventricular pressure load (pulmonary embolism or pulmonic stenosis), or to delayed pulmonic valve closure because of right ventricular volume overload associated with diminished impedance of the pulmonary vascular bed and a prolonged hangout time (atrial septal defect). In pulmonary hypertension, P_2 is increased in intensity and splitting of the second heart sound may be diminished, normal, or accentuated, depending on the cause of the pulmonary hypertension, the pulmonary vascular resistance, and the presence or absence of right ventricular decompensation. Early aortic valve closure, occurring with mitral regurgitation or a ventricular septal defect, may also produce splitting that persists during expiration. It may also occur with constrictive pericarditis. In patients with large atrial septal defects the proportion of right atrial filling contributed by the left atrium and the venae cavae varies reciprocally during the respiratory cycle so that right atrial inflow remains relatively constant. Therefore, the volume and duration of right ventricular ejection are not significantly increased by inspiration, and there is little inspiratory exaggeration of the splitting of S_2. This phenomenon, termed "fixed splitting" of the second heart sound, is of considerable diagnostic value.

A delay in aortic valve closure causing P_2 to precede A_2 results in so-called reversed (paradoxic) splitting of S_2. Splitting is then maximal in expiration, and decreases during inspiration with the normal delay of pulmonic valve closure. The commonest causes of reversed splitting of S_2 are left bundle branch block and delayed excitation of the left ventricle from a right ventricular ectopic beat. Mechanical prolongation of left ventricular systole, resulting in reversed splitting of S_2, may be caused by severe aortic outflow obstruction, a large aorta-to-pulmonary artery shunt, systolic hypertension, and ischemic heart disease or cardiomyopathy with left ventricular failure. P_2 is normally softer than A_2 in the second left intercostal space; when P_2 is greater than A_2 in this area, it suggests pulmonary hypertension, except in patients with atrial septal defect.

The *third heart sound* is a low-pitched sound produced in the ventricle 0.14 to 0.16 s after A_2, at the termination of rapid filling. This sound is frequent in normal children and in patients with high cardiac output. However, in patients over 40 years of age, an S_3 usually indicates ventricular decompensation, AV valve regurgitation, or other conditions which increase the rate or volume of ventricular filling. The left-sided S_3 is best heard with the bell piece of the stethoscope at the left ventricular apex during expiration and with the patient in the left lateral position. The right-sided S_3 is best heard at the left sternal border or just beneath the xiphoid and is increased with inspiration. Often it is accompanied by the systolic murmur of functional tricuspid regurgitation. Third heart sounds often disappear with treatment of heart failure.

An earlier (0.10 to 0.12 s after A_2), higher-pitched third heart sound (pericardial knock) often occurs in patients with constrictive pericarditis; its presence is dependent upon the restrictive effect of the adherent pericardium, which halts diastolic filling abruptly.

The *opening snap* (OS) is a brief, high-pitched, early diastolic sound which is usually due to stenosis of an AV valve, more commonly the mitral valve. It is usually heard best at the lower left sternal border and radiates well to the base of the heart. The A_2-OS interval during exercise is inversely related to the height of the mean left atrial pressure, and ranges from 0.04 to 0.12 s. At the base an OS is often confused with P_2. However, careful auscultation at the upper left sternal border will reveal both components of the second heart sound, followed by the opening snap. The OS of tricuspid stenosis occurs later in diastole than the mitral OS. Since most patients with tricuspid stenosis also have severe mitral valve disease,

the tricuspid OS is often overshadowed by the diastolic rumble and OS originating in the stenotic mitral valve. An OS also may occur when there is increased flow across an AV valve, such as exists with left-to-right intracardiac shunts and mitral or tricuspid regurgitation.

The *fourth heart sound* is a low-pitched, presystolic sound produced in the ventricle during the ventricular filling associated with an effective atrial contraction, and is heard best with the bell piece of the stethoscope. The sound is absent in patients with atrial fibrillation. The S_4 occurs when diminished ventricular compliance increases the resistance to ventricular filling, and it is present frequently in patients with systemic hypertension, aortic stenosis, hypertrophic cardiomyopathy, coronary artery disease, and acute mitral regurgitation. Most patients with an acute myocardial infarction and sinus rhythm have an audible S_4. The fourth heart sound is frequently accompanied by visible and palpable presystolic distention of the left ventricle. It is maximal in intensity at the left ventricular apex with the patient in the left lateral position, and is accentuated by mild isotonic or isometric exercise in the supine position. The right-sided S_4 is present in patients with right ventricular hypertrophy, secondary to either pulmonic stenosis or pulmonary hypertension, and frequently accompanies a prominent presystolic *a* wave in the JVP.

Audible fourth heart sounds also may be present during increased ventricular filling and normal ventricular compliance such as occurs in patients with severe anemia, thyrotoxicosis, or a peripheral arteriovenous fistula. An S_4 frequently accompanies delayed AV conduction even in the absence of clinically detectable heart disease. The incidence of an audible S_4 increases with increasing age. Whether an audible S_4 in adults without other evidence of cardiac disease is abnormal remains controversial.

The *ejection sound* is a sharp, high-pitched event occurring in early systole closely following the first heart sound. Ejection sounds occur in the presence of semilunar valve stenosis, i.e., opening snaps of the aortic or pulmonic valves, and in conditions associated with dilation of the aorta or pulmonary artery. The aortic ejection sound is usually heard best at the left ventricular apex and the second right interspace; the pulmonary ejection sound is of maximal intensity at the upper left sternal border. The latter, unlike most other right-sided acoustical events, is heard better during expiration.

Nonejection or midsystolic clicks, occurring with or without a late systolic murmur, often denote prolapse of one or both leaflets of the mitral valve. They may also be caused by tricuspid valve prolapse (Chap. 188). They probably result from functionally unequal length of the chordae tendineae of either or both AV valves and are heard best along the lower left sternal border and at the left ventricular apex. Systolic clicks may be single or multiple, and they may occur at any time in systole but usually later than the systolic ejection sound. Frequently the midsystolic click is misinterpreted as S_2, and the actual second heart sound is called an OS or S_3.

HEART MURMURS Cardiac murmurs result from vibrations set up in the bloodstream and the surrounding heart and great vessels as a result of turbulent blood flow, the formation of eddies, and cavitation (bubble formation as a result of sudden decrease in pressure).

The intensity or loudness of murmurs may be graded from I to VI. A grade I murmur is so faint that it can be heard only with special effort, and a grade VI murmur is audible with the stethoscope removed from contact with the chest. The configuration of a murmur may be crescendo, decrescendo, crescendo-decrescendo (diamond-shaped), or plateau. The precise time of onset and time of cessation of a murmur depend on the instant in the cardiac cycle at which an adequate pressure difference between two chambers appears and disappears (Fig. 175-4).

The location on the chest wall where the murmur is best heard and the areas to which it radiates can be helpful in identifying the cardiac structure from which the murmur originates. For example, the murmur of aortic valve stenosis is loudest usually in the second right intercostal space and radiates to the carotid arteries. By contrast, the murmur of mitral regurgitation is most often loudest at the cardiac apex and may radiate to the left sternal border and base of the heart

FIGURE 175-4 Schematic representation of ECG, aortic pressure (AOP), left ventricular pressure (LVP), and left atrial pressure (LAP). HSM is a holosystolic murmur; PSM, a presystolic murmur; MDM, a middiastolic murmur; MSM, a midsystolic murmur; EDM, an early diastolic murmur; LSM, a late systolic murmur; and CM, a continuous murmur.

when the posterior mitral leaflet is predominantly involved or to the axilla and back when the anterior leaflet is more severely affected. In the former case, the regurgitant blood is directed toward the posterior left atrial wall.

Often, it is difficult to classify with certainty a cardiac murmur based on its timing, configuration, location, radiation, pitch, or intensity. However, by noting changes in the characteristics of the murmur during maneuvers that alter cardiac hemodynamics, the auscultator often can identify its correct origin and significance (Table 175-1).

Accentuation of a murmur during inspiration which augments systemic venous return implies that it originates on the right side of the circulation; expiratory exaggeration has less significance. Prolonged expiratory pressure against a closed glottis, the Valsalva maneuver, reduces intensity of most murmurs by diminishing both right and left ventricular filling. The systolic murmur associated with *hypertrophic cardiomyopathy* and the late systolic murmur due to a *mitral valve prolapse* are exceptions and may be accentuated during the Valsalva maneuver. Murmurs due to flow across a normal or obstructed semilunar valve increase in intensity in the cycle following a premature ventricular beat or a long RR interval in atrial fibrillation. In contrast, murmurs due to AV valve regurgitation or a ventricular septal defect do not change appreciably during the beat following a prolonged diastole. Standing, which decreases heart size, accentuates the murmur of hypertrophic cardiomyopathy and occasionally the murmur due to mitral valve prolapse. Squatting, which increases both venous return and systemic arterial resistance, increases most murmurs, except those due to hypertrophic cardiomyopathy and mitral regurgitation due to a prolapsed mitral valve, which often decrease. Sustained handgrip exercise, which increases systemic arterial pressure and heart rate, often accentuates the murmurs of mitral regurgitation, aortic regurgitation, and mitral stenosis but usually diminishes those due to aortic stenosis or hypertrophic cardiomyopathy. Pharmacologic interventions include inhalation of amyl nitrite, which reduces systemic arterial pressure and increases blood flow, thereby increasing the intensity of murmurs due to valvular stenosis while diminishing those due to aortic or mitral regurgitation (Table 175-1). Transient external arterial occlusion by the inflation of bilateral arm cuffs to 20 mmHg (2.66 kPa) above systolic blood pressure for 5 s has been shown to intensify murmurs due to left-sided regurgitant lesions; this method is applicable to almost all patients and does not require administration of any drug.

Systolic murmurs *Holosystolic (pansystolic) murmurs* are generated when there is a flow between two chambers which have widely different pressures throughout systole, such as the left ventricle and

either the left atrium or the right ventricle. The pressure gradient is established early in contraction and lasts until relaxation is almost complete. Therefore, holosystolic murmurs begin before aortic ejection, and at the area of maximal intensity they begin with S_1 and end after S_2. Holosystolic murmurs accompany mitral or tricuspid regurgitation, ventricular septal defect, and under certain circumstances, aortopulmonary shunts. Although the typical high-pitched murmur of mitral regurgitation usually continues throughout systole, the shape of the murmur may vary considerably. The holosystolic murmurs of mitral regurgitation and ventricular septal defect are augmented by transient exercise and are diminished by lowering the left ventricular systolic pressure by inhalation of amyl nitrite. The murmur of tricuspid regurgitation associated with pulmonary hypertension is holosystolic and frequently increases during inspiration, a feature of diagnostic importance. Not all patients with mitral or tricuspid regurgitation or ventricular septal defect have holosystolic murmurs (Chap. 188).

Midsystolic murmurs, often crescendo-decrescendo in shape, occur when blood is ejected across the aortic or pulmonic outflow tracts. The murmur starts shortly after S_1 when the ventricular pressure rises sufficiently to open the semilunar valve. Ejection then begins and with it the onset of the murmur; as ejection increases, the murmur is augmented, and as ejection declines, it diminishes. The murmur ends before the ventricular pressure falls enough to permit closure of the aortic or pulmonic leaflets. In the presence of normal semilunar valves an increased flow rate, as occurs in states of elevated cardiac output, ejection into a dilated vessel beyond the valve, or increased transmission of sound through a thin chest wall, may be responsible for the production of this murmur. Most benign, functional murmurs are midsystolic and originate from the pulmonary outflow tract. Valvular or subvalvular obstruction to either ventricle may also cause such a midsystolic murmur, the intensity being related to the flow.

The murmur of aortic stenosis is the prototype of the left-sided midsystolic murmur. The location and radiation of this murmur are influenced by the direction of the high-velocity jet within the aortic root. In *valvular aortic stenosis* the murmur is usually maximal in the second right intercostal space, with radiation into the neck. In *supravalvular aortic stenosis* the murmur is occasionally loudest even higher, with disproportionate radiation into the right carotid artery. In hypertrophic cardiomyopathy, the murmur originates within the left ventricular cavity, and is usually maximal at the lower left sternal edge and apex, with relatively little radiation to the carotids. When the aortic valve is immobile (calcified), the aortic closure sound (A_2) may be soft and inaudible so that the length and configuration of the murmur are difficult to determine. Midsystolic murmurs also occur in patients with mitral regurgitation or, less frequently, tricuspid regurgitation resulting from papillary muscle dysfunction. Murmurs due to mitral regurgitation are often confused with those originating in the aorta, particularly in elderly patients.

The patient's age and the area of maximal intensity aid in determining the significance of midsystolic murmurs. Thus, in a young adult with a thin chest and high velocity of blood flow, a faint or moderate midsystolic murmur heard only in the pulmonic area is usually without clinical significance, while a somewhat louder murmur in the aortic area may indicate congenital aortic stenosis. In elderly patients pulmonic flow murmurs are rare, while aortic systolic murmurs are frequent and may be due to aortic dilatation, to a significant degree of valvular aortic stenosis, or to nonstenotic deformity of the aortic valve. Midsystolic aortic and pulmonic murmurs are intensified by amyl nitrite inhalation and during the cardiac cycle following a premature ventricular beat, while those due to mitral regurgitation are unchanged or softer. Aortic systolic murmurs are diminished by interventions which increase aortic impedance, such as intravenous phenylephrine. Echocardiography or cardiac catheterization may be necessary to separate a prominent and exaggerated functional murmur from one due to congenital semilunar valve stenosis.

Early systolic murmurs begin with the first heart sound and end in midsystole. They may be due to a very small *ventricular septal defect, a large defect with pulmonary hypertension,* or *severe acute mitral* or *tricuspid regurgitation.* In large ventricular septal defects with pulmonary hypertension, the shunting at the end of systole may be small or absent, resulting in an early systolic murmur. A similar murmur may occur with very small muscular ventricular septal defects, the shunt being interrupted in late systole. An early systolic murmur is a feature of tricuspid regurgitation occurring in the absence of pulmonary hypertension. This lesion is common in drug addicts with infective endocarditis, in whom a tall regurgitant right atrial *v* wave reaches the level of the normal right ventricular pressure in late systole, confining the murmur to early systole. In patients with acute mitral regurgitation and a large *v* wave in a noncompliant left atrium, a loud early systolic murmur is frequently heard which diminishes as the pressure gradient between left ventricle and left atrium decreases in late systole (Chap. 188).

Late systolic murmurs are faint or moderately loud high-pitched apical murmurs, which start well after ejection and do not mask either heart sound. They are probably related to papillary muscle dysfunction caused by infarction or ischemia of these muscles or to their distortion by left ventricular dilatation. They may appear only during angina but are common in patients with myocardial infarction or diffuse myocardial disease. Late systolic murmurs following midsystolic clicks are associated with late systolic mitral regurgitation caused by prolapse of the mitral valve into the left atrium (Chap. 188).

Diastolic murmurs *Early diastolic murmurs* begin with or shortly after the second heart sound as soon as the corresponding ventricular pressure falls sufficiently below that in the aorta or pulmonary artery. The high-pitched murmurs of aortic regurgitation or pulmonic regurgitation due to pulmonary hypertension are generally decrescendo, since there is a progressive decline in the volume or rate of regurgitation during diastole. Faint, high-pitched murmurs of aortic regurgitation are difficult to hear unless they are specifically sought by applying firm pressure with the diaphragm over the left midsternal border while the patient sits, leans forward, and holds a breath in full expiration. The diastolic murmur of aortic regurgitation is enhanced by an acute elevation of the arterial pressure such as occurs with handgrip exercise; it diminishes with a decrease in arterial pressure as with amyl nitrite inhalation. The diastolic murmur of congenital pulmonic regurgitation without pulmonary hypertension is low- to medium-pitched. The onset of this murmur is delayed because at the onset of pulmonic valve closure the regurgitant flow is minimal, since the reverse pressure gradient responsible for the regurgitation is negligible at this time.

Middiastolic murmurs usually arise from the AV valves, occur during early ventricular filling, and are due to disproportion between valve orifice size and flow rate. Such murmurs may be loud despite only slight AV valve stenosis when there is normal or increased blood flow. Conversely, the murmur may be soft or even absent despite severe obstruction if the cardiac output is markedly reduced. When stenosis is marked, the diastolic murmur is prolonged and the duration of the murmur is more reliable than its intensity as an index of the severity of valve obstruction.

The low-pitched, middiastolic murmur of mitral stenosis characteristically follows the opening snap. It should be specifically sought by placing the bell of the stethoscope at the site of the left ventricular impulse, which is best localized with the patient on the left side. Frequently the murmur of mitral stenosis is present only at the left ventricular apex, and it may be increased in intensity by mild supine exercise or by inhalation of amyl nitrite. In tricuspid stenosis the middiastolic murmur is localized to a relatively limited area along the left sternal edge and may increase in intensity during inspiration.

Middiastolic murmurs may be generated across the mitral valve in ventricular septal defect, patent ductus arteriosus, or mitral regurgitation, and across the tricuspid valve in atrial septal defect or tricuspid regurgitation. These murmurs are related to the torrential flow across an AV valve, usually follow a third heart sound, and tend to occur with large left-to-right shunts or severe AV valve regurgitation.

A soft middiastolic murmur may sometimes be heard in patients with acute rheumatic fever (Carey-Coombs murmur). It has been attributed to inflammation of the mitral valve cusps or excessive left atrial blood flow as a consequence of mitral regurgitation.

In acute aortic regurgitation, the left ventricular diastolic pressure may exceed the left atrial pressure, resulting in a middiastolic murmur due to "diastolic mitral regurgitation." In severe chronic aortic regurgitation a murmur is frequently present which may be either middiastolic or presystolic (Austin Flint murmur). This murmur appears to originate at the anterior mitral valve leaflet when blood simultaneously enters the left ventricle from both the aortic root and the left atrium.

Presystolic murmurs begin during the period of ventricular filling that follows atrial contraction and therefore occur in sinus rhythm. They are usually due to AV valve stenosis and have the same quality as the middiastolic filling rumble but are usually crescendo, reaching peak intensity at the time of a loud S_1. The presystolic murmur corresponds to the AV valve gradient, which may be minimal until the moment of right or left atrial contraction. It is the presystolic rather than the middiastolic murmur which is most characteristic of tricuspid stenosis and sinus rhythm. A right or left *atrial myxoma* may occasionally cause either middiastolic or presystolic murmurs that resemble the murmurs of mitral or tricuspid stenosis.

Continuous murmurs begin in systole, peak near S_2, and continue into all or part of diastole. These murmurs signify continuous flow due to communication between high- and low-pressure areas which persists through the end of systole and the beginning of diastole. A *patent ductus arteriosus* causes a continuous murmur as long as the pressure in the pulmonary artery is much below that in the aorta. The murmur is intensified by elevation of the systemic arterial pressure and is reduced by amyl nitrite inhalation. When pulmonary hypertension is present, the diastolic portion may disappear, leaving the murmur confined to systole. A continuous murmur is uncommon in aortopulmonary septal defects, since this malformation is generally associated with severe pulmonary hypertension. Surgically produced aortopulmonary connections and the subclavian–pulmonary artery anastomosis result in murmurs similar to that of a patent ductus.

Continuous murmurs may result from congenital or acquired *systemic arteriovenous fistula, coronary arteriovenous fistula,* anomalous origin of the left coronary artery from the pulmonary artery, and communications between the *sinus of Valsalva and the right side of the heart.* Continuous murmurs may also occur when high left atrial pressure results in continuous flow across a small defect in the atrial septum. Murmurs associated with *pulmonary arteriovenous fistulas* may be continuous but are usually only systolic. Continuous murmurs may also be due to disturbances of flow pattern in constricted systemic (e.g., renal) or pulmonary arteries when marked pressure differences between the two sides of the narrow segment persist; a continuous murmur in the back may be present in *coarctation of the aorta; pulmonary embolism* may cause continuous murmurs in partially occluded vessels.

In nonconstricted arteries continuous murmurs may be due to rapid flow through a tortuous bed. Such murmurs typically occur within the bronchial arterial collateral circulation in cyanotic patients with severe pulmonary outflow obstruction. The "mammary souffle," an innocent murmur heard during late pregnancy and early postpartum, may be systolic or continuous. The innocent cervical venous hum is a continuous murmur usually heard over the medial aspect of the right supraclavicular fossa with the patient upright. The hum is usually louder during diastole and can be instantaneously abolished by digital compression of the ipsilateral internal jugular vein. Transmission of a loud venous hum to the area below the clavicles may result in a mistaken diagnosis of patent ductus arteriosus.

The *pericardial friction rub,* which may have presystolic, systolic, and early diastolic scratchy components, may be confused with a murmur or extracardiac sound when heard only in systole. It is best appreciated with the patient upright and leaning forward and may be accentuated during inspiration.

REFERENCES

BARAGAN J et al (eds): *Dynamic Auscultation and Phonocardiography*. Maryland, Charles Press Publishers, 1979

BRAUNWALD E: Physical examination, in *Heart Disease*, 3d ed, E Braunwald (ed). Philadelphia, Saunders, 1988, p. 13.

CRAIGE E: Echophonocardiography and other noninvasive techniques to elucidate heart murmurs, in *Heart Disease*, 3d ed, E Braunwald (ed). Philadelphia, Saunders, 1988, p 65

————: Heart Sounds: Phonocardiography, carotid, apex and jugular venous pulse tracings; and systolic time intervals, in *Heart Disease*, 3d ed, E Braunwald (ed). Philadelphia, Saunders, 1988, p 41

DELL ITALIA LJ et al: Physical examination for exclusion of hemodynamically important right ventricular infarction. Ann Intern Med 99:608, 1983

EILEN SD, CRAWFORD MH, O'ROURKE RA: Accuracy of precordial palpation for detecting increased left ventricular volume. Ann Intern Med 99:628, 1983

EWY GA: The abdominojugular test: Technique and hemodynamic correlates. Ann Intern Med 109:456, 1988

FOWLER NO: Cardiac auscultation, in *Cardiac Diagnosis and Treatment*, 3d ed, NO Fowler (ed). Hagerstown, Harper & Row, 1980, p 62

LEMBO NJ et al: Bedside diagnosis of systolic murmurs. N Engl J Med 318:1572, 1988

PERLOFF JK (ed): *Physical Examination of the Heart and Circulation, 2d ed*. Philadelphia, Saunders, 1990

REDDY PS et al: Normal and abnormal heart sounds in cardiac diagnosis, Part II: Diastolic sounds. Curr Probl Cardiol 10(4):1, 1985

ROTHMAN A, GOLDBERGER AL: Aids to cardiac auscultation. Ann Intern Med 99:346, 1983

SHAVER JA et al: Normal and abnormal heart sounds in cardiac diagnosis, Part I: Systolic sounds. Curr Probl Cardiol 10(3):1, 1985

TAVEL ME: *Clinical Phonocardiography and External Pulse Recordings*, 4th ed. Chicago, Year Book, 1985

176 ELECTROCARDIOGRAPHY

ROBERT J. MYERBURG

INTRODUCTION The electrocardiogram (ECG) is a graphic description of the electrical activity of the heart, recorded from the body surface by electrodes positioned to reflect activity from a variety of spatial perspectives. The source of cardiac electrical activity resides within the working (contracting) myocardial cells, as well as within the specialized conducting tissue (SCT), as described in Chap. 184. However, only that activity generated by atrial and ventricular working muscle is recorded on the standard surface ECG. Electrical activity of the SCT can be deduced from features of the surface ECG, or recorded by signal averaging on the body surface or by intracardiac electrode catheters (see Chap. 185).

The magnitude and direction of the electrical activity recorded on the body surface are instantaneous averages of cumulative cell depolarizations or repolarizations occurring at a point in time. Although much of the electrical activity from individual cells is canceled out before reaching the body surface by opposing forces from other cells, the resultant recording is a reasonably reproducible and accurate approximation of net cardiac electrical activity. However, the signals recorded at the body surface do not identify specific sites of origin because a given vector at the body surface can be accounted for by innumerable combinations of cellular signals at their source in the heart.

Early in the development of the ECG, Einthoven popularized the concept that the human body represents a large volume conductor having the source of cardiac electrical activity at its center. While this theory is not strictly accurate, it provides the clinician with a practical point from which to work. As an extension of this concept, the *net* electrical activity at any instant in the cardiac cycle may be viewed as originating from a polarized point source at a theoretical "electrical center" of the heart. Since this "equivalent dipole" would have direction and magnitude, one might then extend the pattern into a sequence of instantaneous vectors recordable from the body surface. The application of this concept to ECG analysis is discussed below.

LEAD SYSTEMS The ECG lead system is composed of five electrodes, one on each of the four limbs and one placed at various sites on the precordium. Each lead is a continuous recording of the change in electrical potential during the cardiac cycle between two of the electrodes, or between one electrode and a combination of the others. The right-leg electrode is an inactive ground electrode in all leads.

The original lead system developed by Einthoven is based on assumptions of (1) the homogeneity of the body volume conductor, (2) the symmetry of the leads, and (3) a single equivalent dipole at the center of the volume conductor. The *standard limb leads* (I, II, and III) are composed of three bipolar permutations of the right arm (RA), left arm (LA), and left leg (LL) electrodes [Fig. 176-1A (1)]. Lead I records the potential difference between the LA and the RA,

FIGURE 176-1 Lead systems. *A.* Standard limb leads, showing (1) electrode positions, (2) the equilateral triangle of Einthoven, and (3) the conversion of the triangle to a triaxial reference system with positive (+) and negative (−) polarity. *B.* The unipolar chest leads, showing (1) the central terminal of Wilson (CTW) (or the indifferent electrode, i) and the chest electrode (C) (or the exploring electrode, E). The 5000 Ω between CTW and each limb electrode is not shown. The relationship between CTW and V_1 to V_6 in the horizontal plane is shown in part 2. *C.* The augmented unipolar limb leads, using the modified CTW. *D.* The hexaxial frontal plane reference system. Normal ranges are described in the text, and applications are derived in Figs. 176-5 and 176-6. RA, right arm; LA, left arm; LL, left leg; RL, right leg.

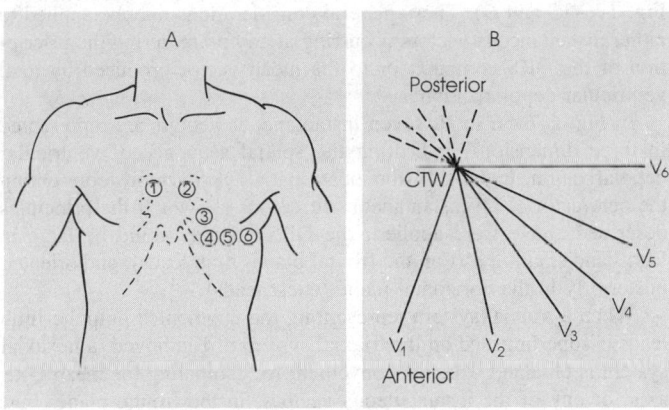

FIGURE 176-2 The unipolar chest leads. *A.* The position of the chest electrode for V₁ to V₆. *B.* The relationship between the CTW and the chest electrode (C) in the horizontal plane.

FIGURE 176-3 Standardization of the ECG. Standard time calibration is 1 mm = 0.04 s or 5 mm = 0.20 s. Standard voltage is 0.1 mV/mm. A repetitive event occurring every 5 mm (A) on time axis (0.20 s) is occurring at 300 per minute. A repetitive event occurring every 10 mm (B) (0.40 s) is occurring at 150 per minute. C, D, and E indicate that repetitive events at 0.60, 0.80, and 1.00 s are occurring at rates of 100, 75, and 60 per minute, respectively.

the positive electrode on the LA and the negative electrode on the RA [Fig. 176-1*A* (2)]. Lead II records the potential difference between the electrodes on the RA and the LL, the positive electrode on the LL. Lead III records the potential difference between the LA and the LL, with the positive electrode on the LL. It is likely that Einthoven arbitrarily selected the relationships between positive and negative electrodes in the three leads in order to have the major deflection of the QRS complex (see below) moving in an upward (positive) direction in most normal individuals.

The central terminal of Wilson (CTW) is constructed by connecting the RA, LA, and LL electrodes through 5000-Ω resistances, in order to cancel out the potentials from these three points. With the forces canceled out, the CTW theoretically remains inactive during the entire cardiac cycle, and an exploring electrode will function as a unipolar lead [Fig. 176-1*B* (1)]. The selection of the positions for the six *unipolar chest leads* [Figs. 176-1*B* (2) and 176-2] was based on the concept that the proximity of the heart to the anterior chest wall resulted in the unipolar chest leads functioning as "semidirect" leads, being influenced primarily by the tissue immediately beneath the electrode. While this concept does not have the quantitative significance originally desired, and the recordings do reflect the activity of the total heart, there is weighting of the voltages recorded by the tissue closest to the exploring electrode. The six standard chest leads (V₁ to V₆) are recorded by positioning the exploring chest electrode as follows: V₁ in the fourth intercostal space (4ICS) at the right sternal border; V₂ in the 4ICS at the left sternal border; V₄ in the 5ICS at the midclavicular line; V₃ midway between V₂ and V₄; V₅ at the left anterior axillary line at the level of V₄ horizontally; and V₆ at the left midaxillary line at the level of V₄ horizontally (Fig. 176-2). The exploring chest electrode is occasionally used in nonstandard positions for special purposes. V₄R, the equivalent position of V₄ on the *right* side of the chest, may be helpful in diagnosing right ventricular myocardial infarction (see below and Chap. 189) and right-sided leads (V₃R to V₆R) can be used to record ECGs in patients with dextrocardia (see Chap. 186). V₇ (left posterior axillary line) and V₈ to V₁₀ (back) are used rarely to explore the left ventricle. The CTW is the indifferent electrode, and the exploring chest electrode is the active electrode for all chest leads.

Unipolar limb leads may be recorded by a system in which the CTW constitutes the indifferent electrode and the exploring electrode is one of the three active limb electrodes. These leads are referred to as VR, VL, and VF. By disconnecting the input to the CTW from the extremity being explored, the voltage of the unipolar limb leads is augmented by as much as 50 percent. This modification is universally used for clinical ECGs, and the leads are labeled aVR, aVL, and aVF (Fig. 176-1*C*).

In recent years, the clinical value of chest wall mapping has been studied by a number of investigators. Multiple electrodes (32 to 192)

are used for simultaneous recording, and computer processing for data reduction and display. This procedure yields information not available from the standard 12-lead ECG. New insights into normal and abnormal depolarization and repolarization patterns are evolving, and the value of sequential changes in ST segments during acute myocardial infarction is being studied.

ELECTROCARDIOGRAPHIC WAVEFORMS, DURATIONS, AND INTERVALS Clinical ECGs are recorded on paper having a graphic background (Fig. 176-3) to permit rapid measurement of standardized time intervals and voltages. Time lines are 1 mm apart, with every fifth line intensified. Standard paper speed is 25 mm/s. Thus, 1 mm = 0.04 s (lighter lines), and 5 mm = 0.20 s (heavier lines). The horizontal lines, 1 mm apart, permit calibration of the voltage deflections of the ECG. Usual standardization is ↑ 10 mm = +1 mV (Fig. 176-3).

The P wave reflecting atrial depolarization is normally the initial wave of activity during the cardiac cycle (Fig. 176-4). Ventricular muscle depolarization is represented by the *QRS complex.* A Q wave is an initial negative wave; an R wave is an initial positive wave or a positive wave following a Q wave; and an S wave is a negative deflection following an R wave (Fig. 176-4). A QRS complex having a Q wave which returns to the baseline but does not produce a positive wave is labeled a QS complex, and the second R wave in a QRS complex having more than one R wave is labeled R′. The T wave represents ventricular muscle repolarization and is sometimes followed by a small wave, the U wave, the mechanism of which remains uncertain. Repolarization of atrial muscle is represented by the Tₐ (or Tₚ) wave, which occurs during the PR interval and QRS complex, and is usually difficult to identify. The interval between the end of the QRS complex and the onset of the T wave is the ST segment, representing the period of time between depolarization of the ventricles and the period of rapid repolarization of ventricular muscle.

The interval between the P wave and the QRS complex is the PR (or PQ) interval, measured from the *onset* of atrial depolarization (P) to the *onset* of ventricular depolarization (Q or R) (Fig. 176-4). The

FIGURE 176-4 The waves of the electrocardiogram—P, QRS, T, and U—are indicated. The measurements of the PR interval, QRS complex, ST segment, and QT interval are identified on the right.

duration is 0.12 to 0.20 s in the adult. Since AV nodal activation begins before the end of depolarization of atrial muscle, the PR interval may be used as a rough approximation of AV conduction time.

The duration of the QRS complex (normal = 0.04 to 0.10 s) reflects the time required for depolarization of ventricular muscle. It may be slightly prolonged by regional block in a portion of the intraventricular SCT or by delayed conduction in a region of ventricular muscle. Block in a bundle branch prolongs the QRS to a greater extent. An approximation of the refractory period of the ventricles may be obtained by measuring the QT interval (from the onset of the QRS to the end of the T wave) (Fig. 176-4). The QT interval is rate-dependent, and may be altered by numerous pathophysiologic or pharmacologic influences. Bazett's formula may be used to calculate the QT interval corrected for heart rate (QT$_c$). The formula is:

$$QT_c = \frac{QT}{\sqrt{R\text{-}R}}$$

where R-R is the interval between two successive QRS complexes. QT$_c$ is prolonged when it is $\geq$0.40 s in men and $\geq$0.45 s in women.

THE VECTOR CONCEPT AND ELECTRICAL AXIS The representation of a force by a graphic description of its direction and magnitude is referred to as a *vector*. In specific reference to cardiac electrical activity, a vector may be projected onto a two-dimensional plane as a scalar vector (Fig. 176-5A to D), or considered in three dimensions as a spatial vector (Fig. 176-5E to H). It may be used to represent instantaneous forces in the sequence of the cardiac electrical cycle (Fig. 176-5A and E), or it may represent either the mean or maximum axis during the cardiac cycle (Fig. 176-5H). Mean, maximum, and instantaneous vectors are most commonly applied to the analysis of the QRS complex, but the same principles may be applied to the P wave, ST segment, or T wave.

When an instantaneous electrical force recorded from the body surface is oriented in a direction perpendicular (or nearly so) to one of the leads (Fig. 176-5C, vector 6), the potential recorded by that lead at that instant will be minimum or isoelectric (Fig. 176-5D, point 6). Conversely, if the lead system is oriented parallel to the direction of an instantaneous electrical force (Fig. 176-5C, vector 4), the potential recorded by that lead will be maximum (Fig. 176-5D, point 4). An intermediate direction will record an intermediate voltage (for example, Fig. 176-5C and D, vector 2). If the instantaneous electrical force is oriented to the positive side of the lead, the deflection will be positive (4 in Fig. 176-5C and D); if the direction is oriented to the negative side, the deflection will be negative (1 in

Fig. 176-5C and D). These general considerations may be applied to either instantaneous vectors occurring at any point during the inscription of the QRS complex, or to the mean vector produced by total ventricular depolarization.

In Fig. 176-5E to H, seven instantaneous vectors are represented in three dimensions, indicating the spatial sequence of ventricular depolarization. In panel H, the mean spatial QRS vector, representing the net vector of all instantaneous forces, is shown. If the principles described above were applied, the QRS voltage would be large in lead I and small in aVF in the frontal plane (limb leads), and oriented posteriorly in the horizontal plane (chest leads).

When a triaxial system representing the augmented unipolar limb leads is superimposed on the triaxial system of Einthoven, a hexaxial system is obtained which is convenient for estimating the mean QRS axis, or any of the instantaneous vectors, in the frontal plane (Fig. 176-1D). When the appropriate positive and negative voltage orientations are assigned to each of the leads, the hexaxial reference system becomes a simple means of scalar vector analysis, requiring a

FIGURE 176-5 *A.* Frontal plane scalar projection of six instantaneous QRS vectors. *B.* Vectors originating from a point source at the electrical center of the heart. *C.* Projection of the vectors on the lead I axis. *D.* Lead I QRS produced by the instantaneous vectors in panel *C* (see text). *E.* Spatial representation of ventricular depolarization. Seven instantaneous vectors in the sequence of depolarization indicated in spatial orientations. *F.* Spatial vectors originating from the electrical center of the heart. *G.* A line drawn through the terminations of the spatial vectors produces a spatial QRS loop (vector loop). *H.* The mean spatial QRS vector, average of all the instantaneous vectors—to the left, slightly inferiorly, and posteriorly. (See text.) *(From JW Hurst, RJ Myerburg, Introduction to Electrocardiography, 2d ed, New York, McGraw-Hill, 1973; modified and reproduced by permission of the publisher.)*

FIGURE 176-6 Three normal ECGs demonstrating: (*A*) horizontal, (*B*) intermediate, and (*C*) vertical mean frontal plane QRS axes constructed on the hexaxial system. In addition, the horizontal plane vector in *C* is constructed on an axial system and is posteriorly oriented. T-wave vectors are similarly constructed.

minimum of two leads for estimation of the mean axis. An ECG which reveals a maximum positive QRS deflection in lead I and an isoelectric deflection in aVF has a mean QRS vector oriented at 0°. Conversely, if the QRS voltage is positive and maximum in lead II and isoelectric in aVL, the mean vector is oriented at +60°. The mean QRS axis in the frontal plane in normal adults ranges from −30 to +110°. Overlap between normal and abnormal occurs in the range of +90 to +110°. Generally, an axis > +90° is referred to as *right axis deviation*, and more negative than −30° as *abnormal left axis deviation*. The determination of the mean QRS axis in the horizontal plane (Fig. 176-2*B*) is similarly derived, normal orientation being to the left and posteriorly.

Three normal ECGs are shown in Fig. 176-6. Analysis of the mean QRS axis in the *frontal plane* (I, II, III, aVR, aVL, aVF) reveals the axis of *A* to be oriented horizontally, of *C* to be oriented vertically, and of *B* to be oriented in an intermediate range. In *A* the net voltage of the QRS complex is largest in lead I, almost isoelectric in lead III, and low in aVF, placing the mean axis in a direction almost perpendicular to lead III. In *B*, the voltages in lead I and aVF are almost identical, and maximum in lead II and aVR. The mean QRS axis is between lead II (+) and aVR (−). In *C*, net voltage is largest in leads II and aVF and almost isoelectric in lead I, placing the mean QRS axis almost perpendicular to lead I. A similar approach is applied to QRS axis determination in the *horizontal plane*. In *C*, the lead in which the net forces are isoelectric is V₃. Therefore, as shown in the axial representation of the horizontal plane of tracing *C*, the QRS vector is oriented to the left and posteriorly. If this information is added to that obtained from the frontal plane axis, it is apparent that the mean QRS vector of electrocardiogram *C* is oriented inferiorly, to the left, and posteriorly. Similar principles may be applied to the analysis of the mean T-wave axis, which is normally oriented in the same general direction as the QRS axis. An angle between the QRS and T axes >45° in the frontal plane, or >60° in the horizontal plane, is abnormal.

ELECTRICAL ACTIVITY OF THE ATRIA The mean P-wave vector is normally directed to the left, inferiorly, and slightly anteriorly; the frontal plane P axis is usually oriented between +30 and +60°. Right atrial enlargement causes tall, peaked P waves (≥0.25 mV), most prominent in standard leads II and V₁ (Fig. 176-7). Left atrial enlargement causes broad, notched P waves in lead II, and inverted or biphasic P waves (with the inverted portion of the biphasic P wave broader and deeper than the upright portion) in lead V₁. The upper limit of normal for P-wave duration is 0.11 s, and the broad P wave of left atrial enlargement usually is ≥0.12 s. However, criteria for left atrial enlargement are nonspecific, similar changes occurring in intraatrial conduction disturbances (Fig. 176-7), and the two must be distinguished by techniques other than ECG.

ABNORMALITIES OF VENTRICULAR DEPOLARIZATION: QRS COMPLEX Since the QRS complex is the ECG representation of the sequence, time, and synchronization of total ventricular muscle depolarization, focal or diffuse abnormalities in ventricular muscle or in the SCT may cause changes in QRS form. Abnormalities may be confined to initial depolarization (Fig. 176-8*B*), terminal depolarization (Fig. 176-8*C*), or mid and late depolarization (Fig. 176-8*D*), or they may be diffuse (Fig. 176-8*E* to *G*).

The normal earliest site of activation is in the midportion of the left side of the interventricular septum, followed closely by a site on the lower portion of the right side of the interventricular septum and

FIGURE 176-7 P waves of right atrial enlargement (RAE) and left atrial enlargement (LAE).

FIGURE 176-8 QRS complexes. The lead is indicated above each example. *A.* Normal. *B.* Prolongation due to initial QRS delay between arrows (1→2) in Wolff-Parkinson-White syndrome (see Chap. 184). *C.* Prolongation due to terminal delay (1→2) in right bundle branch block. *D.* Prolongation due to mid (1→2) and late (2→3) delay in left bundle branch block. *E.* Minor uniform prolongation (1→2) in left ventricular hypertrophy. *F.* Distortion of total QRS pattern (1→2) in a cardiomyopathy. *G.* Uniform prolongation (1→2) in an electrolyte abnormality. *H.* Pathologic Q wave (1→2) in myocardial infarction. Intrinsicoid deflection = 2→3 in *D* and S→2 in *E.*

the adjacent free wall endocardium. The dominant wavefront is that one arising on the left septum, which results in a small initial R wave in V_1 (anterior movement), and a small initial Q wave in I, aVL, and/or V_6 (rightward movement). Small initial Q waves in II, III, and aVF may be observed as an indication of a small superior movement of the initial wavefront. Normal septal Q waves are ≤0.02 s and of low amplitude. A normal R in V_1 is ≤0.4 mV.

After septal depolarization has been initiated, rapid endocardial propagation occurs through both ventricles. In the normal heart, the greater mass of the left ventricle predominates, and the magnitude and direction of the electrical vectors reflect this fact (Fig. 176-6). During normal depolarization, the sequence of instantaneous vectors rotates from rightward and anterior to leftward, posterior, and superior (Fig. 176-5E to G). Most individuals will have maximum QRS duration (i.e., the lead having the longest measurable QRS) of 0.05 to 0.08 s (normal range is 0.04 to 0.10 s). A QRS duration of 0.09 or 0.10 s may be a normal variant or may represent a conduction delay to limited regions of either ventricle (Fig. 176-8). QRS durations ≥0.12 s represent left or right bundle branch block or severe degrees of diffuse intraventricular conduction delay (Fig. 176-13).

Abnormal initial Q waves or an abnormal initial R in V_1 usually represents (1) a loss of muscle mass; (2) abnormal sequence of depolarization; or (3) a change in the relative muscle mass in the two ventricles.

The *intrinsicoid deflection* of the QRS complex is the major deflection *returning* to the baseline in a left (for example, 2→3 in Fig. 176-8D) or a right (S wave→2, Fig. 176-8E) precordial lead. Its *onset* should not exceed 0.035 s from the *onset* of the QRS complex in V_1, or 0.055 s from the *onset* of the QRS in V_5 or V_6. Delayed onset of the intrinsicoid deflection may indicate hypertrophy or intraventricular conduction abnormalities (see Fig. 176-8).

The AV node and His bundle constitute the one normal pathway for impulse conduction from atria to ventricles. However, *accessory pathways* are present in some hearts. These are bands of muscle parallel to the AV junction, named Kent bundles, which form the anatomic substrate for the Wolff-Parkinson-White syndrome (see Chap. 185). The ECG manifestation is the *delta wave* (Fig. 176-8B).

ABNORMALITIES OF VENTRICULAR RE-POLARIZATION: ST SEGMENT, T WAVE, AND U WAVE In the normal ECG, the ST segment is "isoelectric," resting at the same potential as the interval between the T wave and the next P wave. Deviations of the ST segment from the baseline may occur as a result of injury to cardiac muscle, changes in the synchronization of ventricular muscle depolarization, overload or strain on ventricular muscle, or drug or electrolyte influences. Elevations of the ST segment, in association with an elevation of the takeoff point of the ST segment from the QRS complex (the J point), may occur as a normal variant, especially in young individuals (Fig. 176-9A). The most common pathologic causes of ST-segment elevation are acute myocardial infarction and pericarditis (Fig. 176-9B to F), and the normal variant must be differentiated from these. Horizontal depression or a downsloping ST segment merging into the T wave occurs as a result of ischemia, ventricular strain, changes in the pattern of ventricular depolarization, or drug effects (Fig. 176-9H, I, M, N, Q, and R).

Since the sequence of ventricular muscle *de*polarization is from endocardium to epicardium, and *re*polarization represents an electrical process opposite in direction to depolarization, the T wave would be in the opposite direction to the QRS complex if the sequence of repolarization were in the same direction as depolarization. However, T waves assume the same general direction as the major deflection of the QRS complex (see Fig. 176-6). It is assumed, therefore, that the direction of normal repolarization is opposite to the wave of depolarization—from epicardium to endocardium. T waves are considered abnormal when they are of low voltage, flat, or inverted in leads in which they are normally upright, or when they are abnormally tall and peaked. T-wave inversions are reflected vectorially by a widening of the angle between the QRS vector and the T vector (Fig. 176-6). Common causes of abnormalities of the T waves include ischemic heart disease, ventricular hypertrophy and strain, primary muscle disease, abnormal sequences of depolarization, electrolyte abnormalities, and drug influences (see Fig. 176-9C, D, F, I, K, L, and N to R), but the changes are often not specific.

The U wave is usually positive in leads in which the QRS complex is positive. The abnormal U wave is manifested as either an exaggeration of U-wave voltage, the appearance of a U wave in leads in which it is not normally seen, or inversion of a U wave. U-wave abnormalities occur in ischemic heart disease, left ventricular strain, and electrolyte disturbances. Unfortunately, the information they provide is usually nonspecific.

ECG MANIFESTATIONS OF VENTRICULAR HYPERTROPHY The normal dominance of the left ventricle on the features of the QRS complex is decreased or reversed in right ventricular hypertrophy (RVH) and exaggerated in left ventricular hypertrophy (LVH) (Fig. 176-10). RVH causes a shift of the net forces of depolarization from the left and posterior toward the right and anteriorly. On the ECG, this produces tall R waves in V_1 (≥0.5 mV), with an abnormal S wave in V_5 or V_6 (≥0.7 mV). In the frontal plane, the mean QRS axis shifts to the right of vertical (usually >110°). Less extreme

FIGURE 176-9 ST-segment and T-wave changes. Arrows in each panel indicate the major features of each complex. *A*. Early repolarization (J-point elevation), normal variant. *B*. Acute pericarditis: (1) depressed T_a; (2) elevated ST; (3) normal T. *C*. Early acute myocardial infarction (AMI): (1) elevated ST; (2) tall, peaked T wave; steep angle between 1 and 2. *D*. AMI: (1) small Q wave; (2) elevated ST segment; (3) tall, peaked T wave with steep 2→3 angle. *E*. AMI: (1) pathologic Q wave; (2) elevated ST segment. *F*. AMI: (1) Q wave; (2) elevated ST segment; (3) terminal T-wave inversion. *G*. Angina pectoris (Prinzmetal variant) with ST elevation during pain. *H* and *I*. Angina pectoris (usual form) with horizontal or downward sloping ST segment during pain or exercise. *J*. J-point depression with upsloping ST segment during exercise, normal response. *K*. Primary T-wave inversion (2) in ischemia or primary muscle disease. *L*. Myocardial infarction (healed): (1) pathologic Q; (2) ST returning to baseline; (3) symmetrically inverted T wave. *M*. Digitalis effect: (1) downward coving of ST segment, merging into (2) an upright T wave. *N* to *P*. Nonspecific ST-segment and T-wave changes often seen in chronic ischemic heart disease. *Q*. Left ventricular strain pattern with (1) downsloping ST segment and (2) asymmetrically inverted (secondary) T wave. *R*. Downsloping ST segment merging into a deeply inverted T wave in ventricular conduction abnormality.

degrees of RVH may result in preservation of a moderately deep S wave in V_1, with an R-wave voltage exceeding the S-wave voltage, or a normal R wave with a shallow S wave and prominent terminal S waves in V_5 and V_6. The primary QRS manifestation of LVH is an increase in voltage in those leads which reflect the electrical activity of the left ventricle. R waves in the standard limb leads may increase beyond the normal limit of 2.0 mV. Concomitantly, there is a tendency for a shift of the frontal plane QRS axis to the left. It is not likely that LVH alone will cause a shift in the QRS axis beyond $-30°$, but it commonly causes a shift in the range of 0 to $-30°$ (Fig. 176-10). LVH causes a deep S wave in lead V_1 or V_2 (>2.5 mV) or an abnormal R wave in lead V_5 or V_6 (>2.5 mV). When T waves are normal, the presence of voltage criteria for LVH must be interpreted in terms of body habitus of an individual. Young, healthy, thin-chested individuals will frequently exceed the QRS voltage criteria for LVH in its absence. However, when the ST-segment and T-wave changes associated with "strain" are present (Figs. 176-9*Q*

and 176-10), the diagnosis of LVH is clarified. Similarly, borderline voltage criteria are more specific for LVH when associated with the ST-segment and T-wave changes of left ventricular strain.

ACUTE MYOCARDIAL INFARCTION Three pathophysiologic events occur, either in sequence or simultaneously, in an acute myocardial infarction—ischemia, injury, and infarction. The ECG manifestations of these processes include changes in the T waves (ischemia), ST segments (injury), and QRS complexes (infarction). The earliest T-wave changes of acute myocardial ischemia are tall, peaked T waves ("hyperacute") (Fig. 176-9*C* and *D*), followed later by symmetrically inverted T waves (Fig. 176-9*F* and *K*). When the electrical integrity of the cell membranes is affected, currents of injury develop. The injury pattern on ECG during evolution of a transmural infarction is an elevation of the ST segments in the leads facing the infarcting area (Fig. 176-9*C* and *F*). The combination of ischemia and injury causes elevated ST segments, followed by either tall, peaked T waves (in the very early stages) or inverted T waves

FIGURE 176-10 Ventricular hypertrophy. Left ventricular hypertrophy and strain with R wave >2.0 mV in limb leads; R >2.5 mV in V_5 and V_6, and S in V_1 >2.5 mV. The sum of S-V_1 or S-V_2 and R-V_5 or R-V_6 exceeds 3.5 mV. Strain is indicated by the downsloping ST segments and asymmetrically inverted T waves, especially in the lateral chest leads. The QRS-T vector angle is abnormally wide. Right ventricular hypertrophy is indicated by right axis deviation in the frontal plane and abnormal anterior forces in the horizontal plane. The former is indicated by a small R and deep S wave in lead I, and the latter by tall R waves in V_1 and V_2 with deep S waves in V_5 and V_6. The QRS-T angle is wide (strain).

(Fig. 176-11). In leads opposite the region of the acute infarction, reciprocal changes occur: depressed ST segments and upright or isoelectric T waves (Figs. 176-11 and 176-12). There is some controversy about the distinction between "reciprocal changes" and nearly identical changes reflecting coexistent ischemia in a vascular bed remote from the infarction, i.e., "ischemia at a distance." It is likely that remote ST depressions could be due to either. As the period of active injury resolves, the ST segments return to the baseline, but the inverted T waves may persist for days, months, or permanently (Fig. 176-9L). Pathologic Q waves are the QRS manifestation of a transmural myocardial infarction. Q waves are pathologic when they appear in a lead in which Q waves were previously not present, or when the Q waves of normal septal depolarization become exaggerated (>20 ms; >0.2 mV).

The ECG in an acute inferior wall myocardial infarction is shown in Fig. 176-11. Leads II, III, and aVF, which face the inferior surface of the left ventricle (see Fig. 176-1D), demonstrate the direct patterns of infarction (pathologic Q waves), injury (elevated ST segments), and ischemia (inversion of the T waves). Reciprocal changes (depressed ST, tall T) are demonstrated in aVL. The evolution of an acute anterior myocardial infarction is demonstrated in Fig. 176-12. The most obvious direct changes occur in aVL, V_2, and V_3, and reciprocal changes in II, III, and aVF. In the tracing of 4/11, ST elevations (most prominent in aVL, V_2, and V_3) are accompanied by "hyperacute" peaked T waves in V_2 and V_3. On 4/12, deeper Q waves are present in aVL and V_1 to V_3, and T waves have inverted in aVL and V_2 to V_5. ST elevations persist but less prominently. On 4/25, the pattern of a healing infarction—pathologic Q waves and

FIGURE 176-11 Acute inferior wall myocardial infarction. The ECG of 11/29 shows minor nonspecific ST-segment and T-wave changes. On 12/5 an acute myocardial infarction occurred. There are pathologic Q waves (1), ST-segment elevation (2), and terminal T-wave inversion (3) in leads II, III, and aVF indicating the location of the infarct on the inferior wall (see text). Reciprocal changes in aVL (small arrow). Increasing R-wave voltage with ST depression and increased voltage of the T wave in V_2 is characteristic of true posterior wall extension of the inferior infarction.

FIGURE 176-12 Acute anterior wall myocardial infarction. On 4/11, changes of a very early acute myocardial infarction in leads I, aVL, V_2, and V_3, with reciprocal changes in II, III, and aVF. On 4/12, ST segments remain elevated in the anterior leads, but T waves are inverted. On 4/25, a completed large anterior myocardial infarction is recorded—Q in I, aVL, V_1 to V_4, ischemic T waves—is present. Eventually, the T waves might become partially or completely normal, with persistence of the Q waves. An infarction of the true posterior wall of the left ventricle causes ECG changes opposite to those of an anterior infarction. Instead of Q waves, ST elevation, and T-wave inversion in the anterior precordial leads (V_1 and V_2), true posterior infarction is characterized by tall R waves, ST depression, and upright T waves in these leads. These infarctions usually occur in combination with inferior wall infarctions. Right ventricular myocardial infarction occurs infrequently and is almost always associated with inferior and/or posterior infarction of the left ventricle. Right ventricular infarction has no specific pattern on the standard 12-lead ECG; however, ST elevations on special right sided precordial leads (V_1R to V_6R) may identify acute RV infarcts.

A nontransmural (subendocardial or subepicardial) myocardial infarction may cause persistent ST-segment and T-wave changes similar to those seen in transmural infarctions. However, abnormal Q waves do not appear in the QRS complex, although R-wave and/or S-wave voltages may change. The Q-wave criterion for distinguishing transmural and subendocardial infarctions is a useful ECG tool, but pathologic data have shown that exceptions do occur. It is clear that non-Q-wave patterns may reflect more than a subendocardial infarct. Large areas of intramural infarction, with only a shell of epicardium surviving, may not result in Q-wave formation. Thus, it is more accurate to distinguish between Q-wave and non-Q-wave infarctions, rather than transmural and subendocardial infarctions. The ST-segment and T-wave changes of non-Q-wave infarction are common in leads I, II, III, aVL, aVF, and/or V_4 to V_6. Similar, but transient, changes may occur during the pain of angina pectoris, in shock, after pulmonary embolism, and secondary to acute central nervous system lesions.

CHRONIC ISCHEMIC HEART DISEASE Other than Q waves of prior myocardial infarction, the ECG in chronic ischemic heart disease is often nonspecific. The patterns of chronic myocardial ischemia are intrinsically variable, and this fact is compounded by the problem of coexistent ECG changes related to pharmacologic interventions and/or LVH. Chronic ischemic heart disease causes a broad range of ST-segment and T-wave changes (Fig. 176-9G to I, K, L, and N to P). There may be moderate degrees of horizontal ST-segment depression or a downward sloping ST segment, flattening or inversion of T waves, and prominent U waves. It is difficult to define an abnormal ST-segment depression in precise quantitative terms. However, if the J point is more than 0.5 mm below the isoelectric line, the ST segment is horizontal or downsloping, and there is an associated T-wave abnormality, myocardial ischemia should be considered. The common clinical expression of chronic ischemic heart disease, angina pectoris, may be accompanied by a normal resting ECG or nonspecific ST-segment and T-wave changes. However, during spontaneous or exercise-induced pain, the ECG may demonstrate the horizontal or downward sloping ST-segment depressions shown in Fig. 176-9H and I, or rarely the variant pattern of spontaneous transient ST elevations (Prinzmetal variant) (Fig. 176-9G).

INTRAVENTRICULAR CONDUCTION DISTURBANCES The complex anatomy of the specialized conducting system of the ventricles, in conjunction with the focal nature of most cardiac diseases, is reflected in the multiplicity of ECG patterns which result from disorders of the sequence of activation of the ventricles. Disease of both the SCT and ventricular myocardium plays a role in the various patterns. The universal feature of ventricular conduction disturbances is a prolongation of the time required for depolarization of a portion of a ventricle, an entire ventricle, or both ventricles. Delayed or slow conduction may be diffuse or may be confined to a portion of the QRS complex (Fig. 176-8). Prolongation of the QRS may be modest, as in left ventricular hypertrophy, or extreme, as in cardiomyopathies or metabolic abnormalities (Fig. 176-8).

The classic bundle branch block patterns are associated with specific lesions in the left or right bundle branch in the majority of cases. Complete right bundle branch block (RBBB) (Fig. 176-13) is

FIGURE 176-13 Intraventricular conduction abnormalities. Illustrated are right bundle branch block (RBBB); left bundle branch block (LBBB); left anterior hemiblock (LAH); right bundle branch block with left anterior hemiblock (RBBB + LAH); and right bundle branch block with left posterior hemiblock (RBBB + LPH) (see text).

characterized by prolongation of the QRS complex (≥ 0.12 s) with the delayed activation of the right ventricle accounting for a terminal delay on the ECG. Since septal activation from the left bundle branch system normally precedes right ventricular activation, *the initial forces of ventricular depolarization are not disturbed in RBBB*, and the ability to identify coexistent pathologic Q waves is not hindered. The delayed activation of the right ventricle is reflected by the presence of terminal forces directed anteriorly and to the right. The rightward direction of the slow terminal forces is indicated by the broad terminal S wave in leads I, aVL, and V_6 (Fig. 176-13). The anterior orientation of these forces is indicated by a large terminal R wave (R') in V_1. Since initial forces are not disturbed, the normal initial R wave in V_1 persists, followed by an S wave. Incomplete RBBB is present when the waveform criteria for RBBB (rSR') are present, but the QRS duration is <0.12 s.

Left bundle branch block (LBBB) is also characterized by a QRS duration ≥ 0.12 s. However, since normal initial ventricular depolarization is dependent upon the LBB to deliver the impulses of initial depolarization to the left septum, the patterns produced by LBBB are more complex. Normal septal depolarization is disturbed, and delay of the normally dominant left ventricular forces produces a more generalized disturbance of QRS morphology. The septal Q wave in standard leads I, aVL, and V_6 is typically lost. In addition, the initial anterior force reflected by the small R wave in lead V_1 may be lost because of a less anterior orientation of the initial forces. The delay in left ventricular activation produces the greatest degree of slowing in the mid and late portion of the QRS complex. This often results in notching at the peak of the upstroke in leads I and V_6 (see Figs. 176-8D and 176-14), with a late intrinsicoid deflection (>0.055 s) in V_5 and V_6. Most cases of LBBB produce secondary T-wave abnormalities as demonstrated in Fig. 176-14. Because of the changes in the initial forces, and the secondary ST-segment and T-wave changes, it is usually difficult to evaluate the QRS-complex, ST-segment, and T-wave changes of coexistent ischemic heart disease. When the intrinsicoid deflection is delayed in leads V_5 or V_6, but the QRS duration is <0.12 s, incomplete LBBB may be present. LBBB may be associated with either a normal QRS axis (Fig. 176-13) or left axis deviation. Those with left axis deviation usually have more extensive conducting system disease and left ventricular dysfunction. As a group, they are older, have higher mortality rates, and more advanced structural disease.

FIGURE 176-14 *A.* Acute pericarditis with ST-segment elevations in all leads except III, aVR, and V$_1$. *B.* Myocarditis: diffuse ST-segment and T-wave changes, with low-voltage T waves in the limb leads and primary T-wave changes in the chest leads. *C.* Cardiomyopathy: gross distortion of the QRS complex.

The ECG patterns referred to as the *left hemiblocks* must be distinguished from infarction or LVH patterns and from LBBB. *Left anterior hemiblock* (LAH) has been proposed to result from disease in the anterior radiation of fibers referred to as the anterior division of the LBB. *Left posterior hemiblock* (LPH) has been assumed to result from disease in the left posterior radiation. The complex nature of the LBB system has thus far defied a determination of whether focal proximal disease or diffuse distal disease in the distribution of these portions of the LBB is the mechanism responsible for the hemiblock patterns, although it is known that the pathologic process tends to be diffuse in those cases studied at autopsy.

LAH results in a moderate delay of activation of the superior portion of the left ventricular free wall, causing a modest prolongation of the QRS complex and shift of the front plane axis to the left. Initial septal depolarization is undisturbed (Fig. 176-13), and the QRS complex rarely exceeds 0.09 to 0.10 s. The differentiation between LAH and left ventricular hypertrophy (LVH) may occasionally be difficult. In general, LVH alone will not produce a left axis shift beyond $-30°$, and LAH will often produce left axis deviation $\geq -60°$. The key QRS features in left anterior hemiblock include small Q waves in leads I and aVL, with small initial R waves and deep S waves in leads II, III, and aVF.

LPH results in a moderate delay of activation of the posterior-inferior portion of the left ventricular free wall. Again, there is a modest prolongation of the QRS complex, but a shift of the frontal plane QRS axis to the *right*. Thus, the initial septal forces, though generally undisturbed, may be oriented more superiorly, producing small initial Q waves in leads II, III, and aVF. Since the specificity of the ECG manifestations of LPH is not very reliable, many clinicians will not make a diagnosis of isolated LPH without demonstrating a right axis shift on serial ECGs, plus definite exclusion of other causes of right axis shift. Of all the intraventricular conduction disturbances, isolated LPH is the most difficult to diagnose on ECG.

The hemiblocks frequently coexist with disease in the RBB system. The combination of RBBB, plus LAH or LPH, is referred to as *bifascicular block*—implying that two fascicles of the trifascicular model of the intraventricular SCT are diseased. This probably represents a pathophysiologic oversimplification, but it is useful for clinical purposes. Since RBBB alone does not produce abnormal left axis deviation, the coexistence of RBBB with abnormal left axis deviation (Fig. 176-13) is usually interpreted as LAH plus RBBB. Similarly, abnormal right axis deviation in association with RBBB is usually interpreted as the coexistence of LPH with RBBB, when the QRS criteria for LPH are met (Fig. 176-13). As is the case in isolated LPH, the diagnosis of LPH plus RBBB is difficult because a number of clinical settings may cause abnormal right axis deviation in conjunction with RBBB.

Trifascicular block describes abnormal conduction in all three divisions of the intraventricular SCT. The ECG diagnosis can be made only by inference when a patient has bifascicular block and a prolonged PR interval. Confirmation can be achieved only by intracardiac recordings (Chap. 184).

PERICARDITIS, MYOCARDITIS, AND THE CARDIOMYOPATHIES

Acute pericarditis causes elevation of the ST segments in many leads without the reciprocal changes seen in acute myocardial infarction (Fig. 176-14*A*). ST-segment elevation may occur in all leads except aVR and rarely is present in V$_1$. After a period of days, the diffuse ST elevations return to the baseline, and T-wave inversions may occur. Coexistent ST elevations and T-wave inversions do not occur as often as they do in myocardial infarction (compare Figs. 176-11 and 176-14*A*). T-wave abnormalities may persist for weeks or months after the acute episode of pericarditis. If the pericarditis is accompanied by significant degrees of pericardial effusion, electrical alternans may occur. On alternate beats, ECG voltage shifts in magnitude. There also may be low voltage of the QRS complexes and T waves in all leads. Finally, the T$_a$ waves may be transiently depressed because of atrial involvement by the inflammatory process [see Fig. 176-9*B* (1)].

The ECG changes of myocarditis (Chap. 192 and Fig. 176-14*B*) are often difficult to differentiate from the late phase of pericarditis, in which symmetric T-wave inversions are present. However, myocarditis may occur in many other settings, and an appreciation of the range of the ECG changes is important. Almost all systemic infections may produce minor myocardial involvement. Measles, mumps, influenza, hepatitis, infectious mononucleosis, and scarlet fever, just to name a few diseases, may be associated with ECG abnormalities and with histopathologic evidence of myocardial inflammation. When the myocardial involvement is subclinical, the ECG changes are usually subtle and nonspecific. There are minor T-wave changes, manifested as flattening or shallow inversion of the T waves in multiple leads (Fig. 176-9*O* and *P*). The conducting system may be involved, and prolongation of the PR interval may be noted. Resolution of these ECG changes over time is usual.

In clinically evident myocarditis, the ECG demonstrates symmetrically inverted T waves in most of the standard limb leads and in the lateral precordial leads (Fig. 176-14*B*). When the specialized conducting system is involved, bundle branch block or patterns of nonspecific intraventricular conduction defects may occur. Arrythmias are common. Resolution of ECG changes often lags behind clinical resolution of myocarditis.

The ECG may be helpful in distinguishing types of cardiomyopathies (Chap. 192). In the hypertrophic cardiomyopathies, the most common ECG pattern is LVH and strain (Fig. 176-10). When asymmetric septal hypertrophy is present, abnormal septal depolarization may be indicated by the presence of deep abnormal Q waves in leads I, aVL, V$_5$, and/or V$_6$, and a tall initial R wave may be present in V$_1$. In the congestive cardiomyopathies, nonspecific intraventricular conduction abnormalities, indicated by broad, notched QRS complexes without a specific bundle branch block pattern, are common (Fig. 176-14*C*). Nonspecific ST-segment and T-wave abnormalities are almost universal in congestive cardiomyopathies. In the restrictive cardiomyopathies, intraventricular conduction defects, low-voltage QRS complexes, or loss of R-wave progression across the precordium may occur.

ECG ABNORMALITIES IN METABOLIC AND ELECTROLYTE DISTURBANCES

The electrically active tissues of the heart are particularly sensitive to changes in the extracellular concentration of K$^+$, and dramatic ECG changes may accompany abrupt changes in [K$^+$]. The initial effect of acute *hyper*kalemia is the appearance of tall, peaked T waves (Fig. 176-15). As the severity of hyperkalemia increases, the QRS complex widens and blends into the tall, peaked T waves, P-wave voltage decreases and may disappear entirely, and the PR interval is prolonged. As these changes evolve, there is marked prolongation of the QRS complex (Fig. 176-15) with the evolution of continuity between the S wave and T wave, ultimately producing a sine wave configuration. This pattern is a very late and

FIGURE 176-15 Electrolyte disturbances. *Hyperkalemia* (K^+ − 6.8) with tall, peaked T waves. Severe hyperkalemia (K^+ = 9.1) with (1) flattening of the P wave, and ↑ PR interval (1→2), (2) marked widening of the QRS complex (2→3), and (3) merging of the S wave into the T wave. *Hypokalemia* produces flat or inverted T waves with prominent U waves, causing prolonged "QU" interval, while hypocalcemia produces true prolongation of the ST segment with marked QT prolongation.

ominous manifestation of hyperkalemia. Equally dangerous is the occurrence of severe *hypo*kalemia, which also produces characteristic ECG changes. Instead of the tall, peaked T waves of hyperkalemia, hypokalemia produces a flattening or inversion of the T wave with concomitant prominence of the U wave. In its fully developed state, the ECG gives the appearance of a very long QT interval. Careful analysis reveals that the QT interval is not so prolonged, and the U wave has assumed the appearance of the T wave (Fig. 176-15). Thus, the major prolongation is a "QU" prolongation. This ECG manifestation of hypokalemia may forewarn of the occurrence of serious ventricular arrhythmias, especially in the presence of digitalis or class IA antiarrythmic drugs such as quinidine. One must be careful to differentiate the ECG effects of hypo*calcemia* from hypo*kalemia*. Whereas hypokalemia may produce the appearance of a long ST segment and late T wave because of flattening of the T wave and prominence of the U wave, hypocalcemia does, in fact, produce prolongation of the ST segment with a late T wave (Fig. 176-15). Hypocalcemia is not as immediately ominous as hypokalemia in regard to potentially serious ventricular arrhythmias. Most of the other electrolyte imbalances produce ECG changes too nonspecific to be clinically useful.

Abnormalities of metabolism, such as hyper- or hypothyroidism, Addison's disease, diabetic ketoacidosis, and infiltrative diseases, such as amyloidosis and hemochromatosis, all may produce ECG abnormalities which may be helpful in the recognition of the disease process but are often nonspecific.

Many drugs, especially the antiarrhythmics and psychotropics, can influence the ECG. The most common effects are on the AV junction (prolonged PR interval) and on repolarization (ST-T wave changes and prolonged QT intervals).

VECTORCARDIOGRAPHY

A vectorcardiogram (VCG) is a continuous loop representing the sequence of instantaneous electrical vectors in a two-dimensional plane (shown diagrammatically in Fig. 176-5G). This form of recording, requiring simultaneous voltage information from two leads, is achieved by recording one ECG lead on the vertical axis and replacing time by a second lead on the horizontal axis. The resulting loop is photographed on an oscilloscope screen. Most VCG systems today employ an XYZ lead system in which X is analogous to lead I (left-right), Y is analogous to lead aVF (superoinferior), and Z represents a lead in the anteroposterior orientation, most closely analogous to lead V_2. The XY plane records a vectorial loop in the frontal plane, projected on the hexaxial reference in Fig. 176-1D. The XZ plane records the horizontal loop in which the left-right orientation is plotted against the anteroposterior orientation on a

reference system similar to that in Fig. 176-2B. In the YZ plane, the loop is in the sagittal orientation—the anteroposterior orientation (Z) plotted against the superoinferior orientation (Y). Recording in three planes provides information about spatial vectors, as in Fig. 176-5F. Loops consist of comma-shaped dots, the orientation of the comma indicating the direction of rotation, and the frequency of interruption providing a measurement of time. Closely grouped dots indicate a slow change in the magnitude and direction of the vector, while widely spread dots indicate rapid changes. Vectorial information of P waves, QRS complexes, ST segments, and T waves may be obtained.

The greatest value of the VCG today lies in the analysis of Q waves of uncertain significance and of certain intraventricular conduction abnormalities. When normal septal Q waves are absent in lead I or V_6, and no other evidence of septal infarction is present, the VCG may demonstrate either that the normal Q loop in the horizontal plane is absent, indicating a septal infarction or scarring, or conversely that the Q loop in the horizontal plane is morphologically normal but oriented directly anteriorly, accounting for the absence of the initial rightward forces. Similarly, the VCG can be helpful in assessing confusing initial forces or poor R-wave progression in the anterior precordial leads.

The VCG is particularly useful in identifying inferior wall myocardial infarctions. When the ECG is equivocal, the VCG may show the superior displacement of initial forces in the frontal plane and the clockwise rotation that is characteristic of inferior wall myocardial infarction. Furthermore, the difficulty in differentiating inferior wall infarctions from left anterior hemiblock on ECG, or recognizing their coexistence, may be aided by a VCG. In left anterior hemiblock, the initial forces are often normal, but there is superior displacement of the major portion of the frontal plane loop. However, the rotation is counterclockwise, in contrast to the clockwise rotation of inferior wall myocardial infarction. When the combination of inferior wall myocardial infarction and left anterior hemiblock is present, the infarction may be masked on the ECG; but the VCG may show the distinctly abnormal superiorly displaced initial forces of inferior wall myocardial infarction plus the counterclockwise rotation in the frontal plane characteristic of left anterior hemiblock.

REFERENCES

CASTELLANOS A, MYERBURG RJ: The resting electrocardiogram, in *The Heart*, 7th ed, JW Hurst et al (eds). New York, McGraw-Hill, 1990, p 265

COOKSEY JD et al: *Clinical Vectorcardiography and Electrocardiography*, 2d ed. Chicago, Year Book, 1977

FISCH C (ed): *Cardiovascular Clinics*, vol 5, no 3: *Complex Electrocardiography I*. Philadelphia, Davis, 1973

————: Electrocardiography and vectorcardiography, in *Heart Disease*, 3d ed, E Braunwald (ed). Philadelphia, Saunders, 1988, p 180

GOLDMAN MJ: *Principles of Clinical Electrocardiography,* 12th ed. Los Altos, California, Lange Medical Publishers, 1986

HOFFMAN BF, CRANEFIELD PF: *Electrophysiology of the Heart.* New York, McGraw-Hill, 1960

JOSEPHSON RA et al: Can serial exercise testing improve the prediction of coronary events in asymptomatic individuals? Circulation 81; 1:20, 1990

SILVERMAN ME et al: *Electrocardiography: Basic Concepts and Clinical Application.* New York, McGraw-Hill, 1983

177 NONINVASIVE METHODS OF CARDIAC EXAMINATION
Roentgenography, echocardiography, and radionuclide techniques

PATRICIA C. COME / JOSHUA WYNNE / EUGENE BRAUNWALD

ROENTGENOGRAPHY

The chest roentgenogram provides pathoanatomic information about the size and configuration of the heart and great vessels and pathophysiologic information about pulmonary arterial and venous pressures and flow. Chamber dilatation usually produces changes in cardiac size and contour. Myocardial hypertrophy, in contrast, often results in wall thickening at the expense of cavity size, producing only a slight alteration of the cardiac silhouette. Although standard 6-ft posteroanterior (PA) and lateral chest roentgenograms are routinely obtained, a cardiac series (Fig. 177-1) permits better assessment of chamber sizes and shapes. Image-intensification fluoroscopy may be used to detect calcification, recognize pericardial effusion or thickening if epicardial fat can be identified, assess movement of radiopaque valvular prostheses, or define further the size and motion of cardiac chambers and great vessels.

CARDIAC SILHOUETTE The *right atrium* is the most difficult chamber to evaluate. Enlargement, however, may cause bulging of the heart to the right and an increased curvature of the right heart border on PA and left anterior oblique views. The *right ventricle* is best seen on the lateral view, where its anterior wall lies behind the lower third of the sternum. As it enlarges, it displaces lung tissue, filling in the upper retrosternal space. Further dilatation may passively displace other chambers, particularly the left ventricle.

Enlargement of the *left atrial appendage* may be suspected by a bulge beneath the pulmonary artery on the PA film. Dilatation of the body of the *left atrium* is best demonstrated by posterior displacement of the barium-filled esophagus in the lateral or right anterior oblique view. As the left atrium dilates further, its right border contacts right lung posteriorly, forming a second border or "double density" adjacent to the right atrial wall. The left bronchus may be displaced posteriorly and superiorly. The *left ventricle* enlarges inferiorly, posteriorly, and to the left, often increasing the cardiothoracic ratio (maximal cardiac diameter divided by maximal internal thoracic diameter, normally less than 0.50). The chest roentgenogram is a useful screening or initial test, but other imaging techniques, such as echocardiography, provide more definitive assessment of individual cardiac chambers.

PULMONARY VASCULATURE Since pulmonary vessel size is proportional to flow, vessels normally taper from central to peripheral

FIGURE 177-1 Posteroanterior (*A,B*), lateral (*C,D*), right anterior oblique (*E,F*), and left anterior oblique (*G,H*) views of the heart, demonstrating the positions of the cardiac chambers, valves, and interatrial and interventricular septa. AV = azygos vein; SVC = superior vena cava; RA = right atrium; IVC = inferior vena cava; TV = tricuspid valve; RV = right ventricle; MPA = main pulmonary artery; RPA = right pulmonary artery; LPA = left pulmonary artery; AO = aorta; LA = left atrium; LAA = left atrial appendage; LV = left ventricle; MV = mitral valve; IVS = interventricular septum; IAS = interatrial septum; RAA = right atrial appendage. [*From PC Come (ed), Diagnostic Cardiology. Reprinted with permission of Robert E. Dinsmore, M.D., and J.B. Lippincott Company.*]

and from dependent to nondependent portions of the lungs. Increased flow, as with left-to-right shunts, results in enlargement and tortuosity of all vessels. Regional or global reduction of flow, due to pulmonary emboli, emphysematous blebs, or a right-to-left shunt, results in decreased vessel caliber.

Increases in pulmonary venous pressure produce perivascular edema in the dependent portions of the lungs, causing loss of vessel wall definition and redistribution of flow to nondependent areas. Further increases cause interstitial edema, with peribronchial cuffing, perihilar and peripheral lung haziness, and linear densities (Kerley B lines) perpendicular to the pleura. They represent fluid collection in the dependent interlobular septa. Alveolar pulmonary edema, with air bronchograms, may ultimately develop. There may be considerable temporal delay between hemodynamic changes and roentgenographic findings.

Pulmonary artery hypertension produces dilatation of the main pulmonary artery and its central branches. When associated with conditions increasing pulmonary arteriolar resistance, such as primary pulmonary hypertension, the distal pulmonary arteries often appear small ("pruned").

SPECIALIZED RADIOGRAPHIC METHODS *Digital subtraction angiography* (DSA) uses computer processing to digitize high-resolution fluoroscopic images. An image of the region of interest is subtracted from images obtained following intravenous, intracardiac, or intraarterial injection of contrast medium. Elimination of radiographic densities resulting from soft tissues and bone permits excellent definition of vascular structures using a concentration of contrast medium lower than that necessary for routine angiography. Vascular applications include recognition of vascular tumors, pulmonary emboli, and abnormalities of the aorta or of peripheral, cerebral, and renal arteries. Study of the heart permits assessment of ventricular function, intracardiac shunts, other congenital abnormalities, and bypass graft patency.

Computed tomography, *magnetic resonance imaging*, and *positron emission tomography* are also used to provide information about the heart and vessels. These techniques are discussed in Chap. 178.

ECHOCARDIOGRAPHY

Echocardiography uses ultrasound to image the heart and great vessels. A transducer containing a piezoelectric crystal, which interconverts electrical and mechanical (i.e., sound) energy, functions both as the transmitter of sound and as the receiver of reflected waves. Three types of studies are performed: M-mode, two-dimensional, and Doppler. In *M-mode echocardiography*, a single transducer, emitting 1000 to 2000 pulses per second along a single line, provides an "ice-pick" view of the heart, with excellent *temporal* resolution. When beam direction is changed, the heart can be scanned from the ventricles to the aorta and left atrium (Fig. 177-2). *Two-dimensional echocardiography* (Figs. 177-3 and 177-4) produces an image in two distance dimensions by steering the sound beam through an arc of up to 90° some 30 times per second. It provides excellent *spatial* resolution, permitting analysis of structural movement in real time from multiple transducer positions on the chest and upper abdomen. It is also possible to obtain imaging and Doppler echocardiographic studies via the esophagus, using a probe mounted at the tip of a flexible gastroscope. Transesophageal echocardiography appears most valuable in the assessment of prosthetic mitral valve function and in the detection of left atrial thrombus, aortic dissection, and complications of infective endocarditis.

Doppler echocardiography (Fig. 177-5) detects blood flow velocity and turbulence. When sound encounters moving red blood cells, the frequency of its reflected signal is altered. The magnitude of the change *(Doppler shift)* indicates the velocity *V* of blood flow with respect to the sound beam:

$$V = \frac{C \times (\text{Doppler shift})}{(2 \times \text{emitted frequency}) \cos \theta}$$

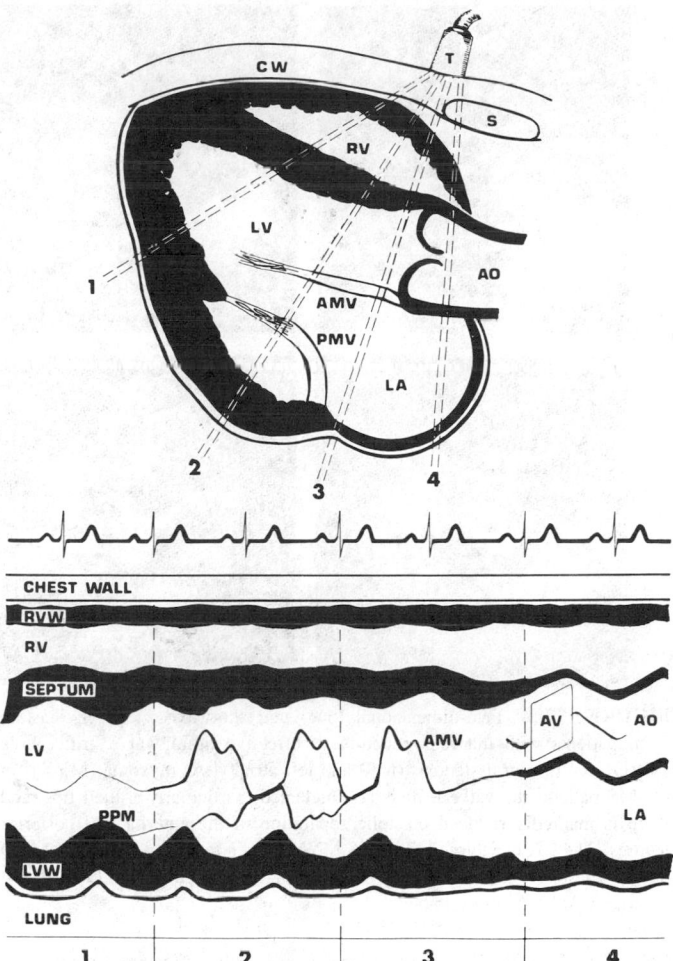

FIGURE 177-2 Schematic diagrams of an M-mode echocardiographic scan through a normal heart. A long-axis section of the heart is depicted in the upper diagram. The echocardiographic movement patterns that arise from the corresponding anatomic structures are illustrated in the bottom diagram. CW = chest wall; T = echocardiographic transducer; S = sternum; RV = right ventricle; LV = left ventricle; AO = aortic root; AMV = anterior mitral leaflet; PMV = posterior mitral leaflet; LA = left atrium; RVW = right ventricular wall; AV = aortic valve; PPM = posterior papillary muscle; LVW = left ventricular wall. [*From PC Come, Echocardiography in diagnosis and management of cardiovascular disease, Compr Ther 6(5):58, 1980. Courtesy of The Laux Company, Inc., Ayer, MA.*]

where *C* is the speed of sound in tissue, and θ is the angle between the Doppler beam and the mean axis of blood flow. An upward shift (increased frequency of the reflected sound) indicates blood motion toward the transducer and a downward shift, motion away. There are several types of Doppler studies, all of which can be performed using a single probe. Pulsed Doppler echocardiography, which uses a single crystal to assess flow velocity and turbulence within operator-selected areas of interest in the heart and great vessels, permits excellent spatial localization of flow disturbances resulting from valvular stenosis and regurgitation and from shunts. Quantitation of high-flow velocity requires a continuous wave transducer with two separate, adjacent crystals, one that continuously transmits sound and one that continuously receives reflected sound. Since continuous wave transducers cannot spatially localize flow disturbances, optimal assessment of flow within the heart and vessels generally requires both pulsed and continuous wave technology. Pressure gradients (*P*) across restrictive orifices such as cardiac valves can be calculated using the modified Bernoulli equation, $P = 4V^2$, where *P* is the pressure gradient in mmHg and *V* the velocity in m/s. Doppler color flow imaging is a complicated, combined imaging and Doppler technique in which blood flow direction, relative velocity, and turbulence are

FIGURE 177-3 Two-dimensional long- and short-axis views in diastole from patients with marked reduction of effective mitral valve orifice area (MVO) due to mitral stenosis (MS) and left atrial (LA) myxoma (MYX). In the MS patient, the valve leaflets are thickened, particularly at their tips, and there is markedly reduced diastolic separation of the anterior and posterior leaflets. The LA is enlarged. The LA MYX is seen to prolapse into the MVO during diastole, causing obstruction. RV = right ventricle; LV = left ventricle; AoV = aortic valve.

FIGURE 177-4 Long-axis parasternal views of the left ventricle in diastole and systole in a normal individual and in patients with dilated cardiomyopathy (CM) and hypertrophic cardiomyopathy (HCM). Normal diastolic wall thicknesses and normal systolic wall thickening and excursion are illustrated in the left panels. In the patient with dilated CM, left ventricular (LV) and left atrial

depicted by various colors superimposed upon a two-dimensional image of the heart. The spatial information permits easier detection of shunts and of valvular regurgitation, especially of the periprosthetic type, and it may facilitate positioning of the sound beam for optimal pulsed and continuous wave Doppler interrogation of flow jets. Temporal resolution is limited by the low frame rate required for analysis. Combined Doppler and imaging techniques permit calculation of cardiac output. Unfortunately, not all patients can be successfully studied by echocardiography. Sound penetration may be suboptimal in many elderly, obese, and emphysematous patients.

VALVULAR HEART DISEASE Imaging echocardiography can detect abnormalities of valve thickness and movement responsible for stenosis and regurgitation. In addition, the heart's response to pressure or volume overload can be assessed in terms of chamber dilatation, hypertrophy, and wall movement. Doppler techniques permit evaluation of regurgitation and stenosis. (See also Chap. 188.)

Mitral stenosis The echocardiographic appearance of a restricted valve opening, due to leaflet thickening and commissural fusion, and of shortened, thickened chordae is virtually diagnostic of rheumatic deformity (Fig. 177-3, left). Planimetry of the mitral area in the diastolic short axis view and evaluation of the rate of falloff of the estimated transmitral diastolic pressure gradient by Doppler permit quite reliable estimation of valve area. Using the Doppler technique, mitral valve area (MVA) in square centimeters can be estimated with the equation, MVA = 220 divided by duration of time (in milliseconds) necessary for the peak diastolic pressure gradient to decrease by 50 percent. Other causes of inflow obstruction, such as atrial myxoma (Fig. 177-3, right) or thrombus, massive annular calcification, supravalvular ring, cor triatriatum, and parachute mitral valve may also be detected.

Mitral regurgitation Systolic mitral competence depends upon normal function of the mitral leaflets and their supporting structures, including the annulus, chordae tendineae, papillary muscles, and surrounding myocardium. Two-dimensional techniques are preferable

(LA) diameters are increased, and there is markedly reduced systolic thickening and excursion of the septum (SEP) and posterior wall (PW). In the patient with HCM, the SEP is abnormally thick and highly echogenic. The LV cavity is small in diastole and almost disappears during systolic contraction. RV = right ventricle; MV = mitral valve; AoV = aortic valve.

FIGURE 177-5 Continuous wave Doppler studies, performed with the probe positioned at the apex, from one patient (*A, B*) with aortic stenosis (AS), aortic insufficiency (AI), and mitral regurgitation (MR) and from another patient (*C, D*) with mital stenosis (MS), severe MR, and AI. Flow away from the transducer, in the AS and MR jets, is depicted below the center (zero flow) line, while flow toward the transducer, in the AI and MS jets, is depicted above the center line. Flow velocity (*V*) in meters per second is given on the right side of each panel. As expected from knowledge of points of crossover between aortic, left ventricular, and left atrial pressures, the AS signal is shorter in duration than the MR signal and has a lower velocity. The AI signal is of longer duration than the MS signal. Instantaneous pressure gradients (*P*) across the valves can be calculated using the equation, $P = 4V^2$. Peak *V* of 5.1 m/s in the AS jet indicates a peak left ventricular to aortic *P* of 104 mmHg, while the peak *V* of 6.8 m/s in the MR jet indicates a left ventricular to left atrial systolic *P* of 185 mmHg. Peak aortic to left ventricular diastolic *P* in the AI jet is 81 mmHg, and peak left atrial to left ventricular *P* in the MS jet is 40 mmHg. Mean gradient, calculated using an off-line computer system, in the MS jet was markedly elevated at 26 mmHg.

to M-mode in recognizing etiologies of mitral regurgitation, which include rheumatic disease, prolapse, flail leaflets resulting from chordal or papillary muscle rupture, annular calcification, atrioventricular canal defects, myxomas, endocarditis, hypertrophic cardiomyopathy, and ventricular dysfunction. Doppler mapping provides a gross estimate of the severity of regurgitation.

Aortic stenosis Subvalvular, valvular, and supravalvular obstruction can generally be detected by two-dimensional echocardiography. Systolic leaflet doming and an unusual number or size of cusps (two in a bicuspid valve) suggest congenital valve disease. Acquired fibrosis and calcification cause valve thickening. Normal leaflet separation excludes critical acquired aortic stenosis, but decreased separation is not specific for stenosis. Doppler detection of high-flow velocity across the valve, corresponding to a high transvalvular gradient, supports stenosis. Lesser flow velocities do not, however, exclude stenosis because both reduced stroke volume and inability to position the Doppler beam parallel to flow may appreciably decrease measured velocities. If velocity can be reliably measured, aortic valve area (AVA) can be quantitated using a continuity equation which assumes equal volume flow across the aortic valve and left ventricular (LV) outflow tract:

$$AVA = \frac{(LV \text{ outflow tract area})(LV \text{ outflow tract velocity})}{\text{velocity in aortic stenotic jet}}$$

Aortic regurgitation Aortic root dilatation and dissection can be distinguished from valve abnormalities causing regurgitation, including congenital disease, sclerosis, endocarditis, prolapse, and flail cusps. Two-dimensional techniques best define structural pathology, but M-mode techniques more readily detect both diastolic vibrations of the anterior mitral leaflet, a very sensitive sign of aortic regurgitation, and premature mitral closure, produced by the marked elevation of left ventricular diastolic pressure which may accompany severe, acute regurgitation. The presence and spatial extent of regurgitation is evaluated by Doppler study.

Tricuspid and pulmonary valve disease Two-dimensional scanning has improved visualization of right-sided valves. Changes in structure and movement may permit detection of rheumatic deformity, Ebstein's malformation, prolapse, flail cusps, endocarditis, congenital dysplasia, and thickening due to carcinoid, amyloid, Loeffler's endocarditis, or endocardial fibrosis. Systolic doming of the pulmonic valve is characteristic of pulmonic stenosis. Stenosis and regurgitation are assessed by Doppler techniques. The flow velocity in a tricuspid regurgitant jet can be used to estimate right ventricular and pulmonary arterial systolic pressures, permitting identification of pulmonary hypertension.

Prosthetic valves Mechanical prostheses are difficult to evaluate, because their intrinsically high echogenicity interferes with the recognition of vegetations and thrombi. Abnormal timing of valve opening and closure, best assessed using combined phonocardiography and M-mode techniques, and abnormalities on Doppler study may suggest dysfunction, but angiography and hemodynamic assessment are often necessary for full evaluation. Abnormalities of bioprostheses, including fibrosis, calcification, vegetations, and tears, are more easily recognized.

Endocarditis Valvular vegetations, characterized by masses of shaggy-appearing echoes, are evident in over half of patients with endocarditis. While their detection is associated with an increased risk of complications, many patients recover uneventfully with antibiotic therapy alone. (See also Chap. 90.)

Left ventricle M-mode echocardiography is widely used to measure left ventricular size, wall thickness, and function. The rate of wall thinning in diastole may permit assessment of diastolic function, and the percentage of shortening of the minor axis, normally greater than 28 percent, and the mean velocity of circumferential fiber shortening are useful measurements of systolic performance. These indexes of systolic performance are influenced, however, by preload and afterload as well as by myocardial contractility. Analyses of end-systolic pressure-dimension relations, which are independent of preload and incorporate afterload, provide better information regarding contractile function. Estimates of global ventricular performance, based on ice-pick M-mode views, are useful, however, only when ventricular shape is normal and systolic movement relatively symmetric in extent and timing. Two-dimensional echocardiography, which images the ventricle in a number of different planes, improves assessment of volumes and function, particularly in patients with asymmetric contraction resulting from ischemic heart disease. The left ventricular apex, the most common site of wall movement abnormalities and thrombi, can be adequately visualized only by two-dimensional techniques.

Echocardiography permits recognition of *cardiomyopathy* and classification into dilated, hypertrophic, and restrictive-obliterative types (Fig. 177-4). In dilated cardiomyopathy, both ventricles are generally enlarged and poorly contracting, and wall thicknesses are normal or only slightly increased. In contrast, appreciable ventricular hypertrophy, usually involving the septum asymmetrically, small ventricular size, enhanced systolic performance and impaired diastolic relaxation, characterize hypertrophic cardiomyopathy. Systolic anterior movement of the mitral valve to abut the septum and partial midsystolic closure of the aortic valve correlate with dynamic obstruction. Increased wall thickness also characterizes infiltrative disorders. In amyloidosis, the thick walls often appear "speckled" and there is diminished voltage on electrocardiogram (ECG).

Pericardial effusion Echocardiography can detect effusions as small as 15 to 20 mL, while certain findings, such as diastolic compression of the right atrium and ventricle, may suggest tamponade.

Cardiac masses   Most masses involving the heart and pericardium are easily recognized. They include myxomas (Fig. 177-3), other primary and secondary tumors, and thrombi. The left atrium and its appendage are best studied by transesophageal echocardiography.

Congenital heart disease   Since valvular abnormalities and relationships of atria, valves, ventricles, and great vessels can easily be recognized by two-dimensional echocardiography, this technique has revolutionized the diagnosis of congenital heart disease. Contrast and Doppler echocardiography, especially color flow mapping, facilitate detection of shunts and of valvular stenosis and regurgitation.

RADIONUCLIDE IMAGING OF THE HEART

There are four major clinical indications for radionuclide study of the heart: (1) assessment of systolic and diastolic ventricular function using radionuclide ventriculography; (2) identification and quantification of intracardiac shunts using radioangiocardiography; (3) assessment of myocardial perfusion using ionic tracers, principally thallium 201; and (4) detection of acute myocardial infarction with infarct-avid radionuclides.

VENTRICULAR PERFORMANCE   Radionuclide ventriculography (RVG) uses a radioactive intravascular indicator to delineate heart chambers and great vessels (Fig. 177-6). The radionuclide, usually technetium 99m, is generally attached to red blood cells. RVGs may be performed using two different methods. In the *first-pass* technique, radiotracer is injected intravenously, and a scintillation camera tracks its transit through the right heart, lungs, and left heart. In the *equilibrium*, or *gated, method*, counts are recorded from several hundred cardiac cycles following uniform distribution of radiotracer throughout the blood pool. The scintigraphic information in each cycle is divided into multiple frames (often 30 or more),

FIGURE 177-6   End-diastolic and end-systolic gated blood pool images from a normal individual (with estimated left and right ventricular ejection fractions of 69 and 45 percent, respectively) and from a patient with idiopathic dilated cardiomyopathy and marked, global reduction of left ventricular systolic function (left ventricular ejection fraction of 23 percent). In the patient with cardiomyopathy, there is very little change in left ventricular cavity size or count density from diastole to systole. The right ventricle, however, shows normal function, with an ejection fraction of 57 percent. RV = right ventricle; LV = left ventricle.

using the ECG as a timing reference. Counts from corresponding frames of each cycle are then summed by computer to provide images of the spatial distribution and density of counts over time. Images are generally obtained in at least two views [anterior and left anterior oblique (LAO)]. Gated scans are frequently obtained after first-pass scans, since no additional injection of radionuclide is required. Because detected counts, after background subtraction, are proportional to blood volume, equilibrium studies permit estimation of chamber volumes, enabling calculation of left and right ventricular ejection fractions, left-to-right ventricular stroke volume ratios, and rates of ventricular ejection and filling. Agreement with standard catheterization methods has been excellent. Repeated scans can be obtained up to 20 h after injection, permitting assessment of the effects of interventions, such as exercise and medications, on ventricular performance.

RVG may be used to detect patients with chronic ischemic heart disease. Since resting function may be normal, exercise is often used to provoke ischemia. Scans are obtained at rest and at peak exercise. Failure to increase left ventricular ejection fraction by at least 5 percent and development of one or more regional wall movement abnormalities have a sensitivity and specificity of approximately 90 and 60 percent, respectively, for detection of significant coronary disease. The test is most helpful in patients with an intermediate pretest probability of disease. Low resting ejection fractions after acute infarction have been correlated with increased short- and long-term morbidity and mortality. Mitral regurgitation, septal rupture, and aneurysms resulting from infarction may also be detected. RVG can assess systolic and diastolic function in patients with cardiomyopathy (Fig. 177-6) or volume overload. A reduced resting ejection fraction correlates with a poor prognosis in patients with mitral or aortic regurgitation, even after valve replacement. The added value of exercise RVG in detecting reduced myocardial reserve due to volume overload remains controversial. Thrombi and other tumors may be recognized, but RVG is less sensitive than echocardiography.

SHUNT SCINTIGRAPHY   Assessment of left-to-right shunts utilizes a modification of the first-pass RVG in which the "region of interest" is focused over an area of lung. Following rapid injection of radiotracer into a large vein, usually the external jugular, the pulmonary time-activity curve is recorded by a gamma camera-computer system. Normally, counts increase sharply as the bolus reaches the lung underlying the detector. Following peak activity, there is a smooth descent and a later, smaller increase in counts representing normal recirculation of the radiotracer following systemic circulation. Left-to-right shunts cause premature interruption of the descent, due to early reappearance of radioactivity within the lung. Computer analysis of the areas under the curve permits reliable determination of the ratio of pulmonic-to-systemic blood flow. Right-to-left shunts may also be recognized and quantified.

MYOCARDIAL PERFUSION IMAGING   Certain radiolabeled monovalent cations, especially the potassium analogue thallium 201 (half-life of 72 h), are widely used to assess myocardial perfusion since their active uptake by normal myocardial cells is proportional to regional blood flow. Areas of myocardial necrosis, fibrosis, and ischemia show reduced thallium accumulation ("cold spots") on images obtained soon after injection. Following its initial accumulation within cells, however, thallium 201 continues to exchange with the systemic pool. After several hours, all viable myocardial cells with intact membrane function will contain nearly equal concentrations.

Thallium 201 scintigraphy is most commonly used to detect exercise-induced ischemia (Fig. 177-7). Thallium is injected intravenously at peak exercise, and images are obtained in several projections 5 to 10 min later. Normal scans show relatively homogeneous distribution of activity, while those of patients with infarction or ischemia typically demonstrate one or more "cold spots." Due to continued exchange of thallium between viable cells and the systemic pool, however, initial defects due to ischemia "fill in" on repeat imaging several hours later. Areas of infarction demonstrate persistent reduction of uptake. Compared to routine exercise electrocardiogra-

FIGURE 177-7 Serial thallium 201 scintigrams obtained in the 45° LAO projection in a patient undergoing exercise testing for evaluation of chest pain. The immediate postexercise image (*left*) demonstrates decreased perfusion of the septum. The 1- and 2-h delayed images (*middle and right*) demonstrate "filling in" of the defect, reflecting redistribution. The computer-derived time-activity curves (*bottom*) confirm the significant reduction in initial counts in the septum, relative to the posterolateral wall, and demonstrate near equalization of activity by 2 h. S = septum; PL = posterolateral wall. [*From PC Come (ed), Diagnostic Cardiology. Reprinted with permission of George A. Beller, M.D., and J.B. Lippincott Company.*]

phy, exercise thallium scintigraphy increases the sensitivity for detection of coronary disease from approximately 60 to 80 percent and increases specificity slightly from about 80 to 90 percent. It is most useful in patients with atypical chest pain in whom the exercise ECG is nondiagnostic or uninterpretable due to left bundle branch block, ventricular hypertrophy, or drug and electrolyte effects; in patients who fail to achieve 85 percent of predicted maximal heart rate; and in patients with a high likelihood of a false-positive exercise ECG study. Thallium scanning improves localization of ischemia and provides prognostic information, since the presence and number of redistributing defects correlate with the incidence of future cardiac events. Thallium scintigraphy has also been used to detect ischemia during pacing, dipyridamole-induced coronary vasodilatation, or spontaneous pain.

Thallium scanning does not distinguish new from old infarcts and is less accurate than serum enzyme analysis in detecting acute necrosis. It does, however, offer prognostic information. Patients with smaller defects have better survival rates. On submaximal exercise thallium tests following infarction, the presence of multiple or redistributing defects or increased lung uptake of thallium (probably representing transudation into the lung during periods of high pulmonary capillary pressure) identifies patients at higher risk for postinfarction morbidity and mortality.

Computed tomography using positron-emitting isotopes of potassium analogues permits quantitative assessment of radiotracer uptake. The short half-lives of such isotopes permit multiple studies over short periods of time, allowing assessment of changes in myocardial perfusion induced by therapeutic interventions.

POSITRON EMISSION TOMOGRAPHY   See Chap. 178.

ACUTE INFARCT SCINTIGRAPHY   Pyrophosphate appears to bind to calcium and organic macromolecules in irreversibly damaged myocardial cells. If coronary flow is sufficient for its delivery to necrotic myocardium (10 to 40 percent of normal flow is required), technetium 99m stannous pyrophosphate will bind there, producing an image with increased uptake ("hot spot"). Scans are most likely to be positive when injections are performed 48 to 72 h after suspected

infarction, when the elevated creatine kinase activity has often returned to normal. The major clinical indication is the detection of acute infarction in those rare patients in whom traditional diagnostic methods cannot be interpreted or have provided equivocal results. Sensitivity and specificity for transmural infarcts are both about 90 percent. Uptake is often fainter and more poorly localized in subendocardial infarcts, and myocardial damage from causes other than coronary disease may result in a positive scan.

REFERENCES

COME PC (ed): *Diagnostic Cardiology. Noninvasive Imaging Techniques.* Philadelphia, Lippincott, 1985

FEIGENBAUM H: *Echocardiography*, 4th ed. Philadelphia, Lea & Febiger, 1986

GERSON MC (ed): *Cardiac Nuclear Medicine.* New York, McGraw-Hill, 1987

HATLE H, ANGELSEN B (eds): *Doppler Ultrasound in Cardiology: Physical Principles and Clinical Applications*, 2d ed. Philadelphia, Lea & Febiger, 1985

HOLMAN BL: Nuclear cardiology, in *Heart Disease*, 3d ed, E Braunwald (ed). Philadelphia, Saunders, 1988, pp 83–139

NANDA NC (ed): *Doppler Echocardiography.* New York, Igaku-Shoin, 1985

SEWARD JB et al: Transesophageal echocardiography: Technique, anatomic correlations, implementation, and clinical applications. Mayo Clin Proc 63:649, 1988

178   NEW CARDIAC IMAGING TECHNIQUES

CHARLES B. HIGGINS

The strategy for applying cardiac imaging techniques for the diagnosis of cardiovascular disease is currently in transition. Echocardiography and cardiac scintigraphy (Chap. 177) have been used with increasing frequency during the past decade. Initially, these techniques were used for preliminary diagnosis but definitive therapy was generally based upon cardiac catheterization and angiography. Echocardiographic findings now have been accepted as sufficiently reliable and definitive for preoperative evaluation of some cardiac lesions. The emergence of the new noninvasive tomographic techniques, which include cine-computed tomography (cine-CT), magnetic resonance imaging (MRI), and positron emission tomography (PET), should encourage further the trend away from catheterization as a requisite for definitive therapy. The strength of cine-CT and MRI lies in their being comprehensive cardiac imaging techniques for evaluation of both cardiac anatomy and function. Because of the good contrast and spatial resolution and the capacity to image the entire heart in a tomographic fashion, quantitation of dimensions and function is achieved by cine-CT and MRI to a degree even exceeding that possible with cardiac angiography. Myocardial metabolism can now be assessed with positron emission tomography and magnetic resonance spectroscopy (MRS). Because these new techniques are still in the stage of development and evaluation, they are not available at many hospitals at the current time. The most readily available of the new techniques is MRI, but many of these instruments are still not fully adapted for cardiac diagnosis.

FAST COMPUTED TOMOGRAPHY (CINE-CT)

The unique design of the cine-CT scanner accomplishes the x-ray exposure for a complete tomogram in 50 ms. This short exposure time vitiates the degrading effects of cardiac motion. Moreover, tomograms at the same level can be obtained sequentially after a delay of only 8 ms and initiated by, as well as related precisely to, the time in the cardiac cycle. The multiple sequential images can all be obtained within a single cardiac cycle and thus provide a true real

TABLE 178-1   Principal indications for the new imaging modalities for cardiovascular diagnosis

Fast computed tomography
1 Thoracic aortic diseases
  a Dissection
  b Aneurysm
2 Pericardial disease
  a Constrictive diseases
  b Pericardial cysts, tumors
3 Paracardiac and intracardiac masses
  a Primary tumors
  b Secondary tumors
  c Intracardiac thrombus
4 Coronary artery bypass graft patency
5 Complications of myocardial infarctions
  a Left ventricular aneurysms
  b Left ventricular thrombus
6 Analysis of ventricular function
  a Global and regional left ventricular function (volume and wall thickness)
  b Global right ventricular function (volume and wall thickness)
  c Distribution of ventricular hypertrophy (assessment of hypertrophic cardiomyopathy)
  d Ventricular function during interventions (exercise, drug interventions)
  e Regional myocardial perfusion (under evaluation)

Magnetic resonance imaging
1 Thoracic aortic diseases
  a Dissection
  b Aneurysm
  c Thrombus
  d Aortitis
  e Aortic hemorrhage
2 Pericardial diseases
  a Constrictive disease
  b Effusion, hemorrhagic vs. nonhemorrhagic
  c Pericardial cyst, tumor
3 Paracardiac and intracardiac masses
  a Primary tumors (myxoma, etc.)
  b Secondary tumors (lung, mediastinal, metastatic)
  c Intracardiac thrombus
4 Hypertrophic cardiomyopathy
  a Variant forms (distribution of hypertrophy)
5 Complications of myocardial infarction
  a Left ventricular aneurysm and pseudoaneurysm
  b Left ventricular thrombus
6 Congenital heart disease
  a Thoracic aortic anomalies
    (1) Arch anomalies
    (2) Coarctation
  b Pulmonary arterial anomalies
    (1) Pulmonary atresia (presence and size of central pulmonary arteries)
    (2) Unilateral absence (atresia)
    (3) Peripheral pulmonary stenoses
  c Complex lesions
    (1) Univentricular atrioventricular connections
    (2) Volume of ventricles
    (3) Presence and size of ventricular septum
    (4) Status of extracardiac operative procedures: Fontan, Rastelli, Jatene, etc.
7 Analysis of ventricular function
  a Ventricular volumes and mass
  b Regional left ventricular function
  c Detection and quantitation of valvular regurgitation

Positron emission tomography
1 Ischemic heart disease
  a Recognition of viable myocardium
  b Regional myocardial perfusion

time image; these images are laced together in a closed-loop cinematic format, termed a *cine-CT display.*

The tomograms are approximately 10 mm in thickness, so that 12 to 14 adjacent tomograms are required to encompass the average adult heart. Eight tomographic levels can be acquired during a single imaging sequence. The maximum number of images is 80 per sequence. When tomographic images encompassing the entire heart are required, cine-CT becomes a three-dimensional imaging technique. Consequently, highly accurate and reproducible measurements of ventricular volume are possible. Such precision is possible because chamber volumes can be measured directly by planimetry of the blood pool on each tomogram encompassing the various cardiac chambers, rather than estimating volumes through assumed geometric models derived from measurements in one or two planes.

The blood pool is distinguished from the myocardium after the intravenous injection of iodinated contrast medium. Since the latter and ionizing radiation are used, cine-CT is not a true noninvasive cardiac imaging technique, like echocardiography and MRI. While cine-CT is effective for the diagnosis of many congenital and acquired abnormalities, its role in anatomic diagnosis is limited because of the high diagnostic yield achieved by other totally noninvasive techniques.

INDICATIONS   The principal indications for fast CT in the diagnosis of heart disease are given in Table 178-1. In ischemic heart disease, cine-CT demonstrates regional wall thinning and absence of systolic wall thickening at the site of prior myocardial infarction. It is most effective for demonstrating complications of infarction such as mural thrombi and true or false aneurysms of the left ventricle. A mural thrombus produces a filling defect projecting into the left ventricular blood pool; it is usually attached to the wall thinned by prior infarction. An aneurysm produces a regional evagination of the left ventricular wall in diastole and paradoxical motion during systole.

Cine-CT has a diagnostic accuracy of greater than 90 percent in the determination of patency of coronary arterial bypass grafts (Fig. 178-1). After intravenous injection of contrast medium, scans are exposed sequentially; the bypass grafts are opacified simultaneously with the ascending aorta. The technique is not usually capable of identifying stenosis of the graft or adequacy of blood flow through the graft, but there is hope that flow abnormalities might be detectable by analysis of contrast-dilution curves or contrast transit times in the grafts.

Cine-CT can be used in the evaluation of hypertrophic and congestive cardiomyopathies by quantitating ventricular volumes and myocardial mass. Because of the wide field of view and three-dimensional scope of this technique, it can depict the distribution of ventricular hypertrophy. This is particularly useful for definitive

FIGURE 178-1   Cine-CT images at the level of the proximal ascending aorta acquired on sequential heart beats during passage of contrast medium throughout the central cardiovascular structures. The bypass grafts to the right (arrow) and left anterior descending (arrow) coronary arteries opacify simultaneously with the ascending aorta (A). Images from upper left to lower right display sequential opacification from pulmonary artery to the aorta.

FIGURE 178-2 CT image shows calcification (arrow) and thickening of the pericardium in a patient with constrictive pericarditis.

assessment of the various forms of hypertrophic cardiomyopathy (Chap. 192).

The role of cine-CT in valvular heart disease is limited when compared to echo Doppler, with or without color flow mapping (Chap. 177) and cine-MRI. While both cine-MRI and echo Doppler can demonstrate the regurgitant flow and estimate its volume, cine-CT can evaluate only indirectly the severity of regurgitation (see below).

For the evaluation of pericardial disease, standard CT or cine-CT can be used to visualize and measure the thickness of the pericardium. The diagnosis of constrictive pericarditis is supported by demonstrating pericardial thickness exceeding 4 mm and, sometimes, calcification (Fig. 178-2). Other indirect signs of this disease shown by CT are: (1) dilated atria and inferior vena cava; (2) small ventricular chambers; and (3) a sigmoid-shaped ventricular septum. Pericardial thickening is also observed for a variable period of time after cardiac surgery and in patients experiencing the postpericardiotomy syndrome (Dressler's syndrome). CT can also be used to demonstrate pericardial effusions and pericardial masses. Standard CT has been used to evaluate intracardiac and paracardiac masses and to define possible cardiac involvement by mediastinal and lung tumors. The capability is considerably enhanced by cine-CT, although MRI seems to be superior to both standard and cine-CT for the evaluation of intra- and paracardiac masses.

The role of CT for the evaluation of congenital heart disease is very limited when considered in relation to the availability and success of echocardiography and MRI. While encouraging results have been shown for cine-CT, the results add little to echocardiography in the display of intracardiac anatomy and seem to be inferior to MRI for defining thoracic aortic and pulmonary arterial abnormalities.

Standard CT as well as cine-CT are effective for the diagnosis of diseases of the aorta (Chap. 197). The accuracy of CT for the diagnosis of aortic dissection exceeds 90 percent, and in some series it is nearly 100 percent. The definitive diagnosis of aortic dissection is based upon the demonstration of displacement of the inner portion

of the aortic wall into the lumen (intimal flap) and/or differential enhancement of the true and false aortic channels.

EVALUATION OF CARDIAC FUNCTION WITH CINE-CT The fast CT scanners have the capability for the evaluation of cardiac function. The exposure time of 50 ms attained by cine-CT is adequate for quantitating many aspects of cardiac function. The three-dimensional nature of the technique permits precise measurement of chamber volume. Right and left ventricular volumes can be assessed with equal accuracy. A disparity in the stroke volumes of the two ventricles is caused by shunts and valvular regurgitation, which can be measured by cine-CT. Cine-CT can also be used for monitoring the effect of interventions on the right and left ventricles. Cine-CT performed at peak effort during supine bicycle exercise has been used to identify the *abnormal* response in patients with suspected coronary arterial stenoses. Most patients with severe lung disease and pulmonary arterial hypertension *also* display an abnormal response to exercise. Cine-CT has also been proposed as a method for measuring regional myocardial perfusion at rest and following interventions which increase myocardial blood flow, such as exercise and vasodilators. Perfusion is estimated by monitoring density values of the myocardium over time on CT scans exposed sequentially during peak opacification and wash-out of contrast medium from the myocardium.

MAGNETIC RESONANCE IMAGING (MRI)

This noninvasive technique uses no ionizing radiation or contrast medium for cardiovascular imaging. MR images are based upon the radiofrequency (RF) signal emitted by hydrogen nuclei of tissues after they have been perturbed by RF pulses in the presence of a strong magnetic field. The RF signal emitted has certain characteristics called *relaxation times:* T1 relaxation time (longitudinal magnetization) and T2 relaxation time (transverse magnetization). These properties are variable among tissues and are the predominant factors responsible for contrast among tissues. The signal intensity of one tissue compared to another (contrast) can be manipulated by varying the elapsed time between application of RF pulses (repetition time) and the time between an RF pulse and sampling the emitted signal (echo delay time).

The blood pool is generally a signal void, which provides high contrast between blood and the myocardial wall (Fig. 178-3). When the evaluation of cardiac structure is desired, the ECG gated spin-

FIGURE 178-3 ECG gated MR image acquired using the spin-echo technique in a short axis plane. There is increased thickness of the free wall of the right ventricle, indicating right ventricular hypertrophy. L = left ventricle; R = right ventricle. (*Reproduced with permission from CB Higgins, 1988.*)

FIGURE 178-4   ECG gated spin-echo MR images acquired in transverse plane demonstrate complications of myocardial infarctions. True aneurysm and mural thrombus (T) (*left*). False aneurysm (A) (*right*). The ostium is nearly as wide as the fundus of the true aneurysm, while the ostium is smaller than the fundus for the false aneurysm.

echo technique, which provides static images with high signal-to-noise ratios, is used. When the primary goal is to assess cardiac contractile function, cine-MR imaging is used.

EVALUATION OF PATHOANATOMY   MRI has been shown to be effective and useful in the diagnosis of a wide variety of cardiovascular abnormalities (Table 178-1). Patients with congenital heart disease are evaluated initially with the use of two-dimensional echocardiography, and in many congenital lesions MR is a secondary diagnostic technique in which the anatomy is displayed with the precision of angiography. In anomalies of the aortic arch and coarctation, MR can be considered the procedure of choice. MR imaging is also frequently the most useful study for the demonstration of pulmonary arterial abnormalities and for evaluating the status of the pulmonary arteries after systemic-pulmonary shunts have been surgically produced.

The major use of MRI in ischemic heart disease has been to demonstrate complications of acute myocardial infarction, such as true and false aneurysms of the left ventricle and intraventricular thrombi (Fig. 178-4). However, in the future, MR may assume a broader role in ischemic heart disease by demonstrating: (1) residual viable myocardium in a region involved by a previous infarct; (2) patency (or lack thereof) of coronary artery bypass grafts; and (3) regional perfusion using MR contrast media. MRI has been used to define the extent and distribution of abnormal muscle in patients with hypertrophic cardiomyopathy and for demonstrating a variety of pericardial diseases. It provides direct imaging of the pericardium, so that a diagnosis of abnormal pericardial thickness can be made.

MR imaging has been found to be effective for demonstrating intracardiac thrombi and tumors (Fig. 178-5). The utility of the technique has been shown in the demonstration of primary and metastatic cardiac tumors and tumors within the mediastinum invading or compressing central cardiovascular structures. The most frequent indication for the use of MR imaging in evaluating an intracardiac mass is when echocardiography raises a question regarding abnormal echogenicity within the cardiac chambers.

Thoracic aortic diseases are evaluated best with MR. In patients with aortic dissection, MRI displays the intimal flap and the extent of the dissection within the aorta (Fig. 178-6). It can also identify thrombus in the false channel and involvement of the arch and visceral arterial branches.

EVALUATION OF CARDIAC FUNCTION   Functional evaluation of the cardiovascular system is now practical using cine-MR. By achieving a temporal resolution of 30 images per cardiac cycle, cine-

MR successfully captures end diastole and end systole, such that end-diastolic and end-systolic volumes, stroke volume, and ejection fraction can be calculated accurately. The temporal resolution of cine-MRI does not capture a single cardiac cycle, but rather separates an "average" cycle, acquired over 256 cardiac cycles, into many component images. A good correlation has been found between left ventricular volumes calculated from cine-MRI and those measured by angiography. Measurement of left ventricular mass using MR imaging has shown a close correlation with postmortem measurements in animals and estimates from angiography in human beings. Accurate measurement of left ventricular mass is important, since changes in mass may be the most effective way to monitor the response to therapy in diseases causing left ventricular hypertrophy. Functional

FIGURE 178-5   ECG gated spin-echo MR image in transverse plane shows a mass (arrow) in the left atrium. (*Reproduced with permission from CB Higgins, 1988.*)

FIGURE 178-6 Aortic dissection. Transverse MR image shows intimal flap (arrow) separating true and false channels.

evaluation in ischemic heart disease by MR is achieved by monitoring wall thickening during the cardiac cycle. The site of previous myocardial infarction can be recognized by the absence or diminution of wall thickening during systole.

IDENTIFICATION AND QUANTITATION OF VALVULAR REGURGITATION The blood pool usually has a homogeneous high signal intensity throughout most of the cardiac cycle on cine-MR. Regurgitation through either the atrioventricular or semilunar valves is associated with a high-velocity jet which causes a signal void within the otherwise high-signal-intensity chamber (Fig. 178-7). This void

FIGURE 178-7 Cine-MRI (gradient refocused technique) in the coronal plane in aortic regurgitation. Images acquired in systole (*above*) and diastole (*below*). Note the signal void (arrow) emanating from the closed aortic valve. (*Reproduced from Sechtem et al, 1987.*)

can be used to identify the presence of valvular regurgitation. In aortic regurgitation, the signal void is in continuity with the closed aortic valve, while in mitral regurgitation it is in continuity with the closed mitral valve. Quantitation of the severity of valvular regurgitation can be accomplished by measuring the right and left ventricular stroke volumes and using these measurements to calculate regurgitant fraction or regurgitant volume. The volume of the signal void caused by regurgitation can also be measured on the images and used to estimate the severity of regurgitation.

MR SPECTROSCOPY

MR spectroscopy is a new tool for the evaluation of myocardial metabolism which might eventually be used to assess the early response of the myocardium to various therapeutic and pharmacologic interventions, establish myocardial viability, assess beneficial or detrimental effects of reperfusion on the ischemically injured myocardium, and investigate the link between myocardial function and metabolism.

MR spectroscopy operates upon the same principle as MR imaging in that the nuclei of some atoms (those with an odd number of nuclear particles) resonate when radiofrequency energy is applied at a frequency specific for a particular atom. After this energy is applied, the nuclei resonate at a characteristic frequency so that the presence of a particular atom within a chemical compound or tissue can be identified by MR. In distinction to imaging, which is usually only sensitive to the presence of a certain atom within a compound, MR spectroscopy can provide a map of the various sites where an atom exists within a compound. MR spectroscopy depicts the very slight difference in resonant frequences of the same nuclei when it exists in different compounds. The slight variation in resonant frequencies of the same nuclei in various compounds is called *chemical shift*, and the graphic display of the various frequencies is the MR spectrum of the nuclei. An example of this is the MR spectrum of phosphorus 31 (^{31}P), where the multiple spectral peaks represent ^{31}P in the compounds inorganic phosphate, creatine phosphate, adenosine phosphate, etc. (Fig. 178-8). The MR spectra are displayed in a convention whereby the portion of the peak in the spectrum (horizontal axis) indicates the specific compounds, e.g., creatine phosphate, while the height of the peak (vertical axis) indicates the relative concentration of the compound.

FIGURE 178-8 Phosphorus 31 magnetic resonance spectrum from a normal subject. The important spectral peaks are inorganic phosphate, not seen; creatine phosphate (PCr); and the three for adenosine triphosphate (ATP). The 2,3-diphosphoglycerate (DPG) peak indicates that the signal is partially derived from intracavitary blood as well as from myocardium. PD = phosphodiester.

The nuclei for which MR spectroscopy seems to be the most useful for diagnostic purposes are hydrogen 1, carbon 13, and phosphorus 31. Hydrogen 1 (proton) spectroscopy has been used to detect lactate in ischemic tissue and lipid accumulation in ischemically injured tissue. Metabolism of energy substrates in the myocardium has been approached using carbon 13; the technique has the potential for monitoring the utilization of fat and glucose by the myocardium and the manner in which ischemia influences their utilization. At this time most attention has been devoted to phosphorus 31 MR spectroscopy as a method for studying high-energy phosphate stores in various myocardial disease states and alterations of high-energy phosphate stores in response to therapeutic interventions.

In experimental preparations, phosphorus 31 spectroscopy has been used to evaluate the influence of potentially toxic agents, such as adriamycin and ethanol, on the myocardium. Calcium channel antagonists have been found to enhance recovery of both function and high-energy phosphate stores of the ischemically injured myocardium. Phosphorus 31 MR spectroscopy may be used also in experimental preparations to determine whether ischemic myocardium which is reperfused is reversibly or irreversibly damaged. Abnormal ^{31}P spectra have been observed in patients with myocardial disease (Fig. 178-8). However, the sensitivity, specificity, and, indeed, the clinical utility of ^{31}P MR spectroscopy have yet to be established.

POSITRON EMISSION TOMOGRAPHY (PET)

PET is a technique in which tomographic images are produced in relation to the concentration and position of positron emitters within the heart or any other organ. The positron is a positively charged electron produced during positron decay of a nucleus. After the positron interacts with a neighboring electron, a pair of photons are emitted in opposite directions. Because the photons simultaneously travel at equal speeds along paths at 180° to one another, photon detectors arrayed in a circle around the body can compute the precise site of origin of the pair. A substantial number of positron emitters are available for evaluating blood flow and various aspects of metabolic activity of the myocardium. Blood flow can be measured with oxygen 15 (^{15}O)-, rubidium 82 (^{82}Rb)-, and nitrogen 13 (^{13}N)-labeled ammonia. Glucose utilization, fat utilization and metabolism, and myocardial oxygen consumption can be assessed by fluorine 18 (^{18}F)-labeled deoxyglucose, carbon 11 (^{11}C)-labeled palmitate, and ^{11}C-labeled acetate, respectively.

PET can evaluate regional myocardial blood flow and metabolism. The transverse tomograms provide distinct spatial separation between various regions of the left ventricle, so that the uptake of metabolic markers can be assigned to the various myocardial regions. This technique may provide the capability of distinguishing between reversibly and irreversibly injured ischemic myocardium and predicting its response to reperfusion. By monitoring changes in metabolic patterns or substrate uptake, it may also prove capable of monitoring early response to therapy.

ASSESSMENT OF REGIONAL MYOCARDIAL BLOOD FLOW Since the various regions of the left ventricle are separated from one another on the transverse tomographic images, PET scans using perfusion markers can be used to detect and localize coronary artery disease. Nitrogen 13 ammonia ([^{13}N]H$_3$) has been used to assess regional myocardial blood flow at rest and in a hyperemic state induced by the powerful vasodilator dipyridamole. This technique has shown regional reduction of the positron emitter in the presence of stenoses which reduce luminal diameter by more than 40 to 50 percent.

Myocardial metabolism An unique feature of PET is the capability to measure regional myocardial substrate uptake and metabolic kinetics in a noninvasive and nonperturbing fashion. Specifically, it has been used to (1) measure regional myocardial uptake of exogenous glucose and free fatty acid; (2) quantitate free fatty acid metabolism in the myocardium in various physiologic states; (3) define the preferential myocardial energy source (fatty acid versus glucose) in various physiologic states; and (4) evaluate myocardial chemical receptor sites.

PET employing [^{13}N]H$_3$ and [^{18}F]DG (deoxyglucose) has been used to evaluate simultaneously regional myocardial perfusion and glucose uptake, respectively, in an effort to distinguish regions with a perfusion defect but containing viable myocardium from irreversibly infarcted myocardium. Using the combination of [^{13}N]H$_3$ (blood flow marker) and [^{18}F]DG (glucose uptake), several patterns of segmental myocardial metabolic abnormalities have been described in patients with various forms of ischemic heart disease. One is a "blood flow–metabolism match," in which a defect in the regional myocardial distribution of both isotopes is present. This pattern is usually caused by myocardial scar or nonviable myocardium (Fig. 178-9A). A second pattern is a "blood flow–metabolism mismatch," in which there is a segmental defect in [^{13}N]H$_3$ without a deficit in [^{18}F]DG (Fig. 178-9B). This indicates reduced perfusion to a myocardial region but continued uptake of glucose. Both patterns have been observed in patients with wall motion abnormalities in the left ventricular region displaying the perfusion defects. This mismatch pattern is considered to be associated with ischemic but viable myocardium since surgical revascularization of patients with this pattern causes improved wall motion in a majority of such segments. Moreover, a substantial percentage of patients showing the mismatch pattern after acute

FIGURE 178-9 Positron emission tomograms in two subjects: matched defects (*left*) and mismatched defects (*right*). Images show distribution for [^{13}N]ammonium and [^{18}F]deoxyglucose. The matched defects (arrowheads) in the anterior regions indicate a scar from a transmural infarct. The mismatched defects show reduced perfusion (arrow) but persistent glucose uptake (arrow) consistent with viable (salvageable) myocardium. (*Images provided courtesy of Heinrich Schelbert, MD.*)

myocardial infarction have demonstrated some recovery of regional function. On the other hand, the match pattern has been associated with no recovery of function after revascularization of akinetic segments.

PET using the positron emitter [^{11}C]palmitic acid has identified the consequences of myocardial ischemia and infarction on myocardial free fatty acid metabolism. These studies revealed that exogenous ^{11}C-labeled palmitic acid can enter two metabolic pools within the myocardium: a rapidly metabolized pool in which the fatty acid is immediately oxidized to CO_2 or a storage pool of triglycerides. During myocardial ischemia, myocardial uptake of [^{11}C]palmitic acid and its distribution into the two pools are altered. The free fatty acid pathway most vulnerable to ischemia is β oxidation, and consequently the amount of [^{11}C]palmitic acid entering this pathway is decreased initially.

Prediction of successful salvage of myocardium after thrombolysis has been achieved by PET imaging of [^{11}C]palmitic acid uptake in the jeopardized myocardium. Successful thrombolysis is associated with resumption of uptake of [^{11}C]palmitic acid in the jeopardized region. The principal indications for PET at the current time are to detect ischemic myocardium and to demonstrate potentially salvageable (viable) myocardium in the presence of acute or chronic myocardial ischemia.

REFERENCES

Cine-CT

CAPUTO GR, LIPTON MJ: Evaluation of regional left ventricular function using cine CT, in *New Concepts in Cardiac Imaging*, GM Pohost et al (eds). Chicago, Yearbook Medical, 1988

STANFORD W et al: Sensitivity and specificity of assessing coronary bypass graft patency with ultrafast computed tomography. Results of a multicenter study. J Am Coll Cardiol 12:1, 1988

MR imaging

BARAKOS JA et al: Magnetic resonance imaging of cardiac and paracardiac masses. Pictoral essay. Am J Roentgenol 153:47, 1989

DIDIER D et al: Congenital heart disease. Gated MR imaging in 72 patients. Radiology 158:227, 1986

DOOMS GC, HIGGINS CB: MR imaging of cardiac thrombi. J Comput Assist Tomogr 10:415, 1986

HIGGINS CB: MR of the heart: Anatomy, physiology and metabolism. Am J Roentgenol 151:239, 1988

———— et al: Magnetic resonance imaging in hypertrophic cardiomyopathy. Am J Cardiol 55:1121, 1985

JOHNS JA et al: Quantitation of acute myocardial infarct size by nuclear magnetic resonance imaging. J Am Coll Cardiol 15:1, 1990

SECHTEM U et al: Cine MRI: Potential for the evaluation of cardiovascular function. Am J Roentgenol 148:239, 1987

———— et al: Mitral or aortic regurgitation: Quantification of regurgitant volumes in patients with cine MR imaging. Radiology 167:425, 1988

SOMMERHOFF BA et al: Aortic dissection: Sensitivity and specificity of MR imaging. Radiology 3:651, 1988

WHITE RD et al: Advances in imaging thoracic aortic disease. Invest Radiol 21:761, 1986

WINKLER M, HIGGINS CB: Suspected intracardiac masses. Evaluation with MR imaging. Radiology 165:117, 1987

MR spectroscopy

BUSER PT et al: Post ischemic recovery of mechanical performance and energy metabolism in the presence of left ventricular hypertrophy. A ^{31}P MRS study. Circ Res 1990

RICHARDS T et al: Proton NMR spectroscopy in canine myocardial infarction. Magn Reson Med 4:555, 1987

Positron emission tomography (PET)

SCHELBERT HR, BUXTON D: Insights into coronary artery disease gained from metabolic imaging. Circulation 78:496, 1988

TILLISCH J et al: Reversibility of wall motion abnormalities: Preoperative determination using positron tomography 18 fluorodeoxyglucose and ^{13}NH$_3$. N Engl J Med 314:884, 1986

DIAGNOSTIC CARDIAC CATHETERIZATION AND ANGIOGRAPHY

WILLIAM GROSSMAN

Cardiac catheterization and angiography remain the gold standard for the assessment of both anatomy and physiology of the heart and vasculature. Initially developed in the animal laboratory, cardiac catheterization was first applied to humans in 1929 by Werner Forssmann, who at age 25 performed a right heart catheterization on himself. Forssmann's primary goal was to develop a therapeutic technique for the direct delivery of drugs into the heart. The potential of Forssmann's technique as a diagnostic tool was appreciated by others, especially André Cournand and Dickinson Richards in New York, who shared the Nobel prize with Forssmann in 1956 for the development of cardiac catheterization. Today, cardiac catheterization and angiography are performed as a combined procedure for diagnostic purposes, therapeutic intervention, or both. This chapter deals with cardiac catheterization as a diagnostic tool.

INDICATIONS FOR CARDIAC CATHETERIZATION Cardiac catheterization is recommended when there is a need to confirm the presence of a clinically suspected condition, define its anatomic and physiologic severity, and determine whether important associated conditions are present. This need most commonly arises when a patient is experiencing increased symptoms of cardiac dysfunction, or when objective measures suggest that rapid deterioration, myocardial infarction, or other adverse events are imminent.

There is debate as to whether cardiac catheterization is necessary in all patients being considered for cardiac surgery. Cardiac catheterization is the only technique currently capable of defining coronary anatomy with sufficient precision to provide the data base for decisions regarding coronary surgery or balloon angioplasty. In patients with other forms of heart disease (e.g., dilated cardiomyopathy, valvular heart disease), cardiac catheterization can provide hemodynamic characterization essential to the design of an appropriate medical regimen as well as assessment of prognosis. In some instances, decisions regarding cardiac surgery can be made without cardiac catheterization and angiography. Examples of such instances include children with simple congenital heart disease (e.g., patent ductus arteriosus, atrial septal defect), for whom a definitive noninvasive diagnosis is available.

Relative contraindications to cardiac catheterization are listed in Table 179-1.

A history of *allergic reaction* to radiographic contrast agents, which may range from urticaria to frank anaphylactic reaction, is an important relative contraindication to cardiac catheterization, which requires appropriate pretreatment. Generally, pretreatment with glucocorticoids (prednisone 20 to 40 mg every 6 h), conventional antihistamines (e.g., diphenhydramine 25 mg every 6 h), and H-2

TABLE 179-1 Relative contraindications to cardiac catheterization and angiography

1 Uncontrolled ventricular irritability: increased risk of ventricular tachycardia and fibrillation during catheterization if ventricular irritability is uncontrolled

2 Uncorrected hypokalemia or digitalis toxicity.

3 Uncorrected hypertension: predisposes to myocardial ischemia and/or heart failure during angiography

4 Intercurrent febrile illness

5 Decompensated heart failure: especially acute pulmonary edema, unless catheterization can be done with patient sitting up

6 Anticoagulated state: prothrombin time >18 s

7 Severe allergy to radiographic contrast agent

8 Severe renal insufficiency and/or anuria: unless dialysis is planned to remove fluid and radiographic contrast load

TABLE 179-2 Patient characteristics associated with increased mortality from cardiac catheterization

1 *Age:* Infants (<1 year old) and the elderly (>70 years old) are at increased risk of death during cardiac catheterization. Elderly women appear to be at higher risk than elderly men.

2 *Functional class:* Mortality in class IV patients is more than 10 times greater than in class I-II patients.

3 *Severity of coronary obstruction:* Mortality for patients with left main disease is more than 10 times greater than in patients with one- or two-vessel disease.

4 *Valvular heart disease:* Especially when severe and is combined with coronary disease is associated with a higher risk of death at cardiac catheterization than coronary artery disease alone.

5 *Left ventricular dysfunction:* Mortality in patients with left ventricular ejection <30 percent is more than 10 times greater than in patients with ejection fraction ≥50 percent.

6 *Severe noncardiac disease:* Patients with renal insufficiency, insulin-requiring diabetes, advanced cerebrovascular and/or peripheral vascular disease, and severe pulmonary insufficiency have an increased incidence of death and other major complications from cardiac catheterization.

antagonists (cimetidine 300 mg every 6 h), starting 18 to 24 h prior to the procedure, is adequate. Despite this pretreatment, occasional individuals will still develop anaphylactic reactions during radiographic contrast angiography, and intravenous epinephrine must be immediately available in such instances.

COMPLICATIONS OF CARDIAC CATHETERIZATION Since cardiac catheterization is an invasive technique, it should not be surprising that potential complications include death, myocardial infarction, stroke, perforation of the heart or great vessels, and local vascular problems. Table 179-2 lists those characteristics associated with increased risk of death from cardiac catheterization.

TECHNIQUES

Cardiac catheterization is performed with the patient in the fasting state and awake, although sedated. Typical sedatives include diazepam (Valium, 5 to 10 mg orally) and diphenhydramine (Benadryl, 25 to 50 mg orally). Prophylactic antibiotics are not necessary. If patients have been anticoagulated chronically with warfarin, this agent must be discontinued for at least 48 h prior to the procedure, and the prothrombin time must be less than 18 if the study is to be done safely. The technique of cardiac catheterization today involves either direct exposure of artery and vein (usually the brachial artery and vein in the antecubital fossa) or catheterization by percutaneous approach (usually involving the femoral vessels). Either technique can be used for right and/or left heart catheterization with coronary arteriography. The brachial approach has advantages in the patient with perpipheral vascular disease involving the abdominal aorta, iliac, or femoral arteries and suspected thrombosis of the femoral or iliac vein or inferior vena cava. Advantages of the percutaneous femoral approach are that arteriotomy and arterial repair are not required; the procedure can be performed repeatedly in the same patient at intervals; infection and thrombophlebitis at the catheterization site are quite rare, and no scar is left.

RIGHT HEART CATHETERIZATION This is most commonly performed under fluoroscopic guidance utilizing a balloon flotation catheter which is advanced from a suitable vein (brachial, femoral, subclavian, or internal jugular) into the superior vena cava, where blood is sampled for oximetry. The catheter is then advanced to the right atrium, where pressure is measured. The balloon is inflated with air or carbon dioxide and advanced to the right ventricle, pulmonary artery, and pulmonary artery wedge positions. Pressures are recorded in each position, and the balloon is then deflated so that pulmonary artery pressure is monitored and blood sampled from the catheter tip. With a thermistor-tipped balloon catheter, cardiac output can be measured utilizing cold saline injection and a small computer (thermodilution technique). Comparison of oxygen saturation in the

vena cava, chambers of the right heart, and pulmonary artery blood permits assessment of the presence of a left-to-right shunt at the atrial, ventricular, or pulmonary artery level which will be manifested as an increase ("step-up") in oxygen saturation of blood as it traverses these vessels and chambers.

The experienced operator will be alert for abnormalities in the course of the catheter during its passage through the right heart chambers, potentially providing information concerning the presence of congenital heart disease. For example, the catheter may pass directly from right to left atrium through an atrial septal defect, may enter an anomalous pulmonary vein draining into the right atrium, or may pass from the pulmonary artery directly into the aorta through a patent ductus arteriosus.

LEFT HEART CATHETERIZATION When left heart catheterization is done from the *brachial approach*, surgical cut-down is performed in the right (or left) antecubital fossa, with exposure of the brachial artery. An arteriotomy is made, and an appropriate catheter (e.g., Sones catheter) is advanced under fluoroscopic guidance to the central aorta, where pressure is measured and recorded. In many laboratories, peripheral arterial pressure is monitored by use of a radial artery line, and at this point in the procedure peripheral and central arterial pressures are compared. Next, the catheter is advanced in retrograde fashion across the aortic valve into the left ventricle where pressure is measured. If a right heart catheter is in place, this is an appropriate time for simultaneous measurement and recording of left heart, right heart, and peripheral arterial pressures together with determination of cardiac output by either thermodilution or Fick principle. These measures allow assessment of possible pressure gradients across the mitral and aortic valves, and catheter pullback on the right side permits assessment of possible gradients across pulmonic and tricuspid valves. Simultaneous measurement of pressures and cardiac output provides the data for calculation of systemic and pulmonary vascular resistances.

The *percutaneous femoral approach* to left heart catheterization involves puncture of the right (or left) femoral artery with a Seldinger needle, passage of a J-tipped guidewire retrograde to the abdominal aorta under fluoroscopic guidance, and placement of an intraarterial sheath with a side arm port for flushing. The side arm is attached to a pressure transducer and flush system, allowing continuous monitoring of peripheral arterial pressure. An appropriate catheter (e.g., pigtail catheter) is then advanced over a guidewire to the descending aorta, at which time the guidewire is removed and the catheter aspirated and flushed vigorously. Under pressure monitoring and fluoroscopic guidance, the catheter is advanced to the ascending aorta, where pressure is recorded simultaneously with peripheral arterial (sidearm) pressure. Subsequent steps in the procedure are identical to those listed for the brachial approach.

An additional method of left heart catheterization is the *transseptal approach*. This approach, which is not commonly employed today except for special diagnostic problems or for purposes of therapeutic intervention, involves a controlled puncture of the interatrial septum with a long stainless steel needle and advancement of a Teflon catheter over the needle into the left atrium. Rarely, direct catheterization of the left heart through the chest wall is necessary, by *left ventricular puncture* through a needle directed at the cardiac apex.

CARDIAC ANGIOGRAPHY

Cardiac angiography involves injection of radiopaque contrast agent into a specific cardiac chamber or vessel using either hand injection or power injection through an automated syringe. Contrast agents utilized today are broadly considered to be either nonionic or ionic; the newer, nonionic contrast agents have less myocardial depressant effect but are substantially more expensive than traditional ionic agents. Radiographic contrast injection is usually associated with vasodilatation and a sensation of marked warmth throughout the distribution of the injection.

CORONARY ANGIOGRAPHIC ANATOMY: REPRESENTATION IN STANDARD PRO

FIGURE 179-1 Representation of coronary anatomy relative to the interventricular and atrioventricular valve planes. Coronary branches are indicated as: L Main (left main), LAD (left anterior descending), D (diagonal), S (septal), CX (circumflex), OM (obtuse marginal), RCA (right coronary artery), CB (conus branch), SN (sinus node), AcM (acute marginal), PD (posterior descending, PL (posterolateral left ventricular). RAO, right anterior oblique, LAO, left anterior oblique. (*From DS Baim, W Grossman, in W Grossman, ed., 1986, with permission.*)

CORONARY ANGIOGRAPHY The commonest type of cardiac angiography currently performed involves selective injection of radiographic contrast agent into the coronary arteries. Placement of the catheter tips into the right and left coronary arteries is carried out under fluoroscopic guidance, and contrast agent is injected during recording of the radiographic image. Each coronary artery is usually viewed in several projections, to permit assessment of severity of stenosis and to minimize overlap of adjacent vessels. In addition to the detection of coronary artery stenoses, coronary angiography is useful for the detection of congenital abnormalities of the coronary circulation, coronary arteriovenous fistulas, and patency of coronary artery bypass grafts. Examples of normal and abnormal coronary anatomy are seen in Figs. 179-1 to 179-3.

LEFT VENTRICULOGRAPHY Injection of radiographic contrast directly into the left ventricular chamber is an important part of routine left heart catheterization, and yields important diagnostic information. Usually, a power injector is utilized to inject 30 to 45 mL of radiographic contrast into the left ventricular chamber at an injection rate appropriate for the particular catheter being used. Angiographic assessment of the left ventricular silhouette at end-

FIGURE 179-2 Coronary angiogram showing a right coronary artery (RCA) with a severe (95 percent) stenosis at its midpoint (*arrow*).

FIGURE 179-3 Coronary angiogram of a left coronary artery (LCA) with a tight stenosis in the proximal left anterior descending (LAD) artery (*black arrow*), immediately prior to the origin of a large septal branch. The circumflex artery (CX) has two moderately severe stenoses (*white arrows*).

FIGURE 179-4 Diagrammatic representation of end-diastolic (solid line) and end-systolic (dashed line) silhouettes of left ventricular cineangiograms in various forms of localized wall motion disorder in patients with coronary heart disease. Normal wall motion is symmetric; a patient with *hypokinesis* exhibits reduced contraction, seen here over the anterior and apical surfaces; a patient with *akinesis* exhibits absent wall motion, seen here over the anteroapical surface; the patient with *dyskinesis* exhibits paradoxic bulging of a small portion of the anterior wall with systole.

diastole and end-systole permits calculation of left ventricular chamber volumes and ejection fraction, as well as assessment of regional wall motion abnormalities. The normal left ventricle ejects 50 to 80 percent of its end-diastolic volume with each beat; that is, its *ejection fraction* is 0.50 to 0.80. In adults, normal values for left ventricular volumes are: end-diastolic volume, 72 ± 15 mL/m² (mean ± standard deviation), and end-systolic volume, 20 ± 8 mL/m². Regional abnormalities of wall motion are illustrated in Fig. 179-4 and include diminished inward motion of a myocardial segment (*hypokinesis*), no inward movement of a myocardial segment (*akinesis*), and paradoxical systolic expansion of a regional myocardial segment (*dyskinesis*).

Left ventriculography is usually performed in the right anterior oblique projection, which allows assessment of the mitral and aortic valves. Mitral regurgitation is easily visualized as the appearance of radiographic contrast in the left atrium during left ventricular systole. Its severity can be estimated qualitatively using a grading system of 1+ (mild, radiographic contrast clears with each beat and never opacifies the entire left atrium) to 4+ (severe, opacification of the entire left atrium occurs within one beat and contrast can be seen refluxing into the pulmonary veins). *Regurgitant fraction* can be calculated by determining the total left ventricular stroke volume (left ventricular end-diastolic volume minus end-systolic volume), subtracting the forward stroke volume (determined by Fick or indicator dilution technique), and dividing by the total stroke volume. The etiology of mitral regurgitation, such as myxomatous degeneration of the mitral leaflets and chordal rupture, may sometimes be identified from the left ventricular cineangiogram. Mitral and aortic stenosis can be *detected* by assessment of the speed and completeness with which the mitral and aortic leaflets open. Also important is an assessment of the thickness of the mitral and aortic leaflets, and the presence and extent of calcification. These findings, however, are usually not useful in estimating the *severity* of stenosis.

Left ventriculography also permits detection of abnormal communications such as ventricular septal defect (Chap. 186). In the most common form of hypertrophic cardiomyopathy (Chap. 192)

(idiopathic hypertrophic subaortic stenosis, IHSS) left ventriculography in the left anterior oblique projection shows anterior motion of the anterior leaflet of the mitral valve during systole and bulging of the interventricular septum into the left ventricular cavity, especially in the subaortic region. Mural thrombi within the left ventricular chamber may be well visualized during left ventriculography. They occur most commonly in the left ventricular apex.

AORTOGRAPHY   Rapid injection of radiographic contrast material into the ascending aorta allows detection of abnormality involving the aorta and aortic valve. It permits detection and qualitative assessment of the severity of aortic regurgitation utilizing a 1+ to 4+ scale, as for mitral regurgitation. Abnormal communications between the aorta and right heart such as patent ductus arteriosus or ruptured sinus of Valsalva aneurysm may be visualized. Aortography can permit identification of aortic aneurysm and of aortic dissection (Chap. 197) and may visualize an intimal flap within the aortic lumen.

PRESSURE MEASUREMENTS

Pressures within the cardiac chambers and great vessels are recorded routinely during cardiac catheterization and provide important information concerning function of ventricular myocardium and cardiac valves. Normal values for pressures measured during cardiac catheterization are summarized in Table 179-3.

Simultaneous measurement of pressures in left ventricle, aorta, and left atrium (or pulmonary capillary wedge position) permits assessment of mitral and aortic valve function. As seen in Fig. 179-5, left ventricular and aortic pressures are essentially equal during systole, while left atrial (pulmonary capillary wedge) and left ventricular pressures are equal during diastole in the normal heart. A pressure gradient between the left ventricle and aorta during systole may be due to obstruction at the level of the aortic valve (e.g., *calcific aortic stenosis*) or at the subaortic level (e.g., *hypertrophic obstructive cardiomyopathy*). A gradient between the left atrium (pulmonary capillary wedge) and left ventricle in diastole generally indicates *mitral stenosis*, although it may also be seen in rare conditions such as cor triatriatum and left atrial myxoma. An example of a large diastolic pressure gradient in a patient with mitral stenosis is seen in Fig. 179-6. As seen in Fig. 179-7, a prominent *v* wave in the pulmonary capillary wedge pressure will often increase substantially during modest exercise in a patient with significant mitral regurgitation. Severe *aortic regurgitation* produces a widening of the aortic pulse pressure, with equilibration of aortic and left ventricular

TABLE 179-3   Normal values for hemodynamic parameters

1 Pressures (mmHg)	
A Systemic arterial	
(*1*) Peak systolic/end-diastolic	100–140/60–90
(*2*) Mean	70–105
B Left ventricle	
(*1*) Peak systolic/end-diastolic	100–140/3–12
C Left atrium (or pulmonary capillary wedge)	
(*1*) Mean	2–10
(*2*) *a* wave	3–15
(*3*) *v* wave	3–15
D Pulmonary artery	
(*1*) Peak systolic/end-diastolic	15–30/4–12
(*2*) Mean	9–18
E Right ventricle	
(*1*) Peak systolic/end-diastolic	15–30/2–8
F Right atrium	
(*1*) Mean	2–8
(*2*) *a* wave	2–10
(*3*) *v* wave	2–10
2 Resistances [(dyn·s)/cm⁵]	
(*1*) Systemic vascular resistance	700–1600
(*2*) Pulmonary vascular resistance	20–130
3 Cardiac output [(L/min)/m²]	2.6–4.2
4 Oxygen consumption [(L/min)/m²]	110–150
5 Arteriovenous oxygen difference (mL/L)	30–50

FIGURE 179-6 Pulmonary capillary wedge (PCW) and left ventricular (LV) pressure tracings in a 40-year-old woman with mitral stenosis. This patient also had systemic hypertension and significant elevation of her LV diastolic pressure. *(From BA Carabello, W Grossman, in W Grossman (ed), 1986, with permission.)*

FIGURE 179-5 Left ventricular (LV), radial artery, and pulmonary capillary wedge (PCW) pressures in a patient with normal cardiovascular function. Note the absence of a pressure gradient between the LV and radial artery in systole and between the LV and PCW in diastole.

pressures in diastole (Fig. 179-8). Right-sided pressures exhibit characteristic deformity in the presence of valvular heart disease affecting the tricuspid or pulmonic valves. In patients with severe *tricuspid regurgitation*, right atrial pressure resembles closely in appearance the right ventricular pressure. Mean right atrial pressure

and right ventricular end-diastolic pressure are both elevated in tricuspid regurgitation. In *tricuspid stenosis* there is a diastolic gradient between right atrium and ventricle.

Characteristic deformities of right and left ventricular diastolic pressures occur in patients with *cardiac tamponade* or *pericardial constriction*. In both conditions there is equalization of left and right ventricular diastolic pressures. However, in constrictive pericarditis,

FIGURE 179-7 Hemodynamic findings at rest and during exercise in a patient with mitral regurgitation. Left ventricular (LV), pulmonary capillary wedge (PCW), and radial artery pressure tracings are shown before (*left*) and during (*right*) the sixth minute of supine bicycle exercise. PCW mean pressure and *v* wave increase substantially with exercise. *(From BH Lorell, W Grossman, in W Grossman (ed), 1986, with permission.)*

FIGURE 179-8 Severe aortic regurgitation. There is equilibration between the left ventricular (LV) and aortic or femoral artery (FA) pressures in diastole. Also, LV diastolic pressure exceeds pulmonary capillary wedge (PCW) pressure early in diastole, indicating premature closure of the mitral valve (a characteristic feature of severe aortic regurgitation). *(From W Grossman, in W Grossman (ed), 1986, with permission.)*

nearly all of ventricular filling occurs shortly after mitral and tricuspid valve opening; following this period of rapid filling, ventricular volumes cannot increase further due to the limit of the constricting pericardium. This abnormality produces an abrupt early ventricular diastolic pressure rise with a mid and late ventricular pressure plateau, giving the so-called square root sign (Fig. 179-9). In contrast, in tamponade there is equalization of diastolic pressures with a gradual increase throughout diastole.

Congestive heart failure due to myocardial contractile dysfunction is associated with characteristic alterations in the ventricular pressure waveforms seen at cardiac catheterization. Both isovolumic pressure rise and pressure decline are not nearly as steep as in the normal heart. The reduced slopes of pressure rise and decline are associated with an abbreviated ejection period, giving the left ventricular pressure tracing a triangular appearance (Fig. 179-10). Also, pressure decline does not continue to zero pressure, so that the minimal left ventricular diastolic pressure may be elevated. This hemodynamic finding correlates with an increased ventricular end-systolic volume, which is a sign of depressed contractile function of the left ventricular myocardium.

MEASUREMENT OF FLOW

Systemic and pulmonary blood flows may be measured by either the Fick or indicator-dilution methods. In the normal heart, these flows are equal and are termed *cardiac output*. Specialized techniques have made it possible to measure coronary artery blood flow (catheter-tip-mounted Doppler flowmeter), coronary sinus blood flow (thermodilution technique), and renal, cerebral, and femoral blood flows as well.

Cardiac output is most commonly measured today by the thermodilution technique, but the standard method, against which this technique and others are calibrated, remains the direct Fick oxygen method. In the direct Fick method, O_2 consumption is measured simultaneous with determination of arteriovenous oxygen difference across the lungs. Fick's principle states that

$$Q \text{ (L/min)} = \frac{O_2 \text{ consumption (mL/min)}}{\text{arteriovenous oxygen difference (mL/L)}}$$

In order to compare individuals of different body weights and sizes, O_2 consumption and cardiac output (Q) are commonly divided by body surface area. Normal values for O_2 consumption and cardiac output are given in Table 179-3. Cardiac output is calculated by dividing O_2 consumption by the arteriovenous O_2 difference across the lungs (estimated pulmonary venous–pulmonary arterial O_2 content); this actually measures *pulmonary blood flow* (Q_p). In patients with left-to-right shunts at the atrial, ventricular, or pulmonary artery levels, pulmonary blood flow exceeds systemic blood flow. In such cases, systemic blood flow (Q_s) is calculated by dividing O_2 consumption by the systemic arteriovenous O_2 difference. The latter is calculated as systemic arterial blood O_2 content minus mixed venous blood O_2 content, using blood from the chamber immediately proximal to the level of the shunt. The Fick method is most dependable when the cardiac output is low and the arteriovenous oxygen difference is large.

For indicator-dilution measurement of cardiac output using the thermodilution technique, a thermistor is mounted on the tip of a balloon-flotation catheter, and the catheter is advanced so that the balloon tip and thermistor are located in the pulmonary artery. Cold dextrose solution or saline is injected via a proximal port on the catheter into the vena cava or right atrium, and the change in

FIGURE 179-9 Left ventricular (LV), right ventricular (RV), and pulmonary capillary wedge (PCW) pressure tracings in a patient with severe constrictive pericarditis. Note the diastolic dip and plateau (''square root sign'') pattern for left and right ventricular diastolic pressures left panel.

FIGURE 179-10 Left ventricular (LV) and aortic (Ao) pressures in a patient with advanced dilated cardiomyopathy. Marked slowing of the rates of left ventricular pressure rise and fall (impairment of contractility and relaxation) give the LV pressure pulse a triangular appearance. Also, the minimal value for left ventricular diastolic pressure is markedly elevated, suggesting an increased end-systolic volume and a reduced LV ejection fraction. *(From W Grossman, in W Grossman (ed), 1986, with permission.)*

temperature monitored at the thermistor is integrated mathematically. This integral is inversely proportional to the volume flow rate past the thermistor, and if the temperatures of the injectate and pulmonary artery blood are measured, cardiac output (actually pulmonary blood flow) can be calculated. In contrast to the Fick method, the indicator-dilution method is least reliable when the cardiac output is low.

Valve areas and resistances Using simultaneous measures of pressure and flow, the resistance to blood flow across cardiac valves as well as the pulmonary and systemic arteriolar beds may be estimated. Valve areas are calculated using the Gorlin formula:

$$A = \frac{\text{flow}}{K \sqrt{\Delta P}}$$

where A = valve orifice area (cm²), *flow* is the blood flow (mL/s) across the stenotic valve, ΔP is the mean pressure gradient (mmHg) during the period of blood flow, and K is a constant (44.3 for the aortic valve and 37.7 for the mitral valve).

The resistance to blood flow through the systemic vascular bed is given as

$$SVR = 80(MAP - RA)/SBF$$

where SVR is systemic vascular resistance (dyn·s/cm⁵), MAP and RA are mean aortic and right atrial pressures (mmHg), 80 is a constant for converting to metric units, and SBF is systemic blood flow (L/min).

Resistance to blood flow through the pulmonary vascular bed is given as

$$PVR = 80(PA - PCW \text{ or } LA)/PBF$$

where PVR is pulmonary vascular resistance [(dyn·s)/cm⁵], PA, PCW, and LA are pulmonary artery, pulmonary capillary wedge, and left atrial mean pressures (mmHg), and PBF is pulmonary blood flow (L/min). Normal values for pulmonary and systemic vascular resistances are given in Table 179-3.

REFERENCES

Grossman W, Barry WH: Cardiac catheterization, in *Heart Disease*, 3d ed, E Braunwald (ed). Philadelphia, Saunders, 1988, p 242

——— (ed): *Cardiac Catheterization and Angiography*, 3d ed. Philadelphia, Lea & Febiger, 1986

Kennedy JW et al: Complications associated with cardiac catheterization and angiography. Cathet Cardiovasc Diagn 8:5, 1982

Roberts WC: Reasons for cardiac catheterization before cardiac valve replacement. N Engl J Med 306:291, 1982

180 THERAPEUTIC APPLICATIONS OF CARDIAC CATHETERIZATION

WILLIAM GROSSMAN / DONALD S. BAIM

The development of catheter-based therapies for the treatment of cardiovascular disease has led to the creation of a new field: interventional cardiology. In current practice, interventional cardiology provides a safe and effective alternative to conventional surgery for many patients with coronary, valvular, and congenital heart disease (Table 180-1).

TREATMENT OF CORONARY STENOSES AND OCCLUSIONS WITH CORONARY ANGIOPLASTY

Percutaneous transluminal coronary angioplasty (PTCA) is an important form of therapy for coronary artery disease (see Chap. 189). More than 200,000 PTCA procedures were performed in the United States alone during 1988, nearly equal to the number of coronary bypass operations. Since PTCA is performed using local anesthesia, during a short (2- to 3-day) hospitalization, its use in suitable patients can greatly decrease expense and recovery time compared to coronary bypass surgery, although it carries a 0.4 to 1.0 percent procedure-related mortality, similar to that for elective coronary bypass surgery.

INDICATIONS The main indication for PTCA is the presence of one or more coronary stenoses that are felt to be responsible for a clinical syndrome warranting revascularization and that are approachable by balloon catheters (Fig. 180-1). Moreover, the risks and benefits for revascularization by PTCA should compare favorably to those of conventional surgery. Thus, significant left main stenosis or multivessel disease in which vessels supplying significant areas of viable myocardium are not approachable by PTCA (due to chronic total occlusion or other unfavorable anatomic features) constitute relative contraindications to PTCA if surgery is technically possible.

For most patients, the clinical syndrome being treated is moderately severe, chronic, stable angina that persists despite medical antianginal therapy. Approximately 15 to 20 percent of current PTCA patients, however, have only mild anginal symptoms despite suitable coronary anatomy and objective evidence of ischemia (i.e., an abnormal exercise test). At the other extreme, some patients have more pressing

TABLE 180-1 Therapeutic applications of cardiac catheterization

Techniques currently under clinical evaluation or in general use

Treatment of coronary stenoses and occlusions
  Percutaneous transluminal coronary angioplasty (PTCA)
  Laser techniques
  Intravascular stent
  Atherectomy
Treatment of valvular stenosis
  Balloon valvuloplasty (aortic, mitral, pulmonic)
Treatment of congenital defects
  Atrial septostomy
  Umbrella closure of patent ductus arteriosus and defects in atrial or
    ventricular septum
  Coil closure of undesired collateral vessels

FIGURE 180-1   Right coronary angioplasty in a patient with unstable angina 6 weeks following successful dilatation. The lesion is shown before (*left panel*) and after (*right panel*) inflation of the PTCA balloon catheter.

indications for PTCA revascularization, including unstable angina or acute myocardial infarction (with or without prior thrombolytic therapy).

As the clinical indications for PTCA have broadened, so have its anatomic capabilities. Thus, PTCA is no longer restricted to proximal, discrete, subtotal, concentric, noncalcified lesions as was the case initially. Angioplasty catheters with smaller deflated profiles, controlled by highly steerable guidewires, are now available that can be advanced successfully across severe stenoses located virtually anywhere in the coronary tree. These balloon catheters tolerate inflation pressures up to 300 psi (20 atm), adequate to dilate even calcific lesions. Totally occluded coronary arteries (particularly those which have been occluded for less than 6 months) can be crossed and dilated effectively, although the success rate remains somewhat lower than for subtotal lesions (i.e., 60 percent versus 90 percent for subtotal stenotic lesions). In addition to lesions in the native coronary tree, lesions in saphenous vein or internal mammary artery bypass grafts can also be dilated successfully to treat postbypass angina. If multiple lesions are responsible for the clinical syndrome, most or all such lesions can generally be dilated during a single procedure.

RESULTS   The current PTCA success rate (for reducing a target stenosis to <50 percent of its original diameter without producing an associated complication) exceeds 90 percent. About half of the failures result from inability to cross the target lesion with the guidewire or balloon catheter, particularly when that target lesion is a chronic total occlusion. The remaining failures are due to excessive local dissection (separation of coronary artery intima from media) resulting from attempted dilatation. While some local dissection is present in virtually all successful PTCA procedures, more extensive dissection (particularly in association with local thrombus formation or vasospasm) can lead to abrupt closure of the dilated segment soon after withdrawal of the balloon catheter. Routine use of vasodilators (nitrates and calcium channel antagonists), anticoagulation (heparin 10,000 to 15,000 units during the procedure), and antiplatelet therapy (aminosalicylic acid, 325 mg/d starting at least 24 h prior to PTCA and continued for 3 to 6 months after the procedure) helps to prevent abrupt closure due to spasm and/or thrombus formation. Closure due to dissection can frequently be reopened by repeat dilatation (Fig. 180-2), but if this is unsuccessful, emergency bypass surgery is required to restore blood flow and prevent myocardial infarction. Emergency bypass surgery is needed currently in only 2 percent of PTCA attempts, but this potential difficulty requires that angioplasty be performed only in hospitals where immediate cardiac surgery is available.

FOLLOW-UP   After successful PTCA of all "culprit" lesions, marked improvement or complete resolution of the presenting ischemic syndrome should be evident. In approximately 20 to 30 percent of patients, however, evidence of ischemia returns within 6 months, due to so-called restenosis of the dilated segment. This appears to result from excessive local myointimal hyperplasia, triggered by platelet adhesion to the freshly dilated surface. To date, despite substantial effort, no mechanical or pharmacologic strategy has substantially reduced this restenosis rate. When recurrent ischemia develops more than 6 months after PTCA, this usually reflects progression of disease at another site, rather than restenosis. Repeat PTCA can be used to treat either restenosis or disease progression, so that only about 10 percent of PTCA patients require bypass surgery during the 5 years following a successful PTCA procedure.

NEWER NONBALLOON TECHNIQUES   In an attempt to circumvent the existing limitations of balloon angioplasty, intensive evaluation of a variety of nonballoon techniques is currently under way. One or more of these newer techniques may aid in crossing total occlusions, dilating rigid or elastic lesions, stabilizing dissections, or reducing the incidence of restenosis.

Laser   Laser energy (at wavelengths from the ultraviolet to the infrared) can be delivered to coronary lesions through optical fibers as small as 0.2 mm in diameter. Depending on the specific delivery parameters, this energy can produce direct ablation of an atherosclerotic plaque, associated with various degrees of local thermal injury. To date, however, no ablative laser technologies have proved adequate to distinguish plaque from normal vessel wall, leading to an unacceptable vessel perforation rate for safe application in the coronary arteries.

On the other hand, lasers can be used to deliver controlled thermal energy to the atherosclerotic plaque. Laser heating of a metal cap (the thermal probe) has been used successfully to cross occlusions in the peripheral circulation and is undergoing preliminary testing in the coronary arteries. Laser light can also be transmitted to the vessel wall from a diffusing fiber contained within a special balloon catheter (laser balloon angioplasty). This heats the vessel wall to 100°C, which appears to mold or weld the diseased wall into a desired configuration, so as to prevent or reverse abrupt closure. The smooth intimal surface which is left behind (and/or the thermal damage inflicted on the vascular smooth-muscle cells) has the potential to reduce restenosis, but this has yet to be demonstrated in clinical trials.

Intravascular stents   Permanent metallic endoprostheses (stents) of several designs can be delivered into the peripheral and coronary circulation to aid in maintaining luminal patency. Over a period of weeks, these stents are covered by endothelial cells and incorporated into the vessel wall. Although stenting improves acute luminal

FIGURE 180-2   Abrupt closure of a mid-right coronary artery lesion following attempted dilatation in a patient with recurrent ischemia following rt-PA therapy for inferior wall infarction. The involved lesion is shown before dilatation (*left panel*), during abrupt closure immediately after initial dilatation (*center panel*, arrows indicate local dissection), and after stabilization by redilatation (*right panel*).

appearance and may be of value in managing elastic lesions or abrupt closure, reduction in restenosis has yet to be demonstrated. Moreover, stenting carries potential hazards, particularly local thrombosis and/or vasospasm.

Mechanical atherectomy catheters Unlike balloon angioplasty—which merely redistributes plaque to improve luminal caliber—atherectomy seeks to remove plaque material from the body. Several catheter designs have been developed, and preliminary testing in the peripheral and coronary circulations suggests that safe enlargement of lumen is possible with potentially less restenosis than is seen following balloon angioplasty.

TREATMENT OF VALVULAR STENOSIS: BALLOON VALVULOPLASTY

Following successful balloon dilatation of vascular stenoses, both pediatric and adult cardiologists applied balloon dilatation to the treatment of stenotic cardiac valves. While the initial use was in patients with congenital pulmonic and aortic stenosis, this technique has now been extended to patients with acquired rheumatic and calcific stenosis of the mitral and aortic valves.

PULMONIC VALVULOPLASTY Although congenital pulmonic stenosis is predominantly a pediatric disease, it is sometimes encountered in adult patients (see Chap. 186). Transvalvular gradients >50 mmHg may produce exertional symptoms or lead to progressive right ventricular hypertrophy or failure. Using a guidewire placed into the pulmonary artery from the femoral vein, one or more valvuloplasty balloons with a combined cross-sectional area as much as 20 percent larger than the pulmonic valve annulus are positioned within the stenotic valve and inflated with liquid contrast medium at pressures of 3 to 5 atm. This typically reduces the transvalvular gradient from 75 to 15 mmHg. More than 1000 procedures have been performed to date, and balloon pulmonary valvuloplasty now stands as the preferred therapy for this lesion.

MITRAL VALVULOPLASTY The predominant application of mitral valvuloplasty is in patients with rheumatic mitral stenosis, in whom stenosis results primarily from commissural fusion with associated leaflet thickening. Such patients previously would have undergone open or closed surgical commissurotomy, but are now treated almost exclusively by balloon valvuloplasty. Other patients (with left atrial thrombus, mitral regurgitation, subvalvular disease, or leaflet thickening or rigidity) have less satisfactory results with either surgical commissurotomy or balloon valvuloplasty and are better treated by surgical valve replacement.

The usual approach to mitral valvuloplasty is via transseptal puncture (right atrium to left atrium), followed by passage of a guidewire across the stenotic valve and into the left ventricle. One or more balloon catheters with a dilating area equivalent to a single 23- to 30-mm diameter balloon are advanced over this guidewire, and inflated within the stenotic valve. Successful dilatation separates fused commissures and enhances leaflet compliance, thus increasing the effective diastolic valve area from 0.9 to 2.0 cm² or more (Fig. 180-3). Although this is still restricted compared to the 3.5- to 5-cm² area of a normal mitral valve or the 4.5-cm² area of an inflated 25-mm balloon, this increase in valve area provides excellent symptomatic relief and is equivalent to the increase in orifice size resulting from surgical mitral commissurotomy or prosthetic mitral valve replacement.

The main complications of mitral valvuloplasty relate to the potential for cardiac perforation during transseptal puncture (approximately 2 percent of patients) and the chance of systemic embolization (approximately 1 percent of patients) despite preprocedure echocardiographic exclusion of patients with left atrial thrombus.

AORTIC VALVULOPLASTY Balloon aortic valvuloplasty may be performed in children with congenital aortic stenosis and in adults with rheumatic or acquired calcific aortic stenosis. Some patients with rheumatic aortic stenosis have leaflet fusion, but the problem in

FIGURE 180-3 Hemodynamic results of mitral valvuloplasty in a 38-year-old woman with mitral stenosis. The transmitral [left atrium (LA)–to–left ventricle (LV)] gradient, cardiac output, and calculated mitral valve area are shown before (*left panel*) and after (*right panel*) balloon dilatation.

acquired calcific aortic stenosis is rigidity of the valve leaflets themselves. In this latter group of patients, balloon valvuloplasty fractures leaflet calcium and provides new hinge points along which the valve leaflets can open.

The most prevalent approach to aortic valvuloplasty consists of femoral arterial puncture with retrograde passage of a guidewire and balloon (inflated diameter 18 to 23 mm) across the valve. Overdilatation of the valve annulus may cause leaflet avulsion and is generally avoided. Aortic valvuloplasty typically increases the effective systolic valve area from 0.6 to 1.0 cm². The resultant valve area is still small compared to the area of a normal aortic valve (3 to 4 cm²) or to the effective area of an inflated 20-mm balloon (3.1 cm²), but it does relieve symptoms at rest or during mild to moderate exertion in most patients with critical aortic stenosis. Unfortunately, the relatively small effective orifice achieved and the high incidence of valvular restenosis (up to 40 percent within 1 year after dilatation) make balloon aortic valvuloplasty most applicable to elderly patients who are poor risks for valve replacement, or as a "bridge" to valve replacement.

TREATMENT OF CONGENITAL MALFORMATIONS

Pediatric interventional cardiologists have developed a number of innovative techniques to correct or palliate congenital cardiac lesions. Some techniques are those described above—i.e., balloon dilatation of stenotic pulmonary arteries, surgical shunts, or balloon valvuloplasty—but others are unique to the pediatric population.

ATRIAL SEPTOSTOMY In some patients with cyanotic congenital heart disease, it is desirable to produce or enlarge an atrial septal defect in order to facilitate passage of oxygenated blood into the right heart. This can be achieved by passage of a balloon catheter from right to left atrium across a patent foramen ovale, followed by forceful withdrawal of the inflated balloon. Alternatively, a catheter with a concealed blade can be passed across the septum. The blade can then be deployed in the left atrium to incise the septum as the catheter is withdrawn. The resulting septal incision can be widened by conventional balloon septostomy.

CLOSURE OF UNDESIRED SHUNTS OR COLLATERAL VESSELS A variety of appliances have been developed to close undesired intracardiac shunts, including defects in the atrial or ventricular septum and patent ductus arteriosus. These devices resemble a single or double (back-to-back) umbrella, which can be folded into a cylinder for containment in a catheter. Under fluoroscopic guidance, the delivery catheter can be positioned across the target defect, so that the umbrella can be deployed to block undesired flow.

Smaller vascular shunts can be closed using special coils. These coils can be placed within a catheter and delivered to the undesired vessel. Once in place, the coil interferes with blood flow and promotes local thrombotic occlusion of the target vessel.

REFERENCES

ANDERSON HV et al: Usefulness of coronary angioplasty in asymptomatic patients. Am J Cardiol 65(1):35, 1990

BAIM DS (ed): A symposium: Interventional cardiology. Am J Cardiol 61:1G, 1988

DETRE K et al: Percutaneous transluminal coronary angioplasty in 1985–86 and 1977–81: The NHLBI Registry. N Engl J Med 318:265, 1988

LOCK JE et al: Transcatheter umbrella closure of congenital heart defects. Circulation 75:593, 1987

MCKAY RG: Balloon valvuloplasty for treating pulmonic, mitral, and aortic valve stenosis. Am J Cardiol 61:102G, 1988

PARK SC et al: A new atrial septostomy technique. Cathet Cardiovasc Diagn 1:195, 1975

SAFIAN RD et al: Balloon aortic valvuloplasty in 170 consecutive patients. N Engl J Med 319:125, 1988

SIGWART U et al: Intravascular stents to prevent occlusion and restenosis after transluminal angioplasty. N Engl J Med 316:701, 1987

SIMPSON JB et al: Transluminal atherectomy for occlusive peripheral vascular disease. Am J Cardiol 61:96G, 1988

WEINTRAUB WS et al: Changing use of coronary angioplasty and coronary bypass surgery in the treatment of chronic coronary artery disease. Am J Cardiol 65(3):183, 1990

181 NORMAL AND ABNORMAL MYOCARDIAL FUNCTION

EUGENE BRAUNWALD

CELLULAR BASIS OF CARDIAC CONTRACTION

The *myocardium* is composed of individual striated muscle cells (fibers), normally 10 to 15 μm in diameter and 30 to 60 μm in length (Fig. 181-1A). Each fiber contains multiple cross-banded strands (myofibrils), that run the length of the fiber and are, in turn, composed of serially repeating structures, the sarcomeres. The remainder of the cytoplasm, lying between the myofibrils, contains other cell constituents, such as the single centrally located nucleus, numerous mitochondria, and intracellular membrane system, the sarcoplasmic reticulum.

The *sarcomere*, the structural and functional unit of contraction, is delimited by two adjacent dark lines, the Z lines (Fig. 181-1). The distance between Z lines varies with the degree of contraction or stretch of the muscle and ranges between 1.6 and 2.2 μm. Within the confines of the sarcomere, alternating light and dark bands are seen, giving the myocardial fibers their striated appearance under the light microscope. At the center of the sarcomere is a dark band of constant width (1.5 μm), the A band, which is flanked by two lighter bands, the I bands, which are of variable width. The sarcomere of heart muscle, like that of skeletal muscle, is made up of two sets of myofilaments. Thicker filaments, composed principally of the protein myosin, traverse and are limited to the A band. They are about 10 nm (100 Å) in diameter, with tapered ends, and measure 1.5 to 1.6 μm in length. Thinner filaments, composed primarily of actin, course from the Z line through the I band into the A band. They are approximately 5 nm (50 Å) in diameter and 1.0 μm in length. Thus, there is overlapping of thick and thin filaments only within the A

band, while the I band contains only thin filaments (Fig. 181-1). On electron-microscopic examination, bridges may be seen to extend between the thick and thin filaments within the A band.

THE CONTRACTILE PROCESS The "sliding" model for muscle rests on the fundamental observation that both the thick and thin filaments are constant in overall length, both at rest and during contraction. With activation of the sarcomere, repetitive interactions take place at the bridges between the actin and myosin filaments, and the actin filaments are propelled further into the A band. In the process, the A band remains constant in width, whereas the I band becomes more narrow and the Z lines move toward one another.

The myosin molecule is a complex, asymmetric fibrous protein with a molecular weight of about 500,000; it has a rod-like portion that is about 150 nm (1500 Å) in length with a globular portion at its end. This globular portion of the myosin contains adenosine triphosphatase (ATPase) activity and also forms the bridges between the myosin and actin. In forming the thick myofilament, the rod-like portions of the myosin molecules are laid down in an orderly, polarized manner, leaving the globular portions projecting outward so that they can interact with actin to generate force and shortening (Fig. 181-2A). Actin has a molecular weight of 47,000. The thin filament is composed of a double helix of two chains of actin molecules wound about each other, intimately associated with two regulatory proteins, tropomyosin and troponin (Fig. 181-2B); the latter can be separated into three components, troponins C, I, and T (Fig. 181-2C). In contrast to myosin, actin has no intrinsic enzymatic activity, but it has the ability to combine reversibly with myosin in the presence of ATP and Mg^{2+}, which activates the myosin ATPase. In relaxed muscle this interaction is inhibited by tropomyosin. During activation Ca^{2+} becomes attached to troponin C which results in a conformational change exposing the actin cross-bridge interaction sites. Physical changes in the cross-bridges result in sliding of the actin along the myosin filaments, ultimately causing muscle shortening and/or the development of tension. The splitting of ATP then dissociates the myosin cross-bridge from the actin. Linkages between actin and myosin filaments are made and broken cyclically as long as sufficient Ca^{2+} is present; these linkages are broken when Ca^{2+} concentration falls below a critical level, and the troponin-tropomyosin complex once more prevents interactions between the myosin cross-bridges and the actin filaments. Ionic calcium is a principal mediator of the inotropic state of the heart; most positive inotropic drugs, including the digitalis glycosides and catecholamines, act by increasing the concentrations of Ca^{2+} in the vicinity of the myofilaments.

The *sarcoplasmic reticulum* (Fig. 181-1B), a complex network of anastomosing, membrane-lined intracellular channels, which invests the myofibrils and which is less profuse in cardiac than in skeletal muscle, consists of a series of interconnecting longitudinally disposed membrane tubules closely applied to the surfaces of the individual sarcomeres; it has no direct continuity with the outside of the cell. However, closely related to the sarcoplasmic reticulum, both structurally and functionally, are the transverse tubules or T system, formed by tubelike invaginations of the sarcolemma, which extend into the myocardial fiber, along the Z lines, i.e., the ends of the sarcomeres.

CARDIAC ACTIVATION At rest, the cardiac cell is polarized; i.e., the interior has a negative charge relative to the outside of the cell, with a transmembrane potential of -80 to -100 mV (Chap. 184). The sarcolemma, which in the resting state is largely impermeable to Na^+ and has a Na^+- and K^+-stimulated pump requiring adenosine triphosphate (ATP) that extrudes Na^+ from the cell, plays a critical role in establishing this resting potential. Thus, the inside of the cell has relatively high concentrations of K^+ with far lower concentrations of Na^+, while the extracellular milieu is high in $[Na^+]$ and low in $[K^+]$. At the same time, in the resting state, the extracellular $[Ca^{2+}]$ greatly exceeds the free intracellular $[Ca^{2+}]$.

During the plateau of the action potential (phase 2) there is a slow inward current which reflects primarily a movement of Ca^{2+} into the cell (Fig. 181-3), although the absolute quantity of Ca^{2+} that crosses

FIGURE 181-1   Microscopic structure of heart muscle. *A.* Myocardium as seen under the light microscope. Branching of fibers is evident. Each fiber, or cell, contains a centrally located nucleus. *B.* Myocardial cell, reconstructed from electron micrographs. Each cell is composed of multiple parallel fibrils. Each fibril is composed of serially connected sarcomeres (N, nucleus). *C.* Sarcomere from a myofibril, with diagrammatic representation of myofilaments. Thick filaments (1.5 μm long, composed of myosin) form the A band, and thin filaments (1 μm long, composed primarily of actin) extend from the Z line through the I band into the A band. The overlapping of thick and thin filaments is seen only in the A band. *D.* Cross sections of the sarcomere indicate the specific lattice arrangements of the myofilaments. In the center of the sarcomere only the thick, or myosin, filaments arranged in a hexagonal array are seen. In the distal portions of the A band, both thick and thin, or actin, filaments are found, with each thick filament surrounded by six thin filaments. In the I band only thin filaments are present. *(From Braunwald et al, 1976.)*

the surface membrane is relatively small and in and of itself appears to be incapable of bringing about full activation of the contractile apparatus. However, the depolarizing current not only extends across the surface of the cell but penetrates deeply into the cell by way of the ramifying T system. As a consequence of the transsarcolemmal movement of Ca^{2+}, much larger quantities of Ca^{2+} are released from the sarcoplasmic reticulum, a process termed "regenerative release" of Ca^{2+}.

The Ca^{2+} released from the sarcoplasmic reticulum then diffuses toward the sarcomere, and as already described, combines with troponin C, and, by repressing the inhibitor of contraction, activates

the myofilaments to produce contraction. The sarcoplasmic reticulum then reaccumulates Ca^{2+}, an energy-requiring process, thereby lowering its concentration in the vicinity of the myofibrils to a level that inhibits the actin-myosin interaction which is responsible for contraction, and in this manner leads to relaxation. Thus, the cell membrane, transverse tubules, and sarcoplasmic reticulum, with their ability to transmit an action potential, to release and then reaccumulate Ca^{2+}, appear to play a fundamental role in the rhythmic contraction and relaxation of heart muscle.

The ATP formed from substrate oxidation is the principal source of energy for almost all of the mechanical work of contraction

A

B

C

FIGURE 181-2 Contractile protein interactions and the role of calcium as activator messenger are shown schematically: *A*. Contractile proteins (myosin and actin) and regulatory proteins (troponin complex and tropomyosin) are shown in relative positions on myofilaments. *B*. Contraction takes place when the heads of myosin molecules, which form cross-bridges of thick filament, bind to actin, followed by shift in orientation of cross-bridge that pulls thin filament toward center of sarcomere. Activation requires calcium binding to troponin complex, reversing inhibition of interaction between myosin and actin. In the cycle of chemical reactions underlying contraction, hydrolysis of ATP produces the cross-bridge motion. Relaxation occurs when calcium becomes dissociated from troponin. *C*. Molecular rearrangements at the level of the thin filament involve regulatory proteins (tropomyosin and troponins C, I, T) in an allosteric effect. Calcium binding to troponin C loosens bond linking troponin I to actin; resulting dissociation of troponin T from actin backbone of thin filament displaces tropomyosin, exposing active sites for interaction with myosin. [*Reproduced by permission, from AM Katz, VE Smith, Hosp Prac, 19(1):69, 1984. Illustration by Bunji Tagawa.*]

performed by the myocardial cell. The high-energy phosphate stores in ATP are in equilibrium with those in the form of creatine phosphate. The activity of the myosin ATPase determines the rate of forming and breaking the actin-myosin cross-bridges and ultimately the velocity of muscle contraction.

THE ROLE OF MUSCLE LENGTH In all forms of striated muscle, including cardiac muscle, the force of contraction depends on initial muscle length. The sarcomere length associated with the most forceful contraction is approximately 2.2 μm. At this length the two sets of myofilaments of the sarcomere are most ideally situated to provide the greatest area for their interaction. In support of the sliding-filament hypothesis, force development diminishes in direct proportion to the decrease in the overlap between thick and thin filaments, and the resultant reduction in the number of reactive sites. The length of the sarcomere also appears to regulate the extent of activation of the contractile system, i.e., its sensitivity to Ca²⁺, which is also greatest at approximately 2.2 μm. When sarcomere length is increased to 3.65 μm, the thin filaments are entirely withdrawn from the A band, and no tension can be developed. Similarly, when the sarcomeres are shorter than 2.0 μm, the thin filaments bypass one another, producing a double overlap of the thin filaments, a reduction of sensitivity of the contractile sites to Ca²⁺, and the capacity for force development also declines.

The relation between the initial length of the muscle fibers and the developed force is of prime importance for the function of heart muscle. This forms the basis of the Frank-Starling relation (Starling's law of the heart), which states that, within limits, an augmentation of initial volume of the ventricle, which is a function of the initial length of the cardiac muscle, results in an increase in the force of ventricular contraction. It has been shown for heart muscle that along the ascending limb of the length–active tension curve sarcomere length is directly proportional to muscle length. As muscle length decreases to the point at which sarcomere length approaches 1.5 μm and at which developed tension approaches zero, the I bands at first narrow, then disappear while the A band remains constant in length. At this latter point, the Z lines abut the edges of the A bands. Thus, the sarcomere length–active tension curve forms the ultrastructural basis of Starling's law of the heart.

MYOCARDIAL MECHANICS

THE FORCE-VELOCITY CURVE The mechanical activity of all muscle may be expressed externally in two ways: shortening and the development of tension. Hill showed in skeletal muscle that the velocity of shortening is inversely related to the magnitude of tension development, an expression of the so-called force-velocity relation, now recognized to be a fundamental property of muscle. Expressed

FIGURE 181-3 Calcium fluxes that activate contraction are downhill, and those that cause relaxation are uphill. As depicted in heart muscle at rest, calcium channels in the sarcolemmal membrane are closed, and intracellular calcium is stored in the sarcoplasmic reticulum. With excitation and membrane depolarization, voltage-sensitive sodium channels (not shown) and calcium channels in the sarcolemma open to allow rapid entry of extracellular sodium and calcium. Entry of calcium is now believed to cause release of calcium from the sarcoplasmic reticulum that initiates contraction. Reuptake of calcium by the sarcoplasmic reticulum by an ATP-dependent calcium pump is essential for the heart to relax. Importantly, contraction is activated mainly by passive calcium fluxes from the sarcoplasmic reticulum. By contrast, during diastole calcium must be pumped actively out of the cytosol to accomplish relaxation. Energy also must be expended during diastole to restore sodium and calcium gradients across the sarcolemma, which provide for the depolarizing ionic currents that generate the action potential. Sodium transport is accomplished by the sarcolemmal sodium pump (Na$^+$, K$^+$-ATPase), which utilizes ATP to pump sodium out of the cell in exchange for potassium. The resultant sodium gradient is largely responsible for active transport of calcium out of the cell during relaxation, via sodium-calcium exchange. [*Reproduced by permission from AM Katz, VE Smith, Hosp Prac, 19(1):69, 1984. Illustration by Bunji Taguwa.*]

simply, the greater the load the muscle is called upon to lift, the lower the velocity of shortening and vice versa. The force-velocity relation also applies to cardiac muscle. However, in this respect there is a basic difference between skeletal and cardiac muscle. Skeletal muscle has a single, essentially fixed, force-velocity curve; i.e., at any given muscle length, force and velocity are always related to each other in the same manner. The contractile activity of skeletal muscle is increased by the recruitment of additional muscle fibers, i.e., motor units, and by increasing the frequency of nerve impulses, while the contractile properties of each individual fiber remain constant. Although resting length also influences the characteristics of contraction, this variable remains essentially fixed in vivo because of the skeletal muscles' skeletal attachments. In contrast, the number of cardiac cells and within them the myofibrils and sarcomeres which become activated during each contraction is constant. However, the contractile activity of the myocardium may be readily altered under physiologic conditions by changes in resting fiber length and by changes in the inotropic state, i.e., the contractility, both of which shift the myocardial force-velocity curve.

Variations in myocardial contractile activity may be expressed as displacements of the force-velocity curve in two fundamental ways. Figure 181-4A shows a family of force-velocity curves obtained from an isolated cardiac muscle; each curve was obtained at a different preload, i.e., with a different degree of stretch on the muscle. Note that changing the preload alters the intercept of the force-velocity curve on the horizontal axis; i.e., it increases the isometric force developed by the muscle. However, within limits, these alterations in preload do not appear to alter the velocity of shortening importantly, since all the curves extrapolate to the same intercept on the vertical axis. Thus, a change in initial length of heart muscle shifts the force-velocity curve primarily by altering the total force which can be developed by the muscle, as illustrated by the isometric length-tension curve, shown in the insert of Fig. 181-4A.

This type of shift in the force-velocity curve may be contrasted with that obtained when a positive inotropic agent, such as Ca^{2+}, digitalis, or norepinephrine (which act ultimately by increasing the concentration of Ca^{2+} in the vicinity of the myofilaments) is added to the muscle while the initial length is held constant (Fig. 181-4B). These agents not only increase the force which the muscle is capable of developing, i.e., the intercept of the force-velocity curve on the horizontal axis, therefore shifting the isometric length-tension curve upward, but they also increase the velocity of shortening of the unloaded muscle, i.e., the extrapolated intercept on the vertical axis.

It has been postulated that an increase in initial muscle length up to an optimal length brings about an increase in the number of effective force-generating sites as a consequence of a more advantageous overlap of interdigitating contractile filaments within the sarcomere as well as in the extent of activation of the contractile

FIGURE 181-4 *A.* Effects of increasing initial muscle length on the force-velocity relation of cat papillary muscle. Initial velocity of shortening has been plotted as a function of load for five different muscle lengths. The maximum velocity of shortening is essentially unchanged, whereas the maximum force of contraction is augmented. The insert shows the places sites, i.e., their sensitivity to Ca^{2+}. A change in the inotropic state, along the length-tension curves at which these force-velocity curves were determined. *B.* Effects of norepinephrine on the force-velocity relation of the cat papillary muscle. Both the maximum velocity of shortening and the force of contraction are increased. *(From Braunwald et al, 1976.)*

sites, i.e., their sensitivity to Ca^{2+}. A change in the inotropic state, characterized by an increase in the velocity of shortening of the unloaded muscle, can also result from an increase in the rate of cyclic force-generating processes at the contractile sites, without a change in the number of these sites, i.e., at a constant muscle length. Increased contractility appears to be related primarily to an increased availability of Ca^{2+} within the cell.

CONTRACTION OF THE INTACT VENTRICLE

Analysis of the heart as a pump has classically centered upon the relation between the filling pressure, or diastolic volume, of the ventricle (length of the muscle fibers) and its stroke volume (the Frank-Starling relation). In the heart-lung preparation the stroke volume is a function of diastolic fiber length at any given level of arterial resistance (afterload), and the failing heart delivers a smaller-than-normal stroke volume from a normal or elevated end-diastolic volume. The relation between the mean atrial or the ventricular end-diastolic pressure and the stroke work of the corresponding ventricle (the ventricular function curve) provides a useful definition of the level of the contractile, or inotropic, state of the ventricle. An increase in ventricular contractility is accompanied by a shift of the ventricular function curve upward and to the left, while depression of contractility is identified by downward and rightward displacement of this relation.

It has been observed that during the adrenergic stimulation of the myocardium accompanying a stress such as exercise, relatively little change in ventricular end-diastolic size occurs, while cardiac output, aortic flow velocity, stroke work, and the rate of ventricular pressure development are all augmented, sometimes greatly. Thus, neural and humorally mediated changes in myocardial contractility, heart rate, venous return, and peripheral vascular resistance may be of greater importance in circulatory adaptation than changes in ventricular end-

diastolic volume and may mask the operation of the Frank-Starling mechanism.

The important influence of the adrenergic neurotransmitter substance norepinephrine (Chap. 67) on the mechanical properties of the myocardium has long been recognized. Direct stimulation of the cardiac adrenergic nerves augments ventricular function as a consequence of the release of norepinephrine from adrenergic nerve endings in the heart. These adrenergic effects are evidenced by tachycardia, a reduction in cardiac dimensions, increased velocity of ejection, and an enhanced rate of tension development.

CONTROL OF CARDIAC PERFORMANCE AND OUTPUT

The extent of shortening of mammalian heart muscle and, therefore, the stroke volume of the intact ventricle are, in the final analysis, determined by three influences: (1) the length of the muscle at the onset of contraction, i.e., the preload; (2) the inotropic state of the muscle, i.e., the position of its force-velocity-length relation; and (3) the tension which the muscle is called upon to develop during contraction, i.e., the afterload. Heart rate determines the cardiac output at any stroke volume as long as the other three influences are maintained.

VENTRICULAR END-DIASTOLIC VOLUME (PRELOAD)   At any level of its inotropic state, the performance of the myocardium is influenced profoundly by ventricular end-diastolic fiber length and therefore by diastolic ventricular volume, i.e., by operation of the Frank-Starling mechanism. The following are the major determinants of ventricular preload in the intact organism:

Total blood volume   When depleted, as in hemorrhage or prolonged vomiting, venous return to the heart declines (Chap. 39) and ventricular end-diastolic volume (preload) falls, as does ventricular performance, as reflected in ventricular work.

Distribution of blood volume At any given total blood volume, the ventricular end-diastolic volume is influenced by the distribution of blood between the intra- and extrathoracic compartments. This distribution in turn is influenced by the following:

1 *Body position.* Gravitational forces tend to pool blood in dependent portions. The upright posture augments extrathoracic at the expense of intrathoracic blood volume, and reduces ventricular work.
2 *Intrathoracic pressure.* Normally, mean intrathoracic pressure during the respiratory cycle is negative, a factor that acts to increase thoracic blood volume and ventricular end-diastolic volume and to enhance the return of blood to the heart, particularly during inspiration, when this pressure becomes more negative. Elevation of intrathoracic pressure, as occurs in a tension pneumothorax, during the Valsalva maneuver, in prolonged bouts of coughing, or with positive-pressure ventilation, tends to impede venous return to the heart and diminish intrathoracic blood volume and ultimately reduces stroke volume and ventricular work.
3 *Intrapericardial pressure.* When elevated, as in pericardial tamponade (Chap. 193), there is interference with cardiac filling, and the resultant reduction in ventricular diastolic volume lowers stroke volume and ventricular work.
4 *Venous tone.* The venous system is not a simple system of passive conduits between the systemic capillary bed and the right atrium. Instead, the smooth muscle in the walls of the venules and veins responds to a variety of neural and humoral stimuli. Venoconstriction occurs during muscular exercise, deep respiration, fright, or marked hypotension, tending to diminish extrathoracic and to augment intrathoracic and intraventricular blood volumes and ventricular performance.
5 *The pumping action of skeletal muscle.* During muscular exercise the contracting skeletal muscles squeeze blood out of the venous bed and, with the aid of the venous valves, displace it centrally, thereby increasing intrathoracic blood volume, ventricular end-diastolic volume, and ventricular work.

Atrial contraction Vigorous, appropriately timed atrial contraction augments ventricular filling and end-diastolic volume. The atrial contribution to ventricular filling is of particular importance in patients with ventricular hypertrophy, in whom the loss of atrial systole (as in atrial fibrillation) tends to reduce ventricular end-diastolic pressure and volume, ultimately lowering myocardial performance. The atrial contribution to ventricular filling may be reduced by atrioventricular dissociation, prolongation or abbreviation of the P-R interval, and depression of the inotropic state of the atrium.

INOTROPIC STATE (MYOCARDIAL CONTRACTILITY) A number of factors determine the level of ventricular performance at any given ventricular end-diastolic volume, i.e., the position of the ventricular function curve. These influences may be considered to operate by modifying myocardial force-velocity-length relations.

Adrenergic nerve activity (See also Chap. 67) The quantity of norepinephrine released by adrenergic nerve endings in the heart is, under ordinary circumstances, dependent on the adrenergic nerve impulse traffic, and alterations in the frequency of nerve impulses modify the quantity of norepinephrine released and acting upon the beta-adrenergic receptors in the myocardium. This mechanism is the most important one which acutely modifies the position of the force-velocity and ventricular function curves under physiologic conditions.

Circulating catecholamines (See also Chap. 67) The adrenal medulla and other sympathetic ganglia outside the heart, when stimulated by adrenergic nerve impulses, release catecholamines, which, when they reach the heart, augment the inotropic state and the frequency of contraction.

The force-frequency relation The position of the myocardial force-velocity curve is influenced also by the rate and rhythm of cardiac contraction; e.g., ventricular extrasystoles result in post-extrasystolic potentiation, presumably by increasing the Ca^{2+} which enters the cardiac cell.

Exogenously administered inotropic agents The cardiac glycosides, isoproterenol, dopamine, dobutamine, and other sympathomimetic agents, calcium, caffeine, theophylline, and their derivatives, all improve the myocardial force-velocity relation and therefore may be used therapeutically to augment ventricular performance at any given ventricular end-diastolic volume.

Physiologic depressants Included among these are severe myocardial hypoxia, hypercapnia, ischemia, and acidosis. Acting either singly or in combination, these influences exert a depressant effect on the myocardial force-velocity curve and lower the level of the left ventricular work at any given ventricular end-diastolic volume.

Pharmacologic depressants These include quinidine, procainamide, disopyramide, high doses of certain calcium antagonists, barbiturates, alcohol, and other local and general anesthetics, as well as many other drugs.

Loss of ventricular substance When a sufficiently large portion of ventricular myocardium becomes nonfunctional or necrotic, as occurs transiently during ischemia (Chap. 190) and permanently in myocardial infarction (Chap. 189), total ventricular performance at any given level of end-diastolic volume is depressed, even if the remaining myocardium functions normally or supranormally.

Intrinsic myocardial depression Although the fundamental mechanisms responsible for depression of myocardial contractility in chronic congestive heart failure still remain to be elucidated, it is now apparent that in this condition the inotropic state of each unit of myocardium is depressed and that the level of ventricular performance at any ventricular end-diastolic volume is thereby lowered.

VENTRICULAR AFTERLOAD The stroke volume is ultimately a function of the extent of ventricular fiber shortening. In the intact heart, as in isolated cardiac muscle, the velocity and extent of shortening of ventricular muscle fibers at any given level of diastolic fiber length and myocardial inotropic state are inversely related to the afterload imposed on the muscle. The afterload on the intact heart may be defined as the tension or stress developed in the wall of the ventricle during ejection. Therefore, the afterload on the ventricular muscle fibers also is dependent on the level of aortic pressure as well as on the volume and thickness of the ventricular cavity, since Laplace's law indicates that the tension of the myocardial fiber is a function of the product of the intracavitary ventricular pressure and ventricular radius divided by the wall thickness. Thus, at the same level of aortic pressure, the afterload faced by a dilated left ventricle is higher than that encountered by a ventricle of normal size. Furthermore, at any level of aortic pressure and left ventricular volume the afterload placed on any wall fiber varies inversely with wall thickness. The aortic pressure, in turn, is influenced largely by the peripheral vascular resistance, the physical characteristics of the arterial tree, and the volume of blood it contains at the onset of ejection. At any given ventricular end-diastolic volume and level of the inotropic state, the left ventricular stroke volume is related inversely to the afterload.

The critical role played by the ventricular afterload in cardiovascular regulation is summarized in Fig. 181-5. As already noted, increases in both preload and contractility increase myocardial fiber shortening, while increases in afterload reduce it. The extent of myocardial fiber shortening and left ventricular size are the determinants of stroke volume. Arterial pressure, in turn, is related to the product of cardiac output and systemic vascular resistance, while afterload is a function of left ventricular size and arterial pressure. An increase in arterial pressure induced by vasoconstriction, for example, augments afterload, which through a negative feedback depresses myocardial fiber shortening, stroke volume, and cardiac output; this in turn tends to restore arterial pressure to its previous level.

When left ventricular function becomes impaired and the chamber dilates, i.e., when there is no preload reserve, left ventricular afterload becomes increasingly important in determining cardiac performance. Increases in afterload may result from the influence on the arterial bed of neural, humoral, or structural changes which can occur in

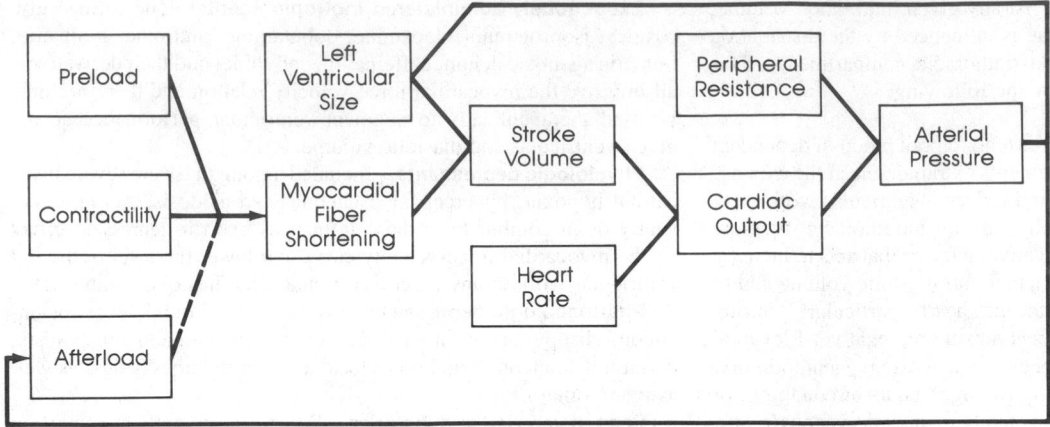

FIGURE 181-5 Scheme of interactions among various components that regulate cardiac activity. Solid lines indicate an augmenting effect; broken line represents an inhibiting effect. *(From Braunwald et al, 1976.)*

response to a fall in cardiac output. This increased afterload may reduce further cardiac output while myocardial oxygen requirements are increased. Treatment with vasodilators (Chap. 182) has the opposite effect. In this way, alterations in the peripheral vascular bed probably play an important role in the hemodynamic and metabolic events which usually are attributed to progressive impairment of the myocardium.

All of the influences acting on cardiac performance enumerated above interact in a complex fashion to maintain cardiac output at a level appropriate to the requirements of the metabolizing tissues, and in a normal person interference with one of these mechanisms may not influence the cardiac output. For example, a moderate reduction of blood volume *or* the loss of the atrial contribution to ventricular contraction can ordinarily be sustained without a reduction in the resting cardiac output. Presumably other factors, such as an increase in the frequency of adrenergic nerve impulses to the heart and an increase in heart rate, will, in a normal individual, augment contractility and sustain cardiac output. Mechanisms are also available that prevent elevation of the cardiac output when there is no physiologic demand for augmented flow. For example, augmentation of myocardial contractility by means of cardiac glycosides does not increase the cardiac output in normal humans. Thus, in analyzing the effect

of an intervention on cardiac output, it is important to recognize that it is the preload, which in turn is related to the volume of blood available for filling the heart, rather than the inotropic state of the myocardium or the afterload which limits cardiac output in the normal individual and that an improvement of myocardial contractility by a drug such as digitalis or the reduction of afterload with nitroprusside would not be expected to elevate the output in a normal subject. On the other hand, in the presence of congestive heart failure, the cardiac output usually is limited by the depressed contractile state of the myocardium, and a positive inotropic drug and/or reduction of afterload would be expected to raise cardiac output, and, indeed, does so (Chap. 182).

EXERCISE   The hemodynamic changes which normally occur during exercise in the upright position are complex (Fig. 181-6). The hyperventilation, the pumping action of the exercising muscles, and the venoconstriction which occur all tend to augment venous return and hence ventricular filling and preload. Simultaneously, the increase in the adrenergic nerve impulses to the myocardium, the increased concentration of circulating catecholamines, and the tachycardia which occur during exercise all combine to augment the contractile state of the myocardium (Fig. 181-6, curves 1 and 2) and lead to an elevation of stroke volume, with no change or even a decrease of end-diastolic

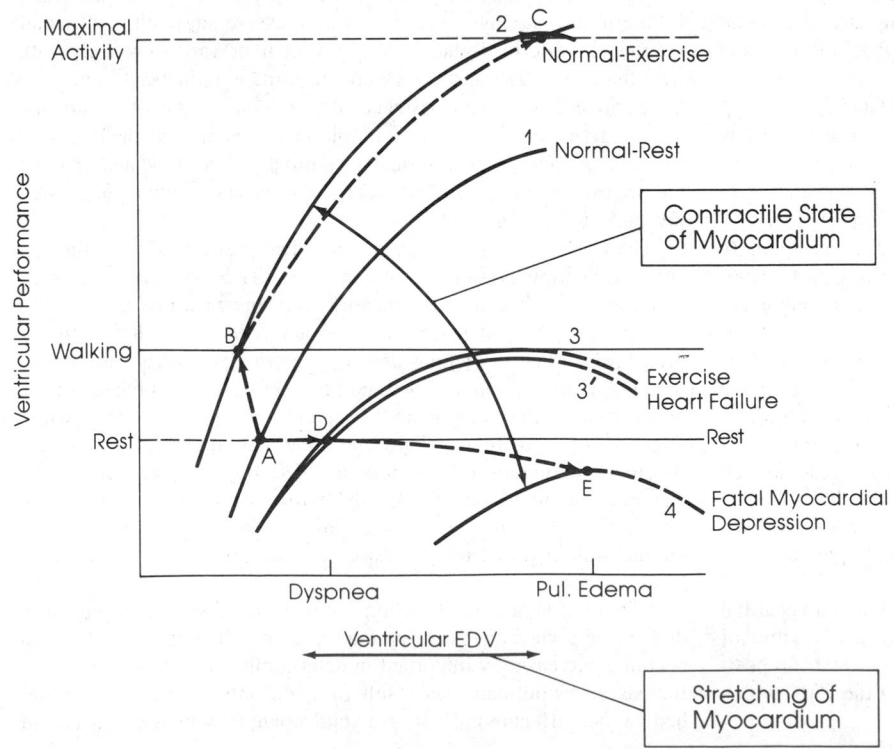

FIGURE 181-6 Diagram showing the interrelations among influences on ventricular end-diastolic volume (EDV) through stretching of the myocardium and the contractile state of the myocardium. Levels of ventricular EDV associated with filling pressures that result in dyspnea and pulmonary edema are shown on the abscissa. Levels of ventricular performance required when the subject is at rest, while walking, and during maximal activity are designated on the ordinate. The dotted lines are the descending limbs of the ventricular-performance curves, which are rarely seen during life but which show the level of ventricular performance if end-diastolic volume could be elevated to very high levels. For further explanation see text. *(From Braunwald et al, 1976.)*

pressure and volume (Fig. 181-6, points A and B). Vasodilatation occurs in the exercising muscles, thus tending to counteract the marked increase in arterial pressure which would otherwise occur as cardiac output rises. This ultimately allows the achievement of a greatly elevated cardiac output during exercise, at an arterial pressure only moderately higher than in the resting state.

THE FAILING HEART

Though heart failure may be readily described as a clinical syndrome, characterized by well-known symptoms and physical signs, a precise physiologic or biochemical definition is far more difficult. However, from the clinical point of view, heart failure may be considered to be the condition in which *an abnormality of cardiac function is responsible for the inability of the heart to pump blood at a rate commensurate with the requirements of the metabolizing tissues and/or can do so only from an abnormally elevated filling pressure.* Abnormalities during systole and/or diastole may be present in heart failure (Fig. 181-7). In so-called *systolic heart failure,* i.e., classic heart failure, an impaired inotropic state causes weakened systolic contraction, which leads, ultimately, to a reduction in stroke volume, inadequate ventricular emptying, cardiac dilatation, and often elevation of ventricular diastolic pressure. Idiopathic dilated cardiomyopathy (Chap. 192) is the prototype of systolic heart failure. In *diastolic heart failure* the principal abnormality involves impaired relaxation of the ventricle and leads to an elevation of ventricular diastolic pressure at a normal diastolic volume. Failure of relaxation can be functional, i.e., as during transient ischemia, or it can be caused by a stiffened, thickened ventricle. Typical conditions in which diastolic failure occurs are restrictive cardiomyopathy secondary to infiltrative conditions, such as amyloidosis or hemochromatosis, as well as hypertrophic cardiomyopathy (Chap. 192). In many patients with cardiac hypertrophy and dilatation, systolic and diastolic failure coexist; the ventricle both empties and fills abnormally. There may be cardiac dilatation, but the ventricle's pressure-volume relation is shifted, raising the ventricular diastolic pressure at any given volume.

Though a defect in myocardial contraction is characteristic of systolic heart failure, this defect may result from a primary abnormality in the heart muscle, as in cardiomyopathy, or it may be secondary to a chronic excessive work load as in hypertension and valvular heart disease, as well as in many forms of congenital heart disease. In ischemic heart disease systolic heart failure results from a loss in the quantity of normally contracting cells. It is important to distinguish heart failure from (1) states of circulatory insufficiency in which myocardial function is not primarily impaired, such as cardiac tamponade or hemorrhagic shock, (2) conditions in which there is circulatory congestion because of abnormal salt and water retention but in which there is no serious disturbance of the heart's function, and (3) conditions in which a normally contracting myocardium is suddenly presented with a load which exceeds its capacity, e.g., accelerated hypertension or rupture of a valve cusp secondary to infective endocarditis.

The intrinsic contractile state of myocardium removed from normal, hypertrophied, and failing animal hearts has been evaluated, and both ventricular hypertrophy and heart failure were shown to reduce the maximum isometric tension and velocity of shortening to subnormal levels; the changes are more marked in the myocardium of animals in which heart failure had been present than in those with hypertrophy alone. Papillary muscles removed from the left ventricles of patients with heart failure have also shown a depression of the maximum degree of active tension which they can develop. Electron-microscopic analysis of failing cat papillary muscles fixed at the apexes of the length–active tension curves revealed sarcomere lengths averaging 2.2 μm. Thus, the abnormalities of contractility do *not* appear to be produced by an alteration in the overlap of filaments within the sarcomere.

The failing ventricle may still eject a normal or nearly normal stroke volume despite considerable depression of function, when its end-diastolic volume increases, i.e., through the operation of the Frank-Starling mechanism. As outlined above, an increase in the initial volume of the ventricle is associated with stretching of the sarcomere, a process that augments the number of sites at which the actin and myosin filaments can interact and/or which increases their sensitivity to Ca^{2+}. Furthermore, the development of ventricular hypertrophy may be considered to provide additional contractile units, and thereby constitutes an important compensatory mechanism when the myocardium's intrinsic inotropic state is depressed.

ASSESSMENT OF CARDIAC PERFORMANCE Several techniques are available for defining impaired cardiac performance in intact humans. With the patient at rest, the cardiac output and stroke volume may be depressed, but not uncommonly these variables are within normal limits. A more sensitive index is the ejection fraction, i.e., the ratio of stroke volume to end-diastolic volume, which may be estimated by standard radiocontrast or radionuclide angiography (Chaps. 177 and 179), and which is frequently depressed in heart failure even when the stroke volume itself is normal. A limitation of the ejection fraction (and of cardiac output) in the assessment of

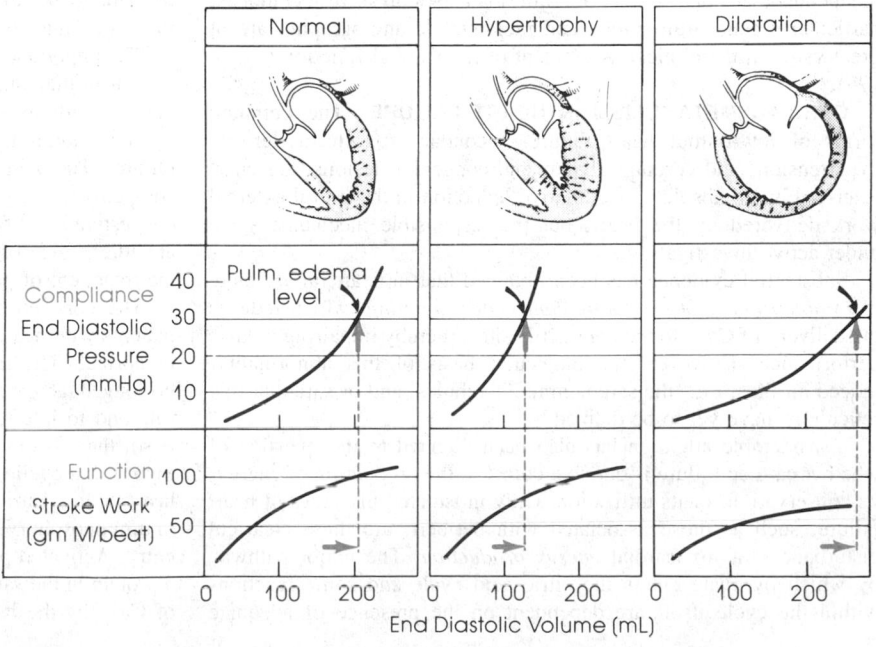

FIGURE 181-7 Relationship between left ventricular end-diastolic volume and (1) end-diastolic pressure (top), describing the *compliance* of the left ventricle, i.e., its *diastolic* properties; and (2) left ventricular stroke work (bottom), describing the ventricle's *systolic* function curve. The normal left ventricle (left) reaches an end-diastolic pressure of 30 mmHg (pulmonary edema level) when its end-diastolic volume is elevated to 200 mL. The concentrically hypertrophied left ventricle (center), exhibits normal systolic function since the relation between left ventricular end-diastolic volume and stroke work is unchanged, but there is "diastolic failure" in that end-diastolic pressure reaches pulmonary edema level (i.e., 30 mmHg) at a lower level than normal (i.e., 130 mL). The dilated ventricle (right) exhibits "systolic failure" in that the maximal stroke work and the stroke volume at any level of end-diastolic volume are depressed. The left ventricle displays increased diastolic compliance, i.e., distensibility, with a higher than normal end-diastolic volume (280 mL) required to reach the pulmonary edema level. (*Reprinted with permission from Gorlin R, Prim Cardiol 6:84, 1980.*)

cardiac function is that these variables are influenced by ventricular loading conditions. Thus, a depressed ejection fraction and lowered cardiac output may be observed in patients with normal ventricular function but reduced preload, as occurs in hypovolemia, or with acutely elevated arterial pressure. An even more sensitive method for detecting impaired ventricular performance is based on the measurement of the circulatory changes occurring during stresses such as exercise or increased afterload. Thus, left ventricular performance may be estimated accurately by measuring the left ventricular end-diastolic pressure, cardiac output, and total body O_2 consumption at rest and during exercise. In normal persons, the cardiac output rises by more than 500 mL/min for each 100-mL increase in minute O_2 consumption. The left ventricular end-diastolic pressure at rest is less than 12 mmHg and rises slightly, remains unchanged, or decreases slightly during exercise, while stroke volume usually rises, especially when exercise is carried out in the upright position. The failing left ventricle, on the other hand, is characterized by an elevation of end-diastolic pressure during exercise, which reaches a value exceeding 12 mmHg, accompanied by either no change or a fall in stroke volume and a subnormal increase in cardiac output related to the increase in minute O_2 consumption. Various degrees of impairment intermediate between the normal response and that of the failing left ventricle during the stress of exercise also have been described.

The potential value of stressing the left ventricle in assessing its performance is emphasized by the fact that the basal values for left ventricular end-diastolic pressure, cardiac index, and ventricular stroke work may be in the same range in patients with depressed ventricular function as in normal persons. The response to stress may prove useful not only in the detection of the impairment of myocardial function, but also in expressing the severity of this impairment quantitatively.

The performance of the left ventricle in humans may also be characterized by examining the instantaneous myocardial force-velocity relations and the extent of shortening during individual cardiac cycles. Angiocardiographic and echocardiographic studies (Chaps. 177 and 179) and analyses of the rate of change of intraventricular pressure (dp/dt) as a function of the simultaneously recorded pressure during isovolumetric contraction have shown that depressions in the velocity of myocardial fiber shortening and of tension development exist in patients with heart failure. In patients with ischemic heart disease these changes are often localized rather than diffuse. Thus, they are manifest by regional wall motion disorders, often in the face of normal global left ventricular function. The end-systolic left ventricular pressure-volume relationship is a particularly useful index of ventricular performance since it is independent of both preload and afterload. Noninvasive techniques, particularly echocardiography and radionuclide angiography, are of great value in the clinical assessment of myocardial function (Chap. 177).

CARDIAC METABOLISM IN HEART FAILURE The common forms of low-output heart failure, secondary to arteriosclerosis, hypertension, and certain valvular and congenital lesions, are characterized by an absolute or a relative reduction in the useful external work delivered by the heart, but the responsible mechanisms are under active investigation.

Substantial evidence has been obtained that in heart failure there is an *abnormality of excitation-contraction coupling,* which reduces the delivery of Ca^{2+} to the contractile sites, thereby impairing cardiac performance. However, the molecular basis of this abnormality, indeed its sites, i.e., the sarcolemma, T tubules, and/or sarcoplasmic reticulum, have yet to be defined.

Considerable attention has also been directed to the question of whether cardiac failure is due to a defect in the production of energy, its conservation, or its utilization. Only in isolated instances of heart failure, such as those associated with beriberi, are there clear-cut disturbances of myocardial *energy production.* The major pathway by which pyruvate enters the citric acid cycle and some reactions within the cycle itself are dependent on the presence of adequate concentrations of thiamine (Chap. 76). Thiamine deficiency results in diminished pyruvic acid utilization by heart slices, and in abnormally low pyruvate extraction coefficients in intact dogs and in humans.

In the second phase of cardiac metabolism, *energy conservation,* the energy of substrate oxidation is converted into the terminal-bond energy of creatine phosphate (CP) and of ATP, the immediate source of chemical energy utilized by heart muscle. This process, known as oxidative phosphorylation, occurs in the mitochondria. The effectiveness of the combined energy production-conservation mechanisms may be studied by measuring the stores of ATP and CP existing in the myocardium, while energy conservation may be evaluated by determining (1) the P/O ratio, i.e., the ratio of high-energy phosphate produced to oxygen consumed in the mitochondria, and (2) the degree of coupling between electron transport and the generation of high-energy phosphate compounds. Although controversy exists concerning the status of this phase of metabolism in heart failure, it now appears that severe impairment of myocardial performance may occur *without* disturbances of mitochondrial function or reduction of high-energy phosphate stores, although abnormalities in these processes have been shown to occur in some forms of experimental (and perhaps of clinical) heart failure.

In the absence of a definitive abnormality of energy liberation or conservation in the failing myocardium, attention has naturally been directed to the possibility that energy *utilization* is abnormal. An abnormality of energy liberation could certainly occur if the contractile proteins themselves were altered. A cardiac myosin isoenzyme characterized by immunologic and electrophoretic properties exhibiting a lower Ca^{2+}-dependent ATPase activity has been shown in some forms of experimentally produced heart failure, particularly those produced by mechanical overloading (Chap. 173). It is possible that this depression may be responsible for a defect in the breakdown of ATP, the process which leads to contraction.

THE ADRENERGIC NERVOUS SYSTEM IN HEART FAILURE In view of the importance of the adrenergic nervous system in stimulating the contractility of the normal myocardium, the activity of this system has also been studied intensively in patients with congestive heart failure. An index of the activity of this system, at rest and during exercise, is provided by measurements of the concentration of norepinephrine (NE) in arterial blood. Relatively small increases in the NE concentration occur during exercise in normal subjects. In patients with heart failure the levels of circulating NE may be markedly elevated at rest, indicating that the activity of the adrenergic nervous system is augmented at rest, and the prognosis varies inversely with the concentration. Also, much greater increments in circulating NE occur when patients with congestive heart failure exercise, again presumably because of an increased activity of the adrenergic nervous system during exercise in these patients.

The importance of the increased activity of the adrenergic nervous system in maintaining ventricular contractility when the function of the myocardium is depressed in congestive heart failure is also shown by the finding that beta-adrenergic blockade may intensify heart failure. The adrenergic nervous system thus plays an important compensatory role in the circulatory adjustments of patients to congestive heart failure, and caution must be exercised in the use of antiadrenergic drugs, particularly beta-adrenergic blocking agents, in the treatment of patients with limited cardiac reserve (Chap. 182).

The concentration and content of the NE in cardiac tissue of patients with heart failure are reduced, sometimes to only 10 percent of normal. The mechanism responsible is not entirely clear, but a prolonged increase in cardiac adrenergic tone appears to play a critical role and to interfere in some manner with the biosynthesis of NE. Also, there is evidence that the beta-adrenergic receptor density and myocardial cyclic AMP concentration are reduced in chronic, severe heart failure. Intracellular cyclic AMP activates protein kinase, which in turn phosphorylates Ca channels, enhancing transarcolemmal Ca^{2+} entry. Activated protein kinase also phosphorylates phospholamban, a protein in the sarcoplasmic reticulum, which enhances the reuptake of Ca^{2+} by the latter and thereby terminates contraction (Fig. 181-

FIGURE 181-8 Schematic representation of influences on intramyocardial Ca^{2+} concentration and excitation-contraction coupling. The action potential is associated with intracellular entry of Na^+ and the extrusion of K^+ (not shown) and the entry of Ca^{2+} (shown). The Na^+-Ca^{2+} exchanger depends on concentration gradients and does not require ATP. Not shown is the energy-dependent sarcolemmal Ca^{2+} pump which extrudes Ca^{2+} from the cell. Isoproterenol and norepinephrine, the latter shown intraneuronally, stimulate the beta-adrenergic receptor in the outer sarcolemma. The beta receptor is coupled to G (guanine nucleotide–binding regulatory) proteins (GR), which in turn activate the catalytic adenylate cyclase (AC). The latter catalyzes the production of cyclic AMP from ATP. AC can be stimulated directly by the administration of *forskolin,* which bypasses both the beta receptor and the G proteins. Cyclic AMP activates protein kinase, which in turn enhances the phosphorylation of the Ca^{2+} channel, increasing transarcolemmal Ca^{2+} influx. Activated protein kinase also phosphorylates phospholamban, which in its phosphorylated form enhances the uptake of Ca^{2+} by the sarcoplasmic tubular network. Phosphodiesterase catalyzes the breakdown of cyclic AMP to AMP while milrinone, caffeine, and isobutylmethylxanthine inhibit phosphodiesterase, thereby augmenting cyclic AMP concentration. Digoxin inhibits the Na^+, K^+-ATPase in the sarcolemma, inhibiting Na^+ efflux from and K^+ influx into the cell. As a consequence the intracellular Na^+ concentration falls and Na^+-Ca^{2+} exchange is reduced, thereby raising intracellular Ca^{2+}. P represents phosphorylation. *(From Feldman MD et al, by permission of the American Heart Association, Inc.)*

8). A deficiency of intracellular cyclic AMP prolongs the action potential and the duration of contraction. The deficiency of intracellular cyclic AMP may be related in part to the "down-regulation" of myocardial beta$_1$ receptors which occurs in heart failure. Changes in the G (guanine regulatory) proteins, which couple the beta receptor to the catalytic adenylate cyclase (which is responsible for the production of cyclic AMP), may also play a role. There is some evidence that increased activity of an inhibitory subunit and reduced activity of the stimulatory subunit of the G proteins occur in heart failure.

In view of the strongly positive inotropic effect exerted by the NE released from these nerves, the adrenergic nervous system may be considered to provide an important potential source of support to the failing myocardium, as long as the number of myocardial beta adrenergic receptors and cyclic AMP concentrations are normal. However, the increments of heart rate and contractile force that occur in animals with experimental heart failure and cardiac NE depletion are abolished or markedly reduced with stimulation of the cardiac adrenergic nerves. Thus, it is likely that when congestive heart failure is accompanied by depletion of cardiac NE stores, the quantity of NE released by the adrenergic nerve endings in the heart is deficient relative to the impulse traffic along these nerves. Furthermore, whatever NE is released may not elicit a normal effect due to reduction of myocardial adrenergic receptor-effector mechanisms.

Cardiac stores of NE are not fundamentally necessary for maintaining the intrinsic contractile state of the myocardium. However, since the reduction of NE stores in heart failure is associated with a diminished release of neurotransmitter, this depletion of NE may be responsible for loss of the much-needed adrenergic support in the failing heart. In the later stages of heart failure, when the levels of circulating catecholamines are elevated and the cardiac NE stores depleted, the myocardium is largely dependent on a more generalized adrenergic stimulation derived from extracardiac sources, presumably the adrenal medulla; this would explain the deterioration of cardiac performance which may occur in patients with heart failure who are treated with beta-adrenergic blocking drugs. This generalized adrenergic stimulation resulting from circulating catecholamines may, however, also exert undesirable side effects, because it elevates vascular resistance and may present the heart with an afterload which is higher than optimal. It may also enhance the likelihood of ventricular arrhythmias. The survival of patients with congestive heart failure varies inversely with the concentration of circulating NE.

In the final analysis, in heart failure, the fundamental abnormality resides in depressions of the myocardial force-velocity relationship and of the length-active tension curve, reflecting reductions in the contractile state of the myocardium (Fig. 181-6, curves 1 to 3). In many instances, cardiac output and external ventricular performance at rest are within normal limits but are maintained at these levels only by an increased end-diastolic fiber length and an elevated ventricular end-diastolic volume, i.e., through the operation of the Frank-Starling mechanism (Fig. 181-6, points A to D). The elevation of left ventricular preload is associated with similar changes in the pulmonary capillary pressure, contributing to the dyspnea experienced by patients with heart failure. The normal improvement of contractility due to augmented adrenergic activity during exercise is attenuated or even prevented by NE depletion which occurs in severe heart failure (Fig. 181-6, curves 3 and 3'). The factors which tend to augment ventricular filling during exercise in the normal subject push the failing myocardium even farther along its flattened length-active tension curve, and although the left ventricle may perform somewhat better, this occurs only as a consequence of an inordinate elevation of ventricular end-diastolic volume and pressure and, therefore, of the pulmonary capillary pressure. The elevation of the latter intensifies dyspnea and therefore plays an important role in limiting the intensity of exercise which the patient can perform. Left ventricular failure becomes fatal when the myocardial length-active tension curve is depressed (Fig. 181-6, curve 4) to the point at which cardiac performance fails to satisfy the requirements of the peripheral tissues even at rest, and/or the left ventricular end-diastolic and pulmonary capillary pressures are elevated to levels which result in pulmonary edema (Fig. 181-6, point E).

REFERENCES

BRAUNWALD E et al (eds): *Congestive Heart Failure: Current Research and Clinical Applications.* New York, Grune & Stratton, 1982

———— et al: *Mechanisms of Contraction of the Normal and Failing Heart,* 2d ed. Boston, Little, Brown, 1976

———— et al: Contraction of the normal heart, in *Heart Disease,* 3d ed, E Braunwald (ed). Philadelphia, Saunders, 1988, pp. 383–425

BRISTOW MR et al: Myocardial α and β-adrenergic receptors in heart failure: Is cardiac-derived norepinephrine the regulatory signal? Eur Heart J 9(Suppl H):35, 1988

COHN JN et al: Plasma norepinephrine as a guide to prognosis in patients with chronic congestive heart failure. N Engl J Med 311:819, 1984

FELDMAN MD et al: Deficient production of cyclic AMP: Pharmacologic evidence of an important cause of contractile dysfunction in patients with end-stage heart failure. Circulation 75:331, 1987

FLEISCHER S, INNUI M: Regulation of muscle contraction and relaxation in heart. Prog Clin Biol Res 273:435, 1988

GROSSMAN W: Evaluation of systolic and diastolic function of the myocardium, in W Grossman (ed): *Cardiac Catheterization and Angiography,* 3d ed. Philadelphia, Lea & Febiger, 1986, p 301

KATZ AM: Cellular mechanisms in congestive heart failure. Am J Cardiol 62:3A, 1988

LOMPRE AM et al: Myosin isoenzyme redistribution in chronic heart overload. Nature 282:105, 1979

MORGAN JP, MORGAN KG: Intracellular calcium and cardiovascular function in heart failure: Effects of pharmacologic agents. Cardiovasc Drugs Ther 3(Suppl 3):959–970, 1989

———— et al: Abnormal intracellular calcium handling: A major cause of systolic and diastolic dysfunction in ventricular myocardium from patients with heart failure. Circulation 81(Suppl III):21–32, 1990

SPIRITO P et al: Noninvasive assessment of left ventricular diastolic function: Comparative analysis of Doppler echocardiographic and radionuclide angiographic techniques. J Am Col Cardiol 7:518, 1986

182 HEART FAILURE

EUGENE BRAUNWALD

Heart failure may be defined as the pathophysiologic state in which an abnormality of *cardiac* function is responsible for the failure of the heart to pump blood at a rate commensurate with the requirements of the metabolizing tissues *and/or* can do so only from an abnormally elevated filling pressure. Heart failure is frequently, but not always, caused by a defect in myocardial contraction, and then the term *myocardial failure* is appropriate. The latter may result from a primary abnormality in the heart muscle, as occurs in the cardiomyopathies (Chap. 192). Myocardial failure may also result from extramyocardial abnormalities, such as coronary atherosclerosis which leads to myocardial ischemia and infarction, as well as from abnormalities of the heart valves in which the heart muscle is damaged by the long-standing excessive hemodynamic burden imposed by the valvular

abnormality, and/or by the rheumatic process (Chap. 187). In patients with chronic constrictive pericarditis, myocardial damage resulting from infiltration of the heart muscle by pericardial inflammation and calcification is common (Chap. 193).

In other patients with heart failure, however, a similar clinical syndrome is present, but without any detectable abnormality of *myocardial* function. In some of these patients the normal heart is suddenly presented with a load that exceeds its capacity, such as an acute hypertensive crisis, rupture of an aortic valve cusp, or massive pulmonary embolism. Heart failure, in the presence of normal myocardial function, also occurs in chronic conditions in which there is impairment of filling of the ventricles due to tricuspid and/or mitral stenosis, constrictive pericarditis without myocardial involvement, endocardial fibrosis, and ventricular hypertrophy.

Heart failure should be distinguished from (1) conditions in which there is circulatory congestion consequent to abnormal salt and water retention but in which there is no disturbance of cardiac function per se (the latter syndrome, termed the *congested state,* may result from the abnormal salt and water retention of renal failure, or from excess parenteral administration of fluids and electrolytes), and (2) from noncardiac causes of inadequate cardiac output, including shock due to hypovolemia and redistribution of blood volume (Chap. 39).

The ventricles respond to a chronically increased hemodynamic burden with the development of hypertrophy. With volume overload when the ventricle is called upon to deliver an elevated cardiac output, as in valvular regurgitation, it develops *eccentric* hypertrophy, i.e., cavity dilatation, with an increase in muscle mass so that the ratio between wall thickness and ventricular cavity size remains relatively constant. With pressure overload when the ventricle is called upon to develop increased pressure, as in valvular aortic stenosis, it develops *concentric* hypertrophy, in which the ratio between wall thickness and ventricular cavity size increases. In both conditions, a stable hyperfunctioning state may exist for many years but myocardial function may ultimately deteriorate, leading to heart failure.

CAUSES OF HEART FAILURE

In evaluating patients with heart failure, it is important to identify not only the *underlying cause* of the heart disease but the *precipitating cause* of heart failure as well. The cardiac abnormality produced by a congenital or acquired lesion such as valvular aortic stenosis may exist for many years and produce no clinical disability. Frequently, however, the manifestations of clinical heart failure appear for the first time in the course of some acute disturbance which places an additional load on a myocardium that chronically is excessively burdened and while compensated has no additional reserves, resulting in further deterioration of cardiac function. Identification of such precipitating causes is of critical importance because their prompt alleviation may be lifesaving. However, in the absence of underlying heart disease these acute disturbances do not usually, by themselves, lead to heart failure.

PRECIPITATING CAUSES

1 *Pulmonary embolism.* Patients with low cardiac output and physical inactivity are at increased risk of developing thrombi in the veins of the lower extremities or the pelvis. Pulmonary embolization may result in further elevation of pulmonary arterial pressure, which in turn may produce or intensify failure of the right ventricle. In the presence of pulmonary vascular congestion, such emboli may also cause infarction of the lung (Chap. 213).

2 *Infection.* Patients with pulmonary vascular congestion are also more susceptible to pulmonary infections, but any infection may precipitate heart failure. The resulting fever, tachycardia, hypoxemia, and the increased metabolic demands may place a further burden on the overloaded, but compensated, myocardium of a patient with chronic heart disease.

3 *Anemia.* In the presence of anemia the oxygen needs of the metabolizing tissues can be met only by an increase in the cardiac

output (Chap. 61); though such an increase in the cardiac output might be sustained by a normal heart, a diseased, overloaded, but otherwise compensated heart may be unable to augment sufficiently the volume of blood which it delivers to the periphery. In this manner the combination of anemia and previously compensated heart disease can lead to inadequate oxygen delivery and precipitate heart failure.

4 *Thyrotoxicosis and pregnancy.* As in anemia and fever, in thyrotoxicosis and pregnancy adequate tissue perfusion requires an increased cardiac output. The development or intensification of heart failure may actually be one of the first clinical manifestations of hyperthyroidism in a patient with underlying heart disease which was previously compensated (Chap. 316). Similarly, heart failure not infrequently occurs for the first time during pregnancy in women with rheumatic valvular disease in whom cardiac compensation may return following delivery.

5 *Arrhythmias.* In patients with underlying but compensated heart disease, arrhythmias are among the most frequent precipitating causes of heart failure. They exert a deleterious effect for a variety of reasons: (*a*) Tachyarrhythmias reduce the time period available for ventricular filling. In patients with coronary artery disease tachyarrhythmias may also cause ischemic myocardial dysfunction. (*b*) The dissociation between atrial and ventricular contractions characteristic of many arrhythmias results in the loss of the atrial booster pump mechanism, thereby tending to raise atrial pressures. (*c*) In any arrhythmia associated with abnormal intraventricular conduction, myocardial performance may become further impaired because of the loss of normal synchronicity of ventricular contraction. (*d*) The marked bradycardia associated with complete atrioventricular block requires a greatly elevated stroke volume if a marked reduction in cardiac output is to be prevented.

6 *Rheumatic and other forms of myocarditis.* Acute rheumatic fever and a variety of infectious or inflammatory processes affecting the myocardium may impair myocardial function in patients with or without preexisting heart disease (Chaps. 187 and 192).

7 *Infective endocarditis.* The additional valvular damage, anemia, fever, and myocarditis which often occur as a consequence of infective endocarditis may, singly or in concert, precipitate heart failure (Chap. 90).

8 *Physical, dietary, environmental, and emotional excesses.* The augmentation of sodium intake, the discontinuation of medications to treat heart failure, physical overexertion, excessive environmental heat or humidity, and emotional crises may all precipitate cardiac decompensation.

9 *Systemic hypertension.* Rapid elevation of arterial pressure, as may occur in some instances of hypertension of renal origin or upon discontinuation of antihypertensive medication, may result in cardiac decompensation (Chap. 196).

10 *Myocardial infarction.* In patients with chronic but compensated ischemic heart disease, a fresh infarct, sometimes otherwise silent clinically, may further impair ventricular function and precipitate heart failure (Chap. 189).

A systematic search for these precipitating causes should be made in every patient with the new development or recent intensification of heart failure, particularly if it is refractory to the usual methods of therapy. If properly recognized, the precipitating cause of heart failure can usually be treated more effectively than the underlying cause. Therefore, the prognosis in patients with heart failure in whom a precipitating cause can be identified, treated, and eliminated is more favorable than in patients in whom the underlying disease process has advanced to the point of producing heart failure.

FORMS OF HEART FAILURE

Heart failure may be described as *high-output* or *low-output*, *acute* or *chronic*, *right-sided* or *left-sided*, *forward* or *backward*, and *systolic* or *diastolic*. These descriptors are often useful in a clinical setting, particularly early in the patient's course, but late in the course the differences between some of these forms often become blurred.

HIGH-OUTPUT VERSUS LOW-OUTPUT HEART FAILURE   It is useful to classify patients with heart failure into those with a low cardiac output, i.e., *low-output heart failure*, and those with an elevated cardiac output, i.e., *high-output heart failure*. The cardiac output is often depressed in patients with heart failure secondary to ischemic heart disease, hypertension, cardiomyopathy, valvular and pericardial disease, but tends to be elevated in patients with heart failure and hyperthyroidism, anemia, pregnancy, arteriovenous fistulas, beriberi, and Paget's disease. In clinical practice, however, low-output and high-output heart failure cannot always be readily distinguished. The normal range of cardiac output is wide [2.5 to 3.8 (liters/min)/m²], and in many patients with so-called low-output heart failure the cardiac output may actually be just within the normal range at rest (although it is lower than it had been previously) and fails to rise normally during exertion. On the other hand, in patients with so-called high-output heart failure the output may not exceed the upper limits of normal (although it would have been found to be so had it been measured before heart failure supervened), but rather it may be close to the upper limit of normal. Regardless of the *absolute* level of the cardiac output, however, cardiac failure may be said to be present when the characteristic clinical manifestations described below are accompanied by a depression of the curve relating ventricular end-diastolic volume to cardiac performance (Fig. 181-6, p. 886).

An integral physiologic component of systolic heart failure (p. 892) is the finding that the heart does not deliver the quantity of oxygen required by the metabolizing tissues. In the absence of peripheral shunting of blood, such inadequate delivery of oxygen to the metabolizing tissues is reflected in an abnormal widening of the normal arterial–mixed venous oxygen difference [35 to 50 mL/L (3.5 to 5.0 mL/dL) in the basal state]. In mild cases, such an abnormality may not be present at rest but becomes evident only during exertion or other hypermetabolic states. In patients with the high-output cardiac states associated with arteriovenous fistula, beriberi, thyrotoxicosis, Paget's disease, etc., the arterial–mixed venous oxygen difference is normal or low. The mixed venous oxygen saturation is raised by the admixture of blood which has been diverted from the metabolizing tissues, and it may be presumed that even in these patients the delivery of oxygen to the latter is reduced despite the normal or even elevated mixed venous oxygen saturation. When heart failure occurs in such patients, the arterial–mixed venous oxygen difference, regardless of the absolute value, still exceeds the level which existed prior to the development of heart failure, and therefore the cardiac output, though normal or elevated, is lower than before heart failure supervened.

The mechanisms responsible for the development of heart failure in patients whose cardiac outputs are initially high are complex and depend on the underlying disease process. In most of these conditions the heart is called upon to pump abnormally large quantities of blood in order to deliver the normal quota of oxygen to the metabolizing tissues. The burden placed on the myocardium by the increased flow load resembles that produced by chronic regurgitant valvular lesions. In addition, thyrotoxicosis and beriberi may also impair myocardial metabolism directly, while severe anemia may interfere with myocardial function by producing myocardial anoxia.

ACUTE VERSUS CHRONIC HEART FAILURE   The prototype of acute heart failure is the patient who suddenly develops a large myocardial infarction or rupture of a cardiac valve, while chronic heart failure is typically observed in patients with dilated cardiomyopathy or multivalvular heart disease which develops or progresses slowly. In acute failure, the sudden reduction in cardiac output often results in systemic hypotension without peripheral edema, while in chronic heart failure, arterial pressure tends to be well maintained, but there is accumulation of edema. Despite these differences in clinical presentation, there is no fundamental distinction between acute and chronic failure. For example, intensive efforts to prevent expansion of blood volume by means of dietary sodium restriction and the administration of diuretics will frequently delay the development of exertional dyspnea and edema in patients with chronic valvular heart disease, i.e., it will mask the clinical manifestations of chronic heart failure, until an acute episode, such as an arrhythmia or infection precipitates acute heart failure. Without intensive efforts to restrict blood volume the same patients would have been considered to have been suffering from chronic heart failure, even though their underlying myocardial disease was no further advanced.

RIGHT-SIDED VERSUS LEFT-SIDED HEART FAILURE Many of the clinical manifestations of heart failure result from the accumulation of excess fluid behind one or both ventricles (Chaps. 36 and 38). This fluid usually localizes upstream to (behind) the specific cardiac chamber which is initially affected. For example, patients in whom the left ventricle is mechanically overloaded (e.g., aortic stenosis) or weakened (e.g., postmyocardial infarction) develop dyspnea and orthopnea as a result of pulmonary congestion, a condition referred to as *left-sided heart failure*. In contrast, when the underlying abnormality affects the right ventricle primarily, e.g., valvular pulmonic stenosis or pulmonary hypertension secondary to pulmonary thromboembolism, symptoms resulting from pulmonary congestion such as orthopnea or paroxysmal nocturnal dyspnea are less common, and edema, congestive hepatomegaly, and systemic venous distention, i.e., clinical manifestations of *right-sided heart failure*, are more prominent. However, when heart failure has existed for months or years, such localization of excess fluid behind the failing ventricle may no longer exist. For example, patients with long-standing aortic valve disease or systemic hypertension may have ankle edema, congestive hepatomegaly, and systemic venous distention late in the course of their disease, even though the abnormal hemodynamic burden initially was placed on the left ventricle, in part because of the secondary pulmonary hypertension and resultant right-sided heart failure, but also because of the persistent retention of salt and water. It is also useful to recall that the muscle bundles composing both ventricles are continuous and both ventricles share a common wall, the interventricular septum. Also, biochemical changes which occur in heart failure and which may be involved in the impairment of myocardial function, such as norepinephrine depletion and alterations in the activity of myosin ATPase, occur in the myocardium of both ventricles, regardless of the specific chamber on which the abnormal hemodynamic burden is placed initially.

BACKWARD VERSUS FORWARD HEART FAILURE For many years a controversy has revolved around the question of the mechanism of the clinical manifestations resulting from heart failure. The concept of *backward heart failure*, propounded by James Hope in 1832, contends that when heart failure occurs, one or the other ventricle fails to discharge its contents normally, the end-diastolic volume of the ventricle rises, the pressures and volumes in the atrium and venous system behind the failing ventricle become elevated, and retention of sodium and water occurs as a consequence of the elevation of systemic venous and capillary pressures and the resultant transudation of fluid into the interstitial space (Chap. 38). In contrast, the proponents of the *forward heart failure* hypothesis, expounded by MacKenzie in 1913, maintain that the clinical manifestations of heart failure result directly from an inadequate discharge of blood into the arterial system. Salt and water retention, then, is a consequence of diminished renal perfusion and excessive proximal tubular sodium reabsorption and of excessive distal tubular reabsorption, through activation of the renin-angiotensin-aldosterone system.

A rigid distinction between *backward* and *forward heart failure* is artificial, since both mechanisms appear to operate to varying extents in most patients with heart failure. However, the rate of onset of heart failure often influences the clinical manifestations. For example, when a large portion of the left ventricle is suddenly destroyed, as in myocardial infarction, although stroke volume is reduced, the patient may die of either acute pulmonary edema, a manifestation of backward failure, or of failure of perfusion of the

systemic tissues. Sometimes both mechanisms operate simultaneously. If the patient survives the acute insult, clinical manifestations resulting from a chronically depressed cardiac output, including the abnormal retention of fluid within the systemic vascular bed, might develop. Similarly, in the case of massive pulmonary embolism, the right ventricle may dilate and the systemic venous pressure may rise to high levels (backward failure), or the patient may develop shock secondary to low cardiac output (forward failure), but this low-output state may have to be maintained for some days before sodium and water retention sufficient to produce peripheral edema occurs.

SYSTOLIC VERSUS DIASTOLIC FAILURE The distinction between these two forms of heart failure, described on p. 887 and in Fig. 181-7, relates to whether the principal abnormality is the inability to expel sufficient blood (systolic failure) or to relax and fill normally (diastolic failure). The major clinical manifestations of systolic failure relate to an inadequate cardiac output with weakness, fatigue, and other symptoms of hypoperfusion, while in diastolic failure they relate principally to an elevation of filling pressures. In many patients, particularly those who have both ventricular hypertrophy *and* dilatation, abnormalities both of contraction and relaxation coexist.

REDISTRIBUTION OF CARDIAC OUTPUT The redistribution of cardiac output serves as an important compensatory mechanism when flow is reduced. This redistribution is most marked when a patient with heart failure exercises, but as heart failure advances, redistribution occurs even in the basal state. Blood flow is redistributed so that the delivery of oxygen to vital organs, such as the brain and myocardium, is maintained at normal or near-normal levels, while flow to less critical areas, such as the cutaneous and muscular beds and splanchnic viscera, is reduced. Vasoconstriction mediated by the sympathetic nervous system is largely responsible for this redistribution, which in turn may be responsible for many of the clinical manifestations of heart failure, such as fluid accumulation (reduction of renal flow), low-grade fever (reduction of cutaneous flow), and fatigue (reduction of muscle flow).

SALT AND WATER RETENTION (See also Chap. 38)

When the volume of blood pumped by the left ventricle into the systemic vascular bed is chronically reduced, and when one or both ventricles fail to expel the normal fraction of their end-diastolic volumes, a complex sequence of adjustments occurs which ultimately results in the abnormal accumulation of fluid. Though, on the one hand, many of the clinical manifestations of heart failure are secondary to this excessive retention of fluid, on the other, this abnormal fluid accumulation and the expansion of blood volume which accompanies it also constitute an important compensatory mechanism which tends to maintain cardiac output and therefore perfusion of the vital organs. Except in the terminal stages of heart failure, the ventricle operates on an ascending, albeit depressed and flattened, function curve (Fig. 181-6), and the augmented ventricular end-diastolic volume and pressure characteristic of heart failure must be regarded as helping to maintain the reduced cardiac output, despite causing pulmonary and/or systemic venous congestion.

In the presence of heart failure, effective filling of the systemic arterial bed is reduced, a condition which initiates the complex hemodynamic, renal, and hormonal adjustments that interact to promote reduced renal sodium and water excretion. Patients with severe heart failure may exhibit a reduced capacity to excrete a water load, which may result in dilutional hyponatremia. These abnormalities may be caused, in part, by excess antidiuretic hormone activity and/or factors that prevent sodium reabsorption in the distal tubule, such as avid proximal tubular reabsorption of sodium or the action of a diuretic acting on the distal tubule.

The importance of elevated systemic venous pressure and of the alterations of renal and adrenal function characteristic of heart failure vary in their relative importance in the production of edema in different patients with heart failure. The renin-angiotensin-aldosterone axis is activated most intensely by acute heart failure, and its activity tends to decline as heart failure becomes chronic. In patients with tricuspid valve disease or constrictive pericarditis the elevated venous pressure and the transudation of fluid from systemic capillaries appear to play the dominant role in edema formation. On the other hand, severe edema may be present in patients with ischemic or hypertensive heart disease, in whom systemic venous pressure is within normal limits or is only minimally elevated. In such patients, the retention of salt and water is probably due primarily to a redistribution of cardiac output and a concomitant reduction in renal perfusion, as well as activation of the renin-angiotensin-aldosterone axis. Regardless of the mechanisms involved in fluid retention, untreated patients with chronic congestive heart failure have elevations of total blood volume, interstitial fluid volume, and body sodium. These abnormalities diminish after clinical compensation has been achieved by treatment.

CLINICAL MANIFESTATIONS OF HEART FAILURE

Dyspnea Respiratory distress which occurs as the result of increased effort in breathing is the most common symptom of heart failure (Chap. 36). In early heart failure, dyspnea is observed only during activity, when it may simply represent an aggravation of the breathlessness which normally occurs under these circumstances. As heart failure advances, however, it appears with progressively less strenuous activity. Ultimately, breathlessness is present even when the patient is at rest. The principal difference between exertional dyspnea in normal persons and in cardiac patients is the degree of activity necessary to induce the symptom. Cardiac dyspnea is observed most frequently in patients with elevations of pulmonary venous and capillary pressures. Such patients usually have engorged pulmonary vessels and interstitial pulmonary edema, which reduces the compliance of the lungs and thereby increases the work of the respiratory muscles required to inflate the lungs. The activation of receptors in the lungs results in the rapid, shallow breathing of cardiac dyspnea. The oxygen cost of breathing is increased by the excessive work of the respiratory muscles. This is coupled with the diminished delivery of oxygen to these muscles, which occurs as a consequence of the reduced cardiac output, and which may contribute to fatigue of the respiratory muscles and the sensation of shortness of breath.

Orthopnea Dyspnea in the recumbent position is often a later manifestation of heart failure than exertional dyspnea. Orthopnea occurs in part because of the redistribution of fluid from the abdomen and lower extremities into the chest causing an increase in the pulmonary capillary hydrostatic pressure, as well as a result of elevation of the diaphragm. Patients with orthopnea generally report that they must elevate their heads on several pillows at night and frequently awaken short of breath or coughing (the so-called nocturnal cough) if their heads slip off the pillows. The sensation of breathlessness usually is relieved by sitting bolt upright, since this position reduces venous return and pulmonary capillary pressure, and many patients report that they find relief from sitting in front of an open window. As heart failure advances, orthopnea may become so severe that patients cannot lie down at all and must spend the entire night in a sitting position. On the other hand, in other patients with long-standing, severe left ventricular failure, symptoms of pulmonary congestion may actually diminish with time as the function of the right ventricle becomes impaired.

Paroxysmal (nocturnal) dyspnea This term refers to attacks of severe shortness of breath and coughing which generally occur at night, usually awaken the patient from sleep, and may be quite frightening. Though simple orthopnea may be relieved by sitting upright at the side of the bed with legs dependent, in the patient with paroxysmal nocturnal dyspnea coughing and wheezing often persist even in this position. The depression of the respiratory center during sleep may reduce ventilation sufficiently to lower arterial oxygen tension, particularly in patients with interstitial lung edema and

reduced pulmonary compliance. Also, ventricular function may be further impaired at night because of reduced adrenergic stimulation of myocardial function. *Cardiac asthma* is closely related to paroxysmal nocturnal dyspnea and nocturnal cough and is characterized by wheezing secondary to bronchospasm—most prominent at night. *Acute pulmonary edema* (Chap. 36) is a severe form of cardiac asthma due to further elevation of pulmonary capillary pressure leading to alveolar edema, associated with extreme shortness of breath, rales over the lung fields, and the transudation and expectoration of blood-tinged fluid. If not treated promptly acute pulmonary edema may be fatal.

Cheyne-Stokes respiration Also known as *periodic* or *cyclic respiration,* Cheyne-Stokes respiration is characterized by diminished sensitivity of the respiratory center to arterial P_{CO_2}. There is an apneic phase, during which the arterial P_{O_2} falls and the arterial P_{CO_2} rises. These changes in the arterial blood stimulate the depressed respiratory center, resulting in hyperventilation and hypocapnia, followed in turn by apnea. Cheyne-Stokes respiration occurs most often in patients with cerebral atherosclerosis and other cerebral lesions, but the prolongation of the circulation time from the lung to the brain which occurs in heart failure, particularly in patients with hypertension and coronary artery disease and associated cerebral vascular disease, also appears to precipitate this form of breathing.

Fatigue and weakness These nonspecific but common symptoms of heart failure are related to the reduction of perfusion of skeletal muscle. Anorexia and nausea associated with abdominal pain and fullness are frequent complaints which may be related to the congested liver and portal venous system.

Cerebral symptoms In severe heart failure, particularly in elderly patients with accompanying cerebral arteriosclerosis, arterial hypoxemia, and reduced cerebral perfusion, there may be alterations in the mental state characterized by confusion, difficulty in concentration, impairment of memory, headache, insomnia, and anxiety. *Nocturia* is common in heart failure and may contribute to insomnia.

PHYSICAL FINDINGS In moderate heart failure the patient appears to be in no distress at rest except that he or she may be uncomfortable when lying flat for more than a few minutes. In more severe heart failure the pulse pressure may be diminished, reflecting a reduction in stroke volume, and occasionally the diastolic arterial pressure may be elevated as a consequence of generalized vasoconstriction. In acute heart failure hypotension may be prominent. There may be cyanosis of the lips and nail beds, sinus tachycardia, and the patient may insist on sitting upright. *Systemic venous pressure* is often abnormally elevated in heart failure and may be recognized by observing the extent of distention of the jugular veins. In the early stages of heart failure the venous pressure may be normal at rest but may become abnormally elevated during and immediately after exertion as well as with sustained pressure on the abdomen (positive abdominojugular reflux).

Third and fourth heart sounds (Chap. 175) are often audible but are not specific for heart failure, and *pulsus alternans*, i.e., a regular rhythm in which there is alternation of strong and weak cardiac contractions and therefore alternation in the strength of the peripheral pulses, may be present. Pulsus alternans may be detected by sphygmomanometry and in more severe instances by palpation; it frequently follows an extrasystole and is observed most commonly in patients with cardiomyopathy or with hypertensive or ischemic heart disease. It is caused by a reduction in the number of contractile units during weak contractions and/or by alternation in the ventricular end-diastolic volume.

Pulmonary rales Moist, inspiratory, crepitant rales and dullness to percussion over the lung bases are common in patients with heart failure and elevated pulmonary venous and capillary pressures. In patients with pulmonary edema, rales may be heard widely over both lung fields; they are frequently coarse and sibilant and may be accompanied by expiratory wheezing. Rales may, however, be caused by many conditions other than left ventricular failure. Patients with long-standing heart failure may have no rales because of increased lymphatic drainage of fluid.

Cardiac edema Cardiac edema is usually dependent, occurring in the legs symmetrically, particularly in the pretibial region and ankles in the evening in ambulatory patients, and in the sacral region of individuals at bed rest. Pitting edema of the arms and face occurs rarely and only late in the course of heart failure.

Hydrothorax and ascites Pleural effusion in congestive heart failure results from the elevation of pleural capillary pressure and transudation of fluid into the pleural cavities. Since the pleural veins drain into *both* the systemic and pulmonary veins, hydrothorax occurs most commonly with marked elevation of pressure in both venous systems, but may also be seen with marked elevation of pressure in either venous bed. It is more frequent in the right pleural cavity than the left. *Ascites* also occurs as a consequence of transudation and results from increased pressure in the hepatic veins and the veins draining the peritoneum (Chap. 48). Marked ascites occurs most frequently in patients with tricuspid valve disease and with constrictive pericarditis.

Congestive hepatomegaly An enlarged, tender, pulsating liver also accompanies systemic venous hypertension and is observed not only in the same conditions in which ascites occurs, but also in milder forms of heart failure from any cause. With prolonged, severe hepatomegaly, as in patients with tricuspid valve disease or chronic constrictive pericarditis, enlargement of the spleen may also occur.

Jaundice This is a late finding in congestive heart failure and is associated with elevations of both the direct- and indirect-reacting bilirubin; it results from impairment of hepatic function secondary to hepatic congestion and the hepatocellular hypoxia associated with central lobular atrophy. Serum transaminase concentrations are frequently elevated. If hepatic congestion occurs acutely, the jaundice may be severe and the enzymes strikingly raised.

Cardiac cachexia With severe chronic heart failure there may be serious weight loss and cachexia because of (1) elevation of the metabolic rate, which results in part from the extra work performed by the respiratory muscles, the increased oxygen needs of the hypertrophied heart, and the discomfort associated with severe heart failure; (2) anorexia, nausea, and vomiting due to central causes, to digitalis intoxication, or to congestive hepatomegaly and abdominal fullness; (3) some impairment of intestinal absorption due to congestion of the intestinal veins; and (4) rarely, in patients with particularly severe failure of the right side of the heart, a protein-losing enteropathy.

Other manifestations With reduction of blood flow the extremities may be cold, pale, and diaphoretic. Urine flow is depressed, and the urine contains protein and has a high specific gravity and a low concentration of sodium. In addition, prerenal azotemia may be present. In patients with long-standing severe heart failure impotence and depression are common.

ROENTGENOGRAPHIC FINDINGS In addition to the enlargement of the particular chambers characteristic of the lesion responsible for heart failure, distention of pulmonary veins is common in patients with heart failure and elevated pulmonary vascular pressures (Chap. 177). Also, pleural effusions may be present and associated with interlobar effusions.

DIFFERENTIAL DIAGNOSIS The diagnosis of congestive heart failure may be established by observing some combination of the clinical manifestations of heart failure, enumerated above, together with the findings characteristic of one of the etiologic forms of heart disease. Since chronic heart failure is often associated with cardiac enlargement, the diagnosis should be questioned, but is by no means excluded, when all chambers are normal in size. Two-dimensional echocardiography is particularly useful in assessing the dimensions of each cardiac chamber. Heart failure may be difficult to distinguish from pulmonary disease, and the differential diagnosis is discussed in Chap. 36. Pulmonary embolism also presents many of the manifestations of heart failure, but hemoptysis, pleuritic chest pain, a right ventricular lift, and the characteristic mismatch between

ventilation and perfusion on lung scan should point to this diagnosis (Chap. 213).

Ankle edema may be due to varicose veins, cyclic edema, or gravitational effects (Chap. 38), but in these patients there is no jugular venous hypertension at rest or with pressure over the abdomen. Edema secondary to renal disease can usually be recognized by appropriate renal function tests and urinalysis and is rarely associated with elevation of the venous pressure. Enlargement of the liver and ascites occur in patients with hepatic cirrhosis, but may also be distinguished from heart failure by normal jugular venous pressure and absence of a positive abdominojugular reflux.

TREATMENT OF HEART FAILURE

The treatment of heart failure may be divided into three components: (1) removal of the precipitating cause, (2) correction of the underlying cause, and (3) control of the congestive heart failure state. The first two are discussed in subsequent chapters together with each specific disease entity or complication. An example is the treatment of pneumococcal pneumonia and acute heart failure followed by mitral valvotomy in a patient with mitral stenosis. In many instances surgical treatment will correct or at least improve the underlying cause. The third component of the treatment of heart failure may, in turn, also be divided into three categories: (1) reduction of cardiac work load, including both the preload and the afterload; (2) control of excessive salt and water retention; and (3) enhancement of myocardial contractility. The vigor with which each of these measures is pursued in any individual patient should depend upon the severity of the heart failure state. Following effective treatment, recurrence of the clinical manifestations of heart failure can often be prevented by continuing those measures that were originally effective. While a simple rule for the treatment of all patients with heart failure cannot be formulated because of the varied etiologies, hemodynamic features, and clinical manifestations of heart failure, insofar as the treatment of chronic congestive failure is concerned, simple measures such as moderate restriction of activity and sodium intake should be tried first. If these are insufficient, therapy with a combination of a diuretic, an angiotensin-converting enzyme inhibitor, and perhaps a digitalis glycoside is then begun. The next step is more rigorous restriction of salt intake and higher doses of loop diuretics sometimes accompanied by other diuretics. If heart failure persists, hospitalization with rigid salt restriction, bed rest, intravenous vasodilators, and positive inotropic agents comes next. In some patients the order in which these measures are applied may be altered.

REDUCTION OF CARDIAC WORK LOAD This consists of reducing physical activity, instituting emotional rest, and reducing afterload. Modest restriction of physical activity in mild cases and rest in bed or in a chair in severe failure remain cornerstones in the treatment of heart failure. Meals should be small in quantity, and every effort should be made to diminish the patient's anxiety. Physical and emotional rest tend to lower arterial pressure, and reduce the load on the myocardium by diminishing the requirements for cardiac output. These influences act in concert to diminish the need for redistribution of the cardiac output, and in many patients, particularly those with mild heart failure, simple bed rest and mild sedation often result in an effective diuresis.

Rest at home or in the hospital should be maintained for 1 to 2 weeks in patients with overt congestive failure and should be continued for several days after the patient's condition has stabilized. The hazards of phlebothrombosis and pulmonary embolism which occur with bed rest may be reduced with anticoagulants, leg exercises, and elastic stockings. In any event, *absolute* bed rest rarely is required, and the patient should be encouraged to sit in a chair and be given toilet privileges unless heart failure is extreme. Heavy sedation should be avoided, but small doses of tranquilizers may be helpful in calming the emotionally disturbed patient through the first few days of therapy and in permitting much-needed sleep. In patients with chronic, mild heart failure, bed rest on weekends will frequently allow continuation of gainful employment. Following recovery from heart failure, the patient's activities must be carefully assessed, and often his or her professional, family, and/or community responsibilities must be reduced. Intermittent rest during the day (e.g., a 1-h nap or enforced rest following lunch) and the avoidance of strenuous exertion are often helpful once compensation has been restored. Weight reduction by restriction of caloric intake in the obese patient with heart failure also diminishes cardiac work load and is an essential component of the therapeutic program.

CONTROL OF EXCESSIVE FLUID RETENTION Many of the clinical manifestations of heart failure result from hypervolemia and expansion of the interstitial fluid volume. By the time fluid retention due to heart failure first becomes clinically evident, most commonly as edema, considerable expansion of the extracellular space has already occurred, and heart failure usually is already advanced. Exertional dyspnea and orthopnea may be caused by displacement of fluid from the systemic to the pulmonary vascular bed. Treatment aimed at reducing extracellular fluid volume is dependent primarily on lowering total body sodium stores, while fluid restriction is of less importance. A negative sodium balance can be achieved by reducing the dietary intake and increasing the urinary excretion of this ion with the aid of diuretics. In severe heart failure mechanical removal of extracellular fluid by means of thoracentesis, paracentesis, and rarely hemodialysis or peritoneal dialysis may also be employed.

Diet In patients with mild heart failure, considerable improvement in symptoms may result from simply reducing the sodium intake, particularly if accompanied by periods of physical rest. In patients with more severe heart failure the sodium intake must be controlled more rigidly, and other measures, such as diuretics, vasodilators, and glycosides, are used. Even following recovery from a bout of heart failure, at least moderate sodium restriction should be maintained. The normal diet contains approximately 6 to 10 g sodium chloride; this intake can be reduced by half simply by excluding salt-rich foods and salt which is added at the table. Reduction of the ordinary dietary intake to approximately one-fourth of normal may be achieved if, in addition, all salt is omitted from cooking. In patients with severe heart failure, in whom the daily sodium chloride intake should be reduced to between 500 and 1000 mg, milk, cheese, bread, cereals, canned vegetables and soups, some salted cuts of meat, and some fresh vegetables, including spinach, celery, and beets, must be eliminated. A variety of fresh fruit, green vegetables, specially processed breads and milk, and salt substitutes are permissible, but it is difficult to keep such diets palatable. Water intake may be ad libitum in all but the most severe forms of congestive heart failure. Late in the course of heart failure, dilutional hyponatremia may develop in patients who are unable to excrete a water load, sometimes because of excessive secretion of antidiuretic hormone. In such cases water intake as well as sodium intake must be restricted.

Attention must also be directed to the caloric content of the diet. Substantial improvement can result from caloric restriction in obese patients with heart failure, in whom weight loss will reduce the load placed on the myocardium. On the other hand, in individuals with severe heart failure and cardiac cachexia, an attempt must be made to maintain nutritional intake and to avoid caloric and vitamin deficiencies.

Diuretics A variety of diuretic agents is available, and in patients with mild heart failure almost all are effective. However, in the more severe forms of heart failure, the selection of diuretics is more difficult, and any existing abnormalities in serum electrolytes must be taken into account. Overtreatment must be avoided, since the resultant hypovolemia may reduce cardiac output, interfere with renal function, and produce profound weakness and lethargy.

THIAZIDE DIURETICS These agents are widely used in clinical practice because of their effectiveness when administered orally. In patients with chronic heart failure of mild or moderate severity the continued administration of chlorothiazide or one of its many ana-

logues abolishes or diminishes the need for rigid dietary sodium restriction, although salty foods and table salt should still be avoided. Thiazides are well absorbed following oral administration; chlorothiazide and hydrochlorothiazide reach their peak action in 4 h, and diuresis persists for approximately 12 h. Thiazide diuretics reduce the reabsorption of sodium and chloride in the first half of the distal convoluted tubule and a portion of the cortical ascending limb of the loop of Henle, and water follows the unreabsorbed salt. Thiazides fail to increase free water clearance, and in some instances reduce it, supporting the hypothesis that these drugs inhibit selective reabsorption of sodium chloride in the distal cortical diluting segment, at a site where the urine is normally diluted (Chap. 222). This may result in the excretion of a hypertonic urine and may contribute to dilutional hyponatremia. As a consequence of increased delivery of sodium to the distal nephron, sodium-potassium ion exchange is enhanced and kaliuresis results. In contrast to the loop diuretics which enhance calcium excretion, the thiazides have the opposite effect. These drugs are effective and useful in the treatment of heart failure as long as the glomerular filtration rate exceeds 50 percent of normal.

Chlorothiazide is administered in doses of up to 500 mg every 6 h. Many derivatives of this compound are available but differ principally in dosage and duration of action and therefore offer few, if any, significant advantages over the parent compound, except for chlorthalidone which may be administered once daily. Potassium depletion and metabolic alkalosis (the latter due to increased H^+ secretion as a substitute for the depleted intracellular stores of potassium and increased proximal tubular reabsorption of filtered HCO_3^- when there is relative depletion of the extracellular fluid volume) are the chief adverse metabolic effects following prolonged administration of the thiazides, of metolazone, and of the loop diuretics. Hypokalemia may seriously enhance the dangers of digitalis intoxication, induce fatigue and lethargy, and may be prevented by the oral supplementation of potassium chloride. However, the solution is not palatable and may be hazardous in patients with renal failure. Therefore, to prevent potassium depletion, in patients receiving thiazide diuretics, intermittent dosage schedules, e.g., omitting the diuretic every third day, and the addition of a potassium-retaining diuretic, such as a spironolactone or triamterene, may be preferable. Other side effects of thiazides include reduction of the excretion of uric acid, which may lead to hyperuricemia, and a hyperglycemic effect, which rarely may precipitate hyperosmolar coma in the poorly regulated diabetic. Skin rashes, thrombocytopenia, and granulocytopenia have also been reported.

METOLAZONE This quinethazone derivative has a site of action and potency similar to that of the thiazides, but has been reported to be effective in the presence of moderate renal failure. The usual dose is 5 to 10 mg/day.

FUROSEMIDE, BUMETANIDE, AND ETHACRYNIC ACID These "loop" diuretics are similar physiologically but differ chemically. These extremely powerful diuretics reversibly inhibit the reabsorption of sodium, potassium, and chloride in the thick ascending limb of Henle's loop, apparently by blocking a cotransport system in the luminal membrane. These agents may induce renal cortical vasodilatation and can produce rates of urine formation which may be as high as one-fourth of the glomerular filtration rate. While other diuretics lose their effectiveness as blood volume is restored to normal levels, the loop diuretics remain effective despite the elimination of excessive extracellular fluid volume. The major side effects of these agents are due to this marked diuretic potency, which on rare occasions may result in contraction of the plasma volume, circulatory collapse, reductions in the renal blood flow and glomerular filtration rate, and the development of prerenal azotemia. Metabolic alkalosis is produced by a large increase in the urinary excretion of chloride, hydrogen, and potassium ions. Hypokalemia (see discussion of thiazides, above) and hyponatremia may occur, and hyperuricemia and hyperglycemia are observed occasionally, as with thiazide diuretics. The reabsorption of free water is decreased.

All three drugs are readily absorbed orally and are excreted in the bile and urine. They are usually effective by mouth and intravenously. Weakness, nausea, and dizziness may complicate the administration of all three loop diuretics; ethacrynic acid has been associated with skin rash and granulocytopenia, as well as with transient or permanent deafness.

These extremely effective diuretics are useful in all forms of heart failure, particularly in otherwise refractory heart failure and pulmonary edema. They have been shown to be effective in patients with hypoalbuminemia, hyponatremia, hypochloremia, hypokalemia, and reductions in the glomerular filtration rate, and to produce a diuresis in patients in whom thiazide diuretics and aldosterone antagonists, alone and in combination, are ineffective.

In patients with refractory heart failure the action of furosemide, bumetanide, and ethacrynic acid may be potentiated by intravenous administration and the addition of thiazide diuretics, carbonic anhydrase inhibitors, osmotic diuretics, and the potassium-sparing diuretics—spironolactone, triamterene, and amiloride. These latter agents act on the cortical collecting ducts, are relatively weak, and therefore are rarely indicated as sole agents. However, their potassium-sparing properties make them particularly useful in conjunction with the more potent kaliuretic agents, the loop diuretics and thiazides. These agents fall into two classes, as noted below.

ALDOSTERONE ANTAGONISTS   The 17-spironolactones resemble aldosterone structurally and act on the distal half of the convoluted tubule and the cortical portion of the collecting duct by competitive inhibition of aldosterone, thereby blocking the exchange between sodium and both potassium and hydrogen in the distal tubules and collecting ducts. These agents produce a sodium diuresis, and, in contrast to the thiazides, ethacrynic acid, and furosemide, they result in potassium retention. Although secondary hyperaldosteronism exists in some patients with congestive heart failure, the spironolactones are effective even in patients in whom the serum aldosterone concentration is within normal limits. Aldactone A may be administered in doses of 25 to 100 mg three to four times daily by mouth. The maximal effect of this regimen is not observed for approximately 4 days. Spironolactones are most effective when administered in combination with thiazide and loop diuretics. The opposing action of these drugs on urine and serum potassium makes possible a sodium diuresis without either hyper- or hypokalemia when spironolactone and one of these other agents are administered in combination. Also, since spironolactone, triamterene, and amiloride act on the distal tubule, they are particularly effective when used in combination with one of these other diuretics which acts more proximally.

Spironolactone, triamterene, and amiloride should not be administered alone to patients with hyperkalemia, renal failure, or hyponatremia. Reported complications include nausea, epigastric distress, mental confusion, drowsiness, gynecomastia, and erythematous eruptions.

TRIAMTERENE AND AMILORIDE   These two drugs exert renal effects similar to those of the spironolactones; i.e., they block sodium reabsorption and secondarily inhibit potassium secretion in the distal tubules. However, their fundamental mechanism of action differs from those of the spironolactones, since they are active in adrenalectomized animals and their action does not depend on the presence of aldosterone. The effective dose of triamterene is 100 mg once or twice daily and that of amiloride is 5 mg daily. Side effects include nausea, vomiting, diarrhea, headache, granulocytopenia, eosinophilia, and skin rash. Both triamterene and the chemically unrelated diuretic amiloride resemble Aldactone A in that their diuretic potency is not great, but they are effective in preventing the hypokalemia characteristic of the administration of thiazides, furosemide, and ethacrynic acid. A number of diuretic preparations contain a combination of a thiazide and either triamterene or amiloride in a single capsule. They may be useful in patients who develop hypokalemia with a thiazide but should not be used in patients with impaired renal function and/or hyperkalemia.

CHOICE OF DIURETICS   Orally administered thiazides or metolazone are the agents of choice in the treatment of chronic cardiac

edema of mild to moderate degree in patients without hyperglycemia, hyperuricemia, or hypokalemia. Spironolactones, triamterene, and amiloride are not potent diuretics when used alone, but they potentiate other diuretics, particularly the thiazides and loop diuretics. However, in patients with heart failure and severe secondary hyperaldosteronism, spironolactone may be quite effective. Ethacrynic acid, bumetanide, or furosemide, given alone or with spironolactone or triamterene, are the agents of choice in patients with severe heart failure refractory to other diuretics. In very severe heart failure the combination of a thiazide, a loop diuretic, and a potassium-sparing diuretic (spironolactone, triamterene, or amiloride) is required.

VASODILATOR THERAPY   In many patients with heart failure, left ventricular afterload is increased as a consequence of the several neural and humoral influences which act to constrict the peripheral vascular bed. These include increased activity of the adrenergic nervous system, elevation of circulating catecholamines, and activation of the renin-angiotensin system, and perhaps of increased circulating antidiuretic hormone as well. In addition to the vasoconstriction, the ventricular end-diastolic volume rises and as a consequence of the operation of Laplace's law, which relates myocardial wall tension to the product of intraventricular pressure and radius, the aortic impedance, i.e., the force which opposes left ventricular ejection, or the ventricular afterload, rises. The maintenance or even the elevation of arterial pressure is generally considered to be a useful compensatory mechanism that allows blood flow to vital organs to persist in the presence of hypovolemia and reduction of the total cardiac output. While this is the case in many forms of shock (Chap. 39), in the presence of severely impaired cardiac function, the increase in afterload may reduce cardiac output further.

As shown in Fig. 181-5, afterload is a major determinant of cardiac function. When cardiac function is normal, a moderate elevation in afterload does not alter stroke volume, because the resultant increase in left ventricular end-diastolic volume, i.e., preload, can be tolerated easily. However, when myocardial function is impaired, such an increase in preload evoked by an elevation of afterload may raise ventricular end-diastolic and pulmonary capillary pressures to levels that may produce severe pulmonary congestion or pulmonary edema. In many patients with heart failure, the ventricle is already operating at the peak, flat portion of its Frank-Starling curve (Fig. 181-6), and any additional increase in aortic impedance (afterload) will reduce stroke volume (p. 886). Conversely, a reduction of afterload will tend to restore hemodynamics to normal by elevating the stroke volume of the failing ventricle, and may reduce the elevated ventricular filling pressure.

The pharmacologic reduction of impedance to left ventricular ejection with vasodilator drugs represents an important adjunct in the management of heart failure. This approach may be particularly helpful but is by no means limited to patients with acute heart failure due to myocardial infarction (Chap. 189), valvular regurgitation, elevated systemic vascular resistance and/or arterial pressure, and marked cardiac dilatation. The reduction of afterload by means of a variety of vasodilators reduces left ventricular end-diastolic pressure, volume, and oxygen consumption, while raising stroke volume and cardiac output and causing only modest reduction in aortic pressure. Vasodilators should not be used in patients with hypotension.

In patients with both acute and chronic heart failure secondary to coronary artery disease, cardiomyopathy, or valvular regurgitation who are treated with vasodilators, cardiac output increases, the pulmonary wedge pressure falls, the signs and symptoms of heart failure are relieved, and a new steady state is achieved in which cardiac output is higher and afterload lower with no or only mild reduction of arterial pressure (Fig. 182-1). Furthermore, the reduction of elevated left end-diastolic pressure may improve subendocardial perfusion.

Vasodilator therapy is useful in the treatment of all forms of heart failure, ranging from the mild, chronic to the severe acute forms.

The several available vasodilators vary in their hemodynamic effects, locus and duration of action, and mode of administration.

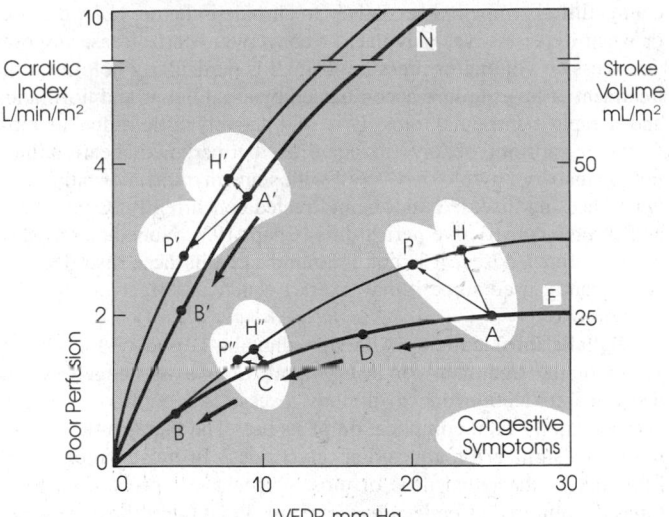

FIGURE 182-1 Effects of various vasodilators on the relationship between left ventricular end-diastolic pressure (LVEDP) and cardiac index or stroke volume in normal (N) and failing (F) hearts. H represents hydralazine or any other pure arterial dilator. It produces only a minimal increase in cardiac index in the normal subject (A′ → H′) or in the patient with heart failure with normal LVEDP (C → H″). In contrast, it elevates output in the patient with heart failure and elevated LVEDP (A → H). P represents a balanced vasodilator, such as sodium nitroprusside or prazosin. It reduces filling pressure in all patients, elevates cardiac output in patients with heart failure and elevated LVEDP (A → P), lowers cardiac output in normal subjects (A′ → P′), and has little effect on cardiac output in heart failure patients with normal filling pressures (C → P″). *(Reprinted with permission from TW Smith et al.)*

Some vasodilators, such as hydralazine, minoxidil, and the alpha-adrenergic blocking agents, act predominantly on the arterial bed and primarily increase stroke volume while others, such as nitroglycerin and isosorbide dinitrate, act almost entirely on the venous side of the circulation; the latter agents cause pooling of blood in the venous bed and act primarily to reduce ventricular filling pressures. Angiotensin-converting enzyme inhibitors, prazosin, and sodium nitroprusside are "balanced vasodilators" which act on both the arterial and venous beds. Some agents, such as sodium nitroprusside, must be administered by continuous intravenous infusion, nitroglycerin requires administration in ointment patch or intravenous forms when a prolonged effect is desired, while isosorbide dinitrate is most effective when it is administered by the sublingual route.

The ideal vasodilator for the treatment of *acute* heart failure should have a rapid onset and brief duration of action when administered by intravenous infusion; sodium nitroprusside qualifies as such a drug, but its use requires careful monitoring of the intraarterial pressure and electrocardiogram, and if possible of the pulmonary artery wedge pressure, in an intensive care unit. For the treatment of chronic congestive heart failure, the agent should be effective on oral administration, and its action should persist for at least 6 h. Angiotensin-converting enzyme inhibitors satisfy these requirements and have become the most useful and widely used vasodilators. It is advisable to commence therapy with very low doses, particularly in patients receiving diuretics, in order to avoid hypotension and gradually increase the dose.

Vasodilators are potent and effective in acutely improving the deranged hemodynamics of heart failure and there is evidence in favor of a beneficial chronic effect as well. Studies with angiotensin-converting enzyme inhibitors have demonstrated a favorable long-term reduction of symptoms and enhancement of exercise tolerance. Importantly, these drugs as well as the combination of hydralazine and isosorbide dinitrate prolong survival of patients with heart failure.

ENHANCEMENT OF MYOCARDIAL CONTRACTILITY—DIGITALIS The improvement of myocardial contractility by means of

cardiac glycosides is an important component in the control of heart failure. The basic molecular structure of the digitalis glycosides is a steroid nucleus to which an unsaturated lactone ring is attached at C-17. These two elements together are called *aglycone* or *genin*, and it is this portion of the molecule which is responsible for the cardiotonic activity. The addition of sugar residues to this basic structure determines water solubility and pharmacokinetic properties for individual glycosides.

Pharmacokinetics In the absence of severe malabsorption, most digitalis glycosides are adequately absorbed from the intestinal tract even in the presence of vascular congestion secondary to heart failure. Oral absorption is close to complete within 2 h. The bioavailability (i.e., percent of intravenous dose) of orally administered glycoside varies. Considerable variability of bioavailability has been found in different commercial preparations of digoxin. The bioavailability of Lanoxin elixir is 70 to 85 percent, Lanoxin tablets 60 to 80 percent, and Lanoxicaps 90 to 100 percent. Digitoxin tablets have a bioavailability of virtually 100 percent. Cholesterol-lowering resins, antidiarrheal agents containing pectin and kaolin, nonabsorbable antacids, and neomycin can reduce the absorption of digoxin and digitoxin. Varying degrees of protein-binding of glycosides occur in the bloodstream (for example, 97 percent for digitoxin and 25 percent for digoxin), and though these differences may account in part for the varying durations of the effect of different glycosides, they are not related to the speed of action of these drugs. The plasma contains only approximately 1 percent of the body stores of digoxin; therefore, digoxin is not effectively removed from the body by dialysis, exchange transfusions, or during cardiopulmonary bypass, presumably because of tissue binding. The major fraction of the glycosides is directly bound by various tissues including the heart, in which the concentration is approximately 30 times that in the plasma for digoxin and 7 times for digitoxin; the latter is less polar and more lipid-soluble than digoxin.

Digoxin, which has a half-life of 1.6 days, is filtered in the glomeruli and secreted by the renal tubules; 85 percent is excreted in the urine, most in unchanged form; only 10 to 15 percent of digoxin is eliminated in the stool through biliary excretion in the presence of normal renal function. The ratio of digoxin clearance to endogenous creatinine clearance is 0.8, and the percentage of the body's total stores of digoxin lost per day can be calculated as (14 ± 0.2) × creatinine clearance in milliliters per minute. In patients with normal renal function a plateau concentration in the blood and tissue is reached after 5 days of daily maintenance treatment without a loading dose (Fig. 65-2). Therefore, significant reductions of the glomerular filtration rate reduce the elimination of digoxin (but not of digitoxin) and, therefore, may prolong digoxin's effect, allowing it to accumulate to toxic levels if it is administered in patients with impaired renal function. The administration of most diuretics does not alter the excretion of digoxin significantly, but spironolactone can inhibit tubular secretion of digoxin, resulting in significant accumulation of the drug. *Digitoxin,* with a half-life of approximately 5 days, is metabolized chiefly in the liver; only 15 percent is excreted in the urine unchanged and an equal fraction in the stool. Drugs such as phenobarbital and phenylbutazone that increase the activity of hepatic microsomal enzymes accelerate the metabolism of digitoxin. To reach a steady state, digitoxin requires maintenance doses for 3 to 4 weeks. *Ouabain* is very rapidly acting, exhibiting an onset of action in 5 to 10 min and a peak effect within 60 min following intravenous injection. It is poorly and irregularly absorbed from the gastrointestinal tract, is excreted by the kidneys, has a half-life of 21 h, and is useful in emergencies.

Mechanism of action The cardiac actions of all digitalis glycosides are alike. The clinical effects result from augmenting myocardial contractility and from prolonging the refractory period of the atrioventricular node, thereby slowing ventricular rate in patients with atrial fibrillation.

The most important effect of digitalis on cardiac muscle is to shift its force-velocity relation upward (Chap. 181). This positive inotropic effect is exhibited in normal, nonfailing hypertrophied as well as in failing hearts. In the absence of heart failure, however, when cardiac output is not limited by cardiac contractility, the drug does not elevate the output.

Excitation-contraction coupling is the membrane and intracellular process most likely involved in producing the positive inotropic effect of digitalis glycosides. These drugs inhibit transmembrane sodium and potassium movement by inhibition of the monovalent cation transport enzyme–coupled Na^+,K^+-ATPase. The latter, localized to the sarcolemma, appears to be the receptor for cardioactive glycosides whose action results in an increase in intracellular sodium content, and this in turn increases intracellular calcium concentration through a Na^+-Ca^{2+} exchange carrier mechanism (see Chap. 173). The increased myocardial uptake of calcium augments calcium released to the myofilaments during excitation (p. 881) and, therefore, invokes a positive inotropic response. There is a correlation between the degree of enzyme inhibition and the inotropic potency of the glycoside.

Cardiac glycosides also produce alterations in the electrical properties of both the contractile cells and the specialized automatic cells. While low concentrations of glycosides produce little effect on the action potential, high concentrations result in a reduction in the resting potential (phase 4, see Fig. 184-1) and an augmented rate of diastolic depolarization. The reduction in the resting potential brings the cell closer to the threshold for depolarization. These two effects lead to increased automaticity and ectopic impulse activity. With the lowering of the resting potential, the rate of rise of the action potential is reduced, resulting in a slowing of conduction velocity, which is conducive to the development of reentry. Thus, the known electrophysiologic effects of digitalis glycosides are capable of explaining the development of both reentry and ectopic foci and the resultant arrhythmias associated with digitalis intoxication.

The glycosides also prolong the effective *refractory period* of the atrioventricular node, largely as a result of an enhanced vagal effect. Digitalis also shortens the refractory period of the atrial and ventricular muscle. Small action potentials are propagated in a decremental fashion in the atrioventricular junction. Most do not reach the ventricles but leave some of the atrioventricular junctional cells in a refractory state. This helps to explain the slowing of ventricular rate produced by digitalis in supraventricular tachycardias. In atrial fibrillation, the slowing of ventricular rate is explained by prolongation of the effective refractory period of the atrioventricular node and increased concealed conduction. These actions reduce the frequency at which impulses penetrate the atrioventricular junction owing to both vagal and possibly direct effects of glycosides on junctional tissue.

Digitalis exerts a clinically significant negative chronotropic action, usually only in the setting of ventricular failure. In heart failure, slowing of the sinus rate following the administration of digitalis results also from withdrawal of sympathetic activity secondary to general improvement in circulatory status due to the positive inotropic effect of the glycoside. In the nonfailing heart the slowing effect is negligible, and digitalis should not be used for the treatment of sinus tachycardia unless heart failure is present. The apparent suppression of pacemaker activity which may take place following large doses of digitalis is probably due not to arrest of the pacemaker but rather to a sinoatrial block related to a depression of conduction of impulses out of the sinus node.

In addition, the digitalis glycosides also exert an action on the peripheral vasculature, causing venous and arterial constriction in normal individuals and reflex dilatation resulting from withdrawal of sympathetic constrictor activity in patients with congestive heart failure.

Use in heart failure   By stimulating myocardial contractility, digitalis improves ventricular emptying; i.e., it increases cardiac output, augments the ejection fraction, promotes diuresis, and reduces the elevated diastolic pressure and volume and end-systolic volume of the failing ventricle with consequent reduction of symptoms resulting from pulmonary vascular congestion and elevated systemic venous pressure. It is most beneficial in patients in whom ventricular

contractility is impaired secondary to chronic ischemic heart disease, or when hypertensive, valvular, or congenital heart disease imposes an excessive volume or pressure load. It is particularly helpful in the treatment of heart failure accompanied by atrial flutter and fibrillation and a rapid ventricular rate. It is of relatively little value in most forms of cardiomyopathy, myocarditis, beriberi with heart failure, mitral stenosis, thyrotoxicosis (all with sinus rhythm), cor pulmonale when the lung disease is not being treated concurrently (Chap. 191), and chronic constrictive pericarditis (Chap. 193). Nonetheless, when used in proper doses, it is not contraindicated in these disorders and is frequently used since it may exert a beneficial effect, albeit not a striking one.

Digitalis intoxication   Although digitalis is one of the cornerstones of the treatment for heart failure, it is a two-edged sword, because intoxication due to digitalis excess is a common, serious, and potentially fatal complication of its use. The therapeutic-to-toxic ratios are similar for all cardiac glycosides. In most patients with heart failure the lethal dose of most glycosides is probably 5 to 10 times the minimal effective dose and only about twice the dose which leads to minor toxic manifestations. In addition, old age, acute myocardial infarction or ischemia, hypoxemia, magnesium depletion, renal insufficiency, hypercalcemia, electrical cardioversion, and hypothyroidism all may reduce the tolerance of the patient to the digitalis glycosides or provoke latent digitalis intoxication. The most common precipitating cause of digitalis intoxication, however, is depletion of potassium stores, which often occurs as a result of diuretic therapy and secondary hyperaldosteronism. Since it is not necessary for a patient to receive a maximally tolerated dose of digitalis to derive a beneficial effect, even small doses provide some therapeutic action; this point should be considered if these drugs are to be used in patients prone to toxicity.

Anorexia, nausea, and vomiting, which are among the earliest signs of digitalis intoxication, are caused by direct stimulation of centers in the medulla and are not of gastrointestinal origin. The most frequent disturbance of cardiac rhythm caused by digitalis is premature ventricular beats, which may take the form of bigeminy because of increased myocardial irritability or facilitation of reentry. Atrioventricular block of varying degrees of severity may occur. Nonparoxysmal atrial tachycardia with variable atrioventricular block is quite characteristic of digitalis intoxication. Sinus arrhythmia, sinoatrial block, sinus arrest, and atrioventricular junctional and multifocal ventricular tachycardia may also occur. These arrhythmias are due to action of the glycoside both on cardiac tissues and on the central nervous system. Chronic digitalis intoxication may be insidious in onset and characterized by exacerbations of heart failure, weight loss, cachexia, neuralgias, gynecomastia, yellow vision, and delirium. Digitalis-toxic cardiac arrhythmias precede extracardiac (gastrointestinal or central nervous system) toxicity in about one-half of cases.

Digitalis intoxication has been reported to occur in as many as 20 percent of hospitalized patients receiving a cardiac glycoside, which emphasizes the importance of recognizing this condition. The administration of quinidine to patients receiving digoxin raises the serum concentration of the latter by reducing both the renal and nonrenal elimination of digoxin and by reducing its volume of distribution and thereby increasing the propensity to digitalis intoxication. The calcium channel antagonist verapamil and the antiarrhythmic agent amiodarone also appear to raise serum digoxin levels. Therefore, serum digoxin concentrations and electrocardiograms should be followed carefully when these drugs are administered to digitalized patients. The radioimmunoassays for digoxin and digitoxin make possible the correlation of serum glycoside levels with the presence of toxicity. In patients receiving standard maintenance doses of digoxin and digitoxin and in whom no sign of intoxication is present, serum concentrations approximate 1 to 1.5 and 20 to 25 ng/mL, respectively. When signs of intoxication are present, serum levels of more than 2 and 30 ng/mL, respectively, of these glycosides are often found. Since many factors other than the serum concentration determine digitalis intoxication, and since there is considerable overlap in serum glycoside concentrations in patients with and without toxicity, these levels cannot be used as a sole guide to digitalis dosage. However, when taken together with findings on the clinical examination and electrocardiogram, they add useful information to the clinical evaluations of digitalis intoxication. In addition they will indicate whether a patient for whom the history of digitalis intake is in doubt has, in fact, been receiving the drug.

Treatment of digitalis intoxication   When tachyarrhythmias result from digitalis intoxication, withdrawal of the drug and treatment with potassium, phenytoin, propranolol, or lidocaine are indicated. Potassium should be administered cautiously and by the oral route whenever possible if hypokalemia is present, but *small* doses may also be helpful when serum potassium levels are normal; *potassium must not be employed in the presence of atrioventricular block or hyperkalemia.* Propranolol should not be used to treat digitalis toxicity in the presence of severe heart failure or atrioventricular block but may be useful otherwise; lidocaine is effective in the treatment of digitalis-induced ventricular tachyarrhythmias in the absence of preceding atrioventricular block. A cardiac pacemaker may be required in digitalis-induced atrioventricular block. Electrical conversion may not only be ineffective in treating these arrhythmias but may induce more serious arrhythmias. However, it may be lifesaving in digitalis-induced ventricular fibrillation. Quinidine and procainamide are of limited value in the treatment of digitalis intoxication. Fab fragments of purified, intact digitalis antibodies represent a potentially lifesaving approach to the treatment of severe intoxication.

SYMPATHOMIMETIC AMINES (See also Chap. 67)   Four sympathomimetic amines which act largely on beta-adrenergic receptors—epinephrine, isoproterenol (isoprenaline), dopamine, and dobutamine—improve myocardial contractility in various forms of heart failure. The latter two agents appear to be most effective; they must be administered by constant intravenous infusion and are useful in patients with intractable heart failure, particularly in those with a reversible component, such as exists in patients who have undergone cardiac surgery, and in some instances of myocardial infarction and shock or pulmonary edema. While they improve the hemodynamics in these conditions, it is not clear that they improve survival. Their administration must be accompanied by careful and continuous monitoring of the electrocardiogram, intraarterial pressure, and if possible pulmonary artery wedge pressure, in an intensive care unit.

Dopamine (p. 387), the naturally occurring immediate precursor of norepinephrine, has a combination of actions which make it particularly useful in the treatment of a variety of hypotensive states and congestive heart failure. At very low doses, that is, 1 to 2 (μg/kg)/min, it dilates renal and mesenteric blood vessels through stimulation of specific dopaminergic receptors, thereby augmenting renal and mesenteric blood flow and sodium excretion. In the range of 2 to 10 (μg/kg)/min, dopamine stimulates myocardial beta receptors but induces relatively little tachycardia, while at higher doses it also stimulates alpha-adrenergic receptors and elevates arterial pressure.

Dobutamine is a synthetic catecholamine which acts on beta$_1$, beta$_2$, and alpha receptors. It exerts a potent inotropic action, has only a modest cardioaccelerating effect, and lowers peripheral vascular resistance, but since it simultaneously raises cardiac output, it has little effect on systemic arterial pressure. Dobutamine, given in continuous infusions of 2.5 to 10 (μg/kg)/min, is useful in the treatment of acute heart failure without hypotension. Like the other sympathomimetic amines it may be particularly valuable in the management of patients requiring relatively short-term inotropic support—up to 1 week—in conditions which are reversible, such as the cardiac depression which sometimes follows open-heart surgery, or in patients with acute heart failure who are being prepared for operation. Adverse effects include sinus tachycardia, tachyarrhythmias, and hypertension.

A major problem with all sympathomimetics is the loss of responsiveness, apparently due to "downregulation" of adrenergic receptors, which becomes evident within 8 h of continuous administration.

Amrinone   This bipyridine, a noncatecholamine, nonglycoside exerts both positive inotropic and vasodilator actions by inhibiting a specific phosphodiesterase. It is suitable for intravenous use only, and by simultaneously stimulating cardiac contractility and dilating the systemic vascular bed it reverses the major hemodynamic abnormalities associated with heart failure. Milrinone, a derivative of amrinone, and several other orally active phosphodiesterase inhibitors are under active investigation for chronic oral administration.

REFRACTORY HEART FAILURE   When the response to ordinary treatment is inadequate, heart failure is considered to be refractory. Before assuming that this state simply reflects advanced, perhaps preterminal, myocardial depression, careful consideration must be given to several possibilities: (1) an underlying and overlooked cause of the heart disease that may be amenable to specific surgical or medical therapy, such as silent aortic or mitral stenosis, constrictive pericarditis, infective endocarditis, hypertension, or thyrotoxicosis; (2) one or a combination of the precipitating causes of heart failure, such as pulmonary or urinary tract infection, recurrent pulmonary emboli, arterial hypoxemia, anemia, or arrhythmia; and (3) complications of overly vigorous therapy, such as digitalis intoxication, hypovolemia, or electrolyte imbalance.

Recognition and proper treatment of the aforementioned complications are likely to make the patient responsive to therapy again. Perhaps the most common complication results from overzealous treatment with diuretics. When administered too rapidly, these drugs can produce sudden hypovolemia before edema fluid can be mobilized to replace the loss of blood volume, the result being a shocklike state with evidence of systemic hypoperfusion in the presence of edema. The chronically excessively diuresed patient may have exchanged the hazards of pulmonary edema and the inconvenience of systemic edema for a persistently depressed cardiac output with its associated weakness, lethargy, prerenal azotemia, and sometimes cardiac cachexia. Temporarily easing up on salt restriction and diuretic administration may overcome this difficulty, but as heart failure worsens, this course of action may lead to increased pulmonary congestion which is equally unacceptable.

Hyponatremia is a late manifestation of refractory heart failure. It, too, may be a complication of overaggressive diuresis leading to reduced glomerular filtration rate and decreased delivery of NaCl to the diluting sites in the distal tubule. Hyponatremia may also result from nonosmotic stimuli for the continued secretion of antidiuretic hormone. Therapy involves improvement of the cardiovascular status, if possible (sometimes requiring the administration of a sympathomimetic amine such as dopamine or dobutamine), as well as temporary cessation of diuretic therapy and restriction of oral water intake. Hypertonic saline is very rarely indicated because total body sodium is usually elevated, not depressed in heart failure.

The combination of an intravenously administered vasodilator, such as sodium nitroprusside, along with a potent sympathomimetic amine, such as dopamine or dobutamine, often results in an additive effect, raising cardiac output and lowering filling pressure. Intravenous amrinone, sometimes accompanied by the administration of a converting enzyme inhibitor, may also be useful in patients with refractory heart failure.

Cardiac transplantation   When patients with heart failure become unresponsive to a combination of all of the aforementioned therapeutic measures, are in New York Heart Association class IV, and are deemed unlikely to survive 1 year, they should be considered for cardiac transplantation (see Chap. 183).

TREATMENT OF ACUTE PULMONARY EDEMA   Pulmonary edema secondary to left ventricular failure or mitral stenosis is described in Chap. 36. It is life-threatening and must be considered a medical emergency. As is the case for the more chronic forms of heart failure, in the treatment of pulmonary edema, attention must be directed to identifying and removing any precipitating causes of decompensation, such as an arrhythmia or infection. However, because of the acute nature of the problem, a number of additional nonspecific measures are necessary. When possible, and if it does not delay treatment unduly, recording pulmonary vascular pressures through a Swan-Ganz catheter and intraarterial pressure directly is advisable. The first six measures listed below are ordinarily applied simultaneously or nearly so.

1 Morphine is administered intravenously repetitively, as needed, in doses from 2 to 5 mg. This drug reduces anxiety, reduces adrenergic vasoconstrictor stimuli to the arteriolar and venous beds, and thereby helps to break a vicious cycle. Naloxone should be available in case respiratory depression occurs.

2 Because the alveolar fluid interferes with oxygen diffusion, resulting in arterial hypoxemia, 100% oxygen should be administered, preferably under positive pressure. The latter increases intraalveolar pressure and therefore reduces transudation of fluid from the alveolar capillaries and impedes venous return to the thorax, reducing pulmonary capillary pressure.

3 The patient should be maintained in the sitting position, with the legs dangling along the side of the bed, if possible, which also tends to reduce venous return.

4 Intravenous loop diuretics, such as furosemide or ethacrynic acid (40 to 100 mg), or bumetanide (1 mg) will, by rapidly establishing a diuresis, reduce circulating blood volume and thereby hasten the relief of pulmonary edema. In addition when given intravenously, furosemide also exerts a venodilator action, reduces venous return, and reduces pulmonary edema even before the diuresis commences.

5 Afterload reduction is achieved with intravenous sodium nitroprusside at 20 to 30 µg/min in patients whose systolic arterial pressures exceed 100 mmHg.

6 If digitalis has not been administered previously, three-fourths of a full dose of a rapidly acting glycoside, such as ouabain, digoxin, or lanatoside C, should be administered intravenously.

7 Sometimes, aminophylline (theophylline ethylenediamine), 240 to 480 mg intravenously, is effective in diminishing bronchoconstriction, increasing renal blood flow and sodium excretion, and augmenting myocardial contractility.

8 If the above mentioned measures are not sufficient, rotating tourniquets should be applied to the extremities.

After these emergency therapeutic measures have been instituted, and the precipitating factors treated, the diagnosis of the underlying cardiac disorder responsible for the pulmonary edema must be established if it is not already known. After stabilization of the patient's condition a long-range strategy for prevention of future episodes of pulmonary edema must be established, and this may require surgical treatment.

PROGNOSIS

The prognosis in heart failure depends primarily on the nature of the underlying heart disease and on the presence or absence of a precipitating factor which can be treated. Also, the long-term prognosis for heart failure is most favorable when the underlying forms of heart disease can be treated. When one of the latter can be identified and removed, the outlook for immediate survival is far better than if heart failure occurs without any obvious precipitating cause. In the latter situation, survival usually ranges between 6 months and 5 years depending on the severity of the heart failure. The prognosis can also be estimated by observing the response to treatment. When clinical improvement occurs with only modest dietary sodium restriction and small doses of diuretics or digitalis, then the outlook is far better than if, in addition to these measures, intensive diuretic therapy and vasodilators are necessary. A large fraction of patients with congestive heart failure die suddenly, presumably of ventricular fibrillation. Unfortunately, there is no evidence that this complication can be prevented by the administration of antiarrhythmic agents.

REFERENCES

ARNOLD SB et al: Long-term digitalis therapy improves left ventricular function in heart failure. N Engl J Med 303:1443, 1980

BERGER BE, WARNOCK DG: Mechanisms of action and clinical use of diuretics, in *The Kidney*, 3d ed, BM Brenner, FC Rector (eds). Philadelphia, Saunders, 1986, p 433

BRAUNWALD E (ed): Newer positive inotropic agents. Circulation 73(Suppl III):1, 1986

—— et al (eds): *Congestive Heart Failure: Current Research and Clinical Applications.* New York, Grune & Stratton, 1982

BRISTOW MR: The adrenergic nervous system in heart failure. N Engl J Med 311:850, 1984

COHN JN (ed): *Drug Treatment of Heart Failure*, 2d ed. Secaucus, NJ, Advanced Therapeutics Communications International, 1988

—— et al (eds): Advances in congestive heart failure. Am J Cardiol (Suppl. A) 62:1, 1988

FIFER MA et al: Hemodynamic and renal effects of atrial natriuretic peptide in congestive heart failure. Am J Cardiol 65(3):211, 1990

FISCH C (guest ed): An account of the foxglove and some of its medical uses: 1785–1985. J Am Coll Cardiol 5 (Suppl A):1A, 1985

GOODMAN LS, GILMAN A (eds): Cardiovascular drugs, in *The Pharmacological Basis of Therapeutics*, 7th ed. New York, Macmillan, 1985, pp 716, 887

ISKANDRIAN AS et al: Predicting left ventricular function: Bedside examination. Prim Cardiol (Suppl) 10:3A, 1984

LEE WH, PACKER M: Prognostic importance of serum sodium concentration and its modification by converting-enzyme inhibition in patients with severe chronic heart failure. Circulation 73:257, 1986

MAKABALI C et al: Dobutamine and other sympathomimetic drugs for the treatment of low cardiac output failure. Semin Anesth 1:63, 1982

SIMON J et al: Pulmonary artery pressure changes during exercise and daily activities in chronic heart failure. J Am Coll Cardiol 15(1):52, 1990

SMITH TW (ed): *Digitalis Glycosides*. New York, Grune & Stratton, 1986

—— et al: Management of heart failure, in *Heart Disease*, 3d ed, E Braunwald (ed). Philadelphia, Saunders, 1988, p 485

SUKI WN et al: Physiology of diuretic action, in *The Kidney: Physiology and Pathophysiology*, 2d ed, DW Seldin, G Giebisch (eds). New York, Raven Press, 1985, p 2127

The Consensus Trial Study Group: Effects of enalapril on mortality in severe congestive heart failure: Results of the Cooperative North Scandinavian Enalapril Survival Study (Consensus). New Engl J Med 316:1429, 1987

183 CARDIAC TRANSPLANTATION

JOHN S. SCHROEDER

Orthotopic allograft cadaver cardiac transplantation as a treatment for end-stage cardiac disease achieved its twentieth anniversary on December 7, 1987. On that day in 1967 Dr. Christiaan Barnard accomplished the first successful cardiac transplant in man, quickly followed by Drs. Norman Shumway and Richard Lower at Stanford University. After an initial early wave of enthusiasm, the problems of immunosuppression slowed application of the procedure until the introduction of cyclosporine in 1980. A subsequent worldwide expansion of cardiac transplantation resulted in approximately 1500 cardiac transplants per year, with further increases limited only by the donor supply. Current 1- and 5-year survival rates of 60 and 70 percent indicate that cardiac transplant is the therapy of choice in patients with end-stage heart disease who are unlikely to survive the next 6 to 12 months. This chapter reviews the procedure, indications, short- and long-term immunosuppressive therapy, and complications.

Since the introduction of cyclosporine in 1980 and the development of "low-dose" triple immunosuppressive regimens using azathioprine and prednisone, 1-year survival is reported at 80 percent and 5-year survival at 60 to 70 percent. The longest survivor has now lived 19 years after transplantation and is functionally well. Therefore, these survival statistics must be compared to those for other medical or surgical therapies in considering alternative therapies for end-stage heart disease.

INDICATIONS AND SELECTION OF CANDIDATES   The limited donor supply and relatively high cost of cardiac transplantation have restricted it to patients most likely to survive and resume a functional life after transplantation. It is estimated that only 2000 potential donors, for a pool of at least 20,000 candidates based on current guidelines, become available yearly in the United States. Attempts to increase donor awareness in both physicians and the public are being made. Optimal candidates for this procedure are those who would be expected to return to a functional life if their hearts were replaced. This requires a mentally vigorous, medically compliant person who has not suffered extensive other end-stage organ damage from cardiac failure or does not have other systemic disease such as severe diabetes mellitus and collagen vascular disease. Long-standing pulmonary hypertension or recurrent pulmonary emboli and infarction may result in irreversible pulmonary hypertension leading to intraoperative death. Several heart transplant centers have initiated cardiac transplantation for newborns with left ventricular hypoplasia, but long-term survival experience is still very limited.

Timing of the recommendation to undergo cardiac transplantation can be difficult and requires assessment of the patient's current disability, stability of course, and likelihood of surviving the next 6 to 12 months. Generally, left ventricular ejection fractions under 15 to 20 percent and presence of serious ventricular arrhythmias indicate a 1-year survival rate of 50 percent or less. Mechanical assistance devices, either a left ventricular assist or a totally implantable device, have been used to "bridge" the critically ill patient until a suitable donor can be found. This approach has been successful, but has been used relatively infrequently because of the potential for infection and the ethical problems of prioritizing distribution of available donor hearts. Tissue cross-matching between donor and recipient has generally not been done because of difficulty in obtaining good matches and lack of correlation between match and outcome. Size, ABO matching, negative lymphocyte cross-match, and avoidance of a transplantation from a cytomegalovirus (CMV)–positive donor to a CMV-negative recipient are more important.

OPERATIVE PROCEDURE The operative technique for orthotopic transplantation developed in animals in the early 1960s by Shumway and Lower remains little changed. In this technique, the surgeon removes the diseased heart but leaves the posterior wall of the right atrium in place and the superior and inferior venae cavae intact. The posterior wall of the left atrium is also left in situ with pulmonary veins intact. The donor heart is then removed in toto with the posterior wall of the right and left atria incised, which allows suturing of left atrial donor rim to recipient rim, and right atrial donor rim to recipient rim, with anastomosis of the aorta and pulmonary artery.

IMMUNOSUPPRESSION AND REJECTION Controlling rejection while avoiding the adverse side effects of immunosuppressive agents is pivotal to successful transplantation. Rejection is characterized by perivascular infiltration of killer T lymphocytes, which migrate into the myocardium and cause cellular necrosis if not checked. Since early rejection can be silent, it is important to detect it before necrosis occurs. Immunologic monitoring of activated T lymphocytes in peripheral blood offers clues to the timing of a rejection process but has not been sufficiently reliable to dictate antirejection therapy. Therefore, repeated percutaneous transvenous right ventricular endomyocardial biopsies via the right internal jugular vein are required for histologic determination of the state of immunosuppression and rejection.

Billingham et al. have graded the stages of rejection as: cannot rule out rejection, mild early rejection, moderate rejection, and severe rejection. Serial biopsies are taken every 1 to 2 weeks early after transplantation, with gradually widening intervals depending on the patient's course and rejection history. Prolongation of isovolumic relaxation time measured by echocardiography may also provide early clues to rejection.

Immunosuppressive therapy regimens vary but usually include triple therapy with cyclosporine, azathioprine, and prednisone. Prophylactic courses of OKT_3 or antithymocyte globulin may also be given early after transplantation. Careful monitoring of the adverse side effects of these agents is extremely important since they include nephrotoxicity, bone marrow suppression, and opportunistic infections.

EARLY COURSE AND COMPLICATIONS It is rare for a cardiac transplant patient to have a completely uncomplicated postoperative

FIGURE 183-1 Electrocardiogram in a patient with a transplanted heart. The arrows denote the P wave generated by the recipient's atrium. The P wave just preceding the QRS complex is generated by the donor heart.

course. In the immediate postoperative period, right heart failure due to pulmonary vascular disease is most life-threatening. During the 2 to 3 weeks after transplantation the patient is hospitalized with meticulous monitoring for evidence of rejection and infections, repeated percutaneous transvenous endomyocardial biopsies, and adjustment of immunosuppressive drugs. During the ensuing 4 to 6 weeks, infectious complications, including bacterial, viral, and protozoan infections, are common. A successful transplant program requires a highly aggressive and sophisticated approach to diagnosis and therapy of infections in the immunocompromised host. Depending on the degree of cardiac cachexia preoperatively, the patient is usually functional at 1 week and discharged from the hospital at 2 to 3 weeks if no major complication occurs.

The average first-year cost ranges from $100,000 to $150,000, depending on the need for repeated hospitalization and cardiac biopsies, and is occasionally much higher. Yearly costs for immunosuppressive agents range from $5,000 to $10,000, in addition to the expense of medical surveillance for rejection or complications.

PHYSIOLOGY AND FUNCTION Since the allografted heart remains denervated, cardiac function differs from that of the innervated heart during both rest and exercise. The electrocardiogram in Fig. 183-1 shows two P waves. The P wave of the recipient's heart reflects the residual sinus node and posterior walls of the remaining native atria but is dissociated from the QRS, since the depolarization impulse does not cross the suture line. Although it does not control donor heart rate, the recipient's sinus node remains innervated and under the influence of the autonomic nervous system. The donor sinus node controls the rate of the transplanted heart. The donor heart's P wave has a regular PR interval, reflecting conduction to the ventricles. Since the controlling sinus node is denervated, it maintains a heart rate of 100 to 110 beats per minute, and rate increase depends on alterations in chronotropic agents perfusing the sinus node.

Ventricular function in response to isometric and isotonic exercise has been studied extensively. The early response to exercise is more dependent on the Frank-Starling mechanism and change in ventricular volume and filling pressure. As exercise proceeds and catecholamines are released with their positive inotropic effects, cardiac output begins to rise. The cardiac transplant recipient can achieve approximately 70 percent of the maximal cardiac output expected for his or her age, easily sufficient for the stresses of everyday life.

LATE COURSE AND COMPLICATIONS Although the rejection process partially subsides, lifelong administration of immunosuppressive drugs, albeit at lower doses, is still required and remains a hazard. Infectious complications and unsuspected rejection continue to occur, requiring ongoing surveillance and monitoring. Cardiac biopsies are performed at 3-month intervals to assess the response to rejection treatment. Table 183-1 shows the causes of death in patients surviving more than 1 year after transplantation in the Stanford program. In addition to the well-known hazards of long-term steroid usage, the immunosuppressed patient is at increased risk for neoplasia.

Accelerated coronary vascular disease appears to be one of the major factors limiting longer-term survival. The process is a fibrointimal hyperplasia which can go undetected by coronary arteriography

TABLE 183-1   Cause of death in patients surviving more than 1 year after cardiac transplantation in the Stanford Program

Cause of death	No. of patients
Graft atherosclerosis	14
Infection	16
Rejection	4
Lymphoproliferative disease	3
Nonlymphoid malignancy	5
Other	6
Cerebrovascular accident	1
Total deaths	49
Total at risk	228

at first and then cause diffuse atherosclerotic changes. Risk factors for its development include number of rejection episodes and elevated lipids, most likely reflecting rejection injury, as well as more commonly accepted causes of atherosclerosis. CMV infections have also been associated with higher frequency of this disease. Uncontrolled trials with anticoagulation, aspirin, and improved immunosuppression with cyclosporine have done little to lower this frequency; 40 to 50 percent of patients show arteriographic evidence of coronary vascular disease 5 years after transplantation. Retransplantation has been employed for some patients with severe graft atherosclerosis.

HEART-LUNG TRANSPLANTATION

Patients with congenital heart disease with Eisenmenger's complex (Chap. 186) or primary pulmonary hypertension (Chap. 212) are now considered for heart-lung transplantation. The surgical technique is similar to that for heart transplantation, except that the pulmonary venous attachments to the left atrium are left intact, and a tracheal anastomosis is required. The postoperative period is more complex, since the lungs may be rejected separately from the heart, requiring repeated endobronchoscopic biopsies when rejection is suspected. The immunosuppressive regimen is similar to that for heart transplants. Long-term survival has in the past been limited by obliterative bronchiolitis due to chronic unrecognized rejection; survival rates have been approximately 50 percent at 1 year and 30 percent at 2 years, but appear to be improving. More recently, heart-lung transplantation has been performed on patients with cystic fibrosis. Single-lung transplants are also potential options for these patients.

REFERENCES

COPELAND JG et al: Orthotopic total artificial heart bridge to transplantation: Preliminary results. J Heart Transplant 8:124, 1989

GAO SZ et al: Clinical and laboratory correlates of accelerated coronary artery disease in the cardiac transplant patient. Circulation 76(suppl V):56, 1987

GRATTAN MT et al: Cytomegalovirus infection is associated with cardiac allograft rejection and atherosclerosis. JAMA 261:3561, 1989

OAKS TE et al: Results of mechanical circulatory assistance before heart transplantation. J Heart Transplant 8:113, 1989

PICANO E et al: Electrocardiographic changes suggestive of myocardial ischemia elicited by dypyridamole infusion in acute rejection early after heart transplantation. Circulation 81(1):72, 1990

SAVIN WM et al: Response of cardiac transplant recipients to static and dynamic exercises. Heart Transplant 1:72, 1981

SCHROEDER JS, HUNT SA: Cardiac transplantation: Update 1987. JAMA 258:3142, 1987

STEVENSON LW et al: Poor survival of patients with idiopathic cardiomyopathy considered too well for transplantation. Am J Med 83:871, 1987

184 THE BRADYARRHYTHMIAS: DISORDERS OF SINUS NODE FUNCTION AND AV CONDUCTION DISTURBANCES

MARK E. JOSEPHSON / FRANCIS E. MARCHLINSKI / ALFRED E. BUXTON

ANATOMY OF THE CONDUCTING SYSTEM   Under normal conditions the pacemaker function of the heart resides in the sinoatrial node, which lies at the junction of the right atrium and superior vena cava. The SA node is approximately $1\frac{1}{2}$ cm long and 2 to 3 mm wide and is supplied by the sinus node artery, which arises from either the right coronary artery (60 percent of cases) or the left circumflex coronary artery (40 percent). Once the impulse exits the sinus node and perinodal tissue, it traverses the atrium until it reaches the atrioventricular node. The blood supply of the AV node is derived from the posterior descending coronary artery (90 percent of cases), which lies at the base of the interatrial septum just above the tricuspid annulus and anterior to the coronary sinus. The electrophysiologic properties of the AV node result in slow conduction, which is responsible for the normal delay in AV conduction, i.e., the PR interval.

The bundle of His emerges from the AV node, enters the fibrous skeleton of the heart, and courses anteriorly across the membranous interventricular septum. It has a dual blood supply from the AV nodal artery and a branch of the anterior descending coronary artery. The branching (distal) portion of the bundle of His gives rise to a broad sheet of fibers that course over the left side of the interventricular septum to form the left bundle branch and a narrow cablelike structure on the right side that forms the right bundle branch. The arborization of both the right and left bundle branches gives rise to the distal His-Purkinje system, which ultimately extends throughout the endocardium of the right and left ventricles.

The sinus node, atrium, and AV node are significantly influenced by autonomic tone. Vagal influences depress automaticity of the sinus node, depress conduction, and prolong refractoriness in the tissue surrounding the sinus node, inhomogeneously decrease atrial refractoriness and slow atrial conduction, and prolong AV nodal conduction and refractoriness. Sympathetic influences exert the opposite effect.

ELECTROPHYSIOLOGIC PRINCIPLES

In the resting state, the interior of most cardiac cells, with the exception of the sinus and AV nodes, is approximately -80 to -90 mV, negative with respect to a reference extracellular electrode. The resting membrane potential is primarily determined by the concentration gradient of potassium across the cell membrane. Activation of cardiac cells results from movement of ions across the cell membrane, causing a transient depolarization known as the *action potential*. The ionic species responsible for the action potential varies among the cardiac tissues, and the configuration of the action potential is therefore unique to each tissue (Fig. 184-1).

The action potential of the His-Purkinje system and ventricular myocardium has five phases (Fig. 184-2). The rapid depolarizing current (phase 0) is mainly determined by an influx of sodium into myocardial cells followed by a secondary (slower) influx of calcium. The repolarization phases of the action potential (phases 1 to 3) are primarily related to outward flux of potassium. The resting membrane potential is phase 4.

The bradyarrhythmias result from abnormalities either of impulse formation, i.e., automaticity, or of conduction. *Automaticity*, which is normally observed in the sinus node, the specialized fibers of the His-Purkinje system, and some specialized atrial fibers, is the property

FIGURE 184-1 Action potential configurations in different regions of the mammalian heart. (*From AM Katz, Physiology of the Heart, New York, Raven, 1977.*)

of a cardiac cell to depolarize spontaneously during phase 4 of the action potential, leading to the generation of an impulse. To exhibit automaticity the resting membrane potential must decrease spontaneously until threshold potential is reached and an all-or-none regenerative response occurs. The ionic components producing spontaneous diastolic depolarization appear to involve the inward current of either sodium or calcium. The velocity of *conduction*, i.e., impulse propagation through cardiac tissues, depends on the magnitude of

FIGURE 184-2 Schematic representation of the action potential in normal ventricle depicting the direction, strength, and period of flow of the ionic currents underlying the action potential. The arrow's direction and size indicate whether current is inward- or outward-directed and the approximate current strength of the ion identified at the arrow's base. The horizontal position of the arrow corresponds to the same moment in the time course of action potential (see text). The five phases of the action potential are indicated by the numerals placed along the waveform. (*From Ten Eick et al; Progress in Cardiovascular Diseases 24(2):157, 1981; used with permission.*)

inward current, which is directly related to the rate of rise and amplitude of phase 0 of the action potential. The more positive the threshold potential and the slower the rate of depolarization toward threshold, the slower the rate of rise of phase 0 of the action potential and the slower the conduction velocity. Disease states or drugs may result in lower rates of rise of phase 0 at any given membrane potential.

Refractoriness is a property of cardiac cells which defines the period of recovery that cells require after being discharged before they can be reexcited by a stimulus. The *absolute refractory period* is defined by that portion of the action potential during which no stimulus, regardless of its strength, can evoke another response. The *effective refractory period* is that part of the action potential during which a stimulus can only evoke a local, nonpropagated response. The *relative refractory period* extends from the end of the effective refractory period to the time that the tissue is fully recovered. During this time a stimulus of greater than threshold strength is required to evoke a response which is propagated more slowly than normal. After completion of the action potential, excitability is recovered, and evoked responses have characteristics similar to the spontaneous normal response.

INTRACARDIAC RECORDINGS OF THE SPECIALIZED CONDUCTING SYSTEM Electrode catheters allow the recording of activation of portions of the specialized conducting system including the bundle of His. To obtain a recording from the bundle of His the electrode catheter is positioned across the tricuspid valve (Fig. 184-3). The interval from local atrial depolarization in the His bundle recording to the onset of depolarization of the His bundle deflection is called the AH interval (normal = 60 to 125 ms) and represents an indirect method of assessing AV nodal conduction time. The interval from the beginning of the His bundle deflection to the earliest onset of ventricular activation, as measured from any of multiple-surface electrocardiogram (ECG) leads or the intracardiac ventricular electrogram, is called the HV interval (normal = 35 to 55 ms) and represents conduction time through the His-Purkinje system. Electrode catheters can be positioned in the area of the sinus node to record high right atrial activity. Left atrial activity may be recorded directly via a catheter placed across a patent foramen ovale, or indirectly using a catheter inserted into the coronary sinus. The atrial activation sequence may be "mapped," and sites of intra- and interatrial conduction abnormalities may be ascertained.

SINUS NODE DYSFUNCTION

The sinus node is normally the dominant cardiac pacemaker because its intrinsic discharge rate is the highest of all potential cardiac pacemakers. Its responsiveness to alterations in autonomic nervous system tone is responsible for the normal acceleration of heart rate during exercise and the slowing that occurs during rest and sleep. Increases in sinus rate normally result from an increase in sympathetic tone acting via beta-adrenergic receptors and/or decrease in parasympathetic tone acting via muscarinic receptors. Slowing of the heart rate is normally due to opposite alterations. In adults, the normal sinus rate under basal conditions is 60 to 100 beats per minute. Sinus bradycardia is said to exist when the sinus rate is less than 60 beats per minute, and sinus tachycardia when it exceeds 100 per minute. However, there is wide variation among individuals, and rates less than 60 per minute do not necessarily indicate pathologic states. For example, trained athletes often exhibit resting rates under 50 beats per minute due to increases in vagal tone. Normal elderly individuals may also show marked sinus bradycardia at rest.

ETIOLOGY Sinus node dysfunction most often is found in the elderly as an isolated phenomenon. Although interruption of the blood supply to the sinus node may produce dysfunction, the correlation between obstruction of the sinus node artery and clinical evidence of sinus node dysfunction is poor. Specific disease states associated with sinus node dysfunction include senile amyloidosis and other

FIGURE 184-3 Normal intracardiac recording. Surface ECG leads I, II, and V₁ are displayed with intracardiac ECGs from the high right atrium (HRA), left atrium from the coronary sinus (CS), and AV junction to obtain a His bundle electrogram (HBE). T = time lines. Atrial activation begins in the high right atrium and spreads inferiorly to the low atrial septum, as recorded in the HBE, and the left atrium, as recorded in the CS. The AH and HV intervals represent AV nodal and His-Purkinje conduction times, respectively. Vertical lines = 0.10 s. (*From ME Josephson, SF Seides: Clinical Cardiac Electrophysiology: Techniques and Interpretations. Philadelphia, Lea & Febiger, 1979.*)

conditions associated with infiltration of the atrial myocardium. Sinus bradycardia is associated with hypothyroidism, advanced liver disease, hypothermia, typhoid fever, and brucellosis; it occurs during episodes of hypervagotonia (vasovagal syncope), severe hypoxia, hypercapnia, acidemia, and acute hypertension. However, in most cases of sinus node dysfunction a specific cause cannot be identified.

MANIFESTATIONS Although marked (≤50 beats per minute) sinus bradycardia may cause fatigue and other symptoms due to inadequate cardiac output, more commonly sinus node dysfunction is manifest as paroxysmal dizziness, presyncope, or syncope. These symptoms usually result from abrupt, prolonged sinus pauses caused by failure of sinus impulse formation (sinus arrest) or block of conduction of sinus impulses to the surrounding atrial tissue (sinus exit block). In either case, the ECG manifestation is a prolonged

period (>3 s) of atrial asystole. In some patients sinus node dysfunction is accompanied by abnormalities in AV conduction. In addition to the absence of atrial activity, lower pacemakers fail to emerge during the sinus pauses, resulting in periods of ventricular asystole and syncope. Occasionally, sinus node dysfunction is manifested initially by the failure of the sinus rate to accelerate in response to conditions such as exercise or fever that normally cause increases in the sinus rate. In some patients sinus node dysfunction may become manifest only in the presence of certain cardioactive drugs: cardiac glycosides, beta-adrenergic blocking drugs, verapamil, quinidine, and other antiarrhythmic agents. These agents, which do not cause sinus node dysfunction in normal people, may unmask evidence of sinus node dysfunction in susceptible individuals.

The *sick sinus syndrome* refers to a combination of symptoms (dizziness, confusion, fatigue, syncope, and congestive heart failure) caused by sinus node dysfunction and manifested by marked sinus bradycardia, sinoatrial block, or sinus arrest. Because these symptoms are nonspecific and because ECG manifestations of sinus node dysfunction are not infrequently intermittent, it may be difficult to prove that such symptoms are actually caused by sinus node dysfunction.

Atrial tachyarrhythmias such as atrial fibrillation, flutter, or atrial tachycardia may be accompanied by sinus node dysfunction. The *bradycardia-tachycardia syndrome* refers to paroxysmal atrial arrhythmia which upon termination is followed by prolonged sinus pauses (Fig. 184-4) or in which there are alternating periods of tachyarrhythmia and bradyarrhythmia. Syncope or presyncope may result from failure of the sinus node to recover function following suppression of automaticity by atrial tachyarrhythmia.

DIAGNOSIS *First-degree sinoatrial exit block* denotes a prolonged conduction time from the sinus node to the surrounding atrial tissue. It cannot be recognized on a standard (surface) ECG but requires invasive intracardiac recordings (see below). *Second-degree sinoatrial exit block* denotes the intermittent failure of conduction of sinus impulses to the surrounding atrial tissue; it is manifested as the intermittent absence of P waves (Fig. 184-5). *Third-degree, or complete, sinoatrial block* is characterized by a lack of atrial activity or by the presence of an ectopic subsidiary atrial pacemaker. On the standard ECG, it cannot be distinguished from sinus arrest, but direct intracardiac recordings of sinus node activity permit this distinction. The *bradycardia-tachycardia syndrome* is manifested on the standard ECG as tachyarrhythmias (Fig. 184-4). Most often these are atrial flutter or fibrillation, although any tachycardia with retrograde conduction to the atria may cause overdrive suppression of the sinus node resulting in clinical appearance of this syndrome.

The most important step in the diagnosis is to correlate symptoms with ECG evidence of sinus node dysfunction. While ambulatory ECG (Holter) monitoring remains a mainstay in evaluating sinus node function, most episodes of syncope are paroxysmal and unpredictable. Single and even multiple 24-h Holter monitor recordings may fail to include a symptomatic episode. Therefore, noting the response to carotid sinus pressure and pharmacologic autonomic "denervation" of the heart is frequently helpful. Carotid sinus pressure is particularly useful in patients in whom paroxysmal dizziness or syncope is compatible with the hypersensitive carotid sinus syndrome (see Chap. 21). In such patients, the response can be dramatic, and sinus pauses in excess of 5 s may occur. Normally a sinus pause of ≤3 s results

FIGURE 184-4 Tachycardia-bradycardia syndrome. Rhythm strip of ECG lead II showing spontaneous cessation of supraventricular tachycardia followed by a 5.6-s pause prior to resumption of sinus activity. The patient was

asymptomatic during supraventricular tachycardia, but the sinus pause caused severe light-headedness.

FIGURE 184-5   Second-degree sinoatrial exit block. Surface ECG denoting abrupt absence of P wave during sinus rhythm. Prior to the pause the sinus rate is regular. The interval of the pause is exactly twice the basal sinus cycle length. The arrow marks the appropriate location for the absent P wave.

from 5 s of unilateral carotid sinus massage. If atropine can prevent the effects of carotid sinus pressure, autonomic dysfunction, not primary (intrinsic) sinus node dysfunction, is responsible. The other noninvasive test of sinus node function involves the use of pharmacologic agents to manipulate the autonomic nervous system and assess the balance of parasympathetic and sympathetic activity on the sinus node. Physiologic or pharmacologic maneuvers which are vagomimetic (Valsalva maneuver or phenylephrine-induced hypertension), vagolytic (atropine), sympathomimetic (isoproterenol or hypotension by nitroprusside), or sympatholytic (beta-adrenergic blocking agents) can be utilized, singly and in combination. These studies are designed to test the response of the sinus node to autonomic stimulation and inhibition and thereby characterize the status of autonomic regulation of the sinus node. Abnormalities of the autonomic control of sinus function are particularly common in patients in whom the only presenting arrhythmia is sinus bradycardia.

Intrinsic heart rate   This is a manifestation of the primary activity of the sinus node, and its determination requires chemical autonomic blockade of the heart. Complete autonomic blockade is achieved with 0.2 mg/kg propranolol intravenously, followed after 10 min by 0.04 mg/kg of atropine sulfate intravenously. Normal values of intrinsic heart rate (in beats per minute) are calculated by the formula $118.1 - (0.57 \times age)$. The use of autonomic blockade can separate patients with asymptomatic sinus bradycardia into a group with primary sinus node dysfunction (slow intrinsic heart rate) and a group with autonomic imbalance (normal intrinsic heart rate). Autonomic blockade is particularly useful when combined with invasive assessment of sinus node function (see below). Autonomic blockade may depress conduction in patients with intrinsic disease of the conduction system and should be carried out only in a setting where arrhythmias can be monitored and rapidly treated.

Sinus node recovery time   Sinus node recovery time is evaluated by assessing the response of the sinus node to rapid atrial pacing (Fig. 184-6). When atrial pacing is discontinued, a pause, the *sinus node recovery time*, occurs prior to resumption of spontaneous sinus rhythm. When the sinus recovery time is prolonged, the results of this test mimic the prolonged sinus pauses seen following termination of atrial tachyarrhythmias in the bradycardia-tachycardia syndrome (see Fig. 184-4). The corrected sinus node recovery time (sinus recovery time − sinus cycle length) normally is less than 550 ms and the uncorrected sinus node recovery time less than 150 percent of the spontaneous cycle length. In patients with symptomatic sinus node dysfunction, prolongation of the sinus node recovery time is often observed. Patients with abnormally slow intrinsic heart rates usually have abnormal sinus node recovery times, while those with normal intrinsic heart rates have normal recovery times.

FIGURE 184-6   Example of sinus node recovery time in a patient with symptomatic sinus node dysfunction. Cessation of atrial pacing at 150 beats per minute (cycle length 400 ms) results in a prolonged sinus pause (2.8 s). Surface ECG leads V_1 and V_6 are shown in addition to intracardiac recordings at the high right atrium (A), which demonstrates atrial pacing rate.

Sinoatrial conduction time   Determination of the conduction time from the sinus node to the atrium allows for the differentiation of abnormalities of sinoatrial conduction from abnormalities of sinus impulse formation. The conduction time equals one-half of the difference between the pause following termination of brief periods of pacing and the sinus cycle length. Alternatively, the sinus node electrogram can be recorded directly by a catheter electrode placed near the sinoatrial node.

EVALUATION   The electrophysiologic investigation of sinus node dysfunction should be undertaken in patients who have had symptoms compatible with sinus node dysfunction and in whom no documentation of the arrhythmia responsible for these symptoms has been obtained by prolonged Holter monitoring. Asymptomatic patients with sinus bradycardia need *not* be tested since no therapy is indicated. Similarly, symptomatic patients with ECG documentation of asystole, sinoatrial block or arrest, or the bradycardia-tachycardia syndrome do not require electrophysiologic tests for diagnosis. However, in symptomatic patients without documentation of an arrhythmia, electrophysiologic assessment of sinus node function can yield information that may be used to guide appropriate therapy. If a pacemaker is indicated, the side of pacemaker implantation for maximum hemodynamic effects can be guided by the results of electrophysiologic investigation. However, the results of tests of sinus node function must be interpreted with caution. Sinus node dysfunction coexists frequently with other disorders such as AV conduction disturbances which may cause symptoms such as syncope. Electrophysiologic evaluation of patients with symptoms such as undiagnosed syncope must not stop with the demonstration of abnormalities of sinus node dysfunction or carotid sinus hypersensitivity. Instead, complete evaluation, including His bundle recordings and programmed atrial and ventricular stimulation (see Chap. 185), is necessary to search for additional electrophysiologic abnormalities which could be responsible for symptoms.

TREATMENT   Permanent pacemakers (page 907) are the mainstay of therapy for patients with symptomatic sinus node dysfunction. Patients with intermittent paroxysms of bradycardia or sinus arrest and with the cardioinhibitory form of the hypersensitive carotid sinus syndrome are usually adequately treated by demand ventricular pacemakers. These devices are reliable, relatively inexpensive, and suffice to prevent episodic symptoms due to abrupt bradycardia. Patients with symptomatic chronic sinus bradycardia or frequent prolonged episodes of sinus node dysfunction may do better with dual-chamber pacemakers that preserve the normal AV activation sequence. Although theoretically an atrial demand pacemaker should be adequate for patients with sinus node dysfunction, the frequent accompaniment of dysfunction in other portions of the cardiac conduction system usually mandates placement of a pacemaker capable of ventricular pacing.

AV CONDUCTION DISTURBANCES

The specialized cardiac conducting system normally ensures synchronous conduction of each sinus impulse from the atria to the ventricles. Abnormalities of conduction of the sinus impulse to the ventricles may portend the development of heart block, which can ultimately lead to syncope or cardiac arrest. In order to evaluate the clinical significance of conduction abnormalities the physician must assess (1) the site of conduction disturbance, (2) the risk of progression to complete block, and (3) the probability that a subsidiary escape rhythm arising distal to the site of block will be electrophysiologically and hemodynamically stable. This latter point is perhaps the most important since the rate and stability of the escape pacemaker determine what symptoms result from heart block. The escape pacemaker following AV nodal block is usually in the His bundle, which generally has a stable rate of 40 to 60 beats per minute and is associated with a QRS complex of normal duration (in the absence of a preexisting intraventricular conduction defect). This contrasts with escape rhythms arising in the distal His-Purkinje system, which have lower intrinsic rates (25 to 45 beats per minute), manifest wide QRS complexes with prolonged duration, and are unstable. Although prolonged QRS complexes are invariable when the distal His-Purkinje pacemakers form the escape mechanism, wide QRS complexes can also coexist with AV nodal block and a His bundle rhythm. Therefore, QRS morphology alone may not be adequate to identify the site of block.

ETIOLOGY The AV node is supplied by the parasympathetic and sympathetic nervous systems and is sensitive to variations in autonomic tone. Chronic slowing of AV nodal conduction may be seen in highly trained athletes who have hypervagotonia at rest. A variety of diseases can also influence AV nodal conduction. These include acute processes such as myocardial infarction (particularly inferior); coronary spasm (usually of the right coronary artery); digitalis intoxication; excesses of beta and/or calcium blockers; acute infections such as viral myocarditis; acute rheumatic fever; infectious mononucleosis; and miscellaneous disorders such as Lyme disease, sarcoidosis, amyloidosis, and neoplasms, particularly cardiac mesotheliomas. AV nodal block may also be congenital.

Two degenerative diseases are commonly responsible for damage to the specialized conducting system and produce AV block usually associated with bundle branch block (see Chap. 176). In *Lev's disease*, there is calcification and sclerosis of the fibrous cardiac skeleton, which frequently involves the aortic and mitral valves, the central fibrous body, and the summit of the ventricular septum. *Lenegre's disease* appears to be a primary sclerodegenerative disease within the conducting system itself with no involvement of the myocardium or the fibrous skeleton of the heart. These two diseases are probably the most common causes of isolated chronic heart block in adults. Hypertension and aortic and/or mitral stenosis are specific disorders that either accelerate the degeneration of the conducting system or have a direct effect by calcification and fibrosis involving the conducting system.

FIGURE 184-7 *A.* Mobitz type I second-degree AV block. Intracardiac recordings demonstrate that the PR prolongation (320, 615 ms) is localized to the AV node (AH 240, 535 ms, respectively). HBE = His bundle electrogram; A = atrium; H = His; V = ventricle. (*From ME Josephson, SF Seides: Clinical Cardiac Electrophysiology: Techniques and Interpretations. Philadelphia, Lea & Febiger, 1979.*) *B.* Mobitz type II second-degree AV block. Intracardiac recordings document block below the His bundle.

(a)

(b)

FIGURE 184-8 Third-degree AV block. Complete heart block with a slow, wide complex escape rhythm is present. Block in this instance is usually intra-His.

First-degree AV block, more properly termed *prolonged AV conduction,* is characterized by a PR interval >0.20 s. Since the PR interval is determined by atrial, AV nodal, and His-Purkinje activation, delay in any one or more of these structures can contribute to a prolonged PR interval. In the presence of a QRS complex of normal duration, a PR interval >0.24 s almost invariably is due to a delay within the AV node. If the QRS is prolonged, delays may be present at any of the levels mentioned above. Delay within the His-Purkinje system is always accompanied by a prolonged QRS duration in addition to a prolonged PR interval. However, as indicated below, it is only with intracardiac recordings that the exact site of delay can be determined.

Second-degree heart block (intermittent AV block) is present when some atrial impulses fail to conduct to the ventricles. Mobitz type I second-degree AV block (AV Wenckebach block) is characterized by progressive PR interval prolongation prior to block of an atrial impulse (Fig. 184-7A). The pause that follows is less than fully compensatory (i.e., is less than two normal sinus intervals), and the PR of the first conducted impulse is shorter than the last conducted atrial impulse prior to the blocked P wave. This type of block is almost always localized to the AV node and associated with a normal QRS duration. It is most often seen as a transient abnormality with inferior wall infarction or with drug intoxication, particularly digitalis, beta blockers, and occasionally calcium channel antagonists. This type of block can also be observed in normal individuals with heightened vagal tone. Although Mobitz type I block can progress to complete heart block, this is uncommon. Even when it does, however, the heart block is usually well tolerated because the escape pacemaker usually arises in the proximal His bundle and provides a stable rhythm. As a result, the presence of Mobitz type I second-degree AV block usually does not mandate aggressive therapy. Therapeutic decisions depend upon the ventricular response and the symptoms of the patient. If the ventricular rate is adequate and the patient is asymptomatic, observation is sufficient.

In Mobitz type II second-degree AV block, conduction fails suddenly and unexpectedly without a preceding change in PR intervals (Fig. 184-7B). It is usually due to disease of the His-Purkinje system and is most often associated with a prolonged QRS duration. It is important to recognize this type of block since it has a high incidence of progression to complete heart block with an unstable, slow, lower escape pacemaker. Therefore, pacemaker implantation is necessary in this condition. Mobitz type II block may occur in the setting of anteroseptal infarction or in the primary or secondary sclerodegenerative or calcific disorders of the fibrous skeleton of the heart. In so-called high-degree AV block there are periods of two or more consecutively blocked P waves. Regardless of the site of origin of the escape rhythm, if it is slow and the patient is symptomatic, a cardiac pacemaker is mandatory.

Third-degree AV block is present when no atrial impulse propagates to the ventricles. If the QRS complex of the escape rhythm is of normal duration, occurs at a rate of 40 to 55 beats per minute, and increases with atropine or exercise, AV nodal block is probable. Congenital complete AV block is usually localized to the AV node (Fig. 184-8). If the block is within the His bundle, the escape pacemaker usually is less responsive to these perturbations. If the escape rhythm of the QRS is wide and associated with rates ≤40, block is usually localized in, or distal to, the His bundle and mandates a pacemaker since the escape rhythm in this setting is unreliable.

AV DISSOCIATION AV dissociation exists whenever the atria and ventricles are under the control of two separate pacemakers and, while present in complete AV block, can occur in the absence of a primary conduction disturbance. AV dissociation unrelated to heart block may occur under two circumstances: First, it may develop with an AV junctional rhythm in response to severe sinus bradycardia. When the sinus rate and the escape rate are similar and the P waves occur just before, in, or following the QRS, *isorhythmic AV dissociation* is said to be present. Treatment usually consists of removal of the offending cause of sinus bradycardia (i.e., discontinuation of digitalis, beta blockers, or calcium antagonists), accelerating the sinus node by vagolytic agents, or insertion of a pacemaker if the escape rhythm is slow and results in symptoms. Second, AV dissociation can be caused by an enhanced lower (junctional or ventricular) pacemaker which competes with normal sinus rhythm and frequently exceeds it. This has been called *interference AV dissociation* because the rapid lower pacemaker results in bombardment of the AV node in a retrograde fashion, rendering it refractory to the normal sinus impulses. Thus, failure of antegrade conduction is a physiologic response in this circumstance. Interference dissociation commonly occurs during ventricular tachycardia accelerated junctional or ventricular rhythms seen with digitalis intoxication, myocardial ischemia and/or infarction, or local irritation following cardiac surgery. The accelerated rhythm should be treated with either antiarrhythmic drugs (see Chap. 185), removal of an offending drug, or correction of the metabolic abnormality or ischemia.

INTRACARDIAC ELECTROCARDIOGRAPHIC RECORDINGS IN DIAGNOSIS AND MANAGEMENT

The main therapeutic decision in patients with AV conduction disturbance is whether or not a permanent pacemaker is required, and a number of circumstances exist in which His bundle electrocardiography can provide a useful diagnostic tool upon which to base this decision. It is unquestionable that patients with *symptomatic* second- or third-degree AV block should be paced, and therefore these patients do not require electrophysiologic study. However, intracardiac ECG recordings can be useful in at least the following three groups of patients:

1 *Patients with syncope and bundle branch or bifascicular block without documentation of AV block.* In such patients the demonstration of marked infra-His conduction disturbances, i.e., a prolonged HV interval (>100 ms) may usually be taken as an indication of the need for the insertion of the permanent pacemaker. With intervals ranging from 60 to 100 ms, the indications for pacing are equivocal. Block below the His bundle developing during atrial pacing at rates of less than 150 beats per minute and the development of an infra-His block or HV prolongation >100 ms following 1 g procainamide intravenously also signify that the patient is at high risk for the development of subsequent AV block and that a pacemaker is indicated. Complete electrophysiologic evaluation, including atrial and ventricular programmed stimulation, is indicated to help identify other possible cardiac etiologies for the syncope. Since the incidence of significant advanced AV block is low in *asymptomatic* patients who have bifascicular block, electrophysiologic evaluation or permanent pacemakers are not cost-effective. In this group observation appears most reasonable.

2 *Patients with 2:1 atrioventricular conduction.* Intracardiac recordings are necessary in order to ascertain the site of the conduction disturbance because the typical ECG features of Mobitz type I or Mobitz type II block cannot be discerned during a 2:1 pattern of AV conduction on the surface ECG. Intracardiac recordings may demonstrate that AV nodal block, intra-His block, infra-His block, or combinations of block may be responsible. A surface electrocardiogram finding that suggests an infra-His lesion is the presence of alternating bundle branch block associated with changing PR intervals. Intracardiac recordings in such patients confirm that the block is almost always in the His-Purkinje system. The finding of infra-His block in patients with asymptomatic second-degree AV block mandates pacemaker therapy because of the high likelihood of their developing symptomatic high-grade AV block and syncope.

3 *Asymptomatic patients with third-degree AV block.* In such patients electrophysiologic studies may be useful in assessing the stability

of the junctional pacemaker. Pacing is indicated when the His bundle escape pacemaker is shown to be unstable by an inadequate response to exercise, atropine, or isoproterenol or by a prolonged junctional recovery time following ventricular pacing.

MANAGEMENT OF BRADYARRHYTHMIAS

PHARMACOLOGIC THERAPY Pharmacologic therapy is usually reserved for acute situations. Atropine (0.05 to 2.0 mg intravenously) and isoproterenol (1 to 4 µg/min intravenously) are useful in increasing heart rate and decreasing symptoms in patients with sinus bradycardia or AV block localized to the AV node. They have an insignificant effect on lower pacemakers. Recently theophylline has been suggested in patients with vasovagal syncope. Long-term therapy of bradyarrhythmias is best accomplished by pacemakers.

PACEMAKERS External energy sources can be used to stimulate the heart when disorders in impulse formation and/or transmission lead to symptomatic bradyarrhythmias. Pacer stimuli can be applied to the atria and/or ventricles. Indications for pacemakers inserted are listed in Table 184-1.

Temporary pacing This is usually instituted to provide immediate stabilization prior to permanent pacemaker placement or to provide pacemaker support when a bradycardia is precipitated by what is presumed to be a transient event such as ischemia or drug toxicity. Temporary pacing is usually achieved by the transvenous insertion of an electrode catheter with the catheter positioned in the right ventricular apex and attached to an external generator. This procedure is associated with a small risk of cardiac perforation, infection at the insertion site, and thromboembolism; the risk of the latter two complications increases markedly if the pacing wire is left in place for more than 48 h. The development of an entirely external transthoracic cardiac pacing system may preclude the need for transvenous pacing in selected patients. However, occasional failure of ventricular capture and significant discomfort related to the large current required for effective transthoracic ventricular stimulation precludes the uniform use of this approach.

Permanent pacing This mode of pacing is instituted for persistent or intermittent symptomatic bradycardia not related to a self-limiting precipitating factor or for documented infranodal second- or third-degree AV block. Permanent pacing leads are usually inserted transvenously through the subclavian or cephalic vein with the leads positioned in the right atrial appendage for atrial pacing and the right ventricular apex for ventricular pacing. The leads are then attached to the pulse generator, which is inserted into a subcutaneous pocket below the clavicle. Epicardial lead placement is used when: (1) transvenous access cannot be obtained; (2) the chest is already open, i.e., in the course of a cardiac operation; and (3) if adequate endocardial lead placement cannot be achieved. Most pacemaker generators are powered by lithium batteries. The life expectancy of the generator is related to (1) current output required for capture; (2) requirement for

---

TABLE 184-1 Indications for pacing

I Symptomatic carotid sinus hypersensitivity
  A Sinus node dysfunction
    1 Symptomatic sinus bradycardia
    2 Sinus pauses > 3 s
  B AV nodal block
    1 Symptomatic second-degree AV block (Mobitz I)
    2 Symptomatic complete heart block
  C Infranodal block
    1 New bifascicular block associated with acute infarction (usually anteroseptal)
    2 Alternating bundle branch block with changing PR
    3 HV > 100 ms in a patient with bifascicular block
    4 Block below the bundle of His with atrial pacing at rates ≤ 150 beats per minute
    5 2 second-degree AV block (Mobitz II)
    6 Complete heart block

incessant or intermittent pacing; and (3) number of cardiac chambers paced. Life expectancy of the simple ventricular demand pacemaker can exceed 10 years.

Pacing code   A code consisting of three to five letters has been developed for describing pacemaker type and function. The first letter indicates the chamber(s) paced and is designated *V* for ventricular pacing, *A* for atrial pacing, or *D* for dual-chamber (both atrial and ventricular) pacing. The second letter indicates the chamber in which electrical activity is sensed and is also indicated by *A*, *V*, or *D*. An additional designation, *O*, has been used when pacemaker discharge is not dependent on a sensed electrical activity. The third letter refers to the response to a sensed electrical signal. The letter *O* represents no response to an underlying electrical signal, usually related to the absence of associated sensing function; *I* represents inhibition of pacing function; *T* represents triggering of pacing function; and *D* indicates a dual response, i.e., spontaneous atrial and ventricular activity inhibiting atrial and ventricular pacing and atrial activity triggering a ventricular response. Additional fourth and fifth letters of the pacing code have been recommended to indicate whether the pacemaker is programmable and whether special antitachycardia functions are available. It follows from the described code that the standard VVI (ventricular demand pacemaker) paces the ventricle, senses the ventricle, and is inhibited by sensed spontaneous ventricular activity, while the DDD pulse generator is capable of sensing and pacing both the atria and ventricles and has a dual response to the sensed atrial and ventricular activity as described above.

Selection of the appropriate pacemaker and pacing mode depends on the clinical condition and the type of bradyarrhythmia being treated. The two most common pacing mode selections are DDD and VVI. DDD, or so-called universal pacing, provides AV sequential pacing, which is ideally suited for the relatively young and active patient who has intact sinus node function or intermittent dysfunction and high-grade persistent or intermittent AV block. The DDD mode will allow for physiologic atrial sensed and ventricular paced rates and improve exercise tolerance. AV synchrony and dual-chamber pacing may also be desirable in patients with borderline hemodynamic reserve who are dependent on atrial contribution to cardiac output and in those patients who develop the pacemaker syndrome (see below) in response to ventricular demand pacing. The DDD pacing mode is contraindicated in chronic atrial fibrillation or flutter, in which case rapid and irregular ventricular pacing will occur to the upper rate limit. In some cases this will produce a more rapid ventricular rate than the patient's own rate in the absence of a pacemaker. Chronotropic insufficiency is another contraindication since the pacemaker will act only as a "fixed rate" pacemaker at the new rate cutoff. In these situations, ventricular demand (VVI) or a rate adaptive pacemaker (see below) is indicated. The DDD pacing mode may also be contraindicated in patients with intermittent or persistent ventriculoatrial (VA) conduction, who may develop pacemaker-mediated tachycardia (see below).

In patients with impaired sinus node function or chronic atrial fibrillation, a sensor-driven, rate-adaptive pacemaker may be implanted. These pacemakers automatically adjust ventricular pacing rates to a sensed indicator of exertion (e.g., body vibration or blood temperature). This positive chronotropic response increases cardiac output and improves exercise tolerance.

Programmability of pacemakers   This allows for modification of pacing function after implantation and for adaptation to changes in clinical needs. Pacemaker programming is accomplished by activation of the programming head positioned over the implanted pulse generator after making the desired changes in programmable parameters (Table 184-2). A radiofrequency system is routinely used to communicate the program to the pacemaker.

Complications   Adverse effects of permanent pacing are usually associated with failure or malfunction of the pacing system. These problems are usually secondary to over- or undersensing, output failure, and/or lead fracture or displacement. Two other problems may occur. The *pacemaker syndrome* consists of fatigue, dizziness,

TABLE 184-2   Programmable pacemaker functions

Rate*	Hysteresis
Energy output	Refractory period
Sensitivity	Mode of function
Lead polarity	AV delay

* Lower and upper rate limits apply to dual-chamber pacing.

syncope, and distressing pulsations in the neck and chest and can be associated with adverse hemodynamic effects. The pathophysiologic contributors to the pacemaker syndrome include (1) loss of atrial contribution to ventricular systole; (2) vasodepressor reflex initiated by cannon *a* waves which are caused by atrial contractions against a closed tricuspid valve observed in the jugular venous pulse (Chap. 175); and (3) systemic and pulmonary venous regurgitation due to atrial contraction against a closed AV valve. The symptoms associated with the pacemaker syndrome can be prevented by maintaining AV synchrony by dual-chamber pacing or, in the case of a ventricular demand pacemaker, by programming a hysteresis escape rate 15 to 20 beats per minute below that of the paced rate. As a result of this programming, sinus activity and thus atrial contraction will be less likely to occur at the same time as ventricular pacing and ventricular contraction. The second major problem peculiar to dual-chamber pacemakers is the development of *pacemaker-mediated tachycardia*, which is caused by ventriculoatrial conduction. In this instance, retrograde depolarization of the atria, resulting from a premature ventricular depolarization or a paced ventricular complex, is sensed and leads to subsequent triggering of ventricular pacing. This, in turn, can result in repetition of the phenomenon of ventriculoatrial conduction with the development of an endless-loop, pacemaker-mediated tachycardia. It may be corrected by programming the atrial refractory period.

REFERENCES

AUSTIN JL et al: Analysis of pacemaker malfunction and complications of temporary pacing in the coronary care unit. Am J Cardiol 49:301, 1982

DULK KD et al: The activitrax rate responsive pacemaker system. Am J Cardiol 61:107, 1988

ELLENBOGEN KA et al: New insights into pacemaker syndrome gained from hemodynamic, humoral and vascular responses during ventriculo-atrial pacing. Am J Cardiol 65(1):53, 1990

HUANG SK et al: Carotid sinus hypersensitivity in patients with unexplained syncope: clinical, electrophysiologic and long-term follow-up observations. Am Heart J 116:989, 1988

LANGENFELD H et al: Course of symptoms and spontaneous ECG in pacemaker patients: a 5-year follow-up study. PACE 11:2198, 1988

LUDMER PL, GOLDSCHLAGER N: Cardiac pacing in the 1980's. N Engl J Med 311:1671, 1984

NICOD P et al: Long-term outcome in patients with inferior myocardial infarction and complete atrioventricular block. J Am Coll Cardiol 12:589, 1988

PARSONETT V et al: Indications for dual chamber pacing. PACE 7:318, 1984

WIRTZFELD A et al: Physiologic pacing: Present status and future develeopments. PACE 10:41, 1984

ZOLL PM et al: External noninvasive temporary cardiac pacing: Clinical trials. Circulation 71:937, 1985

185   THE TACHYARRHYTHMIAS

MARK E. JOSEPHSON / ALFRED E. BUXTON / FRANCIS E. MARCHLINSKI

MECHANISMS OF TACHYARRHYTHMIAS

Tachyarrhythmias may be divided into disorders of impulse propagation and disorders of impulse formation. Disorders of impulse propagation (reentry) are generally considered to be the most common mechanism of sustained paroxysmal tachyarrhythmia. The requirements for initiating reentry include: (1) electrophysiologic inhomogeneity (i.e., differences in conduction and/or refractoriness) in two or more regions of the heart connected with each other to form a potentially closed loop; (2) unidirectional block in one pathway; (3) slow conduction over an alternative pathway, allowing time for the initially blocked pathway to recover excitability; and (4) reexcitation of the initially blocked pathway to complete a loop of activation. Repetitive circulation of the impulse over this loop can produce a sustained tachyarrhythmia. While anatomic obstacles may underlie reentry and provide an inexcitable center around which the impulse can circulate, they are not essential. Reentrant arrhythmias can be reproducibly initiated and terminated by premature complexes and rapid stimulation. The response of these arrhythmias to stimulation can help distinguish them from arrhythmias caused by triggered activity.

Disorders of impulse formation can be subdivided into tachyarrhythmias caused by enhanced automaticity and those caused by triggered activity. In addition to the sinus node, automatic pacemaker activity can be observed in specialized atrial fibers, fibers of the atrioventricular (AV) junction, and Purkinje fibers (see Chap. 184). Myocardial cells do not normally possess pacemaker activity. Enhancement of normal automaticity in latent pacemaker fibers or the development of abnormal automaticity due to partial depolarization of the resting membrane occurs as a consequence of a variety of pathophysiologic states, which include (1) increased endogenous or exogenous catecholamines; (2) electrolyte disturbances (e.g., hyperkalemia); (3) hypoxia or ischemia; (4) mechanical effects (e.g., stretch); and (5) drugs (e.g., digitalis). Tachycardia caused by automaticity cannot be started or stopped by pacing.

Triggered activity has been observed in atrial, ventricular, and His-Purkinje tissue under conditions such as increased local catecholamine concentration, hyperkalemia, hypercalcemia, and digitalis intoxication. All of these conditions produce an accumulation of intracellular calcium which causes depolarizations following the action potential, termed *afterdepolarizations*. With increasing amplitude of the afterdepolarizations, threshold can be reached and repetitive activity produced. In contrast to automatic rhythms, triggered activity

requires preceding activity for initiation and therefore can be initiated by pacing. In contrast to tachyarrhythmias caused by automaticity and reentry, the response of triggered activity to overdrive pacing is acceleration.

The use of electrophysiologic (EP) studies, i.e., intracardiac recordings and programmed stimulation, has greatly expanded our understanding of the mechanisms of tachyarrhythmias. In addition to helping in the diagnosis of arrhythmias, these techniques may be of value in determining the most appropriate types of therapy. EP studies of tachycardias require the positioning of multiple electrode catheters at critical areas within the heart. These electrodes must be capable of both stimulating and recording from multiple sites in the atria and/or ventricles.

PREMATURE COMPLEXES

ATRIAL PREMATURE COMPLEXES (APCs)   APCs can be found on 24-h Holter monitoring in over 60 percent of normal adults. APCs are usually asymptomatic and benign, although at times they may be associated with palpitations. In susceptible patients, they can initiate paroxysmal supraventricular tachycardias. APCs may originate from any location in either atrium, and they are recognized on the ECG as early P waves with a morphology which differs from the sinus P wave (Fig. 185-1A). While APCs usually conduct to the ventricles when they occur late in the cardiac cycle, relatively early APCs may reach the AV conduction system while it is still in its relative refractory period, resulting in a conduction delay manifested by prolonged PR interval following the premature P wave (Fig. 185-1A). Very early APCs may even block in the AV node if this structure is encountered during its effective refractory period. APCs, whether conducted or not, are usually followed by a pause before a return to sinus activity. Most commonly, an APC enters and resets the sinus node, so that the sum of the pre- and postextrasystolic PP intervals is less than the sum of two sinus PP intervals (Fig. 185-1A). In this case the pause is said to be less than fully compensatory. The QRS

FIGURE 185-1 *A*. ECG lead II. Sinus rhythm with two atrial premature complexes (arrows). Note the difference in P-wave configuration between sinus and the premature atrial complexes. In addition, note that the PR interval of the premature complexes is prolonged, due to slowed conduction of the premature impulse through the AV conduction system. *B*. ECG lead V₁. Atrial tachycardia with varying degrees of AV block, typical of digitalis toxicity. *C*. ECG lead II. Atrial flutter. Note the characteristic sawtooth baseline seen in the inferior ECG leads during atrial flutter. Variable degrees of AV conduction block are present. *D*. ECG lead II. Atrial fibrillation. Note the irregular wavy baseline without discrete atrial activity. The ventricular response is irregularly irregular. *E*. ECG leads I, aVR, and V₁. Atrial fibrillation in a patient with Wolff-Parkinson-White syndrome. Note the extremely rapid, grossly irregular ventricular rate with wide, bizarre QRS complexes.

complex following most APCs is normal, although early APCs may be followed by aberrantly conducted QRS complexes.

Since most APCs are asymptomatic, treatment is not required. When they cause palpitations or trigger paroxysmal supraventricular tachycardias (see below), treatment may be useful. Factors that precipitate APCs such as alcohol, tobacco, or adrenergic stimulants should be identified and eliminated, and in their absence mild sedation or the use of a beta blocker may be tried. If this fails, quinidine, procainamide, or a similar agent may be used.

AV JUNCTIONAL COMPLEXES The site of origin of these complexes is thought to be in the bundle of His, since the AV node itself possesses no automaticity (page 906). AV junctional complexes are less common than either atrial or ventricular premature complexes and are more often associated with cardiac disease or digitalis intoxication. Junctional premature impulses can conduct both antegradely to the ventricles and retrogradely to the atrium and, on rare occasions, may fail to conduct in either direction. Premature AV junctional complexes can be recognized by normal-appearing QRS complexes that are not preceded by a P wave. Retrograde P waves (inverted in leads II, III, and aVF) may be observed after the QRS complex.

While often asymptomatic, junctional premature complexes may be associated with palpitations and cause cannon *a* waves which may result in distressing pulsations in the neck. When symptomatic, they should be treated like APCs.

VENTRICULAR PREMATURE COMPLEXES (VPCs) These are among the most common arrhythmias and occur in patients with and without heart disease. Of adult males ≥60 percent will exhibit VPCs during a 24-h Holter monitoring. In patients without heart disease, VPCs have not been shown to be associated with any increased incidence in mortality or morbidity. VPCs may occur in up to 80 percent of patients with previous myocardial infarction, and in this setting, if frequent (>10 per hour) and/or complex (occurring in couplets or triplets), they have been associated with increased mortality. However, cardiac mortality in such patients usually occurs in association with significantly impaired ventricular function. While frequent and complex ventricular ectopy is an independent risk factor, it is not as strong a risk factor as is impaired ventricular function. Moreover, even though ventricular tachycardia and/or fibrillation may be the basis for the sudden death in these patients, this does not a priori establish a cause-and-effect relation between spontaneous ectopy and life-threatening ventricular tachycardia or fibrillation. Very early cycle (R or T) VPCs have been stated by some to increase the risk of sudden death. Although this has been observed during acute ischemia and in the setting of QT prolongation, frequently ventricular tachycardia or fibrillation is precipitated by VPCs which occur after the T wave of the prior beat.

VPCs are recognized by wide (usually >0.14 s), bizarre QRS complexes that are not preceded by P waves (Fig. 185-2A). Often they bear a relatively fixed relationship to the preceding sinus complex and are thus considered fixed coupled VPCs. When fixed coupling is not present and the interval between VPCs has a common denominator, *ventricular parasystole* is said to be present (Fig. 185-3). Under these circumstances the VPCs are a manifestation of abnormal automaticity of a protected ventricular focus; because it is not penetrated by sinus impulses, it is not reset by them and the interectopic intervals remain relatively fixed (≤120 ms variation of mean RR cycle length).

VPCs may occur singly; in patterns of bigeminy, in which every sinus beat is followed by a VPC; in trigeminy, in which two sinus beats are followed by a VPC; in quadrigeminy, etc. Two successive VPCs are termed *pairs* or *couplets*, while three or more consecutive VPCs are termed *ventricular tachycardia*. VPCs may have similar morphologies (monomorphic) or different morphologies (multiformed or polymorphic) (Fig. 185-2C).

Most commonly, VPCs are not conducted retrogradely to the atrium to reset the sinoatrial node. Thus, they produce a fully compensatory pause; i.e., the interval between conducted beats which bracket the VPC equals two basic RR intervals. Ventricular impulses

FIGURE 185-2 *A.* Single ventricular ectopy. During sinus rhythm two premature ventricular complexes (arrows) occur. Note that the QRS configuration is bizarre, different from that during sinus rhythm. The premature ventricular complexes are not preceded by P waves. The QRS width of the premature complexes is approximately 160 ms. The pause surrounding the premature complexes is fully compensatory, the sinus beat after the premature complex occurring on time. *B.* A 5-beat run of nonsustained ventricular tachycardia having a uniform morphology (dots). Although intraventricular conduction during sinus rhythm is slightly prolonged, during the run of ventricular tachycardia the QRS duration is further prolonged. Note that 2:1 VA conduction is present during ventricular tachycardia. Retrograde P waves are denoted by the arrows. *C.* Simultaneous recordings of ECG leads I, aVF, and V₁. A 4-beat run of polymorphic nonsustained ventricular tachycardia is demonstrated. No two consecutive QRS complexes are the same. Polymorphic VT is not associated with a prolonged QT interval in this case.

FIGURE 185-3 Ventricular parasystole. At varying sinus cycle lengths during exercise, interectopic intervals remain constant at 1620–1640 ms. However, the coupling intervals between sinus and ectopic complexes vary between 510 and 310 ms.

may also manifest retrograde conduction to the atrium and cause inverted P waves in leads II, III, and aVF. The pause that results may therefore be less than compensatory. In many instances, the QRS complex will not be associated with retrograde ventriculoatrial (VA) conduction but may block in the AV node. This renders the AV node refractory to the subsequent sinus beat and causes slowed conduction (i.e., prolonged PR interval) or block of the next sinus P wave. This prolonged PR interval is said to be a manifestation of concealed retrograde conduction of the ventricular impulse into the AV node. A VPC that does not produce any manifestation of retrograde concealed conduction and fails to influence the oncoming sinus impulse is termed an *interpolated VPC*.

VPCs can cause palpitations or neck pulsations secondary to either the occurrence of cannon *a* waves or the increased force of contraction due to postextrasystolic potentiation of ventricular contractility. Patients with frequent VPCs or bigeminy may develop syncope because the VPCs do not result in an adequate stroke volume and the cardiac output is reduced due to effective "halving" of the heart rate seen in patients with abnormal ventricular function.

Management In the absence of cardiac disease, isolated asymptomatic VPCs, regardless of configuration and frequency, need no treatment. When arrhythmias are symptomatic, the symptoms should first be addressed by either allaying the patient's anxiety, or if this is not successful, reducing the frequency of the VPCs with antiarrhythmic agents. Beta-adrenergic blockers may be successful in managing VPCs that occur primarily in the daytime or under stressful situations and in specific settings such as mitral valve prolapse and thyrotoxicosis. Quinidine or quinidine-like agents may be tried should this be unsuccessful. In patients with cardiac disease, frequent VPCs are often associated with an increased risk of sudden and nonsudden cardiac death, and many physicians attempt to eliminate or reduce the frequency of these VPCs in an attempt to reduce this risk. However, the cause-and-effect relationship of the VPCs to fatal events has not been established, and it has not been shown definitively that the suppression of VPCs with antiarrhythmic drugs prevents sudden death. In addition, it is important to recognize that the antiarrhythmic agents can also produce the lethal arrhythmias which they are given to prevent. Thus, therapy directed toward VPCs in the setting of chronic cardiac disease may result in an inappropriate and costly use of agents without proven efficacy and with potential side effects in many patients. The high incidence of side effects and the frequent exacerbation of arrhythmias caused by all antiarrhythmic drugs make it mandatory to monitor patients being treated with such agents.

In acute myocardial infarction the greatest incidence of primary ventricular fibrillation occurs within the first 24 h. Temporary prophylactic antiarrhythmic therapy has therefore been recommended for all patients with acute infarction, regardless of the presence or the degree of spontaneous ectopy.

TACHYCARDIAS

Tachycardias refer to arrhythmias with three or more complexes at rates exceeding 100 beats per minute; they occur more often in structurally diseased than in normal hearts. Those paroxysmal tachycardias that are initiated by APCs or VPCs are considered to be due to reentry except some of the digitalis-induced tachyarrhythmias, which are probably due to triggered activity (see below).

If the patient is hemodynamically stable, an attempt should be made to determine the mechanism and origin of the tachycardia since this will usually lead to an appropriate therapeutic decision. Information to be obtained from the ECG includes (1) the presence, frequency, morphology, and regularity of P waves and QRS complexes; (2) the relationship between atrial and ventricular activity; (3) a comparison of the QRS morphology during sinus rhythm and during the tachycardia; and (4) the response to carotid sinus massage or other vagal maneuvers. It is useful first to compare the ECG during the tachycardia with one recorded during sinus rhythm, and it is often

desirable to record long rhythm strips using surface leads with the largest P waves, usually leads II or V_1. One can also utilize the electrodes situated at the end of a flexible pacing catheter inserted into the esophagus behind the left atrium to record atrial activity.

Carotid sinus pressure should only be applied while the patient is electrocardiographically monitored with resuscitative equipment available to manage the rare episode of asystole and/or ventricular fibrillation associated with this procedure. Carotid sinus massage should not be performed in patients with carotid arterial bruits. The patient should be positioned flat with the neck extended. Massage of one carotid bulb at a time should be performed by applying firm pressure just underneath the angle of the jaw for up to 5 s. Alternative vagomimetic maneuvers include the Valsalva maneuver, immersion of the face in cold water, and the administration of 5 to 10 mg edrophonium.

Observation of the jugular venous pulse can provide clues to the presence of atrial activity and its relationship to ventricular ectopy. Intermittent cannon *a* waves suggest AV dissociation, while persistent cannon *a* waves suggest 1:1 VA conduction. Flutter waves may be seen or no atrial activity may be apparent, as in the presence of atrial flutter and fibrillation, respectively. The arterial pulse may also manifest AV dissociation or atrial fibrillation by demonstrating variations in amplitude. A first heart sound of variable intensity during a regular rhythm also suggests AV dissociation or atrial fibrillation.

SINUS TACHYCARDIA In the adult, sinus tachycardia is said to be present when the heart rate exceeds 100 beats per minute; sinus tachycardia rarely exceeds 200 beats per minute and is not a primary arrhythmia; instead, it represents a physiologic response to a variety of stresses, such as fever, volume depletion, anxiety, exercise, thyrotoxicosis, hypoxemia, hypotension, or congestive heart failure. Sinus tachycardia has a gradual onset and offset. The ECG demonstrates P waves with sinus contour preceding each QRS complex. Carotid sinus pressure usually produces modest slowing with a gradual return to the previous rate upon cessation. This contrasts with the response of paroxysmal supraventricular tachycardias, which may slow slightly and terminate abruptly.

Sinus tachycardia should not be treated as a primary arrhythmia, since it is always a physiologic response to a demand placed on the heart. As such, the therapy should be directed to the primary disorder. This may involve institution of digitalis and/or diuretics for heart failure and oxygen for hypoxemia, treatment of thyrotoxicosis, volume repletion, aspirin for fever, or tranquilizers for emotional upset.

ATRIAL FIBRILLATION (AF) This common arrhythmia may occur in paroxysmal and persistent forms. It may be seen in normal subjects, particularly during emotional stress or following surgery, exercise, or acute alcoholic intoxication. It may also occur in patients with heart or lung disease who develop acute hypoxia, hypercapnia, or metabolic or hemodynamic derangements. Persistent AF usually occurs in patients with cardiovascular disease, most commonly rheumatic heart disease, nonrheumatic mitral valve disease, hypertensive cardiovascular disease, chronic lung disease, atrial septal defect, and a variety of miscellaneous cardiac abnormalities. AF may be the presenting finding in thyrotoxicosis. So-called lone AF, which occurs in patients without underlying heart disease, is considered to represent the tachycardia phase of the tachycardia-bradycardia syndrome (p. 904).

The morbidity associated with AF is related to (1) excessive rate of the ventricular response, which in turn may lead to hypotension or angina pectoris in susceptible individuals; (2) the pause following cessation of AF, which can cause syncope; (3) systemic embolization, which occurs most commonly in patients with rheumatic heart disease; (4) loss of the contribution of atrial contraction to cardiac output, which may cause fatigue; and (5) anxiety secondary to palpitations. In patients with severe cardiac dysfunction, particularly those with hypertrophied, noncompliant ventricles, the combination of the loss of the atrial contribution to ventricular filling and the abbreviated filling period due to the rapid ventricular rate in AF can produce marked hemodynamic embarrassment, resulting in hypotension, syncope, or heart failure. In patients with mitral stenosis in whom filling time is critical, development of AF with a rapid ventricular rate may precipitate pulmonary edema (see Chap. 188).

AF is characterized by disorganized atrial activity without discrete P waves on the surface ECG (Fig. 185-1D). Atrial activation is manifested by an undulating baseline or by more sharply inscribed atrial deflections of varying amplitude and frequency ranging from 350 to 600 per minute. The ventricular response is irregularly irregular. This results from the large number of atrial impulses which penetrate the AV node, making it partially refractory to subsequent impulses. This effect of nonconducted atrial impulses to influence the response to subsequent atrial impulses is termed *concealed conduction*. As a result, the ventricular response is relatively slow, considering the actual atrial rate. If AF converts to atrial flutter, which has a slower atrial rate, the effect of concealed conduction may be diminished and a paradoxic increase in the ventricular response may occur. The main factor determining the rate of the ventricular response is the functional refractory period of the AV node or the most rapid paced rate at which 1:1 conduction through the AV node can be observed.

If, in the presence of AF, the ventricular rhythm becomes regular and slow (e.g., 30 to 60 beats per minute), complete heart block is suggested, and if the ventricular rhythm is regular and rapid (≥ 100 beats per minute), a tachycardia arising in the AV junction or ventricle should be suspected. Digitalis intoxication is a common cause of both of these phenomena.

Patients with AF exhibit a loss of *a* waves in the jugular venous pulse and variable pulse pressures in the carotid arterial pulse. The first heart sound usually varies in intensity. On echocardiography the left atrium is frequently enlarged, and in patients in whom the left atrial diameter exceeds 4.5 cm, it may not be possible to convert AF to sinus rhythm or to maintain the latter despite therapy.

Management   In acute AF, a precipitating factor such as fever, pneumonia, alcoholic intoxication, thyrotoxicosis, pulmonary emboli, or pericarditis should be sought. When such a factor is present, therapy should be directed toward the primary abnormality. If the patient's clinical status is severely compromised, electrical cardioversion is the treatment of choice. In the absence of severe cardiovascular compromise, slowing of ventricular rate becomes the initial therapeutic goal. This may be accomplished with digitalis, calcium channel antagonists, or beta-adrenergic blockers, all of which prolong the refractory period of the AV node and slow conduction within it. Intravenous verapamil usually gives the most rapid response. However, in cases where catecholamine levels are likely to be elevated, beta blockers may be favored. Conversion to sinus rhythm may then be attempted, using quinidine or quinidine-like (type IA) agents (Table 185-1). It is important to slow AV node conduction prior to

---

TABLE 185-1   Classification of antiarrhythmic drugs

Type I   Drugs that reduce maximal velocity of phase 0 depolarization ($\dot{V}_{max}$) due to block of inward Na^+ current in tissue with fast response action potentials

   A $\downarrow \dot{V}_{max}$ at all heart rates and $\uparrow$ action potential duration, e.g., quinidine, procainamide, disopyramide

   B Little effect at slow rates on $\dot{V}_{max}$ in normal tissue, $\dot{V}_{max}$ in partially depolarized cells with fast response action potentials
      Effects increased at faster rates
      No change or $\downarrow$ in action potential duration, e.g., lidocaine, phenytoin, tocainide, mexiletine

   C $\downarrow \dot{V}_{max}$ at normal rates in normal tissue
      Minimal effect on action potential duration, e.g., encainide, lorcainide, flecainide

Type II   Antisympathetic agents, e.g., propranolol and other beta-adrenergic blockers: $\downarrow$ SA nodal automaticity, $\uparrow$ AV nodal refractoriness, and $\downarrow$ AV nodal conduction velocity

Type III   Agents that prolong action potential duration in tissue with fast response action potentials, e.g., bretylium, amiodarone

Type IV   Calcium (slow) channel blocking agents: decrease conduction velocity and increase refractoriness in tissue with slow response action potentials, e.g., verapamil, diltiazem

---

administering such drugs because their vagolytic effect and ability to convert AF to atrial flutter may reduce the concealed conduction and lead to an excessively rapid ventricular response. Beta-adrenergic blockers are especially useful in this regard. If medical therapy fails to convert AF, electrical cardioversion is useful; it generally requires 100 to 200 W·s of energy. Anticoagulation should be started at least 2 weeks prior to and continued for 2 weeks following any attempt at cardioversion, either pharmacologic or electrical, in patients with long-standing AF. Anticoagulation appears to decrease the incidence of systemic embolization associated with cardioversion. It is less likely for chronic AF to convert to or remain in sinus rhythm in the presence of long-standing rheumatic heart disease and/or when the atria are markedly enlarged. It is also unlikely for patients with lone AF to be converted to and maintained in sinus rhythm.

If sinus rhythm is restored electrically or pharmacologically, quinidine or related agents may be used to prevent recurrence. In patients in whom cardioversion is unsuccessful or in whom AF is likely to recur, it is probably wisest to allow the patient to remain in AF and to control the ventricular response with calcium antagonists, beta-adrenergic blockers, or digitalis. Since they are always at risk of systemic embolization, chronic anticoagulation must be considered for such patients.

ATRIAL FLUTTER   This arrhythmia occurs most often in patients with organic heart disease. Flutter may be paroxysmal, in which case there is usually a precipitating factor, such as pericarditis or acute respiratory failure, or it may be persistent. Atrial flutter (as well as AF) is very common during the first week following open heart surgery. Atrial flutter is usually less long-lived than is AF, although on occasion it may persist for months to years. Most commonly, if it lasts for more than a week, atrial flutter will convert to AF. Systemic embolization is less common in atrial flutter than AF.

Atrial flutter is characterized by an atrial rate between 250 and 350 beats per minute. Typically, the ventricular rate is half the atrial rate, i.e., approximately 150 beats per minute. If the atrial rate is slowed to <220 per minute by antiarrhythmic agents such as quinidine, which also possess vagolytic properties, the ventricular rate may rise suddenly because of the development of 1:1 AV conduction. Classically, flutter waves are seen as regular sawtooth-like atrial activity, most prominent in the inferior leads (Fig. 185-1C). When the ventricular response is regular and not a simple fraction of the atrial rate, complete AV block is present, which may be a manifestation of digitalis toxicity. Activation mapping suggests that atrial flutter is a form of atrial reentry localized to the low right atrium.

Management   The most effective treatment of atrial flutter is direct current cardioversion, which can be accomplished at low energy (10 to 50 W·s) under mild sedation. In patients who develop atrial flutter following open-heart surgery or recurrent flutter in the setting of acute myocardial infarction, particularly when they are being treated with digitalis, atrial pacing (using temporary pacing wires implanted at the time of operation or a pacing lead inserted into the atrium pervenously) at rates of 115 to 130 percent of the atrial flutter rate can usually convert the atrial flutter to sinus rhythm. Atrial pacing may also result in the conversion of atrial flutter to AF, which allows for easier control of the ventricular response. If immediate conversion of atrial flutter is not mandated by the patient's clinical status, the ventricular response should first be slowed by blocking the AV node with a beta blocker, calcium antagonist, or digitalis; the latter drug occasionally converts atrial flutter into AF. Once AV nodal conduction is slowed with any of these drugs, an attempt to convert flutter to sinus rhythm using quinidine or quinidine-like agents should be made. Increasing doses of the drug selected are administered until the rhythm converts or side effects occur.

Quinidine, quinidine-like drugs, flecainide, and amiodarone (Table 185-2) may be useful in preventing recurrences of both atrial flutter and atrial fibrillation.

PAROXYSMAL SUPRAVENTRICULAR TACHYCARDIAS (PSVT)   In most cases functional differences in conduction and refractoriness in the AV node or the presence of an AV bypass tract provide the substrate for the development of PSVT (previously termed *paroxysmal atrial tachycardia*). Electrophysiologic studies have demonstrated that reentry is the mechanism responsible for the vast majority of cases of PSVT (Fig. 185-4). Reentry has been localized to the sinus node, atrium, AV node, or to a macroreentrant circuit involving conduction in the antegrade direction through the AV node and retrograde through an AV bypass tract. Such a bypass tract may also conduct antegradely, in which case the Wolff-Parkinson-White (WPW) syndrome is said to be present. More frequently, however, the bypass tract manifests only retrograde conduction, and therefore it is termed a *concealed bypass tract* (Fig. 185-4*B*). In the absence of the WPW syndrome, reentry through the AV node or through a concealed bypass tract makes up more than 90 percent of all PSVTs.

AV NODAL REENTRANT TACHYCARDIA There is no age, sex, or disease predisposition for the development of AV nodal reentrant tachycardia, the most common cause of supraventricular tachycardia. It usually presents as a narrow QRS complex with regular rates ranging from 120 to 250 beats per minute. APCs that initiate the arrhythmia are almost always associated with a prolonged PR interval. Retrograde P waves may be absent, buried in the QRS complex, or appear as distortions at the terminal parts of the QRS complex (Fig. 185-4*A*).

AV nodal reentrant PSVT (Fig. 185-5) can be reproducibly initiated and terminated by appropriately timed atrial premature extrastimuli. The onset of the tachycardia is almost always associated with prolongation of the PR interval due to marked AV nodal conduction delay (prolonged AH interval) following the APC that is critical for the genesis of the arrhythmia. The sudden prolongation of the AH interval is consistent with the concept of dual AV nodal pathways: (1) A beta (fast) pathway, which exhibits rapid conduction and a long refractory period, and (2) an alpha (slow) pathway, which has a short refractory period but conducts slowly. During sinus rhythm only conduction over the fast pathway is manifest, resulting in a normal PR interval. The impulse which simultaneously conducts down the slow pathway reaches the His bundle after it has been depolarized and is therefore refractory. Atrial extrastimuli at a critical coupling interval are blocked in the beta pathway because of its longer refractory period and are conducted slowly through the alpha pathway. If conduction down the alpha pathway is slow enough to allow the previously refractory beta pathway time to recover excitability, a single atrial echo or sustained tachycardia ensues. A critical balance between conduction velocity and refractoriness within the node is required to sustain AV nodal reentry. Atrial and ventricular activation occur simultaneously, explaining why P waves may not be apparent on the surface ECG.

Clinical features AV nodal reentry may produce palpitations, syncope, and heart failure, depending on the rate and duration of the arrhythmia and the presence and severity of any underlying heart disease. Hypotension and syncope may occur because of the sudden loss of the atrial contribution to ventricular filling; this can also lead to a marked increase in atrial pressure, acute pulmonary edema, and a reduction in ventricular filling. Simultaneous atrial and ventricular contraction produces cannon *a* waves with each heartbeat.

Treatment In patients without hypotension, vagal maneuvers, particularly carotid sinus massage, can terminate the arrhythmia in 80 percent of cases. If hypotension is present, raising the blood pressure by the cautious use of intravenous phenylephrine may terminate the arrhythmia alone or in combination with carotid sinus pressure. If these maneuvers are unsuccessful, verapamil (2.5 to 10 mg intravenously) is the agent of choice. Propranolol (0.05 to 0.2 mg/kg, intravenously) or other beta blockers may be used to slow or terminate the tachycardia. Digitalis glycosides have a slower onset of action. When these drugs fail to terminate the tachycardia or when the tachycardia is recurrent, atrial or ventricular pacing via a temporary pacemaker inserted pervenously may be used to terminate the arrhythmia. However, if severe ischemia and/or hypotension is caused by the tachycardia, dc cardioversion should be considered.

AV nodal reentry can usually be prevented by the use of drugs

that act primarily on the antegrade slow pathway (such as digitalis, beta blockers, or calcium antagonists) or on the fast pathway (such as quinidine-like agents and newer drugs such as encainide, flecainide, and amiodarone). Drugs most likely to avert recurrences prevent induction of the arrhythmias by programmed stimulation. This technique utilizes temporary pacemaker catheters connected to a physiologic stimulator capable of variable rate pacing and stimulation with one or more precisely timed premature impulses. If episodes of PSVT are frequent and produce disabling symptoms, therapy based on electrophysiologic studies is preferable to empiric drug trials. In symptomatic patients who require therapy, antitachycardia pacemakers may be preferable to the daily administration of antiarrhythmic drugs, particularly if there are long tachycardia-free intervals. Ablation of the AV junction (p. 923) has been developed as a method of controlling AV nodal reentry, but this approach should only be considered as a last resort, since it usually mandates insertion of a permanent ventricular pacemaker.

AV REENTRANT TACHYCARDIA PSVT due to AV reentry incorporates an AV bypass tract that conducts only retrogradely as part of the tachycardia circuit. Thus, the impulse passes antegradely from the atria through the AV node and His-Purkinje system to the ventricles, then retrogradely through the (concealed) bypass tract back to the atrium. Patients with this disorder manifest the same type of PSVT as do patients with the WPW syndrome (see below), but the bypass tract cannot conduct in an antegrade direction during sinus rhythm or other atrial tachyarrhythmias.

AV reentrant tachycardia can be initiated and terminated by either APCs or VPCs. Alternation of the QRS complexes and/or T wave occurs in approximately one-third of such tachycardias. Since atrial activation must follow ventricular activation during AV reentry, the P wave usually occurs after the QRS complex (Fig. 185-4*B*).

Atrial activation mapping is of major value in evaluating the origin of these tachycardias. Most concealed bypass tracts are left-sided. Thus, during supraventricular tachycardia or during ventricular pacing, the earliest activation sequence is recorded in the left atrium, usually via a catheter in the coronary sinus (Fig. 185-6). This eccentric atrial activation is quite distinct from the normal retrograde activation sequence in which the earliest activation of the atria is in the area of the AV junction. The ability of a ventricular stimulus to conduct to the atrium at a time when the bundle of His is refractory and the termination of the tachycardia by a ventricular stimulus that does not reach the atrium are diagnostic of retrograde conduction over a concealed bypass tract.

Treatment is similar to that for AV nodal reentry tachycardia. However, in addition to pharmacologic therapy, patients with reentrant tachycardias involving concealed bypass tracts may be candidates for surgical ablation (p. 923).

SINUS NODE REENTRY AND OTHER ATRIAL TACHYCARDIAS Reentry in the region of the sinus node or within the atria is invariably initiated by APCs. These arrhythmias are less common than AV nodal or AV reentry and are more often associated with underlying cardiac disease. During sinus node reentry the P-wave morphology is identical to that occurring in sinus rhythm, but the PR interval is prolonged. This is in contrast to sinus tachycardia, in which the PR interval tends to shorten. With intraatrial reentry the P-wave configuration differs from that during sinus rhythm, and the PR interval is prolonged (Fig. 185-4*C*).

Treatment Sinus node and atrial reentrant arrhythmias are managed like other reentrant PSVTs.

NONREENTRANT ATRIAL TACHYCARDIAS These may be a manifestation of digitalis intoxication or may be associated with severe pulmonary or cardiac disease, with hypokalemia, or with the administration of theophylline or adrenergic drugs. The latter frequently present as multifocal atrial tachycardias (MAT). By definition, MAT requires ≥3 consecutive P waves of different morphologies at rates greater than 100 bpm. MAT usually has an irregular ventricular rate because of varying A-V conduction. Treatment should be directed at the underlying disorder. The digitalis-induced arrhythmias may be

TABLE 185-2 Drugs used to treat cardiac tachyarrhythmias

Drug	Sinus node	Atrium and ventricle	AV node	His-Purkinje system	Atrioventricular bypass tracts
ELECTROPHYSIOLOGIC EFFECTS					
Digoxin and other cardiac glycosides (also see p. 897)	No change; patients with sinus node disease may develop sinus exit block or arrest	Controversial	Increase in ERP; decreased conduction velocity	No change	No change or decrease in ERP
Propranolol and other beta-adreno-receptor blockers (also see p. 968)	Decreased sinus rate; increased sinus node recovery time	No change	Increase in ERP; decreased conduction velocity	No change	No change
Verapamil	Decreased sinus rate; sinus exit block in patients with sinus node disease	No change	Increase in ERP; decreased conduction velocity	No change	Indirect effects may decrease ERP when given IV
Quinidine	No change; may suppress sinus node in patients with underlying sinus node disease	Increased ERP; decreased conduction velocity	Decrease or no change in ERP, no change in conduction velocity	Decreased automaticity; decreased conduction velocity; increased ERP	Increased ERP may abolish all conduction
Procainamide	No change	Increased ERP; decreased conduction velocity	Decrease or no change in ERP; decrease or no change in conduction velocity	Decreased automaticity; decreased conduction velocity; increased ERP	Increased ERP may abolish all conduction
Disopyramide	No change	Increased ERP; decreased conduction velocity	Decrease or no change in ERP; no change in conduction velocity	Decreased automaticity; increased ERP; decrease conduction velocity	Increased ERP may abolish all conduction
Lidocaine	No change	No change in ERP	No change or decrease in ERP	No change or decrease in ERP	No change, decrease, or increase in ERP
Phenytoin	No change	No change in ERP	No change or decrease in ERP No change or increased conduction velocity	Decrease in ERP; decreased automaticity	
Tocainide	No change	No change	No change	No change; decreased automaticity	Increase in ERP
Bretylium	Initial increase in sinus rate followed by decrease	Increase in ERP	No change	No change	
Amiodarone	Decreased sinus rate	Increased ERP	Increased ERP; decreased conduction velocity	Increased ERP; decreased conduction velocity	Increased ERP
Mexiletine	No change; patients with sinus node disease may develop sinus arrest	No change	Variable and inconsistent effects on conduction and refractoriness	Increased ERP; no change or decreased conduction velocity	
Encainide	No change	Decreased conduction velocity; increase in ERP (oral therapy only)	Decreased conduction velocity; increase in ERP	Decreased conduction velocity	Decreased conduction velocity; increase in ERP; may abolish all conduction
Flecainide	No change; patients with sinus node disease may develop exit block or arrest	Decreased conduction velocity; increase in ERP	Decreased conduction velocity; increase in ERP	Decreased conduction velocity	Decreased conduction velocity; increase in ERP; may abolish all conduction

NOTE: AV = atrioventricular, ERP = effective refractory period, IV = intravenous, SVT = supraventricular tachycardia, VT = ventricular tachycardia, AF = atrial fibrillation, VF = ventricular fibrillation.

TABLE 185-2 Drugs used to treat cardiac tachyarrhythmias (*continued*)

Indications	Side effects and toxicity
CLINICAL EFFECTS	
Slowing of ventricular rate during AF, flutter, and other atrial tachycardias in the absence of preexcitation; SVT due to AV nodal reentry and AV reentry utilizing bypass tracts	Atrial tachycardia, VT, AV nodal block, accelerated junctional rhythms, atrial and ventricular premature depolarizations, VT, VF, anorexia, nausea, vomiting; acceleration of ventricular rate during AF/flutter in the presence of preexcitation causing VF
Slowing of ventricular rate during AF, atrial flutter, and other atrial tachycardias in the absence of preexcitation; SVT due to AV nodal reentry, rentry utilizing bypass tracts; arrhythmias induced by exercise; arrhythmias occurring in the presence of hyperthyroidism; polymorphic VT associated with congenital long QT syndrome	Sinus bradycardia, AV nodal block, congestive heart failure, bronchospasm, masking symptoms of hypoglycemia
Same as digoxin	Sinus arrest in patients with sinus node dysfunction; AV nodal block in patients with AV nodal dysfunction; exacerbation of congestive heart failure (may be potentiated in presence of beta-adrenergic blocking agents); elevation of digoxin levels; hypotension following IV administration; IV administration during AF/flutter in the presence of preexcitation may cause acceleration of ventricular response rate and VF or hemodynamic collapse; IV administration to patients with VT may cause hemodynamic collapse
Atrial and ventricular extrasystoles; atrial and ventricular tachyarrhythmias; all types of SVT; control of ventricular rate in patients with preexcitation and AF and flutter	Anorexia, nausea, vomiting, diarrhea; cinchonism: tinnitus, confusion, hearing and visual changes; thrombocytopenia, hemolytic anemia, rash; drug interactions: elevation of digoxin levels; phenytoin and phenobarbital will decrease quinidine levels; QT prolongation associated with polymorphic VT (torsade de pointes); conversion of nonsustained to sustained VT; acceleration of ventricular response to atrial flutter and fibrillation
Same as quinidine	Anorexia, nausea, confusion, hallucinations; agranulocytosis; lupus erythematosus-like syndrome; QT prolongation associated with polymorphic VT (torsade de pointes); marked elevations in the primary metabolite (NAPA) may be more likely to cause polymorphic VT; conversion of nonsustained into sustained VT; acceleration of ventricular response to atrial flutter and fibrillation
Same as quinidine	Anticholinergic actions including dry mouth, blurred vision, urinary retention or hesitancy, constipation, narrow angle glaucoma; congestive heart failure, especially in patients with abnormal ventricular function; QT prolongation associated with polymorphic VT (torsade de pointes)
VT and VF especially during acute ischemia and myocardial infarction	Dizziness, paresthesias, confusion, delirium, seizures, coma; may depress sinus node in patients with underlying sinus node disease; may suppress escape foci in patients with complete heart block; congestive heart failure or liver disease increase risk of side effects
Tachyarrhythmias induced by digitalis; occasionally effective for ventricular tachyarrhythmias not induced by digitalis alone or in combination with other antiarrhythmic agents; polymorphic VT associated with increased QT	Gingival hypertrophy, rash, blood dyscrasias, nystagmus, ataxia, stupor, coma, lupus erythematosus syndrome, lymph node hyperplasia, peripheral neuropathy, hypocalcemia, hyperglycemia, phlebitis and hypotension during IV administration
VT, VF, frequent VPCs	Ataxia, tremor, paresthesias, light-headedness, nausea, rash, lupus erythematosus syndrome, pulmonary fibrosis, bone marrow suppression; may exacerbate heart failure in patients with ventricular dysfunction
Refractory ventricular VT and VF, especially due to acute ischemia	Initially, transient hypertension; subsequently, hypotension increased in the upright position; the hypotensive effect can be prevented by tricyclic drugs; nausea, vomiting
Refractory atrial and ventricular tachyarrhythmias; refractory SVT due to AV nodal reentry and AV reentry utilizing bypass tracts; not approved by FDA for atrial arrhythmias	Marked sinus bradycardia, complete heart block; IV administration may cause hypotension; increased QT associated with polymorphic VT; increased T_4, hypo- and hyperthyroidism; peripheral neuropathy; proximal myopathy; pulmonary fibrosis; increased liver enzymes, hepatitis; photodermatitis, blue-gray skin discoloration; corneal microdeposits; elevation of digoxin levels; potentiation of oral anticoagulants
Ventricular tachyarrhythmias	Nausea, vomiting, ataxia, tremor, gait disturbances, rash
Refractory atrial and ventricular tachyarrhythmias; SVT due to AV node reentry and AV bypass tracts; not approved by FDA for supraventricular arrhythmias	Refractory polymorphic VT without increased QT if dose is increased too rapidly or in patients with abnormal left ventricular function; AV block in patients with abnormal conduction system; sinus arrest in patients with abnormal sinus node function; nausea, dizziness, blurred vision. May precipitate heart failure in patients with ventricular dysfunction
Same as encainide; not approved by FDA for supraventricular arrhythmias	Same as encainide

FIGURE 185-4 Examples of reentrant PSVT. *A.* AV nodal reentry. No P waves are visible. *B.* AV reentry using a concealed bypass tract. Inverted retrograde P waves are superimposed on the T wave. *C.* Intraatrial reentry. P waves precede the QRS complex.

caused by triggered activity and/or enhanced automaticity. In such atrial tachycardias with AV block secondary to digitalis intoxication (Fig. 185-1B), the atrial rate rarely exceeds 180 per minute, and typically 2:1 block is present. Atrial arrhythmias precipitated by digitalis can usually be treated by withdrawal of the drug.

Automatic atrial tachycardias not caused by digitalis are difficult to terminate, and in such cases the main goal of therapy should be to control the ventricular response, either by drugs which affect the AV node, such as digitalis, beta blockers, or calcium channel antagonists, or by ablation techniques. Surgery has been employed in resistant cases.

PREEXCITATION (WPW) SYNDROME The most frequently encountered type of ventricular preexcitation is that associated with AV bypass tracts. These connections are composed of strands of atrial-like muscle which may occur almost anywhere around the AV rings. The term *Wolff-Parkinson-White (WPW) syndrome* is applied to patients with both preexcitation on the ECG and paroxysmal tachycardias. AV bypass tracts can be associated with certain congenital abnormalities, the most important of which is Ebstein's anomaly.

AV bypass tracts that conduct in an antegrade direction produce a typical ECG pattern of a short PR interval (<0.12 s), a slurred upstroke of the QRS complex (delta wave), and a wide QRS complex. This pattern results from a fusion of activation of the ventricles over both the bypass tract and the AV nodal His-Purkinje system (Fig.

185-7). The relative contribution of activation over each system determines the amount of preexcitation.

During PSVT in WPW the impulse is usually conducted antegradely over the normal AV system and retrogradely through the bypass tract. The characteristics are identical to those described on p. 913. Rarely (approximately 5 percent), tachycardias occurring in patients with WPW will exhibit a reverse pattern with antegrade conduction through the bypass tract and retrograde conduction through the normal AV system. This produces a tachycardia with a wide QRS complex in which the ventricles are totally activated by the bypass tract. Atrial flutter and AF also occur commonly in patients with WPW syndrome. Since the bypass tract does not have the same decremental conducting properties as the AV node, the ventricular responses during atrial flutter or fibrillation may be unusually rapid (Fig. 185-1E) and may cause ventricular fibrillation.

The goals of electrophysiologic evaluation in patients suspected of having the WPW syndrome are (1) to confirm the diagnosis; (2) to localize the bypass tract and determine how many bypass tracts are present; (3) to demonstrate the role of the bypass tract in the genesis of the arrhythmias; (4) to determine the potential for the development of possibly life-threatening rates during atrial flutter or fibrillation; and (5) to evaluate therapeutic options, such as specific pharmacologic agents, pacing therapy, and surgery.

Management This should be aimed at (1) decreasing the occurrence of the APCs and VPCs responsible for the initiation of the

FIGURE 185-5 Mechanism of AV nodal reentry: The atrium, AV node (AVN), and His bundle are shown schematically. The AV node is longitudinally dissociated into two pathways, with different functional properties. The alpha pathway conducts relatively slowly while the beta pathway conducts rapidly (see text). In each panel of this diagram, heavy lines denote excitation in the AV node which is manifest on the surface electrocardiogram, while light lines denote conduction which is concealed and not apparent on the surface electrocardiogram. *A.* During sinus rhythm (NSR) the impulse from the atrium conducts down both pathways. However, only conduction over the fast (beta) pathway is manifest on the surface ECG, producing a normal PR interval of 0.16 s. *B.* An atrial premature depolarization (APD) blocks in the beta

pathway. The impulse conducts over the alpha pathway to the His bundle and ventricles, producing a PR interval of 0.24 s. Because the impulse is premature, conduction over the alpha pathway occurs more slowly than it would during sinus rhythm. *C.* A more premature atrial impulse blocks in the beta pathway, conducting with increased delay in the alpha pathway, producing a PR interval of 0.28 s. The impulse conducts retrogradely up the beta pathway producing a single atrial echo. Sustained reentry is prevented by subsequent block in the alpha pathway. *D.* A still more premature atrial impulse blocks initially in the beta pathway, conducting over the alpha pathway with increasing delay producing a PR interval of 0.36 s. Retrograde conduction occurs over the beta pathway and reentry occurs, producing a sustained tachycardia (SVT).

FIGURE 185-6 Intracardiac recordings during supraventricular tachycardia using a left-sided AV bypass tract. Intracardiac recordings during sinus rhythm (NSR) in supraventricular tachycardia (SVT) are shown. ECG leads I, aVF, and V₁ are displayed with electrograms from the high right atrium (HRA), coronary sinus (CS), His bundle (HBE), and right ventricle (RV). During NSR, the QRS complex and the AH and HV intervals are normal. During SVT the retrograde atrial activation sequence is abnormal. The earliest site of atrial activation is in the CS, which is followed by activation in the HBE and HRA. This activation sequence is diagnostic of a left-sided AV bypass tract conduction retrogradely from ventricle to atrium [From ME Josephson, in Update IV, Harrison's Principles of Internal Medicine, KJ Isselbacher et al (eds), New York, McGraw-Hill, 1983; used with permission.]

tachycardia; (2) increasing the refractory period of the bypass tract (refractory periods <250 ms are associated with rapid ventricular responses during AF); and (3) blocking conduction down the normal AV conduction system. Specific antiarrhythmic therapy can be assessed by electrophysiologic studies, as described on p. 921.

In patients with the WPW syndrome and AF, dc cardioversion should be carried out if there is a life-threatening, rapid ventricular response. Alternatively, lidocaine (3 to 5 mg/kg) or procainamide (15 mg/kg) administered intravenously over 15 to 20 min will usually slow the ventricular response. Caution should be employed when using digitalis or verapamil in patients with the WPW syndrome and AF, since these drugs can shorten the refractory period of the accessory pathway and can increase the ventricular rate, thereby placing the patient at increased risk for ventricular fibrillation. In addition to these drugs, beta blocking agents are of no utility in controlling the ventricular response during AF when conduction proceeds over the bypass tract. Although atrial or ventricular pacing can almost always terminate PSVT in patients with the WPW syndrome, they can induce AF. Successful surgical ablation of bypass tracts is possible in more than 90 percent of cases (p. 923) and offers a permanent cure of SVT and most AF associated with SVT.

Acute management of episodes of PSVT in patients with WPW syndrome is similar to that of PSVT in patients with concealed bypass tracts.

NONPAROXYSMAL JUNCTIONAL TACHYCARDIA
This rhythm usually results from conditions that produce enhanced automaticity or triggered activity in the AV junction and is most commonly due to digitalis intoxication, inferior wall myocardial infarction, myocarditis, endogenous or exogenous catecholamine excess, acute rheumatic fever, or aftereffects of valve surgery.

The onset of nonparoxysmal junctional tachycardia is usually gradual with a "warm-up" period prior to stabilization of the rate, which can range from 70 to 150 per minute, with faster rates usually associated with digitalis intoxication. Nonparoxysmal junctional tachycardia is recognized by a QRS complex identical to that of sinus rhythm. The rate can be influenced by autonomic tone and can be increased by catecholamines, vagolytic agents, or exercise and slowed somewhat by carotid sinus pressure. When this rhythm is due to digitalis intoxication, it usually is associated with AV block and/or dissociation. Early after cardiac surgery, retrograde conduction is more likely to be present due to heightened sympathetic state.

Management This is directed toward elimination of the underlying etiologic factors. Since digitalis is the most common cause of this rhythm, discontinuation of this drug is indicated. If the rhythm is associated with other serious manifestations of digitalis intoxication,

such as ventricular or atrial irritability, active intervention with lidocaine or a beta blocker may be useful, and in some instances use of digitalis antibodies (Fab fragments) should be considered. Cardioversion of this rhythm should not be attempted, particularly in the setting of digitalis intoxication. When AV conduction is intact, atrial pacing can capture and override the junctional focus and provide the AV synchrony necessary to maximize cardiac output. Nonparoxysmal junctional tachycardia usually is not a chronic, recurrent problem, and attention to the acute precipitating events can often resolve the tachycardia.

VENTRICULAR TACHYCARDIA (VT)
Sustained VT is defined as *ventricular tachycardia* that persists for more than 30 s or requires termination because of hemodynamic collapse. VT generally accompanies some form of structural heart disease, most commonly chronic ischemic heart disease associated with a prior myocardial infarction. Sustained VT may also be associated with nonischemic cardiomy-

FIGURE 185-7 ECG in WPW syndrome. There is a short PR interval (0.11s), a wide QRS complex (0.12 s), and slurring on the upstroke of the QRS produced by early ventricular activation over the bypass tract (delta wave, d in lead I). The negative delta waves in V₁ are diagnostic of a right-sided bypass tract. Note the Q wave (negative delta wave) in lead III, mimicking myocardial infarction.

FIGURE 185-8 Ventricular tachycardia with AV dissociation. P waves which are totally dissociated from the underlying ventricular rhythm can be noted in lead III. AV dissociation is highly suggestive of ventricular tachycardia. In V_1 fusion complexes are present, confirming AV dissociation.

opathies, metabolic disorders, drug toxicity, or prolonged QT syndrome, and it occurs occasionally in the absence of heart disease or other predisposing factors. Nonsustained VT (3 beats to 30 s) is also associated with cardiac disease but occurs in its absence more often than the sustained arrhythmia. While nonsustained VT usually does not produce symptoms, sustained VT is almost always symptomatic and is often associated with marked hemodynamic embarrassment and/or the development of myocardial ischemia. A fixed anatomic substrate, not acute ischemia, is responsible for most recurrent episodes of sustained VT. Acute ischemia appears to have little role in the genesis of sustained uniform VT associated with chronic infarction but may play a role in the degeneration of stable VT into ventricular fibrillation (VF). Most episodes of VF begin with VT.

The ECG diagnosis of VT is suggested by a wide-complex tachycardia at a rate exceeding 100 per minute. While the rhythm is usually quite regular, slight irregularity may exist. Atrial activity may be dissociated from ventricular activity (Fig. 185-8), or the atria may be depolarized retrogradely. The onset of the tachycardia is generally abrupt, but in nonparoxysmal tachycardias it can be gradual. The QRS configuration during any episode of VT may be uniform (monomorphic) (Figs. 185-2B and 185-9), or it may vary from beat to beat (polymorphic) (Fig. 185-2C). *Bidirectional tachycardia* refers to VT that shows an alternation in QRS amplitude and direction. Paroxysmal VT is usually initiated by a VPC.

It is important to distinguish supraventricular tachycardia with aberration of intraventricular conduction from VT since the clinical implications and management of these two arrhythmias are totally different. It is always useful to have a 12-lead ECG recorded during

sinus rhythm for comparison with that during the tachycardia. When the tracing obtained during sinus rhythm demonstrates a bundle branch block pattern with the same morphologic features as those during the tachycardia, the diagnosis of supraventricular tachycardia is favored. An infarction pattern on the sinus rhythm tracing suggests the potential presence of the anatomic substrate necessary for VT. Characteristics of the 12-lead ECG during the tachycardia that suggest a ventricular origin for the arrhythmia are (1) a QRS complex >0.14 s in the absence of antiarrhythmic therapy; (2) AV dissociation or variable retrograde conduction; (3) a superior QRS axis; (4) concordance of the QRS pattern in all precordial leads (i.e., all positive or all negative deflections); and (5) other QRS patterns with prolonged duration that are inconsistent with typical right or left bundle branch block patterns. A wide, complex, bizarre tachycardia that is very irregular suggests AF with conduction over an AV bypass tract (p. 916). Similarly, a QRS complex in excess of 0.20 s is uncommon during VT in the absence of drug therapy and is more common with preexcitation. Intravenous verapamil will stop most recalcitrant supraventricular tachycardias involving the AV junction, but it is rarely effective for ventricular tachycardia. Because of this property, verapamil has been utilized to attempt to differentiate supraventricular tachycardia with deviant conduction from ventricular tachycardia. However, this is extremely hazardous, since intravenous verapamil frequently precipitates cardiac arrest in patients with ventricular tachycardias.

The diagnosis of VT can be confirmed by analyzing the relationship between the electrogram recording from the His bundle and ventricular activity. In most cases of VT, the His deflection is not easily seen, but when visible, the interval from the His deflection to the onset of ventricular activation (HV interval) is less than that recorded during sinus rhythm, or negative due to retrograde activation over the His-Purkinje system, or it is dissociated from ventricular activation (Fig. 185-10). During SVT with aberrant conduction the HV interval is greater than or equal to that recorded during sinus rhythm. In patients with a wide QRS complex tachycardia, the diagnosis of VT is confirmed when atrial pacing at rates equal to or greater than that of the tachycardia produces normalization of the QRS complex with a normal HV interval. Regardless of QRS morphology [left or right bundle branch block patterns (Fig. 185-9)], VT due to ischemic heart disease arises from the *left* ventricle, in most instances near the subendocardium.

It has been possible to replicate sustained uniform VT in more than 95 percent of patients with this arrhythmia using programmed stimulation. In most patients the tachycardia is initiated with ventricular premature stimuli. A sustained monomorphic VT with a morphology identical to that of the spontaneous arrhythmia is the rule.

FIGURE 185-9 *A.* Sustained ventricular tachycardia having a uniform morphology. The QRS configuration in V_1 is a right bundle branch block type of configuration. Marked leftward frontal plane axis is present, denoted by the QS complex in lead II. The R/S ratio in lead V_6 is less than 1. The QRS width is greater than 140 ms. Note that 2:1 VA conduction is present with retrograde P waves present after every other QRS complex (best seen in leads I and V_1). *B.* Sustained ventricular tachycardia with a uniform, left bundle branch block type morphology (lead V_1). The QRS width is greater than 160 ms, and there are a Q wave in lead V_6 and a broad initial R wave in V_1, all favoring ventricular tachycardia rather than supraventricular tachycardia with aberrant conduction.

FIGURE 185-10 Intracardiac recordings distinguishing supraventricular tachycardia from ventricular tachycardia. ECG leads I, aVF, and V_1 are shown with a His bundle electrogram (HBE) and time line (TL). Wide QRS complex tachycardia with a right bundle branch block morphology are shown on the left and right panels. On the left, supraventricular tachycardia is diagnosed by the presence of His deflection (H) preceding each QRS complex, with normal HV interval. On the right, during ventricular tachycardia no His bundle deflections can be seen (arrow) and AV dissociation is observed (note single atrial deflection, A). (*From JA Kastor et al, N Engl J Med 304:1004, 1981; reprinted by permission.*)

The clinical significance of polymorphic VT initiated by programmed stimulation is not clear. It has been shown that when more aggressive stimulation is performed (i.e., the use of three or four extrastimuli), polymorphic VT and even VF can be induced in some normal subjects and in patients who have never had a clinical arrhythmia.

Sustained uniform VT can be terminated by programmed stimulation or rapid pacing in at least 75 percent of patients; the remainder require cardioversion. The ability to initiate and terminate a sustained, uniform VT reproducibly permits assessment of pharmacologic and electrical therapy of these arrhythmias. Serial testing of antiarrhythmic agents over a period of several days can be accomplished and predicts the likelihood of success of the agents or devices tested (page 921).

The reproducible termination of VT by programmed stimulation permits evaluation of the effectiveness of antitachycardia pacemakers for long-term therapy of paroxysmal episodes of arrhythmia. Unfortunately, rapid pacing, the most effective form of therapy, can accelerate the tachycardia and/or produce ventricular fibrillation.

Clinical features Symptoms resulting from VT depend on the ventricular rate, duration of the tachycardia, and presence and extent of underlying cardiac disease. When the tachycardia is rapid and associated with severe myocardial dysfunction and cerebrovascular disease, hypotension and syncope are common. However, the presence of hemodynamic stability does not preclude a diagnosis of VT. The loss of the atrial contribution to ventricular filling and an abnormal sequence of ventricular activation are important factors producing a decreased cardiac output during VT.

The *prognosis* of VT depends on the underlying disease state. If sustained VT develops within the first 6 weeks following acute myocardial infarction, the prognosis is poor, with an 85 percent mortality rate at 1 year. Patients with nonsustained VT following myocardial infarction have a threefold greater risk of death than a comparable group of patients without this arrhythmia. However, a cause-and-effect relationship between the nonsustained tachycardia and subsequent sudden death has not been established.

Management The risk-benefit ratio of treating each specific type of VT should be considered before beginning therapy. This is important because antiarrhythmic agents can produce or exacerbate the very arrhythmias which they are given to prevent. In general, patients with VT but without organic heart disease have a benign course; such patients with asymptomatic, nonsustained VT need not be treated since their prognosis will not be affected. Patients with sustained VT in the absence of heart disease usually require therapy because the arrhythmia causes symptoms. These tachycardias may respond to beta blockers, verapamil, or quinidine-like agents. In patients with VT and organic heart disease, if marked hemodynamic embarrassment is present or if there is evidence of ischemia, congestive heart failure, or central nervous system hypoperfusion, the rhythm should be promptly terminated by dc cardioversion (see below). If the patient with organic heart disease tolerates the VT well, pharmacologic therapy may be tried. Procainamide is probably the most effective agent for acute therapy. It may or may not terminate the tachycardia, but almost always slows the rate. In stable patients in whom these drugs do not terminate the arrhythmia, a pacing catheter can be inserted pervenously into the right ventricular apex, and the tachycardia can be terminated by overdrive pacing.

Use of programmed stimulation is probably the most efficacious way to select the appropriate antiarrhythmic agent to prevent recurrent, sustained VT. In a controlled situation, drugs can be serially studied, and the drug that prevents initiation of the tachycardia can be selected; long-term successful prevention of the arrhythmia can then be expected in 90 percent of patients (see p. 921).

Antitachycardia pacing has been used as a means to terminate drug-resistant tachycardia. This usually requires that the tachycardia be stable and slow and the patient be aware of it. No automatic antitachycardia device has been approved for therapy of VT at the time of this writing because pacing during VT may accelerate tachycardia, converting a stable arrhythmia into an unstable one, resulting in severe hemodynamic compromise. However, availability of a new device, the automatic implantable cardioverter defibrillator (AICD) (see below) affords a "backup" means of terminating unstable arrhythmias. Radiofrequency pacemakers, which are best activated by a physician, have been used in occasional patients.

The advent of endocardial catheter and intraoperative mapping has led to the development of new surgical techniques for the management of VT. Activation mapping permits localization of the site of origin of the arrhythmia. In centers in which expertise in mapping is available, operation has been successfully employed to cure tachycardias in the majority of patients in whom it has been undertaken. Even though most patients with VT and ischemic heart disease have markedly impaired left ventricular function and multivessel coronary artery disease, the operative mortality rate has ranged between 8 and 15 percent. Following operation, 85 to 90 percent of survivors are controlled either off (two-thirds of patients) or on (one-third) antiarrhythmic agents that were previously ineffective in controlling these rhythms.

Specific types of VT TORSADE DE POINTES Torsade de pointes ("twisting of the points") (Fig. 185-11) refers to VT characterized by polymorphic QRS complexes that change in amplitude and cycle length, giving the appearance of oscillations around the baseline. This rhythm is by definition associated with QT prolongation. The latter may result from electrolyte disturbances (particularly hypokalemia and hypomagnesemia), use of a variety of antiarrhythmic drugs (especially quinidine), phenothiazines and tricyclic antidepressants, liquid protein diets, intracranial events, and bradyarrhythmias, particularly third-degree AV block. It may also occur as an isolated idiopathic congenital or acquired anomaly.

The electrocardiographic hallmark is polymorphic VT preceded by marked QR prolongation, often in excess of 0.60 s. These patients often have multiple episodes of nonsustained polymorphic VT associated with recurrent syncope, but they may also develop VF and sudden cardiac death.

Therapy should be directed at removing the precipitating factors, i.e., correcting metabolic abnormalities and removing drugs which have induced the prolonged QT interval. In the setting of drug-induced torsade de pointes, atrial or ventricular overdrive pacing and the administration of magnesium have also been useful in terminating and preventing the arrhythmia. For patients with the congenital prolonged QT interval syndrome, beta-adrenergic blocking agents have been the mainstay of therapy; agents which shorten the QT interval may also be useful (e.g., phenytoin). Cervicothoracic sympathectomy has been proposed as a form of therapy for congenital prolonged QT syndrome, but it is not often effective as the sole therapy.

Polymorphic tachycardias associated with normal QT intervals in patients with ischemic heart disease that are initiated by "R-on-T" VPCs are probably caused by reentry, and their treatment is totally different. This is not true "torsade de pointes." In such cases, quinidine-like agents may be the most effective form of therapy and should be administered in full antiarrhythmic doses. However, these arrhythmias may also result from acute, severe ischemia and will only respond to abolition of the ischemia, usually by revascularization.

FIGURE 185-11 Torsade de pointes. During sinus rhythm (lead II) a markedly prolonged QT interval was present. Lead V₁ shows polymorphic VT.

FIGURE 185-12 Ventricular fibrillation. In a patient with coronary disease ventricular fibrillation is initiated by a VPC that produces a rapid polymorphic ventricular tachycardia which rapidly degenerates to ventricular fibrillation (note the undulating baseline with indistinguishable systole and diastole).

ACCELERATED IDIOVENTRICULAR RHYTHM　This arrhythmia, also termed slow VT, with a rate which ranges from 60 to 120 per minute, usually occurs in acute myocardial infarction, often during reperfusion. It may also be seen following cardiac operations, in patients with cardiomyopathy, rheumatic fever, or digitalis intoxication, as well as in patients with no evidence of heart disease. The rhythm is usually transient and rarely causes significant hemodynamic compromise or symptoms.

Treatment is rarely necessary and should usually be considered only if symptoms arise due to impaired hemodynamics, most commonly due to AV dissociation. In most cases, atropine can accelerate the sinus rate to overdrive the ventricular rhythm.

VENTRICULAR FLUTTER AND VENTRICULAR FIBRILLATION (VF)　(Fig. 185-12; see also Chap. 40). Ventricular flutter and VF occur most often in patients with ischemic heart disease. They also occur following administration of antiarrhythmic drugs, particularly those which induce prolonged QT intervals and torsade de pointes (see above), with severe hypoxia or ischemia, and in patients with WPW who develop AF with an extremely rapid ventricular response (page 916). Electrical accidents frequently cause cardiac arrest due to the development of VF. The onset of these arrhythmias is rapidly followed by loss of consciousness and, if untreated, death. Episodes of cardiac arrest recorded during Holter monitoring reveal that approximately three-fourths of the sudden deaths are due to VT or VF.

In patients with VF, the onset almost always begins with a short run of rapid VT, which is initiated by a relatively late coupled VPC. In patients with acute myocardial infarction or ischemia, however, VF is usually precipitated by a single early ventricular complex beat falling on the T wave (the vulnerable period), which produces a rapid VT which degenerates into VF (Fig. 185-9).

The clinical setting in which VF occurs is important, since most patients who have primary VT within the first 48 h of the onset of acute infarction have a good prognosis, with a very low rate of recurrence or sudden cardiac death. In contrast, most patients who experience VF unassociated with the development of acute myocardial infarction have a recurrence rate of 20 to 30 percent in the year following the event (see Chap 40).

Ventricular flutter usually appears as a sine wave with a rate between 150 and 300 beats per minute. These oscillations make it impossible to assign a specific morphology to the arrhythmia and in some cases to distinguish it from rapid VT. VF is recognized by grossly irregular undulations of varying amplitudes, contours, and rates (Fig. 185-12). Electrophysiologic studies have demonstrated that regardless of the apparent gross irregularity on the surface ECG, VF usually starts out with the rapid repetitive sequence of VT which ultimately breaks down into multiple wavelets of reentry.

Electrophysiologic studies have been useful in patients who have been resuscitated from cardiac arrest. Programmed stimulation has demonstrated that in approximately 70 percent of such patients one can reproducibly initiate a sustained VT. Treatment is discussed in Chap. 40.

PHARMACOLOGIC ANTIARRHYTHMIC THERAPY

Prior to initiation of pharmacologic antiarrhythmic therapy, potential aggravating factors such as transient metabolic abnormalities, conges- tive heart failure, or acute ischemia must be corrected and in some cases may suffice to control arrhythmias. In addition, the potential role of drugs as a cause of exacerbating factor in the development of the arrhythmia must be considered.

Antiarrhythmic drugs are used in three principal situations: (1) to terminate an acute arrhythmia, (2) to prevent recurrence of an arrhythmia, and (3) to prevent a life-threatening arrhythmia for which the patient is perceived to be at risk, but which has never occurred.

Most currently available antiarrhythmic agents have a relatively low toxic/therapeutic ratio; all can exert proarrhythmic effects, and therefore they may exacerbate underlying arrhythmias. Serum levels can be determined for most currently available antiarrhythmic agents. Standards for therapeutic and toxic levels can serve only as a rough guide for selecting the appropriate dose in any individual patient. In the final analysis, the therapeutic level in a given patient is that concentration which achieves the desired antiarrhythmic effect, and the toxic level for each patient is that concentration at which undesirable side effects occur. Since many adverse effects are directly related to drug concentrations, the minimal serum level which achieves an effective antiarrhythmic response should be chosen.

In order to determine the therapeutic level for a patient, one must have a standard to judge drug efficacy. For a patient with an incessant arrhythmia, antiarrhythmic drugs may be administered empirically until the arrhythmia is suppressed. If a reproducible precipitating factor such as exercise can be identified, serial drug testing during such a provocative maneuver may be performed. Unfortunately, most arrhythmias are sporadic and occur unpredictably without identifiable precipitating factors. In these cases, if one waits to observe sponta- neous recurrences on each antiarrhythmic drug, assessment of drug efficacy may require months. This type of assessment of efficacy may be adequate for arrhythmias which are not life-threatening. However, this mode of assessment is inadequate for arrhythmias that compromise hemodynamic stability, result in syncope, or cause cardiac arrest. In such cases two methods for determination of arrhythmic drug efficacy have been utilized. The first, which consists of continuous ECG monitoring in the control state and then in the presence of antiarrhythmic drugs, has been used in order to determine the effect that each drug has on spontaneous atrial or ventricular ectopy. This method presupposes that the mechanism responsible for sustained arrhythmias is the same as that causing isolated premature depolarizations (which may or may not be true) and that therefore eradication of isolated ectopy will correlate with prevention of sustained arrhythmias. This method has a number of limitations. First, patients frequently show marked degrees of spontaneous variation in frequency of ectopy, which may mimic antiarrhythmic drug effects. Second, 25 to 30 percent of patients with sustained ventricular arrhythmias such as VT or VF demonstrate only rare spontaneous ectopy. Finally, many patients demonstrate a dissociation between the effects of antiarrhythmic agents on spontaneous ectopy and the effects of the same agent on sustained arrhythmias.

An alternative method to assess drug efficacy is programmed stimulation. Numerous studies have demonstrated that most clinically occurring supraventricular and ventricular tachyarrhythmias may be reproducibly initiated and terminated safely using this technique. Studies are performed initially in a baseline state in the absence of antiarrhythmic drugs (Fig. 185-13). If the patient's clinical arrhythmia can be reproducibly initiated, then the ability of individual anti- arrhythmic drugs to prevent reinduction of the arrhythmia can be

Control **230/min**

Lidocaine 5.1 μg/mL **240/min**

Phenytoin 17.8 μg/mL **230/min**

Procainamide 14.8 μg/mL

Quinidine 4.8 μg/mL

Disopyramide 6.5 μg/mL **190/min**

FIGURE 185-13 Selections of an effective antiarrhythmic drug for ventricular tachycardia by programmed stimulation. From top to bottom, the effects of programmed stimulation during the control state and following administration of several antiarrhythmic agents. During the control state two ventricular extrastimuli initiate the ventricular tachycardia at a rate of 230 per minute. Lidocaine, phenytoin, and disopyramide at the plasma levels shown failed to prevent induction of the tachycardia. Both procainamide and quinidine at the plasma levels shown prevented initiation of sustained tachycardia. Chronic oral quinidine therapy effectively prevented recurrences of the arrhythmia. *(From JA Kastor et al, N Engl J Med 304:1004, 1981; reprinted by permission.)*

assessed either after the drug is administered intravenously or after several days of oral loading in order to achieve a steady state serum concentration. Use of this method assumes that (1) the induced and spontaneous arrhythmias are identical, and (2) prevention of induction of arrhythmias will correlate with prevention or recurrent spontaneous tachycardias on the same drug regimen. This technique has been validated in patients with a variety of reentrant PSVTs, VT, and VF. The technique is safe when carefully performed, the potential complications being those of any intravascular catheterization. Appropriate interpretation of the results of programmed stimulation is critically dependent on correlating the patient's spontaneous arrhythmias with those induced in the laboratory, with regard to rate and morphology.

A number of classifications of antiarrhythmic drugs have been proposed, the most frequently used of which is a modification of that proposed by Vaughn-Williams (Table 185-1). This classification is based in part on the ability of antiarrhythmic drugs to modify the cardiac cellular (1) excitatory currents (Na^+ or Ca^{2+}), (2) action potential duration, and (3) automaticity (phase 4 depolarization). These effects of the drugs on isolated cardiac cells are thought to account for some of the antiarrhythmic properties of the drugs. Thus, depression of excitatory currents by type I and type IV antiarrhythmics results in slowing of conduction velocity and may interrupt arrhythmias by blocking conduction in areas of marginal excitability, where conduction velocity is already slow. Type III antiarrhythmics allegedly exert their action by increasing refractoriness through prolongation of the action potential duration. However, such classifications are limited in that the electrophysiologic effects of these drugs in vivo may differ from their effects on isolated cells. Also the effects of heart rate and fiber geometry are not considered. The uses and actions of currently available antiarrhythmic drugs are summarized in Tables 185-2 and 185-3.

ELECTRICAL THERAPY OF TACHYARRHYTHMIAS

PACEMAKERS Cardiac pacing can be used to terminate and in selected cases prevent recurrent supraventricular and ventricular arrhythmias. Because many tachyarrhythmias appear to be due to a reentrant mechanism with the impulse traveling in a circuit, a properly timed paced impulse can penetrate and prematurely depolarize part of the circuit, rendering it refractory to the next circulating wavefront, thereby interrupting the circus movement. Pacing therapy for arrhythmias is generally reserved for patients whose arrhythmias are refractory to the next circulating wavefront, thereby interrupting the circus movement. Pacing therapy for arrhythmias is generally reserved for patients whose arrhythmias are refractory to drug therapy and who remain hemodynamically stable during the tachycardia. All forms of pacing therapy require repeated demonstration of their effectiveness and reliability in terminating the arrhythmias during electrophysiologic testing prior to implantation of the pacing device.

The type of pacing device and modality selected for arrhythmia termination depend on (1) the rate of the tachycardia (rates >160 per minute are rarely terminated by a single premature stimulus); (2) the type of the arrhythmia (atrial flutter and VT are rarely terminated by single extrastimuli); and (3) concomitant drug therapy. Underdrive pacing, i.e., pacing at a rate slower than the tachycardia, can be used when a single premature stimulus has been demonstrated to reproducibly terminate a tachycardia. It is rarely used today since pacemakers are available which can deliver timed stimuli or an increasing number of stimuli.

Because many tachycardias cannot be terminated by single premature stimuli, pacemakers have been developed which allow for multiple extrastimuli (burst pacing) to be introduced. In reentrant tachycardias involving an accessory AV connection, sequential, near simultaneous activation of the heart from both the atria and the ventricle using a dual-chamber pacemaker will increase the likelihood of bidirectional block and termination of the tachycardia.

Cardiac pacing has also been used to prevent ventricular tachyarrhythmias. Polymorphic VT associated with a long QT interval and bradycardia (torsade de pointes, p. 919) is most likely to respond. Pacing the atrium and/or ventricle at rates between 90 and 120 per minute appears to increase the homogeneity of electrical recovery and markedly reduces the propensity for a recurrence of arrhythmias. Regardless of the arrhythmia being treated and the pacing mode selected, the potential for alterations in pacing requirements for termination of tachycardia and therefore programmability of pacing modes (e.g., underdrive, dual-demand, dual-chamber, burst), as well as rate and coupling interval of introduced extrastimuli, are probably essential features for pacemakers used to terminate tachycardias.

Pacemakers may be self-contained or energized by an external radiofrequency source. The self-contained pacemaker may function

TABLE 185-3   Dose, serum half-life ($t_\frac{1}{2}$) following oral administration, and route of metabolism of drugs used in treatment of arrhythmias

Drug	Mode of administration	$t_\frac{1}{2}$ (oral), h	Route of metabolism
Digoxin	IV, 0.75–1.5 mg Oral, 0.75–1.5 mg loading dose over 12–24 h Maintenance, 0.25–0.50 mg/d	36	Renal
Propranolol	IV, 0.5–1 mg/min to total dose of 0.15–0.2 mg/kg Oral, 10–200 mg q 6 h	3–6	Hepatic
Verapamil	IV, 2.5–10 mg over 1–2 min to total 0.15 mg/kg Oral, 80–120 mg q 6–8 h	3–8	Hepatic
Quinidine	IV, 20 mg/min to total 10–15 mg/kg Oral, 200–400 mg q 6 h	5–9	Hepatic
Procainamide	IV, 40–50 mg/min to total 10–20 mg/kg Oral, 500–1000 mg q 4 h	3–5	Hepatic-renal
Disopyramide	Oral, 100–300 mg q 6–8 h	8–9	Renal
Lidocaine	IV, 20–50 mg/min to total dose of 5 mg/kg loading followed by 1–4 mg/min	1–2	Hepatic
Phenytoin	IV, 20 mg/min total dose to 1000 mg Oral, 1000 mg loading over 24 h Maintenance, 100–400 mg/d	18–36	Hepatic
Tocainide	Oral, 400 to 600 mg q 8–12 h	10–17	Hepatic-renal
Bretylium	IV, 1–2 (mg/kg)/min to total load 5–10 mg/kg Maintenance, 0.5–2 mg/min	8–14	Renal
Amiodarone	IV, 5–10 mg/kg Oral, load 800–1400 mg/d for 1–2 weeks Maintenance, 100–600 mg/d	Unknown	Hepatic
Mexiletine	Oral, 100–300 mg q 6–8 h	9–12	Hepatic
Encainide	Oral, begin at 25 mg tid; at 3 to 5-day intervals may increase to 35 mg tid and then 50 mg tid	1–2 active metabolites: 3–4 and 6–12	Hepatic—active metabolite excreted by kidneys
Flecainide	Oral, begin at 50–100 mg bid; increase by no more than 50 mg not more often than every 4 days to a maximum of 400 mg daily	7–23	Hepatic-renal

automatically [i.e., it incorporates an arrhythmia recognition program (circuit)], or it may be activated by an external magnet. The major advantage of a fully automatic system is that there is no need for the patient to recognize the arrhythmia in order for termination to occur. The advantages of the externally activated system include (1) the decreased risk of unnecessary treatment because of faulty sensing; and (2) the opportunity to initiate monitoring at the time of attempted termination of arrhythmia. This type of monitoring is frequently helpful if pacing techniques are employed to terminate VT, given the risk of acceleration of the arrhythmia by pacing.

The limitations of pacing therapy are primarily related to (1) the changes in the characteristics of the arrhythmia over time such that programmed pacing parameters no longer terminate the tachycardia; and (2) the risk of acceleration of the tachycardia with the development of AF when stimulating the atrium and the development of rapid VT and VF when stimulating the ventricles. Future pacing generators which can also deliver a larger amount of energy and perform cardioversion and defibrillation of accelerated arrhythmias are likely to increase the applicability of pacing therapy for the treatment of arrhythmias.

CARDIOVERSION AND DEFIBRILLATION   Electrical cardioversion and defibrillation remain the most reliable methods for terminating arrhythmias. By depolarizing all or at least a large portion of excitable myocardium in a near homogeneous fashion, the electrical shock can interrupt reentrant arrhythmias. External cardioversion is routinely performed by placing two paddles 12 cm in diameter in firm contact with the chest wall, with one paddle usually located to the right of the sternum at the level of the second rib and the other in the left midclavicular line in the fifth intercostal space. If the patient is conscious, a short-acting barbiturate to act as an anesthetic or an amnesic drug such as diazepam should be administered to prevent patient discomfort. A person skilled in maintaining an airway should be present. Energy is delivered synchronously with the QRS complex for all arrhythmias except ventricular flutter and VF, since asynchron-

ous shocks can produce VF. The amount of energy used will vary with the type of tachycardia being treated. With the exception of AF, supraventricular tachycardias can frequently be terminated with energy levels in the range of 25 to 50 W·s, while AF usually requires ≥100 W·s for termination. For terminating VT, energy levels ≥100 W·s should probably be employed. While energies as low as 25 W·s may be successfully used, they also have a higher incidence of producing VF. At least 200 W·s of energy should be used for initial attempts at terminating VF. If the initial shock fails, all repeated attempts at defibrillation should be with the maximum energy that the defibrillator is capable of delivering (320 to 400 W·s).

Indications for cardioversion depend upon the clinical setting and the patient's general condition. Any tachycardia (except sinus tachycardia) that produces hypotension, myocardial ischemia, or heart failure warrants consideration of prompt termination using external cardioversion. Arrhythmias that fail to terminate with pharmacologic therapy may also be terminated by electrical cardioversion. Transient bradycardias and supraventricular and ventricular irritability following cardioversion are common and usually do not warrant antiarrhythmic intervention.

AUTOMATIC INTERNAL DEFIBRILLATION   An automatic implanted cardioverter-defibrillator device has been developed to allow for prompt recognition and termination of life-threatening ventricular arrhythmias. The device delivers 25 to 33 W·s of energy. Clinical trials testing the function of the device in patients with drug-refractory ventricular arrhythmias have demonstrated survival from sudden death at 1 year ranging between 92 and 100 percent. Based on the results of the initial trials, it appears that an automatic sensing, implanted cardioverter-defibrillator will play an important role in management of life-threatening arrhythmias. At the time of this writing, use of this device should be reserved for patients with VT which is not hemodynamically tolerated or for patients with VF whose arrhythmias are refractory to drug therapy and who are not candidates for surgical intervention (see below). The most frequent problem with the device has been its inappropriate discharge in the absence of sustained ventricular arrhythmias. Additional potential problems include an increase in defibrillation threshold and decrease in tachycardia rates below the rate cut-off of the device in response to many antiarrhythmic drugs. Permanently implanted ventricular pacemakers may interfere with the device's ability to sense VF.

CATHETER ABLATION FOR ARRHYTHMIAS Catheter ablation of tachyarrhythmias, a technique that involves the delivery of large amounts of energy (25 to 400 W·s) through a catheter to effect closed-chest electroablation of the bundle of His, has been primarily used to interrupt AV conduction and prevent a rapid ventricular response to supraventricular arrhythmias. Although not yet approved by the Food and Drug Administration, catheter ablation of the AV junction has become the procedure of choice for creating AV block to control refractory supraventricular arrhythmias. However, the possible introduction of complete heart block necessitating a pacemaker and the small risk of sudden death associated with the procedure make catheter ablation a procedure of "last resort" at this time. This procedure is also under investigation for ablation of ventricular tachycardia and AV bypass tract tachycardia.

SURGICAL TREATMENT OF ARRHYTHMIAS

Programmed stimulation and endocardial activation mapping have provided a better understanding of the mechanisms and sites of origin of many supraventricular and ventricular tachyarrhythmias, so that in selected patients surgical treatment may be considered.

WOLFF-PARKINSON-WHITE SYNDROME Surgery may be preferable to other forms of therapy in some patients, particularly those with recurrent arrhythmias. Advances made in the localization and surgical ablation of bypass tracts now allow for an extremely high success rate with minimal morbidity. As a result, surgery can now be considered not only in patients with drug-refractory arrhythmias but also as a reasonable alternative in (1) patients with symptomatic arrhythmias who require long-term drug therapy; (2) patients with AF and a life-threatening rapid ventricular response; and (3) patients undergoing cardiac surgery for other reasons in whom a bypass tract is present.

SUPRAVENTRICULAR TACHYCARDIA AND OTHER ATRIAL ARRHYTHMIAS Although atrial flutter, AF, and PSVT are usually not life-threatening, they may be refractory to pharmacologic or pacing interventions. In such cases surgery may be considered as a method of removing the abnormal focus, interrupting the reentry circuits, and curing the tachycardia or controlling the ventricular response by creating AV block. In atrial flutter and AF the pathophysiologic substrate cannot be identified; thus, the only surgical option is to destroy the AV node–His bundle region by cryosurgery or transvenous catheter electroablation. Surgery, cryoablation, or electrode catheter ablation requires concomitant implantation of a permanent pacemaker. Focal atrial tachycardias have been treated surgically by discrete resection or ablation by cryothermal injury. Mapping the tachycardia is mandatory if a primary direct approach on the arrhythmia is to be performed. Surgery is for patients with arrhythmias refractory to other treatments and only when the tachycardia has been localized.

VENTRICULAR TACHYCARDIA The demonstration that VT due to ischemic heart disease can often be reliably induced by programmed stimulation and that the arrhythmia is localized to a small region of endocardium in the area of prior infarction has permitted the development of specific surgical techniques for the cure of the arrhythmia.

Preoperatively all morphologically distinct tachycardias that occur spontaneously are induced by programmed stimulation, and their respective sites of origin are determined by catheter activation mapping. Catheter mapping may be supplemented by intraoperative mapping, involving similar techniques. These studies have shown that tachycardias arise in the scar tissue near the endocardium.

Subendocardial resection and endocardial encircling ventriculo-tomy or cryoablation, the surgical techniques that have been applied to the management of ventricular tachycardia, are aimed at removing or isolating the pathophysiologic substrate of the arrhythmia, as identified by mapping. The major criterion for surgical success is the ability to localize the site from which the arrhythmias arise.

REFERENCES

ANDERSON JL: Effectiveness of sotalol for therapy of complex ventricular arrhythmias and comparisons with placebo and Class I antiarrhythmic drugs. Am J Cardiol 65(2):37, 1990

BAR FW et al: Differential diagnosis of tachycardia with narrow QRS complex (shorter than 0.12 seconds). Am J Cardiol 54:555, 1984

BHANDARI AK, SCHEINMAN M: The long QT syndrome. Mod Concepts Cardiovasc Dis 54:45, 1985

BOINEAU JP: Atrial flutter: A synthesis of concepts. Circulation 72:249, 1985

——, COX JL: Rationale for a direct surgical approach to control ventricular arrhythmias. Relation of specific intraoperative techniques for mechanism and location of arrhythmia circuit. Am J Cardiol 49:381, 1982

BREITHARDT G et al: *Nonpharmacological Therapy of Tachyarrhythmias*. Mt Kisco, NY, Futura, 1987

BRUGADA P, WELLENS HJJ (eds): *Cardiac Arrhythmias: Where To Go from Here?* Mt Kisco, NY, Futura, 1987

BURDITT DG, BENSON DW: *Cardiac Preexcitation Syndromes*. Boston, Martinus Nijhoff, 1986

FRAME LN, HOFFMAN BF: Mechanisms of tachycardia, in *Tachycardias*, B Surawicz (ed). Boston, Martinus Nijhoff, 1984

—— et al. Atrial reentry around an anatomic barrier with a partially refractory excitatory gap. Circ Res 58:495, 1986

JOSEPHSON ME: Paroxysmal supraventricular tachycardia: An electrophysiologic approach. Am J Cardiol 41:1123, 1978

——, SEIDES SF: *Clinical Cardiac Electrophysiology: Techniques and Interpretations*. Philadelphia, Lea & Febiger, 1979

——, WELLENS HJJ (eds): *Tachycardias: Mechanisms, Diagnosis, Treatment*. Philadelphia, Lea & Febiger, 1984

KUPPERMANN M, et al: An analysis of the cost effectiveness of the implantable defibrillator. Circulation 81(1):91, 1990

MANOLIS AS, ESTES, NAM III: Value of programmed ventricular stimulation in the evaluation and management of patients with nonsustained ventricular tachycardia associated with coronary artery disease. Am J Cardiol 65(3):201, 1990

WARD DE, CAMM AJ: *Clinical Electrophysiology of the Heart*. Baltimore, Edward Arnold, 1987

WINKLE RA, THOMAS A: The automatic implantable cardioverter defibrillator: The U.S. Experience, in *Cardiac Arrhythmias: Where to Go from Here?* Brugada P, Wellens HJJ (eds). Mt Kisco, NY, Futura, 1987

186 CONGENITAL HEART DISEASE

WILLIAM F. FRIEDMAN / JOHN S. CHILD

Congenital heart disease complicates approximately 1 percent of all live births. Substantial numbers of affected infants reach adulthood because of successful medical and/or surgical management, or because the alteration in cardiovascular physiology caused by the defect is well tolerated.

GENERAL CONSIDERATIONS

ETIOLOGY AND PREVENTION Congenital cardiovascular malformations are generally the result of aberrant embryonic development of a normal structure, or failure of such a structure to progress beyond an early stage of embryonic or fetal development. Malformations are due to complex multifactorial genetic and environmental causes. Recognized chromosomal aberrations and mutations of single genes account for less than 10 percent of all cardiac malformations (Table 186-1).

The presence of a cardiac malformation as one component of the multiple system involvement in Down's, Turner's, and the trisomy 13-15(D₁) and 17-18 (E) syndromes may be anticipated in occasional pregnancies by detection of abnormal chromosomes in fetal cells obtained from amniotic fluid or chorionic villus biopsy. Identification in such cells of the enzyme disorders characteristic of Hurler's

TABLE 186-1 Syndromes with associated cardiovascular involvement

Syndrome	Major cardiovascular manifestations	Major noncardiac abnormalities
HERITABLE AND POSSIBLY HERITABLE		
Ellis–van Creveld	Single atrium or atrial septal defect	Chondrodystrophic dwarfism, nail dysplasia, polydactyly
TAR (thrombocytopenia-absent radius)	Atrial septal defect, tetralogy of Fallot	Radial aplasia or hypoplasia, thrombocytopenia
Holt-Oram	Atrial septal defect (other defects common)	Skeletal upper limb defect, hypoplasia of clavicles
Kartagener	Dextrocardia	Situs inversus, sinusitis, bronchiectasis
Laurence-Moon-Biedl	Variable defects	Retinal pigmentation, obesity, polydactyly
Noonan	Pulmonary valve dysplasia, cardiomyopathy (usually hypertrophic)	Webbed neck, pectus excavatum, cryptorchidism
Tuberous sclerosis	Rhabdomyoma, cardiomyopathy	Phakomatosis, bone lesions, hamartomatous skin lesions
Multiple lentigines (leopard) syndrome	Pulmonic stenosis	Basal cell nevi, broad facies, rib anomalies
Rubenstein-Taybi	Patent ductus arteriosus (others)	Broad thumbs and toes, hypoplastic maxilla, slanted palpebral fissures
Familial deafness	Arrhythmias, sudden death	Sensorineural deafness
Osler-Rendu-Weber	Arteriovenous fistulas (lung, liver, mucous membranes)	Multiple telangiectasia
Apert	Ventricular septal defect	Craniosynostosis, midfacial hypoplasia, syndactyly
Incontinentia pigmenti	Patent ductus arteriosus	Irregular pigmented skin lesions, patchy alopecia, hypodontia
Alagille (arteriohepatic dysplasia)	Peripheral pulmonic stenosis, pulmonic stenosis	Biliary hypoplasia, vertebral anomalies, prominent forehead, deep-set eyes
DiGeorge	Interrupted aortic arch, tetralogy of Fallot, truncus arteriosus	Thymic hypoplasia or aplasia, parathyroid aplasia or hypoplasia, ear anomalies
Friedreich's ataxia	Cardiomyopathy and conduction defects	Ataxia, speech defect, degeneration of spinal cord dorsal columns
Muscular dystrophy	Cardiomyopathy	Pseudohypertrophy of calf muscles, weakness of trunk and proximal limb muscles
Cystic fibrosis	Cor pulmonale	Pancreatic insufficiency, malabsorption, chronic lung disease
Sickle cell anemia	Cardiomyopathy, mitral regurgitation	Hemoglobin SS
Conradi-Hünermann	Ventricular septal defect, patent ductus arteriosus	Asymmetric limb shortness, early punctate mineralization, large skin pores
Cockayne	Accelerated atherosclerosis	Cachectic dwarfism, retinal pigment abnormalities, photosensitivity dermatitis
Progeria	Accelerated atherosclerosis	Premature aging, alopecia, atrophy of subcutaneous fat, skeletal hypoplasia
CONNECTIVE TISSUE DISORDERS		
Cutis laxa	Peripheral pulmonic stenosis	Generalized disruption of elastic fibers, diminished skin resilience, hernias
Ehlers-Danlos	Arterial dilatation and rupture, mitral regurgitation	Hyperextensible joints, hyperelastic and friable skin
Marfan	Aortic dilatation, aortic and mitral incompetence	Gracile habitus, arachnodactyly with hyperextensibility, lens subluxation
Osteogenesis imperfecta	Aortic incompetence	Fragile bones, blue sclera
Pseudoxanthoma elasticum	Peripheral and coronary arterial disease	Degeneration of elastic fibers in skin, retinal angioid streaks
INBORN ERRORS OF METABOLISM		
Pompe's disease	Glycogen storage disease of heart	Acid maltase deficiency, muscular weakness
Homocystinuria	Aortic and pulmonary arterial dilatation, intravascular thrombosis	Cystathionine synthetase deficiency, lens subluxation, osteoporosis
Mucopolysaccharidosis:		
Hurler, Hunter	Multivalvular and coronary and great artery disease, cardiomyopathy	Hurler: Deficiency of α-L-iduronidase, corneal clouding, coarse features, growth and mental retardation Hunter: Deficiency of L-iduranosulfate sulfatase, coarse facies, clear cornea, growth and mental retardation
Morquio, Scheie, Maroteaux-Lamy	Aortic incompetence	Morquio: Deficiency of N-acetylhexosamine sulfate sulfatase, cloudy cornea, normal intelligence, severe bony changes involving vertebrae and epiphyses Scheie: Deficiency of α-L-iduronidase, cloudy cornea, normal intelligence, peculiar facies Maroteaux-Lamy: Deficiency of arylsulfatase B, cloudy cornea, osseous changes, normal intelligence

TABLE 186-1 Syndromes with associated cardiovascular involvement (*continued*)

Syndrome	Major cardiovascular manifestations	Major noncardiac abnormalities
CHROMOSOMAL ABNORMALITIES		
Trisomy 21 (Down's syndrome)	Endocardial cushion defect, atrial or ventricular septal defect, tetralogy of Fallot	Hypotonia, hyperextensible joints, mongoloid facies, mental retardation
Trisomy 13 (D)	Ventricular septal defect, patent ductus arteriosus, double-outlet right ventricle	Single midline intracerebral ventricle with midfacial defects, polydactyly, nail changes, mental retardation
Trisomy 18 (E)	Congenital polyvalvular dysplasia, ventricular septal defect, patent ductus arteriosus	Clenched hand, short sternum, low-arch dermal-ridge pattern on fingertips, mental retardation
Cri-du-chat (short-arm deletion-5)	Ventricular septal defect	Cat cry, microcephaly, antimongoloid slant of palpebral fissures, mental retardation
XO (Turner)	Coarctation of aorta, bicuspid aortic valve	Short female, broad chest, lymphedema, webbed neck
XXXY and XXXXX	Patent ductus arteriosus	XXXY: hypogenitalism, mental retardation, radial-ulnar synostosis XXXXX: small hands, incurving of fifth fingers, mental retardation
SPORADIC DISORDERS		
VATER association	Ventricular septal defect	Vertebral anomalies, anal atresia, tracheo-esophageal fistula, radial and renal anomalies
CHARGE association	Tetralogy of Fallot (other defects common)	Colobomas, choanal atresia, mental and growth deficiency, genital and ear anomalies
Williams	Supravalvular aortic stenosis, peripheral pulmonic stenosis	Mental deficiency, "elfin" facies, loquacious personality, hoarse voice
Cornelia de Lange	Ventricular septal defect	Micromelia, synophrys, mental and growth deficiency
Shprintzen (velocardiofacial)	Ventricular septal defect, tetralogy of Fallot, right aortic arch	Cleft palate, prominent nose, slender hands, learning disability
TERATOGENIC DISORDERS		
Rubella	Patent ductus arteriosus, pulmonic valvular and/or arterial stenosis, atrial septal defect	Cataracts, deafness, microcephaly
Alcohol-induced	Ventricular septal defect (other defects)	Microcephaly, growth and mental deficiency, short palpebral fissures, smooth philtrum, thin upper lip
Phenytoin-induced	Pulmonic stenosis, aortic stenosis, coarctation, patent ductus arteriosus	Hypertelorism, growth and mental deficiency, short phalanges, bowed upper lip
Thalidomide-induced	Variable	Phocomelia
Lithium-induced	Ebstein's anomaly, tricuspid atresia	None

syndrome, homocystinuria, or type II glycogen storage disease may also allow one to predict cardiac disease.

The feasibility of preventive programs will depend upon what is learned in the future about the cause of the majority of cardiovascular anomalies for which no cause is known. An effective rubella vaccine is available, and immunization of children with this vaccine may lessen maternal rubella and its cardiac consequences. Strict testing in animals of new drugs that can be teratogenic when taken early in pregnancy may reduce the chances of another thalidomide tragedy. In this regard, no medications should be taken during pregnancy without prior consultation with a physician. Physicians should be aware of known teratogens, as well as of drugs for which inadequate information exists as to teratogenic potential. Appropriate use of radiologic equipment and techniques for reducing gonadal and fetal radiation exposure should always be employed to reduce the hazards of birth defects.

PATHOPHYSIOLOGY The anatomic and physiologic changes in the heart and circulation due to any specific congenital cardiocirculatory lesion are not static, but rather progress from prenatal life to adulthood. Thus, malformations which are benign, or escape detection in childhood, may become clinically significant in the adult. For example, the functionally normal, congenitally bicuspid aortic valve may thicken and calcify with time, resulting in significant aortic stenosis; or the well-tolerated left-to-right shunt of an atrial septal defect may not result in cardiac decompensation, with or without pulmonary hypertension, until the fourth or fifth decade.

There are issues of particular concern to the *adult* with congenital heart disease that we will discuss separately in this chapter, including pulmonary hypertension and Eisenmenger syndrome of pulmonary vascular obstruction, the hematologic consequences of cyanotic heart disease, the special considerations of pregnancy in the woman with congenital heart disease, and problems involving employability and insurability.

Pulmonary hypertension This is a common accompaniment of many congenital cardiac lesions, and the status of the pulmonary vascular bed is often the principal determinant of the clinical manifestations, the course, and the feasibility of surgical repair. Increases in pulmonary arterial pressure result from elevation of pulmonary blood flow and/or resistance, the latter due sometimes to an increase in vascular tone but usually the result of obstructive, obliterative structural changes within the pulmonary vascular bed. Because pulmonary vascular obstructive disease can be the factor limiting a decision concerning the advisability of operation, it is important to quantify and compare pulmonary to systemic flows and resistances in patients with severe pulmonary hypertension. The causes of pulmonary vascular obstructive disease are unknown, although increased pulmonary blood flow, increased pulmonary arterial blood pressure, elevated pulmonary venous pressure, polycythemia, systemic hypoxemia, acidosis, and the bronchial circulation have been implicated. The designation *Eisenmenger syndrome* is applied to patients with a large communication between the two circulations at the aortopulmonary, ventricular, or atrial levels and bidirectional or predominantly right-to-left shunts because of high-resistance and obstructive pulmonary hypertension. No specific treatment has proved beneficial for obstructive pulmonary vascular disease.

Erythrocytosis This is a physiologic response to chronic hypoxemia. The extremely high hematocrits observed in patients with marked arterial oxygen unsaturation cause a progressive increase in blood viscosity, especially beyond packed red blood cell volumes of 60 percent. Both the hematocrit and the circulating whole blood volume are increased in the polycythemia accompanying cyanotic congenital heart disease; the hypervolemia is the result of an increase in red cell volume. The latter provides an increased oxygen-carrying capacity and enhanced oxygen supply to the tissues. The compensatory polycythemia is often of such severity that it becomes a liability and produces adverse physiologic effects, such as thrombotic lesion in diverse organs and a hemorrhagic diathesis. In this regard, oral steroid contraceptives are contraindicated in the cyanotic female because of the enhanced risk of vascular thrombosis. Red cell volume reduction and replacement with plasma or albumin (erythropheresis) lowers blood viscosity and increases systemic blood flow and oxygen transport and so may be helpful in the management of patients with severe hypoxic polycythemia. Acute phlebotomy without fluid replacement is contraindicated. Repeated phlebotomy may cause depletion of iron stores and excessive production of microcytic erythrocytes that are less deformable, thereby raising blood viscosity and adversely influencing blood flow in the microcirculation, respectively.

PREGNANCY The presence of congenital heart disease or its consequences may pose special problems for the pregnant woman. Thus, pregnant women with pulmonary vascular obstruction, whether pre- or postoperative, are at risk of dying during delivery or in the immediate postpartum period. The cause of the increased mortality rate is poorly understood. A particularly high mortality rate has been reported for those undergoing a cesarean section, although such surgery should cause less cardiovascular stress than that of labor and vaginal delivery. Irrespective of approach to delivery, some simple guidelines include both continuous administration of oxygen and avoidance of inhalant anesthetic agents. Arterial blood gases and, if possible, pulmonary arterial and systemic blood pressure should be monitored serially throughout delivery and the early postpartum period. Some physicians advise early abortion in women with marked pulmonary vascular obstruction because of the risks of pregnancy, and all such women should receive counseling on birth control. Intrauterine devices should be avoided because of the risks of bleeding and infection; oral contraceptive agents are contraindicated because they are associated with a tendency to develop pulmonary vascular or cerebrovascular thrombosis. Use of a barrier method of birth control is preferable. Prevention of pregnancy is safer than any form of management during pregnancy, labor, delivery, and the postpartum period.

In women with regurgitant or obstructive left-side valvular lesions the increased volume and/or pressure load on the left atrium or left ventricle imposed by the augmentation in blood volume during pregnancy may result in pulmonary edema, requiring vigorous cardiac decongestive measures (Chap. 36). With medical control of the pulmonary edema, a normal vaginal delivery with careful local and epidural anesthesia is preferable to nonvaginal delivery.

A unique problem exists in women whose congenital heart disease has been corrected with the use of a prosthetic cardiac valve and/or conduit. Such women are at risk for thromboembolism and/or obstruction of their conduits or valves, and are thus, usually, on anticoagulants. Early in pregnancy coumarin derivatives cause an increase in abortion and stillbirth and in craniofacial, neurologic, and other birth defects. Moreover, the transplacental passage of oral anticoagulants places the fetus at risk of intracranial hemorrhage during delivery. Accordingly, coumarin derivatives should be avoided early (before 10 weeks) and late (after 32 weeks) in pregnancy, and subcutaneous or intravenous heparin should be substituted, although heparin, to a lesser degree, also has been associated with adverse fetal outcome.

INFECTIVE ENDOCARDITIS (See also Chap. 90) Postsurgical patients with prosthetic heterograft or homograft valves or conduits are at particular risk of infective endocarditis. Although routine antimicrobial prophylaxis is recommended for all patients with congenital heart disease and for the majority of patients after operative repair of the lesion, it should be recognized that antibiotic prophylaxis is not uniformly effective. Nonetheless, it is recommended for all dental procedures, gastrointestinal and genitourinary surgery, and diagnostic procedures such as proctosigmoidoscopy and cystoscopy. The risk of endocarditis is undoubtedly related both to the magnitude of bacteremia and to the type of underlying heart disease. Since infection on a prosthetic heart valve or conduit may be devastating, combinations of antibiotics given prophylactically by parenteral route are advisable in these patients.

INSURABILITY Most patients with congenital heart disease must pay significantly more than standard life insurance rates, assuming their anomaly places them in a category that companies have determined is eligible for insurance. There is a paucity of actuarial survival data beyond adolescence for most cardiac lesions that have undergone operative repair. Accordingly, it is often difficult to convince insurance companies to offer insurance at reasonable cost to individual patients whose long term prognosis is quite good.

SPECIFIC CARDIAC DEFECTS

Various classifications of congenital cardiovascular lesions have been proposed, depending on hemodynamic, anatomic, and radiographic factors. Table 186-2 provides a classification of cardiac anomalies that recognizes the general categories of clinical presentation, functional consequences, and site of origin of congenital defects. The text of this section focuses selectively on the more common or important congenital cardiac malformations in adults, whereas Table 186-2 presents a comprehensive list of lesions. Cardiac lesions are organized into those which do or do not result in cyanosis. The acyanotic group is subdivided into malformations with and without a left-to-right shunt. The shunt lesions are segregated by the principal site of communication between the systemic and pulmonary circulations. The acyanotic lesions without a shunt are distinguished by the location of the lesion in the left or right heart and by inflow versus outflow regions on either side of the circulation. Cyanotic lesions are classified with respect to pulmonary blood flow, since the radiographic determination of the magnitude of the latter provides an insight into whether the cyanosis is the result of an obligatory admixture of systemic and pulmonary venous return (increased pulmonary blood flow) or of reduced pulmonary blood flow.

Categorizing the defect(s) in an individual patient requires an answer to a number of basic questions. Is the patient acyanotic or cyanotic? Is pulmonary arterial blood flow increased or not? Does the malformation originate in the left or right side of the heart? Which is the dominant ventricle? Is pulmonary hypertension present or not? With the above information as a foundation, using more refined diagnostic techniques such as echocardiography and Doppler imaging, magnetic resonance imaging, and/or hemodynamic study and angiocardiography leads to a precise anatomic and functional assessment.

TABLE 186-2 Classification of congenital heart disease

GENERAL

Congenitally corrected transposition of the great arteries
The cardiac malpositions
Congenital complete heart block

ACYANOTIC WITH LEFT-TO-RIGHT SHUNT

Atrial level shunt:
  1 Atrial septal defect
    a Ostium primum
    b Ostium secundum
    c Sinus venosus
  2 Atrial septal defect with mitral stenosis (Lutembacher's syndrome)
  3 Partial anomalous pulmonary venous connection

Ventricular level shunt:
  1 Ventricular septal defect
    a Inlet septum
    b Muscular septum
    c Perimembranous septum
    d Infundibular septum
  2 Ventricular septal defect with aortic regurgitation
  3 Ventricular septal defect with left ventricular to right atrial shunt

Aortic root to right heart shunt:
  1 Ruptured sinus of Valsalva aneurysm
  2 Coronary arteriovenous fistula
  3 Anomalous origin of the left coronary artery from the pulmonary trunk

Aortopulmonary level shunt:
  1 Aortopulmonary window
  2 Patent ductus arteriosus

Multiple level shunts:
  1 Complete common atrioventricular canal
  2 Ventricular septal defect with atrial septal defect
  3 Ventricular septal defect with patent ductus arteriosus

ACYANOTIC WITHOUT A SHUNT

Left heart malformations:
  1 Congenital obstruction to left atrial inflow
    a Pulmonary vein stenosis
    b Mitral stenosis
    c Cor triatriatum
  2 Mitral regurgitation
    a Atrioventricular septal (Endocardial cushion)
    b Congenitally corrected transposition of the great arteries
    c Anomalous origin of the left coronary artery from the pulmonary trunk
    d Miscellaneous (double-orifice mitral valve, congenital perforations, accessory commissures with anomalous chordal insertion, congenitally short or absent chordae, cleft posterior leaflet, parachute mitral valve, etc.)
  3 Primary dilated endocardial fibroelastosis
  4 Aortic stenosis
    a Discrete subvalvular
    b Valvular
    c Supravalvular
  5 Aortic valve regurgitation
  6 Coarctation of the aorta

Right heart malformations:
  1 Acyanotic Ebstein's anomaly of the tricuspid valve
  2 Pulmonic stenosis
    a Subinfundibular
    b Infundibular
    c Valvular
    d Supravalvular (stenosis of pulmonary artery and its branches)
  3 Congenital pulmonary valve regurgitation
  4 Idiopathic dilatation of the pulmonary trunk

CYANOTIC

Increased pulmonary blood flow:
  1 Complete transposition of the great arteries
  2 Double-outlet right ventricle of the Taussig-Bing type
  3 Truncus arteriosus
  4 Total anomalous pulmonary venous connection
  5 Single ventricle without pulmonic stenosis
  6 Common atrium
  7 Tetralogy of Fallot with pulmonary atresia and increased collateral arterial flow
  8 Tricuspid atresia with large ventricular septal defect and no pulmonic stenosis
  9 Hypoplastic left heart (aortic atresia, mitral atresia)

TABLE 186-2 Classification of congenital heart disease
(*continued*)

CYANOTIC (*continued*)

Normal or decreased pulmonary blood flow:
  1 Tricuspid atresia
  2 Ebstein's anomaly with right-to-left atrial shunt
  3 Pulmonary atresia with intact ventricular septum
  4 Pulmonic stenosis or atresia with ventricular septal defect (tetralogy of Fallot)
  5 Pulmonic stenosis with right-to-left atrial shunt
  6 Complete transposition of the great arteries with pulmonic stenosis
  7 Double-outlet right ventricle with pulmonic stenosis
  8 Single ventricle with pulmonic stenosis
  9 Pulmonary arteriovenous fistula
  10 Vena caval to left atrial communication

SOURCE: Modified from JK Perloff, in *The Clinical Recognition of Congenital Heart Disease*, 3d ed. Philadelphia, Saunders, 1987.

ACYANOTIC CONGENITAL HEART DISEASE WITH A LEFT-TO-RIGHT SHUNT

ATRIAL SEPTAL DEFECT This is a commonly recognized cardiac anomaly in adults, and occurs more frequently in females than in males. Defects of the *sinus venosus* type occur high in the atrial septum near the entry of the superior vena cava, and are associated frequently with anomalous connection of pulmonary veins from the right lung to the junction of the superior vena cava and right atrium. Sinus venosus defects may also occur low in the atrial septum near the inferior vena cava orifice, associated with anomalous connection of the right inferior pulmonary vein to the right atrium. *Ostium primum* anomalies are a form of atrioventricular septal defect that lie immediately adjacent to the atrioventricular valves, either of which may be deformed and incompetent. Ostium primum defects occur commonly in patients with Down's syndrome, although the more complex atrioventricular septal defects with a common atrioventricular valve and a posterior defect of the basal portion of the interventricular septum are more characteristic of this chromosomal defect. Most often an atrial defect involves the fossa ovalis, is midseptal in location, and is of the *ostium secundum* type. This type of defect should not be confused with a *patent foramen ovale*. Anatomic obliteration of the foramen ovale ordinarily follows its functional closure soon after birth, but residual "probe patency" is a normal variant; atrial septal defect denotes a true deficiency of the atrial septum, and implies functional and anatomic patency. *Lutembacher's syndrome* is the term applied to the rare combination of atrial septal defect and mitral stenosis; this component of the malformation is usually the result of acquired rheumatic valvulitis.

The magnitude of the left-to-right shunt through an atrial septal defect depends on the size of the defect, the diastolic properties of both ventricles, and the relative impedance in the pulmonary and systemic circulations. The left-to-right shunt causes diastolic overloading of the right ventricle, and increased pulmonary blood flow.

Patients with atrial septal defect are usually asymptomatic in early life, although there may be some physical underdevelopment and an increased tendency for respiratory infections; cardiorespiratory symptoms occur in many older patients. Beyond the fourth decade, a significant number of patients develop atrial arrhythmias, pulmonary arterial hypertension, bidirectional and then right-to-left shunting of blood, and cardiac failure. Patients exposed to the chronic environmental hypoxia of high altitude tend to develop pulmonary hypertension at younger ages. In some older patients, left-to-right shunting across the defect increases as progressive systemic hypertension and/or coronary artery disease result in reduced compliance of the left ventricle.

Physical examination   Examination usually reveals a prominent right ventricular cardiac impulse and palpable pulmonary artery pulsation. The first heart sound is normal or split, with accentuation of the tricuspid valve closure sound. Increased flow across the pulmonic valve is responsible for a midsystolic pulmonary ejection murmur. The second heart sound is widely split and is relatively fixed in relation to respiration. A middiastolic rumbling murmur, loudest at the fourth intercostal space and along the left sternal border, reflects increased flow across the tricuspid valve. In patients with ostium primum defects, an apical thrill and holosystolic murmur indicate associated mitral or tricuspid incompetence or a ventricular septal defect.

The physical findings are altered when an increase in the pulmonary vascular resistance results in diminution of the left-to-right shunt. Both the pulmonary and tricuspid murmurs decrease in intensity, the pulmonic component of the second heart sound and a systolic ejection sound are accentuated, the two components of the second heart sound may fuse, and a diastolic murmur of pulmonic incompetence appears. Cyanosis and clubbing accompany the development of a right-to-left shunt.

In adults with atrial fibrillation and an atrial septal defect, the physical findings may be confused with the findings of mitral stenosis with pulmonary hypertension, since the tricuspid flow murmur and widely split second heart sound may be mistakenly thought to represent the diastolic murmur of mitral stenosis and the mitral "opening snap," respectively.

Electrocardiogram   In patients with an ostium secundum defect the ECG usually shows right axis deviation and an rSr′ pattern in the right precordial leads, representing delayed posterobasal activation of the ventricular septum. Right ventricular hypertrophy is common in children but not adults. An ectopic atrial pacemaker or first-degree heart block occurs occasionally in patients with defects of the sinus venosus type. In patients with an ostium primum defect, the right ventricular conduction defect is characteristically accompanied by left axis deviation and by superior orientation and counterclockwise rotation of the QRS loop in the frontal plane. Varying degrees of right ventricular and right atrial hypertrophy may occur with each type of defect, depending on the height of the pulmonary artery pressure; prolongation of the PR interval is most common with ostium primum defects. *Chest roentgenograms* reveal enlargement of the right atrium and ventricle, dilatation of the pulmonary artery and its branches, and increased pulmonary vascular marking. Left atrial enlargement is uncommon in the absence of atrial fibrillation.

Echocardiogram   This shows pulmonary arterial and right ventricular dilatation, and anterior systolic (paradoxical) or flat interventricular septal motion if a significant right ventricular volume overload is present. The defect may be visualized directly from subcostal, right parasternal, or apical echocardiographic windows. In most institutions, two-dimensional echocardiography, supplemented by conventional or color Doppler flow examination, has supplanted cardiac catheterization as the confirmatory test for atrial septal defect. Cardiac catheterization is then employed if inconsistencies exist in the clinical data, if significant pulmonary hypertension or associated malformations are suspected, or if coronary artery disease is a possibility.

Management   Operative repair, ideally in children between 3 and 6 years of age, should be advised for all patients with uncomplicated atrial septal defects in whom there is significant left-to-right shunting, i.e., with pulmonary-to-systemic flow ratios exceeding approximately 2.0:1.0. Excellent results may be anticipated, at low risk, even in patients beyond 40 years of age in the absence of pulmonary hypertension. The defect is closed, usually with a patch of prosthetic material with the patient on cardiopulmonary bypass. In patients with ostium primum defects cleft, deformed, and incompetent valves often require repair. Operation should not be carried out in patients with small defects and trivial left-to-right shunts, or in those with severe pulmonary vascular disease without a significant left-to-right shunt.

Atrioventricular septal defects more complex than the ostium primum defect are associated with failure to thrive, heart failure, and pulmonary hypertension early in life, and require operative correction in infancy. Patients with atrial septal defect of the sinus venosus or ostium secundum types rarely die before the fifth decade. During the fifth and sixth decades the incidence of progressive symptoms, often leading to severe disability, increases substantially. Medical management should include prompt treatment of respiratory tract infections, antiarrhythmic medications for atrial fibrillation or supraventricular tachycardia, and the usual measures for hypertension, coronary disease, or heart failure (see Chap. 182), if these complications occur. Although the risk of infective endocarditis is quite low, antibiotics should be administered prophylactically prior to dental and other indicated diagnostic or surgical procedures (see Chap. 90).

VENTRICULAR SEPTAL DEFECT   Defects of the ventricular septum are common as isolated defects and as one component of a combination of anomalies. The opening is usually single and situated in the membranous portion of the septum. The functional disturbance is dependent primarily on its size and on the status of the pulmonary vascular bed, rather than on the location of the defect. Only small or moderate-size defects are usually seen initially in adulthood since the vast majority of patients with isolated large defects come to medical and, often, surgical attention very early in life.

A wide spectrum exists in the natural history of ventricular septal defect, ranging from spontaneous closure to congestive cardiac failure and death in early infancy. Within this spectrum is the possible development of pulmonary vascular obstruction, right ventricular outflow tract obstruction, aortic regurgitation, and infective endocarditis. Spontaneous closure is more common in patients born with a small ventricular septal defect, and occurs in early childhood in most patients.

Patients with large ventricular septal defects and pulmonary hypertension are those at greatest risk for developing pulmonary vascular obstruction. Thus, large defects should be corrected surgically very early in life when pulmonary vascular disease is still reversible or not yet developed. In patients with severe pulmonary vascular obstruction (Eisenmenger syndrome), symptoms in adult life consist of exertional dyspnea, chest pain, syncope, and hemoptysis. The right-to-left shunt leads to cyanosis, clubbing, and erythrocytosis. In all patients, the degree to which pulmonary vascular resistance is elevated before operation is a critical factor determining prognosis. If the pulmonary vascular resistance is one-third or less of the systemic value, progression of pulmonary vascular disease after operation is unusual. However, if a moderate to severe increase in pulmonary vascular resistance exists preoperatively, either no change or a progression of pulmonary vascular disease is common postoperatively.

Right ventricular outflow tract obstruction develops in approximately 5 to 10 percent of patients who present in infancy with a moderate to large left-to-right shunt. With time, as subvalvular right ventricular outflow tract obstruction progresses, the findings in these patients begin to resemble more closely those of the cyanotic tetralogy of Fallot malformation.

In approximately 5 percent of patients, incompetence of the aortic valve results from insufficient cusp tissue or prolapse of the cusp through the interventricular defect; the aortic regurgitation then complicates and usually dominates the clinical course.

Two-dimensional *echocardiography* with conventional or color Doppler examination can usually define the number and location of defects in the ventricular septum, and detect associated anomalies. Hemodynamic and angiographic study may be employed to assess the status of the pulmonary vascular bed and clarify details of the altered anatomy.

Management   Surgical treatment is not recommended for patients who have normal pulmonary arterial pressures with small shunts (pulmonary-to-systemic flow ratios of less than 1.5 to 2.0:1.0). Operative correction is indicated when there is a moderate to large left-to-right shunt with a pulmonary-to-systemic flow ratio that exceeds

1.5:1.0 or 2.0:1.0, in the absence of prohibitively high levels of pulmonary vascular resistance.

AORTIC ROOT TO RIGHT HEART SHUNTS Three malformations, congenital aneurysm of an aortic sinus of Valsalva with fistula, coronary arteriovenous fistula, and anomalous origin of the left coronary artery from the pulmonary trunk, are the most common causes of aortic root to right heart shunts. *Aneurysm of an aortic sinus of Valsalva,* particularly the right coronary sinus, consist of a separation or lack of fusion between the media of the aorta and the annulus fibrosis of the aortic valve. Rupture usually occurs in the third or fourth decade of life; the receiving chamber of the aortico-cardiac fistula is most often the right ventricle, but occasionally, when the noncoronary cusp is involved, the fistula drains into the right atrium. Abrupt rupture causes chest pain and creates bounding pulses, a continuous murmur accentuated in diastole, and volume overload of the heart. Diagnosis is confirmed by two-dimensional and Doppler echocardiographic studies; cardiac catheterization quantifies the left-to-right shunt, and thoracic aortography visualizes the fistula. Medical management is directed at cardiac failure, arrhythmias, or endocarditis. At operation, the aneurysm is closed and amputated and the aortic wall is reunited with the heart, either by direct suture or with a prosthesis.

Coronary arteriovenous fistula, an unusual anomaly, consists of a communication between a coronary artery and another cardiac chamber, usually the coronary sinus or right atrium or ventricle. The shunt is usually of small magnitude, and myocardial blood flow is not usually compromised. Potential complications include infective endocarditis, thrombus formation with occlusion or distal embolization, rupture of an aneurysmal fistula, and rarely, pulmonary hypertension and congestive failure. The finding of a loud, superficial, continuous murmur at the lower or midsternal border usually prompts a further evaluation of asymptomatic patients. Doppler echocardiography demonstrates the site of drainage; if the site of origin is proximal it may be detectable by two-dimensional echocardiography. Retrograde thoracic aortography or coronary arteriography permits identification of the size and anatomic features of the fistulous tract, which may be closed by suture obliteration.

The third anomaly causing a shunt from the aortic root to the right heart is *anomalous origin of the left coronary artery from the pulmonary artery.* As the elevated pulmonary vascular resistance declines immediately after birth, perfusion of the left coronary artery from the pulmonary artery ceases and the direction of flow in the anomalous vessel reverses. Total myocardial perfusion must pass through the right coronary artery and may be sufficient if adequate collateral channels develop between the two coronary circulations. Myocardial infarction and fibrosis commonly lead to death within the first year, though up to 20 percent of patients survive to adolescence and beyond without surgical correction. In older children or adults mitral regurgitation may result from dysfunction of ischemic or infarcted papillary muscles. The diagnosis of anomalous origin of the coronary artery is supported by the electrocardiographic findings of an anterolateral myocardial infarction. Aortic root or coronary angiography demonstrates the retrograde drainage of the coronary vessel into the pulmonary artery and the presence of a single right coronary artery arising from the aorta. Operative management of adults consists of coronary artery bypass with an internal mammary artery graft or saphenous vein–coronary artery graft. The outcome and prognosis are determined largely by the degree of preoperative myocardial damage.

PATENT DUCTUS ARTERIOSUS The ductus arteriosus is a vessel leading from the bifurcation of the pulmonary artery to the aorta just distal to the left subclavian artery. The vascular channel is open normally in the fetus, but closes immediately after birth. The flow across the ductus is determined by the pressure and resistance relationships between the systemic and pulmonary circulations, and by the cross-sectional area and length of the ductus. In most adults with this anomaly pulmonary pressures are normal and a gradient

and shunt from aorta to pulmonary artery persist throughout the cardiac cycle, resulting in a characteristic thrill and a continuous "machinery" murmur with a late systolic accentuation at the upper left sternal edge. In adults who were born with a large left-to-right shunt through the ductus arteriosus, pulmonary vascular obstruction (Eisenmenger syndrome) with pulmonary hypertension, right-to-left shunting, and cyanosis have usually developed. Severe pulmonary vascular disease results in reversal of flow through the ductus, unoxygenated blood is shunted to the descending aorta, and the toes, but not the fingers become cyanotic and clubbed, a finding termed *differential cyanosis.* The leading causes of death in adults with patent ductus are cardiac failure and infective endocarditis; occasionally severe pulmonary vascular obstruction may cause aneurysmal dilatation, calcification, and rupture of the ductus. In the absence of severe pulmonary vascular disease and predominant left-to-right shunting of blood, the patent ductus should be surgically ligated or divided. Operation should be deferred for several months in patients treated successfully for infective endocarditis, because the ductus may remain somewhat edematous and friable.

ACYANOTIC CONGENITAL HEART DISEASE WITHOUT A SHUNT

CONGENITAL AORTIC STENOSIS Malformations that cause obstruction to left ventricular outflow include congenital valvular aortic stenosis, discrete subaortic stenosis, supervalvular aortic stenosis, and hypertrophic obstructive cardiomyopathy (Chap. 192).

Valvular aortic stenosis Valvular aortic stenosis occurs three to four times more often in males than in females. The congenital bicuspid aortic valve, which is not necessarily stenotic, is one of the most common congenital malformations of the heart, although it may go undetected in early life. Because bicuspid valves may become stenotic with time or be the site of infective endocarditis, the lesion may be difficult to distinguish in adults from acquired rheumatic or degenerative calcific aortic stenosis.

The dynamics of blood flow associated with a congenitally deformed, rigid aortic valve commonly lead to thickening of the cusps and, in later life, to calcification. Hemodynamically significant obstruction causes concentric hypertrophy of the left ventricular wall and dilatation of the ascending aorta.

The hemodynamic abnormalities are discussed in Chap. 188. A peak systolic pressure gradient exceeding 70 mmHg, in association with abnormal cardiac output, or an effective aortic orifice less than 0.6 cm² per square meter of body surface, is considered to represent critical obstruction to left ventricular outflow. In adults, the resting cardiac output is generally normal but often fails to rise normally during muscular exercise.

Many patients with congenital aortic stenosis are asymptomatic. Usually, a murmur is detected on a routine examination. Moderately severe obstruction should be suspected if there is a history of fatigability and exertional dyspnea. With severe obstruction, the inability of the left ventricle to increase its output and maintain cerebral flow during exercise may result in exertional syncope, and the disparity between the oxygen supply and myocardial oxygen requirements may cause angina. The symptomatic patient with valvular aortic stenosis generally has critical stenosis, although a lack of symptoms does not preclude the presence of moderately severe obstruction. Sudden death occurs in patients with critical stenosis, and ventricular arrhythmias, perhaps initiated by acute myocardial ischemia, may be responsible.

Hemodynamically significant obstruction is associated with a left ventricular lift and a precordial systolic thrill over the base of the heart, with transmission to the jugular notch and along the carotid arteries. Presystolic expansion is often palpable. A systolic aortic ejection sound, signifying opening of the aortic valve, is typically heard best at the cardiac apex when the valve is mobile, particularly with mild to moderate stenosis. A fourth heart sound is generally associated with severe obstruction. The systolic murmur starts after the completion of left ventricular isometric contraction, is rhomboid-shaped, loud, harsh, and best heard at the base of the heart. The murmur, like the thrill, radiates to the jugular notch and carotid vessels and to the apex. An early diastolic blowing murmur of aortic regurgitation may be present, but unless the valve has been eroded by infective endocarditis the regurgitation is usually not hemodynamically significant; rarely, in patients with a congenital bicuspid valve, severe aortic regurgitation may be the dominant hemodynamic lesion.

Electrocardiographic evidence of left ventricular hypertrophy tends to reflect the severity of obstruction, although a normal or near-normal electrocardiogram does not exclude severe aortic stenosis. The left ventricular "strain pattern" generally indicates that severe aortic stenosis is present. Two-dimensional echocardiography demonstrates the aortic valve morphology; Doppler echocardiography is the most accurate means of noninvasively estimating the magnitude of obstruction and valvular regurgitation if present. Cardiac catheterization and coronary angiography are indicated particularly if coronary artery disease is suspected.

The medical management of congenital valvular aortic stenosis includes prophylaxis against infective endocarditis and, in patients with diminished cardiac reserve, the administration of digitalis and diuretics and sodium restriction while awaiting operation. If severe aortic stenosis is present, strenuous physical activity should be avoided even when the patient is asymptomatic, and participation in competitive sports should probably be restricted in patients with milder degrees of obstruction. Aortic valve replacement is indicated in asymptomatic adults with severe obstruction, or in patients who are symptomatic with an aortic valve area less than 1.0 cm². If surgery is contraindicated because of a complicating medical problem such as malignancy, or renal or hepatic failure, balloon valvuloplasty may provide short term improvement.

Subaortic stenosis The most common form of subaortic stenosis is the *idiopathic hypertrophic* variety, also termed *hypertrophic cardiomyopathy*, which is present at birth in about one-third of the patients and is discussed in Chap. 192. Both clinically and physiologically, the *discrete* form of subaortic stenosis resembles valvular aortic stenosis. The lesion usually consists of a membranous diaphragm or fibrous ring encircling the left ventricular outflow tract just beneath the base of the aortic valve. Echocardiography demonstrates the subaortic obstruction; Doppler studies show turbulence proximal to the aortic valve and also detect and quantify aortic regurgitation. Treatment consists of excision of the membrane or fibrous ridge.

Supravalvular aortic stenosis This anomaly consists of a localized or diffuse narrowing of the ascending aorta originating just above the level of the coronary arteries at the superior margin of the sinuses of Valsalva. In contrast to other forms of aortic stenosis, the coronary arteries are subjected to the elevated pressures that exist within the left ventricle and are often dilated and tortuous.

COARCTATION OF THE AORTA Narrowing or constriction of the lumen of the aorta may occur anywhere along its length but is most common distal to the origin of the left subclavian artery near the insertion of the ligamentum arteriosum. Coarctation occurs in about 7 percent of patients with congenital heart disease and is twice as common in males as in females, although the lesion occurs frequently in patients with gonadal dysgenesis. Clinical manifestations depend on the site and extent of obstruction and the presence of associated cardiac anomalies, the most common of which is the bicuspid aortic valve. Aneurysmal dilatation within the arterial supply of the circle of Willis produces a high risk of sudden rupture and death.

The majority of children and young adults with isolated, discrete coarctation are asymptomatic. Headache, epistaxis, cold extremities, and claudication with exercise may occur, and attention is usually directed to the cardiovascular system when a heart murmur or hypertension in the upper extremities and absence, marked diminution, or delayed pulsations in the femoral arteries are detected on physical examination. Enlarged and pulsatile collateral vessels may be palpated in the intercostal spaces anteriorly, in the axillae, or posteriorly in the interscapular area. The upper extremities and thorax may be more developed than the lower extremities. A midsystolic murmur over the anterior part of the chest, back, and spinous processes may become continuous if the lumen is narrowed sufficiently to result in a high-velocity jet across the lesion throughout the cardiac cycle. Additional systolic and continuous murmurs over the lateral thoracic wall may reflect increased flow through dilated and tortuous collateral vessels. The electrocardiogram reveals left ventricular hypertrophy of varying degree. Roentgenograms may show a dilated left subclavian artery high on the left mediastinal border and a dilated ascending aorta. Indentation of the aorta at the site of coarctation and pre- and poststenotic dilatation (the "3" sign) along the left paramediastinal shadow are almost pathognomonic. Notching of the ribs, an important radiographic sign, is due to erosion by dilated collateral vessels. Two-dimensional echocardiography from para- or suprasternal windows identifies the site and length of coarctation, while Doppler studies record and quantify the pressure gradient. Magnetic resonance imaging or digital angiography allow visualization of the length and severity of the obstruction and the associated collateral arteries. In adults, cardiac catheterization is indicated primarily to evaluate the status of the coronary arteries.

The chief hazards result from severe hypertension and include the development of cerebral aneurysms and hemorrhage, rupture of the aorta, left ventricular failure, and infective endocarditis. Treatment is surgical; resection and end-to-end anastomosis or subclavian flap angioplasty are employed commonly, although it may be necessary to use a tubular graft, patch, or bypass conduit if the narrowed segment is long. Systemic hypertension postoperatively, in the absence of residual coarctation, appears to be related to the duration of preoperative hypertension.

PULMONARY STENOSIS WITH INTACT VENTRICULAR SEPTUM Obstruction to right ventricular outflow may be localized to the supravalvular, valvular, or subvalvular levels or occur at a combination of these sites. Multiple sites of narrowing of the peripheral pulmonary arteries are a feature of *rubella embryopathy* and may occur with both the familial and sporadic forms of supravalvular aortic stenosis. Valvular pulmonic stenosis is the most common form of isolated right ventricular obstruction.

The severity of the obstructing lesion, rather than the site of narrowing, is the most important determinant of the clinical course. In the presence of a normal cardiac output, a peak systolic transvalvular pressure gradient between 50 and 80 mmHg is considered to be moderate stenosis; levels below and above that range are classified as mild and severe, respectively. Patients with mild pulmonic stenosis are generally asymptomatic and demonstrate little or no progression in the severity of obstruction with age. In patients with more significant stenosis, the severity may increase with time. Symptoms vary with the degree of obstruction. Fatigue, dyspnea, right ventricular failure, and syncope may limit the activity of older patients, in whom moderate or severe obstruction may prevent an augmentation of cardiac output with exercise. In patients with severe obstruction, the systolic pressure in the right ventricle may exceed that in the left ventricle, since the ventricular septum is intact. Right ventricular ejection is prolonged with moderate or severe stenosis, and the sound of pulmonary valve closure is delayed and soft. Right ventricular hypertrophy reduces the compliance of that chamber, and a forceful right atrial contraction is necessary to augment right ventricular filling. A fourth heart sound, prominent *a* waves in the jugular venous pulse, and occasionally, presystolic pulsations of the liver reflect vigorous atrial contraction. The clinical diagnosis is supported by a right parasternal lift and harsh systolic ejection murmur and thrill at the upper left sternal border, typically preceded by a systolic ejection sound, if the obstruction is valvular. The holosystolic decrescendo murmur of tricuspid regurgitation may accompany severe pulmonic stenosis, especially in the presence of congestive heart failure. Cyanosis usually reflects venoarterial shunting through a patent foramen ovale or atrial septal defect. In patients with supravalvular or peripheral pulmonary arterial stenosis, the murmur is systolic or continuous and is best heard over the area of narrowing, with radiation to the peripheral lung fields.

The *electrocardiogram* may be helpful in assessing the degree of obstruction to right ventricular output. In mild cases, the electrocardiogram is often normal, whereas moderate and severe stenoses are associated with right axis deviation and right ventricular hypertrophy. A ventricular strain pattern, as well as high-amplitude P waves in leads II and V_1, indicating right atrial enlargement, is associated with severe stenosis. The chest roentgenogram with mild or moderate pulmonic stenosis often shows a heart of normal size and normal vascularity of the lungs. In the presence of valvular stenosis, poststenotic dilatation of the main and left pulmonary arteries may be evident. With severe obstruction and resultant right ventricular failure, right atrial and ventricular enlargement are generally evident. The pulmonary vascularity may be reduced with severe stenosis, right ventricular failure, and/or a venoarterial shunt at the atrial level.

Two dimensional *echocardiography* visualizes pulmonary valve morphology; the outflow tract pressure gradient can be estimated by Doppler ultrasonography. The cardiac catheter technique of balloon valvuloplasty (Chap. 179) is often effective. Direct surgical relief of moderate and severe obstruction may be accomplished at a low risk. Multiple stenosis of the peripheral pulmonary arteries are usually inoperable, but narrowing of a single branch or at the bifurcation of the main pulmonary trunk may be corrected.

CYANOTIC CONGENITAL HEART DISEASE WITH INCREASED PULMONARY BLOOD FLOW

COMPLETE TRANSPOSITION OF THE GREAT ARTERIES In this condition the aorta arises from the right ventricle to the right of and anterior to the pulmonary artery, which emerges from the left ventricle. This results in two separate and parallel circulations, and some communication between the two circulations must exist after birth to sustain life. Most patients have an interatrial communication, two-thirds have a patent ductus arteriosus, and about one-third have an associated ventricular septal defect. Transposition is more common in males and accounts for approximately 10 percent of cyanotic heart disease.

The course is determined by the degree of tissue hypoxia, the ability of each ventricle to sustain an increased work load in the presence of reduced coronary arterial oxygenation, the nature of the associated cardiovascular anomalies, and the status of the pulmonary vascular bed. Severe morphologic alterations develop in the pulmonary vascular bed by 1 to 2 years of age in most patients who also have an associated large ventricular septal defect or large patent ductus arteriosus in the absence of obstruction to left ventricular outflow.

Surgical treatment The creation or enlargement of an interatrial communication is the simplest procedure for providing increased intracardiac mixing of systemic and pulmonary venous blood; it may be achieved surgically or, preferably, by rupturing the valve of the foramen ovale with a balloon catheter during cardiac catheterization (Rashkind's procedure). Systemic-pulmonary artery anastomosis may be indicated in the patient with severe obstruction to left ventricular outflow and diminished pulmonary blood flow. Intracardiac repair may be accomplished by rearranging the venous returns so that the systemic venous blood is directed to the mitral valve and thence to the left ventricle and pulmonary artery, while the pulmonary venous blood is diverted through the tricuspid valve and right ventricle to the aorta (Mustard or Senning operation). Many surgeons now prefer to correct this malformation in infancy by transposing both coronary

arteries to the posterior artery and transecting, contraposing, and anastomosing the aorta and pulmonary arteries (Jatene or arterial switch operation). For those patients with a ventricular septal defect in whom it is necessary to bypass a severely obstructed left ventricular outflow tract, corrective operation employs an intracardiac ventricular baffle and extracardia prosthetic conduit to replace the pulmonary artery (Rastelli's procedure). Patients with a large ventricular septal defect require closure of the ventricular septal defect and the atrial switch operation early in infancy. There are now many adults who underwent venous switch repair early in life who are experiencing the long-term complications of that operation, including arrhythmias, baffle leaks, or obstruction and reduced performance of the systemic right ventricle.

TOTAL ANOMALOUS PULMONARY VENOUS CONNECTION In this malformation all the pulmonary veins connect either to the right atrium directly or to the systemic veins or their tributaries. Because all venous blood returns to the right atrium, an interatrial communication is an integral part of this malformation. Most unoperated patients surviving to adult life have pulmonary vascular obstructive disease, a reduction in pulmonary blood flow, and cyanosis.

SINGLE VENTRICLE This designation applies to a family of complex lesions with both atrioventricular valves or a common atrioventricular valve opening to a single ventricular chamber. In most patients, the single ventricle morphologically resembles a left ventricular chamber that is separated from an infundibular outlet chamber by a bulboventricular septum; in these cases the anomaly is often referred to as double-inlet left ventricle. Associated anomalies are common and include abnormal great artery positional relationships, pulmonic valvular or subvalvular stenosis, and subaortic stenosis.

Depending upon the associated anomalies, the clinical presentation of single ventricle mimics other conditions in which cyanosis and decreased (or increased) pulmonary blood flow coexist, e.g., tetralogy of Fallot in the former instance and complete transposition of the great arteries in the latter. Survival to adolescence and adulthood depends upon a relatively normal pulmonary blood flow and good ventricular function. Correction of the defect usually consists of creation of a right atrial–pulmonary conduit (the Fontan procedure); some patients are candidates for a septation operation, in which the single ventricle is partitioned with a prosthetic patch.

CYANOTIC CONGENITAL HEART DISEASE WITH DECREASED PULMONARY BLOOD FLOW

TRICUSPID ATRESIA Atresia of the tricuspid valve, an interatrial communication, and, frequently, hypoplasia of the right ventricle and pulmonary artery exist in this malformation. Because of the small or nearly absent right ventricle, this anomaly is basically a "univentricular" heart with a single inlet (mitral) to the left ventricle. The clinical picture is usually dominated by severe cyanosis as a result of obligatory admixture of systemic and pulmonary venous blood in the left ventricle. The electrocardiogram characteristically shows right atrial enlargement, left axis deviation, and left ventricular hypertrophy.

Atrial septostomy and palliative operations to increase pulmonary blood flow, often by systemic arterial or venous–pulmonary artery anastomosis may allow survival to the second or third decade. A Fontan atriopulmonary connection may then allow functional correction in those patients with normal or low pulmonary arterial resistance pressure and good left ventricular function.

EBSTEIN'S ANOMALY This malformation is characterized by a downward displacement of the tricuspid valve into the right ventricle, due to anomalous attachment of the tricuspid leaflets. Tricuspid valve tissue is dysplastic; a variable portion of the septal and inferior cusps adhere to the right ventricular wall some distance away from the atrioventricular junction. The abnormally situated tricuspid orifice produces a portion of the right ventricle lying between the atrioventricular ring and the origin of the valve, which is continuous with the right atrial chamber. This proximal segment is "atrialized," and the distal ventricular chamber is small. The degree of impairment of right ventricular function depends primarily on the extent to which the right ventricular inflow portion is atrialized, and on the magnitude of tricuspid valve regurgitation. Most patients survive at least to the third decade. Although the clinical manifestations are variable, some patients come to initial attention because of progressive cyanosis from right-to-left atrial shunting, or symptoms due to tricuspid regurgitation and right ventricular dysfunction, or paroxysmal atrial tachyarrhythmias with or without bypass tracts (type B Wolff-Parkinson-White syndrome is common). Diagnostic findings by two-dimensional echocardiography include the abnormal positional relation between the tricuspid and mitral valves with apical displacement of the septal tricuspid leaflet. Tricuspid regurgitation is detected and quantified by Doppler examination. Surgical approaches have included prosthetic replacement of the tricuspid valve when the leaflets are tethered, or, in patients within elongated mobil anterior leaflet, creation of a competent, unicuspid valve by insertion of the elongated anterior leaflet into the original tricuspid annulus and plication of the atrialized right ventricle. Transection of bypass tracts may be necessary to abolish atrial tachyarrhythmias.

TETRALOGY OF FALLOT This malformation is responsible for about 10 percent of all forms of congenital heart disease and is the most common cause of cyanotic forms. The four components of the tetralogy of Fallot are ventricular septal defect, obstruction to right ventricular outflow, aortic override (straddle) of the ventricular septal defect, and right ventricular hypertrophy. The basic anomaly results from an anterior and superior deviation of the infundibular ventricular septum away from its usual location in the heart between the limbs of the trabecular septum. This displacement causes subpulmonary obstruction, aortic "override," and a large, nonrestrictive, malalignment-type ventricular septal defect.

The severity of obstruction to right ventricular outflow determines the clinical presentation. The severity of hypoplasia of the outflow tract of the right ventricle varies from mild to complete (pulmonary atresia). Pulmonary valve stenosis and supravalvular and peripheral pulmonary arterial obstruction may coexist; rarely there is unilateral absence of a pulmonary artery (usually the left). A right-sided aortic arch and descending aorta occur in about 25 percent of patients with tetralogy. The coronary arteries may have variations that are surgically important. The anterior descending artery sometimes originates from the right coronary artery, which may also give rise to a left branch coursing anterior to the infundibulum; a single left coronary artery may give rise to a branch that crosses the outflow tract of the right ventricle. Associated noncardiac anomalies are present in 20 to 30 percent of patients.

The relationship between the resistance to blood flow from the ventricles into the aorta and into the pulmonary vessels plays a major role in determining the hemodynamic and clinical picture. Thus, the severity of obstruction to right ventricular outflow is of fundamental significance. In many infants and children the obstruction is mild but progressive. When the obstruction is severe, the pulmonary blood flow is reduced markedly, and large volume of desaturated systemic venous blood is shunted from right to left across the ventricular septal defect. Severe cyanosis and polycythemia occur, and symptoms and sequelae of systemic hypoxemia are prominent.

The *electrocardiogram* ordinarily shows right ventricular and, less often, right atrial hypertrophy. Radiologic examination characteristically reveals a normal-sized, boot-shaped heart (*coeur en sabot*) with prominence of the right ventricle and a concavity in the region of the pulmonary conus. The pulmonary vascular markings are typically diminished, and the aortic arch and knob may be on the right side. Two-dimensional echocardiography from the parasternal or subcostal windows demonstrates the malalignment of the ventricular septal defect and the subpulmonary stenosis. The presence or absence of stenoses at the origins of the main branch pulmonary arteries can

also be assessed. Selective angiocardiography with right ventricular injection provides architectural details of the right ventricular outflow tract, pulmonary valve and annulus, and caliber of the main branches of the pulmonary artery; coronary arteriography identifies the anatomy and course of the coronary arteries.

Factors that may complicate the management of patients with tetralogy of Fallot include infective endocarditis, paradoxic embolism, polycythemia, coagulation defects, and cerebral infarction or abscess. Corrective operation is advisable at some point for almost all patients with this anomaly. Successful correction avoids progressive infundibular obstruction, delayed growth, and complications due to hypoxemia and polycythemia. The size of the pulmonary arteries rather than the age or size of the infant or child is the most important determinant in establishing candidacy for primary repair. Pronounced hypoplasia of the pulmonary arteries is a relative contraindication for an early corrective surgical procedure. When this problem is present, a palliative operation, such as creation of a systemic arterial–pulmonary arterial shunt, is carried out and is usually followed by complete correction, which can be carried out at a lower risk later in childhood.

OTHER FORMS OF CONGENITAL HEART DISEASE

CONGENITALLY CORRECTED TRANSPOSITION The two fundamental anatomic abnormalities in this malformation are transposition of the ascending aorta and pulmonary trunk and inversion of the ventricles. This arrangement results in desaturated systemic venous blood passing from the right atrium through the mitral valve to the left ventricle and into the pulmonary trunk; whereas arterialized pulmonary venous blood flows from the left atrium through the tricuspid valve to the right ventricle and into the aorta. Thus, the circulation is corrected functionally. The clinical presentation, course, and prognosis of patients with congenitally corrected transposition vary depending on the nature and severity of any complicating intracardiac anomalies. Ebstein-type anomalies of the left-side tricuspid atrioventricular valve, ventricular septal defect, obstruction to outflow from the venous ventricle, and congenital heart block are often associated with corrected transposition. The diagnosis of the malformation and associated lesions can often be established by two-dimensional echocardiography and Doppler examination.

MALPOSITIONS OF THE HEART Positional anomalies refer to conditions in which the cardiac apex is in the right side of the chest (dextrocardia), or at the midline (mesocardia), or in which there is a normal location of the heart in the left side of the chest but abnormal position of the viscera (isolated levocardia). Knowledge of the position of the abdominal organs and of the branching pattern of the main stem bronchi is important in categorizing these malpositions. When dextrocardia occurs *without* situs inversus, when the *visceral situs is indeterminate*, or if *isolated levocardia* is present, associated, often complex, multiple cardiac anomalies are usually present. In contrast, mirror-image dextrocardia is usually observed in a patient with complete situs inversus, a condition which occurs most frequently in individuals whose hearts are otherwise normal.

SURGICALLY MODIFIED CONGENITAL HEART DISEASE

Because of the enormous strides in cardiovascular surgical techniques that have occurred in the past 15 years, a large number of long-term survivors of corrective operations in infancy and childhood have reached adulthood. These patients are often challenging because of the diversity of anatomic, hemodynamic, and electrophysiologic residua and sequelae of cardiac operations.

TABLE 186-3	Potential late postoperative problems

Residual shunts
Residual ventricular outflow obstruction
Residual valvular anomalies
Systemic arterial hypertension
Pulmonary vascular obstruction
Arrhythmias and conduction defects
Myocardial dysfunction
Prosthetic valve malfunction
Prosthetic conduit obstruction
Infective endocarditis

REFERENCES

Borow KM, Braunwald E: Congenital heart disease in the adult, in *Heart Disease*, 3d ed, E Braunwald (ed). Philadelphia, Saunders, 1988, p 976

Engle MA, Perloff JK (eds): *Congenital Heart Disease After Surgery*, New York, Yorke, 1983

Fixler DE et al: Trends in congenital heart disease in Dallas County births 1971–1984. Circulation 81(1):37, 1990

Friedman WF: Congenital heart disease in infancy and childhood, in *Heart Disease*, 3d ed, E Braunwald (ed). Philadelphia, Saunders, 1988, p 896

Kirklin JW, Barratt-Boyes BG: *Cardiac Surgery*, New York, Wiley, 1986

Lock JE et al: The use of catheter intervention procedures for congenital heart disease. J Am Coll Cardiol 7:1420, 1986

Mitchell JH et al: 16th Bethesda Conference: Cardiovascular abnormalities in the athlete; Recommendations regarding eligibility for competition. J Am Coll Cardiol 6:1200, 1985

Perloff JK et al: From cyanotic infant to acyanotic adult—The odyssey of blue babies. West J Med 139:673, 1983

———: The UCLA Adult Congenital Heart Disease Program. Am J Cardiol 57:1190, 1986

———: *The Clinical Recognition of Congenital Heart Disease*, 3d ed. Philadelphia, Saunders, 1987

——— et al: Adults with cyanotic congenital heart disease: Hematologic management. Ann Intern Med 109:406, 1988

Roberts WC (ed): *Adult Congenital Heart Disease*. Philadelphia, Davis, 1987

Truesdell SC et al: Life insurance in children with cardiovascular disease. Pediatrics 77:687, 1986

The proper care of the survivor of operation for congenital heart disease requires that the clinician understand the details of the malformation prior to operation, pay meticulous attention to the details of the operative procedure, and recognize the postoperative residua (conditions left totally or partially uncorrected), sequelae (conditions caused by surgery), and the complications that may have resulted from the operation. With the exception of ligation and division of an uncomplicated patent ductus arteriosus, almost every other surgical repair of an anomaly leaves behind, or causes, some abnormality of the heart and circulation which may range from trivial to serious. Thus, even with results that are considered clinically to be good to excellent, continued long-term postoperative follow-up is advisable.

Table 186-3 lists the categories of common, late postoperative problems. Several of these residua, sequelae, and complications deserve special mention. Thus, cardiac operations importantly involving the atria, such as closure of atrial septal defect, or repair of total or partial anomalous pulmonary venous return, or venous switch corrections of complete transposition of the great arteries (the Mustard or Senning operations), may be followed years later by sinus node or atrioventricular node dysfunction or by atrial arrhythmias. Intraventricular surgery may also result in electrophysiologic consequences, including complete heart block necessitation pacemaker insertion to avoid sudden death. In addition, valvular problems may arise late after initial cardiac operation. An example is the progressive stenosis of an initially nonobstructive bicuspid aortic valve in the patient who underwent aortic coarctation repair. Such aortic valves may also be the site of infective endocarditis. After repair of the ostium primum atrial septal defect, the cleft mitral valve may become progressively incompetent. Low-pressure pulmonary regurgitation is common and well tolerated in most patients with repaired tetralogy of Fallot. However, in such patients with significant residual peripheral pulmonary arterial stenoses, severe pulmonary valvular regurgitation may result in right ventricular failure and tricuspid regurgitation. Tricuspid regurgitation may also be progressive in the postoperative patient with tetralogy of Fallot if right ventricular outflow tract obstruction was not relieved adequately at initial surgery. In many patients, inadequate relief of an obstructive lesion, or a residual regurgitant lesion, or a residual shunt will cause or hasten the onset of clinical signs and symptoms of myocardial dysfunction. In many patients, particularly those who were cyanotic for many years before operation, a preexisting compromise in ventricular performance is due to the original underlying malformation. A final category of postoperative problems involves the use of prosthetic valves, patches, or conduits in the operative repair. The special risks in such patients include infective endocarditis, thrombus formation, and premature degeneration and calcification of the prosthetic materials. There are many patients in whom extracardiac conduits are required to correct the circulation functionally, and often to carry blood to the lungs from the right atrium or right ventricle. These conduits may develop intraluminal obstruction and, if they incorporate a prosthetic valve, the latter may show progressive calcification and thickening.

187 RHEUMATIC FEVER

GENE H. STOLLERMAN

DEFINITION Rheumatic fever is an inflammatory disease which occurs as a delayed sequel to pharyngeal infection with group A streptococci. It involves principally the heart, joints, central nervous system, skin, and subcutaneous tissues. The usual manifestations in the acute form are migratory polyarthritis, fever, and carditis. Sydenham's chorea, subcutaneous nodules, and erythema marginatum may occur as other typical manifestations. No single symptom, sign, or laboratory test is pathognomonic of rheumatic fever, although several combinations of them are diagnostic. Although the name *acute rheumatic fever* emphasizes involvement of the joints, rheumatic fever owes its importance to the involvement of the heart, which can be fatal during the acute stage or lead to rheumatic heart disease, a chronic condition due to scarring and deformity of the heart valves.

ETIOLOGY AND PATHOGENESIS The etiologic relationship of group A streptococci to rheumatic fever can be summarized briefly, as follows. (1) Numerous clinical and epidemiologic studies have shown a close association of group A streptococcal infections and rheumatic fever. (2) Antecedent streptococcal infection can almost always be demonstrated immunologically in the acute stage of rheumatic fever by increased titers of antibodies to streptococcal antigens. Moreover, in long-term prospective follow-up studies, rheumatic fever recurs only as a result of intercurrent streptococcal infections. (3) Both primary and secondary attacks of the disease can be prevented by prompt treatment or prevention of streptococcal infections with antimicrobial therapy. The pharyngeal route of infection is necessary to initiate the rheumatic process. Streptococcal skin infections do not do so. Furthermore, strains of group A streptococci that have been clearly associated with outbreaks of rheumatic fever have high virulence properties, such as rich content of the type-specific surface M protein and large hyaluronate capsules (responsible for forming "mucoid" colonies). Such properties make them highly resistant to phagocytosis and cause vigorous immune responses. Such rheumatogenic strains have been associated most frequently with certain M serotypes, such as types 3, 5, 18, 19, and 24.

The mechanism by which the group A streptococcus initiates the disease process remains unknown. A relatively small percentage of persons who suffer from streptococcal sore throats subsequently develop rheumatic fever. The organism is not demonstrable in the lesions when rheumatic fever appears several days or weeks after the acute streptococcal infection. No one product of the streptococcus has been incriminated as a cause of the lesions, either as a direct tissue toxin or as an antigen inducing hypersensitivity. Several streptococcal antigens have demonstrated cross-reactivity with cardiac and other tissues. Their direct relationship to pathogenesis is, however, unproven, and streptococcus-induced autoimmunity as a mechanism to explain the rheumatic process remains a popular but unestablished pathogenetic concept.

INCIDENCE AND EPIDEMIOLOGY   Although rheumatic fever may occur at any age, it is extremely rare in infancy; it appears most commonly between the ages of 5 and 15 years, when streptococcal infection is most frequent and intense. Similarly, the geographic distribution, incidence, and severity of rheumatic fever are, in general, a reflection of the frequency and severity of streptococcal pharyngitis. The attack rate of rheumatic fever following exudative streptococcal pharyngitis in epidemics averages approximately 3 percent. When streptococcal pharyngitis is sporadic and mild or due to strains of lesser rheumatic potential, the attack rate of rheumatic fever may be very much lower. Strains of group A streptococci that cause epidemics of streptococcal pharyngitis are most likely to be rheumatogenic. Following such infections, the attack rate of rheumatic fever is directly correlated with the magnitude of the streptococcal immune response. Analysis of reported epidemics of acute rheumatic fever caused by a variety of serotypes shows some, such as type 5, to be overrepresented, and others to be conspicuously absent. In some populations, such as in Trinidad, strains responsible for rheumatic fever and acute glomerulonephritis are serotypically distinct.

Environmental, bacterial, and host factors which appear to play a role in the development of rheumatic fever are important primarily as they are related to the incidence and severity of preceding streptococcal infection. Such factors as latitude, altitude, dampness, economic factors, and age all affect the incidence of rheumatic fever because they are related to the incidence of streptococcal infection in general. Crowding is, however, the major environmental factor relating to the occurrence of this disease because, regardless of other variables, it promotes interpersonal spread of the most virulent group A streptococcal strains. Such crowding as occurs in military barracks, closed institutions, large families in small quarters, and those massed in the densely populated core of major urban centers is most likely to be associated with an increase in incidence of rheumatic fever.

The attack rate of rheumatic fever following streptococcal infections in patients who have had previous attacks of rheumatic fever is increased to as high as 5 to 50 percent and is also related to the virulence of the reactivating infection. Furthermore, the frequency of rheumatic recurrences following streptococcal infection is consistently greater in those with rheumatic heart disease than in those who escaped cardiac injury during prior attacks. The tendency to suffer recurrences of rheumatic fever following streptococcal infections declines with the passage of years since the preceding attack. It appears, therefore, that certain host variables, as well as probable qualitative and quantitative differences in the nature of the antecedent streptococcal infection, also influence the development of rheumatic fever. To what extent such variables are genetic or acquired has not been settled. It is common to obtain a family history of rheumatic fever as well as to encounter multiple cases among siblings of a single family. However, the concordance of rheumatic fever in identical twins is approximately 20 percent, suggesting only a limited penetrance of genetic predisposition to rheumatic fever. Although investigations of the distribution of haplotypes in rheumatic hosts have been limited in scope and number, there has been so far no consistent association of rheumatic fever, or any of its major manifestations, with any predominant histocompatibility locus antigens. Recently a B-lymphocyte allotypic antigen has been found to be strikingly overrepresented in patients with rheumatic heart disease. Its nature and relation to pathogenesis, however, is not yet known.

The mortality of acute rheumatic fever has been declining steadily for the past 30 years. It is still, however, a major cause of death and disability in children and adolescents in socioeconomically depressed areas of the world. The incidence of rheumatic fever has been decreasing dramatically in countries where housing and economic conditions have been improving steadily. The rate of decrease may have been accelerated by the wide use of antimicrobial therapy. The decrease also may be due to a change in the prevalence of rheumatogenic streptococcal strains. In the past few years, however, local outbreaks of rheumatic fever have occurred in the United States in two military populations, one at the San Diego Naval Base, California, and the other at Fort Leonard Wood, Missouri. Outbreaks have occurred also among schoolchildren in Utah, Ohio, and Pennsylvania. Middle class communities with relatively high standards of living and medical care have been affected. Further investigations of the streptococcal strains causing pharyngitis in these communities have resulted in the recovery of "mucoid" strains of group A streptococci belonging to M-types 3 and 18. These strains were once prevalent in well-studied epidemics of rheumatic fever in the 1940s and 1950s, particularly in military populations. They have rarely been seen since then. The explanation for the reappearance of these strains in middle class communities and in widely separated military bases is unclear and has caused a resurgence of interest in proper diagnosis and treatment of streptococcal sore throat. Rheumatic fever remains, however, a worldwide disease having its greatest incidence wherever poor economic conditions, overcrowding, and substandard housing are most common, and where such conditions promote the transmission of rheumatogenic streptococci.

PATHOLOGY   The lesions of rheumatic fever are disseminated widely throughout the body, with special predilection for connective tissues. Focal inflammatory lesions occur particularly around small blood vessels.

Cardiovascular lesions   The heart is the site of the most characteristic and consequential involvement, and all its layers—endocardium, myocardium, and pericardium—may be involved. This generalized involvement gives rise to the term *rheumatic pancarditis*. The most characteristic and specific pattern of rheumatic inflammation is found in the *myocardial Aschoff body,* a submiliary granuloma. This lesion, when present in its classic form, is generally considered to be pathognomonic of rheumatic fever. In many areas the inflammatory lesion is accompanied by swelling and fragmentation of the collagen fibers and alteration in the staining properties of the ground substances of the connective tissues. This change is described as *fibrinoid degeneration of collagen,* but its chemical basis has not been established. Aschoff bodies with less exudative and more productive changes may persist for many years as the lingering traces of chronic rheumatic inflammation in patients with rheumatic heart disease, long after rheumatic fever has become clinically quiescent. The persistence of such lesions is most common in patients who develop severe mitral stenosis. Eventually the Aschoff body is converted into a spindle-shaped or triangular scar lying between the muscle bundles and surrounding blood vessels.

Rheumatic endocarditis produces the verrucous valvulitis of acute rheumatic fever which leads to the most serious permanent cardiac damage. It may heal with fibrous thickening and adhesion of the valve commissures and chordae tendineae, leading to variable degrees of valvular regurgitation and stenosis. Deformity resulting in functional impairment of the heart occurs most commonly in the mitral and aortic valves, less frequently in the tricuspid, and almost never in the pulmonic valves. *Rheumatic pericarditis* (Chap. 193) produces a serofibrinous effusion, with the deposit of shaggy elements of fibrin on the surface of the heart. The pericardium may become calcified, but pericardial constriction does not occur.

Extracardiac lesions   Involvement of the *joints* is characterized by exudative rather than proliferative changes, and healing of these structures occurs without significant scarring or deformity. *Subcutaneous nodules,* seen during the acute phase of the disease, are composed of granulomas with localized areas of "fibrinoid" swelling of subcutaneous collagen bundles, and perivascular collections of large cells with pale nuclei and prominent nucleoli. Synovitis is usually mild and nonspecific. *Pulmonary* and *pleural* lesions are less definite and less characteristic. Fibrinous pleurisy and rheumatic pneumonitis may occur with exudative and proliferative lesions but without definite Aschoff bodies. Patients with active *chorea* rarely die. The pathologic findings which have been reported in the central nervous system are not consistent, and no characteristic lesion has been reported to explain this clinical manifestation. During active chorea the spinal fluid remains normal, being free of cells, with no increase in total protein and no change in the relative concentration of various proteins.

CLINICAL FEATURES The major clinical manifestations by which rheumatic fever can be recognized are polyarthritis, carditis, chorea, erythema marginatum, and subcutaneous nodules.

Arthritis The classic attack of rheumatic fever appears as an acute migratory polyarthritis accompanied by signs and symptoms of an acute febrile illness. The large joints of the extremities are most frequently affected, but no joint is impervious to the inflammatory process; one may find arthritis of the hands and feet but only rarely of the spine or of the sternoclavicular or temporomandibular joints. Joint effusions occur but are not persistent. As pain and swelling subside in one joint, others tend to become involved. Although such "migratory" involvement is characteristic, it is not invariable, and several large joints may be inflamed at one time. To be acceptable as a criterion for the diagnosis of rheumatic fever, the polyarthritis should involve two or more joints, should be associated with at least two minor manifestations such as fever and elevation of sedimentation rate, and should be associated with high titer of antistreptolysin O or some other streptococcal antibody (Table 187-1). There is nothing distinctive about the arthritis of rheumatic fever, and other causes of migratory polyarthritis that may be associated only fortuitously with high streptococcal antibody levels must, of course, be excluded.

Acute rheumatic carditis Acute rheumatic carditis first manifests itself by the appearance of the heart murmurs of either mitral or aortic regurgitation, the former most frequently. Signs and symptoms of pericarditis and of congestive heart failure may supervene in more severe cases. Death may result from heart failure during the acute stage of the disease, or permanent valvular damage may be sustained which results ultimately in serious disability. Carditis may vary from a fulminating, fatal course to a low-grade, inapparent inflammation. *It is well to bear in mind that the vast majority of patients with carditis do not have symptoms referable to the heart.* The latter occur only in more severe cases when heart failure or pericardial effusions produce characteristic symptoms. For this reason, unless extracardiac manifestations, such as polyarthritis and chorea, are present, patients whose rheumatic fever is manifested only by carditis are frequently not diagnosed and in later life may be discovered to have rheumatic heart disease without a definite history of rheumatic fever.

When carditis is manifest, there is usually tachycardia disproportionate to the degree of fever, gallop rhythms are often heard, and the heart sounds may become fetal or "tic-tac" in quality. Occasionally, arrhythmias and/or a pericardial friction rub may be present.

TABLE 187-1 Jones criteria (revised)

Major manifestations	Minor manifestations
Carditis	Fever
Polyarthritis	Arthralgia
Chorea	Previous rheumatic fever or rheumatic heart disease
Erythema marginatum	Elevated ESR or positive CRP
Subcutaneous nodules	Prolonged PR interval

Two major criteria or one major and two minor criteria indicate a high probability of the presence of rheumatic fever with supporting evidence of preceding streptococcal infection: history of recent scarlet fever; positive throat culture for group A streptococcus; increased ASO titer or other streptococcal antibodies.

SOURCE: American Heart Association, 1965.

Prolongation of the conduction time may lead to dropped beats with varying degrees of heart block. Prolongation of the PR interval and other changes in the electrocardiogram are very common, but these findings, in the absence of clinical manifestations of carditis, have a benign prognosis. Therefore, changes in the electrocardiogram alone, unassociated with significant murmurs or cardiac enlargement, do not by themselves constitute an acceptable criterion for the diagnosis of rheumatic carditis. Pericarditis may cause precordial pain, and a friction rub may be audible.

A definite clinical diagnosis of carditis can be made if one or more of the following can be demonstrated: (1) the appearance of, or change in the character of, organic heart murmurs; (2) definite increase in heart size demonstrated by radiogram or fluoroscopy; (3) pericardial friction rub or effusion best demonstrated by echocardiography; or (4) signs of congestive heart failure. Rheumatic carditis is almost always associated with a significant murmur.

Subcutaneous nodules These are usually small, pea-sized, painless swellings over bony prominences and therefore frequently go unnoticed by the patient. The skin moves freely over them. Characteristic locations are the extensor tendons of the hands and feet, the elbows, margins of the patellae, the scalp, over the scapulae, and over the spinous processes of the vertebrae.

Chorea (Sydenham's chorea, chorea minor, Saint Vitus' dance) This is a disorder of the central nervous system characterized by sudden, aimless, irregular movements, often accompanied by muscle weakness and emotional instability. Chorea is a delayed manifestation of rheumatic fever, and other manifestations may or may not still be present at the time it appears. Polyarthritis, when part of the same attack, always subsides before chorea appears. Carditis is often discovered for the first time when the presenting feature of rheumatic fever is chorea. Chorea usually appears after a long latent period (up to several months) from the antecedent streptococcal infection and at a time when all other manifestations of rheumatic fever have abated. When no previous rheumatic manifestations are noted, such cases are called *pure chorea*.

The clinical onset of chorea is often gradual. Patients may be unusually nervous and fidgety and may have difficulty in writing, drawing, and handiwork. They may stumble or fall, drop things, and grimace. As symptoms become more severe, spasmodic movements extend to all parts of the body, and muscular weakness may become so marked that patients cannot walk, talk, or sit up. Often the weakness is severe enough to simulate paralysis. The irregular, jerky, spasmodic movements may become so violent that cribs and beds must be padded to prevent injury. Symptoms are exaggerated by excitement, effort, or fatigue but subside during sleep. Emotional instability is almost invariable in patients with chorea. All degrees of speech disturbance are seen. Central nervous system stimulants exacerbate and sedatives suppress choreiform activity.

Erythema marginatum This evanescent pink rash is characteristic of rheumatic fever. The erythematous areas often have clear centers and round or serpiginous margins. They vary greatly in size and occur mainly on the trunk and proximal part of the extremities, never on the face. The erythema is transient, migratory, and may be brought out by the application of heat; it is nonpruritic, not indurated, and blanches on pressure.

Minor clinical criteria These are clinical features which occur frequently in rheumatic fever but are also common to many other diseases and are therefore of minor diagnostic value. They include fever, arthralgia, abdominal pain, tachycardia, and epistaxis.

LABORATORY FINDINGS There is no specific laboratory test to indicate the presence of rheumatic fever. The appraisal of rheumatic activity by laboratory findings is, however, of value, since various tests may indicate *continued* rheumatic inflammation when clinical features are not apparent.

Streptococcal antibody tests to disclose preceding streptococcal infection Streptococcal antibody titers differentiate preceding streptococcal from other acute respiratory infections and are increased following asymptomatic as well as symptomatic streptococcal infections. These antibody levels are increased in the early stages of acute rheumatic fever. They may be declining, or low, if the interval between the acute streptococcal infection and the detection of rheumatic fever has been longer than 2 months, a situation which occurs most often in patients whose presenting rheumatic manifestation is chorea. However, patients whose only major manifestation is rheumatic carditis also may have low antibody titers when first seen. Their rheumatic attack may have been in progress several months before becoming symptomatic and recognized. Except in these two instances, *one should be reluctant to make the diagnosis of acute rheumatic fever in the absence of serologic evidence of a recent streptococcal infection.* The antistreptolysin O test (ASO) is the most widely used and best-standardized streptococcal antibody test. In general, single titers of at least 250 Todd units in adults and at least 333 units in children over 5 years of age are considered to be increased. Depending on the general prevalence of streptococcal infections, a varying percentage of the normal population may show titers of this magnitude.

About 20 percent of patients in the early stages of acute rheumatic fever, and most patients who present with chorea, have a low or borderline ASO titer. In these instances, it is advisable to obtain a different streptococcal antibody test such as anti-DNase B, or antihyaluronidase (AH). The antistreptozyme test (ASTZ) is a hemagglutination reaction to a concentrate of extracellular streptococcal antigens absorbed to red blood cells. It is a very sensitive indicator of recent streptococcal infection; virtually all patients with acute rheumatic fever have titers greater than 200 units per milliliter. The real value of the ASTZ test is in *ruling out* rheumatic fever when the titer is low in patients with isolated polyarthritis. To date, the specific antigens involved in the ASTZ test remain unidentified and therefore the test has not yet been adequately standardized. A rise in titer of two dilution tubes or more can be demonstrated for at least one of the specific streptococcal antibodies in almost all recurrent as well as primary attacks of rheumatic fever. Increased streptococcal antibodies, however, do not reflect rheumatic activity per se, and their rate of decline is independent of the course of the rheumatic attack.

Isolation of group A streptococci   Some patients continue to harbor group A streptococci at the onset of acute rheumatic fever, but these organisms are usually present in small numbers and may be difficult to isolate by a single throat culture. The administration of penicillin or other antibiotics may also result in failure to isolate the infecting organism. In addition, a significant number of *normal* individuals, particularly children, may harbor group A streptococci in the upper respiratory tract. For these reasons, throat cultures are less satisfactory than antibody tests as supporting evidence of recent streptococcal infection.

Acute phase reactants   These tests offer objective but nonspecific confirmation of the presence of an inflammatory process. *The erythrocyte sedimentation rate* (ESR) and the test for *C-reactive protein* (CRP) in serum are used most commonly. Unless the patient has received glucocorticoids or salicylates, these reactions are almost always abnormal in patients presenting with polyarthritis or acute carditis, whereas they are often normal in patients with chorea. Other laboratory findings which reflect inflammation include reactions such as leukocytosis, and increases in serum complement, mucoproteins, and alpha$_2$ and gamma globulins. Prolongation of the PR interval of the electrocardiogram, although neither specific for rheumatic fever nor diagnostic of serious cardiac involvement, is frequent in acute rheumatic fever (about 25 percent of all cases), and other nonspecific electrocardiographic changes are also common. Anemia, due to the suppression of erythropoiesis characteristic of chronic inflammatory diseases, is another feature of rheumatic activity.

COURSE AND PROGNOSIS   The course of rheumatic fever varies greatly and is impossible to predict at the onset of the disease. In general, however, approximately 75 percent of acute rheumatic attacks subside within 6 weeks, 90 percent within 12 weeks, and less than 5 percent persist more than 6 months. These last usually consist of severe, intractable forms of rheumatic carditis or stubborn, prolonged attacks of Sydenham's chorea, both of which may persist for as long as several years. Once acute rheumatic fever has subsided and more than 2 months has elapsed after withdrawal of treatment with salicylates or glucocorticoids, rheumatic fever does not recur in the absence of new streptococcal infections. Recurrences are most common within the first 5 years of the initial attack and tend to decline with increasing duration of freedom from rheumatic activity. The frequency of recurrences is dependent upon the frequency and severity of streptococcal infection, the presence or absence of rheumatic heart disease following an attack, and the duration of freedom from the last attack.

Approximately 70 percent of patients who develop carditis do so within the first week of the disease, 85 percent within the first 12 weeks of the disease, and almost all within 6 months from the onset of the acute attack. Thereafter, if significant murmurs have not appeared, the prognosis for a patient in whom recurrences are prevented is excellent.

Chronic rheumatic carditis and the course of rheumatic heart disease   The remarkable variability in the course of rheumatic carditis and rheumatic valvular disease stems from several factors: (1) the variability in the duration and severity of the rheumatic inflammation; (2) the amount of scarring of the valves and myocardium following the abatement of the acute inflammation; (3) the location and severity of the hemodynamic lesion due to valvular insufficiency or stenosis; (4) the frequency of recurrent bouts of carditis; and (5) the progression of valvular calcification and sclerosis, which occurs as a secondary phenomenon in a deformed or injured valve without recurrent or persistent rheumatic inflammation (as seen in congenital valvular disease or following healed acute bacterial endocarditis). These factors, and possibly others not yet appreciated, produce striking variations in the clinical syndromes of rheumatic heart disease.

Chronic rheumatic myocarditis   In this syndrome, the presenting picture is one of chronic heart failure in a patient with a markedly dilated heart and with physical, roentgenographic, and electrocardiographic findings of mitral and/or aortic and sometimes tricuspid regurgitation. The differentiation of this syndrome from other forms of chronic myocarditis may be very difficult, if not impossible, when the associated extracardiac features of rheumatic fever (chorea, polyarthritis, and so forth) are not present (Chap. 192). Although rheumatic fever does not produce *isolated* myocarditis, and is almost invariably a pancarditis, the pericardial inflammation may not be clearly evident, and the mitral valvulitis may not be distinguishable from mitral regurgitation due to dilation of the mitral ring. In such cases one must search diligently for an evanescent friction rub, evidence of pericardial effusion, appearance of a soft aortic regurgitation murmur, and extracardiac clues such as fever responding promptly to salicylates, arthralgias, transient subcutaneous nodules, evanescent erythema marginatum, and subtle signs of chorea.

The course of chronic rheumatic carditis may be intractable and end fatally after months or even several years. Often, however, the patient improves rather suddenly and even recovers cardiac reserve dramatically in association with the disappearance of systemic manifestations of the inflammatory process. The heart may remain large, may decrease somewhat in size, or in occasional instances may return to normal size with varying degrees of residual valvular deformity. Such a course signals the termination of the "toxic" phase of the rheumatic process, and thereafter the course of rheumatic heart disease depends on the variables in healing cited above.

DIFFERENTIAL DIAGNOSIS   Early cases of rheumatic fever may be confused with other diseases which begin with acute polyarthritis. It is wise to exclude *bacteremia* by blood cultures, particularly because such infections may be masked by penicillin given for presumed acute rheumatic fever. Polyarthritis due to *infective endocarditis* in a patient with preexisting rheumatic heart disease may be mistaken for a recurrence of acute rheumatic fever. If streptococcal antibodies are not increased, polyarthritis should be attributed to some cause other than rheumatic fever. Gonococcal polyarthritis may be distinguished from rheumatic fever by the dramatic response of the former to a therapeutic trial of penicillin. In rheumatoid arthritis, joint involvement will persist and characteristic joint deformities may appear. The latter are not seen in rheumatic fever. The rheumatoid factor so characteristic of rheumatoid arthritis is not present in rheumatic fever. Antibodies against nuclear components and other autoantibodies are absent in rheumatic fever. Rheumatic pericarditis and myocarditis, associated with cardiac enlargement and heart failure, are both almost invariably associated with valvular lesions which produce significant murmurs.

Overdiagnosis of rheumatic fever is a danger. Unless ill-defined febrile syndromes are clearly associated with a major manifestation of rheumatic fever, the diagnosis of rheumatic fever should not be made. A common error is the premature, vigorous administration of glucocorticoids or salicylates before the signs and symptoms of rheumatic fever are unmistakable. In the absence of a curative agent, one should not suppress the signs and symptoms of rheumatic fever until they are clearly expressed.

Particularly confusing in the differential diagnosis of rheumatic fever is the drug sensitivity with fever and polyarthritis which may occur after administration of penicillin for a previous pharyngitis. Urticaria or angioedema, if present, helps identify penicillin sensitivity in such cases. The abdominal pain of rheumatic fever may be mistaken for appendicitis, and the crisis of sickle cell anemia may also be associated with joint pain, enlargement of the heart, and cardiac murmurs. The rapidity with which the arthritis symptoms of rheumatic fever are controlled with salicylates is characteristic of this disease. Dramatic response to salicylates does not in itself, however, establish a diagnosis of rheumatic fever.

In order to help clarify the diagnosis of rheumatic fever, the American Heart Association has accepted and modified criteria usually referred to as the *Jones criteria* (Table 187-1). They are not to be used as a substitute for good medical judgment but are recommended as a guide for careful study of questionable cases. The finding of two major criteria, or of one major and two minor criteria, indicates a high probability of the presence of rheumatic fever if supported by evidence of a preceding streptococcal infection. The absence of the latter should always make the diagnosis questionable, except in the situation in which rheumatic fever is first discovered after a long latent period from the antecedent infection (Sydenham's chorea or low-grade carditis). Because the prognosis may differ according to the major manifestations, for recording purposes the diagnosis of rheumatic fever should be followed by a list of the major manifestations present, e.g., rheumatic fever manifested by polyarthritis and carditis (Table 187-2). An indication of the severity of carditis in terms of presence or absence of congestive heart failure and cardiomegaly is also advisable.

TREATMENT   There is no specific cure for rheumatic fever, and no known measures change the course of the attack. Good supportive therapy, however, can reduce the mortality and morbidity of the disease.

Chemotherapy   After rheumatic fever is first diagnosed, a course of penicillin should be given to eliminate group A streptococci. This course is advisable even if bacteriologic examination yields throat cultures negative for streptococci, since the organisms may be present in areas inaccessible to swabs. It is preferable to administer penicillin parenterally. An effective course is a single injection of 1.2 million units of benzathine penicillin intramuscularly or 600,000 units of procaine penicillin intramuscularly daily for 10 days. Attempts to reduce ultimate heart damage by administering penicillin early in the acute rheumatic attack in larger doses have not been successful. After completion of the therapeutic course of penicillin, continuous protection from reinfection with streptococci should be provided by instituting one of the prophylactic regimens described below.

Suppressive therapy   For patients without carditis, treatment with glucocorticoids is unnecessary. Acute arthritis can be relieved with codeine or with salicylate, the latter being preferable to reduce fever and joint inflammation. When salicylate is used in the therapy of rheumatic fever, the dosage should be increased until the drug produces either a clinical effect or systemic toxicity characterized by tinnitus, headache, or hyperpnea. A starting dose of 100 to 125 mg/kg per day in children and 6 to 8 g in adults given in four or five divided doses is recommended. Of the various salicylate preparations ordinary aspirin is cheapest and most effective.

Many physicians prefer glucocorticoids to salicylates for the treatment of carditis, despite the lack of a demonstrated advantage of these adrenal hormones in controlled clinical trials. Glucocorticoids are more potent anti-inflammatory agents but are more likely to be followed by posttherapeutic "rebounds," and they have the additional disadvantage of more frequent side effects, particularly acne, hirsutism, and cushingoid changes in facies and habitus. For this reason it is preferable to begin treatment of patients who have carditis with salicylates; if these drugs fail to reduce fever and to ameliorate heart failure, therapy with glucocorticoids may be initiated promptly. Prednisone is administered in doses of 60 to 120 mg or higher when necessary in four divided doses daily. After the inflammation has been brought under control by either salicylates or glucocorticoids, treatment should be continued until the sedimentation rate approaches near-normal values and should be maintained for several weeks thereafter. To prevent poststeroid rebounds, an "overlap" course of salicylate therapy may be added when steroids are tapered off over a 2-week period. A useful method for tapering steroids is outlined in Chap. 317. Salicylates may then be continued for an additional 2 to 3 weeks. Rebounds of rheumatic activity are usually of short duration and, when mild, are best managed without resuming anti-inflammatory treatment, because a second or even a third rebound may occur when suppressive therapy is discontinued. About 5 percent of rheumatic attacks persist for 6 months or longer, either in the form of spontaneous acute recrudescences or as posttherapeutic rebounds. These "chronic" attacks are most likely to occur in patients with cardiac damage and with previous rheumatic episodes. Weekly tests for C-reactive protein in blood and for erythrocyte sedimentation rate are useful in following the healing process, particularly while treatment with glucocorticoids or salicylates is gradually withdrawn.

Treatment of chorea   The signs and symptoms of chorea usually do not respond well to treatment with antirheumatic agents. Because the patient with chorea is frequently emotionally unstable and because the manifestations of chorea may be exaggerated by emotional trauma, complete mental and physical rest is essential. Patients with chorea should be kept in a quiet room and cared for by sympathetic attendants. Glucocorticoids or salicylates have little or no effect on chorea. Sedatives and tranquilizers, particularly diazepam and chlorpromazine, are useful. Chorea, no matter how severe, disappears during sleep, which should therefore be ensured by adequate sedation. Padded sideboards for the bed may be necessary to avoid injury to the patient. In the absence of other evidence of acute rheumatic disease, it is advisable to allow gradual resumption of physical activity when improvement is apparent rather than waiting for all choreiform movements to disappear, which may require many months.

Because of the great variability in the course of chorea, evaluating the effectiveness of various therapeutic measures is difficult. It is well to remember that chorea is a self-limited disease which is usually

TABLE 187-2   Ninety-nine cases of acute rheumatic fever indicated by three major manifestations of Jones Criteria

Major manifestations*	Percent
Carditis	14
Polyarthritis	14
Chorea	4
Carditis and polyarthritis	44
Carditis and chorea	14
Carditis, chorea, and polyarthritis	6
Polyarthritis and chorea	4
Total	**100**

*Categories are mutually exclusive.

SOURCE: Acute rheumatic fever—Utah. Morb Mort Week Rep 36:109, 1988 not followed by significant neurologic sequelae and that good results are almost invariably obtained by patient, attentive nursing care and by conservative medical management.

PREVENTION OF RECURRENCE   The resurgence of localized outbreaks of rheumatic fever in the United States in recent years has been blamed, in part, upon less than faithful adherence to conventional recommendations for rigorous penicillin regimens known to be highly effective in the prevention of both primary and secondary rheumatic attacks. It is recommended, therefore, that these regimens continue to be employed. The most efficient regimen for continuous prophylaxis against group A streptococci is a monthly intramuscular injection of 1.2 million units of benzathine penicillin G. The disadvantages and discomfort of this regimen have to be weighed against the individual patient's susceptibility to recurrences. Those with rheumatic heart disease, recent rheumatic fever, and exposure to an environment in which the incidence of streptococcal infection is frequent deserve the most effective protection. As a second choice, prophylaxis may be administered orally with either 1 g sulfadiazine daily in a single dose or 200,000 units of penicillin given twice daily on an empty stomach. The duration of continuous prophylaxis cannot be fixed arbitrarily. Certainly, those under the age of 18 years should receive a continuous prophylactic regimen. A minimum period of 5 years is recommended for patients who develop rheumatic fever without carditis over the age of 18 years. The decision to continue prophylaxis beyond this period should take into account a number of variables. Patients with rheumatic heart disease are more susceptible to reactivation of rheumatic fever if they contract a streptococcal infection. Moreover, patients who have had carditis in a previous attack are much more likely to suffer carditis again in a subsequent attack. Climate, age, occupation, household situation, cardiac status, and length of time since the previous attack are all significant variables which influence the risk of recurrence. The decline in recurrence rates with increasing age is due to (1) decreased rate of streptococcal infection and (2) decrease in the rate of rheumatic reactivation following streptococcal infection in older rheumatic subjects. Despite this decreased rate, however, the risk of rheumatic recurrence in adults remains relatively high when the streptococcal disease encountered is severe or epidemic and particularly when rheumatic fever is known to be extant in the population to which a rheumatic subject is exposed.

PREVENTION OF INITIAL RHEUMATIC ATTACKS   Early and adequate treatment of pharyngeal infection due to group A streptococci will prevent initial attacks of rheumatic fever. If clinical streptococcal disease were properly detected by throat cultures and adequately treated, the spread of infection in a given population would be prevented, the epidemiology of streptococcal disease would be modified markedly, and the incidence of rheumatic fever in the community would be diminished. In communities where group A streptococcal disease has been diagnosed early and treated well and where socioeconomic standards are high, the group A organisms cultured frequently from schoolchildren's throats may be of relatively low virulence and may cause rheumatic fever less frequently than do more virulent strains prevalent in many epidemics. The appearance of rheumatic fever in a community, however, signals the presence of rheumatogenic streptococci whose spread must be interrupted by use of effective penicillin regimens. In a closed population, such as a military base or an institution, an outbreak of rheumatic fever is best treated by mass penicillin prophylaxis, that is, treatment of all exposed individuals, whether or not symptomatic.

Streptococcal pharyngitis is adequately treated by a single intramuscular injection of 600,000 units of benzathine penicillin in children less than 10 years of age or 1.2 million units in older children and adults. Any alternate plan of parenteral therapy or combined parenteral and oral therapy should provide for treatment over a period of 10 days. If oral penicillin is employed, at least 800,000 units per day in four divided doses must be given for no less than 10 days to achieve results comparable with a single injection of benzathine penicillin. Erythromycin in daily doses of 1 g for 10 days may be substituted in penicillin-sensitive individuals. Tetracycline is not recommended because some strains of group A streptococci have acquired resistance to it. All group A streptococci have so far remained extremely sensitive to penicillin. When erythromycin has been used extensively in place of penicillin, as in Japan, erythromycin-resistant group A streptococci have emerged with high frequency. Penicillin therefore remains the treatment of choice for streptococcal sore throat.

REFERENCES

CENTERS FOR DISEASE CONTROL: Acute rheumatic fever—Utah. Morb Mort Week Rep 36:108, 1987
————: Acute rheumatic fever at a navy training center—San Diego, CA. Morb Mort Week Rep 37:101, 1988
————: Acute rheumatic fever among army trainees—Fort Leonard Wood, MO 1987–1988. Morb Mort Week Rep 37:519, 1988
AHA COMMITTEE ON RHEUMATIC FEVER AND BACTERIAL ENDOCARDITIS: Prevention of rheumatic fever. Circulation 70:1118A, 1984
AMERICAN HEART ASSOCIATION: Jones criteria (revised) for guidance in the diagnosis of rheumatic fever. Circulation 69:204A, 1984
BISNO AL et al: Contrasting epidemiology of acute rheumatic fever and acute glomerulonephritis. Nature of the Antecedent streptococcal infection. N Engl J Med 283:561, 1970
HOSIER DM et al: Resurgence of acute rheumatic fever. Am J Dis Child 141:730, 1987
JOINT REPORT OF UK-US COOPERATIVE STUDY: The natural history of rheumatic fever and rheumatic heart disease. 10 year report of a cooperative clinical trial of ACTH, cortisone and aspirin. Circulation 32:457, 1965
KAPLAN EL et al: Group A streptococci serotypes isolated from patients and sibling contacts during the resurgence of rheumatic fever in the United States in the mid-1980s. J Infect Dis 159:101, 1989
KHANNA AK et al: Presence of a non-HLA-B cell antigen in rheumatic fever patients and their families as defined by a monoclonal antibody. J Clin Invest 83:1710, 1989
LAND MA, BISNO AL: Acute rheumatic fever: A vanishing disease in suburbia. JAMA 249:895, 1983
MASSELL BF et al: Penicillin and the marked decrease in morbidity and mortality from rheumatic fever in the United States. N Eng J Med 318:280, 1988
READ S, ZABRISKIE JB (eds): Streptococcal Diseases and the Immune Response. New York, Academic, 1980
STOLLERMAN GH: The relative rheumatogenicity of strains of group A streptococci. Modern Concept Cardio Dis 44:35, 1975
————: Rheumatogenic group A streptococci and the return of rheumatic fever, in Advances in Internal Medicine, Vol. 35, Chicago, Year Book Medical Publishers, 1990

188   VALVULAR HEART DISEASE

EUGENE BRAUNWALD

The role of physical examination in the evaluation of patients with valvular disease is also considered in Chap. 175; of roentgenography, echocardiography, and other noninvasive techniques in Chap. 177; of electrocardiography in Chap. 176; of cardiac catheterization and angiography in Chap. 179; and of balloon valvuloplasty in Chap. 180.

MITRAL STENOSIS

ETIOLOGY AND PATHOLOGY   Two-thirds of all patients with mitral stenosis (MS) are females. MS is generally rheumatic in origin. Pure or predominant MS occurs in approximately 40 percent of all patients with rheumatic heart disease. The valve leaflets are diffusely thickened by fibrous tissue and/or calcific deposits. The mitral commissures fuse, the chordae tendineae fuse and shorten, the valvular cusps become rigid, and these changes in turn lead to narrowing at the apex of the funnel-shaped valve. While the initial insult to the mitral valve is rheumatic, the later changes may be a nonspecific process resulting from trauma to the valve caused by altered flow patterns due to the initial deformity. Calcification of the stenotic mitral valve immobilizes the leaflets and narrows the orifice. Thrombus formation and arterial embolization may arise from the calcific valve itself. Rarely, MS is congenital in origin.

PATHOPHYSIOLOGY In normal adults the mitral valve orifice is 4 to 6 cm^2. In the presence of significant obstruction, i.e., when the orifice is less than one-half of normal, blood can flow from the left atrium to the left ventricle only if propelled by an abnormally elevated left atrioventricular pressure gradient (Fig. 196-6), the hemodynamic hallmark of MS. When the mitral valve opening is reduced to 1 cm^2, a left atrial pressure of approximately 25 mmHg is required to maintain a normal cardiac output. The elevated left atrial pressure in turn raises pulmonary venous and capillary pressures, reducing pulmonary compliance and causing exertional dyspnea. The first bouts of dyspnea are usually precipitated by clinical events which increase the rate of blood flow across the mitral orifice, which results in further elevation of the left atrial pressure (see below). In order to assess the severity of obstruction, it is essential to measure both the transvalvular pressure gradient and the flow rate (Chap. 179). The latter is dependent not only on the cardiac output but on the heart rate as well. An increase in heart rate shortens diastole proportionately more than systole, and diminishes the time available for flow across the mitral valve. Therefore, at any given level of cardiac output tachycardia augments the transvalvular gradient and elevates further the left atrial pressure.

The left ventricular diastolic pressure is normal in isolated MS; coexisting mitral regurgitation, aortic valve disease, the residua of damage produced by rheumatic myocarditis, systemic hypertension, or ischemic heart disease are sometimes responsible for elevations which reflect impaired left ventricular function and/or reduced left ventricular compliance. Left ventricular dysfunction, as reflected in reduced ejection fraction and circumferential fiber shortening rate, occurs in about one-fourth of patients with MS. This is a consequence of chronic reduction of preload and extension of the scarring from the valve into the adjacent myocardium. In pure MS and sinus rhythm, the mean left atrial and pulmonary artery wedge pressures are usually elevated and the pressure pulse shows a prominent atrial contraction (*a* wave) and a gradual pressure decline after mitral valve opening (*y* descent). In patients with mild to moderate MS without elevation of the pulmonary vascular resistance, the pulmonary arterial pressure may be near the upper limits of normal at rest and may rise with exercise. In severe MS and whenever the pulmonary vascular resistance is significantly increased, the pulmonary arterial pressure is elevated even when the patient is at rest, and in extreme cases it may exceed the systemic arterial pressure. Further elevations of left atrial, pulmonary capillary, and pulmonary arterial pressures occur during exercise. When the pulmonary arterial systolic pressure exceeds approximately 50 mmHg in patients with MS, or for that matter with any valvular lesion, the increased right ventricular afterload impedes the emptying of this chamber, and right ventricular end-diastolic pressure and volume usually rise as a compensatory mechanism.

Cardiac output This varies considerably. Thus, the hemodynamic response to a given degree of mitral obstruction may be characterized by a normal cardiac output at rest and a high left atrioventricular pressure gradient or, at the opposite end of the hemodynamic spectrum, by a reduced cardiac output and low transvalvular pressure gradient. In a small fraction of patients with moderately severe MS, the cardiac output is normal at rest and rises normally during exertion; under these circumstances, the high atrioventricular pressure gradient elevates the left atrial and pulmonary capillary pressures markedly, and this elevation is responsible for symptoms of relatively severe pulmonary congestion. In the majority of patients with moderate MS, however, the cardiac output is normal at rest but rises subnormally during exertion. In patients with severe MS, particularly those in whom the pulmonary vascular resistance is strikingly elevated, the cardiac output is subnormal at rest and may fail to rise or may even decline during activity. The depressed cardiac output in patients with MS is related primarily to the obstruction of

the mitral orifice but may also be due to the impairment of the function of either ventricle.

Pulmonary hypertension The clinical and hemodynamic features of MS are influenced importantly by the level of the pulmonary artery pressure. Pulmonary hypertension results from (1) the passive backward transmission of the elevated left atrial pressure, (2) pulmonary arteriolar constriction, which presumably is triggered by left atrial and pulmonary venous hypertension (reactive pulmonary hypertension), and (3) organic obliterative changes in the pulmonary vascular bed. The elevation of pulmonary vascular resistance may be considered to be a complication of long-standing and severe MS; in time, the resultant severe pulmonary hypertension results in tricuspid and pulmonary incompetence as well as right sided heart failure. However, the changes in the pulmonary vascular bed may also be considered to exert a protective effect; the elevated precapillary resistance reduces the likelihood of symptoms of pulmonary congestion by reducing the surge of blood into the pulmonary capillary bed which then dams up behind the stenotic mitral valve during activity. However, this protection occurs at the expense of a decreased cardiac output.

SYMPTOMS AND COMPLICATIONS In temperate climates the latent period between the initial attack of rheumatic carditis (in the increasingly rare circumstances in which a history of one can be elicited) and the development of symptoms due to MS is generally on the order of two decades; most patients begin to experience disability in the fourth decade. Once a patient with MS becomes seriously symptomatic, continuous progression of the disease to death usually occurs in 2 to 5 years unless the stenosis is relieved. In economically deprived areas, particularly on the Indian subcontinent, in Central America, and the Middle East, MS tends to progress more rapidly and frequently causes serious symptoms before the age of 20 years. On the other hand, slowly progressive MS in the elderly is being recognized with increasing frequency in the United States and western Europe.

When valvular obstruction is mild, many of the physical signs of MS may be present in the absence of any symptoms. However, even in those patients whose mitral orifices are large enough to accommodate a normal blood flow with only mild elevations of left atrial pressure, extreme exertion, excitement, fever, severe anemia, paroxysmal tachycardia, sexual intercourse, pregnancy, and thyrotoxicosis all may precipitate elevations of pulmonary capillary pressure and lead to dyspnea and cough. As stenosis progresses, the stresses that precipitate dyspnea become less severe, and the patient becomes limited in his or her daily activities. Redistribution of blood from the dependent portions of the body to the lungs, which occurs when the recumbent position is assumed, leads to orthopnea and paroxysmal nocturnal dyspnea. *Pulmonary edema* develops when there is a sudden surge in flow across a markedly narrowed mitral orifice (Chap. 36). When moderately severe MS has existed for several years, *atrial arrhythmias*—premature contractions, paroxysmal tachycardia, flutter, and fibrillation—occur with increasing frequency. The rapid ventricular rate associated with untreated or inadequately treated atrial fibrillation is frequently responsible for acute exacerbations of dyspnea. The development of permanent atrial fibrillation often marks a turning point in the patient's course and is generally associated with acceleration of the rate at which symptoms progress.

Hemoptysis (Chap. 35) results from rupture of pulmonary-bronchial venous connections secondary to pulmonary venous hypertension. It occurs most frequently in patients who have elevated left atrial pressures *without* markedly elevated pulmonary vascular resistances and is almost never fatal. True hemoptysis must be distinguished from the bloody sputum that occurs with pulmonary edema, pulmonary infarction, and bronchitis, three conditions that occur with increased frequency in the presence of MS.

As the condition progresses and the pulmonary vascular resistance rises or when tricuspid stenosis or regurgitation develops, symptoms secondary to pulmonary congestion may diminish, and the episodes of acute pulmonary edema and hemoptysis become reduced in frequency and severity. Elevation of pulmonary vascular resistance further increases right ventricular systolic pressure, leading to right ventricular failure, fatigue, abdominal discomfort due to hepatic congestion, and edema.

Recurrent pulmonary emboli, sometimes with infarction (Chap. 213), are an important cause of morbidity and mortality late in the course of MS, occurring most frequently in patients with right ventricular failure. *Pulmonary infections*, i.e., bronchitis, bronchopneumonia, and lobar pneumonia, commonly complicate untreated MS. *Infective endocarditis* (Chap. 90) is rare in *pure* MS but is not uncommon in patients with combined stenosis and regurgitation. *Chest pain* occurs in about 10 percent of patients with severe MS; it may be due to pulmonary hypertension or myocardial ischemia secondary to coronary atherosclerosis; often the cause cannot be discovered.

Pulmonary and pulmonary vascular changes   In addition to the aforementioned changes in the pulmonary vascular bed, fibrous thickening of the walls of the alveoli and pulmonary capillaries occurs commonly in MS. The vital capacity, total lung capacity, maximal breathing capacity, and oxygen uptake per unit of ventilation are reduced (Chap. 201), and in patients with severe MS the latter fails to rise normally during exertion. The reduction of pulmonary compliance that occurs generally correlates directly with the severity of the dyspnea and with the heightened pulmonary capillary pressure, and these changes are intensified during exercise. In some patients airway resistance is abnormally increased. These alterations in pulmonary mechanics contribute to an increase in the work of breathing and play an important role in the genesis of dyspnea. The changes in the lungs are due, in part, to increased transudation of fluid from the pulmonary capillaries into the interstitial and alveolar spaces as a consequence of the elevated pulmonary capillary pressure. The distribution of blood flow and ventilation may be uneven; as in other conditions in which left atrial pressure is elevated, pulmonary blood flow in the erect position is displaced from the basal to the superior segments of the lung (Chap. 201). The diffusing capacity may be reduced, particularly during exertion, as a result of structural changes in the diffusing surface and reduction of the pulmonary capillary blood volume. The thickening of the alveolar and capillary walls impedes the transudation of fluid into the alveoli and the development of pulmonary edema at times when the pulmonary capillary pressure exceeds the plasma oncotic pressure. The increased capacity of the pulmonary lymphatic system to drain excess fluid also retards the development of pulmonary edema.

Thrombi and emboli   *Thrombi* may form in the left atria, particularly in the enlarged atrial appendages of patients with MS. If they embolize, they do so most commonly to the brain, kidneys, spleen, and extremities. *Embolization* occurs much more frequently in patients with atrial fibrillation or unstable rhythms, in older patients, and in those with a reduced cardiac output, and it is seen in patients with relatively mild, as well as in those with severe, obstruction. Thus, systemic embolization may be the presenting complaint in otherwise asymptomatic patients with mild MS. At operation, thrombi are *not* found more frequently in the left atria of patients with a past history of embolization than in those without this complication, indicating that it is usually the freshly formed clots that dislodge. Patients who have had one or more systemic emboli have an increased predilection for further embolic episodes compared with patients with stenosis of comparable severity without previous embolization. Rarely, a large pedunculated thrombus or a free-floating clot may suddenly obstruct the stenotic mitral orifice. Such "ball valve" thrombi produce syncope, angina, and changing auscultatory signs with alterations in position, findings that resemble those produced by a left atrial myxoma (Chap. 194).

PHYSICAL FINDINGS   (See also Chap. 175)   **Inspection**   Peripheral and facial *cyanosis* may occur in patients with extremely severe MS. In advanced cases there is a malar flush and the facies appear pinched and blue. The jugular venous pulse reveals prominent *a* waves due to vigorous right atrial systole in patients with sinus rhythm who

have severe pulmonary hypertension or associated tricuspid stenosis. When atrial fibrillation is present, the jugular pulse reveals only a single expansion during systole (*c-v* wave). The systemic arterial pressure is usually normal or slightly low.

Palpation   A right ventricular tap is present along the left sternal border, signifying an enlarged right ventricle. The first heart sound may be palpable in patients with pliable valve leaflets. In patients with pulmonary hypertension, the impact of pulmonary valve closure can usually be felt in the second and third left intercostal spaces just left of the sternum; the left ventricle is not palpable in severe, pure MS. A diastolic thrill is frequently present at the cardiac apex, particularly if the patient is turned into the left lateral recumbent position.

Auscultation   The first heart sound (S_1) is generally accentuated and snapping, and since the mitral valve does not close until the left ventricular pressure reaches the level of the elevated left atrial pressure, this sound is often slightly delayed on phonocardiography, particularly in patients with severe stenosis. In patients with pulmonary hypertension, the pulmonary component of the second heart sound (P_2) is often accentuated, and the two components of the second heart sound are closely split. A pulmonary systolic ejection click may be heard in patients with severe pulmonary hypertension and marked dilatation of the pulmonary artery. The opening snap (OS) of the mitral valve is most readily audible in expiration at, or just medial to, the cardiac apex but may also be easily heard along the left sternal edge or at the base of the heart. This sound generally follows the sound of aortic valve closure (A_2) by 0.06 to 0.12 s, that is, it follows P_2. Since the OS occurs when the left ventricular pressure falls below the left atrial pressure, the time interval between A_2 closure and OS varies inversely with the severity of the MS. It tends to be short, that is, 0.06 to 0.07 s, in patients with severe obstruction and long, that is, 0.10 to 0.12 s, in patients with mild MS. The intensities of the OS and S_1 correlate with the mobility of the anterior mitral leaflet.

The OS usually ushers in a low-pitched, rumbling, diastolic murmur, heard best at the apex with the patient in the left lateral recumbent position and often accentuated by exercise carried out just before auscultation. In general, the duration of this murmur correlates with the severity of the stenosis. In patients with sinus rhythm the murmur often reappears or becomes reaccentuated during atrial systole, as atrial contraction reelevates the rate of blood flow across the narrowed orifice. Soft (grade I or II/VI) systolic murmurs are commonly heard at the apex or along the left sternal border in patients with pure MS and do not necessarily signify the presence of mitral regurgitation. Hepatomegaly, ankle edema, ascites, and pleural effusion, particularly in the right pleural cavity, may occur in patients with MS and right ventricular failure.

Associated lesions   With severe pulmonary hypertension a loud pansystolic murmur produced by functional tricuspid regurgitation may be audible along the left sternal border. This murmur may be accentuated by inspiration, diminishes during forced expiration or during performance of the Valsalva maneuver, diminishes or disappears as compensation is restored, and must not be confused with the apical pansystolic murmur of mitral regurgitation, since management is quite different if mitral regurgitation is present.

The recognition of associated mitral regurgitation is of considerable clinical importance in patients with MS. A presystolic murmur and an accentuated first heart sound speak against the presence of serious associated mitral regurgitation, but when the first heart sound and/or the opening snap are soft or absent in a patient with mitral valve disease who also has an apical systolic murmur, it is likely that significant mitral regurgitation and/or serious calcification of the deformed mitral valve leaflets are present. A third heart sound at the apex often signifies that the mitral regurgitation is serious; this sound is generally duller and lower pitched and follows the opening snap. Occasionally, in patients with pure MS, physical signs may falsely suggest mitral regurgitation. Thus, in the presence of severe pulmonary hypertension and right ventricular failure, a third heart sound may originate from the right ventricle. The enlarged right ventricle may rotate the heart in a clockwise direction and form the cardiac apex, giving the examiner the erroneous impression of left ventricular enlargement. Under these circumstances the rumbling diastolic murmur and the other auscultatory features of MS become less prominent or may even disappear and be replaced by the systolic murmur of functional tricuspid regurgitation which is mistaken for mitral regurgitation. When cardiac output is markedly reduced in a patient with MS the typical auscultatory findings, including the diastolic rumbling murmur (silent MS), may not be detectable, but they may reappear as compensation is restored. Associated tricuspid stenosis also tends to obscure many of the physical signs of MS.

The Graham Steell murmur of pulmonary regurgitation, a high-pitched, diastolic, decrescendo blowing murmur along the left sternal border, results from dilatation of the pulmonary valve ring and occurs in patients with mitral valve disease and severe pulmonary hypertension. This murmur may be indistinguishable from the more common murmur produced by mild aortic regurgitation except that it is rarely audible at the second right intercostal space, and may disappear following successful surgical treatment of the MS.

Electrocardiogram   In MS and sinus rhythm the P wave usually suggests left atrial enlargement (Chap. 176). It may become tall and peaked in lead II and upright in lead V_1 when severe pulmonary hypertension or tricuspid stenosis complicates MS and right atrial enlargement occurs. The QRS complex may be normal, even in patients with critical MS. However, with severe pulmonary hypertension, right axis deviation and right ventricular hypertrophy are usually found. When left ventricular hypertrophy is present in patients with MS, it generally indicates that an additional lesion which places a significant burden on the left ventricle, such as mitral regurgitation, aortic valve disease, or hypertension, is present.

Echocardiogram   (See also Chap. 177)   The echocardiogram is the most sensitive and specific noninvasive method for diagnosing MS. The M-mode tracing reveals that the anterior and posterior mitral leaflets do not separate widely in early diastole (i.e., less than 15 mm) and they maintain a fixed relation to each other throughout diastole. However, two-dimensional, color Doppler flow echocardiographic imaging and Doppler echocardiography provide critical information (see Figs. 177-3 and 177-5), including an estimate of the transvalvular gradient and of mitral orifice size, the presence and severity of accompanying mitral regurgitation, the extent of restriction of valve leaflets, their thickness, and the degree of distortion of the subvalvular apparatus. In addition, echocardiography provides an assessment of the size of the cardiac chambers, an estimation of the pulmonary artery pressure, and an indication of the presence and severity of associated tricuspid and pulmonic regurgitation.

Roentgenogram   (Chap. 177)   The earliest changes are straightening of the left border of the cardiac silhouette, prominence of the main pulmonary arteries, dilatation of the upper lobe pulmonary veins, and backward displacement of the esophagus by an enlarged left atrium. In patients with mild or moderate MS, the heart is not grossly enlarged. In severe MS, however, all chambers and vessels upstream to the narrowed valve are prominent, including the two atria, the pulmonary arteries and veins, right ventricle, and superior vena cava. Kerley B lines are fine, dense, opaque, horizontal lines which are most prominent in the lower and midlung fields and which result from distention of interlobular septa and lymphatics with edema when the resting mean left atrial pressure exceeds approximately 20 mmHg. As the pulmonary arterial pressure rises, the smaller pulmonary arteries become attenuated, at first in the lower, then in the mid-, and finally in the upper lung fields. Deposits of hemosiderin occur in the lungs of patients who have had multiple hemoptyses; the hemosiderin-containing macrophages fill the air spaces, and if they become confluent, result in a fine, diffuse nodulation most prominent in the lower lung fields.

DIFFERENTIAL DIAGNOSIS   Significant mitral regurgitation may be associated with a prominent diastolic murmur at the apex, but this murmur commences slightly later than in patients with MS, and there is often clear-cut evidence of left ventricular enlargement on physical examination, roentgenography, and electrocardiography. In addition, an apical pansystolic murmur of at least grade III/VI intensity as well as a third heart sound should arouse the suspicion of significant associated regurgitation. Similarly, the apical middiastolic murmur associated with aortic regurgitation (Austin Flint murmur) may be mistaken for MS. However, in a patient with aortic regurgitation the absence of an opening snap or of presystolic accentuation if sinus rhythm is present points to the *absence* of MS. Tricuspid stenosis, a valvular lesion that occurs very rarely in the absence of MS, may mask many of the clinical features of MS. Echocardiography is particularly useful in detecting MS in patients who have or are suspected of having other valve lesions and in defining the severity of the various lesions.

Exertional dyspnea and recurrent pulmonary infections may be falsely ascribed to pulmonary emphysema in patients with both *chronic lung disease* and MS. Careful auscultation, however, will generally reveal the characteristic opening snap and rumbling diastolic murmur. Similarly, the hemoptysis that occurs in many otherwise asymptomatic patients with MS may be improperly attributed to bronchiectasis or tuberculosis. Actually, the latter condition is uncommon in patients with significant mitral obstruction.

Primary pulmonary hypertension (Chap. 212) results in a number of the clinical and laboratory features observed in MS. It occurs most frequently in young women; however, the OS and diastolic rumbling murmur are absent, there is no left atrial enlargement, and the pulmonary artery wedge and left atrial pressures are *normal*, as is the size of the left atrium on echocardiography. *Atrial septal defect* (Chap. 186) may also be mistaken for MS; in both conditions there is often clinical, electrocardiographic, and roentgenographic evidence of right ventricular enlargement and accentuation of the pulmonary vascularity. The widely split S_2 of atrial septal defect may be confused with the mitral OS, and the diastolic flow murmur across the tricuspid valve mistaken for the mitral diastolic murmur. However, the absence of left atrial enlargement and of Kerley B lines and the demonstration of fixed splitting of S_2 favor atrial septal defect over MS. *Cor triatriatum* is an unusual congenital malformation that consists of a fibrous ring within the left atrium. It results in elevation of the pulmonary venous, capillary, and arterial pressures. This lesion can be recognized most readily by means of left atrial angiography.

Left atrial myxoma (Chap. 194) may obstruct left atrial emptying, resulting in dyspnea, a diastolic murmur, and hemodynamic changes resembling those of MS. However, patients with left atrial myxoma often demonstrate findings suggestive of a systemic disease, with weight loss, fever, anemia, systemic emboli, and elevated erythrocyte sedimentation rate and serum IgG concentration. Usually an OS is not audible, there is no clinical evidence of associated aortic valve disease, and the auscultatory findings frequently change with body position. The diagnosis can be established by demonstrating a characteristic echo-producing mass in the left atrium by two-dimensional echocardiography and a lobulated filling defect by angiocardiography.

CARDIAC CATHETERIZATION AND ANGIOCARDIOGRAPHY
Catheterization of the left side of the heart (Chap. 179) is extremely helpful in deciding whether valvulotomy is necessary in patients in whom it is difficult to estimate the severity of obstruction by clinical means and noninvasive tests. When combined with aortography and left ventricular angiocardiography, this procedure serves as the ultimate method for detecting and estimating associated mitral regurgitation and coexisting lesions such as aortic stenosis and regurgitation as well as left ventricular dysfunction. Left atrial thrombi and tumors may be detected or excluded by angiocardiography, particularly when the contrast medium is injected directly into the left atrium. These "invasive" methods are also helpful in the detection of accompanying conditions, such as coronary artery disease, that impair left ventricular function and would thereby contraindicate or reduce the effectiveness of mitral valvulotomy. Catheterization is not usually necessary to aid in the decision regarding surgery in young (<45 years for males; <50 for females) patients with typical findings

of severe obstruction on clinical examination and echocardiography. In older patients coronary angiography is usually advisable preoperatively, in order to detect patients with critical coronary obstructions which should be bypassed at the time of operation. Catheterization and left ventricular angiography are also indicated in most patients who have undergone previous mitral valve operations and who have redeveloped serious symptoms; in such patients clinical assessment may be particularly difficult, and the hemodynamic studies allow determination of the severity of the lesion, intelligent planning of the operative procedure when it is indicated, and a more accurate estimate of the risk.

MANAGEMENT In the asymptomatic adolescent with mitral valve disease, penicillin prophylaxis of beta-hemolytic streptococcal infections (Chap. 187), prophylaxis for infective endocarditis (Chap. 90), and vocational counseling are important; physically strenuous occupations should be avoided so that premature retirement will not be necessary should symptoms develop later. In symptomatic patients some improvement usually occurs with restriction of sodium intake and maintenance doses of oral diuretics. Digitalis glycosides do not alter the hemodynamics and usually do not benefit patients with pure stenosis and sinus rhythm, but they are necessary for slowing the ventricular rate of patients with atrial fibrillation and for reducing the manifestations of right-sided heart failure in the advanced stages of the disease. Small doses of beta blockers (e.g., atenolol 25 to 50 mg qd) may be added when cardiac glycosides fail to control ventricular rate in patients with atrial fibrillation or flutter. Particular attention should be directed to detecting and treating any accompanying anemia and infections. Hemoptysis is treated by measures designed to diminish pulmonary venous pressure, including bed rest, the sitting position, salt restriction, and diuresis. Anticoagulants should be administered for at least 1 year in patients with MS who have suffered systemic and/or pulmonary embolization and those with atrial fibrillation.

If atrial fibrillation is of relatively recent origin in a patient whose MS is not severe enough to warrant surgical treatment, reversion to sinus rhythm pharmacologically or by means of electrical countershock is indicated. Usually this should be undertaken following 4 weeks of anticoagulant treatment. Conversion to sinus rhythm is rarely helpful in patients with severe MS, particularly those in whom the left atrium is especially enlarged or in whom atrial fibrillation has been present for more than 1 year, since reversion to atrial fibrillation is common.

Mitral valvulotomy Unless there is a specific contraindication, mitral valvulotomy is indicated in the symptomatic patient with pure MS whose effective orifice is less than approximately 1.2 cm². Operation not only usually results in striking symptomatic and hemodynamic improvement but also prolongs survival. In uncomplicated cases, the surgical mortality rate should be 0 to 2 percent. However, there is no evidence that surgical treatment improves the prognosis of patients with slight or no functional impairment. Therefore, unless recurrent systemic embolization has occurred, valvulotomy is *not* recommended for patients who are entirely asymptomatic, regardless of hemodynamic findings. When there is little symptomatic improvement following valvulotomy, it is likely that the procedure was ineffective, that it induced mitral regurgitation, or that associated valvular or myocardial disease was present. The recurrence of symptoms several years after what appeared to be a satisfactory initial result is usually due to an inadequate valvulotomy, but progression of other valvular lesions, the development of myocardial disease, restenosis of the mitral valve, or some combination of these conditions may also be responsible. In the *pregnant patient* with MS operative treatment should be carried out if pulmonary congestion occurs despite intensive medical treatment.

Percutaneous balloon valvuloplasty, described on p. 879, is an alternative to surgical mitral valvuloplasty in patients with pure or predominant rheumatic mitral stenosis. Young patients without extensive valvular calcification or subvalvular deformity are the optimal candidates for this procedure; in them the results approach those of closed surgical commissurotomy. It is particularly useful in pregnant women but may also be used in older patients with severe valvular

deformity with serious extracardiac disease who are poor operative candidates.

An "open" operation using cardiopulmonary bypass is usually preferable to closed commissurotomy for patients with pure MS who have not been operated upon previously. In addition to opening the valve commissures, it is important to loosen any subvalvular fusion of papillary muscles and chordae tendineae and to remove large deposits of calcium, thereby improving valvular function, and to remove atrial thrombi. In patients with significant associated mitral regurgitation, those in whom the valve has been severely distorted by previous operative manipulation, or those in whom the surgeon does not find it possible to improve valve function significantly, the valve may have to be replaced with a prosthesis or a heterograft. Since the operative mortality of replacement of the mitral valve is still approximately 5 to 8 percent and since there are long-term complications of valve replacement, patients in whom preoperative evaluation suggests the possibility that replacement may be required should be operated on only if they have *critical* mitral stenosis, i.e., an orifice <1.0 cm², and are in the New York Heart Association class III, i.e., symptomatic with ordinary activity, despite optimal medical therapy.

VALVE REPLACEMENT The results of replacement of any valve are dependent primarily on (1) the patient's myocardial function at the time of operation, (2) the technical abilities of the operative team and the quality of the postoperative care, and (3) the durability, hemodynamic characteristics, and thrombogenicity of the prosthesis. Increased operative mortality is associated with the degree of preoperative functional disability and pulmonary hypertension. Late complications of replacement of any valve, which fortunately are declining in incidence, include paravalvular leakage, thromboemboli, bleeding due to anticoagulants, mechanical dysfunction of the prosthesis, and infective endocarditis.

The considerations regarding the choice between a bioprosthetic and artificial mechanical valve are similar in the mitral and aortic positions and in the treatment of stenotic, regurgitant, or mixed lesions. All patients who have undergone replacement of any valve with a mechanical prosthesis must be maintained permanently on anticoagulants. The primary advantage of bioprostheses (tissue valves) over mechanical prostheses is the reduction of thromboembolic complications and, except for patients with chronic atrial fibrillation, few such instances have been associated with their use. Bioprosthetic valves are *contraindicated* in younger patients (<35 years) because of accelerated deterioration and are particularly useful in the elderly (>65 years), in whom there is more concern about chronic anticoagulation than about long-term (>15 years) valve durability. These valves are also indicated in women who expect to become pregnant as well as others in whom anticoagulation may be contraindicated. In patients without such contraindications, particularly those under 60 years, a mechanical prosthesis may be preferable. Many surgeons now select the St. Jude prosthesis, a double-disk tilting prosthesis, for replacement of both aortic and mitral valves because of somewhat more favorable hemodynamic characteristics and a suggestion of lower thrombogenicity.

The overall 10-year survival of operative survivors following mitral valve replacement is approximately 60 percent. Long-term prognosis is worse in subgroups of older patients and those with marked disability and striking depression of the cardiac index preoperatively.

MITRAL REGURGITATION

ETIOLOGY Chronic rheumatic heart disease is the cause of severe mitral regurgitation (MR) in about one-third of cases. In contrast to MS, pure or predominantly rheumatic MR occurs more frequently in males. The rheumatic process produces rigidity, deformity, and retraction of the valve cusps and commissural fusion, as well as shortening, contraction, and fusion of the chordae tendineae.

MR may also occur as a congenital anomaly (Chap. 186), most commonly as (1) a defect of the endocardial cushions or in association with (2) corrected transposition, (3) endocardial fibroelastosis, and (4) the "parachute" mitral valve deformity. MR may occur with fibrosis of a papillary muscle in patients with healed myocardial infarction as well as in patients with a ventricular aneurysm involving the base of a papillary muscle. Transient regurgitation may also occur during periods of ischemia involving a papillary muscle or the adjacent myocardium and may accompany bouts of angina pectoris. MR may occur with marked left ventricular enlargement of any cause in which dilatation of the mitral annulus and lateral displacement of the papillary muscles interfere with coaptation of the valve leaflets. In hypertrophic cardiomyopathy the anterior leaflet of the mitral valve is displaced anteriorly during systole, leading to regurgitation (Chap. 192). Massive calcification of the mitral annulus of unknown cause, presumably degenerative, which occurs most commonly in elderly women, can also be responsible for significant MR. Systemic lupus erythematosus, rheumatoid arthritis, and ankylosing spondylitis are less common causes. *Acute* MR may occur secondary to infective endocarditis involving the valve or chordae tendineae, in acute myocardial infarction with rupture of a papillary muscle or one of its heads, as a consequence of trauma, or as a complication of cardiac surgery.

Abnormal elongation of chordae tendineae and/or redundant posterior cusps of the mitral valve with prolapse of the cusps into the left atrium, the so-called floppy valve, leading to the syndrome of midsystolic click and midsystolic murmur, also referred to as the *prolapsing mitral valve leaflet syndrome* (see below), is another important cause of MR.

Regardless of etiology, serious MR tends to be progressive, since enlargement of the left atrium places tension on the posterior mitral leaflet, pulling it away from the mitral orifice, thereby aggravating the valvular dysfunction. Similarly, the dilatation of the left ventricle increases the regurgitation, which in turn enlarges further the left atrium and ventricle, resulting in a vicious cycle; hence the aphorism, "mitral regurgitation begets mitral regurgitation."

PATHOPHYSIOLOGY The regurgitant mitral orifice may be considered to be in parallel with the aortic orifice, and therefore the resistance to left ventricular emptying is reduced in patients with MR. As a consequence, the left ventricle is decompressed into the left atrium during ejection, and with the reduction in left ventricular size there is a rapid decline in left ventricular tension i.e., a progressive reduction in left ventricular afterload, allowing a greater proportion of the contractile activity of the left ventricle to be expended in shortening. The initial compensation to MR consists of more complete systolic emptying of the left ventricle. However, a progressive increase in left ventricular end-diastolic volume occurs as the severity of the regurgitation increases and the function of the left ventricle deteriorates. The atrial contraction wave in the left atrial pressure pulse (*a* wave) is usually not as prominent as it is in MS, but the *v* wave is often much taller, since it is inscribed during ventricular systole, when the left atrium fills from the pulmonary veins as well as from the left ventricle. During early diastole, as the distended left atrium suddenly empties, there is a particularly rapid *y* descent as long as there is no associated MS (Fig. 179-7, p. 875). Left ventricular end-diastolic pressure may be slightly elevated. However, in chronic MR, there is often an increase in left ventricular compliance, so that ventricular volume may be increased with little elevation in end-diastolic pressure. The effective cardiac output usually declines in seriously symptomatic patients. Although a left atrioventricular pressure gradient persisting throughout diastole signifies the presence of significant associated MS, a brief, early diastolic gradient may occur in patients with pure regurgitation as a result of the torrential flow of blood across a normal-sized mitral orifice.

The prompt appearance of contrast material in the left atrium following its injection into the left ventricle signifies the presence and can be useful in the diagnosis of MR. The regurgitant volume can be measured by determining the difference between the total left ventricular stroke volume estimated angiocardiographically and the effective forward stroke volume determined by the Fick method (Chap. 179). The results of such studies suggest that the regurgitant volume may be of the same magnitude as the effective forward stroke volume or may even exceed it in patients with severe regurgitation. Qualitative, but clinically useful, estimates of the severity of regurgitation may be made by Doppler echocardiography, color Doppler flow echocardiographic imaging, and by observation on cineangiograms of the degree of left atrial opacification following the injection of contrast material into the left ventricle.

Patients with *severe* MR may be divided into three subgroups, depending on the compliance, i.e., the pressure-volume relationship, of the left atrium and pulmonary venous bed.

Group 1 *Normal or reduced compliance.* These patients usually have *acute* MR. There is little enlargement of the left atrium, but marked elevation of the left atrial pressure, particularly of the *v* wave. In these patients MR has usually developed suddenly, as when it follows rupture of chordae tendineae, infarction of one of the heads of a papillary muscle, or tear of a mitral leaflet. Pulmonary edema is common. After several months the pulmonary vascular resistance may become markedly elevated, presumably as a consequence of the left atrial hypertension, and right-sided heart failure may also occur; sinus rhythm is usually present.

Group 2 *Marked increase in compliance.* At the opposite end of the spectrum from group 1 are those patients with severe long-standing severe MR, massive enlargement of the left atrium, and normal or only slightly elevated left atrial pressure, pulmonary artery pressure, and pulmonary vascular resistance. These patients usually complain of severe fatigue and exhaustion secondary to a low cardiac output, while symptoms resulting from pulmonary congestion are less prominent; atrial fibrillation is almost invariably present. The association of a near-normal left atrial pressure with a markedly enlarged, thin-walled left atrium indicates that this chamber is far more compliant than normal. Thus, long-standing MR may, in some instances, alter the physical properties of the left atrial wall and thereby displace the atrial pressure-volume curve, allowing a greatly enlarged left atrium to have a normal atrial pressure.

Group 3 *Moderate increase in compliance.* By far the most common group are patients whose clinical and hemodynamic features are between those in the other two groups with variable degrees of enlargement of the left atrium and with significant elevation of the left atrial pressure. Symptoms are secondary to both reduced cardiac output and pulmonary congestion.

SYMPTOMS Only a fraction of patients with chronic MR ever experience any reduction of cardiac reserve, but in those who do become symptomatic, fatigue, exertional dyspnea, and orthopnea may be prominent complaints. Symptoms resulting from pulmonary congestion tend to be less episodic in nature in patients with chronic severe MR than MS, since fluctuations of the mean pulmonary capillary pressure are less marked. Indeed, acute paroxysmal pulmonary edema is quite rare in patients with chronic MR. Hemoptysis and systemic embolism also occur far less frequently in MR than in MS. On the other hand, fatigability, weakness, exhaustion, weight loss, and even cachexia are more prominent and occur most frequently in patients with MR and marked reduction of cardiac output. Right-sided heart failure, with painful hepatic congestion, ankle edema, distended neck veins, ascites, and tricuspid regurgitation, may be observed in patients with MR who have associated pulmonary vascular disease and marked pulmonary hypertension. In patients with *acute* severe MR, left ventricular failure with acute pulmonary edema and/or cardiovascular collapse is common.

PHYSICAL FINDINGS The arterial pressure is usually normal, and in severe MR the arterial pulse is often characterized by a sharp upstroke. The jugular venous pulse shows abnormally prominent *a* waves in patients with sinus rhythm and marked pulmonary hypertension and prominent *v* waves in those with severe accompanying tricuspid regurgitation.

Palpation A systolic thrill is often palpable at the cardiac apex, the left ventricle is hyperdynamic with a brisk systolic impulse and a palpable rapid-filling wave, and the apex beat is often displaced laterally. When the left atrium is markedly enlarged, it may extend anteriorly, and its expansion may be palpable along the sternal border late during ventricular systole, resembling a right ventricular lift. The combination of the retraction of the left ventricle and expansion of the left atrium during systole may produce a characteristic rocking motion of the chest with each cardiac cycle. A right ventricular tap and the shock of pulmonary valve closure may be palpable in patients with marked pulmonary hypertension.

Auscultation The first heart sound is generally absent, soft, or buried in the systolic murmur, and an accentuated mitral closure sound is useful in excluding severe regurgitation. A pulmonary ejection sound is often audible in patients with associated pulmonary hypertension. Splitting of the second heart sound is usually normal, but in patients with severe MR, the aortic valve may close prematurely, resulting in wide splitting of the second heart sound. An OS indicates associated MS but does not exclude predominant regurgitation. A low-pitched third heart sound (S_3) occurring 0.12 to 0.17 s after the aortic valve closure sound, at the completion of the rapid-filling phase of the left ventricle, is believed to be caused by the sudden tensing of the papillary muscles, chordae tendineae, and valve leaflets and is an important auscultatory feature of severe MR. The absence of an S_3 indicates that if MR exists, it may not be severe. The S_3 may be followed, often after a brief interval, by a short, rumbling, diastolic murmur, even in the absence of MS. A fourth heart sound is often audible in patients with acute severe MR of recent onset who are in sinus rhythm. A presystolic murmur is not ordinarily heard in patients with pure MR and sinus rhythm but is present when there is significant associated MS.

A systolic murmur, grade III/VI in intensity or louder, is the most characteristic auscultatory finding in severe MR. It is usually holosystolic (Chap. 175), but it may be decrescendo when the tall *v* wave in the left atrial pressure pulse results in a reduced late systolic left ventricular–atrial pressure gradient in patients with acute severe MR. (The murmur commences in early to midsystole in mitral valve prolapse, see below.) Although the systolic murmur usually radiates into the axilla, in a minority of patients, particularly those with ruptured chordae tendineae or primary involvement of the posterior mitral leaflet, the regurgitant jet strikes the left atrial wall adjacent to the aortic root, and the systolic murmur is referred to the base of the heart and therefore may be confused with the murmur of aortic stenosis. In patients with ruptured chordae tendineae the systolic murmur may have a cooing or "sea gull" quality; in patients with a flail leaflet the murmur may have a musical quality.

Electrocardiogram In patients with sinus rhythm there is evidence of left atrial enlargement, but right atrial enlargement may also be present when pulmonary hypertension is extreme. Chronic, severe MR with left atrial enlargement is generally associated with atrial fibrillation. In many patients there is no clear-cut electrocardiographic evidence of enlargement of either ventricle. In others the signs of left ventricular hypertrophy are often present, although in patients with pulmonary hypertension combined ventricular hypertrophy or rarely pure right ventricular hypertrophy may be noted.

Echocardiogram The left atrium is usually enlarged and/or exhibits increased pulsations; the left ventricle may be hyperdynamic. With ruptured chordae tendineae or a flail leaflet coarse, erratic motion of the involved leaflets may be noted. Vegetations associated with infective endocarditis may be recognized. Incomplete coaptation of the anterior and posterior mitral leaflets, annular calcification, left ventricular dilatation, aneurysm, or dyskinesis, all of which may be of etiologic importance, can often be identified. Doppler echocardiography and color Doppler flow echocardiography imaging are the most accurate noninvasive techniques for the detection and estimation

of MR (Fig. 177-5). The echocardiogram in patients with mitral valve prolapse is described below.

Roentgenogram The left atrium and left ventricle are the dominant chambers; in chronic cases the latter may be enlarged to aneurysmal proportions and forms the right border of the cardiac silhouette. Marked calcification of the mitral leaflets occurs commonly in patients with long-standing combined MR and MS but is uncommon in patients with pure MR. Contrast left ventriculography is useful in the quantification of MR.

TREATMENT Medical The nonsurgical management of MR is directed toward restricting those physical activities that regularly produce extreme fatigue and dyspnea, reducing sodium intake, and enhancing sodium excretion with the appropriate use of diuretics (Chap. 182). Vasodilators and digitalis glycosides increase the forward output of the failing left ventricle. Intravenous nitroprusside (p. 896) or nitroglycerin to reduce afterload and thereby the volume of regurgitant flow are useful in stabilizing patients with acute and/or severe MR. The same considerations as in patients with MS apply to the reversion of atrial fibrillation to sinus rhythm. In the late stages of heart failure anticoagulants and leg binders are used to diminish the likelihood of venous thrombi and pulmonary emboli.

Surgical In the selection of patients for surgical treatment, the chronic, often slowly progressive nature of the disease must be balanced against the immediate risks and long-term uncertainties attendant upon valve reconstruction or replacement. Patients with MR who are asymptomatic or who are limited only during strenuous exertion are not considered to be candidates for surgical treatment, since they may live for many years with little deterioration. On the other hand, unless there are contraindications, surgical treatment should be offered to patients with severe MR whose limitations do not allow them to work full time or to perform normal household activities despite optimal medical management. The risks of surgery rise sharply, the recovery of impaired left ventricular function is incomplete, and the long-term survival is reduced in patients with congestive heart failure. However, conservative management has little to offer these patients, so that operative treatment may be indicated even at these advanced stages of the disease, and occasionally the clinical and hemodynamic improvement following surgical treatment is dramatic. It is likely that the results of surgical treatment will continue to improve and will lead to recommendations of operative treatment for selected patients with MR before they become severely disabled. Though most patients who survive operation appear to be greatly improved, some degree of myocardial dysfunction may persist.

When surgical treatment is contemplated, right- and left-sided heart catheterization and selected left ventricular angiocardiography are generally indicated. These studies are helpful in confirming the presence of severe regurgitation and aid in the identification of patients with primary myocardial disease and relatively mild, functional MR, who usually do not benefit from operation. Hemodynamic studies are also helpful in detecting and assessing the severity of any associated valve lesions, which may have to be dealt with at the time of operation or which might limit the patient's ultimate improvement if they are left untreated. Coronary angiography identifies patients who require concomitant coronary revascularization.

Surgical treatment of MR, especially that caused by valves that are markedly deformed, with shrunken, calcified leaflets secondary to rheumatic fever, requires replacement of the valve with a prosthesis, although in an increasing fraction of patients, particularly those with severe annular dilatation, flail leaflets, mitral valve prolapse, ruptured chordae, or infective endocarditis, reconstruction of the mitral valve apparatus (mitral valvuloplasty) and/or mitral annuloplasty may be successful. Valve reconstruction should be carried out whenever feasible since it spares the patient the long-term adverse consequences of valve replacement (i.e., thromboembolic and hemorrhagic complications in the case of mechanical prostheses and late valve failure necessitating repeat valve replacement in the case of bioprostheses). Also, by preserving the integrity of the papillary muscles and subvalvular apparatus, mitral valvuloplasty maintains left ventricular function.

MITRAL VALVE PROLAPSE

Mitral valve prolapse (MVP) is also variously termed the *systolic click-murmur syndrome, Barlow's syndrome, floppy-valve syndrome,* and *billowing mitral leaflet syndrome,* a common, but highly variable, clinical syndrome resulting from diverse pathogenic mechanisms of the mitral valve apparatus. Among these are excessive or redundant mitral leaflet tissue, which is commonly involved with myxomatous degeneration and greatly increased concentration of acid mucopolysaccharide. It is a frequent finding in patients who have the typical features of Marfan's syndrome or cystic medial necrosis (Chap. 197), although in most patients myxomatous degeneration is confined to the mitral valve leaflets without other clinical or pathologic manifestations of disease; the posterior leaflet is usually more affected than the anterior, and the mitral valve annulus is often greatly enlarged. In many patients, elongated redundant chordae tendineae cause or contribute to the regurgitation. There are probably several subsets of these patients, who differ in regard to the etiology and hemodynamic and clinical sequelae of abnormal mitral valve function. In the majority of patients, the etiology is unknown, but MVP may be a genetically determined collagen tissue disorder. Fragmentation of collagen has been noted and an abnormality in the production of type III collagen has been incriminated in the etiology of the syndrome. MVP may be associated with thoracic skeletal deformities similar to but not as severe as those in Marfan's syndrome, including a high arched palate and alterations of the chest and thoracic spine. MVP may also occur as a sequel of acute rheumatic fever, in chronic rheumatic heart disease and following mitral valvulotomy, in ischemic heart disease, and cardiomyopathies, as well as in 20 percent of patients with ostium secundum atrial septal defect.

MVP is usually a benign abnormality that may progress to a stage involving significant regurgitation and ventricular dilatation in some individuals. In these, prolapse of the valve leads to excessive stress on the papillary muscles, which in turn leads to dysfunction and ischemia of the papillary muscles and subjacent ventricular myocardium; rupture of chordae tendineae and progressive annular dilatation also contribute to valvular regurgitation which then places more stress on the diseased mitral valve apparatus, thereby creating a vicious cycle. The electrocardiographic changes (see below) and ventricular arrhythmias appear to result from regional ventricular dysfunction related to increased stress placed on the papillary muscles.

MVP is more common in females and has been noted in a wide age range but most commonly between the ages of 14 and 30. Echocardiographic surveys have suggested that it may occur in as many as 7 percent of this group. There is an increased familial incidence suggesting an autosomal dominant form of inheritance. In many patients the echocardiographic abnormality is not accompanied by any other clinical manifestation of cardiac disease, and the significance of this finding is uncertain.

MVP encompasses a broad spectrum of severities, ranging from patients with only a systolic click and murmur and mild prolapse of the posterior leaflet of the mitral valve to those with severe MR due to chordal rupture and massive prolapse of both leaflets. In many patients, this condition progresses over years or decades.

Most of the patients are asymptomatic and remain so for their entire lives. Although severe MR is a relatively uncommon complication of MVP, the latter has become the most common cause of isolated *severe* MR. Arrythmias, most commonly ventricular premature contractions and paroxysmal supraventricular and ventricular tachycardia, have been reported and may cause palpitations, lightheadedness, and syncope. Sudden death is a very rare complication. Many patients have chest pain which is difficult to evaluate. It is often substernal, prolonged, poorly related to exertion, and rarely resembles typical angina pectoris. Transient cerebral ischemic attacks

secondary to emboli from the roughened surface of the valve have been reported. Infective endocarditis may occur in patients with MR associated with MVP.

PHYSICAL EXAMINATION Auscultation The most common finding is the mid- or late (nonejection) systolic click, which occurs 0.14 s or more after the first heart sound and is thought to be generated by the sudden tensing of slack, elongated chordae tendineae or by the prolapsing mitral leaflet when it reaches its maximum excursion; systolic clicks may be multiple and are often followed by a high-pitched late systolic crescendo-decrescendo murmur, occasionally "whooping" or "honking," which is heard best at the apex. The click and murmur occur earlier with standing, the Valsalva maneuver, or inhalation of amyl nitrate, interventions which decrease left ventricular volume, exaggerating the propensity of mitral leaflet prolapse. Conversely, squatting and isometric exercise, which increase left ventricular end-diastolic volume, diminish the propensity for the mitral valve leaflets to prolapse, and the click-murmur complex is delayed and may even disappear. Some patients have a midsystolic click without the murmur; others have the murmur without a click.

LABORATORY EXAMINATION The *electrocardiogram* most commonly shows biphasic or inverted T waves in leads II, III, and aVF. The M-mode *echocardiogram* characteristically shows an abrupt posterior displacement of the posterior or sometimes of both mitral valve leaflets in mid- to late systole, immediately after the click, and during the systolic murmur. Two-dimensional echocardiography is particularly useful in identifying the abnormal position and prolapse of the mitral valve leaflets; a useful echocardiographic definition of MVP is systolic displacement of one or both mitral valve leaflets into the left atrium beyond the plane of the mitral annulus and imaged in the parasternal view. Thickening of the mitral valve leaflets identifies a subgroup of patients at higher risk of infective endocarditis and the development of severe MR. Doppler studies are helpful in revealing and evaluating accompanying MR. *Angiocardiography* generally shows prolapse of the posterior and sometimes of both mitral valve leaflets and, rarely, severe MR. Many patients have bulging of the posteroinferior wall of the left ventricle into the left ventricular cavity during systole and/or hypokinesis of the anterolateral left ventricular wall. Others display prolapse of other valves, particularly the tricuspid, in addition to the mitral.

TREATMENT The management of patients with MVP consists of reassurance of the asymptomatic patient, the prevention of infective endocarditis with antibiotic prophylaxis in patients with asystolic murmur and/or the typical echocardiographic features, and the relief of the atypical chest pain; beta blockers have been found to be helpful in this regard, although their use is empiric. Antiarrhythmic agents may be administered if frequent ventricular premature contractions or tachyarrhythmias have caused symptoms. If the patient is symptomatic secondary to severe MR, mitral valve repair or replacement is usually indicated. Antiplatelet aggregation agents (aspirin and dipyridamole) should be given to patients with transient ischemic attacks, and if these are not effective, anticoagulants should be employed.

AORTIC STENOSIS

Aortic stenosis (AS) occurs in about one-fourth of all patients with chronic valvular heart disease; approximately 80 percent of adult patients with symptomatic valvular AS are male.

ETIOLOGY AS may be congenital in origin, it may be secondary to rheumatic inflammation of the aortic valve, or it may be due to degenerative calcification of the aortic cusps of unknown cause. The *congenitally affected valve* may already be stenotic at birth (Chap. 186) and may gradually become more fibrotic and calcified during the first three decades of life, becoming progressively more stenotic. In others, the valve may also be congenitally bicuspid without serious narrowing of the aortic orifice during childhood; its abnormal architecture makes its leaflets susceptible to otherwise ordinary hemodynamic stresses, which ultimately lead to valvular thickening, calcification, increased rigidity, and narrowing of the aortic orifice.

Rheumatic endocarditis of the aortic leaflets produces commissural fusion, resulting sometimes in a bicuspid valve. This, in turn, also makes the leaflets more susceptible to trauma, and ultimately leads to calcification and further narrowing. By the time the obstruction to left ventricular outflow causes serious clinical disability, the valve is usually a rigid calcified mass, and careful examination may make it difficult or even impossible to determine whether the underlying process was rheumatic or congenital. Rheumatic AS is almost always associated with rheumatic involvement of the mitral valve. A rheumatic etiology is also favored by a history of active rheumatic fever and by associated severe aortic regurgitation.

Idiopathic calcific AS occurs most often in the elderly and is occasionally associated with fibrosis and fusion of the valve cusps; the pathologic process is considered to be a degenerative one—a "wear-and-tear" phenomenon. It may produce many of the characteristic physical signs of AS. However, the valvular obstruction is usually relatively mild and of little if any hemodynamic significance; it may, however, on occasion, produce critical obstruction.

OTHER FORMS OF OBSTRUCTION TO LEFT VENTRICULAR OUTFLOW Besides valvular AS, three other lesions may be responsible for obstruction to left ventricular outflow.

1 *Hypertrophic cardiomyopathy*. This is the most common of these conditions. It is characterized by marked hypertrophy of the left ventricle, involving in particular the interventricular septum of the left ventricular outflow tract, and may cause subaortic obstruction, as described in Chap. 192.
2 *Discrete congenital subvalvular AS*. This condition is produced by either a membranous diaphragm or a fibrous ridge just below the aortic valve (Chap. 186).
3 *Supravalvular AS*. This uncommon congenital anomaly is produced by narrowing of the ascending aorta or by a fibrous diaphragm with a small opening just above the aortic valve (Chap. 186).

PATHOPHYSIOLOGY The primary hemodynamic abnormality is obstruction to left ventricular outflow which leads to a systolic pressure gradient between the left ventricle and aorta. When severe obstruction is suddenly produced experimentally, the left ventricle responds by dilatation and reduction of stroke volume. However, in patients the obstruction may be present at birth and/or increase gradually over the course of many years, and left ventricular output is maintained by the presence of left ventricular hypertrophy. This serves as a useful compensatory mechanism since it reduces toward normal the systolic stress developed by each segment of myocardium. A large transaortic valvular pressure gradient may exist for many years without a reduction of cardiac output, left ventricular dilatation, or the development of any symptoms. As AS progresses in severity, the left ventricular systolic pressure continues to rise, but rarely exceeds 300 mmHg.

A peak systolic pressure gradient exceeding 50 mmHg in the face of a normal cardiac output or an effective aortic orifice less than 0.5 cm² per square meter of body surface area, i.e., less than approximately one-third of the normal orifice, is generally considered to represent critical obstruction to left ventricular outflow. The left ventricular pressure pulse exhibits a rounded summit as the contraction of this chamber becomes progressively more isometric. The elevated left ventricular end-diastolic pressure observed in many patients with severe AS does not necessarily signify the presence of left ventricular dilatation or failure, but may reflect diminished compliance of the hypertrophied left ventricular wall.

A large *a* wave in the left atrial pressure pulse is usually present with severe AS. Loss of an appropriately timed, vigorous atrial contraction, as occurs in atrial fibrillation or atrioventricular dissociation, may result in a rapid aggravation of symptoms.

Although the cardiac output at rest is within normal limits in the majority of patients with severe AS, it may fail to rise normally during exercise. Late in the course the cardiac output and left ventricular–aortic pressure gradient decline, and the mean left atrial, pulmonary artery wedge, pulmonary arterial, and right ventricular pressures become elevated.

The hypertrophied left ventricular muscle mass elevates myocardial oxygen requirements. In addition, even in the absence of obstructive coronary artery disease, there may be interference with coronary blood flow, because the pressure compressing the coronary arteries exceeds the coronary perfusion pressure. Metabolic evidence of myocardial ischemia, i.e., lactate production, can be demonstrated in patients with AS both in the presence and in the absence of coronary arterial narrowing, when myocardial oxygen needs are stimulated by isoproterenol.

A significant fraction of patients with rheumatic AS has associated mitral valve disease. AS intensifies the severity of mitral regurgitation by increasing the pressure driving blood from the left ventricle to the left atrium.

SYMPTOMS AS is rarely of hemodynamic or clinical importance until the valve orifice has narrowed to approximately one-third of normal. Severe AS may exist for many years without producing any symptoms because of the ability of the hypertrophied left ventricle to generate the elevated intraventricular pressures and the presence of a competent mitral valve behind the left ventricle.

Most patients with pure or predominant AS have gradually increasing obstruction for years but do not become symptomatic until the fifth to seventh decades. Exertional dyspnea, angina pectoris, and syncope are the three cardinal symptoms. Often there is a history of insidious progression of fatigue and dyspnea associated with gradual curtailment of activities. *Dyspnea* results primarily from elevation of the pulmonary capillary pressures, which in turn is caused by elevations of left atrial and left ventricular end-diastolic pressures, which are due in turn to left ventricular dilatation and/or reduced compliance. *Angina pectoris* usually develops somewhat later and reflects an imbalance between the augmented myocardial oxygen requirements and reduced oxygen availability; the former results from the increased myocardial mass and intraventricular pressure, while the latter may result from accompanying coronary artery disease which is not uncommon in patients with AS, as well as from compression of the coronary vessels by the hypertrophied myocardium. Therefore, angina may occur in severe AS without organic coronary obstruction; the *absence* of angina in such patients usually signifies that severe coronary obstructive disease is unlikely. *Exertional syncope* may result from a decline in arterial pressure caused by vasodilatation in the exercising muscles and inadequate vasoconstriction in nonexercising muscles in the face of a fixed cardiac output, or from a sudden fall in cardiac output produced by an arrhythmia.

Since the cardiac output at rest is usually well maintained until late in the course, marked fatigability, weakness, peripheral cyanosis, and other clinical manifestations of a low cardiac output are usually not prominent until this stage is reached. Orthopnea, paroxysmal nocturnal dyspnea, and pulmonary edema, i.e., symptoms of left ventricular failure, also occur only in the advanced stages of the disease. Severe pulmonary hypertension leading to right ventricular failure and systemic venous hypertension, hepatomegaly, atrial fibrillation, and tricuspid regurgitation are usually preterminal findings.

When AS and MS coexist, the latter lesion masks many of the clinical findings of the former. The reduction of cardiac output induced by MS lowers the pressure gradient across the aortic valve, diminishes the frequency of anginal episodes, and retards the development of severe left ventricular hypertrophy. On the other hand, symptoms considered more characteristic of MS, such as pulmonary congestion and hemoptysis, may be present. Physical, electrocardiographic, radiologic, and echocardiographic examinations in patients with combined AS and MS generally reveal more evidence of left ventricular enlargement than in patients with pure MS, and left heart catheterization is helpful in defining the relative importance of each valvular abnormality.

PHYSICAL FINDINGS AND GRAPHIC TRACINGS   The systemic arterial pressure is usually within normal limits. In the late stages, however, when stroke volume declines, the systolic pressure may fall and the pulse pressure narrow. Systemic hypertension is unusual in patients with marked AS, and a basal systolic arterial pressure exceeding 200 mmHg practically excludes severe narrowing of this valve. The peripheral arterial pulse, as palpated in the carotid or brachial arteries, rises slowly to a delayed sustained peak. Indirect recordings of the carotid pulse exhibit a gradually ascending limb, often with a prominent anacrotic notch or shoulder on the upstroke, as well as a delayed peak, with coarse systolic vibrations. The left ventricular ejection period is prolonged, the preejection period is abbreviated, and the ratio of these two, i.e., the preejection period/systolic ejection period, is characteristically reduced. Late in the course of the disease, in the presence of heart failure, the ratio may be normal. A palpable double systolic arterial pulse, the so-called bisferiens pulse, excludes pure or predominant AS and signifies dominant or pure aortic regurgitation or obstructive hypertrophic cardiomyopathy (Chap. 192). In the late stages of valvular AS, when the pulse pressure is reduced, the pulse amplitude may be so small that the anacrotic nature of the pulse and the delay in its upstroke may become more difficult to appreciate. The jugular venous pulse may be normal, although in many patients the *a* wave is accentuated. This results from the diminished distensibility of the right ventricular cavity caused by the bulging, hypertrophied interventricular septum and/or the presence of pulmonary hypertension.

Palpation   The apex beat is usually active and displaced inferiorly and laterally, reflecting the presence of left ventricular hypertrophy. A double apical impulse may be appreciated, particularly with the patient in the left lateral recumbent position; the first outward expansion occurs during atrial systole and reflects the important contribution made by atrial contraction to ventricular filling, while the second occurs during ventricular systole and usually is forceful and sustained during ejection. The right ventricle is usually palpable only when pulmonary hypertension develops in the late stages of the disease. A systolic thrill is generally present at the base of the heart, in the jugular notch, and along the carotid arteries, but occasionally it is palpable only during expiration and with the patient leaning forward. In patients who do not have marked pulmonary emphysema, a thick chest wall, thoracic deformity, or heart failure, the absence of a systolic thrill suggests that the aortic stenosis is relatively mild.

Auscultation   The rhythm is generally regular until very late in the course; at other times, atrial fibrillation should suggest the possibility of associated mitral valve disease. An early systolic ejection sound, actually the OS of the aortic valve, is frequently audible in children and adolescents with congenital noncalcific valvular AS. This sound usually disappears when the valve becomes calcified and rigid. The sound of aortic valve closure can also be identified most frequently in patients with AS who have pliable valves, and calcification diminishes the intensity of this sound as well. As AS increases in severity, left ventricular systole may become prolonged so that the aortic valve closure sound no longer precedes the pulmonic valve closure sound, and the two components may become synchronous, or aortic valve closure may even follow pulmonic valve closure, causing paradoxic splitting of the second heart sound (Chap. 175). In patients with AS without a left intraventricular conduction defect, this finding usually signifies severe obstruction to left ventricular outflow. A fourth heart sound is audible at the apex in many patients with severe AS, and reflects the presence of left ventricular hypertrophy and an elevated left ventricular end-diastolic pressure; a third heart sound generally occurs when the left ventricle dilates and fails.

The murmur of AS is characteristically an ejection systolic murmur which commences shortly after the first heart sound, increases in intensity to reach a peak toward the middle of the ejection period, and diminishes progressively thereafter to end just before aortic valve closure (Chap. 175). The murmur is usually low-pitched, rough, and rasping in character and is loudest at the base of the heart, most commonly in the second right intercostal space. It is transmitted to the jugular notch and upward along the carotid arteries. In patients with mild degrees of obstruction or in those with severe stenosis with heart failure in whom the stroke volume and therefore the transvalvular flow rate is reduced, the murmur may be relatively soft and brief. However, in almost all patients with severe obstruction, the murmur is at least grade III/VI. Occasionally, the murmur is transmitted downward and to the apex and may be confused with the systolic murmur of MR; however, the latter is usually holosystolic.

Electrocardiogram   This reveals left ventricular hypertrophy in the majority of patients with severe AS (Chap. 176). In advanced cases, ST-segment depression and T-wave inversion (left ventricular "strain") in standard leads I and aVL and in the left precordial leads are evident. However, there is no close correlation between the electrocardiogram and the hemodynamic severity of obstruction, and the absence of electrocardiographic signs of left ventricular hypertrophy does not exclude severe obstruction. Atrioventricular and intraventricular conduction defects, usually caused by infiltration with calcium and/or diffuse fibrotic involvement of the myocardium, are observed in 5 to 10 percent of patients. The presence of left atrial enlargement should suggest the possibility of associated mitral valve disease.

Echocardiogram   This reveals left ventricular hypertrophy and in patients with valvular calcification, multiple, bright, thick, echoes from within the aortic root. While cusp calcification does not necessarily indicate significant valve stenosis, its absence can usually be used to *exclude* such a diagnosis after the age of 25. Eccentricity of the aortic valve cusps is characteristic of congenitally bicuspid valves. Left ventricular dilatation and reduced systolic shortening reflecting impairment of left ventricular function can be recognized. The transaortic valvular gradient can be estimated by Doppler echocardiography. Echocardiography is particularly useful for identifying valvular abnormalities such as MS and aortic regurgitation which sometimes accompany AS (Fig. 177-5), and for differentiating valvular from obstructive hypertrophic cardiomyopathy.

Roentgenogram   The chest roentgenogram may show no or little overall cardiac enlargement for many years, since the development of concentric left ventricular hypertrophy is the initial response to obstruction to left ventricular outflow. Hypertrophy without dilatation may produce some rounding of the cardiac apex in the frontal projection and slight backward displacement in the lateral view; critical AS is often associated with poststenotic dilatation of the ascending aorta. Aortic calcification is usually readily apparent on fluoroscopic examination with an image intensifier or by echocardiography; *the absence of valvular calcification in an adult suggests that severe valvular AS is not present.* In later stages of the disease as the left ventricle dilates, there is increasing evidence of left ventricular enlargement, and there may also be roentgenographic signs of pulmonary congestion, as well as enlargement of the left atrium, pulmonary artery, right ventricle, and right atrium.

Catheterization and angiocardiography   Catheterization of the left side of the heart and coronary arteriography should generally be carried out in patients suspected of having severe AS, particularly before a final decision concerning operative treatment is made. The goals are to (1) determine the severity of the aortic obstruction, often previously estimated by Doppler echocardiography, (2) assess the status of left ventricular function, and (3) determine the location of the left ventricular outflow obstruction. These investigations are especially indicated in the following:

1 Young, asymptomatic patients with noncalcific congenital AS (Chap. 186), in order to define the severity of obstruction to left ventricular outflow, since operation may be indicated in them even in the absence of symptoms if severe AS is present.
2 Patients in whom it is suspected that the obstruction to left ventricular outflow may not be at the aortic valve, but rather in the sub- or supravalvular regions.
3 Patients with clinical signs of AS and symptoms of myocardial ischemia, in whom associated coronary artery disease is suspected.

An effort should be made to determine whether aortic stenosis or coronary atherosclerosis is primarily responsible for the symptoms, and coronary arteriography should be carried out in addition to catheterization of the left side of the heart.

4 Patients with multivalvular disease, in whom the role played by each valvular deformity must be defined before operative treatment is planned.

Angiographic studies are helpful in defining the size of the left ventricular cavity, the thickness of the wall, the site of obstruction, the degree of deformity and mobility of the aortic valve cusps, the diameter of the ascending aorta, and the presence and degree of accompanying mitral and aortic regurgitation and of obstructive coronary disease. In patients with severe narrowing, a jet of contrast substance passing through the aortic orifice is readily visualized.

NATURAL HISTORY   Death in patients with severe AS occurs most commonly in the seventh decade. Based on data obtained at postmortem examination, the average duration of various symptoms in patients *not treated surgically* was as follows: angina pectoris, 3 years; syncope, 3 years; dyspnea, 2 years; and congestive heart failure, 1.5 to 2 years. Moreover, in more than 80 percent of patients who died with AS, symptoms had existed for less than 4 years. Congestive heart failure was considered to be the cause of death in one-half to two-thirds of patients. Among adults dying with valvular AS, sudden death, which presumably results from an arrhythmia, occurred in 10 to 20 percent, and at an average age of 60 years.

TREATMENT   Strenuous physical activity should be avoided even in the asymptomatic stage in patients with *severe* AS. Digitalis glycosides, sodium restriction, and the cautious administration of diuretics are indicated in the treatment of congestive heart failure, but care must be taken to avoid volume depletion. While nitroglycerin is helpful in relieving angina pectoris, vasodilator therapy for heart failure is usually of little value. The most critical decision in the management of AS, indeed of any valvular lesion, concerns the advisability of surgical treatment. The indications and results of operation, as well as the techniques, differ considerably, depending on the patient's age and the nature of the valvular deformity.

In children and adolescents with noncalcific congenital AS, considerable hemodynamic improvement can be anticipated from simple commissural incision under direct vision. This operation is recommended not only for symptomatic patients but also for asymptomatic children and adolescents with hemodynamic evidence of severe obstruction to left ventricular outflow, with a peak systolic pressure gradient exceeding 50 mmHg when the cardiac output is normal, or a calculated effective orifice less than 0.6 cm² per square meter of body surface area.

In the majority of adults with calcific AS, replacement of the valve is necessary. In most instances, it is prudent to postpone operation in patients with severe calcific AS who are asymptomatic, since their future course is difficult to predict and they may continue to do well for many years. However, they should be followed carefully by clinical examination for the development of symptoms and by the various noninvasive tests, such as echocardiograms and/or radionuclide angiograms (Chap. 177), for evidence of deteriorating left ventricular function; operation is generally indicated in patients with severe AS and left ventricular dysfunction, even if they are only mildly symptomatic. It is likely that as the results of surgical replacement of the aortic valve continue to improve, many asymptomatic patients with severe AS will become candidates for operation before their left ventricular function deteriorates. At the present, replacement of the aortic valve should be undertaken in patients with symptoms, even when relatively mild, that are believed to result primarily from AS and who have hemodynamic evidence of severe obstruction. In such patients the operative risk is relatively low (<5 percent) in centers with experience.

When angina pectoris, syncope, or left ventricular decompensation develops in adults with severe valvular AS, the outlook, despite medical treatment, is very poor and can be improved significantly by replacement of the aortic valve with a mechanical or bioprosthetic valve. Therefore, the risk entailed by operation in this group of patients although relatively high is still considerably lower than the risk involved by nonoperative treatment; moreover, the symptomatic improvement in many survivors of operation has been remarkable.

Operation should, if possible, be carried out before frank left ventricular failure supervenes; at this late stage, the operative risk is high (approximately 15 percent) and evidence of myocardial disease may persist even when the operation is technically successful. Furthermore, long-term postoperative survival also correlates inversely with preoperative functional disability. Nonetheless, in view of the very poor prognosis of such patients when they are treated medically, there is usually little choice but to advise immediate surgical treatment. In patients in whom severe AS and coronary artery disease coexist, relief of the AS and revascularization of the myocardium by means of aortocoronary bypass grafting may result in striking clinical and hemodynamic improvement. Since many patients with calcific AS are elderly, particular attention must be directed to the adequacy of hepatic, renal, and pulmonary function before valve replacement is recommended. The mortality rate depends to a substantial extent on the patient's preoperative clinical and hemodynamic state. The 10-year survival rate of operative survivors following aortic valve replacement is approximately 67 percent. Approximately 15 percent of bioprosthetic valves evidence primary valve failure in 10 years, requiring re-replacement, and an approximately equal percentage of patients with mechanical prostheses develop significant hemorrhagic complications as a consequence of treatment with anticoagulants. Fortunately, there is evidence that regression of left ventricular hypertrophy may occur following relief of obstruction.

Percutaneous balloon aortic valvuloplasty, described in Chap. 180, is an alternative to surgery in children and young adults with congenital aortic stenosis and in elderly patients with severe calcific aortic stenosis. Although the restenosis rate is high in the latter, the procedure may be useful in patients who are too ill or frail to undergo surgery, in patients with severe aortic stenosis and advanced extracardiac disease, as well as a "bridge to surgery" in patients with severe left ventricular dysfunction. The improvement in their left ventricular function following balloon valvuloplasty may make them suitable candidates for definitive operation, i.e. valve replacement.

AORTIC REGURGITATION

ETIOLOGY   Approximately three-fourths of all patients with pure or predominant aortic regurgitation (AR) are males; however, females predominate among patients with AR who have associated mitral valve disease. In approximately two-thirds of patients with AR the disease is rheumatic in origin, resulting in a chronic form of the disorder with thickening, deformation, and shortening of the individual aortic valve cusps, changes which prevent their proper closure during diastole. A rheumatic etiology is less common in patients with isolated AR. Acute AR may also result from infective endocarditis, which may attack a valve previously affected by rheumatic disease, a congenitally deformed valve, or rarely a normal aortic valve, and may result in the perforation or erosion of one or more of the leaflets. Patients with discrete membranous subaortic stenosis often develop thickening of the aortic valve leaflets, which in turn leads to mild or moderate degrees of AR and makes these valves particularly susceptible to endocarditis. Aortic regurgitation may also occur in patients with congenital bicuspid aortic valves. Prolapse of an aortic cusp, resulting in progressive chronic AR, occurs in approximately 15 percent of patients with ventricular septal defect (Chap. 186). Congenital fenestrations of the aortic valve occasionally produce mild AR. Although traumatic rupture of the aortic valve is an uncommon cause of acute AR, it does represent the most frequent serious lesion observed in patients surviving nonpenetrating cardiac injuries. In patients with AR due to primary valvular disease, dilatation of the aortic annulus may occur secondarily and intensify the regurgitation.

AR, both acute and chronic, may also be due entirely to marked aortic dilatation, without primary involvement of the valve leaflets; widening of the aortic annulus and separation of the aortic leaflets are responsible for the aortic regurgitation. Syphilis and ankylosing rheumatoid spondylitis may be associated with cellular infiltration and scarring of the media of the thoracic aorta, leading to aortic dilatation, aneurysm formation, and severe regurgitation. In syphilis of the aorta (Chap. 197), the involvement of the intima may narrow the coronary ostia, which in turn may be responsible for myocardial ischemia. Cystic medial necrosis of the ascending aorta, which may or may not be associated with other manifestations of the Marfan syndrome, idiopathic dilatation of the aorta, and severe hypertension all may also widen the aortic annulus and lead to progressive AR. Occasionally, retrograde dissection of the aorta involving the aortic annulus produces aortic regurgitation.

The coexistence of hemodynamically significant AS with AR usually excludes all of the rarer forms of AR because it occurs almost exclusively in patients whose aortic regurgitation is on a rheumatic or congenital basis.

PATHOPHYSIOLOGY The total stroke volume expelled by the left ventricle (i.e., the sum of the effective forward stroke volume and the volume of blood which regurgitates back into the left ventricle) is increased in AR. In patients with wide-open (*free*) AR the volume of regurgitant flow may equal the effective forward stroke volume. In contrast to MR, in which a fraction of the left ventricular stroke volume is delivered into the low-pressure left atrium, in AR the entire left ventricular stroke volume must be ejected into a high-pressure zone, the aorta. The low aortic diastolic pressure (low afterload) facilitates ventricular emptying. However, an increase of the left ventricular end-diastolic volume (increased preload) constitutes the major hemodynamic compensation to aortic regurgitation. The dilatation of the left ventricle allows this chamber to expel a larger stroke volume without requiring any increase in the relative shortening of each myofibril. Therefore, severe AR may occur with a normal effective forward stroke volume and a normal ejection fraction [total (forward plus regurgitant) stroke volume/end-diastolic volume], together with an elevated left ventricular end-diastolic pressure and volume. However, through the operation of Laplace's law (which indicates that myocardial wall tension is the product of intracavitary pressure and left ventricular radius), left ventricular dilatation increases the left ventricular systolic tension required to develop any given level of systolic pressure. As left ventricular function deteriorates, the end-diastolic volume and the ejection fraction and forward stroke volume decline. Deterioration of left ventricular function often precedes the development of symptoms. Considerable thickening of the left ventricular wall also occurs with chronic AR, and at autopsy the hearts of these patients may be among the largest encountered, occasionally exceeding 1000 g in weight.

The reverse pressure gradient from aorta to left ventricle, which is responsible for the aortic regurgitant flow, falls progressively during diastole, accounting for the decrescendo nature of the diastolic murmur. Equilibration between aortic and left ventricular pressures may occur toward the end of diastole in patients with severe AR, particularly when the heart rate is slow, and the left ventricular end-diastolic pressure may be elevated, occasionally to extremely high levels (>40 mmHg). Rarely, the left ventricular pressure exceeds the left atrial pressure toward the end of diastole, and this reversed pressure gradient closes the mitral valve prematurely, or may cause diastolic mitral regurgitation.

In patients with free AR the effective forward cardiac output usually is normal or only slightly reduced at rest, but often it fails to rise normally during exertion. Early signs of left ventricular dysfunction include reductions of the fraction of systolic shortening and of the ejection fraction determined by echocardiography or radionuclide or contrast angiography. In advanced stages there may be considerable elevation of the left atrial, pulmonary artery wedge, pulmonary arterial, and right ventricular pressures, and lowering of the forward cardiac output at rest.

Myocardial ischemia may occur in patients with AR because both left ventricular dilatation and the elevated left ventricular systolic tension tend to augment myocardial oxygen requirements. However, the major portion of coronary blood flow occurs during diastole, when arterial pressure is subnormal, thereby reducing coronary perfusion pressure. The combination of increased oxygen demand and reduced supply may cause myocardial ischemia.

HISTORY A family history may frequently be elicited from patients with AR associated with the Marfan syndrome, and a history of a heart murmur heard early in life may be obtained from patients with congenital AR with or without a ventricular septal defect. Patients with AR of obscure cause should also be questioned about a positive serologic test for syphilis, and about prior chest trauma; a history compatible with infective endocarditis may sometimes be elicited from patients with rheumatic or congenital involvement of the aortic valve, and the infection often precipitates or seriously aggravates preexisting symptoms. Ankylosing spondylitis is usually self-evident.

The interval between the first episode of acute rheumatic fever and the development of hemodynamically significant AR averages approximately 7 years, and this period is followed by an asymptomatic interval of approximately 10 to 20 years, during which the severity of the AR usually increases. Thus, patients with severe AR may remain asymptomatic for many years.

In chronic severe AR, uncomfortable awareness of the heartbeat, especially on lying down, may be an early complaint. Sinus tachycardia during exertion or with emotion, or premature ventricular contractions, may produce particularly uncomfortable palpitations, as well as head pounding. These complaints may persist for many years before the development of exertional dyspnea, usually the first symptom of diminished cardiac reserve. This is followed by orthopnea, paroxysmal nocturnal dyspnea, and excessive diaphoresis. Chest pain occurs frequently, even in younger patients, and it is not necessary to invoke the presence of coronary artery disease to explain this symptom in patients with AR. It may be due to myocardial ischemia, or it may originate from excessive cardiac pounding on the chest wall. Anginal pain may develop at rest as well as during exertion. Nocturnal angina may be a particularly troublesome symptom, and it may be accompanied by marked diaphoresis. The anginal episodes may be prolonged and often do not respond satisfactorily to sublingual nitroglycerin. Late in the course of the disease, evidence of systemic fluid accumulation, including congestive hepatomegaly, ankle edema, and ascites, may develop. Patients with severe AR tolerate high fevers, infections, or cardiac arrhythmias poorly, and may die in pulmonary edema as a result of one of these complications.

In patients with acute severe AR, as may occur in trauma or infective endocarditis, the left ventricle rapidly exhausts its ability to dilate, and left ventricular diastolic pressure rises rapidly with associated elevations of left atrial and pulmonary capillary pressures.

PHYSICAL FINDINGS Even prior to the examination of the heart of the patient with free AR, the jarring of the entire body and the bobbing motion of the head with each systole can be appreciated, and the abrupt distention and collapse of the larger arteries are easily visible. The examination should be directed toward the detection of conditions predisposing to AR, such as the Marfan syndrome, rheumatoid spondylitis, syphilis, essential hypertension, and ventricular septal defect.

Arterial pulse A rapidly rising "water-hammer" pulse, which collapses suddenly as arterial pressure falls rapidly during late systole and diastole (Corrigan's pulse), and capillary pulsations (Quincke's pulse), an alternate flushing and paling of the skin at the root of the nail while pressure is applied to the tip of the nail, are characteristic of free AR. A booming, "pistol-shot" sound can be heard over the femoral arteries, and a to-and-fro murmur (Duroziez's sign) is audible if the femoral artery is lightly compressed with a stethoscope. The arterial pulse pressure is widened, with an elevation of the systolic pressure, sometimes to as high as 300 mmHg, and a depression of the diastolic arterial pressure. The measurement of arterial diastolic pressure with a sphygmomanometer may be complicated by the fact that systolic sounds are frequently heard with the cuff completely deflated. However, the level of cuff pressure at the time of muffling of the Korotkoff sounds generally corresponds fairly closely to the true intraarterial diastolic pressure. The severity of AR does not always correlate directly with the arterial pulse pressure, and severe regurgitation may exist in patients with arterial pressures in the range of 140/60. As the disease progresses, and the left ventricular end-diastolic pressure rises markedly, the arterial diastolic pressure may actually rise also, since the aortic diastolic pressure cannot fall below the left ventricular end-diastolic pressure.

Palpation   The apex beat is displaced laterally and inferiorly. The left ventricle is hyperdynamic in patients with free AR, and the systolic expansion and subsequent retraction of the apex are prominent and contrast sharply with the sustained systolic thrust characteristic of severe AS. A diastolic thrill is often palpable along the left sternal border, and a prominent systolic thrill may be palpable in the jugular notch and transmitted upward along the carotid arteries. This thrill and the accompanying systolic murmur are due to the markedly increased blood flow across the aortic orifice, and do not necessarily signify the coexistence of AS. In many patients with pure AR, or with combined AS and AR, palpation, or indirect recording of the carotid arterial pulse, reveals it to be bisferiens, i.e., with two systolic waves separated by a trough.

Auscultation   In patients with severe regurgitation the aortic valve closure sound is usually diminished or absent. A third heart sound is common, and occasionally a fourth heart sound may also be heard. A loud systolic ejection sound is frequently audible; presumably it results from the sudden dilatation of the aorta by a greatly increased stroke volume. The murmur of AR is typically a high-pitched, blowing, decrescendo diastolic murmur which is usually heard best in the third left intercostal space. In patients with mild regurgitation this murmur is brief, but as the severity increases, the murmur generally becomes louder and longer, and in patients with free AR it is usually holodiastolic. When the murmur is soft, it can be heard best with the diaphragm of the stethoscope and with the patient sitting up, leaning forward, and with the breath held in forced expiration. As it increases in intensity it tends to radiate widely, particularly down the lower sternal edge. In patients in whom the regurgitation is caused by primary valvular disease, the diastolic murmur is usually louder along the left than the right sternal border. However, when the decrescendo diastolic murmur is heard best along the right sternal border, it suggests that the aortic regurgitation is caused by dilatation or an aneurysm of the aortic root. "Cooing" or musical diastolic murmurs suggest eversion of an aortic cusp vibrating in the regurgitant stream. A diastolic blowing murmur along the left sternal border is much more commonly caused by aortic than by pulmonic regurgitation. Unless it is trivial in magnitude, the AR is usually accompanied by peripheral signs such as a widened pulse pressure or a collapsing pulse. On the other hand, with the Graham Steell murmur of pulmonary regurgitation there usually is clinical evidence of severe pulmonary hypertension, including a loud and palpable pulmonary component of the second heart sound. In addition, the phonocardiogram reveals that the murmur of AR begins with the aortic second sound and therefore commences somewhat before the murmur of pulmonary regurgitation.

A midsystolic ejection murmur is frequently audible in AR. It is generally heard best at the base of the heart and is transmitted to the jugular notch and along the carotid vessels. This murmur may be as loud as grade V/VI without indicating the presence of organic obstruction; it is often higher pitched, shorter, and less rasping in quality than the ejection systolic murmur heard in patients with predominant AS. A third murmur which is frequently heard in patients with AR is the Austin Flint murmur, a soft, low-pitched, rumbling middiastolic or presystolic bruit. It is probably produced by the displacement of the anterior leaflet of the mitral valve by the aortic regurgitant stream but does not appear to be associated with hemodynamically significant obstruction to left ventricular filling; earlier onset of and longer Austin Flint murmurs correlate with more severe AR. Both the Austin Flint murmur and the rumbling diastolic murmur of MS are loudest at the apex, but the murmur of MS is usually accompanied by a loud first heart sound and immediately follows the opening snap of the mitral valve, while the Austin Flint murmur is often shorter in duration than the murmur of MS, and in patients with sinus rhythm the latter more frequently is characterized by presystolic accentuation. The auscultatory features of AR are intensified by isometric exercise such as strenuous handgrip, which augments systemic resistance, and reduced by inhalation of amyl nitrite, which evokes the opposite effect. A blowing holosystolic murmur at the apex, which is transmitted to the axilla, may also be heard in patients with aortic regurgitation who have marked left ventricular dilatation and functional mitral regurgitation.

In *acute* severe AR, the elevation of left ventricular end-diastolic pressure may lead to early closure of the mitral valve, an associated middiastolic sound, a soft or absent S_1, a pulse pressure that is not particularly wide, and a soft, short diastolic murmur.

Electrocardiogram   In patients with mild AR there may be no electrocardiographic abnormalities, but with severe chronic AR the electrocardiographic signs of left ventricular hypertrophy become manifest (Chap. 176). In addition to the abnormally tall R waves over the left precordium and deep S waves over the right precordium, patients with severe aortic regurgitation frequently exhibit ST-segment depressions and T-wave inversions in leads I, aVL, V_5, and V_6 ("left ventricular strain"). Left axis deviation and/or QRS prolongation denote diffuse myocardial disease, generally associated with patchy fibrosis, and usually denote a poor prognosis.

Echocardiogram   This reveals increased systolic excursion of the posterior left ventricular wall; the extent and velocity of wall motion are normal or even supernormal, until myocardial contractility declines. A rapid, high-frequency fluttering of the anterior mitral leaflet produced by the impact of the aortic regurgitant jet is a characteristic finding. The echocardiogram is also useful in detecting dilatation of the aortic annulus, and of the left atrium. Thickening of the aortic valve and failure of coaptation of the leaflets may also be noted. Color Doppler flow echocardiographic imaging is very sensitive in the detection of AR, and Doppler echocardiography is helpful in assessing its severity (Fig. 177-5).

Roentgenogram   Moderate or severe degrees of chronic AR are associated with varying degrees of left ventricular enlargement. The apex is displaced downward and to the left in the frontal projection, and frequently the cardiac shadow extends below the left diaphragm. Left ventricular enlargement may also be apparent in the left anterior oblique and lateral projections, in which the left ventricle is displaced posteriorly and encroaches on the spine. In patients in whom primary valvular disease is responsible for the AR, the ascending aorta and aortic knob may be moderately dilated. When AR is caused by primary disease of the aortic wall, aneurysmal dilatation of the aorta may be noted roentgenographically, and the aorta may fill the retrosternal space in the lateral view.

Cardiac catheterization and angiography   These tests should be carried out to aid in the decision regarding surgical treatment. In addition to providing an accurate measurement of the magnitude of regurgitation and the status of left ventricular function, the condition of the coronary arterial bed may be evaluated.

TREATMENT   In deciding upon the advisability and proper timing of surgical treatment, two points should be kept in mind: (1) patients with chronic AR usually do not become symptomatic until *after* the development of myocardial dysfunction; and (2) surgical treatment often does not restore normal left ventricular function. Therefore, careful clinical follow-up and noninvasive testing, with echocardiography or radionuclide angiography, at approximately 6-month intervals, are necessary if operation is to be undertaken at the optimal time, i.e., with the onset of left ventricular dysfunction but prior to the development of severe symptoms. Operation can be deferred as long as the patient remains asymptomatic *and* retains normal left ventricular function.

Replacement of the aortic valve with a suitable mechanical or tissue prosthesis is generally necessary in patients with rheumatic AR and in many patients with other forms of regurgitation. Rarely, when a leaflet has been perforated during an episode of infective endocarditis, or torn from its attachments to the aortic annulus, surgical repair may be possible. When AR is due to aneurysmal dilatation of the annulus and ascending aorta, rather than to primary valvular involvement, it may be possible to reduce the regurgitation by narrowing the annulus or by excising a portion of the aortic root without replacing the valve. More frequently, however, regurgitation can be eliminated only by replacing the aortic valve, excising the aneurysm responsible for the regurgitation, and replacing the latter with a graft. This formidable procedure entails a higher risk than aortic valve replacement alone.

As in patients with other valvular abnormalities, both the operative risk of aortic valve replacement and late mortality are largely dependent on the stage of the disease and on myocardial function at the time of operation; patients with marked cardiac enlargement and prolonged left ventricular dysfunction have a late mortality of approximately 5 percent per year despite a technically satisfactory operation.

Although operation constitutes the principal treatment of aortic regurgitation, and should be carried out before the development of heart failure, the latter usually does respond initially to treatment with digitalis glycosides, salt restriction, diuretics, and vasodilators, especially angiotensin-converting enzyme inhibitors. Digitalis may also be indicated in patients with severe regurgitation and dilated left ventricles without symptoms of frank left ventricular failure. Cardiac arrhythmias and infections are poorly tolerated in patients with free AR, and must be treated promptly and vigorously. Although nitroglycerin and long-acting nitrates are not as helpful in relieving anginal pain as in patients with coronary artery disease or aortic stenosis, they are worth a trial. Patients with syphilitic aortitis should receive a full course of penicillin therapy (Chap. 128).

ACUTE AORTIC REGURGITATION Infective endocarditis, aortic dissection, and trauma are the most common causes of severe, acute AR. Since the left ventricle has not had time to dilate, stroke volume declines and ventricular diastolic pressure rises markedly; the arterial pulse pressure is often not markedly widened and the physical signs characteristic of severe chronic AR may be absent. Premature closure of the mitral valve is common and can be recognized by echocardiography. The first heart sound is soft or absent; the aortic diastolic murmur is characteristically brief. Patients present with pulmonary congestion and edema, and hypotension secondary to a low cardiac output. Acute, severe regurgitation requires prompt surgical treatment, which may be lifesaving.

TRICUSPID STENOSIS

Tricuspid stenosis (TS), a relatively uncommon valvular lesion, is generally rheumatic in origin and is much more common in women than in men. It does not usually occur as an isolated lesion or in patients with pure MR, but most commonly is observed in association with MS, and sometimes with combined MS and AS. Hemodynamically significant TS occurs in 5 to 10 percent of patients with severe MS; rheumatic TS is commonly associated with some degree of regurgitation.

PATHOPHYSIOLOGY A diastolic pressure gradient between the right atrium and ventricle is present. This gradient can be recorded most accurately and conveniently with a double-lumen cardiac catheter. It is augmented when the transvalvular blood flow increases during inspiration, and reduced during expiration. A *mean* diastolic pressure gradient exceeding 4 mmHg is usually sufficient to elevate the mean right atrial pressure to levels which result in systemic venous congestion and, unless sodium intake has been restricted or diuretics have been given, is associated with ascites and edema. In patients

with sinus rhythm, the right atrial *a* wave may be extremely tall and may even approach the level of the right ventricular systolic pressure. The resting cardiac output is usually quite low and fails to rise during exercise. The low cardiac output is responsible for the normal or only slightly elevated left atrial, pulmonary arterial, and right ventricular systolic pressures despite the presence of even moderately severe MS.

SYMPTOMS Since MS generally precedes the development of TS, many patients initially have symptoms of pulmonary congestion. Amelioration of the latter should raise the possibility that TS may be developing. Characteristically, patients complain of relatively little dyspnea for the degree of hepatomegaly, ascites, and edema which they present. Weakness secondary to a low cardiac output and discomfort due to refractory edema, ascites, and marked hepatomegaly are common in patients with TS and/or regurgitation. In some patients TS may be suspected for the first time when symptoms of right ventricular failure persist after an adequate mitral valvulotomy.

PHYSICAL FINDINGS Since TS usually occurs in the presence of other obvious valvular disease, the diagnosis is often missed unless it is specifically considered and searched for. Severe TS is associated with marked hepatic congestion, often resulting in cirrhosis, jaundice, serious malnutrition, severe edema, and ascites. Congestive hepatomegaly and, in cases of severe tricuspid valve disease, splenomegaly are present. The jugular veins are distended, and in patients with sinus rhythm there may be giant *a* waves. The *v* waves are less conspicuous, and since tricuspid obstruction impedes right atrial emptying during diastole, there is a slow *y* descent. In patients with sinus rhythm there may be prominent presystolic pulsations of the enlarged liver as well.

The right ventricle and the shock of pulmonic valve closure are usually not easily palpable. Indeed, a giant *a* wave in the jugular venous pulse without palpatory evidence of pulmonary hypertension or right ventricular enlargement should immediately suggest the possibility of TS. On auscultation, the pulmonic closure sound is not accentuated, and occasionally an OS of the tricuspid valve may be heard or recorded phonocardiographically approximately 0.06 s after pulmonic valve closure. The diastolic murmur of TS has many of the qualities of the diastolic murmur of MS, and since TS almost always occurs in the presence of MS, the less-common valvular lesion may be missed. However, the tricuspid murmur is generally heard best along the left lower sternal margin and over the xiphoid process and is most prominent during presystole in sinus rhythm. In patients with sinus rhythm the presystolic component is often loudest. The murmur is augmented during inspiration, and it is reduced during expiration and particularly during the Valsalva maneuver, when tricuspid blood flow is reduced. This finding (Carvallo's sign) is often most easily elicited when the patient is in the erect position. The diastolic murmur is reduced in amplitude as the stethoscope is inched laterally, only to intensify or reappear as the mitral murmur at the apex.

Noninvasive examinations The features of right atrial enlargement (Chap. 176) include tall, peaked P waves in lead II, as well as prominent, upright P waves in lead V_1. The *absence* of electrocardiographic evidence of right ventricular hypertrophy in a patient with right-sided heart failure who is believed to have MS should suggest associated tricuspid valve disease. The chest roentgenograms in patients with combined TS and MS show particular prominence of the right atrium and superior vena cava without much enlargement of the pulmonary artery and with less evidence of pulmonary vascular congestion than occurs in patients with pure mitral valve disease. On echocardiographic examination the tricuspid valve is usually thickened; the transvalvular gradient can be estimated by Doppler echocardiography.

TREATMENT Patients with TS generally exhibit marked systemic venous congestion; intensive salt restriction and diuretic therapy are required during the preoperative period. Such a preparatory period may diminish hepatic congestion and thereby improve hepatic function sufficiently so that the risks of operation are diminished. Surgical treatment of the tricuspid valve is not ordinarily indicated at the time of mitral valve surgery in patients with *mild* TS. On the other hand, definitive surgical relief of the TS should be carried out, preferably at the time of mitral valvulotomy, in patients with moderate or severe TS who have mean diastolic pressure gradients exceeding 4 to 5 mmHg and tricuspid orifices less than 1.5 to 2.0 cm². TS is almost always accompanied by significant tricuspid regurgitation. Open-heart operations utilizing cardiopulmonary bypass may permit substantial improvement of tricuspid valve function. If this cannot be accomplished, the tricuspid valve may have to be replaced with a prosthesis, preferably a tissue valve.

TRICUSPID REGURGITATION

Most commonly, tricuspid regurgitation (TR) is functional and secondary to marked dilatation of the right ventricle and the tricuspid valve ring. Functional TR may complicate right ventricular enlargement of any cause, including inferior wall infarcts that involve the right ventricle, and it is commonly seen in the late stages of heart failure due to rheumatic or congenital heart disease with severe pulmonary hypertension, as well as in ischemic heart disease, cardiomyopathy, and cor pulmonale. It is in part reversible if pulmonary hypertension is relieved. Rheumatic fever may produce organic TR, often associated with TS. Less commonly, regurgitation results from congenitally deformed tricuspid valves, and it occurs with defects of the atrioventricular canal, as well as with Ebstein's malformation of the tricuspid valve (Chap. 186). Infarction of right ventricular papillary muscles, tricuspid valve prolapse, carcinoid heart disease, endomyocardial fibrosis, infective endocarditis, and trauma may also produce TR.

As is the case for TS, the clinical features of TR result primarily from systemic venous congestion and reduction of cardiac output. With the onset of TR in patients with pulmonary hypertension, as cardiac output declines, symptoms of pulmonary congestion diminish, but the clinical manifestations of right-sided heart failure become intensified. The neck veins are distended, with prominent *v* waves and marked hepatomegaly, ascites, pleural effusions, edema, systolic pulsations of the liver, and positive hepatojugular reflux are common. A prominent right ventricular pulsation along the left parasternal region and a blowing holosystolic murmur along the lower left sternal margin which is generally intensified during inspiration and reduced during expiration or the Valsalva maneuver are characteristic findings; atrial fibrillation is usually present.

The electrocardiogram usually shows changes characteristic of the lesion responsible for the enlargement of the right ventricle which leads to this form of valvular dysfunction. In the rare instances of isolated TR the electrocardiogram often shows incomplete right bundle branch block. Roentgenographic examination usually reveals enlargement of both the right atrium and ventricle. Echocardiography may be helpful by demonstrating right ventricular dilatation and prolapsing or flail tricuspid leaflets; the diagnosis of tricuspid regurgitation can be made by color flow echocardiography and the severity estimated by Doppler examination. The latter is also useful in estimating pulmonary artery pressure.

The cardiac output is usually markedly reduced, and the right atrial pressure pulse may exhibit no *x* descent during early systole, but a prominent *c-v* wave, with a rapid *y* descent. The mean right atrial and the right ventricular end-diastolic pressures are often elevated.

Isolated TR, without pulmonary hypertension, such as that occurring as a consequence of infective endocarditis or trauma, is usually well tolerated and does not require operation. Indeed, even total excision of an infected tricuspid valve is often well tolerated if the pulmonary artery pressure is normal. Treatment of the underlying cause of heart failure usually reduces the severity of functional TR. In patients with mitral valve disease and TR due to pulmonary hypertension and massive right ventricular enlargement, effective surgical correction of the mitral valvular abnormality results in lowering of the pulmonary vascular pressures and gradual reduction or disappearance of the TR without direct treatment of the tricuspid valve. However, recovery may be much more rapid in patients with severe secondary TR if, at the time of mitral valve replacement, tricuspid annuloplasty or, if necessary, tricuspid valve replacement is performed. Surgical treatment of the TR, consisting of either valve replacement or narrowing of the annulus, should be carried out in patients with severe regurgitation secondary to deformity of the tricuspid valve due to rheumatic fever, particularly those *without* severe pulmonary hypertension.

PULMONIC VALVE DISEASE

The pulmonic valve is affected by rheumatic fever far less frequently than the other valves and is uncommonly the seat of infective endocarditis. The most common acquired abnormality affecting the pulmonic valve is regurgitation secondary to dilatation of the pulmonic valve ring as a consequence of severe pulmonary hypertension of any cause. This produces the Graham Steell murmur, a high-pitched, decrescendo, diastolic blowing murmur along the left sternal border, which is difficult to differentiate from the far more common murmur produced by aortic regurgitation. It is of little hemodynamic significance; indeed surgical removal or destruction of the pulmonic valve by infective endocarditis does not produce heart failure unless serious pulmonary hypertension is also present.

Congenital pulmonic stenosis is discussed in Chap. 186.

REFERENCES

BOUDOULAS H, WOOLEY CF (eds): *The Mitral Valve Prolapse Syndrome*. Futura, Mount Kisco, NY 1988

BRAUNWALD E: Valvular heart disease, in *Heart Disease*, 3d ed, E Braunwald (ed). Philadelphia, Saunders, 1988, p 1023

COHEN SR et al: Tricuspid regurgitation in patients with acquired, chronic, pure mitral regurgitation: 1. Prevalence, diagnosis and comparison of preoperative clinical and hemodynamic features in patients with and without tricuspid regurgitation. J Thorac Cardiovasc Surg 94:481, 1987

CRAWFORD MH, KOUCHOUKOS NT (eds): Valvular heart disease. Current Opinion in Cardiology 4:189, 1989

FRANKL WS, BREST AN (eds):*Valvular Heart Disease: Comprehensive Evaluation and Management*. Philadelphia, FA Davis, 1986

FUSTER V et al: Prevention of thromboembolism induced by prosthetic heart valves. Semin Thromb Hemost 14:50, 1988

GALLOWAY AC et al: Current concepts of mitral valve reconstruction for mitral insufficiency. Circulation 78:1087, 1988

GREENBERG BH et al: Arterial dilators in mitral regurgitation: Effects on rest and exercise, hemodynamics and long-term clinical follow-up. Circulation 65:181, 1982

IONESCU MI, COHN LH (eds): *Mitral Valve Disease: Diagnosis and Treatment*. London, Butterworths, 1985

KIRKLIN JW, BARRATT-BOYES BG: Part III. Acquired valvular heart disease, in *Cardiac Surgery*, JW Kirklin, BG Barratt-Boyes (eds). New York, Wiley, 1986, p 323

LINGAMENI R et al: Tricuspid regurgitation: Clinical and angiographic assessment. Cath Cardiovasc Diag 5:7, 1979

MAHAPATRA RK et al: Rheumatic tricuspid stenosis. Indian Heart J 30:1381, 1978

MARKS AR et al: Identification of high-risk and low-risk subgroups of patients with mitral valve prolapse. N Engl J Med 320:1031, 1989

MASUYAMA T et al: Noninvasive evaluation of aortic regurgitation by continuous-wave Doppler echocardiography. Circulation 73:460, 1986

NAIR CK et al: Ten-year results with the St. Jude Medical Prosthesis. Am J Cardiol 65(3):217, 1990

OH JK et al: Prediction of the severity of aortic stenosis by Doppler aortic valve area determination: Prospective Doppler-catheterization correlation in 100 patients. J Am Coll Cardiol 11:1227, 1988

SAFIAN RD et al: Percutaneous aortic valvuloplasty in 170 connective patients. N Engl J Med 319:125, 1988

VAHANIAN A et al: Results of percutaneous mitral commissurotomy in 200 patients. Am J Cardiol 63:847, 1989

189   ACUTE MYOCARDIAL INFARCTION

RICHARD C. PASTERNAK / EUGENE BRAUNWALD

Myocardial infarction is one of the commonest diagnoses occurring in hospitalized patients in western countries. In the United States, approximately 1.5 million myocardial infarctions occur each year. Mortality with acute infarction is approximately 25 percent, with slightly more than half of the deaths occurring before the stricken individual reaches the hospital. Although survival following hospitalization has improved over the last decade and a half, an additional 5 to 10 percent of survivors die in the first year following myocardial infarction. Risk of excess mortality and recurrent nonfatal myocardial infarction persists in patients who recover.

CLINICAL PRESENTATION

Pain is the most common presenting complaint in patients with myocardial infarction. In some instances, the discomfort may be severe enough to be described as the worst pain the patient has ever experienced (Chap. 16). The pain of myocardial infarction is deep and visceral; adjectives commonly used to describe it are *heavy,* *squeezing,* and *crushing.* It is similar in character to the discomfort of angina pectoris but is usually more severe and lasts much longer. Typically the pain involves the central portion of the chest and/or epigastrium, and in about 30 percent of cases it radiates to the arms. Less common sites of radiation include the abdomen, back, lower jaw, and neck. The location of the pain beneath the xiphoid and patients' denial that they may be suffering a heart attack are chiefly responsible for the mistaken diagnosis of indigestion. The pain of myocardial infarction may radiate as high as the occipital area but not below the umbilicus. The pain is often accompanied by weakness, sweating, nausea, vomiting, giddiness, and anxiety. The discomfort usually commences with the patient at rest and exhibits circadian periodicity, occurring more commonly in the morning than at any other time of the day. Less than one-third of the time does the pain begin during a period of exertion; when it does, in contrast to angina pectoris, it does not usually subside with cessation of activity. Approximately one-half of patients with myocardial infarction exhibit the prodrome of unstable angina (Chap. 190).

Although pain is the most common presenting complaint, it is by no means always present; a minimum of 15 to 20 percent of myocardial infarcts are *painless.* The incidence of painless infarcts is greater in patients with diabetes mellitus, and it increases with age. In the elderly, myocardial infarction may present as sudden-onset breathlessness, which may progress to pulmonary edema. Other less common presentations, with or without pain, include sudden loss of consciousness, a confusional state, a sensation of profound weakness, the appearance of an arrhythmia, evidence of peripheral embolism, or merely an unexplained drop in arterial pressure. The pain of myocardial infarction can be similar to pain from acute pericarditis (Chap. 193), pulmonary embolism (Chap. 213), acute aortic dissection (Chap. 197), or costochondritis. These conditions should be considered in the differential diagnosis.

Patients at increased risk of developing acute myocardial infarction include those with unstable angina, multiple coronary risk factors (p. 239), and coronary artery spasm. Less common etiologic factors include hypercoagulability, coronary emboli, collagen vascular disease, coronary artery anomalies, and cocaine abuse.

PHYSICAL FINDINGS   Most patients are anxious and restless, attempting to relieve the pain by moving about in bed, squirming, stretching, belching, or even inducing vomiting. Pallor is common and is often associated with perspiration and coolness of the extremities. The combination of substernal chest pain persistent for more than 30 min and diaphoresis strongly suggests acute myocardial infarction. Although many patients have a normal pulse rate and blood pressure, within the first hour of infarction about one-fourth of patients with anterior infarction have manifestations of sympathetic nervous system hyperactivity (tachycardia and/or hypertension), and up to one-half with inferior infarction show evidence of parasympathetic hyperactivity (bradycardia and/or hypotension).

The precordium is usually quiet, and the apical impulse may be difficult to palpate. In about one-fourth of patients with anterior wall infarction, an abnormal systolic pulsation develops in the periapical area within the first days of the illness and then may resolve. Other physical signs of ventricular dysfunction that may be present include, in decreasing incidence, fourth (S_4) and third (S_3) heart sounds, decreased intensity of heart sounds, and, rarely, paradoxical splitting of the second sound (Chap. 175). A transient apical systolic murmur, presumably due to mitral regurgitation secondary to papillary muscle dysfunction during acute infarction, may be midsystolic or late systolic in timing. A pericardial friction rub is heard in many patients with transmural myocardial infarction at some time in their course if they are examined frequently. Jugular venous distention occurs commonly in patients with right ventricular infarction. The carotid pulse is often slightly decreased in volume despite a normal upstroke. Temperature elevations in the range of 37 to 38°C may be observed during the first week following acute myocardial infarction; however, a temperature exceeding 38°C should prompt a search for other causes. The arterial pressure is variable; in most patients with transmural infarction systolic pressure declines approximately 10 to 15 mmHg from the preinfarction state.

LABORATORY FINDINGS

The laboratory tests of value in confirming the diagnosis of myocardial infarction may be divided into three groups: (1) nonspecific indexes of tissue necrosis and inflammation, (2) the electrocardiogram, and (3) serum enzyme changes.

The *nonspecific reaction* to myocardial injury is associated with polymorphonuclear leukocytosis, which appears within a few hours after the onset of pain, persists for 3 to 7 days, and often reaches levels of 12,000 to 15,000 leukocytes per microliter. The erythrocyte sedimentation rate rises more slowly than the white blood cell count, peaking during the first week, and sometimes remaining elevated for 1 or 2 weeks.

The *electrocardiographic manifestations* of acute myocardial infarction are described in Chap. 176. Although electrocardiographic/pathologic correlations are not excellent, transmural infarction is often diagnosed if the electrocardiogram demonstrates Q waves or loss of R waves; nontransmural infarction is considered to be present if the electrocardiogram shows only transient ST-segment and sustained T-wave changes. However, the latter changes are variable and nonspecific and should not form the sole basis for the diagnosis of infarction. Therefore, a more rational nomenclature for designating electrocardiographic infarction is now commonly in use, with the terms *Q-wave* or *non-Q-wave infarction* in place of the terms *transmural* or *nontransmural infarction,* respectively.

SERUM ENZYMES   Enzymes are released in large quantities into the blood from necrotic heart muscle following myocardial infarction. The rate of liberation of specific enzymes differs following infarction, and the temporal pattern of enzyme release is of diagnostic importance. Creatine phosphokinase (CK) rises within 8 to 24 h, and generally returns to normal by 48 to 72 h, except in the case of large infarctions, when CK clearance is delayed. Lactic dehydrogenase (LDH) rises later (24 to 48 h) and remains elevated for as long as 7 to 14 days. The serum aminotransferase enzymes, AST and ALT (previously designated SGOT and SGPT), were utilized in the diagnosis of myocardial infarction for many years, but have fallen out of favor because it has been recognized that their time course of elevation is intermediate between CK and LDH, thus offering little advantage, and because of lack of tissue specificity. The MB isoenzyme of CK has the advantage over CK and LDH in that it is not present in significant concentrations in extracardiac tissue, and therefore it is more specific. CK-MB isoenzymes are particularly useful when skeletal muscle and/or brain damage are suspected since both of these tissues contain large quantities of the enzyme but none of the MB isoenzyme. The myocardial specificity of the MB isoenzyme determination depends on the technique used for measurement. Radioimmunoassay techniques are most specific, but the more commonly employed gel electrophoresis technique is significantly less specific and therefore prone to more frequent false positives. Five common LDH isoenzymes may be separated by starch-gel electrophoresis. Tissues differ with respect to the specific isoenzyme patterns; the rapidly migrating isoenzyme which predominates in the heart is referred to as LDH_1, while the slowly migrating components predominate in liver and skeletal muscle. LDH_1 rises before total LDH in patients with myocardial infarction and may rise when there is no change in total LDH. Therefore, increased LDH_1 is a more sensitive indicator of myocardial infarction than total LDH; sensitivity exceeds 95 percent. However, measurements of the LDH isoenzymes should be obtained only when the initial CK or CK-MB elevation might have been missed (after 48 h), for they are not more sensitive than CK-MB and therefore only increase cost without increasing diagnostic accuracy.

A two- to threefold elevation of total CK (not CK-MB) may follow an intramuscular injection. This may lead to the erroneous diagnosis of myocardial infarction in a patient who has been given an intramuscular injection of a narcotic for chest pain of noncardiac origin. Other potential sources of total CK elevation worthy of note are (1) muscular diseases including muscular dystrophy, myopathies, and polymyositis, (2) electrical cardioversion, (3) cardiac catheterization, (4) hypothyroidism, (5) stroke, (6) surgery, and (7) skeletal muscle damage secondary to trauma, convulsions, and prolonged immobilization. Cardiac surgery, myocarditis, and electrical cardioversion often result in elevation of serum levels of MB isoenzyme.

While it has long been recognized that the *total* quantity of enzyme released correlates with the size of the infarct, the *peak* enzyme concentration is only weakly correlated with infarct size. It has been demonstrated that the mass of heart muscle infarcted can be estimated from analysis of the concentration-time curve of the enzyme only if the kinetics of the release, degradation, disposal, etc., of the enzyme are known. Thus, while the *area* under the CK-MB time curve is related to infarct size, the *absolute* value of the peak CK-MB and its time to peak are related to the kinetics of CK-MB washout from myocardium. The opening of a coronary artery occlusion (either spontaneously, or by mechanical or pharmacologic means) in the early hours of myocardial infarction will cause early and higher peaking (at about 8 h following reperfusion) of the CK-MB time curve.

Characteristic rises occur in serum enzyme concentration in more than 95 percent of patients with clinically proven myocardial infarction. CK and LDH levels generally do not rise in unstable angina. Many patients with suspected infarction have baseline enzyme levels that are normal and increase threefold in a pattern consistent with infarction, although the absolute level of enzyme in the blood never exceeds the upper limits of normal. These have been termed "microinfarctions," and such patients have a prognosis intermediate between that of unstable angina and that of proven myocardial infarction. Isoenzyme studies are particularly helpful in this situation.

Several radionuclide imaging techniques are of value in the diagnosis or assessment of the patient with acute myocardial infarction (Chap. 178). Acute infarct scintigraphy ("hot-spot" imaging) is carried out with an infarct-avid imaging agent such as [^{99m}Tc] stannous pyrophosphate. Scans are usually positive 2 to 5 days after infarction, particularly in patients with transmural infarcts; although they aid in *localizing* infarcts and provide a measure of infarct size (chap. 177); these scans are less sensitive than CK determination for making the *diagnosis* of myocardial infarction. Myocardial perfusion imaging with thallium 201, which is taken up and concentrated by viable myocardium, reveals a defect ("cold spot") in most patients during the first few hours after development of a transmural infarct (p. 864). However, since it is not possible to distinguish acute infarcts from chronic scars, thallium scanning, although extremely *sensitive*, is not *specific* for *acute* myocardial infarction. Radionuclide ventriculography, carried out with ^{99m}Tc-labeled red blood cells (p. 864), frequently demonstrates wall motion disorders and reduction in ventricular ejection fraction in patients with acute myocardial infarction. While of value in assessing the hemodynamic consequences of infarction, and in aiding in the diagnosis of right ventricular infarction when the right ventricular ejection fraction is depressed, this technique is also quite nonspecific, since many cardiac abnormalities other than myocardial infarction alter the radionuclide ventriculogram. Two-dimensional echocardiography (Chap. 178) can also be of value in patients with acute myocardial infarction. Abnormalities of wall motion, particularly of the septal and inferior-posterior walls, are readily detectable. Although acute infarction cannot be distinguished from old myocardial scar or from acute severe ischemia, the ease and safety of the procedure make its use appealing as a screening tool. Echocardiography may be particularly useful in the diagnosis of right ventricular infarction, ventricular aneurysm, and left ventricular thrombus. Additionally, Doppler echocardiography is useful in the detection of a ventricular septal defect and mitral regurgitation, complications of acute myocardial infarction.

MANAGEMENT

Two general classes of complications have been defined: (1) electrical (arrhythmias) and (2) mechanical ("pump failure"). Ventricular fibrillation is the most common form of arrhythmic death in acute myocardial infarction. The vast majority of deaths due to ventricular fibrillation occur within the first 24 h of the onset of symptoms, and of these deaths, over half occur in the first hour. Although ventricular premature beats or ventricular tachycardia may precede an episode of ventricular fibrillation, the latter may occur without warning arrhythmias. Over the last 25 years, with careful monitoring and prompt attention to arrhythmias, the in-hospital mortality for acute myocardial infarction has been reduced from about 30 to less than 15 percent.

With the incidence of sudden in-hospital arrhythmic deaths markedly reduced, attention has turned to other major complications of acute myocardial infarction, i.e., pump failure and its prevention by attempts to limit infarct size. Nevertheless, pump failure remains the primary cause of in-hospital death from acute myocardial infarction. The extent of ischemic necrosis correlates well with the degree of pump failure and with mortality, both early, i.e., within 10 days of infarction, and later as well. A clinical classification dependent on the status of cardiac pump function originally proposed by Killip divides patients into four groups as follows: class I, no signs of pulmonary or venous congestion; class II, moderate heart failure as evidenced by rales at the lung bases, S_3 gallop, tachypnea, or signs of failure of the right side of the heart including venous and hepatic congestion; class III, severe heart failure, pulmonary edema; class IV, shock with systolic pressure less than 90 mmHg and evidence of peripheral constriction, diaphoresis, peripheral cyanosis, mental confusion, and oliguria. The expected hospital mortality rate of patients in these clinical classes when this classification was established was as follows: class I, 0 to 5 percent; class II, 10 to 20 percent; class III, 35 to 45 percent; and class IV, 85 to 95 percent. With recent advances in management, mortality has fallen, perhaps by as much as one-third, in each class.

GENERAL CONSIDERATIONS   Given the information summarized above, the principal objectives of management of the patient with myocardial infarction are to prevent death from arrhythmia and to minimize the mass of infarcted tissue.

Arrhythmias can usually be managed successfully if trained personnel and appropriate equipment are available when this complication develops. Since mortality from arrhythmia is greatest during the first few hours after infarction, it is obvious that the effectiveness of treatment relates directly to the speed with which patients come under medical observation. The biggest delay usually is not in transportation to the hospital but rather between the onset of pain and the patient's decision to call for help. This delay can best be reduced by education of the public concerning the significance of chest pain and the importance of seeking early medical attention. Increasingly, monitoring and treatment are carried out by trained personnel in the ambulance, shortening even further the time between the onset of the infarction and appropriate care.

A number of "common sense" rules in the management of acute myocardial infarction deserve particular emphasis. It is essential to maintain an optimal balance between myocardial oxygen supply and demand in order to salvage as much of the jeopardized myocardium as possible. Therapeutic strategies that help to attain this goal include rest, analgesia, mild sedation, and a quiet atmosphere in order to reduce anxiety and thereby lower heart rate, a major determinant of myocardial oxygen consumption.

Marked sinus bradycardia (heart rate less than approximately 45 beats per minute) should be treated by leg elevation and atropine or by electrical pacing, particularly if the bradycardia is associated with a fall in blood pressure or with worsening ventricular arrhythmias. However, routine administration of atropine, with resultant increase in heart rate, to patients without serious bradycardia is not recommended. Patients with acute myocardial infarction who have a hyperdynamic state, i.e., tachycardia and elevation of arterial pressure, should be treated with a beta-adrenergic blocking agent. Initially, 0.1 mg/kg propranolol or 15 mg metoprolol given intravenously in three divided doses is safe, if there are no contraindications, such as heart failure, AV block, or history of asthma. All forms of tachyarrhythmias require prompt and direct treatment. Drugs that exert a positive inotropic effect, such as digitalis glycosides and cardioactive sympathomimetics, should be administered only if there is evidence of pronounced heart failure with a low cardiac output due to systolic dysfunction; they should not be given prophylactically. Of the various sympathomimetic amines available, isoproterenol with its chronotropic and vasodilator effects is the least desirable. Dobutamine (p. 899) and amrinone, which have less effect on heart rate and systemic vascular resistance, are more desirable when it is necessary to augment cardiac contractility. However, these drugs have vasodilating potential and may not be tolerated in patients with borderline or frank hypotension. Dopamine (p. 899) is useful in patients with left ventricular failure and systemic hypotension (systolic pressure <90 mmHg. Diuretics are indicated in the presence of pulmonary congestion and should, in fact, be used prior to cardiac stimulants unless the patient is hypovolemic or hypotensive.

All patients should inhale oxygen-enriched air (see below). Particular attention must be paid to preserving arterial oxygenation in patients with hypoxemia, as occurs in patients with chronic pulmonary disease, pneumonia, or left ventricular failure. Severe anemia, which can also extend the area of ischemic injury, should be corrected by cautious administration of packed red blood cells, sometimes accompanied by a diuretic. Associated conditions, particularly infections with accompanying tachycardia and elevated myocardial oxygen demand, require immediate attention. Systolic arterial pressure should not be allowed to deviate by more than 25 to 30 mmHg from the patient's usual level, unless untreated hypertension has been present, in which case a greater fall in arterial pressure is desirable.

CORONARY CARE UNITS These have resulted in improved care of patients with myocardial infarction, reduction in mortality rates, and major increases in knowledge about myocardial infarction. The unit should be equipped with a system which permits continuous monitoring of the cardiac rhythm of *each* patient and hemodynamic monitoring in *selected* patients. Defibrillators, respirators, and facilities for introducing pacing catheters and flow-directed balloon-tipped catheters should be available. Equally important is the organization

of a highly trained team of nurses who can recognize arrhythmias, adjust the dosage of antiarrhythmic drugs, and perform cardiac resuscitation, including electroshock, when necessary.

The policies and procedures for admission to a coronary care unit should ensure that patients are admitted early in their illness when they may expect to derive maximum benefit from the care provided. In the past, all patients with suspected myocardial infarction were admitted to the coronary care unit. Currently, however, several factors have led to a change in this rule. The availability of electrocardiographic monitoring and trained personnel in "intermediate care units" has allowed admission of lower-risk patients (e.g., those not hemodynamically compromised or without active arrhythmias) to such units. For economic reasons, and to utilize limited facilities optimally, many institutions have developed guidelines to aid in triaging patients with suspected myocardial infarction. While most such patients in the United States are admitted to the hospital, in other countries, such as the United Kingdom, the patients at lowest risk may be cared for at home. Once admitted to the hospital the fraction of patients actually admitted to the coronary care unit may depend on a balance between the clinical status of the patient and bed availability. In some units beds are utilized primarily for patients with a complicated course, particularly those who require hemodynamic monitoring. Mortality rates for myocardial infarction treated in coronary care units vary from 5 to 20 percent, according to variations in admission policies, type of population served, nature of the hospital (tertiary care center versus community hospital), and other as yet unidentified factors.

REPERFUSION One of the most important developments in the care of patients with acute myocardial infarction derives from the recognition that early reperfusion of ischemic myocardium can potentially salvage tissue before it becomes irreversibly injured. Since most infarctions are caused by a relatively sudden thrombotic occlusion adjacent to an atherosclerotic plaque in a major epicardial coronary vessel, recent attention has been appropriately directed at techniques to pharmacologically or mechanically recanalize the "culprit" vessel. The thrombolytic agents, streptokinase, and tissue plasminogen activator (tPA) produced by recombinant DNA technology (Chap. 6), have been approved by the Federal Drug Administration for intravenous use in the setting of acute myocardial infarction. These agents, as well as other investigational ones, have been extensively studied in many clinical trials from which emerge important conclusions about the management of patients with acute myocardial infarction. Thrombolytic therapy can reduce in-hospital mortality for myocardial infarction by up to 50 percent when administered within the first hour of the onset of symptoms, with much of this benefit maintained for one or more years. Appropriately employed thrombolytic therapy appears to reduce infarct size and limit left ventricular dysfunction as well. Since salvage of myocardium can only occur before the myocardium is irreversibly injured, timing of thrombolytic therapy is of extreme importance in achieving maximum benefit. While an upper time limit has not been established, it is clear that "every minute counts" and that patients treated within 1 to 3 h of the onset of symptoms stand to benefit most. Although the reduction of mortality is more modest, institution of therapy remains of benefit in many patients seen 3 to 6 h after the onset of infarction, and some benefit appears possible up to 12 h (and perhaps even to 24 h) after, especially if chest discomfort is ongoing and ST segments remain elevated in electrocardiographic leads that do not yet demonstrate new Q waves. In addition to the possibility of early treatment, clinical factors that favor proceeding with thrombolytic therapy include: anterior wall injury, hemodynamically complicated infarction, widespread ECG evidence of myocardial jeopardy, and younger patient.

When compared directly, tPA is more effective than streptokinase at restoring coronary artery flow, but a difference in mortality has not been demonstrated. The current recommended total dose of tPA is 100 mg given as 60 mg intravenously over the first hour, beginning with a 5- to 10-mg bolus, followed by 20 mg each in the second and third hours. Streptokinase is administered as 1.5 million units intravenously over 1 h. Although the optimum adjunctive anticoagulant and antiplatelet regimen has not yet been firmly established, recent studies suggest that 80 to 325 mg of aspirin and 5000 units of heparin should be given with the institution of thrombolytic therapy. This should be followed by 325 mg of aspirin daily and a continuous infusion of heparin for 2 to 5 days.

Clear contraindications to the use of thrombolytic agents include a history of cerebrovascular accident, a recent (within 2 weeks) invasive or surgical procedure (or prolonged cardiopulmonary resuscitation), marked hypertension (systolic arterial pressure greater than 180 mmHg and/or diastolic pressure greater than 100 mmHg) at any time during the acute presentation, and active peptic ulcer disease. Other clinical reasons for an increased risk of bleeding (such as advanced age) should be sought for and the potential benefit of such therapy weighed against expected risk before the decision to administer a thrombolytic agent is made. Following thrombolytic therapy cardiac catheterization and coronary angiography should be carried out if there is evidence of coronary artery reocclusion (reelevation of ST segments, and/or recurrent chest pain) or if recurrent ischemia develops (such as recurrent angina in the early hospital course or a positive exercise stress test prior to discharge). Under these circumstances, and if the coronary anatomy is suitable, coronary angioplasty should be performed. Coronary artery bypass surgery should be reserved for a small minority of patients whose coronary anatomy is unsuitable for angioplasty but in whom revascularization appears to be advisable because of extensive jeopardized myocardium or recurrent ischemia.

Repeat administration of a thrombolytic agent is an alternative to early mechanical revascularization. Although there is little to suggest how this might be best undertaken, one reasonable strategy is to give a half dose of tPA (50 mg over 4 h) if reocclusion occurs 12 to 24 h after the agent is initially given and a repeat full dose (100 mg over 3 h) if such an event occurs more than 24 h later.

Acute primary percutaneous transluminal coronary angioplasty (PTCA), i.e., without preceding thrombolysis, has also been reported to be effective in restoring effective reperfusion in acute myocardial infarction, but this technique is very expensive in terms of personnel and facilities and probably should be limited to inpatients whose coronary anatomy is already known, e.g., in the setting of a post-cardiac catheterization coronary occlusion, and to patients in cardiogenic shock who can be brought to the catheterization laboratory within 3 h of the onset of symptoms.

The amount of myocardial tissue which becomes necrotic secondary to a coronary artery occlusion is determined by factors other than just the site of occlusion. One such important factor is the status of collateral blood supply to ischemic tissue. Myocardium well supplied by collaterals clearly has the capacity to survive hours longer than poorly collateralized areas. Infarct size is now known to vary with time and be affected by a number of therapeutic agents currently in use. The balance between myocardial oxygen supply and demand in areas rendered ischemic determines the ultimate fate of these areas of jeopardized myocardium. While no routine therapeutic approach to reduce infarct size in all patients is currently recommended, the realization that infarct size may be increased by interventions which adversely alter the supply-demand balance has prompted the reevaluation of previously accepted therapeutic maneuvers in the management of patients with acute infarction. Cardioactive sympathomimetic amines are used sparingly and only for clear-cut indications. The early administration of beta blockers, with or without thrombolytic therapy, appears to be of benefit.

TREATMENT OF THE PATIENT WITH AN UNCOMPLICATED INFARCTION

ANALGESIA Since myocardial infarction usually presents with severe pain, one of the important initial therapeutic objectives is the relief of pain. Morphine is an extremely effective analgesic for the pain associated with myocardial infarction. However, it may reduce sympathetically mediated arteriolar and venous constriction. The resultant venous pooling may produce a reduction in cardiac output and arterial pressure. This must be recognized but does not necessarily contraindicate its use. Hypotension associated with venous pooling usually responds promptly to elevation of the legs, but in some patients volume expansion with intravenous saline is required. The patient may experience diaphoresis and nausea, but these events usually pass and are replaced by a feeling of well-being associated with the relief of pain. Morphine also has a vagotonic effect and may cause bradycardia or advanced degrees of heart block, particularly in patients with posteroinferior infarction. These side effects of morphine usually respond to atropine (0.4 mg intravenously). Morphine is routinely administered by repetitive (every 5 min) intravenous injection of small doses of drug (2 to 4 mg) rather than by administration of a larger quantity by the subcutaneous route, by which absorption may be unpredictable. Meperidine hydrochloride or hydromorphone hydrochloride may be effectively employed in place of morphine.

Prior to administering morphine, sublingual nitroglycerin can be given safely to most patients with myocardial infarction. As long as hypotension does not occur, up to three 0.3-mg doses should be administered at about 5-min intervals. In addition to diminishing or abolishing chest discomfort, this form of therapy, once considered contraindicated in the setting of acute myocardial infarction, may be capable of both decreasing myocardial oxygen demand (by lowering preload) and increasing myocardial oxygen supply (by dilating infarct-related coronary vessels or collateral vessels). However, therapy with nitrates should be avoided in patients who present with a low systolic arterial pressure (<100 mmHg). The potential for an idiosyncratic reaction to nitrates, consisting of sudden marked hypotension and bradycardia, should be recognized. This problem, occurring more frequently in patients with inferior wall infarction, can usually be promptly reversed by the rapid administration of intravenous atropine. In patients whose initially favorable response to sublingual nitroglycerin is followed by the return of chest pain, particularly if accompanied by other evidence of ongoing ischemia such as further ST-segment or T-wave shifts, the use of intravenous nitroglycerin should be considered.

Intravenous beta blockers are also useful in the control of the pain of acute myocardial infarction. These drugs have been shown to control pain effectively in some patients, presumably by diminishing ischemia consequent to lowering myocardial oxygen demand. More importantly, there is some evidence that intravenous beta blockers reduce in-hospital mortality, particularly in high-risk patients. Dosing similar to that used to treat the hyperdynamic state (see above) may be utilized.

Glucocorticoids and nonsteroidal anti-inflammatory agents, with the exception of aspirin, should generally be avoided in the setting of acute myocardial infarction. They can impair infarct healing and increase the risk of myocardial rupture, and may produce a larger infarct scar. Additionally, they can increase coronary vascular resistance, thereby potentially reducing flow to ischemic myocardium.

OXYGEN The routine use of oxygen is supported by the observation that the arterial P_{O_2} is reduced in many patients with myocardial infarction and that oxygen inhalation reduces the area of ischemic injury in experimental animals. Although oxygen therapy has been associated with theoretically deleterious effects such as elevation of systemic vascular resistance and slight reduction of cardiac output, the weight of evidence favors its administration. It should be administered by face mask or nasal prongs for the first day or two after infarction.

ACTIVITY Factors which increase the work of the heart may increase the size of the infarct. Circumstances in which heart size, cardiac output, or myocardial contractility are increased should be avoided. It has been demonstrated that 6 to 8 weeks are required for complete healing, i.e., replacement of the infarcted myocardium by scar tissue. The purpose of reduced physical activity is to provide the most favorable possible circumstances for this healing.

Most patients with myocardial infarction should be admitted to a coronary care unit or suitable monitoring facility and remain there for 2 days under constant observation by trained personnel utilizing continuous electrocardiographic monitoring. A catheter should be introduced into a peripheral vein, firmly fixed so that it is not easily dislodged, and be kept open either by the slow infusion of isotonic glucose solution or by a closed heparin lock. In the absence of heart failure or other complications during the first 2 to 3 days, the patient should be in bed most of the day, with one or two periods of 15 to 30 min in a bedside chair. The patient may use a bedside commode and should be bathed but may eat unassisted. Bedside commode privileges are given to all hemodynamically stable patients with a stable rhythm from the first day. The bed should be equipped with a footboard, against which the patient should push both feet regularly to prevent venous stasis and thromboembolism and to maintain muscle tone in the legs.

By the third or fourth day the patient with an uncomplicated course should be spending at least 30 to 60 min in a chair twice a day. At this time the patient's blood pressure should be measured when standing in order to be aware of postural hypotension, which may be a problem when ambulation is begun. Standing and gradual ambulation are usually begun between the third and fifth days post infarction in patients with uncomplicated myocardial infarction. Ambulation is progressively increased, eventually including walks about the hospital floor. In many hospitals a cardiac rehabilitation program with progressive exercise is initiated in the hospital and continued after discharge. The total duration of hospitalization in uncomplicated cases is usually 6 to 11 days, but some physicians still hospitalize patients with Q-wave infarction for 2 weeks. Patients in clinical class II or higher may require 2 or more weeks of hospitalization, depending upon the rapidity with which heart failure resolves and the home situation to which the patient is returning. Many physicians perform a heart rate–limited exercise tolerance test just prior to discharge in selected patients with myocardial infarction. Such testing identifies high-risk patients as those who develop angina, ST-segment change, hypotension, or serious ventricular ectopic activity during or immediately following exercise. These patients require special attention, including measures such as antiarrhythmic drugs for ectopic activity, and beta-adrenergic blockers, long-acting nitrates, and/or calcium channel blocking agents for evidence of ischemia. If ischemia occurs at rest, or if during limited exercise ischemia and/or hypotension occur, coronary arteriography should be carried out. If a large quantity of viable myocardium, perfused by critically narrowed vessel(s), is found at angiography, then revascularization (either by angioplasty or by operation) may be required. Exercise tests also aid in formulating an individualized exercise prescription, which can be much more vigorous in patients who tolerate exercise without any of the above-mentioned adverse signs. Additionally, predischarge stress testing may provide an important psychological benefit related to building the patient's confidence through the demonstration of reasonable exercise tolerance. Furthermore, particularly when no arrhythmias or signs of ischemia are identified, the patient benefits by the physician's reassurance that objective evidence suggests no immediate jeopardy.

The remainder of the convalescent phase of myocardial infarction may be accomplished at home. From 2 to 6 weeks, the patient should be encouraged to increase activity by walking about the house and outdoors in good weather. Patients should still spend 8 to 10 h in bed each night. Additional rest periods in the morning and afternoon may be advisable for selected patients. Normal sexual activity may be resumed during this period.

From 6 to 8 weeks onward, the physician must regulate the patient's activity on the basis of his or her exercise tolerance. It is during this period of increasing activity that the patient may become aware of profound fatigue. Postural hypotension may still be a problem. Most patients will be able to return to work after 12 weeks, and many patients much earlier. A maximal exercise test is frequently performed after 6 to 8 weeks or prior to returning to work. A trend toward earlier ambulation, hospital discharge, and resumption of full activity for patients recuperating from acute myocardial infarction has developed in recent years.

DIET During the first 4 or 5 days, a low-calorie diet divided into multiple small feedings is preferred. Cardiac output increases following ingestion of food, and therefore the quantity of individual feedings should be kept low. If heart failure is present, sodium intake should be restricted. Since constipation is common, it is reasonable to give average or even increased amounts of bulk in the diet. In addition, the ingestion of potassium-rich foods should be encouraged in patients receiving diuretics. During the second week, increasing amounts of food may be introduced into the diet. At this time, the importance of restriction of calories, cholesterol, and saturated fat may be explained to the patient, and he or she can be started on an appropriate diet. Willingness to accept dietary restriction and to discontinue cigarette smoking is usually never greater than it is during this early period of convalescence.

BOWELS Bed rest of 3 to 5 days and the effect of the narcotics utilized for the relief of pain often lead to constipation. A bedside commode, rather than a bed pan, a diet rich in bulk, and the routine use of a stool softener such as dioctyl sodium sulfosuccinate, 200 mg daily, are recommended. If the patient remains constipated despite these measures, a laxative can be safely used. It is safe to perform a gentle rectal examination on patients with acute myocardial infarction.

SEDATION Most patients require sedation during hospitalization in order to withstand the period of enforced inactivity with tranquility. Diazepam 5 mg, oxazepam 15 to 30 mg, or lorazepam 0.5 to 2 mg, given three or four times daily, is usually effective. An additional dose of any of the above medications may be given at night to ensure adequate sleep. Temazepam 15 to 30 mg can also be used to induce sleep. Attention to this problem is especially important during the first few days in the coronary care unit, where the atmosphere of 24-h vigilance may interfere with the patient's sleep. However, sedation is no substitute for reassuring, quiet surroundings.

ANTICOAGULANTS AND ANTIPLATELET AGENTS Few topics have been more controversial than the use of anticoagulants in the routine treatment of acute myocardial infarction. The use of anticoagulant therapy to retard the process of coronary occlusion during the initial phases of the illness has undergone renewed interest as a result of the recognition that thrombosis plays an important role in the pathogenesis of acute myocardial infarction. Recent data from trials employing aspirin and/or thrombolytic agents have led to increased consensus about the appropriate treatment regimens. At the time of thrombolytic therapy, unless contraindications exist, most patients with possible or probable myocardial infarction should be started on aspirin, 160 or 325 mg daily. In the patient who is to receive a thrombolytic agent, a 5000-unit bolus of intravenous heparin should be administered, followed by a constant intravenous infusion beginning at 1000 units per hour adjusted to keep the partial thromboplastin time (PTT) at 1.5 to 2 times normal. Patients with acute myocardial infarction not undergoing thrombolytic therapy should also generally receive aspirin. This strategy has been shown to prevent some patients who present with unstable angina from progressing to myocardial infarction, and data suggest that in-hospital mortality is lowered even among patients who do develop myocardial infarction if they are given aspirin early in their course. Additionally, in order to prevent venous thrombosis, in patients *not* treated with thrombolytic therapy, small subcutaneous doses of heparin (5000 units every 8 to 12 h) should be employed as well. Once the patient is out of the intensive care area, oral anticoagulants should be reserved for patients with congestive heart failure which persists for more than 3 to 4 days or for those with large anterior infarctions in whom the risk of developing a left ventricular thrombus is greater.

The incidence of arterial embolism from a clot originating in the ventricle at the site of an infarction is small but definite. Two-dimensional echocardiography allows for the early detection of left ventricular thrombi in about one-third of patients with anterior wall infarction but rarely in patients with inferior or posterior infarction.

Arterial embolism often presents as a major complication, such as hemiparesis when the cerebral circulation is involved, or hypertension if the renal circulation is compromised. The low incidence of these complications, contrasted with their severity, renders it impractical to establish firm guidelines for the use of anticoagulant drugs as prophylaxis against arterial embolism in acute myocardial infarction. The likelihood of arterial embolism appears to increase with the extent of infarction and the resultant inflammation and endocardial stasis due to akinesis. Therefore the indication for anticoagulation as prophylaxis against arterial embolism increases with the extent of infarction. When a thrombus has been clearly demonstrated by echocardiographic or other techniques, systemic anticoagulation should be undertaken (in the absence of contraindications), for the incidence of embolic complications appears to be markedly lowered by such therapy. The appropriate duration of therapy is unknown, but probably should be carried out for 3 to 6 months.

BETA-ADRENERGIC BLOCKERS The chronic routine use of oral beta-adrenergic blockers for at least 2 years following acute myocardial infarction is supported by several well-conducted placebo-controlled trials which have demonstrated reductions in total mortality, sudden death, and in some instances, the reinfarction rate. While beta blockers are of benefit, even when started as late as 28 days following the acute event, additional benefit probably accrues to those patients who are started earlier, including patients receiving thrombolytic therapy. For patients presenting with the clear picture of a hyperdynamic state, in the absence of contraindications such as congestive heart failure, hypotension, bradycardia, atrioventricular block, or a history of asthma (p. 968), an intravenous dose of a beta blocker such as metoprolol may be given (5 mg every 5 to 10 min three times for a total dose of 15 mg, stopping between doses if any complications arise). This is usually followed by an oral dose regimen of metoprolol (50 to 100 mg bid). Later in the hospital course, a more slowly acting beta blocker, such as atenolol (50 to 100 mg qid) can be prescribed. Beta blocker therapy is probably indicated for most patients after myocardial infarction, except those for whom its use is specifically contraindicated (patients with heart failure, heart block, orthostatic hypotension, or severely compromised left ventricular function, but without symptoms of heart failure) and perhaps those whose excellent long-term prognosis (defined as mortality less than 1 percent per year) markedly diminishes any potential benefit (patients with normal ventricular function, no complex ventricular ectopy, no angina, and a negative maximal exercise stress test).

TREATMENT

ARRHYTHMIAS (See also Chaps. 184 and 185) The improved management of arrhythmias constitutes a most significant advance in the treatment of myocardial infarction.

Ventricular premature systoles Infrequent, sporadic ventricular premature depolarizations occur in almost all patients with infarction and do not require therapy. Suggested indications for suppression of ventricular ectopic beats are generally considered to be the following: (1) the presence of more than five isolated ectopic beats per minute, (2) the occurrence of consecutive or multifocal ventricular extrasystoles, and (3) the occurrence of ectopic ventricular beats early in diastole and hence superimposed on the T wave of the preceding beat (the so-called R-on-T phenomenon). Intravenous lidocaine has become the treatment of choice for such ventricular premature beats and other ventricular tachyarrhythmias because it acts rapidly and side effects disappear soon (15 to 20 min) after its administration is discontinued. Lidocaine is given as an intravenous bolus of 1 mg/kg to establish adequate blood levels quickly. This initial dose usually eliminates the ectopic activity, if present, and is followed by an infusion of 2 to 4 mg/min. An additional bolus of 0.5 mg/kg is given 10 min after the initial bolus if ectopy is still present. The dose should be reduced by half in patients with congestive heart failure, shock, or hepatic

disease. Usually, ventricular premature beats spontaneously disappear after 72 to 96 h. If significant ventricular ectopic activity persists past this time, chronic antiarrhythmic therapy is often initiated although such therapy has not yet been demonstrated to improve survival. Prophylactic antiarrhythmic therapy, in the absence of clinically important ventricular ectopy, is contraindicated as such therapy may actually increase late mortality.

Procainamide, mexiletine, and quinidine are commonly used for the treatment of persistent ventricular ectopic activity. Several other agents are also available for suppression of ventricular ectopy; the choice must be based upon a physician's familiarity with the particular drug and upon patient tolerance. Beta-adrenergic blocking agents are also effective in abolishing ventricular ectopic activity in infarction patients. The latter agents should be used with great care in patients with left ventricular failure since they have a significant negative inotropic action. If the usual doses of these drugs (Chap. 185), singly or in combination, are not effective, blood levels should be measured to ensure that adequate blood concentrations are being obtained. Frequent clinical and electrocardiographic assessment of the patient for signs of drug toxicity is mandatory when higher doses of these agents are employed.

Ventricular tachycardia and ventricular fibrillation Within the first 24 h of myocardial infarction, ventricular tachycardia and fibrillation can occur without prior warning arrhythmias. The occurrence of such primary arrhythmias can be reduced by prophylactic administration of intravenous lidocaine. However, use in this manner has never been shown to reduce overall mortality with acute myocardial infarction. With earlier treatment of active ischemia, more frequent use of beta blocking agents, and the nearly universal success of electrical cardioversion or defibrillation, prophylactic antiarrhythmic drug therapy can no longer be routinely recommended. It should be reserved for patients who cannot reach a hospital or those treated in hospitals that lack the constant presence in the coronary care unit of a physician or nurse trained in the recognition and treatment of ventricular fibrillation. Sustained ventricular tachycardia is treated first with lidocaine, and if it cannot be terminated by one or two 50- to 100-mg doses, electroconversion should be employed (Chap. 185). Electroshock is used immediately in patients with ventricular fibrillation, or when ventricular tachycardia causes hemodynamic deterioration. If fibrillation has persisted for more than a few seconds, the first shock may be unsuccessful, and in this situation it is advisable to administer closed-chest massage and mouth-to-mouth respiration before attempting electroconversion again. Improvement of oxygenation and perfusion increase the likelihood of successful defibrillation. Bretylium is useful in the treatment of both refractory ventricular fibrillation and ventricular tachycardia. For ventricular fibrillation, bretylium is given as a 5-mg/kg bolus and defibrillation is again attempted. If the latter fails, a second bolus of 10 mg/kg is given to facilitate electroconversion of ventricular fibrillation. Ventricular tachycardia can be treated with bretylium 5 to 10 mg/kg injected slowly over 10 min. In either situation, the initial dose of bretylium may be followed by a continuous infusion of 2 mg/min if the arrhythmia is recurrent. Severe postural hypotension occurs after intravenous bretylium administration; therefore, patients should always be supine when and immediately after the drug is given, and intravenous fluids should be available for rapid administration if needed. Ventricular arrhythmias, including the unusual form of ventricular tachycardia known as *torsade de pointes* (Chap. 185), may occur in infarct patients as a consequence of other concurrent problems (such as hypoxia or hypokalemia) or due to the toxic effects of agents already being administered to the patient (such as digoxin or quinidine). A search for such secondary causes should always be undertaken.

Long-term survival is good in patients with *primary* ventricular fibrillation, i.e., ventricular fibrillation resulting as a primary response to acute ischemia and not associated with predisposing factors such as congestive heart failure, shock, bundle branch block, or ventricular aneurysm. In one series, 87 percent of patients with primary ventricular fibrillation left the hospital alive. This prognosis is in sharp contrast to that for patients who develop ventricular fibrillation *secondary* to severe pump failure. Only 29 percent of patients in this group survived.

In patients who develop ventricular tachycardia late in their hospital course, the mortality in 1 year may be as high as 85 percent. Such patients may warrant electrophysiologic study (Chap. 185).

Accelerated idioventricular rhythm   Accelerated idioventricular rhythm (AIVR, "slow ventricular tachycardia"), a ventricular rhythm with a rate of 60 to 100 beats per minute, occurs in 25 percent of patients with myocardial infarction. It is especially frequent in inferoposterior infarction, where it is usually associated with sinus bradycardia. It often occurs transiently during thrombolytic therapy at the time of reperfusion. The rate of AIVR is usually similar to that of the sinus rhythm which precedes and follows it, and this similarity of rate and the relatively minor hemodynamic effects make this rhythm difficult to detect other than by electrocardiographic monitoring. For the most part, this rhythm is benign and does not presage the development of classic ventricular tachycardia. Most AIVR does not require treatment if the patient is monitored carefully since degeneration into a more serious arrhythmia is rare, and if it occurs, the AIVR can generally be readily treated with a drug which decreases the ventricular escape rate, such as mexiletine, and/or one that increases the sinus rate (atropine).

Supraventricular arrhythmias   Sinus tachycardia is the most common arrhythmia of this type. If it occurs secondary to other causes (such as anemia, fever, heart failure, or a metabolic derangement), the primary problem should be treated first. However, if sinus tachycardia appears to be due to sympathetic overstimulation, such as is seen as part of a hyperdynamic state, then treatment with a relatively short acting beta blocker, such as propranolol, should be considered. Other common arrhythmias in this group are junctional rhythm and tachycardia, atrial tachycardia, atrial flutter, and atrial fibrillation. These rhythm disturbances are often secondary to left ventricular failure. The administration of digoxin is usually the treatment of choice for supraventricular arrhythmias if heart failure is present. If heart failure is absent, verapamil (p. 968) is an ideal alternative, as this agent may also help control ischemia. If the abnormal rhythm persists for more than 2 h with a ventricular rate in excess of 120 beats per minute, or at any time when tachycardia induces heart failure, shock, or ischemia (as manifested by recurrent pain or ECG changes), electroshock should be utilized.

Junctional arrhythmias are of diverse etiology, are not indicative of any specific abnormality, and from a therapeutic viewpoint must be considered on an individual basis. Digitalis excess must be ruled out as a cause of junctional tachycardia. In some patients with severely compromised left ventricular function, the loss of appropriately timed atrial systole results in a marked decrease in cardiac output. Right atrial or coronary sinus pacing is indicated in such instances.

Sinus bradycardia   The significance of bradycardia as a factor predisposing to ventricular fibrillation in acute myocardial infarction is controversial. While the incidence of ventricular tachycardia in patients with sustained bradycardia is twice that observed in patients with normal heart rates, sinus bradycardia has also been identified in hospitalized patients as an index of a favorable prognosis. Treatment of sinus bradycardia is indicated if significant ventricular ectopic activity is present or if hemodynamic compromise results from the slow heart rate. Elevation of the legs and/or the foot of the bed is frequently helpful in the treatment of sinus bradycardia. Atropine is the most useful drug for increasing heart rate and should be given intravenously in doses of 0.4 to 0.6 mg. If the rate remains below 60 beats per minute, additional doses of 0.2 mg, up to a total of 2.0 mg, may be given in divided doses. Persistent bradycardia (< 40 beats per minute) despite atropine may be treated with electrical pacing. Isoproterenol should be avoided.

Conduction disturbances   Failure of conduction may develop at three different levels in the conduction system: the atrioventricular (AV) node, the bundle of His, or the more peripheral portions of the conduction system (Chap. 184). If the block occurs in the AV node, the escape rhythm usually originates in the AV junction and the QRS complexes are usually of normal duration; but when the block occurs distal to the AV node, the escape site is ventricular and the QRS configuration is abnormal and its duration is prolonged. Disturbances of conduction may occur in any one or two of the three peripheral branches (fascicles) of the conduction system (p. 858), and their recognition is of value in identifying patients at risk of developing complete heart block. When block occurs in any two of the three fascicles, bifascicular block is said to exist; complete AV block often develops in such patients. Thus, patients who develop the combination of right bundle branch block and either left anterior or left posterior hemiblock or patients with new left bundle branch block have a particularly high risk of progression to complete heart block.

The mortality rate of patients with complete AV block in association with anterior infarction (75 percent) is almost three times that of patients who develop AV block with inferior infarction (25 percent), and the risk of subsequent death in those who survive to leave the hospital is also increased in the former group. This difference is related to the fact that heart block in inferior infarction is usually caused by AV nodal ischemia. The AV node is a small discrete structure, and thus a small amount of ischemia or necrosis can result in AV nodal dysfunction. In anterior wall infarction, heart block is usually related to ischemic malfunction of all three fascicles of the conduction system and thus commonly results only from extensive myocardial necrosis.

Electrical pacing provides an effective means of increasing the heart rate of patients with bradycardia due to AV block, but it is not possible to be sure that such acceleration is always beneficial. For example, in patients with anterior wall infarction and complete heart block, the large size of the infarct is the major factor determining the outcome, and correction of the conduction deficit may not improve the poor prognosis in this group. Pacing does appear to be beneficial, however, in patients with inferoposterior infarction who have complete heart block associated with heart failure, hypotension, marked bradycardia, or significant ventricular ectopic activity. A subgroup of these patients, those with right ventricular infarction, often respond poorly to ventricular pacing because of the loss of the atrial "kick." In such patients, dual chamber, atrioventricular sequential pacing may be required.

In the past, prophylactic placement of a pacing catheter has been advocated for patients with conduction disturbances known to be precursors of complete heart block. However, the recent availability of reliable noninvasive (external) temporary pacing devices makes it possible to pace conscious patients without insertion of a transvenous pacemaker lead. Therefore, routine use of prophylactic pacing is no longer necessary in most situations. Permanent pacing has been advocated for patients who develop the combination of persistent bifascicular and transient third-degree heart block during the acute phase of myocardial infarction. Retrospective studies in such patients suggest that the incidence of sudden death is decreased in those in whom permanent pacing was instituted.

HEART FAILURE   Some degree of transient impairment of left ventricular function occurs in over half of patients with myocardial infarction. The most common clinical signs are pulmonary rales and S_3 and S_4 gallop rhythms. Pulmonary congestion is also frequently seen on the chest roentgenogram. Elevation of left ventricular filling pressure and pulmonary artery pressure are the characteristic hemodynamic findings, but it should be appreciated that these findings may result from a reduction of diastolic ventricular compliance (diastolic failure) and/or a reduction of stroke volume with secondary cardiac dilatation (systolic failure) (Chap. 181). The therapy of heart failure in association with myocardial infarction is similar to that of heart failure secondary to other forms of heart disease, with a few exceptions (Chap. 182). The major difference concerns the use of cardiac glycosides. The benefit following the administration of digitalis in acute myocardial infarction is unimpressive. This is not surprising since the function of the noninfarcted tissue may be normal and digitalis would not be expected to improve the systolic or diastolic dysfunction of infarcted or ischemic tissue. On the other hand, diuretic agents are extremely effective in the treatment of heart failure following myocardial infarction, since they diminish pulmonary congestion in the presence of systolic and/or diastolic heart failure. A fall in left ventricular filling pressure and an improvement in orthopnea and dyspnea follow the intravenous administration of furosemide. This drug should be used with caution, however, as it can result in a massive diuresis with associated decrease in plasma volume, cardiac output, systemic blood pressure, and hence coronary perfusion. Nitrates in various forms may be used to decrease preload and congestive symptoms. Oral isosorbide dinitrate, topical nitroglycerin ointment, or, in patients with severe pulmonary congestion or pulmonary edema, intravenous nitroglycerin, all have the advantage over a diuretic of lowering preload through venodilatation without decreasing the total plasma volume. Additionally, nitrates may improve ventricular compliance if concurrent ischemia is present, since ischemia causes an elevation of left ventricular filling pressure. The patient with pulmonary edema is treated in the manner described in Chap. 182. Studies with vasodilators to reduce cardiac afterload indicate that the reduction in cardiac work, which results from the lowered afterload, may significantly improve left ventricular performance with a reduction of ventricular filling pressure and pulmonary congestion concomitant with an elevation of cardiac output.

Ventricular remodeling   Soon after myocardial infarction, the left ventricle begins to dilate. Acutely, this occurs as the result of expansion of the infarct. Later, lengthening of the noninfarcted segments occurs as well. Overall chamber enlargement is related to the size of the infarction, with greater degrees of dilatation causing more marked hemodynamic impairment, more frequent heart failure, and a poorer prognosis as well. Recent data suggest that progressive dilatation, and its clinical consequences, may be attenuated by afterload-reducing therapy such as vasodilatation induced by the angiotensin converting enzyme inhibitor captopril. Thus, in patients with a depressed ejection fraction (less than 45%), particularly if signs of heart failure are present, consideration should be given to the institution of captopril therapy (beginning with 6.25 mg tid and advancing to 25 to 50 mg tid as tolerated).

Hemodynamic monitoring   Hemodynamic evidence of abnormal left ventricular function becomes apparent when contraction is seriously impaired in 20 to 25 percent of the left ventricle. Infarction of 40 percent or more of the left ventricle usually results in the syndrome of cardiogenic shock (see below). Pulmonary capillary wedge pressure and pulmonary artery diastolic pressure correlate well with left ventricular diastolic pressure and are therefore often referred to as left ventricular filling pressures. Positioning of a balloon flotation catheter in the pulmonary artery enables the physician to monitor left ventricular filling pressure constantly, a technique which is useful in patients who exhibit clinical evidence of hemodynamic abnormalities or instability. However, in view of the complications that can occur, insertion of a pulmonary artery catheter should be limited to those patients with hemodynamic instability. Cardiac output can also be determined with a pulmonary artery catheter. With the addition of intraarterial pressure monitoring, systemic vascular resistance can be calculated as a guide to adjusting vasopressor and vasodilator therapy. Some patients with acute myocardial infarction have markedly elevated left ventricular filling pressures (>22 mmHg) and normal cardiac indexes [>2.6 and <3.6 (L/min)/m²], while others have relatively low filling pressures (<15 mmHg) and reduced cardiac indexes. The former usually benefit from diuresis, while the latter respond to volume expansion by means of intravenous administration of colloid-containing solutions.

Cardiogenic shock—power failure   In recent years efforts to reduce infarct size and prompt treatment of ongoing ischemia and other complications of myocardial infarction have reduced the incidence of cardiogenic shock.

It is useful to consider cardiogenic shock as a form of severe left ventricular failure. This syndrome is characterized by marked hy-

potension with systolic arterial pressure <80 mmHg and a marked reduction of cardiac index [<1.8 (L/min)/m²] in the face of elevated left ventricular filling (pulmonary capillary wedge) pressure >18 mmHg. Hypotension alone is not a basis for the diagnosis of cardiogenic shock, because many patients who make an uneventful recovery will have serious hypotension (systolic pressure <80 mmHg) for several hours. Such patients often have low left ventricular filling pressures, and their hypotension usually resolves with the administration of intravenous fluids. The following *clinical* criteria for cardiogenic shock define a population of patients with a mortality rate of >70 percent: (1) systolic arterial blood pressure <90 mmHg which has declined by at least 30 mmHg below the previous level; (2) clinical signs of peripheral circulatory insufficiency, e.g., cold, moist skin and cyanosis; (3) dulled sensorium; (4) oliguria with urine flow of less than 20 mL/h; and (5) failure of improvement following relief of pain and administration of oxygen. Specifically *excluded* are patients with hypotension secondary to vasovagal reaction, hypovolemia, arrhythmia, drug reaction, or sepsis.

Cardiogenic shock may develop during the first hours of the infarct and be present at the time of initial hospitalization. Alternatively, it may appear after hospitalization—most commonly during the first day but sometimes as late as the sixth day. Risk factors for the in-hospital development of shock include advanced age, depressed left ventricular ejection fraction on admission, large infarct, history of diabetes mellitus, and previous myocardial infarction. Patients with several of these risk factors may be considered for cardiac catheterization and mechanical reperfusion (angioplasty or surgery) *before* the development of shock.

Pathophysiology of pump failure   Marked reduction in the quantity of contracting myocardium is the cause of cardiogenic shock in myocardial infarction, although all organ systems are ultimately involved. The function of the heart is impaired by the initial insult; this results in a decrease in arterial pressure and hence in coronary blood flow because of its dependence on aortic perfusion pressure (Fig. 189-1). The reduction in coronary perfusion pressure and myocardial blood flow further impairs myocardial function and may increase the size of the myocardial infarction. Arrhythmias and metabolic acidosis also contribute to this deterioration because they

FIGURE 189-1   The sequence of events in the vicious cycle in which coronary artery obstruction leads to cardiogenic shock and progressive circulatory deterioration.

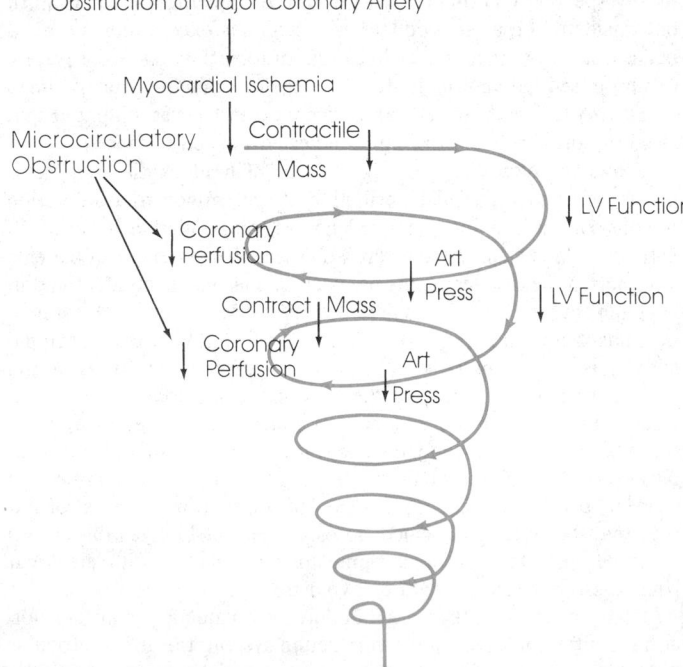

are the result of inadequate perfusion. It is this positive feedback loop which accounts for the high mortality rate associated with the shock syndrome.

Arterial blood pressure is a function of two factors—cardiac output and systemic vascular resistance—and a decrease in either without a compensatory rise in the other will result in a fall in arterial blood pressure. Cardiac output is lower in a population of patients with myocardial infarction and shock. However many patients with myocardial infarction without shock have cardiac outputs in the same range as those in patients with shock, and therefore it is not possible to characterize these patients on the basis of reductions of cardiac output alone. Systemic vascular resistance, the other factor important in determining blood pressure, may be either normal or increased in myocardial infarction. Normally, a fall in cardiac output is accompanied by a compensatory rise in systemic vascular resistance, but in patients with shock due to myocardial infarction, the appropriate elevation in resistance may fail to occur.

A simple schematic diagram depicting the relationship between left ventricular work and filling pressure is seen in Fig 189-2 The upper curve represents the familiar Frank-Starling relationship in the normal heart; the lower curve shows the relation which might be expected in the patient with shock secondary to myocardial infarction. It is obvious that, at all levels of end-diastolic pressure, the left ventricular work of the patient with myocardial infarction is depressed. At point C, the end-diastolic pressure is elevated, but at point B, it may be normal despite the fact that myocardial work is well below that expected of the normal heart at this diastolic pressure, as indicated by point A.

Treatment of pump failure   The physiology and ominous prognosis associated with this condition dictate that all patients with shock should, if possible, have continuous monitoring of arterial pressure and of left ventricular filling pressure (as reflected in the pulmonary capillary wedge pressure measured with a pulmonary artery balloon catheter) as well as frequent determinations of cardiac output. All patients with the shock syndrome should receive oxygen continuously to help combat the hypoxemia which is universally present. When pulmonary edema coexists, endotracheal intubation may be necessary to ensure oxygenation. The relief of pain is important, as some vasodepressor reflex activity may be a response to severe pain. However, narcotics should be used cautiously in view of their propensity to lower arterial pressure.

The primary objective of treatment is to avoid the sequence depicted in Fig. 189-1, by attempting to maintain coronary perfusion by raising the arterial blood pressure with vasopressors (see below), intraaortic balloon counterpulsation, and manipulation of blood volume to a level that ensures an optimum left ventricular filling pressure (approximately 20 mmHg). The latter may require either infusion of crystalloid or diuresis.

FIGURE 189-2   Schematic representation of the Frank-Starling relationship as applied to patients with the shock syndrome in myocardial infarction.

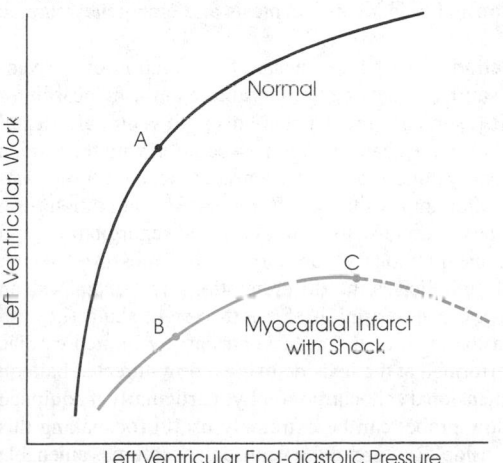

In patients seen within the first 4 h of the onset of infarction, reperfusion by thrombolytic therapy and/or PTCA (p. 877) may improve left ventricular function dramatically, thereby interrupting the cycle of hemodynamic deterioration.

Hypovolemia   This is an easily corrected condition which may contribute to the hypotension and vascular collapse associated with myocardial infarction in some patients. Hypovolemia may be secondary to previous diuretic use, to reduced fluid intake during the early stages of the illness, and/or to vomiting associated with pain or medications. In addition, a state of *relative* hypovolemia may exist; i.e., with the acute reduction in contractile function and ventricular compliance resulting from infarction an increase in vascular volume is needed to maintain cardiac output. Owing to the acute nature of the process, there is insufficient time for compensatory fluid retention to accommodate this need, and relative hypovolemia in a normally hydrated patient results. Consequently, hypovolemia should be identified and corrected in patients with acute myocardial infarction and hypotension before embarking upon more vigorous forms of therapy. If left ventricular filling pressure is in the normal range, fluid should be administered until the cardiac output is maximized. This usually occurs at a left ventricular filling pressure of approximately 20 mmHg. However, the optimal left ventricular filling or pulmonary artery wedge pressure may vary considerably among different patients. Each patient's ideal level is reached by cautious fluid administration during careful monitoring of oxygenation and cardiac output. When the cardiac output plateaus (Fig. 189-2, point C), further increases in left ventricular filling pressure will only increase congestive symptoms and decrease systemic oxygenation. Central venous pressure measurements reflect right rather than left ventricular filling pressure and are inadequate in this situation, since left ventricular function is almost always affected much more adversely than is right ventricular function in acute myocardial infarction.

Vasopressors   A variety of intravenous drugs may be used to augment arterial pressure and cardiac output in patients with cardiogenic shock. Unfortunately, all have important disadvantages or problems associated with their use, and none have been shown to change the outcome in patients with established shock. *Isoproterenol* is a synthetic sympathomimetic amine which is now rarely used in the treatment of shock due to myocardial infarction. Although this agent increases contractility, it also produces peripheral vasodilatation and increases heart rate. The resultant increase in myocardial oxygen consumption and reduction of coronary perfusion pressure may extend the area of ischemic injury. *Norepinephrine* is a potent alpha-adrenergic agent with powerful vasoconstrictive properties. It also possesses beta-adrenergic activity and therefore enhances contractility. Because the increase in afterload and contractility associated with its use causes a marked increase in myocardial oxygen consumption, it should be reserved for relatively desperate situations or for patients with cardiogenic shock and lowered systemic vascular resistance. It should be started at 2 to 4 μg/min. If pressure cannot be maintained with a dosage of 15 μg/min, it is unlikely that a further increase will be beneficial.

Dopamine (Chap. 67) is useful in many patients with power failure. At low doses [2 to 10 (μg/kg)/min] the drug has positive chronotropic and inotropic effects as a consequence of beta receptor stimulation. At higher doses, a vasoconstrictive effect results from alpha receptor stimulation. At lower doses dopamine [≤2 (μg/kg)/min] also has the unique effect of dilating the renal and splanchnic vascular beds and apparently has little effect on myocardial oxygen consumption. Intravenous dopamine is started at an infusion rate of 2 to 5 (μg/kg)/min with increments in dosage every 2 to 5 min up to a maximum of 20 to 50 (μg/kg)/min. Systolic arterial blood pressure should be maintained at approximately 90 mmHg. *Dobutamine* is a synthetic sympathomimetic amine with positive inotropic action and minimal positive chronotropic or peripheral vasoconstrictive activity in the usual dosage range [2.5 to 10 (μg/kg)/min]. It should not be employed when a vasoconstrictor effect is required. However, in patients with less profound degrees of hypotension, dobutamine may be an extremely useful agent, particularly if positive chronotropy is to be avoided.

Amrinone (see p. 899) is a positive inotropic agent without catecholamine structure or activity. It resembles dobutamine in its pharmacologic activity, although it has a potent vasodilating action. Initially a loading dose of 0.75 mg/kg is given over 2 to 3 min. If effective, this is followed by an infusion of 5 to 10 (μg/kg)/min, followed if necessary 30 min later by an additional bolus of 0.75 mg/kg. If necessary, the dose may then be increased up to 15 (μg/kg)/min for short periods.

Patients with global left ventricular ischemia as the cause of power failure and profound hypotension, such as those with critical left main coronary artery obstructive disease, may benefit from brief treatment with a pure vasoconstrictor in preference to a positive inotropic agent. In such cases coronary perfusion may be improved by the vasoconstrictor-induced increase in arterial pressure, whereas a positive inotropic agent may only increase ischemic injury in muscle that is incapable of performing more work. In this situation a pure vasoconstrictor such as *neosynephrine*, 10 to 100 μg/min, should be used, as briefly as possible, usually only as interim therapy while preparations are made for counterpulsation with an intraaortic balloon pump and/or emergency coronary artery surgery.

Cardiac glycosides (Chap. 182)   Controlled studies have failed to demonstrate significant beneficial effects of cardiac glycoside therapy in the early phases (0 to 48 h) of acute myocardial infarction. Hemodynamic improvement has been documented at later times, but this effect, too, is marginal. Since cardiac glycosides cannot improve the function of necrotic myocardium and since pump failure is thought to be related to the total mass of infarcted tissue, digitalis therapy does not usually result in dramatic improvement in patients with acute myocardial infarction and sinus rhythm.

Aortic counterpulsation   In cardiogenic shock mechanical assistance with an intraaortic balloon pumping system capable of augmenting both diastolic pressure and cardiac output can provide circulatory support. A sausage-shaped balloon at the end of a catheter is introduced percutaneously into the aorta via the femoral artery, and the balloon is inflated during early diastole, thereby enhancing both coronary blood flow and peripheral perfusion. The balloon collapses in early systole, thereby reducing the afterload against which left ventricular ejection takes place. Improvement in hemodynamic status has been observed with balloon pumping in a large number of patients, but long-term survival following this mode of therapy in patients with cardiogenic shock is still disappointing. The balloon counterpulsation system may best be reserved for patients whose condition merits mechanical (surgery or angioplasty) intervention (e.g., continuing ischemia, ventricular septal rupture, or mitral regurgitation) and in whom a successful result is likely to result in the reversal of cardiogenic shock. Intraaortic balloon pumping is contraindicated if aortic regurgitation is present or if aortic dissection is possible or suspected. The catheter introduced for balloon counterpulsation is large and frequently produces limb ischemia, particularly if peripheral vascular disease is present or if the catheter is inserted into a relatively small vessel (e.g., as would be present in an elderly female).

There is reason to believe that results of therapy of the shock syndrome secondary to myocardial infarction, while improving gradually as a result of meticulous attention to the details of therapy outlined above, will continue to be disappointing overall because a large fraction of patients with the syndrome have large areas of infarcted myocardium with severe, diffuse coronary atherosclerosis. Although occasional dramatic results have been reported with emergency revascularization surgery or coronary angioplasty, the overall results with these approaches, too, have been disappointing. It is hoped that the widespread and early application of thrombolytic therapy will reduce the amount of myocardium which becomes necrotic and thereby reduce the incidence of this syndrome. Also, revascularization in patients at high risk of developing shock in the hospital may have a similar effect.

Other complications   MITRAL REGURGITATION   Apical systolic murmurs of mitral regurgitation appear in more than one-fourth of patients during the first 5 days after the onset of a myocardial infarction, but mitral regurgitation is of hemodynamic importance in only a minority of these patients. In most patients the murmur is present during the acute phase of infarction, disappearing with recovery. The most common cause of mitral regurgitation following myocardial infarction is dysfunction of the papillary muscles of the left ventricle due to ischemia or infarction.

Mitral regurgitation may also be the result of alteration in the size or shape of the ventricle due to impaired contractility or to aneurysm formation. Either papillary muscle may rupture, the posterior one twice as frequently as the anterior. Left ventricular function may deteriorate dramatically with superimposition of mitral regurgitation. The differential diagnosis includes perforation of the ventricular septum (see below), and the differentiation from mitral regurgitation is conveniently made at the bedside by echocardiography and/or with a flow-directed balloon catheter. Large *v* waves may be recorded in the pulmonary capillary wedge position in patients with hemodynamically significant mitral regurgitation, and there is no oxygen "step up" as the catheter is advanced from the right atrium to the right ventricle. Surgical repair or replacement of the mitral valve may be followed by dramatic improvement in patients in whom acute heart failure results primarily from severe mitral regurgitation due to papillary muscle rupture or dysfunction and in whom myocardial function is relatively well preserved.

If aortic systolic pressure is lowered in patients with mitral regurgitation, a greater fraction of the left ventricular output will be ejected antegrade, thus lessening the regurgitant fraction. To this end, both intraaortic balloon counterpulsation, which lowers the aortic systolic pressure mechanically, and the infusion of sodium nitroprusside or nitroglycerin, which reduce systemic vascular resistance, have been used with success for the interim management of patients with severe mitral regurgitation in the setting of acute myocardial infarction. Ideally, definitive operative treatment should be postponed for 4 to 6 weeks after the infarct. However, if the patient's hemodynamic and/or clinical condition does not improve or stabilize, surgical treatment should be undertaken, even in the acute stage.

Cardiac rupture   Myocardial rupture is a dramatic complication of myocardial infarction most likely to occur during the first week after the onset of symptoms; its frequency increases with the age of the patient. First infarction, no history of angina pectoris, and relatively large Q-wave infarcts are associated with a higher incidence of cardiac rupture. The clinical presentation may often be that of a sudden disappearance of the pulse, blood pressure, and consciousness while the electrocardiogram continues to show sinus rhythm (*apparent* electromechanical dissociation). The myocardium continues to contract, but forward flow is not maintained as blood escapes into the pericardium. Cardiac tamponade (Chap. 193) ensues, and closed-chest massage is ineffective. Although almost universally fatal, there have been instances in which cardiac rupture has been recognized and successfully treated by pericardiocentesis and emergency cardiac surgery.

Septal perforation   The pathogenesis of perforation of the ventricular septum is similar to that of external rupture of the myocardium, but the therapeutic potential is greater. Patients with ventricular septal rupture present with severe heart failure in association with the sudden appearance of a pansystolic murmur, often accompanied by a parasternal thrill. It is often impossible to differentiate this condition from rupture of a papillary muscle with resultant mitral regurgitation, and a tall *v* wave in the pulmonary capillary wedge pressure in both conditions further complicates the differentiation. The diagnosis can be established by the demonstration of a left-to-right shunt (i.e., an oxygen step-up at the level of the right ventricle) by limited cardiac catheterization performed at the bedside using a flow-directed balloon catheter. Two-dimensional echocardiography, particularly if equipped with a Doppler flow probe, can be extremely useful for making this diagnosis at the bedside. Rupture of the ventricular septum is amenable to immediate surgical treatment, albeit at a significant risk, but this form of therapy is ordinarily indicated on an urgent basis in patients whose condition cannot be stabilized rapidly. A prolonged period of hemodynamic compromise may produce end-organ damage and other complications that can be avoided by early intervention including nitroprusside infusion and intraaortic balloon counterpulsation.

The physiology of acute mitral regurgitation and acute ventricular septal perforation are similar in that the level of aortic systolic pressure determines in part the regurgitant volume, the principal difference being the chamber into which the regurgitant fraction is ejected. In septal perforation, a fraction of left ventricular output is ejected into the right ventricle. In a manner analogous to mitral regurgitation, lowering of aortic systolic pressure by mechanical (intraaortic balloon counterpulsation) and/or pharmacologic (nitroglycerin or nitroprusside) means can decrease the hemodynamic compromise caused by perforation.

Ventricular aneurysm The term *ventricular aneurysm* is usually used to describe *dyskinesis* or local expansile paradoxical wall motion. Normally functioning myocardial fibers must shorten more if stroke volume and cardiac output are to be maintained in patients with ventricular aneurysm, and if they are unable to do so, overall ventricular function is impaired. Aneurysms are composed of scar tissue and neither predispose to nor are associated with cardiac rupture.

The complications of left ventricular aneurysm do not usually occur for weeks to months following myocardial infarction; they include congestive heart failure, arterial embolism, and ventricular arrhythmias. Apical aneurysms are the most common and the most easily detected by clinical examination. The physical finding of greatest value is a double, diffuse, or displaced apical impulse. The electrocardiographic finding of ST-segment elevation at rest is present in precordial leads in 25 percent of patients with either apical or anterior aneurysms. Ventricular aneurysms are readily detectable by two-dimensional echocardiography, which may also reveal a mural thrombus in aneurysms involving the anterior wall and/or apex. Rarely, myocardial rupture may be contained by a local area of pericardium, along with organizing thrombus and hematoma. Over time this *pseudoaneurysm* enlarges, maintaining communication with the left ventricular cavity via a narrow neck. Because spontaneous rupture of a pseudoaneurysm often occurs, if recognized, it should be surgically repaired.

Right ventricular infarction Approximately one-third of patients with inferoposterior infarction demonstrate at least a minor degree of right ventricular necrosis. An occasional patient with inferoposterior left ventricular infarction also has extensive right ventricular myocardial infarction. These patients often present with signs of severe right ventricular failure (jugular venous distention, Kussmaul's sign, hepatomegaly) with or without hypotension. ST-segment elevations of the right-sided precordial electrocardiographic leads, particularly lead V_4R, are present in the majority of patients with right ventricular infarction. Radionuclide ventriculography and two-dimensional echocardiography are also sensitive in the detection of right ventricular damage associated with acute myocardial infarction. Catheterization of the right side of the heart often reveals a distinctive hemodynamic pattern resembling cardiac tamponade or constrictive pericarditis (Chap. 193). Volume expansion is often successful in treating low cardiac output and hypotension associated with extensive right ventricular infarction.

Postinfarction ischemia and extension Recurrent angina develops in approximately 25 percent of patients hospitalized for acute myocardial infarction. This percentage is even higher in patients undergoing successful thrombolysis. Since recurrent or persistent ischemia often heralds extension of the original infarct and is associated with a doubling of risk following acute myocardial infarction, patients with these symptoms should be considered for prompt coronary arteriography and mechanical revascularization.

Infarct extension occurs in 5 to 10 percent of patients in the first 10 days following acute myocardial infarction, increasing to as many as 20 percent of patients following thrombolytic therapy. Hospital mortality is as much as four times greater in patients with infarct extension compared with those free of this complication. Careful monitoring for signs or symptoms of recurrent ischemia and early submaximal stress testing should be undertaken in order to identify patients at risk for extension [particularly those presenting with non-Q-wave infarction, with postinfarction angina, with a previous myocardial infarction, or with an early peaking CK-MB curve (less than 15 h)]. Early catheterization with coronary angiography should be considered for most patients with one or more risk factors for infarct extension. In such patients, revascularization (angioplasty or surgery) should be considered in order to prevent infarct extension.

Thromboembolism Clinically apparent thromboembolism complicates myocardial infarction in approximately 10 percent of cases, but embolic lesions are found in 45 percent of patients in necropsy series, suggesting that thromboembolism is often clinically silent. Thromboembolism is considered to be at least an important contributing cause of death in 25 percent of infarct patients who die following admission to the hospital. Arterial emboli originate from left ventricular mural thrombi, while most pulmonary emboli arise in the leg veins. Thromboembolism most commonly occurs in association with large infarcts in the presence of heart failure. Thromboembolism occurs extremely commonly in patients with echocardiographic evidence of a left ventricular thrombus, but only rarely if a thrombus is not present on the echocardiogram. Although well-controlled trials do not exist, the incidence of embolization appears to be decreased by anticoagulation.

Pericarditis (See also Chap. 193) Pericardial friction rubs and/or pericardial pain are frequently encountered in patients with acute transmural myocardial infarction. This complication can usually be managed with aspirin (650 mg qid). It is important to diagnose the chest pain of pericarditis accurately, since failure to appreciate it may lead to the erroneous diagnosis of recurrent ischemic pain and/or infarct extension with resultant inappropriate use of anticoagulants, nitrates, beta blockers, or coronary arteriography. No definite cause and effect relationship between administration of anticoagulants and pericarditis or tamponade has been proved. Nonetheless, the possibility that anticoagulants can cause tamponade in the presence of acute pericarditis is sufficiently high to contraindicate their use in patients with pericarditis, as manifested by either pain or persistent rub, unless there is a compelling indication.

Post-myocardial infarction syndrome—Dressler's syndrome (See also Chap. 193) This syndrome, characterized by fever and pleuropericardial chest pain, is thought to be due to an autoimmune pericarditis, pleuritis, and/or pneumonitis. It may begin from a few days to 6 weeks after myocardial infarction. The occurrence of Dressler's syndrome may be etiologically related to the early use of anticoagulants and appears to have decreased markedly in the last decade as long-term anticoagulants are used less frequently in acute myocardial infarction. The syndrome usually responds promptly to therapy with salicylates. On occasion, corticosteroids may be required to relieve discomfort of an unusual, refractory nature. Effusions associated with Dressler's syndrome may become hemorrhagic if anticoagulants are administered.

REFERENCES

ANTMAN EM, RUTHERFORD JD (eds): *Coronary Care Medicine: A Practical Approach.* Boston, Martinus Nijhoff, 1986

COLLER BS: Platelets and thrombolytic therapy. *N Engl J Med* 322(1):33, 1990

CUNNINGHAM MJ, PASTERNAK RC: Acute myocardial infarction: In-hospital diagnostic decisions, in *Manual of Clinical Evaluation: Strategies for Cost-Effective Care,* MD Aronson, TL Delbanco (eds). Boston, Little, Brown, 1988

DAVIES MJ, THOMAS AC: Plaque fissuring—The cause of acute myocardial infarction, sudden ischaemic death, and crescendo angina. *Br Heart J* 53:363, 1985

GOLDMAN L et al: A computer protocol to predict myocardial infarction in emergency department patients with chest pain. *N Engl J Med* 318:797, 1988

JAIN D et al: Clinical and prognostic significance of lung thallium uptake on rest imaging in acute myocardial infarction. *Am J Cardiol* 65(3):154, 1990

Krone RJ et al and the Multicenter Postinfarction Research Group: Low level exercise testing after myocardial infarction: Usefulness in enhancing clinical risk stratification. Circulation 71:80, 1985

Lee TH, Goldman L: The coronary care unit turns 25: Historical trends and future directions. Ann Intern Med 108:887, 1988

———, ———: Serum enzyme assays in the diagnosis of acute myocardial infarction. Ann Intern Med 105:221, 1986

Muller JE et al: Circadian variation in the frequency of onset of acute myocardial infarction. N Engl J Med 313:1315, 1985

——— et al and the MILIS Study Group: Myocardial infarct extension: Occurrence, outcome, and risk factors in the multicenter investigation of limitation of infarct size. Ann Intern Med 108:1, 1988

Ong L et al: Early prediction of mortality in patients with acute myocardial infarction: A prospective study of clinical and radionuclide risk factors. Am J Cardiol 57:33, 1986

Pasternak RC et al: Acute myocardial infarction, in *Heart Disease*, 3d ed, E Braunwald (ed). Philadelphia, Saunders, 1988, p 1222

Pfeffer MA et al: Effect of captopril on progressive ventricular dilatation after anterior myocardial infarction. N Engl J Med 310:80, 1988

Roig E et al: In-hospital mortality rates from acute myocardial infarction by race in U.S. hospitals: Findings from the National Hospital Discharge Survey. Circulation 76:280, 1987

Siegel D et al: Risk factor modification after myocardial infarction. Ann Intern Med 109:213, 1988

Silver MD, Goldschlager N: Temporary transvenous cardiac pacing in the critical care setting. Chest 93:607, 1988

Schulman SP et al: Prognostic cardiac catheterization variables in survivors of acute myocardial infarction: A five year prospective study. J Am Coll Cardiol 11:1164, 1988

Stack RS et al: Survival and cardiac event rates in the first year after emergency coronary angioplasty for acute myocardial infarction. J Am Coll Cardiol 11:1141, 1988

Stone PH et al and the MILIS Study Group: Prognostic significance of location and type of myocardial infarction: Independent adverse outcome associated with anterior location. J Am Coll Cardiol 11:453, 1988

The Steering Committee of the Physicians' Health Study Research Group: Final report on the aspirin component of the ongoing Physicians' Health Study. N Engl J Med 19:129–35, 1989

TIMI Study Group: Comparison of invasive and conservative strategies after treatment with intravenous tissue plasminogen activator in acute myocardial infarction. Results of the Thombolysis in Myocardial Infarction (TIMI) Phase II Trial. N Engl J Med 320:618, 1989

———: Immediate versus delayed catheterization and angioplasty following thrombolytic therapy for acute myocardial infarction. TIMI IIA Results. JAMA 260:2849, 1988

Topol EJ et al and the Thrombolysis and Angioplasty in Myocardial Infarction Study Group: A randomized trial of immediate versus delayed elective angioplasty after intravenous tissue plasminogen activator in acute myocardial infarction. N Engl J Med 317:581, 1987

Volpi A et al: In-hospital prognosis of patients with acute myocardial infarction complicated by primary ventricular fibrillation. N Engl J Med 317:257, 1987

Wall TC et al: Results of high dose intravenous urokinase for acute myocardial infarction. Am J Cardiol 65(3):124, 1990

190 ISCHEMIC HEART DISEASE

ANDREW P. SELWYN / EUGENE BRAUNWALD

Ischemia refers to a lack of oxygen due to inadequate perfusion. Ischemic heart disease is a condition of diverse etiologies, all having in common a disturbance of cardiac function due to an imbalance between oxygen supply and demand.

ETIOLOGY AND PATHOPHYSIOLOGY

The most common cause of ischemia is atherosclerotic disease of epicardial coronary arteries. By reducing the lumen of these vessels, atherosclerosis causes an absolute decrease in myocardial perfusion in the basal state or limits appropriate increases in perfusion when the demand for flow is augmented. Coronary blood flow can also be limited by arterial thrombi, spasm, and rarely coronary emboli as well as by ostial narrowing due to luetic aortitis. Congenital abnormalities, such as anomalous origin of the left anterior descending coronary artery from the pulmonary artery, may cause myocardial ischemia and infarction in infancy, but this cause is very rare in adults. Myocardial ischemia can also occur if myocardial oxygen demands are abnormally increased, as in severe ventricular hypertrophy due to hypertension or aortic stenosis. The latter can present with angina that is indistinguishable from that caused by coronary atherosclerosis. A reduction in the oxygen-carrying capacity of the blood, as in extremely severe anemia or in the presence of carboxyhemoglobin, is a rare cause of myocardial ischemia. Not infrequently, two or more causes of ischemia will coexist, such as an increase in oxygen demand due to left ventricular hypertrophy and a reduction in oxygen supply secondary to coronary atherosclerosis.

The normal coronary circulation is dominated and controlled by the myocardial requirements for oxygen. This need is met by the heart's ability to vary coronary vascular resistance (and therefore blood flow) considerably while the myocardium extracts a high and relatively fixed percentage of oxygen (Chap. 16). Normally, intramyocardial resistance arterioles demonstrate an immense capacity for dilation. With exercise and emotional stress, the changing oxygen needs affect coronary vascular resistance and in this manner regulate the supply of blood and oxygen (metabolic regulation). These same vessels adapt to physiologic alterations in blood pressure in order to maintain coronary blood flow at levels appropriate to myocardial needs (autoregulation). Although the large epicardial coronary arteries are capable of constriction and relaxation, in healthy persons they serve as conduits and are referred to as *conductance vessels*, while the intramyocardial arterioles normally exhibit striking changes in tone and are therefore referred to as *resistance vessels*.

CORONARY ATHEROSCLEROSIS (See also Chap. 195) Epicardial coronary arteries are a major site of atherosclerotic disease. Dysfunction of vascular endothelium and an abnormal interaction with blood monocytes and platelets lead to subintimal collections of abnormal fat, cells, and debris (i.e., atherosclerotic plaques), which develop at irregular rates in different segments of the epicardial coronary tree and lead eventually to segmental reductions in cross-sectional area. The relationship between pulsatile flow and luminal stenosis is complex, but experiments have shown that when a stenosis reduces the cross-sectional area by approximately 75 percent, a full range of increases in flow to meet increased myocardial demand is not possible. When the luminal area is reduced by more than approximately 80 percent, blood flow at rest may be reduced, and further minor decreases in the stenotic orifice can reduce coronary flow dramatically and cause myocardial ischemia.

Segmental atherosclerotic narrowing of epicardial coronary arteries is caused most commonly by the formation of a plaque, which is subject to fissuring, hemorrhage, and thrombosis. Any of these events can temporarily worsen the obstruction, reduce coronary blood flow, and cause clinical manifestations of myocardial ischemia, as described below. In addition, the location of the stenosis will influence the quantity of myocardium rendered ischemic and thus determine the severity of the clinical manifestations. Severe coronary narrowing and myocardial ischemia are frequently accompanied by the development of collateral vessels, especially when the narrowing develops gradually. When well developed, such vessels can provide sufficient blood flow to sustain the viability of the myocardium at rest but not during circumstances of increased demand.

Once severe stenosis of a proximal epicardial artery has reduced the cross-sectional area by more than approximately 70 percent, the distal resistance vessels will dilate to reduce vascular resistance and maintain coronary blood flow. A pressure gradient develops across the proximal stenosis, and poststenotic pressure falls. When the resistance vessels are maximally dilated, myocardial blood flow becomes dependent on the pressure in the coronary artery distal to the obstruction. In these circumstances alterations in myocardial oxygenation can be caused by changes in myocardial oxygen demand and changes in the caliber of the stenosed coronary artery due to physiologic vasomotion, pathologic spasm, or small platelet plugs. All these transient events can upset the critical balance between oxygen supply and demand and thus precipitate myocardial ischemia.

EFFECTS OF ISCHEMIA The inadequate oxygenation induced by coronary atherosclerosis may cause transient disturbances of the mechanical, biochemical, and electrical function of the myocardium. The abrupt development of ischemia usually affects a segment of left ventricular myocardium with almost instantaneous failure of normal muscle relaxation and contraction. The relatively poor perfusion of the subendocardium causes more intense ischemia of this portion of the wall. Ischemia of large segments of the ventricle will cause transient left ventricular failure, and if the papillary muscles are involved, mitral regurgitation can complicate this event. When ischemic events are transient, they may be associated with angina pectoris; if prolonged, they can lead to myocardial necrosis and scarring with or without the clinical picture of acute myocardial infarction (see Chap. 189). Coronary atherosclerosis is a focal process that causes nonuniform ischemia. As a result, focal disturbances of ventricular contractility cause segmental bulging or dyskinesia and can greatly reduce the efficiency of myocardial pump function.

Underlying these mechanical disturbances are a wide range of abnormalities in cell metabolism, function, and structure. When oxygenated, the normal myocardium metabolizes fatty acids and glucose to carbon dioxide and water. With severe oxygen deprivation, fatty acids cannot be oxidized, and glucose is broken down to lactate; intracellular pH is reduced as are the myocardial stores of high-energy phosphates, adenosine triphosphate (ATP), and creatine phosphate. Impaired cell membrane function leads to potassium leakage and the uptake of sodium by myocytes. The severity and duration of the imbalance between myocardial oxygen supply and demand will determine whether the damage is reversible or whether it is permanent, with subsequent myocardial necrosis.

Ischemia also causes characteristic electrocardiographic changes such as repolarization abnormalities, as evidenced by inversion of the T wave and later by displacement of the ST segment (Chap. 176). Transient ST-segment depression often reflects subendocardial ischemia, while transient ST-segment elevation is thought to be caused by more severe transmural ischemia. Another important consequence of myocardial ischemia is electrical instability, since this may lead to ventricular tachycardia or ventricular fibrillation (Chap. 185). Most patients who die suddenly from ischemic heart disease do so as a result of ischemia-induced malignant ventricular arrhythmias (Chap. 40).

CLINICAL MANIFESTATIONS

ASYMPTOMATIC VERSUS SYMPTOMATIC CORONARY ARTERY DISEASE Postmortem studies on accident victims and military casualties in western countries have shown that coronary atherosclerosis often begins to develop prior to age 20 and is widespread among adults who were asymptomatic during life. In addition, exercise stress tests in asymptomatic persons may show evidence of silent myocardial ischemia, i.e., exercise-induced electrocardiographic changes not accompanied by angina; coronary angiographic studies of such persons frequently reveal obstructive coronary artery disease. Postmortem examination of patients with obstructive coronary artery disease who had no history of any clinical manifestations of myocardial ischemia often shows macroscopic scars of myocardial infarction in regions supplied by diseased coronary arteries. According to population studies, approximately 25 percent of patients with acute myocardial infarction may not reach medical attention, and these patients carry the same adverse prognosis as those who present with the classic clinical syndrome (Chap. 189). Sudden death may be unheralded and is a common presenting manifestation of coronary disease (Chap. 40). Patients can also present with cardiomegaly and heart failure secondary to ischemic damage of the left ventricular myocardium that caused no symptoms prior to the development of heart failure; this condition is referred to as *ischemic cardiomyopathy*. In contrast to the asymptomatic phase of ischemic heart disease, the symptomatic phase is characterized by chest pain due to either angina pectoris or acute myocardial infarction (Chap. 189). Having entered the symptomatic phase, the patient may exhibit a stable or progressive course, revert to the asymptomatic stage, or suddenly die.

CHRONIC STABLE ANGINA PECTORIS This episodic clinical syndrome is due to transient myocardial ischemia. Various diseases that cause myocardial ischemia as well as the numerous pain syndromes with which it may be confused are discussed in Chap. 16. Males constitute approximately 80 percent of all patients with angina pectoris and an even greater fraction of those younger than 50 years of age. The typical patient with angina is a 50- to 60-year-old man who seeks medical help for troublesome or frightening chest discomfort, usually described as heaviness, pressure, squeezing, smothering, or choking and only rarely as frank pain. When the patient is asked to localize the sensation, he or she will typically press on the sternum, sometimes with a clenched fist, to indicate a squeezing, central, substernal discomfort. This symptom is usually crescendo-decrescendo in nature and lasts 1 to 5 min. Angina can radiate to the left shoulder and to both arms, and especially to the ulnar surfaces of the forearm and hand. It can also arise in or radiate to the back, neck, jaw, teeth, and epigastrium.

Although episodes of angina are typically caused by exertion (e.g., exercise, hurrying, or sexual activity) or emotion (e.g., stress, anger, fright, or frustration) and are relieved by rest, they may also occur at rest (see "Unstable Angina Pectoris," below) and at night while the patient is recumbent (angina decubitus). The patient may be awakened at night distressed by typical chest discomfort and dyspnea. The pathophysiology of nocturnal angina may be similar to that of paroxysmal nocturnal dyspnea (Chap. 182), i.e., the expansion of the intrathoracic blood volume that occurs with recumbency causes an increase in cardiac size and myocardial oxygen demand that lead to ischemia and transient left ventricular failure.

The threshold for the development of angina pectoris may vary by time of day and emotional state. A patient may report symptoms upon minor exertion in the morning (a short walk or shaving) yet by midday may be capable of much greater effort without symptoms. Angina may be precipitated by unfamiliar tasks, a heavy meal, or exposure to cold.

Sharp, fleeting chest pain or prolonged, dull aches localized to the left submammary area are rarely due to myocardial ischemia. However, angina pectoris may be atypical in location and may not be strictly related to provoking factors. In addition, this symptom may exacerbate and remit over days, weeks, or months, and its occurrence can be seasonal.

Systematic questioning of the patient with suspected ischemic heart disease is important to uncover a positive family history of ischemic heart disease, diabetes, hyperlipidemia, hypertension, cigarette smoking, and other risk factors for coronary atherosclerosis.

In *variant (Prinzmetal's) angina,* the chest discomfort characteristically occurs at rest or awakens the patient from sleep. It may be accompanied by palpitations or severe shortness of breath, explosive in onset, severe, and frightening. It may also be brought on by effort, although the workload at which it is precipitated usually varies considerably. Variant angina is caused by focal spasm of proximal epicardial coronary arteries; in approximately three-fourths of the patients atherosclerotic coronary artery obstruction is present, in which case the vasospasm occurs near the stenotic lesion.

Physical examination The physical examination is often normal. The patient's general appearance may reveal signs of risk factors associated with coronary atherosclerosis such as xanthelasma, xanthomas (Chap. 195), or diabetic skin lesions. There may also be signs of anemia, thyroid disease, and nicotine stains on the fingertips from cigarette smoking. Palpation can reveal thickened or absent peripheral arteries, signs of cardiac enlargement, and abnormal contraction of the cardiac impulse (left ventricular akinesia or dyskinesia). Examination of the fundi may reveal increased light reflexes and arteriovenous nicking as evidence of hypertension (an important risk factor for ischemic heart disease), while auscultation can uncover arterial bruits, a third and/or fourth heart sound, and, if acute ischemia or previous infarction has impaired papillary muscle function, a late apical systolic murmur due to mitral regurgitation. These auscultatory signs are best appreciated with the patient in the left decubitus position. Aortic stenosis, aortic regurgitation (Chap. 188), and hypertrophic cardiomyopathy (Chap. 192) must be excluded, since these disorders may cause angina even in the absence of coronary artery disease. Examination during an anginal attack is useful, since ischemia can cause transient left ventricular failure with the appearance of a third and/or fourth heart sound, a dyskinetic cardiac apex, mitral regurgitation, and even pulmonary edema.

Laboratory examination Although the diagnosis of ischemic heart disease can be made with confidence from a typical history, a number of simple laboratory tests can be most helpful. The urine should be examined for evidence of diabetes mellitus and renal disease, since both these conditions may accelerate atherosclerosis. Similarly, examination of the blood should include measurements of lipids (cholesterol—total, low density, and high density), glucose, creatinine, hematocrit, and, if indicated based on the physical examination, thyroid function. A chest x-ray is important, since it may show the consequences of ischemic heart disease, i.e., cardiac enlargement, ventricular aneurysm, or signs of heart failure. Calcification of the coronary arteries can sometimes be identified on chest fluoroscopy. These signs can support the diagnosis of coronary artery disease and are important in assessing the degree of cardiac damage and the effects of treatment for heart failure.

Electrocardiogram A normal ECG does not exclude the diagnosis of ischemic heart disease; however, certain characteristic abnormalities in tracings obtained at rest can confirm it. A 12-lead ECG recorded at rest is normal in about half the patients with typical angina pectoris, but there may be signs of an old myocardial infarction (Chap. 176). Serial tracings are particularly useful to look for past or evolving myocardial infarction. Although repolarization abnormalities, i.e., T-wave and ST-segment changes and intraventricular conduction disturbances at rest, are suggestive of ischemic heart disease, they are nonspecific, since they can also occur in pericardial, myocardial, and valvular heart disease or with anxiety, changes in posture, drugs, or esophageal disease. Typical ST-segment and T-wave changes that accompany episodes of angina pectoris and disappear thereafter are more specific. The most characteristic changes include displacement of the ST segment that is similar in every way to that induced during a stress test (see below). The ST segment is usually depressed during angina but may be elevated—sometimes strikingly so—as in the early stages of myocardial infarction and in Prinzmetal's angina.

Stress testing The most widely used test in the diagnosis of ischemic heart disease involves recording the 12-lead ECG before, during, and after exercise on a treadmill or using a bicycle ergometer. The test consists of a standardized incremental increase in external workload while the patient's ECG, symptoms, and arm blood pressure are continuously monitored. Performance is usually symptom-limited and the test is discontinued upon evidence of chest discomfort, severe shortness of breath, dizziness, fatigue, ST-segment depression of greater than 2 mm, a fall in systolic blood pressure exceeding 15 mmHg, or the development of ventricular tachyarrhythmias. This test seeks to establish the relationship between chest discomfort and the typical electrocardiographic signs of myocardial ischemia. The ischemic ST-segment response is generally defined as flat depression of the ST segment of more than 0.1 mV below the baseline (i.e., the PR segment) and lasting longer than 0.08 s. This type of depression is designated ''square wave'' or ''plateau'' and is flat or downsloping. Upsloping or junctional ST-segment changes are not considered characteristic of ischemia and do not constitute a positive test. Although T-wave abnormalities, conduction disturbances, and ventricular arrhythmias that develop during exercise should be noted, they are also not diagnostic. Negative exercise tests in which the target heart rate (85 percent of maximal heart rate for age and sex) is not achieved are considered to be nondiagnostic.

Based on the above criteria, the rate of false-positive diagnoses, using the coronary arteriogram as the gold standard, is approximately 15 percent, and a similar percentage of patients with severe, multivessel coronary artery disease will not have a positive test (false-

negative). According to Bayes' theorem, the probability that ischemic heart disease exists in the patient or population under study (pretest probability) must be considered in light of the diagnostic features of the test in order to interpret a positive or negative test result (Fig. 2-3, p. 7). For example, a positive result on exercise indicates that the likelihood of coronary artery disease is 98 percent in patients with typical angina pectoris, 88 percent in those with atypical chest pain, 44 percent in those with nonanginal chest pain, and 33 percent in asymptomatic persons. The incidence of false-positive tests is increased in patients taking cardioactive drugs such as digitalis and quinidine, or in those with conduction disturbances, resting abnormalities of the ST segment and the T wave, myocardial hypertrophy, or abnormal serum potassium levels. It should be noted that the posterior surface of the heart is less accessible to the ECG and therefore more silent clinically.

The physician should be present throughout the exercise test, and it is important to measure total duration of exercise, the time to the onset of ischemic ST-segment change and chest discomfort, the external work performed, and the internal cardiac work performed; the last is represented by the heart rate–blood pressure product. The depth of the ST-segment depression and the time needed for recovery of these electrocardiographic changes are also important. Because the risks of exercise testing are small but real—estimated at one fatality and two nonfatal complications per 10,000 tests—equipment for resuscitation should be available. Modified (heart rate–limited rather than symptom-limited) exercise tests can be performed safely in patients as early as 10 days after myocardial infarction.

The normal response to exercise includes a progressive increase in heart rate and blood pressure. Failure of the blood pressure to increase or an actual decrease in blood pressure with signs of ischemia during the test is an important adverse prognostic sign, since it may reflect ischemia-induced global left ventricular dysfunction. The presence of pain or severe ST-segment depression at a low workload and ST-segment depression that persists for more than 5 min after the termination of exercise will increase the specificity of the test and indicate severe ischemic heart disease.

The exercise test can be enhanced by the intravenous administration of a radioisotope such as thallium 201 to assess regional myocardial perfusion by means of a gamma camera (p. 865). Images are recorded immediately after exercise (to identify acute ischemia) and 2 to 4 h later to discriminate between reversible ischemia and infarction (Fig. 177-7). Another radioisotope, most often technetium 99m, can be used to label the blood pool for gated radioisotope angiography. This technique (Fig. 177-6) can provide a measure of ventricular volume, ejection fraction, and regional myocardial wall motion at rest and during exercise, and can identify transient global and regional left ventricular dysfunction due to myocardial ischemia. A reduction in ejection fraction during exercise with the appearance of regional wall motion abnormalities is an important sign and suggests the presence of severe ischemia and/or multivessel coronary disease.

Although these tests were developed to detect myocardial ischemia and by inference coronary artery disease, the relationship between the presence and severity of these two conditions is complex. More recently, the severity of signs of ischemia in all the tests described above has been shown to correlate with risk for future adverse coronary events (myocardial infarction and death).

Two-dimensional echocardiography records cross-sectional images of the left ventricle and can identify regional wall motion abnormalities due to myocardial infarction (Chap. 177). In this way, this test can also be used as an aid in the diagnosis of ischemic heart disease.

Coronary arteriography (Chap. 179) This invasive diagnostic method outlines the coronary anatomy and can be used to detect important evidence of coronary atherosclerosis or to exclude this condition. By this means, one can assess the severity of obstructive lesions and both global and regional function of the left ventricle. Coronary arteriography is indicated in (1) patients with chronic stable or unstable angina pectoris who are refractory to medical therapy and who are being considered for revascularization, i.e., percutaneous transluminal coronary angioplasty or coronary artery bypass graft surgery; (2) patients with troublesome symptoms that present diagnostic difficulties in whom there is need to confirm or rule out the diagnosis of coronary artery disease; and (3) patients suspected of having left main stem or three-vessel coronary artery disease based on signs of severe ischemia on noninvasive testing, regardless of the presence or severity of symptoms.

Examples of other possible clinical situations include:

1 Patients with chest discomfort suggestive of angina pectoris but a negative exercise test who require a definitive diagnosis for guiding medical management, alleviating psychological stress, career or family planning, or insurance purposes.
2 Patients who have been admitted to the hospital several times for suspected acute myocardial infarction but in whom this diagnosis has not been established and in whom the presence or absence of coronary artery disease should be determined.
3 Patients with careers that involve the safety of others (e.g., airline pilots) who have questionable symptoms, suspicious or positive noninvasive tests, and in whom there are reasonable doubts about the state of the coronary arteries.
4 Patients with aortic stenosis or hypertrophic cardiomyopathy and angina in whom the pain could be due to coronary artery disease.
5 Male patients aged 45 and females aged 55 years of age or older who will undergo valve replacement and who may or may not have clinical evidence of myocardial ischemia.
6 Patients who are at high risk after myocardial infarction because of the recurrence of angina, heart failure, frequent ventricular premature contractions, or signs of ischemia in the stress test.
7 Patients with angina pectoris, regardless of severity, in whom noninvasive testing reveals signs of severe ischemia, i.e., early and/or marked (>2 mm) ST-segment depression, large or multiple perfusion defects and/or increased lung uptake on thallium-201 scintigrams following exercise, global left ventricular dysfunction precipitated by exercise, and/or exercise-induced hypotension.

PROGNOSIS

The principal prognostic indicators in patients with ischemic heart disease are the functional state of the left ventricle, the location and severity of coronary artery narrowing, and the severity or activity of myocardial ischemia. Angina pectoris of recent onset, unstable angina, angina unresponsive to medical therapy, or symptoms of congestive heart failure all indicate an increased risk for adverse coronary events. The same is true for physical signs of heart failure, episodes of pulmonary edema, or roentgenographic evidence of cardiac enlargement. An abnormal resting ECG or positive evidence of myocardial ischemia during a stress test also indicate increased risk. Most importantly, the following signs during noninvasive testing indicate a high risk for coronary events: a strongly positive exercise test showing onset of myocardial ischemia at low workloads, large or multiple perfusion defects or increased lung uptake during stress thallium scanning, a decrease in left ventricular ejection fraction during exercise on radionuclide ventriculography, hypotension with ischemia during stress testing, and episodes of asymptomatic ischemia recorded during continuous monitoring of the ECG in patients with unstable or stable angina pectoris and coronary artery disease.

On cardiac catheterization, elevations in left ventricular end-diastolic pressure and ventricular volume and a reduced ejection fraction are the most important signs of left ventricular dysfunction and are associated with a poor prognosis. Patients with chest discomfort but normal left ventricular function and normal coronary arteries have an excellent prognosis. In patients with normal left ventricular function and mild angina but with critical stenoses (≥ 70 percent luminal diameter) or one, two, or three epicardial coronary arteries, the 5-year mortality rates are approximately 2, 8, and 11 percent, respectively. Obstructive lesions of the proximal left anterior

descending coronary artery are associated with a greater risk than are lesions of the right or left circumflex coronary artery, since the former vessel usually perfuses a greater quantity of myocardium. Critical stenosis of the left main coronary artery is associated with a mortality of about 15 percent per year.

With any degree of obstructive coronary artery disease, mortality is greatly increased when left ventricular function is impaired; conversely, at any level of left ventricular function, the prognosis is influenced importantly by the extent of myocardium perfused by the critically obstructed vessels. It is useful to consider that coronary atherosclerosis demonstrates its harmful potential by causing transient myocardial ischemia and characteristically destroys myocardium, thereby reducing cardiac reserve at an unpredictable rate. The larger the amount of myocardial necrosis, the less the heart is able to withstand additional damage and the poorer the prognosis. In this light, the various indices of ischemic damage, such as the ECG showing evidence of an old infarction and symptoms or signs of heart failure or cardiac enlargement, should be taken as indications of myocardial damage.

The segmental atherosclerotic plaques in epicardial arteries go through phases of cellular activity, degeneration, endothelial instability, abnormal vasomotion, platelet aggregation, and fissuring or hemorrhage. These factors can also temporarily worsen the stenosis and cause abnormal reactivity of the vessel wall thus exacerbating the manifestations of ischemia. The development of unstable angina and/or severe ischemia during stress testing reflects rapid progression.

MANAGEMENT

Each patient must be evaluated individually with respect to life patterns, risk factors, control of symptoms, and prevention of damage to left ventricular myocardium. The degree of the patient's disability and the specific physical and emotional stresses that precipitate pain must all be carefully recorded in order to set the proper goals for treatment. The management plan should consist of (1) explanation and reassurance, (2) reduction of risk factors in an attempt to slow the progression of coronary atherosclerosis, (3) treatment of coexisting conditions capable of aggravating angina, (4) sensible adaptations of activities to minimize anginal attacks, (5) a program of drug therapy, and (6) definition of end points that will indicate the need to consider mechanical revascularization.

EXPLANATION AND REASSURANCE Patients with ischemic heart disease need to understand their condition as best they can and to realize that a long and useful life is possible even though they suffer from angina pectoris or have experienced and recovered from an acute myocardial infarction. Offering case histories of persons in public life who have lived with coronary disease can be of great value when encouraging patients to resume or maintain activity and return to their occupation.

REDUCTION OF RISK FACTORS (SECONDARY PREVENTION) (See also Chap. 195) Clinical trials in selected patients seem to indicate that effective modification of risk factors (e.g., plasma lipid levels) can slow the growth of coronary atherosclerosis. Ideal weight should be attained and maintained, hypertension treated if present, and cigarette smoking forbidden. Diabetes mellitus and hyperlipidemia, when present, should be treated. Unless angina is provoked by strenuous activity, the patient should be encouraged to engage in steady, dynamic exercise such as walking; isometric exercise may be hazardous. By maintaining good physical condition, the patient will be able to perform physical work more efficiently and at a lower pulse rate, thus reducing the frequency of angina pectoris. Patients in good physical condition may also have a better chance of surviving a myocardial infarction.

ELIMINATION OF COEXISTING ILLNESS A number of illnesses that are not primarily cardiac in nature may either increase oxygen demand or decrease oxygen supply to the myocardium and may precipitate or exacerbate angina. In the former category, hypertension and hyperthyroidism may be treated successfully in order to reduce the frequency of anginal attacks. Decreased myocardial oxygen supply may be due to reduced oxygenation of the blood (e.g., in intrinsic pulmonary disease or, when carboxyhemoglobin is present, due to cigarette or cigar smoking) or decreased oxygen-carrying capacity (e.g., in anemia). Correction of these abnormalities, if present, may reduce or even eliminate anginal symptoms.

ADAPTATION OF ACTIVITIES   Therapy of ischemic heart disease consists of eliminating the discrepancy between the demand of the heart muscle for oxygen and the ability of the coronary circulation to meet this demand. Most patients will understand this fundamental concept and utilize it in the rational programming of activity. Many tasks that ordinarily evoke angina may be accomplished without symptoms simply by reducing the speed at which they are performed. Patients must appreciate the diurnal variation in their tolerance of certain activities and should reduce their energy requirements in the morning and immediately after meals. Sometimes it is helpful to alter the eating pattern, taking small and more frequent meals.

It may be necessary to recommend a change in employment or residence to avoid physical stress; however, with the exception of manual laborers, most patients with ischemic heart disease can usually continue to function merely by allowing more time to complete each task. In some patients, anger and frustration may be the most important factors precipitating myocardial ischemia. If these cannot be avoided, training in stress management can be useful. A treadmill exercise test to determine the approximate heart rate at which ischemic electrocardiographic changes or symptoms develop may be helpful in the development of a specific exercise program. Ambulatory electrocardiography during daily activities may also be helpful in this regard.

DRUG THERAPY Nitrates   This is the most valuable class of drugs in the management of angina pectoris. Nitrates act by causing systemic venodilation, thereby reducing myocardial wall tension and oxygen requirements, as well as by dilating the epicardial coronary vessels and increasing blood flow in collateral vessels. The activity of these agents depends on their absorption, which is most rapid and complete through the mucous membranes. For this reason, nitroglycerin is administered sublingually in tablets of 0.4 or 0.6 mg. Patients with angina should be instructed to take the medication both to relieve an attack and also in anticipation of stress that is likely to induce an attack. When the patient experiences discomfort on exertion, he or she should cease activity and place a tablet under the tongue. The discomfort generally disappears more rapidly with nitroglycerin than would be expected if the drug were not administered. Walking up a hill or flight of stairs or sexual intercourse may produce angina consistently, so that discomfort can often be prevented by the anticipatory use of nitroglycerin. The value of this prophylactic use of the drug cannot be overemphasized.

The dose of nitroglycerin should be sufficient to relieve discomfort but not so large as to produce hypotension, headache, or a feeling of pulsating fullness in the head. The last is the most common side effect of nitroglycerin and fortunately only rarely becomes disturbing at the doses usually required to relieve or prevent angina. Nitroglycerin deteriorates with exposure to air, moisture, and sunlight, so that if the drug neither relieves discomfort or headache nor produces a slight sensation of burning at the sublingual site of absorption, the preparation may be inactive and a fresh supply should be obtained. If relief is not achieved after the first dose of nitroglycerin, a second or third dose may be given, but the patient should be instructed not to continue to take the medication if the first few doses are ineffective. If discomfort continues for more than 7 to 10 min despite treatment, the patient should consult his or her physician or report promptly to a hospital emergency room for evaluation of possible unstable angina or acute myocardial infarction (Chap. 189).

Asking the patient with recently diagnosed angina pectoris to record the occurrence of pain relative to activity and other precipitating factors as well as nitroglycerin consumption is often helpful to the physician attempting to tailor a management program. Such a diary

may also be valuable for detecting changes in the frequency or severity of discomfort that may signify the development of unstable angina pectoris and/or herald an impending myocardial infarction.

Unfortunately, none of the long-acting nitrates is as effective as sublingual nitroglycerin for the relief of angina. These preparations can be swallowed, chewed, or administered as a patch or paste by the transdermal route. They can provide effective plasma levels for up to 24 h, but the therapeutic response is highly variable, and tolerance often develops. Different preparations and/or administration during the daytime only should be tried in an attempt to relieve discomfort in the individual patient while avoiding side effects such as headache and dizziness. Individual dose titration is important in order to prevent side effects. Useful preparations include isosorbide dinitrate (5 to 20 mg sublingually every 3 h or 4 to 40 mg PO tid), nitroglycerin ointment (0.5 to 2.0 inches qid), or sustained-release transdermal patches (5 to 25 mg per day). Long-acting nitrates are relatively safe and can be used together with intermittent sublingual nitroglycerin to relieve discomfort and prevent attacks of angina.

Beta-adrenoceptor blockade (See also Chap. 67) Beta-adrenoceptor blockade represents an important component of the pharmacologic treatment of angina pectoris. These drugs reduce myocardial oxygen demand by inhibiting the increase in heart rate and myocardial contractility caused by adrenergic activity. Beta blockade reduces these variables most strikingly during exercise while causing only small reductions in heart rate, cardiac output, and arterial pressure at rest. Propranolol is usually administered in an initial dose of 20 to 40 mg four times a day and is increased as tolerated to 320 mg per day in divided doses; sometimes higher doses are required. Long-acting beta-blocking drugs (atenolol, 50 to 100 mg per day, and nadolol, 40 to 80 mg per day) offer the advantage of once-a-day dosage (see Table 67-1). The therapeutic aims include relief of angina and effective inhibition of exercise-induced increases in heart rate. These drugs can produce fatigue, impotence, cold extremities, intermittent claudication, and bradycardia and can worsen disturbed cardiac conduction, left ventricular failure, and bronchial asthma or intensify the hypoglycemia produced by oral hypoglycemic agents and insulin. Reducing the dose or even discontinuation of the drug may be necessary if these side effects develop and persist.

Calcium channel antagonists   Nifedipine (10 to 40 mg qid), verapamil (80 to 120 mg tid), and diltiazem (30 to 90 mg qid) are all coronary vasodilators that produce variable and dose-dependent reductions in myocardial oxygen demand, contractility, and arterial pressure. These combined pharmacologic effects are of advantage and make these agents quite effective in the treatment of angina pectoris. Verapamil and diltiazem may produce symptomatic disturbances in cardiac conduction and bradyarrhythmias, exert negative inotropic actions, and are more likely to worsen left ventricular failure, particularly when used in combination with beta-adrenergic blockers in patients with underlying left ventricular dysfunction. Although useful effects are usually achieved when calcium channel antagonists are combined with beta-adrenoceptor blockers and nitrates, careful individual titration of dose is essential with these potent combinations. Variant (Prinzmetal's) angina responds particularly well to calcium channel antagonists, supplemented when necessary by nitrates. Population studies in asymptomatic adults have shown that aspirin (325 mg orally on alternate days) can decrease the incidence of myocardial infarction. Although this has not been established in all patients with known coronary disease, this prescription seems reasonable in the absence of side effects or contraindications.

Treatment of angina and heart failure   Patients with angina pectoris and coronary artery disease may also have evidence of elevated ventricular diastolic pressures and volumes due to transient ischemia. This transient left ventricular failure with angina can be controlled by the judicious use of nitrates, calcium channel antagonists, and even beta blockers. For patients with established congestive heart failure the increased left ventricular wall tension raises myocardial oxygen demand. Treatment of congestive heart failure with digitalis and diuretics (Chap. 182) can help to decrease heart size, wall tension, and myocardial oxygen demands, which will help to control angina and ischemia. Nocturnal angina can often be relieved by these agents; however, there is no benefit—and possibly aggravation of angina—when these drugs are used in patients with a normal heart size and no evidence of heart failure. Nitrates are particularly useful and can improve the disturbed hemodynamics of congestive heart failure and relieve angina by preventing or reversing myocardial ischemia. The combination of congestive heart failure and angina in patients with coronary artery disease usually indicates a poor prognosis and warrants serious consideration of cardiac catheterization and mechanical revascularization, if possible.

Aspirin This should be given in a dose of 160 to 325 mg/d.

MECHANICAL REVASCULARIZATION

It is important to appreciate that the basic management of patients with a lifelong condition such as ischemic heart disease is medical. The years of medical management may be punctuated by mechanical revascularization procedures, as described below, but these interventions should not replace the continuing need to ease symptoms and modify risk factors.

PERCUTANEOUS TRANSLUMINAL CORONARY ANGIOPLASTY (PTCA) PTCA is a widely used method to achieve revascularization of the myocardium in patients with symptomatic ischemic heart disease and suitable proximal stenoses of epicardial coronary arteries. Whereas patients with stenosis of the left main coronary artery and those with distal three-vessel coronary artery disease who require revascularization are best treated with coronary artery bypass surgery, PTCA is widely employed in patients with symptoms due to proximal stenoses of one or two vessels, and even selected patients with three-vessel disease, and may offer many advantages over surgery.

The method is described in Chap. 179. After a flexible guidewire is advanced into a coronary artery and across the stenosis to be dilated, a miniature balloon catheter is advanced over the guidewire and into the stenosis followed by repeated inflations until the stenosis is decreased or relieved. The development of a range of steerable guidewires, low-profile balloon catheters, and the use of high inflation pressures have all helped to decrease complications, reach more distal lesions, and dilate more complex stenoses.

Indications and patient selection The most common clinical indication for PTCA is angina pectoris, stable or unstable, which should be accompanied by evidence of ischemia in an exercise test. This symptom should be sufficiently severe to warrant the consideration of bypass graft surgery. Some physicians will perform angioplasty on asymptomatic or mildly symptomatic patients with suitable stenosis of the left anterior descending coronary artery and severe ischemia on an exercise test, but the value of this procedure in improving outcome has not been established. PTCA can also be used to dilate stenoses in native coronary arteries and in bypass grafts in patients who have recurrent angina following coronary artery surgery. This is an important indication when considering the technical difficulties and the increased mortality that accompanies reoperation. Angioplasty has also been carried out in patients with recent total occlusion (within 3 months) of a coronary artery and severe angina; in this group the primary success rate is decreased to approximately 50 percent.

Risks Two and three vessels can be dilated in sequence with only a modest increase in risk. Female gender, left ventricular damage, stenosis of an artery perfusing a large segment of myocardium without collaterals, long eccentric or irregular stenoses, and calcified plaques all increase the likelihood of complications. The major complications are usually due to dissection or thrombosis with vessel occlusion, uncontrolled ischemia, and ventricular failure. In experienced hands, the overall mortality rate should be less than 1 percent, the need for emergency coronary surgery 3 to 5 percent, and myocardial infarction in approximately 3 percent of cases. Minor

complications occur in 5 to 10 percent of patients and include occlusion of a branch of a coronary artery and complications of arterial catheterization.

Efficacy Primary success, i.e., adequate dilation with relief of angina, is achieved in 85 to 90 percent of cases. Recurrent stenosis of the dilated vessels occurs in 20 to 40 percent of cases within 6 months of the procedure, and angina will recur within 6 to 12 months in 25 percent of cases. This recurrence of symptoms and restenosis is more common in patients with unstable angina or with incomplete dilation of the stenosis. It is usual clinical practice to administer aspirin, and a calcium channel antagonist for months after the procedure. Although aspirin may help prevent acute coronary thrombosis during and immediately following PTCA, there are no controlled clinical trials that have demonstrated that these medications reduce the incidence of restenosis.

If patients do not develop restenosis or angina within the first year after angioplasty, the prognosis for maintaining improvement over the subsequent 4 years is excellent. If restenosis occurs, PTCA can be repeated with the same success and risks but the likelihood of restenosis increases with the third or more attempt.

Between 30 and 50 percent of patients with symptomatic coronary artery disease who require revascularization can be treated by PTCA and need not undergo coronary artery bypass grafting. Successful angioplasty is less invasive and expensive than coronary artery surgery, requires only 2 to 3 days in the hospital, and permits considerable savings in the cost of care. Successful PTCA also allows earlier return to work and the resumption of an active life.

CORONARY ARTERY BYPASS GRAFTING In this procedure, a section of a vein (usually the saphenous) is used to form a connection between the aorta and the coronary artery distal to the obstructive lesion. Alternatively, anastomosis of one or both of the internal mammary arteries to the coronary artery distal to the obstructive lesion may be employed.

Although some indications for coronary artery bypass surgery are controversial, certain areas of agreement exist:

1 The operation is relatively safe, with mortality rates less than 1 percent when the procedure is performed by an experienced surgical team in selected patients with normal left ventricular function.

2 Intraoperative and postoperative mortality increases with the degree of ventricular dysfunction and surgical inexperience. The effectiveness and risk of coronary artery bypass grafting vary widely depending on case selection and the skill and experience of the surgical team, so that the latter must be taken into account when a patient is being considered as a candidate for this procedure.

3 Occlusion is observed in 10 to 20 percent of *vein grafts* during the first year, the incidence is approximately 2 percent per year during 5- to 7-year follow-up and 5 percent per year thereafter. Long-term patency rates are considerably higher for internal mammary artery implantations; in patients with left anterior descending coronary artery obstruction, survival is better when coronary bypass involves the internal mammary artery rather than a saphenous vein.

4 Angina is abolished or unequivocally reduced in approximately 85 percent of patients following complete revascularization. Although this is usually associated with graft patency and restoration of blood flow, the pain may also have been alleviated as a result of infarction of the ischemic segment or a placebo effect.

5 Coronary artery bypass grafting does not appear to reduce the incidence of myocardial infarction in patients with chronic ischemic heart disease; perioperative myocardial infarction occurs in 5 to 10 percent of cases, but in most instances these infarcts are small.

6 Mortality is reduced by operation in patients with stenosis of the left main coronary artery. Some reduction in mortality is also achieved in patients with three-vessel coronary artery disease and impaired left ventricular function. However, there is no evidence that coronary artery surgery improves survival in patients with one- or two-vessel disease who have chronic stable angina and normal left ventricular function or in patients with one-vessel disease and impaired left ventricular function. Evidence is conflicting concerning the effects of operation on survival in patients with impaired left ventricular function and obstructive disease of two coronary arteries, one of which is the proximal left anterior descending artery.

7 Other important considerations affecting outcome include the age and gender of the patient as well as accompanying medical problems such as diabetes mellitus, obesity, and renal disease.

Indications for coronary artery bypass grafting are usually based on the severity of symptoms, coronary anatomy, and ventricular function. The ideal candidate is male, less than 70 years of age, has no other complicating disease, has troublesome or disabling symptoms that are not adequately controlled by medical therapy, wishes to lead a more active life, and has severe stenoses of several epicardial coronary arteries with objective evidence of myocardial ischemia as a cause of the chest discomfort. Great symptomatic benefit can be anticipated in such patients. When the patient also has a disturbance of left ventricular function, coronary artery bypass grafting may, in addition, prolong life.

UNSTABLE ANGINA PECTORIS

The following three patient groups may be said to have unstable angina pectoris: (1) patients with new onset (<2 months) angina that is severe and/or frequent (≥3 episodes per day); (2) patients with accelerating angina, i.e., those with chronic stable angina who develop angina that is distinctly more frequent, severe, longer, or precipitated by less exertion than previously; (3) those with angina of any duration that occurs at rest. Unstable angina may be primary, i.e., occur in the absence of an extracardiac condition that has intensified myocardial ischemia, or it may be precipitated by a condition extrinsic to the coronary vascular bed that has intensified myocardial ischemia, such as anemia, fever, infection, tachyarrhythmias, emotional stress, or hypoxemia. Unstable angina may also develop shortly after myocardial infarction. Unstable angina, particularly when it is characterized by rest pain or occurs in the postinfarction state, carries an adverse prognosis, with significant risk of acute myocardial infarction or the development of intractable chronic stable angina.

When unstable angina is accompanied by objective electrocardiographic evidence of transient myocardial ischemia (ST-segment changes and/or T-wave inversions during episodes of chest pain), it is almost always associated with critical stenoses in one or more major epicardial coronary arteries. Less than 10 percent of patients with unstable angina have normal coronary arteries on arteriography. The atherosclerotic lesions may have a complicated morphology, with evidence of superimposed thrombosis in approximately 25 to 60 percent of cases. Segmental spasm in the vicinity of atherosclerotic plaques may also play a role in the development of unstable angina.

MANAGEMENT   The patient should be admitted promptly to the hospital for observation, further diagnosis, and treatment. It is important to identify and treat concomitant conditions that can intensify ischemia, such as uncontrolled tachycardia, hypertension and diabetes mellitus, cardiomegaly, heart failure, arrhythmias, thyrotoxicosis, and any acute febrile illness. Acute myocardial infarction should be ruled out by means of serial ECGs and measurements of plasma cardiac enzyme activity.

Continuous electrocardiographic monitoring should be carried out and the patients should receive reassurance and sedation. Thrombus formation frequently complicates this condition. Therefore, intravenous heparin should be given for 3 to 5 days to maintain the partial thromboplastin time at 2 to 2.5 times control, followed by oral aspirin at a dose of 325 mg/d. Beta-adrenergic blocking drugs and calcium channel antagonists should be administered, but with caution and an awareness of all the possible side effects discussed above. Dosages must be titrated to avoid bradycardia, heart failure, and hypotension. Nitroglycerin should be given by the sublingual route. In addition, intravenous nitroglycerin is quite effective, although it requires continuous monitoring of intraarterial pressure. It is begun at a dosage of 5 μg/min and is raised in 5-μg/min increments to a level at which chest pain is abolished but systolic arterial pressure is maintained or reduced only slightly and other side effects are avoided.

The majority of patients improve with such treatment. However, the clinical outcome is highly variable. If angina and/or electrocardiographic evidence of ischemia do not diminish within 24 to 48 h of the comprehensive treatment described above in patients with no obvious contraindications for revascularization, then cardiac catheterization and coronary arteriography should be performed. If the anatomy is suitable, PTCA can be performed with surgical standby. If angioplasty cannot be done, coronary artery bypass grafting should be considered to relieve symptoms and myocardial ischemia and as a means of preventing myocardial damage. If the patient's symptoms and signs are controlled on medical therapy, a diagnostic exercise ECG should be obtained near the time of hospital discharge. If there is obvious evidence of myocardial ischemia, serious consideration should be given to catheterization and revascularization. It should be recognized that severe coronary artery disease is usually present in patients with unstable angina who respond to medical therapy, and although the unstable state may be controlled, it is often converted to severe chronic stable angina and ultimately requires mechanical revascularization.

ASYMPTOMATIC (SILENT) ISCHEMIA

Obstructive coronary artery disease, acute myocardial infarction, and transient myocardial ischemia are frequently asymptomatic. During continuous ambulatory electrocardiographic monitoring, the majority of ambulatory patients with typical chronic stable angina are found to have objective evidence of myocardial ischemia (ST-segment deviation) during episodes of chest discomfort while they are active outside the hospital, but many of these patients also appear to have more frequent episodes of asymptomatic ischemia. In addition, there is a large (but as yet unknown) number of totally asymptomatic people with severe coronary atherosclerosis who exhibit ST-segment changes during activity. Evidence of frequent episodes of ischemia (symptomatic and asymptomatic) during daily life appears to indicate an increased likelihood of adverse coronary events such as death and myocardial infarction. The widespread use of exercise electrocardiography during routine examinations has also defined some of these heretofore unrecognized patients with asymptomatic coronary artery disease. Longitudinal studies have demonstrated an increased incidence of coronary events (sudden death, myocardial infarction, and angina) in asymptomatic patients with positive exercise tests. In addition, patients who are asymptomatic after suffering a myocardial infarction are nonetheless at far greater risk for a second coronary event than is the general population. Patients who seek evaluation and who have asymptomatic ischemia should be subjected to a detailed noninvasive examination, utilizing stress electrocardiography and radionuclide scintigraphy.

MANAGEMENT   The management of patients with asymptomatic ischemia must be individualized. Thus, the physician should consider the following: (1) the degree of positivity of the exercise test, particularly the stage of exercise at which electrocardiographic signs of ischemia appear, the magnitude and number of the perfusion defect(s) on thallium scintigraphy, and the change in left ventricular ejection fraction which occurs during ischemia and/or during exercise on radionuclide ventriculography; (2) the electrocardiographic leads showing a positive response, with changes in the anterior precordial leads indicating a less favorable prognosis than changes in the inferior leads; and (3) the patient's age, occupation, and general medical condition. Most would agree that an asymptomatic 45-year-old commercial airline pilot with 4-mm ST-segment depression in leads V_1 to V_4 during mild exercise should undergo coronary arteriography, whereas the asymptomatic, sedentary 75-year-old retiree with 1-mm ST-segment depression in leads II and III during maximal activity need not. However, there is no consensus about the appropriate procedure in the large majority of patients for whom the situation is less extreme. Patients with evidence of severe ischemia on noninvasive testing (as outlined earlier) should undergo coronary arteriography. Asymptomatic patients with three-vessel coronary disease and impaired left ventricular function may be considered appropriate candidates for coronary artery bypass surgery.

While the incidence of asymptomatic ischemia can be reduced by treatment with beta blockers, calcium channel antagonists, and long-acting nitrates it is not clear whether this is necessary or desirable in patients who have not suffered a myocardial infarction. However, there is evidence that beta-adrenoceptor blockade begun 7 to 35 days after acute myocardial infarction improves survival (Chap. 189). This therapy is recommended in asymptomatic patients as long as there are no contraindications such as heart failure, bradycardia, heart block, or asthma.

REFERENCES

ADAMS PC et al: Platelet/vessel wall interactions, rheologic factors and thrombogenic substrate in acute coronary syndromes: Preventive strategies. Am J Cardiol 60:9G, 1987

BELLER GA et al: Sensitivity, specificity and prognostic significance of noninvasive testing for occult or known coronary disease. Prog Cardiovasc Dis 24:241, 1987

BRAUNWALD E: Unstable angina—A classification. Circulation 80:410, 1989

BRAUNWALD E, SOBEL BE et al: Coronary blood flow and myocardial ischemia, in *Heart Disease*, 3d ed, E Braunwald (ed). Philadelphia, Saunders, 1988, p 1191

HEUSCH G: Alpha-adrenergic mechanisms in myocardial ischemia. Circulation 71(1):1, 1990

KING SB et al: Percutaneous transluminal angioplasty: The second decade. Am J Cardiol 62:2K, 1988

LADENHEIM ML et al: Incremental prognostic power of clinical history, exercise electrocardiography and coronary artery disease. Am J Cardiol 59:270, 1987

ROCCO MB et al: Prognostic importance of myocardial ischemia detected by ambulatory monitoring in patients with stable coronary artery disease. Circulation 78:877, 1988

RUTHERFORD JD et al: Chronic ischemic heart disease, in *Heart Disease,* 3d ed, E Braunwald (ed). Philadelphia, Saunders, 1988, p 1314

RYAN TJ et al: Guidelines for percutaneous transluminal coronary angioplasty. A report of the American College of Cardiology/American Heart Association Task Force on assessment of diagnostic and therapeutic cardiovascular procedures (Subcommittee on Percutaneous Transluminal Coronary Angioplasty). Circulation 78:486, 1988

SELWYN AP, GANZ P et al: Myocardial ischemia in coronary disease. N Engl J Med 318:1058, 1988

THEROUSE P et al: Aspirin, heparin or both to treat acute unstable angina. N Engl J Med 319:1105, 1988

VALLE GA: Silent ischemia: A clinical update. Chest 97(1):186, 1990

VARNAUSKAS E et al: Twelve-year follow-up of survival in the randomized European Coronary Surgery Study. N Engl J Med 319:332, 1988

191 COR PULMONALE

JOHN BUTLER

DEFINITIONS *Cor pulmonale* is the enlargement of the right ventricle due to the increase in its afterload that occurs in diseases of the thorax, lung, and pulmonary circulation; the presence of right ventricular failure is not necessary for cor pulmonale to be present. In this chapter, *right heart failure* is defined as a chronic increase in the end-diastolic transmural pressure of the right ventricle that is not expected from an increase in pulmonary blood flow. Since this definition specifies a sustained rise in transmural pressure, transient changes that normally occur with breathing and changes in posture are excluded. Right ventricular *preload* is defined as the end-diastolic transmural pressure of the ventricle; right ventricular *afterload* as the transmural pressure during systolic ejection.

NORMAL FUNCTION OF THE PULMONARY CIRCULATION

The pulmonary circulation is interposed between the right and the left ventricles for the purpose of gas exchange, the filtering out of

particles, and the chemical "conditioning" of the blood (such as the conversion of angiotensin I to angiotensin II). It is an extraordinarily efficient, low-resistance system. Normally, flow through the pulmonary vascular bed depends not only on the right ventricle but also on respiratory movements and the contraction of the left ventricle. *Respiratory motion* facilitates pulmonary blood flow by aspirating blood into the thorax on inhalation; the blood is then propelled forward by the positive pressure of exhalation acting on a one way valved system. *Left ventricular systole* assists pulmonary blood flow because the left ventricular contraction augments ejection by tensing the right ventricular wall against the bulging ventricular septum; the driving pressure across the pulmonary circulation is increased because the left ventricular end-diastolic pressure and, therefore, the downstream pulmonary vascular pressure are reduced by an effective left ventricle; the systemic venous pressure, which causes venous return, is raised by the left ventricular output; and an efficient small left ventricle reduces the total volume of blood in the cardiac fossa and lowers the right atrial pressure to aid the returning systemic venous inflow.

The right ventricle ejects blood by a milking movement in contrast to the pumping action of the left ventricle. The stroke volume of the right ventricle, as of the left (Chap. 181), depends on its afterload, preload, rate, and myocardial contractility. The afterload due to the pulmonary artery pressure is low. It depends on alterations of pulmonary blood volume as much as on changes in pulmonary blood flow. The pulmonary artery pressure normally rises when blood is displaced into the chest at the start of exercise, on assuming recumbency, or with cold, anxiety, or pain. It is astonishing that a driving pressure of only about 0.5 kPa (5 cmH$_2$O) between the pulmonary artery [average 1.5 kPa (15 cmH$_2$O)] and the left atrium [average 1.0 kPa (10 cmH$_2$O)] drives the entire cardiac output of 6 L/min or more at rest, and up to 30 L/min during exercise, through a network of such minute capillary vessels in the pulmonary vasculature.

The vascular resistance R of the pulmonary circulation (p. 877) is calculated as the intravascular driving pressure [DP = pulmonary artery pressure minus downstream intravascular pressure] divided by flow rate $\dot{Q}$. The caliber of a distensible vessel depends on its transmural pressure. R increases when vessels collapse, narrow, or lengthen, or when the viscosity of the blood increases.

$$R = \frac{Kl\mu}{r^4}$$

where K = constant
l = length
r = radius
μ = viscosity

A single value of R is obviously misleading because the relationship between driving pressure and flow is not linear through zero. There is an apparently decreasing "resistance" as flow increases because vessels are distended and recruited (Fig. 191-1).

The preload of the right ventricle is determined by the systemic venous return in relation to its contractility. Since the right ventricle constitutes a compliant reservoir for the heart, acute changes in venous return (e.g., its rise on inhalation and fall on exhalation) are accommodated with little change in pressure.

PATHOPHYSIOLOGY Sustained marked elevations in intrathoracic pressure, associated with mechanical ventilation and especially positive end-expiratory pressure (PEEP) cause intrathoracic vessels to narrow and can lead to such reductions in cardiac output as to endanger life.

Chronic dysfunction of the right ventricular myocardium is rarely a cause of right heart failure, since normally it is so thin-walled, and so much of its muscle function is provided by the left ventricle. It could be important when the muscle is hypertrophied in cor pulmonale because it can be affected by ischemic coronary artery disease. Acute right ventricular infarction, usually accompanying infarction of the inferior wall of the left ventricle (Chap. 189) but occasionally occurring

FIGURE 191-1 Relationship between flow and driving pressure ("vascular resistance") in the pulmonary circulation. Note that it does not pass through zero at the origin since an opening pressure must be overcome before flow starts. Thus the calculated vascular resistance (reciprocal of relationship of flow to pressure, dashed lines) falls (1 → 2) as flow increases. *(Modified from Graham et al., 1983.)*

as an isolated event, is one of the causes of acute right ventricular failure.

The amount of right ventricular enlargement in cor pulmonale ranges from slight to severe depending on the increase of afterload and its duration. When there is pulmonary vascular or parenchymal lung disease and the resistance to pulmonary blood flow is increased, a periodic rise in cardiac output and afterload occurs with exercise which can elevate pulmonary artery pressure markedly. Afterload is chronically augmented when lung volume is enlarged, as in obstructive airflow disease, due to the lengthening of the pulmonary vessels and the flattening of the alveolar capillaries. Afterload can also increase when lung volume is reduced in restrictive lung diseases because pulmonary vessels are compressed and distorted. Right ventricular afterload rises with hypoxic vasoconstriction, an important cause of pulmonary hypertension. Hypoxic vasoconstriction in regions of the lung affected by disease is useful in distributing blood flow to normally ventilated regions. However, the elevation in pulmonary artery pressure becomes a significant stress when the lung disease is diffuse or when the entire lung becomes hypoxic due to hypoventilation. Hypoxic vasoconstriction results from alveolar, rather than intravascular hypoxia in the adult and is made worse by hypercarbia, probably because of the associated acidosis. When the hematocrit is markedly elevated, as in cyanotic congenital heart disease, an increase in blood viscosity can intensify the pulmonary hypertension.

CLINICAL SYNDROMES

The diseases causing cor pulmonale comprise those in which the pulmonary vasculature is primarily involved, and those in which the impediment to blood flow is secondary to diseases of the lung. The main syndromes and their physiologic responses are summarized in Table 191-1.

It has been estimated that about 50,000 people die each year from embolic pulmonary vascular disease in the United States (Chap. 213). Probably half die within the first hour from acute heart failure due to massive, or multiple, emboli. Chronic cor pulmonale due to recurrent emboli or to other vascular causes is rare. More than half of patients with severe obstructive lung diseases have cor pulmonale, so this may constitute 6 or 7 percent of all adult heart diseases in the

TABLE 191-1	Cor pulmonale	
Mechanisms	Responses	Characteristics
PULMONARY VASCULAR DISEASES		
I Emboli, large or multiple	Fall in output due to acute obstruction	Acute cor pulmonale Right ventricular distention Shock
II Emboli, small; vasculitis; widespread lung damage (ARDS)	Pulmonary hypertension due to widespread hypoxia and microvascular obstruction High output	Subacute cor pulmonale Right ventricular distention Breathlessness and fever
III Emboli, medium and recurrent; primary pulmonary hypertension; diet or drug vasopathy	Pulmonary hypertension due to vascular obstruction Low or normal output	Chronic cor pulmonale Right heart hypertrophy Breathlessness
RESPIRATORY DISEASES		
I Obstructive *A* Chronic bronchitis and emphysema; chronic asthma	Pulmonary hypertension due to hypoxia, vascular stretching and loss Heart beat impeded externally by lung hyperinflation Normal or high output	Chronic cor pulmonale "Blue bloater" Underventilation
II Restrictive *A* Intrinsic: interstitial fibrosis, lung resection	Hypertension due to hypoxia, vascular distortion and loss Normal or low output	Chronic cor pulmonale Breathlessness Overventilation
B Extrinsic: obesity, myxedema, muscle weakness, kyphoscoliosis, upper airway obstruction, diminished respiratory drive, high altitude	Hypertension due to alveolar hypoxia Normal or high output	Chronic cor pulmonale Peripheral edema Underventilation

United States. It constitutes a higher percentage of all forms of heart disease in countries such as the United Kingdom, where the incidence of obstructive lung disease is higher.

PULMONARY VASCULAR DISEASES In these conditions the right ventricular afterload is elevated as a consequence of the pulmonary vascular restriction to blood flow. The pulmonary hypertension may be severe, unlike the mild rise in pressure found in parenchymal pulmonary diseases. This form of chronic cor pulmonale usually results from repeated pulmonary emboli. Sometimes it is caused by pulmonary hypertension due to vasculitis, sometimes there is a chemically induced vasospasm, and sometimes it is due to unknown causes, when it is referred to as *primary pulmonary hypertension* (Chap. 212).

Thromboembolic pulmonary vascular hypertension is quite rare because of (1) the enormous capacity of the pulmonary vascular bed, so that when some vessels are obstructed, others are recruited; and (2) the normal rapid lysis of pulmonary emboli. The right ventricle begins to fail at systolic pressures exceeding approximately 40 to 45 mmHg. However, when emboli are recurrent, or when pulmonary vascular resistance rises gradually and right ventricular hypertrophy develops, higher pressures, sometimes above systemic arterial levels, may be generated.

Cor pulmonale due to pulmonary emboli This condition is associated with three distinct syndromes, depending on whether the emboli are very numerous and large, less numerous and medium-sized, or very small.

Acute cor pulmonale due to very numerous or large emboli causes a dramatic, low-output state, quite unlike chronic cor pulmonale. It can also occur with a moderate-sized embolism if the pulmonary circulation is critically compromised by previous pulmonary vascular disease. In acute cor pulmonale, there is frequently a marked fall in cardiac output since the right ventricle is unable to generate the pressure necessary to drive blood through the compromised pulmonary vascular bed. Acute cor pulmonale is suggested by the history of a sudden onset of severe dyspnea and collapse in a patient with, or predisposed to, venous thrombosis. The low cardiac output causes pallor, sweating, hypotension, and a rapid pulse of small amplitude. The neck veins are distended and often exhibit the prominent *v* waves of tricuspid regurgitation. The liver may also be pulsatile, distended, and tender. A systolic murmur of tricuspid regurgitation at the left sternal border may be accompanied by a presystolic (S$_4$) gallop rhythm. Blood gases frequently show hypoxemia due to ventilation/perfusion mismatching and a low Pa$_{CO_2}$ due to hyperventilation. If sufficient blood flow is sustained over the critical first two or three hours, the natural thrombolytic response usually results in fragmentation of the clot to a sufficient extent that the patient can survive. Although it has been shown that treatment with thrombolytic agents lyses clots more rapidly than heparin (Chap. 213), this therapy is probably indicated only when blood flow is critically reduced and not improving.

Subacute cor pulmonale This condition is characterized by right ventricular distention and is associated with moderate pulmonary hypertension, most often due to multiple small emboli, pulmonary vascular obstruction caused by vasculitis, and/or hypoxia. Patients may present with malaise, dyspnea, and cyanosis. When septic microvascular embolization, or endotoxemia, occurs, an inflammatory edema develops, and hypoxic vasoconstriction is added to the embolic and thrombotic obstructions. In the adult respiratory distress syndrome (ARDS), the elevation in pulmonary artery pressure is usually not marked and cor pulmonale is not present. Because of the positive intrathoracic pressures of mechanical ventilation, the right ventricle is frequently small. However, sometimes the ventricle may be distended due to myocardial depression or because cardiac output is increased by hypoxia or the fever of sepsis.

Chronic cor pulmonale This condition can be caused by recurrent, medium-sized emboli that fail to lyse, particles from intravenous drug abuse, parasites, tumor tissue, or, rarely, pulmonary vascular compression caused by neoplastic diseases. *Primary pulmonary hypertension* (Chap. 212) causes chronic cor pulmonale, typically in young adult females. Chronic cor pulmonale can also be caused by any chronic widespread vasculitis such as occurs in association with the collagen vascular disorders, particularly the CREST syndrome (Chap. 271), or, occasionally, widespread radiation pneumonitis. Very rarely it is due to a vasoconstrictor arteriopathy associated with chemicals such as crotalaria, ingested as food, or drugs such as aminorex.

Symptoms and signs Breathlessness is a characteristic feature of pulmonary hypertension due to pulmonary vascular disease. In contrast to the orthopnea of left ventricular failure, it is particularly distressing during even mild exertion, and it is *not* relieved by sitting up. An unproductive cough is another frequent complaint. Occasionally there can be episodes with the production of pink, frothy sputum and radiologic changes suggestive of a patchy pulmonary edema. Anterior chest pain, due to acute dilation of the root of the pulmonary artery, can occur. The elevation in systemic venous pressure can cause hepatomegaly and ankle edema.

The patient has tachypnea that is evident on mild exertion and at rest; it may even persist during sleep. Occasionally there is cyanosis due to arterial hypoxemia and a low cardiac output. A right ventricular heave is felt in the epigastrium and a high-pitched pulmonary ejection click to the left of the upper sternum. There can be a soft midsystolic ejection murmur preceding a loud pulmonary second sound that is often palpable. The second (pulmonary) component of the second heart sound is intensified. Rarely, a diastolic murmur of pulmonary valve regurgitation is heard. There is a prominent *a* and a recognizable *v* wave in the jugular venous pulse and a systolic murmur of tricuspid regurgitation is common. The onset of right ventricular failure is reflected by an increase of venous pressure, the development of larger *v* waves associated with worse tricuspid regurgitation, a hepatojugular reflux, and a gallop rhythm with third and fourth heart sounds.

Special studies Noninvasive methods of cardiac diagnosis developed for the left heart are less useful when applied to the right side of the heart. The right ventricle is often hidden on the postero-anterior x-ray. Normally its cavity is so irregular that its volume cannot be quantitated angiographically or echocardiographically, and its muscle may be so thin that it has little influence on the ECG.

In pulmonary hypertension due to pulmonary vascular obstructions, *arterial blood gases* show hypoxia due to ventilation/perfusion mismatching and an increase in anatomic shunt. However, frequently the outstanding feature is the hypocarbia (due to the alveolar hyperventilation) that accompanies pulmonary artery hypertension. Usually there are no abnormalities on spirometry, but the ratio of dead space to tidal volume may be high, particularly when there are large vessel obstructions. The diffusing capacity of the lung is characteristically reduced when the vascular disease is severe enough to cause a capillary vasculitis and loss of capillary blood volume. Typically, exercise causes severe dyspnea with a marked fall in Pa$_{O_2}$. In practice, exercise testing may be a useful way to follow changes in the pulmonary hypertension of these patients because exercise ability is limited by cardiac output and the latter, in turn, by the severity of the pulmonary vascular obstruction.

The pulmonary trunk and hilar vessels are enlarged on *radiologic examination*. Widening of the hilum is judged from the ratio of the distance between the start of the first divisions of the right and left main pulmonary arteries divided by the transverse diameter of the thorax. A ratio >0.36 suggests pulmonary hypertension. Another indicator is simple widening of the descending right pulmonary artery shadow, usually under 16 mm, to over 20 mm. Ventilation and perfusion lung scans, and systemic venography showing deep vein thrombosis are helpful in confirming the diagnosis of embolic pulmonary vascular disease. The ECG is relatively insensitive, but is much more reliable in cor pulmonale due to pulmonary vascular diseases (in which the lung size and the position of the heart are normal) than in obstructive airflow disease. The usual findings are P pulmonale and right axis deviation.

Echocardiography allows the measurement of thickness of the right ventricular wall and, although volume changes cannot be measured, this technique can show enlargement of the right ventricular cavity in relation to that of the left ventricle. If the pulmonary valve can be imaged, its late opening, early closure, and tenseness during diastole may be used in estimating pulmonary artery pressure. Greater precision comes from the measurement of peak regurgitant tricuspid flow and pulmonic regurgitant flow with Doppler echocardiography, from which right ventricular systolic pressure can be calculated (Chap. 177).

Failure of the right ventricular ejection fraction (measured by radionuclide angiography) to increase normally on exercise appears to be a good indicator of pulmonary hypertension and/or intrinsic right ventricular dysfunction. Thallium 201 scintigraphy is also useful for diagnosing cor pulmonale, since the hypertrophied right ventricle is imaged (normally there is no visible right ventricular myocardium in relation to the marked uptake by the left ventricle).

Cardiac catheterization is necessary for the precise measurement of the pulmonary artery pressure, the calculation of pulmonary vascular resistance, and the response to oxygen and vasodilators. It is sometimes indicated to exclude congenital and left heart diseases and, in some instances, because angiography must be carried out to confirm the nature of the pulmonary vascular obstruction. Measurements of pressure and flow should be made during exercise to look for abnormal pressure increments or poor responses of cardiac output.

Lung biopsy can be useful in showing vasculitis in some types of specific pulmonary vascular disease such as the collagen vascular diseases, rheumatoid arthritis, and Wegener's granulomatosis.

RESPIRATORY DISEASES   Cor pulmonale may be caused by both obstructive and restrictive lung diseases. In these syndromes the cor pulmonale is usually associated with only modest increments of pulmonary artery pressure. Cor pulmonale is much more commonly due to obstructive than to restrictive disease, partly because restrictive lung disorders have a much lower life expectancy once they reach the stage of cor pulmonale. Respiratory diseases are usually associated with local or generalized distortions of lung volume which affect the position and, perhaps, function of the heart, so that physical signs and special studies in this type of cor pulmonale tend to be blurred by noncardiac factors.

CHRONIC OBSTRUCTIVE LUNG DISEASE (COLD) (See Chap. 210)   This is the most common cause of chronic cor pulmonale. The enlargement of the right ventricle is attributed to the mild-to-moderate pulmonary hypertension which is common in severe obstructive bronchitis and emphysema and rare (though not unknown) in asthma. Pulmonary artery systolic pressure is typically in the range of 30 to 50 mmHg, far below the systemic levels which appear to be tolerated in congenital heart disease and in normal people native to high altitudes.

The pulmonary hypertension is due to the generalized pulmonary vasoconstriction caused by the alveolar hypoxia and hypercarbia, the mechanical effects of the high lung volume on the pulmonary vessels, the loss of small vessels in the vascular bed in regions of emphysema, and the increased blood viscosity caused by the frequently associated polycythemia. Of these, the first is undoubtedly the most important. Pulmonary artery pressure rises further on exercise. The pulmonary artery pressure is decreased acutely by oxygen breathing, but not to normal, so chronic (home) oxygen therapy is often helpful. Cardiac output tends to be high in the absence of heart failure if hypoxia and hypercarbia are present. Because of the importance of hypoxic pulmonary vasoconstriction in causing pulmonary hypertension, the hypoventilating "blue bloater" patient with alveolar hypoxia and hypercarbia is characterized by cor pulmonale, while the emphysematous "pink puffer," without alveolar hypoxia, is less affected. Ischemic left heart disease is a frequent complication in these cigarette-smoking patients and there could be a rise in pulmonary artery pressure secondary, in part, to the increase in left atrial pressure resulting from left heart dysfunction. Almost half of all patients who die with cor pulmonale due to obstructive airflow disease also have left ventricular hypertrophy.

Right ventricular failure may be difficult to diagnose in obstructive lung disease. It appears to complicate cor pulmonale in the stage of ventilatory failure with hypoxia and hypercarbia. When there is a worsening of the airflow due to an increasing obstruction or asthmatic deterioration, the hypoxia and hypercarbia increase cardiac output by their direct vasodilator effects on systemic arterioles. Hypoxic pulmonary vasospasm is intensified, arrhythmias are common complications, and right heart failure ensues. The liver becomes palpable and tender because it is both swollen and displaced by the low diaphragm. A hepatojugular reflux is present. There is also a "square-wave" response to the Valsalva maneuver, a prolonged expiratory pressure against a closed glottis. This square wave response is a sustained rise in systemic blood pressure, with no bradycardia on releasing the positive pressure, rather than the normal rise and then fall in pressure with a characteristic bradycardia on release.

Any exacerbation of obstructive lung disease leads to a mechanical impediment to venous return which causes a difficult diagnostic problem in deciding whether or not right heart failure is present. The increase in obstruction to airflow is associated with prolonged exhalation, during which all of the intrathoracic pressures are more positive, and a high functional residual capacity that raises pressure around the heart relative to the normal subcostal pressures. The raised pressure around the heart impedes venous return and leads to a raised jugular venous pressure and peripheral edema. Yet this is not right

ventricular failure since the transmural filling pressure and pulmonary blood flow response to a sustained stress are normal.

Pathology   In obstructive airflow disease the right ventricular hypertrophy increases with time. The main pulmonary arteries are enlarged and the muscular pulmonary arteries show the development of prominent longitudinal muscle, together with prominent fibrosis and elastic changes, that continues into the arterioles, where the media also becomes muscularized. The small vessels and capillaries are distorted or disappear in regions of hyperinflation which sometimes greatly reduces the vascular bed.

Symptoms and signs   The history of a productive cough and dyspnea, perhaps with wheezing, frequently reflects the severity of the addiction to cigarette smoking. Breathlessness limits the patient's ability in the minor stresses of daily living. Frequently there is a history of emergency hospital admissions because of respiratory infection, sometimes necessitating mechanical ventilation. There may have been increasing somnolence on breathing oxygen, or other symptoms of hypercarbia such as recurring headaches, confusion, and even vomiting which, combined with blurred optic discs (also due to cerebral vasodilation), constitutes the "pseudo tumor cerebri" syndrome. Hypoxia due to hypoventilation is usually worse at night, particularly when severe snoring leads to episodes of obstructive apnea (Chap. 217).

Physical findings   These are of the obstructive airflow disease, together with a raised jugular venous pressure, a palpable liver, and ankle edema. Often there is nicotine staining of the fingers. The skin may be warm and the arterial pulse bounding in the high cardiac output state induced by hypoxia and hypercarbia. The chest distention due to the obstructive airflow and the rhonchi and wheezes due to the chronic bronchitis usually makes cardiac auscultation difficult. However, a protodiastolic (third) heart sound and a systolic murmur of tricuspid regurgitant may be audible. Signs of right heart failure are, as discussed above, difficult to separate from those due to severe airflow obstruction. However, a sudden worsening of peripheral edema and rise of systemic venous pressure when atrial fibrillation occurs or when pulmonary infection supervenes is usually considered as showing heart failure. This may be confirmed by the positive hepatojugular reflux and Valsalva responses described above. The distinction is important since patients can survive for years with the high systemic venous pressure and edema that are part of the airflow obstruction syndrome, yet usually have a poor prognosis after right heart failure develops.

Special studies   *Pulmonary function studies* show marked airflow obstruction with severe hypoxemia and hypercarbia. Exercise is limited by ventilatory rather than cardiac dysfunction until right ventricular failure develops.

The *chest roentgenogram* reveals an increased total lung capacity (hyperinflation) which makes the degree of right heart enlargement difficult to assess. The central pulmonary arteries are large but the vessels are narrowed and disappear at the periphery, particularly in regions of the lungs which are markedly emphysematous. The ECG is relatively insensitive because the enlarged lungs characteristic of obstructive airflow disease are poor electrical conductors and the inspiratory position of the chest is associated with a vertical and leftwardly rotated position of the heart. If it does show right axis deviation, right ventricular hypertrophy, and right atrial enlargement as P pulmonale, with inferior shift of the P vector, there can be little doubt that cor pulmonale is present. Arrhythmias, particularly atrial fibrillation and multifocal atrial tachycardia, are common.

Echocardiographic imaging is often difficult because of the air in the distended lungs and the closeness of the densely reflective sternum, but may reveal an increased cross section of the right ventricular cavity and a greater thickness of the right ventricular wall. Myocardial scintigraphy shows an abnormally high ratio of right to left ventricular ^{201}Tl uptake; at present this is probably the most accurate noninvasive way of documenting an increased right ventricular muscle mass.

Right heart catheterization is usually unnecessary. It can be done at the bedside with a balloon-tipped, flow-directed, multichannel catheter fitted with thermocouples for measuring cardiac output by thermodilution (Chap. 179). The "balloon wedge" pressure measured through the catheter shows a normal left atrial pressure at rest in patients with uncomplicated cor pulmonale. However, cardiac catheterization is useful in assessing left ventricular function, the severity of the pulmonary hypertension and its response to oxygen breathing. An exercise study is helpful, particularly in excluding left heart dysfunction when a possible left heart abnormality has been found, for instance, by echocardiography.

Treatment This is aimed at correcting the alveolar hypoxia by judiciously increasing the inspired O_2 concentration (FI_{O_2}) (ventilation is, in part, driven by hypoxia in these patients) and by improving alveolar ventilation by relieving the airflow obstruction. When the lung disease improves and hypoxic vasospasm due to the alveolar hypoxia and hypercarbia are corrected, tachypnea, and thus overdistension due to gas trapping, lessens. The signs attributed to right heart failure are relieved. Bronchodilators and antibiotics lessen the airflow obstruction and diuretics relieve the edema.

In view of the possibility that part of the afterload of the ventricles is due to the external load from the necessary systolic distortion of the surrounding distended lungs, it is particularly interesting that recent studies have shown that the severity of the cor pulmonale in these patients is related more to the mechanical abnormalities of the lung function than the height of the pulmonary artery pressure.

RESTRICTIVE LUNG DISEASES Cor pulmonale in restrictive lung disease is associated with two different clinical syndromes: (1) hyperventilation in patients with "intrinsic" restrictive diseases or space-occupying intrathoracic lesions; and (2) hypoventilation in patients with "extrinsic" diseases, such as obesity, myxedema, or severe neuromuscular dysfunction. Pulmonary hypertension is due to the hypoxemia and to the increased pulmonary vascular resistance resulting from compression of the pulmonary circulation. Again, oxygen is the main treatment, but specific therapy may be available for some of the underlying lung diseases.

Combined obstructive airflow and restrictive lung disease has a particularly grim outlook. It frequently occurs in patients with a restrictive disease who smoke cigarettes.

PROGNOSIS Although prognosis in cor pulmonale is based on the degree of pulmonary hypertension, the presence of cor pulmonale is difficult to relate to the distress and morbidity of patients with obstructive airflow disease. However, it appears that death due to right ventricular failure per se is very rare compared with death due to the underlying pulmonary disease in these patients.

REFERENCES

GRAHAM R et al: Dopamine, Dobutamine and Phenotolamine effects on pulmonary vascular mechanics. J Appl Physiol 54:1277, 1983

MATHAY RA et al: Pulmonary artery hypertension in chronic obstructive pulmonary disease: Determination by chest radiography. Invest Radiol 16:95, 1981

McDONALD IG, BUTLER J: Distribution of vascular resistance in the isolated, perfused dog lung. J Appl Physiol 23:463, 1967

McFADDEN FR, BRAUNWALD E: Cor pulmonale and pulmonary thromboembolism, in Heart Disease, E Braunwald (ed). Philadelphia, Saunders, 1988, 3d ed, pp 1597–1616

PERMUTT S et al: Interaction between the circulatory and ventilatory pumps, in Thorax, Part 3, vol 29: Lung Biology in Health and Disease, C Roussos, PT Macklem (eds). New York, Marcel Dekker, 1985, pp 701–735

WIDIMSKY J: Non-invasive diagnosis of pulmonary hypertension in chronic lung diseases. Prog Resp Res 20:69, 1985

WILKINSON M et al: A pathophysiological study of 10 cases of hypoxic cor pulmonale. Q J Med, N.S. 66, 249:65, 1988

192 THE CARDIOMYOPATHIES AND MYOCARDITIDES

JOSHUA WYNNE / EUGENE BRAUNWALD

CARDIOMYOPATHY

The cardiomyopathies are diseases that involve the myocardium primarily and are not the result of hypertension or congenital, valvular, coronary, arterial, or pericardial abnormalities.[1] When the cardiomyopathies are classified on an etiologic basis, two fundamental forms are recognized: (1) a primary type, consisting of heart muscle disease of unknown cause; (2) a secondary type, consisting of myocardial disease of known cause, or associated with a disease involving other organ systems (Table 192-1). In many cases it is not possible to arrive at an etiologic diagnosis on clinical grounds, and thus it is often more desirable to classify the cardiomyopathies on the basis of differences in their pathophysiology and clinical presentation (Tables 192-2 and 192-3). The distinction between the functional categories is not absolute, however, and there is often some overlap.

DILATED (CONGESTIVE) CARDIOMYOPATHY Left and/or right ventricular systolic pump function is impaired, leading to cardiac enlargement and often producing symptoms of congestive heart failure. Mural thrombi are often present, particularly in the left ventricular apex. Histologic examination reveals extensive areas of interstitial and perivascular fibrosis, with minimal necrosis and cellular infiltration. Although no cause is apparent in many cases, dilated cardiomyopathy (formerly called congestive cardiomyopathy) is probably the end result of myocardial damage produced by a variety of toxic, metabolic, or infectious agents. There is increasing evidence to suggest that in at least some patients dilated cardiomyopathy may be the late sequel of acute viral myocarditis, possibly mediated through an immunologic mechanism. Although most commonly a disease of middle-aged men, it may occur in any patient population. A reversible form of dilated cardiomyopathy may be found with selenium deficiency, hypophosphatemia, hypocalcemia, and chronic uncontrolled tachycardia. A small number of patients have familial forms of the disease; in some, there is evidence of X-linked inheritance. *Right ventricular dysplasia* is a unique cardiomyopathy marked by progressive replacement of the right ventricular wall with adipose tissue. Often associated with ventricular arrhythmias, the clinical course is variable; sudden death is a constant threat.

Clinical manifestations Symptoms of left- and right-sided congestive failure, manifested by dyspnea on exertion, fatigue, orthopnea, paroxysmal nocturnal dyspnea, peripheral edema, and palpitations, develop gradually in most patients. Some patients have left ventricular dilatation for months or even years before becoming symptomatic. Although vague chest pain may be present, typical angina pectoris is unusual and suggests the presence of concomitant coronary artery disease.

Physical examination Variable degrees of cardiac enlargement and findings of congestive heart failure are noted. In patients with advanced disease, the pulse pressure is small, and the jugular venous pressure is elevated. Third and fourth heart sounds are common, and mitral or tricuspid regurgitation may occur. Diastolic murmurs, valvular calcification, hypertension, and changes of vascular disease in the optic fundi militate *against* the diagnosis of cardiomyopathy.

Laboratory examinations The chest roentgenogram demonstrates left ventricular enlargement, although generalized cardiomegaly is often seen, sometimes due to a concomitant pericardial effusion.

---

[1] Diffuse myocardial fibrosis secondary to multiple myocardial scars produced by extensive coronary arterial narrowing and occlusion can impair left ventricular function and is frequently referred to as ischemic cardiomyopathy. According to the definition given above, however, the term *cardiomyopathy* should be restricted to a condition *primarily* involving heart muscle. In ischemic "cardiomyopathy" the *primary* involvement is in the coronary vessels.

TABLE 192-1   Etiologic classification of cardiomyopathies

I Primary myocardial involvement
  A Idiopathic (D,R,H)
  B Familial (D,H)
  C Eosinophilic endomyocardial disease (R)
  D Endomyocardial fibrosis (R)
II Secondary myocardial involvement
  A Infective (D)
    1 Viral myocarditis
    2 Bacterial myocarditis
    3 Fungal myocarditis
    4 Protozoal myocarditis
    5 Metazoal myocarditis
  B Metabolic (D)
  C Familial storage disease (D,R)
    1 Glycogen storage disease
    2 Mucopolysaccharidoses
  D Deficiency (D)
    1 Electrolytes
    2 Nutritional
  E Connective tissue disorders (D)
    1 Systemic lupus erythematosus
    2 Polyarteritis nodosa
    3 Rheumatoid arthritis
    4 Progressive systemic sclerosis
    5 Dermatomyositis
  F Infiltrations and granulomas (R,D)
    1 Amyloidosis
    2 Sarcoidosis
    3 Malignancy
    4 Hemochromatosis
  G Neuromuscular (D)
    1 Muscular dystrophy
    2 Myotonic dystrophy
    3 Friedreich's ataxia (H,D)
    4 Refsum's disease
  H Sensitivity and toxic reactions (D)
    1 Alcohol
    2 Radiation
    3 Drugs
  I Peripartum heart disease (D)
  J Endocardial fibroelastosis (R)

NOTE: The principal clinical manifestation(s) of each etiologic grouping is denoted by D (dilated), R (restrictive), or H (hypertrophic) cardiomyopathy.
SOURCE: Adapted from the WHO/ISFC task force report on the definition and classification of cardiomyopathies, 1980.

TABLE 192-2   Clinical classification of cardiomyopathies

1 Dilated (congestive): Left and/or right ventricular enlargement, impaired systolic function, congestive heart failure, arrhythmias, emboli

2 Restrictive: Endomyocardial scarring or myocardial infiltration resulting in restriction to left and/or right ventricular filling

3 Hypertrophic: Disproportionate left ventricular hypertrophy, typically involving septum more than free wall, with or without an intraventricular systolic pressure gradient; usually of a nondilated left ventricular cavity

The lung fields may demonstrate evidence of pulmonary venous hypertension and interstitial or alveolar edema. The electrocardiogram often shows sinus tachycardia or atrial fibrillation, ventricular arrhythmias, left atrial enlargement, diffuse nonspecific ST-T-wave abnormalities, and sometimes intraventricular conduction defects. Echocardiography (Fig. 177-4) and radionuclide ventriculography (Fig. 177-6) show left ventricular enlargement, with normal or minimally thickened or thinned walls, and systolic dysfunction (reduced ejection fraction); a pericardial effusion is often noted. Radioisotopic imaging with gallium 67 may identify patients with dilated cardiomyopathy and myocarditis.

Hemodynamic studies reveal a cardiac output that may be normal, or moderately to severely reduced at rest; it does not increase normally with exercise. The left ventricular end-diastolic, left atrial, and pulmonary capillary wedge pressures usually are elevated; when failure of the right side of the heart supervenes, the right ventricular end-diastolic, right atrial, and central venous pressures are also elevated. Angiography reveals a dilated, diffusely hypokinetic left ventricle, often with some degree of mitral regurgitation; the coronary arteries are normal, thereby excluding so-called ischemic cardiomyopathy. Transvenous endomyocardial biopsy (Chap. 179) may be helpful in excluding certain conditions such as myocardial infiltration by amyloid; in some patients there is biopsy evidence of myocardial round cell inflammation, suggesting an inflammatory etiology and compatible with previous viral myocarditis.

Treatment   Most patients pursue an inexorably downhill course, and the majority, particularly those over 55 years of age, die within 2 years of the onset of symptoms, but spontaneous improvement or stabilization occurs in a minority. Death is due to either congestive heart failure or ventricular arrhythmia; sudden death, presumably arrhythmic in etiology, is a constant threat. Systemic embolization is common, and all patients without contraindications should receive anticoagulants. Strenuous exertion should be interdicted. Treatment of heart failure in dilated cardiomyopathy primarily is directed toward improvement in symptoms; a modest improvement in longevity is achieved with specific vasodilator therapy (hydralazine-nitrate combination and enalapril). Standard therapy of heart failure with salt restriction, diuretics, digitalis, and vasodilators may produce symptomatic improvement, at least in the initial phases of the illness; however, these patients appear to be at increased risk of digitalis toxicity. Some patients with dilated cardiomyopathy who have evidence of myocardial inflammation have been treated with corticosteroids, often in association with azathioprine; others have been treated cautiously with gradually increasing doses of beta-adrenergic blockers. However, the indications and value of such experimental therapy remain controversial. Antiarrhythmic agents may be used to

TABLE 192-3   Laboratory evaluation of the cardiomyopathies

	Dilated (congestive)	Restrictive	Hypertrophic
Chest roentgenogram	Moderate to marked cardiac enlargement Pulmonary venous hypertension	Mild cardiac enlargement	Mild to moderate cardiac enlargement
Electrocardiogram	ST-segment and T-wave abnormalities	Low-voltage Conduction defects	ST-segment and T-wave abnormalities Left ventricular hypertrophy Abnormal Q waves
Echocardiogram	Left ventricular dilatation and dysfunction	Increased left ventricular wall thickness Normal systolic function	Asymmetric septal hypertrophy (ASH) Systolic anterior motion (SAM) of the mitral valve
Radionuclide studies	Left ventricular dilatation and dysfunction (RVG)	Normal systolic function (RVG)	Vigorous systolic function (RVG) Asymmetric septal hypertrophy (RVG or ^{201}Tl)
Cardiac catheterization	Left ventricular dilatation and dysfunction Elevated left- and often right-sided filling pressures Diminished cardiac output	Normal systolic function Elevated left- and right-sided filling pressures	Vigorous systolic function Dynamic left ventricular outflow obstruction Elevated left- and right-sided filling pressures

NOTE: RVG = radionuclide ventriculogram; ^{201}Tl = thallium 201.

treat symptomatic or serious arrhythmias, although they may be extremely resistant to the usual as well as investigational agents. Because of this, alternative experimental therapies, such as surgical interruption of the arrhythmic circuit or implantation of an automatic internal defibrillator, have gained favor. In patients with advanced disease who are refractory to medical therapy and who have no contraindications to the procedure, cardiac transplantation should be considered (Chap. 183).

Alcoholic cardiomyopathy Individuals who consume large quantities of alcohol over many years may develop a clinical picture identical to idiopathic dilated cardiomyopathy; indeed, alcoholic cardiomyopathy is the major form of secondary dilated cardiomyopathy in the western world. Ceasing alcohol consumption before severe heart failure has developed may halt the progression, or even reverse the course of this disease, unlike the idiopathic variety, which is marked by progressive deterioration. Alcoholics with advanced heart failure have a poor prognosis, particularly if they continue to drink; less than one-quarter survive 3 years. The key to the treatment of alcoholic cardiomyopathy is total and permanent abstinence. Although thiamine deficiency may be present in some of these patients, alcoholic cardiomyopathy is associated with a low cardiac output and systemic vasoconstriction. In contrast, beriberi heart disease (Chaps. 76 and 194) is characterized by elevated cardiac output and diminished peripheral vascular resistance, so that thiamine deficiency per se does not appear to cause alcoholic cardiomyopathy. A second presentation of alcoholic cardiotoxicity may be found in individuals without overt heart failure, and consists of recurrent supraventricular or ventricular tachyarrhythmias. Termed the "holiday heart syndrome," it typically appears after a drinking binge; atrial fibrillation is seen most frequently, followed by atrial flutter and ventricular premature depolarizations. Some patients develop left ventricular hypertrophy, perhaps related to concomitant systemic hypertension; they may present with symptoms of pulmonary congestion due to abnormal diastolic stiffness (diminished compliance) of the left ventricle.

Peripartum cardiomyopathy Cardiac dilatation and congestive heart failure of unexplained cause may develop during the last month of pregnancy or within the first few months after delivery. The etiology of this disorder is unknown but may relate to a preexisting cardiomyopathy that was not apparent prior to pregnancy. Necropsy shows cardiac enlargement, often with mural thrombi, along with histologic evidence of myocardial degeneration and fibrosis. The patient who develops peripartum cardiomyopathy is typically multiparous, black, and over the age of 30. While some patients are malnourished, there is no conclusive evidence that dietary deficiencies are etiologically involved. The symptoms, signs, and treatment are similar to those in patients with idiopathic dilated cardiomyopathy; pulmonary and systemic emboli are particularly common. The mortality rate may be as high as 25 to 50 percent. The prognosis in these patients appears to be closely related to whether the heart size returns to normal after the first episode of congestive heart failure. If it does, subsequent pregnancies may sometimes be well tolerated; if the heart remains enlarged, however, further pregnancies frequently produce increasing myocardial damage, ultimately leading to refractory congestive heart failure and death. Those who recover should be encouraged to avoid further pregnancies, particularly if cardiomegaly persists.

Neuromuscular disease (See also Chap. 365) Cardiac involvement is common in many of the muscular dystrophies. In *Duchenne's progressive muscular dystrophy*, myocardial involvement is most frequently indicated by a distinctive and unique electrocardiographic pattern consisting of tall R waves in right precordial leads with an R/S ratio greater than 1.0, often associated with deep Q waves in the limb and lateral precordial leads, and is not found in other forms of muscular dystrophy. These electrocardiographic abnormalities appear to result from selective transmural necrosis of the posterobasal left ventricle and associated papillary muscle. A variety of supraventricular and ventricular arrhythmias is frequently found. Rapidly progressive congestive heart failure may develop despite extended periods of

apparent circulatory stability during which the only detectable abnormalities are in the electrocardiogram. *Myotonic dystrophy* is characterized by a variety of electrocardiographic abnormalities, especially disorders of impulse formation and particularly conduction, but other overt clinical evidence of heart disease is uncommon. Because of the abnormalities of impulse generation and conduction, syncope and sudden death are major hazards; in appropriate patients, insertion of a permanent pacemaker may be efficacious. In *limb-girdle* and *fascioscapulohumeral dystrophy,* cardiac involvement is uncommon and seldom severe. Involvement of the heart is very common in *Friedreich's ataxia* (manifested by abnormal electrocardiographic or echocardiographic findings), with as many as half of the patients developing cardiac symptoms. The electrocardiogram most commonly demonstrates ST-segment and T-wave abnormalities. The echocardiogram may demonstrate left ventricular hypertrophy, with either symmetric or asymmetric hypertrophy of the left ventricular septum compared with the free wall. Although morphologically similar to some cases of hypertrophic cardiomyopathy, cellular disarray is lacking.

Drugs A variety of pharmacologic agents may damage the myocardium acutely, producing a pattern of inflammation (myocarditis), or they may lead to chronic damage of the type seen with idiopathic dilated cardiomyopathy. Certain drugs produce only electrocardiographic abnormalities, while others may precipitate fulminant congestive heart failure and death. The anthracycline derivatives, particularly *doxorubicin* (Adriamycin), are powerful antineoplastic agents, which, when given in high doses (more than 550 mg/m^2 for doxorubicin), may produce fatal heart failure. The incidence of heart failure is related not only to the dose of the drug but to the presence or absence of several risk factors (cardiac irradiation, age greater than 70 years, underlying heart disease, hypertension, treatment with cyclophosphamide); at any dose patients with these risk factors have an eight- to tenfold greater frequency of developing heart failure than do patients lacking them. Radionuclide ventriculography (Chap. 177) may document preclinical deterioration of left ventricular function and allow appropriate dose adjustments; by so monitoring left ventricular function, it is often possible to continue doxorubicin even in patients at high risk for developing heart failure. Recent efforts to modify the dose schedule by giving the drug more slowly have further reduced the risk of cardiotoxicity. Some patients with congestive heart failure, even those with severe depression of left ventricular function, have demonstrated recovery of cardiac function with aggressive management with digitalis, diuretics, and vasodilators. High-dose *cyclophosphamide* may produce congestive heart failure acutely or within 2 weeks of administration; a characteristic histopathologic feature is myocardial edema and hemorrhagic necrosis. Rarely, patients treated with *5-fluorouracil* will develop chest pain and electrocardiographic changes of myocardial ischemia or infarction. Electrocardiographic changes and arrhythmias may result from treatment with tricyclic antidepressants, the phenothiazines, emetine, lithium, and various acrosol propellants. *Cocaine abuse* is associated with a variety of life-threatening cardiac complications, including sudden death, myocarditis, and acute myocardial infarction (resulting from coronary spasm and/or thrombosis with or without underlying coronary artery stenosis).

RESTRICTIVE CARDIOMYOPATHY The hallmark of the restrictive cardiomyopathies is abnormal diastolic function; the ventricular walls are excessively rigid and impede ventricular filling. Myocardial fibrosis, hypertrophy, or infiltration secondary to a variety of etiologies is usually responsible. The infiltrative diseases, which represent important etiologies for secondary restrictive cardiomyopathy, may also show some impairment of systolic function. Myocardial involvement with *amyloid* is a common cause of secondary restrictive cardiomyopathy, although restriction is also seen in hemochromatosis, glycogen deposition, endomyocardial fibrosis, fibroelastosis, the eosinophilias, neoplastic infiltration, and myocardial fibrosis of diverse causes. In many of these conditions, particularly those with substantial concomitant endocardial involvement, partial obliteration of the ventricular cavity by fibrous tissue and thrombus contributes to the abnormally increased resistance to ventricular filling. As a result of persistently elevated venous pressure these patients commonly have dependent edema, ascites, and an enlarged, tender liver. The jugular venous pressure is elevated and does not fall normally, or it may rise with inspiration (Kussmaul's sign). The heart sounds may be distant, and third and fourth heart sounds are common. In contrast to constrictive pericarditis, which these diseases resemble, the apex impulse is usually easily palpable. The electrocardiogram shows low-voltage, nonspecific ST-T-wave changes and various arrhythmias. Pericardial calcification on x-ray, which would suggest constrictive pericarditis, is absent. Echocardiography typically reveals symmetrically thickened left ventricular walls and normal or slightly reduced systolic function. Cardiac catheterization shows a decreased cardiac output, elevation of the right and left ventricular end-diastolic pressures, and a dip-and-plateau configuration of the diastolic portion of the ventricular pressure pulse resembling that seen in constrictive pericarditis.

Differentiation from constrictive pericarditis, at the bedside and even after cardiac catheterization, may be difficult or impossible (Chaps. 179 and 193). This distinction is of importance because the latter condition is potentially curable by operation. Helpful in the differentiation of these two diseases are right ventricular transvenous endomyocardial biopsy (by revealing interstitial infiltration or fibrosis in restrictive cardiomyopathy) and computed tomography or magnetic resonance imaging (by demonstrating a thickened pericardium in constrictive pericarditis).

Endomyocardial fibrosis   This is a progressive disease of unknown etiology that occurs most commonly in children and young adults residing in tropical and subtropical Africa, particularly Uganda and Nigeria. The disease is characterized by fibrous endocardial lesions of the inflow portion of the right or left ventricle (or both) and often involves the atrioventricular valves, producing valvular regurgitation. The apex of the ventricles may be obliterated by a mass of thrombus and fibrous tissue. In many ways this disease resembles eosinophilic endomyocardial disease, although they occur in quite different geographic areas and age groups. Endomyocardial fibrosis is a frequent cause of heart failure in Africa, accounting for up to one-quarter of deaths due to heart disease.

The clinical picture depends upon which ventricle and atrioventricular valve show predominant involvement; left-sided involvement results in symptoms of pulmonary congestion, while predominant right-sided disease presents features of a restrictive cardiomyopathy. Medical treatment is often disappointing, and surgical excision of the fibrotic endocardium and replacement of the involved atrioventricular valve has led to substantial symptomatic improvement in a small number of patients.

Eosinophilic endomyocardial disease   Also called *Loeffler's endocarditis* and *fibroplastic endocarditis*, this disease appears to be a subcategory of the hypereosinophilic syndrome in which the heart is predominantly involved. Typically, the endocardium of either or both ventricles thickens markedly, with involvement of the underlying myocardium. Large mural thrombi may develop in either ventricle, thereby compromising the size of the ventricular cavity and serving as a source of pulmonary and systemic emboli. Hepatosplenomegaly and localized eosinophilic infiltration of other organs are usually present. Routine management with digitalis, diuretics, afterload-reducing agents, and anticoagulation as indicated, in conjunction with glucocorticoids and cytotoxic drugs (hydroxyurea in particular), appears to have improved survival substantially.

Differential diagnosis   Involvement of the heart is the most frequent cause of death in *primary amyloidosis* (Chap. 266), while clinically significant cardiac involvement is uncommon in the secondary form. Focal deposits of amyloid in elderly patients (*senile cardiac amyloidosis*) is common and usually clinically insignificant. In a minority of patients the clinical cardiac findings are identical to those of primary amyloidosis, the principal difference being the structural composition of the amyloid protein. Biopsy of the rectal mucosa, gingiva, liver, kidney, and myocardium permits the diagnosis to be made before death in over three-quarters of cases. The heart is firm, rubbery, and noncompliant, and four clinical presentations (alone or in combination) are seen: (1) diastolic dysfunction (restrictive cardiomyopathy); (2) systolic dysfunction; (3) arrhythmias; and (4) orthostatic hypotension. The two-dimensional echocardiogram may be helpful in making the diagnosis of amyloidosis and may show a thickened myocardial wall with a distinctive "speckled" appearance. *Hemochromatosis* (Chap. 327) should be suspected if cardiomyopathy occurs in the setting of diabetes mellitus, hepatic cirrhosis, and increased skin pigmentation. Phlebotomy may be of some benefit if employed early in the course of the disease. Continuous subcutaneous administration of deferoxamine may reduce body iron stores in advanced cases, but whether this produces clinical improvement is unclear. Myocardial *sarcoidosis* (Chap. 277) is generally associated with other manifestations of systemic disease and may have restrictive as well as congestive features, since cardiac infiltration by sarcoid granulomas results not only in increased stiffness of the myocardium but also in diminished systolic contractile function. A variety of arrhythmias, including atrioventricular block, have been noted. *Endocardial fibroelastosis* is a disease seen in infants, characterized by a thickened endocardium that shows proliferation of elastic tissue. It is most unusual in adult patients, although small patches of it may be found in patients with endomyocardial fibrosis.

HYPERTROPHIC CARDIOMYOPATHY   This disease is characterized by left ventricular hypertrophy, typically of a nondilated chamber, without obvious antecedent cause. The hypertrophy is thus not secondary to a cardiovascular or systemic disease, such as hypertension or aortic stenosis, that places a hemodynamic burden on the left ventricle. Two commonly found features of the disease have attracted the greatest attention: (1) heterogeneous left ventricular (LV) hypertrophy, often with asymmetric septal hypertrophy (ASH), wherein the upper portion of the interventricular septum is preferentially hypertrophied compared to the posterobasal left ventricular free wall; and (2) a dynamic left ventricular outflow tract pressure gradient, related to narrowing of the subaortic area as a consequence of the midsystolic apposition of the anterior mitral valve leaflet against the hypertrophied septum, i.e., systolic anterior motion of the mitral valve (SAM). Initial studies of this disease emphasized the dynamic "obstructive" features, and it has been termed idiopathic hypertrophic subaortic stenosis (IHSS), hypertrophic obstructive cardiomyopathy (HOCM), and muscular subaortic stenosis. It has become clear, however, that only about one-quarter of patients with hypertrophic cardiomyopathy demonstrate an outflow tract gradient. The ubiquitous pathophysiologic abnormality is not systolic but rather *diastolic* dysfunction, characterized by increased stiffness of the hypertrophied muscle. This results in elevated diastolic filling pressures and is present despite a hyperdynamic left ventricle.

The pattern of hypertrophy is distinctive in hypertrophic cardiomyopathy and differs from that seen in secondary hypertrophy (as in hypertension). Most patients have striking regional variations in the extent of hypertrophy in different portions of the left ventricle, and the majority demonstrate a ventricular septum whose thickness is disproportionately increased when compared with the free wall. Other patients may demonstrate disproportionate involvement of the apex or left ventricular free wall; 10 percent or more of patients have concentric involvement of the ventricle. All, however, show a bizarre and disorganized arrangement of cardiac muscle cells in the septum, whether or not a gradient is present, along with a variable degree of myocardial fibrosis and abnormalities of the small intramural coronary arteries.

About half of all cases of hypertrophic cardiomyopathy appear to be transmitted as autosomal dominants with a variable degree of expression and penetrance; there is considerable variability in the extent of hypertrophy and symptoms even in close relatives. The remainder of cases appear to occur sporadically, but some may represent new mutations. Echocardiographic studies have confirmed that about one-third of the first-degree relatives (i.e., parents, siblings, and children) of patients with familial hypertrophic cardiomyopathy have evidence of the disease, although in many of these patients the extent of hypertrophy is mild, no outflow tract pressure gradient is present, and symptoms are not prominent. Since the hypertrophic characteristics may not be apparent in childhood and only first appear in adolescence, a single normal echocardiogram in a child does not entirely exclude the presence of the disease.

In contrast to the obstruction produced by a fixed narrowed orifice, such as valvular aortic stenosis, the pressure gradient in hypertrophic cardiomyopathy, when present, is dynamic and may change between examinations and even from beat to beat. Obstruction appears to result from further narrowing of an already small left ventricular outflow tract by systolic anterior motion of the mitral valve against the hypertrophied septum. While SAM may be found in a variety of other conditions besides hypertrophic cardiomyopathy, it is *always* found when obstruction is present in hypertrophic cardiomyopathy. Three basic mechanisms are involved in the production of the dynamic pressure gradient: (1) increased left ventricular contractility, which reduces left ventricular systolic volume and increases the ejection velocity of the blood moving through the outflow tract, thus drawing the anterior mitral valve leaflet against the septum as a result of reduced distending pressure; (2) decreased ventricular volume (preload), which reduces further the size of the outflow tract; and (3) decreased aortic impedance and pressure (afterload), which increases the velocity of flow through the subaortic area and also reduces ventricular systolic volume. Interventions that increase myocardial contractility, such as exercise, isoproterenol, and digitalis glycosides, and those that reduce ventricular volume, such as the Valsalva maneuver, sudden standing, nitroglycerin, amyl nitrite, or tachycardia, all may cause an increase in the gradient and the murmur. Conversely, elevation of arterial pressure by phenylephrine, squatting, sustained handgrip, augmentation of venous return by passive leg raising, and expansion of the blood volume all increase ventricular volume and ameliorate the gradient and murmur. Sometimes the hypertrophied septum bulges into the outflow tract of the right ventricle, thereby impeding the ejection of blood from this chamber as well.

Clinical features   Many patients with hypertrophic cardiomyopathy are asymptomatic and may be relatives of patients with known disease. Unfortunately, the first clinical manifestation of the disease may be sudden death, frequently occurring in children and young adults, often during or after physical exertion. In symptomatic patients the most common complaint is dyspnea, largely due to increased stiffness of the left ventricular walls, which impairs ventricular filling and leads to elevated left ventricular diastolic and left atrial pressures. Other symptoms include angina pectoris, fatigue, syncope, and near syncope ("graying-out spells"). Symptoms are not related to the presence or severity of an outflow gradient. Most patients with gradients demonstrate a double or triple apical impulse, a rapidly rising carotid arterial pulse, and a fourth heart sound. The hallmark of obstructive hypertrophic cardiomyopathy is a systolic murmur, which is typically harsh, diamond-shaped, and usually begins well after the first heart sound, since ejection is unimpeded early in systole. The murmur is best heard at the lower left sternal border as well as at the apex, where it is often more holosystolic and blowing in quality, no doubt due to the mitral regurgitation that usually accompanies obstructive hypertrophic cardiomyopathy.

Laboratory evaluation   The *electrocardiogram* commonly shows left ventricular hypertrophy and widespread, deep, broad Q waves that suggest an old myocardial infarction but apparently result from the abnormal electrophysiologic properties of the hypertrophied septum. Many patients demonstrate arrhythmias, both atrial (supraventricular tachycardia or atrial fibrillation) as well as ventricular (ventricular tachycardia) during ambulatory (Holter) monitoring. *Chest roentgenography* may be normal, although a mild to moderate increase in the cardiac silhouette is common. The mainstay of the diagnosis of hypertrophic cardiomyopathy is the *echocardiogram*, which demonstrates left ventricular hypertrophy, often with the septum 1.3 or more times the thickness of the high posterior left ventricular

free wall. The septum may demonstrate an unusual ground-glass appearance, probably related to its abnormal cellular architecture and myocardial fibrosis. Systolic anterior motion of the mitral valve is found in patients with pressure gradients. The left ventricular cavity is typically small in hypertrophic cardiomyopathy, with vigorous posterior wall motion, but reduced septal excursion. A rare form of hypertrophic cardiomyopathy, found principally in Japan, is characterized by massive apical hypertrophy, often associated with giant negative T waves on the electrocardiogram and a "spade-shaped" left ventricular cavity on angiography. The two-dimensional *echocardiogram* is particularly useful in identifying all of the characteristic changes, including the size and shape of the left ventricular cavity. The indirectly recorded *carotid arterial pulse* tracing rises unusually rapidly and often displays a "spike-and-dome" configuration when an outflow pressure gradient is present. *Radionuclide scintigraphy* with thallium 201 frequently reveals evidence of myocardial perfusion defects even in asymptomatic patients.

The two typical *hemodynamic* features are an elevated left ventricular diastolic pressure due to diminished left ventricular compliance and, when obstruction is present, a systolic pressure gradient between the body of the left ventricle and the subaortic region. When a gradient is not present, it often can be induced by provocative maneuvers such as infusion of isoproterenol, inhalation of amyl nitrite, or the Valsalva maneuver.

Treatment   Beta-adrenergic blockers are often used and may ameliorate to some degree the symptoms of angina pectoris and syncope in one-third to one-half of patients. Resting intraventricular pressure gradients are usually unchanged, although these drugs may limit the increase in the gradient that occurs during exercise. It is not known whether beta-adrenergic blockers offer any protection against sudden death, which is presumably arrhythmic in origin. It is not established whether any antiarrhythmic agent is efficacious in this setting. However, the experimental agent amiodarone appears to be effective in reducing the frequency of supraventricular as well as life-threatening ventricular arrhythmias. The calcium channel antagonists are agents that may reduce the stiffness of the ventricle, reduce the elevated diastolic pressures, increase exercise tolerance, and, in some instances, reduce the severity of outflow tract gradients, although adverse side effects occur in about one-quarter of patients. Disopyramide has been used in some patients to reduce left ventricular contractility and the outflow gradient. Surgical myotomy/myectomy of the hypertrophied septum may result in lasting symptomatic improvement in about three-quarters of operated patients, but the mortality of approximately 5 percent limits the operation to severely symptomatic patients with large pressure gradients who are unresponsive to medical management. Digitalis, diuretics, nitrates, and beta-adrenergic agonists are best avoided if possible, particularly in patients with known left ventricular outflow tract pressure gradients.

Prognosis   The natural history of hypertrophic cardiomyopathy is variable, although many patients demonstrate an improvement or stabilization of symptoms with time. Atrial fibrillation is common late in the course of the disease; its onset usually leads to a striking increase in symptoms, presumably due to loss of the atrial contribution to filling of the thickened ventricle. This rhythm, when sustained, is associated with a poor prognosis. Infective endocarditis occurs in less than 10 percent of patients, and endocarditis prophylaxis is indicated, particularly in patients with resting obstruction and mitral regurgitation. Progression of hypertrophic cardiomyopathy to left ventricular dilatation and dysfunction without an outflow gradient has been reported but is unusual; in about 5 to 10 percent of patients, however, some degree of left ventricular systolic impairment, wall thinning, and chamber enlargement occurs over time. The major cause of mortality in hypertrophic cardiomyopathy is sudden death, which may occur in asymptomatic patients or interrupt an otherwise stable course in symptomatic ones. Predictors of sudden death include: age less than 30 years, ventricular tachycardia on ambulatory monitoring, and a family history of sudden death. There is no correlation between the risk of sudden death and the severity of symptoms or the presence or severity of an outflow tract pressure gradient. Since sudden death often occurs during or just after physical exertion, strenuous exercise should be avoided in all patients, regardless of symptoms. Although hemodynamic factors may play a role, it is likely that most deaths, particularly those that are sudden, are due to ventricular arrhythmias.

MYOCARDITIS

Myocarditis is said to be present when the heart is involved in an inflammatory process. Most commonly the result of an infectious process, myocarditis may also be present in hypersensitivity states such as acute rheumatic fever (Chap. 187) or may be caused by radiation, chemicals, physical agents, and drugs. Myocarditis may be acute or chronic. In an unknown number of cases, acute myocarditis progresses to chronic dilated cardiomyopathy. While almost every infectious agent is capable of producing myocarditis, clinically significant acute myocarditis in the United States is caused most commonly by viruses. Coxsackievirus B is the most frequent cause of viral myocarditis, but coxsackievirus A, influenza, rubeola, rubella, polio-, adeno-, and echoviruses also cause the disease. In most cases, the presence of myocarditis is inferred only by the finding of transient electrocardiographic ST-T-wave abnormalities, but arrhythmias, heart failure, and death may occur in fulminant cases, particularly in infants and pregnant women. Myocarditis is frequently associated with acute pericarditis, particularly when it is caused by coxsackievirus B strains or echoviruses (Chap. 145).

Physical examination may be normal in patients who have only electrocardiographic abnormalities, although more severe cases may show a muffled first heart sound, along with a third heart sound and a murmur of mitral regurgitation. A pericardial friction rub may be audible in patients with associated pericarditis.

Experimental studies suggest that exercise may be deleterious in patients with myocarditis, and strenuous activity should be proscribed until the electrocardiogram has returned to normal. Prolonged bed rest has been advocated for more severe cases, although its efficacy remains to be established. Patients who develop congestive heart failure respond to the usual measures (digitalis, diuretics, salt restriction), but they appear to be unusually sensitive to digitalis. Arrhythmias are common and are occasionally difficult to manage. Deaths attributed to heart failure, tachyarrhythmias, and heart block have been reported, and it seems prudent to monitor the electrocardiogram of patients with arrhythmias, especially during the acute illness.

Though viral myocarditis is most often self-limited and without sequelae, active disease may recur, and it is likely that acute viral myocarditis occasionally progresses to a chronic form. Patients with viral myocarditis often give a history of a preceding upper respiratory febrile illness, and viral nasopharyngitis or tonsillitis may be evident clinically. The isolation of virus from the stool, pharyngeal washings, or other body fluids, and changes in specific antibody titers are helpful clinically. Some instances of apparent *idiopathic* dilated cardiomyopathy (page 975) appear to arise from mild or subclinical episodes of myocarditis. While corticosteroids may exacerbate heart damage in animals with acute viral myocarditis, a small number of humans with congestive heart failure and inflammatory myocarditis appear to respond to an experimental protocol utilizing immunosuppression with prednisone and azathioprine. Serial right ventricular endomyocardial biopsies have shown regression of inflammatory infiltrates in some patients so treated. However, the effects of this treatment program have not been rigorously compared to a comparable control group.

Bacterial myocarditis Bacterial involvement of the heart is uncommon, but when it does occur, it is usually as a complication of bacterial endocarditis (typically due to *Staphylococcus aureus* and enterococci). Myocardial abscess formation may involve the valve rings and interventricular septum. *Diphtheritic myocarditis* develops in over one-quarter of the patients with diphtheria, is one of the most serious complications, and is the most common cause of death due to diphtheria (Chap. 102). Cardiac damage is due to the liberation of a toxin that inhibits protein synthesis, and leads to a dilated, flabby, hypocontractile heart; the conducting system is frequently involved as well. Cardiomegaly and severe congestive heart failure typically appear after the first week of illness. ST-segment and T-wave abnormalities on the electrocardiogram are the rule, but atrial and ventricular arrhythmias, bundle branch block, and abnormalities of atrioventricular conduction are also common. Prompt therapy with antitoxin is crucial; antibiotic therapy is also indicated but is of less urgency.

Chagas' disease Chagas' disease, caused by the protozoan *Trypanosoma cruzi* and transmitted by an insect vector (Chap. 161), produces an extensive myocarditis that typically becomes evident years after the initial infection. It is one of the most common causes of heart disease encountered in Central and South America; in rural areas up to 20 percent of the population may be affected. Although only a minority of infected individuals have an acute illness, upwards of one-third develop chronic myocardial damage. Electrocardiographic evidence of cardiac involvement may appear in adolescence, although symptoms often do not appear until adulthood. The chronic form is characterized by dilatation of several cardiac chambers, fibrosis and thinning of the ventricular wall, aneurysm formation in the areas of thinning (especially at the apex), and mural thrombi. Chronic progressive heart failure, often predominantly right-sided, is the rule. The electrocardiogram typically shows right bundle branch block and left anterior hemiblock, which may progress to complete atrioventricular block. The echocardiogram may reveal a unique pattern of hypokinesis of the posterior left ventricular wall and relatively preserved septal motion. Ventricular arrhythmias are common and are seen particularly during and after exertion; oral amiodarone appears to be particularly effective in treating ventricular tachyarrhythmias. The cause of death is either intractable congestive heart failure or an arrhythmia. Therapy is directed toward amelioration of the congestive heart failure and arrhythmias; the latter may require implantation of a pacemaker. Medical therapy is often unsatisfactory or unavailable, however, and a more promising tactic has been the institution of public health measures, particularly the use of insecticides to eliminate the vector.

Toxoplasmic myocarditis (See also Chap. 162) This uncommon form of protozoal myocardial involvement occurs most frequently in immunosuppressed adults; congenital toxoplasmal infections are much more common, but myocarditis is not a prominent feature. Myocardial involvement may lead to cardiac dilatation, pericarditis, and pericardial effusion. Heart failure, arrhythmias, and conduction abnormalities may be seen. Because of the difficulty in diagnosing this condition, it may be a more common problem than is usually appreciated. Treatment is with pyrimethamine and sulfonamides, but the response to treatment is variable.

Giant cell myocarditis This rare myocarditis of unknown cause is characterized by the presence of multinucleated giant cells in the myocardium. It usually causes rapidly fatal congestive heart failure and arrhythmia in young to middle-aged adults. At necropsy, the distinctive features include cardiac enlargement, ventricular thrombi, grossly visible serpiginous areas of myocardial necrosis in both ventricles, and microscopic evidence of giant cells within an extensive inflammatory infiltrate. The cause of giant cell myocarditis remains obscure, although it occurs in association with thymoma, systemic lupus erythematosus, and thyrotoxicosis. No therapy has been shown to be efficacious.

Lyme carditis (See also Chap. 132) Lyme disease is caused by a tick-borne spirochete and is most common in the northeastern United States during the summer months. About 10 percent of patients develop symptomatic cardiac involvement, with conduction abnormalities the most common manifestations. Concomitant myopericarditis is not uncommon, and mild asymptomatic left ventricular dysfunction may occur. Penicillin is used to treat the accompanying skin rash, arthritis, and neurologic abnormalities. A temporary pacemaker may be needed for symptomatic heart block; the utility of glucocorticoids in reversing heart block is uncertain, but they are usually employed.

Human immunodeficiency virus myocarditis In addition to myocardial opportunistic infections by a wide variety of organisms and metastatic involvement by Kaposi's sarcoma, cardiac involvement in the acquired immunodeficiency syndrome (AIDS) (Chap. 264) often consists of a mild focal myocarditis. An occasional patient demonstrates advanced congestive heart failure with four-chamber cardiac enlargement. Therapy has been uniformly unsuccessful.

Radiation myocarditis A variety of acute and chronic cardiac complications may result from the use of ionizing radiation in the treatment of carcinoma of the lung or breast, lymphoma, or Hodgkin's disease. Only an occasional patient manifests acute cardiac abnormalities; typically such an abnormality consists of acute pericarditis. The most common presentation is that of chronic pericardial effusion or constriction occurring months or years after exposure (in rare cases up to 10 years) (Chap. 193). Myocardial fibrosis, resulting from damage to the microvasculature, often with formation of atherosclerotic plaques of the epicardial coronary arteries, is also common.

REFERENCES

Braunwald E: Hypertrophic cardiomyopathy—continued progress. N Engl J Med 320:800, 1989

Chaudary S, Jaski BF: Fulminant mumps myocarditis. Ann Intern Med 110:569, 1989

Coplan NL, Bruno MS: Acquired immunodeficiency syndrome and heart disease: The present and the future. Am Heart J 117:1175, 1989

Heilbrunn SM et al: Increased beta-receptor density and improved hemodynamic response to catecholamine stimulation during long-term metoprolol therapy in heart failure from dilated cardiomyopathy. Circulation 79:483, 1989

Jarcho JA et al: Mapping a gene for familial hypertrophic cardiomyopathy to chromosome 14ql. N Engl J Med 321:1372, 1990

Karam R et al: Hypertensive hypertrophic cardiomyopathy or hypertrophic cardiomyopathy with hypertension? A study of 78 patients. J Am Coll Cardiol 13:580, 1989

Karch SB, Billingham ME: The pathology and etiology of cocaine-induced heart disease. Arch Pathol Lab Med 112:225, 1988

Kounis NG et al: Hypersensitivity myocarditis. Ann Allergy 62:71, 1989

McAlister HF et al: Lyme carditis: An important cause of reversible heart block. Ann Intern Med 110:339, 1989

Olshausen KV et al: Long-term prognostic significance of ventricular arrhythmias in idiopathic dilated cardiomyopathy. Am J Cardiol 61:146, 1988

Popma JJ et al: Diagnostic and prognostic utility of right-sided catheterization and endomyocardial biopsy in idiopathic dilated cardiomyopathy. Am J Cardiol 63:955, 1989

Rezkalla SH, Kloner RA: Management strategies in viral myocarditis. Am Heart J 117:706, 1989

Romeo F et al: Predictors of sudden death in idiopathic dilated cardiomyopathy. Am J Cardiol 63:138, 1989

Spirito P et al: Clinical course and prognosis of hypertrophic cardiomyopathy in an outpatient population. N Engl J Med 320:749, 1989

Stewart JM et al: Symptomatic cardiac dysfunction in children with human immunodeficiency virus infection. Am Heart J 117:140, 1989

Sunnerhagen KS et al: Regional left ventricular wall motion abnormalities in dilated idiopathic cardiomyopathy. Am J Cardiol 65(1):364, 1990

Surgical treatment of hypertrophic obstructive cardiomyopathy. Lancet 1:358, 1989

Thiene G et al: Right ventricular cardiomyopathy and sudden death in young people. N Engl J Med 318:129, 1988

Webb JG et al: Apical hypertrophic cardiomyopathy: Clinical follow-up and diagnostic correlates. J Am Coll Cardiol 15(1):83, 1990

Wynne J, Braunwald E: The cardiomyopathies and myocarditides, in *Heart Disease*, 3d ed, E Braunwald (ed). Philadelphia, Saunders, 1988, pp 1410–1469

193   PERICARDIAL DISEASE

EUGENE BRAUNWALD

NORMAL FUNCTIONS OF THE PERICARDIUM The visceral pericardium is a serous membrane, separated by a small amount of fluid, an ultrafiltrate of plasma, from a fibrous sac, the parietal pericardium. The pericardium prevents sudden dilatation of the cardiac chambers during exercise and hypervolemia, and as the result of the development of a negative intrapericardial pressure during ejection it facilitates atrial filling during ventricular systole. The pericardium also restricts the anatomic position of the heart, minimizes friction between the heart and surrounding structures, prevents displacement of the heart and kinking of the great vessels, and probably retards the spread of infections from the lungs and pleural cavities to the heart. Notwithstanding the foregoing, total absence of the pericardium does not produce obvious clinical disease. In partial left pericardial defects the main pulmonary artery and left atrium may bulge through the defect; rarely herniation and subsequent strangulation of the left atrium may cause sudden death.

ACUTE PERICARDITIS

It is useful to classify the types of pericarditis both clinically and etiologically (Table 193-1), as this disorder is by far the most common pathologic process involving the pericardium.

Pain, a pericardial friction rub, electrocardiographic changes, and pericardial effusion with cardiac tamponade and paradoxic pulse are cardinal manifestations of many forms of acute pericarditis and will be considered prior to a discussion of the most common forms of the disorder.

TABLE 193-1   Classification of pericarditis

I Clinical classification
  A Acute pericarditis (<6 weeks)
    1 Fibrinous
    2 Effusive (or bloody)
  B Subacute pericarditis (6 weeks to 6 months)
    1 Constrictive
    2 Effusive-constrictive
  C Chronic pericarditis (>6 months)
    1 Constrictive
    2 Effusive
    3 Adhesive (nonconstrictive)
II Etiologic classification
  A Infectious pericarditis
    1 Viral
    2 Pyogenic
    3 Tuberculous
    4 Mycotic
    5 Other infections (syphilitic, parasitic)
  B Noninfectious pericarditis
    1 Acute myocardial infarction
    2 Uremia
    3 Neoplasia
      a Primary tumors (benign or malignant)
      b Tumors metastatic to pericardium
    4 Myxedema
    5 Cholesterol
    6 Chylopericardium
    7 Trauma
      a Penetrating chest wall
      b Nonpenetrating
    8 Aortic aneurysm (with leakage into pericardial sac)
    9 Postirradiation
    10 Associated with atrial septal defect
    11 Associated with severe chronic anemia
    12 Infectious mononucleosis
    13 Familial Mediterranean fever
    14 Familial pericarditis
      a Mulibrey nanism*
    15 Sarcoidosis
    16 Acute idiopathic
  C Pericarditis presumably related to hypersensitivity or autoimmunity
    1 Rheumatic fever
    2 Collagen vascular disease
      a Systemic lupus erythematosus
      b Rheumatoid arthritis
      c Scleroderma
    3 Drug-induced
      a Procainamide
      b Hydralazine
      c Other
    4 Postcardiac injury
      a Postmyocardial infarction (Dressler's syndrome)
      b Postpericardiotomy

* An autosomal recessive syndrome, characterized by growth failure, muscle hypotonia, hepatomegaly, ocular changes, enlarged cerebral ventricles, mental retardation, and chronic constrictive pericarditis.

Pain is an important but not invariable symptom in various forms of acute pericarditis; it is usually present in the acute infectious types and in many of the forms presumed to be related to hypersensitivity or autoimmunity. Pain is often absent in a slowly developing tuberculous, postirradiation, neoplastic or uremic pericarditis. The pain of pericarditis is often severe (Chap. 16). It is characteristically in the center of the chest, referred to the back and the trapezius ridge. Often the pain is pleuritic, i.e., sharp and aggravated by inspiration, coughing, and changes in body position, but sometimes it is a steady, constrictive pain, which radiates into either arm or both arms and resembles that of myocardial ischemia; confusion with myocardial infarction is common. Characteristically, however, the pericardial pain may be relieved by sitting up and leaning forward. The differentiation of acute myocardial infarction from acute pericarditis becomes even more perplexing when, with acute pericarditis, the serum transaminase and creatine kinase levels rise, presumably because of concomitant involvement of the epicardium. However, these enzyme elevations, if they occur, are quite modest, given the extensive electrocardiographic ST-segment elevation in pericarditis.

The *pericardial friction rub* is the most important physical sign; it may have up to three components per cardiac cycle, as described in Chap. 175, and can sometimes be elicited only when firm pressure with the diaphragm of the stethoscope is applied to the chest wall. It is heard most frequently during expiration with the patient in the sitting position, but an independent pleural friction rub may be audible during inspiration, with the patient leaning forward or in the left lateral decubitus position. The rub is often inconstant and transitory, and a loud to-and-fro leathery sound may disappear within a few hours, possibly to reappear the following day.

Moderate elevations of the MB fraction of creatine phosphokinase may occur and reflects accompanying myocarditis.

The *electrocardiogram* in acute pericarditis without massive effusion usually displays changes secondary to acute subepicardial inflammation (Fig. 176-14, p. 858). There is widespread elevation of the ST segments, involving two or three standard limb leads and V_2 to V_6, with reciprocal depressions only in aVR and sometimes V_1 and without significant changes in QRS complexes, except occasionally for some reduction in voltage. After several days, the ST segments return to normal and only then do the T waves become inverted. In contrast, in acute myocardial infarction, reciprocal depression of ST segments is usually more prominent; QRS changes occur, particularly the development of Q waves, and notching and loss of the amplitude of R waves; and T-wave inversions usually occur within hours *before* the ST segments have become isoelectric. Sequential electrocardiograms are useful in distinguishing acute pericarditis from acute myocardial infarction. Early repolarization is a normal variant and may also cause widespread ST-segment elevation, most prominent in left precordial leads. However, in this condition the T waves are usually tall and the ST/T ratio is under 0.25, but exceeds this number in acute pericarditis. Depression of the PQ segment (below the TP segment) also is common and reflects atrial involvement. With large pericardial effusions, the QRS voltage is reduced; atrial premature beats and atrial fibrillation are sometimes noted.

PERICARDIAL EFFUSION   Usually associated with one or more of the above-mentioned manifestations of pericarditis and an enlargement of the cardiac silhouette, pericardial effusion is especially important clinically when it develops within a relatively short time, since it may lead to cardiac tamponade. Differentiation from cardiac enlargement may be difficult, but heart sounds tend to become faint; the friction rub may disappear or remain clearly audible, and the apex impulse may vanish, but sometimes it is palpable well medial to the left border of cardiac dullness. The chest roentgenogram may show a "water bottle" configuration of the cardiac silhouette, but it may also be normal or almost so. Lucent pericardial fat lines may be seen deep within the cardiopericardial silhouette. Fluoroscopic examination may show the ventricular pulsations to be diminished. When the effusion is large, an area of dullness and tubular breath sounds is often encountered at the angle of the left scapula, probably caused by compression of the lung (Ewart's sign).

Diagnosis of pericardial effusion   Echocardiography (Chap. 177) is the most effective diagnostic laboratory technique available, since it is sensitive, specific, simple, innocuous, and noninvasive, and may be performed at the bedside. The presence of pericardial fluid is recorded as a relatively echo-free space between the posterior pericardium and left ventricular epicardium in patients with small effusions and such a space between the anterior right ventricle and the parietal pericardium just beneath the anterior chest wall with larger effusions (Fig. 193-1). In patients with large effusions the heart may swing freely within the pericardial sac; when severe, the extent of this motion alternates and may be associated with electrical alternans. Two-dimensional echocardiography allows localization and estimation of the quantity of pericardial fluid. In tamponade, during inspiration, right ventricular diameter increases while left ventricular diameter and mitral valve opening decrease. Often the right ventricular cavity is reduced and there is late diastolic inward motion (collapse) of the right ventricular free wall, and of the right atrium. The diagnosis

FIGURE 193-1   Two-dimensional (upper panel) and short-axis (lower panel) parasternal scans in systole in a patient with a large pericardial effusion surrounding the entire heart. Fluid is seen to extend behind the left atrium (white arrowhead) and anterior to the descending thoracic aorta (DA). AoV = aortic valve; LA = left atrium; LV = left ventricle; PE = pericardial effusion; RV = right ventricle. *(Modified from PC Come (ed), Diagnostic Cardiology: Noninvasive imaging techniques, Philadelphia, Lippincott, 1985.)*

of pericardial fluid or thickening may be confirmed by one of the following:

1 *Cardiac catheterization.* A catheter is introduced into the right atrium and rotated so that its tip makes contact with the lateral right atrial wall. In the presence of an effusion, or pericardial thickening, the tip of the catheter is separated from the radiolucent lungs by an opaque band.

2 *Angiocardiography.* Contrast medium is injected rapidly into the right atrium; again the lateral wall is separated from the edge of the cardiac silhouette.

When it is deemed desirable to remove pericardial fluid for diagnostic and/or therapeutic purposes, a needle attached to a properly grounded electrocardiographic lead is inserted into the pericardial space, usually through a subxiphoid approach, and if possible using echocardiographic control. Intrapericardial pressure should be measured before fluid is withdrawn. Pericardial effusion nearly always has the physical characteristics of an exudate. Bloody fluid is commonly due to tuberculosis or tumor, but it may also be found in the effusion of rheumatic fever or in the post-cardiac injury syndrome (see below). Occasionally, bloody fluid may be found in the effusion of uremic pericarditis and in the hemopericardium following myocardial infarction, especially following the administration of anticoagulants.

CARDIAC TAMPONADE The accumulation of fluid in the pericardium in an amount sufficient to cause serious obstruction to the inflow of blood to the ventricles results in cardiac tamponade. The amount of fluid necessary to produce this critical state may be as small as 250 mL, when the fluid develops rapidly, or over 2000 mL in slowly developing effusions when the pericardium has had the opportunity to stretch and adapt to the increasing volume of fluid. The volume of fluid required to produce tamponade varies directly with the thickness of the ventricular myocardium and inversely with the thickness of the parietal pericardium. Tamponade results most often from bleeding into the pericardial space following cardiac operations, trauma (including cardiac perforation during diagnostic procedures), tuberculosis, tumor (most commonly carcinoma of the lung and breast and lymphoma), and aortic dissection, but it may occur in acute viral or idiopathic pericarditis, postirradiation pericarditis, renal failure during dialysis, and hemopericardium which may result when a patient with any form of acute pericarditis is treated with anticoagulants.

The clinical manifestations are due to the fall in cardiac output and to systemic venous congestion. However, the classic findings of falling arterial pressure, rising venous pressure, and a small quiet heart with faint heart sounds usually are seen only with severe tamponade usually occurring within minutes, as happens with cardiac trauma or rupture. More frequently, tamponade develops more slowly and the clinical manifestations, resembling those of heart failure, include dyspnea, orthopnea, hepatic engorgement, and jugular venous hypertension. A high index of suspicion is required, since, in many instances, no obvious cause for pericardial disease is apparent, and tamponade should be considered in any patient with hypotension and elevation of jugular venous pressure with a prominent *x* descent; often the *y* descent is diminutive or absent. A widening of the area of flatness to percussion across the anterior aspect of the chest wall, a paradoxical pulse (see below), relatively clear lung fields, diminished pulsations of the cardiac silhouette on fluoroscopy, enlargement of the cardiac silhouette in subacute or chronic tamponade, reduction in amplitude of the QRS complexes, and *electrical alternans* of the P, QRS, and T waves should raise the suspicion of cardiac tamponade.

A positive Kussmaul's sign (see below) is rare in cardiac tamponade, as is a pericardial knock. Their presence suggests that an organizing process and epicardial constriction are present in addition to effusion. Since immediate treatment of tamponade may be lifesaving, prompt measures to establish the diagnosis definitely, i.e., echocardiography followed by cardiac catheterization, should be undertaken. The latter reveals elevation of the right atrial pressure with prominence of the *x* but not of the *y* descent. When measured, the pericardial pressure is also elevated and equal to the right atrial pressure. There is "equalization" of pressures, i.e., the pulmonary artery wedge is equal, or close, to right atrial, right ventricular, and pulmonary artery diastolic pressures. The "square root" sign in the ventricular pressure pulses and the prominent *y* descent in atrial and jugular venous pressure are characteristic of constrictive pericarditis (see below) and are usually absent in tamponade. In an emergency, pericardiocentesis may be carried out without cardiac catheterization but preferably after confirmation of the clinical diagnosis by echocardiography.

Paradoxical pulse This important clue to the presence of cardiac tamponade consists of *a greater than normal (10 mmHg) inspiratory decrease in systolic arterial pressure.* When severe, it may be detected by palpating weakness or disappearance of the arterial pulse during inspiration, but usually sphygmomanometric measurement of systolic pressure during slow respiration is required (Fig. 193-2).

The mechanism of paradoxical pulse in cardiac tamponade is complex. Normally, the inspiratory decline in intrathoracic pressure enhances right ventricular filling by virtue of the increased pressure gradient between the extrathoracic veins and the chambers of the right side of the heart. As a consequence right ventricular diastolic volume and stroke output increase, and this increase is transmitted to the left side of the heart several cardiac cycles later, leading to an increase in systemic arterial pressure during the following expiration. Therefore, normally a small fall in left ventricular stroke volume and pressure occur during inspiration. Also, left ventricular afterload rises during inspiration as intrapericardial pressure falls, contributing to

FIGURE 193-2 Simultaneous recording of electrocardiogram (ECG), blood flow velocity in the superior vena cava (SVC), brachial arterial pressure (BA), and the pneumogram (Pneumo) in a patient with cardiac compression and paradoxical pulse. A downward deflection of the pneumogram denotes inspiration, when SVC blood velocity rises and arterial pressure falls (paradoxical pulse). Arterial pressure is maintained during prolonged expiratory pause.

the small inspiratory decline in left ventricular stroke volume and arterial pressure. In cardiac tamponade, since both ventricles share a tight incompressible covering, i.e., the pericardial sac, the inspiratory increase in right ventricular volume compresses and reduces left ventricular volume substantially; leftward bulging of the interventricular septum further reduces the left ventricular cavity as the right ventricle enlarges during inspiration. Thus, in cardiac tamponade the inspiratory augmentation of right ventricular volume causes an exaggerated reciprocal reduction in left ventricular volume. Also, respiratory distress increases the fluctuations in intrathoracic pressure, which exaggerates the mechanism just described.

Low-pressure tamponade refers to mild tamponade in which the intrapericardial pressure is increased from its slightly subatmospheric levels to +5 to +10 mmHg; in some instances hypovolemia coexists. As a consequence the central venous pressure is normal or only slightly elevated while arterial pressure is unaffected. The patients are asymptomatic or complain of mild weakness and dyspnea. The diagnosis is aided by echocardiography, and both hemodynamic and clinical manifestations improve following mild pericardiocentesis.

Paradoxical pulse, a hallmark of cardiac tamponade, occurs in only approximately one-third of patients with *constrictive pericarditis*. It is important to bear in mind that paradoxical pulse is not pathognomonic of pericardial disease because it may be observed in various forms of restrictive cardiomyopathies (Chap. 192) and, in some cases of hypovolemic shock, chronic obstructive airways disease, and severe bronchial asthma.

TREATMENT All patients with acute pericarditis should be observed frequently and carefully for the possibility of a developing effusion or, if effusion is already present, for signs of tamponade. In the presence of an effusion, arterial and venous pressures and heart rate should be monitored continuously or followed carefully and serial echocardiograms obtained. When a diagnostic pericardiocentesis of a large effusion is carried out, an attempt should be made to remove as much fluid as possible. If manifestations of tamponade appear, pericardiocentesis must be carried out at once, since relief of the intrapericardial pressure may be lifesaving. A small catheter advanced over the needle inserted into the pericardial cavity may be left in place to allow draining of the pericardial space if fluid reaccumulates.

VIRAL OR IDIOPATHIC FORM OF ACUTE PERICARDITIS This disorder is an important clinical entity because of its frequency and because it may be confused with other more serious illnesses. In some cases an A or B coxsackievirus or the virus of influenza, echovirus type 8, mumps, herpes simplex, chickenpox, or adenovirus has been isolated from pericardial fluid and/or appropriate elevations in viral antibody titers have been noted; in other instances, acute pericarditis has occurred in association with illnesses of known viral origin and, presumably, was caused by the same agent. More commonly there is an antecedent infection of the respiratory tract, but in many patients such an association is not evident and viral isolation and serologic studies are negative. Most frequently, a viral causation cannot be established nor can it be excluded; the term *acute idiopathic pericarditis* is then appropriate. However, regardless of the specific causative factor, the clinical manifestations are similar. This form of acute pericarditis occurs at all ages but is more frequent in young adults; it is often associated with pleural effusions and pneumonitis. The appearance of fever and precordial pain at about the same time, often 10 to 12 days after a presumed viral illness, constitutes an important feature in the differentiation of acute pericarditis from myocardial infarction, in which pain precedes fever. The constitutional symptoms are usually mild to moderate, but occasionally the initial symptoms are stormy, the temperature rising to 40°C. The disease ordinarily runs its course in a few days to 2 weeks, but occasionally after the patient has apparently recovered he or she may have one or several recurrences, weeks or even months later. Tamponade is unusual and constrictive pericarditis develops rarely, although accumulation of some pericardial fluid is common. A pericardial friction rub is often audible. The ST segment alterations

in the electrocardiogram are usually transitory, but the abnormal T waves may persist for several years or indefinitely and be a source of confusion in persons without a clear history of pericarditis. Pleuritis and pneumonitis frequently accompany pericarditis. The erythrocyte sedimentation rate is elevated. Granulocytosis followed by lymphocytosis is common.

There is no specific therapy, but anti-inflammatory treatment with aspirin, if necessary up to 900 mg qid, may be given. If this is ineffective, one of the nonsteroidal anti-inflammatory agents, such as indomethacin (25 to 75 mg qid) or a glucocorticoid (e.g., prednisone, 20 to 80 mg daily) effectively suppresses the clinical manifestations of the acute illness and may be useful in patients in whom the purulent and tuberculous forms of pericarditis have been excluded. After the patient has been asymptomatic and afebrile for about 1 week, the dose of the anti-inflammatory agent is gradually tapered. Occasionally progression to chronic constrictive pericarditis occurs. Recurrences occur in about one-fourth of patients, but the tendency to relapse decreases within 2 years after the initial episode. When recurrences continue beyond this period and are frequent, prolonged, and disabling, pericardiectomy may be effective in terminating the illness.

POST-CARDIAC INJURY SYNDROME An acute form of pericarditis may appear under a variety of circumstances which have one common feature: previous injury to the myocardium, with blood in the pericardial cavity. The syndrome has been observed when the injury has been induced in the course of a cardiac operation (postpericardiotomy syndrome). It may also follow myocardial infarction (Dressler's syndrome) (Chap. 189) or develop after trauma of the heart (Chap. 194), for example a stab wound, contusions after a nonpenetrating blow to the chest, or perforation of the heart with a pacemaker catheter.

The principal symptom is the pain of acute pericarditis, which usually develops 1 to 4 weeks following the cardiac injury but sometimes appears only after a lapse of months. Recurrences are common and may occur up to 2 years or more after the injury. Fever to 40°C, pericarditis, pleuritis, and pneumonitis are the outstanding features, the bout of illness usually subsiding in 1 or 2 weeks. The pericarditis, which appears to be the most constant lesion, may be of the fibrinous variety, or it may be a pericardial effusion, which is often serosanguineous and sometimes causes tamponade. Rarely, the pericarditis may be accompanied by arthralgias. Leukocytosis, an increased sedimentation rate, and electrocardiographic changes typical of acute pericarditis may also occur.

The mechanisms responsible for the clinical manifestations have not been identified, but there is a likelihood that they are the result of a hypersensitivity reaction in which the antigen originates from injured myocardial tissue and/or pericardium; the suggested designation of post-cardiac injury syndrome for this group of disorders implies that they may have a common pathogenetic mechanism. Circulating autoantibodies to myocardium occur frequently, but their precise role in this syndrome has not been defined. Viral infection may also play an etiologic role, since antiviral antibodies are often elevated in patients who develop this syndrome following cardiac surgery.

The clinical picture mimics acute viral or acute idiopathic pericarditis. Moreover, it is possible that the recurrences that occur so frequently in the latter condition are not always caused by an exacerbation of the original (presumably viral) infection, but that the original injury may have initiated the sequence of events that culminates in the post-cardiac injury syndrome.

Often no treatment is necessary aside from aspirin and analgesics. The management of pericardial effusion and tamponade has already been discussed. When the illness is followed by a series of disabling recurrences, therapy with a nonsteroidal anti-inflammatory agent or a glucocorticoid is usually effective.

DIFFERENTIAL DIAGNOSIS Differential diagnosis of *acute idiopathic pericarditis* is primarily one of exclusion, as there is no specific test for this disorder. Consequently all other disorders that may be associated with acute fibrinous pericarditis must be considered. When associated with *acute myocardial infarction,* acute fibrinous pericarditis may be confused with acute viral or idiopathic pericarditis; this complication of infarction, described on p. 963, is characterized by the occurrence of fever, pain, and a friction rub in the first 4 days following the development of the infarct (to be distinguished from the pericarditis in Dressler's syndrome, which occurs a week or two following myocardial infarction). Electrocardiographic abnormalities (such as the appearance of Q waves, brief ST-segment elevations with reciprocal changes, and earlier T-wave changes in myocardial infarction), the extent of the elevations of myocardial enzymes, and the total clinical picture are helpful in relating pericarditis to acute myocardial infarction. A common diagnostic error is assuming that acute viral or idiopathic pericarditis represents acute myocardial infarction and vice versa.

Acute pericarditis occurring as a component of the *post-cardiac injury* syndrome is most likely to be confused with acute idiopathic pericarditis. Pericarditis secondary to post-cardiac injury is differentiated from acute idiopathic pericarditis chiefly by timing. If it occurs within a few weeks of a myocardial infarction or a chest blow, it may be justified to conclude that the two are probably related. If the infarct has been silent or the chest blow forgotten, the relationship to the pericarditis may not be recognized.

It is important to distinguish *pericarditis due to collagen disease* from acute idiopathic pericarditis. Most important in the differential diagnosis is the pericarditis due to systemic lupus erythematosus (Chap. 269); often pain is present, sometimes the pericarditis appears as an asymptomatic effusion and rarely tamponade develops. Very rarely, when pericarditis occurs in the absence of other evidence of any underlying disorder, differentiation from acute viral and idiopathic pericarditis or tuberculous pericarditis may be made on discovery of lupus erythematosus (LE) cells, a rise in antinuclear antibodies, or by the specific methods for diagnosing tuberculosis (see below). Acute pericarditis is also an occasional complication of *rheumatoid arthritis, scleroderma,* and *polyarteritis nodosa,* but again, other evidence of these diseases is usually obvious. Asymptomatic pericardial effusion is also frequent in these disorders. It is important to question every patient with acute pericarditis about the ingestion of procainamide, hydralazine, isoniazid, cromolyn, and minoxidil, since these drugs can cause this syndrome.

The pericarditis of *acute rheumatic fever* is generally associated with evidence of severe pancarditis and with cardiac murmurs (Chap. 187). *Pyogenic (purulent) pericarditis* is usually secondary to cardiothoracic operations, immunosuppressive therapy, rupture of the esophagus into the pericardial sac, and rupture of a ring abscess in a patient with infective endocarditis and with septicemia complicating aseptic pericarditis. It is now uncommonly due to pneumococcal pneumonia and pleuritis, previously the most common cause. *Tuberculous pericarditis* (see Chap. 125) may present as an acute pericarditis, associated with fever, weight loss, and other clinical manifestations of active systemic tuberculosis; the diagnosis may be aided by a positive tuberculin test and evidence of pulmonary or mediastinal tuberculosis. Tubercle bacilli can be cultured from the pericardial space only infrequently, and a biopsy of the pericardium with bacteriologic and histologic examination may be required. Alternatively, tuberculous pericarditis may present as a chronic asymptomatic effusion, as subacute effusive-constrictive pericarditis, or frank chronic constrictive pericarditis (see below). *Uremic pericarditis* (Chap. 224) occurs in up to one-third of patients with chronic uremia, and is seen most frequently in patients undergoing chronic hemodialysis. It may be fibrinous or associated with a bloody effusion. A friction rub is common, but pain is usually absent. Treatment with an anti-inflammatory agent and intensification of hemodialysis are usually adequate therapy. Occasionally, tamponade occurs and pericardiocentesis is required. When uremic pericarditis is recurrent or persistent, pericardiectomy is necessary. Pericarditis due to *neoplastic diseases* results from irradiation or extension of primary or metastatic tumors (most commonly carcinoma of the lung and breast, malignant

melanoma, and lymphoma) to the pericardium or from invasion by a lymphomatous or leukemic process; pain, atrial arrhythmias, and tamponade are complications which occur occasionally. *Mediastinal irradiation* for neoplasm may cause pericarditis after eradication of the tumor. Unusual causes of acute pericarditis include syphilis, fungus infection (histoplasmosis, blastomycosis, aspergillosis, and candidiasis), and parasitic infestation (amebiasis, toxoplasmosis, echinococcosis, trichinosis).

CHRONIC PERICARDIAL EFFUSIONS   Chronic pericardial effusions are not infrequently encountered in patients without an antecedent history of acute pericarditis. They may cause few symptoms per se, and may be suspected by finding an enlarged cardiac silhouette on chest roentgenogram which may be obtained in the course of the workup of a patient with symptoms related to the underlying illness.

Tuberculosis   This is a common cause of chronic pericardial effusion, although less so in the United States than in other parts of the world (Chap. 125). The symptoms are often those of a chronic, systemic illness in an individual with effusion. It is important to bear this condition in mind when a middle-aged or elderly person with fever has apparent enlargement of the cardiac silhouette of undetermined origin, with or without elevation of venous pressure. Weight loss, fever, and fatigability are sometimes observed. Inasmuch as effective specific methods of therapy have now reduced strikingly the mortality rate from the previous figures of about 70 percent, overlooking a tuberculous pericardial effusion is a serious error. Consequently, no method of examination should be omitted to establish this diagnosis. Included are chest roentgenograms for pulmonary tuberculosis and a search for tuberculosis in other organs; tuberculin skin tests, repeated after several weeks; cultures and smears of gastric washings and of pleural and pericardial fluid. Finally, if the diagnosis is still obscure, a pericardial biopsy, preferably by a limited thoracotomy, should be performed. If definitive evidence is then still lacking, but the specimen shows caseation necrosis, anti-tuberculous chemotherapy for at least 24 months is justified (Chap. 125). Pericardiectomy should be carried out in order to prevent the development of constriction if the biopsy specimen shows a thickened pericardium.

Other causes of chronic pericardial effusion   *Myxedema* may be responsible for a pericardial effusion that is sometimes massive but rarely, if ever, causes cardiac tamponade. The other manifestations of myxedema should clarify the diagnosis, but unfortunately, even when they are present, the diagnosis is frequently overlooked. It is important, therefore, to carry out appropriate tests for thyroid function (Chap. 316) in patients with an enlarged cardiac outline of undetermined origin. The cardiac silhouette is markedly enlarged and an echocardiogram is necessary to distinguish cardiomegaly from pericardial effusion. *Cholesterol pericardial disease* produces large pericardial effusions with a high cholesterol content, which may induce an inflammatory response and constrictive pericarditis.

Neoplasms, systemic lupus erythematosus, rheumatoid arthritis, mycotic infections, radiation therapy, pyogenic infections, severe chronic anemia, and chylopericardium may also cause chronic pericardial effusion and should be considered and specifically looked for in such patients.

Aspiration and analysis of the pericardial fluid are often helpful in diagnosis. In infections the organism can often be identified by smear or culture. Grossly sanguineous pericardial fluid results most commonly from a neoplasm, tuberculosis, uremia, or slow leakage from an aortic aneurysm.

CHRONIC CONSTRICTIVE PERICARDITIS

This disorder results when the healing of an acute fibrinous or serofibrinous pericarditis or a chronic pericardial effusion is followed by obliteration of the pericardial cavity with the formation of granulation tissue. This gradually contracts and forms a firm scar, encasing the heart and interfering with filling of the ventricles. In some reports, a high percentage of all cases has been of tuberculous origin. In other series, particularly those reported in the United States in the last two decades, tuberculosis has been an infrequent cause. The condition also may follow purulent infection, trauma, cardiac operation of any type, mediastinal irradiation, histoplasmosis, neoplastic disease, and acute viral or idiopathic pericarditis, rheumatoid arthritis, lupus erythematosus, and chronic renal failure with uremia treated by chronic dialysis. In many patients the cause of the pericardial disease is undetermined, and in them it is presumed that an asymptomatic or forgotten bout of viral pericarditis, acute or idiopathic, was the inciting event. Rarely, routine radiographic examination may reveal calcification of the pericardium in a person who is free of all symptoms referable to the heart. The heart may also be constricted and compressed by malignant tumors or organized blood clot in the pericardial cavity.

The basic physiologic abnormality in symptomatic patients with chronic constrictive pericarditis, as in those with cardiac tamponade, is the inability of the ventricles to fill adequately during diastole because of the limitations imposed by the rigid, thickened pericardium or the tense pericardial fluid. However, in constrictive pericarditis, ventricular filling is unimpeded during early diastole but is reduced abruptly when the elastic limit of the pericardium is reached; in cardiac tamponade, ventricular filling is impeded throughout diastole. Stroke volume is reduced, and the end-diastolic pressures in both ventricles, as well as the mean pressures in the atria, pulmonic veins, and systemic veins, are all elevated to about the same levels. Despite these hemodynamic changes myocardial function may be normal; instead, the ventricles may be considered to be underloaded. In constrictive pericarditis the central venous and right and left atrial pressure pulses display an M-shaped contour, with prominent x and y descents; the y descent is the most prominent deflection and is interrupted by a rapid rise in pressure during early diastole, when ventricular filling is impeded by the constricting pericardium. In cardiac tamponade the pressure contour differs in that the most prominent deflection is the x trough, while the y descent in the jugular venous pulse and the "square root" sign in the ventricular pressure pulse during diastole are usually absent. These characteristic changes are transmitted to the jugular veins, where they may be recognized by inspection or recorded. In constrictive pericarditis, both ventricular pressure pulses exhibit characteristic "square root" signs during diastole. These hemodynamic changes, although characteristic, are not pathognomonic of constrictive pericarditis but may also be observed in cardiomyopathies characterized by restriction of ventricular filling, as discussed in Chap. 192.

CLINICAL FINDINGS   Weakness, fatigue, weight loss, and anorexia are common. The patients often appear to be chronically ill with decreased muscle mass and a protuberant abdomen; ankle edema may or may not be prominent. Contrary to a widely held impression, dyspnea, though absent or slight at rest, is often present on exertion, and orthopnea is common in chronic constrictive pericarditis, although it is not severe. Attacks of acute left ventricular failure (acute pulmonary edema) practically never occur. The cervical veins are distended and may remain so even after intensive diuretic treatment, and venous pressure may fail to decline during inspiration (Kussmaul's sign). In about one-third of the cases a paradoxical pulse may be observed. Congestive hepatomegaly is pronounced and may impair hepatic function; ascites is common and is usually more prominent than dependent edema. In about half of the patients, the heart is normal in size; if it is enlarged, the enlargement is rarely extreme. The apical pulse is reduced in intensity, retracts in systole, and moves outward in diastole. The heart sounds may be distant, an early third heart sound, i.e., a pericardial knock, occurring 0.06 to 0.12 s after aortic valve closure which coincides with a sudden deceleration in ventricular filling, is often conspicuous, and murmurs are usually absent. The apex beat is poorly defined, and cardiac pulsations under fluoroscopic examination are diminished. Because of the high sustained venous pressure, congestive splenomegaly may make the spleen palpable. In the absence of infective endocarditis or tricuspid

valve disease, splenomegaly in a patient with congestive heart failure should arouse suspicion of constrictive pericarditis. Protein-losing gastroenteropathy due to impaired lymphatic drainage from the small intestine, and the nephrotic syndrome, or sometimes only marked proteinuria or hypoalbuminemia, may complicate chronic constrictive pericarditis. The electrocardiogram frequently displays low voltage of the QRS complex and diffuse flattening or inversion of the T waves. P mitrale may be present in patients with sinus rhythm; atrial fibrillation is present in about one-third of patients.

Systemic and/or pulmonary venous congestion is initially the result of impaired filling of the ventricles caused by the restrictive action of the inelastic pericardium. However, the fibrotic process may extend into the myocardium and cause myocardial scarring, and venous congestion may then be due to the combined effects of the myocardial and pericardial lesions. The interference with filling reduces the work of the heart and perhaps this leads to myocardial atrophy. The latter probably accounts for the delayed beneficial effects of operative treatment observed in some patients with advanced disease.

Inasmuch as the usual physical signs of cardiac disease (murmurs, cardiac enlargement) may be inconspicuous or absent in chronic constrictive pericarditis, hepatic enlargement and dysfunction associated with intractable ascites may lead to a mistaken diagnosis of cirrhosis of the liver. This error should be avoided if the neck veins are inspected carefully in all patients with ascites and hepatomegaly. *Given a clinical picture resembling that of cirrhosis, but with the added feature of distended neck veins, careful search for calcification of the pericardium by chest roentgenograms, fluoroscopy, and echocardiography should be carried out and may disclose a curable or remediable form of heart disease.* Calcification occurs in only about one-half of these patients and usually in those with longstanding pericardial constriction. Most patients with chronic constrictive pericarditis show pericardial thickening on echocardiographic examination. However, echocardiography cannot definitively exclude the diagnosis. Magnetic resonance imaging (MRI) is more precise in establishing or excluding the presence of a thickened pericardium (Chap. 178). Pericardial thickening and even pericardial calcification, however, are not synonymous with constrictive pericarditis since they may occur without seriously impairing ventricular filling. Very rarely, surgical exploration of the pericardium is necessary to establish the diagnosis.

DIFFERENTIAL DIAGNOSIS   Like cor pulmonale (Chap. 191), chronic constrictive pericarditis may be associated with severe systemic venous hypertension but with little or no pulmonary congestion; the heart may not appear to be enlarged, and a striking inspiratory fall in arterial pressure may be present. However, in cor pulmonale advanced parenchymal pulmonary disease is usually evident and venous pressure *falls* during inspiration, i.e., Kusmaul's sign is negative. *Tricuspid stenosis* (p. 951) may also simulate the picture of chronic constrictive pericarditis; congestive hepatomegaly, splenomegaly, and ascites may be equally prominent, and the manifestations of left-sided heart failure may be inconspicuous. However, in tricuspid stenosis, the characteristic murmur, the almost universal coexistence of mitral stenosis, the absence of a paradoxic pulse, as well as the absence, in the jugular venous pulse, of the steep, deep y descent followed by a rapid ascent (manifested by the diastolic shock on palpation and its audible equivalent, the pericardial knock), facilitates the clinical differentiation.

It is of the greatest importance, though often difficult, to distinguish chronic constrictive pericarditis from various forms of heart disease which are characterized by a similar physiologic abnormality, i.e., restriction of ventricular filling, leading to a similar clinical picture. Described in Chap. 192, these include endomyocardial fibrosis; infiltrative cardiomyopathies such as amyloidosis, hemochromatosis, sarcoidosis, and scleroderma; and idiopathic myocardial hypertrophy. In the latter the marked thickening of the ventricular wall is responsible for the diminished compliance.

The features favoring the diagnosis of one of the above forms of cardiomyopathy are a well-defined apex beat, conspicuous enlargement of the heart, and pronounced orthopnea with attacks of acute left ventricular failure, left ventricular hypertrophy, gallop sounds (in place of a pericardial knock), bundle branch block, and in some cases significant Q waves in the electrocardiogram. The echocardiogram shows ventricular thickening, sometimes with a granular sparkling appearance. At catheterization, patients with chronic constrictive pericarditis usually have left atrial or pulmonary arterial wedge pressure equaling right atrial pressure, the latter often exceeding 15 mmHg despite intensive medical treatment for heart failure; the pulmonary artery systolic pressure is often less than 50 mmHg, and the right ventricular end-diastolic pressure often reaches one-third of the systolic pressure; the cardiac output is slightly depressed. In contrast, in patients with cardiomyopathy, the left atrial usually exceeds the right atrial pressure by more than 5 mmHg, the mean right atrial pressure often falls to below 15 mmHg following intensive treatment with diuretics, the pulmonary artery systolic pressure often exceeds 50 mmHg, and the right ventricular end-diastolic pressure is usually less than one-third of the systolic pressure, while the cardiac output is markedly depressed. The volumes of both ventricles, as determined by angiography or echocardiography, are characteristically reduced or normal in constrictive pericarditis, and the ejection fractions are normal or almost so; the left ventricular end-diastolic volume may also be normal in some cardiomyopathies but it is frequently elevated in others in which the ejection fraction is markedly reduced; the latter finding militates strongly against the diagnosis of constrictive pericarditis. The echocardiogram in chronic constrictive pericarditis characteristically shows pericardial thickening, i.e., a distinct echo posterior to the left ventricular wall, and paradoxical septal motion. The left ventricular wall moves sharply outward in early diastole and then remains flat. The definitive diagnosis of restrictive cardiomyopathy, when it is due to an infiltrative disease such as amyloidosis, can often be established by endomyocardial biopsy. MRI is very useful in distinguishing between restrictive cardiomyopathy and chronic constrictive pericarditis (p. 978).

It is important to emphasize that when a patient has progressive, disabling, and unresponsive congestive failure, and if he or she displays any of the phenomena of constrictive heart disease, the most careful and detailed clinical and laboratory studies must be carried out in order to detect or exclude constrictive pericarditis, which is potentially a curable condition. In some instances cardiac catheterization, selective angiocardiography, coronary arteriography, endomyocardial biopsy, and MRI may be required. However, in the rare instance when even these examinations do not yield a definitive diagnosis, surgical exploration of the pericardium is the only decisive method of determining whether constrictive pericarditis is responsible for the clinical manifestations of heart failure.

Occult constrictive disease Patients with this condition may have unexplained fatigue, dyspnea, and chest pain. No overt manifestations of pericardial disease are present, but following the rapid intravenous infusion of 1 liter of saline solution, the atrial and ventricular pressure pulses and diastolic equilibration of intracardiac pressures found in overt constrictive pericarditis occur. Although symptomatic improvement may follow pericardiectomy, this procedure should not be carried out in asymptomatic persons.

TREATMENT Pericardial resection is the only definitive treatment of constrictive pericarditis, but dietary sodium restriction and diuretics are useful during preoperative preparation. Digitalis may be beneficial in the prevention of heart failure when resection of the thickened pericardium permits an increased inflow into the ventricles and hence places an enhanced burden on an atrophic myocardium. The benefits derived from a complete cardiac decortication are often striking, and frequently the improvement, though slight at first, is progressive over a period of many months. The risk of this operation depends on the extent of penetration of the myocardium by the calcific process, by the severity of myocardial atrophy, and by the extent of secondary impairment of hepatic and/or renal function. Operative mortality is in the range of 7 to 10 percent. Therefore, surgical treatment should be carried out relatively early in the course.

Many instances of constrictive pericarditis are of tuberculous origin. Antituberculous therapy during the phase of effusion may prevent the development of constriction, and such therapy should be carried out before and after operation, if a tuberculous origin is suspected or cannot be excluded in a patient with chronic constrictive pericarditis (Chap. 125).

SUBACUTE EFFUSIVE-CONSTRICTIVE PERICARDITIS This form of pericardial disease is characterized by a combination of a tense effusion in the pericardial space, as well as constriction of the heart by thickened pericardium. It shares a number of features both with pericardial effusion producing cardiac compression and with pericardial constriction. It may be caused by tuberculosis, multiple attacks of acute idiopathic pericarditis, radiation, traumatic pericarditis, uremia, and scleroderma. The heart is generally enlarged, and there are a paradoxical pulse and a prominent x descent in the atrial pressure pulse. Following pericardiocentesis, the physiologic findings may change from those of cardiac tamponade to those of pericardial constriction, with a "square root" sign in the ventricular pressure pulse and a prominent y descent in the atrial and jugular venous pressure pulses. Furthermore, the intrapericardial pressure and the central venous pressure may decline, but not to normal. In many patients the condition progresses to the chronic constrictive form of the disease. Wide excision of both the visceral and parietal pericardium is usually effective.

OTHER DISORDERS OF THE PERICARDIUM

Pericardial cysts appear as rounded or lobulated deformities of the cardiac silhouette, most commonly at the right cardiophrenic angle. They do not cause symptoms, and their major clinical significance lies in the possibility of confusion with a tumor, ventricular aneurysm, or massive cardiomegaly. *Tumors* involving the pericardium are most commonly secondary to malignant neoplasms originating in or invading the mediastinum, including carcinoma of the bronchus and breast, lymphoma, and melanoma. The most common *primary* malignant tumor is the mesothelioma. The usual clinical picture of malignant pericardial tumor is an insidiously developing, often bloody, pericardial effusion. Surgical exploration is required to establish a definitive diagnosis and to carry out definitive or, more commonly, palliative treatment.

REFERENCES

BUSH CA et al: Occult pericardial disease. Circulation 56:924, 1977

FOWLER NO et al: Cardiac tamponade: A comparison of right versus left heart compression. J Am Coll Cardiol 12:187, 1988

GOLD RG: Post-viral pericarditis. Eur Heart J 9:(G):175, 1988

HANCOCK EW: Subacute effusive-constrictive pericarditis. Circulation 43:183, 1971

HATLE LK et al: Differentiation of constrictive pericarditis and restrictive cardiomyopathy by Doppler echocardiography. Circulation 79:357, 1989

LORELL B, BRAUNWALD E: Pericardial disease, in *Heart Disease,* 3d ed, E Braunwald (ed). Philadelphia, Saunders, 1988, pp 1484–1534

McCAUHGAN BC et al: Early and late results of pericardiectomy for constrictive pericarditis. J Thorac Cardiovasc Surg 89:340, 1985

NISHIMURA RA et al: Constrictive pericarditis: Assessment of current diagnostic procedures. Mayo Clin Proc 60:397, 1985

RIBEIRO P et al: Constrictive pericarditis as a complication of coronary artery bypass surgery. Br Heart J 51:205, 1984

SAGRISTA-SAULEDA J et al: Tuberculosis pericarditis: Ten year experience with a prospective protocol for diagnosis and treatment. J Am Coll Cardiol 11:724, 1988

SHABETAI R: Pericardial and cardiac pressure. Circulation 77:1, 1988

194   CARDIAC TUMORS, CARDIAC MANIFESTATIONS OF SYSTEMIC DISEASES, AND TRAUMATIC CARDIAC INJURY

WILSON S. COLUCCI / EUGENE BRAUNWALD

TUMORS OF THE HEART

PRIMARY TUMORS   Primary tumors of the heart are rare and are often classified as "benign" histologically (Table 194-1). However, since all cardiac tumors have the potential for causing life-threatening complications, and many are now curable by surgery, it is important that this diagnosis be made whenever possible. Approximately three-quarters are *histologically* benign, and the remainder are malignant, in almost all cases sarcomas.

Clinical presentation   Cardiac tumors may present with a wide array of cardiac and noncardiac manifestations. There may be signs and symptoms of all the more common forms of heart disease, including chest pain, syncope, heart failure, murmurs, arrhythmias, conduction disturbances, and pericardial effusion or tamponade. The specific signs and symptoms produced are most closely related to the location of the tumor.

Myxoma   Myxomas are the most common type of primary cardiac tumor, accounting for one-third to one-half of all cases. They occur at all ages and show no sex preference. Although the large majority of myxomas are sporadic, some are familial with autosomal dominant transmission or are part of a syndrome that involves a complex of abnormalities including lentigines or pigmented nevi, primary nodular adrenal cortical disease with or without Cushing's syndrome, myxomatous mammary fibroadenomas, testicular tumors, and/or pituitary adenomas with gigantism or acromegaly. Certain constellations of findings have been referred to as the *NAME syndrome* (nevi, atrial myxoma, myxoid neurofibroma, and ephelides) or the *LAMB syndrome* (lentigines, atrial myxoma, and blue nevi). Approximately 7 percent of cardiac myxomas are familial or part of the "complex myxoma" syndrome described above.

Most authorities consider the myxoma a true neoplasm, while others have suggested that it is formed by organization of an intracardiac thrombus attached to the endocardium. The large majority of sporadic myxomas are solitary and located in the atria, particularly the left, where they arise from the interatrial septum in the vicinity of the fossa ovalis. Sporadic myxomas may also occur in the ventricles or may be found in multiple locations. In contrast to sporadic myxomas, familial or "complex" myxomas tend to occur in younger individuals, are more often multiple in location, and are more likely to have postoperative recurrences, probably reflecting their multicentric nature (Table 194-2). Most are pedunculated on a fibrovascular stalk and average 4 to 8 cm in diameter. The most common clinical presentation resembles that of mitral valve disease, either stenosis as a result of tumor prolapse into the mitral orifice during diastole or regurgitation as a consequence of injury to the valve by tumor-induced trauma. Ventricular myxomas may cause outflow obstruction and may therefore mimic subaortic or subpulmonic stenosis. Characteristically, the symptoms and signs are highly dependent on position, intermittent, and sudden in onset as a result of changes in tumor position with gravity. On auscultation, a characteristic low-pitched sound, termed a "tumor plop," is audible during early or middiastole and is thought to result from the tumor abruptly stopping as it strikes the ventricular wall. Myxomas may also present with peripheral or pulmonary emboli, or any of several noncardiac signs and symptoms including fever, weight loss, cachexia, malaise, arthralgia, rash, clubbing, Raynaud's phenomenon, hypergamma-globulinemia, anemia, polycythemia, leukocytosis, elevated erythrocyte sedimentation rate, thrombocytopenia, or thrombocytosis. Not surprisingly, myxomas are frequently misdiagnosed as endocarditis, collagen vascular disease, or noncardiac tumor.

Both M-mode and two-dimensional echocardiography (Fig. 177-3, p. 862) are useful in the diagnosis of cardiac myxoma, the latter having the advantage of allowing determination of the site of tumor attachment and tumor size, important considerations in the planning of surgical excision. Computed tomography and magnetic resonance imaging may provide important information regarding the size, shape, and surface characteristics of the tumor. Because myxomas may be familial, echocardiographic screening of first-degree relatives is appropriate, particularly if the patient is young or has multiple tumors. While cardiac catheterization and angiography are often performed prior to surgery, catheterization of the chamber from which the tumor originates is attended by the risk of dislodgment of tumor emboli. In many centers catheterization is no longer considered mandatory when adequate noninvasive information is available.

Surgical excision utilizing cardiopulmonary bypass is indicated in all patients and is generally curative. Occasional reports of tumor recurrence are most likely due to inadequate excision of multiple tumor sites.

Other benign tumors   Cardiac *lipomas*, although relatively common, are usually incidental findings at postmortem examination and seldom result in symptoms. However, they may grow as large as 15 cm and present with symptoms due to mechanical interference with cardiac function, arrhythmias, or conduction disturbances, or as an

TABLE 194-1   Relative incidence of primary tumors of the heart

Type	Percent
BENIGN	
Myxoma	30.5
Lipoma	10.5
Papillary fibroelastoma	9.9
Rhabdomyoma	8.5
Fibroma	4.0
Hemangioma	3.5
Teratoma	3.3
Mesothelioma of the AV node	2.8
Other benign tumors	2.1
Total	75.1
MALIGNANT	
Sarcomas	18.6
Lymphoma	1.6
Other malignant tumors	4.7
Total	24.9

SOURCE: Modified from HA McAllister, JJ Fenoglio, in *Atlas of Tumor Pathology*, Washington, Armed Forces Institute of Pathology, 1978, fasc 15, 2d series.

TABLE 194-2   Comparison of clinical features of sporadic myxoma and syndrome myxoma

Feature	Sporadic	Syndrome
Age (yr) (range)	56 (39–82)	25 (10–56)
Female/male ratio	2·7:1	1·8:1
Patients (no.)	70	44
Cardiac myxomas (no.)	72	103
Distributions of myxomas (%):		
Atrial/ventricular	100/0	87/13
Single/multiple	99/1	50/50
Biatrial	0	23
Recurrent	0	18
Familial	0	27
Freckling (%)	0	68
Noncardiac tumors (%)	0	57
Endocrine neoplasm (%)	0	30
Familial (%)	0	14

SOURCE: From HJ Vidaillet et al.

abnormality of the cardiac silhouette on chest x-ray. *Papillary fibroelastomas,* similarly, are relatively common findings on cardiac valves or the adjacent endothelium but seldom result in clinical symptoms. Occasionally, these growths may cause mechanical interference with valvular function. *Rhabdomyomas* and *fibromas,* the most frequent tumors in infants and children, most commonly occur in the ventricles, and therefore produce signs and symptoms by mechanical obstruction which may mimic valvular stenosis, congestive heart failure, restrictive or hypertrophic cardiomyopathy, and pericardial constriction. Rhabdomyomas are probably hamartomatous growths, are multiple in about 90 percent of cases, and may be associated with tuberous sclerosis, adenoma sebaceum, and benign kidney tumors. *Hemangiomas* and *mesotheliomas* are generally small tumors, most often intramyocardial in location, and may cause atrioventricular (AV) conduction disturbances and even sudden death as a result of their propensity for location in the region of the AV node.

Sarcomas Cardiac sarcomas may be of several histologic types, but in general are characterized by a rapidly downhill course leading to the patient's death in weeks to months from the time of presentation as a result of hemodynamic compromise, local invasion, or distant metastases. Sarcomas commonly involve the right side of the heart, and because of their rapid growth, invasion of the pericardial space and obstruction of the cardiac chambers or venae cavae are common. At the time of presentation these tumors have often spread too extensively for surgical excision. While there are scattered reports of palliation with surgery, radiotherapy, and/or chemotherapy, the overall experience with cardiac sarcomas is poor. The one exception to this appears to be cardiac lymphosarcomas, which may respond to a combination of chemo- and radiotherapy.

TUMORS METASTATIC TO THE HEART Tumors metastatic to the heart are several times more common than primary tumors, and as the life expectancy of patients with various forms of malignant neoplasms is extended by more effective therapy, it is likely that the frequency of cardiac metastases will also increase. Although cardiac metastases occur in 1 to 20 percent of all tumor types, the incidence is especially high in malignant melanoma, and to a somewhat lesser extent in leukemia and lymphoma. In absolute numbers, cardiac metastases are most common in carcinoma of the breast and lung, reflecting the high incidence of these cancers. Cardiac metastases almost always occur in the setting of widespread primary disease, and most often there is either primary or metastatic disease elsewhere in the thoracic cavity. Nevertheless, occasionally a cardiac metastasis may be the initial presentation of a tumor elsewhere in the body.

Cardiac metastases reach the heart via the bloodstream, lymphatics, or direct invasion and generally are small, firm nodules; although diffuse infiltrations may also occur, especially with sarcomas or hematologic neoplasms. The pericardium is most often involved, followed by myocardial involvement of any chamber, and, rarely, by involvement of the endocardium or cardiac valves.

Cardiac metastases result in clinical manifestations only about 10 percent of the time, and rarely are they the cause of death. In most patients they are *not* the cause of the presenting clinical features but occur in the setting of a previously recognized malignant neoplasm. While cardiac metastases may present a large number of nonspecific signs and symptoms, the most common are dyspnea, signs of acute pericarditis, cardiac tamponade, a rapid increase in the cardiac silhouette on chest x-ray, the new onset of an ectopic tachyarrhythmia, AV block, and congestive heart failure. As with primary cardiac tumors, the clinical presentation is more closely related to the location and size of the tumor than to its histologic type. Many of these signs and symptoms may also occur with myocarditis, pericarditis, or cardiomyopathy resulting from radiotherapy or chemotherapy.

The electrocardiographic findings are entirely nonspecific and may include ST-T-wave changes, decreased QRS voltage, arrhythmias, and conduction disturbances. On chest roentgenography the cardiac silhouette is most often normal but may reveal a pericardial effusion or bizarre contour. Echocardiography is useful for the diagnosis of pericardial effusion and the visualization of larger metastases. Computed tomography, magnetic resonance imaging, and radionuclide imaging with gallium or thallium may provide useful anatomic information. Angiography may delineate discrete lesions, and pericardiocentesis can allow a specific cytologic diagnosis. Since most patients with cardiac metastases have widespread disease, therapy generally consists of pericardiocentesis when there is hemodynamic compromise and treatment directed at the primary tumor. The removal of a malignant effusion by pericardiocentesis with or without concomitant instillation of a sclerosing agent (e.g., tetracycline) may palliate symptoms and delay or prevent reaccumulation of the effusion.

CARDIAC EFFECTS OF CANCER THERAPY See Chap. 192.

CARDIOVASCULAR MANIFESTATIONS OF SYSTEMIC DISEASES

DIABETES MELLITUS (See Chap. 319) In patients with insulin-dependent diabetes mellitus there is an increased incidence of large-vessel atherosclerosis and myocardial infarction, and diabetics are more likely to have an abnormal or absent pain response to myocardial ischemia, probably as a result of generalized autonomic nervous system dysfunction. Diabetic patients may also have myocardial dysfunction characteristic of a restrictive cardiomyopathy in the absence of large-vessel coronary artery disease, as evidenced by elevated left ventricular filling pressures. Histologically, these patients have increased amounts of collagen, glycoprotein, triglycerides, and cholesterol in the myocardial interstitium, and in some cases intimal thickening, hyaline deposition, and inflammatory changes have been observed in small intramural arteries. While these changes alone seldom result in clinical heart failure, it is likely that they contribute to the excessive cardiovascular morbidity and mortality of diabetics. There is some evidence that insulin therapy results in an amelioration of the myocardial dysfunction.

MALNUTRITION AND THIAMINE DEFICIENCY (BERIBERI) Malnutrition (See Chap. 71) In patients whose intake of protein, calories, or both is severely deficient, the heart may become thin, pale, and flabby with myofibrillar atrophy and interstitial edema. The systolic pressure and cardiac output are low and the pulse pressure narrow. Generalized edema is common and is due to a combination of factors, including reduced serum oncotic pressure and myocardial dysfunction. Such profound states of malnutrition, termed *marasmus* in the case of caloric deficiency or *kwashiorkor* in the case of relative protein deficiency, are most common in underdeveloped countries. However, significant nutritional heart disease may also occur in developed nations, particularly in patients with severe cardiac failure in whom gastrointestinal hypoperfusion and venous congestion may cause anorexia and malabsorption. Open-heart surgery poses an increased risk in such patients, who may benefit from preoperative intensive hyperalimentation. Deficient nutrients and minerals should be replaced gradually since rapid expansion of the intravascular space may stress the weakened heart and result in overt congestive heart failure.

Thiamine deficiency (See Chap. 76) In many cases, malnutrition is accompanied by thiamine deficiency, although this hypovitaminosis may also occur in the presence of an adequate protein and caloric intake, particularly in the Far East, where polished rice deficient in thiamine may be a major dietary component. The widespread use of thiamine-enriched flour in western nations confines this disease primarily to alcoholics and food faddists. Clinically, there is usually evidence of generalized malnutrition, peripheral neuropathy, glossitis, and anemia. The characteristic cardiovascular syndrome is that of high-output heart failure with tachycardia, increased cardiac output, and often elevated filling pressures in the left and right sides of the heart. It appears that the major cause of the high-output state is vasomotor depression, the precise mechanism of which is not understood, but which leads to a reduced systemic vascular resistance. The cardiac examination reveals a wide pulse pressure, tachycardia, a third heart sound, and, frequently, a systolic murmur at the apex. The electrocardiogram may show decreased voltage, a prolonged QT interval, and T-wave abnormalities; the chest x-ray generally shows a large heart with signs of congestive heart failure. The response to thiamine is often dramatic, with an increase in systemic vascular resistance, decrease in cardiac output, clearing of pulmonary congestion, and a reduction in heart size often occurring in 12 to 48 h. Although the response to digitalis and diuretics may be poor prior to thiamine therapy, these agents may be important *after* thiamine is given, since the left ventricle may not be capable of dealing with the increased workload presented by the return of vascular tone.

OBESITY (See Chap. 72)   Although not defined as a disease per se, severe obesity is associated with an increase in cardiovascular morbidity and mortality, due in part to hypertension, glucose intolerance, and atherosclerotic coronary artery disease, all of which are more prevalent in obese patients. In addition, these patients have a distinct abnormality of the cardiovascular system characterized by increases in total and central blood volumes, cardiac output, and left ventricular filling pressure. It appears that cardiac output is elevated in order to help supply the metabolic needs of the excessive adipose tissue. Left ventricular filling pressure is often at the upper limits of normal and rises excessively with exercise. As a result of chronic volume and pressure overload, eccentric cardiac hypertrophy with cardiac dilation and abnormal ventricular function may develop. Pathologically, there is left and, in some cases, right ventricular hypertrophy and generalized cardiac enlargement, which is not due simply to fatty infiltration of the myocardium. Clinically, these patients may develop pulmonary congestion, peripheral edema, and exercise intolerance, findings which may be difficult to recognize in massively obese patients. Weight reduction is the most effective therapy and results in reduction in blood volume and in return of cardiac output toward normal. Digitalis, sodium restriction, and diuretics may also be useful. This form of heart disease should be distinguished from the Pickwickian syndrome (Chap. 217), which may share several of the cardiovascular features but, in addition, frequently has components of central apnea, hypoxemia, pulmonary hypertension, and cor pulmonale.

THYROID DISEASE (See Chap. 316)   Thyroid hormone exerts a major influence on the cardiovascular system by a number of direct and indirect mechanisms, and not surprisingly, cardiovascular effects are prominent in both hypo- and hyperthyroidism. Thyroid hormone causes increases in total-body metabolism and oxygen consumption that indirectly place an increased workload on the heart. In addition, although the exact mechanism has not been defined, thyroid hormone exerts direct inotropic, chronotropic, and dromotropic effects that are similar to those seen with adrenergic stimulation (e.g., tachycardia, increased cardiac output). It has been shown that thyroid hormone increases the synthesis of myosin and of Na^+,K^+-ATPase, as well as the density of myocardial beta-adrenergic receptors.

Hyperthyroidism   Excess thyroid hormone results in increases in heart rate, cardiac output, stroke volume, pulse pressure, and measures of left ventricular contractility. Patients may present with palpitations, systolic hypertension, fatigue, or, in patients with underlying heart disease, angina or heart failure. Sinus tachycardia is found in about 40 percent of patients, and atrial fibrillation in about 15 percent. Other findings include a hyperactive precordium, an increase in the intensity of the first heart sound and the pulmonic component of the second heart sound, and a third heart sound. An increased incidence of mitral valve prolapse has been associated with hyperthyroidism, and in some cases there may be a midsystolic murmur heard best at the left sternal border with or without a systolic ejection click. A systolic scratchy sound, the *Means-Lerman scratch*, may occasionally be heard at the left second intercostal space during expiration and is thought to result from the rubbing of the hyperdynamic pericardium against the pleura. Elderly patients with hyperthyroidism may present with only the cardiovascular manifestations of thyrotoxicosis, which may be resistant to therapy until the hyperthyroidism is controlled. Although there is some evidence that

hyperthyroidism per se can result in myocardial dysfunction, angina pectoris and congestive heart failure are unusual, unless there is coexistent underlying heart disease, and in many cases will resolve with therapy of the hyperthyroidism.

Hypothyroidism   There is a reduction in cardiac output, stroke volume, heart rate, blood pressure, and pulse pressure. In about one-third of patients there is a pericardial effusion which only rarely results in tamponade. Increased capillary permeability results in pleural and pericardial effusions, but only rarely results in tamponade. Other clinical signs include cardiomegaly, bradycardia, weak arterial pulses, and distant heart sounds. As a result of earlier detection and treatment of hypothyroidism, these overt signs are commonly absent, and the major findings may be exertional dyspnea and easy fatigability. Although the signs and symptoms of myxedema may suggest the diagnosis of congestive heart failure, in the absence of other cardiac disease, myocardial failure is uncommon. Biochemical abnormalities, including elevations of creatine kinase, serum glutamic oxaloacetic transaminase, and lactic dehydrogenase, may lead to a mistaken diagnosis of myocardial infarction. The electrocardiogram generally shows sinus bradycardia and low voltage and may show prolongation of the QT interval, decreased P-wave voltage, prolonged AV conduction time, intraventricular conduction disturbances, and nonspecific ST-T-wave abnormalities. Chest x-ray may show cardiomegaly, often with a "water bottle" configuration, pleural effusions, and, in some cases, evidence of congestive heart failure. Pathologically, the heart is pale, dilated, and flabby, often with myofibrillar swelling, loss of striations, and interstitial fibrosis.

Patients with hypothyroidism frequently have elevations of cholesterol and triglycerides and severe atherosclerotic coronary artery disease. Prior to treatment with thyroid hormone, patients with hypothyroidism frequently do not have angina pectoris, presumably because of the low metabolic demands made by their condition. However, such patients, especially when elderly, are prone to angina and myocardial infarction during replacement of thyroid hormone, and this should always be done with extreme care, starting with very low doses which are increased gradually.

MALIGNANT CARCINOID (See Chap. 262)   These tumors elaborate a variety of vasoactive amines (e.g., serotonin), kinins, indoles, and other substances which are believed to be responsible for the diarrhea, flushing, and labile blood pressure seen in these patients. The cardiac lesions due to gastrointestinal carcinoids are almost exclusively in the right side of the heart and occur only when there are hepatic metastases, suggesting that the substance responsible for the cardiac lesions is inactivated by passage through the liver and lungs. Similar lesions occur in the left side of the heart when there is a right-to-left shunt or the tumor is located in the lungs. Fibrous plaques are found on the endothelium of the cardiac chambers, valves, and great vessels. These plaques, which result in distortion of the cardiac valves, consist of smooth muscle cells imbedded in a stroma of acid mucopolysaccharide and collagen, and presumably result from healing of endothelial injury. The clinical syndrome is most often that of tricuspid regurgitation, pulmonic stenosis, or both. In some cases a high-output state may occur, presumably as a result of a decrease in systemic vascular resistance due to a vasoactive substance released by the tumor. Progression of the cardiac lesions does not appear to be affected by treatment with serotonin antagonists, and in some severely symptomatic patients valve replacement is indicated. Coronary artery spasm, presumably due to a circulating vasoactive substance, may occur in patients with carcinoid syndrome.

PHEOCHROMOCYTOMA (See Chap. 318)   In addition to causing hypertension, which may be labile or sustained, the high circulating levels of catecholamines may also cause direct myocardial injury. Focal myocardial necrosis and inflammatory cell infiltration are seen in about 50 percent of patients who die with pheochromocytoma and may contribute to clinically significant left ventricular failure and pulmonary edema. In addition, hypertension results in left ventricular hypertrophy.

RHEUMATOID ARTHRITIS AND THE COLLAGEN VASCULAR DISEASES Rheumatoid arthritis (See Chap. 270) There may be inflammation of any or all parts of the heart in patients with rheumatoid arthritis. *Pericarditis* is the most common cause of clinically apparent disease and may be found in 30 to 50 percent of all patients with rheumatoid arthritis, particularly those with subcutaneous nodules, if carefully searched for by echocardiography or at postmortem examination. However, only a small fraction of these patients will have clinical evidence of pericarditis, which usually follows a benign course, but occasionally may progress to cardiac tamponade or constrictive pericarditis. The pericardial fluid is generally an exudate, with decreased concentrations of complement and glucose and elevated cholesterol. Treatment is directed at the underlying rheumatoid arthritis and may include glucocorticoids. Pericardiectomy is usually required in cases of tamponade or persistent effusion. *Coronary arteritis* with intimal inflammation and edema is present in about 20 percent of cases but only rarely results in angina pectoris or myocardial infarction. The cardiac valves, most often the mitral and aortic, may be involved by inflammation and granuloma formation which in some cases may cause clinically significant regurgitation due to valve deformity. Myocarditis rarely results in cardiac dysfunction.

Seronegative arthropathies The seronegative arthropathies (Chaps. 274 and 283), ankylosing spondylitis, Reiter's syndrome, psoriatic arthritis, and the arthritides associated with ulcerative colitis and regional enteritis may be accompanied by a pancarditis and proximal aortitis; the latter may result in aortic regurgitation and may extend into the anterior mitral valve ring and/or AV node. Both aortic regurgitation and AV block are more common in patients with peripheral joint involvement and long-standing disease; and treatment with aortic valve replacement and permanent pacemaker placement may be required. Up to one-fifth of patients with peripheral joint involvement and disease for more than 30 years have significant aortic regurgitation. Occasionally, aortic regurgitation precedes the onset of arthritis, and, therefore, the diagnosis of a seronegative arthritis should be considered in young males with isolated aortic regurgitation.

Systemic lupus erythematosus (SLE) (See Chap. 269) Pericarditis is common, occurring in about two-thirds of patients, and generally pursues a benign course, although rarely tamponade or constriction may result. The characteristic *endocardial lesions* of SLE, described by Libman and Sacks, consist of wartlike lesions most often located at the angles of the AV valves or on the ventricular surface of the mitral valve. Hemodynamically important valvular regurgitation is rare. Myocarditis generally parallels the activity of the disease, and although common histologically, seldom results in clinical heart failure unless associated with hypertension. Although arteritis of large coronary arteries may rarely result in myocardial ischemia, there is also an increased frequency of coronary atherosclerosis which may be related to hypertension or glucocorticoid therapy.

TRAUMATIC HEART DISEASE

Cardiac damage may be due to both penetrating and nonpenetrating injuries. The most frequent cause of a *nonpenetrating injury* is impact of the chest against the steering wheel of an automobile. Serious injury of the heart may ensue even though no external sign of thoracic trauma is evident. Although the commonest injury is myocardial contusion, any structure of the heart may be affected by the trauma. If the valvular apparatus is ruptured, a loud heart murmur produced by valvular regurgitation may appear, followed by the development of rapidly progressive heart failure. The most serious consequence of nonpenetrating injury is rupture, either of the atria or of the ventricles, which is generally fatal. Hemopericardium may also follow tearing of a pericardial vessel or coronary artery.

Myocardial contusion may cause arrhythmias, bundle branch block, or electrocardiographic abnormalities resembling those of infarction, and so it is important to bear trauma in mind as a cause of otherwise unexplained electrocardiographic changes. Similarly, myocardial contusion may produce positive radionuclide scans and regional impairment of ventricular function, as occurs in myocardial infarction (Chap. 177). Pericardial effusion may occur weeks or even months after the accident. In these cases, the pericardial effusion is a manifestation of the postcardiac injury syndrome, which resembles the postpericardiotomy syndrome (Chap. 193).

Acute myocardial failure resulting from rupture of a valve usually requires operative correction. Myocardial infarction due to trauma is treated similarly to that due to ischemic heart disease (Chap. 189). Pericardial hemorrhage often leads to constriction which must be treated by decortication.

Penetrating injuries of the heart, produced by bullets or stab wounds, usually result in immediate or very rapid death because of hemopericardium or massive hemorrhage. However, sometimes the patient survives the acute incident and presents with a cardiac murmur and congestive heart failure. A left-to-right shunt due to traumatic ventricular septal defect, aortopulmonary artery fistula, or coronary arteriovenous fistula may be suspected and confirmed by cardiac catheterization and angiocardiography. Operation is indicated if hemodynamically significant abnormalities are present or if a foreign body, e.g., a bullet, is lodged in the heart. Immediate thoracotomy should be carried out if there is cardiac tamponade and/or shock, whether the trauma was penetrating or nonpenetrating. Pericardiocentesis may be helpful in patients with tamponade, but usually only as a holding maneuver. Patients who suffer penetrating injuries of the heart should be carefully examined several weeks after the event to rule out a ventricular septal defect or mitral regurgitation that may have gone undetected at the time of emergency surgery.

Rupture of the aorta is a common consequence of chest trauma. Indeed, rupture of the aorta at the isthmus or just above the aortic valve is the most common vascular deceleration injury. The clinical presentation is similar to that in aortic dissection (Chap. 197). The arterial pressure and pulse amplitude may be increased in the upper extremities and decreased in the lower extremities, and on chest roentgenogram there may be widening of the mediastinum. Occasionally, the rupture is limited by the aortic adventitia and results in a silent false aneurysm that may be discovered months or years after the injury. When great vessel rupture is due to a penetrating injury, there is usually a hemothorax and, less often, a hemopericardium. Hematoma formation may compress major vessels, and arteriovenous fistulae may be formed, sometimes resulting in high-output congestive heart failure.

REFERENCES

AYZENBERG O et al: Beriberi heart disease. S Afr Med J 68:263, 1985

COHN PF, BRAUNWALD E: Traumatic heart disease, in *Heart Disease*, 3d ed, E Braunwald (ed). Philadelphia, Saunders, 1988, p 1535

COLUCCI WS, BRAUNWALD E: Primary tumors of the heart, in *Heart Disease*, 3d ed, E Braunwald (ed). Philadelphia, Saunders, 1988, p 1470

DOHERTY NE, SIEGEL J: The cardiovascular manifestations of systemic lupus erythematosus. Am Heart J 110:1257, 1985

FEIN FS, SONNENBLICK EH: Diabetic cardiomyopathy. Progr Cardiovasc Dis 27:255, 1985

FYKE FE et al: Primary cardiac tumors: Experience with 30 consecutive patients since the introduction of two-dimensional echocardiography. J Am Coll Cardiol 5:1465, 1985

KLEIN I, LEVEY GS: New perspectives on thyroid hormone, catecholamines, and the heart. Am J Med 76:167, 1984

LOCKWOOD WB, BROGHAMER WL JR: The changing prevalence of secondary cardiac neoplasms as related to cancer therapy. Cancer 15:2659, 1980

MATTOX K et al: Cardiac evaluation following heart injury. J Trauma 25:758, 1985

ROSS EM, ROBERTS WC: The carcinoid syndrome: Comparison of 21 necropsy subjects with carcinoid heart disease to 15 necropsy subjects without carcinoid heart disease. Am J Med 79:339, 1985

VIDAILLET HJ et al: "Syndrome myxoma": A subset of patients with cardiac myxoma associated with pigmented skin lesions and peripheral and endocrine neoplasms. Br Heart J 57:247, 1987

STOLLERMAN E: Rheumatic fever, connective tissue disorders and heart disease, in *Heart Disease*, 2d ed, E Braunwald (ed). Philadelphia, Saunders, 1988, p 1641

section 2 Disorders of the vascular system

ATHEROSCLEROSIS AND OTHER FORMS OF ARTERIOSCLEROSIS

EDWIN L. BIERMAN

Arteriosclerosis, a generic term for thickening and hardening of the arterial wall, is responsible for the majority of deaths in the United States and most westernized societies. One type of arteriosclerosis is *atherosclerosis*, the disorder of the larger arteries that underlies most *coronary artery disease*, *aortic aneurysm*, and *arterial disease of the lower extremities* and also plays a major role in *cerebrovascular disease*. Atherosclerosis is by far the leading cause of death in the United States, both above and below age 65 (Table 195-1).

Other types of arteriosclerosis include focal calcific arteriosclerosis (*Mönckeberg's sclerosis*) and *arteriolosclerosis*. The major arterial diseases other than arteriosclerosis include *congenital structural defects*, *inflammatory* or *granulomatous diseases* (e.g., syphilitic aortitis), and disorders affecting mainly the smaller vessels, such as *hypersensitivity* or autoimmune diseases.

THE NORMAL ARTERY

STRUCTURE The normal artery wall consists of three reasonably well-defined layers: the intima, the media, and the adventitia.

Intima A single continuous layer of *endothelial cells* lines the lumen of all arteries. The intima is delimited on its outer aspect by a perforated tube of elastic tissue, the *internal elastic lamina*. This tube of elastic tissue is particularly prominent in the large elastic arteries and the medium-caliber muscular arteries, and it disappears in capillaries. The endothelial cells are attached to one another by a series of junctional complexes and are also attached, apparently somewhat tenuously, to an underlying meshwork of loose connective tissue, the *basal lamina*. These lining endothelial cells normally form a barrier that controls the entry of substances from the blood into the artery wall. Such substances usually enter the cells by specific transport systems. Normally, no other cell type is present in the intima of most arteries.

Media The media consists of only one cell type, the *smooth-muscle cell*, arranged in either a single layer (as in small muscular arteries) or multiple lamellae (as in elastic arteries). These cells are surrounded by small amounts of collagen and elastic fibers, which they elaborate, and usually take the pattern of diagonal concentric spirals through the vessel wall. They are closely apposed to one another and may be attached by junctional complexes. The smooth-muscle cell appears to be the major connective tissue–forming cell of the artery wall, producing collagen, elastic fibers, and proteoglycans. In that sense it is analogous to the fibroblast in skin, the osteoblast in bone, and the chondroblast in cartilage. The media is bounded on the luminal side by the *internal elastic lamina* and on the abluminal side by a less continuous sheet of elastic tissue, the *external elastic lamina*. In *elastic arteries*, like the aorta and the major pulmonary arteries, elastic lamellae are prominent. Such arteries expand and increase their elastic tension with the pulse of systole. In diastole, the elastic fibers recoil, helping to propel the blood distally and progressively damping the pulsatile character of flow toward more terminal vessels. In *muscular arteries*, in which smooth-muscle cells predominate, peripheral flow is regulated, particularly in arterioles, by contraction (vasoconstriction) and relaxation (vasodilatation). Located about midway through the media of most arteries is a "nutritional watershed." The outer portion is nourished from the small blood vessels (vasa vasorum) in the adventitia; the inner layers receive their nutrients from the lumen.

Adventitia The outermost layer of the artery is the adventitia, which is delimited on the luminal aspect by the external elastic lamina. This external coat consists of a loose interwoven admixture of collagen bundles, elastic fibers, smooth-muscle cells, and fibroblasts. This layer also contains the vasa vasorum and nerves.

METABOLISM AND FUNCTION The artery wall is a metabolically active organ that must meet a steady demand for energy to maintain smooth-muscle tension and endothelial cell function and to repair and replenish tissue constituents. The mechanical forces on the arterial wall are complex, and considerable tensile stresses are imposed on it, mainly by hydraulic force. Shear or frictional stresses are especially prominent near the entrance regions of branches. The form and manner in which these forces are dissipated depend upon flow, the amount of elastic tension developed, and the tethering or external support provided by surrounding structures. Arteries are also permeable pipes, which constantly exchange fluid and solutes with the blood they carry.

Maintenance of the endothelial cell lining is critical. Endothelial cell turnover occurs at a slow rate but may be accelerated in focal areas by changing patterns of flow along the vessel wall. When intact, these cells selectively control the passage of circulating substances by active transport (endocytosis and exocytosis) through their cytoplasm, and they elaborate connective tissue components to form their own substratum. In addition, intact endothelial cells function to prevent clotting partly by elaboration of a particular prostaglandin (prostacyclin or PGI_2) that inhibits platelet function, thereby enhancing unimpeded flow of blood. When the lining is damaged, platelets adhere to it, in part as the result of production of a different class of prostaglandins, the thromboxanes, and form a clot; endothelial cells function in the clotting process by elaboration of key substances, including factor VIII.

The metabolism of arteries reflects the biochemistry of smooth-muscle cells. Arterial smooth-muscle cells form abundant collagen,

TABLE 195-1 Deaths by cause in the United States, 1986

| Causes of death | No. of deaths, thousands | | | |
| | Below age 65 | | Age 65 and above | |
	Male	Female	Male	Female
All causes	396	222	709	779
All cardiovascular diseases	119	54	357	438
Ischemic heart disease	71	25	203	222
Cerebrovascular disease	11	10	48	81
Hypertensive disease*	1	1	3	4
All infectious disease	5	3	1	2
All cancer	86	75	165	143
Accidents	52	17	13	12

* A substantial proportion of deaths of hypertensive persons occurs with ischemic heart disease or cerebrovascular disease; such deaths are classified in those categories.
SOURCE: National Center of Health Statistics, *Vital Statistics Report, Final Mortality Statistics, 1986.*

elastic fibers, soluble and insoluble elastin, and glucosaminoglycans (mainly dermatan sulfate). Multiple anabolic and catabolic pathways are present. These cells metabolize glucose by both anaerobic and aerobic glycolysis. A variety of catabolic enzymes are present including fibrinolysins, mixed-function oxidases, and lysosomal hydrolases. Because of the prominence of lipids in atherosclerotic lesions, much attention has been directed to lipid metabolism in arteries. Arterial wall cells can synthesize fatty acids, cholesterol, phospholipids, and triglycerides from endogenous substrates to satisfy their structural needs (membrane replenishment), but smooth-muscle cells appear preferentially to utilize lipids from plasma lipoproteins transported into the wall. Circulating lipoproteins traverse endothelial cells in pinocytotic vesicles. Smooth-muscle cells possess specific high-affinity surface receptors for certain apoproteins on the surface of lipid-rich lipoproteins, thus facilitating the entry of lipoproteins into the cell by adsorptive endocytosis. As has been shown for cultured skin fibroblasts, in arterial smooth-muscle cells these vesicles fuse with lysosomes, resulting in catabolism of lipoprotein components (Chap. 326). Free cholesterol entering the cell in this manner inhibits endogenous cholesterol synthesis, facilitates its own esterification, and partially limits further entry of cholesterol by regulating the number of lipoprotein receptors. However, lipoprotein cholesterol can gain entry into arterial smooth muscle cells by receptor-independent pathways, potentially causing cholesterol ester accumulation.

Thus, many complex and interrelated metabolic processes are present in arterial wall cells. Although some of these may play a role in the production of arteriosclerosis, no one biochemical reaction can be singled out as culpable. Physiologic factors, such as transfer processes across the endothelial lining, the flux of oxygen and substrates from both the luminal and adventitial sides of the wall, and the reverse flow of catabolic products, need to be considered as well. The ability of the arterial wall to maintain the integrity of its endothelium, prevent platelet aggregation, prevent adherence of blood mononuclear cells, prevent cholesterol accumulation, and ensure the nutrition of its middle portion may be the critical determinants of the arteriosclerotic process.

CHANGES WITH AGING   The major change that occurs with normal aging in the arterial wall in humans is a slow, apparently continuous, symmetric increase in the thickness of the intima. This intimal thickening results from a gradual accumulation of smooth-muscle cells (presumably resulting from migration of these cells from the media and their subsequent proliferation) surrounded by additional connective tissue. In the nondiseased artery wall, lipid content, mainly cholesterol ester and phospholipid (particularly sphingomyelin), also progressively increases with age. Phospholipid synthesis rises with aging (perhaps in response to the need for more membrane formation for plasma membranes, vesicles, lysosomes, and other intracellular organelles) followed by a compensatory increase in activity of all phospholipases except sphingomyelinase. While most of the phospholipid in the normal artery wall appears to be derived from in situ synthesis, the cholesterol ester that accumulates with aging appears to be derived from plasma, since it contains principally linoleic acid, the major plasma cholesterol ester fatty acid. Furthermore, low-density lipoproteins (LDL) are immunologically detectable in the intima of normal arteries in direct relation to their concentration in plasma. It has been estimated that between the second and sixth decade, the normal intima accumulates approximately 25 μmol (10 mg) cholesterol per gram of tissue. Thus, as the normal artery ages, smooth-muscle cells and connective tissue accumulate diffusely in the intima, leading to progressive thickening of this layer, coupled with progressive accumulation of sphingomyelin and cholesterol linoleate. This diffuse age-related intimal thickening is to be distinguished from focal discrete raised fibromuscular plaques, a characteristic feature of atherosclerosis.

Functionally, these changes with aging result in gradually increasing rigidity of vessels. The larger arteries may become dilated, elongated, and tortuous, and aneurysms may form in areas of an encroaching degenerating arteriosclerotic plaque. Such "wear-and-tear" changes are frequently proportional to the vessel diameter and correlated with branching, curvature, and anatomic points of attachment. The amount of external support also determines the ability of vessels, weakened by loss of elasticity, to withstand hydrostatic pressure. The unsupported cerebral arteries may be particularly vulnerable in this regard. Although senescence is accompanied by the intimal thickening that is a feature of localized atheromatosis, the changes of aging and arteriosclerosis appear to be separate and distinct processes.

NONATHEROMATOUS FORMS OF ARTERIOSCLEROSIS

Atherosclerosis involves primarily the intimal layer and occurs most commonly in the abdominal aorta and its large renal and lower extremity branches, the coronary arteries, and the cerebral vasculature. It may accompany or accelerate the other major forms of arteriosclerosis, *focal calcification* and *arteriolosclerosis* (Table 195-2).

FOCAL CALCIFICATION   Not to be confused with atherosclerosis is focal calcification of the media, particularly in the medium-sized muscular arteries. This type of arteriosclerosis is called *Mönckeberg's sclerosis* and is common in the lower extremities, upper extremities, and the arterial supply of the genital tract in both sexes. This disorder is rare in individuals below age 50 and affects both sexes indiscriminately. The process involves degeneration of smooth-muscle cells, followed by calcium deposition. The vessels become hard and tortuous, so that palpable vessels such as the radial artery can be felt as rigid tubes. Its characteristic radiologic appearance consists of regular concentric calcifications in cross section and a railroad track in longitudinal section, commonly seen in vessels in the pelvis, legs, and feet. The medial changes alone do not narrow the lumen, have little effect on the circulation, and have relatively little clinical significance. However, in the lower extremities, medial arterial calcification is often associated with atherosclerosis, leading to arterial occlusion. These changes are common in the elderly and in patients on long-term corticosteroid therapy, but in individuals with diabetes mellitus, focal calcification may be accelerated and severe. It is much more common in diabetics with neuropathy, and sympathetic denervation of medial smooth muscle has been implicated in its etiology.

Focal calcification also can produce the arteriosclerotic aortic valve in the elderly. Progressive calcium deposition occurs on the aortic surface of normal trileaflet aortic valves with age, resulting in a spectrum of clinical findings ranging from an innocent systolic murmur to severe calcific aortic stenosis (Chap. 188).

ARTERIOLOSCLEROSIS   This disorder involves hyaline and degenerative changes affecting both the intima and media of small

---

TABLE 195-2   Disorders associated with early arteriosclerosis

ATHEROSCLEROSIS

Diabetes mellitus
Hypertension
Familial hypercholesterolemia
Familial combined hyperlipidemia
Familial dysbetalipoproteinemia
Hypothyroidism
Werner's syndrome
Cholesterol ester storage disease
Systemic lupus erythematosus

NONATHEROMATOUS ARTERIOSCLEROSIS

Diabetes mellitus
Chronic renal insufficiency
Chronic vitamin D intoxication
Pseudoxanthoma elasticum
Idiopathic arterial calcification in infancy
Aortic valvular calcification in the elderly
Werner's syndrome
Homocystinuria

arteries and arterioles, particularly in the spleen, pancreas, adrenal, and kidney. In the kidney, but not necessarily elsewhere, arteriolosclerosis is almost invariably associated with hypertension. Lesser degrees of sustained hypertension characteristically cause *hyalinization* of renal arterioles; more severe or malignant hypertension produces a typical *fibrous and elastic hyperplasia*, and even necrosis, of the media and intima.

ATHEROSCLEROSIS

LESIONS **Morbid anatomy** Atherosclerosis is a patchy nodular type of arteriosclerosis. The lesions are commonly classified as *fatty streaks*, *fibrous plaques*, and *complicated lesions*. *Fatty streaks* may be the earliest lesions of atherosclerosis. They are characterized by an accumulation of lipid-filled smooth-muscle cells and macrophages (foam cells) and fibrous tissue in focal areas of the intima. They are stained distinctly by fat-soluble dyes but may be visible without staining as yellowish or whitish patches on the intimal surface. The lipid is mainly cholesterol oleate, partly derived from synthesis in situ. The fatty streak is usually sessile and causes little obstruction and no symptoms. The lesion is universal, appearing in various segments of the arterial tree at different ages beginning in the aorta in infancy. In all children, regardless of race, sex, or environment, fatty streaks are present in the aorta by age 10 and increase to occupy as much as 30 to 50 percent of the aortic surface by age 25, but they do not appear to extend further with aging. Despite a presumed relation between fatty streaks and fibrous atherosclerotic plaques, aortic fatty streaks are not correlated with the location and extent of fibrous lesions. In the coronary arteries, the extent of fatty streaks may be a better indicator of the development of clinically significant raised lesions later in life. They are usually observed by age 15 and continue to involve more surface area with increasing age. Fatty streaks in the cerebral arteries are also present in all populations, develop during the third and fourth decade, and are more extensive in those populations having a higher incidence of cerebrovascular disease. It is generally believed that fatty streaks may be reversible, but the evidence is inconclusive.

Fibrous plaques, also called raised lesions or pearly plaques, are palpably elevated areas of intimal thickening and represent the most characteristic lesion of advancing atherosclerosis. They do not share with fatty streaks the ubiquitous distribution among populations. These plaques first appear in the abdominal aorta, coronary arteries, and carotid arteries in the third decade and increase progressively with age. They appear in men before women, in the aorta before the coronary arteries, and much later in the vertebral and intracranial cerebral arteries. Reasons for the difference in susceptibility of various segments of the arterial tree and the nonuniform distribution of lesions are not known. Typically, the fibrous plaque is firm, elevated, and dome-shaped, with an opaque glistening surface that bulges into the lumen. It consists of a central core of extracellular lipid and necrotic cell debris ("gruel") covered by a fibromuscular layer or cap containing large numbers of smooth-muscle cells, macrophages, and collagen. Thus the plaque is much thicker than is normal intima. Although the lipid, like that of fatty streaks, is mainly cholesterol ester, the principal esterified fatty acid is linoleic rather than oleic. Thus plaque cholesterol ester composition differs from fatty streaks but resembles plasma lipoproteins.

The *complicated lesion* is a calcified fibrous plaque containing various degrees of necrosis, thrombosis, and ulceration. These are the lesions frequently associated with symptoms. With increasing necrosis and accumulation of gruel, the arterial wall progressively weakens, and rupture of the intima can occur, causing aneurysm and hemorrhage. Arterial emboli can form when fragments of plaque dislodge into the lumen. Stenosis and impaired organ function result from gradual occlusion as plaques thicken and thrombi form.

Localization Although the term *generalized atherosclerosis* is commonly used clinically, lesions are actually irregularly distributed;

different vessels are involved at different ages and to varying degrees. The aorta, especially its abdominal portion, is involved earliest and most severely by atherosclerotic lesions, and it is the bellwether of lesions elsewhere. The *aorta* is usually most heavily involved in its abdominal portion, about the orifices of its branches (particularly at the level of the coronary and intercostal arteries), in the aortic arch, and frequently at its bifurcation into the iliac arteries. There is more atherosclerosis in the lower than in the upper limbs. In the legs, the incidence decreases peripherally, as the musculoelastic vessels give way to large muscular arteries and these become smaller vessels, such as the plantar or digital arteries. Plaques and thromboses are particularly common in the *femoral* artery, in Hunter's canal, and in the *popliteal* artery just above the knee joint. The *anterior* and *posterior tibial* arteries are often occluded together, but in different sites—the posterior where it rounds the internal malleolus and the anterior where it is superficial and becomes the dorsalis pedis artery. The peroneal artery, which is well embedded in muscle, often escapes when other major vessels are occluded, and it may be the main blood supply to the extremity (*peroneal leg*). Atherosclerosis in abdominal branches, except for the renal and mesenteric arteries, causes less difficulty than in coronary and cerebral vessels.

In the *coronary arteries*, raised lesions are most prominent in the main stems, the highest incidence being a short distance beyond the ostia. Atherosclerosis is nearly always found in the epicardial (extramural) portions of the vessels, while the intramural coronary arteries are spared. Coronary atherosclerosis is often diffuse. The degree to which the lumen is narrowed varies, but once the process is present, all the intima of the extramural portions of the vessel is usually involved. A single tiny plaque occluding an otherwise normal coronary artery is rare. Selective involvement of the coronary arteries may relate to the unique hemodynamic forces, unlike those of other major arteries, resulting from greater flow in diastole than systole. The implications of these flow patterns for atherogenesis are as yet unknown. Typical atheromatous fibrous plaques also develop in saphenous vein aortocoronary bypass grafts.

In the cervical and cerebral arteries the distribution of atherosclerosis is patchy, as it may be in other arteries. It first appears in the base of the brain in the carotid, basilar, and vertebral arteries. The proximal portion of the internal carotid artery in the neck is a site of special predilection. There is a concentration of lesions near bifurcations. Atherosclerosis in the *pulmonary artery* bears no relation to the severity of the disease in the aorta or other systemic arteries. There is some involvement in about half of adults over 50 years of age who have no reason to have pulmonary hypertension. Pulmonary hypertension per se, however, is associated with medial hypertrophy, intimal thickening, and great acceleration of atheroma formation.

THEORIES OF ATHEROGENESIS One generally accepted theory for the pathogenesis of atherosclerosis consistent with a variety of experimental evidence is the *reaction to injury* hypothesis. According to this idea the endothelial cells lining the intima are exposed to repeated or continuing insults to their integrity. The injury to the endothelium may be subtle or gross, resulting in a loss of the ability of the cells to function normally or to attach to one another and to the underlying connective tissue. In the extreme, the cells may desquamate. Examples of types of "injury" to the endothelium include chemical injury, as in chronic hypercholesterolemia or homocystinemia, mechanical stress associated with hypertension, and immunologic injury, as may be seen after cardiac or renal transplantation. Loss of functional endothelial cells at susceptible sites in the arterial tree would lead to exposure of the subendothelial tissue to increased concentrations of plasma constituents and a sequence of events including platelet adherence, platelet aggregation and formation of microthrombi, and release of platelet granular components, including a potent mitogenic factor. This platelet factor, in conjunction with other plasma constituents, including lipoproteins and hormones such as insulin, could stimulate both the migration of medial smooth-muscle cells into the intima and their proliferation at these sites of injury. These proliferating smooth-muscle cells would deposit a connective tissue matrix and accumulate lipid, a process that would be particularly enhanced with hyperlipidemia. Macrophages derived from circulating blood monocytes can also accumulate lipid.

Adherence of monocytes to altered endothelial cells and their migration into the arterial wall to become resident macrophages may be the earliest cellular abnormality in atherogenesis. Thus repeated or chronic injury could lead to a slowly progressing lesion involving a gradual increase in smooth-muscle cells, macrophages, connective tissue, and lipid. Areas where the shearing stress on endothelial cells is increased, such as branch points or bifurcation of vessels, would be at greater risk. As the lesions progress and the intima becomes thicker, blood flow over the sites will be altered and will potentially place the lining endothelial cells at even greater risk for further injury, leading to an inexorable cycle of events culminating in the complicated lesion. However, a single or a few injurious episodes may lead to a proliferative response that could regress, in contrast to continued or chronic injury. This hypothesis of reaction to injury thus is consistent with the known intimal thickening observed during normal aging, would explain how many of the etiologic factors implicated in atherogenesis might enhance lesion formation, might explain how inhibitors of platelet aggregation could interfere with lesion formation, and fosters some optimism regarding the possibility of interrupting progression or even producing regression of these lesions.

Other theories of atherogenesis are not mutually exclusive. The *monoclonal hypothesis* suggests, on the basis of single isoenzyme types found in lesions, that the intimal proliferative lesions result from the multiplication of single, individual smooth-muscle cells, as do benign tumors. In this manner, mitogenic, and possibly mutagenic, factors that might stimulate smooth-muscle cell proliferation would act on single cells. Focal *clonal senescence* may explain how intrinsic aging processes contribute to atherosclerosis. According to this theory, the intimal smooth-muscle cells that proliferate to form an atheroma are normally under feedback control by diffusible agents (mitosis inhibitors) formed by the smooth-muscle cells in the contiguous media, and this feedback control system tends to fail with age as these controlling cells die and are not adequately replaced. This is consistent with the recent observation that cultured human arterial smooth-muscle cells, like fibroblasts, show a decline in their ability to replicate as a function of donor age. If this loss of replicative potential applies to a controlling population of smooth-muscle cells, then cells that are usually suppressed would be able to proliferate.

The *lysosomal theory* suggests that altered lysosomal function might contribute to atherogenesis. Since lysosomal enzymes can accomplish the generalized degradation of cellular components required for continuing renewal, this system has been implicated in cellular aging and the accumulation of lipofuscin or "age pigment." It has been suggested that increased deposition of lipids in arterial smooth-muscle cells may be related in part to a relative deficiency in the activity of lysosomal cholesterol ester hydrolase. This would result in increased accumulation of cholesterol esters within the cells, perhaps accentuated by lipid overloading of lysosomes, eventually leading to cell death and extracellular lipid deposition. Consonant with this idea, patients with the rare cholesterol ester storage disease, caused by a defect in lysosomal cholesterol ester hydrolase, may have accelerated atherosclerosis. However, lipid droplets in foam cells are often cytoplasmic rather than lysosomal.

RECOGNITION OF ATHEROSCLEROSIS Angiographic visualization of deformity in the lumen of a vessel remains the best presumptive test of silent atherosclerosis. Coronary angiography now permits visualization and assessment of arteries as small as 0.5 mm in diameter. Several sophisticated noninvasive techniques have been developed for demonstrating its presence. Doppler probes for measuring velocity and amount of blood flow have been used noninvasively and adapted to determine vessel outlines. Ultrasonic techniques are not yet clinically useful for detection of plaques in the coronary arteries.

Functional tests based on pathophysiologic or metabolic effects of a narrowed arterial lumen often give indirect clues. Assessment of electrocardiographic changes induced after standardized exercise is a relatively simple noninvasive aid to the diagnosis of coronary atherosclerosis with significant narrowing. Similarly, myocardial perfusion defects demonstrable with imaging techniques using radionuclides are usually attributable to atherosclerosis (Chap. 178). Digital plethysmography with exercise often unmasks significant atherosclerotic involvement of lower extremity arteries.

Radiographic demonstration of calcification in the location of arteries does not always indicate the presence of atherosclerosis. Although calcified coronary vessels usually indicate atherosclerosis, complete luminal obstruction may occur in the absence of any calcification. Calcification or beading of peripheral arteries is not correlated directly with atherosclerosis, but more likely reflects medial sclerosis. Abnormalities in retinal arterioles evident upon funduscopic examination are not well correlated with atherosclerosis in arteries. Thus despite the availability of a variety of tests, detection of atherosclerosis usually awaits one of the clinical complications attending a critical decrease of blood flow in an involved vessel. As yet there is no blood test for atherosclerosis. Knowledge of the prevalence and incidence of arteriosclerosis and most of the inferences concerning its causes are derived from tabulations of the appearance of its complications.

Ischemic heart disease (IHD), synonymous with *coronary heart disease* or *arteriosclerotic heart disease* (Chap. 190), is the most reliable indicator of atherosclerosis available today. Practically all patients with myocardial infarction, as defined by electrocardiographic and enzyme changes, have coronary atherosclerosis. Rare exceptions are due to congenital anomalies of the coronary vessels, emboli, or ostial occlusion due to other types of cardiac or vascular disease. Nontraumatic *sudden death* (Chap. 40) makes up a sizable portion of all deaths eventually certified as due to IHD. At autopsy, evidence of fresh myocardial infarction or of *coronary thrombosis* is usually absent. While ventricular fibrillation may have been due to sudden closure of a partially compromised vessel by a small thrombus or embolus, or to *spasm*, none of these need have preceded a fatal arrhythmia. The majority of victims of sudden death have had a previous diagnosis of IHD; the number who had diabetes or hypertension is also significant. In epidemiologic studies of IHD, *angina pectoris* and electrocardiographic changes attributable to ischemia without infarction are considered "softer end points" and treated separately.

Cerebrovascular disease (stroke) is a less reliable criterion for the presence of atherosclerosis. It includes *cerebral hemorrhage* and *cerebral thrombosis* (Chap. 351). Cerebral thrombosis, including infarction or softening without evidence of embolus, is usually due to atherosclerosis. On the other hand, cerebral hemorrhage is most often the result of congenital aneurysms or of vascular defects peculiar to hypertension and diabetes. Dissections of the aorta (Chap. 197), *peripheral vascular disease* (Chap. 198), thrombosis of other major vessels, and ischemic renal disease (Chap. 230) likewise are not used to determine the prevalence of atherosclerosis in a population or as an index of atherosclerosis elsewhere. Therefore, from an epidemiologic standpoint, consideration of atherosclerosis focuses on IHD.

INCIDENCE AND PREVALENCE According to the National Health Examination Survey, about 5 million Americans have IHD. It is the leading cause of death in males after age 35 and in all persons after age 45. Premature deaths from IHD, arbitrarily defined as those appearing before age 65, occur preponderantly in men, and a third of all deaths from IHD in males occur before age 65. In fact nearly all the excess premature mortality in American males is due to IHD. Between the ages of 35 and 55 the death rate is five times higher in white men than in white women in the United States. The exceptions are women with hypertension, diabetes, hyperlipidemia, or premature (usually iatrogenic) menopause, who are at increased risk and often share the risk of the male. For both sexes, there is more than a fivefold increase in the average annual incidence of myocardial infarction between ages 40 and 60. A distressing higher mortality rate in younger nonwhite women is probably due mainly

TABLE 195-3   Age-adjusted death rates by cause in the United States, 1968 and 1986

Cause of death	Rate per 100,000 population		Percent change
	1968	1986	
All deaths	744	542	−27
All cardiovascular diseases	362	175	−52
Ischemic heart disease	242	119	−51
Cerebrovascular disease	71	31	−56
Rheumatic heart disease	7	2	−69
Cancer	129	133	+3

SOURCE: The National Center for Health Statistics, *Vital Statistics Report, Final Mortality Statistics, 1986.*

TABLE 195-4   Risk factors for atherosclerosis

Male sex
Family history of premature IHD (before age 55 in a parent or sibling)
Hyperlipidemia
Cigarette smoking (currently smoking more than 10 cigarettes per day)
Hypertension
Low HDL-cholesterol [below 0.9 mmol/L (35 mg/dL)]
Diabetes mellitus
Personal history of cerebrovascular disease or occlusive peripheral vascular disease
Severe obesity (>30% overweight)
High lipoprotein (a)

to a greater incidence of hypertension in blacks. There is less difference between men and women in the prevalence of angina pectoris than in that of myocardial infarction; after age 65 more women than men have angina without a history of infarction.

Changing death rates   Death rates in the United States from IHD rose appreciably between 1940 and 1960. Mortality peaked in 1963 and started to decline, with the rate of decline accelerating in recent years for all ages, for both sexes, and for whites and nonwhites. This recent decline in mortality from coronary atherosclerosis (Table 195-3) is the first recorded in American history and is almost unique among industrialized countries. In other parts of the world, including the Soviet Union and many countries in Eastern Europe, IHD death rates are still climbing. By 1986 the reduction in IHD death rate averaged more than 30 percent. The trend cannot be attributed to a single cause, but there has been a concurrent change in living habits including reduced cigarette smoking among middle-aged men, decreased consumption of animal fats and cholesterol, better control of hypertension, and improved treatment of IHD.

International comparisons   In most industrialized countries, IHD is the major single cause of premature cardiovascular deaths. There are, however, marked differences in premature death rates among them. The seven having the highest rates in men between 35 and 74 years of age are Finland, Scotland, Northern Ireland, Australia, New Zealand, England, and the United States. Much lower age-adjusted death rates from IHD are found in Latin America and Japan. The rates in Japan are about one-sixth of those in the United States. Subsamples obtained in many countries convey the strong impression that upper socioeconomic classes that have adopted the culture of western industrialized countries have far more IHD than do lower socioeconomic classes. Among the most obvious cultural differences between these groups are total calories, fat content of the diet, and amount of physical work. Extensive epidemiologic studies have not revealed the reasons for differences between cultures that are superficially similar. Migrants to the United States tend to have a higher risk of death from premature IHD than do age-matched relatives who remain at home. Although there are many instances in which different ethnic groups in the same locality have widely differing prevalences of IHD, the available data suggest that cultural factors are more important than genetic determination of IHD. Nevertheless, genetic heterogeneity undoubtedly underlies many of the striking differences in susceptibility seen among individuals sharing the same ethnic and cultural setting.

ETIOLOGIC FACTORS   A number of conditions and habits present more frequently in individuals who develop atherosclerosis than in the general population; these factors have been termed *risk factors*. The majority of people below age 65 afflicted with atherosclerosis have one or more identifiable risk factors other than aging per se (Table 195-4). The risk factor concept implies that a person with at least one risk factor is more likely to develop a clinical atherosclerotic event and is likely to do so earlier than a person with no risk factors. The presence of multiple risk factors further accelerates atherosclerosis. They vary in terms of importance in the population

of the United States. Hypercholesterolemia, hypertension, and cigarette smoking may be the most potent factors involved in causation of atherosclerosis. Risk factors also vary in terms of their potential reversibility with current techniques of preventive management.

Thus age, gender, and genetic factors are currently considered to be irreversible risk factors, whereas continually emerging evidence suggests that elimination of cigarette smoking and treatment of hypertension reverses the high risk for atherosclerosis attributable to those factors. A major multicenter trial has shown that reduction of hypercholesterolemia reduces the risk of IHD. Life insurance policyholder data suggest that reduction of marked obesity reduces total mortality, presumably by diminishing the sequelae of atherosclerosis. Other potentially reversible factors are currently under study.

These factors are not mutually exclusive since they clearly interact. For example, obesity, particularly of the abdominal type (assessed by the waist/hip circumference ratio), appears to be causally associated with hypertension, hyperglycemia, hypercholesterolemia, and hypertriglyceridemia. Genetic factors may play a role by exerting direct effects on arterial wall cell structure and metabolism, or they may act indirectly via such factors as hypertension, hyperlipidemia, diabetes, and obesity. Aging appears to be one of the more complex factors associated with the development of atherosclerosis, since many of the risk factors in themselves are related to aging, e.g., elevated blood pressure, hyperglycemia, and hyperlipidemia. Thus in addition to the possible involvement of intrinsic aging in atherogenesis (perhaps through effects on arterial wall metabolism), a variety of associated metabolic factors are also age-dependent.

Hyperlipidemia   Both *hypercholesterolemia* and *hypertriglyceridemia* appear to be important risk factors for atherosclerosis. While there is no absolute quantitative definition of hyperlipidemia, statistical definitions, based on the upper 5 or 10 percent of the distribution of plasma lipid levels within a population, are often used. Such definitions are likely to detect affected individuals from families with one of the familial hyperlipidemias or having hyperlipidemia associated with other diseases or drugs; they also are useful for prediction of emergence of premature atherosclerosis and institution of preventive measures. However, these upper limits of "normality" are too high for defining those cholesterol and triglyceride levels that are correlated with increasing risk of IHD in whole populations. Thus, correlations between the cholesterol concentrations in young men in North America and the incidence of premature IHD indicate that an increasing risk can be detected when the cholesterol level is higher than 5.20 mmol/L (200 mg/dL), a value close to the median for men from 40 to 49 years of age in this population. Extrapolation of similar data from other populations suggests that a cholesterol level at birth averages 1.5 mmol/L (60 mg/dL). Within a month the average has risen to about 3 mmol/L (120 mg/dL) and by the first year to 4.5 mmol/L (175 mg/dL). A second rise begins in the third decade and continues to about age 50 in men and somewhat later in women.

A similar age-related increase in plasma triglyceride levels is also observed. The increases in cholesterol are associated mainly with a rise in *low-density lipoprotein* (LDL) concentrations, the increases in triglyceride with a rise in *very low density lipoproteins* (VLDL). Adiposity may play a key role in this age-associated rise in triglyceride and cholesterol levels since the increases in triglyceride, cholesterol, and body weight with age in whole populations occur concurrently. In primitive people who remain thin throughout adulthood, plasma lipids do not increase with age. Metabolic mechanisms have been postulated whereby abdominal obesity, which is associated with insulin resistance of peripheral tissues and compensatory hyperinsulinemia, promotes enhanced production of triglyceride- and cholesterol-rich lipoproteins by the liver. Current concepts of plasma lipoprotein transport suggest that accumulation of cholesterol in the circulation may in part be secondary to excessive production of triglyceride-rich lipoproteins.

Hypercholesterolemia is associated unequivocally with increased incidence of premature IHD; however, its importance varies in relation to age. In the Framingham Study, cholesterol levels in men below age 40 were closely related to the future development of IHD; this relation was much less pronounced in older individuals. In the Multiple Risk Factor Intervention Trial (MRFIT), men with cholesterol levels above about 6 mmol/L (240 mg/dL) had more than a threefold increase in risk of IHD death compared to men with cholesterol levels below about 5 mmol/L (200 mg/dL). There is a continuous gradient of risk as the cholesterol level ascends. These data are supported by comparisons of the prevalence of IHD and cholesterol (or LDL) in many other populations. The relationship of triglycerides and VLDL to IHD is confounded by a rise in cholesterol as VLDL increases. Nevertheless, in several, but not all, population studies, increased triglycerides (or VLDL) are independently correlated with premature IHD.

Hypertriglyceridemia may be associated with premature atherosclerosis in some specific disorders; this association may not be apparent in studies of whole populations. Patients with high VLDL who come from families with familial combined hyperlipidemia appear to be at the same increased risk as those affected members of these families with elevated LDL levels. In contrast, patients with comparably elevated VLDL levels who come from families with pure monogenic familial hypertriglyceridemia do not appear to have an increased risk. In addition, high VLDL may increase the risk for premature atherosclerosis when associated with other risk factors for coronary artery disease, such as in diabetics, and in patients on chronic hemodialysis who smoke and are hypertensive. Individuals in whom remnant lipoproteins accumulate, with resulting elevations in both cholesterol and triglycerides (Chap. 326), also seem to be at risk for early development of atherosclerosis.

Some of these relationships were clarified in a comprehensive study in Seattle of the role of the genetics of hyperlipidemia in clinical atherosclerosis in which 500 consecutive survivors of myocardial infarction were tested. Hyperlipidemia was present in about one-third of the group. Approximately one-half of the males and two-thirds of the females below age 50 had either hypertriglyceridemia, hypercholesterolemia, or both. On the other hand, in individuals over age 70 the prevalence of atherosclerotic coronary disease was very high, yet virtually no males (and only about one-fourth of the females) had hyperlipidemia. Thus, in both sexes there appeared to be a progressive decline with age in the association of hyperlipidemia with myocardial infarction. More than half of the hyperlipidemic atherosclerotic survivors appeared to have simple monogenic familial disorders inherited as an autosomal dominant trait (*familial combined hyperlipidemia, familial hypertriglyceridemia,* and *familial hypercholesterolemia,* in descending order of frequency, Table 195-5). These simply inherited hyperlipidemias (particularly hypercholesterolemia) were more frequent in myocardial infarction survivors below age 60 than in those who were older. In contrast, nonmonogenic forms of hyperlipidemia occurred with equal frequency above and below age 60. Thus it appears that genes associated with the simply inherited hyperlipidemias accelerate changes seen with age, leading to atherosclerosis at an earlier age than usual. All studies indicate that hyperlipidemia is a more meaningful risk factor below age 50 and that it operates independently of, and in addition to, hypertension, diabetes, obesity, and other factors. For men and women over age 65, there is no evidence of a correlation between hyperlipidemia and atherosclerosis or its complications.

TABLE 195-5 Frequency of hyperlipidemia in survivors of myocardial infarction

Disorder	% of total myocardial infarction survivors		
	Under age 60	Over age 60	Ratio
1 Monogenic hyperlipidemias	20.6	7.5	—
a Familial hypercholesterolemia	4.1	0.7	6:1
b Familial hypertriglyceridemia	5.2	2.7	2:1
c Familial combined hyperlipidemia	11.3	4.1	3:1
2 Polygenic hypercholesterolemia	5.5	5.5	1:1
3 Sporadic hypertriglyceridemia	5.8	6.9	1:1

SOURCE: Goldstein et al. 1973.

When the screening of individuals for hyperlipidemia occurs after a myocardial infarction, it is several decades too late, although interruption of further progression of atherosclerosis may be possible. Screening at birth or in childhood for genetic hyperlipidemia is not practical or useful except in the instance of familial hypercholesterolemia, which may affect about 1 in 1000 children. This is detectable by LDL elevations in cord blood when one already knows that a parent is affected. Other genetic or nongenetic primary hyperlipidemia is often not apparent until the third decade. *Today, screening measurement of blood cholesterol levels (nonfasting) is recommended for all adult patients. It is especially important in all young persons who have a family history of premature IHD.*

Hyperlipidemia is best confirmed by measurement of the concentration of total cholesterol and triglycerides and of high-density lipoprotein cholesterol in serum or plasma in a sample obtained after an overnight fast. The measurements should be made by a reliable laboratory that follows a program of standardization. Routine use of lipoprotein electrophoresis provides little additional information, is nonspecific, and is not recommended for screening or for management. In adults less than 65 years of age, a cholesterol concentration (C) greater than 6 mmol/L (240 mg/dL) or a triglyceride concentration (TG) greater than 2.8 mmol/L (250 mg/dL) clearly indicates hyperlipidemia sufficient to require some attention by the physician to the items listed in Table 195-6. Less severe degrees of hypercholesterolemia nevertheless can impart some degree of risk for IHD. The National Cholesterol Education Program has suggested that total cholesterol (C) > 6.2 mmol/L (240 mg/dL) is "high risk" and should prompt careful evaluation (Table 195-6), estimation of LDL cholesterol, and some approach to cholesterol lowering. Cholesterol between 5.2 and 6.1 mmol/dL (200 and 239 mg/dL) is borderline high. The presence of two or more risk factors (independent of C or TG levels) listed in Table 195-4, or preexisting IHD, puts these patients in the

TABLE 195-6 Factors to consider in patients with hyperlipidemia

1 Disorders to which hyperlipidemia is secondary
  a Uncontrolled diabetes mellitus (insulin deficiency)
  b Hypothyroidism
  c Uremia
  d Nephrotic syndrome (hypoproteinemia)
  e Obstructive liver disease
  f Dysproteinemia (multiple myeloma, lupus erythematosus)
2 Drugs producing or aggravating hyperlipidemia
  a Oral contraceptives
  b Estrogens
  c Glucocorticoids
  d Antihypertensives
3 Dietary factors
  a Caloric intake (recent weight gain)
  b Content of saturated fats and cholesterol
  c Alcohol intake
4 Genetic disorders (primary hyperlipidemias)
  a Family history of hyperlipidemia or xanthomas
  b History of pancreatitis or recurrent abdominal pain

TABLE 195-7   Guidelines for treatment of high blood cholesterol in adults

Decision	Basis	Cholesterol, mmol/L (mg/dL)		
		Desirable	Borderline-high	High
LDL estimation	Total C	<5.2 (200)	5.2–6.1 (200–239)*	>6.2 (240)
Treatment				
Diet	LDL-C	<3.4 (130)	3.4–4.1 (130–159)*	>4.2 (160)
Drug†	LDL-C			>5.1 (190) or >4.2 (160)*

* Becomes high-risk if definite IHD or >2 risk factors (see Table 195-4) are present.
† After a trial of diet alone.
SOURCE: National Cholesterol Education Program.

high-risk category. For treatment decisions, and when TG < 4.5 mmol/L (400 mg/dL), LDL cholesterol (LDL-C) levels can be estimated as total C − HDL-C − TG/5. Patients considered at high risk for IHD should be aggressively treated to lower blood cholesterol out of the high-risk range (Table 195-7). If C < 5 mmol/L (200 mg/dL), the tests need not be repeated for several years in an adult who maintains body weight and does not otherwise change in health or life-style. If causes of *secondary hyperlipidemia* or offending drugs are absent, attention to the origin of *primary hyperlipidemia* turns mainly to diet and genetic causes. Severe hyperlipidemia [C > 7.8 mmol/L (300 mg/dL) or TG > 5.6 mmol/L (500 mg/dL)] usually reflects a genetic disorder; when xanthomas are present, it practically always does. Diagnosis always includes examination of first-degree relatives and proceeds according to information contained in Chap. 326.

Reduction of hypercholesterolemia results in a decrease in progression of atherosclerosis in humans and other primates. Several controlled trials of different diets which have been accompanied by fall in mean cholesterol levels in small test populations have shown a favorable effect on incidence of the overall complications of IHD. The drug clofibrate given to a normal population reduced the incidence of nonfatal myocardial infarctions and was associated with a reduction of cholesterol levels; however, total mortality was not lowered. In the Lipid Research Clinics trial, the drug cholestyramine given to hypercholesterolemic asymptomatic men reduced morbidity and mortality from myocardial infarction in direct relation to the degree of cholesterol lowering; again, however, total mortality was not reduced. Lipid lowering by means of bile acid binding resins (with niacin and diet therapy) also decreases progression and even induces regression of coronary lesions as demonstrated by angiography in patients who have had coronary artery bypass graft surgery. Another fibric acid drug, gemfibrozil, has been shown to reduce mortality from IHD (but not total mortality) in association with lowered TG and C and raised HDL-C. Thus, the weight of evidence strongly favors conservative measures to reduce cholesterol levels in patients through middle age and aggressive measures in patients who are frankly hypercholesterolemic and are at high risk for progression of IHD.

The first step in treatment of primary hyperlipidemia is attention to diet. All patients with mild to moderate hyperlipidemia should first be brought to normal weight if they exceed it and then be maintained on a diet emphasizing decreases in intake of saturated fat and cholesterol. If hypertriglyceridemia is present, alcohol intake should be limited or eliminated. A single dietary approach to all forms of hyperlipidemia, including reduced intake of calories, cholesterol, and saturated fat, is appropriate for most patients. The degree of dietary restriction would be proportional to the degree and nature of the hyperlipidemia. The maximum effect of such a regimen will be observed within 3 months after body weight has stabilized. If at that time LDL-C is greater than 4.9 mmol/L (190 mg/dL), drugs such as a bile acid–binding resin (cholestyramine or colestipol) or nicotinic acid should be considered. If TG remains greater than 3.4 mmol/L (300 mg/dL), a fibric acid derivative (clofibrate or bezafibrate)

may be tried. These two types of drugs may be used simultaneously if both C and TG are high. In patients with familial hypercholesterolemia (Chap. 326) combined therapy with a resin and nicotinic acid has achieved dramatic normalization of LDL cholesterol levels. New cholesterol synthesis inhibitors (e.g., lovastatin), which are more potent than resins, are currently being studied. However, further studies are needed to define the long-term efficiency of various hypolipidemic agents in the prevention of atherosclerosis and its sequelae in specific disorders. The long-term effects of these drugs used before puberty are unknown, and their use during pregnancy is not advocated. There is a paucity of data to justify their use in the elderly.

High-density lipoproteins (HDL)   The level of HDL, a complex family of particles that carry about 20 percent of the total plasma cholesterol, is inversely associated with the development of premature atherosclerosis and therefore can be considered an "antirisk factor." HDL levels can be assessed simply by measurement of cholesterol in the supernatant fluid after the other lipoproteins in plasma have been precipitated. Thus individuals whose HDL cholesterol is elevated may be less likely to develop IHD; conversely, low HDL cholesterol is associated with increased risk of IHD. In the Framingham Study, low HDL cholesterol was a more potent lipid risk factor than was high cholesterol or LDL. At least five diverse population studies have confirmed a close correlation between IHD and low HDL, independent of other factors.

Consistent with differences in risk between the sexes, HDL cholesterol averages about 25 percent higher in women than in men. Estrogens tend to raise and androgens tend to lower HDL levels. In women, low HDL, particularly when associated with diabetes and obesity, markedly raises the risk of IHD. Octogenarians tend to have high HDL, which may be partly familial. Of interest for preventive measures, cigarette smoking decreases and regular strenuous exercise increases HDL cholesterol. Regular exercise increases HDL even in individuals after myocardial infarction. A small daily intake of alcohol has been associated with both reduced risk of IHD and high HDL levels. Mechanisms for these effects remain unknown.

The utility of HDL cholesterol measurements in individuals is limited since the analytical error in most laboratories exceeds the differences in HDL levels associated with risk. HDL measurements are most helpful for estimation of LDL cholesterol. Because of the close inverse relationship between plasma triglycerides (or VLDL) and HDL, HDL in most hypertriglyceridemic persons, with or without hypercholesterolemia, will be predictably low. Low HDL cholesterol is one of the factors that can place patients in a high-risk category for IHD (Table 195-7).

Hypertension (See Chap. 196)   High blood pressure is an important risk factor for atherosclerosis, mainly IHD and cerebrovascular disease. The risk increases progressively with increasing blood pressure; in the Framingham Study, IHD incidence in middle-aged men with blood pressures exceeding 160/95 was more than five times that in normotensive men (blood pressure 140/90 or less). Hypertensive men and women are both affected, with the diastolic pressure perhaps being more important. In industrialized populations, blood pressure appears to increase inexorably with age; however, the nature of this age relation varies among populations, since there are remote primitive populations that age without any changes in blood pressure levels. The age-associated blood pressure increase might be related to physical activity or dietary factors, particularly sodium and total caloric content. In contrast to the other age-related risk factors, hypertension appears to increase atherosclerosis throughout the age span.

Conversely, the risk for atherosclerosis appears diminished by therapeutic reduction of blood pressure. Recent intervention studies have shown convincingly that reduction of diastolic levels that had been greater than 105 mmHg significantly reduces the incidence of strokes, IHD, and congestive heart failure in men. Even when patients with diastolic pressures between 90 and 105 mmHg are similarly maintained on adequate treatment, the incidence of some of these complications may be reduced. Special urgency for relief of hypertension obtains when hyperlipidemia, diabetes, or other risk factors are present.

Cigarette smoking Not only is cigarette smoking one of the more potent risk factors for atherosclerosis, it is also one of the factors that when reduced or eliminated clearly decreases the risk of developing atherosclerosis. Ample statistical evidence supports a mean increase of about 70 percent in the death rate, and a three- to fivefold increase in risk of IHD, in men who smoke one pack of cigarettes per day compared with nonsmokers. In general, the increase in death rate is proportional to the amount smoked and decreases with age. Excess morbidity from myocardial infarction is also present in women smokers, but the relationship is somewhat less firm than in men. However, there is an impressive accentuation of IHD mortality in women over age 35 taking oral contraceptives who in addition smoke cigarettes. In some atherosclerosis-prone populations, such as patients maintained on long-term hemodialysis, cigarette smoking interacts with other risk factors, resulting in a marked enhancement of atherosclerosis mortality. Such interaction is also likely for diabetic and hypertensive populations.

The association of smoking and increased IHD remains unexplained. Pipe and cigar smokers have a lesser increase in risk of IHD, presumably because less smoke is inhaled. Smokers dying of causes other than IHD have been found at autopsy to have more coronary atherosclerosis than nonsmokers. The major influence of smoking is upon the incidence of sudden death, however. Those who stop smoking show a prompt decline in risk and may reach the risk level of nonsmokers as early as after 1 year of abstention.

Hyperglycemia and diabetes mellitus (See Chap. 319) Studies in a variety of populations have shown an association of hyperglycemia with clinically evident atherosclerotic disease, suggesting a role of hyperglycemia in atherogenesis. In known diabetics, both insulin-dependent and non-insulin-dependent types, there is at least a twofold increase in incidence of myocardial infarction compared with nondiabetics. This risk is markedly increased in younger diabetics, and diabetic women are even more prone to IHD than are diabetic men. There is an increased tendency toward cerebral thrombosis and infarction but not toward cerebral hemorrhage in diabetes. Gangrene of the lower extremities has been variously estimated to be from 8 to 150 times as frequent in diabetics as in nondiabetics and is most often found in diabetics who smoke. Diabetes mellitus is associated with an increase in atherosclerosis observed at autopsy in a variety of populations worldwide, whether the prevalence of atherosclerosis in a particular population is high or low. The approximately twofold increase in the frequency of hypertension among diabetics, particularly adult females, may accentuate the risk. This relationship is presumably associated with abdominal obesity.

The risk for atherosclerotic disease, however, does not appear to be grossly related to the degree of hyperglycemia among diabetics. Results in the University Group Diabetes Program Study have suggested that reduction of blood glucose by insulin does not appear to influence mortality from established atherosclerosis during a 5-year period. Thus, hyperglycemia and atherosclerosis are associated, since there is an increased prevalence of large-vessel disease in known diabetics and, conversely, an increased prevalence of hyperglycemia in association with atherosclerotic disease. These associations remain unexplained and reversibility undocumented. Clinical and experimental studies also support a role for high circulating insulin levels in IHD. The capillary microangiopathy, pathognomonic of diabetes mellitus and causing important dysfunction of the kidneys and retina, has unknown clinical significance in relation to atherosclerotic disease in larger arteries.

Obesity In general, morbidity and mortality from IHD are higher in direct relation to the degree of overweight beyond about 30 percent. Furthermore, from data obtained in the Framingham Study, it appears that obesity may accelerate atherosclerosis since its effect is more apparent before age 50. Nevertheless, some of the major epidemiologic studies of coronary heart disease have not demonstrated an independent relationship between this condition and anything less than very severe

obesity. Recent studies have shown a close relation between type of obesity (i.e., abdominal) and IHD. Furthermore, obesity is a disorder closely associated with four other potent risk factors, i.e., hypertriglyceridemia, hypercholesterolemia, hyperglycemia, and hypertension. The relationship between obesity and atherosclerosis is thus multifaceted; since in practice obesity does not occur "independently," it is of considerable importance as a risk factor.

Physical inactivity Study of the relationship of the prevalence of IHD to daily (occupational) physical activity is made difficult because so many variables are involved. Among prospective studies the Framingham data do indicate that the less sedentary an individual is, the less susceptible that individual is to sudden death. Physical work may be the major determinant of greatly differing incidences of IHD in southern black and white males in the United States and in populations that move from rural areas to urbanized environments. How physical activity may operate to decrease death from IHD, or possibly to decrease atherogenesis, is not known. Beyond the amelioration of hyperlipidemia by increasing caloric expenditure, no mechanism has been demonstrated. The meaning of the physical activity–induced increase in HDL, the antirisk factor for IHD, remains mysterious. Physical training has been shown to improve exercise performance in patients with IHD and angina pectoris. Regular physical activity is supported as a desirable element in a program of preventive health maintenance.

Stress and personality There is a valid clinical impression that psychic or emotional stress and anxiety are associated with precipitation of overt IHD and sudden death. Debate continues as to whether there may be distinct personality types prone to or relatively immune to premature IHD (the so-called personality types A and B) and whether the presumably more deleterious type is amenable to correction beyond elimination of cigarette smoking, adverse dietary patterns, and avoidance of stressful life situations. Many social and demographic analyses have so far failed to reach any agreement about the etiologic relationships of occupation and similar situational factors and the incidence of IHD.

Genetic factors Premature atherosclerosis often appears to be familial. In many instances this can be attributed to the inheritance of risk factors such as hypertension, diabetes mellitus, and hyperlipidemia. Occasionally, families with excessive premature vascular disease can be found in which none of the known risk factors appears to be operating. Genetic determinants of protective factors, such as HDL, and of nonlipid risk factors, such as apolipoprotein B, and lipoprotein (a), need to be understood; undoubtedly other important determinants remain to be discovered. Nevertheless, family history is one of the more important factors to be weighed in assessment of risk in helping the physician to avoid missing treatable risk factors and in institution of appropriate preventive measures.

ROLE OF DIET IN RISK FOR ATHEROSCLEROSIS The relationship of diet to IHD remains an area of intense interest and persistent controversy. In epidemiologic studies, no population habitually subsisting on a diet low in saturated fat and cholesterol has an appreciable amount of IHD. These populations also tend to have lower plasma lipid concentrations. There is a general upward shift of average cholesterol and triglyceride levels in highly developed countries, which is an effect of change in total culture and life-style as well as in diet. Dietary changes in migrant populations who move from more primitive to more industrialized societies commonly include increased intake of total calories, animal fats, cholesterol, and salt, leading to a diet-accentuated emergence of risk factors such as obesity, hyperlipidemia, diabetes, and hypertension. There is no question that the plasma cholesterol (and LDL) level is sensitive to the amount of saturated fat and cholesterol in the diet. The "average" adult male in the United States eats about 140 g fat per day and about 0.1 mmol (400 mg) cholesterol. The mixture of fats ingested usually contains about three times as much saturated fatty acids (mainly palmitic and stearic) as polyunsaturated fatty acids (mainly linoleic and linolenic). If a healthy young adult switches from this diet to one containing the same amount of total fat in which the ratio of polyunsaturates to saturates is closer to unity and the cholesterol content is less than 0.07 mmol (300 mg) per day, the cholesterol concentration will usually drop by 10 to 15 percent within 2 weeks and remain depressed on continuation of the diet.

The average cholesterol level in most populations is most closely related to the amount of animal fats (meat, eggs, and milk products, major sources of long-chain saturated fatty acids and cholesterol) in the diet. Increased animal fat consumption also tends to be correlated with a greater proportion of dietary fats being saturated and with lesser intake of complex carbohydrates and vegetable fibers; these are dietary changes that may lead to a rise in plasma cholesterol levels. The average triglyceride level is more sensitive to total caloric balance and to alcohol intake. It is important to note that physical activity, emotional stress, smoking, and intake of coffee or tea have only weak or indirect influences on total cholesterol and triglyceride concentrations.

In experimental animals added dietary cholesterol and fat are essential for the production of atherosclerosis. Typical American diets fed to nonhuman primates produce aortic and coronary atherosclerosis which is reversible when a cholesterol-free diet is fed. Controlled metabolic studies in humans show a direct relation between dietary and plasma cholesterol below intakes of about 0.15 mmol (600 mg) per day; no relation is observed at higher intakes when plasma cholesterol is already high. There appear to be marked genetic variations in the ability of dietary cholesterol to influence plasma cholesterol among individuals and among populations. The relation between dietary polyunsaturated/saturated fat ratio (P/S) and both cholesterol and triglyceride levels also has been amply established. The unique triglyceride-lowering effects of the particular long-chain polyunsaturated fatty acids in large ocean fish are currently under study.

A definitive prospective study of the effect of diet on IHD in the general population has never been undertaken. Nevertheless, preliminary reports of newer studies of alterations of diet in high-risk populations, coupled with published findings of studies in selected populations, provide strong evidence of a reversible relation among diet, plasma lipids, and IHD. On this basis, numerous authoritative nutrition councils have recommended prudent dietary modifications for the general population of western countries to be instituted early in life and to include a caloric intake adjusted to achieve and maintain ideal body weight, a reduction in total fat calories to 30 to 35 percent of total calories achieved by a substantial reduction in dietary saturated fat to less than 10 percent of total calories, and a reduction in cholesterol intake to less than 300 mg per day. Although a causal relationship in humans between sodium intake and hypertension has not been firmly established, avoidance of excessive dietary sodium also has been recommended.

RISK FACTORS AND MECHANISMS OF ATHEROGENESIS

Adiposity produces insulin resistance in peripheral tissues (mainly muscle and adipose), which leads to compensatory hyperinsulinemia. The liver is not resistant to some effects of insulin, and enhanced production of triglyceride-rich lipoproteins results, leading to elevated plasma triglyceride and cholesterol levels. Thus it has been demonstrated that body weight is related not only to triglyceride levels but also to cholesterol levels. Concomitantly, obesity is associated with increased total-body cholesterol synthesis. Obesity, particularly the abdominal type, produces higher circulating levels of insulin, both in the basal state and after stimulation with glucose or other secretagogues. Since obesity is related to atherosclerosis—both directly and via hypertension, hypertriglyceridemia, hypercholesterolemia, and hyperglycemia—it is not surprising that many studies show a relationship between serum insulin levels, particularly after oral glucose intake, and atherosclerotic disease of the coronary and peripheral arteries. A few studies, however, suggest that this association between insulin and atherosclerosis occurs independently of obesity. It has been postulated that insulin may directly affect arterial wall metabolism, leading to increased endogenous lipid synthesis and thus predisposing to atherosclerosis. Insulin has been shown to stimulate proliferation of arterial smooth-muscle cells, enhance binding of LDL and VLDL, and decrease binding of HDL to cells; it therefore may be one of the plasma factors involved in atheroma formation.

Hypertension may enhance atherogenesis by directly producing injury via mechanical stress on endothelial cells at specific high-pressure sites in the arterial tree. This would allow the sequence of events in the chronic injury hypothesis of atherogenesis to take place. In addition, hypertension might allow more lipoproteins to be transported through intact endothelial lining cells by altering permeability. Hypertension markedly increases lysosomal enzyme activity, presumably owing to stimulation of the cellular disposal system by the internalization of increased amounts of plasma substances. This might lead to increased cell degeneration and release of the highly destructive enzymes (within the lysosomes) into the arterial wall. Experimental hypertension also increases the thickness of the intimal smooth-muscle layer in the arterial wall and increases connective tissue elements. It is still not known if continued high pressure within the artery produces changes in the ability of smooth-muscle cells or stem cells to proliferate.

Diabetes could provide a unique contribution to atherogenesis. Although the fundamental genetic abnormality in human diabetes mellitus remains unknown, it has been suggested that genetic diabetes in humans represents a primary cellular abnormality intrinsic to all cells, resulting in a decreased life span of individual cells, which in turn results in increased cell turnover in tissues. If arterial endothelial and smooth-muscle cells are intrinsically defective in diabetes, accelerated atherogenesis can be readily postulated on the basis of any one of the current theories of pathogenesis. Platelet dysfunction in diabetes might also play a role.

The role of glucose in atheroma formation, if any, is poorly understood. Hyperglycemia is known to affect aortic wall metabolism. Sorbitol, a product of the insulin-independent aldose reductase pathway of glucose metabolism (the polyol pathway) accumulates in the arterial wall in the presence of high glucose concentrations, resulting in osmotic effects including increased cell water content and decreased oxygenation. Increased glucose also appears to stimulate proliferation of cultured arterial smooth-muscle cells. Glycosylation of apolipoproteins and other key proteins intrinsic to arterial wall cell function might also be involved.

The development of atherosclerosis accelerates in approximate quantitative relation to the degree of *hyperlipidemia*. A long-established theory suggests that the higher the circulating levels of lipoprotein, the more likely they are to gain entrance to the arterial wall. By an acceleration of the usual transendothelial transport, large concentrations of lipoproteins within the arterial wall could overwhelm the ability of smooth-muscle cells and monocyte-derived macrophages to metabolize them. Lipoproteins have been immunologically identified in atheroma, and in humans there is a close relationship between plasma cholesterol and arterial lipoprotein cholesterol concentration. Chemically modified or oxidized lipoproteins, possibly produced in hyperlipidemic disorders, could gain access to the scavenger arterial wall macrophages, leading to formation of foam cells as in xanthomas. It is possible that the lipid that accumulates in the arterial wall with increasing age results from infiltration of plasma lipoproteins. However, atheromatous lesions are associated with a more marked increase in arterial wall lipids, which may result in part from injury to the endothelium possibly produced by chronic hyperlipidemia, as demonstrated in cholesterol-fed monkeys. A further mechanism for accelerated atherogenesis in hyperlipidemia is related to the ability of LDL to stimulate proliferation of arterial smooth-muscle cells.

The effect of *chronic smoke inhalation* from cigarettes could result in repetitive injury to endothelial cells, thereby accelerating atherogenesis. Hypoxia stimulates proliferation of cultured human arterial smooth-muscle cells; thus, since cigarette smoking is associated with high levels of carboxyhemoglobin and low oxygen delivery to tissues, another mechanism for atherogenesis is suggested. Hypoxia could produce diminished lysosomal enzyme degradative ability, as evidenced by impaired degradation of LDL by smooth-muscle cells, causing LDL to accumulate in the cells. Consistent with this suggestion is the fact that aortic lesions that resemble atheroma have been produced in experimental animals by systemic hypoxia, and lipid accumulation in the arterial wall of cholesterol-fed rabbits and monkeys appears to be increased by hypoxia.

RISK FACTOR REVERSAL AND REGRESSION OF ATHERO-SCLEROSIS Although the emergence of clinical consequences of atherosclerosis can be lessened, no convincing instance of regression or interruption of progression of atherosclerosis in asymptomatic individuals, determined by direct or indirect examination of lesions, by removal or reversal of any single risk factor or group of risk factors has yet been proved in humans. Nevertheless, feasibility of such demonstrations is now established, and the recent angiographic evidence in patients who have had coronary bypass surgery of interruption of lesion progression and even regression associated with lipid lowering is encouraging. Through mass-media educational efforts, whole communities can be influenced to reduce smoking, change diet, and lower blood pressure levels. Adult males in the United States have lowered cigarette consumption, although increases among teenage girls have kept total usage high. There has been a trend toward lower cholesterol and saturated fat consumption in the United States, coupled with increasing attention to reducing overweight and the use of exercise programs. Concomitantly, and perhaps causally, there has been the noted decline in IHD mortality. Treatment of hyperlipidemia in some instances has been shown to reduce atherosclerotic involvement of peripheral vessels by both invasive and noninvasive measurement. There is also some encouraging evidence in animals, most notably in primates, that relatively complicated plaques induced by hyperlipidemia will regress, and that further progression of atherosclerosis will cease when hyperlipidemia is removed. Therefore efforts to prevent atherogenesis, to interrupt progression, and perhaps to promote regression of existing lesions by risk factor reduction seem warranted.

PREVENTION Although premature IHD is overall the most costly and common of the untimely complications of atherosclerosis, preoccupation with IHD should not obscure the fact that angina pectoris and myocardial infarction are expressions of late-stage atherosclerotic lesions. Factors precipitating these clinical events may be independent of those leading to initiation of plaque formation or its progression to a complicated lesion. Steps taken to prevent recurrence of myocardial infarction or fatal arrhythmia, termed *secondary prevention,* will not necessarily be the same as those taken to delay or prevent formation of atherosclerosis (*primary prevention*). Since atherosclerotic plaques have been detected in the coronary arteries of American males as early as the second decade in autopsy studies of Korean and Vietnam war deaths, primary prevention of atherosclerosis must begin early in life, long before there is any suspicion of IHD.

Thus, *prevention of atherosclerosis, rather than treatment, is the goal.* Although an effective program has not been established with certainty, enough is known to act as a guide both in identification of those with a higher risk and in development of conservative measures that probably will reduce that risk. Thus prevention currently is equated with risk factor reduction.

The decline of American death rates from premature IHD today coincides with two trends in health practices. One is the increasing acceptance of the importance of detecting and attempting to correct some of the risk factors correlated with atherosclerosis. The other is a greater awareness of the dietary sources of cholesterol and saturated fats and a tendency of the public to restrict their intake somewhat. Whether these trends are causally related to the decline in death rate is not known. While a rigorous approach to changes in life-style for the general population may be debatable, it is desirable to continue finding and helping those most susceptible to early atherosclerosis. The physician's role in risk factor reduction involves treatment of hypertension and advice regarding diet, body weight, smoking, and exercise. Drug treatment of hyperlipidemia should be limited to those individuals at high risk who do not respond adequately to dietary

management. Although preliminary trials are encouraging, the long-term value of antiplatelet drugs in reducing either the mortality rate or incidence of myocardial infarction in individuals with IHD remains unproved, and trials are continuing.

TREATMENT There is no agent proven to have any value in "treatment" of atherosclerosis unless it clearly reduces severe hyperlipidemia or obvious hypertension. In fact, there is no treatment of atherosclerosis, only of its complications. While end-stage treatment technology has reduced morbidity (Chap. 190), prevention remains the long-term goal of both research and medical practice.

REFERENCES

BIERMAN EL: Aging and atherosclerosis, in *Principles of Geriatric Medicine,* 2d ed, WR Hazzard et al (eds). New York, McGraw-Hill, 1990, Chap 45, pp 458–465

EVERHART JE et al: Medical arterial calcification and its association with mortality and complications of diabetes. Diabetologia 31:16, 1988

GORDON T et al: Diabetes, blood lipids, and the role of obesity in coronary heart disease risk for women. The Framingham Study. Ann Intern Med 87:393, 1977

KANNEL WB et al: Cholesterol in the prediction of atherosclerotic disease. New perspectives based on the Framingham Study. Ann Intern Med 90:85, 1979

LEAF A: Management of hypercholesterolemia: Are preventive interventions indicated? N Engl J Med 321(10):680, 1989

LEVY RI: Declining mortality in coronary heart disease. Arteriosclerosis 1:312, 1981

MARTIN MJ et al: Serum cholesterol, blood pressure, and mortality: Implications from a cohort of 361,662 men. Lancet 2:933, 1986

McGILL HC: Persistent problems in the pathogenesis of atherosclerosis. Arteriosclerosis 4:443, 1984

NATIONAL CHOLESTEROL EDUCATION PROGRAM: Report of the National Cholesterol Education Program Expert Panel on Detection, Evaluation and Treatment of High Blood Cholesterol in Adults. Arch Intern Med 148:36, 1988

PELL S, FAYERWEATHER WE: Trends in the incidence of myocardial infarction and in associated mortality and morbidity in a large employed population, 1957–1983. N Engl J Med 312:1005, 1985

ROSS R: The pathogenesis of atherosclerosis—an update. N Engl J Med 314:488, 1986

STEINBERG D: Lipoproteins and atherosclerosis: A look back and a look ahead. Arteriosclerosis 3:283, 1983

196 HYPERTENSIVE VASCULAR DISEASE

GORDON H. WILLIAMS

An elevated arterial pressure is probably the more important public health problem in developed countries—being common, asymptomatic, readily detectable, usually easily treatable, and often leading to lethal complications if left untreated. As a result of extensive educational programs in the late 1960s and 1970s by both private and governmental agencies, the number of undiagnosed and/or untreated patients has been significantly reduced to a level of less than 20 percent. This factor may be the most important one responsible for the decline in cardiovascular mortality which has taken place during the past 20 years (Chap. 195). Although our understanding of the pathophysiology of an elevated arterial pressure has increased, in 90 to 95 percent of cases the etiology (and thus potentially the prevention or cure) is still largely unknown. As a consequence, in most cases the hypertension is treated nonspecifically, resulting in a large number of minor side effects and a relatively high (~50 percent) noncompliance rate.

DEFINITION

Since there is no dividing line between normal and high blood pressure, arbitrary levels have been established to define those who have an increased risk of developing a morbid cardiovascular event and/or will clearly benefit from medical therapy. These definitions should consider not only the level of diastolic pressure but also systolic pressure, age, sex, and race. For example, patients with a diastolic pressure greater than 90 mmHg will have a significant reduction in morbidity and mortality with adequate therapy. These, then, are patients who have hypertension and who should be considered for treatment.

The level of *systolic* pressure is also important in assessing arterial pressure's influence on cardiovascular morbidity. Males with normal diastolic pressures (<82 mmHg) but elevated systolic pressures (>158 mmHg) have a 2½-fold increase in their cardiovascular mortality rates when compared with individuals with similar diastolic pressures but whose systolic pressures are normal (<130 mmHg). However, reduction in mortality and morbidity with treatment has not been definitively documented in these patients. Other significant factors which modify blood pressure's influence on the frequency of morbid cardiovascular events are age, race, and sex with young black males being most adversely affected by hypertension.

When hypertension is suspected, blood pressure should be measured at least twice on two separate examinations. In adults, a *diastolic* pressure below 85 mmHg is considered to be normal; between 85 and 89 is high normal; 90 to 104 is mild hypertension; 105 to 114 moderate hypertension; 115 or greater is severe hypertension. When the diastolic pressure is below 90 mmHg, a *systolic* pressure below 140 mmHg indicates normal blood pressure; between 140 and 159 is borderline isolated systolic hypertension; 160 or higher is isolated systolic hypertension. Increasing use of 12- or 24-h blood pressure monitoring may provide additional useful information in patients who are difficult to classify. However, normal values for this procedure are not currently available.

Arterial pressure fluctuates in most persons, whether they are normotensive or hypertensive. Those who are classified as having *labile* hypertension are patients who sometimes, but not always, have arterial pressures within the hypertensive range. These patients are often considered to have borderline hypertension.

Sustained hypertension can become accelerated or enter a malignant phase. Though a patient with *malignant hypertension* often has a blood pressure above 200/140, it is papilledema, usually accompanied by retinal hemorrhages and exudates, and not the absolute pressure level, that defines this condition. *Accelerated hypertension* signifies a significant recent increase over previous hypertensive levels associated with evidence of vascular damage on funduscopic examination but without papilledema.

FREQUENCY   The prevalence of hypertension depends on both the racial composition of the studied population and the criteria used to define the condition. In a white suburban population as used in the Framingham Study, nearly one-fifth have blood pressures greater than 160/95, while almost one-half have pressures greater than 140/90. An even higher prevalance has been documented in the nonwhite population.

ETIOLOGY

The cause of elevated arterial pressure is unknown in most cases. The prevalence of various forms of secondary hypertension depends on the nature of the population studied and how extensive the evaluation is. There are no available data to define the frequency of secondary hypertension in the general population, although in middle-aged males it has been reported to be 6 percent. On the other hand, in referral centers where patients undergo an extensive evaluation, it has been reported to be as high as 35 percent. The various forms of hypertension are outlined in Table 196-1, and their relative frequencies are given in Table 196-2.

ESSENTIAL HYPERTENSION   Patients with arterial hypertension and no definable cause are said to have *primary*, *essential*, or *idiopathic hypertension*. Undoubtedly, the primary difficulty in uncovering the mechanism(s) responsible for the hypertension in these patients is attributable to the variety of systems that are involved in

TABLE 196-1   Classification of arterial hypertension

I Systolic hypertension with wide pulse pressure
  A Decreased compliance of aorta (arteriosclerosis)
  B Increased stroke volume
    1 Aortic regurgitation
    2 Thyrotoxicosis
    3 Hyperkinetic heart syndrome
    4 Fever
    5 Arteriovenous fistula
    6 Patent ductus arteriosus
II Systolic and diastolic hypertension (increased peripheral vascular resistance)
  A Renal
    1 Chronic pyelonephritis
    2 Acute and chronic glomerulonephritis
    3 Polycystic renal disease
    4 Renovascular stenosis or renal infarction
    5 Most other severe renal disease (arteriolar nephrosclerosis, diabetic nephropathy, etc.)
    6 Renin-producing tumors
  B Endocrine
    1 Oral contraceptives
    2 Adrenocortical hyperfunction
      a Cushing's disease and syndrome
      b Primary hyperaldosteronism
      c Congenital or hereditary adrenogenital syndromes (17α-hydroxylase and 11β-hydroxylase defects)
    3 Pheochromocytoma
    4 Myxedema
    5 Acromegaly
  C Neurogenic
    1 Psychogenic
    2 "Diencephalic syndrome"
    3 Familial dysautonomia (Riley-Day)
    4 Polyneuritis (acute porphyria, lead poisoning)
    5 Increased intracranial pressure (acute)
    6 Spinal cord section (acute)
  D Miscellaneous
    1 Coarctation of aorta
    2 Increased intravascular volume (excessive transfusion, polycythemia vera)
    3 Polyarteritis nodosa
    4 Hypercalcemia
  E Unknown etiology
    1 Essential hypertension (>90% of all cases of hypertension)
    2 Toxemia of pregnancy
    3 Acute intermittent porphyria

the regulation of arterial pressure—peripheral and/or central adrenergic, renal, hormonal, and vascular—and to the complexity of the relationships of these systems to one another. Several abnormalities have been described in patients with essential hypertension, often with a claim that one or more of these are primarily responsible for the hypertension. While it is still uncertain whether these individual abnormalities are primary or secondary, varying expressions of a single disease process or reflective of separate disease entities, the accumulating data increasingly support the latter hypothesis. Thus, just as pneumonia is caused by a variety of infectious agents, even though the clinical picture observed may be similar, so essential hypertension likely has a number of distinct causes. Therefore, the

TABLE 196-2   Prevalence of various forms of hypertension in the general population and in specialized referral clinics*

Diagnosis	General population, %	Specialty clinic, %
Essential hypertension	92–94	65–85
Renal hypertension:		
Parenchymal	2–3	4–5
Renovascular	1–2	4–16
Endocrine hypertension:		
Primary aldosteronism	0.3	0.5–12
Cushing's syndrome	<0.1	0.2
Pheochromocytoma	<0.1	0.2
Oral contraceptive–induced	2–4	1–2
Miscellaneous	0.2	1

* Estimates based on a number of reports in the literature.

distinction between primary and secondary hypertension has become blurred, and the approach to both the diagnosis and therapy of hypertensive patients has been modified. For example, as a group of patients with essential hypertension are separated into a distinct subset (e.g., low-renin essential hypertension), they have not been reclassified as a form of secondary hypertension but rather remain in the essential hypertensive group. In this chapter, we define those individuals with a specific organ defect responsible for hypertension as having a *secondary* form of hypertension. In contrast, individuals who may have generalized or functional abnormalities causing their hypertension are defined as having *essential* hypertension.

Heredity   Genetic factors have long been assumed to be important in the genesis of hypertension. Data supporting this view can be found in animal studies as well as population studies in humans. One approach has been to assess the correlation of blood pressures within families (familial aggregation). From these studies the minimum size of the genetic factor can be expressed by a correlation coefficient of approximately 0.2. However, the variation in the size of the genetic factor in different studies reemphasizes the likely heterogeneous nature of the essential hypertensive population. Additionally, most studies support the concept that the inheritance is probably multifactorial or that a number of different genetic defects each have as one of their phenotypic expressions an elevated blood pressure.

Environment   A number of environmental factors have been specifically implicated in the development of hypertension including salt intake, obesity, occupation, family size, and crowding. These factors have all been assumed to be important in the increase in blood pressure with age in more affluent societies, in contrast to the decline in blood pressure with age in more primitive cultures.

SALT-SENSITIVITY   The environmental factor which has received the greatest attention is salt intake. Even this factor illustrates the heterogeneous nature of the essential hypertensive population in that the blood pressure in only approximately 60 percent of hypertensives is particularly responsive to the level of sodium intake. The etiologic basis for this special sensitivity to salt varies, with primary aldosteronism, bilateral renal artery stenosis, renal parenchymal disease, or low-renin essential hypertension accounting for about half of the patients. In the remainder, the pathophysiology is still uncertain, but recent postulated contributing factors include chloride, calcium, a generalized cellular membrane defect, and "nonmodulation" (see below).

Most studies assessing the role of salt in the hypertensive process have assumed that it is the sodium ion which is important. However, some investigators have suggested that the chloride ion may be equally important. This suggestion is based on the observation that feeding chloride-free sodium salts to salt-sensitive hypertensive animals fails to increase arterial pressure. Calcium has also been implicated in the pathogenesis of some forms of essential hypertension. A low calcium intake has been associated with an increase in blood pressure in epidemiologic studies; an increase in leukocyte cytosolic calcium levels has been reported in some hypertensives; and finally calcium entry blockers are effective antihypertensive agents. Several studies have reported a potential link between the salt-sensitive forms of hypertension and calcium. It has been postulated that with salt loading and a defect in the kidney's ability to excrete it, a secondary increase in circulating natriuretic factors may occur. One of these, the so-called digitalis-like natriuretic factor, inhibits ouabain-sensitive sodium-potassium ATPase and thereby leads to intracellular calcium accumulation and a hyperreactive vascular smooth muscle.

A third postulated explanation for salt-sensitive hypertension is a generalized membrane defect. This hypothesis derives most of its data from studies on circulating blood elements, particularly red blood cells, in which abnormalities in the transport of sodium across the cell membrane have been documented. Since both increases and decreases in the activity of different transport systems have been reported, it is likely that some abnormalities are primary and some secondary processes. It has been assumed that this abnormality reflects a defect in the cellular membrane and that this defect occurs in many,

perhaps all cells of the body, particularly the vascular smooth muscle. Because of this defect, there is then an abnormal accumulation of calcium within vascular smooth muscle, resulting in a heightened vascular responsivity to vasoconstrictor agents. This defect has been proposed to be present in 35 to 50 percent of the essential hypertensive population based on studies using red cells. Other studies suggest that the abnormality in the red cell sodium transport is not a fixed abnormality but can be modified by environmental factors. Finally, the mechanisms underlying salt sensitivity in some patients may be a defect in the kidney's ability to excrete sodium appropriately, secondary to an abnormality in the control of the renal circulation and aldosterone secretion with changes in sodium intake. Sodium intake normally modulates adrenal and renal vascular responses to angiotensin II. With dietary sodium restriction, the adrenal response is enhanced and the renal vascular response reduced. Sodium loading has the opposite effect. In this subset of hypertensives this adjustment is absent, thus leading to the term "nonmodulators" to describe those patients in whom the excretion of a sodium load is impaired.

Each of these hypotheses has as a common final pathway an increase in cytosolic calcium resulting in increased vascular reactivity. However, as described above, several mechanisms might produce the increase in calcium accumulation.

Factors modifying the course of essential hypertension   Age, race, sex, smoking, serum cholesterol, glucose intolerance, and weight may all alter the prognosis of this disease. The younger the patient when hypertension is first noted, the greater the reduction in life expectancy if left untreated. In the United States, urban blacks have about twice the prevalence rate for hypertension as whites and more than four times the hypertension-induced morbidity rate. At all ages and in both white and nonwhite populations, females with hypertension fare better than males. Yet, females with hypertension run the same relative risk of a morbid cardiovascular event compared with their normotensive counterparts as males do. Accelerated atherosclerosis is an invariable companion of hypertension. Thus, it is not surprising that independent risk factors associated with the development of atherosclerosis, e.g., an elevated serum cholesterol, glucose intolerance, and/or cigarette smoking, significantly enhance the effect of hypertension on mortality rates regardless of age, sex, or race (Chap. 195). There also is no question that there is a positive correlation between obesity and arterial pressure. A gain in weight is associated with an increased frequency of hypertension in subjects with normal pressures, and weight loss in obese subjects with hypertension lowers their arterial pressure and, if they are being treated, the intensity of therapy required to maintain them normotensive. However, there are no convincing data that obesity adversely affects the hypertension-associated mortality rate.

Natural history   Because essential hypertension is a heterogeneous disorder, variables in addition to the level of arterial pressure modify its course. Thus, the probability of developing a morbid cardiovascular event with a given arterial pressure may vary by as much as twentyfold depending on whether associated risk factors are present (Table 196-3). Although exceptions have been reported, most untreated adults with hypertension will develop further increases in their arterial pressure with time. Furthermore, both from actuarial data and from experience in the era prior to effective therapy, it has been documented that untreated hypertension is associated with a shortening of life by 10 to 20 years, usually related to an acceleration of the atherosclerotic process, with the rate of acceleration in part related to the severity of the hypertension. Even individuals with relatively mild disease, i.e., without evidence of end organ damage, left untreated for 7 to 10 years have a high risk of developing significant complications. Nearly 30 percent will exhibit atherosclerotic complications, and more than 50 percent will have end organ damage related to the hypertension itself, e.g., cardiomegaly, congestive heart failure, retinopathy, a cerebrovascular accident, and/or renal insufficiency. Thus, even in its mild forms, hypertension is a progressively lethal disease, if left untreated.

TABLE 196-3   Factors indicating an adverse prognosis in hypertension

I   Black race
II   Youth
III Male
IV   Persistent diastolic pressure >115 mmHg
V   Smoking
VI   Diabetes mellitus
VII Hypercholesterolemia
VIII Obesity
IX   Evidence of end organ damage
   A Cardiac
      1 Cardiac enlargement
      2 ECG changes of ischemic or left ventricular strain
      3 Myocardial infarction
      4 Congestive heart failure
   B Eyes
      1 Retinal exudates and hemorrhages
      2 Papilledema
   C Renal: impaired renal function
   D Nervous system: cerebrovascular accident

SECONDARY HYPERTENSION

As noted earlier, in only a small minority of patients with an elevated arterial pressure can a specific cause be identified. Yet, they should not be ignored for at least two reasons: (1) with correction of the cause their hypertension may be cured, and (2) the secondary forms may provide insight into the etiology of essential hypertension. Nearly all the secondary forms are related to an alteration in hormone secretion and/or renal function and are discussed in detail in other chapters.

RENAL HYPERTENSION (See also Chap. 230)   Hypertension produced by renal disease is the result of either (1) a derangement in the renal handling of sodium and fluids leading to volume expansion or (2) an alteration in renal secretion of vasoactive materials resulting in a systemic or local change in arteriolar tone. The main subdivisions of renal hypertension are renovascular hypertension, including pre-eclampsia and eclampsia, and renal parenchymal hypertension. A simple explanation for *renal vascular hypertension* is that decreased perfusion of renal tissue due to stenosis of a main or branch renal artery activates the renin-angiotensin system, described in Chap. 317. Circulating angiotensin II elevates arterial pressure by direct vaso-constriction, by stimulation of aldosterone secretion with resultant sodium retention, and/or by stimulating the adrenergic nervous system. In actual practice only about one-half of patients with renovascular hypertension have absolute elevations in renin activity in peripheral plasma, although when renin measurements are referenced against an index of sodium balance, a much higher fraction have inappropriately high values. The use of the competitive angiotensin antagonist, saralasin (1-sar, 8-ala, angiotensin II), has further clarified the role of angiotensin in the genesis of the hypertension in this disease. Nearly all patients with surgically correctable disease have exhibited a reduction of arterial pressure when given this agent in the sodium- or volume-depleted state.

Activation of the renin-angiotensin system also has been offered as an explanation for the hypertension in both acute and chronic *renal parenchymal disease*. In this formulation the only difference between renovascular and renal parenchymal hypertension is that the decreased perfusion of renal tissue in the latter case results from inflammatory and fibrotic changes involving multiple small intrarenal vessels. There are enough differences between the two conditions, however, to suggest that there are other mechanisms active in renal parenchymal disease: (1) peripheral plasma renin activity is elevated far less frequently in renal parenchymal than in renovascular hypertension; (2) cardiac output is said to be normal in the renal parenchymal type (unless uremia and anemia are present), but slightly elevated in renovascular hypertension; (3) circulatory responses to tilting and to the Valsalva maneuver are exaggerated in the latter condition; and (4) blood volume tends to be high in patients with severe renal parenchymal disease and low in patients with severe renovascular

hypertension. Alternative explanations for the hypertension in renal parenchymal disease include the possibilities that the damaged kidneys (1) produce an unidentified vasopressor substance other than renin, (2) fail to produce a necessary humoral vasodilator substance (perhaps prostaglandin or bradykinin), (3) fail to inactivate circulating vaso-pressor substances, and/or (4) are ineffective in disposing of sodium, and the retained sodium is responsible for the hypertension as outlined earlier. Though all these explanations, including participation of the renin-angiotensin system, probably have some validity in individual patients, the hypothesis involving sodium retention is particularly attractive. It is supported by the observation that those patients with chronic pyelonephritis or polycystic renal disease who are salt wasters do not develop hypertension, and by the observation that removal of salt and water by dialysis or diuretics is effective in controlling arterial pressure in the majority of patients with renal parenchymal disease.

A rare form of renal hypertension results from the excess secretion of renin by juxtaglomerular cell tumors or nephroblastomas. The initial presentation is similar to that of hyperaldosteronism with hypertension, hypokalemia, and overproduction of aldosterone. However, in contrast to primary aldosteronism, peripheral renin activity is *elevated instead of subnormal*. This disease can be distinguished from other forms of secondary aldosteronism by the presence of normal renal function and with unilateral increases in renal vein renin concentration without a renal artery lesion.

ENDOCRINE HYPERTENSION   Adrenal hypertension   Hypertension is a feature of a variety of adrenal cortical abnormalities. In *primary aldosteronism* (Chap. 317) there is a clear relationship between the aldosterone-induced sodium retention and the hypertension. Normal individuals given aldosterone develop hypertension only if they also ingest sodium. Since aldosterone causes sodium retention by stimulating renal tubular exchange of sodium for potassium, hypokalemia is a prominent feature in most patients with primary aldosteronism, and therefore the measurement of serum potassium provides a simple screening test. The effect of sodium retention and volume expansion in chronically suppressing plasma renin activity is critically important for the definitive diagnosis. In most clinical situations plasma renin activity and plasma or urinary aldosterone levels parallel each other, but in patients with primary aldosteronism, aldosterone levels are high and relatively fixed because of autonomous aldosterone secretion, while plasma renin activity levels are suppressed and respond sluggishly to sodium depletion. Primary aldosteronism may be secondary either to a tumor or bilateral adrenal hyperplasia. It is important to distinguish between these two conditions preoperatively, as usually the hypertension in the latter is not modified by operation.

The sodium-retaining effect of large amounts of glucocorticoids also offers an explanation for the hypertension in severe cases of Cushing's syndrome (Chap. 317). Moreover, increased production of mineralocorticoids also has been documented in some patients with Cushing's syndrome. However, the hypertension in many cases of Cushing's syndrome does not seem volume-dependent, leading investigators to speculate that it may be secondary to glucocorticoid-induced production of renin substrate (angiotensin-mediated hypertension) or a steroid-induced change in vascular reactivity. In the forms of the adrenogenital syndrome due to C-11 or C-17 hydroxylase deficiency (Chap. 317) deoxycorticosterone accounts for the sodium retention and the resultant hypertension, which is accompanied by suppression of plasma renin activity.

In patients with pheochromocytoma (Chap. 318) increased secretion of epinephrine and norepinephrine by a tumor most often located in the adrenal medulla causes excessive stimulation of adrenergic receptors, which results in peripheral vasoconstriction and cardiac stimulation. This diagnosis is confirmed by demonstrating increased urinary excretion of epinephrine and norepinephrine or their metabolites.

Acromegaly (See also Chap. 313)   Hypertension, coronary atherosclerosis, and cardiac hypertrophy are frequent complications of this condition.

Hypercalcemia (See also Chap. 339) The hypertension which occurs in up to one-third of patients with hyperparathyroidism ordinarily can be attributed to renal parenchymal damage due to nephrolithiasis and nephrocalcinosis. However, increased calcium levels can also have a direct vasoconstrictive effect. In some cases, the hypertension disappears when the hypercalcemia is corrected. Thus, paradoxically the increased serum calcium level in hyperparathyroidism raises blood pressure, while epidemiologic studies suggest that a high calcium intake lowers blood pressure. To further confuse the issue, calcium entry blocking agents are effective antihypertensive agents. Additional studies are needed to resolve these seemingly conflicting observations.

Oral contraceptives The most common cause of endocrine hypertension is that resulting from the use of estrogen-containing oral contraceptives. Indeed, this may be the most common form of secondary hypertension. The mechanism producing the hypertension is likely to be secondary to activation of the renin-angiotensin-aldosterone system. Thus, both volume (aldosterone) and vasoconstrictor (angiotensin II) factors are important. The estrogen component of oral contraceptive agents stimulates the hepatic synthesis of the renin substrate angiotensinogen, which in turn favors the increased production of angiotensin II and secondary aldosteronism. Women taking oral contraceptives have increased plasma concentrations of angiotensin II and aldosterone with some increase in arterial pressure. However, only about 5 percent actually have an increase in arterial pressure greater than 140/90, and in about half of these the hypertension will remit within 6 months of stopping the drug.

Why some women taking oral contraceptives develop hypertension and others do not is unclear but may be related to (1) increased vascular sensitivity to angiotensin II, (2) the presence of mild renal disease, (3) familial factors (over one-half have a positive family history for hypertension), (4) age (hypertension is significantly more prevalent in women over age 35), and/or (5) obesity. Indeed some investigators have suggested that the oral contraceptives are simply unmasking patients with essential hypertension.

COARCTATION OF THE AORTA (See also Chap. 186) The hypertension associated with coarctation may be caused by the constriction itself, or perhaps by the changes in the renal circulation which result in an unusual form of renal arterial hypertension. The diagnosis of coarctation is usually evident from physical examination and routine x-ray findings.

LOW-RENIN ESSENTIAL HYPERTENSION Approximately 20 percent of patients who by all other criteria have essential hypertension have suppressed plasma renin activity. This occurs more frequently in black than in white patients. Though these patients are not hypokalemic, they have been reported to have expanded extracellular fluid volumes, and it is tempting to implicate sodium retention and renin suppression due to excessive production of an unidentified mineralocorticoid. Involvement of the adrenal cortex is suggested by the observation that large doses of spironolactone, the mineralocorticoid antagonist, and the inhibition of steroidogenesis by aminoglutethimide can result in sodium loss and lowering of blood pressure in these patients. A search for other mineralocorticoids occasionally reveals increased secretion of 18-hydroxy-11-deoxycorticosterone, or 16-hydroxydehydroepiandrosterone, or 19-hydroxyandrostenedione in some patients. However, the frequency of these abnormalities is no greater than in patients with normal renin hypertension. Some studies have suggested that many of these patients have an increased sensitivity of their adrenal cortex to angiotensin II which may be the underlying mechanism. Since this altered sensitivity has been reported even in patients with normal renin hypertension, it is likely that patients with low-renin hypertension are not a distinct subset but rather form part of a continuum of patients with essential hypertension.

HIGH-RENIN ESSENTIAL HYPERTENSION Approximately 15 percent of patients with essential hypertension have plasma renin levels elevated above the normal range. It has been suggested that plasma renin plays an important role in the pathogenesis of the elevated blood pressure in these patients. However, most studies have documented that saralasin significantly reduces blood pressure in less than half of these patients. This has led some investigators to postulate that the elevated renin levels and blood pressure may both be secondary to an increased activity of the adrenergic system. It has been proposed that, in those patients with angiotensin-dependent high-renin hypertension whose arterial pressures are lowered by saralasin, the mechanism responsible for the increased renin and, therefore, the hypertension is a compensatory hyperreninemia secondary to a decreased adrenal responsiveness to angiotensin II. Additional studies have documented that patients with high-renin hypertension are the same as the nonmodulators described on p. 1003.

EFFECTS OF HYPERTENSION

Patients with hypertension die prematurely; the most common cause of death is heart disease, with stroke and renal failure also frequent, particularly in those with significant retinopathy.

EFFECTS ON HEART Cardiac compensation for the excessive work load imposed by increased systemic pressure is at first sustained by concentric left ventricular hypertrophy, characterized by an increase in wall thickness. Ultimately, the function of this chamber deteriorates, the cavity dilates, and the symptoms and signs of heart failure appear (Chap. 182). Angina pectoris may also occur because of the combination of accelerated coronary arterial disease and increased myocardial oxygen requirements as a consequence of the increased myocardial mass (Chap. 190). On physical examination the heart is enlarged and has a prominent left ventricular impulse. The sound of aortic closure is accentuated, and there may be a faint murmur of aortic regurgitation. Presystolic (atrial, fourth) heart sounds appear frequently in hypertensive heart disease, and a protodiastolic (ventricular, third heart) sound or summation gallop rhythm may be present. Electrocardiographic changes of left ventricular hypertrophy (Chap. 176) are common; evidence of ischemia or infarction may be observed late in the disease. The majority of deaths due to hypertension result from myocardial infarction or congestive heart failure.

NEUROLOGIC EFFECTS The neurologic effects of long-standing hypertension may be divided into retinal and central nervous system changes. Because the retina is the only tissue in which the arteries and arterioles can be examined directly, repeated ophthalmoscopic examination provides the opportunity to observe the progress of the vascular effects of hypertension (Table 196-4). The Keith-Wagener-Barker classification of the *retinal changes* in hypertension has provided a simple and excellent means for serial evaluation of hypertensive patients. Increasing severity of hypertension is associated with focal spasm and progressive general narrowing of the arterioles, as well as the appearance of hemorrhages, exudates, and papilledema. These retinal lesions often produce scotomata, blurred vision, and even blindness, especially in the presence of papilledema or hemorrhages of the macular area. Hypertensive lesions may develop acutely and, if therapy results in significant reduction of blood pressure, may show rapid resolution. Rarely, these lesions resolve without therapy. In contrast, retinal arteriolosclerosis results from endothelial and muscular proliferation, and it accurately reflects similar changes in other organs. Sclerotic changes do not develop as rapidly as hypertensive lesions, nor do they regress appreciably with therapy. As a consequence of increased wall thickness and rigidity, sclerotic arterioles distort and compress the veins as they cross within their common fibrous sheath, and the reflected light streak from the arterioles is changed by the increased opacity of the vessel wall.

Central nervous system dysfunction also occurs frequently in patients with hypertension. Occipital headaches, most often in the morning, are among the most prominent early symptoms of hypertension. Dizziness, lightheadedness, vertigo, tinnitus, and dimmed vision or syncope may also be observed, but the more serious manifestations are due to vascular occlusion, hemorrhage, or encephalopathy (Chap. 351). The pathogenesis of the former two disorders are quite different. *Cerebral infarction* is secondary to the

TABLE 196-4   Classification of hypertensive and arteriolosclerotic retinopathy

Degree	Hypertension — Arterioles — General narrowing AV ratio*	Focal spasm†	Hemor-rhages	Exudates	Papilledema	Arteriolosclerosis — Arteriolar light reflex	AV crossing defects‡
Normal	3:4	1:1	0	0	0	Fine yellow line, red blood column	0
Grade I	1:2	1:1	0	0	0	Broadened yellow line, red blood column	Mild depression of vein
Grade II	1:3	2:3	0	0	0	Broad yellow line, ''copper wire,'' blood column not visible	Depression or humping of vein
Grade III	1:4	1:3	+	+	0	Broad white line, ''silver wire,'' blood column not visible	Right-angle deviation, tapering, and disappearance of vein under arteriole. Distal dilatation of vein
Grade IV	Fine, fibrous cords	Obliteration of distal flow	+	+	+	Fibrous cords, blood column not visible	Same as grade III

* This is the ratio of arteriolar to venous diameters.
† This is the ratio of diameters of region of spasm to proximal arteriole.
‡ Arteriolar length and tortuosity increase with severity.

increased atherosclerosis observed in hypertensive patients, while *cerebral hemorrhage* is the result of both the elevated arterial pressure and the development of cerebral vascular microaneurysms (Charcot-Bouchard aneurysms). Only age and arterial pressure are known to influence the development of the microaneurysms. Thus, it is not surprising that the association of arterial pressure with cerebral hemorrhage is much better than with either cerebral or myocardial infarction.

Hypertensive encephalopathy consists of the following symptom complex: severe hypertension, disordered consciousness, increased intracranial pressure, retinopathy with papilledema, and seizures. The pathogenesis is uncertain but probably not related to arteriolar spasm or cerebral edema. Focal neurologic signs are infrequent, and if present, suggest that infarction, hemorrhage, or transient ischemic attacks are more likely diagnoses. Although some investigators have suggested that prompt lowering of arterial pressure in these patients may adversely affect cerebral blood flow, most studies indicate that this is not the case.

RENAL EFFECTS (See also Chap. 230)   Arteriolosclerotic lesions of the afferent and efferent arterioles and the glomerular capillary tufts are the most common renal vascular lesions in hypertension and result in decreased glomerular filtration rate and tubular dysfunction. Proteinuria and microscopic hematuria occur because of glomerular lesions, and approximately 10 percent of the deaths secondary to hypertension result from renal failure. Blood loss in hypertension occurs not only from renal lesions; epistaxis, hemoptysis, and metrorrhagia also occur frequently in these patients.

APPROACH TO THE PATIENT WITH HYPERTENSION

In evaluating patients with hypertension, the initial history, physical examination, and laboratory tests should be directed at (1) uncovering correctable secondary forms of hypertension (Table 196-1), (2) establishing a pretreatment baseline, (3) assessing factors which may influence the type of therapy or which may be adversely modified by therapy, and (4) determining whether other risk factors for the development of arteriosclerotic cardiovascular disease are present (Chap. 195). Ideally, this evaluation would also determine the underlying mechanism(s) in essential hypertension, particularly if such information leads to a more specific therapeutic program. Unfortunately, at the present time this aspect of the evaluation is limited either by lack of knowledge of the underlying mechanisms, uncertainty as to the specificity of therapy for a distinct subset even

if the underlying mechanisms are known, or the prohibitive expense in defining a subset of hypertensive patients even if specific therapy were available. However, with the accumulation of additional information a fifth component in the evaluation of patients with hypertension may become increasingly more important.

SYMPTOMS AND SIGNS   The majority of patients with hypertension have no specific symptoms referable to their blood pressure elevation and will be identified only in the course of a physical examination. When symptoms do bring the patient to the physician, they fall into three categories. They are related to (1) the elevated pressure itself, (2) the hypertensive vascular disease, and (3) the underlying disease in the case of secondary hypertension. Though popularly considered a symptom of elevated arterial pressure, headache is characteristic only of severe hypertension; most commonly it is localized to the occipital region, is present when the patient awakens in the morning, and subsides spontaneously after several hours. Other possibly related complaints include dizziness, palpitations, easy fatigability, and impotency. Complaints referable to vascular disease include epistaxis, hematuria, blurring of vision owing to retinal changes, episodes of weakness or dizziness due to transient cerebral ischemia, angina pectoris, and dyspnea due to cardiac failure. Pain due to dissection of the aorta or to a leaking aneurysm is an occasional presenting symptom.

Examples of symptoms related to the underlying disease in secondary hypertension are polyuria, polydipsia, and muscle weakness secondary to hypokalemia in patients with primary aldosteronism, or weight gain and emotional lability in patients with Cushing's syndrome. The patient with a pheochromocytoma may present with episodic headaches, palpitations, diaphoresis, and postural dizziness.

CLINICAL EVALUATION   History   A strong family history of hypertension, along with the reported finding of intermittent pressure elevation in the past, favors the diagnosis of essential hypertension. Secondary hypertension often develops before the age of 35 or after the age of 55 years. The history of use of adrenal steroids or estrogens is of obvious significance. A history of repeated urinary tract infections suggests chronic pyelonephritis, although this condition may occur in the absence of symptoms; nocturia and polydipsia suggest renal or endocrine disease, while trauma to either flank or an episode of acute flank pain may be a clue to the presence of renal injury. A history of weight gain is compatible with Cushing's syndrome, and weight loss with pheochromocytoma. A number of aspects of the history aid in determining whether vascular disease has progressed to dangerous stages. These include angina pectoris and symptoms of cerebrovascular insufficiency, of congestive heart failure, and/or of peripheral vascular insufficiency. Other risk factors that should be elicited include cigarette smoking, diabetes mellitus, lipid disorders, and a family history of early deaths due to cardiovascular disease.

Physical examination The physical examination starts with the patient's general appearance. For instance, are the round face and trunkal obesity of Cushing's syndrome present? Is muscular development in the upper extremities out of proportion to that in the lower extremities, suggesting coarctation of the aorta? The next step is to compare the blood pressures and pulses in both upper extremities and in the supine and standing positions. A rise in diastolic pressure when the patient goes from the supine to the standing position is most compatible with essential hypertension; a fall, in the absence of antihypertensive medications, suggests secondary forms of hypertension. Detailed examination of the ocular fundi is mandatory, since funduscopic findings provide one of the best indications of the duration of hypertension and of prognosis. The Keith-Wagener-Barker classification of funduscopic changes (Table 196-4) is useful; the specific changes in each fundus should be recorded and a grade assigned. Palpation and auscultation of the carotid arteries for evidence of stenosis or occlusion are important; narrowing of a carotid artery may be a manifestation of hypertensive vascular disease, and it may also be a clue to the presence of a renal arterial lesion, since these two lesions may occur together. In examination of the heart and lungs, one should search for evidence of left ventricular hypertrophy and cardiac decompensation. Is there a left ventricular lift? Are third and fourth heart sounds present? Are there pulmonary rales? Chest examination also includes a search for extracardiac murmurs and palpable collateral vessels that may result from coarctation of the aorta.

The most important part of the abdominal examination is auscultation for bruits originating in stenotic renal arteries. Bruits due to renal arterial narrowing nearly always have a diastolic component or may be continuous and are best heard just to the right or left of the midline above the umbilicus, or in the flanks; they are present in many patients with renal artery stenosis due to fibrous dysplasia and in 40 to 50 percent of those with functionally significant stenosis due to arteriosclerosis. The abdomen also should be palpated for abdominal aneurysm and for the enlarged kidneys of polycystic renal disease. The femoral pulses must be carefully felt, and, if they are decreased and/or delayed in comparison to the radial pulse, the blood pressure in the lower extremities must be measured. Even if the femoral pulse is normal to palpation, arterial pressure in the lower extremities should be recorded at least once in patients in whom hypertension is discovered before the age of 30 years. Finally, examination of the extremities for edema and a search for evidence of a previous cerebrovascular accident and/or other intracranial pathology should be performed.

Laboratory investigation Controversy exists as to what laboratory studies should be performed in patients presenting with hypertension. In general, the disagreement resides in how extensively to evaluate the patient for secondary forms of hypertension or subsets of essential hypertension. In the following discussion laboratory studies are divided into those which should be performed in all patients with sustained hypertension (basic studies) and those which should be added if (1) from the initial evaluation a secondary form of hypertension is suggested and/or (2) arterial pressure is not controlled after initial therapy (secondary studies).

BASIC STUDIES Renal status is evaluated by assessing the presence of protein, blood, and glucose in the urine and measuring serum creatinine and/or blood urea nitrogen (BUN). Microscopic examination of the urine is also helpful. A serum potassium level is needed both as a screen for mineralocorticoid-induced hypertension and as a baseline prior to initiating diuretic therapy.

Other blood chemistries may also be useful, particularly since they can often be ordered as a battery of automated tests at minimal cost to the patient. For example, a blood glucose is helpful both because diabetes mellitus may be associated with accelerated arteriosclerosis, renal vascular disease, and diabetic nephropathy in patients with hypertension, and because primary aldosteronism, Cushing's

syndrome, and pheochromocytoma all may be associated with hyperglycemia. Furthermore, since antihypertensive therapy with diuretics, for example, can raise the blood glucose level, it is important to establish a baseline. The possibility of hypercalcemia may also be investigated. Serum uric acid is useful because of the increased incidence of hyperuricemia in patients with renal and essential hypertension and because, as with blood glucose, the level subsequently may be raised by treatment with diuretics. Serum cholesterol and triglycerides may be measured to identify other factors which predispose to the development of arteriosclerosis. An electrocardiogram should be obtained in all cases as an assessment of cardiac status, particularly if left ventricular hypertrophy is present, and as a baseline. The chest roentgenogram may also be helpful by providing the opportunity to identify aortic dilatation or elongation and the rib notching that occurs in coarctation of the aorta.

SECONDARY STUDIES (Table 196-5) Certain clues from the history, physical examination, and basic laboratory studies may suggest an unusual cause for the hypertension and dictate the need for special studies. For example, the abrupt onset of severe hypertension and/or the onset of hypertension of any severity under the age of 25 or after the age of 50 years should lead to laboratory tests to exclude renovascular hypertension and pheochromocytoma. A history of headaches, palpitations, anxiety attacks, unusual sweating, hyperglycemia, and weight loss should also lead to tests to exclude pheochromocytoma. The presence of an abdominal bruit should lead to workup for renovascular hypertension, and the finding of bilateral upper abdominal masses on physical examination, consistent with polycystic renal disease, to the performance of an intravenous pyelogram. An elevated creatinine or blood urea nitrogen, associated with proteinuria and hematuria, should initiate a detailed workup for renal insufficiency (Chap. 222). Special studies for secondary hypertension are also indicated if there is therapeutic failure with the initial drug program. The specific diagnostic measures depend on the most likely causes of secondary hypertension.

Pheochromocytoma (See also Chap. 318) The easiest and best screening procedure for pheochromocytoma is the measurement of catecholamines or their metabolites in a 24-h urine collected during the time the patient is hypertensive. Measurement of plasma catecholamine levels may also be useful. These tests may be indicated even in patients who do not have episodic hypertension, since over half the patients with pheochromocytoma have fixed hypertension. Provocative tests are seldom if ever indicated, although occasionally a suppressive test may be useful.

Cushing's syndrome (See also Chap. 317) A 24-h urine test for cortisol or the administration of 1 mg dexamethasone at bedtime, followed by measurement of plasma cortisol at 7 to 10 A.M. is the best test for the presence of this condition. A urine cortisol less than 2750 nmol (100 μg) or suppression of the plasma cortisol level to below 140 nmol/L (5 μg/dL) effectively rules out Cushing's syndrome.

TABLE 196-5 Laboratory tests and special studies for evaluation of hypertension

I Basic studies
  A Always included
    1 Urine for protein, blood, and glucose
    2 Hematocrit
    3 Serum potassium
    4 Serum creatinine and/or blood urea nitrogen
    5 Electrocardiogram
  B Usually included, depending on cost and other factors
    1 Microscopic urinalysis
    2 White blood cell count
    3 Plasma/blood glucose, cholesterol, and triglycerides
    4 Serum calcium, phosphate, and uric acid
    5 Chest x-ray
II Special studies to screen for secondary hypertension
  A Renovascular: digital subtraction angiogram or rapid sequence IVP
  B Pheochromocytoma: 24-h urine for creatinine, metanephrines, and catecholamines or plasma catecholamines
  C Cushing's syndrome: overnight dexamethasone suppression test or 24-h urine cortisol

Renovascular hypertension (See also Chap. 230) The standard screening test for renal vascular hypertension has been the rapid-sequence intravenous pyelogram (IVP). Features suggestive of renal ischemia include (1) unilateral delayed appearance and excretion of contrast material, (2) a difference in kidney size greater than 1.5 cm, (3) irregular contour of the renal silhouette, suggesting partial infarction or atrophy, (4) indentations on the ureter or renal pelvis, possibly due to dilated ureteral arteries (collateral notching), and (5) hyperconcentration of contrast medium in the collecting system of the smaller kidney. When these criteria are used, the false-positive rate is 11 percent and the false-negative rate 12 percent. The digital subtraction angiogram has been received with considerable enthusiasm as a more precise screening test for renal vascular disease. Its ultimate place as a screening test is unclear, however, because of its relatively high cost and the need for an arterial rather than a venous injection. The isotope renogram and saralasin infusion test, both enthusiastically endorsed in the past as screening procedures, are now used infrequently either because of lower sensitivity and specificity or limited availability.

The definitive test of surgically correctable renal disease is the combination of a renal angiogram and renal vein renin determinations. The renal arteriogram both establishes the presence of a renal arterial lesion and aids in determining whether the lesion is due to atherosclerosis or to one of the fibrous or fibromuscular dysplasias. It does not, however, prove that the lesion is responsible for the hypertension, nor does it permit prediction of the chances of surgical cure; it must be noted that (1) renal artery stenosis is a frequent finding by angiography and at postmortem in normotensive individuals, and (2) essential hypertension is a common condition and may occur in combination with renal arterial stenosis which actually may not be responsible for the hypertension. Bilateral renal vein catheterization for measurement of plasma renin activity is, therefore, used to assess the functional significance of any lesion noted on arteriography. When one kidney is ischemic and the other is normal, all the renin released comes from the involved kidney. In the most straightforward situation, the ischemic kidney has a significantly higher venous plasma renin activity than the normal kidney by a factor of 1.5 or more. Moreover, the renal venous blood draining the uninvolved kidney exhibits levels similar to those in the inferior vena cava below the entrance of the renal veins. Significant benefit from operative correction may be anticipated in at least 80 percent of patients with the findings described above if care is taken to prepare the patient properly prior to renal vein blood sampling, i.e., discontinuing renin-suppressing drugs, such as beta blockers, for at least 10 days, placing the patient on a low sodium intake for 4 days, and/or giving a converting enzyme inhibitor for 24 h. When obstructing lesions in the *branches* of the renal arteries are demonstrated by arteriography, an attempt to obtain blood samples from the main *branches* of the renal vein should be made in an effort to identify a localized intrarenal arterial lesion responsible for the hypertension.

Primary aldosteronism (See also Chap. 317) These patients almost always exhibit hypokalemia. Diuretic therapy often complicates the picture when the hypokalemia is first observed and needs to be assessed. Given hypokalemia, the relation between plasma renin activity and the aldosterone level becomes the key to the diagnosis of primary aldosteronism. The aldosterone concentration or excretion is high and plasma renin activity is low in primary aldosteronism, and these levels are relatively unaffected by changes in sodium balance. A critical part of the evaluation after primary aldosteronism has been established is to determine whether unilateral or bilateral disease is present since surgical removal of the lesion usually reduces arterial pressure only in those with unilateral disease.

Plasma renin activity measurements Some studies have suggested that most hypertensive patients should have a plasma renin level measured and related to a 24-h urine sodium excretion rate to assess whether high, low, or normal levels are present. It has been proposed that this information may be important for both therapeutic and prognostic reasons. However, it is unclear, on the basis of presently available data and treatment programs, that these random measurements are really useful except in patients with findings suggestive of renal vascular disease or mineralocorticoid excess in whom lateralizing renal vein renin levels or suppressed peripheral renin levels may be of diagnostic and/or therapeutic significance.

TREATMENT

Virtually every patient with a diastolic arterial pressure which persistently exceeds 90 mmHg is a candidate for diagnostic studies and for subsequent treatment. Furthermore, at any given level of blood pressure elevation, the ultimate risk of developing hypertensive vascular complications is greater in men than in women, and in younger than in older persons. It may be argued, then, that it is hard to justify producing the uncomfortable side effects of therapy in, for example, an asymptomatic woman over 70 years of age with a diastolic pressure of 90 mmHg. On the other hand, it is easy to justify side effects in a man of 30 with a diastolic pressure exceeding 110 mmHg, because such a person may be expected to receive the greatest benefit from therapy. Fortunately, the choice of treatment is such that a satisfactory program to control arterial pressure with minimal side effects can be developed for most patients, particularly as more studies assessing the impact of specific therapeutic agents on the patient's quality of life are reported. A reasonable guideline would be that all patients with diastolic pressure repeatedly above 90 mmHg should be treated unless specific contraindications exist. There is controversy regarding the advisability of treating isolated *systolic* hypertension. Until the results of a well-controlled prospective study provide evidence to the contrary, treatment of isolated systolic hypertension may not be indicated. Patients with labile hypertension or isolated systolic hypertension who are not treated should have regular follow-up examinations at 6-month intervals, because of the frequent development of progressive and/or sustained hypertension.

The identification of an operable form of secondary hypertension does not automatically mean that surgical treatment is indicated. The decision depends upon the age and general health of the patient, the natural history of the lesion, and the response of the pressure to drug therapy. In patients with renovascular hypertension the feasibility of renal angioplasty, surgical repair versus nephrectomy, and the degree of overall renal function impairment must be considered. Age and general health are important in patients with renovascular hypertension due to arteriosclerosis, because there is no evidence that repair of the stenosis increases life expectancy in the elderly patient with other evidence of vascular disease. Knowledge of the natural history of the disease is especially important when approaching the decision in the young patient with renal-artery stenosis due to fibrous dysplasia. If the arteriographic appearance suggests that the stenosis is due to intimal or subadventitial fibroplasia, the lesion may be expected to progress and operation or angioplasty is required. Medial fibroplasia, on the other hand, often remains stable, and operation or angioplasty may not be necessary if pressure can be controlled by drug therapy. The decision regarding operation should also be considered carefully in patients with primary aldosteronism when bilateral adrenal venography does not demonstrate a tumor, because such patients may prove to have multinodular hyperplasia. This means that bilateral adrenalectomy would be required to eliminate the aldosterone excess, and, even then, hypertension usually persists. If hypokalemia can be controlled by spironolactone or other drug therapy, and arterial pressure lowered with antihypertensive agents, then it is reasonable to withhold operative treatment.

GENERAL MEASURES Nondrug therapeutic intervention is probably indicated in all patients with sustained hypertension and probably most with labile hypertension. The general measures employed include (1) relief of stress, (2) diet, (3) regular exercise, and (4) control of other risk factors contributing to the development of arteriosclerosis. Relief of emotional and environmental stress is one of the reasons for the improvement in hypertension that occurs when a patient is hospitalized. Though it is usually impossible to extricate the hypertensive patient from all internal and external stresses, he or she should be advised to avoid any unnecessary tensions. In rare instances, it may be appropriate to recommend a change of job or of life-style. Recently it has been suggested that relaxation techniques may also lower arterial pressure. However, it is uncertain that these techniques alone have much long-term effect.

Dietary management has three aspects:

1 Because of the documented efficacy of sodium restriction and volume contraction in lowering blood pressure, patients previously were instructed to curtail sodium intake drastically. Some investigators have suggested this is no longer necessary. They base their conclusion on two observations: (1) In many patients the blood pressure is not sensitive to the level of sodium intake, and (2) diuretics provide another method of decreasing body sodium stores in those individuals whose blood pressure may be sodium-sensitive. However, a number of reports have documented that while mild sodium restriction has little, if any, direct action on blood pressure, it significantly potentiates the efficacy of nearly all antihypertensive agents and thus, by allowing blood pressure control with lower doses of drugs, side effects are reduced. In addition, it is quite clear that in some hypertensive patients, as noted above, the level of sodium intake does influence the blood pressure. Thus, since there is no apparent risk to mild sodium restriction, the most practical approach now is to advise mild dietary sodium restriction (up to 5 g NaCl per day), which can be achieved by eliminating all additions of salt to food which is prepared normally. Some studies have also reported lowering of arterial pressure by *increasing* calcium intake. While the advisability of this form of dietary alteration is still controversial, since a moderately high calcium intake probably also reduces the extent of age-related osteoporosis, it is probably a useful adjunct.

2 Caloric restriction should be urged for the patient who is overweight. Some obese patients will show a significant reduction in pressure simply as a consequence of weight loss.

3 A restriction in intake of cholesterol and saturated fats is recommended since such a diet may diminish the incidence of arteriosclerotic complications. Regular exercise is indicated within the limits of the patient's cardiovascular status. Not only is exercise helpful in controlling weight, but in addition there is evidence that physical conditioning itself may lower arterial pressure. Isotonic exercises (jogging, swimming) are better than isometric exercises (weight lifting) since, if anything, the latter raises arterial pressure. The dietary management outlined above is aimed at the control of other risk factors. Probably the most significant additional step that could be taken in this area would be to convince the smoker to give up cigarettes.

DRUG THERAPY (Table 196-6) To make rational use of antihypertensive drugs, the sites and mechanisms of their action must be understood. In general, there are five classes of drugs: diuretics, antiadrenergic agents, vasodilators, calcium entry blockers, and angiotensin-converting enzyme (ACE) inhibitors.

Diuretics (See also Chap. 182) The thiazides are the most frequently used and most extensively investigated members of this group, and their early effect certainly is related to sodium diuresis and volume depletion. A reduction in peripheral vascular resistance also has been reported by some workers to be important in the long term. Traditionally, thiazide diuretics have formed the cornerstone of most therapeutic programs designed to lower arterial pressure and are usually effective within 3 to 4 days. However, in recent years increasing resistance to their routine use has occurred primarily because of their adverse metabolic effects, which include hypokalemia due to renal potassium loss, hyperuricemia due to uric acid retention, carbohydrate intolerance, and hyperlipidemia. The more potent loop-acting diuretics, furosemide and bumetanide, also have been shown to be antihypertensive but have been less extensively used for this purpose primarily because of their shorter duration of action. Spiro-

nolactone causes renal sodium loss by blocking the effect of endogenous mineralocorticoids, and therefore it may be more effective in patients whose mineralocorticoids are present in excess, e.g., primary or secondary aldosteronism. Although they do not compete directly with aldosterone, triamterene and amiloride act at the same site as spironolactone to impede sodium reabsorption and are effective in the same situations as spironolactone, except triamterene has little intrinsic antihypertensive effect. Their major disadvantage is that they can produce hyperkalemia, particularly in patients with impaired renal function. Any of these three potassium-sparing diuretics can also be given along with thiazide diuretics to minimize renal potassium loss.

Antiadrenergic agents (See also Chap. 67) These drugs act at one or more sites either centrally on the vasomotor center, in peripheral neurons modifying catecholamine release, or by blocking adrenergic receptor sites on target tissue. Drugs that appear to have predominant *central actions* are *clonidine, methyldopa, guanabenz,* and *guanfacine*. These drugs and their metabolites are predominantly alpha-receptor agonists. Stimulation of alpha$_2$ receptors in the vasomotor centers of the brain *reduces* sympathetic outflow, thereby reducing arterial pressure. Usually a fall in cardiac output and heart rate also occurs, more commonly with clonidine and guanabenz, but the baroreceptor reflex is intact. Thus, postural symptoms are absent. However, rebound hypertension may rarely occur when these drugs, particularly clonidine and guanabenz, are stopped. This is probably secondary to the increase in norepinephrine release which had been inhibited by these agents secondary to their agonist effect on presynaptic alpha receptors.

Another class of antiadrenergic agents is the *ganglionic blocking* drugs, which have little effect when the patient is supine but prevent reflex vasoconstriction in the upright position. Ganglionic blocking agents interfere with parasympathetic as well as sympathetic function, and this results in such side effects as impairment of visual accommodation, paralytic ileus, retention of urine, and failure of erection and ejaculation. Because of these problems, ganglionic blocking agents are now usually reserved for the rapid lowering of arterial pressure by parenteral administration of the short-acting agent *trimethaphan* in patients with severe hypertension.

Various drugs act at *postganglionic adrenergic nerve endings*. The *rauwolfia alkaloids* such as reserpine are the oldest members of the group; their long-term effect results from their ability to inhibit the storage of norepinephrine within the vesicles in adrenergic nerve endings, thus leading to depletion of catecholamine stores. The frequent side effects including depression, nasal congestion, diarrhea, impairment of sexual function, and increased gastric secretion have limited the use of these drugs. Reserpine is contraindicated in patients with current or past depression. *Guanethidine* and its shorter-acting analogue guanadrel block the release of norepinephrine from adrenergic nerve endings. They usually reduce cardiac output and lower systolic more than diastolic blood pressure. They also produce a greater postural effect than the other drugs that act at the nerve endings, and orthostatic hypotension is a frequent side effect particularly if other factors promoting vasodilation are present, e.g., heat, exercise, alcohol ingestion. However, centrally mediated side effects (sedation, depression) are infrequently observed since these drugs are poorly soluble in lipids and, therefore, do not readily enter the central nervous system.

The last group of drugs affecting the adrenergic system are those which block the *peripheral adrenergic receptors*, alpha, beta, or both (see also Chap. 67). *Phentolamine* and *phenoxybenzamine* block the action of norepinephrine at *alpha*-adrenergic receptor sites. While the above two compounds block both presynaptic (alpha$_2$) and postsynaptic (alpha$_1$) alpha receptors, the former action accounts for the tolerance which develops, while *prazosin* is more effective because it selectively blocks only *postsynaptic alpha* receptors, i.e., alpha$_1$ receptors. Thus, presynaptic alpha activity remains, suppressing norepinephrine release, and tolerance only infrequently occurs. Accordingly, prazosin produces less tachycardia but more postural

TABLE 196-6   Drugs used in treatment of hypertension—listed according to site of action

Site of action	Drug	Dosage	Indications	Contraindications	Frequent or peculiar side effects
DIURETICS					
Renal tubule	Thiazides: e.g., hydrochlorothiazide	Depends on specific drug Oral: 25 mg daily or twice daily	Mild hypertension, as adjunct in treatment of moderate to severe hypertension	Diabetes mellitus, hyperuricemia, primary aldosteronism	Potassium depletion, hyperglycemia, hyperuricemia, hypercholesterolemia, dermatitis, purpura, depression, hypercalcemia
	Loop acting: e.g., furosemide	Oral: 40–80 mg 2 or 3 times a day	Mild hypertension, as adjunct in severe or malignant hypertension particularly with renal failure	Hyperuricemia, primary aldosteronism	Potassium depletion, hyperuricemia, hyperglycemia, hypocalcemia, blood dyscrasias, rash, nausea, vomiting, diarrhea
	Potassium-sparing: Spironolactone	Oral: 25 mg 2 to 4 times daily	Hypertension due to hypermineralocorticoidism, adjunct to thiazide therapy	Renal failure	Hyperkalemia, diarrhea, gynecomastia, menstrual irregularities
	Triamterene	Oral: 50–100 mg 1 or 2 times daily	Hypertension due to hypermineralocorticoidism, adjunct to thiazide therapy	Renal failure	Hyperkalemia, nausea, vomiting, leg cramps, nephrolithiasis, GI disturbances
	Amiloride	Oral: 5–10 mg daily			
ANTIADRENERGIC AGENTS					
Central	Clonidine	Oral: 0.05–0.6 mg twice daily	Mild to moderate hypertension, renal disease with hypertension		Postural hypotension, drowsiness, dry mouth, rebound hypertension after abrupt withdrawal, insomnia
	Guanabenz	Oral: 4–16 mg twice daily			
	Guanfacine	Oral: 1–3 mg daily			
	Methyldopa (also acts by blocking sympathetic nerves)	Oral: 250–1000 mg twice daily IV: 250–1000 mg every 4–6 h (tolerance may develop)	Mild to moderate hypertension (oral), malignant hypertension (IV)	Pheochromocytoma, active hepatic disease (IV), during MAO inhibitor administration	Postural hypotension, sedation, fatigue, diarrhea, impaired ejaculation, fever, gynecomastia, lactation, positive Coombs tests (occasionally associated with hemolysis), chronic hepatitis, acute ulcerative colitis, lupuslike syndrome
Autonomic ganglia	Trimethaphan	IV: 1–6 mg/min	Severe or malignant hypertension	Severe coronary artery disease, cerebrovascular insufficiency, diabetes mellitus (on hypoglycemic therapy), glaucoma, prostatism	Postural hypotension, visual symptoms, dry mouth, constipation, urinary retention, impotence
Nerve endings	Rauwolfia alkaloids: Reserpine	Oral: 0.05–0.25 mg daily	Mild to moderate hypertension in young patient	Pheochromocytoma, peptic ulcer, depression, during MAO inhibitor administration	Depression, nightmares, nasal congestion, dyspepsia, diarrhea, impotence
	Guanethidine	Oral: 10–150 mg daily	Moderate to severe hypertension	Pheochromocytoma, severe coronary artery disease, cerebrovascular insufficiency, during MAO inhibitor administration	Postural hypotension, bradycardia, dry mouth, diarrhea, impaired ejaculation, fluid retention, asthma
	Guanadrel	Oral 5–75 mg twice daily			
Alpha receptors	Phentolamine	IV: 1–5 mg	Suspected or proved pheochromocytoma	Severe coronary artery disease	Tachycardia weakness, dizziness, flushing
	Phenoxybenzamine	Oral: 10–50 mg once or twice daily (tolerance may develop)	Proven pheochromocytoma		Postural hypotension, tachycardia, miosis, nasal congestion, dry mouth
	Prazosin	Oral: 1–10 mg twice daily	Mild to moderate hypertension	Use with caution in the elderly	Sudden syncope, headache, sedation dizziness, tachycardia anticholinergic effect, fluid retention
	Terazosin	Oral: 1–20 mg daily			

(continued)

hypotension than direct-acting vasodilators, e.g., hydralazine, and rarely can produce substantial hypotension following the first dose.

A variety of effective *beta-adrenergic receptor blocking agents* are available which block sympathetic effects on the heart and should be most effective in reducing cardiac output and in lowering arterial pressure when there is increased cardiac sympathetic nerve activity. In addition, they block the adrenergic nerve-mediated release of renin

from the renal juxtaglomerular cells, and this action may be an important component of their blood pressure–lowering action. Beta-adrenergic blockers are particularly useful when employed in conjunction with vascular smooth-muscle relaxants, which tend to evoke a reflex increase in myocardial contractility, and with diuretics, the administration of which often results in an elevation of circulating renin activity. In practice, beta blockers appear to be effective even

TABLE 196-6   Drugs used in treatment of hypertension—listed according to site of action *(continued)*

Site of action	Drug	Dosage	Indications	Contraindications	Frequent or peculiar side effects
ANTIADRENERGIC AGENTS *(continued)*					
Beta receptors	Propranolol	Oral: 10–120 mg 2 to 4 times daily	Mild to moderate hypertension (especially with evidence for hyperdynamic circulation), adjunct to hydralazine therapy	Congestive heart failure, asthma, diabetes mellitus (on hypoglycemic therapy), during MAO inhibitor administration, COPD, sick sinus syndrome, 2d or 3d degree heart block	Dizziness, depression, bronchospasm, nausea, vomiting, diarrhea, constipation, heart failure, fatigue, Raynaud's phenomenon, hallucinations, hypertriglyceridemia, hypercholesterolemia, psoriasis; sudden withdrawal may precipitate angina or myocardial injury in patients with heart disease
	Metoprolol	Oral: 25–150 mg twice daily			
	Nadolol	Oral: 20–120 mg daily			
	Atenolol	Oral 25–100 mg daily			
	Timolol	Oral: 5–15 mg twice daily			
	Pindolol	Oral: 5–30 mg twice daily			Less resting bradycardia than other beta blockers
	Acebutolol	Oral: 200–600 mg twice daily			
	Labetalol	Oral: 100–600 mg twice daily IV: 2 mg/min			
VASODILATORS					
Vascular smooth muscle	Hydralazine	Oral: 10–75 mg 4 times daily IV or IM: 10–50 mg every 6 h (tolerance may develop)	As adjunct in treatment of moderate to severe hypertension (oral), malignant hypertension (IV or IM), renal disease with hypertension	Lupus erythematosus, severe coronary artery disease	Headache, tachycardia, angina pectoris, anorexia, nausea, vomiting, diarrhea, lupus-like syndrome, rash, fluid retention
	Minoxidil	Oral 2.5–40 mg twice daily	Severe hypertension	Severe coronary artery disease	Tachycardia, aggravates angina, marked fluid retention, hair growth on face and body, coarsening of facial features, possible pericardial effusions
	Diazoxide	IV: 1–3 mg/kg up to 150 mg rapidly	Severe or malignant hypertension	Diabetes mellitus, hyperuricemia, congestive heart failure	Hyperglycemia, hyperuricemia, sodium retention
	Nitroprusside	IV:0.5–8 (μg/kg)/min	Malignant hypertension		Apprehension, weakness, diaphoresis, nausea, vomiting, muscle twitching
ANGIOTENSIN-CONVERTING ENZYME INHIBITORS					
Converting enzyme	Captopril	Oral: 12.5–75 mg twice daily	Mild to severe hypertension, renal artery stenosis	Renal failure (reduction of dose), bilateral renal artery stenosis, pregnancy	Leukopenia, pancytopenia, hypotension, cough, angioedema, urticarial rash, fever, loss of taste, acute renal failure in bilateral renal artery stenosis
	Enalapril	Oral: 2.5–40 mg daily			Same as captopril, but little evidence for leukopenia, but increased frequency of cough and angioedema
	Enalaprilat	IV: 0.625–1.25 mg over 5 minutes every 6–8 hrs			
	Lysinopril	Oral: 5–40 mg daily			
CALCIUM CHANNEL ANTAGONISTS					
Vascular smooth muscle	Nifedipine	Oral: 10–30 mg 4 times daily	Mild to moderate hypertension	Heart failure, 2d or 3d degree heart block	Tachycardia, flushing, gastrointestinal disturbances, hyperkalemia, edema, headache
	Diltiazem	Oral: 30–90 mg 4 times daily			Same as nifedipine, except no tachycardia, but can cause heart block, constipation, and liver dysfunction
	Verapamil	Oral: 30–120 mg 4 times daily or as SR form 120–480 mg daily			

when there is no evidence of increased sympathetic tone with about one-half or more of all hypertensive patients showing a fall in pressure. However, these agents can precipitate congestive heart failure and asthma in susceptible individuals and must be used with caution in diabetics receiving hypoglycemic therapy because they inhibit the usual sympathetic responses to hypoglycemia. Cardioselective beta-blocking agents (so-called beta$_1$ blockers) have been developed (metoprolol, atenolol) which may be superior to nonselective beta blockers such as propranolol and timolol in patients with bronchospasm. Nadolol, a nonselective beta blocker, unlike other drugs of this class is excreted unchanged in the urine and has a half-life of 14 to 20 h. Therefore, only one dose a day is required. Atenolol also usually only needs to be given once a day. Pindolol and acebutolol are nonselective beta blockers with partial agonist activity and, therefore, produce less bradycardia. Labetalol exerts both alpha- and beta-adrenergic blocking actions. Thus, it lowers arterial pressure by the same complex actions as do beta blockers, but also directly by reducing systemic vascular resistance. Usually it has a more rapid onset of action but produces more postural symptoms and chronic sexual dysfunction than the other beta blockers.

Vasodilators   *Hydralazine* is the most versatile of the drugs that cause direct relaxation of vascular smooth muscle; it is effective both orally and parenterally, acting mainly on arterial resistance, rather than on venous capacitance vessels, as evidenced by lack of postural changes. Unfortunately, the effect of hydralazine on peripheral resistance is partly negated by reflex increases in sympathetic discharge that raise heart rate and cardiac output. This limits the usefulness of hydralazine, especially in patients with severe coronary artery disease. However, the efficacy of hydralazine can be increased if it is given in conjunction with beta blockers or drugs such as methyldopa or clonidine, all of which block reflex sympathetic stimulation of the heart. A serious side effect of doses of hydralazine exceeding 300 mg per day has been the production of a lupus erythematosus-like syndrome.

Minoxidil is even more potent but unfortunately produces significant hirsutism and fluid retention and, therefore, is mainly limited to patients with severe hypertension and renal insufficiency.

Diazoxide, a thiazide derivative, is restricted in its application to acute situations. It is not a diuretic; in fact, it causes sodium retention. However, like other thiazides, it reduces carbohydrate tolerance. It must be given rapidly intravenously to guarantee effect. It begins to act immediately to lower blood pressure, and its effects may last for several hours. *Nitroprusside* given intravenously also acts as a direct vasodilator, with onset and offset of actions that are almost immediate. These latter two drugs are useful only for the treatment of hypertensive emergencies (Table 196-7).

Angiotensin-converting enzyme (ACE) inhibitors   Drugs from several of the categories discussed above have been shown to possess an additional action resulting in inhibition of renin secretion. These include clonidine, reserpine, methyldopa, and beta blockers. A second group of drugs in this class are those which inhibit the enzyme converting angiotensin I into angiotensin II, e.g., captopril, enalapril, and lysinopril. These agents are useful because they not only inhibit the generation of a potent vasoconstrictor (angiotensin II) but also may retard the degradation of a potent vasodilator (bradykinin), alter prostaglandin production (most notably with captopril), and can modify the activity of the adrenergic nervous system. They are especially useful in renal or renovascular hypertension, as well as in accelerated and malignant hypertension. They are also as effective in mild, uncomplicated hypertension as beta blockers and thiazides—probably with fewer side effects, particularly those that adversely affect the patient's quality of life.

These drugs should be used with caution when the renin system is activated, e.g., with severe heart failure, prior diuretic therapy, or substantial salt restriction, in order to avoid profound hypotension. Usually diuretics are stopped 2 to 3 days before starting an ACE inhibitor and added back later if needed.

Calcium channel antagonists   These drugs (diltiazem, nifedipine, and verapamil) modify the entry of calcium into cells by blocking the slow or voltage-dependent calcium channels, resulting in vasodilatation and in the case of nifedipine, usually reflex tachycardia. Diltiazem and verapamil both can slow atrioventricular conduction—a feature not observed with nifedipine. While calcium channel antagonists are also useful in angina pectoris (see Chap. 189), because of their negative inotropic actions they should be used with caution in hypertensive patients with heart failure.

APPROACH TO DRUG THERAPY (Fig. 196-1)   The aim of drug therapy is to use the agents just described, alone or in combination, to return arterial pressure to normal levels with minimal side effects. Ideally, one would choose a therapeutic program which specifically corrects the underlying defect resulting in the elevated blood pressure, e.g., spironolactone for patients with primary aldosteronism. As our knowledge of the mechanisms underlying the hypertension in individual patients increases, more specific drug programs will become available. This presumably will result in normalization of blood pressure with fewer side effects. In the absence of that information an empiric approach is used, which takes into consideration efficacy, safety, impact on the quality of life, and ease of administration. When used in combination, drugs are chosen for their different sites of action. However, except for those patients with severe hypertension (average diastolic blood pressure greater than 130 mmHg) in whom intensive therapy with several agents simultaneously usually is required, most patients should *initially* be treated with a single agent. Since many effective antihypertensive agents are available, a number of useful therapeutic regimens have been developed, with the ideal program still unclear. Initial therapy with a diuretic or beta blocker has been the usual first approach. However, the Joint National Committee on Detection, Evaluation, and Treatment of Hypertension has recently added ACE inhibitors and calcium channel antagonists as first-line therapy, thus replacing the old stepped-care approach.

TABLE 196-7   Therapeutic agents used to treat malignant hypertension

| Drug | Route | Time course of action | | | Oral preparation available |
		Onset	Peak	Duration	
IMMEDIATE ONSET					
Diazoxide	IV bolus	1–3 min	2–4 min	4–12 h	No
Nitroprusside	Continuous IV	<1 min	1–2 min	2–5 min	No
Trimethaphan	Continuous IV	<1 min	1–2 min	2–5 min	No
DELAYED ONSET					
Enalaprilat	IV	10–15 min	3–4 h	6–24 h	Yes
Hydralazine	IV, IM	10–20 min	20–40 min	4–12 h	Yes
Labetalol	IV	5 min	20–30 min	3–6 h	Yes
Methyldopa	IV	1–3 h	3–5 h	2–12 h	Yes
Nifedipine	SL	5–15 min	30–60 min	3–6 h	Yes
Reserpine	IM	2–3 h	3–4 h	6–24 h	Yes

Continue
Therapy ← Controlled ← Low-dose ACE Inhibitor,
Calcium Entry Blocker, or
Beta Blocker

↓ Uncontrolled

Continue
Therapy ← Controlled ← Double Dose

↓ Uncontrolled

Reduce Dose
of Initial
Drug ← Controlled ← Add Low-dose Thiazide

↓ Uncontrolled

Continue
Therapy ← Controlled ← Full-dose Initial Drug
and Low-dose Thiazide

↓ Uncontrolled

Sequential Withdrawal
of Beta Blocker or
Calcium
Antagonist, ← Controlled ← 1. Assess Compliance; Search
for Secondary Causes
Then Thiazide
as Long as Pressure
Is Controlled
2. Add Converting Enzyme Inhibitor
If Not Initially Used

↓ Uncontrolled

1. Add Another Antiadrenergic
Agent (e.g., Clonidine), Peripheral
Vasodilator (e.g., Hydralazine),
or Calcium Antagonist
(If Not Initially Used),
or Combinations Thereof
2. When Controlled, Sequential
Withdrawal of Drugs Initially Used,
as Long as Pressure is Controlled

FIGURE 196-1 Schematic approach to the treatment of the patient with hypertension in whom a specific form of therapy is unavailable or unknown.

The physician is, therefore, required to choose from four classes of agents for initial therapy with little evidence that one is more effective than another. Because of their reduced side effects, some have suggested that an ACE inhibitor or calcium channel blocker be used first, with a slight preference for ACE inhibitors because of their longer duration of action and potentially less severe adverse effects. We agree with this suggestion. The reason for choosing one drug over the others is empiric although, in general, older individuals and blacks may be particularly responsive to diuretics while younger individuals and whites respond well to beta blockers, ACE inhibitors, and calcium channel antagonists.

The schema outlined in Fig. 196-1 takes into account the presently available data on effectiveness, adverse reactions, compliance, impact on quality of life, and economic impact (including cost, usage of health care resources, quality and quantity of work performance) in deciding when to use a given agent. This approach is applicable to all patients in whom an indication for a specific form of therapy is lacking. Because of its lower cost, low-dose thiazide therapy, e.g., 25 mg of hydrochlorothiazide (or its equivalent) daily, often has been the first choice. However, three major concerns with widespread thiazide usage have arisen: relatively poor compliance rates (approximately 80 percent) probably reflecting an adverse effect on the patient's quality of life; adverse metabolic effects (hypokalemia, hypomagnesemia, hyperglycemia, and possibly hypercholesterol-

emia); and potentially an increased frequency of cardiac arrhythmias including sudden death, probably secondary to the electrolyte disturbances. These concerns coupled with the eight- to tenfold increase in cost associated with the frequent need for potassium supplementation or a potassium-sparing diuretic have caused some to suggest that thiazides should play a more restricted role in initial antihypertensive therapy, limited to those individuals who are volume expanded. Thus, ACE inhibitors, beta blockers, and calcium channel antagonists are probably the preferred first line therapy for hypertension, with beta blockers being particularly useful in patients with a hyperactive hemodynamic state, e.g., hypertension with an elevated heart rate.

Under any circumstance, the agent should be started at a low dose, e.g., 25 mg of atenolol, 25 mg of captopril, 5 mg of enalapril, or 120 mg of diltiazem (or their equivalents) in divided doses as needed (Table 196-6). If arterial pressure is lowered to less than 140/90 with any of these agents, no further therapy is indicated (Fig. 196-1). If it is not, the next step is to double the dose of the primary agent. If still not controlled, then 25 mg of hydrochlorothiazide (or its equivalent) daily should be added. Thiazides potentiate the action of ACE inhibitors and probably of beta blockers and at least are additive to the antihypertensive effect of calcium channel antagonists. Combining diuretics with ACE inhibitors is particularly appealing since the adverse metabolic effects of the thiazide, in part, will be ameliorated by the ACE inhibitor. This is not true for beta blockers or calcium antagonists. Indeed, beta blockers and thiazides may actually potentiate each other's adverse effects insofar as electrolytes (hypokalemia) and metabolic actions (hypercholesterolemia) are concerned.

If therapy with two drugs does not achieve blood pressure control, the primary agent should be increased to full dose, e.g., 100 mg of captopril or atenolol, 20 mg of enalapril, or 360 mg of diltiazem. While larger doses than these can be used, it is probably advisable to switch to another medication rather than increase the dose further. Occasionally, increasing the thiazide to the equivalent of 50 mg of hydrochlorothiazide daily may bring about control of the hypertension; however, thiazide doses higher than this are seldom, if ever, warranted since they almost invariably produce significant side effects. If the blood pressure is still not controlled, then a detailed search for a secondary cause of hypertension as outlined above is indicated. If none is found, then a dietary assessment often will reveal a high sodium intake. With reduction in salt intake to 5 g per day or less, blood pressure often is controlled. If the blood pressure is still not controlled, then the primary agent should be switched, maintaining the thiazide. Caution should be used if an ACE inhibitor was not the original agent, since administration of such an agent to a patient who already is taking a diuretic may lead to profound hypotension. If none of the changes produce better control of arterial pressure, then the combination of a calcium channel antagonist and an ACE inhibitor or triple therapy usually with a diuretic, ACE inhibitor, and hydralazine may be effective.

If the blood pressure is controlled, then there should be stepwise reduction in the dose and/or withdrawal of some of the agents in order to determine the minimal therapeutic program that will maintain the blood pressure at 140/90 mmHg or less.

Fewer than 5 percent of patients will still be hypertensive at this point. In them, one first should consider the reasons for therapeutic failure as shown in Table 196-8. If none can be identified, then one of the other agents such as a vasodilator listed in Table 196-6 (e.g., hydralazine) or an antiadrenergic agent (e.g., prazosin or clonidine) should be added. If blood pressure is controlled, previous drugs are sequentially withdrawn in order to determine the minimal therapeutic program that maintains a normal blood pressure.

While the recommendations outlined above are satisfactory for a large majority of patients, it is important to use a flexible approach since individual patients may respond differently to individual drugs and drug combinations. For those patients requiring multiple drugs, once the appropriate combination has been found, the use of a single formulation with the appropriate combination of drugs may simplify

TABLE 196-8　Reasons for poor therapeutic response in patients with hypertension

1 Inadequate patient compliance
2 Volume expansion
　a Excessive sodium intake
　b Secondary to nondiuretic antihypertensive agent
3 Excessive weight gain
4 Inadequate doses
5 Drug antagonism
　a Cold remedies
　b Sympathomimetics
　c Oral contraceptives (estrogens)
　d Adrenal steroids
6 Secondary forms of hypertension

the regimen and thereby increase compliance. Every effort should be made to reduce the number of times each day the patients must interrupt his or her schedule for the medication. Pharmacologic treatment of essential hypertension is usually lifelong, and since most patients are asymptomatic, compliance with a complex regimen may be a serious problem, particularly if the therapeutic regimen has a negative impact on the quality of the patient's life.

Special considerations　Four groups of patients with hypertension require special consideration because of associated conditions.

RENAL DISEASE　Reduction of arterial pressure in hypertensive patients with impaired renal function is often accompanied initially by an increase in serum creatinine. This change does not represent further structural renal damage and should not deter continuation of therapy, since achievement of blood pressure control may eventually reduce the value toward normal. However, if serum creatinine increases in patients treated with a converting enzyme inhibitor, care needs to be exercised since these patients may have bilateral renal artery disease. Their renal function will continue to deteriorate as long as the converting enzyme inhibitor is given. Thus, converting enzyme inhibitors should be used cautiously in patients with impaired renal function and renal function should be assessed frequently (every 4 to 5 days) for the first 3 weeks. While converting enzyme inhibitors are contraindicated in patients with bilateral renal artery stenosis, these are the drugs of choice in patients with unilateral renal artery stenosis and a normally functioning contralateral kidney and perhaps in patients with chronic renal failure.

CORONARY ARTERY DISEASE　In these patients who may also be taking cardiac glycosides, thiazides should be used judiciously and a reduction in serum potassium levels should be looked for and if found, should be corrected rapidly. Beta blockers should be withdrawn carefully, if at all, in these patients. Finally, calcium channel antagonists and converting enzyme inhibitors may be particularly useful in these patients since they minimize a number of potential adverse reactions accompanying other therapeutic agents, particularly nonspecific vasodilators.

DIABETES MELLITUS　The diabetic patient with hypertension is particularly challenging since many of the agents used to lower blood pressure can affect glucose metabolism adversely. Converting enzyme inhibitors may be particularly useful in these individuals. They have no known adverse effects on glucose or lipid metabolism and may actually minimize the development of diabetic nephropathy by reducing renal vascular resistance and renal perfusion pressure—the primary factor underlying renal deterioration in these patients.

PREGNANCY　The patient who is pregnant and hypertensive or who develops hypertension during pregnancy (pregnancy-induced hypertension, preeclampsia, eclampsia) is particularly difficult to treat. Because it is uncertain that autoregulation of uterine blood flow occurs, lowering blood pressure in the pregnant hypertensive may result in reduced placental and fetal perfusion. Thus, a conservative approach to lowering blood pressure is usually indicated. In the second and third trimesters, antihypertensives often are not indicated unless the diastolic pressure exceeds 95 mmHg. In general, severe salt restriction and/or diuretics are not given because of the associated

increase in fetal wastage. Beta blockers need to be used cautiously for similar reasons. Methyldopa and hydralazine are the most frequent antihypertensives used since they have no known adverse effects on the fetus. Little is known about the safety of other antihypertensives in pregnancy except that nitroprusside and converting enzyme inhibitors may cause adverse effects on the fetus and should be avoided.

Probably fewer than one-third of hypertensive patients in the United States are being treated effectively. Only a small number of these failures is related to drug unresponsiveness. The majority is related to (1) failure to detect hypertension, (2) failure to institute effective treatment of the asymptomatic hypertensive subject, and (3) failure of the asymptomatic hypertensive subject to adhere to therapy. In order to improve this deficiency, patients must be educated to continue treatment once an effective regimen has been identified. Side effects and inconveniences of treatment must be minimized or counteracted in order to obtain the patient's continued cooperation.

MALIGNANT HYPERTENSION

In addition to marked blood pressure elevation in association with papilledema and retinal hemorrhages and exudates, the full-blown picture of malignant hypertension may include manifestations of hypertensive encephalopathy, such as severe headache, vomiting, visual disturbances (including transient blindness), transient paralyses, convulsions, stupor, and coma. These have been attributed to spasm of cerebral vessels and to cerebral edema. In some patients who have died, multiple small thrombi have been found in the cerebral vessels. Cardiac decompensation and rapidly declining renal function are other critical features of malignant hypertension. Oliguria may, in fact, be the presenting feature. The vascular lesion characteristic of malignant hypertension is fibrinoid necrosis of the walls of small arteries and arterioles, and this can be reversed by effective antihypertensive therapy.

The pathogenesis of malignant hypertension is unknown. However, at least two independent processes, dilatation of cerebral arteries and generalized arteriolar fibrinoid necrosis, contribute to the associated signs and symptoms. The cerebral arteries dilate because the normal autoregulation of cerebral blood flow decompensates secondary to the markedly elevated arterial pressure. As a result, cerebral blood flow is excessive, producing the encephalopathy associated with malignant hypertension. Many patients also show evidence of a microangiopathic hemolytic anemia; this secondary phenomenon could contribute to the deterioration of renal function. Most patients also have elevated levels of peripheral plasma renin activity and increased aldosterone production, and these may be involved in causing vascular damage.

About 1 percent of hypertensive patients develop the malignant phase, which occurs in the course of both essential and secondary hypertension. Rarely it is the first recognized manifestation of the blood pressure problem. The average age at diagnosis is 40, and men are more often affected than women. Prior to the availability of effective therapy, life expectancy after diagnosis of malignant hypertension was less than 2 years, with most deaths being due to renal failure, cerebral hemorrhage, or congestive heart failure. With the advent of effective antihypertensive therapy, at least half of the patients survive for more than 5 years.

Malignant hypertension is a medical emergency and requires immediate therapy. The initial aim of therapy should be to reduce diastolic pressure by one-third, but not below 95 mmHg. The drugs available for treatment of malignant hypertension can be divided into two groups on the basis of time of onset of action (Table 196-7). Those in the first group act within a few minutes but are not satisfactory for long-term management. If the patient is having convulsions, if arterial pressure must be reduced rapidly, then one from the immediate-acting group should be used. *Diazoxide* is the easiest to administer, for no individual titration of dosage is required. It primarily effects arteriolar and not venous tone. A dose of 300 mg is given rapidly intravenously, and the antihypertensive effect is noted in 1 to 3 min. The same dose can be repeated when the pressure begins to rise, usually after several hours. In an occasional patient, pressure may drop below normal levels after diazoxide administration. Because of this, some physicians use a modified program, giving 150 mg rather than 300 mg initially, followed by a second 150-mg dose in 5 min if the blood pressure response has been minimal. It should not be used in patients in whom aortic dissection or myocardial infarction is suspected. Because it can increase the force of myocardial contraction, often a beta blocker is given concomitantly. The other two agents in this group require continuous infusion and close monitoring. *Nitroprusside* is given by continuous intravenous infusion at a dose of 0.5 to 8.0 (μg/kg)/min. It is probably the agent of choice in this condition. It has the advantage over the ganglionic blockers of not being associated with the development of tachyphylaxis and can be utilized for days with few side effects. The dosage must be controlled with an infusion pump. *Trimethaphan*, a ganglionic blocker, is given at a rate of 1 to 15 mg/min. The patient should be in the sitting position, and the pressure should be monitored closely, preferably in an intensive care unit. Monitoring may be more complex than with nitroprusside, but trimethaphan may be better therapy in acute aortic dissection. An intravenous form of one ACE inhibitor, *enalaprilat*, has also proven effective in preliminary studies. Finally, intravenous *labetalol* may be particularly useful in patients with a myocardial infarct or angina since it prevents an increase in heart rate. However, it may be ineffective in patients previously treated with beta blockers and is contraindicated in patients with heart failure, asthma, bradycardia, or heart block.

Patients given any of these agents should also receive other medications effective for long-term control. Those in the second group in Table 196-7 require 30 min or more to obtain full effect but have the advantage of being satisfactory for subsequent oral administration and for long-term management of the patient's hypertension. If such a delay in attainment of full effect is acceptable, intravenous *methyldopa* is an effective drug with which to begin therapy if symptoms of encephalopathy are absent. A dose of 500 mg in 100 to 200 mL 5% dextrose in water is given intravenously over 30 min; if the effect is inadequate in 2 to 4 h, a second dose of 500 to 1000 mg is given. Additional intravenous doses may then be given every 6 h until the pressure is stabilized. Intravenous *hydralazine* is effective in many patients within 10 min; an effective protocol involves giving 10-mg doses intravenously every 10 to 15 min until the desired effect has been obtained or until a total of 50 mg has been administered. The total required for response may then be repeated intramuscularly or intravenously every 6 h. Hydralazine should be used with caution in patients with significant coronary artery disease and should be avoided in patients evidencing myocardial ischemia or aortic dissection. Sublingual *nifedipine* recently has been reported to be useful in some cases, although it may produce tachycardia and success has not been uniform.

Furosemide is an important adjunct to the therapy just discussed. Given either orally or intravenously, it serves to maintain sodium diuresis in the face of a falling arterial pressure and thus will speed recovery from encephalopathy and congestive heart failure as well as maintain sensitivity to the primary antihypertensive drug. Digitalis (Chap. 182) also is indicated if there is evidence of cardiac decompensation.

In patients with malignant hypertension in whom the existence of pheochromocytoma is suspected, urine should be collected for measurement of the products of catecholamine metabolism, and drugs which might release additional catecholamines, such as methyldopa, reserpine, and guanethidine, must be avoided. The parenteral drug of choice in these patients is phentolamine, administered with care to avoid a precipitous reduction in arterial pressure.

There is hope even for patients who fail to respond sufficiently to any of the forms of therapy and who show progressive deterioration in renal function. In some, a period of peritoneal dialysis or hemodialysis to deplete extracellular fluid has resulted in better blood pressure control and eventual improvement in renal function. In other patients with refractory hypertension and renal failure who do not respond to volume depletion or hypotensive therapy, including minoxidil, particularly those with marked elevation of plasma renin activity, bilateral nephrectomy has resulted in amelioration of hypertension; subsequently these patients have been maintained on chronic dialysis or have received renal homografts. However, bilateral nephrectomy should be avoided where possible since (1) the loss of renal erythropoietin will contribute to the associated anemia, (2) vitamin D metabolism may be adversely affected, and (3) all residual renal function will be lost.

REFERENCES

AMERY A et al: Mortality and morbidity results for the European working party on high blood pressure in the elderly trial. Lancet 1:1349, 1985

BERGLUND G et al: Prevalence of primary and secondary hypertension: Studies in a random population sample. Br Med J 2:554, 1976

BLAUSTEIN MP: Role of natriuretic factor in essential hypertension: An hypothesis. Ann Intern Med 98:785, 1983

BOUDOULAS H et al: Left ventricular mass and systolic performance in chronic systemic hypertension. Am J Cardiol 57:232, 1986

COOPE J, WARRENDER TS: Randomized trial of treatment of hypertension in elderly patients in primary care. Br Med J 293:1145, 1986

CURB JD et al: Antihypertensive drug side effects in the hypertension detection and follow-up program. Hypertension 11:51, 1988

DANNENBERG AL et al: Incidence of hypertension in the Framingham study. Am J Public Health 78:676, 1988

GOTTDIENER JS et al: Left ventricular hypertrophy in men with normal blood pressure: Relation to exaggerated blood pressure response to exercise. Ann Intern Med 112(3):161, 1990

HOLME I et al: Treatment of mild hypertension with diuretics. The importance of ECG abnormalities in the Oslo study and in MRFIT. JAMA 251:1298, 1984

JOINT NATIONAL COMMITTEE ON DETECTION, EVALUATION AND TREATMENT OF HIGH BLOOD PRESSURE: 1988 report. Arch Intern Med 148:1023, 1988

KAPLAN NM: Systemic hypertension: Therapy, in *Heart Disease*, 3d ed, E Braunwald (ed). Philadelphia, Saunders, 1988, p 862

KOTCHEN TA et al: Effect of chloride on renin and blood pressure responses to sodium chloride. Ann Intern Med 98:817, 1983

LITTENBERG B et al: Screening for hypertension. Ann Intern Med 112(3):192, 1990

MCCARRON DA: Calcium in the pathogenesis and therapy of human hypertension. Am J Med 78:27, 1985

OBERMAN A et al: Pharmacologic and nutritional treatment of mild hypertension: Changes in cardiovascular risk status. Ann Intern Med 112(2):89, 1990

SUBCOMMITTEE OF NON-PHARMACOLOGIC THERAPY OF THE JOINT NATIONAL COMMITTEE ON DETECTION, EVALUATION AND TREATMENT OF HIGH BLOOD PRESSURE: Non-pharmacological approaches to the control of high blood pressure: Final report. Hypertension 8:444, 1986

WEINBERGER MH et al: Definitions and characteristics of sodium sensitivity and blood pressure resistance. Hypertension 8:127, 1986

WILLIAMS GH: Quality of life and its impact on hypertensive patients. Am J Med 82:98–105, 1987

————: Converting enzyme inhibitors in the treatment of hypertension. New Engl J Med 319:1517–1525, 1989

————, HOLLENBERG NK: Pathophysiology of essential hypertension, in *Cardiology*, WW Parmley, J Chatterjee (eds). Philadelphia, Lippincott, 1987

WOODS JW: Oral contraceptives and hypertension. Hypertension 11:1, 1988

WORKING GROUP ON HYPERTENSION IN DIABETES: Statement on hypertension in diabetes mellitus: Final report. Arch Intern Med 147:830, 1987

WORKING GROUP ON HYPERTENSION IN THE ELDERLY, NATIONAL HIGH BLOOD PRESSURE EDUCATION PROGRAM: Statement on hypertension in the elderly. JAMA 256:70, 1986

197 DISEASES OF THE AORTA

VICTOR J. DZAU / MARK A. CREAGER

The aorta is the conduit through which the blood ejected from the left ventricle is delivered to the systemic arterial bed. In adults, its diameter is approximately 3 cm at the origin and 2.5 cm in the descending portion in the thorax. The aortic wall consists of a thin intima, a thick media, and an adventitia of smooth muscle cells, collagen, and elastic tissue. In addition to its conduit function, the viscoelastic and compliant properties of the aorta also subserve a

TABLE 197-1   Diseases of the aorta: classification and etiology

Aneurysm
  Atherosclerosis
  Cystic medial necrosis
  Syphilitic infection
  Mycotic infection
  Rheumatic aortitis
  Trauma
Aortic dissection
  Cystic medial necrosis
  Systemic hypertension
  Atherosclerosis
Aortic occlusion
  Atherosclerosis
  Thromboembolism
Aortitis
  Syphilitic aortitis
  Rheumatic aortitis
  Takayasu's arteritis and aortic arch syndromes
  Giant cell arteritis

buffering function. The aorta is distended during systole to enable a portion of the stroke volume to be stored and it recoils during diastole so that blood continues to flow to the periphery during diastole. Because of its continuous exposure to high pulsatile pressure and shear stress, the aorta is particularly prone to injury and disease resulting from mechanical trauma (Table 197-1).

ANEURYSMS

An aneurysm is defined as a pathologic dilatation of a segment of a blood vessel. A *true* aneurysm involves all three layers of the vessel wall and is distinguished from a *pseudoaneurysm* in which the intimal and medial layers are disrupted and the dilatation is lined by adventitia only and sometimes by perivascular clot. Aneurysms may also be classified according to their gross appearance. A *fusiform* aneurysm affects the entire circumference of a segment of the vessel resulting in a diffusely dilated lesion. In contrast, a *saccular* aneurysm involves only a portion of the circumference, resulting in an outpouching of the vessel wall.

The most common cause of aortic aneurysm is atherosclerosis. Other etiologies include cystic medial necrosis, syphilis or other bacterial infections, rheumatic aortitis, and trauma. Aortic aneurysms are also classified according to location, i.e., abdominal vs. thoracic. Those in the abdominal aorta are almost always due to atherosclerosis. Aneurysms of the ascending thoracic aorta may be caused by cystic medial necrosis, atherosclerosis, syphilis, bacterial infections, or rheumatoid arthritis. Aneurysms of the descending thoracic aorta are usually contiguous with infradiaphragmatic aneurysms and, as with the latter, are usually due to atherosclerosis.

Aortic aneurysms usually do not produce symptoms. However, as they expand they may become painful. Compression or erosion of adjacent tissue by aneurysms may also cause symptoms. The formation of mural thrombi within the aneurysm may predispose to peripheral embolization. Occasionally an aneurysm may leak, leading to extravasation of blood into the vessel wall and the periadventitial area and causing acute pain and local tenderness. This is usually a harbinger of rupture and represents a medical emergency. More often, acute rupture occurs without any prior warning and is always life-threatening.

ATHEROSCLEROTIC ANEURYSMS Seventy-five percent of atherosclerotic aneurysms are located in the distal abdominal aorta below the renal arteries. An abdominal aneurysm commonly produces no symptoms and is usually detected on routine examination as a palpable, pulsatile, and nontender mass or is an incidental finding on abdominal x-ray or ultrasound performed for other reasons. Some patients may complain of strong pulsations in the abdomen, others of low back pain. Rarely leakage of the aneurysm may result in severe pain and tenderness. Acute pain and hypotension occur with rupture of the aneurysm, requiring emergency operation.

Abdominal radiography may demonstrate the calcified outline of the aneurysm. The *diagnosis* is generally confirmed by ultrasound which can delineate the transverse and longitudinal dimensions of the aneurysm; mural thrombus may be detected. Ultrasound is useful for serial documentation of aneurysm size. Both computed tomography (CT) with contrast and magnetic resonance imaging (MRI) have been introduced for the detection and follow-up of aortic aneurysm. These relatively expensive techniques provide higher resolution than ultrasound and have replaced the latter in some centers. However, abdominal aortography remains the gold standard in evaluating patients with aneurysm for surgery. This technique is useful in documenting the extent of the aneurysm, especially its upper and lower limits, and the extent of associated atherosclerotic vascular disease. However, aortography may underestimate the diameter of an aneurysm since the presence of mural clots may reduce the luminal size.

The location and the severity of associated atherosclerotic vascular disease influence the overall prognosis. Frequently it is the severity of coronary artery and cerebral vascular diseases that determines the long-term prognosis in these patients. The most common cause of death of patients with aneurysms is rupture. The risk of rupture increases with the size of the aneurysm. The mortality of patients with abdominal aneurysms exceeding 6 cm in diameter is approximately 50 percent in 2 years, while in those with lesions between 4 and 6 cm, it is 25 percent.

Operative excision with replacement with a graft is indicated for patients with abdominal aneurysms greater than 6 cm in diameter, as well as in symptomatic patients and in those with rapidly expanding aneurysms irrespective of the absolute diameter. Except for patients with exceptionally high operative risk, operation is also usually recommended in patients with aneurysm diameter 5 to 6 cm. Serial noninvasive follow-up of smaller (<5 cm) aneurysms is an alternative to immediate surgery. In surgical candidates, a careful preoperative cardiac and general medical evaluation followed by appropriate therapy of complicating conditions are essential. With careful preoperative cardiac evaluation and postoperative care, which includes Swan-Ganz catheterization, operative mortality approximates 1 to 5 percent. Following acute rupture, the mortality of emergency operation is generally greater than 50 percent.

CYSTIC MEDIAL NECROSIS This is due to the degeneration of collagen and elastic fibers in the media of the aorta, which are replaced by multiple clefts of mucoid material. Cystic medial necrosis characteristically affects the proximal aorta, results in circumferential weakness and dilatation, and leads to the development of fusiform aneurysms involving the ascending aorta and the sinuses of Valsalva. This condition is particularly prevalent in patients with the Marfan syndrome (Chap. 333), but is also seen in pregnancy and hypertension and sometimes as an isolated condition in patients without any other condition. The clinical manifestations include expanding aneurysms, rupture, and aortic regurgitation. Operative repair is indicated to prevent rupture. Control of arterial pressure is an important part of the long-term management of this condition.

MYCOTIC ANEURYSM This rare condition develops as the result of staphylococcal, streptococcal, or salmonella infections of the aorta, usually at an atherosclerotic plaque. Blood cultures are usually positive and reveal the nature of the infecting agent. The aneurysms are usually saccular. Treatment requires parenteral antibiotics and surgical excision.

TRAUMA Aortic rupture may develop following penetrating injury or blunt trauma. Deceleration injury may tear the aortic isthmus at the site of insertion of the ligamentum arteriosum.

Other causes of aortic aneurysm, such as syphilitic infection and rheumatic vasculitis, are discussed later under aortitis.

AORTIC DISSECTION

Aortic dissection is caused by a circumferential or transverse tear of the intima, usually at the right lateral wall of the ascending aorta where the hydraulic shear is high. It has been speculated that the

FIGURE 197-1 Classification of aortic dissections. Stanford classification: Top panels illustrate type A dissections that involve the ascending aorta independent of site of tear and distal extension; type B dissections (bottom panels) involve transverse and/or descending aorta without involvement of the ascending aorta. DeBakey classification: Type I dissection involves ascending to descending aorta (top left); type II dissection is limited to ascending or transverse aorta, without descending aorta (top center + top right); type III dissection involves descending aorta only (bottom left). *(From DC Miller, in RM Doroghazi, EE Slater (eds). Aortic Dissection. New York, McGraw-Hill, 1983, with permission.)*

initiating event is a medial hemorrhage that disrupts the intima. Another common site is the descending thoracic aorta just below the ligamentum arteriosum. The pulsatile aortic flow then dissects along the elastic lamellar plates of the aorta and creates a false lumen. The dissection usually propagates distally down the descending aorta and into its major branches, but it may also propagate proximally. In some cases a secondary distal intimal disruption occurs, resulting in the reentry of blood from the false to the true lumen.

DeBakey and coworkers classified aortic dissections as: type I, in which an intimal tear occurs in the ascending aorta and the dissection extends into the descending aorta; type II, in which the dissection is limited to the ascending aorta; and type III, in which the intimal tear is located in the descending area with distal propagation of the dissection (Figure 197-1). Another classification (Stanford) is that of type A, in which the dissection involves the ascending aorta, and type B, in which it is limited to the descending aorta.

The factors that predispose to aortic dissection include systemic hypertension, a coexisting condition in 70 percent of patients, and cystic medial necrosis. Aortic dissection is the major cause of morbidity and mortality in patients with the Marfan syndrome. The incidence is increased in patients with congenital aortic valve anomalies (e.g., bicuspid valve), coarctation of the aorta, and, in otherwise normal women, during the third trimester of pregnancy.

Clinical manifestations Acute aortic dissection presents with the sudden onset of pain (Chap. 16), which is often described as very severe and tearing, associated with diaphoresis. The pain may be localized to the front or back of the chest, often the interscapular region, and typically migrates with the propagation of the dissection. Other symptoms include syncope, dyspnea, and weakness. Physical findings may include hypertension or hypotension, loss of pulses, aortic regurgitation, pulmonary edema, and neurologic findings due to carotid artery obstruction (hemiplegia, hemianesthesia) or spinal cord ischemia (paraplegia). These clinical manifestations reflect complications resulting from the dissection occluding the major arteries. Bowel ischemia, hematuria, and myocardial ischemia have all been observed. Furthermore, clinical manifestations may result from the compression of adjacent structures (such as superior cervical ganglia, superior vena cava, bronchus, esophagus) by the expanding dissecting aneurysm and include Horner's syndrome, superior vena caval syndrome, hoarseness, dysphagia, and airway compromise. Hemopericardium and cardiac tamponade may complicate a type A lesion with retrograde dissection.

In dissections involving the ascending aorta, the chest x-ray often reveals a widened superior mediastinum. A pleural effusion (usually left-sided) may also be present. The electrocardiogram usually excludes acute myocardial ischemia unless a coronary artery is involved in the dissection. In dissections of the descending thoracic aorta, a widened mediastinum may also be observed on chest x-ray. In addition, the descending aorta may appear to be wider than the ascending portion. The diagnosis of aortic dissection is established by aortography which should be performed as soon as the diagnosis is seriously considered. It is important to identify the entry point, the intimal flap, and the false and true lumina and to establish the extent of dissection into the major arteries. Magnetic resonance imaging (Chap. 178) and CT with contrast have also been shown to be highly accurate in detecting aortic dissection. Two-dimensional echocardiography has also been helpful in some cases.

Treatment Medical therapy should be initiated as soon as the diagnosis is considered. The patient should be closely monitored. Unless hypotension is present, therapy should be aimed at reducing cardiac contractility and systemic arterial pressure, and thereby shear stress. Immediate parenteral administration of a beta-adrenergic blocker, unless contraindicated, should be accompanied by nitroprusside infusion. Recently, labetalol (p. 1011) has also been introduced as a parenteral agent in the acute therapy of dissection. If there is a contraindication to the use of beta blockers, parenteral reserpine may be substituted. Direct vasodilators, such as diazoxide and hydralazine, are contraindicated as these agents can increase hydraulic shear and may propagate dissection.

For ascending aortic dissection (type A), surgical correction, which includes reconstruction of the aortic wall, is the preferred treatment. Emergency operation carries a high operative mortality (up to 45 percent). Thus, if possible, stabilization of the patient's clinical status with semielective surgery 14 days or later is preferred. However, with continued pain and evidence of continuing dissection, despite medical therapy, emergency surgery is indicated. The major causes of perioperative mortality and morbidity include myocardial infarction, paraplegia, renal failure, tamponade, hemorrhage, and sepsis. In general, medical therapy is the preferred treatment for uncomplicated and stable distal dissection (type B) unless there is clinical evidence of propagation, compromise of major branches of the aorta, or continued pain.

Overall, the prognosis of aortic dissection is poor. Long-term therapy should include control of blood pressure and cardiac output with the use of beta-adrenergic blockers and other agents.

AORTIC OCCLUSION

CHRONIC ARTERIOSCLEROTIC OCCLUSIVE DISEASE
Chronic occlusive disease usually involves the distal abdominal aorta below the renal arteries. The disease extends frequently to the common iliac arteries but may spare the external iliac arteries. Because of the slowly progressive nature of the atherosclerotic process, the natural history of aortic occlusion is usually chronic and insidious. Claudication characteristically involves the lower back, buttocks, and thighs and may be associated with impotence in males (Leriche syndrome). The severity of the symptoms depends on the adequacy of collaterals.

With sufficient collateral blood flow a complete occlusion of the abdominal aorta may occur in some cases without the development of ischemic symptoms. The physical findings include absence of femoral and other distal pulses bilaterally and the detection of an audible bruit over the abdomen (usually at or below the umbilicus) and the common femoral arteries. Atrophic skin, loss of hair, and coolness of lower extremities are usually observed. In advanced ischemia, rubor on dependency and pallor on elevation can be seen.

The diagnosis is usually established by the physical examination and noninvasive testing, including leg pressure measurements, Doppler velocity analysis, and pulse volume recordings. The anatomy may be defined by abdominal aortography prior to revascularization. Operative treatment is indicated in patients with debilitating symptoms and/or with the development of leg ischemia.

ACUTE OCCLUSION The complication of acute occlusion occurring in the distal abdominal aorta represents a medical emergency as it threatens the viability of the lower extremities. It usually occurs as the result of an occlusive embolus that almost always originates from the heart. Rarely acute occlusion may occur as the result of in situ thrombosis in a preexisting severely narrowed segment of the aorta, or plaque rupture and hemorrhage into such an area.

The clinical picture is one of acute ischemia of the lower extremities. Severe rest pain, coolness, and pallor of the lower extremities and the absence of distal pulses bilaterally are the usual manifestations. Diagnosis should be established rapidly by aortography. Emergency thrombectomy or revascularization is indicated.

AORTITIS

Aortitis frequently affects the ascending aorta and may result in aneurysmal dilatation and aortic regurgitation; it occasionally obstructs branch vessels of the aorta.

SYPHILITIC AORTITIS This late manifestation of luetic infection (Chap. 128) usually affects the proximal ascending aorta, particularly the aortic root, resulting in aortic dilatation and aneurysm formation. Syphilitic aortitis may occasionally involve the aortic arch or the descending aorta. The aneurysms may be saccular or fusiform and are usually asymptomatic, but compression of and erosion into adjacent structures may result in symptoms; rupture may also occur.

The initial lesion is an obliterative endarteritis of the vasa vasorum, especially in the adventitia. This is an inflammatory response to the invasion of the adventitia by the spirochetes. Destruction of the aortic media occurs as the spirochetes spread into this layer, usually via the lymphatics of the vasa vasorum. Destruction of collagen and elastic tissues leads to dilatation of the aorta, scar formation, and calcification. These changes account for the characteristic radiographic appearance of a calcified ascending aortic aneurysm.

The disease typically presents as an incidental radiographic finding 15 to 30 years after initial infection. Symptoms may result from aortic regurgitation, from narrowing of coronary ostia due to syphilitic aortitis, from compression of adjacent structures (e.g., esophagus), or from rupture. Diagnosis is established by a positive serologic test, i.e., VDRL or fluorescent treponemal antibody (see Chap. 128). Treatment includes penicillin and surgical excision and repair.

RHEUMATIC AORTITIS Rheumatoid arthritis (Chap. 270), ankylosing spondylitis (Chap. 274), psoriatic arthritis (Chap. 283), Reiter's syndrome (Chap. 274), Behçet's syndrome (Chap. 275), relapsing polychondritis, and inflammatory bowel disorders may all be associated with aortitis involving the ascending aorta. The inflammatory lesions usually involve the ascending aorta, and may extend to the sinuses of Valsalva, the mitral valve leaflets, and adjacent myocardium. The clinical manifestations are aneurysm, aortic regurgitation, and involvement of the cardiac conduction system.

TAKAYASU'S ARTERITIS AND OTHER AORTIC ARCH SYNDROMES Inflammatory diseases of the aortic arch resulting in obstruction of the aorta and its major arteries characterize this major group of diseases. Takayasu's arteritis is also termed *pulseless disease*

because of the frequent occlusion of the large arteries of the aorta. It may also involve the descending thoracic and abdominal aorta and occlude large branches such as the renal arteries. The pathology is a panarteritis with marked intimal hyperplasia, medial and adventitial thickening, and, in the chronic form, fibrosis. The disease is most prevalent in young females of Asian descent. During the acute stage, fever, malaise, weight loss, and other systemic symptoms may be evident. An elevation of the erythrocyte sedimentation rate is common. The chronic stages of the disease present with symptoms related to large artery occlusion, including upper extremity claudication, cerebral ischemia, syncope, etc. The chronic disease is intermittently active. Since the process is progressive and there is no definitive therapy, the prognosis is usually poor. Glucocorticoids and immunosuppressive agents have been reported to be effective in some patients during the acute phase. Occasionally anticoagulation prevents thrombosis and complete occlusion of a large artery. Surgical bypass of a critically stenotic artery may be necessary.

GIANT CELL ARTERITIS (See Chap. 276) This affects primarily large- and medium-sized arteries. The pathology is that of focal granulomatous lesions involving the entire arterial wall. It may be associated with polymyalgia rheumatica (Chap. 27). Obstruction of medium-sized arteries (e.g., temporal and ophthalmic arteries) and of major branches of the aorta and the development of aortitis and aortic regurgitation are some of the complications of the disease. High-dose corticosteroid therapy may be effective when given early.

REFERENCES

BULKLEY BH, ROBERTS WC: Ankylosing spondylitis and aortic regurgitation. Circulation 48:1014, 1973

DeSanctis RW et al: Medical progress: Aortic dissection. N Engl J Med 317:1060, 1987

Estes JE Jr: Abdominal aortic aneurysm: A study of one hundred and two cases. Circulation 11:258, 1950

Larsen EW, Edwards WD: Risk factors for aortic dissection: A necropsy study of 161 cases. Am J Cardiol 53:849, 1984

Szilagyi DE et al: Contribution of abdominal aortic aneurysmectomy to prolongation of life. Ann Surg 164:678, 1966

Whittemore AD et al: Aortic aneurysm repair: Reduced operative mortality associated with maintenance of optimal cardiac performance. Ann Surg 192:414, 1980

198 VASCULAR DISEASES OF THE EXTREMITIES

MARK A. CREAGER / VICTOR J. DZAU

ARTERIAL DISORDERS

ATHEROSCLEROSIS OF THE EXTREMITIES Atherosclerosis (arteriosclerosis obliterans) is the leading cause of occlusive arterial disease of the extremities in patients over 40 years old; the highest incidence occurs in the sixth and seventh decades of life. As in patients with atherosclerosis of the coronary and cerebral vasculature, there is an increased prevalence of peripheral atherosclerotic occlusive disease in individuals with hypertension, hypercholesterolemia, diabetes mellitus, and in cigarette smokers. Atherosclerosis of the extremities is seen most frequently in elderly males.

Pathology (See Chap. 195) Segmental lesions causing stenosis or occlusion are usually localized in large- and medium-sized vessels. The pathology of the lesions includes atherosclerotic plaques with calcium deposition, thinning of the media, patchy destruction of muscle and elastic fibers, fragmentation of the internal elastic lamina, and thrombi comprised of platelets and fibrin. The primary sites of involvement are the abdominal aorta and iliac arteries in 30 percent of symptomatic patients, the femoral and popliteal arteries in 80 to 90 percent of patients, and the more distal vessels (including the tibial and peroneal arteries) in 40 to 50 percent of patients. Atherosclerotic lesions occur preferentially at arterial branch points, sites of increased turbulence, altered shear stress, and intimal injury. Involvement of the distal vasculature is most common in elderly individuals and patients with diabetes mellitus.

Clinical evaluation The most common symptom is intermittent claudication, which is defined as a pain, ache, cramp, numbness, or sense of fatigue in the muscles; it occurs during exercise but is relieved with rest. The site of claudication is distal to the location of the occlusive lesion. For example, buttock, hip, and thigh discomfort occur in patients with aortoiliac disease (Leriche syndrome), whereas calf claudication develops in patients with femoral-popliteal disease. Symptoms are far more common in the lower than in the upper extremities because of the higher incidence of obstructive lesions. In patients with severe arterial occlusive disease, rest pain may develop. Patients will complain of pain or a feeling of cold or numbness in the foot and toes. Frequently these symptoms occur at night when the legs are in a ''neutral'' position and improve when the legs are in a dependent position. With severe ischemia, rest pain may be persistent.

Important physical findings of chronic arterial insufficiency include decreased or absent pulses distal to the obstruction, the presence of bruits over the narrowed artery, and muscle atrophy. With more severe disease, hair loss, thickened nails, smooth and shiny skin, reduced skin temperature, and pallor or cyanosis are frequent physical signs. In addition, ulcers or gangrene may occur. Elevation of the legs and repeated flexing of the calf muscles produces pallor of the soles of the feet whereas rubor, secondary to reactive hyperemia, may develop when the legs are dependent. The duration of time for rubor to develop or for the veins in the foot to fill when the patient's legs are transferred from an elevated to a dependent position is related to the severity of the ischemia and the presence of collateral vessels. Patients with severe ischemia may develop peripheral edema, because frequently they keep their legs in a dependent position. Ischemic neuritis can result in numbness and hyporeflexia.

Noninvasive testing The history and physical examination are usually sufficient to establish the diagnosis of peripheral arterial occlusive disease. Objective assessment of the severity of disease is obtained by noninvasive techniques. These include digital pulse volume recordings, Doppler blood flow velocity, wave-form analysis, segmental pressure measurements, stress testing (usually using a treadmill), and tests of reactive hyperemia. In the presence of significant arterial occlusive disease, the volume displacement in the leg is decreased with each pulse and the Doppler velocity contour becomes progressively flatter.

Arterial pressure can be recorded noninvasively along the legs by serial placement of sphygmomanometric cuffs and use of a Doppler device to auscultate or record blood flow. Normally, blood pressures in the legs and arms are similar. Indeed, ankle pressures may be slightly higher than arm pressures due to pulse wave reflection. In the presence of hemodynamically significant stenoses the arterial pressure in the leg is decreased. Thus, if one were to obtain a ratio of the ankle and brachial artery pressures, it would be >1.0 in normal individuals and <1.0 in patients with arterial occlusive disease. A ratio of <0.5 is consistent with severe ischemia.

Treadmill testing allows the physician to assess functional limitations objectively. Decline of the ankle-brachial systolic pressure ratio immediately after exercise may provide further support for the diagnosis of arterial occlusive disease in patients with equivocal symptoms and findings on examination. Exercise testing also allows simultaneous evaluation for the presence of coronary artery disease.

Angiography should not be used for routine diagnostic testing, but is performed prior to potential revascularization. It is useful for defining the anatomy to assist operative planning and is also indicated if nonsurgical interventions are being considered, such as percutaneous transluminal angioplasty or thrombolysis.

Prognosis The natural history of patients with peripheral arterial occlusive disease is influenced primarily by the extent of coexistent coronary artery and cerebral vascular disease. Studies utilizing coronary angiography have estimated that approximately one-half of patients with symptomatic peripheral arterial occlusive disease also have significant coronary artery disease. Life table analysis has indicated that patients with claudication have a 72 percent 5-year and a 50 percent 10-year survival rate. The majority of deaths are either sudden or secondary to myocardial infarction. The likelihood of symptomatic progression of peripheral arterial occlusive disease appears less than the chance of succumbing to coronary artery disease. Approximately 70 percent of nondiabetic patients who present with mild to moderate claudication remain symptomatically stable. Improvement may occur in 10 to 15 percent of these patients; deterioration is likely to occur in the remainder with approximately 5 percent of the group ultimately undergoing amputation. Prognosis is worse in those patients who continue to smoke cigarettes or have diabetes mellitus.

Treatment Therapeutic options include supportive measures, pharmacologic treatment, nonoperative interventions, and surgery. Supportive measures include meticulous care of the feet. The feet should be kept clean and excessive drying should be prevented with the use of moisturizing creams. Well-fitting and protective shoes are advised to reduce trauma. Sandals and shoes made of synthetic materials that do not ''breathe'' should be avoided. Elastic support hose should be avoided since these reduce blood flow to the skin. In patients with ischemia at rest, shock blocks under the head of the bed together with a canopy over the feet may improve perfusion pressure and ameliorate some of the rest pain.

Treatment of associated factors that contribute to the development of atherosclerosis should be initiated. The importance of discontinuing cigarette smoking cannot be overemphasized. The physician must assume a major role in this lifestyle modification. It is important to control blood pressure in hypertensive patients but to avoid hypotensive levels. Treatment of hypercholesterolemia is advocated, although reduction in cholesterol levels has not been shown unequivocally to reverse peripheral atherosclerotic lesions. However, it has been shown to prevent or to slow progression of the disease. Patients with claudication should also be encouraged to exercise regularly and to progressively increasing levels. Daily walking to the onset of claudication may improve muscle efficiency and prolong walking distance. Patients should be advised not to walk ''through their claudication,'' but to rest until the symptoms resolve before resuming ambulation. Other forms of exercise, such as bicycle riding and swimming, provide overall cardiovascular and psychologic benefit and often are tolerated better than walking.

PHARMACOLOGIC MANAGEMENT This form of treatment of patients with peripheral arterial occlusive disease has not been as successful as the medical treatment of coronary artery disease (Chap. 190). In particular, vasodilators, as a class, have not proven to be beneficial. During exercise, peripheral vasodilation occurs normally distal to sites of significant arterial stenoses. As a result, perfusion pressure falls, often to levels less than that generated in the interstitial tissue by the exercising muscle. Unless vasodilators are able to improve collateral blood flow, it is unlikely that they would improve perfusion pressure and thereby increase blood supply to the exercising muscle. Drugs such as alpha-adrenergic blocking agents, calcium channel antagonists, papaverine, and other vasodilators have not been shown to be effective in patients with occlusive arterial disease. Pentoxifylline, a substituted xanthine derivative, is reported to decrease blood viscosity and to increase red cell flexibility, thereby increasing blood flow to the microcirculation and enhancing tissue oxygenation. One placebo-controlled study demonstrated that pentoxifylline increased duration of exercise on the treadmill in patients with claudication. Additional studies are required to confirm this drug's efficacy in patients with peripheral arterial occlusive disease.

Platelet inhibitors, particularly aspirin, have been reported to decrease progression of atherosclerosis in patients with peripheral arterial occlusive disease. However, no study with aspirin has demonstrated any improvement in exercise capacity. The anticoagulants heparin and warfarin have not been shown to be effective in patients with *chronic* arterial occlusive disease but may be useful in *acute* arterial obstruction secondary to thrombosis or systemic embolism. Similarly, thrombolytic intervention using drugs such as streptokinase, urokinase, or recombinant tissue plasminogen activator may have a role in the treatment of acute arterial occlusion, but is not effective in patients with chronic arterial occlusion secondary to atherosclerosis.

REVASCULARIZATION   Such procedures, including nonoperative as well as operative interventions, are usually reserved for patients with progressive, severe or disabling symptoms, ischemia at rest, and for those individuals who must be symptom-free because of their occupation. Angiography should be performed principally in those patients who are being considered for a revascularization procedure. Nonoperative interventions include percutaneous transluminal angioplasty (PTA) and the experimental procedures of laser angioplasty and atherectomy. PTA of the iliac artery is associated with a higher success rate than PTA of the femoral and popliteal arteries. Approximately 90 percent of iliac PTAs are initially successful and the 3-year patency rate is in excess of 70 percent. The initial success rate for femoral-popliteal PTA is approximately 80 percent with a 50 percent 3-year patency rate.

Several operative procedures are available for treating patients with aortoiliac and femoral-popliteal artery disease. The preferred operative procedure depends on the location and extent of the obstruction(s) and the general medical condition of the patient. Operative procedures for aortoiliac disease include aorto-bifemoral bypass, axillo-femoral bypass, femoral-femoral bypass, and aortoiliac endarterectomy. The most commonly utilized procedure is the aorto-bifemoral bypass, using knitted dacron grafts. Operative mortality ranges from 2 to 5 percent, mostly due to ischemic heart disease. Immediate graft patency approaches 99 percent and 5- and 10-year graft patency in survivors is in excess of 90 and 80 percent respectively. Operative complications include myocardial infarct and stroke, infection of the graft, peripheral embolization, and sexual dysfunction from interruption of autonomic nerves in the pelvis.

Operative therapy for femoral-popliteal artery disease includes in situ and reverse autogenous saphenous vein bypass grafts, polytetrafluoroethylene (PTFE) or other synthetic materials, and thromboendarterectomy. Operative mortality ranges from 1 to 3 percent. Long-term patency rate is dependent on the type of graft utilized, the location of the distal anastomosis, and the patency of run-off vessels beyond the anastomosis. Patency rates of femoral-popliteal saphenous vein bypass grafts at 1 year approach 90 percent and at 5 years 70 to 80 percent. In contrast, 5-year patency rates of infrapopliteal PTFE grafts are less than 30 percent. Lumbar sympathectomy alone or as an adjunct to aortofemoral reconstruction has fallen into disfavor. While this procedure may increase blood flow to the skin, it does not increase blood flow to muscle. There is no good clinical evidence that lumbar sympathectomy increases graft patency or improves limb survival.

THROMBOANGIITIS OBLITERANS   Thromboangiitis obliterans (Buerger's disease) is an inflammatory occlusive vascular disorder involving small- and medium-sized arteries and veins in the distal upper and lower extremities. Cerebral, visceral, and coronary vessels may also be affected. This disorder develops most frequently in men under the age of 40. The prevalence is high in Asians and individuals whose lineage originates in eastern Europe. While the cause of thromboangiitis obliterans is not known, there is a definite relationship to cigarette smoking and an increased incidence of HLA-B5 and -A9 antigens in patients with this disorder.

In the initial stages of thromboangiitis obliterans, polymorphonuclear leukocytes infiltrate the wall of the small- and medium-sized arteries and veins. The internal elastic lamina is preserved and thrombus may develop in the vascular lumen. As the disease progresses, mononuclear cells, fibroblasts, and giant cells replace the neutrophils. Later stages are characterized by perivascular fibrosis and recanalization.

The clinical features of thromboangiitis obliterans often include a triad of claudication of the affected extremity, Raynaud's phenomenon (see below), and migratory superficial vein thrombophlebitis. Claudication is usually confined to the lower calves and feet or forearms and hands because this disorder primarily affects distal vessels. In the presence of severe digital ischemia, trophic nail changes, ulcerations and gangrene may develop at the tips of the fingers. The physical examination shows normal brachial and popliteal pulses, but reduced or absent radial, ulnar, and/or tibial pulses. Arteriography is helpful in making the diagnosis. Smooth tapering segmental lesions in the distal vessels are characteristic, as are collateral vessels at sites of vascular occlusion. Proximal atherosclerotic disease is usually absent. The diagnosis can be confirmed by excisional biopsy and pathologic examination of an involved vessel.

There is no specific treatment except abstention from tobacco. The prognosis is worse in individuals who continue to smoke but results are discouraging even in those who do stop smoking. Arterial bypass of the larger vessels may be used in selected instances, as well as local debridement, depending on symptoms and severity of ischemia. Antibiotics may be useful; anticoagulants and corticosteroids are not helpful. If these measures fail, amputation may be required.

ACUTE ARTERIAL OCCLUSION   This results in the sudden cessation of blood flow to an extremity. The severity of ischemia and the viability of the extremity are dependent upon the location and extent of the occlusion and the presence and subsequent development of collateral blood vessels. There are two principal causes of acute arterial occlusion: embolism and thrombus in situ.

The most common sources of arterial emboli are the heart, aorta, and large arteries. Cardiac disorders that cause thromboembolism include atrial fibrillation, both chronic and paroxysmal, and acute myocardial infarction, ventricular aneurysm, cardiomyopathy, infectious and marantic endocarditis, prosthetic heart valves, and atrial myxoma. Emboli to the distal vessels may also originate from proximal sites of atherosclerosis and aneurysms of the aorta and large vessels. Less frequently, an arterial occlusion may result paradoxically from a venous thrombus that has entered the systemic circulation via a patent foramen ovale or other septal defect. Arterial emboli tend to lodge at the bifurcation of vessels because the caliber of the vessel decreases at these sites; in the lower extremities, emboli lodge most frequently in the femoral artery, followed by the iliac artery, aorta, and popliteal and tibioperoneal arteries.

Acute arterial thrombosis in situ occurs most frequently in atherosclerotic vessels at the site of a stenosis or aneurysm, and in arterial bypass grafts. Trauma to an artery may also result in the formation of an acute arterial thrombus. Arterial occlusion may complicate arterial punctures and placement of catheters. Less frequent causes include the thoracic outlet compression syndrome, causing subclavian artery occlusion, and entrapment of the popliteal artery by abnormal placement of the medial head of the gastrocnemius muscle. Polycythemia and hypercoagulable disorders (Chaps. 289 and 297) are also associated with acute arterial thrombosis.

Clinical features   The symptoms of the acute arterial occlusion depend upon the location, duration, and severity of the obstruction. Often severe pain, paresthesias, numbness, and coldness develop in the involved extremity within 1 hour. Paralysis may occur with severe and persistent ischemia. Physical findings include loss of pulses distal to the occlusion; cyanosis or pallor; mottling; decrease in skin temperature; muscle stiffening; loss of sensation; weakness; and/or absent deep tendon reflexes. If acute arterial occlusion occurs in the presence of an adequate collateral circulation, as is often the case in acute graft occlusion, the symptoms and findings may be less impressive. In this situation, the patient complains about an abrupt decrease in the distance walked before claudication occurs, or of modest pain and paresthesias. Pallor and coolness are evident, but sensory and motor functions are generally preserved. The diagnosis of acute arterial occlusion is usually apparent from the clinical presentation. Arteriography is useful for confirming the diagnosis and demonstrating the location and extent of occlusion.

Treatment Once the diagnosis is made the patient should be anticoagulated with intravenous heparin to prevent propagation of the clot. In cases of severe ischemia of recent onset and particularly when limb viability is jeopardized, immediate intervention to ensure reperfusion is indicated. Surgical thromboembolectomy or arterial bypass procedures are used to restore blood flow to the ischemic extremity promptly, particularly when a large proximal vessel is occluded.

Intraarterial thrombolytic therapy is effective when acute arterial occlusion is caused by a thrombus in an atherosclerotic vessel or arterial bypass graft. Thrombolytic therapy also may be indicated when the patient's overall condition contraindicates surgical intervention or when smaller distal vessels are occluded, thus preventing surgical access. Intraarterial streptokinase is administered as a bolus injection of 25,000 to 250,000 IU followed by a continuous infusion of 5000 to 15,000 IU/h. One approach for administering intraarterial urokinase is to give a bolus of 60,000 to 120,000 IU followed by 240,000 IU/h for 2 h, 120,000 IU for 2 h, and then 60,000 IU/hour. Clinical trials are now in progress to assess the efficacy of intraarterial recombinant tissue plasminogen activator (rtPA). Meticulous observation for hemorrhagic complications is required during intraarterial thrombolytic therapy.

If the limb is not in jeopardy, a more conservative approach that includes observation and administration of anticoagulants may be taken. Anticoagulation prevents recurrent embolism and reduces the likelihood of thrombus propagation. It can be initiated with intravenous heparin and followed by oral warfarin. Recommended dosages are the same as those used in deep vein thrombosis (see p. 1024). Emboli resulting from infectious endocarditis, prosthetic heart valves, or atrial myxoma often require surgical intervention to remove the cause.

ATHEROEMBOLISM Atheroembolism constitutes a subset of acute arterial occlusion. In this condition, multiple small deposits of fibrin, platelet, and cholesterol debris embolize from proximal atherosclerotic lesions or aneurysmal sites. Atheroembolism may occur after intraarterial procedures. Since the emboli tend to lodge in the small vessels of the muscle and skin and may not occlude the large vessels, distal pulses usually remain palpable. Patients complain of acute pain and tenderness at the site of embolization. Digital vascular occlusion may result in ischemia and the "blue toe" syndrome; digital necrosis and gangrene may develop. Localized areas of tenderness, pallor, and livido reticularis (see later) occur at sites of emboli. Skin or muscle biopsy may demonstrate cholesterol crystals.

Ischemia resulting from atheroemboli is notoriously difficult to treat. Usually neither surgical revascularization procedures nor thrombolytic therapy are helpful because of the multiplicity, composition, and distal location of the emboli. Some evidence suggests that platelet inhibitors prevent atheroembolism. Surgical intervention to remove or bypass the atherosclerotic vessel or aneurysm that causes the recurrent atheroemboli may be necessary.

THORACIC OUTLET COMPRESSION SYNDROME This refers to a symptom complex resulting from compression of the neurovascular bundle at the thoracic outlet (artery, vein, or nerves) as it courses through the neck and shoulder. Cervical ribs, abnormalities of the scalenus anticus muscle, the proximity of the clavicle to the first rib, or abnormal insertion of the pectoralis minor muscle may compress the subclavian artery and brachial plexus as these structures pass from the thorax to the arm. Patients may develop shoulder and arm pain, weakness, paresthesias, claudication, Raynaud's phenomenon, and even ischemic tissue loss and gangrene. Examination is often normal unless provocative maneuvers are performed. Occasionally distal pulses are decreased or absent and digital cyanosis and ischemia may be evident. Tenderness may be present in the supraclavicular fossa. Several maneuvers are used to confirm the diagnosis of vascular compression and suggest the location of the abnormality. These include the scalene, costoclavicular, and hyperabduction maneuvers which may cause subclavian bruits and loss of pulses in the

arm. A chest x-ray will indicate the presence of cervical ribs. The electromyogram will be abnormal if the brachial plexus is involved.

Most patients can be managed conservatively. They should be advised to avoid those positions that cause symptoms. Many patients benefit from shoulder girdle exercises. Surgical procedures such as removal of the first rib or resection of the scalenus anticus muscle are necessary occasionally for relief of symptoms or treatment of ischemia.

ARTERIOVENOUS FISTULA These abnormal communications between an artery and a vein, bypassing the capillary bed, may be congenital or acquired. Congenital arteriovenous fistulas are the result of persistent embryonic vessels that fail to differentiate into arteries and veins; these may be associated with birth marks, are located in almost every organ of the body, and frequently occur in the extremities. Acquired arteriovenous fistulas are either created to provide vascular access for hemodialysis or occur as a result of a penetrating injury such as a gunshot or knife wound or as a complication of arterial catheterization or surgical dissection. An infrequent cause of arteriovenous fistula is rupture of an arterial aneurysm into a vein.

The clinical features depend on the location and size of the fistula. Frequently a pulsatile mass is palpable, and a thrill and bruit lasting throughout systole and diastole are present over the fistula. With longstanding fistulas, clinical manifestations of chronic venous insufficiency, including peripheral edema, large tortuous varicose veins, and stasis pigmentation, become apparent because of the high venous pressure. Evidence of ischemia may occur in the distal portion of the extremity. Skin temperature is higher over the arteriovenous fistula. Large arteriovenous fistulas may result in an increased cardiac output with consequent cardiomegaly and high-output heart failure (Chap. 182).

Diagnosis is often evident from the physical examination. Compression of a large arteriovenous fistula may cause reflex slowing of the heart rate (Nicoladoni-Branham sign). Arteriography can confirm the diagnosis and is useful in demonstrating the site and size of the arteriovenous fistula. *Treatment* may involve surgery, radiotherapy, or embolization. Congenital arteriovenous fistulas are often difficult to treat because the communications may often be numerous and extensive and new ones frequently develop after ligation of the most obvious ones. Many of these lesions are best treated conservatively using elastic support hose to reduce the consequences of venous hypertension. Occasionally, embolization with autologous material, such as fat or muscle, or with hemostatic agents, such as gelatin sponges or silicon spheres, are used to obliterate the fistula. Acquired arteriovenous fistulas are usually amenable to surgical treatment that involves division or excision of the fistula. Occasionally this requires autogenous or synthetic grafting to reestablish continuity of the artery and vein.

RAYNAUD'S PHENOMENON Raynaud's phenomenon is characterized by episodic digital ischemia, manifested clinically by the sequential development of digital blanching, cyanosis, and rubor of the fingers or toes following cold exposure and subsequent rewarming. Emotional stress may also precipitate Raynaud's phenomenon. The color changes are usually well demarcated and are confined to the fingers or toes. Typically, one or more digits will appear white when the patient is exposed to a cold environment or touches a cold object. The blanching, or pallor, represents the ischemic phase of the phenomenon and is secondary to vasospasm of digital arteries. During the ischemic phase capillaries and venules dilate, and cyanosis results from the deoxygenated blood that is present in these vessels. Sensation of cold, numbness, or paresthesias of the digits often accompany the phases of pallor or cyanosis.

With rewarming, the digital vasospasm resolves, and blood flow into the dilated arterioles and capillaries increases dramatically. This "reactive hyperemia" imparts a bright red color to the digits. In addition to rubor and warmth, patients often experience a throbbing, painful sensation during the hyperemic phase. Although the triphasic color response is typical of Raynaud's phenomenon, some patients

TABLE 198-1 Classification of Raynaud's phenomena

Primary or idiopathic Raynaud's phenomenon: Raynaud's disease
Secondary Raynaud's phenomenon
  Collagen vascular diseases:
    Scleroderma, systemic lupus erythematosus, rheumatoid arthritis, dermatomyositis, polymyositis
  Arterial occlusive diseases:
    Atherosclerosis of the extremities, thromboangiitis obliterans, acute arterial occlusion, thoracic outlet syndrome
  Pulmonary hypertension
  Neurologic disorders
    Invertebral disc disease, syringomyelia, spinal cord tumors, stroke, poliomyelitis, carpal tunnel syndrome
  Blood dyscrasias
    Cold agglutinins, cryoglobulinemia, cryofibrinogenemia, myeloproliferative disorders, Waldenström's macroglobulinemia
  Trauma
    Vibration injury, hammer hand syndrome, electric shock, cold injury, typing, piano playing
  Drugs
    Ergot derivatives, methysergide, β-adrenergic receptor blockers, bleomycin, vinblastin, cisplatin

may develop only pallor and cyanosis; others may experience only cyanosis.

Pathophysiology Raynaud originally proposed that cold-induced, episodic digital ischemia was secondary to exaggerated reflex sympathetic vasoconstriction. This theory is supported by the fact that adrenergic-blocking drugs as well as sympathectomy decrease the frequency and severity of Raynaud's phenomenon in some patients. An alternative hypothesis is that there is enhanced digital vascular responsiveness to cold or to normal sympathetic stimuli. It is also possible that normal reflex sympathetic vasoconstriction is superimposed on local digital vascular disease, or that there is enhanced adrenergic neuroeffector activity.

Raynaud's phenomenon is broadly separated into two categories: the idiopathic variety termed *Raynaud's disease* and the secondary variety, which is associated with other disease states or known causes of vasospasm (Table 198-1).

Raynaud's disease This appellation is applied when the secondary causes of Raynaud's phenomenon have been excluded. Over 50 percent of patients with Raynaud's phenomenon have Raynaud's disease. Women are affected about five times more often than men and the age of presentation is usually between 20 and 40 years. The fingers are involved more frequently than the toes. Initial episodes may involve only one or two fingertips, but subsequent attacks may involve the entire finger and may include all of the fingers. The toes are affected in 40 percent of patients. Although vasospasm of the toes usually occurs in patients with symptoms in the fingers, it may happen alone. Rarely, the earlobes and the tip of the nose are involved. Raynaud's phenomenon occurs frequently in patients who also have migraine headaches or variant angina. These associations suggest that there may be a common predisposing cause for the vasospasm.

The physical examination is often entirely normal; the radial, ulnar, and pedal pulses are normal. The fingers and toes may be cool between attacks and may perspire excessively. Thickening and tightening of the digital subcutaneous tissue, i.e., *sclerodactyly,* develops in 10 percent of patients. Angiography of the digits for diagnostic purposes is not indicated.

Patients with Raynaud's disease, in general, appear to have the milder forms of Raynaud's phenomenon. Less than 1 percent of these patients lose a part of a digit. After the diagnosis is made the disease spontaneously improves in approximately 15 percent of patients and progresses in about 30 percent.

Secondary causes of Raynaud's phenomenon Raynaud's phenomenon occurs in 80 to 90 percent of patients with systemic sclerosis (scleroderma) and is the presenting symptom in 30 percent (Chap. 271). It may be the only symptom of scleroderma for many years. Abnormalities of the digital vessels may contribute to the development of Raynaud's phenomenon in this disorder. Ischemic fingertip ulcers

may develop and progress to gangrene and autoamputation. About 20 percent of patients with systemic lupus erythematosus (SLE) have Raynaud's phenomenon (Chap. 269). Occasionally, persistent digital ischemia develops and may result in ulcers or gangrene. In most severe cases, the small vessels are occluded by a proliferative endarteritis. Raynaud's phenomenon occurs in about 30 percent of patients with dermatomyositis or polymyositis (Chap. 364). It frequently develops in patients with rheumatoid arthritis and may be related to the intimal proliferation that occurs in the digital arteries.

Atherosclerosis of the extremities is a frequent cause of Raynaud's phenomenon in men over 50 years of age. Thromboangiitis obliterans is an uncommon cause of Raynaud's phenomenon but should be considered in young men, particularly in those who are cigarette smokers. The development of cold-induced pallor in these disorders may be confined to one or two digits of the involved extremity. Occasionally, Raynaud's phenomenon may occur following acute occlusion of large- and medium-sized arteries by a thrombus or embolus. Embolization of atheroembolic debris may cause digital ischemia. The latter often involves one or two digits and should not be confused with Raynaud's phenomenon. In patients with the thoracic outlet syndrome, Raynaud's phenomenon may result from diminished intravascular pressure, stimulation of sympathetic fibers in the brachial plexus, or a combination of both. Raynaud's phenomenon occurs frequently in patients with primary pulmonary hypertension (Chap. 212); this is more than coincidental and may reflect a neurohumoral abnormality that affects both the pulmonary and digital circulations.

A variety of blood dyscrasias may be associated with Raynaud's phenomenon. Cold-induced precipitation of plasma proteins, hyperviscosity, and aggregation of red cells and platelets may occur in patients with cold agglutinins, cryoglobulinemia, or cryofibrinogenemia. Hyperviscosity syndromes that accompany myeloproliferative disorders and Waldenström's macroglobulinemia should also be considered in the initial evaluation of patients with Raynaud's phenomenon.

Raynaud's phenomenon occurs often in patients whose vocations require the use of vibrating hand tools such as chain saws or jackhammers. The frequency of Raynaud's phenomenon also seems to be increased in pianists and typists. Electric shock injury to the hands and frostbite may lead to the later development of Raynaud's phenomena.

Several drugs have been causally implicated in Raynaud's phenomenon. These include ergot preparations, methysergide, beta-adrenergic receptor antagonists, and the chemotherapeutic agents bleomycin, vinblastine, and cisplatin.

Treatment Most patients with Raynaud's phenomenon experience only mild and infrequent episodes. These patients need reassurance and should be instructed to dress warmly and avoid unnecessary cold exposure. In addition to gloves and mittens, patients should protect the trunk, head, and feet with warm clothing in order to prevent cold-induced reflex vasoconstriction. Tobacco use is contraindicated.

Drug treatment should be reserved for the severe cases. Adrenergic blocking agents have been the most frequently prescribed; reserpine, in doses of 0.25 to 0.5 mg orally once a day has been shown to increase nutritional blood flow to the fingers. A single infusion of intraarterial reserpine, 0.5 mg, into the brachial or radial artery has been reported to reduce pain and promote healing of ulcerations. Some but not all patients achieve satisfactory results with long-term reserpine therapy. Moreover, systemic use of the drug is limited by side effects of nasal stuffiness, lethargy, and depression. The postsynaptic alpha$_1$-adrenergic antagonist prazosin has been used with favorable responses. Other sympatholytic agents such as methyldopa, guanethidine, and phenoxybenzamine may be useful in some patients. The calcium channel antagonists, especially nifedipine (10 to 30 mg tid) and diltiazem (30 to 90 mg tid), have also been found to decrease the frequency and severity of Raynaud's phenomena. Occasionally surgical sympathectomy is helpful in patients who are unresponsive to medical therapy, but benefit is often transient.

ACROCYANOSIS In acrocyanosis there is arterial vasoconstriction and secondary dilatation of the capillaries and venules with resulting persistent cyanosis of the hands and, less frequently, the feet. Cyanosis may be intensified by exposure to a cold environment. Women are affected much more frequently than men and the age of onset is usually less than 30 years. Generally patients are asymptomatic but seek medical attention because of the discoloration. Examination reveals normal pulses, peripheral cyanosis, and moist palms. Trophic skin changes and ulcerations do *not* occur. The disorder can be distinguished from Raynaud's phenomenon because it is persistent and not episodic, the discoloration extends proximally from the digits, and blanching does not occur. Ischemia secondary to arterial occlusive disease can usually be excluded by the presence of normal pulses. Central cyanosis and decreased arterial oxygen saturation are not present. Patients should be reassured, and advised to dress warmly and avoid cold exposure. Pharmacologic intervention is not indicated.

LIVEDO RETICULARIS In this condition, localized areas of the extremities develop a mottled or net-like appearance of reddish to blue discoloration. The mottled appearance may be more prominent following cold exposure. The idiopathic form of this disorder occurs equally in men and women and the most common age of onset is in the third decade. Patients with the idiopathic form usually are asymptomatic and seek attention for cosmetic reasons. Livedo reticularis also occurs following atheroembolism (see above). Rarely, skin ulcerations develop. Patients should be reassured and advised to avoid cold environments. No drug treatment is indicated.

PERNIO (CHILBLAINS) Pernio is a vasculitic disorder that is associated with exposure to cold; acute forms have been described. Raised erythematous lesions develop on the lower part of the legs and feet in cold weather. These are associated with a pruritic and burning sensation and they may blister and ulcerate. Pathologic examination demonstrates angiitis characterized by intimal proliferation and perivascular infiltration of mononuclear and polymorphonuclear leukocytes. Giant cells may be present in the subcutaneous tissue. Patients should avoid exposure to cold, and ulcers should be kept clean and protected with sterile dressings. Sympatholytic drugs may be effective in some patients.

ERYTHROMELALGIA (ERYTHERMALGIA) This disorder is characterized by burning pain and erythema of the extremities. The feet are involved more frequently than the hands, and males are affected more frequently than females. Erythromelalgia may occur at any age but is most common in middle age. It may be primary or secondary to disorders such as polycythemia vera and hypertension. Patients complain of burning in the extremities, precipitated by exposure to a warm environment and aggravated by the dependent position. The symptoms are relieved by exposing the affected area to cool air or water or by elevation. Erythromelalgia can be distinguished from ischemia secondary to arterial occlusive disorders and peripheral neuropathy because the peripheral pulses are present and the neurologic examination is normal. There is no specific treatment; aspirin may produce relief. Treatment of associated disorders in secondary erythromelalgia may be helpful.

VENOUS DISORDERS

Veins in the extremities can be broadly classified as either superficial or deep. In the lower extremity, the superficial venous system includes the greater and lesser saphenous veins and their tributaries. The deep veins of the leg accompany the major arteries. Perforating veins connect the superficial and the deep systems at multiple locations. Bicuspid valves are present throughout the venous system to direct the flow of venous blood centrally.

VENOUS THROMBOSIS The presence of thrombus within a superficial or deep vein and the accompanying inflammatory response in the vessel wall is termed venous thrombosis or thrombophlebitis. Initially the thrombus is composed principally of platelets and fibrin. Red cells become interspersed with fibrin and the thrombus tends to propagate in the direction of blood flow. The inflammatory response in the vessel wall may be minimal or characterized by granulocyte infiltration, loss of endothelium, and edema.

The factors that predispose to venous thrombosis were initially described by Virchow in 1856 and include stasis, vascular damage, and hypercoagulability. Accordingly, a variety of clinical situations are associated with an increased risk of venous thrombosis (Table 198-2). Venous thrombosis may occur in more than 50 percent of patients having orthopedic surgical procedures, particularly those involving the hip or knee, and in 10 to 40 percent of patients who undergo abdominal or thoracic operations. The prevalence of venous thrombosis is particularly high in patients with cancer of the pancreas, lungs, genitourinary tract, stomach, and breast. Risk of thrombosis is increased following trauma, such as fractures of the spine, pelvis, femur, and tibia. Immobilization, regardless of the underlying disease, is a major predisposing cause of venous thrombosis. This may account for the relatively high incidence in patients with acute myocardial infarction or congestive heart failure. The incidence of venous thrombosis is increased during pregnancy and in individuals who use estrogens. A variety of clinical disorders that produce systemic hypercoagulability, including antithrombin III, protein C, and protein S deficiencies; systemic lupus erythematosus; myeloproliferative diseases; dysfibrinogenemia; and disseminated intravascular coagulation, may cause venous thrombosis. Venulitis occurring in thromboangiitis obliterans, Behçet's disease, and homocysteinuria also may cause venous thrombosis.

DEEP VENOUS THROMBOSIS The most important consequences of this disorder are pulmonary embolism (Chap. 213) and the syndrome of chronic venous insufficiency. Deep thrombosis of the iliac, femoral, or popliteal veins is suggested by unilateral leg swelling, warmth, and erythema. Tenderness may be present along the course of the involved veins, and a cord may be palpable. There may be increased tissue turgor, distention of superficial veins, and the appearance of prominent venous collaterals. In some patients, deoxygenated hemoglobin in stagnant veins imparts a cyanotic hue to the limb, a condition called *phlegmasia cerulea dolens*. In markedly edematous legs, the interstitial tissue pressure may exceed the capillary perfusion pressure, causing pallor, a condition designated *phlegmasia alba dolens*.

The diagnosis of deep venous thrombosis of the calf is often difficult to make at the bedside. This is because only one of the multiple veins may be involved, allowing adequate venous return through the remaining patent vessels. The most common complaint is calf pain. Examination may reveal posterior calf tenderness, warmth, increased tissue turgor or modest swelling, and rarely, a cord. Increased resistance or pain during dorsiflexion of the foot, *Homan's sign,* is an unreliable diagnostic sign.

Deep venous thrombosis occurs less frequently in the upper extremity than in the lower extremity, but the incidence is increasing

---

TABLE 198-2 Conditions associated with an increased risk for development of venous thrombosis

Surgery
  Orthopedic, thoracic, abdominal, and genitourinary procedures
Neoplasms
  Pancreas, lung, ovary, testes, urinary tract, breast, stomach
Trauma
  Fractures of spine, pelvis, femur, tibia
Immobilization
  Acute myocardial infarction, congestive heart failure, stroke, postoperative convalescence
Pregnancy
Estrogen use (for replacement or contraception)
Hypercoagulable states
  Deficiencies of antithrombin III, protein C, or protein S; circulating lupus anticoagulant; myeloproliferative diseases; dysfibrinogenemia; disseminated intravascular coagulation
Venulitis
  Thromboangiitis obliterans, Behçet's disease, homocysteinuria
Previous deep vein thrombosis

because of the greater utilization of subclavian vein catheters. The clinical features and complications are similar to those described for the leg.

Diagnosis Deep venous thrombosis can be diagnosed by venography. Contrast medium is injected into a superficial vein of the foot and directed to the deep system by the application of tourniquets. The presence of a filling defect or absence of filling of the deep veins is required to make the diagnosis.

A variety of noninvasive tests can also diagnose deep venous thrombosis at less discomfort and cost. Plethysmographic techniques used to measure changes in venous capacitance during physiologic maneuvers include impedance plethysmography (IPG) and phleborheography (PRG). The IPG uses skin electrodes and the PRG uses a series of air-filled cuffs to detect changes in leg volume. Venous obstruction blunts the normal changes in venous capacitance that occur during respiration or following inflation and deflation of a thigh cuff. The predictive value of these tests for detecting occlusive thrombi in proximal veins is approximately 90 percent. However, these tests are much less sensitive in the detection of deep venous thrombosis of the calves. A combination of ultrasonographic techniques, Doppler ultrasonography and B-mode (two-dimensional) imaging, termed duplex ultrasonography, is often useful. The Doppler ultrasound measures the velocity of blood flow in veins. This velocity is normally affected by respiration and by manual compression of the foot or calf. Flow abnormalities occur when deep venous obstruction is present. By imaging the deep veins using B-mode ultrasonography, the presence of thrombus can be detected by direct visualization or by inference when the vein does not collapse with compressive maneuvers. The positive predictive value of this diagnostic test approaches 95 percent for *proximal* deep vein thrombosis.

^{125}I-fibrinogen scanning is occasionally used for the diagnosis of deep venous thrombosis. Since this isotope is actively taken up by propagating venous thrombi, increases in radioactivity detected with a counter imply the presence of a thrombus. Fibrinogen scans detect more than 90 percent of calf vein thrombi but are less specific for proximal venous thrombi. A serious limitation of the technique is that it may take 48 to 72 h after administration of the isotope for a fibrinogen scan to become positive.

Deep vein thrombosis must be differentiated from a variety of disorders that cause unilateral leg pain or swelling, including muscle trauma or hemorrhage, ruptured popliteal cyst, and lymphedema. It may be difficult to distinguish swelling caused by the postphlebitic syndrome from that due to acute recurrent deep venous thrombosis. Leg pain may also result from nerve compression syndromes, arthritis, tendinitis, fractures, and arterial occlusive disorders. A careful history and physical examination can usually determine the cause of these symptoms.

Treatment Prevention of pulmonary embolism is the most important reason for treating patients with deep vein thrombosis, since in the early stages the thrombus may be loose and poorly adherent to the vessel wall. Patients should be placed in bed and the affected extremity should be elevated above the level of the heart until the edema and tenderness subside. Anticoagulants prevent thrombus propagation and allow the endogenous lytic system to operate. Heparin should be administered intravenously as an initial bolus of 5000 to 10,000 IU, followed by a continuous infusion of 1000 IU/h. The rate of the heparin infusion should be adjusted so that the activated partial thromboplastin time (APTT) is approximately twice the control value. Intermittent intravenous and subcutaneous injections of heparin have been used as alternative forms of therapy. In less than 5 percent of patients, heparin therapy may cause thrombocytopenia. Infrequently, these patients develop arterial thrombosis and ischemia. Heparin treatment should be maintained for at least 7 to 10 days. It is important to overlap heparin treatment with oral anticoagulant therapy for at least 4 to 5 days because the full anticoagulant effect of warfarin is delayed. The dose of warfarin should be adjusted to maintain the prothrombin time by 4 to 7 s beyond control values.

The use of anticoagulants for isolated deep vein thrombosis of the calf is controversial because the incidence of pulmonary embolism is very low. However, approximately 20 percent of calf thrombi propagate to the thigh, thereby increasing the risk of pulmonary embolism. Therefore, patients with calf vein thrombosis should either receive anticoagulants or be followed with serial noninvasive tests to determine whether proximal propagation has occurred.

Anticoagulant treatment should be continued for 3 to 12 months for patients with acute proximal deep vein thrombosis to decrease the chance of recurrence. The duration of anticoagulant treatment for patients with calf vein thrombosis should be at least 6 weeks. The duration of treatment is indefinite for patients with *recurrent* deep vein thrombosis and for those in whom associated causes, such as malignancy or hypercoagulability, have not been eliminated. If treatment with anticoagulants is contraindicated because of a bleeding diathesis or risk of hemorrhage, protection from pulmonary embolism can be achieved by mechanically interrupting the flow of blood through the inferior vena cava. Inferior vena cava plication generally has been replaced by percutaneous insertion of a filter.

Thrombolytic drugs such as streptokinase, urokinase, and tissue plasminogen activator also may be used, but there is no evidence that thrombolytic therapy is more effective than anticoagulants in preventing pulmonary embolism. However, early administration of thrombolytic drugs may preserve venous valves and decrease the potential for developing postphlebitic syndrome.

Prophylaxis should be considered in clinical situations where the risk of deep vein thrombosis is high. Low-dose heparin (5000 units 2 h prior to surgery and then 5000 units every 8 or 12 h postoperatively), often supplemented with dihydroergotamine (0.5 mg), warfarin, dextran, and external pneumatic compression are all useful. Low-dose heparin, however, does not reduce the risk of deep vein thrombosis following hip or knee surgery. Instead, warfarin, in doses that increase the prothrombin time to 1.5 to 2 times control values, is effective and can be started 48 to 72 h after surgery. External pneumatic compression devices applied to the legs are used to prevent deep vein thrombosis when even low doses of heparin may cause serious bleeding, such as during neurosurgery or transurethral resection of the prostate.

SUPERFICIAL VEIN THROMBOSIS Thrombosis of the greater or lesser saphenous veins or their tributaries, i.e., superficial vein thrombosis, does not result in pulmonary embolism or chronic venous insufficiency. It is associated with intravenous catheters and infusions, occurs in varicose veins, and may develop in association with deep vein thrombosis. Migrating superficial vein thrombosis is often a marker for a carcinoma and may also occur in patients with vasculitides, such as thromboangiitis obliterans. The clinical features of superficial vein thrombosis are easily distinguishable from those of deep vein thrombosis. Patients complain of pain localized to the site of the thrombus. Examination reveals a reddened, warm, and tender cord extending along a superficial vein. The surrounding area may be red and edematous.

Therapy is primarily supportive. Initially, patients can be placed at bed rest with leg elevation and application of warm compresses. Nonsteroidal anti-inflammatory drugs may provide analgesia, but also may obscure clinical evidence of thrombus propagation. If a thrombosis of the greater saphenous vein develops in the thigh and extends towards the saphenofemoral vein junction, it is reasonable to consider anticoagulant therapy to prevent extension of the thrombus into the deep system and a possible pulmonary embolism.

VARICOSE VEINS These are dilated tortuous superficial veins that result from defective structure and function of the valves of the saphenous veins, from intrinsic weakness of the vein wall, or rarely from arteriovenous fistulas. Varicose veins can be categorized as primary or secondary. Primary varicose veins originate in the superficial system and occur twice as frequently in women as men. Approximately half of patients have a family history of varicose veins. Secondary varicose veins result from deep venous insufficiency and incompetent perforating veins, or from deep venous occlusion causing enlargement of superficial veins that are serving as collaterals.

Patients with venous varicosities are often concerned about the cosmetic appearance of their legs. Symptoms consist of a dull ache or pressure sensation in the legs after prolonged standing; it is relieved with leg elevation. The legs feel heavy and occasionally mild ankle edema develops. Extensive venous varicosities may cause skin ulcerations near the ankle. Superficial venous thrombosis may be a recurring problem and rarely a varicosity ruptures and bleeds. Visual inspection of the legs in the dependent position usually confirms the presence of varicose veins.

Varicose veins can usually be treated with conservative measures. Symptoms often decrease when the legs are elevated periodically, when prolonged standing is avoided, and when elastic support hose are worn. External compression stockings provide a counterbalance to the hydrostatic pressure within the veins. Small symptomatic varicose veins may be treated with sclerotherapy in which a sclerosing solution is injected into the involved varicose vein and a compression bandage is applied. Surgical therapy usually involves extensive ligation and stripping of the greater and lesser saphenous veins and should be reserved for those patients who are very symptomatic, suffer recurrent superficial vein thrombosis, and/or develop skin ulceration. Surgical therapy may be indicated for cosmetic reasons.

CHRONIC VENOUS INSUFFICIENCY This may result from deep vein thrombosis and/or valvular incompetence. Following deep vein thrombosis, the delicate valve leaflets become thickened and contracted so that they are incapable of preventing retrograde flow of blood; the vein becomes rigid and thick-walled. Although most veins recanalize after an episode of thrombosis, the large proximal veins may remain occluded. Secondary incompetence develops in distal valves because high pressures distend the vein and separate the leaflets. Primary deep venous valvular dysfunction also may occur without previous thrombosis. Patients with venous insufficiency often complain of a dull ache in the leg that worsens with prolonged standing and resolves with leg elevation. Examination demonstrates increased leg circumference, edema, and superficial varicose veins. Erythema, dermatitis, and hyperpigmentation develop along the distal aspect of the leg, and skin ulceration may occur near the medial and lateral malleoli. Cellulitis may be a recurring problem.

Patients should be advised to avoid prolonged standing or sitting; frequent leg elevation is helpful. Graduated compression stockings should be worn during the day. These efforts should be intensified if skin ulcers develop. Ulcers should be treated with applications of wet to dry dressings and occasionally dilute topical antibiotic solutions. An Unna paste boot often is effective. Recurrent ulceration and severe edema may be treated by surgical interruption of incompetent communicating veins. Rarely surgical valvuloplasty and bypass of venous occlusions are employed.

LYMPHATIC DISORDERS

Lymphatic capillaries are blind-ended tubes formed by a single layer of endothelial cells. The absent or widely fenestrated basement membrane of lymphatic capillaries allows greater access to interstitial proteins and particles. Lymphatic capillaries merge to form larger vessels which contain smooth muscle and are capable of vasomotion. Small- and medium-sized lymphatic vessels empty into progressively larger channels which drain into the thoracic duct. The lymphatic circulation is involved in the absorption of interstitial fluid and in the response to infection.

LYMPHEDEMA Lymphedema may be categorized as primary or secondary (Table 198-3). The prevalence of primary lymphedema is approximately 1 per 10,000 individuals. Primary lymphedema may be secondary to agenesis, hypoplasia, or obstruction of the lymphatic vessels. It may be associated with Turner's syndrome, Noonan's syndrome, the yellow nail syndrome, the intestinal lymphangiectasia syndrome, and with lymphangiomyomatosis. Women are affected more frequently than are men. There are three clinical subtypes: *congenital lymphedema* which appears shortly after birth, *lymphedema*

TABLE 198-3   Classification of lymphedema
Primary
Congenital (includes Milroy's disease)
Lymphedema praecox (includes Meige's disease)
Lymphedema tarda
Secondary
Recurrent lymphangitis
Filariasis
Tuberculosis
Neoplasm
Surgery
Radiation therapy

praecox which has its onset at the time of puberty, and *lymphedema tarda* which usually begins after the age of 35. Familial forms of congenital lymphedema (Milroy's disease) and lymphedema praecox (Meige's disease) may be inherited in an autosomal dominant manner with variable penetrance; autosomal or sex-linked recessive forms are less common.

Secondary lymphedema is an acquired condition resulting from damage to, or obstruction of, previously normal lymphatic channels (Table 198-3). Recurrent episodes of bacterial lymphangitis, usually caused by streptococci, are a very common cause of lymphedema. The most common cause of secondary lymphedema worldwide is filariasis (Chap. 169). Tumors, such as prostate cancer and lymphoma, also can obstruct lymphatic vessels. Both surgery and radiation therapy for breast carcinoma may cause lymphedema of the upper extremity. Less common causes include tuberculosis, contact dermatitis, lymphogranuloma venereum, rheumatoid arthritis, pregnancy, and self-induced or factitious lymphedema following application of tourniquets.

Lymphedema is generally a painless condition but patients may experience a chronic dull, heavy sensation in the leg and most often patients are concerned about the appearance of the leg. Lymphedema of the lower extremity, initially involving the foot, gradually progresses up the leg so that the entire limb becomes edematous. In the early stages of lymphedema, the edema is soft and pits easily with pressure. In the chronic stages of lymphedema, the limb has a woody texture and the tissues become indurated and fibrotic. At this stage, the edema may no longer be pitting. The limb loses its normal contour and the toes appear square. Lymphedema should be distinguished from other disorders that cause unilateral leg swelling, such as deep vein thrombosis and chronic venous insufficiency. In the latter, edema is softer and there is often evidence of a stasis dermatitis, hyperpigmentation, and superficial venous varicosities.

The evaluation of patients with lymphedema should include diagnostic studies to clarify the etiology. Abdominal and pelvic ultrasound and computed tomography can be used to detect obstructing lesions such as neoplasms. Lymphoscintigraphy and lymphangiography are rarely indicated but either can be used to confirm the diagnosis or differentiate primary from secondary lymphedema. Lymphoscintigraphy involves the injection of radioactively labeled technetium-containing colloid into the distal subcutaneous tissue of the affected extremity. Lymphangiography requires the isolation and cannulation of a distal lymphatic vessel and subsequent injection of contrast material. In primary lymphedema, lymphatic channels are absent, hypoplastic, or ectatic. In secondary lymphedema, lymphatic channels *usually* are dilated and the level of obstruction may be determined.

Treatment Patients with lymphedema of the lower extremities must be instructed to take meticulous care of their feet to prevent recurrent lymphangitis. Skin hygiene is important and emollients can be used to prevent drying. Prophylactic antibiotics are often helpful and fungal infection should be treated aggressively. Patients should be encouraged to participate in physical activity; frequent leg elevation can reduce the amount of edema. Patients can be fitted with graduated compression hose to reduce the amount of lymphedema that develops with upright posture. Occasionally, intermittent pneumatic compression devices can be applied at home to facilitate reduction of the edema. Diuretics are contraindicated and may cause depletion of intravascular volume and metabolic abnormalities. Recently, microsurgical lymphovenous anastomotic procedures have been performed to rechannel lymph flow from obstructed lymphatic vessels into the venous system.

REFERENCES

BERNSTEIN EF: *Noninvasive Diagnostic Techniques in Vascular Disease*, 3d ed. St. Louis, Mosby, 1985

BROWSE NL: The diagnosis and management of primary lymphedema. J Vasc Surg 3:181, 1986

COFFMAN JD: Intermittent claudication and rest pain. Physiologic concepts and therapeutic approaches. Prog Cardiovasc Dis 22:59, 1979

————: *Raynaud's Phenomenon*. New York, Oxford, 1989

DOUBILET P, ABRAMS HL: The cost of underutilization. Percutaneous transluminal angioplasty for peripheral vascular disease. N Engl J Med 310:95, 1984

FAIRBAIRN JF II et al: *Peripheral Vascular Diseases*, 5th ed. Philadelphia, Saunders, 1980

FOGLE MA et al: A comparison of in situ and reversed saphenous vein grafts for infra inguinal reconstruction. J Vasc Surg 5:46, 1987

HIRSH J et al: *Venous Thromboembolism*. New York, Grune & Stratton, 1981

HULL R et al: Adjusted subcutaneous heparin vs warfarin sodium in the long term treatment of venous thrombosis. N Engl J Med 306:189, 1982

KAKKAR VV et al: Prevention of fatal postoperative pulmonary embolism by low doses of heparin. An international trial. Lancet 1:567, 1977

LOSCALZO J et al: *The Textbook of Vascular Medicine and Biology*. Boston, Little, Brown, in press

MARDER VJ, SHERRY S: Thrombolytic therapy: Current status. N Engl J Med 318:1512, 1988

MOSER KM, LeMOINE JR: Is embolic risk conditioned by location of deep venous thrombosis. Ann Intern Med 94:439, 1981

VAN BREDA A et al: Urokinase vs. streptokinase in local thrombolysis. Radiology 165:109, 1987

LABORATORY VALUES OF CLINICAL IMPORTANCE

INTRODUCTORY COMMENTS

In preparing the Appendix, the editors have taken into account the fact that the system of international units (SI, système international d'unités) is now used in most countries and in virtually all medical and scientific journals including those in the United States.[1] However, many or most clinical laboratories in the United States continue to report values in traditional units. Therefore, in this book we utilize both systems for the Appendix and for the text itself. Values in SI units appear first, and *traditional units appear in parentheses* after the SI units. This dual approach is also used for the large part in the text. In those instances in which the numbers remain the same but only the terminology is changed (mmol/L for meq/L or IU/L for mIU/mL) only the SI units are given. In all other instances the SI unit is followed by the traditional unit in parentheses. The SI base units, SI derived units, other units of measure referred to in the Appendix, and SI prefixes are listed in Tables A-1 to A-3 at the end of the Appendix. Conversions from one system to another can be made as follows:

$$mmol/L = \frac{mg/dL \times 10}{atomic\ weight}$$

$$mg/dL = \frac{mmol/L \times atomic\ weight}{10}$$

ASCITIC FLUID

See Table 48-1, p. 270.

BODY FLUIDS AND OTHER MASS DATA

Body fluid, total volume: 50 percent (in obese) to 70 percent (lean) of body weight
  Intracellular: 0.3–0.4 of body weight
  Extracellular: 0.2–0.3 of body weight
Blood:
  Total volume:
    Males: 69 mL per kg body weight
    Females: 65 mL per kg body weight
  Plasma volume:
    Males: 39 mL per kg body weight
    Females: 40 mL per kg body weight
  Red blood cell volume:
    Males: 30 mL per kg body weight (1.15–1.21 L/m² body surface area)
    Females: 25 mL per kg body weight (0.95–1.00 L/m² body surface area)

[1] Young DS: Implementation of SI Units for Clinical Laboratory Data. Ann Intern Med 106:114, 1987

[2] Since cerebrospinal fluid concentrations are equilibrium values, measurements of the same parameters in blood plasma obtained at the same time is recommended. However, there is a time lag in attainment of equilibrium, and cerebrospinal levels of plasma constituents that can fluctuate rapidly (such as plasma glucose) may not achieve stable values until after a significant lag phase.

CEREBROSPINAL FLUID[2]

		Conversion factor (CF) (C × CF = SI)
Osmolality	292–297 mosmol/kg (292–297 mosmol/L)	—
Electrolytes:		
Sodium	137–145 mmol/L (137–145 meq/L)	—
Potassium	2.7–3.9 mmol/L (2.7–3.9 meq/L)	—
Calcium	1–1.5 mmol/L (2.1–3.0 meq/L)	0.5
Magnesium	1–1.2 mmol/L (2.0–2.5 meq/L)	0.5
Chloride	116–122 mmol/L (116–122 meq/L)	—
CO_2 content	20–24 mmol/L (20–24 meq/L)	—
P_{CO_2}	6–7 kPa (45–49 mmHg)	0.1333
pH	7.31–7.34	—
Glucose	2.2–3.9 mmol/L (40–70 mg/dL)	0.05551
Lactate	1–2 mmol/L (10–20 mg/dL)	0.1110
Total protein:	0.2–0.4 g/L (20–40 mg/dL)	0.01
Prealbumin	2–6 percent	—
Albumin	56–75 percent	—
Alpha$_1$ globulin	2–7 percent	—
Alpha$_2$ globulin	4–12 percent	—
Beta globulin	8–16 percent	—
Gamma globulin	3–12 percent	—
IgG	0.01–0.014 g/L (1–1.4 mg/dL)	0.01
IgA	0.001–0.003 g/L (0.1–0.3 mg/dL)	0.01
IgM	0.0001–0.00012 g/L (0.01–0.012 mg/dL)	0.01
Ammonia	15–47 μmol/L (25–80 μg/dL)	0.5872
Creatinine	44–168 μmol/L (0.5–1.9 mg/dL)	88.40
Myelin basic protein	<4 μg/L	—
CSF pressure	50–180 mmH$_2$O	—
CSF volume (adult)	100–160 mL	—
Leukocytes:		
Total	<4 per mL	—
Differential:		
Lymphocytes	60–70 percent	—
Monocytes	30–50 percent	—
Neutrophils	1–3 percent	—

CHEMICAL CONSTITUENTS OF BLOOD

See also "Function Tests," especially "Metabolic and Endocrine."

	Conversion factor (CF) (C × CF = SI)
Acetoacetate, plasma: <100 μmol/L (<1 mg/dL)	97.95
Albumin, serum: 35–55 g/L (3.5–5.5 g/dL)	10
Aldolase: 0–100 nkat/L (0–6 U/L)	16.67
Alpha₁ antitrypsin, serum: 0.8–2.1 g/L (85–213 mg/dL)	0.01
Alpha fetoprotein (adult), serum: <30 μg/L (<30 ng/mL)	—
Aminotransferases, serum:	
Aspartate (AST, SGOT): 0–0.58 μkat/L (0–35 U/L)	0.01667
Alanine (ALT, SGPT): 0–0.58 μkat/L (0–35 U/L)	0.01667
Ammonia, whole blood, venous: 47–65 μmol/L (80–110 μg/dL)	0.5872
Amylase, serum: 0.8–3.2 μkat/L (60–180 U/L)	0.01667
Arterial blood gases:	
[HCO₃⁻]: 21–28 mmol/L (21–28 meq/L)	—
P_CO₂: 4.7–5.9 kPa (35–45 mmHg)	0.1333
pH: 7.38–7.44	—
P_O₂: 11–13 kPa (80–100 mmHg)	0.1333
Ascorbic acid (vitamin C), serum: 23–57 μmol/L (0.4–1.0 mg/dL)	56.78
Barbiturates, serum: normal, nondetectable	
Phenobarbital, "potentially fatal" level: approximately 390 μmol/L (9 mg/dL)	43.06
Most short-acting barbiturates, "potentially fatal" levels: approximately 150 μmol/L (35 mg/L)	4.419
Base, total, serum: 145–155 mmol/L (145–155 meq/L)	—
β-Hydroxybutyrate, plasma: <300 μmol/L (<3 mg/dL)	96.05
Bilirubin, total, serum (Malloy-Evelyn): 5.1–17 μmol/L (0.3–1.0 mg/dL)	17.10
Direct, serum: 1.7–5.1 μmol/L (0.1–0.3 mg/dL)	17.10
Indirect, serum: 3.4–12 μmol/L (0.2–0.7 mg/dL)	17.10
Bromides, serum: nondetectable	
Toxic levels: >17 mmol/L (>17 meq/L)	—
Bromsulphalein, BSP (5 mg per kg body weight, intravenously): 5 percent or less retention after 45 min	—
Calciferols (vitamin D), plasma:	
1,25-dihydroxyvitamin D [1,25(OH)₂D]: 5–14 nmol/L (20–60 pg/mL)	0.2400
25-hydroxyvitamin D [25(OH)D]: 20–100 nmol/L (8–42 ng/mL)	2.496
Calcium, ionized: 1.1–1.4 mmol/L (2.3–2.8 meq/L; 4.5–5.6 mg/dL)	0.2495
Calcium, plasma: 2.2–2.6 mmol/L (9–10.5 mg/dL)	0.2495
Carbon dioxide content, plasma (sea level): 21–30 mmol/L (21–30 meq/L)	—
Carbon dioxide tension (P_CO₂), arterial blood (sea level): 4.7–6.0 kPa (35–45 mmHg)	0.1333
Carbon monoxide content, blood: symptoms with over 20 percent saturation of hemoglobin	
Carotenoids, serum: 0.9–5.6 μmol/L (50–300 μg/dL)	0.01863
Ceruloplasmin, serum: 270–370 mg/L (27–37 mg/dL)	10
Chlorides, serum (as Cl⁻): 98–106 mmol/L (98–106 meq/L)	—
Cholesterol: see Table A-4	
Complement, serum:	
C3: 0.55–1.20 g/L (55–120 mg/dL)	0.01
C4: 0.20–0.50 g/L (20–50 mg/dL)	0.01

	Conversion factor (CF) (C × CF = SI)
Copper, serum: 11–22 μmol/L (70–140 μg/dL)	0.1574
Creatine phosphokinase, serum (total):	
Females: 0.17–1.17 μkat/L (10–70 U/L)	0.01667
Males: 0.42–1.50 μkat/L (25–90 U/L)	0.01667
Creatinine, serum: <133 μmol/L (<1.5 mg/dL)	88.40
Digoxin serum:	
Therapeutic level: 0.6–2.8 nmol/L (0.5–2.2 ng/mL)	1.281
Toxic level: >3.1 nmol/L (>2.4 ng/mL)	1.281
Ethanol, blood:	
Mild to moderate intoxication: 17–43 mmol/L (80–200 mg/dL)	0.2171
Marked intoxication: 54–87 mmol/L (250–400 mg/dL)	0.2171
Severe intoxication: >87 mmol/L (>400 mg/dL)	0.2171
Fatty acids, free (nonesterified), plasma: <180 mg/L (<18 mg/dL)	10
Ferritin, serum: 15–200 μg/L (15–200 ng/mL)	—
Fibrinogen, plasma: see "Platelets and Coagulation"	—
Fibrinogen split products: see "Platelets and Coagulation"	—
Folic acid, red cell: 340–1020 nmol/L cells (150–450 ng/mL cells)	2.266
Gastrin, serum: 40–200 ng/L (40–200 pg/mL)	—
Globulins, serum: 20–30 g/L (2.0–3.0 g/dL)	10
Glucose (fasting), plasma:	
Normal: 4.2–6.4 mmol/L (75–115 mg/dL)	0.05551
Diabetes mellitus: >7.8 mmol/L [>140 mg/dL (on more than one occasion)]	0.05551
Glucose, 2 h postprandial, plasma:	
Normal: <7.8 mmol/L (<140 mg/dL)	0.05551
Impaired glucose tolerance: 7.8–11.1 mmol/L (140–200 mg/dL)	0.05551
Diabetes mellitus: >11.1 mmol/L on more than one occasion (>200 mg/dL)	0.05551
Hemoglobin, blood (sea level):	
Male: 140–180 g/L (14–18 g/dL)	10
Female: 120–160 g/L (12–16 g/dL)	10
Hemoglobin A₁c: up to 6 percent of total hemoglobin	—
Immunoglobulins, serum:	
IgA: 0.9–3.2 g/L (90–325 mg/dL)	0.01
IgD: 0–0.08 g/L (0–8 mg/dL)	0.01
IgE: <0.00025 g/L (<0.025 mg/dL)	0.01
IgG: 8.0–15.0 g/L (800–1500 mg/dL)	0.01
IgM: 0.45–1.5 g/L (45–150 mg/dL)	0.01
Iron, serum: 14–32 μmol/L (80–180 μg/dL)	0.1791
Iron-binding capacity, serum: 45–82 μmol/L (250–460 μg/dL)	0.1791
Saturation: 0.2–0.45 (20–45 percent)	
Lactate dehydrogenase, serum:	
200–450 units/mL (Wrobleski)	—
60–100 units/mL (Wacker)	—
0.4–1.7 μkat/L (25–100 units/L)	0.01667
Lactic dehydrogenase isoenzymes, serum (agarose):	
Fraction 1 (of total): 0.14–0.25 (14–26 percent)	0.01
Fraction 2: 0.29–0.39 (29–39 percent)	0.01
Fraction 3: 0.20–0.25 (20–26 percent)	0.01
Fraction 4: 0.08–0.16 (8–16 percent)	0.01
Fraction 5: 0.06–0.16 (6–16 percent)	0.01
Lactate, venous plasma: 0.6–1.7 mmol/L (5–15 mg/dL)	0.1110
Lead, serum: <1.0 μmol/L (<20 μg/dL)	0.04826
Lipids: see Table A-4	—
Lipids, triglyceride, serum: see "Triglycerides"	

Conversion
factor (CF)
(C × CF = SI)

Lipoprotein: see Table A-4 —
Lithium, serum:
  Therapeutic level: 0.6–1.2 mmol/L (0.6–1.2 meq/L) —
  Toxic level: >2 mmol/L (>2 meq/L) —
Magnesium, serum: 0.8–1.2 mmol/L (2–3 mg/dL) 0.4114
Osmolality, plasma: 285–295 mosmol per kg serum water —
Oxygen content:
  Arterial blood (sea level): 17–21 volume percent —
  Venous blood, arm (sea level): 10 to 16 volume percent —
Oxygen percent saturation (sea level):
  Arterial blood: 0.97 mol/mol (97 percent) 0.01
  Venous blood, arm: 0.60–0.85 mol/mol (60–85 percent) 0.01
Oxygen tension (P_{O_2}) blood: 11–13 kPa (80–100 mmHg) 0.1333
pH, blood: 7.38–7.44 —
Phenytoin, plasma:
  Therapeutic level: 40–80 μmol/L (10–20 mg/L) 3.964
  Toxic level: >120 μmol/L (>30 mg/L) 3.964
Phosphorus, inorganic, serum: 1.0–1.4 mmol/L (3–4.5 mg/dL) 0.3229
Potassium, serum: 3.5–5.0 mmol/L (3.5–5.0 meq/L) —
Proteins, total, serum: 55–80 g/L (5.5–8.0 g/dL) 10
Protein fractions, serum:
  Albumin: 35–55 g/L [3.5–5.5 g/dL (50–60 percent)] 10
  Globulin: 20–35 g/L [2.0–3.5 g/dL (40–50 percent)] 10
  Alpha$_1$: 2–4 g/L [0.2–0.4 g/dL (4.2–7.2 percent)] 10
  Alpha$_2$: 5–9 g/L [0.5–0.9 g/dL (6.8–12 percent)] 10
  Beta: 6–11 g/L [0.6–1.1 g/dL (9.3–15 percent)] 10
  Gamma: 7–17 g/L [0.7–1.7 g/dL (13–23 percent)] 10
Pyruvate, venous, plasma: 60–170 μmol/L (0.5–1.5 mg/dL) 113.6
Quinidine, serum:
  Therapeutic range: 4.6–9.2 μmol/L (1.5–3 mg/L) 3.082
  Toxic range: 15.4–18.5 μmol/L (5–6 mg/L) 3.082
Salicylate, plasma: 0 mmol/L —
  Therapeutic range: 1.4–1.8 mmol/L (20–25 mg/dL) 0.07240
  Toxic range: >2.2 mmol/L (>30 mg/dL) 0.07240
Sodium, serum: 136–145 mmol/L (136–145 meq/L) —
Steroids: see "Metabolic and Endocrine" under "Function Tests" —
Triglycerides: <1.8 mmol/L (<160 mg/dL) 0.01129
Urea nitrogen, serum: 3.6–7.1 mmol/L (10–20 mg/dL) 0.3570
Uric acid, serum:
  Men: 150–480 μmol/L (2.5–8.0 mg/dL) 59.48
  Women: 90–360 μmol/L (1.5–6.0 mg/dL) 59.48
Vitamin A, serum: 0.7–3.5 μmol/L (20–100 μg/dL) 0.03491
Vitamin B$_{12}$, serum: 148–443 pmol/L (200–600 pg/mL) 0.7378
Zinc, serum: 11.5–18.5 μmol/L (75–120 μg/dL) 0.1530

FUNCTION TESTS

Circulation

Arteriovenous oxygen difference: 30–50 mL/L
Cardiac output (Fick): 2.5–3.6 L/m² body surface area per min

Conversion
factor (CF)
(C × CF = SI)

Contractility indexes:
  Maximum left ventricular dp/dt: 1650 ± 300 mmHg/s
  Maximum $(dp/dt)/p$: 44 ± 8.4 s^{-1}
  (dp/dt)/DP at DP = 40 mmHg: 37.6 ± 12.2 s^{-1} (DP = diastolic press.)
  Mean normalized systolic ejection rate (angiography): 3.32 ± 0.84 end-diastolic volumes per second
  Mean velocity of circumferential fiber shortening (angiography) 1.66 ± 0.42 circumferences per second
Ejection fraction, stroke volume/end-diastolic volume (SV/EDV):
  Normal range: 0.55–0.78; average: 0.67
End-diastolic volume: 75 ± 15 mL/m²
End-systolic volume: 25 ± 8 mL/m²
Left ventricular work:
  Stroke work index: 30–110 (g·m)/m²
  Left ventricular minute work index: 1.8–6.6 [(kg · m)/m²]/min
  Oxygen consumption index: 110–150 mL
Pressures, intracardiac and intraarterial: see Table A-5
Pulmonary vascular resistance: 2–12 (kPa·s)/L [20–120 (dyn·s)/cm⁵]
Systemic vascular resistance: 77–150 (kPa·s)/L [770–1500 (dyn·s)/cm⁵]
Systolic time intervals: see Table A-6

Gastrointestinal See also "Stool."

Absorption tests:
  D-Xylose absorption test: After an overnight fast, 25 g xylose is given in aqueous solution by mouth. Urine collected for the following 5 h should contain 33–53 mmol (5–8 g) (or >20 percent of ingested dose). Serum xylose should be 1.7–2.7 mmol/L 1 h after the oral dose (25–40 mg per 100 mL).
  Vitamin A absorption test: A fasting blood specimen is obtained and 200,000 units of vitamin A in oil is given by mouth. Serum vitamin A levels should rise to twice fasting level in 3–5 h.
Bentiromide test (pancreatic function): 500 mg bentiromide (chymex) orally; p-aminobenzoic acid (PABA) measured in plasma and/or urine
  Plasma: >3.6(±1.1) mg/L at 90 min
  Urine: >50 percent recovered as PABA in 6 h
Gastric juice:
  Volume:
    24 h: 2–3 L
    Nocturnal: 600–700 mL
    Basal, fasting: 30–70 mL/h
  Reaction:
    pH: 1.6–1.8
    Titratable acidity of fasting juice: 4–9 μmol/s (15–35 meq/h) 0.261
  Acid output:
    Basal:
      Females (mean ± 1 SD): 0.6 ± 0.5 μmol/s (2.0 ± 1.8 meq/h) 0.2778
      Males (mean ± 1 SD): 0.8 ± 0.6 μmol/s (3.0 ± 2.0 meq/h) 0.2778
    Maximal (after subcutaneous histamine acid phosphate 0.004 mg/kg body weight and preceded by 50 mg promethazine or after betazole 1.7 mg/kg body weight or pentagastrin 6 μg/kg body weight):
      Females (mean ± 1 SD): 4.4 ± 1.4 μmol/s (16 ± 5 meq/h) 0.2778
      Males (mean ± 1 SD): 6.4 ± 1.4 μmol/s (23 ± 5 meq/h) 0.2778
  Basal acid output/maximal acid output ratio: 0.6 or less

	Conversion factor (CF) (C × CF = SI)
Gastrin, serum: 40–200 ng/L (40–200 pg/mL)	—
Secretin test (pancreatic exocrine function): 1 unit per kg body weight, intravenously	
Volume (pancreatic juice): >2.0 mL/kg in 80 min	—
Bicarbonate concentration: >80 mmol/L (>80 meq/L)	—
Bicarbonate output: >10 mmol in 30 min (>10 meq in 30 min)	—

Metabolic and endocrine

	Conversion factor (CF) (C × CF = SI)
Adrenocorticotropin (ACTH) plasma, 8 A.M.: <18 pmol/L (<80 pg/mL)	0.2202
Adrenal cortex function tests: see Chap. 317	
Adrenal medulla function tests: see Chap. 318	
Adrenal steroids, plasma:	
Aldosterone, 8 A.M.: <220 pmol/L (patient supine, 100 meq Na and 60–100 meq K intake) (<8 ng/dL)	27.74
Cortisol:	
8 A.M.: 140–690 nmol/L (5–25 μg/dL)	27.59
4 P.M.: 80–330 nmol/L (3–12 μg/dL)	27.59
Dehydroepiandrosterone (DHEA): 7–31 nmol/L (2–9 μg/L)	3.467
Dehydroepiandrosterone sulfate (DHEA sulfate): 1.3–6.7 μmol/L (500–2500 μg/L)	0.002714
11-Deoxycortisol (compound S): <30 nmol/L (<1 μg/dL)	28.86
17-Hydroxyprogesterone:	
Women: follicular phase, 0.6–3 nmol/L (0.20–1 μg/L); luteal phase, 1.5–10.6 nmol/L (0.5–3.5 μg/L)	3.026
Men: 0.2–9 nmol/L (0.06–3 μg/L)	3.026
Adrenal steroids, urinary excretion:	
Aldosterone: 14–53 nmol/d (5–19 μg/d)	2.774
Cortisol, free: 55–275 nmol/d (20–100 μg/d)	2.759
17-Hydroxycorticosteroids: 5.5–28 μmol/d (2–10 mg/d)	2.759
17-Ketosteroids:	
Men: 24–88 μmol/d (7–25 mg/d)	3.467
Women: 14–52 μmol/d (4–15 mg/d)	3.467
Angiotensin II, plasma, 8 A.M.: 10–30 nmol/L (10–30 pg/mL)	—
Arginine vasopressin (AVP), plasma:	
Random fluid intake: 2.3–7.4 pmol/L (2.5–8 ng/L)	0.92
Calcitonin, plasma: <50 ng/L (<50 pg/mL)	—
Catecholamines, urinary excretion:	
Free catecholamines: <590 nmol/d (<100 μg/d)	5.911
Epinephrine: <275 nmol/d (<50 μg/d)	5.458
Metanephrines: <7 μmol/d (<1.3 mg/d)	5.458
Vanillylmandelic acid (VMA): <40 μmol/d (<8 mg/d)	5.046
Glucagon, plasma: 50–100 ng/L (50–100 pg/mL)	—
Gonadal function tests: see Chaps. 321 and 322	—
Gonadal steroids, plasma:	
Androstenedione:	
Women: 3.5–7.0 nmol/L (1–2 ng/ml)	3.492
Men: 3.0–5.0 mmol/L (0.8–1.3 ng/ml)	3.492
Estradiol:	
Women: 70–220 pmol/L (20–60 pg/mL), higher at ovulation	3.671
Men: <180 pmol/L (<50 pg/mL)	3.671
Progesterone:	
Men, prepubertal girls, preovulatory women, and postmenopausal women: <6 nmol/L (2 ng/mL)	3.180
Women, luteal, peak: >16 nmol/L (>5 ng/mL)	3.180

	Conversion factor (CF) (C × CF = SI)
Testosterone:	
Women: <3.5 nmol/L (<1 ng/mL)	3.467
Men: 10–35 nmol/L (3–10 ng/mL)	3.467
Prepubertal boys and girls: 0.17–0.7 nmol/L (0.05–0.2 ng/mL)	3.467
Gonadotropins, plasma:	
Women, mature, premenopausal, except at ovulation:	
FSH: 5–20 IU/L (5–20 mIU/mL)	
LH: 5–25 IU/L (5–25 mIU/mL)	
Ovulatory surge:	
FSH: 12–30 IU/L (12–30 mIU/mL)	
LH: 25–100 IU/L (25–100 mIU/mL)	
Postmenopausal women:	
FSH: >12–30 IU/L (>12–30 mIU/mL)	
LH: >50 IU/L (>50 mIU/mL)	
Men, mature:	
FSH: 5–20 IU/L (5–20 mIU/mL)	
LH: 5–20 IU/L (5–20 mIU/mL)	
Children of both sexes, prepubertal:	
FSH: <5 IU/L (<5 mIU/mL)	
Growth hormone, after 100 g glucose by mouth: <5 μg/L (<5 ng/mL)	
Human chorionic gonadotropin, β subunit (β-hCG), plasma:	
Men and nonpregnant women: <3 IU/L (<3 mIU/mL)	—
Insulin, serum or plasma, fasting: 43–186 pmol/L (6–26 μU/mL)	7.175
Insulin-like growth factor 1 (somatomedin C, IGF-1/SM-C): see Chap. 314	—
Oxytocin:	
Random: 1–4 pmol/L (1.25–5 ng/L)	0.80
Ovulatory peak in women: 4–8 pmol/L (5–10 ng/L)	0.80
Pancreatic islet function tests: see Chap. 319	—
Parathyroid function tests: see Chap. 340	—
Pituitary function tests: see Chaps. 313 to 315	—
Pregnancy tests: see Chap. 322	—
Prolactin, serum: 2–15 μg/L (2–15 ng/mL)	—
Renin-angiotensin function tests: see Chap. 317	—
Semen analysis: see Chap. 321	—
Thyroid function tests:	
Dynamic tests of thyroid function: see Chap. 316	—
Radioactive iodine uptake, 24 h: 5–30 percent (range varies in different areas due to variations in iodine intake)	
Resin T_3 uptake: 0.25–0.35 (25–35 percent) (varies among laboratories; for calculation of indexes of resin T_3 uptake, see Chap. 316)	0.01
Reverse triiodothyronine (rT_3), plasma: 0.15–0.61 nmol/L (10–40 ng/dL)	0.01536
Thyroid-stimulating hormone (TSH): 0.4–5 mU/L (0.4–5 μU/mL)	—
Thyroxine (T_4), serum radioimmunoassay: 64–154 nmol/L (5–12 μg/dL)	12.86
Triiodothyronine (T_3), plasma: 1.1–2.9 nmol/L (70–190) ng/dL)	0.01536

Pulmonary See Tables A-9 and A-10.

Renal

	Conversion factor (CF) (C × CF = SI)
Clearances (corrected to 1.72 m² body surface area):	
Measures of glomerular filtration rate:	
Inulin clearance (C1):	
Males (mean ± 1 SD): 2.1 ± 0.4 mL/s (124 ± 25.8 mL/min)	0.01667

	Conversion factor (CF) (C × CF = SI)
Females (mean ± 1 SD): 2.0 ± 0.2 mL/s (119 ± 12.8 mL/min)	0.01667
Endogenous creatinine clearance: 1.5–2.2 mL/s (91–130 mL/min)	0.01667
Urea: 1.0–1.7 mL/s (60–100 mL/min)	0.01667
Measures of effective renal plasma flow and tubular function:	
p-Aminohippuric acid clearance (Cl_{PAH}):	
Males (mean ± 1 SD): 10.9 ± 2.7 mL/s (654 ± 163 mL/min)	0.01667
Females (mean ± 1 SD): 9.9 ± 1.7 mL/s (594 ± 102 mL/min)	0.01667
Concentration and dilution test:	
Specific gravity of urine:	
After 12-h fluid restriction: 1.025 or more	—
After 12-h deliberate water intake: 1.003 or less	—
Protein excretion, urine: <0.15 g/d (<150 mg/d)	0.001
Males: 0–0.06 g/d (0–60 mg/d)	0.001
Females: 0–0.09 g/d (0–90 mg/d)	0.001
Specific gravity, maximal range: 1.002–1.028	—
Tubular reabsorption, phosphorus: 79–94 percent of filtered load	—

HEMATOLOGIC EXAMINATIONS
See also "Chemical Constituents of Blood."

Bone marrow   See Table A-12.

Erythrocytes and hemoglobin   See also Table A-12.

	Conversion factor (CF) (C × CF = SI)
Carboxyhemoblogin:	
Nonsmoker: 0–0.023 (0–2.3 percent)	0.01
Smoker: 0.021–0.042 (2.1–4.2 percent)	0.01
Erythrocyte "life span":	
Normal survival: 120 days	—
Chromium-labeled, half-life (t_1): 28 days	—
Glucose-6-phosphate dehydrogenase: 12.1 ± 2 IU/gHb (WHO)	—
Ham's test (acid serum): negative	—
Haptoglobin, serum 0.5–2.2 g/L (50–220 mg/dL)	0.01
Hemoglobin, plasma: 0.01–0.05 g/L (1–5 mg/dL)	0.01
Hemoglobin A_2 (HbA₂): 0.015–0.035 (1.5–3.5 percent)	0.01
Hemoglobin, fetal (HbF): <0.02 (<2 percent)	0.01
Hemoglobin H prep: negative	—
Methemoglobin: <0.017 (<1.7 percent)	0.01
Osmotic fragility:	
Slight hemolysis: 0.45–0.39 percent	—
Complete hemolysis: 0.33–0.30 percent	—
Plasma iron turnover: 20–42 mg/d or 0.45 mg/kg body weight per day	—
Protoporphyrin, free erythrocyte (FEP): 0.28–0.64 μmol/L of red blood cells (16–36 μg/dL of red blood cells)	0.0177
Red cell distribution width (Coulter): 13 ± 1.5 percent	
Sedimentation rate:	
Westergren, <50 years of age:	
Males: 0–15 mm/h	
Females: 0–20 mm/h	
Westergren, >50 years of age:	
Males: 0–20 mm/h	
Females: 0–30 mm/h	
Sucrose hemolysis: negative	

Leukocytes   See Table A-13.

Platelets and coagulation

	Conversion factor (CF) (C × CF = SI)
Alpha₂ antiplasmin: 70–130 percent	
Antithrombin III: 80–120 percent	
Bleeding time:	
Duke method: <4 min	
Simplate: <7 min	
Clot retraction, qualitative: apparent in 60 min, complete <24 h, usually <6 h	
Euglobulin lysis time: >2 h	
Factor II: 60–100 percent	
Factor V: 60–100 percent	
Factor VII: 60–100 percent	
Factor IX: 60–100 percent	
Factor X: 60–100 percent	
Factor XI: 60–100 percent	
Factor XII: 60–100 percent	
Factor XIII: clot stable in urea	
Fibrinogen: 2.0–4.0 g/L (200–400 mg/dL)	0.01
Fibrin split products: <10 mg/L (<10 μg/mL)	—
Plasminogen: 2.4–4.4 CTA U/mL	
Protein C (antigenic assay): 58–148 percent	
Protein S (antigenic assay): 58–148 percent	
Partial thromboplastin time (activated PTT): comparable to control	
Prothrombin time (quick one-stage): control ± 1 s	
Protamine paracoagulation (3P) test: negative	
Platelets: 130,000–400,000 per microliter	
Thrombin time: control ± 3 s	
von Willebrand's antigen: 60–150 percent	

Miscellaneous

	Conversion factor (CF) (C × CF = SI)
Leukocyte alkaline phosphatase (LAP): 0.2–1.6 μkat/L (13–100 U/L)	0.01667
Lysozyme (muramidase), serum: 5–25 mg/L (5–25 μg/mL)	—
Lysozyme, urine: <2 mg/L (<2 μg/mL)	—
Schilling test: excretion in urine of orally administered radioactive vitamin B_{12}: 7–40 percent	—
Viscosity, plasma: 1.7–2.1	—
Viscosity, serum: 1.4–1.8	—

STOOL

	Conversion factor (CF) (C × CF = SI)
Bulk:	
Wet weight: <197.5 (115 ± 41) g/d	—
Dry weight: <66.4 (34 ± 15) g/d	—
Alpha₁ antitrypsin: 0.98 (±0.17) mg/g dry weight stool	—
Coproporphyrin: 600–1500 nmol/d (400–1000 μg/d)	1.527
Fat (on diet containing at least 50 g fat): <6.0 (4.0 ± 1.5) g/d when measured on a 3-day (or longer) collection	
Percent of dry weight: <0.30 (<30.4 percent)	0.01
Coefficient of fat absorption: >0.95 (>95 percent)	0.01
Fatty acid:	
Free: 0.01–0.10 (1–10 percent of dry matter)	0.01
Combined as soap: 0.005–0.12 (0.5–12 percent of dry matter)	0.01
Nitrogen: <1.7 (1.4 ± 0.2) g/d	—
Protein content: minimal	—
Urobilinogen: 68–470 μmol/d (40–280 mg/d)	1.693
Water: 0.65 (approximately 65 percent)	0.01

URINE

Conversion factor (CF)
(C × CF = SI)

See also "Metabolic and Endocrine" under "Function Tests."

Acidity, titratable: 20–40 mmol/d (20–40 meq/d)	—
Ammonia: 30–50 mmol/d (30–50 meq/d)	—
Amylase: 35–260 Somogyi units/h	
Amylase/creatinine clearance ratio [(Cl$_{am}$/Cl$_{cr}$) × 100]: 1–5	—
Bentiromide (pancreatic function): 50 percent excreted in 6 h as p-amino benzoic acid (PABA) after 500 mg oral bentiromide	—
Calcium (10 meq/d or 200-mg/d calcium diet): <3.8 mmol/d (<7.5 meq/d)	0.5
Catecholamines: <600 nmol/d (<100 μg/d)	5.911
Copper: 0–0.4 μmol/d (0–25 μg/d)	0.01574
Coproporphyrins (types I and III): 150–460 nmol/d (100–300 μg/d)	1.527
Creatine, as creatinine:	
Adult males: <380 pmol/d (<50 mg/d)	7.625
Adult females: <760 pmol/d (<100 mg/d)	7.625
Creatinine: 8.8–14 mmol/d (1.0–1.6 g/d)	8.840
Glucose, true (oxidase method): 0.3–1.7 mmol/d (50–300 mg/d)	0.5551
5-Hydroxyindoleacetic acid (5-HIAA): 10–47 μmol/d (2–9 mg/d)	5.230
Lead: <0.4 μmol/d (<80 μg/d)	0.004826
Protein: <0.15 g/d (<150 mg/d)	0.1
Porphobilinogen: none	—
Potassium: 25–100 mmol/d [25–100 meq/d (varies with intake)]	—
Sodium: 100–260 mmol/d [100–260 meq/d (varies with intake)]	—
Urobilinogen: 1.7–5.9 μmol/d (1–3.5 mg/d)	1.693
Vanillylmandelic acid (VMA): <40 μmol/d (<8 mg/d)	5.046
D-Xylose excretion: 5 to 8 g within 5 h after oral dose of 25 g	—

TABLE A-1 SI and other units

Quantity	Name of unit	Symbol for unit	Derivation of units
SI BASE UNITS			
Length	meter	m	
Mass	kilogram	kg	
Time	second	s	
Thermodynamic temperature	Kelvin	K	
Amount of substance	mole	mol	
SI DERIVED UNITS			
Area	square meter	m^2	
Force	newton	N	(m·kg)/g^2
Pressure	pascal	Pa	N·m^2
Work, energy	joule	J	N·m
Celsius temperature	degree Celsius	°C	K
OTHER UNITS RETAINED FOR USE			
Time	minute	min	
	hour	h	
	day	d	
Volume	liter	L	

TABLE A-2 Radiation derived units

Quantity	Old unit	SI unit	Name for SI unit (and abbreviation)	Conversion
Activity	curie (Ci)	Disintegrations per second (dps)	becquerel (Bq)	1 Ci = 3.7 × 10^{10} Bq 1 mCi = 37 mBq 1 μCi = 0.037 MBq or 37 GBq 1 Bq = 2.703 × 10^{-11} Ci
Absorbed dose	rad	joule per kilogram (J/kg)	gray (Gy)	1 Gy = 100 rad 1 rad = 0.01 Gy 1 mrad = 10^{-3} cGy
Exposure	roentgen (R)	coulomb per kilogram (C/kg)	—	1 C/kg = 3876 R 1 R = 2.58 × 10^{-4} C/kg 1 mR = 258 pC/kg
Dose equivalent	rem	joule per kilogram (J/kg)	sievert (Sv)	1 Sv = 100 rem 1 rem = 0.01 Sv 1 mrem = 10 μSv

TABLE A-3 SI prefixes and their symbols

Factor	Prefix	Symbol for prefix
10^9	giga	G
10^6	mega	M
10^3	kilo	k
10^2	hecto	h
10^1	deka	da
10^{-1}	deci	d
10^{-2}	centi	c
10^{-3}	milli	m
10^{-6}	micro	μ
10^{-9}	nano	n
10^{-12}	pico	p
10^{-15}	femto	f
10^{-18}	alto	a

TABLE A-4 Classification of total cholesterol and LDL-cholesterol values

	Total plasma cholesterol	LDL-cholesterol	Conversion factor (C to SI)
Desirable	<5.20 mmol/L (<200 mg/dL)	<3.36 mmol/L (<130 mg/dL)	0.02586
Borderline high	5.20–6.18 mmol/L (200–239 mg/dL)	3.36–4.11 mmol/L (130–159 mg/dL)	0.02586
High	≥6.21 mmol/L (≥240 mg/dL)	≥4.14 mmol/L (≥160 mg/dL)	0.02586

SOURCE: The Expert Panel. Report of the National Cholesterol Education Program Expert Panel on Detection, Evaluation, and Treatment of High Blood Cholesterol in Adults. Arch Intern Med 148:36, 1988

TABLE A-5 Hemodynamic values

Pressures (mmHg):
Systemic arterial:	
Peak systolic/end-diastolic	100–140/60–90
Mean	70–105
Left ventricle:	
Peak systolic/end-diastolic	100–140/3–12
Left atrium (or pulmonary capillary wedge):	
Mean	2–12
a wave	3–10
v wave	3–15
Pulmonary artery:	
Peak systolic/end-diastolic	15–30/4–14
Mean	9–17
Right ventricle:	
Peak systolic/end-diastolic	15–30/2–7
Right atrium:	
Mean	2–6
a wave	2–8
v wave	2–7
Resistances [(dyn·s)/cm⁵]:	
Systemic vascular resistance	700–1600
Total pulmonary resistance	100–300
Pulmonary vascular resistance	30–130
Flows:	
Cardiac index (liters per minute per square meter)	2.4–3.8
Stroke index (milliliters per beat per square meter)	30–65
Oxygen consumption (liters per minute per square meter)	110–150
Arteriovenous oxygen difference (milliliters per liter)	30–50

TABLE A-6 Systolic time intervals in normal individuals (in milliseconds)

Regression equation		SD of index
QS₂ (M)	= −2.1 HR + 546	14
QS₂ (F)	= −2.0 HR + 549	14
PEP (M)	= −0.4 HR + 131	13
PEP (F)	= −0.4 HR + 133	11
LVET (M)	= −1.7 HR + 413	10
LVET (F)	= −1.6 HR + 418	10

NOTE: QS₂ = total electromechanical systole, PEP = preejection phase, LVET = left ventricular ejection time, HR = heart rate, M = male, F = female, SD = standard deviation of the systolic time interval index. Systolic ejection period = 220–320 ms per beat; diastolic filling period = 380–500 ms per beat.
SOURCE: AM Weissler, CL Garrard, Mod Concepts Cardiovasc Dis 40:1, 1971.

TABLE A-7 Normal values of echocardiographic measurements in adults*

	Range, cm	Mean, cm	Number of subjects
Age (years)	13 to 54	26	134
Body surface area (m²)	1.45 to 2.22	1.8	130
RVD—flat	0.7 to 2.3	1.5	84
RVD—left lateral	0.9 to 2.6	1.7	83
LVID—flat	3.7 to 5.6	4.7	82
LVID—left lateral	3.5 to 5.7	4.7	81
Posterior LV wall thickness	0.6 to 1.1	0.9	137
Posterior LV wall amplitude	0.9 to 1.4	1.2	48
IVS wall thickness	0.6 to 1.1	0.9	137
Mid IVS amplitude	0.3 to 0.8	0.5	10
Apical IVS amplitude	0.5 to 1.2	0.7	38
Left atrial dimension	1.9 to 4.0	2.9	133
Aortic root dimension	2.0 to 3.7	2.7	121
Aortic cusps' separation	1.5 to 2.6	1.9	93
Percentage of fractional shortening†	34 to 44%	36%	20
Mean rate of circumferential shortening (Vcf)‡, or mean normalized shortening velocity	1.02 to 1.94 circ/s	1.3 circ/s	38

* RVD = right ventricular dimension; LVID = left ventricular internal dimension; d = end diastole; s = end systole; LV = left ventricle; IVS = interventricular septum.

† $\dfrac{LVIDd - LVIDs}{LVIDd}$

‡ $\dfrac{LVIDd - LVIDs}{LVIDd \times \text{ejection time}}$

SOURCE: From H Feigenbaum, Echocardiography, in *Heart Disease—A Textbook of Cardiovascular Medicine,* E Braunwald (ed), Philadelphia, Saunders, 1980.

TABLE A-8 Amplitude of Q, R, S, and T waves in scalar electrocardiogram of 100 normal adults*

	I	II	III	aV_R	aV_L	aV_F	V₁	V₅	V₆
Patients with Q wave	38%	41%	50%	—	38%	40%	0%	60%	75%
Q amplitude:									
Mean	0.4	0.6	0.9	—	0.4	0.7	0	0.3	0.3
Range	0 to 0.10	0 to 1.6	0 to 2.3	—	0 to 1.1	0 to 1.7	0	0 to 1.8	0 to 1.8
R amplitude:									
Mean	5.6	8.9	4.5	1.3	3.4	6.0	1.9	12.6	10.2
Range	1.0 to 10.0	2.0 to 16.9	1.0 to 12.1	0 to 2.9	0 to 8.2	0 to 13.8	1.0 to 6.0	7.0 to 21.0	5.0 to 18.0
S amplitude:									
Mean	2.0	2.1	2.4	7.0	2.6	—	8.0	2.5	1.3
Range	0 to 5.0	0 to 3.7	0 to 6.4	2.2 to 11.8	0 to 5.8	—	3.0 to 13.0	0 to 5.0	0 to 2.0
T amplitude:									
Mean	1.9	2.3	1.0	—	0.3	1.7	1.0	3.3	1.0
Range	1.0 to 3.0	1.0 to 4.0	−2.0 to 2.0	—	−1.0 to 2.0	0 to 4.0	−2.0 to 2.0	2.0 to 7.0	1.0 to 4.0

* Values of Q, R, S, and T amplitudes are in millimeters (1 mm = 0.1 mv).
SOURCE: From J D Cooksey et al, *Clinical Vectorcardiography and Electrocardiography,* 2d ed, Chicago, Year Book Medical Publishers, 1977. Used by permission.

TABLE A-9   Summary of values useful in pulmonary physiology

	Symbol	Typical values Men	Women
PULMONARY MECHANICS			
Spirometry—volume-time curves:			
Forced vital capacity	FVC	$\geq$4.0 liters	$\geq$3.0 liters
Forced expiratory volume in 1 s	FEV_1	>3.0 liters	>2.0 liters
FEV_1/FVC	FEV_1%	>60%	>70%
Maximal midexpiratory flow	MMF (FEF 25–27)	>2.0 liters per second	>1.6 liters per second
Maximal expiratory flow rate	MEFR (FEF 200–1200)	>3.5 liters per second	>3.0 liters per second
Spirometry—flow-volume curves:			
Maximal expiratory flow at 50% of expired vital capacity	$\dot{V}_{max}$ 50 (FEF 50%)	>2.5 liters per second	>2.0 liters per second
Maximal expiratory flow at 75% of expired vital capacity	$\dot{V}_{max}$ 75 (FEF 75%)	>1.5 liters per second	>1.0 liters per second
Resistance to airflow:			
Pulmonary resistance	RL (R_L)	<3.0 cmH$_2$O/s per liter	
Airway resistance	Raw	<2.5 cmH$_2$O/s per liter	
Specific conductance	SGaw	>0.13 cmH$_2$O/s	
Pulmonary compliance:			
Static recoil pressure at total lung capacity	Pst TLC	25 $\pm$ 5 cmH$_2$O	
Compliance of lungs (static)	CL	0.2 L/cmH$_2$O	
Compliance of lungs and thorax	C(L + T)	0.1 L/cmH$_2$O	
Dynamic compliance of 20 breaths per minute	C dyn 20	0.25 $\pm$ 0.05 liters per cmH$_2$O	
Maximal static respiratory pressures:			
Maximal inspiratory pressure	MIP	>90 cmH$_2$O	>50 cmH$_2$O
Maximal expiratory pressure	MEP	>150 cmH$_2$O	>120 cmH$_2$O
LUNG VOLUMES			
Total lung capacity	TLC	6–7 liters	5–6 liters
Functional residual capacity	FRC	2–3 liters	2–3 liters
Residual volume	RV	1–2 liters	1–2 liters
Inspiratory capacity	IC	2–4 liters	2–4 liters
Expiratory reserve volume	ERV	1–2 liters	1–2 liters
Vital capacity	VC	4–5 liters	3–4 liters
GAS EXCHANGE (SEA LEVEL)			
Arterial O$_2$ tension	Pa$_{O_2}$	95 $\pm$ 5 mmHg	
Arterial CO$_2$ tension	Pa$_{CO_2}$	40 $\pm$ 2 mmHg	
Arterial O$_2$ saturation	Sa$_{O_2}$	97 $\pm$ 2%	
Arterial blood pH	pH	7.40 $\pm$ 0.02	
Arterial bicarbonate	HCO$_3^-$	24 $\pm$ 2 mmol/L	
Base excess	BE	0 $\pm$ 2 mmol/L	
Diffusing capacity for carbon monoxide (single breath)	DL$_{CO}$	25 mL CO/min/mmHg	
Dead space volume	V$_D$	50 $\pm$ 25 mL	
Physiologic dead space: dead space-tidal volume ratio (rest) (exercise)	V$_D$/V$_T$	$\leq$35% V$_T$ $\leq$20% V$_T$	
Alveolar-arterial difference for O$_2$	A-a D$_{O_2}$	$\leq$20 mmHg	

TABLE A-10 Prediction equations for spirometric tests, lung volumes, and gas exchange in adults

Variable	Sex	Age (A)	Height (H)	Weight (W)	Constant (C)	Standard deviation (SD)
PULMONARY MECHANICS						
Spirometry—volume-time curves* (H in inches):						
FVC	M	−0.025	+0.148	—	−4.241	0.74
	F	−0.024	+0.115	—	−2.852	0.52
FEV$_1$	M	−0.032	+0.092	—	−1.260	0.55
	F	−0.025	+0.089	—	−1.932	0.47
MEFR	M	−0.047	+0.109	—	+2.010	1.66
(FEF 200–1200)	F	−0.036	+0.145	—	−2.532	1.19
MMF	M	−0.045	+0.047	—	+2.513	1.12
(FEF 25–75)	F	−0.030	+0.060	—	+0.551	0.80
Spirometry—flow-volume curves† (H in centimeters):						
$\dot{V}_{max}$ 50	M	−0.015	+0.069	—	−5.400	1.422
(FEF 50%)	F	−0.013	+0.035	—	−0.444	1.22
$\dot{V}_{max}$ 75	M	−0.012	+0.044	—	−4.143	1.026
(FEF 75%)	F	−0.014	—	—	+3.042	0.936
Lung volumes‡ (H in meters; W in kilograms):						
TLC	M	—	+6.92	−0.017	−4.30	0.67
	F	−0.015	+6.71	—	−5.77	0.48
FRC	M	+0.015	+5.30	−0.037	−3.89	0.56
	F	—	+5.13	−0.028	−4.50	0.41
RV	M	+0.022	+1.98	−0.015	−1.54	0.38
	F	+0.007	+2.68	—	−3.42	0.32
VC	M	−0.020	+4.81	—	−2.81	0.50
	F	−0.022	+4.04	—	−2.35	0.40
Gas exchange§ (H in meters; W in kilograms):						
DL$_{CO}$	M	−0.20	+32.5	—	−17.6	5.1
	F	−0.16	+21.2	—	−2.66	3.6

NOTE: Answer = (A × age) + (H × height) + (W × weight) + C ± 2 SD. Example: The normal value and lower limit for the FEV$_1$ are sought in a man, age 40 years, height 183 cm, and weight 91 kg. The following equation gives the normal value:

FEV$_1$ = (−0.032 × 40) + (0.092 × 72) + (−1.260) = 4.08 liters

The lower limit of normal:

4.08 − (2 × SD) = 4.08 − (2 × 0.55) = 2.98 liters

Only 2.5% of a normal population will fall below this value (2 SD below the mean).

For other abbreviations, see Table A-9.

* Morris et al, Am Rev Respir Dis 103:57, 1971.
† Knudson et al, Am Rev Respir Dis 113:587, 1976.
‡ Grimby G, Söderholm B, Acta Med Scand 173:199, 1963.
§ Coates JE, *Lung Function and Application in Medicine*, Philadelphia, Davis, 1965.

TABLE A-11 Differential nucleated cell counts of bone marrow

	Normal, mean%*	Range, %†
Myeloid:	56.7	
Neutrophilic series:	53.6	
Myeloblast	0.9	0.2–1.5
Promyelocyte	3.3	2.1–4.1
Myelocyte	12.7	8.2–15.7
Metamyelocyte	15.9	9.6–24.6
Band	12.4	9.5–15.3
Segmented		
Eosinophilic series	3.1	1.2–5.3
Basophilic series	<0.1	0–0.2
Erythroid:	25.6	
Pronormoblasts	0.6	0.2–1.3
Basophilic normoblasts	1.4	0.5–2.4
Polychromatophilic normoblasts	21.6	17.9–29.2
Orthochromatic normoblasts	2.0	0.4–4.6
Megakaryocytes	<0.1	
Lymphoreticular	17.8	
Lymphocytes	16.2	11.1–23.2
Plasma cells	2.3	0.4–3.9
Reticulum cells	0.3	0–0.9

* From MM Wintrobe et al, *Clinical Hematology*, 8th ed, Philadelphia, Lea & Febiger, 1981.
† Range observed in 12 healthy men.

TABLE A-12 Erythrocytes and hemoglobin: Normal values at various ages

Age	Red blood cell count,* 10^{12}/L	Hemoglobin,* g/L (g/dL)	Vol. packed RBCs,* mL/dL	Corpuscular values MCV, fL	MCH, pg	MCHC, g/L (g/dL)	MCD, μm
Days 1–13	5.1 ± 1.0	195 ± 50 (19.5 ± 5)	54.0 ± 10.0	106–98	38–33	340–360 (36–34)	8.6
Days 14–60	4.7 ± 0.9	140 ± 33 (14 ± 3.3)	42.0 ± 7.0	90	30	330 (33)	8.1
3 months to 10 years	4.5 ± 0.7	122 ± 23 (12.2 ± 2.3)	36.0 ± 5.0	80	27	340 (34)	7.7
11–15 years	4.8	131 (13.14)	39.0	82	28	340 (34)	
Adults:							
Females	4.8 ± 0.6	140 ± 20 (14 ± 2)	42.0 ± 5.0	90 ± 7	29 ± 2	340 ± 20 (34 ± 2)	7.5 ± 0.3
Males	5.4 ± 0.9	160 ± 20 (16 ± 2)	47.0 ± 5.0	90 ± 7	29 ± 2	340 ± 20 (34 ± 2)	7.5 ± 0.3

* The range of values represents almost the extremes of observed variations (93 percent or more) at sea level. The blood values of healthy persons should fall well within these mean ± SD figures.
NOTE: MCV = mean corpuscular volume, MCH = mean corpuscular hemoglobin, MCHC = mean corpuscular hemoglobin concentration, MCD = mean corpuscular diameter.
SOURCE: MM Wintrobe et al, *Clinical Hematology,* 8th ed, Philadelphia, Lea & Febiger, 1981.

TABLE A-13 Normal leukocyte count, differential count, and hemoglobin concentration at various ages

Age	Leukocytes, total	Neutrophils Total	Band	Segmented	Eosinophils	Basophils	Lymphocytes	Monocytes
12 mo	11.4(6.0–17.5)	3.5(1.5–8.5)	0.35	3.2	0.3(0.05–0.7)	0.05(0–0.20)	7.0(4.0–10.5)	0.55(0.05–1.1)
		_31_	_3.1_	_28_	_0.4_	_0.4_	_61_	_4.8_
4 yr	9.1(5.5–15.5)	3.8(1.5–8.5)	0.27(0–1.0)	3.5(1.5–7.5)	0.25(0.02–0.65)	0.05(0–0.20)	4.5(2.0–8.0)	0.45(0–0.8)
		_42_	_3.0_	_39_	_2.8_	_0.6_	_50_	_5.0_
6 yr		4.3(1.5–8.0)	0.25(0–1.0)	4.0(1.5–7.0)	0.23(0–0.65)	0.05(0–0.20)	3.5(1.5–7.0)	0.40(0–0.8)
		_51_	_3.0_	_48_	_2.7_	_0.6_	_42_	_4.7_
10 yr	8.1(4.5–13.5)	4.4(1.8–8.0)	0.24(0–1.0)	4.2(1.8–7.0)	0.20(0–0.60)	0.04(0–0.20)	3.1(1.5–6.5)	0.35(0–0.8)
		_54_	_3.0_	_51_	_2.4_	_0.5_	_38_	_4.3_
21 yr	7.4(4.5–11.0)	4.4(1.8–7.7)	0.22(0–0.7)	4.2(1.8–7.0)	0.20(0–0.45)	0.04(0–0.20)	2.5(1.0–4.8)	0.30(0–0.8)
		_59_	_3.0_	_56_	_2.7_	_0.5_	_34_	_4.0_

NOTE: Values are expressed as "cells × 10⁹/L." The numbers underlined are percentages.
SOURCE: WJ Williams et al (eds), *Hematology,* 3d ed, New York, McGraw-Hill, 1983. By permission.

INDEX

(Page numbers in **boldface** indicate major discussions; numbers preceded by *A* indicate Atlas plates.)

TOPICAL TABLE OF CONTENTS